PSYCHIATRIC CARE OF THE MEDICAL PATIENT

THIRD EDITION

EDITED BY

Barry S. Fogel, MD

CLINICAL PROFESSOR OF PSYCHIATRY

HARVARD MEDICAL SCHOOL; AND

CENTER FOR BRAIN/MIND MEDICINE

BRIGHAM AND WOMEN'S HOSPITAL

BOSTON, MA

EDITED BY

Donna B. Greenberg, MD

ASSOCIATE PROFESSOR OF PSYCHIATRY

HARVARD MEDICAL SCHOOL; AND

MASSACHUSETTS GENERAL HOSPITAL

BOSTON, MA

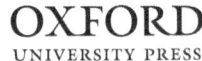

OXFORD

UNIVERSITY PRESS

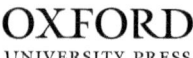

Oxford University Press is a department of the University of
Oxford. It furthers the University's objective of excellence in research,
scholarship, and education by publishing worldwide.

Oxford   New York
Auckland   Cape Town   Dar es Salaam   Hong Kong   Karachi
Kuala Lumpur   Madrid   Melbourne   Mexico City   Nairobi
New Delhi   Shanghai   Taipei   Toronto

With offices in
Argentina   Austria   Brazil   Chile   Czech Republic   France   Greece
Guatemala   Hungary   Italy   Japan   Poland   Portugal   Singapore
South Korea   Switzerland   Thailand   Turkey   Ukraine   Vietnam

Oxford is a registered trademark of Oxford University Press
in the UK and certain other countries.

Published in the United States of America by
Oxford University Press
198 Madison Avenue, New York, NY 10016

Library of Congress Cataloging-in-Publication Data
Psychiatric care of the medical patient / edited by Barry S. Fogel and Donna B. Greenberg.—Third edition.
p. ; cm.
Includes bibliographical references and index.
ISBN 978–0–19–973185–5 (hardcover : alk. paper); 978–0–19–063680–7 (paperback : alk. paper)
I. Fogel, Barry S. editor.   II. Greenberg, Donna B. (Donna Beth), editor.
[DNLM: 1. Mental Disorders—complications.   2. Mental Disorders—diagnosis.   3. Mental Disorders—therapy.
4. Psychophysiologic Disorders.   5. Stress, Psychological.   WM 140]
RC454.4
616.89—dc23
2014015217

1 3 5 7 9 8 6 4 2
Printed in the United States of America
on acid-free paper

BF: I dedicate this book to my wife Xiaoling and my children Susanna, Juliana, and William James.

DG: This book is dedicated with gratitude for my family and dear friends with a focus on the new generation just walking.

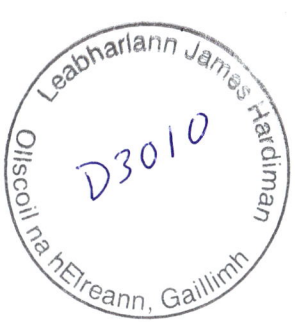

CONTENTS

PART IV

MAJOR SYMPTOMS AND SYNDROMES

PART V

NEUROPSYCHIATRIC DISORDERS

PART VI

MEDICAL SPECIALTIES

PREFACE

This third edition of *Psychiatric Care of the Medical Patient* reflects changes in medicine, psychiatry, and the healthcare system over the two decades since the first edition was published. Medical psychiatry—the medical subspecialty that applies psychiatric knowledge and skills to the problems of patients with general medical problems—is continually evolving. What remains constant is the primacy of the sacred relationship between the patient and the physician, and the psychiatrist's knowledge and experience of medicine as a basis of that relationship.

Medical psychiatrists like general psychiatrists have expertise in the diagnosis and treatment of primary mental disorders, appreciating the relevance to health of patients' developmental histories, family relationships, and social and occupational environments, and understanding how the physician–patient relationship can be an aid or an impediment to a favorable outcome of medical care. In addition, medical psychiatrists have detailed knowledge of one or more specific general medical or surgical specialties, as well as familiarity with aspects of neurology, endocrinology, and clinical pharmacology that are particularly relevant to the interaction of mental disorders with general medical conditions and their respective treatments. In addition medical psychiatrists are highly aware of healthcare system issues and relationships among different physicians, specialties, and disciplines.

These differences can be seen as a matter of degree, as all good general psychiatrists should have some of the knowledge and skills we attribute to medical psychiatrists. General psychiatrists can become medical psychiatrists, beginning by focusing their practices on patient populations with general medical issues. Even so, there really is a qualitative difference in the attitudes and professional identity of medical psychiatrists. Medical psychiatrists view themselves as physicians above all, not as mental health professionals with medical training. Their aims are not limited to diagnosing and managing primary mental disorders or differentiating between "functional" and "organic" etiologies for symptoms. When they evaluate patients they aim to understand patients' adaptations to their existential predicaments, which include whatever diseases afflict them or threaten them, be those categorized as "mental" or otherwise. This understanding often is accompanied by the psychiatrist's empathy and the patient's trust. Along these lines, a motivated physician who is not a psychiatrist but who is psychologically minded and emotionally intelligent can effectively function as a medical psychiatrist for many of his or her own patients with the aid of ongoing consultation and mentorship from a psychiatrist.

The patient who sees a medical psychiatrist might begin the relationship with tentativeness, skepticism, or ambivalence. Ideally these feelings give way to trust and confidence. Highly specific knowledge of the medical issues the patient faces can be an important factor in bringing about the change. It can be transformative when a patient senses—or concludes—that the medical psychiatrist can grasp without excessive explanation the details of the patient's symptoms and functional impairments, drug side effects, burdens in adhering to treatment, difficult treatment-related decisions, and more.

We believe there are many patients who need what medical psychiatrists can offer and who don't get it, usually because the need isn't recognized and sometimes because resources don't permit it. The need is greater than ever because of specific changes and trends in medicine and the healthcare system. We offer an illustrative and far from exhaustive list:

1. People are living longer and accumulating more chronic diseases and impairments. These conditions make increasing demands for adaptation at the same time as patients' physical and/or mental capacity to adapt can be diminished by illness.

2. The healthcare system demands more standardization, care according to evidence-based practice guidelines, and rules-based recordkeeping that severely limits discussion of subjective, synthetic, speculative, and holistic perspectives. At the same time we are increasingly recognizing how different patients can be, based on their age and gender, their genetics, their ethnic origins and family environments, their personalities, their social and economic circumstances, their personal preferences, and their particular combination of comorbid conditions. It is a sometimes daunting challenge to respect this diversity and effectively advocate for appropriate individualization of care within the current context.

3. Electronic health records, rapidly becoming the norm, can be an impediment to patient care. When a physician's eyes and attention are focused on a screen, they are not focused on the patient. When records are full of cut-and-pasted routine information, and when medical notes are filled-in templates, auditors can check boxes to ensure that coding rules are followed—but it can be difficult for physicians to see what is distinctive about a patient, to convey important subjective perceptions, and to effectively message their colleagues through the record. Alerts about potential drug–drug and drug–disease

interactions can be triggered too often—or not often enough—for physicians to depend on them. The time spent dealing with the electronic record may not be offset by the time saved or adverse events averted—with the patient thus losing valuable face time with the physician or the physician losing time for reflection, research, and recreation. (As information technology advances, these issues eventually will be resolved: better voice recognition, better processing of free text and other unstructured data, more intelligent machines, and effective deployment of hypertext will help.)

4. The Internet has had profound—and mixed—effects on patients' health and their adaptation to illness. Patients are better informed but sometimes misinformed by what they find online. Through social media patients can find others with similar problems, but time spent online is time not spent in direct face-to-face interaction. It remains to be seen for whom online social support works as well as the traditional kind.

5. Hospitalizations are shorter, and people now receive care in community settings who would not have just 20 years ago. Care rendered in a hospital for a serious illness involves many people of different specialties and disciplines, whose efforts often are not optimally coordinated. The team of physicians and other health professionals who get to know a patient in the hospital or emergency room is different from the team caring for the patient outside the hospital. The outpatient team has different resources and a different time frame for action, and it may have different goals and incentives. Communication failures are common—and even with good communication there can be failures of coordination of care.

6. Patient autonomy has become a dominant principle—usually but not always for the best. Competent patients are expected to give or withhold informed consent for medical procedures and to give advance directives for their care in hypothetical life-or-death circumstances. Despite current pressures to "get advance directives" or "get informed consent" from patients, taking informed consent and advance directives seriously requires much more than getting patients' signatures on long and detailed printed forms. How questions are asked, when they are asked, and who asks them all will affect answers to the questions on those forms.

7. While physicians have less control over what happens to their patients, they are no less accountable for medical outcomes. Physicians must teach and persuade, suggest and motivate, rather than simply order and prescribe.

8. Patients' expectations for care are greater because more conditions can be treated. Because of the Internet and direct-to-patient advertising, patients know what is available and may request or even demand particular treatments. At the same time costs are escalating and physicians are pressed to limit the use of expensive treatments.

9. Consumption of psychotropic drugs—mostly by people who have never received even an evaluation by a psychiatrist—is endemic in the United States. For example, the *point*—not lifetime—prevalence of antidepressant use in a recent Mayo Clinic community survey was 13%, and among women aged 50–64 years the rate was 24%. By the time patients see psychiatrists they usually have experienced one or more psychotropic drugs, or they currently are taking one or more. This alters the presentation of mental disorders to psychiatrists as well as often affects the attitude a patient has when a new psychotropic drug prescription is proposed.

10. Attention to pain as "the fifth vital sign" has increased, with mixed effects. While fewer patients are suffering from untreated severe pain, the misuse, abuse, and ineffective use of prescription opiates clearly has increased. Pain research has advanced, with better understanding of neuropathic pain, more specific treatment for many painful conditions, greater recognition of unusual pain syndromes, and improved methodology for rehabilitation. All chronic pain is now appreciated as having a neuropathic aspect. Tools for recognition of addiction and new treatment options such as buprenorphine have evolved as well. Dissemination of these advances to date has been uneven, as is typical of medical innovations.

11. Cognitive impairment disorders have increased in prevalence with the aging of the population, and there is much greater differentiation of the diseases that cause them. The distinctions among dementia syndromes and their underlying neurodegenerative diseases are widely appreciated in the neurological community. Symptomatic treatments are used both for neurodegenerative diseases and for their neuropsychiatric complications such as depression and psychosis. Diagnostic practice, which just a few decades ago was typically the identification of a "chronic organic brain syndrome" and "ruling out a treatable dementia", has moved toward broader appreciation of distinct neurodegenerative diseases that elicit physicians' intellectual interest.

12. Some highly prevalent mental disorders including depression, generalized anxiety, and ADHD are less stigmatized than they once were. Nonetheless, many disorders including schizophrenia, borderline personality, and drug dependence continue to carry stigma. An unfortunate consequence is a tendency toward diagnosis of nonstigmatized conditions when the diagnosis of a stigmatized condition, either as an alternative or as comorbidity, would be more accurate and helpful in planning treatment.

13. Brain imaging has captured the public's imagination with positive effects like broader public support for brain research. There are, however, some prevalent misconceptions. For example, some patients believe that normal brain imaging rules out neurodegenerative disease. In cases of traumatic brain injury, defense lawyers have essentially argued that normal anatomic brain imaging means that an injury will not lead to prolonged disability, while plaintiffs' lawyers have argued that abnormal functional brain imaging means that it will; neither inference is necessarily correct.

14. Complementary and alternative medicine (CAM), including the use of herbal remedies and nutritional supplements, has moved toward the mainstream of practice, but it is not quite there. Many popular treatments have weak evidentiary support, and the use of complementary and alternative treatments can delay access to evidence-based conventional treatments or can interact adversely with them. For specific patients the consideration of evidence-based CAM treatments that are potentially superior to conventional treatments is almost random, depending on the physician's personal knowledge and experience.

15. Perceptions are changing of what is normal function later in life and what losses of function are acceptable. More people than in the past believe that they should continue in their occupations, remain as athletic as they were when they were younger, and have an active sexual life well into their 70s and 80s.

16. There are an ever-increasing number of circumstances where medical situations that once had to be accepted are now potentially changeable, although often with pain, inconvenience, and/or expense. For example, an aging face can be made to look younger with Botox or aesthetic surgery. A postmenopausal woman can conceive and bear a healthy child with the aid of IVF, using donor eggs or her own eggs or embryos frozen at an earlier time. Bionic devices can partially alleviate losses in vision or hearing; prosthetic limbs can be attached to nerves and function more like natural ones.

17. Long-term psychodynamic therapy is not as central to general psychiatric practice as it once was. At the same time, the evidence base supporting psychodynamic concepts of defense mechanisms, attachment styles, and personality organization has increased. Psychodynamic understanding has particular value in helping patients adapt to general medical illnesses, their symptoms and impairments, and the demands of their treatments. Ironically, psychodynamic theory and practice might find broader application in medical psychiatry than in the treatment of primary mental disorders.

18. Organized religion is important to a smaller proportion of the population, but it is essential to the lives of believers. Many people are "spiritual but not religious," and many have deeply felt ethical principles and transpersonal motivations not based on belief in a higher power or transcendent being. Faced with illness-related existential challenges, patients turn to their principles, but without conventional religious affiliations they may not have an obvious source of assistance in applying them. Medical psychiatrists sometimes can help patients discover and utilize their spiritual or religious resources.

19. The population in the United States—and in several other upper-income and middle-income countries—is getting fatter, with steadily increasing rates of overweight and obesity and the syndromes associated with excessive weight, including Type 2 diabetes and obstructive sleep apnea. Medical, surgical, and cognitive-behavioral therapies for obesity have an increasing evidence base, but the majority of people with medically significant overweight and even morbid obesity are not effectively treated.

20. Sleep disturbance, sleep disorders, and sleep deficits are highly prevalent, and their pervasive impact on physical and mental health is increasingly recognized. Even so, sleep does not yet get the attention it deserves, and therapies for sleep disorders that are efficacious in controlled studies are less effective in actual practice. Principles of sleep hygiene are known to the field but not necessarily taught to patients or followed by patients even when they are known. The critical sleep-related questions are changing. Where two decades ago the question might have been, "Could this patient have obstructive sleep apnea?" it might now be, "Is this patient using his CPAP machine, and if not, why not?"

21. Questionnaire-based screening tests and patient-reported outcome measures have become mainstream and in some contexts mandatory.

The editors of this volume have selected chapter authors whom we regard as medical psychiatrists or as key members of medical-psychiatric teams. Many of them have training in neurology, internal medicine, obstetrics and gynecology, or another nonpsychiatric specialty. In our editorial dialogue with them we have asked them questions from our own medical-psychiatric perspective. This perspective, and, implicitly, the attitudes and identity of the medical psychiatrist, are conveyed by the first three sections of this book, which describe the evaluation of medical-psychiatric patients and a comprehensive approach to assessing major symptoms and syndromes.

The potential of healthcare to prolong life and to enhance the quality of life has never been greater. Yet, there often are gaps between the potential of 21st-century medicine, patients' expectations from their healthcare, and the reality of patients' healthcare experiences, clinical outcomes, and health-related quality of life. Medical psychiatrists participate in efforts to identify and close such gaps. In doing so they begin with the legacy of the physician–patient relationship; they draw upon know-how and wisdom developed and articulated by 20th-century psychiatrists, and they apply 21st-century medical knowledge. The editors' hope is that this third edition of *Psychiatric Care of the Medical Patient* will support—and memorialize—this effort.

Barry S. Fogel, MD
Donna B. Greenberg, MD
Boston, Massachusetts
April 2015

ACKNOWLEDGMENTS

We deeply appreciate the work of our contributing authors, whose chapters reflect the time and care given to this project. In the academic world book chapters may not 'count' as much as peer-reviewed journal articles, but in the real world the clinical wisdom found in a good medical textbook can stick in a physician's mind and durably improve practice.

We acknowledge David D'Addona, our editor at Oxford University Press. He's the best of the many editors we have worked with in over 30 years of writing for medical publications. David has a great sense of what would make someone want to read—or even buy—a medical textbook when so much information is instantly and freely available online. In addition, no one could do a better job of making a tardy contributor—or editor—feel guilty and understood at the same time.

We remember our late colleague Dr. Alan Stoudemire, a wonderful physician, prolific writer, and tireless proponent of medical psychiatry, who collaborated with us and inspired us from the early 1980s until his death shortly after the second edition of this book was published. We also remember Dr. W. Victor ("Vic") Vieweg, a cardiologist-psychiatrist who co-wrote our cardiology chapter. Vic was an outstanding teacher and scholar of both psychiatry and cardiology, whom we were honored to have as a contributor to this volume.

BF: Above all I must acknowledge the contribution of my wife, Xiaoling Jiang, PhD. Xiaoling is a trilingual literary scholar who has lived in China, Japan, and the United States; she has observed the changes of the last two decades in medicine and psychiatry from outside the medical profession and from a global perspective, deconstructing them with her usual acuity. Answering her many questions about the content of the book and my own contributions to it evoked many new insights. She encouraged me to pursue the project and helped me protect the time to complete it. And, she inspires me in general.

I also would like to thank the many fellows and junior faculty in neuropsychiatry and behavioral neurology whom I have mentored over the past 17 years at the Brigham and Women's Hospital. Several have contributed chapters to this volume; all have contributed to the evolution of my thinking about how neurological, psychiatric, and general medical perspectives can be better integrated. It has given me joy to see them succeed in their scientific and clinical work.

DG: I am indebted to many of my medical and psychiatric colleagues at Massachusetts General Hospital. They set a high standard of clinical reasoning, dedication, and curiosity, and their passion for medicine is infectious! Further inspiration comes from the psychiatrists and psychologists, nationally and internationally, who express their creativity at the bedside of the medically ill, challenging all of us to do better.

CONTRIBUTORS

Ruchi Aggarwal, MD
Department of Psychiatry and
Behavioral Sciences
University of Oklahoma Health Sciences Center
Oklahoma City, OK

Sherese Ali, MD
Consultant Neuropsychiatrist
Toronto, ON

Stephanie Assuras, PhD
Assistant Professor of Neuropsychology
Department of Neurology
Columbia University Medical Center
New York, NY

David J. Axelrod, MD, JD
Department of Medicine
Division of Internal Medicine
Jefferson Internal Medicine Associates
Philadelphia, PA

Aditya Bardia, MD, MPH
Department of Medicine
Harvard Medical School; and
Massachusetts General Hospital Cancer Center
Boston, MA

Scott R. Beach, MD
Department of Psychiatry
Harvard Medical School; and
Massachusetts General Hospital
Boston, MA

Madeleine Becker, MD, FAPM
Associate Director, Division of Consultation-Liaison
Psychiatry
Director, Psychosomatic Medicine Fellowship
Thomas Jefferson University Hospital
Department of Psychiatry and Human Behavior
Philadelphia, PA

Philip A. Bialer, MD
Memorial Sloan Kettering Cancer Center
Department of Psychiatry; and
Weill Cornell Medical College
New York, NY

Donald R. Bodner, MD
Department of Urology
University Hospitals Case Medical Center and
Cleveland Department of Veterans Affairs Medical Center
Case Western University School of Medicine
Cleveland, Ohio

Robert J. Boland, MD
Department of Psychiatry
Brigham and Women's Hospital/Harvard Medical School
Boston, MA

David Borsook, MD, PhD
Departments of Anesthesia and Radiology
Boston Childrens Hospital
Department of Psychiatry, Massachusetts General Hospital
Harvard Medical School
Boston, MA

Megan Moore Brennan, MD
Assistant Clinical Professor
Columbia University College of Physicians and Surgeons
Assistant Dean for Education at Bassett
Bassett Medical Center
Cooperstown, NY

Harold Bronheim, MD
Departments of Psychiatry and Medicine
Icahn School of Medicine at Mount Sinai
New York, NY

Richard P. Brown, MD
Department of Psychiatry
Columbia University College of Physicians
and Surgeons
New York, NY

Thomas Markham Brown, MD
Audie L. Murphy Memorial Veterans
Administration Medical Center
South Texas Veterans Health Care System
San Antonio, TX

T. H. Eric Bui, MD, PhD
Department of Psychiatry
Harvard Medical School; and
Massachusetts General Hospital
Boston, MA

Lucienne A. Cahen, MD
Department of Psychiatry
Harvard Medical School; and
Massachusetts General Hospital and
Division of Behavioral and Mental Health
Spaulding Rehabilitation Hospital
Boston, MA

Deborah A. Cahn-Weiner, PhD
Department of Neurology
University of California-San Francisco
San Francisco, CA

Gayun Chan-Smutko, MS, CGC
Center for Cancer Risk Assessment
Massachusetts General Hospital Cancer Center
Boston, MA

Meredith E. Charney, PhD
Massachusetts General Hospital; and
Department of Psychiatry
Harvard Medical School
Boston, MA

Keira Chism, MD
Department of Psychiatry and
Human Behavior
Thomas Jefferson University Hospital
Philadelphia, PA

Eva H. Chittenden, MD
Director of Education
Palliative Care Division, Department of Medicine
Massachusetts General Hospital
Assistant Professor of Medicine
Harvard Medical School
Boston, MA

Harvey Max Chochinov, MD, PhD, FRCPC
Distinguished Professor of Psychiatry
University of Manitoba
Canada Research Chair in Palliative Care
Manitoba Palliative Care Research Unit CancerCare
Manitoba
Winnipeg, Canada

Amit Chopra, MD
Department of Psychiatry
West Penn Allegheny Health System
Pittsburgh, PA

Heidi Christianson, PhD
Department of Psychiatry and
Behavioral Medicine
Medical College of Wisconsin
Milwaukee, WI

Lewis M. Cohen, MD
Department of Medicine
Tufts University School of Medicine; and
Baystate Medical Center
Springfield, MA

Ariel Dalfen, MD, FRCPC
Assistant Professor
Department of Psychiatry
University of Toronto Faculty of Medicine; and
Head Perinatal Mental Health Program
Mount Sinai Hospital
Toronto, Ontario, Canada

Hillary G. D'Amato
Department of Psychiatry
Harvard Medical School; and
Massachusetts General Hospital
Boston, MA

**Diane de Camps Meschino,
MD, BSc(H), FRCPC**
Department of Psychiatry
University of Toronto Faculty of Medicine; and
Women's College Hospital
Toronto, Ontario, Canada

Lex Denysenko, MD, FAPM
Department of Psychiatry and Human Behavior
Thomas Jefferson University Hospital
Philadelphia, PA

Kimiko Domoto-Reilly, MD
Department of Neurology
University of Washington
Seattle, WA

Robert L. Doyle, MD
Department of Psychiatry
Massachusetts General Hospital
Boston, MA

Amelia Dubovsky, MD
Psychiatry Consultation Service
Harborview Medical Center
Psychiatry and Behavioral Sciences
University of Washington
Washington, WA

Stanley H. Ducharme, PhD
Professor of Urology
Boston University Medical Center
Clinical Psychologist
Boston Medical Center
Boston, MA

Margaret Dundon, PhD
Veterans Health Administration
National Center for Health Promotion and Disease
Prevention
Durham, NC

Shawn Fagan, MD
Burn and Reconstructive Surgery
Critical Care Medicine
Joseph M Still Burn Centers, Inc
Boston, MA

Marc D. Feldman, MD
Department of Psychiatry and Behavioral Medicine
The University of Alabama
Tuscaloosa, AL

Howard Field, MD
Department of Psychiatry and
Human Behavior
Thomas Jefferson University Hospital
Philadelphia, PA

Barry S. Fogel, MD, MBA
Department of Psychiatry
Harvard Medical School; and
Brigham and Women's Hospital
Boston, MA

Gregory L. Fricchione, MD
Assistant professor of Surgery
Division of Burns Surgery
Massachusetts General Hospital
Harvard Medical School
Boston, MA

Wendy Froehlich-Santino, MD
Departments of Psychiatry & Behavioral
Science and Pediatrics
Stanford University School of Medicine
Stanford, CA

Anna M. Georgiopoulos, MD
Department of Psychiatry
Harvard Medical School; and
Massachusetts General Hospital
Boston, MA

Patricia L. Gerbarg, MD
Department of Psychiatry
New York Medical College
Valhalla, NY

Michael J. Germain, MD
Department of Medicine
Tufts University School of Medicine; and
Baystate Medical Center
Springfield, MA

Richard J. Goldberg, MD, MS
Professor, Department of Psychiatry and Human Behavior
Warren Alpert School of Medicine at
Brown University
Providence, RI

Richard T. Goldberg, EdD
Department of Psychiatry
Harvard Medical School; and
Massachusetts General Hospital and
Division of Behavioral and Mental Health
Spaulding Rehabilitation Hospital
Boston, MA

Michael G. Goldstein, MD
Veterans Health Administration National Center
for Health Promotion and Disease Prevention
Providence, RI

Jeffrey S. Gonzalez, PhD
Departments of Medicine and Epidemiology &
Population Health
Albert Einstein College of Medicine
Bronx, NY

Cheryl Gore-Felton, PhD
Department of Psychiatry and Behavioral Sciences
Stanford University School of Medicine
Stanford, CA

Tristan Gorrindo, MD
Department of Psychiatry
Harvard Medical School; and
Massachusetts General Hospital
Boston, MA

Jeremy Goverman, MD
Assistant professor of Surgery
Division of Burns Surgery
Massachusetts General Hospital
Harvard Medical School
Boston, MA

Stephen A. Green, MD
Department of Psychiatry
Georgetown University School
of Medicine
Washington, DC

Donna B. Greenberg, MD
Department of Psychiatry
Harvard Medical School; and
Massachusetts General Hospital
Boston, MA

Joseph A. Greer, PhD
Center for Psychiatric Oncology &
Behavioral Sciences,
Massachusetts General Hospital Cancer Center
Department of Psychiatry,
Harvard Medical School
Boston, MA

Gregory M. Gressel, MD
Department of Obstetrics
Gynecology & Reproductive Sciences
Yale University School of Medicine
New Haven, CT

Sophie Grigoriadis, MD, MA, PhD, FRCPC
Head Women's Mood and Anxiety Clinic:
Reproductive Transitions
Fellowship Director
Department of Psychiatry
Sunnybrook Health Sciences Centre Scientist
Sunnybrook Research Institute
Adjunct Scientist
Women's College Research Institute
Associate Professor
Department of Psychiatry
University of Toronto
Toronto, Canada

Tracey M. Guthrie, MD
Department of Psychiatry and Human Behavior
Warren Alpert School of Medicine at
Brown University
Providence, RI

Scott D. Haltzman, MD
David Lawrence Center
Naples, FL

James C. Hamilton, PhD
Associate Professor of Psychology
Clinical Affiliate Associate Professor of Internal Medicine
University of Alabama
Tuscaloosa, AL

Ashley S. Hart, PhD
Veteran's Administration Boston Healthcare System
Boston, MA

Mehrul Hasnain, MD
Department of Psychiatry
Memorial University
Waterford Hospital
St. John's, Newfoundland,
Canada

Eric P. Hazen, MD
Department of Psychiatry
Harvard Medical School; and
Massachusetts General Hospital
Boston, MA

Krystal A. Hedge
Department of Psychology
University of Alabama
Tuscaloosa, AL

Thomas W. Heinrich, MD
Department of Psychiatry and Behavioral
Medicine; and
Department of Family and Community Medicine
Medical College of Wisconsin
Milwaukee, WI

Paul J. Helmuth, MD
Valley Medical Associates
Springfield, MA

Seth D. Herman, MD
Department of Physical Medicine & Rehabilitation
Spaulding Rehabilitation Hospital; and
Massachusetts General Hospital
Boston, MA

Douglas H. Hughes, MD
Department of Psychiatry
Boston University School of Medicine
Boston, MA

Daniel P. Hunt, MD
Department of Medicine
Harvard Medical School; and
Massachusetts General Hospital
Boston, MA

Alana Iglewicz, MD
Department of Psychiatry
University of California-San Diego; and
VA San Diego Healthcare System
San Diego, CA

Kelly Irwin, MD
MGH Psychiatric Oncology and Behavioral Sciences
MGH Cancer Center; and
MGH Schizophrenia Program
Harvard Medical School
Boston, MA

Mary Lou Jackson, MD
Massachusetts Eye and Ear Infirmary
Department of Ophthalmology
Harvard Medical School
Boston, MA

Natalie L. Jacobowski, MD
Department of Psychiatry
Vanderbilt University School of Medicine
Nashville, TN

Andres M. Kanner, MD
Department of Neurology
University of Miami Miller School of Medicine
Miami, FL

Nasser Karamouz, MD
Department of Psychiatry
Harvard Medical School; and
Massachusetts General Hospital and
Division of Behavioral and Mental Health
Spaulding Rehabilitation Hospital
Boston, MA

Suzanne R. Karl, DO
Department of Psychiatry
The Zucker Hillside Hospital
North Shore-LIJ Health System
Glen Oaks, NY

Gabor I. Keitner, MD
Department of Psychiatry
The Warren Alpert School of Medicine at Brown
University; and
Rhode Island Hospital
Providence, RI

Shahram Khoshbin, MD
Associate Professor of Neurology
Harvard Medical School
Department of Neurology
Brigham and Women's Hospital
Boston, MA

Phillip M. Kleespies, PhD
Department of Psychiatry
Boston University School of Medicine; and
Veteran's Administration Boston Healthcare System
Boston, MA

Danielle N. Ko, MBBS, LLB
Department of Medicine
Harvard medical School; and
Massachusetts General Hospital
Boston, MA

Robert M. Kohut Jr, MD
Department of Urology
Case Western Reserve University
School of Medicine
Cleveland, OH

Richard Kradin, MD
Director of Dyspnea Clinic
Pulmonary and Critical Care Unit
Center for Psychoanalytical Studies
Massachusetts General Hospital and
Associate Professor of Medicine and Pathology
Harvard Medical School
Boston, MA

M. Alexandra Kredlow
Department of Psychiatry
Massachusetts General Hospital
Boston, MA

Elisabeth J. Shakin Kunkel, MD
Vice Chair for Clinical Affairs
Department of Psychiatry and Human Behavior
Thomas Jefferson University
Philadelphia, PA

W. Curt LaFrance Jr, MD, MPH
Departments of Psychiatry
and Neurology
The Warren Alpert School of Medicine at
Brown University; and
Rhode Island Hospital
Providence, RI

Norman B. Levy, MD
Professor Emeritus
Psychiatry
SUNY, Downstate Medical Center; and
Director of Psychiatry
Southern California Mental Health Associates
Los Angeles, CA

Joseph A. Locala, MD
Division of Medicine and Psychiatry
University Hospitals Case Medical Center; and
Department of Psychiatry
Case Western Reserve University School
of Medicine
Cleveland, OH

Steven E. Locke, MD
Department of Psychiatry
Harvard Medical School; and
Beth Israel Deaconess Medical Center
Boston, MA

Elizabeth W. Loder, MD, MPH
Department of Neurology
Harvard Medical School; and
Brigham and Women's Hospital
Boston, MA

Joseph Z. Lux, MD
Department of Psychiatry
New York University School of Medicine; and
Bellevue Hospital Center
New York, NY

José R. Maldonado, MD, FAPM, FACFE
Associate Professor of Psychiatry, Internal Medicine,
Surgery, Emergency Medicine & Law
Medical Director
Psychosomatic Medicine Service
Stanford University School of Medicine
Stanford, CA

Paul Malloy, PhD
Department of Psychiatry & Human Behavior
The Warren Alpert Medical School of Brown University
Brown University
Providence, RI

Vaughn L. Mankey, MD
West Lake Hills, TX

Michael Marcangelo, MD
Department of Psychiatry and
Behavioral Neurosciences
Pritzker School of Medicine at the
University of Chicago
Chicago, IL

Christine Marchionni, MD
Psychiatry
Temple University Hospital
Philadelphia, PA

Dimitri Markov, MD
Department of Psychiatry and Human Behavior
Thomas Jefferson University Hospital
Philadelphia, PA

Jeevendra Martyn, MD
Department of Anesthesiology
Harvard Medical School; and
Massachusetts General Hospital
Boston, MA

Cynthia A. Gutierrez, PharmD
South Texas Veterans Health Care System
San Antonio, TX

Scott McGinnis, MD
Department of Neurology
Harvard Medical School; and
Brigham and Women's Hospital; and
Massachusetts General Hospital
Boston, MA

Mario F. Mendez, MD, PhD
Department of Psychiatry & Biobehavioral Sciences; and
Department of Neurology
David Geffen School of Medicine
University of California-Los Angeles
Los Angeles, CA

Cynthia W. Moore, PhD
Department of Psychiatry
Harvard Medical School; and
Massachusetts General Hospital
Boston, MA

George T. Moses, DO, MA, FAPA
Family Care Behavioral Health, INC.
Zanesville, OH

Shamim H. Nejad, MD
Director, Burns and Trauma Psychiatry
Medical Director, Addiction Consultation Team
Division of Psychiatry and Medicine
Department of Psychiatry
Massachusetts General Hospital
Assistant Professor of Psychiatry,
Harvard Medical School
Boston, MA

Aaron P. Nelson, PhD
Department of Psychiatry
Harvard Medical School;
Department of Neurology
Brigham and Women's Hospital
Boston, MA

Christian J. Nelson, PhD
Department of Psychiatry and Behavioral Sciences
Memorial Sloan-Kettering Cancer Center
New York, NY

Caitlin M. Nevins
The California School of Professional Psychology
San Francisco, CA

Patricia J. O'Malley, MD
Assistant Professor in Pediatrics
Department of Pediatrics primary,
Emergency Medicine secondary
Harvard Medical School; and
Medical Director, Pediatric Palliative Care
MassGeneral Hospital for Children and
Massachusetts General Hospital
Boston, MA

Laura Ortiz-Terán, MD, PhD
Department of Neurology
Harvard Medical School; and
Beth Israel Deaconess Medical Center
Boston, MA

Gregory J. O'Shanick, MD, DLFAPA
Center for Neurorehabilitation Services
Richmond, VA
Adjunct Clinical Professor of Psychiatry and
the Behavioral Sciences
Keck School of Medicine
University of Southern California
Los Angeles, CA

Olu Oyesanmi, MD, MPH
Economic Cycle Research
Plymouth Meeting, PA

Lawrence Park, MD
Food and Drug Administration
Washington, DC

David L. Perez, MD
Departments of Neurology and Psychiatry
Harvard Medical School; and
Brigham and Women's Hospital
Massachusetts General Hospital
Boston, MA

Pedro E. Pérez-Cruz, MD, MPH
Department of Medicine
Harvard Medical School; and
Massachusetts General Hospital
Boston, MA; and
Departamento Medicina Interna, Facultad de Medicina
Pontificia Universidad Católica de Chile
Santiago, Chile

John R. Peteet, MD
Department of Psychiatry
Harvard Medical School;
Brigham and Women's Hospital; and
Dana Farber Cancer Institute
Boston, MA

Donn A. Posner, PhD
Department of Psychiatry and Human Behavior
The Warren Alpert School of Medicine at
Brown University
Providence, RI

Terry Rabinowitz, MD, DDS
Professor, Departments of Psychiatry and Family Medicine,
University of Vermont College of Medicine
Medical Director, Division of Consultation
Psychiatry and Psychosomatic Medicine
Medical Director, Telemedicine
Burlington, VT

Shreya Raj, MD
Departments of Psychiatry and Neurology
Harvard Medical School; and
Brigham and Women's Hospital
Boston, MA

David B. Reuben, MD
Multicampus Program in Geriatric Medicine and
Gerontology
Director
Division of Geriatrics
Chief
Archstone Professor of Medicine
David Geffen School of Medicine at UCLA
Los Angeles, CA

Jarrett W. Richardson, MD
Department of Psychiatry & Psychology
Center for Sleep Medicine
Mayo Clinic College of Medicine
Rochester, MN

David Ring, MD, PhD
Chief of Hand Surgery, Massachusetts
General Hospital
Department of Orthopaedic Surgery,
Harvard Medical School
Massachusetts General Hospital
Boston, MA

Fernando A. Rivera, MD, FACP
Assistant Professor of Medicine, Mayo College of Medicine
Consultant Division of Diagnostic and
Consultative Medicine
Mayo Clinic
Jacksonville, FL

Gail Erlick Robinson, MD, DPsych, FRCPC
Departments of Psychiatry and Obstetrics/Gynecology
University of Toronto Faculty of Medicine; and
Women's Mental Health Program
University Health Network
Toronto, Ontario, Canada

Andrew J. Roth, MD
Department of Psychiatry and Behavioral Sciences
Memorial Sloan-Kettering Cancer Center and
Professor Clinical Psychiatry
Weill Cornell Medical College
New York, NY

Steven A. Safren, PhD
Department of Psychiatry
Harvard Medical School; and
Massachusetts General Hospital
Boston, MA

Shirlene Sampson, MS, MD
Associate Professor in Psychiatry
Department of Psychiatry and Psychology
Mayo Clinic College of Medicine
Rochester, MN

Rani A. Sarkis, MD, MSc
Department of Neurology
Harvard Medical School; and
Brigham and Women's Hospital
Boston, MA

David B. Sarwer, PhD
Departments of Psychiatry and Surgery
The Edwin and Fannie Gray Hall Center for Human
Appearance and
Center for Weight and Eating Disorders; and
Perelman School of Medicine at the University of
Pennsylvania
Philadelphia, PA

Jeremiah M. Scharf, MD, PhD
Departments of Neurology and Psychiatry
Harvard Medical School
Brigham and Women's Hospital; and
Massachusetts General Hospital
Boston, MA

Lidia Schapira, MD
Associate Professor of Medicine
Harvard Medical School
Associate Physician
Massachusetts General Hospital Cancer Center
Boston, MA

Allen D. Seftel, MD
Departments of Surgery and Urology; and
MD Anderson Cancer Center at Cooper University
Health Care
Marlton, NJ

Lawrence F. Selter, MD
Department of Psychiatry
Massachusetts General Hospital
Boston, MA

Kristen M. Shannon, MS, CGC
Center or Cancer Risk Assessment
Mass General Hospital Cancer Center
Boston, MA

Richard J. Shaw, MD
Departments of Psychiatry and Behavioral
Science and Pediatrics
Stanford University School of Medicine
Stanford, CA

Robert L. Sheridan, MD
Department of Surgery
Harvard Medical School
Shriners Hospital for Children; and
Massachusetts General Hospital
Boston, MA

John L. Shuster, MD
Chief Medical Officer
MindCare Solutions Group, Inc.; and
Clinical Professor of Psychiatry
Vanderbilt University School of Medicine
Nashville, TN

David A. Silbersweig, MD
Department of Psychiatry and
Institute for the Neurosciences
Brigham and Women's Hospital; and
Harvard Medical School
Boston, MA

Naomi M. Simon, MD
Department of Psychiatry
Harvard Medical School; and
Massachusetts General Hospital
Boston, MA

Christopher L. Sola, DO
Department of Psychiatry and Psychology
Mayo Clinic College of Medicine
Rochester, MN

David Spiegel, MD
Department of Psychiatry and
Behavioral Sciences
Stanford University School of Medicine
Stanford, CA

Jacqueline C. Spitzer, MSEd
Center for Weight and Eating Disorders; and
Department of Psychiatry
Perelman School of Medicine at the University of
Pennsylvania
Philadelphia, PA

Hans Steiner, MD
Departments of Psychiatry & Behavioral Science
and Pediatrics
Stanford University School of Medicine
Stanford, CA

Erin Sterenson, MD
Department of psychiatry and psychology
Olmsted Medical Center
Rochester, MN

Frederick J. Stoddard Jr., MD
Professor
Harvard Medical School
Boston, MA

Kimberly Stoner, MD
Departments of Medicine and Psychiatry
Medical College of Wisconsin
Milwaukee, WI

Alan Stoudemire, MD†
Department of Psychiatry
Emory University School of Medicine
Atlanta, GA

Craig B. H. Surman, MD
Scientific Coordinator, Adult ADHD Research Program
Massachusetts General Hospital;
Assistant Professor of Psychiatry
Harvard Medical School
Boston, MA

Robert Swift, MD, PhD
Department of Psychiatry and Human Behavior
The Warren Alpert Medical School of Brown
University; and
The Center for Alcohol and Addiction Studies; and
The Providence VA Medical Center
Providence, RI

Jennifer J. Thomas, PhD
Department of Psychiatry
Harvard Medical School; and
Massachusetts General Hospital
Boston, MA

Mayanka Tickoo, MD
Department of Medicine
Tufts University School of Medicine
Boston, MA

---

†deceased

Lara Traeger, PhD
Department of Psychiatry
Harvard Medical School; and
Massachusetts General Hospital
Boston, MA

Hong-Phuc T. Tran, MD
Department of Geriatric Medicine
UCLA Medical Center
Santa Monica, CA

Nils R. Varney, PhD, ABPP
United States Naval Beaufort Hospital
Port Royal, SC

W. Victor R. Vieweg, MD†
Department of Psychiatry and Internal Medicine
Virginia Commonwealth University School of Medicine
Richmond, VA

Ana-Maria Vranceanu, PhD
Assistant Professor in Psychology
Department of Psychiatry
Harvard Medical School; and
Clinical Psychologist
Behavioral Medicine Service
Massachusetts General Hospital
Boston, MA

Jennifer Wallis, PhD
Department of Ophthalmology
Harvard Medical School; and
Massachusetts Eye and Ear Infirmary
Boston, MA

Tal E. Weinberger, MD
Clinical Assistant Professor
Sidney Kimmel Medical Center at
Thomas Jefferson University
Department of Psychiatry and Human Behavior
Philadelphia PA

Sarah R. Weintraub, PhD
Veteran's Administration Boston Healthcare System
Boston, MA

C. Donald Williams, MD, CGP
Academy of Organizational and Occupational Psychiatry
Yakima, WA

Linda L. M. Worley, MD
Mental Health Chief Physician Consultant,
VISN 16 Veterans Health Administration
Adjunct Professor of Medicine Vanderbilt University
Adjunct Professor of Psychiatry University of
Arkansas for Medical Sciences
Fayetteville, AR

Monique V. Yohanan, MD, MPH
Milliman Care Guidelines
San Francisco, CA

Mary C. Zeng, MD
Department of Psychiatry
Harvard Medical School; and
Massachusetts General Hospital
Boston, MA

Sidney Zisook, MD
Distinguished Professor
Department of Psychiatry
University of California-San Diego and
San Diego VA Healthcare System
La Jolla, CA

†deceased

PART I

DIAGNOSTIC METHODS

1.

PRINCIPLES OF MEDICAL PSYCHIATRY

Donna B. Greenberg and Barry S. Fogel

INTRODUCTION

Medical psychiatry is a medical specialty concerned with patients' mood, thinking, and behavior in the context of general medical or neurological conditions, surgery, and/or trauma. Medical psychiatrists view the longitudinal course of a medical illness in a full context of genetic, developmental, social, and environmental factors, and as a chapter in a life narrative. It is concerned with patients (1) who have medically unexplained physical symptoms or physical symptoms disproportionate to apparent pathology, (2) who have pain or other distressing symptoms that remain after their underlying medical condition has been treated, (3) who do not adhere to medically prescribed treatment, (4) whose high risk for medical conditions or complications can be reduced by behavioral changes, (5) whose chronic medical conditions have a course that is influenced by emotional factors, or (6) who have primary mental disorders concurrently with general medical conditions, where the treatment of the mental disorder must be modified in consideration of the medical conditions and their treatments or the general medical treatment must be modified in consideration of the mental disorder and its treatment. In all of these situations an integration of the perspectives of psychiatry, behavioral neurology, internal medicine, and health psychology can be useful.

THE CULTURAL ENVIRONMENT OF MEDICAL PSYCHIATRIC PRACTICE

Over the past few decades, general psychiatry has become more "medical," cognitive and behavioral neurology has burgeoned as a neurological subspecialty that shares a common certification process with the psychiatric subspecialty of neuropsychiatry, and general internal medicine has increasingly focused attention on behavior change and treatment adherence to close the gap between treatment efficacy and treatment effectiveness. Neuropsychologists have become essential partners to neurologists in the practice of cognitive and behavioral neurology, and psychologists specializing in behavioral medicine have established an important role in medical clinics. Thus, many disciplines have concerns overlapping with those of medical psychiatrists, and many individual practitioners in those disciplines have overlapping skills. However, medical psychiatrists have a distinctive combination of knowledge, skills, and perspectives drawn from general psychiatry, general internal medicine, neuropsychiatry and behavioral neurology, and health psychology. They have the capacity to take into consideration the biological implications of medical treatment and to consider the existential and moral issues faced by the patient and family as well as the neuropsychiatric elements of the patient's presentation. This book embodies the perspectives of the editors: one is a psychiatrist and neurologist and the other a psychiatrist and internist.

The advent of the serotonin reuptake inhibitor (SSRI) antidepressant drugs and second-generation neuroleptic drugs has made it easier for nonpsychiatrist physicians to undertake treatment of major depression and even some psychotic conditions. Tricyclic antidepressants, monoamine oxidase inhibitors, first-generation antipsychotic drugs, and lithium all have side-effect profiles and/or dosing issues that made their use especially challenging for nonpsychiatrists. At this time, the patients seen by medical psychiatrists often are already taking a psychotropic drug when they come for their first consultation. The medical psychiatrist becomes the specialist evaluating the therapeutic and adverse effects of already-present psychotropic agents in the context of medical illness. The dynamic is somewhat different in the medical-psychiatric context than it might be if the patient were independently coming to the psychiatrist for psychiatric diagnosis and treatment.

Advances in diagnostic technology, including new blood tests and new imaging procedures, have reduced the number of grossly missed diagnoses in patients with medically unexplained symptoms. It is now unusual to find patients diagnosed as hysterical who turn out to have their symptoms totally explained by a missed diagnosis like multiple sclerosis, lupus, or a slow-growing brain tumor. We more often encounter symptom amplification, a patient's nonacceptance of a diagnosis that is supported by valid diagnostic data, a patient's attachment to a diagnosis not supported by scientific evidence, or valid disagreements between the physician and the patient about how a known condition should be managed.

Advances in brain imaging, genetics, and psychopharmacology have brought about a change in the perception of mental disorders in the general population and among nonpsychiatric physicians. It is now widely accepted that most mental disorders are related to brain dysfunction, even in cases when they are initiated by or exacerbated by life events. Nevertheless, the psychiatrist is not yet seen by the general public as a type of clinical neuroscientist. Psychiatrists' training still emphasizes the ability to listen with empathy to patients' narratives, to perceive subtle emotional communication, and to understand patients' existential predicaments as well as their diagnoses. Nonpsychiatrists—both patients and health professionals—still perceive psychiatrists as in some way different from other physicians. These perceptions may include the attribution of esoteric skill, as well as less admirable attributes.

As more medical conditions are treatable, as life expectancy has increased, and as the cost of care escalates, the medical profession and the healthcare system in general have focused more on quality of life. Function and well-being are more often now explicitly described and measured. A focus on the patient's quality of life in the face of chronic illness or disability fits well with the tradition of integrating humanistic and physiologic perspectives on illnesses of all kinds. The medical psychiatrist asks, "How can I be helpful to this patient?" in the broadest sense, to increase function and quality of life as well as life expectancy and freedom from distressing symptoms. Some medical psychiatrists even venture to touch upon the meaning of life in their interactions with patients.

Ironically, another tradition in twentieth-century psychiatry—one that has been codified in the *Diagnostic and Statistical Manual* of the American Psychiatric Association and in the *International Classification of Diseases*—gives primacy to the classification of mental disorders by characteristic symptoms. This allows treatment, research, and reimbursement for care to be based on categorical diagnosis. This tradition of diagnostic classification by characteristic symptoms was motivated in part by the aim of making psychiatric diagnoses more reliable and thereby improving the quality of psychiatric research. This methodology is necessarily reductionist; in the absence of definitive biologic markers, it can convey specious precision in diagnosis. Nevertheless, formal psychiatric diagnosis by consensus criteria is essential to evidence-based practice. It is necessary but rarely sufficient for optimizing the overall outcomes of care in patients with multiple comorbidities.

Electronic medical records, the adoption of which in the United States has been heavily promoted by the federal government, have increased the standardization of clinical data and have improved the availability of such data to consultants. These records also permit the systematic application of decision support tools and predictive analytics at the point of care. At the same time, the use of such records for documenting physician services for billing and compliance purposes has filled electronic records with content of little clinical interest or professional perceptiveness; promiscuous cutting and pasting can propagate errors. Decision-making prompts such as drug interaction warnings, if generated too frequently and without priorities, tend to be ignored by busy clinicians. The care of patients with multiple and complex chronic conditions will generate huge volumes of data which can be opaque without systematic, intelligent data reduction and summarization. It frequently falls to the medical psychiatrist to put a surfeit of data into a patient-centered context, summarizing the present and past history in a way that acknowledges its meaning and import to the patient, sets priorities for action, weeds out erroneous and obsolete data, and highlights what is most important going forward.

The Internet has profoundly changed medical practice in ways that are especially relevant to medical psychiatrists. Getting information about medical conditions is now very easy for patients and families. Patients and families frequently come to visits with preformed ideas about the clinical situation rather than with completely open minds. In order to provide information about treatment options, the physician often must start with correcting misinformation. Sometimes online clinical information relieves patients' anxiety, but often it increases it. Specialists, including medical psychiatrists, are no longer gatekeepers controlling access to arcane knowledge. Instead they are interpreters, critics, and expert users of information that increasingly is available to all. Medical psychiatrists have an important role in summarizing and clarifying the data that exist and in using their expert communication skills to elicit and address patients' beliefs, including those arising from online self-study.

THE EVOLVING ROLE OF THE MEDICAL PSYCHIATRIST

Other aspects of the contemporary environment of medical practice affect what medical psychiatrists do and the challenges they face. These include (1) a trend toward institutional medical practice, with most physicians employed by hospitals, clinics, or group practices; (2) greater reliance on practice guidelines and other explicit and usually evidence-based standards of care; (3) greater use of screening tests and rating scales in routine practice, with quantitative measurement of care outcomes; (4) greater legitimacy of complementary and alternative medicine, with wider use of vitamins, herbs, and bodywork; and (5) devolution of most psychotherapy and psychosocial treatments to nonmedical disciplines.

The current system of physician payment in the United States has complex effects on medical-psychiatric practice. The current regulatory requirement that health plans cover mental health and substance abuse services potentially increases the supply of services. However, as long as such services are managed separately ("carved out") from general medical services, they create barriers to the integration of psychiatric and general medical care. Physician payment schedules do provide more compensation for longer visits with patients, but the requirements for documentation of longer visits bias the use of the physician's time toward broader scope rather than greater depth of interaction. Medicare and some other health plans pay individual physicians for coordination of care but don't usually cover interdisciplinary conferences. Some health plans engage in "gain sharing" with physician groups who make the care of chronic diseases more efficient; the physician group receives a percentage of the amount by which the total cost of caring for a clinical population was less than expected. Integrating medical and psychiatric care for patients with complex medical and psychiatric comorbidities can reduce overall costs and improve outcomes, but health systems have difficulty attributing benefits and rarely pay for medical-psychiatric services based on their economic value to the healthcare system. Overall, there is increasing recognition that patients with a combination of medical and psychiatric issues tend to be high utilizers of healthcare services, and that there would be financial as well as clinical benefits from more intensive management of their care. The editors believe that medical psychiatrists should have a major role in designing solutions for managing such patients, and that they will always have a direct role in finding individual solutions for the most complex and difficult of them.

The foregoing circumstances imply that the medical psychiatrist plays a range of different roles, addresses a range of different questions, and operates within a range of financial and organizational constraints. The traditional roles of the medical psychiatrist are (1) consulting to the patient's attending physician; (2) serving as a liaison between the psychiatry service and a nonpsychiatric specialty service, typically assisting with mental health screening, training of clinic staff on relevant psychiatric issues, program development, and interdisciplinary rounds and conferences; (3) engaging in ongoing treatment of individual patients' mental disorders, concurrent with the referring physician's treatment of the nonpsychiatric condition; and (4) when the medical psychiatrist is also fully trained in a general medical specialty, providing principal care to patients with problems within both psychiatry and their other specialty. More recently, some additional roles have emerged: (5) providing principal care to patients with comorbid psychiatric and medical problems when the latter are relatively stable and are less complex and demanding than the mental disorder(s); (6) managing and/or training multidisciplinary teams treating patients with medical-psychiatric comorbidities, especially those with depression and general medical illness (von Korff, 2011); and (7) serving as utilization reviewers or care managers on behalf of health plans or other payer organizations.

THE MIND–BODY PROBLEM

Throughout the entire literature of medical psychiatry, psychosomatic medicine and related disciplines, there is a residue of dualistic thinking. For example, major depression, which clearly comprises significant disturbances of brain metabolism, neurotransmission, endocrine regulation, and chronobiology, is called a "mental disorder," while migraine, a condition with no greater physiologic disturbance than major depression and equally great emotional accompaniments, is a called a (general) medical condition. Major depression frequently is associated with physical pain. Stress and sleep problems contribute to migraine attacks and to relapses of depression. Primary care physicians treat both depression and heart failure. The former is nonetheless called a "psychiatric problem," but the latter is not called a "cardiologic problem"; heart failure is described in relation to an organ system affected and not in relation to a specialty that frequently treats it.

There is some utility in grouping conditions in which disturbances of mood, thinking, and/or behavior are the exclusive or greatly predominant expressions of disease, such as obsessive-compulsive disorder or schizophrenia. Yet these conditions are not purely "mental" either. Neurologists do not treat them—not because they are not brain diseases but because historically they were not viewed as brain diseases and because caring for such patients requires skills not ordinarily taught in neurology residency. These conditions might usefully be viewed as "brain diseases with predominant behavioral symptoms" or as "brain diseases that typically present with behavioral symptoms."

The characterization of chronic pain illustrates further problems of nomenclature. In patients with chronic pain, the central nervous system has "learned to feel pain." Is the condition neurological if the learning takes place in the spinal cord and psychiatric if it takes place above the tentorium?

George Engel, by teaching medical students and physicians to focus on the patient's personal story and the experience of illness, highlighted the psychological and social context in the practice of medicine. With appreciation for the interaction of the psychological with the somatic, he described the "biopsychosocial" model of medical practice (Engel, 1977). More than 30 years later, "biopsychosocial" would be viewed for the most part by nonpsychiatric physicians as a psychiatric term of art. References to "psychiatric comorbidity" would be widely understood, but such terminology does not overcome the dualism of separating the psyche and the soma, the brain and the mind.

Nevertheless, diagnoses must be made and coded even when they rest on a shaky philosophical foundation. In this volume, contributing authors will refer to psychiatric illnesses, (primary) mental disorders, "mental and behavioral symptoms and syndromes," and "disorders of mood, cognition, and/or behavior." These are distinguished from "general medical illnesses," which are conditions typically within the ambit of nonpsychiatric specialties. Medical psychiatrists must be aware that patients, families, nonpsychiatric physicians, and nonmedical health professionals might think that "mental" illness is somehow in the mind rather than in the brain, or think of chronic pain that exceeds visible pathology as usually and primarily due to emotional disturbance. These viewpoints should be recognized as the prejudices that they are—ones to be elicited and then challenged if they interfere with a more constructive understanding of a patient's clinical problem.

THE MEDICAL-PSYCHIATRIC ENCOUNTER

CONTEXT

In its classic form a clinical encounter begins with a chief complaint, followed with a history of the present illness, prior medical history, developmental history, social and occupational history, family history, review of systems, and finally a physical examination. However, the medical-psychiatric encounter always takes place within a specific context and under specific constraints and expectations that will critically affect how the clinical work is done. The following outline describes what should be considered—explicitly or implicitly—prior to the first encounter with a medical-psychiatric patient.

1. Define the context of the encounter:
   a. Who are the interested parties?
   b. Will there be collateral sources of information?
   c. Are there caregivers, and how will they be involved?
   d. What is the purpose of the encounter?
   e. What is the definition of success?
   f. Is this a single encounter or the beginning of a relationship?
   g. How much time is available for the encounter, including both time with the patient and time needed for documentation and communication activities?

2. Assemble relevant background data:
   a. From the clinical record
   b. From outside clinical records
   c. Nonclinical data relevant to the problem
   d. Primary data (e.g., diagnostic images) rather than interpretive reports

3. Determine constraints on follow-up:
   a. Organizational (e.g., related to the site of care)
   b. Financial (e.g., related to what a health plan covers and what a patient would be willing to pay for uncovered services)
   c. Circumstantial (e.g., how long a patient will be in the hospital; where the patient usually lives)

4. Specify the work products:
   a. A note in the medical record
   b. A specific oral or written communication with a specific person or agency
   c. A specific oral or written communication with the patient
   d. Prescriptions, test requisitions, and other direct orders

While these considerations should precede the encounter with the patient, most of them need not be documented. In fact, more precise conception of the purpose of a medical-psychiatric encounter and the audience for the record of it sometimes can inspire shorter but more effective clinical records and communications.

DISTINCTIVE ASPECTS OF THE MEDICAL-PSYCHIATRIC HISTORY

The medical-psychiatric history contains the same elements as a general medical history, but there are different points of emphasis and differences in the scope and depth of the interview. It is most detailed in the areas necessary for the success of the clinical encounter.

Chief Complaint

The *chief complaint* in medical psychiatry often is not a complaint of the patient. In this situation someone else—for example, a physician encountering noncompliance with treatment or a family member unable to manage a patient's care at home—is the person with a problem to be solved with the medical psychiatrist's help. When the chief complaint is from the patient, it may be a complaint about the treatment rather than a complaint of a symptom of disease. It is perhaps best to replace "chief complaint" with an alternative term like "presenting problem" or "main issue"—implicitly if not explicitly.

History of the Present Illness and Its Three Dimensions

The *history of the present illness* in medical psychiatry has three dimensions. One dimension is the *history of the presenting problem*—one typically related to mood, cognition, and/or behavior, including health-related behavior. A second dimension is the history of *the patient's known general medical conditions* and how they are related in time to the presenting problem. The third dimension concerns the *impact of the predicament*—both the presenting problem and medical conditions—on the patient's life. This includes changes in functional capacity, in actual life activities, and in the meaning and enjoyment of life.

Past Medical History and Life History

The *past medical history* describes discrete illnesses, surgeries, and traumatic events as well as chronic or relapsing-remitting medical conditions. The special focus in medical psychiatry is on the *interaction* between general medical conditions, symptoms related to mood, cognition, and behavior (whether or not diagnosed as mental disorders), and functional performance. General medical conditions can be precipitated or aggravated by emotional stress. On the other hand, general medical conditions are themselves sources of emotional stress. General medical illness can precipitate or aggravate mental disorders, either via emotional stress or via direct physiological effects of the illness or its treatment. The general medical illness, the mental disorder, or the combination of the two can impair physical, instrumental, and/or social function. Functional impairment in turn can have both physical and emotional consequences, both directly and indirectly. The medical-psychiatric history comprises at least parallel histories of the patient's general medical, behavioral, and functional problems; at best it describes the interplay of the three (Viederman, 1984).

The *life history* is the biographical sketch on which the history of illness is superimposed. Relating the history of illness to the life history is relevant both for objectively gauging the severity of the patient's illness and for appreciating the subjective meaning of the illness to the patient. For example, a highly educated person with a neurodegenerative disease will fail simple bedside memory tests at a more advanced stage of brain disease than one with poor education and below-average intellect. And the loss of memory, when it comes, can be a more fundamental blow to the former individual's self-concept. Similarly, a talented athlete with a general medical illness who is now capable of only an average physical performance may be showing disease-related functional impairment, and the emotional impact of that impairment may be great if the patient's self-esteem or income are related to his athletic prowess.

The life history typically surveys family background, formal education, work, avocations, friendships, intimate relationships, current family relationships, and episodes of trauma, illness, financial problems, or other challenges and how they affected physical health, mental health, and relationships. It also touches on areas of success and accomplishment, and on what gives meaning and joy to the patient's life.

The agenda of obtaining a comprehensive life history can help the physician–patient relationship develop. A full life history is rarely obtained in an initial clinical encounter; it tends to be filled in gradually as a relationship develops between the clinician and the patient. Some elements come to the foreground on their own schedule when there is greater trust. As the relationship develops, the clinician "listens with the third ear" (Reik, 1948) for the emotional dimension of the patient's experience.

Social History: Relationships and Work

The *social history* places the patient in a nexus of relationships—intimate and nonintimate, related and unrelated to the care of the patient's illness. The medical psychiatrist is interested in (1) positive relationships that enhance the patient's life, (2) relationships that cause trouble for the patient, (3) relationships that have changed for the better or the worse in the time period of interest for the evaluation, and (4) relationships that are potential resources for helping the patient. Changes in relationships can be causes or effects of illness or can be unrelated.

The *occupational history* can be conceived in terms of time scales. The lifetime occupational history with information about finding and losing work, moving or changing jobs, relationships with employers, and so forth, can in many cases provide a "personality biopsy," particularly if the patient provides information about his health, activities, and emotional state while doing various jobs and while undergoing job transitions. The occupational history provides evidence related to all five major personality factors: extraversion, neuroticism, openness to experience, conscientiousness, and agreeableness (Costa & Widiger, 2002).

The *recent occupational history* can shed light on how the patients' illnesses have affected their occupational performance and how they have or have not adapted to their symptoms and impairments in physical and/or mental function. Discrepancies in severity between biological markers of disease, symptoms, functional impairments, and occupational performance lead to identification of both diagnostic issues and therapeutic opportunities.

The patient's *current work situation* should be considered as a physical environment, a social environment, and a set of performance requirements. The medical psychiatrist should attempt to build a mental picture of the patient's workplace. Exposure to toxic substances should be considered, although often the toxic personality of a boss or coworker is more relevant to the patient's health. The physical demands of the patient's work should be elicited by detailed questions if the clinician is not highly familiar with the patient's job. People with similar job titles can face different physical and emotional demands. Overtime, shift work, frequent travel across time zones, and other chronobiologic stresses are important given the medical significance of sleep quality and quantity. Falling asleep on a day job is likely to be noticed and is a virtually pathognomonic sign of excessive daytime sleepiness.

All patients should be asked if they have traveled abroad. A *geographical history* should be taken if there is any reason to believe the patient has traveled to places where unusual infectious diseases or parasitic infestations are prevalent. Patients involved in international business, those in the military, immigrants, family members of immigrants, and patients with international travel as an avocation fall into this category. In this context it is noteworthy that the anxieties of undocumented immigrants and their families about the risk of deportation can impede the development of trust and full disclosure of relevant information.

Substance Use History

The *substance use history* in general medicine usually comprises a few questions about alcohol and tobacco and a perfunctory question about illicit drugs. Medical psychiatrists can bring greater precision to the substance abuse history by considering the following:

1. Misuse of prescription drugs, especially opiates but also stimulants and benzodiazepines, is common. Medical patients, including those receiving concurrent psychiatric treatment, often are prescribed drugs that can be misused. Patients who have been prescribed these drugs should be questioned about how they use them, how frequently they refill their prescriptions, and whether more than one doctor or pharmacy is involved in providing their prescriptions. Suspicious, guarded, evasive, or inconsistent replies should be followed up with a fact check.

2. *How* substances are used, and not just the quantity used, matters. This is particularly important in medical-psychiatric patients, who can be more sensitive—or more tolerant—to the pharmacological effects of particular substances than an average person with no medical illness. Patients should be asked about the physical and mental effects of their usual dose of a substance and whether the substance is used in order to get a particular effect.

3. The illicit drugs most commonly used, the route of administration, and what the drugs are called vary between communities. Inquiry about illicit drugs is more productive when the questions asked are more specific.

4. Patients often come to medical settings having recently discontinued or cut down on their use of a substance, or having been forced to do so once they have begun medical treatment in an institutional setting. They may have given up a substance because they no longer tolerate it, because a physician told them to, or because they fear its adverse effects on their medical condition. Or, illness-related disability interferes with their ability to obtain their former drug of choice. Patients should be asked about discontinuation of substance use or changes in substance use as well as what they are using currently.

Functional History and Activity History

The *functional history* and *activity history* are concerned with what the patient is able to do—either alone, with supervision, with assistive devices, or with human assistance—and with what the patient actually does. Questions in this area, to be time efficient, should be centered on functions that are threatened by the patient's medical conditions. Functions reviewed comprise the following: (1) basic physical activities of daily living (ADLs) such as eating, bed mobility, transferring, walking, using the toilet, dressing, bathing, and grooming; (2) instrumental activities of daily living (IADLs) such as shopping, driving or using public transportation, communicating by telephone, mail, texting, or email, paying bills and managing money, and household maintenance; (3) parenting and caregiving activities appropriate to the patient's age and family situation; (4) social activities both individual and group; and (5) recreational activities.

The history often will include corroborating history from a collateral source such as a family member, friend, or nurse. Discrepancies between the patient's report and a collateral source report of functional capacity raise the issue of potential cognitive impairment or of minimization or amplification of symptoms—either by the patient or by collateral source. Discrepancies between what the patients can potentially do and what they actually do raise concerns about apathy, fatigue, or impaired executive cognitive function (see chapter 86).

Sexual History

The *sexual history,* like the occupational history, can be taken in relation to different time scales. The *lifetime sexual history* provides insight into gender identity and gender preference and into personality. It gives an indication of the patient's overall level of libido and in general how important sex is in the patient's life. It can indicate whether the patient's sexuality is oriented toward emotional intimacy, physical pleasure, or procreation, whether the patient has used sex manipulatively, and whether there are themes of dominance and submission or unusual sexual interests.

The *recent* or *illness-related* sexual history focuses on how the patient's sexual life has changed or not changed in connection with the illness and with contemporaneous changes in life situation and relationships. Illness-related changes in sexual activity can be either causes or effects. Given the wide variability of baseline sexual activity in the general population, the sexual history should include both the patient's current sexual activity and whether it represents a change from baseline. Also, how the patient feels about any change should be explored.

Medication History

The *medication history* should include details of nutritional supplements, herbs, and other complementary and alternative treatments. It should include any medications or supplements recently discontinued or changed in dosage, why the medications or supplements were changed, and whether there were symptoms associated with the change. It should include the history of any adverse reaction to a drug or supplement, especially adverse reactions that were either medically serious or emotionally disturbing. In addition to adverse reactions, patients should be asked about unusual reactions to medications even if they were not adverse; for example, did they have a euphoric reaction to a drug, or find that a tiny dose of a particular medication was nonetheless effective. Finally, the medication history should elicit differences if any between how medicines were prescribed and how they actually were taken. Patients frequently adjust dosages of medications to optimize effects and minimize side effects. They also may reduce the dosage or frequency of a medication if they cannot afford it. And, patients can think they are taking a medication as prescribed, while a subsequent pill count may show they were not.

Family History

An essential *family history* includes the health history and salient behavioral facts about all first-degree relatives, often expressed as a genogram. Because many mental disorders are not diagnosed, it is important to know if family members have had unusual symptoms or impairments that are potentially due to mental disorders, particularly focusing on familial mental disorders with symptoms related to those displayed by the patient. Hypomanic behavior often is recognized but not diagnosed as a mental disorder if it has some adaptive aspects. Likewise, depression that is apparently reactive to life circumstances may be viewed as normal by the patient or other informant. Also, nonprofessionals may lump chronic mental disorders with personality traits; a patient with generalized anxiety disorder may be seen as a nervous and worried person rather than someone with a chronic mental illness.

The timing of deaths in the family and the causes of death are data that can that can suggest a genetic predisposition to a disease that can shorten life expectancy. The early death of a parent can be a strong influence on a patient's emotional development. The death of a family member just before a new medical problem or flare-up of an old one suggests a potential causal relationship—typically one of contribution rather than sole causation. Concerns for children are an important dimension of the experience of illness for parents and grandparents. Family histories can change over time, with new diagnoses arising in family members as time passes.

Review of Systems

The *review of systems* in medical psychiatry differs from a generic review of systems in two ways. First, it explores the details of sleep and the details of eating in greater depth. Second, it reviews the status of chronic or relapsing-remitting conditions that are not actively symptomatic at the time of the interview. Such conditions are relevant to a holistic understanding of the patient and to comprehensive treatment planning. One common example is when a patient has no symptoms in a particular system because he avoids activities that provoke symptoms. The patient with COPD who stops walking outside the home because of fear of dyspnea can be more impaired by COPD than one who continues an active life but frequently complains of respiratory symptoms.

The review of systems conducted as a rapid series of closed-ended questions is not, in general, a good use of clinical time. When patients' cognitive and behavioral status permits, screening questionnaires followed up by targeted questions may be a more efficient route to the relevant facts. This topic is discussed at length in chapter 4.

Physical and Neurological Examination

The next chapter describes in detail the *physical and neurological examination* of the medical-psychiatric patient. Emphasis is placed on selected elements of the examination that will screen for dysfunction in an important system, quantify the severity of dysfunction by challenging the patient, or test diagnostic hypotheses.

Formulation and Intervention

The *formulation* builds toward a conclusion of how to be helpful to the patient. It begins with the listing of known and probable diagnoses and the current status of the patient's diseases and disorders. Current treatment, treatment options, and expected treatment results are delineated in the areas relevant to the presenting issue. Functional limitations are defined, and there is an appraisal of the severity of critical symptoms. These are understood in the context of the life history and coping strategies of the patient. With this background, the medical psychiatrist suggests *interventions* to address the presenting problem and, to the extent relevant in the given context, to improve the patient's function, well-being, symptom control, and medical prognosis. In moving from the assessment to a suggested intervention, the medical psychiatrist draws upon the base of specific knowledge and therapeutic principles described throughout this volume. Some principles are specific to particular medical specialties and clinical contexts, while some concepts apply to a range of settings and situations. These concepts are now described.

EXCESSIVE ILLNESS BEHAVIOR

Contemporary medical psychiatry has moved away from dichotomizing patients into those with "legitimate" or "organic" conditions and those with primarily "mental" problems. The concept of *excessive illness behavior* makes room for the complexity of person–disease interactions and medical–psychiatric comorbidity. It also comprises behavior ranging from normal expressions of distress to florid somatization. Principles of assessing and treating excessive illness behavior are similar across the spectrum of severity and complexity (see chapter 37).

Begin with Communication and Building Trust

In treating excessive illness behavior, the first principle is good communication. This begins with an interview that builds trust with the patient. The medical psychiatrist aims to understand who the patient is, what he cares about, and the meaning of the illness to the patient as a human being. The clinician must, to some extent, join the patient's reality as a precondition for leading him out of it.

Understand the Medical Realities

In order to engage productively with a patient who is displaying excessive illness behavior, medical psychiatrists must be personally satisfied that they know what is true about their patients' general medical conditions. This often requires assembling, reviewing, and if necessary reassessing the data; communicating with other physicians; and pursuing additional data and/or expert opinions. They can then clarify for the patient and/or concerned caregivers what is true, what is uncertain, and what is simply not so.

Facilitate Tolerance of Uncertainty

Since uncertainty provokes anxiety, the medical psychiatrist must acknowledge and facilitate the patient's coping with uncertainty. How this is done will depend on the actual level of uncertainty, the consequences of being wrong, the patient's personality, and the interpersonal context. Sometimes it is appropriate for a physician to act as an authority and be unequivocal; on other occasions it may be more useful to acknowledge uncertainty and to commit to close follow-up and frequent communication.

Link Stressors and Symptoms When Supported by the Data

Often the optimal intervention for a medical-psychiatric patient involves educating the patient about the connection between physical symptoms and psychosocial stressors. While this often appears obvious to clinicians, it is surprising how often patients do not make the connection until it is pointed out.

Apply Systematic Behavioral Analysis

For patients with excessive illness behavior, the behavior itself may amplify and sustain chronic illness or interfere with adherence to medically appropriate treatment and thus the chance of cure. Psychological, interpersonal, social, economic, and even political factors affect how episodes of illness are precipitated, sustained, experienced, and reported. In order to interrupt vicious circles of illness and maladaptive illness-related behavior, clinicians must first identify them, analyzing the antecedents and consequences of illness-related behavior and applying the results of the analysis to planning treatment—or, in some cases, to inform a decision *not* to pay attention to particular symptoms, complaints, and requests for help. This book's chapters on treatment adherence, on excessive illness behavior, and on personality and the physician–patient relationship present specific tactics for implementing this strategy.

Don't Expect the Patient to Accept a Psychiatric Diagnosis

Patients with excessive illness behavior can have obvious depression or anxiety but be resistant to seeing themselves as having any "mental disorder." The medical psychiatrist often sees clearly how depression or anxiety produce actual physical symptoms in addition to worsening the emotional experience of whatever other physical symptoms the patient might have. While psychiatrists can easily see the value of treating depression or anxiety if it is present, patients who view such treatment as delegitimizing their complaints will just say no—or perhaps find any treatment offered to be intolerable, inconvenient, or otherwise undesirable. Resolving the problem with empathic connection and a trusting physician–patient relationship is nice work if one can get it, but open-ended psychotherapeutic engagement often is not feasible in a busy clinical setting. For this reason it is well worth considering techniques for overcoming patients' resistance to treatment that have shown effectiveness in everyday practice settings, including motivational interviewing techniques, structured patient education, regularly scheduled general medical appointments not contingent on having complaints, and treatments with antidepressant drugs for an explicitly recognized nonpsychiatric indication.

Be Alert to Potentially Inappropriate Treatments

Patients with excessive illness behavior often get inappropriate treatments with adverse effects that cause or provoke a new illness or condition. In evaluating such patients and reviewing their medication lists, diagnostic procedures, hospitalizations, and surgeries, the medical psychiatrist should begin with skepticism and curiosity. After satisfying themselves as to the accuracy of the information provided, they should consider whether particular interventions were medically necessary or were deviations from standard practice. Such deviations can arise not only from direct or indirect pressures from patients, but also from countertransference. Physicians sometimes do too much when confronted with patients whom, in their hearts, they would prefer not to treat at all.

CIRCULAR PROCESSES

In most general medical conditions, and particularly those with frequent psychiatric accompaniments, the patient's behavior influences the course of illness. In addition to treatment adherence, the patient's diet, activities, and sleep patterns may affect clinical outcomes. These relationships can give rise to circular processes—positive feedback loops that make matters ever worse until the processes are interrupted by events, circumstances, or therapeutic interventions. These processes include:

1. Pain → Inactivity → Physiologic changes due to inactivity (e.g., cardiovascular deconditioning, joint contractures) → Increased pain

2. Pain → Treatment with opiates → Opiate tolerance and dependence → Increased pain

3. Chronic general medical disease → Nocturnal symptoms → Sleep disruption → Physiologic changes due to inadequate sleep → Worsening of general medical illness

4. Chronic general medical disease → Depression → Increased cortisol secretion, decreased sleep, irregular food intake, decreased physical activity → Worsening of general medical illness

5. Chronic general medical disease → Apathy → Nonadherence to treatment → Worsening of general medical disease

6. General medical disease → Toxic-metabolic encephalopathy → Cognitive impairment → Nonadherence to treatment → Worsening of general medical illness

7. Alcohol addiction → Alcohol-related diseases and conditions (e.g., cirrhosis, pancreatitis, traumatic brain injury) → Impaired executive cognitive function → Poor judgment → Increased drinking

8. Excessive illness behavior → Inappropriate tests, procedures, and treatments →Adverse reactions → Iatrogenic diseases and conditions → Increased illness-related behavior

9. Hostile, suspicious, and potentially litigious behavior → Defensive medicine → Anger over cost, inconvenience, discomfort and/or adverse effects of unnecessary or excessive procedures or treatments → Increased hostility and mistrust

10. General medical illness → Moods and behavior difficult for significant others → Deterioration or loss of important relationships → Emotional and physiological changes related to separation and to loss of social support → Worsening of general medical illness or its symptoms

NEUROPSYCHIATRIC PERSPECTIVES

Neuropsychiatry is a subspecialty distinguished both by the kind of patients and conditions it treats and by its perspective on symptoms and conditions—one that is particularly attentive to alterations in brain function associated with symptoms and conditions that are subjective or historically viewed as "mental." Since the late 1990s the neuropsychiatric perspective has been increasingly evident in medical psychiatry, applied not only to the psychiatric aspects of neurological diseases but also to the psychiatric aspects of other general medical illnesses. This neuropsychiatric perspective is applied not only to mental disorders but also to pain and to such symptoms as sleep disturbance, apathy, and fatigue.

As basic neuroscience progresses and the general public is more aware of the brain, physicians of all specialties are more open to the idea that chronic distress can change the anatomy, physiology, and chemistry of the brain in a way that contributes to future suffering. What is recurrent or persistent can become chronic, whether it be anxiety, depression, pain, the experience of trauma, or the craving for a mind-altering substance. Understanding this impels clinicians to intervene vigorously to reduce distressing symptoms and addictive behaviors. The medical psychiatrist keeps the hypothesis of persistent changes in brain function in mind when considering the patient's history of illness. The full story of a patient's illness, including what goes on when symptoms are not at their worst, is a basis for inferring that persistent changes in the brain have taken place. Reduction of symptoms and full remission of symptoms can have very different prognostic implications. With these considerations in mind, we introduce a neuropsychiatric viewpoint on some specific symptoms and syndromes that will be recurrent topics throughout this volume.

LONGITUDINAL PERSPECTIVE IS ESSENTIAL FOR ACCURATE DIAGNOSIS AND FORMULATION

Many neuropsychiatric conditions can only be accurately diagnosed by reference to their course over time; the choice among diagnostic alternatives cannot be made based on a single examination of the patient. These include the degenerative dementias, the spectrum of schizophrenia, and the spectrum of bipolar disorder. The medical psychiatrist may have the role of reminding other physicians of remaining diagnostic uncertainty or of seeking information about patients' past histories from outside records or collateral sources. Alternatively, they sometimes have to clarify for patients or families that a lack of diagnostic certainty is not the same thing as diagnostic ignorance or lack of useful understanding.

Consider the patient who presents with mild cognitive impairment, who probably has frontotemporal degeneration or Alzheimer-type pathology and whose cognition is getting worse but has not yet reached the point of frank dementia. When talking to the patient and family, the conclusion should not be "we're not sure what's wrong" or "we'll need to follow the patient over time to make a diagnosis." The patient and family need to know that the patient has a degenerative brain disease and has a prognosis of progressive loss of function. Life decisions and care decisions need to be made at a point where the prediction of prognosis is more certain than the prediction of postmortem brain pathology.

Conversely, a pathological diagnosis can be certain—as it would be in a case of Huntington's disease—yet there might be considerable uncertainty about prognosis in areas of great importance to life decisions and needs for care. The estimation of prognosis will combine data from genetic analysis with assessment of the rate of change in the signs of disease, comparing multiple data points. A question like "Will I need institutional care 2 years from now?" or "When will I have to stop driving?" has no definite answer. But medical psychiatrists, by integrating multiple longitudinal observations—clinical, imaging, neuropsychological—can do better than "I don't know."

When a patient with a general medical illness presents with a specific symptom or syndrome such as difficult-to-treat pain, excessive illness behavior, anxiety, depression, or resistance to treatment, it is useful whenever feasible to review the patient's response earlier in life to stresses similar to the current one. These stresses might be previous flare-ups of the current active medical problem, a different illness, or physical or psychological trauma. Some patients get anxious when they are physically sick, others get depressed, and still others get angry. Such dispositions are likely to be "hard-wired." Time relationships and potential causal relationships are variable and go well beyond a naïve concept of emotional reaction to illness. Episodes of clinical depression can precede and perhaps trigger episodes of relapsing-remitting general medical conditions; they can accompany them and possibly share an underlying neuroimmunologic basis or they may follow them, linked in various potential ways. Emotional reactions to the symptoms of illness, to the prognosis of the illness, or to actual or feared illness-associated functional, social, or occupational consequences, all are possible—as are psychiatric side effects of general medical treatments. There can be much to disentangle; knowing what happened on other similar occasions can be a guide.

DEPRESSION IS A DISEASE AND REMISSION IS THE GOAL OF TREATMENT

We view clinical depression as a relapsing condition that involves neurologic, endocrine, and chronobiologic dysfunction, and often has a somatic presentation. The longitudinal course of that disorder may track with the ups and downs of a comorbid chronic general medical disease, making everything less bearable. As further chapters document, a trial of antidepressant medication is appropriate in patients with chronic pain and/or distress from chronic unexplained symptoms whether or not they meet diagnostic criteria for major depression or they accept a diagnosis of depression. Optimal care of clinical depression entails the serious pursuit of remission of symptoms—not merely a measurable reduction in them. Before accepting that patients must reconcile themselves to chronic depression, a psychiatrist should ensure that the patient has had adequate trials of several different pharmacologic regimens—some of which involve multiple drugs, concurrent psychotherapy when feasible, and consideration of electroconvulsive therapy and repetitive transcranial magnetic stimulation. Medical psychiatrists specifically should add consideration of whether concurrent general medical conditions or their treatments, issues with treatment adherence, or genetic variations imply that an apparently adequate trial of a treatment actually was not adequate, or that a promising treatment was aborted for reasons that could have been avoided if the patient's specific circumstances had been appreciated. For example, patients might not tolerate an antidepressant drug at a usual dose because they are slow metabolizers of that drug. If the drug were given at a lower dose, it might be tolerated and effective. Medical psychiatrists' experience gives them a profound understanding of how bad depression can be—especially when combined with general medical illness—and how seriously its treatment must be taken.

ANGER CAN BE A CLINICAL PHENOMENON

A state of excessive and dysfunctional anger can accompany general medical illness in some patients. While it can be an enduring personality trait manifesting clinically because the patient is in a clinical setting, it also can truly be an illness-linked affect just like sadness or worry. While clinical anger in general medical populations can be measured by rating scales, it is has been much less well studied than depression and anxiety. Anger can be part of the syndrome of depression, or, like apathy, it can occur independently of it. It is worsened by physiological arousal—sympathetic activation—and by conditions that impair inhibition. Because it impairs patients' relationships with both clinical professionals and informal caregivers, anger deserves the medical psychiatrist's systematic consideration. The psychiatrist should consider whether the anger is a new problem or an old one; whether it is synchronized in some way with fluctuations in the general medical course; and whether it is associated with another neuropsychiatric syndrome. Also, clinicians should consider whether anger is part of an unfortunate circular process, where the physiologic accompaniments of anger, its impact on treatment adherence, and/or its impact on caregiving relationships make the medical outcome worse—and the patient angrier.

CHRONIC PAIN IS A CENTRAL NERVOUS SYSTEM DISORDER

The central nervous system (CNS) is altered by chronic exposure to a painful stimulus in ways that can sustain the experience of pain when the noxious stimulus is no longer present. For this reason chronic pain can be viewed as a disorder of the CNS. This disorder involves chronic sensitization—changes in neurons and synapses that make them more excitable by normal, nonnoxious stimuli (Woolf, 2011). These changes are persistent but not necessarily irreversible. Furthermore, long-term exposure to painful stimuli causes changes in limbic and cerebellar circuits that can give rise to depressive symptoms and avoidance behavior. Persistent pain impairs executive cognitive function, with consequences for organization, planning, resistance to distraction, persistence, judgment, and self-awareness. Sleep architecture and endocrine function can be disrupted as well. The depressed mood and apparently self-defeating behavior of many patients with chronic pain is rooted in widespread alterations in brain function. Effective treatment and restoration of normal health and function will require far more than analgesics, and problems with treatment adherence early in the process can be anticipated.

ADDICTION IS A BRAIN DISEASE THAT AFFLICTS THE WILL

The neuropsychiatric viewpoint on addiction is that it is a chronic disorder of brain function with frequently severe social complications. Addressing addiction requires that the physician face and make peace with the duality of mind and brain. Addicts are afflicted by a condition that is not entirely under their control, but at the same time they must exert their will to do something about it. Like people with many other kinds of maladaptive behavior, addicts have trouble "bringing the future into the present"—being aware at the point of temptation of the future harm of indulging their addictions and being able to translate that awareness into effective inhibition of the addictive behavior. Medical conditions and their symptoms can increase motivation for addictive behavior—for example, pain can lead to a desire to take narcotics—and they can decrease self-awareness or inhibitory capacity, especially when the conditions or their treatments impair the function of the frontal lobes or their connections. Completing a potentially vicious circle, addictive behavior—especially the abuse of alcohol or drugs—can cause or exacerbate medical conditions that increase the patient's vulnerability to future addictive behavior (see chapter 38).

Given the potential harm that addiction to narcotics can bring, physicians treating persistent pain can face a conflict between the imperative to take pain seriously and the imperative to prevent the suffering of addiction. As there is no definitive test for determining vulnerability to addiction, analysis of the patient's biography—how the patient has adapted to illness, stress, and other challenges over the life course—can aid in the judgment of which reports by the patient can be trusted and which must be independently verified. Instruments for measuring cognitive, instrumental, social, and occupational functioning can have a role, as can the critical review of records and timely interviews with collateral sources. All of this data gathering and consideration typically falls between the acute phase of pain treatment—when relief is the highest priority—and the commitment to longer-term therapy with or without agents that can become substances of abuse.

CHRONIC FATIGUE AND APATHY ARE MAJOR SYMPTOMS SEPARABLE FROM DEPRESSION

Fatigue and fatigability are subjective experiences. Apathy, a tripartite phenomenon comprising a lack of concern, a lack of feeling, and a lack of motivation, is more directly apparent in its more severe forms. Both have the objective consequence of decreased activity—a consequence that can worsen the prognosis of many diseases and conditions via physical deconditioning, decreased treatment adherence, and/or direct metabolic consequences such as insulin resistance. Both fatigue and apathy reflect neurophysiological disturbances, apathy being exclusively a CNS phenomenon while fatigue has a neuromuscular dimension as well. Gross brain diseases, neuromuscular diseases, and the indirect effects of endocrine dysfunction, systemic inflammation, and sleep disturbance can cause apathy and/or fatigue. Drugs prescribed for either psychiatric or general medical indications can have apathy and/or fatigue as side effects.

Depression and anxiety can have apathy and/or fatigue as accompaniments. However, many patients have the latter without the former and might reject the diagnosis of depression or anxiety if it were proposed by the physician. Treatment directed at relieving fatigue generally is well received by patients. Identifying apathy and/or fatigue as a focus of intervention stimulates the exploration of the underlying causes, which usually include physiologic as well as strictly emotional factors (see chapter 34).

SLEEP DESERVES MORE ATTENTION THAN IT OFTEN GETS

People sleep for between a quarter and a third of their lives. The quality and quantity of a patient's sleep is strongly related to his overall well-being, and sleep has—like several of the other cardinal neuropsychiatric symptoms—a reciprocal relationship with health, function, activity, and well-being. Detailed inquiry about the subjective and objective features of sleep is always relevant and sometimes crucial to optimal formulation and treatment planning. Both primary and secondary sleep disorders are common in the medical-psychiatric population; a typical situation is the obese patient with depression, hypertension, the metabolic syndrome, and obstructive sleep apnea. Recognition and effective treatment of the sleep apnea is crucial to a favorable long-term outcome.

While an adequate amount of restful sleep is essential, helping medical-psychiatric patients obtain it often is difficult. For example, many patients with obstructive sleep apnea do not wear their continuous positive airway pressure (CPAP) masks all night. The key point is that it is really worth trying to get the patient's sleep right because doing so will necessarily help many other things, and finding the reasons for poor sleep is likely to be otherwise useful. Furthermore, patients find inadequate sleep to be unacceptable, and forming an alliance with a physician around sleep improvement can be easier than forming one that is explicitly *psycho*therapeutic (see chapters 9 and 33).

COGNITIVE IMPAIRMENT IS EVERYWHERE

It is increasingly appreciated that cognitive impairment without delirium or frank dementia is widespread in general medical contexts. Examples include patients with prolonged stays in intensive care units, those who have had open heart surgery with hours on cardiopulmonary bypass, those who have had intensive cancer chemotherapy, and those with persistent attention deficit hyperactivity disorder; there are dozens more. The nondementia cognitive impairments seen in general medical contexts are more evident on

neuropsychological testing or on high-sensitivity bedside examinations than they are on brief informal mental status testing or on instruments like the Mini-Mental State Examination (Folstein et al., 1975) interpreted with its usual cutoff scores. They are functionally significant—causing patients and their families concern and sometimes distress, affecting performance in work both at formal occupations and at home, and altering the quality of interpersonal relationships. The medical psychiatrist is often the first physician to appreciate the extent and relevance of illness-associated cognitive impairment. A factually informed empathic connection with the patient and/or caregivers concerning the cognitive impairment and associated changes in mood and behavior can be a great relief to those who are worried. Follow-up includes steps to limit the adverse effect of the cognitive impairment on treatment adherence and to promote the avoidance (when feasible) of treatments that might make it worse. Depending on the severity of the impairment and its prognosis, the medical psychiatrist might need to help with issues ranging from disability status to driving safety to legal competence.

As in other medical-psychiatric contexts, the cognitive impairments associated with general medical illness occur on top of a "cognitive life story." Lifelong learning disabilities or intellectual gifts can affect the relationship between the magnitude of the insult to the brain and clinically observed performance; they also change the meaning and significance of cognitive impairment to the patient. A mathematician who loses the ability to calculate because of a brain disease is likely to have far more brain damage than a patient with the same current impairment who had difficulty with math before dropping out of high school. And, the former patient probably will have greater awareness of the loss and will suffer more from it. Patients in an early stage of a degenerative brain disease with at most mild cognitive impairment can suddenly become demented when illness-associated cognitive impairment is superimposed. Sometimes the syndrome is one of delirium evolving into dementia, but in other cases the patient never has an altered sensorium. When an older patient develops obvious cognitive impairment from a medical illness or treatment-related brain insult that usually causes mild or minimal cognitive symptoms, the pre-illness history should be reviewed in depth for evidence of prodromal dementia.

PHYSICIAN–PATIENT RELATIONSHIPS AND TREATMENT ADHERENCE CAN BE NEUROPSYCHIATRIC ISSUES

Optimal physician–patient relationships require that the patient show active participation, attention, concentration and memory, expressive language and accurate comprehension, short-term memory, and executive cognitive function, along with the ability to trust, to confide, and to accept care. Adherence to treatment requires the same things, with the added challenge in most cases of carrying out the plan of treatment amidst all of the distractions of real life in an environment that may lack cues and controls that reduce executive demands. There are many ways in which these prerequisites for optimal treatment relationships can be disrupted by a wide range of gross brain diseases and by primary mental disorders. An attention deficit, a paranoid psychosis, a subtle deficit in comprehension of orally presented material, or amnestic mild cognitive impairment (and these are just a very few examples) can cause a patient to miss an appointment or not to take medication as prescribed. Personality conflicts, miscommunication, and practical barriers also play a role, but these have always been considered by psychiatrists asked to assist when general medical treatment is not working. What is new is a greater emphasis on the neuropsychiatric possibilities.

DISABILITY SHOULD BE DECONSTRUCTED

Neuropsychiatric conditions can interact with general medical illness to produce functional disability; the combination of the two can disable a patient when neither the general medical illness nor the neuropsychiatric problem would be disabling in itself. Because of their perspective, medical psychiatrists often are effective advocates for such patients when they are seeking disability benefits, accommodations at the workplace, or simply the understanding of their loved ones (see chapter 86).

While explanation and advocacy are useful, they occasionally conflict with the agenda of treatment, particularly when the goal is to eliminate or mitigate the disability. For example, the clinician may want to convince an insurance company that a bad back plus a major depression make a full day's work impossible, while at the same time wanting to convince the patient that effective treatment of the depression and progressive mobilization can restore function even if the anatomy of the lumbar spine doesn't change.

THE IMPORTANCE OF SPECIALIZED MEDICAL KNOWLEDGE

Many chapters of this book educate readers about specific medical conditions, their usual treatments, and what patients with them suffer. When doing psychotherapy with patients going through rigorous treatments of serious medical conditions, it is essential to know what the treatments are like and what experiences the patient might still have in store. When working with patients with somatoform disorders or excessive illness behavior, it is essential to know the details of the symptoms, diagnosis, and treatment of the "organic" medical disease along with the symptoms that are amplified or mimicked.

KNOW THE MEDICAL FACTS AND APPRECIATE THE SUBJECTIVE EXPERIENCE OF THE ILLNESS

For example, the neurological evaluation of patients with nonepileptic seizures (NES) is much like the evaluation of patients with epileptic seizures. Once NES has been diagnosed and a decision has been made to discontinue antiepileptic drugs now thought unnecessary, the approach to discontinuing the antiepileptic drug is much like the one that would be taken in a patient with epilepsy. Since many patients have both epileptic and nonepileptic seizures, medical psychiatrists treating patients with NES must be equipped to detect any emerging evidence for epilepsy—or other neurological disorders—even as they help patients to identify and deal with stressors differently and to accept diagnosis and treatment for any primary mental disorder they also have. Familiarity with electroencephalography and its limits, antiepileptic drugs and their pharmacology, side effects, interactions with psychotropic drugs, and the symptomatology of unusual types of epileptic seizures are all needed to provide optimal *psychiatric* care for such patients.

The discussion of NES illustrates a perspective that applies to many other medical specialty contexts. Whether it is working with burn victims or patients with end-stage renal failure, an effective medical psychiatrist must understand the symptoms and the treatments the patient with the illness will experience—the subjective dimension—as well as the objective facts of how the disease and its treatments affect the brain and how psychotropic medications affect the disease and interact with its treatments.

COMPREHENSIVELY ANALYZE MEDICATION ACTIONS AND INTERACTIONS

Comprehensive review of the medication list has always been critical in medical-psychiatric consultation. The medical psychiatrist may be the first physician to collect all of the relevant data—especially when complementary and alternative treatments, borrowed medications, or drugs taken not as prescribed are involved, or when there are issues of substance abuse. Psychiatrists may be more assiduous in pursuing collateral source information or in gaining their patients' confidence so that they disclose additional facts; the greater legal protection for the confidentiality of psychiatric data can be relevant as well. Medications recently discontinued can have as much impact on the brain as those recently started—so the recent history of medication changes must be included when the medication list is considered. Information about potential drug interactions and side effects is extremely easy to obtain over the Internet or through databases linked to electronic medical records, but deciding what information is truly significant is nontrivial. The time sequence of medication changes and symptom changes helps, but the medical psychiatrist can bring some additional assets: (1) consideration of individual differences, such as differences in the genetics of drug metabolism and differences in the tolerability of different types of side effects; (2) elicitation of the patients' subjective experience of medications and of the meaning to them of relying upon—or simply of taking—certain medications; (3) detailed and structured observation of the patient's cognitive and affective mental status—often a sensitive indicator of medication toxicity; and (4) collaborative dialogue about the relative importance of taking, risks of taking, and risks of not taking particular medications.

CONSIDER FUNCTION AS WELL AS SYMPTOMS

A recurrent theme in medical psychiatry is that in chronic diseases, the goal of treatment cannot be presumed: once cure is off the table, goals may differ among patients and between patients and their physicians. For some patients relief of particular symptoms is paramount, but for others the preservation of particular functions or continuation of particular activities matters more. Physical and mental activity promotes health, as does positive emotional engagement in both intimate and nonintimate relationships. Functional impairments can lead to changes in social and/or economic status that worsen the prognosis for both physical and mental conditions. The issue of functional versus symptomatic outcomes is salient for some patients with chronic pain: inactivity and narcotic analgesics can bring them short-term reduction in pain at the cost of greater chronic impairment.

HELP PATIENTS ADDRESS GENETIC INFORMATION

As the cost of genotyping falls rapidly and the association of genes with diseases is better understood, patients and their families will get ever more information about their genetic differences and their genetic risks. For major conditions determined by a single gene or chromosomal abnormality, it is likely that genetic testing will be clinically motivated, the results will be unambiguous, and genetic counseling will be readily available. The task of genetic counselors has been to interpret family and medical histories to assess the chance of a disease, educate about inheritance, genetic testing, management, and prevention and to promote informed choices about the condition (see chapter 64). The broad availability of genotyping will necessarily change what genetic counselors do, as they will increasingly have to help patients make sense of their genotypes in situations where there are statistical associations of genes with diseases, but the precise pattern of inheritance isn't known. Analysis of the family tree will provide an initial estimate of risk of a condition that does not manifest until later in life, such as vulnerability to cancer or dementia; knowing the genotype will help refine it. Knowing that one is at risk for a particular disease may be least emotionally burdensome when it points the way to an action that will reliably prevent the disease, even if that action is an unpleasant one. It is most burdensome when nothing can be done to prevent an awful illness like Huntington's disease. At all points on the continuum, powerful emotions like fear, guilt, anger, and the pain of loss can occur and can be helped by the medical psychiatrist's informed empathy; and here, as elsewhere, the clinician can help patients tolerate unavoidable uncertainty. Realizing that misconceptions and overinterpretation of genetic data are always possible, solid knowledge of the specialized medical facts is the point of departure. In clinical genetics, the facts will change from year to year as the big data from widespread genotyping are successfully analyzed, challenging clinicians to stay informed about the genetic issues relevant to their long-term patients.

PUT PRACTICE GUIDELINES IN THEIR PROPER PLACE

Evidence-based practice guidelines are rapidly finding a place in American medicine, moving from statements of ideals to criteria for performance evaluation and payment of clinicians. For many years physicians have resisted practice guidelines because of a conviction that medicine is an art as well as a science, and that patients can have crucial individual differences from statistical norms on which the much of the evidence behind guidelines is based. However, most patients are *not* outliers, and a universal and generic objection to practice guidelines is merely an excuse. Most patients will do better if their physicians follow guidelines rather than improvise (see chapter 88).

Medical psychiatrists, however, specialize in seeing exceptions to rules. Medical-psychiatric patients have multiple comorbid conditions, and the guidelines for one condition can be incompatible with the guidelines for another. Drug interactions, genetic variations, and behavioral differences, all can make a guideline inappropriate for a particular patient.

The broad multispecialty perspective of medical psychiatry is useful in framing the case that a particular patient should be treated outside of guidelines and excluded from the calculation of aggregated outcomes. Nonetheless, medical psychiatrists encounter patients treated outside of practice guidelines who would clearly do better if their physicians followed the guidelines and did not view them as exceptions. Whether the reason for the physician's inappropriate deviation from standards is related to countertransference, misdiagnosis, or lack of skill, the medical psychiatrist can effectively advocate for patients to get the standard treatment they need and to avoid the ill effects of inappropriate treatment. For medical psychiatrists working in smaller medical communities where physicians must get along even when they disagree, advocacy of this kind calls upon skills in diplomatic and tactful communication. On occasion it is helpful to suggest that a practice guideline be followed "to relieve the patient's anxiety."

UNDERSTAND WHY SPECIALIST OPINIONS MAY DIFFER

Medical psychiatrists can become adept at recognizing when patients are outliers or special cases who will need nonstandard treatment or modification of how standard treatment is delivered. In addition to patients with complex comorbidities and genetic differences, mental and behavioral factors including personality can also be good reasons for deviation from guidelines. When medical psychiatrists suspect that the treatment of a general medical condition needs to change to improve its outcome—whether the change is toward greater or lesser compliance with practice guidelines and local customs—a second opinion is likely to be part of the strategy. Whether they give, receive, or interpret second opinions, medical psychiatrists should appreciate that when the second opinion does not confirm the first there is a conflict to be resolved, and they can assist with that resolution. A tie-breaking third opinion usually is not the answer.

A basic approach to reconciling conflicting second medical opinions is to begin with the question of whether the two physicians were working with the same facts—for example, accessing the same set of records, images, laboratory results, and medical history. Next is the question of whether particular facts were interpreted differently—for example, whether a particular image was read as normal or abnormal. If facts and their interpretations are aligned, the medical psychiatrist questions whether different inferences and judgments from the facts are based on different supplementary information and different principles of inference, for example, whether the two physicians applied different diagnostic criteria. Finally, different recommendations for action may be based on different presumptions about the goals and constraints of treatment or different knowledge about the patient's preferences. When the reasons for a difference of opinion are elucidated, it often becomes clear which opinion is more applicable in the given case (see chapter 82).

THE RELATIONAL PERSPECTIVE

Just as a patient's illness occurs within a life story, it occurs within a nexus of relationships—intimate and nonintimate, familial, social and professional. A vast literature of social psychology has established the relevance of adequate and healthy social relationships to optimal physical health. While the main focus of most medical psychiatrists—like most general psychiatrists—is individual patient encounters, it has always been known that changes in the social network can greatly help or harm patients.

Not only are social relationships important to health and to healthcare, but function within relationships is an essential expression of human existence that can be altered for better or worse by illness. Relevant factors include (1) the predicament of illness, with issues ranging from financial stress, disruption of daily routines by caregiving, competing loyalties and obligations, and the fear of loss; (2) changes in cognitive function due to the illness or its treatment, which in turn influence interpersonal communication and social behavior; (3) the patient's emotional reaction to illness; (4) empathy or the lack of empathy on the part of others for the patient or on the part of the patient for others; (5) where the patient is in the course of life; and (6) the expectations and needs of others from the patient.

Direct intervention in family and other interpersonal relationships—for example, family or couples therapy or a caregivers' support group—is an appealing option when it is obvious that such relationships are a locus of distress or are adversely affecting treatment outcomes. However, one can only treat nonpatients when they agree to be treated. Referrals to nonmedical family therapists or to support groups may not be accepted even when offered very appropriately.

In general medical settings it is routine for physicians to talk with concerned family members, and it is usual for this to be done with the informal assent of the patient, especially if the patient is acutely ill. When medical psychiatrists are knowledgeable about the patient's general medical issues and have a strong working relationship with the patient's principal physician or specialty service, they can be in a particularly strong position for engaging family members in dialogue. If medical psychiatrists are a regular part of a specialty service team, they might even be sought out spontaneously by family members interested in their advice and opinions. In all circumstances when the patient is competent, it is essential to seek the patient's unambiguous consent first and to define both with the patient and the family the scope and the aims of the conversation.

In formulating a case and contemplating intervention, consideration should be given to several types of relationships and how they might facilitate a better outcome or relieve the patient's distress: physician–patient relationships, family relationships, nonfamilial social relationships, and spiritual/religious relationships whether with clergy, other believers, or the divine.

The medical psychiatrist should consider how the patient's illness affects what he does for others. When illness makes a patient less able to care for a spouse or a child, feelings of anxiety and guilt can be more distressing to the patient than physical pain. Similarly, while impaired occupational function due to illness can cause distress because of its financial implications, the more salient loss for many patients is the social context of work and the existential meaning of being productive.

PHYSICIAN RELATIONSHIP TO PATIENT-FORMS A CONTINUUM FROM EXPERT TO HEALER

The role of a medical psychiatrist ranges from that of a technical expert to that of a healer. Physical illness and its discomforts, losses, and threats can induce psychological regression and intensify transference, for better or for worse. In typical medical-psychiatric contexts, transference is recognized and managed or utilized but rarely interpreted. In particular the discussion of negative transference is interpreted only to the extent helpful in reducing disruption of treatment. Medical-psychiatric consultations in the hospital are intense brief encounters, where positive transference, if present, can be used to promote a better adaptation to illness. Ongoing involvement of the medical psychiatrist in the care of a chronic disease is a less intense but more open-ended relationship in which, at best, the patient feels the psychiatrist is a part of his life and potentially available to help at times of distress or challenge, offering empathic companionship and expert advice as the patient faces the existential challenge of illness. In long-term treatment, medical psychiatrists build the patient's trust through repeated demonstrations of skill and empathy. Once trust is established, clinicians can positively influence even those patients who did not have a positive transference to them at the outset.

Medical psychiatrists can make therapeutic use of the power of positive transference only when such transference is present and when their own feelings toward a patient are positive. When either transference or countertransference is negative, it is usually best to assume the role of the technical expert and aim to limit the intensity of the physician–patient relationship. Referral to another psychiatrist sometimes is an option; when it is not, one should consider whether there is a preexisting positive relationship with a general medical physician that could be an effective psychotherapeutic channel if that physician is willing and is appropriately advised.

BRIEF INDIVIDUAL PSYCHOTHERAPY IS POWERFUL

A significant part of many medical psychiatrists' practices comprise patients without major Axis I or Axis II disorders, who, under the extraordinary stress of general medical illness or physical trauma, develop mental and behavioral symptoms and seek psychotherapeutic help. Many such patients get great benefit from relatively brief psychotherapy. The therapist's activities include some combination of educating the patient on the facts of the general medical condition, identifying and explaining the patient's emotional and behavioral responses to the sick role, analyzing changes in important personal relationships, and assisting the patient in solving life problems associated with the illness. The medical psychiatrist is flexible and pragmatic, deciding at any given time whether introspection, empathy, emotional support, or practical assistance is most appropriate. Negative transference is addressed only when it directly interferes with treatment and is interpreted in a circumscribed manner so as to overcome the patient's resistance without mobilizing intense affects that could be potentially disorganizing. The conceptual framework and therapeutic language can be that of psychodynamics or that of cognitive-behavioral therapy; the essential work is the same either way. Patients are helped to understand their situations more clearly, to face them with less anxiety and more thoughtfulness, and to identify and utilize their inner and external resources (see chapter 10).

FAMILY THERAPY CAN HELP FAMILIES MEET THE CHALLENGE OF ILLNESS

Serious general medical illness or trauma challenges families to face new practical demands while coping with their emotional reactions to the illness or injury of someone they love. Families' habits of communication, ways of dividing work, and consensus (or lack of consensus) about familial obligations that may have been acceptable prior to the medical event can emerge as dysfunctional in the new context. If a family didn't see their usual ways as a problem before the medical event, they are unlikely to suddenly become introspective and self-aware just because there is a medical crisis. The medical psychiatrist's identification of issues of problematic family functioning must be gradual and tactful when the family has not yet granted the psychiatrist a license to treat anyone except for, possibly, the patient with the medical illness. Often the most acceptable place to start is by providing information to the family if this is acceptable to the patient. Assessing and attempting to improve communication within the family around illness-related issues is a relatively nonthreatening next step. Moving on to more sensitive issues concerning obligations, loyalties, and conflicts is conditional on establishing

trust and family consensus on a common agenda. If the latter do not develop after a few meetings with a family, it is probably better to focus on the individual rather than attempt to persuade or entice a family into conjoint treatment (see chapter 11).

CONSIDER THE PATIENT'S ROLE AS A PARENT

When patients are parents of dependent children, the parental role is almost always one of their most important concerns along with their occupation and their intimate relationships. It is thus curious that while physicians virtually always ask patients about their work, they sometimes do not ask them about their children and parental relationships. Even when a medical-psychiatric patient does not present with a problem related to parenting, the medical psychiatrist should routinely ask all adult patients if they are parents and, if so, to try to learn a bit about each of their children in terms of age, temperament, functioning, coping abilities, specific challenges, and so forth. Parents usually like discussing their children. An open-ended inquiry such as "Tell me about your children" often can enhance the relationship between the clinician and the patient while eliciting important information. When the patient is a less-experienced parent of children under the age of 6 years, the clinician might make the point that very young children feel more secure and cope better with stress when routines and nonparental caregivers are as consistent as possible. Clinicians can think creatively with parents about how to engage supports and utilize resources to increase consistency for their children.

When children are old enough to understand the parent's illness and anticipate potential future events such as medical emergencies, the clinician can help parents plan how they will talk with their children about what is wrong and what might happen. When the children are adolescents or young adults, they can be of significant practical help to their parents; helping a sick parent can be a positive experience if it is not so demanding as to completely disrupt other aspects of the child's life. In this situation the clinician can help parents figure out what it is reasonable to ask of their children and how to effectively communicate their condition, their needs, and their concerns for their children's welfare (see chapter 12).

GROUP THERAPY HAS A SPECIAL PLACE IN MEDICAL PSYCHIATRY

Group therapy, which actually had its origins in support groups for patients with general medical illness, can be preferable to individual psychotherapy for some medical-psychiatric patients. These include patients who are anxious and uneasy with the one-on-one context of individual psychotherapy, preferring to hear others talk about their issues before speaking up about their own. They also include patients who see individual psychotherapy as stigmatizing or as a sign of weakness, but who wouldn't have the same negative view of a "support group" for people with the same illness. Group therapy for patients with general medical illness and associated emotional issues has empirically demonstrated benefits for mood, pain, and life adjustment. While evidence that group therapy affects longevity or the course of a major medical illness like cancer is inconclusive (though suggestive), there is better evidence for psychiatric benefits. The greatest constraint on the effectiveness of group therapy for medical-psychiatric patients is the availability of a suitable group at the point in a patient's course of illness when emotional concerns are in the foreground and the patient is motivated to accept the referral. In a large metropolitan area there is likely to be a suitable group when it is needed, but if it is not associated with the same hospital, doctors, or provider network, a referral might not be feasible. It is not known whether groups for people with varied medical conditions are as effective in general as groups for people who all have the same illness, but more homogeneous groups are more likely to provide patients with practical suggestions for coping with the specific challenges of an illness like breast cancer or lupus. In the end, starting with the belief that group therapy for medically ill patients is a good idea and using local experts and online social networking, the patient or the physician often can find a resource. Those who believe in the special virtues of group therapy for the medically ill note the following: (1) group therapy allows patients access to emotional support, and to learn new interpersonal and coping skills without identifying themselves as abnormal; (2) patients discover they are not unique in their predicaments, and this can relieve feelings of existential isolation and personal misfortune; (3) as patients see how others cope with the challenges of illness they come to respect others' efforts, leading to greater respect for their own; (4) listening to others' accounts of their experiences, patients may feel that their own experiences are understood and validated; and (5) patients have the opportunity to help others, an activity that is intrinsically satisfying and meaningful. Some patients will be comforted by knowing that others are worse off. Meeting and getting to know and coming to care about another patient with a worse case of the same illness can have a different and more positive emotional effect than merely knowing that such patients exist.

SPIRITUAL EXPERIENCE IS UNIVERSAL AND WORTH EXPLORING

All human beings are capable of an experience and viewpoint that might be called "spiritual"; the experience of spirituality does not require religious belief or affiliation. The spiritual state of mind is a peaceful one of secure attachment and "remembered wellness"; some patients can attain it despite current pain, anxiety, and actual separation from or loss of loved ones. Medical psychiatrists work with their patients to find internal and external resources for facing the emotional challenges of illness. In this context they should elicit information about patients' spiritual experiences and orientation. The clinicians who simply show openness to and interest in their patients' spirituality can encourage them to make use of it; shared belief is not necessary (see Waldfogel & Wolpe, 1993, and chapter 18).

SUMMARY

Medical psychiatry might be described as a specialty in which outliers are the norm and exceptions are the rule. While general medical illness and ultimately mortality are universals of the human condition, most people cope with illness without psychiatric assistance. Patients come to us—or are sent to us—because they are different in some way. The differences medical psychiatrists encounter in the practice comprise a broad range that includes comorbid primary mental disorders, gross brain lesions in regions that affect emotional experience or emotional communication, CNS side effects of general medical drugs, genetically based variations in drug metabolism, challenging family circumstances, past trauma, substance abuse, and personality traits that impede coping with a particular illness. Beginning with the differences that create problems, we then look for differences that might help with solutions, a search that also covers a broad range.

The specialty requires that clinicians know at the outset a little bit about a lot of things—so they can quickly grasp the gist of the patient's problem and formulate the right questions. The clinician also must know about the patient's specific conditions and treatments in great detail, with appreciation of their nuances and subjective aspects.

The perspective of medical psychiatry is simultaneously episodic and longitudinal. The problem at hand usually is related to the patient's present coping with a current medical situation, but both the problem and the solution are best understood in relation to the patient's course of illness and personal biography. The patient's history and examination are never complete, as new information emerges and new observations are made with every clinical encounter. The top priority for treatment can change in response both to medical events and to life events.

Medical psychiatrists live in a real world of preemptive medical events, a complex and imperfect healthcare system, changing psychiatric nosology, and the continuing stigma of mental illness and the psychiatric profession. What enables us to be effective is that we are *physicians* above all.

Overall, the healthcare system is in the process of moving from *delivering services* to *pursuing outcomes*. Diagnosing and treating diseases, and the procedures and services used to do that, increasingly are viewed as means to an end. Medical psychiatry has *always* focused on the outcomes of care, attending to functional and subjective dimensions of medical illness.

Medical psychiatrists face a challenge similar to the one faced by many of our patients: how to be confident and calm in the face of uncertainty. Evidence-based medicine teaches us rules, but we see exceptions every day. Whether following guidelines or intentionally deviating from them, we are rarely certain in advance whether the treatment we choose will work as we hope and expect. Even so, we want our patients to know and to feel that the decisions we have made were good ones: well informed, rational, and responsive to their individual differences and specific circumstances and preferences. This challenge of combining confidence and humility, extensive and detailed knowledge, curiosity, and skepticism in appropriate proportions is faced by all good physicians at times; medical psychiatrists face it more often than most.

Medical psychiatry is an especially satisfying specialty to practice, for two main reasons. The first is that medical psychiatrists have more time with their patients than most other specialists. The second is that the field brings rigor, discipline, and specialized knowledge to the psychological and relational aspects of medical care, while also assimilating the detail and precision of its biomedical aspects.

DISCLOSURE STATEMENTS

Dr. Fogel is Chief Scientific Officer of Synchroneuron Inc., Managing Director of Anal-Gesic LLC, and Executive Vice President of PointRight Inc. He is the sole inventor or lead inventor on several pharmaceutical patents. In his opinion these affiliations do not entail any conflict of interest with regard to the editing of this book or his personal contributions to it. He has no other potential conflicts, direct or indirect, financial or otherwise, to disclose in connection with the editing of this book or his personal contributions to it.

Dr. Greenberg has no conflicts of interest to disclose.

REFERENCES

Costa, P. T. Jr., & Widiger, T. A., eds. (2002). *Personality disorders and the five-factor model of personality. 2.* Washington, DC: American Psychological Association.

Engel, G. L. (1977). The need for a new medical model: A challenge for biomedicine. *Science, 196*, 129–136.

Folstein, M. F., Folstein, S. E., & McHugh, P. R. (1975). "Mini-mental state". A practical method for grading the cognitive state of patients for the clinician. *Journal of Psychiatric Research, 12*(3), 189–198.

Reik, T. (1948). *Listening with the third ear: The inner experience of a psychoanalyst.* New York: Grove Press.

Viederman, M. (1984).The active dynamic interview and the supportive relationship. *Comprehensive Psychiatry, 29*, 147–157.

Von Korff, M., Katon, W. J., Lin, E. H., Ciechanowski, P., Peterson, D., Ludman, E. J., et al. (2011). Functional outcomes of multi-condition collaborative care and successful ageing: results of randomised trial. *British Medical Journal, Nov 10; 343*, d6612.

Waldfogel, S., & Wolpe, P. R. (1993). Using awareness of religious factors to enhance interventions in consultation psychiatry. *Hospital and Community Psychiatry, 44*(5), 473–477.

Woolf, C. J. (2011). Central sensitization: implications for the diagnosis and treatment of pain. *Pain, 152*, S2–15, 2011.

2.

PHYSICAL AND NEUROLOGICAL EXAMINATION

Barry S. Fogel

INTRODUCTION

In general medical patients, the physical examination typically comprises a combination of *hypothesis testing* driven by the chief complaint and medical history and *screening for physical signs* related to various organ systems. The latter is driven by customary practice and often by the need to comply with practice guidelines and/or billing regulations, and it may be perfunctory. In any case, it would not be feasible to routinely examine each organ system at the level of completeness and detail typical of a specialist in that system. This is often the case with the neurological examination, as a complete neurological examination is time consuming, and the level of neurological knowledge and skill can vary considerably among accomplished physicians who are not neurologists. Furthermore, examinations of other organ systems often are abbreviated when the system is outside the scope of the presenting complaint. The generalist's examination of the skin often is less meticulous and complete than that of a dermatologist; physicians outside of orthopedics, physical medicine, or rheumatology tend to be less complete and quantitative in their examination of joints.

No physician would regard a computed tomography (CT) scan of the brain as ruling out all brain disease, though it could be definitive in ruling out hydrocephalus, or a sufficiently large brain tumor or intracerebral hemorrhage. If demyelinating disease were suspected, magnetic resonance imaging (MRI) would have fewer false negatives than a CT scan. Different types of physical examination are like different imaging procedures or different laboratory test panels—their sensitivity and specificity and ultimate diagnostic value depend on what conditions are to be diagnosed or ruled out and on the prior probability that the patient has one of the conditions of interest. If a physical examination is done purely for screening or for "medical clearance" without any diagnostic hypothesis or list of conditions to be excluded, it is likely to have many false negatives if considered in the light of specific diagnostic hypotheses formed after careful consideration of the patient's presenting problem, its context, and findings on laboratory tests and diagnostic imaging.

PURPOSES AND TYPES OF PHYSICAL EXAMINATIONS

There are several situations in which physical examinations conducted by medical psychiatrists—or at their behest—can add special value to the care of the patient:

1. *Narrowing a differential diagnosis prior to ordering diagnostic tests and imaging procedures.* For example, patients with depression, anxiety, fatigue, multiple somatic complaints, and weight loss frequently will have both a chronic general medical disease and a mood disorder. In this situation, characteristic physical findings suggestive of adrenal hyperactivity or adrenal insufficiency would trigger the measurement of plasma cortisol and follow-up provocative tests if there were even a borderline abnormality. In the absence of physical findings or a history of endocrine disease, it is unlikely that a plasma cortisol level would be obtained as part of a general "medical screen" in such a patient.

2. *Looking for physical signs supporting the diagnosis of a specific condition that often has symptoms or functional impairment in excess of findings on a nonfocused, general physical examination.* Conditions ranging from vulvodynia to many of the focal neuropathies due to nerve entrapment or compression have characteristic physical findings that would not be detected or not be adequately characterized without a specialized examination.

3. *Quantifying the severity of a known physical condition to better assess its relationship to the patient's subjective distress and functional impairments.* For example, measuring changes in vital signs and auscultating the heart and the chest following mild exertion can help the clinician understand why a patient with cardiac or pulmonary disease might be unmotivated to exercise. Anxiety about exercise might be commensurate with changes in vital signs and objective signs of dyspnea or be disproportionate to them, and the approach to the psychological dimension of rehabilitation will differ accordingly.

4. *Getting a subjective sense of the patient's condition to better understand its emotional impact.* This is most obvious in the case of skin lesions or physical deformities, or when the patient is in evident distress from pain or dyspnea, but it is also helpful when the patient is asked to perform a task during the physical examination and does it with unusual effort or excessive timidity.

5. *Enhancing positive transference through appropriate touching of the patient.* Patients who are dying, patients with a poor prognosis, patients in pain, and patients with stigmatized conditions can in many cases be comforted and reassured by the physician's touch during the examination. Psychiatrists are well aware of the potential problem of boundary violations and evocation of anxiety or negative transference in individuals predisposed by their history or their diagnosis. Notwithstanding, even the limited touch involved in taking vital signs can have positive effects in contexts where a more extensive physical examination by the psychiatrist would be unwise.

6. *Communicating across disciplinary lines to stimulate a fresh look at a patient's problem.* Citing a specific physical sign that is unequivocally present yet not previously noted on another physician's examination can be an effective way to request a second look at the patient with a fresh perspective. Many specialists find an inquiry about a physical sign more welcome and less meddlesome than the medical psychiatrist's expressing a concern that there might be a missed or underappreciated diagnosis.

Physical examinations by medical psychiatrists are of four general types (see Table 2.1). The *first type* is essentially the same as the examination by a primary care physician. A patient, for example one with delirium, is thought to have an acute medical illness, which, if present, is likely to show manifest physical signs that will be found on examination, such as the signs of heart failure, pneumonia, or an acute abdomen. Or, a homeless and medically neglected patient with chronic mental illness is admitted to hospital and screened for comorbid medical conditions that, though apparent when a general medical history and physical are done, went unrecognized because the patient was not receiving regular medical care. The *second type* of examination is performed when a patient has medically unexplained symptoms or an obscure diagnosis after examination by a primary care physician, examination in an emergency room, or even examination by other medical specialists. In this case, *specialized, focused examinations of greater depth and scope* than typical of a general medical examination are needed. These are *hypothesis-driven*, based on the patient's symptoms, medical history, context, and results of prior diagnostic investigations and laboratory tests. This type also includes a careful redo of a screening examination that might have been done rapidly and with low sensitivity in the context of "medically clearing" a patient for admission to a psychiatric inpatient service. The *third type* of examination is performed when a patient has a known disease—such as an autoimmune disease, cancer, or chronic organ failure—that is relapsing-remitting, progressive, or subject to recurrence, and the medical psychiatrist aims to determine *whether the disease has relapsed or progressed,* as this will have impact on the interpretation of symptoms and on treatment planning. In this situation the examination is focused on assessing the *presence and severity—the latter sometimes quantitatively—of specific*

Table 2.1 TYPES OF PHYSICAL EXAMINATION IN MEDICAL PSYCHIATRY

EXAMINATION TYPE	PURPOSE	SCOPE AND DEPTH	SPECIAL FEATURES
Screening for general medical diseases	Identify conditions missed because of lack of recent medical care or brevity of recent medical visits	Similar to a primary care physician's comprehensive examination	Focus on acute diseases or chronic diseases depending on context and setting
Investigating poorly explained symptoms	Determine cause of symptoms not well explained by diagnoses to date; identify potentially missed diagnoses	Focus on conditions that could better explain the patient's symptoms; deep and detailed examination of relevant organ systems	Hypothesis-driven; methodology similar to subspecialist examination
Assessing status of a known disease	Assess current activity (e.g., exacerbation, remission, or relapse) and severity; screen for complications of the disease and its treatments	Organ system focus; thorough assessment of disease-specific signs	Quantitate results using specialty-specific scales
Functionally-focused examination	Evaluate for disability and/or assess for symptom amplification or excessive illness behavior	Do simultaneous physical examination, functional assessment, and observation of patient behavior during the examination	Quantitate physical findings, functional impairments, and symptoms; note inconsistencies

physical signs. The methodology is that of the relevant medical specialty. Further, if the patient is receiving treatments such as immunosuppressive drugs known to predispose to serious adverse effects or complications, the examination might also include screening for such problems. The *fourth type* of examination focuses on *physical function* and is typical of the examinations done for disability evaluation and for assessment of suspected symptom amplification and excessive illness behavior. The examination specifically aims to observe function and to relate physical signs and other measures of disease severity to the symptoms and impairments reported by the patient and to observed performance. Examination methodology draws from several specialties, notably including physical medicine, geriatrics, neurology and orthopedics.

The analysis of physical examinations by type is applicable not only to the examinations conducted personally by medical psychiatrists but also to medical psychiatrists' reviews of the examinations done by other physicians. It aids in recognizing when a particular part of an examination should be repeated or expanded, either by the medical psychiatrist or by another specialist whose examination will be responsive to the issues raised by the medical psychiatrist.

With this background we offer suggestions for the examination that take into account the organ system and the purpose of the examination.

SETTING OF THE EXAMINATION AND DEMOGRAPHICS

Examination findings in hospitalized patients and other acutely ill patients can change from hour to hour, and neurological symptoms, especially mental status findings, can be context-dependent. These considerations are of particular relevance in the assessment of delirium. If it will not be self-evident from the medical record, the examiner should note the time and place of the examination and, if applicable, whether there was anything unusual about environmental conditions, such as an unusually high environmental temperature or a particularly noisy and distracting environment such as that of a busy emergency room or intensive care unit (ICU).

The age and gender of the patient will of course be indicated on every page of the medical record, but it is worth noting whether the patient looks younger or older than his or her chronological age. Many of the diseases and impairments associated with aging correlate more strongly with biological rather than chronological age. While there is a no generally accepted definition for biological age, experienced clinicians usually will agree when a patient looks significantly older or younger than his or her years. The holistic perception of age by clinicians integrates diverse items including rate of movement, mental acuity, skin condition, and oral health. A Danish longitudinal study of 1826 same-sex twins aged 70 or older examined the relationship between age as perceived by assessors of various backgrounds looking at passport-style photographs and a range of health outcomes including physical function, cognitive function, and mortality; some twin pairs also had analyses of leukocyte telomere length. Perceived age was correlated in the expected direction with all of the health outcomes and was inversely associated with leukocyte telomere length (Christensen et al., 2009). Judgments of apparent age by people without clinical training had nearly as strong an associations with health outcomes as judgments of apparent age by geriatric nurses.

Primary care physicians' judgments of apparent age significantly exceeding chronological age, although relatively insensitive to patients' health status, can be remarkably specific. In a primary care population of patients aged 30–70, Hwang et al. (2011) showed that a physician's judgment of apparent age 5 or more years older than chronological age was 82% specific for poor general health as assessed by the SF-12 questionnaire; apparent age 10 or more years greater than chronological age was 99% specific for poor health.

Note also should be made of the patient's ethnicity, which is not always evident from the patient's surname. Particular nationalities are associated not only with genetic diseases but also with a higher prevalence of cytochrome P450 variants that imply slow or fast metabolism of commonly prescribed psychotropic and general medical drugs, or a greater vulnerability to particular medically serious drug interactions.

GENERAL APPEARANCE, HEIGHT AND WEIGHT

The general appearance of the patient, including how the patient is dressed and groomed, can give important clues to the patient's functional capacities and to whether there is impairment of executive cognitive function due to problems with the frontal lobes and/or their connections. These clues will be absent if the patient has been dressed and groomed by caregivers prior to the examination. Note should be taken of signs of physical abuse; often bruises will be covered by garments, and so the entire skin should be checked at some point in the examination. Muscle bulk should be noted; its significance will depend on demographics. Increased muscle bulk due to athletic activities will be associated with an increased serum creatinine; this can lead to underestimation of renal function if it is not taken into account. Disproportionately increased muscle bulk associated with excessive hair and testicular atrophy raises a suspicion of anabolic steroid use. Diminished muscle bulk has a broad differential diagnosis including deconditioning due to immobility, nerve or muscle disease, and catabolic states such as those due to cancer. In addition, patients with diminished muscle bulk can have a serum creatinine level within normal limits in the presence of moderate renal insufficiency.

The distribution of body fat should be noted. Excess abdominal fat is more strongly correlated with the metabolic syndrome than excess fat in the buttocks, hips, and thighs; a patient with a waist circumference of 40 inches or more has an increased risk of the metabolic syndrome even if he or she has a normal body mass index (BMI) (Chen et al., 2013). Neck circumference is an independent risk factor for the metabolic syndrome; it is significantly associated even when waist circumference and BMI are taken into account (Zhou et al., 2013). Central obesity with peripheral wasting is typical of hypercortisolism, whether the latter is associated with adrenal hyperplasia or with exogenous corticosteroids.

A medical outpatient's height should be measured on the first encounter and his/her weight measured at the first and subsequent visits. Height should be measured on admission and weight should be measured on a regular basis for patients in hospitals or institutional settings, and the BMI should be calculated and recorded. Changes in weight are of obvious diagnostic relevance and often can be detected earlier with routine weighing than with casual observation alone.

VITAL SIGNS

Vital signs comprise temperature, pulse, blood pressure, and respiratory rate. The measurement of each has nuances that are relevant in medical-psychiatric contexts.

TEMPERATURE

People with depression, apathy, delirium, or subacute cognitive impairment can have systemic diseases—for example, infection, cancer, or autoimmune disease—that are associated with low-grade fever. If the fever is recognized it triggers a medical assessment, and the involvement of the psychiatrist usually is limited to managing symptoms and the psychiatric comorbidities of the medical problem responsible for the fever. However, low-grade fevers can be missed, or erroneously diagnosed, because of errors in the measurement or interpretation of body temperature data. The normal range for mean oral temperature is 98.2 ± 0.7°F (36.8 ± 0.4°C). Axillary temperatures are lower; rectal and tympanic temperatures are higher; the difference in temperature between sites is not consistent either within or between individuals (Sund-Levander & Grodzinski, 2013). Circadian variation in body temperature is approximately 1.4°F (0.77°C) between the daily minimum (typically in the early morning hours) and the daily maximum (typically in the early evening). Twenty-four-hour monitoring of body temperature in hospitalized patients with recent fever showed that 16% had temperatures exceeding 38°C at some point during the day that were not detected by routine monitoring of vital signs (Varela et al., 2011).

Older people tend to have baseline body temperatures toward the lower end of the normal range; those who are obese or who are impaired in cognitive and/or physical function are more likely to have low baseline body temperature (Lu et al., 2009). Physiologic amounts of progestins—whether endogenous or exogenous—raise body temperature by 1.1°F (0.6°C). While it is obvious that hot and cold foods and drinks can influence oral temperature, it is less appreciated that mouth breathing, such as that due to nasal obstruction or sleep apnea, can reduce oral temperature. In patients who habitually mouth breathe a rectal or tympanic temperature measurement may be more accurate.

A patient with a baseline oral temperature of 97.5°F could be febrile with an oral temperature of 98.9°F taken in the morning. On the other hand, a young woman taking oral contraceptives could have an evening oral temperature of 99.8°F without fever. This is another reason why the time of the physical examination is important to record.

A baseline body temperature usually can be found in a patient's primary care record or hospital chart. A record of the baseline body temperature should be sought when the patient has a high normal temperature and the clinical setting suggests a significant probability of a condition associated with a low-grade fever.

PULSE

In the physician's office and at the bedside, the patient's pulse often is measured by a nurse or medical assistant using the same automated device used to measure blood pressure. However, valuable additional data are obtained by determining the pulse by traditional palpation of an artery. Irregularity of the pulse suggests cardiac arrhythmia; excessive regularity of the pulse, without the expected variation in rate associated with respiration, suggests cardiopulmonary disease. Palpation of the pulse for a full minute is far more sensitive to these abnormalities than the 15-second palpation that is commonly done at the bedside. Changes in pulse with changes in posture—or the lack thereof—give insight into hydration status and autonomic function. When a patient changes from the supine to the standing position there is a transient increase in pulse associated with the transient drop in venous return to the heart. The absence of this increase suggests autonomic dysfunction. A large increase in pulse associated with a drop in blood pressure is seen in dehydration and also in the presence of drugs that cause orthostatic hypotension by alpha-adrenergic antagonism; lower-potency first-generation antipsychotic drugs lower blood pressure by this mechanism. Checking the pulse when the patient is experiencing acute anxiety can identify patients whose anxiety is associated with significant tachycardia. Complete lack of variability of the pulse rate in a patient with tachycardia suggests paroxysmal atrial tachycardia or atrial flutter, which can be either the primary cause of the anxiety or a complication of anxiety related to an anxiety-induced increase in sympathetic tone and decrease in vagal tone. Tachycardia with some variability but not pronounced irregularity is more likely to be sinus tachycardia, and in that case the anxiety is more likely primary and the tachycardia secondary. Tachycardia with an irregularly irregular rhythm most often is due to atrial fibrillation; paroxysmal atrial fibrillation can either trigger anxiety or be triggered by it. In patients with paroxysmal arrhythmias, a careful palpation of the pulse when the patient is symptomatic is diagnostically useful and is feasible not only in inpatient settings but in outpatient settings when there is an observer—potentially a family member—at hand. If the examiner or the patient has one, a mobile phone attachment (e.g., one marketed by AliveCor) can be used to record a one-lead ECG rhythm strip up to 5 minutes long, sufficient to allow a more confident assessment of the heart rhythm accounting for a rapid or irregular pulse palpated at the bedside.

BLOOD PRESSURE

The accurate measurement of blood pressure is essential to the accurate diagnosis of numerous conditions of medical-psychiatric interest, beginning with hypertension—a widely prevalent condition that is both a risk factor for cardiovascular and cerebrovascular disease and a sign of endocrine disorders or medication side effects. The American Heart Association publishes extremely detailed guidelines for measuring blood pressure; actual practice in clinics deviates from guidelines, yielding different results that often lead to different conclusions about diagnosis and the need for treatment (Pickering et al., 2005; Ray, Nawarskas, & Anderson, 2011; Minor et al., 2012). Because a number of commonly prescribed psychotropic drugs can raise blood pressure, the detection of hypertension can be critical for management of treatment-related cardiovascular risk. A borderline blood pressure on a prior examination deserves follow-up using rigorous methodology. Several points are relevant:

1. The patient's arm should be supported at the level of the patient's right atrium when the blood pressure is taken. This is halfway between the bed or examining table and the sternum if the patient is supine. If the arm is lower, the measured pressure will be higher, and if it is higher, the measured pressure will be lower, by approximately 2 mmHg per inch above or below the ideal level.

2. A cuff of adequate size must be used; given the high prevalence of obesity, many patients will require a "large adult" cuff for an accurate reading. Using a cuff that is too small is a common cause of erroneously high blood pressure measurements. Specifically, if the arm circumference is 35 cm or greater the standard adult size cuff is too small; in this situation a large adult cuff should be used if the arm circumference is between 35 cm and 44 cm, and an adult thigh cuff should be used if the arm circumference is 45 cm or greater.

3. The cuff must be deflated slowly—not faster than 2 mmHg per second. If the cuff is deflated too rapidly the systolic blood pressure will be underestimated and the diastolic blood pressure will be overestimated.

4. Blood pressure is influenced by the patient's position. Diastolic pressure is approximately 5 mmHg higher sitting as opposed to supine; systolic pressure is approximately 8 mmHg higher supine as opposed to standing. Sitting with the back unsupported—as on an examining table—can increase the diastolic pressure by approximately 6 mmHg.

5. Ambulatory patients typically have higher blood pressures when measured by the physician than when measured by a nurse; the mean difference in one large study was 6.3 mmHg in the systolic pressure and 7.9 mmHg in the diastolic pressure.

6. 24-hour ambulatory blood pressure recording is the most reliable and valid way to determine whether a patient has high blood pressure.

7. Normal blood pressure is lower at night than in the daytime. A nighttime blood pressure of greater than 125 mmHg systolic or 75 mmHg diastolic is abnormal.

8. Orthostatic hypotension, whether due to dehydration, autonomic dysfunction, or an endocrine disorder, can present as anxiety or panic when standing or walking, as phobic avoidance of standing or walking, or as a tendency to fall. This is especially true in older patients with cognitive impairment or in others who cannot precisely describe their problem. Orthostatic hypotension due to dehydration usually is immediate, but orthostatic hypotension due to autonomic dysfunction can be delayed, coming on a few minutes after the patient stands up. If a patient with suspicious symptoms does not show a blood pressure drop immediately on standing up, the blood pressure should be measured again after he or she has been standing for at least five minutes.

9. The standard context for measuring blood pressure in the clinic is after five minutes at rest. Exercise or anxiety can raise the blood pressure, and recovery with relaxation can take a few minutes.

RESPIRATORY RATE

Respiratory rate can be accurately measured by counting breaths over a minute or more; in the authors' experience this is not consistently done by clinicians, despite evidence that in adults an abnormally high respiratory rate (over 20 breaths per minute) is a valid indicator of illness severity and poor prognosis (Cretikos et al., 2008; Bianchi et al., 2013). Periodic breathing—breathing that cyclically oscillates between shallow and deep with a cycle length of 1–2 minutes—should be noted; it can reflect a primary problem either in the cardiovascular system or in the central nervous system (CNS). Its most severe form is Cheyne-Stokes respiration, in which there is actual apnea at the nadir of the cycle. Periodic breathing is worse with exercise in patients with heart failure. In heart failure patients, periodic breathing both correlates with severity of disease and carries independent weight as an indicator of poor prognosis (Dhakal et al., 2012; McGee, 2013).

Patients with recurrent functional hyperventilation—with or without associated panic attacks—do not necessarily have tachypnea; their breathing may be deeper than normal rather than more rapid than normal; this pattern is common in younger patients (Han et al., 1997). Thus, a normal respiratory rate, even during a panic attack, does not rule out episodic functional hyperventilation as the basis of somatic symptoms of anxiety.

SKIN, HAIR, AND NAILS

The critical question concerning skin examination in medical psychiatry is whether the entire skin was examined. Outpatient physical examinations and emergency room triage examinations that do not include a complete examination of the skin can miss valuable and occasionally critical diagnostic information. Many of the systemic diseases that can present with psychiatric symptoms have early dermatologic manifestations; lupus and Addison's disease are two examples. The medical psychiatrist can promote earlier diagnoses of such conditions by suggesting that psychiatric and dermatologic conditions might have a common cause and make (or suggest) a referral to a dermatologist. (For a comprehensive review of the topic see Goldsmith et al., 2012.) Skin diseases, including those that signify systemic diseases, can look different in patients of color (Kelley & Taylor, 2009). For example, while lupus is more common in people of color, the characteristic facial rash is more difficult to see on a dark skin. The skin findings of greatest interest in examining a patient with a psychiatric presentation depend, as usual, on the clinical context and the prevalence of particular diseases in the population from which the patient comes. For example, a subacute mental status change with multiple somatic symptoms would warrant a careful look for a rash in any case, but one might think of Lyme disease in a hiker from New England, lupus in an African-American woman with a positive family history, and syphilis in a sex worker. Hair pulling (trichotillomania) and skin picking (dermatillomania) are impulse-control disorders with a number of associated psychiatric comorbidities including obsessive–compulsive disorder and depression. Hair pulling and skin picking can occur in areas ordinarily covered by clothing. For example, patients may pull underarm hair or pubic hair. Trichotillomania can be distinguished from alopecia areata by testing hair adjacent to the bald area; in trichotillomania this hair has normal resistance to being pulled, while in alopecia areata the hair can be easily pulled out. The differential diagnosis of hair loss is facilitated by trichoscopy, the examination of the scalp and hairs with a surface microscope with 10x to 70x magnification (Pedrosa, Morais, Lisboa, & Azevedo, 2013). "Tele-trichoscopy" would be a consideration for physicians with microscope attachments for their mobile phones; such attachments are widely available with magnification in a suitable range. Patients sometimes use cosmetics, style their hair, or cover their heads in order to conceal areas on the scalp or the face where hair has been pulled out. Concealment measures of this kind will be noted on a careful examination of the integument that considers the possibility.

Skin picking that meets diagnostic criteria for a mental disorder—including subjective distress or functional impairment as well as skin damage not explained by a general medical condition—affects 1%–2% of the general population. Patients with the disorder can pick at the skin virtually anywhere they can reach—so only a complete skin examination can rule out the condition (Grant et al., 2012).

Nail biting (onychophagia) can be distinguished from intrinsic nail disease and, like other self-inflicted dermatologic problems, it should be noted because of its association with other psychiatric disorders including anxiety disorders, attention deficit-hyperactivity disorder (ADHD), and Tourette syndrome.

In patients with impaired mobility and/or impaired somatic sensation, including frail and debilitated patients with poor nutrition, there is a high risk of skin breakdown in areas subjected to pressure or shearing forces; in patients near the end of life there can be "skin failure," with skin breakdown in the face of trivial and unavoidable stresses to the skin. Patients at risk for skin breakdown should be examined frequently, focusing on areas such as the sacrum, buttocks, and heels that are subject to pressure when the patient lies in bed. Abnormal erythema of the skin often precedes actual breakdown of the skin, though this may be difficult to see in people with dark skins. Abnormal skin temperature—either warmer or cooler than the surrounding skin—is another sign of impending skin breakdown. This phenomenon sometimes can be appreciated on palpation; it can be confirmed using a noncontact infrared thermometer (Sprigle et al., 2001; Rapp et al., 2009). The clinical reality is that pressure ulcers, which can develop literally in hours, frequently are missed by clinicians at their early stages and then present with involvement of subcutaneous tissues or even damage to underlying muscle. One reason they are missed is that the physicians and nurses involved in the patient's care don't examine skin areas at risk with sufficient frequency. When patients are acutely ill, the clinician's focus usually is elsewhere than the skin. The issue of unnoticed skin breakdown can present to medical psychiatrists when they evaluate patients for delirium; if there is a significant area of skin breakdown, the associated inflammation (and often infection) can be a factor that causes or contributes to delirium. Skin breakdown in areas where more attention (e.g., frequent repositioning and pressure-relieving devices) could easily have prevented the problem raises questions of quality of care and/or the appropriateness of the setting of care relative to the patient's vulnerabilities and functional impairments. Several other observations on complete skin examination of special interest to psychiatrists are presented in Table 2.2. In practice, they may not be recorded or even noticed on physical examinations that do not pay special attention to the skin.

Typically the write-up of a general physical examination with no detail about the skin leaves the medical psychiatrist uncertain whether skin conditions of interest were present but not seen, seen and not noted, or simply not looked for. If any of the above diagnostic considerations are applicable to the patient, skin condition is not fully described, and the examiner's usual procedures are not known, the medical psychiatrist must consider recommending (or personally conducting) a new, complete, and hypothesis-driven examination of the skin.

HEAD, EYES, EARS, NOSE, AND THROAT

HEAD

The examination of the head in an adolescent or young adult with a history suggestive of a developmental disorder should include notes on the shape of the head and a measurement of

Table 2.2 SKIN FINDINGS OF MEDICAL-PSYCHIATRIC INTEREST

SKIN CONDITION	PSYCHIATRIC SIGNIFICANCE
"Tracks"	Intravenous drug use
Tattoos, piercings, and other body art	The nature, location, and content of the body art can reveal psychodynamic or psychosexual issues. Poorly implemented body art can raise concerns of infection.
Unexplained (or non-credibly explained) bruises, cuts, scratches or burns, particularly in atypical places for accidental injury	Differential diagnosis includes abuse by a caregiver or intimate, impulsive or deliberate self-injury, and sadomasochistic sexual behavior
Razor cuts on the arms, legs, or trunk	Self-injurious behavior; often associated with borderline personality disorder
Unusually heavy makeup, particularly when visiting a physician	Differential diagnosis includes histrionic personality and efforts to conceal a revealing skin lesion.

head circumference. Specific congenital and developmental conditions are associated with microcephaly, macrocephaly, and/or abnormalities of the shape of the head. Pediatricians routinely note head circumference, but this is not the rule with their nonpediatric colleagues. When a patient has chronic cognitive impairment, either developmental or acquired, and the patient has had a recent change in behavior or mental status, the head should be carefully checked for *signs of trauma.* Signs of head trauma without a credible history to explain them raise the issue of abuse.

EYES

Examination of the eyes offers a window into the body's interior. General ophthalmology texts extensively cover ocular manifestations of systemic diseases (e.g., Friedman et al., 2009). Systemic conditions with psychiatric presentations can have eye signs at presentation; on occasion the eye signs are diagnostic (like Kayser-Fleischer rings in Wilson's disease) or point to a category of disease (like dry eyes in Sjögren's syndrome). Other systemic conditions with prominent psychiatric accompaniments, for example diabetes or lupus, can be complicated by eye involvement that increases the challenge of illness by threatening a loss of vision. A typical general physical examination will look for evident disease of the conjunctiva and sclera, measure the pupils and test them for reactivity to light and accommodation, test extraocular movements, look for cataracts, confirm that the optic nerve head is not swollen, and assess the retina and its blood vessels to the extent that these are visible without dilating the eye. Visual fields, if tested at all, typically will be tested with moving fingers for gross intactness of peripheral vision in four quadrants. This should be done separately for each eye. In the author's experience, visual acuity is not consistently tested.

The hypothesis-driven examination of the eyes has broader scope and addresses specific questions. Visual acuity is tested in good light with a pocket vision screener, with patients wearing glasses or contact lenses if they ordinarily do so to read. Visual acuity of 20/200 or worse in the better eye, with optimal correction of refractive error, is regarded as functional blindness. Patients with poor cognitive function or with poor communication due to psychotic illness can have severe visual impairment but not complain of it. Instead they can display avoidance behaviors, have falls or other accidents, or experience hallucinations and visual misperceptions. Identifying the presence of significant visual impairment leads to ophthalmologic consultation, diagnosis, and intervention. If the patient is unable to participate in bedside visual acuity testing, a visual evoked potential study can be done.

More detailed evaluation of the visual fields is indicated when the clinical history, the mental status examination, or the sensorimotor examination suggests a tumor, stroke, or other focal cerebral lesion. A reasonable bedside evaluation can be done by confrontation testing with the examiner 18–24 inches away from the patient, looking at the patient eye-to-eye, and testing each eye separately. Testing with small finger movements—about 2mm—at the extreme periphery of the visual field, checking both outer quadrants, is a highly sensitive screening test for temporal field defects. Testing with both eyes open the patient's ability to perceive simultaneous movements in the left and the right visual fields screens for extinction, a phenomenon that is a sign of contralateral parietal lobe disease. Extinction is present when the patient can see a stimulus when it is presented alone, but fails to see it when it is presented simultaneously with a stimulus on the opposite side. Confrontation testing with a small object such as the tip of a cotton swab, one eye at a time, can approximately map the visual field and can, in a cooperative patient, measure the patient's blind spots. A red pinhead is more sensitive to subtle defects than a white object. As with the testing of visual acuity, the aim of testing visual fields is to identify defects suggesting primary diseases of the eye or the brain that require diagnostic follow-up, as well as to identify visual problems of significance to the patient's everyday function, safety, and well-being.

A very quick, simple test for gross visual field defects and for the extinction phenomenon is the finger counting test. The examiner tests one eye at a time, having the patient block the other one with his or her hand. The examiner simultaneously presents one or two fingers at the periphery of the right upper quadrant and one or two fingers at the periphery of the left upper quadrant and asks the patient to state the *total* number of fingers the examiner is holding up. The process is repeated with fingers at the periphery of the left lower quadrant and the right lower quadrant. If the patient has a quadrant or more of field defect in either or both eyes, or has extinction in any quadrant, he or she will undercount the sum of fingers. This identifies a potential defect that can be examined further (Anderson et al., 2009).

Evidence of conjunctivitis is obvious when the entire conjunctiva is involved; the condition can be missed or underestimated if there is disproportionate involvement of the conjunctiva of the eyelids (the palpebral conjunctiva). If the patient complains of a foreign body sensation or of eye irritation, and the conjunctiva are not obviously inflamed, the examiner should flip the eyelid and look at the palpebral conjunctiva.

In the medical-psychiatric context, abnormally small or abnormally large pupils most often are due to the effects of drugs: opiates give small pupils, and anticholinergic and sympathomimetic drugs give large ones. However, some patients with anticholinergic side effects, including many patients of advanced age, do not show widely dilated pupils but instead show medium-sized pupils that are poorly reactive to light and accommodation. Patients with large pupils due to sympathomimetic drugs typically do not show impaired pupillary reactivity. Patients with diseases affecting the optic nerves, such as glaucoma or retinitis pigmentosa, can have impaired function of the afferent limb of the pupillary light reflex (an "afferent pupil"): both pupils react normally to light shined into the unaffected eye while both pupils react slowly, incompletely, or not at all to light shined into the affected eye. A practical bedside procedure for identifying an afferent pupillary defect in the presence of an intact efferent limb of the reflex is the swinging flashlight test. The examiner shines a flashlight into each eye, alternately. When the flashlight shines into the eye with the afferent defect, the pupil dilates since the afferent stimulus from the affected eye is less than the afferent stimulus from the unaffected eye. The defect can be quantitated by determining what density of neutral-density filter placed in front of the better eye will make the test negative. A meta-analysis of studies of pupillary light reflexes in glaucoma diagnosis showed that the swinging flashlight test was highly *specific* for optic nerve disease, though not as *sensitive* as infrared pupillometry (Chang et al., 2013). Patients with autonomic disorders, including those with Parkinson's disease or Lewy body dementia and also including some adults with autism spectrum disorders, can show pupillary light reflexes that are slow and delayed in onset (Giza et al., 2012). These findings, when present, can help in differential diagnosis.

Screening examination of ocular movements attempts to verify that extraocular movements are full and conjugate. When they are not, there is either a primary problem with the extraocular muscles, a cranial nerve palsy, or dysfunction of the brainstem oculomotor control system. Patients with myasthenia gravis—another condition of medical-psychiatric interest because of its sometimes delayed diagnosis and puzzling symptoms—can have a breakdown of full and conjugate movements on an intermittent basis; in untreated patients, eye movements get worse with fatigue. In patients treated for myasthenia with cholinesterase inhibitors, eye movements will get worse as their drugs wear off. Having a patient with ocular myasthenia open and forcefully close their eyes repeatedly for a minute or more sometimes can elicit weakness in one or more of the ocular muscles. Full and conjugate movements, of course, do not rule out all impairments of oculomotor control. Patients with fully normal oculomotor function are able to shift their gaze from one target to another rapidly and accurately without overshooting or undershooting the target. The inability to generate a targeted eye movement at all implies significant cerebral dysfunction. Recurrent overshooting or undershooting the target—ocular dysmetria—indicates impaired function of the cerebellar motor control system. The most common neurological conditions in which ocular dysmetria is encountered are multiple sclerosis and cerebellar stroke, particularly a stroke due to occlusion of the posterior inferior cerebellar artery (Grimaldi & Manto, 2012). Eye movements are discussed further below in connection with the examination of the cranial nerves.

EARS

Physical examination of the ears might reveal impacted ear wax, important as an indicator of neglect or self-neglect as well as an explanation for communication problems. The eardrums once visualized might show evidence of prior trauma or infections. Most important from the medical psychiatric standpoint is the ears' functional performance in hearing and balance.

Hearing loss of over 25 dB (mild loss) if the speech frequencies are involved and, even more, any hearing loss of over 40 dB (moderate to severe loss) can impair communication and social functioning and can worsen the functional consequences of cognitive impairments. Functionally significant hearing loss has greater than 40% prevalence in the population over 65 (Gates & Mills, 2005) and a similarly high prevalence among younger people with excessive noise exposure The latter include people who regularly listen to loud music and those who work in noisy environments or use noisy machines without wearing ear protection. Because of the stigma associated with hearing loss and with wearing hearing aids, many patients do not complain of their hearing loss. Screening at the bedside is simple, but, as with other elements of the physical examination, the medical psychiatrist should know—either from the documentation or from personal knowledge of the examiner's practice—how the examiner did the screening. Two well-validated bedside tests of hearing are the rubbing finger test (hearing two fingers rubbed together 6 inches away from each ear) and correctly repeating a sequence of three digits whispered two feet away from each ear (Chou et al., 2011). The tests have similar sensitivity and specificity for detecting hearing loss of 30 dB or more; repeating digits is sensitive to impaired speech discrimination as well as pure tone loss in the speech frequencies. Selective low-frequency or high-frequency hearing loss will not be detected by these screening procedures, but it may be relevant to auditory symptoms like tinnitus. Quantitative screening of hearing loss between 500 Hz and 4000 Hz is feasible with a bedside otoscope/audiometer (e.g., the Welch-Allyn AudioScope®); evaluating hearing loss outside that range requires formal audiometry.

Perception of an auditory signal conducted through the air versus through the bone is tested using a 512Hz tuning fork and comparing the hearing threshold when the tuning fork is held a few inches from the ear with that when it is held against the mastoid process. Normally the sound will be louder when presented to the ear than to the bone, because the former presentation takes advantage of the amplification of sound by the middle ear. Reversal of the normal pattern implies middle ear disease such as otosclerosis or a perforated eardrum, or blockage of the ear canal. Comparing air with bone conduction using a 128Hz tuning fork (the kind used to test vibration sense) can give a false-positive result; low frequencies are conducted better by bone and are amplified less by the middle ear than are higher frequencies. Testing of vestibular function is addressed in the section on the neurological examination.

NOSE

Examination of the nose focuses on allergic rhinitis and nasal obstruction. Nasal allergy often is associated with other allergic phenomena including asthma, and nasal obstruction leads to snoring and mouth breathing and sometimes to obstructive sleep apnea. Swollen, boggy mucosa over the turbinate cartilage is a characteristic sign, which can be seen with or without erythema. Damage to the nasal septum from cocaine or other snorted drugs of abuse should be looked for in appropriate contexts, though it is not necessarily seen on a general physical examination even when it is present on a specialist examination because the damage may be further up the nose than can be seen with an otoscope speculum. Testing of the sense of smell, discussed further below, has a role in the assessment of traumatic brain injury, dementia, limbic epilepsy, and multiple sclerosis, and in the assessment of nasal damage due to snorted drugs of abuse.

MOUTH

The mouth warrants a systematic look for signs of oral cancer and precancerous changes in patients who smoke; those patients' risk is even higher if they also abuse alcohol. The oral cancer examination includes grasping the tongue with a gloved hand or piece of gauze and flipping the tongue over to see its underside and the floor of the mouth. This step, routine in the dentist's office, often is omitted on physicians' screening physical examinations. Loss of lingual papillae is associated with vitamin deficiency. The mouth is a usual site of candidiasis and other mycotic infections in immunosuppressed patients. Oral mycoses can take a variety of forms; acute candidiasis can be erythematous or pseudomembranous; chronic candidiasis can present as leukoplakia, a hyperplastic condition (Muzyka & Epifanio, 2013). Patients with serious systemic illness may not complain of symptoms when they have oral candidiasis, especially when there is impairment of cognition or communication; the condition manifests instead with diminished oral intake. Also, the brunt of the condition may be in the inferior pharynx so that a cursory look in the oral cavity may miss it. Nonspecialists usually do not carry mirrors or fiberoptic devices for fully visualizing the pharynx; what is important is considering when the condition is likely in a given context of disease, drug therapy, and symptoms, and knowing that looking in the mouth and only the part of the throat that is visible without aids can lead to a false negative.

The condition of the teeth and gums tends to be mentioned in passing if at all, unless the patient has a gross problem like a dental abscess or multiple missing teeth. If problems typically in the domain of dentistry are not mentioned in the report of a physical examination, it does not mean they were not present. The common lack of attention to dental and periodontal status is unfortunate, because periodontal disease is endemic worldwide and has both general medical and neuropsychiatric implications. Periodontal disease can (1) cause a systemic inflammatory state, (2) increase blood levels of C-reactive protein, and (3) increase the risk of coronary artery disease. The increase in proinflammatory cytokines associated with periodontal disease can contribute to neuropsychiatric symptoms including depression and apathy (Kronfol & Remick, 2000; Van Dyke, 2008). There is a reciprocal relationship as well: depression worsens the prognosis and treatment outcome of periodontal disease (Rosania et al., 2009). When a patient has significant periodontal disease on a screening examination assessment, the medical psychiatrist often can find valuable information by asking whether the patient is aware of it and if so, what if anything is being done about it. Lack of awareness and/or lack of apparent concern about obvious gum disease can be evidence of apathy, denial of illness, dental phobia, or problems accessing or paying for dental care.

Halitosis—clinically significant "bad breath"—is a condition that affects approximately 25% of the world's population. It has implications for patients' social and marital interactions, and ultimately for their self-confidence and self-esteem. Even patients who are generally self-aware may be unaware of their halitosis, especially if they live alone. However, lack of awareness of *severe* halitosis can be clue to defects in self-awareness and self-monitoring.

The differential diagnosis of halitosis is of medical-psychiatric interest. Approximately 85% of cases are of oral origin—due to periodontal disease and/or to coating of the posterior tongue by a film rich in anaerobic bacteria. In about 10% the foul odor originates from the nose or the oropharynx (e.g., from rhinosinusitis or tonsiliths), and in the remaining 5% the source is gastrointestinal or systemic. Of the latter type, fruity odors due to diabetes probably are the most common; end-stage liver failure and end-stage kidney failure also have characteristic odors. Halitosis due to systemic conditions or nasal conditions can be differentiated from the more usual oral cases because they give a foul odor to breath expired through the nose; the latter cause a foul odor from the mouth only.

Halitosis is common in patients with mouth breathing because it is made worse by a dry mouth; thus it is associated with sleep apnea. It is exacerbated by drugs with anticholinergic effects because the latter inhibit saliva production (Bollen & Beikler, 2012).

NECK AND SPINE

The ability to feel the contents of the neck depends in part on its size and shape. It is easier to palpate a thyroid gland, appreciate the filling of neck veins, or hear a carotid bruit in a long and thin neck. When the patient has a short thick neck, the absence of a sign on neck examination related to the thyroid, vascular system, or lymph nodes is more likely to be a false negative. In addition, patients with short thick necks are more likely to have obstructive sleep apnea, and, as noted above, abnormally high neck circumference is a risk factor for the metabolic syndrome that adds incrementally to the risk associated with increased waist circumference and elevated BMI.

Careful auscultation for carotid bruits—at multiple locations along the carotid arteries—is worthwhile in patients at high risk for atherosclerosis affecting large blood vessels. While carotid bruits are not always present in patients with large vessel disease, there are few false positives.

The neck is a good place to check for rigidity in patients who may have extrapyramidal motor disease or extrapyramidal side effects of psychotropic drugs. Neck rigidity can be unequivocal in patients who lack "cogwheel rigidity" of the upper extremities. Evaluation of the passive range of motion of the neck can show limitations related to degenerative disease of the cervical spine—a highly prevalent condition in later life that can be associated with cervical radiculopathy (and often neck or arm pain) as well as with impairment in gait and balance due chronic spinal cord impingement.

The spine examination is of evident relevance to understanding back pain, the most common type of disabling chronic pain of benign cause. Generalized spasm of the lumbar paravertebral muscles can be seen with back pain regardless of its cause; but localized, unilateral, segmental spasm of lumbar muscles points to impingement on the corresponding lumbar nerve roots, or pain in a body part innervated by those nerve roots. When there is disease of the vertebrae themselves, for example, from bony metastases or from osteoporosis of the spine with compression fractures, palpation or general percussion of the spinous processes in the midline can show localized tenderness. If vertebrae have collapsed, the spinous processes will be unusually close together, and review of long-term medical records may show that the patient has lost height.

Posture should be noted; abnormal posture can be the cause of muscle strain, and it can be a characteristic sign of a disease. Patients with Parkinson's disease are stooped; those with progressive supranuclear palsy stand erect. Significant scoliosis in a young or middle-aged adult typically is due to a neurodevelopmental problem, and the presence of one such problem increases the likelihood of another one—making it more likely that there will be data in the developmental and educational history potentially relevant to a presenting psychiatric issue.

CHEST

In the medical-psychiatric context the most common reasons for examination of the chest are (1) as part of a general screen for systemic diseases that can affect mood or cognition, (2) to understand the cause of shortness of breath, and (3) to assess the severity of a known pulmonary disease. The question often arises whether an individual's disease-related emotional distress and his or her impairments in physical, social, and/or occupational function are commensurate with the objective severity of pulmonary disease. When symptoms or disabilities are disproportionate to findings on pulmonary examination it suggests that psychiatric or non-pulmonary medical comorbidities are contributing to the distress and dysfunction.

Dyspnea is of particular interest to medical psychiatrists because of its circular relationship with anxiety. Dyspnea often is the most distressing symptom experienced by a patient with heart or lung disease, and its presence can trigger anxiety even when the patient knows its cause and is not worried about it. Anxiety attacks, regardless of their cause, can present with subjective shortness of breath and/or with sighing or hyperventilation. Frequent sighing and greater reliance for breathing on the chest wall muscles rather than the diaphragm suggest that anxiety is contributing to tachypnea and/or dyspnea, in the absence of disease that directly affects the muscular function or the range of motion of the diaphragm. A contribution from anxiety does not, of course, rule out the simultaneous presence of pulmonary disease, since both dyspnea and the lack of oxygen can induce anxiety.

The chest examination should include observation of the qualitative aspects of respiration, particularly in patients who suffer from anxiety, dyspnea, or both. These qualitative aspects include the apparent effort the patient makes to breathe, retractions of the intercostal muscles, changes in position the patient makes to improve breathing, and the relative involvement of the chest wall muscles in comparison with the diaphragm in respiration.

When observing the patient's breathing and counting respirations, sighing should be noted. Sighing in a social context typically implies frustration or boredom, while private sighing is more often associated with sadness (Teigen, 2008). Deep sighing is strongly correlated with depression in patients with chronic disease, as was shown rigorously in a recent study of patients with rheumatoid arthritis (Robbins et al., 2011). When dyspnea is associated with frequent sighing, it is likely that anxiety contributes to the subjective perception of dyspnea and that relief of anxiety will at least partially relieve the dyspnea.

Recurrent attacks of dyspnea in a person without known or apparent lung disease raises the issue of panic attacks with prominent respiratory symptoms or of a functional hyperventilation syndrome. However, the differential diagnosis also includes recurrent small pulmonary emboli. In that condition a meticulous examination of the chest, listening systematically in many locations, sometimes reveals friction rubs or other abnormal breath sounds, *if the examination is done when the patient has recently become short of breath.* A standard auscultation of the chest when the patient is not symptomatic is unlikely to be positive. When chest examination findings together with the patient's history suggest the diagnosis of recurrent pulmonary embolism, the medical psychiatrist's response will depend on the context of his or her practice. In some contexts the medical psychiatrist will directly order a timely lung scan; in others the order must come from the patient's primary care doctor or general medical specialist. When the psychiatrist communicates with a general medical physician, mentioning a localized friction rub or abnormal breath sounds can facilitate the latter's consideration of the diagnosis and willingness to order an imaging procedure to confirm it or rule it out. Mentioning that a patient does not have prominent anxiety despite significant dyspnea can similarly motivate a more intensive evaluation by the general medical physician.

HEART

As diagnostic technology for evaluating cardiac disease has advanced, the diagnostic importance of physical examination of the heart has diminished. Nonetheless, by finding abnormalities on physical examination of the heart, the medical psychiatrist can motivate a further evaluation of cardiac disease by laboratory, physiological, or imaging procedures, and can prompt reconsideration of heart disease by a cardiologist or general medical physician who has seen the patient in the past. Further, by recognizing the limitations of physical examination of the heart, medical psychiatrists can better appreciate what cardiac conditions might still be present in a psychiatric patient who has been "medically cleared" utilizing a routine physical examination and a non individualized battery of laboratory tests.

The limitations of physical examination of the heart are greater in obese patients. The accumulation of fat in the chest wall attenuates abnormal heart sounds and also makes it harder to estimate the size of the heart by percussion.

A full cardiac examination includes an assessment of the size of the heart by percussion (if feasible given the patient's anatomy), palpation of the cardiac impulse at the apex, and auscultation at the base of the heart and the apex of the heart, in the sitting and supine positions—and in some contexts with the patient lying on the left side—both at rest and after vigorous exercise. Auscultation around the entire area of the heart would be added if pericarditis were under consideration. Attention is paid to the splitting of the second heart sound and the variation of the two components of the second heart sound with respiration, whether there is a third and/or fourth heart sound, and whether there are murmurs, clicks, or friction rubs. Murmurs are characterized by their amplitude, pitch, location, variation in amplitude with body position and with exercise, and whether they are constant throughout systole or diastole or rapidly diminish in amplitude.

The cardiac component of a typical physical examination—even one by an internist or cardiologist—typically includes a proper subset of the above observations, although the written record examination typically does characterize any abnormal sounds that were heard. In reviewing the record of a physical examination of the heart, the medical psychiatrist should consider whether some part of the ideal full examination was omitted and whether the missing part would be specifically relevant to a current diagnostic hypothesis. If medical psychiatrists do their own examinations, the scope and focus should be hypothesis-driven—for example, when the hypothesis is one of heart failure, they should listen carefully for a third heart sound and examine the patient lying down and after exercise. The interpretation of examination findings should consider whether they are inconclusive or potentially falsely negative for the suspected condition. The documentation of the hypothesis, the physical findings, and their interpretation, all are useful in communicating diagnostic concerns to a primary care physician or cardiologist and in prompting more conclusive diagnostic studies.

When a chronically ill patient has heart failure among his or her diagnoses, it may be known to—or at least knowable by—the medical psychiatrist how the findings on physical examination of the patient's heart differ when the heart failure is optimally compensated and when it is decompensated. While physical signs elsewhere in the body, such as those of pulmonary edema or venous congestion, might also be present when the heart failure is decompensated, there may be consistent cardiac findings such as a loud third heart sound or a palpably enlarged heart. If the medical psychiatrist knows, from the medical record or from discussion with the primary care physician or cardiologist, the patient's personal "signature" of heart failure, the psychiatrist can utilize this perspective to improve his or her assessment if the particular patient shows an acute change in mental status or loss of function. A brief cardiac examination focusing on the patient-specific signs will suggest whether a change in mood, cognition, behavior, or physical functioning is likely to be associated with worsening heart failure.

The limitations of the bedside cardiac examination can be reduced greatly with technology. Electronic stethoscopes that both amplify and record heart sounds bring consistency to the description of murmurs; applications are available for mobile devices that offer graphical representation of heart sounds that can be transmitted online to a consultant. Point-of-care pocket-sized ultrasound devices enable even internal medicine residents with only 2 or 3 hours of training to make highly specific diagnoses of left ventricular dysfunction or pericardial effusion (Alexander et al., 2004; Ruddox et al., 2013).

ABDOMEN

The main issue for medical psychiatrists on the abdominal examination is the problem of false negatives. It is unlikely that a finding of an acute abdomen will turn out to be a false positive; specialist examination and diagnostic procedures will virtually always make possible a specific diagnosis. An optimal abdominal examination—something that can be impossible if the patient has significant abdominal obesity or if a patient is delirious and agitated—would provide information on:

1. The presence or absence of peritonitis and, if present, whether it is localized or generalized;

2. The presence or absence of ascites, and, if present, the amount

3. The approximate size of the liver, whether the liver is tender, and whether the liver is unusually hard or soft

4. Whether the spleen is enlarged

5. Whether there is an abdominal aortic aneurysm

6. Whether there are normal bowel sounds

7. Whether there are any abnormal masses or areas of localized tenderness

8. Whether there are any hernias or defects in the abdominal wall

9. Whether there is lower abdominal fullness suggesting fecal impaction

When a patient is cooperative and sufficiently thin, it is possible for an experienced examiner to provide this information. If the patient's behavior, body type, or corpulence prevents a confident answer in any of these areas and the patient is acutely ill, the physician typically must resort to laboratory tests and diagnostic imaging to settle any outstanding questions. The medical psychiatrist, reviewing the findings of the physical examination of the abdomen in a chronically ill patient, can identify what is not known by keeping in mind the limitations of the abdominal examination as performed and recorded. Together with diagnostic hypotheses, this guides the orders for further investigations and/or the communication with the general medical physician(s) involved.

When the patient has a relapsing-remitting or fluctuating gastrointestinal condition with known and variable physical signs, a targeted abdominal examination by the medical psychiatrist can help establish the contribution of the medical condition to an acute change in mental status. For example, in an institutionalized patient with moderate dementia and a tendency toward fecal impaction, discovery on examination that the patient's lower abdomen feels full but soft—as it did the last time the patient had fecal impaction—would identify fecal impaction as a likely cause of an acute agitated delirium superimposed on the dementia. Or, in a patient receiving palliative chemotherapy for widely disseminated ovarian cancer, the examination finding of a reaccumulation of ascites might help link an increase in depressed mood and pain complaints to progression of the cancer rather than to an emotional reaction to the cancer diagnosis.

On occasion, the medical psychiatrist will attend to an abdominal sign that is particularly meaningful in the medical-psychiatric context. An borderline-enlarged spleen can prompt a more thorough search for chronic low-grade infection or autoimmune disease in a patient with a syndrome of chronic fatigue thought most likely to reflect a somatoform disorder. A small, hard liver typical of alcoholic cirrhosis can encourage the medical psychiatrist to further question the validity of a patient's denial of a drinking problem, and to order or suggest additional diagnostic tests such as a coagulation panel, an ammonia level, or an abdominal ultrasound. Further, the physical finding of a grossly abnormal liver might be mentioned to a patient and family when confronting a denial of alcoholism.

PELVIS AND GENITALS

The examination of the pelvis in women, and of the external genitalia in patients of either gender, usually is not done directly by the medical psychiatrist because of concerns about perceived boundary violations. This can create a problem, however, if the general medical physician responsible for "medical clearance" has omitted or deferred the physical examination of the pelvis and genitals. Patients presenting with recent-onset medical–psychiatric issues, such as depression or anxiety with prominent somatic symptoms, need thorough evaluation for infectious diseases and for cancer, and there are both common infections and common neoplasms that affect the reproductive system. Some specific conditions that can be diagnosed by physical examination and have important medical-psychiatric dimensions include polycystic ovary syndrome, ovarian cancer, pelvic inflammatory disease, testicular cancer, and testicular atrophy due to anabolic steroid abuse; in addition, several common sexually-transmitted diseases (STDs) have characteristic physical findings on genital examination. Thus an essential point for the medical psychiatrist is that someone should examine the reproductive system in connection with the current evaluation if it hasn't been done recently and at a time when the patient was symptomatic.

The qualitative dimension of the pelvic examination is valuable information not necessarily recorded in the medical record but potentially available through the medical psychiatrist's directly communication with the examiner. The medical psychiatrist should consider inquiring in greater detail about a female patient's history of sexual and intimate relationships if it is known that she had intense discomfort during the pelvic examination or had an intense emotional reaction to the examination. In this situation there could be a history of trauma or abuse, or the patient might suffer from a primary gynecologic condition that causes significant dyspareunia that is secondarily affecting sexual relationships, marital satisfaction, and/or self-esteem.

ANORECTAL REGION

The same considerations about potential boundary issues and the risk of missing important diagnoses apply to the examination of the perianal skin and to the digital rectal examination (DRE), and they are applicable to general medical physicians, many of whom omit the DRE when they do general physical examinations because of concerns about patients' modesty or a feeling that the DRE is too invasive for a routine examination (Wong et al., 2012). Medical psychiatrists will at times encounter patients who have not had a DRE even when they saw a general medical physician for a condition such as chronic constipation for which a DRE would obviously be informative.

Diagnoses that are potentially detectable on DRE include prostatic hyperplasia, prostate cancer, and rectal cancer; hemorrhoids, anal fissures, perianal abscesses, anal cancer, and other anal pathology; and fecal impaction. In female patients DRE can aid in the diagnosis of pelvic inflammatory disease.

Of particular medical-psychiatric interest is the sensitivity of the DRE to disorders of anal sphincter control and to pelvic floor dysfunction. Abnormally low anal sphincter tone suggests autonomic neuropathy or sacral cord injury. A missing anal wink reflex suggests sensory or autonomic neuropathy. Pelvic floor dyssynergia is a major cause of chronic constipation that responds in the majority of cases to biofeedback training, eliminating the need for long-term laxative use.

A complete DRE comprises the following 10 steps (Talley, 2008): (1) reassuring the patient and explaining the purpose of the examination; (2) positioning the patient in the left lateral decubitus position; (3) inspecting the perineum; (4) asking the patient to strain while watching the perineum; (5) testing the anal wink reflex; (6) beginning palpation of the anus itself to assess tenderness and prompt relaxation of the sphincter; (7) assessing resting sphincter tone; (8) palpating the rectal walls, including palpation of the prostate gland through the anterior wall; (9) evaluating pelvic floor function; and (10) removing the finger and examining the feces for blood, pus, or mucus. To evaluate pelvic floor function the examiner asks the patient to strain and push the examiner's finger out; when function is normal the anal sphincter relaxes and the perineum descends by 1 cm to 3.5 cm. Nondescent of the perineum coupled with external anal sphincter contraction implies pelvic floor dyssynergia. The patient is then asked to squeeze the examiner's finger. If the pelvic muscles and anal sphincter are functioning properly the finger will be squeezed and lifted toward the umbilicus. This tests the muscle functions needed to ensure fecal continence.

In patients with delirium or dementia with agitation, the diagnosis of acute anal disease may explain a recent change in mental status. In cognitively intact patients with chronic mental illness and no constipation or specific anal or pelvic complaint, the main function of DRE is screening for prostate cancer and colorectal cancer. While DRE is underutilized as a tool for identifying dysfunction of the anal sphincter and pelvic floor, the historical emphasis on the DRE in prostate cancer screening has not been supported by rigorous studies. DRE identifies few prostate cancers that have not already caused elevated levels of prostate-specific antigen. Those that are found by DRE alone are not necessarily aggressive ones, and there is no convincing evidence that finding prostate cancers on DRE (or on PSA screening) reduces prostate cancer mortality (Ilic et al., 2013). As to screening for colon cancer, fecal occult blood testing is less sensitive than colonoscopy, and testing for blood at the time of a DRE is less sensitive than testing spontaneously passed stool. In particular, bleeding from an advanced premalignant lesion is more likely to be detected by testing of spontaneously passed stool (Ashraf et al., 2012). Notwithstanding, testing stool from a DRE is better than no testing at all, so it should be considered when examining patients unlikely to comply with home-based stool collection or to have a screening colonoscopy. As with women and pelvic examination, when a man shows unusual discomfort or emotional distress related to a rectal examination it raises the issue of history of sexual trauma or physical abuse—a topic to be explored sensitively at an appropriate time. There may be relevance to ongoing intimate relationships when the patient is a man who has sex with other men.

Finally, as noted in the discussion of the abdominal examination, fecal impaction sometimes is the explanation for acute changes in behavior or mental status in institutionalized, cognitively impaired patients. Rectal examination can be the key to this diagnosis in some cases, though when the impaction is higher in the colon an imaging procedure—sometimes just a plain abdominal X-ray—will confirm the diagnosis even though the rectal examination is negative.

NEUROLOGICAL EXAMINATION

There are three overlapping purposes of the neurological examination: (1) to detect deviations from normal function, (2) to test hypotheses about the systems or anatomic loci responsible for the deviation from normal function, and (3) to measure the severity of dysfunction. Most of the neurological examination involves stimulating the patient in some way and observing a response. An absent or abnormal response can result from impaired perception of the stimulus, failed execution of a response, or ineffective linkage between the perception of the stimulus and execution of the response. A neurological examination can be incomplete for diagnostic purposes when it fails to detect dysfunction that is present, when it does not convincingly rule out dysfunction that is not present, or when it gathers insufficient data to explain whether the problem is with perception, execution of the response, the connection between the two, or some combination.

NEUROLOGICAL MENTAL STATUS EXAMINATION

In contrast to the psychiatric mental status examination, which aims to detect and characterize disorders of mood, thought process and content, and behavior, the neurological mental status examination focuses on detection and characterization of disorders of the level of consciousness, cognition (including attention and orientation, memory, language, and learned cognitive skills such as calculation), perception, executive function, and praxis (execution of skilled motor performances). The neurological mental status examinations performed in general medical contexts for screening purposes typically are brief and limited, leaving several domains of mental status unexamined. The medical psychiatrist's neurological mental status examination should be broader in scope; but to be practical, it must be focused and hypothesis-driven. Hypotheses are suggested by some combination of the history, findings on the general physical and neurological examination, laboratory and/or imaging abnormalities, and demographic and environmental circumstances such as coming from an area in which an infectious disease that frequently causes brain dysfunction is endemic. In bedside or office assessment for the presence of cognitive or perceptual dysfunction, the critical concern is test *sensitivity*. The two most common reasons for insensitivity of such assessments are that (1) functions that ought to be evaluated are not tested at all, and (2) the items covering an area of function are too easy to detect abnormality in patients with high baseline function and/or mild impairment. An example of the former is not testing visual memory in a patient with temporal lobe lesion of the right hemisphere; an example of the latter is testing memory in an alcoholic practicing lawyer by asking him to recall three common words after three minutes.

Both types of test insensitivity can be avoided by beginning with a hypothesis about how a specific impairment would be likely to affect the specific patient. In tests to *characterize* or *measure the severity* of a cognitive or perceptual impairment, the clinician should aim for a level of difficulty that will put the patient's performance in the middle of the range, avoiding both the "floor" and the "ceiling." The components of the neurological mental status examination are now discussed in detail.

General Behavior

The patient's comportment, attention to the examiner's questions, effort devoted to answering them, and response to potential distractions in the environment should be described unless they are normal throughout the entire examination. Lack of engagement in the examination, if not obviously reflecting conscious or intentional refusal to be examined, can be a sign of a diminished or fluctuating level of consciousness, impaired executive function, or apathy. A lack of persistence in answering questions can indicate impaired attention. Distraction during the examination by ordinary environmental stimuli (e.g., a nurse walking past on her way to another patient) can be a sign of impaired attention or impaired executive function. Undue silliness and jocularity during the examination is usually due to defective inhibition, a form of executive impairment.

Orientation and Attention

The phenomenon of orientation is related to level of consciousness, perception of the environment, and memory; being oriented is expressed by behavior as well as by the spoken word. A hospitalized patient calling the nurse "waiter" and demanding that the dinner menu be brought at 3:00 a.m. is disoriented in a different way than one who behaves appropriately and knows the day, time, and name of the hospital but doesn't know what county the hospital is in. Orientation to place is indicated in one way by behavior typical of being in that place; in another way it is indicated by verbalization of the location's complete address. The latter depends on memory and language in addition to knowing where one is. Orientation to day and time similarly is expressed both by behavior and by verbalizations, the latter dependent partially on memory and language. Disoriented behavior is common in delirium and in the later stages of dementia; patients with mild cognitive impairment might misstate the date but behave in a way that shows awareness of the season, day versus night, and so on.

A severely inattentive person would be unable to focus on the task of a formal mental status examination and be unable to consistently answer the examiner's questions.

The record of the examination should cite an example of the patient's distractibility and/or lack of persistence. Less severe impairment in attention often can be demonstrated by having a patient count backwards from 20 to 1, recite the months of the year in reverse, or repeatedly take 7 or 3 from 100. Doing the second task requires sufficient language function to retrieve the names of the months; doing the third task requires basic ability to calculate. The indicator of impaired attention is the inability to complete the task even if it is begun correctly. A typical way for a patient to fail the months in reverse task is to get part way through the months and then complete the task by naming the months in forward order.

Another option for bedside testing of attention is having the patient alternate numbers and letters, for example, 1-A-2-B-3-C, and so on. If the patient's attention wanders, he or she may continue the task by simply counting or reciting the alphabet. The requirement for maintaining mental set is greater for the alternating condition than for a simple count. For patients unable to talk, a similar test of attention would be asking them to tap an alternating rhythm with their fingers: one tap, two taps, one tap, two taps, and so on. An inattentive patient would be likely either to stop tapping or to tap without alternating.

Visual attention can be impaired when simple attention is intact. Since visual attention is critical to driving or operating dangerous machinery, it is an important function to test when the examiner might be asked to comment on the patient's ability to drive or to return to work. A simple bedside task is to give the patient a sheet of paper full of randomly oriented and randomly spaced letters and numbers, and to ask them to cross out a defined subset of them—for example the even numbers and the vowels. A specific problem with visual attention is suggested if the patient misses the targets in one half or one quadrant of the page, or if targets are missed that are oriented in a particular direction. When visual fields are tested by confrontation, visual inattention might be shown by the patient's missing some but not all small finger movements at the periphery of vision but not larger movements or larger static objects. The fact that the stimulus is seen some of the time rules out a gross visual field defect.

Auditory attention can be tested by presenting a series of numbers and asking the patient to signal when he or she hears an odd number or hears one specific number. Or, a patient can be presented with a series of tones that may be either high or low and asked to signal when he or she hears a high tone but not a low one.

People with more severe general impairments of attention will have trouble with both tests of visual and of auditory attention; people with milder impairments may show problems with one sensory modality or type of task but not with another. When the purpose of the examination is to show that attention is not intact, any unequivocally abnormal test result will suffice. Giving several tests of different types makes sense when the goal is to determine the scope and severity of impairment or to identify areas in which function is relatively preserved.

Memory

When the objective in memory testing is to identify delirium or dementia—the latter as a syndrome diagnosis as distinct from the diagnosis of a neurodegenerative disease that will eventually produce the syndrome of dementia—the typical procedure of testing recall of three or four unrelated words after a five minute delay usually is sufficient. Memory testing as part of the clinical neurological examination acquires subtlety when the question is one of memory loss *from the patient's baseline*, or when the disease or condition suspected can have differential effects on a particular kind of memory such as visual memory or memory for spoken as opposed to written language. The medical psychiatrist who evaluates previously obtained information on the patient's memory must determine what exactly was tested, decide whether the testing was sufficient to address the current hypothesis, and consider whether the patient's memory performance might be different now from what it was when last tested by a prior clinician.

A cognitively intact, literate adult should be able to accurately repeat four unrelated words after the words are presented no more than three times; once they have been accurately repeated (registered) the patient should be able to recall, after a few minutes, at least three of the four words without aid, and the fourth with a cue (e.g., the first letter of the word or the category to which the word belongs). If the patient cannot register the words, there is likely a problem with motivation or cooperation, attention, or language. If the patient cannot recall even three of four correctly registered words without aid but can recall all four with cues or with multiple choice, there is a memory problem that involves the recall process but does not involve complete forgetting of the material. Verbal memory deficits that disappear with cueing and/or multiple choice questions are likely to involve problems with executive function (frontal lobes and their connections) and/or with language (e.g., word-finding problems). Complete forgetting of material that was accurately registered suggests dysfunction of the primary memory circuits that comprise the hippocampus, medial thalamus, and mammillary bodies and their connections. Regardless of the specific memory test done or the modality of presentation, comparison of registration (repetition), free (unaided) recall, and cued recall helps to identify the nature of memory loss when it is present.

For detecting subtle deficits or mild impairment in individuals with high premorbid functioning, two alternative bedside tests of verbal memory should be considered. These are more difficult than recalling four unrelated words yet not too difficult for a literate adult of normal intelligence, even one with limited formal education. The first is the two-sentence logical memory test. The patient is given two unrelated sentences to remember, and is asked to recall as many details of each as possible, without mixing them up. The two sentences are presented three times, stopping after the first or second trial if the patient recalls the sentences perfectly. Then, after a few minutes of intervening activity—for example, testing other cognitive functions—the patient is asked to recall the details of the first sentence and then the details of the second one. If the first sentence has five details and the second has

eight, a normal adult will be able to recall at least 10 of the 13 details by the third try, and will be able to keep the sentences separate. On recall five minutes later, the patient should lose no more than two of the details that were recalled on the last attempted repetition of the sentences.

For example, the first sentence is "A hunter killed a wolf at the edge of the forest," and the second is "In an orchard, behind a tall fence, there were trees with many ripe apples." The five details from the first sentence would be hunter, killed, wolf, edge, and forest, and the eight details from the second sentence would be orchard, behind, tall, fence, trees, many, ripe, and apples.

If the two-sentence memory test does not show definite abnormality, but a deficit in verbal memory is suspected from the patient's history or other clinical data, the possibility of a verbal memory deficit can be further investigated with a six-item paired associate learning task. Here the patient is presented with six pairs of words—five of which are not obviously associated with each other. For example, the six pairs might be rain–clouds, hammer–stairs, up–left, shoe–right, blanket–car, wood–dress. The examiner then presents the first word in each of the six pairs and asks the patient to recall the second. The word pairs are presented up to three times with the words presented in the recall condition in a different order each time; if the patient gets all six pairs correct on the first or second try, the pairs are not presented again. If the patient is able to learn at least four of the six pairs by the third try, recall is tested one more time after a few minutes with an intervening distraction. An adult of normal intelligence without a verbal memory deficit should be able to learn at least five of the six pairs by the third try and should lose no more than one of the associations after a five minute interval with an intervening distraction. When the two-sentence memory test and the six paired associates were used to test verbal memory as part of a 20-minute high-sensitivity bedside cognitive screening test, qualitative judgments of the nature and severity of memory impairment from the bedside assessment were highly correlated with those based on comprehensive neuropsychological testing (Faust & Fogel, 1989). Patients with hearing loss or with central auditory processing problems may require words to be presented in writing rather than spoken. Patients with impaired speech but intact writing should be asked to perform memory tasks in writing. Those with impairments of expressive language can be asked to point to pictures of items to be recalled. A neuropsychologist or behavioral neurologist can assist with the distinction of memory deficits from other types of cognitive impairments when there are multifocal cognitive deficits such as might be found in patients with multiple strokes, multiple sclerosis, or multiple brain metastases.

Patients suspected of having with selective impairment of visual memory must be tested in the visual modality. The direct equivalent of the typical verbal memory test is having the patient copy three simple shapes, then draw the same shapes immediately after the originals have been removed, and finally to draw them from memory after a few minutes delay with an intervening distraction. As with verbal memory, multiple choice can be used to identify patients in whom memory loss is due to executive cognitive dysfunction rather than true forgetting. A simpler yet face-valid bedside or office test of visual memory is hiding three dollar bills around the bedside or the office while the patient watches, having him or her immediately point to where they were hidden, and then having the patient point out after a delay where the money was hidden. A cooperative patient with normal visual memory should have no problem finding the money.

Language

Language functions include spontaneous speech, comprehension, repetition, naming and word finding; in addition, there are nonverbal aspects related to transmitting and receiving emotion through the rate, rhythm, volume, and intonation of speech. Because of the complexity of language, there are several ways in which it can fail. The distinctions are psychiatrically relevant as well as helpful in localizing the brain dysfunction within the dominant hemisphere, and in determining whether there is a contribution of nondominant hemisphere dysfunction to the patient's communication impairment. Anatomic brain imaging, despite its ever-improving spatial resolution and wide availability, does not necessarily answer all relevant questions about impairment of function, so precision and specificity in the assessment of language is neurologically as well as psychiatrically useful.

The detailed examination of language goes beyond the scope of this chapter, but several fundamental points related to specific language disorders will be mentioned:

1. *Transcortical motor aphasia.* Patients with left-hemisphere medial frontal dysfunction, including those with hypotensive infarcts at the border zone of the anterior cerebral and middle cerebral arteries, can show transcortical motor aphasia, a disorder in which there is very little spontaneous speech and in which speech is initiated with great difficulty, but comprehension and repetition are intact. In addition to being able to repeat sentences, patients with this type of aphasia can complete familiar phrases such as "Roses are red, violets are (blue)." Such patients are of special interest to medical psychiatrists for three reasons. First, their occurrence with border zone (aka "watershed") infarction means that they will appear in intensive care units and in acute medical-surgical environments where they might be seen by a consulting psychiatrist before they are seen by a neurologist. Second, because of their difficulty initiating speech they can appear uncooperative, apathetic, or electively mute before the language disorder is appreciated. Third, patients with transcortical motor aphasia have an especially good prognosis for recovering language function within 18 months when the aphasia was caused by a stroke (Cauquil-Michon et al., 2011; Flamand-Roze et al., 2011). If a comprehensive language examination confirms the diagnosis of transcortical motor aphasia, the patient and family can be offered realistic hope of improvement that can improve morale and enhance motivation for speech therapy.

2. *Broca's aphasia.* Patients with Broca's aphasia (aka *non-fluent aphasia*), typically due to a left middle cerebral artery stroke, have a lesion in the frontal lobe anterior to the part of the motor strip that controls the movements of the mouth. They speak with great effort and poor accuracy and are not better with repetition. Comprehension is relatively intact. The typical emotional response is depression but not suspiciousness or paranoia.

3. *Wernicke's aphasia.* Patients with Wernicke's aphasia (aka *fluent aphasia*), typically due to an embolic infarction of the posterior superior temporal lobe, easily generate large amounts of abnormal speech and continually misunderstand what others are saying to them. They are often unaware of their deficit, particularly early on, and this contributes to suspiciousness or even frank paranoia. The abnormal speech is on occasion misdiagnosed as a manifestation of delirium or of a primary psychosis; demonstration of markedly impaired comprehension and repetition should be sufficient to differentiate the condition.

4. *Anomia.* Patients with *nominal aphasia* or *anomia* due to a dominant posterior parietal lesion cannot accurately name items, whether they are presented visually or they are described in words; their spontaneous speech can show word substitutions, letter substitutions, or circumlocutions, the latter including elaborate descriptions of things for which the patient cannot find the right word. Impaired naming is seen not only in focal lesions but also in diffuse or multifocal processes such as toxic encephalopathy, encephalitis, or neurodegenerative diseases. Impaired naming can show a circular relationship with anxiety. Patients become anxious because they cannot find the words they are looking for; as anxiety increases, they have more trouble finding a suitable alternative for conveying their thought.

5. *Impairment of prosody.* Patients with lesions or dysfunction in the nondominant hemisphere can show problems with the production and/or interpretation of prosody: the tempo, rhythm, pitch, and loudness of speech that convey emotion, distinguish statements, questions, and commands, and indicate whether speech is to be taken seriously or ironically or facetiously. Varieties of aprosodia—expressive and receptive, with and without impairment of repetition—parallel the varieties of aphasia. Posterior lesions such as those involving the non-dominant posterior superior temporal region impair comprehension of prosody, and anterior lesions such as those involving the non-dominant anterior perisylvian region or the medial frontal region impair expression of prosody (Heilman et al., 2004; Wildgruber et al., 2006). Prosodic impairment is of obvious medical-psychiatric interest because of its functional implications; it can be occupationally disabling, and it can bring conflict and frustration to caregiving relationships. Testing for prosodic impairment parallels testing for aphasia. The patient is asked to name the emotions conveyed by sentences spoken by the examiner and to say

whether sentences are meant as questions, statements, or commands; to read sentences to convey different emotions and intentions; and to repeat sentences with the same words that differ in prosody.

The examiner can assess prosody at the bedside by giving the following tests: (1) asking the patient to read a sentence—for example, "My friend is moving to a beautiful new house"—in an angry, sad, happy, ironic/facetious, or questioning tone; (2) reading a sentence to the patient with prosody conveying different emotions or meanings and asking him or her what emotion or meaning is conveyed; and (3) asking the patient to repeat sentences presented by the examiner with prosody expressing the same emotion or meaning.

6. *Dyslexia and dysgraphia.* Almost all dominant hemisphere brain lesions that significantly affect spoken language will also affect reading and/or writing. Thus, having the patient hand-write a one-paragraph summary of his or her own recent illness can be a time-efficient and sensitive (albeit nonspecific) way to screen for language problems in those with medical or epidemiologic risk factors for brain diseases that might affect language. The converse is not true; focal brain lesions in certain specific locations can impair writing and/or reading without impairing spoken language.

Understanding the precise nature of a patient's language dysfunction is useful in determining the relationship of that dysfunction to the patient's mental and behavioral symptoms—causal, concurrent, or coincidental. If the language dysfunction has not been previously characterized, there may be opportunities to improve the patient's relationships with caregivers by doing so and explaining the findings to them.

Calculation

Questions about very simple arithmetical facts are more a test of long-term memory than of calculation itself. Obviously wrong answers to over-learned arithmetical facts—for example, "two plus two equals five"—suggest malingering, conversion, or elaboration of cognitive symptoms. Multistep calculations or calculations involving numbers with two or more digits are true tests of calculation. When they are failed, they suggest dysfunction of the dominant parietal lobe. However, the usual principle of analysis of cognitive deficits applies. To ascribe a cognitive deficit to a specific brain region or system, one must establish that the input pathway and output pathway are not cause of the problem: the patient must be sufficiently motivated and attentive, must understand the calculation to be done, and must be able to express the answer verbally, in writing, or by indication of a choice among alternatives.

Visual-Spatial Functions

Visual-spatial functions involve the visual association areas in the anterior occipital lobes, posterior inferior temporal lobes, and the parietal lobes, the latter especially on the nondominant side. These functions are sometimes neglected in routine bedside mental status examination, and in themselves they contribute so little to the score of standard bedside cognitive screening instruments that patients can get passing scores despite severe impairment in the visual-spatial domain.

The quickest and most practical bedside test of visual-spatial function is the clock drawing task (CDT). The patient is given a sheet of paper and is asked to draw the face of a clock and to set the hands at a specific time, commonly "ten after eleven". Patients with disturbances of visual-spatial functions may draw a circle that is not round, that is incomplete, or that is too small to accommodate the numbers of the clock. The numbers may be misplaced, either found outside the circle or incorrectly distributed within the circle. If there is neglect of half of the visual field (typically the left half) or of a quadrant (typically the left upper or left lower quadrant), this will be reflected by the absence of numbers in the given half or quarter of the clock. Hands may be misplaced or of the wrong length.

If the clock drawing is not executed perfectly, the patient can be asked to copy a clock that is correctly drawn. The copying task rules out contributions of memory impairment and/or poor planning to errors in the drawing—continued failure suggests problems either with visual perception, with the task of drawing (constructional praxis), or both. Impairment in visual perception can be distinguished from impairment in drawing performance by having the patient distinguish correctly from incorrectly drawn clocks, stating what is wrong about the ones that are incorrect.

There are more than 20 published systems for administering and scoring the CDT, but none has been accepted as a standard. They were comprehensively reviewed by Mainland et al. (2014). They concluded that for *identifying* cognitive impairment, simpler systems using only a spontaneous clock drawing worked as well as more complex and time-consuming ones. More complex systems can help determine whether CDT errors are related to visual-spatial deficits, impaired praxis, impaired executive function, impaired attention, and so forth. Specific types of errors on the CDT deficits have been correlated with specific regional abnormalities on functional brain imaging. Regardless of the administration procedure and scoring system, impairment on the CDT has been shown by numerous studies to correlate with impairment on longer and more systematic tests of visual-spatial function and with functional impairment such as poor driving ability (Freund et al., 2005).

A basic scoring system for the CDT applied to 536 patients in a memory disorder clinic identified dementia with 71% sensitivity and 88% specificity; patients were scored abnormal if they had any of the following errors on the spontaneous CDT: (1) refusal to do the drawing, (2) inaccurate time setting, (3) no hands, (4) missing numbers, (5) number substitutions, or (6) number repetitions (Lessig et al., 2008). The CDT has been successfully applied as a brief cognitive screener in general medical patient populations ranging from those with cancer to those with fibromyalgia, and it has been used to identify which elderly patients undergoing femoral fracture repair were at highest risk for postoperative delirium

(Meziere et al., 2013). *Minor* errors on the CDT are commonly seen in elderly patients without cognitive impairment; these have been systematically characterized (Hubbard et al., 2008).

In addition to its remarkable psychometric properties, the CDT has practical utility in communicating the physician's concern about a patient's cognitive impairment. A badly drawn clock has face validity in making the case with a caregiver or other physician that there is a functionally significant problem.

Another test of visual perception that is feasible whenever language is intact is scene analysis. A picture with rich content in both the background and the foreground is shown to the patient, who is asked to describe what is seen. As a follow-up, the patient can be asked to point out specific details or identify particular elements in the picture. Like the clock drawing, scene analysis tasks have appealing face validity. Caregivers can easily understand there is a problem when the patient looks at a picture and neglects its left half or is unable to distinguish the main figure from the background.

Praxis

Praxis refers to the ability to execute a complex motor activity, assuming gross motor and sensory function adequate to physically complete the task. Apraxia typically results from parietal lobe and/or frontal lobe dysfunction. One or both hemispheres may be involved depending on the task. To test for praxis the patient is asked to demonstrate how he or she would do various tasks, usually involving a tool, such as cutting with scissors, hammering a nail, or swinging a baseball bat. The patient with intact praxis will demonstrate the use of the imaginary tool; one with impaired praxis either will use the body part as if it were the tool or will fail to do the task at all. A patient who fails an initial test of praxis can be asked to imitate the action when it is performed by the examiner. If the action can be copied accurately, the patient's ability to organize and execute the motor performance is intact but the ability to conceive it is impaired. It is unusual to see apraxia without other cognitive and/or perceptual problems.

Medical psychiatrists sometimes are asked to evaluate patients who claim to be—or who are said to be—unable to do certain physical tasks despite apparently intact motor function. This problem, when due to apraxia, occasionally is misunderstood as reflecting malingering, conversion, or symptom amplification. A more detailed neurological examination with an extended cognitive evaluation will resolve the issue.

Executive Function

Executive functions comprise goal-setting, organization and planning, persistence, resistance to distraction, understanding the significance of environmental cues, self-regulation and self-control, inhibition of socially inappropriate behavior, abstract reasoning, insight, and judgment. They are often thought of as "frontal lobe" functions; however, the neural circuits involved in executive functions also include the basal ganglia, thalamus and cerebellum, and they are influenced by neuromodulators originating in brainstem, thalamus, and basal forebrain nuclei. The tasks used to test executive function rely upon inputs from and outputs to other brain regions. Executive functions are the last cognitive functions to reach maturity and usually the first to be impaired by diffuse encephalopathy or neurodegenerative disease.

Executive functions can be classified into three groups with anatomical associations. Inhibition and self-control are related to the orbital frontal region and its connections; abstract reasoning, organization and planning, judgment, and interpretation of environmental cues are associated with the dorsolateral frontal lobe and its connections; initiation, motivation, and persistence are associated with the medial frontal lobe and its connections. The frontal lobe functions that typically are tested as part of a neurological examination in the office or at the bedside are mainly—or entirely—those of the dorsolateral frontal systems. Thus, typically, dysfunction of the orbital frontal or medial frontal system is inferred from the history and from observation of the patient's behavior during the examination. A well-documented neurological mental status examination describes any elements of the patient's behavior during the examination that offer remarkable evidence of apathy or disinhibition, a typical example of the latter being the production of vulgar language when the patient is asked to list words beginning with the letters f, a, and s. Patients with impairment in executive function perform better on cognitive tests when the patient's executive function is augmented by cues from or the physical or social environment, and when there are few potential distractions. Thus, a patient with impaired executive function might be well oriented and pass basic bedside memory tests when at home, but be disoriented and fail memory tests when examined in the setting of an intensive care unit. For this reason the context of the examination is especially relevant when assessing executive function. When the findings on cognitive examination are unexpected given the patient's diagnosis and condition, documentation of mental status should note the time and place of the examination and anything remarkable about the environment at that time.

The CDT is an excellent screening test for dorsolateral frontal function when visual-spatial function is intact. When visual-spatial function is intact and executive function is impaired, a free-drawn clock is incorrect but a copied clock is correct. The free-drawn clock typically shows poor planning and organization. Numbers may be poorly spaced, duplicated, or omitted. If the clock is to be set at "ten after eleven" the patient might point the large hand toward the ten rather than the two. If the patient can copy a clock drawing perfectly, a poor performance on the free clock drawing cannot be attributed to visual-spatial dysfunction or to impaired praxis.

Other useful and common bedside tests of dorsolateral frontal function include:

1. Listing items that belong to a given category, such as vegetables, fruits, tools, or pieces of furniture. This task requires organization and persistence and the ability to maintain the mental set to stick with a single category.

2. Listing words that begin with a specific letter of the alphabet, such as a, f, s, or t. A person with intact frontal lobe function and intact naming will be able to name at least eight items in 30 seconds that begin with any of those letters. Production of vulgar language on this task suggests impaired orbital-frontal function.

3. Explaining what pairs of words have in common when there is something obviously different about them: for example, hammer and screwdriver, school and prison, president and dictator, love and hate. The patient with intact language and dorsolateral frontal function will easily name the common category; patients with impaired function will be unable to shift their mental focus from the differences. Patients with impaired orbital frontal function occasionally will produce bizarre responses that they have failed to inhibit.

4. Sorting cards by color, by number, and by shape. Patients with impaired dorsolateral frontal function can have difficulty shifting from one sorting rule to another.

5. Writing a short account of the present illness. Patients with impaired frontal function but no language impairment will write grammatical sentences but will give an incomplete, poorly organized, or perseverative account or one that includes irrelevant or even inappropriate content.

Formal testing of orbital frontal inhibitory functions has been done in the neuropsychology laboratory, for example, using the Iowa Gambling Task (IGT; Bechara, 2010). The Executive Interview Test (Royall et al., 1992) is a bedside screening test with several items related to inhibitory functions. For example, the examiner asks the patient not to shake his hand and then stretches his hand out to the patient. Patients with impaired frontal lobe functions often are unable to inhibit their response to the cue and will reach for the examiner's hand. However, the test can be failed because of either dorsolateral frontal dysfunction or orbital frontal dysfunction. Findings that point more specifically to the orbital frontal system are those related to lack of inhibition of inappropriate responses to emotionally salient cues.

The following points concerning executive function are of special interest to the medical psychiatrist:

1. Deficits in executive function underlie functional impairment in many cases of brain diseases or traumatic brain injury, and they can be disproportionate to other kinds of cognitive impairment.

2. Schizophrenia, bipolar disorder, and severe depression all are associated with impaired executive function, and this feature can contribute to disability they cause.

3. Drugs and alcohol can impair executive function disproportionately to other cognitive functions.

4. Patients with impaired executive function may present with complaints about their memory; their caregivers' initial complaints often concern inappropriate or irresponsible behavior, bad judgment, or resistance to care.

Metacognition

Metacognition—"knowing about knowing"—comprises patients' awareness of their own cognitive and mnemonic capabilities and defects, and also their judgments about whether particular judgments or memories are valid or should be questioned. Dementing diseases affect both cognition and metacognition, but cognitive and metacognitive dysfunctions need not be highly correlated early in the course of illness. Some drugs, notably alcohol and benzodiazepines, impair cognition and metacognition in parallel, so that individuals are unaware of the extent of their drug-induced impairment. Others, notably anticholinergic agents, can impair cognition to a similar extent while leaving the patient aware that his or her cognition has been affected by a drug (Mintzer & Griffiths, 2003). This may account for a greater propensity of patients to complain of the cognitive side effects of anticholinergic drugs than to complain of the cognitive side effects of benzodiazepines. Patients with relatively intact metacognition will be less disabled for a given degree of cognitive impairment. For example, if metamemory is intact, a patient with an early dementia will take notes, use technology-based reminders, and ask for directions rather than forget important tasks, miss appointments, or get lost while perhaps blaming others for their mistakes. Metacognition can be assessed by asking the patient to evaluate his/her own cognitive performance and comparing the patient's self-evaluation with the examiner's observations and history provided from collateral sources.

GAIT AND BALANCE

The observation of gait and the testing of gait and balance can reveal much about CNS function, but they sometimes are omitted when the patient is examined in bed. Impaired gait and balance are related to the risk of falls with injury, a significant threat to patients in hospitals and in long-term care settings. Fear of falling is an important factor in social withdrawal and functional decline in frail old people. And, determining the underlying reason for impaired gait and/or balance can lead to a new, psychiatrically relevant neurological or general medical diagnosis.

The basic observation of gait requires simply that the patient get up from a chair or from a bed, stand in place briefly, then walk across the room, turn around, return to the bed or chair, and finally sit down or lie down. The examiner observes the speed and the difficulty with which the steps are executed and whether movements are symmetrical, steps are of normal length, and the arms swing as expected. Unusual postures or hand positions are noted, as are any adventitious movements of the hands, fingers, or face.

If the patient feels faint and must sit down shortly after arising from bed or chair, orthostatic hypotension should be suspected. If the arm does not swing on one side but it does on the other, the patient should be examined for hemiparesis and for lateralized spasticity or rigidity. Very small steps with a stooped posture and difficulty stopping and/or turning around suggest a diagnosis of Parkinson's disease. A shuffling gait with feet "glued to the floor" suggests hydrocephalus. While difficulty turning around is typical of Parkinson's disease the sign is nonspecific.

A specific gait-related performance—getting up from a chair and walking 10 feet—can be timed with a stopwatch and used as a repeatable measure for tracking a patient's response to a treatment such as physical therapy, levodopa therapy of Parkinson's disease, or the placing of a shunt to treat hydrocephalus.

When basic observations of gait are normal but problems with the motor system (including coordination) are a concern, there are several options for making walking more difficult and thereby unmasking asymmetries, coordination problems, or adventitious movements. These include walking on heels or on tiptoes, walking on the sides of the feet, or walking on a narrow line touching heel to toe. In some contexts asking the patient to hop in place on one foot may be appropriate. When observations of gait are normal but the history suggests a concern about gait stability, the examiner should try to reproduce conditions associated with the reported problems, such as dim lighting or the need to circumvent obstacles.

Standing balance can be given a stress test in order to assess balance-related complaints or to test hypotheses about the systems for standing balance—the vestibular system, the midline cerebellum and its connections, the visual system, and the proprioceptive system. If the patient can stand stably with eyes open, he or she can be asked to close the eyes; this removes the stabilizing effect of visual input and can cause a loss of balance if lower-extremity position sense is impaired. Standing on the toes or on the heels, or with one foot in front of the other heel to toe, makes an additional demand on balance-related systems. A patient who is stable on two feet can be asked to stand on one foot; marked asymmetry of performance is abnormal.

When gait is said to be normal on a reported examination, or no comment at all is made about gait in the report of an office examination of an ambulatory patient, it can be inferred that casual observation of the patient's walking into and out of the office showed no evident abnormality. If there are open hypotheses that can be tested by a more thorough examination of the patient's gait, the patient should be reexamined with those hypotheses in mind. Abnormalities are documented; if the patient is normal on all bedside tests of gait that were given, the examiner should indicate which tests were done unless the examination was done in a clinic specializing in gait and balance problems that follows a consistent and known routine.

CRANIAL NERVES

The examination of the cranial nerves is interwoven with the physical examination of the head, eyes, ears, nose, and throat. The items most often omitted on routine screening neurological examinations are testing of the senses of smell and taste. When cranial nerves II through XII are reported as intact, it is explicit that smell was not tested, and it can be assumed that taste was not tested if taste was not mentioned specifically.

CRANIAL NERVE I: OLFACTORY NERVE

The primary pathway for the sense of smell—the olfactory tract—begins in the olfactory bulb and ends in the ipsilateral medial temporal lobe. The olfactory bulb can be damaged by trauma to the nose or inhalation of toxic substances. The olfactory tract can be damaged by traumatic brain injury, particularly when the injury affects the orbital frontal region; the tract can be demyelinated in multiple sclerosis. The olfactory cortex and its connections are vulnerable to a broad range of brain diseases, including both Alzheimer's disease and Parkinson's disease. Loss of olfactory sense implies diminished ability to discriminate tastes. It entails safety risks, particularly for individuals who live alone; a person with complete anosmia cannot smell smoke in case of fire or tell by smell that food has spoiled. Several types of patients encountered by medical psychiatrists have specific indications for olfactory testing: (1) patients with complaints of memory loss, (2) patients with a history of traumatic brain injury, (3) patients with suspected multiple sclerosis, (4) patients with motor symptoms suggesting Parkinson's disease, (5) patients with complaints of altered taste or smell, and (6) patients who have weight loss and/or diminished appetite.

Loss of olfactory function in degenerative brain diseases can occur early in their course—even before the other characteristic signs of the disease are fully manifest. Unequivocal defects in olfactory function are seen in patients with very early Parkinson's disease and in patients with mild cognitive impairment who will go on to develop Alzheimer's disease (Casjens et al., 2013; Sun et al., 2012). The finding of an olfactory deficit raises the risk of dementia incrementally after controlling for findings on neuropsychological testing and brain imaging. Loss of olfaction helps distinguish early Parkinson's disease from motor symptoms due to vascular disease or severe depression. Olfactory testing determines three features of olfaction: olfactory thresholds, discrimination of different scents, and identification (naming) of scents. Comprehensive formal testing of olfaction is time consuming and requires relatively expensive standardized olfactory stimuli. The University of Pennsylvania Smell Identification Test (UPSIT) (Doty, 1995) and Sniffin' Sticks (Hummel et al., 1997) are the two olfactory test kits most often cited in the neurological and ear, nose, and throat literature; they deserve consideration when there are research issues or forensic issues that warrant the time and expense of quantifying and fully characterizing deficits. For clinical diagnostic purposes, practical bedside tests usually suffice.

For quantitative determination of olfactory threshold at the bedside, the following procedure can be followed using a standard alcohol wipe as the stimulus (Davidson & Murphy, 1997). One nostril is tested at a time; the patient closes the eyes and mouth and occludes one nostril. A metric ruler is held touching the open nostril at one end and pointing straight down. The stimulus is placed 30 cm from the nostril and moved one centimeter closer to the nostril with each breath. The patient signals when he or she can smell the stimulus; the distance in centimeters from the nostril is the threshold. A variation of the test using a 14g cup of peanut butter as the stimulus was used by Stamps et al. (2013) to identify patients in a memory clinic who had probable Alzheimer's disease. In contrast to normal controls or patients with mild cognitive impairment (MCI) or non-Alzheimer dementias, the patients with probable Alzheimer's disease showed marked asymmetry of the olfactory threshold, at least 5 cm worse on the left in all cases and >10 cm worse on the left in all of the mild cases.

Testing of olfactory discrimination and olfactory naming can be done, one nostril at a time, using commonly recognized and easily available odorants such as instant coffee, extracts of vanilla, almond, or lemon, and common spices like cinnamon or clove. Patients with bilaterally occluded nostrils can be tested retronasally by presenting the stimulus orally, having the patient rinse the mouth after each odorant is presented (Croy et al., 2013). Three or four different scents are sufficient to screen for olfactory discrimination and olfactory naming deficits. Patients are asked to name each scent presented; if unable to do so, they are asked to pick from among four choices. Scratch-and-sniff screening cards with three scents are commercially available.

CRANIAL NERVE II: OPTIC NERVE

The neurologist's examination of the optic nerve focuses on the appearance of the optic nerve head, visual acuity, and the visual fields. A pale, flat optic disk is a sign of optic atrophy, most often as a result of a prior episode of optic neuritis. A swollen optic disk with fuzzy margins, accompanied by absent venous pulsations, is a sign of increased intracranial pressure from hydrocephalus, an intracranial mass, or pseudotumor cerebri. Visual acuity usually is tested with a pocket screening card; to be meaningful, patients must be tested with corrective lenses or reading glasses if they are ordinarily used. Geriatric psychiatrists who frequently must assess visual acuity in patients who need reading glasses but don't have them at hand can benefit from keeping a few different strengths of reading glasses in their examining rooms or medical bags. Visual fields are tested at the bedside by confrontation. Peripheral fields are tested using minimal finger movements at the extremes of the fields. This procedure can easily identify loss of peripheral vision. or the loss of a half or a quarter of the visual field from damage to an optic tract or occipital cortex. Using a red or white push pin a few millimeters in diameter (or the tip of a long cotton swab), it is possible to map the patient's blind spots and thus determine whether they are enlarged, as they might be by glaucoma. The optic nerve is the afferent limb of the pupillary reflex response to light. Shining a light in one eye normally leads to constriction of both pupils. If either pupil constricts, the afferent limb is intact. If one pupil does not constrict but the other does, there is a problem with the non-constricting pupil or with its innervation. For example, if the right pupil constricts when a light is shined into the left eye but then dilates when the light is shined into the right eye the function of the right optic nerve is impaired. This might be seen following optic neuritis on the right. If the right pupil constricts when the light is shined into the right eye but not when it is shined into the left eye, and the left eye constricts when light is shined into the left eye, the two optic nerves are intact and the nerve supply to the right pupil is intact, but the connection across the midline from the left pretectal region to the right Edinger-Westphal nucleus nucleus is impaired. This situation might be seen with demyelinating disease or small-vessel cerebrovascular disease that is damaging white matter tracts in the midbrain.

Pupils, although reactive, can be larger or smaller than normal because of drug effects. Large pupils despite bright light suggest a cholinergic deficit. The examination of the optic fundus and testing of the pupillary light reflex should be done in dim light. Excessively small pupils in dim light suggest a sympathetic deficit; they also can be due to the use of opiates. The fact that a patient has normal peripheral vision does not imply a quick and consistent response to a stimulus anywhere in the patient's field of vision—especially an unexpected stimulus or one embedded within a field of distractors. The useful field of view (UFOV), defined as the visual field over which information can be rapidly extracted without head or eye movements, can be markedly smaller than the visual fields as assessed by confrontation. When this is the case there can be major functional consequences, notably a significant impairment in the ability to drive safely. Reduction in UFOV has been linked to an increased rate of at-fault motor vehicle crashes (Ball et al., 2006). The test, which is computer-administered, evaluates the patient's ability to perceive a centrally presented visual stimulus while simultaneously attending to a peripheral one and to identify a target stimulus amidst distractors (Visual Awareness, 2013). When UFOV is impaired despite normal visual fields, the cause of the problem is impairment in the cortical processing of visual information rather than in the eyes, optic nerves, optic tracts, or primary visual cortex. While UFOV is not tested routinely, the literature on the test highlights an important limitation of bedside visual field testing—or even traditional optometry—in testing a dimension of visual function of great importance to everyday life.

CRANIAL NERVES III, IV, AND VI—OCULOMOTOR, TROCHLEAR AND ABDUCENT NERVES

The third cranial nerve innervates the pupillary muscles as well as the extraocular muscles apart from the superior oblique and lateral rectus. The fourth cranial nerve innervates the superior oblique muscle, and the sixth cranial nerve innervates the lateral rectus. The routine examination tests the extraocular motor functions of cranial nerves III, IV, and VI by having the patient follow a moving finger up, down, left, and right. The third cranial nerve's control of the pupil is assessed by observing the size of the pupils at rest, and the reactions of the pupils to accommodation and to a light shined separately into the right eye and the left eye. The pupillary light reflex is discussed above in connection with testing the optic nerve. Accommodation is tested by having the patient focus on the examiner's finger as it is moved in from a distance toward the patient's nose. The normal response is brisk constriction of the pupils as both eyes move medially to maintain focus on the examiner's finger. Accommodation depends on the cholinergic innervation of the pupil and is disrupted by the anticholinergic effects of drugs; impaired accommodation is a common reason for a complaint of blurred vision when it occurs as a medication side effect. Even without a complaint of blurred vision, impairment of accommodation supports a suspicion of anticholinergic excess as a reason for or contributor to an alteration of mental status.

The function of the third cranial nerve apart from controlling the pupil, and the sole function of the fourth and sixth cranial nerves, is eye movement. The examination of eye movements is an extensive subject beyond the scope of this chapter. We will, however, mention three eye movement disorders with special interest to medical psychiatrists:

1. *Internuclear ophthalmoplegia.* To turn the eyes to the left, a signal from the left paramedian pontine reticular formation goes to the nucleus of the left abducent nerve and, via the right medial longitudinal fasciculus (MLF), to the nucleus of the right oculomotor nerve. If the right MLF is disrupted by infarction, demyelination, or inflammation, the effect of the patient's attempting to look left will be that the left eye will abduct, the right eye will not adduct, and the left eye will show nystagmus with a quick component to the left, as if the abducting eye were returning toward the midline again and again to coax the recalcitrant right eye to move. Lesions of the left MLF will have the corresponding impact on attempted rightward gaze. Because the third nerves and medial rectus muscles themselves are unaffected in this condition, both eyes will adduct when accommodation is tested. Causes of internuclear ophthalmoplegia include multiple sclerosis, brainstem strokes, and spirochete infections including neurosyphilis and neuroborreliosis.

2. *Ocular dysmetria.* Precisely and rapidly shifting one's gaze from one point to another requires accurate saccades (rapid conjugate eye movements between fixation points). When medial cerebellar structures (or their connections) that are associated with eye movements are disrupted the result is ocular dysmetria, a condition where saccades are either too short or too long. The eye undershoots or overshoots the target and there must be a corrective saccade to bring it to the correct fixation point. The bedside test is having the patient rapidly shift gaze from a finger on one of the examiner's hands to a finger on the other hand; this is done repeatedly, with the examiner repositioning the target finger before each shift in fixation point. Ocular dysmetria is an unambiguous sign of cerebellar system dysfunction, unlike nystagmus which has several alternative explanations.

3. *Diplopia.* Subjectively experienced double vision can occur any time the patient's gaze is not conjugate, but it does not necessarily do so because patients can suppress the image from one of the two eyes. Diplopia can be fixed or can be variable according to the direction of gaze or the level of fatigue or CNS drug side effects. Diplopia present only when looking in specific directions can arise from monocular weakness or impairment of gaze in a particular direction, whether on a muscular or neural basis, or from intranuclear ophthalmoplegia. Diplopia dependent on the level of fatigue can occur when the patient has a phoria (latent mal-alignment of binocular vision that is suppressed by fixation of gaze). In this situation the eyes are not aligned if one eye is covered, but binocular fixation is sufficient to line them up. When the patient is fatigued or the CNS is depressed by medications, the eyes may be unable to attain full alignment even when binocular vision is attempted. Drugs such as anticholinergics that impair accommodation can cause diplopia when the patient looks at near objects because the eyes do not converge sufficiently. Ocular myasthenia gravis causes diplopia that first appears or gets worse after the patient exercises the eyes; repeated forceful blinking may be enough to provoke diplopia in many patients with ocular myasthenia.

CRANIAL NERVE V: TRIGEMINAL NERVE

One of the thickest nerves in the body, the trigeminal nerve provides sensory innervation to the face and motor innervation to the muscles of mastication. It has three branches—ophthalmic, maxillary, and mandibular. Testing of its sensory functions typically is limited to testing light touch with a cotton swab, pain with a sharp object like a toothpick, and temperature with a cool object like a tuning fork. Position and vibration senses in the face usually are not tested. Sensation is tested in areas served by each of the three branches of the nerve, since diseases around the skull and face can disrupt branches of the nerve selectively. The ophthalmic branch of the trigeminal nerve is the afferent limb of the corneal reflex—blinking of the eyes when the cornea on one side is stroked lightly with a wisp of cotton. The cotton is presented from the side to avoid confounding of the tactile stimulus with visual threat. The motor functions are tested by palpating the masseter muscles while the patient clenches the teeth, then having the patient move the jaw from side to side against resistance.

From the medical-psychiatric viewpoint, the trigeminal nerve is important because of its role in facial pain: trigeminal neuralgia, or tic douloureux, is the classic example of paroxysmal neuropathic pain. Like other types of neuropathic pain, trigeminal neuralgia can present with symptoms disproportionate to signs, thus sometimes raising the issue of a somatoform disorder. Signs are not entirely absent, however, sensory examination of one or more branches of the trigeminal nerve on the affected side will be abnormal. As a large nerve, the trigeminal nerve is more likely than smaller ones to be affected by systemic diseases that cause cranial nerve damage, such as chronic meningitis or autoimmune vasculitis. These conditions also are potential causes of mental status changes.

Assessment of the trigeminal nerve is important in evaluating cases of dizziness or vertigo because of the proximity of the trigeminal nerve to the acoustic nerve at the cerebellopontine angle. Tumors of that region can present with vertigo—a condition in which psychosomatic factors sometimes are suspected. A tumor of that region large enough to cause vertigo often is large enough to impinge on the trigeminal nerve and cause either partial unilateral facial sensory loss or a unilaterally decreased corneal reflex.

CRANIAL NERVE VII: FACIAL NERVE

The facial nerve provides motor innervation to the muscles of the face and also is the afferent pathway for the sense of taste from the anterior two-thirds of the tongue. The facial nerve is tested by having the patient move the face in various ways—close the eyes forcibly, smile, or blow through pursed lips. Asymmetry of the face is observed as well; total dysfunction of the facial nerve on one side—Bell's palsy—causes a drooping of the face on one side, incomplete eye closure, and a widened palpebral fissure. The input to the facial nerve motor nuclei from the cerebral hemispheres is bilateral; specifically, the upper motor neurons for upper face are bilateral while the upper motor neurons for the lower face are contralateral only. A hemispheric stroke will affect the lower face and not the forehead—immediately indicating facial weakness of central origin as distinguished from facial weakness due to a facial nerve lesion. Asymmetry of the face when smiling spontaneously can occur in patients whose deliberate smile is symmetrical; this finding points to dysfunction of the contralateral temporal lobe. This is of medical-psychiatric interest because acquired temporal lobe lesions, such as those due to embolic stroke or tumor, can present with changes in mood or behavior without changes in motor function that would immediately suggest gross brain disease.

Testing the sense of taste often is omitted from general physical examinations. However, the sense of taste is of special medical-psychiatric interest because its impairment can influence appetite, weight, and eating behavior. Some patients with a loss of taste lose their appetite. Others increase their salt or sugar intake because they cannot adequately taste the saltiness or sweetness of their food; this can adversely affect patients' general medical conditions. The sense of taste usually is tested using a salt or sugar solution on a cotton swab, testing on the front of the tongue, one side at a time. Sour, bitter, and umami (savory) stimuli are less consistently available at the bedside, and many of the potential choices have smells that potentially confound the testing process. However, non-odorous sour and umami stimuli are readily available at a grocery store, namely citric acid (sour salt) and monosodium glutamate. Most common causes of taste loss affect all of the primary tastes, although not necessarily equally; small lesions of the brainstem can produce dissociation of sensation for different primary tastes. Anatomical lesions of the facial nerve usually affect both taste and motor function, although a selective lesion of the chorda tympani nerve can impair taste without producing facial weakness. When weakness in the face is accompanied by a loss of the sense of taste it confirms a neural rather than (or in addition to) a muscular or cerebral cause for facial weakness. Loss of the sense of taste also can occur as a side effect of medication (notably cancer chemotherapy agents) or due to zinc deficiency; in this case the loss of taste is bilateral and applies to the posterior as well as the anterior tongue, and there is no associated facial motor deficit.

CRANIAL NERVE VIII: VESTIBULOCOCHLEAR OR AUDITORY VESTIBULAR NERVE

The vestibulocochlear nerve runs from two parts of the inner ear—the labyrinth and the cochlea—through the petrous bone to join the brainstem at the cerebellopontine angle. Dysfunction of the eighth nerve and/or its connections can present with any combination of hearing loss, tinnitus, impaired balance, and/or vertigo (a subjective sensation of motion). The bedside or office examination of the eighth nerve comprises testing of hearing, testing of balance, and observation for nystagmus on testing of extraocular movements. The testing of hearing was discussed above in connection with the examination of the ears, and the testing of balance was discussed in connection with testing of gait. Intactness of the vestibular division of the eighth nerve and its connections can be assessed by caloric testing; irrigating the ear canal with cold water produces lateral nystagmus with a quick component moving away from the stimulated ear; irrigating it with warm water produces nystagmus with a quick component toward the stimulated ear The Barany maneuver (see below) can be used to evoke the characteristic nystagmus of benign positional vertigo—nystagmus that typically is unidirectional (or at least asymmetrical) and has both a lateral and a rotatory component.

Abnormalities on testing of the vestibulocochlear nerve can be related to dysfunction of the sensory organ, a lesion in the nerve (most often an acoustic neuroma), or problems with the central connections of the nerve, of which the most common causes are brainstem strokes and demyelinating disease. While brain imaging procedures, especially MRI, are the mainstay of differential diagnosis, brainstem auditory evoked potentials can provide complementary information that is at times essential, because small lesions of the central auditory pathways can be beneath the resolution of MRI.

Several issues concerning testing of the eighth nerve are of special interest to medical psychiatrists:

1. Hearing loss can significantly increase the functional impairment associated with mild cognitive impairment or early dementia. Even when a patient has a neurodegenerative disease, identifying and mitigating hearing loss can in effect improve memory, and it can increase the executive functional resources available for instrumental activities by reducing the cognitive demand associated with resolving ambiguous auditory perceptions. Since adaptation to the use of a hearing aid requires memory and executive function, and adaptation is most effortful at the beginning, hearing aids are more likely to be useful when started at the stage of mild cognitive impairment rather than later in the course of a dementing illness. Auditory misperceptions can contribute to suspiciousness and paranoid ideation as well. However, remediation of hearing loss is rarely

useful in reversing paranoid delusions once they are established, even if misheard communications have contributed to them.

2. Because by age 80 more than half of all individuals have hearing loss, every elderly patient should be screened for it.

3. Younger patients who present with mental or behavioral symptoms but have no complaint of hearing loss should nonetheless be screened for hearing loss if have any of the following: (a) tinnitus, (b) vertigo, (c) a family history of deafness, (d) a developmental disorder associated with hearing loss, (e) a history of multiple ear infections, (f) severe head injury, and/or (g) occupational or avocational exposure to loud noise (barotrauma). People working on construction sites, at airports, and at rock concerts are all exposed to potentially injurious levels of noise, and they will develop hearing loss in time if they do not wear ear protection. Similarly, people who spend several hours a day listening to loud music using headphones are at risk for barotrauma-related hearing loss. Hearing loss from barotrauma disproportionately affects the perception of higher frequencies, with maximum loss around 4000 Hz. Audiometry or audioscopy can demonstrate the characteristic pattern of barotrauma-induced hearing loss, thus supporting a specific etiology as well as confirming the presence of impairment.

4. Patients with tinnitus may have the condition on a cerebral basis or because of dysfunction of the cochlea, the eighth nerve, or the brainstem auditory pathways. When a patient with tinnitus and episodic vertigo has unilateral hearing loss that disproportionately affects lower frequencies, the diagnosis of Meniere's disease is likely (Stapleton & Mills, 2008). This is a condition of particular interest to medical psychiatrists because it is associated both with depression and with autoimmunity (Gasquez et al., 2011).

5. Dizziness, usually a lightheaded feeling but occasionally true vertigo, can be an expression of anxiety of any cause. In old age the symptom can present with reluctance to walk or fear of falling, or with an actual history of falls. Among the medical conditions to be excluded before ascribing dizziness to anxiety are disorders of the vestibular system and its connections via the eighth nerve to brainstem nuclei associated with balance and eye movement. The standard neurological examination includes observation for nystagmus on gaze in different directions. The nystagmus associated with vestibular dysfunction, which usually has some rotatory component, can escape casual observation if it is of low amplitude. It can help the examiner to focus attention on a scleral blood vessel while having the patient look up, down, left, and right; the high contrast of the red blood with the white sclera highlights the rotatory movement.

If the patient's history suggests vertigo or dizziness greatest with changes in position, the examination should include efforts to provoke nystagmus by movements of the head and body such as the Barany maneuver (aka Dix-Hallpike test), which tests for benign positional vertigo due to dysfunction of the posterior semicircular canal of the inner ear on one side (Fife et al., 2008). The patient sits on an examination table positioned so that he or she can be moved into the supine position with the head hanging down over the edge of the table. As the patient is moved from the sitting to the supine position with the head extended, the head is gently rotated 45 degrees toward the side of the ear that will be tested. The patient's eyes are kept open and observed for combined vertical and torsional (rotatory) nystagmus that is accompanied by reproduction of the patient's symptoms of vertigo. Nystagmus begins after a latency of a few seconds, decreases and stops within a minute, reverses direction when the patient is returned to the upright seated position, and fatigues and ultimately disappears on repeated trials. The facts that the positional nystagmus can reliably be provoked by a well-defined maneuver and that it diminishes with repetition of the maneuver supports the diagnosis of a condition that is both physiologically based and of benign significance. Nystagmus and vertigo of other, less benign causes also can be provoked by the Barany maneuver. However, in most of these cases the nystagmus will not diminish with repetition and/or there will be other neurologic or otologic signs.

There are several other useful bedside tests of neuro-vestibular function, which are helpful in evaluating dizziness, vertigo, and unsteady gait, which frequently are caused by disease of the inner ear or eighth nerve, but also can reflect injury to the pons or the cerebellar system by a stroke or demyelinating disease. They are thoughtfully reviewed by Newman-Toker (2014), whose syllabus on neuro-vestibular testing is available for download on the Internet. One valuable example is the horizontal head impulse test, which evaluates the vestibulo-ocular reflex (VOR), in particular the function of the horizontal semicircular canals of the inner ear and their connections in the brainstem. Patients with acute onset imbalance and vertigo due to cerebellar strokes have a normal VOR, while those with an eighth nerve lesion or inner ear disease usually have an abnormal one. A normal VOR raises concerns about a central cause of vertigo and imbalance, potentially one involving the cerebellum and/or its connections, such as MS or a posterior circulation stroke. Two other unequivocal signs that vertigo is central rather than peripheral are pure vertical nystagmus and pure rotatory nystagmus with no lateral component.

The horizontal head impulse test requires a patient to maintain fixation on the examiner's finger while the examiner rapidly rotates the patient's head 10–20 degrees laterally with a "flicking" motion. The patient should be told in advance what the examiner plans to do, and the examiner should rotate the head slowly once or twice to illustrate. When the head is rapidly rotated toward the side of a vestibular lesion the patient will be unable to maintain fixation and will require a corrective saccade after the head movement stops. This test has been nicknamed "dolls eyes on steroids": It serves much the same purpose as caloric testing but is more convenient. Adaptations to test the other semicircular canals and the utricle and saccule of the labyrinth have been described (Halmagyi et al., 2001).

CRANIAL NERVE IX: GLOSSOPHARYNGEAL NERVE

The glossopharyngeal nerve supplies sensory innervation to the posterior oral cavity and pharynx and the sense of taste to the posterior third of tongue. It is the route to the brainstem for signals from carotid body baroreceptors and carotid glomus chemoreceptors. It is the afferent limb of the gag reflex. On the efferent side it supplies parasympathetic (cholinergic) innervation of the parotid gland. On screening examinations the ninth nerve is evaluated by testing the gag reflex; this is done by stimulating the posterior palate with a tongue blade or cotton swab. Ideally this is done one side at a time, to enable detection of unilateral ninth nerve lesions. Similarly to the blink reflex, stimulation of the gag reflex on one side produces contraction of the palatal muscles bilaterally. Thus, if the context suggests the possibility of a unilateral ninth nerve lesion and a screening neurological examination described the ninth nerve as intact, it would be worth rechecking the gag reflex, one side at a time. If the gag reflex is absent or markedly hypoactive, which it can be on a central basis, finding intact taste on the posterior third of the tongue supports the cause being central and not peripheral.

Of particular interest to medical psychiatrists is that lesions of the ninth nerve can produce unusual and distressing symptoms that are easily diagnosed if, and only if, the physician is familiar with the syndrome. Glossopharyngeal neuralgia, a syndrome similar to trigeminal neuralgia, presents with paroxysmal lancinating pains at the base of the tongue or around the palate. Attacks can be accompanied by vagally mediated syncope.

CRANIAL NERVE X: VAGUS NERVE

The vagus nerve provides motor and sensory function to the gastrointestinal tract from the palate and pharynx through the ileum, and also innervates the respiratory tract—larynx, trachea, and lungs—and the heart. It is the afferent pathway for the baroreceptors and chemoreceptors of the aorta and the carotid artery. Autonomic symptoms—cardiovascular or gastrointestinal—frequently accompany vagus nerve lesions. On the screening neurological examination, the tenth nerve is tested in its role as the efferent limb of the gag reflex If the soft palate is stimulated on either side, the palatal muscles should contract on both sides. The palate will fail to contract and rise normally on the side of a tenth nerve lesion; complete paralysis of the palate is more likely to occur with nuclear or infranuclear lesions. Lesions of the recurrent laryngeal nerves—the branches of the vagus nerves that supply the larynx—present with hoarseness, but visualization of the vocal cords with a mirror or fiberoptics is necessary to confirm which side is affected. The vagus nerve—one of the longest in the body—is vulnerable to any of the systemic diseases that cause polyneuropathy, such as diabetes or amyloidosis, and to toxins such as lead or solvents that cause polyneuropathy. Many of these conditions also have neuropsychiatric dimensions and can present with prominent mental and behavioral symptoms.

Identification of a previously unsuspected neuropathy can significantly affect the differential diagnosis of the presenting symptoms.

CRANIAL NERVE XI: ACCESSORY NERVE

The accessory nerve is the motor nerve supplying the trapezius and sternomastoid muscles. It is tested by having the patient shrug the shoulders and turn the face to the side, against resistance. Medical psychiatrists evaluating patients for suspected motor conversion symptoms can, on occasion, note nonphysiological patterns of weakness that arise from patients being unaware that contraction of a sternomastoid muscle turns the face to the opposite side, or being unaware that the trapezius muscle has a different nerve supply than the other muscles of the shoulder area. Trapezius weakness on a central basis is on the opposite side from sternomastoid weakness; when caused by an accessory nerve lesion, the weakness of the two muscles obviously is ipsilateral.

CRANIAL NERVE XII: HYPOGLOSSAL NERVE

The hypoglossal nerve is the motor efferent to all but one of the intrinsic muscles of the tongue. It is tested by having the patient protrude the tongue with the mouth open and by having him or her push the tongue against each cheek against external resistance. Because contraction of the tongue muscles pushes the tongue forward, unilateral weakness of the tongue will cause the tongue to point toward the weak side. When the weakness is due to upper motor neuron dysfunction—for example, when it is due to a cerebral stroke—the tongue will not be atrophic. Prominent atrophy of the tongue is indicative of disease of the lower motor neuron—either in the twelfth nerve nucleus or the hypoglossal nerve itself. Fasciculations of the tongue indicate disease affecting the hypoglossal nerve nuclei, most often amyotrophic lateral sclerosis (ALS). ALS can present with neuropsychiatric symptoms, and fasciculations of the tongue may precede more prominent bulbar signs and symptoms. Careful inspection of the tongue for fasciculations is particularly relevant in patients suspected of having frontotemporal dementia, as this is the type of dementia specifically associated with ALS.

MOTOR FUNCTIONS

The basic motor examination comprises assessment of muscle tone and bulk, testing of muscle strength, observation of involuntary movements including tics, tremors, dystonia and dyskinesia, and noting of fasciculations if they are present. Because it is not practical to test every muscle in the body, the screening motor examination typically tests a set of proximal and distal muscles bilaterally, looking for asymmetry and for a proximal–distal gradient—proximal weakness being typical of myopathy and distal weakness typical of polyneuropathy. While examiners do not typically record exactly which muscles they have screened, a conservative assumption for the medical psychiatrist is that a nonspecialized examination of the motor system might have a "blind spot," with positive examination findings to be found if one looks in the right place. In particular, the motor aspects of damage to a specific nerve—whether from trauma, entrapment, or another cause such as vascular or autoimmune disease—can only be assessed by testing the muscles innervated by the nerve involved.

Motor disorders can be of neuropsychiatric import but go unnoticed or be minimized by the patient; tardive dyskinesia is a poignant example. In these cases the patient might not complain of the problem, and the physicians might not notice it unless they are looking for it. In addition, involuntary movements, tremors, and fasciculations can fluctuate in intensity over time and simply not be present at the time of a specific neurological examination. Thus they cannot be ruled out for all time by a single examination, no matter how expertly performed and carefully documented. Some specific points deserve mention:

1. Increased muscle tone in limbs can be thought of as unidirectional (spastic) or bidirectional (rigid), the latter implying simultaneous contraction of agonist and antagonist muscles. The former is a sign of pyramidal tract dysfunction, the latter of extrapyramidal dysfunction. Rigidity can be accompanied by tremor; this is a characteristic finding in Parkinson's disease, drug-induced parkinsonism, and malignant extrapyramidal reactions to neuroleptics. Parkinsonian tremor, whether due to Parkinson's disease or due to antipsychotic drugs, has a lower frequency than the tremor of patients with malignant neuroleptic reactions. Tremulous rigidity need not feel like a cogwheel or ratchet, and for this reason the author prefers the term "tremulous rigidity" to "cogwheel rigidity."

2. In addition to spasticity and rigidity, medical psychiatrists often encounter two other types of abnormality of muscle tone. The first one, *paratonia*, can take one or both of two forms: oppositional paratonia ("gegenhalten") and facilitatory paratonia ("mitgehen"). In the former condition the patient resists passive movement of a limb by the examiner. In the latter condition the patient assists, augments, or extends the passive movement. Both types of paratonia are associated with cognitive and motor signs of frontal lobe dysfunction (Beversdorf & Heilman, 1998). The examiner can test for both types of paratonia by holding the patient's arm, asking him or her to relax, and then holding the patient's hand and passively flexing and extending the elbow three times, ending with the elbow extended, then letting of the patient's hand. If oppositional paratonia is present, the patient will resist passive movement in both directions; if facilitatory paratonia is present, the patient will flex the elbow after the hand is released.

The second type of abnormal tone of special interest is the *waxy flexibility of catatonia*. The syndrome of catatonia involves multiple behaviors, one of which is offering slight and even resistance to passive movement of the patient's limbs by the examiner. (The mildness of the resistance distinguishes it from most cases of oppositional paratonia.) Waxy flexibility often is accompanied by

catalepsy, the maintenance against gravity of the limbs in a position into which they were placed by the examiner. The other motor phenomena of catatonia are stereotypies (frequent repetitive non–goal-directed movements), mannerisms (caricatures of normal behaviors), and grimacing. Catatonia, once associated primarily with schizophrenia, has increasingly been recognized as a syndrome that can also arise from mood disorders and even from general medical conditions (Tandon et al., 2013). It is important to recognize because it responds to treatment with benzodiazepines and/or electroconvulsive therapy, and it is potentially dangerous if not treated. In a case series of patients with catatonia in the ICU, Saddawi-Konefka et al. (2014) reported two patients with premorbid chronic anxiety who developed catatonia in the ICU in the context of benzodiazepine withdrawal. This calls attention to yet another potential cause of catatonia in the medical-psychiatric context, important because long-term benzodiazepine treatment often is discontinued, either deliberately or inadvertently, when patients are hospitalized.

3. The rigidity of malignant catatonia or neuroleptic malignant syndrome feels more intense than the rigidity of Parkinson's disease or drug-induced Parkinsonism.

4. Loss of muscle bulk can be disproportionate to loss of strength. For example, atrophy of the thenar eminence in carpal tunnel syndrome or of the hypothenar eminence in ulnar nerve entrapment can be noted even when the strength of the intrinsic hand muscles is near normal.

5. Loss of muscle strength, like loss of cognitive function, should be assessed with respect to the patient's pre-illness baseline. Athletes and patients with highly physical occupations can have strength that is within normal limits for the general population despite their having had a significant loss of function due to neuromuscular disease.

6. Myasthenia gravis, an autoimmune disease of the neuromuscular junction, is characterized by maximal muscle strength at the beginning of exercise followed by loss of strength as exercise continues and reserves of acetylcholine are depleted. While patients with severe myasthenia will have weakness at the outset, those with less severe disease can have a normal motor examination unless they are tested following exercise of the muscles involved.

7. Tremors should be characterized by frequency, amplitude, the most involved muscle groups, and the circumstances that bring them out; essential tremor is made worse by action, while the alternating or "pill-rolling" tremor of Parkinson's disease is worse at rest. Many psychotropic drugs can cause or worsen tremors; neuroleptics and antidepressants (of all classes) can produce fine tremors and can exacerbate action tremors or the rest tremor of Parkinsonism. The distinction between drug-induced tremors is clinically important because they should be treated differently. A beta blocker can help an action tremor, but it is of no use for Parkinsonian tremor.

8. The predominant frequency of a tremor in Hz is the single most useful quantitative datum in differential diagnosis. It can be reliably measured at the bedside using the built-in accelerometer of a smartphone, employing the iSeismo application, one originally developed to measure and report seismic activity (www.iseismometer.com; the application is available for both iOS and Android operating systems). The phone is strapped to the tremulous limb; the application records motion on three axes, plots the motion on a graph with time markers, and calculates the frequency spectrum of the motion (Joundi et al., 2011). Another smartphone application for monitoring tremor, the Lift Pulse (www.liftlabdesigns.com) assesses the fluctuation in tremor amplitude over time as well as measuring its predominant frequency.

9. An unusual tremor syndrome, orthostatic tremor, is a high-frequency (13 Hz–18 Hz) tremor in the leg muscles elicited by standing up and relieved by sitting or walking. Patients with this rare disorder sometimes are misdiagnosed and are seen by psychiatrists because of their secondary depression and anxiety. Confirming a high-frequency tremor in the legs, for example by using a smartphone app, can expedite a correct diagnosis. Many movement disorders—including tics and dyskinesia—fluctuate over time and are responsive both to the environment and to what the patient is doing at the time. It is thus possible to judge an involuntary movement as mild or even absent, when at a different time it is moderate or even severe. The history in these situations is one of flurries or attacks of involuntary movements alternating with quiet periods with few or no involuntary movements. The clustering of involuntary movements shows fractal symmetry; clusters of discrete involuntary movements within a flare-up of the movement disorder are spaced proportionally to the pattern of flare-ups over the course of time.

10. Environmental responsiveness of involuntary movements does not imply a "psychogenic" origin. In neuroleptic-induced vacuous chewing movements (VCM), a rat model of tardive dyskinesia, higher levels of environmental noise are associated with a significantly greater frequency of abnormal movements.

11. There are a number of movement disorders in which involuntary movements are associated with or triggered by voluntary ones. Chief among these are the occupational dystonias such as writer's cramp. These conditions are regarded as involuntary and based in dysfunction of motor control systems. Patients with these conditions usually have subtle abnormalities of somatic sensation as well; patients with writer's cramp have an impaired ability to localize touch on the affected and the unaffected hand. (Lin & Hallett, 2009). This movement disorder and other occupational dystonias will be found on neurological examination only if the patient is asked to perform the action that ordinarily triggers it; the sensory disorder will be found only if it is looked for specifically, as touch localization is not part of the screening sensory examination.

12. Some common movement disorders, notably tardive dyskinesia and Tourette syndrome, have multiple and varied manifestations. For such patients, a video recording of the patient's typical involuntary movements is a valuable supplement to a verbal description of them. Video recording is standard in many movement disorder clinics. Informal video recording with the medical psychiatrist's smartphone can capture essential features of a movement disorder that then can be reviewed with a neurologic subspecialist.

13. The clinical import of involuntary movements can be great even when the movements themselves are mild and functionally insignificant. For example, a patient born to a parent with Huntington's disease has a 50% chance of getting the condition. Such a patient showing even very mild chorea—if there is no other explanation for it—establishes that he or she has inherited a neurodegenerative disease.

14. While mild fasciculations can be seen in normal individuals and in patients with nerve root inflammation, pronounced fasciculations strongly suggest disease of motor neurons, most often due to ALS. ALS is associated with neurodegenerative conditions that can present with changes in mental status, particularly one of the variants of frontotemporal degeneration (FTD). Fasciculations can occur at a point in the disease where weakness and atrophy are still mild. When the fasciculations are themselves mild, they may be seen only if specifically sought. The small, discrete movements of fasciculations are best detected in the examiner's peripheral vision. As in the examples just given for chorea and dyskinesia, fasciculations of little functional consequence in themselves can be clinically important in a context of suspected ALS.

COORDINATION (CEREBELLAR FUNCTION)

Coordination is disturbed by dysfunction—whether due to a drug or metabolic state or due to an anatomical lesion—of the cerebellum and its connections in the brainstem, thalamus, frontal lobes, and spinal cord. Impaired coordination in the limbs is associated with dysfunction of the lateral cerebellum—the cerebellar hemispheres—while impaired gait and impaired standing or sitting balance are associated with dysfunction of the midline cerebellum—the cerebellar vermis. The standard screening examination for limb coordination is done on the left and the right separately, in the upper and the lower extremities. The patient puts the index finger on the nose, then touches the examiner's finger, then touches the nose, and then touches the examiner's finger, which has moved to a different location. If the patient significantly overshoots or undershoots the mark when touching the examiner's finger, cerebellar dysfunction is suspected. The other usual test of upper extremity coordination is the performance of rhythmic alternating movements, typically having the patient tap the knee, the thigh, or a tabletop with, alternately, the palm of the hand and the back of the hand. Clumsiness or irregular rhythm in performing the task is a sign of impaired coordination, with an irregular rhythm particularly suggestive of cerebellar system dysfunction.

The lower extremity is tested by having the patient touch the heel to the contralateral shin just below the knee, and then slide the heel straight down the shin toward the ankle. If the heel wobbles from side to side, impaired coordination is suspected. Rhythmic alternating movements are tested by having the patient alternately tap the floor with the heel and with the toes.

The interpretation of failure on tests of coordination should take into account vision, position sense, and noncerebellar aspects of the motor system. A particularly common issue in interpretation is whether a wobble on heel-to-shin testing or missed targets on finger-nose-finger testing is due to an action-induced tremor rather than to the inaccurate targeting of directed movement—dysmetria—that is characteristic of cerebellar system dysfunction. Follow-up observations can help make the distinction. Action tremors are present any time the patient makes an intentional movement, so they will be present if the patient slowly tracks the examiner's finger movement with his or her own finger—an activity that would not require precise targeting of a single movement. Having the patient move his or her fingertip quickly back and forth between the examiner's left index finger and right index finger requires precise targeting of the upper extremity movement and can reveal undershooting or overshooting that can be clear-cut even if there is an action tremor superimposed upon it. The same tasks carried out with the patient's big toe touching the examiner's index finger(s) can be useful in making the same distinction.

SENSORY FUNCTIONS

The sensory examination evaluates the patient's perception of light touch (typically tested with a wisp of cotton), pain (typically tested with a sharp object like a pin or toothpick), temperature (typically tested with a cool metal tuning fork), vibration (typically tested with 128 Hz tuning fork), and position sense (typically tested with small movements of the fingers and toes). Less consistently tested is discriminative sensation, such as touch localization, two-point discrimination, stereognosis (the ability to identify an object placed into the hand when the eyes are closed), and graphesthesia (the ability to identify a letter or number traced on the skin). Obviously, an exhaustive examination of all forms of sensation is not feasible; screening and hypothesis testing are the realistic options.

Sensory screening most often fails because of insensitivity when the examiner presents stimuli too strong to reveal the deficit, which is usually a partial loss of sensation rather than total anesthesia. For example, a defect in position sense in the feet is missed because the toe movements made by the examiner are too large. The other main error on sensory testing is not doing the specific testing needed to assess the relevant diagnostic hypothesis. For example, a patient with a parietal lobe lesion may have marked deficits in discriminative

sensation without any deficit in the primary sensation of touch, pain, temperature, position, or vibration. Such a patient must be specifically tested for touch localization, stereognosis, graphesthesia, and/or extinction of the stimulus on the affected side when both sides are stimulated simultaneously.

Sensory thresholds can be quantitated using specialized instruments. Quantitative sensory data can be used to assess the course of a disease affecting the peripheral nerves and to measure treatment response.

Several points on the sensory examination are of particular interest to medical psychiatrists:

1. Many toxic, metabolic, and autoimmune conditions that also cause neuropsychiatric symptoms are accompanied by polyneuropathy. Polyneuropathy is a common neurological side effect of drugs and is virtually universal with cisplatin and carboplatin, drugs commonly used in the chemotherapy of solid tumors. It also can be an early sign of nervous system damage from alcohol abuse, or of recurrent hyperglycemia that has not developed into frank diabetes. The early stage of polyneuropathy can be asymptomatic, or the patient can be unconcerned about symptoms of neuropathy because of the CNS effects of the disease. Careful testing of pain and temperature sense in the fingers and toes will detect early signs of axonal neuropathies, as these conditions first affect the small-diameter nerve fibers that carry pain and temperature sense. Moving from the toes or fingers proximally, there will be a gradient of increasing sensation. The sensory loss will be uniform across the fingers and across the toes.

2. Demyelinating neuropathies, most due to either autoimmune or vascular disease, differentially affect large-diameter myelinated nerve fibers. These conditions first affect position and vibration sense and, at the outset, pain and temperature sense can be relatively spared. This distinctive pattern of sensory loss aids in the differential diagnosis of the neuropathy.

3. A common reason for medical psychiatric consultation is pain in excess of apparent physical signs. One cause of this phenomenon is localized nerve or nerve root compression which, by differentially affecting large fiber signals that modulate pain sensation, can cause pain and dysesthesia disproportionate to motor weakness, muscle atrophy, or gross sensory loss. Of these conditions the carpal tunnel syndrome is the best known, but there are many other syndromes entrapment neuropathies, some of them occupational. Nerve root impingement by osteoarthritic bony deformities or by herniated intervertebral disks also can at times produce disproportionate pain and dysesthesia. The key to the diagnosis is precisely mapping the area of altered or diminished sensation—which, in the case of a nerve entrapment, should closely follow the known territory of a specific nerve. Some of these territories show minor variability, but for practical purposes they are consistent: the sensory territory of the median nerve might not split the fourth finger, but it will always include the middle finger and never include the fifth

finger. Corroborating data from the physical examination include atrophy of the muscles in the same territory—which can occur with or without obvious weakness—and tenderness of the nerve over the point of entrapment.

Occasionally an entrapment neuropathy will present with a well-defined trigger point that will reproduce the patient's pain if pressed on but without a well-defined zone of sensory loss. These neuropathies are particularly likely to be misdiagnosed because of the almost negative neurological examination. A prime example is the anterior cutaneous nerve entrapment syndrome (ACNES) of the abdomen (Akhnikh et al., 2013; van Assen et al., 2013). In this condition the anterior cutaneous branch of one of the intercostal nerves (most often T11) gets entrapped as it passes through the rectus abdominis muscle just medial to its lateral edge. Patients have episodic abdominal pain—sometimes severe enough to provoke surgical consultation, imaging procedures, or even laparoscopy—or chronic abdominal pain misdiagnosed as irritable bowel syndrome or a somatoform disorder. The disorder can be diagnosed with great confidence by a targeted physical examination alone. When ACNES is present, there is a tender spot over the rectus abdominis muscle point no more than 2 cm in diameter, pressure on which produces the characteristic pain. The patient, lying supine on the examination table, is asked to lift his or her head off the examining table. This tenses the rectus abdominis and exacerbates the pain; if the cause of the pain were visceral no increase in pain would be expected. There might be some sensory alteration in the vicinity of the trigger point, but clear-cut sensory loss with a well-defined boundary is not the rule. The majority of patients with this disorder respond well to local injections with a local anesthetic and a corticosteroid. If injections are not sufficient, surgery to release the entrapment usually will permanently alleviate the pain.

In addition to getting entrapped by normal anatomic structures, cutaneous nerves can be entrapped by scar tissue. In the inguinal region, entrapments of the ilioinguinal and genitofemoral nerves are a common cause of persistent postoperative pain. Patients with these disorders can be misdiagnosed as having psychosomatic problems or analgesic dependency. The presence of sensory loss in a pattern consistent with the territory of the entrapped nerve supports the diagnosis; blocking the pain with an injection of local anesthetic at the presumed site of entrapment will confirm it. Table 2.3 lists some

Table 2.3 COMMON ENTRAPMENT NEUROPATHIES

NEUROPATHY	EARLY SYMPTOMS	MOTOR SIGNS	SENSORY SIGNS
Median nerve at the wrist (carpal tunnel)	Pain in wrist radiating proximally; paresthesias in thumb and index finger	Thumb weakness and/or atrophy of thenar muscles (later than symptoms and sensory signs)	Sensory loss on palmar side of medial 3.5 fingers; palm is spared
Ulnar nerve at the elbow (cubital tunnel)	Deep ache around the elbow; tingling in ring and little fingers	Grip weakness and/or hypothenar atrophy (later than symptoms and sensory signs)	Sensory loss on *both palmar and dorsal* sides of ulnar 1.5 fingers; palm is spared
Ulnar nerve at the wrist (compression in Guyon's canal)	Pain and numbness of ulnar 1.5 fingers, or painless atrophy of hypothenar and interosseous muscles	Hypothenar and interosseous weakness and/or atrophy	Sensory loss on palmar side of ulnar 1.5 fingers
Radial nerve in proximal forearm (posterior interosseous nerve syndrome)	Dull aching pain over front of elbow	Weakness of extension of third and fourth fingers early; weakness of extension of all fingers and of thumb adduction later	None
Suprascapular nerve entrapment	Poorly circumscribed dull aching pain in posterior shoulder	Supraspinatus and/or infraspinatus weakness and/or atrophy	None
Lateral femoral cutaneous nerve (meralgia paresthetica)	Numbness, tingling, and painful hypersensitivity in anterolateral thigh	None	Decreased pinprick sensation accompanied by hypersensitivity to light touch
Common peroneal nerve entrapment	Pain radiating from knee to dorsal foot; sensory loss on dorsum of foot	Foot drop (may come later than sensory symptoms)	Sensory loss on dorsum of foot
Tarsal tunnel syndrome	Burning pain and tingling of plantar region; pain triggered by pressing or rubbing plantar surface of foot	Weak flexors of great toe; clawing of other toes due to weak flexors (later than sensory symptoms)	Sensory loss over one or both sides of the plantar surface of the foot, depending on site of entrapment
Lower trunk of brachial plexus (thoracic outlet syndrome)	Pain and paresthesia of ulnar aspect of forearm, hand, and ulnar two fingers	Usually none; rarely atrophy and weakness of intrinsic hand muscles	None

common entrapment neuropathies encountered in patients with localized pain and an unremarkable routine physical examination. The common entrapment neuropathies illustrate several important points relevant to the problem of missed or inaccurate diagnoses by physicians unfamiliar with them:

a. Pain can be disproportionate to findings on sensory and motor examination.

b. Pain usually comes before muscle weakness, even when the nerves involved have primarily motor functions.

c. Pain can be poorly localized.

d. Decreased pinprick sensation can be accompanied by *hypersensitivity and discomfort* with light touch stimulation.

e. Muscular weakness and muscle atrophy are *partially* correlated; one can be much more prominent than the other.

f. Patterns of motor and/or sensory findings are highly specific; findings *not* present help distinguish entrapment neuropathies from nerve root lesions such as those associated with herniated disks.

There are many rare entrapment neuropathies; many are associated with particular occupations, hobbies, or sports, or with pregnancy. When patients present localized nonvisceral pain or sensory symptoms unexplained, or unconvincingly explained, by the physicians they have seen to date, it is worth considering whether the pattern of symptoms fits one of the entrapment neuropathies and whether the history suggests activities, injuries, or systemic risk factors that would predispose to that particular entrapment.

Closely related to entrapment neuropathies, and raising similar diagnostic issues, are compression neuropathies; like entrapment neuropathies, these involve a localized insult to a peripheral nerve. These are of particular medical-psychiatric interest because they can be caused by pressure from medical devices and can occur in the context of anesthesia, surgery, and/or rehabilitation. Crutches, walkers, and self-powered wheelchairs all are associated with compression neuropathies, which can be due to pressure directly from a device or from muscle hypertrophy related to using it.

4. Nerve root impingement ideally would produce sensory loss precisely following a dermatome from the associated spine around to the front of the body. However, the sensory dermatomes of adjacent nerve roots overlap somewhat, so the width of the band of sensory alteration is variable.

5. The finding of a sensory loss in a dermatome also can aid in the diagnosis of herpes zoster and post-herpetic neuralgia, conditions that can cause severe pain with minimal physical signs apart from the sensory examination, since these conditions are based on infection of dorsal root ganglia and do not affect motor function at all. The diagnosis is obvious when the acute attack of herpes zoster is accompanied by a prominent rash, but this is not always the case, and on occasion the rash was present and not noticed by the patient.

6. Limb weakness or paralysis are common neurologic conversion symptoms. Patients with conversion weakness or paralysis often also show sensory changes in the affected limbs, just as do patients with weakness or paralysis on an "organic" basis. However, the sensory changes, if carefully mapped, often are incompatible with those expected from the lesion location inferred from the pattern of motor deficits. Dermatomes on the arms and legs follow precise patterns that the patient may not know; for example, the territory of S1 goes from the low back down the back of the leg but does not include the anterior leg, and the territory of L5 includes the big toe but not the little toe.

7. Patients with traumatic spinal cord injuries or spinal cord infarcts usually have clear-cut "sensory levels" below which there is absent or diminished sensation and above which sensation is intact. However, in patients where the spinal cord is impinged upon by a slowly progressive extrinsic mass or is affected by an intramedullary tumor, there may not be a clear-cut sensory level, and the areas of normal and diminished sensation can follow an irregular pattern. This can happen because the lesion does not totally destroy normal spinal cord neurons and axons and/or because it extends up and down the cord for several levels. These patients are ones in whom neurological conversion symptoms may be suspected. Notwithstanding, the patient with a genuine spinal cord lesion will have some areas of diminished sensation below the lowest level of the lesion and no areas of diminished sensation above the highest level of the lesion.

8. Patients with parietal lobe damage, most often due to a tumor or stroke but occasionally due to other conditions such as demyelinating disease, arteriovenous malformations, or parasitic infestation, can show a combination of sensory and motor symptoms suggestive of neurological conversion because primary sensory modalities may be relatively intact, and motor strength on direct testing may be normal as well. Nonetheless, the patient may be incapable of many simple voluntary motor actions because of apraxia and may *experience* grossly abnormal sensation in the affected areas because of the lack of discriminative sense. In this situation a sensory examination that includes testing of stereognosis (identification of an object placed in the hand without looking at it), two-point discrimination, discrimination of textures, graphesthesia, and extinction on simultaneous bilateral stimulation will identify "parietal lobe" sensory loss. Formal testing of praxis will also support the diagnosis of parietal lobe dysfunction. If the lesion is on the nondominant side, there will be impaired visual-spatial function; if it is on the dominant side, there usually will be an impaired ability to calculate.

REFLEXES

The reflex examination has always had particular interest for psychiatrists because, in contrast to the sensory and motor examinations, it requires less patient cooperation and because it is difficult for patients with malingered illness or conversion symptoms to precisely mimic abnormal reflexes. Apart from their continued utility in assessing potential symptoms of conversion or malingering, abnormal reflex findings continue to be valuable despite advances in brain imaging for several reasons. First, in progressive brain diseases like tumors, dementing diseases, and hydrocephalus, focal abnormalities in the function of the nervous system can appear before there are changes visible with the usual anatomic imaging procedures. Second, reflexes provide evidence as to whether anatomic or biochemical abnormalities seen on testing are functionally significant. Third, in relapsing-remitting diseases like multiple sclerosis, abnormal reflexes can provide evidence of disease activity prior to obvious changes in the patient's symptoms.

A typical screening neurological examination tests the deep tendon jerks at the biceps, triceps, brachioradialis, patellar, and Achilles tendons, and tests the plantar reflex by stroking the lateral sole from the heel towards the toe. When brain disease is suspected, this is augmented by testing primitive reflexes or "frontal release signs"—reflexes present in normal infants but not usually present in adults without frontal system dysfunction. These are discussed below.

Reflexes can be scored on a scale of a scale of 1+ to 4+ or a scale of 0.5+ to 5+. The four-point scale is encountered more often; the six-point scale adds the score of 0.5+ to indicate that reflexes are present only with facilitation and the score of 5+ to indicate the presence of sustained clonus. Reflexes are scored zero only if they are absent even when something is done to enhance them (facilitation)—typically the voluntary contraction of other muscles, as when the knee jerks are enhanced by clenching the fists. On the four-point scale, reflexes are scored 1+ if they are spontaneously present but of low amplitude or if they are present only with facilitation. Brisker than average reflexes that are possibly (but not necessarily) abnormal limits are scored 3+; those viewed as unequivocally beyond normal limits are scored 4+. Any reflex accompanied by unsustained clonus would be at least 3+, and one accompanied with sustained clonus would always be 4+.

Markedly increased reflexes suggest a central nervous system problem that affects the pyramidal motor system; something prevents descending inhibition of reflex loops in the spinal cord. When reflexes are *extremely* increased, with sustained clonus, dramatic extensor plantar responses and proximal spread of reflex muscle contractions, brainstem or spinal cord rather than purely cerebral dysfunction should be suspected. *Mild* reflex asymmetry can potentially reflect a longstanding developmental variation; for this reason, finding a record of a single reliable and complete baseline neurological examination can be very helpful diagnostically. The presence of mild reflex asymmetry in the past when the patient was well can reassure the clinician that its current presence doesn't necessarily signify new CNS disease; on the other hand, if

reflexes were unequivocally symmetrical at an earlier time, present mild asymmetry suggests an acquired neurological disorder. A significant asymmetry in the size of the extremities suggests a congenital or early acquired reason for a mild asymmetry in reflexes. Such asymmetries can be present and yet never be noted on recorded physical examinations until they are specifically sought.

Generalized hyperreflexia can be due to bilateral anatomic lesions of the brain or upper cervical spinal cord; in general medical settings, it more often represents increased CNS excitability or lack of inhibition on the basis of a toxic-metabolic encephalopathy or withdrawal from drugs or alcohol. Patients with generalized hyperreflexia from toxic-metabolic causes may or may not have extensor plantar reflexes.

The range of normal for deep tendon jerks is broad. Present but hypoactive (1+) reflexes can be seen occasionally in people without neurological disease; they are seen commonly in patients with cerebellar disorders and patients with systemic or muscular conditions that cause generalized weakness without significant CNS dysfunction. Hypothyroidism is classically associated with a delayed relaxation phase of the ankle, knee, and biceps reflexes; the *intensity* of the delayed reflex can be normal, increased, or decreased in this situation. Relaxation time over 320 msec is abnormal; this time interval of approximately one-third of a second is long enough to be judged clinically. While hypothyroidism is the most common cause of delayed relaxation of deep tendon jerks, and 75% of patients with clinical hypothyroidism will have it, there are other diagnostic possibilities with medical-psychiatric implications including anorexia nervosa, pernicious anemia, and sarcoidosis (Marinella, 2004). While patients with truly *subclinical* hypothyroidism would not be expected to have them, the presence of such "hung-up" reflexes would increase the likelihood that thyroid dysfunction, despite only borderline abnormal laboratory tests, was contributing to the patient's mental condition, as it would be direct evidence of altered CNS function due to the endocrine disease. When a specific deep tendon reflex is totally absent, the usual reason is damage or dysfunction of a nerve or nerve root involved in the reflex; for example, a missing ankle jerk usually is due to dysfunction of either the sciatic nerve or the first sacral root.

Polyneuropathy—as opposed to mononeuropathy multiplex—affects the longest nerves earliest and most severely. Patients with polyneuropathy can lose both ankle jerks, have diminished knee jerks, and have normal biceps and triceps reflexes. The particular relevance of polyneuropathy to medical psychiatrists is that polyneuropathy is a common expression of neurotoxicity that also can affect the brain, and patients can have polyneuropathy demonstrable on examination without complaining of symptoms.

Deep tendon reflexes can aid in identifying neurological conversion symptoms or in demonstrating neuropathology in a patient with an obvious mental disorder who also has a complaint of pain or sensorimotor dysfunction. Deep tendon reflex responses are not as subjective as sensory testing, they are less dependent on patients' cooperation than motor testing, and they are difficult to simulate by volitional movements. In addition, they should bear a consistent relationship to the putative anatomy of the neurological condition that the patient would have if his or her complaints were based a neurological disorder. In this connection, some reflexes seldom tested routinely occasionally can be diagnostically valuable. For example, neither the knee jerk nor the ankle jerk test the L5 root, but the less-known medial hamstring reflex does, and a study correlating surgical findings with the preoperative neurological examination showed the medical hamstring reflex to be as accurate in localizing the level of a herniated lumbar disk to L5 as the ankle jerk is in localizing it to S1 (Esene et al., 2012). The report of the study presents the psychometric properties of the different lower extremity deep tendon jerks and describes the technique for eliciting the reflex.

The extensor plantar reflex, or Babinski sign, is regarded by many physicians as virtually pathognomonic of CNS dysfunction involving the pyramidal motor system. The finding is accepted by physicians of all specialties as evidence that there is "something organic" and as such, it is of particular use to the medical psychiatrist lobbying for consideration or reconsideration of a patient's general medical diagnosis. Unlike voluntary withdrawal in response to noxious stimulation of the sole, the Babinski sign is consistent and repeatable. When the extensor plantar reflex is due to cortical disease, it typically involves only the big toe. Lesions lower down the neuraxis usually also involve extension and sometimes abduction of the other toes, and spinal lesions virtually always do so (Deng et al., 2013). Inter-rater reliability of the Babinski sign is highly dependent on examiners' skills, which can be improved by education and training (Morrow & Reilly, 2011). The latter authors provide excellent guidance in eliciting and interpreting the plantar response:

1. Correct interpretation of the response is more important to reliability than the precise details of stimulation of the sole. When it is not feasible to stimulate the sole because of either impaired access or excessive ticklishness, the sign can be elicited by other forms of stimulation, including firmly stroking the medial surface of the tibia from proximal to distal (Chaddock sign), firmly compressing the lower calf muscles (Gordon sign), or firmly stroking the skin beneath the lateral malleolus from proximal to distal (Oppenheimer sign).

2. Extension of the big toe due to contraction of the extensor hallucis longus (EHL) muscle is essential to the extensor response. Extension or abduction of the other toes need not be present. Extension of the big toe should be synchronous with activity of other flexor muscles of the lower extremity, usually as the flexors of the knee and/or the ankle. (This synchronous muscle flexion need not be accompanied by joint movement.)

3. Extension of the big toe relative to the other toes can mimic the appearance of an extensor response, but if it does not involve contraction of the EHL such an event

is not a Babinski sign. For example, this can occur if all toes might flex followed by the big toe relaxing before the other toes, or if all of the other toes flex while the big toe remains motionless.

It is well-recognized that toxic-metabolic encephalopathy can produce extensor plantar reflexes. Less frequently, the extensor reflex is unilateral even though the cerebral dysfunction is bilateral. Notwithstanding, the most likely cause of a unilateral extensor plantar response is unilateral or at least asymmetrical pyramidal tract disease, and an assessment for anatomical lesions is warranted.

Equivocal or absent plantar reflexes do occur and generally are uninterpretable unless reflexes are markedly asymmetrical. An equivocal plantar response sometimes can be converted into a clear-cut extensor response by stroking the sole more laterally, or converted into a clear-cut flexor response by stroking the sole more medially.

Primitive reflexes, otherwise known as frontal release signs, involve more complex responses to stimulation than the deep tendon jerks. The method for eliciting and interpreting the primitive reflexes has been nicely reviewed by Schott and Rossor (2003).

Two groups of primitive reflexes—grasping reflexes and primitive oral reflexes—are familiar to generalist physicians. When properly assessed, they can contribute incrementally to neuropsychiatric diagnosis.

GRASPING REFLEXES

There are two types of grasping reflex, one elicited by movement of the examiner's fingers across the palm and the other elicited by prolonged touch in one spot. The first grasping reflex is elicited by first applying deep pressure to the palmar surface of the hand and then stroking distally toward the fingers. When the reflex is present, the hand will grasp the examiner's fingers and will continue hold on firmly as the examiner moves his or her fingers. The grasp will persist as long as the examiner pulls the fingers away; stroking the dorsum of the patient's hand may release the reflex. The second grasping reflex is initially elicited by light, static pressure (rather than movement) by the examiner's fingers on the radial part of the hollow of the hand. This elicits a gradual closing of the patient's hand on the examiner's fingers. When the second grasping reflex is strong the stimulus can be given anywhere on the patient's palm; the patient will reposition his or her hand to get a good grasp. In severe cases, the examiner can remove his or her fingers from the patient's hand and the patient will pursue the examiner's moving fingers, attempting to grasp them again, demonstrating a "groping reflex". Both types of grasping reflex suggest frontal system dysfunction; they are especially common in degenerative dementia. A unilateral grasp reflex implies unilateral or at least asymmetrical disease; however, a bilateral grasp reflex sometimes can be seen with unilateral lesions. Two examples of interpreting the sign are as follows: (1) the occurrence of a new unilateral grasp reflex in a patient with multiple sclerosis can be a sign of disease relapse or progression, or (2) the occurrence of a grasp reflex in a patient with mild cognitive impairment would increase the probability that the impairment will evolve into dementia.

PRIMITIVE ORAL REFLEXES

Primitive oral reflexes represent vestiges of infant feeding behavior. The suck reflex, when present, can be elicited by putting something into the mouth—typically a tongue depressor. The rooting reflex is a turning of the mouth toward a stimulus that gently strokes the cheek; in more severe cases the mouth moves toward anything nearby brought into the field of view. The snout reflex is a puckering of the lips elicited by gentle pressure on the nasal philtrum. It should be distinguished from the pouting reflex, which is elicited by pressure on the lips or around the mouth and reflects pyramidal tract dysfunction rather than specifically frontal system dysfunction. The primitive oral reflexes are not lateralized. Their occurrence is diagnostically nonspecific beyond suggesting cerebral disease. The presence of two or three of the primitive oral reflexes could be helpful in distinguishing between a degenerative dementia and a dementia syndrome due to conversion or to another primary mental disorder.

THE EVOLVING ROLE OF THE PHYSICAL EXAMINATION

Increasingly, imaging and laboratory tests have become the primary standard for diagnosis in general medicine with the physical examination acquiring a less central role. While in some primary care settings the traditional general physical examination will remain relevant, the physical examination in secondary and tertiary care will continue to evolve. The authors expect several trends to continue:

1. The physical examination will be more hypothesis-driven and more individualized.

2. Individual components of the physical examination will be approached from a psychometric viewpoint, with population-specific and examiner-specific assessments of reliability, validity, and sensitivity and specificity for specific diagnoses.

3. Clinicians will make greater use of point-of-care technology to augment their senses when examining patients. Electronic stethoscopes are now common; handheld ultrasound units may become standard tools for bedside (or at least emergency room) cardiac and abdominal examinations.

4. The ubiquity of smartphones implies that digital images and audio and video recordings will become a standard way to record physical findings and share them with specialist colleagues. Smartphone accessories such as magnifying lenses and couplers to diagnostic instruments (e.g., ophthalmoscopes and stethoscopes) will facilitate this process. Devices intrinsic to smartphones, such as accelerometers and cameras, will be used to collect physiologic information. Ultimately, the ease of transmitting physical findings between physicians and obtaining near real-time specialist advice may alter patterns of referral and payment for subspecialty care.

5. Specific parts of the physical examination will be the focus of structured training and objective competency assessment.

6. During the transition toward a more individualized, psychometrically informed, hypothesis-driven, and technologically assisted physical examination, there will be considerable variation in examination technique and in the validity and value of findings. The medical psychiatrist will need to consider the qualitative and methodological aspects of the physical examinations a patient has had to date—not just their nominal scope—to decide whether they answer the diagnostic questions at hand.

CLINICAL PEARLS

- The physical exam has a number of distinct purposes: (1) narrowing a differential diagnosis prior to ordering diagnostic tests; (2) looking for physical signs to support the diagnosis of a specific condition that often has symptoms or functional impairment in excess of findings on a nonfocused, general physical examination; (3) quantifying the severity of a known physical condition to better assess its relationship to the patient's subjective distress and functional impairments; (4) getting a subjective sense of the patient's condition to better understand its emotional impact; (5) enhancing positive transference through appropriate touching of the patient; and (6) communicating across disciplinary lines to stimulate a fresh look at a patient's problem.

- If a patient with suspicious symptoms for orthostatic hypotension due to autonomic dysfunction does not show a blood pressure drop immediately on standing up, the blood pressure should be measured again after the patient has been standing for at least 5 minutes.

- Patients with recurrent functional hyperventilation—with or without associated panic attacks—do not necessarily have tachypnea; their breathing may be deeper than normal rather than more rapid than normal. This may be the case more often in younger patients (Han et al., 1997).

- *Visual* attention can be impaired when simple attention and (static) visual acuity are intact. Visual attention is critical to driving or operating dangerous machinery. A simple bedside task is to give the patient a sheet of paper full of randomly oriented and randomly spaced letters and numbers and ask the patient to cross out a defined subset—for example, the even numbers and the vowels.

- The patient with transcortical motor aphasia, associated with border zone infarcts and paucity of speech, can repeat sentences and can complete familiar phrases such as "Roses are red, violets are (blue)."

- Patients with Wernicke's aphasia may be suspicious and paranoid early on, before they are aware of their deficits. Lack of comprehension and inability to repeat support the diagnosis.

- Almost all dominant-hemisphere brain lesions that significantly affect spoken language will also affect reading and/or writing. Thus, having the patient hand-write a one paragraph summary of the recent illness can be a time-efficient and sensitive (albeit nonspecific) way to screen for language problems in patients with medical or epidemiologic risk factors for brain diseases that might affect language.

- The clock drawing test (CDT) is an excellent screening test for dorsolateral frontal function when visual-spatial function is intact. When visual-spatial function is intact and executive function is impaired, the spontaneous drawing of the clock typically shows poor planning and organization. Numbers may be poorly spaced, duplicated, or omitted; if the clock is to be set at "ten after eleven" the patient might point the large hand toward the ten rather than the two. If the patient can then copy a clock drawing perfectly, the poor performance on the spontaneous clock drawing cannot be attributed to visual-spatial dysfunction or to impaired praxis.

DISCLOSURE STATEMENT

Dr. Fogel is Chief Scientific Officer of Synchroneuron Inc., Managing Director of Anal-Gesic LLC, and Executive Vice President of PointRight Inc. He is the sole inventor or lead inventor on several pharmaceutical patents. In his opinion these affiliations do not entail any conflict of interest with regard to the editing of this book or his personal contributions to it. He has no other potential conflicts to disclose, direct or indirect, financial or otherwise, in connection with the editing of this book or his personal contributions to it.

REFERENCES

Akhnikh, S., deKorte, N., & deWinter, P. (2013). Anterior cutaneous nerve entrapment syndrome (ACNES): the forgotten diagnosis. *European Journal of Pediatrics*,

Alexander, J. H., Peterson, E. D., Chen, A. Y., Harding, T. M., Adams, D. B., & Kisslo, J. A. Jr. (2004). Feasibility of point-of-care echocardiography by internal medicine house staff. *American Heart Journal, 147*(3), 476–481.

Anderson, A. J., Shuey, N. H., & Wall, M. (2009). Rapid confrontation screening for visual field defects and extinction. *Clinical and Experimental Optometry, 92*(1), 45–48.

Ashraf, I., Paracha, S. R., Arif, M., Choudhary, A., Matteson, M. L., Clark, R. E., et al. (2012). Digital rectal examination versus spontaneous passage of stool for fecal occult blood testing. *Southern Medical Journal, 105*(7), 357–361.

Ball, K. K., Roenker, D. L., Wadley, V. G., Edwards, J. D., Roth, D. L., McGwin, G. Jr., et al. (2006). Can high-risk older drivers be identified through performance-based measures in a department of motor vehicles setting? *Journal of the American Geriatrics Society, 54*, 77–84.

Bechara, A. (2010). *Iowa Gambling Test Professional Manual*. Lutz, FL: Psychological Assessment Resources.

Beversdorf, D. Q., & Heilman, K. M. (2008). Facilitatory paratonia and frontal lobe functioning. *Neurology, 51*(4), 968–761.

Bianchi, W., Dugas, A. F., Hsieh, Y. H., Saheed, M., Hill, P., Lindauer, C., et al. (2013). Revitalizing a vital sign: improving detection of tachypnea at primary triage. *Annals of Emergency Medicine, 61*(1), 37–43.

Bollen, C. M. L., & Beikler, T. (2012). Halitosis: the multidisciplinary approach. *International Journal of Oral Science, 4*(2), 55–63.

Casjens, S., Eckert, A., Woitalla, D., Ellrichmann, G., Turewicz, M., Stephan, C., et al. (2013). Diagnostic value of the impairment of olfaction in Parkinson's disease. *PLoS ONE, 8*(5), e64735.

Cauquil-Michon, C., Flamand-Roze, C., & Denier, C. (2011). Border zone strokes and transcortical aphasia. *Current Neurology and Neuroscience Reports, 11*(6), 570–577.

Chang, D. S., Xu, L., Boland, M. V., & Friedman, D. S. (2013). Accuracy of the pupil assessment for the detection of glaucoma: a systematic review and meta-analysis. *Ophthalmology, 120*, 2217–2225.

Chen, S., Chen, Y., Liu, X., Li, M., Wu, B., Li, Y., et al. (2013). Insulin resistance and metabolic syndrome in normal-weight individuals. *Endocrine*, DOI 10.1007/s12020-013-0079-8; published online November 5, 2013.

Chou, R., Dana, T., Bougatsos, C., Fleming, C., & Beil, T. (2011). *Screening for hearing loss in adults ages 50 years and older. A review of the evidence for the U.S. Preventive Services Task Force*. Rockville, MD: Agency for Health Care Research and Quality: March, 2011.

Christensen, K., Thinggaard, M., McGue, M., Rexbye, H., Hjelmborg, J. V., Aviv, A., et al. (2009). Perceived age as a clinically useful biomarker of aging: cohort study. *British Medical Journal, 339*, b5262.

Cretikos, M. A., Bellomo, R., Hillman, K., Chen, J., Finfer, S., & Flabouris, A. (2008). Respiratory rate: the neglected vital sign. *Medical Journal of Australia, 188*, 657–659.

Croy, I., Hoffmann, H., Philpott, C., Rombaux, P., Welge-Luessen, A., Vodicka, J., et al. (2014). Retronasal testing of olfactory function: an investigation and comparison in seven countries. *European Archives of Otorhinolaryngology, 271*(5), 1087–1095.

Davidson, T. M., & Murphy, C. (1997). Rapid clinical evaluation of anosmia—the alcohol sniff test. *Archives of Otolaryngology—Head and Neck Surgery, 123*(6), 591–594.

Deng, T., Jia, J. P., & Guo, D. (2012). Cortical versus non-cortical lesions affect expression of Babinski sign. *Neurological Science, 34*(6), 855–859.

Dhakal, P. D., Murphy, R. M., & Lewis, G. D. (2012). Exercise oscillatory ventilation in heart failure. *Trends in Cardiovascular Medicine, 22*, 185–191.

Doty, R. L. (1995). *The Smell Identification Test Administration Manual*. Haddon Heights, NJ: Sensonics Inc.

Esene, I. N., Meher, A., Elzoghby, M. A., El-Bahy, K., Kotb, A., & El-Hakim, A. (2012). Diagnostic performance of the medial hamstring reflex in L5 radiculopathy. *Surgical Neurology International, 3*, 104.

Faust, D., & Fogel, B. S. (1989). The development and initial validation of a sensitive bedside cognitive screening test. *Journal of Nervous and Mental Disease, 177*(1), 25–31.

Fife, T. D., Iverson, D. J., Lempert T., Furman, J. M., Baloh, R. W., Tusa, R. J., et al. (2008). Practice parameter: therapies for benign paroxysmal positional vertigo (an evidence-based review): Report of the Quality Standards Subcommittee of the American Academy of Neurology. *Neurology, 70*, 2067–2074.

Flamand-Roze, C., Cauquil-Michon, C., Roze, E., Souillard-Scemama, R., Maintigneux, L., Ducreux, D., et al. (2011). Aphasia in border-zone infarcts has a specific initial pattern and good long-term prognosis. *European Journal of Neurology, 18*(12), 1397–1401.

Freund, B., Gravenstein, S., Ferris, R., Burke, B. L., & Shaheen, E. (2005). Drawing clocks and driving cars: Using brief tests of cognition to screen driving competency in older adults. *Journal of General Internal Medicine, 20*, 240–244.

Friedman, N. J., Kaiser, P. K., & Pineda R. (2009). *The Massachusetts Eye and Ear Infirmary Illustrated Manual of Ophthalmology,* 3rd edition. New York: Saunders Elsevier.

Gasquez, I., Soto-Varela, A., Aran, I., Santos, S., Batuecas, A., Trinidad, G., et al. (2011). High prevalence of systemic autoimmune diseases in patients with Meniere's disease. *PLoS ONE, 6*(10), e26759.

Gates, G. A., & Mills, J. H. (2005). Presbyacusis. *Lancet, 366*(9491), 1111–1120.

Giza, E., Fotiou, D., Bostantjopoulou, S., Katsarou, Z., Gerasimou, G., Gotzamani-Psarrakou, A., et al. (2012). Pupillometry and 123I-DaTSCAN imaging in Parkinson's Disease: a comparison study. *International Journal of Neuroscience, 122,* 26–34.

Goldsmith, L., Katz, S., Gilchrest, B., Paller, A. S., Leffell, D. J., & Wolff, K. (2012). *Fitzpatrick's Dermatology in General Medicine.* New York: McGraw-Hill.

Grant, J. E., Odlaug, B. L., Chamberlain, S. R., Keuthen, N. J., Lochner, C., & Stein, D. J. (2012). Skin picking disorder. *American Journal of Psychiatry, 169*(11), 1143–1149.

Grimaldi, G., & Manto, M. (2012). Topography of cerebellar deficits in humans. *Cerebellum, 11,* 336–351.

Halmagyi, G. M., AW, S. T., Cremer, P. D., Curthoys, I. S., & Todd, M. J. (2001). Impulsive testing of individual semicircular canal function. *Annals of the New York Academy of Sciences, 942,* 192–200.

Han, J. N, Stegen, K., Simkens, K., Cauberghs, M., Schepers, R., Van den Bergh, O., et al. (1997). Unsteadiness of breathing in patients with hyperventilation syndrome and anxiety disorders. *European Respiratory Journal, 10,* 167–176.

Heilman, K., Leon, S. A., & Rosenbek, J. C. (2004). Affective aprosodia from a medial frontal stroke. *Brain and Language, 89,* 411–416.

Hubbard, E. J., Santini, V., Blankevoort, C. G., Volkers, K. M., Barrup, M. S., Byerly, L., et al. (2008). Clock drawing performance in cognitively intact elderly. *Archives of Clinical Neuropsychology, 23*(3), 295–327.

Hummel, T., Sekinger, B., Wolf, S. R., Pauli, E., & Kobal, G. (1997). 'Sniffin' sticks': olfactory performance assessed by the combined testing of odor identification, odor discrimination and olfactory threshold. *Chemical Senses, 22,* 39–352.

Hwang, S. W., Atia, M., Nisenbaum, R., Pare, D. E., & Joordens, S. (2011). Is looking older than one's actual age a sign of poor health? *Journal of General Internal Medicine, 26*(2), 136–141.

Ilic, D., Neuberger, M. M., Djulbegovic, M., & Dahm, P. (2013). Screening for prostate cancer. *Cochrane Database, Jan 31,* 1, CD004720.

Joundi, R. A., Brittain, J. S., Jenkinson, N., Green, A. L., & Aziz, T. (2011). Rapid tremor frequency assessment with the iPhone accelerometer. *Parkinsonism and Related Disorders, 17,* 288–290.

Kelley, A. P., & Taylor, S. (2009). *Dermatology for Skin of Color.* New York: McGraw-Hill.

Kronfol, Z., & Remick, D. G. (2000). Cytokines and the brain: implications for clinical psychiatry. *American Journal of Psychiatry, 157,* 683–694.

Lessig, M. C., Scanlan, J. M., Nazemi, H., & Borson, S. (2008). Time that tells: critical clock-drawing errors for dementia screening. *International Psychogeriatrics, 20*(3), 459–470.

Lin, P. T., & Hallett, M. (2009). The pathophysiology of focal hand dystonia. *Journal of Hand Therapy, 22*(2), 109–114.

Lu, S., Leasure, R., & Dai, Y. (2009). A systematic review of body temperature variations in older people. *Journal of Clinical Nursing, 19,* 4–16.

Mainland, B. J., Amodeo, S., & Shulman, K. I. (2014). Multiple clock drawing scoring systems: simpler is better. *International Journal of Geriatric Psychiatry, 29*(2), 127–136.

Marinella, M. A. (2004). Woltman's sign of hypothyroidism. *Hospital Physician, 40*(1), 31–32.

McGee, S. (2013). Cheyne-Stokes breathing and reduced ejection fraction. *American Journal of Medicine, 126*(6), 536–540.

Meziere, A., Paillaud, E., Belmin, J., Pariel, S., Herbaud, S., Canouï-Poitrine, F., et al. (2013). Delirium in older people following proximal femoral fracture repair: role of a preoperative cognitive screening test. *Annales Francaises de Anesthesie et de Reanimation, 32*(9), e91–e96.

Minor, D. S., Butler, K. R., Artman, K. L., et al. (2012). Evaluation of blood pressure measurement and agreement in an academic health sciences center. *Journal of Clinical Hypertension, 14,* 222–227.

Mintzer, M., & Griffiths, R. R. (2003). Lorazepam and scopolamine: A single-dose comparison of effects on human memory and attentional processes. *Experimental and Clinical Psychopharmacology, 11*(1), 56–72.

Morrow, J. M., & Reilly, M. M. (2011). The Babinski sign. *British Journal of Hospital Medicine, 72*(10), M157–M159.

Muzyka, B. C., & Epifanio, R. N. (2013). Clinical approaches to oral mucosal disorders, Part I: Update on oral fungal infections. *Dental Clinics of North America, 57*(4), 561–581.

Newman-Toker, D. E. (2014). Neuro-vestibular examination. http://content.lib.utah.edu/cdm/ref/collection/ehsl-dent/id/9, accessed June 17.

Pedrosa, A. G., Morais, P., Lisboa, C., & Azevedo, F. (2013). The importance of trichoscopy in clinical practice. *Dermatology Research and Practice, 2013,* 986970.

Pickering, T. G., Hall, J. E., Appel, L. J., Falkner, B. E., Graves, J., Hill, M. N., et al. (2005). Recommendations for blood pressure measurement in humans and experimental animals: Part I: Blood pressure measurement in humans: A statement for professionals from the subcommittee of professional and public education of the American Heart Association Council on High Blood Pressure Research. *Hypertension, 45,* 142–161.

Rapp, M. P., Bergstrom, N., & Padhye, N. S. (2009). Contribution of skin temperature regularity to the risk of developing pressure ulcers in nursing facility residents. *Advances in Skin Wound Care, 22,* 506–513.

Ray, G. M., Nawarskas, J. J., & Anderson, J. R. (2011). Blood pressure monitoring technique impacts hypertension treatment. *Journal of General Internal Medicine, 7,* 623–629.

Robbins, M. L., Mehl, M. R., Holleran, S. E., & Kasle, S. (2011). Naturally observed sighing and depression in rheumatoid arthritis patients: a preliminary study. *Health Psychology, 30*(1), 129–133.

Rosania, A. E., Low, K. G., McCormick, C. M., & Rosania, D. A. (2009). Stress, depression, cortisol and periodontal disease. *Journal of Periodontology, 80*(2), 260–266.

Royall, D. R., Mahurin, R. K., & Gray, K. F. (1992). Bedside assessment of executive cognitive impairment: the executive interview. *Journal of the American Geriatrics Society, 40*(12), 1221–1226.

Ruddox, V., Stokke, T. M., Edvardsen, T., Hjelmesæth, J., Aune, E., Bækkevar, M., et al. (2013). The diagnostic accuracy of pocket-size cardiac ultrasound performed by unselected residents with minimal training. *International Journal of Cardiovascular Imaging, 29,* 1749–1757.

Saddawi-Konefka, D., Berg, S. M., Nejad, S. H., & Bittner, E. A. (2014). Catatonia in the ICU, an important and underdiagnosed cause of altered mental status: a case series and review of the literature. *Critical Care Medicine, 42*(3), e234–e241.

Schott, J. M., & Rossor, M. N. (2003). The grasp and other primitive reflexes. *Journal of Neurology, Neurosurgery and Psychiatry, 74,* 558–560.

Sprigle, S., Linden, M., McKenne, D., Davis, K., & Riordan, B. (2001). Skin temperature measurement to predict incipient pressure ulcers. *Advances in Skin Wound Care, 14,* 133–137.

Stamps, J. J., Bartoshuk, L. M., & Heilman, K. M. (2013). *Journal of the Neurological Sciences, 333,* 19–24.

Stapleton, E., & Mills, R. (2008). Clinical diagnosis of Meniere's disease: how useful are the American Academy of Otolaryngology Head and Neck Surgery Committee on Hearing and Equilibrium guidelines? *Journal of Laryngology and Otology, 122,* 773–779.

Sun, G. H., Raji, C. A., MacEachern, M. P., & Burke, J. F. (2012). Olfactory identification testing as a predictor of the development of Alzheimer's dementia: a systematic review. *Laryngoscope, 122*(7), 1455–1462.

Sund-Levander, M., & Grodzinski, E. (2013). Assessment of body temperature measurement options. *British Journal of Nursing, 22*(16), 942–950.

Talley, N. J. (2008). How to do and interpret a rectal examination in gastroenterology. *American Journal of Gastroenterology, 103,* 820–822.

Tandon, R., Heckers, S., & Bustillo, J. (2013). Catatonia in DSM-5. *Schizophrenia Research, 150,* 26–30.

Teigen, K. H. (2008). Is a sigh "just a sigh"? Sighs as emotional signals and responses to a difficult task. *Scandinavian Journal of Psychology, 49*(1), 49–57.

van Assen, T., Jenneke, W., de Jager-Kievit, A. J., & Roumen, R. M. (2013). Chronic abdominal wall pain misdiagnosed as functional abdominal pain. *Journal of the American Board of Family Medicine, 26,* 738–744.

Van Dyke, T. E. (2008). Resolution of inflammation: Unraveling mechanistic links between periodontitis and cardiovascular disease. *Journal of Dentistry, 37,* S582–S583.

Varela, M., Ruiz-Esteban, R., Martinez-Nicolas, A., Cuervo-Arango, J. A., Barros, C., & Delgado, E. G. (2011). "Catching the spike and tracking the flow": Holter-temperature monitoring in patients admitted in a general internal medicine ward. *International Journal of Clinical Practice, 65*(12), 1283–1288.

Visual Awareness. (2013). Home page, http://www.visualawareness.com.

Wildgruber, D., Ackermann, H., Kreifelts, B., & Ethofer, T. (2006). Cerebral processing of linguistic and emotional prosody: fMRI studies. *Progress in Brain Research, 156,* 249–268.

Wong, R. K., Drossman, D. A., Bharucha, A. E., Rao, S. S., Wald, A., Morris, C. B., et al. (2012). The digital rectal examination: a multicenter survey of physicians' and students' perceptions. *American Journal of Gastroenterology, 107,* 1157–1163.

Zhou, J., Ge, H., Zhu, M., Wang, L. J., Chen, L., Tan, Y. Z., et al. (2013). Neck circumference as an independent predictive factor to cardiometabolic syndrome. *Cardiovascular Diabetology, 12,* 76. Published online at http://www.cardiab.com/content/12/1/76.

3.

NEUROPSYCHOLOGICAL ASSESSMENT

Aaron P. Nelson and Stephanie Assuras

INTRODUCTION

Neuropsychology is the science of human behavior based on the function of the brain. Clinical neuropsychology is an applied discipline that uses principles of brain–behavior relationships to evaluate and diagnose abnormality in the realm of behavior and cognition. This process of evaluation and diagnosis, termed *neuropsychological assessment*, involves obtaining information about an individual's history and current functioning as well as administering a variety of behavioral measures designed to probe specific cognitive functions. A clinical neuropsychologist analyzes and integrates information collected during the assessment process with the aim of providing diagnostic clarification or helping to guide treatment planning.

HISTORICAL PERSPECTIVE

Clinical neuropsychology traces its roots to the confluence of three major tributaries of psychological science: psychophysics, the psychometric method, and the lesion method in behavioral neuroanatomy. New methodologies for viewing the brain, both structurally and functionally, continue to illuminate the everyday miracles of thought, memory, and emotion. The integration of clinical work with experimental discoveries has reached a new zenith in cross-fertilization of both endeavors. The phenomenal growth of clinical neuropsychology over the past half century owes much to contemporaneous work in clinical neuroscience.

Although it is not possible to pinpoint the date of its establishment as a discipline, Arthur Benton points out that clinical neuropsychology lacked the usual trappings of a coherent specialty prior to 1960 (Benton, 1992). There were no professional organizations, journals, or training programs. In its earliest form, neuropsychology was practiced in medical settings in association with departments of neurology and neurosurgery. Psychologists with expertise in psychological measurement and a special interest in behavior effects of brain injury designed tests to assess various abilities in their patients.

Although theories of brain function can be traced back to the writings of the ancients, the term *neuropsychology* came into use only relatively recently. The ancient Egyptians originally localized the seat of human thought in the heart. This notion remained largely unchallenged until some 3000 years later, when a Greek student of Pythagoras proposed that the brain was responsible for sensation and thought and advanced the notion that specific aspects of mental function were represented in specific regions of the brain. This approach to thinking about the brain was later termed *localization* and became the center of great controversy 2000 years later. Hippocrates, writing in the fourth century BC, claimed the brain as the organ of intellect, sensation, and emotion. Furthermore, he posited that mental illness was rooted in abnormal brain function. Along this line, he advanced the hypothesis that epilepsy was not the result of demonic possession but rather an organic ailment.

Beginning in the middle of the 19th century, psychophysics comprised a refined approach to the precise measurement of various human attributes. Galton's studies of individual differences in sensory and psychomotor responses epitomized this approach, as did the early work of Ebbinghaus on "individual memory curves of retention" (Ebbinghaus, 1885/1913). At the beginning of the 20th century, Binet and Simon (1916) and others introduced the revolutionary concept of measurable intelligence, a notion that continues to have a profound and controversial impact on human society. The psychometric method was employed to design and construct measurement methods possessing validity and reliability, which are crucial underpinnings of all psychological and neuropsychological tests.

The lesion method has its origins in early case reports of brain–behavior effects in injury and illness. The famous case of Phineas Gage in 1848 involved a railroad worker who survived a catastrophic injury in which an iron spike was blasted through his head, essentially disconnecting the anterior portion of his brain (Harlow, 1868). The resulting pattern of spared and affected functions in Gage gave rise to an early understanding of the functional role of the frontal lobes in human behavior. The pioneering work of Paul Broca, a French neurologist who described his patient "Tan" in 1861 (Broca, 1861), was instrumental in unveiling the role of the dominant hemisphere in human language function. In the 1950s, Scoville and Milner's studies of patient "HM" shed new light on the role of the limbic system in anterograde memory function (Scoville & Milner, 1957).

The advent of World War I saw the first period in history when modern American medicine had to cope with the tragedy of "industrial" warfare. Legions of combatants returned from Europe with life-altering brain injuries. Assessing the cognitive consequences of such injuries spurred the growth of early assessment methodologies. The aftermath of World War II marked the establishment of modern clinical psychology, with an emphasis on the special skill of psychological testing. Measurement of intelligence was the venue in which early testing applications were most significant.

The earliest codification of neuropsychological examination methods can be attributed to Dr. Ralph Reitan. A pioneering neuropsychologist, Reitan and his colleagues assembled a battery of test measures in which specific patterns of scores were linked to dysfunction of associated brain regions (Reitan & Wolfson, 1993). Later approaches diverged from a reliance on a set battery of tests and instead used a more dynamic method, the "process" approach to neuropsychological assessment developed by Dr. Edith Kaplan in her work at the Boston Veterans Administration Hospital (Kaplan, 1990). This technique entails ongoing in situ hypothesis testing in which particular attention is paid to the qualitative aspects of a patient's test response. Although quantitative data are also important, the patient's route to solving a particular cognitive problem often reveals an underlying process that can be reflective of spared and affected brain regions. In contemporary practice, both of these methods rely on a vast body of knowledge about characteristic syndromes that are associated with underlying disease states.

The current practice of clinical neuropsychology concerns itself with assessment of cognitive functions, through the use of test instruments, for the purpose of understanding the functional integrity of the brain. By relying on knowledge of brain–behavior relationships and characteristic syndromes, the results of assessment are useful for diagnosis and treatment of brain-related injuries and illness.

FUNDAMENTAL ASSUMPTIONS

The study of clinical neuropsychology is firmly rooted in the larger field of neuroscience and therefore rests on the assumption that the nervous system impacts behavior and cognition. Conversely, inferences can be made about the integrity of the brain based on observable behavior. The ability to make accurate and meaningful inferences is predicated on a thorough understanding of two streams of knowledge: (a) the neural infrastructure underlying normal human cognition and behavior, and (b) the characteristic profiles of neurocognitive and neurobehavioral syndromes.

Observable behavior is frequently the most sensitive manifestation of brain pathology. Such behavior can range from subtleties of social comportment to performance on a specific neuropsychological test. A competent neuropsychologist will sample multiple domains of behavior. Observable behavior, including "test behavior," reflects an interaction between the domains of person and environment. Variables from each domain must be considered in order to arrive at an understanding of the clinical significance of a given behavior.

Individual tests used in neuropsychological practice focus on measurement of particular cognitive processes. In order to be useful, each test must be constructed according to sound psychometric principles and possess adequate validity and reliability. In addition, there must be appropriate normative data with which to compare a single patient's performance. The neuropsychologist relies on a comprehensive understanding of test construction and standardization in order to select and interpret measures for a given clinical context. This includes choosing tests with normative data derived from subjects of similar age, education, and nationality to the patient currently being tested (Attix et al., 2009).

The interpretation of test results depends on an understanding of the component processes involved in any given test response. For example, the ability to name an object to visual confrontation depends on multiple processes that are mediated by different brain systems. The individual must first orient and attend to the stimulus. Second, the stimulus must be accurately registered at the level of visual perception. Third, the neural pathway that links the visual percept to meaningful recognition must be patent. Fourth, the ability to assign a phonemic/lexical label to the object must be intact. Finally, the individual must be able to convey a response through speech. Because a complex cognitive action, such as naming a simple object, can be undermined by perturbation at any point within the network linking multiple functions, a neuropsychologist must understand the component processes involved in each behavior. By examining the patient's function in multiple domains with multiple measures, the neuropsychologist can determine which processes and associated neural circuits are functioning abnormally.

Performance on a single test is not sufficient to make a diagnostic inference. A common misconception is that a poor score on a particular test denotes an impairment in the domain that the test is nominally designed to assess. For example, if a patient performs poorly on a "memory" test, this does not necessarily signify impairment in memory but could indicate difficulties with attention or language. A neuropsychologist will evaluate a profile of test results in a dynamic, interactive fashion in order to arrive at a diagnostic formulation.

Neuropsychological testing is simply one means of obtaining a sample of behavior. A neuropsychologist must proceed with caution in using test data to predict behavior. The testing environment is, by necessity, contrived to promote a standard approach to test administration. This contrivance constitutes a challenge in understanding how test performance corresponds to "real life" behavior. For example, a patient who complains of difficulty with concentration and memory at work may perform quite normally in the context of the quiet, distraction-free examination room. Discrepancy between "test behavior" and "real-life" behavior is the source of ongoing challenge for the design of an ecologically valid assessment environment.

CLINICAL APPLICATIONS

The overall purpose of the neuropsychological evaluation is the creation of a dynamic portrait of the patient in cognitive, psychological, and functional terms. Characterizing cognitive strengths and weaknesses is a critical goal of the neuropsychological evaluation, as this contributes to an understanding of the underlying etiology and clarification of the differential diagnosis. Precise quantitative measurement of cognitive functions also yields data that can be useful for establishing a baseline of cognitive functioning against which to calibrate degree of change in patients over time. This involves systematically monitoring cognitive functioning to determine response to a specific treatment intervention, or to characterize the course of a symptomatic pattern for the purpose of further clarifying a diagnosis or prognosis. For example, with objective quantitative data, neuropsychologists are in a unique position to evaluate the efficacy of treatment interventions (e.g., pharmacotherapy, electroconvulsive therapy, neurosurgery) by reevaluating after initiation of therapy.

As Americans live longer and become more aware of the relationship between aging and dementia, they are more likely to notice subtle changes in cognitive function in themselves and in family members. This awareness is particularly heightened in individuals with a family history of neurodegenerative disease. Detection of subtle cognitive dysfunction in aging is even more challenging in individuals of high baseline intellectual ability. Neuropsychological assessment can be useful in identifying abnormalities of cognitive function that may not be evident on casual observation, within a standard office mental status examination, or through the use of common brief screening measures (e.g., Mini Mental State Examination, Montreal Cognitive Assessment).

Because of its knowledge base in behavioral neuroscience, neuropsychology has an important role in treatment planning. Enumeration of cognitive strengths and intact abilities can be used to design real-world adaptive or compensatory strategies that a patient may employ to circumvent deficits. Neuropsychologists make specific and detailed recommendations for rehabilitation in cases of brain injury, tumor, and stroke, and are central to the planning process for patients and families confronting dementing illnesses. Recommendations for supplementary diagnostic procedures (e.g., imaging, electroencephalogram, polysomnography) and/or referral for additional specialty consultation (e.g., neurology, ophthalmology) can be indicated to round out the diagnostic process. Referral to psychiatry may be indicated for consideration of the potential benefits of pharmacological intervention (e.g., treatment with antidepressant, stimulant, cognitive-enhancing, or mood-stabilizing medication).

Prescribed treatment recommendations may include compensatory strategies and skill acquisition programs to address cognitive weaknesses. Behavioral strategies to enhance planning and organization can be implemented via post-evaluation consultation with the neuropsychologist or through the use of structured workbooks and guides. If more intensive or ongoing treatment is indicated, a referral can be made to a clinician or program specializing in cognitive rehabilitation. Health-related behavioral modifications are often recommended. For example, a patient with insomnia resulting in suboptimal daytime cognitive function will benefit from learning about sleep hygiene factors that can lead to improved, restorative sleep. Modification of environmental factors can be effective for enhancing patient safety and caregiver confidence; the use of tracking devices for wandering patients (e.g., GPS-enabled shoes and bracelets) can be practical solutions for a common problem in elderly individuals with neurodegenerative illness.

The neuropsychological exam can be "negative" in a range of scenarios. The "worried well" may be relieved to learn that their occasional word-finding hesitancy does not bespeak the onset of a dementia; recommendations for maintaining optimal brain health going forward are often appreciated. Interestingly, not all patients are relieved to learn that their cognitive symptoms do not have an underlying organic etiology. Discussion of this type of patient is beyond the scope of our chapter. However, a recommendation for individual psychotherapy is often more "acceptable" to the patient after he or she has been through a comprehensive evaluation process or if it is contextualized as a means of enhancing cognitive health.

Neuropsychological assessment can delineate the potential impact of brain pathology on venues of real-life functioning, ranging from the most rudimentary human activities (bathing and dressing) to work life and the complexities of intimate relationships. Neuropsychologists can provide an explanatory context for a patient's cognitive, social, or behavioral difficulties. In addition, in the case of progressive disease, neuropsychologists can provide education about how the patient's changing condition will impact day-to-day functioning differently over time. It is not unusual for an otherwise sensitive spouse to blame an affected husband or wife for a particular behavior, which had been assumed to be under voluntary control. Learning that the behavior is part and parcel of a disease process dramatically alters this attribution and allows both patient and spouse to work together on the problem.

Neuropsychological consultation is frequently pivotal in cases involving adjudication of criminal or civil matters. Neuropsychologists with special training and experience in forensics play an important role in determination of competency in matters ranging from criminal responsibility to guardianship. There has been significant increased appreciation of the utility of neuropsychological knowledge for assisting the courts in understanding functional consequences of neurological disorder in personal injury cases ranging from product liability to accidental injury. Neuropsychology is becoming central to determination of competency and medical decision making in end-of-life care. Neuropsychologists have pioneered the development of specialized and embedded measures of effort and symptom validity for use in cases in which motivational factors are important (cf., Bianchini et al., 2001).

APPROACH TO NEUROPSYCHOLOGICAL ASSESSMENT

Three major approaches to neuropsychological assessment have emerged during the last half century.

FIXED BATTERY APPROACH

The fixed battery approach to neuropsychological assessment was developed primarily by Ralph Reitan and his colleagues (cf., Reitan & Wolfson, 1992). This approach to assessment was formulated in the 1950s, two decades before the advent of widely available structural brain imaging. At that time, this type of assessment was relied upon as a first-line diagnostic method in patients with stroke, brain tumor, or traumatic injury. Relying strictly on quantitative scores and indices, the Halstead-Reitan battery yields information regarding lesion laterality, localization, and extent of overall neuropsychological impairment. As the name suggests, practitioners of this approach typically utilize a standard set of tests in the context of assessment and do not vary this battery, if possible. The battery is designed to assess each major cognitive domain and therefore ensure a comprehensive assessment of every patient. A clear advantage of this approach is the ability to detect deficits that are unsuspected or not otherwise evident. Another advantage is that practitioners of this method become very familiar with the subtleties of the battery and develop a greater sensitivity to slight variations in the performance of component tasks. Disadvantages of this approach include inefficiency (i.e., a time-consuming battery is administered in all cases, including those for whom more focused assessment would be sufficient) and lack of flexibility. Some have also criticized the most widely used fixed-battery approach for insufficient assessment of key functions, including memory (Lezak, 1995).

PROCESS APPROACH

Another major neuropsychological methodology is the Boston Process approach, primarily developed by Edith Kaplan and colleagues (Milberg et al., 1986). This approach proceeds in a hypothesis-driven manner and uses the patient's test performance to guide and inform an evolving and dynamic assessment strategy. The process-oriented evaluation is individually tailored to each patient and uses specific tests for the purpose of answering particular questions. As answers to these questions emerge during the evaluation, the neuropsychologist moves through a series of decision points, probing particular cognitive functions as needed; test selection occurs in real time. In addition, this approach stresses qualitative aspects of test performance, examining the process by which the patient solves a problem rather than exclusively relying on test scores as quantitative data. Tests are administered in a standardized fashion but can also be modified to test the limits of cognitive function and to produce richer qualitative data. Task performance is analyzed across multiple measures to parse out component processes and identify specific cognitive deficits.

FLEXIBLE BATTERY APPROACH

In current practice, most neuropsychologists utilize the so-called "flexible battery" approach (Sweet et al., 2001). Just as the name implies, a select battery of tests may be the starting point for assessing a particular case type. For example, a specific set of test measures is used for evaluating elderly individuals referred with a question of dementia. However, the clinician can modify the battery either beforehand or during the course of the assessment depending upon specifics of the case, including questions that emerge during the administration of other test measures. This approach has the virtue of generating a substantial repository of core common data on similar cases that can be pooled for both clinical and academic benefit, while allowing for latitude in the individual case.

CLINICAL METHOD

Clinical neuropsychological assessment comprises a series of activities during which information is elicited and analyzed in the service of diagnosis and treatment planning. This process is illustrated in Figure 3.1. Although test administration is the most time-consuming component of the process, it is often the case that some of the most valuable information emerges while discussing a patient's history and current life situation. The information obtained during the initial interview is important for differential diagnosis and frequently guides the remainder of the assessment.

REFERRAL QUESTION AND CHIEF COMPLAINT

The first task of a neuropsychological assessment is to clarify the reason for referral. Patients are typically referred for neuropsychological assessment by other clinicians involved in their care, often for assistance in diagnostic clarification and treatment planning. After the referral question is ascertained, the patient is seen and a chief complaint is elicited including a clear description of the onset and course of the complaint (e.g., symptoms, concerns) as well as information regarding the medical and social context in which the problem(s) emerged. The patient's overall understanding of the rationale for the consultation and appreciation of his/her current circumstances is also sought.

HISTORY

Information is obtained from a variety of sources including the patient's self-report, observations of family members or close friends, medical records, and prior evaluations from academic or work situations. Information is obtained regarding (1) past medical history including illnesses, injuries, surgeries, medications, hospitalizations, substance abuse, and relevant family medical history; (2) past psychiatric history including hospitalizations, medications and outpatient treatment; (3) developmental background including circumstances of gestation, birth and delivery, acquisition of developmental milestones, and early socialization skills; (4) social development including major autobiographical events and relationships (a three-generational geneogram is highly useful in gaining relevant family information); (5) educational background including early school experiences and academic performance during high school, college, postgraduate study, and other educational and technical training (the presence of

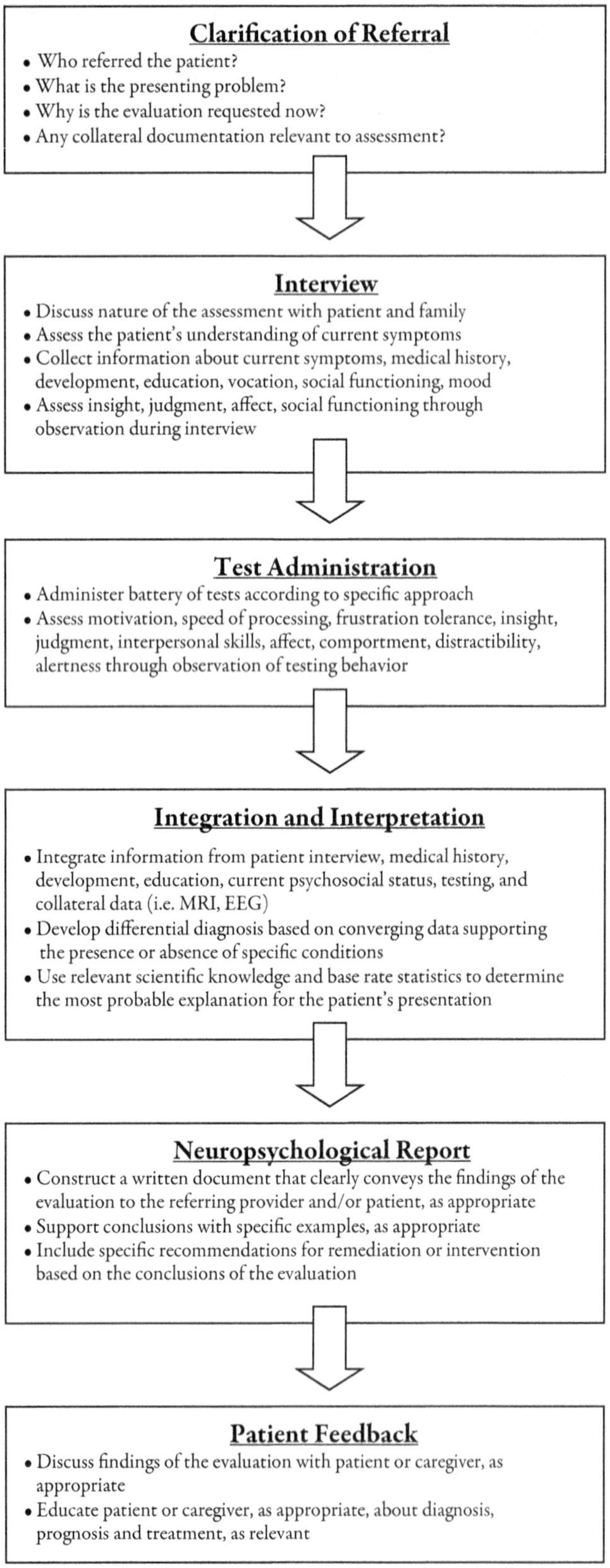

Clarification of Referral

- Who referred the patient?
- What is the presenting problem?
- Why is the evaluation requested now?
- Any collateral documentation relevant to assessment?

Interview

- Discuss nature of the assessment with patient and family
- Assess the patient's understanding of current symptoms
- Collect information about current symptoms, medical history, development, education, vocation, social functioning, mood
- Assess insight, judgment, affect, social functioning through observation during interview

Test Administration

- Administer battery of tests according to specific approach
- Assess motivation, speed of processing, frustration tolerance, insight, judgment, interpersonal skills, affect, comportment, distractibility, alertness through observation of testing behavior

Integration and Interpretation

- Integrate information from patient interview, medical history, development, education, current psychosocial status, testing, and collateral data (i.e. MRI, EEG)
- Develop differential diagnosis based on converging data supporting the presence or absence of specific conditions
- Use relevant scientific knowledge and base rate statistics to determine the most probable explanation for the patient's presentation

Neuropsychological Report

- Construct a written document that clearly conveys the findings of the evaluation to the referring provider and/or patient, as appropriate
- Support conclusions with specific examples, as appropriate
- Include specific recommendations for remediation or intervention based on the conclusions of the evaluation

Patient Feedback

- Discuss findings of the evaluation with patient or caregiver, as appropriate
- Educate patient or caregiver, as appropriate, about diagnosis, prognosis and treatment, as relevant

Figure 3.1 Schematic of Neuropsychological Evaluation.

a learning disability should be assessed); (6) vocational history including work performance, work satisfaction, and relationships with supervisors and coworkers; and (7) recreational interests and hobbies.

BEHAVIORAL OBSERVATIONS

Physical appearance is inspected including symmetry of anatomical features, facial expression, manner of dress, and attention to personal hygiene. The patient is asked specific questions regarding unusual sensory or motor symptoms. Affect and mood are assessed with respect to range and modulation of felt and expressed emotions and their congruence with concurrent ideation and the contemporaneous situation. Interpersonal comportment is assessed in the context of the interview. Specifically, attention is paid to whether the patient's behavior reflects a normal awareness of self and other in the interaction, along with whether the patient is motivated and complies with examination requests, instructions, and test procedures. An appreciation of the patient's level of motivation to participate in the evaluation and comply with examination instructions is crucial to assessing the validity of the test data. General level of arousal or alertness is determined by observing the patient's degree of drowsiness, tendency to yawn or fall asleep during the interview, level of interpersonal engagement, and speed of response in conversation. Environmental and diurnal factors can modify arousal, and an attempt should be made to assess whether this is relevant in the case of a particular patient by inquiring about consistency of arousal level and any fluctuations that the patient or caregiver has observed.

EXAMINATION

A sufficiently broad range of neuropsychological functions is evaluated using tests and other assessment techniques. The major domains to be surveyed include general intellectual ability, attention, executive function and comportment, memory, language, visuospatial abilities, motor functioning, and mood/personality. As a prelude to test administration, it is imperative to establish the integrity of sensation and perception because impairments in these areas can invalidate the results of examination. For example, it would be incorrect to conclude that a patient has a receptive language impairment when, in fact, there is a primary hearing deficit.

DIAGNOSTIC FORMULATION

Data from the history, observation, and testing of the patient are analyzed collectively to produce a concise understanding of the patient's symptoms and neuropsychological diagnosis. A configuration of abilities and limitations is developed and used both diagnostically and as a framework through which to address the goals of treatment. When possible, the diagnostic formulation should identify the neuropathological factors that give rise to the patient's clinical presentation, including underlying anatomy and disease process.

RECOMMENDATIONS AND FEEDBACK

Consultation concludes with the process of feedback, through which the findings of the evaluation and treatment recommendations are reviewed with relevant individuals (i.e., referring physician, the patient, family, treatment team members). As discussed earlier in the chapter, a variety of treatment plans may be advised including neurological evaluation, psychiatric consultation, psychotherapy, cognitive/behavioral remediation, and vocational guidance. Recommendations should be pragmatic and individually tailored to each patient's specific needs. Strategies for optimizing performance in personal, educational, occupational, and relational spheres are identified and discussed in lay language that the patient and family member(s) can understand. When possible, the clinician outlines concrete strategies to facilitate remediation of identified problems. Appropriate neuropsychological follow-up is also arranged when indicated.

DOMAINS OF NEUROPSYCHOLOGICAL FUNCTION

The fractionation of neuropsychological functions into specific domains is a somewhat arbitrary organizational contrivance. In reality, there is considerable overlap within and between cognitive domains. For example, working memory shares much common ground with aspects of attention and language.

GENERAL INTELLECTUAL ABILITY

Determining an individual's level of intellectual functioning is a fundamental component of the neuropsychological assessment. Intelligence encompasses a broad range of capacities, many of which are not directly assessed in the traditional clinical setting. The estimate of general intellectual ability is based on both formal assessment methods and a survey of demographic factors and life accomplishments. Information regarding the patient's educational background and longstanding

difficulties (e.g., learning disability, repeated grades), occupational history, and special abilities is used to establish an estimate of baseline intellectual functioning. Once established, general level of intelligence serves as a point of reference from which to evaluate performance in other domains. Test performance should always be compared with an estimate of premorbid level of functioning, which is critical in establishing whether there has been a change in cognitive status. However, it is important to note that an individual's profile of cognitive abilities can range considerably from domain to domain; variable capability across diverse neuropsychological functions is often the rule rather than the exception in normal human development (Schretlen, 2003). While superior intelligence may obscure the detection of cognitive deficits, low baseline intelligence may appear to represent a cognitive decline when no change from a previous level of functioning has occurred.

Formal measures of general intellectual function typically assess a broad range of functions through multiple subtests (e.g., WAIS-IV, WASI-II, WISC-IV) and yield an "intelligence quotient" as well as other derived index scores. Other test instruments obtain high correlations with IQ measures and have been used to estimate overall intellectual ability (e.g., Ravens Progressive Matrices). In cases of known or suspected impairment, premorbid ability can also be surmised from performance on measures presumed less sensitive to cerebral dysfunction (e.g., vocabulary). Single-word reading tests (e.g., WTAR) have been used to estimate baseline verbal intelligence in patients with early degenerative conditions. In addition, so-called "best performance methods" can be used. This method assumes that the patient's highest level of performance can be used to set a reference point for optimal baseline ability (Table 3.1).

Table 3.1 GENERAL INTELLECTUAL ABILITY

TEST NAME	DESCRIPTION
Wechsler Intelligence Scales	The Wechsler Adult Intelligence Scale (WAIS-IV) is composed of 13 individual subtests. Administration of all subtests generates Full-Scale IQ and four different performance indices: Verbal Comprehension Index, Perceptual Reasoning Index, Working Memory Index, and Processing Speed Index.
	The Wechsler Abbreviated Scale of Intelligence (WASI) is designed to be a short and reliable measure of intelligence that produces Indices that are similar to those obtained with the WAIS-IV.
	The Wechsler Intelligence Scale for Children (WISC-IV) is used for testing children and adolescents ranging in age from 6–17 years.
	The Wechsler Preschool and Primary Scale of Intelligence (WPPSI) is used for testing children ranging in age from 4–6.5 years.
Wechsler Test of Adult Reading (WTAR)	The WTAR is a measure of recognition vocabulary requiring oral reading of 50 phonetically "irregular" words. It is used to estimate premorbid baseline intellectual ability in patients with known or suspected dementia. Similar measures include the NART, NART-Revised and ANART. Errors consist of word mispronunciations.
Raven's Standard and Colored Progressive Matrices	These are standardized measures of nonverbal analogical reasoning widely used both within and outside the United States as a "culture fair" measure of general intellectual ability. Both tests require the patient to demonstrate an understanding of the logic underlying visual patterns by selecting the missing component of the pattern from a series of choices. The Standard Matrices contain 60 black and white items ranging from simple to extremely difficult, while the Colored Matrices consist of 36 colored items that span a limited range of complexity. Errors consist of incorrect identification of the missing component of the visual pattern.

Table 3.2 ATTENTION AND EXECUTIVE FUNCTIONING

FUNCTION	TEST	DESCRIPTION
ATTENTION SPAN	Digit Span	The examiner reads increasingly long strings of numbers aloud. The examinee must repeat the numbers aloud in the same order, first forward and then in the reverse order.
	Spatial Span	The examiner taps a series of blocks in fixed locations. The examinee must repeat this series in the same order, and then in the reverse order.
SUSTAINED ATTENTION & VIGILANCE	Auditory & Visual Continuous Performance Test (CPT)	Basic auditory vigilance is tested by having the patient listen to a series of letters read serially and responding to a single target letter or series of letter configurations. Visual vigilance can be tested by showing a series of single numbers on a computer screen and requires responding to a target stimulus, but not to nontarget stimuli.
	Paced Auditory Serial Addition Test (PASAT)	The patient hears a tape-recorded voice reading numbers at various rates, ranging from every 2.4 seconds to every 1.2 seconds. The objective of the task is to sum the last two numbers heard and voice the sum aloud (e.g., if the numbers from the tape were "5, 2, 8, 4", the patients responses would be the following (in italics): "5, 2, *7*, 8, *10*, 4, *12*," etc.). The process of voicing the sum aloud serves as interference, which must be overcome in order to attend to the following number. In total, 60 numbers are read in each of the four trials and every subsequent trial is faster than the one preceding it.
SET-SHIFTING	Trail Making Test A & B	This measures of visual scanning, visuomotor tracking, and response set flexibility. Trails A involves connecting consecutively numbered circles, from 1 to 25. Trails B requires the patient to continually shift set, alternating between letters and numbers (i.e., 1, A, 2, B, etc.). Both tasks must be performed as quickly as possible and without lifting the writing utensil from the paper.
	Wisconsin Card Sorting Test	A measure of nonverbal concept formation, response set flexibility, sustained attention, and ability to integrate corrective feedback. The patient must sort cards according to underlying principles (color, form, number), which must be deduced and which are shifted at set intervals.
	Luria Graphomotor Sequencing	Involves using a pencil to copy a series of patterns (i.e., m-n-m-n, peaks and plateaus, and multiple loops) without lifting the pencil. Errors consist of failing to alternate (i.e., m-n-m-m-m-m)
	Luria Motor Sequences	Involves performing repeated sequences of hand movements. Errors consist of failure to maintain the order of movements within each sequence.
RESPONSE INHIBITION	Stroop Color-Word Interference Test	Composed of 3 parts that require (1) reading a series of black and white color words (red, blue, green), (2) identifying the color of red, blue and green 'Xs', and (3) identifying the ink color of incongruent color words (i.e., the correct response to the word 'red' printed in blue ink would be 'blue'). In all conditions the patient is asked to perform as quickly as possible.
	Motor Go-No-Go	Involves responding to a target signal (1 loud knock) by lifting a finger, but not to a second signal (2 loud knocks). The tendency to respond to the second signal must be inhibited. The examiner produces a series of 1 or 2 knocks and observes the patient's responses. Each hand is tested separately.
PLANNING	Delis-Kaplan Executive Function System (DKEFS) Tower Test	Involves ordering 4 colored beads within a set of constraints. Only one bead may be moved at a time, and beads moved from their initial placement may not be returned. Similar tests include Tower of Hanoi and Tower of London.
PERSEVERANCE	Verbal & Design Fluency	Letters: the examinee must recite as many words as possible that start with a particular letter, with the exception of proper nouns, numbers, and more than one iteration of the same root word. This is repeated with three different letters in total. Categories: the examinee must recite as many words as possible from a particular category. This is repeated with three different categories in total. Design: the examinee must create as many unique designs as possible by connecting lines between dots laid out in a grid.

ATTENTION AND EXECUTIVE FUNCTION

Attention

Many cognitive capacities are inherently predicated on a fundamental ability to attend to the surrounding environment. For example, an individual cannot effectively name an object if the object is not first attended to and visually processed. Because attention is a prerequisite for other aspects of cognitive function, disruption of attention can generally skew the results of a neuropsychological assessment. Early assessment of attention is vital for informing the scope of the examination and the analysis of test data (Table 3.2).

Attention is a general term that encompasses a number of different component processes. Attention span refers to the number of unrelated "bits" of information that can be held on line at a given moment in time. Assessment of attention span is typically accomplished through the recall of progressively longer series of information bits, such as numbers (digit span) or spatial locations (spatial span). Sustained attention, also called vigilance, refers to the capacity to maintain active attention over time. The most common method of assessing vigilance utilizes a target detection paradigm. Here the patient is instructed to respond to an infrequently occurring target stimulus. For example, on a measure of auditory vigilance, the patient hears a series of letters of the alphabet and must signal by pressing a response key each time a particular target is presented (see CPT, PASAT). Selective attention is similar to sustained attention, but requires a response only to a particular class of stimuli and not other stimuli. Set-shifting refers to the capacity to relinquish an existing procedural strategy in favor of a new response, based on recognition of a change in reward contingencies. It is typically measured with tasks requiring the patient to shift focus among stimulus features of a test display (see Trail Making A and B, Wisconsin Card Sorting Test, Luria Graphomotor Sequences). Resistance to interference, also called response inhibition, refers to the ability to sustain a given response even in the face of a salient distraction designed to undermine the target response. This is assessed with tasks requiring the patient to inhibit overlearned responses or other distractions that could undermine a desired response (see Stroop Interference Test, Trail Making Test).

Executive Functioning

Executive functions require the capacity to process information in a planful, organized, and contextually appropriate manner. Formal tests of executive function assess a number of different capacities including some functions mentioned above (set-shifting, overcoming interference, response inhibition) and also planning, perseverance, initiation, reasoning, and abstraction. Planning involves thinking several steps ahead of one's current circumstances for the purpose of informing and altering a course of action. Tests measuring planning ability often require subjects to determine the correct series of steps needed to successfully reach a particular goal (see DKEFS Tower Test). Perseverance is the ability to sustain a particular course of action, even in the absence of an external prompt. Measurement of perseverance often begins with both examiner and subject performing the same task, but involves the subject continuing the task even after the examiner has stopped (see Luria Motor Sequences, Verbal and Design Fluency). Initiation refers to the ability to spontaneously commence an action in the absence of a direct prompt from the external environment. This function is measured with presentation of a task followed by a period of time during which the subject is expected to respond independently (see Verbal Fluency, Go-No-Go). Reasoning involves using a system of logic to solve a particular problem or task. This can be measured in a variety of ways, including using visual puzzles and verbal analogies (see Ravens Progressive Matrices, WAIS-IV Comprehension). Abstraction is the ability to articulate shared attributes of dissimilar objects (e.g., WAIS-IV Similarities, Wisconsin Card Sorting Test) (Table 3.2).

COMPORTMENT, INSIGHT, AND JUDGMENT

Although few tests probe these functions in a formal manner, they are important components of neuropsychological function and are frequently disturbed in cases of neurological and neuropsychiatric illness. Comportment refers to the ability to behave in a contextually appropriate manner. Disturbances often manifest as socially inappropriate behaviors that suggest insensitivity to accepted cultural norms. Examples might include making offensive comments, crossing interpersonal boundaries, interrupting during conversation, or failing to attend to personal hygiene. In the context of neuropsychological assessment, insight involves an accurate perception of one's mental and physical condition as well as appreciation of the impact of one's behavior on others. Cognitively impaired individuals often lack one or both of these components of insight. Judgment involves the capacity to perceive and assess one's environment accurately and to make decisions that reflect sensitivity to preserving the safety and integrity of oneself, one's resources, and one's environment.

A neuropsychologist can assess these functions informally through naturalistic observation, reports from individuals familiar with the patient, and also by inquiring about any accidents or legal infractions involving the patient. Formal measures of these functions exist primarily in the form of questionnaires that quantify the degree to which the patient manifests disturbances in these general areas. The Frontal Systems Behavior Scale (FrSBe) comprises descriptions of various behaviors that are characteristic of patients with frontal lobe damage. Each behavior is assigned a severity rating by the patient and by a family member, and the overall severity rating is thought to reflect the degree of behavioral disturbance present. The Neuropsychiatric Inventory (NPI) is another self-report rating scale that is completed by a family member or caregiver. Both the extent of the patient's behavior and the degree of subsequent familial distress are rated.

LEARNING AND MEMORY

The assessment of learning and memory function is perhaps the most complex endeavor of the neuropsychological examination. Working memory involves holding a stimulus or set of stimuli in mind in order to either produce it after a delay (e.g., looking up a telephone number and remembering it until it is successfully dialed) or use it in a mental procedure involving manipulation of information (e.g., carrying out mental arithmetic). The simpler aspect of working memory, also called maintenance of information, can be tested by requiring a subject to hold information in mind and reproduce it after a short delay (see Digit Span Forward). The more complex component of working memory can be tested in a number of ways, all of which entail online maintenance and manipulation of information (see Tests of Mental Control, WAIS-IV Letter-Number Sequencing, WAIS-IV Arithmetic, PASAT). Memory is assessed with respect to modality of presentation (auditory vs. visual), material (linguistic vs. figural), and locus of reference (personal vs. nonpersonal). Also important is the time of initial exposure, namely whether information was learned before the onset of brain damage (retrograde memory; see Boston Retrograde Memory Test, Transient Events Test) or after (anterograde memory; see WMS-IV, RAVLT, Bushke SRT, Three Words/Three Shapes, Warrington RMT). The evaluation of memory should include measures that allow the dissociation of component processes entailed in the acquisition and later recall of information, namely encoding, consolidation, and retrieval. To this end, measures are used to assess performance with respect to length of interval between exposure to information and demand for recall (immediate vs. short vs. long delay) and extent of facilitation required to demonstrate retention (free recall vs. cued recall vs. recognition). The assessment of retrograde memory function poses a special problem insofar as it is difficult to know with certainty what information was previously registered in the remote memory of a particular patient. Although there are a number of formal tests that can be used for this purpose (e.g., Boston Remote Memory Battery, Transient Events Test), we also assess this aspect of memory function by asking for personal information which presumably is well known, or had been well known at one time, by the patient (i.e., names of family members, places of prior employment). In these instances it is helpful to obtain confirmation of the accuracy of this information from family members or friends, if possible (see Table 3.3).

LANGUAGE

Language is the medium through which much of the neuropsychological examination is accomplished. Language function is assessed both opportunistically, as during the interview, and via formal test instruments (Table 3.4). Conversational speech is observed with respect to fluency, articulation, and prosody. The patient's capacity to respond to interview questions and test instructions provides an

Table 3.3 LEARNING AND MEMORY

FUNCTION	TEST	DESCRIPTION
WORKING MEMORY	Tests of Mental Control	The examinee is asked to recite familiar sequences such as the alphabet, days of the week, months of the year, and numbers from 1–20 as quickly as possible. The examinee then must recite all sequences, except the alphabet, in reverse order. Serial subtractions involve subtracting a particular number until a predetermined point is reached.
	WAIS-IV Letter-Number Sequencing	The patient hears a series of alternating numbers and letters and is required to reconfigure them so that all of the numbers are recited first, in ascending order, and then letters in alphabetical order.
	WAIS-IV Arithmetic	Involves mental calculation of aurally presented arithmetic problems of increasing difficulty.
	See also **Digit Span Forward** and **PASAT** in Table 3.2.	
RETROGRADE MEMORY	Boston Retrograde Memory Test	Involves showing a series of black and white photos of famous persons from the 1920s to the 1980s. If the patient cannot spontaneously generate the correct name, the examiner can give a semantic cue (i.e., "he was a singer in the 1920s") and then a phonemic cue (i.e., first name). This test assumes that the patient has been exposed to the information in the first place.
	Transient Events Test (TET)	This is a measure of memory for popular news events from the 1950s through the 1990s. Items were selected by way of the *New York Times* index according to the criteria that they were mentioned at least 250 times during a particular year and less than five times over the subsequent 2 years. Hence, all items were of transient notoriety thereby minimizing confounding effects of overexposure. Free recall and recognition are tested.

(continued)

Table 3.3 (CONTINUED)

FUNCTION	TEST	DESCRIPTION
ANTEROGRADE MEMORY	Wechsler Memory Scale (WMS-IV)	This is a composite battery of tests assessing orientation, attention, learning, and memory for verbal and visual information across immediate and delayed intervals. It yields a series of index scores.
	Rey Auditory Verbal Learning Test	This measure of verbal encoding, learning, and retention involves drilling the examinee on a series of 15 unrelated words over five successive trials. Learning is followed by an interference trial, immediate recall, and 30-minute delayed recall and recognition. Various comparisons yield information regarding sensitivity to proactive and retroactive interference and rate of forgetting.
	Bushke Selective Reminding Test	This is a special type of list-learning test that is most helpful in cases where encoding is intact, but there may be a question of impairment at the level of consolidation or storage. A list of 12 words is read, and the patient must repeat as many words as possible. However, different from the previous list-learning tasks, the examiner then reads only the words that the patient did not recall. This continues across 6 trials, and each time the patient must try to recite as many words as possible but only hears the words not recalled on the preceding trial. There are immediate and delayed recall trials followed by visual multiple choice recognition paradigms.
	Three Words Three Shapes Memory Test	The patient is instructed to copy three words and three shapes, after which incidental recall is tested. The patient is drilled on the words and shapes until criterion is reached, and recall is tested after intervals of 5, 15, and 30 minutes. Recognition is tested using distracter shapes and words.
	Warrington Recognition Memory Test	Involves the visual presentation of single words and faces at the rate of one every 3 seconds. The patient is instructed to reach each word silently and make and report a judgment regarding his association (pleasant or unpleasant) to it. Immediately afterward, the patient is shown a pair of words, each containing a target word and a distracter, with the instruction to identify the one presented previously. Memory for faces is tested in the same way.

informal index of receptive language ability or comprehension. Visual confrontation naming is carefully assessed so that word-finding problems and paraphasic errors may be elicited. Repetition is measured with phrases of varying length and phonemic complexity. Auditory comprehension is evaluated by asking the patient questions that range in length and grammatical complexity. Reading measures include identification of individual letters, common words, irregularly spelled words, and nonwords, as well as measures of reading speed and comprehension. Spelling can be assessed in both visual and auditory modalities. A narrative handwriting sample can be obtained by instructing the patient to describe a standard stimulus scene.

VISUOSPATIAL FUNCTIONS

After establishing the integrity of basic visual acuity, the spatial distribution of visual attention is evaluated. The presence of visual neglect is assessed through the use of tasks that require scanning across all quadrants of visual space. Assessment of left/right orientation involves directing patients to point to specific body parts, either on themselves or the examiner. Topographical orientation can be tested by instructing the patient to indicate well-known locales on a blank map. Graphic reproduction of designs and assembly of patterns using sticks, blocks, or other media are used to assess visual organization and constructional abilities. Facial recognition represents a special component perceptual process and can be measured using Benton's Facial Recognition Test. The Judgment of Line Orientation Test assesses perceptual accuracy in judging the angular displacement of lines. Warrington's Visual Object Space Perception Battery is an example of a collection of measures designed to assess various aspects of perceptual function (see Table 3.5).

MOTOR FUNCTIONS

Naturalistic observations of the patient's gait and upper and lower extremity coordination are an important part of the motor examination. Hand preference should be assessed either through direct inquiry or a formal handedness questionnaire (Table 3.6). Motor speed, dexterity, and programming are tested with timed tasks, some of which involve repetition of a specific motor act (e.g., finger tapping, peg placement) and others that involve more complex motor movements (e.g., finger sequencing, sequential hand

Table 3.4 LANGUAGE FUNCTION

TEST NAME	DESCRIPTION
Boston Diagnostic Aphasia Examination (BDAE)	This is composed of measures that assess all aspects of expressive and receptive language function including naming, comprehension, repetition, reading, writing, praxis, and prosody.
Boston Naming Test	One component of the BDAE, this measure of confrontation naming is often administered independently. It consists of a series of 60 black and white line drawings of objects. Naming difficulty increases as the objects progress from high frequency to low frequency. Stimulus cues are provided in the event of perceptual difficulty. Phonemic cues are used to distinguish between retrieval difficulties and lack of knowledge of a particular object name.
Nelson Denny Reading Test	This test contains two multiple-choice measures that assess vocabulary and reading comprehension. Reading speed is also computed. Reading comprehension can be scored on the basis of both a standard and extended length of time.
Wide Range Achievement Test (WRAT-4)	This standardized battery of acquired scholastic skills includes measures of spelling, written arithmetic, and single word reading.
Wechsler Individual Achievement Test (WIAT-II)	This Wechsler test assesses the academic achievement of children, adolescents, and adults, aged 4 through 85 years. The test enables the assessment of a broad range of academic skills or only a particular area of need within the areas of reading, written language, oral language, and math.

Table 3.5 VISUOSPATIAL FUNCTIONING

TEST NAME	DESCRIPTION
Benton Facial Recognition Test	This task is composed of two parts. The first involves matching a target face with one of six faces. The target stimulus is always identical to the correct answer. The second part of the task involves choosing the three photographs, out of the array of six, that contain the same face as the target photograph. Increasing use of camera angle and shadow contribute to the progressive difficulty of the task.
Benton Line Orientation Test	This task involves judging the spatial orientation of sets of line segments by comparing them to a grid composed of 11 radii. It is sensitive to visuoperceptual deficits associated with posterior right hemisphere lesions.
Visual Object Space Perception Battery	This battery contains eight individual tests that each probe a specific component of object or space perception. Individual subtests are untimed and can be given in isolation or within the context of the full battery. Normative data are based on healthy control subjects as well as patients with right- and left-hemisphere lesions.
Visual Cancellation	The objective of this task is to circle each instance of a target letter or symbol from among a field of similar stimuli. There are a total of 60 targets evenly distributed among the four quadrants of the 8-1/2 × 11 inch page. Errors of omission involve failing to respond to the target stimulus. Errors of commission involve responding to stimuli other than the target stimulus.
Hooper Visual Organization Test	This task involves examining line drawings of objects that have been broken into fragments and rotated. The objective is to mentally reorganize each set of fragments and subsequently identify the corresponding coherent whole.
Complex Figure Drawing	This task involves copying a complex line drawing, usually the Rey-Osterreith complex figure or Taylor complex figure. Ability to reproduce the gestalt as well as the internal details of the design facilitate the detection of various perceptual deficits. Significant distortion of or failure to copy one side of the figure can indicate the presence of hemispatial neglect.

Table 3.6 MOTOR FUNCTIONING

TEST NAME	DESCRIPTION
Finger Oscillation Test	Finger tapping speed is measured by having the patient tap a key as quickly as possible over a period of 10 seconds, using the index finger. Each hand is tested a number of times and trial totals are averaged. Poor performance consists of slow tapping speed. Unilateral motor weakness can be assessed by comparing tapping speeds of each hand. Bilateral weakness is assessed through comparison with age-matched norms.
Hand Dynamometer	Grip strength is measured in each hand by having the patient squeeze a pressure-calibrated instrument. Unilateral motor weakness can be assessed by comparing performance with each hand. Bilateral weakness is assessed through comparison with age-matched norms.
Grooved Pegboard	Measures of fine motor speed and dexterity, entailing placement of pegs in a pegboard, are obtained with each hand separately. Poor performance consists of difficulty grasping and manipulating the pegs, resulting in slowed performance.
Reitan-Klove Sensory-Perceptual Examination	Collection of measures of tactile, auditory, and visual perception using unilateral and double simultaneous stimulation. Fingertip number writing, visual fields, and tactile finger recognition are tested.

positions). Manual grasp strength can be assessed with a hand dynamometer.

AFFECT, MOOD, AND PSYCHOLOGICAL FUNCTIONING

Standardized measures of mood, personality, and psychopathology can be used to assess the contribution of psychiatric illness to the patient's presentation and diagnosis (Table 3.7). However, it is important to understand that many neurological illnesses can cause disorders of affect and mood. In addition, certain neurological illnesses can produce symptoms that overlap with particular psychiatric disorders. Therefore, neuropsychologists must possess a thorough understanding of the psychiatric profiles associated with various neurobehavioral

syndromes and proceed with caution when evaluating psychiatric symptoms in the presence of neurological or medical illness.

DEMENTIA SCREENING TOOLS

Because detection of age-related cognitive impairment and dementia plays a significant role in neuropsychological evaluation, a number of specific screening tools have been developed (Table 3.8). Many of these measures are designed to quickly assess gross level of functioning in major cognitive domains and can be administered in a matter of minutes (see Blessed Dementia Scale, MMSE). The Mattis Dementia Rating Scale is a more comprehensive set of items designed to stage severity of impairment in patients with known dementia.

Table 3.7 PSYCHOLOGICAL FUNCTIONING AND MOOD

TEST NAME	DESCRIPTION
Beck Depression Inventory	This instrument is used to assess depression severity based on self-reported ratings of a number of different relevant symptoms. Higher scores indicate greater severity of symptoms.
Beck Anxiety Inventory	This instrument is used to assess anxiety severity based on self-reported ratings of a variety of somatic, cognitive, and psychological symptoms of anxiety. Higher scores indicate greater severity of symptoms.
Personality Assessment Inventory (PAI)	This test contains 344 questions with a scale ranging from false, not at all true, to very true. It consists of 22 non-overlapping scales that assess constructs relevant to personality and psychopathology. Validity, treatment, and interpersonal scales are also included.
Minnesota Multiphasic Personality Inventory-2 (MMPI-2)	This series of 537 true/false questions load on to a number of different subscales that correspond to various personality traits or types of psychopathology. Scores on each subscale are standardized. Combinations of high and low scores on individual subscales correspond differentially to the presence or absence of various psychopathologies. Careful interpretation of subscale scores is crucial to the accurate use of this measure.

Table 3.8 DEMENTIA SCREENING TOOLS

TEST NAME	DESCRIPTION
Blessed Dementia Scale	Consists of two parts: (1) a rating scale of Activities of Daily Living to be completed by a caregiver other independent rater, and (2) a brief screening measure of orientation, concentration, and memory. Higher scores indicate greater severity of dementia.
Mini Mental Status Exam (MMSE)	This is a set of brief tasks that can be administered at the bedside and used to screen for obvious cognitive impairment. Includes items that assess attention, orientation, language, memory, and construction. Lower scores indicate greater severity of dementia.
Montreal Cognitive Assessment (MoCA)	This brief screening measures assesses multiple cognitive domains, including short-term and long-term memory recall, visuospatial abilities, language, attention and concentration, and aspects of executive functioning.
Mattis Dementia Rating Scale (DRS-2)	This scale assesses a wide range of neuropsychological domains including attention, initiation and perseverance, construction, conceptualization, and memory. It is used for grading and tracking overall degree of dementia. Lower scores indicate greater severity of dementia.

CONTENDING WITH SPECIAL CIRCUMSTANCES

EXAMINING THE PATIENT WITH SENSORY OR MOTOR DEFICITS

Patients with limitations in primary sensory or motor function present special challenges for assessment. Visual problems are highly common within the aging population, including presbyopia, glaucoma, and cataracts. Since a considerable amount of typical testing procedures entails visual processing of various stimuli and materials, patients should be examined while using their usual corrective lenses. Keeping several pairs of reading glasses of varying diopter strength on hand as part of testing equipment is always a good idea. When evaluating the blind patient, tests requiring visual processing are simply excluded from the test battery.

Acquired visual impairment is often observed in individuals with traumatic brain injury, stroke, tumor, or different types of neurodegenerative disease. It is important to distinguish between peripheral and central causes of impaired performance in the neuropsychological examination, as these etiologies have different diagnostic significance and will respond to different types of treatment interventions. This determination can be difficult in some cases and require additional specialty evaluation by ophthalmology or neuro-ophthalmology.

As is the case with visual impairment, diminished hearing is an exceedingly common problem in the elderly patient.

Interestingly, many older patients are either reluctant to acknowledge or unaware of problems with diminished hearing acuity. Furthermore, a significant number of patients with identified hearing loss are unwilling to utilize hearing aids. When examining the hearing-impaired patient, the clinician must speak clearly, slowly, and loudly. It can be helpful and informative to have the patient repeat back questions to ensure apprehension. Ideally, a clinician with American Sign Language (ASL) expertise will be available to examine patients with congenital or acquired deafness. As this is frequently not possible, the neuropsychologist will adapt testing methods to the situation.

Adaptation of patient response modality is necessary in individuals with disorders of expressive speech or motor function. Various forms of assistive technology have been developed for use with both aphasic and paralyzed patients. However, it is often advantageous to utilize tests in which recognition responses (as opposed to expressive language, figure drawing, or motor enactment) are required. It is important to consider both the efficiency and tolerability of a testing method with the patient in the service of establishing and maintaining an empathic connection throughout what can be an emotionally arduous process.

Lateralized sensory deficits can be partially accommodated by presenting information to the relatively spared side. For example, directing spoken instruction to the preferred ear or presenting visual information to the relatively spared hemifield. Using visual stimuli in vertical arrays can be helpful as well. Various authors have considered the sensory and/or motoric demands of many commonly used neuropsychological tests and proposed alternative administration approaches (cf., Caplan & Schechter, 1995).

Hill-Briggs et al. (2007) provide a comprehensive review of issues pertaining to neuropsychological test administration, accommodations, modifications, specialized test development, and disability-related factors that influence test interpretation across the spectrum of disabled individuals. Bylsma and Doninger (2004) review the assessment of individuals with significant visual loss.

EXAMINING PATIENTS FROM DIVERGENT LINGUISTIC/CULTURAL BACKGROUNDS

Neuropsychologists are increasingly involved in the evaluation of individuals from divergent cultural backgrounds and for whom English is not the primary language. It is naïve to assume that simply translating the examiner's instructions and test items from standard English to the native language of the examinee will overcome a huge gulf in cultural experience and all that comes with it. People from different parts of the world are acculturated with widely varying attitudes toward the very notion of testing and assessment. Neuropsychologists must be highly sensitive to these deeply ingrained and pervasive differences and take them into account when endeavoring to examine individuals of different nationality.

The optimal approach is to have access to a network of practitioners with varying cultural and linguistic competencies, armed with tests that have been developed and standardized within the cultural/linguistic context of patients of different nationality. Although neuropsychology is making headway in this regard, we are truly only at the beginning of the beginning in this work. Given realistic constraints extant in most healthcare settings, it is usually necessary to compromise by using professional interpreters and adopt a highly conservative approach to test data generated in this fashion.

SUMMARY

Although clinical neuropsychology is a relatively new discipline, it traces its roots back to the ancients who wondered about the "seat of the soul" and the source of human thought. Drawing from the earliest studies of brain–behavior relationships in patients with naturally acquired lesions, and the accumulating body of literature in cognitive neuroscience, neuropsychologists have created a diverse collection of test instruments and other assessment methods which permit the precise measurement of specific components of human thinking. Together with a comprehensive knowledge of neuropathologic syndromes and functional neuroanatomy, the results of neuropsychological examination provide both descriptive and diagnostic information regarding the condition of the brain. As in all venues of medicine, diagnostic precision is a prerequisite for sound therapy. Because of its relative newness as a clinical discipline, several applied paradigms currently exist and there is some debate regarding preferred methods. Neuropsychologists in the 21st century face the challenge of establishing and promulgating an approach to assessment and treatment that unifies clinical practice and embraces the need for progressively refined normative information suited to diverse patient populations.

CLINICAL PEARLS

- A competent neuropsychologist will sample multiple domains of behavior. Observable behavior, including "test behavior," reflects an interaction between the domains of person and environment. Variables from each domain must be considered in order to arrive at an understanding of the clinical significance of a given behavior.

- Performance on a single test is not sufficient to make a diagnostic inference

- Discrepancy between "test behavior" and "real life" behavior is the source of ongoing challenge for the design of an ecologically valid assessment environment.

- Neuropsychologists have pioneered the development of specialized and embedded measures of effort and symptom validity for use in cases in which motivational factors are important.

- The Boston Process approach proceeds in a hypothesis-driven manner and uses the patient's test performance to guide and inform an evolving and dynamic assessment strategy. The process-oriented evaluation is individually tailored to each patient and uses specific tests for the purpose of answering particular questions. Test selection occurs in real time.

- The information obtained during the initial interview is important for differential diagnosis and frequently guides the remainder of the assessment.

- The first task of a neuropsychological assessment is to clarify the reason for referral.

- The fractionation of neuropsychological functions into specific domains is a somewhat arbitrary organizational contrivance. In reality, there is considerable overlap within and between cognitive domains. For example, working memory shares much common ground with aspects of attention and language.

- Variable capability across diverse neuropsychological functions is often the rule rather than the exception in normal human development (Schretlen, 2003).

- Premorbid ability can also be surmised from performance on measures presumed less sensitive to cerebral dysfunction (e.g., vocabulary). Single-word reading tests (e.g., WTAR) have been used to estimate baseline verbal intelligence in patients with early degenerative conditions.

- Early assessment of attention is vital for informing the scope of the examination and the analysis of test data.

- Sustained attention, also called vigilance, refers to the capacity to maintain active attention over time. The most common method of assessing vigilance utilizes a target detection paradigm. Here the patient is instructed to respond to an infrequently occurring target stimulus, for instance a sound or word, as a measure of auditory vigilance.

- Resistance to interference, also called response inhibition, refers to the ability to sustain a given response even in the face of a salient distraction designed to undermine the target response.

- Planning involves thinking several steps ahead of one's current circumstances for the purpose of informing and altering a course of action. Tests measuring planning ability often require subjects to determine the correct series of steps needed to successfully reach a particular goal (see DKEFS Tower Test).

- Perseverance is the ability to sustain a particular course of action even in the absence of an external prompt.

- Comportment refers to the ability to behave in a contextually appropriate manner.

- Working memory involves holding a stimulus or set of stimuli in mind in order to either produce it after a delay (e.g., looking up a telephone number and remembering it until it is successfully dialed) or use it in a mental procedure involving manipulation of information (e.g., carrying out mental arithmetic).

DISCLOSURE STATEMENTS

Dr. Nelson has no conflicts to disclose.

Dr. Assuras has no conflicts to disclose.

REFERENCES

Attix, D. K., Story, T. J., Chelune, G. J., Ball, J. D., Stutts, M. L., Hart, R. P., & Barth, J. T. (2009). The prediction of change: normative neuropsychological trajectories. *The Clinical Neuropsychologist, 23*(1), 21–38.

Benton, A. (1992). Clinical neuropsychology: 1960-1990. *Journal of Clinical and Experimental Neuropsychology, 14*(3), 407–417.

Bianchini, K. J., Mathias, C. W., & Greve, K. W. (2001). Symptom validity testing: A critical review. *The Clinical Neuropsychologist, 15*(1), 19–45.

Binet, A., & Simon, T. (1916). *The development of intelligence in children: The Binet-Simon Scale.* Publications of the Training School at Vineland New Jersey Department of Research No. 11. E. S. Kite (Trans.). Baltimore: Williams & Wilkins.

Broca, P. (1861). Perte de la parole, ramollissement chronique et destruction partielle du lobe antérieur gauche. *Bulletin de la Société d'Anthropologie, 2*, 235–238.

Bylsma, F. D., & Doninger, N. (2004). Neuropsychological assessment in individuals with severe visual impairment. *Topics in Geriatric Rehabilitation, 20*(3), 196–203.

Caplan, B., & Schechter, J. (1995). The role of nonstandard neuropsychological assessment in rehabilitation: History, rationale, and examples. In L. Cushman & M. Scherer (Eds.), *Psychological assessment in medical rehabilitation. Measurement and instrumentation in psychology* (pp. 359–392). Washington, DC: American Psychological Association.

Ebbinghaus, H. 1913. *Memory: A Contribution to Experimental Psychology.* (H. Ruger, & C. Bussenius, Trans.) New York, NY: Teachers College.

Harlow, J. M. (1868). Recovery from the passage of an iron bar through the head. Published 1868 in *Bulletin of the Massachusetts Medical Society.* Reprinted in *History of Psychiatry, 4*(14), 274–281 (1993). 10.1177/0957154X9300401407.

Hill-Briggs, F., Dial, J. G., Morere, D. A., & Joyce, A. (2007). Neuropsychological assessment of persons with physical disability, visual impairment or blindness, and hearing impairment or deafness. *Archives of Clinical Neuropsychology, 22*(3), 389–404.

Kaplan, E. (1990). The process approach to neuropsychological assessment of psychiatric patients. *Journal of Neuropsychiatry and Clinical Neuroscience, 2*(1), 72–87.

Lezak, M. D. 1995. *Neuropsychological Assessment* (3rd ed). New York: Oxford University Press.

Milberg W.P., Hebben N.A., & Kaplan, E. (1986). The Boston process approach to neuropsychological assessment. In I. Grant & K. Adams (Eds.), *Neuropsychological Assessment of Neuropsychiatric Disorders* (pp. 58–80). New York: Oxford University Press.

Reitan, R.M., & Wolfson, D. 1993. *The Halstead-Reitan Neuropsychological Test Battery: Theory and clinical interpretation* (2nd ed). Tucson, AZ: Neuropsychology Press.

Schretlen, D. J., Munro, C. A., Anthony, J. C., Pearlson, G. D. (2003). Examining the range of intraindividual variability in neuropsychological test performance. *Journal of the International Neuropsychological Society, 9*(6), 864–870.

Scoville, W. B., & Milner, B. (1957). Loss of recent memory after bilateral hippocampal lesions. *Journal of Neurology, Neurosurgery, and Psychiatry, 20*(1), 11–21.

Sweet, J. J., Moberg, P. J., & Suchy, Y. (2001). Ten-year follow-up survey of clinical neuropsychologists: Part I. Practices and beliefs. *The Clinical Neuropsychologist, 14*(1), 18–37.

4.

RATING SCALES AND SCREENING TESTS

Barry S. Fogel

SUMMARY

Rating scales and screening procedures derived from them have become an essential component of medical-psychiatric practice. Familiarity with the psychometric properties of a rating scale and understanding of the specific construct the scale was designed to measure can protect the clinician against misinterpretation of scores. Medical psychiatrists make daily use of widely-known scales for anxiety, depression, cognition, and functional status; important differences between commonly-used measures for these constructs are noted. Beyond these general-purpose scales there are instruments designed to measure psychiatric constructs specific to medical conditions such as fear of movement or fear of hypoglycemia; these have a special role in assessing patients who have no primary mental disorder but who have cognitive or behavioral issues significantly affecting general medical treatment outcomes. In a multidisciplinary or multi-specialty context rating scales can provide an efficient and effective common language. Simultaneous monitoring of multiple scales can help in the management of patients with multiple interacting comorbidities, impairments, and treatments. Systematic use of self-rated scales can make medical psychiatrists more efficient. Online test administration and computerized adaptive testing are enabling ever more subtle assessments to be convenient and scalable. At best, rating scales can enable assessments to be more complete and reliable, can improve communication between clinicians, can allow more objective and quantitative assessment of treatment outcomes, and can permit a more rigorous analysis of tradeoffs between wanted and unwanted effects of treatments. On the other hand, over-reliance on a handful of specific rating scales can lead clinicians to neglect important symptoms because they are not measured well by their customary instruments.

INTRODUCTION

As medical practice increasingly becomes evidence-based, quantitative rating scales and standardized screening tests that once were common only in research settings have become customary in clinical care. Symptom rating scales were adopted early in psychiatric research because for most primary mental disorders there are no generally accepted physiological measures of disease severity and treatment response. Screening tests to help general medical physicians and other clinicians identify mental disorders have been widely promoted because such conditions historically have been underdiagnosed in general medical practice. Rating scales have also been employed to *screen out* patients who are *not* at significant risk for particular adverse events: for example, patients with very low suicide risk may not need intensive observation even though they are severely depressed. Screening tests—especially those that involve self-rating or rating by a briefly trained nonclinician—take up little physician time. Utilization of rating scales and screening tests in routine clinical practice has evolved from the exception to the norm during the author's career in medicine.

The existence of a generally accepted rating scale for a symptom or syndrome has become an essential prerequisite for the symptom or syndrome to be a focus for clinical attention. All clinical trials of drug treatments must have measurable, quantitative end points to be acceptable to the Food and Drug Administration (FDA). Furthermore, if a medical psychiatrist wants to focus the attention of a general medical physician on a specific mental, behavioral, or functional issue, mentioning a rating-scale score (or its verbal equivalent) can be a very efficient way to do it.

This chapter aims to make the medical psychiatrist a better-informed user of screening tests and rating scales. After reviewing some basic psychometric terminology, it will focus on how the clinical populations and settings of medical psychiatry should affect the selection and interpretation of these instruments. Specific rating scales are discussed to illustrate particular issues in the selection, use, and interpretation of such scales in medical psychiatry. The reader is referred to standard references for full reviews of psychiatric rating scales and general health rating scales (Rush et al., 2008; McDowell, 2006). Websites that provide resources for measurement of health status and health-related quality of life, and, where applicable, websites operated by scale authors or publishers, offer further details. For example, cdc.gov/hrqol describes health-related quality of life scales that currently enjoy wide acceptance in the United States. The National Institutes of Health maintains a website entirely devoted to its Patient Reported Outcome Measure Information System (PROMIS). The instruments described, which include measures of medical-psychiatric interest, take advantage of contemporary methodologies of item response theory and computer adaptive testing (National Institutes of Health, 2014).

WHAT MEDICAL-PSYCHIATRIC RATING SCALES MEASURE

General psychiatric rating scales measure mental and behavioral symptoms and syndromes. In medical-psychiatric settings, general psychiatric rating scales have their place—but they are complemented by scales relevant to the relationship and interaction of psychiatric and general medical conditions. These include (1) scales for rating specific symptoms and syndromes like pain, sleep disturbance, or sexual dysfunction that can reflect either primary mental disorders, general medical disorders, or the combination of the two; (2) scales that directly assess cognitive function; (3) scales that measure general health status; (4) scales of functional performance; and (5) scales for quantifying the psychosocial impact of general medical illness.

In acute medical-psychiatric contexts, scales for risk assessment—specifically of the risks of suicide or violence—have a special place. In the care of chronic general medical conditions, scales that measure impediments to treatment adherence or to optimal treatment outcomes are especially relevant.

RELATIONSHIP OF RATING SCALES TO SCREENING TESTS

Rating scales can be used as screening tests for specific diagnoses. Based on a rating scale score, a patient is identified as probably having a particular disease, disorder, syndrome, or condition. The actual diagnosis is made by a clinician, who combines the data from the rating scale (often the items and not just the score) with some combination of elements from the medical history, clinical examination, and diagnostic tests. Psychometric properties like sensitivity and specificity are applied to the concept that patients with scores above a threshold have the diagnosis, and all others do not. In practice, patients with scores near the cutoff score often are viewed probabilistically—more likely than not to have the diagnosis, but not as certainly as those well above the threshold (or well below it, when the diagnostic criterion is a low score on the rating scale). Less commonly, a rating scale is made into a screening test by applying Boolean logic, a regression equation, a decision tree, or a neural net algorithm, using individual item scores as the independent variables.

In the context of general medical illness, psychiatric rating scale items that are typical of a particular primary mental disorder might instead be attributable to a general medical illness. The diagnosis of a syndrome (e.g., clinical depression) is independent of the attribution of specific symptoms, but the diagnosis of a *primary* mental disorder (e.g., major depressive disorder) is not. The attribution issue reduces the certainty of a diagnosis of a *primary mental disorder* made using a rating scale criterion. Nonetheless, using rating-scale item responses as a point of departure in a psychiatric interview can make the interview more productive. Furthermore, summing scale items, or applying a validated algorithm for combining relevant items, complements the more subjective clinical process

of synthesizing clinical data, and in some situations the standardized approach is superior. Once a diagnosis is made, rating scales—if they are sufficiently sensitive to changes—can be used to track the course of illness and measure the patient's response to treatment.

TYPES OF RATING SCALES

Rating scales measure the severity of a disease, syndrome, condition, symptom, functional impairment, or disability. They are quantitative and usually ordinal rather than truly continuous. Points on an ordinal scale can be represented as words and/or pictures; the 0–10 rating scale for pain (Fig. 5.1) is a familiar example. Rating scales can be have a single factor or dimension, or can be multifactorial. The score on a single dimension is the sum of a specific subset of item scores.

Rating scales are completed by the patient, by a caregiver or other collateral source, by a trained rater who is not a clinician, or by a clinician who might or might not require specialized training on the scale. Some patient-completed scales require only that the patient answer specific factual questions, while others require the patient to make judgments or self-assessments. The latter type of scale will be insensitive in the face of impaired metacognition or denial of illness. Patient-completed scales that refer to a time other than the immediate present rely on the patient's memory, and if they ask the patient to count events or summarize experiences during an interval, some degree of executive function is required as well. For this reason the validity of such scales decreases in the face of cognitive impairment. Note in this connection that scales of binary items like symptom checklists impose less cognitive demand than scales with ordinal items, and frequency-based ordinal items impose a greater cognitive demand on the patient than severity-based ones.

Some clinician-rated scales require the clinician to have specialized training in psychology or psychiatry. Clinician-rated scales that draw heavily on clinical expertise will be less reliable with less experienced clinicians. All of the above issues deserve consideration when determining whether a published measure of scale's reliability is applicable in a specific clinical situation.

When there are self-rated, caregiver-rated, and clinician-rated versions of the same scale, agreement of scores among the versions strengthens confidence in the rating. On the other hand, disagreement between self-ratings and caregiver/family ratings and/or clinician ratings is diagnostically valuable information. Disagreement between self-ratings and clinician ratings can represent impaired metacognition, unawareness of deficits or denial of illness, symptom amplification by the patient, clinician underestimation of the patient's distress, or, if the self and clinician ratings are done at different times, fluctuation of the condition. When ratings of symptoms by family members or other caregivers are more severe than patients' self-ratings, the discrepancy can reflect patients' denial or families' distress. Discrepancies between family/caregiver ratings and clinician ratings have implications similar to those of discrepancies between self-ratings and clinician ratings. Ultimately, reconciling the difference between the clinician's ratings and the patient's ratings can be an important part of building a therapeutic relationship.

Symptom rating scales assign a numerical score to one specific physical or emotional symptom such as pain, dyspnea, or anxiety. The symptom can be either reported by the patient or inferred from observations.

Disease and syndrome rating scales are sums—often weighted by severity and/or frequency over a specified time period—of the symptoms and signs that are characteristic of a disease or syndrome. Getting a scale score by summing item scores is most reliable and valid if all items are measuring the same underlying construct, items are scaled similarly, and the clinical significance of the items is similar. These assumptions do not necessarily apply to scales commonly used in clinical practice. For example, most clinicians would agree that a patient's having mild and intermittent depressive symptoms of four different kinds is of lesser concern than having severe and persistent suicidal ideation alone. Yet, both might contribute 4 points to the total score on a depression rating scale comprising items that rate the severity of individual depressive symptoms on a 4-point scale and sum the item scores to get an overall depression rating.

Functional assessment scales assess patients' level of independence in performing each of a set of physical, instrumental, and/or social activities. Functional assessment scales sometimes include an indication of how much help is required by a patient who is not independent in an activity. Results can be reported as a description of the dependencies identified, a count of activities in which the patient is dependent, or a score that weights dependencies according to how much help is required to do each activity requiring assistance. Functional ratings can refer either to capabilities at the time of the rating or to activities actually performed or attempted over a specified time interval. The result of a functional assessment scale that refers to a specific period can be different if the rater is asked to describe the patient's worst function, best function, or usual function during the period. When the functional assessment is done to assess improvement in a patient getting rehabilitation, it is important to track the patient's best level of function and usual level of function; when it is done to assess caregiving needs, an assessment of the patient's worst function is essential.

Functional assessments can either be historical—based on reported observations or on the patient's recall—or can be based on direct observation of the patient attempting to do each activity being rated. Observed functioning will be no worse than the patient's worst functioning and no better than the patient's best functioning, but it may not be representative of the patient's usual functioning. In particular, the circumstances of observation are important for patients with brain dysfunction who have become reliant on environmental cues to carry out activities properly. When such patients are tested in an unfamiliar hospital or clinic environment, they may appear more impaired than when tested in a home full of cues.

Cognitive performance scales are sums of item scores, where each item tests a specific cognitive capability and gives the patient's performance a binary or ordinal score. When something as complex as cognition is reduced to a single dimension, there necessarily will be tradeoffs between sensitivity and specificity, and important areas of function will be assessed perfunctorily or not at all. For patients with severe cognitive impairment, there are scales that test residual cognitive capacity based on inference of cognitive function from observed behavior. Cognitive performance scale scores usually are reported as a single number, although clinicians often characterize cognitive deficits by adding a note about specific test items missed, or about the patient's approach to the item. For example, on a cognitive rating scale patients' scores on memory items might depend only on whether they can recall all of the words on a list previously presented to them. A clinician's note—for example, that the words could be recalled by a patient when he was cued with the categories to which the words belonged—would be valuable in interpreting the score, because it would indicate that memory storage was intact even though free recall was impaired. This could help in the differential diagnosis of the cognitive impairment identified by the scale.

Behavior rating scales and psychopathology rating scales rate patients for the presence and severity of each of a list of symptoms and signs applicable to many different psychiatric diagnoses. As with functional assessment, results can be reported qualitatively or quantitatively—which specific items were present, or the sum of scores across all items. The former is more commonly done when the scale is used primarily as a structure for conducting and reporting a clinical assessment; the latter is done when the scale is used to characterize illness severity or measure treatment response.

Burden of illness scales are designed to quantify the overall load of disease carried by a patient. These are especially relevant in populations like frail elderly people, those with severe developmental disorders, and victims of severe trauma in which patients typically have multiple disease diagnoses, several of which are severe enough to cause distress, impair function, or shorten life expectancy. Such scales typically are counts of diseases or conditions weighted by their severity, symptomatic or functional impact, or implications for life expectancy or future healthcare utilization.

Predictive scales are sums of item scores, or results of algorithms applied to item scores, that are designed to predict a specific health outcome such as a fall or other injury, hospitalization, mortality, or service utilization. They are based on predictive models. They are used to identify patients at risk, to assist with making prognoses, to risk-adjust outcome-based healthcare performance measures, and to identify addressable risk factors in high-risk patients.

Adverse event or side-effect rating scales can be either general or specific to a particular drug or class of drugs. The latter are particularly relevant when a useful drug has a very high incidence of side effects; and quantifying the burden of side effects helps assess the risk versus the benefit for the treatment. For example, the Columbia Suicide Rating Scale

(C-SSRS; Posner et al., 2011), discussed further below, was originally developed to measure suicidal ideation as a potential side effect of initiating antidepressant drug treatment.

Global assessment scales are single-item scales that ask a clinician or other expert assessor to assign a numerical score to how sick, how symptomatic, or how impaired a patient is. The most useful global assessment scales are *anchored* by detailed descriptions of cases that would get various specific scores along the scale.

Generic rating scale items—which by themselves can serve as single-item rating scales—include the following:

1. *The simple one-directional ordinal scale.* For a 5-point scale, several examples are:
   a. 0, 1, 2, 3, 4
   b. None, minimal, mild, moderate, severe
   c. A, B, C, D, E
   d. Poor, Fair, Good, Very Good, Excellent
   e. Never, rarely, occasionally, frequently, all the time

An ordinal scale will be more comparable between patients if all raters are given a common set of examples corresponding to the different possible responses to the item. Without such anchors, an ordinal scale can still be valuable in comparing the condition of the same patient from one time to another, if the ratings at the two different times are performed by the same person.

2. *The bidirectional, symmetric ordinal scale* (aka Likert scales, after the psychologist Rensis Likert, who described them). There are several items, usually eight or more. Items are ordinal, bidirectional, and typically expressed in words: for example, patients are given a statement and is asked whether they strongly agree, agree, neither agree nor disagree (or are not sure), disagree, or strongly disagree. Positive or negative numerical scores are assigned to each item; the assignment of scores to responses can differ by item. The sum of the numerical item scores is the scale score. Likert scales in which item scores have five options and those in which item scores have seven options are the most common. One species of Likert scale utilizes items with an even number of response choices, forcing patients to choose to either agree or disagree with each item, even if their agreement or disagreement is mild.

3. *The visual analog scale.* In this scale, the patient is asked to mark on a line segment a place corresponding to the severity of the symptom being assessed. The line segment can be either horizontal or vertical. If the segment is horizontal, the left end means the symptom is absent; the right end means the symptom is present with maximum possible severity. If the segment is vertical, the bottom means the symptom is absent and the top means the symptom is present with maximum severity. A common set of anchoring examples make scores more comparable between patients. The visual analog scale can be converted into a numerical 0–100 scale by measuring the distance from the left (or bottom) of the line segment to the patient's mark, dividing that distance by the length of the entire segment, and multiplying by 100.

4. *A numerical scale.* The usual range is 0–10 or 0–100. In contrast to ordinal scales, there usually is a presumption that the scale is homogeneous—that for example the difference between a 10 and a 20 and that between a 60 and a 70, have similar clinical significance.

Frequency-severity or duration-severity scales are combinations of two or more single-item ordinal scales that together capture the time course of a symptom (or syndrome). Patients typically are asked to rate how often (or for how long) they have the symptom and what is the average severity (or the worst severity). The combination of scales often is valuable in understanding a patient's experience of the symptom. However, simply adding frequency and severity scales to make a single score requires an assumption that severity and duration are of equal weight in determining the overall negative valence of the symptom.

USES OF RATING SCALES

The potential medical-psychiatric uses of a rating scale include the following:

1. Framework for structuring a clinical assessment;
2. Screening test;
3. Support for a diagnosis;
4. Aid to treatment-related decisions;
5. Aid to prognosis;
6. Measurement of clinical course;
7. Measurement of treatment response;
8. Aid to prediction of future course or treatment response;
9. Rigorous measurement of an area of function that is important to the understanding of medical-psychiatric conditions but is poorly covered by routine medical and psychiatric histories (e.g., measurement of sleepiness/wakefulness and measurement of apathy/motivation);
10. Communication between clinicians, including communication across disciplines and standardization of medical records;
11. Broadening the scope of patient assessment within practical time constraints, by facilitating reliable and structured input from patients, family caregivers, and clinicians of various disciplines; and
12. Inquiring via patient questionnaires about areas patients might be reluctant to discuss in face-to-face interviews, including sexuality and substance use.

CONSIDERATIONS IN CHOOSING RATING SCALES AND SCREENING TESTS

A rating scale or screening test should be considered in relation to the patient population being rated, the purpose of the scale, who will be obtaining the data, who will utilize the score, and the direct and indirect costs of utilization. Specific considerations include the following:

1. *The patient population.* The scale should be easy to administer within the contexts in which the patients are usually treated. If the scale involves self-rated items, the questions should be appropriate to the educational and cultural background of the patients. The time needed to do the rating should be compatible with the typical length of the clinical encounter, and the procedure for rating should be compatible with the typical process of the clinical encounter and with the usual environment in which the patient is seen. The scale should be sensitive enough to detect variability within the patient population. Cutoff scores for identifying cases should be adjusted if necessary for differences in population norms for non-cases.

2. *The purpose of the scale.* If the scale will be used to follow longitudinal course or treatment response it must be suitable for repeated administration. For scales that measure cognitive performance, learning effects must be taken into account and alternate forms used if necessary. If the scale is used as a screening test in a non-psychiatric setting it should be easily utilized by people without training in psychiatry or another mental health profession.

3. *Who will be receiving and utilizing the score.* If the score will be placed in a common medical record used by various disciplines, widely known scales usually are preferable even if they are not optimal. When using a scale likely to be unfamiliar to most users of the medical record, a brief explanatory note on the scale should be included in the record that describes what the scale measures and whether there is a cutoff score for identification of a case. If the score will be used within a multidisciplinary service where there are joint conferences or rounds at which a scale can be introduced and explained, it usually is better to select the scale with optimal characteristics for the patient population treated and the specific purpose.

4. *Direct and indirect costs of utilization.* Some rating scales are explicitly in the public domain. However, many of the most useful and most broadly accepted scales are subject to copyrights held by a copyright owner that requires a fee to be paid for each test administration. Intermediate between them are tests subject to copyrights held by a copyright owner who permits free clinical use of the scale but charges a licensing fee when the test is used in funded research. When scales are used in funded clinical research the cost of licensing a specific proprietary scale usually is negligible in relation to the cost of the study as a whole. When this is the case, one should choose the scale with the optimal characteristics for the patient population and the purpose of the study.

The main indirect cost of administering a scale is the professional time involved; this gives a big advantage to brief scales and to scales based on patient or caregiver questionnaires, those that can be administered by non-clinical staff, and those that can be administered by computer. Most third-party payers do not pay clinicians extra for using rating scales, so the net financial effect is negative unless the rating scale can replace some part of the traditional clinical history and examination and/or the test score or item responses can replace text in a medical record that would take the clinician significant time to write.

5. *Psychometric optimality versus regulatory requirements and clinical custom.* When a rating scale is rarely used in clinical practice, clinicians reading study results based on measurements with that scale might be reluctant to rely upon them to guide treatment decisions. When a scale is used to measure the outcome of treatment with an investigational drug or device, the FDA may mandate the use of a particular standard scale for measuring the primary endpoint, and other standard scales for measuring potential adverse events. Researchers may need to compromise between a practical need to use a standard, commonly accepted rating scale for a particular purpose and the scientific ideal of a using a less-familiar rating scale that is optimal from a the point of view of content, psychometric properties, and adaptation to the specific patient population and clinical context at hand. The usual solution is to use both scales if this can be done without excessive burden on study subjects. In the case of a treatment trial, the score on the standard scale is used to define the primary endpoint of the study and the optimal scale is used to define a secondary endpoint. Both primary and secondary endpoints are reported when the study results are published.

GENERIC VERSUS SPECIALTY-SPECIFIC RATING SCALES

Medical psychiatrists are concerned with the interrelation of general medical conditions, trauma, and surgery; the patient's mood, thinking, and behavior; and the patient's functional status and well-being. Most of the variables of medical-psychiatric interest can be measured by instruments like depression rating scales, cognitive screening tests, and assessments of physical and instrumental function, that are applicable to patients with a wide range of diseases and conditions. Specialty-specific tests, or tests applicable only to patients with specific underlying medical conditions, are most useful when the pattern of psychiatric symptoms or functional impairments seen in a particular context differs significantly from those seen in relation to medical illness in general. For example, military veterans who have suffered repeated blast injuries can show a characteristic combination of neuropsychiatric and general medical complaints that differ from those of patients who have suffered other kinds of trauma. Similarly, patients with spinal cord injuries or with radical pelvic surgery have distinctive types of sexual problems. In specialty clinics for blast injury survivors, or for patients with spinal cord injuries, symptom rating scales tailored to these patient populations might be more useful than general-purpose instruments. When a medical psychiatrist begins working in a liaison capacity with a medical, surgical, or rehab specialty service, the use of specialized rating scales should be part of a discussion of how different specialists will work together.

SOME BASIC PSYCHOMETRIC TERMINOLOGY

Several terms are ubiquitous in discussions of rating scales and screening tests. Their definitions are straightforward, but their usage in the medical-psychiatric context raises specific issues that will be noted.

RELIABILITY

Reliability refers to the consistency of a scale score or categorical test result between two different raters (inter-rater reliability) or between two different ratings or test administrations (test-retest reliability).

Reliability Issues

Inter-rater reliability for many scales is high when both raters are highly trained and experienced, but considerably lower when raters do not have scale-specific training and experience. The incorporation of a rating scale within the clinical routine of a specialty service tends to increase its inter-rater reliability (when used on that service, with its typical patient population). When scales are based on a clinical assessment by interview or examination, there can be high inter-rater reliability for the *scoring* of assessment—for example, how two different raters would score the same video recording of an interview—but lower inter-rater reliability when two raters separately interview or examine the patient. Furthermore, when each rater does a separate interview or examination, there is confounding with test-retest reliability.

Test-retest reliability depends on the interval between the two test administrations and what is being rated. When there is circadian variation in the thing being measured, ratings a few hours apart can be significantly different. Learning effects and fatigue can change scores if two ratings are done on the same day. If the raters are different for the first and second rating, there is confounding with inter-rater reliability.

For these reasons test-retest reliability is context-dependent. It is valuable to confirm reliability of a rating scale within one's specific clinical context before using it in research or relying upon it for important clinical decision making. In addition, steps can be taken to improve the reliability of a rating scale to be used for a specific purpose. For example, consider the use of the Abnormal Involuntary Movement Scale (AIMS; see (Munetz & Benjamin, 1988) to assess a young female patient's response to a new drug treatment of tardive dyskinesia (TD). It is known that inter-rater reliability of the AIMS is lower with inexperienced raters, and that TD can

show circadian fluctuation and fluctuation linked to the menstrual cycle. To improve the reliability of the AIMS, the investigator could perform the AIMS procedure during morning clinic visits scheduled during the first week of the patient's menstrual cycle each month. The standard examination for AIMS scoring would be videotaped, and all recordings would be scored by the same experienced rater. With this strategy, reliability of measuring TD would be maximized, as would the likelihood of seeing therapeutic effects of the new drug if they were indeed present.

INTERNAL CONSISTENCY

Internal consistency refers to the extent to which the different items of a multi-item scale, test, or questionnaire are measuring the same construct. If a rating scale counts symptoms that are not consistently associated with one another, internal consistency will be lower. Internal consistency is measured with specialized statistics, of which *Cronbach's alpha* is the most widely used. An alpha of 0.9 or greater is excellent; one between 0.7 and 0.9 usually is acceptable.

Internal Consistency Issues

Cronbach's alpha can be inflated when a test has many items that are very similar to each other; it will be spuriously low if the scale is tested on a clinical population in which there is little variation in the construct to be measured. When rating scales are used as screening tests to identify potential cases of a condition, their internal consistency may be less important than when they are used to measure the condition's severity or to track its response to a treatment. For example, if the goal of an alcohol use disorder rating scale is to identify patients with drinking problems of any kind, it may not matter that the various manifestations of problem drinking included in the scale are not highly correlated with one another.

VALIDITY

Validity refers to the relationship between the scale score or screening test result and some other determination of the same construct—typically one that is widely recognized and accepted. Types of validity include the following:

Face validity—obvious association of scale items with the thing being tested;

Criterion validity—correlation of scale scores with a "gold standard" measure of the same thing, such as a laboratory test result or the score on a rating scale that is deemed more definitive, for example because it is more detailed, broader in scope, and/or obtained under more rigorous conditions;

Convergent validity—correlation of scale scores with other scales that measure the same construct;

Divergent validity—*lack* of correlation of the scale with scales thought to measure a distinct construct;

Predictive validity—ability of the scale score to predict a clinical outcome or other future event; and

Construct validity—an integrated judgment of whether the scale measures the underlying concept of interest. A judgment of construct validity includes consideration of the other types of validity.

Validity Issues

When a scale measuring a mental or behavioral construct is used to communicate with patients and families, the *face validity* of scale items helps in convincing them that the scale score is meaningful as the basis for a diagnosis, a treatment decision, or medical advice. For example, if a patient with dementia failed a test of reading and understanding road signs, it would be relatively easy to convince a family that it was time for the patient to stop driving; this might be more convincing than a score on a test of calculation or word-list memory that has no direct relationship with driving ability, even if the latter actually is more highly correlated with the likelihood of car crashes over the coming year. When a rating scale is used for communication with a non-psychiatric physician, it will work better if the scale has validity with respect to a *criterion* the physician already accepts, or *convergent validity* with respect to a scale the physician already uses. Thus it is helpful to know whether the recipient of a communication is familiar with the construct that the scale measures, and to know what he or she currently understands as appropriate ways to assess it.

SENSITIVITY, SPECIFICITY, AND RELATED CONCEPTS

When evaluating a screening test, which may be a rating scale used in conjunction with a specified cutoff score for identifying a case, the ideal is a test that identifies all patients with the condition and rules out the condition in everyone else. A test can fall short of the ideal either by failing to detect the condition when it is present, or by misidentifying unaffected patients as cases, or both. Which of the two potential shortcomings of a test is the greater problem depends on the purpose of the test, on the costs and consequences of different types of error, on the rate of the condition of interest in the patient population to be tested, and on the way the condition of interest manifests in the population to be tested. How closely a screening test attains the ideal is captured by two ratios: sensitivity and specificity. These two ratios are determined by the combination of the properties of the test *and* the specific population to which the test is applied. The ratios are defined in terms of the counts of patients in each of four mutually exclusive and comprehensive categories:

True Positive (TP): Patients who are positive on the screening test and has the condition of interest;

True Negative (TN): Patients who are negative on the screening test and do not have the condition of interest;

False Positive (FP): Patients who are positive on the screening test but do not have the condition of interest; and

False Negative (FN): Patients who are negative on the screening test but have the condition of interest.

Sensitivity (TP/(TP+FN))

Sensitivity is the proportion of patients with the condition of interest that are positive on the test. While sensitivity often is thought of as a property of a test, it is really a property of a test *in a specific clinical context.* For example, a screening test for dementia might be highly sensitive when applied to detect moderate dementia in a population of high school graduates, but insensitive when applied to detect mild dementia in a population with graduate degrees.

Sensitivity Issues

When a screening test is based on applying a cutoff score to the summary score on a rating scale, sensitivity can be increased simply changing the criterion used to determine whether the test is "positive". Taken to the extreme, it is true for any rating scale used as a screening test that the criterion for identifying cases can be set so that everyone who takes the test will meet the criterion and the test is 100% sensitive. In this case there are no false negatives because there are no negatives at all. However, sensitivity is meaningless without simultaneous consideration of specificity, which in the extreme case just given would be quite low unless most or all of the population had the condition, making the screening test unnecessary in the first place. A measure of a test's sensitivity is most meaningful if it is calculated on a sample of patients typical of the clinical population in which the test will be used, the sample contains a sufficient number of patients with and without the condition of interest, and the patients in the sample who have the condition are representative of the clinical population with respect to the severity of the condition of interest and the range of symptoms and signs they display.

High sensitivity is essential in situations where the test is used to rule out a condition which, if present, would urgently require management or treatment. For example, screening tests for the risk or suicide or violence must be highly sensitive if they are used to determine when a psychiatric inpatient is safe to discharge. Furthermore, to be useful such tests should show high sensitivity *in the specific population in which they will be used,* for a example a chronically-disabled population, a population of combat veterans, or an incarcerated population of violent offenders.

SPECIFICITY (TN/(FP+TN))

Specificity is the proportion of patients who don't have the condition of interest who are negative on the test. In other words, specificity is the sensitivity of the test for detecting *non*-cases.

Specificity Issues

The considerations mirror those for sensitivity. When a screening test is based on reaching a threshold score on a rating scale, raising the threshold will increase the test's specificity at the expense of its sensitivity. High specificity is desirable in situations where being wrong about calling a patient a "case" entails unnecessary cost, risk, or stigma. The diagnosis of psychogenic non-epileptic seizures (PNES) offers a useful medical-psychiatric example; the diagnosis of HIV infection is a good general medical one. A common approach to clinical situations where both high sensitivity and high specificity are needed is a two stage screening approach, where a highly sensitive and moderately specific test is given first, and those who screen positive are given a more specific test to validate the diagnosis–often one that is more expensive or less convenient.

PREDICTIVE VALUE

Positive Predictive Value (PPV) is the proportion of patients who test positive that actually have the condition of interest. Expressed as a formula, PPV = TP/(TP+FP).

Negative Predictive Value (NPV) is the proportion of patients who test negative test that in fact not have the condition of interest. Expressed as a formula, NPV = TN/(TN+FN).

Predictive Value Issues

Like sensitivity and specificity, PPV and NPV are attributes of *a test and a population*, not attributes of a test in itself. A test with high sensitivity and high specificity can have a low PPV if the condition of interest is very rare in the population tested. For, example, suppose a test is 99% sensitive and 95% specific for a condition with a prevalence of 1% in the population tested. Its PPV will be approximately 20%, since out of every 100 people in the population approximately 1 will be a true positive and 4 will be false positives (that is, negatives to which the test was insensitive). In this situation five patients who "screened in" would have to undergo further evaluation to identify one patient who truly had the condition of interest. When the implications of a diagnosis are weighty and the condition of interest is relatively rare in the population to be tested, a test must have very high specificity to be clinically useful.

Like PPV, NPV is always relative to a specific population, and the considerations for NPV mirror those for PPV, just as the considerations for specificity mirror those for sensitivity. A very high prevalence of the condition of interest in the test population will imply a low NPV unless a test is extremely sensitive.

The relationship of sensitivity, specificity, PPV and NPV is illustrated in Figure 4.1.

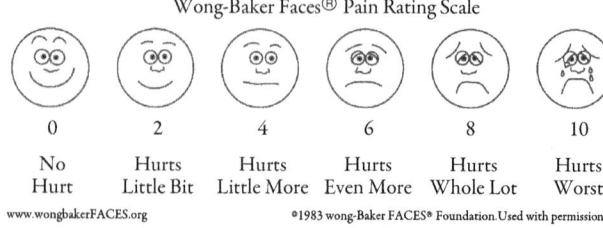

Figure 4.1 Wong-Baker FACES® Pain Rating Scale.

RECEIVER OPERATING CHARACTERISTIC

The receiver operating characteristic (ROC) is a curve that illustrates the tradeoff of sensitivity and specificity for a screening test that is based on a rating scale with various options for the cutoff score (criterion level) for determining that a patient has the condition of interest. The ROC curve is drawn within a box where the x-axis is the rate of false positives and the y-axis is the rate of true positives. Each point on the curve is determined by a cutoff score for the test on the underlying rating scale. Note that the cutoff scores themselves do not appear on either the x-axis or the y-axis. It sometimes makes an ROC curve more comprehensible to label a few points on the curve that correspond to specific cutoff scores.

Figure 4.3, from an article on diagnostic test interpretation (Tape, 2013) illustrates the ROC curve for serum T4 as a screening test for hypothyroidism, the latter diagnosed clinically. The three points on the curve represent three different cutoff points for the serum concentration of thyroxine (T4): 5, 7, and 9 μg/dL.

The ROC curve for a test with no predictive value would be a line with slope 1—the diagonal of the square in which the ROC curve is drawn. When a test has such a ROC curve, higher sensitivity can only be had by reducing specificity. The ROC curve for an ideal test would be a vertical line along the y-axis plus a horizontal line at y = 100%. With an ideal test there is a cutoff score at which false positives are zero and true positives are 100%. With a very good but not ideal test the rate of true positives will approach 100% at a cutoff score that implies only a very small number of false positives.

ROC Issues

A test of no value whatever would have an ROC of 50%; a test with an ROC of 90% or higher would have outstanding value;

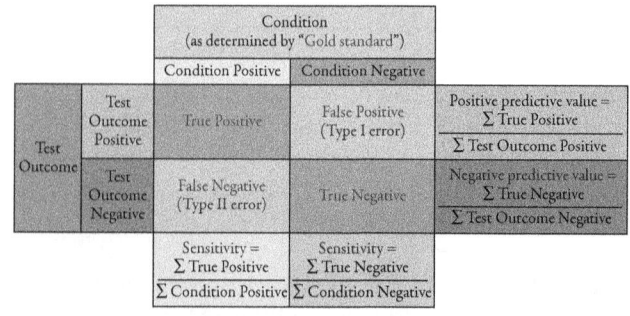

Figure 4.2 Relationship of Test Attributes.

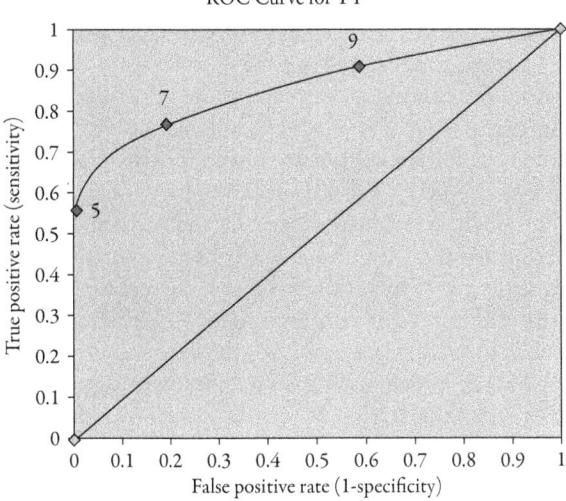

Figure 4.3 ROC Curve for Serum T4 as a Test for Hypothyroidism.

most clinical purposes require an ROC of at least 70%. The usual tradeoff is between the cost of a test (including burden on clinicians and patients) and the ROC.

One way to attain high specificity while maintaining high sensitivity is to utilize a two-stage testing procedure where the first screening test, one with high sensitivity, identifies patients with high risk of having the condition, and the second test, one with high specificity, is used to determine whether a high-risk patient actually does have it. In psychiatric contexts, the usual two-stage procedure begins with a scale based on a patient or family/caregiver questionnaire. A subset of patients is identified as comprising probable cases based on application of a cutoff score to the questionnaire-based scale. Each probable case undergoes an examination by a clinician to rate him or her on a second scale. Only patients that meet a specified criterion for the clinician-rated scale score are identified as positive (probable cases) by this two-stage screening procedure.

BIAS IN SELF-RATINGS

All self-rating scales are subject to various types of *response bias*. Some patients will tend to answer yes/no questions positively and to agree more often than they disagree; this is called *acquiescence bias*. The reverse bias—a tendency to answer negatively and to disagree—is less common in the general population, but can be shown by angry or hostile patients. Acquiescence bias and its reverse can be mitigated by balancing the wording of scale items equally as positive and negative statements.

Social desirability bias is shown when patients answer questions in a conventional, "proper" way. Patients may be reluctant to honestly answer questions related to alcohol or drug use, tolerance of unlawful behavior, personal prejudices, or symptoms commonly associated with mental illness.

Central tendency bias is shown when patients rarely show strong agreement or disagreement with statements and rarely characterize a symptom as severe. It is common in the general population, and its prevalence may vary by ethnicity, family background, and personality type.

Acquiescence bias can be mitigated by test design; social acceptability bias can be more difficult to resolve if the condition being rated is stigmatized and widely viewed as unacceptable. Central tendency bias can be adjusted for at the individual patient level when a scale is used to follow the course of illness or measure the effects of treatment. In theory, central tendency bias could be assessed with a set of nonclinical items and the bias estimate used to adjust the interpretation of the clinical self-rating (e.g., choice of a cutoff score for identifying a patient as probably having a particular disorder). However, this is not done in practice.

Response biases have cultural correlates; specific ethnic groups may be less willing to express strong opinions or to admit to having socially undesirable attitudes or behavior. Cultural issues should be considered when using rating scales in multicultural clinical populations and when choosing from among rating scale options for use in a specific cultural group.

Clinicians can increase the utility of serial self-ratings of a particular symptom or syndrome by doing one or more simultaneous clinician ratings early on to "anchor" the scale. For example, a clinician might note that a self-rating of 10 on a depressive symptom questionnaire such as the PHQ-9 (Kroenke et al., 2001) corresponds to a rating of 15 on the clinician version of the same scale given on the same occasion, and that a self-rating of 20 corresponds to a clinician rating of 30. The patient would be regarded by the clinician as someone who tends to under-rate symptoms of depression, and the clinician might then interpret a subsequent self-rating of 5 as equivalent to a clinician rating of 7 or 8.

Visual analog scales (VAS) and ordinal scales for same condition yield similar results and they have similar clinical utility. However, the continuous nature of the VAS pain scale and its lack of intermediate anchoring points can produce paradoxical results when the scale is used to measure day-to-day changes in acute pain. In the short term, scores on the VAS and on an ordinal pain scale can even change in opposite directions (DeLoach et al., 1998). The visual analog scale can be problematic for neurological patients with impaired visual perception; this is most dramatic for patients with right-hemisphere lesions and left hemineglect, where a horizontal visual analog scale will always be marked toward the right side. Arranging the visual analogue scale vertically mitigates the problem of hemi-inattention, but other visual perceptual difficulties can make the test less valid nonetheless. On the other hand, scales that rely on verbal definitions can be affected by language problems—a virtue of a visual analog pain scale that is anchored by emoticons depicting pain and suffering is that it works without regard to language; it can be valid even for patients with aphasia.

The continuous nature of scores on a visual analog scale facilitates the use of parametric statistics in analyzing outcomes in the research context. This can increase statistical power to capture a significant difference in outcomes between patient groups.

An underlying tacit assumption of many ordinal scales is that there is uniform scaling; for example, a score of 20 is twice as bad as a score of 10 on a scale measuring a distressing symptom or syndrome. However, this assumption is impossible to prove because there is no standard criterion of "badness" of symptoms. Of greater concern is that when using rating scales with many items of diverse content, there can be major clinical differences between patients with the same summary score. Often it is important to know which specific items on a scale the patient endorsed. For this reason it is useful for clinicians to review item-level responses and for staff to keep self-rating forms together with the clinical record, at least until they can be reviewed by the clinician. Of particular importance to medical psychiatrists is the review of patients' responses to items describing physical symptoms that can be either due to the patient's general medical illness or due to depression, anxiety, or another disorder conventionally viewed as "mental." If symptoms of general medical illness account for much of a patient's score on a rating scale for depression or anxiety, this should be noted in the medical record to help future readers of the record to understand the meaning of the score.

RATING SCALES AND COGNITIVE IMPAIRMENT

Many rating scales rely on the patient's recall of thoughts, behavior, and mood over a specified period such as the past week, the past month, or the interval since the last visit. Patients with impairment of memory may be unable to recall accurately their mental state and behavior in the recent past, reducing the validity of the scale. Other cognitive impairments that can alter rating scales based on patient interviews or questionnaires include impairments of attention and concentration, impairment of comprehension, and impaired self-awareness. When cognitive impairment limits the validity of scales based on patient interview or questionnaires, alternatives are scales based on caregiver interviews or questionnaires, or on observation of the patient's behavior by clinical staff. Discrepancies between self-ratings and observer-based ratings can raise the suspicion of cognitive impairment, or denial or unawareness of symptoms. Several of the scales designed for rating mental and behavioral symptoms in patients with gross brain diseases come in self-rated, caregiver-rated, and clinician-rated versions.

THE COPYRIGHT ISSUE

While some well known and very useful rating scales are in the public domain, for example, the Hamilton Depression Scale and the Visual Analog Scale for pain, many standard psychiatric rating scales are copyrighted. In some cases a test will be in the public domain but a particular way of scoring the test will be copyrighted: the CLOX scoring system for the neuropsychological interpretation of clock drawings (Royall et al., 1998) is an example. When scales or scoring systems are copyrighted, the copyright owner must be paid a royalty if the test is used in sponsored research. Whether use of a scale in an individual physician's clinical practice constitutes "fair use" or requires payment of a fee depends on the scale. The obligation to pay a significant fee per use for a rating scale makes it less appealing for routine clinical use unless the administration and interpretation of the test is a billable procedure—as it is for some tests designed for use by clinical psychologists—or the use of the test is subsidized by a care management organization such as a health plan. In the medical-psychiatric context, it usually is not feasible to charge a separate fee for a rating scale that is incorporated into a clinical evaluation; for this reason, most clinicians will prefer tests that either are in the public domain or are usable royalty-free under fair use conditions. Some widely used rating scales with enforced copyrights offer the offsetting benefit of extensive support of the scale by the copyright holder. Support for scales may include online training, user groups, durable educational materials, test administration forms, and maintenance of databases of references and norms for various populations.

A REPERTOIRE OF RATING SCALES

Medical psychiatrists tend to encounter a similar set of problems regardless of the underlying general medical condition: depression, anxiety, cognitive impairment, pain, apathy, sleep disturbance, sexual dysfunction, and so on. Ratings of mental and behavioral symptoms, syndromes, and conditions that are based on questioning a patient—whether by a questionnaire, via computer, or by a clinical interview—can be complicated in the medical-psychiatric context by the effects of general medical illnesses and their treatments on self-awareness, memory, cognition, and communication. When this is the case, scales based on direct observations by a family member or professional caregiver may be more valid. A more subtle point is that mental and behavioral symptoms that are consistently associated in patients with a particular primary mental disorder may not be consistently associated in patients with the same major symptom in the context of a general medical condition. A rating scale designed for a primary psychiatric population can have different psychometric properties when used in a medical-psychiatric population. For example, in primary major depression, vegetative symptoms, apathy, anhedonia, depressed mood, and depressive thoughts tend to be correlated; in depression due to some general medical conditions the correlation does not apply. A patient with mood changes due to a frontal lobe glioma might have severe apathy and anhedonia but have few depressive thoughts. The patient's summary score on a standard depression rating scale would understate the severity of the patient's mental disorder, because the usual thoughts associated with severe depression would be absent or minimized.

Pragmatic considerations of time and cost are relevant to the choice of rating scales for use in general medical settings. Finally, the time available for psychiatric activities—including doing rating scales—can be tightly constrained in general medical settings, so even a few minutes' difference in time to complete a scale can be decisive in choosing it over one with similar psychometric properties.

With these considerations in mind the author offers a basic repertoire of rating scales with proven feasibility and clinical utility in medical-psychiatric settings.

DEPRESSION RATING SCALES

The *Patient Health Questionnaire-9 Questions* (PHQ-9) has emerged as a widely accepted screening test and rating scale for depression in general medical and in community settings. Based on the *Diagnostic and Statistical Manual of Mental Disorders-IV* (DSM-IV) diagnostic criteria for depression, the test sums the scores of nine ordinal items rated 0–3 based on how often in the past 2 weeks the patient has experienced various symptoms of depression. A tenth question, not included in the summary score, is a 4-point ordinal self-rating of impairment due to depressive symptoms. The PHQ-9 takes less than 5 minutes to complete, even when patients take time to consider their answers. A modified version—the PHQ-9-OV (observational version)—is designed to be completed by a caregiver familiar with the patient, in situations where cognitive or communication problems preclude the use of a questionnaire-based scale (Saliba et al., 2012). Pfizer holds a copyright on the scale but permits it to be used by clinicians royalty-free. It is available in over 30 languages.

In a validation study of the PHQ-9, the authors studied 580 patients in community primary care settings who both completed a PHQ-9 and had structured diagnostic interviews by mental health professionals (Kroenke et al., 2001). The study report includes an ROC analysis that shows the sensitivity–specificity tradeoff for different choices of cut point. In the reported primary care population, with a cutoff of ≥9 the test is 95% sensitive and 84% specific for a diagnosis of major depression, To attain 95% specificity, a cutoff of ≥15 is needed; at that level the sensitivity drops to 68%. Overall, the ROC curve supports the value of the PHQ-9 rating scales as the basis of a screening test in community primary care settings for major depression as defined by DSM-IV. The PHQ-9-OV was tested with dementia patients in skilled nursing facilities and was shown to be highly correlated with the Cornell Scale for Depression in Dementia (Phillips, 2012).

The PHQ-9 is both *scored* and *interpreted*; it is possible to exceed the cut point on the test but yet not receive a clinical diagnosis of major depression. Making a diagnosis of any depressive disorder requires both a total score greater than or equal to the cut point, and either loss of pleasure, depressed mood, or both, at least half of the days in the past 2 weeks. A diagnosis of *major* depression requires that five or more items were present on at least half of the days in the past 2 weeks, or that at four items were present on at least half of the days and that on several days the patient had thoughts of self-harm or of being better off dead.

Four of the PHQ-9 items concern symptoms that frequently accompany significant general medical illnesses in the absence of any primary or secondary mental disorder: sleep disturbance, altered appetite, decreased energy, and impaired concentration. The PHQ-9 is sensitive to depressive disorders that might respond to antidepressant treatment. As noted elsewhere in this volume, medical psychiatrists usually find it more productive to focus on the choice of optimal treatment rather than on the question of whether to attribute symptoms to the general medical illness, to a comorbid primary mental disorder, or to a discrete process—"secondary depression"—that is different from the general medical illness in itself, but is not exactly the same as primary depression in its symptoms, course, prognosis, and/or treatment response. Patients scoring in the range of primary major depression on the PHQ-9 frequently will respond to treatment for depression.

THE BECK DEPRESSION INVENTORY

The Beck Depression Inventory (BDI; see Beck et al., 1988, 1996) is a 21-item questionnaire that, like the PHQ-9, asks the patient to rate individual items on a scale on a scale of 0–3. In keeping with the DSM-IV, the scale asks about symptoms in the past 2 weeks. However, the patient is asked to rate the *severity* of each individual symptom rather than its frequency. Like the PHQ-9, the BDI is copyrighted. The copyright owner, Pearson, does not grant royalty-free duplication rights, and it sells BDI test forms for approximately $2.00 each. The test has been translated into numerous languages. The BDI takes 5–10 minutes if completed by the patient and somewhat longer if the questions are asked by an interviewer. Cut points for mild, moderate, and severe depression are ≥14, ≥20, and ≥29, respectively.

While the BDI has been exhaustively validated, the additional time required for its administration, the cost of the test, and lack of an observer-based version favor the PHQ-9 over the BDI for routine clinical use. However, the BDI has special strengths relevant to the *understanding* of patients' depressive symptoms in addition to measuring them, and to the measurement of change in symptom severity with treatment: (a) It has 21 items rather than 9; (b) Items measure symptom severity rather than symptom frequency, and (c) The BDI captures two discrete dimensions of depression—the affective (8 items) and the somatic (13 items; see Steer et al., 1999). While the two dimensions are moderately correlated (correlation coefficient = 0.57), one would expect the correlation to be weaker in patients with general medical illness, in whom some of the somatic items could be due to the medical condition.

HAMILTON DEPRESSION RATING SCALE

The Hamilton Depression Rating Scale (HAM-D or HDRS; see Hamilton, 1980) is a 17-item clinician-rated scale for depression that was specifically developed to measure the severity of the symptoms of primary depressive illness and to follow their change with treatment. It was not designed to be a diagnostic test, let alone a test to screen for depression in general medical settings. It takes 20–30 minutes to conduct the structured clinical interview upon which the scale scores are based (see Williams, 1988, for details of the interview). The 17 ordinal items all rate the *current* presence and/or severity of depressive symptoms; frequency of symptoms over an interval is not measured. Item scores range from 0–2 or from 0–4; the maximum score on the 17-item scale is 50 points. Cut points for mild, moderate, and severe depression are ≥8, ≥14, and ≥19, respectively. The 31-point range of scores associated with severe depression implies that the scale will not show ceiling effects and will thus be able to measure relative change even in patients who remain severely depressed. The items give considerable weight to somatic symptoms: scores indicating severe depression can be reached from symptoms of medical illness alone, and somatic improvements can substantially reduce the HDRS score even if a patient remains severely depressed and actively suicidal. Overall, the HDRS is not as well suited for use in general medical settings as the BDI or the PHQ-9.

GERIATRIC DEPRESSION SCALE

The Geriatric Depression Scale (GDS; see Yesavage et al., 1982) originally was 30-item questionnaire with yes–no items concerning the patient's symptoms at the present time; it is now most widely used in a 15-item version that comprises a subset of the original items (Sheikh & Yesavage, 1986). When the GDS refers to the recent past, the time frame is indeterminate—for example, "Are you in good spirits most of the time?" There are no items concerning the frequency or severity of particular symptoms. The scale is in the public domain, it is available in many languages, and there are smartphone versions for both the iOS and Android operating systems. It takes a typical patient about 5 minutes to complete the 15-item version. Items are phrased both positively and negatively, but the phrasing is not balanced; for the 15-item version, the answers to 10 questions are more likely to be answered "yes" if the patient is depressed. The scale's author recommends that if items are not completed, the sum on the items that are complete should be scaled up proportionally and rounded up to the next integer. A score 5 or greater on the 15-item version suggests that a patient should be evaluated clinically for depression. Wancata and colleagues (2006) concluded from a review of 42 publications on the GDS that with its usual cutoff scores (5 on the 15-item version and 10 on the 30-item version) and a validity criterion of a clinical diagnosis of major depression by a psychiatrist, the scale's sensitivity and specificity are, respectively, 0.805 and 0.750 for the 15-item version and 0.753 and 0.770 for the 30-item version. Marc et al. (2008) tested the 15-item GDS against a clinical consensus diagnosis of DSM-IV major depression in an ethnically diverse elderly homecare population in New York and found that with an optimal cutoff score of 5, the sensitivity and specificity were 0.718 and 0.782. The test performed equally well in men and women, and in various ethnic groups.

The GDS has some obvious benefits for screening in medical-psychiatric settings. It requires little time, the respondent burden is low, there are smartphone versions, and it can give valid information even about patients with moderate cognitive impairment. However, it is better for use as a screening test than as a tool for following the clinical course of a patient already diagnosed with depression, because the severity and frequency of the individual items are not rated. Also, it will not capture the severity of a depression in which two or three symptoms are very severe and others are not present or not acknowledged. It also should be noted that more than 20% of cases of major depression will *not* be identified by the GDS with its usual cutoff score. Thus, it is more helpful in case-finding than it is in ruling out clinically significant depression.

Like the BDI, the GDS has a factor structure, although exploratory factor analyses give different results depending on the clinical population studied and the language in which the scale was administered. The most consistent factors to appear in factor analyses of the GDS are dysphoria, positive mood (or its absence), and a factor capturing apathy, cognitive impairment, and social withdrawal (Kim et al., 2013).

CORNELL SCALE FOR DEPRESSION IN DEMENTIA

The Cornell Scale for Depression in Dementia (CSDD; see Alexopoulos et al., 1998) is a depression rating scale optimized for use in patients with moderate to severe cognitive impairment. It is based on answers to interview questions that are given to a caregiver of the patient—typically a family member, nurse, or aide. Depressive symptoms identified by the caregiver interview are then confirmed in a brief interview with the patient, which uses questions that are phrased more simply. If the caregiver and the patient interviews are discrepant, the clinician is instructed to re-interview both and then make a clinical judgment. Ultimately the score on each item is a clinical judgment rather than the answer of either the caregiver or the patient to a specific question. Items on the CSDD refer to the week prior to the interview, and item scores range from 0–2, where 1 corresponds to mild or intermittent symptoms and 2 corresponds to severe and presumably persistent ones. There are 19 items covering five domains: mood (sadness, anxiety, irritability, and lack of emotional reactivity), behavior (agitation, retardation, multiple somatic complaints, and loss of interest in activities), physical symptoms (changes in appetite, weight, or energy), cyclic functions (diurnal variation and various attributes of sleep), and ideation (suicidal thinking, self-deprecation, pessimism, and mood-congruent delusions). Rating several of the items requires a judgment that the symptoms are not long-standing and due to chronic general medical illness. The CSDD requires administration by a skilled clinician and takes between 20–30 minutes to complete. The scale is copyrighted; permission for clinical use can be obtained from the scale's authors.

Both the CSDD and the PHQ-9-OV are suitable tests for quantifying depression in patients with moderate to severe cognitive impairment. The CSDD, with 10 more items and a medically oriented perspective on sleep disturbance, diurnal variation, and somatic symptoms, offers a better qualitative understanding of the patient's symptoms; but, asking the rater to judge whether somatic symptoms are due to chronic medical illness rather than depression can be problematic. Both the CSDD and the PHQ-9-OV can be used to follow change over time, although neither one includes an assessment of symptom severity not confounded by symptom frequency.

RATING SUICIDE RISK: THE COLUMBIA SUICIDE SEVERITY RATING SCALE

The assessment of suicide risk is a crucial part of the psychiatric assessment of any patient with depression. Notwithstanding, it is only recently that a standardized measure of suicide risk has emerged that has predictive validity and wide international acceptance. The Columbia Suicide Severity Rating Scale (C-SSRS; see Posner et al., 2011) was originally developed to screen adolescents in antidepressant clinical trials for suicide risk, after it was recognized that a significant minority of depressed adolescents treated with SSRIs developed suicidal ideation as a treatment-emergent side effect. The US FDA essentially mandated the use of the C-SSRS in antidepressant clinical trials, and soon it became a standard component of side-effect monitoring in all psychotropic drug trials. The C-SSRS is a copyrighted instrument that is available for clinical use without a fee; substantial royalties must be paid for the use of the scale in funded research. It has been translated into over 100 languages. A website, www.cssrs.columbia.edu, provides downloadable copies of the scale, links to references on the scale's psychometric properties, and links to training resources.

The C-SSRS is an interview-based scale that is administered by a person who has had basic training on how to conduct the interview; Columbia provides educational materials for this training. The interviewer need not be a mental health professional. The longest version of the interview takes no more than 10 minutes to administer, and the six-question screening version can be completed in about 2 minutes. It comes in several versions for clinical use: (1) lifetime and past month, (2) since last visit, (3) risk assessment, (4) clinical practice screener, (5) pediatric lifetime, and (6) pediatric since last visit. Items are either binary (yes/no or checklist), ordinal measures of severity or frequency, or counts of suicidal or self-injurious actions. All versions of the scale elicit history of death wishes, suicidal ideation, suicidal intent, and suicidal behavior. A risk-assessment version adds a clinical status checklist, a treatment history, and questions about potentially activating events and protective factors.

The count of "yes" answers to five questions on suicidal intent yields a scale score ranging from 0–5; suicidal behavior is scored similarly, and the sum of the two scores gives a score from 0–10 measuring suicidal intent or behavior. Higher scores on these scales have been shown to predict suicide attempts during antidepressant drug trials. The scale items concerning the severity of past attempts, clinical status, activating events, and protective factors are used qualitatively to guide further clinical assessment and decision making.

Neither the C-SSRS nor a psychiatric evaluation can predict whether or when a specific individual will attempt suicide. However, the C-SSRS can help guide decisions about the intensity of supervision needed to protect a patient and the level of psychiatric care that might be appropriate. When depressed patients have both a low lifetime C-SSRS score and a low recent C-SSRS score, they rarely will require hospitalization to mitigate the risk of self-harm. In the medical-psychiatric context, a low C-SSRS score can be used to support a recommendation against an expensive and intrusive "suicide watch." The use of a well-recognized suicide risk scale can aid interdisciplinary communication and also can mitigate concerns about legal risk.

For distressed patients—whether the primary condition is depression or a painful somatic condition—monitoring of the C-SSRS from one visit to the next can aid in the determination of whether interventions such as antidepressant treatment or intensive pain management are working. The alleviation of suicidal thoughts and wishes to be dead is a face-valid indicator that a patient is in less overall emotional distress.

Prior to the C-SSRS, there were several other published suicide-risk rating scales, but none attained the broad acceptance of the C-SSRS, which has been administered to millions of patients. As previously existing scales are not psychometrically superior or more suitable for routine clinical use, the medical psychiatrist should consider using the C-SSRS if a suicide rating scale is going to be used at all. The brief screening version of the C-SSRS—which consists of only six yes/no questions with a follow-up on timing if the patient reports suicidal behavior—is sufficiently simple that it was successfully incorporated into the initial nursing assessment of *all* patients in a general hospital, and a version administered by telephone via an automated voice response system is under development (Mundt et al., 2010). When it is applied universally in this way, it will identify patients not previously suspected of having suicide risk, thus triggering a more timely psychiatric evaluation.

ASSESSMENT OF VIOLENCE RISK

Concern about the potential for violence is a common reason for psychiatric consultation in medical settings. There is an extensive literature on instruments and algorithms for assessment of violence risk, summarized in recent comparative reviews and meta-analyses (McDermott et al., 2008; Fazel et al., 2012). At this time, no rating scale for violence risk has attained the same level of broad acceptance as the C-SSRS has attained for suicide risk. This may be due in part to the fact that violence risk has different determinants in incarcerated or recently released criminals, chronically mentally ill patients, residents of long-term care facilities, general hospital inpatients, and medical or psychiatric outpatients. A critical distinction is among impulsive, predatory, and psychotic aggression. A clinician would be concerned about the former in a delirious patient and the latter in a paranoid patient, and violence risk assessment tools designed for predicting predatory aggression in prior offenders would be of relatively little value in either of those situations. A practical question faced by the medical psychiatrist is what must be done to ensure the safety of the staff and other patients during the clinical encounter, and what must be done to ensure the safety of others afterward. As with suicide, serious violent behavior is a relatively rare event, and many patients will require hospitalization or other intrusive treatment in order to prevent one bad outcome. However, employing standardized rating scales for violence risk can make care more efficient and less intrusive by identifying patients very *un*likely to be violent, because such scales do have reasonable *negative* predictive value.

Medical psychiatrists called upon to assess violence risk in general medical settings should consider five contributors to risk: (1) antisocial personality traits with an associated history of violence, paranoid ideation, anger, and/or coercive sexuality; (2) neurological conditions that can impair impulse control, such as delirium or frontal system dysfunction; (3) loss of inhibition due to the effects alcohol or drugs such as benzodiazepines; (4) increased arousal due to stimulant drugs or to withdrawal of alcohol or opiates; (5) current life circumstances such as financial, legal, or marital problems arousing strong negative emotions. Each of these factors can be rated, but there is no established algorithm for combining them into a validated summary index of risk. The extensive literature on prediction of violence has primarily concerned recidivism in individuals with a history of violence or criminal behavior, not the prediction of violence in general medical contexts. Nonetheless it can be valuable to know, in the longer-term management of patients with chronic general medical conditions, whether a patient has strong antisocial traits and to know whether they are "clinically angry."

While personality inventories in general measure psychopathy as a dimension, the most valid evaluation of antisocial traits comes from synthesizing the patient's documented history (and thus the observations of others) and the results of a structured interview. The Hare Psychopathy Checklist (PCL-R; see Hare, 2003) is a widely used instrument for doing this. Like the C-SSRS, it is supported with a website and extensive training materials. Unlike the C-SSRS there is a fee for its routine clinical use, and it is designed for use only by mental health professionals. The PCL-R comprises 20 items, each a 3-point ordinal scale rating how strongly various personality traits or historical descriptions apply to the patient. It can take over an hour to complete because of the need to collect and synthesize data. It is thus impractical for the assessment of the potential for violence in acute medical situations. Its potential value in medical psychiatry is a contribution to understanding why a patient with a chronic illness might have chronic problems in relationships with physicians and institutions, such as making unreasonable demands, seeking inappropriate compensation or disability status, and so on. It has two factors, one reflecting interpersonal style (e.g., manipulative, shallow, grandiose) and the other reflecting a history of antisocial behavior and lifestyle (irresponsible behavior, parasitic lifestyle). The inter-rater reliability of the test depends on the raters' skill. The ability of the test specifically to predict violence depends on context. When the issue of psychopathy and the potential for violence is central to long-term treatment planning, the medical psychiatrist might consider requesting a PCL-R as part of a battery of psychological tests that would also include screening for psychotic phenomena and for executive cognitive impairment.

Anger is the affect most strongly associated with violence. Patients' level of anger can be practically assessed and quantitated with the Clinical Anger Scale (CAS; see Snell et al., 1995). The CAS comprises 21 self-reported 4-point ordinal items; these are summed to produce a score of 0–63. Items cover both specific angry thoughts and the effects of anger on general health, sleep, appetite, sexual interest, and decision making. There is a specific question about the desire to hurt others because of anger. Most of the questions refer to how the patient is feeling at the time of the test; references to the effect of anger on health and function refer to an indefinite time period including the present. A score of 20 is the threshold for moderate clinical anger; 30 is the threshold for severe clinical anger. The scale has high internal consistency and positive correlations with other scales measuring anger. Of interest, the test authors' research group found little effect of social desirability bias on the test score.

The CAS has not been extensively studied in general medical settings; it is worth noting that several questions concern physical symptoms, cognitive complaints, and functional impairments possibly due to general medical illness but also potentially due to the sympathetic arousal and neuropsychological effects of anger. While this can be viewed as confounding the interpretation of the test and limiting its usefulness, the CAS offers a valuable perspective on the patient's attribution of symptoms. In fact, if a patient feels too angry to sleep it is likely that addressing the patient's anger may improve sleep—even if there are also general medical conditions that also influence sleep onset or sleep quality. When a medical-psychiatric patient is preoccupied with anger, the clinician's adopting anger as a focus of treatment can be more acceptable to the patient than labeling the problem as depression, even when antidepressants will be part of the prescription.

ANXIETY RATING SCALES

The distinctions between affective, cognitive, and somatic dimensions of anxiety, and between anxiety as a personality trait and anxiety as a symptom, can make the measurement of anxiety challenging. The overlap of anxiety symptoms with the symptoms of general medical illness adds a further complication. Conditions like phobias, obsessive compulsive disorder, and posttraumatic stress disorder (PTSD) have prominent cognitive aspects; generalized anxiety disorder and panic disorder have a more somatic emphasis. Finally, the symptoms of anxiety and those of depression appear to converge later in life; anxiety is often a prominent symptom of late-onset major depression. This phenomenon may explain the historical overutilization of antianxiety drugs in primary care as the sole treatment of patients with primary major depression and associated anxiety. Separately reviewing the lifetime history of anxiety symptoms and depressive symptoms with the patient can help deconstruct the problem.

Anxiety scales widely used in medical settings include the Generalized Anxiety Disorder Assessment, the Beck Anxiety

Inventory, the Hamilton Anxiety Rating Scale, and the State-Trait Anxiety Inventory. In addition, there are specialized scales used to rate the symptoms of obsessive compulsive disorder, PTSD, and phobias.

THE GENERALIZED ANXIETY DISORDER ASSESSMENT

The Generalized Anxiety Disorder Assessment (GAD-7; see Spitzer et al., 2006) is for generalized anxiety what the PHQ-9 is for major depression. The scale consists of seven questions about cognitive and emotional symptoms of anxiety (but not autonomic symptoms), each of which is self-rated by the patient according to the frequency with which it occurs: not at all (0), several days (1), more than half of days (2), or nearly every day (3). The total score is the sum of the item scores; it thus ranges from 0–21. Cutoff scores for mild, moderate, and severe generalized anxiety are ≥5, ≥10, and ≥15, respectively. The threshold score of 10 gives 89% sensitivity and 82% specificity for generalized anxiety disorder. Scores of 10 or higher are seen in 74% of cases of panic disorder, 72% of patients with social anxiety disorder, and 66% of patients with PTSD. The GAD-7 is thus useful for screening and measuring symptom severity, but in itself it cannot serve as the basis for a diagnosis. Of particular interest to medical psychiatrists: the GAD-7 does not include somatic symptoms such as palpitations, dyspnea, dizziness, numbness and tingling, and so forth. It is thus very unlikely to be confounded by general medical conditions with symptoms that overlap those of anxiety-based autonomic arousal.

THE BECK ANXIETY INVENTORY

The Beck Anxiety Inventory (BAI; see Beck et al., 1988) is a 21-item self-report questionnaire concerning symptoms of anxiety. Each item is rated for severity and associated distress on a scale of 0–3; the overall scale score is the sum of the item scores. In its initial validation study in patients with anxiety disorders or depression the scale showed high internal consistency and test–retest reliability of 0.75 over 1 week. Patients with severe anxiety scored higher on the BAI than patients with primary depression, and, on a group basis, patients with a primary anxiety diagnosis (with or without depression) scored higher than patients with a primary depression diagnosis (with or without anxiety). The scale was decomposed into two factors: one measuring somatic symptoms of anxiety such as numbness and tingling, dizziness, and shakiness, and the other measuring subjective symptoms of anxiety and panic, such as feeling terrified, scared, or being afraid of dying. The BAI can be completed in a few minutes by a cognitively intact patient.

THE HAMILTON ANXIETY SCALE

The Hamilton Anxiety Scale (HAM-A or HARS; see Hamilton, 1959) is a clinician-rated scale comprising 14 ordinal items, each rated for severity on a scale of 0–4; the scale takes 15–30 minutes to complete. Unlike many of the other commonly used anxiety rating scales, it is in the public domain. Items cover anxious mood, tension, fears, insomnia, concentration and memory problems, depressed mood, muscular symptoms, sensory symptoms, cardiovascular symptoms, respiratory symptoms, gastrointestinal symptoms, genitourinary symptoms, autonomic symptoms, and anxious behavior at the interview. The symptoms rated in each organ system are those that can be caused by anxiety alone in the absence of primary organ system pathology—for example, palpitations and sinus tachycardia but not atrial fibrillation, or dyspnea and sighing but not wheezing. The score on the HAM-A is the sum of items; it thus ranges from 0–56. Patients with scores of ≥14 are likely to have clinically relevant anxiety; those with scores of 30 or higher are severely anxious. While they may have clinically relevant anxiety, they do not necessarily have anxiety *disorders*, because patients with depression can have equally high scores on the HAM-A.

The emphasis of the HAM-A on somatic symptoms of anxiety is a mixed blessing for the medical psychiatrist. A patient with multisystem disease can have a high score on the HAM-A solely from symptoms of his or her general medical illness. On the other hand, if a patient has symptoms confined to a single organ system that could be due either to anxiety or to a general medical condition, and the HAM-A shows somatic symptoms potentially due to anxiety in multiple organ systems along with fear and anxious mood, anxiety is supported as a cause—or at least an aggravating factor—of the symptom of interest.

Because the HAM-A is heavily weighted on somatic symptoms that are not specific for anxiety, it is not well suited for diagnosis or screening, particularly in general medical patients. It is more appropriately used to measure change over time in symptoms of anxiety in response to psychiatric treatment or to changes in a patient's general medical condition.

SPIELBERGER STATE–TRAIT ANXIETY INVENTORY

The State-Trait Anxiety Inventory (STAI; see Spielberger et al., 1970) in its most commonly administered form is a 20-item self-rated scale that measures both long-term anxious traits and current anxious feelings (state). It produces two scores—one rating trait anxiety, and the other rating state anxiety. All items are 4-point ordinal items; the items measuring traits are bidirectional and related to frequency ("almost never" to "almost always"), while the state items are unidirectional and related to intensity. Items are balanced, with some indicating more anxiety and other indicating less anxiety. The STAI was originally developed on a non-patient population, and perhaps for this reason it is often used in studies of non-patients such as family caregivers and in studies of general medical patients without known anxiety disorders. The state anxiety scale is sensitive to changes in anxious mood with changes in circumstances or with treatment. The STAI takes about 5 minutes to complete and requires a sixth-grade reading level, making it suitable for a broad range of clinical populations.

Overall, the STAI is weighted less on the physical dimensions of anxiety and more on the emotional and cognitive dimensions. Medical psychiatrists might find the test particularly useful in medical-patient populations with a high prevalence of general medical symptoms that can also be caused by anxiety alone. The STAI has the additional benefit of putting the patient's current anxiety in the context of the patient's past emotional style. A patient with high state anxiety and low trait anxiety might be facing more severe situational stresses than a patient with a similar level of state anxiety but high trait anxiety. The probability that an underlying medical condition is contributing to the anxiety symptoms is greater in the former case, as well. Further, when a patient with low trait anxiety develops high state anxiety in an acutely stressful situation, supportive psychotherapy can draw upon the defenses and coping skills that kept the patient's anxiety low in the past. The patient also can be reassured that antianxiety drug treatment is likely to be short term, as the state anxiety symptoms are likely to abate when the acute stress has resolved.

Like the HAM-A and the BAI, the state scale of the STAI can be used to monitor the response of anxiety symptoms to psychiatric treatment or to changes in the patient's general medical status. It offers the advantage of self-rating; however, the HAM-A would appear to be preferable for patients in whom the main issue is multiple somatic complaints linked to an anxiety disorder.

RATING SCALES FOR SPECIFIC ANXIETY DISORDERS

Obsessive-compulsive disorder (OCD), various phobias, and PTSD have historically been classified as anxiety disorders, though the latter clearly has many symptoms unrelated to anxiety that can account for much of the patient's distress and disability. These conditions all have characteristic mental and behavioral symptoms that can overshadow anxious mood and somatic manifestations of anxiety, and for that reason they are best rated with syndrome-specific scales. Following are selected examples of such scales, with comments on their use in medical-psychiatric contexts.

YALE–BROWN OBSESSIVE COMPULSIVE SCALE

The Yale–Brown Obsessive Compulsive Scale (Y-BOCS; see Goodman et al., 1989a, Goodman et al., 1989b) has, in the past 25 years, become the standard instrument for clinician assessment of symptom severity in OCD. Its particular virtue is that it works regardless of the specific obsessions and compulsions from which the patient suffers. It comprises 10 clinician-rated items, each rated on a 5-point ordinal scale from 0 (no symptoms) to 4 (extreme symptoms). Subscales for obsessions and for compulsions are defined. The administration of the Y-BOCS is a two-stage process. The patient and clinician first review a checklist of obsessions and compulsions and identify the ones from which the patient suffers; the patient then chooses the three that he or she finds most prominent or distressing. The 10 ordinal items then refer to the occurrence of the three target symptoms. The five items

related to obsessions are time occupied by obsessive thoughts, interference with activities due to obsessive thoughts, distress associated with obsessive thoughts, resistance against obsessions, and degree of control over obsessive thoughts. The five items concerning compulsive behaviors are homologous. The Y-BOCS has acceptable internal consistency and inter-rater reliability, and it has been shown to be sensitive to clinically relevant changes in OCD symptoms with treatment. A self-rated version and a computer-administered version are available.

Of particular interest to medical psychiatrists is the sensitivity of the Y-BOCS to obsessions and compulsions that can present as general medical problems or that can become impediments to medical treatment adherence. The former comprise somatic obsessions, contamination obsessions, and potentially self-injurious compulsions like excessive handwashing. The latter include checking compulsions, cleaning and washing compulsions, ritualized eating, and repetition compulsions. These specific symptoms are identified on the symptom checklist and then become the basis of the quantitative score.

THE OBSESSIVE COMPULSIVE INVENTORY

An alternative to the Y-BOCS specifically designed for self-rating of OCD symptoms in general medical contexts is the Obsessive Compulsive Inventory (OCI; see Foa et al., 1998). The full OCI comprises 42 items relating to different types of obsessions and compulsions, each rated on a scale of 0–4 for how much distress the symptom caused the patient during the previous month. Distress ratings are calculated for six domains: washing, checking, ordering, obsessions, hoarding, and neutralizing. An 18-item version has similar content and psychometric properties (Foa et al., 2002). The OCI provides less detail than the Y-BOCS on the patient's psychopathology; in particular, it focuses on distress caused by symptoms rather than frequency, ability to resist, and so on, and it combines ratings of obsessive thoughts and compulsive behaviors in its scoring. Its virtue is that is it a self-rated instrument that surveys all main types of obsessive compulsive symptoms, making it well suited for screening and initial diagnosis (Abramowitz & Deacon, 2006). Once a patient has been diagnosed and begun treatment, the Y-BOCS appears more suitable for measuring treatment response, because it assesses multiple aspects of severity and not just distress, and after the initial assessment all Y-BOCS scale items will focus on the obsessions and compulsions most relevant to the patient.

PHOBIA RATING SCALES

Clinically significant phobias involve a combination of two factors: physiological arousal (fear or anxiety) in the presence of or contemplation of the phobic stimulus, and avoidance behavior. Rating scales for phobia are either for phobias in general, or specific scales for specific phobias such as agoraphobia, social phobia, or blood injury phobia. The IAPT Phobia Scale (Improving Access to Psychological Therapies, 2013) is a 3-item self-rated screening test for phobias in general. Each item asks the patient to rate on a scale of 0–8 how much they would avoid particular circumstance: The questions concern the following: (1) "Social situations due to a fear of being embarrassed or making a fool of myself"; (2) "Certain situations because of a fear of having a panic attack or other distressing symptoms (such as loss of bladder control, vomiting or dizziness)"; and (3) "Certain situations because of a fear of particular objects or activities (such as animals, heights, seeing blood, being in confined spaces, driving or flying)". A score of 4 (marked avoidance) on any specific item suggests the clinical diagnosis of a phobic disorder.

Virtually all rating scales for specific phobias measure both arousal and avoidance behavior. In medical settings the most relevant phobias are of three kinds: (1) those that interfere with medical treatment, prominently including blood injury phobias (fears of injections, venipuncture, or surgery), dental phobia, and disease-specific fears such as fear of hypoglycemia in insulin-dependent diabetics; (2) those that interfere with patients coming to a hospital, clinic, or doctor's office, including agoraphobia, severe social phobia, and specific fears of clinical settings; and (3) phobias with panic attacks or other autonomic symptoms severe enough to present as medical problems in their own right.

In addition to the usual benefits of rating symptoms, the quantitative rating of phobias can help in gauging the relative severity of physiological symptoms versus avoidant behavior. For example, premedication prior to a feared procedure is likely to be an effective solution when autonomic symptoms are severe and avoidant behavior is not.

Most commonly used phobia scales are self-rating instruments, although many of them could be completed by a proxy and give clinically useful scores. However, psychometric properties should not be presumed to be the same if an informant is filling out the questionnaire on the patient's behalf.

The medical psychiatrist addressing issues of medical fears and associated avoidance can utilize either general scales for rating medical fears and avoidance or scales that are specific for a particular disease and clinical situation. Representing the former are two self-rated omnibus scales, the Medical Fear Survey (MFS) and the Medical Avoidance Survey (MAS) (Kleinknecht et al., 1996). The MFS comprises a set of 5-point ordinal items (originally 70, subsequently 50 or 25) on which specific feared situations are rated on a scale of 1 (no fear or concern at all) to 5 (terror); the shorter versions use 4-point items that eliminate "terror" as an option. Typical items are "giving blood" or "seeing wounds." The MAS comprises 21 items relating to reasons why a person might avoid seeing a doctor or seeking treatment, ranging from fear that blood will be drawn to concern about cost; they are rated on an ordinal scale of 0 ("I wouldn't avoid treatment for that reason") to 4 ("I have avoided treatment for that reason in the past and I would continue to do so now"). The MFS can be decomposed into seven factors that are related to fears of mutilation, deformed persons, cutting objects, medical/dental examinations, hypodermic injections, blood draws, and physical symptoms. The MAS can be decomposed into three factors that are related to fear that serious illness will be discovered, fear of blood draws or injections, and concerns about logistics and costs. Both instruments have been used extensively in research, and,

notably, a subscale of the MFS specifically dealing with fears of blood and injections has been used as a brief and practical measure of blood injection injury phobia. Medical psychiatrists encountering patients who frequently miss, cancel, or reschedule appointments, or who do not follow through with medical treatment recommendations, might consider these scales as an efficient way to determine whether phobic avoidance is critical, instead of or in addition to logistical problems, personality issues, or problems with physician–patient relationships.

In addition to general fears related to medical care, patients can have *condition-specific fears* that involve both anxiety and avoidance behavior. These fears can have major effects on treatment adherence and on clinical outcomes. Three illustrative examples are *fear of falling* in people with disorders of gait or balance (e.g., vestibular disorders), *fear of movement* in people with painful musculoskeletal conditions (e.g., osteoarthritis or low back pain), and *fear of hypoglycemia* in patients with insulin-dependent diabetes. For each of these fears there is at least one widely accepted rating scale that is brief enough to be used in clinical practice and psychometrically sound enough to be used in research.

The Short Falls Efficacy Scale–International (FES–I) is a 7-item questionnaire assessing a patient's fear of falling in connection with various activities. Each item is a 4-point ordinal scale ranging from 1 (not at all concerned) to 4 (very concerned). The seven activities are getting dressed or undressed, taking a bath or shower, getting in or out of a chair, going up or down stairs, reaching for something above the head or on the ground, walking up or down a slope, and going out to a social event. The scale, which has very high internal consistency (Cronbach's alpha = 0.92) nicely and efficiently captures, characterizes, and quantitates fear of falling.

The Tampa Kinesiophobia Scale (TSK; see Kori et al.,1990) is a self-rated questionnaire that measures fears and avoidance behavior related to body movement and pain. It comprises 11, 13, or 17 four-point bidirectional ordinal (Likert-type) items rated from 1 (strongly disagree) to 4 (strongly agree), referring to statements like "Pain always means I have injured my body" and "Simply being careful that I do not make any unnecessary movements is the safest thing I can do to prevent my pain from worsening". The scale has gained wide acceptance by specialists in physical medicine and rehabilitation (Woby et al., 2005; Damsgard et al., 2007; Roelofs et al., 2011). Although it was developed for use with low back pain patients, it has subsequently been applied to diverse pain populations including those with neck pain, osteoarthritis (Shelby et al., 2012), fibromyalgia (Burwinkle et al., 2005), and chronic fatigue syndrome (Silver et al., 2002). For the medical psychiatrist, the TSK score offers a measurable target for improvement with cognitive-behavioral and/or pharmacological treatment that is not based on diagnosing a "mental disorder".

The Hypoglycemia Fear Survey–II (HFS–II; see Cox et al., 1987; Irvine et al., 1994; Gonder-Frederick et al., 2011) is exemplary of a highly specific scale for a medical phobia that is prevalent, treatable, and relevant to medical outcome. It rates two dimensions of fear of hypoglycemia: worry about hypoglycemia and behavior aimed at avoiding hypoglycemia. The test comprises 33 ordinal items, each self-rated or informant-rated, for frequency on a scale of 0 (never) to 4 (always) in reference to the past 6 months. There are 15 items concerning specific avoidant or precautionary behaviors and 18 items concerning specific hypoglycemia-related worries. Factor analyses of data from various diabetic populations have confirmed the distinctness and internal consistency of the two factors. Fear of hypoglycemia, as measured by the scale, is associated with having had hypoglycemic attacks requiring assistance; it is also associated with worse glycemic control. Diabetic patients' scores on the HFS–II can be used to compare the impact of different treatments on their health-related quality of life. Clinically, medical psychiatrists can identify patients with a disproportionate fear of hypoglycemia that *is in itself* a relevant mental health outcome that *can lead to* a worse general medical outcome.

Social phobia (social anxiety disorder) and *agoraphobia* clearly can affect patients' participation in medical treatment. Each is treatable and each is measurable. The reader is referred to textbooks and review articles on these disorders for details on available rating scales and screening tests.

RATING POSTTRAUMATIC STRESS DISORDER

Posttraumatic stress disorder (PTSD) appears frequently in medical contexts, where it sometimes is an unrecognized yet functionally significant comorbidity with a major impact on health-related quality of life. PTSD is especially prevalent following catastrophic medical events like burns, multiple trauma, and spinal cord injury, or following injuries associated with assault, abuse, rape, or combat (Roberts et al., 2010). These are all populations in which screening for PTSD would have a high yield and could, if followed up and treated effectively, improve ultimate clinical outcomes. Furthermore, medical and surgical treatments and hospitalization can, for individual patients, be traumatic events that give rise to subsequent PTSD. PTSD is amenable to self-rating, because patients with PTSD are painfully aware of their symptoms and usually do not deny them if asked about them specifically.

Two similar self-rated scales of PTSD symptoms have been used widely in general medical-surgical populations to assess posttraumatic symptoms both in patients and in family caregivers. One is the *PTSD Checklist—Civilian Version* (PCL-C; see Blanchard et al., 1996) and the other is the *Davidson Trauma Scale* (DTS; see Davidson et al., 1997). Both have 17 items corresponding to DSM criteria for PTSD. The PCL-C asks the patient to rate distress from each symptom over the past month on a 4-point ordinal scale (from 0–4). The DTS asks the patient to rate the frequency of each symptom over the past week and, separately, the severity of each symptom over the past week, on a 5-point ordinal scale. Both tests have excellent psychometric properties and can be used either for screening or for following patients' response to treatment.

Self-rated scales for PTSD are more practical for use as screening tests or tools for epidemiologic study than the standard Clinician-Administered PTSD Scale (CAPS; see Blake et al., 1990 and Blake et al., 1995), which takes 45–60 minutes to administer and is viewed as the definitive instrument against which the self-rated scales are validated. The self-rated scales refer to the "event". In most general medical contexts, the identity of the event is self-evident; if it is not, the clinician will need to clarify with the patient just what the event of interest is.

The CAPS has a two-stage structure much like the Y-BOCS. The patient first reviews a list of potentially traumatizing events and, together with the clinician, selects up to three based on their severity or how recently they occurred. Then, with these events in mind, the clinician questions the patient about the 17 symptoms covered in the PCL and the DTS, rating each on 5-point scales for severity and for frequency. The clinician can add specific behavioral descriptions and can note if he/she thinks the patient is amplifying or minimizing a symptom. As on the DTS, the total score is the sum of the frequency and severity scores for the 17 items. The CAPS can be utilized to assess PTSD symptoms over the past week, the past month, or the lifetime of the patient. The lifetime score can relate the symptoms of PTSD to up to three separate events.

Both the CAPS and the self-rated tests give not only an overall rating of the severity of posttraumatic symptoms but also establish whether criteria for a formal diagnosis of PTSD are present, and profile the qualitative aspect of the syndrome—whether, for example, intrusive reexperiencing phenomena predominate over emotional numbing and avoidance.

GENERAL AND NEUROPSYCHIATRIC PSYCHOPATHOLOGY SCALES

For the medical psychiatrist, a general psychopathology rating scale can serve several specific purposes: (1) It can organize the data collection and synthesis of a psychiatric evaluation and ensure that ever-important areas like psychotic phenomena are considered and recorded; (2) It can provide a quick quantitative measure of "how mentally ill is this patient"— potentially useful in communicating with other professionals and in making judgments about change over time or with treatment; and (3) It can provide a simple tool for monitoring whether a stressful or neurotoxic general medical treatment (e.g., cancer chemotherapy) is causing clinically significant mental and behavioral side effects.

The Brief Psychiatric Rating Scale (BPRS; see Overall & Gorham, 1962) is a venerable and still widely used general psychopathology measure that was originally developed to monitor the course of patients with schizophrenia. It is a clinician-rated scale that combines information obtained from the patient in a 15–30-minute diagnostic interview with observations made during the interview. It has 18 items, all rated on a scale of 1 (not present) to 7 (very severe), with the ratings referring to the 2 or 3 days immediately before the evaluation. The scale items cover somatic concern, anxiety, emotional withdrawal, conceptual disorganization, guilt feelings, tension, mannerisms and posturing, grandiosity, depressive mood, hostility, suspiciousness, hallucinatory behavior, motor retardation, uncooperativeness, unusual thought content, blunted affect, excitement, and disorientation. The BPRS is in the public domain.

For rating psychopathology related to dementia and other gross brain diseases, the Neuropsychiatric Inventory (NPI; see Cummings, 1997) serves a purpose similar to that of the BPRS for general psychopathology. The NPI comprises 10 or 12 items that are scored by the clinician after interviewing a caregiver of the patient. For each item the clinician asks a yes/no question to determine whether a particular symptom has been observed over the past 4 weeks. If yes, the clinician asks follow-up questions to rate frequency on a scale of 1 (less than once a week) to 4 (every day) and severity on a scale of 1 (mild) to 3 (severe). The item score is the product of the frequency and severity scores. In addition, the caregiver's distress about the patient's symptom is rated on a scale of 0 (no distress) to 5 (very severe or extreme distress). The overall score on the NPI is the sum of the item scores; the sum of distress scores is reported separately. The NPI comes in three alternate versions: a questionnaire version for caregivers (the NPI-Q), a version based on a clinician interview of nursing home staff (the NPI-NH), and a version that incorporates direct observations by the clinician during a structured examination of the patient (the NPI-C). The NPI is a copyrighted instrument that is licensed royalty-free to clinicians; a fee must be paid to license the test for use in funded research.

The 12 symptom areas covered by the NPI are delusions, hallucinations, agitation/aggression, depression/dysphoria, anxiety, elation/euphoria, apathy/indifference, disinhibition, irritability/lability, aberrant motor behavior, sleep disturbance, and appetite and eating disorders.

Thus there are several salient differences in the NPI that make it more useful than the BPRS for assessing dementia patients and other medical-psychiatric patients with similar issues: (1) It makes use of input from caregivers; (2) It covers a four-week period, and therefore counts infrequently occurring but potentially severe symptoms; (3) It covers eating and sleeping-related problems; (4) It captures neuropsychiatric symptoms more precisely; the apathy and indifference seen in many patients with early Alzheimer's disease are not the same symptom as the emotional withdrawal and blunted affect seen in patients with schizophrenia; (5) It specifically measures caregiver distress, and (6) It separately measures the frequency and the severity of symptoms.

The broad coverage of the NPI makes it less sensitive than a more specialized scale for measuring and monitoring specific neuropsychiatric symptoms or syndromes that might be the focus of medical-psychiatric concern. An example is the syndrome of apathy. In neuropsychiatric disorders including Parkinson's disease, effects of medial frontal lesions, and vascular dementia, the syndrome of apathy—a pathological lack of motivation, affect, or interest—can be a prominent symptom that is distinguishable from depression. It is important to recognize it, because it can be treated specifically and because its misdiagnosis as depression can lead to its treatment with

antidepressants that in some cases make apathy worse. While behavioral neurologists have always distinguished apathy from depression, wider recognition of apathy as a discrete symptom clearly was facilitated by the development of rating scales specific for that condition. Apathetic patients can be unable to care for themselves yet be unconcerned about their disability; this is a challenge to clinicians and to family caregivers. Yet, even severe apathy might contribute only slightly to the total score on the BPRS and only modestly to the total score on the NPI.

The use of a specialized rating scale focused on apathy is best for measuring the severity of apathy and for following changes in apathy in response to treatment. Moreover, the use of an apathy rating scale sensitizes the user—and the consumers of scale scores—to the issue of apathy. After rating several patients with an apathy rating scale and seeing apathy scale scores reported by their colleagues, physicians will recognize more patients with apathy in their clinical practice.

The Apathy Evaluation Scale (AES; see Marin et al., 1991) is an 18-item instrument with self-rated, informant-rated and clinician-rated versions that covers all three aspects of the syndrome of apathy: cognitive (lack of interest), affective (lack of feeling or concern), and motivational (lack of will or drive). Each item describes an aspect of behavior. In the clinician version, the item is given a score from 1 (behavior not characteristic of the patient) to 4 (behavior very characteristic of the patient), all with respect to the patient's behavior over the past 4 weeks. The self-rated and informant-rated versions use a differently-worded description of the 4-point scale. The AES has been shown to measure apathy as a phenomenon distinct from depression and has demonstrated favorable psychometric properties in a range of medical and psychiatric patient populations (Clarke et al., 2011).

The AES can be especially useful in assessing and following patients who have lost their interest and drive in connection with severe general medical illness and its treatment—for example, patients with cancer who have just undergone rigorous and exhausting chemotherapy—but do not show the syndrome of major depression. It is also applicable to assessing apathy as a residual syndrome in patients who have been treated for depression with antidepressant drugs, yet remain passive and disengaged despite relief of their dysphoric mood. The AES was used in this way in a recent multicenter drug trial reported by Raskin et al. (2012). The investigators identified 483 patients who had been treated with an SSRI other than escitalopram for 3 months or more, with relief of depressive symptoms but persistence of apathy as indicated by AES scores >30. Eight weeks of treatment with a different antidepressant drug—either escitalopram or duloxetine—reduced apathetic symptoms by an average of 14 points.

For measuring behavioral symptoms of frontal systems dysfunction apart from apathy, and not mixing them with various symptoms of primary psychoses, the Frontal Systems Behavior Scale (FrSBe; see Grace et al., 2001) can serve similarly to the AES in the measurement of apathy. The FsSBe measures three factors, corresponding to executive dysfunction, disinhibition, and apathy (Stout et al., 2003).

FUNCTIONAL ASSESSMENT

Functional assessment scales rate patients' ability to perform physical activities (e.g., walking or dressing) or instrumental activities (e.g., shopping, handling money, or using public transportation). Patients are rated as to whether they can perform specific activities independently, with supervision, or with assistance, or cannot perform them at all. Depending on the scale, scores may also reflect *how much* assistance is needed; for example, if the assistance required involves weight-bearing or not, and if it requires one person or two. The physical activities of daily living (ADL) conventionally comprise eating, mobility in bed, transferring from bed to chair, walking, using the toilet, bathing, grooming, and dressing. The instrumental activities of daily living (IADL) include shopping, driving or using public transportation, keeping one's living quarters in order, managing one's money, taking medications, and communicating by telephone, by mail, or via electronic media. The most widely used scale for measuring ADLs is the Katz Index of Activities of Daily Living (Katz et al., 1963), and the most widely used scale for measuring IADL is the Lawton Scale of Instrumental Activities of Daily Living (Lawton & Brody, 1969). Both of these scales were originally designed to be clinician-rated, but the scale items permit rating by the patient or by the patient's informal caregivers. Performance on the ADL index frequently is reported as a count of dependencies rather than as a summary score. It is also common to simply indicate the specific activities in which the patient is not independent. When scored as originally described, the Lawton IADL scale does not distinguish subtle from severe dependencies in IADLs; a patient who could dial only a few familiar numbers would get full credit for use of the telephone. For this reason it is most helpful in answering questions related to the need for assisted living or supportive services rather than questions about decision-making competence.

A summary scale that comprises physical and instrumental functions, specifically adapted for measurement of rehabilitation outcome, is the Functional Independence Measure (FIM; see Granger et al., 1993; Granger, 1998). The FIM has become an international standard for its purpose; it is supported, much as the C-SSRS, by a large academically-affiliated organization that warehouses normative data, investigates the scale's psychometric properties in various populations, provides training materials, runs user groups, and so on. Its particular virtue is its sensitivity to the kinds of change that take place in post–acute rehabilitation programs following trauma, surgery, or stroke. The measure comprises 18 items, each measured on a 7-point scale. Thirteen items relate to physical functions of self-care, continence, transfers, and locomotion; five items relate to cognitive functions of comprehension, expression, social interaction, problem solving, and memory. A score of 7 corresponds to complete independence; 6 corresponds to independence using a device, 5 corresponds to requiring supervision only, and 4 through 1 correspond to a progressively greater need for physical assistance. The FIM has very high inter-rater reliability when the two raters are comparably trained therapists. Its virtue is its high sensitivity to changes during rehabilitation, which mainly derives from its subdivision of physical dependence into four levels.

Ratings of ADLs and IADLs are used to assess clinical course and treatment response, as well as to determine eligibility for compensation or supportive services. ADL independence is a critical criterion for physical therapy outcome, and IADL independence is a critical criterion for occupational therapy outcome. Several considerations in the use of these scales are especially relevant to medical psychiatrists:

1. ADLs and IADLs may be rated differently by patients, caregivers, and clinicians. Overestimation of independence by patients can reflect denial of illness or bad judgment due to frontal systems dysfunction. Underestimation of independence can reflect depression, demoralization, or delusional beliefs. Overestimation of independence by a family member may reflect denial or simply a lack of familiarity with the patient's challenges, particularly when patient and the relative do not live together; underestimation of independence may reflect an overprotective attitude or a conscious or unconscious intent to infantilize the patient. In any case, discrepancies in judgments of dependence among clinicians, patients, and families can cause interpersonal conflicts that should be resolved to optimize the outcome of care. Medical psychiatrists can be helpful in these situations because they can appreciate the medical basis of a patient's disability as well as the cognitive, emotional, and interpersonal issues involved.

2. When neuropsychiatric factors strongly influence ADL performance, a patient can perform independently at one time in one context while requiring supervision or physical assistance at a different time in a different context. An 85-year-old patient with mild dementia, who is independent in basic self-care while living in her home of 50 years, might be unable to use the toilet or walk safely while in the hospital for an acute medical condition.

3. Ratings of ADLs are the usual basis of entitlements to supportive services, for example, reimbursements from long-term care insurance and eligibility for Medicaid-funded nursing home care or home care services. Patients with inconsistent ADL independence due to neuropsychiatric conditions can truly require residential care or supportive services, yet pass a specific one-time test of ADL performance. The medical psychiatrist who appreciates this point can at times be an essential advocate for such patients.

4. ADL and IADL performance are affected by motivational state. Drugs and mental disorders that affect motivation can affect ratings of function, often reversibly.

5. The FIM's sensitivity to incremental changes in performance during the early stages of rehabilitation enables therapists and other clinicians to know when patients are making progress toward independence even though they

still require help or supervision. The medical psychiatrist can infer from increasing FIM scores that a patient is making progress, and provide realistic encouragement to a patient or caregiver. In later stages of rehabilitation, instrumental function can be much more impaired than physical function. In these cases the score on the FIM might be near maximal while the patient is still functioning well below baseline. When this is so the medical psychiatrist often can provide useful information or advocacy. If cognitive, emotional, or behavioral factors prevent a patient from being truly independent in life, he or she usually will need continuing treatment that addresses those factors and a supportive environment in the interim.

6. In the author's experience, judgments of functional independence by clinicians vary by the clinician's role and training. Specifically, therapists tend to focus on patients' best performance and what proportion of a task they can do independently; nurses providing supportive care tend to focus on how much assistance patients needs at the time they need the most help. For example, a patient might progress in rehabilitation from continually needing help with transfers to needing help just once a day, when getting into bed at night. If, however, that one transfer required a two-person assist and the patient lived alone, home care still might not be feasible. Discrepant views of the meaning of "improvement" among patients, family caregivers, therapists, and physicians can produce conflicts that present to the medical psychiatrist, just as do differences in perceptions of functional independence.

COGNITIVE RATING SCALES

Brief quantitative rating scales for testing of cognition during clinical encounters occupy a middle ground between the unstandardized assessment that is part of a psychiatric mental status examination and the extensive assessments performed by neuropsychologists. Cognitive rating scales are used to detect dementia and delirium, to quantify the scope and severity of cognitive deficits, and, to a lesser extent, to characterize the nature of any deficits found. Commonly used scales all have acceptable reliability, but their validity depends on the purpose for which they are used. This is especially the case when scales are used as screening tests for dementia or mild cognitive impairment, where the usual tradeoff between sensitivity and specificity exists. Relatively high cutoff scores will lead to some poorly-educated patients being misclassified as cognitively impaired. Relatively low cutoff scores will lead to missing actual cognitive impairment in patients with high premorbid intelligence or mild impairment. Another common feature of brief cognitive rating scales is their greater sensitivity to generalized, diffuse, or multifocal cognitive deficits than to focal cognitive deficits, particularly when the latter involve nonverbal functions.

As disease-modifying therapy for dementing illnesses become available, the emphasis on cognitive screening will shift toward sensitivity rather than specificity. Clinicians will not want to miss opportunities to intervene in patients with borderline or mild dementia who have not yet lost their functional independence.

For many years the most widely used brief bedside cognitive rating scale has been the Mini-Mental State Examination (MMSE) (Folstein et al., 1975). While the drawbacks of the instrument are widely known, the enormous literature on the scale and its widespread familiarity among clinicians have maintained its place in clinical practice. In the author's view, however, the aims of the MMSE are better attained by the Montreal Cognitive Assessment (MoCA) (Nasreddine et al., 2005), a scale of similar length and scope that addresses several of the shortcomings of the MMSE.

Both the MMSE and the MoCA are clinician-administered scales of general cognitive performance that yield scores between 0 and 30 based on the patient's performance on a standardized clinical examination that tests attention, concentration, memory, language, praxis, and some visuospatial functions. Table 4.1 compares the two scales.

Medical psychiatrists should be aware that "normal" scores on the MMSE or the MoCA, or even perfect scores on those scales, can rule out delirium or frank dementia, but they cannot rule out cognitive impairment in general. Many patients with functionally significant deficits will have a normal MMSE because their deficits are in areas that the MMSE does not test, or that account for only a point or two of the MMSE score. A patient with a large right-hemisphere stroke could have left hemineglect and severely impaired visual memory and score 29 out of 30 on the MMSE, losing a point only for the drawing item. Furthermore, patients with degenerative brain diseases develop mild cognitive impairment (MCI) before they develop dementia, and, at the stage of MCI, total cognitive rating scale scores usually fall at the lower end of the "normal" range.

When either the MMSE or the MoCA is used to follow changes in patients' cognitive performance over time, the words used to test memory should be changed to mitigate potential learning effects. Both the MoCA and the second edition of the MMSE (MMSE-II) have alternate forms with different lists. If the clinician is using the original MMSE, the lack of alternate forms can be compensated by keeping at hand a set of different 3-word lists of comparable difficulty that can be substituted for the test's usual items each time the test is repeated.

The numerical score on the MMSE or the MoCA concisely conveys the degree of a patient's cognitive impairment to any clinician with training in the clinical neurosciences, as these tests are ubiquitous. The "message" of an MMSE score can be articulated further by noting the reason a patient lost points—for example, "the patient got 29/30 on the MMSE, losing a point on the drawing of the intersecting pentagons."

Two significant "blind spots" of the MMSE and, to a lesser extent, the MoCA are visuospatial functions and executive cognitive function. Relatively isolated deficits in visuospatial function can occur as a consequence of right hemisphere lesions. Executive cognitive dysfunction has a wide range of potential causes including degenerative brain diseases,

COGNITIVE FUNCTION OR TEST FEATURE	MMSE	MOCA
Attention and Concentration	Serial 7s *or* spelling "world" backwards	Repeating 5 digits forward and 3 digits backward, signaling to the letter "A," serial 7s
Language	Naming a pencil and a watch; repeat "no ifs, ands, or buts"; following a 3-stage spoken command; following a 1-step written command	Naming of three pictured animals; listing words starting with "f" in 60 seconds (verbal fluency); repetition of two sentences
Orientation	Date, day, season, state, county, town, hospital, floor	Date, day, place, city
Memory	3-word list presented, immediate recall scored, list presented up to six times until learned, then delayed recall after an intervening test item	5-word list presented twice for immediate recall; delayed recall at end of test
Abstract Reasoning	—	Similarities: two word pairs are presented
Executive Function	—	Alternating trail-making (connecting 1-A-2-B, etc.)
Visual-Spatial	Copy intersecting pentagons	Copy 3-D cube, draw clock
Time to Administer	10 minutes	10 minutes
Alternate Forms	Examiner can change the three words for the memory test	Original plus two alternates
Copyright status	Publisher expects fees for clinical or research	Free for clinical use; license needed for commercial research

toxic-metabolic encephalopathy, medication side effects, and major primary mental disorders including bipolar disorder and schizophrenia. Establishing that executive cognitive function is impaired can be particularly useful when the medical psychiatrist is called upon to explain why instrumental function is much worse than physical function in a patient who otherwise has grossly intact memory, orientation, and so on.

Two practical and empirically validated bedside scales for executive cognitive function are the Clock Drawing Test (CDT; described in Chapter 2, with additional comments below; see also Royall et al., 1999) and the Executive Interview Test (EXIT; see Royall et al., 1992). The EXIT gives a score of 0–50 based on a 25-item structured clinical examination that takes about 15 minutes. Each item is an ordinal item scored 0 if the response is normal and scored 1 or 2 if the item is abnormal, according to severity of abnormality. The examination is designed to elicit signs of executive dysfunction including perseveration, imitation behavior, intrusions, lack of spontaneity, disinhibited behaviors, and utilization behavior; it also checks for the presence of a grasp reflex and a snout reflex. Mentioning which items were responsible for a high EXIT score adds to its value as a tool for communicating with other clinicians.

The unique value of the EXIT to the medical psychiatrist is that it contains items—and tests for signs—that are not usually included in other bedside examinations. For example, one item presents the patient with anomalous sentences (e.g., "Mary fed a little lamb") and asks the patient to repeat them. The mildly impaired patient will spontaneously correct the phrase despite the examiner's instructions; a grossly impaired one might continue with the second phrase in the

familiar verse. Either type of error shows impairment in working memory—the ability to keep an instruction in mind despite a distracting stimulus. Executive functions like working memory are provably important to self-care and occupational function, yet are not directly tested by typical brief cognitive screens.

The CDT has both literal and figurative "face validity"—when a caregiver or clinician sees a grossly disorganized clock face produced by an educated adult, it is not hard to convince the person that there is an issue with brain function. Moreover, neglect of the left half or one of the left quadrants of the clock strongly suggests a structural lesion of the right hemisphere. Though they perhaps communicate less than an image of the drawing, there are over 20 different ordinal rating scales for clock drawings that measure just how bad the drawing is. No specific scoring system has become a de facto standard. Royall, the co-developer of the EXIT, devised a scoring system for the clock drawing, the CLOX (Royall et al., 1998) that is especially focused on errors due to executive dysfunction. The CLOX comprises two tasks: CLOX1 is a free drawing of a clock, and CLOX2 is a copy of a clock drawn in front of the patient by the examiner. CLOX1 is highly sensitive to executive cognitive dysfunction; both CLOX1 and CLOX2 will be impaired in cases of constructional apraxia or global dementia.

The patient's score on CLOX1 ranges from 0–15, with 15 representing a perfect performance and a score less than 10 suggesting executive cognitive dysfunction. The clock drawing task is presented in a way that increases the likelihood of failure if the patient has impaired executive function. The patient is shown a blank sheet of paper and is asked by the examiner to "Draw me a clock that says 1:45. Set the hands and numbers on the face so a child could read them." The opposite side of the blank sheet of paper has a circle printed in its left lower corner, and it is intended the paper be placed on a light colored surface so that the printed circle will slightly show through. The patient is thus presented with several confusing cues and distractors: the words "hands" and "face," the number 45, and the circle showing through slightly from the opposite side. Patients with impaired executive function will make errors of organization and planning or errors related to distractibility and lack of inhibition; for example, drawing a hand or a face, pointing one clock hand to the 4 and one to the 5, writing the time in digits, or tracing the small circle showing through from the other side of the page.

Low scores on CLOX1 are strongly associated with poor scores on the EXIT25 and other tests of executive function (Royall et al., 1998). They are also associated with functional defects in brain areas associated with executive function (Shon et al., 2013).

SCALES FOR PAIN, SLEEP DISTURBANCE, AND SEXUAL DYSFUNCTION

Pain, sleep disturbance, and sexual dysfunction are three somatic expressions of general medical illness that often come to psychiatrists' attention because of their relationship to mental symptoms, especially depression and anxiety. These symptoms are especially likely to cause emotional distress. They can be caused or exacerbated by mental disorders and by transient emotional states. And, they are often helped by cognitive-behavioral or other psychotherapeutic interventions.

With the exception of simple quantitative measures of pain intensity, the most useful rating scales for these three symptomatic domains involve multidimensional or qualitative characterization of symptoms as well as some form of quantitative summary. The former aspect of the scales guides diagnosis and choice of treatment; the latter aspect is used to categorize symptom severity and quantify the outcome of treatment.

PAIN

The 0–10 Numerical Rating Scale (NRS), the Pain Faces (Figure 4.3), and the Visual Analog Scale (VAS) are all simple one-dimensional measures of current pain intensity. The first two scales are explicitly ordinal scales; the last is continuous, but because the scaling is not uniform it is essentially an ordinal scale as well. (Uniform scaling means that a difference of a specific number means the same thing at any point on the scale. This is not the case: for most patients a difference between 10 and 30 does not have the same subjective significance as a difference between 60 and 80.) These scales are useful in an acute care setting to inform a decision as to whether acute pain treatment with an opiate or other major analgesic is necessary, and to decide whether such treatment has been adequate. They are, in the author's opinion, less useful in evaluating and developing treatment strategy for chronic or recurrent pain.

Pain rating scales differ in the *process* of gathering information from the patient and in the breadth and specificity of scale *content*. Information about a patient's pain can be elicited in a primarily verbal or primarily visual channel (e.g., verbal pain descriptors or the NRS versus Pain Faces or the VAS). It can be elicited from the patient, from a proxy such as a family member, or from a clinical observer, usually a nurse. It can be responsive to a fixed set of questions, or interactive with a software application that presents questions based on responses to previous ones. Content can comprise any combination of ratings of frequency, severity, and intensity, and it can include a checklist of qualitative attributes of the pain—for example, shooting, aching, burning, and so on. Some pain rating scales include measurements of pain-associated depression, anxiety, fear, catastrophic thinking, self-perceived coping adequacy, and/or other pain-associated emotions and cognitions. Pain-associated distress and pain-associated functional impairment can be rated.

Pain rating scales can be generic or can be designed for specific clinical populations such as those with low back pain, neck pain, or upper extremity pain. Pain rating scales for specific patient populations can be more sensitive to changes with treatment, because the scale consists entirely of items actually encountered in the clinical context for which the scale was designed. The medical psychiatrist working in liaison with a specific medical or surgical subspecialty should consider using such scales.

THE BRIEF PAIN INVENTORY

The Brief Pain Inventory (BPI) (Cleeland & Ryan, 1994) addresses the limitations of single-item pain ratings. It is a self-rated instrument that takes 5 minutes to complete in its short form and 10 minutes in its long form. It is copyrighted but is available royalty-free for clinical use (there is a charge for use in funded research). It has been translated into numerous languages and has been psychometrically validated in many of them.

The long form of the BPI rates pain on the 11-point NRS (i.e., 0-10), but asks four questions: the status of the pain now, at its worst in the past week, at its best in the past week, and on average in the past week. There are seven questions about different kinds of functional impairment, each rated on a similar 11-point scale. The use of analgesics is covered, including the frequency of use, the degree of relief obtained, and the duration of relief. There is a set of yes/no questions about the qualitative nature of the pain, e.g., shooting, throbbing. Finally, the patient is asked to what he or she attributes the pain. The short form of the BPI asks only about the past 24 hours and includes the same four questions about pain severity and seven questions about pain-related impairment. There is a single question about degree of relief obtained from pain medication.

The BPI has been accepted by the US Food and Drug Administration as a primary patient-reported outcome measure in studies of analgesic treatments. It frequently is included as the pain measure in controlled studies of treatments of conditions that cause pain. Pain issues typically encountered by medical psychiatrists include functional impairment due to pain or the fear of pain, tolerability of pain, erroneous attribution of pain, emotional reactions to specific pain treatment modalities, and use of pain medications other than as prescribed. In addition, medical psychiatrists occasionally encounter intractable pain with a neuropathic origin that has not been appreciated or fully addressed. The qualitative description of the pain included in the long form of the BPI can provide clues to neuropathic mechanisms. Overall, the BPI is the pain questionnaire best suited for use in medical psychiatry.

Some additional points can be made:

1. Among patients with brain diseases, those with left hemisphere lesions may prefer to rate pain using a visual method; those with right hemisphere lesions may prefer a verbal method.

2. Ordinal pain scales such as the NRS can be calibrated for individual patients by anchoring the numbers with the patient's rating of nearly universal pain experiences such as muscle aches from a flu-like illness, heartburn, a muscle strain or sprain, menstrual cramps, or a tension headache.

3. Neuropathic pain often involves symptoms in excess of obvious signs, and thus can raise concerns about somatization until a correct diagnosis is made. Neuropathic pains have distinguishing characteristics like "shooting" and "burning" and association with unpleasant numbness. These will be picked up by a scale like the long form of the BPI, with its checklist of pain adjectives. The structured characterization of pain quality is done more extensively by the McGill Pain Questionnaire (MPQ), also available in long and short forms, which strongly emphasizes the qualitative characteristics of the pain (Melzack, 1987). For example, on the short form of the MPQ the patient is given 15 descriptors of pain - 11 sensory and 4 affective - and asked to rate each of them for intensity as 0 = none, 1 = mild, 2 = moderate or 3 = severe.

4. Rating scales like the BPI usefully distinguish pain intensity/severity from pain interference, the latter comprising the impact of the pain on mood, sleep, relations with others, daily activities, and enjoyment of life. They do not usually distinguish intensity of pain – a purely sensory dimension – from *severity* of pain, a dimension that comprises the unpleasantness (hurtfulness) of pain. While these are highly correlated they are not identical, Brain lesions and primary mental disorders can lead to dissociation of pain intensity from degree of hurt; treatments like hypnosis for pain control deliberately induce such a dissociation. When pain and hurt are dissociated in a given patient and pain is rated with a scale like the BPI that treats intensity/severity as a unitary construct, the patient should be instructed to rate "how bad the hurting is" rather than how strong the sensation is.

5. The distress and impairment ("interference") associated with pain often can be modified even when pain continues as a sensory experience. When distress and impairment become the focus of treatment, they should be separately measured. This can be done using the 7 interference items of the BPI.

6. Pain is a major factor in provoking agitation and other behavioral symptoms in individuals with moderate or severe dementia, especially when the patient is too cognitively impaired to describe the pain or request relief. Pain rating scales for patients with dementia rely on nonverbal expressions of discomfort and distress as observed by caregivers. An example of such a scale is the Pain Assessment in Advanced Dementia scale (PAINAD; see Warden et al., 2003). The PAINAD produces a pain score of 0–10 by summing five items, each rated on a 0–2 scale, that capture nonverbal signs of pain and discomfort: breathing (labored breathing or hyperventilation), vocalization (moaning, groaning, or crying), facial expression (sad, frightened, or grimacing), body language (tenseness of the body or agitation), and consolability. It has good psychometric properties and has been cross-validated with similar scales.

SLEEP DISTURBANCE

Sleep has both quantitative and qualitative dimensions. In the setting of general medical illness, patients often feel their sleep is inadequate because it is insufficiently restorative even though time spent asleep might be close to what it was when the patient was in better general health. Non-restorative sleep usually is due to disruption of sleep architecture, with insufficient time spent in the deeper stages of sleep. Another reason sleep can be qualitatively inadequate is that it comes at the wrong time, out of phase with the patient's schedule of activity. Two obvious consequences of nonrestorative sleep are fatigue and excessive daytime sleepiness. Impairment of daytime cognitive and motor performance is another, important because it can lead to poor occupational or academic performance and to motor vehicle accidents. Less obviously, poor-quality sleep can cause or exacerbate depression, and it can impede a patient's response to antidepressant treatment.

Rating sleep is valuable for determining to what extent poor sleep might be affecting a patient's physical and emotional health. If the rating scale has suitable dimensions of measurement, it also can screen patients for specific, treatable sleep disorders.

Sleep can be rated based on a patient and/or an observer's historical account, or it can be comprehensively recorded in a sleep laboratory. More recently, sleep quantity and quality can be measured by inexpensive and widely available technology. Home-based sleep measurement technology adds a quantitative and objective component to sleep ratings.

Sleep rating scales are of two general types: comprehensive scales, and scales designed for screening for specific sleep disorders such as obstructive sleep apnea.

PITTSBURGH SLEEP QUALITY INDEX

The Pittsburgh Sleep Quality Index (PSQI; see Buysse et al., 1989) is a 19-item questionnaire that probes seven domains related to sleep quality: subjective sleep quality, sleep latency, sleep duration, habitual sleep efficiency, sleep disturbances, use of sleeping medication, and daytime dysfunction. Each domain is rated on a scale of 0–3; the sum of domain scores gives an overall sleep quality index that ranges from 0–21. The PSQI is a combination of multiple choice and fill-in-the-blanks items. The scale has high internal consistency within each domain but only moderate correlation of domain scores with the overall scores, compatible with the clinical observation that poor sleep quality is a multidimensional issue. The scale is copyrighted but may be used by clinicians without a royalty; it has been used in over 500 published studies. Cognitively impaired individuals may find it difficult to complete the questionnaire, as the fill-in-the-blanks items require reasonably intact memory function and writing ability.

The PSQI is helpful in describing what is wrong with patients' sleep in a standardized, quantitative format. Its broad scope is useful when evaluating sleep in medical-psychiatric patients with multiple comorbidities that can affect sleep in a variety of ways and can cause daytime impairments that overlap with those caused by sleep disorders. However, it is not designed to screen for any specific sleep disorder or to distinguish between common causes of insomnia or excessive daytime somnolence.

THE INSOMNIA SYMPTOM QUESTIONNAIRE

The Insomnia Symptom Questionnaire (ISQ; see Okun et al., 2009) is a self-rated instrument that focuses on diagnosing and measuring the severity of chronic insomnia. It comprises 13 items, all referring to the patient's experience over the past month. The first five items ask about difficulty falling asleep, difficulty staying asleep, frequent awakenings, feeling that sleep is not sound, and feeling that sleep is unrefreshing. If the patient has any of these complaints, they are asked to rate its frequency on a scale of 1 (don't know) to 2 (less than once a week) to 5 (every night) and indicate how long they have had the problem in weeks, months, or years. If patients have any sleep problems, they complete the next eight questions, which refer to effects of sleep disturbance on daily life, including daytime sleepiness, irritability, fatigue, and so on. These are scored for severity on a scale of 0–4. The rule for identifying cases of insomnia is not a simple score, but rather an algorithm based on item response theory. Patients screen in for chronic insomnia if they have symptoms that include difficulty initiating or maintaining sleep or having nonrefreshing sleep, at least one of the symptoms occurs three or more times a week, symptoms have persisted for 4 weeks or more, and at least one of the eight aspects of daily life has been affected "quite a bit" (3) or "extremely" (4). With this scoring algorithm, the ISQ is more than 90% sensitive to a clinical diagnosis of insomnia, and cases identified with the ISQ show significant differences on polysomnographic indices of sleep quality from non-cases.

EPWORTH SLEEPINESS SCALE

The Epworth Sleepiness Scale (ESS; see Johns, 1991) is a patient questionnaire with eight ordinal items, all concerned with the likelihood of dozing off or falling asleep in particular situations like sitting and reading or riding in a car as a passenger. The patient rates each situation on a scale of 0–3, with 3 signifying a high probability of falling asleep. A score of 9 or higher implies a high probability of a diagnosable sleep disorder. The scale is available in several languages. It is copyrighted but can be used by clinicians without a royalty.

Medical psychiatrists should consider giving patients the ESS not only when they present with sleep complaints but also when (1) there is cognitive impairment that fluctuates during the day, involves mainly attention and memory, and is not explained by delirium or dementia; (2) the patient is taking a medication with the potential to cause sleepiness as a side effect, such as a benzodiazepine or opiate analgesic; (3) the patient has had an at-fault motor vehicle accident; or (4) the patient has had an otherwise-unexplained decline in occupational performance.

THE FATIGUE SEVERITY SCALE

Patients with poor quality sleep can suffer more from fatigue than from sleepiness; fatigue is also a prominent feature of many neurological, autoimmune and infectious diseases that have prominent medical-psychiatric dimensions. Treatment of comorbid or consequential anxiety or depression can alleviate some of the fatigue caused by these conditions; at the same time, many psychotropic medications can exacerbate fatigue.

The Fatigue Severity Scale (Krupp, 1989) is a validated self-assessment instrument for quantifying fatigue. It comprises 9 bidirectional Likert-type ordinal items such as "I am easily fatigued" and "Fatigue interferes with my physical functioning." These are rated from 1 (strongly disagree) to 4 (neutral) to 7 (strongly agree). It has excellent psychometric properties (Valko et al., 2008).

SCREENING FOR OBSTRUCTIVE SLEEP APNEA

Patients identified as having excessive daytime sleepiness or significant fatigue can have disordered nighttime sleep or can be sleepy or fatigued for other reasons. Screening tests for specific common conditions like obstructive sleep apnea (OSA) can aid in the diagnosis. The psychiatric and general medical benefits of treating OSA are large, but polysomnography, the gold standard for OSA diagnosis, is expensive and often difficult to arrange. Screening tests for OSA help avoid polysomnography in patients very unlikely to have the condition, while justifying the expense (and in some cases facilitating third-party payment) of polysomnography or a trial of therapy with continuous positive airway pressure (CPAP) for patients who screen in. Fortunately, screening for moderate to severe OSA utilizing information from the history and physical examination alone has both high sensitivity and high specificity. This can be done with the a four-item screening tool (Takegami et al., 2009). This tool utilizes only four variables: gender, BMI, blood pressure, and the frequency of snoring (from the patient's history). Item scores are 4 if the patient is male, 0 if female; a score of 1–6 based on the patient's body mass index, a score of 1–4 based on the patient's blood pressure, 4 if the patient reports snoring every day or often, and 0 otherwise. The sum is thus between 2 and 18. The authors' screening strategy is interesting: patients with scores of 8 or below are screened out, as they have less than 9% chance of having moderate OSA and no chance of having severe OSA. Patients with scores of 14 or above are referred for polysomnography and CPAP titration because they have a greater than 91% chance of having severe OSA. Those with scores between 9 and 13 inclusive are referred for overnight home pulse oximetry, with a decision about polysomnography based on the results. The two-stage strategy adopted by the authors for OSA screening should be considered for use with other medical-psychiatric conditions where the clinician would like to be conservative, both about ruling out a diagnosis and about investing in an expensive or otherwise difficult diagnostic procedure or treatment.

REAL-TIME RECORDING OF SLEEP DATA

The Fitbit (www.fitbit.com), a personal monitor of sleep and activity that is worn as a wristband, synchronizes with a smartphone to produce a daily log of time in bed, sleeping and waking times, number of awakenings, total sleep time, and restless time during the night. It can be used to corroborate information obtained from rating scales like the ISQ, and to complement them in following the patient's response to treatment. Continuous nighttime pulse oximetry using a fingertip sensor is also available in the consumer market from multiple vendors; it can be utilized to make a decision about the need for polysomnography and sleep apnea treatment in borderline cases.

SEXUAL DYSFUNCTION

The prevalence of sexual dysfunction—and, more broadly, changes in sex life for patients and their spouses or partners—is extremely high in patients with serious chronic diseases. Loss of desire is common, with both endocrine and interpersonal mechanisms involved. Patients with heart disease and/or their sexual partners may fear that sexual activity will be harmful or even fatal. In patients with brain diseases that have altered personality or emotional communication, spouses or partners may feel that the person they once desired no longer exists, even while feelings of non-sexual attachment and caring are stronger than ever. Despite their prevalence and emotional importance, sexual issues often are avoided in physician–patient–caregiver dialogues. They are a routine part of the conversation when the patient is a young man with a spinal cord injury, but not as consistently in the case of a breast cancer patient in her 60s or a man in his 70s with mild Alzheimer's disease.

Incorporation of an adequate sexual history into a medical-psychiatric consultation can be difficult, either because of constraints of time or because of the timing of the interview. Self-rated scales of sexual function offer a way to cover this important area outside of the interview, at a time that is suitable for the patient. Responding in private to a questionnaire evokes less anxiety than being questioned face to face, and responses are less confounded by the physician–patient relationship. The emphasis of sexual dysfunction scales ranges from the mechanical—focused on male erectile dysfunction—to the predominantly interpersonal. The medical psychiatrist using a sexual dysfunction scale should choose a scale with the appropriate emphasis for the patient and the clinical situation.

While there are special scales available for measuring sexual function in specific medical conditions, this chapter will describe three characteristic scales for use in general medical populations. One, the Arizona Sexual Experiences Scale (ASEX) (McGahuey et al., 2000), is a very brief, convenient tool for screening patients for sexual dysfunction and quantifying its change, applicable to both men and women. The other two scales are gender-specific scales that provide deeper insight into the nature of patients' sexual issues, separate objective from subjective dimensions, and give clues to diagnosis.

THE ARIZONA SEXUAL EXPERIENCE SCALE

The Arizona Sexual Experience Scale (ASEX; see McGahuey et al., 1990) comprises five 7-point unidirectional ordinal items constructed so that higher scores are associated with more difficulty. Four items apply to both men and women: overall sex drive, ease of sexual arousal, ease of reaching orgasm, and satisfaction with orgasms. There is a single question for men about ease of getting and maintaining erections and a single question for women about vaginal lubrication. Questions all relate to the prior week, and the questions about orgasm are to be answered only if the patient was sexually active in the prior week. The scale is copyrighted by the University of Arizona, which asks that clinicians seek permission for its use.

The virtues of the ASEX for medical psychiatrists are its brevity, its applicability to both men and women, and the 1-week time frame for recall, which makes it more relevant to patients with fluctuating sexual function, and less demanding on patients with cognitive or emotional issues that would make it difficult for them to accurately summarize a month's experience. The 7-point design gives the scale relatively high sensitivity to incremental changes associated with treatment for sexual dysfunction or the course of the patient's illness.

THE BRIEF SEXUAL FUNCTION INVENTORY

The Brief Sexual Function Inventory (BSFI; see O'Leary et al., 1995) is an 11-item survey of male sexual function comprising 5-point unidirectional ordinal self-ratings of sex drive, erections, ejaculation, the patient's subjective concern over his sexual function, and overall satisfaction. All questions refer to the prior 30 days. The scale, which is in the public domain, has acceptable psychometric properties. It separately measures the objective and subjective dimensions of specific symptoms, and provides more detail than the ASEX on specific functional issues. For example, it has four questions about erections: frequency of having them, their firmness, difficulty of getting them, and the extent to which they are perceived as a problem. The BSFI is well suited for the assessment of male patients with relatively stable chronic conditions. Its focus on the prior 30 days makes it less useful for patients with sexual problems that fluctuate in connection with medical treatments or their level of general medical symptoms. While the BSFI screens for sexual dysfunction, measures it, and describes it, it does not diagnose its cause. Further, the subjective dimensions of sexuality are strongly influenced by a patient's intimate relationships; a sexual partner's response to a man's physical sexual dysfunction can make it a greater or lesser problem for the patient, with a greater or lesser effect on the patient's overall satisfaction.

THE FEMALE SEXUAL FUNCTION INDEX

The Female Sexual Function Index (FSFI; see Weigel et al., 2005) comprises 19 unidirectional ordinal items assessing female sexual function over the prior 4 weeks. Items have either five or six levels. Domains covered are frequency and intensity of desire; frequency, intensity, confidence, and satisfaction with physical and emotional arousal; frequency, difficulty initiating, and difficulty maintaining lubrication; frequency, difficulty reaching, and satisfaction with orgasm; satisfaction with emotional closeness during sexual relations, with sexual relations per se, and with overall sexual life; and pain during or after intercourse. A great virtue of the FSFI is its level of detail—dissecting the issues of frequency, intensity, and subjective experience, and its identification of sexually-associated pain when it is an issue. The 4-week recall period raises issues in patients with unstable medical status, changing treatments, or cognitive difficulties in summarizing 28 days of experience. On the other hand, the longer recall period increases the chances of capturing relevant information from patients who have sexual relations infrequently—a not-uncommon situation in people with significant general medical problems.

The first two questions in the FSFI concern sexual desire, and by themselves they can be used as a screen for hypoactive sexual desire. The first item asks how often the patient felt sexual desire or interest over the previous 4 weeks; the second asks how the patient would rate her level of sexual desire or interest over that period. The frequency and intensity items are summed, yielding a score between 2 and 10. A score of 5 or less identified women with Hypoactive Sexual Desire Disorder with >85% sensitivity and >90% specificity across four different validation studies (Gerstenberger et al., 2010). A particular benefit of this two-question screen is that it does not require that the patient have a sexual partner or be sexually active.

SCALAR SUMMARIES OF HEALTH, FUNCTION, AND THE NEED FOR CARE

Summary measures of the overall functional impact of physical or mental illness have been used in treatment outcome studies for decades. Such measures can be one-dimensional or multidimensional, clinician-rated or self-rated.

Medical psychiatrists can make use of scores on these scales in several ways. Clinician-rated, scalar measures of physical health, function, and the need for care are used to answer the question of "how sick is this patient." They can also be used to provide a global judgment of the outcome of general medical or psychiatric treatment. Two examples are offered here, the Karnofsky Scale (Karnofsky & Burchenal, 1949) and the Global Assessment of Function (Endicott et al., 1976).

KARNOFSKY PERFORMANCE STATUS

The Karnofsky Performance Status (KPS) or "Karnofsky scale" (Karnofsky & Burchenal, 1949; Péus et al., 2013), widely used in palliative care, is a percentage between 0% and 100% that combines an assessment of disease severity and functional impairment due to disease. While it is expressed as a number between 0 and 100, it is not truly a continuous scale; it is better understood as three contiguous scales joined together. It is shown in Table 4.2.

Table 4.2 KARNOFSKY PERFORMANCE STATUS

Able to carry on normal activity and to work; no special care needed.	100	Normal no complaints; no evidence of disease
	90	Able to carry on normal activity; minor signs or symptoms of disease
	80	Normal activity with effort; some signs or symptoms of disease
Unable to work; able to live at home and care for most personal needs; varying amount of assistance needed.	70	Cares for self; unable to carry on normal activity or to do active work
	60	Requires occasional assistance, but is able to care for most personal needs
	50	Requires considerable assistance and frequent medical care
Unable to care for self; requires equivalent of institutional or hospital care; disease may be progressing rapidly.	40	Disabled; requires special care and assistance
	30	Severely disabled; hospital admission is indicated although death not imminent
	20	Very sick; hospital admission necessary; active supportive treatment necessary
	10	Moribund; fatal processes progressing rapidly
	0	Dead

The scale's apparent value is in its efficient communication among different clinicians and specialties when discussing patient populations such as those with pancreatic cancer or ALS that usually follow a progressive and ultimately fatal course, with potentially some periods of improvement or stabilization.

GLOBAL ASSESSMENT OF FUNCTIONING

The Global Assessment of Functioning (GAF; see Endicott et al., 1976; Hilsenroth et al., 2000) combines symptoms and functional impairment differently from the Karnofsky Scale, in keeping with its ultimate focus on the need for treatment and the outcome of treatment of mental illness. In the GAF, either more severe symptomatology or greater functional impairment implies a lower score; significant suicidal behavior implies a score of 20 or below, regardless of the severity of other symptoms or impairments. The GAF focuses on social, occupational, and, where applicable, academic functioning rather than on physical function, and on mental and behavioral symptoms both in themselves and as causes of functional impairment. The interpretation of a GAF score can be complicated by symptoms and impairments due to physical illness, since the GAF is based on the assumption that social and occupational impairments are due to mental illness (Yamauchi et al., 2001). The integration of symptomatic and functional aspects of the GAF is not standardized, and in general there are many open issues about how to optimize its value as a diagnostic tool. In any case, it is insufficiently sensitive to reliably measure small changes in a patient's mental health (Aas, 2011). Despite its very broad acceptance as a scalar summary measure of mental illness, the GAF will rarely be a scale of choice for the medical psychiatrist.

MULTIDIMENSIONAL HEALTH AND HEALTH-RELATED QUALITY OF LIFE MEASURES

Multidimensional scales of health and health-related quality of life usually are questionnaire-based and self-rated. In addition to their use in epidemiological and clinical research, they have clinical utility in two specific areas. By rating several dimensions of symptoms and function, they help clinicians see the tradeoffs of positive and negative effects of treatments, and secondary benefits of treatments for quality of life and well-being. And, by covering a broad scope of issues, they expand the scope of the medical psychiatrist's consideration beyond the issues that feasibly can be covered in an initial consultation. They can thus help direct the evaluation of the patient at follow-up visits. Multidimensional instruments like the World Health Organization Health Related Quality of Life Scale–Brief Version (WHOQOL-BREF) and the SF-36 have particularly broad scope and thus are especially useful for this purpose.

THE SF-36 (36-ITEM SHORT FORM HEALTH SURVEY)

The 36-Item Short Form Health Survey (SF-36; version 2 the SF-36v2) (Ware et al., 2000) is a brief but comprehensive self-rated questionnaire concerning a patient's overall health and function, developed by the RAND Corporation for use in the Medical Outcomes Study and subsequent epidemiological research. While it remains popular in outcomes research, it is less frequently encountered in routine clinical use. Its particular value is its focus on the *functional consequences* of physical and mental illness. Medical psychiatrists working in settings where time limitations make it infeasible to elicit the biographical narrative that puts the present illness into context can use the SF-36 as a shortcut to contextual understanding. The questionnaire takes 5–10 minutes to complete and refers to the patient's health status in the previous 4 weeks; there is a variant available that addresses health status in the past week. Individual items are of several different types: binary; unidirectional ordinal with three, five, or six points; and bidirectional ordinal with five points. Items relate variously to the presence, severity, and frequency of symptoms. Domains are (1) physical functioning, (2) role limitations because of physical health problems, (3) bodily pain, (4) social functioning, (5) general mental health, (6) role limitations because of emotional problems, (7) vitality, and (8) general health perceptions. While the RAND Corporation holds the copyright to the original SF-36, it allows it to be used without charge in both clinical and research contexts as long as any publication based on SF-36 data properly attributes the instrument and notes any modifications made by the user. The instrument is available in numerous languages and has an extensive literature establishing its construct validity, and its sensitivity to changes in health status and differing outcomes of different medical treatments and systems of care. The combination of minimal cost, self-rating with low respondent burden, extensive validation, and broad scope make the SF-36 an instrument of choice for the medical psychiatrist. A revised and somewhat improved version of the instrument is available from a private copyright holder and is subject to a licensing fee, even for clinical use.

THE WORLD HEALTH ORGANIZATION HEALTH RELATED QUALITY OF LIFE SCALE–BRIEF VERSION

The World Health Organization Health Related Quality of Life Scale—Brief Version (WHOQOL Group, 1998) consists of 26 items, each a unidirectional 5-point ordinal scale that covers a very broad range of health-related issues covering domains of overall health and quality of life, physical health, psychological health, social relationships, and environment. In contrast to the SF-36, it includes extensive coverage of social and environmental issues related to health and health care. It is available for clinical use without a fee. There are distinctive questions in the WHOQOL-BREF that can open up productive lines of inquiry concerning the patient's social and environmental history, an area of medical-psychiatric relevance that often has a low priority in evaluations focused on diagnosing and treating acute conditions. Some examples of these questions are:

1. How satisfied are you with the support that you get from your friends?

2. How satisfied are you with the conditions of your living place?

3. To what extent do you have the opportunity for leisure activities?

4. How safe do you feel in your everyday life?

5. Do you have enough money to meet your needs?

COMPREHENSIVE ASSESSMENT INSTRUMENTS FOR POST-ACUTE CARE: THE MINIMUM DATA SET AND THE OUTCOME AND ASSESSMENT INFORMATION SET

Post-acute care, which comprises facility-based care in skilled nursing facilities (SNFs), independent rehabilitation facilities (IRFs), and assisted living facilities (ALFs), as well as formal and informal home health care, is partially reimbursed in the United States by the Medicare and Medicaid systems. With this reimbursement comes regulation, a key component of which is a requirement that the care provider electronically submit standardized clinical assessments as a condition of reimbursement. These standardized assessments are used both for determining reimbursement rates and for measuring the quality of care provided. The standardized assessment for SNFs is called the Minimum Data Set (MDS; see Center for Medicare and Medicaid Services, 2013). The standardized assessment for Medicare-covered skilled home care (as distinguished from home assistance with basic activities of daily living) is the Outcome and Assessment Information Set (OASIS; Center for Medicare and Medicaid Services, 2012). The MDS is of particular interest to medical psychiatrists because its scope includes assessments of mood, cognition, behavior, and pain, along with indicators of the use of psychotropic drugs—particularly antidepressants, antipsychotics, and antianxiety and hypnotic drugs. The neuropsychiatric section of the OASIS is mainly useful for identifying the presence of a mental or behavioral problem and roughly estimating its severity and/or frequency; it provides less support than the MDS for the diagnosis of depression, dementia, or delirium. Both the MDS and the OASIS have their origin in tools for assessing functional dependency and needs for care and supervision, rather than for medical diagnosis; this might explain why some items of natural interest to a psychiatrist are missing. For example, the MDS does not have items dealing with patients' sleep.

An SNF patient's first MDS is based on an assessment that must be completed by day 8 of the SNF stay for patients covered by traditional, fee-for-service Medicare, and by day 14 for all patients regardless of the source of payment. For traditional Medicare patients who remain in the facility less than 8 days, the facility must submit a combined admission/discharge MDS. For patients with other payers who remain in the facility for less than 14 days, the facility must submit a combined admission/discharge MDS unless the patient had an "unplanned discharge." Patients discharged to the community would always have planned discharges unless the discharge was against medical advice. After the initial MDS, follow-up assessments must be submitted on a specified schedule if the patient remains in the facility. In addition, a significant change in a patient's condition, or the start or end of physical and/or occupational therapy, would be an occasion for a required MDS update. Thus, if a medical psychiatrist is called to consult on a patient in an SNF, there is likely to be an MDS available; and if an outpatient or hospital inpatient has recently been in an SNF, MDS data usually can be obtained, although not necessarily immediately.

The OASIS assessment must be completed for all home care patients—regardless of the payer—within 5 days of the start of care, if the home care agency is to be eligible for Medicare reimbursement for *any* of its patients. Thus, if a patient has received formal home care from a Medicare-certified agency for a least 1 week, there will be OASIS data available from the home care agency that cared for the patient. The only exceptions allowed are pediatric patients, obstetrical patients, and those who are receiving no nursing care but only support with instrumental activities such as housecleaning or shopping.

The medical-psychiatric content of the MDS comprises the following:

1. A cognitive assessment. This is done by interview using the Brief Interview for Mental Status (BIMS). If the patient is unable to complete the BIMS, the nursing staff perform an observation-based rating of the patient's memory and "cognitive skills for daily decision making"—essentially executive function.

2. Screening for delirium using the Confusion Assessment Method (Inouye et al., 1990).

3. Screening for depression using the PHQ-9 or PHQ-9-OV.

4. A single-item assessment of the risk of self-harm.

5. A pain interview; if a patient cannot complete the pain interview, there is a pain rating based on observation of behavioral signs of distress and discomfort.

6. Ratings of the frequency of each of several problem behaviors including wandering, verbal or physical abuse of others, and resistance to care.

7. Binary items concerning the presence of hallucinations or delusions.

8. The number of days in the past week the patient received any drug in each of several classes of psychotropic drug: antidepressant, antipsychotic, antianxiety, and hypnotic.

9. Whether the patient has a history of chronic mental illness or mental retardation; there are specific questions about

depression, bipolar disorder, schizophrenia, anxiety, substance abuse, and post-traumatic stress disorder.

Curiously, the MDS does not include a sleep history apart from the item on the PHQ-9 relating to changes in sleep pattern.

The OASIS provides a much smaller number of neuropsychiatric items, with the effect that it is a relatively nonspecific screen for psychiatric conditions not yet explicitly diagnosed. This is in contrast to the MDS, which actually can be used to make reasonably confident new diagnoses of depression, delirium, or cognitive impairment. OASIS item responses are clinical judgments based on all data available to the clinician, including medical records, interviews of the patient, observations of the patient, communications from other clinicians, and interviews of caregivers. The relevant content comprises the following:

1. A composite rating of level of consciousness, attention, orientation, comprehension, and immediate memory on the day of the evaluation, using a single-item 5-point scale ranging from 0 (intact) to 4 (totally dependent due to delirium, persistent vegetative state, stupor, or coma).

2. A single-item 5-point scale rating the temporal pattern of a patient's confusion over the last 14 days, ranging from 0 (not confused) to 1 (confused in new situations only) to 4 (constantly confused).

3. A single-item 5-point scale rating the frequency with which a patient has felt anxious (or shown signs of anxiety) during the past 14 days.

4. A complex item concerning depression screening. The item asks if the patient has been screened for depression by the agency using a standardized instrument—one that has been validated for use in a community-dwelling home care population—and if so, whether the instrument indicated a need for further evaluation for depression. One option is to complete the PHQ-2, a two-item version of the PHQ-9 with questions about the frequency of low mood and the frequency of loss of pleasure or interest in the last 14 days.

5. A checklist of six behavioral symptoms; items are checked if they occurred at least once in the prior week. The items are memory deficit, impaired decision making, verbal disruption, physical aggression, "disruptive, infantile, or socially inappropriate behavior," and "delusional, hallucinatory, or paranoid behavior."

6. A 6-point scale rating the frequency of disruptive or dangerous behavior.

While the medical-psychiatric content of the OASIS is much less rich than that of the MDS, it is still valuable in several ways. It is helpful in setting the context of the first encounter with a patient currently receiving home care. And, when a patient receiving home care has a change in mental, behavioral, or functional status, the scales of the OASIS provide a standardized way for the nursing staff to communicate what has changed.

WHAT'S NEXT: THE PATIENT-REPORTED OUTCOME MEASUREMENT SYSTEM

Over the years since many currently-used questionnaire-based rating scales were developed there have been substantial advances in psychometric theory and technology. The National Institutes of Health (NIH) in 2002 began an initiative to develop new methods for patient-reported healthcare outcome measurement—one that emphasized a rigorous and methodical approach to developing and validating new measures and that took full advantage of computerized adaptive testing. Computerized adaptive testing permits the patient's responses to current questions to determine the choice of future questions. This enables a scale to be simultaneously broader in scope and richer in detail, without compromising efficiency and user-friendliness. All scales developed under the initiative are in the public domain, though private entities are involved in developing related software and in providing fee-based services to users. Extensive information about the Patient-Reported Outcome Measurement System (PROMIS) initiative and the scales developed under it are available from the NIH website www.nihpromis.org.

Areas tested by PROMIS instruments include the following:

Emotional distress: anger, anxiety, and depression

Applied cognition: abilities and general concerns

Psychosocial illness impact: positive and negative

Alcohol: positive effects, negative effects, positive expectancies, and negative expectancies

Fatigue: general and cancer-specific

Pain: behavior, interference, and intensity, general and cancer-specific

Physical function: mobility and upper extremity, general and cancer-specific

Sleep: sleep disturbance and sleep-related impairment

Sexual function: satisfaction, interest, lubrication, vaginal pain, erectile function, orgasm, therapeutic aids, sexual activities, anal discomfort, and interfering factors

Social roles: satisfaction with social roles, ability to participate in them and actual participation in them; satisfaction with discretionary social activities; companionship, instrumental support, informational support, and emotional support; and social isolation

PROMIS is a source of forms for paper-based administration, items for constructing customized scales, and Web-based testing with automated scoring. It remains to be seen when and how the PROMIS resources will replace well-established scales. The familiarity of a scale can trump its psychometric properties, especially if one of the purposes of the scale is communication across specialties and disciplines.

COMBINING RATING SCALES TO ADDRESS PATIENT-SPECIFIC ISSUES: "THE INSTRUMENT PANEL"

Patients seen in medical-psychiatric contexts typically have multiple comorbid conditions—several medical conditions and at least one mental disorder—and are taking multiple medications. When efforts are made to treat one disease, syndrome, or symptom, it is not unusual to make another one worse. If the symptoms that get worse cause more distress or functional impairment than the ones that are relieved, the patient may feel globally worse and may reject the treatment—even if it is effective for its specific indication. Simply asking patients about side effects is not enough, since a treatment-induced problem might not be linked by the patient to that treatment, and because patients often do not complain about negative symptoms such as apathy or loss of function.

Patients in general are concerned about six goals, variably emphasizing one or another:

1. Longevity, including preventing disease and removing threats to life;

2. Relief of pain and other unpleasant symptoms;

3. Avoiding side effects of treatment;

4. Positive well-being, vigor, and ability to enjoy life;

5. Ability to function in physical, social, and occupational realms; and

6. Quality of familial and intimate relationships.

From the patient's viewpoint, the doctor's priority of diagnosing and treating diseases is merely a means to the above ends. And, when one of the six concerns must be traded off against another, different patients will have different preferences. For example, some patients would prefer to die sooner or to suffer cognitive impairment rather than live in severe pain, while others will tolerate great discomfort in order to live a bit longer and to retain their intellectual function.

The medical-psychiatric evaluation should give the psychiatrist a good picture of a patient's goals and their relative importance. Review of the medical history and knowledge of the patient's specific medical conditions and treatments inform the prediction of potential tradeoffs between desirable goals across the course of illness. The psychiatrist can then create an "instrument panel" of rating scales that can be followed from one visit to the next, helping to identify when improvement in one area is associated with decline in another and leads to an overall negative effect from the patient's viewpoint. When this happens, changes in either the psychiatric or general medical treatment strategy may be helpful.

A basic instrument panel might include a measure of the severity of symptoms of the patient's most important medical condition, with a second condition included if there are two of equal importance; a pain rating scale if pain has been a symptom of the general medical illness; a depression rating scale; another psychiatric rating scale if there is a history of a specific psychiatric illness; a cognitive rating scale; and a broad-scope functional assessment measure such as the SF-36. If the patient's cognitive status and motivation permit the use of self-rated scales, he or she can be given a set of questionnaires to be completed prior to the next visit. The burden on the patient is relatively small, and the benefits are several. The visit is not excessively taken up by closed-ended questions, leaving more time for the patient's agenda and for answering questions. The scope of topics covered is more complete than would be feasible in an interview. Documentation is improved. And, patterns of simultaneous changes can be appreciated that might go unnoticed without seeing change in scale scores side by side.

RATING SCALES AS A TOOL FOR PATIENT EDUCATION AND ALLIANCE-BUILDING

When patients and their caregivers come to understand that mental disorders are well defined, that they have been extensively and rigorously studied, and that recommended therapies are evidence-based, they are more likely to accept the idea of psychiatric treatment and more likely to adhere to treatment once it is started. Prejudice and stigma persist, and while a rating scale may not be as destigmatizing as a blood test or a brain image, its quantitative nature can engage a more objective view by the patient. The Intelligence Quotient, which is a score on a psychometric rating scale, is widely accepted—perhaps excessively so—by the general public as a valid measurement of something real and important. Further, the Internet has widely disseminated quantitative collective consumer ratings of hotels, restaurants, films, and even prescription drugs. In the current social context, the performance of a rating scale and the discussion of the meaning of the items and the scores can enhance the relationship between the patient and the clinician.

USE OF RATING SCALES TO ESTABLISH REMISSION

In medical-psychiatric contexts it is common to encounter patients who have been started on psychotropic drugs—typically SSRI antidepressants or benzodiazepines—by nonpsychiatric physicians and have remained on them for months or even years while continuing to have significant mental symptoms. General medical physicians may not see complete remission of depression as realistic in the context of serious chronic medical illness—but in fact, many patients cope well with illness, maintaining a positive affect and taking pleasure in living. When a patient was not depressed prior to developing a general medical illness, the goal for antidepressant treatment should be remission, not merely relief, unless it becomes clear after serious and persistent treatment—including trials of different antidepressants and psychotherapy—that remission is not a feasible goal. A significantly elevated score on a depression rating scale or an anxiety rating scale can establish—and effectively communicate to general medical physicians, patients, and caregivers—that psychotropic drug treatment to date has not resolved the problem and that the diagnosis, drug, and/or dosage need to be revisited. In this connection it is very helpful for all physicians practicing in a particular setting to be familiar with at least one common depression rating scale such as the PHQ-9 or the BDI.

CLINICAL PEARLS

- Rating scales and screening tests should be a routine part of the practice of medical psychiatry.

- Questionnaire-based tests—whether completed by the patient or by caregivers or other informants—are the most efficient way to quantify symptoms and to expand the scope of medical-psychiatric evaluation without increasing the length of clinical encounters.

- Impairment of cognition, metacognition, or self-awareness can reduce the validity of self-rated scales. Relationship issues—or neuropsychiatric issues in the informant—can reduce the validity of scales rated by a caregiver or other informant.

- Discrepancies between symptom ratings by the patient, the caregiver, and the clinician are valuable diagnostic data; the clinician should analyze them.

- Clinicians should select for routine use a set of rating scales that are well suited to the patient populations they usually see.

- Specialized scales for medical-psychiatric problems such as kinesiophobia or sleep apnea work better than generic rating scales developed primarily for patients with primary mental disorders without general medical comorbidity.

- The choice of a cognitive screening test should be patient-specific and selected to avoid floor and ceiling effects; the appropriate cut point for abnormality will vary according to the patient's educational level and premorbid functioning.

- For patients with multiple conditions and/or adverse effects of medications, the use of a multiscale "instrument panel" can help both the clinician and the patient to understand tradeoffs between the benefits and adverse effects of treatment, and to appreciate how psychiatric and general medical issues interact to affect function and well-being.

- Scores on widely known rating scales such as the Numerical Rating Scale for pain or the MMSE can be used to efficiently and effectively communicate the presence and severity of symptoms and syndromes across disciplinary lines.

- When rating scales are used as screening tests there is always a tradeoff between sensitivity and specificity. Criteria for identifying cases should be set according to the clinical purpose of the test, and results should not be over-interpreted. The C-SSRS with a low cut point can identify patients who definitely *do not* need intensive suicide precautions; those just above the threshold aren't necessarily at high risk, they just need further clinical assessment. Similarly, the MMSE with a cut point of 24 can identify patients who are cognitively impaired and definitely need further assessment for the cause, but it does not rule out cognitive impairment in patients with higher scores.

- A two-stage approach to screening can reconcile issues of sensitivity and specificity. One cut point is used to identify definite cases, and another one is used to definitely rule out the diagnosis. Patients with scores between the two cut points are assessed with a second method that has the power to discriminate cases from non-cases among patients with such intermediate scores. The use of nighttime monitoring of PaO_2 in patients with intermediate scores on the four-question test for obstructive sleep apnea is an excellent example of this approach.

DISCLOSURE STATEMENT

Dr. Fogel is Chief Scientific Officer of Synchroneuron Inc., Managing Director of Anal-Gesic LLC, and Executive Vice President of PointRight Inc. He is the sole inventor or lead inventor on several pharmaceutical patents. In his opinion these affiliations do not entail any conflict of interest with regard to the editing of this book or his personal contributions to it. He has no other potential conflicts, direct or indirect, financial or otherwise, to disclose in connection with the editing of this book or his personal contributions to it.

REFERENCES

Aas, I. H. M. (2011). Guidelines for rating global assessment of functioning. *Annals of General Psychiatry*, 10, 2.

Abramowitz, J. S., & Deacon, B. J. (2006). Psychometric properties and construct validity of the Obsessive-Compulsive Inventory-Revised: replication and extension with a clinical sample. *Anxiety Disorders*, 20, 1016–1035.

Alexopoulos, G. A., Abrams, R. C., Young, R. C., et al. (1988). Cornell scale for depression in dementia. *Biological Psychiatry*, 23, 271–284.

Beck, A. T., Epstein, N., Brown, G., & Steer, R. A. (1988). An inventory for measuring clinical anxiety: psychometric properties. *Journal of Consulting and Clinical Psychology*, 56(6), 893–897.

Beck, A. T., Steer, R. A., Brown, G. K. (1996). *Beck Depression Inventory-II Manual*. San Antonio, TX: Psychological Corporation.

Beck, A. T., Steer, R. A., & Garbin, M. G. (1988). Psychometric properties of the Beck Depression Inventory: twenty-five years of evaluation. *Clinical Psychology Review*, 8, 776–100.

Blake, D. D., Weathers, F. W., Nagy, L. M., et al. (1990). A clinician rating scale for assessing current and lifetime PTSD: The CAPS-1. *The Behavior Therapist*, 13, 187–188.

Blake, D. D., Weathers, F. W., Nagy, L. M., et al. (1995). The development of a clinician-administered PTSD scale. *Journal of Traumatic Stress, 8*, 75–90.

Blanchard, E. B., Jones-Alexander J., Buckley, T. C., et al. (1996). Psychometric properties of the PTSD checklist (PCL). *Behaviour Research and Therapy, 34*, 669–673.

Burwinkle T., Robinson, J. P., & Turk, D. C. (2005). Fear of movement: factor structure of the Tampa Scale of Kinesiophobia in patients with fibromyalgia syndrome. *Journal of Pain, 6*(6), 384–391.

Buysse, D. J., Reynolds, C. F., Monk, T. H., Berman, S. R., & Kupfer, D. J. (1989). The Pittsburgh Sleep Quality Index: A new instrument for psychiatric practice and research. *Psychiatry Research, 28*, 193–213.

Center for Medicare and Medicaid Services. (2012). OASIS-C Guidance Manual. Available at: http://www.cms.gov/Medicare/Quality-Initiatives-Patient-Assessment-Instruments/HomeHealthQualityInits/HHQIOASISUserManual.html.

Center for Medicare and Medicaid Services. MDS 3.0 RAI Manual. Available at: http://www.cms.gov/Medicare/Quality-Initiatives-Patient-Assessment-Instruments/NursingHomeQualityInits/MDS30RAIManual.html.

Clarke, D. E., Ko, J. Y., Kuhl, E. A., van Reekum, R., Salvador, R., & Marin, R. S. (2011). Are the available apathy measures reliable and valid? A review of the psychometric evidence. *Journal of Psychosomatic Research, 70*, 73–97

Cox, D. J., Irvine A., Gonder-Frederick L., Nowacek, G., & Butterfield, J. (1987). Fear of hypoglycemia: quantification, validation and utilization. *Diabetes Care, 10*, 617–621.

Cummings, J. (1997). The Neuropsychiatric Inventory: Assessing psychopathology in dementia patients. Neurology 48 (Suppl. 6): S10-S16.

Damsgard, E., Fors, T., Anke, A., & Røe, C. (2007). The Tampa Scale of Kinesiophobia: a Rasch analysis of its properties in low back and more widespread pain. *Journal of Rehabilitation Medicine, 39*(9), 672–678.

Davidson, J. R.T., Book, S. W., Colket, J. T., Tupler, L. A., Roth, S., David, D., et al. (1997). Assessment of a new self-rating scale for post-traumatic stress disorder. *Psychological Medicine, 27*, 153–160.

DeLoach, L. J., Higgins, M. S., Caplan, A. B., & Stiff, J. L. (1998). The visual analog scale in the immediate postoperative period: intrasubject variability and correlation with a numeric scale. *Anesthesia and Analgesia, 86*(1), 102–106.

Endicott, J., Spitzer, R. L., Fleiss, J. L., & Cohen, J. (1976). The Global Assessment Scale: a procedure for measuring overall severity of psychiatric disturbance. *Archives of General Psychiatry, 33*, 766–771.

Fazel, S., Singh, J. P., Doll, H., & Grann, M. (2012). Use of risk assessment instruments to predict violent and antisocial behaviour in 73 samples involving 24,827 people: systematic review and meta-analysis. *British Medical Journal, 345*, e4692

Foa, E. B., Huppert, J. D., Leiberg S, Langner, R., Kichic, R., Hajcak, G., et al. (2002). The Obsessive-Compulsive Inventory: development and validation of a short version. *Psychological Assessment, 14*(4), 485–496.

Foa, E. B., Kozak, M. J., Salkovskis, P. M., Coles, M. E., & Amir, N. (1998). The validation of a new obsessive-compulsive disorder scale: the obsessive-compulsive inventory. *Psychological Assessment, 10*, 206–214.

Gerstenberger, E. P., Rosen, R. C., Brewer, J. V., Meston, C. M., Brotto, L. A., Wiegel, M., & Sand, M. (2010). Sexual desire and the female sexual function index (FSFI): a sexual desire cutpoint for clinical interpretation of the FSFI in women with and without Hypoactive Sexual Desire Disorder. *Journal of Sexual Medicine, 7*, 3096–3103.

Gonder-Frederick, L. A., Schmidt, K. M., Vajda, K. A., Greear, M. L., Singh, H., Shepard, J. A., et al. (2011). Psychometric properties of the Hypoglycemia Fear Survey-II for adults with type I diabetes. *Diabetes Care, 34*, 801–806.

Goodman, W. K., Price, L. H., Rasmussen, S. A., Mazure, C., Delgado, P., Heninger, G. R., & Charney, D. S. (1989a). The Yale-Brown Obsessive Compulsive Scale– II. Validity. *Archives of General Psychiatry, 46*, 1012–1016.

Goodman, W. K., Price, L. H., Rasmussen, S. A., Mazure, C., Fleischman, R. L., Hill, C. L., et al. (1989b). The Yale-Brown Obsessive Compulsive Scale–I. *Development, use, and reliability. Archives of General Psychiatry, 46*, 1006–1011.

Grace, J., & Malloy, P. (2001). *Frontal Systems Behavior Scale (FrSBe): Professional Manual.* Lutz, PL: Psychological Assessment Resources.

Granger, C. V., Hamilton, B. B., Linacre, J. M., Heinemann A. W., & Wright, B. D. (1993). Performance profiles of the Functional Independence Measure. *American Journal of Physical Medicine & Rehabilitation, 72*(2), 84–89.

Granger, C. V. (1998). The emerging science of functional assessment: our tool for outcomes analysis. *Archives of Physical Medicine & Rehabilitation, 79*(3), 235–240.

Hamilton, M. (1959). The assessment of anxiety states by rating. British *Journal of Medical Psychology, 32*(1), 50–55.

Hamilton, M. (1980). Rating depressive patients. *Journal of Clinical Psychiatry, 41*, 21–24.

Hare, R. D. (2003). *Manual for the Revised Psychopathy Checklist*, 2nd ed. Toronto, ON: Multi-Health Systems.

Hilsenroth, M. J., Ackerman, S. J., Blagys, M. D., Baumann, B. D., Baity, M. R., Smith, S. R., et al. (2000). Reliability and validity of DSM-IV Axis V. *American Journal of Psychiatry, 157*, 1858–1863.

Improving Access to Psychological Therapies. (2013). The IAPT Phobia Scale. Available at: http://www.patient.co.uk/doctor/IAPT-Phobia-Scale.

Irvine, A., Cox, D. J., & Gonder-Frederick, L. (1994). The Fear of Hypoglycemia Scale. In Bradley, C. (Ed.). *Handbook of psychology and diabetes: a guide to psychological measurement in diabetes research and practice* (pp. 133–158). New York: Psychology Press (reprinted 2013).

Karnofsky, D. A., & Burchenal, J. H. (1949). The clinical evaluation of chemotherapeutic agents in cancer. In C. M. McLeod (Ed.) *Evaluation of chemotherapeutic agents* (pp. 191–205). New York: Columbia University Press.

Katz, S., Ford, A. B., Moskowitz, R. W., Jackson, B. A., & Jaffe, M. W. (1963). Studies of illness in the aged: the Index of ADL, a standardized measure of biological and psychological function. *JAMA, 185*, 914–919.

Kim, G., DeCoster., J, Huang, C. H., & Bryant, A. N. (2013). A meta-analysis of the factor structure of the Geriatric Depression Scale (GDS): the effects of language. *International Psychogeratrics, 25*(1), 71–81.

Kleinknecht, R. A., Thorndike, R. M., & Walls, M. M. (1996). Factorial dimensions and correlates of blood, injury, injection and related medical fears: cross validation of the medical fear survey. *Behavioral Research and Therapy, 34*(4), 323–331.

Kori, S. H., Miller, R. P., & Todd, D. D. (1990). Kinesiophobia: a new view of chronic pain behavior. *Pain Management, 3*, 35–42.

Kroenke, K., Spitzer, R. L., & Williams, J. B. W. (2001). The PHQ-9: Validity of a brief depression severity measure. *Journal of General Internal Medicine, 16*, 606–613.

Krupp, L. B. (1989). The fatigue severity scale: Application to patients with multiple sclerosis and systemic lupus erythematosus. *Archives of Neurology, 46*, 1121–1123.

Lawton, M. P., & Brody, E. M. (1969). Assessment of older people: Self-maintaining and instrumental activities of daily living. *Gerontologist, 9*, 179–186.

Marc, L. G., Raue, P. J., & Bruce, M. L. (2008). Screening performance of the geriatric depression scale (GDS-15) in a diverse elderly home care population. *American Journal of Geriatric Psychiatry, 16*(11), 914–921.

Marin, R. S., Biedrzycki, R. C., & Firinciogullari, S. (1991). Reliability and validity of the Apathy Evaluation Scale. *Psychiatry Research, 38*(2), 143–162.

McDermott, B. E., Quanbeck, C. D., Busse D., Yastro, K., & Scott, C. L. (2008). The accuracy of risk assessment instruments in the prediction of impulsive versus predatory aggression. *Behavioral Sciences & the Law 26*(6), 759–77.

McDowell, I. (2006). *Measuring health: a guide to rating scales and questionnaires.* New York: Oxford University Press.

McGahuey, C. A., Gelenberg, A. J., Laukes, C. A., Moreno, F. A., Delgado, P. L., McKnight, K. M., et al. (2000). The Arizona Sexual Experience Scale (ASEX): reliability and validity. *Journal of Sex & Marital Therapy, 26*, 25–40.

Mundt, J. C., Greist, J. H., Gelenberg, A. J., Katzelnick, D. J., Jefferson, J. W., Modell, J. G., et al. (2010). Feasibility and validation of a computer-automated Columbia-Suicide Severity Rating Scale using interactive voice response technology. *Journal of Psychiatric Research, 44*(16), 1224–1228.

Munetz, M. R., & Benjamin, S. (1988). How to examine patients using the Abnormal Involuntary Movement Scale. *Hospital & Community Psychiatry 39*(11), 1172–1177.

Nasreddine, Z. S., Phillips, N. A., Bédirian, V., Charbonneau, S., Whitehead, V., Collin, I., et al. (2005). The Montreal Cognitive Assessment, MoCA: a brief screening tool for mild cognitive impairment. *Journal of the American Geriatric Society, 53*(4), 695–659.

National Institutes of Health. (2010). *Healthy People 2020 Foundation Health Measure Report: Health-Related Quality of Life and Well-Being.* Bethesda MD: National Institutes of Health.

National Institutes of Health (2014). www.nihpromis.org. Accessed June 22, 2014.

O'Leary, M. P., Fowler, F. J., Lenderking, W. R., Barber, B., Sagnier, P. P., Guess, H. A., et al. (1995). A brief male sexual function inventory for urology. *Urology, 465*, 697–706.

Okun, M. L., Krayvitz, H. M., Sowers, M. F., Moul, D. E., Buysse, D. J., Hall, M., et al. (2009). Psychometric evaluation of the insomnia symptom questionnaire: a self-report measure to identify chronic insomnia. *Journal of Clinical Sleep Medicine, 5*(1), 41–51.

Overall, J. E., & Gorham, D. R. (1962). The Brief Psychiatric Rating Scale. *Psychological Reports, 10*, 799–812.

Péus, D., Newcomb, N., & Hofer, S. A. (2013). Appraisal of the Karnofsky Performance Status and proposal of a simple algorithmic system for its evaluation. *BMC Medical Informatics and Decision Making, 13*(1), 72. [Epub ahead of print, July 19.]

Phillips, L. J. (2012). Measuring symptoms of depression: comparing the Cornell Scale for Depression in Dementia and the Patient Health Questionnaire-9-Observation Version. *Research in Gerontological Nursing, 5*(1), 34–42.

Posner, K., Brown, G. K., Stanley, B., Brent, D. A., Yershova, K. V., Oquendo, M. A., et al. (2011). The Columbia-Suicide Severity Rating Scale: Initial validation and internal consistency findings from three multi-site studies with adolescents and adults. *American Journal of Psychiatry, 168*, 1266–1277.

Raskin, J., George, T., Granger, R. E., et al. (2012). Apathy in currently nondepressed patients treated with an SSRI for a major depressive episode: outcomes following randomized switch to either duloxetine or escitalopram. *Psychiatric Research, 46*(5), 667–674.

Roberts, J. C., deRoon-Cassini, T. A., & Brasel, K. J. (2010). Posttraumatic stress disorder: a primer for trauma surgeons. *Journal of Trauma, 69*, 231–237.

Roelofs, J., van Breukelen, G., Sluiter, J., et al. (2011). Norming of the Tampa Scale for Kinesiophobia across pain diagnoses and various countries. *Pain, 152*(5), 1090–1095.

Royall, D. R., Cordes, J. A., & Polk, M. (1998). CLOX: an executive clock drawing task. *Journal of Neurology, Neurosurgery and Psychiatry, 64*(5), 588–594.

Royall, D. R., Mahurin, R. K., & Gray, K. F. (1992). Bedside assessment of executive cognitive impairment: the executive interview. *Journal of the American Geriatrics Society, 40*(12), 1221–1226.

Royall, D. R., Mulroy, A. R., Chiodo, L. K., & Polk, M. J. (1999). Clock drawing is sensitive to executive control: a comparison of six methods. *The Journals of Gerontology Series B: Psychological Sciences and Social Sciences, 54*(5), P328–P333.

Rush, A. J., First, M. B., & Blacker, D. (Eds.). (2008). *Handbook of psychiatric measures* (2nd edition). Washington, DC: American Psychiatric Publishing, Inc.

Saliba, D., DiFilippo, S., Edelen, M. O., Kroenke, K., Buchanan, J., & Streim, J. (2012). Testing the PHQ-9 interview and observational versions (PHQ-9-OV) for MDS 3.0. *Journal of the American Medical Directors Association, 13*(7), 618–625.

Sheikh, J. I., & Yesavage, J. A. (1986). Geriatric Depression Scale (GDS): Recent evidence and development of a shorter version. In Brink, T. L., (Ed.). *Clinical gerontology: a guide to assessment and intervention.* (pp. 165–173). London: Routledge.

Shelby, R. A., Somers, T. J., Keefe, F. J., DeVellis, B. M., Patterson, C., Renner, J. B., et al. (2012). Brief fear of movement scale for osteoarthritis. *Arthritis Care Research, 64*(6), 862–871.

Shon, J. M., Lee, D. Y., Seo, E. H., Sohn, B. K., Kim, J. W., Park, S. Y., et al. (2013). Functional neuroanatomical correlates of the executive clock drawing task (CLOX) performance in Alzheimer's disease: an FDG-PET study. *Neuroscience, 246*, 271–280.

Snell, W. E., Gum, S., Shuck, R. L., Mosley, J. A., & Hite, T. L. (1995). The Clinical Anger Scale: preliminary reliability and validity. *Journal of Clinical Psychology, 51*(2), 215–216.

Spielberger, C. D., Gorsuch, R. R., & Luchene, R. E. (1970). *State-Trait Personality Inventory.* Palo Alto, CA: Consulting Psychologists Press.

Spitzer, R. L., Kroenke K, Williams, J. B., & Löwe, B. (2006). A brief measure for assessing generalized anxiety disorder: the GAD-7. *Archives of Internal Medicine, 166*(10), 1092–1097.

Steer, R. A., Ball, R., Ranieri, W. F., & Beck, A. T. (1999). Dimensions of the Beck depression inventory-II in clinically depressed outpatients. *Journal of Clinical Psychology, 55*(1), 117–128.

Stout, J. C., Ready, R. E., Grace, J., Malloy, P. F., & Paulsen, J. S. (2003). Factor analysis of the frontal systems behavioral scale (FrSBe). *Assessment, 10*(1), 79–85.

Takegami, M., Hayashino, Y., Chin, K., Sokejima, S., Kadotani, H., Akashiba, T., et al. (2009). Simple four-variable screening tool for identification of patients with sleep-disordered breathing. *Sleep, 32*(7), 939–948.

Tape, T. G. (2013). Interpreting Diagnostic Tests. Available at: http://gim.unmc.edu/dxtests/

Valko, P. O., Bassetti, C. L., Bloch, K. E., Held, U., & Baumann, C. R. (2008). Validation of the fatigue severity scale in a Swiss cohort. *Sleep, 31*(11), 1601–1607.

Wancata, J., Alexandrowicz, R., Marquart, B., Weiss, M., & Friedrich, F. (2006). The criterion validity of the Geriatric Depression Scale: a systematic review. *Acta Psychiatrica Scandinavica, 114*(6), 398–410.

Warden, V., Hurley, A. C., & Volicer, L. (2003). Development and psychometric validation of the pain assessment in advanced dementias (PAINAD) scale. *Journal of the American Medical Directors Association, 4*, 9–15.

Ware, J. E., Kosinski, M., & Dewey, J. E. (2000). *How to score version two of the SF-36 health survey.* Lincoln, RI: QualityMetric, Incorporated.

Weigel, M., Meston, C., & Rosen, R. (2005). The female sexual function index (FSFI): cross-validation and development of clinical cutoff scores. *Journal of Sex and Marital Therapy, 31*(1), 1–20.

Wikipedia: Sensitivity and Specificity. Available at: www.wikipedia.org/sensitivity_and_specificity.

Williams, J. B. (1988). A structured interview guide for the Hamilton Depression Rating Scale. *Archives of General Psychiatry, 45*, 742–747.

Woby, S. R., Roach, N. K., & Urmston, M. (2005). Psychometric properties of the TSK-11: a shortened version of the Tampa scale for kinesiophobia. Pain 117(1–2), 137–144.

WHOQOL Group. (1998). Development of the World Health Organization WHOQOL-BREF quality of life assessment. Psychol. Med. 28, 551–5458

Yamauchi, K., Ono, Y., Baba, K., & Ikegami, N.(2001). The actual process of rating the Global Assessment of Functioning scale. *Comprehensive Psychiatry 42*(5), 403–409.

5.

LABORATORY TESTS

Kimberly Stoner

INTRODUCTION

Nearly a century ago, William J. Mayo wrote in *Surgery, Gynecology, and Obstetrics*, "I have been surprised to note the readiness with which high-grade young men, graduates from medical institutions which are models of our time, yield to the temptation of machine-made diagnoses." (Huth & Murray, 2000, p. 354). If Dr. Mayo was concerned about overreliance on technology in 1923, one can only imagine what he would think of medical practice today. Countless biomarkers of disease states have been discovered and are measured in laboratories daily. MRI centers have appeared in shopping malls and billboards encouraging drivers to come in for a variety of screening CT scans. Computer-savvy people search websites in an effort to find a diagnosis that explains their symptoms, albeit with a reported average success rate of only 22.1% (Siempos et al., 2008). "Machine-made diagnoses" are abundant.

Despite the increased availability, laboratory testing is not a substitute for a thorough patient history and physical exam for clinicians to diagnose and manage patients (Hampton, et al., 1975). Decades later this sentiment persists. While laboratory testing is important, reviewing the history thoroughly and conducting a clinical interview remain the "cornerstones" (Hendren & He, 2006) in the diagnosis and treatment of psychiatric conditions. Symptoms elicited during the history and physical exam findings allow clinicians to generate a differential diagnosis, with laboratory tests and imaging studies then confirming or refuting their hypotheses. Several factors have led to the shift away from widespread use of screening comprehensive metabolic profiles, toward more hypothesis-driven, selective testing. Skyrocketing healthcare costs have led some insurers to stop reimbursing for laboratory tests drawn without clear indication (Staver, 1979). Concerns have been raised about the risks of radiation exposure for patients who undergo repeated imaging studies (Hendrick, 2010). Research has led to the revision of clinical practice guidelines, upon the determination that not all patients will benefit from screening. In addition to the lack of survival benefit for certain age groups or the lack of cost-effectiveness of screening in low-risk populations, there is increasing recognition of potential harm to patients with false-positive test results (Salz, Richman, & Brewer, 2010).

While an increased emphasis on evidence-based medical practice and cost-containment measures have led to more judicious use, patients continue to undergo many laboratory tests annually. It is critically important for psychiatrists who provide consultative or collaborative care to medical patients to be cognizant of the indications for laboratory testing and to be competent in the interpretation of test results. There are many clinically sound reasons for psychiatrists to order laboratory tests in medically ill patients. Diagnostic criteria for many psychiatric diseases require that general medical conditions be excluded as the primary cause of patients' symptoms. Certain psychiatric populations are at higher risk for having lab abnormalities including geriatric patients, patients with alcohol dependence, and eating disorder patients. Some psychiatric medications may lead to lab abnormalities (see chapter 23, Medically Significant Side Effects of Psychotropic Drugs, to review these medications) or require monitoring for toxicities. Laboratory testing may help psychiatrists detect when patients with addiction have relapsed, or if patients have not been compliant with taking prescribed medications. This chapter reviews general principles of laboratory testing and identifies laboratory tests that may be part of an appropriate evaluation for patients presenting with some psychiatric syndromes.

PRINCIPLES OF LABORATORY MEDICINE

"NORMAL" VALUES AND THEIR SIGNIFICANCE

Laboratory test results are considered "abnormal" when they fall outside of the reference range employed by the laboratory performing the test. Normal values are usually established by determining the average value and including two standard deviations above and below the mean (Edwards & Baird, 2005). This statistical approach will identify 95% of test results as being "normal" with the 2.5% of highest values and 2.5% of lowest values deemed "abnormal." However, statistical significance does not always portend clinical significance. The distinction between disease and health is seldom a well-demarcated line lying two standard deviations from the mean. A hypoglycemic patient with a blood glucose of 69 mg/dl may experience fewer symptoms of hypoglycemia than a poorly controlled diabetic patient with a "normal" glucose of 70 mg/dl. Similarly, a statistically insignificant lab test result that falls within the reference range may still be clinically important. Patients who have a baseline creatinine of 0.6 mg/dl have acute kidney injury warranting intervention when their creatinine rises to a level of 1.2 mg/dl, but both of these values may fall within the normal reference range. Reference ranges themselves may vary in difference patient populations. Most reference ranges are established by sampling healthy 20–40-year-olds (Edwards & Baird, 2005) and may not represent the true normal range for patients of different ages, gender, or ethnicity. Furthermore, what is statistically normal may not be physiologically normal. If there is a high prevalence of iron deficiency in a population, the reference range for mean corpuscular volume (MCV) in asymptomatic patients may be low relative to that in a typical Western population in which iron deficiency is less common.

PATIENT SAFETY AND SOURCES OF LABORATORY ERROR

Sometimes abnormal lab values are statistically and clinically significant but go unnoticed by providers. By convention, abnormal values are usually highlighted in some manner when documented. Despite efforts to flag abnormal lab results, it has been reported that physicians do not always note or respond appropriately to important laboratory findings (Nykanen et al., 1993). This may be due to an increasing amount of laboratory data generated by more efficient methodology and computer automation, without a corresponding increase in medical professionals' abilities to sort through a barrage of test results (Mayer et al., 1998). Abnormal laboratory results fail to elicit an appropriate clinical response in up to 30% of cases (Altshuler, 1994). Some laboratories have instituted reporting policies mandating that extremely abnormal values must be communicated directly to a care provider to decrease the risk of their being overlooked. However, the manner in which abnormal lab results are flagged continues to be potentially problematic. A value that is 20 units outside of the normal range may be highlighted no differently than a value that is 1 unit outside of the normal range. For tests such as gamma-glutamyl-transferase (GGT), an abnormally low value has no clinical significance, but the results are flagged in the same manner as an abnormally high value. By chance alone, 5% of laboratory test results will be abnormal, implying that a physician with a large patient panel who orders many tests will be overwhelmed with abnormal test flags. Many laboratories have responded to the problem with protocols for directly notifying physicians of abnormal test results that may imply serious short-term medical consequences, such as a potassium level >6 mEq/mL.

Laboratory errors are responsible wholly or in part for a significant proportion of diagnostic errors in medicine (Graber, 2005). Laboratory errors can be divided into preanalytical, analytical and postanalytical errors. Preanalytical errors occur prior to the sample being analyzed and include the timing of the phlebotomy, improper filling of the specimen tube, patient hydration status, duration of tourniquet application, and elapsed time before analysis of the specimen (Ritchie, Ledue, & Craig, 2007). Studies suggest most errors occur in the preanalytical phase (Bonini, Plebani, Ceriotti, & Rubboli, 2002). Errors can also occur during specimen analysis, if reagents are degraded or a machine is improperly calibrated. Postanalytical errors occur after specimen analysis, such as the test result being entered with a missing decimal point or into a different patient's chart. These preanalytic, analytic, and postanalytic sources of error have been the focus of attention for personnel working in clinical labs. "Pre-pre" and "post-post" analytical errors have also been described (Laposata & Dighe, 2007) and are of concern to the ordering physician. "Pre-pre" analytical errors occur when a physician decides to order the wrong test for the clinical question at hand. "Post-post" analytical errors occur when the accurate test results are misinterpreted.

One reason patients see medical psychiatrists is that they have physical symptoms and a "negative work-up" for "organic causes." Sometimes the psychiatrist must function as an advocate to reopen consideration of a missed medical diagnosis. When the "normal" lab test results do not fit with the history, it is time to reconsider whether there is laboratory error using the framework above to distinguish different types of potential errors. One particularly common error of interpretation is to regard a single normal test result as ruling out a disease that tends to fluctuate—where lab values sometimes are normal and sometimes are not. This is the case, for example, in prediabetes or early type 2 diabetes, where the fasting plasma glucose may be normal but the postprandial glucose is not. In Hashimoto's thyroiditis, there may be euthyroid periods alternating with periods of clinical hypothyroidism (see chapter 6 on endocrine testing).

BIOSTATISTICAL TERMS USED IN EVALUATING DIAGNOSTIC TESTS

Characterization of test performance is helpful in interpreting test results. Standard terminology has evolved to describe the performance of tests utilized to make a yes/no decision about the presence of a disease or condition. This terminology is applicable to laboratory tests, physiological tests, imaging procedures, and psychological tests. Table 5.1 offers definitions of terms frequently used to describe the properties of diagnostic tests.

All test characteristics are a function of both the test and the clinical context in which it is applied. When the test involves converting a continuous quantity into a binary decision, the cut point for diagnosis may also affect test characteristics. Sensitivity and specificity are the best known test characteristics. 100% sensitivity means that every patient in the population examined who tests negative will not have the disease. 100% specificity means that every patient in the population examined who tests positive will have the disease. Typically, a test will approach 100% sensitivity only by sacrificing specificity, and conversely. For this reason a single laboratory test seldom suffices to make a definitive diagnosis. Likelihood ratios are an extension of the sensitivity and specificity concepts that specifically concern how test results modify diagnostic impressions formed without them (Lawrence & Gyorkos, 1996). By definition, likelihood ratios describe how

Table 5.1 TERMINOLOGY USED IN THE EVALUATION OF DIAGNOSTIC TESTS

TERM	DEFINITION
Clinical significance	Test results that are important enough to alter the management plan for a patient
False negative	Patients with disease who have a normal or negative test.
False positive	Patients without disease who have an abnormal or positive test.
Likelihood ratio of a negative test (LR−)	Calculated as (1−sensitivity)/specificity or false negative rate divided by true negative rate. The amount by which the pretest probability of disease is reduced in patients with a negative test.
Likelihood ratio of a positive test (LR+)	Calculated as sensitivity/(1−specificity) or true positive rate divided by false positive rate. The amount by which the pretest probability is increased in patients with a positive test.
Mean	Mathematical average of a sample of test results.
Negative predictive value (NPV)	The proportion of people with a negative test result who do not have the disease.
Positive predictive value (PPV)	The proportion of people with a positive test result who have the disease.
Pretest probability	The probability of disease before a test is run which is equal to the prevalence of the disease.
Prevalence	Proportion of persons who have the disease at a specified time.
Receiver operator characteristic (ROC)	Curve generated by plotting sensitivity on the y axis vs. 1−specificity (false positive rate) on the x axis to demonstrate a progressive trade off between sensitivity and specificity as a function of the decision level distinguishing disease and health.
Reference ranges or intervals	Values that are considered "normal" for a laboratory test, generally two standard deviations around the mean. 95% of values will fall within this interval.
Sensitivity	The proportion of people with the disease who test positive.
Specificity	The proportion of people without the disease who test negative.

much a positive test result increases or negative test result decreases the risk relative to the estimated risk prior to the test being done. A likelihood ratio value of 1 implies that a test is useless in improving the distinction of diseased patients from healthy ones (Mayer, et al., 1998). Tests with high likelihood ratios significantly improve diagnostic accuracy. When there is a low baseline suspicion of disease in a particular patient, a test must have a very high likelihood ratio to be the basis of a confident diagnosis. For example, if a patient's baseline risk of having HIV infection is less than 1%, the likelihood ratio for an HIV screening test would have to exceed 100 for it to be the basis of even a tentative diagnosis.

Receiver operating characteristic (ROC) curves provide a graphical illustration of the balance between sensitivity and specificity. ROC curves provide information on test performance at all cut points for determining abnormality (Obuchowski, Lieber, & Wians, 2004). A diagonal line with a slope of 1 going through the origin of the graph would be the ROC of a test result that had no value in discriminating disease—in other words, one where sensitivity can only be gained by sacrificing specificity to an equal extent. The area under the ROC curve is referred to as either the "area under the curve" (AUC) or as the "receiver operating characteristic" (ROC), and it represents the overall value of a test in distinguishing the presence or absence of a disease or condition. The AUC of the diagonal line representing a worthless test is 0.5; the AUC of a perfect test would be 1.0 (Klee, 2004; Mayer et al., 1998). Tests with AUC values of less than 0.7 are rarely useful in clinical contexts; those with values between 0.7–0.9 represent tests that may be useful in specialized contexts, and those with values >0.9 are candidates for more general clinical use (Wians, 2009). While generally tests with a higher ROC are better, other considerations are also relevant in selecting tests. The prevalence of the disease in the population to be tested, the cost of the test, and relative consequences of false-positive and false-negative test results can sometimes argue for the choice of a test with a lower ROC as the initial test for a disease in a specific clinical setting (Boyd, 1997).

DETERMINING WHICH LAB TESTS ARE INDICATED

Medical psychiatrists may be called upon to review laboratory tests already done or to suggest tests not yet done. The former case is typical when many physicians have already seen a patient for medically unexplained symptoms, or when a patient is emotionally distressed and disappointed with the care (McGorm et al., 2010) The latter case is typical when medical psychiatrists want to initiate a treatment with medical contraindications or precautions, or when they are encountering a patient with a psychiatric syndrome from a demographic group likely to have unrecognized or untreated medical comorbidity.

The increased morbidity and mortality of psychiatric patients compared to the general population was first described a century ago (Bonhoeffer, 1912) and it still persists (Green et al., 2003) despite advances in medical care. Some excess medical morbidity may be attributable to the difficulty that mentally ill persons have with access to care or with adherence to recommended medical treatment. Side effects of commonly prescribed psychotropic drugs—especially atypical antipsychotic drugs—also contribute. Nearly a quarter of psychiatric outpatients do not have a regular source of general medical care (Tanielian et al., 1999). Even after a patient has entered a general medical care setting, the stigma of mental illness may interfere with receiving optimal care (Kim et al., 2007; Kuey, 2008). Even clinicians free from any biases against people with mental illness may find it difficult to do a comprehensive history and examination on a patient with cognitive impairment, agitation, or paranoid ideation. In a study of 102 psychiatric inpatients transferred to an acute medical ward, only 23% could communicate the nature of their illness or location of their pain, and 78% of the medical diagnoses that were ultimately made were unrelated to the patient's description of the problem (Bunce et al., 1982). It is important that medical psychiatrists review the medical evaluations of their patients and do not assume that all appropriate laboratory tests have already been ordered by other providers, or that the results have been correctly interpreted in context. One reason is that patients with serious mental illness often have undiagnosed or inadequately treated general medical conditions. The second reason is that patients—particularly those with primary mental disorders, personality problems, or tendencies toward symptom amplification and dramatic self-expression—may be perceived by nonpsychiatric physicians as having medically unexplained symptoms on the basis of false-negative laboratory tests. The false negatives may be due to any of the error types described above. Probably the most frequent false negatives in this context are conclusions based on tests insufficient to rule out the most likely medical diagnosis, or application of criteria for abnormal results that are inappropriate for the patient's demographics and/ or clinical context. The first step in the process that leads to an interpretation of laboratory data is deciding which, if any, laboratory tests should be obtained on a particular patient. While clinicians are advised to "order the test for patients in whom it is indicated, not order it when it is not indicated, and interpret the test results appropriately in light of other clinical factors" (Jackson, 2007, p. 733), how to do this is not always obvious or simple in specific clinical situations. Ironically, studies aiming to determine the prevalence of inappropriate laboratory test utilization may use methodologically unsound criteria for "inappropriateness" (van Walraven & Naylor, 1998). Studies investigating the prevalence of lab abnormalities and the rates of significant undetected medical illness in patients with psychiatric conditions have yielded divergent results. While one reason is the wide variability in the demographics and settings in which psychiatric patients are seen, another is the variability in the choice of tests used to detect or to confirm particular medical conditions. Determining which laboratory tests to request may prove more difficult than interpreting their results.

THE PREVALENCE OF MEDICAL DISEASE IN PATIENTS WITH PSYCHIATRIC SYMPTOMS

As just noted, the prevalence of previously unrecognized medical illness in patients presenting to psychiatrists with mental and behavioral symptoms varies enormously between studies, and it depends upon whether the question concerns the presence of any undiagnosed medical illness or an undiagnosed medical illness *responsible for the*

psychiatric symptoms. Thirty-six years ago, a study of 636 psychiatric patients using the diagnostic methodology current at the time failed to find a single case in which an undetected medical illness was responsible for the patient's psychiatric symptoms (Willett & King, 1977). A recent review of 1340 psychiatric admissions in the Veterans Affairs system found that medical disease was responsible for causing the psychiatric symptoms in only 2.8% of cases (Reeves et al., 2010). In contrast, 63% of patients presenting to an emergency department with new psychiatric symptoms were found to have an organic condition responsible for them (Henneman, Mendoza, & Lewis, 1994). The prevalence of undiagnosed medical disease causing psychiatric symptoms has been reported to be 46% in state psychiatric hospital inpatients (Hall et al., 1981) and 16%–17% in outpatients at community health centers (Bartch et al., 1990; Koran et al., 1989). A 1992 review of 21 studies including different psychiatric populations concluded that about half of patients had significant medical disease, and the disease likely contributed to the psychiatric symptoms in over a quarter of them (Koranyi and Potoczny, 1992).

The literature thus provides estimates ranging from zero to 63% for "organic" etiology of mental and behavioral symptoms in clinical populations evaluated by psychiatrists. This extraordinarily wide range of estimates can be accounted for by several factors: (1) differences in the demographics of the samples and the prevalence of general medical conditions in the sampled populations; (2) differences in the presenting symptoms and syndromes—obviously, an acute change in mental status is more likely to have a general medical cause than a stable chronic psychosis; (3) differences in the patients' access to and utilization of general medical care; (4) sensitivity and scope of the medical evaluations performed; and (5) whether the estimate includes only medical conditions that are the primary or sole cause of the psychiatric problem, or also includes medical conditions responsible for aggravating the psychiatric problem or triggering a relapse of a previously stable mental disorder.

For the same reasons, it is difficult to prescribe a single universal standardized evidence-based medical evaluation of a patient presenting to a psychiatrist with mental and/ or behavioral symptoms (Zun, 2005). However, standardized approaches to general medical evaluation of psychiatric patients can be created for specific clinical populations in specific treatment settings.

A RATIONAL APPROACH TO LABORATORY TEST SELECTION

The prevalence of the condition is a critically important factor in determining whether or not laboratory testing for the condition should be performed. Prevalence is the foundation of the concept of "testing threshold," which is defined as the probability of disease above which physicians should test before initiating treatment for that disease, and below which physicians should neither treat nor test (Mayer, 2004). J. E. Hardison wrote in *The New England Journal of Medicine* in 1979, "The less the indication there is for a test, the more likely a positive result is falsely positive" (cited in Huth & Murray, 2000, p. 354). The positive predictive value of a laboratory test increases considerably as the prevalence of the disease increases. (Wians, 2009).

Laboratory test results influence up to 70% of medical decision making (Forsman, 1996); and because they may be perceived as more objective than a history and examination, such tests can carry disproportionate weight in clinicians' minds. Laboratory tests should be chosen thoughtfully, because tests can be harmful: false positives can lead to unnecessary and sometimes injurious treatments and procedures; false negatives can lead to delays in diagnosis and treatment; and waiting for irrelevant test results can delay the initiation of treatment.

The first question to ask in deciding whether or not to order a test is, *How likely is this test to be truly abnormal—a true positive—in this patient?* Factors that have been reported to increase the likelihood that a psychiatric symptom is attributable to a medical illness include lack of prior psychiatric history, very rapid onset, onset before age 12 or after age 40 years, disorientation, depressed level of consciousness, abnormal vital signs, focal neurologic deficits, and the presence of visual or tactile hallucinations (Reeves et al., 2000).

Of course, if the diagnosis is obvious and the test result is expected to be positive, the test might not be necessary.

Kamp and Rosse concluded in 1990 after reviewing over 2000 test results on a group of psychiatric inpatients that admission testing was not justified because the abnormal test results were "predictable." A test with a result expected to be abnormal would be appropriate if it was useful in quantifying the severity of the disease or condition, and such quantification would be useful in planning treatment and/or following the outcome of treatment. Another situation in which a "predictably abnormal" test would be warranted is when the clinical diagnosis, though highly likely, could be wrong, the test in question would help rule out a diagnostic error, and the consequences of a wrong diagnosis would be costly, dangerous, and/or irreversible.

The second question to ask when deciding whether or not to order a laboratory test is, *How will the test result change the treatment plan for the patient?* If an intoxicated-appearing patient reports that he has been consuming vodka, it is not necessary to measure a blood alcohol level to diagnose alcohol intoxication. If the episode of intoxication represents a relapse in a patient known to be alcohol dependent, the blood alcohol level is unlikely to change the treatment plan. However, if the patient is new to the healthcare system, finding a blood alcohol level of 300 mg/dl in a patient who was awake and ambulatory would clinch a new diagnosis of alcohol dependence and thus be quite valuable in planning the next steps in treatment.

The third question to ask when deciding whether or not to order a laboratory test is, *When will the test results be available?* The required turnaround time for results should be considered when determining whether or not to order a test, because it impacts the clinical utility (Pannall et al., 1996). For example, ordering a carbohydrate deficient transferrin (CDT) to help confirm a diagnosis of alcohol dependence in a recently admitted inpatient may not be rational if the report would take 10 days to arrive and the patient, if alcohol dependent, would start exhibiting symptoms of alcohol withdrawal on the second hospital day. When a test will be used to inform a decision on the treatment of a chronic disease, the turnaround time is less important.

LABORATORY TESTS USED IN THE EVALUATION OF PSYCHIATRIC SYMPTOMS AND THEIR INTERPRETATION

LABORATORY TESTS

There are over 3,000 laboratory tests currently available, and only a small fraction of them are described in the following section. For additional strategies on selecting and interpreting laboratory tests or for information on lab tests not covered in this chapter, a free website for physicians can be found at http.//www.arupconsult.com. Following is a selection of commonly conducted laboratory tests, in alphabetical order, with guidelines for interpretation of particular relevance to medical psychiatrists.

Alanine aminotransferase (ALT) is found primarily in hepatocytes, but is also found in lower concentrations in cardiac and skeletal muscle. Elevated ALT may signify hepatitis, but inflammation or damage in other tissues may also cause ALT elevation. Clinicians monitoring ALT in patients taking potentially hepatotoxic drugs generally do not consider an ALT elevation clinically significant until it is at least 3 times above the upper limit of normal, with some physicians classifying an ALT elevation of up to 5 times the upper limit of normal as "mild" (Musana, Yale, & Abdulkarim, 2004). Low ALT values may signify starvation, but often patients with low ALT are asymptomatic. The take-home is that you don't necessarily diagnose hepatitis or drug-induced hepatotoxicity if the ALT is 2–3x normal—you do monitor, and you may get consultation.

Albumin is synthesized in the liver and usually accounts for the majority of protein in the blood. Abnormal albumin levels are usually of clinical concern, since the action of many medications, hormones, and calcium levels are affected by protein binding. Low levels are associated with increased mortality. (Fried et al., 1998). Elevated albumin levels are generally due to volume depletion. Low albumin levels may be related to poor nutritional intake, impaired production in patients with cirrhosis, chronic inflammation or loss of albumin into the urine in nephrotic syndrome. **Prealbumin** has a shorter half life than albumin, making low levels a more sensitive marker of acute nutritional compromise (Beck and Rosenthal, 2002). Serum levels decline in protein malnutrition states such as malignancy or cirrhosis and with zinc deficiency. Production decreases after 14 days of consuming a diet that provides only 60% of required proteins (Le Moullac, Gouache, & Bleiberg-Daniel, 1992). Prealbumin has been used to assess nutrition in elderly patients admitted to the hospital. (Nutritional Care Consensus Group, 1995) While alcoholics may have elevated levels of prealbumin after binge drinking, an assessment of nutrition by prealbumin level may be assessed after one week (Staley, 1984).

Alkaline phosphatase is found in liver, intestines, and bones, and elevated levels may occur in liver or gallbladder disease, healing fractures, or cancers involving bone. Laboratories can fractionate alkaline phosphatase in order to determine if the elevation is from a gastrointestinal source or bone. Low alkaline phosphatase levels are generally not of direct clinical concern but can occur in vitamin B12 deficiency, vitamin D intoxication, hypothyroidism, or hypophosphatemia (Chernecky & Berger, 2008).

Ammonia is a waste product of nitrogen breakdown in protein metabolism. Elevated levels are most often seen in patients with cirrhosis, but can also occur in patients on valproic acid or those who are consuming high-protein diets. Elevated ammonia has been associated with hepatic encephalopathy, but there is poor correlation between the level of ammonia and the degree of confusion in patients. This is perhaps because the concentration of ammonia in the brain may correlate poorly with the concentration of ammonia in the blood (Butterworth, 2002). Ammonia levels will be increased if the specimen is not on ice or there is a delay in processing the specimen (Chernecky & Berger, 2008). Low ammonia levels are generally not of clinical concern.

Amylase is found in the pancreas and salivary glands, so inflammation in either tissue can cause an elevated level. Laboratories can fractionate amylase to determine if it is from a pancreatic or salivary source, which may be useful in diagnosing—and in confronting denial in—eating disorder patients with frequent self-induced vomiting. (Please see chapter 32 for more information on eating disorders.) Low amylase levels are not clinically significant. Amylase is renally cleared, so levels can be falsely elevated in patients with renal failure (Chernecky & Berger, 2008).

Antinuclear antibodies (ANA) are produced by the immune system against one's own DNA in autoimmune diseases such systemic lupus erythematosus, but can also occur with certain medications such as carbamazepine. The cutoff for distinguishing normal from abnormal is usually 1:20 dilution. Higher titers such as 1:320 are indicative of a more strongly positive test. Steroids and other immunosuppressive agents may cause false-negative results. The likelihood of having a positive ANA increases with age, and nearly a quarter of women over age 65 years will test positive in the absence of disease (Goroll & Mulley, 2009). One third of healthy first-degree relatives of lupus patients have a positive ANA (Chernecky & Berger, 2008). However, a high-titer ANA may be a clue to the physician that an autoimmune disease might develop, and the patient should be followed. A negative ANA in a patient without a clear pattern of symptoms of connective tissue disease argues against the diagnosis. In patients with systemic lupus erythematosus (SLE), 93% have a positive ANA; since ANA is nonspecific, antibody to double-stranded DNA would clarify the diagnosis (Reichlin, 2013). ANA is typically present many years before the diagnosis of SLE. In one sample of patients with SLE, 78% had a positive ANA at a dilution of 1:120 or more 2 years before symptoms and 9 years

before diagnosis (Arbuckle, 2003). Chapter 61 discusses rheumatic diseases.

Arterial blood gases (ABGs) measure oxygen and carbon dioxide content in arterial blood, as well as measuring pH. Carbon dioxide levels can be increased in patients with lung disease; they are decreased with hyperventilation. Hypercarbia has been associated with induction of panic symptoms, but either high carbon dioxide or low oxygen content can produce anxiety. The partial pressure of arterial oxygen (PaO_2) decreases with age and in lung conditions including pulmonary embolus and pneumonia. Oxygen and pH results will be lower if the specimen is not placed on ice and processed promptly (Chernecky & Berger, 2008). The patient's temperature must be recorded when the ABG is drawn, since fever raises the oxygen content. ABGs should be considered in patients with episodic dyspnea suggesting panic attacks when there is something atypical about the presentation. The patient who hyperventilates because of a panic attack will have a low $PaCO_2$ and a high PaO_2; the patient with recurrent pulmonary emboli will have a low $PaCO_2$ and a low PaO_2. Estimating the PaO_2 by measuring oxygen saturation with a pulse oximeter is a noninvasive aid to diagnosis in situations where obtaining an arterial blood sample is not feasible. However, it will not offer information about low carbon dioxide or dangerous hypercarbia in chronic lung disease. Chapter 54 discusses pulmonary diseases.

Aspartate aminotransferase (AST) is found in liver as well as cardiac and skeletal muscle. Elevated levels may indicate hepatitis, but they can also signify a myocardial infarction or rhabdomyolysis. Alcoholic hepatitis is classically taught to cause elevations in both AST and ALT, with an AST to ALT ratio greater than 2 to 1. This pattern of enzyme elevation implies liver disease and is not present in heavy drinkers without liver damage (Nyblom et al., 2004). Low AST levels are not usually of clinical concern but are sometimes found in patients with cirrhosis. AST levels can be falsely decreased in patients with elevated blood urea nitrogen levels (Chernecky & Berger, 2008).

Bicarbonate regulates the pH of body fluids. Levels increase in patients with lung disease who have chronic retention of carbon dioxide. Levels fall in eating disorder patients with vomiting, or with abuse of laxatives and/or diuretics.

Bilirubin is the product of hemoglobin breakdown during red blood cell degradation in the spleen. The indirect bilirubin is then sent to the liver where it is conjugated to form direct bilirubin. Blood tests measure total and direct bilirubin levels, and indirect bilirubin is calculated by their difference. Direct bilirubin increases in biliary obstruction, while indirect bilirubin is increased in hemolytic anemias. The bilirubin must be significantly elevated before a jaundiced appearance becomes obvious. Scleral icterus is associated with bilirubin at 3 or above.

Blood alcohol level or blood toxicology screens (unlike urine toxicology screens) indicate a specific level of the substance such as alcohol, acetaminophen, or aspirin, rather than just the absence or presence of the substance or its metabolites (McPherson & Pincus, 2006). Knowing the blood level can be clinically important for the management of patients who have overdosed. Also, unusually high levels of alcohol or a sedative-hypnotic drug in a patient who is awake imply pharmacologic tolerance, a useful fact in confirming a suspected diagnosis of substance dependence as opposed to episodic substance abuse.

Blood urea nitrogen (BUN) measures the concentration of urea nitrogen from the breakdown of protein in the blood. It is produced by the liver and eliminated by the kidneys. Increased levels (known as azotemia) may cause confusion, agitation or coma. Levels increase with renal insufficiency, volume depletion and upper gastrointestinal bleeding. Low BUN values typically occur in a setting of decreased muscle mass, protein-calorie malnutrition or volume overload.

Calcium is stored in bone and is involved in muscle contraction and nerve conduction. High levels of calcium are seen in volume depletion, vitamin D toxicity, hyperparathyroidism, cancer, immobilization, and fractures. Hypercalcemia can cause altered mental status; typically, mild to moderate hypercalcemia causes fatigue or depression while moderate to severe hypercalcemia is associated with cognitive impairment, delirium, and, at the highest levels, stupor or coma. Abnormally low levels of calcium occur in vitamin D deficiency, hypoparathyroidism, and with high pH (Haist & Robbins, 1997). Calcium is largely protein-bound in the blood. To correct the total calcium because of an abnormal albumin level, subtract 0.8 mg/dL from the total calcium for every 1.0 g/dL by which the serum albumin concentration is >4 g/dL. Conversely, when albumin levels are low, total calcium can be corrected by adding 0.8 mg/dL for every 1.0 g/dL by which the albumin is <4 g/dL. For a direct measure of calcium in the setting of high or low albumin, an **ionized calcium level** is the preferred test.

Carbohydrate deficient transferrin (CDT) is used to detect alcohol abuse, although in some institutions results may take 1–2 weeks to obtain, limiting its usefulness. CDT is best reported as percentage of transferrin. It has moderate sensitivity and specificity as a longer-term marker of heavy ethanol use (Ingall, 2012; Center for Substance Abuse Treatment, 2006). An elevated CDT level is best used in combination with other markers of alcohol abuse (Neumann & Spies, 2003). The specificity of the test is decreased in patients with liver disease, and false negatives may occur in patients with iron overload (Chernecky & Berger, 2008). It is especially useful as a marker of abstinence because it returns to baseline levels 2–5 weeks after ethanol cessation. Declining CDT values support abstinence (Ingall, 2012).

Carboxyhemoglobin forms in the blood when carbon monoxide binds to hemoglobin. Carbon monoxide (CO) binds to hemoglobin more strongly than oxygen. Carboxyhemoglobin levels are above 3% in nonsmokers, and levels of 10% in smokers are normal. Carbon monoxide poisoning leads to elevated carboxyhemoglobin levels with acute symptoms of headache, dizziness, fatigue, flu-like malaise, blurred vision, nausea, and vomiting. If the exposure is more severe, confusion, syncope, seizures, and stroke-like syndromes can be seen. When CO poisoning is suspected due to faulty furnaces, poor ventilation of flame-based heating sources, or exposure to internal combustion engine exhaust, a carboxyhemoglobin level should be obtained immediately, performed by spectrophotometric CO oximetry. Pulse oximetry is unreliable to assess oxygenation, as most pulse oximeters cannot distinguish oxyhemoglobin and COHb (Guzman, 2012).

Ceruloplasmin is a protein involved in the transport of copper and iron. It is most often ordered to assess for Wilson's disease, which is distinguished by low ceruloplasmin levels and high urine copper levels (Czaja et al., 1987). Malabsorption, as in patients with celiac disease, can also cause low ceruloplasmin levels. The majority (85%–90%) of patients with Wilson disease have <20 mg/dL; however, in Wilson's disease, ceruloplasm is sometimes normal or elevated. Low ceruloplasm is also seen in liver disease (Cauza, Maier-Dobersberger, & Polli, 1997) or conditions of kidney or intestinal protein loss. Ceruloplasmin is an acute-phase reactant, and its synthesis is stimulated by estrogens (Brewer, 1992). Diseases associated with high ceruloplasmin levels are too numerous for the test to be specific enough to be of clinical value. In patients with neurological symptoms suggestive of Wilson's disease, low serum ceruloplasmin, bolstered by Kayser-Fleisher rings by slit lamp eye exam, and elevated urinary copper excretion suggest the diagnosis.

C peptide is formed in the pancreas when proinsulin is converted to insulin. Decreased levels are seen in type 1 diabetics. The test is most often performed for the evaluation of factitious hypoglycemia by surreptitious insulin injection. Patients who are hypoglycemic because of self-administration of insulin (factitious hypoglycemia) will have high serum insulin levels and undetectable C peptide (Threatte & Henry, 1996).

Creatine phosphokinase (CK or CPK) is found in cardiac and skeletal muscle and in the brain. Laboratories can measure myocardial and skeletal muscle CK, specifically helping to distinguish acute myocardial infarction from rhabdomyolysis; measurement of brain CK is not clinically relevant. Significant elevations of skeletal muscle CK imply skeletal muscle breakdown that is of clinical concern because of the renal toxicity of the myoglobin that is released at the same time as the CK (Sauret, Marnides, & Wang, 2002). Situations associated with such elevations of skeletal muscle CK include alcohol abuse, extreme exertion, immobility (e.g., due to stroke) with pressure injury to muscles, and the neuroleptic malignant syndrome or malignant catatonia. Low CK levels are seen in patients with reduced muscle mass and do not provide information of incremental diagnostic value. Elevations of CK occur after an intramuscular injection is administered.

Creatinine is produced in muscle and renally excreted. Elevated values are indicative of kidney failure. Values may be 20%–40% higher when drawn in the late afternoon (Chernecky & Berger, 2008). Low creatinine values are seen in patients with decreased muscle mass, including frail elderly people, malnourished patients, and those who have been immobile for prolonged periods. The significance is that when such patients develop renal insufficiency, the creatinine may not be elevated beyond the normal range for healthy young adults. Chapter 59 discusses kidney disease and dialysis.

Epstein-Barr virus antibodies (EBV ABs) develop and persist in patients who have been infected with the virus that causes infectious mononucleosis, whether or not they are clinically symptomatic. Twenty percent of patients with acute infection have a negative Monospot test, the heterophile antibody latex agglutination test to horse red cells (Chernecky & Berger, 2008). This test can be negative particularly in the first month, and once positive may persist for a year. Cytomegalovirus or toxoplasmosis are a consideration in heterophile negative patients with mono-like symptoms and signs (Ebell, 2004). High EBV antibody titers have been reported in patients with chronic fatigue syndrome, but there is poor correlation between titers and symptoms. EBV antibodies are common given the high prevalence of exposure to the virus and cannot be used reliably to diagnose chronic fatigue syndrome (Koo, 1989). See chapter 34 for a discussion of fatigue and chapter 60 for a discussion of EBV infection.

Folate or vitamin B9 is formed in the intestine, stored in the liver, and involved in blood cell function and neuronal function. Elevated levels may occur in patients taking supplements and in patients with hepatic insufficiency. Low levels occur in patients with protein-calorie malnutrition, patients with malabsorption syndromes, and in severe alcoholics who do not eat regularly. Clinically significant folate deficiency is usually associated with macrocytosis of red blood cells (elevated MCV). Some antiepileptic drugs, such as phenytoin, cause folate deficiency as indicated by a low serum folate. Other antiepileptic drugs interfere with the conversion of folate into tetrahydrofolate, its active form. These patients can have central nervous system (CNS) dysfunction due to folate deficiency without a decreased serum folate. Sulfasalazine and trimethoprim/sulfamethoxazole are also associated with folate deficiency.

Gamma glutamyl transpeptidase (GGT) is an enzyme found mainly in the cells of the biliary tract. Patients with even mild alcoholic hepatitis will show elevations of GGT, but elevation of GGT alone does not establish a diagnosis of hepatitis or of alcoholism (Neumann & Spies, 2003). A number of mildly hepatotoxic drugs can elevate GGT without affecting other "liver enzymes" or causing clinical symptoms. An isolated elevation of GGT is not a reason for discontinuing a drug that is clinically valuable, but it does imply a need for follow-up monitoring of the GGT, AST, ALT, and bilirubin to rule out a progressive problem that eventually will become clinically significant and require discontinuation of the drug.

Glucose is a monosaccharide that is the main source of cellular energy. Levels are elevated in diabetic patients and also increase with cortisol levels. Due to the brain's reliance on glucose, hypoglycemia can cause confusion, anxiety, and may even present with focal neurologic findings mimicking a stroke (Haist & Robbins, 1997). Hypoglycemia is most often a side effect of diabetic medications, but it can occur in fasting patients with severe liver disease due to impaired gluconeogenesis. Hypoglycemia can occur in patients with insulinomas or with self-administration of insulin to produce a factitious illness. Patients with prediabetes or mild diabetes can have a normal fasting glucose with an elevated 2-hour postprandial glucose, or an elevated fasting glucose with a normal 2-hour

postprandial glucose; the latter case is most likely to occur when the meal is not a standardized high-carbohydrate meal or glucose challenge.

Glycosylated hemoglobin (HbA1c) is proportional to the average plasma glucose over 4 weeks to 3 months, with more weight on the last 4 weeks. Once a red blood cell is glycosylated, it remains so for the remainder of its 120-day life span. While previously only approved to monitor glycemic control in diabetics, a high glycosylated hemoglobin level can now be used to make the diagnosis of diabetes or prediabetes (insulin resistance). Hemoglobin A1c does have some ethnic and racial differences and may be altered in the setting of shorter red cell survival.

In order to identify who is at risk for diabetes, the American Diabetes Association has set the threshold for prediabetes as HbA1c 5.7–6.4 and the threshold for full diagnosis of diabetes as HbA1c ≥6.5. Parallel criteria for prediabetes are fasting plasma glucose of 100 to 125 mg/dl, or a 2-hour plasma glucose of 140 mg/dl (7.8 mmol/l to 199 mg/dl) after a 75 g oral glucose tolerance test. Parallel criteria for full diagnosis of diabetes is fasting plasma glucose ≥126 mg/dl or a 2-hour plasma glucose of 200 mg/dl during an oral glucose tolerance test. Classic symptoms of hyperglycemia or hyperglycemic crisis with a random plasma glucose >200 mg/dl also makes the diagnosis (Selvin et al., 2010; American Diabetes Association, 2013). In the psychiatric context, the HbA1c is useful in monitoring patients on second-generation antipsychotic drugs for the development of insulin resistance. Low levels are not clinically significant (American Diabetes Association, 2013).

Hemoglobin is the protein in red blood cells that carries oxygen. Blood hemoglobin is the concentration of the hemoglobin in gm/dL and **hematocrit** is the percentage of blood volume that consists of red blood cells. Levels of both are elevated when plasma volume is depleted and when there is an increased number of red blood cells produced, as when patients live at high altitude, smoke heavily, or have polycythemia vera. Both the hemoglobin and the hematocrit are decreased in anemia, whether due to bleeding, hemolysis, or a chronic disease such as chronic renal failure that is associated with decreased secretion of erythropoietin, the endogenous stimulant of red cell production.

Human immunodeficiency virus (HIV) testing is generally performed as two tests. A more sensitive enzyme immunoassay (ELISA) is performed first, and positive test results then are confirmed with a more specific Western blot or immunofluorescence test (Owen, Yang, & Spira, 2008). The rationale behind the two-step process of testing is that the risk of missing the diagnosis, as well as the risk of diagnosing a healthy patient with HIV, are both clinically unacceptable. When the two tests are used in conjunction, less than 0.1% of test results are inaccurate. However, false negatives can still occur if testing is performed soon after the infection occurs. A measure of viral load HIV RNA by the reverse transcriptase polymerase chain reaction test may be more informative in the first 6 weeks after exposure (Sax & Bartlett, 2013). The Centers for Disease Control (CDC) modified its recommendations for screening in 2006 to include all persons ages 13–64 years, rather than limiting the test to patients with certain high-risk behaviors. Chapter 63 discusses HIV and sexually transmitted infections.

Lipase is a pancreatic enzyme that breaks down fats and triglycerides. Most often, elevated levels are a marker of acute pancreatitis, with levels of 3 times the upper limit of normal considered clinically significant (Lankisch, Burchard-Reckert, & Lehnick, 1999). Levels may not be elevated in patients with chronic pancreatitis.

Lyme IgG and IgM are antibodies to *Borrelia burgdorferi*. IgM levels peak about 1 month after infection, so a low level does not exclude disease. IgG rises 2–6 weeks after signs of illness and can remain elevated for decades after the infection has resolved. These tests have no value at the time of the tick bite. Many other infectious and autoimmune diseases will cause false-positive tests for Lyme disease, including infectious mononucleosis, syphilis, rheumatoid arthritis, and systemic lupus erythematosus. Serology testing does not make the diagnosis of Lyme nor does it exclude the diagnosis. It is not useful for screening asymptomatic individuals in endemic areas, as the false positives can be greater than true positives. These tests have a place for patients who may have been exposed to ticks and who have signs of disseminated disease. Diagnostic testing usually begins with an enzyme linked immunosorbent assay (ELISA). If the ELISA is positive, then a Western blot is sent. If Western blot is negative, the serology is deemed negative. The patient has not been exposed to *Borrelia burgdorferi*. Serum *Borrelia burgdorferi* C6 peptide antibody (VlsE C6 peptid ELISA) becomes positive earlier and has greater specificity—96% alone and 99% with two-step testing (Chernecky & Berger, 2008; Hu & Steere, 2013). Chapter 60 details infectious diseases.

Magnesium located in bone and cartilage and is found universally within the cells of the body. High levels occur in renal failure, and iatrogenically in pregnant women being treated for preterm labor or eclampsia with intravenous magnesium. Magnesium may be used orally in antacids or as an element of enemas in older patients. Hypermagnesemia can present with decreased consciousness and slurred speech; however, mildly elevated levels are usually asymptomatic. Hyperbilirubinemia will decrease magnesium levels (Chernecky & Berger, 2008). Hypermagnesemia with hyponatremia can follow intoxication with amphetamine or cathinones (Prosser & Nelson, 2012). Lithium overdose is associated with high levels of magnesium, as are tumor lysis syndromes and other catabolic states in the setting of renal insufficiency such as rhabdomyolysis, seen in neuroleptic malignant syndrome, and malignant catatonia.

Magnesium levels should be checked in patients with hypocalcemia, as the two typically are associated. Hypomagnesemia can occur in dehydrated patients, particularly those with diarrhea; in eating disorder patients who abuse laxatives and/or diuretics; and in malnourished chronic alcoholics. Repletion of body fluids and electrolytes with intravenous solutions that do not contain magnesium can aggravate the problem. Hypomagnesemia can present with psychosis, agitation, or depression, and is particularly dangerous in patients with prolonged QT intervals because of increased risk of cardiac arrhythmias (Haist & Robbins, 1997). One context in which it is essential to check magnesium levels is antidepressant overdose. In this situation the risk of QT prolongation and associated arrhythmia is high, and either the depression itself or a period of stupor or coma due to the overdose can be associated with dehydration. Hypomagnesemia is a consideration whenever the QT interval is prolonged, particularly in the setting of medications that prolong the QT interval, due to the greater danger of serious arrhythmia. See chapter 52.

Mean corpuscular volume (MCV) is the calculated volume of erythrocytes. Elevated levels are seen in alcoholics, vitamin B12 and/or folate deficiency, patients with malabsorption, cigarette smokers, and patients with high reticulocyte counts. Because an elevated MCV can have diverse causes, it is unacceptably nonspecific with respect to the diagnosis of alcohol abuse or dependence, even in clinical settings where the baseline prevalence of alcoholism is high (Neumann & Spies, 2003).

Abnormally low MCVs occur in patients with iron deficiency anemia (commonly seen in menstruating females and in patients with chronic gastrointestinal bleeding) and in patients with inherited disease of the red blood cells such as sickle cell disease and thalassemia. In clinical contexts—for example, recent immigrants from countries with a high prevalence of parasitic diseases and travelers recently returned from such countries—parasitic infestations associated with blood loss should be included in the differential diagnosis.

Phosphate is stored in bones and is elevated in patients with renal failure. Patients with hyperphosphatemia should be evaluated for possible hypocalcemia. Low phosphate levels can lead to irritability, encephalopathy, and seizures if extreme. Most commonly, low levels occur in the setting of inadequate oral nutrition; but patients with alcoholism, vitamin D deficiency, and treatment for diabetic ketoacidosis are also at risk (Haist & Robbins, 1997). Hypophosphatemia can also develop in patients treated for dehydration with intravenous solutions that do not contain phosphate.

Platelets are produced in the bone marrow and are involved in blood clotting. Low platelets may be due to decreased production in patients with cancer, alcoholism, or nutritional compromise; destruction in autoimmune conditions; or sequestration in patients with an enlarged spleen. Thrombocytopenia is not associated with increased bleeding risk until the platelet count falls below 20,000 per microliter (Haist & Robbins, 1997). Thus, spontaneous bleeding with lesser degrees of thrombocytopenia implies an additional cause of abnormal bleeding such as a colon lesion, drugs or inherited diseases that impair blood clotting, impaired hepatic synthesis of clotting factors, or qualitative platelet dysfunction such as that seen in von Willenbrand's disease. Thrombocytosis can occur in patients with acute inflammation or infection, and is associated with an increased risk of thrombosis when the platelet count exceeds 1,000,00/microL (Buss, Stuart, & Lipscomb, 1985). Patients with thrombocytosis due to a clonal abnormality causing increased production are at risk for both bleeding and clotting (Schafer, 2006).

Potassium is an intracellular cation that affects cardiac repolarization and cardiac conduction, rendering it very clinically significant because it predisposes to cardiac arrhythmias.

It is excreted by the kidneys and by the colon via the stool. The most common cause of hyperkalemia is renal failure, but it can occur in other diseases such as Addison's and with medications such as ACE inhibitors and potassium-sparing diuretics such as amiloride (Haist & Robbins, 1997). Severe hyperkalemia can lead to cardiac arrest, especially if the onset is acute. Electrocardiogram changes associated with hyperkalemia are peaked T-waves and shortened QT interval. Hypokalemia usually occurs in patients with vomiting or diarrhea, or those taking diuretics. In collecting the blood sample, using a tourniquet and having the patient pump the hands can raise venous potassium levels by up to 20% (Chernecky & Berger, 2008). Potassium levels are higher in the afternoon and early evening and may be falsely elevated if the blood specimen hemolyzes prior to analysis.

Rapid plasma reagin (RPR) is a nontreponemal serologic test for syphilis in which the serum reacts to a cardiolipin-cholesterol-lecithin antigen. The test has greater sensitivity during the secondary rather than the primary stage of syphilis. Consuming alcohol within 24 hours prior to testing can lead to a false-negative result (Chernecky & Berger, 2008). False-positive results are very common in autoimmune and other infectious diseases. However, the RPR is still preferred over the nontreponemal Venereal Disease Research Laboratory test for syphilis, because it is more sensitive. If there is a history of previously treated syphilis, the nonreactive RPR suggests that no further treatment is warranted as there is no sign of active infection. A sign of new infection in someone who had been treated in the past would be a fourfold increase in titer. If there is no history of treatment, syphilis has a low prevalence, and the RPR is positive, then the next step would be the Treponema pallidum-particle agglutination assay, a specific treponemal test. For economic reasons, some laboratories are now beginning with a specific treponemal ELISA. The harm of potentially treating a patient with penicillin unnecessarily is much less than the harm of allowing the disease to progress to later stages and the risk of the patient transmitting infection to others. Chapter 63 discusses HIV and sexually transmitted infections.

Sodium is a cation in extracellular fluid which is elevated in patients with volume depletion and diabetes insipidus, and can be decreased for any of a wide range of conditions associated with increased secretion of antidiuretic hormone (ADH). Hypernatremia can present with depressed sensorium and disorientation; in fact, it often occurs because the patient who has lost water is not alert, responding to thirst, and replacing the losses. Diabetes insipidus—decreased secretion of ADH by the hypothalamus or insensitivity of the kidney to ADH—is the principal cause of hypernatremia. In psychiatric contexts, this side effect of lithium is an important consideration. Hyponatremia, particularly when acute, can cause psychiatric symptoms including anxiety, confusion, or sedation, and can cause seizures. A serum sodium of 110 mEq/L will cause CNS dysfunction in virtually all patients; a level of 125 can cause symptoms if acute, but may be asymptomatic if it has developed over several weeks. The list of possible causes of low sodium is lengthy, and the differential diagnosis varies based on the volume status of the patients. Hypervolemic hyponatremia is due to heart, liver, or kidney failure. Euvolemic hyponatremia is due to hypothryroidism or the syndrome of inappropriate antidiuretic hormone (ADH) secretion. Hypovolemic hyponatremia occurs when both sodium and water are depleted because of vomiting or diarrhea, or renal tubular loss (Haist & Robbins, 1997). Volume status can be assessed by measuring orthostatic blood pressure changes and by noting an increase or decrease in the levels of blood constituents such as the hematocrit or BUN. A number of psychiatric medications have been reported to cause SIADH; a list of common ones is found in Box 5.1). Psychiatric patients with polydipsia, beer potomania, and eatingdisorder patients who water-load prior to a weigh-in are at risk for hyponatremia. Patients with severe hyperglycemia can have hyponatremia because the ADH system regulates serum osmolality, and glucose can substitute for sodium in determining serum osmolality. Chronic hyponatremia, particularly in patients who are not symptomatic, should be corrected slowly (e.g., over days) to avoid central pontine myelinolysis.

Thyroid stimulating hormone (TSH) is released by the anterior pituitary to regulate secretion of thyroxine (T4) and triiodothyronine (T3) by the thyroid gland. Elevated levels are seen in hypothyroidism—and rarely in patients with TSH-secreting pituitary adenomas—and low levels are seen in patients with hyperthyroidism, and rarely in patients with hypopituitarism or with suppression of TSH secretion by a prolactin-secreting or nonsecreting pituitary tumor. TSH will also become low in patients on levothyroxine who are taking excessive doses of thyroid replacement or are deliberately ingesting thyroid hormones to lose weight or produce a factitious illness. TSH levels take 6–8 weeks to reach a steady level after a levothyroxine dose is adjusted (Hueston, 2001). Patients with a TSH <10 micro units per milliliter do not have more physical or neuropsychiatric symptoms than healthy controls (Jorde et al., 2006); nonetheless, individual patients may have a history and other laboratory findings suggesting a clinically relevant disturbance of thyroid function. (This is discussed further in chapters 6 and 55, which deal with endocrine testing and endocrine diseases.) Current practice guidelines recommend screening all women over age 50 years for thyroid disorders because of the high prevalence

---

Box 5.1 **PSYCHIATRIC DRUGS ASSOCIATED WITH SIADH**

amantadine, amitriptyline, aripiprazole, carbamazepine, chlorpromazine, clomipramine, desipramine, doxepin, duloxetine, escitalopram, fluoxetine, fluvoxamine, fluphenazine, haloperidol, imipramine, lorazepam, nortriptyline, olanzapine, paroxetine, perphenazine, pramipexole, protriptyline, sertraline, thioridazine, thiothixene, tranylcypromine, trimipramine, valproic acid, venlafaxine.

Source: www.micromedexsolutions.ocm/micropmedex2 (copyright 1974–2013) of primary hypothyroidism in that population. Secondary hypothyroidism due to lack of TSH release from the pituitary will present with low TSH and low free T4, but accounts for less than 5% of cases of clinical hypothyroidism (Hueston, 2001). Medical psychiatrists may see low TSH from a pituitary or a hypothalamic cause in patients who have had radiation to the brain.

Free thyroxine (Free T4) is a measure of active, nonprotein–bound thyroid hormone. Levels are high in hyperthyroidism and low in hypothyroidism. Free T4 also decreases with age (Kennedy-Malone, Fletcher, & Plank, 2004) and it may be transiently decreased in the context of acute, severe illness. Clinical situations of chronic inflammation in which there is an excess of thyroid-binding globulin can lead to spurious elevation of total T4, and situations of malnutrition or hepatic dysfunction with low levels of thyroid-binding globulin can lead to a spurious low value of total T4. Determination of free T4 is particularly helpful in these situations. Within the normal range of free T4, there is no association of low T4 levels with clinical depression (Williams et al., 2009).

Urinalyses are most often ordered to look for evidence of urinary tract infections, but can also reveal hematuria suggesting urinary tract cancer or a bleeding disorder, or proteinuria suggesting kidney disease. Diabetic nephropathy is the most common kidney disease associated with proteinuria. Urine specific gravity—which, when low, suggests low urine osmolality—can be a clue to SIADH, diabetes insipidus, or water intoxication. The urine dipstick has high sensitivity but poor specificity for hematuria and pyuria, while the microscopic evaluation of urine is both sensitive and specific (Simerville, Maxted, & Pahira, 2005). Weakly positive leukocyte esterase or nitrites on dipstick are not as reliable a marker for infection as increased white blood cell counts on microscopy.

Urine catecholamines are measured in the evaluation of patients for pheochromocytoma. Due to the infrequent incidence of this disease (less than 1% of hypertensive patients), this test is less valuable when suspicion is low. Fractionated metanephrines in a 24-hour urine can be used to rule out pheochromocytoma when suspicion is low, but is only part of an evaluation to make the diagnosis when clinical suspicion for pheochromocytoma is very high (Young & Kaplan, 2013). Suspicion would be high in a patient with headaches, generalized sweating, and tachycardia, or in patients with episodes of hypertension, resistant hypertension, an episode of hypertension during a procedure, history of familial syndromes like neurofibromatosis 1, von Hippel-Lindau disease, multiple endocrine neoplasia 2 (with medullary thyroid cancer and hyperparathyroidism), or an incidental adrenaloma. Fractionated catecholamines (dopamine, norepinephrine, epinephrine) and metanephrines (metanephrine and normetanephrine) in a 24-hour urine collection with creatinine measured to document adequate sample is a sensitive test. Fractionated plasma metanephrines can be added when suspicion is high. It is practical, and some feel a specific test for first-line diagnostic testing, as patients with pheochromocytomas can experience panic attacks. Elevated urine catecholamine levels may also occur with heavy consumption of bananas, beer, chianti wine, cheese, walnuts, and coffee (Chernecky & Berger, 2008).

Human chorionic gonadotropin (HCG) is a highly sensitive and specific test for pregnancy. Within 2 weeks of conception, HCG is elevated in the blood but not necessarily in the urine; after 2 weeks a urinary HCG is as sensitive as a blood HCG. Urinary HCG is the basis of home pregnancy test kits (Haist & Robbins, 1997). HCG-secreting tumors are virtually the only reason for a false positive HCG-based pregnancy test. Blood HCG measurement is of particular value in psychiatric contexts when female patients of reproductive age have had unprotected sexual intercourse and are taking medications highly associated with birth defects.

Urine toxicology screens are used to check for suspected substance abuse. The sensitivity of the test relates to how long after ingestion of the substance the urine sample is obtained. The time limits for detection are as follows: alcohol, 3–10 hours; amphetamines, 24–48 hours; barbiturates, up to 6 weeks; benzodiazepines, up to 6 weeks; cocaine, 2–4 days but up to 10–22 days with heavy use; phencyclidine (PCP), 1–8 days (ketamine may cause a false-positive PCP test); tetrahydrocannabinol (THC), 6–11 weeks with heavy use (McPherson & Pincus, 2006). Opiate detection depends on the half life of opiate used, but not all opiates are tested for in a routine urine drug screen panel. While morphine is noted, oxycodone is not usually detected. Fentanyl is not found because it has no metabolites. It can be difficult to distinguish between heroin, codeine, or morphine use among patients with low morphine and codeine concentrations. Many panels do not routinely screen for methadone; verapamil metabolites can contribute to false positives (Moeller, Lee, & Kissack, 2008). Amphetamine assays are complicated by false positives attributed to many prescription stimulants, and bupropion, phenothiazines, and tricyclic antidepressants may interfere with the immunoassay (see Box 5.2).

***Box 5.2* THE TIME LIMITS FOR DETECTION IN URINE TOXIC SCREENS**

Alcohol: 3 to 10 hours

Amphetamines: 24 to 48 hours

Barbiturates: up to 6 weeks

Benzodiazepines: up to 6 weeks

Cocaine: 2 to 4 days but up to 10 to 22 days with heavy use

Phencyclidine (PCP): 1 to 8 days (ketamine may cause a false positive PCP test)

Tetrahydrocannabinol (THC): 6 to 11 weeks with heavy use

Box 5.2 reproduced by permission, from Moeller, 2008, Table 3. Summary of Agents Contributing to Positive Results by Immunoassay (p. 69).

Vitamin B12, or cyanocobalamin levels, reflect absorption of B12 from dietary sources. Normal B12 absorption requires gastric acid, intrinsic factor (secreted by the stomach), and normal ileal function. Levels are low in patients with B12 malabsorption due to ileal disease, lack of intrinsic factor on an autoimmune basis (pernicious anemia), or chronically low gastric acidity related to advanced age or to chronic use of proton pump inhibitor drugs or H2 blocking drugs that chronically suppress gastric acid secretion. Due to the amount of B12 stored in the liver, patients with impaired B12 absorption or with little or no B12 dietary intake (as in severely malnourished patients or in vegans who do not take B12 supplements) will not develop a deficiency for months to years after B12 intake and/or absorption is inadequate. In patients with borderline low levels, a **methylmalonic acid** level that is abnormally high will confirm that the low B12 level is clinically significant (Antony, 2007). B12 levels can be elevated in patients taking large doses of B12 supplements or with acute hepatitis, since it is stored in the liver and released when hepatocytes are damaged.

LABORATORY TESTS USED IN THE EVALUATION OF PSYCHIATRIC SYNDROMES

Table 5.2 lists laboratory tests that physicians should consider ordering as a component of a comprehensive evaluation of a patient evaluated in a medical psychiatric context. As noted above, this panel of tests should be modified based on the clinical setting and the characteristics of the patient population to be evaluated. Medical psychiatrists might begin by considering this panel of tests and then adding or subtracting tests based on the specifics of the case. Efforts should be made to obtain the results of tests recently done elsewhere. If the results of a recent test are normal and credible, and the patient's status with respect to the relevant condition has not changed, the test may be omitted. Borderline abnormal tests done elsewhere typically are repeated.

SUMMARY

A single abnormal test result may have no clinical significance, particularly when the abnormality is mild and the result has been obtained in the context of multiple screening tests. On average, one in 20 test results will be a statistical outlier in a completely healthy patient. Individual tests done to test clinical hypotheses and tests with markedly abnormal values with potentially severe clinical consequences should be treated differently, with the patient promptly evaluated for conditions related to the laboratory abnormality. Moreover, many laboratory abnormalities associated with CNS dysfunction will have much greater import if they develop rapidly than if they develop gradually. For this reason the degree of abnormality of test results must be interpreted in temporal context. Overall, physicians need to treat patients, not lab values, and should aim to confirm diagnoses through a convergence of history, examination, and laboratory tests and, where appropriate, diagnostic procedures. "Ruling out" diagnoses through individual laboratory tests and "ruling in" diagnoses through laboratory findings alone is frequently expensive and occasionally dangerous.

Table 5.2 SUMMARY OF LABORATORY WORKUP OF COMMON PSYCHIATRIC SYNDROMES

PSYCHIATRIC SYNDROME	LABORATORY TESTS TO INVESTIGATE POTENTIAL MEDICAL CAUSES OF PSYCHIATRIC SYMPTOMS	FOR FURTHER INFORMATION
Anxiety	Hgb & Hct, TSH and free T4, blood and urine toxicology screen, glucose, ABG, sodium, calcium, magnesium, phosphate, urine catecholamines	See chapter 33
Delirium	Glucose, ABG, sodium, phosphate, calcium, BUN, magnesium, urinalysis, blood and urine toxicology screen, electroencephalogram, brain imaging, liver function tests including ammonia, WBC, albumin and prealbumin	See chapter 31
Depression	Hgb & Hct, liver function tests, TSH and free T4, sodium, BUN, creatinine, urinalysis, cortisol	See chapter 29
Fatigue	WBC, Hgb & Hct, calcium, sodium, BUN, creatinine, potassium, phosphate, TSH and free T4, liver function,	See chapter 36
Mania/Psychosis	TSH and free T4, sodium, vitamin B12, ceruloplasmin and urine copper, RPR, HIV, blood and urine toxicology screen, WBC, BUN, creatinine, iron, liver function tests, urinalysis, calcium, phosphate, glucose, folate, cortisol	
Alcohol abuse and dependence	ALT, AST, CDT, MCV, GGT, blood alcohol level, albumin, lipase, glucose, bilirubin direct and total	
Dementia	ABG, blood & urine toxicology screens, Hgb & Hct, WBC, glucose, BUN, calcium, magnesium, TSH and free T4, vitamin B12, folate, urinalysis, RPR, heavy metal in 24 hour urine, sodium, liver function test, brain imaging, lumbar puncture, phosphate, creatinine	See chapter 32
Eating Disorders	Hgb & Hct, WBC, platelet, glucose, BUN, creatinine, calcium, magnesium, TSH and free T4, vitamin B12, folate, sodium, liver function test, cholesterol profile, FSH and LH, DEXA scan, amylase, potassium, bicarbonate, phosphate	See chapter 34

CLINICAL PEARLS

- A statistical approach will identify 95% of test results as being "normal," with 2.5% of highest values and 2.5% of lowest values deemed "abnormal." However, statistical significance does not always portend clinical significance.

- "Pre-pre" analytical errors occur when a physician decides to order the wrong test for the clinical question at hand.

- "Post-post" analytical errors occur when the test involves converting a continuous quantity into a binary decision. The cut point for diagnosis may also affect test characteristics.

- Sensitivity and specificity are the best known test characteristics. 100% sensitivity means that every patient in the population examined who tests negative will not have the disease. 100% specificity means that every patient in the population examined who test positive will have the disease. Typically, a test will approach 100% sensitivity only by sacrificing specificity, and conversely.

- Factors that have been reported to increase the likelihood that a psychiatric symptom is attributable to a medical illness include lack of prior psychiatric history, very rapid onset, onset before age 12 or after age 40 years, disorientation, depressed level of consciousness, abnormal vital signs, focal neurological deficits, and the presence of visual or tactile hallucinations (Reeves et al., 2000).

- The three questions to ask in deciding whether or not to order a test are as follows:

  1. How likely is this test to be truly abnormal—a true positive—in this patient?
  2. How will the test result change the treatment plan for the patient?
  3. When will the test results be available?

- Prealbumin has a shorter half life than albumin, making low levels a more sensitive marker of acute nutritional compromise (Beck & Rosenthal, 2002).

- Many laboratory abnormalities associated with CNS dysfunction will have much greater import if they develop rapidly than if they develop gradually.

- Medical psychiatrists may see low TSH from a pituitary or a hypothalamic cause in patients who have had radiation to the brain.

- Amphetamine assays are complicated by false positives attributed to many prescription stimulants.

- In patients with borderline low levels of B12, a methylmalonic acid level that is abnormally high will confirm that the low B12 level is clinically significant (Antony, 2007).

DISCLOSURE STATEMENT

Dr. Stoner has no conflicts of interest to disclose.

REFERENCES

Altshuler, C. H. (1994). Data utilization, not data acquisition, is the main problem. *Clinical Chemistry, 40*, 1616–1620.

American Diabetes Association. (2013). Diagnosis and classifications of diabetes mellitus. *Diabetes Care, 36*(Suppl 1), S67–S74.

Antony, A. C. (2007). Megaloblastic anemias. In L. Goldman & D. Ausiello (Eds.) *Cecil's Medicine.* (23rd ed.) (pp. 1231–1240). Philadelphia, PA: Saunders Elsevier.

Arbuckle, M. R., McClain, M. T., Rubertone, M. V., Scofield, R. H., et al. (2003). Development of autoantibodies before the clinical onset of systeic lupus erythematosus. *New England Journal of Medicine, 349*, 1526–1533.

Bartch, D. A., Shern, D. L., Feinberg, L. E., Fuller, B. B., & Willet, A. B. (1990). Screening CMHC outpatients for physical illness. *Hospital and Community Psychiatry, 41*, 786–790.

Beck, F. K., & Rosenthal, T. C. (2002). Prealbumin: A marker for nutritional evaluation. *American Family Physician, 65*, 1575–1579.

Bonhoeffer, K. (1912). Die Psychosen im Gefolge von akuten Infektionen Allgemeiner Krankungen. *Handbuch der Psychiatrie*, Aschaffenburg, GL (ed.) Leipzig, Germany: Deuticke, *3*, 1–60.

Bonini, P. A., Plebani, M., Ceriotti, F., & Rubboli, F. (2002). Errors in laboratory medicine. *Clinical Chemistry, 48*, 691–698.

Botto, L. D., Lisi, A., Robert-Gnansia, E., Erickson, J. D., Vollset, S. E., et al. (2005). International retrospective cohort study of neural tube defects in relation to folic acid recommendations: are the recommendations working? *British Medical Journal, 330*, 571.

Boyd, J. C. (1997). Mathematical tools for demonstrating the clinical usefulness of biochemical markers. *Scandinavian Journal of Clinical and Laboratory Investigation, 227*(Suppl), 46–63.

Brewer, G. J., & Yuzbasiyan-Gurkan V. (1992). Wilson disease. *Medicine (Baltimore), 71*, 1139.

Buss, D. H., Stuart, J. J., & Lipscomb, G. E. (1985). The incidence of thrombotic and hemorrhagic disorders in association with extreme thrombocytosis: An analysis of 129 cases. *American Journal of Hematology, 20*(4), 365.

Bunce, D. F. M., Jones, R., Badger, L. W., & Jones, S. E. (1982). Medical illness in psychiatric patients: barriers to diagnosis and treatment. *Southern Medical Journal, 75*, 941–944.

Butterworth, R. F. (2002). Pathophysiology of hepatic encephalopathy: A new look at ammonia. *Metabolic Brain Disease, 17*, 221–227.

Cauza, E., Maier-Dobersberger, T., Polli, C., et al. (1997). Screening for Wilson's disease in patients with liver diseases by serum ceruloplasmin. *Journal of Hepatology, 27*, 358.

Center for Substance Abuse Treatment. (2006). The role of biomarkers in the treatment of alcohol use disorders. *Substance Abuse Treatment Advisory, 5*(4). Available at: http://www.kap.samhsa.gov/products/manuals/advisory /pdfs/0609_biomarkers.pdf.

Chernecky, C. C., & Berger, B. J. (Eds.). (2008). *Laboratory tests and diagnostic procedures.* St Louis, MO: Saunders Elsevier.

Czaja, M. J., Weiner, F. R., Schwarzenberg, S. J., Steinlieb, H., Scheinberg, I. H., et al. (1987). Molecular studies of ceruloplasmin deficiency in Wilson's disease. *Journal of Clinical Investigation, 80*, 1200–1204.

Ebell, M. H. (2004). Epstein Barr virus infectious mononucleosis. *American Family Physician, 70*, 1279.

Edwards, N., & Baird, C. (2005). Interpreting laboratory values in older adults. *Medsurg Nursing, 14*, 220–230.

Forsman, R. W. (1996). Why is the laboratory an afterthought for managed care organizations? *Clinical Chemistry, 42*, 813–816.

Fried, L. P., Kronmal, R. A., Newman, A. B., Bild, D. E., Mittelmark, M. B., et al. (1998). Risk factors for 5-year mortality in older adults. *Journal of the American Medical Association, 279*, 585–592.

Goroll, A. H., & Mulley, A. G. (Eds.). (2009). Evaluation of polyarticular complaints. In in *Primary care medicine: Office evaluation and management of the adult patient.* 6th ed. (pp. 1012–1022). Philadelphia, PA: Lippincott, Williams and Wilkins.

Graber, M. L. (2005). The physician and the laboratory: partners in reducing diagnostic error related to laboratory testing. *American Journal of Clinical Pathology, 124*(Suppl. 1), S1–S4.

Green, A. I., Canuso, C. M., Brenner, M. J., & Wojcik, J. D. (2003). Detection and management of comorbidity in patients with schizophrenia. *The Psychiatric Clinics of North America, 26*(1), 115–139.

Guzman, J. A. (2012). Carbon monoxide poisoning. *Critical Care Clinics, 28*(4), 537–548.

Haist, S. A., & Robbins, J. B. (Eds.). (1997). *Internal medicine on call.* (2nd ed., pp. 156–203). Stamford, CT: Appleton and Lange.

Hall, R C., Gardner, E. R., Popkin, M. K., Lecann, A. F., Stickney, S. K. (1981). Unrecognized physical illness prompting psychiatric admission: a prospective study. *American Journal of Psychiatry, 138*, 629–635.

Hampton, J. R., Harrison, M. J. G., Mitchell, J. R. A., et al. (1975). Relative contributions of history-taking, physical exam, and laboratory investigation to diagnosis and management of medical outpatients. *British Medical Journal, 2*, 486–489.

Hendren, R. L., & He, X. Y. (2006). Laboratory and diagnostic testing. In M. K. Dulcan & J. M. Wiener (Eds.). *Essentials of child and adolescent psychiatry* (pp. 99–111). Arlington, VA: American Psychiatric Publishing, Inc.

Hendrick, R. E. (2010). Radiation doses and cancer risks from breast imaging studies. *Radiology, 257*(1), 246–253.

Henneman, P. L., Mendoza, R., & Lewis, R. J. (1994). Prospective evaluation of emergency department medical clearance. *Annals of Emergency Medicine, 24*, 672–677.

Hueston, W. J. (2001). Treatment of hypothyroidism. *American Family Physician, 64*, 1717–1725.

Hu L. Steere, & A. C. Steere (2013). Diagnosis of Lyme Disease. Up to Date. http://www.uptodate.com/contents/diagnosis-of-lyme-disease?source=search_result&search=lyme+disease+diagnosis&selectedTitle=1%7E150

Huth, E. J., & Murray, T. J. (Eds.). (2000). *Medicine in quotations: Views of health and disease through the ages* (p. 354). Hanover, PA: The Sheridan Press.

Ingall, G. B. (2012). Alcohol biomarkers. *Clinics in Laboratory Medicine, 32*, 391–406.

Jackson, B. R. (2007). Managing laboratory test use: principles and tools. *Clinics in Laboratory Medicine, 27*, 733–748.

Jorde, R., Waterloo, K., Storhaug, H., Nyrnes, A., Sundsfjord, J., et al. (2006). Neuropsychological function and symptoms in subjects with subclinical hypothyroidism and the effect of thyroxine treatment. *Journal of Clinical Endocrinology & Metabolism, 91*, 145–153.

Kamp, P., & Rosse, R. B. (1990). Benefits of routine laboratory investigations. *British Journal of Psychiatry, 157*, 620–621.

Kennedy-Malone, L., Fletcher, K., & Plank, L. (2004). *Management guidelines for nurse practitioners working with older adults.* Philadelphia, PA: FA Davis.

Kim, M. M., Swanson, J. W., Swartz, M. S., et al. (2007). Healthcare barriers among severely mentally ill homeless adults: Evidence from the Five-site Health and Risk Study. *Administration and Policy in Mental Health, 34*, 363–375.

Klee, G. G. (2004). Clinical interpretation of reference intervals and reference limits: A plea for assay harmonization. *Clinical Chemistry and Laboratory Medicine, 42*, 752–757.

Koo, D. (1989) Chronic fatigue syndrome: A critical appraisal of the role of Epstein-Barr virus. *Western Journal of Medicine, 150*, 590–596.

Koran, L. M., Sox, Jr., H. C., Marton, K. I., Moltzen, S., Sox, C. H., et al. (1989). Medical evaluation of psychiatric patients: Results in a state mental health system. *Archives of General Psychiatry, 46*, 733–740.

Koranyi, E. K., & Potoczny, W. M. (1992) Physical illnesses underlying psychiatric symptoms. *Psychother and Psychosomatics, 58*(3–4), 155–160.

Kuey, L. (2008). The impact of stigma on somatic treatment and care for people with comorbid mental and somatic disorders. *Current Opinion in Psychiatry, 21*, 403–411.

Lankisch, P. G., Burchard-Reckert, S., & Lehnick, D. (1999). Underestimation of acute pancreatitis: Patients with only a small increase in amylase/lipase levels can also have or develop severe acute pancreatitis. *Gut, 44*, 542–544.

Lawrence, J., & Gyorkos, T. W. (1996). Inferences for likelihood ratios in the absence of a "gold standard." *Medical Decision Making, 16*, 412–417.

Laposata, M., & Dighe, A. (2007). "Pre-pre" and "post-post" analytical error: High-incidence patient safety hazards involving the clinical laboratory. *Clinical Chemistry and Laboratory Medicine, 45*, 712–719.

Le Moullac, B. M., Gouache, P. M., & Bleiberg-Daniel, F. (1992). Regluation of hepatic transthyretin messenger RNA levels during moderate protein and food restriction in rats. *Journal of Nutrition, 122*(4), 864–870.

Mayer, D. (2004). *Essential evidence-based medicine* (pp. 350–360). Cambridge, UK: Cambridge University Press.

Mayer, M., Wilkinson, I., Heikkinen, R., Orntoft, T., & Magid, E. (1998). Improved laboratory test selection and enhanced perception of test results as tools for cost-effective medicine. *Clinical Chemistry and Laboratory Medicine, 36*, 683–690.

McGorm, K., Burton, C., Weller, D., Murray, G., & Sharpe, M. (2010). Patients repeatedly referred to secondary care with symptoms unexplained by organic disease: Prevalence, characteristics and referral pattern. *Family Practice, 27*, 479–486.

McPherson, R. A., & Pincus, M. R. (2006). Toxicology and therapeutic drug monitoring. In R. A. McPherson, & M. R. Pincus (Eds.). *Henry's Clinical Diagnosis and Management by Laboratory Methods* (21st ed.) (pp. 147–169), chapter 23. Philadelphia, PA: Saunders Elsevier.

Moeller, K. E., Lee, K. C., & Kissack, J. C. (2008). Urine drug screening: Practical guide for clinicians. *Mayo Clinic Proceedings, 83*(1), 66–76.

Musana, K. A., Yale, S. H., & Abdulkarim, A. S. (2004) Tests of liver injury. *Clinical Medicine & Research, 2*, 129–131.

Neumann, T., & Spies, C. (2003). Use of biomarkers for alcohol use disorders in clinical practice. *Addiction, 98*(Suppl 2), 81–91.

Nutritional Care Consensus Group. (1995). Measurement of visceral protein status in assessing protein and energy malnutrition: Standard of care. *Nutrition, 11*, 169–171.

Nyblom, H., Berggren, U., Balldin, J., & Olsson, R. (2004). High AST/ALT ratio may indicate advanced alcoholic liver disease rather than heavy drinking. *Alcohol and Alcoholism, 39*, 336–339.

Nykanen, P, Boran, G. Pince, H., et al. (1993). Interpretative reporting and alarming based on laboratory data. *Clin Chim Acta, 222*, 33–48.

Obuchowski, N. A., Lieber, M. L., & Wians, F. H. Jr. (2004). ROC curves in clinical chemistry: Uses, misuses, and possible solutions. *Clinical Chemistry, 50*, 1118–1125.

Owen, S. M., Yang, C., Spira, T., Ou, C. Y., Pau, C. P., Parekh, B. S., et al. (2008). Alternative algorithms for human immunodeficiency virus infection diagnosis using tests that are licensed in the United States. *Journal of Clinical Microbiology, 46*, 1588–1595.

Panall, P., Marshall, W., Jabor, A., & Magid, E. (1996). A strategy to promote the rational use of laboratory tests. *Journal of the International Federation of Clinics, 8*, 16–19.

Prosser, J. M., & Nelson, L. S. (2012). The toxicology of bath salts: A review of synthetic cathinones. *Journal of Medical Toxicology, 8*, 33–42.

Reeves, R. R. Parker, J. D., Loveless, P., Burke, R. S., & Hart, R. H. (2010). Unrecognized physical illness prompting psychiatric admission. *Annals of Clinical Psychiatry, 22*, 180–185.

Reeves, R. R., Pendarvis, E. J., & Kimble, R. (2000). Unrecognized medical emergencies admitted to psychiatric units. *American Journal of Emergency Medicine 18*, 390–393.

Reichlin M. (2013). Measurement and clinical significance of anti-nuclear antibodies. *Up to Date*, http://www.uptodate.com/contents/measurement-and-clinical-significance-of-antinuclear-antibodies?source=search_result&search=ana&selectedTitle=1%7E150

Ritchie, R. F., Ledue, T. B., & Craig, W. Y. (2007). Patient hydration: a major source of laboratory uncertainty. *Clinical Chemistry and Laboratory Medicine, 45*, 158–166.

Salz, T., Richman. A. R., & Brewer, N. T. (2010). Meta-analyses of the effect of false-positive mammograms on generic and specific psychosocial outcomes. *Psycho-Oncology, 19,* 1026–1034.

Sauret, J., Marnides, G., & Wang, G. K. (2002) Rhabdomyolysis. *American Family Physician, 65,* 907–913.

Sax, P., & Bartlett, J. (2013). Acute and early HIV, clinical manifestations and diagnosis. *UptoDate,* http://www.uptodate.com/contents/acute-and-early-hiv-infection-clinical-manifestations-and-diagnosis?source=search_result&search=hiv&selectedTitle=1%7E150

Schafer, A. I. (2006). Thrombocytosis: When is an incidental finding serious? *Cleveland Clinic Journal of Medicine, 73,* 767–774.

Selvin, E., Steffes, M. W., Zhu, H., Matsushita, K., Wagenknecht, L., et al. (2010). Glycated hemoglobin, diabetes, and cardiovascular risk in nondiabetic adults. *New England Journal of Medicine, 362,* 800–811.

Siempos, I. I., Spanos, A., Issaris, E. A., Rafailidis, P.I, & Falagas, M. E. (2008). Non-physicians may reach correct diagnoses by using Google: a pilot study. *Swiss Medical Weekly, 138*(49–50), 741–745.

Simerville, J. A., Maxted, W. C., & Pahira, J. J. (2005). Urinalysis: A comprehensive review. *American Family Physician, 71,* 1153–1162.

Staley, M. J., Naidoo, D., & Pridmore, S. A. (1984). Concentrations of transthyretin (prealbumin) and retinol-binding protein in alcoholics during alcohol withdrawal [Letter]. *Clinical Chemistry, 30,* 1887.

Staver, S. (1979). Blue Cross-Shield act to halt reimbursement for routine tests. *American Medical News, 22*(7), 1.

Tanielian, T. L., Cohen, H. L., Marcus, S. C., & Pincus, H. A. (1999). General medical care for psychiatric patients. *Psychiatric Services, 50*(5), 637.

Threatte, G. A., & Henry, J. B. (1996). Carbohydrates. In J. B. Henry (Ed.). *Clinical Diagnosis and Management by Laboratory Methods* (19th ed.). Philadelphia, PA: W. B. Saunders Co.

Van Walraven, C., & Naylor, D. (1998). Do we know what inappropriate laboratory utilization is? A systematic review of laboratory clinical audits. *Journal of the American Medical Association, 280,* 550–558.

Wians, F. H. (2009). Clinical laboratory tests: Which, why and what do the results mean? *Lab Medicine, 40,* 105–113.

Willett, A. B., & King, T. (1977). Implementation of laboratory screening procedures on a short-term psychiatric inpatient unit. *Diseases of the Nervous System, 38,* 867–870.

Williams, M. D., Harris, R., Dayan, C. M., Evans, J., Gallacher, Y., et al. (2009). Thyroid function and the natural history of depression: findings from the Caerphilly Prospective Study(CaPS) and a meta-analysis. *Clinical Endocrinology, 70,* 484–492.

Young, W. F., & Kaplan, N. M. (2013).Clinical presentation and diagnosis of pheochromocytoma. *UpToDate.* http://www.uptodate.com/contents/clinical-presentation-and-diagnosis-of-pheochromocytoma?source=search_result&search=pheochromocytoma&selectedTitle=1%7E150

Zun, L. S. (2005). Evidence-based evaluation of psychiatric patients. *Journal of Emergency Medicine, 28*(1), 35–39.

6.

LABORATORY EVALUATION OF ENDOCRINE DISORDERS IN PATIENTS WITH NEUROPSYCHIATRIC SYMPTOMS

Fernando A. Rivera, Shirlene Sampson, and Christopher L. Sola

INTRODUCTION

Whether an endocrine disorder is contributing to the presentation of neuropsychiatric symptoms is an important question for medical psychiatrists. It has long been known that hormonal disorders include cognitive, affective, and behavioral changes. These symptoms often precede or present simultaneously with the somatic signs and symptoms of endocrine disease and may confuse even the most astute diagnostician. Hormonal symptoms may be mislabeled during early stages as neurotic or somatoform; during more advanced stages, endocrine disorders may be misdiagnosed as dementia or primary psychosis. Endocrine disorders are more likely to present with neuropsychiatric symptoms in older patients and in children, who may be more sensitive to disruption of brain function by hormones.

In this chapter we focus on endocrine evaluation of patients who present with neuropsychiatric signs and symptoms, either alone or in combination with other nonpsychiatric symptoms. Chapter 55 will provide further detail on the psychiatric dimensions of specific primary endocrine disorders. Here we will deal with testing of the endocrine functions of the thyroid, adrenal, pituitary, and testes, and also with diabetes mellitus, hypoglycemia, and pheochromocytoma. Female reproductive endocrinology is covered in chapter 67.

When patients with known endocrine disorders are referred to medical psychiatrists for concurrent psychiatric syndromes, they are likely to be treated specifically for psychiatric syndromes whether or not the symptoms are thought to be secondary to the endocrine condition or merely comorbid. Similarly, when an endocrine disorder develops during the course of treatment of a chronic psychiatric illness, treatment of the endocrine disorder typically will be added to the ongoing psychiatric treatment. When a patient newly presents with neuropsychiatric symptoms, and a previously undiagnosed endocrine condition is identified, many endocrinologists would suggest treating the endocrine condition and following the patient to see if the psychiatric disorder resolves. A more nuanced approach would draw on the experience of the endocrinologist and his or her colleagues with other patients who had the same endocrine disorder, to assess whether the presenting patient's psychiatric symptoms are disproportionate to the endocrine abnormality. If so, it is likely that the endocrine condition is a contributing or provocative factor in the psychiatric disorder and not its sole cause. Concurrent treatment of the endocrine and the psychiatric condition would be preferable in such cases, as it would be when patients are suffering greatly from mental symptoms or when their behavior poses a risk to their health and safety or to the safety of other people.

LABORATORY TESTS OF THE THYROID

Thyroid disease can produce neuropsychiatric symptoms in two ways—through the effects of an excess or deficiency of thyroid hormones on metabolism and neurotransmission, and through autoimmune inflammatory processes affecting the brain directly. Autoimmune diseases can result in the release of cytokines with neuropsychiatric effects or can affect other endocrine organs such as the adrenals and ovaries. Hypothyroidism and hyperthyroidism are remarkable because neuropsychiatric symptoms can be their most prominent manifestation, so thyroid disease may be discovered in working up the symptoms of brain dysfunction. By contrast, the implications of antibodies directed at the thyroid are considered more often after a patient has already been diagnosed with thyroid disease.

A combination of two tests—the serum thyroid stimulating hormone (TSH) and serum free thyroxine (T4)—is highly sensitive and specific in detecting thyroid hormone excess or deficiency. The test results often point to the underlying cause of the thyroid dysfunction, most often due to disease of the thyroid itself and much less often due to pituitary or hypothalamic dysfunction.

THYROID STIMULATING HORMONE

The serum TSH level should be performed (or checked if recently done) in all medical-psychiatric patients in whom there is any suspicion of thyroid dysfunction, and in all female patients over 50 with psychiatric disorders whether or not there are signs and symptoms specifically pointing to the thyroid. Thyroid dysfunction should be suspected when neuropsychiatric symptoms occur that are potentially due to too much or too little thyroid hormone, in combination with typical physical symptoms or signs on physical examination. The neuropsychiatric and general somatic symptoms and signs of hypothyroidism and thyrotoxicosis are summarized in Table 6.1.

Like other pituitary hormones, TSH is released in a pulsatile manner, but its serum level varies smoothly because the serum half-life of TSH is 50 minutes. In normal individuals the serum level of TSH has a circadian rhythm, with a peak level at 2 a.m. to 4 a.m. and a nadir between 4 p.m. and 8 p.m. The recommended time for drawing a diagnostic TSH level is first thing in the morning (Sviridonova, Fadeyev, Sych, & Melnichenko, 2013). A spot TSH level drawn in the late afternoon can be in the normal range, slightly higher than the morning reading—a false negative in patients with mild hypothyroidism. Apart from the circadian rhythm, changes in TSH from hour to hour and from day to day are relatively small, so that a single serum TSH drawn in the morning is sufficient for diagnostic purposes.

TSH IN MONITORING THYROID HORMONE REPLACEMENT FOR HYPOTHYROIDISM

TSH Is Elevated, Free T4 Is Low

TSH is elevated in primary hypothyroidism. Free T4 is low. After treatment for clinical hypothyroidism is initiated, the dose of levothyroxine is adjusted to bring TSH levels into the lower half of the normal range.

TSH responses to levothyroxine replacement are gradual and should be measured at about 2 months after initiating treatment and a similar period after any subsequent change in dosage.

Data from recent studies, including the National Health and Nutrition Examination Survey of the Centers for Disease Control (NHANES III, 2013), are challenging the validity of the traditional TSH reference range of 0.5 μU/mL to 5.0 μU/mL (0.5–5.0 mU/L). When patients with a family history of thyroid disease or the presence of thyroid antibodies are excluded from the reference population, the TSH normal range appears to be more narrow (0.5–2.5 μU/mL

Table 6.1 CLINICAL SIGNS AND SYMPTOMS OF THYROID HORMONE EXCESS AND DEFICIENCY

CONDITION	NEUROPSYCHIATRIC SYMPTOMS AND SIGNS	OTHER SOMATIC SYMPTOMS AND SIGNS
Hypothyroidism	Apathy	Cold intolerance
	Depressed mood or depressive syndrome	Edema (nonpitting)
	Irritability	Weight gain
	Cognitive impairment	Constipation
	Delirium (in severe cases)	Amenorrhea or irregular periods
	Psychosis (in severe cases)	Hair loss
	Slow speech	Cool skin
	Mania (rarely)	Hoarse voice
	Fatigue	
	Weakness	
	Muscle stiffness	
	Hypersomnia or sleepiness	
	Worsening of sleep apnea	
	Delayed relaxation phase of reflexes	
	Increased sedative and anticholinergic effects of CNS drugs	
Thyrotoxicosis (usually due to hyperthyroidism)	Anxiety	Heat intolerance
	Increased activity	Warm skin
	Impaired attention and concentration	Weight loss
	Rapid speech	Frequent bowel movements
	Mixed affective state	Amenorrhea or irregular periods
	Psychosis (in severe cases)	Dyspnea
	Delirium (in "thyroid storm")	Hair loss
	Fatigue	Tachycardia and palpitations
	Weakness	Lid retraction and lid lag
	Proximal myopathy with muscle wasting (in advanced cases)	Atrial fibrillation
	Insomnia	Heart failure
	Hyperactive reflexes	

SOURCES: Brent, 2008; Nayak & Hodak, 2007; DeGroot et al. (2009) in *Endocrinology*, 2007.

[0.5–2.5 mu/L]). Therefore, a target range of approximately 1.0 μU/mL to 2.5 μU/mL (1.0–2.5 mU/L) seems appropriate for patients with defined thyroid disease receiving replacement levothyroxine. Whether patients without known thyroid disease or risk factors whose serum TSH levels are between 2.5 μU/mL and 5.0 μU/mL (2.5–5.0 mIU/L) should be treated remains less clear, especially for older patients.

The mainstay of thyroid hormone replacement is levothyroxine therapy, which should always be taken on an empty stomach one hour before or 2 to 3 hours after intake food or other medications. Although much attention has recently been focused on therapy with liothyronine or combination T3/T4 therapy using either thyroid hormone extract or synthetic T3/T4 combinations, most evidence to date shows no clinical advantage of combined T3/T4 therapy over traditional levothyroxine treatment.

SUBCLINICAL HYPOTHYROIDISM

TSH Is Elevated, Free T4 Is Normal

Subclinical hypothyroidism is defined as the presence of an above-normal TSH with simultaneous free T4 and free T3 levels in the normal range (Surks et al., 2004). A patient with a TSH greater than 10.0 mIU/L would be treated for hypothyroidism despite a normal free T4 and free T3 and the lack of the typical clinical syndrome.

There are no generally accepted recommendations for subclinical hypothyroidism (Biondi & Cooper, 2008; Garber, 2012). While endocrinologists would not *routinely* treat *asymptomatic* patients with a TSH <10.0 mIU/L they might differ on whether to regard major depression poorly responsive to standard antidepressant drugs as a symptom of hypothyroidism for the purpose of deciding whether a patient was "asymptomatic." The identification of additional non-psychiatric symptoms or signs of hypothyroidism—for example, cold intolerance or slow deep tendon jerks—would be relevant to a consulting endocrinologist and special effort to elicit them is worthwhile. Subclinical hypothyroidism may be associated with an increased risk of atherosclerosis and cardiac events, but reversal of these effects with T4 therapy has not been systematically studied (Kratzsch & Pulzer, 2008; Cooper, 2007).

TSH IN SECONDARY OR TERTIARY HYPOTHYROIDISM

TSH Is Normal, Free T4 Is Low

With rare exceptions a normal TSH rules out a primary abnormality of thyroid function. A TSH level with a free T4 level should be done when the clinical context and the combination of neuropsychiatric and other somatic symptoms increases the probability that secondary thyroid dysfunction is present; for instance, when there is a history of head trauma or brain radiation. The addition of a free T4 to TSH level will improve diagnostic sensitivity. When the TSH is normal or below the normal range and the free T4 level is low, the patient is diagnosed with hypothyroidism due to pituitary (secondary) or hypothalamic (tertiary) dysfunction

TSH IN DIAGNOSING AND MONITORING TREATMENT OF THYROTOXICOSIS

TSH Is Low, Free T4 Is High

The TSH levels currently available from clinical laboratories are determined by immunoradiometric assays. They are either third generation assays that can measure levels as low as 0.01 mIU/L, or fourth generation assays that can measure levels down to 0.004 mIU/L. Either one is sufficiently sensitive to the presence of hyperthyroidism, which is diagnosed when the level of TSH is below the normal range and a free T4 or free T3 is above the normal range. The normal range of TSH varies between laboratories; a range of 0.3 mIU/L–0.5 mIU/L on the low end to 4.00 mIU/L–5.00 mIU/L on the high end would be typical, although, as has been noted, below a range of 0.5 mIU/L–2.5 mIU/L might more accurately capture the range of values for individuals with no thyroid disease whatever (DeGroot et al., 2009).

With either the third-generation or fourth-generation TSH assay, the sensitivity is high enough to make unnecessary the TRH stimulation test for the diagnosis of hyperthyroidism, because in hyperthyroidism there is a very strong correlation between a low baseline TSH and a blunted TSH response to exogenous TRH.

TSH remains suppressed for several months after treatment for hyperthyroidism (Brent, 2008).

TSH Is Low, Free T4 Normal, Free T3 High

If TSH is low and free T4 is normal, free T3 should be checked. T3 may be elevated in certain cases of Graves' disease or if T3 is given exogenously.

Central or Secondary Thyrotoxicosis

TSH Is Normal or High, Free T4 High, Free T3 High

When the TSH is normal or above the normal range and the free and total T4 and free and total T3 level is high—a rare situation—the patient may be diagnosed with secondary hyperthyroidism, which is usually due to a TSH-secreting pituitary adenoma (Nayak & Hodak, 2007).

Subclinical Hyperthyroidism

TSH Low, Free T4 Normal, Free T3 Normal

Subclinical hyperthyroidism is defined as the presence of a below-normal serum TSH with simultaneous free T4 and free T3 levels in the normal range. Specifically, a patient with a TSH <0.1 mIU/L would be treated for hyperthyroidism even if the free T4 and free T3 were normal and the patient did not show the typical clinical syndrome of thyrotoxicosis.

AUTOANTIBODIES AND AUTOIMMUNE DISEASE

There are two common autoimmune thyroid diseases: Hashimoto's disease, which usually causes hypothyroidism, and Graves' disease, which usually causes hyperthyroidism

(Pearce, Farwell, & Braverman, 2003; Brent, 2008). These conditions are associated with antithyroid antibodies, of which five specific types are measured by clinical laboratories: antithyroid peroxidase antibodies, antithyroglobulin antibodies, anti–TSH receptor antibodies, thyroid-stimulating immunoglobulins, and thyrotropin-binding inhibitory immunoglobulins.

Thyrotoxicosis means an abnormally high level of thyroid hormone in the serum. It is most frequently due to hyperthyroidism—overactivity of the thyroid gland (Nayak & Hodak, 2007). Other cases are due to extrathyroidal sources of thyroid hormone or due to consumption of exogenous thyroid hormone, the latter being much more common than the former. The most common cause of hyperthyroidism is Graves' disease; other common causes are subacute thyroiditis, postpartum thyroiditis, toxic (hormone-secreting) thyroid adenomas, and toxic multinodular goiter. In most cases of thyrotoxicosis, the free T4 is elevated. The incidence is highest in women between 20 and 40 years old (Brent, 2008).

Graves' disease is a systemic autoimmune disorder that prominently involves the thyroid gland, but also affects the eyes and the skin. The thyroid in Graves' disease is diffusely enlarged. The diagnosis usually can be made clinically, and three of the five antithyroid antibodies mentioned above are characteristic of the disease. Their presence is diagnostically helpful when the patient has typical skin and/or eye changes of Graves' disease but does not have an elevated level of T4 or T3. These three antibodies are antithyrotropin stimulating hormone receptor (TSH-R), thyroid-stimulating immunoglobulin (TSI), and TSH receptor binding inhibitor immunoglobulin (TBII). TSH-R is seen in the large majority of patients with Grave's disease (Barbesino & Tomer, 2013). TBII misses milder forms of Grave's disease. While patients with Graves' disease can also have anti thyroid peroxidase antibodies (anti-TPO) and antithyroglobulin (anti-TG) antibodies, these are more common in Hashimoto's disease than Graves' disease and can occur in some patients without thyroidal illness.

The special relevance of anti-TSH-Rs, TSIs, and TBIIs to medical psychiatrists is that some patients with autoimmune thyroid disease alternate between hypothyroid and hyperthyroid states, producing a clinical picture that can be confusing, especially when the main symptoms of the thyroid disease are neuropsychiatric. Knowledge of the presence of antibodies that can stimulate or inhibit T4 production by binding to T4-secreting cells can explain a fluctuating clinical course and can prompt the clinician to consider that changes in neuropsychiatric symptoms could be due to a switch between thyroid hormone excess and deficiency.

These tests are not routine, and are generally reserved for the evaluation of the patient with typical ophthalmologic signs of Graves' disease but with normal or borderline thyroid function and minimal or no thyroid enlargement; pregnancy complicated by Graves' disease; or atypical fluctuating hypohyperthyroidism (Pearce et al., 2003).

Patients with other systemic autoimmune diseases including rheumatoid arthritis (RA), systemic lupus erythematosus (SLE), and idiopathic thrombocytopenic purpura (ITP) have one or more antithyroid antibodies in a minority of cases. These patients are at greater risk of developing hypothyroidism than patients with similar demographics who do not have antithyroid antibodies. These systemic autoimmune disorders are associated with neuropsychiatric symptoms. When new neuropsychiatric symptoms present in patients with RA or SLE, reevaluation of thyroid status and testing for anti-TPO and anti-TG should be considered.

FACTITIOUS THYROTOXICOSIS

TSH Low, Free T4 High, Thyroglobulin Low or Low Normal

Factitious thyrotoxicosis due to self-administration of T4 or T3 can be established by measurement of the serum thyroglobulin (TG) level. In hyperthyroidism, the level of TG is elevated or high normal because it is secreted along with T4 and T3. When exogenous thyroid hormone is taken, secretion of T4 and T3 by the thyroid decreases and hence serum TG will be low or low normal. Thyroglobulin is a glycoprotein integral in follicular storage of thyroid hormone; it is normally present in serum, and the serum level is increased in hyperthyroidism, in some cases of thyroiditis, and in papillary and follicular cancer of the thyroid, where it is a useful marker of tumor recurrence following thyroidectomy or radiation therapy (Brent, 2008; Mariotti, Martino, Cupini, et al., 1982).

ELEVATED T4 IN SEVERE PSYCHIATRIC DISORDER

TSH Normal, Free T4 Transiently Elevated

Transient elevation of T4 can be seen in patients with acute, severe psychiatric disorders such as acute schizophrenia or mania (Spratt, Pont, & Miller, 1982). In these patients, TSH is not suppressed and occasionally it is elevated. The T4 level returns to normal in less than a month. The presumptive cause is a stress-related alteration in activity of the hypothalamic-pituitary-thyroid axis; if the cause were intrinsic, thyroid overactivity (hyperthyroidism) the TSH level would be decreased.

EUTHYROID SICK SYNDROME

TSH Normal, Free T4 Normal or Low, Free T3 Low

Any acute severe medical illness or trauma can cause a decrease in the level of T3, and sometimes also T4, in the absence of underlying thyroid gland pathology and with a normal TSH level. This condition is called the "sick euthyroid" or "euthyroid sick" syndrome. The more common form consists of a reduction in total T3 and free T3 with normal levels of TSH and T4. The reduction of the T3 level is proportional to the severity of the patient's medical illness, and it is thought to reflect impaired conversion of T4 to T3. Other very sick patients can present with significant reductions in total T4 and free T4 as well. This variant has a worse clinical outcome than the one in which only T3 levels are low. The diagnosis can only be confirmed by resolution of the thyroid hormone abnormality when the patient recovers from the acute medical condition. The present consensus of endocrinologists is not to give supplementary thyroid hormone to euthyroid sick patients unless there is independent evidence to suggest they are actually hypothyroid.

The euthyroid sick syndrome is the result of complex mechanisms that combine the effect of some drugs, cytokines, nutritional, and endocrine factors at all levels of the thyrotropic axis from the hypothalamus to the cellular transporters and nuclear receptors of thyroid hormones. The pattern of this condition depends on the underlying disease and its severity. Thirty-five years after the initial description, the pathophysiological significance of these anomalies remains controversial. It remains unclear whether the hormone responses of the euthyroid sick syndrome represent an adaptive and normal physiologic response to conserve energy and protect against a catabolic state, or whether it is a maladaptive response contributing to a worsening of the patient's condition (Luca, Goichot, & Brue, 2010).

LITHIUM-INDUCED HYPOTHYROIDISM

TSH High, Free T4 Low

Among psychotropic drugs, lithium is the only one associated with alteration of thyroid function. Lithium induces a decrease in production of T4 from the thyroid gland, as well as interference with the conversion of T4 to T3. The American Psychiatric Association Practice Guidelines for the Treatment of Patients with Bipolar Disorder conclude that hypothyroidism will develop in 5% to 35% of patients with that disorder, usually within 6 to 18 months of lithium treatment initiation. The wide range of reported prevalence rates has been attributed to methodological differences across studies such as variable sample sizes, durations of lithium exposure, assays of varying sensitivity, and different cutoff points for diagnosis. The risk is higher in women (American Psychiatric Association, 2002).

Baseline thyroid function tests should be measured prior to starting lithium therapy to ensure that previously undetected thyroid dysfunction is not contributing to mood symptoms. Pertinent thyroid function tests include TSH and free T4 levels, as well anti-TPO and anti-TG antibodies if the TSH is elevated; presence of the latter implies a higher risk for clinical hypothyroidism and thus a need for closer monitoring. Subsequent monitoring of thyroid function tests is usually conducted 3 months after starting lithium and every 6–12 months thereafter; in addition, patients should be questioned regularly at outpatient visits about physical symptoms suggestive of hypothyroidism. The development of hypothyroidism in a patient on lithium is a reason to begin thyroid hormone supplementation, but not necessarily to discontinue lithium if the patient has done very well on it. Current practice guidelines do not specify criteria for managing thyroid replacement therapy in patients with lithium-induced hypothyroidism; a reasonable target for T4 supplementation is bringing the TSH into the lower half of the normal range.

In the presence of elevated TSH levels without clinical signs of hypothyroidism, some societies recommend checking serum TSH levels every 3 months, without giving adjunctive thyroid hormone therapy unless TSH levels rise above 10 mU/L. Others advise thyroid supplementation whenever TSH levels rise above normal, particularly when mood symptoms are not in full remission. When lithium is discontinued, thyroid function can return to normal but it does not always do so, and even when it does it may take up to 2 years. If a patient is begun on T4 replacement and lithium is discontinued, the patient's need for thyroid replacement, and the appropriateness of the dose of T4, should be reassessed annually and whenever a change in symptoms suggests the possibility of thyroid excess or deficiency (American Psychiatric Association, 2002; Cowdry et al., 1983).

EFFECTS OF DEPRESSION ON THYROID FUNCTION TESTS

Depression can be accompanied by subtle thyroid dysfunction. Patients presenting with depression rarely have frank clinical hypothyroidism—the maximum reported prevalence is 4%; in a specific clinical population the rate will be higher if patients are relatively older and there is a higher proportion of women in the sample. However, subclinical hypothyroidism has been found in as many as 40% of patients presenting with depression, depending on the clinical population sampled. Depression has been linked to an abnormal diurnal TSH rhythm as well, with an absent nocturnal increase, and in one study, patients with major depression (as opposed to nonmajor depression) had a lower basal TSH. About 25%–30% of patients with depression have a blunted TSH response to exogenous TRH. A possible explanation is that chronic TRH hypersecretion associated with depression leads to downregulation of pituitary TRH receptors. Supporting this hypothesis are reports of elevated Cerebrospinal fluid (CSF) concentrations of TRH in depressed patients (Wolkowitz & Rothschild, 2003; Bauer, Goetz, Glenn, & Whybrow, 2008). The blunting of TSH response to TRH occurs in a minority of cases, making it unsuitable as a diagnostic test for depression. Subtyping patients with depression according to their response to TRH stimulation has not proved helpful in predicting patients' response to antidepressant treatments (Bauer et al., 2008).

LABORATORY TESTS OF THE ADRENAL

The adrenal cortex produces two types of steroid hormones which are regulated by two different feedback loops. Glucocorticoids, of which cortisol is most important; is regulated by a hypothalamic-pituitary-adrenal loop involving corticotropin releasing hormone (CRH) from the hypothalamus and adrenocorticotropic hormone (ACTH) from the pituitary. Mineralocorticoids, of which aldosterone is most important, is regulated by a feedback loop involving the kidneys and the lungs, renin and angiotensin.

While neuropsychiatric symptoms as the sole manifestation of adrenal disorders is a rare occurrence, excess or deficiency of glucocorticoids usually entails mental and behavioral symptoms. When patients present with a combination of neuropsychiatric symptoms and general somatic symptoms and signs compatible with excess or deficiency of adrenal hormones, the laboratory evaluation of adrenal function is indicated. Measurement of serum cortisol is not, however, part of the routine laboratory screening of patients who present with changes in mood, behavior, or cognition; the presence of general somatic symptoms or physical signs characteristic of an adrenal disorder is the prompt for laboratory investigation. If a serum cortisol level has been recently measured, and it is known that it was drawn between 8 a.m. and 9 a.m., it can be compared with a normal range of 7 µg/mL to 25 µg/mL. Values <7 µg/mL suggest adrenal insufficiency, and values >25 µg/mL raise a concern of glucocorticoid excess. Table 6.2 lists the neuropsychiatric and general somatic manifestations of glucocorticoid excess and of adrenal insufficiency.

CUSHING'S SYNDROME (GLUCOCORTICOID EXCESS)

Cushing's syndrome is the clinical disorder that comes from prolonged exposure to inappropriately elevated plasma glucocorticoid levels. While glucocorticoids are often administered chronically for the treatment of allergic, autoimmune, inflammatory, or neoplastic disorders, the causes of endogenous excess of cortisol are rare. The differential diagnosis of endogenous Cushing's syndrome includes (1) excessive pituitary ACTH secretion, usually due to a pituitary adenoma (Cushing's disease); (2) adrenocortical carcinoma and other adrenal tumors; and (3) ectopic production of ACTH by malignancies (most commonly, small-cell carcinoma of the lung). In adults, Cushing's disease accounts for 60% to 70% of all cases, adrenal tumors for approximately 20%, and the ectopic ACTH syndrome for the remaining 10% to 20% (Ioachimescu & Hamrahian, 2013; Loriaux, 1990; Nieman et al., 2008).

Laboratory diagnosis of Cushing's syndrome is based on a combination of three findings: (1) excessive secretion of cortisol over a 24-hour period as indicated by an above-normal value of a 24-hour urinary free cortisol; (2) loss of normal diurnal variation in cortisol secretion as indicated by an elevated late-night salivary cortisol level; and (3) loss of feedback inhibition of the hypothalamic-pituitary-adrenal axis as indicated by failure of exogenous dexamethasone given at 11 p.m. to reduce the morning cortisol level (the low-dose

Table 6.2 CLINICAL SIGNS AND SYMPTOMS OF ADRENAL HORMONE EXCESS AND DEFICIENCY

NEUROPSYCHIATRIC SYMPTOMS	SOMATIC SYMPTOMS/SIGNS
Adrenal insufficiency	
Weakness	*Weight loss*
Fatigue	*Abdominal pain*
Anorexia	*Nausea, vomiting*
	Diarrhea, constipation
	Hyperpigmentation
Salt craving	*(palmar creases, extensor surfaces inside of cheeks)*
	Vitiligo
Postural dizziness	*postural hypotension*
	Hyponatremia
	Hypoglycemia
	Anemia
	Eosinophilia
Adrenal Hyperfunction (Schneider, 2012)	
Depression	Central obesity
	Buffalo hump
Difficulty climbing stairs	Rounded face
or getting up from chair	Recurrent infection
without using arms	Proximal myopathy
Loss of Libido	acne
Manic-like, (exogenous)	Diabetes
Irritability, insomnia	Edema
Short-term memory loss	Facial plethora
Psychosis	Wide purple striae
	Osteoporosis
	Change in photos
	Hypokalemia
	Amenorrhea
	Hirsutism
	Hypertension

SOURCE: Nieman et al., 2012.

overnight dexamethasone suppression test (DST)). The relevant threshold values are (1) urinary free cortisol >200 µg/24 hours (551nmol/24h); (2) midnight salivary cortisol based on assay norms; and (3) 8 a.m. cortisol >50 nmol/L (or >2 µg/dL) the morning after 1 mg of oral dexamethasone at 11 p.m. the previous evening. Salivary cortisol is in equilibrium with the free cortisol in the circulation. Thus, the finding of an elevated midnight salivary cortisol level on at least two separate occasions should raise concern about the possibility of Cushing's syndrome if the saliva sample was taken on a quiet, restful night. When values are on the borderline, or in situations where one of the three tests is abnormal and another is normal, the diagnosis can be confirmed by a standard low-dose dexamethasone suppression test; this is done by giving 0.5 mg of dexamethasone orally every 6 hours for 2 days, then measuring the 8 a.m. cortisol on the third day. The threshold value for abnormality is the same.

Once hypercortisolism is established, further tests are needed to determine the cause. These begin with measurement of serum ACTH. If the ACTH level is low or undetectable, the cause is in the adrenal itself, usually an adrenal adenoma. If the ACTH level is elevated or normal (which would be inappropriate if cortisol were high) the cause is either hypersecretion of ACTH by the pituitary or ectopic ACTH secretion, as by a hormone-secreting cancer. Excessive secretion of ACTH by a pituitary adenoma usually can be suppressed by giving dexamethasone 2 mg every 6 hours for 48 hours (the high-dose dexamethasone suppression test). ACTH secretion by malignant extrapituitary tumors is not suppressible by dexamethasone even at a high dose.

Some patients with major depression and some alcohol-dependent patients have adrenal test profiles indistinguishable from those of patients with mild Cushing's disease (i.e., Cushing's syndrome of pituitary origin), They have elevated cortisol levels and show suppression of cortisol production with high-dose dexamethasone but not with low-dose dexamethasone. Their endocrine abnormalities resolve with remission of their depression or with abstinence from alcohol. Further workup to establish whether the patient has Cushing's disease is done in collaboration with an endocrinologist; identification of a pituitary adenoma by an imaging procedure establishes the diagnosis.

ADDISON'S DISEASE
(ADRENOCORTICAL INSUFFICIENCY)

Inadequate production of adrenal corticosteroids may result from a variety of primary adrenal disorders (Addison's disease) or be secondary to inadequate ACTH secretion (secondary adrenal insufficiency) (Dorin, Qualls, & Crapo, 2003). Addison's disease refers to insufficiency of glucocorticoids and mineralocorticoids and the associated clinical syndrome, rather than to a specific cause of adrenal damage or dysfunction. Destructive inflammation of the adrenal gland on an autoimmune basis is the leading cause, accounting for the majority of cases in developed countries. Other causes of adrenal insufficiency include infiltration of the adrenal with metastatic cancer; infections such as TB, syphilis, HIV, or disseminated fungal infections; and drugs such as ketoconazole, fluconazole, rifampin, and megestrol. Adrenal insufficiency keeps company with other autoimmune endocrine disorders like hypothyroidism, premature ovarian failure, Type I diabetes mellitus, and hypoparathyroidism. The

neuropsychiatric and general somatic symptoms and signs of adrenal insufficiency are shown in Table 6.2 above. Most are due to deficiency of glucocorticoids. Hypokalemia, which is secondary to mineralocorticoid deficiency, would be seen only in cases of Addison's disease but no in cases of secondary adrenal insufficiency. Hyperpigmentation of the skin, due to secretion of melanocortin synchronously with ACTH, is also exclusively of Addison's disease, in which ACTH secretion is mainly decreased.

Initial laboratory screening for adrenal insufficiency begins with an 8 a.m. serum cortisol level. If this is <7 μg/dL, further assessment is warranted. If the 8 a.m. serum cortisol is borderline low, or if there is there is reason to suspect atypical chronobiology of cortisol secretion (e.g., night shift work), a 24-hour urinary free cortisol should be obtained. A value of <4 μg/24 hours suggests adrenal insufficiency. Other laboratory tests that can help define adrenal status are (1) plasma ACTH, which is low in primary adrenal insufficiency and high in secondary adrenal insufficiency; (2) serum aldosterone, which is low in primary adrenal insufficiency but normal in secondary adrenal insufficiency; (3) plasma renin activity, which is high in primary adrenal insufficiency but normal in secondary adrenal insufficiency; and (4) DHEA and DHEA-S, which are low in both primary and secondary adrenal insufficiency.

The definitive diagnosis of primary adrenal insufficiency is based on proving that the adrenal gland does not adequately secrete cortisol even when vigorously stimulated by the pituitary. To do this, the patient is challenged in the morning with an intravenous dose of 250 μg of synthetic 1-24 ACTH (generic name *cosyntropin*, trade name Cortrosyn®). Serum cortisol is measured prior to the injection and at 30 and 60 minutes afterward. A normal adrenal gland will secrete sufficient cortisol to raise the serum concentration to >20 μg/dL (550nmol/L) over baseline; if this does not happen the adrenal function is insufficient.

Confirmation of the diagnosis of secondary adrenal insufficiency and determination of its cause requires a specialist endocrine evaluation that includes anatomic imaging (MRI unless there is a contraindication) of the pituitary-hypothalamic region. Depending on the context, it may be important in cases of central adrenal insufficiency to determine that the adrenal would be normally responsive to ACTH if secretion of the latter were normal. This can be confirmed with a low-dose cosyntropin test, which is performed in the same way as the cosyntropin test for Addison's disease except with a 1μg dose of cosyntropin rather than with a 250μg dose. A normal adrenal gland that has been underproducing cortisol solely because of insufficient ACTH will immediately secrete cortisol, producing a significant rise in the serum cortisol from baseline.

Treatment of Addison's disease usually requires both glucocorticoid and mineralocorticoid replacement. A typical glucocorticoid replacement regimen would be hydrocortisone, 20 mg in the morning and 10 mg in the late afternoon. A single morning dose of a more potent, longer-acting glucocorticoid such as prednisone (5.0–7.5 mg) is also effective. The only available oral mineralocorticoid preparation is fludrocortisone (Florinef); the dose of this agent is adjusted for the individual patient based on blood pressure and serum potassium determinations. Patients with secondary adrenal insufficiency require only glucocorticoid replacement.

LABORATORY ASSESSMENT OF ADRENAL SUPPRESSION BY EXOGENOUS GLUCOCORTICOIDS

Exposure to supraphysiologic doses of glucocorticoids—more than 20 mg per day of prednisone or equivalent—for 2 weeks or more can cause clinically relevant suppression of the hypothalamic-pituitary-adrenal axis. While frank Addison's disease is unusual when exogenous glucocorticoids are withdrawn, exposure to long-term high-dose glucocorticoids causes a loss of adrenal reserve. This can cause a relative deficiency of glucocorticoids if the patient is challenged by acute illness, surgery, or trauma. This relative deficiency can manifest as hypotension, hypoglycemia, weakness and cognitive impairment, or even life-threatening adrenal crisis. It is unknown whether an episode of acute psychosis represents a stress that can precipitate signs of adrenal insufficiency in this context.

Adrenal reserve is assessed in the laboratory with a cosyntropin stimulation test; the procedures are identical to those used in assessing a patient for Addison's disease. If serum cortisol does not increase with a 250μg dose of cosyntropin, the adrenal gland is virtually unresponsive to ACTH and exogenous glucocorticoids will be necessary to cover periods of severe physiological stress. If the serum cortisol increases with a 250μg dose but not with a 1μg dose, there is a lesser degree of adrenal suppression; this would be seen in a recovering adrenal gland. While glucocorticoid supplementation at times of stress would still be indicated, the cortisol increase with the higher dose of cosyntropin is a positive prognostic sign. A cosyntropin stimulation test should be repeated every 3 months in a patient with adrenal insufficiency caused by exogenous glucocorticoids who is no longer receiving supraphysiologic doses or who has been switched to alternate-day therapy to permit recovery of adrenal function. Once the test normalizes, the patient will no longer need glucocorticoid supplementation.

LABORATORY ASSESSMENT OF CALCIUM METABOLISM

Too much or too little calcium can alter mental status, all the more if the change in calcium is rapid. Because serum calcium is measured routinely as part of blood chemistry screening panels, it is unusual for diagnoses of parathyroid disorders to be missed in patients receiving regular medical care. Extreme values of calcium are encountered in two situations: (1) patients with rapidly increasing calcium, for example, cancer patients with multiple bony metastases; and (2) patients with hyperparathyroidism who have not received general medical care, for example, homeless patients with chronic mental illness who have deliberately avoided health professionals. Medical psychiatrists typically see patients with mild to moderate abnormalities of serum calcium and parathyroid hormone (PTH) and are asked to assess the relevance of those abnormalities to the patient's current mental and behavioral symptoms.

Primary hyperparathyroidism is characterized by hypercalcemia and low phosphate due to excessive PTH secretion, usually due to a parathyroid adenoma, more often in women than men. Fifteen percent of cases are due to parathyroid hyperplasia. Cancer causes hypercalcemia when osteoclastic metastases leach calcium from bone or when a PTH-like substance is produced by the tumor. The most common cancers associated with hypercalcemia are lung, breast, multiple myeloma, renal, cervix, and head and neck.

Other causes include hyperthyroidism, sarcoidosis (and other granulomatous diseases), vitamin A and vitamin D intoxication, immobilization, drugs (thiazides, lithium), Addison's disease, familial hypocalciuric hypercalcemia, and acute renal failure with rhabdomyolysis (Inzucchi, 2004).

SYMPTOMS AND SEVERITY OF HYPERCALCEMIA

The severity of the symptoms of hypercalcemia parallels the severity of the serum calcium level, the rate of the increase, and the overall health condition of the patient. A screening serum calcium often calls attention to this diagnosis; there should be a low threshold in patients presenting with the symptoms and signs in Table 6.3.

The clinical symptomatology is minimal for most of the patients with mild hypercalcemia (levels greater than the normal serum calcium level but <12 mg/dL [3.0 mmol/L]), although some report mild fatigue, depression, constipation, mild polyuria, mild increase in thirst, or vague changes in cognition.

Typical manifestation of hypercalcemia are more common with serum calcium levels of 12 mg/dL to 14 mg/dL [3.0–3.5 mmol/L] and include anorexia, nausea, abdominal pain, muscle weakness, and depressed mental status.

At serum calcium levels greater than 14 mg/dL (3.5 mmol/L), lethargy, disorientation, and coma may occur.

EVALUATION OF ETIOLOGY OF HYPERCALCEMIA

The diagnosis of hypercalcemia would require a comprehensive medical history, physical exam, laboratory work and occasionally imaging studies. Blood tests include: serum calcium, serum PTH, ionized calcium, phosphorus, and serum creatinine levels (Sheppard & Smith, 2007).

Relation of Calcium to Albumin

It is always appropriate and standard of care to calculate serum calcium corrected for the hypoalbuminemia level, especially in patients with conditions such as malnutrition, nephritic syndrome, cirrhosis, chronic obstructive pulmonary disease, or chronic congestive heart failure. The measured serum calcium level should be corrected for a low albumin level by adding 0.8 mg/dL (0.2 mmol/L) of calcium for each 1 g/dL (10 g/L) of albumin that a patient's serum is <4 g/dL. An accurate ionized calcium measurement will help on these cases; however,

Table 6.3 NEUROPSYCHIATRIC AND SOMATIC SYMPTOMS/SIGNS OF HIGH AND LOW CALCIUM

CONDITION	NEUROPSYCHIATRIC SYMPTOMS	SOMATIC SYMPTOMS/SIGNS
Hypercalcemia		
Mild	Fatigue	Acid indigestion
	Nausea	Musculoskeletal pain
	Anorexia	Pancreatitis
	Thirst	Constipation
		Polyuria
	Lack of initiative	
	Cognitive decline	
Moderate	Depressive	
	Apathy	
	Poor concentration	
	Confusion,	Dehydration
	disorientation	Renal stones
	Visual and auditory hallucinations	
	Catatonia	
	Delusions	
	Hallucinations	
Severe	Stupor, coma	
Hypocalcemia		
Mild	Asymptomatic	Neck irradiation
Moderate	Paresthesias, tetany	Muscle cramps
	Carpopedal spasm	Poor oral nutrition
	Seizure	Renal tubular loss
	Anxiety, panic attacks, phobia	
	Depression	
	Cognitive decline	Stigmata of alcoholism
Severe	Confusion	Laryngeal strider
	Hallucination	
	Delirium	

ionized calcium samples must be drawn under anaerobic conditions and kept on ice for accurate results. Additionally, the availability and cost of this test somewhat limit this decision.

FACTITIOUS HYPERCALCEMIA

Total Calcium Elevated, Ionized Calcium Normal

When an elevated serum calcium is detected, factitious hypercalcemia caused by elevated levels of the plasma proteins that bind calcium (such as in HIV infection, chronic hepatitis, and multiple myeloma) is a consideration. The ionized calcium level is normal on these patients.

FURTHER EVALUATION OF HYPERCALCEMIA

After the first test confirms hypercalcemia, the following recommendation is the simultaneously measurement of serum PTH and serum plasma ionized calcium levels. In the absence of plasma protein abnormalities, obtaining a total serum calcium level is usually adequate; ionized calcium samples must be drawn under anaerobic conditions and kept on ice for accurate results.

Serum Calcium High, PTH High or Normal

With normal parathyroid glands, hypercalcemia will suppress PTH. If the serum calcium level is elevated and the PTH level is high or inappropriately normal, the diagnosis of PTH-mediated hypercalcemia or primary hyperparathyroidism is made.

There are indications for surgical intervention in patients with primary hyperparathyroidism: increase in serum calcium level >1 mg/dL (0.25 mmol/L) above upper limit of normal in otherwise asymptomatic patients; creatinine clearance <60 ml/min (0.06 L/min) in asymptomatic patients; T-score (Bone Density Scan [DXA] or bone densitometry) of −2.5 or worse at the lumbar spine, total hip, femoral neck, or distal radius; or age <50 years. Surgery is also indicated in patients in whom medical surveillance is neither desired nor possible, including those with significant bone, kidney, gastrointestinal, or neuro-muscular symptoms typical of primary hyperparathyroidism (Bilezikian, Khan, & Potts, 2009; Inzucchi, 2004).

HYPOPARATHYROIDISM

Low Calcium, High Phosphate, Low PTH, Normal Albumin

Hypoparathyroidism occurs most commonly due to surgical damage to the parathyroids during surgery for head and neck cancer or thyroid surgery, or neck irradiation. Other causes are rare and include parathyroid aplasia; infiltration by amyloid, sarcoid, or hemochromatosis; and autoimmune disease.

Low Calcium, Low Magnesium

Magnesium facilitates function of the parathyroid hormone, so conditions associated with magnesium deficiency such as poor nutrition, malabsorption, alcoholism, or renal tubular wasting from cisplatin treatment may be contributing factors.

Low Vitamin D

Vitamin D deficiency contributes to hypocalcemia. The vitamin deficiency may be due to chronic renal failure, inadequate sunlight, or intake.

Acute Pancreatitis Is Associated with Low Calcium

Acute symptomatic hypocalcemia should be treated with intravenous calcium gluconate. Chronic hypocalcemia due to hypoparathyroidism is treated by administration of oral calcium and if unsuccessful, vitamin D supplementation.

DISORDERS OF GLUCOSE METABOLISM

DIABETES MELLITUS

Diabetes mellitus, a chronic metabolic disease characterized by increased circulating blood glucose levels, results from the inadequate supply or action of insulin. Several distinct types of diabetes mellitus are caused by a complex interaction of genetics and environmental factors. Diabetes mellitus is diagnosed in most patients on the basis of their fasting glucose level. The more sensitive oral glucose tolerance test is less frequently performed, although it remains a standard way to diagnosed diabetes during gestation. A diagnosis of diabetes also can be made if a random plasma glucose level equals or exceeds 200 mg/dL (11.1 mmol/L) in the setting of symptomatic hyperglycemia, such as polyuria, polydipsia, or blurred vision. The hemoglobin A1c value is a long-term (2–3 months) marker of glycemic control. The American Diabetes Association additional *criteria for diagnosis of diabetes* is A1c ≥6.5, fasting plasma glucose ≥126 mg/dL. The patients at increased risk for diabetes who meet criteria for prediabetes have a fasting plasma glucose of 100 mg/dL to 125 mg/dL or a Hgb A1c

5.7–6.4. With an oral glucose tolerance test, prediabetes as defined by the plasma glucose may be 140 mg/dl (7.8 mmol/L to 199 mg/dL (American Diabetes Association, 2013).

HYPOGLYCEMIA

Hypoglycemia is a syndrome best defined by the following triad of clinical findings (Whipple's triad): (1) characteristic symptoms, (2) plasma or serum glucose concentration <50 mg/dL, and (3) reversal of symptoms by glucose administration. As a general rule, this means glucose levels <55 mg/dL (3.0 mmol/L) with clinical symptomatology that is relieved promptly after the glucose level is raised (Cryer et al., 2009). The symptoms of hypoglycemia are described in Table 6.4.

FACTITIOUS HYPOGLYCEMIA

The presence of anti-insulin antibodies or low C-peptide levels at the time of hypoglycemia strongly suggests a factitious etiology like surreptitious injection of insulin (Horwitz, 1989). Insulin from the pancreas is secreted as proinsulin and broken into insulin and C-peptide. C-peptide has no biological activity. Screening of urine or blood for sulfonylureas is available for patients suspected of surreptitious oral hypoglycemic agent ingestion.

In the 1970s and 1980s, hypoglycemia was overdiagnosed (Cahill & Soeldner, 1974; Gastineau, 1983; Nelson, 1985). Reactive hypoglycemia became a fashionable diagnosis to account for a variety of poorly defined physical and psychological ills including depression, anxiety, fatigue, sexual dysfunction, and overall loss of vitality (Yager & Young, 1974).

Table 6.4 NEUROPSYCHIATRIC AND SOMATIC MANIFESTATIONS OF HYPERGLYCEMIA AND HYPOGLYCEMIA

Hyperglycemia	Neuropsychiatric Symptoms	Somatic Symptoms/ Signs
	fatigue, anorexia,	Polyuria
	weakness, cognitive impairment, blurred vision	Excessive thirst
	delirium, depression,	Sweet craving
	neuropathic pain	Dehydration
	coma	Infection
Hypoglycemia	Cognitive impairment, somnolence, anxiety, tremor, weakness, hunger, irritability, feeling faint, lethargy, confusion, dizziness, weakness, incoordination, bizarre behavior, change in personality, seizures, coma	Sweating Hyperventilation Palpitations Headache, Blurred Vision Slurred speech Hemiparesis

Although most common in type 1 diabetes mellitus, severe hypoglycemia also can occur in type 2 diabetes in patients who are taking insulin or drugs (such as sulfonylureas and meglitinides) that stimulate the release of insulin. Patients may be taking too large a dose of insulin, delaying or skipping a meal, eating fewer carbohydrates than normally, or exercising more than usual. The sulfonylureas vary mostly in dose and half-life. Those with long half-lives, such as glipizide extended release and glyburide, can cause profound, prolonged hypoglycemia, especially in older patients and patients with impaired renal function.

Hypoglycemia is rare in non-diabetic individuals because healthy persons have adequate mechanisms for maintaining glucose homeostasis (metabolism). Alcohol ingestion is a potential factor for hypoglycemia because affects hepatic glycogen stores directly. At the same time, alcohol intoxication can make the symptoms of hypoglycemia harder to recognize.

An important issue in the psychopharmacological management of patients with hypoglycemia is the risk of beta-blocker therapy. Early misdiagnosis of an anxiety disorder and treatment with agents whose action blocks the normal response to hypoglycemia may prevent subjective experience of potentially lethal hypoglycemia.

Fasting hypoglycemia has other less common causes including insulin-secreting islet cell tumors of the pancreas, large non–islet-cell tumors, severe liver or renal disease, adrenal insufficiency, hypopituitarism, severe inanition, autoimmune disorders associated with antibodies to insulin or to the insulin receptor, and drugs or toxins (Cryer et al., 2009).

DISORDERS OF PITUITARY FUNCTION

Both the excess and deficiency of pituitary hormones are associated with neuropsychiatric as well as general somatic symptoms. Disturbances in the secretion of ACTH have neuropsychiatric effects through an influence on adrenal hormones, and TSH has its influence on thyroid hormone secretion. Similarly, luteinizing hormone (LH) and follicle stimulating hormone (FSH) influence the production of sex hormones by the ovary and testis; growth hormone influences the production of IGF-1 (somatomedin C) by the liver. For this reason, laboratory testing of levels of pituitary hormones is typically accompanied by testing of the associated hormones in the target organs. Prolactin is the only exception.

The most common causes of pituitary hypersecretion are hormone-secreting tumors, mostly histologically benign adenomas. Adenomas secrete only one pituitary hormone; it is thus possible for a patient with a pituitary adenoma to have an excess of one pituitary hormone and a deficiency of another one. Nonsecreting pituitary adenomas can cause deficiencies in pituitary hormones by displacing normal secreting cells. Panhypopituitarism, a simultaneous deficiency of all of the pituitary hormones, can be caused by a vascular insult to the entire pituitary.

ACROMEGALY

Age-matched and sex-matched serum IGF-1 levels are elevated in acromegaly. Consequently, an IGF-1 level provides a useful laboratory screening measure when clinical features raise the possibility of acromegaly. Due to pulsatility of GH secretion, measurements of a single random GH level is not useful for the diagnosis or exclusion of acromegaly and does not correlate with disease severity (Molitch et al., 2006; Webb et al., 2012; Melmed, 2006).

HYPERPROLACTINEMIA

Prolactin, the pituitary hormone that stimulates breast development and lactation, is the hormone most commonly secreted by hormone-secreting pituitary adenomas. Prolactin secretion is tonically inhibited by dopamine; it is stimulated by TRH. Dopamine antagonist drugs raise prolactin levels, with first-generation antipsychotic drugs like haloperidol and fluphenazine having particularly potent effects and risperidone the most likely of the atypical antipsychotics to raise prolactin. Metoclopramide, a dopamine agonist used for gastrointestinal rather than psychiatric indications, also raises prolactin levels. Other drugs associated with increased prolactin levels include opiates, verapamil, cimetidine, and estrogen-containing oral contraceptives. In a minority of cases, primary hypothyroidism increases prolactin levels presumably because of increased hypothalamic TRH secretion. Moderate elevation of prolactin levels can be seen in liver failure and in renal failure.

Prolactin levels rise following convulsive seizures and may double from baseline in the 10–20 minutes after a suspected event. This test may be a useful adjunct to differentiate generalized tonic-clonic or complex partial seizure from psychogenic nonepileptic seizure among adults and older children. It does not distinguish seizure from syncope (Chen, So, & Fisher, 2005). Finally, prolactin levels are elevated during lactation (initially as high as 300 when the mother has maximum estrogen priming, but later in lactation only minimally elevated)—and can be elevated by frequent nipple stimulation even in the absence of lactation (Snyder & Cooper, 2013).

Although there are many potential causes of an elevated prolactin, extremely high prolactin levels are virtually always due to pituitary tumors. An increase in prolactin level beyond the range explainable by any of a patient's current drug and medical conditions, (about 200 mg/L) is strongly suggestive of a pituitary tumor and should trigger a full work-up including imaging of the pituitary and testing of the other pituitary hormones.

Hyperprolactinemia is considered the most common pituitary hormone hypersecretion syndrome in both men and women. The pituitary adenomas (prolactinomas) are the most common cause of elevated serum prolactin levels (PRL levels >200 ug/L) Other etiologies include pregnancy, lactation, sleep, stress, systemic disorders, and drug-induced hypersecretion. Hyperprolactinemia in women is manifested by galactorrhea, irregular menses, and infertility. Men usually have no physical symptoms but both genders may experience reduced libido, depression, and anxiety (Levenson, 2006).

The decrease in serum prolactin levels with treatment in women with prolactinomas is usually associated with a return of normal ovulatory menstrual cycles and cessation of galactorrhea. Fertility is generally restored, and many of these women experience perfectly normal term pregnancies. Careful monitoring for symptoms of pituitary expansion during pregnancy is essential, although complication rates in women with microadenomas are low. Normalization of serum prolactin concentrations in men similarly results in restoration of normal gonadal function, assuming there is no impairment of gonadotropin secretion from the primary pituitary tumor.

In most centers, initial therapy for prolactinomas is medical, with either bromocriptine or cabergoline. Transsphenoidal surgery is usually reserved for patients with rapidly enlarging pituitary tumors or patients not responding to or unable to tolerate the side effects of ergot alkaloid therapy.

GONADOTROPINS

Hormone-secreting pituitary tumors rarely secrete the gonadotropins LH and FSH; pituitary tumors are more likely to cause a decrease in these hormones. In women the most common reason for significant elevation of FSH is ovarian failure, whether due to menopause, surgical removal of the ovaries, or autoimmune disease. The most common reason for elevation of LH is the LH surge associated with ovulation. In men, elevation of FSH and elevation of LH occur together as a response to primary testicular failure, an age-associated condition. Low values of LH and FSH are seen in various conditions that affect fertility, including polycystic ovary syndrome. These conditions are discussed in detail in chapter xx. The neuropsychiatric and general somatic effects of these hormones are via their effects on the ovaries and testes rather than direct ones. Alterations in gonadotropin secretion are suggested by changes in the female menstrual cycle and by changes in libido and/or fertility in either sex.

When testing pituitary gonadotropins in menstruating women, it is optimal to draw the sample on day 5–7 of the menstrual cycle prior to the LH surge associated with ovulation. Levels of LH and FSH can be tested at any time in men or in postmenopausal women. In men, measurement of the LH and FSH should be accompanied by a free testosterone level. A low testosterone level with an elevated LH and FSH suggests primary testicular failure; if both LH and testosterone are low, there is dysfunction of either the hypothalamus or the pituitary. The distinction can be made by challenging the patient with a 50mg oral dose of clomiphene, a drug that stimulates the secretion of gonadotropin-releasing hormone by the hypothalamus. If pituitary gonadotropin secretion is intact, the LH level will rise significantly.

MALE HYPOGONADISM

The measurement of the serum total testosterone, free plus protein-bound and typically ranging from 300 ng/dL (10.4 nmol/liter) to 800 ng/dL, is the usual measure of this hormone. It is best drawn at 8 a.m. and repeated once or twice if not declarative, in order to guide the evaluation of male hypogonadism (Brambilla, Matsumoto, Araujo, & McKinlay, 2009). Testosterone levels can vary quite a bit from day to day, and the level, especially in young men, is higher in the morning.

Free testosterone is suggested if the measurement is at the lower limit of normal or if there is a condition likely to alter sex hormone–binding globulin. Conditions which change the concentration of sex hormone–binding globulin and make the free testosterone level more valuable include liver disease, severe systemic illness, and corticosteroid treatment (Manni et al., 1985; Mayo, 2013). Testosterone binding is reduced in proportion to obesity. Older men may have slightly increased binding to sex hormone–binding globulins.

The equilibrium dialysis method in dedicated laboratories is the standard for measuring free testosterone. Free testosterone by an analog method, commonly offered in hospitals and commercial laboratories, is not reliable; and indirect calculations of free testosterone should be checked against norms of the measuring laboratory (Snyder, Matsumoto, Kirkland, & Martin, 2013).

An understanding of male hypogonadism requires a review of the two major functions of the testes: secretion of testosterone and production of sperm. Hypogonadism refers to a deficiency of either or both of these essential functions. Inadequate sperm production alone usually presents as infertility, whereas the consequences of testosterone deficiency depend on the stage of sexual development of the patient. An excellent review of this complex area has been published (Bhasin et al., 2006).

Hypogonadal disorders in men can generally be grouped into those associated with diseases involving the testes directly (primary hypogonadism) and those associated with disorders of the hypothalamic-pituitary axis (secondary hypogonadism). In teenage boys, testosterone deficiency is characterized by failure of normal secondary sexual characteristics to develop (i.e., delayed puberty). In postpubertal males, testosterone deficiency is accompanied by symptoms including decreased libido and energy, sexual dysfunction, and decreased body hair and muscle mass.

Primary gonadal failure is typically associated with elevated serum gonadotropin concentrations and is therefore referred to as hypergonadotropic hypogonadism. The testosterone is low, and FSH and LH are high. The most common cause of this disorder in young men is Klinefelter's syndrome, associated with an abnormal chromosomal constitution of 47,XXY. Other causes of primary gonadal failure include myotonic dystrophy, mumps orchitis, testicular trauma or irradiation, and autoimmune testicular failure. Uremia and chronic alcohol abuse have features suggestive of both primary and secondary hypogonadism.

Hypogonadotropic hypogonadism may be due to either primary pituitary or hypothalamic pathology. Pituitary causes include destructive pituitary tumors, prolactinomas (see above), hemochromatosis, sarcoidosis, therapeutic irradiation or surgery, and severe systemic illness. The classic hypothalamic cause of hypogonadotropic hypogonadism is Kallmann's syndrome. This syndrome is characterized by a deficiency of the hypothalamic peptide gonadotropin-releasing hormone (GnRH). Patients with Kallman's syndrome present as prepubertal eunuchs with minimal development of secondary sexual characteristics. Associated features may include anosmia or hyposmia and cleft palate and lip. The treatment of prostate cancer with GnRH analogs such as leuprolide is another etiology for secondary hypogonadism. Hypogonadism can follow anabolic-androgenic steroid dependence.

Male hypogonadism of any etiology may cause significant psychological distress and impaired social adjustment. Low self-esteem and self-confidence and feelings of inadequacy, isolation and alienation are common. Male patients with recently acquired loss of libido and drive not explained by major depression or drugs deserve a screening testosterone level and attention paid to gonadal size on physical examination. If these screening measures suggest hypogonadism, further workup is indicated.

An appropriate *initial* diagnostic evaluation of a patient with suspected hypogonadism should include a careful history and physical examination, focusing on the disorders outlined above. The degree of sexual development, testicular size, and evidence of pituitary dysfunction should be the focus of the physical examination.

Laboratory studies should include a serum testosterone, gonadotropin levels (LH and FSH), and a serum prolactin level. The results of these studies should define the level of the primary pathologic disturbance (i.e., a primary testicular disorder versus a central abnormality in hypothalamic-pituitary function). Patients falling into the latter category usually require radiographic imaging of the pituitary either by CT scanning or MRI. All patients with hypogonadism should be referred for further endocrinologic investigation. Appropriate therapy for testosterone deficiency is either a long-acting injectable testosterone preparation such as testosterone enanthate, or one of the new transdermal testosterone patches, gel and buccal mucosa lozenges Bolona, 2007). Oral androgens are not the agents of choice for hypogonadal men, as they are less effective in restoring normal virilization and have considerably greater toxicity (see below). Hypogonadotropic hypogonadal men desiring fertility should be treated with clomiphene, gonadotropins or pulsatile GnRH rather than with androgens.

Androgen/testosterone replacement therapy in men should be initiated only after the possibility of occult prostate cancer has been eliminated.

The amount of testosterone required to maintain lean mass, fat mass, strength and sexual function varies widely in men. The diagnosis of androgen deficiency had been based on a single laboratory criterion: a testosterone level more that two standard deviations below the mean in normal young men; however, the dose required to prevent adverse changes varies considerably. Most of the estradiol of men (80%) results from aromatization of testosterone. It turns out that both deficiency of testosterone and deficiency of estradiol contribute to decline of sexual function in men. Estrogen deficiency also contributes to an increase in fat accumulation (Finkelstein et al., 2013).

Recent guidelines for testosterone therapy in adult men with androgen deficiency syndromes by the Endocrine Society suggest that only men with consistent symptoms and signs and unequivocally low serum testosterone levels be treated. The treatment is based on an initial test of morning total testosterone level, and in some patients free testosterone level. Testosterone in these cases improves sense of well being, muscle mass and strength, bone mineral density, and sexual function. Contraindications are breast or prostate cancer, a prostate nodule or PSA greater than 3 ng/ml if without urologic intervention, erythrocytosis, hyperviscosity, obstructive sleep apnea, lower urinary symptoms, or class III or IV heart failure. The goal is a mid-normal range testosterone incorporating the patient's preference and managed with a standardize plan of follow-up (Bhasin et al., 2006).

The relationship between aging-related testosterone deficiency and late-onset hypogonadism has been unclear. A recent study has suggested that late-onset hypogonadism may be defined by the presence of at least three sexual symptoms associated with a total testosterone level of less than 11 nmol per liter (3.2ng per ml) and a free testosterone level of less than 220 pmol per liter (64pg per ml) (Wu et al., 2010). Psychological symptoms do not parallel testosterone level, but loss of physical vigor does. This study suggested that the requirement of the presence of at least three sexual symptoms with a total testosterone level of less than 11 nmol per liter and a free testosterone level of less than 220 pmol per liter was appropriate for testosterone replacement, as had been suggested in practice guidelines.

PANHYPOPITUITARISM

A number of medical conditions (tumor like craniopharyngioma, macroadenoma, breast metastases, infarct, infiltrative diseases such as hemochromatosis,) can cause diffuse damage to the pituitary gland, with decreased secretion of all of the pituitary hormones. This leads to hypothyroidism, hypoadrenalism, hypogonadism, and growth hormone deficiency all at once. Patients with panhypopituitarism have a chronically ill appearance and show the neuropsychiatric symptoms of apathy, dysphoric mood, and cognitive impairment. A presentation of a patient with multiple somatic symptoms and prominent apathy in the context of one of the predisposing conditions should lead to laboratory testing for panhypopituitarism. An adequate screening test panel would include serum levels of TSH and free T4, cortisol (drawn at 8–9 a.m.), and, if the patient is male, a free testosterone. A low cortisol level would be followed up with an ACTH level, and a low testosterone would be followed up with an LH level to confirm a problem at the level of the pituitary or above. Anatomic imaging of the pituitary-hypothalamic region would then help identify the cause of the problem.

Hormone replacement in panhypopituitarism conventionally has included replacement of T4, cortisol, and testosterone or estrogen. Replacement of growth hormone is done less consistently. Measuring the serum level of IGF-1 can be useful in making the decision about growth hormone replacement. A very low or absent level of IGF-1 and residual mental and physical symptoms after replacement of thyroid, adrenal, and gonadal hormones suggests value in a trial of GH replacement with careful monitoring of symptoms potentially attributable to GH deficiency.

PHEOCHROMOCYTOMA

Pheochromocytomas are rare catecholamine-secreting tumors that arise most often from chromaffin tissue of the adrenal medulla. While most patients with pheochromocytomas are hypertensive, hypertension is endemic and pheochromocytomas are rare; routine testing of hypertensive patients for pheochromocytoma is not warranted. Patients with hypertension should have a laboratory evaluation for pheochromocytoma if they have one or more conditions that raise the likelihood of their having the condition well above the population base rate. These conditions are (1) hypertension refractory to standard, stepped antihypertensive drug therapy and not explained by renal artery stenosis or by another endocrine disorder; (2) paroxysmal hypertension accompanied by headache, sweating, tremor, and other signs of sympathetic overactivity; (3) hypertension associated with hypermetabolism (e.g., weight loss despite increased caloric intake); (4) a personal history of associated disorders such as neurofibromatosis, tuberous sclerosis, Sturge-Weber syndrome, or multiple endocrine neoplasia; or (5) pheochromocytoma or an associated condition in a first-degree relative. About 10% of patients with pheochromocytomas do not have hypertension at all but do have discrete episodes of symptoms of sympathetic overactivity, including paroxysmal sweating and paroxysmal atrial tachycardia or fibrillation or ventricular tachycardia.

The most sensitive test for pheochromocytoma is a random plasma free metanephrine level. Because it is less specific than 24-hour urine studies, it is best done in patients where the clinical suspicion is already high. A less sensitive but more specific test should be used when clinical suspicion is low, or to confirm the diagnosis when the plasma metanephrine level is somewhat elevated but is inconclusive. That test is a 24-hour urine for catecholamines and metabolites (Pacak et al., 2007).

Table 6.5 NEUROPSYCHIATRIC AND SOMATIC SYMPTOMS OF PHEOCHROMOCYTOMA

NEUROPSYCHIATRIC SYMPTOMS	SOMATIC SIGNS
Panic attacks	Refractory hypertension
Headaches	Orthostatic hypertension
Palpitations	Paroxysmal hypertension
Visual blurring	Pallor and flushing
Especially as episodes (Spells)	
	Atrial tachycardia or fibrillation

Once the chemical diagnosis of pheochromocytoma is made, the tumor(s) must be located. Most can be found on an MRI of the adrenal region. Tumors not found on MRI will be picked up on scintigraphy using radiolabeled metaiodobenzylguanidine.

ENDOCRINE SCREENING IN PATIENTS WITH WEIGHT LOSS AND FAILURE TO THRIVE

Weight loss in *hyperthyroidism* is due primarily to increased catabolism, but other causes include increased intestinal motility and malabsorption. Most patients have hyperphagia. In older patients, however, hyperthyroidism often causes anorexia with accelerated weight loss. The average weight loss in a patient with hyperthyroidism is 16% of usual body weight (Hoogwerf & Nuttall, 1984). Weight gain occurs quickly with treatment.

Uncontrolled diabetes mellitus is a common cause of weight loss with increased appetite, particularly with new-onset type 1 diabetes mellitus. There is a loss in lean body mass as well as loss of extracellular and cellular water due to the osmotic diuresis from glucosuria. The etiology of weight loss in uncontrolled diabetes is likely multifactorial—a combination of anorexia, depression, pain, malabsorption, gastroparesis, and enteropathy. Some reports describe persons who intentionally undertreat their diabetes in order to lose weight (Rodin & Daneman, 1992). Although patients with poorly controlled or undiagnosed type 2 diabetes can occasionally present with weight loss, weight gain is much more common. However, some patients with type 2 diabetes can occasionally present with diabetic neuropathic cachexia, an unusual and poorly understood syndrome characterized by profound weight loss (as much as 60% of body weight) and often severe neuropathic pain of the anterior thighs (Neal, 2009). The pathophysiology is not clear, especially since there is no strong relationship between glucose control and resolution of weight loss, which usually happens spontaneously after months or years.

Chronic *primary adrenal insufficiency* often presents with significant weight loss, although other associated signs and symptoms are more prominent: dehydration, anorexia, lassitude, fatigue, and weakness. Adrenal insufficiency that is acute or due to hypothalamic or pituitary dysfunction is usually not associated with weight loss (Dorin, Qualls, & Crapo, 2003).

Anorexia, nausea, constipation, and polyuria may account for weight loss in patients with the classic clinical manifestations of *hyperparathyroidism*. However, the majority of patients with primary hyperparathyroidism are asymptomatic and do not have weight loss (Bolland, Grey, Gamble, & Reid, 2005).

The hyperadrenergic state among patients with *pheochromocytoma* would theoretically cause weight loss with increased appetite, but only 5% of patients with pheochromocytomas report weight loss (Goldstein et al., 1999).

Table 6.6 BASIC PSYCHIATRIC SYNDROMES THAT CAN BE CAUSED BY ENDOCRINE ABNORMALITIES

	DEPRESSION	MANIA	PSYCHOSIS	DELIRIUM	DEMENTIA	WEIGHT LOSS
TSH	X	X	X	X	X	
Calcium	X	X	X	X	X	
PTH	X	X	X			
Cortisol	X	X	X	X		X
ACTH	X	X	X	X		X
Glucose	X	X		X		
IGF-1	X	X	X			
Prolactin	X					
Testosterone	X					

Delirium, depression, and dementia are the most common conditions affecting cognitive status in older adults. The evaluation of any patient with failure to thrive (FTT) should include an evaluation to identify signs or symptoms of delirium, dementia, and depression. These conditions may result from medical comorbidities and medication effects; each may also contribute to the development of disability, malnutrition, and frailty. Dementia and depression were among the five leading causes of FTT in a case series of inpatients admitted with FTT (Hildebrand, Joos, & Lee, 1997).

BASIC ENDOCRINE SCREENING TESTS

There is scant empirical cost-benefit evidence to inform the laboratory work-up for depression. For patients at higher risk of underlying medical illness, consideration should be given to assessing TSH sensitive level and fasting serum glucose level.

Psychosis could be secondary to a medical condition. A large number and variety of medical conditions (Patkar, Mago, & Masand, 2004) and endocrine dysfunctions may lead to psychotic symptoms, including thyroid, parathyroid, or adrenal abnormalities. Screening tests should include TSH sensitive, PTH, serum calcium level, cortisol and ACTH levels.

A number of endocrine laboratory tests may be considered in the patient with delirium. However, the desire for diagnostic completeness can increase costs and possibly delay the prompt treatment of more obvious disorders. Targeted testing is appropriate in most instances, especially in the elderly: glucose, calcium and thyroid function tests could be initially included in the preliminary assessment.

The American Academy of Neurology (AAN) recommends screening for hypothyroidism in patients with dementia (Knopman et al., 2001). There are no clear data to support or refute ordering "routine" laboratory studies such as a complete blood count, electrolytes, glucose, and renal and liver function tests. The cost effectiveness of obtaining multiple laboratory studies in all patients is questioned because the yield is low (Weytingh, Bossuyt, & van Crevel, 1995) (see Table 6.6).

CLINICAL PEARLS

- TSH responses to levothyroxine replacement are gradual and should be measured at about 2 months after initiating treatment and a similar period after any subsequent change in dosage.

- A patient with a TSH >10.0 mIU/L would be treated for hypothyroidism despite a normal free T4 and free T3 and the lack of the typical clinical syndrome.

- A TSH level with a free T4 level should be done when the clinical context and the combination of neuropsychiatric and other somatic symptoms increases the probability that secondary thyroid dysfunction is present; for instance, when there is a history of head trauma or brain radiation.

- A target range of approximately 1.0 μU/mL to 2.5 μU/mL (1.0–2.5 mU/L) seems appropriate for patients with defined thyroid disease receiving replacement levothyroxine.

- Factitious thyrotoxicosis due to self-administration of T4 or T3 can be established by measurement of the serum thyroglobulin (TG) level.

- Some patients with major depression and some alcohol-dependent patients have adrenal test profiles indistinguishable from those of patients with mild Cushing's disease (i.e., Cushing's syndrome of pituitary origin)

- The presence of anti-insulin antibodies or low C-peptide levels at the time of hypoglycemia strongly suggests a factitious etiology like surreptitious injection of insulin (Horwitz, 1989).

- The most sensitive test for pheochromocytoma is a random plasma free metanephrine level. Because it is less specific than 24-hour urine studies, it is best done in patients where the clinical suspicion is already high.

- Exposure to supraphysiological doses of glucocorticoids—namely, more than 20 mg per day of prednisone or equivalent—for 2 weeks or more can cause clinically relevant suppression of the hypothalamic-pituitary-adrenal axis.

- Hypogonadism can follow after patients stop anabolic-androgenic steroids taken for some time for body building.

DISCLOSURE STATEMENTS

Dr. Fernando Rivera has no conflicts to disclose, no extramural funding, no patients, and no direct or indirect financial or personal relationships, interests, or affiliations, whether or not directly related to the subject of the chapters.

Dr. Christopher Sola has no conflicts to disclose, no extramural funding, no patients, and no direct or indirect financial or personal relationships, interests, or affiliations, whether or not directly related to the subject of the chapters.

Dr. Sampson is transcranial magnetic stimulation equipment loan for research and educational purposes by Neuronetics, Inc. No personal financial income from any company.

REFERENCES

American Diabetes Association. (2011). *Diabetes Care, 34,* S11–S61.

American Diabetes Association. (2013). Diagnosis and classification of diabetes mellitus. *Diabetes Care, 36*(Suppl 1), S67–S74.

American Psychiatric Association. (2002). Practice guideline for the treatment of patients with bipolar disorder (revision). *American Journal of Psychiatry, 159,* 1–50.

Barbesino, G., & Tomer, Y. (2013). Clinical utility of TSH receptor antibodies. *Journal of Clinical Enocrinology & Metabolism, l98,* 2247–2255.

M. Bauer, Goetz, T. Glenn, T., & Whybrow, P. C. (2008). The thyroid-brain interaction in thyroid disorders and mood disorders. *Journal of Neuroendocrinology, 20,* 1101–1114.

Fagin, J. A., & Mitsiades, N. (2008). Molecular pathology of thyroid cancer: Diagnostic and clinical implications. *Best Practice Research of Clinical Endocrinolology and Metabolism, 22*(6), 955–969. doi:10.1016/j.beem.2008.09.017.

Bhasin, S., Cunningham, G. R., Hayes, F. J., et al. (2006). Testosterone therapy in adult men with androgen deficiency syndromes: An Endocrine Society clinical practice guideline. *Journal of Clinical Endocrinology & Metabolism, 91,* 1995–2010.

Bilezikian, J. P., Khan, A. A., & Potts, J. T. Jr. (2009). Third international workshop on the management of asymptomatic primary hyperparathyroidism. *Journal of Clinical Endocrinology & Metabolism, 94*(2), 335–339.

Bolland, M. J., Grey, A. B., Gamble, G. D., & Reid, I. R. (2005). Association between primary hyperparathyroidism and increased body weight: A meta-analysis. *Journal of Clinical Endocrinology & Metabolism, 90*(3), 1525–1530.

Bolona, E. R. (2007). Testosterone use in men with sexual dysfunction. A systematic review and metaanalysis of randomized placebo controlled studies. *Mayo Clinic Proceedings, 82,* 20.

Brambilla, D. J., Matsumoto, A. M., Araujo, A. B., & McKinlay, J. B. (2009). The effect of diurnal variation on clinical measurement of serum testosterone and other sex hormone levels in men. *Journal of Clinical Endocrinology & Metabolism, 94,* 907–913.

Brent, G. A. (2008). Graves' disease: Clinical practice. *New England Journal of Medicine, 358,* 2594–2605.

Cahill, G. F. Jr., & Soeldner, J. S. (1974). A non-editorial on non-hypoglycemia. *New England Journal of Medicine, 291,* 904–905.

Chen, D. K., So, Y. T., & Fisher, R. S. (2005). Use of serum prolactin in diagnosing epileptic seizures: Report of the therapeutics and technology assessment subcommittee of the American Academy of Neurology. *Neurology, 65,* 668–675.

Cooper, D. S. (2007). Approach to the patient with subclinical hyperthyroidism. *Journal of Clinical Endocrinology & Metabolism, 92*(1), 3–9.

Cryer, P. E., Axelrod, L., Grossman, A. B. Heller, S. R. Montori, V. M., Seaquist, E. R., Service, F. J., & Endocrine Society. (2009). Clinical practice guideline: Evaluation of hypoglycemic disorders. *Journal of Clinical Endocrinology & Metabolism, 94,* 709–728.

DeGroot, L. J., et al. (2009). *Thyroid gland, in Endocrinology* (6th ed.). In J. L. Jameson, L. J. DeGroot (Eds), Philadelphia, Elsevier Saunders.

Dorin, R. I., Qualls, C. R., & Crapo, L. M. (2003). Diagnosis of adrenal insufficiency. *Annals of Internal Medicine, 138*(3), 194–214.

Finkelstein, J. S., Lee, H., Burnett-Bowie, S. M., et al. (2013). Gonadal steroids and body composition, strength, and sexual function in men. *New England Journal of Medicine, 369,* 1011–1022.

Gastineau, C. F. (1983). Is reactive hypoglycemia a clinical entry? *Mayo Clinic Proceedings, 58,* 545–549.

Goldstein, R. E., O'Neill, J. A. Jr., Holcomb, G. W. 3rd, Morgan, W. M. 3rd, Neblett, W. W. 3rd, et al. (1999). Clinical experience over 48 years with pheochromocytoma. *Annals of Surgery, 229*(6), 755.

Hildebrand, J. K., Joos, S. K., & Lee, M. A. (1997). Use of the diagnosis "failure to thrive" in older veterans. *Journal of the American Geriatrics Society, 45*(9), 1113.

Hoogwerf, B. J., & Nuttall, F. Q. (1984). Long-term weight regulation in treated hyperthyroid and hypothyroid subjects. *American Journal of Medicine, 76*(6), 963.

Horwitz, D. L. (1989). Factitious and artifactual hypoglycemia. *Endocrinology and Metabolism Clinics of North America, 18,* 203–210.

Ioachimescu, A. G., & Hamrahian, A. H. (2013). Diseases of the adrenal gland. In: *Cleveland Clinic: Current Clinical Medicine* (2nd ed.). Elsevier Saunders; 2010:sec 4.

Inzucchi, S. E. (2004). Management of hypercalcemia. Diagnostic workup, therapeutic options for hyperparathyroidism and other common causes. *Postgraduate Medicine, 115*(5), 27–36.

Knopman, D. S., DeKosky, S. T., Cummings, J. L., Chui, H., Corey-Bloom, J., Relkin, N., et al. (2001). Practice parameter: diagnosis of dementia (an evidence-based review). Report of the Quality Standards Subcommittee of the American Academy of Neurology. *Neurology, 56*(9), 1143–1153.

Kratzsch, J., & Pulzer F. (2008). Thyroid gland development and defects. *Best Practice Research of Clinical Endocrinology Metabolism, 22,* 57–75.

Levenson, J. L. (2006). Psychiatric issues in endocrinology. *Primary Psychiatry, 13*(4), 27–30.

Loriaux, D. L. (1990). Cushing's syndrome. In K. L. Becker (Ed.), *Principles and practice of endocrinology and metabolism* (pp. 595–600). Philadelphia: Lippincott.

Luca, F., Goichot, B., & Brue, T. (2010). Non thyroidal illnesses. *Annals of Endocrinology (Paris), 71*(Suppl 1), S13–S24.

Mariotti, S., Martino, E., Cupini, C., et al. (1982). Low serum thyroglobulin as a clue to the diagnosis of thyrotoxicosis factitia. *New England Journal of Medicine, 307,* 410–412.

Manni, A., Pardridge, W. M., Cefalu, W., et al. (1985). Bioavailability of albumin-bound testosterone. *Journal of Clinical Endocrinology & Metabolism, 61,* 705.

Melmed S. (2006). Acromegaly: Medical progress. *New England Journal of Medicine, 355,* 2558–2573.

Molitch, M. E., Clemmons, D. R., Malozowski, S., Merriam, G. R., Shalet, S. M., Vance, M. L., Endocrine Society's Clinical Guidelines Subcommittee, Stephens, P. A. (2006). Evaluation and treatment of adult growth hormone deficiency. *Journal of Clinical Endocrinology & Metabolism, 91,* 1621–1634.

Nayak, B., & Hodak, S. P. (2007). Hyperthyroidism. *Endocrinology and Metabolism Clinics of North America, 36*(3), 617–656.

Neal, J. M. (2009). Diabetic neuropathic cachexia: A rare manifestation of diabetic neuropathy. *Southern Medical Journal, 102*(3), 327.

Nelson, R. L. (1985). Hypoglycemia: Fact or fiction? *Mayo Clinic Proceedings, 60,* 844–850.

NHANES III. (2013). National Health and Nutrition Examination Survey of the Centers for Disease Control. http://wwwn.cdc.gov/nchs/nhanes/search/nhanes13_14.aspx

Nieman, L. K., Biller, B. M., Findling, J. W., Newell-Rice J, Savage, M. O., Stewart, P. M., et al. (2008). The diagnosis of Cushing's syndrome: an Endocrine Society clinical practice guideline. *Journal of Clinical Enocrinology & Metabolism; 93,* 1526–1540.

Pacak, K., Eisenhofer, G., Ahlman, H., Bornstein, S. R., Gimenez-Roqueplo, A. P., et al. (2007). Pheochromocytoma: Recommendations for clinical practice from the First International Symposium. *Nature Clinical Practice. Endocrinology and Metabolism, 3,* 92–102.

Patkar, A. A., Mago, R., & Masand, P. S. (2004). Psychotic symptoms in patients with medical disorders. *Current Psychiatry Reports, 6*(3), 216.

Pearce, E. N., Farwell, A. P., & Braverman, L. E. (2003). Thyroiditis. *New England Journal of Medicine, 348*(26), 2646–2655.

Rodin, G. M., & Daneman, D. (1992). Eating disorders and IDDM. A problematic association. *Diabetes Care, 15*(10), 1402.

Sheppard, M. M., & Smith, J. W. 3rd. (2007). Hypercalcemia. *American Journal of Medical Science, 334*(5), 381–385.

Snyder, P. J., Matsumoto, A. M., Kirkland, J. L., & Martin, K. A. (2013). Clinical features and diagnosis of male hypogonadism. Wolters Kluwer Health, www.uptodate.com Sep 2012; *7462*(9), 1–20.

Snyder, P. J., & Cooper, D. S. (2013). Causes of hyperprolactinemia. New England Journal of Medicine, *369,* 2012.

Surks, M. I., Ortiz, E., Daniels, G. H., et al. (2004). Subclinical thyroid disease: scientific review and guidelines for diagnosis and management. *Journal of the American Medical Association, 291*(2), 228–238.

Sviridonova, M. A., Fadeyev, V. V., Sych, Y. P., & Melnichenko, G. A. (2013). Clinical significance of TSH circadian variability in patients with hypothyroidism. *Endocrinology Research, 38*(1), 24–31. doi:10.3109/07435800.2012.710696. Epub 2012 Aug 2.

Spratt, D. I., Pont, A., & Miller, M. B. (1982). Hyperthyroxinemia in acute psychiatric disorders. *American Journal of Medicine, 73,* 41–48.

Webb, E. A., O'Reilly, M. A., Clayden, J. D., Seunarine, K. K., Chong, W. K., Dale, N., et al. (2012). Effect of growth hormone deficiency on brain structure, motor function and cognition *Brain, 135*(Pt 1), 216–227. doi:10.1093/brain/awr305. Epub 2011 Nov 26.

Weytingh, M. D., Bossuyt, P. M., & van Crevel, H. (1995). Reversible dementia: More than 10% or less than 1%? A quantitative review. *Journal of Neurology, 242*(7), 466.

Wolkowitz, O. M., & Rothschild, A. J. (2003). *Psychoneuroendocrinology: The scientific basis of clinical practice.* Washington, DC: American Psychiatric Association.

Wu, F. C. W., Tajar, A., Beynon, J. M., et al. (2010). Identification of late-onset hypogonadism in middle-aged and elderly men. *New England Journal of Medicine, 363,* 123–135.

Yager, J., & Young, R. T. (1974). Non-hypoglycemia is an epidemic condition. *New England Journal of Medicine, 291,* 907–908

7.

NEUROIMAGING IN PSYCHIATRY
THE CLINICAL-RADIOGRAPHIC CORRELATE

David L. Perez, Laura Ortiz-Terán, and David A. Silbersweig

INTRODUCTION

Clinical psychiatry is a rapidly evolving field. Diagnostically, psychiatrists are trained to recognize symptoms such as negative affect, impulsivity, grandiosity, and thought disorder, and subsequently determine if symptoms "fit" into established diagnoses. Over the next few decades, structural and functional neuroimaging techniques currently used to research the neural correlates of psychiatric symptoms will likely identify adjunct neural biomarkers to confirm diagnosis and, more importantly, identify predictors of prognosis and treatment response. Furthermore, neuroimaging techniques help detect medical and/or neurological conditions that exhibit prominent behavioral, affective, and/or cognitive symptoms that resemble primary mental disorders.

In this chapter we review structural and functional neuroimaging techniques and discuss the clinical-radiographic correlates of common medical and neurological differential diagnoses with prominent neuropsychiatric symptoms. The neural circuits frequently implicated in psychiatric and neuropsychiatric conditions are also detailed, and the structural and functional neuroimaging abnormalities commonly found in schizophrenia, major depressive disorder (MDD), and posttraumatic stress disorder (PTSD) are briefly summarized. Lastly, the potential for neuroimaging to aid prognosis, treatment selection, and identify targets for neuromodulation are explored.

STRUCTURAL NEUROIMAGING TECHNIQUES

COMPUTED TOMOGRAPHY

Computed Tomography (CT) of the brain was the first modern neuroimaging technique, available for research in the late 1960s and used clinically by the 1970s. This technique utilizes an ionizing X-radiation tube that rotates axially around a patient with detectors positioned on the opposite side measuring the amount of radiation transmitted. Data acquired by the detectors is digitized to create an axial tomographic 2D image of the body. Importantly, bodily tissues have varying densities and differ in their ability to attenuate radiation. Distinct tissue densities are represented on a black-and-white scale (see Table 7.1). The use of an iodinated contrast agent aids detection of vascular pathology and disorders that disrupt the blood brain barrier (i.e., metastatic tumors). Brain CT scans can be rapidly performed, are readily available, and may be particularly useful in identifying acute hemorrhage and bony lesions, but have limited spatial resolution, expose patients to radiation (0.5–8 mSv), and are prone to artifacts, particularly in the posterior fossa. Also, CT scans are relatively insensitive to acute ischemic stroke detection; a well visualized hypodensity may not be appreciable until more than 24 hours after symptom onset. Subtle ischemic changes such as sulcal effacement and loss of gray-white matter differentiation may be seen within the first few hours of stroke onset. Hyperdensity of the middle cerebral artery (MCA), known as a "dense MCA sign," may indicate intra-arterial clot and provides supportive evidence of an acute ischemic stroke.

MAGNETIC RESONANCE IMAGING

The physical properties of hydrogen, one the most abundant elements in the human body, provide the basis for magnetic resonance imaging (MRI). Hydrogen has a single spinning proton with a positive charge that generates a magnetic field along its north/south axis. Normally the field surrounding a given hydrogen proton is oriented randomly in relation to neighboring hydrogen protons; however, when an external magnetic field (B_0) such as that from a MRI magnet is applied, protons align with the direction of the field in a parallel or antiparallel direction. In addition to this realignment, the individual hydrogen protons precess (change in the alignment of the rotational axis) at a frequency called the *Larmor frequency*. If a radiofrequency pulse is then directed into the tissue, spinning protons that are in a position of low energy or in parallel move into a position of high energy or antiparallel. This repositioning generates a transverse magnetic field. When the radio frequency pulse is switched off, protons reorient back to the original position and induce an electromagnetic field that is detected by a coil outside the tissue. This response is measured and analyzed to produce MR-based images. Variations in the Larmor frequency of individual protons enable the spatial characterization that distinguishes MRI from nuclear magnetic spectroscopy (Grossman & Yousem, 2003).

Table 7.1 BRAIN TISSUE CHARACTERISTICS ON COMPUTED TOMOGRAPHY (CT) AND MAGNETIC RESONANCE IMAGING (MRI)

	CT	T1	T2	DWI	FLAIR
Air	black	black	black	white (artifact)	black
Water/Cerebrospinal Fluid	black	black	white	black	black
Fat	black	white	black	**	black
Calcium	white	black	black	**	black
Blood (hyperacute <7 hours)	white	dark gray	light gray–white	white	light gray–white
Blood (acute 7–72 hours)	white	dark gray-gray	dark gray	dark gray	dark gray
Blood (subacute >72 hours)	light gray–gray	light gray–white	dark gray	dark gray	dark gray
Gray Matter	gray	gray	light gray	light gray	light gray
White Matter	dark gray	white	dark gray	gray	dark gray
Edema	dark gray–black	dark gray	white	white	white
Infarction hyperacute (0–6 hours)	*	gray	light gray	white	light gray
Infarction acute (6 hours–4 days)	dark gray	dark gray	white	white	white
Infarction subacute (4–14 days)	dark gray–black	dark gray	white	light gray–white	white
Infarction chronic	black	black	dark gray–black	gray	dark gray–black

DWI indicates diffusion weighted image; FLAIR, fluid attenuated inversion recovery.

*Indirect signs of infarction such as hyperdense arteries and loss of gray/white differentiation.

**indicates not consistently appreciated.

The appearance of the brain on MRI is dependent on acquisition properties that are described using parameters such as echo times and time repetition. These parameters create different sequences referred as *T1* and *T2* (see Table 7.2). On T1 sequences, white matter consisting mainly of fat-rich myelinated axons appears white; gray matter structures such as cerebral cortex and the nuclei of the brainstem and diencephalon appear gray. T2 sequences display as white brain regions with a high water content; a normal brain will show a pattern of gray and white inverse to that seen on T1 sequences. Fluid attenuated inversion recovery (FLAIR) is a T2-based image that uses an inversion recovery pulse sequence to block cerebrospinal fluid signal. While T2-based sequences are useful at detecting parenchymal pathology such as prior infarcts, mass lesions, edema, and white matter demyelinating plaques, FLAIR images particularly aid the detection of periventricular abnormalities that may be obscured by cerebrospinal fluid signal on T2 images. T1 sequences are most useful in delineating brain anatomy (i.e., regional atrophy). The addition of gadolinium, a paramagnetic heavy metal that decreases the T1 relaxation times of tissues when injected intravenously as a contrast agent, enhances lesions that disrupt the blood–brain barrier including acute demyelinating white matter lesions, vascular lesions, and high-grade glial tumors. In addition, susceptibility weighted imaging (SWI) is an magnetic resonance technique that employs a gradient echo pulse sequence that is particularly sensitive to venous blood, hemorrhage, and iron deposition (although insensitive to hyperacute blood). When ordering a clinical MRI, while there are variations across institutions, standard brain MRI orders will almost always include T1, T2, and FLAIR sequences; however, the use of contrast, SWI, or diffusion sequences (discussed below) should be specifically requested based on the differential diagnosis.

Clinical radiologists, neurologists, and neuropsychiatrists mainly rely on visual inspection to identify pathology on CT or MRI brain scans. However, quantitative techniques for MRI interpretation originally devised for research are beginning to be used in clinical practice. *Manual volumetry* is a technique that combines manual tracing of regions of interest (ROIs) with calculations that estimate the volume of structures based on cross-sectional areas. While this technique is widely available, it is time consuming, operator dependent, and requires that operators have an exquisite familiarity with the neuroanatomy of the region(s) being imaged. A more convenient, automated approach is *Voxel-based morphometry* (VBM). In VBM, T1-based MRI sequences for a given cohort of subjects are spatially normalized to the same stereotactic space. During spatial normalization, distinct brains are deformed to correspond regionally to one another and enable cross-subject comparisons. Following normalization, an automated segmentation procedure subdivides the ROIs into voxels (cubes of brain tissue) and characterizes each voxel as comprised of gray or white matter. Thereafter, voxel-wise *statistical parametric mapping* (SPM) techniques are applied across groups to detect group differences (Ashburner & Friston, 2000). Analyses that label all of the voxels within a

Table 7.2 RELATIONSHIPS OF T1 AND T2 MRI SEQUENCES AND TIME REPETITION (TR) AND ECHO TIME (TE) ACQUISITION PARAMETERS

	TR	TE
T1	Short	Short
T2	Long	Long

brain image according to statistical test outcomes, called a *statistical parametric map,* may include whole brain comparisons or may be limited to a priori ROIs. In addition to volumetric analyses, techniques have also been devised to quantify variations in morphology (shape) as a complement to volumetric analyses (Csernansky et al., 1998). Clinically, since the specificity and sensitivity of these techniques are not yet well validated at the individual subject level, quantitative structural analyses currently only allow for the detection of significant group differences. However, technical advancements under investigation may allow these analyses to be applied to specific individuals in the future.

More recently, techniques have been developed to measure the cerebral cortex, a highly folded structure that does not lend itself well to manual tracings. Automated software aids the measurement of cortical gray matter thickness through the creation of inflated surface representations (Fischl & Dale, 2000) and has been validated against histological analysis (Rosas et al., 2002) and manual regional MRI measurements (Kuperberg et al., 2003; Salat et al., 2004).

DIFFUSION WEIGHTED IMAGING/DIFFUSION TENSOR IMAGING

Diffusion weighted imaging (DWI) and diffusion tensor imaging (DTI) are T2-weighted scans that rely on the detection and quantification of the random movement of water, also known as *Brownian movement.* While the displacement induced by one hydrogen molecule is not appreciable, their collective impact generates a significant and quantifiable displacement of a chaotic nature. In biological tissues, since molecular movement may be influenced by multiple variables including capillary microcirculation that cannot be readily measured, the term *apparent diffusion coefficient* (ADC) is used to describe diffusion-based images.

Diffusion weighted images are acquired in X, Y, and Z planes and are combined to produce DWI and ADC sequences. These sequences provide a diffusivity calculation without qualifying the direction of tissue water movement, termed *isotropic diffusion.* For example, decreases in ADC values (and corresponding increases in DWI) reflect restricted diffusion and serve as an indirect measure of gray or white matter disintegrity. DWI can be understood as an index of tissue permeability difference and is measured in terms of mean diffusivity (MD). DWI sequences aid the identification of acute ischemic strokes, and provide adjunct information in the radiographic evaluation of neoplasms, traumatic brain injury, and demyelinating processes (Schaefer, Grant, & Gonzales, 2000). Clinically, in cases of a

suspected acute stroke where a hypodensity is not well delineated on a CT scan, a brain MRI with diffusion sequences should be specifically requested. Furthermore, a hyperintensity on DWI should correspond to a hypointensity on ADC; otherwise, a T2-shine-through effect may cause false positive interpretations of an acute stroke if an abnormality is seen only on DWI. If a brainstem stroke is suspected, clinicians may also request thin sections through the brainstem to improve test sensitivity.

DTI-based imaging relies on the principle that when the diffusion in a structured system, such as the brain, is quantified, molecular displacement may be limited by physical barriers. Displacement that is direction dependent (i.e., axonal) is called *anisotropic.* The processing of diffusion values limited by structural anatomy (i.e., axons) in each voxel is called *tensor.* A tensor can be defined as a set of coexisting magnitudes dependent upon direction and coordinates (eigenvector and eigenvalues [λ]). DTI-enabled tractography permits the reconstruction and 3D visualization of the neural column structure. DTI maps are typically displayed as color maps representing the whole brain connectivity, with the direction of tracks indicated by distinct colors. Red typically indicates the X-axis, green the Y-axis, and blue the Z-axis. If applied to white matter axonal fibers, tractography provides structural connectivity information, including delineating pathology such as fiber deviation/destruction caused by tumors or infarctions.

An important DTI measurement to consider is the anisotropic fraction (AF). AF quantifies microstructure integrity of the white matter and is obtained by recording water diffusivity along white matter tracts (Ries et al., 2008). This measure has the advantage of detecting microstructural abnormalities with high sensitivity. Loss of tissue organization causes a decrease in anisotropy (and an increase in AF). It is theorized that reduced water diffusion parallel to axonal tracts, measured by the AF, is indicative of axonal degeneration, disruption and partial breakdown of cytoarchitecture (Beaulieu, 2002), or demyelination (Song et al., 2002).

At present, there is no consensus on the optimal method to analyze DTI data clinically. An early devised method was the *fiber assignment by continuous tracking* (FACT) technique using the selection of multiple ROIs. Using FACT, either voxels within a ROI are manually placed within a tract of interest, or every voxel above a certain threshold anisotropy value is examined. The latter method is considered superior, as it may find tracts omitted by only inspecting select ROIs; however, this approach is also more computationally demanding (Mukherjee, Berman, Chung, Hess, & Henry, 2008).

An alternative approach is the application of voxel-based analyses using SPM or similar techniques. Achieving adequate coregistration of DTI images across subjects, however, can be challenging given individual differences in brain shape, size, and white matter anatomy. *Tract-based spatial statistics* (TBSS) is an automated method to detect group-wise changes in diffuse metrics from the white matter of the entire brain (Smith et al., 2006). Anisotropic fraction (AF) images for each subject in a cohort are registered to construct a mean AF map. This map is skeletonized to identify core white matter tracts containing the highest AF values. AF values from individual subjects are then projected onto the AF skeleton, and voxel-wise statistics are applied to identify significant differences. Importantly, the TBSS method can detect changes in AF simultaneously throughout the white matter of the brain, while DTI fiber tracking derives results only from preselected white matter tracts. At the present time, there is no specific routine clinical indication for DTI imaging; however, a DTI scan may be requested and used to augment and/or clarify radiographic findings.

MAGNETIC RESONANCE SPECTROSCOPY

Magnetic resonance spectroscopy (MRS) is used to measure the average amount of distinct metabolites in brain tissue over the duration of an approximately 15-minute scan. It detects and quantifies resonance signals of molecules present at much lower concentrations and differentiates molecules based on their magnetic resonance properties. This technique relies in part on chemical-shift imaging which takes into account the effect of the local chemical environment on particular nuclei. The metabolic profile of a region can be obtained through single voxel MRS (SVMRS) or multivoxel MRS imaging. SVMRS provides a metabolic average score within the selected voxel, while multivoxel MRS provides, within a unique image acquisition, various molecular images indicating the spatial distribution of different metabolites. The major limitation of SVMRS is the lack of spatial information due to limited sampling, although voxel size across single voxel and multivoxel MRS is typically similar.

The central nervous system metabolites measured with MRS are outlined in Table 7.3 and Figure 7.1. Commonly detected metabolites include N-acetyl aspartate (NAA), a marker of neuronal integrity; choline (Cho), an indicator of

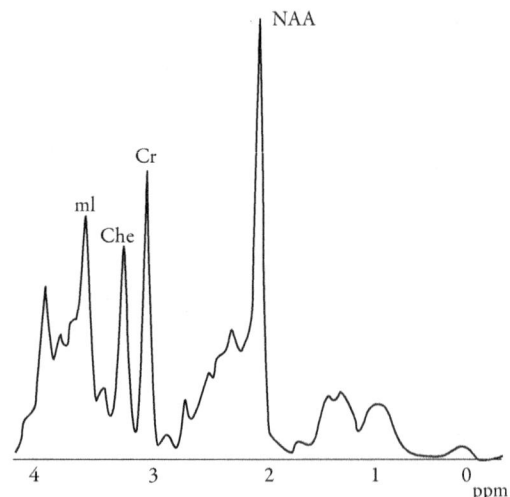

Figure 7.1 Magnetic resonance spectroscopy illustration. The number of signals represented corresponds to the number of different metabolites sampled within a specified voxel. The position of distinct peaks on the horizontal axis is proportional to the intensity of the magnetic field, normally called *chemical-shift*, and measured in parts per million (ppm). The area under the curve for each signal provides a relative concentration of each metabolite. mI indicates Myoinositol; Cho, Choline; Cr, Creatine; NAA, N-Acetyl-Aspartate.

cell membrane synthesis; and creatine (Cr), associated with cellular energy metabolism. MRS, thus far, is the only readily available technique enabling in vivo sampling of metabolic information and is used clinically to aid diagnosis of metabolic disorders (i.e., leukodystrophies), distinguish neoplasms from other abnormal brain signals (high-grade brain tumors characterized by high Cho and low NAA), and assess the effects of chemotherapeutics on brain tumors by helping to distinguish between necrosis and neoplasm recurrence.

FUNCTIONAL NEUROIMAGING TECHNIQUES

SINGLE PROTON EMISSION COMPUTED TOMOGRAPHY

Brain single proton emission computed tomography (SPECT) is a functional neuroimaging technique that detects gamma ray projections, produced as radionuclide decay, with a scintillation camera. The camera is rotated around a patient's head 360 degrees over an approximately 20-minute period to gather whole brain data. This technique measures regional cerebral blood flow (rCBF), which indirectly reflects neuronal activity in different brain regions and allows for the detection of functional brain abnormalities. The injected tracers currently used in the clinical practice are ^{99m}Tc-hexamethyl-propylene-amine-oxime (^{99m}Tc-HMPAO) and ^{99m}Tc-ethyl cysteinate dimer (^{99m}Tc-ECD). These tracers are lipophilic, cross the cell membrane, and remain intracellular following their conversion to hydrophilic compounds. Their incorporation is proportional to rCBF in the first few minutes after injection. The SPECT image does not change

Table 7.3 COMMONLY DETECTED METABOLITES IN MAGNETIC RESONANCE SPECTROSCOPY (MRS)

METABOLITE	ABBREVIATION	ACTION
N-Acetyl-Aspartate	NAA	Neuronal marker
Choline	Cho	Membrane turnover marker
Creatine/Phosphocreatine	Cr/PCr	Index of energetic metabolism
Lactate	Lac	Product of anaerobic metabolism
Myoinositol	mI	Astrocyte marker
Lipids	Lip	Cell membrane/myelin sheath marker
Glutamine	Gln	Involved in synaptic processes
Glutamate	Glu	Involved in synaptic processes

following subsequent modifications in blood flow, since the tracer is "locked in" to the cells that have taken it up (Farid, Caillat-Vigneron, & Sibon, 2011). This characteristic has made SPECT imaging particularly clinically useful for seizure foci detection if the tracer is injected in close temporal proximity to seizure onset (Knowlton, Lawn, Mountz, & Kuzniecky, 2004). Of note, the tracer takes approximately 30 seconds to reach the brain, and the switch from ictal hyperperfusion to postictal hypoperfusion occurs approximately in 1–2 minutes following seizure termination in temporal regions and sooner in extratemporal regions. Ictal SPECT imaging thus requires tracer injection within seconds of seizure onset (Van Paesschen, 2004). SPECT tracers have longer half-lives and are less expensive to manufacture than those used in positron emission tomography (PET). The main limitation of SPECT imaging apart from exposing the patient to ionizing radiation (approximately 6–10 mSv) is its relatively limited spatial resolution, although recent technical advancements, including coregistration of SPECT images on MRI rather than CT scans, have improved resolution.

POSITRON EMISSION TOMOGRAPHY

Brain PET is a nuclear medicine technique for the visualization of physiological and biochemical brain changes by a scintillation camera that detects gamma rays produced when positrons released from a tracer compound collide with ambient electrons. The release of diametrically opposed gamma rays produces a more spatially accurate image compared to SPECT. This information is converted into a 3D brain image. There are several radionuclides commonly used, including carbon-11, nitrogen-13, oxygen-15, and fluorine-18. Fluorine-18 has the longest half-life, and fluorodeoxyglucose (^{18}F-FDG), an analogue of glucose labeled with fluorine-18, is used frequently as a marker of brain function. Measuring regional cerebral glucose metabolism via ^{18}F-FDG PET has become a standard technique to detect regional hypometabolism in neurodegenerative diseases (and often times the preferred technique to SPECT for regional hypometabolism detection, given greater spatial resolution). An example of a well-recognized regional hypometabolism finding is bilateral parietal-temporal hypometabolism in Alzheimer's disease (Herholz, Carter, & Jones, 2007). PET can also be utilized with antibody-radionuclide compounds to determine the distribution of particular molecules in the brain, and with ligand-radionuclide compounds to determine the distribution of neurotransmitter receptors. Pittsburgh Compound B allows *in vivo* detection of amyloid in the diagnostic work-up of Alzheimer's disease (Klunk et al., 2004). The radiolabeled dopamine receptor ligand ^{11}C-raclopride has been used to quantify dopamine receptors in patients with schizophrenia and early Parkinson's disease (Brooks et al., 1992; Farde et al., 1990). Use of interictal PET (with ^{18}F-FDG) to detect regional hypometabolism aids in determining seizure foci in patients undergoing epilepsy surgery evaluations (Ho et al., 1995). While the need for a cyclotron to manufacture PET tracers increases test expense (approximately 1500–5000 USD for PET, roughly 1000 USD for SPECT) and exposes subjects to radiation (4–8 mSV), the spatial resolution and the superior quantitative aspects of PET make it frequently the procedure of choice in most clinical situations requiring the aid of a nuclear medicine brain scan. To aid clinical-radiographic interpretations across functional neuroimaging techniques, particularly PET and SPECT, clinicians should provide specific clinical symptoms (and suspected affected brain regions if possible) in their test requisitions to guide neuroradiologists.

FUNCTIONAL MRI

Functional MRI (fMRI) is a noninvasive, non–radiation-based neuroimaging technique, which uses the inherent magnetic properties of hemoglobin to provide a proxy for neuronal activity. Red blood cells contain hemoglobin molecules with centrally positioned iron atoms. The binding and unbinding of oxygen to hemoglobin results in conformational changes, with oxyhemoglobin (diamagnetic) and deoxyhemoglobin (paramagnetic) having distinct magnetic properties. Deoxyhemoglobin configurations create a surrounding inhomogeneous magnetic field leading to decreased signal. In healthy individuals, regional brain activations coincide with local vasodilation so that venous blood draining from active neurons is *more* oxygenated than if the neurons were less active. Therefore, less deoxyhemoglobin (and more oxyhemoglobin) due to increased neural demand for oxygen and parallel compensatory blood flow that exceeds the regional metabolic demand in a given functionally active region leads to increased blood oxygen level dependent (BOLD) signal (Logothetis, Pauls, Augath, Trinath, & Oeltermann, 2001). While BOLD fMRI provides a proxy for neural activity based on venous blood flow patterns, more recently developed methods such as *arterial spin labeling* (ASL) provide an arterial phase measure of cerebral blood flow with the potential for improved spatial and temporal resolution. If the regulation of vascular tone in response to downstream neuronal demand is impaired, as with cerebral atherosclerotic disease, flow-related fMRI activation patterns may not change as expected in the context of increased neuronal activity.

Overall, fMRI provides high spatial resolution but has limitations in temporal resolution based on the hemodynamic response (1–2 seconds). Techniques combining fMRI with electroencephalogram recordings may provide complementary spatial and temporal information; similarly, dual use of fMRI and magnetoencephalography (MEG) may also serve as complementary techniques. fMRI is exquisitely sensitive to small head movements and respiratory artifacts. Compared to SPECT and PET, fMRI has improved spatial and temporal resolution and does not expose subjects to ionizing radiation. However, subjects with metallic implants, including surgically implanted devices such as cardiac pacemakers, are unable to participate in MRI-based investigations. The MRI environment itself is also confining and may cause patients with claustrophobia to not participate; fMRI technology has not yet been extended to the increasingly popular "open MRI" whereby data is acquired in a less confined environment.

FUNCTIONAL NEUROIMAGING METHODS

Functional neuroimaging evaluations probing neuropsychiatric symptoms have utilized a broad array of paradigm and nonparadigm experimental designs and analysis techniques. Most broadly, paradigm-based experimental design may be subdivided into techniques that naturalistically "capture" symptoms or techniques that ask subjects to participate in tasks in order to examine active neural circuits. The symptom capture method has been used to characterize neural activations in phenomena such as hallucinations in patients with schizophrenia and tics in patients with Tourette syndrome (Silbersweig et al., 1995; Stern et al., 2000). For example, in a study probing visual hallucinations in a cohort of patients with paranoid schizophrenia and prominent auditory verbal hallucinations, subjects were placed in a PET scanner following the injection of a $H_2 {}^{15}O$ tracer and instructed to relax, close their eyes, and press a button each time auditory hallucinations were experienced. Group analyses identified activations in bilateral thalamus, hippocampus/parahippocampal gyrus, right ventral striatum, anterior cingulate cortex, and left orbitofrontal cortex. Furthermore, in a unique case study of an unmedicated patient with paranoid schizophrenia experiencing dual auditory and visual hallucinations (perceiving colored scenes with rolling, disembodied heads, and hearing the heads verbalize command instructions), hallucinations were associated with visual association and auditory-linguistic association cortex activations and relative absence of prefrontal cortex activity (see Figure 7.2). Studies

of this type approximate a naturalistic identification of neural circuits active during acute symptom occurrence.

The more commonly used method in functional neuroimaging studies of patients with psychiatric disease has been the use of paradigm-based tasks to probe underlying neural circuit differences. Examples include using working memory tasks to probe dorsolateral prefrontal cortex function in patients with schizophrenia (Callicott et al., 2000), the presentation of war-related images and sounds to patients with Vietnam War related PTSD (Bremner et al., 1999), and displaying affectively valenced faces to patients with major depressive disorder (Sheline et al., 2001). Task-based fMRI paradigms are currently used clinically in language and memory lateralization evaluations for presurgical planning in patients awaiting neurosurgical intervention, particularly those requiring epilepsy surgeries (Tharin & Golby, 2007).

The two major types of paradigm design are block and event-related designs. In *block designs*, similar conditions are grouped together to form discrete experimental blocks. Within each block, multiple stimuli of the same subtype are presented consecutively within each block, and an output of interest (i.e., BOLD signal) is averaged across the entire block. At a minimum, blocks are divided into control blocks and condition-of-interest blocks. An example of this would be the presentation of trauma-related words to patients with PTSD compared to healthy controls as the condition-of-interest block, and the subsequent presentation of neutral words during control blocks (Protopopescu et al., 2005; see Figure 7.3).

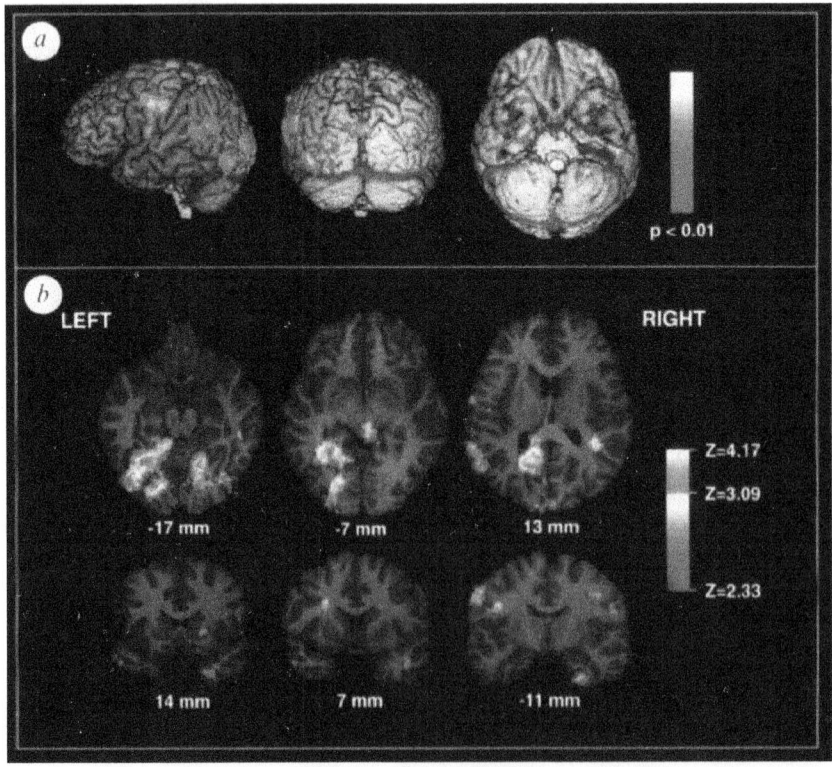

Figure 7.2 Functional activation pattern in a patient with schizophrenia experiencing dual auditory and visual hallucinations, recorded using a symptom capture paradigm with the patient also utilized as his own control. Reprinted by permission from Macmillan Publishers Ltd: *Nature*. Silbersweig DA, Stern E, Frith C, Cahill C, Holmes A, Grootoonk S, et al. A functional neuroanatomy of hallucinations in schizophrenia. 1995;378:176–9.

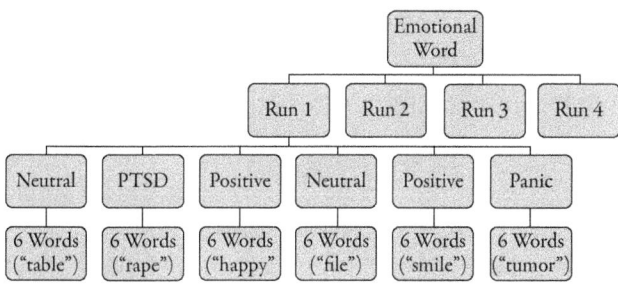

Figure 7.3 Sample diagram of a block design developed to probe the neural correlates of affective word processing. In this particular experiment, each run is composed of six distinct blocks, with each block containing six similarly affectively valenced words. Each affectively valenced block (i.e., PTSD-specific words) across runs would contain six different words that are similarly affectively valenced. The order of blocks across runs is typically randomized. Adapted from Protopopescu X, Pan H, Tuescher O, Cloitre M, Goldstein M, Engelien W, et al. Differential time courses and specificity of amygdala activity in post-traumatic stress disorder subjects and normal control subjects. *Biological Psychiatry* 2005;57:464–73.

Block design use improves signal detection power and simplifies analyses, but is limited by relative temporal insensitivity.

In *event-related designs*, stimuli are presented in discrete, short-duration events with the potential to randomize timing and stimuli order. Stimuli may be presented at intervals ranging from 2 and 20 seconds apart, depending on the specifics of the experiment. Also, stimuli across conditions (i.e., negative vs. neutral words) are randomized rather than consecutively displayed. While event-related designs lack the statistical power of block designs, this strategy enables the detection of changes in neural activity from baseline and allows for more sophisticated analytic methodology (Huettel, Song, & McCarthy, 2004).

In evaluating functional neuroimaging findings, it is important to also consider if "state" or "trait" characteristics are being evaluated at the time of the experiment. In state evaluations, disease-specific symptoms of interest are actively experienced by participants and probed during a functional neuroimaging study. An example is the previously described symptom capture experiment in hallucinating patients with paranoid schizophrenia. In trait investigations, the neural correlates of functions hypothesized to be related to disease pathophysiology are probed (i.e., fear conditioning and extinction learning experiments in PTSD patients), but the disease-specific symptomatology are not necessarily experienced during data acquisition.

Over the last decade, a shift has occurred in the exploration of functional activation patterns. Most early functional neuroimaging studies compared task-of-interest activation patterns to control conditions by performing subtraction-based analyses ("subtracting" out control or baseline activation patterns) to identify regions specifically implicated in task performance. This approach is also known as a *univariate* analysis. While this technique continues to prove useful in delineating structure–function relationships, brain function is now recognized as organized into spatially distributed regions that form discrete networks that coactivate (or deactivate) during task and rest (nontask) conditions. These functional connectivity investigations are *multivariate* analyses that probe coherent activation patterns within and across neural networks. In

multivariate analyses, distinct functional connectivity patterns across groups are descriptively detailed rather than the result of computed subtraction-based analyses. Functional connectivity may be examined during the performance of particular tasks, or while subjects rest and allow their minds to wander without focusing on any given thought or task. Resting state, task-free paradigms provide a powerful alternative approach to delineate neural circuit differences across psychiatric conditions (including default mode network disturbances), and may have an emerging role in a broad array of applications including presurgical mapping and the early detection of neurodegenerative disease (Greicius et al., 2007; Liu et al., 2009).

One commonly used method to probe functional connectivity are *regions of interest based methods* that select "seeds" and subsequently examine whole brain functional activation patterns in relation to these predetermined regions (Zhang & Raichle, 2010). *Component-based multivariate analyses* offer a distinct approach whereby advanced computational statistical methods decompose functional data into statistically distinct connectivity maps, or components. Components are suggested to represent functionally bound neural networks. Independent component analysis and principal component analyses are two of the more commonly used methods of this type. Advances in *graph theory* have also recently been applied to functional activation patterns to define the relationship between regions (nodes) based on their functional connectivity strengths. In particular, the brain's functional connections exhibit small-world properties (Watts & Strogatz, 1998), whereby a limited number of temporally and spatially interconnected regions form distinct networks rather than being constructed as a network of random connections. Specific sites within a network that exhibit particularly robust connectivity are termed *modules* and *hubs*, and the strength of functional connections between nodes may be depicted by vectors of varying thickness (Pan, Epstein, Silbersweig, & Stern, 2011; Sepulcre et al., 2010; Zhang & Raichle, 2010).

NEUROIMAGING AND DIFFERENTIAL DIAGNOSIS

When evaluating a patient with behavioral, affective, and/or cognitive complaints, accessory features of the clinical history and physical examination help determine the need for neuroimaging. A history of previously diagnosed psychiatric disease, age of symptom onset, known neurologic and medical conditions, and family history all aid in determining if a patient's psychiatric symptoms are primary or secondary to a medical/neurological condition. If psychiatric symptoms are suspected to be secondary manifestations based on aspects of the history, laboratory tests, and/or clinical examination, it is useful to systematically consider diseases across broad diagnostic categories including infection, cerebrovascular disease, oncologic, paraneoplastic, demyelinating, neurodegenerative, trauma-related, and rheumatologic/inflammatory conditions (see Table 7.4, Figure 7.4). Neuroimaging evaluations may either help refine the differential diagnosis, or guide diagnosis itself.

For example, a primary central nervous system (CNS) infection should be considered in a patient presenting with

Table 7.4 SAMPLE OF MEDICAL AND NEUROLOGIC CONDITIONS WITH POTENTIALLY PROMINENT PSYCHIATRIC SYMPTOMS

DISEASE CATEGORIES	SUPPORTIVE HISTORY	SELECT RADIOGRAPHIC SCANS OF PARTICULAR DIAGNOSTIC UTILITY
Infection		
Herpes Simplex Virus, Varicella Zoster Virus	Fever, meningeal irritation, delirium, seizures	MRI: High T2WI signal in the temporal lobe(s). Restricted diffusion/gyriform edema. Meningeal enhancement.
Human Immunodeficiency Virus (HIV) Dementia	Opportunistic infections, subcortical cognitive deficits	MRI: Generalized atrophy. Nonspecific T2WI WM lesions. CT: Generalized atrophy.
Neurosyphilis	Neuropsychiatric symptoms, meningeal irritation, focal deficits	MRI: Generalized cerebral atrophy and ventricular dilatation. Strokes. Meningeal enhancement.
Cerebrovascular		
Small Vessel Disease/ Binswanger's Disease	Subcortical cognitive deficits	MRI: Periventricular/subcortical T2WI hyperintense WM lesions. CT: Subcortical hypoattenuation.
Large Vessel Strokes	Cortical deficits: aphasia, neglect, visual field loss	MRI: T2WI hyperintensities. Mass effect. DWI high, ADC low. CT: Hypoattenuation.
Lacunar Strokes	Motor/somatosensory deficits	MRI: T2WI hyperintensities. DWI high, ADC low. CT: Punctate hypoattenuation.
Posterior Reversible Encephalopathy Syndrome	Hypertension, headache, seizures, vision loss	MRI: Posterior predominant T2WI hyperintensities. CT: Hypoattenuation.
Cerebral Amyloid Angiopathy	Dementia	MRI: Hypointense SWI lesions.
Oncologic		
Malignant Primary CNS Tumor	Headache, focal deficits, seizures	MRI (preferred) and CT: Mass effect +/- post-contrast enhancement.
Benign CNS Tumor (i.e. orbital groove meningioma)	Seizures, cognitive/affective deficits	MRI (preferred) and CT: Variable mass effect and post-contrast enhancement.
Carcinomatous Meningitis	Meningeal irritation, delirium	MRI: Sulcal enhancement.
Metastatic CNS Tumor	Focal deficits, headache, known malignancy	MRI (preferred) and CT: Enhancing mass lesions at the gray-white junction.
Limbic Paraneoplastic		
Anti-NR1/NR2 of N-methyl-D-aspartate (NMDA) receptor	Ovarian teratoma	MRI: High signal mainly in the temporal lobe(s) in T2WI. Restricted diffusion, gyriform edema.
Anti-Hu (ANNA-1)	Small cell lung cancer	MRI: High signal mainly in the temporal lobe(s) in T2WI. Restricted diffusion, gyriform edema.
Anti-Voltage-Gated Potassium Channels (VGKC)	Thymoma, small cell lung cancer	MRI: High signal mainly in the temporal lobe(s) in T2WI. Restricted diffusion, gyriform edema.
Demyelinating		
Multiple Sclerosis	Optic neuritis, relapsing-remitting deficits	MRI: T2WI WM hyperintense lesions, enhancing acute WM lesions.
Neurodegenerative		
Alzheimer's Disease	Progressive amnesia, anomia	MRI (preferred) and CT: Medial temporal lobe atrophy.
Frontal Temporal Dementia Behavioral Variant	Progressive impulsivity, apathy, personality change	MRI (preferred) and CT: Frontotemporal atrophy.

(continued)

Table 7.4 (CONTINUED)

DISEASE CATEGORIES	SUPPORTIVE HISTORY	SELECT RADIOGRAPHIC SCANS OF PARTICULAR DIAGNOSTIC UTILITY
Diffuse Lewy Body Disease	Visual hallucinations, fluctuating delirium, parkinsonism	MRI: Brain stem, substantia nigra, and cortical atrophy on T1WI.
Sporadic Creutzfeldt-Jakob Disease (CJD)	Myoclonus, ataxia, rapidly progressive cognitive decline	MRI: High signal on T2WI and DWI in the striatum and posterior cortical ribbon.
Inflammatory		
Systemic Lupus Erythematosus	Rash, arthritis, headache, constitutional symptoms	MRI: High T2WI signal in WM, non specific.
Primary Angitis of the CNS	Headache, focal neurologic deficits	MRI: Restricted diffusion on DWI and ADC. High intensity T2WI lesions.
Neurosarcoidosis	Cough, mediastinal adenopathy	MRI: Dural/leptomeningeal enhancement. Hypothalamus/pituitary and intraparenchymal lesions.
Traumatic Brain Injury		
Diffuse Axonal Injury	Variable deficits but includes coma	MRI: High intensity T2WI lesions +/- hemorrhage on SWI. CT: Focal high density with surrounding low-density edema.
Acute Subdural Hemorrhage	Brief lucid period prior to loss of consciousness, herniation	CT (preferred): Crescent-shaped high density fluid collection. MRI: Isointense on T1WI, hypointense on T2WI.
Other		
Toxic Leukoencephalopathy (i.e. Antineoplastic Drugs)	Subcortical cognitive deficits	MRI: Variable T2WI WM hyperintensities.
Thiamine Deficiency: Wernicke-Korsacoff Syndrome	Alcoholism, nystagmus, ataxia, confabulation, amnesia	MRI: mammillary body atrophy on T1WI, hyperintensity on T2WI. Enhancement.
Normal Pressure Hydrocephalus	Magnetic gait, urinary incontinence, subcortical dementia	MRI: Hydrocephalus, periventricular T2WI hyperintensities. CT: Hydrocephalus and periventricular hypoattenuation.

NOTE: CT scan abnormalities are delineated based on changes in "density" while MRI-based abnormalities are described by delineating lesional "intensity." Gadolinium may be used as an intravenous contrast for T1WIs and iodinated contrast is available for use in CT scans. Also, similar findings are typically denoted in both T2WIs and FLAIR sequences with the except that FLAIR sequences improve delineation of periventricular pathologies. T2WI indicates T2-weighted image; WM, white matter; DWI, diffusion weighted image; SWI, susceptibility weighted image; CSF, cerebrospinal fluid; CT, computed tomography.

acute-subacute mental status change, fever, and meningeal irritation (photophobia, nuchal rigidity). The additional presence of focal neurologic signs, including papilledema or lateralizing weakness, numbness or cortical deficits including aphasia, neglect, or visual field deficits, suggest parenchymal involvement and warrant a CT brain scan prior to cerebral spinal fluid sampling. FLAIR/T2 and T1 post-gadolinium MRI sequences can also help confirm if an infection extends to the brain parenchyma, as in a meningoencephalitis, or aid the diagnosis of a limbic encephalitis (i.e., herpes simplex virus) presenting with fever and mental status change without definitive meningeal irritation.

Patients with cerebrovascular disease may also present with underrecognized affective and behavioral symptoms. One such example is apathy in patients with an anterior cerebral artery stroke. If a detailed neurologic examination screening for corticospinal tract involvement (i.e., leg weakness, numbness, Babinski sign, increased reflexes) along with either a CT scan or DWI and ADC MRI sequences are not performed, an anterior cerebral artery stroke could be mistaken for a hypoactive delirium.

Increasing characterized paraneoplastic phenomena may present with prominent limbic symptoms, and can be investigated using cerebral spinal fluid sampling, antibody testing, oncologic screening, and MRI brain imaging (Dalmau & Rosenfeld, 2008). A well characterized example is the case of anti-N-methyl-D-aspartate (NMDA) receptor antibodies presenting with psychosis, memory deficits, altered mental status, seizures, dyskinesias, and autonomic disturbances in young women with undetected ovarian teratomas. FLAIR, T2, and T1post-gadolinium sequences may identify medial temporal lobe and prefrontal cortical inflammation supportive of limbic encephalitis.

Screening for vascular disease, and particularly small vessel (microangiopathic) white matter disease, is an important component of the diagnostic work-up for geriatric patients presenting with progressive subcortical cognitive impairments (diminished processing speed, retrieval deficits with relatively

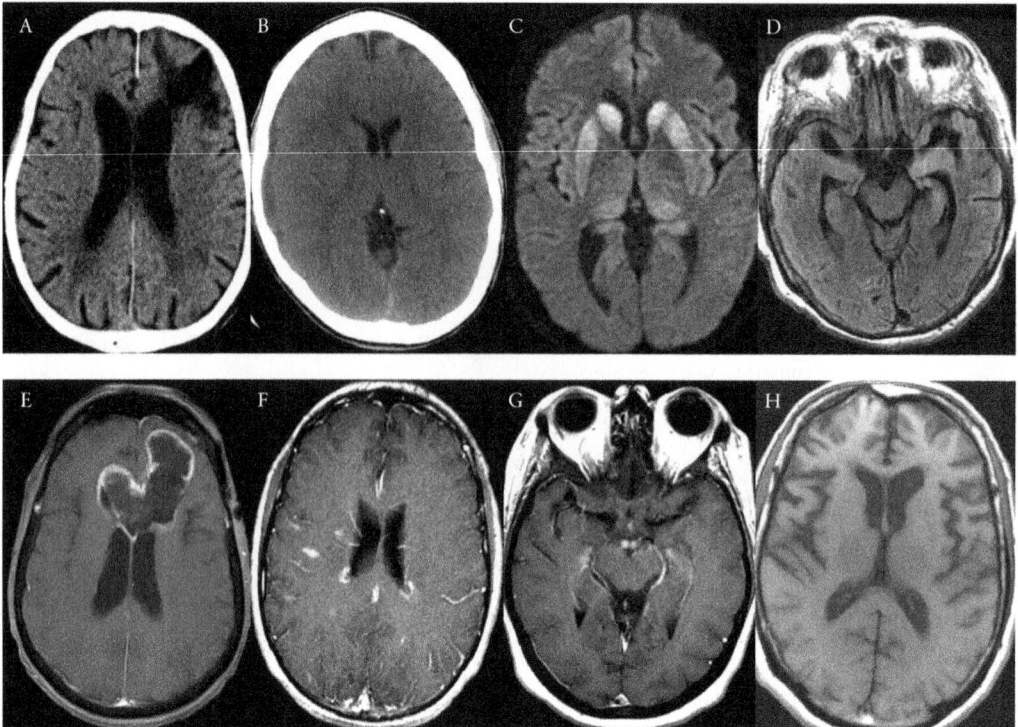

Figure 7.4 Sample diagnoses aided by radiographic findings. **A.** Computed tomography (CT) scan of an elderly man with impulsivity and disinhibition revealing hypoattenuation in the left frontal region consistent with a prior stroke. **B.** Noncontrast CT scan of a young woman with recent blunt head trauma demonstrating a right frontotemporal subacute subdural hemorrhage. **C.** Diffusion weighted image (DWI) of a woman with mood lability and myoclonus showing bilateral caudate and putamen restricted diffusion consistent with prion disease. **D.** Fluid attenuated inversion recovery (FLAIR) scan in an elderly woman with medically refractory seizures demonstrating increased left hippocampal FLAIR signal related to anti-HU paraneoplastic antibodies. **E.** T1 post-gadolinium scan of a woman with marked apathy demonstrating a heterogeneously enhancing intraparenchymal mass lesion consistent with a high-grade glioma. **F.** T1 post-gadolinium scan of a young man presenting with right-sided weakness found to have multifocal periventricular and subcortical enhancing white matter lesions consistent with an acute multiple sclerosis flare. **G.** T1 post-gadolinium scan of a middle-aged woman with alcohol dependence presenting with gait instability, amnesia, nystagmus, and bilateral gaze palsy, demonstrating bilateral mamillary body enhancement consistent with Wernicke-Korsakoff syndrome. **H.** T1 MRI of a man with progressive personality change and apathy revealing bilateral frontal, anterior temporal, and peri-insular atrophy with sulcal widening, consistent with frontotemporal dementia. Adapted from Perez DL, Larvie M, Acar D, Daffner K. Teaching NeuroImage: Apathetic variant of frontotemporal dementia, *Neurology* 2011;77(20):e117. Note: all images are displayed using radiographic conventions (i.e., right hemisphere displayed on the left side of the scan).

preserved retention/recognition on memory testing) and/or late-onset mood disturbance. Extensive hypoattenuation of the periventricular and subcortical white matter on CT scan, or T2/FLAIR hyperintensity on MRI, would support cerebrovascular disease, particularly in patients with a known history of hypertension, hyperlipidemia, and/or diabetes mellitus. Structural and functional imaging also aids in the diagnosis of neurodegenerative disorders through detection of lobar patterns of atrophy with associated sulcal widening (i.e., medial temporal or frontal) and focal hypometabolism (temporal/parietal or frontal/anterior temporal/insular) as present in Alzheimer's disease and frontotemporal dementia. Ventricular enlargement frequently accompanies neurodegenerative disease (hydrocephalus *ex vacuo*) and can be discerned from other forms of hydrocephalus, including normal pressure hydrocephalus, by concurrently detecting sulcal widening and a lack of periventricular signal abnormality suggestive of transependymal flow.

When evaluating potentially abnormal structural neuroimaging findings, it is also useful to consider the effects of normal aging (Fox & Schott, 2004). Assessing the extent to which atrophic changes are within the normal limits for age is a sophisticated clinical judgment, with the potential for differences of opinion even among experienced neuroradiologists;

unfortunately there are not yet well-accepted guidelines to assist clinicians in these determinations. Despite this, comparative analyses show that the aging brain loses volume in nonlinear and region-dependent fashion, and prefrontal cortical volume decreases more rapidly than other brain regions. Reductions in cortical volume, particularly in prefrontal and temporal regions, have been estimated to be approximately 0.5% per year in patients over 60 years of age (Fjell et al., 2009). Furthermore, volumetric reductions in aging populations are thought to reflect reductions in synaptic spine density rather than actual neuronal loss. Physical exercise and cognitively stimulating activities may also modulate the trajectory of normal age-related brain changes by promoting successful cognitive aging and enhanced neuroplasticity (Daffner, 2010). Thus, patient age is an important, heterogeneously presenting variable to consider when evaluating neuroimaging findings.

In general, a common problem in daily clinical practice is the extent to which brain imaging findings may be overinterpreted or underinterpreted. Radiographic misinterpretation can be partially avoided by familiarizing ordering physicians with the limitations of the individual neuroimaging techniques as previously discussed. Examples of this include the limitation of CT scans to appreciate even subtle ischemic stroke changes only on the order of several hours post stroke, while DWI imaging may capture early ischemic change within 30 minutes of stroke onset. Therefore, when performing clinical-radiographic interpretations, particularly in diagnostically challenging cases, we urge ordering clinicians to collaborate closely with neuroradiologists and like-minded neuropsychiatrists.

NEURAL CIRCUITS IMPLICATED IN PSYCHIATRIC DISEASE

After obtaining structural and/or functional imaging in the neuropsychiatric evaluation of a patient, clinicians are left with the task of performing clinical-radiographic interpretations. A given radiographic finding (i.e., evidence of acute demyelination on T1-weighted post-gadolinium MRI imaging) may be incidental to a psychiatric complaint or may mediate, at least in part, the clinical symptomatology. An example of this clinical dilemma is increased anxiety in a patient accumulating lesions in prefrontal white matter pathways secondary to relapsing-remitting multiple sclerosis. An understanding of neural circuits mediating affect, behavior, and cognition helps determine whether particular neuroimaging findings are directly related to the patient's symptomatology (see Table 7.5).

Three nonmotor prefrontal-subcortical parallel circuits initially characterized by Alexander, DeLong, and Strick (1986) aid in understanding prefrontal neural circuits; these include orbitofrontal, anterior cingulate, and dorsolateral prefrontal cortex–subcortical pathways (see Figure 7.5). The orbitofrontal-subcortical pathway participates in inhibition of socially inappropriate behavior and in empathic behavior; its dysfunction is associated with personality change, impulsivity, utilization/imitation behavior, mania, and obsessive compulsive disturbances (Mega & Cummings, 1994). The anterior cingulate–subcortical pathway is involved in motivated behavior, affective regulation, and conflict monitoring, and dysfunction has been linked to akinetic mutism, apathy, and impaired response inhibition among other deficits (Devinsky, Morell, & Vogt, 1995; Etkin, Egner, & Kalisch, 2011). The dorsolateral prefrontal–subcortical circuit participates in higher order executive functions, and dysfunction may manifest as poor organization and planning, environmental dependency, working memory deficits, and impaired set shifting.

The amygdala and related prefrontal, ventral striatal, and brainstem connections are important in understanding the neural correlates of fear responses, emotional processing, and emotional memories (Cahill, Babinsky, Markowitsch, & McGaugh, 1995; LeDoux, 2007; Phelps & LeDoux, 2005). The amygdala, an almond-shaped structure in the anterior medial temporal lobe, is composed of distinct nuclei. Afferents from sensory thalamus and cortex, the hippocampal formation, and multimodal association cortices project to the lateral nucleus (LeDoux, 2007). Medial prefrontal regions project to the basal nucleus, intercalated cells, and central nucleus. The central nucleus, the major output structure of the amygdala, has efferent projections to brainstem structures including neuromodulatory systems (norepinephrine, dopamine, serotonin, and acetylcholine), periaqueductal gray, hypothalamus, and parasympathetic nuclei. The basal nucleus of the amygdala

sends efferent projections to the ventral medial prefrontal cortex, ventral striatum, and multimodal association cortices. These connections enable reciprocal interactions between the amygdala and the medial prefrontal cortex; the amygdala, in turn, functions as a major node in central autonomic pathways that are frequently dysfunctional in patients with affective disorders (see Figures 7.6 and 7.7). Disruptions of prefrontal efferents projecting onto the amygdala may result in unregulated amygdalar activity (impaired top-down inhibition) and subsequent heightened affective symptoms and fear responses.

The cortical-hippocampal system for declarative memory (including episodic and semantic memory) comprises a widely distributed neural network involved in the conscious recollection of past experiences and factual information (Eichenbaum, 2000). Neocortical association cortices, the parahippocampal region, and the hippocampus comprise three major components of this circuit. Neocortical regions including the ventromedial prefrontal, anterior cingulate, dorsolateral prefrontal, posterior parietal, and temporal cortices provide afferent cognitive, motor, or perceptual information to subregions of the parahippocampus. The parahippocampal region serves as a convergence site for cortical information and projects to the hippocampus, where subsequently individual elements of a memory are linked to one another. The outcome of hippocampal processing returns to the parahippocampal region and to neocortical regions via reciprocal connections. Additional regions in the declarative memory circuit include the fornix, mammillary bodies, and anterior nuclei of the thalamus; the thalamus projects to the anterior cingulate cortex as part of the previously described prefrontal–subcortical loop.

Circuits implicated in the modulation of reward, addiction, and pleasure involve both cortical and subcortical structures. Dopaminergic projections from the ventral tegmental area in the midbrain to the nucleus accumbens in the ventral striatum (mesolimbic pathway) are implicated in reinforcing the effects of drugs of abuse. Mesolimbic dopamine, while initially thought to encode reward, has been more closely linked to reward prediction and salience (Volkow & Li, 2004). Behaviors commonly seen in patients with addiction disorders, including compulsion and disinhibition, are associated with hypoactivity of the orbitofrontal and anterior cingulate cortices. Hypofunction of the ventral striatum has also been linked to anhedonia, particularly in patients with major depressive disorder (Epstein et al., 2006).

Another neural system of emerging importance in psychiatric and neuropsychiatric diseases is the brain's default mode network (DMN; See Figure 7.8). This widely distributed network consists of regions that co-deactivate during a broad array of task performances and subsequently coactivate when individuals are allowed to rest and self-reflect without specific instructions (Buckner, Andrews-Hanna, & Schacter, 2008; Raichle et al., 2001). The core regions associated with the DMN include ventral and dorsal medial prefrontal cortex, posterior cingulate cortex/precuneus, inferior parietal lobule, lateral temporal cortex, and the hippocampal formation.

Lastly, widely distributed neuromodulatory monoamine pathways should also be considered when deducing if clinical symptoms may be explained by radiographic findings. These

Table 7.5 COMMONLY IMPLICATED CIRCUITS IN PSYCHIATRIC AND NEUROPSYCHIATRIC CONDITIONS

COMMONLY IMPLICATED CIRCUITS IN NEUROPSYCHIATRIC CONDITIONS	COMPONENTS	HEALTHY FUNCTION	DYSFUNCTION
Orbitofrontal–Subcortical Pathway	OFC	Socially Appropriate	Personality Change
	VM Caudate	&	Impulsivity
	MDM Globus Pallidus	Empathic Behavior	Utilization/Imitation Behavior
	MD & VA Thalamic Nuclei	Value-Based Decision-Making	Mania
			Obsessive Compulsive Disturbances
Anterior Cingulate–Subcortical Pathway	ACC	Motivated Behavior	Akinetic Mutism
	NA and VM Striatum	Affect Regulation	Apathy
	Ventral Globus Pallidus	Conflict Monitoring	Impaired Response Inhibition
	MD & VA Thalamic Nuclei		
Dorsolateral Prefrontal–Subcortical Pathway	DLPFC	Working Memory	Environmental Dependency
	DL Caudate	Organization	Impaired Working Memory
	LDM Globus Pallidus	Planning	Poor Planning/Organization
	MD & VA Thalamic Nuclei		Impaired Set Shifting
Prefrontal–Amygdala–Subcortical–Brainstem Pathways	Multimodal Association Cortex	Fear Responses	Abnormal Affective Processing
	Hippocampal Formation	Emotional Processing	&
	Sensory Thalamus	Emotional Memory	Impaired Emotional Regulation
	Sensory Cortex		
	Medial Prefrontal Cortex		
	Amygdala		
	Brainstem/Periaqueductal Gray		
	Ventral Striatum		
	Hypothalamus		
Cortical-Hippocampal Pathways	Neocortical Association Cortices	Declarative Memory	Amnesia
	Parahippocampus	Contextual Emotional	
	Hippocampus	Memory	
	Fornix		
	Mammillary Bodies		
	Anterior Thalamic Nuclei		
Reward Pathways	Ventral Tegmental Area	Reward Prediction	Addiction
	NA and Ventral Striatum	Salience	Anhedonia
	Orbitofrontal Cortex		
	Anterior Cingulate Cortex		

(continued)

Table 7.5 (CONTINUED)

COMMONLY IMPLICATED CIRCUITS IN NEUROPSYCHIATRIC CONDITIONS	COMPONENTS	HEALTHY FUNCTION	DYSFUNCTION
Default Mode Network	Ventral and Dorsal Medial PFC	Self Referential Processing	Under Investigation
	Posterior Cingulate Cortex		
	Precuneus		
	Inferior Parietal Lobule		
	Lateral Temporal Cortex		
	Hippocampal Formation		

OFC indicates orbitofrontal cortex; VM, ventral medial; MDM, medial dorsomedial; MD, mediodorsal; VA, ventral anterior; ACC, anterior cingulate cortex; NA, nucleus accumbens; DLPFC, dorsolateral prefrontal cortex; DL, dorsolateral; LDM, lateral dorsomedial; PFC, prefrontal cortex.

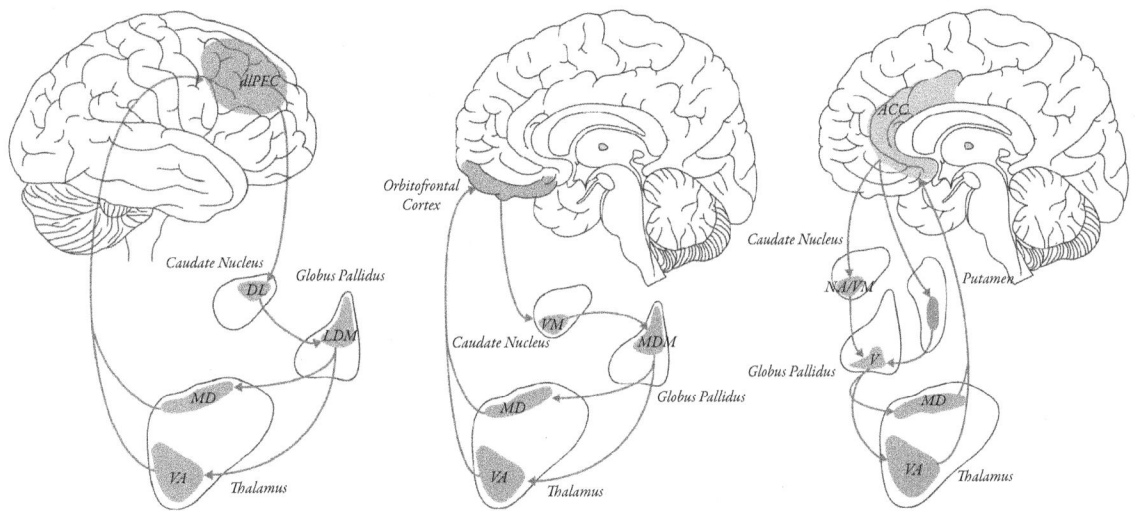

Figure 7.5 Graphic depiction of dorsolateral, orbitofrontal, and anterior cingulate prefrontal–subcortical circuits. dlPFC indicates dorsolateral prefrontal cortex; DL, dorsolateral; LDM, lateral dorsomedial; MD, mediodorsal; VA, ventral anterior; VM, ventromedial; MDM, medial dorsomedial; NA, nucleus accumbens; V, ventral; ACC, anterior cingulate cortex. Adapted from Perez DL, Catenaccio E, Epstein J (2011) Confusion, hyperactive delirium, and secondary mania in right hemispheric strokes: A focused review of neuroanatomical correlates. *Journal of Neurology and Neurophysiology* S1. doi:10.4172/2155-9562. S1-003.

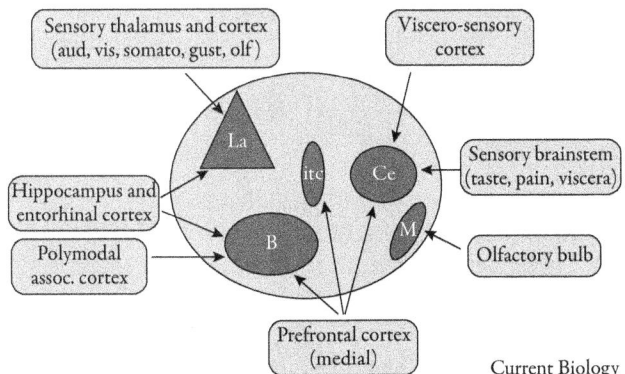

Figure 7.6 Inputs into specific amygdala nuclei. B indicates basal nucleus; Ce, central nucleus; ict, intercalated cells; La, lateral nucleus; M, medial nucleus; aud, auditory; vis, visual; somato, somatosensory; gust, gustatory; olf, olfactory; assoc, association. Reprinted from publication *Current Biology*, 17(20), Joseph LeDoux, The Amygdala, R868-74., 2007, with permission from Elsevier.

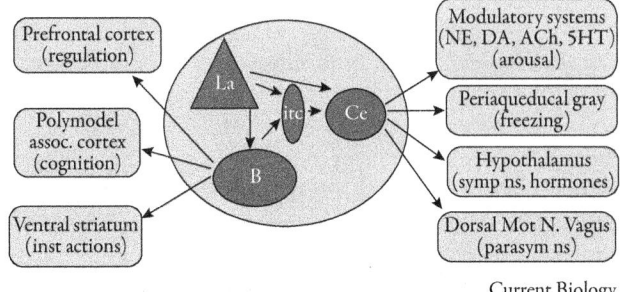

Figure 7.7 Output from amygdala nuclei. B indicates basal nucleus; Ce, central nucleus; itc, intercalated cells; La, lateral nucleus; NE, norepinephrine, DA, dopamine; Ach, acetylcholine; 5HT, serotonin; parasym ns, parasympathetic nervous system; symp ns, sympathetic nervous system; assoc, association; inst, instinctual. Reprinted from publication *Current Biology*, 17(20), Joseph LeDoux, The Amygdala, R868-74, 2007, with permission from Elsevier.

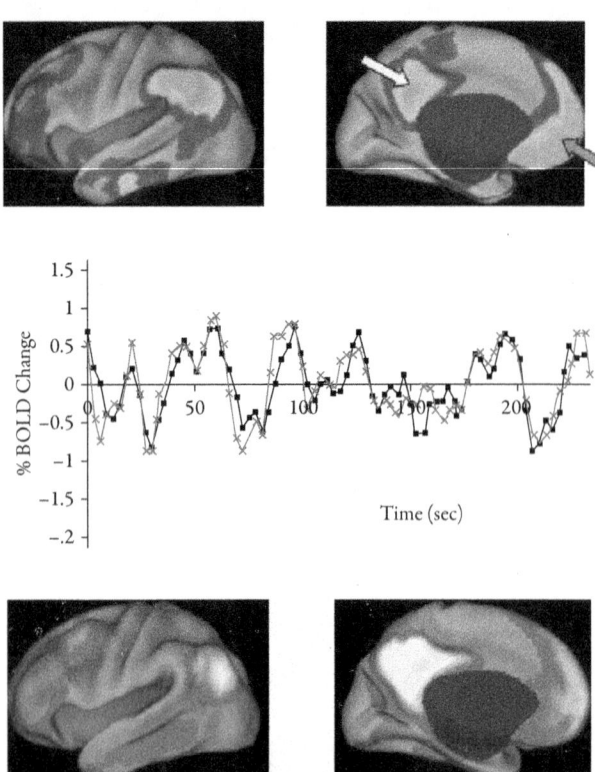

Figure 7.8 Default mode network (DMN). Performance of a wide variety of tasks leads to decreased activity in broadly distributed regions including dorsal medial prefrontal cortex and posterior cingulate cortex/precuneus referred to as the DMN (top row). This distributed network can be appreciated by capturing low-frequency oscillations in the blood oxygen level dependent (BOLD) signal (middle row). The same regions that deactivate with task increase in activity when subjects allow their minds to freely wander and self-reflect (bottom row). Reprinted from *Trends in Cognitive Sciences*, 14: Raichle ME. Two views of brain function. 180–90, 2010 with permission from Elsevier.

include dopamine pathways (mesolimbic and mesocortical circuits), serotonergic projections from the raphe nuclei, norepinephrine projections from the locus coeruleus, and cholinergic output from the basal forebrain/Nucleus Basalis of Meynert. Having reviewed neural circuits implicated across psychiatric diseases, the following section briefly outlines the neural correlates of schizophrenia, MDD, and PTSD.

FUNCTIONAL NEUROANATOMY OF SCHIZOPHRENIA, MDD, AND PTSD

Schizophrenia is a chronic disintegrative thought disorder where patients frequently experience auditory hallucinations and bizarre or paranoid delusions. While a neural basis for schizophrenia has been suspected for over a century, advances in structural and functional neuroimaging techniques over the last 30 years have greatly advanced our understanding of this condition. Structural studies first using CT scans, and more recently utilizing automated methods such as VBM applied to T1 MRI scans, have commonly identified diminished whole brain volume, increased ventricular size, and regional atrophy in hippocampal, prefrontal, superior temporal, and inferior parietal cortices in patient with schizophrenia compared to control groups (Keshavan, Tandon, Boutros, & Nasrallah, 2008; Pearlson & Marsh, 1999; Shenton, Dickey, Frumin, &

McCarley., 2001; see Table 7.6). A reversal of or diminished hemispheric asymmetry has also been characterized. Functional neuroimaging studies have commonly identified hypoactivity of the prefrontal cortex (including the dorsolateral prefrontal cortex associated with executive dysfunction) and temporal lobe dysfunction (Brunet-Gouet & Decety, 2006; Keshavan et al., 2008). Also, while the clinical phenotype of schizophrenia only infrequently poses a diagnostic challenge, clinicians are not yet able to predict treatment response based on clinical phenotype. In promising preliminary research, a positive correlation has been identified between activity of the dorsolateral prefrontal cortex and response to atypical antipsychotic drugs or cognitive behavioral therapy (Kumari et al., 2009; van Veelen et al., 2011). Leftward shifts in frontal cortical asymmetry have also been associated with a positive response to atypical antipsychotic drugs (Szeszko et al., 2010).

MDD is a frequently encountered mental disorder characterized by depressed mood, diminished sense of self-worth, anhedonia, and apathy among other features. Structural studies in patients with MDD have frequently identified volumetric reductions in prefrontal regions including the subgenual anterior cingulate cortex, orbitofrontal cortex, hippocampus, and striatum. Functional neuroimaging studies using PET, SPECT, and fMRI–based techniques have demonstrated increased activity in the subgenual cingulate, amygdala, and mediodorsal thalamus, and diminished activity in dorsal anterior cingulate cortex, dorsolateral prefrontal cortex, and ventral striatum (Drevets, Price, & Furey, 2008; Lorenzetti, Allen, Fornito, & Yucel., 2009; Vago, Epstein, Catenaccio, & Stern, 2011). From a symptom domain perspective, specific neural circuit disturbances have been linked to particular symptoms of MDD (i.e., anhedonia and ventral striatum hypoactivity, impaired working memory and dorsolateral prefrontal cortex hypoactivity) but the neural systems mediating phenotypic subtypes, such as patients with or without suicidal ideation, are not yet well understood. Emerging research suggests increased anterior cingulate cortex activity/volume and hippocampal size may predict antidepressant treatment response (Chen et al., 2007; MacQueen, 2009; Mayberg et al., 1997).

PTSD is a disorder characterized by reexperiencing phenomena, hyperarousal, emotional numbing, and avoidance in the setting of previously experienced or witnessed life-endangering trauma. Volumetric analyses conducted in patients with PTSD compared to control populations have primarily identified hippocampal and anterior cingulate cortex atrophy (Karl et al., 2006; Woon & Hedges, 2009). Functional neuroimaging studies, mainly using univariate approaches to date, have identified prefrontal (anterior cingulate and orbitofrontal cortices) and hippocampal hypoactivity, and parallel amygdalar hyperactivity (Lanius, Bluhm, Lanius, & Pain, 2006; Liberzon & Sripada, 2008). In limited studies to date, rostral anterior cingulate cortex volume and diminished amygdala and ventral (subgenual) anterior cingulate cortex activity in response to an aversive visual task may predict a positive response to cognitive behavioral therapy (Bryant et al., 2008a; 2008b).

In addition to identifying neural predictors of prognosis and treatment response, delineating the neural correlates of psychiatric symptoms through neuroimaging techniques may

Table 7.6 COMMON STRUCTURAL AND FUNCTIONAL ABNORMALITIES IN PATIENTS WITH SCHIZOPHRENIA, MAJOR DEPRESSIVE DISORDER (MDD) AND POSTTRAUMATIC STRESS DISORDER (PTSD)

DISEASE	COMMON VOLUMETRIC FINDINGS	COMMON FUNCTIONAL FINDINGS	PRELIMINARY PREDICTORS OF TREATMENT RESPONSE
Schizophrenia	↓ Total brain volume	↓ Prefrontal (i.e., dlPFC) activity during rest and cognitive challenge studies	↓ dlPFC activity during a working memory task → ↓atypical antipsychotic response
	↑ Ventricular size		
	↓ Hippocampal volume	Temporal lobe dysfunction during rest and cognitive challenge studies	↑ dlPFC activity during a working memory task → ↑ CBT response
	↓Reversal of cerebral asymmetry		
	↓ STG, IPL, dlPFC		↑ Frontal structural asymmetry → ↑ atypical antipsychotic response
	↑ Basal Ganglia (related to typical antipsychotic drugs)		
	↓ Basal Ganglia (related to atypical antipsychotic drugs)		
MDD	↓ Prefrontal (sgACC, OFC)	↑ sgACC	↑ ACC activity (during rest and affective challenge studies) and volume → ↑ antidepressant response
	↓ Hippocampal volume	↑ AMG	
	↓ Striatum	↑ Mediodorsal thalamus	↑ Hippocampal volume → ↑ antidepressant response
		↓ dorsal ACC	
		↓ dlPFC	
		Insular dysfunction	
PTSD	↓ Hippocampal volume	↓ Hippocampus	↓ AMG and ventral ACC activity during an affective challenge task → ↑ CBT response
		↓ Medial prefrontal (ACC, OFC)	
	↓ ACC	↑ AMG	↑ Rostral ACC volume → ↑ CBT response

Preliminary structural and functional predictors of treatment response are also highlighted. Also, unless otherwise specified, functional findings reflect primarily task-driven abnormalities.

STG indicates superior temporal gyrus; IPL, inferior parietal lobule; dlPFC, dorsolateral prefrontal cortex; sgACC, subgenual anterior cingulate cortex; OFC, orbitofrontal cortex, ACC, anterior cingulate cortex; AMG, amygdala; CBT, cognitive behavioral therapy.

help identify potential targets for neuromodulatory interventions. Two of the more targeted neuromodulatory approaches are transcranial magnetic stimulation (TMS) and deep brain stimulation (DBS). Medication-resistant MDD has been the most well studied condition, with hypoactivity of the dorsolateral prefrontal cortex and hyperactivity of the subgenual cingulate cortex targeted using TMS and DBS respectively (Mayberg et al., 2005; Pascual-Leone, Rubio, Pallardo, & Catala, 1996). Ongoing research will likely broaden the use of these techniques for the treatment of additional affective and psychotic disorders.

across psychiatric diseases. Furthermore, additional novel targets will be identified for neuromodulation and biofeedback techniques such as real-time fMRI. Overall, this endeavor will help clarify final common pathways through which medical/neurological disorders and primary psychiatric disorders produce behavioral, affective, perceptual, and cognitive symptoms.

In summary, physicians treating psychiatric disorders will increasingly make use of structural and functional neuroimaging techniques. Proficiency in the use and interpretation of neuroimaging findings will become the norm for psychiatrists, and a working knowledge of function–structure relationships will enable future advancement in the field.

SUMMARY

This chapter has outlined the emerging role for neuroimaging in the diagnosis and management of patients with psychiatric and neuropsychiatric conditions. Ongoing translational research endeavors will help link neuroimaging advances with genetic and epigenetic information to clarify endophenotypes

CLINICAL PEARLS

- Computed tomography (CT) scans are relatively insensitive to acute ischemic stroke detection; a well visualized hypodensity may not be appreciable until more than 24 hours after symptom onset. Subtle ischemic changes such as sulcal effacement and loss of gray/white matter differentiation may be seen within the first few hours of stroke onset.

- Hyperdensity of the middle cerebral artery (MCA), known as a "dense MCA sign," may indicate intra-arterial clot and provides supportive evidence of an acute ischemic stroke.

- On brain MRI: while T2-based sequences are useful at detecting parenchymal pathology such as prior infarcts, mass lesions, edema, and white matter demyelinating plaques, fluid attenuated inversion recovery (FLAIR) images particularly aid the detection of periventricular abnormalities which may be obscured by cerebrospinal fluid signal on T2 images. T1 sequences are most useful in delineating brain anatomy (i.e., regional atrophy).

- The addition of gadolinium, a paramagnetic heavy metal that decreases the T1 relaxation times of tissues when injected intravenously as a contrast agent, enhances lesions that disrupt the blood–brain barrier including acute demyelinating white matter lesions, vascular lesions, and high-grade glial tumors.

- Clinically, in cases of a suspected acute stroke where a hypodensity is not well delineated on a CT scan, a brain MRI with diffusion sequences should be specifically requested.

- A T2-shine-through effect may cause false positive interpretations of an acute stroke if an abnormality is seen only on diffusion weighted images (DWI).

- If a brainstem stroke is suspected, clinicians may also request thin sections through the brainstem to improve test sensitivity.

- Anisotropic fraction (AF) quantifies microstructure integrity of the white matter and is obtained by recording water diffusivity along white matter tracts (Ries et al., 2008). This measure has the advantage of detecting microstructural abnormalities with high sensitivity.

- Magnetic resonance spectroscopy (MRS), thus far, is the only readily available technique enabling *in vivo* sampling of metabolic information. Clinically it is used to aid diagnosis of metabolic disorders (i.e., leukodystrophies); to distinguish neoplasms from other abnormal brain signals (high-grade brain tumors characterized by high choline, an indicator of cell membrane synthesis, and low N-acetyl aspartate, a marker of neuronal integrity; and to assess the effects of chemotherapeutics on brain tumors by helping to distinguish between necrosis and neoplasm recurrence.

- SPECT imaging is particularly clinically useful for seizure foci detection if the tracer is injected in close temporal proximity to seizure onset (Knowlton et al., 2004). Of note, the tracer takes approximately 30 seconds to reach the brain, and the switch from ictal to postictal hypoperfusion occurs approximately in 1–2 minutes following seizure termination in temporal regions and sooner in extratemporal regions.

- Measuring regional cerebral glucose metabolism via 18F-FDG PET has become a standard technique to detect regional hypometabolism in neurodegenerative diseases.

- While increased blood oxygen level dependent (BOLD) signal (Logothetis et al., 2001) in fMRI provides a proxy for neural activity based on venous blood flow patterns, more recently developed methods such as *arterial spin labeling* (ASL) provide an arterial phase measure of cerebral blood flow with the potential for improved spatial and temporal resolution. In evaluating functional neuroimaging findings, it is important to also consider if "state" or "trait" characteristics are being evaluated at the time of the experiment.

- Reductions in cortical volume, particularly in prefrontal and temporal regions, have been estimated to be approximately 0.5% per year in patients over 60 years of age (Fjell et al., 2009).

- Diffusion weighted imaging (DWI) may capture early ischemic change within 30 minutes of stroke onset.

- Emerging research suggests increased anterior cingulate cortex activity/volume and hippocampal size may predict antidepressant treatment response (Chen et al., 2007; MacQueen, 2009; Mayberg et al., 1997).

DISCLOSURE STATEMENTS

Dr. David L. Perez has no conflicts of interest or disclosures to report.

Dr. Laura Ortiz-Terán has no conflicts of interest or disclosures to report.

Dr. David A. Silbersweig has no conflicts of interest or disclosures to report.

REFERENCES

Alexander, G. E., DeLong, M. R., & Strick, P. L. (1986). Parallel organization of functionally segregated circuits linking basal ganglia and cortex. *Annual Review of Neuroscience, 9*, 357–381.

Ashburner, J., & Friston, K. J. (2000). Voxel-based morphometry—the methods. *Neuroimage, 11*, 805–821.

Beaulieu, C. (2002). The basis of anisotropic water diffusion in the nervous system—a technical review. *NMR in Biomedicine, 15*, 435–455.

Bremner, J. D., Staib, L. H., Kaloupek, D., Southwick, S. M., Soufer, R., & Charney, D. S. (1999). Neural correlates of exposure to traumatic pictures and sound in Vietnam combat veterans with and without posttraumatic stress disorder: a positron emission tomography study. *Biological Psychiatry, 45*, 806–816.

Brooks, D. J., Ibanez, V., Sawle, G. V., Playford, E. D., Quinn, N., Mathias, C. J., et al. (1992). Striatal D2 receptor status in patients with Parkinson's disease, striatonigral degeneration, and progressive supranuclear palsy, measured with 11C-raclopride and positron emission tomography. *Annals of Neurology, 31*, 184–192.

Brunet-Gouet, E., & Decety, J. (2006). Social brain dysfunctions in schizophrenia: a review of neuroimaging studies. *Psychiatry Research*, *148*, 75–92.

Bryant, R. A., Felmingham, K., Kemp, A., Das, P., Hughes, G., Peduto, A., et al. (2008a). Amygdala and ventral anterior cingulate activation predicts treatment response to cognitive behaviour therapy for post-traumatic stress disorder. *Psychological Medicine*, *38*, 555–561.

Bryant, R. A., Felmingham, K., Whitford, T. J., Kemp, A., Hughes, G., Peduto, A., et al. (2008b). Rostral anterior cingulate volume predicts treatment response to cognitive-behavioural therapy for post-traumatic stress disorder. *Journal of Psychiatry and Neuroscience*, *33*, 142–146.

Buckner, R. L., Andrews-Hanna, J. R., & Schacter, D. L. (2008). The brain's default network: anatomy, function, and relevance to disease. *Annals of the NY Academy of Sciences*, *1124*, 1–38.

Cahill, L., Babinsky, R., Markowitsch, H. J., & McGaugh, J. L. (1995). The amygdala and emotional memory. *Nature*, *377*, 295–296.

Callicott, J. H., Bertolino, A., Mattay, V. S., Langheim, F. J., Duyn, J., Coppola, R., et al. (2000). Physiological dysfunction of the dorsolateral prefrontal cortex in schizophrenia revisited. *Cerebral Cortex*, *10*, 1078–1092.

Chen, C. H., Ridler, K., Suckling, J., Williams, S., Fu, C. H., Merlo-Pich, E., et al. (2007). Brain imaging correlates of depressive symptom severity and predictors of symptom improvement after antidepressant treatment. *Biological Psychiatry*, *62*, 407–414.

Csernansky, J. G., Joshi, S., Wang, L., Haller, J. W., Gado, M., Miller, J. P., et al. (1998). Hippocampal morphometry in schizophrenia by high dimensional brain mapping. *Proceedings of the National Academy of Sciences USA*, *95*, 11406–1111.

Daffner, K. R. (2010). Promoting successful cognitive aging: a comprehensive review. *Journal of Alzheimer's Disease*, *19*, 1101–1122.

Dalmau, J., & Rosenfeld, M. R. (2008). Paraneoplastic syndromes of the CNS. *Lancet Neurology*, *7*, 327–340.

Devinsky, O., Morrell, M. J., & Vogt, B. A. (1995). Contributions of anterior cingulate cortex to behaviour. *Brain*, *118*(Pt 1), 279–306.

Drevets, W. C., Price, J. L., & Furey, M. L. (2008). Brain structural and functional abnormalities in mood disorders: implications for neurocircuitry models of depression. *Brain Structure & Function*, *213*, 93–118.

Eichenbaum, H. (2000). A cortical-hippocampal system for declarative memory. *Nature Reviews, Neuroscience*, *1*, 41–50.

Epstein, J., Pan, H., Kocsis, J. H., Yang, Y., Butler, T., Chusid, J., et al. (2006). Lack of ventral striatal response to positive stimuli in depressed versus normal subjects. *American Journal of Psychiatry*, *163*, 1784–1790.

Etkin, A., Egner, T., & Kalisch, R. (2011). Emotional processing in anterior cingulate and medial prefrontal cortex. *Trends in Cognitive Science*, *15*, 85–93.

Farde, L., Wiesel, F. A., Stone-Elander, S., Halldin, C., Nordstrom, A. L., Hall, H., et al. (1990). D2 dopamine receptors in neuroleptic-naive schizophrenic patients. A positron emission tomography study with [11C]raclopride. *Archives of General Psychiatry*, *47*, 213–219.

Farid, K., Caillat-Vigneron, N., & Sibon, I. (2011). Is brain SPECT useful in degenerative dementia diagnosis? *Journal of Computer Assisted Tomography*, *35*, 1–3.

Fischl, B., & Dale, A. M. (2000). Measuring the thickness of the human cerebral cortex from magnetic resonance images. *Proceedings of the National Academy of Sciences USA*, *97*, 11050–11055.

Fjell, A. M., Walhovd, K. B., Fennema-Notestine, C., McEvoy, L. K., Hagler, D. J., Holland, D., et al. (2009). One-year brain atrophy evident in healthy aging. *Journal of Neuroscience*, *29*, 15223–15231.

Fox, N. C., & Schott, J. M. (2004). Imaging cerebral atrophy: Normal ageing to Alzheimer's disease. *Lancet*, *363*, 392–394.

Greicius, M. D., Flores, B. H., Menon, V., Glover, G. H., Solvason, H. B., Kenna, H., et al. (2007). Resting-state functional connectivity in major depression: Abnormally increased contributions from subgenual cingulate cortex and thalamus. *Biological Psychiatry*, *62*, 429–437.

Grossman, R. I., & Yousem, D. M. (2003). *Neuroradiology: The requisites*. Philadelphia, PA: Elsevier.

Herholz, K., Carter, S. F., & Jones, M. (2007). Positron emission tomography imaging in dementia. *British Journal of Radiology*, *80*(Spec No 2), S160–S167.

Huettel, S. A., Song, A. W., & McCarthy, G. (2004). *Functional magnetic resonance imaging*. Sunderland, MA: Sinauer Associates, Inc.

Ho, S. S., Berkovic, S. F., Berlangieri, S. U., Newton, M. R., Egan, G. F., Tochon-Danguy, H. J., et al. (1995). Comparison of ictal SPECT and interictal PET in the presurgical evaluation of temporal lobe epilepsy. *Annals of Neurology*, *37*, 738–745.

Karl, A., Schaefer, M., Malta, L. S., Dorfel, D., Rohleder, N., & Werner, A. (2006). A meta-analysis of structural brain abnormalities in PTSD. *Neuroscience & Biobehavioral Reviews*, *30*, 1004–1031.

Keshavan, M. S., Tandon, R., Boutros, N. N., & Nasrallah, H. A. (2008). Schizophrenia, "just the facts": What we know in 2008 Part 3: neurobiology. *Schizophrenia Research*, *106*, 89–107.

Klunk, W. E., Engler, H., Nordberg, A., Wang, Y., Blomqvist, G., Holt, D. P., et al. (2004). Imaging brain amyloid in Alzheimer's disease with Pittsburgh Compound-B. *Annals of Neurology*, *55*, 306–319.

Knowlton, R. C., Lawn, N. D., Mountz, J. M., & Kuznicky, R. I. (2004). Ictal SPECT analysis in epilepsy: subtraction and statistical parametric mapping techniques. *Neurology*, *63*, 10–15.

Kumari, V., Peters, E. R., Fannon, D., Antonova, E., Premkumar, P., Anilkumar, A. P., et al. (2009). Dorsolateral prefrontal cortex activity predicts responsiveness to cognitive-behavioral therapy in schizophrenia. *Biological Psychiatry*, *66*, 594–602.

Kuperberg, G. R., Broome, M. R., McGuire, P. K., David, A. S., Eddy, M., Ozawa, F., et al. (2003). Regionally localized thinning of the cerebral cortex in schizophrenia. *Archives of General Psychiatry*, *60*, 878–888.

Lanius, R. A., Bluhm, R., Lanius, U., & Pain, C. (2006). A review of neuroimaging studies in PTSD: heterogeneity of response to symptom provocation. *Journal of Psychiatric Research*, *40*, 709–729.

LeDoux, J. (2007). The amygdala. *Current Biology*, *17*, R868–R874.

Liberzon, I., & Sripada, C. S. (2008). The functional neuroanatomy of PTSD: a critical review. *Progress in Brain Research*, *167*, 151–169.

Liu, H., Buckner, R. L., Talukdar, T., Tanaka, N., Madsen, J. R., & Stufflebeam, S. M. (2009). Task-free presurgical mapping using functional magnetic resonance imaging intrinsic activity. *Journal of Neurosurgery*, *111*, 746–754.

Logothetis, N. K., Pauls, J., Augath, M., Trinath, T., & Oeltermann, A. (2001). Neurophysiological investigation of the basis of the fMRI signal. *Nature*, *412*, 150–157.

Lorenzetti, V., Allen, N. B., Fornito, A., & Yucel, M. (2009). Structural brain abnormalities in major depressive disorder: a selective review of recent MRI studies. *Journal of Affective Disorders*, *117*, 1–17.

MacQueen, G. M. (2009). Magnetic resonance imaging and prediction of outcome in patients with major depressive disorder. *Journal of Psychiatry and Neuroscience*, *34*, 343–349.

Mayberg, H. S., Brannan, S. K., Mahurin, R. K., Jerabek, P. A., Brickman, J. S., Tekell, J. L., et al. (1997). Cingulate function in depression: a potential predictor of treatment response. *Neuroreport*, *8*, 1057–1061.

Mayberg, H. S., Lozano, A. M., Voon, V., McNeely, H. E., Seminowicz, D., Hamani, C., et al. (2005). Deep brain stimulation for treatment-resistant depression. *Neuron*, *45*, 651–660.

Mega, M. S., & Cummings, J. L. (1994). Frontal-subcortical circuits and neuropsychiatric disorders. *Journal of Neuropsychiatry and Clinical Neurosciences*, *6*, 358–370.

Mukherjee, P., Berman, J. I., Chung, S. W., Hess, C. P., & Henry, R. G. (2008). Diffusion tensor MR imaging and fiber tractography: theoretic underpinnings. *American Journal of Neuroradiology*, *29*, 632–641.

Pan, H., Epstein, J., Silbersweig, D. A., & Stern, E. (2011). New and emerging imaging techniques for mapping brain circuitry. *Brain Res Rev*, *67*, 226–251.

Pascual-Leone, A., Rubio, B., Pallardo, F., & Catala, M. D. (1996). Rapid-rate transcranial magnetic stimulation of left dorsolateral prefrontal cortex in drug-resistant depression. *Lancet*, *348*, 233–237.

Pearlson, G. D., & Marsh, L. (1999). Structural brain imaging in schizophrenia: a selective review. *Biological Psychiatry, 46,* 627–649.

Phelps, E. A., & LeDoux, J. E. (2005). Contributions of the amygdala to emotion processing: from animal models to human behavior. *Neuron, 48,* 175–187.

Protopopescu, X., Pan, H., Tuescher, O., Cloitre, M., Goldstein, M., Engelien, W., et al. (2005). Differential time courses and specificity of amygdala activity in posttraumatic stress disorder subjects and normal control subjects. *Biological Psychiatry, 57,* 464–473.

Raichle, M. E., MacLeod, A. M., Snyder, A. Z., Powers, W. J., Gusnard, D. A., & Shulman, G. L. (2001). A default mode of brain function. *Proceedings of the National Academy of Sciences USA, 98,* 676–682.

Ries, M. L., Carlsson, C. M., Rowley, H. A., Sager, M. A., Gleason, C. E., Asthana, S., et al. (2008). Magnetic resonance imaging characterization of brain structure and function in mild cognitive impairment: a review. *Journal of the American Geriatrics Society, 56,* 920–934.

Rosas, H. D., Liu, A. K., Hersch, S., Glessner, M., Ferrante, R. J., Salat, D. H., et al. (2002). Regional and progressive thinning of the cortical ribbon in Huntington's disease. *Neurology, 58,* 695–701.

Salat, D. H., Buckner, R. L., Snyder, A. Z., Greve, D. N., Desikan, R. S., Busa, E., et al. (2004). Thinning of the cerebral cortex in aging. *Cerebral Cortex, 14,* 721–730.

Schaefer, P. W., Grant, P. E., & Gonzalez, R. G. (2000). Diffusion-weighted MR. imaging of the brain. *Radiology, 217,* 331–345.

Sepulcre, J., Liu, H., Talukdar, T., Martincorena, I., Yeo, B. T., & Buckner, R. L. (2010). The organization of local and distant functional connectivity in the human brain. *PLoS Computational Biology, 6,* e1000808.

Sheline, Y. I., Barch, D. M., Donnelly, J. M., Ollinger, J. M., Snyder, A. Z., & Mintun, M. A. (2001). Increased amygdala response to masked emotional faces in depressed subjects resolves with antidepressant treatment: an fMRI study. *Biological Psychiatry, 50,* 651–658.

Shenton, M. E., Dickey, C. C., Frumin, M., & McCarley, R. W. (2001). A review of MRI findings in schizophrenia. *Schizophrenia Research, 49,* 1–52.

Silbersweig, D. A., Stern, E., Frith, C., Cahill, C., Holmes, A., Grootoonk, S., et al. (1995). A functional neuroanatomy of hallucinations in schizophrenia. *Nature, 378,* 176–179.

Smith, S. M., Jenkinson, M., Johansen-Berg, H., Rueckert, D., Nichols, T. E., Mackay, C. E., et al. (2006). Tract-based spatial statistics: Voxelwise analysis of multi-subject diffusion data. *Neuroimage, 31,* 1487–1505.

Song, S. K., Sun, S. W., Ramsbottom, M. J., Chang, C., Russell, J., & Cross, A. H. (2002). Dysmyelination revealed through MRI as increased radial (but unchanged axial) diffusion of water. *Neuroimage, 17,* 1429–1436.

Stern, E., Silbersweig, D. A., Chee, K. Y., Holmes, A., Robertson, M. M., Trimble, M., et al. (2000). A functional neuroanatomy of tics in Tourette syndrome. *Archives of General Psychiatry, 57,* 741–748.

Szeszko, P. R., Narr, K. L., Phillips, O. R., McCormack, J., Sevy, S., Gunduz-Bruce, H., et al. (2012). Magnetic Resonance imaging predictors of treatment response in first-episode, schizophrenia. *Schizophrenia Bulletin, 38,* 569–578.

Tharin, S., & Golby, A. (2007). Functional brain mapping and its applications to neurosurgery. *Neurosurgery, 60,* 185–201; discussion, 201–202.

Vago, D. R., Epstein, J., Catenaccio, E., & Stern, E. (2011). Identification of neural targets for the treatment of psychiatric disorders: the role of functional neuroimaging. *Neurosurgery Clinics of North America, 22,* 279–305, x.

Van Paesschen, W. (2004). Ictal SPECT. *Epilepsia, 45*(Suppl 4), 35–40.

van Veelen, N. M., Vink, M., Ramsey, N. F., van Buuren, M., Hoogendam, J. M., & Kahn, R. S. (2011). Prefrontal lobe dysfunction predicts treatment response in medication-naive first-episode schizophrenia. *Schizophrenia Research, 129,* 156–162.

Volkow, N. D., & Li, T. K. (2004). Drug addiction: the neurobiology of behaviour gone awry. *Nature Reviews Neuroscience, 5,* 963–970.

Watts, D. J., & Strogatz, S. H. (1998). Collective dynamics of "small-world" networks. *Nature, 393,* 440–442.

Woon, F. L., & Hedges, D. W. (2009). Amygdala volume in adults with posttraumatic stress disorder: a meta-analysis. *Journal of Neuropsychiatry and Clinical Neurosciences, 21,* 5–12.

Zhang, D., & Raichle, M. E. (2010). Disease and the brain's dark energy. *Nature Reviews Neurology, 6,* 15–28.

8.

CLINICAL NEUROPHYSIOLOGY IN MEDICAL PSYCHIATRY

Rani A. Sarkis and Shahram Khoshbin

Clinical neurophysiology comprises electroencephalography (EEG), evoked potential (EP) studies, electromyography (EMG), nerve conduction studies, and specialized investigations such as electrical testing of specific reflex arcs (e.g., the blink reflex). It can be critical in the differentiation of neurological conditions with similar phenomenology but different brain mechanisms, and its objective nature gives it a special place in the investigation of somatoform neurological symptoms. This chapter will describe the most commonly used procedures of clinical neurophysiology and highlight points of special interest to medical psychiatrists.

ELECTROENCEPHALOGRAPHY (EEG)

The surface electroencephalogram is a neurophysiological tool which measures brain activity with the aid of surface scalp electrodes. The exact source of this brain activity is the result of a complex interplay of large populations of neurons and surrounding glia, with the majority of the activity generated by dendritic synaptic potentials in gray matter pyramidal cells (Schaul, 1998). On a larger scale, the corticocortical and thalamocortical connections are also an important contributor to the EEG signal. For example, the thalamocortical connections are known to be essential in the generation of a number of sleep rhythms such as the sleep spindle (Speckmann & Caspers, 1979).

The standard EEG consists of electrodes placed according to the 10-20 international electrode system (Jasper, 1958). The *10* and *20* refer to the percentage of the distance, used to guide placement, from nasion (the craniometric point at the bridge of the nose where the frontal and nasal bones of the skull meet) to inion (the projecting part of the occipital bone at the base of the skull) anteroposteriorly, and then left to right preauricular points (Figure 8.1). In total, 19 electrodes are placed in addition to a ground and reference electrode. Electrode nomenclature consists of the following: C for central, F for frontal, Fp for frontopolar, O for occipital, P for parietal, T for temporal. Odd numbers refer to electrodes on the left and even numbers on the right. All central electrodes have a "z" subscript.

The electrical activity is then measured between 2 electrode pairs as a voltage difference. The electrodes can be paired in two different ways (montages) and then amplified. In the referential montage, all the electrodes are referred to the same electrode, for example, one attached to an earlobe. In contrast, the bipolar montage consists of pairs of successively numbered electrodes: electrode 1 linked to electrode 2, electrode 2 to 3, and so forth. With the current digital technology the EEG reviewer can easily switch between montages to better assess the brain activity in question.

The electrical activity once recorded can be characterized by its amplitude in microvolts (5-200 μV) and its frequency. Surface EEG frequencies include Delta (0–4 Hz), Theta (4–8Hz), alpha (8–13 Hz), and beta (>13 Hz) (Table 8.1). By convention, any upward deflection on EEG is termed *negative* and any downward deflection is termed *positive*.

THE NORMAL EEG DURING WAKEFULNESS AND SLEEP

The "normal" adult EEG consists of a prominent alpha rhythm predominantly located in the posterior head regions, and low voltage faster frequencies (LVF) in the frontal regions (Figure 8.2). Alpha rhythm and posterior dominant rhythm are sometimes used interchangeably; however, under certain circumstances a person's posterior dominant rhythm may consist of lower frequencies. When the posterior dominant rhythm attenuates with eye opening and reappears with eye closure, it is considered *reactive*. The normal 8–13 Hz posterior background rhythm/alpha rhythm is achieved in the majority of cases at the age of 3 years. The normal alpha rhythm is reactive to eye opening and is maintained throughout life in healthy individuals. However, 10% of normal individuals do not have an appreciable posterior dominant rhythm on standard EEG, due to its having a very low amplitude when measured at the scalp (<15uV). The frequency of the rhythm seems to be closely related to cerebral blood flow.

As the person transitions to drowsiness (stage I sleep), slow roving eye movements are noted on EEG, the posterior alpha rhythm gradually disappears, and the brain activity consists of fronto-centro-temporal theta activity alongside prominent frontocentral beta activity (Figure 8.3). With deeper levels of

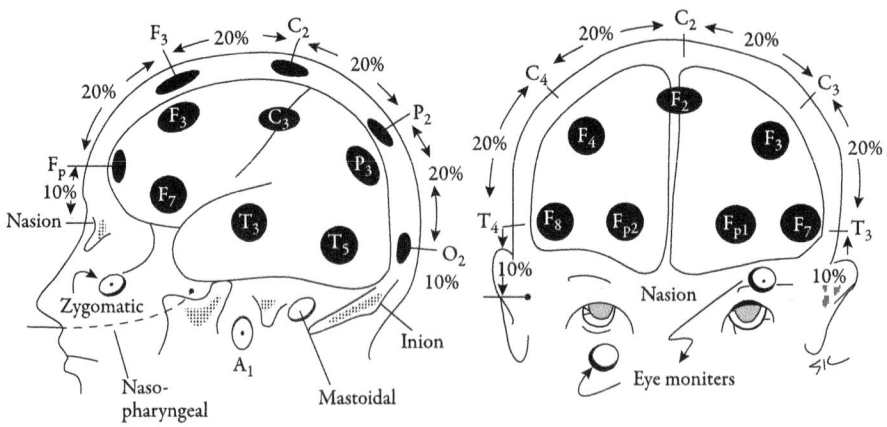

Figure 8.1 EEG electrode set up. Scalp EEG electrodes are placed according to the 10–20 system. Occasionally, extra electrodes are placed for monitoring of eye movements.

Table 8.1 FREQUENCY BANDS OF INTEREST CAPTURED WITH SCALP EEG

FREQUENCY TERM	RANGE
Alpha α	8–13 Hz
Beta β	>13 Hz
Theta θ	4–8 Hz
Delta δ	0–4 Hz

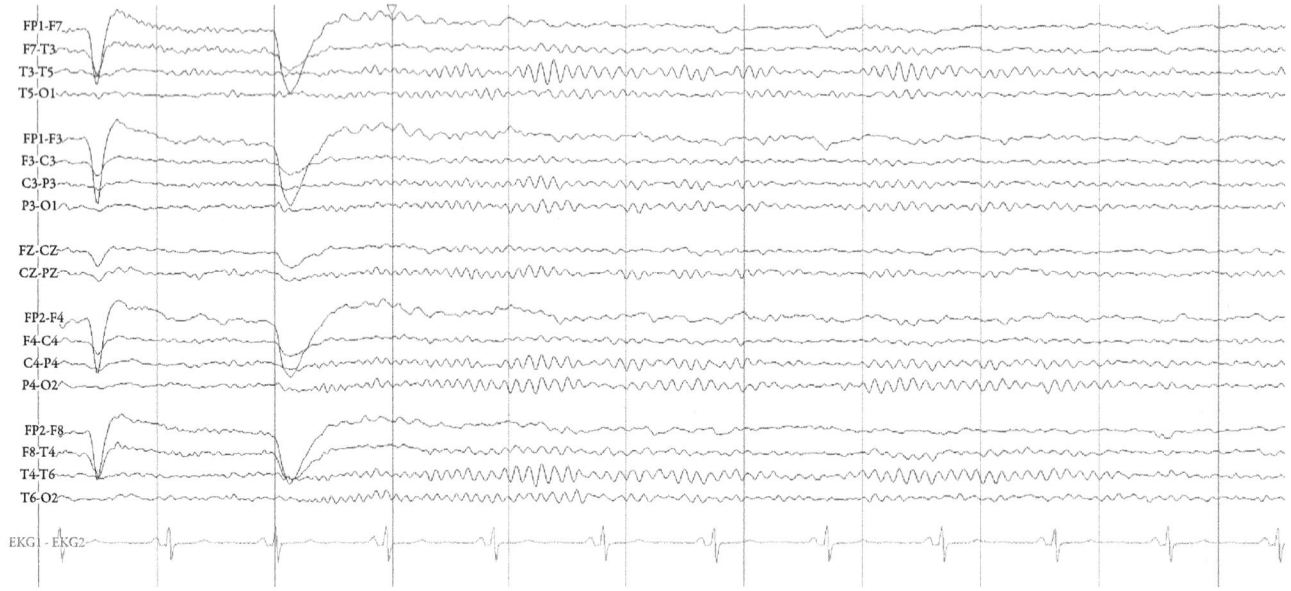

Figure 8.2 Normal adult EEG. A double banana montage is used with the left temporal chain on top, then left parasagittal chain, then midline electrodes, then right parasagittal chain, then the right temporal chain. A 10-second EEG sample is shown with the distance between each bar representing 1 second. The prominent positive deflections (downward) are due to artifact from the eye blink. During the first 2 seconds the patient has the eyes open, then upon eye closure an 11 Hz posterior alpha rhythm is seen; indicating that it is reactive. Lower voltage faster activity is noted in the anterior electrodes.

sleep, vertex waves appear. These waves are prominent negative waves, best appreciated in the midline electrodes, and can occur in isolation or in trains. Stage II sleep is characterized by the persistence of vertex waves and the appearance of 12–14 Hz frontocentral, sinusoidal rhythms termed *sleep spindles* (Figure 8.4). In addition to the sleep spindles, K complexes can also be seen, which are characterized by an initial negativity, a slow positivity, and then another negativity seen prominently in the frontal or midline regions. Stages III and IV sleep are lumped together and termed *slow-wave sleep* and consist of higher voltage theta and delta activity. REM (rapid eye movement sleep) is characterized by rapid eye movements, intermittent alpha activity, and the appearance of sawtooth waves over the central regions.

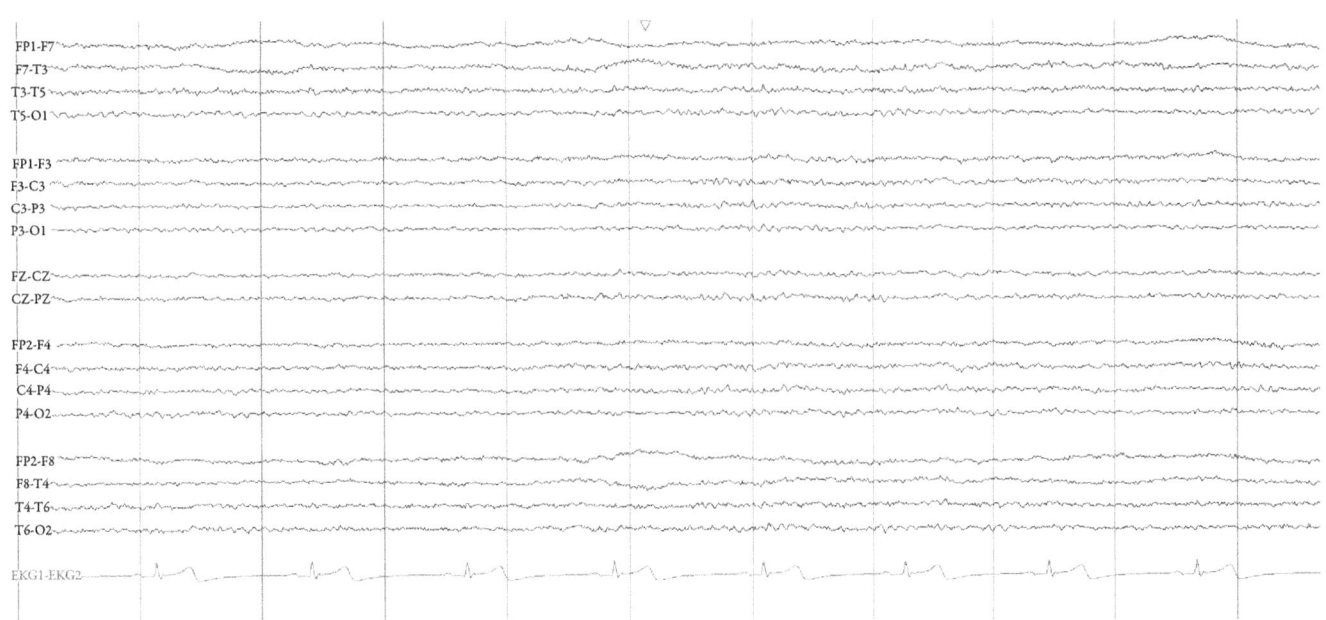

Figure 8.3 Normal EEG during drowsiness. As the patient transitions to drowsiness (stage I sleep), roving eye movements are noted (white arrow indicates artifact due to roving eyes). The voltage of the background becomes attenuated and the alpha rhythm noted during wakefulness dissipates.

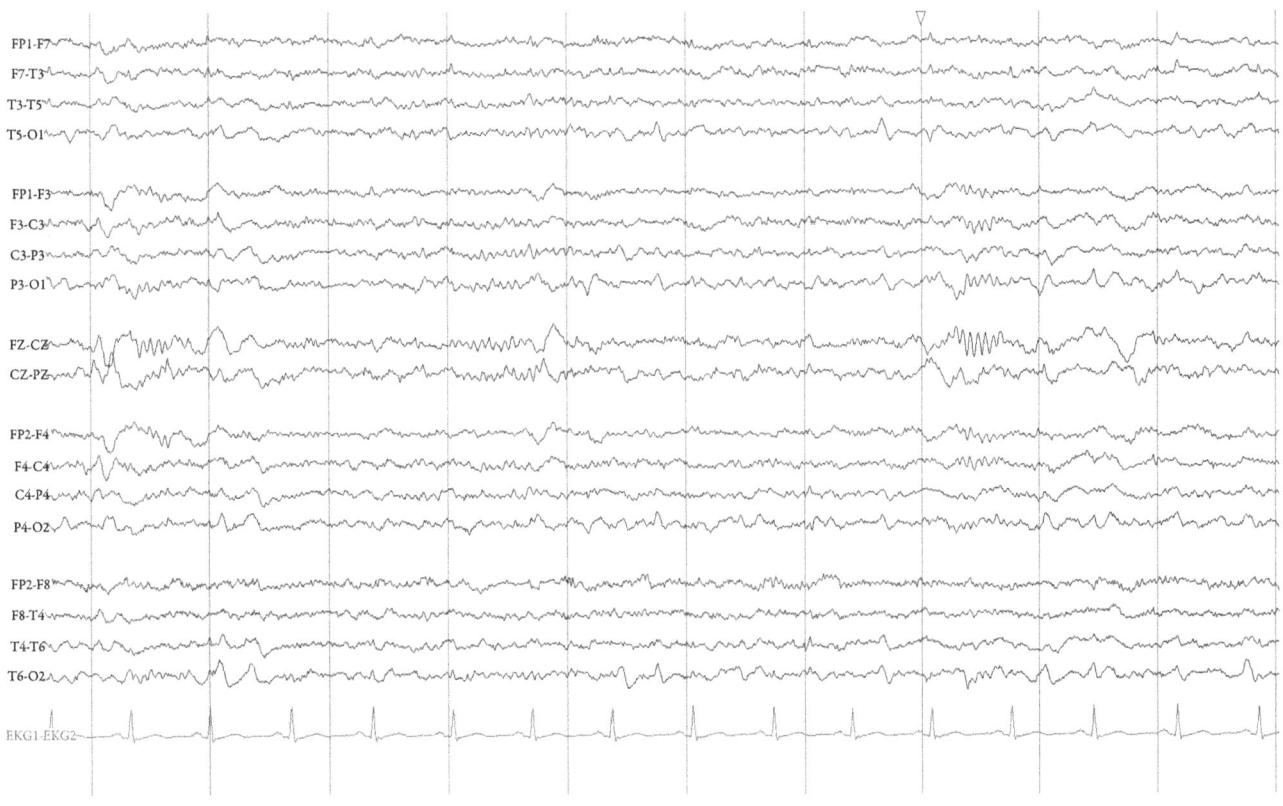

Figure 8.4 EEG during stage II sleep. The record consists of bilateral slowing predominantly in the theta range. In this EEG sample several vertex waves and sleep spindles can be seen, which are most prominent in the midline electrodes.

EEG ABNORMALITIES

EEG abnormalities can be broadly divided into slow-wave abnormalities and epileptiform abnormalities. Slow-wave abnormalities are documented when activity in the theta and delta range is seen (Figure 8.5) beyond what is expected for a normal EEG. For example, any slowing during wakefulness is usually abnormal. Based on the location of the slowing on EEG, it can further be classified into focal or generalized. Other descriptors of the slowing also include whether it is continuous or intermittent. In general, focal cerebral abnormalities cause focal slowing on EEG, while more diffuse processes such as metabolic derangements cause diffuse slowing

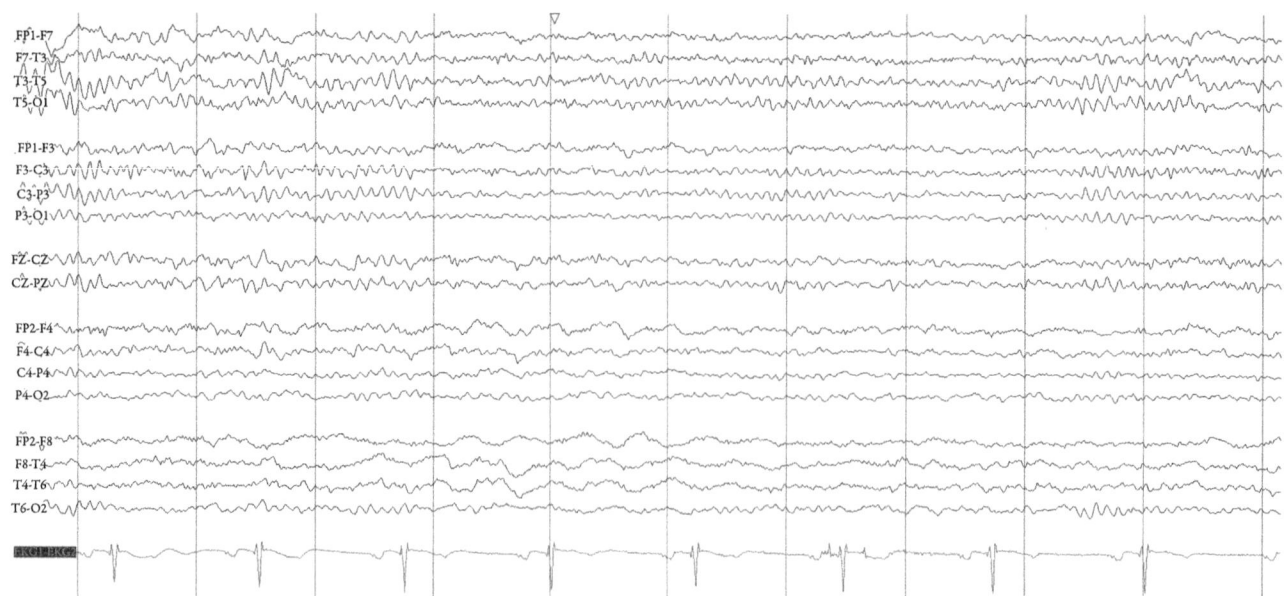

Figure 8.5 EEG with focal slowing. EEG of a 68-year-old patient with a prior right middle cerebral artery stroke and a transient episode of confusion. The EEG during wakefulness shows focal slowing in the delta range in the right temporal chain, likely due to the prior stroke.

on EEG. Certain slowing patterns can be readily distinguishable. Continuous polymorphic delta activity is a pattern suggestive of a structural cerebral lesion with disruption of white matter tracts in the majority of the cases. In the absence of any structural lesion on imaging, continuous slowing may represent a postictal state and should resolve with time. Frontal intermittent delta activity (FIRDA) is a nonspecific pattern seen in metabolic encephalopathy and raised intracranial pressure. FIRDA can also be seen in normal drowsy individuals, and as a result is not necessarily pathological (Accolla, Kaplan, Maeder-Ingvar, Jukopila, & Rossetti, 2011).

Epileptiform abnormalities include spikes and sharp waves. A spike is defined as a transient (i.e., *transient wave*) that is distinguishable from the background activity, with duration of 20 to less than 70 milliseconds (Chatrian et al., 1974). A sharp wave is similar, but its duration is 70 to 200 milliseconds (Figure 8.6). Spikes and sharp waves are often followed by a slow wave, and can also be classified as focal or generalized.

When the spikes or sharp waves are periodic and lateralized to one hemisphere, they are termed *PLEDs*: periodic lateralized epileptiform discharges (Figure 8.7). PLEDs are seen under different circumstances; they can represent an injury pattern seen with an acute insult (Garcia-Morales et al., 2002) and resolve with time, or ongoing ictal activity (there are cases where clinical findings are correlated with each discharge, such as clonic movements), or a postictal state.

THE ROUTINE INPATIENT AND OUTPATIENT EEG

The standard routine EEG consists of 20–40 minutes of recording with the EEG technologist at bedside. During the procedure the patient is asked to open and close the eyes to assess for reactivity. Ideally, stage II sleep should be captured during the recording, as abnormalities may arise or become more prominent during this stage. Slow-wave sleep and REM sleep are rarely seen during the routine EEG.

Other activation procedures are also performed depending on the circumstances. The purpose of the activation procedures is to "bring out" focal or epileptiform activity not apparent in the record. During the hyperventilation procedure, the patient is asked to hyperventilate for 3 minutes. Hyperventilation is of higher yield in young adults, and is contraindicated during pregnancy and in patients with asthma, cardiovascular disease, or cerebrovascular disease, due to theoretical concerns regarding bronchospasm or ischemia. Photic stimulation is another activation procedure, where flickering lights of variable frequencies are shined into the patients' eyes. In rare circumstances, the activation procedures themselves may trigger a nonepileptic seizure. In the inpatient setting, the activation procedures may not be performed unless specifically requested by the ordering physician. When dealing with a comatose individual, verbal and noxious stimuli are often given by the technologist to assess for reactivity on EEG.

THE EEG REPORT

A complete report should include the following:

- The patient's posterior background and whether it is reactive
- A description and characterization of beta activity
- Stages of sleep noted
- Response to activation methods
- Single lead EKG rhythm
- Presence of any asymmetries
- Documentation of any slowing or epileptiform discharges
- A comparison of the current EEG to any prior EEGs

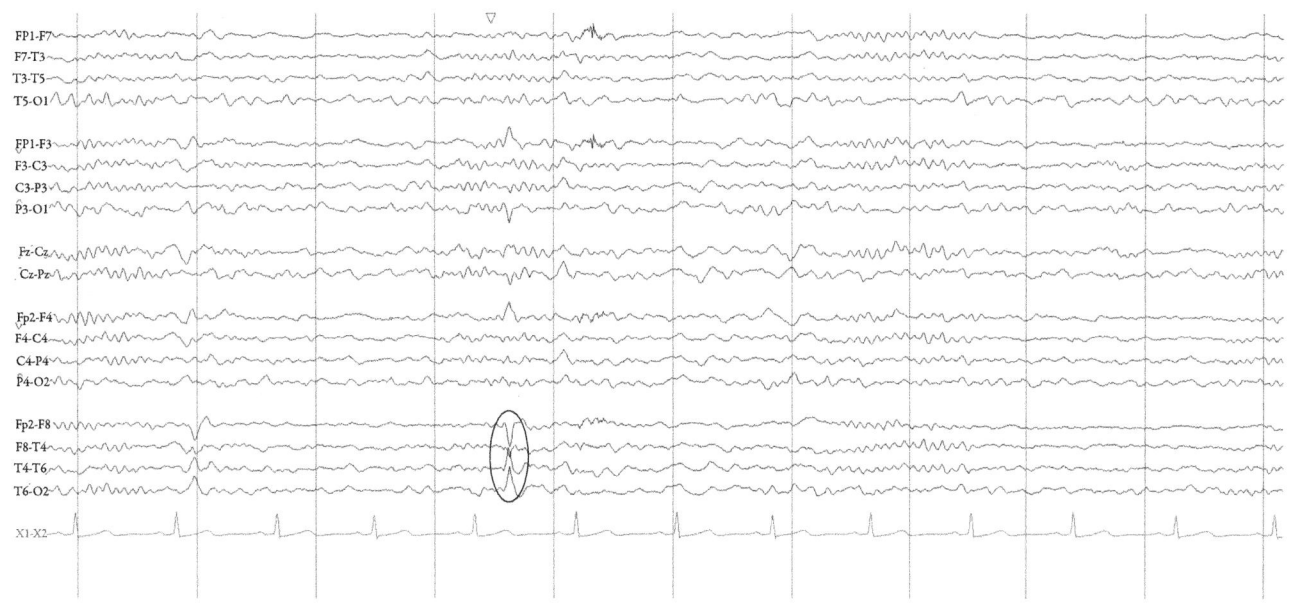

Figure 8.6. EEG with sharp wave. EEG of a 29-year-old woman with a history of epilepsy. The EEG shows stage II sleep with prominent sleep spindles and focal right temporal sharp waves (encircled).

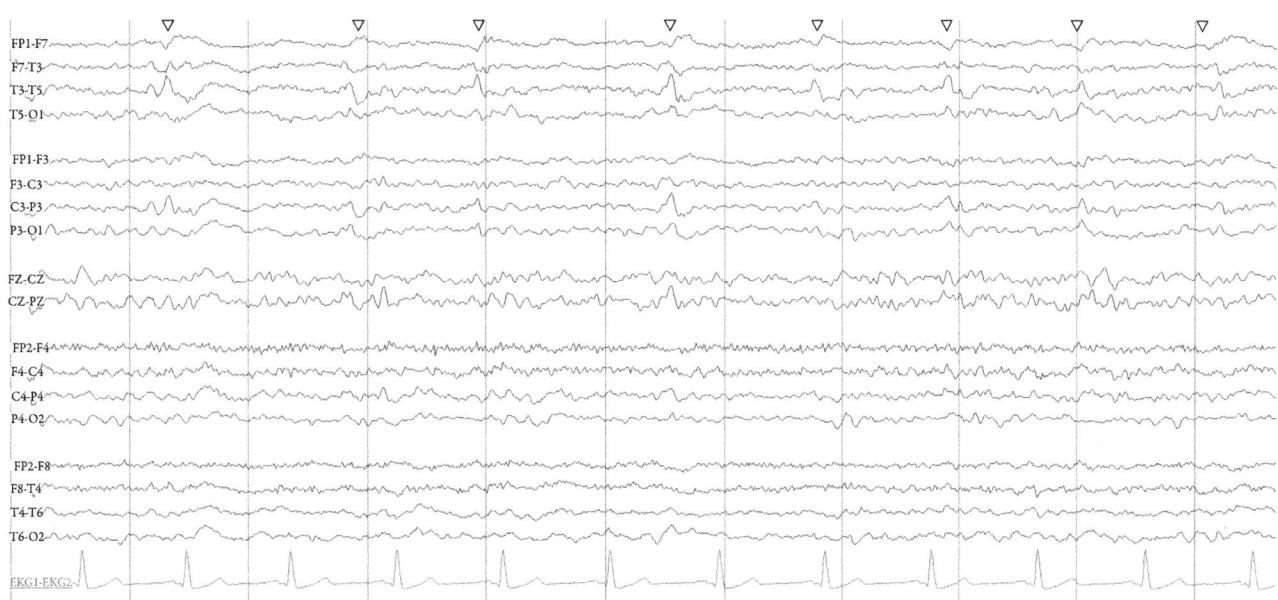

Figure 8.7 EEG with PLEDs (periodic lateralized epileptiform discharges). EEG of a 72-year-old man with a history of head trauma, a left subdural hematoma, and altered mental status. The EEG shows periodic sharp waves (arrows) in the left hemisphere at a frequency of ~1 Hz.

As can be clearly seen above, the EEG report includes important information not limited to epileptiform activity. The body of the report should always be scrutinized by the treating physician and not rely solely on the electroencephalographer's conclusions. For example, REM sleep noted on a routine EEG is suggestive of medication effect or possibly narcolepsy. Due to the complexities involved in EEG interpretation, it is always advisable to consult with the EEG reader when in doubt.

It also has to be kept in mind that an EEG is always interpreted in the context of the patient's age. Certain degrees of temporal slowing, for example, are allowed in the elderly.

Comparisons to prior EEGs are invaluable, as it may show new epileptiform activity or may establish the progression of an encephalopathy or degenerative brain disease. Finally, there are certain EEG waveforms that are suspicious but do not fulfill criteria for epileptiform activity; these may be labeled as "sharply contoured" discharges. When these are reported and the clinical suspicion of epileptic seizures is high, a repeat routine EEG, a more prolonged study, and/or a provocative procedure such as sleep deprivation is advised. In addition, a spike/sharp wave noted on EEG does not automatically mean a patient has epilepsy. In fact, studies have documented the presence of interictal abnormalities in 0.3%–0.9% of healthy controls (Gibbs, Gibbs, & Lennox, 1943; Thorner, 1942).

A common dilemma facing the treating physician is the determination of the number and length of EEGs required in a given clinical setting. The first limitation is the number of machines available at the EEG lab, and the number of technicians. Under these circumstances it is best to consult with the EEG lab first. The other factors to consider are the level of consciousness of the patient and the question being asked. In the majority of cases a routine 20–30-minute EEG is usually obtained to rule out nonconvulsive status epilepticus, assess the level of encephalopathy, or screen for epileptiform abnormalities. However, it is known that comatose patients may require more than 24 hours of monitoring to capture subclinical seizures on EEG, while in awake patients with altered mentation 24 hours is usually enough. The yield of nonconvulsive seizure detection in the ICU rises from 61% in one hour to 88% by 24 hours in the noncomatose patient with altered mental status (Claassen, Mayer, Kowalski, Emerson, & Hirsch, 2004). The threshold should be low for undertaking longer EEG monitoring periods in any patient with a history of epilepsy for whom there is a question of current disease activity. In patients with suspected nonepileptic seizures, video with simultaneous EEG telemetry is the gold standard, and the time of monitoring to capture the event is variable depending on the patient. It should be long enough to capture at least one typical seizure. (See chapter 43 on epilepsy for further detail).

EEG IN THE AWAKE PATIENT WITH ALTERED MENTAL STATUS

The terms delirium and encephalopathy are often used interchangeably to describe the condition of the awake patient with altered mental status. When faced with this clinical scenario, the EEG can aid the physician with the differential diagnosis. The EEG is a very sensitive tool for the detection of encephalopathy; however, it has low specificity with regards to determining the etiology. The degree of EEG abnormality tends to correlate with the severity of the encephalopathy and tends to improve with its resolution.

A general rule of thumb is that abnormalities limited to the cortex will cause slowing of the posterior background frequency, while abnormalities involving subcortical structures lead to increased polymorphic delta activity, triphasic waves, or FIRDA.

EEG in Toxic and Metabolic Encephalopathies

A number of metabolic derangements can lead to abnormalities on EEG including electrolyte disturbances, hypo/hyperglycemia, osmotic changes, endocrine dysfunction, and organ failure (Kaplan, 2004). The degree of abnormalities is associated with the rate of change of the CNS level of the metabolite or toxin, with more acute changes causing the most severe abnormalities.

Hypoglycemia may lead to focal slowing on EEG, which goes along with focal neurologic deficits noted on examination. The EEG of a hyperthyroid patient may show a slight increase in the alpha frequency and excessive beta activity. Hypothyroidism shows lower alpha frequencies.

Other than patterns of slowing, hypoglycemia and hypocalcemia have been associated with epileptiform discharges on EEG, while nonketotic hyperglycemia may be a cause of PLEDs (Hennis, Corbin, & Fraser, 1992; Honigsberger, 1999).

Even at therapeutic levels certain medications may cause EEG abnormalities. Drugs such as carbamazepine, gabapentin, clozapine, lithium, and tricyclic antidepressants cause slowing of the background rhythm. Clozapine is notorious for causing spike and wave discharges in patients without a known history of epilepsy and is implicated in lowering seizure threshold (Freudenreich, Weiner, & McEvoy, 1997). Meanwhile, lithium can enhance epileptiform discharges in patients with known epilepsy.

At toxic levels lithium may cause a confusional state secondary to an encephalopathy or subclinical seizure activity; in this case the EEG is helpful to distinguish between the two, and to determine the need for benzodiazepines (Kaplan & Birbeck, 2006). EEG abnormalities noted in lithium toxicity include diffuse slowing, spikes, and triphasic waves. In general, at toxic doses, medications and toxins are expected to produce generalized slowing and a decrease in the frequency of the posterior background. Epileptiform discharges including PLEDs have been described with toxic doses of baclofen, mercury, manganese, isoniazid, tricyclics, penicillin, and aminophylline (Yamada & Meng, 2009). A different pattern, where generalized periodic epileptiform discharges with a low frequency <0.25 Hz are noted, can be seen with ketamine and PCP intoxication (Stockard et al., 1976).

Benzodiazepines, barbiturates, and cocaine cause increases in beta activity in the 20–25 Hz range termed *excessive beta* (Figure 8.8). The finding of excessive beta on EEG is suggestive of the patient using one of these drugs, and is clinically useful. Excessive beta is more pronounced in younger individuals and with acute intake of the drug.

One of the common abnormalities first described in hepatic and renal encephalopathy is the presence of *triphasic waves* (Figure 8.9). These are theta waves with an initial negativity, a large amplitude positivity, and then another negativity, providing it with the "tri-phasic" morphology. They occur in a periodic fashion with a frequency of 1–2 Hz. The occurrence of triphasic waves has been documented in up to 25% of patients with hepatic encephalopathy, and in some series has been associated with worse outcome and increased mortality (Karnaze & Bickford, 1984). They are frequently seen in patients with mild to moderate encephalopathy but have also been documented in patients who are awake with no apparent encephalopathy. Of note, in some instances it is difficult to distinguish triphasic waves from epileptiform discharges, and, in a patient with no clear etiology of altered mental status, a trial of benzodiazepines is warranted.

Although the triphasic waves were initially described in patients with liver disease, they were later found to occur in

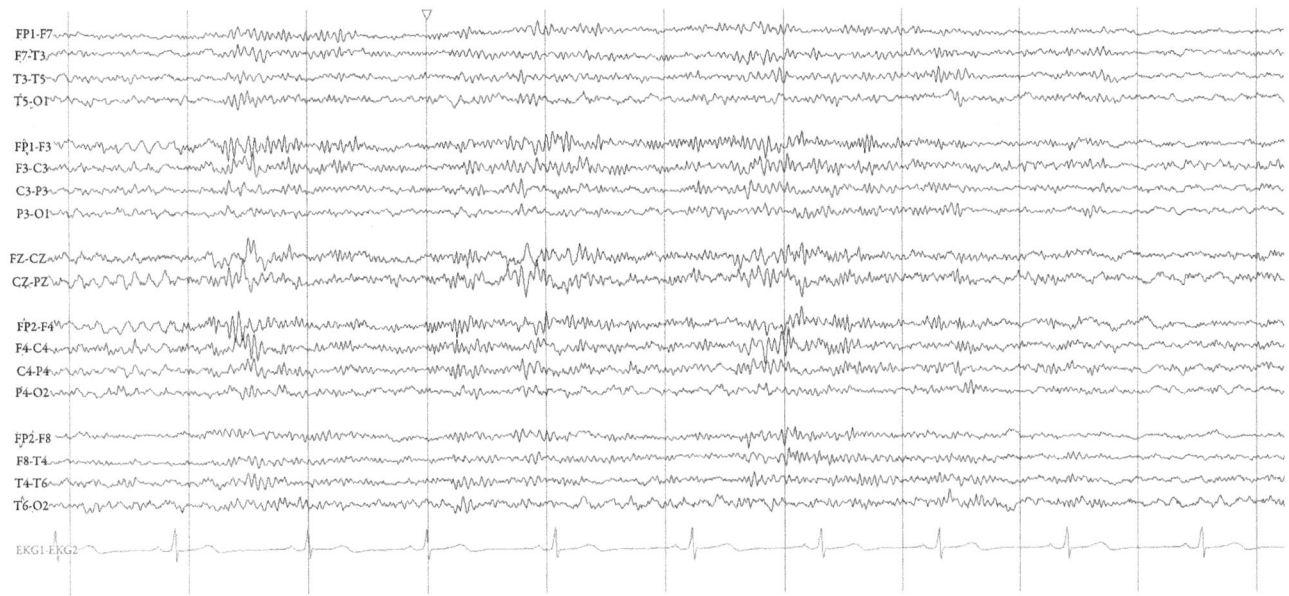

Figure 8.8 EEG with excessive beta. A 27-year-old woman with anxiety and headaches, currently on diazepam. The EEG shows excessive beta activity throughout the record, which is a result of the diazepam.

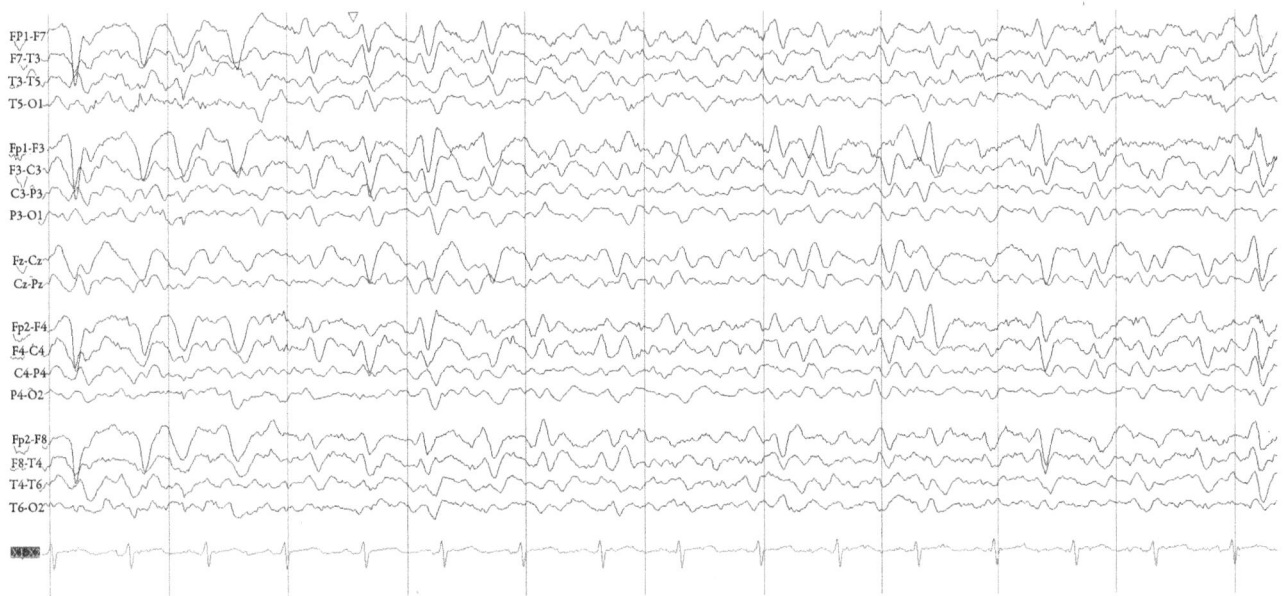

Figure 8.9 EEG with triphasic waves. EEG of a 30-year-old patient with meningitis, renal failure, and agitation. The EEG sample during wakefulness shows bilateral, frontally predominant theta waves which have a triphasic morphology (arrow), commonly referred to as "triphasic waves." The record also shows bilateral slowing in the theta>delta range.

patients with uremia, electrolyte imbalances, anoxic brain injury, and medication intoxications (Kaplan, 2004).

The EEG in chronic alcoholics is also nonspecific; however, a higher percentage of these patients have a low voltage EEG as compared to the normal population.

EEG in Autoimmune and Infectious Encephalopathies

Other important causes of alterations in mental status include the autoimmune and infectious encephalopathies. With acute viral or bacterial encephalitis, the EEG changes are nonspecific with diffuse slowing. Herpes encephalitis is an exception

where characteristic EEG findings can be seen. The virus has a predilection for the temporal lobes, and subsequently after a few days of clinical symptoms; characteristic PLEDs are noted in the temporal regions, sometimes independently, a phenomenon termed *bi-PLEDs*. The PLEDs are transient in nature and resolve within 3–4 days (Lai & Gragasin, 1988). Similarly characteristic EEG findings are also seen in subacute sclerosing panencephalitis (SSPE) and Creutzfeld-Jakob disease (CJD). SSPE is the result of chronic measles infection and is characterized by the appearance of high voltage spike and wave discharges occurring every 4–15 seconds. In CJD early changes on EEG are nonspecific, while later stages of the disease are characterized by periodic discharges occurring at a frequency near 1 Hz. In patients with clinically suspected CJD these periodic discharges had sensitivity, specificity, and positive and negative predictive values were 64%, 91%, 95%, and 49% with respect to an autopsy diagnosis of the disease (Steinhoff et al., 1996).

In HIV infection the EEG is an early and sensitive indicator of HIV-associated encephalopathy. In a study published before anti-retroviral therapy was available, 30% of patients initially presenting with HIV infection and normal cognitive function had abnormal EEGs, showing slowing and diminished reactivity of awake background rhythms; follow-up EEGs six to nine months later were abnormal in 40% of patients (Koralnik et al., 1990). EEG abnormalities are reduced significantly by antiretroviral therapy, with benefits observed after as little as four weeks of therapy, with greater benefit in patients with more rapid normalization of CD4 counts (Babiloni et al., 2014). Patients with AIDS dementia or with opportunistic infections of the CNS display more dramatic EEG abnormalities, such as severe diffuse or focal slowing, or epileptiform abnormalities. Because of its high sensitivity to encephalopathies of various kinds the EEG is valuable in the differential diagnosis of HIV-positive patients with mental status changes, especially when there is potential confounding of the symptoms of primary mental disorder and the symptoms of gross brain disease due to HIV or associated with it.

Autoimmune encephalitides are another important category of causes leading to altered mental status. They can be broadly divided into paraneoplastic and nonparaneoplastic. The nonparaneoplastic group includes Hashimoto's encephalitis and systemic lupus erythematosus (Flanagan & Caselli, 2011). Patients with Hashimoto's encephalopathy findings typically show bilateral slowing, but there are case reports of focal temporal seizures (Arain et al., 2001). EEG slowing from this condition is expected to resolve with treatment (Rodriguez et al., 2006). EEG findings are also common in patients with SLE and seem to have a predilection for the left hemisphere (Glanz, Laoprasert, Schur, Robertson-Thompson, & Khoshbin, 2001).

Similar EEG findings are also noted in the paraneoplastic syndromes and are based on the area of the brain involved. With limbic encephalitis, all patients tend to have temporal abnormalities including slowing and/or epileptiform discharges. Clinically a high proportion of these patients also exhibit neuropsychiatric symptoms, and the disorder may present with such symptoms. (Rosenfeld & Dalmau, 2010). A recently described EEG finding in patients with limbic encephalitis is the *extreme delta brush,* which resembles a pattern seen in premature infants (Schmitt et al., 2012).

EEG in Nonconvulsive Status Epilepticus

One of the most important indications to order an immediate EEG in the inpatient setting is to rule out nonconvulsive status epilepticus (NCSE).

Nonconvulsive seizures have been documented in around 21.5% of patients with altered mental status admitted to the hospital. Nonconvulsive status epilepticus is defined when the seizure activity is prolonged (there is no consensus on duration but a time period of >30 minutes is usually accepted). NCSE is difficult to diagnose because it is not accompanied by any tonic or clonic motor activity and is indistinguishable clinically from delirium or secondary psychosis not associated with NCSE. It is imperative to diagnose it early, as treatment has been associated with favorable outcomes. The EEG is the gold standard to diagnose NCSE and should be prioritized if the clinical suspicion is high. Circumstances where suspicion should be high include the abrupt onset of alteration in mental status, waxing and waning course, and clinical signs such as subtle automatisms (lip smacking, fumbling, etc.) (Chang & Shinnar, 2011). In those circumstances intravenous antiepileptic drugs (AEDS) are needed to try to abort the seizure activity (benzodiazepines, fosphenytoin, phenobarbital, levetiracetam, valproic acid, or lacosamide). Ultimately, any patient with altered mental status of unclear cause requires an EEG.

EEG in the Setting of Head Trauma

Traumatic brain injury (TBI) is classified into mild, moderate, and severe based on the duration of loss of consciousness or of posttraumatic amnesia. As discussed in detail elsewhere in this book, patients with mild traumatic brain injury do not necessarily have insignificant residual impairment in brain function, and a significant minority of such patients continue to experience neuropsychiatric symptoms months after the injury. In this patient population an acute EEG may reveal slowing with attenuation of the posterior background voltage. These changes tend to resolve with time as the patient recovers. However, most patients with residual symptoms following mild TBI will have normal EEGs, so the test is of limited diagnostic value except when the patient has symptoms suggestive of epilepsy such as episodic alterations of consciousness (Arciniegas, 2011) Patients with more severe degrees of injury may experience early posttraumatic seizures or late posttraumatic seizures. Early posttraumatic seizures may not necessarily recur, and, as a result, long-term antiepileptic drugs are not needed. The EEG is useful in aiding prognostication, as evidence of epileptiform activity would place the patient at higher risk of recurrence.

EEG in Patients with Cognitive Complaints

Before discussing EEG changes in dementia, one has to become familiar with EEG changes in normal aging. Common changes include a decrease in frequency of the posterior dominant rhythm by 0.5–1 Hz, although authorities in the field still consider any frequency less than 8 Hz during the waking state to be abnormal regardless of age. In addition, focal temporal theta slowing can be seen and may be a signature of subclinical cerebrovascular disease. There is no clear cutoff for how much theta slowing is allowed in the elderly, with quoted ranges between 10%-15% of the record. EEG changes in Alzheimer's disease are nonspecific and include slowing in the theta range and bursts of frontotemporal delta (Figure 8.10). In Parkinson's disease, theta and delta slowing

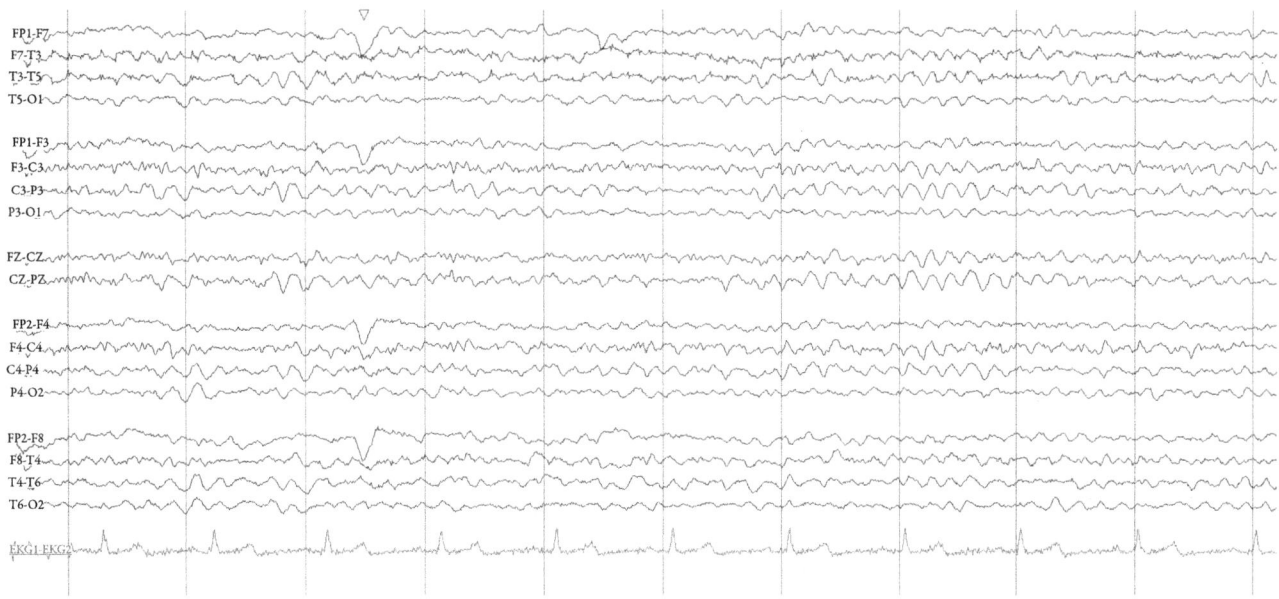

Figure 8.10 EEG in dementia. This EEG is from a 90-year-old woman with Alzheimer's disease and confusion. The white arrow shows an eye blink. The posterior background rhythm is in the theta range (6–7 Hz in this case).

may be seen over the posterior head regions. In frontotemporal dementia, the alpha seems to be preserved and frontotemporal slowing is expected (Jenssen, 2005).

The EEG can be useful in a patient who is exhibiting apparently severe cognitive deficits and has a history or examination atypical for dementia. In this setting a normal EEG would be evidence against the diagnosis of a dementing process (Holschneider & Leuchter, 1999). However, an EEG with a posterior background rhythm of 8–8.5 Hz—at the lower end of the normal range—could represent significant change from the patient's baseline. As such, it would be weaker evidence against a dementing process than one with an alpha rhythm between 10 Hz and 12 Hz.

EEG IN PATIENTS WITH ANXIETY DISORDERS AND PSYCHOSIS

Differentiating panic attacks from simple partial seizures can be difficult on clinical grounds due to the common symptomatology and similar brain regions involved (Hurley et al., 2006). The two conditions may also exist within the same patient (Mintzer & Lopez, 2002). There are also a few case reports of patients incorrectly diagnosed with panic disorder who in fact had a new onset of focal epilepsy (Gallinat, Stotz-Ingenlath, Lang, & Hegerl, 2003; Scalise, Placidi, Diomedi, De Simone, & Gigli, 2006); the latter diagnosis would not only influence treatment but would be an indication to work up the patient to exclude a focal lesion such as a tumor. EEG in this clinical situation is most valuable when it shows an ictal pattern simultaneous with the patient experiencing his or her typical symptoms. Interictal epileptiform discharges suggestive of epilepsy are less diagnostically specific, but would support a trial of antiepileptic drugs. The caveat is that in some patients with only simple partial seizures, the scalp EEG may be negative both ictally and interictally; in these cases a high

clinical suspicion should drive more extensive neuroimaging and electrophysiologic testing.

The EEG in a patient with a history of diagnosed epilepsy who is presenting with new psychotic symptoms is useful in corroborating the clinical impression of the relationship of the psychosis to the seizure disorder. If discrete, repetitive, stereotypic mental or behavioral symptoms are ictal, one would expect the EEG to show seizure discharges coincident with the symptoms; video recording with EEG telemetry can demonstrate such a relationship. Psychotic symptoms occurring as part of recurrent episodes of delirium lasting minutes to hours at a time would most likely be postictal, and the EEG usually will show focal or diffuse slowing coincident with the symptoms. A persistent psychosis with gradual onset in a patient with several years' history of limbic epilepsy is likely to be an interictal psychosis—one related to the patient's persistent abnormal brain electrical activity, but with symptoms not synchronous with seizures or postictal states. In this case the EEG in the symptomatic patient usually shows temporal sharp wave or spike activity but not frank seizure discharges or focal slowing. On the other hand, EEG is not routinely recommended in the assessment of a patient with first-episode schizophrenia and no known history of epilepsy. Some studies have shown that patients with normal EEG were more likely to remit after one year of treatment (Freudenreich et al., 2007).

EEG IN EPILEPSY AND PSYCHOGENIC NONEPILEPTIC SEIZURES

Psychogenic nonepileptic seizures (PNES) are characterized by involuntary repetitive episodes of movement, behavior, and/or alteration of consciousness, sensation, or memory (Alsaadi & Marquez, 2005) without ictal or postictal changes on EEG consistent with the pattern of symptoms seen (Figures 8.11 and 8.12). Patients may present with generalized or unilateral

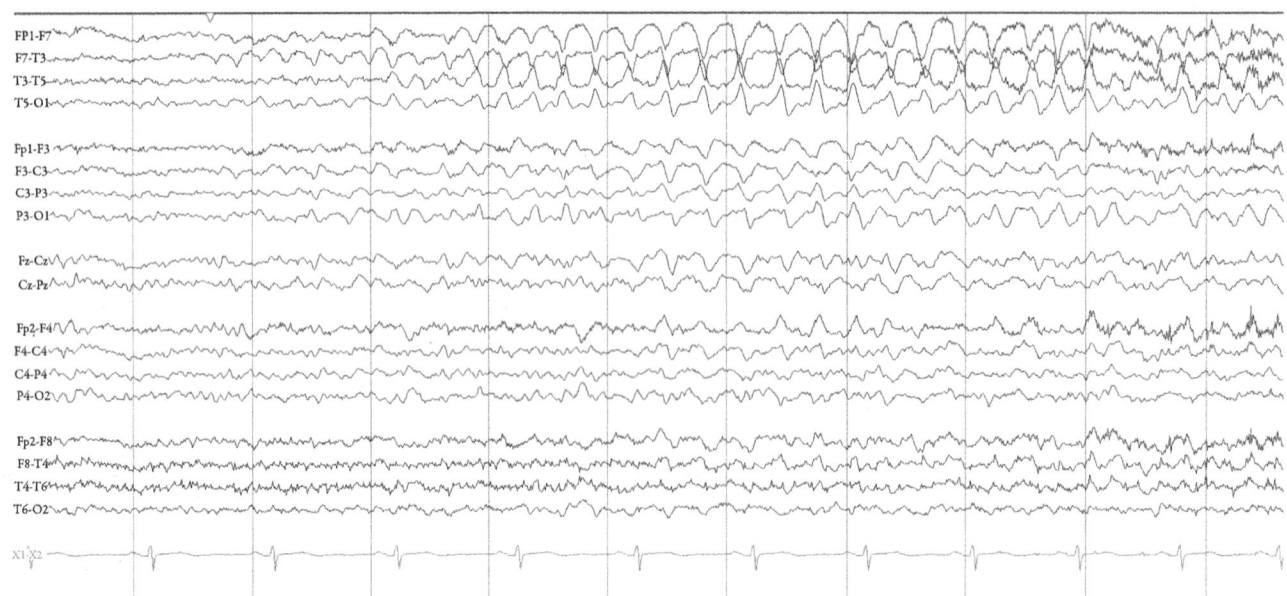

Figure 8.11 EEG of a seizure. This EEG of a 40-year-old man with a history of epilepsy shows a focal left temporal seizure during sleep. The seizure starts with rhythmic theta activity in the left temporal region, which changes in amplitude and morphology.

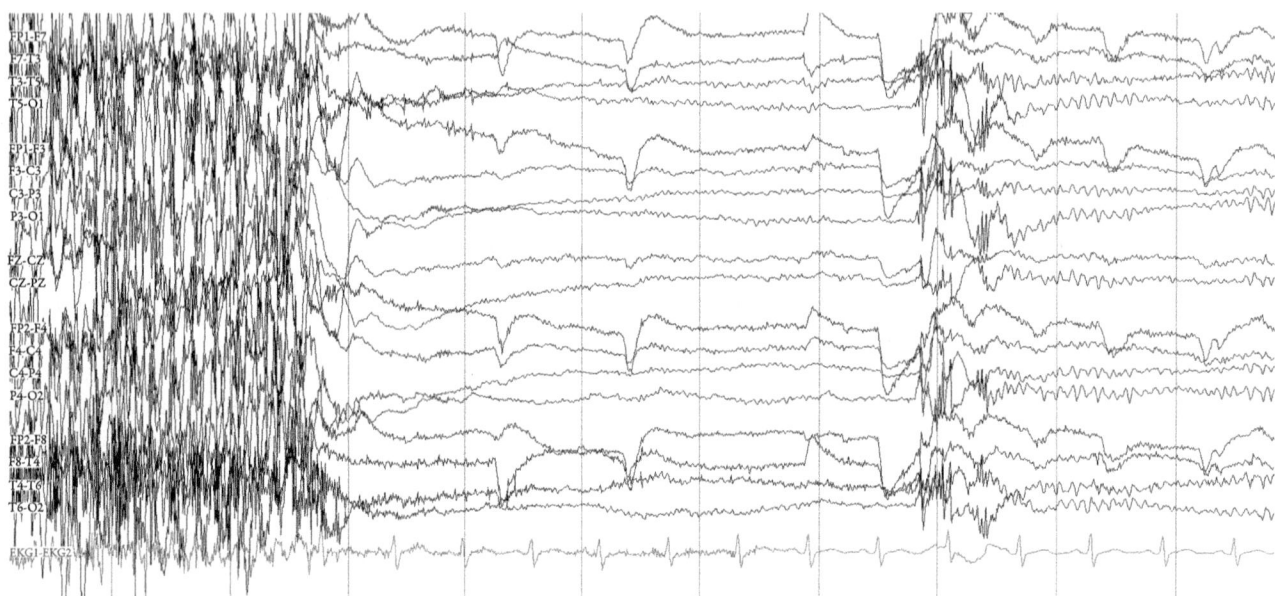

Figure 8.12 EEG in PNES (psychogenic nonepileptic seizures). A 30-year-old patient with spells of generalized shaking. At the beginning of the recording there is a lot of EEG artifact due to the shaking. A few seconds afterwards, a posterior alpha rhythm is appreciated after an eye blink.

shaking, unresponsiveness, bizarre behavior, weeping, pelvic thrusting, or forceful eye closure, among others. PNES is discussed in detail in chapter 43.

Patients with PNES frequently have genuine epilepsy as well. In this patient population, video EEG is the gold standard for diagnosis, as it is the best way to determine whether the mental and behavioral symptoms are simultaneous with seizure discharges or immediately follow them. Video EEG is definitive when the suspected PNES include loss or alteration of consciousness or bilateral tonic–clonic movements, as alterations in the EEG at the brain surface are inevitably present during epileptic seizures with such symptoms. More

complex but stereotyped and repetitive behavior, without major alteration of consciousness, can result from seizure discharges deep in the frontal lobe that do not spread to the brain surface. Seizures of this type can yield a video EEG suggestive of PNES—showing the typical symptomatic behavior with no coincident EEG change. Clinical suspicion should be high if the spells are stereotypic in nature, cluster, and tend to occur out of sleep. In rare circumstances, invasive electrode placements may be necessary to definitively settle the issue. They are undertaken when clinical suspicion of frontal lobe epilepsy is high because of the patient's history or findings of anatomic or functional brain imaging.

A NOTE ON QUANTITATIVE EEG AND EEG MODIFICATIONS

The standard EEG setup relies on electrodes placed on the scalp; however, there are a number of additional electrodes (Table 8.2) which are thought to increase the detection of epileptiform activity from the mesial temporal lobes, which is distant from the scalp. The placement of these electrodes should be discussed with the electrophysiologist, as different centers seem to favor different types of electrodes.

Advances in technology now permit the quantitative analysis of EEG signals in real time. In the ICU, quantitative EEG often is used in patients who are stuporous, comatose, or intubated. In these patients it provides semiautomated detection of changes in brain function related to hypoxia, ischemia, or seizure activity. Outside the ICU, quantitative EEG has as yet no established place in routine clinical practice. Applications of quantitative EEG have been limited to the research setting in psychiatric patients, and attempts have even been made to try to predict response to treatment (Coutin-Churchman et al., 2003; Hunter, Muthen, Cook, & Leuchter, 2010; Knott, 2000).

EVOKED POTENTIALS

An evoked potential (EP) consists of an electrical response elicited by presenting a patient with a sensory stimulus (auditory, sensory, or visual). Typically the stimulus is presented repeatedly and responses are summed, so that signals linked to the stimulus are augmented and background activity unrelated to the stimulus cancels out. Unlike the EEG, which captures spontaneous electrical activity, evoked potentials are dependent on the stimulus and are time-locked to it. Evoked potentials are used to assess the integrity of the sensory pathway, from the sense organ to the sensory cortex. In the medical-psychiatric context, EPs are used for two purposes: (1) to determine whether complaints of sensory loss are accompanied by and are proportionate to changes in the relevant parts of the nervous system; and (2) to detect demyelinating diseases that may not be diagnosable by anatomic brain imaging and that may have neuropsychiatric complications or comorbidities.

The setup of the test depends on the sensory stimulus being given. In general, a few scalp electrodes are placed to measure cortical responses if the stimulus is visual or auditory.

For visual evoked potentials (VEPs), electrodes are placed bilateral occipital, bilateral temporal, midline occipital, and midline frontal.

For auditory evoked potentials (AEPs), electrodes are placed on the left or right earlobes or mastoid process and vertex.

If the stimulus is sensory, then electrodes are placed at a location between C3 and P3 or C4 and P4, midline frontopolar, over Erb's point (angle between the clavicular head of the sternocleidomastoid muscle and the clavicle, thus placing it above the brachial plexus), cervical spine at C5, thoracic spine T12, and iliac crest.

VEPs assess the integrity of the visual system by stimulating each eye with a black and white checkerboard pattern repetitively (Figure 8.13). The expected signal is a positive wave measured by the occipital scalp electrodes at 100 milliseconds after the stimulus is given. The interval between the stimulus and the positive wave is the *latency* of the VEP. Normal ranges are determined by each laboratory, and are usually between 90–110 milliseconds. The finding of a prolonged latency is not specific for demyelinating disease, as it can also be seen in ocular disease (glaucoma), compressive lesions of the optic tract (tumors), and lesions of the occipital cortex. The test itself relies on patient cooperation and an experienced technologist.

VEPs are useful in confirming a diagnosis of hysterical blindness. If a patient has a visual acuity of 20/120 or better, the routine VEP stimulus will produce a definite positive wave at approximately 100 msec after the stimulus (Figure 8.14); this is true even if the patient does not focus on the stimulus, which a hysterically blind person obviously would not do (Howard & Dorfman, 1986). The VEP can be used in a more subtle way to diagnose patients complaining of impairment in visual acuity that is apparently disproportionate to ophthalmological and neurological findings. The stimulus for the VEP is a checkerboard of black and white squares that rhythmically alternates, black squares becoming white and white becoming black. If the patient's visual acuity is sufficient to resolve the squares, the alternation will be an effective repetitive stimulus and will produce a definite positive wave at 100 msec. If the acuity is too poor to resolve the squares, the patient will not perceive a changing stimulus and there will be no positive wave. Delay of the positive wave of the VEP suggests demyelination of the optic nerve or optic tract. This is most often due to optic neuritis; 30% of patients with optic neuritis will develop (or already have) multiple sclerosis (MS). Vitamin B12 deficiency also is associated with prolonged

Table 8.2 ADDITIONAL ELECTRODES WHICH CAN BE PLACED IN ADDITION TO THE STANDARD EEG SETUP

TYPE OF ELECTRODE	LOCATION	DEGREE OF INVASIVENESS
Anterior temporal	Between external auditory meatus and outer canthus of the eye	Noninvasive
Sphenoidal	Through mandibular notch	Minimally invasive, done at bedside.
Nasopharyngeal	Through nasal cavity	Minimally invasive, done at bedside.
Foramen ovale	Through foramen ovale	Invasive, placed by neurosurgeon

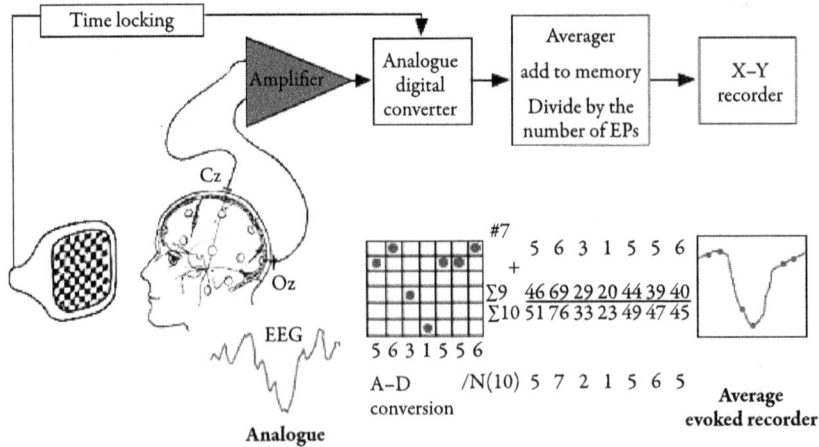

Figure 8.13 Diagram representing steps used in recording visual evoked potentials. The patient is asked to concentrate on a checkerboard pattern and the brain activity is then amplified and digitally converted. The repeated stimuli are then averaged.

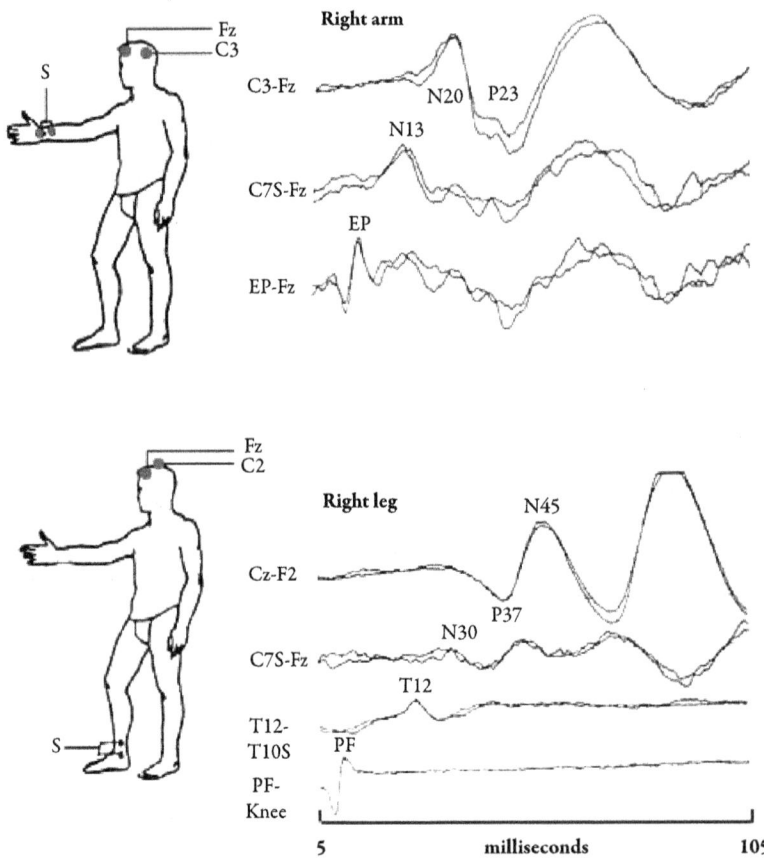

Figure 8.14 Examples of arm and leg somatosensory evoked potentials. Several stimulations of the median nerve (above), or posterior fibular (nerve below) are averaged between a pair of electrodes (C7S= 7th cervical spine, EP = Erb's point, T12: 12th thoracic spine, PF = popliteal fossa). The signals obtained are labeled P for positive and N for negative.

latency of the VEP. VEPs can be abnormal early in the course of MS at a time when the MRI is normal or nondiagnostic. The test should be considered when the patient is suspected of MS on clinical grounds, has a history of visual symptoms, and has a normal or nondiagnostic MRI.

AEPs, also known as *brainstem auditory evoked potentials* (BAEPs) assess the integrity of the auditory pathways, which connect the cochlea on each side with its primary auditory

cortex in the contralateral superior temporal lobe. In this test, a patient is presented with an auditory stimulus consisting of brief clicks. A complex signal of 6 waveforms is generated as the signal travels from the cochlear nerve, up the brainstem, and then reaches the cortex. Each wave represents a location on the way from the inner ear to the auditory cortex (Figure 8.15). If the time between one wave and the next is prolonged over the normal interval, there is demyelination

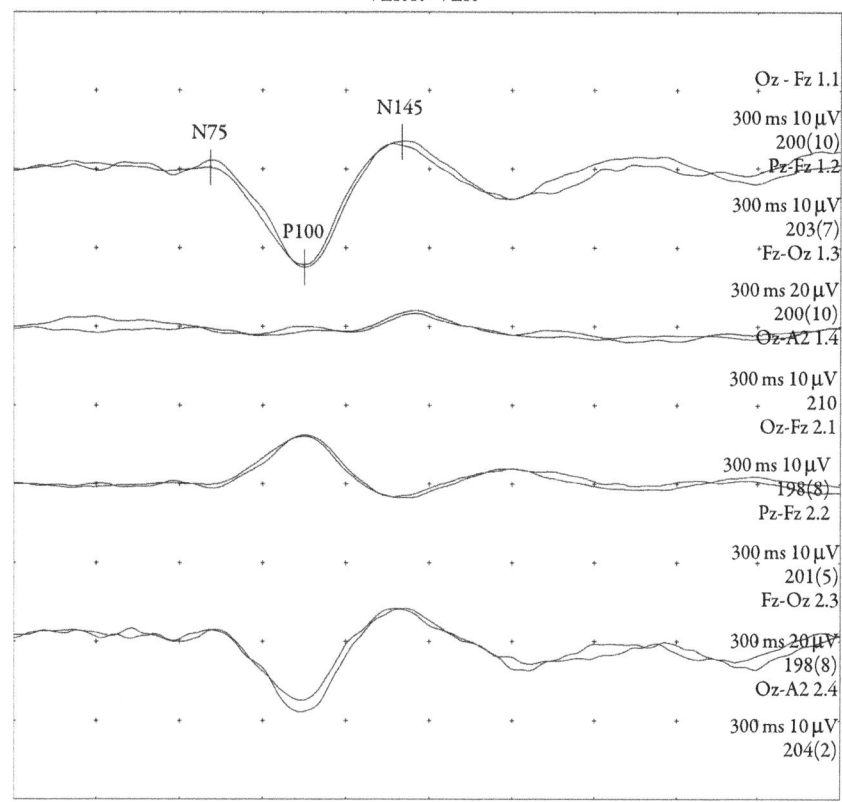

Figure 8.15 Normal visual evoked potentials tracing. The interval between crosses corresponds to 300 milliseconds. A positive deflection is noted at around 105 milliseconds corresponding to the P100 waveform.

of the auditory pathway between the two corresponding locations, a partial lesion of the pathway. or anatomic impingement on the pathway.

As with VEPs, the AEPs may provide evidence of demyelination in a patient clinically suspected of MS at a time when the MRI is normal or nondiagnostic. It would be particularly sensitive in this setting if the patient had complaints of vertigo or impaired balance, or if the neurological examination showed nystagmus or unsteady gait.

Just as the VEPs can be used to assess alleged loss of visual acuity, the AEPs can be used to assess the magnitude of genuine hearing loss. The stimulus for the AEP is a series of clicks. If the clicks are above the threshold for hearing they will produce an AEP; if they are below the threshold they will not. If a patient has a normal AEP at a volume at which they deny hearing, it can be concluded that the patient's deafness is of cerebral origin—due either to conversion, malingering, or a disorder of higher cortical function. In the last case there would always be evidence of cerebral cortical damage on an anatomic image.

Somatosensory evoked potentials (SSEPs) assess the transmission of a sensory signal from peripheral nerves to the contralateral somatosensory cortex (Figure 8.16). The three nerves stimulated in a standard SSEP test are the median nerves and, in the lower extremities, either the posterior tibial nerves (at the ankles), or the peroneal nerves at the fibular heads. The signal is then measured at the brachial plexus (for the median nerve) and at the lumbar spine (for the posterior tibial or peroneal nerve), the cervical spine, and the contralateral cerebral cortex. Delayed latency of the SSEP is evidence for demyelination of the sensory pathway; the differential diagnosis includes demyelinating neuropathies and myelopathies as well as encephalopathies. Completely normal SSEPs would suggest a diagnosis of conversion in a patient complaining of severe sensory loss in a limb. An SSEP study would be appropriate when MS is suspected in a patient with prominent sensory symptoms but a normal MRI. Both the AEP and the SSEP can be used in confirming—or disconfirming—a diagnosis of brain death in a patient who might conceivably be "locked in"—alive and conscious but unable to respond to stimuli because of motor system damage. If a cortical potential can be evoked by an auditory or somatosensory stimulus, the patient is alive.

ELECTROMYOGRAPHY AND NERVE CONDUCTION STUDIES

Electromyography (EMG) is the study of the electrical activity of muscle fibers. This is typically done using a needle inserted into the muscle of interest, though the EMG is recorded on the surface of the skin in some contexts. It is useful in diagnosing three types of problems: (1) intrinsic diseases of muscle; (2) disturbances in the nerve supply to muscle;

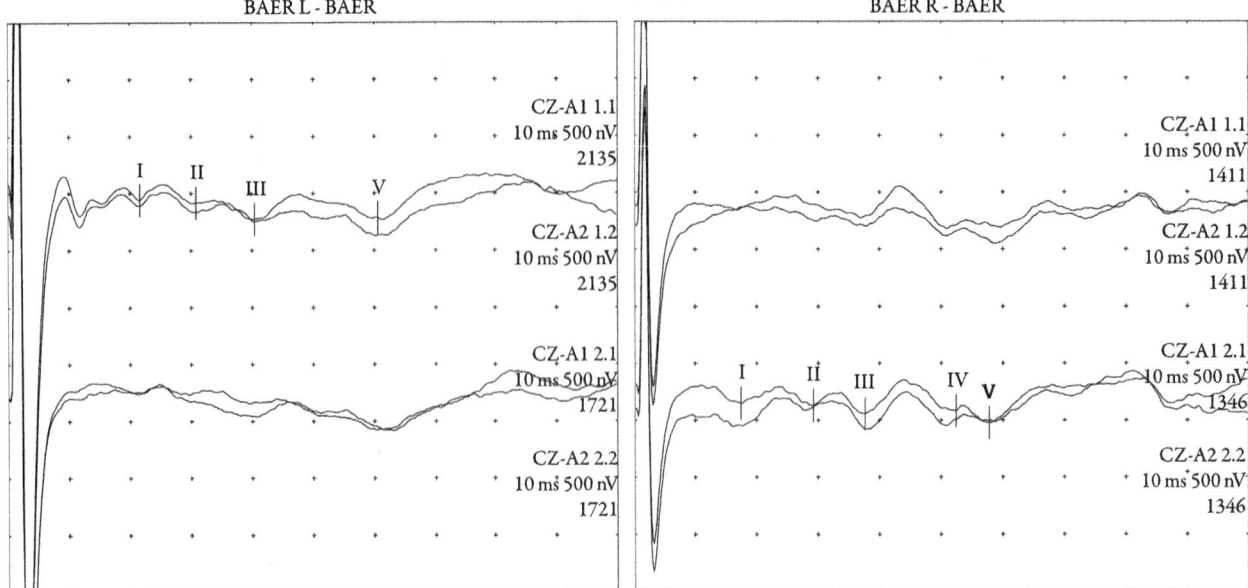

Figure 8.16 Left and right brainstem auditory evoked potentials showing the normal latency for waves I, II, II, IV, and V. The distance between the small crosses corresponds to 10 milliseconds.

(3) disorders of the neuromuscular junction; and (4) disturbances in motor control. Electromyography requires a skilled operator and can involve technical subtleties, depending on the muscles of interest. A medical psychiatrist would be most likely to initiate an EMG study in a patient with a complaint of weakness that is ascribed by the patient and/or other physicians to either systemic illness or depression, but might actually involve primary disease of muscle (e.g., polymyositis) or the neuromuscular junction (e.g., myasthenia gravis or Lambert-Eaton syndrome). Disproportionate involvement of proximal muscles is a clue to myopathy; dramatic decline in strength with continued exertion of a single muscle group is typical of myasthenia. Neither of these is typical of the general weakness and asthenia of systemic disease nor of the anergia and fatigability of depression.

Nerve conduction studies involve the application of a discrete, standardized electrical stimulus to a specific nerve distally and measuring the voltage over a specified proximal part of the nerve. There are well-established normal ranges for the amplitude of the proximal signal and for the interval between the distal stimulus and the proximal response—or, considering the distance as well as the time, the nerve conduction velocity. Nerve conduction tests can establish damage to specific nerves, as from trauma, demyelination, ischemia, compression, or entrapment, as well as polyneuropathy—diffuse damage to nerves throughout the body with the greatest effect on the long nerves to the extremities.

The second special use of nerve conduction tests in medical psychiatry is in establishing the diagnosis of an entrapment neuropathy with severe symptoms—usually of pain—that has been underappreciated or misdiagnosed by the patient's other physicians. In the medical-psychiatric context, nerve conduction studies have two special uses. One is to establish that

patient has polyneuropathy. This may be valuable when the patient's neuropsychiatric symptoms may be due to a drug or toxin that is known to affect the peripheral nerves as well as the brain. A patient with significant cerebral problems may not complain of neuropathic symptoms like numbness and tingling but may nonetheless have polyneuropathy, and the presence of the polyneuropathy may be useful in the differential diagnosis. For example, a patient with mental-status changes potentially due to heavy metal exposure would be expected to show polyneuropathy as well, if the heavy metal exposure were severe enough to explain their neuropsychiatric symptoms. A test proving neuropathy may be useful in confronting a patient who abuses alcohol or drugs; some patients are more effectively motivated by test results they find more "objective" than a psychological or psychiatric examination.

The second special use of nerve conduction tests in medical psychiatry is in establishing the diagnosis of an entrapment neuropathy with severe symptoms—usually of pain—that has been underappreciated or misdiagnosed by the patient's other physicians, leading to the patient's experiencing significant emotional distress. Entrapment neuropathies, which include the common carpal tunnel syndrome as well as some unusual entrapments, such as that of the infrascapular nerve associated with holding an infant when breastfeeding, can cause pain and dysesthesia disproportionate to any obvious physical sign. In such cases the nerve conduction study is virtually always abnormal, often markedly so. Specific treatment to decompress the nerve usually follows the nerve conduction study, frequently leading to relief of both physical and mental distress.

Special EMG techniques using repetitive nerve stimulation may also be used to assess the neuromuscular junction and diagnose myasthenia gravis. These patients may complain of vague weakness, which at times is discarded as psychogenic. In the patient with chronic back pain, the EMG may reveal objective signs of radiculopathy and aid in the diagnosis. The test is also useful in assessing the integrity of the muscles and nerves in the setting of neurotoxins. Alcoholic patients may experience a sensory polyneuropathy in addition to thiamine deficiency, which in itself can cause a motor and sensory neuropathy as well (Morrison & Chaudhry, 2012). Unlike the previous neurophysiological tests, the EMG test may cause patients significant discomfort from the needle insertion or nerve stimulation. In addition, the EMG is a very dynamic test, as the examiner will have to decide which muscles to sample based on real-time findings; hence significant expertise is needed.

CLINICAL PEARLS

- Frontal intermittent delta activity (FIRDA) is a nonspecific pattern seen in metabolic encephalopathy and raised intracranial pressure, but also in normal drowsy individuals and is not necessarily pathological (Accolla et al., 2011).

- A general rule of thumb is that abnormalities limited to the cortex will cause slowing of the posterior background frequency, while abnormalities involving subcortical structures lead to increased polymorphic delta activity, triphasic waves, or FIRDA.

- REM sleep noted on a routine EEG is suggestive of medication effect or possibly narcolepsy.

- Interpretation of EEG is related to age; certain degrees of temporal slowing, for example, are allowed in the elderly.

- When "sharply contoured" discharges are reported and the clinical suspicion of epileptic seizures is high, a repeat routine EEG, a more prolonged study, and/or a provocative procedure such as sleep deprivation is advised.

- EEG abnormalities noted in lithium toxicity include diffuse slowing, spikes, and triphasic waves.

- In the medical-psychiatric context, EPs are used for two purposes: (1) to determine whether complaints of sensory loss are accompanied by and are proportionate to changes in the relevant parts of the nervous system, and (2) to detect demyelinating diseases that may not be diagnosable by anatomic brain imaging and that may have neuropsychiatric complications or comorbidities.

- The test should be considered when the patient is suspected of MS on clinical grounds, has a history of visual symptoms, and has a normal or nondiagnostic MRI.

- The VEP should be considered when the patient is suspected of MS on clinical grounds, has a history of visual symptoms, and has a normal or nondiagnostic MRI.

- There are two special uses of nerve conduction studies in medical psychiatry. One is to establish that a patient has

polyneuropathy. This may be valuable when the patient's neuropsychiatric symptoms might be due to a drug or toxin that is known to affect the peripheral nerves as well as the brain. The second special use of nerve conduction tests is in establishing the diagnosis of an entrapment neuropathy with severe symptoms—usually of pain—that has been underappreciated or misdiagnosed by the patient's other physicians.

DISCLOSURE STATEMENTS

Dr. Khoshbin has no disclosures.

Dr. Sarkis has received travel funding for an investigator's meeting from Sunovion pharmaceuticals.

REFERENCES

Accolla, E. A., Kaplan, P. W., Maeder-Ingvar, M., Jukopila, S., & Rossetti, A. O. (2011). Clinical correlates of frontal intermittent rhythmic delta activity (FIRDA). *Clinical Neurophysiology*, 122(1), 27–31.

Alsaadi, T. M., & Marquez, A. V. (2005). Psychogenic nonepileptic seizures. *American Family Physician*, 72(5), 849–856.

Arain, A., Abou-Khalil, B., & Moses, H. (2001). Hashimoto's encephalopathy: Documentation of mesial temporal seizure origin by ictal EEG. *Seizure*, 10(6), 438–441.

Arciniegas, D. B. (2011). Clinical electrophysiologic assessments and mild traumatic brain injury: State-of-the-science and implications for clinical practice. *International Journal of Psychophysiology*, 82(1), 41–52.

Chang, A. K., & Shinnar, S. (2011). Nonconvulsive status epilepticus. *Emergency Medicine Clinics of North America*, 29(1), 65–72.

Claassen, J., Mayer, S. A., Kowalski, R. G., Emerson, R. G., & Hirsch, L. J. (2004). Detection of electrographic seizures with continuous EEG monitoring in critically ill patients. *Neurology*, 62(10), 1743–1748.

Coutin-Churchman, P., Anez, Y., Uzcategui, M., Alvarez, L., Vergara, F., Mendez, L., et al. (2003). Quantitative spectral analysis of EEG in psychiatry revisited: Drawing signs out of numbers in a clinical setting. *Clinical Neurophysiology*, 114(12), 2294–2306.

Flanagan, E. P., & Caselli, R. J. (2011). Autoimmune encephalopathy. *Seminars in Neurology*, 31(2), 144–157.

Freudenreich, O., Holt, D. J., Cather, C., & Goff, D. C. (2007). The evaluation and management of patients with first-episode schizophrenia: A selective, clinical review of diagnosis, treatment, and prognosis. *Harvard Review of Psychiatry*, 15(5), 189–211.

Freudenreich, O., Weiner, R. D., & McEvoy, J. P. (1997). Clozapine-induced electroencephalogram changes as a function of clozapine serum levels. *Biological Psychiatry*, 42(2), 132–137.

Gabuzda, D. H., Levy, S. R., & Chiappa, K. H. (1988). Electroencephalography in AIDS and AIDS-related complex. *Clinical Electroencephalography*, 19(1), 1–6.

Gallinat, J., Stotz-Ingenlath, G., Lang, U. E., & Hegerl, U. (2003). Panic attacks, spike-wave activity, and limbic dysfunction. A case report. *Pharmacopsychiatry*, 36(3), 123–126.

Garcia-Morales, I., Garcia, M. T., Galan-Davila, L., Gomez-Escalonilla, C., Saiz-Diaz, R., Martinez-Salio, A., et al. (2002). Periodic lateralized epileptiform discharges: Etiology, clinical aspects, seizures, and evolution in 130 patients. *Journal of Clinical Neurophysiology*, 19(2), 172–177.

Gibbs, F., Gibbs, E., & Lennox, W. (1943). Electroencephalographic classification of epileptic patients and control subjects. *Archives of Neurology & Psychiatry*, 50, 111–128.

Glanz, B. I., Laoprasert, P., Schur, P. H., Robertson-Thompson, A., & Khoshbin, S. (2001). Lateralized EEG findings in patients with neuropsychiatric manifestations of systemic lupus erythematosus. *Clinical Electroencephalography, 32*(1), 14–19.

Chatrian, G. E., Bergamini, L., Dondey, M., Klass, D. W., Lennox-Buchthal, M., & Petersen, I. (1974). A glossary of terms most commonly used by clinical electroencephalographers. *Electroencephalography and Clinical Neurophysiology, 37*(5), 538–548.

Hennis, A., Corbin, D., & Fraser, H. (1992). Focal seizures and non-ketotic hyperglycaemia. *Journal of Neurology, Neurosurgery, and Psychiatry, 55*(3), 195–197.

Holschneider, D. P., & Leuchter, A. F. (1999). Clinical neurophysiology using electroencephalography in geriatric psychiatry: Neurobiologic implications and clinical utility. *Journal of Geriatric Psychiatry and Neurology, 12*(3), 150–164.

Honigsberger, L. (1969). Blood calcium and the EEG. *Electroencephalography and Clinical Neurophysiology, 26*(5), 539–540.

Howard, J. E., & Dorfman, L. J. (1986). Evoked potentials in hysteria and malingering. *Journal of Clinical Neurophysiology, 3*(1), 39–49.

Hunter, A. M., Muthen, B. O., Cook, I. A., & Leuchter, A. F. (2010). Antidepressant response trajectories and quantitative electroencephalography (QEEG) biomarkers in major depressive disorder. *Journal of Psychiatric Research, 44*(2), 90–98.

Hurley, R. A., Fisher, R., & Taber, K. H. (2006). Sudden onset panic: Epileptic aura or panic disorder? *The Journal of Neuropsychiatry and Clinical Neurosciences, 18*(4), 436–443.

Jasper, H. (1958). Report of the committee on methods of clinical examination in electroencephalography. *Electroencephalography and Clinical Neurophysiology, 10*, 370–375.

Jenssen, S. (2005). Electroencephalogram in the dementia workup. *American Journal of Alzheimer's Disease and Other Dementias, 20*(3), 159–166.

Kaplan, P. W. (2004). The EEG in metabolic encephalopathy and coma. *Journal of Clinical Neurophysiology, 21*(5), 307–318.

Kaplan, P. W., & Birbeck, G. (2006). Lithium-induced confusional states: Nonconvulsive status epilepticus or triphasic encephalopathy? *Epilepsia, 47*(12), 2071–2074.

Karnaze DS, Bickford RG (1984). Triphasic waves: a reassessment of their significance. Electroencephalography and Clinical Neurophysiology, 57(3), 193–198.

Knott, V. J. (2000). Quantitative EEG methods and measures in human psychopharmacological research. *Human Psychopharmacology, 15*(7), 479–498.

Lai, C. W., & Gragasin, M. E. (1988). Electroencephalography in herpes simplex encephalitis. *Journal of Clinical Neurophysiology, 5*(1), 87–103.

Mintzer, S., & Lopez, F. (2002). Comorbidity of ictal fear and panic disorder. *Epilepsy & Behavior, 3*(4), 330–337.

Pogarell, O., Mulert, C., & Hegerl, U. (2007). Event-related potentials in psychiatry. *Clinical EEG and Neuroscience, 38*(1), 25–34.

Rodriguez, A. J., Jicha, G. A., Steeves, T. D., Benarroch, E. E., & Westmoreland, B. F. (2006). EEG changes in a patient with steroid-responsive encephalopathy associated with antibodies to thyroperoxidase (SREAT, hashimoto's encephalopathy). *Journal of Clinical Neurophysiology, 23*(4), 371–373.

Rosenfeld, M. R., & Dalmau, J. (2010). Update on paraneoplastic and autoimmune disorders of the central nervous system. *Seminars in Neurology, 30*(3), 320–331.

Santamaria, J., & Chiappa, K. H. (1987). The EEG of drowsiness in normal adults. *Journal of Clinical Neurophysiology, 4*(4), 327–382.

Scalise, A., Placidi, F., Diomedi, M., De Simone, R., & Gigli, G. L. (2006). Panic disorder or epilepsy? A case report. *Journal of the Neurological Sciences, 246*(1–2), 173–175.

Schaul, N. (1998). The fundamental neural mechanisms of electroencephalography. *Electroencephalography and Clinical Neurophysiology, 106*(2), 101–107.

Schmitt, S. E., Pargeon, K., Frechette, E. S., Hirsch, L. J., Dalmau, J., & Friedman, D. (2012). Extreme delta brush: A unique EEG pattern in adults with anti-NMDA receptor encephalitis. *Neurology, 79*(11), 1094–1100.

Speckmann, E., & Caspers, H. (Eds.). (1979). *Origin of cerebral field potentials.* Stuttgart: Thieme.

Steinhoff, B. J., Racker, S., Herrendorf, G., Poser, S., Grosche, S., Zerr, I., et al. (1996). Accuracy and reliability of periodic sharp wave complexes in Creutzfeldt-Jakob disease. *Archives of Neurology, 53*(2), 162–166.

Stockard, J. J., Werner, S. S., Aalbers, J. A., & Chiappa, K. H. (1976). Electroencephalographic findings in phencyclidine intoxication. *Archives of Neurology, 33*(3), 200–203.

Thorner, M. (1942). Procurement of electroencephalograph tracings in 1000 flying cadets for evaluating the Gibbs technique in relation to flying ability. USAD School of Aviation Medical Research Report, No. 7–1.

Yamada, T., & Meng, E. (2009). Diffuse EEG abnormalities. In T. Yamada, & E. Meng (Eds.), *Practical guide for clinical neurophysiologic testing: EEG* (pp. 219–248). Philadelphia, PA: Lippincott Williams and Wilkins.

9.

NEUROPSYCHIATRY OF PRIMARY SLEEP DISORDERS

Amit Chopra and Jarrett W. Richardson

INTRODUCTION

Sleep disorders are commonly observed in psychiatric populations, and detailed exploration of sleep complaints is key to comprehensive psychiatric evaluation. Primary sleep disorders must be differentiated from sleep disorders secondary to mental illnesses for appropriate referral and optimal treatment outcomes in psychiatric patients. This chapter covers clinical features, diagnosis, and treatment of common primary sleep disorders and their comorbidity with psychiatric disorders.

PHYSIOLOGY OF NORMAL SLEEP

Human sleep comprises alternating cycles of non–rapid eye movement (NREM) sleep and rapid eye movement (REM) sleep. NREM sleep is further divided into three stages of increasing depth of responsiveness including N1–N3 stages. Healthy young adults typically have four to six sequential cycles of NREM sleep followed by REM sleep. Approximately two-thirds of sleep time is spent in NREM sleep, and another quarter consists of REM sleep in adults. Table 9.1 summarizes the characteristics and percentage of the night spent in each sleep stage for healthy adults, which serves as a useful reference. In the elderly, the relative percentage of time spent in "deep sleep" decreases, and sleep is generally more shallow and fragmented.

During N1 sleep, a person can easily be awakened by environmental stimuli. N2 sleep is characterized by sleep spindles and K complexes on electroencephalogram (EEG). N3 is referred to as *slow-wave sleep*, and it is characterized by more than 20% delta wave sleep on EEG. Environmental stimuli must be significant to awaken a patient from slow-wave sleep. The transition from NREM to REM sleep usually occurs through N2, and REM is characterized by high frequency EEG, episodic bursts of vertical eye movements, penile tumescence, and muscle atonia. The first REM episode is often only 1–5 minutes in duration and occurs 70–100 minutes after sleep begins. There is marked interindividual variability in arousal threshold in REM sleep. In general, slow-wave or deep sleep is more common early in the night and REM periods more common toward morning because of progressively longer REM episodes. Due to this phenomenon, people commonly better recall dreams that occur just before their morning awakening, and men experience morning erections. Patients with disrupted sleep often spend the majority of the night in stages N1 and N2, with little slow-wave or REM sleep. The exact role that slow-wave and REM sleep play in a refreshing night's sleep is not well understood, but it is clear that significant reductions in either state lead to undesirable results including daytime somnolence, depressed mood, and cognitive impairment. In animal studies, prolonged absolute sleep deprivation has resulted in death attributed to sepsis (Bergmann et al., 1996).

SLEEP EVALUATION

Comprehensive clinical interview and physical examination along with appropriate investigations are key to diagnostic sleep evaluation. Clinicians need to focus on medical and

Table 9.1 **SLEEP STAGES IN HEALTHY ADULTS**

STAGE	PERCENTAGE	EEG CHARACTERISTICS	PHYSIOLOGIC CHANGES
Stage 1	2%–5%	Slow eye movements	Easy to arouse
Stage 2	45%–55%	Spindles, K complexes	More difficult to arouse
Stage 3\4	13%–23%	Slow EEG frequency	Difficult to arouse
REM	20%–25%	Rapid eye movements	Variable arousal threshold
		Muscle atonia	Penile engorgement
		Increased EEG frequency	

psychiatric history with a particular emphasis on sleep complaints. Acute and chronic pain should be assessed in the medically ill, as they are important causes of sleep disturbances. Questionnaires such as the Stanford Sleepiness Scale and Epworth Sleepiness scale should be used in patients to assess the severity of daytime somnolence. Box 9.1 lists the important areas of assessment for thorough evaluation and diagnosis of underlying sleep disorders.

Patients are often unaware of their nighttime breathing complaints, such as snoring, apneic spells, or behavioral events such as dream enactment behaviors. Therefore, collateral history from a bed partner is vital to gain information about nighttime respiratory and behavioral events. It is not uncommon for bed partners to have moved out of the bedroom because of intolerable snoring or dream-enactment behaviors, so collateral information may not be available. Further laboratory investigation should likely be pursued for adequate evaluation of sleep complaints in these circumstances.

The physical examination should focus on body mass index, neck circumference, nasal and oropharyngeal abnormalities, cervical/supraclavicular lymphadenopathy, and thyroid examination. Thorough pulmonary and cardiovascular examination allows assessment of the cardiopulmonary sequelae of sleep-disordered breathing. Neurological examination should be done to assess level of alertness, cognition, and to rule out neuromuscular disorders that may lead to

Box 9.1 ESSENTIAL ISSUES IN A SLEEP DIAGNOSTIC
INTERVIEW OF PATIENTS AND BED PARTNERS

Presenting complaint
Previous sleep evaluations
Sleep schedule—parenting issues?
Work schedule—rotating shifts?
Nap schedule—frequent? prolonged?
Exercise schedule—late in evening?
Sleep environment—bright light? noisy? too hot/cold?
Initial/middle/insomnia
Nocturnal movements
Sleepwalking/somnambulism/enuresis
Excessive daytime somnolence
Motor vehicle accidents
Cataplexy/sleep paralysis/ hallucinogenic experiences
Snoring
Observed apneas
Sleep position
GI reflux—diagnosed? partially treated?
Pain—chronic? acute? medications wear off?
Erectile problems
Alcohol/street drug/caffeine use/abuse/dependence
Depression/mania/panic attacks
Vivid dreams/nightmares
Prescription drug use/abuse/dependence
Family sleep history

Childhood sleep history.

sleep-disordered breathing. Detailed mental state examination should be done to rule out psychiatric issues such as mood and anxiety disorders.

INVESTIGATIONS

OVERNIGHT PULSE OXIMETRY

Overnight pulse oximetry can be a useful initial screening tool to detect repetitive oxygen desaturations >4% in patients at risk of sleep-disordered breathing. It measures only one variable; without other data the clinician cannot correlate the oxygen saturation with the corresponding sleep stage, heart rhythm, or body position (Svanborg et al., 1990); therefore, it should not be used as a definitive diagnostic method. Normal findings on oximetry do not rule out sleep apnea, as younger patients may not have significant oxyhemoglobin desaturations with apneic episodes or, alternatively, the patient may not have slept during the oximetry study. Patients with positional (supine-dependent) apnea who happen to sleep on their sides may have normal oximetry study results.

POLYSOMNOGRAPHY

At present, the overnight polysomnographic (PSG) study conducted in an accredited sleep disorders center remains the state of the art diagnostic procedure for evaluation of sleep disorders. The standard procedure involves multiple monitors including electroencephalogram, surface electromyogram, electro-oculogram, electrocardiogram, pulse oximetry, respiratory airflow, and respiratory effort (Phillipson & Remmers, 1989). Continuous videotaping is helpful for assessing possible parasomnias or unusual nocturnal movements. Sleep technologists can record body position and describe snoring intensity. Under these circumstances patients are observed to sleep for at least one sleep cycle with NREM and REM sleep in the supine and nonsupine positions.

PSG is the gold standard for diagnostic investigations for assessment of sleep-disordered breathing (SDB) including obstructive or central sleep apnea syndromes. PSG is conducted in a split-night fashion where the first half of the night is utilized to assess the nature and severity of SDB and, during second half of the night, a positive airway pressure (PAP) trial is applied to determine optimal PAP pressure settings for adequate control of SDB. Other indications for PSG study include excessive daytime somnolence, parasomnias, and periodic limb movements of sleep. PSG is not indicated for diagnosis of restless legs syndrome.

Portable monitoring can be used to assess obstructive sleep apnea, and it is usually performed in the home without a sleep technician in attendance. Portable monitoring includes overnight oximetry, partial cardiorespiratory studies, and a fully portable PSG with monitoring of EEG, EOG, and EMG. Portable equipment that monitors EEG is often prone to malfunction due to displacement during sleep without sleep technologists available to rectify a faulty signal. The American Academy of Sleep Medicine recommends that portable monitoring may be acceptable for assessment of OSA in certain carefully defined conditions, including patients with high pretest probability of moderate to severe OSA and absent medical comorbidities; nonambulatory or medically unstable patients; or to assess response to therapy in previously diagnosed OSA (Collop et al., 2007).

MULTIPLE SLEEP LATENCY TEST

The multiple sleep latency test (MSLT) is used to identify disorders of excessive daytime somnolence including narcolepsy. Patients must first have an overnight PSG study to exclude other sleep disorders causing disrupted nocturnal sleep. If patients have at least 6 hours of sleep, then an MSLT can be conducted the next day. Patients are asked to take four to five 20-minute scheduled naps, 2 hours apart. Patients wear electroencephalographic, electromyographic, electro-oculographic, and electrocardiographic leads. The MSLT test measures the initial sleep latency and REM latency if applicable. Patients are asked to stay awake between naps, refrain from stimulants like caffeine, and, if clinically indicated, undergo drug testing to detect occult sedative use.

Mean sleep latency over four or five naps is obtained, with a value <5 minutes suggestive of excessive daytime sleepiness; a value >10 minutes is considered to be normal. Values between 5 and 10 minutes should be considered on a continuum of sleepiness, with lower values indicating greater sleepiness. Patients with narcolepsy have sleep latency <8 minutes. Presence of REM sleep occurring within 15 minutes of sleep onset (SOREMP) during naps is also recorded. SOREMPs in two or more naps is considered abnormal and is thought to be neurophysiological marker of narcolepsy, although other causes, including abrupt withdrawal of REM-suppressant medications (antidepressants, stimulants), moderate to severe OSA, and sleep deprivation should be ruled out.

MAINTENANCE OF WAKEFULNESS TEST

The maintenance of wakefulness test (MWT) measures the ability of the patient to stay awake. This test is not used to diagnose sleep disorders, but it can be helpful in assessing the response to stimulants or a patient's fitness to drive. Patients are asked to sit in a comfortable recliner or bed in a dimly lit room and instructed to stay awake rather than to sleep. Each trial lasts until patient goes to sleep, or after 40 minutes if no sleep occurs. Normal sleep latency for this study is 30.4 minutes, and a sleep latency of 19 minutes or less correlates with driving impairment.

ACTIGRAPHY

An actigraph is a small watch-like device to be worn on the wrist of the nondominant hand that interprets periods of relative absence of wrist movements as sleep, and periods of high activity as wakefulness. There seems to be good correlation between total sleep time recorded by actigraphy and polysomnography. However, since this equipment counts limb movements and does not record EEG activity, specific sleep stages cannot be identified. One distinct advantage of actigraphy is that the compact device is worn 24 hours per day for 1 to 2 weeks. This permits identification of irregular sleep/wake patterns in the patient's unique work/home environment. Actigraphy can be used to assist in diagnosis of sleep disorders including circadian rhythm disorders, insomnia, and hypersomnia.

DIAGNOSIS AND TREATMENT OF PRIMARY SLEEP DISORDERS

Primary sleep disorders can be broadly organized by the patient's most common presenting sleep complaint—excessive daytime sleepiness or insomnia. Many medical, neurological, and psychiatric conditions cause sleep disruption leading to insomnia or excessive daytime drowsiness (Boxes 9.2 and 9.3).

Box 9.2 CAUSES OF EXCESSIVE DAYTIME SOMNOLENCE

Primarily Neurological

Idiopathic narcolepsy
Narcolepsy caused by sarcoidosis
Narcolepsy caused by lesion near the third ventricle
Idiopathic hypersomnia
Recurrent hypersomnia
Traumatic brain injury
Restless legs syndrome
Periodic limb movement disorder
Restless legs syndrome/periodic limb movement disorder caused by uremia
Restless legs syndrome/periodic limb movement disorder caused by peripheral Neuropathy
Restless legs syndrome/periodic limb movement disorder caused by Medication (tricyclic antidepressants, etc.)
Sleeping sickness
Increased intracranial pressure
Delirium
Kleine-Levin syndrome

Primarily Medical

Obstructive sleep apnea
Obstructive sleep apnea caused by acromegaly
Obstructive sleep apnea caused by hyperthyroidism
Central sleep apnea
COPD
Asthma
Gastroesophageal reflux
Hypoventilation syndrome
Periodic limb movements caused by chronic renal failure
Periodic limb movements caused by hyperthyroidism
Periodic limb movements caused by hepatic encephalopathy

(continued)

SLEEP RELATED BREATHING DISORDERS

Sleep related breathing disorders (SRBD) describes a group of disorders characterized by apneas (complete cessation of airflow), hypopneas (partial cessation of airflow), or the quantity

of ventilation during sleep. Apneic events are categorized as obstructive (inspiratory effort present during cessation of airflow), central (inspiratory effort absent during cessation of airflow), and mixed (both central and obstructive). The apnea/hypopnea index (AHI) refers to number of apnea/hypopnea events per hour, and it is used to quantify the severity of obstructive and central sleep apnea syndromes.

OBSTRUCTIVE SLEEP APNEA

CLINICAL FEATURES

Obstructive sleep apnea (OSA) is the most common sleep-disordered breathing disorder. It is characterized by the repetitive collapse or partial collapse of the pharyngeal airway during sleep and the need to arouse to resume ventilation. Sleep apnea is defined as a period of 10 seconds or more with no respiratory movement. Hypopnea is a similar period of abnormally slow or shallow respiration, insufficient for normal gas exchange. OSA can occur at any age, with a greater prevalence in males than in females (4% vs. 2%). The steepest prevalence increase is in the transition from middle to old age. At younger ages it is more common in African-American patients.

High-risk patients for OSA include those who are obese or being considered for bariatric surgery, those with treatment-resistant hypertension, diabetes mellitus type II, atrial fibrillation, pulmonary hypertension, congestive heart failure, and stroke (Epstein et al., 2009). Box 9.4 summarizes the diagnostic criteria of this common disorder. Box 9.5 outlines the medical complications of OSA.

DIAGNOSIS

Comprehensive sleep history in a suspected OSA patient includes assessment of symptoms including snoring, witnessed apneas, gasping/choking episodes, and daytime drowsiness. Subjective assessment of daytime sleepiness can be done by using scales including the Epworth sleepiness scale and the Stanford sleepiness scale. Physical examination findings in OSA patients include increased neck circumference, BMI >30 kg/m2, modified Mallampati score on the oropharyngeal exam of 3 or 4, presence of retrognathia, macroglossia, enlarged tonsils, elongated/enlarged uvula, and nasal abnormalities (polyps, septum deviation).

The accepted objective measures of OSA diagnosis include in-laboratory polysomnography (PSG) and home testing with portable monitors (PM). PM is not indicated in patients with major medical comorbidities including, but not limited to, congestive heart failure, moderate to severe pulmonary disease, neuromuscular disease, and those with a comorbid sleep disorder such as narcolepsy or nocturnal myoclonus (Collop et al., 2007). Respiratory events in OSA comprise primarily obstructive apneas and hypopneas, which are characterized by cessation or reduction in airflow with ongoing respiratory effort. Based on the apnea/hypopnea index (AHI) derived from diagnostic study, OSA is divided into categories of severity: mild (AHI=5–15 events per hour), moderate (AHI=15–30 events per hour) and severe (AHI>30 events per hour).

TREATMENTS

OSA is a chronic disease which requires long term multidisciplinary management. Patients with OSA need to be treated because the cardiovascular complications of OSA are potentially fatal, excessive daytime sleepiness puts patients at risk of accidents, cognitive problems compromise daytime performance, and effective treatment exists. Treatment options should be discussed in the context of the severity of OSA, associated risk factors, and the patient's expectations. The treatments of OSA can be broadly classified under positive airway pressure (PAP) and non-PAP therapies.

POSITIVE AIRWAY PRESSURE THERAPY

PAP therapy is the treatment of choice for mild, moderate, and severe OSA and should be offered as an option for all patients. PAP may be delivered in continuous (CPAP), bilevel (BPAP), and auto (APAP) modes. PAP is applied through nasal, oral, and oronasal interface. The treatment for OSA has been revolutionized by the use of CPAP therapy in the last few decades. This treatment involves delivering pressurized air (ranging typically from 5 to 20 cm of water pressure) to the sites of upper airway blockage (generally oropharynx, less commonly nasopharynx) and forcing the airway open. Apneas and snoring are eliminated, allowing the patient to sleep continuously without arousals. The CPAP device is generally introduced during overnight polysomnography (PSG) study in the sleep lab, where staff can adjust the CPAP pressures appropriately.

Bilevel (BPAP) therapy represents a modification of CPAP where the positive pressure fluctuates depending on whether airflow is inspiratory or expiratory (Hillberg & Johnson, 1997). Bilevel pressure is considerably more expensive and is reserved for patients who cannot tolerate CPAP. Automated positive airway pressure(APAP)devices, which can continually optimize positive airway pressure, can be used in self-adjusting mode for unattended treatment of moderate to severe OSA in the absence of medical comorbidities (Morgenthaler et al., 2006). Supplemental oxygen alone is inadequate for OSA, and patients with both OSA and intrinsic lung disease who have persisting hypoxia despite CPAP may benefit from supplemental oxygen delivered via the CPAP mask.

PAP treatment ideally involves a multidisciplinary care team including a sleep specialist, referring physician, nursing staff, sleep technologist, and respiratory specialist. Patients should be educated about the function and the benefits of PAP treatment, care of the equipment, and potential problems including leakage through the PAP interface, claustrophobia due to the PAP interface, and dry mouth or nasal congestion which may lead to PAP noncompliance. Close follow-up in the first few weeks with trained healthcare providers is indicated to establish effective PAP usage patterns and remediate problems if needed. After initial PAP set up, long-term follow-up is recommended on a yearly basis and as needed to troubleshoot PAP-related issues (Kushida et al., 2006a).

CPAP effectively treats OSA in the majority of people, but despite its efficacy in ameliorating symptoms CPAP usage has been reported as 65%–80% in OSA patients. According to a review study, short-course educational interventions were not particularly successful, although cognitive behavioral therapy (CBT) led to a significant improvement in average nightly CPAP usage (Smith et al., 2009).

NON-PAP THERAPIES

Non-PAP therapies include behavioral treatments, oral appliances, nasal expiratory positive airway devices, and surgical treatments of OSA. Behavioral treatments for OSA include weight loss (BMI <25), exercise, positional therapy, and avoidance of alcohol or sedatives at bedtime. Weight loss through diet and exercise is an important element of the treatment plan for any overweight patient with OSA, which can be successful with motivated patients. For patients who develop apneas only when lying supine, positional therapy may be effective, and this may include having them use a device such as a t-shirt with an attached cloth tube of tennis balls that keeps them off their backs. Little data are available regarding long-term adherence with this practical intervention.

Promising studies examine the role of oral appliance devices that pull the tongue or the mandible forward in treatment of mild to moderate OSA (Kushida et al., 2006b). Patients with abnormalities of the soft tissue or skeletal structures surrounding the upper airway, or poor response to PAP therapy, may consider surgery. Surgical procedures that may be considered for management of OSA include tonsillectomy, uvulopalatopharyngoplasty, maxillary mandibular advancement (MMA) and tracheostomy. MMA improves PSG parameters comparable to CPAP in majority of OSA patients. Most of the other surgical treatments of OSA are rarely curative but may improve clinical outcomes (Caples, Rowley, & Prinsell, 2010). Tonsillectomy may be considered as the first line of treatment in children with moderate to severe OSA.

OSA AND PSYCHIATRIC COMORBIDITY

OSA needs to be included in the differential diagnosis of patients with mood and behavioral issues, since OSA patients may demonstrate symptoms including depressed mood, irritability, personality changes, and cognitive impairment. Studies have noted variable prevalence of depression from 17.6% to 45% in OSA patients.

A recent study of depression in OSA patients has reported a statistically significant correlation between Epworth sleepiness scale (ESS) scores and Hamilton depression rating scores (HDRS), suggesting that depression improves after improvement in daytime sleepiness in OSA patients (El-Sherbini, Bediwy, & El-Mitwalli, 2011). This finding supports the hypothesis that sleep fragmentation and daytime sleepiness due to OSA may have an important role in the generation of depression in these patients. Higher depression scores, and not the severity of sleep apnea, were predictive of daytime sleepiness and poor quality of life in patients with REM-related OSA in a recent study (Pamidi et al., 2011). Patients with OSA may report improvement in their mood and energy within days, and this positive reinforcement leads to good CPAP compliance (Berthon-Jones, Lawrence, Sullivan, & Grunstein, 1996).

CENTRAL SLEEP APNEA SYNDROMES

Central sleep apnea syndromes are characterized by recurrent cessation of respiration due to apneas with no associated ventilatory effort. Different etiologies include primary CSA, Cheyne-Stokes breathing pattern, high-altitude periodic breathing, and CSA due to drug or substance use (long-acting opiates such as methadone, morphine, hydrocodone).

CLINICAL FEATURES

Recurrent apneas can lead to sleep fragmentation, excessive daytime sleepiness, or insomnia. A high ventilatory response to CO_2 seems to be a predisposing factor in development of CSA. Central apneas occur primarily during NREM sleep and less commonly during REM sleep. Oxygen desaturations are minimal in CSA, and arterial $PaCO_2$ less than 40 mmHg is typically observed during wakefulness.

Cheyne-Stokes breathing pattern is characterized by recurrent apneas/hypopneas alternating with prolonged hyperpneas, during which tidal volume waxes and wanes in a crescendo–decrescendo pattern. It is more commonly observed in elderly males with medical conditions such as congestive heart failure and stroke. CSA due to opiate use occurs due to respiratory suppression mediated through the action of opiates on mu receptors on the ventral surface of medulla, and it is typically seen after opiate use for at least 2 months.

DIAGNOSIS

Polysomnographic findings in primary CSA show five or more central apneas per hour of sleep. Cheyne-Stokes breathing pattern is characterized by at least 10 central apneas and hypopneas per hour of sleep in which hypopnea has a crescendo–decrescendo pattern of tidal volume during polysomnography study. Central apneas are associated with arousals from sleep leading to sleep fragmentation.

TREATMENT

After central sleep apnea (CSA) has been differentiated from obstructive sleep apnea by means of an overnight sleep study, treatments consisting of supplemental oxygen to reduce hypoxia and PAP therapies including CPAP, adaptive-servo ventilation (ASV) device, and BPAP (spontaneous timed-ST mode) can be effective in treatment of central sleep apnea syndromes (Aurora et al., 2012).

CSA AND PSYCHIATRIC COMORBIDITY

CSA has been found in 30% of the stable methadone maintenance treatment patients and in patients prescribed time-release opioid analgesic management (Wang D et al.,

2005). CSA symptoms tend to improve upon reduction of opiate dosage if possible.

RESTLESS LEGS SYNDROME AND PERIODIC LIMB MOVEMENTS

CLINICAL FEATURES

Restless legs syndrome (RLS) is a sensorimotor disorder characterized by characterized by an irresistible urge to move the legs, which is often accompanied by uncomfortable paresthesias felt deep inside the legs. These symptoms are made worse by rest (lying or sitting) and are at least partially and temporarily relieved by walking or moving the legs. The urge to move the legs worsens in the evening or night, with relative relief in the morning. The term *periodic limb movements* (PLM) describes the objective leg movements, while *restless legs syndrome* describes the subjective discomfort. PLMs occur in 80% to 90% patients with RLS but are not specific for RLS. Boxes 9.6 and 9.7 outline the diagnostic criteria of these overlapping disorders.

Between 5% and 15% of patients have RLS, with higher rates in those with uremia (15%–20%) and rheumatoid arthritis (30%). Periodic limb movements are more common with up to 34% of persons over 65 having this condition (Lugaresi et al., 1986). RLS occurs 1.5–2 times more commonly in women than in men. Clinicians need to carefully check whether the patient is taking any of the medications shown in Box 9.8 that can cause or exacerbate periodic limb movements (Ware et al., 1984). The differential diagnosis of RLS/PLMs is outlined in Box 9.9.

DIAGNOSIS

An overnight sleep study is not essential, since the diagnosis of restless legs syndrome can be made based on the patient's history. However, this approach can lead to a clinician overlooking possible periodic limb movements that are not associated with a restless feeling. A sleep study is valuable when a patient may have a coexisting sleep disorder like sleep apnea, or if the patient fails to respond to treatment for presumed restless legs syndrome. Helpful lab tests include complete blood count,

---

Box 9.6 DIAGNOSTIC CRITERIA: PERIODIC LIMB MOVEMENT DISORDER

1. Insomnia or excessive sleepiness. The patient can be symptomatic with the movements noted by an observer.

2. Repetitive, highly stereotyped movements usually involving extension of the big toe with partial flexion of the ankle, knee, and sometimes hip.

Adapted from American Sleep Disorders Association (1997), *The International Classification of Sleep Disorders, Revised: Diagnostic and coding manual*. Rochester, MN.

Box 9.7 DIAGNOSTIC CRITERIA: RESTLESS LEGS SYNDROME

Essential Signs/Symptoms

1. Unpleasant nocturnal sensation in the legs or difficulty falling asleep.

2. "Creeping" sensation of the calves often associated with generalized aches and pains.

3. The discomfort is relieved by movement of the limbs.

Essential Polysomnographic Findings

1. Repetitive episodes of muscle contractions (0.5–5 seconds in duration) separated by an interval of 20–40 seconds.

2. An arousal or awakening may be associated with the movement.

Adapted from American Sleep Disorders Association (1997), *The International Classification of Sleep Disorders, Revised: Diagnostic and coding manual*. Rochester, MN.

---

ferritin (since restless legs can be triggered by anemia), and low cobalamin and folate levels.

TREATMENT

The non–ergot dopamine (DA) agonists pramipexole (0.125–0.75 mg) and ropinirole (0.25–2 mg) are FDA-approved medications with proven efficacy in treatment of RLS. DA agonists are effective, but their use is limited by adverse effects—especially augmentation and impulse-control disorders (Early & Silber, 2010).

Augmentation refers to an earlier onset of symptoms in the evening following long-term treatment with dopaminergic drugs (mainly L-DOPA). Other characteristic features include an increase in symptom severity, a shorter latency to RLS symptoms while at rest, and an expansion of symptoms to other parts of the body. Among impulse-control disorders

---

Box 9.8 CONDITIONS/MEDICATIONS THAT CAN CAUSE OR EXACERBATE PERIODIC LIMB MOVEMENTS

Conditions

Barbiturate withdrawal
    Anticonvulsant withdrawal
    Benzodiazepine withdrawal
    Iron deficiency anemia

Medications

Tricyclic antidepressants
    Caffeine
    Lithium
    Phenothiazines

Selective serotonin reuptake inhibitors.

(ICD), pathological gambling, compulsive shopping, and hypersexuality have been noted in 7%–17% of RLS patients taking dopaminergic medications (Early & Silber, 2010). ICDs secondary due to dopaminergic medications usually resolve or substantially improve after discontinuation of these medications.

Alternative treatment options for treatment of RLS include clonazepam, gabapentin, pregabalin, and low and high potency opioids. Benzodiazepines and opioids are controlled agents that require monitoring for tolerance and addiction and are therefore not first-line treatment choices.

RLS AND PSYCHIATRIC COMORBIDITY

Studies have shown increased prevalence of depression and anxiety disorders in RLS patients. These patients can develop irritability, depressed mood, or cognitive disturbance due to disrupted sleep, although symptoms including anhedonia, loss of appetite, weight gain or loss, low self-esteem, and suicidal thoughts are not typical of RLS. Psychotropic medications including antipsychotics (both typical and atypical), antidepressants (TCAs, SSRIs, mirtazapine, venlafaxine) and lithium have been linked to exacerbation of RLS.

The pathophysiology of antidepressant-induced worsening of RLS remains unclear, but dopaminergic hypofunction combined with serotonergic and noradrenergic hyperfunction have been suggested as a possible etiology. In contrast, bupropion, due to primarily dopaminergic action, appears to reduce the periodic leg movements of sleep (PLMS) and RLS symptoms.

If poor sleep is a major factor in the depressive phenotype, then screening for RLS should be considered. A positive RLS screen warrants consideration of such nonpharmacological measures as physical exercise, sleep hygiene, and CBT along with optimization of RLS treatment. Such an approach may eliminate or reduce depressive symptoms, but should be considered as an initial step only if depressive symptoms are mild (Chopra, Pendergrass, & Bostwick, 2011).

RLS patients already taking serotonergic antidepressants for treatment of depression may complain of the paradox of continued sleepiness and resultant fatigue, and poor motivation despite mood improvement and reduced irritability. RLS exacerbation should be suspected, and RLS and PLMS therapy optimized as the initial approach with a goal of achieving 6–8 hours of restful sleep per night. If the response is only partial, the serotonergic antidepressant medication may need to be reduced or switched to a different antidepressant drug. Alternatives to serotonergic agents include bupropion, with the addition of benzodiazepines or buspirone in patients with comorbid or persistent anxiety (Chopra et al., 2011).

PARASOMNIAS

Parasomnias are undesirable physical events during entry into sleep, within sleep, or during arousals from sleep (American Academy of Sleep Disorders, 2001; Vignatelli et al., 2005). Parasomnias can be broadly classified in to NREM parasomnias (disorders of arousal) and REM parasomnias including REM sleep behavior disorder (RBD). Psychiatrists can be called to evaluate medically ill patients who have nocturnal agitation, sleepwalking, and unusual behaviors.

NREM PARASOMNIAS

The common disorders of arousal arising from NREM sleep include confusional arousals, sleep terrors, sleepwalking (somnambulism) and sleep-related eating disorders (SRED).

CLINICAL FEATURES

Confusional arousals consist of mental confusion or confusional behavior during or following arousals, typically from slow-wave sleep and usually in the first part of the night. Sleep terrors consist of arousals from slow-wave sleep accompanied by crying and behavioral manifestations of intense fear, with autonomic symptoms including tachycardia, tachypnea, diaphoresis, flushing of skin, and increased muscle tone. Amnesia for episodes of confusional arousals and sleep terrors is usually present, and these disorders tend to occur more commonly in children. Genetic factors play an important role in causation of 65% cases of sleepwalking.

Sleepwalking consists of complex behaviors that are usually initiated during slow-wave sleep and characterized by walking in an altered state of consciousness. Sleepwalking usually arises from first third or half of night, and amnesia is usually present for these episodes. Sleepwalking can involve routine behaviors, although inappropriate, agitated, belligerent, and violent behaviors can occur, particularly in men. The prevalence of sleepwalking in childhood has been noted to be as high as 17% (peaking at ages 8–13 years) and it is considered to be normal developmental sleep phenomenon except in those patients with clinical consequences. However, if sleepwalking persists beyond adolescence or into adulthood, it may deserve clinical attention. Polysomnography findings of multiple arousals from slow-wave sleep can support the clinical diagnosis of sleepwalking.

Sleep-related eating disorders (SRED) consist of recurrent episodes of involuntary eating (multiple times per night), typically during partial arousals from sleep with subsequent partial recall. The problematic consequences of SRED may include consumption of peculiar forms or combinations of food or ingestion of inedible and toxic substances such as raw/frozen foods, animal food, and cleaning solutions. The patients complain of early morning anorexia and abdominal distension, along with adverse health consequences including weight gain and obesity. SRED is most commonly associated with sleepwalking disorder, and it is more prevalent in young females (up to 83% of the cases). Medication-induced SRED has been noted with psychotropic medications including zolpidem, triazolam and lithium carbonate. SRED must be differentiated from night eating syndrome (NES), which is characterized by overeating between the evening meal and nocturnal sleep onset, eating during complete awakenings from sleep with full recall, and absence of peculiar or bizarre eating behaviors.

DIAGNOSIS

In addition to detailed clinical history, polysomnography (PSG) findings of multiple arousals from slow-wave sleep with video recordings of accompanying sleep-related behaviors can help confirm the diagnosis of NREM parasomnias. PSG can be helpful to rule out other causes of arousals from sleep such as OSA and can also confirm REM with normal atonia to exclude REM sleep behavior disorder (RBD).

TREATMENT

NREM parasomnias deserve further clinical evaluation and treatment in cases where the behaviors are potentially injurious or violent or disruptive to others in the household, while mild cases may need reassurance only. Medications such as clonazepam or imipramine may be effective. Avoidance of sleep deprivation and techniques for self-hypnosis may be effective as well.

NREM PARASOMNIAS AND PSYCHIATRIC COMORBIDITY

There is no significant association between childhood sleepwalking and psychiatric disorders, although adults with sleepwalking may have a current or past history of nonpsychotic depressive and anxiety disorders. Violence and homicide leading to legal consequences has been reported, along with accidental self-harm and pseudo-suicides. Increased incidence of SRED has been noted in patients with eating disorders (inpatient group 16.7% and outpatient group 8.7%) as compared to 4.6% in controls (Winkelman, Herzog, & Fava, 1999).

REM PARASOMNIAS

CLINICAL FEATURES

RBD is the parasomnia of most interest to the medical psychiatrist. Patients with this condition appear to "act out their dreams," as they lack muscle atonia during REM sleep. Patients and their bed partners can be seriously injured by hitting, kicking, rolling, and other more complex behaviors. Although no good epidemiologic data are available, REM behavior disorder is likely the most common parasomnia behavior.

RBD is a male-predominant disorder, and the major predisposing factors are male sex, age 50 years or older, and underlying neurological disorders—particularly Parkinson's disease, Lewy body dementia, narcolepsy, and stroke. Idiopathic RBD is diagnosed in the absence of comorbid neurological conditions.

DIAGNOSIS

Polysomnographic findings in RBD include an excessive amount of sustained EMG activity, intermittent loss of REM atonia, or excessive phasic muscle twitch activity of the submental or limb EMG during REM sleep. Signs of autonomic nervous system activation such as tachycardia are uncommon during REM sleep activation in RBD as compared to the disorders of arousal.

TREATMENT

Treatment includes modifying the bedroom environment to reduce injury to the patient and bed partner. Recommended measures include placing a mattress on the floor, padding corners of furniture, window protection, and removing potentially dangerous items such as guns or sharp objects from the bedroom.

Clonazepam is suggested for the treatment of RBD but should be used with caution in patients with dementia, gait disorders, or concomitant OSA (Schenck & Mahowald, 1990). Its use should be monitored carefully over time, as RBD in some patients appears to be a precursor to neurodegenerative disorders with dementia. Clonazepam has been associated with reduction in sleep-related injurious (SRI) behaviors (Aurora et al., 2010). Melatonin may be considered due to fewer side effects (Aurora et al., 2010). RBD patients on psychotropic medications, particularly antidepressants, should be closely monitored for worsening of RBD symptoms.

REM PARASOMNIAS AND PSYCHIATRIC COMORBIDITY

An acute form of RBD emerges during intense REM rebound states, such as during withdrawal from alcohol and sedative-hypnotics or with drug intoxication. Use of most antidepressants with the exception of bupropion has been recognized as a precipitating factor for RBD. Psychiatric disorders are not considered as predisposing factors, with the exception of PTSD.

HYPERSOMNIAS OF CENTRAL ORIGIN

Hypersomnias of central origin include a group of disorders with the primary symptom of excessive daytime drowsiness when the underlying cause of the primary symptom is not due to circadian rhythm disorder, sleep-related breathing disorder, or another cause of disturbed nocturnal sleep. These disorders include narcolepsy, recurrent hypersomnia (Kleine-Levin syndrome), and idiopathic hypersomnia.

NARCOLEPSY

CLINICAL FEATURES

Narcolepsy is characterized by a pentad of symptoms including excessive daytime sleepiness, disturbed nocturnal sleep, cataplexy, hypnagogic hallucinations, and sleep paralysis; the later three are manifestations of REM intrusion into wakefulness. Narcolepsy can be associated with or without cataplexy, which is defined as abrupt muscle atonia associated with a powerful emotional trigger (such as laughing) without loss of consciousness. Cataplexy occurs in 70% of the patients, and its presence is virtually diagnostic of narcolepsy. The associated symptoms include REM sleep behavior disorder, automatic behaviors, and obesity.

The prevalence rate of narcolepsy is about 1 in 4,000 in North America and Europe with equal male to female prevalence. Symptoms usually appear in the teens or twenties, and onset after age 55 and before age 10 is rare.

DIAGNOSIS

Detailed clinical interview in combination with PSG (to rule out other causes of sleepiness) and MSLT remain the current gold standard in the diagnosis of narcolepsy in adults. Mean sleep latency <8 minutes with two or more SOREMPs are observed on MSLT following sufficient nocturnal sleep (minimum of 6 hours). HLA antigen DQB1*602 is specifically associated with narcolepsy (almost all patients) although it is positive in 12%–38% of the general population. Low CSF hypocretin levels <110 pg/ml have been found in more than 90% of the patients with narcolepsy and never in controls.

TREATMENT

Narcolepsy is a lifelong disorder, with chronic sleepiness being the most disabling symptom. General strategies include patient and family education, counseling regarding good sleep hygiene, discussion of safety issues including driving recommendations, and vocational counseling. Behavioral techniques that have been found to be helpful in treatment of narcolepsy include avoidance of sleep deprivation, maintaining a constant sleep/wake cycle, and taking two 15-minute scheduled daytime naps to reduce daytime drowsiness.

The main goal of pharmacological treatment is to improve daytime alertness and reduction in episodes of cataplexy in narcolepsy patients. Treatment of excessive daytime sleepiness involves use of modafinil and stimulants. Modafinil at a starting dose of 200 mg in the morning is considered to be first-line treatment of excessive sleepiness in narcolepsy patients. An additional 200 mg can be added the morning dose or in the afternoon to extend the alerting effects of modafinil. Mild side effects of modafinil include headache, nervousness, insomnia, and dry mouth. Rare but serious side effects include Stevens-Johnson's syndrome, aggression, suicidality, and psychosis.

Psychostimulants including methylphenidate, amphetamine/dextroamphetamines, and methamphetamine have been used effectively to treat sleepiness in narcolepsy patients. Combination of sustained release stimulants in the morning, with additional immediate acting stimulants in the afternoon, have been found to be effective in patients complaining of sleepiness in the afternoon or late evening. There is little evidence of abuse and addiction of stimulant medications in narcolepsy patients.

Sodium oxybate, the sodium salt of gamma hydroxybutyrate (GHB), may be the drug of choice in patients with both excessive daytime sleepiness and cataplexy. It is only available in liquid form and is prescribed twice during the night, with the second dose taken 2.5–4 hours later than the bedtime dose. Mild to moderate side effects of sodium oxybate include dizziness, headache, nausea, pain, somnolence, sleep disorder, confusion, infection, vomiting, enuresis, and night terrors. Respiratory depression, bradycardia, delirium, myoclonus, hypothermia, and coma can occur in sodium oxybate overdose.

Stimulant medications often do not provide significant relief from cataplexy despite improvement in daytime sleepiness. Patients with significant cataplexy symptoms need additional medications with anticataplectic activity. REM suppressant medications including tricyclic antidepressants, SSRIs, reboxetine, and venlafaxine have efficacy in treating cataplexy associated with narcolepsy, but these medications do not improve excessive daytime sleepiness (Morgenthaler et al., 2007).

NARCOLEPSY AND PSYCHIATRIC COMORBIDITY

Higher levels of anxiety, depression, and impulsivity have been noted in narcolepsy patients with cataplexy as compared to controls (Dimitrova et al., 2011). Increased prevalence of binge-eating disorders and sleep-related eating disorders has also been noted in narcolepsy patients.

Due to the presence of hypnagogic or hypnopompic hallucinations, narcolepsy patients may be misdiagnosed with psychotic disorders such as schizophrenia. According to a recent case control study, no indication for an increased prevalence of schizophrenia or any other psychotic disorders has been reported in narcolepsy patients compared to population controls (Fortuyn HA et al., 2009). Stimulant induced psychosis may be a more likely diagnostic possibility in narcolepsy patients presenting with psychotic symptoms (Fortuyn et al., 2009).

IDIOPATHIC HYPERSOMNIA

CLINICAL FEATURES

Idiopathic hypersomnia is characterized by constant and severe day time sleepiness with features of nonrefreshing prolonged naps and post-awakening confusion (sleep drunkenness). It is categorized as idiopathic hypersomnia with (>10 hours) or without (<10 hours) long sleep time. The onset of idiopathic hypersomnia usually occurs before 25 years of age. This disorder is stable in severity and long lasting, with complications including social and occupational impairment.

DIAGNOSIS

Nocturnal polysomnography (to exclude other causes of daytime drowsiness) and MSLT are done to establish diagnosis of idiopathic hypersomnia. Mean sleep latency of less than 8 minutes and fewer than 2 SOREMPs are recorded on MSLT in patients with idiopathic hypersomnia.

TREATMENT

Idiopathic hypersomnia is usually a lifelong disease, although recent series suggest that hypersomnia may spontaneously disappear in 14% to 25% patients. Modafinil and stimulant medications are the mainstay of treatment of idiopathic hypersomnia (Morgenthaler et al., 2007).

IDIOPATHIC HYPERSOMNIA AND PSYCHIATRIC COMORBIDITY

A prospective cohort study of 75 patients with idiopathic hypersomnia, who were compared with 30 healthy controls, showed slightly higher but nonsignificant levels of anxiety and depression in patients as compared to controls (Vernet & Arnulf, 2009). During clinical assessment, depression (unipolar or bipolar) should always be considered in patients presenting with idiopathic hypersomnia.

RECURRENT HYPERSOMNIA: KLEINE-LEVIN SYNDROME

CLINICAL FEATURES

Kleine-Levin syndrome is characterized by recurrent episodes of hypersomnia, often associated with cognitive and behavioral symptoms, that typically occur weeks or months apart. Episodes usually last for a few days to several weeks and are often preceded by prodromal symptoms of fatigue and headache. Patients may sleep as long as 16–18 hours per day. Sleep and behavior are normal between episodes, which may occur 1–10 times per year. Kleine-Levin syndrome is a rare disorder, and approximately 200 cases have been reported to date in the literature with 4:1 male to female ratio. The frequency of HLA DQB1*02 has been noted to be increased in patients with Kleine-Levin syndrome.

DIAGNOSIS

Head imaging including CT and MRI scans are normal, although EEG findings are significant for generalized slowing of background with paroxysmal bursts of bisynchronous high amplitude theta-delta waves. CSF fluid cytology and protein are normal.

TREATMENT

Stimulant medications may be used to with some success in treating hypersomnia in patients with Kleine-Levin syndrome. Lithium treatment has not been shown to decrease the number of relapses, but it has been associated with shorter duration of recurrent hypersomnia episodes with absence of behavioral symptoms in a small case series (Poppe et al., 2003).

KLEINE-LEVIN SYNDROME AND PSYCHIATRIC COMORBIDITY

Associated symptoms may include cognitive symptoms such as feelings of unreality, confusion, hallucinations, and behavioral symptoms including hyperphagia, hypersexuality, irritability, and aggression. In a large case series of 339 patients with Kleine-Levin syndrome, depression was more frequently reported in women than in men. A few cases of recurrent hypersomnia have been reported to have an alternation between hypersomniac episodes and manic depressive episodes.

CIRCADIAN RHYTHM SLEEP DISORDERS

Circadian rhythm sleep disorders (CSRDs) are characterized by persistent and recurrent pattern of sleep disturbance caused primarily by alterations of the circadian timing system, misalignment between endogenous circadian rhythm, and exogenous factors that affect timing or duration of sleep. CSRDs are associated with insomnia and/or excessive daytime sleepiness leading to social or occupational impairment. CSRDs include advanced sleep phase disorder, delayed sleep phase disorder, free-running disorder, irregular sleep/wake rhythm, shift work disorder, and jet lag disorder.

CLINICAL FEATURES

Advanced sleep phase disorder (ASPD) is characterized by habitual sleep onset and wake-up times that are several hours earlier relative to conventional or desired times. Individuals typically complain of excessive evening sleepiness and early morning insomnia. The prevalence of ASPD is noted to be 1% in middle-aged and older adults and increases with age.

Delayed sleep phase disorder (DSPD) is characterized by habitual sleep/wake times that are delayed (usually >2 hours) relative to conventional or socially acceptable times. Individuals typically have difficulty falling asleep at socially acceptable times, and attempts to fall asleep earlier are often unsuccessful, leading to secondary conditioned insomnia. Affected individuals prefer late wake-up times and report sleep drunkenness in the morning. The exact prevalence of DSPD in the general population is unknown, and it is more commonly noted in adolescents and young adults with a reported prevalence of 7%–16%.

Free-running disorder (FRD) is characterized by sleep symptoms that occur due to intrinsic circadian rhythm being not entrained to a 24-hour period (usually slightly longer), leading to quite variable sleep patterns that can be congruent to a free-running circadian pacemaker. Most individuals with FRD are totally blind due to lack of photic input to their circadian pacemakers. The actual incidence of FRD is unknown, and rare cases have been reported in sighted people.

Irregular sleep/wake rhythm disorder (ISWD) is characterized by lack of clearly defined circadian rhythm of sleep and wake. The sleep/wake cycle is disorganized so that sleep and wake are variable through out the 24-hour period.

Shift work disorder (SWD) is characterized by complaints of insomnia or excessive sleepiness that occur in relation to work hours that are scheduled during the usual sleep period. The sleep disturbances are most commonly noted in night shifts and early morning shifts. This condition usually persists for the duration of shift work.

Jet lag disorder (JLD) is a circadian rhythm disorder characterized by mismatch between the timing of the endogenous circadian clock and the sleep/wake pattern generated by a change in time zone. Affected individuals complain of disturbed sleep, decreased alertness, and impaired daytime function. The severity of symptoms is dependent on the number of time zones traveled and direction, with eastward travel being more difficult to adjust to than westward travel.

DIAGNOSIS

Thorough clinical interview, sleep diaries/logs, and actigraphy are used to confirm diagnosis of CSRD. Polysomnography (PSG) is not indicated in the diagnosis of CSRD; however, it may be helpful to rule out additional primary sleep disorders in patients with CSRD.

TREATMENTS

Recommended treatments of ASPD include sleep/wake scheduling and bright light exposure in the evening after 8 p.m. to phase-delay circadian rhythms and reduce evening sleepiness. Hypnotic medications may be used to maintain sleep in the early morning (Reid & Zee, 2011). Treatment of DSPD aims at shifting the affected individual to sleep at an earlier, socially acceptable time. The treatment modalities for DSPD include chronotherapy, timed exogenous melatonin administration, and morning bright light exposure.

The therapeutic approaches to FRD are focused on entraining the intrinsic pacemaker. Timed light exposure, fixed sleep/wake schedules, and timed exogenous melatonin administration can help entrain the intrinsic circadian pacemaker. Physical activity, behavioral techniques to improve

sleep hygiene, timed exogenous melatonin, and bright light exposure are available therapeutic options for ISWR.

Treatment of SWD aims to phase-shift (usually delay) the circadian clock so that the patient is alert at night and sleeps during the day. Different options include bright light exposure during the first part of the night shift (leading to phase delay) and avoiding bright light on the commute home from work (leading to phase advance). Timed light exposure is key to management of JLD, minimizing morning light and maximizing afternoon light on eastward flights and staying awake till the lights are out on westward flights. Medication options include melatonin (2–5 mg) before bedtime upon arrival (repeat up to 4 nights) or hypnotics (zolpidem 10 mg) up to 3 nights.

CSRD AND PSYCHIATRIC COMORBIDITY

CSRDs are chronic disorders associated with social/occupational impairment and psychiatric sequelae. DSPD has been associated with increased incidence of depressive symptoms, depressive disorders, and schizoid and avoidant personality disorders. Affected individuals' use of sedatives/hypnotics, alcohol, and stimulants to treat symptoms of insomnia and sleepiness may lead to substance use issues in ASPD and DSPD. ISWR is more commonly noted in children with mental retardation and institutionalized elderly with dementia, and FRD in sighted people is associated with increased incidence of psychiatric and personality disorders.

PRIMARY INSOMNIA

As outlined in Box 9.3, insomnia can be caused by a variety of medical, neurologic, psychiatric, and environmental conditions. If possible, any factors that cause or exacerbate insomnia can be corrected. However, in many patients with primary insomnia no specific trigger exists.

CLINICAL FEATURES

Primary insomnia disorder is defined as a subjective report of sleep initiation, duration, consolidation, or quality that occurs despite adequate opportunity for sleep, leading to some daytime impairment. Insomnia symptoms occur in approximately 33%–50% of the adult population, with specific insomnia disorders in 5%–10%. Risk factors for insomnia include increasing age, female sex, comorbid disorders (medical, psychiatric, primary sleep disorders), shift work, and possibly unemployment and lower socioeconomic status. Patients with chronic pain and psychiatric disorders have insomnia rates as high as 50%–75%.

Careful history including characterization of main complaint (difficulty with sleep initiation and/or sleep maintenance, poor sleep quality), past and current precipitants, duration, frequency (nights per week), daytime symptomatology and distress, course (intermittent, progressive), aggravating and alleviating factors, and previous treatments and responses are key to insomnia evaluation. The clinician must ascertain that the patient's sleep and time complaints occur despite adequate time available for sleep, in order to differentiate insomnia from behaviorally induced insufficient sleep. Attention should be paid to sleep onset time, as unusual sleep onset and wake times may indicate circadian rhythm disorders such as delayed or advance sleep phase syndrome. Cognitive distortions and negative behaviors associated with insomnia should be explored, including use of alcohol, sedatives, and hypnotic medications. Common daytime consequences of insomnia include fatigue, sleepiness, mood and cognitive complaints, poor quality of life, and exacerbation of comorbid illnesses such as mood disorders.

Patients with primary insomnia can generally be subdivided into three major types. Those with "psychophysiologic" or "conditioned" insomnia learn to associate sleeplessness with certain circumstances, like their own bedroom. These patients become progressively tense as bedtime approaches, which can be detected with surface electromyography (Hauri & Fisher, 1986). In contrast, patients with idiopathic insomnia typically have lifelong difficulties sleeping. The cause of this syndrome is unknown, although neurochemical abnormalities of the arousal or sleep-regulating areas have been suggested (Hauri, 1994). Sleep state misperception or paradoxical insomnia is a rare type of primary insomnia. Patients with this disorder complain of subjective sleep disturbance that is not consistent with objective data. In order to meet criteria for this diagnosis, polysomnography needs to demonstrate normal duration and quality of sleep.

TREATMENTS

Treatment of insomnia includes behavioral, psychological, and pharmacological therapies. The goals of insomnia treatment include reduction of sleep and waking symptoms, improvement of daytime function, and reduction of distress. Behavioral/psychological treatments and pharmacological treatments can be used alone or in combination to treat insomnia. Treatment outcome can be monitored longitudinally with clinical evaluation, questionnaires, and sleep logs.

SLEEP HYGIENE

Among the best studied and most readily available tools for improving sleep disturbance in medical patients are environmental and behavioral management (Hauri & Fisher, 1986; Hauri, 1994). More specific behavioral studies have led to some basic information about sleep habits that can be helpful to patients that have disturbed sleep. These sleep hygiene techniques have been found to have particular efficacy in patients who have chronic insomnia complaints.

Establishing a regular awakening time, essentially every day of the week, optimizes resetting the circadian clock. Unfortunately, the "clock" tends to drift rapidly back to the old schedule as soon as there is variability in rising times, so persistence and consistency are important. When regular exercise is an option, doing it in the late afternoon several hours before bedtime may improve sleep to some degree, because of the association of falling body temperature and

sleep. Avoiding clock watching can help reduce the arousal effects of becoming aggravated by checking the seemingly interminable hours through the night. Most people recall only the periods of wakefulness at night, so clock watching can reinforce the irritating perception that no sleep occurred.

Patients should avoid alcohol, nonprescribed sedatives, and stimulants (such as caffeine and nicotine any time during the day). They should not sleep on a full stomach (particularly if the patient is prone to gastroesophageal reflux reflux). Introducing "unwinding" stimuli as pre-bedtime routines can be helpful to most patients with sleep complaints. Treating GE reflux with an antacid and H_2-blocking medication prior to the hour of sleep can be beneficial.

COGNITIVE BEHAVIORAL THERAPY FOR INSOMNIA

Cognitive behavioral therapy for insomnia (CBT-I) is a combination of cognitive therapy coupled with behavioral techniques (sleep restriction, stimulus control) with or without relaxation therapy. CBT-I uses a psychotherapeutic approach to reconstruct cognitive distortions with positive and appropriate concepts about sleep and its effects.

Stimulus control technique is designed to extinguish the negative association between the bed and undesirable outcomes such as wakefulness, frustration, and worry. These negative states are frequently conditioned, in response to efforts to sleep, as a result of prolonged periods of time in bed awake. The objectives of stimulus control therapy are for the patient to form a positive and clear association between the bed and sleep and to establish a stable sleep/wake schedule. Patients are instructed to go to bed only when sleepy, and use the bed for sleep only. If unable to fall asleep within 20 minutes, then patients are instructed to leave the bed and engage in a relaxing activity until drowsy, then return to bed—and repeat if necessary.

Sleep restriction is intended to improve sleep continuity by limiting time in bed to the total sleep time in order to enhance sleep drive. As sleep drive increases and the window of opportunity for sleep remains restricted, with daytime napping prohibited, sleep becomes more consolidated. When sleep continuity substantially improves, time in bed is gradually increased to provide sufficient sleep time for the patient to feel rested during the day, while preserving the newly acquired sleep consolidation. In addition, the approach is consistent with stimulus control goals in that it minimizes the amount of time spent in bed awake, helping to restore the association between bed and sleeping.

Relaxation training includes progressive muscle relaxation, deep breathing, or guided imagery, and it is designed to lower cognitive and somatic arousal states that may interfere with sleep. It can be especially helpful in patients with hyperarousal states, and it is often combined with cognitive therapy.

PHARMACOLOGICAL TREATMENTS

The pharmacological treatments for insomnia aim to improve sleep quantity and quality, reduce sleep latency and wake after sleep onset, and reduce daytime impairment. Current

FDA-approved medications for treatment of insomnia include benzodiazepine receptor agonists (BzRAs) and melatonin receptor agonist (Schutte-Rodin, Broch, Buysse, Dorsey, & Sateia, 2008). Other medications that are used off-label to treat insomnia include antidepressant and antiepileptic drugs. Over-the-counter drugs including antihistamines, melatonin, and valerian have been used to treat insomnia, although evidence regarding the efficacy and safety of these agents is limited (Schutte-Rodin et al., 2008).

BENZODIAZEPINE RECEPTOR AGONISTS

Examples of short/intermediate-acting benzodiazepine receptor agonists (BzRAs) include zaleplon, zolpidem, and eszopiclone. All of these agents have been shown to have positive effects on sleep latency, total sleep time (TST), and/or waking after sleep onset (WASO) in placebo-controlled trials. Factors including symptom pattern, past response, cost, and patient preference should be considered in selecting a specific hypnotic agent (Schutte-Rodin et al., 2008).

Medications with short half life (zaleplon) are likely to reduce sleep latency but have little effect on WASO, and are less likely to result in residual daytime sedation. Whereas eszopiclone has a relatively longer half life, it is more likely to improve sleep maintenance and also more likely to produce residual sedation. Benzodiazepines (BZDs) such as lorazepam and clonazepam are not specifically approved for insomnia, although they might be used if appropriate for the patient's symptoms and comorbid conditions.

Potential adverse effects of BzRAs include residual sedation, memory and performance impairment, falls, undesired behaviors during sleep (including sleepwalking, sleep eating, and sleep driving), somatic symptoms, and drug interactions (Schutte-Rodin et al., 2008). A few cases of serious amnestic behaviors, with suicidal and parasuicidal gestures in patients with access to firearms, have been reported in patients taking zolpidem with alcohol (Gibson & Caplan, 2011; Chopra et al., 2013). These cases highlight the importance of discussing undesired sleep-related behaviors associated with zolpidem use and advising patients to take precautions, such as firearm safety and not mixing alcohol with hypnotic medications, in order to prevent untoward events. There seems to be a consensus that triazolam carries the highest rates of reported amnesia, dissociative episodes, and rebound insomnia and anxiety. BZDs should be used with caution in patients with compromised respiratory function (COPD, sleep apnea).

Empirical data supports both daily and intermittent usage in terms of frequency of hypnotic medications. In clinical practice, hypnotics are often used over duration of 1–12 months. Randomized controlled studies of medications including zolpidem/eszopiclone have demonstrated continued efficacy without significant side effects. Patients should be followed up at 6-month intervals if hypnotic medications are used on long-term basis to monitor efficacy, side effects, tolerance, or abuse. Gradual tapering of both dosage and frequency of hypnotic medications is recommended to prevent rebound insomnia and withdrawal symptoms (Schutte-Rodin et al., 2008).

RAMELTEON

Ramelteon is a melatonin receptor agonist which is FDA approved for treatment of insomnia. It is a short-acting medication administered at bedtime, and it is primarily used for sleep onset insomnia.

ANTIDEPRESSANTS

Sedating low-dose antidepressants may be tried if insomnia is accompanied with comorbid depression or prior trial of BzRAs or ramelteon has been unsuccessful. Examples of these drugs include trazodone, mirtazapine, doxepin, and amitriptyline. Factors such as treatment history, coexisting psychiatric and medical conditions, specific side effect profile, cost, and pharmacokinetic profile may guide the selection of a specific agent. These medications are not FDA approved for insomnia, and their efficacy for this indication is not well established (Schutte-Rodin et al., 2008).

OTHER MEDICATIONS

Medications including gabapentin, quetiapine, and olanzapine may be used in clinical practice, although evidence of efficacy for these drugs for the treatment of chronic primary insomnia is insufficient (Schutte-Rodin et al., 2008).

SLEEP AND PSYCHIATRIC DISORDERS

SLEEP AND ANXIETY DISORDERS

Patients with anxiety disorders often complain of difficulty initiating and maintaining sleep. PSG findings in patients with anxiety disorders comprise longer sleep latency, increased wake time after sleep onset, increased arousals leading to sleep disruption, reduced SWS, reduced sleep efficiency, and reduced total sleep time.

Generalized anxiety disorder patients demonstrate impaired sleep initiation and maintenance as compared to healthy controls along with normal latency to REM sleep, unlike depressed patients. Patients with panic disorder experience at least one nocturnal sleep-related panic attack, and one-third of the patients experience nocturnal panic attacks that preferentially occur in NREM sleep during transition to slow-wave sleep. Symptoms of nocturnal panic attacks are similar to daytime panic attacks. There is usually no reported dreaming before the panic attack.

Patients with posttraumatic stress disorder (PTSD) experience insomnia and recurrent distressing dreams of the traumatic event. Excessive motor activity and awakenings with somatic anxiety symptoms are sleep manifestations of heightened arousal in PTSD.

SLEEP AND MOOD DISORDERS

Patients with clinical depression almost uniformly complain of sleep disturbances, with a majority (80%) of them having insomnia and the rest complaining of hypersomnia. PSG abnormalities in major depression include prolonged sleep latency, sleep fragmentation, increased wake time, early morning awakenings, decreased SWS, shortened REM latency, increased REM density, and increased overall REM as well as reduced TST and SE.

Improvement in these sleep parameters has been observed after treatment with both cognitive behavioral therapy and pharmacological treatment with antidepressants. Most antidepressants suppress REM sleep; many affect SWS and sleep continuity measures. Residual sleep disturbances have been associated with increased relapse rates in depressed patients in remission.

Patients with mania invariably have decreased need for sleep, and severe insomnia may be an early symptom and trigger for a manic episode. PSG findings in mania are similar to those found in major depression, including poor sleep continuity, reduced SWS, short latency to REM sleep, and increased eye movements during REM sleep.

SLEEP AND SCHIZOPHRENIA

Schizophrenia is associated with sleep disturbances including insomnia, disturbed circadian rhythm, and daytime sleepiness. PSG findings in schizophrenic patients include increased sleep latency, decreased sleep efficiency, decreased SWS, and decreased REM latency. Strong correlation has been demonstrated between insomnia and positive symptoms of schizophrenia including delusions, hallucinations, and disorganization.

Disruption of circadian rhythm patterns has also been noted in schizophrenia, with predisposition to delayed sleep phase pattern and increased daytime sleep. Poor sleep hygiene and substance abuse may further contribute to worsening of sleep patterns in schizophrenic patients.

Use of low-potency sedating antipsychotics has been associated with improved sleep continuity in schizophrenic patients, but this may occur at the expense of daytime sedation. The role of antipsychotics leading to sleep disturbances including REM or slow-wave abnormalities in schizophrenic patients is unclear, as these agents have been associated with both improvement and worsening of REM and slow-wave sleep parameters.

The side effects of neuroleptics that may affect sleep quality include akathisia and worsening of restless legs syndrome or periodic limb movements of sleep. Metabolic side effects of neuroleptic medications such as weight gain may also place schizophrenic patients at increased risk of obstructive sleep apnea and resultant day time sleepiness.

SLEEP AND ATTENTION DEFICIT HYPERACTIVITY DISORDER

The estimated prevalence of sleep problems in children with attention deficit hyperactivity disorder (ADHD) is 5 times higher as compared to healthy controls. The sleep problems in ADHD children may be attributed to ADHD itself, or ADHD comorbidities such as mood disorders, anxiety disorders, and substance abuse. Stimulant medications frequently used to treat ADHD have insomnia as a common side effect. Polysomnography findings in children with ADHD include increased rates of periodic limb movements of sleep and sleep-related breathing disorders. Inattention and hyperactivity may improve upon adequate treatment of sleep-related breathing disorders in children with ADHD.

SLEEP AND ALCOHOL DEPENDENCE

Alcohol dependence is associated with sleep disturbances including insomnia, obstructive sleep apnea, and circadian rhythm disturbances. Decreased sleep efficiency and total sleep time, decreased REM latency, and decreased SWS has been noted on PSG. The suppression of SWS has been linked to growth hormone suppression in alcoholic patients and linked to poor quality of sleep. Nonrestorative sleep in alcoholics has been associated with increased alcohol consumption. OSA patients with alcohol abuse pose a special challenge, because alcohol is believed to decrease the neuromuscular tone of the upper airway. These patients often require higher CPAP settings to prevent apneas, and, if the sleep study is done when the patient is sober, often the pressure setting is inadequate.

CLINICAL PEARLS

- Questionnaires such as the Stanford Sleepiness Scale and Epworth Sleepiness Scale can assess the severity of daytime somnolence.

- From bed partners, collateral information can offer what patients don't know about their nighttime breathing complaints, such as snoring, apneic spells, or behavioral events such as dream enactment behaviors.

- Polysomnographic study is not indicated for diagnosis of restless legs syndrome.

- The American Academy of Sleep Medicine recommends that portable monitoring may be acceptable for assessment of obstructive sleep apnea (OSA) in certain carefully defined conditions including patients with high pretest probability of moderate to severe OSA and absent medical comorbidities, nonambulatory, or medically unstable patients, or to assess response to therapy in previously diagnosed OSA (Collop et al., 2007).

- The Maintenance of Wakefulness Test can be helpful in assessing the response to stimulants or a patient's fitness to drive.

- Supplemental oxygen alone is inadequate for OSA, and patients with both OSA and intrinsic lung disease who have persisting hypoxia despite CPAP may benefit from supplemental oxygen delivered via their CPAP masks.

- Clinical follow-up of potential problems once CPAP is instituted—including leakage through the PAP interface, claustrophobia due to the PAP interface, and dry mouth or nasal congestion—heads off PAP noncompliance.

- For patients who develop apneas only when lying supine, positional therapy may be effective. This may include having them use a device such as a t-shirt with an attached cloth tube of tennis balls that keeps them off their backs.

- Patients with OSA may report improvement in their mood and energy within days, and this positive reinforcement leads to good CPAP compliance (Berthon-Jones et al., 1996).

- Central sleep apnea (CSA) has been found in 30% of the stable methadone maintenance treatment patients and in patients prescribed time-release opioid analgesic management (Wang et al., 2005). CSA symptoms tend to improve upon reduction of opiate dosage.

- While dopamine agonists can treat restless leg syndrome (RLS), augmentation of the syndrome and an increase in impulse control disorders like gambling can be side effects.

- Bupropion, due to its primarily dopaminergic action in contrast to SSRIs, appears to reduce the periodic leg movements of sleep and RLS symptoms.

- If poor sleep is a major factor in the depressive phenotype, then screening for RLS should be considered.

- Delayed sleep phase disorder has been associated with increased incidence of depressive symptoms, depressive disorders, and schizoid and avoidant personality disorders.

- In patients with panic disorder, nocturnal panic attacks preferentially occur in NREM sleep during transition to slow-wave sleep.

- Polysomnography abnormalities in major depression include prolonged sleep latency, sleep fragmentation, increased wake time, early morning awakenings, decreased SWS, shortened REM latency, increased REM density, and increased overall REM, as well as reduced TST and SE.

- There is a strong correlation between insomnia and positive symptoms of schizophrenia, including delusions, hallucinations, and disorganization.

- OSA patients with alcohol abuse pose a special challenge, because alcohol is believed to decrease the neuromuscular tone of the upper airway. These patients often require higher CPAP settings to prevent apneas, and, if the sleep study is done when the patient is sober, often the pressure setting is inadequate.

DISCLOSURE STATEMENTS

Dr. Chopra has no conflict of interest to disclose.

Dr. Richardson has no conflict of interest to disclose.

REFERENCES

American Academy of Sleep Medicine (2001). *International classification of sleep disorders, revised: Diagnostic and coding manual* (pp. 141–214). Chicago, Illinois: American Academy of Sleep Medicine.

Aurora, R. N., Zak, R. S., Maganti, R. K., et al. (2010). Best practice guide for the treatment of REM sleep behavior disorder (RBD). Standards of Practice Committee, American Academy of Sleep Medicine. *Journal of Clinical Sleep Medicine, 6*(1), 85–95.

Aurora, N., Chowdhuri, S., Ramar, K., et al. (2012). The treatment of central sleep apnea syndromes in adults: Practice parameters with an evidence-based literature review and meta-analyses. *Sleep, 35*(1), 17–40.

Bergmann, B. M., Gilliland, M. A., Feng, P. F., et al. (1996). Are physiologic effects of sleep deprivation in the rat mediated by bacterial invasion? *Sleep, 19*(7), 554–562.

Berthon-Jones, M., Lawrence, S., Sullivan C. E., & Grunstein, R. (1996). Nasal continuous positive airway pressure treatment: current realities and future. *Sleep, 19*(9 Suppl), S131–S135.

Caples, S. M., Rowley, J. A., & Prinsell, J. R. (2010). Surgical modifications of the upper airway for obstructive sleep apnea in adults: A systematic review and meta-analysis. *Sleep, 33*(10), 1396–1407.

Chopra, A., Pendergrass, D. S., & Bostwick, J. M. (2011). Mirtazapine-induced worsening of restless legs syndrome (RLS) and ropinirole-induced psychosis: Challenges in management of depression in RLS. *Psychosomatics, 52*(1), 92–94.

Chopra, A., Selim, B., Silber, M. H., & Krahn, L. H. (2013). Para-suicidal amnestic behavior associated with chronic zolpidem use: Implications for patient safety. *Psychosomatics, 54*(5), 498–501.

Collop, N. A., Anderson, W. M., Boehlecke, B., et al. (2007). Clinical guidelines for the use of unattended portable monitors in the diagnosis of obstructive sleep apnea in adult patients. Portable Monitoring Task Force of the American Academy of Sleep Medicine. *Journal of Clinical Sleep Medicine, 3*(7), 737–747.

Dimitrova, A., Fronczek, R., Van der Ploeg, J., et al. (2011). Reward-seeking behavior in human narcolepsy. *Journal of Clinical Sleep Medicine, 7*(3), 293–300.

Earley, C. J., & Silber, M. H. (2010). Restless legs syndrome: understanding its consequences and the need for better treatment. *Sleep Medicine, 11*(9), 807–815.

El-Sherbini, A. M., Bediwy, A. S., & El-Mitwalli, A. (2011). Association between obstructive sleep apnea (OSA) and depression and the effect of continuous positive airway pressure (CPAP) treatment. *Neuropsychiatric Disease and Treatment, 7,* 715–721.

Epstein, L. J., Kristo, D., Strollo, P. J. Jr., et al. (2009).Clinical guideline for the evaluation, management and long-term care of obstructive sleep apnea in adults. Adult Obstructive Sleep Apnea Task Force of the American Academy of Sleep Medicine. *Journal of Clinical Sleep Medicine, 5*(3), 263–276.

Fortuyn, H. A., Lappenschaar, G. A., Nienhuis, F. J., et al. (2009). Psychotic symptoms in narcolepsy: phenomenology and a comparison with schizophrenia. *General Hospital Psychiatry, 31*(2), 146–154. Epub Jan 24.

Gibson, C. E., Caplan, J. P. (2011). Zolpidem-associated parasomnia with serious self-injury: a shot in the dark. *Psychosomatics, 52*(1), 88–91.

Hillberg, R. E., & Johnson, D. C. (1997). Noninvasive ventilation. *New England Journal of Medicine, 337*(24), 1746–1752.

Hauri, P. J. (1994). Primary insomnia. In M. H. Kryger, T. Roth, & W. C. Dement (Eds.), *Principles and practice of sleep medicine* (2nd ed., pp. 497–498). Philadelphia: W. B. Saunders.

Hauri, P., & Fisher, J. (1986). Persistent psychophysiologic (learned) insomnia. *Sleep, 9*(1), 38–53.

Kushida, C. A., Littner, M. R., & Hirshkowitz, M. (2006a). Practice parameters for the use of continuous and bilevel positive airway pressure devices to treat adult patients with sleep-related breathing disorders. American Academy of Sleep Medicine. *Sleep, 29*(3), 375–380.

Kushida, C. A., Morgenthaler, T. I., Littner, M. R., et al. (2006b). Practice parameters for the treatment of snoring and obstructive sleep apnea with oral appliances: An update for 2005. American Academy of Sleep Medicine. *Sleep, 29*(2), 240–243.

Lugaresi, E., Cirignotta, F., Coccagna, G., et al. (1986). Nocturnal myoclonus and restless legs syndrome. *Advances in Neurology, 43*, 295–307.

Morgenthaler, T. I., Aurora, R. N., Brown, T., et al. (2006). Practice parameters for the use of autotitrating continuous positive airway pressure devices for titrating pressures and treating adult patients with obstructive sleep apnea syndrome: An update for 2007–evidence tables. *Sleep, 29*(8), 1031–1035.

Morgenthaler, T. I., Kapur, V. K., Brown, T., et al. (2007). Practice parameters for the treatment of narcolepsy and other hypersomnias of central origin. Standards of Practice Committee of the American Academy of Sleep Medicine. *Sleep, 30*(12), 1705–1711.

Pamidi, S., Knutson, K. L., Ghods, F., et al. (2011). Depressive symptoms and obesity as predictors of sleepiness and quality of life in patients with REM-related obstructive sleep apnea: cross-sectional analysis of a large clinical population. *Sleep Medicine, 12*(9), 827–831.

Phillipson, E. A., & Remmers, J. E. (1989). American Thoracic Society Consensus Conference on Indications and Standards for Cardiopulmonary Sleep Studies. *American Review of Respiratory Disease, 139*, 559–568.

Poppe, M., Friebel, D., Reuner, U., et al. (2003). The Kleine-Levin syndrome—effects of treatment with lithium. *Neuropediatrics, 34*(3), 113–119.

Reid, K. J., & Zee, P. C. (2011). Circadian disorders of the sleep-wake cycle. In M. H. Kryger, T. Roth, & W. C. Dement (Eds.), *Principles and Practice of Sleep Medicine, 5th Edition* (pp. 691–701). St. Louis: Elsevier Saunders.

Schenck, C. H., & Mahowald, M. W. (1990). Polysomnographic, neurologic, psychiatric and clinical outcome report on 70 consecutive cases with the REM behavior disorder (RBD), sustained clonazepam efficacy in 89.5% of 57 treated patients. *Cleveland Clinic Journal of Medicine, 57*, S10–S24.

Schutte-Rodin, S., Broch, L., Buysse, D., Dorsey, C., & Sateia, M. (2008). Clinical guideline for the evaluation and management of chronic insomnia in adults. *Journal of Clinical Sleep Medicine, 4*(5), 487–504.

Smith, I., Nadig, V., & Lasserson, T. J. (2009). Educational, supportive and behavioural interventions to improve usage of continuous positive airway pressure machines for adults with obstructive sleep apnoea. *Cochrane Database System Reviews, (2)*, CD007736.

Svanborg, E., Larssson, H., Carlsson-Nordlander, B., Pirskanen, R. (1990). A limited diagnostic investigation for obstructive sleep apnea syndrome. Oximetry and static charge sensitive bed. *Chest, 98*(6), 1341–1345.

Vernet, C., & Arnulf, I. (2009). Idiopathic hypersomnia with and without long sleep time: a controlled series of 75 patients. *Sleep, 32*(6), 753–759.

Vignatelli, L., Bisulli, F., Zaniboni, A., Naldi, I., Fares, J. E., Provini, F., et al. (2005). Interobserver reliability of ICSD-R minimal diagnostic criteria for the parasomnias. *Journal of Neurology, 252*(6), 712–717.

Wang, D., Teichtahl, H., Drummer, O. et al. (2005). Central sleep apnea in stable methadone maintenance treatment patients. *Chest, 128*(3), 1348–1356.

Ware, J. C., Brown, F. U., Moorad, P. J., et al. (1984). Nocturnal myoclonus and tricyclic antidepressants. *Sleep Research, 13*, 72.

Winkelman, J. W., Herzog, D. B., & Fava, M. (1999). The prevalence of sleep-related eating disorder in psychiatric and non-psychiatric populations. *Psychological Medicine, 29*(6), 1461–1466.

PART II

THERAPEUTIC MODALITIES

10.

PSYCHOTHERAPEUTIC PRINCIPLES AND TECHNIQUES

PRINCIPLES OF MEDICAL PSYCHOTHERAPY

Stephen A. Green

INTRODUCTION

The interaction between many physicians and patients remains an impersonal, if not mechanistic, encounter. Symptomatic individuals present themselves for diagnosis and treatment with the expectation that they will be cured, or at least significantly relieved of their particular suffering. Because of this cause-and-effect mindset, the *intellectual* activity of problem solving has become the basis of medical practice for many practitioners. Obviously, considerable empathy and concern is involved in this process, as the particular problems under consideration affect the physical and mental health of individuals. However, treating illness is generally considered an exercise of determining etiology, prescribing the indicated therapeutic regimen, and meticulously monitoring the treatment response and course of the illness. This approach is based on the biomedical model, a parochial standard that compromises patient care by embracing the inaccurate notion of a mind-body dichotomy and perpetuating the reductionistic notion that complex phenomena are ultimately explained by a single principle (Engel, 1977).

Given the evolution of medicine into a highly specialized world that utilizes increasingly sophisticated—and impersonal—technology, a major impact of the biomedical model has been to dissect the patient into more and more composite parts. It isolates individuals from their daily environment of psychosocial supports and stressors, thereby promoting "the physician's preoccupation with the body and disease and the corresponding neglect of the patient as a person." It fails to consider "how the patient behaves and what he reports about himself and his life" because "it does not include the patient and his attributes as a person, a human being" (Engel, 1980). In sum, the biomedical model suggests that treating a patient's specific physical pathology is synonymous with treating the patient, which ignores the fundamental truth that all illness simultaneously affects one's mind and body. Rigid adherence to this model thereby compromises patient care in a significant way: it prevents requisite attention to abnormal emotional states of medical patients that may derive from a psychological reaction to the illness or reflect concurrent psychopathology that is often unrecognized. For example, approximately 50% of patients who present to primary care physicians with depressive disorders remain undiagnosed (Regier et al., 1988), despite studies demonstrating that two-thirds of the top 10% utilizers of primary care physicians have diagnosed recurrent major depression (Katon et al., 1990) and the fact that depression is possibly the most common illness presenting to primary care physicians (Katon, 1987).

The biopsychosocial model highlights the inextricable link between mind-body interaction and, consequently, enhances understanding of the pathogenesis, clinical course, and treatment of diverse disease processes, as well as mechanisms of death (Engel, 1968; 1971; Greene, Goldstein, & Moss, 1972; Lown, Verrier, & Rabinowitz, 1977; Reich et al., 1981). While Engel, an internist with psychoanalytic training, is credited with coining the term *biopsychosocial*, the concept that multiple genetic, physiologic, psychodynamic, environmental, and social factors all interact in a systems model to influence the onset and outcome of medical illness had been stated early in the 20th century by psychiatrists Franz Alexander and Adolph Meyer. The theories of Meyer, Alexander, and Engel in this respect have received extensive validation (Stoudemire, 1995; Stoudemire & McDaniel, 1999). The biopsychosocial model is now an established paradigm that recognizes how disturbances in physiologic functioning influence, and are in turn affected by, one's psychological functioning; it thereby emphasizes the clinical reality that optimal medical treatment requires a comprehensive appreciation of the interplay between patients' organic pathology, their intrapsychic lives, and the positive and negative impact of their social environment.

This biopsychosocial treatment approach, as discussed by Engel (1980), is conceptualized by interposing the patient between two hierarchies that combine to form an overall hierarchy of natural systems. The person is at the same time at the highest level of an organismic hierarchy, which ranges from subatomic particles through the nervous system, and the lowest stratum of a social hierarchy, which ranges from a two-person system to the biosphere. These two hierarchies are in a dynamic equilibrium, since every system (e.g., cells or two-person) within each hierarchy is a distinctive whole that is simultaneously interrelated with every other system. Consequently, disturbances at any system level can alter any other system level; through feedback controls, they may modify or aggravate the system originally affected.

According to the biopsychosocial model, pathologic mood states that exist concurrently with medical illness may be predominantly biological or psychological in origin. For example, the biological model advocates that depression is the symptomatic and behavioral expression of abnormalities associated with central nervous system biogenic amines, and that appropriate treatment requires use of pharmacological agents that influence neurotransmission. The psychological paradigm suggests that dynamic interaction of unconscious, preconscious, and conscious thoughts and feelings produce psychic conflict that may result in depression, and that treatment rests heavily on a comprehensive study of the patient's *illness dynamics* (Green, 1985)—that is, the varied psychosocial factors affecting, and affected by, the patient's organic pathology—information which is then incorporated into an individualized psychotherapeutic approach.

As this chapter discusses, psychotherapy is generally classified as a *supportive* or *introspective* treatment. The former attempts to minimize emotional distress; one such treatment is a patient support group. Introspective therapy, on the other hand, seeks to compel patients to actively confront and grapple with disturbing feelings in an effort to gain better affective control; insight-oriented psychotherapy is the prototype intervention. There are many variants of these therapeutic approaches (American Psychiatric Association, 1996), each emphasizing different methods for resolving distressing psychological states. For example, cognitive therapy attempts to modify irrational beliefs and distorted perceptions toward the self and the environment, while interpersonal therapy seeks to define and explore specific stressors, such as social isolation, in order to minimize their regressive impact. However, *all* psychotherapies ultimately are based in a supportive or introspective orientation, which can be administered on an individual basis or in broader settings such as couples, family, or group therapy. How individuals react emotionally to their illness determines whether supportive or introspective psychotherapy is indicated for the treatment of pathologic mood states that exist concurrently with a medical illness.

RESPONSES TO ILLNESS

Impaired health, whether it takes the form of a mild upper respiratory infection or a life-threatening cerebrovascular accident, is a universal condition that precipitates a predictable emotional response: *illness is experienced as a loss—specifically, the loss of health—because it diminishes one's level of functioning.* This is most obvious when serious ailments permanently and profoundly change an individual's physical status, such as the severe restrictions caused by blindness. However, even a limited illness may precipitate considerable feelings of loss due to the symbolic significance to the patient. In addition to challenging omnipotent wishes—highlighting one's vulnerability to physical ailments whose onset, course, and response to treatment are often unexplainable and unpredictable—an episode of ill health conveys specific symbolic meaning that derives from the highly personalized interplay between patients' physical pathology, intrapsychic life, and

social environment. This determines how, and to what extent, they react affectively to a particular loss of health.

Whether illness is experienced in the literal sense, as a result of concrete physical restrictions, or more symbolically, due to implied or anticipated limitations, it promotes the same psychological response—*a grief reaction during which patients mourn the loss of their previous state of health.* The process is akin to bereavement. Illness obliges one to acknowledge and confront a diminished level of functioning, causing individuals to progress through a series of feeling states—denial, anxiety, anger, depression, helplessness—before resolving the various emotions precipitated by their loss.

This is most obvious during a medical emergency, such as an acute appendicitis. The gravity of the initial pain caused by an inflamed appendix, which may be quite severe, is often dismissed as indigestion or the effects of an enterovirus. Other feelings supplant the early denial as the significance of the symptoms becomes clearer. Anxiety emerges as patients ruminate about the morbidity (and possible mortality) of surgery, as well as their need to abdicate considerable responsibility for their well-being and comfort to anonymous caretakers. This anxiety can persist during the recuperative period, focused on such issues as the restrictions and length of convalescence; however, emerging resentments usually predominate during this stage, prompting patients to discharge their anger on family members, friends, and even medical personnel who provide succor and support. These feelings eventually give way to a period of helplessness and overt depression, characterized by mood, behavioral, and cognitive changes, when one is most aware of the losses brought on by a surgical emergency that has relegated all other activities (e.g., professional and social responsibilities) to positions of secondary importance. Most patients emerge from this phase, progressively reestablishing an emotional equilibrium by working through all of the feelings precipitated by illness. This requires their appropriate assessment of the specific limitations caused by their disease, as well as a general acknowledgment of their vulnerability and ultimate mortality.

An abnormal emotional response to illness occurs when one is unable to effectively grieve the losses caused by ill health. For a variety of reasons idiosyncratic to a particular individual during a particular period of life, the patient may be unable to recognize, experience, and put into proper perspective some or all of the feelings precipitated by illness. That individual may completely deny all emotions, or, more commonly, experience a specific mood to the relative exclusion of all others. In effect, the patient becomes mired in some phase of the grief process, preoccupied with the feelings characteristic of that stage. This forestalls attainment of an emotional resolution regarding the loss of health, a situation that can evolve into an emotional state similar to pathological grief whose symptomatic expression may take the form of a mood disturbance (e.g., excessive anxiety and/or depression), a behavioral disturbance (e.g., compulsive eating or substance abuse), or impaired object relationships (Brown & Stoudemire, 1983). Subsequent effects on somatic functioning—which may aggravate the initial organic pathology—derive from mind-body interactions. Because of this interdependence, *affective resolution of the loss of health is essential for physical, as well as psychological well-being.* Absent this grief work, a pathologic illness response emerges, characterized by a psychobiological disequilibrium generally more disabling than that caused by the initial illness. The most frequent abnormal psychological reactions to illness include pathologic degrees of denial, anxiety, anger, depression, and dependency.

THE DENIAL RESPONSE

Denial, the refusal to perceive or accept external reality, is a common ego mechanism that enables a person to partially or completely ablate distressing cognitions and/or moods. If a patient's denial is absolute in the presence of a serious illness, that primitive behavior is classified as a *psychotic ego mechanism* (Vaillant 1977). Less pronounced denial, however, may have an adaptive purpose by enabling individuals to temporarily ignore the overwhelming impact of a stressor that might otherwise threaten psychological integrity. For example, it is often invoked when specific circumstances limit the effectiveness of higher level ego functioning in emotionally healthy individuals (e.g., the conviction that one will certainly survive in battle). Similarly, it is associated with better short-term psychological adjustment following a myocardial infarction (Hackett & Cassem, 1974), and diminished morbidity and mortality during hospitalization (Levenson et al., 1989).

Denial becomes maladaptive when it is so excessive that it prevents accurate assessment and acceptance of the realities of life. At this point it is exclusively defensive, providing illusory comfort by prompting actions that promote a false sense of well-being, or insure inactivity such that a patient's reaction to illness is actually a nonresponse. Denial may be present throughout the course of illness, from the moment of onset, during the period of initial treatment and convalescence, and extending into the rehabilitative phase. The long-standing cardiac patient who attributes cramping in his left arm to "overwork," or the woman who decides to have her breast mass evaluated "in a few months," exemplifies acute denial of illness. Noncompliance with one's therapeutic regimen often reflects continued denial. This can apply to the period of initial hospitalization, illustrated by the patient who refuses to remain at bedrest (Reichard, 1964) as well as chronic care, seen in the individual with diabetes mellitus who repeatedly ignores dietary restrictions. It may also be observed in the terminal patient who adamantly refuses to acknowledge impending death. An excessive unconscious rejection of illness may therefore ultimately complicate accurate diagnosis and interfere with definitive treatment.

THE ANXIETY RESPONSE

Signal anxiety alerts one to danger and subsequently prompts purposeful, self-protective behavior. The onset of illness is always accompanied by heightened anxiety, as patients question the extent and degree of their ailments. Common concerns, such as whether or not symptoms signal the beginning of a fatal illness, usually give way to speculation about the diagnostic work-up, course of treatment, and ultimate prognosis. Patients may wonder how they will be perceived by others, and how they will regard themselves if they become disfigured or chronically debilitated. They ruminate about the toll of their illness on family relationships, professional responsibilities, friendships, and day-to-day functioning. In short, they attempt to assess the impact of illness on the overall quality of life in the near and distant future. Although a difficult and disconcerting exercise, this is usually an adaptive response to illness, spurring them to seek timely medical attention and adhere to prescribed treatments.

Illness can also precipitate pathologic levels of anxiety that cause patients undue concern about their physical status. As a consequence, patients become hypersensitive to all aspects of care from diagnostic procedures to therapeutic interventions, a preoccupation that has diverse detrimental effects. A new sign or symptom may take on considerable significance, interfere with the patient's ability to provide an accurate medical history, significantly augment the apprehension accompanying routine examination and treatment, and generally distract the individual from the pleasures and responsibilities of daily life. If this evolves into a chronic anxiety, patients become burdened with unpleasant moods in addition to the discomfort of their physical pathology. Moreover, continued demands for reassurance from family, friends, and health professionals may progressively alienate supportive persons, ultimately isolating the patient from fundamental sources of emotional support. In this fashion, pathologic anxiety can compromise every phase of medical treatment and decrease the patient's potential for returning to optimal functioning.

THE ANGER RESPONSE

Patients who demonstrate anger as the predominant response to loss of health express the affect in the same way one grieves the death of a loved one—focusing feelings of frustration, resentment, and overt hostility in several directions. They may rage at the gods with a diffuse, globally expressed anger, cursing their bad luck and wondering, "Why me?" Alternatively, they may direct that anger toward themselves; the individual who herniates a lumbar disc while moving furniture holds himself most responsible for the painful disruption of his life. Anger is also focused on family members and friends, whose various behaviors are often implicated as contributors to the development or exacerbation of an illness; a patient may view the demands of her spouse as the primary cause of her hypertension or migraine headaches. Patients may judge members of their social network as insensitive to their plight, or resent family members because of their greater dependence on them. Patients may even blame ancestors for a defective gene pool that predisposes them to a particular illness. Finally, health personnel frequently bear the brunt of a patient's hostility. In addition to providing succor and support, caretakers exert considerable control over the patient's life, which often takes the form of deprivation and discomfort. They subject patients to unpleasant diagnostic tests, restrict diets, limit activity levels, and prescribe medications that cause unpleasant, sometimes dangerous side effects. Moreover, practitioners may fail to cure disease, and often bear grim news about an individual's welfare and mortality. For these reasons, physicians are prime targets for patients' angry feelings.

The hallmark of an anger response is *conflict*. Instead of working through feelings evoked by illness, patients engage in a variety of struggles with the people in their lives. These struggles may be obvious, such as debate surrounding the refusal to submit to a diagnostic procedure or refusal to agree to rehabilitative therapy. The impotent pleas of family members urging reconsideration, as well as the frustration of healthcare providers, mirror the patient's considerable hostility. Struggles may also be covert. They can take the form of passive-aggression, such as ignoring dietary restrictions or irresponsible adherence to a medication regimen, behaviors that afford patients the pleasure of secret control over their caretakers by undermining efforts to help them. Displacement is an additional mechanism with which to disguise true anger about the loss of health. For example, an individual angry about the need for orthopedic surgery that will significantly restrict his physical activity for weeks may start struggling with his wife over long-standing marital difficulties as a way of discharging his feelings about the upcoming surgery and subsequent convalescence.

In sum, the anger response promotes a generalized non-compliance with the treatment, progressively transforming the patients' supportive alliances—including those with their caretakers—into adversarial relationships. In addition to detracting from the level of medical care, this reaction often isolates patients from a support system that could help them negotiate the stressful life situation of ill health.

THE DEPRESSION RESPONSE

Individuals who react to physical illness in this fashion manifest affective, cognitive, and behavioral changes characteristic of a clinical depression (Klerman, 1981; Rodin & Voshart, 1986). These changes vary in degree, depending on factors particular to individuals and their disease process; as a consequence, the intensity of the depression response may range from a relatively mild adjustment disorder to a major depressive episode. The clinical presentation encompasses four general areas of objective and subjective signs and symptoms.

First, alterations of affect occur. This usually presents as a *sustained lowering of mood accompanied by pronounced sadness, tearfulness, and anhedonia*, though affective changes may also include irritability, agitation, and hypomania. Second, the physiological sequelae of depression are manifest in *wide-ranging somatic symptoms* that can affect any organ system (Lindemann, 1944). Third, depression causes changes in usual patterns of behavior beyond those resulting from restrictions imposed by the illness state. This behavior change often takes the form of a *generalized withdrawal*—physically and psychologically—from one's environment. Mounting preoccupation with the loss of health causes patients to invest less and less energy into family matters, social relationships, and professional responsibilities. As this isolation grows, the patient's world becomes increasingly joyless. Finally, as with all types of depression, a prominent aspect of this illness response is *diminished self-esteem*. The effects of physical

impairment, aggravated by the patient's subsequent mood disturbance, raise considerable fear and doubt about the prospect of regaining the premorbid state of health. This negativism fosters self-criticism characterized by feelings of weakness, self-reproach, and worthlessness.

This depressive response to illness affects medical treatment in a variety of ways. Psychophysiological symptoms of depression complicate the diagnosis of a physical illness (e.g., when attempting to differentiate between a dementia and cognitive dysfunction caused by depression), making ongoing evaluation and treatment a difficult task. Depression has the capacity to suppress the immunological response (Schindler, 1985; Schleifer, Keller, Meyerson, et al., 1984), with obvious adverse effects on the body's ability to battle an illness, and can become so severe that it poses a greater threat to the patient than the physical pathology. Neurovegetative symptoms, such as extreme anorexia, may progress to the point of *passive self-destructive behavior; purposeful suicidal actions* also occur (Slaby & Glicksman, 1985). Finally, the withdrawal that is characteristic of the depression response progressively isolates patients from the usual supports of their environment. This subverts the therapeutic alliance with various healthcare personnel, alienates family and friends, and may become so extreme that the individual may essentially abandon the will to live (Engel, 1968).

THE DEPENDENCY RESPONSE

Illness limits autonomy because of factors internal to individual patients (e.g., restrictions caused by specific symptoms, general preoccupation with the disease), as well as external issues (e.g., limitations imposed by the structured hospital routine or requirements of a therapeutic regimen). The adaptive aspect of this regression permits patients to revert to more passive behaviors characteristic of early childhood. *This allows caretakers to take a necessary degree of control of the treatment, and simultaneously provides patients with the comfort and familiarity of diminished responsibility.* The defensive aspect of regression helps patients contend with the distressing emotions precipitated by illness by assigning to others concern and accountability for their welfare.

Although regression helps maintain emotional equilibrium during periods of illness, it can interfere with medical treatment if the dependency becomes too great, too intense, or does not diminish as the physical disorder improves. This danger is addressed in Parsons's (1951) description of the "sick role," which emphasizes the collaborative aspect of medical treatment. During the early phase of illness, functional impairment is legitimized by healthcare personnel who identify affected persons as *patients* and, consequently, exempt them from various societal responsibilities. Patients' dependency on their caretakers is acknowledged and accepted as caretakers labor to make them well. With improvement, however, individuals are expected to assume increasing levels of independent functioning. Parsons envisions this collaborative process as a "common task" between patient and healthcare provider and underscores the fact that individuals bear definite responsibility for aspects of their care (e.g., active participation in long-term rehabilitation). This transition period of the sick role has particular relevance to the dependency response. Patients may find the ministrations of others so gratifying that they are disinclined to strive toward the autonomy of their premorbid life. They abdicate increasing responsibility to family, friends, and healthcare personnel, and savor the nurturing pleasures of dependency. Unfortunately, this decline to greater levels of helplessness compromises patients' physical and emotional well-being.

Excessive dependency is often manifested as noncompliance with medical treatment. This may cause an individual to continue harmful habits (e.g., smoking), to be irresponsible with medications, or to allow known symptoms to get worse before seeking medical attention. Whether these motivations are purposeful or unconscious, they yield the same results—prolonged dependency on health personnel who are obliged to provide the care necessitated by the patient's neglect. In addition to possibly aggravating the patient's physical status, pathologic dependency often subverts supportive relationships. The prevailing dynamics within a family may be considerably disrupted by a patient's continued regression, altering established roles in a manner that undermines the emotional welfare of all concerned. In a similar fashion, relationships with professional colleagues may suffer, and medical personnel may come to view the regressed individual as a "hateful patient" (Groves, 1978), a realistic and understandable countertransference response often triggered by increasingly annoying dependent demands. All these behaviors—which reflect evolution into the role of "professional patient," in which a person becomes more concerned with being cared for than with discharging the responsibilities of adult life—may be overt or covert. It is particularly important for health providers to appreciate a dependency response that might be disguised by seeming compliance. The longer the patient's wish to remain in the sick role goes unrecognized, the likelier it is that the collaborative doctor–patient relationship will degenerate into an adversarial conflict harmful to each member.

MEDICAL PSYCHOTHERAPY

Reasoned attention by medical personnel to the heightened emotions precipitated by an individual's ill health can help facilitate an adaptive adjustment to illness, and thereby prevent the onset of an abnormal illness response. However, all therapeutic measures must be carefully tailored to each patient based on a comprehensive understanding of the patient's illness. Interventions designed to facilitate the grief work accompanying the loss of health are required for some individuals, but contraindicated in patients so overwhelmed by their affective state that they require support of adaptive ego functioning (e.g., by supplying obsessional patients with considerable information about their day-to-day condition, or prescribing psychoactive medications). Unfortunately, many patients become increasingly encumbered by the distressing feelings and harmful behaviors that characterize a particular pathologic reaction to illness. Continued negative impact on their physical and emotional well-being signals the need for

medical psychotherapy, a specialized form of psychotherapeutic intervention. Medical psychotherapy is based on "the communicated understanding between physician and patient concerning the biologic, psychologic and social aspects" of an individual's illness, as discussed by Goldberg and Green (1985). The treatment, which can be utilized for crisis situations (e.g., acute onset of illness) or chronic conditions (e.g., persisting illness), can take either a supportive or introspective approach.

The correlation between grief work and the usual emotional reaction to illness suggests that patients should routinely be guided toward working through feelings about their loss of health. However, that course is sometimes contraindicated, as insight-oriented therapy rests on their ability to tolerate the heightened anxiety attending exploratory work, and certain patients have characteristic personality features that render anxiety-provoking psychotherapy ineffective and/or harmful. Clinicians' expert knowledge concerning the substantive and temporal course of grief work is counterproductive if it prompts them to doggedly confront the defensive structure and maladaptive behaviors in these individuals. For example, patients who exhibit alexithymia, a relative inability to express psychological distress by direct verbal means (Sifneos, 1972–73), are more likely to regress if the clinician attempts to pressure them to confront affects associated with the stages of grieving. Their diminished capacity for self-examination, due to a fundamentally concrete style of perceiving, evaluating, and discussing life events (Nemiah & Sifneos, 1970), often impedes the grief process associated with loss of health.

When treating medical and surgical patients unable to contend with the emotions precipitated by illness, the clinician's most important decision concerns a clear delineation of therapeutic goals. The physician must choose between commending and encouraging the patient's usual style of emotional functioning, or pursuing a more introspective analytic path. The former approach attempts to foster an atmosphere of support and reassurance that can then be exploited to enhance the clinician's positive influence; the latter course attempts to help the patient work through conflictual feelings precipitated by illness. Correct treatment of a patient's abnormal illness response requires the physician to choose between a supportive, anxiety-suppressing approach or an introspective, anxiety-provoking stance as the appropriate form of medical psychotherapy. That clinical decision is based on understanding patients' *illness dynamics*, as well as conjointly assessing their physical state and emotional needs at any given time during their illness.

ILLNESS DYNAMICS

Everyone lives within a distinctive context of supports and stressors that influence day-to-day functioning and interpersonal relationships. *Illness dynamics* refers to those diverse factors as they affect an individual's response to a specific disease at a particular time in life (Green, 1985). Supports and stressors derive from conscious and unconscious determinants that converge in one's mind, causing the patient to perceive, assess, and defend against the loss of health in a highly subjective manner (Box 10.1). Illness dynamics cause patients to evaluate all illness-related information in a fashion that reflects particular values, needs, wishes, and fears, thereby shaping a distinctive perception of ill health. This idiosyncratic biopsychosocial profile may help them accommodate to the emotions precipitated by loss of health or, alternatively, impede that effort.

Illness fosters regression when it affects major sources of gratification for an individual (e.g., an injury that impedes the activity of a vigorous athlete). It may also cause regression by promoting the emergence of unconscious fears (e.g., requiring a Type A individuals to become considerably dependent on caretakers). These types of reactions have widespread impact on the total organism as a result of diffuse mind-body interactions. Reiser (1975) discusses how the brain translates idiosyncratic symbolic meanings of events into physiological changes that may promote the onset of illness and/or aggravate its clinical course, or help maintain a healthy homeostasis. As an illustrative example, he posits the reaction of two individuals with comparable coronary artery disease to the final desperation play of a football game that determines its outcome. The excitement of victory for one individual *or* the disappointment of defeat for the other might precipitate an adverse cardiac event in *either* fan—depending on how each transforms his psychological reaction into a physiological reaction. In the extreme, Reiser suggests that "major life experiences, such as bereavement, can influence even the capacity to sustain the life process itself." This thesis is supported by considerable laboratory and clinical data that include investigation of immunologic responses and cardiovascular functioning (Henry, 1975).

Illness dynamics also affect the doctor–patient relationship as well as sources of support in an individual's social network. According to Lipowski (1975), the process of evaluating the state of ill health

... influences the patient's perceptions and mood as well as the content and form of what he communicates concerning his illness, how, to whom, and when. It affects his decision to seek or delay medical consultation, his degree of compliance with medical advice and management, as well as his relationship with his family, employers, health professionals and other concerned people.

These interactions significantly influence an individual's ability to contend with illness. Engel has discussed the day-to-day impact of these interacting factors on clinical care in both theoretical (1977) and practical (1980) terms. A classic case report of the clinical application of the biopsychosocial model demonstrated how treatment of a middle-aged man suffering an acute myocardial infarction was compromised by inattention to his characterologic structure and style of interpersonal relationships (Engel, 1971). Heightened anxiety, which precipitated neurogenic responses that augmented a potentially fatal arrhythmia, may have been averted had the patient's caretakers been familiar with his illness dynamics—specifically, his need to be obsessively informed about medical procedures in order to satisfy a fundamental need for control.

In sum, *illness dynamics derive from the interplay between the components of one's biological, psychological, and social existence, transforming an episode of ill health into a highly subjective experience. By shaping its meaning in this fashion, these interacting factors can convert the same disease into very different illness experiences in two individuals who require the identical diagnostic assessment, acute treatment, and ongoing care.* Illness dynamics span an enormous and complex range—given the breadth of psychosocial factors influencing and being influenced by a specific organic pathology—causing patients to define their particular ailments in highly idiosyncratic terms. If this results in an abnormal illness response, the clinician must then decide if supportive or introspective psychotherapy is indicated for its treatment.

DETERMINING THE INITIAL THERAPEUTIC APPROACH

The decision of whether patients suffering from an abnormal illness response require introspective (anxiety-provoking) investigation of their emotions, or are more in need of supportive (anxiety-suppressing) treatment—and whether either approach should be supplemented by pharmacotherapy—is founded on the systematic assessment of objective clinical findings. The most fundamental component is an

---

Box 10.1 ILLNESS DYNAMICS

Biological

Nature, severity, and time course of disease
    Affected organ system, body part, or body function
    Baseline physiologic functioning and physical resilience

Psychological

Maturity of ego functioning and object relationships
    Personality type
    Stage in the life cycle
    Interpersonal aspects of the therapeutic relationship
        (e.g., counter transference of health care providers)
    Past psychiatric history
    Effect of medical history on attitudes toward treatment
        (e.g., history of postoperative complications)

Social

Dynamics of family relationships
    Family attitudes toward illness
    Level of interpersonal functioning (e.g., educational and
        occupational achievements; ability to form and maintain
        friendships)
    Cultural attitudes

accurate DSM multi-axial psychiatric diagnosis, particularly as it applies to major mental illness. Psychosis, for example, demands intensive support in the form of highly structured psychosocial and pharmacological interventions. This applies whether the cause is physical (e.g., due thyroid dysfunction) or secondary to acute regression in an individual with a chronic mental illness (e.g., schizophrenia).

When patients do not exhibit evidence of major Axis I pathology, their general level of *ego functioning* and maturity of *object relationships* are the most useful criteria for determining the appropriate type of medical psychotherapy. More specific parameters are the selection criteria for brief psychotherapy proposed by Sifneos (1972), such as the level of sexual development and adjustment, intellectual skills, educational and occupational achievements, and the degree of autonomy and ability to assume responsibility. These criteria broadly assess psychological strengths and weaknesses and measure a person's ability to pursue self-selected goals while simultaneously contending with exceptional stresses of life, such as ill health.

Vaillant (1977) provides a more detailed evaluation of *ego functioning* in his excellent study of basic adaptational styles as determined by *prevailing ego defense mechanisms*. Anxiety-provoking work is definitely contraindicated in an individual who relies heavily on psychotic defense mechanisms (e.g., denial, delusional projection, and distortion). A middle-aged diabetic woman who responds to the recent amputation of her lower leg by acting as if the limb were still intact is ill-suited for introspective work. That individual requires considerable ego support, provided in the form of psychopharmacologic treatment and consistent reality testing. Although immature mechanisms (e.g., schizoid withdrawal, projection, passive-dependent and passive-aggressive behavior, acting-out, and hypochondriasis) may not cause such severe regression, they typify a personality structure that is generally unresponsive to an anxiety-provoking approach because of limitations on the patient's capacity to modulate mood and control impulses. Conversely, the presence of neurotic mechanisms (e.g., intellectualization, repression, displacement, reaction formation, and dissociation) and the more sophisticated mechanisms (e.g., suppression, humor, anticipation, altruism, and sublimation) reflect flexibility and resilience of ego functioning sufficient to tolerate the heightened anxiety of intensive emotional self-scrutiny.

The quality of an individual's *object relationships* provides a general measure of interpersonal functioning, another important barometer of one's ability to tolerate anxiety. This information helps define the patient's motivation and ability to be involved in a productive and gratifying manner with others, important data when assessing capacity for the emotional intensity and mutuality of a therapeutic relationship. The pattern of interaction with family members, friends, and professional colleagues may yield a picture of marked passivity, characterized by a patient's dependency on most of the people in that individual's life. Other maladaptive modes of relating, such as fight–flight behavior or a series of short-lived superficial encounters involving fluctuating idealization and unreasonable denigration of partners, may reflect the extreme anxiety emanating from unresolved issues of separation and individuation. These patterns of object relationships suggest the necessity of a supportive psychotherapeutic approach, one which would be supplemented by pharmacotherapy in more extreme instances such as the inability to differentiate self from nonself. Conversely, patients' object relationships may reveal important criteria for introspective therapy, such as the importance they ascribe to independent functioning, their ability to abdicate autonomy when they recognize the need to rely on the support of others, and a history of at least one meaningful relationship reflecting basic trust and a shared emotional involvement.

Determining the appropriateness of anxiety-suppressing or anxiety-provoking psychotherapy is also influenced by the *patient's willingness for self-scrutiny and desire for emotional change*. These are predicated on a requisite degree of intelligence and psychological-mindedness, often evidenced in people's insights into their reactions to their own illness. *Attention to the therapeutic relationship* can supply other indicators for introspective work, including the patient's realistic expectations concerning the expertise of the therapist and the anticipated goals of treatment, the patient's ability to be affectively and cognitively involved in psychotherapy, and the patient's ability to relate consistently to the therapist throughout encouraging and disheartening phases of both the medical illness and the psychiatric treatment. An individual's responsiveness to trial interpretations provides data concerning each of these indicators for introspective work. Malan (1976), Sifneos (1972), and Davanloo (1980) discuss the diagnostic value of these interventions, and Viederman (1984) describes how communicating to patients an empathic and accurate understanding of their plight enhances a sense of trust that facilitates the psychotherapy.

All factors noted in this section help establish what Karasu and Skodol (1980) call a "psychotherapy diagnosis," a judgment concerning "the psychotherapeutic approach by which the patient is likely to derive maximal benefit" not exclusively determined by diagnostic criteria.

ANXIETY-SUPPRESSING PSYCHOTHERAPY

Ever since Freud (1919) praised the "gold" of psychoanalytic interpretations, supportive psychotherapy has erroneously been considered an "inferior" form of treatment as compared to insight-oriented work. This negative, and unfair, reputation derives from a variety of factors, ranging from the long-standing belief that characterologic change is the primary goal of psychotherapy to the frustration of practitioners who struggle to successfully implement this treatment modality (Wallace, 1983). The relative inattention afforded anxiety-suppressing psychotherapy over the years reflects this bias and may explain why it remains a somewhat nebulous form of treatment. Divergent conceptualizations confuse basic therapeutic issues, such as the distinction between supportive therapy and supportive relationships; and consequently, anxiety-suppressing therapy has frequently been explicated via "negative definitions" that declare *what it is not* (Buckley, 1986).

Winston, Pinsker, and McCullough's (1986) review of the literature significantly clarified the fundamental goals and techniques of this treatment modality, which highlighted its relevance to medical psychotherapy. *Anxiety-suppressing psychotherapy requires the clinician to be active and supportive in ways that contain the patient's anxiety within limits that were acceptable premorbidly and allowed the patient to function.* The overall treatment is focused on symptomatic relief as opposed to structural intrapsychic change, an approach based on concrete, sometimes controlling, therapeutic directives. The major goal of treatment is to dissipate the powerful emotions that negatively affect the patient's psychological well-being. The patient is not guided toward discovery of unconscious motivations and conflicts that may have crystallized into an abnormal illness response. Rather, therapists offer consistent encouragement and support intended to maximize their influence by exploiting a working alliance solidified by trust and cooperation (Werman, 1984). The clinician attempts to curtail emotional dysfunction precipitated by illness by altering factors external to the individual, such as effecting changes in living arrangements or prescribing psychoactive medication. The therapeutic maneuvers most often used to achieve this end are *abreaction, suggestion,* and *manipulation,* as classically described by Bibring (1954).

Abreaction involves catharsis of intense, often unconscious, emotions. Acknowledging and expressing these warded-off feelings brings at least a temporary sense of relief to individuals who, for example, previously resorted to unhealthy behaviors (e.g., social isolation) in order to avoid the impact of unrecognized yet intense affects. Absent the opportunity for such expression these feelings can build up and eventually overwhelm an individual (e.g., with uncontrollable anxiety or morbid depression), akin to a flooded stream overflowing its banks. *Suggestion,* according to Bibring, involves "the induction of ideas, impulses, emotions, actions . . . by the therapist (an individual in authoritative position) in the patient (an individual in dependent position) independent of, or to the exclusion of, the latter's rational or critical (realistic) thinking." He is describing a process of change effected by direct inculcation of beliefs, attitudes, or behavior; for a patient in the throes of an abnormal illness response, this might include insisting on better communication with family members or urging participation in a rehabilitation regimen. *Manipulation* is defined as the therapist's use of words or attitudes to "neutralize certain emotional systems in the patient, mobilize others and utilize them for technical purposes or curative aims." For example, a therapist may attempt to mute the hypochondriasis exacerbating a patient's dependency response by mobilizing healthier obsessional behaviors, such as keeping him apprised of laboratory data that indicate clinical gains.

Because anxiety-suppressing psychotherapy rests on the clinician's ability to influence and guide the patient, *eliciting and maintaining a positive transference* are primary goals of treatment. Careful attention to unconscious issues embodied in an individual's psychodynamics and illness dynamics identifies doctor–patient interactions that may by used by the therapist whose inherent power (Frank, 1961) can be enhanced

in a manner that parallels Alexander's studied manipulation of the transference (1946). Techniques used to foster the positive transference, summarized by Winston, Pinsker, and McCullough (1986), emanate from clinicians' basic posture of presenting themselves as real, objective, and analytic. They offer advice and reassurance (e.g., opinions concerning the patient's response to a given therapeutic regimen), as well as praise when warranted (e.g., when individuals engage in meaningful discussions about their illness with family members or progress in a rehabilitative program). Therapists provide "an auxiliary ego" to their patients, which may take the form of educating them to the facts of their illness, identifying and justifying their affective and behavioral responses to the sick role, explaining changes in interactions with friends and family members, and problem-solving life issues caused by ill health. Therapists communicate all this in a style more personally conversational than clinical, which at times might reveal some of their own feelings and values. The negative transference is addressed only when it directly interferes with treatment, and is interpreted in a circumscribed manner so as to overcome the patient's resistance without mobilizing intense affects that could be potentially disorganizing.

Supporting and enhancing a patient's defensive structure is another major goal of anxiety-suppressing psychotherapy. The therapist must identify and maintain those mechanisms that provide the basis of an individual's ego functioning. This knowledge is useful in helping to reinforce the patient's reality testing, particularly if the patient is observed to utilize projection and distortion. It also highlights important defenses that should not be challenged by the clinician. For example, primitive ego defense mechanisms can be adaptive under some circumstances, such as the denial following a myocardial infarction (Hackett & Cassem, 1974), and prevent a patient from becoming overwhelmed by emotional distress and/or acting out in a self-destructive fashion. In addition to preserving a patient's fundamental defenses, the therapist should attempt to discover and mobilize healthier ego functioning. For example, the reality testing of an individual with diabetes mellitus preoccupied with "slipping into coma," despite excellent control of the illness, might be enhanced by working with the patient's obsessional defenses (e.g., regular, detailed discussion of insulin needs and blood sugars).

Attending to an individual's diminished self-esteem is the third goal of supportive psychotherapy. When stressed by life events that limit the ability to cope with a variety of intensely painful affects, patients often become demoralized and begin to doubt their self-worth. The medical patient needs protection from the isolation attending the sick role and, consequently, benefits significantly from interventions that bolster self-esteem. The therapist's active interest and attention, which communicates concern and respect, can offset feelings of helplessness and hopelessness. Specifically, the clinician is reassuring (e.g., *validating the normalcy of a patient's feeling state),* and offers advice, (e.g., *recommending actions that have helped others plagued by the same illness).* The interventions provide support and educate patients as to the legitimacy of their emotional distress.

Two related aspects of supportive psychotherapy that are particularly relevant to treatment of abnormal illness responses are attention to a specific focus and a defined structure of the therapeutic environment. The *"benign neglect" afforded unconscious material (e.g., fantasies, dreams, and transference distortions)* helps to contain the patient's level of anxiety, which permits him or her to concentrate psychic energies on the "here-and-now." Treatment of individuals in the throes of severe anxiety responses, for example, would *address worries concerning the potentially debilitating effects of their illness* and not explore possible dynamic roots of their considerable separation anxiety. This focus is mirrored in the structure of the therapeutic interaction, which is predominantly characterized by an active *give-and-take* between the two participants, as opposed to the open-ended communication of introspective work and its characteristic intervals of silence. This helps the patient concentrate fully on concrete treatment goals.

ANXIETY-PROVOKING PSYCHOTHERAPY

Insight-oriented psychotherapy seeks to *promote psychological maturation by therapeutically exploiting the turmoil of an emotional upheaval.* The fundamental task is to help patients acknowledge, bear, and *put into proper perspective painful feelings that adversely affect their lives* (Semrad, 1969). This conceptualization of the treatment highlights its relationship to the grief process. The patient is first made aware of previously unrecognized emotions that have been kept out of consciousness by various defensive maneuvers. Patients then experience those affects within the therapeutic environment, as well as in the context of important relationships. Finally, *by recognizing the intensity, diversity, and ambivalence of these feelings, patients come to achieve some resolution of the conflicts such feelings arouse.*

Several disciples of the analytic school have tailored the anxiety-provoking model into a variety of brief psychotherapies well suited for the treatment of an abnormal illness response (Alexander & French, 1946; Davanloo, 1980; Malan, 1976; Mann, 1973; and Sifneos, 1972). Despite conceptual and technical differences, all these approaches share several characteristics: (1) *persistent pursuit of unconscious material (instinctual drives, as well as ego defenses);* (2) *active, confronting interventions by the therapist; and* (3) *attention to a central focus that helps limit the degree of clinical regression.* The goal of such treatment is *working through,* a therapeutic process that guides the patient toward insight and self-understanding so as to effect significant and lasting behavioral change (Greenson, 1967). Except for time limitations—and the fact that the focus of treatment is circumscribed (e.g., to the emotional reaction to physical illness) —the process of these therapies is identical to long-term insight-oriented psychodynamic work.

Anxiety-provoking therapy is studied attention to the interrelationship between two general areas of individuals' lives: first, *their libidinal impulses, the anxiety they provoke, and the defenses utilized to contain them;* and second, *lifelong patterns of object relationships that characterize each person's historical past, current existence, and the transference relationship.* Elucidating the dynamic interaction between these two triads provides patients with meaningful insights that help liberate them from long-standing repetitive maladaptive patterns. Although introspective therapy continually challenges defenses that contain unacknowledged affects, it periodically employs supportive techniques when the level of therapeutic tension threatens the treatment. *Consequently, all the technical maneuvers discussed by Bibring (1954) come into play, though clarification and interpretation are most often used.*

Clarification is a technique in which the therapist restates the patient's observations in a manner that helps define those issues more clearly. In Bibring's words, it refers to aspects of the therapeutic process ". . .which assist the patient to reach a higher degree of self-awareness, clarity and differentiation of self-observation . . ." As an example he describes how a patient's feelings are clarified when the therapist "shows him that what he describes as fatigue. . .is actually an expression of depression" or that certain patterns of conduct reflect typical responses to distinctive situations. *Interpretation*, on the other hand, attempts to bring to awareness one's unrecognized thoughts and emotions. This usually requires prior therapeutic maneuvers, such as manipulation or clarification, in preparation for an appropriately timed interpretative observation that "makes conscious the unconscious meaning, source, history, mode or course of a given psychic event" (Greenson, 1967). That is, interpretations provide insight that helps patients understand unconscious forces that motivate a specific behavior, and thereby afford them an opportunity to modify it.

THE ART OF MEDICAL PSYCHOTHERAPY

As noted, medical psychotherapy generally conforms to an anxiety-suppressing or anxiety-provoking approach. However, focusing only on the theoretical underpinnings and techniques of these two treatments neglects some realities of the clinical environment. The actual implementation of supportive and introspective interventions, within the context of a comprehensive treatment plan, requires *flexibility and pragmatism* on the part of the clinician. The task, which is fundamentally guided by constant attention to the patient's illness dynamics, may be facilitated by the following guidelines.

First, although a specific type of medical psychotherapy is *predominant* in the treatment of an abnormal illness response, a *specific therapy rarely occurs in an isolated form* because of the ever-present interrelationship between anxiety-suppressing and anxiety-provoking techniques. Psychoanalysis, for example, places a premium on therapeutic neutrality and abstinence. However, even Freud acknowledged the importance of supportive maneuvers, most notably as they pertain to maintaining the working therapeutic alliance (Freud, 1913; Greenson, 1967). Alternatively, Winston, Pinsker, and McCullough (1986) discuss "a continuum of supportive therapies" that incorporate expressive (anxiety-provoking) work to a degree determined by the patient's level of ego strength. Pine (1986) emphasizes this point, describing techniques for achieving "interpretive content" in the context of supportive therapy. He outlined specific maneuvers that enable individuals "generally characterized by a fragility of defense" to tolerate this anxiety-provoking intervention. These observations do not blur the distinction between the supportive and introspective approaches as much as they indicate a positive interaction between aspects of each approach, such as the need to interpret negative transference feelings that arise during anxiety-suppressing therapy. In Pine's words, "supportive and insight therapies are not *counterposed*, in some *opposition* to one another, but are *counterpoised*, in some *balance* with one another." The degree to which this occurs in the treatment of an individual's abnormal illness response is guided by the particulars of the patient's illness dynamics.

Second, supportive and introspective treatment have been discussed within the context of a single episode of ill health. However, most illness is chronic, and its elongated time course has implications for the practice of medical psychotherapy, both for the patient and clinician. *The onset of a long-term illness may so overwhelm individuals that they initially can only tolerate an anxiety-suppressing approach; however, this does not suggest that patients will require support throughout the entire clinical course.* Slaby and Glicksman (1985) observe that coping mechanisms appropriate to one stage of life-threatening illness are not necessarily appropriate at later stages. While some patients repeatedly require anxiety-suppressing work during the prolonged course of a disease, others might regress with that approach, since supportive treatment can help reestablish one's emotional equilibrium in a way that eventually fosters a sense of mastery. In this way it can protect against the recurrence of an abnormal illness response during subsequent bouts of ill health, as well as generally enhance adaptive ego function via a positive ripple effect. In this sense, supportive care can parallel the work of crisis intervention as described by Caplan (1964), which promotes the acquisition of new coping mechanisms, increases self-esteem, and diminishes fear about the recurrence of a particular stressor. That same adaptation can derive from a patient's assessment of illness over time, and can replace feared fantasies with the reality of symptomatic relief, loving support from family and friends, and a level of functioning that affords some sense of control over the illness. Such responses can minimize the emotional turmoil accompanying future progression of disease and may even facilitate subsequent anxiety-provoking work designed to help grieve a further decline in health.

Third, consultation-liaison psychiatrists are concerned with the *diagnosis and treatment of psychiatric disorders in the medically ill.* As a result, the practitioner must constantly deal with the interaction between psychic and physical events, which may be overt (e.g., delirium) or subtle (e.g., a "masked" depression). These problems are mind-body in origin, and their treatment frequently utilizes biological interventions in conjunction with psychotherapy. The use of psychoactive medications is often an integral aspect of medical psychotherapy, supplying structure and support the patient lacks because of the physical and/or psychological impact of illness.

Pharmacotherapy provides acute relief of symptoms and, with certain individuals, facilitates continued remission via treatment with maintenance medication. When the treatment goals of an abnormal illness response are concerned with interpersonal relationships, family issues, or occupational and social adjustment, then treatment predominantly shifts to *psychotherapy focused on resolving traumatic and painful emotions associated with the loss of health.*

The interactive effects of psychotherapeutic and biological treatments have been intensively studied. Klerman (1975) demonstrated that the patient's level of affective distress influences their accessibility and response to psychosocial interventions, a powerful argument for the use of medications to facilitate and/or optimize psychotherapy. *Subsequent investigation disproved long-standing hypotheses concerning negative interactions between medications and psychotherapy* (Rounsaville, Klerman, & Weissman, 1981), and further suggested the benefits of combining these therapeutic approaches (Luborsky, Singer, & Luborsky, 1976; Muskin, 1990). As a result, practitioners more readily accept that psychosocial and biological therapeutic interventions are complementary, and that in major mental disorders combined therapy is almost always superior to the exclusive use of one or another treatment as a single modality (Cohen-Cole & Stoudemire, 1987).

The combined approach has been conceptualized as a means of tailoring treatment to the particular state and trait issues affecting an individual (Extein & Bowers, 1979). Van Praag (1979) describes the combination of "tablets and talking"—the former directed toward neurochemically mediated issues (e.g., vegetative symptoms of depression; mania), the latter targeting psychosocial issues (e.g., intrapsychic and interpersonal events). When personality traits form the basis of an individual's pathologic illness response, then medical psychotherapy alone, either as supportive or introspective work, is the indicated treatment. However, pronounced disease-related symptoms often dominate a patient's illness response. For example, up to 20% of general medical inpatients have an anxiety disorder (Strain, Leibowitz, & Klein, 1981); panic disorder is present up to seven times more often in patients in medical settings than in the general population (Rosenbaum & Pollack, 1989); and depression is present in up to 30% of medical inpatients (Rodin & Voshart, 1986). When a patient's symptoms are severe, practitioners must rely on somatic therapies to alleviate affective turmoil as well as to strengthen the therapeutic alliance (Klerman, 1976), as severe agitation or psychomotor retardation can impede collaborative work between patients and caretakers and thereby undermine the effectiveness of psychotherapy.

Some general points concerning combined therapy should be noted. *First, practitioners must be particularly wary of the side effects of psychoactive medications.* Some, which are little more than an annoyance in fundamentally healthy patients, can seriously complicate treatment of the medically ill and sometimes be life-threatening. Also, because many patients who require medical psychotherapy are already taking a variety of other medications, clinicians must be particularly *mindful of drug interactions* when prescribing psychoactive substances (Brown & Stoudemire, 1998). Finally, a particular medication within a general class of psychoactive medications may be indicated for specific medical conditions; for example, because the 2-keto-benzodiazepines (e.g., diazepam,) are metabolized via oxidation in the liver, their clinical effects are subject to the status of hepatic enzymes that may be affected by liver disease or concurrent medications.

Relief from state-related symptoms permits subsequent psychotherapy, which may be predominantly anxiety-provoking or anxiety-suppressing. There are several schools of brief psychotherapy within each of these broad categories, and consequently there is debate as to the therapeutic efficacy of each particular approach. Burke, White, and Havens (1979), for example, argue for the utility of matching a particular patient with a specific form of brief therapy based on the individual's psychosexual development. Utilizing an Ericksonian framework Erickson (1963), they suggest that Mann's (1973) time-limited, existential technique, which focuses on mastery of separation, is most effective for passive-dependent individuals who have not resolved the adolescent conflict of "identity versus role confusion." In contrast, patients with an Oedipal orientation struggling with issues of "intimacy versus isolation" are better served by the more confronting analytic approach of Malan (1976) or Sifneos (1972) that seeks to promote insight. Ursano and Hales (1986), on the other hand, believe that the spectrum of psychotherapies substantially overlap in selection criteria, technique, duration, and goals of treatment, and differ more in types of interventions. This lends support to Bennet's (1984) caution that the clinician refrain from seeking "perfectionism" in trying to fit a patient with a particular form of brief psychotherapy. Ursano and Hales (1986) also underscore how the distinction between brief psychodynamic psychotherapy, interpersonal psychotherapy, and cognitive techniques has more to do with perspective and emphasis of specific aspects of treatment than with fundamental differences in the treatment approach. For example, much of the cognitive therapist's work helping an individual identify faulty perceptions that evolve into maladaptive defenses is quite similar to the clarification and interpretation of defenses in brief psychodynamic psychotherapy.

Fourth, although anxiety-suppressing and anxiety-provoking therapy are founded on a psychodynamic understanding of the patient, each of these treatment modalities has distinctive cognitive and behavioral attributes. For example, clarification and interpretation of defenses and unconscious material remains the foundation of insight-oriented work; however, behavioral interventions (e.g., limit-setting maneuvers) complement the exploratory process. And supportive work can occur within a clinical framework completely apart from psychodynamic psychotherapy. Moos and Schaefer (1984), for example, utilize a cognitive approach based on crisis theory when treating patients unable to cope with the impact of physical illness. They outline two sets of treatment goals for these individuals—illness-related tasks (e.g., dealing with pain and incapacitation, dealing with the hospital environment, and developing adequate relationships with healthcare staff) and general tasks (e.g., preserving a reasonable emotional balance, preserving a satisfactory self-image and maintaining a sense of competence

and mastery, sustaining relationships with family and friends, and preparing for an uncertain future)—and describes the major types of coping skills employed to deal with these various tasks. The treatment includes fundamental interventions of supportive therapy such as education, reassurance, and abreaction, which are effected via cognitive problem-solving techniques. Anxiety-suppressing therapy can also take the form of behavioral interventions, such as relaxation protocols and desensitization (e.g., to treat excessive anxiety) or positive and negative reinforcement (e.g., to deal with excessive regression).

Fifth, although supportive and insight-oriented therapy have been discussed in terms of individual treatment, medical psychotherapy is effected in a variety of clinical formats. An individual's abnormal illness response can be treated in the context of family therapy, couples work, or group psychotherapy. Each approach may be anxiety-suppressing or anxiety- provoking depending on the prevailing illness dynamics. When the psychological well-being of a family is adversely affected by the illness of one of its members (Borden, 1962; Binger, Alblin, Feuerstein, et al., 1969; Livsey, 1972), supportive work can facilitate the family's accommodation to the illness and may actually be part of the individual's treatment (Rosman, Minuchin, & Leibman, 1975). Couples work is indicated when an individual's abnormal illness response causes increasing distance in the relationship and threatens its viability. The psychological health of each member, their dynamic interaction, and the particular losses incurred by the patient's ill health (e.g., decreased sexual function) determine if a supportive or introspective intervention is indicated. The same decision making applies to group therapy. Several attributes of the group process (e.g., diffusion of the transference and greater interpersonal contact) bolster impaired ego functioning and, consequently, favor group therapy as a supportive form of medical psychotherapy. Group therapy patients benefit from information sharing (Bilodeau & Hackett, 1971) and a generalized acceptance of emotional expression (Adsett & Bruhn, 1968; Stein, 1971), as well as the mutual support derived from discussing common medical experiences such as amputation, myocardial infarction, and the impact of a mastectomy or colostomy (Slaby & Glicksman, 1985). As for insight-oriented groups, they have traditionally been used in the treatment of the so-called *classic psychosomatic illnesses* (Stein, 1971) and have been effective in helping patients adjust to terminal illness (Yalom & Greaves, 1977; Spiegel, 1979).

Moos and Schaefer (1984) points out that "a patient may deny or minimize the seriousness of a crisis while talking to a family member, seek relevant information about prognosis from a physician, [and] request reassurance and emotional support from a friend." Because one's illness response can take on such a complexity, varied therapeutic modalities are often used in combination to effect a medical psychotherapy that targets the patient's distinctive needs.

Sixth, mention should be made of the implications for the clinician when a patient's long-term illness necessitates ongoing medical psychotherapy, *particularly when the patient fails to adapt to the loss of health.* That circumstance can readily promote a negative countertransference, which is often related to patients' character pathology (Groves, 1978; Kahana & Bibring, 1964; Lipsitt, 1970) or to specific clinical issues, such as hypochondriasis (Adler, 1981; Brown & Vaillant, 1981). In these instances health providers may become increasingly frustrated and resentful, as they respond to patients' overt and covert negativism by experiencing a corresponding helplessness and hopelessness of their own. When this type of countertransference remains unrecognized, clinicians are more likely to act out their anger as opposed to using it constructively. Sternbach (1974) describes how this destructive cycle sadly produces a multitude of patients derogatorily labeled "crocks," and how antagonism toward them promotes a progressive dissolution of the therapeutic alliance.

SUMMARY

All medical illness produces emotional responses that form an integral part of the disease process. Although many patients successfully accommodate to their particular impairment, others suffer abnormal illness responses because they cannot negotiate the affective turmoil precipitated by ill health. Medical personnel who ignore these psychological reactions provide suboptimal, if not detrimental, treatment. Effective medical care is founded on *understanding what a particular disease means to a particular patient at a particular time in life*. This requires a full understanding of illness dynamics. The patient's illness dynamics define a distinctive biopsychosocial environment that guides clinicians to the specific psychological needs to be addressed during the course of treatment. If this approach fails to abort an abnormal illness response, intensive focused attention via medical psychotherapy should be offered to the patient. *The form of the treatment* is also based on patients' illness dynamics, which measure their ability to tolerate anxiety by providing information concerning the maturity of their ego functioning and object relationships. The psychotherapeutic approach may be supplemented with pharmacotherapy when the patient's affective distress is extreme. This comprehensive biopsychosocial approach is the only acceptable medical model if "one is to treat the whole patient and not merely characterize the nature of an illness and impede biological deterioration" (Slaby & Glicksman, 1985). *The biopsychosocial approach to patient assessment and treatment is the cornerstone philosophy of this entire textbook.*

CLINICAL PEARLS

- When patients do not exhibit evidence of major Axis I pathology, their general level of *ego functioning* and maturity of *object relationships* are the most useful criteria for determining the appropriate type of medical psychotherapy.

- The presence of neurotic ego mechanisms (e.g., intellectualization, repression, displacement, reaction formation, and dissociation) and the more sophisticated ego mechanisms (e.g., suppression, humor, anticipation, altruism, and sublimation) reflect flexibility and resilience of ego functioning sufficient to tolerate the heightened anxiety of intensive emotional self-scrutiny.

- The quality of an individual's *object relationships* provides a general measure of interpersonal functioning, another important barometer of one's ability to tolerate anxiety.

- Viederman (1984) describes how communicating to patients an empathic and accurate understanding of their plight enhances a sense of trust that facilitates the psychotherapy.

- The major goal of supportive treatment is to dissipate the powerful emotions that negatively affect the patient's psychological well-being. The patient is not guided toward discovery of unconscious motivations and conflicts that may have crystallized into an abnormal illness response.

- *Abreaction* involves catharsis of intense, often unconscious, emotions. Acknowledging and expressing these warded-off feelings brings at least a temporary sense of relief to individuals who, for example, previously resorted to unhealthy behaviors (e.g., social isolation) in order to avoid the impact of unrecognized, yet intense, affects.

- Therapists provide "an auxiliary ego" to their patients, which may take the form of educating them to the facts of their illness, identifying and justifying their affective and behavioral responses to the sick role, explaining changes in interactions with friends and family members, and problem-solving life issues caused by ill health.

- The negative transference is addressed only when it directly interferes with treatment, and is interpreted in a circumscribed manner so as to overcome the patient's resistance without mobilizing intense affects that potentially could be disorganizing. In insight-oriented psychotherapy, by recognizing the intensity, diversity, and ambivalence of these feelings, patients come to achieve some resolution of the conflicts such feelings arouse.

- The actual implementation of supportive and introspective interventions, within the context of a comprehensive treatment plan, requires flexibility and pragmatism on the part of the clinician.

- Much of the cognitive therapist's work, helping an individual identify faulty perceptions that evolve into maladaptive defenses, is similar to the clarification and interpretation of defenses in brief psychodynamic psychotherapy

DISCLOSURE STATEMENT

Dr. Green has no conflicts of interest to disclose.

REFERENCES

Adler, G. (1981). The physician and the hypochondriacal patient. *New England Journal of Medicine*, 304(23), 1394–1396.

Adsett, C., & Bruhn, J. (1968). Short-term group psychotherapy for myocardial infarction patients and their wives. *Canadian Medical Association Journal*, 99, 577–581.

Alexander, F., & French, T. (1946). *Psychoanalytic therapy*. New York: Ronald Press.

American Psychiatric Association (1996). *Practice Guidelines*. (pp. 91–96), Washington, DC: American Psychiatric Press.

Bennett, M. (1984). Brief psychotherapy in adult development. *Psychotherapy: Theory, Research, and Practice*, 21, 171–177.

Bibring, E. (1954). Psychoanalysis and the dynamic psychotherapies. *Journal of the American Psychoanalytical Association*, 2, 745–770.

Bilodeau, C., & Hackett, T. (1971). Issues raised in a group setting by patients recovering from myocardial infarction. *American Journal of Psychiatry*, 128, 73–78.

Binger, C. Alblin, A. Feuerstein, R., et al. (1969). Childhood leukemia: emotional impact on patient and family. *New England Journal of Medicine*, 280, 414–418.

Borden, W. (1962). Psychological aspects of a stroke: patient and family. *Annals of Internal Medicine*, 57, 689–692.

Brown, H., & Vaillant, G. (1981). Hypochondriasis. *Archives of General Psychiatry*, 141, 723–726.

Brown, J., & Stoudemire, G. (1983). Normal and pathological grief. *Journal of the American Medical Association*, 250(3), 378–382.

Brown, T. M., & Stoudemire, A. (1998). *Psychiatric side effects of prescription and over the counter medications*. Washington, DC: American Psychiatric Press.

Buckley, P. (1986). Supportive psychotherapy: a neglected treatment. *Psychiatric Annals*, 16(9), 515–521.

Burke, J., White, H., & Havens, L. (1979). Which short-term therapy? *Archives of General Psychiatry*, 36, 177–187.

Caplan, G. (1964). *Principles of preventive psychiatry*. New York: Basic Books.

Cohen-Cole, S., & Stoudemire, A. (1987). Major depression and physical illness. *Psychiatric Clinics of North America*, 10(1), 1–17.

Davanloo, H. (Ed.). (1980). *Short term dynamic psychotherapy*. New York: Aronson.

Engel, G. (1968). A life-setting conducive to illness: the giving-up-given-up complex. *Annals of Internal Medicine*, 69, 293–298.

Engel, G. (1971). Sudden and rapid death during psychological stress. *Annals of Internal Medicine*, 74, 771–782.

Engel, G. (1977). The need for a new medical model: a challenge for biomedicine. *Science*, 196, 129–136.

Engel, G. (1980). The clinical application of the biopsychosocial model. *American Journal of Psychiatry*, 137, 535–544.

Erickson, E. (1963). *Childhood and society*. New York: W.W. Norton.

Extein, I., & Bowers, M. (1979). State and trait in psychiatric practice. *American Journal of Psychiatry*, 136, 690–693.

Frank, J. (1961). *Persuasion and healing*. Baltimore: Johns Hopkins University Press.

Freud, S. (1913). On beginning the treatment. In J. Strachey (Trans. & Ed.). *The standard edition of the complete psychological works of Sigmund Freud* (Vol. 12, pp. 121–144). London: Hogarth Press, 1955.

Freud, S. (1919). Lines of advance in psychoanalytic therapy. In J. Strachey (Trans. & Ed.). *The standard edition of the complete psychological works of Sigmund Freud* (Vol. 17; pp. 157–168). London: Hogarth Press, 1955.

Goldberg, R., & Green, S. (1985). Medical psychotherapy. *American Family Physician*, 31(1), 173–178.

Green, S. (1985). *Mind and body: The psychology of physical illness*. Washington, DC: American Psychiatric Press.

Greene, W., Goldstein, S., & Moss, A. (1972). Psychosocial aspects of sudden death. *Archives of Internal Medicine*, 129, 725–731.

Greenson, R. (1967). *The technique and practice of psychoanalysis* (Vol. I). New York: International Universities Press.

Groves, J. (1978). Taking care of the hateful patient. *New England Journal of Medicine*, 298, 883–887.

Hackett, T., & Cassem, N. (1974). Development of a quantitative rating scale to assess denial. *Journal of Psychosomatic Research*, 18, 93–100.

Henry, J. (1975). The induction of acute and chronic cardiovascular disease in animals by psychosocial stimulation. *International Journal of Psychiatry in Medicine*, 6, 147–158.

Kahana, R., & Bibring, G. (1964). Personality types in medical management. In N. Zinberg (Ed.). *Psychiatry and medical practice in a general hospital* (pp. 108–123). New York: International Universities Press.

Karasu, T., & Skodol, A. (1980). VIth axis for DSM-III: psychodynamic evaluation. *American Journal of Psychiatry*, 137, 607–610.

Katon, W. (1987). The epidemiology of depression in medical care. *International Journal of Psychiatry in Medicine*, 17, 93–112.

Katon, W. Von Korff, M. Lin, E. et al. (1990). Distressed high utilizers of medical care: *DSM-III-R* diagnosis and treatment needs. *General Hospital Psychiatry*, 12, 355–362.

Klerman, G. (1975). Combining drugs and psychotherapy in the treatment of depression. In M. Greenblatt (Ed.). *Drugs in combination with other therapies* (pp. 213–228). New York: Grune & Stratton.

Klerman, G. (1976). Combining drugs and psychotherapy in the treatment of depression. In J. Cole, A. Schatzberg, & S. Frazier (Eds.), *Depression: Biology, psychodynamics and treatment* (pp. 213–227). New York: Plenum Press.

Klerman, G. (1981). Depression in the medically ill. *Psychiatric Clinics of North America*, 4(2), 301–318.

Levenson, J. L., Mishra, A. Hamer, R., et al. (1989). Denial and medical outcome in unstable angina. *Psychosomatic Medicine*, 51, 27–35.

Lindemann, E. (1944). Symptomatology and management of acute grief. *American Journal of Psychiatry*, 101, 141–146.

Lipowski, Z. (1975). Psychiatry of somatic disease: epidemiology, pathogenesis, classification. *Comprehensive Psychiatry*, 16, 105–124.

Lipsitt, D. (1970). Medical and psychological characteristics of "crocks." *Psychiatry in Medicine*, 1, 15–25.

Livsey, C. (1972). Physical illness and family dynamics. *Advances in Psychosomatic Medicine*, 8, 237–251.

Lown, B. Verrier, R., & Rabinowitz, S. (1977). Neural and psychologic mechanisms and the problem of sudden cardiac death. *American Journal of Cardiology*, 39, 890–902.

Luborsky, L. Singer, B., & Luborsky, L. (1976). Comparative studies of psychotherapies. In R. Spitzer & D. Klein (Eds.). *Evaluation of psychological therapies*. Baltimore: Johns Hopkins University Press.

Malan, D. (1976). *The frontier of brief psychiatry*. New York: Plenum.

Mann, J. (1973). *Time-limited psychotherapy*. Cambridge: Harvard University Press.

Moos, R., & Schaefer J. (1984). The crisis of physical illness: an overview and conceptual approach. In R. Moos (Ed.), *Coping with physical illness, 2, new perspectives* (pp. 3–26). New York: Plenum.

Muskin, P. (1990). The combined use of psychotherapy and pharmacotherapy in the medical setting. *Psychiatric Clinics of North America*, 13(2), 341–353.

Nemiah, J., & Sifneos, P. (1970). Psychosomatic illness: a problem of communication. *Psychotherapy and Psychosomatics*, 18, 154–160.

Parsons, T. (1951). *The social system*. Glencoe, IL: The Free Press.

Pine, F. (1986). Supportive psychotherapy: a psychoanalytic perspective. *Psychiatric Annals*, 16(9), 526–529.

Regier, D., Hirschfeld, R., Goodwin, F., et al. (1988). The NIMH Depression Awareness, Recognition and Treatment Program: structure, aims, and scientific basis. *American Journal of Psychiatry*, 145, 1351–1357.

Reich, P., DeSilva, R., Lown, B., et al. (1981). Acute psychological disturbances preceding life-threatening ventricular arrhythmias. *Journal of the American Medical Association*, 246, 233–235.

Reichard, J. (1964). Teaching principles of medical psychology to medical house officers: methods and problems. In N. Zinberg (Ed.). *Psychiatry and medical practice in a general hospital* (pp. 169–204). New York: International Universities Press.

Reiser, M. (1975). Changing theoretical concepts in psychosomatic medicine. In M. Reiser (Ed.). *American handbook of psychiatry.* (Vol. 4, pp. 477–500). New York: Basic Books.

Rodin, G., & Voshart, K. (1986). Depression in the medically ill: overview. *American Journal of Psychiatry, 143,* 696–705.

Rosenbaum, J., & Pollack, M. (1989). Anxiety. In T. Hackett & N. Cassem (Eds.). *Massachusetts General Hospital Handbook of General Hospital Psychiatry* (2nd ed., pp. 154–183). Littleton, MA: PSG Publishing Company.

Rosman, B., Minuchin, S., & Leibman, R. (1975). Family lunch session: an introduction to family therapy in anorexia nervosa. *American Journal of Orthopsychiatry, 45,* 846–853.

Rounsaville, B. Klerman, G., & Weissman, M. (1981). Do psychotherapy and pharmacotherapy of depression conflict? *Archives of General Psychiatry, 38,* 24–29.

Schindler, B. (1985). Stress, affective disorders, and immune function. *Medical Clinics of North America, 69,* 585–597.

Schleifer, S. Keller, S. Meyerson, A., et al. (1984). Lymphocyte function in major depressive disorder. *Archives of General Psychiatry, 41,* 484–486.

Semrad, E. (1969). A clinical formulation of the psychoses. In E. Semrad & D. van Buskirk (Eds.). *Teaching psychotherapy of psychotic patients* (pp. 17–30). New York: Grune & Stratton.

Sifneos, P. (1972). *Short-term psychotherapy and emotional crisis.* Cambridge: Harvard University Press.

Sifneos, P. (1972–73). Is dynamic psychotherapy contraindicated for a large number of patients with psychosomatic diseases? *Psychotherapy and Psychosomatics, 21,* 133–136.

Sifneos, P. (1973). The prevalence of "alexithymic" characteristics in psychosomatic patients. *Psychotherapy and Psychosomatics, 22,* 255–262.

Slaby, A., & Glicksman, A. (1985). *Adapting to life-threatening illness.* New York: Praeger.

Spiegel, D. (1979). Psychological support for women with metastatic carcinoma. *Psychosomatics, 20,* 780–787.

Stein, A. (1971). Group therapy with psychosomatically ill patients. In H. Kaplan & B. Sadock (Eds.). *Comprehensive group psychotherapy* (pp. 581–601). Baltimore: Williams & Wilkins.

Sternbach, R. (1974). Varieties of pain games. *Advances in Neurology, 4,* 423–430.

Stoudemire, A. (Ed.). (1995). *Psychological factors affecting medical conditions.* Washington, DC: American Psychiatric Press.

Stoudemire, A., & McDaniel, J. S. (1999). History, classification, and current trends in psychosomatic medicine. In B. Sadock & V. Sadock (Eds.). *Comprehensive textbook of psychiatry* (7th ed.). Baltimore: Williams & Wilkins (in press).

Strain, J., Leibowitz, M., & Klein, L. (1981). Anxiety and panic attacks in the medically ill. *Psychiatric Clinics of North America, 4,* 333–350.

Ursano, R., & Hales, R. (1986). A review of brief individual psychotherapies. *American Journal of Psychiatry, 143,* 1507–1517.

Vaillant, G. (1977). *Adaptation to life.* Boston: Little, Brown.

Van Praag, H. (1979). Tablets and talking: a spurious contrast in psychiatry. *Comprehensive Psychiatry, 20,* 502–510.

Viederman, M. (1984). The active dynamic interview and the supportive relationship. *Comprehensive Psychiatry, 25,* 147–157.

Wallace, E. (1983). *Dynamic psychiatry in theory and practice.* Philadelphia: Lea & Febiger.

Werman, D. (1984). *The practice of supportive psychotherapy.* New York: Brunner/Mazel.

Winston, A., Pinsker, H., & McCullough, L. (1986). A review of supportive psychotherapy. *Hospital and Community Psychiatry, 37*(11), 1105–1114.

Yalom, I., & Greaves, C. (1977). Group therapy with the terminally ill. *American Journal of Psychiatry, 134,* 396–400.

11.

FAMILY THERAPY IN CHRONIC MEDICAL ILLNESS

Gabor I. Keitner

Advances in healthcare technology, more medical treatment options, and more choices for improved lifestyle have contributed to longevity and more patients living with chronic illness and disability. The extended period of time spent with disability or chronic illness has profound effects on the lives of loved ones caring for and living with such patients (Schulz & Beach, 1999). The ways in which a patient's family of caregivers, in turn, deal with illness has a significant impact on the course and outcome of that illness. It is important to understand this reciprocal relationship between illness and family coping in order to assess the patient and social situation and to provide appropriate family interventions.

The goals of this chapter are to provide an overview of the impact of illness on families, to provide evidence for the benefit of family intervention for medially ill patients and families, to describe a model of family assessment that can guide relevant treatment options, and to present a family intervention approach that is applicable in a wide range of clinical circumstances.

THE IMPACT OF ILLNESS ON THE FAMILY

Numerous studies have evaluated the impact of a wide range of illnesses on families and caregivers. These include cardiovascular disease (Coyne et al., 2001; Gallo et al., 2003; Rohrbaugh, Shoham, & Coyne, 2006), diabetes (Fisher, Chesla, Skaff, Mullen, & Kanter, 2002) cancer (Cliff & MacDonagh, 2000; Manne, Norton, Winkel, Ostroff, & Fox, 2007; Northouse, Mood, Templin, Mellon, & George, 2000; Rolland, 2003; KL Weihs, Enright, T., & Simmens, 2008), gastrointestinal disorders (Baanders & Heijmans, 2007), fibromyalgia (Bigatti & Cronan, 2002), neurological disorders (De Ridder, Schreurs, & Bensing, 1998; Helder et al., 2002), rheumatoid arthritis (Riemama, Taal, & Rasker, 1999), chronic pain (Margolis, Merkel, Tait, & Richardson, 1991), hemodialysis (Kimmel et al., 2000), and dementia (Vitaliano et al., 2001).

Instead of detailing the unique problems associated with each of such a wide range of disorders, it is more useful to find common factors that most families experience while dealing with illness. Understanding the nature of such general stresses should allow for thinking of commonalities in family treatment approaches.

Research on families and health has led to the following general conclusions: (1) family relationships have a powerful influence on health, as great as that of well-known biomedical risk factors; (2) marriage is the family relationship with the greatest impact on health for adults; (3) the most important type of support provided by families is emotional support; and (4) the adverse effects on health of critical or hostile family relationships are of greater magnitude than the beneficial effects of positive or supportive relationships (Campbell, 2003).

Families influence health by a variety of different pathways. In addition to sharing genes that are risk factors for diseases or influences on the effectiveness of treatment, families that live together share exposure to infectious agents, noxious environments, or toxic substances. Behavioral patterns relevant to health such as smoking, eating habits, exercise, and adherence to prescribed medical treatments tend to be shared within families. Finally, family relationships also can affect physical health via neuroendocrine and psychoimmunologic mechanisms (Campbell, 2003).

There are a wide variety of responses by family members to chronic illness in their loved ones, ranging from functional adaptation to significant dysfunction. More than one-half of families caring for the chronically ill manage the burden effectively (Rabins, Fitting, Eastham, & Fetting, 1990). Such families are able to adapt to changing circumstances and are able to balance the needs of individuals and the family system so as to ensure the family's well being. A family's response to the illness of a member depends more on that family's functioning than on the nature of the illness. In general, the perceived impact of the illness on significant others is not dependent on the type of chronic disease (Baanders & Heijmans, 2007). More important is the adequacy of the fit between the psychosocial demands of the illness, the family's coping style, and the availability of adequate resources.

A biopsychosocial perspective of the family's situation ensures that the biological, psychological, and social components impacting the family are sufficiently evaluated. Biological parameters include the nature of the illness, physical limitations, and current pharmacological treatments. Psychological parameters include the meaning of the illness and its specific symptoms to the patient and to the family, habitual ways of coping with difficulties, personality styles, frustration tolerance and impulse control, intellectual functioning, insight, and spirituality. Social parameters include interpersonal and family relationships, social connections and support systems, work functioning, and other situational stresses. Such a comprehensive evaluation leads to a biopsychosocial formulation that is shared with the patient and family as a foundation for developing an appropriate treatment plan.

A basic task for families dealing with chronic disorders is to create ways of understanding the illness that allows the family to retain a sense of competence and mastery (Rolland, 2003). Rolland (2003) has described a family systems health model for the assessment of and intervention with families facing chronic and life-threatening disorders. This model identifies three dimensions: psychosocial types of disorders, major phases in the natural history of the illness, and key family system variables.

Psychosocial types of illness refer to the demands on the family made by the varying nature of disorders. Some illnesses have an acute or gradual onset. Illnesses can be progressive, constant, or relapsing -remitting. Outcomes can be hopeful or terminal. Different phases of illness (crisis, chronic, terminal) also impose their own demands on the family requiring different adaptations. Key family variables that impact on the family's capacity to cope effectively include the family and individual life cycle, multigenerational legacies related to illness and loss, and belief systems.

A family is best understood and helped by utilizing such a broad conceptual framework, which takes into consideration the demands of the illness and the coping capacities of the family.

A number of family characteristics have been demonstrated by multiple studies to influence illness outcomes. Protective factors include good communication, adaptability, clear roles, achieving family development tasks, support for individual members, expression of appreciation, commitment to the family, social connectedness, spending time together, and religious/spiritual orientation (Weihs et al., 2002). Conversely, many risk factors for detrimental illness outcome have also been identified. These include low cohesion/closeness, poor family organization, inconsistent structure, poor conflict resolution, lack of agreement about disease beliefs and expectations, low relationship satisfaction, high conflict, high criticalness, poor problem solving, and high hostility (Fisher, 2006).

It is helpful to understand such protective and risk factors in order to develop and implement family treatment approaches that modify the risk factors and enhance those that are effective.

EVIDENCE FOR BENEFIT OF FAMILY INTERVENTIONS IN MEDICAL ILLNESS

A wide variety of family interventions have been developed and tested for many medical illnesses, including dementia, cardiovascular diseases, cancer, diabetes, arthritis, stroke, chronic pain, traumatic brain injury, systemic lupus erythematosis, and AIDS (Chesla et al., 2004). In spite of differences, most family approaches can be divided into two broad

categories: psycho-educational and relationship-focused. The goals of psycho-educational interventions are to increase knowledge about the illness and to teach patients and family members more effective ways of managing it. Skills training includes lifestyle modifications relating to diet and exercise, learning skills to monitor the illness such as blood pressure monitoring, and supporting adherence to prescribed medical treatment (DiMatteo, 2004). Relationship-focused interventions attempt to directly improve family functioning by helping families to communicate more effectively, solve problems, resolve conflicts, and develop a greater sense of cohesiveness. These interventions also include some degree of education about the illness and discussion of more effective illness-related coping skills.

Two meta-analyses of family/psychosocial interventions for adult patients with chronic illnesses have been published (Hartmann, Bazner, Wild, Eisler, & Herzog, 2010; Martire, Lustig, Schultz, & Miller, 2004). Martire et al. (2004) used meta- analysis to focus on the benefits of interventions that involved a family member, for patients and for family members. Patient outcomes examined included depressive symptoms, anxiety, relationship satisfaction, physical disability, and mortality. Family member outcomes included depressive symptoms, anxiety, relationship satisfaction, and caregiving burden. Family psychosocial interventions were defined as nonmedical interventions that were psychologically, socially, or behaviorally oriented and that involved a member of an adult patient's family or both the patient and the family member. All studies had to be randomized controlled trials and all had to include a comparison of the family intervention with a usual medical treatment. Of 235 studies identified, 70 met criteria for inclusion in this analysis. The majority of the family interventions consisted of a combination of different types of psychosocial and behavioral approaches. Most commonly these included education with emotional support or emotional support with skills training. Family members included spouses, children, or siblings. The most common illness groups studied were individuals suffering from dementia, cardiovascular disease, osteoarthritis, pulmonary disease, Parkinson's, and cancer.

Overall results showed the strongest evidence of efficacy for benefits to family members, with lesser evidence for an effect on the outcome of the patient's disease. Family interventions led to family members feeling less depressed and less burdened. The interventions also led to reduced anxiety in family members when the therapeutic focus was on relationship issues between the patient and the family member. Interestingly, the interventions did not appear to enhance the family member's satisfaction in his or her relationship with the patient. The family interventions led to a reduction in depressive symptoms in the patient only when the interventions focused on spouses or couples. Family interventions also enhanced patients' survival, particularly for patients with cardiovascular disease. This was more likely to happen when the interventions did not address relationship issues. There was no evidence that the family interventions reduced anxiety or disability in patients or that they increased their relationship satisfaction. Changes in patients were not dependent on whether the patient was or was not included in the intervention. Family interventions were not associated with negative outcomes for either the patient or his/her family members (Martire et al., 2004).

Hartmann et al. (2010) also conducted a meta-analysis of randomized clinical trials evaluating the effects of family-based interventions for adult patients compared to standard treatment. Family interventions were categorized as being psycho-educational or those that addressed relationships and attempted to improve family functioning directly. The family was defined as any significant person with a close relationship to the patient. This meta-analysis focused on three outcomes: the physical health of the patient, including level of functional dependency, clinical symptoms, self-rated physical health status, and disease management; the mental health of the patient, including degree of depression, degree of anxiety, quality of life, general mental health, and self efficacy; and the health of family members, including caregiver burden, depression, anxiety, general mental health, and self efficacy in the family member. Sub-analyses were conducted to identify possible moderators such as types of disease, types of interventions, and types of family members involved in the treatment. Fifty-two randomized clinical trials involving over 8,000 patients (52% women) were chosen from over 4,000 potentially eligible studies. The diseases studied included cardiovascular diseases and stroke, cancer, arthritis, diabetes, AIDS, and systemic lupus erythematosus. All family interventions led to significantly better physical health of patients compared to standard treatment. Both psycho-educational and relationship-focused interventions showed a significant positive effect. The overall effect was greater when the family member involved in the treatment was a spouse rather than another type of significant other.

Family interventions also led to improved mental health of the patient compared to standard treatment. In this case it did not matter whether the involved family member was a spouse or another type of family member. Again, both psycho-educational and relationship-focused interventions showed similarly significant positive effects. Family members' health, such as caregiver burden, depression, anxiety, quality of life, and self-efficacy, were all improved by family interventions. In this case, relationship-focused interventions were more effective than those focused on psycho-education.

The results of this meta-analysis showed that family-oriented interventions in chronic illnesses were more effective for improving health outcomes and reducing mental health problems in both patient and caregivers than were commonly used treatments (Hartmann et al., 2010). Although the results were small, if statistically significant, effects, they corresponded to an OR of 1.7 to 1.84, meaning the patients receiving the family intervention had a 72%–84% greater chance of improved health compared to those receiving usual care. Family interventions also produced a more sustained improvement then standard care alone. There was also a tendency toward greater benefits from a longer course of family treatment, and a greater patient benefit when the family treatment focused on spouses as opposed to other family members.

These reviews show that many different types of family interventions are effective in helping to deal with a wide range of medical illnesses. They do not provide information on what specific interventions may be the most helpful for a given illness at a particular point in time, nor what are the mechanisms that lead to change. It is impractical to try to learn many different types of family therapies for different disorders, particularly when there is not any evidence to suggest such a need. It makes more clinical sense to become familiar with a family approach that lends itself to application in a wide variety of situations. The key to effective family treatments is a comprehensive evaluation of the family's needs and functioning, so that the intervention can be adjusted to meet those needs.

The first essential step in family therapy is an assessment of the family.

FAMILY ASSESSMENT

The essential task in meeting with families for the first time is to evaluate and assess their functioning in the context of understanding their problem. The family assessment is the first step in determining both the need for further interventions and the specific areas of family life that might need to be addressed. The family assessment provides more information about the problem as well as the social system. The family social system is the substrate for the evolution of the problem and may be contributing to improving or maintaining it. Family assessment should focus on (a) adjustments related to the diagnosis of the medical illness, (b) clarification of treatment options, and (c) collaboration in carrying out a treatment plan. The assessment should also identify family strengths.

There are many different ways to assess a family and many different kinds of information that can be gathered. Some assessments begin with a long history of the family's life, past connections, and evolution as a family unit. This can include information on families of origin and the construction of a family genogram. Other assessments focus mainly on process issues in the family during the assessment. The focus is on observations of current family interactional patterns, with the assumption that these are representative of the way in which the family deals with issues outside of the assessment session. All of these approaches have merit, and they are not mutually exclusive. The challenge for a clinician is to integrate various aspects of these different approaches in such a way as to meet the goals of the evaluation without becoming sidetracked by peripheral issues or too much detail, and taking so long to complete the evaluation that the family loses interest.

The most important step in meeting with a family for the first time is to establish connection with the family. The family needs to feel understood, respected and validated. The clinician needs to put the family members at ease and make them feel comfortable enough to participate openly in the assessment process. Family members should not be blamed for their loved one's problems and should not be judged for perceived deficiencies in managing an illness. The assessment is used to gain a better understanding of how everybody sees the problems at hand, to gather information to allow for a more comprehensive treatment plan, to provide an opportunity for all members involved in trying to cope with the illness to ask questions and to solicit the help of all involved in setting up a meaningful treatment plan. It is useful to have as many family members and significant others as possible attend an initial assessment. Significant others can include extended family members, good friends, coworkers, other healthcare providers, and spiritual counselors.

GOALS OF THE FAMILY ASSESSMENT

There are three overriding goals when conducting a family assessment. The first is to orient the family to the assessment process by establishing an open and collaborative relationship with those present. The second goal is to have all family members identify current problems and concerns. The third goal is for the clinician to identify the family's transactional style, which may be relevant for understanding the way the family deals with illness in one of the family members. Dysfunctional transactional patterns are repetitive interactional processes that prevent effective resolution of ongoing interpersonal problems. The assessment can take from 1 to 2 hours depending on the nature of the family's problems and the skill level of the clinician (see Box 11.1).

MODEL OF FAMILY ASSESSMENT

A comprehensive family assessment should be focused and systematic. The McMaster Model of Family Functioning (MMFF) is one of the more developed and validated family assessment and treatment models available (Ryan, Epstein, Keitner, Miller, & Bishop, 2005). It provides a framework for evaluating multiple dimensions of family functioning, leading to a structured treatment program as indicated. The assessment process consists of four identifiable components: orientation, data gathering, problem description, and problem clarification (see Box 11.2).

Box 11.1 GOALS OF THE FAMILY ASSESSMENT

1. Establish an open and collaborative relationship to orient family

2. Have all family members identify current problems and concerns

3. Opportunity for clinician to identify family's transactional style

---

Box 11.2 COMPONENTS OF FAMILY ASSESSMENT

A. Orientation

B. Data Gathering

C. Problem Description

D. Problem Clarification

The *orientation* explains the purpose of the evaluation and establishes goals for the assessment process. It is helpful to normalize the assessment process by explaining that family meetings are a regular component of the assessment and treatment of most patients. The clinician explains that the goal of the meeting is to provide an opportunity for all family members to identify what they see as problems and to bring up any areas of concern. They should also be assured that they will have an opportunity to ask questions and that they will be included in the development of ongoing treatment plans.

During the *data gathering stage,* the clinician should clarify the family members' names, ages, relationships within the family, and living arrangements. It is also helpful to find out what family members do for a living and the phase of the family's life cycle. The clinician should then ask each family member what he or she perceives are the problems. Each family member should be given sufficient time to be able to *identify problems,* and all family members should be helped to express their concerns without being interrupted by others. The challenge for the clinician is to gather sufficient information so as to be able to understand the problems but not to get so bogged down in details that there is no time for the exploration of other problems and concerns. Once the presenting problems are clearly outlined and there is consensus between the clinician and the family that its problems are understood and agreed upon, the clinician then moves on to assess *broader dimensions of family functioning.* These include problem-solving, communications, roles, affective responsiveness, affective involvement, and behavior control (see Box 11.3).

Problem-solving refers to a family's ability to resolve problems to a level that maintains effective family functioning. Family problems can be affective or instrumental. *Affective problems* refer to difficulties in dealing with emotions such as anger or sadness. *Instrumental problems* refers to problems of everyday life, such as managing resources and dealing with daily obstacles. Questions about family problem-solving skills can be general, or the family can be asked to think of recent problems that they have dealt with to use as an example. The following questions may be helpful in exploring problem-solving skills: **Who noticed the problem? What was done after the problem was noticed? Did you discuss the problem together? What did you decide to do about the problem? Did you follow through on the decision that**

Box 11.3 BROADER DIMENSIONS OF FAMILY FUNCTIONING

a) Problem-solving

b) Communications

c) Roles

d) Affective responsiveness

e) Affective involvement

f) Behavioral control

---

was made about the problem? Did you review whether the solution to the problem worked or not? Do you deal with emotional and practical problems in the same way?

Communication refers to verbal exchange of information within the family. Nonverbal communication is obviously also very important but much more difficult to assess reliably. Communications can also be affective or instrumental. Families can have marked difficulties in affective communications but can communicate very well about instrumental issues. Families with poor functioning tend to have unclear and indirect forms of communication. The following questions may be helpful in exploring how the family communicates: **How much time to do spend talking with each other? Can you talk about practical things with each other? Can you talk about your feelings with each other? Do you feel that you can say what you want to, or do you have to be guarded about what you say? Can you talk to each other directly, or do you have to go through someone else to let each other know how you think or feel?**

Roles are repetitive patterns of behavior by which family members fulfill family functions such as the provision of resources, nurturance and support, sexual gratification, personal development, and maintenance and management of the family system including decision making, boundaries, and household finances. The following questions may be helpful in exploring family roles: **How do you divide family responsibilities? Who does the cooking? Who does the shopping? Who cleans the house? Who handles the money? Who looks after the home and cars? Who gets involved with the children's education? Who is involved in major decisions? Are responsibilities fairly shared between family members?**

Affective responsiveness refers to whether family members are able to respond to the full spectrum of feelings experienced in emotional life, and whether the emotion experienced is appropriate for the situation. It refers to a person's capacity to experience particular types of emotions. It assesses whether family members tend to be overcome with feelings or are not sufficiently capable of experiencing them. Two types of feelings are assessed. *Welfare emotions* consist of affection, warmth, tenderness, support, and happiness. *Emergency emotions* include fear, anger, sadness, and disappointment. The following questions can be helpful in eliciting information regarding emotional responsiveness: **Does anyone in the family seem to be overly emotionally responsive? Are there some family members who do not seem to respond with enough feelings? Do some people feel too happy or sad or angry, or not enough?**

Affective involvement refers to the extent to which the family shows interest in and values the activities of individual family members. Do family members show an appropriate amount of interest and concern for each other? Are they involved with each other? Do they support each other, or are they disconnected? The following questions can help explore aspects of affective involvement: **Does anybody care about what is important to you? Do you feel that your family is there for you? Do you think that they are really concerned about you, or are they just going through the motions? Do you think that your family intrudes too much into your life?**

Behavior control refers to the ways in which a family establishes rules about acceptable behavior related to physically dangerous situations, situations involving meeting and expressing psychological needs and drives, and situations involving socializing behavior between family members and people outside the family. It concerns parental discipline toward children as well as standards and expectations of behavior that adults set for each other. The following questions can be used to explore behavior control in the family: **Do you have rules in the family about how to handle different situations? Do you allow hitting or yelling at each other? Do you have rules about drinking? About driving too fast? Do you have rules about letting each other know where you are when you are away from home? Are the rules clear? Are they consistent? Do you know what to expect if the rules are broken? How do you deal with a disagreement about rules?**

ADDITIONAL INVESTIGATIONS

A comprehensive family assessment should not preclude a diagnostic workup that also includes psychological and biological information. For adults this may include a psychosocial history, psychiatric examination, medical history, and physical examination. Laboratory and radiology tests as well as neurological and psychological assessments should be ordered as indicated. Information from any of these sources may add to the understanding of what the family is dealing with.

PROBLEM DESCRIPTION

After an assessment, the problems that a family faces and the family's ways of dealing with the problems should be clear to both the clinician and the family. It is helpful to try to group problems into related clusters to avoid getting bogged down with excessive detail or to have such a large problem list that it makes the family feel overwhelmed. What may seem to be many different problems often emanate from a few core problems.

PROBLEM CLARIFICATION

The final step in the assessment process is to obtain agreement between the clinician and family members on the problems identified. If the clinician has been careful to listen to each family member and has checked out the understanding of the problems with the family, there should be good agreement on the final problem list. If there are disagreements about the problem list, these should be resolved before proceeding to recommendations for treatment.

TOOLS FOR FAMILY ASSESSMENT

There are family assessment instruments that allow for a quantifiable evaluation of family functioning, to track change over time, make comparisons with other families, and to carry out quantitative research.

SUBJECTIVE FAMILY RATING SCALES

Subjective family rating scales are self-report paper-and-pencil or computer touchscreen instruments filled out by individual family members to reflect their views of their family's functioning. These scales are cost effective, as they can be filled out in less than 30 minutes and do not require trained interviewer time. The disadvantage to their use is that they are restricted to an internal perspective of family functioning and may not reflect ways that a family may appear to function to an outside observer. Different scales also emphasize different aspects of family functioning or measure the same concept differently. Family members can fill out these instruments in the waiting room or at home before the first session, as well as during the course of treatment as a way of monitoring progress. The following are examples of commonly used instruments.

Family Assessment Device (Epstein, Baldwin, & Bishop, 1983): Assesses the dimensions of the McMaster model of family functioning—problem-solving, communication, roles, affective responsiveness, affective involvement, behavior control, and general functioning.

Dyadic Adjustment Scale (Spanier, 1976): Measures satisfaction, cohesion, consensus, and affectional expression in couples.

Family Environment Scale (Moos & Moos, 1981): Assesses relationship (cohesion, expressiveness, conflict), personal growth (independence, achievement, mortality/religion), and system maintenance (organization, control).

Family Adaptability and Cohesion Evaluation Scale III (Olson et al., 1989): Measures of adaptability (rules, power structure, roles) and cohesion (emotional bonding, autonomy, boundaries).

Self-Report Family Inventory (Beavers & Hampson, 1990): Assesses conflict resolution, styles of relating, intergenerational boundaries, and family competence.

EXTERNALLY RATED INSTRUMENTS OF FAMILY FUNCTIONING

These instruments are administered by trained interviewers and provide a more "objective" view of a family's functioning. They modify the tendency on a family's part to want to see themselves in a particular way. A disadvantage of these instruments is that they are relatively expensive to use, as they take longer to administer and require trained interviewers to rate the family reliably. The following are some of the commonly used instruments.

The Global Assessment of Relational Functioning (GARF) scale is similar to the individual based Global Assessment of Functioning but focuses instead on relational adjustment and on the quality of the family environment (Rosen et al., 1997). The GARF measures relational functioning on a scale of 1–99. Scores of 1–28 apply to a family that is too dysfunctional to be able to function together; scores of 21–40 describe a family that is seriously dysfunctional; scores of 41–60 define a family that has occasional times of satisfactory functioning, but dysfunction predominates; scores of 61–80 define the family that is functioning with some dissatisfaction; and scores of 81–99 define a family where family functioning is satisfactory. Areas assessed include problem solving, organization, and emotional climate.

The McMaster Clinical Rating Scale is a semistructured interview that assesses family dimensions including communications, problem solving, affective involvement, affective responsiveness, roles, behavior control, and general functioning (Miller et al., 1994).

The Beavers Interactional Styles Scale evaluates a family's competence and style. It also assesses power, parental coalitions, clarity of expression, conflict, negotiation, responsibility, and empathy (Beavers & Hampson, 1990).

The Camberwell Family Interview measures expressed emotion, the amount of criticism expressed by family members about each other, emotional overinvolvement, and the extent to which family members are involved in each others lives (Brown & Rutter, 1966).

The Psychosocial Adaptation to Illness Scale is a semistructured interview that evaluates patient and family adjustment to illness (Derogatis, 1986).

There is no absolute advantage to either an external or internal perspective on family functioning. Both perspectives are important, and each may be relatively more useful to answer different kinds of questions. A discrepancy between an outside evaluator and family members' perception of their family's functioning, as well as differences between individual family member's views of their own family's functioning, may provide particularly useful clinical information about the family's problems. Information from both kinds of assessments can be complimentary. Which one is used will depend on the questions being asked and the time and resources available to undertake the evaluation.

A systematic assessment of the family is central to understanding the relevant issues in the family and their potential role in influencing the patient's presenting problems. A good family assessment can be therapeutic in and of itself, as it provides an opportunity for family members to express and listen to concerns in a safe, nonjudgmental environment. The assessment of the family is part of a comprehensive biopsychosocial formulation that should be the foundation for a treatment plan that deals with the medical illness.

FAMILY THERAPY

There are many different schools of family therapy. These include strategic family therapy, structural family therapy, experiential family therapy, narrative therapy, cognitive behavioral family therapy, solution-focused therapy, emotionally focused family therapy, integrative family therapy, and problem-centered family therapy (Gurman & Jacobson, 2002; Nichols, 2010; Pisani & McDaniel, 2005). There is reasonable empirical evidence at this time that family interventions, as adjuncts to medical treatment, provide benefits to patients and family members above and beyond what they receive from usual medical treatment. There have not been any studies to date that compare the relative effectiveness of different types of family therapy. One cannot say with any degree of assurance that any particular type of family therapy is better than another for any particular type of disorder or any particular type of family problem. Therapists tend to practice the kind of family therapy that they are familiar with, regardless of the problems they are presented with. How can a clinician interested in learning family therapy techniques to help families deal with the impact of medical illness know what to do, given this undefined state of affairs?

The large numbers of family therapies can be broadly divided into two groupings, *psycho-educational interventions* and *relationship-focused interventions*. Psycho-educational interventions educate patients and family members about disease processes, what is required for the best care for these diseases, information about how individuals and families are affected by the disease, and ways in which family interactions and behaviors can influence the course and outcome of that disease. Psycho-educational interventions assume that increased knowledge by family members will lead to better disease management and treatment outcome. Psycho-educational interventions can be provided to individual families or in a multifamily group format (Gonzalez et al., 1989).

Relationship-focused family interventions focus on the quality of intrafamilial life, the nature of interpersonal relationships in the family, and processes that prevent family members from being able to work together in such a way as to feel connected with each other and effective in dealing with demands being placed on them. Relationship-focused interventions involve attempts to improve communications, ways of solving problems, managing conflicts, setting realistic expectations, and increasing mutual support. Relationship-focused family interventions may also involve educating the family about the illness.

It is very unlikely that any one therapist can become proficient in a number of different types of family therapy. It may be useful to integrate different elements from different schools of family therapy for a given family, but there is a risk of losing focus and confusing families when the therapist does not have an internally consistent therapeutic framework. It is probably less confusing for therapists and their patients if the therapist is proficient in and practices, at most, one or two types of family therapy. A therapist may best be served by learning a family therapy model that is not rigid, one that encourages a broad assessment of the family's needs, and one that enlists the open collaboration of the family in working toward mutually agreed goals in treatment.

The Problem Centered Systems Therapy of the Family (PCSTF) (Ryan et al., 2005) is one such model of family treatment. The PCSTF was developed to help families clearly identify their needs and concerns, to assess obstacles in the way of addressing their concerns, and to work with them to develop more effective ways of functioning as a family. It is a generic family treatment model that addresses a wide range of family problems.

Problems in the family as they deal with a medical illness may come to the attention of clinicians in a variety of ways. Patients may be continually noncompliant with treatment. There may be lack of improvement in spite of following treatment recommendations. Patients may show signs of anxiety

and sadness along with feelings of being left alone to deal with their illness, feeling that they are not receiving sufficient support, or feeling blamed. There may be persistent disagreements and misunderstandings between the patient, family members, and treatment providers. Patients may also directly express concern about relationship problems at home when asked (see Box 11.4).

Particularly problematic times for the family in the course of a patient's illness are at the time of acute symptoms and diagnosis, during the acute treatment period (particularly if symptom control takes time), and during the maintenance phase when patients and families need to adjust to the reality of persistent symptoms with a chronic illness. Although the kinds of problems presented by these different phases of the illness may vary, the family's ways of dealing with the problem are likely to be consistent over time. It is largely for that reason that it is most useful to focus on the family's usual coping skills, ways of functioning, and problem-solving processes rather than attempting to tailor a particular family approach to a particular illness at a particular period of time. The goal should be to help a family identify its strengths and weaknesses in order to be able to make decisions about what they want to do, and, if they are willing, to help them to learn to deal with problems more effectively. Learning more effective ways of dealing with problems will put a family in the best position to deal with a variety of unforeseen problems in the future.

PROBLEM CENTERED SYSTEMS THERAPY OF THE FAMILY

The PCSTF is a problem-focused, behaviorally directed family therapy model that empowers families to work effectively on resolving distressing situations (Keitner, Heru, & Glick, 2010). A unique feature of the PCSTF is that it focuses on stages of treatment rather than on specific intervention skills or particular personality characteristics of the therapist. These stages are referred to as *macro stages of treatment* and differ from *micro-family techniques*, which occur within the macro stages. The major value attached to this treatment model is that optimal family functioning is most likely to be achieved when there is open, direct, and clear communication among family members. Apart from this expectation, the model leaves it up to the family to determine which aspects of their family's lives they are content with and which they wish to see change, regardless of how an external evaluator may see the family's problems. The only exception to this norm is when there is evidence of dangerous behavior in the family, such as physical and emotional abuse of any family members. The PCSTF has been empirically validated as a useful adjunct in the treatment of patients with mood disorders (Miller et al., 2005, 2008; Solomon, Keitner, Ryan, Kelley, & Miller, 2008).

The PCSTF emphasizes the need for a comprehensive understanding of the family system, including its problems and strengths. In addition to the presenting problems, the assessment includes understanding the structure, organization, and transactional patterns within the family. The assessment process includes reviewing multiple dimensions of family life as described above in the assessment section. The presenting problem may not necessarily be the most important one. Focusing prematurely on the presenting problem, without understanding the broader context in which it is embedded, may lead to a preoccupation with peripheral issues and to missing a problem that might be generating the most distress. A thorough assessment also reassures family members that they are being understood, and helps them take a step back to understand their problems from a broader perspective.

It is preferable to include as many family members as possible, at least for the initial assessment. Having all family members present gives a clear signal that everybody is involved in the process and that each person may have an impact on outcome. It can also encourage family members to participate actively in the treatment process. Subsequent meetings can be more limited in the number of participants, depending on the issues being discussed and logistics concerning the ability of different family members to participate in the available time.

The emphasis is on the macro or major stages of treatment. These stages are *assessment, contracting, treatment, and closure. Micro moves* refers to specific techniques such as labeling, clarifying communication patterns, or focusing the family on a particular problem. Macro and micro moves are different from a therapist's particular personality style, which may include qualities such as choice of wording, use of gestures, and ways of helping families to look at difficult situations. A number of schools of family therapy have become well known because of the particular personality style and skills of a charismatic family therapist. The PCSTF focuses on these stages and steps in therapy and depends less on the particular personality of the therapist. It accommodates therapists with a variety of clinical styles.

The therapist models open and direct communication with the family by explaining his or her formulations and actions with the family along each step of the therapy process, and makes sure that family members clearly understand and agree. The PCSTF assumes that family members understand their problems and are interested in changing them and that they have the capacity to do so with support and guidance.

Active collaboration with all family members reinforces the therapeutic alliance between the therapist and the family. The family needs to be an active and willing participant in each step of the treatment. There needs to be agreement between the therapist and family members about the formulation of the presenting problem and about the steps that are likely to be helpful in resolving them. The family also has to be committed to following through on the steps agreed upon to bring about the desired change in the family. The therapeutic contract is based on this mutual commitment to work at therapy.

The family's strengths are recognized and fostered during treatment. It is much easier and more helpful to the family to reinforce its strengths rather than trying to eliminate its weaknesses. Too much focus on pathology may bring about more pathology. The therapist helps the family recognize its own capacities to address and deal with difficult situations.

Family members are directly involved in identifying, clarifying, and resolving their difficulties. The role of the therapist is that of a catalyst, clarifier, and facilitator. The therapist provides a safe environment in which family members can be more open with each other, communicate more clearly with each other, and be more active in their problem solving. The goal is to help families develop effective problem-solving methods that can be generalized to resolve future difficulties.

The PCSTF focuses mostly on the current problems. When appropriate, it may be necessary to review past issues to obtain a full understanding of how the current problems came about, what it means to the individual family members, and what attempts have been made at resolution; but once the meaning of the problem is understood, the focus is on what the family wants to do about it now.

Changing attitudes, beliefs, and opinions is important, but the PCSTF emphasizes change primarily in observable behaviors. Such changes in behavior are the defined goals of treatment. Cognitions and affect are important, but behavioral change is more measurable and manifest. It is much easier to change what one does than what one thinks and feels.

Treatment is generally time-limited, taking six or eight sessions spaced over a period of weeks or months. The length of each individual session or the time between them will vary depending on the issues involved, the stage of treatment, and the urgency of the situation. The assessment session(s) may take longer (up to an hour or an hour and a half) while a later task-setting treatment session may range from 15 minutes to 45 minutes. Imposing time limitations on therapy sessions tends to stimulate therapist and families to be more actively involved in the treatment process, thereby facilitating change.

STAGES OF TREATMENT

The stages of treatment are assessment, contracting, treatment, and closure. Each stage contains a sequence of sub-stages, the first of which is always orientation. Orientation at each stage of the process is a critical component. Family members need to be oriented as to what to expect. Their agreement and permission to proceed needs to be obtained before treatment can begin, and again during the treatment process. It models a way of approaching potentially difficult situations and can be useful in minimizing resistance that may emerge in later stages, reminding families of their agreement to collaborate in the treatment goals.

ASSESSMENT

The assessment stage is made up of orientation, data gathering, problem description, and problem clarification. The assessment stage is the most important of the macro stages. It is the stage during which information and observations are gathered so as to be able to develop a comprehensive and meaningful biopsychosocial formulation, which is the roadmap for effective treatment. The assessment stage has three main goals. First, the therapist orients the family to the treatment process and establishes an open collaborative relationship with family members. Second, the therapist, with the help of family members, identifies all current problems in the family including the presenting problem. Third, the therapist identifies to families dynamic interactional patterns that appear to be related to the family's problems. The therapist's formulation is presented to the family for acceptance as accurate or for revision as needed. The assessment stage should not be rushed. Extra time taken at this point may well reduce the number of task-oriented treatment sessions that will be required later in the treatment process. The process of identifying, clarifying, and understanding various family members' perspectives of the problems are often therapeutic in and of themselves.

The therapist should orient the family by letting them know the purpose of the meeting and by finding out what each expects will happen during the session and what they hope the outcome will be. The orientation should normalize the meeting by explaining that this is common practice with most patients, as a way of avoiding the implication that there is something wrong with this particular family. The therapist should also empower the family by letting them know that not only will they be asked questions but they will also have the opportunity to ask questions of the therapist and will be included in any decisions about treatment options. If the family has no questions and is in agreement, then the next step is to gather the necessary data.

During the data-gathering stage, information is collected about the presenting problems, overall family functioning, additional investigations that may be indicated, and other potential problems. The therapist asks each family member what he or she thinks are the problems in the family. During this process the family learns to focus on specific issues, to communicate concerns clearly, and to listen. It is important to give each family member time to articulate concerns. Once the presenting problems have been sufficiently and clearly delineated, the family's overall functioning needs to be assessed. At this point the therapist can assess the family along the dimensions of the McMaster Model of Family Functioning (communications, problem solving, affective involvement, affective responsiveness, roles, behavior control) as outlined earlier in this chapter. The assessment should focus on detailing strengths and difficulties in each of these areas of family life to determine their impact on the family's ability to cope with illness. The emphasis should be on strengths, because this will be central to the therapeutic planning that will follow.

Throughout the assessment stage the therapist needs to be aware of and recognize potentially dysfunctional transactional patterns. Dysfunctional patterns tend to occur in association with the presenting problems and can be dealt with once the problem is more comprehensively understood.

Additional investigations may be helpful to be able to arrive at a comprehensive biopsychosocial assessment. The therapist should gather appropriate information concerning medical history, physical examination findings, and related laboratory and radiological tests. Much of this information may need to be gathered outside of the assessment session itself, but it is information that needs to be incorporated into a proper understanding of what the family is trying to deal with.

The purpose of the problem-description step is to summarize the identified difficulties and to develop a list of problems to be addressed. The family and the therapist need to come to mutual agreement about the problem list. Any disagreements need to be resolved before the treatment process can proceed. With clarification and agreement on the problems, the family can move on to the stage of contracting.

CONTRACTING

The goal of this stage is to prepare a contract between family members and the therapist that delineates the expectations, goals, and commitments regarding therapy. The steps in this stage include orientation, outlining options, negotiating expectations, and drawing up a contract. The therapist orients the family to the stage of deciding what they want to do about the problems and solicits their agreement to move forward.

Although there are many options for how to deal with a variety of different problems, in fact there are generally four broad options that family members can choose in dealing with any problem. The family can continue to function as before, without attempting to bring about any change. The family can attempt to work out their problems on their own, without the help of the therapist. The family can choose another type of treatment. The family can agree to engage with the therapist in the current treatment format.

The likelihood of a successful outcome for therapy will be greatly enhanced if family members proactively, out of their own free will, agree to engage in the treatment process and in defining their own goals. The therapist should not try to persuade or entice the family into treatment. The only exception to this general rule is when a dangerous situation exists such as physical abuse, suicidality, or a behavior pattern that can significantly worsen illness in a family member.

The goal of the contracting stage is to formulate a set of expectations that each family member wants to see occur in order for the problems to be resolved successfully. The expectations should be stated in concrete behavioral terms to allow for clearly identifying and assessing change. The behaviors should be observable to all family members. The therapist and family should take each of the problems outlined in the assessment and negotiate a set of behavioral goals related to those problems—which, in fact, if carried out, will give the family a sense that they are making changes. The main technique for establishing treatment goals is that family members negotiate what they would like from each other and how they want each other to change. The therapist's primary role during this process is to facilitate the interaction between family members to ensure that clear, behaviorally defined expectations of change are established. The therapy should also make sure that expectations are realistic for the time frame the family has designated to make the changes. The therapist may also need to raise additional problems that are not addressed by the family during the negotiating process, particularly if the therapist feels those problems may be central to the ongoing difficulties the family is experiencing. It is useful to limit, to two or three at a time, the number of changes that any family member expects from others. It is helpful to write down the list of expectations from each family member in order to decrease the likelihood of misunderstandings in subsequent meetings.

TREATMENT

The goals of the treatment stage are to develop and employ problem-solving strategies to change the identified problems. Two therapeutic techniques are used to accomplish these goals. The first is focused on producing behavioral change in the family through task setting. The therapist helps the family to set tasks that they can work on between meetings. Evaluation of the success or failure of the family in accomplishing these tasks becomes the main focus of the work in subsequent family sessions. The second set of techniques promotes cognitive and behavioral changes that are likely to increase the family's ability to address their problems successfully. The treatment stage consists of orientation, clarifying priorities, setting tasks, and task evaluation.

The first step, as usual, is to orient the family to this new stage and to obtain their permission and collaboration to proceed. Clarifying priorities involves listing problems in order of importance. In general, priorities should be given to problems that involve communications and behavioral control because problems in these areas can lead to difficulties in solving other problems. If families cannot communicate about issues, it is going to be difficult for them to negotiate expectations. Similarly, if chaotic behavior is allowed to proceed, this is likely to disrupt treatment.

When setting tasks, the therapist asks the family to negotiate with each other what changes they would like from each other that, if carried out, would represent a move in the direction of meeting their expectations of change. The problem to be worked on is taken from the priority list. Such behavioral changes are the tasks the family will be working on during the course of treatment. If family members are unable to come up with reasonable tasks and expectations from each other, the therapist may have to make some suggestions, checking with the family to ensure that these are agreeable to everyone. When negotiating and assigning tasks, the therapist should consider the following general principles.

The therapist should be open and direct with the family about the purpose of the assigned tasks. Often it is not a specific task that is important, but the fact that family members are making an effort to meet each other's needs in a way that is different from their usual patterns. The task should be direct and purposeful and not paradoxical. The idea is not to back the family into change, but to have them move toward it in a proactive and purposeful manner. Tasks should be directed toward bringing about change in those dimensions of family functioning that had been identified as problematic during the assessment process.

Tasks should be directed at changing dysfunctional family transactional patterns. The initial tasks should be simple and achievable to increase the potential for success. As the family gains confidence in themselves and are empowered by the process of change, more complicated tasks can be negotiated. Tasks should be reasonable with regard to age, gender, and sociocultural norms for that family. Tasks should be oriented toward increasing positive behaviors rather than decreasing negative ones. Tasks should be behavioral and concrete enough to be understood and evaluated by family members.

Tasks should be meaningful and important to the family. Family members should feel that they could accomplish the tasks assigned to them, making it likely that they will commit themselves to carrying them out. Emotionally oriented tasks should emphasize positive, not negative, feelings. Tasks should fit reasonably into the family's schedule of activities.

A maximum of two tasks per session is usually reasonable in order not to overload the family. Assignment of tasks to family members should be balanced so that major responsibility for completing tasks does not reside with one or two members. Vindictiveness and rehashing of the past should be avoided, and focus should be placed on constructive ways of dealing with the current situation. These principles of task setting are made explicit to the family when tasks are being negotiated (see Box 11.5).

Task evaluation is a critical process. This is the crux of the therapeutic work. It is in the review of the family's success or failure in carrying out the tasks that the real issues in the family become manifest. The tasks, apart from their intrinsic value, are a stimulus for core family issues to emerge and become more evident, not only to the therapist but also to the family members through the eyes of the therapist. Obstacles in carrying out agreed tasks become stimuli and catalysts for bringing about

---

Box 11.5 PRINCIPLES OF TASK SETTING

1. Reasonable in regard to age, gender, sociocultural norms

2. Oriented to increasing positive behaviors

3. Behavioral and concrete so everyone can assess outcome

4. Meaningful and important

5. Feasible

6. If emotional, focused on positive emotions not negative

7. Fit into family schedule

8. Maximum of 2 tasks per session

9. Balance assignment of tasks among family members

10. Focused on constructive solutions (avoid vindictive rehashing)

subsequent changes. The ways in which families have difficulty accomplishing tasks provide the best immediate evidence of what the family needs to work on. Failure to accomplish tasks should not be seen by the therapist or the family as an obstacle to change, but as an opportunity to gain a much clearer insight into the problems of the family in a more immediate, nonintellectual and affective manner. If the family is committed to the change process, awareness of the particular ways in which they run into obstacles in carrying out their tasks allows them to make more constructive and effective changes.

If the agreed upon tasks are accomplished, the therapist provides positive reinforcement, reviewing and highlighting the positive aspects of the family's performance to ensure that the family members understand what worked so they can continue to resolve problems in the future. If the tasks are not accomplished or only partially accomplished, the therapist needs to go through the particular steps in some detail to find out what went wrong. Failure to accomplish a task provides important information about difficulties that may not have been fully understood during the assessment process.

In addition to reviewing the specifics of the family's attempt to accomplish a failed task, it is also important to determine whether the task was too difficult for that particular family at that particular time. If the task was too difficult, a simpler task, broken down into smaller, more manageable pieces, may be needed. A task may have failed owing to difficulties that were not apparent during the previous assessment. In this case, knowledge of the new difficulties can be incorporated into the formulation of the family's problems and into the setting of new tasks.

A failed task may also mean that the family is not interested in working to bring about change. They may have changed their minds about their commitment to therapy, or they may decide that the amount of effort involved is too great. If noncompliance is a key reason for the failure of tasks, this needs to be addressed with the family directly to determine if they are invested enough in the treatment process to make treatment succeed. In general, unless there is a dangerous situation involved, it should be more important for the family to obtain good results in therapy than it is for the therapist. If they are not ready to commit to the treatment process, they should be offered the opportunity to return to the therapist at some future date if and when they decide they are ready to make the effort they will need to put into the treatment. This perspective can be offered in a supportive way, indicating that success comes with true commitment when the family has the time and energy to apply themselves to the process.

During the treatment stage, the major part of each session is devoted to reviewing previously assigned tasks and developing and negotiating new tasks. There are, however, other specific intervention tools that can help the therapist and family negotiate their way through the process of bringing about meaningful change. The therapist can be helpful by clarifying problems and can provide feedback on the perception of family functioning. Clarification of problems helps families become aware of processes in the family patterns of organization and problem solving of which they may not have been aware. It is assumed that with sufficient knowledge, changes

will more readily take place. The therapist can also label and interpret transactional processes and unacknowledged affect. Labeling and interpreting of process is based on observable behaviors that occur during the therapy sessions, therefore making them more immediate and real. By learning to understand the transactional patterns, families can modify them to be less destructive. The therapist can also provide education to modify incorrect assumptions, expectations, and information about the illness, its consequences, and treatment options. Providing the family with information about the illness, its etiology, course, and treatment may help to eliminate misunderstandings and empower the family to develop better coping skill for managing the illness.

CLOSURE

The final macro stage of closure consists of orientation, summary of treatment, long-term goals, and follow-up. During the orientation step, the therapist points out to the family that the goals of treatment have been met. If the family wants to continue with further therapy, this needs to be renegotiated. It is expected that families should be able to resolve new issues that come up using their newly learned coping skills. They should return for treatment only if they run into significant problems that they could not resolve on their own. It is important not to make professional patients out of families by keeping them too dependent on the therapist. Family members should be asked to summarize what they have learned during treatment. The therapist confirms or elaborates on their perceptions and adds any insights that may have been overlooked. The family is encouraged to discuss and set long term goals. They should identify issues they anticipate might come up or prove problematic in the future. The family is supported by recognizing that they have been able to make significant gains and that they have developed effective ways of identifying and dealing with family problems. The therapy ends at this point, although for some families an intermittent follow-up schedule may be appropriate. This could be at 3, 6, or 9 months. If needed, the follow-up session should support and monitor progress rather than rehash issues that have already been dealt with.

SUMMARY

There is increasing evidence that involving the families of patients with a wide range of medical illnesses improves the management of the illness as well as the functioning of the ill patients' family members. Recognition of this evidence should lead to greater attempts at routinely involving the families of medically ill patients in their care. In reality, this does not happen commonly. Involving families will only happen when clinicians not only recognize the importance of doing so, but also feel competent to engage, assess, and treat families. Training in family assessments and family interventions are not standard components of most healthcare training programs. The goal of this chapter is to present a model of assessment and treatment that can be readily implemented.

Most families cope very well with adversity and do not require family therapy. Even families that are coping well, however, can benefit from further support and education as a way of helping them to sustain their efforts. Other families have a more difficult time in adapting to and dealing with the onset and course of an illness in one of their family members. It is becoming increasingly clear that it is in the patient's and family's best interest to address difficulties with a knowledgeable healthcare provider. The clinician's job in helping to manage an illness can also be made easier if families are included as collaborators in the disease management process. Recognition of this reality will, it is hoped, encourage clinicians to become trained in how to provide family assessment and interventions.

CLINICAL PEARLS

- A basic task for families dealing with chronic disorders is to create ways of understanding the illness that allows the family to retain a sense of competence and mastery (Rolland, 2003).

- The key to effective family treatments is a comprehensive evaluation of families' needs and their functioning so that the intervention can be adjusted to meet those needs.

- What may seem to be many different problems often emanate from a few core problems.

- A good family assessment can be therapeutic in and of itself.

- Optimal family functioning is most likely to be achieved when there is open, direct, and clear communication among family members.

- The presenting problem may not necessarily be the most important one.

- This model assumes that family members understand their problems and are interested in changing them, and that they have the capacity to do so with support and guidance.

- It is much easier and more helpful to the family to reinforce its strengths rather than trying to eliminate its weaknesses.

- It is much easier to change what one does than what one thinks and feels.

- The process of identifying, clarifying, and understanding various family members' perspectives of the problems are often therapeutic in and of themselves.

- The therapist should not try to persuade or entice the family into treatment.

- It is useful to limit, to two or three at a time, the number of changes that any family member expects from others.

- Often it is not a specific task that is important but the fact that family members are making an effort to meet each other's needs in a way that is different from their usual patterns.

- Tasks should be oriented toward increasing positive behaviors rather than decreasing negative ones.

- It is in the review of the family's success or failure in carrying out the tasks that the real issues in the family become manifest.

- Unless there is a dangerous situation involved, it should be more important for the family to obtain good results in therapy than it is for the therapist.

DISCLOSURE STATEMENT

Dr. Keitner has no conflicts to disclose.

REFERENCES

Baanders, A., & Heijmans, M. (2007). The impact of chronic diseases. *Family and Community Health*, *30*(4), 305–317.

Beavers, R., & Hampson, R. B. (1990). *Successful families: Assessment and intervention*. New York: Norton.

Bigatti, M., & Cronan, T. (2002). An examination of the physical health, healthcare use, and psychological wellbeing of spouses of people with fibromyalgia syndrome. *Health Psychology*, *21*(2), 157–166.

Brown, G. W., & Rutter, M. (1966). The measurement of family activities and relationships: A methodological study. *Human Relations*, *19*, 241–263.

Campbell, T. L. (2003). The effectiveness of family interventions for physical disorders. *Journal of Martial and Family Therapy*, *29*(2), 263–281.

Chesla, C., Fisher, L., Mullan, J., Skaff, M., Gardiner, P., & Chum, K. (2004). Family and disease management in African-American patients with type 2 diabetes. *Diabetes Care*, *27*, 2850–2855.

Cliff, A. M., & MacDonagh, R. P. (2000). Psychosocial morbidity in prostate cancer: II. A comparison of patients and partners. *BJU International*, *86*(7), 834–839.

Gurman, A. S., & Jacobon, N. S. (Eds.). (2002). *Clinical handbook of couple therapy* (3rd edition) New York: The Guilford Press.

Coyne, J. C., Rohrbaugh, M. J., Shoham, V., Sonnega, J. S., Nickles, J. M., & Cranford, J. A. (2001). Prognostic importance of martial quality for survival of congestive heart failure. *American Journal of Cardiology*, *88*, 526–529.

De Ridder, D., Schreurs, K., & Bensing, J. (1998). Adaptive tasks, coping and quality of life of chronically ill patients. The case of Parkinson's disease and the chronic fatigue syndrome. *Journal of Health Psychology*, *3*, 87–101.

Derogatis, L. (1986). Psychosocial adaptation to illness scale. *Psychosomatics*, *30*, 77–91.

DiMatteo, M. (2004). Variations in patients' adherence to medical recommendations: A quantitative review of 50 years of research. *Medical Care*, *43*(3), 200–209.

Epstein, N. B., Baldwin, L. M., & Bishop, D. S. (1983). The McMaster family assessment device. *Journal of Marital and Family Therapy*, *9*(2), 171–180.

Fisher, L. (2006). Research on the family and chronic disease among adults: Major trends and directions. *Families, Systems, and Health*, *24*(4), 373–380.

Fisher, L., Chesla, C., Skaff, M., Mullen, J., & Kanter, R. (2002). Depression and anxiety among partners of European-American and Latino patients with type 2 diabetes. *Diabetes Care, 25*, 1564–1570.

Gallo, L. C., Troxel, W. M., Matthews, K. A., & Kuller, L. H. (2003). Martial status and quality in middle-aged women: Associations with levels and trajectories of cardiovascular risk factors. *Health Psychology, 22*(5), 453–463.

Gonzalez, S., Steinglass, P., & Reiss, D. (1989). Putting the illness in its place. *Family Process, 28*(1), 69–87.

Hartmann, M., Bazner, E., Wild, B., Eisler, I., & Herzog, W. (2010). Effects of interventions involving the family in the treatment of adult patients with chronic physical diseases: A meta-analysis. *Psychotherapy and Psychosomatics, 79*(3), 136–148.

Helder, D., Kaptein, A., Van Kempen, G., Weinman, J., Van Houwelingen, J., & Roos, R. (2002). Living with Huntington's disease: Illness perceptions, coping mechanisms, and spouses' quality of life. *International Journal of Behavioral Medicine, 9*(1), 37–52.

Keitner, G. I., Heru, A. M., & Glick, I. D. (2010). Family assessment. In *Clinical manual of couples and family therapy* (pp. 63–92). Washington: American Psychiatric Publishing.

Kimmel, P., Peterson, R., Weihs, K., Shidler, N., Simmens, S., & Alleyne, S. (2000). Dyadic relationship conflict, gender, and mortality in urban hemodialysis patients. *Journal of the American Society of Nephrology, 11*, 1518–1525.

Manne, S., Norton, T., Winkel, G., Ostroff, J., & Fox, K. (2007). Protective buffering and psychological distress among couples coping with breast cancer: The moderating role of relationship satisfaction. *Journal of Family Psychology, 21*(3), 380–388.

Margolis, R., Merkel, W., Tait, R., & Richardson, W. (1991). Evaluating patients with chronic pain and their families: How you can recognize maladaptive patterns. *Canadian Family Physician, 37*, 429–435.

Martire, L., Lustig, A., Schultz, R., Miller, G., & VS, H. (2004). Is it beneficial to involve a family member? A meta-analysis of psychosocial interventions for chronic illness. *Health Psychology, 23*, 599–611.

Miller, I. W., Kabacoff, R. I., Epstein, N. B., Bishop, D. S., Keitner, G. I., Baldwin, L. M., et al. (1994). The development of clinical rating scale for the McMaster model of family functioning. *Family Process, 33*, 53–69.

Miller, I. W., Keitner, G. I., Ryan, C. E., Solomon, D. A., Cardemil, E. V., & Beevers, C. G. (2005). Treatment matching in the post hospital care of depressed patients. *American Journal of Psychiatry, 162*, 2131–2138.

Miller, I. W., Keitner, G. I., Ryan, C. E., Uebelacker, L. A., Johnson, S. L., & Solomon, D. A. (2008). Family treatment for bipolar disorder: Family impairment by treatment interactions. *Journal of Clinical Psychiatry, 69*(5), 732–740.

Moos, R., & Moos, B. (1981). *Family environment scale manual*. Palo Alto, California: Consulting Psychologists Press.

Nichols, M. (2010). *Family therapy concepts and methods* (9th edition). Boston, MA: Allyn & Bacon.

Northouse, L. L., Mood, D., Templin, T., Mellon, S., & George, T. (2000). Couples' patterns of adjustment to colon cancer. *Social Science & Medicine, 50*(2), 271–284.

Olson, D. H., Russell, C. S., & Sprenkle, D. H. (1989). *Circumplex model: Systemic assessment and treatment of families*. New York: Haworth Press.

Pisani, A., & McDaniel, S. (2005). An integrative approach to health and illness in family therapy. In J. L. Lebow (Ed.), *Handbook of clinical family therapy* (pp. 569–590). Hoboken, NJ: John Wiley & Sons, Inc.

Rabins, P. V., Fitting, M. D., Eastham, J., & Fetting, J. (1990). The emotional impact of caring for the chronically ill. *Psychosomatics, 31*(3), 331–336.

Riemama, R., Taal, E., & Rasker, J. (1999). The burden of care for informal caregivers of patients with rheumatoid arthritis. *Psychology & Health, 14*, 773–794.

Rohrbaugh, M. J., Shoham, V., & Coyne, J. C. (2006). Effect of marital quality on eight-year survival of patients with heart failure. *American Journal of Cardiology, 98*(8), 1069–1072.

Rolland, J. (2003). Mastering family challenges in serious illness and disability. In F. Walsh (Ed.), *Normal family process growing diversity and complexity* (pp. 460–489). New York: Guilford.

Rosen, K. H., McCollum, E. E., Middletown, K., Looke, L., & Bird, K. (1997). Interrater reliability and validity of the global assessment of relational functioning (GARF) scale in a clinical setting: A preliminary study. *American Journal of Family Therapy, 25*(4), 357–360.

Ryan, C. E., Epstein, N., Keitner, G. I., Miller, I., & Bishop, D. (2005). *Evaluating and treating families: The McMaster approach*. New York: Routledge Taylor & Francis Group.

Schulz, R., & Beach, S. R. (1999). Caregiving as a risk factor for mortality: The caregiver health effects study. *Journal of the American Medical Association, 282*(23), 2215–2219.

Solomon, D. A., Keitner, G. I., Ryan, C. E., Kelley, J., & Miller, I. W. (2008). Preventing recurrence of bipolar 1 mood episodes and hospitalizations: Family psychotherapy plus pharmcotherapy versus pharmacotherapy alone. *Bipolar Disorders, 10*(7), 798–805.

Spanier, G. B. (1976). Measuring dyadic adjustment: New scales for assessing the quality of marriage and similar dyads. *Journal of Marriage and the Family, 38*, 15–28.

Vitaliano, P., Scanlan, J., Zhang, J., Savage, M., Brunnett, B., & Barefoot, J. (2001). Are the salutogenic effects of social supports modified by income? A test of an "added value hypothesis." *Health Psychology, 20*, 155–165.

Weihs, K., Enright, T., & Simmens, S. (2008). Close relationships and emotional processing predict decreased mortality in women with breast cancer: Preliminary evidence. *Psychosomatic Medicine, 70*, 117–124.

Weihs, K., Fisher, L., & Baird, M. A. (2002). Families, health, and behavior: A section of the commissioned report by the committee on health and behavior: Research, practice and policy, division of neurosciences and behavioral health and division of health promotion and disease prevention, institute of medicine. *National Academy of Sciences Families, Systems, and Health, 20*(1), 7–47.

12.

PARENT GUIDANCE FOR MEDICALLY ILL PARENTS

Vaughn L. Mankey and Cynthia W. Moore

INTRODUCTION

The challenges experienced as a result of a serious illness are usually not isolated to the individual with the illness alone. Often the innermost sphere of relationships is very much affected in both emotional and practical ways, typically including the nuclear family. Mounting evidence documents the distress that both adult family members and dependent children experience when a loved one is sick and/or going through rigorous treatment (Armistead, Klein, & Forehand, 1995; Braun, Mikulincer, Rydall, Walsh, & Rodin, 2007; Northouse et al., 2007).

A number of serious, sometimes fatal, conditions can affect individuals in their childbearing and child-rearing years, and parents may actually experience greater distress than nonparents with the same conditions (Bloom & Kessler, 1994; Rauch & Moore, 2010). After all, parents must contend with the stress of the illness and treatment as well as the ongoing responsibilities of caring for dependent children. By considering the number of serious illnesses that afflict adult patients at child-rearing age, the scale of illness' impact on families is more clearly seen. Examining a few illnesses and some associated statistics helps bring the issue to life more concretely.

CANCER

At least 18% of recently diagnosed cancer patients, and 14% of all cancer survivors, are parenting minor children. This translates to more than 1.5 million cancer survivors having close to 3 million children at home (Weaver, Rowland, Alfano, & McNeel, 2010). Over half a million of these children are living with a parent in the early stages of cancer treatment and recovery. These data underestimate the numbers of affected children, most notably by omitting noncustodial parents and children who have already experienced a parent's death from cancer. Furthermore, the cutoff of 18 years that defines minors does not reflect the ongoing need for substantial parenting support for older adolescents and young adults (Rauch & Moore, 2010).

DIABETES

The Center for Disease Control and Prevention's most recent National Diabetes Fact Sheet (2007) reports that there are 23.5 million adults over 20 years of age that have diabetes in the United States alone. If we subtract the 12.2 million U.S. adults over 60 years old with diabetes we see that roughly 11.3 million U.S. adults between the ages of 20 and 60 have diabetes. This age group includes the most common ages for having and raising children. According to Halle (2002) and collaborators, data from the National Health Interview Survey of 2000 indicates that 84% of males and 86% of females over 45 years old have had at least one biological child. Although these numbers are not specific to males/females with diabetes, it is safe to assume that there are millions of parents with diabetes in the U.S.

HIV/AIDS

Schuster et al. (2000) also describe that an estimated 28% of US adults with HIV have dependent children. An even larger proportion of adults with HIV are parents generally speaking, as this estimate does not include parents who have young adult children.

Looking only at these three illness categories quickly demonstrates that a significant number of parents and their families are affected by serious illnesses. If all serious illnesses were to be considered, the number of parents whose families must contend with the challenges of illness is certainly in the millions—just in the United States alone. Clearly this is a large public health issue, as the effects on parents, children, and family units can be several and severe at times.

CLINICAL GUIDANCE FOR THE PARENT

Parents with serious illnesses often worry about how their children could be affected by their illness almost immediately after diagnosis. In fact, for some ill parents, worries about their children are pronounced, distressing, and may even affect treatment decisions (Duric & Stockler, 2001; Yellen & Cella, 1995; Muriel et al., 2010).

As healthcare providers, learning more about these parental concerns is the first step to caring for this aspect of a patient's psychosocial needs. Providers can begin by routinely asking all adult patients if they are parents and, if so, learning a bit about each of their children in terms of age, temperament, functioning, coping abilities, specific challenges, and so forth. Parents usually like discussing their children. A provider's open-ended inquiry, such as, "Tell me about your children," can often enhance the relationship between provider and patient while eliciting important information. Asking parents directly if they have any concerns about how their illness may affect their children can elicit the parents' primary concerns and can potentially identify children at risk of needing additional support. Once the parent's concerns are understood, customized interventions can be designed and implemented. Clinical experience suggests that there is no simple formula to predict the effects of an individual's illness on loved ones; therefore, there is no one-size-fits-all intervention that can be broadly applied. However, some of the variables that influence and mitigate the effects of an illness within a family can be considered for each family, allowing for personally relevant assistance. Some of these variables relate to features of the illness itself, and others to the families and family members affected. Many of these variables are discussed in this chapter, as are ways in which the healthcare team can consider them when providing personalized assistance.

CASE EXAMPLES

Throughout this chapter, two case examples will be used to illustrate many of the illness and family variables, along with the guiding principles for clinicians. The basic histories of the two patients and their families are described below, and additional information will be provided throughout the chapter as relevant.

PANCREATIC CANCER

Kelly O'Brien is a 45-year-old female diagnosed 2 months ago with unresectable stage III pancreatic cancer after evaluation for back pain and a 15-pound unintended weight loss. She and her husband Jim have three children: an 8-year-old son, Connor; a 6-year-old daughter, Brianna; and a 3-year-old son, Michael. Kelly has received two rounds of chemotherapy with gemcitabine and experienced some nausea, fatigue, and thinning hair. She knows that her lowered white blood cell count leaves her particularly susceptible to infections.

Kelly works part-time as a bookkeeper for Jim's business from home, but she sees caring for their children as her primary job. She notes that Connor has had "challenges" in school since kindergarten, and was recently diagnosed with ADHD and a reading disorder at the beginning of this school year, making him eligible to receive supportive services at school. Brianna is "like a little mother" sometimes, both bossing her brothers around and looking for ways to "make Mom feel better." Michael is "all boy," loud, active, exuberant, and increasingly difficult for Kelly to manage.

DIABETES

David is a 50-year-old male with a 15-year history of diabetes. He and his wife Irene have two children: a 17-year-old daughter, Monica, and a 13-year-old son, Jason. Monica is creative, expressive, and involved in drama club and advanced art classes. Jason is the star soccer player of his team, generally active, athletic, and a "doer instead of a talker." David's diabetes was of insidious onset and was discovered by his primary care provider (PCP) after presenting with polyuria. David tried to check his blood sugars regularly from the beginning, and usually did so at least once a day. Despite some small improvements in diet and beginning intermittent exercise a few times a week, his sugars remained fairly high. He had frequent follow-up appointments with his PCP, and about 12 years ago he was placed on Metformin, which he took regularly twice a day. However, his blood glucose levels tended to remain high.

About 10 years ago he was referred to an endocrinologist who specializes in diabetes, and he was started on insulin injections 3 times a day. He has had a number of appointments with other specialists over the years for monitoring of other possible sequelae of diabetes. He sees an ophthalmologist regularly, and more recently he had several appointments with a podiatrist after a small foot ulcer was slow to heal. He often has low energy and feels sluggish. He recently had a seizure that was witnessed by both children after he took insulin before breakfast, which was then unexpectedly delayed.

It can be helpful to have an organizing framework when considering the impact of a parent's serious illness on the family system and the children. The same framework can also guide interventions with parents to support family functioning and children's normal development. Rolland's Family Systems illness model (1999), which emphasizes the goodness of fit between the psychosocial demands of the disorder and the strengths and vulnerabilities of the family, provides such a framework and will guide the following discussion. Rolland describes three lenses through which families facing medical illness can be helpfully assessed: the developmental stage of the family, the developmental phase of the illness, and the psychosocial aspects of the illness. The developmental stage of the family refers to the relative age of the family—from pre-parenthood, through the ascending ages of children, into their young adulthood. The developmental phase of the illness is delineated into the crisis, chronic, terminal, and survivorship phases. Psychosocial aspects of the illness include acuity of onset; a progressive, constant, or relapsing course; the degree of incapacitation; the illness outcome; and the predictability of the illness. Each lens interacts with the others and, considered together, they create a nuanced description of the family's challenges.

DEVELOPMENTAL STAGE OF THE FAMILY

Parent guidance is most helpful when the uniqueness of a family's identity is considered. The family's current stage along the life cycle affects the developmental tasks and important issues the family faces. For example, some stages require intense bonding and high cohesion, while others call for loosening the external family boundary as personal identity and autonomy become more important (McGoldrick & Carter, 2003). In all stages, family cohesion, open communication among all family members, and a clear family identity apart from the illness are markers of good functioning.

HOPEFUL OR EXPECTANT PARENTS

Young couples dealing with a chronic illness may find that decisions about starting a family are affected by the medical picture. For example, a young adult with cancer may have to decide whether to bank eggs or sperm prior to beginning treatment, whether to delay attempts to become pregnant, or whether to have any, or additional, children. Other chronic illnesses can complicate fertility or a couple's confidence that starting a family is a good idea. A medical illness overlaid on a pregnancy may heighten anxiety about a range of possibilities, such as the effects of the pregnancy on the mother's health and/or the effects of the parent's medical condition on the pregnancy and eventually the child. Most expectant parents plan for the new baby's physical needs and arrange the surrounding environment to accommodate the new family member. These arrangements may require more creativity if a parent's medical needs must also be considered, for example, to limit trips up and down stairs or to minimize lifting and carrying. In addition, parents may spend a lot of time fantasizing about what changes the new baby will bring. For example, parents may wonder how the baby will affect other relationships and how time and tasks will be divided.

Clinicians can support couples as they prepare for, and adjust to, parenthood in a number of ways:

1. Encourage couples to build or broaden support networks.

2. Help couples anticipate the likely changes and practical needs they will have.

3. Emphasize communicating about and preparing for the added workload of parenthood.

FAMILIES WITH YOUNG CHILDREN

New parents and families with young children are typically in a stage of higher cohesion and bonding, as adults learn to provide consistent and responsive care for their wholly dependent children. Parents must learn about their children's unique personalities and temperaments and begin to create consistent routines. Infants and toddlers are forming trusting attachments that provide them with the security to explore the world, and comfort when they experience distress. Young children must also learn to communicate their needs, while adults learn to perceive them before language is fully developed. Once verbal, preschool children require time and guidance to use language effectively to get what they need and want.

Introducing a parent's medical illness into young families in which children are so dependent on parents for all their needs poses some particular challenges. Parents may find that effects of the illness make the physical demands of their children hard to manage—the diaper changes in awkward positions, lifting and carrying a tired or tantruming toddler, diminished sleep due to a child's being unable to settle himself at night. A child's access to one or both parents may be intermittently disrupted with hospital stays, doctor's appointments, or symptoms causing a parent's inability to manage the physical challenges of childcare. Even such young children are

likely to be aware of a parent's absence, without understanding the reasons for the absence. Additionally, infants and toddlers may recognize parents' anxiety and distress and feel (and act) distressed as a result.

Clinicians should emphasize that very young children feel more secure and thrive when consistent routines and caregivers are maintained. Clinicians can think creatively with parents about how to engage supports and utilize resources to increase consistency for the children. For example, if parental illness necessitates having additional caregivers, parents may try to write down the child's routine and preferences so that others can recreate a consistent environment.

Kelly described her 3-year-old son, Michael, as becoming hard for her to manage, primarily because of his high activity level and her exhaustion. Her patience with his efforts to do things "by myself!" was much less than she remembered with her other two children. Until recently, she and Michael had stayed busy during the school day with a preschool gym program, swimming lessons, and a play group. We discussed the fact that her fatigue and concern about contagious illnesses were obstacles to her providing Michael with the physical and social stimulation on which he thrived. She and Jim decided that they would look into preschool programs for Michael and also try to have her treatments occur during preschool time. This was not an easy decision, given the value Kelly placed on caring for her children during their early years, but made sense in terms of providing a predictable schedule for Michael and some unscheduled time for her.

FAMILIES WITH SCHOOL-AGED CHILDREN

Although elementary school-aged children spend many hours a week in school and after-school activities, family cohesion remains critically important to their well-being. Between ages 6–12 years, children rely on parents to help them achieve in school, connect with friends, and master skills that allow them to be competent and confident. Parents must support children's increasingly complex routines, negotiate limits and discipline, and discern when a child is impeded in meeting developmental challenges and what the impediments are. Thus, while the physical demands of parenting may be somewhat less intense, the emotional demands can feel just as challenging when medical illness is part of the picture. Fatigue, anxiety and depression, and frequent medical appointments can interfere with all these aspects of parenting.

In addition, school-aged children are capable of making comparisons—among peers who are fast and slow runners, fluent and challenged readers, "popular" and socially invisible—and among parents who look or function differently than others. Clinicians can encourage parents to engage in open, honest, and ongoing communication about the parent's medical condition with their children so they can understand and adjust to the ways their family may differ from others. Honest conversations about the illness itself and the changes it may bring can also allow a family to retain a sense of itself apart from the impact of the illness, as the differing needs and wishes of all family members can be discussed and negotiated.

Once again, clinicians can help parents think through how to spend limited energy. Frequently, parents' focus is on maintaining the routine—providing rides, procuring supplies, getting groceries, and doing laundry. While completing these tasks helps keep a household running smoothly, parents may not have enough energy left over to spend time talking with children, enjoying time together, or noticing a child's altered behavior or mood. Clinicians may help parents determine what tasks can be delegated to friends, family, or paid helpers, and what functions only they themselves can fulfill in their children's lives.

Kelly and Jim described their relief at having 8-year-old Connor finally receiving services at school to address his reading disability and ADHD, but Kelly noted that homework could still take far longer than Connor could sustain focus. She was accustomed to coaching him through homework daily, but found it more difficult to do so for several days after chemotherapy treatments. Without her calming presence, Connor could erupt in frustration or simply give up after only a halfhearted attempt to finish. Kelly and Jim were able to talk with Connor about why Kelly was not helping him on some days but was on others, how much his efforts in school mattered to them, and what he thought would help with homework on the days Kelly was not available. Connor surprised them by asking if a high school boy who lived nearby could help when his mother could not, and then practice baseball with him. This would give him the opportunity to spend time with an older youth he admired, and allow him to finish homework early in the afternoon while his focus was best.

FAMILIES WITH ADOLESCENTS

Families with adolescents enter a phase in which family cohesion and individual autonomy must be rebalanced. Adolescents are developing a clearer sense of their own identities—strengths, challenges, beliefs, and values—and practicing skills that will allow them to function as independent adults. Parents sometimes struggle to decide how much freedom to allow adolescents, how much to trust their impulse control (especially when with peers), and how to maintain a feeling of connection with teens who increasingly want to spend time with friends.

Although the way parents monitor their adolescents' behavior looks different from the more hands-on approach used with younger children, the function and importance of parents' monitoring does not change. When medical illness intrudes on family life, parents may be tempted to respond in ways that may not be in their teenagers' best interest. Parents might reduce their monitoring of teens' activities due to fatigue or side effects, physical absence necessitated by treatment, and adolescents' own pushback against needing to be "babysat" by other adults. Additionally, teens may be asked to "step up to the plate" and take on a variety of new roles to help out at home such as caring for younger siblings, household tasks, even caring for the ill parent. While an increase in expectations is not always problematic, a balance must be maintained between adult needs and expectations and age-appropriate adolescent needs for socializing and down-time (Pedersen & Revenson, 2005).

In addition, as adolescents approach the end of high school they typically engage in conversations about their next step toward adulthood—whether college, trade school, or a job. Parents have an enormously important role in supporting this "launch," one that requires time, energy, and patience. All three of these qualities can be in short supply when illness is also part of the picture. In addition, worrying about a parent can make it more difficult for an adolescent to feel comfortable leaving home. He or she may feel guilty for pulling away at a difficult time, responsible for taking care of family members, or anxious about making the adjustment to life away from home.

Clinicians can help parents think about how much they are expecting of adolescents, how this has changed because of the medical illness, and what are the benefits and disadvantages to the teen, and the family, of this arrangement. Ongoing, open communication is particularly important so that adolescents do not feel overly burdened or excluded from decision making.

David's need for three-times-daily insulin and frequent blood sugar testing are embarrassing and irritating to his 13-year-old son Jason, who wishes his father could be physically active or eat out at restaurants "without all the drama." When David suffered from his foot ulcer, he stopped coaching Jason's soccer team. Both of them miss the "guy time" together and David describes feeling a little less connected to Jason. When asked why he thought this was the case, David replied that coaching allowed him one-on-one time with his son when they drove to practices and games together, as well as a window into his son's friendships. When he couldn't think of any other activities that would keep him as well connected to his adolescent son, he decided to see if he could continue as an assistant coach and minimize as best he could the time standing when his foot was bothering him.

FAMILIES WITH YOUNG ADULTS

Once children are functioning independently, the tasks for the family change yet again. Young adult children are proving themselves in new careers, often searching for or sustaining intimate relationships, and taking on adult tasks such as saving money, buying a car, signing a lease, perhaps even starting a family. Although families vary widely, many young adults continue to rely on their parents for support, advice, and encouragement as they negotiate these new challenges. Parents' titrated involvement can enhance confidence as well as promote better decision making. Medical illness in a parent can disrupt this process. Some young adult children may feel pulled to stay very involved in family life, such as when parents consistently rely on young adult offspring for care or support. In other families, parents may not remain involved enough in the young adult's life at critical times.

Young adults are often better able to communicate directly with their parents about the impact the illness is having on their lives. However, clinicians should still encourage parents to invite their adult children to engage in this communication and even to discuss how the communication is going. Is the family talking too much, too little, or just the right amount about the illness? Are people discussing the various aspects of the illness and its consequences that are important to everyone?

PHASE OF ILLNESS

Along with the family developmental phase, considering the developmental phase of the illness itself can elucidate some of the specific effects the illness can have on a family.

CRISIS PHASE

The *crisis phase* often occurs in the initial stages of the illness—when symptoms are first noticed, a new diagnosis given, or when the initial treatment options are presented. However, there can be additional crisis moments at any point in a serious illness. Factors contributing to a sense of crisis may include shock about what the patient is experiencing, the threat of disability or death, a fear of lasting loss or drastic change, and worry that the patient or family cannot cope with the situation. Individuals may openly display their sense of fear, shock, or sadness, or use other coping strategies such as intellectualization, problem solving, or denial that make it more difficult for physicians to notice the underlying sense of crisis.

Even well-meaning parents may have difficulties explaining the crisis to children and commonly try to "protect" them by hiding the ill parent's symptoms or limiting shared information. Some parents tell partial truths or even overt untruths, hoping to shelter the children from the tumult of emotions that the parents themselves may be experiencing. However, children are often keen observers, especially in regards to their parents on whom they depend for the provision of their needs and wants. Children may sense that there is a significant problem through even small cues, such as a change in the day's schedule, a different tone of voice, or a decrease in the parent's attention. When children notice changes, they often wonder why they have occurred. Without accurate information about what is actually occurring, children are left to worry alone. They attempt to piece together the bits of information they have gathered to arrive at an explanation that makes sense to them. Depending on the developmental stage and temperament of the children (among other variables), many of these assumptions can be inaccurate, and some are even self-blaming and illogical. Some explanations may cause significant guilt or anxiety in children. In fact, Rosenheim and Reicher (1985) have described that children who know about a parent's cancer diagnosis are less anxious than those who were not told. The wish to protect children by withholding information is actually an error of kindness that has the potential to do harm instead of good.

Clinicians can encourage parents to provide open, honest, and age-appropriate information to all children in the family. Euphemisms, like "booboo" and "ouchy" should be avoided, and specific illness names should be used because this will decrease confusion and the possible concern that the children themselves may experience similar symptoms the next time they have a booboo. Providing information about the illness and the preliminary plan to deal with the crisis is helpful. A clear, definitive plan is not always available, though, and is not necessary. Clinicians can suggest that parents inform their children that the ill parent is getting good care, getting the proper tests, and the immediately appropriate treatment (if applicable). This is often sufficient information to help children feel like things are under control.

During the crisis phase when emotions are running high, parents are encouraged to temper strong displays of emotion while discussing information with children. It is certainly acceptable for parents to show and discuss that they are upset, worried, or sad, but efforts should be made not to project a sense of being completely overwhelmed, helpless, or out of control. Children often take their cues from parents, and a parent's strong distress may be unsettling and internalized by the children. Compas and colleagues (1996) found that perceived stress predicted an adolescent's anxiety, depression, and stress response syndrome in families where a parent has cancer.

Prior to her formal diagnosis, Kelly and Jim had shared the news of her feeling ill with the children, as they needed an explanation for why she seemed tired and less able to do things she had always done for them and the household. They had told the children that "Mommy's back has been hurting, and she has been pretty tired. We're going to the doctor to find out what is wrong and to help her feel better." Once Kelly and Jim received the specific diagnosis, they were understandably very upset, tearful, and nervous. When they were able to be calmer, they brought the kids together and told them, "We found out what is causing Mommy's back to hurt. It's called pancreatic cancer, and it is causing pain because it is growing in Mommy's belly and pushing on things inside where it should not be. We are talking with the doctors now about how to help Mommy feel better and to see if we can make the cancer stop growing. We will let you know more as we learn more. Do you have any questions right now?"

In addition to sharing information, parents in the crisis phase of an illness are often required to disrupt normal family routines and reorganize in order to meet the immediate needs of the ill parent and ongoing needs of the family. Supports are often summoned, and a host of well-wishers may descend upon a family. This outside support is often necessary but may be experienced by children as a disruption. Clinicians can encourage parents to minimize this sense of disruption, as structure, routine, and predictability is often stabilizing and comforting for children. Parents may consider designating a "Captain of Kindness" outside the nuclear family who can organize the efforts of volunteers. This will allow the family to receive the needed support without being responsible for all the administrative work that can come with organizing it. In addition, an outside "Minister of Information" can be appointed to relay news updates to supports, without intrusion into family time (Rauch & Muriel, 2006).

Sometimes, even in the crisis phase, it is immediately clear that an illness will have lasting effects throughout the parent's life. Parents may immediately realize that life has irrevocably changed, and they will be dealing with uncertainty in the days and years ahead. It can be a challenge to integrate this information into expectations of the ill parent, the couple's relationship, and the family's future. At times this involves an immediate sense of grief, as the "new normal" is imagined and the pre-illness identities and expectations begin to feel lost. While preparing children for the immediate realities is important, sharing all of these types of concerns at an early stage of illness can be overwhelming for some children. Younger children will not think immediately about many of these longer-term changes, and time will allow for step-wise explanations and realizations. However, adolescents in particular may have some of the same worries as adults and should be encouraged to bring all of their questions and concerns to the parents for discussion. Parents need not have all the answers, but the power of a parent's listening to and thinking with a child is immense. It is perfectly acceptable for a parent to respond to a perplexing question with, "That is a great question, and I'm really glad you asked. I'm not sure of the answer right now, but I will think about it, talk to the doctor (nurse, social worker, etc.) and get back to you." This builds trust and mutual respect and facilitates communication. It also helps the child to not worry alone or go seeking answers elsewhere, which is important given the host of inaccurate and personally irrelevant information that is abundantly available to them from other sources.

CHRONIC PHASE ("THE LONG HAUL")

The *chronic phase* of an illness occurs in conditions that are more prolonged and chronic in nature, as the name suggests. In these illnesses, both the course of symptoms and treatment can be marked by a sense of ongoing constancy, steady or step-wise progression, or drastic episodic changes.

During the chronic phase, family roles and relationships may remain stuck in patterns developed in the crisis phase. However, solutions that worked in the short term may not be adequate for the long-term nature of a chronic illness. For example, an adolescent daughter may have prepared dinner every night, cared for siblings, and done all the laundry during the week her mother was hospitalized, but this level of effort will be difficult to sustain for months. Parents should be encouraged to be thoughtful about the role changes that occur, to openly acknowledge them, and to talk about them in an ongoing way. Some role changes may be welcomed by all parties, while others may be resisted or felt to be inappropriate or burdensome. Therefore, when possible, children should be included in conversations about role changes. Often adolescents are asked to take on more responsibilities for the family to help "pick up the slack," but they may be resistant to doing so based on the historical roles of family members as well as their own current needs. Socialization, identity exploration, school achievement, and extracurricular activities, among others, are all developmentally appropriate tasks for a teen. Clinicians can remind parents of these normal developmental tasks for teens, and how the appropriate navigation of these tasks is important for their teens' long-term healthy development. Parents should be encouraged to remain mindful of the multiple tasks teens are juggling as they seek to divide up

new roles and tasks within the family. Often a balance can be struck between helping the family, coping with the illness, and normal adolescent activities. Again, ongoing honest communication typically facilitates attaining and maintaining this balance.

For children, maintaining as much of a "normal" life as possible under the "abnormal" conditions of a serious illness in a parent can be a challenging yet important endeavor. Clinicians can think with parents about how they can facilitate this relative normalcy by maintaining structure and routines, protecting family time, designating illness-free time (when the illness is not a topic of discussion or focus of activity), and anticipating changes and preparing for them.

When David had his seizure, he was afraid to drive for a while because he worried he could have another seizure at any time. Although he knew this was unlikely if he took good care of his blood sugar, he was hesitant nonetheless. This meant that Irene had to juggle more than her usual heavy load and was now responsible for taking Monica to play practice and voice lessons, as well as Jason to soccer practice—not to mention driving for all other household errands and social events. This was a significant change in role for Irene, because she and David had always shared the transportation of children and running errands, and she struggled to manage the new demands. She was able to share with David that she understood his concerns and that she felt it was important that he also understand the additional time the increased driving was taking her, as well as the challenges she was having in keeping up with everything as a result. They were able to commit to working together to find a solution that was agreeable to both. They decided to talk with the doctor about David's fears and, if need be, to obtain help with driving from a close family friend. They decided they would only change the children's schedules as a last resort.

With open communication and thoughtful consideration of each family member's needs, along with the collective needs of the family unit, a balance can be struck to maximize autonomy while maintaining intimacy and appropriate family cohesion. The challenge of living with the illness can be seen as a family struggle that affects all members as well as the unit, and is best faced and managed collectively. Clinicians may share the image that family members stand together as a team with interlinked arms—facing the opponent of chronic illness. This image not only highlights the cohesion of the family, but also identifies the true cause of the challenges, which is the illness itself. It is normal that all family members have negative feelings about the difficult circumstances that an illness can bring. Some of these feelings may seem shameful or be a source of guilt for family members, including children. Sometimes members may wish another family was dealing with the illness instead of their own. They may wish the ill person would die quickly to end suffering or to end the burden of caregiving. They may wish to escape and wonder about leaving the family. Clinicians can facilitate the sensitive expression, normalization, and validation of these feelings, which can be important for family members. When these feelings are shared in a format with everyone being "on the same team," with the illness as the true adversary and the focus of negative feelings, family members can come together in support of one another instead of directing the feelings toward one another.

That being said, all families have typical ups and downs, and when a parent is sick, a common interpretation of distress is that it is caused by the illness. When parents share that their children are changing, clinicians can suggest that parents:

1. Consider whether the change is due to normal development rather than the illness.

2. Ask healthy adults if they have noted similar changes in their children.

3. Speak to the child directly about the observed changes and exploring the child's own observations and explanations.

An open-ended, nonjudgmental approach is usually most appreciated by the children and can garner significant information.

TERMINAL PHASE

The *terminal phase* of the illness involves a family's recognizing the impending loss of a loved one and coming to terms with the loss of what is, and could be. Parents and children alike may consider the future milestones that will be celebrated without the dying parent. Grief can be profound for all involved, but thoughtful preparation can be helpful.

If the terminal phase provides enough time, many families take the opportunity to discuss unresolved issues in hopes that no one will be left holding regrets. In addition, parents can plan ahead for the ongoing care and support of children. If the dying parent has a custodial co-parent already, then the two may brainstorm about what sorts of resources (both human and otherwise) could be helpful as the remaining parent continues raising the children. Some parents may opt to designate a close family member or lifelong friend who knows the dying parent well to be a guiding mentor, support, and a living legacy who can share a life history of the dying parent with a child. Thoughtful choosing of a supportive adult that has a good rapport and "fit" with a child is important, and a different adult might be selected for each child in the family. Similar considerations may be relevant in choosing a custodial guardian if the dying parent is single, with the important additional component of legal arrangements being required. Obtaining legal counsel to help with these arrangements should be advised by clinicians to ensure a smooth transition in the custody and care of children losing their only parent. Parents might also consider making appropriate financial plans for their children.

Other types of legacies may also be considered and prepared by the dying parent, such as letters, scrapbooks, videos, or voice recordings. These can be tangible ways in which children feel connected to a parent as they continue to grow and develop even after the parent is gone. Through such legacies, parents can be encouraged to reflect on and share favorite memories and moments with the child, their love and pride for the child, and their intimate knowledge of the child. However, it is best if parents do not include critical materials (even with the good intention to spur self-improvement) or specific expectations for the child. Children will likely revisit these legacies many times at different stages of their lives. Material that could be viewed as critical, or parental expectations that have gone unfulfilled, could be a source of significant shame or guilt for a child later in life. Legacy leaving is discussed more in depth by Rauch and Muriel (2006).

During the terminal phase of the illness, parents often reach a point where a decision has to be made regarding treatment goals. Individuals vary widely in what types of treatment they accept and for how long. Parents of children at home are often willing to trade quality of life to gain a survival advantage (Yellen & Cella, 1995). However, at some point in the terminal phase, a parent's healthcare team will likely advise the parent that pursuing active treatment will no longer provide an additional survival benefit. Recommendations may include transitioning the course of treatment towards palliative care. Clinicians can help parents to share the news of the transition to palliative care with children by thinking with them about age-appropriate explanations. For example, parents may say that even after receiving the best treatments available, the illness is not responding the way everyone hoped it would, and more medicine cannot make the illness go away. For some medications, there may even be negative side effects that could make the parent feel worse if continued. Parents can describe how the new treatment goals are to improve the quality of life for the parent, to decrease pain and suffering, and to sustain functionality as much as possible. Parents can also describe their goal as being to live as well as they can, for as long as they can.

Once a parent requires significant care from others, which can be both physically and emotionally challenging, a decision may need to be made about whether this care should occur at home or at a hospice facility. Clinicians can help parents to think about the many variables involved in making this decision. Sometimes the dying parent wishes to spend the last days in the comfort of home, and this can be accomplished for many, even with children there. When a dying parent is quite ill at home, the location and setup of the space should be considered. Children may want to frequently see the dying parent, but may be distressed by some aspects of the terminal illness such as moments of great pain, agitation, or confusion. It is helpful for children to have space at home that serves as a reprieve from exposure to emotionally difficult situations.

Hospice care in a setting outside the home can be an appropriate choice for other families, as the healthy parent may not be able to adequately care for the dying parent, or some children may feel extremely anxious knowing the parent is going to die soon in the room down the hall. A thoughtful approach to either scenario can help children be resilient even in the final stages of a parent's serious illness. Clinicians can guide parents to help children say goodbye in ways that foster a minimizing of regrets both in the present and in the future. For each child this may mean the goodbye is quite different, but addressing unfinished business, sharing important feelings and sentiments, and spending time together in meaningful ways can diminish future regrets.

SURVIVORSHIP PHASE

While survivorship can mean many things, including the time following diagnosis, it is used here to describe the phase of illness encompassing remission or cure from a serious illness that has the threat of future return in some form. Not all illnesses have this phase, as sometimes remission or cure is not possible. However, when remission has occurred the threat of recurrence is a unique challenge.

A parent who has survived a serious illness knows first-hand the toll such an illness can take on the body, mind, and family unit. Thus, the *survivorship phase* may be colored by a sense of anxiety—less intense than in the crisis phase, yet still significant in its effects. Many parents who have had cancer may worry about the cancer's potential return and feel uncertain about the future (Lee-Jones et al., 1997). Anxiety may peak at various points of survivorship, such as before a check-up, while awaiting scan or other test results, or on the anniversary of the initial diagnosis. Some parents describe feeling like their emotions are "on a roller coaster" during this phase in the illness.

Children can be sensitive to these ups and downs and have their own interpretations and feelings about them. Some children may worry more, for example, when a parent ends treatment because they feel like less is being done for the parent proactively. Clinicians can recommend that parents reassure their children that the ill parent is still being actively monitored, and that the children will remain in the communication loop. If children know they will be informed about important news, it may allow them to resume daily living without feeling they have to monitor the parent for signs of relapse. Children may have input as to what type of news they would like to hear, as well as when, how, and by whom it is shared. Often a brief discussion of these variables when there is only good news to share can help parents properly set the stage should bad news arise.

For some parents who have experienced a serious illness, survivorship feels like a new lease on life, and significant life changes are made. Children may have various reactions to these changes, so preparation and explanations can be helpful. In addition, the skew in relationship roles that existed during the crisis and chronic phases may begin to rebalance. This transition can bring its own challenges as some family members resist relinquishing new roles, while others may want to hoist all prior responsibilities onto the now healthier parent who is not quite ready to return to the premorbid level of functioning. Honest yet gentle and respectful sharing of feelings can help families re-navigate roles.

After David's seizure he grew more concerned than ever about his health. He decided to commit to a strict regimen of exercise, healthy eating, and adherence to his doctor's recommendations about medication. He sought the help of his physician, a nutritionist, and a personal trainer, and lost over 100 pounds, getting close to his ideal body weight. His blood glucose stabilized significantly, and regular insulin injections were no longer necessary. He felt more energetic, engaged, and happier, and became more active in his children's and family's activities. He also took up some hobbies of his own, like long-distance running. While very glad about David's new energy and optimism, his daughter Monica had some difficulties with his increased interest

---

in her personal life. She had come to value having more independence as a 17-year-old, and they began to have more heated discussions about his "intrusiveness." After Irene noticed that Monica became upset when David asked more personal questions, they were able to sit down and discuss ways to balance David's interest with Monica's privacy, and what boundaries felt comfortable to both of them.

PSYCHOSOCIAL ASPECTS OF ILLNESS

The third lens through which an illness can be viewed, Rolland's "psychosocial" aspects of the illness, can be thought of as its unique fingerprint. The acuteness of onset, typical course, likely outcomes, incapacitation, and overall predictability comprise this fingerprint and predict elements of the family's experience.

ACUTENESS OF ONSET

Medical conditions with an acute onset, such as stroke, heart attack, or injuries from a motor vehicle accident often feel shocking and frightening at first. Their "out of the blue" nature means that family members are unprepared and often overwhelmed. Parents may want help in quickly finding age-appropriate language to describe what has occurred to their children, to reassure children that the immediate danger is over, and to explain what steps must now be taken to help the ill parent heal. A clinician knowledgeable about child development can be an invaluable resource to parents in these situations. Such a clinician can advise parents about age-appropriate language and concepts, which can be used when describing the acute medical circumstances to children.

Illnesses like cancer and diabetes often have a more gradual onset, where symptoms are noticed over time and diagnosis is not immediate. Parents may have some choice about how and when they will talk to children and thus can be better prepared. However, the ambiguity of the period leading up to a firm diagnosis often leaves parents feeling anxious and not ready to talk openly with their children about unconfirmed worries. Children are frequently aware that something is amiss but feel reluctant to ask questions, a combination that can lead to distress.

Clinicians can think with parents about what children are noticing about the ill parent at home, the changes the illness has caused in the family's daily life, and how they can begin to talk about a still-uncertain diagnosis. Parents can continue to ask children what they are noticing so that parents can continue to explain any observed changes to their children.

Kelly and Jim describe telling their children about her diagnosis of pancreatic cancer as one of the hardest things they have ever done. They worried about how much each child would understand and how they would react, predicting that Brianna would "cry for days" and that Connor would not say much, but be "a bear to live with." They were reluctant to use the word "cancer" for fear of scaring the children, but realized that they had probably already overheard it mentioned in phone conversations. After some thought, they were able to sit down with all three children and explain that Kelly's string of recent doctor's appointments had been to help figure out why her back was hurting so much, and that the doctors had just told them that Kelly has an illness called pancreatic cancer. They clarified that cancer is not the kind of illness that anyone else can catch just by being near her, and that nothing she or the children did or didn't do, gave her cancer. They also described how she would begin receiving a special, strong medicine to treat the cancer, called "chemotherapy."

Kelly and Jim went on to elicit the children's questions and reactions, to normalize their fear and sadness and acknowledge their own, and to talk concretely about how Kelly's diagnosis and treatment would affect each of the children's day-to-day lives. Michael, their 3-year-old, had a predictably shorter attention span than Connor or Brianna, but did hear explanations for a number of new words, and the message that some things would change but a lot would stay the same. Later that day, and regularly thereafter, both parents checked in with each child individually to help ensure that questions were clearly answered, and no child was worrying alone.

COURSE

Expectations about how a parent's illness will affect the family in the near and distant future are influenced by the typical course of the illness. Rolland suggests that it is useful to think about three types, including progressive, constant, or relapsing illness courses. A medical event such as a stroke or spinal cord injury may be thought of as having a fairly constant course. Major adjustments will likely need to be made almost immediately but, once accomplished, daily life may be fairly consistent and predictable over the longer term. A relapsing course, as with cancer, may feel more like a roller coaster with uncertainty about daily functioning, unpredictable changes that contribute to loss of control, and more frequent family reorganizing. A progressive illness is one that becomes gradually worse, necessitating incremental adjustments over time. Although changes may be fairly predictable and gradual, the fact that the future will certainly be more difficult makes a progressive course quite challenging.

Parents may benefit from having their experience described by such a framework, with an emphasis on identifying areas that continue to be controllable for them and their children. Clinicians can think with parents about how to make sure that the balance of responsibilities in the family is allowing each member's continued normal development; they can also discuss key points in the illness course where that balance should be reassessed. For example, changes in roles typically occur when the functional status of the ill parent changes due to new or worsening symptoms. Clinicians can help families anticipate and prepare for the changes at home that are likely to occur with a new limitation. Clinicians may ask about or suggest ways the parent's previous roles, which are now compromised, might be filled by other family members, friends, or community resources. Again, it is important for children's normal developmental needs and perspectives to be included in such planning.

Kelly's family had finally adjusted to the rigors of her chemotherapy schedule when she had to be admitted to the hospital on an emergency basis due to vomiting and abdominal bloating and pain. She underwent

stent placement to bypass a blockage in her small intestine. When she returned home, the routine had to change, again. Kelly was unable to manage the household tasks that she had fiercely insisted on doing, and was not supposed to drive right away. Their 6-year-old, Brianna, struggled a great deal with these new changes although her parents had described her as being so "flexible compared to her brothers" up until this point. When they talked with Brianna, she could only say that she wanted "the old Mommy" back. With a little more encouragement, she said that she missed her "Mommy–daughter" time. Initially confused, after some thought Kelly realized that Brianna had spent quite a bit of time with her as she completed household tasks—folding laundry, cooking dinner—and that Kelly's ability to allow her daughter to feel helpful was one of the things that gave Brianna a sense of control.

INCAPACITATION

Illness incapacitation includes the sorts of treatments required, and changes to the patient's and family's quality of life. For children, the impact of incapacitation is partly mediated by parents' coping styles as well as by their own developmental stage. For example, a parent's 5-day hospitalization may cause significant separation anxiety in a preschooler but be easily tolerated by an adolescent who is reassured that the parent will be better after the hospital stay. An elementary school–aged child who is told only that the parent is "having some tests" may have a harder time adjusting to a weak, postsurgery parent than a child who was told that "the doctors are going to remove the part of Mom's intestine that has cancer, and when she gets home she'll need a few weeks to really rest in bed."

Clinicians can guide parents to anticipate changes in the ill parent, so that parents can in turn prepare children. Parents can be encouraged to think about all the ways they can keep life as normal as possible for the family while dealing with a variety of symptoms. The medical team may need to remind parents of the importance of optimizing support networks and asking for help, redistributing roles in an equitable, flexible way, and checking in regularly with children about what are the best and worst parts of home life recently.

Certain changes are more salient to children than others, and should be explicitly discussed. These include side effects of many chemotherapy treatments like nausea, fatigue, and hair loss; gross physical changes following surgery, such as large scars, amputations, colostomy bags; mood changes and irritability common with steroid use; and changes in eating or feeding habits. Particularly confusing are some of the cognitive changes that occur as a result of brain injury or disease—word-finding difficulties, short-term memory deficit, lack of organization or focus in someone who previously "kept everyone on track."

David and his wife Irene noticed that 13-year-old Jason was more withdrawn and irritable than usual. Both asked him what was bothering him, but didn't get far. A light bulb went off for Irene when she was signing off on Jason's homework and noticed that his science class was doing a unit on hormonal systems, which included a discussion of diabetes. She asked him about what had been presented, and he shared that the teacher had mentioned that "frequently uncontrolled diabetes leads to foot or partial leg amputation." He was terrified that his father's recent return to coaching would hasten such an outcome. Knowing this, David and Irene were able to describe for him all the ways that David was working to prevent such a serious problem, as well as to clarify the likelihood for most diabetics of needing an amputation.

When a parent has such significant changes in functioning that they seem "not themselves," each family member will need to grapple with how to redefine his or her relationship to the parent. There may be aspects of the relationship that are unaffected by the illness and can still be enjoyed. For example, a father and 12-year-old son shared a love of astronomy—they frequently visited a local observatory, as well as programs at a science museum relating to space. After this father became bedridden, his son was crushed that their field trips were no longer possible. After talking together about how much they missed the trips, they hit on the idea of watching Nova episodes online and talking about them together. It wasn't as exciting as using the observatory telescope, but preserved their capacity to bond over a common interest.

OUTCOME

Illness outcome describes the likely effect of the illness on the patient's expected lifespan. Whether an illness is life-threatening or not usually has a substantial impact on how it is experienced by the family. However, sometimes the seriousness of this threat is not obvious to children. In our case study, David's adolescents had not realized prior to his seizure that uncontrolled blood sugar levels could be a medical emergency and even fatal. When an illness worsens quality of life but is not life-threatening, parents should make this point clearly to children. A younger child whose mother experienced severe fatigue from rheumatoid arthritis worried that she might come home and find her mother "asleep forever in bed." What seems more difficult to many parents is how to talk about an illness that is life-threatening or likely to be fatal.

In regard to the possibility of a parent's dying, clinicians may remind parents that children are often focused much more on the here and now. A question like, "Is Mom going to die?" often reflects worry about losing a parent in the near future (weeks to months). Parents, however, tend to think many years ahead and thus struggle with how to answer honestly while not worrying children needlessly. When possible, parents can create a "safety zone" for their children, as Kelly tried to do shortly after her diagnosis when asked by 8-year-old Connor, "Can't you die from cancer?":

"I'm glad you asked that tough question. You're right, people can die from cancer. But, right now no one is worrying about my dying . . . my doctors are focused on treating this disease and helping me feel better. I'm hoping that the next 4 months of treatment will leave me feeling well enough to take our usual summer trip. If anything changes, I'll let you know, ok?"

PREDICTABILITY

The predictability of an illness guides the family's expectations for what the near future will look like. Predictability is somewhat in the eye of the beholder, as patients and families vary in how much they want to know about what *could* happen, and the same event may surprise some families but not others. While some families feel as though the best they can do is "expect the unexpected," frequently there are patterns in certain aspects of the illness that become familiar and thus can be discussed and experienced as more controllable. For example, it is not uncommon for a patient who is very anxious at the start of chemotherapy to complete the final round feeling as though it is almost routine. Children may never be happy about a parent's needing to stay in bed for 2 days after treatment, but knowing which 2 days the parent will be less available can help.

Some families are also experienced at preparing for the unexpected, and these skills can be useful in the context of an unpredictable medical illness. Clinicians can help parents to anticipate events that might affect the children, such as emergency hospitalization, an ambulance at the home, the possibility of a seizure, and the potential of abrupt schedule changes. Parents can then consider whether there are plans to make that would minimize disruptions for children. For example, the family might discuss who would be available to come over in the middle of the night to care for children if needed, or post a list of important phone numbers, or review how to call an ambulance and what to say to the operator. When a family does get taken by surprise by some new development, it can help to discuss their response and what worked well and less well. This may enhance their sense of control about the possibility of managing something similar in the future.

David's diabetes had seemed fairly stable to his children for quite a while when they witnessed his seizure. Both were frightened by what they saw, and his daughter Monica later told her parents that she couldn't stop worrying that it would happen again. In hindsight, David and his wife Irene wished they had mentioned to their children that a seizure was a possibility, and what to do in response. Monica had called 911 while Jason stayed with his father, but neither knew the signs of the oncoming seizure or were aware that a sugary snack was what he needed in time to prevent it. Once the family discussed this information, both Monica and Jason felt more confident that they could help their father in the future.

SUMMARY

There are millions of parents in the United States and around the world who are living with serious illnesses and caring for children at home. Given that a serious illness can affect the physical and psychological functioning of a parent, the effects on the family (and children within the family) can be significant. As outlined throughout this chapter, and summarized in Table 12.1, there are a number of variables related to both the family and the illness than can modify the family's response to the illness. With thoughtful consideration of these variables, clinicians can provide parents with guidance that enhances the resiliency of children as they anticipate and experience some of the challenges an illness can bring.

Table 12.1 SUGGESTIONS TO CLINICIANS

	CRISIS PHASE	CHRONIC AND SURVIVORSHIP PHASES	TERMINAL PHASE
Parent of:	Focus on maintaining children's sense of safety and security. • Consistent rules and routines when possible • Identify readily available supports	Promote a sense of the family as a team, with more in common than just the illness. Be mindful of how role changes impact each person's development.	Focus on making the most of the time together for as long as possible, and on leaving children tangible reminders of the parent's love. Consider setting of end-of-life care from both adult and child perspectives.
Toddler (1–3)	• Familiar caregivers • Consistent routines and micro-environment (portable crib and blankets) • Transitional objects available (blankie, stuffed rabbit)	• Honest assessment of what additional help with child may be required, how often, and who is available • Written routines for caregivers • Prepare for toddler distress with parental absence • Be patient with regression	• Preverbal, will have few memories of the parent • Consider letters, videotaping, annotated photos from parent • Identify people who can tell stories about the parent as child gets older
Pre-schooler (3–5)	• Provide basic information (who and what) • Confirm the child's lack of responsibility for the illness • Specify immediate impact on child • Minimize displays of strong parental emotion to child • Name child's emotions • Familiar caregivers, the fewer the better	• Be understanding about egocentric concerns and requests • Emerging anxieties about the world (e.g., fear of the dark, monsters) are developmentally normal but may be heightened; be prepared to seek help if they are very distressing or long-lived • Be patient with regression but keep expectations consistent (e.g., use your words, not your hands) • Encourage teachers to maintain preschool's normalcy • Correct misperceptions and self blame about parent's mood or functioning	• Consider letters, videotaping, annotated photos from parent • Provide notice of an imminent death, when known, so child has the option of a last visit • Many strangers in the home may be upsetting • Be clear that adult distress is not the child's fault
Grade-schooler (6–12)	• Provide simple, age-appropriate information about diagnosis and treatment • Clarify risk of contagion • Specify short-term impact on child • Ask what has been noticed and explain child's observations • Minimize displays of strong parental emotion to child • Elicit, discuss, normalize child's emotions • Emphasize areas of control	• Separate treatment side effects from illness progression • Clarify risk of contagion • Child's distress will often be unrelated to parental illness; remember to inquire about child's own individual challenges • Consider what the ill parent uniquely provides the child and save time and energy for those functions • Maintain consistent school routine and expectations • Protect family time not focused on the illness	• Begin to discuss the idea that the parent will not get better • Plan how to answer, "Will you die?" • Help child express love, in ways that are comfortable to child • Consider impact of setting of parent's care on child's access to parent and exposure to suffering • As above, consider leaving a written legacy to child • If death is imminent, may discuss how child wants to be notified
Adolescent (13–18)	• Provide age-appropriate information about who, what, when, where and why • Specify impact on child • Ask what has been noticed and explain child's observations • Elicit, discuss, normalize child's emotions while respecting privacy • Emphasize areas of control • Encourage reliance on friends, trusted adults for additional support	• Include adolescent in discussions about role changes and new responsibilities; find a fair balance • Monitor teens, watch for risk-taking behavior • Provide enough information about expected changes so teens can make informed decisions about the future • Protect family time not focused on the illness, while respecting the adolescent's need for time with peers	• Suggestions for grade-schoolers apply • Acknowledge the love underlying conflictual relationships • Demonstrate that surviving parent has ample support from other adults • Help adolescent make choices that will minimize regrets, without suggesting that they will or should have regrets

CLINICAL PEARLS

- As couples prepare for parenthood:
  - Encourage couples to build or broaden support networks.
  - Help couples anticipate the likely changes and practical needs they will have.
  - Emphasize communicating about and preparing for the added workload of parenthood

- For patients with young children: Clinicians can think creatively with parents about how to engage supports and utilize resources to increase consistency of routines for the children.

- For school age children: Encourage ongoing communication about the parent's medical condition with the children so children can understand and adjust to the ways their family may differ from others. Clinicians may help parents determine what tasks can be delegated to friends, family, or paid helpers, and what functions only they themselves can fulfill in their children's lives.

- For adolescents: Clinicians can help parents support their adolescents' friendships and "launch" into the world, while maintaining reasonable expectations for teens providing help at home.

- For young adult children: Clinicians should encourage parents to invite their adult children to engage in this communication and even to discuss how the communication is going.
  - Is the family talking too much, too little, or just the right amount about the illness?
  - Are people discussing the various aspects of the illness and its consequences that are important to everyone?

- At points in illness: Clinicians can suggest that parents inform their children that the ill parent is getting good care, getting the proper tests, and the immediately appropriate treatment (if applicable).

- Parents need not have all the answers, but the power of a parent's listening to and thinking with a child is immense.

- In the time after acute treatment, when things are better: Clinicians can recommend that parents reassure their children that the ill parent is still being actively monitored and that the children will remain in the communication loop.

- Children may have input as to what type of news they would like to hear, as well as when, how, and by whom it is shared. Often a brief discussion when there is only good news to share can help parents properly set the stage should bad news arise.

- Clinicians can think with parents about how to make sure that the balance of responsibilities in the family is allowing each member's continued normal development; they can also discuss key points in the illness course where that balance should be reassessed.

DISCLOSURE STATEMENTS

Dr. Moore Nothing to disclose.

Dr. Mankey has no disclosures or conflicts to report.

REFERENCES

Armistead, L., Klein, K., & Forehand, R. (1995). Parental physical illness and child functioning. *Clinical Psychology Reviews, 15*(5), 409–422.

Bloom, J. R., & Kessler, L. (1994). Risk and timing of counseling and support interventions for younger women with breast cancer. *Journal of the National Cancer Institute, Monograph 16*, 199–206.

Braun, M., Mikulincer, M., Rydall, A., Walsh, A., & Rodin, G. (2007). Hidden morbidity in cancer: spouse caregivers. *Journal of Clinical Oncology, 25*(30), 4829–4834.

Compas, B. E., Worsham. N. L., Ey, S., & Howell, D. S. (1996). When Mom or Dad has cancer: II. Coping, cognitive appraisals, and psychological distress in children of cancer patients. *Health Psychology, 15*(3), 167–175.

McGoldrick, M., & Carter, B. (2003). The family life cycle. In F. Walsh (Ed.), *Normal family processes: Growing diversity and complexity* (3rd ed., pp. 375–398). New York, NY: Guilford Press.

Northouse, L. L., Mood, D. W., Montie, J. E., Sandler, H. M., Forman, J. D., Hussain, M., et al. (2007). Living with prostate cancer: patients' and spouses' psychosocial status and quality of life. *Journal of Clinical Oncology, 25*(27), 4171–4177.

Duric, V., & Stockler, M. (2001). Patients' preferences for adjuvant chemotherapy in early breast cancer: a review of what makes it worthwhile? *Lancet Oncology, 2*, 691–697.

Halle, T. (2002). Charting parenthood: a statistical portrait of fathers and mothers in America. Report by Child Trends, Washington DC. http://www.childtrends.org/wp-content/uploads/2013/03/ParenthoodRpt2002.pdf

Lee-Jones, C., Humphris, G., Dixon, R., & Hatcher, M. B. (1997). Fear of cancer recurrence—a literature review and cognitive formulation to explain exacerbation of recurrence fears. *Psycho-Oncology, 6*(2), 95–105.

Muriel, A.C., Moore, C., Baer, L., Park, E.R., Kornblith, A.B., Prigerson, H et al. (2010). Psychosocial distress and parenting concerns among adults with cancer. *Psycho-Oncology, 19*(S2), A470.

Centers for Disease Control and Prevention. (2007). *National Diabetes Fact Sheet*. Washington, DC: Department of Health and Human Services.

Pedersen, S., & Revenson, T. A. (2005). Parental illness, family functioning, and adolescent well-being: A family ecology framework to guide research. *Journal of Family Psychology, 19*(3), 404–409.

Rauch, P. K., & Moore, C. W. (2010). Editorial: A population-based estimate of the number of US cancer survivors residing with their minor children. *Cancer, 116*, 4218–4220.

Rauch, P. K., & Muriel, A. C. (2006). *Raising an emotionally healthy child when a parent is sick*. New York, NY: McGraw-Hill.

Rolland, J. S. (1999). Parental illness and disability: a family systems framework. *Journal of Family Therapy, 21*, 242–266.

Rosenheim, E., & Reicher, R. (1985). Informing children about a parent's terminal illness. *Journal of Child Psychology & Psychiatry, 26*, 995–998.

Schuster, M., Kanouse, D., Morton, S., Bozzette, S., Miu, A., Scott, G., Shapiro, M. (2000). HIV-infected parents and their children in the United States. *American Journal of Public Health, 90*(7), 1074–1081.

Weaver, K., Rowland, J., Alfano, C., & McNeel, T. (2010). Parental cancer and the family: a population-based estimate of the number of US cancer survivors residing with their minor children. *Cancer, 116*, 4395–4401.

Yellen, S. B., & Cella, D. F. (1995). Someone to live for: social well-being, parenthood status, and decision-making in oncology. *Journal of Clinical Oncology, 13*, 1255–1264.

13.

GROUP PSYCHOTHERAPY FOR MEDICALLY ILL POPULATIONS

Cheryl Gore-Felton and David Spiegel

INTRODUCTION

Decades of research has resulted in compelling evidence for the efficacy of group psychotherapy in reducing psychiatric and physical symptoms, as well as increasing social support among medically ill patients (Blake-Mortimer et al., 1999; Reuter et al., 2010). The diagnosis of an acute, chronic, or life-threatening illness poses challenges to individuals and their families that have considerable impact on psychosocial functioning. Patients are confronted with the sense of their own mortality, which often causes acute stress and, in some cases, chronic stress with substantial disturbance in psychiatric functioning that can be quite disabling (Blake-Mortimer et al., 1999; Evans et al., 2005).

Using group psychotherapy to treat medically ill populations has its origins at the beginning of the 20th century when social workers and physicians began co-leading groups of tuberculosis patients (Fobair, 1997). The focus of these groups was on providing patients with information, education, and support to deal with their illness. Groups developed specifically for cancer patients were first reported in the 1970s (Franzino et al., 1976; Yalom & Greaves, 1977).

Although individual psychotherapy has demonstrated efficacy in reducing psychological distress, group psychotherapy has particular advantages over individual therapy, in that it provides validation for normative processes that would otherwise be seen as abnormal, emotional support, exposure to new interpersonal and coping skills, symptom relief, and enhanced competence (Yalom, 1995). Moreover, there is burgeoning evidence of biobehavioral mechanisms that help to explain why groups are effective in enhancing psychosocial functioning. For example, Taylor et al. (2000) put forth a theoretical model of stress response in females that relies heavily on the influence of the hormone oxytocin to explain affiliative responses under duress. She also noted that such groups provide opportunities for "downward comparisons," finding ways to feel fortunate in relation to others with similar problems. In addition, groups offer an opportunity for people to consolidate their own sense of competence in coping with problems by helping others with similar problems (Yalom & Greaves, 1977; Ferlic et al., 1979; Cummings & VandenBos, 1981; Mumford et al., 1984; Fawzy et al., 1990; Greer, 1991; Strain et al., 1991; Spiegel, 1993; Mittelman et al., 1996; Edelman et al., 1999; Block, 2001).

Although few would disagree that there is a robust empirical literature indicating the positive effects of group therapy on psychological well-being, there remains disagreement about whether or not group therapy can enhance health by altering disease processes. Indeed, people often ask, "Do groups help cancer patients live longer?" In this chapter we describe the rationale for group therapy among medically ill populations; the effects of group therapy on psychosocial, biomedical, and survival outcomes; different methods of group therapy; and group leadership issues. We emphasize intervention with patients diagnosed with cancer, human immunodeficiency virus (HIV), and acquired immune deficiency syndrome (AIDS). In this chapter we quote statements made by participants in therapy groups for patients with chronic general medical conditions that we have led personally. All patient quotes not otherwise attributed are from participants in our own groups.

RATIONALE FOR GROUP THERAPY

As the treatments for life-threatening illnesses such as cancer and AIDS continue to improve, individuals are living longer and healthier lives. This has resulted in these illnesses being thought of as chronic instead of terminal. The management of chronic illnesses poses challenges for patients and physicians, often requiring approaches that enhance the quality of survivorship. Indeed, the impact of chronic, serious illness on social, psychological, and physical demands faced by patients and their families can be profound and may require assistance to make adaptive changes (see chapter 11 on family therapy).

Although the treatments for cancer and AIDS have resulted in more life years, these medical treatments often contribute to survival at considerable cost. For instance, the physiological long-term and late effects of therapies for adult cancer can cause a variety of problems. These problems can include energy loss, sexual dysfunction, cognitive impairment, (Kesler et al., 2009) lymphedema, physical disfigurement, and major physiological complications that impair organ systems and can cause death (Loescher et al., 1989). Similarly, among patients with AIDS, long-term use of highly active antiretroviral therapy (HAART) has resulted in a wide range of disorders that include metabolic (Moyle, 2007) and dermatological disorders (Luther & Glesby, 2007) and alterations in serum lipids (Riddler et al.,

2003). These physiological impairments can have significant adverse effects on psychological as well as social functioning.

EFFECTS OF CHRONIC ILLNESS ON MOOD

Mood disorders are prevalent among the medically ill and occur at much higher rates than the general population. The lifetime prevalence rate of major depression in the US general population is estimated at 16%, while the prevalence among medically ill patients ranges from 20%–50% (Kessler et al., 2003). Moreover, there is evidence suggesting that depression significantly contributes to the progression of medical illness, worsening prognosis (Evans et al., 2005).

CANCER PATIENTS

Depression among cancer patients is associated with poor prognosis (Giese-Davis et al., 2011) and increased morbidity (Evans et al., 2005). The exact mechanism of this relationship remains unclear, resulting in no empirically validated standardized approach to treat depression among such patients. In recent years, research to develop efficacious interventions that ameliorate depression has increased. Researchers have also begun to examine pathways other than neurotransmitters to explain symptoms of depression. Psychiatric illnesses like depression were once thought to be solely brain disorders, but there is a growing body of research which asserts that an activated immune system that secretes cytokines is responsible for depression and explains the association of depression with disease (Capuron & Dantzer, 2003). Cytokines can cross the blood–brain barrier, and once in the brain they can cause all of the symptoms found in depression (e.g., fatigue, depressed mood, lack of interest; see Capuron & Dantzer, 2003). Indeed, a complex relationship between psychosocial factors, endocrine activation, circadian rhythms, immune defenses, and tumor progression suggests that interventions that enhance psychological functioning may influence biological functioning, thereby bolstering survival (Sephton & Spiegel, 2003). For instance, it has been asserted that the disruption of sleep/wake rhythms and corresponding sleep debt may suppress the cancer fighting immune response (Vgontzas & Chrousos, 2002). If this is true, then psychotherapy that focuses on reducing stress and regulating sleep patterns using sleep hygiene protocols (for review, see Stepanski & Wyatt, 2003) may be a very effective, noninvasive treatment that improves cancer survival.

Psychotherapeutic intervention can be beneficial at any time during diagnosis and treatment; however, there are indications that treatment may be particularly beneficial immediately following diagnosis. For example, patients' patterns of coping with a cancer diagnosis (Dunkel-Schetter et al., 1992) and the types of psychosocial needs expressed (Liang et al., 1990) usually do not change significantly after the initial diagnosis. Moreover, newly diagnosed patients are particularly vulnerable to severe emotional distress. A study of newly diagnosed patients with breast, colorectal, head and neck, lung, and prostate carcinomas, as well as skin cancers other than malignant melanoma, found that almost all (96%) reported current symptoms of fatigue (66%), worry (61%), difficulty sleeping (48%), and pain (42%) (Whelan et al., 1997). For women, breast cancer is the most prevalent type of cancer, accounting for almost one-quarter of all cancer cases (Parkin et al., 2005). Treatment advances have resulted in women surviving longer, and with that comes treatment-related problems that are often persistent (e.g., vasomotor symptoms, body image, & fatigue), resulting in decreased quality of life (Duijts et al., 2011).

HIV/AIDS PATIENTS

Similar to breast cancer patients, newly diagnosed HIV or AIDS patients often experience severe emotional distress. Notification of positive HIV serostatus can be accompanied by depression, fear, anxiety, anger (Naar-King et al., 2007), and feelings associated with stigma (Alonzo & Reynolds, 1995). There is a growing body of evidence that indicates that depression, stressful life events, and trauma influence the course of HIV disease (Leserman, 2008). While the causal pathways of this relationship continue to be explored, there is evidence suggesting that behavioral mechanisms may account for part of the relationship: namely, depression, mood disturbance, and poor coping strategies to deal with stress predict noncompliance with antiretroviral therapy in HIV-positive patients, which has deleterious effects on health outcomes (Gore-Felton & Koopman, 2008). Interestingly, there is evidence that suggests that a positive psychosocial factor such as optimism is associated with better health behaviors and slower HIV disease progression (Ironson & Hayward, 2008).

The emotions that accompany life-threatening diagnosis and treatment are necessary responses to multiple problems that accompany the diagnosis. Typical emotional responses include a radical alteration in one's sense of self, which is frequently followed by a decrease in self-esteem, fear of abandonment, uncertainty about disease progression, and fear of dying and death. The distress can be chronic for some patients. There is evidence that less social support is associated with disease progression in breast cancer and HIV-positive patients. In a prospective study of 2,835 women diagnosed with stages 1 to 4 breast cancer, social isolation was associated with a 66% increased risk of all-cause mortality and a twofold increased risk of breast cancer mortality (Kroenke et al., 2006). Similarly, in a sample of 96 men followed prospectively for up to 9 years, higher cumulative average stressful life events and lower cumulative average social support predicted faster progression to AIDS (Leserman et al., 2002).

IMPACT OF CHRONIC ILLNESS ON SOCIAL SUPPORT

Despite the positive influence of social support on health, individuals suffering from chronic medical problems often find themselves with diminished social resources (White et al., 1992). Part of the explanation for this may be the amount of pain and suffering that is associated with the illness. For example, cancer-related pain is associated with decreased physical and social activity (Strang, 1992). Additionally, the psychosocial impact of the illness on family members can be so overwhelming that their ability to be a source of support to the patient is diminished.

When a spouse is diagnosed with cancer, the threat of possible death and disability coupled with the financial burden of surgery and treatment can cause long-term loss of stability in family roles (Northouse, 1988). Moreover, existing family problems are often intensified, which creates a fragile family structure in which members are less capable of providing much-needed support (Cohen & Wellisch, 1974).

Distress increases among family members as the dying process ensues (Gotay, 1984; Northouse, 1988). The ability of the family to openly communicate about the probability of dying has been linked to positive adjustment, cohesion, and decreased conflict during terminal illness (Spiegel et al., 1983; Northouse, 1988; Block, 2001), and it has also been linked to better adjustment for the bereaved following the patient's death (Cohen & Wellisch, 1974; Northouse, 1988). When communication is poor, family members may restrict their expression of feelings as they attempt to protect one another from awareness of death. Also, family members may experience a sense of social isolation as those closest to the family find it difficult to visit the patient because of confusion about how much to say (Cohen & Wellisch, 1974; Northouse, 1988). Furthermore, excessive focus on aggressive medical treatment with apparent curative intent rather than hospice care is associated with poor end-of-life care (Earle et al., 2003), more depression, and even shorter survival. (Temel et al., 2010).

Understandably, significant others have difficulty coping with the patient's illness. As a woman diagnosed with AIDS stated in group: "My husband is acting like he is the one who is sick. I feel like I have to take care of him, and it should be the other way around."

Family and friends generally share the patient's anxiety, fear, and feelings of powerlessness, but they also struggle with accepting the physiological as well as psychological changes that accompany their loved one's diagnosis. The patient is likely to experience a pervasive sense of loss of control, often accompanied by feelings of isolation, and is in need of support. However, because of the psychological distress that the support system experiences, the patient may find that the support system is inadequate. Moreover, any conflict or unresolved issues that were part of the family before the patient became ill will complicate the family's as well as the patient's ability to adapt to the impending physical and psychological changes. In addition, patients with young children often experience considerable anxiety about how their illness will affect their children's lives. This is particularly true for single mothers who do not have adequate support systems to take care of their children if they become incapacitated or die.

Furthermore, loved ones often experience helplessness, which may manifest itself as feelings of inadequacy. These emotions frequently translate into cognitions such as, "I can't fix it," as family members and friends withdraw into silence or actually physically distance themselves. The impact of this withdrawal on patients can be devastating. For example, in one group an HIV-positive woman sobbed:

> "We are having a family reunion next month, and I called my grandmother to tell her when I would arrive. She told me I would have to stay in a motel because she didn't want me using her bathroom. Part of me thinks she is scared of getting something, but most of me thinks she just doesn't want to be bothered."

The overwhelming sense of rejection catapulted this patient into depression and a marked awareness of abandonment and aloneness.

The negative psychosocial impact on individuals and family members provides a rationale for group intervention for the medically ill. Moreover, group psychotherapy is a highly effective and efficient treatment modality that provides immediate social support, a "social laboratory" for assessing problems and trying out solutions, and a means of finding commonalities and differences (Spiegel, 1993; Yalom, 1995).

INDIVIDUAL VERSUS GROUP THERAPY

There is evidence that individuals benefit from individual psychotherapy (Cain et al., 1986); however, group therapy has been shown to be at least as effective (Cain et al., 1986; Fawzy et al., 1996; Hosaka, 1996). Moreover, group therapy offers unique advantages as a psychotherapeutic intervention, and many studies have demonstrated positive effects of group therapy for cancer patients. These positive outcomes include beneficial effects on mood, adjustment, and pain (Gustafson & Whitman, 1978; Wood et al., 1978; Ferlic et al., 1979; Spiegel et al., 1981; Spiegel & Bloom, 1983; Fawzy et al., 1990; Butler et al., 2009).

Group psychotherapy offers four unique advantages over individual therapy:

1. *Universality.* Many patients are socially isolated from others who are suffering from the same illness. Thus, the power of a group allows patients the opportunity to experience others who are facing the same problems. This realization assists patients in disconfirming their feelings of uniqueness, which is often experienced as relief (Yalom, 1995). Individual therapy also assists patients in normalizing their feelings and behaviors, but there is no opportunity for patients to experience consensual validation and at the same time develop interpersonal intimacy with others who have suffered similar experiences. When patients come to realize that problems they thought were the result of their own poor coping also happen to others, it becomes clear that the problems are inherent to the disease process rather than to their particular personality and life situation. This realization helps patients accept their situation while at the same time assists them in overcoming feelings of stigmatization that occur with diseases such as cancer and HIV/AIDS. In learning to like and

respect others who are coping with similar problems, they come to like and respect themselves.

2. *Helper-therapy principle.* The helper-therapy principle is the process through which patients gain enhanced self-efficacy through their ability to help others (Riessman, 1965). Having cancer or AIDS is a meaningless tragedy to patients. But using that experience to be able to help others going through a similar situation enhances one's sense of competence and helps to develop a renewed sense of meaning in life; in other words, something genuinely good emerges from a bad situation. Helping others has been extremely beneficial to women attending a support group for women living with HIV/AIDS. For example, a woman in a HIV/AIDS support group stated:

> "There are times when I'm so sick of being sick and tired, then I come to group and something I say is helpful to someone else. It makes me think that I'm good for something and my life is not so meaningless after all."

Group therapy increases the likelihood of constructive compassion with other patients (Yalom, 1995). The group format allows patients to give unique support to one another and provides an expanded social network, role models for coping with various aspects of the illness, and an opportunity to enhance self-esteem by giving concrete help to others in a similar situation.

3. *Social support.* An often-noted benefit of attendance at support groups is that members can relate to each other in special ways that counter the social isolation they often experience after a diagnosis (Tracy & Gussow, 1976; Toseland & Hacker, 1982). Being part of a group can afford patients a sense of community necessary for successful coping and provide opportunities to learn from one another (Spiegel, 1993). Members come to feel part of a new and accepting social group in which their common bond is the very thing that makes them feel excluded in the outside world (Spiegel, 1993). They can contact one another outside group meetings and thereby develop a new support network.

4. *Cost effectiveness.* Group therapy is clearly more cost effective than individual therapy, in that it makes limited professional resources available to many more people. Economically, group therapy may be up to four times more affordable for patients and for institutions (Hellman et al., 1990; Yalom & Yalom, 1990). Two well-conducted meta-analytic studies demonstrate that psychoeducational (Devine, 1992) and psychotherapeutic (Mumford et al., 1984) interventions produce cost savings in medical treatment. Mumford et al. (1984) examined 58 cost-offset studies and found that there was a significant reduction in inpatient costs (e.g., reduction in hospitalization) following outpatient psychotherapy. Devine (1992) analyzed 191 studies that examined the effects of psychoeducational care on recovery, postoperative pain, and psychological distress in surgical patients. Across studies, psychoeducational care resulted in faster postoperative recovery, less postoperative pain, and less psychological distress. Moreover, there is evidence indicating that psychosocial intervention in medically ill patients results in shorter hospital stays (Mumford et al., 1984; Devine, 1992) and reduced distress-related outpatient visits to doctors (Cummings & VandenBos, 1981; Lorig et al., 1985; Browne et al., 1990). Thus, as a method of improving adaptive coping, improving adherence to complex and difficult medical treatments, preventing clinically significant anxiety and depression, and treating more serious psychiatric comorbidities, group psychotherapies are both effective and cost effective. Such interventions are far less expensive than other routine medical and surgical treatments for cancer and HIV, and the risk-benefit ratio is highly favorable. While growing healthcare costs are a problem, this is not a rational place to economize. Indeed, with the growing body of research suggesting that a viable pathway to tumor suppression is through psychosocial factors, it would seem prudent for medical health centers and hospitals to explore methods of delivering psychosocial interventions as adjuvant treatment to individuals with serious medical illnesses as the standard of care.

EFFECTIVENESS OF GROUP THERAPY AS ADJUNCTIVE TREATMENT

There have been a number of research studies that have assessed the effectiveness of group psychotherapy for cancer patients. There is also a growing body of literature examining the effects of group psychotherapy for people living with HIV/AIDS. The range of intervention types has increased over the past decade to include cognitive behavioral, psychoeducational, cognitive existential, and mindfulness approaches. The literature illuminates several psychosocial domains that have shown improvement with group psychotherapy: psychological distress, interpersonal functioning, quality of life, and survival.

PSYCHOLOGICAL DISTRESS

One of the first published studies examining the effects of group therapy was conducted by (Bloom et al., 1978). This important research revealed that patients who received group therapy had significantly higher levels of personal control compared to patients who received only standard medical care. The study was limited by small sample size and nonrandomization, making it difficult to generalize the results to the general population.

Building on several studies (Spiegel & Yalom, 1978; Bloom et al., 1978; Wood et al., 1978; Ferlic et al., 1979; Maisiak et al., 1981; Cain et al., 1986; Spiegel et al., 1981) Spiegel and colleagues conducted a one year prospective study examining the effects of support groups for metastatic breast cancer patients. Oncologists referred 109 women to the study, and each participant was randomly assigned to either a weekly support group or a control group who received standard medical care. The group was facilitated by a psychiatrist and a social worker. Evaluations at 4 and 8 months showed no significant differences between the groups; however, at 12 months patients in the support group had significantly better coping styles, fewer phobias, and less confusion and fatigue compared to the control group. Furthermore, additional research has supported the finding that group psychotherapy is effective in improving overall mood, anxiety, and coping (Cunningham et al., 1993; Fawzy et al., 1990). This reduction in distress has been replicated in a new sample involving 125 women with metastatic breast cancer (Classen et al., 2001). In this study, the dependent variable was a reduction in scores on the Impact of Event Scale. The intervention group in this randomized trial also experienced a significant reduction in pain compared to the control group (Butler et al., 2009).

Various group interventions provide psychological benefits to cancer patients, independent of stage of diagnosis or type of treatment (Bottomley, 1997). Specifically, there is clear evidence that group psychotherapy for cancer patients is effective in reducing anxiety and depression (Gustafson & Whitman, 1978; Wood et al., 1978; Ferlic et al., 1979; Spiegel et al., 1981; Spiegel & Bloom, 1983; Mulder et al., 1992) and improving coping skills (Fawzy et al., 1990).

Group therapy has an opportunity to prevent full anxiety and depressive syndromes in cancer patients. The idea of preventing rather than treating anxiety and depression among cancer patients was tested in a large individual intervention trial (N = 465; see Pitceathly et al., 2009). The brief intervention, a cognitive behavioral format with two telephone sessions following the initial visit shortly after cancer diagnosis, was effective in reducing the incidence of anxiety and depression among high-risk but not low-risk patients. Clearly, there is a continuum from normal fear to anxiety and from sadness to depression. Some adverse affective response can be expected with the diagnosis and treatment of cancer. Interventions in the medical setting may help people manage their normal emotional responses to adverse medical conditions, and reduce or in some cases prevent the development of clinically significant symptoms of anxiety and depression. There is a continuum also between disease-related stress and clinical psychopathology. Often patients and their families are more receptive to receiving help with stress management than with psychiatric problems. Group interventions have the advantage of "normalizing" stress responses and potentially reducing the risk of developing more serious emotional problems. This intermediate zone of psychopathology is often diagnosed within the domain of "adjustment disorders" (American Psychiatric Association, 2000). While a substantial minority of cancer patients meet diagnostic criteria for clinical anxiety and depression (Derogatis et al., 1983; Breitbart et al., 1995; Grassi & Rosti, 1996), the majority have adjustment problems that may well benefit from group and individual psychotherapeutic intervention.

Meta-analyses of the psychosocial effects of group psychotherapies for cancer patients have generally concluded that there are robust treatment effects. One analyzing for three dependent outcomes among breast cancer patients—anxiety, depression, and quality of life, (Naaman et al., 2009)—concluded that there was a moderate effect for anxiety and a moderate to strong effect for depression. More severely affected patients showed a stronger improvement in quality of life with group intervention. The researchers also concluded that short-term interventions emphasizing coping skills seemed more effective for those with early-stage disease, while those with more advanced breast cancer benefitted more from longer interventions emphasizing support. A *Cochrane Database* meta-analysis of psychotherapy (most in group format) for patients with advanced cancer showed significant reductions in depression with a moderate effect size. The authors note that the moderate effect size found in their meta-analysis differed from the weak effect size found in the extant literature, and this difference was likely because most of the trials included in previous studies did not select patients with clinically diagnosed depression or advanced stages of cancer (Akechi et al., 2008).

However, some randomized trials have shown little or no psychological benefit. In one study involving 210 women recently diagnosed with breast cancer, the intervention consisted of an unusual combination of two weekly 6-hour sessions of psychoeducation and eight weekly 2-hour sessions of group psychotherapy. There were no significant effects of the intervention on psychological outcome, although patients in both treatment and control samples who were on antidepressants improved over time (Boesen et al., 2011). Another trial providing a 6-day cancer rehabilitation course shortly after diagnosis reported no significant differences between treatment and control groups at 6-month follow-up (Ibfelt et al., 2011).

Indeed, one meta-analysis that concluded there was little evidence for psychological benefit from psychosocial intervention for cancer patients (Newell et al., 2002) eliminated three-quarters of the published trials (from 327 to 82) based on criteria that included whether caregivers were blinded to the treatment condition, which is hard to imagine. Furthermore, they assessed a wide array of outcomes ranging from the psychosocial to treatment side effects to immune function. Thus, their surprising null conclusion seems to have more to do with the methods of the meta-analysis than the content of the studies reviewed. On balance, however, the bulk of studies and reviews conclude that group intervention improves quality of life and reduces distress for cancer patients.

Among HIV-positive homosexual/bisexual men, social support has been significantly and positively related to active behavioral coping (Wolf et al., 1991). Furthermore, brief group therapy for depressed persons with HIV infection effectively reduced symptoms of emotional distress (Cacioppo et al., 1992; Kelly et al., 1993), especially when it included a supportive/expressive approach which emphasized emotional expression and dealing with existential concerns.

INTERPERSONAL FUNCTIONING

The type of isolation experienced by patients with catastrophic illness reinforces death anxiety because death is often conceptualized as being alone, separated from family and friends (Spiegel, 1990). A support group has the beneficial effect of moderating the patient's sense of isolation by providing a new social network. The group becomes a powerful medium for restoring patients' homeostasis, in that the very experience that separates them from the rest of the world is what bonds them with others in the group (Spiegel, 1990). Being with others who have the same illness and who share similar experiences mitigates the anxiety of facing the illness on one's own and normalizes disease-related feelings and experiences. Involvement in a group also allows patients to better mobilize their existing resources, as well as to develop new coping strategies and sources of support.

QUALITY OF LIFE AND SURVIVAL

Support groups and other psychosocial interventions play an important role in enhancing the quality of life for HIV-positive persons (Beckett & Rutan, 1990; Markowitz et al., 1992) and cancer patients (Spiegel & Glafkides, 1983; Spiegel & Wissler, 1983; Forester et al., 1985). Moreover, there is surprising evidence that group psychotherapy may affect the quantity as well as the quality of life. A randomized clinical trial of palliative care for non–small cell lung cancer patients published in the *New England Journal of Medicine* (Temel et al., 2010) produced a clear but apparently paradoxical finding: "Despite receiving less aggressive end-of-life care, patients in the palliative care group had significantly longer survival than those in the standard care group (median survival 11.65 vs. 8.9 months; P = 0.02)." The palliative care condition reduced depression as well. The intervention involved an average of four visits that focused on choices about resuscitation preferences, pain control, and quality of life. The study demonstrates that at the end of life, the most aggressive treatments may not be the most effective—not only psychologically but also medically.

Eight of 15 published clinical trials demonstrate an effect of psychotherapeutic support on cancer survival time, and none show a worsening of outcome. Spiegel and colleagues (1989) first conducted a prospective randomized trial on the effect of group psychotherapy of patients with metastatic breast cancer in the 1970s and published the survival results in 1989. Fifty women with metastatic breast cancer were randomly assigned to a year of weekly support groups with training in self-hypnosis for pain control. Forty-eight months after the study had begun, all of the control patients had died but one-third of the treatment sample were still alive. Surprisingly, the treatment group survived an average of 18 months longer than 36 control patients who had been randomly assigned to routine care.

A decade later a replication study from the same investigators showed no overall effect of a similar group therapy intervention on breast cancer survival, but a significant interaction with tumor type such that those with estrogen receptor negative cancers who were randomized to group therapy lived significantly longer than did ER-negative patients receiving standard

care alone (Spiegel et al., 2007) While this failed to confirm the main hypothesis that facing death together could improve survival, major advances in hormonal and chemotherapies had improved overall survival for women with metastatic breast cancer in the interim (Peto et al., 2000); however, women with ER-negative tumors do not benefit from the major improvement in treatment outcome associated with anti-estrogen treatments (Peto et al., 2000). A randomized trial of psycho-educational groups for women with primary breast cancer found significantly reduced rates of relapse and longer survival (Andersen et al., 2008). In addition to this, our original study (Spiegel et al., 1989), our replication trial (Spiegel et al., 2007), the recent palliative care study (Temel et al., 2010), three other randomized trials (Richardson et al., 1990; Fawzy et al., 1993; Kuchler et al., 1999; Kuchler et al., 2007), and one matched cohort trial (McCorkle et al., 2000) have found that psychosocial treatment for patients with a variety of cancers results in both psychological and survival benefit. However, seven other published studies (Linn et al., 1982; Ilnyckyj et al., 1994; Cunningham et al., 1998; Edelman et al., 1999; Goodwin et al., 2001; Kissane et al., 2007 Kissane et al., 2004), six involving breast cancer patients (Edelman et al., 1999; Ilnyckyj et al., 1994; Goodwin et al., 2001; Kissane et al., 2007, 2004; Cunningham et al., 1998) found no survival benefit for those treated with psychotherapy. Three of these seven studies showed no emotional benefit of the intervention (Ilnyckyj et al., 1994; Cunningham et al., 1998; Edelman et al., 1999), making any survival benefit unlikely. In a fourth study, the treatment group was more depressed than the control group at baseline (Goodwin et al., 2001), which gave them a poorer medical prognosis based on recent research (Giese-Davis et al., 2011). Furthermore, no studies show that such attention to emotion and mortality shortens survival (Spiegel, 2002).

Thus, there is growing evidence that group psychotherapy may influence survival time as well as adjustment to serious chronic medical illness. The mechanisms underlying such an effect are yet to be determined but may involve diet, exercise, sleep, adherence to medical treatment, or changes in endocrine and immune function (Spiegel, 1991; Sephton et al., 2000; Sephton & Spiegel, 2003; McDonald et al., 2005; Antoni et al., 2006; Innominato et al., 2010).

It should be mentioned that caregivers of patients with a chronic illness suffer a great deal of stress, which can impact the health of the patient. For example, Taerk (1983) found that groups for oncology nurses resulted in improvement in patient care and ward atmosphere. Moreover, among caregivers of Alzheimzer's patients, support groups have been effective at delaying the onset of nursing home care for the patients (Mittelman et al., 1993).

DIFFERENT METHODS OF GROUP PSYCHOTHERAPY

Group interventions for chronically ill patients employ various strategies. Some of the groups are structured with more of an educational focus, while others are unstructured and more affectively oriented.

Educational groups have as a goal the dissemination of information. They can be very helpful to patients who have been newly diagnosed with a disease. Educational groups can also be effective in teaching prevention tools. For example, at-risk populations such as teenagers engaging in unprotected sexual behavior may modify risky sexual behavior after becoming informed through an educational group (Mansfield et al., 1993; Magura et al., 1994). Furthermore, educational groups can reduce feelings of helplessness and inadequacy by giving patients a sense of mastery and control (Fawzy et al., 1995).

Cognitive behavioral groups typically employ problem-focused skills-building and coping strategies. These groups have been successful at improving quality of life through better coping and increased medical compliance for chronically ill patients suffering from diabetes, asthma, HIV/AIDS, and cancer (Kelly et al., 1993). Many of the psychotherapies that have shown promise in improving emotional adjustment and influencing survival time involve encouraging open expression of emotion and assertiveness in assuming control over the course of treatment, life decisions, and relationships (Spiegel & Yalom, 1978; Spiegel et al., 1981, 1989; Fawzy et al., 1990).

Recently, as noted above, the range of interventions has grown. An existential group intervention known as *meaning-centered group psychotherapy* was designed to help cancer patients facing death to develop a sense of meaning, peace, and purpose in their lives (Breitbart et al., 2010). In a small randomized trial comparing this approach to supportive group psychotherapy, those in the meaning-centered intervention reported greater improvements in spiritual well-being and meaning and reductions in anxiety and desire for death. This finding is consistent with an important randomized trial of *dignity therapy*, an existentially oriented individual intervention designed for people with advanced disease. In that trial, 165 of 441 patients were assigned to dignity therapy, 140 to palliative care, and 136 to client-centered care. While improvements were noted in all conditions, dignity therapy proved superior in reducing depression and improving quality of life and spiritual well-being (Chochinov et al., 2011).

SUPPORTIVE-EXPRESSIVE THERAPY

Supportive-expressive therapy is group therapy option that deals with emotional, existential and practical issues of cancer patients. Its combination of components makes it relevant to cancer patients at different stages of illness, with different sources of psychosocial distress. Supportive-expressive therapy comprises:

1. *Social support.* Psychotherapy, especially in groups, can provide a new social network with the common bond of facing similar problems (Spiegel, 1993). There is strong evidence that social contact has positive emotional effects and reduces overall mortality risk (House et al., 1988). Social isolation has been shown to be as strongly related to age-adjusted mortality as serum cholesterol levels or smoking. Indeed, being married predicts better medical

outcome with cancer (Goodwin et al., 1987), while social stress such as divorce, loss of a job, or bereavement is associated in some studies with a greater likelihood of a relapse of cancer (Ramirez et al., 1989).

2. *Emotional expression.* The expression of emotion is important in reducing social isolation and improving coping. Moreover, emotional suppression and avoidance are associated with poorer coping (Greer et al., 1979; Greer, 1991). However, group and individual psychotherapies can facilitate the expression of emotion appropriate to the disease. Doing so seems to reduce the repressive coping strategy that reduces expression of positive as well as negative emotion. Emotional suppression also reduces intimacy in families, limiting opportunities for direct expression of affection and concern. Indeed, there is evidence that those who are able to ventilate strong feelings directly cope better with cancer (Derogatis et al., 1979; Greer et al., 1979; Pettingale, 1984; Temoshok et al., 1985; Greer, 1991).

3. *Detoxifying dying.* This component of the therapy involves examining the threat of death in a straightforward manner rather than avoiding it. The goal is to help those facing the threat of death by reducing their anxiety about it as well as exploring fears associated with the process of dying. This exploration enables patients to think about what they control. These discussions often lead patients into making positive life changes while reducing their overwhelming fears and anxieties. One woman with metastatic breast cancer described her experience in this way:

   "What I found is that talking about death is like looking down into the Grand Canyon (I don't like heights). You know that if you fell down, it would be a disaster, but you feel better about yourself because you're able to look. I can't say I feel serene, but I can look at it now" (Spiegel, 1993).

4. *Reordering life priorities.* When cure is not possible, a realistic evaluation of the future can help those with life-threatening illness make the best use of remaining time. One of the costs of unrealistic optimism is the loss of time for accomplishing life projects, communicating openly with family and friends, and setting affairs in order. Facing the threat of death can aid in making the most of life (Spiegel et al., 1981). Discussing these issues directly can help patients take control of those aspects of their lives they can influence while grieving and relinquishing those they cannot.

5. *Family support.* Psychotherapeutic interventions can also be quite helpful in improving communication, identifying needs, increasing role flexibility, and adjusting to new medical, social, vocational, and financial realities. There is evidence that an atmosphere of open and shared problem solving in families results in reduced anxiety and depression among cancer patients (Spiegel & Wissler, 1983).

Thus, facilitating the development of such open addressing of common problems is a useful therapeutic goal. Groups can also help family members to ventilate feelings that tend to be brushed aside in the face of those affecting the medically ill. As one husband of a metastatic breast cancer patient put it: *"This group is a place where I come to feel better about feeling bad."* Group members also learn role flexibility, rearranging family duties and decreasing the tendency to reassure rather than discuss serious problems. Group interventions may help to augment family support by helping to improve communication and to help patients practice ways of both giving to, and seeking help from, family members. At times, however, especially when there is resistance to facing and dealing with disease-related issues, family consultation or treatment may be important.

6. *Communication with physicians.* Support groups are useful tools for facilitating better communication with physicians and other healthcare providers. Groups provide mutual encouragement to get questions answered, to participate actively in treatment decisions, and to consider alternatives carefully. Groups must be careful not to interfere with medical treatment and decisions; rather, the goal is to encourage patients to be assertive in getting clear information that will assist in reaching informed decisions.

7. *Symptom control.* Many treatment approaches involve teaching cognitive techniques to manage anxiety, anticipatory nausea and vomiting, and pain. Cognitive techniques include learning to identify emotions as they develop, to analyze sources of emotional response, and to move from emotion-focused to problem-focused coping. Behavioral techniques include specific self-regulation skills such as self-hypnosis, meditation, biofeedback, and progressive muscle relaxation (Burish & Lyles, 1981; Morrow & Morrell, 1982; Zeltzer & LeBaron, 1982; Spiegel & Bloom, 1983; Spiegel, 1990).

ROLE OF SELF-HELP GROUPS

There is evidence suggesting that self-help groups are beneficial in assisting patients to modify behaviors, (e.g., Alcoholics Anonymous) and reduce psychological distress. In post-mastectomy patients, those who attended self-help groups experienced less psychological distress compared to patients who did not attend self-help groups (Silverman-Dresner, 1989–1990). Moreover, self-help members tend to utilize the services of professionals more than people who do not attend self-help groups and were more likely to use more than one source for support.

Self-help groups may be particularly helpful for newly diagnosed individuals who not only require social support but are in need of information. Self-help groups often have information on professional referrals in the community and surrounding areas. For a patient who is overwhelmed by a recent diagnosis of a severe illness, having a self-help group manage

the wealth of information and provide support during the process can be extremely beneficial. However, the complexity of medical problems and treatments facing patients with cancer and HIV infection, along with the array of frequently intense emotional responses, often requires the help of a well-trained therapist.

Simply "stirring the pot" by raising emotionally-laden issues without working them through to the point of active coping and mastery can proliferate problems, making group leadership by a professional therapist crucial. In one study comparing unstructured peer discussion groups to educational groups for women with early-stage breast cancer, those in the unstructured groups actually showed evidence of worsening self-esteem, body image, and intrusive thoughts about the illness (Helgeson et al., 1999). This study underscores the importance of well-trained group leaders and a clear and clinically tested theoretical orientation to treatment.

As people have growing access to the internet, online support groups will become more popular. This provides access to support for those too far from treatment centers or too physically impaired to attend groups regularly (Owen et al., 2004). There are few systematic studies, but there is evidence that such virtual interaction can be surprisingly effective in reducing distress (Lieberman et al., 2003; Lieberman & Goldstein, 2005).

GROUP MEMBERSHIP

The population of the group is an important question, because issues related to gender, sexuality, diagnosis, prognosis, age, culture, and so on, can be extremely important in terms of group cohesiveness. Heterogeneous groups are often educational. They meet for a brief period and do not require a great deal of group cohesiveness to function. As groups become more long term and require more group interaction to function properly, it is best to constitute the group to be as homogeneous as possible, especially in regard to prognosis. At the same time, if a woman in a group of primary breast cancer patients suffers a relapse, it is crucial for her and for the morale of all group members that she be made to feel welcome and supported in that group.

For HIV/AIDS populations, people will have very different issues to deal with in relation to their HIV infection. For example, issues arising for HIV-infected heterosexuals will not be identical with those arising for infected gay men. Moreover, individuals infected through intravenous substance use and struggling with recovery issues have unique needs. Additionally, people of color confront another set of issues stemming from their minority status within society and the specific cultural mores of their own ethnic communities. Furthermore, women, as a group, may be defined by their own set of issues including the gender-specific manifestations of HIV/AIDS infection. Age range within a specific group also needs to be considered. Young adults are typically grappling with adult developmental issues, which are significantly different from the issues faced by older adults.

The socioeconomic background of the population will vary. It is important to note that the majority of increase of HIV infection is in low-income minority communities. Because of this, the efforts to reach out to these populations require special innovation. The social demands put upon this particular population affect their ability to adequately seek and maintain medical treatment for their illness. To address some of these issues and encourage treatment compliance, it may be necessary for treatment services to provide some of the group participants with assistance such as travel vouchers and childcare subsidies. Although treatment providers may feel this is expensive, it is considerably more costly to do nothing and to continue to allow this segment of the AIDS population to go untreated.

LEADERSHIP ISSUES

Groups are often led by two therapists. This is crucial for new therapists. Ideally, new therapists should be matched with a more experienced group facilitator (Yalom, 1995). Besides allowing the newer leader to learn from the veteran, the presence of co-leaders decreases anxiety and allows therapists to fully attend to the group process. Once the group is over, the co-leaders can debrief regarding the session. This provides valuable information about each therapist's behavior and deepens the understanding of the group process. Depending upon the specific group population and their collective issues and needs, each therapist should possess clinical expertise in that group's unique and defining issues. There are issues that define a group more specifically than simply sharing an HIV/AIDS diagnosis; for example, substance abuse, gay issues, heterosexual issues, issues regarding race or ethnicity, and issues specific to women infected with HIV/AIDS.

Therapists should have training and experience in psychotherapy or group therapy, as well as training and experience in psychosocial support for patients with life-threatening illness or medical management of HIV disease. In addition, they should also have at least minimal knowledge of the disease that is the focus of the group, such as HIV infection or cancer. This knowledge is crucial—not so much because the therapist can impart it to group members, but rather because it enhances the therapist's own understanding of living with this disease. Co-leaders should ideally complement one another's abilities. For example, a group may have one leader who is a psychiatrist and the other a social worker. This interdisciplinary approach allows for a broader context in which to place the group members' experience. This is particularly important when working with underserved populations who may need a great deal of support in accessing social services as well as medical services. For example, an African-American woman diagnosed with AIDS stated:

> "I've got my two kids at home, but no one to watch them while I go to all my doctor appointments and I can't afford to pay anyone. So, when I run out of my meds I've been taking my friends' meds."

One of the co-facilitators of this group was a social worker who was able to refer this patient to a preschool program in the community. This intervention not only allowed the woman to attend her medical appointments, but it also gave her a much needed reprieve from the stressful tasks and duties of being a single parent.

The training of group leaders is an important part of developing effective group interventions. For example, therapists who were trained in supportive/expressive group therapy improved in four areas: (1) facilitating the expression of affect; (2) facilitating exploration of personal and specific cancer-related issues in the here and now; (3) facilitating supportive group interaction; and (4) facilitating active coping strategies (Classen et al., 1997). Interestingly, these dimensions represent the areas that are thought to be associated with positive patient outcome.

It is not uncommon for therapists leading supportive/expressive therapy groups to feel uncomfortable with the emphasis on facilitating difficult and painful discussions about such topics as fears of disease progression, dying, and death. It may seem counterintuitive to encourage the discussion of "negative" topics, especially with most patients believing they should be thinking "positively." Indeed, one common concern about groups for the medically ill is that they will demoralize patients by exposing them to disease progression or death among other members. When a death of a group member occurs, the therapists are challenged with facilitating the grieving process among the group members.

In supportive/expressive therapy, the therapists facilitate the emotions of the group members, which are typically sadness, anger, and fear. While processing their emotions, many group members express a desire to attend memorial or funeral services. The therapists' role is to allow the group members to grieve in their own ways. Some group members may want to attend services, while others decide not to. Each group copes with the loss of a member in its own unique way. For example, in a women's HIV group one of the members died quite suddenly. This particular woman had a wonderful sense of humor and the uncanny ability to bring the group into full laughter effortlessly. The group members along with the therapists decided to attend the memorial service together. This shared experience of grief was processed in subsequent group meetings. One of the group members stated, "I know that if she could have seen us all there, she would have loved the attention and cracked a joke!"

This prompted the other group members to begin to share memories, funny anecdotes, and humorous moments related to the deceased group member. Amidst the laughter and the tears, the group members were able to accept the death and explore its effect on them in a therapeutic environment. This appeared to be extremely beneficial to the group members. There is evidence consistent with our clinical observation from a variety of studies indicating that patients feel better about themselves to the extent that they can face what may lie ahead (Fawzy et al., 1990). During the grieving process, group members are faced with the seriousness of their illness and often begin to explore spiritual issues related to faith and hope. Moreover, cultivating a fighting spirit (Greer et al., 1979), a kind of realistic optimism, seems to help those with serious illness accept the worst but hope for the best.

Training programs for therapists must be cognizant of an initial reaction to avoid the topic of death and dying. It is extremely important to assist therapists in tolerating their own emotional reactions to the worsening of illness and death of group members.

SUMMARY

Studies of psychotherapeutic treatments for cancer patients, both group and individual, have reported a variety of positive effects ranging from reduction in anxiety and depression to a number of recent studies suggesting increases in survival time.

There is substantial evidence of a need for psychotherapeutic intervention among cancer and HIV/AIDS patients, including those without a psychiatric diagnosis. Such interventions are effective in reducing distress, improving coping, improving adherence to treatment regimens, and enhancing interaction with healthcare professionals. In addition, groups provide social support, which has been shown to decrease disease progression among cancer and HIV patients. As health reform gets underway, psychotherapy may be seen as too costly. However, psychotherapy techniques have shown themselves in the medical arena to be needed, effective, and cost efficient. Psychosocial support for medically ill patients should be integrated into standard medical care and practice.

CLINICAL PEARLS

- Group therapy has a long track record of reducing psychiatric symptoms and increasing social support in the medically ill.

- Compared to individual psychotherapy, group therapy allows patients access to emotional support and to learn new interpersonal and coping skills without seeming to be abnormal.

- Patients get to help others and to see that others may have more troubles than they do.

- Group therapy has beneficial effects on mood, adjustment, and pain (Gustafson & Whitman, 1978; Wood et al., 1978; Ferlic et al., 1979; Spiegel et al., 1981; Spiegel & Bloom, 1983; Fawzy et al., 1990; Butler et al., 2009).

- Advantages of group therapy are as follows:
  - Patients discover that they are not unique in their predicament.
  - Patients can have intimate experiences and consensual validation with others suffering the burden of similar illness.
  - As they respect others coping with illness, they learn to respect themselves.
  - The opportunity to help others in a similar situation enhances the patient's sense of competence and ability to develop a renewed sense of meaning in life.

- Members come to feel part of a new and accepting social group in which their common bond is the very thing that makes them feel excluded in the outside world (Spiegel, 1993).

- Group therapy is cost effective.

- Breast cancer patients who received group therapy had significantly higher levels of personal control

- Eight of 15 published clinical trials demonstrate an effect of psychotherapeutic support on cancer survival time, and none show a worsening of outcome.

- Many of the psychotherapies that have shown promise in improving emotional adjustment and influencing survival time involve encouraging open expression of emotion and assertiveness in assuming control over the course of treatment, life decisions, and relationships (Spiegel & Yalom, 1978; Spiegel et al., 1981, 1989; Fawzy et al., 1990).

- Beneficial foci of supportive/expressive therapy are social support, detoxifying dying, emotional expression, reordering life priorities, family support, communication with physicians, and symptom control.

DISCLOSURE STATEMENTS

Drs. Gore-Felton and Spiegel have no conflicts to disclose. Grant Support: Dr. Gore-Felton receives support for research on a health monitoring device (Vital Connect, Inc.) and Dr. Spiegel receives research support from NIH/NIMH (R01 MH074849-06) and NIH/NCCAM (5P30AT005886-02).

REFERENCES

Akechi, T., Okuyama, T., et al. (2008). Psychotherapy for depression among incurable cancer patients. *Cochrane Database of Systematic Reviews*, (2), CD005537.

Alonzo, A. A., & Reynolds, N. R. (1995). Stigma, HIV and AIDS: an exploration and elaboration of a stigma trajectory. *Social Science & Medicine*, 41(3), 303–315.

Andersen, B. L., Yang, H. C., et al. (2008). Psychologic intervention improves survival for breast cancer patients: a randomized clinical trial. *Cancer*, 113(12), 3450–3458.

Antoni, M. H., Lutgendorf, S. K., et al. (2006). The influence of bio-behavioural factors on tumour biology: pathways and mechanisms. *Nature Reviews Cancer*, 6(3), 240–248.

American Psychiatric Association. (2000). *Diagnostic and Statistical Manual of Mental Disorders, Fourth Edition, Text Revision.* Washington, DC: American Psychiatric Press.

Beckett, A., & Rutan, J. S. (1990). Treating persons with ARC and AIDS in group psychotherapy. *International Journal of Group Psychotherapy*, 40(1), 19–29.

Blake-Mortimer, J., Gore-Felton, C., et al. (1999). Improving the quality and quantity of life among patients with cancer: a review of the effectiveness of group psychotherapy. *European Journal of Cancer*, 35(11), 1581–1586.

Block, S. D. (2001). Perspectives on care at the close of life. Psychological considerations, growth, and transcendence at the end of life: the art of the possible. *Journal of the American Medical Association*, 285(22), 2898–2905.

Bloom, J. R., Ross, R. D., et al. (1978). The effect of social support on patient adjustment after breast surgery. *Patient Counselling and Health Education, 1*(2), 50–59.

Boesen, E. H., Karlsen, R., et al. (2011). Psychosocial group intervention for patients with primary breast cancer: a randomised trial. *European Journal of Cancer, 47*(9), 1363–1372.

Bottomley, A. (1997). Where are we now? Evaluating two decades of group interventions with adult cancer patients. *Journal of Psychiatric and Mental Health Nursing, 4*(4), 251–265.

Breitbart, W., Bruera, E., et al. (1995). Neuropsychiatric syndromes and psychological symptoms in patients with advanced cancer. *Journal of Pain and Symptom Management, 10*(2), 131–141.

Breitbart, W., Rosenfeld, B., et al. (2010). Meaning-centered group psychotherapy for patients with advanced cancer: a pilot randomized controlled trial. *Psycho-Oncology, 19*(1), 21–28.

Browne, G. B., Arpin, K., et al. (1990). Individual correlates of health service utilization and the cost of poor adjustment to chronic illness. *Medical Care, 28*(1), 43–58.

Burish, T. G., & Lyles, J. N. (1981). Effectiveness of relaxation training in reducing adverse reactions to cancer chemotherapy. *Journal of Behavioral Medicine, 4*(1), 65–78.

Butler, L. D., Koopman, C., et al. (2009). Effects of supportive-expressive group therapy on pain in women with metastatic breast cancer. *Health Psychology, 28*(5), 579–587.

Cacioppo, J. T., Uchino, B. N., et al. (1992). Relationship between facial expressiveness and sympathetic activation in emotion: a critical review, with emphasis on modeling underlying mechanisms and individual differences. *Journal of Personality and Social Psychology, 62*(1), 110–128.

Cain, E. N., Kohorn, E. I., et al. (1986). Psychosocial benefits of a cancer support group. *Cancer, 57*(1), 183–189.

Capuron, L., & R. Dantzer, R. (2003). Cytokines and depression: the need for a new paradigm. *Brain, Behavior, and Immunity, 17*(Suppl 1), S119–S124.

Chochinov, H. M., Kristjanson, L. J., et al. (2011). Effect of dignity therapy on distress and end-of-life experience in terminally ill patients: a randomised controlled trial. *Lancet Oncology, 12*(8), 753–762.

Classen, C., Abramson, S., et al. (1997). Effectiveness of a training program for enhancing therapists' understanding of the supportive-expressive treatment model for breast cancer groups. *Journal of Psychotherapy Practice and Research, 6*(3), 211–218.

Classen, C., Butler, L. D., et al. (2001). Supportive-expressive group therapy and distress in patients with metastatic breast cancer: a randomized clinical intervention trial. *Archives of General Psychiatry, 58*(5), 494–501.

Cohen, C. I., & Wellisch, D. K. (1974). Living in limbo: psychosocial intervention in families living with a cancer patient. *American Journal of Psychotherapy, 34*, 561–571.

Cummings, N. A., & VandenBos, G. R. (1981). The twenty years Kaiser-Permanente experience with psychotherapy and medical utilization: implications for national health policy and national health insurance. *Health Policy Quarterly, 1*(2), 159–175.

Cunningham, A. J., Edmonds, C. V., et al. (1998). A randomized controlled trial of the effects of group psychological therapy on survival in women with metastatic breast cancer. *Psycho-Oncology, 7*(6), 508–517.

Cunningham, A. J., Lockwood, G. A., et al. (1993). Which cancer patients benefit most from a brief, group, coping skills program? *International Journal of Psychiatry & Medicine, 23*(4), 383–398.

Derogatis, L. R., Abeloff, M. D., et al. (1979). Psychological coping mechanisms and survival time in metastatic breast cancer. *Journal of the American Medical Association, 242*(14), 1504–1508.

Derogatis, L. R., Morrow, G. R., et al. (1983). The prevalence of psychiatric disorders among cancer patients. *Journal of the American Medical Association, 249*(6), 751–757.

Devine, E. C. (1992). Effects of psychoeducational care for adult surgical patients: a meta-analysis of 191 studies. *Patient Education and Counseling, 19*(2), 129–142.

Duijts, S. F., Faber, M. M., et al. (2011). Effectiveness of behavioral techniques and physical exercise on psychosocial functioning and health-related quality of life in breast cancer patients and survivors—a meta-analysis. *Psycho-Oncology, 20*(2), 115–126.

Dunkel-Schetter, C., Feinstein, L. G., et al. (1992). Patterns of coping with cancer. *Health Psychology, 11*(2), 79–87.

Earle, C. C., Park, E. R., et al. (2003). Identifying potential indicators of the quality of end-of-life cancer care from administrative data. *Journal of Clinical Oncology, 21*(6), 1133–1138.

Edelman, S., Lemon, J., et al. (1999). Effects of group CBT on the survival time of patients with metastatic breast cancer. *Psychooncology, 8*(6), 474–481.

Evans, D. L., Charney, D. S., et al. (2005). Mood disorders in the medically ill: scientific review and recommendations. *Biological Psychiatry, 58*(3), 175–189.

Fawzy, F. I., Cousins, N., et al. (1990). A structured psychiatric intervention for cancer patients. I. Changes over time in methods of coping and affective disturbance. *Archives of General Psychiatry, 47*(8), 720–725.

Fawzy, F. I., Fawzy, N. W., et al. (1995). Critical review of psychosocial interventions in cancer care. *Archives of General Psychiatry, 52*(2), 100–113.

Fawzy, F. I., Fawzy, N. W., et al. (1993). Malignant melanoma. Effects of an early structured psychiatric intervention, coping, and affective state on recurrence and survival 6 years later. *Archives of General Psychiatry, 50*(9), 681–689.

Fawzy, F. I., Fawzy, N. W., et al. (1996). A post-hoc comparison of the efficiency of a psychoeducational intervention for melanoma patients delivered in group versus individual formats: An analysis of data from two studies. *Psycho-Oncology, 5*(2), 81–89.

Ferlic, M., Goldman, A., et al. (1979). Group counseling in adult patients with advanced cancer. *Cancer, 43*(2), 760–766.

Fobair, P. (1997). Cancer support groups and group therapies. Part I. Historical and theoretical background and research on effectiveness. *Journal of Psychosocial Oncology, 15*, 63–81.

Forester, B., Kornfeld, D. S., et al. (1985). Psychotherapy during radiotherapy: effects on emotional and physical distress. *American Journal of Psychiatry, 142*(1), 22–27.

Franzino, M. A., Geren, J. J., et al. (1976). Group discussion among the terminally ill. *International Journal of Group Psychotherapy, 26*(1), 43–48.

Giese-Davis, J., Collie, K., et al. (2011). Decrease in depression symptoms is associated with longer survival in patients with metastatic breast cancer: a secondary analysis. *Journal of Clinical Oncology, 29*(4), 413–420.

Goodwin, J. S., Hunt, W. C., et al. (1987). The effect of marital status on stage, treatment, and survival of cancer patients. *Journal of the American Medical Association, 258*(21), 3125–3130.

Goodwin, P. J., Leszcz, M., et al. (2001). The effect of group psychosocial support on survival in metastatic breast cancer. *New England Journal of Medicine, 345*(24), 1719–1726.

Gore-Felton, C., & Koopman, C. (2008). Behavioral mediation of the relationship between psychosocial factors and HIV disease progression. *Psychosomatic Medicine, 70*(5), 569–574.

Gotay, C. C. (1984). The experience of cancer during early and advanced stages: the views of patients and their mates. *Social Science & Medicine, 18*(7), 605–613.

Grassi, L., & Rosti, G. (1996). Psychosocial morbidity and adjustment to illness among long-term cancer survivors. A six-year follow-up study. *Psychosomatics, 37*(6), 523–532.

Greer, S. (1991). Psychological response to cancer and survival. *Psychological Medicine, 21*(1), 43–49.

Greer, S., Morris, T., et al. (1979). Psychological response to breast cancer: effect on outcome. *Lancet, 2*(8146), 785–787.

Gustafson, J., & Whitman, H. (1978). Towards a balanced social environment on the oncology service. *Social Psychiatry and Psychiatric Epidemiology, 13*(3), 147–152.

Helgeson, V. S., Cohen, S., et al. (1999). Education and peer discussion group interventions and adjustment to breast cancer. *Archives of General Psychiatry, 56*(4), 340–347.

Hellman, C. J., Budd, M., et al. (1990). A study of the effectiveness of two group behavioral medicine interventions for patients with psychosomatic complaints. *Behavioral Medicine, 16*(4), 165–173.

Hosaka, T. (1996). A pilot study of a structured psychiatric intervention for Japanese women with breast cancer. *Psycho-Oncology*, 5(1), 59–64.

House, J. S., Landis, K. R., et al. (1988). Social relationships and health. *Science*, 241(4865), 540–545.

Ibfelt, E., Rottmann, N., et al. (2011). No change in health behavior, BMI or self-rated health after a psychosocial cancer rehabilitation: Results of a randomized trial. *Acta Oncologica*, 50(2), 289–298.

Ilnyckyj, A., Farber, J., et al. (1994). A randomized controlled trial of psychotherapeutic intervention in cancer patients. *Annals of the Royal College of Physicians and Surgeons of Canada*, 27(2), 93–96.

Innominato, P. F., Palesh, O., et al. (2010). Regulation of circadian rhythms and hypothalamic-pituitary-adrenal axis: an overlooked interaction in cancer. *Lancet Oncology*, 11(9), 816–817.

Ironson, G., & Hayward, H. (2008). Do positive psychosocial factors predict disease progression in HIV-1? A review of the evidence. *Psychosomatic Medicine*, 70(5), 546–554.

Kelly, J. A., Murphy, D. A., et al. (1993). Outcome of cognitive-behavioral and support group brief therapies for depressed, HIV-infected persons. *American Journal of Psychiatry*, 150(11), 1679–1686.

Kesler, S. R., Bennett, F. C., et al. (2009). Regional brain activation during verbal declarative memory in metastatic breast cancer. *Clinical Cancer Research*, 15(21), 6665–6673.

Kessler, R. C., Berglund, P., et al. (2003). The epidemiology of major depressive disorder: results from the National Comorbidity Survey Replication (NCS-R). *Journal of the American Medical Association*, 289(23), 3095–3105.

Kissane, D. W., Grabsch, B., et al. (2004). Supportive-expressive group therapy: the transformation of existential ambivalence into creative living while enhancing adherence to anti-cancer therapies. *Psychooncology*, 13(11), 755–768.

Kissane, D. W., Grabsch, B., et al. (2007). Supportive-expressive group therapy for women with metastatic breast cancer: survival and psychosocial outcome from a randomized controlled trial. *Psycho-Oncology*, 16(4), 277–286.

Kroenke, C. H., Kubzansky, L. D., et al. (2006). Social networks, social support, and survival after breast cancer diagnosis. *Journal of Clinical Oncology*, 24(7), 1105–1111.

Kuchler, T., Bestmann, B., et al. (2007). Impact of psychotherapeutic support for patients with gastrointestinal cancer undergoing surgery: 10-year survival results of a randomized trial. *Journal of Clinical Oncology*, 25(19), 2702–2708.

Kuchler, T., Henne-Bruns, D., et al. (1999). Impact of psychotherapeutic support on gastrointestinal cancer patients undergoing surgery: survival results of a trial. *Hepato-Gastroenterology*, 46(25), 322–335.

Leserman, J. (2008). Role of depression, stress, and trauma in HIV disease progression. *Psychosomatic Medicine*, 70(5), 539–545.

Leserman, J., Petitto, J. M., et al. (2002). Progression to AIDS, a clinical AIDS condition and mortality: psychosocial and physiological predictors. *Psychological Medicine*, 32(6), 1059–1073.

Liang, L. P., Dunn, S. M., et al. (1990). Identifying priorities of psychosocial need in cancer patients. *British Journal of Cancer*, 62(6), 1000–1003.

Lieberman, M. A., Golant, M., et al. (2003). Electronic support groups for breast carcinoma: a clinical trial of effectiveness. *Cancer*, 97(4), 920–925.

Lieberman, M. A., and B. A., Goldstein (2005). Self-help on-line: an outcome evaluation of breast cancer bulletin boards. *Journal of Health Psychology*, 10(6), 855–862.

Linn, M. W., Linn, B. S., et al. (1982). Effects of counseling for late stage cancer patients. *Cancer*, 49(5), 1048–1055.

Loescher, L. J., Welch-McCaffrey, D., et al. (1989). Surviving adult cancers. Part 1: Physiologic effects. *Annals of Internal Medicine*, 111(5), 411–432.

Lorig, K., Lubeck, D., et al. (1985). Outcomes of self-help education for patients with arthritis. *Arthritis and Rheumatism*, 28(6), 680–685.

Luther, J., & Glesby M. J. (2007). Dermatologic adverse effects of antiretroviral therapy: recognition and management. *American Journal of Clinical Dermatology*, 8(4), 221–233.

Magura, S., Kang, S. Y., et al. (1994). Outcomes of intensive AIDS education for male adolescent drug users in jail. *Journal of Adolescent Health*, 15(6), 457–463.

Maisiak, R., Cain, M., et al. (1981). Evaluation of TOUCH: an oncology self-help group. *Oncology Nursing Forum*, 8(3), 20–25.

Mansfield, C. J., Conroy, M. E., et al. (1993). A pilot study of AIDS education and counseling of high-risk adolescents in an office setting. *Journal of Adolescent Health*, 14(2), 115–119.

Markowitz, J. C., Klerman, G. L., et al. (1992). Interpersonal psychotherapy of depressed HIV-positive outpatients. *Hospital & Community Psychiatry*, 43(9), 885–890.

McCorkle, R., Strumpf, N. E., et al. (2000). A specialized home care intervention improves survival among older post-surgical cancer patients. *Journal of the American Geriatrics Society*, 48(12), 1707–1713.

McDonald, P. G., Antoni, M. H., et al. (2005). A biobehavioral perspective of tumor biology. *Discovery Medicine*, 5(30), 520–526.

Mittelman, M. S., Ferris, S. H., et al. (1996). A family intervention to delay nursing home placement of patients with Alzheimer disease. A randomized controlled trial. *Journal of the American Medical Association*, 276(21), 1725–1731.

Mittelman, M. S., Ferris, S. H., et al. (1993). An intervention that delays institutionalization of Alzheimer's disease patients: treatment of spouse-caregivers. *Gerontologist*, 33(6), 730–740.

Morrow, G. R., & Morrell, C. (1982). Behavioral treatment for the anticipatory nausea and vomiting induced by cancer chemotherapy. *New England Journal of Medicine*, 307(24), 1476–1480.

Moyle, G. (2007). Metabolic issues associated with protease inhibitors. *Journal of Acquired Immune Deficiency Syndromes*, 45(Suppl 1), S19–S26.

Mulder, C. L., Pompe, G. V. D., et al. (1992). Do psychosocial factors influence the course of breast cancer? A review of recent literature, methodological problems and future directions. *Psycho-Oncology*, 1(3), 155–167.

Mumford, E., Schlesinger, H. J., et al. (1984). A new look at evidence about reduced cost of medical utilization following mental health treatment. *American Journal of Psychiatry*, 141(10), 1145–1158.

Naaman, S. C., Radwan, K., et al. (2009). Status of psychological trials in breast cancer patients: a report of three meta-analyses. *Psychiatry*, 72(1), 50–69.

Naar-King, S., Bradford, J., et al. (2007). Retention in care of persons newly diagnosed with HIV: outcomes of the Outreach Initiative. *Aids Patient Care and Standards*, 21(Suppl 1), S40–S48.

Newell, S. A., Sanson-Fisher, R. W., et al. (2002). Systematic review of psychological therapies for cancer patients: overview and recommendations for future research. *Journal of the National Cancer Institute*, 94(8), 558–584.

Northouse, L. L. (1988). Family issues in cancer care. *Advances in Psychosomatic Medicine*, 18, 82–101.

Owen, J. E., Klapow, J. C., et al. (2004). Improving the effectiveness of adjuvant psychological treatment for women with breast cancer: the feasibility of providing online support. *Psycho-Oncology*, 13(4), 281–292.

Parkin, D. M., Bray, F., et al. (2005). Global cancer statistics, 2002. *Ca: A Cancer Journal for Clinicians*, 55(2), 74–108.

Peto, R., Boreham, J., et al. (2000). UK and USA breast cancer deaths down 25% in year 2000 at ages 20–69 years. *Lancet*, 355(9217), 1822.

Pettingale, K. W. (1984). Coping and cancer prognosis. *Journal of Psychosomatic Research*, 28(5), 363–364.

Pitceathly, C., Maguire, P., et al. (2009). Can a brief psychological intervention prevent anxiety or depressive disorders in cancer patients? A randomised controlled trial. *Annals of Oncology*, 20(5), 928–934.

Ramirez, A. J., Craig, T. K., et al. (1989). Stress and relapse of breast cancer. *British Medical Journal*, 298(6669), 291–293.

Reuter, K., Scholl, I., et al. (2010). Implementation and benefits of psychooncological group interventions in german breast centers: a pilot study on supportive-expressive group therapy for women with primary breast cancer. *Breast Care*, 5(2), 91–96.

Richardson, J. L., Shelton, D. R., et al. (1990). The effect of compliance with treatment on survival among patients with hematologic malignancies. *Journal of Clinical Oncology*, 8(2), 356–364.

Riddler, S. A., Smit, E., et al. (2003). Impact of HIV infection and HAART on serum lipids in men. *Journal of the American Medical Association, 289*(22), 2978–2982.

Riessman, F. (1965). The helper therapy principle. *Social Work, 10*, 27–32.

Sephton, S., & Spiegel, D. (2003). Circadian disruption in cancer: a neuroendocrine-immune pathway from stress to disease? *Brain, Behavior, and Immunity, 17*(5), 321–328.

Sephton, S. E., Sapolsky, R. M., et al. (2000). Diurnal cortisol rhythm as a predictor of breast cancer survival. *Journal of the National Cancer Institute, 92*(12), 994–1000.

Silverman-Dresner, T. (1989–1990). Self-help groups for women who have had breast cancer. *Imagination, Cognition and Personality, 9*(3), 237–242.

Spiegel, D. (1990). Facilitating emotional coping during treatment. *Cancer, 66*(6 Suppl), 1422–1426.

Spiegel, D. (1991). Psychosocial aspects of cancer. *Current Opinion in Psychiatry, 4*, 889–897.

Spiegel, D. (1993). *Living Beyond Limits: New hope and help for facing life-threatening illness.* New York: Times Books/ Random House.

Spiegel, D. (2002). Effects of psychotherapy on cancer survival. *Nature Reviews Cancer, 2*(5), 383–389.

Spiegel, D., & Bloom, J. R. (1983). Group therapy and hypnosis reduce metastatic breast carcinoma pain. *Psychosomatic Medicine, 45*(4), 333–339.

Spiegel, D., Bloom, J. R., et al. (1983). Family Environment as a Predictor of Adjustment to Metastatic Breast Carcinoma. *Journal of Psychosocial Oncology, 1*(1), 33–44.

Spiegel, D., Bloom, J. R., et al. (1989). Effect of psychosocial treatment on survival of patients with metastatic breast cancer. *Lancet, 2*(8668), 888–891.

Spiegel, D., Bloom, J. R., et al. (1981). Group support for patients with metastatic cancer. A randomized outcome study. *Archives of General Psychiatry, 38*(5), 527–533.

Spiegel, D., Butler, L. D., et al. (2007). Effects of supportive-expressive group therapy on survival of patients with metastatic breast cancer: a randomized prospective trial. *Cancer, 110*(5), 1130–1138.

Spiegel, D., & Glafkides, M. C. (1983). Effects of group confrontation with death and dying. *International Journal of Group Psychotherapy, 33*(4), 433–447.

Spiegel, D., & Wissler, T. (1983). Perceptions of family environment among psychiatric patients and their wives. *Family Process, 22*(4), 537–547.

Spiegel, D., & Yalom, I. D. (1978). A support group for dying patients. *International Journal of Group Psychotherapy, 28*(2), 233–245.

Stepanski, E. J., & Wyatt J. K. (2003). Use of sleep hygiene in the treatment of insomnia. *Sleep Medicine Reviews, 7*(3), 215–225.

Strain, J. J., Lyons, J. S., et al. (1991). Cost offset from a psychiatric consultation-liaison intervention with elderly hip fracture patients. *American Journal of Psychiatry, 148*(8), 1044–1049.

Strang, P. (1992). Emotional and social aspects of cancer pain. *Acta Oncologica, 31*(3), 323–326.

Taerk, G. (1983). Psychological support of oncology nurses: a role for the liaison psychiatrist. *Canadian Journal of Psychiatry, 28*(7), 532–535.

Taylor, S. E., Klein, L. C., et al. (2000). Biobehavioral responses to stress in females: tend-and-befriend, not fight-or-flight. *Psychological Review, 107*(3), 411–429.

Temel, J. S., Greer, J. A., et al. (2010). Early palliative care for patients with metastatic non-small-cell lung cancer. *New England Journal of Medicine, 363*(8), 733–742.

Temoshok, L., Heller, B. W., et al. (1985). The relationship of psychosocial factors to prognostic indicators in cutaneous malignant melanoma. *Journal of Psychosomatic Research, 29*(2), 139–153.

Toseland, R. W., & Hacker, L. (1982). Self-help groups and professional involvement. *Social Work, 27*(4), 341–347.

Tracy, G. S., & Gussow, Z. (1976). Self-Help Health Groups: A Grass-Roots Response to a Need for Services. *the Journal of Applied Behavioral Science, 12*(3), 381–396.

Vgontzas, A. N., & Chrousos, G. P. (2002). Sleep, the hypothalamic-pituitary-adrenal axis, and cytokines: multiple interactions and disturbances in sleep disorders. *Endocrinology and Metabolism Clinics of North America, 31*(1), 15–36.

Whelan, T. J., Mohide, E. A., et al. (1997). The supportive care needs of newly diagnosed cancer patients attending a regional cancer center. *Cancer, 80*(8), 1518–1524.

White, N. E., Richter, J. M., et al. (1992). Coping, social support, and adaptation to chronic illness. *Western Journal of Nursing Research, 14*(2), 211–224.

Wolf, T. M., Balson, P. M., et al. (1991). Relationship of coping style to affective state and perceived social support in asymptomatic and symptomatic HIV-infected persons: implications for clinical management. *the Journal of Clinical Psychiatry, 52*(4), 171–173.

Wood, P. E., Milligan, M., et al. (1978). Group counseling for cancer patients in a community hospital. *Psychosomatics 19*(9), 555–561.

Yalom, I. (1995). *the theory and Practice of Group Psychotherapy Edition 4*, Basic Books.

Yalom, I. D., & Greaves, C. (1977). Group therapy with the terminally ill. *the American Journal of Psychiatry 134*(4), 396–400.

Yalom, V., & Yalom, I. (1990). Brief interactive group psychotherapy. *Psychiatric Annals, 20*: 362–367.

Zeltzer, L., & LeBaron, S. (1982). Hypnosis and nonhypnotic techniques for reduction of pain and anxiety during painful procedures in children and adolescents with cancer. *the Journal of Pediatrics, 101*(6), 1032–1035.

14.

COGNITIVE BEHAVIORAL THERAPIES

Lara N. Traeger and Joseph A. Greer

INTRODUCTION

Cognitive behavioral therapy (CBT) refers to a diverse group of psychotherapies that share a set of fundamental assumptions: cognitions (e.g., interpretations and beliefs) affect behaviors, and cognitive activity can be monitored and altered to mediate behavior change. CBT interventions are applicable to medical patients, who may benefit from enhancing skills for health risk reduction or chronic disease management. Treatment models can be adapted to address associations of cognitions, health behaviors, emotions, and patient health outcomes, with an emphasis on the role of self-regulation. Common treatment goals include improving health behaviors such as medical adherence, reducing psychological symptoms that may exacerbate medical disability, and/or directly improving functional status.

CBT interventions have evolved over the past several decades through the convergence of behavioral and cognitive theories of change. Behavior therapy is considered a precursor to CBT; methods emerged as a response to psychodynamic therapies and through clinical applications of classical and operant conditioning theories (Eysenck, 1966; Wolpe, 1958). In comparison to psychodynamic treatment models, behavior therapy is time-limited and problem-oriented, with a focus on symptom reduction. Albert Ellis (1957) and Aaron T. Beck (1963, 1964) were among the first to formalize clinical models that emphasized the primacy of cognitions in therapeutic change. Ellis's rational emotive therapy introduced a directive therapeutic approach for changing irrational beliefs, whereas Beck elaborated specific cognitive patterns associated with depression (i.e., negative thinking about the self, world, and others) as targets for change. These approaches integrated cognitive mechanisms into existing behavioral models and, consequently, could be used to explain a broader range of psychopathology. Current models vary in the extent to which behaviors or cognitions are primary targets of change. However, since the early success of CBT to treat depression, support for CBT approaches has grown, and applications have expanded to diverse psychiatric and medical conditions. The CBT literature reflects a commitment to empirical validation of treatment methods (Dobson & Dozois, 2010).

COGNITIVE BEHAVIORAL MODEL

CBT emphasizes that a person's interpretations of a situation influence emotional reactions and behaviors used to cope with or adapt to the situation. Cognitions, behaviors, and emotions continually reinforce each other via multidirectional paths. We highlight these associations and their implications in the following case study.

CASE STUDY 1

Patient K. B. is a 45-year-old woman who has recently returned to full-time employment despite residual fatigue following radiation therapy for an early-stage breast cancer. During K. B.'s first week, her supervisor noted a few errors in her work and asked her to correct them. Since then, K. B. has become increasingly worried that her work is noticeably suffering. Consequently, K. B.'s anxiety has escalated. She has started drinking more coffee, skipping exercise to reduce risk of worsening fatigue, and avoiding additional contact with her supervisor. K. B. is also frustrated that despite her daytime fatigue, she is having increasing problems with insomnia at night. K. B.'s sensitivity to fatigue appears to be increasing, triggering long-standing worries about incompetence, unemployment, and financial instability, and new ruminations about cancer recurrence.

This scenario demonstrates the cognitive, behavioral, and emotional cycle that can be triggered by a situational interpretation (i.e., the meaning of the supervisor's actions). Alternatively, K. B. could have interpreted the supervisor's actions as hostile, supportive, or of an unclear nature, leading to different outcomes. However, interpretations and coping often reflect existing patterns or styles of thinking and behaving—such as exaggerated fears of failure and behavioral avoidance in the case of K. B. When life stressors occur, these patterns can appear entrenched or rigid, leading to clinically significant distress. Identifying maladaptive cognitive and behavioral responses is a fundamental task in CBT that informs the therapeutic approach.

In medical populations, the confounding of psychological factors, disease symptoms, and treatment side effects highlights the importance of comprehensive assessment and consultation with patients' other providers. Several factors could be associated with K. B.'s fatigue and sleep concerns, including residual effects of radiotherapy, uncontrolled pain symptoms, misinformation about sleepiness versus fatigue, psychological distress, and compensatory behaviors that may further disrupt sleep/wake cycles (e.g., increasing caffeine intake or reducing daytime activity). In an ongoing downward spiral, fatigue and insomnia may then interfere with the ability to appraise accurately and problem-solve current stressors. This case formulation highlights potential treatment targets for symptom reduction. The next section describes the basic characteristics of CBT and the key interventions that may be integrated into CBT treatment plans.

ELEMENTS OF COGNITIVE BEHAVIORAL INTERVENTIONS

CBT interventions reflect a problem-oriented, skills-based approach to therapeutic change. The first one to two sessions may be dedicated to collecting information about a patient's presenting problems, sharing and revising the CBT case formulation, and using this formulation to establish tailored treatment goals. At each subsequent therapy session, the therapist and patient review progress via informal feedback and relevant symptom inventories (e.g., Hospital Anxiety and Depression Scale [Zigmond & Snaith, 1983]), and set the current session agenda.

Throughout treatment, the therapist encourages active collaboration with the patient serving as cotherapist. Socratic questioning is used to guide patients in their own discovery of problematic patterns in thoughts and behaviors. Sessions typically focus on building skills that address these patterns. Patient self-efficacy is a critical concept in CBT, particularly for medical patients who may be facing some uncontrollable aspects of a disease or its treatment. Between-session assignments are used to practice and problem-solve the skills in real-life situations. Most interventions are time-limited, with the intention for patients to become increasingly independent in their use and application of CBT skills. Interventions typically conclude with a focus on relapse prevention by anticipating and problem-solving potential obstacles to the ongoing use of CBT skills.

In the following sections, we describe common CBT strategies and other methods that may be combined with CBT. Rather than simply strung together, strategies are selectively integrated into a cohesive treatment plan that is directly informed by the CBT case formulation. We also provide recommendations throughout this chapter for adapting treatment plans to incorporate factors associated with medical conditions.

PSYCHOEDUCATION

Psychoeducation is a core feature of CBT interventions. At the start of treatment, a critical aim for the therapist is to engage patients in understanding the CBT model and collaborating to identify how the model applies specifically to them. The model is an important road map to help patients discover and evaluate associations between their thoughts, feelings, and behaviors that may be impacting health and quality of life. Additionally, the model may be a tool for reinforcing areas in which patients may have personal responsibility or control over chronic disease management. For instance, a patient on long-acting pain medications may benefit from

reviewing the impact of missed or delayed doses on pain control. Among adults with asthma, a review of optimal inhaler use and education about associations of anxiety with asthma physiology may improve both disease knowledge and commitment to specific symptom management goals. Finally, given the goal-oriented and active nature of CBT, therapists must often employ treatment motivation strategies, which we further address in the next section.

MOTIVATIONAL ENHANCEMENT

Throughout treatment, CBT therapists commonly incorporate techniques for monitoring and enhancing motivation for therapeutic change. Motivation is a key element in complex health behavior change, such as cessation of tobacco use, changes in physical activity and dietary patterns, and improvements in medical treatment adherence. Ambivalence may be prominent in patients who are experiencing depression-related anhedonia or hopelessness, or anxiety-related avoidance. Patients also may be relying on health risk behaviors (e.g., smoking or overeating) to cope with negative affect. Examples of motivational techniques include collaborative treatment goal-setting, information provision, encouragement, feedback on goal progress, and treatment contracting.

In comparison to basic techniques, motivational interviewing (MI) is a brief (generally 1–2 sessions) evidence-based communication method that was developed to enhance personal commitment to behavior change (Miller & Rollnick, 2002). This method is based on assumptions of personal autonomy. A variety of strategies may be used to elicit a patient's own intrinsic arguments for change and to use these arguments as the source of motivation. MI is goal-oriented but does not involve teaching specific skills (Miller & Rollnick, 2009). In practice, MI is sometimes combined with CBT or used to enhance entry into an intensive behavior change program. For instance, Safren and colleagues include MI communication strategies as a prelude to their CBT intervention for improving depression and adherence to medical treatments in adults with a chronic illness (Safren, Gonzalez, & Soroudi, 2008).

BEHAVIORAL ACTIVATION

Behavioral activation (BA [Martell, Addis, & Jacobson, 2001]) is a straightforward, empirically supported intervention that was developed for depression treatment and relapse prevention, which is also a core component of CBT. BA does not simply encourage patients to become more active. Rather, the intervention represents a collaborative effort between the therapist and patient to identify specific activities that may be personally rewarding and that may interrupt current behavior/environment contingencies (e.g., impact of a patient's social avoidance on sadness and sense of isolation). The patient is encouraged to schedule meaningful and achievable activities and then monitor progress throughout each week. When working with medical patients, therapists must consider complicating factors such as medication regimens, functional status, symptoms (e.g., dyspnea, pain), and daily fatigue patterns in order to plan and adapt rewarding activities. Activity pacing can help modulate daily activities according to current level of energy. Careful planning is necessary to maintain patient motivation and, in turn, promote patient confidence (Carney & Freedland, 2008).

GUIDED EXPOSURE

Exposure is a core component in many CBT interventions for anxiety (Craske, Antony, & Barlow, 2006; Craske & Barlow, 2006; Foa, Hembree, & Rothbaum, 2010). Patients learn to interrupt behavior/environment contingencies associated with anxiety through use of imaginal or in vivo (real life) exposures to feared situations. Interventions may also incorporate interoceptive exposure, the intentional induction of fear sensations such as hyperventilation. During treatment, the therapist and patient collaborate to plan systematic, graded exposure exercises that will provoke conditioned fear responses in the short term, so that patients accumulate evidence disconfirming their inaccurate appraisals and ultimately extinguish the conditioned responses in the long term.

In medical populations without clinically significant anxiety, exposure principles nevertheless may be relevant for cases in which subclinical anxiety is interfering with adherence to medical treatment or exacerbating disability (e.g., exaggerated fear-avoidance of physical activity in patients with fatigue or pain). Duhamel and colleagues (2010) included an exposure component in their pilot trial of CBT for patients who underwent hematopoietic stem cell transplantation and were experiencing subsequent symptoms of posttraumatic stress. Guided exposure to stimuli that were associated with posttraumatic stress was combined with psychoeducation, cognitive restructuring, social support skills, and relaxation training. Patients who completed the treatment reported fewer posttraumatic stress symptoms related to their illness, including fewer intrusive thoughts and avoidance behaviors, relative to patients in a no-therapy control condition.

ADAPTIVE THINKING

Cognitive techniques represent a cornerstone of CBT interventions for reducing emotional distress and optimizing coping with current and future stressors. Patients are taught to identify inaccurate and unhelpful thoughts (e.g., "I bet my doctor has not returned my call yet because she has bad news to share") that may be occurring automatically in stressful situations. Over time, patients may be able to identify cognitive distortions or problematic patterns of thinking (in this case, "fortune telling") that frequently characterize their automatic thoughts. Several common cognitive distortions and example automatic thoughts are shown in Table 14.1.

Table 14.1 DEFINITIONS AND EXAMPLES OF 11 COMMON COGNITIVE ERRORS

COGNITIVE DISTORTIONS	DEFINITIONS	EXAMPLES
All-or-nothing thinking	Placing experiences in one of two opposite categories	"I missed my medication dose this morning. I simply can't take care of myself."
Discounting the positives	Deciding that if a good thing has happened, then it couldn't have been very important	"I've been so fatigued since I started chemotherapy. Being able to play with my nieces today without feeling exhausted was just an aberration."
Jumping to conclusions	Focusing on one aspect of a situation in deciding how to understand it	"The reason my doctor hasn't yet returned my call is because she has bad news to tell me."
Mind reading	Believing one knows what another person is thinking, with very little evidence	"That person is staring at me because they can tell that I'm sick."
Fortune telling	Believing one knows what the future holds, while ignoring other possibilities	"I am never going to be able to change my eating habits."
Magnifying/minimizing	Evaluating the importance of a negative event, or the lack of importance of a positive event, in a distorted manner	"Being diagnosed with diabetes has limited my whole life."
Making "should" statements	Telling oneself that one should do—or should have done—something, when it is more accurate to say that one would like to do—or wishes one had done—the preferred thing	"My surgery was weeks ago. I should be back to work by now."
Labeling	Using a label to describe a behavior, then imputing all the meanings the label carries	"I can't seem to push myself to go to physical therapy. I must be lazy."
Inappropriate blaming	Using hindsight to determine what one "should have done"	"I should have had my cough checked by a doctor a long time ago."

Adapted from DeRubeis, R. J., Webb, C. A., Tang, T. Z., & Beck, A. T. (2010). Cognitive therapy. In K. S. Dobson (Ed.), *Handbook of cognitive-behavioral therapies*. New York, NY: The Guilford Press.

After learning to identify and label automatic thoughts, patients are then taught to challenge them (e.g., "What is the evidence that this thought is true?" or "What would I say to a good friend in the same situation?") and replace them with new thoughts that are more rational and adaptive. The patient then tests the new thoughts to determine whether they help reduce distress and frame situations in a more helpful light. Skills are reinforced through the practice of monitoring and challenging automatic negative thoughts throughout the week.

A key challenge in applying adaptive thinking skills in medical populations is that patients with severe or advancing illness may indeed face realistic progression toward feared events. Greer and colleagues (2009) have adapted a decisional model to help patients evaluate the extent to which negative thoughts may contain both biased and realistic elements. Adaptive thinking skills may be supplemented with acceptance-oriented coping skills (e.g., mindfulness) when thoughts are deemed realistic, or with information seeking when more "data" are needed.

PROBLEM SOLVING

Problem-solving therapy (PST) is a CBT intervention that focuses on developing and strengthening attitudes and skills for resolving current problems (D'Zurilla & Nezu, 2007). In PST, attention is focused on evaluating and addressing each patient's problem orientation (e.g., optimistic versus doubtful) and problem-solving style (e.g., constructive versus impulsive or avoidant). Patients learn to use a practical, systematic approach in which problems are viewed as solvable challenges. This approach emphasizes four main skills: articulating problems, generating potential solutions, evaluating each solution with regard to advantages and disadvantages, and executing and monitoring a plan of action. The primary aims of PST are to reduce psychological distress and improve quality of life among patients. Evidence supporting PST to improve symptom management and treatment adherence has been generated across a range of complex medical conditions, such as diabetes and cancer (Hill-Briggs & Gemmell, 2007; Lee, Chiou, Chang, & Hayter, 2010; Nezu, Nezu, Friedman, Faddis, & Houts, 1998).

RELAXATION

Relaxation training is frequently integrated into CBT for a wide range of psychiatric and medical conditions. A key aim of relaxation training is to promote resilience and optimal coping in the context of life stressors. Pioneering work by Herbert Benson and colleagues documented reductions in several physiologic stress indices following a brief meditation session among long-term practitioners (Wallace, Benson, & Wilson, 1971). Relaxation increasingly has been applied in therapeutic settings to elicit a state of downregulated sympathetic nervous system activity and upregulated parasympathetic activity, through attention to a variety of different stimuli (e.g., abdominal breathing, progressive muscle relaxation, yoga sequences, or imagery). Relaxation training typically includes psychoeducation about stress symptoms and the purpose of relaxation practice, introduction to a relaxation exercise, monitoring of effects on current stress symptoms, and problem-solving regular relaxation practice. For patients with a medical comorbidity, stress symptoms should be discussed with the patient's medical providers to rule out confounding conditions prior to initiation of relaxation training. Current symptom profiles should also be considered when selecting an appropriate relaxation exercise (e.g., imagery instead of muscle tensing/relaxing exercises in patients with chronic pain). The brief, portable nature of relaxation interventions supports delivery in medical treatment settings. For instance, relaxation training has shown anxiolytic benefits in adults undergoing intensive anticancer chemotherapy (Jacobsen et al., 2002) and radiotherapy (Decker, Cline-Elsen, & Gallager, 1992) regimens.

BIOFEEDBACK

Biofeedback therapy refers to procedures that facilitate real-time observation and measurement of physiologic stress responses. A core assumption of biofeedback methods is that by increasing awareness of these responses, which are usually hidden, patients may be able to exercise more psychological or behavioral control over them. For instance, biofeedback can be combined with relaxation training so that patients may observe in vivo effects of relaxation on indices of peripheral autonomic activity. Demonstrations of mind–body connections may promote uptake of and adherence to CBT strategies for managing stress and stress-induced symptoms. Proposed outcomes of biofeedback will depend on the specific medical population and the type of physiological process that is monitored.

Diverse biofeedback protocols have been tested in a range of medical conditions, including epilepsy (Nagai, 2011), incontinence and constipation (Enck, Van der Voort, & Klostherhalfen, 2009), hypertension (Greenhalgh, Dickson, & Dundar, 2010), and Raynaud's disease (Malenfant, Catton, & Pope, 2009), with mixed effects. Electromyographic and temperature feedback combined with relaxation have shown promise in reducing migraine headache frequency and severity (Nestoriuc & Martin, 2007). Biofeedback methods have also been integrated with other CBT strategies to treat conditions such as temporomandibular disorders (Crider, Glaros, & Gervitz, 2005).

SELECTIVE INTEGRATION OF COGNITIVE BEHAVIORAL TECHNIQUES

Many chronic medical conditions are associated with elevated risk for psychological problems such as depression. Depressed individuals, in turn, have difficulties with motivation, interest, and problem solving, and are therefore less likely to practice self-care behaviors such as physical activity, healthy eating, and adherence to medical regimens. The following case study illustrates some of these relationships and the selective integration of treatment methods to address them.

J. M. is a 32-year-old male who has been taking daily HIV medications for several years. He understands that the medications are needed to control his disease, but he sometimes skips doses to avoid this nagging reminder that all is not right in his life. He has not had a close, intimate relationship with anyone since he was diagnosed, and he can find few reasons to continue fighting for his health. J. M. volunteers at a local HIV center and is very good at mentoring others to take their medications on time and to seek social support from others. Other HIV-infected adults look to him for guidance. But when J. M. feels particularly down, his words seem hollow, and he avoids the HIV center in favor of staying at home in bed. On those days, even simple chores or a walk around the block feel overwhelming, so he reasons that he could not be of use to anyone else.

Despite J. M.'s careful efforts to hide his depressed moods, a case worker at the center takes note of his struggles and refers him for mental health services. By the time he meets with a CBT therapist for treatment evaluation, he has refused antidepressant medication and is maintaining an ambivalent stance toward "opening wounds" in talk therapy. The CBT therapist expresses her appreciation for his honesty. She provides some brief psychoeducation about the general purpose and rationale for CBT and also for antidepressant medications. They agree to have two trial CBT sessions and then revisit J. M.'s thoughts about continuing with the treatment.

The first session focuses on exploring J. M.'s current experiences. The therapist reviews the CBT model to help organize and illustrate associations between specific thoughts (perceived self-worth), feelings (despondence) and behaviors (social avoidance) that are elicited during the discussion. Socratic questioning is used to help J. M. critically examine his own cycles of depression and poor HIV self-care. Based on the model, the therapist and J. M. work together to identify realistic treatment goals. J. M.'s goals focus on improving depression and adherence, with a long-term aim of developing meaningful social relationships. The therapist shares her own diagnostic impressions and introduces CBT techniques that could help J. M. learn or enhance skills for meeting his goals. Given the initial ambivalence that J. M. expressed, the therapist also uses motivational interviewing to elicit J. M.'s motivation for engaging in therapy. Throughout treatment, this method is revisited as needed to reinforce J.M's personal autonomy and inherent desire to improve his quality of life. J. M. also regularly completes validated self-report inventories of depression symptoms and medication adherence, which provide continual feedback on goal progress.

Together, the therapist and J. M. generate a treatment plan based on the CBT model of J. M.'s depression. The therapist provides psychoeducation about depression and HIV. J. M. begins considering that medication adherence and self-care could be a step toward enjoying meaningful relationships with others (rather than a reminder of failure or loss). Behavioral activation is introduced to help J. M. increase engagement in activities that he considers personally rewarding, such as spending time with his uncle and helping the HIV center with creative projects. The therapist and J. M. also brainstorm a variety of activities for times when energy level or HIV medication side effects may fluctuate.

Weekly logs of activities and mood ratings allow the therapist and J. M. to pinpoint days in which enjoyable activities did not improve mood. This information facilitates a transition into adaptive thinking skills. Through identification of automatic negative thoughts, J. M. begins to realize that he is engaging in a negative internal dialog with himself, focused on perceptions of low self-worth, especially when he is in group social situations. This pattern leads to sadness, shame, and the urge to isolate during social events. J. M. learns to monitor, challenge, and modify these thoughts through both in-session work and homework assignments. He continues to describe the exercises as awkward, but the therapist has noticed that J. M. has become increasingly able to recognize his own patterns of unhelpful cognitive and behavioral responses during setbacks—namely, angry self-talk and avoidance. The therapist and J. M. continue to problem-solve the use of adaptive thinking skills over the next few sessions. As J. M. engages in more helpful self-talk, his acceptance of living with HIV begins to increase. He has expressed more commitment to problem-solving the expansion of his social connections and to testing his old beliefs that he is not worthy of an intimate relationship.

CBT APPROACHES AND OUTCOMES IN MEDICAL POPULATIONS

CBT protocols that have been established in the general population commonly target specific psychiatric outcomes (e.g., worry in patients with generalized anxiety, or depression and anhedonia in patients with major depressive disorder). In comparison, research studies of CBT for medical patients are more likely to focus on individuals who are homogeneous with respect to medical illness. Interventions often comprise a combination of CBT strategies with multiple targets including psychological adjustment, health behaviors, disability, and/or disease-specific quality of life. Protocols that comprise this literature have varied in the extent to which they are based on theoretical principles for improving symptoms and/or facilitating complex health behavior changes (Eccleston, Williams, & Morley, 2009). The following section describes CBT approaches and supporting evidence for improving several common concerns in medical patients.

DEPRESSION

Across diverse medical populations, evidence supports the use of CBT to reduce depression symptoms, with larger effects in studies that limit participation to adults who meet criteria for clinical depression (Beltman, Oude Voshaar, & Speckens, 2010). Common treatment elements include psychoeducation, behavioral activation, adaptive thinking skills, and problem solving, with attention to associations between depression symptoms and aspects of disease-specific quality of life. A comparative review of nonpharmacological interventions for patients with chronic heart disease (education, relaxation, behavioral strategies, and cognitive strategies) demonstrated that both cognitive and behavioral strategies may reduce depression severity (Welton, Caldwell, Adamopoulos, & Vedhara, 2009). While older adults are typically underrepresented in CBT trials (Wilson, Mottram,

& Vassilas, 2008), reviews of CBT for depression in medical illnesses that are primarily diagnosed in older adulthood, such as chronic obstructive pulmonary disease (Fritzsche, Clamor, & von Leupoldt, 2011), suggest that CBT is feasible and potentially effective in this age group. Among patients, the long-term benefits of CBT have not yet been established.

ANXIETY

Common anxiety treatment strategies include psychoeducation, self-monitoring, exposure, adaptive thinking, and relaxation training. Specific protocols vary in the extent to which each strategy is emphasized. For instance, guided exposure to feared situations may be used to treat anxiety related to specific triggers (e.g., blood/injection/injury phobias), whereas this strategy is less relevant for nonspecific (generalized) anxiety. In the general population, CBT is efficacious for reducing anxiety severity within different anxiety disorders (Hofmann & Smits, 2008; Hunot, Churchill, de Lima, & Teixeira, 2007) and has also shown a potential advantage over pharmacological treatments for panic disorder in particular (Roshanaei-Moghaddam et al., 2011).

In medical populations, CBT interventions often address triggers for illness-related anxiety (such as fear of cancer recurrence) and typically adopt a generalist approach toward anxiety as a symptom. Anxiety is also often a secondary endpoint in treatments that target other problems such as depression or medical disability. Consequently, interventions vary in the extent to which they include theoretically based anxiety treatment strategies, and evidence for improvements in anxiety is mixed. CBT has shown promise in preventing or reducing anxiety in patients coping with a range of conditions such as cancer (Greer et al., 2012; Osborn, Demoncada, & Feuerstein, 2006), chronic obstructive pulmonary disease (Hynninen, Bjerke, Pallesen, Bakke, & Nordhus, 2010), and spinal cord injury (Mehta et al., 2011).

INSOMNIA

The objective of CBT for primary insomnia (Smith & Neubauer, 2003) is to improve sleep through changes in sleep hygiene practices and cognitions about sleep. Common strategies include psychoeducation, relaxation training, and cognitive restructuring (e.g., of catastrophic thinking related to sleep loss). Patients monitor sleep/wake patterns through daily sleep diaries, daytime activity records, and/or the use of an actigraph unit (a portable measure of gross motor activity) throughout the treatment period. These data provide feedback that can be reviewed at each treatment session. CBT approaches for optimizing sleep include stimulus control (facilitating sleep initiation) and sleep restriction (limiting actual time in bed to the amount of sleep time). In medical patients, primary insomnia versus insomnia secondary to a medical condition may be difficult to distinguish. CBT can be adapted to address unique sleep challenges among specific patient populations, such as disruptions in daytime activity and sunlight exposure, nocturnal dyspnea, or swallowing problems, and disease-related or treatment-related pain and fatigue.

CBT for insomnia has shown promise among medical patients, including those with HIV, cancer, and chronic pain (Smith, Huang, & Manber, 2005). Among older adults, limited data suggest that this treatment may lead to mild improvements in nighttime awakenings in particular (Montgomery & Dennis, 2003). CBT approaches to insomnia may also have a small to moderate effect on reducing comorbid anxiety, and very limited evidence supports that this effect may be comparable between patients with or without medical comorbidity (Belleville, Cousineau, Levrier, & St-Pierre-Delorme, 2011).

CHRONIC DISEASE MANAGEMENT

CBT protocols have been developed to treat or reduce disability associated with a range of medical concerns. These treatments emphasize that for patients with a chronic illness, disease self-management plays a critical role in effective patient care. CBT treatment targets and proposed outcomes may be multifold, including medical adherence, medical symptom reduction, optimal healthcare utilization, and disease-specific quality of life. Typically, treatments combine health education with CBT strategies to increase patient skills for engaging in self-care. For instance, CBT for adult asthma may integrate psychoeducation (e.g., about inhaler use and/or the link between anxiety and asthma physiology) with strategies for changing inaccurate thoughts (e.g., underemphasizing or overemphasizing respiratory symptoms) that provoke suboptimal inhaler use and/or worsen asthma attacks. CBT for chronic heart disease may combine education about cardiovascular function with strategies for promoting heart-healthy behaviors (e.g., physical activity, healthy eating behaviors) and adaptive thinking about the challenges of making such lifestyle changes.

Typically, CBT protocols for disease self-management have been tested in medical participants who do not necessarily meet criteria for clinical depression or anxiety. Rather, these studies reflect the assumption that all patients could benefit from additional skills for coping with the sequelae of their condition. Results of a small number of studies of CBT for adult asthma suggested that compared to control conditions, CBT may improve disease-specific quality of life but not depression symptoms or excess healthcare utilization (e.g., emergency room visits or hospitalizations [Yorke, Fleming, & Shuldham, 2006]). On the other hand, results from one of the largest psychological treatment trials in post–myocardial infarction (MI) adults suggests that CBT may improve both depression severity and quality of life among participants, in the absence of improving medical outcomes (Berkman et al., 2003). A comparative review of common psychological intervention elements for chronic heart disease identified that behavioral strategies in particular may improve depression and also reduce risk of both nonfatal cardiac events and mortality (Welton, Caldwell, Adamopoulos, & Vedhara, 2009). A small number of trials of CBT for adult epilepsy have examined diverse outcomes, with no reliable evidence to support benefits for seizure frequency, depression, or quality of life (Ramaratnam, Baker, & Goldstein, 2011).

PAIN

For patients experiencing chronic pain, CBT commonly targets the role of cognitions and behaviors that exacerbate pain intensity, distress, and disability. Strategies such as education, mental distraction from pain, relaxation training (e.g., muscle relaxation or deep breathing), and behavioral goal setting are used to improve pain management. Adaptive thinking skills may be used to modify unhelpful expectations about pain control (e.g., "my medications should completely cure my pain") and beliefs about the meaning of pain symptoms. Through these methods, CBT participants learn to elucidate and interrupt cycles of behavioral inactivity (e.g., fearful avoidance of physical activity that could trigger pain) and physiological overactivity (e.g., anxious arousal and muscular tension) that lead to poorer pain outcomes.

Trials of CBT for patients with chronic pain commonly focus on altering pain severity, disability, and mood. It should be noted, however, that most trials have identified disability and mood as the primary outcomes. Findings suggest that CBT may be moderately effective in controlling low back pain intensity (Chou & Hoyt Huffman, 2007), with mixed evidence for improving disability (Hoffman, Papas, Chatkoff, & Kerns, 2007; Henschke et al., 2010). Results from a small number of studies also suggest that CBT alone or in combination with biofeedback has the potential to reduce orofacial pain intensity, as well as depression and interference of orofacial pain in usual activities (Aggarwal et al., 2011). Combined findings across different types of chronic pain (except headaches) have suggested small effects of CBT on pain severity and disability at 6-month follow-up (Eccleston, Williams, & Morley, 2009).

FATIGUE

As in the case of chronic pain, medical patients with fatigue symptoms may attempt to restrict physical activity, leading to unintended consequences such as increased sensitivity to transient fatigue symptoms and catastrophizing about the consequences of such symptoms. CBT interventions for fatigue commonly integrate basic CBT strategies (e.g., behavioral activation, adaptive thinking) with physical rehabilitation goals. Contingency planning (e.g., what to do on a day when fatigue is elevated versus relatively low) can facilitate the use of behavioral activation and promote patient confidence in engaging in meaningful activities (Carney & Freedland, 2008). Providers may also guide patients in planning "experiments" in which they incrementally increase exposure to physical activity while monitoring and challenging negative cognitions during each activity.

Fatigue is a common endpoint in trials of CBT for diverse medical populations. These interventions vary in the extent to which they include specific strategies to reduce fatigue. A randomized controlled trial of CBT for persistent fatigue in cancer survivors showed that CBT improved fatigue and functional status (Gielissen, Verhagen, Witjes, Bleijenberg, 2006), with sustained benefits at long-term follow-up (Gielissen, Verhagen, & Bleijenberg, 2007). Trials of CBT

specifically for patients with chronic fatigue syndrome suggest that CBT is moderately effective in reducing fatigue in this population (Malouff, Thorsteinsson, Rooke, Bhullar, & Schutte, 2008) and may be superior to other types of treatment (e.g., relaxation, counseling, activity pacing therapy [limiting stress and avoiding exacerbation of fatigue], and education [Price, Mitchell, Tidy, & Hunot, 2008; White et al., 2011]). Results from a parallel randomized trial of activity pacing, graded exercise (incremental increases in activity) and CBT showed that graded exercise and CBT interventions were both safe and moderately efficacious in improving fatigue and physical functioning relative to activity pacing or standard medical care alone (White et al., 2011). Incremental benefits of combining CBT with other types of treatment for fatigue have not been established.

PRACTICAL CONSIDERATIONS: ADAPTING CBT IN MEDICAL POPULATIONS

CBT interventions have been incorporated into clinical practice guidelines for a wide range of psychiatric disorders. Multicomponent approaches have been adapted to address how cognitions and behaviors can influence psychological adjustment, health behaviors, and functional status among medical patients. In practice, medical conditions introduce unique aspects to consider during CBT evaluation and delivery.

SYMPTOM OVERLAP

Psychiatric symptoms can overlap with or mask disease symptoms and treatment side effects (e.g., fatigue, dyspnea, appetite disturbances, and uncontrolled pain). Patient cognitions and emotional distress levels may also fluctuate over time in response to uncertain disease course or certain disease progression. Assessment and treatment planning should include collaboration with a patient's other medical providers, and attention to complicating factors such as medication overuse, psychiatric comorbidity, stress and poor coping, and sleep disturbance (Lipchik, Smitherman, Penzien, & Holroyd, 2006). Contextual factors, including financial stressors and deficits in social support, may further reduce patient resources for accessing available resources and should be part of the initial assessment. In many cases, CBT approaches will be useful whether the symptoms are due to psychological factors, medical factors, or both.

PATIENT PREFERENCES, EXPECTATIONS, AND NEEDS

Patient histories play an important role in the acceptability of CBT for managing medical conditions. For individuals with idiopathic or poorly controlled symptoms, a long history of searching for proper diagnosis or symptom relief can lead to profound discouragement. On the other hand, patients who expect immediate symptom relief from CBT may become disillusioned soon after therapy initiation (Lipchik, Smitherman, Penzien, & Holroyd, 2006). Motivations for talk therapy must be clarified at CBT entry; finding an appropriate balance between hope and realistic expectations is a critical step toward maintaining patient engagement in treatment.

Currently, the accessibility and acceptability of CBT and of talk therapies in general vary widely across geographic and clinic settings and individual patients. When available, CBT may be appealing to medical patients and healthcare providers for a number of reasons. For one, CBT interventions are unlikely to have side effects and contraindications relative to pharmacological agents. Patients may prefer talk therapy due to already complicated medication schedules or personal preferences. CBT interventions also largely rely on patients' personal efforts. Some conditions (e.g., chronic pain) may not be cured or completed controlled by medication or physical therapies, and CBT can help patients enhance their quality of life in the presence of residual symptoms. The CBT focus on learning and maintaining practical skills is also designed to reduce risk of relapse as stressors change over time.

CLINICAL PEARLS

- CBT strategies emphasize self-regulation (e.g., a patient with chronic fatigue may work on identifying and planning activities that correspond with daily level of fatigue)

- A situational interpretation (e.g., "My oncologist probably has not returned my call yet because she has bad news to tell me.") can trigger a cycle of negative cognitions, emotions and unhelpful behaviors.

- By developing a CBT model of the patient's symptoms, the therapist and patient may identify areas in which the patient can take personal responsibility or control over chronic disease management.

- Socratic questioning is an interview technique used to help a patient discover problematic patterns in thoughts or behaviors.

- Motivational interviewing is a method assuming patient autonomy, which elicits a patient's own intrinsic arguments for change and uses these arguments as the source of motivation.

- Behavioral activation represents a collaborative effort between the therapist and patient to identify specific activities that may be personally rewarding.

- Adaptive thinking skills may be supplemented with acceptance-oriented coping skills when thoughts are deemed realistic, or with information seeking when more "data" are needed.

- Problem-solving therapy emphasizes four main skills: articulating problems, generating potential solutions, evaluating each solution with regard to advantages and disadvantages, and executing and monitoring a plan of action.

- Interventions typically conclude with a focus on relapse prevention by anticipating and problem-solving potential obstacles to the ongoing use of CBT skills.

- CBT in medical settings can help patients enhance quality of life in the presence of residual symptoms and related stressors that may change over time.

DISCLOSURE STATEMENTS

Dr. Traeger served as an independent consultant on a single advisory board meeting for Novartis Oncology. Her research has been funded through grants from the National Cancer Institute and the American Cancer Society.

Dr. Greer has no conflicts to disclose. His research is funded through grants from the National Cancer Institute and the American Cancer Society as well as institutional support from the Massachusetts General Hospital Cancer Center.

REFERENCES

Aggarwal, V. R., Lovell, K., Peters, S., Javidi, H., Joughin, A., & Goldthorpe, J. (2011). Psychosocial interventions for the management of chronic orofacial pain. *Cochrane Database of Systematic Reviews*, CD008456.

Beck, A. T. (1963). Thinking and depression. *Archives of General Psychiatry, 9*, 324–333.

Beck, A. T. (1964). Thinking and depression, II: theory and therapy. *Archives of General Psychiatry, 10*, 561–571.

Belleville, G., Cousineau, H., Levrier, J., & St-Pierre-Delorme, M. E. (2011). Meta-analytic review of the impact of cognitive-behavior therapy for insomnia on concomitant anxiety. *Clinical Psychology Review, 31*, 638–652.

Beltman, M. W., Oude Voshaar, R. C., & Speckens, A. E. (2010). Cognitive–behavioural therapy for depression in people with a somatic disease: meta-analysis of randomised controlled trials. *The British Journal of Psychiatry, 197*, 11–19.

Berkman, L. F., Blumenthal, J., Burg, M., Carney, R. M., Catellier, D., Cowan, M. J., et al. (2003). Effects of treating depression and low perceived social support on clinical events after myocardial infarction: the Enhancing Recovery in Coronary Heart Disease Patients (ENRICHD) Randomized Trial. *Journal of the American Medical Association, 289*, 3106–3116.

Carney, R. M., & Freedland, K. E. (2008). Depression in patients with coronary heart disease. *The American Journal of Medicine, 121*(11B), S20–S27.

Chou, R., & Hoyt Huffman, L. (2007). Nonpharmacologic therapies for acute and chronic low back pain: a review of the evidence for an American Pain Society/American College of Physicians clinical practice guideline. *Annals of Internal Medicine, 147*, 492–504.

Craske, M., Antony, M., & Barlow, D. H. (2006). *Mastery of your fears and phobias: Therapist guide* (2nd ed.). New York: Oxford University Press.

Crider, A., Glaros, A. G., & Gervirtz, R. (2005). Efficacy of biofeedback-based treatments for temporomandibular disorders. *Applied Psychophysiology and Biofeedback, 30*, 333–345.

Decker, T. W., Cline-Elsen, J., & Gallagher, M. (1992). Relaxation therapy as an adjunct in radiation oncology. *Journal of Clinical Psychology, 48,* 388–393.

Dobson, K. S., & Dozois, D. J. A. (2010). Historical and philosophical bases of the cognitive-behavioral therapies. In K. S. Dobson (Ed.), *Handbook of cognitive-behavioral therapies* (pp. 1–38). New York, NY: The Guilford Press.

Duhamel, K. N., Mosher, C. E., Winkel, G., Labay, L. E., Rini, C., Meschian, Y. M., et al. (2010). Randomized clinical trial of telephone-administered cognitive-behavioral therapy to reduce post-traumatic stress disorder and distress symptoms after hematopoietic stem-cell transplantation. *Journal of Clinical Oncology, 28,* 3754–3761.

D'Zurilla, T. J., & Nezu, A. M. (2007). *Problem-solving therapy: A positive approach to clinical intervention* (3rd ed.). New York, NY: Springer Publishing Co.

Eccleston, C., Williams, A. C. D. C., & Morley, S. (2009). Psychological therapies for the management of chronic pain (excluding headache) in adults. *Cochrane Database of Systematic Reviews,* CD007407.

Ellis, A. (1957). Rational psychotherapy and individual psychology. *Journal of Individual Psychology, 13,* 38–44.

Enck, P., Van der Voort, I. R., & Klosterhalfen. S. (2009). Biofeedback therapy in fecal incontinence and constipation. *Neurogastroenterology and Motility, 21*(11), 1133–1141.

Eysenck, H. J. (1966). *The effects of psychotherapy.* New York, NY: International Science Press.

Foa, E., Hembree, E., & Rothbaum, B. (2010). Prolonged exposure therapy for PTSD: *Emotional processing of traumatic experiences. Therapist guide.* (2nd ed.). USA: Oxford University Press.

Fritzsche, A., Clamor, A., & von Leupoldt, A. (2011). Effects of medical and psychological treatment of depression in patients with COPD—a review. *Respiratory Medicine, 105*(10), 1422–1433.

Gielissen, M. F., Verhagen, C. A., & Bleijenberg, G. (2007). Cognitive behaviour therapy for fatigued cancer survivors: long-term follow-up. *British Journal of Cancer, 97*(5), 612–618.

Gielissen, M. F., Verhagen, S., Witjes, F., & Bleijenberg, G. (2006). Effects of cognitive behavior therapy in severely fatigued disease-free cancer patients compared with patients waiting for cognitive behavior therapy: a randomized controlled trial. *Journal of Clinical Oncology, 24*(30), 4882–4887.

Greer, J. A., Traeger, L., Bemis, H., Solis, J., Hendriksen, E. S., Park, E. R., et al. (2012). A pilot randomized controlled trial of brief cognitive-behavioral therapy for anxiety in patients with terminal cancer. *The Oncologist, 17*(10), 1337–1345.

Greenhalgh, J., Dickson, R., & Dundar, Y. (2010). Biofeedback for hypertension: a systematic review. *Journal of Hypertension, 28*(4), 644–652.

Greer, J. A., Graham, J. S., & Safren, S. A. (2009). Resolving treatment complications associated with comorbid medical conditions. In M. Otto & S. Hofmann (Eds.), *Avoiding treatment failure in anxiety disorders* (pp. 317–346). New York: Springer.

Henschke, N., Ostelo, R. W., van Tulder, M. W., Vlaeyen, J. W., Morley, S., Assendelft, W. J., et al. (2010). Behavioural treatment for chronic low-back pain. *Cochrane Database of Systematic Reviews,* CD002014.

Hill-Briggs, F., & Gemmell, L. (2007). Problem solving in diabetes self-management and control: a systematic review of the literature. *Diabetes Education, 33*(6), 1032–1050.

Hoffman, B. M., Papas, R. K., Chatkoff, D. K., & Kerns, R. D. (2007). Meta-analysis of psychological interventions for chronic low back pain. *Health Psychology, 26,* 1–9.

Hofmann, S. G., & Smits, J. A. J. (2008). Cognitive-behavioral therapy for adult anxiety disorders: a meta-analysis of randomized placebo-controlled trials. *Journal of Clinical Psychiatry, 69*(4), 621–632.

Hunot, V., Churchill, R., Silva de Lima, M., & Teixeira, V. (2007). Psychological therapies for generalised anxiety disorder. *Cochrane Database of Systematic Reviews,* CD001848.

Hynninen, M. J., Bjerke, N., Pallesen, S., Bakke, P. S., Nordhus, I. H. (2010). A randomized controlled trial of cognitive behavioral therapy for anxiety and depression in COPD. *Respiratory Medicine, 104*(7), 986–994.

Jacobsen, P. B., Meade, C. D., Stein, K. D., Chirikos, T. N., Small, B. J., Ruckdeschel, J. C. (2002). Efficacy and costs of two forms of stress management training for cancer patients undergoing chemotherapy. *Journal of Clinical Oncology, 20,* 2851–2862.

Lipchik, G. L., Smitherman, T. A., Penzien, D. B., & Holroyd, K. A. (2006). Basic principles and techniques of cognitive-behavioral therapies for comorbid psychiatric symptoms among headache patients. *Headache, 46,* S119–S132.

Lee, Y.-H., Chiou, P.-Y., Chang, P.-H., & Hayter, M. (2010). A systematic review of the effectiveness of problem-solving approaches towards symptom management in cancer care. *Journal of Clinical Nursing, 20,* 73–85.

Malenfant, D., Catton, M., & Pope, J. E. (2009). The efficacy of complementary and alternative medicine in the treatment of Raynaud's phenomenon: a literature review and meta-analysis. *Rheumatology, 48*(7), 791–795.

Malouff, J. M., Thorsteinsson, E. B., Rooke, S. E., Bhullar, N., & Schutte, N. S. (2008). Efficacy of cognitive behavioral therapy for chronic fatigue syndrome: a meta-analysis. *Clinical Psychology Review, 28*(5), 736–745.

Martell, C. R., Addis, M. E., & Jacobson, M. S. (2001). *Depression in context: Strategies for guided action.* New York, NY: Norton.

Mehta, S., Orenczuk, S., Hansen, K. T., Aubut, J. A. L., Hitzig, S. L., Legassic, M., et al. (2011). An evidence-based review of the effectiveness of cognitive behavioral therapy for psychosocial issues post spinal cord injury. *Rehabilitation Psychology, 56*(1): 15–25.

Miller, W. R., & Rollnick, S. (2002). *Motivational interviewing: Preparing people for change* (2nd ed.). New York, NY: Guilford Press.

Miller, W. R., & Rollnick, S. (2009). Ten things that motivational interviewing is not. *Behavioural and Cognitive Psychotherapy, 37,* 129–140.

Montgomery, P., & Dennis, J. A. (2003). Cognitive behavioural interventions for sleep problems in adults aged 60+. *Cochrane Database of Systematic Reviews,* CD003161.

Nagai, Y. (2011). Biofeedback and epilepsy. *Current Neurology and Neuroscience Reports, 11,* 443–450.

Nestoriuc, Y., & Martin, A. (2007). Efficacy of biofeedback for migraine: a meta-analysis. *Pain, 128,* 111–127.

Nezu, A. M., Nezu, C. M., Friedman, S. H., Faddis, S., & Houts, P. S. (1998). *Helping cancer patients cope: a problem-solving approach.* Washington, DC: American Psychological Association.

Osborn, R. L., Demoncada, A. C., & Feuerstein, M. (2006). Psychosocial interventions for depression, anxiety, and quality of life in cancer survivors: meta-analyses. *International Journal of Psychiatry in Medicine, 36,* 13–34.

Price, J. R., Mitchell, E., Tidy, E., & Hunot, V. (2008). Cognitive behaviour therapy for chronic fatigue syndrome in adults. *Cochrane Database of Systematic Reviews,* CD001027.

Ramaratnam, S., Baker, G. A., & Goldstein, L. H. (2011). Psychological treatments for epilepsy. *Cochrane Database of Systematic Reviews,* CD002029.

Roshanaei-Moghaddam, B., Pauly, M. C., Atkins, D. C., Baldwin, S. A., Stein, M. B., & Roy-Byrne, P. (2011). Relative effects of CBT and pharmacotherapy in depression versus anxiety: is medication somewhat better for depression, and CBT somewhat better for anxiety? *Depression and Anxiety, 28,* 560–567.

Safren, S. A., Gonzalez, J. S., & Soroudi, N. (2008). *Coping with chronic illness: A cognitive-behavioral therapy approach for adherence and depression: Therapist guide.* New York, Oxford: Oxford University Press.

Smith, M. T., Huang, M. I., & Manber, R. (2005). Cognitive behavior therapy for chronic insomnia occurring within the context of medical and psychiatric disorders. *Clinical Psychology Review, 25,* 559–592.

Smith, M. T., & Neubauer, D. N. (2003). Cognitive behavior therapy for chronic insomnia. *Clinical Cornerstone, 5,* 28–40.

Wallace, R. K., Benson, H., & Wilson, N. F. (1971). A wakeful hypometabolic physiologic state. *American Journal of Physiology, 221*(3), 795–799.

Welton, N. J., Caldwell, D. M., Adamopoulos, E., & Vedhara, K. (2009). Mixed treatment comparison meta-analysis of complex interventions: psychological interventions in coronary heart disease. *American Journal of Epidemiology, 169*, 1158–1165.

White, P. D., Goldsmith, K. A., Johnson, A. L., Potts, L., Walwyn, R., DeCesare, J. C., et al. (2011). Comparison of adaptive pacing therapy, cognitive behaviour therapy, graded exercise therapy, and specialist medical care for chronic fatigue syndrome (PACE): a randomised trial. *Lancet, 377*, 823–836.

Wilson, K., Mottram, P. G., & Vassilas, C. (2008). Psychotherapeutic treatments for older depressed people. *Cochrane Database of Systematic Reviews*, CD004853.

Wolpe, J. (1958). *Psychotherapy by reciprocal inhibition*. Stanford, CA: Stanford University Press.

Yorke, J., Fleming, S. L., & Shuldham, C. (2006). Psychological interventions for adults with asthma. Cochrane Database of Systematic Reviews, CD002982.

Zigmond, A. S., & Snaith, R. P. (1983). The hospital anxiety and depression scale. *Acta Psychiatrica Scandinavica, 67*, 361–370.

15.

NONADHERENCE TO TREATMENT

Joseph A. Greer, Paul J. Helmuth, Jeffrey S. Gonzalez, and Steven A. Safren

INTRODUCTION

Prescribing physicians generally practice assuming a complex, though tacit, agreement with their patients under which they strive to listen carefully to the presenting symptoms, undertake appropriate testing and examination, provide a thoughtful diagnosis, and recommend a course of treatment. Patients, in turn, are expected to take medications as prescribed and return for follow-up care at some predetermined interval to report any progress or problems. Of course, this general approach to medical care, which derives from modern medical education and training, can break down for any number of reasons. For example, a patient may have insufficient trust in her doctor, may be unable to obtain the medication for financial or insurance reasons, may be frightened by potential dangers of taking the medication, may experience unacceptable side effects, or she may simply forget the doses. In any case, given the heavy reliance of physicians on regular dosing of prescription medications for the treatment of chronic illnesses, patient nonadherence represents a significant challenge because of the potential for poor medical outcomes. In this chapter we will focus on adherence to medications among patients with chronic medical conditions, with attention to the scope of the problem, causes and correlates of nonadherence, methods to assess adherence, and efficacious interventions to improve adherence.

When describing and discussing the extent to which patients take medications as prescribed, researchers and public health officials have employed a number of different terms. Starting in the 1950s, the term *compliance* has been used in the medical literature. However, the World Health Organization and National Institutes of Health now prefer the term *adherence*, given the pejorative implications of the word *noncompliance* with its connotation of a passive role for patients in receiving medical advice that seems to assign blame for patients' willful and deviant rejection of that advice. The term *adherence* is thought to imply a more active and collaborative role for patients in medical treatment decisions that includes an element of trust with the physician, and mutual agreement on the choice of medication and expectations for dosing (National Council on Patient Information and Education, 2007).

MEDICATION NONADHERENCE: PREVALENCE, COST, AND ADVERSE OUTCOMES

An extensive scholarly literature documents widespread problems with medication adherence across a number of disease states. According to a report by the World Health Organization, adherence to long-term therapies for chronic conditions averages 50% in developed countries, with even lower rates in developing nations (Sabaté & World Health Organization, 2003). However, deriving reliable estimates for adherence rates to medical recommendations is challenging given the variability of measurements, diseases, and thresholds for defining adherence. For example, DiMatteo conducted a meta-analysis of published studies over a 50-year period and observed much higher mean rates of treatment adherence among patients with HIV (88.3%) compared to those with pulmonary diseases (68.8%) or diabetes (67.5%). With respect to the type of medical recommendation, the mean rate for adherence to prescribed medications was 79.4% based on the average of 328 studies (DiMatteo, 2004).

While the prevalence rates vary widely in the literature, the problem of nonadherence is clearly costly to the healthcare system. Researchers estimated the total direct and indirect costs for failing to adhere to prescription drug therapy in the United States at approximately $177 billion in 2000 (Ernst & Grizzle, 2001), while others have suggested that the figure may be much higher and closer to $300 billion (DiMatteo, 2004). The costs incurred result from increased outpatient visits, emergency department visits, hospital admissions, and inpatient stays, as well as overall healthcare expenditures (Pittman, Chen, Bowlin, & Foody, 2011). For example, one study showed that patients who were less adherent to imatinib for chronic myeloid leukemia had more all-cause inpatient days (14.8 vs. 1.8 days, p < .001) and higher total healthcare spending ($107,341 vs. $58,278, p < .05) compared to those with better adherence to the oral chemotherapy (E. Q. Wu et al., 2010). Similar trends have also been observed for patients taking medications for HIV, hypertension, type-2 diabetes, and asthma (Bender & Rand, 2004; Dragomir et al., 2010; Nachega et al., 2010; Wu, Seiber, Lacombe, Nahata, & Balkrishnan, 2011). Efforts to improve patient adherence thus represent a useful investment for the US healthcare system, as the increased pharmacy costs for treating chronic conditions are easily offset by savings related to decreased healthcare expenditures (Sokol, McGuigan, Verbrugge, & Epstein, 2005).

For most clinicians, the dramatic association between poor prescription medication adherence and adverse medical outcomes creates even greater concern than the substantial costs to the healthcare system. In general, patients who have low adherence to medical treatment recommendations (both prescription and nonprescription) experience 26% worse outcomes, according to a meta-analysis of the scholarly literature over the past three decades (DiMatteo, Giordani, Lepper, & Croghan, 2002). Patients with hypertension or coronary artery disease, for example, who are adherent to prescription medications experience decreased risk of stroke, heart failure, and cardiovascular events, as well as all-cause mortality (Bailey, Wan, Tang, Ghani, & Cushman, 2010; Dragomir, et al., 2010; Ho, Magid, Shetterly, Olson, Maddox, et al., 2008; Jackevicius, Li, & Tu, 2008). In fact, increasing adherence to a daily antihypertensive drug regimen by one pill per week appears to decrease stroke risk by 8%–9% and mortality by 7% over a 5-year period (Bailey, et al., 2010). Additionally, medication nonadherence helps to account for failures of patients to achieve lower blood pressures after physicians prescribe increased intensity of the antihypertensive regimens (Ho, Magid, Shetterly, Olson, Peterson, et al., 2008) and may in part explain the differential survival among African-American patients with heart failure as compared to Caucasians (J. R. Wu et al., 2010). Similarly, a number of adverse clinical outcomes are associated with nonadherence to antiviral medications among patients with HIV, such as disease progression, treatment resistance, and worse survival (Bangsberg et al., 2001; Harrigan et al., 2005; Hogg et al., 2002; Lima et al., 2007; Nachega et al., 2007). Taken together, these data underscore the importance of optimizing adherence to prescribed regimens as clinicians consider salient factors to reduce the risk of morbidity, and in some cases mortality, for patients with chronic conditions.

BARRIERS TO MEDICATION ADHERENCE

A variety of patient, provider, and system-level factors potentially compromise adherence to medications. Given the complex underlying causes of nonadherence, clinicians ideally would want to assess and consider the different types of barriers patients experience in order to tailor their interventions accordingly (Sabaté & World Health Organization, 2003). Using the case example below, we illustrate some of the various obstacles to medication adherence that patients experience and present strategies for identifying these barriers.

CASE STUDY

Ms. R is a 61-year-old, divorced woman of Puerto Rican descent who receives federal disability benefits for psychiatric reasons (depression and anxiety). She meets with her primary care physician quarterly to manage her chronic medical problems, including hypertension, diabetes, and coronary artery disease. During a routine visit, Ms. R's blood pressure readings were higher than normal, and her blood sugar was also elevated. The patient became tearful during the clinical interview, noting that she had been feeling very stressed recently due to assuming the care of her grandchildren when her daughter had an accident. Initially, Ms. R attributed the elevated blood pressure readings to her increased psychosocial stress. However, upon further probing, the primary care physician learned that the patient was unable to provide the names and doses of her prescribed antihypertensive medications. Moreover, although Ms. R had been regularly refilling her insulin and diabetic supplies, her prescriptions for antihypertensive medications had lapsed for more than 2 months.

Patient Factors. To understand the reasons for nonadherence, a clinician working with a patient such as Ms. R may want to begin with an assessment of factors that are potentially within the patient's control. Indeed, researchers have observed that common barriers to adherence include issues ranging from simple forgetfulness and concerns about possible side effects to more subtle, underlying attitudes and beliefs regarding the severity of illness, effectiveness of the medication, need for ongoing therapy, and one's confidence in following through with complex regimens (Bartlett, 2002; National Council on Patient Information and Education, 2007; Osterberg & Blaschke, 2005). Moreover, Ms. R's comorbid psychiatric problems may be contributing to her difficulty in adhering to prescribed regimens. Several meta-analyses have documented the strong association between depression and poor treatment adherence in patients with various chronic conditions, including hypertension, diabetes, and HIV, both at clinical and subthreshold levels for mood symptoms (J. S. Gonzalez, Batchelder, Psaros, & Safren, 2011; J. S. Gonzalez et al., 2008; Grenard et al., 2011). Compounding these potential barriers are concerns about English language skills and health literacy. Many patients with chronic medical conditions may lack the ability to comprehend information and instructions regarding the frequency, dosing, side effects, and course of therapy (Kalichman, Pope, et al., 2008; Osborn et al., 2011).

Provider Factors. The provider–patient relationship has the potential to mitigate or exacerbate problems with medication nonadherence. A recent meta-analysis showed that patients whose physicians communicate poorly have a 19% higher risk of nonadherence than those whose physicians communicate well (Zolnierek & Dimatteo, 2009). Time pressures during clinic encounters, lack of expressed empathy and inclusion of patients in the decision-making process, as well as overestimation of adherence are key issues that may impair communication about prescription medications. In particular, physicians often fail to consider the complexity and costs of regimens or sufficiently describe the benefits and risks of therapy, potential side effects, and relevant dosing information (Choudhry et al., 2011; Ingersoll & Heckman, 2005; Osterberg & Blaschke, 2005). Writing instructions down on paper, while helpful, is simply not enough to ensure proper adherence. In the case of Ms. R, had her physician accepted the patient's explanation for the elevated blood pressure reading without pursuing follow-up questions about the names and doses for the antihypertensive agents or calling the pharmacy, Ms. R's nonadherence would likely have been overlooked. Patient-centered approaches to care that solicit individual patients' reasons for missing doses, as well as motivations and supports for maximizing adherence, not only improve communication but also build trust in the therapeutic relationship. Studies show that both quality of communication and level of trust in providers predict adherence to prescribed medications (Piette, Heisler, Krein, & Kerr, 2005; Schoenthaler et al., 2009).

Healthcare System Factors. Patient–provider interactions, of course, occur in the broader context of the healthcare system, which may serve as another salient barrier to accessing treatment and optimizing adherence. Specifically, in response to rising healthcare costs, third-party payers have sought to limit pharmacy expenditures by introducing restrictive formularies, increasing medication copayments, employing monthly prescription caps, and applying high deductibles to patient benefits. These efforts at cost reduction are especially problematic for individuals with chronic conditions, such as those with congestive heart failure, diabetes, or schizophrenia, who are more likely to utilize emergency department and inpatient medical services when faced with higher copayments, benefit caps, or other cost-sharing measures. In fact, for each 10% increase in cost-sharing overall, prescription drug spending on behalf of patients decreases by 2%–6% (Goldman, Joyce, & Zheng, 2007). In addition, older patients with chronic diseases and mood disorders are at increased risk of cost-related medication nonadherence (Briesacher, Gurwitz, & Soumerai, 2007).

Ms. R's Reasons for Nonadherence. As with many patients in clinical settings, Ms. R's reasons for medication nonadherence are complex and multifactorial. On further questioning, her physician discovered that she was experiencing a benefit cap in the form of the "donut hole" with respect to her Medicare prescription drug benefit. Ms. R then revealed that she felt that her diabetes was "the most important medical problem" she had. Given her limited resources, she had prioritized the purchase of insulin but felt she could forego her antihypertensive medications until after her prescription benefit resumed in the next calendar year. Although her language skills and known mood disorder may have contributed to her challenges with medication adherence at other times in the course of her illnesses, they were not relevant for the time period of the present vignette. She and her primary care provider then reviewed her medication regimen to incorporate some lower cost generic drugs that would most likely keep her yearly expenses below the benefit cap for the following year. Additionally, they reviewed the clinical importance of treating hypertension, as well as strategies for maintaining her drug therapy and improving communication about the costs and side effects of her medications.

METHODS FOR ASSESSING MEDICATION ADHERENCE

Accurate assessment of adherence to drug therapy is the first step in reducing the medical risks and associated costs resulting from prescription medication nonadherence. However, no single "gold standard" exists to evaluate this health behavior in either clinical or research contexts, with all forms of assessment possessing various biases or errors in measurement (J. S. Gonzalez & Schneider, 2011; Hansen et al., 2009). Even the most reliable and direct assessments, such as patient observation or laboratory measurements of drug metabolites in body fluids, are imperfect. In the case of directly observed therapy, patients may hold pills in their mouths without ingesting.

Although testing blood or urine samples may help overcome this concern, laboratory results only provide information about the use of the medication at one time point rather than over a sustained period (Farmer, 1999). In certain situations, direct assessment methods can be quite valuable, such as when a clinician tests for the presence of narcotics in urine to confirm that a patient is using the prescription opioids for a chronic medical condition rather than diverting doses. Nonetheless, these direct approaches are costly, time consuming, and generally impractical in clinical settings. Table 15.1 details common methods for assessing medication adherence and potential sources of measurement error (J. S. Gonzalez & Schneider, 2011).

Table 15.1 METHODS FOR ASSESSING MEDICATION ADHERENCE AND POTENTIAL THREATS TO VALIDITY

METHOD	POTENTIAL SOURCES OF MEASUREMENT ERROR
Direct patient observation	• No significant source of error for observed doses
Medication level in biologic fluids	• Metabolism and other ingested substances may affect accuracy • Laboratory errors
Biologic markers	• Metabolism and other ingested substances may affect accuracy • Laboratory errors
Healthcare provider estimates	• Healthcare provider has limited information on which to base estimate, and this may be biased by inaccurate patient reports and/or biologic markers as indicators of adherence
Pharmacy claims data	• No information about ingestion of medication • Patient may use more than one pharmacy or may share medications with family and friends • Documentation errors
Electronic monitoring	• No information about ingestion of medication • Does not document pocketed doses or pills taken from other sources (e.g., pill box) • Device errors/malfunctions
Pill count	• Potential for medication dumping before assessment if not unannounced • No information about ingestion of medication • Human errors in counting
Self-reported adherence (patient interviews, diaries and self-report measures)	• Inaccuracies relating to patient memory • Report bias (patient may purposely overestimate adherence) • Characteristics of the question and how they are administered (e.g., interview vs. questionnaire) may affect how patients respond • Incomplete recording is common for diaries • Numeracy and literacy issues could influence reporting

Adapted from Gonzalez & Schneider, 2011.

Due to ease of implementation, clinicians often prefer to use indirect methods for evaluating adherence to drug therapy. Such methods include estimates from the healthcare provider, pharmacy claims data, electronic monitoring devices, pill counts, and self-report by patients. Multiple studies show that, across disease states, physicians overestimate their patients' adherence to prescribed medications, and their assessments often fail to correlate with other measures of adherence (Daniels et al., 2011; Trindade, Ehrlich, Kornbluth, & Ullman, 2011; Walshe et al., 2010). Therefore, clinicians would be better served by relying on alternative methods that provide a more valid and reliable estimate of patient adherence.

Pharmacy refill data may be used in a number of clinical and research scenarios. Traditionally, researchers have examined medical records and claims data from large databases to determine rates of prescription refills, noting that the proportion of days covered for filled prescriptions is strongly associated with medical outcomes and healthcare utilization patterns. Although the findings from investigations of large epidemiological studies that incorporate claims data are meaningful in demonstrating the potential clinical effects of nonadherence at the population level, such methods offer limited value in discerning an individual patient's use of a prescribed medication. Recently, in tandem with trends to provide incentives for improved disease management to providers and medical care organizations, both pharmacies and health insurers are using individual patient refill data to alert patients and clinicians directly about potential nonadherence to medications (Bambauer et al., 2006). While these initiatives may prove useful in improving patient adherence, some caution is warranted. Specifically, physicians do not routinely inform pharmacies and insurers when they advise patients to discontinue particular medication regimens. Such gaps in communication among medical providers, pharmacists, and insurers may lead to serious medication errors and adverse outcomes.

Electronic monitoring devices are an alternate, objective measure of medication adherence, most commonly used for research purposes. For example, the Medication Event Monitoring System (MEMS™, Aardex; Zurich, Switzerland) consists of a standard pill bottle with a specialized cap containing an electronic microprocessor that records the exact date and time the bottle was opened, thus providing researchers with detailed information about medication-taking behaviors over time. Although this method of assessment has many strengths and correlates well with pharmacy refill data (Hansen, et al., 2009), opening of a MEMS pill bottle may underestimate the true rate of adherence because patients can remove pills for multiple doses at one time. For example, in a study of 128 HIV-infected individuals treated with at least three antiretroviral agents, 41% of the sample reported taking out more than one dose at a time (Bova et al., 2005). The converse is also a possibility, as patients perhaps may open the pill bottle without actually ingesting the medication. While MEMS devices have generally served more as a tool for assessment than for intervention, recent innovations have adapted electronic pill caps with a wireless technology that sends audiovisual signals to cue patients when to take their medications. Still, these products are not only expensive but also may interfere with use of other strategies for improving adherence to prescribed medications, such as weekly pillbox organizers (Kalichman, Cain, Cherry, Kalichman, & Pope, 2005). For these reasons, their application in clinical settings is limited.

Another method of assessment for adherence commonly used in clinical trials involves counting pills and calculating the ratio of the number of pills remaining in the bottle compared to the total number of pills that should have been consumed during a specified time period. To use this approach, patients are generally asked to bring their medication bottles to the study assessment or medical visit, which has the potential to introduce significant error in measurement (Choo et al., 1999; Farmer, 1999). Since patients often transfer medications to other containers, such as pillboxes, they may unintentionally invalidate the pill count. Others may directly manipulate the number of pills in advance of an assessment in order to appear more adherent to the physician or researcher. To overcome these issues, investigators who study medication adherence in patients with HIV, for example, have begun to examine the feasibility, reliability, and validity of conducting unannounced pill counts over the telephone. This approach is unobtrusive and demonstrates very high concordance (>90%) with unannounced home-visit pill counts, even among patients of low socioeconomic status (Kalichman et al., 2010; Kalichman, Amaral, et al., 2008; Kalichman et al., 2007). Although pill counts have fallen out of favor somewhat with the advent of other objective measures, such as electronic monitoring devices, unannounced pill counts over the telephone may represent an acceptable, valid, and cost-effective measure of medication adherence that could be generalized to clinical settings.

Given their practical application, ease of administration, and low burden to patients, self-report assessments are the most popular tools for measuring medication adherence among individuals with chronic illnesses. Various interviews, diaries, questionnaires, scales, and single-item measures exist, some of which can be generally applied while others are disease-specific. More importantly, these measures tend to overestimate rates of adherence due to their susceptibility to response bias from poor memory or social desirability, and they may vary with respect to their validity and reliability in correlating with other, more objective measures of adherence (Shi, Liu, Fonseca, et al., 2010; Wagner & Miller, 2004). Nonetheless, in the case of HIV disease, for which adherence to antiretroviral therapy is especially important to clinical outcomes, investigators have found that responses on self-report questionnaires of medication adherence are significantly associated with virologic response to treatment (Nieuwkerk & Oort, 2005). Among the most common instruments is the Adult AIDS Clinical Trial Group (AACTG) adherence measure, which asks patients whether they have missed any prescribed doses within certain time frames (e.g., past 2 days, 7 days, 2 weeks, 1 month, etc.), along with reasons for nonadherence (Chesney et al., 2000). Otherwise, general medication adherence instruments that are widely used and possess adequate validity include the Morisky Medication Adherence

Scale, the Brief Medication Questionnaire, and the visual analogue scale (Morisky, Green, & Levine, 1986; Svarstad, Chewning, Sleath, & Claesson, 1999). While these measures appear to show moderate concordance with electronic monitoring devices, their correlation with pharmacy refill records is somewhat weaker (Cook, Wade, Martin, & Perri, 2005; Shi, Liu, Koleva, et al., 2010).

Despite the abundant literature on medication adherence for patients with chronic illnesses ranging from cancer and HIV to hypertension and diabetes, no single self-report measure has emerged as the optimal tool for predicting nonadherence or adverse clinical outcomes. Nonetheless, some general principles can be derived that may inform clinical practice. First, single-item global assessments of adherence, with which individuals rate their ability to take all medications as prescribed for the past month using either a visual analogue scale, percentage-base response, or qualitative assessment (i.e., very poor to excellent), perform very well when correlated with electronic medication monitoring methods (J. S. Gonzalez & Schneider, 2011; Lu et al., 2008; Schneider, Gonzalez, & Psaros, 2011). In addition, such global tools may be more accurate than asking patients to recall the number of missed doses and are especially useful for minority patients who are non–native English speakers or who may have limited health literacy and numeracy (i.e., the ability to process and respond to numerical and quantitative information) (Buscher, Hartman, Kallen, & Giordano, 2011; Giordano, Guzman, Clark, Charlebois, & Bangsberg, 2004; Golbeck, Ahlers-Schmidt, Paschal, & Dismuke, 2005). Finally, at least in the case of HIV medication adherence, studies suggest that both the reliability and predictive validity of measurements can be maximized by evaluating adherence across multiple time points and combining multiple methods of assessment (Liu et al., 2001; Llabre et al., 2006).

INTERVENTIONS TO IMPROVE MEDICATION ADHERENCE

Despite the accumulation of evidence underscoring the need to assess and address medication nonadherence in patients with chronic medical conditions, clinical and research efforts aimed at improving this health behavior have been disappointing to date. A meta-analysis of 78 intervention trials for enhancing medication adherence published by the Cochrane Collaboration reveals mixed results for both short-term and long-term adherence treatments (Haynes, Ackloo, Sahota, McDonald, & Yao, 2008). Specifically, less than half of the tested interventions led to significant improvement in medication adherence, and even fewer had effects on clinical outcomes. The target patient populations and diseases were diverse and included individuals with HIV, diabetes, asthma, chronic obstructive pulmonary disease, hypertension, rheumatoid arthritis, dyslipidemia, heart disease, and psychological disorders, among others. Moreover, treatment approaches varied considerably, ranging from simple educational and reminder systems to more complex combinations of psychotherapy, self-monitoring, reinforcement, telephone follow-up,

and supportive care. Unfortunately, the poor methodological rigor, small sample sizes, limited statistical power, imprecise measurement of adherence, diversity of interventions, and inconsistent clinical effects of the studies prohibit any conclusions about the overall utility and generalizability of any single approach. Two other recent meta-analyses highlight the potential promise of reinforcement and reminder systems (i.e., "reminder packaging") for increasing adherence to medications (Mahtani, Heneghan, Glasziou, & Perera, 2011; Schedlbauer, Davies, & Fahey, 2010). Nonetheless, based on the studies to date, further high-quality research is undeniably needed to develop innovative, efficacious, and clinically relevant approaches for improving medication adherence over the long term, along with related medical outcomes.

In the following section, we describe two novel approaches for improving medication adherence among patients with various chronic medical conditions. Based on our federally funded research studies, the first depicts a cognitive behavioral therapy intervention tailored to patients with type 2 diabetes and depression (NIH 1R01 MH078571; Principal Investigators: Safren and Gonzalez); and the second details a Web-based disease management program for asthma in adult primary care patients (NIH 1R43 HL096244; Principal Investigators: Helmuth and Greer). We illustrate the principles of the different intervention strategies using clinical case examples.

COGNITIVE BEHAVIORAL THERAPY FOR ADHERENCE AND DEPRESSION (CBT-AD) IN TYPE 2 DIABETES

CASE STUDY

Mr. M is a 60-year-old, non-Hispanic White male who was diagnosed with type 2 diabetes 3 years ago. His other medical problems include hypertension, coronary artery disease, and obesity (BMI of 45). Additionally, he meets criteria for recurrent major depressive disorder and has been seeing a counselor for many years. Upon most recent testing, his diabetes was in poor control with a hemoglobin A1C of 10.2% (goal is less than 7.0%). Mr. M admits to poor adherence to his oral hypoglycemic medications, noting that his travel schedule for work interferes with his ability to take his daily doses on time. Similarly, he does not exercise and often eats out at restaurants due to his variable work schedule. Stating that he is "completely overwhelmed" by stressors in his job and marriage, the patient believes that he does not have the time or energy to focus on his diabetes care. Yet, he does report considerable shame and guilt about his health behavior patterns and his weight, noting that his wife continually pressures him to eat better, take his medications, and begin an exercise program.

Mr. M is a good candidate for CBT-AD given his presenting concerns, though his low motivation and negative thought processes about his self-efficacy may compromise his participation. CBT-AD is a 10–12 session treatment consisting of five core modules that focus on improving medication adherence and depression symptoms, given the strong comorbidity between the two in patients with type 2 diabetes (J. Gonzalez et al., 2010; J. S. Gonzalez et al.,

2007). To begin, Mr. M would meet with the CBT therapist to discuss and address his problems in managing his oral hypoglycemic medications. This first session is entitled *Life Steps* and comprises 11 informational, problem-solving, and cognitive-behavioral steps that target a range of self-care behaviors, namely medication adherence (Safren, Otto, & Worth, 1999; Safren et al., 2001). For example, these steps include educating the patient about adherence, scheduling doses, using stimulus control to cue taking medication such as alarms and visual reminder systems, reframing thoughts to be more adaptive regarding adherence, and improving communication with medical providers. The goal of the Life Steps session is to clarify and problem-solve obstacles to self-care by identifying barriers to optimal adherence, generating possible solutions, and developing targeted action plans. In the case of Mr. M, a key feature of Life Steps would be to address his concerns about missing doses because of his work schedule. Considering his frequent use of a calendar feature on his smart phone to manage his many work-related appointments, he could reasonably add medication dosage times to his electronic schedule. By doing so, he would not only increase the likelihood of remembering doses but also symbolically elevate the importance of medication adherence relative to his other daily priorities. In the subsequent sessions, Mr. M and his CBT therapist would spend the first few minutes reviewing these strategies to enhance medication adherence prior to learning and practicing new skills also aimed at treating comorbid depression symptoms.

After the first Life Steps session, the treatment turns to the first core module: *Education and Motivational Enhancement.* Spanning two sessions, in this module, Mr. M would learn about the principles of cognitive-behavioral therapy, including a discussion of the complex interactions among thoughts, behaviors, and physical symptoms in exacerbating depression. In addition, since Mr. M had spent many years in supportive, psychodynamic psychotherapy, he would benefit from an overview of the process of CBT including the goal-oriented nature of treatment, collaborative focus, and use of "homework assignments" to practice skills learned in session. Finally, the CBT therapist and Mr. M would work together to increase his motivation by clarifying his goals for treatment and examining the pros and cons of working on his mood symptoms and self-care behaviors versus maintaining the status quo. Mr. M might identify his desire to feel better about his body and improve his quality of life, or his wish to avoid having another heart attack, as salient factors motivating him to change.

The next module (approximately one session) focuses on behavioral activation and scheduling of pleasant events, while monitoring fluctuations in mood within and across days. Given the utility of identifying and engaging in meaningful and reinforcing activities to improve mood (Hopko, Lejuez, Ruggiero, & Eifert, 2003), Mr. M would want to examine the relationship between his stress level (i.e., "feeling overwhelmed") and predominant focus on work-related activities at the exclusion of pleasurable events. In discussion with his CBT therapist, Mr. M might reveal that he had previously enjoyed taking ballroom dance lessons with his wife when they were younger. Capitalizing on this prior experience, he could perhaps reinitiate this activity and schedule weekly dance classes, which would not only help his mood but also increase his physical activity level and potentially enhance his relationship with his wife. Other key components of this module pertain to tracking of blood glucose levels, exercise, and dietary behaviors.

Given the role that negative thoughts and self-talk play in perpetuating depression, the third module of CBT-AD involves training in cognitive restructuring the maladaptive thought processes that worsen mood and compromise self-care behaviors, including adherence to medications. Specifically, the aims of these sessions are to elicit patients' negative automatic thoughts, examine potential distortions in perception, and reframe these thoughts to be more realistic and adaptive (A. Beck, 1987; J. Beck & Beck, 1995). For example, like many patients with type 2 diabetes, Mr. M may avoid checking his blood sugars because the readings remind him of how badly he is managing his disease, prompting negative thoughts such as, "This is useless; I'll never be able to get my blood sugars down." Recognizing that such extreme thoughts only make him feel ineffective and more depressed, Mr. M could work with his CBT therapist to challenge this distortion by identifying past exceptions to the perception or by taking a less judgmental approach, using the reading as one data point for understanding the factors associated with blood sugar control rather than as a measure of self-worth.

The problem-solving module covers the next two sessions and incorporates skills for overcoming behavioral avoidances and challenges to self-care. Drawing on the principles of problem-solving therapy (D'Zurilla, 1986; Nezu & Perri, 1989), patients work on deconstructing daunting tasks into a series of manageable steps by first brainstorming possible courses of action, evaluating those potential decisions, and executing a straightforward behavioral plan. For example, Mr. M might realize that successful weight loss will require reducing his work hours to allow for sufficient time to plan meals and participate in regular physical activity. To address this problem, he and his CBT therapist would explore possible solutions for modifying his schedule, rate each solution's potential for resolving the problem, and then choose the optimal course of action that will help him move forward, recognizing that most solutions have salient advantages and disadvantages. In essence, these problem-solving skills aid patients like Mr. M to overcome ambivalence and avoidance in the face of challenging life decisions.

The final module consists of two sessions focused relaxation training, including diaphragmatic breathing and progressive muscle relaxation. Given Mr. M's tendency to feel overwhelmed by multiple life stressors, such techniques may help him learn to identify the physiological triggers of his mood symptoms and to practice simple methods for calming his body. Also, as he builds mastery in these skills he may gain confidence in his ability to manage stress, which may improve his overall self-efficacy and generalize to other health behaviors.

CBT-AD is an evidenced-based treatment that was first tested in samples of patients with HIV disease and comorbid depression (Safren et al., 2009), now undergoing efficacy study for use in individuals with type 2 diabetes with medication adherence and depression symptoms as primary outcomes (J. Gonzalez, et al., 2010). The client treatment manual, along with therapist guide, has been published (Safren, Gonzalez, & Soroudi, 2007a; Safren, Gonzalez, & Soroudi, 2007b). Yet, we recognize that broad dissemination of CBT-AD may be challenging, particularly for clinicians practicing in resource-poor communities who don't have access to psychotherapists possessing the necessary training and expertise in both CBT and management of medication adherence. Therefore, in the following section, we present a novel approach to caring for patients with chronic medical conditions that utilizes automated Web-based tools to enhance medication adherence, self-management of disease, and patient–provider communication.

A WEB-BASED MODULE FOR ASTHMA MANAGEMENT IN PRIMARY CARE

CASE STUDY

Mrs. D is a 45-year-old African-American woman who has a lifelong history of asthma. She has had a recent increase in her symptoms of asthma with breathlessness, cough, and decreased exercise tolerance over the last 6 months. She attributes some of her symptoms to cigarette smoking. She had previously quit smoking at age 25 at the time of her first pregnancy and reports that she started smoking again in the past year because of stress related to her pending divorce. Furthermore, she has had problems with symptoms of increased worry regarding finances since her daughter is planning to go to college, and she recently lost her job as a rental property manager. Mrs. D uses her albuterol "rescue" inhaler two or three times per day and feels that it is "the only thing" that helps with her symptoms of breathlessness. Her primary care doctor has prescribed multiple controller medications in the past, but she doesn't feel that they help sufficiently and has never continued taking them because "they don't work well enough to be worth the copay amount." She frequently uses all of her rescue inhaler doses before the prescription is due for renewal at the pharmacy.

At the time of enrolling in the Web-based asthma management program through her primary care physician's office, Mrs. D was feeling especially frustrated with her symptoms of shortness of breath and insomnia. She attributed some of her sleep problems to anxiety, but admitted that she frequently wakes from sleep with coughing and needs to use her inhaler in the middle of the night. Mrs. D is a good candidate for use of the online disease management module because it would provide her with needed patient educational information as well as tools for self-management, among other resources.

When enrolling in the program, Mrs. D would be given a password and introduced to the online version of the Web-based asthma management module by a medical assistant in her primary care doctor's office. She would learn about the two major functions of the program: (1) online questionnaires to assess her asthma control, medication adherence, and behavioral comorbidities; and (2) self-management tools to assist her in taking better care of herself with respect to her asthma. With her primary care doctor, she would review her symptoms and her office spirometry report and would be classified as having "moderate, persistent asthma." Since patients with moderate asthma are noted to benefit from daily measurement of their peak flow rate using a simple handheld device, her doctor will give her a prescription to obtain her own peak flow meter. Also, at this enrollment visit Mrs. D and her doctor would work together to develop an online *Asthma Action Plan* (AAP), with instructions on what actions to take should she have an asthma attack. For example, if her peak flow reading is low, it would place her in the "red zone" or the "yellow zone" as calculated as a percentage of her personal best peak flow reading. She would then follow the AAP instructions that she and her doctor decided upon regarding use of her inhalers, addition of prednisone, and instructions for when to go to the emergency department or call the medical office. Finally, at the initial visit, Mrs. D would complete baseline questionnaires in their online format. The self-report questionnaires in the asthma management program include the following:

- Asthma Control Test: A 5-item self-report questionnaire to determine asthma control over the past month (Nathan et al., 2004).
- Morisky Medication Adherence Questionnaire: A 4-item questionnaire to assess adherence to medications, in this case controller medications for treating asthma (Morisky et al., 1986).
- Smoking Questionnaire: Up to three items to clarify if the patient is a present smoker, former smoker, or never smoker (Centers for Disease Control and Prevention, 2008).
- Hospital Anxiety and Depression Scale: A 14-item tool for measuring symptoms of anxiety and depression during the past week in medical patient populations (Zigmond & Snaith, 1983).
- Stage of Change Questionnaire: Single-item instrument to assess patient readiness to make changes in taking medications as prescribed, with five possible stages including pre-contemplation, contemplation, preparation, action, and maintenance (Marcus, Selby, Niaura, & Rossi, 1992).

The self-report questionnaires are brief (26 items total), which Mrs. D would be able to complete in less than 10 minutes. The Web-based program immediately calculates the results of the questionnaires and provides a tailored response that is sent to the individual patient as well as to the medical provider. Thus, both Mrs. D and her doctor would receive concise messages similar to the one below. For Mrs. D's physician, the results of the questionnaires would transfer into the electronic medical record in a similar manner as laboratory results. Her doctor would then be able to address the concerns raised by the results of the self-report questionnaires, although Mrs. D would have already received feedback herself in the following format:

Below are results from your asthma questionnaires. Please use the link to educational materials at the bottom of the screen to learn more about your asthma or other related conditions.

Asthma Control Score: Low
Your asthma control test results indicate that your asthma is not well controlled at this time. Please call your doctor's office to arrange for a visit or to discuss your asthma medications.

Adherence to Asthma Medications: Low
You appear to be having difficulty using your asthma controller medications as prescribed. Please consider what may be interfering with your ability to use these medications on a daily basis. You and your doctor may discuss ways to improve your adherence at your next office visit.

Smoking Status: Current Smoker, daily. Has tried to quit.
Consider what might increase your chances of success when you try to quit smoking again. Please click on the educational links below to view information on resources to help you quit smoking.

Anxiety Symptoms: Mild
Your test for anxiety suggests that you have mild symptoms of anxiety. You may review links to information on anxiety below. Please also discuss your symptoms with your doctor.

Depression Symptoms: Mild
Your test for depression suggests that you have mild symptoms of depression. You may review links to information on depression below. Please also discuss your symptoms with your doctor.

Stage of Change (for improving use of controller medications): Contemplation
It seems that you are thinking about taking your asthma medications more regularly. Please consider the pros and cons of changing this behavior in order to help motivate you to take your medications on a daily basis. You may discuss this with your doctor at your next visit.

In addition to completing the Asthma Control Test, our comprehensive approach also assesses for the various behavioral and psychological correlates to asthma control such as medication adherence, psychological distress, and smoking status, using online self-report measures. The complex associations between asthma symptoms, psychological distress, and adherence to asthma medications remain incompletely elucidated, although symptoms of anxiety and depression are common among individuals with asthma (Goodwin, Jacobi, & Thefeld, 2003; Goodwin et al., 2003; Heaney, Conway, Kelly, & Gamble, 2005). Moreover, symptoms of depression have been associated with increased asthma severity, as well as functional impairment, increased number of visits to physicians and emergency departments, and impairments in health-related quality of life (Dahlen & Janson, 2002; Mancuso et al., 2008; Strine, Mokdad, Balluz, Berry, & Gonzalez, 2008). Anxiety and depression are also associated with poor adherence to asthma treatment (Bosley, Fosbury, & Cochrane, 1995; Cluley & Cochrane, 2001; Smith et al., 2006).

Because the Asthma Control Test score for Mrs. D was low on the initial questionnaire, she will receive email requests to complete the questionnaires again in one month. The results of repeat testing will come to her and to her doctor, with concise interpretations and instructions for both. Ideally, because her asthma control was poor, she should receive information from her doctor and from the website about the importance of using controller medications even though they do not offer quick relief of symptoms. As she monitors her lung function at home by obtaining her daily peak flow rate and documenting it in the asthma management website, Mrs. D would see steady improvements in her lung function as she becomes more adherent to use of her controller medication. Moreover, the online patient educational materials about smoking cessation might help to improve her motivation for quitting cigarette smoking. After her asthma control improves, Mrs. D would receive less frequent email contact. The patient contact for the Web-based module is determined using an algorithm that prioritizes those patients with poor asthma control for more intensive intervention (see Figure 15.1 below).

At one of her subsequent follow-up visits, Mrs. D might discuss her symptoms of anxiety with her primary care doctor, noting that she has been feeling more stressed recently because of her divorce and her finances. She might have some questions about anxiety after being informed that her screening test was positive on the asthma control website. After discussing the overlap in symptoms of anxiety and asthma, especially breathlessness and chest tightness, she and her doctor could determine a plan of care for addressing her symptoms of worry and insomnia. Similarly, she might raise her concerns about cigarette smoking and ask for information about medications to help her quit, having read some online information about the options for prescription drugs that could improve her chances of quitting.

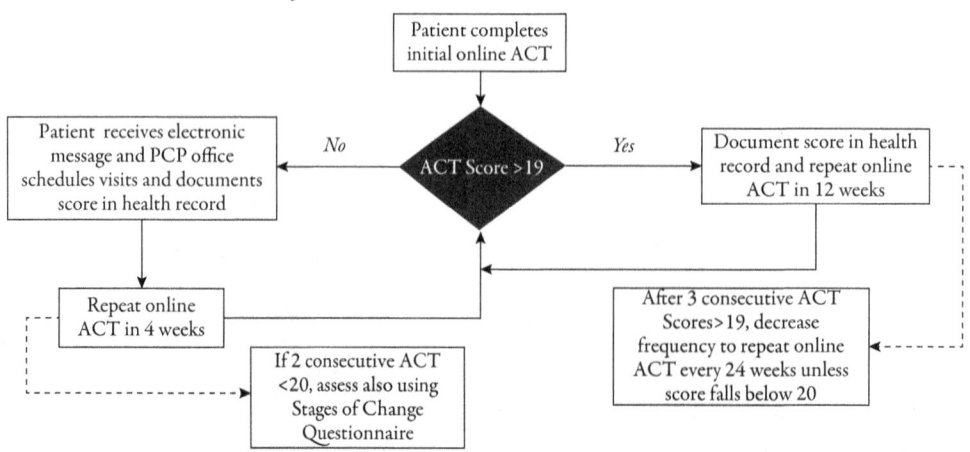

Figure 15.1 Web-based Asthma Management Algorithm.

If Mrs. D were to fail to complete a questionnaire, she would receive a second email message reminding her to do so. If she failed to respond to the second message, a notification would automatically go to her doctor indicating that Mrs. M is no longer adherent to the online program. The triage nurse from her primary care doctor's office would then try to contact her by phone to encourage her to continue using the online asthma management program.

Because medication adherence is the most proximal factor for asthma control, our tool applies Prochaska's transtheoretical behavior change methods to improve medication adherence (James O. Prochaska, 1979). Interventions derived from the transtheoretical model have also been used in diverse populations to improve health risk behaviors, including alcohol and substance abuse, smoking, poor medication adherence, and physical inactivity (Johnson et al., 2006; J. M. Prochaska et al., 2004; J. O. Prochaska, Velicer, Prochaska, & Johnson, 2004; Sarkin, Johnson, Prochaska, & Prochaska, 2001). We assess stage of behavioral change for improving adherence to asthma controller medications (e.g., pre-contemplation, contemplation, preparation, action, maintenance, or termination) in those patients who report poor adherence to medications. For example, patients who are in the contemplation stage are planning to change their health behaviors in the next 6 months, and although they are aware of both the pros and cons of changing they remain ambivalent. These patients are not yet ready for "action-oriented" programs, so clinicians should focus on enhancing motivation for change during office visits (J. O. Prochaska & DiClemente, 1983). Our tool provides such relevant data to clinicians, with suggestions for tailoring interventions to individual patients based on their current stage of change.

Our Web-based asthma management program is designed to help patients improve overall control of asthma, including medication adherence. The assessment of adherence is within the context of a comprehensive program to manage chronic diseases, consistent with recent trends in medical care that prioritize a patient-centered approach. Care management activities that provide services to patients with chronic illnesses are now required for physician practices to receive recognition in newer models of care such as the *Patient-Centered Medical Home* (NCQA, 2011). Moreover, through these programs and ongoing payment reform underway with public and private insurers, disease management activities, including assessment and support for medication adherence, will be increasingly tied to physician reimbursement (Rosenthal, 2008). Thus, physicians and their patients will benefit from greater access to cost-effective tools that provide patient-centered disease management programs that include patient educational materials, self-management tools, assessment and support for medication adherence, and resources for undertaking health behavior change.

SUMMARY

Nonadherence to self-administered medications remains a critical concern that compromises medical care and results in increased healthcare costs and utilization of services. Multiple patient, provider, and system factors contribute to the problem of nonadherence, necessitating clear communication during clinical encounters as well as tailored interventions to maximize patient self-care behaviors and understanding of the importance of taking prescribed medications consistently. Although the scholarly literature on patient adherence to medications is vast and continually evolving, the following recommendations can be gleaned, which may offer some guidance to clinicians seeking to address this important problem with their patients:

1. When prescribing a new medication, communicate clearly the purpose of the drug, potential side effects, likely outcomes, and plan for follow-up care should questions or concerns arise.

2. Simplify complex medication regimens to utilize once-daily dosing with as few pills and dietary restrictions as possible.

3. Encourage patients to invite caregivers and family members to be present when giving instructions, in order to support and reinforce patients' efforts to take medications as prescribed.

4. Inquire about medication adherence at each medical visit in a patient-centered and nonjudgmental manner. (For example, "Many individuals have problems remembering to take their doses of medication exactly as prescribed. Has this been difficult for you over the past month?").

5. Probe about various factors related to the patient (i.e., forgetfulness, health beliefs, depression, motivation, side effects, etc.) and healthcare system (i.e., medical insurance problems, high copayments, inadequate access to follow-up care) that may be contributing to nonadherence.

6. To assess medication adherence, try to gather data from multiple sources when possible, such as patient self-report, pharmacy refill data, and/or unannounced telephone pill counts.

7. Consider using simple, global assessments or ratings of self-reported adherence, which may be most feasible, generalizable, and cost-effective in diverse clinical settings.

8. For patients not ready to make a positive change in their adherence behaviors, utilize motivational enhancement strategies to encourage progress from contemplation to action (i.e., defining patient goals, examining the pros and cons of improving adherence versus maintaining the status quo, exploring and problem-solving obstacles to self-efficacy and confidence, etc.).

9. When appropriate and available, make use of evidence-based interventions such as CBT-AD to provide support for patients seeking to improve medication adherence and comorbid depression.

10. Provide patient-centered resources for comprehensive disease management that integrate medication adherence, access to patient education materials, support for health behavior change (e.g., weekly pillbox organizers, diaries, reminder systems), and self-management tools (i.e., action plans for home-based monitoring of blood pressure, blood sugars, peak expiratory flow rate, etc.).

CLINICAL PEARLS

- Patients who have low adherence to medical treatment recommendations (both prescription and nonprescription) experience 26% worse outcomes.

- To understand the reasons for nonadherence by a patient, a clinician may want to begin with an assessment of factors that are potentially within the patient's control.

- Unannounced pill counts over the telephone may represent an acceptable, valid, and cost-effective measure of medication adherence that could be generalized to clinical settings.

- Among the most common instruments is the Adult AIDS Clinical Trial Group (AACTG) adherence measure, which asks patients whether they have missed any prescribed doses within certain time frames (e.g., past 2 days, 7 days, 2 weeks, 1 month, etc.), along with reasons for nonadherence (Chesney et al., 2000).

- A meta-analysis of 78 intervention trials for enhancing medication adherence published by the Cochrane Collaboration reveals mixed results for both short-term and long-term adherence treatments (Haynes, Ackloo, Sahota, McDonald, & Yao, 2008).

- Encourage patients to invite caregivers and family members to be present when giving instructions in order to support and reinforce patients' efforts to take medications as prescribed.

- Inquire about medication adherence at each medical visit in a patient-centered and nonjudgmental manner. (For example, "Many individuals have problems remembering to take their doses of medication exactly as prescribed. Has this been difficult for you over the past month?")

DISCLOSURE STATEMENTS

Dr. Safren is funded through various NIH grants, and no industry support. He, however, receives royalties from book publishers, including Oxford University Press and Guilford Press.

Dr. Greer has no conflicts to disclose. His research is funded through grants from the National Cancer Institute and the American Cancer Society, as well as institutional support from the Massachusetts General Hospital Cancer Center.

REFERENCES

Bailey, J. E., Wan, J. Y., Tang, J., Ghani, M. A., & Cushman, W. C. (2010). Antihypertensive medication adherence, ambulatory visits, and risk of stroke and death. *Journal of General Internal Medicine, 25*(6), 495–503.

Bambauer, K. Z., Adams, A. S., Zhang, F., Minkoff, N., Grande, A., Weisblatt, R., et al. (2006). Physician alerts to increase antidepressant adherence: fax or fiction? *Archives of Internal Medicine, 166*(5), 498–504.

Bangsberg, D. R., Perry, S., Charlebois, E. D., Clark, R. A., Roberston, M., Zolopa, A. R., et al. (2001). Non-adherence to highly active antiretroviral therapy predicts progression to AIDS. *AIDS, 15*(9), 1181–1183.

Bartlett, J. A. (2002). Addressing the challenges of adherence. *Journal of Acquired Immune Deficiency Syndrome, 29 Suppl 1*, S2–S10.

Beck, A. (1987). *Cognitive therapy of depression*. New York: The Guilford Press.

Beck, J., & Beck, A. (1995). *Cognitive therapy*. New York: The Guilford Press.

Bender, B. G., & Rand, C. (2004). Medication non-adherence and asthma treatment cost. *Current Opinion in Allergy and Clinical Immunology, 4*(3), 191–195.

Bosley, C. M., Fosbury, J. A., & Cochrane, G. M. (1995). The psychological factors associated with poor compliance with treatment in asthma. *European Respiratory Journal, 8*(6), 899–904.

Bova, C. A., Fennie, K. P., Knafl, G. J., Dieckhaus, K. D., Watrous, E., & Williams, A. B. (2005). Use of electronic monitoring devices to measure antiretroviral adherence: practical considerations. *AIDS and Behavior, 9*(1), 103–110.

Briesacher, B. A., Gurwitz, J. H., & Soumerai, S. B. (2007). Patients at-risk for cost-related medication nonadherence: a review of the literature. *Journal of General Internal Medicine, 22*(6), 864–871.

Buscher, A., Hartman, C., Kallen, M. A., & Giordano, T. P. (2011). Validity of self-report measures in assessing antiretroviral adherence of newly diagnosed, HAART-naive, HIV patients. *HIV Clinical Trials, 12*(5), 244–254.

Centers for Disease Control and Prevention. (2008). *Behavioral Risk Factor Surveillance System Survey Questionnaire*. Atlanta, Georgia: U.S. Department of Health and Human Services.

Chesney, M. A., Ickovics, J. R., Chambers, D. B., Gifford, A. L., Neidig, J., Zwickl, B., et al. (2000). Self-reported adherence to antiretroviral medications among participants in HIV clinical trials: the AACTG adherence instruments. Patient Care Committee & Adherence Working Group of the Outcomes Committee of the Adult AIDS Clinical Trials Group (AACTG). *AIDS Care, 12*(3), 255–266.

Choo, P. W., Rand, C. S., Inui, T. S., Lee, M. L., Cain, E., Cordeiro-Breault, M., et al. (1999). Validation of patient reports, automated pharmacy records, and pill counts with electronic monitoring of adherence to antihypertensive therapy. *Medical Care, 37*(9), 846–857.

Choudhry, N. K., Fischer, M. A., Avorn, J., Liberman, J. N., Schneeweiss, S., Pakes, J., et al. (2011). The implications of therapeutic complexity on adherence to cardiovascular medications. *Archives of Internal Medicine, 171*(9), 814–822.

Cluley, S., & Cochrane, G. M. (2001). Psychological disorder in asthma is associated with poor control and poor adherence to inhaled steroids. *Respiratory Medicine, 95*(1), 37–39.

Cook, C. L., Wade, W. E., Martin, B. C., & Perri, M., 3rd. (2005). Concordance among three self-reported measures of medication adherence and pharmacy refill records. *Journal of American Pharmacists Association (2003), 45*(2), 151–159.

D'Zurilla, T. J. (1986). *Problem solving therapy: A social competence approach to clinical interventions*. New York: Springer.

Dahlen, I., & Janson, C. (2002). Anxiety and depression are related to the outcome of emergency treatment in patients with obstructive pulmonary disease. *Chest, 122*(5), 1633–1637.

Daniels, T., Goodacre, L., Sutton, C., Pollard, K., Conway, S., & Peckham, D. (2011). Accurate assessment of adherence: self-report and clinician report vs electronic monitoring of nebulizers. *Chest*, *140*(2), 425–432.

DiMatteo, M. R. (2004). Variations in patients' adherence to medical recommendations: a quantitative review of 50 years of research. *Medical Care*, *42*(3), 200–209.

DiMatteo, M. R., Giordani, P. J., Lepper, H. S., & Croghan, T. W. (2002). Patient adherence and medical treatment outcomes: a meta-analysis. *Medical Care*, *40*(9), 794–811.

Dragomir, A., Cote, R., Roy, L., Blais, L., Lalonde, L., Berard, A., et al. (2010). Impact of adherence to antihypertensive agents on clinical outcomes and hospitalization costs. *Medical Care*, *48*(5), 418–425.

Ernst, F. R., & Grizzle, A. J. (2001). Drug-related morbidity and mortality: updating the cost-of-illness model. *Journal of American Pharmacists Association (Washington)*, *41*(2), 192–199.

Farmer, K. C. (1999). Methods for measuring and monitoring medication regimen adherence in clinical trials and clinical practice. *Clinical Therapeutics*, *21*(6), 1074–1090; discussion 1073.

Giordano, T. P., Guzman, D., Clark, R., Charlebois, E. D., & Bangsberg, D. R. (2004). Measuring adherence to antiretroviral therapy in a diverse population using a visual analogue scale. *HIV Clinical Trials*, *5*(2), 74–79.

Golbeck, A. L., Ahlers-Schmidt, C. R., Paschal, A. M., & Dismuke, S. E. (2005). A definition and operational framework for health numeracy. *American Journal of Preventive Medicine*, *29*(4), 375–376.

Goldman, D. P., Joyce, G. F., & Zheng, Y. (2007). Prescription drug cost sharing: associations with medication and medical utilization and spending and health. *Journal of the American Medical Association*, *298*(1), 61–69.

Gonzalez, J., McCarll, L., Cagliero, E., Delahanty, L., Soper, T., Goldman, V., et al. (2010). Cognitive-behavioral therapy for adherence and depression (CBT-AD) in type 2 diabetes. *Journal of Cognitive Psychotherapy: An International Quarterly*, *24*, 329–343.

Gonzalez, J. S., Batchelder, A. W., Psaros, C., & Safren, S. A. (2011). Depression and HIV/AIDS treatment nonadherence: a review and meta-analysis. *Journal of Acquired Immune Deficiency Syndrome*, *58*(2), 181–187.

Gonzalez, J. S., Peyrot, M., McCarl, L. A., Collins, E. M., Serpa, L., Mimiaga, M. J., et al. (2008). Depression and diabetes treatment nonadherence: a meta-analysis. *Diabetes Care*, *31*(12), 2398–2403.

Gonzalez, J. S., Safren, S. A., Cagliero, E., Wexler, D. J., Delahanty, L., Wittenberg, E., et al. (2007). Depression, self-care, and medication adherence in type 2 diabetes: relationships across the full range of symptom severity. *Diabetes Care*, *30*(9), 2222–2227.

Gonzalez, J. S., & Schneider, H. E. (2011). Methodological issues in the assessment of diabetes treatment adherence. *Current Diabetes Report*, *11*(6), 472–479.

Goodwin, R. D., Jacobi, F., & Thefeld, W. (2003). Mental disorders and asthma in the community. *Archives of General Psychiatry*, *60*(11), 1125–1130.

Goodwin, R. D., Olfson, M., Shea, S., Lantigua, R. A., Carrasquilo, O., Gameroff, M. J., et al. (2003). Asthma and mental disorders in primary care. *General Hospital Psychiatry*, *25*(6), 479–483.

Grenard, J. L., Munjas, B. A., Adams, J. L., Suttorp, M., Maglione, M., McGlynn, E. A., et al. (2011). Depression and medication adherence in the treatment of chronic diseases in the United States: a meta-analysis. *Journal of General Internal Medicine*, *26*(10), 1175–1182.

Hansen, R. A., Kim, M. M., Song, L., Tu, W., Wu, J., & Murray, M. D. (2009). Comparison of methods to assess medication adherence and classify nonadherence. *Annals of Pharmacotherapy*, *43*(3), 413–422.

Harrigan, P. R., Hogg, R. S., Dong, W. W., Yip, B., Wynhoven, B., Woodward, J., et al. (2005). Predictors of HIV drug-resistance mutations in a large antiretroviral-naive cohort initiating triple antiretroviral therapy. *Journal of Infectious Diseases*, *191*(3), 339–347.

Haynes, R. B., Ackloo, E., Sahota, N., McDonald, H. P., & Yao, X. (2008). Interventions for enhancing medication adherence. *Cochrane Database of Systematic Reviews*(2), CD000011.

Heaney, L. G., Conway, E., Kelly, C., & Gamble, J. (2005). Prevalence of psychiatric morbidity in a difficult asthma population: relationship to asthma outcome. *Respiratory Medicine*, *99*(9), 1152–1159.

Ho, P. M., Magid, D. J., Shetterly, S. M., Olson, K. L., Maddox, T. M., Peterson, P. N., et al. (2008). Medication nonadherence is associated with a broad range of adverse outcomes in patients with coronary artery disease. *American Heart Journal*, *155*(4), 772–779.

Ho, P. M., Magid, D. J., Shetterly, S. M., Olson, K. L., Peterson, P. N., Masoudi, F. A., et al. (2008). Importance of therapy intensification and medication nonadherence for blood pressure control in patients with coronary disease. *Archives of Internal Medicine*, *168*(3), 271–276.

Hogg, R. S., Heath, K., Bangsberg, D., Yip, B., Press, N., O'Shaughnessy, M. V., et al. (2002). Intermittent use of triple-combination therapy is predictive of mortality at baseline and after 1 year of follow-up. *AIDS*, *16*(7), 1051–1058.

Hopko, D. R., Lejuez, C. W., Ruggiero, K. J., & Eifert, G. H. (2003). Contemporary behavioral activation treatments for depression: procedures, principles, and progress. *Clinical Psychology Review*, *23*(5), 699–717.

Ingersoll, K. S., & Heckman, C. J. (2005). Patient-clinician relationships and treatment system effects on HIV medication adherence. *AIDS and Behavior*, *9*(1), 89–101.

Jackevicius, C. A., Li, P., & Tu, J. V. (2008). Prevalence, predictors, and outcomes of primary nonadherence after acute myocardial infarction. *Circulation*, *117*(8), 1028–1036.

Johnson, S. S., Driskell, M. M., Johnson, J. L., Prochaska, J. M., Zwick, W., & Prochaska, J. O. (2006). Efficacy of a transtheoretical model-based expert system for antihypertensive adherence. *Disease Management*, *9*(5), 291–301.

Kalichman, S. C., Amaral, C., Swetsze, C., Eaton, L., Kalichman, M. O., Cherry, C., et al. (2010). Monthly unannounced pill counts for monitoring HIV treatment adherence: tests for self-monitoring and reactivity effects. *HIV Clinical Trials*, *11*(6), 325–331.

Kalichman, S. C., Amaral, C. M., Cherry, C., Flanagan, J., Pope, H., Eaton, L., et al. (2008). Monitoring medication adherence by unannounced pill counts conducted by telephone: reliability and criterion-related validity. *HIV Clinical Trials*, *9*(5), 298–308.

Kalichman, S. C., Amaral, C. M., Stearns, H., White, D., Flanagan, J., Pope, H., et al. (2007). Adherence to antiretroviral therapy assessed by unannounced pill counts conducted by telephone. *Journal of General Internal Medicine*, *22*(7), 1003–1006.

Kalichman, S. C., Cain, D., Cherry, C., Kalichman, M., & Pope, H. (2005). Pillboxes and antiretroviral adherence: prevalence of use, perceived benefits, and implications for electronic medication monitoring devices. *AIDS Patient Care and STDS*, *19*(12), 833–839.

Kalichman, S. C., Pope, H., White, D., Cherry, C., Amaral, C. M., Swetzes, C., et al. (2008). Association between health literacy and HIV treatment adherence: further evidence from objectively measured medication adherence. *Journal of the International Association of Physicians in AIDS Care (Chicago)*, *7*(6), 317–323.

Lima, V. D., Geller, J., Bangsberg, D. R., Patterson, T. L., Daniel, M., Kerr, T., et al. (2007). The effect of adherence on the association between depressive symptoms and mortality among HIV-infected individuals first initiating HAART. *AIDS*, *21*(9), 1175–1183.

Liu, H., Golin, C. E., Miller, L. G., Hays, R. D., Beck, C. K., Sanandaji, S., et al. (2001). A comparison study of multiple measures of adherence to HIV protease inhibitors. *Annals of Internal Medicine*, *134*(10), 968–977.

Llabre, M. M., Weaver, K. E., Duran, R. E., Antoni, M. H., McPherson-Baker, S., & Schneiderman, N. (2006). A measurement model of medication adherence to highly active antiretroviral therapy and its relation to viral load in HIV-positive adults. *AIDS Patient Care and STDS*, *20*(10), 701–711.

Lu, M., Safren, S. A., Skolnik, P. R., Rogers, W. H., Coady, W., Hardy, H., et al. (2008). Optimal recall period and response task for self-reported HIV medication adherence. *AIDS and Behavior*, *12*(1), 86–94.

Mahtani, K. R., Heneghan, C. J., Glasziou, P. P., & Perera, R. (2011). Reminder packaging for improving adherence to self-administered long-term medications. *Cochrane Database of Systematic Reviews, 9,* CD005025.

Mancuso, C. A., Wenderoth, S., Westermann, H., Choi, T. N., Briggs, W. M., & Charlson, M. E. (2008). Patient-reported and physician-reported depressive conditions in relation to asthma severity and control. *Chest, 133*(5), 1142–1148.

Marcus, B. H., Selby, V. C., Niaura, R. S., & Rossi, J. S. (1992). Self-efficacy and the stages of exercise behavior change. *Research Quarterly for Exercise and Sport, 63*(1), 60–66.

Morisky, D. E., Green, L. W., & Levine, D. M. (1986). Concurrent and predictive validity of a self-reported measure of medication adherence. *Medical Care, 24*(1), 67–74.

Nachega, J. B., Hislop, M., Dowdy, D. W., Chaisson, R. E., Regensberg, L., & Maartens, G. (2007). Adherence to nonnucleoside reverse transcriptase inhibitor-based HIV therapy and virologic outcomes. *Annals of Internal Medicine, 146*(8), 564–573.

Nachega, J. B., Leisegang, R., Bishai, D., Nguyen, H., Hislop, M., Cleary, S., et al. (2010). Association of antiretroviral therapy adherence and health care costs. *Annals of Internal Medicine, 152*(1), 18–25.

Nathan, R. A., Sorkness, C. A., Kosinski, M., Schatz, M., Li, J. T., Marcus, P., et al. (2004). Development of the asthma control test: a survey for assessing asthma control. *Journal of Allergy and Clinical Immunology, 113*(1), 59–65.

National Council on Patient Information and Education. (2007). Enhancing prescription medicine adherence: A national action plan. Retrieved from http://www.talkaboutrx.org/documents/enhancing_prescription_medicine_adherence.pdf

NCQA. (2011). *Standards and Guidelines for NCQA's Patient-Centered Medical Home (PCMH) 2011.* Washington, DC: NCQA.

Nezu, A. M., & Perri, M. G. (1989). Social problem-solving therapy for unipolar depression: an initial dismantling investigation. *Journal of Consulting and Clinical Psychology, 57*(3), 408–413.

Nieuwkerk, P. T., & Oort, F. J. (2005). Self-reported adherence to antiretroviral therapy for HIV-1 infection and virologic treatment response: a meta-analysis. *Journal of Acquired Immune Deficiency Syndrome, 38*(4), 445–448.

Osborn, C. Y., Cavanaugh, K., Wallston, K. A., Kripalani, S., Elasy, T. A., Rothman, R. L., et al. (2011). Health literacy explains racial disparities in diabetes medication adherence. *Journal of Health Communication, 16*(Suppl 3), 268–278.

Osterberg, L., & Blaschke, T. (2005). Adherence to medication. *New England Journal of Medicine, 353*(5), 487–497.

Piette, J. D., Heisler, M., Krein, S., & Kerr, E. A. (2005). The role of patient-physician trust in moderating medication nonadherence due to cost pressures. *Archives of Internal Medicine, 165*(15), 1749–1755.

Pittman, D. G., Chen, W., Bowlin, S. J., & Foody, J. M. (2011). Adherence to statins, subsequent healthcare costs, and cardiovascular hospitalizations. *American Journal of Cardiology, 107*(11), 1662–1666.

Prochaska, J. M., Prochaska, J. O., Cohen, F. C., Gomes, S. O., Laforge, R. G., & Eastwood, A. L. (2004). The transtheoretical model of change for mutli-level interventions for alcohol abuse on campus. *Journal of Alcohol and Drug Education, 47*(3), 34–50.

Prochaska, J. O. (1979). *Systems of psychotherapy: a transtheoretical analysis.* Homewood, IL: Dorsey Press.

Prochaska, J. O., & DiClemente, C. C. (1983). Stages and processes of self-change of smoking: toward an integrative model of change. *Journal of Consulting and Clinical Psychology, 51*(3), 390–395.

Prochaska, J. O., Velicer, W. F., Prochaska, J. M., & Johnson, J. L. (2004). Size, consistency, and stability of stage effects for smoking cessation. *Addictive Behaviors, 29*(1), 207–213.

Rosenthal, M. B. (2008). Beyond pay for performance—emerging models of provider-payment reform. *New England Journal of Medicine, 359*(12), 1197–1200.

Sabaté, E., & World Health Organization. (2003). *Adherence to long-term therapies: evidence for action.* Geneva: World Health Organization.

Safren, S. A., Gonzalez, J. S., & Soroudi, N. (2007a). *Coping with chronic illness: A cognitive-behavioral therapy approach for adherence and depression: Therapist guide.* New York: Oxford University Press.

Safren, S. A., Gonzalez, J. S., & Soroudi, N. (2007b). *Coping with chronic illness: A cognitive-behavioral therapy approach for adherence and depression: Workbook.* New York: Oxford University Press.

Safren, S. A., O'Cleirigh, C., Tan, J. Y., Raminani, S. R., Reilly, L. C., Otto, M. W., et al. (2009). A randomized controlled trial of cognitive behavioral therapy for adherence and depression (CBT-AD) in HIV-infected individuals. *Health Psychology, 28*(1), 1–10.

Safren, S. A., Otto, M. W., & Worth, J. L. (1999). Life-Steps: Applying cognitve behavioral therapy to patient adherence in HIV medication treatment. *Cognitive and Behavioral Practice, 6*, 332–341.

Safren, S. A., Otto, M. W., Worth, J. L., Salomon, E., Johnson, W., Mayer, K., et al. (2001). Two strategies to increase adherence to HIV antiretroviral medication: life-steps and medication monitoring. *Behavior Research and Therapy, 39*(10), 1151–1162.

Sarkin, J. A., Johnson, S. S., Prochaska, J. O., & Prochaska, J. M. (2001). Applying the transtheoretical model to regular moderate exercise in an overweight population: validation of a stages of change measure. *Preventive Medicine, 33*(5), 462–469.

Schedlbauer, A., Davies, P., & Fahey, T. (2010). Interventions to improve adherence to lipid lowering medication. *Cochrane Database of Systematic Reviews*(3), CD004371.

Schneider, H., Gonzalez, J., & Psaros, C. (2011). *Validating self-report adherence in type 2 diabetis [abstract B-044].* Paper presented at the Society of Behavioral Medicine Conference.

Schoenthaler, A., Chaplin, W. F., Allegrante, J. P., Fernandez, S., Diaz-Gloster, M., Tobin, J. N., et al. (2009). Provider communication effects medication adherence in hypertensive African Americans. *Patient Education and Counseling, 75*(2), 185–191.

Shi, L., Liu, J., Fonseca, V., Walker, P., Kalsekar, A., & Pawaskar, M. (2010). Correlation between adherence rates measured by MEMS and self-reported questionnaires: a meta-analysis. *Health Qual Life Outcomes, 8*, 99.

Shi, L., Liu, J., Koleva, Y., Fonseca, V., Kalsekar, A., & Pawaskar, M. (2010). Concordance of adherence measurement using self-reported adherence questionnaires and medication monitoring devices. *Pharmacoeconomics, 28*(12), 1097–1107.

Smith, A., Krishnan, J. A., Bilderback, A., Riekert, K. A., Rand, C. S., & Bartlett, S. J. (2006). Depressive symptoms and adherence to asthma therapy after hospital discharge. *Chest, 130*(4), 1034–1038.

Sokol, M. C., McGuigan, K. A., Verbrugge, R. R., & Epstein, R. S. (2005). Impact of medication adherence on hospitalization risk and healthcare cost. *Medical Care, 43*(6), 521–530.

Strine, T. W., Mokdad, A. H., Balluz, L. S., Berry, J. T., & Gonzalez, O. (2008). Impact of depression and anxiety on quality of life, health behaviors, and asthma control among adults in the United States with asthma, 2006. *J Asthma, 45*(2), 123–133.

Svarstad, B. L., Chewning, B. A., Sleath, B. L., & Claesson, C. (1999). The Brief Medication Questionnaire: a tool for screening patient adherence and barriers to adherence. *Patient Education and Counseling, 37*(2), 113–124.

Trindade, A. J., Ehrlich, A., Kornbluth, A., & Ullman, T. A. (2011). Are your patients taking their medicine? Validation of a new adherence scale in patients with inflammatory bowel disease and comparison with physician perception of adherence. *Inflammatory Bowel Diseases, 17*(2), 599–604.

Wagner, G., & Miller, L. G. (2004). Is the influence of social desirability on patients' self-reported adherence overrated? *Journal of Acquired Immune Deficiency Syndrome, 35*(2), 203–204.

Walshe, L., Saple, D. G., Mehta, S. H., Shah, B., Bollinger, R. C., & Gupta, A. (2010). Physician estimate of antiretroviral adherence in India: poor correlation with patient self-report and viral load. *AIDS Patient Care and STDS, 24*(3), 189–195.

Wu, E. Q., Johnson, S., Beaulieu, N., Arana, M., Bollu, V., Guo, A., et al. (2010). Healthcare resource utilization and costs associated with non-adherence to imatinib treatment in chronic myeloid leukemia patients. *Current Medical Research and Opinion*, *26*(1), 61–69.

Wu, J., Seiber, E., Lacombe, V. A., Nahata, M. C., & Balkrishnan, R. (2011). Medical utilization and costs associated with statin adherence in Medicaid enrollees with type 2 diabetes. *Annals of Pharmacotherapy*, *45*(3), 342–349.

Wu, J. R., Lennie, T. A., De Jong, M. J., Frazier, S. K., Heo, S., Chung, M. L., et al. (2010). Medication adherence is a mediator of the relationship between ethnicity and event-free survival in patients with heart failure. *J Card Fail*, *16*(2), 142–149.

Zigmond, A. S., & Snaith, R. P. (1983). The hospital anxiety and depression scale. *Acta Psychiatrica Scandinavica*, *67*(6), 361–370.

Zolnierek, K. B., & Dimatteo, M. R. (2009). Physician communication and patient adherence to treatment: a meta-analysis. *Medical Care*, *47*(8), 826–834.

16.

HYPNOSIS IN PSYCHOSOMATIC MEDICINE

José R. Maldonado

INTRODUCTION

Hypnosis is a psychophysiological state of attentive, receptive concentration, with a relative suspension of peripheral awareness. Hypnotic phenomena occur spontaneously, and the alteration of consciousness that hypnotized individuals experience has a variety of therapeutic applications.

Hypnosis is a natural state of attentive, focused concentration. As such, most individuals are able to experience variable trance-like states at different times in their daily lives. The hypnotic capacity or hypnotizability of a given subject (i.e., the degree of natural ability to enter a trance state) will determine the degree of assistance required to enter trance states. Highly hypnotizable individuals enter trance states with ease, on many occasions even without being fully aware of it. Individuals with moderate hypnotizability require more direction or help from a therapist who facilitates the trance experience, while those with low hypnotizability may not be able to benefit much from hypnosis as a treatment tool.

The ability to enter a trance state is widely and naturally distributed throughout the general population. Therefore, some patients may experience trance states or inadvertently take suggestions without planning. This may have potential positive or negative consequences depending on the patient and the circumstances of the interaction. For example, moderately to highly hypnotizable individuals may use hypnotic techniques to enhance pain management, stop the use of nicotine, diminish chemotherapy side effects, assist in managing the psychological and physical discomfort of intraoperative and postoperative procedures and childbirth, and assist in the management of various psychosomatic conditions (e.g., asthma, irritable bowel syndrome, warts). Similarly, high hypnotic capacity may actually become a liability to patients who are unaware of their hypnotic capacity or of their unconscious use of this mechanism, as in the case of individuals suffering from a dissociative and somatoform disorder or nocebo (i.e., negative placebo) effect.

BACKGROUND

The oldest written record of cures by hypnosis was obtained from the Ebers Papyrus, which gives us an idea about some of the theory and practice of Egyptian medicine before 1552 BC

(Joachim, 1890; Ebbell, 1937). In the Ebers Papyrus, a treatment was described in which the physician placed his hands on the head of the patient and, claiming superhuman therapeutic powers, gave forth with strange remedial utterances that were suggested to the patients and that resulted in cures.

The Egyptians are thought to have originated the "Sleep Temples," in which the priests gave similar treatment to their patients through the use of suggestion. These temples became very popular in Egypt and spread throughout Greece and Asia Minor (Okasha, 1993). Trance experiences were described by ancient Greeks, often as vehicles for treatment of mental or physical illness. Hippocrates is known to have discussed the phenomenon, saying, "the affliction suffered by the body, the soul sees quite well with the eyes shut" (Chadwick, 1950).

Hypnosis was identified as a formal phenomenon of psychotherapeutic usefulness in the 18th century. Franz Anton Mesmer (1734–1815) employed it as an alternative treatment for many ills that now would be labeled as stress-related or psychosomatic (Lopez, 1993). His work is credited with being the first Western conceptualization of a psychotherapy, a therapeutic talking interaction between doctor and patient (Ellenberger, 1970). Yet, the results of a Royal Commission in France concluded that the effects of hypnosis were the result of the "pure gold of imagination."

Jean-Martin Charcot (1825–1893), chief of neurology at the Salpêtrière Hospital in Paris, rehabilitated hypnosis as a subject for scientific study (Charcot, 1890). One of his disciples, Pierre Janet (1859–1947), a general practitioner and psychologist, laid the early foundation for dissociative reactions and ego states (Janet, 1887, 1889, 1904, 1907). In fact, the First International Congress for Experimental and Therapeutic Hypnotism was held in Paris, France, August 8–12, 1889.

More recently, interest in hypnosis seemed to wax and wane depending on the needs of the times. The extreme symptoms observed in patients with dissociative syndromes prompted the writings of William James (1902), Boris Sidis (Sidis & Goodhart, 1905), and Morton Prince (1906), who went on to found the *Journal of Abnormal Psychology*. The early use of hypnosis in the treatment of physical illness was championed by James Braid (1843) and James Esdaile (Esdaile, 1957; Ernst, 1995), including hypnoanalgesia.

Interest in hypnosis revived during World War II, when army psychiatrists found the technique helpful in treating what was then called "traumatic neurosis" (Kardiner & Spiegel, 1947). This was followed by an era of serious scientific exploration and the development of various hypnotizability scales (e.g., Stanford Hypnotic Susceptibility Scales (Hilgard, 1965; Weitzenhoffer & Hilgard, 1959; Weitzenhoffer, 1962) in an attempt to measure the presence and depth of the hypnotic experience. Later on, shorter hypnotizability scales were developed for use in clinical settings. Investigations included studies of the relationships among hypnotizability, placebo response, and acupuncture, studies of the differential hypnotizability of patients with psychosis and other psychiatric disorders, and investigations used in determining neurophysiological correlates of the hypnotic state and hypnotic capacity.

It was not until the second part of the 20th century, though, that the various professional associations in Europe and North America officially recognized hypnosis as a valuable therapeutic intervention (i.e., British Medical Association, 1955; American Medical Association, 1958; American Psychological Association, 1960; American Psychiatric Association, 1960). Since then, two professional hypnosis societies have emerged in North America: the Society for Clinical and Experimental Hypnosis (SECH, 1949), which emphasizes research in the field, and the American Society for Clinical Hypnosis (ASCH, 1957). A division of the American Psychological Association (Division 30, 1968; also known as the Society of Psychological Hypnosis) is devoted to the study of hypnosis in the field of psychology. In 1959 the International Society for Clinical and Experimental Hypnosis was founded. A more detailed account of the history of hypnosis is beyond the scope of this chapter and may be found elsewhere (Maldonado & Spiegel, 2008)

COMPONENTS OF THE HYPNOTIC PROCESS

The hypnotic experience may be understood as involving three interconnecting factors: absorption, dissociation, and suggestibility.

ABSORPTION

Absorption refers to the tendency to engage in self-altering and highly focused attention with complete immersion in a central experience at the expense of contextual orientation (Hilgard, 1970; Tellegen & Atkinson, 1974; Tellegen, 1981). Hypnotized individuals can become so intensely absorbed in their trance experience that they often choose to ignore the environmental context and other peripheral events. It facilitates complete immersion in a central experience at the expense of contextual orientation and peripheral awareness. As a person becomes absorbed in a central focus of attention, more peripheral perceptions, thoughts, and memories become less important. During the hypnotic process, individuals can become so intensely absorbed in their trance experience that they tend to, or are better able to, ignore many somatic (e.g., pain) and/or environmental stimuli (e.g., medical procedures).

DISSOCIATION

Dissociation refers to the ability to separate mental processes so they seem to occur independently from each other. The process of dissociation is complementary to absorption. During hypnosis, the intense absorption characteristic of the hypnotic state permits keeping out of conscious awareness many routine experiences that would ordinarily be conscious, by the process of nonpathological dissociation. When working properly in our daily lives, dissociation allows us to carry out several complex tasks simultaneously. There are a wide variety of dissociated states that range from the normal ability to carry out simultaneous tasks to a number of psychiatric disorders. An example of a rather common form of dissociation is the ability to perform a high-complexity task (i.e., a surgical procedure) while carrying out a conversation regarding one's political views or a recent sport event. In fact, not only motor activities can be dissociated but also rather complex emotional states and sensory experiences as well.

Dissociated affect and memories can elicit complex motor or pseudoneurologic dysfunction, as in the case of conversion disorder (Maldonado & Spiegel, 2000; Maldonado, 2007). Complex forms of dissociation can prevent access to memory, resulting in dissociative amnesia, dissociative fugue, or dissociative identity disorder (Maldonado, Butler, & Spiegel, 2000).

Another, more common, example of how dissociated memories affect patients is the hyperemesis experienced by some chemotherapy patients who experience nausea and vomiting just with the sight, or sometimes the thought, of the hospital (conditioned nausea and emesis). Memories that are dissociated at the time of the traumatic experience may reemerge when they are triggered by external cues, as in flashbacks associated with posttraumatic stress disorder that are often seen in cases of traumatic experiences such as motor vehicle accidents or traumatic surgical procedures or interventions.

SUGGESTIBILITY

Suggestibility implies the ability to influence someone's beliefs or behaviors by suggestion. Owing to the intense absorption experienced during trance, hypnotized individuals have a heightened responsiveness to social cues, including suggestions (formal or not) given by the therapist. This enhanced suggestibility allows hypnotized subjects to accept instructions more easily. Hypnotized individuals are not deprived of their will, but they do have a tendency to accept instructions in an uncritical way when under trance, a process that may be aided by the phenomenon of "source amnesia." Thus a hypnotized individual receives a suggestion, internalizes it, forgets the source of origin, then believes s/he generated the idea to which s/he now responds, thus lowering critical thinking about its validity.

This does not mean that the subject is deprived of will. Nevertheless, highly suggestible individuals do have a tendency to suspend the usual conscious curiosity that makes us question the reason for our actions and to respond to suggested ideas in a less critical fashion. Because of this, highly hypnotizable individuals are more prone to accept some suggestions or ideas no matter how irrational or illogical they might appear to be. A conscientious physician may use this aspect of the hypnotic experience to bypass the patient's defenses and facilitate change or symptom relief. On the other hand, because of their decreased awareness, highly hypnotizable individuals are less likely to identify a physician's mistakes, and may be misguided and confused by comments or instructions (whether given under hypnosis or not) that are negative, vague, or misguided.

ASSESSMENT OF HYPNOTIZABILITY OR HYPNOTIC CAPACITY

There are definitive advantages associated with knowing a patient's level of hypnotic capacity. As previously mentioned, patients' hypnotizability levels vary considerably. The use of formal hypnotizability assessments allows physicians to objectively determine their patient's level of hypnotic capacity. Thus, while moderate and highly hypnotizable patients may be offered hypnosis as a treatment option, those with low capacity may be referred to more appropriate techniques (e.g., progressive relaxation, biofeedback). Data suggests that hypnotizability is a rather stable trait. The only long-term study published to date demonstrated that the initial hypnotizability assessment (i.e., SHSS) correlated highly with scores at a 10-year, 15-year, and 25-year retest, with obtained correlations of .64, .82, and .71, respectively (Piccione, Hilgard, et al.,1989) As stated by the study authors: "the flux in subjects' lives over a quarter of a century, through marriage and child-rearing, occupational shifts, traumas associated with illness, death of loved ones, and loss by divorce, cannot be assumed to be trivial"(Piccione , et al.,1989).

These findings compared favorably with other studies of similar sample size and duration, of measures of individual differences over time. These include the stability over time of IQ scores (i.e., test–retest correlations were 0.73 for the full scale IQ, 0.70 for Verbal IQ, and 0.57 for Performance IQ [Kangas & Bradway, 1971]), personality assessment (i.e., a retest correlation of 0.50 [Huntley & Davis, 1983]), and occupational interests (i.e., a 20-year test–retest correlation of 0.72 for men 22–25 years old at first testing and 0.64 for those 19–21 years old at first testing [Campbell & Hansen, 1981]). Standardized hypnotizability assessments can provide therapists with clinical data that allows for rational predictions about patients' expected responses. For instance, the relative ability, or lack thereof, to restructure one's inner experience aided by the use of hypnosis may provide information about a subject's interpersonal style.

From a therapeutic perspective, these data may help provide clues about likely response to intervention (i.e., hypnotic suggestibility predicted differences in responding to the hypnotic and imaginative analgesia suggestions, with higher hypnotizability associated with greater response to hypnoanalgesia suggestions). Hypnotizability levels may even facilitate the differential diagnosis. For example, we would expect patients suffering from dissociative disorders, PTSD, and conversion disorder to score high on hypnotizability measures while those experiencing psychosis and OCD would be expected to score low; discrepancies from these predictions may make a practitioner rethink the diagnosis.

Brief scales have been designed for quick assessment in the clinical setting— for example, the Hypnotic Induction Profile (HIP [Spiegel & Spiegel, 1987, 2004), the Stanford Hypnotic Clinical Scale (SHCS [Hilgard & Hilgard, 1975]). They are brief—about 5 to 10 minutes are required for the HIP, and 20 minutes for the SHCS—and extremely accurate. An even briefer test is the use of the Eye Roll Sign (ERS) and its relation to innate trance capacity (Spiegel, 1972; Frischholz & Nichols, 2010) This is part of the more formal HIP assessment scale.

There are even group hypnotizability measures, which can be administered to larger groups of individuals at the same time and rated at the end of the experience to allow for assessments of larger groups. These scales are usually used in the screening of large groups for study rather than clinical purposes (Shor & Orne, 1962). All scales involve a structured hypnotic induction, followed by an assessment of the subject's response to a variety of suggestions.

The HIP is a brief (5–7 minutes) standardized assessment designed to measure the patients' natural ability to tap into and use their hypnotic capacity (Spiegel & Spiegel, 1987). It consists of a rapid hypnotic induction instruction for an upward gaze, quickly followed by lowering of the eyelids, and suggestions for physical relaxation and a floating sensation. The induction process is followed by a structured set of instructions. The individual's response to them, during and shortly after the test (posthypnotic suggestion), predicts hypnotic capacity and future response to treatment with hypnosis.

Subjects are rated on five important items that assess cognitive and behavioral aspects of the hypnotic experience: (1) hand dissociation; (2) hand levitation, after formal end of trance state; (3) unconscious compliance with posthypnotic suggestion; (4) response to the cutoff signal; and (5) sensory alteration (see Appendix A for a copy of the HIP and instructions for administration). At least one study suggests that the HIP compares favorably with longer (about 20–25 minutes) assessments such as the Stanford Hypnotic Clinical Scale for Adults (SHCS:A), with a 0.41 correlation (p<.01) (Gritzalis, Oster, et al., 2009).

NEUROBIOLOGY OF HYPNOSIS

There has always been some mystery regarding how hypnosis works. In ancient times it was blamed on spirits or gods. In medieval times it was believed to be caused by demonic possession. Mesmer believed it was elicited by manipulation of the body's energies or "magnetic fluid." The biggest dichotomy occurred early on between those like Charcot (1825–1893), who believed hypnosis to be the result of a diseased nervous system and argued that normal people could not be hypnotized (Charcot, 1890), and those like Bernheim (1840–1919) at the School of Nancy, who believed hypnosis to be a trait mediated by suggestion and exhibited to different degrees by normal individuals (Berheim, 1889/1964; Widlocher & Dantchev, 1994).

Since those early days, various research efforts have attempted to correlate the hypnotic experience with actual physiological changes, which has prompted many theories. Rudolf Heidenhain (1880) explained it by the physiological mechanism of cortical inhibition (Windholz, 1996). Pavlov (1910) believed it was mediated via partial cortical inhibition (Windholz, 1996). Yet, to date, the "seat of hypnosis" has not been found in the brain, although recent research points toward involvement of the frontal and anterior cingulate cortex (Kropotov, Crawford, et al., 1997; Rainville, Hofbauer, et al., 2002; Spiegel, 2003). There is ample clinical and research experience indicating that the hypnotic process affects both electrical and metabolic processes in the brain. Similarly, as we have observed in clinical experience, hypnotic activity is capable of causing various physiological changes.

Hypnotizability has been found to be significantly correlated with cerebrospinal fluid levels of homovanillic acid, a metabolite of dopamine (Spiegel & King, 1992). This finding provides additional evidence suggesting the involvement of the frontal cortex in the hypnotic process. Further dispelling the myth of a link between hypnosis and sleep, studies have shown that the administration of psychostimulants (e.g., amphetamine) may enhance hypnotizability (Sjoberg & Hollister, 1965), while GABAergic agents and opioids may cause sedation, decrease absorption and attention, and thus interfere with the hypnotic process. Some have postulated that the automaticity observed in hypnotic motor behavior could represent an activation of the basal ganglia, which is involved in both implicit memory and routine motor activity (Graf & Schacter, 1985; Schacter, 1987, 1992; Mishkin & Murray, 1994).

Similarly, the brain electrical pattern of a hypnotized subject actually resembles that of a fully awake and attentive individual more than the pattern of a person who is asleep. In fact, power spectral analysis of brain electrical activity has found increased alpha activity among highly hypnotizable individuals, and an alpha laterality difference favoring the left hemisphere among highly hypnotizable individuals (Morgan, Macdonald, et al., 1974; Edmonston & Grotevant, 1975). Finally, some have demonstrated that highly susceptible subjects show more electric power in the right parietotemporal region than the left, while those with low susceptibility have left-side predominance or equilibrated power in all derivations (Meszaros & Szabo, 1999). Yet, not all studies support the right hemispheric dominance theory of the hypnotic process, suggesting that data analysis techniques led to misinterpretations of previously obtained data (Edmonston & Moscovitz, 1990).

Meanwhile, others have suggested that hemispheric activation on hypnotic challenge may depend in large part on the kind of task the challenge involves, and several general aspects of the hypnotic process may more appropriately be understood to be mediated by the left hemisphere, including concentrated attentional focus and the role of language in the establishment of hypnotic experience (Jasiukaitis, Nouriani, et al., 1997).

There may also be frontal versus posterior topographical differences among highly and poorly hypnotizable individuals.

In fact, more recent studies of power spectral analysis suggest that theta power, especially in the frontal region, best differentiates highly hypnotizable from poorly hypnotizable individuals. These studies found greater theta power in the more frontal areas of the cortex for highly hypnotizable subjects. During the actual hypnotic induction, theta power increased markedly for both groups in the more posterior areas of the cortex, whereas alpha activity increased across all sites. In the period just preceding and following the hypnotic induction, poorly hypnotizable subjects displayed an increase in theta activity, whereas highly hypnotizable subjects displayed a decrease. Finally, power spectral analysis studies found that theta power, especially in the frontal region, best differentiates highly hypnotizable from poorly hypnotizable individuals, suggesting that anterior/posterior cortical differences may be more important than hemispheric laterality for understanding the hypnotic processes (Sabourin, Cutcomb, et al., 1990; Graffin, Ray, et al., 1995).

Event-related potentials (ERPs) have been used to study the effects of hypnotic hallucination on brain electrical activity. These studies are based on the premise that hypnotically induced changes in perception should be reflected in alterations in ERP amplitude. Several studies have found that highly hypnotizable subjects who experience a visual hallucination obstructing visual contact with the target exhibited significant reductions in P_{300} amplitude throughout the scalp and in N_{200} in the occipital region (Spiegel, Cutcomb, et al., 1985; Jasiukaitis, Nouriani, et al., 1996)

Hypnotic auditory hallucination studies (using auditory evoked potentials, or AEPs) have yielded similar results, suggesting P_{300} differences among highly hypnotizable individuals hallucinating a reduction or increase in tones, while subjects with low hypnotizability did not show such a change (Sigalowitz, Dywan, et al., 1991). Others have confirmed these findings, backing the hypothesis that hypnotic susceptibility is associated with efficient attentional processing, such that highly hypnotizable subjects can more effectively partition attention toward relevant stimuli and away from irrelevant stimuli than can poorly hypnotizable subjects (Crawford, Corby, et al., 1996; Lamas & Valle-Inclan, 1998)

Postulating that somatic conversion disorders may represent a form of selective attention, we studied a group of patients presenting with lateralized (i.e., unilateral) motor deficits (i.e., motor conversion) using somatosensory event-related potentials (SERPs) (Maldonado, 1997, 2001) We found that subjects exhibited a "normal N_{140}" on the unaffected side (as expected in all "normal controls"), but an *enhanced* N_{140} on the affected side (Maldonado, 2007) Even more remarkably, when we provided hypnotic suggestions for time regression (e.g., some time prior to the onset of symptoms), subjects experienced complete normalization of the SERP's response. These findings suggest the possibility of an unconscious autohypnotic model used by patients suffering from conversion disorder in order to create their symptoms.

Similarly, others have examined the effects of positive obstructive and negative obliterating instructions on simultaneous visual and auditory ERPs—P_{300} signals. They found that highly hypnotizable subjects showed greater ERP amplitudes while experiencing negative hallucinations and lower ERP amplitudes while experiencing positive obstructive hallucinations, suggesting a rather robust physiological marker of hypnosis—an alteration in consciousness that corresponds to participants' subjective experiences of perceptual alteration (Barabasz, Barabasz, et al.,1999)

Hypnoanalgesia may be similarly explained physiologically by a mechanism by which hypnotic suggestions facilitate the filtering of somatosensory (electrical) stimulation affecting ERP amplitude. Thus, suggestions of a tingling, cool, numbing sensation can be given with the idea that it would filter out any other sensations in the area by a process such as competitive inhibition. In fact, studies of moderately to highly hypnotizable adults with chronic low back pain have found that hypnotic analgesia led to significant mean reductions in perceived sensory pain and distress, suggesting that this was an active process that required inhibitory effort, dissociated from conscious awareness, where the anterior frontal cortex participates in a topographically specific inhibitory feedback circuit that cooperates in the allocation of thalamocortical activities (Crawford, Knebel, et al.,1998)

Finally, brain imaging studies (i.e., positron emission tomography [PET] scan studies) have demonstrated a global increase in cerebral perfusion during hypnosis (Ulrich, Meyer, et al., 1987). Further PET studies have suggested that during hypnosis there is specific activation of the anterior attentional systems involving focusing (anterior cingulate) and arousal (frontal, especially on the right) (Posner and Petersen, 1990). Similarly, PET scans were used to measure regional cerebral blood flow (rCBF) of highly hypnotizable subjects asked to produce vivid auditory hallucinations (Szechtman, Woody, et al.,1998). Studies found that subjects capable of producing the hallucinations had increased rCBF in the right anterior cingulate gyrus. Of interest, the "externality" and "clarity" of the hallucinations were highly correlated with blood flow in this region.

Subsequent PET studies found that among highly hypnotizable individuals, the hypnotic state was accompanied by significant increases in both occipital rCBF and delta EEG activity, which were highly correlated with each other ($r = 0.70$, $P < 0.0001$) (Rainville, Hofbauer, et al.,1999; Rainville, Hofbauer, et al., 2002). Peak increases in rCBF were also observed in the caudal part of the right anterior cingulate sulcus and bilaterally in the inferior frontal gyri. Hypnosis-related decreases in rCBF were found in the right inferior parietal lobule, the left precuneus, and the posterior cingulate gyrus. Hypnosis with suggestions produced additional widespread increases in rCBF in the frontal cortices, predominantly on the left side. Moreover, the medial and lateral posterior parietal cortices showed suggestion-related increases overlapping partly with regions of hypnosis-related decreases. Results support a state theory of hypnosis in which occipital increases in rCBF and delta activity reflect the alteration of consciousness associated with decreased arousal and possible facilitation of visual imagery. Frontal increases in rCBF that are associated with suggestions for altered perception might reflect the verbal mediation of the suggestions, working memory, and top-down processes involved in the reinterpretation of the perceptual experience.

PET scans studies using $^{15}O\text{-}CO_2$ in highly hypnotizable subjects who were asked to "see changes in color patterns" in a number of visual stimuli found both the left and right hemisphere color areas were activated when they were asked to perceive color, whether they were actually shown the color or the gray-scale stimulus; moreover, these brain regions had decreased activation when subjects were told to see the gray scale, whether they were actually shown the color or gray scale stimulus (Kosslyn, Thompson, et al., 2000) Thus, the observed changes in subjective experience achieved while in a hypnotic state are reflected by changes in brain function similar to those that occur in perception. These findings suggest that hypnotic alteration of perception is more than mere compliance with suggestion; rather, it involves alteration in sensory experience.

APPLICATION OF HYPNOSIS IN PSYCHOSOMATIC MEDICINE

The literature on the usefulness of hypnosis in the treatment of medical conditions is limited. Most papers are based on single case reports or small size samples, thus limiting the interpretation of the findings. Nevertheless, numerous studies are underway, and the number of rigorous scientific studies and publication is growing. We suggest that practitioners interested in the use of hypnosis for the treatment of medical conditions continue to monitor the literature for newer and more rigorous studies on the subject. Already published studies that merit discussion will be summarized in the sections to follow.

SUGGESTIONS WITHOUT TRANCE: A POTENTIAL TRAP FOR THE HIGHLY HYPNOTIZABLE

As mentioned before, hypnosis is a natural phenomenon that most patients can experience to a certain degree. For better or worse, highly hypnotizable individuals can enter trance states with ease and, on occasion, without even being fully aware of it. Thus, it is important for physicians to know that some patients may experience trance states even without formal induction. Highly hypnotizable individuals are extremely receptive to suggestions given by a person in a position of authority (i.e., nurse, physician), and thus their attitude and comments may have profound effects, both positive and negative, in these individuals. This "hypnotic phenomenon" may augment the placebo effect in either a positive or negative way, as demonstrated by the following case study.

CASE STUDY 1: UNREMITTING PAIN

A 75-year-old woman was referred to me for treatment of pain with hypnosis. The patient had been diagnosed with metastatic breast cancer that now was invading her hip bone, which was the source of her pain. When she came for her hypnotic sessions it was evident that she was a highly hypnotizable individual. In fact, she scored highly in objective hypnotizability measure (9 out of 10).

During her first session she entered the trance state with ease, and during it she was able to experience complete pain relief. Even with such success during trance, we were disappointed at the fact that as soon as she exited the trance state, the pain immediately returned. The same occurred during the second session. Thus, during the third session instead of working on the issue of pain control we did some hypnotic exploratory work to address the "reasons why she couldn't let go of the pain."

Under a hypnotic regression the patient was asked to "return to the moment when "this pain started." Immediately the patient recalled a meeting with her oncologist a few months back. At the time of that meeting, the patient had just begun to experience pain and brought it to her oncologist's attention. After discussing with her the "dangers of addiction if opioid medications were used," he inadvertently suggested that she will live the rest of her life with pain. His words were forever "imprinted" in her mind: "I'm sorry, but there is nothing I can do. You will be in pain until the day you die." To a highly hypnotizable patient this meant a lot. In her mind, she made "being in pain" equal to "being alive."

Once the "source" of her pain was clarified, the session focused on the meaning of her pain. To her, it served as a reminder that she was still alive; as long as she could feel the pain at its most severe, even at night, when it sometimes seemed endless, she knew she was alive. So, her discomfort was a "painful reminder that she was alive" and thus her need to hold on to the pain.

Her high level of suggestibility allowed her to "take" the initial suggestion. Thus our strategy then was to use this same hypnotic capacity to reverse the initial damage and help the patient conquer her pain. In her case, we used hypnosis to alter her perception of pain for a tingling sensation on the affected site. This tingling "continued to provide her reassurances about her life" without the need for her to experience the pain. The suggestion was to have a constant "tingling sensation which would filter the hurt out of the pain." She was able to master self-hypnotic techniques, which she continued to practice at home with great success. She later used her newly learned skills to help control symptoms of nausea and vomiting associated with chemotherapy.

ANXIETY RESPONSES TO MEDICAL PROCEDURES

The hypnotic experience can be used to produce a state of relaxation. Therefore, hypnotic techniques can be used to reduce the anxiety associated with a number of medical procedures (Deyoub, 1980; Covino & Frankel, 1993). Once patients have been trained in the use of self-hypnosis, they can use it in preparation for both a hospital visit and for medical tests or interventions, and while in the clinic or the hospital.

Hypnotic techniques have been successfully used to assist phobic patients to undergo a number of medical/surgical and diagnostic procedures, thus diminishing the need for excessive anesthesia or antianxiety medication, improving compliance, and eliminating trauma to patients (Covino & Frankel, 1993; Cadranel, Benhamou, et al.,1994; Ellis & Spanos, 1994;

Rape & Bush, 1994; Chandler, 1996; Kessler & Dane, 1996; Lambert, 1996; Lang, Joyce, et al.,1996; Mize, 1996).

Among patients undergoing colonoscopic examination, for whom other forms of anesthesia were not available, those able to benefit from hypnotic intervention reported less intense pain than patients in whom hypnosis was unsuccessful (Cadranel, Benhamou, et al., 1994) In addition, the hypnosis group reported a much better rate of successfully completed colonoscopies (100% versus 50%) and were more compliant with further testing later on (100% versus 2%, p < 0.001).

Phobic responses to modern imaging studies (i.e., magnetic resonance imaging [MRI], PET scans, and computerized tomography [CT] scans) are among the most common types of phobias we encounter. Hypnosis has been highly successful in facilitating the performance of imaging procedures such as MRI and CT scans (Friday & Kubal, 1990; Phelps, 1990; Chandler, 1996; Simon, 1999).

CASE STUDY 2: CLAUSTROPHOBIA

Take for example the case of a 43-year-old woman who suffered from convulsions that were resistant to treatment with conventional anticonvulsant therapy. Appropriately, her neurologist wanted to obtain a brain MRI to assess for the presence of a possible source of irritation that could explain the onset and maintenance of the seizures. Nevertheless, the patient repeatedly refused the MRI scan because of claustrophobia. On two occasions the patient presented to the MRI suite. The first time she took a look at the machine and walked away. The second time she was premedicated with diazepam (30 mg), but was unable to tolerate the procedure after just a few minutes and had to stop. Finally, she had a psychiatric evaluation.

In my office she proved to be highly hypnotizable (9 out of 10). Under hypnosis we explored the associations between the scanner and her anxiety. Images of a coffin came to mind. These were followed by memories of her father lying in the funeral home. He had died suddenly, without prior history or warning, of a massive hemorrhagic stroke associated with a congenital aneurysm. We then explored her anxiety as it related to fears of what the test might show. This included the possibility of a malformed blood vessel or other pathology that might affect her brain, as happened to her father. Once this was discussed she felt that it "was better to know than to avoid." She was trained in self-hypnosis. After inducing a relaxed state, she was instructed to "create in your mind's eye a place where you can feel safe and comfortable, knowing that sounds and people in the room will not disturb you." We also "practiced" going to the MRI scanner room by having her imagine that she was both the patient in the room and the technician operating the machine. In this fashion she felt more "in control" of the situation. The next day, we met her at the scanner room. Once she was on the imaging table she induced a self-hypnotic trance. When the test began I left the room with the agreement that the technician would let her know when the test was over. She imagined herself walking through a forest and crossing a river. As she walked to the riverbank, instead of floating she saw herself slowly sinking as she followed the contours of the river, walking down to the bottom of the river. Once on the bottom she held on to some algae. When she exhaled, her breath formed a gigantic bubble or "cocoon" that allowed her to breathe under water and be safe. As the magnets in the MRI shifted in position she imagined that the sound was the clanking sound of motorboat engines on the surface. She remained in this state for approximately 2 hours, while both noncontrast and contrast tests were performed. She tolerated the procedure well and easily came out of the trance state once the signal was given.

Hypnosis has been successfully used to help anxious patients tolerate procedures that otherwise would not be performed, or the patient might need to be exposed to larger than normal doses of antianxiety medications due to needle phobia. These include needle injections and phlebotomy (Dash, 1981; Zeltzer & LeBaron, 1982; Bell, Christian, et al., 1983; Kellerman, Zeltzer, et al., 1983; Morse & Cohen, 1983; Nugent, Carden, et al., 1984; Cyna, Tomkins, et al., 2007; Robertson, 2007; Abramowitz & Lichtenberg, 2009), needle biopsy and aspiration (Usberti, Grutta d'Auria, et al., 1984; Adams & Stenn, 1992; Ellis & Spanos, 1994; Lang, Berbaum, et al., 2006), bone marrow aspiration (Hageman-Wenselaar, 1988; Ellis & Spanos, 1994; Liossi & Hatira, 1999), and lumbar punctures (Hageman-Wenselaar, 1988; Ellis & Spanos, 1994; Simon & Canonico, 2001; Kellerman, Zeltzer, Ellenberg, et al., 1983).

CASE STUDY 3: NEEDLE PHOBIA

One of our patients, a 47-year-old, married, successful businessman was referred for "inability to participate in medical treatment." The patient had recently been diagnosed with esophageal cancer, after presenting to the emergency room with a 3-month history of weight loss, chills, shortness of breath, chest pains, and difficulty swallowing. Imaging studies revealed a large mass. Because of the size and location of the mass, and the stage of the disease, he was turned down for treatment in his previous hospital. He was presented to the tumor board of our institution where the gastrointestinal surgeons decided to take his case.

There was only one problem. The patient had experienced "terror of needles" from the age of 7. At that time he was receiving immunizations at school when he panicked and moved abruptly, causing a needle to break off the syringe and remain deep in his arm. He required surgery to remove it. From that moment on he did everything possible to "stay far from them."

In fact, while at the previous hospital institution he experienced an event which reinforced his fears. He was asleep when a phlebotomist entered his room. She placed her tray filled with syringes, collection tubes, and (of course) needles on his bed. As she began to explore his arm veins, he suddenly woke up, saw the needles, and fled. That was the end of his admission.

He now faced two (and according to him equally difficult) problems: the tumor and his phobia to needles. The proposed cancer treatment involved an aggressive course of high-dose chemotherapy and radiation. If this approach was successful at reducing the tumor size, surgery would follow. He discussed his phobia with his surgeon, who assured the patient that "every possible precaution would be taken." Nevertheless, the patient refused to enter the hospital. Finally, a psychiatric consultation was requested.

I saw the patient in my office. After reviewing his medical and psychiatric history it was obvious that aggressive treatment (both physical and psychological) was required if he was

to survive. He already had delayed his chemotherapy and surgical intervention because of his phobia. His surgeon had placed him on benzodiazepine medications, but despite his level of sedation, the phobia was still preventing him from obtaining the urgently needed treatment. I suggested the addition of a selective serotonin reuptake-inhibitor (SSRI), but realized that we might not have the time to wait for the medication to take effect. Therefore we decided to supplement his treatment with hypnosis.

The patient underwent his first hypnotic trance during the first session. Like many phobic patients, he proved to be highly hypnotizable with an HIP of 8.5 out of 10. He was trained in self-hypnotic techniques. His medications were rearranged. He was started on an SSRI, his short-acting benzodiazepine was switched to a longer-acting drug, and he was ordered to practice his self-hypnotic exercise six times a day. On the third day after our first session, he called to say that he thought he was "ready." I met him in the surgical clinic. With the patient under hypnosis, a central line was placed to administer his chemotherapy. After 3 weeks of aggressive chemotherapy and local radiation treatment, the patient was admitted to the hospital for surgical excision of the mass.

He was able to tolerate every treatment aspect with only minimal discomfort. Unfortunately, his course was difficult and filled by numerous complications including infections, the creation of several fistulas, and the development of a pneumothorax requiring bilateral chest tube and drainage placements. Nevertheless, he continued to manage his phobia well. Certainly, given his complications he required multiple needle sticks and even blood transfusions, but tolerated them well. In fact, the nursing staff was amazed and fascinated by his "little ritual" prior to injections or blood draws while he "self-induced a hypnotic trance." Certainly, we believe that medications helped his overall anxiety and phobic condition. The patient said, "I could not have gone through this without hypnosis."

The concomitant use of hypnosis and medications is common practice in the psychosomatic medicine service. Certainly, as in many other aspects of psychiatry and medicine, the combined used of multiple complementary treatment modalities is the norm. Sometimes hypnosis is used alone because it is the patient's preference, the patient is an extremely good (highly hypnotizable) candidate, there are medical contraindications to the use of central nervous system depressant agents (i.e., respiratory depression, intraoperative EEG monitoring), or the clinician is dealing with a relatively simple procedure. Other times, as in case study 3, the complexity of the situation requires more aggressive and prompt intervention. In that case, we needed to move so quickly that we didn't have much time for medication (the SSRI) to work. Hypnosis played a key role in the patient's accepting and going through treatment. It became an invaluable adjunct to his overall treatment.

DERMATOLOGICAL CONDITIONS

Psychogenic factors have been implicated in essentially all skin disorders (Cheek, 1961; Kellner, 1975; Manferto, 1975; Medansky & Handler, 1981; Tobia, 1982; Arone di Bertolino,

1983; Elitzur & Brenner, 1986; Tsushima, 1988; Haustein & Seikowski, 1990; Gherardi, Fabrizio, et al.,1993; Bellini, 1998; Shenefelt, 2000, 2002, 2003)

Hypnosis has been helpful for several specific skin disorders: pruritus (Arone di Bertolino, 1983; Ament & Milgrom, 1967; Shertzer & Lookingbill, 1987; Sampson, 1990; Mitchell, 1995; Rucklidge & Saunders, 1999, 2002; Tuerk & Koo, 2008; Tsiskarishvili, Eradze, et al., 2010), eczema (Faure & Burger, 1954; Vlarsky & Janousek, 1960; Goodman, 1962; Zheltakov, IuK, et al., 1963; Kierland, 1965; Mirvish, 1978; Hajek, Jakoubek, et al., 1989; Hajek, Jakoubek, et al., 1990; Hajek, Radil, et al., 1991; Mantle, 1999; Ersser, Latter, et al., 2007), scleroderma (Surwit, Allen, et al., 1982; Freedman, Ianni, et al., 1984; Haustein, Weber, et al., 1995; Seikowski, Weber, et al., 1995), atopic dermatitis (West, Kierland, et al., 1961; Stewart & Thomas, 1995), genital herpes simplex virus (Putilin, 1961; Arone di Bertolino, 1981; Gould & Tissler, 1984; Elitzur & Brenner, 1986; Surman & Crumpacker, 1987; Fox, Henderson, et al., 1999; Pfitzer, Clark, et al., 2005), psoriasis (Novotny, 1962; Secter & Barthelemy, 1964; Frankel & Misch, 1973; Waxman, 1973; Winchell & Watts, 1988; Kantor, 1990; Zachariae, Oster, et al., 1996; Tausk & Whitmore, 1999), chronic urticaria (Shertzer & Lookingbill, 1987), chronic plaque-type psoriasis (Tausk & Whitmore, 1999) and warts, even though they result from viral agents such as human papillomavirus (Vollmer, 1946; Mc, 1949; Sinclair-Gieben & Chalmers, 1959; Ullmann, 1959; Wendel, 1959; Seeman, 1960; Ullman & Dudek, 1960; Clarke, 1965; Lyell, 1966; Dudek, 1967; Stankler, 1967; Leidman Iu, 1968; Konig, 1969; Nasemann, 1969; Tenzel & Taylor, 1969; Surman, Gottlieb, et al., 1972; French, 1973; Leidman Iu, 1973; Surman, Gottlieb, et al., 1973; Fischer, 1974; Clawson & Swade, 1975; Skalicanova, Nagyova, et al., 1977; Tasini & Hackett, 1977; Cohen, 1978; Dreaper, 1978; Johnson & Barber, 1978; Sheehan, 1978; Wilkening, 1978; Johnson, 1980; Rowe, 1982; Straatmeyer & Rhodes, 1983; Morris, 1985; Noll, 1988; Spanos, Stenstrom, et al., 1988; Steele & Irwin, 1988; Spanos, Williams, et al., 1990; Bolton, 1991; Esman, 1992; Ewin, 1992; Ferreira & Duncan, 2002; Herold, 2002; Meineke, Reichrath, et al., 2002; Phoenix, 2007; Ewin, 2011; Kekecs & Varga, 2011).

In chronic urticaria and atopic dermatitis, hypnosis has led to long-term improvements.

In chronic urticaria, remissions of 7 years duration as measured by three self-report parameters were achieved by hypnosis (Shertzer & Lookingbill, 1987). Of interest, highly hypnotizable subjects had fewer hives and more frequently related stress as a causative factor of their outbreaks. Improvements were maintained during a 2-year follow-up in a group of patients suffering from atopic dermatitis resistant to conventional treatment, who experienced statistically significant subjective and objective benefit (p < 0.01) after treatment with hypnosis (Stewart & Thomas, 1995).

A 3-month randomized, single-blind, controlled trial used hypnosis in adults with stable, chronic, plaque-type psoriasis. Highly or moderately hypnotizable subjects were randomized to receive either hypnosis with active suggestions of improvement or neutral hypnosis with no mention of their disease

process. The results demonstrated that highly hypnotizable subjects showed significantly greater improvement than did moderately hypnotizable subjects, independent of treatment group assignment (Tausk & Whitmore, 1999).

Published controlled studies on the use of hypnosis to cure warts are confined to using direct suggestion in hypnosis (DSIH), with cure rates of 27% to 55% (Johnson, 1980). Prepubertal children respond to DSIH almost without exception, but adults often do not. Clinically, many adults (80%) who fail to respond to DSIH will heal with individual hypnoanalytic techniques that cannot be tested against controls (Ewin, 1992).

A study comparing the effects of hypnotic suggestions versus topical salicylic acid and placebo found that subjects in all groups developed equivalent expectations of treatment success, but only the hypnotic subjects had lost significantly more warts than the no-treatment controls at the 6-week follow-up (Spanos, Williams, et al., 1990).

At least one carefully controlled study demonstrated that simple hypnotic instructions to the effect that the warts would "tingle and disappear" resulted in a rate of improvement that was significantly better than the spontaneous rate of remission of warts (Surman, et al., 1973).

The ability of highly hypnotizable individuals to control peripheral skin temperature and blood flow has been replicated in several well-controlled experiments (Zimbardo, Maslach, et al., 1970; Grabowska, 1971; Kistler, Mariauzouls, et al., 1999). Some have demonstrated plethysmographic measure changes caused by hypnotically mediated rapid vasodilatation after direct suggestion in cases of Raynaud's disease treated with hypnosis (Conn & Mott, 1984).

GASTROINTESTINAL CONDITIONS

Gastrointestinal conditions helped by hypnosis include inflammatory bowel disease such as ulcerative colitis, Crohn's disease, and related conditions (Susmano, Feldfeber, et al., 1960; Grumiller & Strotzka, 1973; Freiwald, Liedtke, et al., 1975; Snape, 1994; Schafer, 1997; Mawdsley, Jenkins, et al., 2008), irritable bowel syndrome (Byrne, 1973; Whorwell, Prior, et al., 1984; Whorwell, Prior, et al., 1987; Whorwell, 1989, 1991; Snape, 1994; Francis & Houghton, 1996; Houghton, Heyman, et al., 1996; Galovski & Blanchard, 1998, 2002; Vidakovic-Vukic, 1999; Forbes, MacAuley, et al., 2000; Gonsalkorale, Houghton, et al., 2002; Palsson, Turner, et al., 2002; Gonsalkorale, Miller, et al., 2003; Gonsalkorale & Whorwell, 2005; Tan, Hammond, et al., 2005; Whorwell, 2005, 2008, 2009; Barabasz & Barabasz, 2006; Palsson, 2006; Palsson, Turner, et al., 2006; Roberts, Wilson, et al., 2006; Simren, 2006; Whitehead, 2006; Wilson, Maddison, et al., 2006; Al Sughayir, 2007; Vlieger, Menko-Frankenhuis, et al., 2007; Webb, Kukuruzovic, et al., 2007; Hefner, Rilk, et al., 2009; Miller & Whorwell, 2009; Carruthers, Morris, et al., 2010; Shinozaki, Kanazawa, et al., 2010), dysphagia (Magonet, 1961; Black, 1980; Gurian, 1981; Kopel & Quinn, 1996), vocal cord dysfunction (Anbar & Hehir, 2000), esophageal achalasia/cardiospasm (Schneck, 1958; Jones,

Cooper, et al., 2006), irritable bowel syndrome (Houghton, Heyman, et al., 1996), and peptic and duodenal ulcer disease (Bick, 1958; Zane, 1966; Montera, 1968; Kanishchev & Shutova, 1974; Bishay, Stevens, et al., 1984, 1988; Colgan, Faragher, et al., 1988; Whorwell, 1991; Francis % Houghton, 1996; Soo, Moayyedi, et al., 2005).

The clinical relevance of these studies was illustrated by a controlled trial of hypnosis in relapse prevention of duodenal ulcers (Colgan, Faragher, et al., 1988). In this study, 30 patients with rapidly relapsing ulcer disease were randomly assigned after ranitidine treatment to hypnosis or no further treatment. On follow-up, 100% of the control subjects but only 53% of the hypnosis patients experienced relapse.

A randomized controlled trial demonstrated that IBS-patients treated with hypnosis reported significant improvement in pain, abdominal distension, and diarrhea, as well as emotional well-being compared with a control group. Absenteeism from work was reduced. These improvements continued during the 18-month follow-up period (Houghton, Heyman, et al., 1996).

A randomized study comparing the use of "gut-directed hypnotherapy" versus a specially devised audiotape intervention demonstrated a reduction in median symptom score, from 14.0 to 8.5, in hypnotherapy patients compared with an unchanged score of 13 in audiotape patients ($P < 0.05$) (Forbes, MacAuley, et al., 2000).

Hypnosis has been repeatedly used with great success for symptomatic control in emesis, regardless of the cause, in both children (Keller, 1995) and adults (Covino & Frankel, 1993; Faymonville, 1995). In an excellent example of how hypnosis actually exerts direct physiologic changes, researchers monitored the gastric acid secretion among 28 highly hypnotizable subjects (Klein & Spiegel, 1989). When subjects were hypnotized and instructed to eat an imaginary meal, basal acid output rose 89%. Similarly, when instructed to use hypnosis to experience deep relaxation they exhibited a significant (39%) drop in basal acid output.

CARDIAC CONDITIONS

In the treatment of cardiovascular problems, applications of hypnosis have been discussed in angina pectoris (Kobayashi, Ishikawa, et al., 1970; Wilkinson, 1981; Zaitsev, Shafikova, et al., 1990), essential hypertension (Friedman & Taub, 1977, 1978; Gay, 2007), and recovery from myocardial infarction and cardiac surgery (Gruen, 1972; Kavanagh, Shephard, et al., 1974; Zaitsev, Shafikova, et al., 1990; Greenleaf, Fisher, et al., 1992; Kosov, Zamotaev Iu, et al., 1997; Baglini, Sesana, et al., 2004).

Hypnosis can affect the patient's perception of exertion and influence the relation between the sympathetic and vagal systems. Gemignani et al. (2000) studied the physiological and EEG responses of highly hypnotizable volunteers suffering from simple phobia. Under hypnotic suggestion, subjects exposed to aversive stimuli experienced significant increases in heart rate (HR) and respiratory rate (RR), with a shift of the sympathovagal indexes toward a sympathetic predominance.

These subjects also experienced a significant increase in the EEG gamma band with left frontocentral prevalence.

Finally, Williamson and colleagues (2001), using healthy, highly hypnotizable volunteers, demonstrated dramatic changes in ratings of perceived exertion (RPE) when asked to imagine themselves in an uphill bicycle grade. They found significant increases in RPE, HR, mean blood pressure (BP), rCBF in the right insular cortex, and right thalamic activation. Conversely, when subjects were asked to imagine themselves on a perceived downhill grade they observed decrements in both the ratings of perceived exertion RPE and rCBF in the left insular cortex and anterior cingulate cortex, but it did not alter exercise HR or BP responses.

PULMONARY CONDITIONS

Hypnosis has been useful for asthma (Herraiz Ballestero, Rodriguez Fontela, et al., 1952; Magonet, 1952; White, 1961; Maher-Loughnan, Mason, et al., 1962; Fry, Mason, et al., 1964; Brown, 1965, 1968; Gilder, 1968; Luparello, Lyons, et al., 1968; Maher-Loughnan, 1970; Smith, Colebatch, et al., 1970; Moorefield, 1971; Aronoff, Aronoff, et al., 1975; Collison, 1975; Ben-Zvi, Spohn, et al., 1982; Neinstein & Dash, 1982; Lewis, Lewis, et al., 1983; Zamotaev, Sultanova, et al., 1983; Ewer & Stewart, 1986; Pastorello, Codecasa, et al., 1987; Morrison, 1988; Spector & Kinsman, 1988; Murphy, Lehrer, et al., 1989; Wilkinson, 1989; Isenberg, Lehrer, et al., 1992; Kohen & Wynne, 1997; Hackman, Stern, et al., 2000; Anbar, 2003; Brown, 2007), hay fever (Langewitz, Izakovic, et al., 2005), and hyperventilation (Clarke & Gibson, 1980).

Patients can learn to use self-hypnotic techniques rather than medication when they begin to feel an anxiety-precipitated asthmatic attack coming on. This may help interrupt the vicious cycle of anxiety and bronchoconstriction (Aronoff, Aronoff, et al., 1975; Collison, 1975; Gluzman & Ziselson, 1987; Kohen, 1987; Kohen & Wynne, 1997)

A common technique is to have asthmatic patients enter a state of self-hypnosis and imagine that they are somewhere they naturally breathe easily, such as breathing cool ocean spray (Spiegel & Spiegel, 1987). In asthmatic patients, hypnotizability is correlated with treatment response (Collison, 1975). A study of 120 adult asthma patients experienced significant benefit from the use of hypnosis (Collison, 1975). The authors described that 21% of subjects had an "excellent response" to treatment, becoming completely free from asthma and requiring no drug therapy. An additional 33% had a "good response" with "worthwhile decrease in frequency and severity of the attacks of asthma" or a decrease in drug requirements. Furthermore, about half of the 46% who did not respond had a marked subjective improvement in general well-being. Others have reported similar results in children (Aronoff, Aronoff, et al., 1975; Kohen, Olness, et al., 1984; Gluzman & Zisel'son, 1987; Kohen, 1987).

A randomized controlled trial including 39 adults with mild to moderate asthma demonstrated that after brief treatment with hypnosis, patients with a high susceptibility score showed marked improvement (74.9%) in the degree of bronchial hyperresponsiveness to a standardized methacholine challenge test, and a reduction in the use of bronchodilators by 26.2% (Ewer & Stewart, 1986).

Another study found that after self-hypnotic treatment and training, patients with treatment-resistant asthma reported a two-thirds decline in the number of hospital admissions (due to complications of asthma), decreased need for the use of PRN-steroid medications, reduced length in hospital stay, and an overall improvement in their perception of illness (Morrison, 1988). A retrospective analysis of 121 asthmatic patients who were treated by hypnotherapy showed that 21% of the subjects had an excellent response to treatment, becoming completely free from asthma and requiring no drug therapy (Collison, 1975). And an additional 33% had a good response, with worthwhile decrease in frequency and severity of the attacks of asthma or a decrease in drug requirements.

ONCOLOGICAL CARE

Hypnosis improves the tolerance of treatments such as chemotherapy (Hilgard & LeBaron, 1982; Zeltzer, Kellerman, et al., 1983; Zeltzer, LeBaron, et al., 1984; Katz, Kellerman, et al., 1987; Syrjala, Cummings, et al., 1992; Jacknow, Tschann, et al., 1994; Genuis, 1995; Steggles, Damore-Petingola, et al., 1997; Renouf, 1998; Marchioro, Azzarello, et al., 2000; Richardson, Smith, et al., 2006; Figueroa-Moseley, Jean-Pierre, et al., 2007; Neron & Stephenson, 2007; Richardson, Smith, et al., 2007; Jakubovits, 2011), anticipatory anxiety and side effects (Hoffman, 1982; Redd, Andresen, et al., 1982; Axelrod, Vinciguerra, et al., 1988; Marchioro, Azzarello, et al., 2000), external beam radiation therapy (Bertoni, Bonardi, et al., 1999; Steggles, 1999), interventional radiology (Lang, Joyce, et al., 1996; Lang, Benotsch, et al., 2000; Spiegel, 2006), and surgery, its recovery, and painful procedures (Kessler & Dane, 1996; Lambert, 1996; Spiegel & Moore, 1997; Wild & Espie, 2004).

As discussed before, hypnosis may be of assistance in the management of the discomfort and anxiety associated with many of the procedures needed in the treatment of cancer, such as chemotherapy, radiation therapy, claustrophobia, and the need for repeated diagnostic tests.

OBSTETRICS AND GYNECOLOGY

Hypnosis has multiple applications in the field of obstetrics and gynecology (Mun, 1964; Ferraris, 1975; Goldman, 1992; Oster, 1994; Baram, 1995; Schauble, Werner, et al., 1998; Brown & Hammond, 2007; VandeVusse, Irland, et al., 2007). These include assistance in obstetrical delivery and pain management during labor (Winkelstein, 1958; Werner, 1959; Rodger, 1961; Gueguen, 1962; Gross & Posner, 1963; Roden, 1970; Johnson, 1980; Freeman, Macaulay, et al., 1986; Oster, 1994; Schauble, Werner, et al., 1998; Brown & Hammond, 2007; VandeVusse, Irland, et al., 2007; Landolt & Milling, 2011), management of premature contractions (Omer, Friedlander, et al., 1986), hypnotic breech to cephalic

conversion (Mehl, 1994; Boog, 2004; Tiran, 2004), hyperemesis gravidarum (Kroger & De, 1946; Giorlando & Mascola, 1957; Mun, 1964; Piscicelli, 1968; Muzelak, 1974; Savel'ev, 1974; Fuchs, Paldi, et al., 1980; Smith, 1982; Poliakov, 1989; Frankel, 1994; Iancu, Kotler, et al., 1994; Torem, 1994; Simon, 1999; Simon & Schwartz, 1999; Brent, 2002; Buckwalter & Simpson, 2002; McCormack, 2010), pregnancy-induced hypertension (Smith, 1989), sexual dysfunction (Baram, 1995), urinary incontinence (Baram, 1995), condylomata acuminata (Straatmeyer & Rhodes, 1983; Klapper, 1984), chronic pelvic pain (Baram, 1995), and functional infertility (Mun, 1964; Gravitz, 1995).

Authors have reported the use of hypnotic preparation for labor and delivery, suggesting various advantages over Lamaze techniques (Oster, 1994). Among the advantages of using hypnosis are an improvement in the mother's psychological comfort, a heightened sense of involvement in the birth process, a diminished level of anxiety, and improved pain management.

A study of the effect of hypnotic relaxation as an adjunct to pharmacological treatment of premature contractions demonstrated that the rate of pregnancy prolongation was significantly higher for the hypnotic-relaxation group than for the medication-alone group (Omer, Friedlander, et al., 1986).

Unfortunately, most of the writings in this area are in the form of case reports or small series.

A prospective case series comparing 100 pregnant women whose fetuses were in breech position at 37 to 40 weeks' gestation and a matched comparison group of women with similar obstetric and sociodemographic parameters derived from clinical databases showed that 81% of the fetuses in the hypnotic intervention group converted to vertex presentation compared with only 48% of those in the comparison (control) group (Mehl, 1994). Others have further commented on the topic, but no other studies have been published (Boog, 2004; Tiran, 2004).

PAIN MANAGEMENT

The experience of pain does not exist in isolation. It is usually interpreted within the context of the subjective distress associated with a major medical illness or somatic trauma and in the context of the patient's life experiences and temporal social circumstances. The "pain experience" represents a combination of both tissue damage and the emotional reaction to it. There is ample evidence suggesting that psychological factors greatly influence the pain experience in either positive or negative ways (Beecher, 1956). In fact, the intensity of pain is directly associated with its meaning. Hypnosis, by the mechanisms of dissociation and absorption, can mediate an alteration in the subjective experience of pain.

Various well designed studies have described the usefulness of hypnotic intervention as adjunct to analgesia (Moskowitz, 1996). The use of hypnosis has been shown to increase tolerance to the procedure among angioplasty patients (Weinstein & Au, 1991). Similarly, patients on the hypnosis group reported lower levels of intraoperative pain scores during surgery compared to patients receiving conscious intravenous sedation (control group [Faymonville, Fissette, et al., 1995]). Both studies found that hypnotized patients required less narcotic pain medication during the procedure compared to controls.

A randomized clinical trial of metastatic breast cancer patients demonstrated that a combination of hypnosis and group psychotherapy resulted in a 50% reduction in pain, which was accompanied by similarly significant reduction in mood disturbance (Spiegel, Bloom, et al., 1981).

Among subjects undergoing interventional radiologic procedures, the use of hypnosis was associated with a significant reduction in the need of anesthesia in the form of intravenous conscious sedation or patient-controlled anesthesia (Lang, Joyce, et al., 1996). The hypnosis group used less drug (0.28 vs. 2.01 drug units; p < .01) and reported less pain (median pain rating 2 vs. 5 on a 0–10 scale; p < .01). In addition, significantly more control patients exhibited oxygen desaturation and/or needed interruptions of their procedures for hemodynamic instability, thus suggesting that self-hypnotic relaxation can reduce the need for sedative medications and improve the safety of the procedure.

A study of moderately to highly hypnotizable adults with chronic low back pain demonstrated that they were able to significantly reduce pain perception following hypnotic analgesia instructions during cold-pressor pain training (Crawford, Knebel, et al., 1998). During the hypnotic condition there was evidence of an enhanced N_{140} in the anterior frontal region, suggesting inhibitory processing; reduced amplitudes of P_{200} (bilateral midfrontal and central, and left parietal) and P_{300} (right midfrontal and central), suggesting decreased spatiotemporal perception. Meantime, subjects reported highly significant mean reductions in perceived sensory pain and distress, reduction in chronic pain, increased psychological well-being, and increased sleep quality.

Most hypnoanalgesia treatment techniques involve the creation of a state of physical relaxation coupled with visual or somatic imagery, which allows a substitute focus of attention away from the physical sensation of pain. The technique to be used depends on the patient's hypnotic capacity. Highly hypnotizable individuals are much better at dissociating body parts or moving the pain to another part of the body or even away from the body. They can use fairly simple and direct imagery such as "seeing the pain melting away" or "being washed away by the river's waters." Some highly hypnotizable individuals may create a sensation of numbing at the affected area just by suggesting it.

Meanwhile, poorly suggestible patients may need more assistance from the therapist—for instance, more direct or concrete suggestions such as imagining injection of a local anesthetic into the affected area accompanied by its associated tingling numbness. A useful suggestion is to have subjects remember what a Novocain shot felt like the last time they went to the dentist. Then remind them of how slowly the gum, then the cheeks and the tongue became numb and "went to sleep." Once they can hold the image on their mind, they can imagine "the same shot" being administered "wherever it is needed in your body. Then slowly imagine the progressive numbing that follows as the medication spreads through the . . . (skin, nerves, muscle, or whatever the patient needs)."

Other images, such as changes in temperature, either warmth or coolness, of the area may also be helpful. Like "imagine the feeling of immersing your hand in cold water or snow until it is numb."

The images or metaphors that are selected for pain control may be used to filter the hurt or to transform the painful experience. Most patients who use hypnoanalgesia can still feel the pain, but may be unable to distinguish between the signal of pain and the discomfort caused by the signal. Thus, patients are taught not to fight but to transform painful signals into less uncomfortable ones. Fighting pain may only enhance it by focusing attention on the pain and increasing physical tension, which can place traction on painful body parts thereby increasing the sense of discomfort in adjacent tissues.

Regardless of any specific induction or metaphor use, there are four specific steps in the use of hypnosis that can make psychotherapy for pain management briefer, more goal-oriented, and efficient: (1) the assessment of hypnotizability; (2) the induction of hypnoanalgesia and development of individualized pain coping strategies; (3) the use of direct suggestion, cognitive reframing, hypnotic metaphors, and pain relief imagery; and (4) brief psychodynamic reprocessing, during the trance state, of emotional factors in the patient's experience of chronic pain (Eimer, 2000).

The precise mechanisms that mediate hypnotic analgesia are not known. Some time ago it was believed that hypnoanalgesia somehow involved the release or production of endogenous opioids (Frid & Singer, 1979). By now, several studies have not only failed to prove this theory but have proven that hypnotic analgesia is completely unaffected by the administration of opioid antagonist agents such as naloxone (Goldstein & Hilgard, 1975; Spiegel & Albert, 1983; Moret, Forster, et al., 1991). Despite lack of definitive explanation regarding its mechanism of action, there is no doubt that hypnotic analgesia works (DeBenedittis, Panerai, et al., 1989).

Studies have shown the superiority of hypnotic analgesia over placebo (McGlashan, Evans, et al., 1969) and acupuncture (Knox & Shum, 1977). In fact, a study using hypnosis as a method of analgesia reported significant increases of tolerance of pain and distress during hypnosis as compared to the waking state, thus hypothesizing that highly hypnotizable subjects were able to experience a hypnotically induced dissociation between the sensory/discriminative and the affective/motivational dimensions of pain (DeBenedittis, Panerai, et al., 1989). After measuring plasma concentrations of beta-endorphin and adrenocorticotropic hormone (ACTH), they concluded that hypnotic analgesia was not mediated either by endorphins or by ACTH.

A number of studies have proposed new potential biological mechanisms mediating hypnoanalgesia. One study examined the changes in motor neuron excitability to electrical stimulus during conditions of resting wakefulness (not hypnotic) and suggestions for hypnotic analgesia. Its findings suggest that hypnotic sensory analgesia was, at least in part, (Kiernan, Dane, et al., 1995) mediated by either descending spinal cord antinociceptive mechanisms or by diminished nociceptive awareness mediated by other brain mechanisms.

Other studies utilizing SERP measures to noxious stimuli seem to confirm the presence of active inhibitory processes during cognitive strategies in hypnotic analgesia, and to confirm that these inhibitory processes also regulate the autonomic activities in pain perception (De Pascalis, Magurano, et al., 2001). For example, 33 subjects' neural responses (EEG) were measured during the 40–540 ms period following phasic electrical stimulations to the right hand, under control and hypnosis conditions (Croft, Williams, et al., 2002). Resultant amplitudes were computed and grouped into seven scalp topographies, and for each frequency relations between these topographies and pain ratings, performance, and stimulus intensity measures were assessed. Gamma activity (32–100 Hz) over prefrontal scalp sites predicted subject pain ratings in the control condition (r=0.50, P=0.004), and no other frequency/topography combination did. This relation was unchanged by hypnosis in the poorly hypnotizable subjects but was not present in the highly hypnotizable subjects during hypnosis, suggesting that hypnosis interferes with this pain/gamma relation.

In a group of patients with fibromyalgia, hypnoanalgesia studied using PET scans found that patients experienced less pain during hypnosis than at rest. At the same time, the cerebral blood flow was bilaterally increased in the orbitofrontal and subcallosal cingulate cortices, the right thalamus, and the left inferior parietal cortex, and was decreased bilaterally in the cingulate cortex, supporting the notion of the multifactorial nature of hypnotic analgesia with contributions from cortical and subcortical brain regions (Wik, Fischer, et al., 1999).

Another PET study compared brain images of subjects in a hypnotic resting state with mental imagery and a hypnotic state with stimulation; namely, warm non-noxious versus hot noxious stimuli applied to right thenar eminence (Faymonville, Laureys, et al., 2000). Statistical parametric mapping demonstrated that noxious stimulation caused an increase in rCBF in the thalamic nuclei, anterior cingulate, and insular cortices, while the hypnotic state induced a significant activation of a right-sided extrastriate area and the anterior cingulate cortex. The interaction analysis showed that the activity in the anterior (mid-) cingulate cortex was related to pain perception and unpleasantness differently in the hypnotic state than in control situations. Hypnosis decreased both pain sensation and the unpleasantness of noxious stimuli, which suggests that hypnotic analgesia with an instruction that the pain will not be bothersome (rather than literally reduced in intensity) is mediated by reduced activity in the anterior cingulate cortex (Faymonville, Laureys, et al., 2000).

A follow-up study among highly hypnotizable right-handed volunteers using H2(15)O-PET found that hypnosis, compared to the resting state, reduced pain perception by 50%, while the pain perception during rest and mental imagery was not significantly different (Faymonville, Roediger, et al., 2003). Analysis of PET data showed that the hypnotic state compared to normal alertness (i.e., rest and mental imagery) significantly enhanced the functional modulation between midcingulate cortex and a large neural network encompassing bilateral insula, pregenual anterior cingulate cortex, pre-supplementary motor area, right prefrontal cortex, and

striatum, thalamus, and brainstem. These findings point to a critical role for the midcingulate cortex in the modulation of a large cortical and subcortical network underlying its influence on sensory, affective, cognitive, and behavioral aspects of nociception in the specific context of hypnosis.

More recently, PET imaging studies have confirmed that hypnosis, when used to produce hypnotic analgesia, can modulate the cerebral network involved in noxious perception (Faymonville, Boly, et al., 2006). In fact, when compared to the resting state, hypnosis reduced pain perception in somatosensory cortex by approximately 50%. In these subjects, hypnoanalgesia-induced reduction of affective and sensory responses to noxious thermal stimulation was modulated by the activity in the midcingulate cortex (area 24a'). Also, compared to normal alertness (i.e., rest and mental imagery) the hypnotic state significantly enhanced the functional modulation between midcingulate cortex and a large neural network involved in sensory, affective, cognitive, and behavioral aspects of nociception.

After determination of the heat pain threshold of 12 healthy volunteers, fMRI scans were performed during repeated painful heat stimuli (Schulz-Stubner, Krings, et al., 2004). Subjects under the hypnosis paradigm exhibited less activation in the primary sensory cortex, the middle cingulate gyrus, precuneus, and the visual cortex when compared with responses without hypnosis. An increased activation was seen in the anterior basal ganglia and the left anterior cingulate cortex. There was no difference in activation within the right anterior cingulate gyrus in our fMRI studies, and no activation was seen within the brainstem and thalamus under either condition. These findings suggest that clinical hypnosis may prevent nociceptive inputs from reaching the higher cortical structures responsible for pain perception.

The development of "neurosignatures of pain" can influence subsequent pain experiences (Melzack, 1991; Coderre, Katz, et al., 1993; Melzack, 1993) and may be expanded in size and easily reactivated (Melzack, 1991, 1993; Elbert, Flor, et al., 1994). Therefore, hypnosis and other psychological interventions need to be introduced early as adjuncts in medical treatments for onset pain before the development of chronic pain (Crawford, Knebel, et al., 1998).

APPLICATION OF HYPNOSIS IN PSYCHIATRIC DISORDERS PERTINENT TO PSYCHOSOMATIC MEDICINE

The use of hypnosis in the management of psychiatric disorders in general is beyond the scope of this chapter and has been discussed elsewhere. (Maldonado & Spiegel, 2002, 2008). Yet, there are some specific psychiatric disorders that are particularly pertinent for the psychosomatic medicine specialist, such as the management of traumatic events related to posttraumatic stress disorder (Maldonado & Spiegel, 1994, 1998, 2002, 2008; Cardeña, Maldonado, et al., 2008), acute phobic reactions interfering with medical care (e.g., claustrophobia or needle phobia), behavioral modification (e.g., smoking and weight management, sleep disturbances), and treatment of some somatoform disorders (i.e., conversion disorder [Maldonado & Spiegel, 2000; Maldonado, 2007).

POSTTRAUMATIC STRESS DISORDER

Initially, the principal role for hypnosis in the psychotherapy of trauma was limited to abreaction, based on Freud's cathartic method. The idea was that some intense affect associated with the traumatic event needed to be released, and that simply repeating the event with its associated emotion in the trance state would suffice to resolve the symptoms. However, it became clear to Freud that conscious cognitive work must be done on the material for it to be successfully worked through (Freud, 1914/1958).

A number of studies among individuals suffering from posttraumatic stress disorder (PTSD) have demonstrated that these patients usually score in the high hypnotizability range (Stutman & Bliss, 1985; Spiegel, Hunt, et al., 1988; Cardeña, Maldonado, et al., 2008). Reports also suggest high hypnotizability scores among children who were victims of severe punishment during childhood (Nash, Lynn, et al., 1984; Spiegel & Cardeña, 1991). Some researchers in the field suggest a possible explanation, that the impact of the stress suffered during trauma encourages a more effective use of dissociative defenses and self-hypnotic abilities, thus enhancing or mediating symptomatology (Spiegel, Detrick, et al., 1982; Kluft, 1984, 1992). If this hypothesis is correct, then the controlled use of hypnosis in the clinical setting may assist in modulating and managing symptoms associated with PTSD and, over time, help to integrate memories of trauma (Maldonado & Spiegel, 1994).

In fact, the major categories of symptoms in PTSD are similar to the components of the hypnotic process (American Psychiatric Association, 1994; Maldonado & Spiegel, 1994, 2007; Maldonado, Page, et al., 2002). Hypnotic absorption is similar to the intrusive reliving of traumatic events. When in a flashback, trauma victims become so absorbed in reexperiencing the traumatic event that they lose touch with their present surroundings and even forget that the events took place in the past. Similarly, patients suffering from PTSD may dissociate feelings to the extent of experiencing the so-called "psychic numbing," which allows them to disconnect current affects from their everyday experience in an attempt to avoid emotions triggering memories associated with the trauma. Finally, suggestibility is comparable to hyperarousal. The heightened sensitivity to environmental cues observed in patients suffering from PTSD is similar to that experienced by a hypnotized individual who responds to suggestions of coldness by shivering.

For therapy to be effective in cases of traumatic stress, cognitive restructuring, emotional expression, and relationship management must accompany the patient's controlled reexperiencing of the traumatic events. To that effect, the therapeutic environment must provide the patient with an enhanced sense of control over the memories of the experience. One of the ways to accomplish that is through symbolic restructuring of the traumatic experiences during work with hypnosis (Spiegel & Spiegel, 1987) and the use of a grief work model (Spiegel, 1981). Hypnosis can be used to provide controlled and safe access to the dissociated or repressed memories of the traumatic experience at a pace the patient can tolerate, and then can assist patients to restructure their memories of the events.

Given the growing evidence that many people enter a dissociated state during physical trauma (Spiegel & Cardeña, 1991; Cardeña & Spiegel, 1993; van der Kolk, Hostetler, et al., 1994; van der Kolk & Fisler, 1995; Butler, Duran, et al., 1996; Cardeña, Maldonado, et al., 2008) and the principle of state-dependent memory (Bower, 1981; Bremner, Krystal, et al., 1996; Butler, Duran, et al., 1996), it makes sense that enabling patients to enter a structured dissociative state in therapy would facilitate their access to memories of the traumatic experience—memories that can be worked through to resolve the posttraumatic symptomatology. In the more immediate context of the medical setting, the use of hypnosis can help to control the dissociative symptoms and traumatic flashbacks, help manage anxiety symptoms, and improve sleep. Over the long term, though, hypnosis can be helpful in allowing the victim to review aspects of the trauma in a controlled manner. Memories can be experienced or reviewed for a time with the assurance that they can be put aside afterward. In the context of hypnotic facilitated psychotherapy, patients can be quickly taught how to produce a state of physical relaxation despite whatever psychological stress they experience, thereby dissociating the somatic reaction from the psychological preoccupation and allowing for modulation of the traumatic memory and an enhanced sense of control over the experience. Patient and therapist can then find a condensation image that symbolizes some aspect of the trauma.

The Split Screen Technique

It is often helpful to have patients project the images of the traumatic event on an imaginary screen, which gives them some sense of distance from the event. It is also useful to divide the screen in half, having the patient picture on one side some aspect of the event (e.g., a trauma victim's image of the accident) and on the other side of the screen some positive aspect of the event (e.g., having survived and being able to be with the family; veering the car into a divider in order to prevent hurting someone else). This exercise enables the patient to restructure his or her view of the incident—facing it, but not simply in the familiar terms of the powerlessness, victimization, pain, and fear with which it was initially associated. Patients can then be taught a self-hypnosis exercise in which they grieve and work through traumatic memories while enhancing their sense of control over the process (Spiegel, 1981).

CASE STUDY 4: TREATMENT-RELATED POSTTRAUMATIC STRESS DISORDER

Hypnosis can also be very effective in the management of patients who may have phobia due to previous bad medical experiences or have PTSD secondary to previous past procedures or treatment.

One of our patients was a 75-year-old married woman who had been recently diagnosed with breast cancer. She had discovered a "lump" in her breast a few months earlier, which she brought to her primary care physician's attention. He suspected breast cancer and immediately referred her to a surgeon in our institution. She was soon scheduled to undergo a needle biopsy. She informed him that she had suffered from claustrophobia all her life and didn't know whether she could tolerate a surgical procedure. He reassured her that "You will be sound asleep and will notice nothing."

She was admitted to the one-day surgical suite thinking, "Everything has been taken care of." Soon after arriving, she received her first "shock" when a nurse came into her area to place an IV line. The patient thought that someone would "give me something to take care of my anxiety." After the IV was in place, someone injected a "sedative" but she didn't feel any anxiety relief. Soon afterward her stretcher was wheeled to the surgical suite and before she had time to protest, her arms and legs were placed in restraints, she was draped, her face was covered, and then "the mask was placed." She recalls that as "the most traumatic experience in my life." For whatever reason she did not respond to the anesthesia well and remembers being conscious "most of the time."

After surgery she was shaken. In fact, she exhibited many symptoms of PTSD. One thing was clear in her mind: "I will never go through this again." A few days later, when she went to the surgeon's office to get the results of her biopsy, she was informed that she had cancer and would need further treatment. Her options were a lumpectomy followed by radiation therapy or a radical mastectomy. She knew two things: she didn't want to have further surgery. But if she needed surgery, she wanted to "preserve the breast if she could," so she decided to explore the first option.

She made an appointment with the radiation oncology clinic for an evaluation as part of the lumpectomy/XRT treatment plan. When she arrived at the hospital she found that the XRT Clinic was in the basement of the building. It took her over three hours of pain and agony in the lobby "trying to force myself to get down there." Finally, the social worker for the oncology service found her and brought her down. As she walked through the unit the patient had a panic attack. Frightened and anxious, she ran out of the building and decided she could not go through the treatment. Her surgeon was notified of the events and he quickly called her. She informed him that she "couldn't do it."

After much talking over the phone, the patient agreed to "think about it for a while." When 2 months had passed with no news from the patient, the surgeon called her again and stressed the need to do something quickly. The patient asked for some more time. The surgeon gave her one more week to think about it. A week later, the surgeon called her again to find out her decision. If she could not undergo radiation therapy (XRT), she needed to do the radical mastectomy as soon as possible. She dreaded this alternative as much as the XRT, so she agreed to try the presurgical meeting with the radiation therapy group again. During her second visit to the XRT suite, the patient was greeted and escorted by a social worker and a nurse, who stayed with her the entire time. Nevertheless, once again the patient had a panic attack and left the unit before she could complete the necessary

pretreatment measurements. Finally a psychiatric consult was requested. It took her about 4 weeks to find the courage to make an appointment with my office.

I received her in the waiting room of our office building. It took her about 10 minutes to walk from the receiving area to the end of the hallway leading to my office. This walk usually takes me one minute or less. During this walk her anxiety and discomfort were evident. Once in my office she insisted that the door and the window blinds remain open. Similarly, she requested that the blinds to my windows be wide open. During my initial interview with her she made clear that she had suffered from claustrophobia all her life, but had always managed it by altering her life in a way that she was always able to avoid claustrophobic situations. For example, she had never taken an elevator in her life, and her husband did all the shopping.

Nevertheless, she remained very functional, managing a small 3-storey apartment building. She reported a remarkably small number of panic attacks given her extreme agoraphobia and claustrophobia. She had managed to do so well because, "I knew what to do. I would never force myself into those situations." This was the first time in her life when she found herself completely "out of control." She also described classic PTSD symptoms following her painful experience during her last operation. She had experienced flashbacks, recurrent dreams, and autonomic reactivity by just thinking of a radiation machine or lying on a medical table.

We discussed her biopsy, the XRT suite, and the events leading to the referral. She made it clear that she would like to "preserve the breast," but "I don't think I could go through it again." Worse yet, she not only would not go back to the XRT suite but she had up made her mind that she couldn't go through surgery, either. We discussed her treatment options including the use of medication, psychotherapy, and/or hypnosis. Given the fact that it had taken so much time to get to me, we were running out of time. Her surgeon had made it clear during our conversation that she should have initiated treatment weeks ago. She expressed a terrifying fear of medication side effects, "especially those that control the mind."

Finally, she agreed to try hypnosis as an alternative. We discussed how hypnosis might help control some of her anxiety and at the same time allow her to regain some of the control she felt she had lost over her mind, her body, and her life. Like many phobic patients she proved to be a highly hypnotizable subject. She scored a 10 on the 10-point HIP scale. Over the following 3 weeks I saw her four times. During those sessions she learned to use self-hypnosis and to dissociate from unpleasant environments. In fact, she used self-hypnotic exercises to "practice going through surgery and being in the XRT suite."

During the third and fourth weeks we worked on the surgery phobia. She had multiple unpleasant memories of her first surgery. The idea of been placed on the operating room table was unbearable. She could not even conceive the idea of being tied to the table and placed under anesthesia. A new phobia, to be intubated, had been developed.

She practiced under hypnosis coming to the hospital, sitting in the waiting room, changing into the hospital gown, going into the surgical suite, and inducing a self-hypnotic trance before "being put to sleep." Under hypnosis she put herself into a trance.

She also imagined that she played the role of the anesthetist. In her mind, she intubated herself and she operated the gas and drips. Thus she had complete control over what was going on. Finally, toward the end of the fourth week, she underwent a lumpectomy. We worked in concert with the anesthesiologist who was fully aware of what we were doing. He allowed her time to put herself under. After she gave him the signal that she was ready, as we had discussed, he walked her through the procedure. The patient did beautifully in surgery.

After surgery we were faced with the real test, a prolonged course of XRT. By now the patient had mastered the use of self-hypnosis, but now she had to deal with confined spaces, loud machines, and prolonged periods of isolation for the next 3 months. During weeks 5 to 7 while she was recovering from the surgery, we had time to prepare, and we worked intently on her claustrophobia and panic attacks. She was then able to use her self-hypnosis exercise to undergo the first treatment of the 3-month, five-times-a-week radiation therapy course.

Not only did she do well during this surgery and subsequent course of radiation treatment, but about a year later this patient was faced with an additional surgical procedure when a follow-up mammogram revealed another mass. Once again, after a single hypnosis session, the patient was able to undergo the biopsy procedure without any difficulty. Fortunately, the mass was benign and no further treatment was required.

CONVERSION DISORDERS

As first suggested by Janet (1907), it is our belief that the symptoms of conversion disorder can be understood in part as reflecting the presence of uncontrolled hypnotic states. Studies have already reported that conversion patients are very hypnotizable (an average 9.7 on the HIP 12-point scale [Bliss, 1984]) Others have corroborated that conversion patients are more highly hypnotizable than the population at large (Maldonado, 1996, 1997; Maldonado & Jasiukaitis, 2003). For example, studies suggest that the percentage of the general population that is highly hypnotizable is between 20%–30% compared to about 69% in patients suffering from psychogenic seizures (Peterson, Sumner, et al., 1950; Peterson, Sumner & Jones, 1950). Maldonado and colleagues have hypothesized that patients suffering from a conversion disorder may indeed be using their own capacity to dissociate in order to displace the uncomfortable feelings or affects into a chosen part of the body, which then becomes dysfunctional (Maldonado, 1996, 1997; Maldonado & Jasiukaitis, 2003).

Even though most patients are not aware of it, highly hypnotizable individuals have an unusual capacity to control (albeit unconsciously) somatic functions. This is evident by the high hypnotizability levels observed in subjects experiencing psychosomatic disorders and conversion reactions. Years ago, Charcot correctly reported an association between conversion disorder and high hypnotic capacity (1890). However, he incorrectly assumed that they both indicated similar central nervous system dysfunction. The symptoms of conversion disorder can be understood in part as reflecting the presence of uncontrolled hypnotic states. Indeed, hypnosis may be useful in both the diagnosis and treatment of many psychosomatic

illnesses and conversion symptoms (Maldonado, 1996, 2007; Maldonado & Spiegel, 2000; Maldonado & Jasiukaitis, 2003)

Hypnosis by itself is not treatment. It should always be used as an adjuvant to, rather than in lieu of, medical treatment. In cases of conversion symptoms and psychosomatic processes, hypnosis is used not to treat but to allow patients to control the effects on their bodies of their emotional stress and mind states. It is not advised to force a cure in a patient. Rather, patients are trained in the use of self-hypnotic techniques and then allowed to improve at a pace that feels comfortable, while the clinician provides suggestions for improved control and mastery and explores the unconscious psychological reasons behind the presence of symptoms, including the possibility of secondary gain.

When considering the treatment of conversion disorders, hypnosis may be useful in two ways. First, it may assist in confirming the diagnosis. Second, it may be therapeutic (i.e., part of a comprehensive treatment plan that includes therapy to help the patient develop more mature and adaptive defense mechanisms; see (Maldonado, 2007). Clinicians treating patients with conversion symptoms must pay attention to verbal and nonverbal cues given to the patient. It is also not unusual for patients with conversion to present wide variations of symptoms during the course of a session. In fact, during a hypnotic induction the clinician may bring on symptoms, worsen, or ameliorate them. Even though it may be tempting to "cure your patient," you must be aware that premature "cures" (i.e., before the patient feels safe and has developed the necessary tools to deal with whatever emotional distress caused the conversion to begin with) usually are followed by the development of symptom substitution. Also, educate the professionals for whom you are consulting to make certain they do not give the patient the message that the problem is "all in your head." There are several steps to be considered (Maldonado, 2007) in the comprehensive treatment of patients with conversion disorder (see Box 16.1). The first step is a thorough neurological and medical evaluation, given the high comorbidity between conversion diagnoses and organic conditions (Krumholz & Niedermeyer, 1983; Barsky, 1989). The second step is timely diagnosis. Studies show a 6-year to 8-year delay before the diagnosis of conversion disorder is made (Bowman, 1993), usually because of previous misdiagnosis of and treatment for medical, neurological, or other psychiatric conditions. The failure to make a timely diagnosis and the use of excessive diagnostic tests or inappropriate treatments may lead to iatrogenic problems or may "validate" the patient's perceived deficits. Some treatments, particularly psychoactive medications (e.g., anticonvulsants, benzodiazepines, barbiturates, antipsychotics) may worsen conversion symptoms by causing neurological side effects (e.g., balance problems, memory deficits) and promote dissociative states (e.g., depersonalization, derealization, mental slowing).

The third step involves the therapeutic reassurance by both sets of doctors (i.e., internist or neurologist and therapist) that there is a good level of certainty that the symptoms are not due to a deadly medical or neurological condition (e.g., "you don't have a brain tumor," "you don't have a seizure disorder") but are secondary to underlying psychological factors. Usually, an explanation of the mind/body interaction and how unconscious and psychological processes may affect the body in more common medical conditions is of help. Patients often feel reassured when physicians explain that psychological factors, pressures, and stress can create havoc in the body and be as serious nevertheless, thus in need of prompt attention.

The fourth step involves the development of a coordinated effort by both sets of clinicians that ensures the patient does not fall through the cracks, that no unnecessary tests and procedures are performed, medications that may worsen symptoms are not prescribed, and the mind/body connection is continuously reinforced. The fifth step is continuous surveillance to accurately diagnose and aggressively treat any comorbid psychiatric disorder. This is particularly important given the high comorbidity between conversion disorder and other Axis-I disorders (especially mood, anxiety, dissociative, and other somatoform disorders). The most common psychiatric diagnoses are major depressive disorder and dissociative disorders, both of which have been found in about 85% of acute conversion cases (Ziegler, Imboden, et al., 1960; Roy, 1980; Bowman, 1993).

The sixth (and last step) involves working through the patients' defenses and helping them develop more mature and adaptive defense mechanisms to prevent the development of future conversion episodes. The ultimate goal is the development of an appropriate level of control and mastery. This can be achieved with any number of psychotherapeutic modalities, but hypnotically facilitated psychotherapy is particularly useful and effective (Maldonado, 2007).

The use of hypnosis in the treatment of conversion disorder itself involves several phases (Maldonado & Spiegel, 2002; Maldonado, 2007). The first phase involves exploring the meaning of the symptoms: it is important never to eliminate a symptom fully without understanding its purpose and replacing it with a more mature and adaptive defense. The second phase involves symptom alteration—that is, taking the patient's mind away from the presenting symptoms while allowing him or her to find more appropriate ways to cope with anxiety. This may be accomplished by *prescribed symptom substitution,* in which a given symptom is exchanged for another that is less impairing or pathological until the patient is ready to give up the original symptom (e.g., changing the perception of intense cancer pain to a numbing, tingling sensation in the same area), or by *symptom extinction,* in which the patient agrees to "give up" the symptom after working through the problem in psychotherapy. The third phase involves maximizing the patient's level of functioning. Hypnosis may be used to increase the patient's motivation, enhance his or her sense of mastery, and strengthen his or her defenses.

BEHAVIOR MODIFICATION

PRIMARY INSOMNIA

Even though the word *hypnosis* literally means sleep, hypnosis is not a form of sleep and it is not related to sleep. In fact, if you fall asleep you come out of trance. Nevertheless, because hypnosis can be helpful in inducing a state of physical relaxation and because by focusing intently on a pleasant scene you can avoid your mind wandering about the many problems causing sleep disturbance, it may facilitate a state of physiological sleep. In fact, the hypnotic experience can create a state of physical relaxation which in turn may diminish sympathetic tone. The hypnotic trance may provide patients a structured way of managing preoccupation with anxiety-producing problems, thereby facilitating entrance into a restful sleep.

After inducing a state of self-hypnosis, patients are taught to create a sensation of buoyancy, floating, or any other sensation that they associate with physical relaxation. Images such as floating on an inflatable mattress in a pool, or floating down the river on an inner tube could be rather effective. After patients are successful at this exercise they may proceed to put their worries or thoughts on hold for tonight, knowing that they can always deal with them tomorrow. There are a number of imagery techniques that patients can use to put problems on hold. For example, patients can project these thoughts onto an imaginary screen, and then imagine either changing the content of the screen (as you would change television channels), putting the podcast on pause, or simply turning it off.

Subjects can also imagine themselves sitting by a riverbank observing leaves flowing down the stream. They can then imagine themselves placing their thoughts over the leaves and watching them floating away, not holding on to any particular thought, while allowing the body to feel progressively relaxed; or they may imagine themselves lying restfully in a comfortable and safe place while they see themselves placing the disturbing thoughts onto the clouds, watching the breeze slowly carrying them away.

It is important to point out that any hypnotic approach should be accompanied by sound sleep hygiene practices.

These include going to bed always at the same time, avoiding large meals or exercise just prior to bedtime, keeping the bedroom as a place to sleep, avoiding doing work or reading in bed, and avoiding looking at the clock when awakened. It is important to trace the source of the problem, differentiating primary insomnia from sleep disturbances that occur secondary to physiological disorders such as sleep apnea, or serious psychiatric conditions such as major depression or anxiety disorders.

There are very few research data available on the efficacy of hypnosis in the treatment of sleep disorders (Bauer & McCanne, 1980; Stanton, 1989; Nielsen, 1990; Becker, 1993). Most of the literature is limited to case reports, or studies with such a small sample that it is difficult to interpret the results. Yet, they have reported that 50% of patients suffering from chronic dyssomnia experienced improvement in their sleep patterns lasting over 16 months after a simple 2-session treatment course (Becker, 1993). The largest reported study included 45 patients treated with hypnosis, stimulus control, or placebo (Staton, 1989). It demonstrated significant improvement in early insomnia in the hypnosis group compared to comparators. Few formal studies have been reported, but most case reports suggest that hypnosis is useful in the treatment not only of primary insomnia but other sleep disturbances as well (Bauer & McCanne, 1980; Schenck & Mahowald, 1995).

SMOKING CESSATION

Effective smoking cessation consists of pharmacotherapy and behavioral support. Counseling increases abstinence rates parallel to the intensity of support. Nearly 100 articles dealing with the topic can be found in the published literature, all suggesting that hypnosis is useful in assisting in nicotine abstinence. Nearly half have been published in the last decade.

A meta-analysis demonstrated that unassisted smoking cessation (i.e., "cold turkey") has been reported to have a low success rate of as little as 7.3% at 10-month follow-up (Baillie, Mattick, et al., 1995) A *Cochrane* review examined pooled data from 17 trials of brief advice versus no advice (or usual care) and found an unassisted quit rate of 2% to 3%, and that a brief advice intervention can increase quitting by a further 1% to 3% (Stead, Bergson, et al., 2008).

First-line pharmacological drugs for smoking cessation include nicotine replacement therapies (i.e., patch, gum, inhaler, nasal spray, lozenge/tablets), the nicotinic acetylcholine receptor partial agonist (i.e., varenicline) and antagonists (i.e., bupropion) with scientifically well documented efficacy when used for 2–3 months and mostly mild side effects. Nicotine replacement therapy has a 12%–25% efficacy after 16 weeks on active treatment, but the abstinent rate drops to 17% at 1-year follow-up off active treatment (Tonnesen, Norregaard, et al., 1991). The newer agents have results. For weeks 9 through 12, the 4-week continuous abstinence rates were 44.0% for varenicline versus 17.7% for placebo (*P*<.001) and versus 29.5% for bupropion SR (*P*<.001). But for weeks 9 through 52, the continuous abstinence rates were 21.9% for varenicline versus 8.4% for placebo (*P*<.001) and versus 16.1%

for bupropion SR (Gonzales, Rennard, et al., 2006). In summary, the data suggests that at present, with the most optimal drugs and counseling, a 1-year abstinence rate is approximately 25% (Tonnesen, 2009).

Studies show that the success rate in cigarette cessation after hypnotic treatment ranges from 20% to 64% (Crasilneck & Hall, 1968; Spiegel, 1970; Hyman, Stanley, et al., 1986; Schwartz, 1987; Williams & Hall, 1988). These abstinence rates are superior to the rates of unassisted quitting (Gritz & Bloom, 1987). The success rate depends on a number of factors, including the patient's motivation and hypnotizability as well as the therapist's expertise. A variation of the single-session treatment approach, consisting of one to five sessions with or without the use of audiotapes or self-hypnotic training, as needed, is widely used in medical settings (Dengrove, Nuland, et al., 1970; Spiegel, 1970; Pederson, Scrimgeour, et al., 1975; Watkins, 1976; Stanton, 1978, 1991; Berkowitz, Ross-Townsend, et al., 1979; Javel, 1980; Rabkin, Boyko, et al., 1984; Barabasz, Baer, et al., 1986; Frank, Umlauf, et al., 1986; Hyman, Stanley, et al., 1986; Neufeld & Lynn, 1988; Williams & Hall, 1988; Elkins & Rajab, 2004)

The single-session approach (Spiegel, 1970) emphasizes training a susceptible subject on the use of self-hypnosis rather than relying on endless hypnotic sessions induced by a physician. The goal is to teach individuals to tap into their ability to enter a self-hypnotic trance, then provide them with a strategy that is intrinsically self-reinforcing (Spiegel & Spiegel, 1987). This allows patients to practice the technique whenever the urge to smoke comes. It uses cognitive restructuring to emphasize how the act of smoking is destructive to the body and how the effects of smoking limit what one can do with one's life due to a shortened life span and deteriorating quality of life. Repetitive self-hypnotic experiences are used to emphasize patients' commitment to protect their bodies from the poison in cigarettes.

The approach is based on the cognitive restructuring model. It involves emphasizing that smoking is destructive specifically to the patient's body and thereby limits what he or she can do. The focus during hypnosis is then placed on protecting the patient's body from poison in the same way that the patient would protect an infant or a pet from ingesting noxious food. This approach enables the patient to balance the urge to smoke against the urge to protect the body from damage. In other words, the focus is on what the patient is *for* rather than what he or she is *against* (Spiegel, 1970).

This method also reinforces the idea of self-control. The patient is trained in self-hypnosis and on how to think, rather than to avoid thinking about smoking. Once the technique has been learned, it is up to the patient to use it or not. Initially patients are asked to practice the technique a few times a day at prescribed times, plus at any other time the patient experiences nicotine cravings. Later on, as patients become more proficient and have less craving they are instructed to use the technique whenever they feel the urge to smoke. This approach requires that patients examine their priorities and balance their urge to smoke against the need to protect the body from the damage caused by further smoking. Smokers are instructed to focus on what they are for (i.e., protecting their bodies) rather than what they are against (i.e., smoking). Thus, while there is no evidence that treatments using hypnosis are more effective than other interventions for smoking, they may well be more efficient in that they enable patients to employ self-hypnosis to reinforce a cognitive restructuring strategy, while at the same time providing an episode of physical relaxation. Strategies for smoking cessation, including the use of medications, are discussed in chapter 53.

WEIGHT MANAGEMENT

Unlike the case of hypnosis intervention for smoking cessation, there are few data on the long-term effects of hypnosis for weight control. Clinical experience suggests that patients who are within 20% of their ideal body weight may obtain the most benefit from restructuring techniques that use self-hypnosis in combination with a medical regimen.

A meta-analysis performed on 18 studies in which a cognitive behavioral therapy (CBT) was compared with the same therapy supplemented by hypnosis indicated that the addition of hypnosis substantially enhanced CBT's outcome (Kirsch, Montgomery, et al., 1995) In fact, the analysis suggested that the average client receiving cognitive behavioral hypnotherapy showed greater improvement than at least 70% of clients receiving nonhypnotic treatment. Effects seemed particularly pronounced for treatments of obesity, especially at long-term follow-up, indicating that unlike those in nonhypnotic treatment, clients to whom hypnotic inductions had been administered continued to lose weight after treatment ended.

Similarly, various studies suggested a significant correlation between hypnotizability scores and weight reduction (Andersen, 1985; Kirsch, Montgomery, et al., 1995; Kirsch, 1996) A meta-analysis of the effects of CBTs and hypnosis for weight reduction found that the mean weight loss in the group using CBT plus hypnosis was twice that of the group treated with CBT alone—in other words, the mean weight loss was 6.03 lbs. (2.74 kg) in the CBT/nonhypnosis and 14.88 lbs. (6.75 kg) in the CBT plus hypnosis, with an effect size of of 0.98 SD (Kirsch, 1996). Correlational analyses suggested that the benefits of hypnosis increased substantially over time (r = .74). For example, in a study of 109 subjects who completed a behavioral treatment with or without hypnosis, the hypnosis group experienced significant additional weight loss at the 8-month and 2-year follow-ups, while those in the behavioral treatment exhibited little further change. Moreover, the subjects who used hypnosis were better able to achieve and maintain their personal weight goals (Bolocofsky, Spinler, et al., 1985).

When hypnosis is used for weight management, it must be applied within the context of a comprehensive medical treatment plan that includes sensible eating habits and an exercise program tailored to the patient's needs and capabilities. Just as in the case of smoking cessation, the goal of hypnosis is to restructure the patient's experience around food and eating practices. The intent is that the patient will modify his or her perception of food and understand what new approaches are for (e.g., lower body weight, healthier lifestyle, better controlled blood sugars and blood pressure) and not what they

are against (e.g., food). In addition, hypnosis can be used to help patients provide positive self-reinforcement for compliance with a revised eating regimen (Crasilneck & Hall, 1985).

During the course of psychotherapy, in and out of hypnotic trance, patients are asked to examine their relationship with food and their food intake practices and to consider the damaging effects of overeating or starvation on their bodies. The ultimate purpose is to restructure the eating experience so that it becomes an exercise about learning to eat with respect for one's body. Once again, the emphasis is on what the patient is for rather than what he or she is against.

When used as part of a weight loss program, the most important component of this approach consists in teaching patients how to use self-hypnosis to control their eating patterns. Patients are asked to prepare a list of foods that are consistent with their goals and their commitment to eating with respect for their bodies. Patients are then asked to compare their craving to eat with their stated goals and the healthy items they placed in their list. If the desired food is on the list, the patient is encouraged to eat it like a gourmet, focusing intently on all aspects of the eating experience and enjoying it. If the food is not on the list, the patient is asked to recognize the desire for it rather than to fight it or ignore it. At that point, the patient uses self-hypnosis to examine this urge in light of the commitment to protect and treat the body with respect and, therefore, to eat with respect.

Using this method, patients see their desire to eat not as an occasion to feel deprived, but rather as an occasion to enhance their mastery over their urges by choosing to protect their bodies. The use of self-hypnosis also allows patients to learn to respond in a planned way rather than to react to somatic signals of hunger and satiety—to eat when they are hungry but stop eating as soon as they are satisfied. But hypnotic capacity may play an even deeper role.

The literature suggests that aspects of hypnotizability may be involved in the etiology and maintenance of self-defeating eating. There may be further relationships between weight, shape, dietary concerns, hypnotizability, dissociative capacity, and fantasy proneness that are not fully understood (Hutchinson-Phillips, Gow, et al., 2007). A study of 102 female college students (mean age 21) completed the Eating Attitudes Test and the Goldfarb Fear-of-Fat Scale and were assessed for hypnotizability on the Harvard Group Scale of Hypnotic Susceptibility (Groth-Marnat & Schumaker, 1990). The results indicated that level of hypnotizability was related to attitudes toward food intake and the fear of becoming overweight, and support the thesis that hypnotizability may be one of a variety of predisposing factors in the development and maintenance of extreme attitudes toward eating and weight regulation.

One thing to consider is that the approach to all forms of disordered eating should not be the same. For example, patients suffering from bulimia have been found to be significantly more hypnotizable than control subjects (p < .003; Covino, Jimerson, et al., 1994). Not surprisingly, they have also scored higher on self-report scales of dissociative experiences (p <.02). These results are consistent with previous reports on hospitalized patients and college students and suggest that psychological factors associated with hypnotizability might play a role in the etiology and treatment of bulimia nervosa (Kranhold, Baumann, et al., 1992). In that regard, a psychotherapeutic regimen that includes hypnotic exploration and training in self-hypnosis to promote self-control would be recommended. Chapter 32 outlines a comprehensive approach to weight control and reduction.

DENTISTRY

Hypnosis has long been used to advantage in dentistry as (1) an adjunct to dental procedures and in the management of dental phobia (Lu, 1994; Rustvold, 1994; Wilks, 1994; Hammarstrand, Berggren, et al., 1995; Moore, Abrahamsen, et al., 1996; Peretz, 1996; Robb & Crothers, 1996; Shaw & Niven, 1996; Shaw & Welbury, 1996; Kroll, 1962; Seidner, 1967; Gall, 1969; Smith, 1969; McAmmond, Davidson, et al., 1971; Newman, 1973; 1974; Benson, 1974, 1975; Lucas, 1975; Schey, 1976; Weyandt, 1976; Kevesater, 1977; Kisby, 1977, 1978; Romanson & Clark, 1981; Fassbind, 1983; Reis e Almeida, 1983; Katcher, Segal, et al., 1984; Smith, 1986; Forgione, 1988; Schmierer & Schmierer, 1990; Moore, Brodsgaard, et al., 2002; Gaspar, Linninger, et al., 2003); (2) an analgesic (or adjuvant to analgesic) for minor dental procedures (Herod, 1995; Enqvist, Bjorklund, et al., 1997); (3) the sole method of analgesia for patients with a history of hypersensitivity to local anesthetic agents (Kleinhauz & Eli, 1993); and (4) for the treatment of associated painful conditions such as temporomandibular dysfunction (Golan, 1989; Oakley, McCreary, et al., 1994; Simon & Lewis, 2000) and bruxism (LaCrosse, 1994).

It has been helpful for periodontal disease (Wood & Zadeh, 1999), promotion of routine flossing (Kelly, McKinty, et al., 1988), excessive gagging (Morse, Hancock, et al., 1984), placement of dental implants (Gheorghiu & Orleanu, 1982), dental extractions (McCay, 1963; Lucas, 1965), and psychogenic oral pain (Golan, 1997).

HYPNOSIS IN PEDIATRIC CARE

All children are highly hypnotizable, and hypnotic interventions can be very useful in the care of the pediatric patient. Several authors have also reported on the usefulness of hypnotic interventions in a variety of pediatric problems (Dikel & Olness, 1980; Olness, 1981; Olness & MacDonald, 1981; Place, 1984; Lambert, 1996, 1999).

Various researchers have described their experiences treating a large number of adolescents and children (n = 505) with hypnosis (Kohen, Olness, et al., 1984; Kohen, 1986, 1987; Kohen & Wynne, 1997). The problems treated included enuresis, acute pain, chronic pain, asthma, habit disorders, obesity, encopresis, and anxiety. In this population, half of the sample (51%) achieved complete resolution of the presenting symptom after hypnotic intervention (Kohen, Olness, et al., 1984). In addition, another third (32%) achieved significant improvement. Hypnotic interventions were used with

children as young as 3 years old. Impressively, their results suggest that maximum benefit was achieved after only four visits.

Similarly, others have described the usefulness of hypnosis in the management of side effects associated with the treatment of cancer in pediatric patients such as nausea and vomiting, fear, and discomfort (Olness, 1981; Gardner & Lubman, 1982; Hall, 1982; Hilgard & LeBaron, 1982; Redd, Andresen, et al., 1982; Zeltzer & LeBaron, 1982; Kellerman, Zeltzer, et al., 1983; Zeltzer, Kellerman, et al., 1983; Kaye, 1984; Hockenberry & Cotanch, 1985; Katz, Kellerman, et al., 1987; Fortuin, 1988; Hageman-Wenselaar, 1988; Feldman & Salzberg, 1990; Zeltzer, Dolgin, et al., 1991; Morrow & Hickok, 1993; Ellen & Burrows, 1994; Ellis & Spanos, 1994; Jacknow, Tschann, et al., 1994; Genuis, 1995; Keller, 1995; Spiegel & Moore, 1997; Steggles, Damore-Petingola, et al., 1997; Bertoni, Bonardi, et al., 1999; Liossi & Hatira, 1999; Lynch, 1999; Marchioro, Azzarello, et al., 2000; Wild & Espie, 2004; Richardson, Smith, et al., 2006). In pediatric cancer patients, hypnosis has been demonstrated to be useful as adjunct in invasive procedures, such as bone marrow aspirations and lumbar punctures (Hageman-Wenselaar, 1988; Ellis & Spanos, 1994; Rape & Bush, 1994; Liossi & Hatira, 1999). The use of hypnosis in these cases lowered pediatric morbidity by removing exposure to sedative hypnotic and anxiolytic agents. It also diminished later anxiety to multiple invasive examinations common in patients suffering from hematologic and malignant diseases. The use of imagery and hypnotic techniques with suggestions for a favorable postoperative course has been associated with significantly lower postoperative pain ratings and shorter hospital stays (Lambert, 1996, 1999).

Several randomized controlled studies on behavioral intervention for chemotherapy in children with cancer have found that children in the hypnosis group had the greatest reduction of both anticipatory and post-chemotherapy symptoms compared to controls (Zeltzer & LeBaron, 1982; Zeltzer, Kellerman, et al., 1983; Zeltzer, LeBaron, et al., 1984; Zeltzer, Dolgin, et al., 1991; Steggles, Damore-Petingola, et al., 1997). The cognitive distraction/relaxation intervention appeared to have a maintenance effect in which symptoms did not get much worse or much better, while children in the control group had symptoms that consistently became worse over time.

A prospective randomized and controlled single-blind trial of pediatric patients among cancer patients receiving chemotherapy found that those randomized to the hypnosis group used less PRN antiemetic medication than control subjects (p < .02). In addition, the hypnosis group experienced less anticipatory nausea than the control group at 1 to 2 month after diagnosis (p < .02; Jacknow, Tschann, et al., 1994).

Hypnosis has been used successfully in children to significantly reduce the pain associated with invasive procedures (Hilgard & LeBaron, 1982; Rape & Bush, 1994). In fact, hypnosis was superior to an attentional control condition for analgesia among children undergoing painful procedures (Zeltzer & LeBaron, 1982). A prospective randomized study assigned 44 children scheduled for an upcoming voiding cystourethrography (VCUG) to receive hypnosis (n = 21) or routine care (n = 23) while undergoing the procedure (Butler, Symons, et al., 2005). Eligible children and parents met with the research assistant (RA) before the day of the scheduled procedure for an initial assessment. Immediately after this assessment, those who were randomized to the hypnosis condition were given a 1-hour training session by a trained therapist in self-hypnotic visual imagery. Parents and children were instructed to practice using the imaginative self-hypnosis procedure several times a day in preparation for the upcoming procedure. The therapist was also present during the procedure to conduct similar exercises with the child. Results indicate significant benefits for the hypnosis group compared with the routine care group in the following 4 areas: (1) parents of children in the hypnosis group compared with those in the routine care group reported that the procedure was significantly less traumatic for their children compared with their previous VCUG procedure; (2) observational ratings of typical distress levels during the procedure were significantly lower for children in the hypnosis condition compared with those in the routine care condition; (3) medical staff reported a significant difference between groups in the overall difficulty of conducting the procedure, with less difficulty reported for the hypnosis group; and (4) total procedural time was significantly shorter—by almost 14 minutes—for the hypnosis group compared with the routine care group. Moderate to large effect sizes were obtained on each of these four outcomes.

Among 75 children with urological diseases (i.e., in patients with total epispadias, exstrophy, and trauma of the urinary bladder), postoperative hypnotherapy helped in training and restoration of micturition, as a result of which a second operative intervention was not needed (Shulman, 1995).

Because children are highly hypnotizable and are easily absorbed in images, the main focus for children undergoing painful procedures is on imagery rather than relaxation. Images can be as simple as suggesting that they are playing an imaginary baseball game, picturing themselves going to another room in the house, or imagining themselves watching a favorite cartoon or television show. This enables them to restructure their experience of what is going on and dissociate themselves psychologically from pain and fear of the procedure.

Hypnosis has been long reported as a useful tool in the management of asthma and dyspnea in children (Aronoff, Aronoff, et al., 1975; Kohen, Olness, et al., 1984; Kohen, 1987; Kohen and Wynne, 1997; Anbar, 2000, 2001, 2003). Like their adult counterparts, asthmatic children treated with hypnosis reported a significant (50%) improvement in their symptoms (Aronoff, Aronoff, et al., 1975). Others have described that 20% of asthma patients (children between the ages of 2 and 5 years) experienced "complete symptom resolution" and an additional 33% experienced a "considerable improvement in symptoms" after hypnotic treatment and training (Collison, 1975; Kohen, Olness, et al., 1984; Gluzman & Ziselson, 1987; Kohen, 1987; Kohen & Wynne, 1997). Yet others reported that hypnosis use (n = 303 children) was associated with improvement in 80% of patients with persistent asthma, chest pain/pressure, habit cough, hyperventilation, shortness of breath, sighing, and vocal

cord dysfunction (Anbar, 2002). No patients' symptoms worsened, and no new symptoms emerged following hypnotherapy.

Several authors have described the utility of hypnosis training in the management of chronic dyspnea (Anbar, 2001). On a small retrospective study, 16 patients were taught to use self-hypnosis in one session. A second session was provided to three patients within 2 months. Thirteen of 16 subjects reported their dyspnea and any associated symptoms had resolved within one month of their final hypnosis instruction session. Eleven believed that resolution of their dyspnea was attributable to hypnosis, because their symptoms cleared immediately after they received hypnosis instruction or with its regular use. The remaining three reported that their dyspnea had improved. Patients were followed for a mean 9 months (range: 2–15 months) after their final hypnosis session. Ten of the 16 regularly used self-hypnosis at home for at least one month after the final hypnosis session. There was no recurrence of dyspnea, associated symptoms, or onset of new symptoms in patients in whom the dyspnea resolved. Under supervision of the pediatric pulmonologist, two of seven patients discontinued their chronic antiinflammatory therapy when they became asymptomatic after hypnosis.

Others have reported on the use of hypnosis in children with cystic fibrosis (Belsky & Khanna, 1994). The experimental group demonstrated significant changes in locus of control, health locus of control, self-concept, and trait anxiety, and significantly increased peak expiratory flow rates using an air flow meter immediately after self-hypnosis when compared to the control group.

Hypnosis has also been used for the treatment of nocturnal enuresis (Krupnova, 1985; Banerjee, Srivastav, et al., 1993). When compared with imipramine, hypnotic suggestions for the management of functional nocturnal enuresis had equally positive response (i.e., all dry beds, with 76% on imipramine vs. 72% in the hypnosis group). Nevertheless, during a 9-month follow-up, 68% of patients in the hypnosis group maintained a positive response whereas only 24% of the imipramine group did (Banerjee, Srivastav, et al., 1993).

Hypnosis has been reported to be successful with various childhood dermatological disorders such as eczema (Mantle, 1999) and psoriasis (Winchell & Watts, 1988). There have been reports of a 95% "immediate improvement" of severe resistant atopic dermatitis with the use of hypnosis, which was maintained for up to 18 months after treatment (Stewart & Thomas, 1995).

The use of hypnosis for the treatment of warts in children has long been established (Mc, 1949; Wendel, 1959; Seeman, 1960; Dudek, 1967; Leidman Iu, 1968, 1973; Tasini & Hackett, 1977; Wilkening, 1978; Noll, 1988). An intriguing case reported the use of hypnosis for the treatment a 7-year-old female with 82 common warts. The lesions had been present for 12–18 months and were refractory to routine dermatologic treatment. Hypnotic suggestions were given for the facial warts to disappear before warts from the rest of the body. After 2 weeks, eight of 16 facial warts were gone, with no other changes. After three additional biweekly sessions, all 82 warts were gone (Noll, 1988).

A prospective randomized controlled study found that children could be trained in self-hypnosis with specific suggestions for control of salivary IgA (p < .01), although there were no significant changes in salivary IgG (Olness, Culbert, et al., 1989). Several papers have reported on beneficial hypnosis treatment in the management of other medical disorders in pediatric patients including headaches management (Kuttner, 1993) and migraine (Olness & MacDonald, 1981), functional abdominal pain, and irritable bowel syndrome (Vlieger, Menko-Frankenhuis, et al., 2007).

FURTHER INFORMATION, TRAINING, CERTIFICATION, AND REFERRALS

The two factors to consider are (1) does your patient suffer from a condition amenable to hypnotic intervention, and (2) is your patient hypnotizable? If the answer to both questions is positive, the next question is, should you use hypnosis? If you are trained in the use of hypnosis within the context of psychotherapy or your psychosomatic training, you are on your way to assisting your patients to develop mastery over their symptoms by providing them with a valuable tool to explore and control what they experience.

If, on the other hand, you are not skilled in the use of hypnotic skills you may need to refer the patient to a practitioner or therapist who is. And you are not alone. Unfortunately, the number of clinicians and psychiatrists well trained in hypnosis is very small. In a study of 400 physicians in central Texas, the majority of physicians (79%) and residents (67%) had received no prior training, and even fewer had experienced hypnosis themselves (Elkins & Wall, 1996). This study highlighted the need for patient and physician education, given the high rate of endorsed misconceptions about hypnosis held by patients and medical practitioners alike. On the other hand, it was somewhat encouraging to find that 85% of medical practitioners expressed interest in learning more about hypnosis.

Unfortunately, hypnosis training is widely variable within psychiatric residency programs and is dependent on the faculty and training director interests within each individual training program (Walling & Baker, 1996; Walling, Baker, et al., 1996). In a nationwide survey of all psychiatric residency directors in the United States, 63% of responding program directors report offering either required or elective courses in hypnosis. Yet, of the programs offering hypnosis training, the mean number of hours provided was 8 over the course during the 4-year residency program. This would suggest that many psychiatrists have only rudimentary understanding and training, and a very limited exposure to hypnosis during their formative years. The limited training is not standardized and likely inadequate to allow psychiatric trainees to be proficient or comfortable in the use of hypnosis in their clinical practice.

Despite the limited availability during residency, psychiatric residents seem to be interested in the topic. Studies show that 50% of interviewed psychiatric residents have sought additional hypnotherapy training beyond the standard lectures and seminars offered during by their residency programs, and almost 30% had attended external hypnosis workshops or presentations.

In the U.S. there are two reputable professional organizations providing training and fostering research in clinical hypnosis: the Society for Clinical and Experimental Hypnosis, which emphasizes research in the field, and the American Society for Clinical Hypnosis. Each of these organizations holds annual scientific meetings, publishes a journal, and offers well-organized regional and national workshops providing basic training seminars and advanced training courses. ASCH offers a board examination and certification in clinical hypnosis. Faculty members from Stanford University offer basic and advanced workshops in clinical hypnosis during the annual meeting of the American Psychiatric Association and the Academy of Psychosomatic Medicine. For more information, contact Jose Maldonado, MD, course director (650-725-5599), or call one of the professional organizations listed. There are many similar professional organizations in Europe and throughout the world, including the International Society for Hypnosis, the European Society of Hypnosis, the British Society of Clinical Hypnosis, and the Australian Society of Hypnosis.

There are many excellent books and chapters devoted to providing practitioners basic training in clinical hypnotic techniques, and specific instructions and hypnotic suggestions (Erickson, 1967; Crasilneck & Hall, 1985; Spiegel & Spiegel, 1987; Watkins, 1987; Hammond, 1990; Maldonado & Spiegel, 1996, 2002, 2008; Spiegel & Spiegel, 2004) Despite how comprehensive these may be, they are no substitute for hands-on training and professional supervision.

SUMMARY

Hypnosis is a natural human trait that can be measured, taught, and mastered. The ability to use this hypnotic capacity varies throughout the population. This natural capacity to enter hypnosis may be a liability in certain cases, such as phobic and conversion disorders, pain syndromes, and certain psychosomatic and medical conditions. Nevertheless, hypnosis may also be used during the medical therapeutic process to help patients deal with a number of psychological, psychosomatic, and medical conditions. Patients may learn this technique during brief sessions and continue to derive long-lasting benefits through the ongoing use of self-hypnosis exercises.

Hypnosis may enhance other therapeutic processes, such as physical therapy, that can speed recovery and response to treatment. Thus, aided by the use of hypnosis patients may gain a different perspective on the relationship between psychological and physical states. Physicians using hypnosis as adjuncts to their primary treatment modalities are encouraged to train their patients in the use of self-hypnosis. This facilitates an enhanced sense of mastery and independence in patients. It allows patients to use their hypnotic capacity, rather than be used by it.

CLINICAL PEARLS

- The hypnotic capacity or hypnotizability of a given subject (i.e., the degree of natural ability to enter a trance state) will determine the degree of assistance required to enter trance states.

- High hypnotic capacity may actually become a liability to patients who are unaware of their hypnotic capacity or of their unconscious use of this mechanism, as is the case of individuals suffering from a dissociative and somatoform disorder, or nocebo (i.e., negative placebo) effect.

- The hypnotic experience may be understood as involving three interconnecting factors: absorption, dissociation, and suggestibility.

    - **Absorption** refers to the tendency to engage in self-altering and highly focused attention with complete immersion in a central experience at the expense of contextual orientation (Hilgard, 1970; Tellegen & Atkinson, 1974; Tellegen, 1981).
    - **Dissociation** refers to the ability to separate mental processes so they seem to occur independently from each other.
    - **Suggestibility** implies the ability to influence someone's beliefs or behaviors by suggestion.

- Formal assessments of hypnotizability allow physicians to objectively determine the patient's level of hypnotic capacity.

- Hypnotizability is a rather stable trait.

- The Hypnotic Induction Profile (HIP) is a brief (5–7 minutes), standardized assessment designed to measure patients' natural ability to tap into and use their hypnotic capacity (Spiegel & Spiegel, 1987).

- For better or worse, highly hypnotizable individuals can enter trance states with ease and, on occasion, without even being fully aware of it. Thus it is important for physicians to know that some patients may experience trance states even without formal induction.

- A common technique is to have asthmatic patients enter a state of self-hypnosis and imagine that they are somewhere where they naturally breathe easily, such as breathing cool ocean spray (Spiegel & Spiegel, 1987).

- Most patients who use hypnoanalgesia can still feel the pain but may be unable to distinguish between the signal of pain and the discomfort caused by the signal. Thus, patients are taught not to fight but to transform painful signals into less uncomfortable ones.

- Regardless of any specific induction or metaphor use, there are four specific steps in the use of hypnosis that can make psychotherapy for pain management briefer, more goal-oriented, and efficient:

    - the assessment of hypnotizability;
    - the induction of hypnoanalgesia and development of individualized pain coping strategies;
    - the use of direct suggestion, cognitive reframing, hypnotic metaphors, and pain relief imagery; and
    - brief psychodynamic reprocessing, during the trance state, of emotional factors in the patient's experience of chronic pain. (Eimer, 2000).

- In the specific context of hypnosis, the midcingulate cortex appears to have a critical role in the modulation of a large cortical and subcortical network underlying its influence on sensory, affective, cognitive, and behavioral aspects of nociception.

- It is unlikely that opioid neurotransmission underlies the midcingulate activation or the mechanism of hypnosis.

- The development of "neurosignatures of pain" can influence subsequent pain experiences (Melzack, 1991, 1993; Coderre, Katz, et al., 1993) and may be expanded in size and easily reactivated (Melzack, 1991, 1993; Elbert, Flor, et al., 1994). Therefore, hypnosis and other psychological interventions need to be introduced early, before the development of chronic pain, as adjuncts in medical treatments (Crawford, Knebel, et al., 1998).

- Individuals suffering from PTSD usually score in the high hypnotizability range (Stutman & Bliss, 1985; Spiegel, Hunt, et al., 1988; Cardeña, Maldonado, et al., 2008).

- The major categories of symptoms in PTSD are similar to the components of the hypnotic process (American Psychiatric Association, 1994; Maldonado & Spiegel, 1994, 2007; Maldonado, Page, et al., 2002)

- For therapy to be effective in cases of traumatic stress, cognitive restructuring, emotional expression, and relationship management must accompany the patient's controlled reexperiencing of the traumatic events.

- Many people enter a dissociated state during physical trauma (Spiegel & Cardeña, 1991; Cardeña & Spiegel, 1993; van der Kolk, Hostetler, et al., 1994; van der Kolk & Fisler, 1995; Butler, Duran, et al., 1996; Cardeña, Maldonado, et al., 2008).

- Clinicians treating patients with conversion symptoms must pay attention to verbal and nonverbal cues given to the patient.

- It is often helpful to have patients project the images of the traumatic event on an imaginary screen which gives them some sense of distance from the event.

- As first suggested by Janet (1907), the symptoms of conversion disorder can be understood in part as reflecting the presence of uncontrolled hypnotic states.

- Even though most patients are not aware of it, highly hypnotizable individuals have an unusual capacity to control (albeit unconsciously) somatic functions.

- In cases of conversion symptoms and psychosomatic processes, hypnosis is used not to treat but to allow patients to control the effects on the body of their emotional stress and mind states. It is not advised to force a cure on a patient.

- Hypnosis may first assist in confirming the diagnosis of conversion disorder. Second, it may be therapeutic—part of a comprehensive treatment plan that includes therapy to help the patient develop more mature and adaptive defense mechanisms (Maldonado, 2007).

- Educate professionals caring for the patient to make certain they do not give the patient the message that the problem is "all in their head."

- Even though the word *hypnosis* literally means sleep, hypnosis is not a form of sleep and it is not related to sleep. In fact, if you fall asleep, you come out of trance.

- The ultimate purpose of hypnosis for weight management is to restructure the eating experience so that it becomes an exercise about learning to eat with respect for one's body. The emphasis is on what the patient is *for*, rather than *against*.

DISCLOSURE STATEMENT

Dr. Maldonado has no actual or potential conflict of interest to disclose, including any financial, personal or other relationships with other people or organizations within twelve years of the submission of this work that could inappropriately influence, or be perceived to influence the concept discussed in this chapter.

REFERENCES

(1968). "Hypnosis for asthma—a controlled trial. A report to the Research Committee of the British Tuberculosis Association." *Br Med J* 4(5623): 71–76.

(1974). "[Hypnosis—against dental phobias]." *Tid Tann* 35(3): 150–151.

(1978). "Study finds hypnosis is more effective than acupuncture in dental pain relief." *J Am Soc Psychosom Dent Med* 25(1): 35–36.

(1988). "Hypnotherapy for duodenal ulcer." *Lancet* 2(8603): 159–160.

Abramowitz, E. G., & Lichtenberg, P. (2009). Hypnotherapeutic olfactory conditioning (HOC), case studies of needle phobia, panic disorder, and combat-induced PTSD. *International Journal of Clinical and Experimental Hypnosis, 57*(2), 184–197.

Adams, P. C., & Stenn, P. G. (1992). Liver biopsy under hypnosis. *Journal of Clinical Gastroenterology, 115*(2), 122–124.

Al Sughayir, M. A. (2007). Hypnotherapy for irritable bowel syndrome in Saudi Arabian patients. *Eastern Mediterranean Health Journal = La revue de sante de la Mediterranee orientale = al-Majallah al-sihhiyah li-sharq al-mutawassit, 13*(2), 301–308.

Ament, P., & Milgrom, H. (1967). Effects of suggestion on pruritus with cutaneous lesions in chronic myelogenous leukemia. *Journal of the American Society of Psychosomatic Dentistry and Medicine, 14*(4), 122–125.

Anbar, R. D. (2000). Self-hypnosis for patients with cystic fibrosis. *Pediatric Pulmonology, 30*(6), 461–465.

Anbar, R. D. (2001). Self-hypnosis for management of chronic dyspnea in pediatric patients. *Pediatrics, 107*(2), E21.

Anbar, R. D. (2002). Hypnosis in pediatrics: applications at a pediatric pulmonary center. *BMC Pediatrics, 2*, 11.

Anbar, R. D. (2003). Self-hypnosis for anxiety associated with severe asthma: a case report. *BMC Pediatrics, 3*, 7.

Anbar, R. D., & Hehir, D. A. (2000). Hypnosis as a diagnostic modality for vocal cord dysfunction. *Pediatrics, 106*(6), E81.

Andersen, M. S. (1985). Hypnotizability as a factor in the hypnotic treatment of obesity. *International Journal of Clinical and Experimental Hypnosis, 33*(2), 150–159.

APA (2013). *Diagnostic and Statistical Manual of Mental Disorders, 5th Ed*. Washington, D.C., American Psychiatric Association.

Arone di Bertolino, R. (1981). [Psychosomatic treatment of recurrent herpes simplex]. *Minerva Medica, 72*(19), 1207–1212.

Arone di Bertolino, R. (1983). [Hypnosis in dermatology]. *Minerva Medica, 74*(51–52), 2969–2973.

Aronoff, G. M., Aronoff, S., & Peck, L. W. (1975). Hypnotherapy in the treatment of bronchial asthma. *Annals of Allergy, 34*(6), 356–362.

Axelrod, A., Vinciguerra, V., Brennan-O'Neill, E, & Moore, T. (1988). A preliminary report on the efficacy of hypnosis to control anticipatory nausea and vomiting caused by cancer chemotherapy. *Progress in Clinical and Biological Research, 278*: 147–150.

Baglini, R., Sesana, M., et al. (2004). Effect of hypnotic sedation during percutaneous transluminal coronary angioplasty on myocardial ischemia and cardiac sympathetic drive. *American Journal of Cardiology, 93*(8), 1035–1038.

Baillie, A. J., Mattick, R. P., & Hall, W. (1995). Quitting smoking: estimation by meta-analysis of the rate of unaided smoking cessation. *Australian Journal of Public Health, 19*(2), 129–131.

Banerjee, S., Srivastav, A., & Palan, B. M. (1993). Hypnosis and self-hypnosis in the management of nocturnal enuresis: a comparative study with imipramine therapy. *American Journal of Clinical Hypnosis, 36*(2), 113–119.

Barabasz, A., & Barabasz, M. (2006). Effects of tailored and manualized hypnotic inductions for complicated irritable bowel syndrome patients. *International Journal of Clinical and Experimental Hypnosis, 54*(1), 100–112.

Barabasz, A., Barabasz, M., Jensen, S., Calvin, S., Trevisan, M., & Warner, D. (1999). Cortical event-related potentials show the structure of hypnotic suggestions is crucial. *International Journal of Clinical and Experimental Hypnosis, 47*(1), 5–22.

Barabasz, A. F., Baer, L., Sheehan, D. V., & Barabasz, M. (1986). A three-year follow-up of hypnosis and restricted environmental stimulation therapy for smoking. *International Journal of Clinical and Experimental Hypnosis, 34*(3), 169–181.

Baram, D. A. (1995). Hypnosis in reproductive health care: a review and case reports. *Birth, 22*(1), 37–42.

Barsky, A. J. (1989). Somatoform disorders. In H. I. Kaplan, & B. Sadock. Baltimore (Eds.), *Comprehensive textbook of psychiatry* (pp. 1009–1027). MD: Williams & Wilkins.

Bauer, K. E., & McCanne, T. R. (1980). An hypnotic technique for treating insomnia. *International Journal of Clinical and Experimental Hypnosis, 28*(1), 1–5.

Becker, P. M. (1993). Chronic insomnia: outcome of hypnotherapeutic intervention in six cases. *American Journal of Clinical Hypnosis, 36*(2), 98–105.

Beecher, H. K. (1956). Relationship of significance of wound to pain experienced. *Journal of the American Medical Association, 161*(17), 1609–1613.

Bell, D. S., Christian, S. T., & Clements, R. S., Jr. (1983). Acuphobia in a long-standing insulin-dependent diabetic patient cured by hypnosis. *Diabetes Care, 6*(6), 622.

Bellini, M. A. (1998). Hypnosis in dermatology. *Clinics in Dermatology, 16*(6), 725–726.

Belsky, J., & Khanna, P. (1994). The effects of self-hypnosis for children with cystic fibrosis: a pilot study. *American Journal of Clinical Hypnosis, 36*(4), 282–292.

Ben-Zvi, Z., Spohn, W. A., Young, S. H., & Kattan, M. (1982). Hypnosis for exercise-induced asthma. *American Review of Respiratory Disease, 125*(4), 392–395.

Benson, P. (1975). The role of suggestion and hypnosis in dental practice. *Dental Anaesthesia and Sedation, 4*(3), 23–28.

Benson, P. E. (1974). The role of suggestion and hypnosis in dental practice. *The Articulator, (Syd), 12*–15.

Berheim, H. (1889/1964). *Hypnosis and suggestion in psychotherapy: A treatise on the nature of hypnotism (1889).* New Hyde Park, NY, University Books.

Berkowitz, B., Ross-Townsend, A., & Kohberger, R. (1979). Hypnotic treatment of smoking: the single-treatment method revisited. *American Journal of Psychiatry, 136*(1), 83–85.

Bertoni, F., Bonardi, A., Magno, L., Mandracchia, S., Martinelli, L., Terraneo, F., & Tonoli, S. (1999). Hypnosis instead of general anaesthesia in paediatric radiotherapy: report of three cases. *Radiotherapy and Oncology: Journal of the European Society for Therapeutic Radiology and Oncology, 52*(2), 185–190.

Bick, H. (1958). [Study of hypnosis in therapy of gastric and duodenal ulcers.]. *Hippokrates, 29*(6), 182–183.

Bishay, E. G., Stevens, G., & Lee, C. (1984). Hypnotic control of upper gastrointestinal hemorrhage: a case report. *American Journal of Clinical Hypnosis, 27*(1), 22–25.

Black, S. (1980). Dysphagia of pseudobulbar palsy successfully treated by hypnosis. *New Zealand Medical Journal, 91*(656), 212–214.

Bliss, E. L. (1984). Hysteria and hypnosis. *Journal of Nervous and Mental Disease, 172*(4), 203–206.

Bolocofsky, D. N., Spinler, D., & Coulthard-Morris, L. (1985). Effectiveness of hypnosis as an adjunct to behavioral weight management. *Journal of Clinical Psychology, 41*(1), 35–41.

Bolton, R. A. (1991). Nongenital warts: classification and treatment options. *American Family Physician, 43*(6), 2049–2056.

Boog, G. (2004). [Alternative methods instead of external cephalic version in the event of breech presentation. Review of the literature]. *Journal de gynecologie, obstetrique et biologie de la reproduction, 33*(2), 94–98.

Bower, G. H. (1981). Mood and memory. *Am Psychol, 36*(2), 129–148.

Bowman, E. S. (1993). Etiology and clinical course of pseudoseizures. Relationship to trauma, depression, and dissociation. *Psychosomatics, 34*(4), 333–342.

Braid, J. (1843). *Neurohypnology, or the rationale of nervous sleep considered in relation with animal magnetism, illustrated by numerous cases of its successful application in the relief and cure of disease* London: John Churchill.

Bremner, J. D., Krystal, J. H., Charney, D. S., & Southwick, S. M. (1996). Neural mechanisms in dissociative amnesia for childhood abuse: relevance to the current controversy surrounding the 'false memory syndrome'. *American Journal of Psychiatry, Jul;153*(7 Suppl), 71–82.

Brent, R. (2002). Medical, social, and legal implications of treating nausea and vomiting of pregnancy. *American Journal of Obstetrics and Gynecology, 186*(5 Suppl Understanding), S262–S266.

Brown, D. (2007). Evidence-based hypnotherapy for asthma: a critical review. *International Journal of Clinical and Experimental Hypnosis, 55*(2), 220–249.

Brown, D. C., & Hammond, D. C. (2007). Evidence-based clinical hypnosis for obstetrics, labor and delivery, and preterm labor. *International Journal of Clinical and Experimental Hypnosis, 55*(3), 355–371.

Brown, E. A. (1965). The treatment of bronchial asthma by means of hypnosis as viewed by the allergist. *Journal of Asthma Research, 3*(2), 101–119.

Buckwalter, J. G., & Simpson, S. W. (2002). Psychological factors in the etiology and treatment of severe nausea and vomiting in pregnancy. *American Journal of Obstetrics and Gynecology, 186*(5 Suppl Understanding), S210–S214.

Butler, L. D., Duran, R. E., Jasiukaitis, P., Koopman, C., & Spiegel, D. (1996). Hypnotizability and traumatic experience: a diathesis-stress model of dissociative symptomatology. *American Journal of Psychiatry, 153*(7 Suppl), 42–63.

Butler, L. D., Symons, B. K., Henderson, S. L., Shortliffe, L. D., & Spiegel, D. (2005). Hypnosis reduces distress and duration of an invasive medical procedure for children. *Pediatrics, 115*(1), e77–e85.

Byrne, S. (1973). Hypnosis and the irritable bowel: case histories, methods and speculation. *American Journal of Clinical Hypnosis, 15*(4), 263–265.

Cadranel, J. F., Benhamou, Y., Zylberberg, P., Novello, P., Luciani, F., Valla, D., & Opolon, P. (1994). Hypnotic relaxation: a new sedative tool for colonoscopy? *Journal of Clinical Gastroenterology, 18*(2), 127–129.

Campbell, D. P. & Hansen, J. C. (1981). *Manual for the Strong-Campbell interest inventory.* Palo Alto, CA, Consulting Psychologists Press.

Cardeña, E., Maldonado, J. R., van der Hart, O., & Spiegel, D. (2008). In E. Foa, T. Keane, & M. Friedman (Eds.), .*Hypnosis. Effective treatments for PTSD* (pp. 427–457). New York, NY, Guilford.

Cardeña, E. & Spiegel, D. (1993). Dissociative reactions to the San Francisco Bay Area earthquake of 1989. *American Journal of Psychiatry, 150*(3), 474–478.

Carruthers, H. R., Morris, J., Tarrier, N., & Whorwell, P. J. (2010). Mood color choice helps to predict response to hypnotherapy in patients with irritable bowel syndrome. *BMC Complementary and Alternative Medicine, 10,* 75.

Chadwick, J. M., W. (1950). *The medical works of hippocrates.* Springfield, IL, Charles C. Thomas.

Chandler, T. (1996). Techniques for optimizing MRI relaxation and visualization. *Administrative Radiology Journal, 15*(3), 16–18.

Charcot, J. M. (1890). *Oeuvres Completes de JM Charcot.* Paris, Lecrosnier et Babe.

Cheek, D. B. (1961). Possible uses of hypnosis in dermatology. *Medical Times, 89,* 76–82.

Clarke, G. H. (1965). The charming of warts. *Journal of Investigative Dermatology, 45,* 15–21.

Clarke, J. H. (1996). Teaching clinical hypnosis in U.S., & Canadian dental schools. *American Journal of Clinical Hypnosis, 39*(2), 89–92.

Clarke, P. S., & Gibson, J. R. (1980). Asthma hyperventilation and emotion. *Australian Family Physician, 9*(10), 715–719.

Clawson, T. A., Jr., & Swade, R. H. (1975). The hypnotic control of blood flow and pain: the cure of warts and the potential for the use of hypnosis in the treatment of cancer. *American Journal of Clinical Hypnosis, 17*(3), 160–169.

Coderre, T. J., Katz, J., Vaccarino, A. L., & Melzack, R. (1993). Contribution of central neuroplasticity to pathological pain: review of clinical and experimental evidence. *Pain, 52*(3), 259–285.

Cohen, S. B. (1978). Editorial: warts. *American Journal of Clinical Hypnosis, 20*(3), 157–159.

Colgan, S. M., Faragher, E. B., & Whorwell, P. J. (1988). Controlled trial of hypnotherapy in relapse prevention of duodenal ulceration. *Lancet, 1*(8598), 1299–1300.

Collison, D. R. (1975). Which asthmatic patients should be treated by hypnotherapy? *Medical Journal of Australia, 1*(25), 776–781.

Conn, L., & Mott T., Jr., (1984). Plethysmographic demonstration of rapid vasodilation by direct suggestion: a case of Raynaud's disease treated by hypnosis. *American Journal of Clinical Hypnosis, 26*(3), 166–170.

Covino, N. A., & Frankel, F. H. (1993). Hypnosis and relaxation in the medically ill. *Psychotherapy and Psychosomatics, 60*(2), 75–90.

Covino, N. A., Jimerson, D. C., Wolfe, B. E., Franko, D. L., & Frankel, F. H. (1994). Hypnotizability, dissociation, and bulimia nervosa. *Journal of Abnormal Psychology, 103*(3), 455–459.

Crasilneck, H. B., & Hall, J. A. (1968). The use of hypnosis in controlling cigarette smoking. *Southern Medical Journal, 61*(9), 999–1002.

Crasilneck, H. B., & Hall, J. A. (1985). *Clinical hypnosis: principles and applications.* New York, NY, Grune & Stratton.

Crawford, H. J., Corby, J. C., & Kopell, B. S. (1996). Auditory event-related potentials while ignoring tone stimuli: attentional differences reflected in stimulus intensity and latency responses in low and highly hypnotizable persons. *International Journal of Neuroscience, 85*(1–2), 57–69.

Crawford, H. J., Knebel, T., Kaplan, L., Vendemia, J. M., Xie, M., Jamison, S., & Pribram, K. H. (1998). Hypnotic analgesia: 1. Somatosensory event-related potential changes to noxious stimuli and 2. Transfer learning to reduce chronic low back pain. *International Journal of Clinical and Experimental Hypnosis, 46*(1), 92–132.

Croft, R. J., Williams, J. D., Haenschel, C., & Gruzelier, J. H. (2002). Pain perception, hypnosis and 40 Hz oscillations. *International Journal of Psychophysiology, 46*(2), 101–108.

Cyna, A. M., Tomkins, D., Maddock, T., & Barker, D. (2007). Brief hypnosis for severe needle phobia using switch-wire imagery in a 5-year old. *Paediatric Anaesthesia, 17*(8), 800–804.

Dash, J. (1981). Rapid hypno-behavioral treatment of a needle phobia in a five-year-old cardiac patient. *Journal of Pediatric Psychology, 6*(1), 37–42.

De Pascalis, V., Magurano, M. R., Bellusci, A., & Chen, A. (2001). Somatosensory event-related potential and autonomic activity to varying pain reduction cognitive strategies in hypnosis. *Clinical Neurophysiology, 112*(8), 1475–1485.

DeBenedittis, G., Panerai, A. A., & Villamira, M. A. (1989). Effects of hypnotic analgesia and hypnotizability on experimental ischemic pain. *International Journal of Clinical and Experimental Hypnosis, 37*(1), 55–69.

Dengrove, E., Nuland, W., & Wright, M. E. (1970). A single-treatment method to stop smoking using ancillary self-hypnosis: discussion. *International Journal of Clinical and Experimental Hypnosis, 18*(4), 251–256.

Deyoub, P. L. (1980). Hypnosis for the relief of hospital-induced stress. *Journal of the American Society of Psychosomatic Dentistry and Medicine, 27*(4), 105–109.

Dikel, W., & Olness, K. (1980). Self-hypnosis, biofeedback, and voluntary peripheral temperature control in children. *Pediatrics, 66*(3), 335–340.

Dreaper, R. (1978). Recalcitrant warts on the hand cured by hypnosis. *Practitioner, 220*(1316), 305–310.

Dudek, S. Z. (1967). Suggestion and play therapy in the cure of warts in children: a pilot study. *The Journal of Nervous and Mental Disease, 145*(1), 37–42.

Ebbell, B. (1937). *The Papyrus Ebers. The greatest Egyptian medical document.* Copenhagen, Levin&Munksgaard.

Edmonston, W. E., Jr., & Grotevant, W. R. (1975). Hypnosis and alpha density. *American Journal of Clinical Hypnosis, 17*(4), 221–232.

Edmonston, W. E., Jr., & Moscovitz, H. C. (1990). Hypnosis and lateralized brain functions. *International Journal of Clinical and Experimental Hypnosis, 38*(1), 70–84.

Eimer, B. N. (2000). Clinical applications of hypnosis for brief and efficient pain management psychotherapy. *American Journal of Clinical Hypnosis, 43*(1), 17–40.

Elbert, T., Flor, H., Knecht, S., Hampson, S., Larbig, W., & Taub, E. (1994). Extensive reorganization of the somatosensory cortex in adult humans after nervous system injury. *Neuroreport, 5*(18), 2593–2597.

Elitzur, B., & Brenner, S. (1986). [Treatment of infectious skin diseases by hypnosis]. *Harefuah, 110*(2), 73–74.

Elkins, G. R., & Rajab, M. H. (2004). Clinical hypnosis for smoking cessation: preliminary results of a three-session intervention. *International Journal of Clinical and Experimental Hypnosis, 52*(1), 73–81.

Elkins, G. R., & Wall, V. J. (1996). Medical referrals for hypnotherapy: opinions of physicians, residents, family practice outpatients, and psychiatry outpatients. *American Journal of Clinical Hypnosis, 38*(4), 254–262.

Ellen, S., & Burrows, G. D. (1994). The use of alternative therapies by children with cancer. *Medical Journal of Australia, 161*(2), 170–171.

Ellenberger, H. (1970). *The discovery of the unconscious: The history and evolution of dynamic psychiatry.* New York, NY, Basic Books.

Ellis, J. A., & Spanos, N. P. (1994). Cognitive-behavioral interventions for children's distress during bone marrow aspirations and lumbar punctures: a critical review. *Journal of Pain and Symptom Management, 9*(2), 96–108.

Enqvist, B., Bjorklund, C., Engman, M., & Jakobsson, J. (1997). Preoperative hypnosis reduces postoperative vomiting after surgery of the breasts. A prospective, randomized and blinded study. *Acta Anaesthesiologica Scandinavica, 41*(8), 1028–1032.

Erickson, M. H. (1967). *Advanced techniques of hypnosis and therapy: Selected papers of Milton H. Erickson, M.D.,* New York, NY, Grune & Stratton.

Ernst, W. (1995). 'Under the influence' in British India: James Esdaile's mesmeric hospital in Calcutta, and its critics. *Psychological Medicine, 25*(6), 1113–1123.

Ersser, S. J., Latter, S., Sibley, A., Satherley, P. A., & Welbourne, S. (2007). Psychological and educational interventions for atopic eczema in children. *Cochrane Database of Systematic Reviews,* (3), CD004054.

Esdaile, J. (1957). *Hypnosis in medicine and surgery (1846).* New York, NY, Julian Press.

Esman, A. H. (1992). Warts and all. *Journal of the Royal Society of Medicine, 85*(6), 366.

Ewer, T. C., & Stewart, D. E. (1986). Improvement in bronchial hyper-responsiveness in patients with moderate asthma after treatment with a hypnotic technique: a randomised controlled trial. *British Medical Journal, (Clin Res Ed), 293*(6555), 1129–1132.

Ewin, D. M. (1992). Hypnotherapy for warts (verruca vulgaris), 41 consecutive cases with 33 cures. *American Journal of Clinical Hypnosis, 35*(1), 1–10.

Ewin, D. M. (2011). Treatment of HPV with hypnosis-psychodynamic considerations of psychoneuroimmunology: A brief communication. *International Journal of Clinical and Experimental Hypnosis, 59*(4), 392–398.

Fassbind, O. (1983). [Dental indications for hypnosis]. *SSO Schweiz Monatsschr Zahnheilkd, 93*(5), 375–376.

Faure, H., & Burger, A. (1954). [Refractory eczema cured in 2 sessions of hyphosis]. *Le Progres Medical, 82*(17), 339–340.

Faymonville, M. E., Boly, M., & Laureys, S. (2006). Functional neuroanatomy of the hypnotic state. *Journal of Physiology, Pairs, 99*(4-6), 463–469.

Faymonville, M. E., Fissette, J., Mambourg, P. H., Roediger, L., Joris, J., & Lamy, M. (1995). Hypnosis as adjunct therapy in conscious sedation for plastic surgery. *Reginal Anesthesia, 20*(2), 145–151.

Faymonville, M. E., Laureys, S., Degueldre, C., DelFiore, G., Luxen, A., Franck, G., . . . Maquet, P. (2000). Neural mechanisms of antinociceptive effects of hypnosis. *Anesthesiology, 92*(5), 1257–1267.

Faymonville, M. E., Roediger, L., Del Fiore, G., Delgueldre, C., Phillips, C., Lamy, M., . . . Laureys, S. (2003). Increased cerebral functional connectivity underlying the antinociceptive effects of hypnosis. *Brain Research. Cognitive Brain Research, 17*(2), 255–262.

Feldman, C. S., & Salzberg, H. C. (1990). The role of imagery in the hypnotic treatment of adverse reactions to cancer therapy. *Journal of the South Carolina Medical Association, 86*(5), 303–306.

Ferraris, G. (1975). [Hypnosis in obstetrics]. *Minerva Medica, 66*(74), 3914–3920.

Ferreira, J. B., & Duncan, B. R. (2002). Biofeedback-assisted hypnotherapy for warts in an adult with developmental disabilities. *Alternative Therapies in Health and Medicine, 8*(3), 144, 140–142.

Figueroa-Moseley, C., Jean-Pierre, P., Roscoe, J. A., Ryan, J. L., Kohli, S., Palesh, O. G., Ryan, E. P., Carroll, J., & Morrow, G. R. (2007). Behavioral interventions in treating anticipatory nausea and vomiting. *Journal of the National Comprehensive Cancer Network, 5*(1), 44–50.

Fischer, T. (1974). [Methods of treating warts]. *Lakartidningen, 71*(41), 3917–3918.

Forbes, A., MacAuley, S., & Chiotakakou-Faliakou, E. (2000). Hypnotherapy and therapeutic audiotape: effective in previously unsuccessfully treated irritable bowel syndrome? *International Journal of Colorectal Disease, 15*(5-6), 328–334.

Forgione, A. G. (1988). Hypnosis in the treatment of dental fear and phobia. *Dental Clinics of North America, 32*(4), 745–761.

Fortuin, A. A. (1988). Hypnotherapy as antiemetic treatment in cancer chemotherapy. *Recent Results in Cancer Research. Fortschritte* der Krebsforschung. Progres dans les Recherches sur le Cancer, 108: 112–116.

Fox, P. A., Henderson, D. C., Barton, S. E., Champion, A. J., Rollin, M. S., Catalan, J., McCormack, S. M., & Gruzelier, J. (1999). Immunological markers of frequently recurrent genital herpes simplex virus and their response to hypnotherapy: a pilot study. International Journal of STD & AIDS, 10(11), 730–734.

Francis, C. Y., & Houghton, L. A. (1996). Use of hypnotherapy in gastrointestinal disorders. European Journal of Gastroenterology and Hepatology, 8(6), 525–529.

Frank, R. G., Umlauf, R. L., Wonderlichm, S. A., & G. S. Ashkanazi (1986). Hypnosis and behavioral treatment in a worksite smoking cessation program. Addictive Behaviors, 11(1), 59–62.

Frankel, F. H. (1994). Comment on Torem's 'Hypnotherapeutic techniques in the treatment of hyperemesis gravidarum'. American Journal of Clinical Hypnosis, 37(2), 160.

Frankel, F. H., & Misch, R. C. (1973). Hypnosis in a case of long-standing psoriasis in a person with character problems. International Journal of Clinical and Experimental Hypnosis, 21(3), 121–130.

Freedman, R. R., Ianni, P., & Wenig, P. (1984). Behavioral treatment of Raynaud's phenomenon in scleroderma. Journal of Behavioral Medicine, 7(4), 343–353.

Freeman, R. M., Macaulay, A. J., Eve, L., Chamberlain, G. V., & Bhat, A. V. (1986). Randomised trial of self hypnosis for analgesia in labour. British Medical Journal, 292(6521), 657–658.

Freiwald, M., Liedtke, R., & Zepf, S. (1975). [The imagination of the diseased organ in patients with ulcerative colitis and functional heart disorders in experimental catathymic experiences (author's transl)]. Psychotherapie, Medizinische Psychologie, 25(1), 15–24.

French, A. P. (1973). Treatment of warts by hypnosis. American Journal of Obstetrics and Gynecology, 116(6), 887–888.

Freud, S. (1914/1958). Remembering, repeating and working-through (further recommendations on the technique of psycho-analysis II) (1914). In J. Strachey (Ed.), The Standard Edition of the Complete Psychological Works of Sigmund Freud (pp. 145–156). London, Hogarth Press.

Frid, M., & Singer, G. (1979). Hypnotic analgesia in conditions of stress is partially reversed by naloxone. Psychopharmacology (Berlin), 63(3), 211–215.

Friday, P. J., & Kubal, W. S. (1990). Magnetic resonance imaging: improved patient tolerance utilizing medical hypnosis. American Journal of Clinical Hypnosis, 33(2), 80–84.

Friedman, H., & Taub, H. A. (1977). The use of hypnosis and biofeedback procedures for essential hypertension. International Journal of Clinical and Experimental Hypnosis, 25(4), 335–347.

Friedman, H., & Taub, H. A. (1978). A six-month follow-up of the use of hypnosis and biofeedback procedures in essential hypertension. American Journal of Clinical Hypnosis, 20(3), 184–188.

Frischholz, E. J., & Nichols, L. E. (2010). A historical context for understanding An eye roll test for hypnotizability by Herbert Spiegel, M.D. American Journal of Clinical Hypnosis, 53(1), 3–13.

Fry, L., Mason, A. A., et al. (1964). Effect of hypnosis on allergic skin responses in asthma and hay-fever. British Medical Journal, , 1(5391), 1145–1148.

Fuchs, K., Paldi, E., Abramovici, H., & Peretz, B. A. (1980). Treatment of hyperemesis gravidarum by hypnosis. International Journal of Clinical and Experimental Hypnosis, 28(4), 313–333.

Gall, J. (1969). Hypnosis—dental hypnotherapy. Glasgow Dental Journal, 1(1), 29–33.

Galovski, T. E., & Blanchard, E. B. (1998). The treatment of irritable bowel syndrome with hypnotherapy. Applied Psychophysiology and Biofeedback, 23(4), 219–232.

Galovski, T. E., & Blanchard, E. B. (2002). Hypnotherapy and refractory irritable bowel syndrome: a single case study. American Journal of Clinical Hypnosis, 45(1), 31–37.

Gardner, G. G., & Lubman, A. (1982). Hypnotherapy for children with cancer: some current issues. American Journal of Clinical Hypnosis, 25(2-3), 135–142.

Gaspar, J., Linninger, M., Kaan, B., Balint, M., Fejerdy, L., & Fabian, T. K. (2003). [Effectiveness of standardized direct suggestions in dental hypnosis]. Fogorv Sz, 96(5), 205–210.

Gay, M. C. (2007). Effectiveness of hypnosis in reducing mild essential hypertension: a one-year follow-up. International Journal of Clinical and Experimental Hypnosis, 55(1), 67–83.

Gemignani, A., Santarcangelo, E., Sebastiani, L., Marchese, C., Mammoliti, R., Simoni, A., & Ghelarducci, B. (2000). Changes in autonomic and EEG patterns induced by hypnotic imagination of aversive stimuli in man. Brain Research Bulletin, 53(1), 105–111.

Genuis, M. L. (1995). The use of hypnosis in helping cancer patients control anxiety, pain, and emesis: a review of recent empirical studies. American Journal of Clinical Hypnosis, 37(4), 316–325.

Gheorghiu, V. A., & Orleanu, P. (1982). Dental implant under hypnosis. American Journal of Clinical Hypnosis, 25(1), 68–70.

Gherardi, D., Fabrizio, E., Chirillo, S., & Garzia, P. (1993). [Psychiatric aspects in dermatology. Clinical contribution]. Minerva Psichiatr, 34(1), 19–23.

Gilder, S. S. (1968). Hypnosis for asthma. Canadian Medical Association Journal, 99(24), 1212.

Giorlando, S. W., & Mascola, R. F. (1957). The treatment of hyperemesis gravidarum with hypnotherapy. American Journal of Obstetrics and Gynecology, 73(2), 444–447.

Gluzman, S. A., & Zisel'son, A. D. (1987). [Psychotherapy of bronchial asthma in children]. Pediatriia, (5), 107–108.

Golan, H. P. (1989). The role of hypnosis. Journal of the Massachusetts Dental Society, 38(2), 92–93.

Golan, H. P. (1989). Temporomandibular joint disease treated with hypnosis. American Journal of Clinical Hypnosis, 31(4), 269–274.

Golan, H. P. (1997). The use of hypnosis in the treatment of psychogenic oral pain. American Journal of Clinical Hypnosis, 40(2), 89–96.

Goldman, L. (1992). The use of hypnosis in obstetrics. Psychiatric Medicine, 10(4), 59–67.

Goldstein, A., & Hilgard, E. R. (1975). Failure of the opiate antagonist naloxone to modify hypnotic analgesia. Proceedings of the National Academy of Sciences of the United States of America, 72(6), 2041–2043.

Gonsalkorale, W. M., Houghton, L. A., & Whorwell, P. J. (2002). Hypnotherapy in irritable bowel syndrome: a large-scale audit of a clinical service with examination of factors influencing responsiveness. American Journal of Gastroenterology, 97(4), 954–961.

Gonsalkorale, W. M., Miller, V., Afzal, A., & Whorwell, P. J. (2003). Long term benefits of hypnotherapy for irritable bowel syndrome. Gut, 52(11), 1623–1629.

Gonsalkorale, W. M., & Whorwell, P. J. (2005). Hypnotherapy in the treatment of irritable bowel syndrome. European Journal of Gastroenterology and Hepatology, 17(1), 15–20.

Gonzales, D., Rennard, S. I., Nides, M., Oncken, C., Azoulay, S., Billing, C. B., Watsky, E. J., Gong, J., Williams, K. E., & Reeves, K. R. (2006). Varenicline, an alpha4beta2 nicotinic acetylcholine receptor partial agonist, vs sustained-release bupropion and placebo for smoking cessation: a randomized controlled trial. Journal of the American Medical Association, 296(1), 47–55.

Goodman, H. P. (1962). Hypnosis in prolonged resistant eczema: a case report. American Journal of Clinical Hypnosis, 5, 144–145.

Gould, S. S., & Tissler, D. M. (1984). The use of hypnosis in the treatment of herpes simplex II. American Journal of Clinical Hypnosis, 26(3), 171–174.

Grabowska, M. J. (1971). The effect of hypnosis and hypnotic suggesion on the blood flow in the extremities. Polish Medical Journal, 10(4), 1044–1051.

Graf, P., & Schacter, D. L. (1985). Implicit and explicit memory for new associations in normal and amnesic subjects. Journal of Experimental Psycology. Learning, Memory, and Cognition, 11(3), 501–518.

Graffin, N. F., Ray, W. J., & Lundy, R. (1995). EEG concomitants of hypnosis and hypnotic susceptibility. Journal of Abnormal Psychology, 104(1), 123–131.

Gravitz, M. A. (1995). Hypnosis in the treatment of functional infertility. American Journal of Clinical Hypnosis, 38(1), 22–26.

Greenleaf, M., Fisher, S., Miaskowski, C., & DuHamel, K. (1992). Hypnotizability and recovery from cardiac surgery. *American journal of Clinical Hypnosis, 35*(2), 119–128.

Gritz, E., & Bloom, J. (1987). *Psychosocial sequelae of cancer in long-term survivors and their families.* Western Regional Conference of the American Cancer Society, Los Angeles, CA.

Gritzalis, N., Oster, M., & Frischholz, E. J. (2009). A concurrent validity study between the Hypnotic Induction Profile (HIP) and the Stanford Hypnotic Clinical Scale for Adults (SHCS:A) in an inpatient sample: a brief report. *American Journal of Clinical Hypnosis, 52*(2), 89–93.

Gross, H. N., & Posner, N. A. (1963). An evaluation of hypnosis for obstetric delivery. *American Journal of Obstetrics and Gynecology, 87*: 912–920.

Groth-Marnat, G., & Schumaker, J. F. (1990). Hypnotizability, attitudes toward eating, and concern with body size in a female college population. *American Journal of Clinical Hypnosis, 32*(3), 194–200.

Gruen, W. (1972). A successful application of systematic self-relaxation and self-suggestions about postoperative reactions in a case of cardiac surgery. *International Journal of Clinical and Experimental Hypnosis, 20*(3), 143–151.

Grumiller, I., & Strotzka, H. (1973). [Psychosomatic aspects of ulcerative colitis]. *Fortschritte auf dem Gebiete der Rontgenstrahlen und der Nuklearmedizin, 0*(0), suppl:328–330.

Gueguen, J. (1962). [Delivery under hypnosis. (Method and results)]. *Gynecologie et obstetrique, 61*: 92–113.

Gurian, B. (1981). Hypnosis in the treatment of dysphagia. *Journal of Oral Medicine, 36*(4), 99–101.

Hackman, R. M., Stern, J. S., & Gershwin, M. E. (2000). Hypnosis and asthma: a critical review. *Journal of Asthma, 37*(1), 1–15.

Hageman-Wenselaar, L. H. (1988). [Hypnosis for pain control during lumbar puncture and bone marrow aspirations in children with cancer]. *Tijdschr Kindergeneeskd, 56*(3), 120–123.

Hajek, P., Jakoubek, B., & Radil, T. (1990). Gradual increase in cutaneous threshold induced by repeated hypnosis of healthy individuals and patients with atopic eczema. *Perceptual and Motor Skills, 70*(2), 549–550.

Hajek, P., Jakoubek, B., Radil, T., & Adamovska, E. (1989). Pain threshold in patients with atopic eczema influenced by hypnosis. *Activitas Nervosa Supierior, 31*(3), 222–223.

Hajek, P., Radil, T., & Jakoubek, B. (1991). Hypnotic skin analgesy in healthy individuals and patients with atopic eczema. *Homeostasis in Health and Disease: International Journal Devoted to Integrative Brain Functions and Homeostatic Systems, 33*(3), 156–157.

Hall, H. R. (1982). Hypnosis and the immune system: a review with implications for cancer and the psychology of healing. *American Journal of Clinical Hypnosis, 25*(2-3), 92–103.

Hammarstrand, G., Berggren, U., & Hakeberg, M. (1995). Psychophysiological therapy vs. hypnotherapy in the treatment of patients with dental phobia. *European Journal of Oral Sciences, 103*(6), 399–404.

Hammond, D. C., Ed. (1990). *Handbook of hypnotic suggestions and metaphors.* New York, NY, W. W. Norton & Company.

Haustein, U. F., & Seikowski, K. (1990). [Psychosomatic dermatology]. *Dermatologische Monatschrift, 176*(12), 725–733.

Haustein, U. F., Weber, B., & Seikowski, K. (1995). [Substance P and vasoactive intestinal peptide in patients with progressive scleroderma. Determination of plasma level before and after autogenic training]. *Der Hautarzt; Zeitschrift fur Dermatologie, Venerologie, und Verwandte Gebiete, 46*(2), 102–106.

Hefner, J., Rilk, A., Herbert, B. M., Zipfel, S., Enck, P., & Martens, U. (2009). [Hypnotherapy for irritable bowel syndrome—a systematic review]. *Zeitschrift fur Gastroenterologie, 47*(11), 1153–1159.

Herod, E. L. (1995). Psychophysical pain control during tooth extraction. *General Dentistry, 43*(3), 267–269.

Herold, D. A. (2002). [Suggestion—salicylic acid—travel. What really helps control warts? (interview by Dr. Thomas Meissner)]. *MMW Fortschritte der Medizin, 144*(43), 16.

Herraiz Ballestero, L., Rodriguez Fontela, C., Simkin, B., & Mesones, H. (1952). [Spirometric registration of the effect of deep hypnosis in bronchial asthma.]. *Prensa Med Argent, 39*(52), 3299–3301.

Hilgard, E. R. (1965). *Hypnotic susceptibility.* New York, Harcourt, Brace & World.

Hilgard, E. R., & Hilgard, J. R. (1975). *Hypnosis in the relief of pain.* Los Altos, CA, William Kaufmann.

Hilgard, J. R. (1970). *Personality and hypnosis: A study of imaginative involvement.* Chicago, IL, University of Chicago Press.

Hilgard, J. R., & LeBaron, S. (1982). Relief of anxiety and pain in children and adolescents with cancer: quantitative measures and clinical observations. *International Journal of Clinical and Experimental Hypnosis, 30*(4), 417–442.

Hockenberry, M. J., & Cotanch, P. H. (1985). Hypnosis as adjuvant antiemetic therapy in childhood cancer. *Nursing Clinics of North America, 20*(1), 105–107.

Hoffman, M. L. (1982). Hypnotic desensitization for the management of anticipatory emesis in chemotherapy. *American Journal of Clinical Hypnosis, 25*(2–3), 173–176.

Houghton, L. A., Heyman, D. J., & Whorwell, P. J. (1996). Symptomatology, quality of life and economic features of irritable bowel syndrome—the effect of hypnotherapy. *Alimentary Pharmacology & Therapeutics, 10*(1), 91–95.

Huntley, C. W., & Davis, F. (1983). Undergraduate Study of Values scores as predictors of occupation 25 years later. *Journal of Personality and Social Psychology, 45*: 1148–1155.

Hutchinson-Phillips, S., Gow, K., & Jamieson, G. A. (2007). Hypnotizability, eating behaviors, attitudes, and concerns: a literature survey. *International Journal of Clinical and Experimental Hypnosis, 55*(1), 84–113.

Hyman, G. J., Stanley, R. O., Burrows, G. D., & Horne, D. J. (1986). Treatment effectiveness of hypnosis and behaviour therapy in smoking cessation: a methodological refinement. *Addictive Behaviors, 11*(4), 355–365.

Iancu, I., Kotler, M., Spivak, B., Radwan, M., & Weizman, A. (1994). Psychiatric aspects of hyperemesis gravidarum. *Psychotherapy and Psychosomatics, 61*(3–4), 143–149.

Isenberg, S. A., Lehrer, P. M., & Hochran, S. (1992). The effects of suggestion and emotional arousal on pulmonary function in asthma: a review and a hypothesis regarding vagal mediation. *Psychosomatic Medicine, 54*(2), 192–216.

Isenberg, S. A., Lehrer, P. M., & Hochran, S. (1992). The effects of suggestion on airways of asthmatic subjects breathing room air as a suggested bronchoconstrictor and bronchodilator. *Journal of Psychosomatic Research, 36*(8), 769–776.

Jacknow, D. S., Tschann, J. M., Link, M. P., & Boyce, W. T. (1994). Hypnosis in the prevention of chemotherapy-related nausea and vomiting in children: a prospective study. *Journal of Developmental and Behavioral Pediatrics, 15*(4), 258–264.

Jakubovits, E. (2011). [Possibilities of hypnosis and hypnosuggestive methods in oncology]. *Magyar onkologia, 55*(1), 22–31.

James, W. (1902). *Varieties of religious experiences.* New York, NY: Random House.

Janet, P. (1887). L'anesthésie systématisée et la dissociation des phénomènes psychologiques. *Revue Philosophique, 23*, 449–472.

Janet, P. (1889). *L'automatisme psychologique.* Paris, Félix Alcan.

Janet, P. (1904). L'amnésie et la dissociation des souvenirs par l'émotion. *Journal de Psychologie, 1*, 417–453.

Janet, P. (1907). *Major symptoms of hysteria: Fifteen lectures given in the medical school of Harvard University.* New York, NY: Macmillan.

Jasiukaitis, P., Nouriani, B., Hugdahl, K., & Spiegel, D. (1997). Relateralizing hypnosis: or, have we been barking up the wrong hemisphere? *International Journal of Clinical and Experimental Hypnosis, 45*(2), 158–177.

Jasiukaitis, P., Nouriani, B., & Spiegel, D. (1996). Left hemisphere superiority for event-related potential effects of hypnotic obstruction. *Neuropsychologia, 34*(7), 661–668.

Javel, A. F. (1980). One-session hypnotherapy for smoking: a controlled study. *Psychological Reports, 46*(3 Pt 1), 895–899.

Joachim, H. (1890). *Papyros Ebers. Das älteste Buch über Heilkunde. Aus dem Ägyptischen zum erstenmal vollständig übersetzt.* Berlin.

Johnson, J. M. (1980). Teaching self-hypnosis in pregnancy, labor, and delivery. *American Journal of Maternal Child Nursing, 5*(2), 98–101.

Johnson, R. F. (1980). Warts, blisters, and stigmata: role of suggestions in some unusual skin changes. *Journal of the American Society of Psychosomatic Dentistry and Medicine, 27*(3), 72–86.

Johnson, R. F., & Barber, T. X. (1978). Hypnosis, suggestions, and warts: an experimental investigation implicating the importance of 'believed-in efficacy'. *American Journal of Clinical Hypnosis, 20*(3), 165–174.

Jones, H., Cooper, P., Miller, V., Brooks, N., & Whorwell, P. J. (2006). Treatment of non-cardiac chest pain: a controlled trial of hypnotherapy. *Gut, 55*(10), 1403–1408.

Kangas, J., & Bradway, K. (1971). Intelligence at middle age: A thirty-eight year follow-up. *Developmental Psychology, 5,* 333–337.

Kanishchev, P. A., & Shutova, T. M. (1974). [Treatment of neuroses in patients with ulcer disease and chronic gastritis]. *Vrachebnoe delo, 0*(7), 61–65.

Kantor, S. D. (1990). Stress and psoriasis. *Cutis, 46*(4), 321–322.

Kardiner, A., & Spiegel, H. (1947). *War stress and neurotic illness.* New York, NY, Paul Hoeber, Inc.

Katcher, A., Segal, H., & Beck, A. (1984). Comparison of contemplation and hypnosis for the reduction of anxiety and discomfort during dental surgery. *American Journal of Clinical Hypnosis, 27*(1), 14–21.

Katz, E. R., Kellerman, J., & Ellenberg, L. (1987). Hypnosis in the reduction of acute pain and distress in children with cancer. *Journal of Pediatric Psychology, 12*(3), 379–394.

Kavanagh, T., Shephard, R. J., & Doney, H. (1974). Hypnosis and exercise. A possible combined therapy following myocardial infarction. *American Journal of Clinical Hypnosis, 16*(3), 160–165.

Kaye, J. M. (1984). Hypnotherapy and family therapy for the cancer patient: a case study. *American Journal of Clinical Hypnosis, 27*(1), 38–41.

Kekecs, Z., & Varga, K. (2011). [Positive suggestion techniques in somatic medicine]. *Orvosi hetilap, 152*(3), 96–106.

Keller, V. E. (1995). Management of nausea and vomiting in children. *Journal of Pediatric Nursing, 10*(5), 280–286.

Kellerman, J., Zeltzer, L., Ellenberg, L., & Dash, J. (1983). Adolescents with cancer. Hypnosis for the reduction of the acute pain and anxiety associated with medical procedures. *Journal of Adolescent Health Care, 4*(2), 85–90.

Kellner, R. (1975). Psychotherapy in psychosomatic disorders. *Archives of General Psychiatry, 32*(8), 1021–1028.

Kelly, M. A., McKinty, H. R., & Carr, R. (1988). Utilization of hypnosis to promote compliance with routine dental flossing. *American Journal of Clinical Hypnosis, 31*(1), 57–60.

Kessler, R., & Dane, J. R. (1996). Psychological and hypnotic preparation for anesthesia and surgery: an individual differences perspective. *International Journal of Clinical and Experimental Hypnosis, 44*(3), 189–207.

Kevesater, R. (1977). [Hypnosis against dental phobias]. *Tandlakartidningen, 69*(1), 28–29.

Kierland, R. R. (1965). Vascular Reactions of the Skin in Eczema. *Journal of Pediatrics, 66,* (Suppl), 203–206.

Kiernan, B. D., Dane, J. R., Phillips, L. H., & Price, D. D. (1995). Hypnotic analgesia reduces R-III nociceptive reflex: further evidence concerning the multifactorial nature of hypnotic analgesia. *Pain, 60*(1), 39–47.

Kirsch, I. (1996). Hypnotic enhancement of cognitive-behavioral weight loss treatments—another meta-reanalysis. *Journal of Consulting and Clinical Psychology, 64*(3), 517–519.

Kirsch, I., Montgomery, G., & Sapirstein, G. (1995). Hypnosis as an adjunct to cognitive-behavioral psychotherapy: a meta-analysis. *Journal of Consulting and Clinical Psychology, 63*(2), 214–220.

Kisby, L. (1977). The use of hypnosis on the anxious pediatric dental patient. *Journal of Pedodontics, 1*(4), 310–317.

Kistler, A., Mariauzouls, C., Wyler, F., Bircher, A. J. & Wyler-Harper, J. (1999). Autonomic responses to suggestions for cold and warmth in hypnosis. *Forschende Komplementarmedizin, 6*(1), 10–14.

Klapper, M. (1984). Condylomata acuminata and hypnosis. *Journal of the American Academy of Dermatology, 10*(5 Pt 1), 836–839.

Klein, K. B., & Spiegel, D. (1989). Modulation of gastric acid secretion by hypnosis. *Gastroenterology, 96*(6), 1383–1387.

Kleinhauz, M., & Eli, I. (1993). When pharmacologic anesthesia is precluded: the value of hypnosis as a sole anesthetic agent in dentistry. *Special Care in Dentistry: Official Publication of the American Association of Hospital Dentists, the Academy of Dentistry for the Handicapped, and the American Society for Geriatric Dentistry, 13*(1), 15–18.

Kluft, R. P. (1984). Treatment of multiple personality disorder. A study of 33 cases. *Psychiatric Clinics of North America, 7*(1), 9–29.

Kluft, R. P. (1992). The use of hypnosis with dissociative disorders. *Psychiatric Medicine, 10*(4), 31–46.

Knox, V. J., & Shum, K. (1977). Reduction of cold-pressor pain with acupuncture analgesia in high- and low-hypnotic subjects. *Journal of Abnormal Psychology, 86*(6), 639–643.

Kobayashi, T., Ishikawa, H., & Tawara, I. (1970). Psychosomatic aspects of angina pectoris. *Scandinavian Journal of Rehabilitation Medicine, 2*(2), 87–91.

Kohen, D. P. (1986). Applications of relaxation/mental imagery (self-hypnosis) in pediatric emergencies. *International Journal of Clinical and Experimental Hypnosis, 34*(4), 283–294.

Kohen, D. P. (1987). A biobehavioral approach to managing childhood asthma. *Child Today, 16*(2), 6–10.

Kohen, D. P., Olness, K. N., Colwell, S. O., & Heimel, A. (1984). The use of relaxation-mental imagery (self-hypnosis) in the management of 505 pediatric behavioral encounters. *Journal of Developmental and Behavioral Pediatrics, 5*(1), 21–25.

Kohen, D. P., & Wynne, E. (1997). Applying hypnosis in a preschool family asthma education program: uses of storytelling, imagery, and relaxation. *American Journal of Clinical Hypnosis, 39*(3), 169–181.

Konig, K. J. (1969). [The treatment of the common wart]. *Zeitschrift fur Haut- und Geschlechtskrankheiten, 44*(7), 247–254.

Kopel, K. F., & Quinn, M. (1996). Hypnotherapy treatment for dysphagia. *International Journal of Clinical and Experimental Hypnosis, 44*(2), 101–105.

Kosov, V. A., Zamotaev Iu, N., Mandrykin Iu, V., & Papikian, II (1997). [The significance of drug-free psychotherapeutic methods in the rehabilitation of patients after aortic-coronary shunting]. *Klinicheskaia meditsina, 75*(9), 33–35.

Kosslyn, S. M., Thompson, W. L., Costantini-Ferrando, M. F., Alpert, N. M., & Spiegel, D. (2000). Hypnotic visual illusion alters color processing in the brain. *American Journal of Psychiatry, 157*(8), 1279–1284.

Kranhold, C., Baumann, U., & Fichter, M. (1992). Hypnotizability in bulimic patients and controls: A pilot study. *European Archives of Psychiatry and Clinical Neurosciences, 242:* 72–76.

Kroger, W. S., & De, L. S. (1946). The psychosomatic treatment of hyperemesis gravidarum by hypnosis. *American Journal of Obstetrics and Gynecology, 51,* 544–552.

Kroll, R. G. (1962). Hypnosis for the poor risk dental patient. *American Journal of Clinical Hypnosis, 5:* 142–144.

Kropotov, J. D., Crawford, H. J., & Polyakov, Y. I. (1997). Somatosensory event-related potential changes to painful stimuli during hypnotic analgesia: anterior cingulate cortex and anterior temporal cortex intracranial recordings. *International Journal of Psychophysiology: Official Journal of the International Organization of Psychophysiology, 27*(1), 1–8.

Krumholz, A., & Niedermeyer, E. (1983). Psychogenic seizures: a clinical study with follow-up data. *Neurology, 33*(4), 498–502.

Krupnova, M. S. (1985). [Clinical picture and treatment of nocturnal enuresis in children]. *Zhurnal nevropatologii i psikhiatrii imeni S.S. Korsakova 85*(3), 427–430.

Kuttner, L. (1993). Managing pain in children. Changing treatment of headaches. *Canadian Family Physician Medecin de Famille Canadien, 39,* 563–568.

LaCrosse, M. B. (1994). Understanding change: five-year follow-up of brief hypnotic treatment of chronic bruxism. *American Journal of Clinical Hypnosis, 36*(4), 276–281.

Lamas, J. R., & Valle-Inclan, F. (1998). Effects of a negative visual hypnotic hallucination on ERPs and reaction times. *International Journal of Psychophysiology, 29*(1), 77–82.

Lambert, S. A. (1996). The effects of hypnosis/guided imagery on the postoperative course of children. *Journal of Developmental and Behavioral Pediatrics, 17*(5), 307–310.

Lambert, S. A. (1999). Distraction, imagery, and hypnosis. Techniques for management of children's pain. *Journal of Child and Family Nursing, 2*(1), 5–15; quiz 16.

Landolt, A. S., & Milling, L. S. (2011). The efficacy of hypnosis as an intervention for labor and delivery pain: a comprehensive methodological review. *Clinical Psychology Review, 31*(6), 1022–1031.

Lang, E. V., Benotsch, E. G., Fick, L. J., Lutgendorf, S., Berbaum, M. L., Berbaum, K. S., Logan, H., & Spiegel, D. (2000). Adjunctive non-pharmacological analgesia for invasive medical procedures: a randomised trial. *Lancet, 355*(9214), 1486–1490.

Lang, E. V., Berbaum, K. S., Faintuch, S., Hatsiopoulou, O., Halsey, N., Li, X., Berbaum, M. L., Laser, E., & Baum, J. (2006). Adjunctive self-hypnotic relaxation for outpatient medical procedures: a prospective randomized trial with women undergoing large core breast biopsy. *Pain, 126*(1-3), 155–164.

Lang, E. V., Joyce, J. S., Spiegel, D., Hamilton, D., & Lee, K. K. (1996). Self-hypnotic relaxation during interventional radiological procedures: effects on pain perception and intravenous drug use. *International Journal of Clinical and Experimental Hypnosis, 44*(2), 106–119.

Langewitz, W., Izakovic, J., Wyler, J., Schindler, C., Kiss, A., & Bircher, A. J. (2005). Effect of self-hypnosis on hay fever symptoms—a randomised controlled intervention study. *Psychotherapy and Psychosomatics, 74*(3), 165–172.

Leidman Iu, M. (1968). [Experience in the treatment of warts in children by suggestion]. *Vestnik dermatologii i venerologii, 42*(2), 86–89.

Leidman Iu, M. (1973). [Hypnospsychotherapy as a means of treating warts in children under ambulatory conditions]. *Voprosy okhrany materinstva i detstva, 18*(12), 57–59.

Lewis, R. A., Lewis, M. N., & Tattersfield, A. E. (1983). Asthma and suggestion: psychological or physical? *Agents and Actions. Supplements, 13*, 71–79.

Liossi, C., & Hatira, P. (1999). Clinical hypnosis versus cognitive behavioral training for pain management with pediatric cancer patients undergoing bone marrow aspirations. *International Journal of Clinical and Experimental Hypnosis, 47*(2), 104–116.

Lopez, C. A. (1993). Franklin and Mesmer: an encounter. *Yale Journal of Biology and Medicine, 66*(4), 325–331.

Lu, D. P. (1994). The use of hypnosis for smooth sedation induction and reduction of postoperative violent emergencies from anesthesia in pediatric dental patients. *ASDC Journal of Denistry for Children, 61*(3), 182–185.

Lucas, O. N. (1965). Dental extractions in the hemophiliac: Control of the emotional factors by hypnosis. *American Journal of Clinical Hypnosis, 69*: 301–307.

Lucas, O. N. (1975). The use of hypnosis in hemophilia dental care. *Annals of the New York Academy of Sciences, 240*: 263–266.

Luparello, T., Lyons, H. A., Bleecker, E. R., & McFadden, E. R., Jr. (1968). Influences of suggestion on airway reactivity in asthmatic subjects. *Psychosomatic Medicine, 30*(6), 819–825.

Lyell, A. (1966). Management of warts. *British Medical Journal, 2*(5529), 1576–1579.

Lynch, D. F., Jr. (1999). Empowering the patient: hypnosis in the management of cancer, surgical disease and chronic pain. *American Journal of Clinical Hypnosis, 42*(2), 122–130.

Magonet, A. P. (1952). Hypnosis in asthma. *Medical World, 76*(4), 93–97.

Magonet, A. P. (1961). Hypnosis in dysphagia. *International Journal of Clinical and Experimental Hypnosis, 9*: 291–295.

Maher-Loughnan, G. P. (1970). Hypnosis and autohypnosis for the treatment of asthma. *International Journal of Clinical and Experimental Hypnosis, 18*(1), 1–14.

Maher-Loughnan, G. P., Mason, A. A., Macdonald, N., & Fry, L. (1962). Controlled trial of hypnosis in the symptomatic treatment of asthma. *British Medical Journal, , 2*(5301), 371–376.

Maldonado, J. (1996). Psychological and physiological factors in the production of conversion disorder. *Society for Clinical and Experimental Hypnosis Annual Meeting.* Tampa, FL.

Maldonado, J. (2001). Reviews in Psychiatry: Conversion Disorders. *154th annual meeting of the American Psychiatric Association.* New Orleans, LA, APPI.

Maldonado, J., Butler, L., & Spiegel, D. (2000). Treatment of dissociative disorders. In P. Nathan, & J. Gorman(Eds.), *A guide to treatments that work, 2nd Edition,* (pp. 463–496). New York, NY: Oxford University Press.

Maldonado, J., & Jasiukaitis, P. (2003). Selective attention as possible mechanism of symptom production in conversion disorders. *Journal of Psychosomatic Research, 55,* 140.

Maldonado, J., & Spiegel, D. (1994). Treatment of post traumatic stress disorder. In S. Lynn, & J. Rhue (Eds.). *Dissociation: Clinical, Theoretical and Research Perspectives,* (pp. 215–241). New York, NY, Guilford Press:.

Maldonado, J., & Spiegel, D. (1996). Hypnosis for psychiatric disorders. In D. Dunner (Ed.). *Current Psychiatric Therapy II,* (pp. 600–608). Philadelphia, PA: W. B. Saunders Company.

Maldonado, J., & Spiegel, D. (1998). Trauma, dissociation and hypnotizability. In R. Marmar and D. Bremmer (Eds.). *Trauma, Memory and Dissociation.* Washington, DC: American Psychiatric Press.

Maldonado, J., & Spiegel, D. (2000). Conversion disorder. In K. Phillips (Ed). *Review of Psychiatry: Somatoform and Factitious Disorders,* (*20*: pp. 95–128). Washington DC: American Psychiatric Press.

Maldonado, J., & Spiegel, D. (2002). Hypnosis. In J. Talbot, & S. Yudosky (Eds.). *Textbook of Psychiatry, Fourth Edition* (pp. 1461–1516). Washington, DC: American Psychiatric Press.

Maldonado, J. R. (1996). The psychophysiology of conversion disorders. *Psychosomatics, 37*(2), 216–217.

Maldonado, J. R. (1997). Conversion disorder: Are the symptoms the result of pure psychology or true physiological changes? *Psychosomatics, 38*(2), 190–191.

Maldonado, J. R. (2007). Conversion Disorder. In G. Gabbard, & K. Phillips (Eds.). *Treatments of psychiatric disorders* (4th ed., pp. 443–456). Washington, DC: American Psychiatric Press.

Maldonado, J. R., & Jasiukaitis, P. (2003). Selective attention as possible mechanism of symptom production in conversion disorders. *Journal of Psychosomatic Research, 55,* 140–141.

Maldonado, J. R., Page, K., Koopman, C., Stein, H., & Spiegel, D. (2002). Acute stress reactions following the assassination of Mexican presidential candidate Colosio. *Journal of Traumatic Stress, 15*(5), 401–405.

Maldonado, J. R., & Spiegel, D. (2007). Dissociative disorders. In J. Talbot, & S. Yudosky (Eds.). *Textbook of Psychiatry* (5th ed., pp. 759–804). Washington, DC: American Psychiatric Press.

Maldonado, J. R., & Spiegel, D. (2008). Hypnosis. In A. Tasman, J. Kay, J. A. Lieberman, M. B. First, & M. Maj (Eds.). *Psychiatry, 2* (pp. 1982–2026). Chichester, England: Wiley-Blackwell.

Manferto, G. (1975). [Hypnosis in dermatology]. *Minerva Med66*(73), 3864–3865.

Mantle, F. (1999). Hypnosis in the management of eczema in children. *Paediatric Nursing, 11*(5), 24–26.

Marchioro, G., Azzarello, G., Viviani, F., Barbato, F., Pavanetto, M., Rosetti, F., Pappagallo, G. L., & Vinante, O. (2000). Hypnosis in the treatment of anticipatory nausea and vomiting in patients receiving cancer chemotherapy. *Oncology, 59*(2), 100–104.

Mawdsley, J. E., Jenkins, D. G., Macey, M. G., Langmead, L., & Rampton, D. S. (2008). The effect of hypnosis on systemic and rectal mucosal measures of inflammation in ulcerative colitis. *American Journal of Gastroenterology, 103*(6), 1460–1469.

Mc, D. M. (1949). Juvenile warts removed with the use of hypnotic suggestion. *Bulletin of the Menninger Clinic, 13*(4), 124–126.

McAmmond, D. M., Davidson, P. O., & Kovitz, D. M. (1971). A comparison of the effects of hypnosis and relaxation training on stress reactions in a dental situation. *American Journal of Clinical Hypnosis, 13*(4), 233–242.

McCay, A. R. (1963). Dental extraction under self-hypnosis. *Medical Journal of Australia, 50*(1), 820.

McCormack, D. (2010). Hypnosis for hyperemesis gravidarum. *Journal of Obstetrics and Gynaecology: The Journal of the Institute of Obstetrics and Gynaecology, 30*(7), 647–653.

McGlashan, T. H., Evans, F. J., & Orne, M. T. (1969). The nature of hypnotic analgesia and placebo response to experimental pain. *Psychosomatic Medicine, 31*(3), 227–246.

Medansky, R. S., & Handler, R. M. (1981). Dermatopsychosomatics: classification, physiology, and therapeutic approaches. *Journal of the American Academy of Dermatology, 5*(2), 125–136.

Mehl, L. E. (1994). Hypnosis and conversion of the breech to the vertex presentation. *Archives of Family Medicine, 3*(10), 881–887.

Meineke, V., Reichrath, J., Reinhold, U., & Tilgen, W. (2002). Verrucae vulgares in children: successful simulated X-ray treatment (a suggestion-based therapy). *Dermatology, 204*(4), 287–289.

Melzack, R. (1991). Sensory and pharmacological modulation of pain. *Canadian Journal of Physiology and Pharmacology, 69*(5), 695–696.

Melzack, R. (1993). Pain: past, present and future. *Canadian Journal of Experimental Psychology = Revue Canadienne de Psychologie Experimentale, 47*(4), 615–629.

Meszaros, I., & Szabo, C. (1999). Correlation of EEG asymmetry and hypnotic susceptibility. *Acta Physiologica Hungarica, 86*(3-4), 259–263.

Miller, V., & Whorwell, P. J. (2009). Hypnotherapy for functional gastrointestinal disorders: a review. *International Journal of Clinical and Experimental Hypnosis, 57*(3), 279–292.

Mirvish, I. (1978). Hypnotherapy for the child with chronic eczema. A case report. *South African Medical Journal = Suid-Afrikaanse Tydskrif vir Geneeskunde, 54*(10), 410–412.

Mishkin, M., & Murray, E. A. (1994). Stimulus recognition. *Current Opinion in Neurobiology, 4*(2), 200–206.

Mitchell, C. W. (1995). Effects of subliminally presented auditory suggestions of itching on scratching behavior. *Perceptual and Motor Skills, 80*(1), 87–96.

Mize, W. L. (1996). Clinical training in self-regulation and practical pediatric hypnosis: what pediatricians want pediatricians to know. *Journal of Developmental and Behavioral Pediatrics, 17*(5), 317–322.

Montera, A. (1968). [Hypnosis: complement to the management of peptic ulcer]. *Hospital (Rio J), 74*(1), 270–289.

Moore, R., Abrahamsen, R., & Brodsgaard, I. (1996). Hypnosis compared with group therapy and individual desensitization for dental anxiety. *European Journal of Oral Sciences, 104*(5-6), 612–618.

Moore, R., Brodsgaard, I., & Abrahamsen, R. (2002). A 3-year comparison of dental anxiety treatment outcomes: hypnosis, group therapy and individual desensitization vs. no specialist treatment. *European Journal of Oral Sciences, 110*(4), 287–295.

Moorefield, C. W. (1971). The use of hypnosis and behavior therapy in asthma. *American Journal of Clinical Hypnosis, 13*(3), 162–168.

Moret, V., Forster, A., Laverriere, M. C., Lambert, H., Gaillard, R. C., Bourgeois, P., Haynal, A., Gemperle, M., & Buchser, E. (1991). Mechanism of analgesia induced by hypnosis and acupuncture: is there a difference? *Pain, 45*(2), 135–140.

Morgan, A. H., Macdonald, H., & Hilgard, E. R. (1974). EEG alpha: lateral asymmetry related to task, and hypnotizability. *Psychophysiology, 11*(3), 275–282.

Morris, B. A. (1985). Hypnotherapy of warts using the Simonton visualization technique: a case report. *American Journal of Clinical Hypnosis, 27*(4), 237–240.

Morrison, J. B. (1988). Chronic asthma and improvement with relaxation induced by hypnotherapy [see comments]. *Journal of the Royal Society of Medicine, 81*(12), 701–704.

Morrow, G. R., & Hickok, J. T. (1993). Behavioral treatment of chemotherapy-induced nausea and vomiting. *Oncology, 7*(12), 83–89; discussion 93–84, 97.

Morse, D. R., & Cohen, B. B. (1983). Desensitization using meditation-hypnosis to control needle phobia in two dental patients. *Anesthesia Progress, 30*(3), 83–85.

Morse, D. R., Hancock, R. R., & Cohen, B. B. (1984). In vivo desensitization using meditation-hypnosis in the treatment of tactile-induced gagging in a dental patient. *International Journal of Psychosomatics, 31*(3), 20–23.

Moskowitz, L. (1996). Psychological management of postsurgical pain and patient adherence. *Hand Clinics, 12*(1), 129–137.

Mun, C. T. (1964). Some Uses of Hypnosis in Gynecology. *Medical Journal of Malaysia, 18,* 223–225.

Murphy, A. I., Lehrer, P. M., Karlin, R., Swartzman, L., Hochron, S., & McCann, B. (1989). Hypnotic susceptibility and its relationship to outcome in the behavioral treatment of asthma: some preliminary data. *Psychological Reports, 65*(2), 691–698.

Muzelak, R. (1974). [Hypnotherapy of hyperemesis gravidarum (author's transl)]. *Ceskoslovenska Gynekologie, 39*(3), 201–202.

Nasemann, T. (1969). [Clinical aspects and virology of warts and condylomas]. *Munchener Medizinische Wochenschrift, 111*(1), 47–56.

Nash, M. R., Lynn, S. J., & Givens, D. L. (1984). Adult hypnotic susceptibility, childhood punishment, and child abuse: a brief communication. *International Journal of Clinical and Experimental Hypnosis, 32*(1), 6–11.

Neinstein, L. S., & Dash, J. (1982). Hypnosis as an adjunct therapy for asthma: case report. *Journal of Adolescent Health Care, 3*(1), 45–48.

Neron, S., & Stephenson, R. (2007). Effectiveness of hypnotherapy with cancer patients' trajectory: emesis, acute pain, and analgesia and anxiolysis in procedures. *International Journal of Clinical and Experimental Hypnosis, 55*(3), 336–354.

Neufeld, V., & Lynn, S. J. (1988). A single-session group self-hypnosis smoking cessation treatment: a brief communication. *International Journal of Clinical and Experimental Hypnosis, 36*(2), 75–79.

Newman, M. (1973). Dental hypnosis. *Journal of the American Dental Association, 86*(1), 36.

Nielsen, G. (1990). Brief integrative dynamic psychotherapy for insomnia. Systematic evaluation of two cases. *Psychotherapy and Psychosomatics, 54*(4), 187–192.

Noll, R. B. (1988). Hypnotherapy of a child with warts. *Journal of Developmental and Behavioral Pediatrics, 9*(2), 89–91.

Novotny, F. (1962). [Autosuggestive psychotherapy of psoriasis]. *Ceskoslovenska dermatologie, 37:* 108–112.

Nugent, W. R., Carden, N. A., & Montgomery, D. J. (1984). Utilizing the creative unconscious in the treatment of hypodermic phobias and sleep disturbance. *American Journal of Clinical Hypnosis, 26*(3), 201–205.

Oakley, M. E., McCreary, C. P., Clark, G. T., Holston, S., Glover, D., & Kashima, K. (1994). A cognitive-behavioral approach to temporomandibular dysfunction treatment failures: a controlled comparison. *Journal of Orofacial Pain, 8*(4), 397–401.

Okasha, A. (1993). Psychiatry in Egypt. *Psychiatric Bulletin, 17:* 548–551.

Olness, K. (1981). Hypnosis in pediatric practice. *Current Problems in Pediatrics, 12*(2), 1–47.

Olness, K. (1981). Imagery (self-hypnosis) as adjunct therapy in childhood cancer: clinical experience with 25 patients. *American Journal of Pediatric Hematology/Oncology, 3*(3), 313–321.

Olness, K., Culbert, T., & Uden, D. (1989). Self-regulation of salivary immunoglobulin A by children. *Pediatrics, 83*(1), 66–71.

Olness, K., & MacDonald, J. (1981). Self-hypnosis and biofeedback in the management of juvenile migraine. *Journal of Developmental and Behavioral Pediatrics, 2*(4), 168–170.

Omer, H., Friedlander, D., & Palti, Z. (1986). Hypnotic relaxation in the treatment of premature labor. *Psychosomatic Medicine, 48*(5), 351–361.

Oster, M. I. (1994). Psychological preparation for labor and delivery using hypnosis. *American Journal of Clinical Hypnosis, 37*(1), 12–21.

Palsson, O. S. (2006). Standardized hypnosis treatment for irritable bowel syndrome: the North Carolina protocol. *International Journal of Clinical and Experimental Hypnosis*, *54*(1), 51–64.

Palsson, O. S., Turner, M. J., Johnson, D. A., Burnelt, C. K., & Whitehead, W. E. (2002). Hypnosis treatment for severe irritable bowel syndrome: investigation of mechanism and effects on symptoms. *Digestive Diseases and Sciences*, *47*(11), 2605–2614.

Palsson, O. S., Turner, M. J., & Whitehead, W. E. (2006). Hypnosis home treatment for irritable bowel syndrome: a pilot study. *International Journal of Clinical and Experimental Hypnosis*, *54*(1), 85–99.

Pastorello, E. A., Codecasa, L. R., Gerosa, A., Buonocore, E., Sillano, V., & Zanussi, C. (1987). The role of suggestion in asthma. II. Effects of a bronchoconstrictor drug on bronchial reactivity under bronchoconstrictor or bronchodilator suggestion. *Annals of Allergy*, *59*(5), 339–340.

Pastorello, E. A., Codecasa, L. R., Pravettoni, V., Zara, C., Incorvaia, C., Froldi, M., & Zanussi, C. (1987). The role of suggestion in asthma. I. Effects of inactive solution on bronchial reactivity under bronchoconstrictor or bronchodilator suggestion. *Annals of Allergy*, *59*(5), 336–338.

Pederson, L. L., Scrimgeour, W. G., & Lefcoe, N. M. (1975). Comparison of hypnosis plus counseling, counseling alone, and hypnosis alone in a community service smoking withdrawal program. *Journal of Consulting and Clinical Psychology*, *43*(6), 920.

Peretz, B. (1996). Relaxation and hypnosis in pediatric dental patients. *Journal of Clinical Pediatric Denistry*, *20*(3), 205–207.

Peterson, D. B., Sumner, J. W., Jr., & G. A. Jones (1950). Role of hypnosis in differentiation of epileptic from convulsive-like seizures. *American Journal of Psychiatry*, *107*(6), 428–433.

Pfitzer, B. E., Clark, K., & Revenstorf, D. (2005). [Medical hypnosis in cases of herpes labialis improves resistance for recurrence. A pilot study]. *Der Hautarzt; Zeitschrift fur Dermatologie, Venerologie, und verwandte Gebiete*, *56*(6), 562–568.

Phelps, L. A. (1990). MRI and claustrophobia. *American Family Physician*, *42*(4), 930.

Phoenix, S. L. (2007). Psychotherapeutic intervention for numerous and large viral warts with adjunctive hypnosis: a case study. *American Journal of Clinical Hypnosis*, *49*(3), 211–218.

Piccione, C., Hilgard, E. R., & Zimbardo, P. G. (1989). On the degree of stability of measured hypnotizability over a 25-year period. *Journal of Personality and Social Psychology*, *56*(2), 289–295.

Piscicelli, U. (1968). [Hypnosis therapy in hyperemesis gravidarum]. *Minerva Med*, *59*(27), 1555–1565.

Place, M. (1984). Hypnosis and the child. *Journal of Child Psychology and Psychiatry, and Allied Disciplines*, *25*(3), 339–347.

Poliakov, V. V. (1989). [Treatment of hyperemesis gravidarum by hypnosis]. *Akush Ginekol (Mosk)*(5), 57–58.

Posner, M. I., & Petersen, S. E. (1990). The attention system of the human brain. *Annual Review of Neuroscience*, *13*, 25–42.

Prince, M. (1906). *The dissociation of personality*. New York, Longmans-Green.

Putilin, S. A. (1961). [Hypnotherapy of severe herpetiform dermatosis in pregnancy]. *Voprosy okhrany materinstva i detstva 6*: 90–91.

Rabkin, S. W., E. Boyko, Shane, F., & Kaufert, J. (1984). A randomized trial comparing smoking cessation programs utilizing behaviour modification, health education or hypnosis. *Addictive Behaviors*, *9*(2), 157–173.

Rainville, P., Hofbauer, R. K., Bushnell, M. C., Duncan, G. H., & Price, D. D. (2002). Hypnosis modulates activity in brain structures involved in the regulation of consciousness. *Journal of Cognitive Neuroscience*, *14*(6), 887–901.

Rainville, P., Hofbauer, R. K., Paus, T., Duncan, G. H., Bushnell, M. C., & Price, D. D. (1999). Cerebral mechanisms of hypnotic induction and suggestion. *Journal of Cognitive Neuroscience*, *11*(1), 110–125.

Rape, R. N., & Bush, J. P. (1994). Psychological preparation for pediatric oncology patients undergoing painful procedures: a methodological critique of the research. *Child Health Care*, *23*(1), 51–67.

Redd, W. H., Andresen, G. V., & Minagawa, R. Y. (1982). Hypnotic control of anticipatory emesis in patients receiving cancer chemotherapy. *Journal of Consulting and Clinical Psychology*, *50*(1), 14–19.

Reis e Almeida, F. S. (1983). [Dental hypnosis]. *Rev Port Estomatol Cir Maxilofac*, *24*(2), 183–197.

Renouf, D. (1998). Hypnotically induced control of nausea: a preliminary report. *Journal of Psychosomatic Research*, *45*(3), 295–296.

Richardson, J., Smith, J. E., McCall, G., & Pilkington, K. (2006). Hypnosis for procedure-related pain and distress in pediatric cancer patients: a systematic review of effectiveness and methodology related to hypnosis interventions. *Journal of Pain and Symptom Management*, *31*(1), 70–84.

Richardson, J., Smith, J. E., McCall, G., Richardson, A., Pilkington, K., & Kirsch, I. (2007). Hypnosis for nausea and vomiting in cancer chemotherapy: a systematic review of the research evidence. *European Journal of Cancer Care*, *16*(5), 402–412.

Robb, N. D., & Crothers, A. J. (1996). Sedation in dentistry. Part 2: Management of the gagging patient. *Dental Update*, *23*(5), 182–186.

Roberts, L., Wilson, S., Singh, S., Roalfe, A., & Greenfield, S. (2006). Gut-directed hypnotherapy for irritable bowel syndrome: piloting a primary care-based randomised controlled trial. *British Journal of General Practice: The Journal of the Royal College of General Practitioners*, *56*(523), 115–121.

Robertson, J. (2007). Review: distraction, hypnosis, and combined cognitive-behavioural interventions reduce needle related pain and distress in children and adolescents. *Evidence-Based Nursing*, *10*(3), 75.

Roden, R. G. (1970). Management of delivery under hypnosis. *Canadian Family Physician Medecin de Famille Canadien*, *16*(5), 77–78.

Rodger, B. P. (1961). Hypnosis as an adjunct to delivery room anesthesia: benefits of a psychologic approach. *Anesthesia and Analgesia*, *40*, 206–209.

Romanson, P. C., & Clark, J. B. (1981). Hypnosis—a dental perspective. *Ontario Dentist*, *58*(7), 17–18.

Rowe, W. S. (1982). Hypnotherapy and plantar warts. *Australian and New Zealand Journal of Psychiatry*, *16*(4), 304.

Roy, A. (1980). Hysteria. *Journal of Psychosomatic Research*, *24*(2), 53–56.

Rucklidge, J. J., & Saunders, D. (1999). Hypnosis in a case of long-standing idiopathic itch. *Psychosomatic Medicine*, *61*(3), 355–358.

Rucklidge, J. J., & Saunders, D. (2002). The efficacy of hypnosis in the treatment of pruritus in people with HIV/AIDS: a time-series analysis. *International Journal of Clinical and Experimental Hypnosis*, *50*(2), 149–169.

Rustvold, S. R. (1994). Hypnotherapy for treatment of dental phobia in children. *General Dentistry*, *42*(4), 346–348.

Sabourin, M. E., Cutcomb, S. D., Crawford, H. J., & Pribram, K. (1990). EEG correlates of hypnotic susceptibility and hypnotic trance: spectral analysis and coherence. *International Journal of Psychophysiology*, *10*(2), 125–142.

Sampson, R. N. (1990). Hypnotherapy in a case of pruritus and Guillain-Barre syndrome. *American Journal of Clinical Hypnosis*, *32*(3), 168–173.

Savel'ev, A. A. (1974). [Treatment of hyperemesis gravidarum by hypnosis]. *Akush Ginekol (Mosk)*(3), 69–70.

Schacter, D. L. (1987). Implicit expressions of memory in organic amnesia: learning of new facts and associations. *Human Neurobiology*, *6*(2), 107–118.

Schacter, D. L. (1992). Understanding implicit memory. A cognitive neuroscience approach. *American Psychologist*, *47*(4), 559–569.

Schafer, D. W. (1997). Hypnosis and the treatment of ulcerative colitis and Crohn's disease. *American Journal of Clinical Hypnosis*, *40*(2), 111–117.

Schauble, P. G., Werner, W. E., Rai, S. H., & Martin, A. (1998). Childbirth preparation through hypnosis: the hypnoreflexogenous protocol. *American Journal of Clinical Hypnosis*, *40*(4), 273–283.

Schenck, C. H., & Mahowald, M. W. (1995). Two cases of premenstrual sleep terrors and injurious sleep-walking. *Journal of Psychosomatic Obstetrics and Gynaecology*, *16*(2), 79–84.

Schey, L. (1976). Effectiveness of hypnosis on reducing dental anxiety. *Dental Hygiene*, *50*(3), 115–119.

Schmierer, A., & Schmierer, G. (1990). [Possibilities for hypnosis in dental practice]. *Zahnarztl Prax*, *41*(5), 178–181.

Schneck, J. M. (1958). Hypnotherapy for achalasia of the esophagus (cardiospasm). *American Journal of Psychiatry, 114*(11), 1042–1043.

Schulz-Stubner, S., Krings, T., Meister, I. G., Rex, S., Thron, A., & Rossaint, R. (2004). Clinical hypnosis modulates functional magnetic resonance imaging signal intensities and pain perception in a thermal stimulation paradigm. *Reginal Anesthesia and Pain Medicine, 29*(6), 549–556.

Schwartz, J. (1987). *Smoking Cessation Methods: United States and Canada, 1978–85* (USPHS NIH 87–2940). N. C. I. Division of Cancer Prevention and Control.

Secter, II, & Barthelemy, C. G. (1964). Angular chelosis and psorasis as psychosomatic menifestations. *American Journal of Clinical Hypnosis, 7*, 79–81.

Seeman, W. (1960). Hypnotic wart treatment: a report of treatment of warts in an eleven year old child. *Journal of the Kansas Medical Society, 61*, 151.

Seidner, S. (1967). [Hypnosis in the dental practice]. *Quintessenz, 18*(1), 115–116.

Seikowski, K., Weber, B., & Haustein, U. F. (1995). [Effect of hypnosis and autogenic training on acral circulation and coping with the illness in patients with progressive scleroderma]. *Hautarzt, 46*(2), 94–101.

Shaw, A. J., & Niven, N. (1996). Theoretical concepts and practical applications of hypnosis in the treatment of children and adolescents with dental fear and anxiety. *British Dental Journal, 180*(1), 11–16.

Shaw, A. J., & Welbury, R. R. (1996). The use of hypnosis in a sedation clinic for dental extractions in children: report of 20 cases. *ASDC Journal of Denistry for Children, 63*(6), 418–420.

Sheehan, D. V. (1978). Influence of psychosocial factors on wart remission. *American Journal of Clinical Hypnosis, 20*(3), 160–164.

Shenefelt, P. D. (2000). Hypnosis in dermatology. *Archives of Dermatology, 136*(3), 393–399.

Shenefelt, P. D. (2002). Complementary psychotherapy in dermatology: hypnosis and biofeedback. *Clinics in Dermatology, 20*(5), 595–601.

Shenefelt, P. D. (2003). Applying hypnosis in dermatology. *Dermatology Nursing, 15*(6), 513–517, 538; quiz 518.

Shenefelt, P. D. (2003). Biofeedback, cognitive-behavioral methods, and hypnosis in dermatology: is it all in your mind? *Dermatologic Therapy, 16*(2), 114–122.

Shertzer, C. L., & Lookingbill, D. P. (1987). Effects of relaxation therapy and hypnotizability in chronic urticaria. *Archives of Dermatology, 123*(7), 913–916.

Shinozaki, M., Kanazawa, M., Kano, M., Endo, Y., Nakaya, N., Hongo, M., & Fukudo, S. (2010). Effect of autogenic training on general improvement in patients with irritable bowel syndrome: a randomized controlled trial. *Applied Psychophysiology and Biofeedback, 35*(3), 189–198.

Shor, R. E., & Orne, E. C. (1962). *Harvard group scale of hypnotic susceptibility.* Palo Alto, CA, Consulting Psychologist Press.

Shul'man, S. A. (1995). [Use of hypnosis in multimodal treatment of children with urologic diseases]. *Khirurgiia,* (4), 30–31.

Sidis, B., & Goodhart, S. (1905). *Multiple personality.* New York : Appleton-Century-Crofts.

Sigalowitz, S., Dywan, J., & Ismailos, L. (1991). Electrocortical evidence that hypnotically-induced hallucinations are experienced. *Society for Clinical and Experimental Hypnosis.* New Orleans, LA.

Simon, E. P. (1999). Hypnosis in the treatment of hyperemesis gravidarum. *American Family Physician, 60*(1), 56, 61.

Simon, E. P. (1999). Hypnosis using a communication device to increase magnetic resonance imaging tolerance with a claustrophobic patient. *Military Medicine, 164*(1), 71–72.

Simon, E. P. (1999). Improving tolerance of MR imaging with medical hypnosis. *American Journal of Roentgenology, 172*(6), 1694–1695.

Simon, E. P., & Canonico, M. M. (2001). Use of hypnosis in controlling lumbar puncture distress in an adult needle-phobic dementia patient. *International Journal of Clinical and Experimental Hypnosis, 49*(1), 56–67.

Simon, E. P., & Lewis, D. M. (2000). Medical hypnosis for temporomandibular disorders: treatment efficacy and medical utilization outcome. *Oral Surgery, Oral Medicine, Oral Pathology, Oral Radiology, and Endodontics, 90*(1), 54–63.

Simon, E. P., & Schwartz, J. (1999). Medical hypnosis for hyperemesis gravidarum. *Birth, 26*(4), 248–254.

Simren, M. (2006). Hypnosis for irritable bowel syndrome: the quest for the mechanism of action. *International Journal of Clinical and Experimental Hypnosis, 54*(1), 65–84.

Sinclair-Gieben, A. H., & Chalmers, D. (1959). Evaluation of treatment of warts by hypnosis. *Lancet, 2*, 480–482.

Sjoberg, B. M., Jr., & Hollister, L. E. (1965). The effects of psychotomimetic drugs on primary suggestibility. *Psychopharmacologia, 8*(4), 251–262.

Skalicanova, M., Nagyova, H., & Koradova, E. (1977). [Suggestive and group psychotherapy in some children's somatic diseases (author's transl)]. *Ceskoslovenska psychiatrie, 73*(3), 174–177.

Smith, B. J. (1982). Management of the patient with hyperemesis gravidarum in family therapy with hypnotherapy as an adjunct. *Journal of the New York State Nurses' Association, 13*(1), 17–26.

Smith, C. H. (1989). Acute pregnancy-associated hypertension treated with hypnosis: a case report. *American Journal of Clinical Hypnosis, 31*(3), 209–211.

Smith, M. M., Colebatch, H. J., & Clarke, P. S. (1970). Increase and decrease in pulmonary resistance with hypnotic suggestion in asthma. *American Review of Respiratory Disease, 102*(2), 236–242.

Smith, R. (1986). Hypnosis—adjuvant in dental treatment. *British Dental Journal, 160*(10), 344.

Smith, S. R. (1969). Hypnosis in general dental practice. 1. *Probe, 11*(1), 5–6 passim.

Smith, S. R. (1969). Hypnosis in general dental practice. 2. *Probe, 11*(2), 43–45 concl.

Snape, W. J., Jr. (1994). Current concepts in the management of the irritable bowel syndrome. *Revista de Gastroenterologia de Mexico, 59*(2), 127–132.

Soo, S., Moayyedi, P., Deeks, J., Delaney, B., Lewis, M., & Forman, D. (2005). Psychological interventions for non-ulcer dyspepsia. *Cochrane Database of Systematic Reviews,* (2), CD002301.

Spanos, N. P., Stenstrom, R. J., & Johnston, J. C. (1988). Hypnosis, placebo, and suggestion in the treatment of warts. *Psychosomatic Medicine, 50*(3), 245–260.

Spanos, N. P., Williams, V., & Gwynn, M. I. (1990). Effects of hypnotic, placebo, and salicylic acid treatments on wart regression. *Psychosomatic Medicine, 52*(1), 109–114.

Spector, S. L., & Kinsman, R. H. (1988). The role of suggestion in asthma. *Annals of Allergy, 61*(2), 157–158.

Spiegel, D. (1981). Vietnam grief work using hypnosis. *American Journal of Clinical Hypnosis, 24*(1), 33–40.

Spiegel, D. (2003). Negative and positive visual hypnotic hallucinations: attending inside and out. *International Journal of Clinical and Experimental Hypnosis, 51*(2), 130–146.

Spiegel, D. (2006). Wedding hypnosis to the radiology suite. *Pain, 126*(1–3), 3–4.

Spiegel, D., & Albert, L. H. (1983). Naloxone fails to reverse hypnotic alleviation of chronic pain. *Psychopharmacology, 81*(2), 140–143.

Spiegel, D., Bloom, J. R., & Yalom, I. (1981). Group support for patients with metastatic cancer. A randomized outcome study. *Archives of General Psychiatry, 38*(5), 527–533.

Spiegel, D., & Cardeña, E. (1991). Disintegrated experience: the dissociative disorders revisited. *Journal of Abnormal Psychology, 100*(3), 366–378.

Spiegel, D., Cutcomb, S., Ren, C., & Pribram, K. (1985). Hypnotic hallucination alters evoked potentials. *Journal of Abnormal Psychology, 94*(3), 249–255.

Spiegel, D., Detrick, D., & Frischholz, E. (1982). Hypnotizability and psychopathology. *American Journal of Psychiatry, 139*(4), 431–437.

Spiegel, D., Hunt, T., & Dondershine, H. E. (1988). Dissociation and hypnotizability in posttraumatic stress disorder. *American Journal of Psychiatry, 145*(3), 301–305.

Spiegel, D., & King, R. (1992). Hypnotizability and CSF HVA levels among psychiatric patients. *Biological Psychiatry, 31*(1), 95–98.

Spiegel, D., & Moore, R. (1997). Imagery and hypnosis in the treatment of cancer patients. *Oncology, 11*(8), 1179–1189; discussion 1189–1195.

Spiegel, H. (1970). A single-treatment method to stop smoking using ancillary self-hypnosis. *International Journal of Clinical and Experimental Hypnosis, 18*(4), 235–250.

Spiegel, H. (1970). Termination of smoking by a single treatment. *Archives of Environmental Health, 20*(6), 736–742.

Spiegel, H. (1972). An eye-roll test for hypnotizability. *American Journal of Clinical Hypnosis, 15*(1), 25–28.

Spiegel, H., & Spiegel, D. (1987). *Trance and treatment: Clinical uses of hypnosis.* Washington, DC: American Psychiatric Press.

Spiegel, H., & Spiegel, D. (2004). *Trance and treatment: Clinical uses of hypnosis.* Washington, DC: American Psychiatric Press.

Stankler, L. (1967). A critical assessment of the cure of warts by suggestion. *The Practitioner, 198*(187), 690–694.

Stanton, H. E. (1978). A one-session hypnotic approach to modifying smoking behavior. *International Journal of Clinical and Experimental Hypnosis, 26*(1), 22–29.

Stanton, H. E. (1989). Hypnosis and rational-emotive therapy—a de-stressing combination: a brief communication. *International Journal of Clinical and Experimental Hypnosis, 37*(2), 95–99.

Stanton, H. E. (1991). Smoking cessation in a single session: an update. *International Journal of Psychosomatics, 38*(1-4), 84–88.

Stead, L. F., Bergson, G., & Lancaster, T. (2008). Physician advice for smoking cessation. *Cochrane Database of Systematic Reviews*(2), CD000165.

Steele, K., & Irwin, W. G. (1988). Treatment options for cutaneous warts in family practice. *Family Practice, 5*(4), 314–319.

Steggles, S. (1999). The use of cognitive-behavioral treatment including hypnosis for claustrophobia in cancer patients. *American Journal of Clinical Hypnosis, 41*(4), 319–326.

Steggles, S., Damore-Petingola, S., Maxwell, J., & Lightfoot, N. (1997). Hypnosis for children and adolescents with cancer: an annotated bibliography, 1985–1995. *Journal of Pediatric Oncology Nursing: Official Journal of the Association of Pediatric Oncology Nurses, 14*(1), 27–32.

Stewart, A. C., & Thomas, S. E. (1995). Hypnotherapy as a treatment for atopic dermatitis in adults and children. *British Journal of Dermatology, 132*(5), 778–783.

Straatmeyer, A. J., & Rhodes, N. R. (1983). Condylomata acuminata: results of treatment using hypnosis. *Journal of the American Academy of Dermatology, 9*(3), 434–436.

Stutman, R. K., & Bliss, E. L. (1985). Posttraumatic stress disorder, hypnotizability, and imagery. *American Journal of Psychiatry, 142*(6), 741–743.

Surman, O. S., & Crumpacker, C. (1987). Psychological aspects of herpes simplex viral infection: report of six cases. *American Journal of Clinical Hypnosis, 30*(2), 125–131.

Surman, O. S., Gottlieb, S. K., & Hackett, T. P. (1972). Hypnotic treatment of a child with warts. *American Journal of Clinical Hypnosis, 15*(1), 12–14.

Surman, O. S., Gottlieb, S. K., Hackett, T. P., & Silverberg, E. L. (1973). Hypnosis in the treatment of warts. *Archives of General Psychiatry, 28*(3), 439–441.

Surwit, R. S., Allen, L. M., 3rd, Gilgor, R. S., & Duvic, M. (1982). The combined effect of prazosin and autogenic training on cold reactivity in Raynaud's phenomenon. *Biofeedback and Self-Regulation, 7*(4), 537–544.

Susmano, A., Feldfeber, B., & Meeroff, M. (1960). [Ulcerative colitis and hypnosis. Apropos of a case.]. *Med Panam, 14,* 235–241.

Syrjala, K. L., Cummings, C., & Donaldson, G. W. (1992). Hypnosis or cognitive behavioral training for the reduction of pain and nausea during cancer treatment: a controlled clinical trial. *Pain, 48*(2), 137–146.

Szechtman, H., Woody, E., Bowers, K. S., & Nahmias, C. (1998). Where the imaginal appears real: a positron emission tomography study of auditory hallucinations. *Proceedings of the National Academy of Sciences of the United States of America, 95*(4), 1956–1960.

Tan, G., Hammond, D. C., & Joseph, G. (2005). Hypnosis and irritable bowel syndrome: a review of efficacy and mechanism of action. *American Journal of Clinical Hypnosis, 47*(3), 161–178.

Tasini, M. F., & Hackett, T. P. (1977). Hypnosis in the treatment of warts in immunodeficient children. *American Journal of Clinical Hypnosis, 19*(3), 152–154.

Tausk, F., & Whitmore, S. E. (1999). A pilot study of hypnosis in the treatment of patients with psoriasis. *Psychotherapy and Psychosomatics, 68*(4), 221–225.

Tellegen, A. (1981). Practicing the two disciplines for relaxation and enlightenment: comment on role of the feedback signal in electromyograph biofeedback: the relevance of attention by Qualls and Sheehan. *Journal of Experimental Psychology. General, 110*(2), 217–231.

Tellegen, A., & Atkinson, G. (1974). Openness to absorbing and self-altering experiences (absorption), a trait related to hypnotic susceptibility. *Journal of Abnormal Psychology, 83*(3), 268–277.

Tenzel, J. H., & Taylor, R. L. (1969). An evaluation of hypnosis and suggestion as treatment for warts. *Psychosomatics, 10*(4), 252–257.

Tiran, D. (2004). Breech presentation: increasing maternal choice. *Complementary Therapies in Nursing & Midwifery, 10*(4), 233–238.

Tobia, L. (1982). [Hypnosis in dermatology]. *Minerva Med, 73*(10), 531–537.

Tonnesen, P. (2009). Smoking cessation: How compelling is the evidence? A review. *Health Policy, 9*(Suppl 1), S15–S25.

Tonnesen, P., Norregaard, J., Simonsen, K., & Sawe, U. (1991). A double-blind trial of a 16-hour transdermal nicotine patch in smoking cessation. *The New England Journal of Medicine, 325*(5), 311–315.

Torem, M. S. (1994). Hypnotherapeutic techniques in the treatment of hyperemesis gravidarum. *American Journal of Clinical Hypnosis, 37*(1), 1–11.

Tsiskarishvili, N. V., Eradze, M., & Tsiskarishvili Ts, I. (2010). [Psychophysical and physical methods in treatment of dermatoses, accompanied by skin dryness and itching]. *Georgian Medical News,* (181), 28–32.

Tsushima, W. T. (1988). Current psychological treatments for stress-related skin disorders. *Cutis, 42*(5), 402–404.

Tuerk, M. J., & Koo, J. (2008). A practical review and update on the management of pruritus sine materia. *Cutis, 82*(3), 187–194.

Ullman, M., & Dudek, S. (1960). On the psyche and warts. II. Hypnotic suggestion and warts. *Psychosomatic Medicine, 22,* 68–76.

Ullmann, M. (1959). On the psyche and warts. I. Suggestion and warts: a review and comment. *Psychosomatic medicine, 21,* 473–488.

Ulrich, P., Meyer, H. J., Diehl, B., & Meinig, G. (1987). Cerebral blood flow in autogenic training and hypnosis. *Neurosurgical Review, 10*(4), 305–307.

Usberti, M., Grutta d'Auria, C., Borghi, M., Pecchini, F., Pecoraro, C., & Dal Canton, A. (1984). Usefulness of hypnosis for renal needle biopsy in children. *Kidney International, 26*(3), 351–352.

van der Kolk, B. A., & Fisler, R. (1995). Dissociation and the fragmentary nature of traumatic memories: overview and exploratory study. *Journal of Traumatic Stress, 8*(4), 505–525.

van der Kolk, B. A., Hostetler, A., Herron, N., & Fisler, R. E. (1994). Trauma and the development of borderline personality disorder. *Psychiatric Clinics of North America, 17*(4), 715–730.

VandeVusse, L., Irland, J., Healthcare, W. F., Berner, M. A., Fuller, S., & Adams, D. (2007). Hypnosis for childbirth: a retrospective comparative analysis of outcomes in one obstetrician's practice. *American Journal of Clinical Hypnosis, 50*(2), 109–119.

Vidakovic-Vukic, M. (1999). Hypnotherapy in the treatment of irritable bowel syndrome: methods and results in Amsterdam. *Scandinavian Journal of Gastroenterology Supplement, 230,* 49–51.

Vlarsky, J., & Janousek, B. (1960). [Our experience with the treatment of eczema with hypnosis]. *Ceskoslovenska Dermatologie, 35,* 86–89.

Vlieger, A. M., Menko-Frankenhuis, C., Wolfkamp, S. C., Tromp, E., & Benninga, M. A. (2007). Hypnotherapy for children with functional abdominal pain or irritable bowel syndrome: a randomized controlled trial. *Gastroenterology, 133*(5), 1430–1436.

Vollmer, H. (1946). Treatment of warts by suggestion. *Psychosomatic Medicine, 8*, 138–142.

Walling, D. P., & Baker, J. M. (1996). Hypnosis training in psychology intern programs. *American Journal of Clinical Hypnosis, 38*(3), 219–223.

Walling, D. P., Baker, J. M., & Dott, S. G. (1996). A national survey of hypnosis training—its status in psychiatric residency programs: a brief communication. *International Journal of Clinical and Experimental Hypnosis, 44*(3), 184–188.

Watkins, H. H. (1976). Hypnosis and smoking: a five-session approach. *International Journal of Clinical and Experimental Hypnosis, 24*(4), 381–390.

Watkins, J. G. (1987). *Hypnotherapeutic technique: The practice of clinical hypnosis. Volume Two.* New York: Irvington Publishers.

Waxman, D. (1973). Behaviour therapy of psoriasis—a hypnoanalytic and counter-conditioning technique. *Postgraduate Medical Journal, 49*(574), 591–595.

Webb, A. N., Kukuruzovic, R. H., Catto-Smith, A. G., & Sawyer, S. M. (2007). Hypnotherapy for treatment of irritable bowel syndrome. *Cochrane Database of Systematic Reviews*, (4), CD005110.

Weinstein, E. J., & Au, P. K. (1991). Use of hypnosis before and during angioplasty. *American Journal of Clinical Hypnosis, 34*(1), 29–37.

Weitzenhoffer, A. M. (1962). Estimation of hypnotic susceptibility in a group situation. *American Journal of Clinical Hypnosis, 5*, 115–126.

Weitzenhoffer, A. M. (1962). The significance of hypnotic depth in therapy. *International Journal of Clinical and Experimental Hypnosis, 10*, 75–78.

Weitzenhoffer, A. M., & Hilgard, E. R. (1959). *Stanford hypnotic susceptibility scale, forms A & B.* Palo Alto, CA: Consulting Psychologists Press.

Wendel, K. (1959). [Again: suggestion therapy of warts]. *Hippokrates, 30*(3), 148.

Werner, W. E. (1959). Hypnosis from the viewpoint of obstetrics and clinical demonstration of the training of patients for delivery under hypnosis. *New York State Journal of Medicine, 59*(8), 1561–1566.

West, J. R., Kierland, R. R., & Litin, E. M. (1961). Atopic dermatitis and hypnosis. Physiologic stigmata before, during, and after hypnosis. *Archives of Dermatology, 84*, 579–588.

Weyandt, J. A. (1976). Hypnosis in a dental patient with allergies. *American Journal of Clinical Hypnosis, 19*(2), 123–125.

White, H. C. (1961). Hypnosis in bronchial asthma. *Journal of Psychsomatic Research, 5*, 272–279.

Whitehead, W. E. (2006). Hypnosis for irritable bowel syndrome: the empirical evidence of therapeutic effects. *International Journal of Clinical and Experimental Hypnosis, 54*(1), 7–20.

Whorwell, P. J. (1989). Hypnotherapy in irritable bowel syndrome. *Lancet, 1*(8638), 622.

Whorwell, P. J. (1991). Use of hypnotherapy in gastrointestinal disease. *British Journal of Hospital Medicine, 45*(1), 27–29.

Whorwell, P. J. (2005). Review article: The history of hypnotherapy and its role in the irritable bowel syndrome. *Alimentary Pharmacology & Therapeutics, 22*(11–12), 1061–1067.

Whorwell, P. J. (2008). Hypnotherapy for irritable bowel syndrome: the response of colonic and noncolonic symptoms. *Journal of Psychosomatic Research, 64*(6), 621–623.

Whorwell, P. J. (2009). Behavioral therapy for IBS. *Nature Clinical Practice. Gastroenterology & Hepatology, 6*(3), 148–149.

Whorwell, P. J., Prior, A., & Colgan, S. M. (1987). Hypnotherapy in severe irritable bowel syndrome: further experience. *Gut, 28*(4), 423–425.

Whorwell, P. J., Prior, A., & Faragher, E. B. (1984). Controlled trial of hypnotherapy in the treatment of severe refractory irritable-bowel syndrome. *Lancet, 2*(8414), 1232–1234.

Widlocher, D., & Dantchev, N. (1994). [Charcot and hysteria]. *Revue Neurologique (Paris), 150*(8-9), 490–497.

Wik, G., Fischer, H., Bragee, B., Finer, B., & Fredrikson, M. (1999). Functional anatomy of hypnotic analgesia: a PET study of patients with fibromyalgia. *European Journal of Pain, 3*(1), 7–12.

Wild, M. R., & Espie, C. A. (2004). The efficacy of hypnosis in the reduction of procedural pain and distress in pediatric oncology: a systematic review. *Journal of Developmental and Behavioral Pediatrics, 25*(3), 207–213.

Wilkening, K. (1978). [Therapy of juvenile warts]. *Deutsche medizinische Wochenschrift, 103*(7), 317.

Wilkinson, J. B. (1981). Hypnotherapy in the psychosomatic approach to illness: a review. *Journal of the Royal Society of Medicine, 74*(7), 525–530.

Wilkinson, J. B. (1989). Chronic asthma and hypnotherapy. *Journal of the Royal Society of Medicine, 82*(11), 694–695.

Wilks, C. G. (1994). 'The use of hypnosis in the management of 'gagging' and intolerance to dentures'. *British Dental Journal, 176*(9), 332.

Williams, J. M., & Hall, D. W. (1988). Use of single session hypnosis for smoking cessation. *Addictive Behaviors, 13*(2), 205–208.

Williamson, J. W., McColl, R., Mathews, D., Mitchell, J. H., Raven, P. B., & Morgan, W. P. (2001). Hypnotic manipulation of effort sense during dynamic exercise: cardiovascular responses and brain activation. *Journal of Applied Physiology, 90*(4), 1392–1399.

Wilson, S., Maddison, T., Roberts, L., Greenfield, S., & Singh, S. (2006). Systematic review: the effectiveness of hypnotherapy in the management of irritable bowel syndrome. *Alimentary Pharmacology & Therapeutics, 24*(5), 769–780.

Winchell, S. A., & Watts, R. A. (1988). Relaxation therapies in the treatment of psoriasis and possible pathophysiologic mechanisms. *Journal of the American Academy of Dermatology, 18*(1 Pt 1), 101–104.

Windholz, G. (1996). Hypnosis and inhibition as viewed by Heidenhain and Pavlov. *Integrative Physiological and Behavioral Science, 31*(2), 155–162.

Winkelstein, L. B. (1958). Routine hypnosis for obstetrical delivery; an evaluation of hypnosuggestion in 200 consecutive cases. *American Journal of Obstetrics and Gynecology, 76*(1), 152–160.

Wood, G. J., & Zadeh, H. H. (1999). Potential adjunctive applications of hypnosis in the management of periodontal diseases. *American Journal of Clinical Hypnosis, 41*(3), 212–225.

Zachariae, R., Oster, H., Bjerring, P., & Kragballe, K. (1996). Effects of psychologic intervention on psoriasis: a preliminary report. *Journal of the American Academy of Dermatology, 34*(6), 1008–1015.

Zaitsev, V. P., Shafikova, A. G., et al. (1990). [The efficacy of the hypnosuggestive psychotherapy of myocardial infarct patients]. *Terapevticheskii arkhiv, 62*(10), 97–100.

Zamotaev, I. P., Sultanova, A., & Vorob'eva, Z. V. (1983). [Effect of hypnotic suggestion in bronchial asthma]. *Sovetskaia meditsina*, (2), 7–10.

Zane, M. D. (1966). The hypnotic situation and changes in ulcer pain. *International Journal of Clinical and Experimental Hypnosis, 14*(4), 292–304.

Zeltzer, L., Kellerman, J., Ellenberg, L., & Dash, J. (1983). Hypnosis for reduction of vomiting associated with chemotherapy and disease in adolescents with cancer. *Journal of Adolescent Health Care, 4*(2), 77–84.

Zeltzer, L., & LeBaron, S. (1982). Hypnosis and nonhypnotic techniques for reduction of pain and anxiety during painful procedures in children and adolescents with cancer. *Journal of Pediatrics, 101*(6), 1032–1035.

Zeltzer, L., LeBaron, S., & Zeltzer, P. M. (1984). The effectiveness of behavioral intervention for reduction of nausea and vomiting in children and adolescents receiving chemotherapy. *Journal of Clinical Oncology, 2*(6), 683–690.

Zeltzer, L. K., Dolgin, M. J., LeBaron, S., & LeBaron, C. (1991). A randomized, controlled study of behavioral intervention for chemotherapy distress in children with cancer. *Pediatrics, 88*(1), 34–42.

Zheltakov, M. M., IuK, S., & Somov, B. A. (1963). [Combined treatment of patients suffering from neurodermatitis, eczema and other dermatoses with hypnosis, electric sleep and corticosteroid.]. *Soviet Medicine, 27,* 59–63.

Ziegler, F. J., Imboden, J. B., & Meyer, E. (1960). Contemporary conversion reactions: a clinical study. *American Journal of Psychiatry, 116,* 901–910.

Zimbardo, P., Maslach, C., & Marshall, G. (1970). *Hypnosis and the psychology of cognitive and behavioral control.* Stanford, CA: Stanford University Press.

APPENDIX A

HYPNOTIC INDUCTION PROFILE EVALUATION SHEET AND THE CORRESPONDING HYPNOTIC INDUCTION PROTOCOL

Spiegel, H. and D. Spiegel (1978). Trance and treatment: Clinical uses of hypnosis. New York, N.Y., Basic Books.

Spiegel , H. and D. Spiegel (2004). Trance and Treatment: Clinical Uses of Hypnosis (2nd Edition). Washington, DC, American Psychiatric Press.

Hypnotic Induction Profile
Evaluation Sheet

Name _____ Date _____

Age _____ Sequence: Initial _____ Previous _____ When _____

Position of Subject: Chair-Stool _____ Supine _____ Chair _____ Standing _____

Item

A   UP-Gaze   0 - 1 - 2 - 3 - 4

B   Roll: 0 - 1 - 2 - 3 - 4

C   Squint: 0 - 1 - 2 - 3 - 4

D   Eye-Roll Sign (roll and squint)   0 - 1 - 2 - 3 - 4

E   Arm (R-L) Levitation Instruction   0 - 1 - 2 - 3 - 4

F   Tingle   0 -   1 - 2

G ___ Dissociation   0 -   1 - 2

H ___ Levitation
(postinduction)

no reinforcement			3 - 4
I St		2 - 3	
2 nd	1 - 2		
3 rd	1		Smile _____
4 th	0		Surprise _____

I ___ Control Differential   0 -   1   2

J ___ Cut-off   0 -   1   2

K ___ Amnesia to Cut-off   0 -   1   2
       or No-Test

L ___ Floating Sensation   0 -   1   2

Summary Scores:

_____ Induction Score   Profile Score   0 - 1 - 2 - 3 - 4 - 5

                        ____ Soft   ____ Zero   ____ Intact

                        ____ Decrement   ____ Special Zero   ____ Increment

_____ Minutes

Revised from Spiegel H, Spiegel D. "Trance & Treatment", American Psychiatric Press, 1987, Wash., D.C.

HYPNOTIC INDUCTION PROFILE PROTOCOL

UP-GAZE Get as comfortable as possible with your arms resting on the arms of the chair and both feet up. Now look toward me. As you hold your head in that position, look up toward your eyebrows-now toward the top of your head.

UPGAZE: 0 - 1 - 2 - 3 - 4

EYEROLL As you continue to look upward, close your eyelids slowly. That's right close, close, close...

ROLL: 0 - 1 - 2 - 3 - 4   SOUINT: 0 - 1 - 2 - 3 - 4

LEFT ARM LEVITATION Keep your eyelids closed and continue to look upward. Take a deep breath, hold.... Now, exhale, let your eyes relax while keeping the lids closed, and let your body float. Imagine a feeling of floating, floating right down through the chair .... There will be something pleasant and welcome about this sensation of floating. As you concentrate on this floating, I am going to concentrate on your left arm and hand. Touch arm and hand. In a while I am going to stroke the middle finger of your left hand.

Lift hand slightly and put it down again. Leave your right hand resting lightly on person's left hand.

After I do, you will develop movement sensations in that finger. Then the movements will spread, causing your left hand to feel light and buoyant, and you will let it float upward. Ready? Stroke finger and arm.

First one finger, then another. As these restless movements develop, your hand becomes light and buoyant. your elbow bends, your forearm floats into an upright position. You may get a sensation of a magnetic pull on the back of your hand.

If happens right away	**4**
If no response in 5 seconds. This is an exercise in your imagination.	
Just imagine your hand to be a big, buoyant balloon and let it float	
upwards. *If hand goes up now score:*	**3**
If no response in 5 seconds. I'll help you get it Started. Encircle wrist, boost.	
Let your hand be a balloon. Just let it go. *If person takes over, score:*	**2**
If person does not takes over, continue: You have the power to let it float upward.	
If person now takes over, let go and say: That's right. score:	**1**
If person does not take over, continue: Help it along. Just put it up there. score:	**0**
Let go. If arm comes down, this is the end of the test.	
This is rare. Can say: This is not for everyone. *Skip to treatment session.*	

Now I'm going to position your arm in this manner so ... and let it remain in this upright position. (*arm is positioned with the elbow comfortably supported on the arm rest of the chair and the forearm is in an upright position.*) In fact, it will remain in that position even after I give you the signal for your eyes to open. When your eyes are open, even when I put your hand down, it will float right back up to where it is now. You will find something amusing about this sensation. Later, when I touch your left elbow, your usual sensation and control will return.

Now I am going to count backwards. At two, your eyes will again roll upward with your eyelids closed. At one, let them open very slowly.

Ready ... three...two, with your eyelids closed, now roll up your eyes, and one, let them open very slowly.

All right, stay in this position and describe what physical sensations you are aware of now in your left arm and hand. (*let them describe*)

Is it comfortable?	**YES**	**NO**
Are you aware of any tingling sensations?	**YES**	**NO**

DISSOCIATION Does your left hand feel as if it is not as much a part of your body as your right hand?

YES	**2**
YES, A LITTLE BIT	**1**
No. Does your left hand feel as connected to the wrist as your right hand feels connected to the wrist? Are they exactly the same or is there a difference?	
THERE IS A DIFFERENCE	**1**
NO DIFFERENCE	
	0

LEVITATION - POST INDUCTION (each reinforcement is followed by 5 second pause).

Now note this. *Gently lower left hand & wait to see if hand floats upward. If so, score:* **4**

Now turn your head, look at your left hand, and watch what is going to happen. **3**

While concentrating on your left hand, imagine it to be a huge, buoyant balloon. **2**

Now, while imagining it to be a balloon permit it to act out as if it were a balloon.
That's right, be "big' about it. **1**

This is your chance to be a method actor or a ballet dancer. Think of your
left hand as a balloon or as the arm of a ballet dancer and permit it to act
as if it were a balloon. That's right, just put it up there, just the way a
ballet dancer would.

If necessary, fake it, pretend. **0**

CONTROL DIFFERENTIAL   While it remains in the upright position, by way of comparison, raise your right hand. Now put your right arm down. Are you aware of a difference in the sensation in your right arm going up, compared to your left? For example, does one arm feel heavier than the other? Are you aware of a relative difference in your sense of control in one arm compared to the other as it goes up?
On a more or less basis, are you aware of any relative difference in your sense of control in one arm compared to the other as it goes up?

YES. In which arm do you feel more. control? *If difference is reported* **2**

If spontaneously reports "a little bit" **1**

NO. *Circle the '0' and then repeat.* Let's try it again. *Put person's arm down* **0**

Now again. Look at your left hand. Imagine it to be a huge, buoyant balloon. Just like an actor
or an athlete. Now raise your right hand up and put your right arm down. Now this time are you
aware of any relative difference in control in one arm compared to the other as it goes up?

If YES, in which arm do you feel more control?

If difference is reported now, draw square around the '1' **1**

If still NO, draw a square around '0' **0**

CUT-OFF   Now note this.
*Cup person's elbow with your right hand and lower person's arm. Touch person's left hand give direction to
"make a fist. Move your hand up to touch elbow and finally bring your hand down. patient's arm, ending by
firmly pressing patient's hand.)*

Before there was a difference in control between the two forearms. Is that difference still there or is it going away?

YES **2**

NO (or) *It's beginning to go away: 'I still have more control in the right arm,' repeat "cut off" described above.*
Make a fist a few times. That's right. Open your fist and now put your hand down. Shake both hands a few
times and tell me when you feel that your control is equal.

If control becomes equal **1**

If control is still not equal, repeat until control is equal, and score: **0**

AMNESIA TO CUT OFF   You see that relative difference in control that was in your arms is gone. Do you
have any idea why? Is there anything I said or did that might account for it? **0**

If patient says 'NO' or says 'YES' and gives wrong answer score: **2**

If patient mentions 'elbow' say: What about it? If patient can't remember elbow being touched, score: **1**

If patient specifies "elbow touch" and being touched, ask: Are you inferring that I touched your elbow
or do you remember whether or not I did?

If "infers", score: **1**

If "remembers", ask: How many times? If remembers one elbow touch, score: **1**

If patient remembers two elbow touches, score: **0**

FLOATING SENSATION   When your arm went up before, did you feel a physical sensation that you can describe as a
lightness, floating, or buoyancy in your left arm or hand? Were you aware of similar sensations in any other part of your
body-such as your head, neck, chest, abdomen, thighs, legs, or all over--or just in your left hand or arm?

If floating in other parts of body in addition to left hand or arm **2**

If floating in left hand and/or arm only **1**

EYE-ROLL SIGN FOR HYPNOTIZABILITY

17.

MIND–BODY MEDICINE

Gregory L. Fricchione

INTRODUCTION

The National Center for Complementary and Alternative Medicine defines mind–body medicine as an approach that "focuses on the interactions among the brain, mind, body and behavior, and on the powerful ways in which emotional, mental, social, spiritual, and behavioral factors can directly affect health" (NCCAM, 2007). Mind–body medicine may also be conceptualized as the scientifically based dimension of what was once named *complementary and alternative medicine* (CAM). In 2007 close to 40% of Americans were using CAM therapies and spending close to 34 billion dollars in out-of-pocket expenses to pay for them (Barnes, Bloom, & Nahin, 2008; Nahin, Barnes, Stussman, & Bloom, 2009). Mind–body therapies accounted for 17% of this CAM usage (Bertisch, Wee, Phillips, & McCarthy, 2009). However, mind–body medicine was never really "alternative" in the sense of the unresearched use of herbs, folk remedies, and rituals. Mind–body medicine uses the evidence-based effects of thoughts, beliefs, emotions, and behaviors to positively influence physical health.

The field of medicine may be thought of as having three component areas—medications, procedures, and self-care (Benson, 1975). This has been called the *three-legged stool* model. In this schema mind–body medicine may be conceptualized as the self-care leg, comprising information derived from the subspecialty of psychosomatic medicine. To promote healing it employs an array of heterogeneous, researched techniques including relaxation exercises, meditation, biofeedback, guided imagery, hypnosis, yoga, tai chi, qi gong, and autogenic training. In this chapter we will point out the common elements of these techniques and the core elements of the mind–body approach, which can all elicit the relaxation response (RR). The focus on a repetitive activity—such as breathing, or a phrase, word, or prayer—and disruption of the train of everyday thoughts and concerns are the two main features of eliciting the RR: a physiological state of decreased stress characterized by diminished heart rate, blood pressure, respiratory rate, and oxygen consumption, along with peripheral vasodilatation (Benson, 1975).

Mind–body medicine is often seen as a philosophical conception of healing and health as well as a group of techniques. Many techniques originated in ancient Eastern cultural traditions and may have a religious foundation based on a particular conceptualization of human life. However, even though some people will feel attracted by the religious aspects they are not essential for therapeutic effect. Throughout this chapter we will attempt to show how recent research is providing evidence for the effectiveness of these treatments, establishing their scientific value and facilitating their integration into mainstream medicine. There is already enough evidence of the clinical efficacy of the mind–body techniques to make them viable options for patients who want to improve their self-care.

The approaches of mind–body medicine will be mainly complementary to current allopathic therapies, but for some conditions they may also be efficacious when used alone. These approaches reflect a unitary concept of mind–body integration and the more modern terms *integrative medicine* and *whole person medicine* focus attention on caring for the person interpenetrating with the organism. Within this framework mind–body medicine takes center stage as it stresses a multisystem integrative model that best comports with the organic unity that is the human being.

Perhaps mind–body medicine is best described in what Francis Peabody said to graduating medical students some 75 years ago:

> "The good physician knows his patients through and through, and his knowledge is bought dearly. Time, sympathy and understanding must be lavishly dispensed, but the reward is to be found in that personal bond, which forms the greatest satisfaction of the practice of medicine. One of the essential qualities of the clinician is interest in humanity, for the secret of the caring of the patient is in the caring for the patient." (Peabody, 1927)

It is essential for the physician to be interested in and to form a bond with the whole person as patient if true caring is to take place.

STRESS PHYSIOLOGY

DEFINITION OF STRESS AND DISTRESS

Being alive involves *stress* as a stimulus; stress requires biological, psychological, and social adaptations. *Eustress* can be thought of as the normal physiological workings of the living organism. It consists of homeostatic mechanisms called *eustasis,* which can be visualized as a U-shaped curve with suboptimal responsivity on each side of the curve leading to poor adaptation (Chrousos, 2009). *Pathogenic stress* or *distress* occurs when homeostasis is threatened, or perceived to be so, in the setting of overwhelming or sustained external and internal stressors.

Stress as *distress* can thus be defined as a state of disharmony or of threatened homeostasis (Chrousos & Gold, 1992). It refers to a disruption of the dynamic equilibrium among the person's physiological, psychological, and social dimensions as a result of the perceived presence of an external or internal threat. Alterations in the environment may provoke a physiological response mediated by several interconnected physiological networks constituting the so-called *stress response system*. The stress response system is composed of elements of the central nervous system (CNS), the hypothalamus-pituitary-adrenal (HPA) axis, and the immune system. Stressors, the stress system, and the stress response are the three key elements in this process.

Distress is accompanied by overactivity of the stress response system mediated primarily by hypothalamic corticotrophin-releasing hormone (CRH), originally known as *corticotrophin releasing factor* (CRF), and locus coeruleus A1-A2 derived norepinephrine (NE). Walter Cannon in the early 1900s did groundbreaking work on one axis of the stress response system, the autonomic nervous system (ANS; Cannon, 1929). He focused on the sympathetic nervous system (SNS) and its production of "the flight–fight response" and was first to use the term *homeostasis*. Hans Selye, another 20th century stress researcher, focused on the HPA axis (Selye, 1946).

AUTONOMIC NERVOUS SYSTEM

The CNS and the peripheral ANS have sympathetic and parasympathetic components. All these systems constitute a complex matrix with overlapping boundaries under the ultimate top-down control of the brain. This interconnected system maintains homeostasis by modulating different bodily functions and controlling the administration, distribution, and use of energy. In this way the brain adapts the level of functioning of different organs to global bodily demands under each specific circumstance. It is constantly functioning at varying levels of intensity, autoregulated by negative feedback and feed-forward mechanisms. It can also be overactivated by persistent or overwhelming stressors that make adaptation difficult. It is at this point that we talk about *distress*, which can be acute in the face of an enormous stressor or chronic in the setting of persistent unrelenting ones.

When the stress response is activated, some functions can be stimulated, such as metabolism, cardiac output, vascular tone, respiration, and muscle contraction. Other functions can be suppressed, such as the excretory system and gastrointestinal and reproductive activity (Tsigos & Chrousos, 2002). The acute stress response is characterized by an increased heart rate, increased breathing rate, increased metabolism, increased oxygen consumption, and increased beta and reduced alpha brain wave activity. Chronic stress may lead to hypertension, depression, and prolonged inflammatory response.

The efferent pathways from the central nucleus of the amygdala travel to a multiplicity of critical brain structures, including the parabrachial nucleus (resulting in dyspnea and hyperventilation), the dorsomedial nucleus of the vagus nerve and nucleus ambiguous (activating the parasympathetic nervous system/PNS), and the lateral hypothalamus (resulting in SNS activation). Through reciprocal neuronal pathways connecting the amygdala to the medial prefrontal cortex, the specific cognitive experience of the specific anxiety disorder will differ, although fear symptoms may overlap. During panic attacks the fear is of imminent death; in social phobia, the fear is of embarrassment; in posttraumatic stress disorder, the traumatic memory is remembered or reexperienced; in obsessive compulsive disorder, obsessional ideas recur and intrude; and in generalized anxiety disorder, anxiety is "free-floating" (i.e., not conditioned to specific situations or triggers).

The CNS as stated above plays an essential role in the regulation of the stress response. The ANS controls a wide array of functions—cardiovascular, respiratory, gastrointestinal, renal, endocrine, immune, and others—that are affected under conditions of stress (Chrousos, 2007). While the SNS activates the stress response, the PNS can dampen this effect and restore balance in the autonomic response.

The SNS efferent output flows down the intermediolateral cell column in preganglionic fibers to synapse in a bilateral chain of sympathetic ganglia from whence postganglionic mostly NE fibers proceed to enervate vascular smooth muscle, the heart, the gut, the kidney and other organs. The SNS through its enervation of the adrenal medulla has a humoral component resulting in the secretion of circulating epinephrine. The great vagus nerve is the major PNS cholinergic outflow tract. The ANS also contains SNS and PNS subdivisions with neuronal subpopulations that co-locate special peptide transmitters. CRH, Neuropeptide Y (NPY), somatostatin, and galanin are co-localized in NE neurons of this type. Vasoactive intestinal peptide, substance P, and calcitonin gene-related peptide co-localize within cholinergic neurons (Chrousos, 2007).

HYPOTHALAMIC-PITUITARY-ADRENAL AXIS

Activation of the HPA axis results in secretion of glucocorticoids, hormones that act at many levels to modulate the body's energy resources and restore the body to homeostasis after acute disruption (Herman et al., 2003). The medial parvocellular division of the paraventricular hypothalamic nucleus (PVN) houses CRH neurons that release the CRH required for adrenocorticotrophin (ACTH) secretion from the pituitary, along with arginine vasopressin (AVP). CRH is also expressed outside of the hypothalamus in the hippocampus, amygdala, nucleus accumbens, bed nucleus of the stria terminalis (BNST), thalamus, hypothalamus, cerebral cortex cerebellum, and hindbrain (Denver, 2009). There are at least two G-protein-coupled receptors (CRF 1 and CRF 2) that mediate CRH functioning. CRH binds to CRF 1 receptors in the pituitary, where signal transduction involving protein kinase A (PKA) and protein kinase C (PKC) leads to ACTH synthesis and secretion. ACTH moves through the systemic circulation, arriving at the adrenal cortex where it promotes synthesis and secretion of corticosterones like cortisol in the human. The CRH neurons are regulated by direct somatic, visceral, and humoral sensory afferents relayed from nuclei, like the nucleus of the solitary tract (NTS), the raphe, the subfornical organ and lamina terminalis, other parts of the hypothalamus, the BNST, and the thalamus. These "reactive" stimuli are generally excitatory. At the same time, the paralimbic medial prefrontal cortex and limbic forebrain structures such as the hippocampus, amygdala, and lateral septum, along with parts of the hypothalamus and thalamus, are thought to provide indirect "anticipatory" signals through projected connections to select brainstem, hypothalamic, and BNST regions that in turn enervate the PVN. It is thought that paralimbic and limbic areas that service "anticipatory" voluntary stress responses, when integrated with "reactive" reflexive stress responses, can modulate the HPA axis through tuning of the PVN CRH output.

Glucocorticoids can stimulate energy mobilization (glycogenolysis) in the liver, SNS-mediated vasoconstriction, proteolysis, and lipolysis; suppress innate immunity, reproductive function, and bone and muscle growth; and inhibit mood, leading to behavioral depression. This profile can become pathogenic if prolonged. Thus a premium is placed on multiple feedback control mechanisms to shut this response down.

The interaction of the ANS and HPA is shown in Box 17.1 and the modulation of the HPA stress response is outlined in Box 17.2 (Ulrich-Lai & Herman, 2009).

APPRAISAL

Cognitive and emotional appraisal of a stressor is accomplished as an amalgam by the brain (Lewis, 2005). A stressor is most distressing when it is perceived as such. Certain events or experiences are universally threatening, but there is a lot of room

---

Box 17.1 CNS REGULATION OF THE AUTONOMIC STRESS RESPONSE

SNS Activation: infralimbic cortex (IL), the central amygdala (CeA), locus coeruleus (LC) and the ventrolateral medulla (VLM)

PNS Activation: anterior bed nucleus of stria terminalis (aBST), prelimbic cortex (PL), dorsal motor nucleus of the vagus nerve (DMX), nucleus ambiguus (NA)

SNS and PNS Interactivity: nucleus of the solitary tract (NTS), paraventricular nucleus of the hypothalamus (PVN), dorsomedial hypothalamus (DMH),

Mediation: Sympathetic outflow to preganglionic SNS in the intermediolateral cell column occurs via direct innervation from the rostral VLM, LC and PVN, which are thought to initiate sympathetic responses. The NTS in turn receives direct input from neurons in the IL, the CeA, and the PVN. Other hypothalamic regions, most notably the DMH, modulate ANS activation through connections with the PVN (and possibly other descending pathways).

Parasympathetic outflow to postganglionic PNS occurs via effector organs mediated largely by descending outputs from the DMX and the NA and is under the direct influence of the PL, the PVN, and possibly other descending relays.

(Adapted from Ulrich-Lai and Herman, 2009, p. 400)

Box 17.2 MODULATION OF THE HPA AXIS

Modulation of the dorsal part of the medial parvocellular paraventricular nucleus of the hypothalamus (PVNmpd) is key to the HPA stress response and originates in several brain regions:

Stimulation:

1. The PVN receives direct noradrenergic, adrenergic and peptidergic innervation from the nucleus of the solitary tract (NTS).

2. The dorsomedial hypothalamus (dmDMH) and the arcuate nucleus (Arc) provide intrahypothalamic stress excitation.

3. The anterior part of the bed nucleus of the stria terminalis (BST), particularly the anteroventral nucleus of the BST, activates HPA axis stress responses.

4. The PVN also receives a stress-excitatory drive from the dorsal raphe, the tuberomammillary nucleus, the supramammillary nucleus, and the spinal cord, among others.

Inhibition (most of these inputs are GABAergic):

1. Activation of the PVNmpd is inhibited by numerous hypothalamic circuits, including the medial preoptic area (mPOA), the ventrolateral component of the dorsomedial hypothalamus (vlDMH), and local neurons in the peri-PVN region (pPVN), encompassing the PVN surround and the subparaventricular zone.

2. The posterior subregions of the BST provide a prominent forebrain inhibition of HPA responses.

(Adapted from Ulrich-Lai and Herman, 2009, p. 401)

---

for personification of particular threats. Depending on our appraisal, the mediators of the stress response may or may not emerge (Lazarus & Folkman, 1984). In fact, it has recently been shown that anticipatory cognitive appraisal is an important determinant of the cortisol stress response (Gaab, Rohleder, Nater, & Ehlert, 2005). On the other hand, the brain also determines the physiological and behavioral responses to stress. The limbic system is a set of structures related to the control of emotional responses, behavior, and long-term memory. Key structures involved include the hippocampus and the amygdala. The amygdala, which is responsible for fear conditioning, serves as a tripwire for the stress response. It has connections with the prefrontal cortex (PFC), which is related to attention and motivation and can inhibit amygdalar tone, and with the hypothalamus, which regulates endocrine and autonomic system functioning. The hippocampus is a target of stress hormones, and chronically increased levels of cortisol induce a structural remodeling associated with selective atrophy and altered behavioral and physiological responses (McEwen, 1999).

THE VICIOUS CYCLE

The PFC regions (dorsolateral/ DLPFC, dorsomedial/ DMPFC, ventromedial/ vmPFC, and inferior/ iPFC) cooperate to help us plan for the future and manage higher order decision making in concert with the anterior cingulate cortex (ACC). When we are not stressed, the PFC and its extensive connections to cortices and subcortices orchestrate behavior, thought, and emotion in a reasonable, goal-directed, and regulated way. Direct and indirect connections to the aminergic cell bodies in the brainstem allow the PFC to modulate NE flow from the locus coeruleus, dopamine (DA) from the ventral tegmentum, and serotonin from the nucleus raphe. When unstressed, there is the potential for optimal levels of amine releases in the PFC creating what is called a "delicious cycle." This situation potentiates a top-down guidance of attention and thought (DLPFC), error monitoring and reality testing (DMPFC), inhibition of inappropriate actions (iPFC), and regulation of emotions (vmPFC; Arnsten, 2009).

When we are distressed, on the other hand, the amygdala stimulates the stress response pathways in the HPA axis and the brainstem with outpourings of cortisol, NE, and DA. Interaction of the basolateral nucleus (BLA) and central nucleus (CeA) of the amygdala with modulatory regions such as the medial prefrontal cortex (mPFC) is of importance here (Jovanovic & Kessler, 2010; Lanius et al., 2010).

The BLA is thought to compare conditioned stimulus inputs and unconditioned stimulus inputs regulating CeA activation of the hardwired fear and stress circuitry, leading to inhibition or activation of the fear response. Recent research has begun to determine the role of inhibitory neural circuitry in modulating the fear response at the cellular level (Herry et al., 2008; Likhtik et al., 2008; LeDoux & Gorman, 2001). Sensory inputs, as well as associative inputs from the hippocampus and cortex, project directly and indirectly to the CeA. "On" and "off" inhibitory circuits within the CeA are thought to differentially modulate fear output and extinction of fear. Additionally, direct projections from the infralimbic region of the mPFC activate inhibitory neurons in the intercalated region between the BLA and CeA, serving to inhibit, in a top-down manner, the stress-enhancing fear output of the CeA.

The neurochemical environment of highly elevated cortisol and NE may impair PFC top-down regulation and strengthen amygdala-driven bottom-up dynamics. On the other hand, optimal levels of catecholamine release enhance PFC regulation (Arnsten, 2009). In some disorders such as ADHD, an increase in noradrenergic tone back to effective levels is conceptualized to increase selective attention and thus enhance cognition. Stress-induced catecholamine excess impairs PFC higher order functioning in the context of activated amygdalar fear conditioning accompanied by bottom-up sensory hypervigilance and habituated motor responses as opposed to thoughtful, pliant approaches characteristic of top-down PFC control. Stress can thus set up an amygdala-centered "vicious cycle" (see Table 17.1).

IMMUNE SYSTEM

The immune system also plays an important role in the stress response, and it is well integrated in the psychoneuroendocrinology system. A variety of physical as well as psychosocial stressors stimulate the stress response systems, resulting in

Table 17.1 "DELICIOUS" VS. "VICIOUS" CYCLES

	DELICIOUS CYCLE	VICIOUS CYCLE
Anatomy:	DLPFC; rlPFC; VMPFC; DMPFC	CeA→ ++++LC; SN; VTA
	→ + LC; SN; VTA → optimal PFC	→ DLPFC; rlPFC; VMPFC; DMPFC→ impaired PFC
Neurochemistry:	NE, DA, GLU, GABA	NE, DA, GLU, GABA
Physiology:	PFC can regulate its own transmitter input → optimal amine levels enhance PFC functioning including VMPFC control of CeA and nucleus accumbens	Distress activates CeA, which overactivates SNS, HPA and brainstem NE and DA→ impairs PFC regulation and strengthens amygdala function
Neurobehavior:	Attention, thought and action regulation (DLPFC)	Impaired higher order PFC functions
	Inhibition of inappropriate motor response (rlPFC)	Elevated fear conditioning
	Appropriate emotional responses and habits (VMPFC)	Reflexive, hot responder to sensory stimuli
	Error monitoring and reality testing (DMPFC)	"Bottom-up" regulation
	Thoughtful top-down control and selective attention through PFC	

(Adapted from Arnsten, 2009, p. 411)

the output of CRH and catecholamines. It is of interest that postganglionic SNS fibers secrete CRH and that norepinephrine and epinephrine stimulate IL-6 release by immune cells and other peripheral cells through effects on beta-adrenergic receptors (Chrousos, 2009). Stress activates transcription factor NF-kB, which then produces proinflammatory cytokines (Bierhaus, Humpert, & Nawroth, 2004) This signaling molecule is an essential mediator at the blood–brain barrier that translates peripheral immune signals to the CNS. Catecholamines from SNS fibers increase NF-kB DNA nuclear binding in immune cells, including the macrophage predisposing to the inflammatory response syndrome (Miller, Maletic, & Raison, 2008).

During the inflammatory response syndrome, cytokine-induced activation of the monocyte enzyme indoleamine 2, 3 dioxygenase (IDO) leads to catabolism of L-tryptophan into L-kynurenine, which is then metabolized to quinolinic acid and kynurenic acid (Miller, 2009). These latter two metabolites are neuroactive and lead to cellular oxidative stress in the hippocampus and other areas of the brain. A reduction in CNS stores of L-tryptophan can lead to depressive symptoms, while elevations in kynurenine metabolites can produce delirium and cognitive dysfunction. Interferon-alpha as part of an inflammatory response syndrome stimulates IDO and is thought to reduce serotonin function, deplete dopamine, and activate the dorsal ACC, resulting in vulnerability to depression, fatigue, psychomotor slowing, and anxiety and alarm.

Proinflammatory cytokines gain access to the circumventricular region of the brain directly through fenestrated endothelium zones (area postrema, subfornical organ, median eminence, pineal gland) and indirectly through cellular active transport, endothelial cell and perivascular macrophage activation, and peripheral vagal paraganglia stimulation that gets transmitted through the NTS and hypothalamus into the brain and proceeds to interact with neurotransmitter metabolism, neuroendocrine action, and neuroplasticity (Saper & Breder, 1994). This interaction may result in excitotoxicity, oxidative stress, aminergic changes, and trophic factor reductions.

Microglial cells are the primary central targets of proinflammatory signals originating in the periphery. Once activated, they release cytokines, chemokines, and reactive oxygen species, which then initiate a sequence of effects including activation of astroglial cells. The CNS inflammatory response syndrome is amplified as a result. Eventually IL-1, IL-6, and TNF-alpha and interferons stimulate IDO, which, as mentioned, breaks down tryptophan into kynurenine, thus reducing brain serotonin stores and increasing quinolinic acid—a potent NMDA agonist that can produce excitotoxicity and severe oxidative stress (Miller, 2009).

At the same time, oligodendrocytes are also sensitive to this cascade and especially to TNF-alpha, which can have a toxic effect leading to apoptosis and demyelination. Cytokines also stimulate CRH and the HPA axis. In acute stress situations cortisol elevation will, along with PNS vagal stimulation, tend to reduce NF-kB activation. This can shut down the inflammatory response if all goes well.

These aspects of the immune response's physiology hypothetically have relevance in the genesis or progression of multiple diseases. Distress has been related to proneness to viral infections, progression from HIV to AIDS, flares of multiple sclerosis, lupus, and arthritis, and risk of developing coronary heart disease and Alzheimer's disease (Cohen, Tyrrell, & Smith, 1991; Dong et al., 2004; Matthews & Gump, 2002; Mohr, Hart, Julian, Cox, & Pelletier, 2004; Sandberg et al., 2000; Cole et al., 2001).

Catecholamines and glucocorticoids both control the amplitude of immune response through negative feedback mechanisms. In physically threatening situations, inflammatory cytokines, mainly IL-6, stimulate the HPA axis, and the subsequent elevation of cortisol levels will eventually induce the suppression of the immune/inflammatory reaction. Simultaneously, the SNS causes systemic secretion of cytokines, which will eventually suppress the immune system (Stratakis & Chrousos, 1995). Thus, activation of the HPA axis helps to regulate the activity of the immune response

and, in the case of psychological distress, the immune system can be suppressed. However, paradoxically, under conditions of chronic stress such as caregiver burden, marital strife, or even perceived stress, there are increases in acute phase proteins (C-reactive protein- CRP), IL-6, and other inflammatory mediators that can become persistent, leading to a chronic inflammatory response syndrome (G. E. Miller et al., 2009). Maltreatment in early childhood is associated with elevated CRP 20 years later (Danese, Pariante, Caspi, Taylor, & Poulton, 2007). How does one reconcile this longstanding paradox in mind–body research?

PARADOX OF THE STRESS IMMUNE RESPONSE

If chronic stress enhances secretion of immunosuppressive glucocorticoids, why then do chronic stressors accentuate the vulnerability to inflammatory diseases? There is a current hypothesis that reconciles this apparent conflict (G. E. Miller et al., 2008). Under conditions of chronic stress, such as the caregiving of family members with brain cancer, functional resistance of monocyte-macrophages to cortisol negative feedback permits continuation of NF-kB signaling, resulting in the immune response syndrome. Early life stress can leave this same signature of blunted cortisol feedback inhibition of cellular immunity and increased proinflammatory signaling (Miller et al., 2009). It appears that chronic stress such as unemployment or chronic caregiving may result in a biphasic immune response with some reduction of cellular and humoral immune activity coinciding with low-grade, nonspecific inflammation (Segerstrom & Miller, 2004).

SPECIFICITY OF THE STRESS RESPONSE

The modification of the global activity of the immune system also depends on the time and the type of stressor. Stressors differ one from another not only in intensity but also in temporal and qualitative properties. This has been referred to as the *specificity of the stress response* (Pacak & Palkovits, 2001). Different types of stressors will affect the immune response in diverse ways leading to different disorders. A recent meta-analysis suggests that acute stressors are associated with suppression of specific humoral immunity, while brief naturalistic stressors tend to suppress cellular immunity and, as noted above, chronic stressors are associated with both cellular and humoral immune suppression as well as nonspecific inflammation (Segerstrom & Miller, 2004).

This discussion on stressor types leads us to stop and briefly consider the meaning of the flight or fight response. To more fully understand it, we need to adopt an evolutionary developmental perspective. The stress response is an adaptive preservationary phenomenon. Biologically, the "flight or fight response" is a primitive response, a reflection of early stages in our species' development, and thus it is not well suited to deal with the type of stressors we face nowadays. To understand how the stress response, evolutionarily designed to help us survive, can also hurt us, we will employ two useful concepts: allostasis and allostatic load.

ALLOSTASIS AND ALLOSTATIC LOADING

Allostasis, a concept introduced in the field of stress medicine by Sterling and Eyer, is the ability to achieve stability through change (Sterling & Eyer, 1988). It refers to the biological mechanisms that protect the body from internal and external stress and maintain the internal balance of homeostasis. But sometimes the stress system cannot maintain the internal balance for various reasons. Selye (1946) had already described the so-called "general adaptation syndrome" by identifying three stages: the *alarm stage*, in which the acute stress response is activated; the *stage of resistance*, in which the body makes an effort to return to a state of homeostasis, but the perception of a threat is still present, resulting in a persistent stress response; and the *state of exhaustion* in which the stress continues for a long time, the body cannot function normally, and organ systems fail.

In the presence of chronic stress, the persistent overactivation of allostatic systems can lead to a variety of diseases. This long-term effect of the physiologic response to stress has been called *allostatic load* –the metabolic wear and tear on the organism at the cellular level that occurs as the price for maintaining allostasis of physiological systems (McEwen & Stellar, 1993). There are four proposed mechanisms associated with allostatic load (McEwen, 1998): (1) frequent stress or multiple stressors; (2) prolonged exposure to stress and the consequent lack of adaptation; (3) inability to shut off allostatic responses or delayed shutdown once a stressor is terminated; and (4) inadequate (insufficient) response. These burdens on allostatic load lead to an overactivation of other systems in order to compensate for the deficit.

It is now increasingly clear that psychosocial stress can get translated into metabolic activation and be processed at the cellular level as *oxidative stress*. Mental stress reflects a challenge to the organism's allostatic state of "stability through change" (McEwen, 1998). It takes metabolic energy input for the brain to maintain physiological parameters within a normative range in response to external and internal environmental stressors, and this can lead to allostatic loading. It is the brain's stress response systems, consisting of the amygdala/lateral hypothalamus–driven SNS and the HPA axis, that serve as conduits to the body's end organs of what the brain mesocorticolimbic system processes as a challenge or a threat. This stress hormone and transmitter–induced state alerts these target tissues to the need to alter their metabolisms to meet this new state of affairs in order to maintain allostasis. This works well if the challenge or threat is acute and self-limited. However, if the psychosocial stress is chronic, this process can be pathogenic because of cellular oxidative stress (Epel et al., 2006).

Allostatic load can also be conceptualized as a cumulative measure of dysregulation across the regulatory systems. There have been different proposed physiological parameters that reflect levels of physiologic activity of these systems, and allostatic load would be the composite sum of the number of parameters for which the subject was rated in the highest risk quartile. Among these proposed measures are systolic and diastolic blood pressures, overnight urinary cortisol, norepinephrine and epinephrine, ratio of the waist to hip measurement, glycosylated hemoglobin value, high-density lipoprotein cholesterol and ratio to the total serum cholesterol concentration, dihydroepiandrostendione, fibrinogen, C-reactive protein, and Interleukin-6 (Seeman, Singer, Rowe, Horwitz, & McEwen, 1997; Gruenewald, Seeman, Karlamangla, & Sarkisian, 2009).

In one study, frailty defined as weight loss, exhaustion, weak grip, slow gait, and low physical activity correlated with higher allostatic load scores (Gruenewald et al., 2009). In another study of allostatic loading, Epel and her colleagues (2004) were able to show that psychological perceived stress measured on the Perceived Stress Scale, or objective psychological stress measured in chronicity of caregiving in mothers taking care of their chronically ill children, were both associated with peripheral blood mononuclear cell (PBMC) telomere length shortening, low telomerase activity (telomerase maintains telomere length) and oxidative stress. Mindfulness meditation appears to reduce oxidative stress and buffer against the aging effects on telomeres (Epel, Daubenmier, Moskowitz, Folkman, & Blackburn, 2009).

Meditation may impact allostatic loading via epigenetic pathways of gene expression. The genes of interest are involved in oxidative metabolism, apoptosis, activation of NF-kB, and ribosomal functioning. In one study, the cross-sectional PBMC gene expression profile of experienced meditators (M group) was compared with the gene expression profile taken at two times in novices who had never learned the core meditative RR practice. Time 1 is pre–RR training (N1 group) and time 2 is at 8 weeks post–RR training (N2 group). Results showed that certain genes activated and deactivated in the M group and 8 weeks post–RR training (N2 group) were not changed accordingly in the N1 group, suggesting that the N2 group after RR training was moving closer to the gene expression profile of the experienced meditators, all of whom had at least 5 years of experience in a wide variety of RR-eliciting meditative practices including mindfulness-based stress reduction and various yoga techniques (Dusek et al., 2008). The transcriptome changes seen with RR practice relate to more efficient mitochondrial metabolism, with improvement in insulin function and cell aging and reduction in NF-kB immune activation. These effects may relate to the known physiological results of RR elicitation, which include reduction in blood pressure and oxygen consumption. These results receive support from a recent study that employed a similar research methodology (gene expression profiling and bioinformatics analysis of PBMCs) to investigate changes in the leukocyte transcriptomes of highly stressed women undergoing primary treatment for stage III and below breast cancer, who underwent a 10-week course of treatment with cognitive behavioral stress management (CBSM), which includes RR training (Antoni et al., 2012). The authors found that the treatment can reverse anxiety-related upregulation of NF-kB–associated proinflammatory gene regulation.

The metabolic wear and tear and oxidative stress that comes with allostatic loading may be related to the epidemic of metabolic syndrome. This syndrome, which now affects nearly 40% of the US population, is characterized by truncal obesity, insulin receptor insensitivity leading to Type II diabetes, hyperlipidemia, and hypertension (Ford, Li, & Zhao, 2010). It is of interest in this regard that mind–body therapies have shown some effectiveness for the management of metabolic syndrome, perhaps related to the common RR elicited transcriptomic effects of these therapies (Anderson & Taylor, 2011).

OXIDATIVE STRESS AND THE PROINFLAMMATORY TRANSCRIPTION FACTOR NF-KB

Allostatic loading can lead to oxidative stress, with the resultant production of free radicals and stress-sensitive heat shock protein (HSP) gene expression/production (e.g., HSP 40/70/90) as a ligand for the toll-like 4 receptor. Activation of this receptor can stimulate macrophages to produce proinflammatory and cytotoxic mediators (inducible nitric oxide-iNO, TNF-alpha, IL-6, IL-12) through an iNOSynthase/NF-kB/cAMP reactive element binding (CREB) protein/COX-2 mechanism (Billack et al., 2002).

The proinflammatory transcription factor NF-kB is a bridge between stress and oxidative cellular activation (Bierhaus et al., 2004). Activation of NF-kB, evoked by psychosocial stress, may directly target endothelial functioning in the vasculature and thus represent an additional risk factor for cardiovascular, cerebrovascular, and renal disease. At the same time hypertension, obesity, insulin-resistant diabetes mellitus, and hyperlipidemia (metabolic syndrome) can activate NF-kB, as can psychologically produced oxidative stress, cytokines, growth factors, angiotensin II, and advanced glycation end-products (AGEs). Activation then leads to NF-kB nuclear translocation in endothelial, smooth muscle, monocyte/macrophage, and renal glomerular and epithelial cells.

NF-kB then binds to DNA and activates transcription of genes for cytokines, adhesion molecules, coagulation factors, and AGE receptors (RAGEs) setting the stage for endothelial dysfunction, atherosclerotic cardiac and cerebrovascular disease, renal disease, and so forth. In addition, NF-kB stimulates the proliferation of tumor cells and enhances their survival by upregulating anti-apoptotic genes (Schottelius & Dinter, 2006).

The extent of NF-kB activation in PBMCs correlates with oxidative stress (Hofmann et al., 1999). In addition, PBMC NF-kB is activated by psychosocial stress (15-minute Trier Social Stress Test; Bierhaus et al., 2004). For instance, maternal caregiving stress, resulting in oxidative stress–induced telomere shortening in PBMCs, may be related to NF-kB activation. Immobilization stress in rats increases NF-kB activation and dependent gene expression (Madrigal et al., 2002). Lymphocyte NF-kB increases in women who are stressed by breast biopsy (Nagabhushan, Mathews, & Witek-Janusek, 2001). This activation is correlated with a stress-dependent increase in catecholamines and cortisol. And therapeutic interventions that decrease oxidative stress can reduce NF-kB activation (Hofmann et al., 1999).

When stress is removed, NF-kB usually downregulates within 60 minutes. Some individuals are unable to downregulate this quickly, suggesting a variability in stress perception that can be translated into prolonged NF-kB activation. This differential response to stress stimuli may be a product of genomic activation differences. The group of individuals who are unable to downregulate NF-kB quickly may theoretically benefit most from RR training, perhaps through activating effects on the stabilizing Ik-Ba inhibitor complex.

Chronic diseases (coronary artery disease, diabetes mellitus, end stage renal disease, etc.) are associated with elevated allostatic loading. They also have higher levels of depression and anxiety as allostatic load disorders, and may be more susceptible to psychosocial stress. Chronically activated NF-kB states may then be exacerbated by repeated or perpetuated stress states. The so-called RAGE ligands (AGEs, amyloid B-peptides, etc.), already upregulated by NF-kB in chronic diseases, may in turn mediate a perpetuated NF-kB activation by overriding autoregulatory Ik-Ba inhibition.

In this way NF-kB activation by psychosocial stress may be converted into a constant allostatic threat. Psychosocial stress–induced NF-kB activation can now be tracked in accessible PBMCs. Along with measurement of genomic alterations, changes in oxidative metabolites, and telomere dynamics, NF-kB activation measurement will help with research into this potential link between stress and pathology. It will also help with the study of whether stress reduction therapies can influence cellular activities (Bierhaus et al., 2004).

One way to impact the stress-related upregulation of NF-kB is to stabilize the association of Ik-Ba with NF-kB. This reduces the production of protein activators of oxidative stress (Stefano et al., 2001). Mental activities such as RR or belief may be able to effect such stabilization through enhancement of constitutive nitric oxide mechanisms. Perhaps that is why individuals taught the RR had decreased oxygen consumption, which correlated with exhaled nitric oxide (Dusek et al., 2006).

Mechanisms involving oxidative stress and its mediator, NF-kB, constitute a plausible explanation of how stress is implicated in the genesis and progression of multiple disorders. The statistical association between stress and these disorders is clear, and although more research is required to establish unequivocally a causal link, consistent evidence suggests that this causal relation exists (Cohen, Janicki-Deverts, & Miller, 2007). In addition to the importance of stress management for the health of individuals, there are extraordinary socioeconomic implications as reflected in a review of studies showing that at least 60% of medical visits are associated with stress-related conditions (Perkins, 1994).

What does mind-body medicine have to offer? Interventions to reduce stress and enhance resiliency are available to promote health and prevent illness.

RESILIENCY

Resiliency is a term that comes to us from structural engineering and refers to the ability to rebound or to bounce back from a stressor or adversity. Resiliency reflects good adjustment across different domains in the face of significant adversity. It consists of five major capacities: (1) the capacity to experience reward and motivation nested in dispositional optimism and high positive emotionality; (2) the capacity to circumscribe fear responsiveness so that one can continue to be effective through active coping strategies despite fear; (3) the capacity to use adaptive social behaviors to secure support through bonding and teamwork and to provide support through altruism; (4) the ability to use cognitive skills to reinterpret the meaning of negative stimuli in a more positive light; and (5) the integration of a sense of purpose in life along with a moral compass, meaning, and spiritual connectedness (Feder, Nestler, & Charney, 2009) (See Box 17.3).

Over the past decade, more has been learned about the neurobiology of mechanisms of passive resilience (the absence of key molecular susceptibility characteristics) and active resilience (the presence of central molecular promoters of healthy adaptations). (Russo, Murrough, Han, Charney, & Nestler, 2012). Molecular adaptations within the DA reward and motivation circuitries are associated with vulnerability and resiliency (Krishnan et al., 2007). For example, a naturally occurring single nucleotide polymorphism (SNP), G196A Met/Met, promotes insusceptibility to stress by virtue of deficits in activity-dependent Brain Derived Neurotrophic Factor (BDNF) release in the nucleus accumbens. In another study, the ratio of CRH to NPY also seems to reflect a relationship between vulnerability and resiliency. High CRH increase (associated with increased acute stress response + negative affect) with low NPY (associated with decreased anxiolysis) correlates with high allostatic loading and low resilience, and increased propensity to alcohol abuse (Valdez & Koob, 2004). When there is lower haplotype-driven NPY expression (SNPrs 16147 in NPY promoter region) in limbic areas associated with amygdala arousal and emotional valencing, there is higher amygdala activation and diminished resiliency (Zhou et al., 2008). Dihydroepiandrosterone −S over cortisol and NPY over norepinephrine ratios reflect resiliency in Navy Seal commandos exposed to a stressful capture exercise (Southwick, Vythilingam, & Charney, 2005).

Box 17.3 **THE FIVE COMPONENTS OF RESILIENCY**

1. Capacity to experience reward and motivation nested in dispositional optimism and high positive emotionality;

2. Capacity to circumscribe fear responsiveness so that one can continue to be effective through active coping strategies despite fear;

3. Capacity to use adaptive social behaviors to secure support through bonding and teamwork and to provide support through altruism;

4. Capacity to use cognitive skills to reinterpret the meaning of negative stimuli in a more positive light;

5. Capacity to integrate a sense of purpose in life along with a moral compass, meaning, and spiritual connectedness.

(Adapted from Feder, Nestler, & Charney, 2009)

In a human depression study, the serotonin transporter allele 5-HTTLPR with 2 short arms SS, thought to be a risk for depression in and of itself, when combined with maltreatment in childhood plus low social support will be twice as likely to cause depression when compared to those with 5-HTT SS and no maltreatment and low social supports. However, this latter profile is more likely than the 5-HTT SS group with maltreatment and good social supports to cause depression, which in turn is more likely to cause depression than the group with 5-HTT SS plus no maltreatment and good social supports (Kaufman et al., 2004). It should be noted, however, that a recent meta-analysis found no evidence that the 5-HTTLPR conveyed extra risk for depression beyond the stressful life events (Risch et al., 2009).

There are HPA axis–related genes that may interact with resiliency to stress. For example, SNPs of the *CRH type 1* receptor gene may moderate the effects of child maltreatment on susceptibility to depression in adulthood (Bradley et al., 2008). And four SNPs of the gene (*FKBP5*) that codes for a protein chaperone that regulates glucocorticoid receptor (GR) sensitivity modulate the association of child abuse with the risk of PTSD in adulthood (Binder et al., 2008). In addition there is a catechol-O-methyltransferase polymorphism (Val158Met) that has relevance to resiliency. Those with low-activity Met158 develop higher levels of catecholamines in response to stress, resulting in lower resilience to anxiety and negative mood states (Heinz & Smolka, 2006).

There are also epigenetic mechanisms of resiliency in which the environment can change chromatin structure through methylation or acetylation of histones or direct methylation of DNA.

If evolution made us a species that relies on social support for our survival and health, then it had to create a species that had the capacity to give social support, to be prosocial, and to be altruistic. Indeed, altruistic behavior has been associated with good health outcomes as long as stress does not overwhelm the individual's ability to cope (Post, 2009). In the rat model, maternal nurturance has been shown to increase levels of the transcription factor nerve growth factor-inducible protein A (NGFI-A), known as EGR1, in the hippocampus of the nurtured pup. This allows for hypomethylation and stimulation of the hippocampal GR gene. Higher levels of hippocampal GR translates into certain neurobehavioral outcomes in the adult, including lower baseline and post-stress glucocorticoid secretion levels, lower anxiety-like behaviors, and in females improved nurturance of their own offspring (Meaney & Szyf, 2005). In resilient mice, chronic stress activates several potassium channel subunits in VTA DA neurons, and this blocks a stress-induced increase in VTA excitability and downstream release of BDNF in the nucleus accumbens (Krishnan et al., 2007).

CONSCIOUS POSITIVE EXPECTATION AND THE PLACEBO RESPONSE

We have talked about optimism, or conscious positive expectation, as part of resiliency. This leads to a consideration of placebo. The *placebo effect* is not an epithet, even though in medicine it has developed that connotation. It is instead an important part of human self-care, and it stems from the fact that belief in conscious positive expectation aids in the healing process. There is very interesting work in three important human brain disorders—pain, depression, and Parkinson's disease—that establishes the importance of placebo. A possible reason why the placebo is so active in these three very important public health problems is because placebo actually works directly on the brain mesolimbic/mesocortical reward and motivation circuitries (Fricchione & Stefano, 2005). There are neuroimaging studies that point this out. One experiment shows that if you apply a standard heat pain paradigm to subjects, you will see the ACC activate while the DLPFC is relatively deactivated. The ACC is the place that modulates all forms of human pain, so this may represent a pain signature. Then if you do the same experiment but apply a placebo cream prior to the heat stimulus, you will see the opposite pattern–ACC activation goes down, DLPFC activation goes up, and pain is reduced (Zubieta et al., 2005). The endogenous opioid mu receptor system is of importance in placebo pain response, which can be blocked by naloxone. In depression, which is notoriously placebo responsive, functional neuroimaging studies reveal metabolic increases in PFC, posterior insula, inferior parietal cortex, and dorsal ACC, and decreases in the pregenual ACC, thalamus, and hypothalamus with successful placebo treatment (Mayberg et al., 2002). Antidepressant responses occur in similar regions but are more robust, and also included brainstem activation.

In elegant studies with Parkinson's disease (PD) patients, researchers using positron emission tomography with the DA ligand raclopride have been able to show that a placebo of subcutaneous saline can improve PD symptoms coinciding with the displacement of the raclopride, presumably by DA, from the substantia nigra and the ventral tegmentum DA cell bodies (de la Fuente-Fernandez, Schulzer, & Stoessl, 2004).

THE MIND–BODY MEDICINE HYPOTHESES

Four hypotheses of mind–body medicine emerge based on the science summarized above (Fricchione, 2009). The **first hypothesis** is that the mind and body are a unity. Every external and internal experience produced is the result of and results in biological reactions in the brain. These biological reactions change the ecology of the brain, and this transduction of experience unifies what we consider to be mind activity and the body.

The **second hypothesis** is that psychosocial stress gets transduced into cellular stress. This cellular stress is mitochondrial oxidative stress, and every cell has to deal with psychosocial stress in this very physiological way because of the influence of the stress response systems.

The **third hypothesis is** that this cellular oxidative stress is what uncovers disease vulnerability. This is essentially a nonspecificity stress diathesis model. If both of my parents died of coronary artery disease, it is a good bet that I have vulnerability for coronary artery disease. I may not manifest that

vulnerability if I can build my resiliency and hold in check my psychosocial stress and, by extension, my cellular oxidative stress. In short, cellular oxidative stress is a key factor in the elaboration of mind–body effects.

Our genetic endowment is not completely writing the script for us, and this fact is revolutionizing the field of psychosomatic medicine. The environment is having its say in terms of which genes are activated and which genes are inactivated, and this epigenetic transcriptomic effect is essential for the field of medicine in general. Meaney and colleagues (Weaver et al., 2004; Champagne & Meaney, 2007), in a series of experiments mentioned above, have shown that rat pup recipients of high nurturance have an activation of an important promoter gene that leads downstream to the production of an elevation in GR receptors in the hippocampus. It is the process of hypomethylation at the 5-HT7 gene that leads to the increased production of the GR promoter gene. This epigenetic change produces, in those highly nurtured rat pups when they become adults, the resilience to better face a standard stress paradigm in the laboratory. The Meaney lab has extended this exciting work by showing that environmental enrichment can reverse some of the effects of being a rat pup who has had a poorly nurturant upbringing, by causing epigenetic changes at the estrogen receptor that in turn elevates oxytocin functioning, leading to increased attachment behavior in adulthood.

In the human model it is now known that if you perceive a task as stressful, such as taking care of a chronically ill child, telomeres in PBMCs will age 10 times faster than average as measured in number of base pairs lost per year (Epel et al., 2004). This effect is tied to oxidative stress in these PBMCs, as the production of oxidative metabolites is increased along with telomere shortening and the reduced activity of the telomere maintenance enzyme telomerase. Studies like these establish for us the potential for a new field of medicine, which is being called **enviromimetics** (McOmish & Hannan, 2007). Can salugenic environmental changes be reliably mimicked to effectively change gene activation and deactivation so that the changes will have health benefits? This is an area ripe for study.

THE FOURTH HYPOTHESIS

Most of the stress-related challenges we face as human beings are consequences of the fact that we are all mammals. We all are subject to separation stress because, as summarized by John Bowlby, the great English psychiatrist and father of attachment theory, our environments of evolutionary adaptiveness have to be that of secure base attachment (Bowlby, 1982). Stress itself can thus be reframed as a separation challenge (Fricchione, 2011). Illness in this regard can be surmised to be an enormous separation challenge and consequently an enormous source of stress. Distress associated with insecure attachment style will lead to a compounding of the separation challenge associated with illness culminating in poorer coping and worse outcomes (Ciechanowski et al., 2004). Conversely, a secure attachment style nurtured in childhood and persisting in adulthood will make coping with illness more adaptable (Ciechanowski et al., 2002; Thompson & Ciechanowski, 2003; Ciechanowski et al., 2010).

This leads to the **fourth hypothesis**, which we might call the **mind–body medicine equation hypothesis** (Fricchione, 2011). Building on the earlier work of medical sociologist George Albee (1982), it is very simple and heuristic. If one thinks about the numerator as being stress or allostatic loading and about the denominator as being resiliency, a pretty good picture of one's vulnerability to illness in the future will emerge. This might be called an *illness index* or the propensity to illness (see Figure 17.1). Flip the numerator to resiliency and the denominator to stress, and you get the quotient changed to propensity to health—a *health index*. For example, if one studies women with systemic lupus erythematosus, when you populate the variables in the equation and you stratify the groups into low social support leading to a decrease in the denominator, the propensity to a lupus flare will go up. There are many examples of this relationship in the literature (Ward et al., 1999; Sutcliffe et al., 1999; Sewitch et al., 2001; Seeman, 2000; Case, Moss, Case, McDermott, & Eberly, 1992; Horsten, Mittleman, Wamala, Schenck-Gustafsson, & Orth-Gomér, 2000; Ruberman, Weinblatt, Goldberg, & Chaudhary, 1984).

Because of this relationship, it is advisable that doctors and nurses take heed of this equation when they evaluate patients and create treatment plans. There should be some ability in the clinical encounter to get an objective feel for the level of patient stress and the level of patient resiliency. The problem is compounded once illness takes hold because, as mentioned above, illness itself is an enormous stress because it ignites the threat of separation (Fricchione, 2011).

In a classic study in the *New England Journal of Medicine,* over 2,000 men post–myocardial infarction were followed by Ruberman and his colleagues (1984) for a period of 36 months. They stratified the groups into a high numerator group with high life stress. Mortality was increased over those 36 months. Then they looked at the group with low social support or high social isolation, a low denominator, and these subjects also died at a high rate over 36 months. But then, when the researchers looked at a group with combined high numerator and low denominator, the 3-year mortality was enormously high.

So what are the attachment solutions available to relieve the separation stress of illness?

At the Benson-Henry Institute (BHI), we have the RR Resiliency Enhancement Program (3RP), which offers a composite attachment solution strategy (Fricchione, 2011). It begins with individual integrative medicine consultations and management of stress-related conditions performed by our internists. They can then refer patients to our 3RP group interventions, which all start with RR training.

We teach RR first with a component of mindfulness and yoga, because it seems to be an enhancer of the educational component of the REP. We then teach cognitive behavioral skills in the group setting. This is geared toward breaking the negative thinking traps and catastrophizing that can lead to pathogenic stress. Also in the group setting, social support is an important component, as is encouragement of prosocial behavior. Optimism and belief in conscious positive expectation are important parts of the positive psychology aspect of our approach, as is accenting meaning, purpose, gratitude, and life enjoyment. Spirituality, basically defined as a sense of connectedness to something greater than ourselves, is also addressed in the 3RP. In addition, exercise and nutrition education are of course important factors. The 3RP is designed to reduce stress and enhance resiliency, theoretically improving the health index. Results show that 12 out of 23 symptoms on the Medical Symptom Checklist were significantly decreased in frequency, along with improvement in psychological symptoms on the Symptom Checklist-90-Revised and health-promoting lifestyle behaviors on the Health Promoting Lifestyle Profile-II (Samuelson et al., 2010). The improved physical symptoms included headache, visual disturbance, dizziness, nausea, constipation, diarrhea, abdominal pain, back ache, chest pain, palpitations, insomnia, and fatigue.

An example of this heuristic equational effect can be found in the BHI Mind Body Cardiac Wellness programs. In a recently released US Center for Medicaid and Medicare Services report, the BHI cardiac rehabilitation program was found to produce a significant reduction in post–cardiac event mortality and a significantly increased time to rehospitalization over the 3-year study period when compared not only to a noncardiac rehabilitation sample but also to a traditional cardiac rehabilitation control group in a cohort of cardiac patients 65 years old and older (Shepard et al., 2009). We cautiously surmise that this positive outcome results from the ability of our mind–body cardiac rehabilitation program to reduce stress and to increase resiliency, not only through exercise prescription and nutritional guidance but also through RR training, social support and teamwork, cognitive skills training, positive psychology, and conscious positive expectation.

USE AND EFFICACY OF MIND–BODY TECHNIQUES

A significant interest in mind–body medicine among the general population has been documented in national surveys in the United States (Wolsko, Eisenberg, Davis, & Phillips, 2004). Around 20% of the population have used a mind–body intervention of some kind in the last year. Meditation

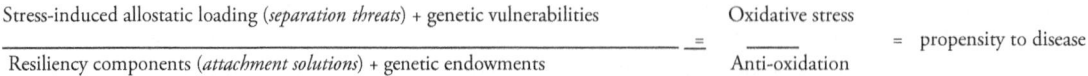

$$\frac{\text{Stress-induced allostatic loading (\textit{separation threats}) + genetic vulnerabilities}}{\text{Resiliency components (\textit{attachment solutions}) + genetic endowments}} = \frac{\text{Oxidative stress}}{\text{Anti-oxidation}} = \text{propensity to disease}$$

Figure 17.1 Mind–Body Medicine Equation. (Fricchione, 2011).

and relaxation techniques were the most highly endorsed. In another study, health professionals manifested higher interest in learning these approaches and lower interest in biofeedback and hypnosis (Sierpina, Kreitzer, Cunningham, Elder, & Bruckner, 2007). Mind–body therapies were most frequently used for different chronic conditions such as anxiety, depression, chronic pain, insomnia, gastrointestinal disorders, and fatigue, for which currently available therapies are not entirely satisfactory. In fact, anxiety and pain have been proposed as the symptoms that best predict the public's search for alternative therapies (Hassed, 2006). However, the main reason why people use these kinds of interventions is not dissatisfaction with conventional medicine but because they have found these interventions to be more congruent with their own values, beliefs, and philosophical orientations toward health and life (Astin, 1998).

The RR-based approaches have been shown to be beneficial in many disorders (Mandle, Jacobs, Arcari, & Domar, 1996). However, not all studies are reliable and caution must be used. Many studies have methodological problems, and statistical significance is not synonymous with efficacy. The use of unblinded "pragmatic trials," which compare a treatment with "usual care" or no additional care, can carry a risk of bias (Power & Hopayian, 2011). The components of an outcome measure must be carefully considered and include not only the specific effect of a mind–body intervention but also nonspecific effects such as placebo, cognitive measurement biases, and the "frustrebo effect," which is the adverse effect in the control group of not receiving the treatment the subject thinks is needed. These confounders may lead to a nonspecific benefit being touted as a specific benefit of the mind–body intervention. Despite the difficulties inherent in this clinical research area, evidence for the efficacy of mind–body interventions is slowly proceeding, although integration within mainstream medicine will likely be more of a marathon than a sprint (Ernst, Pittler, Wider, & Boddy, 2007; Nahin, Pontzer, & Chesney, 2005).

With these caveats in mind, Astin and colleagues (2003) believe there is strong to moderate evidence based on meta-analyses of mind–body intervention efficacy in the following medical conditions: cardiovascular disease (Dusseldorp, van Elderen, Maes, Meulman, & Kraaij, 1999; Linden, Stossel, & Maurice, 1996); cancer treatment tolerance (Meyer & Mark, 1995; Devine & Westlake, 1995); incontinence (Weatherall, 1999); surgical outcomes (Devine, 1992; Johnston & Vogele, 1993); insomnia (NIH Consensus Panel, 1996; Morin, Culbert, & Schwartz, 1994); headache (Haddock et al., 1997; Holroyd & Penzien, 1994); chronic low back pain (van Tulder et al., 2000; NIH Consensus Panel, 1996); arthritis self-care (Astin, Beckner, Soeken, Hochberg, & Berman, 2002; Superio-Cabuslay, Ward, & Lorig, 1996; Lorig & Holman, 1993); and hypertension (Linden & Chambers, 1994; Jacob et al., 1991; Eisenberg et al, 1993; also.

Pelletier (2004) reports that for acute pain (Seers & Carroll, 2004) and fibromyalgia (Hadhazy, Ezzo Creamer, & Berman, 2000) there is also strong evidence, and adds a number of other conditions where research is less definitive but

current RCTs indicate positive efficacy: allergies (Watkins, 1994), asthma (Castes et al., 1999; McQuaid & Nassau, 1999; Smyth, Stone, Hurewitz, & Kaell, 1999), dermatological disorders (Kabat-Zinn et al., 1998), diabetes (Aikens, Kiolbasa, & Sobel, 1997; Jablon, Naliboff, Gilmore, & Rosenthal, 1997; Henry et al., 1997), HIV progression (Cruess et al., 1999; Robinson, Mathews, & Witek-Janusek, 1999), irritable bowel syndrome (Schwarz, Taylor, Scharff, & Blanchard, 1990; Blanchard & Malamood, 1996; Galovski & Blanchard, 1998; Vollmer & Blanchard, 1998), post-stroke rehabilitation (Moreland, Thomson, & Fuoco, 1998), peptic ulcer (Levenstein, Ackerman, & Kiecolt-Glaser, 1999), pregnancy outcomes (Scott, Berkowitz, & Klaus, 1999), chronic obstructive pulmonary disease (Devine & Pearcy, 1996), and tinnitus (Andersson & Lyttkens, 1999). Many other disorders are also likely to respond to mind–body interventions, but sufficient studies have not yet been done.

The role of stress in the presentation of anxiety and depressive symptoms has been widely discussed (Esch, Stefano, Fricchione, & Benson, 2002; Swaab, Bao, & Lucassen, 2005) and mind–body interventions have been shown to be effective (Benson et al., 1978; Kabat-Zinn et al., 1992) in reducing these stress-related symptoms, although there are methodological limitations (Pilkington, Kirkwood, Rampes, & Richardson, 2005; Toneatto & Nguyen, 2007).

In one Cochrane meta-analysis of 11 randomized or quasi-randomized controlled trials of relaxation techniques (progressive muscle relaxation, relaxation imagery, autogenic training) in participants diagnosed with depression or having a high level of depressive symptoms, self-rated and clinician-rated depression scores and response/remission were the primary outcomes (Jorm, Morgan and Hetrick, 2008). Relaxation techniques were more effective at reducing self-rated depressive symptoms than no or minimal treatment, but data on clinician-rated depressive symptoms were less conclusive; overall, they were not as effective as psychological treatments. Meeks et al. (2007) found that mind–body approaches were effective in treating anxiety, depression, and sleep dysfunction in an elderly cohort. And in a pilot study, a 24-week multimodal mind–body group intervention consisting of psychoeducation, lifestyle modification, meditation, and mind/body skills training was shown to be promising in reducing chronic depression and aiding overall health (Little, Kligler, Homel, Belisle, & Merrell, 2009).

Both anxiety and depression play important roles in the prognosis of somatic complaints. While the level of depression is related to the reporting of somatic symptoms (Nakao, Yamanaka, G., & Kuboki, 2001), anxiety improvement is a good indicator for somatic symptom reduction through mind–body interventions (Nakao, Fricchione, et al., 2001).

Some studies are based on multicomponent approaches that include combinations of different interventions, while others are based on one specific intervention. Other studies have focused their attention on specific indications for interventions (Barrows & Jacobs, 2002). Meditation techniques such as mindfulness-based stress reduction appear to be helpful for mental health problems, cardiovascular conditions, insomnia, premenstrual syndrome, psoriasis, and chronic pain. Hypnosis has been used for the treatment of acute and chronic pain, including surgical interventions. Biofeedback can be useful for defecation disorders, enuresis, stroke rehabilitation, and many pediatric conditions; and relaxation therapies are indicated for the treatment of insomnia, hypertension, and headache. These indications do not necessarily indicate specificity for each approach. When one technique shows efficacy for one condition, it is likely that the other techniques will also display some efficacy because of similar underlying mechanisms.

Because they promote self-care, mind–body interventions also appear to be cost effective. It has been documented that these approaches reduce ambulatory visits, postsurgical days in the hospital, unnecessary procedures, and medical costs (Benson, Beary, & Carol, 1974; Sobel, 2000). As part of the cost-effectiveness analysis, mind–body interventions also improve patient satisfaction, sense of control, and quality of life (Sobel, 1995). It should also be stressed that mind–body interventions in most cases are to be used as complementary therapies in combination with conventional medical treatments and procedures (Jacobs, 2001). So, for example, tai chi has been shown to augment escitalopram treatment of geriatric depression in one randomized controlled trial (Lavretsky et al., 2011). Tai chi training also appears to reduce balance impairments in patients receiving usual treatments for mild to moderate Parkinson's disease, with additional benefits of improved functional capacity and reduced falls (Li et al., 2012). And in a study of tai chi for fibromyalgia, of 66 randomly assigned patients receiving usual treatments, the 33 in the tai chi group had clinically important functional improvements in the Fibromyalgia Impact Questionnaire total score and in quality of life (Wang et al., 2010). Research will also be needed to define the role of mind–body medicine in primary prevention as well as in secondary and tertiary prevention, considering that stress plays a role in the onset of many diseases and in their exacerbations (Astin, 2004).

SUMMARY

The heuristic mind–body medicine equation can be derived from the research described above. In this equation the propensity to health and optimal performance is defined by a relationship between the stress burden (allostatic load) and genetic vulnerability as denominator, and the personal resources, which help us to cope with stressors (resiliency), and genetic endowment as numerator. Included in the numerator of the equation are all the mentioned self-management skills regarding the ability to elicit the relaxation response, cognitive skills, social support, prosocial behavior, positive psychology, and spiritual beliefs. Gene expression changes, induced epigenetically, may form the links within the numerator between genes and resiliency and within the denominator between genes and stress. Thus mind–body medicine interventions, by promoting a secure attachment style and enriched environment, are effective in buffering against stress and in building resiliency (Fricchione, 2011). They give the body a better chance to heal.

This kind of approach is important in clinical medicine and in public health. Consideration of mind–body approaches to promote health—not only mental health but physical health as well—and also to prevent illnesses is warranted. Mind–body medicine is an important bridge between clinical medicine and public health.

CLINICAL PEARLS

- Catecholamines and glucocorticoids both control the amplitude of immune response through negative feedback mechanisms. In physically threatening situations, inflammatory cytokines, mainly IL-6, stimulate the HPA axis, and the subsequent elevation of cortisol levels will eventually induce the suppression of the immune/inflammatory reaction. Simultaneously, the SNS causes systemic secretion of cytokines, which will eventually suppress the immune system (Stratakis & Chrousos, 1995).

- It appears that chronic stress such as unemployment or chronic caregiving may result in a biphasic immune response with some reduction of cellular and humoral immune activity coinciding with low-grade, nonspecific inflammation (Segerstrom & Miller, 2004).

- It is now increasingly clear that psychosocial stress can get translated into metabolic activation and processed at the cellular level as *oxidative stress*.

- This long-term effect of the physiologic response to stress has been called *allostatic load* –the metabolic wear and tear on the organism at the cellular level that occurs as the price for maintaining allostasis of physiological systems (McEwen & Stellar, 1993).

- Mindfulness meditation appears to reduce oxidative stress and buffer against the aging effects on telomeres (Epel et al., 2009).

- Meditation may impact allostatic loading via epigenetic pathways of gene expression.

- When stress is removed, NF-kB usually downregulates within 60 minutes. Some individuals are unable to downregulate this quickly, suggesting a variability in stress perception that can be translated into prolonged NF-kB activation.

- Altruistic behavior has been associated with good health outcomes as long as stress does not overwhelm the individual's ability to cope (Post, 2009).

- Environmental enrichment can reverse some of the effects of being a rat pup who has had a poorly nurturant upbringing, by causing epigenetic changes at the estrogen receptor that in turn elevates oxytocin functioning, leading to increased attachment behavior in adulthood.

- Secure attachment style nurtured in childhood and persisting in adulthood will make coping with illness more adaptable (Ciechanowski et al., 2002; Thompson & Ciechanowski, 2003; Ciechanowski et al., 2010).

- There should be some ability in the clinical encounter to get an objective feel for the level of patient stress and the level of patient resiliency.

- We cautiously surmise that mind–body cardiac rehabilitation programs are able to reduce stress and to increase resiliency, not only through exercise prescription and nutritional guidance but also through RR training, social support and teamwork, cognitive skills training, positive psychology, and conscious positive expectation.

- Self-management skills include the ability to elicit the relaxation response, cognitive skills, social support, prosocial behavior, positive psychology, and spiritual beliefs.

- Gene expression changes, induced epigenetically, may form the links between genes and resiliency and between genes and stress.

- Mind–body medicine interventions, by promoting a secure attachment style and enriched environment, are effective in buffering against stress and in building resiliency (Fricchione, 2011). Thus they give the body a better chance to heal.

DISCLOSURE STATEMENT

Dr. Fricchione receives book royalties from The Johns Hopkins University Press.

REFERENCES

Aikens, J. E., Kiolbasa, T. A., & Sobel, R. (1997). Psychological predictors of glycemic change with relaxation training in non-insulin-dependent diabetes mellitus. *Psychotherapy and Psychosomatics, 66*, 302–306.

Albee, G. W. (1982). Preventing psychopathology and promoting human potential. *American Psychologist, 37*, 1043–1050.

Anderson, J. G., & Taylor, A. G. (2011). The metabolic syndrome and mind-body therapies: A systematic review. *Journal of Nutrition and Metabolism, 2011*, 276419. Epub 2011 May 18.

Andersson, G., & Lyttkens, L. (1999). *A meta-analytic review of psychological treatments for tinnitus. British Journal of Audiology, 33*, 201–210.

Antoni, M. H., Lutgendorf, S. K., Blomberg, B., Carver, C. S., Lechner, S., Diaz, A., et al. (2012). Cognitive-behavioral stress management reverses anxiety-related leukocyte transcriptional dynamics. *Biological Psychiatry, 71*, 366–372.

Arnsten, A. F. T. (2009). Stress signalling pathways that impair prefrontal cortex structure and function. *Nature Reviews. Neuroscience, 10*, 410–422.

Astin, J. A., Beckner, W., Soeken, K., Hochberg, M. C., & Berman, B. (2002). Psychological interventions for rheumatoid arthritis: a meta-analysis of randomized controlled trials. *Arthritis and Rheumatism, 47*, 291–302.

Astin, J. A., Shapiro, S. L., Eisenberg, D. M., & Forys, K. L. (2003). Mind-body medicine: state of the science, implications for practice. *Journal of the American Board of Family Practice, 16*, 131–147.

Astin, J. A. (2004). Mind-body therapies for the management of pain. *Clinical Journal of Pain, 20*, 27–32.

Astin, J. A. (1998). Why patients use alternative medicine: results of a national study. *Journal of the American Medical Association, 279*, 1548–1553.

Barnes, P. M., Bloom B., & Nahin, R. L. (2008). Complementary and alternative medicine use among adults and children: United States, 2007. *National Health Statistics Report, Dec 10*(12), 1–23.

Barrows, K. A., & Jacobs, B. P. (2002). Mind-body medicine. An introduction and review of the literature. *Medical Clinics of North America, 86*, 11–31.

Benson, H., Beary, J. F., & Carol, M. P. (1974). The relaxation response. *Psychiatry, 37*, 37–46.

Benson, H., Frankel, F. H., Apfel, R., Daniels, M. D., Schniewind, H. E., Nemiah, J. C., et al. (1978). Treatment of anxiety: a comparison of the usefulness of self-hypnosis and a meditational relaxation technique. An overview. *Psychotherapy and Psychosomatics, 30*, 229–242.

Benson, H. (1975). *The relaxation response*. New York: William Morrow.

Bertisch, S. M., Wee, C. C., Phillips, R. S., & McCarthy, E. P. (2009). Alternative mind-body therapies used by adults with medical conditions. *Journal of Psychosomatic Research, 66*, 511–519.

Bierhaus, A., Humpert, P. M., & Nawroth, P. P. (2004). NF-kappaB as a molecular link between psychosocial stress and organ dysfunction. *Pediatric Nephrology, 19*, 1189–1191.

Billack, B., Heck, D. E., Mariano, T. M., Gardner, C. R., Sur, R., Laskin, D. L., & Laskin, J. D. (2002). Induction of cyclooxygenase-2 by heat shock protein 60 in macrophages and endothelial cells. *American Journal of Physiology – Cell Physiology, 283*, C1267–C1277.

Binder, E. B., Bradley, R. G., Liu W, Epstein, M. P., Deveau, T. C., Mercer, K. B., et al. (2008). BP5 polymorphisms and childhood abuse with risk of posttraumatic stress disorder in adults. *Journal of the American Medical Association, 299*, 1291–1305.

Blanchard, E. B., & Malamood, H. S. (1996). Psychological treatment of irritable bowel syndrome. *Professional Psychology: Research and Practice, 27*, 241–244.

Bowlby, J. (1982). *Attachment and loss, Vol. 1* (2nd ed.). New York: Basic Books.

Bradley, R. G., Binder, E. B., Epstein, M. P., Tang, Y., Nair, H. P., Liu, W., et al. (2008). Influence of child abuse on adult depression: moderation by the corticotrophin-releasing hormone gene. *Archives of General Psychiatry, 65*, 190–200.

Cannon, W. (1929). *Bodily changes in pain, hunger, fear, and rage.* New York: Appleton.

Case, R. B., Moss, A. J., Case, N., McDermott, M., & Eberly, S. (1992). Living alone after myocardial infarction. Impact on prognosis. *Journal of the American Medical Association, 267*, 515–519.

Castes, M., Hagel, I., Palenque, M., Canelones, P., Corao, A., & Lynch, N. R. (1999). Immunological changes associated with clinical improvement of asthmatic children subjected to psychosocial intervention. *Brain, Behavior, and Immunity, 13*, 1–13.

Champagne, F. A., & Meaney, M. J. (2007). Transgenerational effects of social environment on variations in maternal care and behavioral response to novelty. *Behavioral Neuroscience, 121*, 1353–1363.

Chrousos, G. P., & Gold, P. W. (1992). The concepts of stress and stress system disorders. Overview of physical and behavioral homeostasis. *Journal of the American Medical Association, 267*, p. 1244–1252.

Chrousos, G. P. (2007). Organization and integration of the endocrine system. *Sleep Medicine Clinics, 2*, 125–145.

Chrousos, G. P. (2009). Stress and disorders of the stress system. *Nature Reviews. Endocrinology, 5*(7), 374–381.

Ciechanowski, P., Russo, J., Katon, W., Von Korff, M., Ludman, E., Lin, E., et al. (2004). Influence of patient attachment style on self-care and outcomes in diabetes. *Psychosomatic Medicine, 66*, 720–728.

Ciechanowski, P., Russo, J., Katon, W. J., Lin, E. H., Ludman, E., Heckbert, S., et al. (2010). Relationship styles and mortality in patients with diabetes. *Diabetes Care, 33*, 539–544.

Ciechanowski, P. S., Katon, W. J., Russo, J. E., & Dwight-Johnson, M. M. (2002). Association of attachment style to lifetime medically unexplained symptoms in patients with hepatitis C. *Psychosomatics, 43*, 206–212.

Cohen, S., Tyrrell, D. A., & Smith, A. P. (1991). Psychological stress and susceptibility to the common cold. *New England Journal of Medicine, 325*, 606–612.

Cohen, S. D., Janicki-Deverts, & Miller, G. E. (2007). Psychological stress and disease. *Journal of the American Medical Association, 298,* 1685–1687.

Cole, S. W., Naliboff, B. D., Kemeny, M. E., Griswold, M. P., Fahey, J. L., & Zack, J. A. (2001). Impaired response to HAART in HIV-infected individuals with high autonomic nervous system activity. *Proceedings of the National Academy of Sciences, U.S.A., 98,* 12695–12700.

Cruess, D. G., Antoni, M. H., Kumar, M., Ironson, G., McCabe, P., Fernandez, J. B., et al. (1999). Cognitive-behavioral stress management buffers decreases in dehydroepiandrosterone sulfate (DHEA-S) and increases in the cortisol/DHEA-S ratio and reduces mood disturbance and perceived stress among HIV-seropositive men. *Psychoneuroendocrinology, 24,* 537–549.

Danese, A., Pariante, C. M., Caspi, A., Taylor, A., & Poulton, R. (2007). Childhood maltreatment predicts adult inflammation in a life-course study. *Proceedings of the National Academy of Sciences, U.S.A., 104,* 1319–1324.

de la Fuente-Fernández, R., Schulzer, M., & Stoessl, A. J. (2004). Placebo mechanisms and reward circuitry: clues from Parkinson's disease. *Biological Psychiatry, 56*(2), 67–71. Review.

Denver, R. J. (2009). Structural and functional evolution of vertebrate neuroendocrine stress systems. *Annals of the New York Academy of Sciences, 1163,* 1–16.

Devine, E. C., & Pearcy, J. (1996). Meta-analysis of the effects of psychoeducational care in adults with chronic obstructive pulmonary disease. *Patient Education and Counseling, 29,* 167–178.

Devine, E. C., & Westlake, S. K. (1995). The effects of psychoeducational care provided to adults with cancer: a meta-analysis of 116 studies. *Oncology Nursing Forum, 22,* 1369–1381.

Devine, E. C. (1992). Effects of psychoeducational care for adult surgical patients: a meta-analysis of 191 studies. *Patient Education and Counseling, 19,* 367–376.

Dong, M., Giles, W. H., Felitti, V. J., Dube, S. R., Williams, J. E., Chapman, D. P., et al. (2004). Insights into causal pathways for ischemic heart disease: Adverse childhood experiences study. *Circulation, 110,* 1761–1766.

Dusek, J. A., Chang, B. H., Zaki, J., Lazar, S., Deykin, A., Stefano, G. B., et al. (2006). Association between oxygen consumption and nitric oxide production during the relaxation response. *Medical Science Monitor, 12,* CR1–10.

Dusek, J. A., Otu, H. H., Wohlhueter, A. L., Bhasin, M., Zerbini, L. F., Joseph, M. G., et al. (2008). Genomic counter-stress changes induced by the relaxation response. *PLoS One, 3,* e2576.

Dusseldorp, E., van Elderen, T., Maes, S., Meulman, J., & Kraaij, V. (1999). A meta-analysis of psychoeducational programs for coronary heart disease patients. *Health Psychology, 18,* 506–519.

Eisenberg, D. M., Delbanco, T. L., Berkey, C. S., Kaptchuk, T. J., Kupelnick, B., Kuhl, J., & Chalmers, T. C. (1993). Cognitive behavioural techniques for hypertension: are they effective? *Annals of Internal Medicine, 118,* 964–972.

Epel, E., Daubenmier, J., Moskowitz, J. T., Folkman, S., & Blackburn, E. (2009). Can meditation slow rate of cellular aging? Cognitive stress, mindfulness, and telomeres. *Annals of the New York Academy of Sciences, 1172,* 34–53.

Epel, E. S., Blackburn, E. H., Lin, J., Dhabhar, F. S., Adler, N. E., Morrow, J. D., & Cawthon, R. M. (2004). Accelerated telomere shortening in response to life stress. *Proceedings of the National Academy of Sciences, U.S.A., 101,* 17312–17315.

Epel, E. S., Lin, J., Wilhelm, F. H., Wolkowitz, O. M., Cawthon, R., Adler, N. E., et al. (2006). Cell aging in relation to stress arousal and cardiovascular disease risk factors. *Psychoneuroendocrinology, 31,* 277–287.

Ernst, E., Pittler, M. H., Wider, B., & Boddy K. (2007). Mind-body therapies: are the trial data getting stronger? *Alternative Therapies in Health and Medicine, 13,* 62–64.

Esch, T., Stefano, G. B., Fricchione, G. L., & Benson, H. (2002). The role of stress in neurodegenerative diseases and mental disorders. *Neuro Endocrinology Letters, 23,* 199–208.

Feder, A., Nestler, E. J., & Charney, D. S. (2009). Psychobiology and molecular genetics of resilience. *Nature Reviews. Neuroscience, 10,* 446–457.

Ford, E. S., Li, C., & Zhao, G. (2010). Prevalence and correlates of metabolic syndrome based on a harmonious definition among adults in the US. *Journal of Diabetes, 2,* 180–193.

Fricchione, G., & Stefano, G. B. (2005). Placebo neural systems: nitric oxide, morphine and the dopamine brain reward and motivation circuitries. *Medical Science Monitor, 11,* MS54–MS65. Epub 2005 Apr 28.

Fricchione, G. L. (2011). Compassion and healing in medicine and society. On the nature and uses of attachment solutions to separation challenges. Johns Hopkins University Press, Baltimore MD.

Fricchione, G. L. (2009). The "new" science of mind body medicine. In Y. E. Kawachi & M. Nakao (Eds.), *The healthy hospital: maximizing the satisfaction of patients, health workers, and the community.* The Seventh Teikyo-Harvard Symposium, June 26–27, 2009.

Gaab, J., Rohleder, N., Nater, U. M., & Ehlert, U. (2005). Psychological determinants of the cortisol stress response: the role of anticipatory cognitive appraisal. *Psychoneuroendocrinology, 30,* 599–610.

Galovski, T. E., & Blanchard, E. B. (1998). The treatment of irritable bowel syndrome with hypnotherapy. *Applied Psychophysiology and Biofeedback, 23,* 219–232.

Gruenewald, T. L., Seeman, T. E., Karlamangla, A. S., & Sarkisian, C. A. (2009). Allostatic load and frailty in older adults. *Journal of the American Geriatrics Society, 57,* 1525–1531.

Haddock, C. K., Rowan, A. B., Andrasik, F., Wilson, P. G., Talcott, G. W., & Stein, R. J. (1997). Home-based behavioral treatments for chronic benign headache: a meta-analysis of controlled trials. *Cephalalgia, 17,* 113–118.

Hadhazy, V. A., Ezzo J, Creamer, P., & Berman, B. M. (2000). Mind-body therapies for the treatment of fibromyalgia. A systematic review. *Journal of Rheumatology, 27,* 2911–2918.

Hassed, C. (2006). *Mind-Body Medicine: Science, Practice and Philosophy.* Available from: http://www.lifestyleandculturelectures.org/lectures/mindfulness/MindBodyMedicine.pdf.

Heinz, A., & Smolka, M. N. (2006). The effects of catechol O-methyltransferase genotype on brain activation elicited by affective stimuli and cognitive tasks. *Reviews in the Neurosciences, 17,* 359–367.

Henry, J. L., Wilson, P. H., Bruce, D. G., Chisholm, D. J., & Rawling, P. J. (1997). Cognitive-behavioural stress management for patients with non-insulin dependent diabetes mellitus. *Psychology, Health & Medicine, 2,* 109–118.

Herman, J. P., Figueiredo H, Mueller, N. K., Ulrich-Lai, Y., Ostrander, M. M., Choi, D. C., & Cullinan, W. E. (2003). Central mechanisms of stress integration: hierarchical circuitry controlling hypothalamo-pituitary-adrenocortical responsiveness. *Frontiers in Neuroendocrinology, 24,* 151–180.

Herry, C., Ciocchi, S., Senn, V., Demmou, L., Muller, C., & Luthi, A. (2008). Switching on and off fear by distinct neuronal circuits. *Nature, 454,* 600–605.

Hofmann, M. A., Schiekofer, S., Isermann, B., Kanitz, M., Henkels, M., Joswig, M., et al. (1999). Peripheral blood mononuclear cells isolated from patients with diabetic nephropathy show increased activation of the oxidative-stress sensitive transcription factor NF-kappaB. *Diabetologia, 42,* 222–232.

Holroyd, K. A., & Penzien, D. B. (1994). Pharmacological versus non-pharmacological prophylaxis of recurrent migraine headache: a meta-analytic review of clinical trials. *Pain, 42,* 1–13.

Horsten, M., Mittleman, M. A., Wamala, S. P., Schenck-Gustafsson, K., & Orth-Gomér, K. (2000). Depressive symptoms and lack of social integration in relation to prognosis of CHD in middle-aged women. The Stockholm Female Coronary Risk Study. *European Heart Journal, 21,* 1072–1080.

Jablon, S. L., Naliboff, B. D., Gilmore, S. L., & Rosenthal, M. J. (1997). Effects of relaxation training on glucose tolerance and diabetic control in type II diabetes. *Applied Psychophysiological Biofeedback, 22,* 155–169.

Jacob, R. G., Chesney, M. A., Williams, D. M., Ding, Y., & Shapiro, A. P. (1991). Relaxation therapy for hypertension: Design effects and treatment effects. *Annals of Behavioral Medicine, 13,* 5–17.

Jacobs, G. D. (2001). Clinical applications of the relaxation response and mind-body interventions. *Journal of Alternative and Complementary Medicine, 7*(Suppl 1), S93–S164.

Johnston, M., & Vogele, C. (1993). Benefits of psychological preparation for surgery: A meta-analysis. *Annals of Behavioral Medicine, 15,* 245–256.

Jorm, A. F., Morgan, A. J., & Hetrick, S. E. (2008). Relaxation for depression. *Cochrane Database of Systematic Reviews* (4), CD007142 doi: 10.1002/14651858.CD007142.pub2

Jovanovic, T., & Ressler, K. J. (2010). How the neurocircuitry and genetics of fear inhibition may inform our understanding of PTSD. *American Journal of Psychiatry, 167,* 648–662.

Kabat-Zinn, J., Wheeler, E., Light, T., Skillings, A., Scharf, M. J., Cropley, T. G., et al. (1998). Influence of a mindfulness meditation-based stress reduction intervention on rates of skin clearing in patients with moderate to severe psoriasis undergoing phototherapy (UVB) and photochemotherapy (PUVA). *Psychosomatic Medicine, 60,* 625–632.

Kabat-Zinn, J., Massion, A. O., Kristeller, J., Peterson, L. G., Fletcher, K. E., Pbert, L., et al. (1992). Effectiveness of a meditation-based stress reduction program in the treatment of anxiety disorders. *American Journal of Psychiatry, 149,* 936–943.

Kaufman, J., Yang, B. Z., Douglas-Palumberi, H., Houshyar, S., Lipschitz, D., Krystal, J. H., & Gelernter, J. (2004). Social supports and serotonin transporter gene moderate depression in maltreated children. *Proceedings of the National Academy of Sciences, U.S.A., 101,* 17316–17321.

Krishnan, V., Han, M. H., Graham, D. L., Berton, O., Renthal, W., Russo, S. J., et al. (2007). Molecular adaptations underlying susceptibility and resistance to social defeat in brain reward regions. *Cell, 131,* 391–404.

Lanius, R. A., Vermetten, E., Loewenstein, R. J., Brand, B., Schmahl, C., Bremner, J. D., & Spiegel, D. (2010). Emotion modulation in PTSD. Clinical and neurobiological evidence for a dissociative subtype. *American Journal of Psychiatry, 167,* 640–647.

Lavretsky, H., Alstein, L. L., Olmstead, R. E., Ercoli, L. M., Riparetti-Brown, M., Cyr, N. S., & Irwin, M. R. (2011). Complementary use of Tai Chi augments escitalopram treatment of geriatric depression. *American Journal of Geriatric Psychiatry. 19,* 839–850.

Lazarus, R., & Folkman, S. (1984). *Stress, appraisal and coping.* New York: Springer.

LeDoux, J., & Gorman, J. (2001). A call to action: overcoming anxiety through active coping. *American Journal of Psychiatry, 158,* 1953–1995.

Levenstein, S, Ackerman, S., Kiecolt-Glaser, J. K., & Dubois, A. (1999). Stress and peptic ulcer disease. *Journal of the American Medical Association, 281,* 10–11.

Lewis, M. D. (2005). Bridging emotion theory and neurobiology through dynamic systems modeling. *Behavioral and Brain Sciences, 28,* 169–194; discussion 194–245.

Li, F., Harmer, P., Fitzgerald, K., Eckstrom, E., Stock, R., Galver, J., Maddalozzo, G., & Batya, S. S. (2012). Tai chi and postural stability in patients with Parkinson's disease. *New England Journal of Medicine, 366,* 511–519.

Likhtik, E., Popa, D., Apergis-Schoute, J., Fidacaro, G. A., & Pare, D. (2008). Amygdala intercalated neurons are required for expression of fear extinction. *Nature, 454,* 642–645.

Linden, W., & Chambers, L. (1994). Clinical effectiveness of non-drug treatment for hypertension: A meta-analysis. *Annals of Behavioral Medicine, 16,* 35–45.

Linden, W., Stossel, C., & Maurice, J. (1996). Psychosocial interventions for patients with coronary artery disease: a meta-analysis. *Archives of Internal Medicine, 156,* 745–752.

Little, S. A., Kligler, B., Homel, P., Belisle, S. S., & Merrell, W. (2009). Multimodal mind body therapy for chronic depression: A pilot study. *Explore (NY), 5,* 330–337.

Lorig, K., & Holman, H. (1993). Arthritis self-management studies: a twelve-year review. *Health Education Quarterly, 20,* 17–28.

Madrigal, J. L., Hurtado, O., Moro, M. A., Lizasoain, I., Lorenzo, P., Castrillo, A., et al. (2002). The increase in, T.N.F-alpha levels is implicated in NF-kappaB activation and inducible nitric oxide synthase expression in brain cortex after immobilization stress. *Neuropsychopharmacology, 26,* 155–163.

Mandle, C. L., Jacobs, S. C., Arcari, P. M., & Domar, A. D. (1996). The efficacy of relaxation response interventions with adult patients: a review of the literature. *Journal of Cardiovascular Nursing, 10,* 4–26.

Matthews, K., & Gump, B. B. (2002). Chronic work stress and marital dissolution increase risk of posttrial mortality in men from the Multiple Risk Factor Intervention Trial. *Archives of Internal Medicine, 162,* 309–315.

Mayberg, H. S., Silva, J. A., Brannan, S. K., Tekell, J. L., Mahurin, R. K., McGinnis, S., & Jerabek, P. A. (2002). The functional neuroanatomy of the placebo effect. *American Journal of Psychiatry, 159,* 728–737.

McEwen, B. S., & Stellar, E. (1993). Stress and the individual: mechanisms leading to disease. *Archives of Internal Medicine, 153,* 2093–101.

McEwen, B. S. (1998). Protective and damaging effects of stress mediators. *New England Journal of Medicine, 338,* 171–179.

McEwen, B. S. (1999). Stress and hippocampal plasticity. *Annual Reviews in the Neurosciences, 22,* 105–122.

McOmish, C. E., & Hannan, A. J. (2007). Enviromimetics: exploring gene environment interactions to identify therapeutic targets for brain disorders. *Expert Opinion on Therapeutic Targets, 11,* 899–913.

McQuaid, E. L., & Nassau, J. H. (1999). Empirically supported treatments of disease-related symptoms in pediatric psychology: asthma, diabetes, and cancer. *Journal of Pediatric Psychology, 24,* 305–328.

Meaney, M. J., & Szyf, M. (2005). Environmental programming of stress responses through, D.N.A methylation: life at the interface between a dynamic environment and a fixed genome. *Dialogues in Clinical Neuroscience, 7,* 105–125.

Meeks, T. W., Wetherell, J. L., Irwin, M. R., Redwine, L. S., & Jeste, D. V. (2007). Complementary and alternative treatments for late-life depression, anxiety, and sleep disturbance: a review of randomized controlled trials. *Journal of Clinical Psychiatry, 68,* 1461–1471.

Meyer, T. J., & Mark, M. M. (1995). Effects of psychosocial interventions with adult cancer patients: a meta-analysis of randomized experiments. *Health Psychology, 14,* 101–108.

Miller, A. H., Maletic, V., & Raison, C. L. (2008). Inflammation and its discontents: The role of cytokines in the pathophysiology of major depression. *Biological Psychiatry, 65,* 732–741.

Miller, A. H. (2009). Norman Cousins Lecture. Mechanisms of cytokine-induced behavioral changes: psychoneuroimmunology at the translational interface. *Brain, Behavior, and Immunity, 23,* 149–158.

Miller, G. E., Chen, E., Fok, A. K., Walker, H., Lim, Nicholls, E. F., et al. (2009). Low early-life social class leaves a biological residue manifested by decreased glucocorticoid and increased proinflammatory signalling. *Proceedings of the National Academy of Sciences, 106,* 14716–14721.

Miller, G. E., Chen, E., Sze, J., Marin, T., Arevalo, J. M., Doll, R., et al. (2008). Functional genomic fingerprint of chronic stress in humans: blunted glucocorticoid and increased NF-kappaB signaling. *Biological Psychiatry, 64,* 266–272.

Mohr, D. C., Hart, S. L., Julian, L., Cox, D., & Pelletier, D. (2004). Association between stressful life events and exacerbation in multiple sclerosis: a meta-analysis. *British Medical Journal, 328,* 731.

Moreland, J. D., Thomson, M. A., & Fuoco, A. R. (1998). Electromyographic biofeedback to improve lower extremity function after stroke: a meta-analysis. *Archives of Physical Medicine and Rehabilitation, 79,* 134–140.

Morin, C. M., Culbert, J. P., & Schwartz, S. M. (1994). Nonpharmacological interventions for insomnia: a meta-analysis of treatment efficacy. *American Journal of Psychiatry, 151,* 1172–1180.

Nagabhushan, M., Mathews, H. L., & Witek-Janusek, L. (2001). Aberrant nuclear expression of AP-1 and NF-kappaB in lymphocytes of women stressed by the experience of breast biopsy. *Brain, Behavior, and Immunity, 15*, 78–84.

Nahin, R. L., Barnes, P. M., Stussman, B. J., & Bloom, B. (2009). Costs of complementary and alternative medicine (CAM) and frequency of visits to CAM practitioners: United States, 2007. *National Health Statistics Report, July 30* (18), 1–14.

Nahin, R. L., Pontzer, C. H., & Chesney, M. A. (2005). Racing toward the integration of complementary and alternative medicine: A marathon or a sprint? *Health Affairs, 24*, 991–993.

Nakao, M., Yamanaka, G., & Kuboki, T. (2001). *Major depression and somatic symptoms in a mind/body medicine clinic. Psychopathology, 34*, 230–235.

Nakao, M., Fricchione, G., Myers, P., Zuttermeister, P. C., Baim, M., Mandle, C. L., et al. (2001). Anxiety is a good indicator for somatic symptom reduction through behavioral medicine intervention in a mind/body medicine clinic. *Psychotherapy and Psychosomatics, 70*, 50–57.

NCCAM National Institutes of Health. *Mind-Body Medicine: An Overview*. (2007). Available from: http://www.qigonginstitute.org/html/papers/NCCAMmindbody.pdf.

NIH Technology Assessment Panel on Integration of Behavioral and Relaxation Approaches into the Treatment of Chronic Pain and Insomnia. (1996). Integration of behavioural and relaxation approaches into the treatment of chronic pain and insomnia. *Journal of the American Medical Association, 276*, 313–318.

Pacak, K., & Palkovits, M. (2001). Stressor specificity of central neuroendocrine responses: implications for stress-related disorders. *Endocrine Reviews, 22*, 502–548.

Peabody, F. W. (1927). The care of the patient. *Journal of the American Medical Association, 88*, 877–882.

Pelletier, K. R. (2004). Mind-body medicine in ambulatory care: an evidence-based assessment. *Journal of Ambulatory Care Management, 27*, 25–42.

Perkins, A. (1994). Saving money by reducing stress. *Harvard Business Review, 72*, 12.

Pilkington, K., Kirkwood, G., Rampes, H., & Richardson, J. (2005). Yoga for depression: the research evidence. *Journal of Affective Disorders, 89*, 13–24.

Post, S. G. (2009). It's good to be good: science says it's so. Research demonstrates that people who help others usually have healthier, happier lives. *Health Progress, 90*, 18–25.

Power, M., & Hopayian, K. (2011). Exposing the evidence gap for complementary and alternative medicine to be integrated into science-based medicine. *Journal of the Royal Society of Medicine, 104*, 155–161.

Risch, N., Herrell, R., Lehner, T., Liang, K. Y., Eaves, L., Hoh, J., et al. (2009). Interaction between the serotonin transporter gene (5-HTTLPR), stressful life events, and risk of depression: a meta-analysis. *Journal of the American Medical Association, 301*, 2462–2471.

Robinson, F. P., Mathews, H. L., & Witek-Janusek L. (1999). Stress and HIV disease progression: psychoneuroimmunological framework. *Journal of the Association of Nurses in AIDS Care, 10*, 21–31.

Ruberman, W., Weinblatt, E., Goldberg, J. D., & Chaudhary, B. S. (1984). Psychosocial influences on mortality after myocardial infarction. *New England Journal of Medicine, 311*, 552–559.

Russo, S. J., Murrough, J. W., Han M-H, Charney, D. S., & Nestler, E. J. (2012). Neurobiology of resilience. *Nature. Neuroscience, 15*, 1475–1484.

Samuelson, M., Foret, M., Baim, M., Lerner, J., Fricchione, G., Benson, H., et al. (2010). Exploring the effectiveness of a comprehensive mind-body intervention for medical symptom relief. *Journal of Alternative and Complementary Medicine, 16*, 187–192.

Sandberg, S., Paton, J. Y., Ahola, S., McCann, D. C., McGuinness D, Hillary, C. R., et al. (2000). The role of acute and chronic stress in asthma attacks in children. *Lancet, 356*, 982–987.

Saper, C. B., & Breder, C. D. (1994). The neurologic basis of fever. *New England Journal of Medicine, 330*, 1880–1886.

Schottelius, A. J., & Dinter H. (2006). Cytokines, NF-kappaB, microenvironment, intestinal inflammation and cancer. *Cancer Treatment Research, 130*, 67–87.

Schwarz, S. P., Taylor, A. E., Scharff, L., & Blanchard, E. B. (1990). Behaviorally treated irritable bowel syndrome patients: a four-year follow-up. *Behavioral Research and Therapy, 28*, 331–335.

Scott, K. D., Berkowitz, G., & Klaus, M. (1999). A comparison of intermittent and continuous support during labor: a meta-analysis. *American Journal of Obstetrics & Gynecology, 180*, 1054–1059.

Seeman, T. E., Singer, B. H., Rowe, J. W., Horwitz, R. I., & McEwen, B. S. (1997). Price of adaptation—allostatic load and its health consequences. MacArthur studies of successful aging. *Archives of Internal Medicine, 157*, 2259–2268.

Seeman, T. E. (2000). Health promoting effects of friends and family on health outcomes in older adults. *American Journal of Health Promotion, 14*, 362–370.

Seers, K., & Carroll, D. (1998). Relaxation techniques for acute pain management: a systematic review. *Journal of Advanced Nursing, 27*, 466–475.

Segerstrom, SC, & Miller, G. E. (2004). Psychological stress and the human immune system: a meta-analytic study of 30 years of inquiry. *Psychological Bulletin, 130*, 601–630.

Selye, H. (1946). The general adaptation syndrome. *Journal of Clinical Endocrinology, 6*, 177.

Sewitch, M. J., Abrahamowicz, M., Bitton, A., Daly, D., Wild, G. E., Cohen, A., et al. (2001). Psychological distress, social support, and disease activity in patients with inflammatory bowel disease. *American Journal of Gastroenterology, 96*, 1470–1479.

Shepard, D. S., Stason, W. B., Strickler, G. K., Lee, A. J., Bhalotra, S., Ritter, G., et al. (2009). Evaluation of lifestyle modification and cardiac rehabilitation in Medicare beneficiaries. Supported by the Centers for Medicare & Medicaid Services under contract number 500-95-0060, Task Order 02 to Brandeis University and number 500-02-0012-MDBU to the Delmarva Foundation for Medical Care. April 30, 2009.

Sierpina, V. S., Kreitzer, M. J., Cunningham, A. J., Elder, W. G., & Bruckner, G. (2007). Use of mind-body therapies in psychiatry and family medicine faculty and residents: attitudes, barriers, and gender differences. *Explore (NY), 3*, 129–135.

Smyth, J. M., Stone, A. A., Hurewitz, A., & Kaell, A. (1999). Effects of writing about stressful experiences on symptom reduction in patients with asthma or rheumatoid arthritis: a randomized trial. *Journal of the American Medical Association, 281*, 1304–1309.

Sobel, D. S. (1995). Rethinking medicine: improving health outcomes with cost-effective psychosocial interventions. *Psychosomatic Medicine, 57*, 234–244.

Sobel, D. S. (2000). The cost-effectiveness of mind-body medicine interventions. *Progress in Brain Research, 122*, 393–412.

Southwick, S. M., Vythilingam, M., & Charney, D. S. (2005). The psychobiology of depression and resilience to stress: implications for prevention and treatment. *Annual Review of Clinical Psychology, 1*, 255–291.

Stefano, G. B., Murga, J., Benson, H., Zhu, W., Bilfinger, T. V., & Magazine, H. I. (2001). Nitric oxide inhibits norepinephrine stimulated contraction of human internal thoracic artery and rat aorta. *Pharmacological Research, 43*, 199–203.

Sterling, P., & Eyer, J. (1988). Allostasis: A new paradigm to explain arousal pathology. In S. Fisher & J. Reason (Eds.), *Handbook of life stress, cognition and health* (pp. 629–649). New York: John Wiley & Sons.

Stratakis, C. A., & Chrousos, G. P. (1995). Neuroendocrinology and pathophysiology of the stress system. *Annals of the New York Academy of Sciences, 771*, 1–18.

Superio-Cabuslay, E., Ward, M. M., & Lorig, K. R. (1996). Patient education interventions in osteoarthritis and rheumatoid arthritis: a meta-analytic comparison with nonsteroidal anti-inflammatory drug treatment. *Arthritis Care Research, 9*, 292–301.

Sutcliffe, N., Clarke, A. E., Levinton, C., Frost, C., Gordon, C., & Isenberg, D. A. (1999). Associates of health status in patients with systemic lupus erythematosus. *Journal of Rheumatology, 26*, 2352–2356.

Swaab, D. F., Bao, A. M., & Lucassen, P. J. (2005). The stress system in the human brain in depression and neurodegeneration. *Ageing Research Reviews, 4*, 141–194.

Thompson, D., & Ciechanowski, P. S. (2003). Attaching a new understanding to the patient-physician relationship in family practice. *Journal of the American Board of Family Practice, 16*(3), 219–226.

Toneatto, T., & Nguyen, L. (2007). Does mindfulness meditation improve anxiety and mood symptoms? A review of the controlled research. *Canadian Journal of Psychiatry, 52*, 260–266.

Tsigos, C., & Chrousos, G. P. (2002). Hypothalamic-pituitary-adrenal axis, neuroendocrine factors and stress. *Journal of Psychosomatic Research, 53*, 865–871.

Ulrich-Lai, Y. M., & Herman, J. P. (2009). Neural regulation of endocrine and autonomic stress responses. *Nature Reviews in the Neurosciences, 10*, 397–409.

Valdez, G. R., & Koob, G. F. (2004). Allostasis and dysregulation of corticotropin-releasing factor and neuropeptide Y systems: implications for the development of alcoholism. *Pharmacology, Biochemistry, & Behavior, 79*, 671–689.

van Tulder, M. W., Ostelo, R., Vlaeyen, J. W., Linton, S. J., Morley, S. J., & Assendelft, W. J. (2000). Behavioral treatment for chronic low back pain: a systematic review within the framework of the Cochrane Back Review Group. *Spine, 25*, 2688–2699.

Vollmer, A., & Blanchard, E. B. (1998). Controlled comparison of individual versus group cognitive therapy for irritable bowel syndrome. *Behavior Therapy, 29*, 19–33.

Wang, C., Schmid, C. H., Rones, R., Kalish, R., Yinh, J., Goldenberg, D. L., Lee, Y., & McAlindon T. (2010). A randomized trial of tai chi for fibromyalgia. *New England Journal of Medicine, 363*, 743–754.

Ward, M. M., Lotstein, D. S., Bush, T. M., Lambert, R. E., van Vollenhoven, R., & Neuwelt, C. M. (1999). Psychosocial correlates of morbidity in women with systemic lupus erythematosus. *Journal of Rheumatology, 26*, 2153–2158.

Watkins, A. D. (1994). *The role of alternative therapies in the treatment of allergic disease. Clinical and Expimental Allergy, 24*, 813–825.

Weatherall, M. (1999). Biofeedback or pelvic floor muscle exercise for female genuine stress incontinence: a meta-analysis of trials identified in systematic review. *BJU International, 83*, 1015–1016.

Weaver, I. C., Cervoni, N., Champagne, F. A., D'Alessio, A. C., Sharma, S., Seckl, J. R., et al. (2004). Epigenetic programming by maternal behavior. *Nature Neuroscience, 7*, 847–854.

Wolsko, P. M., Eisenberg, D. M., Davis, R. B., & Phillips, R. S. (2004). Use of mind-body medical therapies. *Journal of General Internal Medicine, 19*, 43–50.

Zhou, Z., Zhu, G., Hariri, A. R., Enoch, M. A., Scott, D., Sinha, R., et al. (2008). Genetic variation in human NPY expression affects stress response and emotion. *Nature, 452*, 997–1001.

Zubieta, J. K., Bueller, J. A., Jackson, L. R., Scott, D. J., Xu, Y., Koeppe, R. A., et al. (2005). Placebo effects mediated by endogenous opioid activity on mu-opioid receptors. *Journal of Neuroscience, 25*, 7754–7762.

18.

SPIRITUAL AND RELIGIOUS ISSUES IN MEDICAL ILLNESS

Gregory L. Fricchione and John R. Peteet

Science without religion is lame,
Religion without science is blind.
—*Albert Einstein*

INTRODUCTION

Consideration of healthy religious factors during psychiatric treatment has traditionally been taboo ever since Freud alienated most of psychiatry and psychoanalysis from salutogenic religious behaviors in part due to his adoption of Feuerbach's wish-fulfillment and projection views on the subject (Stepansky, 1986). Within psychiatry itself, those seeking a more religious or spiritually oriented approach initially gravitated toward the psychology of Carl Jung, who tended to turn psychology into a form of mysticism of the self, and religion into a form of mystical psychology. Over the past 30 years, however, some physicians and nurses, as well as pastoral counseling and chaplaincy movements, have attempted to integrate the religious/spiritual and the psychotherapeutic aspects of patient care. In the past 20 years, improved research has validated the association between religion and health, if not the causality, and the positive role that it can play in recovery from illness. One need not be a believer to employ an understanding of the power of spirituality and religion to promote healing in the care of patients with medical illness.

This chapter explores the appropriate role of psychiatrists in dealing with the religious and spiritual concerns of their patients, particularly in the context of medical illness. To begin, we focus on the role of the physician and/or psychiatrist in the emotional crisis of physically ill patients. Then we will focus on the downstream effects of spirituality and religion on physical and mental health (Fricchione, 2011a). We discuss how the neurobiology of religious experience is related to the mammalian anatomy of attachment in the limbic system, and then the clinical approach to understanding a patient's religious beliefs, how to use this knowledge to better treat the patient, when to make a chaplaincy referral, and issues related to the care of Jehovah's Witnesses patients.

Patients encountering severe physical illness face what philosophers call the "limit questions": Who am I? What is the meaning of my life? Where am I going? Will I be separated from my loved ones?—questions that express universal existential concerns in the domains of identity, hope, meaning, purpose, morality, and relationship to ultimate authority. The spiritual answer to each of these existential questions depends on the connection that the individual feels in relation to a reality greater than himself or herself. As our colleagues in medicine and surgery have less and less time to spend with individual patients, psychiatrists and palliative care specialists working in general hospitals are called upon more often than in the past to engage with their patients in a dialogue that bridges life and death, stepping into the anxiety-provoking and often terrifying "intermediate area" between separation and attachment first described by D.W. Winnicott (1953). From an object-relations perspective (Horton, 1981), the physician acts as a transitional object, an object that can be held in the transition, offering solace that comes from "transitional relatedness." The physician becomes a parental figure of protection and guidance, with the capacity to accompany the vulnerable individual facing the threat of separation to a safe place. One such place may be a safer emotional-spiritual world for the patient who holds a belief in such a reality.

Indeed, the origin of caring for all physicians may be traced to the anxiety-ridden separation/attachment experience of the person who is ill and the willingness of the physician to enter into the patient's emotional world by being a consistent, knowledgeable, and caring fellow human being. In the process, medically ill persons derive the solace and confidence required to negotiate their illness-precipitated developmental challenges, including the challenge of facing death (Fricchione, 1993).

While transitional relatedness, or providing an empathic caring presence, can seem like extra duty for physicians already burdened by the technical pressures of providing medical expertise, it is often key to the role played by medical psychiatrists. Nevertheless, it must be stressed that this transitional role is and always will be at the heart of every clinical physician's calling.

As Peabody (1927) said to medical students 70 years ago: "One of the essential qualities of the clinician is interest in humanity, for the secret of the care of the patient is in caring for the patient." Visitors to the Massachusetts General Hospital see these famous words etched in the lobby's marble wall. Alongside it is another famous quote of Dr. Edward Churchill, speaking over 50 years ago: "Charity in the broad spiritual sense, that is our desire to relieve suffering, is the most prized possession of medicine." So a major contention of this chapter is this: that clinicians and patients meet in the most spiritual of all earthly places—the bedside.

Healing is a product not only of curing but of caring, a caring that is spiritually inspired. The word *heal* comes from the old English word *haelen*. It means not only to restore to health by way of a cure but also "to set right; to amend" (American Heritage Dictionary, 1978), as in the phrase "to heal a rift between us." In addition, "to heal" can mean "to restore a person to spiritual wholeness" (American Heritage Dictionary, 1993). This form of healing is the major goal of religion. It is of interest that the root meaning of the word *religion* comes from the Latin word *religio*, which can be translated as "to bind back"; that is, to reattach or to restore.

This theme of restoration and reattachment is at the core of human spirituality—a uniquely human capacity for consolation in response to the awareness of separation and loss. Both religion and medicine are formal human structures within which human spirituality can be given expression by offering care and consolation.

Paul Tillich and T.S. Eliot characterized the 20th century as an "Age of Anxiety," and so far there is little evidence that the 21st century will become anxiety free. Tillich believed modern humanity was marked by a sense of disconnection, of separation from a spiritual source of life's meaning and purpose, from what he called our "Ground of Being," a term he essentially used for God (Tillich, 1951). Nevertheless, most Americans believe in a "Ground of Being." This percentage has remained steady in polls taken over many years at 92% to 96%. While the percentage of Americans who believe institutional religion is essential to their lives has dropped from 75% to 58%, the percentage reporting that spirituality is essential has risen from 58% to 76%. The clear message is that God, spirituality, and even religion remain important sources of understanding and solace for most patients in the United States.

DEFINITIONS OF SPIRITUALITY

One of the obstacles to bringing religious and medical healing together has been the challenge of defining spirituality. One consensus, from the Fetzer Foundation's 2003 conference on Spirituality in Palliative Medicine, has focused on spirituality as a connection to something larger than oneself that gives meaning to one's life (Fetzer Institute, 2003).

The word *spirituality* comes from the Latin word *spiritus*, meaning breath. The Benedictine monk and psychologist Steindl-Rast defined spirituality as "aliveness—super aliveness. . . . It's the breath of all of creation. Whenever we are alive, on every level, we are spiritual, and we are fully spiritual when we come alive on the highest level of our caring for

one another and caring for this planet" (Olsen, 1996). For Steindl-Rast the act of the spirit is caring. Spirituality in this sense is the lifeblood at the heart of medicine as well as religion. It attaches physicians and all of us to that "spark of life that can be felt," to that "Ground of Being," to that breath of all life one might call "the Holy Spirit."

Several years ago, the Swiss theologian Hans Kung gave the annual Oskar Pfister lecture at an American Psychiatric Association meeting. He implored the audience to attend to spiritual life and religious heritage in patient care. Several psychiatrists have since written on the subject. One such psychiatrist was the late Irving M. Rosen, working at the interface of medicine and psychiatry, who came to view spirituality as a "domain, a level of development of the mature and responsible person" (Rosen, 1993). He came to the conclusion that "religion is man acting as the inclusive scientist searching for what is most real and lastingly valuable" (Rosen, 1993). He went on to say:

The whole person is one . . . who can find meaning; come through suffering, commit to trust and love and deal effectively with stress and the stress emotions of anxiety, anger, guilt, shame, and grief. From this matrix there emerges the "Witnessing Self" able to apply the powers of meditation and finally to reach a sense of compassion and unity with the universe, the ultimate goal of meditation. We can help our patients by seeing and affirming these issues or helping the patients to grow in them. The cognitive aspect of spirituality is accessible to our understanding and use. There is also an energy aspect, the 'Spirit' or spark of life that can be felt, but I think we need to learn more about it if it is to be controlled and used in helping (Rosen, 1993 p. 77).

In an effort to integrate spirituality into medical care, a recent consensus conference, *Improving the Quality of Spiritual Care as a Dimension of Palliative Care*, recommended the following definition of spirituality:

Spirituality is the aspect of humanity that refers to the way individuals seek and express meaning and purpose and the way they experience their connectedness to the moment, to self, to others, to nature, and to the significant or sacred (Puchalski et al., 2009, p. 887).

This definition includes the critical elements of connectedness, meaning, and the search for the significant and the sacred in life. These elements have theological, philosophical, empirical, and clinical dimensions. From the clinical and public health points of view, it is important to realize that spirituality thus understood will intersect with modern concepts of health-promoting human resiliency, which emerges from neurobiological substrates in the brain, motivation and reward circuitries, and paralimbic cortices that have the capacity to inhibit amygdalar fear conditioning.

The Consensus Conference recommended implementation of an inpatient spiritual care model that would include a spiritual screening, followed by the possibility of a spiritual history taken by physicians or nurses, which might then lead to a spiritual assessment by board-certified chaplains or multidisciplinary team rounds such that a spiritual treatment plan could be fashioned (see Figure 18.1).

In the outpatient setting, a spiritual history might lead to a chaplaincy or spiritual care provider referral. Existential concerns, particularly at end of life, feelings of abandonment by God or others, anger at God or others, concerns about relationship with deity, conflicted or challenged belief systems, despair/hopelessness, grief/loss, guilt/shame, reconciliation, isolation, religious-specific issues (ritual needs or inability to perform usual practices), and religious/spiritual struggle issues (loss of faith or meaning; disappointment with community aide) are common spiritual *diagnoses* that can trigger a clergy, chaplain, or pastoral counselor consultation (Puchalski et al., 2009, p. 894). It is important to realize that spiritual challenges are really threatened loss of connectedness.

THE NEUROBIOLOGY OF THE CRISIS OF PHYSICAL ILLNESS AND SPIRITUALITY

The emotional center of the brain—the limbic system—is essential to the experience of illness. The limbic system brings emotional valence to the patient's cognitive appraisal of the crisis of illness and its meaning. Genetic endowment and personal factors, physical and social environmental factors, and illness-related factors are all colored by emotion. Indeed, gene expression itself can be altered by social and environmental changes such as nurturance or the lack thereof that is reflected in limbic emotional responses (Champagne, 2010). In Moos and Tsu's model of the crisis of physical illness (1977), the patient cognitively appraises the emotionalized illness challenge and then focuses on adaptive tasks that test coping skills and determine the outcome of the crisis.

The limbic system mediates the basic drives to self and species preservation, attachment behavior, and territoriality (MacLean, 1990). Thus, while the cortex may cognitively appraise the illness and its threat, the limbic system is buffeted by turbulent undercurrents of fear of excessive dependency and the possibility of a final separation from life and loved ones through death. This threat will be appreciated in a fear-conditioned amygdalar response that can then precipitate a lateral hypothalamic stimulation of sympathetic nervous system drive and a paraventricular hypothalamic stimulation of the pituitary-adrenal outpouring of adrenocorticotrophin and cortisol. When persistent and/or overwhelming, this distress response will be pathogenic to end organs. Clinically, this existential condition may give way to symptoms of anxiety and depression, the end-state of which might be conservation-withdrawal with disengagement and inactivity signifying a given-up state (Ironside, 1980). Territoriality is threatened by illness

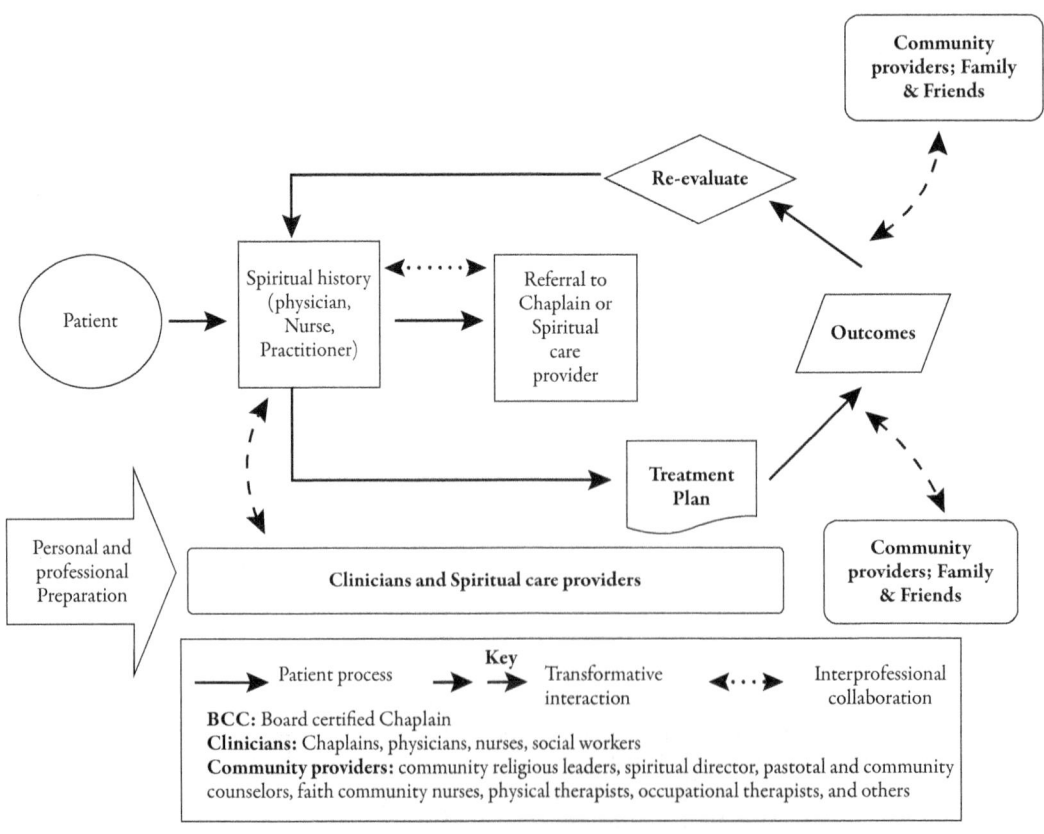

Figure 18.1 Proposed Spiritual Care Implementation Model. (From Puchalski et al., 2009)

when patients are removed from their homes, have their clothes taken away, and are forced to yield an element of control to strangers. The need for basic trust is heightened, while attachments are strained as patients are separated from family members both literally and symbolically. The amygdala, hippocampus, and thalamocingulate areas, among other limbic regions, mediate these experiences (LeDoux, 1996). The emotionality of the illness affects perception of predicament and allocation of cognitive focus, whether as "threat-stress" or as "opportunity-challenge." Spirituality and religion, to the extent that they promote conscious positive expectation and the resiliency of connectedness, may serve to promote healthy adaptation to illness. Human resiliency is a product of the maturity of certain brain regions that can serve as brakes on a runaway amygdala-driven fear conditioning pathway (Charney, 2004). A healthy brain reward and brain motivation pathway, with terminal zones in the hippocampus and nucleus accumbens in the former case and in the anterior cingulate cortex and the dorsolateral prefrontal cortex in the latter case, will afford the individual a better chance of living life with pleasure, happiness, optimism, purpose, meaning, and conscious positive expectation and belief in the future. A healthy anterior cingulate will also provide the necessary feedbacks that encourage social support and prosocial behavior, which are also essential components of human resiliency. And finally, when these prefrontal and paralimbic cortical regions are capable of doing their jobs well, they will be able to modulate amygdalar responses and thus help the individual avoid the metabolic wear and tear of the distress that has its common source in human separation fear. Spirituality is another term for how we can enhance our brain's capacity to achieve resilience through the strengthening of our connectedness to a source(s) of solace and nurturance, resulting in social support and in belief in a more benign future (Fricchione, 2011a,b). Spiritual and religious exercises such as meditations that can provoke an oceanic feeling of loss of self consciousness, coincident with deep connection to something greater than oneself, can enlist other areas of the brain such as the right parietal lobe in addition to prefrontal and paralimbic regions (Newberg & D'Aquili, 2001).

When asked what the worst part of their illness experience is, most patients will give answers that reflect the fear of separation and loss of attachment (Fricchione, 2011a). What seems like anxiety and depression, as described above, is perhaps better understood as a threat to the attachment to loved ones and life itself that all humans share. Family members also share the challenge of this separation. Here is an exchange with the wife of a terminally ill man in the throes of his final struggle with glioblastoma multiforme:

> All three doctors decided I should stop giving John the chemo, for it is not fair to put him through it. I was glad I did not have to make that decision, but all three agreed that was best. No one knows, but they think John has a few weeks. My prayer has always been if the Lord takes him, John will be confused and never have to say goodbye to his girls. It looks as if that prayer will be answered, for he is not aware he is ill but he does feel love all around him. I pray John will go peacefully as if he was going to sleep. We are keeping him at home. The girls and I are heartbroken, but we would never wish for John to suffer, and he can not even hold his head upright. My head hurts from crying, so I will write more tomorrow, but I had to tell my

> best friend.
> Love, Mary

Berlin (1986) has written about the practical implications of this emotional reaction to separation, which links the intellectual and emotional missions of religion and medicine, holding out the hope for an integration of medicine with patients' spiritual lives. He suggests that it is essential that during hospitalization, patients find an atmosphere conducive to the formation of supportive attachments and that with the resultant reduction of distress, the chances of recovery from illness may be enhanced (Querido, 1959). In the same vein, patients who enjoy a sense of spiritual connection may experience a reduction in distress. In the "intermediate area" between separation and attachment that illness creates, spirituality in medical care can thus be examined and nurtured. The power of positive religious belief can be real and indeed may promote healing in some patients. The proinflammatory cytokine interleukin-6 may mediate some of these effects. Its rise correlates with spiritual struggles, and its reduction has been associated with religious attendance (Lutgendorf et al., 2004; Koenig et al., 1997).

From the perspective of what might be called the psychosomatic or mind–body medicine hypothesis, distress in response to a crisis (becoming more pathogenetic when chronic) is processed in limbic and cortical brain areas, resulting in "stress response system" (hypothalamic-pituitary-adrenal axis; locus coeruleus-sympathetic nervous system; vagal complex-visceral nervous system) and immune system changes that may predispose to or exacerbate disease states (Chrousos & Gold, 1992; Reichlen, 1993). Human physiology will seek a state of stability as a result of change, called *allostasis* (McEwen, 1998). To the extent that spiritual and religious behavior on the part of the patient and spirituality in the patient–doctor relationship mollify distress, there may be "downstream" effects that promote health, above and beyond the epidemiologic effects of a healthier lifestyle, better diet, and improved compliance. The placid state achieved through spirituality in the patient, the family, the staff, and the doctor may rekindle the "remembered wellness" of "secure base attachment" in the midst of illness-induced separation anxiety and depression (Benson, 1996; Bowlby, 1969). A less stressed, neurobiologic equilibrium may then promote healing. Human health requires secure attachment because it is part of our mammalian evolutionary heritage. Our brain's reward and motivation circuitries in the setting of secure attachment provide us with survival advantage, which in part results from the more metabolically efficient allostatic mechanisms associated with modulation of the stress and immune response systems.

Freud, to his credit, attempted to address the innate human fear of separation head on, so to speak. He contended that there is a mature "reality principle" according to which one realizes that life has no purpose and that the pain of separation must simply be endured. This endurance can be aided through "powerful deflections" such as scientific endeavors; "substitutive satisfactions" such as the "illusions in contrast to reality" provided by art; and "intoxicating substances" such as narcotics, alcohol, and cocaine (Freud, 1961). Then there is religion, whose technique, to quote Freud, "consists in depressing the value of life and distorting the picture of the real world in a delusional manner—which presupposes an intimidation of intelligence" (Freud, 1961, p. 36).

All of these approaches allow humans to tap into an ability to deny (or at least to hold in abeyance) the idea of their own death with its specter of purposelessness and to limit reflection on the myriad contingencies that may hasten death. Some approaches are more adaptive than others; indeed, pathogenic stress can be reduced by adaptive denial with documented health benefits (Hackett & Cassem, 1968; Levenson et al., 1989). Of course, psychoactive drugs still provide a popular strategy. This is reflected in Sydenham's famous remark: "Among the remedies which it has pleased Almighty God to give to man to relieve his suffering, none is so universal and so efficacious as opium." But drugs have many side effects, not the least of which is the potential for hastening the patient's demise.

Understood in this light, Marx's intended epithet that religion is the "opium of the masses" becomes a compliment. Ultimately, not even science as a powerful deflection or, as Yeats called it, "the opium of the suburbs," can soothe the individual with severe illness who is facing death. In the midst of such an illness-induced threat, the typical patient moves from the suburbs and takes his or her place in an existential ghetto of need and sorrow. This is a corollary to the anecdotal common wisdom, "There are few atheists in a foxhole."

RESEARCH ON RELIGION AND SPIRITUALITY IN HEALTHCARE

We now consider some of the issues that pertain to religion and spirituality in the medical setting.

In the last quarter-century, researchers have focused more attention on the interface of spirituality, religious commitment, and medicine. Matthews (Matthews et al., 1993a, 1993b; Matthews and Larson, 1995; Matthews and Saunders, 1997), Koenig (Koenig et al., 2001), and others (Chatters, 2000) have reviewed what has become a large literature. While the American people are highly religious and even participate in religious healing activities, healthcare providers are frequently less religious, leading to the neglect of religious factors in medical practice and the neglect of religious variables in clinical research (King & Bushwick, 1994; Maugans & Wadland, 1991; Waldfogel, Wolpe, & Shmuely,

1998). Furthermore, research into the provision of spiritual care to patients with advanced illness indicates that a majority do not feel their spiritual needs are being supported by the medical system (Balboni et al., 2007). Balboni et al. (2007) found in a study of 230 advanced cancer patients that most (88%) considered religion to be at least somewhat important. Nearly half (47%) reported that their spiritual needs were minimally or not at all supported by a religious community, and 72% reported that their spiritual needs were supported minimally or not at all by the medical system.

The importance of religious and spiritual needs and resources of 51 psychiatric and 50 medical-surgical patients were described by Fitchett and colleagues in a 1997 study. Three or more specific religious needs (average five), were reported by 88% of the psychiatric and 76% of medical-surgical patients. The most frequently reported needs were (1) expression of caring and support from another person, (2) knowledge of God's presence, (3) prayer, (4) purpose and meaning in life, and (5) a chaplain to visit and pray. This study validates two major themes: illness uncovers existential vulnerability and clarifies for medical and psychiatric patients alike what the real limit questions are, and these questions are considered by most patients to be broadly spiritual in nature. Thus, in the context of the patient's need for purpose and meaning when ill, the solace of relationships with caring individuals (physicians, nurses, and chaplains, as well as family members) and the consoling sense of a divine presence become important attachment resources. A significant majority of both psychiatric (80%) and medical-surgical patients (86%) defined themselves as spiritual, and more than two-thirds of both groups noted that religion was a source of great comfort and support.

There has still been a relative dearth of validated religious variables in clinical research, as noted by Matthews (1997). Over a 5-year period up to 1986, in 2,348 psychiatric studies, only 3% used a religious measure; and this was most often simply denomination. Only one study had used a validated measure of religious commitment (Larson et al., 1986). Of 603 *Journal of Family Practice* articles over a 10-year span up to 1988, only 4% used a religious measure and, again, only one used a validated measure (Craigie et al., 1988). And in a survey of 1666 *Clinical Research* abstracts, only 1% used religious measures and none used a validated tool (Dowell et al., 1993).

SOME SELECTED VALIDATED SCALES OF RELIGIOUS VARIABLES

A number of scales now measure dimensions of religious commitment including worship attendance, prayer, reading of scripture or other religious material, importance and meaning of religion in one's life, intrinsic orientation toward religion, and intimacy with the patient's concept of God (Matthews, 1997). For example, Koenig and his colleagues at the Duke University Center for the Study of Religion/Spirituality and Health devised the Religious Coping Index (RCI; see Koenig et al., 1992, 1995). The RCI studies the extent to which patients use religion to help them cope with the stress induced by illness. The RCI is composed of three items: (1) an open-ended question on how the person copes with stress (a religious response is given a score of 10); (2) a self-rated item where the person rates on a visual analog scale from 0 to 10 the extent to which religion helps adaptation; and (3) an observer-rated item where the interviewer rates the patient on a 0 to 10 scale based on how much the person uses religion to cope. The RCI has a score range of 0 to 30.

While the term *religion* has usually been reserved for the beliefs, practices, and experiences entailed in a person's relationship to a purposeful God, it has in more recent times expanded to include such aspects of spirituality as a search for life's meaning and for answers to questions about human limitations, whether or not one takes part in traditional religious behaviors (Apolito, 1970). Kass developed a questionnaire called the Index of Core Spiritual Experiences (INSPIRIT) that measures experiences of the spiritual core (Kass et al., 1991). Kass went on to develop the Inventory of Positive Psychological Attitudes (IPPA), which assesses life purpose and satisfaction along with self-confidence during perceived stress. Comparing INSPIRIT and IPPA scores allows one to surmise the relationship between spirituality and well-being.

The Systems of Belief Inventory (SBI), developed by Holland and her colleagues, is a validated 54-item scale (Holland et al., 1998). The SBI seeks to combine the strengths of scales such as the RCI in defining aspects of religious behavior with the strengths of the INSPIRIT in measuring spiritual experiences.

One of the few validated instruments to measure existential well-being is the McGill QOL scale (Cohen et al., 1996).

THE EFFECTS OF RELIGIOUS BELIEF AND RELIGIOUS EXPERIENCE ON MEDICAL AND PSYCHIATRIC ILLNESS

Koenig (2001) acknowledges that religion can have negative effects on mental and physical health and cites the Jonestown and Waco tragedies, as well as situations wherein religious beliefs forestalled needed psychiatric care. He comes to the conclusion, nonetheless, that the evidence for positive health effects far outweighs the evidence for negative health effects. See Table 18.1 for a review of selected studies.

Table 18.1 SELECTED STUDIES OF RELIGIOUS EFFECTS ON HEALTH

A. Substance Abuse		
Authors	*Cohort*	*Results*
Desmond, 1981	248 males with opiate Dependence	Those enrolled in long-term religiously based treatment-significantly more abstinence (45% vs. 5%) from addiction to opiates over a year of follow-up, religiosity predicted lower alcohol and tobacco use
Adlaf & Smart, 1985	2066 High school students	More religious, less alcohol use
Amoateng & Bahr, 1986	16,130 High school students	More religious, less alcohol use
Moore et al., 1990	1014 Male med students	Lack of religious affiliation-strongest predictor of subsequent alcoholism in subsequent 16 years
Koenig et al., 1994a	2969 ECA participants	Weekly church attendance led to 29% of the risk of alcoholism during 6 months compared with less frequent attenders
Kendler et al., 1997	1902 White female twins	Religiosity predicted lower alcohol and tobacco use
Craig et al., 1997	101 Male VA patients	85% of those with no religious preference or non-mainstream preference had poor outcomes in a 12-step alcohol rehab program at 1 year follow-up while 63.3% (Protestants) and 70.1% (Catholics) had good outcomes

B. Illness Coping and Life Adjustment		
Authors	*Cohort*	*Results*
Cook & Wimberley, 1983	145 Parents of child cancer victims	80% comforted by religion: 40% with ↑ Religious commitment. Better physiologic and emotional adjustment
Conway, 1985–1986	200 Elderly families	91% used prayer to cope with medical illness; 86% thought of God or religiousbeliefs to cope
Kaczorowski, 1989	114 Advanced cancer	↓ State and trait anxiety correlated with (c/w) patients' spiritual well being (sex, age, use of support groups controlled for)
Burgener, 1994	135 Dementia caregivers	(1) Religious attendance significantly c/w general well-being and social functioning; (2) When spiritual needs met, mental health improved and caregiver stress decreased

(continued)

Table 18.1 (CONTINUED)

C. Psychiatric Illness

Authors	Cohort	Results
Williams et al., 1991	720 Adults	Psychological distress inversely c/w religious attendance (age, sex, education, marital status, gender, race controlled for)
Koenig et al., 1992	850 Hospitalized veterans	Religious coping inversely c/w both self reported and observer measured baseline depression ($p < .001$) and depression risk at future hospitalization
Koenig et al., 1994b	2679 ECA participants	Church attendance c/w ↓ rates of psycho-pathology
Kendler et al., 1997	1902 White female twins	Religiosity predicted a lower risk of current or lifetime depression
Koenig et al., 1998	94 Elderly medical ill	Intrinsic religiosity (religious belief or experience) but not church attendance or private religious activities significantly and independently predicted shorter time to remission of mild to moderate depressive disorder

D. Medical Illness

Authors	Cohort	Results
Hannay, 1980	1344 Outpatients	Monthly religious activity significantly c/w reduced medical ($p < .001$) mental ($p < .001$) and social ($p < .001$) symptoms
Byrd, 1988	393 CCU Patients	192 patients received intercessory prayer from prayer groups; 201 patients were un-prayed-for controls, prayed-for patients had better outcomes with less (1) Cardiac arrest (3 vs. 14, $p < .02$) (2) CHF (8 vs. 20, $p < .03$) (3) Pneumonia (3 vs. 13, $p < .03$) (4) Antibiotics need (3 vs. 17, $p < .005$) (5) Intubation need (0 vs 12, $p < .002$)
Idler & Kasl, 1992	2812 Elderly	Religiosity was inversely c/W subsequent disability ($p < .0013$) and c/w improved function ($p < .0014$) in this prospective study
Harris et al., 1995	40 Cardiac transplant Recipients	At one year post-transplant, religious beliefs and practices preoperatively predicted at the $p > .05$ level (1) Better physical function (2) Reduced health anxiety (3) Better compliance (4) Less overall anxiety (5) Higher self-esteem
Contrada et al., 2004	142 (115 men, 27 women)	Pre op Subjective intrinsic religiosity in patients post cardiac surgery c/w fewer complications and shorter hospital stay, independent of biomedical and psychosocial variables
Benson et al., 2006	post- CABG: 604 (?intercessory prayer->yes) 597 (?intercessory prayer-> no) 601 (known intercessory prayer)	In? of prayer group, complications in 52% of prayed for vs 51% of non prayed for; in 59% of those certain about being prayed for vs 52% uncertain

E. Mortality

Authors	Cohort	Results
Comstock & Partridge, 1972	91,909 Individuals	At least weekly church attendance c/w: (1) 50% fewer deaths from coronary artery disease (CAD) (2) 56% fewer deaths from emphysema (3) 75% fewer deaths from cirrhosis (4) 53% fewer suicides

(continued)

Table 18.1 (CONTINUED)

Enstrom, 1989	Mormon men	Mormons had half the cancer and heart disease rates of control populations
Gardner & Lyon, 1982	Mormon men	Highly observant Mormons had half the rates of cancer and heart disease as less observant Mormons
Berkel & de Waard, 1983	Seventh Day Adventists	Adventist men lived 9 years and women 4 years longer than general population. Adventists had 50% fewer neoplasms, 41% fewer episodes of cardiac disease
Zuckerman et al., 1984	225 Elderly, forced to move	In a 2-year prospective study religiously committed had twice the survival rate
Schoenbach et al., 1986	2059 In church	Participants c/w lower mortality risk from cardiac disease in persons ≥ 60 years of age
Goldbourt et al., 1993	Jews	In a 23-year study, Orthodox Jews had a 20% lower mortality from coronary artery disease than did other Jews
Oxman et al., 1995	232 Elderly patients	Those with strong religious coping leading to comfort more likely to survive 6 months post-operative. Mortality rate three times as high in those without religious strength. Mortality rate 12 times higher in those without religious strength who are also socially isolated
Strawbridge et al., 1997	5286 Individuals	Weekly church attendance over 28 years of study c/w improved survival (demographic, social, health factors controlled for)
Ironson et al., 2002	279 patients w/HIV/AIDS	High scores on a Spirituality/Religiousness Index c/w long-term survival, health behaviors, less distress and lowering urinary cortisol levels

Levin and Schiller (1987) also concluded from their review that religiosity does confer beneficial health effects. This benefit was seen across a wide range of disease and conditions. When comparing religious denominations, a relatively lower risk for cardiovascular disease, high blood pressure, stroke, certain cancers, inflammatory bowel disease, and for overall and specific cause mortality appears to occur in more behaviorally demanding groups such as Seventh Day Adventists, Mormons, Orthodox Jews, and the clergy of all faiths (Levin & Schiller, 1987). And, when individual characteristics of religious commitment such as religious service attendance are studied, there is a trend toward health benefit and reduced morbidity and mortality in those with greater religiosity. Studies of specific diseases support both of these observations. Levin guardedly concludes that there is an association between religion and health.

Some researchers, however, find no association. (Sloan, Bagiella, & Powell, 1999) Sloan and Bagiella (2002) feel many articles cited to support an association between religion and health are methodologically flawed or irrelevant to the association. For example, religiosity and spirituality are value-laden factors usually measured by self-report questionnaires, which are subject to a variety of subjective variables. In the 266 studies they reviewed, 83% included nonpertinent health benefits; for example, those related to lifestyle and not to anything specifically religious. Overlap with community activity and social engagement confounds the religious attendance literature (Sloan, 2005). What is meant by religious behavior and spirituality in these studies is not specific. The lack of consistency in the findings suggests that there is no easy way to operationalize religiosity. Subjects who want to present themselves as religious may be prone to embellish their activity level in interviews. Sloan also takes exception to the host of outcome variables used in many studies because the number of variables makes the study vulnerable to the sharpshooter's fallacy—shoot your bullets into the side of a barn and then draw the bulls-eye. He concludes that there is no empirical basis for the assertions that religious involvement is associated with health benefits (Sloan & Bagiella, 2002; Sloan, 2005; Sloan, Bagiella & Powell, 1999). This is certainly most clear with intercessory prayer (prayers of others on behalf of the patient), which has not been shown effective in any well-designed study. For example, Benson et al. (2006) found no benefit of such prayers for cardiac surgery patients. In this study, some subjects were unaware they were being prayed for after bypass surgery. There was no significant difference between health outcomes in those who actually were being prayed for versus those who were not prayed for. Furthermore, those subjects who knew they were being prayed for showed a slight trend toward more complications.

Most recently, the epidemiologist Lynda H. Powell and her colleagues at Rush-Presbyterian-St. Luke's Medical Center reviewed 150 papers, eliminating those with methodological flaws (Powell et al., 2003). Sloan sees this paper as the most thorough review of the empirical evidence to date (Sloan, 2005). Powell and her colleagues conclude that there is a strong, consistent, prospective and often graded reduction in risk of mortality in church/service attenders. After adjusting for confounding variables, this reduction in overall mortality risk reaches approximately 25%. However, the researchers found no link between religious depth and physical health, and in patients no evidence that religion or spirituality improves recovery; in fact, there is a suggestion that recovery is impeded, although religiosity may increase with severity of illness. More methodologically sound studies are clearly needed.

So, is the association between religion and health due to chance, bias, or confounding, or is it valid? It appears unlikely that the association is due to chance, given the variety and number of studies showing significant health benefits and the fact that large censuses and randomized samples were used in many of them (Levin, 1987, 1994). Levin points out that bias is also unlikely given the fact that prospective and retrospective and cohort and case-control studies with children and adults and a wide variety of denominations and demographics with acute and chronic conditions have been used.

The issue of confounding is another matter. It could be that psychosocial rather than religious factors are at work. Health-related behaviors attendant to religious belief, such as the eschewing of tobacco, alcohol, and drugs, and the adoption of a healthier diet and exercise may be operative in the benefits attributed to religious activity. Social supports must be considered, as they have been shown to buffer the effects of anger and stress (Henry, 1982; House et al., 1988). Belief, ritual, and faith may all produce a sense of calm and harmony and a sense of being loved that not only improve subjective health perceptions but also enhance health based on expectancies, providing a ripe field for placebo response effects.

Thoresen and Harris (2002) have concluded that religious and/or spiritual factors do appear to be associated with physical and overall health, but the relationship is most likely more complex and modest than some contend. Clearly, more research about specific factors at work will be needed. As Chatters (2000) puts it: "Such investigations must appreciate the multi-dimensional nature of religious involvement, reflect an awareness of inter- and intragroup variability that may alter the meaning and significance of religious factors, and use state-of-the-art methods, study designs and analytic procedures." Future research will require a component analysis that explores the features of religion and spirituality that intersect with health variables.

The question of whether religiosity facilitates health is complex and hinges on the potential association's strength (moderate to strong according to Levin (1994) but weak according to Sloan), consistency (repeatedly observed), specificity (a specific disease effect not found, rather general effects on morbidity and mortality), temporality (not conclusively demonstrated that cause [religion] precedes effect [health]), biologic gradient (dose-response relationship suggested but not directly inferable), coherence (difficult to assess how association coheres because of multiplicity of conditions and outcomes), experiment (little evidence available for religious behaviors, attitudes, and affiliations), analogy (exists in that other psychosocial constructs have exhibited causal disease

effects), and plausibility (an effect of religion on health is biologically plausible given what we know of behavioral medicine and neuroimmunology). Using these so-called Hill criteria, Levin concludes that the answer to the question of whether religion causes health is a promising "maybe" (Hill, 1965).

Perhaps the most provocative criterion for causality involves plausibility: is it plausible that religion contributes to health? As Koenig and Levin both argue, the health benefit of religion is not necessarily dependent on supernatural phenomena. What Levin (1994) prefers to call "superempirical discarnate force or power" leaves open the possibility that some currently immeasurable phenomenon (e.g., *prajna*, chi, life force, etc.) might someday become measurable. So while the causal element may be a superempirical natural energy, which is tapped into by religious or spiritual pursuits, we need not invoke this construct to explain a plausible biomedical connection between religion and health. Well-known physiologic pathways linked to psychosocial and behavioral mechanisms (healthier lifestyles, less substance abuse, greater social support) may offer health-enhancing salutary effects that buffer against the pathogenic changes of disease-related high-risk activity and stress. Nevertheless, even when the positive effects of social support are controlled, studies like that of Oxman and colleagues (1995) suggest that there is still a separate benefit attributable to a strong personal religious belief system.

A look at underlying brain mechanisms with special attention to how and why the brain evolved may help clarify these issues. Max Horkheimer (1970) proposed that, in the third millennium, if it is not plausible to have a relationship with "the totally other" then there is no meaning at all in life that transcends self-preservation. While the urge to be cured in medicine may flow from the desire for self-preservation, the urge to be cared for and to care in medicine must have as its wellspring a spiritual source of connectedness to something beyond ourselves.

THE BRAIN AND SPIRITUALITY

Over the last several years there has been interest in neuroimaging studies of spirituality, including both meditative techniques and religious belief. Based on cerebral blood flow studies using single photon positron emission tomography (SPECT), Newberg and his colleagues have assembled a schema to explain the neural circuitry responsible for spiritual and religious experiences reflected in meditation and prayer (Cohen et al., 2009; Newberg et al., 2003; 2001). To summarize, this circuitry is dominated by activation in the dorsolateral prefrontal cortex (DLPFC), anterior cingulate cortex (ACC), basal ganglia and thalamus. The assumption is that the prefrontal cortex (PFC) strengthens focus and attention; the ACC enhances empathy and social awareness; and the basal ganglia add better modulation of movement and emotional tone. The thalamus then can develop a heightened sensory perception of the world and our place in it.

The first functional magnetic resonance imaging (fMRI) study of meditation was undertaken in 2000 and found that this brain motivation circuitry was activated against the background general inactivation of other brain areas (Lazar et al., 2000). Long-term practitioners of meditation compared to controls had significantly more consistent and sustained activation in the DLPFC and the ACC during meditation versus short-term practitioners compared to controls (Baron Short et al., 2010).

Recently, the neural activation patterns that correlated with religious belief and with nonreligious belief using fMRI were studied in 15 committed Christian believers and 15 nonbelievers (Harris et al., 2009). The subjects were asked to evaluate the truth or falsity of both religious and nonreligious propositions. In both groups, belief was associated with activation in the ventromedial PFC. It is of interest that this region is noted to be important for self-representation, emotional associations, reward, and motivational behaviors.

In an earlier fMRI study, researchers described three psychological dimensions of religious belief including perception of God's level of involvement, perception of God's emotion (love vs. anger), and doctrinal/experiential religious knowledge (Kapogiannis et al., 2009). Subjects rated 70 statements on a Likert scale providing conceptual dissimilarity ratings for pairs of statements regarding religious beliefs. Perception of God's involvement activated two right-sided anterior (lateral and medial frontal gyri) posterior networks. Love modulated the right middle frontal gyrus, while anger stimulated the left medial temporal gyrus. Religious knowledge, on the other hand, when doctrinal, modulated right inferior temporal and medial temporal gyri, as well as right inferior parietal, left middle cingulate, and left superior temporal gyri; and, when experiential, modulated bilateral occipital, left fusiform, left precuneus, and left frontal regions.

Thus, religious belief appears to engage neural networks involved with abstract semantic processing, imagery, intention, and emotional *theory of mind* processes, which mediate the cognitive ability to understand mental states in others. The process of adopting religious beliefs seems to somewhat depend on cognition/emotion amalgamation in the anterior insular cortices. Signal in the insula reflects rejection of religious statements deemed false (Harris et al., 2009).

It may help to see the relevance of this new data to our discussion if we briefly survey the neuroscience of this circuitry. Mega and his colleagues (1997) reviewed the anatomy and phylogeny of the limbic system, focusing on the paleocortical and archicortical trends as two "para-limbic belts," to use Mesulam's term (Mesulam, 1985) (see Figure 18.2, Ballantine et al., 1967). The paleocortical trend ending in orbitofrontal cortex is closely linked with development of the amygdala. The archicortical trend ending in the cingulate cortex is closely linked with the hippocampus and its development. While the paleocortical belt is best at analyzing object features, the archicortical belt is best at analyzing object locations. This coincides with the view of Pandya and Yeterian (1990) in their conceptualization of two primordial moieties in brain evolution specialized for "what" (piriform-insular) and "where" (hippocampus) questions.

The paleocortical progression ultimately involves hippocampus–cingulate connections. Area 24 of the anterior cingulate cortex (ACC), with many overlapping reciprocal connections with the medial orbitofrontal cortex (MOFC),

is the intersection or the "nexus in the distributed networks subserving internal motivating drives and externally directed attentional mechanisms" (Mega et al., 1997, p. 323). It is a candidate zone for where the divisions of the limbic system work in concert to unite perceptions, internal relevance, and meaning with external attention to facilitate response selection. Thus, in the ACC we find the integration of paleocortical data, concerned with answering the "what" questions of life, with archicortical data pertaining to the "where" questions. Given the MOFC's intimate overlapping relationship with the ACC, it may be that they work in tandem to synthesize object feature and object location importance.

The limbic basal ganglia–thalamocortical circuit's cortical terminal zones are the ACC and MOFC, from the point of view of the functional neuroanatomic circuits proposed by Alexander and his colleagues (1990). Saver and Rabin (1997) suggested a "limbic marker hypothesis for religious-mystical experience," in which the limbic system signifies certain exteroceptive or interoceptive stimuli as numinous and meaningful. Of course the medial temporal lobe limbic zones have long been cited as important in this regard, due to the deeply felt experiences of those with limbic region seizures. But it would seem that the ACC and MOFC "limbic" cortices would be essential for spirituality given that the integrative "what" and "where" function they subserve could be applied to the larger context of universal concern in order to achieve such sensitivity.

Whether one ascribes to MacLean's "triune brain" or to Butler's "four brains in the forebrain" view of brain evolution, the clearest finding of central importance to the development of spiritual experience is the fact that the mammalian attachment strategy is a product of the evolution of what is called the *lemnothalamic-medial division of the dorsal pallium* (MacLean, 1990; Butler, 1994a,b). This results in the uniqueness of such medial limbic divisions as the thalamocingulate, which, as MacLean points out, is responsible for the mammalian behavioral triad of maternal nurturance, the infant cry of separation, and play.

With this background in brain evolution, we can hypothesize that there was indeed an evolution of basal ganglia–thalamo-"cortical" loops (Fricchione, 2011a). Primitive periallocortical loops were followed by an overlayering of proisocortical loops, culminating in isocortical circuits as afferentation from the thalamus moved into expanding cortical zones with return connections to basal ganglia and thalamus. In this context of evolutionary loop design, one sees a progression in function from earlier, more primitive levels of attachment behavior in terms of attraction to sources of food and repulsion from predators and in terms of attraction to potential sexual mates, on upward to the ACC/MOFC and prefrontal cortical loops and their mediation of familial and social attachments (Schore, 1996). The thalamocingulate connection, based on lesion and morphine experiments, is thought by MacLean to be particularly important for the development of what he calls a "memory of the past," given the key role played by the mammalian behavioral triad in our evolutionary survival strategy.

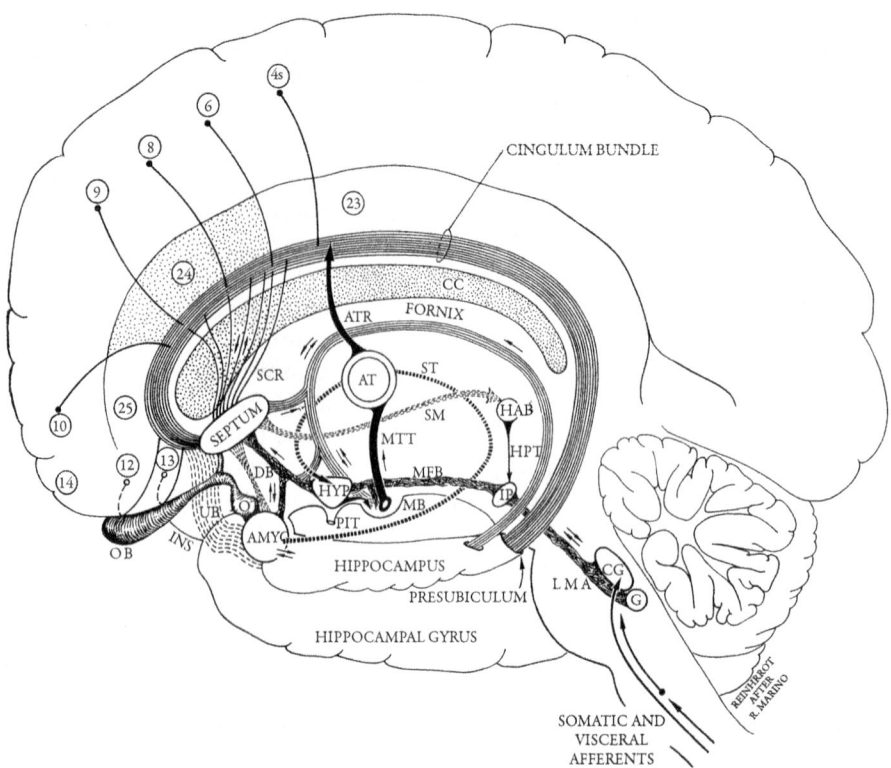

Figure 18.2 A Candidate Neurocircuitry for Spiritual Connectedness. (Adapted from Ballantine HT, Cassidy WL, Flanagan NB, & Marino N. (1967). Stereotaxic anterior cingulotomy for neuropsychiatric illness and intractable pain. *Journal of Neurosurgery, 26*, 488–495, p. 491; see also Fricchione, 2011a, p. 123).

While the ACC/MOFC loop refines brain reward circuitry and its emotional valencing to form a "memory of the past" as it pertains to mammalian behavioral attachment, the dorsolateral prefrontal cortical (DLPFC) loop also makes a major contribution (Fricchione, 2011a). The DLPFC was an outcropping, to a large extent, from both the ACC, which itself developed from the hippocampal moiety, and the insular cortex from the piriform moiety. As such, the DLPFC provides increasingly complex versions of the "where" and "what" questions as they relate to the separation/attachment process. "Where am I?" the organism asks, in relation to an object of attraction/attachment or repulsion/separation. Am I close enough to receive the positive reinforcement of ACC pleasure, or am I too far away, and as a consequence do I feel the negative valence of the pain of separation? Furthermore, what is the object to which I am attracted or repulsed? Is it truly an object to be attached to, or should I separate from it? These essential separation/attachment questions, which even the simplest of organisms must address in terms of sensorimotor behavior, become enhanced and refined in the complexity of the newly evolved basal ganglia thalamocortical loops (Fricchione, 2011a).

The human PFC maintains the *future action programs* for cognition and behavior (Ingvar, 1985). Because these action programs can be stored and retrieved for future use, Ingvar terms them "memories of the future" (Ingvar, 1985, p. 127). In the extensive connections of the DLPFC to the ACC and the connection of them both to the medial temporal lobe memory system (hippocampus) and

association cortices, the network from "memory of the past" to the "now-situation" to "memory of the future" is set (Fricchione, 2011a). The memory of past attachment serves as an attractant in the formation of our memory of the future. Humans tend to long for relationships that are associated with attachment security and solace. Once mammals who have adopted an attachment strategy for survival become conscious of their memory of the past in relation to memory of their mortal future, "paradise" is lost. Conscious mammals will always be beset by the knowledge of the tree of good and evil, namely that what they face is separation from those they love.

Thus, humans with their PFC expansion, which remains intimately connected with the past evolutionary loops associated with amygdala food status (LeDoux, 1996) and sexual reproductive attachment, and moreover with cingulate maternal, familial, and social attachment, can think into the future and gain survival advantage. Humans can also anticipate their exquisitely painful future separations and, by extension, plan how to avoid them.

However, in this evolutionary development a bargain has been joined. The price paid for anticipatory abilities that promote attainment of high attachments is the knowledge that there exists a seemingly final separation: death.

The person suffering with illness feels this *archetypal separation anxiety* (Fricchione, 2011a,b). Ironically, the birth of our spiritual drives derives from our unique ability to contemplate and affectively experience the meaning of separation and attachment.

IMPLICATIONS FOR THE DOCTOR–PATIENT RELATIONSHIP (PRAGMATIC APPLICATIONS FOR MEDICAL PSYCHIATRIC PRACTICE)

A patient's communion with family, friends, doctors, nurses, and other staff, along with religious observances, sacraments and prayer, contemplation, and meditation, facilitate attachment solutions to the separation problem of illness (Fricchione, 2011b).

Understanding brain evolution and the design of increasingly advanced basal ganglia thalamocortical loops enhances the development of a model of how spirituality or "spirito-taxis" can work downstream to alter physiologic functioning at the level of organs and tissues (Fricchione, 2011a). In such a scenario the corticolimbic interrelatedness among the loops exerts an overall modulatory effect on the stress response systems. Stress-system changes will then have important stabilizing regulatory effects on organs like the heart, and tissues like the immune system. The purpose of this control is to ensure metabolic economy in the face of internal and external pressures. While it is healthy to exert energy in the course of an acute illness challenge, it is necessary to have control mechanisms to modulate these energy responses when the acute stressor abates. Perhaps spirituality works downstream to help us make the most of our metabolic flow, improving modulation and the pliancy of stress and immune response potential. For example, Koenig et al. (1997) found an association between higher levels of interleukin-6, a cytokine associated with inflammatory response syndrome, and low church attendance. Others have found a relationship between spiritual struggle and IL-6, with preoperative spiritual distress associated with elevated preoperative IL-6 and post–cardiac surgery depression (Ai et al., 2010). Perhaps enhanced and refined attachment experienced in the spiritual and caring relationship works its way down the evolutionary chain of complexity, establishing a consonance of purpose at each level, thereby reducing the stress associated with isolation and loss of control. This should eventually be testable.

PRACTICAL CLINICAL IMPLICATIONS

To facilitate access to the potential positive aspects of the spiritual experience of connectedness in the midst of illness, physicians, including consultant psychiatrists, need to become more comfortable with exploring this area with their patients. Patients' psychological struggles with their illnesses can be more fully understood only when spiritual aspects of their lives are discussed. For patients who are not "psychologically minded," often to the point of being embarrassed or offended by the prospect of a psychiatric visit, a spiritual discussion can often detoxify the experience and pave the way toward "transitional relatedness" and a healing interaction (Horton, 1981). *Transitional relatedness* refers to the capacity of a caregiver to remain supportively connected to another person who is feeling torn away from all attachments. It requires the commitment to provide loving care by accompanying the patient into an "intermediate area" between threatened separation from and safe attachment to loved ones. This relatedness provides insight into a patient's spirituality and can be used by the physician and consultant psychiatrist to develop treatment approaches that will strengthen coping, enlist the benefit of belief, and improve compliance (Waldfogel & Wolpe, 1993).

It is essential not to predispose patients to a sense of guilt over not "being good at" religious practices and spiritual belief. We must avoid at all costs imparting to them a sense of responsibility for any worsening of their illness process, as if a failure of their spirituality and belief could cause such a downslide. Moreover, spirituality is not a substitute for adherence to mainstream medical and surgical management.

Religion can be maladaptive as well as adaptive in terms of its impact on health (Jarvis & Northcott, 1987). Repression and overcontrol, especially in certain religious cults, can be destructive. Instead of tranquility and peace, such religious narrow-mindedness can lead to fear, prejudice, obsessive-compulsiveness, and even paranoia (Koenig, 1997). Dire physical consequences may ensue when competent members of certain religious groups (e.g., Jehovah's Witnesses and Christian Scientists) decline medical treatment (Coakly & McKenna, 1986). A psychiatric consultant will sometimes be needed to render a medical-legal opinion regarding the capacity of an individual to refuse treatment (Appelbaum & Grisso, 1988). In the case of Jehovah's Witnesses, a common dilemma for physicians and surgeons involves their 1945 decision to refuse blood transfusions on the basis of their communally held beliefs that blood cannot be taken in as nourishment (Panico, Jeng & Brewster, 2011). This belief is based on their interpretation of two biblical passages, one from Genesis and one from Leviticus. They will, however, frequently accept various coagulation factors as well as fractions of plasma such as albumin, cryoprecipitate, or immunoglobulin. Ever since the decision in *Schloendorff v Society of New York Hospital* in 1914, adults who have the capacity to give informed consent have the right to refuse medical treatment, and this legally holds in the case of a Jehovah's Witness who refuses a blood transfusion. When dealing with a Jehovah's Witness patient it is advisable to have extensive conversations about procedures and their risks and benefits and to document them as soon as possible in the chart. Making contingency plans regarding potential acute blood loss situations that can minimize blood loss, increase blood production through the use of erythropoietin stimulating agents, and optimize hemodynamic parameters is essential. After helping to determine if the patient has capacity to refuse, consultation psychiatrists can work with the team to provide support to the patient, family, and staff, and can work together with the Jehovah's Witnesses' Hospital Liaison Committee and Visitation Groups to provide comfort even though the psychiatrist may strongly disagree with the decision that has been made. The team may also work with the church's Hospital Liaison Committee and the church elders when the psychiatrist has questions about whether a particular patient's refusal of treatment is based on religious delusional material that lies outside of the commonly held canon of beliefs.

In a nonemergency, a competent adult patient who refuses blood on religious grounds must sign a Release of Liability for Blood-Free Treatment. If he or she has a minor child or is pregnant, the patient must also complete a Statement Regarding Arrangements for Care of Minor Child, to be used in the event of the patient's death. If the patient does not do so, or if there are questions about the suitability of any person named as caretaker, the hospital counsel should be consulted before treatment proceeds. In an emergency, the physician should honor refusal of blood if an adult patient is able to understand the risks of that refusal.

The decision to let adults make medically harmful decisions does not extend to their making decisions on behalf of their children. Parents of minors are not permitted to refuse lifesaving treatments that their children need, and physicians must alert their legal departments and seek guardianship when this occurs. In emergencies involving minor children, the law has always protected physicians who act to save the child's life regardless of religious opposition of the parents. In nonemergencies, legal counsel should be obtained before ever overriding parental or guardian religious protests.

A pregnant woman presents a complicated legal situation because of the state's interest in the fetus's life. In the latter stages of pregnancy, the administration of blood may be justified to preserve the life of the viable fetus. Before proceeding with treatment, the hospital counsel should be consulted. After delivery, the mother has the right to refuse blood for herself unless any minor child would be abandoned if she died. The courts have stated that the state's interest in the welfare of children will override the parent's or guardian's right to refuse blood on behalf of a child who is under 18 years of age. In an emergency, the hospital will administer blood over parental objection if necessary to preserve the life or health of the child. In other situations, before proceeding with treatment the hospital counsel should be consulted to determine whether court intervention is necessary. The courts have consistently overridden parental refusal of lifesaving medical interventions for children when they are refused by parents on religious grounds. In the emergency treatment of children in urgent life-threatening situations, physicians are essentially immune from liability if they proceed without parental consent.

Parents or guardians, therefore, may not refuse lifesaving treatment on behalf of their minor children. This principle has been defined in cases involving parents who, on religious grounds, refused blood transfusions necessitated by chemotherapy for their child, and parents who treated their son's bowel obstruction with prayer, resulting in the child's death. If parents refuse lifesaving treatment, the physician should consult with the hospital attorney to discuss the advisability of court intervention if time permits. In a medical emergency where death or a serious worsening of the minor's condition will occur without immediate treatment, the physician should always render treatment despite the lack of parental consent.

While overriding the parental decision to refuse treatment of a child based on religiously derived wishes is more clear-cut in acute life-threatening situations, cases in which the child suffers from a chronic, more insidious disease are more problematic. In these latter situations, the consultation psychiatrist might advocate for maintenance of a therapeutic alliance with the family despite this special form of noncompliance. This is in some ways akin to what many diabetologists must do with patients with type I diabetes and their families, forgoing in the early stages of treatment the temptation to demand tight control and high compliance in favor of maintaining a therapeutic alliance. This maintenance of contact may allow for the physician's message, threatening at the outset, to gradually gain some degree of acceptance. It also allows the team to better anticipate impending acute emergencies so that lifesaving medical treatment can be delivered whenever necessary.

Individual adults outside of an organized religious body who suffer from religious delusions—idiosyncratic, fixed, false beliefs, often with an unusual supernatural theme—may be found by the psychiatric consultant to have diminished capacity to refuse treatment (Stotland, 1999).

SPIRITUAL ASSESSMENT

As mentioned in the Consensus Conference on Spiritual Care, all patients can benefit from simple spiritual screening at the point of entry into healthcare systems (Puchalski et al., 2009). This should be followed when appropriate by spiritual history taking and by spiritual assessment, which might then evoke a multidisciplinary spiritual care plan. Spiritual screening can be achieved with simple questions such as, "Is spirituality or religion important in your life" and "how well are these resources working for you in these times?" Next there is spiritual history taking, and there are now several bedside approaches available to clinicians. One that has become popular is the *FICA* method (Puchalski & Romer, 2000). In this approach the patient is asked four questions: "What is your **f**aith or belief?" "Is it **i**mportant in your life and does it influence you?" "Are you part of a religious or spiritual **c**ommunity?" and "How would you like me, your healthcare provider, to **a**ddress these issues in your healthcare?"

In order to examine a patient's inner spiritual life, one may ask questions like these that come from the suggestions of Ned Cassem, former Psychiatrist in Chief at the Massachusetts General Hospital (Cassem, 1997):

- Which books hold special meaning for you?

- How do you want to be remembered?

- How would you rank the common virtues?

- Are there things you are especially proud of?

- Who are your role models?

- Who are your friends . . . and enemies?

- Is there anyone whose interest you would put ahead of your own?

- What are your strongest and weakest qualities?

- What would you like to be free of?

- Who are the people who see you at your best?

- Do you have an ideal sense of who you would like to be?

- Do you have a code or a rule to live by?

- Have you ever had a sense of union or closeness with God?

The enrichment of the patient–doctor relationship that emerges in the dialogue around questions like these adds to the spiritual strength of the "vulnerable self," as Avery Weisman called it, and aids in the search for meaning in the midst of illness.

When spiritual distress—such as existential concern, a sense of abandonment by God, anger at God, challenged belief systems, despair, grief at loss, guilt or shame, need for reconciliation, isolation, ritual needs, and struggle over loss of faith or meaning—is appreciated, a request for a formal spiritual assessment by a board certified chaplain or pastoral counselor may be made.

CHAPLAINCY REFERRAL

In most instances when patients are not critically ill, it will be enough to do a spiritual screening and to gather a religious history, gauging whether these assets and strengths are available to the patient and determining if a chaplaincy visit is required or desired. A hospital chaplain is a cleric or layperson commissioned to provide pastoral care at a healthcare institution. Chaplains at most medical institutions require ecclesiastic endorsement, ordination or commission, and theological training. Many are certified for competency by chaplaincy organizations. By contrast, a pastoral counselor is a minister, priest, or rabbi, presumably with some formal training in counseling. Ideally, pastoral counselors integrate their mission of pastoral care with the behavioral sciences in an outpatient setting. Certification by the American Association of Pastoral Counselors requires religious endorsement, training in theology and the behavioral sciences, and counseling skills. There are some helpful guidelines physicians can follow in making chaplaincy referrals, providing the patient is agreeable (M. Means, personal communication; W. Moczynski, personal communication). Appropriate for referral are requests for:

- Prayer, religious rites, sacraments, a memorial service, devotional literature, prayer books, rosaries, Bibles, and other religious materials, initiated by the patient or family

- Emotional support and comfort

- Notification of local clergy

- Support regarding imminent death of a patient

- Support regarding ethical dilemmas

- Support regarding death of a patient's family member

- Aid in dealing with visiting clergy or a difficult religious group

- Aid when spiritual screening and history gathering reveal spiritual distress or religious issues, or concerns that create problems for patients

The spiritual care specialist can devise a spiritual health intervention that will contain therapeutic communication techniques (compassionate presence, reflective listening, life review, support enhancement, and nonabandonment), therapies (guided visualization, storytelling, dignity-conserving therapy, meaning-oriented therapy) and self-care (spiritual readings, reconciliation, journaling, art, music, relaxation response techniques such as yoga, tai chi, meditation) (Puchalski et al., 2009).

It is important to remember that consultant psychiatrists may sometimes find themselves in the role of gatekeeper, discouraging chaplaincy involvement because certain patients may have their conditions exacerbated in the face of religious hyperstimulation. Such patients may be in the midst of a psychotic episode, or they may be suffering from temporal lobe epilepsy or delirium.

Clearly, chaplains and clergy are often able to help patients deal with concerns about guilt, anger, faith, and family in powerful ways because of the important role well-trained chaplains serve. Given their specialized training, chaplains may see grief as multilayered, with the sense of loss not only emerging from the material life disengagement that serious disease engenders, but also from spiritual estrangement that serious illness may imply to patients with a religious background. But despite their lack of specialized knowledge, physicians should feel comfortable enough, when appropriate, to encourage religious behaviors such as prayer and spiritual exercises such as meditation to reduce stress and enhance resiliency if patients are receptive to these practices. Of course, it is obvious that spiritual and religious beliefs and practices are not for everyone and that the atheistic or agnostic approaches used by certain patients deserve the respect of the physicians and psychiatrists caring for them. Meissner (1984) described prayer as a creative cognitive pursuit that engages the prayor in a close personal relationship with the patient's concept of God, "someone" who will not abandon them no matter how vast and threatening the universe feels. Meditation is a practice that can provide an affective experience of closeness with God and often merges with mystical religious experience. Both prayer and meditation may reinforce a personal attachment to the patient's conception of Divine comfort and confidence.

When physicians ignore patients' religious beliefs, their medical diagnostic assessment may be incomplete (Waldfogel & Wolpe, 1993). Conflicts may emerge in the clinical milieu unless the physician develops a sophisticated understanding of religion's importance in the patient's illness experience (Waldfogel & Wolpe, 1993, p. 474). Having a grasp of the patient's underlying religious structure is therefore not only important to providing solace but also is needed for effective diagnosis and treatment. Toward that end, Waldfogel and Wolpe have adapted Glock's typology of religious issues that includes the five dimensions of ideology, intellect, ritual, experience, and consequence, to which they have added a sixth dimension of support provided by attachment to a religious community (Glock, 1962). Incorporating knowledge of religious beliefs, participation in religious rituals, and affiliation with a religious community in a treatment plan can enhance the work of the consultation psychiatrist and bolster a patient's coping ability. When we seek to understand patients along the spiritual dimensions mentioned, we see them within a larger context. This can facilitate patient movement "closer to a transpersonal source of meaning and to the human community that shares those meanings" (Waldfogel & Wolpe, 1993, p. 476).

When patients are severely ill, the discussion of religious and spiritual issues will often engage doctor and patient in a spiritual exchange. Patients frequently seek information about the physician's religious attitudes. In medical settings, when not contraindicated by the patient's psychiatric diagnosis, rather than being a boundary violation some clinicians consider that providing personal spiritual information may solidify the patient–doctor bond at critical moments, offering the potential for a psychologically healing interaction. I (GF) recall an elderly Sikh man with colon cancer on whom I consulted for the question of depression. I had very little knowledge of the Sikh religion. Nevertheless, we had a dialogue about our spiritual lives and I came away admiring his particular religious commitment, his framework for understanding his predicament. As he came to know me as someone with a spiritual orientation, he seemed more at ease and relieved of the fear that his religious beliefs would be minimized or denigrated. This is a personal strategy, however, that some clinicians would not employ.

Psychiatrists who are not comfortable discussing their personal spiritual leanings, or lack thereof, may help their patients by acknowledging, when appropriate, the pertinence of spirituality in humanity's search for meaning while respectfully declining to discuss their own particular sentiments. Of course, seeing hospitalized patients on the consultation-liaison service is different from dealing with patients longitudinally in insight-oriented psychotherapy. Psychodynamic considerations usually preclude the disclosure of religious beliefs and spiritual orientation on the part of the psychiatrist. This is especially true when psychoanalytic techniques are being used or when working with personality-disordered patients where boundary issues are a particular concern. In our experience, issues of transference and countertransference are not usually significant limiting factors when patients with severe medical illness and their doctors in the hospital discuss spiritual interests. When people empathically face the seriousness of a separation threat, whether they are alike or different, they often come together to form an attachment solution and to discover common ground.

Medical and psychiatric trainees can benefit from education in how religion and spirituality affect the illness experience. To date, 49 medical schools and 32 psychiatric residency programs have received curriculum awards for courses in spirituality and medicine from the Templeton Foundation (GWISH.org).

SUMMARY

As noted earlier, Edward Churchill once said, "Charity in the broad spiritual sense, that is our desire to relieve suffering, is the most prized possession of medicine." Our relief of suffering and thus the carrying out of the spiritual mission of medicine may be strengthened at the bedside by improving our understanding of the multisystem integration of the whole person in terms of the separation/attachment process (Fricchione, 2011b). Treatments can then be devised that enhance the patient's spiritual connectedness.

Regardless of the religious orientation of the consulting psychiatrist, mounting clinical data suggests that integration of religious and spiritual supports into the overall treatment planning of medically ill patients may relieve their suffering and is perhaps associated with improved coping and prognosis (Table 18.1). Religious counseling should be available to those patients who request or seem suitable for such interventions.

The human spiritual imperative or "spirito-taxis" is made possible by the evolutionary maturation of the brain motivation circuitry. Spirituality provides an important attachment solution to the anxiety and dysphoria associated with the separation challenge of illness and death. This is the place in medicine where science and religion have an opportunity to meet in conciliation and wonder.

CLINICAL PEARLS

- Patients encountering severe physical illness face what philosophers call the "limit questions": Who am I? What is the meaning of my life? Where am I going? Will I be separated from my loved ones?—questions that express universal existential concerns in the domains of identity, hope, meaning, purpose, morality, and relationship to ultimate authority.

- From an object-relations perspective (Horton, 1981), the physician acts as a transitional object, an object that can be held in the transition, offering solace that comes from "transitional relatedness."

- *Transitional relatedness* refers to the capacity of a caregiver to remain supportively connected to another person who is feeling torn away from all attachments. It requires the commitment to provide loving care by accompanying the patient into an "intermediate area" between threatened separation from and safe attachment to loved ones.

- Clinicians and patients meet in the most spiritual of all earthly places—the bedside.

- The placid state achieved through spirituality . . . may rekindle the "remembered wellness" of "secure base attachment" in the midst of illness-induced separation anxiety and depression (Benson, 1996; Bowlby, 1969).

- Mammalian attachment strategy is a product of the evolution of what is called the lemnothalamic-medial division of the dorsal pallium (MacLean, 1990; Butler, 1994a,b), resulting in the uniqueness of such medial limbic divisions as the thalamocingulate, which, as MacLean points out, is responsible for the mammalian behavioral triad of maternal nurturance, the infant cry of separation, and play.

- "Where am I?" the organism asks, in relation to an object of attraction/attachment or repulsion/separation. Am I close enough to receive the positive reinforcement of anterior cingulate pleasure, or am I too far away, and as a consequence do I feel the negative valence of the pain of separation? Furthermore, what is the object to which I am attracted or repulsed? Is it truly an object to be attached to, or should I separate from it? These essential separation/attachment questions, which even the simplest of organisms must address in terms of sensorimotor behavior, become enhanced and refined in the complexity of the newly evolved basal ganglia thalamocortical loops (Fricchione, 2011a).

- Ironically, the birth of our spiritual drives derives from our unique ability to contemplate and affectively experience the meaning of separation and attachment.

- Insight into a patient's spirituality and can be used by the physician and consultant psychiatrist to develop treatment approaches that will strengthen coping, enlist the benefit of belief, and improve compliance (Waldfogel & Wolpe, 1993).

- In discussing religious issues, we must avoid at all costs imparting to patients a sense of responsibility for any worsening of their illness process as if a failure of their spirituality and belief could cause such a downslide.

- While overriding the parental decision to refuse treatment of a child based on religiously derived wishes (for instance, in Jehovah's Witnesses) is more clear-cut in acute, life-threatening situations, cases in which the child suffers from a chronic, more insidious disease are more problematic. Here, the consultation psychiatrist might advocate for maintenance of a therapeutic alliance with the family despite this special form of noncompliance.

DISCLOSURE STATEMENTS

Dr. Fricchione has no conflicts of interest to disclose.

Dr. Peteet has no conflicts of interest to disclose.

REFERENCES

Adlaf, E. M.,& Smart, R. G. (1985). Drug use and religious affiliation. *British Journal of Addiction, 80*, 163–171.

Ai, A. L., Pargament, K. I., Appel, H. B., & Kronfol, Z. (2010). Depression following open heart surgery: A path model involving interleukin-6, spiritual struggle, and hope under pre-operative stress. *Journal of Clinical Psychology, 66*, 1057–1075.

Alexander, G. E., Crutcher, M. D., & DeLong, M. R. (1990). Basal ganglia-thalamo-cortical circuits: parallel substrates for motor, oculomotor, "prefrontal" and "limbic" functions. *Progress in Brain Research, 85*, 119–146.

American Heritage Dictionary (1978). Wm. Morris (Ed.), Boston: Houghton Mifflin, p. 607.

American Heritage Dictionary (1993). Robert Costello (Ed.), Boston: Houghton Mifflin, p. 626.

Amoateng, A. Y.,& Bahr, S. J. (1986). Religion, family, and adolescent drug use. *Sociological Perspectives, 29*(1), 53–76.

Apolito, A. (1970). Psychoanalysis and religion. *American Journal of Psychoanalysis, 30*, 115–126.

Appelbaum, P. S.,& Grisso, T. (1988). Assessing patients' capacities to consent to treatment. *New England Journal of Medicine, 319*, 1635–1638.

Balboni, T. A., Vanderwerker, L. C., Block, S. D., Paulk, M. E., Lathan, C. S., Peteet, J. R., & Prigerson, H. G. (2007). Religiousness and spiritual support among advanced cancer patients and associations with end-of-life treatment preferences and quality of life. *Journal of Clinical Oncology, 25*(5), 555–560.

Ballantine, H. T., Cassidy, W. L., Flanagan, N. B., & Marino, N. (1967). Stereotaxic anterior cingulotomy for neuropsychiatric illness and intractable pain. *Journal of Neurosurgery, 26*, 488–495.

Baron Short, E., Kose, S., Mu, Q., Borckardt, J., Newberg, A., George, M. S., & Kozel, F. A.(2010). Regional brain activation during meditation shows time and practice effects: an exploratory, fMRI study. *Evidence Based Complementary & Alternative Medicine, 7*, 121–127.

Benson, H. (1996). *Timeless healing: The power and biology of belief.* New York: Scribner.

Benson, H., Dusek, J. A., Sherwood, J. B., Lam, P., Bethea, C. F., Carpenter, W., et al.(2006). Study of the therapeutic effects of intercessory prayer (STEP) in cardiac bypass patients: a multicenter randomized trial of uncertainty andcertainty of receiving intercessory prayer. *American Heart Journal, 151*, 934–942.

Berkel, J.,& de Waard, F. (1983). Mortality pattern and life expectancy of Seventh Day Adventists in the Netherlands. *International Journal of Epidemiology, 12*(4), 455–459.

Berlin, R. M. (1986). Attachment behavior in hospitalized patients. *Journal of the American Medical Association, 255*, 3391–3393.

Bowlby, J. (1969). *Attachment and loss* (Vols. I and II). New York: Basic Books.

Burgener, S. C. (1994). Caregiver religiosity and well-being in dealing with Alzheimer's dementia. *Journal of Religion & Health, 33*(2), 175–189.

Butler, A. B. (1994a). The evolution of the dorsal thalamus of jawed vertebrates, including mammals: cladistic analysis and a new hypothesis. *Brain Research Reviews, 19*, 29–65.

Butler, A. B. (1994b). The evolution of the dorsal pallium in the telencephalon of ammiotes: a cladistic analysis and a new hypothesis. *Brain Research Reviews, 19*, 66–101.

Byrd, R. D. (1988). Positive therapeutic effects of intercessory prayer in a coronary care unit population. *Southern Medical Journal, 81*, 826–829.

Cassem, N. (1997). Spirituality and Healing Symposium, Academy of Psychosomatic Medicine Annual Meeting, Coronado, CA.

Chatters, L. M. (2000). Religion and health: public health research and practice. *Annual Review of Public Health, 21*, 335–367.

Champagne, F. A.(2010). Epigenetic influence of social experiences across the lifespan. *Developmental Psychobiology, 52*(4), 299–311.

Charney, D. S.(2004). Psychobiological mechanisms of resilience and vulnerability: implications for successful adaptation to extreme stress. *American Journal of Psychiatry, 161*, 195–216.

Chrousos, G. E.,& Gold, P. W. (1992). The concepts of stress and stress system disorders. Overview of physical and behavioral homeo-stasis. *Journal of the American Medical Association, 267*, 1244–1252.

Coakly, D. V.,& McKenna, G. W. (1986). Safety of faith healing. *Lancet, 1*, 444.

Cohen, D. L., Wintering, N., Tolles, V., Townsend, R. R., Farrar, J. T., Galantino, M. L., & Newberg, A. B.(2009). Cerebral blood flow effects of yoga training: preliminary evaluation of 4 cases. *Journal of Alternative and Complementary Medicine, 15*(1), 9–14.

Cohen, S. R., Mount, B. M., Tomas, J. J., & Mount, L. F. (1996), Existential well-being is an important determinant of quality of life. Evidence from the McGill Quality of Life Questionnaire.*Cancer, 77*, 576–586.

Colantonio, A., Kasl, S. V., & Ostefeld, A. M. (1992). Depressive symptoms and other psychosocial factors as predictors of stroke in the elderly. *American Journal of Epidemiology, 136*, 884–894.

Comstock, G. W., & Partridge, K. B. (1972). Church attendance and health. *Journal of Chronic Diseases, 25,* 665–672.

Contrada, R. J., Goyal, T. M., Cather, C., Rafalson, L., Idler, E. L., & Krause, T. J. (2004). Psychosocial factors in outcomes of heart surgery: the impact of religious involvement and depressive symptoms. *Health Psychology, 23,* 227–238.

Conway, K. (1985–1986). Coping with the stress of medical problems among black and white elderly. *International Journal of Aging and Human Development, 21,* 39–48.

Cook, J. A., & Wimberley, D. W. (1983). If I should die before I wake: religious commitment and adjustment to the death of a child. *Journal for the Scientific Study of Religion, 22*(3), 222–238.

Craig, T. J., Krishna, G., & Poniarski, R. (1997). Predictions of successful vs. unsuccessful outcome of a 12-stay inpatient alcohol rehabilitation program. *American Journal on Addictions, 6,* 232–236.

Craigie, F. C., Larson, D. B., & Lyons, J. S. (1988). A systematic analysis of religious variables in the Journal of Family Practice. *Journal of Family Practice, 27*(5), 509–513.

Desmond, D. P., & Maddux, J. F. (1981). Religious programs and careers of chronic heroin users. *American Journal of Drug and Alcohol Abuse, 8*(1), 71–83.

Dowell, E. H., Matthews, D. A., & Larson, D. B. (1993). No room at the inn? Neglect of religious variables by clinical epidemiologists. *Clinical Research, 41,* 516A.

Enstrom, J. E. (1989). Health practices and cancer mortality among active California Mormons. *Journal of the National Cancer Institute, 81,* 1807–1814.

Fetzer Institute. (2003). Multidimensional measurement of religiousness/spirituality for use in health research: A report of the Fetzer Institute/National Institute on Aging Working Group. Kalamazoo, MI.

Fitchett, G., Burton, L. A., & Sivan, A. B. (1997). The religious needs and resources of psychiatric patients. *Journal of Nervous & Mental Disease, 185,* 320–326.

Freud, S. (1961). *Civilization and its discontents.* (Trans. by James Strachey, pp. 23–25). New York: Norton.

Fricchione, G. L. (2011a). *Compassion and healing in medicine and society. On the nature and use of attachment solutions to separation challenges.* Baltimore: Johns Hopkins University Press.

Fricchione, G. L. (2011b). Separation-Attachment Theory in illness and the role of the healthcare practitioner. In T. A. Hutchinson (Ed.), *Whole person care. A new paradigm for the 21st century* (Chapter 5, pp. 45–58). New York: Springer.

Fricchione, G. L. (1993). Illness and the origin of caring. *Journal of Medical Humanities, 24,* 15–21.

Gardner, J. W., & Lyon, J. L. (1982). Cancer in Utah Mormon men by church activity level. *American Journal of Epidemiology, 116,* 243–257.

Glock, C. Y. (1962). On the study of religious commitment. *Religious Education, 57,* S98–S109.

Goldbourt, U., Yaari, S., & Medalie, J. H. (1993). Factors predictive of long-term coronary heart disease mortality among 10,059 male Israeli civil servants and municipal employees. *Cardiology, 82,* 100–121.

Hackett, T. H., & Cassem, N. H. (1968). The coronary care unit: an appraisal of its psychological hazards. *New England Journal of Medicine, 279,* 1365–1370.

Hannay, D. R. (1980). Religion and health. *Social Science & Medicine, 14A,* 683–685.

Casar Harris, R. C., Dew, M. A., Lee, A., Amaya, M., Buches, L., Reetz, D., & Coleman, G. (1995). The role of religion in heart-transplant recipients' long-term health and well-being. *Journal of Religion & Health, 34*(1), 17–32.

Harris, S., Kaplan, J. T., Curiel, A., Bookheimer, S. Y., Iacoboni, M., & Cohen, M. S. (2009). The neural correlates of religious and nonreligious belief. *PLoS One, 4,* e0007272; 1–9.

Henry, J. P. (1982). The relation of social to biological processes in disease. *Social Science & Medicine, 16,* 369–380.

Hill, A. B. (1965). The environment and disease: association or causation? *Proceedings of the Royal Society of Medicine, 58,* 1217–1219.

Holland, J. C., Kash, K. M., Passik, S., Gronert, M. K., Sison, A., Lederberg, M., Russak, S. M., Baider, L., & Fox, B. (1998). A brief spiritual beliefs inventory for use in quality of life research in life-threatening illness. *Psycho-oncology, 7,* 460–469.

Horkheimer, M. (1970). Die Sehsucht nach dem ganz Anderen. Ein Interview mit Kommentar von H. Gumnion. [Hamburg].

Horton, P. C. (1981). *Solace: the missing dimension in psychiatry.* Chicago: University of Chicago Press.

House, J. S., Landis, K. R., & Umberson, D. (1988). Social relationships and health. *Science, 241,* 540–545.

Idler, E. L., & Kasl, S. V. (1992). Religion, disability, depression, and the timing of death. *American Journal of Sociology, 97*(4), 1052–1079.

Ingvar, D. H. (1985). Memory of the future: an essay on the temporal organization of conscious awareness. *Human Neurobiology, 4,* 127–136.

Ironside, W. (1980). Conservation-withdrawal and action-engagement: on a theory of survivor behavior. *Psychosomatic Medicine, 42*(SupplII), 163–175.

Ironson, G., Solomon, G. F., Balbin, E. G., O'Cleirigh, C., George, A., Kumar, M., et al. (2002). Ironson-Woods Spirituality/Religiousness Index is associated with long survival, health behaviors, less distress and low cortisol in people with HIV/AIDS. *Annals of Behavioral Medicine, 24,* 34–38.

Jarvis, G. K., & Northcott, H. C. (1987). Religion and differences in morbidity and mortality. *Social Science & Medicine, 25,* 813–824.

Kaczorowski, J. M. (1989). Spiritual well-being and anxiety in adults diagnosed with cancer. *Hospice Journal, 5*(3/4), 105–116.

Kapogiannis, D., Barbey, A. K., Su, M., Zamboni, G., Krueger, F., & Grafman, J. (2009). Cognitive and neural foundations of religious belief. *Proceedings of the National Academy of Sciences, 106,* 4876–4881.

Kass, J. D., Friedman, R., Leserman, J., Zuttermeister, P., & Benson, H. (1991). Health outcomes and a new index of spiritual experience. *Journal for the Scientific Study of Religion, 30,* 203–211.

Kendler, K. S., Gardner, C. O., & Prescott, C. A. (1997). Religion, psychopathology, and substance use and abuse: a multimeasure, genetic-epidemiologic study. *American Journal of Psychiatry, 154,* 322–329.

King, D. E., & Bushwick, B. (1994). Beliefs and attitudes of hospital inpatients about faith healing and prayer. *Journal of Family Practice, 39*(4), 349–352.

H. G., Cohen, H. J., Blazer, D. G., Pieper, C., Meador, K. G., Shelp, F., Goli, V., & DiPasquale, B. (1992). Religious coping and depression among elderly, hospitalized medically ill men. *American Journal of Psychiatry, 149,* 1693–1700.

Koenig, H. G. (1997). *Is religion good for your health? Effects of religion on physical and mental health.* New York: Haworth Press.

Koenig, H. G., George, L. K., & Peterson, B. L. (1998). Religiosity and remission of depression in medically ill older patients. *American Journal of Psychiatry, 155,* 536–542.

Koenig, H. G., Cohen, H. J., Blazer, D. G., Kudler, H. S., Krishnan, K. R., Sibert, T. E. (1995). Religious coping and cognitive symptoms of depression in elderly medical patients. *Psychosomatics, 36,* 369–375.

Koenig, H. G., George, L. K., Meador, K. G., Blazer, D. G., & Ford, S. M. (1994a). Religious practices and alcoholism in a southern adult population. *Hospital and Community Psychiatry, 45*(3), 225–231.

Koenig, H. G., George, L. K., Meador, K. G., Blazer, D. G., & Dyck, P. B. (1994b). Religious affiliation and psychiatric disorder among Protestant baby boomers. *Hospital and Community Psychiatry, 45*(6), 586–594.

Koenig, H. G., Cohen, H. J., George, L. K., et al. (1997). Attendance at religious services, interleukin-6, and other biological indicators of immune function in older adults. *International Journal of Psychiatry in Medicine, 27,* 233–250.

Koenig, H. G., McCullough, M. E., & Larson, D. B. (2001). *Handbook of religion and health.* New York: Oxford University Press.

Larson, D. B., Pattison, E. M., Blazer, D. G., Omran, A. R., & Kaplan, B. H. (1986). Systematic analysis of research on religious variables in four major psychiatric journals. 1978–1982. *American Journal of Psychiatry, 143*(3), 329–334.

Lazar, S. W., Bush, G., Gollub, R. L., Fricchione, G. L., Khalsa, G., & Benson, H. (2000). Functional brain mapping of the relaxation response and meditation. *Neuroreport, 11*(7), 1581–1585.

LeDoux, J. (1996). *The emotional brain.* New York: Simon & Schuster.

Levenson, J. L., Mishra, A., Hamer, R. M., & Hastillo, A. (1989). Denial and medical outcome in unstable angina. *Psychosomatic Medicine, 51,* 27–35.

Levin, J. S., & Schiller, P. L. (1987). Is there a religious factor in health? *Journal of Religion & Health, 26,* 9–36.

Levin, J. S. (1994). Religion and health: is there an association, is it valid, and is it causal? *Social Science in Medicine, 38,* 1475–1482.

Lutgendorf, S. K., Russell, D., Ullrich, P., Harris, T. B., & Wallace, R. (2004). Religious participation, interleukin-6, and mortality in older adults. *Journal of Health Psychology, 23,* 465–475.

Matthews, D. A. (1997). *The faith factor. Is religion good for your health?* Presented at Harvard Medical School/Mind-Body Medical Institute. Spirituality and Healing in Medicine ConferenceIV, Boston, MA.

Matthews, D. A., Larson, D. B., & Barry, C. P. (1993a). The faith factor: an annotated bibliography of clinical research on spiritual subjects. (Vol. *I*), Rockville, MD: National Institute for Health Care Research.

Matthews, D. A., Larson, D. B., & Barry, C. P. (1993b). The faith factor: an annotated bibliography of clinical research on spiritual subjects. (Vol. *II*), Rockville, MD: National Institute for Health Care Research.

Matthews, D. A., & Larson, D. B. (1995). The faith factor: an annotated bibliography of clinical research on spiritual subjects. (Vol. *III*), Rockville, MD: National Institute for Health Care Research.

Matthews, D. A., & Saunders, D. M. (1997). The faith factor: an annotated bibliography of clinical research on spiritual subjects. (Vol. *IV*), Rockville, MD: National Institute for Health Care Research.

Maugans, T. A., & Wadland, W. C. (1991). Religion and family medicine: a survey of physicians and patients. *Journal of Family Practice, 32*(2), 210–213.

McEwen, B. S. (1998). Protective and damaging effects of stress mediation. *New England Journal of Medicine, 338,* 171–179.

MacLean, P. D. (1990). *The trauma brain in evolution.* New York: Plenum Press.

Mega, M. S., Cummings, J. L., Salloway, S., & Malloy, P. (1997). The limbic system: an anatomic, phylogenetic, and clinical perspective. *Journal of Neuropsychiatry and Clinical Neurosciences, 9,* 315–330.

Meissner, W. W. (1984). *Psychoanalysis and religious experience.* New Haven: Yale University Press.

Mesulam, M.-M. (1985). Patterns in behavioral neuroanatomy: association areas, the limbic system, and hemispheric specialization. In M.-M. Mesulam (Ed.), *Behavioral neurology* (pp. 1–70). Philadelphia: Davis.

Moore, R. D., Mead, L., & Pearson, T. (1990). Youthful precursors of alcohol abuse in physicians. *American Journal of Medicine, 88,* 332–336.

Moos, R. H., & Tsu, V. D. (1977). The crisis of physical illness: an overview. In *Coping with physical illness.* New York: Plenum Press.

Newberg, A., Pourdehnad, M., Alavi, A., & d'Aquili, E. G. (2003). Cerebral blood flow during meditative prayer: preliminary findings and methodological issues. *Perceptual & Motor Skills, 97*(2), 625–630.

Newberg, A., Alavi, A., Baime, M., Pourdehnad, M., Santanna, J., & d'Aquili, E. (2001). The measurement of regional cerebral blood flow during the complex cognitive task of meditation: a preliminarySPECT study. *Psychiatry Research, 106*(2), 113–122.

Newberg, A. B., & D'Aquili, E. (2001). *Why god won't go away.* NY: Ballantine Books.

Olsen, K. (1996). Fully alive. A peak experience with a modern mystic. *Spirituality and Health,* Fall 6–8.

Oxman, T. E., Freeman, D. H., & Manheimer, E. D. (1995). Lack of social participation or religious strength and comfort as risk factors for death after cardiac surgery in the elderly. *Psychosomatic Medicine, 57,* 5–15.

Pandya, D. N., & Yeterian, E. H. (1990). Prefrontal cortex in relation to other cortical areas in rhesus monkey: architecture and connections. *Progress in Brain Research, 85,* 63–94.

Panico, M. L., Jeng, G. Y., & Brewster, U. C. (2011). When a patient refuses life-saving care: issues raised when treating a Jehovah's Witness. *American Journal of Kidney Diseases, 58,* 647–653.

Peabody, F. W. (1927). The care of the patient. *Journal of the American Medical Association, 88,* 877–882.

Powell, L. H., Shahabi, L., & Thoresen, C. E. (2003). Religion and spirituality. Linkages to physical health. *American Psychologist, 58,* 36–52.

Puchalski, C., Ferrell, B., Virani, R., Otis-Green, S., Baird, P., Bull, J., et al. (2009). Improving the quality of spiritual care as a dimension of palliative care: the report of the Consensus Conference. *Journal of Palliative Medicine, 12,* 885–904.

Puchalski, C., & Romer, A. L. (2000). Taking a spiritual history allows clinicians to understand patients more fully. *Journal of Palliative Medicine, 3,* 129–137.

Querido, A. (1959). Forecast and follow-up: An investigation into the clinical, social, and mental factors determining the results of hospital treatment. *British Journal of Prevtive & SocialMedicine, 13,* 33–49.

Reichlen, S. (1993). Neuroendocrine-immune interactions. *New England Journal of Medicine, 329,* 1246–1253.

Rosen, I. M. (1993). Experiences at the interface between psychiatry and religion. *Rhode Island Journal of Medicine, 76,* 75–77.

Saver, J. L., & Rabin, J. (1997). The neural substrates of religious experience. *Journal of Neuropsychiatry and Clinical Neurosciences, 9,* 498–510.

Schoenbach, V. J., Kaplan, B. H., Fredman, L., & Kleinbaum, D. G. (1986). Social ties and mortality. Evans County, Georgia. *American Journal of Epidemiology, 123,* 577–591.

Schore, A. N. (1996). The experience dependent maturation of a regulatory system in the orbital prefrontal cortex and the origin of developmental psychopathology. *Development and Psychopathology, 8,* 59–87.

Sloan, R. P., Bagiella, E., & Powell, T. (1999). Religion spirituality and medicine. *Lancet, 353,* 664–667.

Sloan, R. P., & Bagiella, E. (2002). Claims about religious involvement and health—doneoutcomes. *Annals of Behavioral Medicine, 24,* 14–21.

Sloan, R. P. (2005). Field analysis of the literature on religion, spirituality and health. www.metanexus.net/.../pdf/TARP-Sloan.pdf

Stepansky, P. (1986). Feuerbach and Jung as religious critics, with a note on Freud's psychology of religion. In P. Stepansky (Ed.), *Freud: Appraisals and reappraisals* (Vol. *1,* pp. 215–239). Hillsdale, NJ: Analytic.

Stotland, N. L. (1999). When religion collides with medicine. *American Journal of Psychiatry, 156,* 304–307.

Strawbridge, W. J., Cohen, R. D., Shema, S. J., & Kaplan, G.A. (1997). Frequent attendance at religious services and mortality over 28 years. *American Journal of Public Health, 87,* 957–961.

Thoresen, C. E., & Harris, A. H. (2002). Spirituality and health: what's the evidence and what's needed? *Annals of Behavioral Medicine, 24,* 3–13.

Tillich, P. (1951). *Systematic theology.* Chicago: University of Chicago Press.

Waldfogel, S., & Wolpe, P. R. (1993). Using awareness of religious factors to enhance interventions in consultation-liaison psychiatry. *Hospital and Community Psychiatry, 44,* 473–477.

Waldfogel, S., Wolpe, P. R., & Shmuely, Y. (1998). Religious training and religiosity in psychiatry residency programs. *Academy of Psychiatry, 22*(1), 29–35.

Williams, D. R., Larson, D. B., Buckler, R. E., et al. (1991). Religion and psychological distress in a community sample. *Social Science & Medicine, 32,* 1257–1262.

Winnicott, D. W. (1953). Transitional objects and transitional phenomena. *International Journal of Psychoanalysis, 34,* 89–97.

Zuckerman, D. M., Kasl, S. V., & Ostfeld, A. M. (1984). Psychosocial predictors of mortality among the elderly poor. *American Journal of Epidemiology, 119,* 410–423.

19.

TECHNOLOGY IN TREATMENT AND PHYSICIAN–PATIENT COMMUNICATION

Steven E. Locke and Tristan Gorrindo

Patient: Well, my boyfriend made me come here.
Computer: YOUR BOYFRIEND MADE YOU COME HERE?
Patient: He says I'm depressed much of the time.
Computer: I AM SORRY TO HEAR YOU ARE DEPRESSED.
Patient: It's true. I am unhappy
Computer: DO YOU THINK COMING HERE WILL HELP YOU NOT TO BE UNHAPPY?
Patient: I need some help, that much seems certain.
Computer: WHAT WOULD IT MEAN TO YOU IF YOU GOT SOME HELP?
Patient: Perhaps I could learn to get along with my mother.
–Excerpts from a patient–computer psychotherapy session conducted with ELIZA in 1966

INTRODUCTION

Psychiatry is no stranger to technology. When ELIZA, the computer-based therapist, was unveiled in 1966, many felt that this was the beginning of a new revolution in psychiatry (Weizenbaum, 1966). And while ELIZA's inventor, Joseph Weizenbaum, never meant for it to be a formal treatment tool, computer-assisted therapy would not become widely available for another four decades.

In a specialty devoted to interpersonal relationships, self-awareness, and the human condition, patients and providers have been skeptical about the role of technology in psychiatry. For many, technology doesn't seem a natural fit in psychiatry. And while many providers are now seeing the usefulness of electronic medical records and computer-assisted treatments, technology's greatest influence on psychiatry may actually be the way in which it has influenced the patient–physician relationship.

TECHNOLOGY AS TREATMENT

INTRODUCTION AND OVERVIEW

In 1965, a man walked into a laboratory at the University of Wisconsin and, without understanding the significance of his contribution, opened a new chapter in the history of medicine. Sitting in front of a 3" × 4" sapphire blue screen, he watched the white letters as they spelled out questions: "Are you sitting down?" Using the keyboard of the PDP-9 computer, he typed, "No." The screen flashed, "Why don't you pull up a chair and make yourself comfortable." Using a script prepared by Dr. Slack, the computer inquired about symptoms and the patient responded, mimicking a clinician–patient interview. And so the field of patient–computer dialogue was born.

The introduction of technology into the doctor–patient relationship has always been ambivalently received as an intrusion. Although Laennec's invention of the stethoscope improved the physician's ability to make accurate cardiac diagnoses, this disruptive innovation introduced a lasting change in the doctor–patient relationship. Today a doctor no longer places his ear on the patient's chest to listen to the heart, but performs the auscultative exam in a brief, often perfunctory fashion in anticipation of detailed information captured by modern diagnostic technologies. How has psychiatric practice fared during the transformative onslaught of technology in the era of information-age medicine? Perhaps unsurprisingly, adoption of technology has occurred more slowly in psychiatry than in other specialties. In this chapter we will describe a variety of ways that technology has appeared in psychiatric care, both at the psychiatry/general medicine interface and in behavioral health in other settings.

COMPUTER-BASED PATIENT ASSESSMENT

Medical History Taking

Four years after the publication of Warner Slack's seminal paper on computer–patient dialogue, the computer-assisted medical history was first implemented in clinical care around 1970 by Morris Collen, director of research at Kaiser-Permanente (KP) in Oakland, California. Patients completed a paper history form that was designed to be machine-readable, producing an electronic record that became part of the patient's electronic medical record. The KP standardized history had the advantage of thoroughness and increased the likelihood that often overlooked psychosocial factors and habits would be investigated. Around the same time, Slack and Maultsby programmed a computer to take a psychiatric history from a patient (Maultsby & Slack, 1971). Soon after, John Greist and his colleagues developed a computer-administered psychiatric symptom checklist that measured change in clinical condition by tracking a patient's symptoms over time (Greist, Klein, & Van Cura, 1973). These early pioneers and their collaborators spawned a generation of clinical researchers dedicated to studying the use of computers in psychiatry and mental health.

Mental Health Screening and Assessment of Behavior

The development of computer-based screening tools for behavioral symptoms and mental disorders in the 1970s was soon followed by the introduction of the personal computer (PC). The PC made it possible to not only automate the use of standardized measures of psychopathology for use in mental health screening, but also to efficiently disseminate these tools more widely. The exponential growth of Internet access and broadband availability in recent years has led to the migration of computer-assisted assessment of signs and symptoms of mental disorders, from the personal computer to the Internet. Currently, the widespread availability of Software-as-a-Service (SaaS) providers has made it possible for these assessment programs and their data to be stored in "the Cloud"—secure servers accessible from any Internet-connected device including tablet computers and smartphones. While such programs offer many advantages, including scalability, access, and the potential for linkage with institutional and personal electronic health records as well as use from the "medical home" of the future, remaining questions about privacy, confidentiality, and security must be resolved before adoption can be widespread.

Lee Baer, John Greist, and their collaborators conducted computer-assisted screening for mental disorders beginning in the 1980s using automated telephone interviews to query people about their experience of a standardized list of psychiatric symptoms, with the goal of identifying those individuals who might likely benefit from psychiatric evaluation and treatment(Baer et al., 1995). Since then, the use of automated methods for screening large populations for a variety of mental disorders including depression, alcohol abuse, and eating disorders has become widespread and is used in community, military, college health, and workplace settings (www.mentalhealthscreening.org). Increasingly, automated screening for depression, alcohol and substance abuse, and other behavioral conditions is being deployed by healthcare organizations, insurers, employers, and student health services (Farzanfar et al., 2011).

Computer-assisted assessment of patient behavior can supplement the evaluations done in primary care and specialty care settings, where clinicians are pressed for time and assessment of behavioral and psychosocial issues often is neglected in favor of other priorities. Mental health measures can be completed easily using tablet computers in waiting rooms, secure patient Internet portals, or commercially available automated telephone screening services. Unfortunately, these screening tools are underutilized relative to the scope of the problem of psychiatric comorbidity in general medical illness. Despite the well-established relationship between depression and poorer clinical outcomes in coronary artery disease (CAD), and the recommendation by the American College of Cardiology that CAD patients be screened for depression routinely (American College of Cardiology, 2010), many CAD patients are not screened. Automated, computerized screening for depression could address this deficit. It is not known why this obvious solution isn't utilized; one possible explanation is that while the direct cost of automated screening is low, the indirect costs and systems problems related to following up the patients who screen in for depression discourage its adoption.

Obviously, interactions with machines are not, in general, substitutes for human contact and communication—but there are ways and contexts in which computer-based interviews have advantages over conventional clinical interviews. Computers are more reliable than human interviewers, they pursue questions inexorably without finding it tedious, and the extent of their queries is limited only by patient fatigue. They easily accommodate multiple languages and can be available 24×7 in diverse locations, and computerized services can quickly be scaled to serve large populations at a low incremental cost. Computerized systems can offer information and education using interactive multimedia in a way that continually checks patients' understanding of the material presented; human clinicians are encouraged to verify patients' understanding of their illnesses and treatment, but often do not have the time to do so. Finally, computer–patient dialogue may be of extraordinary value in contexts where patients are asked to disclose information of a sensitive, personal nature that might cause them shame or embarrassment if expressed to a human interviewer. Patients' preferences to make disclosures during a computerized interview have been shown regarding questions about substance abuse, sexual behavior, and sexually transmitted diseases such as HIV (Locke et al., 1992; Richens et al., 2010), suggesting that computers are experienced as less judgmental. For these reasons there is growing interest in systems that augment traditional clinical care by adding well-designed and clinically effective computer-based behavioral technologies, in the belief that such systems will increase access to behavioral healthcare in a variety of resource-poor settings, as well as improve quality and reduce health costs. One website, PsychCentral (www.psychcentral.com) is a frequently updated source of self-assessment tools that can be used with patients. Other websites are emerging, and a search at www.nimh.gov, nida.gov, or va.gov will lead to other useful validated tools that are available online and downloadable for use in clinical practice.

One approach to reach underserved populations without access to computers or the Internet is the use of interactive voice response telephony, or IVR. Robert Friedman and his colleagues at Boston Medical Center have been studying the use of IVR telephony at the intersection of primary care and psychiatry for two decades. Friedman and his team have based their work on the concept of a "virtual visit" in which a computer-based telehealth system (which they call "Technology Linked Care" or "TLC") guides a patient through an interactive interview that (1) collects information via an automated interview, (2) uses algorithms and expert systems to make clinical inferences, and (3) provides automated psychoeducation, care management, and health coaching to guide patients to manage their symptoms or improve health behavior between office visits. This procedure takes place with no human intervention at all—in contrast to applications that screen patients and quantify symptoms, or provide structured psychoeducation, but ultimately rely upon a human interviewer to confirm diagnoses and prescribe interventions. Their research has demonstrated the usefulness of the TLC model in the management of hypertension, promotion of dietary change, increased exercise, medication adherence, help with smoking cessation and abstinence from alcohol, and management of depression and other mental disorders (Friedman, Stollerman, Mahoney, & Rozenblyum, 1997). TLC has screened for depression, dysthymia, bipolar disorder, PTSD, acute stress disorder, generalized anxiety disorder, panic disorder, somatization, social phobia, alcohol and drug abuse, stress, and violence. Usually, after screening, the automated IVR system encourages the person to seek help, provides resources, and monitors adherence using follow-up calls to ensure help has been sought (Farzanfar, Stevens, Vachon, Friedman, & Locke, 2007). The widespread use of smartphones that offer significant computer power in handheld devices broadens the potential scope of phone-based interactive applications. For example, smartphone applications can collect and transmit physiological data as well as self-reports of symptoms. Mobile phone transmissions can offer a high level of security, and the incremental cost of using them is low because most patients already own smartphones and have phone accounts with data transmission capabilities. Low-income patients without computers or other Internet access often own smartphones or have family members who do. For these reasons mobile phones are likely in the near future to become the most widespread personal health appliances. Mobile platforms and smartphones can also be used in technology-supported self-care. A systematic review of five studies found that interventions that used text messaging to provide motivation, support, and tips for quitting smoking delivered by mobile phones can help people stop, though the results varied. Whittaker and colleagues reported that as of November 2012, there are no published studies on smartphone applications designed to help people stop smoking (Whittaker et al., 2012). Nevertheless, there are many new apps for various mobile platforms and smartphones that, despite being untested in clinical trials, claim to be useful adjuncts to a self-care program for reducing tobacco and alcohol use. A common theme in this book, detailed in almost all of the specialty-specific chapters, is that chronic medical conditions and mental disorders are frequently associated both in primary care and in specialty settings. When general medical illness is associated with a mental disorder—particularly with depression or clinical severity—outcomes are likely to be poorer and the cost of care is likely to be higher (Ciechanowski, Katon, & Russo, 2000; Katon, 1996; Katon & Ciechanowski, 2002; Roy-Byrne et al., 2008). The continually widening availability and decreasing cost of Internet-connected mobile devices argues for the routine integration of "behavioral informatics" into clinical practice, facilitating the identification and treatment of comorbid mental disorders in patients with chronic general medical illness. This is an emerging area in both research and development, and there are many product companies that are field testing their mobile devices in partnership with clinical providers and delivery systems.

Psychometrics

Beginning in 1962 the most widely used psychometric ever developed, the Minnesota Multiphasic Personality Inventory (MMPI), was offered in a machine-scorable format (Fowler & Miller, 1969; Pearson, Rome, Swenson, Mataya, & Brannick, 1965). At first, computers were simply used to scan, read, and score multiple-choice forms, but starting in 1986 programs were sold for installations on PCs that could administer the questions, one at a time, to patients sitting in front of a monitor and responding via a keyboard. A proprietary program generated a report that could be printed at the site of care or mailed to the supervising clinician (Biskin & Kolotkin, 1977; Johnson, Giannetti, & Williams, 1978; Russell, Peace, & Mellsop, 1986).

Currently, hundreds of psychometrics can be administered over the Internet or via personal computers or Internet-connected mobile devices. Computers can also administer interactive tests, interviews, and questionnaires via the telephone using IVR (Rose et al., 2010; Turvey, Willyard, Hickman, Klein, & Kukoyi, 2007). Many of these tests, particularly those that have been validated and standardized using reference populations, are protected by copyright and available only through payment of a license or subscription fee. Best-known examples of these are the MMPI-2, the SCL-90R, the MINI, and the Beck Depression Inventory. In contrast, other psychometrics have been validated in clinical trials and are available as computer-administered tests in the public domain with no fee required. Examples of these are the SCL-90, the Hopkins Symptom Checklist, the CIDI, and the Alcohol Use Disorders Identification Test (AUDIT; see http://whqlibdoc.who.int/hq/2001/who_msd_msb_01.6a.pdf). Some widely used psychometrics are copyrighted but have been made available for widespread use without need for prior permission. The PHQ-9 (Kroenke, Spitzer, & Williams, 2001) is the best known example.

Computer-based tests and interviews can be administered for automated clinical assessment, including the use of standardized histories or symptom inventories. Such instruments or clinical assessment tools have the advantages of scalability, affordability, reliability and, ideally, validity. Properly developed, implemented, and deployed, they can be efficient ways to screen for behavioral symptoms or mental disorders in large or at-risk populations. The Patient Protection and Affordable Care Act (2010) mandates that screening for depression in primary care will be a public health requirement for public and private insurers, effective in 2014. This federal mandate presents both an opportunity and a challenge to improve the quality and integration of behavioral health into primary care during the next decade.

Physicians are increasingly interested in developing their own interactive interviews or questionnaires for use with patients over the Internet or collected by a tablet computer or kiosk. Most institutions have policies, procedures, and guidance that address the means for collecting patient-level data using tools such as Survey Monkey and REDCap in a secure and HIPAA-compliant fashion. Many professional societies have telemedicine committees and they may also be a source for guidance.

Psychophysiology

Applied psychophysiological research during the last century led to a variety of computer-based psychodiagnostic tools (EEG, fMRI, evoked potentials, PET scans, etc.) as well as somatic treatments (electroconvulsive therapy, transcranial magnetic stimulation, etc.) in use today. Beginning in the 1970s, however, a new field generally known as *biofeedback* emerged, following Neal Miller's seminal research on operant conditioning of the autonomic nervous system (Chen, Ju, Sun, & Lin, 2009). Biofeedback involved training patients to alter measurable physiological variables such as skin conductance, skin temperature, surface EMG activity, or EEG alpha power. Biofeedback was directed at psychosomatic conditions that seemed poorly responsive to the nonspecific psychodynamic treatments that were highly prevalent at the time. Microprocessor-based systems would amplify electrical signals from physiologic sensors, interpret them, and present the patient with simple graphical or auditory cues that would change in real time. Responding to these cues, patients could acquire control of bodily processes ordinarily outside of their awareness. Ideally this would lead to relief of symptoms associated with the physiological processes modified by the procedure, such as tension headaches or high blood pressure. Biofeedback, with its emphasis on self-regulation rather than the use of drugs, proved to be a practical route for the introduction of behavioral medicine into primary care practices during the 1980s and 1990s (Schwartz, 2005). However, it has not become a fixture in mainstream primary care medicine, probably because of its limited applicability and efficacy. Biofeedback, buoyed by the popularity of complementary and alternative medicine with its emphasis on self-regulation as an alternative to pills, became a beachhead for the introduction of technology into clinical behavioral health practice. Technology-enhanced self-regulation accompanied relaxation training and meditation and became a comfortable modality to facilitate the integration of behavioral medicine into primary care during the 1980s and 1990s.

Wellness and Health Risk Appraisals

Research in behavioral medicine, preventive medicine, and occupational health began to document the "toxic" effects of psychosocial stressors in ordinary life and in the workplace. Since the 1960s it has become more widely accepted that exposure to prolonged or severe acute stressors is often followed by the emergence of physical symptoms (e.g., headache, pain) or even frank medical disorders (e.g., hypertension, myocardial infarction, cardiac arrhythmias). This awareness provoked interest in the use of computer-assisted assessment methods for measuring stress and coping effectiveness, both in the workplace and in medical settings. Health risk appraisals (HRAs), first developed by the CDC in the 1980s to identify individuals with lifestyle factors associated with adverse health change (Centers for Disease Control, 1984), were adapted by employers and "wellness" program vendors for computer administration and later for delivery via the Internet. These self-administered HRA questionnaires took histories that identified modifiable risks that could be addressed through behavior change programs that were designed to facilitate adoption of a healthier lifestyle and reduction of unhealthy habits (e.g., smoking, poor diet, sedentary behavior, misuse of alcohol; Huskamp & Rosenthal, 2009). As research indicated that such workplace stress management programs led to healthier employees and reduced health care costs (Baicker, Cutler, & Song, 2010), pharmaceutical companies began to take notice. Johnson & Johnson has offered its employees the *Live for Life* program (now *Health & Wellness*) since 1979 and has sold it to employers throughout the United States. Today there are scores of such programs: most Fortune 500 companies offer them, either on-site through their employee assistance programs, via contractors, or through community-based services covered by their employee health benefits. The widespread use of computer-assisted HRAs has made it possible to efficiently screen entire populations for symptoms and signs of stress and to refer them to programs that teach and improve coping strategies and techniques (Hyner, 1999). In addition, the use of HRAs with Medicare recipients has been associated with reductions in annual health costs even without subsequent participation in wellness programs (Loeppke, 2011).

Suicide Risk Assessment

A clinician's ability to assess the risk of patient self-injury or suicide is a critically important but often overlooked skill, although it is essential in most clinical settings. All physicians are taught to assess suicide risk during medical school or residency, yet it is a skill often lost as pressing clinical workflow impedes busy clinicians who too frequently wish to avoid probing patients for feelings of hopelessness or thoughts of suicide and risk, opening a Pandora's box. However, because roughly half of the patients who commit suicide are seen by a physician within the month preceding their deaths (Luoma, Martin, & Pearson, 2002; Vannoy et al., 2010) deployment of better methods for screening patients for suicide risk in general medical settings is crucial. As it has been established that patients are more likely to disclose certain types of sensitive information during a computer-administered interview, it warrants consideration that computer interviews have a potential role in suicide risk assessment. Automated assessment provides an opportunity to introduce the screening into a busy clinical setting while minimizing the disruption in workflow. Furthermore, detailed screening can be performed as a second-stage assessment, restricted to use in the minority of patients who have disclosed suicidal thoughts (e.g., thoughts of self-harm or feeling that they or others would be better off if they were dead) during a prior depression screening administered in the waiting room (e.g., following a positive response to item 9 on the PHQ-9). However, the US Preventive Services Task Force assessed the value of routine screening for suicide and concluded, "the evidence is insufficient to recommend for or against routine screening by primary care clinicians to detect suicide risk in the general population" (Gaynes et al., 2004). Despite the lack of a USPSTF recommendation, the report endorsed the assessment of suicidal ideation as the standard of care in the evaluation of depression, and recommended routine depression screening to identify patients with thoughts of suicide. The Task Force further recommended that primary care clinicians will need evidence-based management strategies for the patients who are identified as at risk for suicide.

One of the challenges for computer-based suicide risk detection is that despite the known association with suicide of epidemiologic risk factors such as depression, social isolation, substance abuse, and impulsivity, only rarely do individuals with these risk factors end their lives. Reliance upon these risk factors alone would generate too many false positives unless considered together with a current clinical assessment, and in that way a computer-based interview may be assistive. Depression screening was recommended by the US Preventive Services Task Force, *as long as there are systems in place to enable appropriate treatment.* The expected increase in routine depression screening will therefore require improved methods to follow up patients who report suicidal ideation during self-administered screening (McDowell, Lineberry, & Bostwick, 2011). Computer-based methods have the potential to improve the efficiency and dissemination of this process. The trend toward using computer-assisted screening will lead to the opportunity to study this issue on a population health basis and lead to greater understanding of the role of computer-based or computer-assisted interviewing in the assessment of suicide risk.

As early as 1973, John Greist and his colleagues at the University of Wisconsin developed a computer program that queried patients about their history and psychiatric symptoms and used a predictive model to estimate the risk of a suicide attempt. Not only did they report that the patients preferred the computer interview to talking to a physician, but also, using a retrospective design in a subsequent study, they found that the computer performed better than clinicians in predicting suicide attempts in their small sample of 22 patients. A subsequent larger prospective study (Erdman, Greist, Gustafson, Taves, & Klein, 1987) found that the computer was better at detecting suicide attempters, although clinicians were better at identifying non-attempters. The computer was more sensitive at detecting those at risk, but there were more false positives than the clinicians observed in their assessments. Thus the inference is that computers could be used for screening but would require a follow-up assessment by a clinician. However, wide-scale implementation would depend upon improving the ability of such a screening approach to have both great sensitivity AND specificity for it to be practical. Since then, computer-based screening for suicidal ideation and risk has been used to assess patients with HIV, adolescents with depression, and people with substance abuse. However, ethical considerations and the low frequency of suicide in primary care have limited the practical utility of routine suicide risk screening in general medical settings. Instead, the approach that we recommend is a two-stage screening solution using the PHQ-9 for all patients and a computer-administered approach (i.e., tablet, IVR telephony, or via the Internet using a secure patient web portal), followed by the administration of the P4 Screener, a brief structured interview to assess suicide risk, administered in an office setting where clinical evaluation is available (Dube, Kurt, Bair, Theobald, & Williams, 2010).

Substance Abuse

Computers and the Internet have been used for the identification and treatment of alcohol and substance abuse. Self-administered paper-and-pencil questionnaires have been used for several decades to collect information about substance use from patients, and the National Institute on Drug Abuse and the National Institute on Alcohol Abuse and Alcoholism provide on their websites standardized questionnaires that can be used both to screen for substance abuse behavior and monitor its course (Maisto, Connors, & Allen, 1995). During the past decade, several of these questionnaires have been evaluated for use in computer-based self-assessment by comparing the results of administration of computer-administered versions with the previously validated paper-and-pencil versions. Examples include the Michigan Alcohol Screening Test (MAST; Selzer, 1971) and the Drug Abuse Screening Test (DAST; Gavin, Ross, & Skinner, 1989). These 20-item measures are too long for use in general medical settings for screening, but shorter measures have become widely used: the CAGE four-item screen for alcohol abuse (Gavin, et al., 1989), the Alcohol Use Disorders Identification Test (AUDIT) of 10-items, and the AUDIT-C four-item (Bush, Kivlahan, McDonell, Fihn, & Bradley, 1998) test are excellent screening tools for alcohol misuse. Brief screening for substance abuse other than alcohol is more complex and harder to reduce to ultra-brief screeners, though the two-item Conjoint Screener (TICS) has been validated (Brown, Leonard, Saunders, & Papasouliotis, 2001) and has the sensitivity and specificity suitable for primary care use, if followed up with the AUDIT and the DAST as appropriate. The CRAFFT (**C**ar, **R**elax, **A**lone, **F**orget, **F**riends, **T**rouble) is a six-item screener for use with adolescents that screens for both problem drinking as well as drug use. The CRAFFT asks about behaviors that are reliable indicators of consumption and risk; it also can be self-administered and machine scored (Crum, 2007).

Computer-based approaches to primary care screening and intervention for substance abuse offer the possibility of easily accessible, reliable, efficient, and scalable methods of detection. These methods can leverage motivational interviewing methods, leading to brief interventions that engage patients in behavior change and/or referral for specialty care. Computer-assisted interventions offer advantages in that participants are more likely to disclose substance use to computers than to human interviewers, as previously mentioned. Several computer and/or Internet-based interventions are available and have shown promising results in studies of brief computer-based interventions for smoking and for problem drinking. Those screening tools, whether paper-and-pencil or online, merely alert the patient and the clinician to the existence of a problem. It is left to the patient to discuss the results with his or her clinician. Although there are evidence-based brief interventions for smoking cessation and the reduction of risky drinking for use by primary care providers, there are also programs that integrate automated assessment with self-guided treatment.

Boston University researchers and clinicians have developed two websites that enable individuals to complete anonymous online self-assessments for alcohol and substance abuse problems. The project is based on the Alcohol, Smoking and Substance Involvement Screening Test (ASSIST) developed for the World Health Organization by an international group of substance abuse researchers for the detection and management of substance abuse and related problems in general medical settings. A nonprofit company, Join Together, operates two sibling websites, *DrugScreening.org* and *AlcoholScreening.org*. The latter site provides more intensive assessment and feedback on alcohol consumption and directs users to treatment resources.

Another well-regarded website, *Drinker's Checkup* (www. drinkerscheckup.com), is an evidence-based self-assessment tool and treatment program developed at the University of New Mexico by psychologist Reid Hester with funding from the National Institute of Alcohol Abuse and Alcoholism (NIAAA). A companion program, *Moderate Drinking* (www.moderatedrinking.com) was created to assist individuals who want to reduce their drinking and are interested to learn about moderate drinking or abstaining. Like *Drinker's Checkup* it is also evidence-based, and the modest program fee supports a nonprofit organization that "aims to help people make responsible decisions about their drinking" and to assist those who wish to cut down on their alcohol use.

Advantages of Computer Assessment

Computer-based interviews have been used to assess a wide variety of medical and behavioral factors that are important in the medical care of patients, as summarized in the following chart:

MEDICAL HISTORY/ROS	PSYCHIATRIC HISTORY
Adverse drug reactions	Suicide risk assessment
Compliance monitoring	Symptom monitoring
Sexual abuse/trauma	Eating disorders
HIV risk assessment	Substance abuse
Sexual function	Risky behaviors

Patients have great difficulty disclosing during the medical encounter information related to their behavior or experiences that are private, embarrassing, or shameful, even when the disclosure is vital to their care. The most common examples are matters of sexual behavior, gender identity and orientation, histories of traumatic experiences, substance abuse, and sexually transmitted diseases. Furthermore, the US Preventive Services Task Force is concerned that most clinicians do not do an adequate job collecting this type of information during routine care. In contrast, computers have generally outperformed clinicians in collecting such information when it has been collected using queries delivered by a computer. Despite the widespread bias that machines would not be effective in such sensitive dialogue, it has been shown repeatedly that well-written computer interviews that can establish rapport and provide reasonable assurance about privacy of the information provided can elicit histories from patients indicating greater levels of disclosure (Locke et al., 1992; Richens et al., 2010).

In addition to minimizing the potential for embarrassment, computer-based interviews offer the opportunity for enhanced privacy, anonymity, and greater reliability. In addition, an interview administered by a computer has potential multilingual capability and can even include comprehension checks along with a built-in glossary to increase the likelihood that the information is tailored for the individual patient.

COMPUTER-BASED PATIENT EDUCATION

When Dr. Slack arrived in Boston in 1970, he and his colleagues undertook a series of studies designed to assess the ability of computers not only to take a history but also to assist patients in making informed medical decisions about treatment. In one study, 46 women with symptoms of a urinary tract infection (UTI) were offered interactive computer-based education about the routine treatment for a UTI, including the option of initiating immediate treatment with oral sulfisoxazole while awaiting the results of the urine culture. Provided by the computer with balanced, easy-to-understand information about the options, 35 women decided to take the sulfisoxazole without waiting for the culture results; one decided to wait for the culture (which was negative), and 10 were referred for further evaluation. Of the 35 who elected to take the medication, 30 thought that a program that enabled them to make the decision was "a good thing" and only one thought it "better if left up to someone else."

In the ensuing years the field of informed medical decisionmaking grew, and the role of tailored patient educational materials has expanded into a billion-dollar industry. Early in the dot-com boom, former Surgeon General C. Everett Koop helped to found *DrKoop.com,* which became famous for the tagline "information is the best medicine," which was coined for a patient education media venture. The first consumer education website for mental health was launched in January 1995 as *Psych Central: John Grohol's Mental Health Page;* it got its start by indexing online support groups in the summer of 1991. Psych Central is currently the Internet's oldest independent mental health and psychology network, as well as the largest; it reports having 1.5 million users every month.

Another leading site for consumer and patient health education is Healthwise.org. Founded by Don Kemper in 1975 as a print media producer, Healthwise.org is a nonprofit educational resource dedicated to "helping people make better health decisions [by providing] content that's easy to understand, engaging, and motivating." Healthwise is now a major online provider of both interactive health content and decision support tools; its content is tested with consumers and clinicians for quality, accuracy, and usability, and requires that information provided is evidence-based and reviewed by experts.

WebMD is another major force in online consumer health education, a major provider of health information services for consumers, physicians, healthcare professionals, employers, and health plan providers. Like Healthwise, WebMD has an editorial board and process to ensure the quality of its content. There are other commercial health information websites, of varying quality, too numerous to mention. However, there are also educational websites created and maintained by academic institutions that leverage their faculty and their brand to build consumer confidence in the quality of their information.

Several companies that provide patient and consumer education grew out of the laboratories of academic researchers that leveraged the ability to increase dissemination through the advantages of commercialization. One such example is HealthMedia. Founded in 1998 by Dr. Victor Strecher, HealthMedia focuses on the development of tailored patient education materials. Initially, computers were used to produce tailored print media for patient education; later, technology was developed to assemble tailored videos assembled on the fly for individual patients and shipped to their homes from massive video servers. HealthMedia has developed a technological methodology that effectively emulates a health coaching session without the coach, using interactive media (now delivered over the Internet) that offers the advantages of scalability and economy. The company conducts and publishes outcomes research on their programs to determine the impact on compliance, medical utilization, and productivity. The research is conducted through an exclusive relationship with the Health Media Research Laboratory (HMRL) at the University of Michigan, which provides ongoing research for HealthMedia. In turn, the for-profit company builds commercial digital health coaching programs that are science-based and designed to deliver measurable outcomes. This partnership between a private company and academic institution has been successful and offers a model for other, similar ventures in behavioral medicine.

In addition to HealthMedia, several for-profit companies focus on population health management, and contract with large employers and integrated delivery systems. The degree of customization, personalization, tailoring, and interactivity varies a great deal among the various vendors and providers, with a general trend to move toward greater interactivity and mobile applications ("apps") for smartphones and tablet computing. Behavioral health is increasingly being integrated into population health programs, as its relevance to overall health outcomes is more widely recognized.

In 1959, Ledley and Lusted published in *Science* a rules-based probability model that could be adapted for use in clinical reasoning. During the next decade, Morris Collen at Kaiser Permanente Health Plan instituted a computer-assisted system to aid medical diagnosis, using questions and symptoms on computer punch cards that were sorted by patients into yes and no piles and then tabulated by machine processing. However, the first use of a computer to assist a clinician in diagnosis and to guide management of a patient's condition was the acid–base decision support program developed by Howard Bleich at Beth Israel Hospital in 1969. Since that time computers have become widely used to guide treatment, but only recently have they been introduced into clinical psychiatry.

During the 1970s, the field of artificial intelligence and expert systems provided the tools for the growing integration of decision support tools into general medical care. This was largely driven by the economic incentives of managed care in an effort to control costs. During the 1980s, this wave swept through mental health; managed behavioral healthcare companies ("carve-outs") developed computer-based decision support tools to guide their utilization reviewers and care managers in allocating only that level of treatment that was deemed medically necessary. Thus, for most clinicians, the first introduction to decision support in mental health was more focused on benefit to the payer rather than to the patient or the clinician.

In the same era, however, clinical researchers began to evaluate the usefulness of computers as tools to guide clinicians in the care of their patients. Tools were developed to assist not only in diagnosis but also to suggest treatment strategies using evidence-based algorithms developed by clinical experts (Oquendo et al., 2003; Osser, 1993; Trivedi et al., 1998; Trivedi, Fava, Marangell, Osser, & Shelton, 2006). Patients with major depression treated in the Texas Algorithm Medication Project using a computer-assisted decision support system showed greater improvement in their depression than those who received treatment as usual (Trivedi et al., 2004). However, the real challenge is less likely to be the issue of efficacy or even of cost-efficiency than the need to overcome the barriers to adoption of decision support tools in systems of care (Trivedi et al., 2009). Perhaps the most successful of all the innovations in computer-based decision support for both clinicians and patients has been the widespread availability of online drug–drug and drug–food interaction checkers. Finally, the free online resource from the National Library of Medicine, PubMed, makes it easy for clinicians, patients, and family members to search the Medline database.

PATIENT-CENTERED CARE AND SHARED DECISION MAKING

Reflecting a paradigm shift in healthcare, the concept of "shared decisionmaking" emerged during the 1990s and had a marked impact on the doctor–patient relationship. The revolutionary societal changes in the 1960s caused a mistrust of authority and yearning for autonomy that served as a catalyst in fostering the emergence of a new model, "patient-centered care" (Gerteis & Commonwealth Program for Patient-Centered Care, 1993). As the new paradigm arose, the centuries-old traditional authoritarian or paternalistic model yielded to social pressure, as melodramatically depicted in the film *Patch Adams*. Patient-centered care leveled the playing field for patients and doctors and laid the foundation for the development of decision support tools not only for use by clinicians but also by patients and families. This sea change in healthcare took on the qualities of a social movement, spearheaded by Dartmouth's John Wennberg who coined the term *informed shared medical decisionmaking*, and its tenets became embodied in the influential report of the Institute of Medicine, *Crossing the Quality Chasm* (Institute of Medicine, 2001). The wide dissemination and influence of the IOM report helped to accelerate the development and adoption of new information technologies by legitimizing and endorsing the paradigm shift. Thus emerged patient-centric clinical computing, tailored Internet-based consumer health education, and online tools to assist with personal healthcare decisions (Drake, Cimpean, & Torrey, 2009). Medical information websites for patients as consumers have changed the physician–patient relationship. No longer are physicians the sole providers of guidance to patients. Rather, their role has been to help patients evaluate information, and the emerging paradigm in information age medicine is that of "shared decisionmaking."

Use of technology in Shared Decision Making

The forerunner of modern shared decision-making tools was the *Problem Knowledge Coupler* (PKC) developed in the early 1980s by Lawrence Weed, creator of the problem-oriented medical record. Weed and his followers used computers to assemble structured information about patients from their histories, physical findings, and lab results, and used combinatorial rather than probabilistic or algorithmic logic to discern patterns that guided diagnostic and care management decisions. What was especially revolutionary was that the clinicians who used the PKCs showed the computer screens to the patients and invited them to participate in the clinical reasoning and treatment planning.

Weed's pioneering work on decision aids influenced a generation of health services researchers including John Wennberg, Albert Mulley, and Michael Barry, who created the Foundation for Informed Medical Decision Making (FIMDM) as a joint venture between Dartmouth Medical School and Massachusetts General Hospital. FIMDM was founded to study the role of informed shared medical decision making in helping patients and their doctors to manage important medical conditions, including coronary artery disease, prostate cancer, breast cancer, back pain, osteoarthritis, benign uterine conditions, depression, diabetes, and benign prostatic hyperplasia.

They define shared decisionmaking as "a style of counseling in which the healthcare provider communicates to the patient personalized information about the options, outcomes, probabilities, and scientific uncertainties of available treatment options, and the patient communicates his or her values and the relative importance he or she places on benefits and harms . . . True shared decisionmaking requires three key elements: a patient who is fully informed about the risks and benefits of all viable options, an involved patient (and family members, if appropriate), and a shared process that involves both healthcare provider and patient."

The Foundation has been a leader in using technology to provide high-quality, unbiased, easily understood information to patients about their condition and its treatment so that they can make an informed decision about their treatment options with confidence. In research using interactive media and linear videotapes, FINDM researchers have studied how creating a caring and compassionate learning environment, in which shared decisions can be made by patients in partnership with their doctors, affects the choices that patients make and their satisfaction with the outcomes.

The Foundation's decision aids can be accessed on their website at http://www.informedmedicaldecisions.org/patient_decision_aids.html.

Decision Aid titles that pertain to psychiatry in the general medical setting include the following:

- Acute Lower Back Pain: Managing Your Pain Through Self Care
- Chronic Low Back Pain: Managing Your Pain and Your Life
- Living with Metastatic Breast Cancer: Making the Journey Your Own
- Living Better with Chronic Pain
- Living with Diabetes: Making Lifestyle Changes to Last a Lifetime
- Looking Ahead: Choices for Medical Care When You're Seriously Ill
- Coping with Symptoms of Depression
- Growing Older, Staying Well
- Sleeping Better: Help for Long-Term Insomnia

In the future, there will be cloud-based interactive multimedia platforms that patients can access via the Internet that will deliver informed medical decision-making aids to patients and families that can be "prescribed" by their clinical team to assist them in making medical decisions about treatment. Successful implementation of the shared decisionmaking model requires that the clinician assess the patient's capacity to exercise adequate judgment in clinical decision making.

COMPUTER-GUIDED AND COMPUTER-ADMINISTERED PSYCHOTHERAPIES

Despite the availability of evidence-based behavioral treatments for mental disorders, there are barriers that have prevented them from reaching the majority of the people suffering from mental illness who might benefit from them. These barriers include cost, availability, logistics, stigma, and training. Computer-assisted or online self-guided treatment, under appropriate clinical supervision, has the potential to vastly increase affordability and access to effective treatments. Computer delivery of behavioral therapies represents the possibility for models of care that can be used for population health management and lead to affordable and effective improvements in public health.

The first reported use of computers in psychotherapy was that of Kenneth Colby and his colleagues at Stanford University in 1966. Colby, a maverick psychoanalyst working in the Department of Computer Science at Stanford, created "Overcoming Depression," a program that used an early version of natural language processing to lead a patient through a course of cognitive behavioral therapy for depression (Colby, Watt, & Gilbert, 1966). In 1977, Slack developed a form of computer-guided therapy that he called "soliloquy therapy." Based on the premise that talking about one's problems can be salutary, Slack programmed a computer to ask people in simple language if they felt sad or blue. If a volunteer answered using the keyboard that he did, the program then asked, "Tell me about your sadness." Other prompts were used to engage the patient and reinforce speaking freely. In those days very few computers understood speech, so Slack's program simply "listened" as the subjects spoke into a microphone and when the patient stopped speaking, it encouraged the person to continue. At the conclusion of the preliminary study, Slack noted that the subjects reported that they felt better, and although the design did not permit conclusions about the effectiveness of soliloquy therapy he tucked it away until two decades later, when he and his colleagues conducted a randomized clinical trial that showed that soliloquy therapy reduced anxiety (Slack, Porter, Balkin, Kowaloff, & Slack, 1990).

During the 1980s, computer-based self-help programs made their appearance. A self-help sweepstakes held in 1985 included among its entrants several behavioral programs: Managing Stress, Problem Solving, Stress and Conflict, and Coping with Stress (Turkle, 1995). Roger Gould, a psychiatrist at UCLA, created a stress management program called the *Therapeutic Learning Program*, a problem-solving therapy that used natural language processing to help people identify and solve personal problems. The program was used at Harvard Community Health Plan and at Kaiser Permanente Medical Group in California (Colby, Gould, & Aronson, 1989).

A series of computer-delivered behavior therapy programs were developed in the 1990s by Lee Baer, John Greist, Isaac Marks, and their colleagues in the United States and Great Britain. These international collaborators developed cognitive behavioral therapy (CBT) programs for depression, anxiety, and obsessive compulsive disorder. The programs were tested in clinical trials, and the behavioral program for depression, COPE, was tested in an open trial of patients with mild to moderate depression. COPE consisted of an introductory videotape and 9 booklets, accompanied by 11 telephone calls to an IVR system that made self-help recommendations to patients based on information they entered. The study team reported clinical improvement in the patients that was on the scale of that seen in studies of antidepressant medication. In a randomized clinical trial of patients with obsessive compulsive disorder, these investigators found that computer-guided CBT was more effective than self-guided therapy delivered by IVR, but that both were more effective than a relaxation control (Greist et al., 2002).

Currently, self-guided treatment programs are mostly based upon forms of CBT (Baer, Greist, & Marks, 2007). Most of these programs focus on depression, but some have also focused on anxiety, eating disorders, and substance abuse. Some of these programs are standalone programs that run on a computer; others are available via the Internet. Some programs are merely text on a screen, while others use interactive multimedia. In addition, programs at the intersection of wellness and mental health have addressed smoking cessation, weight loss, risky drinking, and medication adherence. These programs have been used more widely in Great Britain, New Zealand, and Australia, where the health systems make it easier to deploy the programs and the governments support their development. Meta-analyses have shown the field of self-guided, computer-based treatments is still in its infancy. In a recent review of computer-assisted psychotherapy, Cartreine, Locke, and Ahern concluded that some treatments work better than others and that although they are sometimes as effective as face-to-face therapy, they do not appear to be better. They also believed that because of their scalability, and the observation that dropout rates in computer-based CBT is similar to that of face to face treatment, computer-delivered self-guided therapy may have a role in population health management for selected patients or for use in conjunction with clinical care (Cartreine, Ahern, & Locke, 2010).

Another use of computers in psychotherapy is as a therapist-assist technology for in-session use. Programs have been developed for use by a clinician that guides the therapist through the delivery of a structured care program, such as CBT or exposure therapy. Such programs enable nonspecialist clinicians to deliver specialized behavioral healthcare in the office, by telephone, or over the Internet (with appropriate security). This technology can be very advantageous in rural or other resource-poor settings. It also facilitates the development of highly specialized treatments that can be delivered using evidence-based treatments that have been manualized and adapted for delivery by a clinician guided by a computer. These treatments can be delivered either in a supervised clinical setting or in a behavioral health medical home to a select subset of patients screened to ensure that their complexity, symptom severity, and comorbidities do not preclude remote care. Psychotherapy assistive technologies are being studied for use with veterans with PTSD, adolescents with depression, and patients with phobias. As the evidence accrues for their efficacy, safety, and efficiency, it may be possible to have behavioral healthcare managers assigned to clusters of primary care practices and delivering care to some patients remotely.

APPLICATIONS OF ADVANCED BEHAVIORAL TECHNOLOGIES IN HEALTHCARE

Some of psychiatry's most sophisticated technologies leap right off the pages of science fiction comic books and out of futuristic television shows. Virtual reality, in which a user sits inside a simulator or dons a helmet with a small computer screen inside, is routinely used to treat PTSD in veterans. Building on the basic principles of script therapy, virtual reality exposure therapy (Rothbaum, 2010) places the patient back into the warzone environment in which they suffered a trauma. Therapists have the ability to control environmental variables to recreate the precise amount of daylight, smells, background noises, and general setting in which the event occurred. Relaxation coaching and traditional habituation techniques are then practiced within these environments. Similar simulators have been constructed for a number of specific phobias (heights, airplanes, animals), and, more poignantly, for victims of the World Trade Center attacks.

Virtual worlds, such as Linden Labs' *Second Life* (Linden Lab, 2009), offer novel ways for psychiatric engagement and education. In Second Life, users operate avatars to negotiate interactions with other individuals—shopping, hanging out at cafes, conducting research at virtual libraries, and attending virtual seminars. The MGH Benson-Henry institute has offered courses in relaxation within this virtual world; the UC Davis department of psychiatry replicated their clinic within Second Life and developed a psychosis simulator, in which users can walk through a virtual clinic and experience what it must be like to have schizophrenia. Some practitioners are also conducting group and individual therapy sessions within private practice offices (Gorrindo & Groves, 2009).

The "Games for Health" movement largely focuses on the use of video games as a means of engaging and educating patients about disease, compliance, and treatment. Successful games have been used for improving diet, motivating physical activity, increasing asthma regimen compliance, pediatric cancer education, substance abuse education, and facilitating diabetes regimen compliance and understanding (http://www.gamesforhealth.org/). This burgeoning field has gained increasing momentum over the last few years, with annual conferences and a peer-review journal.

BEHAVIORAL TELEMEDICINE

Telemedicine holds the great promise of being able to connect patient and provider over great distance. Using two-way interactive videoconferencing, telepsychiatry (a branch of telemedicine) allows those who have difficulty accessing traditional office-based care to obtain mental health services. Applications of telepsychiatry include prehospitalization assessment and post-hospital follow-up care, scheduled and urgent outpatient visits, medication management, psychotherapy, and consultation. While psychiatric specialists are often located at some distance from the patients they are evaluating, best practice guidelines required that appropriate staff be available to meet patient needs before, during, and after mental health telemedicine encounters (Yellowlees, Shore, & Roberts, 2010). Numerous studies have suggested that clinical outcomes and patient satisfaction are similar when comparing telepsychiatry and in-person based interventions (Sharp, Kobak, & Osman, 2011).

Recent studies have examined the feasibility, utility, and cost-effectiveness of asynchronous telepsychiatry. This novel "store-and-forward" methodology allows clinical data, including video, to be collected by nurse practitioners or other medical specialists using structured or semistructured interviews. The compiled data and video are then forwarded to a psychiatrist for diagnostic review and treatment planning (Butler & Yellowlees, 2011). Recommendations are often returned to primary care providers via letter or email for implementation.

LEGAL, REGULATORY, AND LIABILITY ISSUES

Computer software delivered via desktop computers, the Internet, or mobile platforms will transform healthcare. The programs, services, and devices have the potential for causing both advantageous and harmful effects. Although the federal government's role in protecting the public through the regulation of medical devices has been a subject for political discourse including legislation offered in both the House and Senate, in 2011 the Food and Drug Administration (FDA) announced plans to publish a new guidance document that will define the types of clinical decision support (CDS) software it will regulate. With the growing trend to offer decision support on mobile platforms (smartphones and tablets), the FDA's guidance will shape the future of behavioral telehealth. Even though a few years have passed since the initial announcement, FDA has recently reaffirmed its intention to draft this guidance.

In September 2011, the FDA gave its clearest explanation to date regarding what it expects to include in the CDS category. The agency identified three sources of information as helping to define CDS: (1) that entered into the database either manually or automatically, gathered from any source (including data from a medical device, environmental data, or demographic data); (2) that converted by any means including algorithms, formulae, database look-ups or comparisons, or rules or associations; (3) that which produces actionable information, presumably intended for use in the diagnosis of disease or other conditions, or in the cure, mitigation, treatment, or prevention of disease.

In assessing software for regulatory purposes, it is important to distinguish between software that merely provides support and analysis, and software that actually performs a measurement. FDA sent a warning letter on March 15, 2012, to NeuroTax regarding its product MindStreams. FDA declared the software to be a medical device because the software allowed a physician or psychologist to assess cognitive deficits in patients by having the patient respond to prompts. Software that actually measures cognitive function is not CDS.

UNREGULATED PRODUCTS

As explained in a 2013 guidance that FDA issued on mobile medical applications, FDA does not regulate those manual office functions that are simply automated for the ease of the user (e.g., office automation). But if software is intended to help with any part of cure, mitigation, treatment, or prevention of disease or a medical condition, the FDA may consider it a *device*. For example, a program or website that queries patients about behavioral symptoms and tallies them up and presents the score to a clinician is an unregulated application. If, however, the tallied score is provided to the patient, along with a diagnosis and treatment recommendations, the FDA is likely to regulate it. What is less clear is the use of technology to support self-care, especially in the context of wellness and health promotion.

PREMARKET REVIEWED PRODUCTS

The answer to the question of whether the FDA will require premarket review is a moving target. Experts anticipate that the FDA will provide greater clarity in their forthcoming guidance document. Software functions likely to require review might include real-time or online patient monitoring, alarms and alerts capability, seriousness of the disease intended to be monitored, the device's contribution to the decision-making process, innovation in data output, individualized patient care recommendations, and the transparency of decision mechanisms. Programs that assess suicide or homicide risk raise obvious regulatory as well as liability concerns.

CURRENTLY REGULATED PRODUCTS

In April 2014 the FDA, with guidance from the Office of the National Coordinator (ONC) and the FCC, explained that it does not intend to focus its regulatory oversight on the following products/functionalities, even if they meet the statutory definition of a medical device:

- Evidence-based clinician order sets tailored for a particular condition, disease, or clinician preference
- Drug-drug interaction and drug-allergy contraindication alerts to avert adverse drug events
- Most drug dosing calculations
- Drug formulary guidelines
- Reminders for preventative care (e.g., depression screening, mammography, colonoscopy, immunizations, etc.)
- Facilitation of access to treatment guidelines and other reference material that can provide information relevant to particular patients
- Calculation of prediction rules and severity of illness assessments (e.g., PHQ-9, AUDIT, Montreal Cognitive Assessment, Young Mania Rating Scale, APACHE score, Charlson Index)
- Duplicate testing alerts
- Suggestions for possible diagnoses based on patient-specific information retrieved from a patient's EHR

In that same report, FDA offered examples of CDS it *does* plan to regulate, including:

- Computer-aided detection/diagnostic software
- Remote display or notification of real-time alarms (physiological, technical, advisory) from bedside monitors
- Radiation treatment planning
- Robotic surgical planning and control
- Electrocardiography analytical software (and, by implication, electroencephalographic or fMRI analytic software)

The cost of an FDA premarket review for a small company attempting to develop clinical innovations is considerable and can be an obstacle for healthcare improvement. Consequently, the need to protect the public must be balanced against the need for a business climate that supports innovation. The challenge is to exploit the potential benefits of behavioral telehealth when integrated into general medical care so as to maximize benefit and minimize risk of harm.

TECHNOLOGY IN THE RELATIONSHIP

Psychiatry has often distinguished itself from many other fields within medicine through explicit attention to the rules under which the physician and patient interact, often referred to as *the frame*. It has long been held that psychiatrists should withhold details about their personal lives and avoid interacting with patients outside of the office to protect the treatment relationship. The goal has been to preserve a *tabula rasa* so that traditional psychotherapeutic dynamics (e.g., transference and projections) could be understood and leveraged within treatment. Physicians are taught to avoid revealing too many personal details about their lives and to confine their relationship with the patient to clinical space. Through the eyes of the patient, the modern physician lives and dies within the confines of the exam room, never to leave and encounter the real world pressures of kids, friendships, and hobbies. For most psychiatrists in nonrural settings, this was a pretty straightforward task prior to the Internet age but has become almost impossible in modern times.

It is estimated that that two-thirds of US households have broadband connections to the Internet and that nearly 80% of broadband users have searched for health information online (Fox, 2011). While it is not surprising that most of these Internet searches center on disease and treatment, most providers are surprised to learn that 44% of Internet users look for information about doctors or other health professionals (Fox, 2011). Most patients are likely looking for information pertinent to their care, such as where the doctor went to school or contact information, rather than personal details. However, modern search engines comingle the personal and professional spheres; patients are bound to stumble upon one while looking for the other.

Many physicians have taken an abstinence approach to this problem, electing not to post or publish any personal information on the Internet; almost all physicians, however, now have some digital footprint (Gorrindo & Groves, 2008). Mortgage records, campaign donations, state medical board profiles, and neighborhood newsletters are just a few of the many channels through which easily discoverable information is published to the Internet without explicit approval. The *modern physician* recognizes this fact and chooses not to shy away from the digital world, but rather to embrace it as a way of promoting his public self, managing this tricky negotiation carefully and intentionally.

EMAIL

For physicians who are facile with computers and the Internet, email affords quick communication with patients and it offers the benefit of instant documentation of a conversation. In 2008, it was estimated that approximately 30% of physicians emailed with their patients (Menachemi, Prickett, & Brooks, 2011). Modern search engines have facilitated the ascertainment of physician email addresses for patients; consequently, physicians who have been reluctant to engage in email exchanges with patients may find themselves receiving emails regardless.

The major pitfalls associated with patient–physician emails fall into several categories. First, there are regulatory guidelines surrounding the encryption and integrity of email communication, which is much higher than the regular email systems most physicians use for their personal email accounts. The second regards the mechanics of which types of requests are appropriate for email. Most would argue that medical emergencies should not be conveyed via email, but even mundane tasks such as scheduling may not be appropriate for practices where outside email communication runs the risk of disrupting practice flow. Finally, there is the risk that email communications might be misunderstood or misinterpreted, resulting in an experience where the patient might feel ashamed, confused, or disregarded.

The Federation of State Medical Boards and the AMA have some specific guidelines when it comes to email with patients. Both organizations suggest that:

1. Medical professionals should have written policies that describe the appropriate use of email, the types of transactions that are appropriate for email, and the limitations to privacy that may come with email communication. This process should be treated with the same attention to detail as one might use in obtaining informed consent from a patient for a medication.

2. Medical professionals should use email systems that are encrypted and HIPAA compliant.

3. Medical professionals should establish an appropriate system for inserting email communications into a patient's medical record.

4. Email communications with patients must be secure; ordinary email does not afford this required protection. Most private EHR systems include this functionality. Additionally, there are commercial vendors of secure email and messaging (e.g., Zixcorp and McKesson). Practitioners should avoid anger, sarcasm, harsh criticism, and libelous references to third parties in messages.

5. Practitioners should consider using commercially available encryption software for laptops, smartphones, and tablets. This is especially important for external hard drives and memory sticks (or thumb drives) that may contain protected health information and are easily lost or stolen.

SOCIAL MEDIA

Websites such as Facebook, LinkedIn, and Google Plus are among some of the most common social network sites. A recent trend has been the evolution of support groups for patients with chronic illness from face-to-face meetings to the creation of online communities, leveraging the power of social media to create ways for patients living with chronic conditions to learn from and support each other. One of the

best-know examples is PatientsLikeMe (PatientsLikeMe.com), co-founded in 2004 by three MIT engineers. The team created a consumer-oriented online health data-sharing platform intended to transform the way patients manage their own conditions, as well as to change the way industry conducts research and improves patient care. The power of social networking, though, lies in the connections "between the pages"; Facebook contains powerful search tools that allow a user to find friends or acquaintances and then view their pages. Social networks allow a user to build a virtual web connecting millions of people, where ideas and personal information flow freely. These sites are built to encourage the sharing of personal information including hobbies, favorite music, personal photos, and even birthdays. Privacy settings, when used appropriately, can limit a user's personal information to just friends or acquaintances, but such settings often are left at their default values by users, thus permitting the sites to potentially reveal personal information to anyone on the Internet.

When medical professionals use social networking websites, they need to be mindful of posting personal and unprofessional material. A study in 2008 estimated that 64% of medical students and 13% of residents used Facebook (Thompson et al., 2008). Since that time, use of Facebook and social network technology has grown throughout the general population and has likely grown within medical community as well. Strikingly, in this study only a third of these Facebook profiles were made private, and most accounts shared at least one personal detail.

Medical professionals must always be mindful of how information might be perceived by others, especially if it runs the risk of portraying them as unprofessional. For example, posting pictures from a Halloween party that shows the physician clearly intoxicated while dressed in scrubs might be misconstrued as drinking on the job by a patient who stumbled across the photo.

There are several guidelines for using social networking websites:

1. Physicians should use built-in privacy settings to limit the amount of personal information that is available to the general public and patients. What items are available to the public should support the physician's professional "brand" or identity.

2. Physicians should always ask themselves, "What would a potential patient think about what I'm about to post? Is there a way in which I might be misunderstood?"

3. Physicians should not "friend" patients on their social networking websites, because it implies that it is within their scope of practice to spend time socially with a patient.

BLOGS AND WEBSITES

It has become increasingly common for hospital and clinics to create webpages for their physicians containing basic demographic and clinic-related information. It is not uncommon that a physician might have a personal webpage or a blog, as well. A physician can easily post thoughts or musings on a blog without the technical know-how necessary for building or running an entire website. While only a small number of medical professionals currently use blogs, in a study of blogs written by self-identified medical professionals it was estimated the 40% of blogs described individual patients, sometimes with enough detail that the patient might actually be identifiable (Lagu, Kaufman, Asch, & Armstrong, 2008). And, given the self-reflective nature of what most people post on blogs, it's not uncommon for physicians with blogs to want to write about medicine. But what happens when one also wants to write about events in one's personal life, or even one's political interpretation of current events? As patients search for information on their physicians, they will be pleased to find the medical information posted by their physicians on webpages and blogs—but what will they think of the personal information, and how will that information change their perception of their physicians? Physicians who wish to have webpages or blogs should consider having separate personal and professional web personas as a way of mitigating any conflation that might occur from having medical information intermixed with personal information.

As a corollary, physicians should also have a constant awareness of what is posted about them on the Internet. Physicians should be searching for their own names on a regular basis. In this exercise, the physician should be asking, what would a patient think of me? What if this was the only information they had about me? Physicians should act promptly to remove incorrect, inappropriate, or deceptive information. Online reputation management services may be helpful should physicians have names that could be confused with web content that would lessen a physician's public image.

TWITTER

Twitter is a social networking and microblogging service that allows users to "tweet" by posting short messages (up to 140 characters in length) to followers. Typically, the content of these tweets focuses on whatever is on the user's mind, and often the content of tweets direct people to websites and news stories. The strict limit on the lengths of tweets forces messages to be concise and to the point. However, the brevity of these messages creates the potential for messages to be misunderstood. For example, "What a day today has been," could convey elation, disgust, defeat, or even shame.

Twitter does, however, have utility to medical professionals; when used to promote one's brand or professional identity it can be a particularly engaging way to patient to follow their physician. Appropriate uses of tweets in the context might be, "This month is depression awareness month. Be sure to call us if you would like to learn more," or, "We are pleased to announce the addition of Dr. Smith to our practice," or, "Interesting new study published today reminding us about the importance of Vitamin D," with a link attached. These uses promote professional identity as well as the health of the

patient. They also boost patient engagement in a physician's practice, with little in the way of additional financial or personnel cost to the practice.

GENERAL GUIDANCE

In recent years hospitals, medical schools, and medical societies have created general guidelines for physicians around appropriate online use. The American Medical Association (Shore, Halsey, Shah, Crigger, & Douglas, 2011) provides a few guiding principles for physicians to consider when engaging patients on the Internet and in managing their digital presence:

1. Physicians should maintain an awareness of patient privacy and confidentiality consideration at all times.

2. Physicians should use privacy settings.

3. Physicians should routinely monitor their own Internet presence.

4. Physicians must maintain appropriate boundaries of the patient–physician relationship.

5. Physicians should consider separating personal and professional content online.

6. Physicians should notify colleagues if they see unprofessional material online.

7. Physicians must recognize that actions online and content posted may negatively affect their reputations and can undermine public trust in the medical profession.

It should also be noted that different generations of physicians may require different types of guidance (Gorrindo & Groves, 2011). For those physicians who feel uncomfortable with technology and who simply need enough knowledge to "stay out of trouble," starting with a basic primer about social media may be useful and sufficient. The CDC has published a social media kit (http://www.cdc.gov/healthcommunication/ToolsTemplates/SocialMediaToolkit_BM.pdf) that provides nuts-and-bolts level information about social media technology along with concrete advice for practitioners to embrace social media as a way of building an online presence that supports and enhances an appropriate professional identity. In contrast, physicians who grew up with technology and feel facile within Web 2.0 tools may need guidance that focuses on online professionalism, maintaining boundaries, and balancing the personal and professional when online.

CLINICAL PEARLS

- Patients' preferences to make disclosures during a computerized interview have been shown regarding questions about substance abuse, sexual behavior, and sexually transmitted diseases such as HIV (Locke et al., 1992; Richens et al., 2010), suggesting that computers are experienced as less judgmental.

- One website, PsychCentral (www.psychcentral.com) is a frequently updated source of self-assessment tools that can be used with patients.

- A search at www.nimh.gov, nida.gov, or va.gov will lead to other useful validated tools, available online and downloadable for use in clinical practice.

- Technology Linked Care (TLC) has screened for depression, dysthymia, bipolar disorder, PTSD, acute stress disorder, generalized anxiety disorder, panic disorder, somatization, social phobia, alcohol and drug abuse, stress, and violence. Usually, after screening, the automated IVR system encourages the person to seek help, provides resources, and monitors adherence using follow-up calls to ensure help has been sought (Farzanfar, Stevens, Vachon, Friedman, & Locke, 2007).

- Medical information websites for patients as consumers have changed the physician–patient relationship. No longer are physicians the sole providers of guidance to patients. Rather, their role has been to help patients evaluate information, and the emerging paradigm in information-age medicine is that of "shared decisionmaking."

- Successful implementation of the shared decisionmaking model requires that the clinician assess the patient's capacity to exercise adequate judgment in clinical decision making.

- In a recent review of computer-assisted psychotherapy, Cartreine, Locke, and Ahern concluded that some treatments work better than others, and that though they are sometimes as effective as face-to-face therapy, they do not appear to be better.

- When medical professionals use social networking websites, they need to be mindful of posting personal and unprofessional material.

- The *modern physician* chooses not to shy away from the digital world, but rather to embrace it as a way of promoting his public self, managing this tricky negotiation carefully and intentionally.

- Medical professionals should have written policies that describe the appropriate use of email, the types of transactions that are appropriate for email, and the limitations to privacy that may come with email communication. This process should be treated with the same attention to detail as one might use in obtaining informed consent from a patient for a medication.

- Practitioners should avoid anger, sarcasm, harsh criticism, and libelous references to third parties in messages.

- Physicians should always ask themselves, "What would a potential patient think about what I'm about to post? Is there a way in which I might be misunderstood?"

- Physicians should not "friend" patients on their social networking websites, because it implies that it is within their scope of practice to spend time socially with a patient.

- For those physicians who feel uncomfortable with technology and who simply need enough knowledge to "stay out of trouble," starting with a basic primer about social media may be useful and sufficient. The CDC has published a social media kit (http://www.cdc.gov/health-communication/ToolsTemplates/SocialMediaToolkit_BM.pdf) that provides nuts-and-bolts level information about social media technology.

DISCLOSURE STATEMENTS

Dr. Locke

Dr. Locke is the Chief Medical Officer of iHope Network, Inc. He is also a shareholder. Dr. Locke is also the Chief Medical Officer of Frame Health, Inc. and is also a shareholder. He is also a consulting psychiatrist at Beth Israel Deaconess Medical Center where he is assisting in the development of a telepsychiatry consulting service to primary care practices.

Dr. Gorrindo

Dr. Gorrindo is the Director of Postgraduate Medical Education at Massachusetts General Hospital and has no commercial disclosures to report.

REFERENCES

Baer, L., Greist, J., & Marks, I. M. (2007). Computer-aided cognitive behaviour therapy. *Psychother Psychosom, 76*(4), 193–195.

Baer, L., Jacobs, D. G., Cukor, P., O'Laughlen, J., Coyle, J. T., & Magruder, K. M. (1995). Automated telephone screening survey for depression. *Journal of the American Medical Association, 273*(24), 1943–1944.

Baicker, K., Cutler, D., & Song, Z. (2010). Workplace wellness programs can generate savings. *Health Affairs, 29*(2), 304–311.

Biskin, B. H., & Kolotkin, R. L. (1977). Effects of computerized administration on scores on the Minnesota Multiphasic Personality Inventory. *Applied Psychological Measurement, 1*(4), 543–549.

Brown, R. L., Leonard, T., Saunders, L. A., & Papasouliotis, O. (2001). A two-item conjoint screen for alcohol and other drug problems. *Journal of the American Board of Family Practice, 14*(2), 95–106.

Bush, K., Kivlahan, D. R., McDonell, M. B., Fihn, S. D., & Bradley, K. A. (1998). The AUDIT alcohol consumption questions (AUDIT-C): an effective brief screening test for problem drinking. Ambulatory Care Quality Improvement Project (ACQUIP). Alcohol Use Disorders Identification Test. *Archives of Internal Medicine, 158*(16), 1789–1795.

Butler, T. N., & Yellowlees, P. (2011). Cost Analysis of Store-and-Forward Telepsychiatry as a Consultation Model for Primary Care. *Telemedicine Journal and e-Health,* Jan–Feb;*18*(1), 74–77.

Cartreine, J. A., Ahern, D. K., & Locke, S. E. (2010). A roadmap to computer-based psychotherapy in the United States. *Harv Rev Psychiatry, 18*(2), 80–95.

Centers for Disease Control. (1984). *CDC health risk appraisal user manual.* Atlanta, GA: Centers for Disease Control, Division of Health Education, Center for Health Promotion and Education.

Chen, C. W., Ju, M. S., Sun, Y. N., & Lin, C. C. K. (2009). Model analyses of visual biofeedback training for EEG-based brain-computer interface. *Journal of computational neuroscience, 27*(3), 357–368.

Ciechanowski, P. S., Katon, W. J., & Russo, J. E. (2000). Depression and diabetes: impact of depressive symptoms on adherence, function, and costs. *Archives of Internal Medicine, 160*(21), 3278–3285.

Colby, K. M., Gould, R. L., & Aronson, G. (1989). Some pros and cons of computer-assisted psychotherapy. *Journal of Nervous and Mental Disease, 177*(2), 105–108.

Colby, K. M., Watt, J. B., & Gilbert, J. P. (1966). A computer method of psychotherapy: preliminary communication. *Journal of Nervous and Mental Disease, 142*(2), 148–152.

Crum, R. (2007). Researchers develop and test six-question tool to screen adolescents for substance abuse in health care settings. Retrieved from http://www.rwjf.org/reports/grr/045222.htm.

Drake, R. E., Cimpean, D., & Torrey, W. C. (2009). Shared decision making in mental health: prospects for personalized medicine. *Dialogues in Clinical Neuroscience, 11*(4), 455–463.

Dube, P., Kurt, K., Bair, M. J., Theobald, D., & Williams, L. S. (2010). The p4 screener: evaluation of a brief measure for assessing potential suicide risk in 2 randomized effectiveness trials of primary care and oncology patients. *Primary Care Companion – Journal of Clinical Psychiatry, 12*(6).

Erdman, H. P., Greist, J. H., Gustafson, D. H., Taves, J. E., & Klein, M. H. (1987). Suicide risk prediction by computer interview: a prospective study. *Journal of Clinical Psychiatry, 48*(12), 464–467.

Farzanfar, R., Locke, S. E., Heeren, T. C., Stevens, A., Vachon, L., Thi Nguyen, M. K., & Friedman, R. H. (2011). Workplace telecommunications technology to identify mental health disorders and facilitate self-help or professional referrals. *American Journal of Health Promotion, 25*(3), 207–216.

Farzanfar, R., Stevens, A., Vachon, L., Friedman, R., & Locke, S. E. (2007). Design and development of a mental health assessment and intervention system. *Journal of Medical Systems, 31*(1), 49–62.

Fowler, R. D., Jr., & Miller, M. L. (1969). Computer interpretation of the MMPI. Its use in clinical practice. *Archives of General Psychiatry, 21*(4), 502–508.

Fox, S. (2011, Feb). *Health Topics.* Pew Internet & American Life Project. Pew Research Center, Washington, DC.

Friedman, R. H., Stollerman, J. E., Mahoney, D. M., & Rozenblyum, L. (1997). The virtual visit: using telecommunications technology to take care of patients. *Journal of the American Medical Informatics Association, 4*(6), 413–425.

Gavin, D. R., Ross, H. E., & Skinner, H. A. (1989). Diagnostic validity of the drug abuse screening test in the assessment of DSM-III drug disorders. *British Journal of Addiction, 84*(3), 301–307.

Gaynes, B. N., West, S. L., Ford, C. A., Frame, P., Klein, J., & Lohr, K. N. (2004). Screening for suicide risk in adults: a summary of the evidence for the US Preventive Services Task Force. *Annals of Internal Medicine, 140*(10), 822–835.

Gerteis, M. P., & Commonwealth Program for Patient-Centered Care. (1993). *Through the patient's eyes: understanding and promoting patient-centered care* (1st ed.). San Francisco: Jossey-Bass.

Gorrindo, T., & Groves, J. E. (2008). Web searching for information about physicians. *Journal of the American Medical Association,, 300*(2), 213–215.

Gorrindo, T., & Groves, J. E. (2009). Computer Simulation and Virtual Reality in the Diagnosis and Treatment of Psychiatric Disorders. *Academic Psychiatry, 33*(5), 413–417.

Gorrindo, T., & Groves, J. E. (2011). Medical eProfessionalism: A tale of two Doctors. *Journal of Clinical Ethics, 22*(2), 176–178.

Greist, J. H., Klein, M. H., & Van Cura, L. J. (1973). A computer interview for psychiatric patient target symptoms. *Archives of General Psychiatry, 29*(2), 247–253.

Greist, J. H., Marks, I. M., Baer, L., Kobak, K. A., Wenzel, K. W., Hirsch, M. J., . . . Clary, C. M. (2002). Behavior therapy for obsessive-compulsive disorder guided by a computer or by a clinician compared with relaxation as a control. *Journal of Clinical Psychiatry, 63*(2), 138–145.

Huskamp, H. A., & Rosenthal, M. B. (2009). Health Risk Appraisals: How Much Do They Influence Employees' Health Behavior? *Health Affairs, 28*(5), 1532–1540.

Hyner, G. C. (1999). *SPM handbook of health assessment tools:* The Society of Prospective Medicine.

Institute of Medicine (U.S.); Committee on Quality of Health Care in America. (2001). *Crossing the quality chasm: a new health system for the 21st century.* Washington, D.C.: National Academy Press.

Johnson, J. H., Giannetti, R. A., & Williams, T. A. (1978). A self-contained microcomputer system for psychological testing. *Behavior Research Methods, 10*(4), 579–581.

Katon, W. (1996). The impact of major depression on chronic medical illness. *General Hospital Psychiatry, 18*(4), 215–219.

Katon, W., & Ciechanowski, P. (2002). Impact of major depression on chronic medical illness. *J Psychosom Res, 53*(4), 859–863.

Kroenke, K., Spitzer, R. L., & Williams, J. B. (2001). The PHQ-9: validity of a brief depression severity measure. *Journal of General Internal Medicine, 16*(9), 606–613.

Lagu, T., Kaufman, E. J., Asch, D. A., & Armstrong, K. (2008). Content of weblogs written by health professionals. *Journal of General Internal Medicine, 23*(10), 1642–1646.

Linden Lab. (2009). *Second Life.* Retrieved from www.secondlife.com.

Locke, S. E., Kowaloff, H. B., Hoff, R. G., Safran, C., Popovsky, M. A., Cotton, D. J., et al. (1992). Computer-based interview for screening blood donors for risk of HIV transmission. *Journal of the American Medical Association,, 268*(10), 1301–1305.

Loeppke, R. (2011). CDC HRA briefing. Retrieved from http://prevent. org/data/files/hra/loeppke-cdc%20hra%20briefing%20short%20 version%202-1-11.pdf

Luoma, J. B., Martin, C. E., & Pearson, J. L. (2002). Contact with mental health and primary care providers before suicide: a review of the evidence. *American Journal of Psychiatry, 159*(6), 909–916.

Maisto, S. A., Connors, G. J., & Allen, J. P. (1995). Contrasting self-report screens for alcohol problems: a review. *Alcoholism: Clinical and Experimental Research, 19*(6), 1510–1516.

Maultsby, M. C., Jr., & Slack, W. V. (1971). A computer-based psychiatry history system. *Archives of General Psychiatry, 25*(6), 570–572.

McDowell, A. K., Lineberry, T. W., & Bostwick, J. M. (2011). Practical suicide-risk management for the busy primary care physician. *Mayo Clinic Proceedings, 86*(8), 792–800.

Menachemi, N., Prickett, C. T., & Brooks, R. G. (2011). The use of physician-patient email: a follow-up examination of adoption and best-practice adherence 2005–2008. *Journal of Medical Internet Research, 13*(1), e23.

Oquendo, M. A., Baca-Garcia, E., Kartachov, A., Khait, V., Campbell, C. E., Richards, M., . . . Mann, J. J. (2003). A computer algorithm for calculating the adequacy of antidepressant treatment in unipolar and bipolar depression. *Journal of Clinical Psychiatry, 64*(7), 825–833.

Osser, D. N. (1993). A systematic approach to the classification and pharmacotherapy of nonpsychotic major depression and dysthymia. *Journal of Clinical Psychopharmacology, 13*(2), 133–144.

Pearson, J. S., Rome, H. P., Swenson, W. M., Mataya, P., & Brannick, T. L. (1965). Development of a computer system for scoring and interpretation of Minnesota Multiphasic Personality Inventories in a medical clinic. *Annals of the New York Academy of Sciences, 126*(2), 684–695.

Richens, J., Copas, A., Sadiq, S. T., Kingori, P., McCarthy, O., Jones, V., . . . Pakianathan, M. (2010). A randomised controlled trial of computer-assisted interviewing in sexual health clinics. *Sexually Transmitted Infections, 86*(4), 310–314.

Rose, G. L., Skelly, J. M., Badger, G. J., Maclean, C. D., Malgeri, M. P., & Helzer, J. E. (2010). Automated screening for at-risk drinking in a primary care office using interactive voice response. *Journal of Studies on Alcohol and Drugs, 71*(5), 734–738.

Rothbaum, B. O. (2010). Virtual reality exposure therapy. *The Corsini Encyclopedia of Psychology.* New York: John Wiley & Sons, Inc.

Roy-Byrne, P. P., Davidson, K. W., Kessler, R. C., Asmundson, G. J., Goodwin, R. D., Kubzansky, L., et al. (2008). Anxiety disorders and comorbid medical illness. *General Hospital Psychiatry, 30*(3), 208–225.

Russell, G., Peace, K., & Mellsop, G. (1986). The reliability of a micro-computer administration of the MMPI. *Journal of Clinical Psychology, 42*(1), 120–122.

Schwartz, M. (2005). *Biofeedback: A Practitioner's Guide* (3rd ed.). New York, NY: Guilford Press.

Selzer, M. L. (1971). The Michigan alcoholism screening test: the quest for a new diagnostic instrument. *American Journal of Psychiatry*, *127*(12), 1653–1658.

Sharp, I. R., Kobak, K. A., & Osman, D. A. (2011). The use of videoconferencing with patients with psychosis: a review of the literature. *Annals of General Psychiatry*, *10*(1), 14.

Shore, R., Halsey, J., Shah, K., Crigger, B., & Douglas, S. (2011). Report of the AMA Council on Ethical and Judicial Affairs: Professionalism in the use of social media. *Journal of Clinical Ethics*, *22*(2), 165–172.

Slack, W. V., Porter, D., Balkin, P., Kowaloff, H. B., & Slack, C. W. (1990). Computer-assisted soliloquy as an approach to psychotherapy. *MD Computing*, *7*(1), 37–42, 58.

Thompson, L. A., Dawson, K., Ferdig, R., Black, E. W., Boyer, J., Coutts, J., & Black, N. P. (2008). The intersection of online social networking with medical professionalism. *Journal of General Internal Medicine*, *23*(7), 954–957.

Trivedi, M., Daly, E., Kern, J., Grannemann, B., Sunderajan, P., & Claassen, C. (2009). Barriers to implementation of a computerized decision support system for depression: an observational report on lessons learned in. *BMC Medical Informatics and Decision Making*, *9*(1), 6.

Trivedi, M. H., DeBattista, C., Fawcett, J., Nelson, C., Osser, D. N., Stein, D., & Jobson, K. (1998). Developing treatment algorithms for unipolar depression in Cyberspace: International Psychopharmacology Algorithm Project (IPAP). *Psychopharmacology Bulletin*, *34*(3), 355–359.

Trivedi, M. H., Fava, M., Marangell, L. B., Osser, D. N., & Shelton, R. C. (2006). Use of treatment algorithms for depression. *Primary Care Companion – Journal of Clinical Psychiatry*, *8*(5), 291–298.

Trivedi, M. H., Rush, A. J., Crismon, M. L., Kashner, T. M., Toprac, M. G., Carmody, T. J., et al. (2004). Clinical results for patients with major depressive disorder in the Texas Medication Algorithm Project. *Archives of General Psychiatry*, *61*(7), 669–680.

Turkle, S. (1995). *Life on the Screen: Identity in the Age of the Internet*: Simon and Schuster.

Turvey, C. L., Willyard, D., Hickman, D. H., Klein, D. M., & Kukoyi, O. (2007). Telehealth screen for depression in a chronic illness care management program. *Telemedicine Journal and e-Health*, *13*(1), 51–56.

Vannoy, S. D., Fancher, T., Meltvedt, C., Unützer, J., Duberstein, P., & Kravitz, R. L. (2010). Suicide Inquiry in Primary Care: creating context, inquiring, and following up. *Annals of Family Medicine, 8*, 33–39.

Weizenbaum, J. (1966). ELIZA—a computer program for the study of natural language communication between man and machine. *Communications of the ACM, 9*(1), 36–45.

Whittaker, R., McRobbie, H., Bullen, C., Borland, R., Rodgers, A., & Gu, Y. (2012). Mobile phone-based interventions for smoking cessation. *Cochrane Database Systematic Reviews, 11*, CD006611.

Yellowlees, P., Shore, J., & Roberts, L. (2010). Practice guidelines for videoconferencing-based telemental health—October 2009. *Telemedicine Journal and e-Health*, *16*(10), 1074–1089.

20.

PSYCHIATRY AND PHYSICAL MEDICINE AND REHABILITATION

Nasser Karamouz, Richard T. Goldberg, Lucienne A. Cahen, and Seth D. Herman

INTRODUCTION

Almost all rehabilitation patients have a reactive emotional response to their injuries, and some patients going through rehabilitation may have other chronic psychiatric symptoms as well. The role of the psychiatric team in a rehabilitation hospital is to help the patient and staff to optimally carry on the rehabilitation tasks. This can be accomplished more effectively if the members of the psychiatric team are familiar with the field of physical medicine and rehabilitation (PM&R) and the role of the physiatrist as the leader of the multidisciplinary team.

Physiatrists are physicians who specialize in physical medicine and rehabilitation. Physical medicine and rehabilitation is a subspecialty of medicine that focuses on three major areas of patient care: diagnosis and treatment of musculoskeletal injury and pain, neuromuscular disorders through study of nerve conduction studies and electromyography, and rehabilitation of patients with severe impairments resulting from traumatic brain injury, spinal cord injury, stroke, and other disabling events (www.physiatry.org). Physical medicine and rehabilitation does not adopt one organ system but treats the "whole" person with a focus on enhancing the function and quality of life of the individual. Not only the biological needs but the emotional, social, and even spiritual needs are addressed to ensure optimal recovery and function of the patient.

HISTORICAL BACKGROUND

Howard Rusk is one of the founding fathers of physical medicine and rehabilitation (Rusk, 1972). In 1942 he created a program in an Air Force hospital to promote the recovery of injured soldiers, which he initially named the Army Air Force Reconditioning and Recreation Program; it was later renamed the Army Air Force Convalescent Committee. The program demonstrated that rehabilitation programs enabled injured soldiers to return to active duty and restored disabled soldiers back to a functional level when they returned home (Gritzer & Arluke, 1985). The formal training of doctors of physical medicine and rehabilitation was initiated by Dr. John Stanley Coulter, who eventually promoted physical medicine and rehabilitation to be part of formal medical education. Dr. Frank Krusen is credited as well with contributing to the establishment of physical medicine and rehabilitation in the 1930s and ultimately established the first 3-year residency program in Physical Medicine and Rehabilitation at Mayo Clinic in 1936. He created the term *physiatrist* to identify the physician who treats patients via physical medicine and rehabilitation modalities. Both Drs. Coulter and Krusen were leaders in organizing the American Academy of Physical Medicine in 1938. Further promotion of the specialty occurred when, in 1945, a section on PM&R was established in the American Medical Association. Ultimately, in 1947, Physical Medicine and Rehabilitation was declared a specialty of medicine by the Advisory Board of Medical Specialties. Since that time, the field of physical medicine and rehabilitation has continued to grow and expand, especially with an increased demand for services with the aged population, the disabling effects of war, trauma, and other medical conditions such as neurological disorders like Parkinson's disease and cancer.

THE PHYSIATRIST ROLE

The physiatrist is typically the lead physician who directs the medical and rehabilitation treatment program among a team of healthcare providers such as physical therapists, occupational therapists, speech language pathologists, psychologists, nurses, social workers, and other consulting physicians including psychiatrists and other medical specialties. The aim is to provide an interdisciplinary approach for optimal recovery of the patient. The patient is monitored with regular team meetings that enable all members of the team to discuss the recovery of the patient and to ensure optimal progress. The team establishes functional goals and determines the most appropriate discharge plan, such as to home versus another facility. Ultimately, communication among all members of the rehabilitation team is key to ensuring continued recovery and restoration of the patient with the ultimate goals of independence and quality of life.

Table 20.1 WORLD HEALTH ORGANIZATION (WHO) DEFINITIONS

TERM	DEFINITION
Impairment	Any loss or abnormality of body structure or of physiologic or psychologic function
Disability	Any restriction or lack resulting from an impairment of the ability to perform an activity in the manner or within range considered normal for the human being
Handicap	A disadvantage for a given individual, resulting from an impairment or a disability, that limits or prevents the fulfillment of a role that is normal for that individual
Activity	The nature and extent of functioning at the level of the person
Participation	The nature and extent of a person's involvement in life situations in relationship to impairments, activities, health conditions, and contextual factors

REHABILITATION TERMINOLOGY

The physiatrist's specialized training enables identification of a patient's physical, emotional, and cognitive deficits to develop a treatment plan. Functional assessments rely on an understanding of the distinctions among impairment, disability, and handicap, and, more recently, the new philosophic framework of activity and participation as defined by the World Health Organization (World Health Organization, 1980, 1997). Examples include difficulty with community reintegration, earning a wage, navigating architectural barriers (Author, 1998). The identification of these components of function drives the development of the treatment plan to promote quality of life and independent functioning (see Table 20.1).

EMOTIONAL ASPECTS OF REHABILITATION

PREMORBID FUNCTIONING

Although most injuries or illnesses requiring rehabilitation may cause emotional distress, many of the patient's emotional responses may be secondary to the patient's premorbid psychiatric disorders. Occasionally the psychiatric disorders actually are the *cause* of the initial injury (suicide attempts, drunk driving, violence, psychotic behaviors resulting in injuries). This is an important distinction to consider, especially when the injury is expected to cause emotional or behavioral changes. For instance, in patients with traumatic brain injury we cannot simply *assume* that all the post-injury psychiatric symptoms are secondary to the brain injury.

EMOTIONAL IMPACT OF ILLNESS OR INJURY

Most of the rehabilitation programs provide help for the following conditions:

- Amputations
- Stroke and other Neurological Disorders
- Burn Injuries
- Traumatic Brain Injury
- Spinal Cord Injuries
- Pediatric Rehabilitation

When we look at the above programs, it seems that most frequently the injuries or illnesses for these patients may have happened suddenly. Usually the patient has not had the time for any adequate preparation or development of coping strategies. Frequently the changes are not just an episodic event but will affect the patients for a long time, maybe for the rest of their lives. It may change them personally, financially, vocationally, and in many other ways. The patient is not the only one affected by the injury. In most cases it affects the patient's family members and significant others.

ACUTE STAGE OF INJURY OR ILLNESS

Because of the severity of their condition, patients usually require urgent medical or surgical interventions. During this acute stage, the patient and family do not have the ability or willingness to perceive the long-term effect of such injuries. This is partially due to a defense mechanism of denial and partially because at this stage they are not certain if the patient will survive. They can focus on the bigger picture only after survival is secured. Usually, the emotional issues related to a patient's survival are experienced by patient and his or her family while the patient is in the intensive care unit. To continue to secure such survival, the patient is usually transferred to the medical-surgical units for further stabilization. When the patient and family are no longer worried about the patient's survival, then the patient is usually stable enough to be transferred to a rehabilitation setting. At this point the patient and the family can begin to evaluate the patient's overall impairment. The stage of comparison begins. Patients begin to compare themselves to others as well to their previously healthy selves. The patient and family begin to see the possible problems in the future. This stage of awareness is usually a difficult stage of emotional coping, and mostly occurs at the time that patients are being admitted to the rehabilitation hospital.

PREADMISSION PROCESS

Before the admission to the rehabilitation hospital, the patient and family need to understand what is expected to be accomplished in the rehabilitation setting. If one expects the need for rehabilitation after a planned medical or surgical intervention, it would be beneficial to prepare the patient for the expected rehabilitation process as soon as practically possible. Such preparation can be done in an acute hospital or, if possible, even before the patient is admitted to the acute hospital for such a procedure. Increasing the patient's physical strength via exercise, and adequately treating any underlying possible psychiatric or cognitive disturbances, will better prepare them for the upcoming rehabilitation. Some patients arrive in the rehabilitation setting having unrealistic ideas and expectations about their prognosis or disposition, as well as the length of stay in the rehabilitation facility. These misperceptions are partially due to wishful thinking and partly due to wrong rehabilitation information given to the patient by those who are not fully familiar with the strengths and limitations in the field of PM&R. These misperceptions can cause significant stress for the patient after arrival to the rehab hospital. We can minimize such problems by requesting a consultation from a competent PM&R specialist to evaluate the patient in the acute hospital prior to admission to a rehabilitation facility. Such a consultant has the knowledge to initiate the conversation about the goal of the patient's admission to a rehabilitation hospital. Such consultation and liaison work is extremely helpful to patients and their families and to the staff in the rehabilitation setting. The medical psychiatrist in the acute hospital is able to play a significant role in such patients' emotional preparation. The physiatrists who do PM&R consultations in acute hospitals are best suited to advise the medical and surgical staff about the need for a psychiatric evaluation for emotionally vulnerable patients whom they are asked to see prior to transfer to a rehabilitation hospital. Some patients cannot tolerate the high level of physical, cognitive, and emotional intensity of active rehabilitation. They may respond better if their rehabilitation plan is designed to respect their limitations. We should recommend the "dosage" of rehabilitation in the same manner that we determine the "dosage" of medications for our patients. Some patients may optimally need a higher dosage of a given medication but may not be able to tolerate it, and we need to give them a lower amount to minimize adverse effects. The same is true in the rehabilitation setting, as some patients are unable or unwilling to accept the intensity of their rehabilitation and their treatment plan needs to be modified accordingly. In such cases more rehabilitation does not necessarily result in a better outcome, and may have an "adverse effect."

At the time of transferring patients from the acute hospital to a rehabilitation facility the medical team, including the medical psychiatrist, needs to work with patients to evaluate their physical and emotional status in order to guide them to an appropriate rehabilitation facility. For example, patients who are admitted to an acute rehabilitation hospital should meet the criteria for the need of 3 hours of active rehabilitation therapy per day, while the requirement for admission to a skilled nursing facility is approximately 1.5 hours per day. Some patients who need frequent or daily visits by their physician (PM&R) need to be referred to an active rehabilitation facility, because most skilled nursing facilities allow only for weekly or monthly physician visits. However, going to a skilled nursing facility does not necessarily indicate insufficient rehabilitation—as,

for example, patients with joint replacement from both skilled nursing facilities and inpatient rehabilitation facilities receive considerable amounts of follow-up rehabilitation care (Dejong et al., 2009). Psychiatric services for patients who are in need of active psychiatric care may not be adequate in most skilled nursing facilities, and such patients are better served in an inpatient rehabilitation facility. A long-term acute care hospital is another option for some patients, and their criteria for admission and the extent of their services falls in between that of active rehabilitation and skilled nursing facilities. Patients who are actively suicidal and are under one-to-one supervision are not appropriate for admission to a rehabilitation hospital. Patients who are taking intramuscular or intravenous neuroleptics should be further stabilized before they are admitted to a rehabilitation facility. Patients should also be relatively stable medically and should not be significantly violent, although some agitation and aggressiveness can be expected from some neurologically impaired patients who are confused but in need of rehabilitation.

If there are any significant psychiatric issues, then the discussion between the psychiatry staff at the referring and admitting hospitals can be clinically helpful. Physical and cognitive rehabilitation care should not be denied to the patients who suffer from severe psychiatric illnesses; however, one can reasonably question the clinical appropriateness of such rehabilitation admission if the degree of the psychiatric symptoms is so severe that they would significantly interfere with the rehabilitation process.

ADMISSION TO THE REHABILITATION HOSPITAL

When we consider the admission process, we should be aware that there are two aspects of admission that need to be distinguished—one administrative, the other clinical. This distinction is not usually recognized institutionally. Administratively, we need to determine whether the patients are signing in directly to admit themselves or, alternatively, patients have a legal representative who signs in for the patient so that he or she can be admitted to the rehabilitation hospital. Occasionally, patients who seem incompetent, but are nonetheless competent in the eyes of the law because they do not have a legal representative, arrive in the admissions office at the rehabilitation hospital and are unwilling to be admitted and wish to go home. It would be challenging for a psychiatrist working in the rehabilitation hospital to be called to the admissions office to evaluate such a patient for a safe disposition. In most cases the patient can be encouraged to accept admission for a brief evaluation to see that a safe discharge plan can be designed. Rarely the patient refuses to be admitted and the question of the patient's competency is raised, which is difficult to assess at the time of admission. Patients who are confused should have a heathcare proxy, and patients who are unwilling to be admitted for inpatient rehabilitation should have a legal guardian available or, at a minimum, the process of obtaining guardianship should be initiated prior to their arrival at a rehabilitation hospital.

Once the patient is administratively admitted to the hospital, the all-important process of clinical admission begins. Patients must be evaluated to determine both the nature and severity of their impairments as well as the degree of their understanding of deficits. Patients should be encouraged to think reasonably about the fears, hopes, and expectations that come with rehabilitation. Some patients may minimize their problems while others may be vigilant and unnecessarily focus too much on the possibilities for poor outcomes. The rehabilitation team needs to conduct a full evaluation and come up with a complete rehabilitation care plan. After the primary evaluation and clarification of the expectations of staff and patient (or the patient's formal representatives), a therapeutic contract is designed. When the patient and family agree with such a rehabilitation care plan, then the patient finally can be clinically admitted to the program and the rehabilitation process can begin. Reaching this therapeutic agreement is essential. During the active phase of the rehabilitation process, patients should be reminded of the therapeutic contract if they forget or otherwise undermine the therapeutic care plan and refuse to participate in rehabilitation.

ACTIVE PHASE OF THE REHABILITATION PROCESS

As the rehabilitation process evolves, patients continue to compare themselves to others as well to the previously healthy self. At times the patient may have no adequate cognitive or emotional readiness to make this comparison, but the family begins to compare the patient with who she or he was before the injury. At times, the emotional pain arising from this comparison is so significant and difficult to accept that denial can become the main defense mechanism for the patient and/or the family. If such denial occurs, the patient and family may encounter significant difficulty with the rehabilitation treatment plan—especially since rehabilitation, by its very nature, confronts the patient with the impairment and related deficits. For instance, if a patient uses denial in order to cope with reduced walking ability, it will be impossible for the patient to continue denial while the physical therapist is encouraging the patient to walk. Similarly, if a patient uses denial to overcome the emotional pain arising from expressive aphasia, the patient will be directly confronted while working with the speech therapist. If some patients cannot accept the fact that they are so compromised that they cannot even dress themselves, during their work with their occupational therapist they will be constantly confronted with their deficits. In short, a patient who is in denial will find it difficult to continue to use denial as a defense mechanism when confronted repeatedly while working with the rehabilitation team. As one cannot simultaneously deny and repeatedly be confronted at the same time, a patient may deal with this dilemma by refusing rehabilitation. If such denial continues, the patient will begin to break the previously agreed therapeutic contract. Psychiatry consultation and psychological treatment are usually considered for such patients. If the patient's denial cannot be challenged supportively, then the patient may express wishes to leave prematurely and against medical advice. Some patients are at higher risk for leaving against medical advice—for example, patients with traumatic brain injury who are 24–35 years old, have a history of intentional injury, alcohol, and substance abuse. These patients need to be identified and evaluated by the psychiatric team soon after admission to the rehabilitation hospital to prevent such risks and also to implement a treatment response in case such patients try to leave prematurely (Kim, Colantino, Bayley, & Dawson, 2011). Although these patients may not be considered a danger to themselves from a purely psychiatric point of view, nonetheless at times they can be clearly unsafe for discharge and meet the criteria for involuntary commitment to an appropriate facility. One example would be a patient who has symptoms of left neglect, who can be in immediate and substantial danger if he leaves the hospital and tries to cross a busy road. Patients for whom a psychiatric consult is requested will, at times, refuse psychiatric services. In most cases this is related to the patient's anxiety or lack of understanding of psychiatric services. They may accept help if we initially back off, supportively reassure them about our role, and give them enough time and space to reconsider their initial refusal. If there is any evidence to suggest those patients can be a danger to themselves or others, it is necessary to supportively establish the fact that they are required to talk with us in order to rule out such safety risks.

THE MULTIDISCIPLINARY REHABILITATION TEAM

The treatment plan for most patients and their disposition after discharge is usually a complicated process and based on the recommendations made and approved by the multidisciplinary team members rather than by any individual member of the team. It is crucial that the psychiatrist and psychologist working in a rehabilitation setting become closely familiar with the short-term and long-term goals and disposition for patients and try to resolve any suspected psychiatric symptoms that may interfere with accomplishing the plan of care. Rehabilitation care plans are based on professional standards, evidenced-based practices, and research, as well as the individual needs of patients. The team includes various staff from different specialized clinical backgrounds.

- **Rehabilitation Nurses** are familiar with the profound impact of disability upon patients' lives and try to prevent further complications while educating them in how they should prepare themselves for the next stage of their care. Nurses have significant information about the overall emotional status of their patients, how they are usually coping, and how patients are reacting to their families and friends during their visits. Nurses are in the forefront of the direct patient care at all times and have significant clinical information that can help the psychiatrist in proper psychiatric management of patients.

- **Case Managers** assist patients in setting appropriate goals and begin the challenging task of obtaining the necessary services for patients during their treatment and after discharge. Coordinating the psychiatric care and post-discharge follow-up for patients becomes easier with ongoing communication between the case manager and the psychiatric team. In recent years the work of case managers has become increasingly challenging, primarily because of the limitations on resources available to them while they try to provide the best discharge planning for their patients. These challenges are becoming more intense in light of additional pressure from various sources to discharge patients as soon as possible. Although such pressures are felt by all the team members, case managers are on the front lines in such battles. These opposing forces and resulting challenges should be a focal point for PM&R practitioners in the hospital setting.

- **Physical Therapists** evaluate and treat problems related to mobility, strength, coordination, and endurance. They are helpful in reporting any adverse effect of psychotropic medications on patients, and the psychiatrist is fortunate to have their input while modifying patient's medications.

- **Occupational Therapists** assist patients to further improve their ability to perform everyday tasks such as eating, dressing, personal hygiene, meal preparation, housekeeping, and skills required to rejoin the community. If there is any concern about the functional ability of patients, occupational therapists can evaluate them in the community. With such information in addition to other data and the report by the therapeutic recreation specialist, the psychiatrist can better advise the team in terms of a plan to increase the safety of the patient after discharge.

- **Speech-Language Pathologists** try to improve the patient's ability to speak, swallow, understand, read, write, focus, remember, and solve problems. This can be done individually or in a group setting and with or without computer-assisted techniques. They can recommend the best way to communicate with the patient and review the cognitive ability of patients with the psychiatrist, which is important in patients who cannot be fully examined during the psychiatric interview. They also monitor food intake by patients, which makes them a reliable source for the psychiatrist to get information about the possibility of any swallowing problems secondary to psychotropic medications.

- **Respiratory Therapists** assist with 24-hour coverage for evaluating and treating conditions related to respiratory problems.

- **Therapeutic Recreation (TR) Specialists** evaluate a patient's premorbid leisure interests and lifestyle. Once identified, these interests are combined with basic therapy goals that focus on education, skills teaching, and community reentry. Treatment programs are designed to give patients an opportunity to enjoy activities of choice such as adaptive sports, games, crafts, horticulture, pet therapy, community outings, and, when available, music therapy. The focus of many sessions may be improving specific physical and/or cognitive therapy goals and social skills. Sessions may be conducted individually or in groups. The TR specialist may also provide assistive recreational devices to improve independence with leisure activities. Educating the patient and family about ways to have an active leisure lifestyle after discharge, through home and community resources, is another important component of the TR program. Most patients have significant free time while they are in the hospital, and the TR can be very helpful in designing projects based on the interests of patients to keep their minds off an emotionally painful preoccupation with their condition. Such help from TR has allowed some patients to avoid the use of psychiatric medications and to use nonpharmacological approaches to cope with their emotional conditions. TR specialists may also help coordinating the process for patients to become voluntary visitors to help other patients with similar problems; for some patients, being able to relate to others with the same challenges can provide significant assistance in their own coping. The staff from therapeutic recreation is usually the key element in organizing periodic gatherings for patients who have been discharged from the inpatient rehabilitation programs. During these events, patients can meet with staff members who took care of them during their hospitalizations. Such reunions have had many benefits for patients and their families, while educating staff about the long-term effect of their rehabilitation work. Because of such follow-ups, we can periodically obtain firsthand information and direct knowledge from patients and their families that is useful in rehabilitation and discharge planning for other patients.

- **Dietitians** recommend therapeutic diets, supplements, and special feeding programs, and educate patients and families about guidelines to follow after discharge. Depression, especially when combined with a lack of adequate activity, can cause significant weight gain. Also, some patients who have depression may experience weight loss, and the dietician is helpful to the psychiatrist in monitoring such symptoms of depression and the efficacy of the use of antidepressants. Depending on a patient's individualized needs, other professionals, consulting physicians, neuropsychologists, social workers and counselors, and hospital chaplains may also join the rehabilitation team.

WHO SHOULD DO THE COUNSELING?

During the active phase of rehabilitation, the patient usually receives different levels of counseling from various members of the rehabilitation team. As mentioned earlier, some patients minimize their problems and some have a tendency to exaggerate them. The consultant who is trying to help the patient to deal with deficits should have a good understanding of the actual degree of the patient's impairment and possible prognosis. For instance, if the patient has emotional struggles regarding lack of mobility the physical therapist is the most appropriate counselor to help the patient to express fears and concerns. If the patient is unreasonably concerned about impairment and is not able to be objective about potential outcomes, the physical therapist will have the appropriate knowledge about the patient's condition to offer reassurance. If counseling is to be provided by the psychiatrist or the psychologist, he or she needs to be informed by the rehabilitation team about the details of patient's deficits, rehabilitation needs, and possible prognosis. If the consultant psychiatrist lacks such critical knowledge, the patient's minimization or exaggeration of the problem may cause the counseling to go in the wrong direction.

PATIENT–STAFF INTERACTIONS

As the rehabilitation process continues, the patient and the rehabilitation therapist gradually establish a close therapeutic relationship. For some patients such a supportive relationship is at least as important as the therapist's knowledge and skill. During the rehabilitation process, by definition many emotional and physical boundaries become fragile. Frequently some physical boundaries need to be broken in order to provide effective rehabilitation. For instance, during physical therapy there is a great deal of touching and holding in order to address the patient's ability to sit up and sit down, walk, and maintain balance. Most patients feel comfortable with such approaches, but others may show increased anxiety and discomfort during these kinds of therapeutic interactions. When patients have difficulty with such interactions with rehabilitation staff, the discomfort can negatively impact their participation in physical therapy. In particular, patients diagnosed with schizophrenia need to be cautiously observed for their apprehensive reaction and avoidance behavior during such therapeutic contacts. It is common to observe patients with such diagnoses becoming increasingly anxious when the usual and expected social and physical "boundaries" are broken. Staff respect patients' need for such personal space, but it is not usually possible to keep these boundaries intact when, for example, a physical therapist needs to frequently touch or hold a patient therapeutically or a nurse has to provide personal care. There are also occasions in which other patients may feel "too comfortable" or "too pleased" with such broken boundaries and react personally rather than therapeutically. Patients with a history of affective disorders—for example, those with hypomania—are in this category. Fortunately such patients are usually able to respond to supportive limit-setting when needed. Psychiatrists and counselors working in rehabilitation facilities can use the opportunity to observe some of their patients during rehabilitation sessions to become more familiar with the patient/staff interactions.

SOURCES OF STRESS FOR THE STAFF

The staff working in a rehabilitation hospital may, with or without being fully aware of it, experience a range of emotional disappointments. The psychiatrist and the psychologist working with the team need to be aware of these professional challenges and also monitor their own responses to such stresses. The process of physical rehabilitation can be very slow. At times it is complicated, with no simple solution available to *eliminate* the patient's problem. Rehabilitation may be defined as the optimal outcome for a patient's physical, cognitive, and emotional problems. Although patients who receive rehabilitation can get better, they usually cannot be cured. This outcome is in contrast with a patient who is admitted to a hospital for surgery and at the time of discharge expects to be, and often is, completely cured and on the road to a full recovery. Being "cured" should not typically be expected at the time of discharge from the rehabilitation hospital. The rehabilitation team may have provided exceptionally competent therapeutic services, and the patient may have improved significantly; however, the patient will likely experience some difficulties with thinking, walking, or talking at the time of discharge. This reality can be disappointing to patients and their families as well as to their caregivers who had wishes, consciously or unconsciously, for a complete cure. The rehabilitation staff gradually recognizes that they cannot help everybody no matter how hard they try. During the process of rehabilitation, patients and staff have many close physical and emotional interactions and occasionally, depending on patients' emotional status and possible underlying psychopathology (i.e., borderline personality), some undesirable emotions may be created among the caregivers. The psychiatrist and psychologist working with the team should be aware of these stresses on staff, including themselves, and monitor the possible effect of such emotional perceptions on the patient's care. If such stresses, for various reasons, are felt by the majority of the team members it is beneficial to have a team meeting to discuss the patient–staff emotional interactions and review the plan of care.

Another source of stress is that staff are trained to believe that all patients have a desire to get better. Sometimes the staff are confronted by patients who do not wish to improve and may resist any fair treatment plan or discharge dispositions. At times the patients are not participating in their plan of care because they have limited cognition, and they do not comprehend the need for any rehabilitation. At other times there are patients that are clearly benefitting from their condition due to a primary (unconscious) or a secondary (conscious) gain, which clearly minimizes their interest to actively try to get better. Also, patients who have conversion disorder may become too anxious about getting better because their symptoms are protecting them from an intrapsychic conflict that needs to be addressed before they become ready to give up their symptoms. At times, patients are not interested in getting better simply because they like to be hospitalized. For instance, some patients who live alone and feel lonely and apprehensive at home may report feeling good in the hospital, where they have fair security, are taken care of by dedicated staff, and usually have more frequent visits by family and friends. We cannot motivate such patients by informing them that if they do not work hard in their rehabilitation they cannot get better to go home. Such statements actually indicate to the patients that if they would like to stay longer they should slow down their participation in their rehabilitation activities; however, when such patients are educated that they will become disqualified to stay in the hospital if they do not participate 3 hours a day in their rehabilitation, they may try to qualify and prolong their stay by increasing their participation.

The slow pace of the rehabilitation process can be another source of stress. Frequently, rehabilitation staff cannot find a simple solution to their patients' problems, and there is rarely any immediate success. For patients who have had recent surgical interventions, participation in rehabilitation activities can cause some degree of pain and discomfort. Frequently those patients blame their therapists for causing such pain, and become angry or simply minimize participation in their rehabilitation. Some difficulties may also arise when the rehabilitation team is unable to decide if a patient's lack of optimal participation in rehabilitation is due to the patient's *unwillingness* to participate or by the patient's *inability* to do the task. The rehabilitation team expects the psychiatrist and the psychologist to use his/her expertise to clarify whether the patient cannot or will not fully cooperate, and why.

COPING MECHANISMS

A patient with physical disability arrives at a rehabilitation hospital after initial diagnosis and treatment have been accomplished in an acute care setting. The patient has an expectation of being restored to the baseline that came before acute hospitalization. Every patient comes into rehabilitation with previous strengths and weaknesses. Age, gender, previous illnesses, and socioeconomic background are predictors for outcome.

Culture and social class must be understood by the psychiatrist and psychologist who are undertaking psychotherapy with the patient (Goldberg, 2003). Cultural attitudes toward illness affect the reactions of patients toward disability. For example, patients whose families came from traditional countries where the entire family makes decisions about medical treatment may require more intensive family communication and support in the rehabilitation process. Patient whose families were born and raised in the United States may have more freedom in making individual choices about treatment. Age and gender are important predictors of outcome with specific disabilities. For example, spinal cord injury has a ratio of 8 or 9 to 1 in favor of male to female. Within the male population, there is a bimodal distribution in which there is a large group of young men who have been involved in motor vehicle accidents and sports injuries, and an older population who have been injured at work. Psychological treatment focuses on the specific needs of each age group. Young men may not have completed their educational and vocational training. Older men may have established themselves in an occupation, but they may not be capable of returning to a former job.

A psychiatric assessment, along with psychological screening, the report by the rehabilitation team, and direct observation of patients in their rehabilitation program determines the motivational and cognitive strengths of each patient. For motivational assessment one needs to differentiate between abulia and depression, as well as patient's inability versus unwillingness to participate in their rehabilitation care. Screening for alcohol and drug addiction is necessary in the overall evaluation for success. Family history is important not only for assessment of psychiatric disorders and previous psychiatric hospitalizations, but also to determine familial attitudes toward disability. Illness affects the whole family, and in turn the family's attitude toward illness contributes to a patient's willingness to work toward rehabilitation.

Functional impairments that limit a person's ability to carry out activities of daily living such as managing a house, caring for children, cooking, cleaning, managing personal finances, completing an education, or earning a living are common elements to consider in all disabilities. Disabilities have a profound effect on a person's psychological outlook and psychiatric stability. Persons with previous psychiatric disorders have the additional task of coping with their physical disabilities.

How does one cope with loss? A person with physical disability feels humiliated by a decline in function. An initial strategy may be denial. One pretends that life can proceed as usual until one is faced with insuperable barriers of rejection in the community. In a rehabilitation hospital, a patient is confronted with the tasks of transfer from bed to chair, of using a commode, of standing, balancing, ambulating, ascending and descending stairs. At admission a patient may have a high expectation that he or she will walk out of the hospital at the end of 4 or 5 weeks. When the expectation level is not fulfilled, then comes the hard task of adapting—not just adjusting—to disability.

Adaptation to disability requires a patient to develop the functional skills and cognitive capacity to prepare for return to living independently in the community or semi-independently in an assisted living home. The older term, *adjustment*, meant that a patient had to accept the limitations associated with disability without denial. Although this coping strategy worked for some patients, it did not work for others. Some patients with disability used denial as a healthy mechanism for overcoming disability. A famous example of this strategy was Franklin D. Roosevelt, who became paralyzed from poliomyelitis at the age of 39 (Goldberg, 1981; Oshinsky, 2005). He never accepted the prognosis that he would never walk again, and until his death at age 63 he was planning to return to Warm Springs, Georgia, to complete his rehabilitation. As clinicians we encourage patients to maintain hope that they will improve function with the advent of new technologies while at the same time preparing them to face the realistic challenges of adapting to disability.

Adaptation requires a patient to separate his concept of disability from his concept of himself. Being paraplegic or brain injured or hemiplegic is not the same as being oneself. The person's idea of self as physically disabled may spread to other aspects of self-image. The person with amputation becomes the amputee; the person with blindness becomes the blind man. The phenomenon of spread reaches out to intellectual, emotional, and even spiritual aspects of oneself. By recognizing and learning how to separate the disability from the person, one can adapt to the realistic limitations of disability.

Language is the lattice through which we perceive reality. How we label our patients determines in part how we treat them. When we understand our patients as persons rather than as categorical diseases, then we bring a humane attitude to our work. Before the term *political correctness* came into vogue, the philosophy and principles of rehabilitation distinguished between impairments and persons. Similarly, the term *handicapped* was assigned to specific restrictions imposed by disability at home, school, and work. "The handicapped" should not be used as a general term referring to persons with disability.

Rehabilitation helps a person with disability to appreciate remaining assets rather than dwelling on liabilities. Focusing on loss of physical function to the detriment of preserving remaining assets leads to a patient's negative expectations. Psychiatrists and psychologists help patients to focus on their remaining assets rather than on their limitations. Patients with a stroke or spinal cord injury may find ways to perform their jobs by adapting to their work environment. For example, an architect with left hemiplegia from an embolic stroke who can no longer do architectural drawings may find work inspecting building sites, since his visual perception remains intact. He may walk around construction sites with the use of a cane.

In a culture that idealizes persons with physical wholeness and attractiveness, physical disability is perceived as a disadvantage in school, work, and marriage. Physical disfigurement as a consequence of burns, amputation, or hemiplegia from stroke further complicates the rehabilitation process. Body image affects a person's self-image, which makes social integration into the community more difficult. The task of psychiatry and psychology is to help a person with physical disability to incorporate a change in body image with a patient's former picture of himself or herself.

COPING STRATEGIES

Although coping strategies may vary among different disabilities, there are specific common elements that guide the care of patients coping with all disabilities. First, care of the patient coping with loss and grief requires the utmost sensitivity by psychiatrists and psychologists. Second, clinicians must focus on the positive assets of the person rather than functional limitations imposed by disability (Wright, 1960). Third, a clinician helps to combat the phenomenon of spread—that is, the idea that because a person has a physical, cognitive, or affective disorder, he or she cannot function normally and compete with able-bodied persons. Disability causes physical, cognitive, and emotional limitations that produce specific handicaps at home, school, and work. Rehabilitation services help persons to cope with limitations in order to become less handicapped in activities of daily living.

Fourth, the clinician helps the patient to cope with the inferior social status of persons with disability, which may exist in some societies. Fifth, the clinician helps the patient to cope with the devaluation of a significant segment of persons with disability due to physical disfigurement such as burns, stroke, and amputation. Devaluation of a person with disability is counteracted by focus on a patient's abilities, moral values, and contributions to community. Inferior social status is perceived when a community focuses only on the disability to the exclusion of other assets of the patient.

In the following sections, specific disabilities will be explored as examples in the setting of psychological and psychiatric treatment to cope with limitations and deficits.

COPING WITH AMPUTATION

Amputation is the classic example of loss. The loss of any body part is symbolic of loss of health and ultimately loss of life. Mourning for loss is the first requirement of adaptation to amputation. Mourning for a lost limb is a normal process of grieving. This period may proceed while the patient is in a rehabilitation program, but if untreated it may persist for several years. Mourning may also be a reaction to cumulative losses that occurred prior to amputation. The person who has an amputation may feel victimized by previous life events. A clinician will treat feelings of isolation, guilt, and vulnerability that have existed antecedent to amputation. When a patient feels targeted to suffer, then intervention is required to prevent suicide. Grief may also be prolonged by concurrent events, such as separation, divorce, and loss of income. For men, amputation may mean loss of power, sexuality, physical prowess, and livelihood. For women, in addition to the prior losses, amputation may mean loss of sexual attractiveness, youth, and body integrity. Amputation is a visible disability and thus is an object of curiosity, staring, and stigma.

Coping with amputation requires understanding of loss. An amputee needs time to mourn the loss of a body part while beginning a structured program of physical and occupational therapy. Rehabilitation is structured around 3 hours of therapy daily. A patient needs to be prepared to tolerate long periods of work in therapy. Psychiatry may follow a patient from the admission to the rehabilitation hospital to discharge. Psychology works with a patient in reasserting body image and self-image. A person with amputation may feel that bodily integrity is completely altered. Coping with amputation requires a therapist to help a patient reconstruct a new body image and self-image. In most instances, over 50% of former activities can be engaged. A psychologist draws two circles to represent the patient's values, interests, and family interaction before and after amputation. The patient describes which values, interests, and family activities can still be accomplished after amputation. The two circles are overlapping, and the areas of agreement are shaded in to represent activities that the patient can still perform. Self-image is improved when the patient perceives that former activities can still be performed. Values, interests, family, and religion remain the same. As a patient becomes aware that he or she can still do many activities at home, school, or work, he or she regains hope for the future. (Dembo, 1956).

Disfigurement in amputation may be modified by the early fitting of a prosthesis. The degree of cosmetic disfigurement in women is related to symptoms of avoidance and emotional numbing characterized by posttraumatic stress disorder (Fukunishi, 1999).

Anxiety and depression are common sequelae of amputation (Horgan & MacLachlan, 2004). Anxiety is associated with depression, poorly perceived quality of life, less self-esteem, and previous level of anxiety before amputation. O'Toole,

Goldberg, and Ryan (1985) concluded that below-knee amputees were more likely than above-knee amputees to be depressed due to sensitivity to their difference from able-bodied persons. Whereas patients with above-knee amputation were glad they survived their surgery, those with below-knee amputation were disturbed by the physical and aesthetic changes in their appearance. Prostheses can help reduce anxiety about altered body image.

The presence of phantom pain can further contribute to patient's difficulty with rehabilitation. Phantom limb pain (PLP) is the pain experienced in the limbs than no longer exist. Distortion of body image is associated with phantom pain (Lindesay, 1985). The onset of phantom limb pain in 50% of cases occurs immediately after or within 24 hours following amputations An additional 25% of patients experience such pain within a week of their surgeries (Weeks, Anderson-Barnes, & Tsao,   2010). Various medications including antidepressants, anticonvulsants, clonidine and nonsteroidal antiinflammatory drugs, calcitonin (Wall & Heyneman, 1999), and opioids or other agents have been used to treat PLP. In the rehabilitation setting it is desirable to use some medication that does not cause so much sedation or fatigue that it can interfere with the rehabilitation process. The use of antidepressants or anticonvulsants (e.g., carbamazepine, gabapentin) used alone or in combinations can be helpful. Morphine, gabapentin, and ketamine have short-term analgesic efficacy in patients with phantom limb pain (Alviar, Hale, & Dunoca, 2011). In a patient with PLP who also experienced restless legs syndrome, the use of dopamine agonist agents was reported to be beneficial (Skidmore, Drago, Foster, & Helman, 2009). Nonpharmacological approaches such as mirror therapy (Rothgangel, Braun, Beurskens, Setz, & Wade, 2011), transcutaneous electrical nerve stimulation, and nerve block (Ilfed, 2010) have been helpful in some cases.

COPING WITH STROKE

Stroke is an abrupt, sudden, often unexpected calamity that results in multiple losses of sensation, movement, language, cognition, vision, swallowing, touch, and loss of position. A person who had formerly been able to carry on normal tasks of daily living and other roles such as earning a living, attending school, or being a parent or grandparent, suddenly finds that he or she is limited in one or several of these aspects of life. When a simple skill is learned as a child, we forget about these simple tasks and use our bodies to attain higher goals such as education, work, or homemaking. The sick body requires mental planning and organizational skills. The sick body is felt as strange, alienated, unsafe and insecure. A person with stroke perceives the body as both subject and object. The sick body is also an object of investigation from the outside and is continually being examined by experts who guide the person back to health (Kvigney & Kirkevold, 2003).

The body as viewed from the outside may be beautiful, misshapen, sexual, or ugly. For example, the female body may be viewed as an object of attraction, reproduction, awe, or envy. After stroke, a person is aware that the appearance of the body is changed by paralysis, facial droop, ataxia, or position of the limbs. The loss of an attractive body may lead not only to the uncomfortable gaze of others but also to the experience of suffering from within. Visible contracture of an arm or leg, drooling from the paralyzed side of the mouth, weight gain resulting from inactivity, benign neglect of one side to appear as being inattentive or not caring to engage in direct eye contact, failing to dress appropriately or to maintain an attractive appearance with cosmetics or hair grooming—all of these deficits contribute to the emotional suffering and depression of a person with stroke.

Coping strategies with stroke begin by recognition of the overwhelming devastation and loss of function *within a blink of an eye*. Initially the focus is on survival and medical treatment. When medical and neurological stability is achieved, the patient will be ready for rehabilitation. After a patient has entered a rehabilitation program, physical and cognitive limitations become more apparent. A patient wants to know how much function will return. Some patients begin with an optimistic attitude toward completion of a rehabilitation program. "I'm always going to keep it in my head that someday I'll walk again." However, they usually are informed that the outcome is in doubt and will depend on the degree of physical and mental restoration as well as possible future medical complications. Some patients have to be sent back to the referring hospital for acute care. Following their stay, they return to rehabilitation. The patient is encouraged to optimally participate in rehabilitation despite some physical and emotional barriers. Rehabilitation has its ups and downs, but in the long run there is usually an upward trend. When patients meet an obstacle in the program, they may become depressed and wish to give up. Here is where the effort of psychiatry and psychology is crucial in contributing to a positive outcome. Both psychotherapy and psychopharmacology help to keep patients in the program.

Toward the end of the rehabilitation program, a patient may express optimism of outcome but may have an unrealistic assessment of functional capacities after discharge. A patient with hemianopsia may not be able to drive a car. A patient with hemiplegia or hemiparesis may not be able to return to skilled labor such as plumbing or carpentry or roofing. A patient with professional training in computer science, engineering, medicine, or scientific research may not be able to continue fulltime work. Neuropsychological testing may be helpful in delineating the areas of strength and weakness in a patient's recovery. A realistic assessment of mental capacities and limitations caused by stroke will help to inform a patient and family about future potential for work. Since professional workers are often primarily identified with their vocation, the loss of work may be traumatic. Professionals, small business owners, and self-employed persons may be able to restructure their work rather than give it up entirely. For example, we have treated physicians who could not return to lecturing or to private practice but who could teach and supervise others in a case study. The length and amount of recovery depends on the location of the stroke and the age of the person. Persons who cannot return to work may develop a hobby or perform volunteer work in the community.

Most patients experience some psychological consequences after stroke. Anxiety is seen in almost 20% of stroke patients. There is insufficient evidence to provide a clear pharmacological recommendation to treat such symptoms; however, paroxetine and buspirone have been found to be effective in reducing anxiety symptoms in stroke patients (Campbell Burton et al., 2011). Depression is the most common psychiatric disorder that adversely affects stroke outcome and is often underdiagnosed or inadequately treated (Ramasubbu, 2011). Its reported prevalence varies from 20% to 80% (Tharwani, Yerramsetty, Mannelli, Patkar, & Masand, 2007). At times, the symptoms that family and staff are observing in "depressed" patients may only be related to the stroke symptoms. Those symptoms may be simply due to poststroke fatigue, pseudodepressive manifestations of ischemic stroke, state of indifference, lack of concerns, or suppression of excitement and passion (apathy). Some patients may appear depressed due to lack of variations in normal speech characteristics such as speed and tone (aprosody), or disorders of motivation, loss or reduction of desire and interest, loss of drive or preferences, and may have flat affect without subjective feelings of depression (athymhormia), or fluctuation of emotions and periodic emotional outbursts (pseudobulbar palsy). Selective serotonin reuptake inhibitors (SSRIs) are considered to be the first choice treatment of poststroke depression (Arseniou, Arvaniti, & Samakouri, 2011). There has been no association of SSRIs and the risk of hemorrhagic stroke, regardless of prior history of cerebrovascular events (Douglas I, et al., 2011). After a stroke, initiation or resumption of treatment with SSRIs should be considered, especially if the patient has a history of depression or was taking SSRIs before the stroke (Reid et al., 2011). A patient's history of prestroke depression is a significant predictor of poststroke depression (Reid et al., 2010). The medical psychiatrist who usually sees patients soon after a stroke is in a good position to offer SSRIs. Use of SSRIs such as fluoxetine 5–10 days after an acute ischemic stroke has resulted in an improvement of poststroke motor recovery and overall improvement (Cramer, 2011). The same result has been achieved by treating patients with escitalopram (Jorge, Acion, Moser, Adams, & Robinson, 2010). Stroke patients with depression who started antidepressants while in an inpatient rehabilitation hospital had longer length of stay compared to patients in the same impairment condition who had initiated antidepressants in the acute hospitals or sooner (Weeks et al., 2011). Stroke patients treated with antidepressants had a better recovery from disability even 9 months after stopping their antidepressants, indicating that antidepressants may facilitate the neural mechanism of recovery in patients with stroke (Mikami et al., 2011). Modulation of spontaneous brain plasticity by medications is an encouraging factor in treatment of patients with ischemic stroke who suffer from moderate to severe motor deficit (Chollet et al., 2011).

COPING WITH BURNS

Burns rank as the third leading cause of accidental deaths among adults and children in the United States and as the eighth leading cause of nonfatal injuries in children from age 1–4 years. Children living in circumstances of abuse and neglect are especially vulnerable to burns from a boiling pot on a stove or from touching a faulty electric wire. Adults with drug addiction, mental illness or retardation, dementia, alcoholism, or chronic cigarette smokers are vulnerable to burns either through neglect or through self-inflicted attempts of suicide. In addition, there are adults who practice immolation for a religious or political cause. Burns are a common cause of facial disfigurement, especially among children where the head represents a disproportionate portion of the human body. Among children the head, the neck, and the armpits are the most frequent locations of burns. Posttraumatic stress disorder is one of the common psychiatric disorders following burn injury (Difede, 2002). Although many burn survivors are able to surmount the initial period of acute stress by drawing upon their own psychological and spiritual resources, a significant number of survivors need psychiatric and psychological help during their rehabilitation (Patterson, 2000).

In the acute phase of survival after burns, the survivor is mourning losses of health, physical function, beauty, productivity, and sometimes the loss of a loved one who was victimized by an accident that caused the burns. In the initial stage, the burn survivor is completely devastated and overwhelmed by loss and can think only of survival. When a loved one has died in the fire or explosion, the survivor needs to be monitored for suicidality. A psychiatrist provides empathy, trauma counseling, and expert care. Many survivors respond well to antidepressant medications. After the acute phase has passed, the survivor may be ready to be visited by a SOAR (Survivors Offering Assistance in Recovery) volunteer. The volunteer is not a substitute for good medical, nursing, and psychological care. Reactive depression and grief may respond to a combination of medications, psychological care, and emotional support. Emotional support may be given both to the patient who is the burn survivor and to the patient's family members, who may be undergoing an extraordinary experience of survivor guilt, anger, and helplessness. A wide variety of factors are predictive of psychological adjustment after burn injury. These factors can be summarized under these categories: (1) burn size, site, inhalation injury, pulmonary complications, catabolic state (Herndon & Tomkins, 2004), temperature regulation (Esselman et al., 2007); patient characteristics: age, gender, education, unemployment, loss of occupational status (Klein et al., 2011; Browne et al., 1985); (3) premorbid psychiatric history that may include alcohol and drug use, anxiety, depression, suicidal ideation and attempts, behavioral problems (Schneider, 2010); acute stress disorder during the first 4 weeks after burn injury and posttraumatic stress disorder that may persist for a month or more after burn injury (Ehde et al., 2000; Van Loey et al., 2003; Fauerbach et al., 2009); depression as a common psychiatric disorder after burn injury (Orr, 1989; Fauerbach et al., 2000; Wiechman et al., 2001; Edwards et al., 2007); sleep disturbances (Schneider, 2010); body image and disfigurement (Fukunishi, 1999; Fauerbach et al., 2000).

Treatment interventions for burn patients have included cognitive behavioral therapy, supportive psychotherapy, pharmacologic treatment for anxiety, depression sleep, and pain management, and social support from family, friends, and burn survivors. When patients are admitted to a rehabilitation hospital they have been transferred from an intensive care setting in an acute care hospital. In the acute care setting, the patient may have been sedated in order to increase wound healing, stabilize temperature, prevent and treat wound infections, adjust diet to high carbohydrate and protein intake, and stabilize mental status. For the first month after burn injury the patient is physically devastated and overwhelmed by illness. When the patient enters a rehabilitation hospital, he or she often expresses gladness to be alive.

After the first 1 or 2 weeks the patient becomes aware of contractures of arms and legs, neck and armpits, and pain and difficulty in movement. Superimposed upon the physical disabilities resulting from burns, there is disfigurement. Many patients are afraid to look at their faces in the mirror. They need to be gradually desensitized to their disfigurement by cognitive behavioral therapy and relaxation therapy that emphasizes the positive assets that remain. Pharmacologic treatment is helpful in addressing the anxiety and depression engendered by pain, discomfort, and disfigurement.

The transition point between discharge from the rehabilitation hospital to the community provokes anxiety. Patients with burns are fearful of facing friends, fellow workers, and family who have not seen them in hospital. Psychological counseling addresses the issue of stigma in the community. A preparatory visit home may be helpful. The Phoenix Society provides support through visits by burn survivors.

Special problems arise in the context of patients who have become burned while attempting to immolate themselves or others. Patients who have burned themselves in the setting of uncontrolled rage turned inward or in protest against a societal injustice require close psychiatric monitoring. We have treated suicidal patients in rehabilitation by providing one-to-one supervision and appropriate restraints. A small group of patients may be both suicidal and homicidal. While the patient is under our care, he/she is protected from invasion of privacy. However, the patient is ultimately answerable to the court after discharge.

COPING WITH TRAUMATIC BRAIN INJURY

Traumatic brain injury (TBI) is a brain injury acquired after birth from physical trauma to the brain by events like motor vehicle accidents, falls, gunshot wounds, and other injuries. TBI is the leading cause of death in the United States and in other developed nations among individuals under age 45 years. TBI is also the leading cause of disability among this group (Bruns & Hauser, 2003). TBI is a cause of higher rates of hospitalization among individuals over age 65 than among those in any other age group (Coronado et al., 2005). TBI may vary in severity. Generally, those with moderate and severe TBI are initially seen in an acute care setting and later transferred to an inpatient rehabilitation hospital. Treatment by an interdisciplinary team continues for many weeks and is followed by outpatient treatment in clinics and residential settings. Those with mild TBI are generally treated in an outpatient setting by specialists in neurology, physiatry, psychiatry, psychology,

and other rehabilitation specialists. A further distinction may be made between persons who experience a mild concussion with only transient confusion, brief loss of consciousness, and resolution of clinical symptoms within 15 minutes (Glenn et al., 2008). Cognitive impairment does not usually persist beyond 3 to 6 months after concussion (Mittenberg, 2000; Glenn, 2008).

There are multiple and varied effects of TBI on physical function, cognition, communication, affect, social and community integration, work, and financial stability. Individuals with an acquired brain injury are more vulnerable to psychiatric disorders for many years after injury (Bradbury et al., 2008). Social integration is a long-term problem that persists for 10 years or more after onset of injury (Lefebvre et al., 2008). Quality of life includes acceptance by family and friends of the individual's impairments, integration in a community's social and work life that may include volunteer and part-time paid work, a safe environment tailored to the individual's optimal level of independence, and adaptation of the individual to the impairments.

Damage to specific locations of the brain may cause specific alterations of mood, cognition, attention, concentration, sensation, perception, language, and psychosocial adjustment. Neuropsychology is helpful in discriminating the multiple impairments caused by TBI. Neuropsychology may also make specific recommendations to psychiatry and physical medicine specialists in how to treat the individual with brain injury. Cognitive behavioral therapy (CBT) is the most commonly used psychological technique for addressing the changes in self-image and body image caused by TBI (Whitehouse, 1994; Nochi, 1998; Cantor et al., 2005; Dewar & Gracey, 2007). The threat to an individual's identity is based on changes in thoughts, feelings, social roles, and functions. The individual must integrate the former self with the self that now exists post-TBI. The patient needs to understand that only some aspects of self may have changed but not all aspects. This is a challenging but important task for the psychiatric team in rehabilitation hospitals.

Although CBT is most commonly used, individual supportive as well as insight-oriented psychotherapy may also have a place in treatment of TBI patients (Judd & Wilson, 2005). There has been a presumption that individuals with brain injury are unable to process the conceptual changes necessary for growth and adjustment. Therefore, treatment has focused on concrete and specific changes in behavior. A similar argument has been made with individuals with mental retardation, learning disabilities, and schizophrenia. This line of reasoning infantilizes persons with mental disabilities and restricts them from expression of their innermost feelings of rejection, anger, depression, and estrangement from family and friends. A therapeutic alliance between a therapist and individual with TBI may be more difficult because of the countertransference of feelings of anger and contempt (Lewis, 1991). A therapist has to be aware of her or his own feelings toward brain injury and to be capable of setting realistic goals.

The psychiatric assessment and psychological assistance needs to continue beyond the discharge from a rehabilitation hospital. The vast majority of individuals with mild traumatic brain injury and postconcussive symptoms recover within a period of 6 months from onset of their accident or trauma. However, 10%–20% of patients have persistent symptoms of headache, dizziness, fatigue, loss of memory, loss of concentration, noise intolerance, anxiety, confusion, and depression (Glenn, 2008). Mittenberg (2000) suggests, however, that cognitive impairment does not usually persist beyond 3 months in patients who have sustained a mild head injury. There may also be premorbid cognitive and affective symptoms that might have been ignored prior to injury. Traumatic head injury may activate normal psychological symptoms such as irritability, anxiety, and depression that occur in the range of the general population.

Persistent postconcussive symptoms may have a psychological basis and may be seen in outpatient clinics where patients with mild head injury appear for many months following trauma. Most patients recover in a period of a few months, after which their symptoms resolve. Only a small group of patients recover more slowly and may not return to former activities such as school, work, or homemaking. Previous studies have noted an association between persistent postconcussive symptoms and depression (Glenn et al., 2001), psychiatric disorder including depression, anxiety, and conversion disorder (Mooney & Speed, 2001), mild traumatic brain injury (Rapoport, 2003), child sexual abuse (Raskin, 1997), ongoing litigation (Larrabee, 1997), and polysubstance use (Shahin, Gopinath, & Robertson, 2010).

Coping with mild traumatic brain injury and persistent post-concussive symptoms requires the identification of premorbid experiences that existed before the brain injury. These experiences include history of concussions, child abuse, alcoholism, or drug addiction in the individual's family; chaotic family environment; frequent moves in the family; illness or disease in the individual or in the individual's family; marital stress; bereavement; attitude toward illness and disability; and any other trauma that would have impact on the individual's belief structure. Recent study of two nationwide samples indicates that the scope of TBI as a health concern in young patients is greater than previously documented, and females are more sensitive than males to the effects of mild traumatic brain injuries (Halldorsson et al., 2012). A psychiatrist may enlist the help of a clinical psychologist and social worker to identify family members, friends, and community resources that might support a person's reintegration in the community (McCarthy, 2011).

Recently research has been conducted on the relationship between posttraumatic stress disorder (PTSD) and traumatic brain injury. Jones, Harvey, and Brewin (2005) investigated the relationship between dissociation and PTSD in road traffic accidents. They found that there was no significant difference in the incidence or severity of either Acute Stress Disorder or PTSD between the non-TBI and TBI groups 6 weeks and 3 months post-trauma. Mild TBI patients have significantly more symptoms of PTSD compared with patients who suffered moderate to severe degrees of injury (Jamora et al., 2012).

Stress may result from the effort of coping with the physical and cognitive limitations of TBI. TBI is an overwhelming, devastating experience for individuals who previously have never experienced a severe illness. The stress experienced during the traumatic event and its aftermath may be sufficient to trigger PTSD even though the individual may not remember the details of the trauma. PTSD may also occur when a patient reacts emotionally to the description of the traumatic event as told to him by a witness. This reaction may be due in part to the pain, impairment, unexpected medical procedures, and unfamiliar surroundings associated with the treatment of TBI. Some recent research being conducted by the Veterans Administration on survivors from the Iraq and Afghanistan wars may be helpful in differentiating between the overlapping clinical symptoms of TBI and PTSD.

The family and friends of patients who sustain TBI and are in a coma are specially stressed due to the lack of clear criteria for the prognosis. *Disorders of consciousness* (DoC) are a challenging clinical condition that has not been adequately addressed in the past. Such patients require unique integrated medical and rehabilitation approaches, cyclical assessments, outcome-linked therapeutic interventions, and interdisciplinary monitoring in order to ensure the optimal outcome (McNamee, Howe, Nakase-Richardson, & Peterson, 2012). There has been a perception among most clinicians that if the patient is "unresponsive," he or she is not a candidate for full and ongoing clinical evaluation and possible rehabilitation or other interventions. There has been no standard of care for such patients, although up to 15% of them can show significant recovery up to 3–5 years post-injury. The improvement of responsiveness and regaining consciousness should not be considered as an exception in patients who have remained in vegetative state (VS) for more than 6 months. However, such patients still remain severely disabled and this may have important ethical implications (Estraneo et al., 2010). In contrast to patients in VS, patients in a minimally conscious state (MCS) may have a better prognosis even one year after coma onset. Determining the boundaries between diagnosis of VS and MCS is becoming more possible using repeated clinical evaluation as well as imaging and neurophysiological tools available today (Luauté et al., 2010). With our enhanced knowledge in the pathobiology of TBI, the progress in neuro-diagnostic technologies, and increased clinical interest among experts, we are achieving better results in evaluating and providing rehabilitation to assist such patients (Seel et al., 2010). There are also better scales to assist the clinician in improving the assessment of patients with DoC (Løvstad et al., 2010). Amantadine is reported to promote functional recovery of patients who are experiencing prolonged disorders of consciousness after traumatic brain injury (Giacino et al., 2012). A few studies address the course of recovery from prolonged DoC in patients with TBI. In one particular study, which examined the acute and long-term outcome of persons with DoC, 21% of patients improved sufficiently to be capable of living without in-house supervision. Such findings indicate the need for further studies and revisiting the current criteria for authorization of rehabilitation services for patients with DoC (Nakase-Richardson et al., 2012).

Diagnosis of brain injuries from blasts resulting from various improvised explosive devices in recent wars in Iraq and

Afghanistan can be challenging for some clinicians. These injuries can be caused by initial shock followed by supersonic blast wind and prolonged front of underpressure. Many symptoms, including cognitive impairment and diffuse axonal injuries, can be caused by blast injuries. However, the result of a standard neuroimaging of the brain may not easily reveal structural change (Ropper, 2011). This should be an important factor to consider when the rehabilitation team is comparing the neuroimaging findings to symptomatology of their patients. Some of these patients may be wrongly considered to be only suffering from simple cases of PTSD, or they may be thought to be maximizing their symptomatology for various reasons.

Psychopharmacology and TBI Patients

TBI can cause variety of neuropsychiatric symptomatology such as cognitive impairment, affective disorders, significant anxiety, and sleep disturbances. Agitation, verbal and physical aggressiveness, restlessness, fluctuation of mood, and psychosis as well as other neurobehavioral symptoms can be frequently observed in patients who sustain TBI. The agitation and aggression in TBI patients may seem more frequent or severe in a male population. However, others have found no significant sex differences among these patients in terms of frequency, duration, presentation, or extent of posttraumatic agitation (Kadyan et al., 2004). Some patients may have underlying psychiatric disorders unrelated to their injuries. These illnesses should be treated with appropriate psychotropic medications. Clinicians working with TBI patients have been cautious in using certain psychotropic medications in such populations. The main problem is that most agents that can help psychosis or agitation can probably cause further cognitive impairment and possibly impair neurorehabilitation progress in these already cognitively vulnerable patients. Chronic use of haloperidol and risperidone, for example, could hinder the recovery of TBI patients. This adverse effect cannot simply be attributed to the sedative effect of such agents (Hoffman, Cheng, Zafonte, & Kline, 2008). Despite convincing evidence of adverse effects of some psychotropic medications in the TBI population, however, one cannot simply avoid psychotropic medications in TBI patients altogether. The agitation and severe emotional disturbances in TBI patients, if not treated properly, can clearly interfere with their rehabilitation care plan as well as the safety of the patient and others. A significantly agitated and aggressive patient can cause disruptions in the therapeutic environment which can easily interfere with the care plan of other patients in the rehabilitation program. Such agitation can cause significant emotional pain. Clinicians may also consider the negative impact of untreated emotional and behavioral symptomatology on patients, as well as on family and caregivers. For example, usually a patient's neurological deficits would create sympathy, but the patient's inappropriate or aggressive behaviors may cause discomfort and anger in family members and friends, and possibly in some caregivers. At times, such *behavioral* complications, rather than neurological deficits, have become the main cause of disability in TBI patients, indicating the

need for behavioral and/or cautious psychopharmacological interventions.

Dopamine-enhancing medications (such as amantadine) have been the most consistent agents in helping the cognitive impairment in TBI patients, although acetylcholinesterase inhibitors and antidepressants can also be beneficial for some (Writer & Schillerstrom, 2009). Animal study has indicated that administration of D-amphetamine combined with sensorimotor exercise can produce a steady acceleration of motor recovery, but an alpha 1-NA receptor antagonist drug, such as clonidine or haloperidol, produces negative effect on neurological recovery (Lombardi, 2008). The first-generation or so-called *typical antipsychotics* (haloperidol, thioridazine, fluphenazine, thioxanthenes) can cause adverse effects due to their blockade of D_2 dopamine receptors (Elovic, Lansang, Li, & Ricker, 2003). Patients suffering from TBI may be more vulnerable to the side effects of such psychotropic medications. TBI patients treated with haloperidol reportedly are at greater risk for neuroleptic malignant syndrome compared with the general population (Bellamy, Kane-Gill, Falcione, & Seybert, 2009). Some of the adverse effect, such as extrapyramidal symptoms and Parkinsonism, can further interfere with the patient's optimal progress during the active phase of their physical rehabilitation. At times, even a single administration of haloperidol to a TBI patient in the acute hospital has resulted in progressive disabling motor restlessness, torticollis, urinary symptoms, and confusion for the patient that continued in the rehabilitation hospital (Desai Nierenberg, & Duhaime, 2010).

Atypical antipsychotic medications (AAPs) such as quetiapine, aripiprazole, and olanzapine will not cause as much blockade of D^2 dopamine receptors compared with the first generation of antipsychotics, and are usually tolerated better by these patients. Some AAPs may even have a selected neuroprotective effect, as reported in an animals (Kurosawa et al., 2007). We can consider AAPs as primary agents for the management of psychosis or severe agitation and aggressive behavior that are *not responding to other more "benign" agents*. The AAPs have different mechanisms of actions and a diverse side-effects profile (Elovic et al., 2003). Occasionally they may cause some of the same adverse effects that are usually seen with the use of the typical antipsychotic agents. For example, there is a concern that the use of haloperidol and/or risperidone not only delays behavioral recovery after TBI but also can cause functional impairment in uninjured controls (Kline, Hoffman, Cheng, Zafonte, & Massucci, 2008). The amount of the agents and the length of their use may also contribute to the degree of their adverse effects. Some data suggest that a chronic high dosage of the haloperidol or risperidone can be detrimental in TBI patients, but multiple low dosages of such agents may not cause significant adverse effects (Kline et al., 2007). Overall, the atypical antipsychotics are clinically more appropriate in TBI patients, but side effects need to be monitored closely. The oldest atypical antipsychotic, clozapine, is not usually used in TBI populations due to its significant adverse effects including seizures and agranulocytosis (Michals et al., 1993). Ziprasidone may cause QT prolongation and patients on risperidone need to be watched for orthostatic hypotension which can interfere with rehabilitation.

Clinicians need to be aware of increased risk of sudden cardiac death and stroke in individuals who are recovering from TBI (Glenn, 2010). Experts using antipsychotics are consistently aware of the importance of monitoring their patients for akathisia, neuroleptic malignant syndrome, and tardive dyskinesia. The use of metrics such as the 14-item Agitated Behavioral Scale is useful to reliably monitor the patient's clinical response to the therapeutic interventions (Corrigan, 1989).

In addition to antipsychotic medications, other agents have also been beneficial in helping TBI patients and *should be tried first*. The antidepressant trazodone, which is most frequently used, can help patients' agitation and sleep disturbances, usually without interfering with their rehabilitation process. Trazodone can help underlying depression that the patient with TBI is unable to verbalize. Reportedly almost half of the patients who suffered TBI have depression at one month post injury, and almost one-third of such patients still are experiencing severe depression 3–5 years after their TBI (Dikman, Bombardier, Machamer, Fann, & Tamkin, 2004). The risk of suicide attempts following TBI and during the first 5 years may reach 15% (Silver, Hales, & Yudofsky, 2002). While treating depression in this population, one should remember that patients who had TBI may be more prone to having seizures and more sensitive to the sedative and to the anticholinergic side effects of antidepressants.

Trazodone is also beneficial in treating patients' anxiety, which frequently interferes with their optimal participation in rehabilitation. To reduce patient's anxiety, beta blockers have been used with some success. Propranolol has been used for a long time and is reported to be a good option for the treatment of agitation, especially during the acute stage of recovery (Brook et al., 1992). Use of benzodiazepines and other sedatives are usually avoided, as they may cause further decreases in patients' cognitive ability as well as possibly causing periodic paradoxical reaction.

At times, patients' lack of interest or interaction rather than their agitation or hyperactivity can become a matter of concern for the caregivers. Apathy is mostly related to frontal/subcortical circuitry abnormality, but is also seen in patients experiencing diffuse axonal injury (Paus, 2001). Although the presence of apathy in TBI patients is usually a neurological symptom, other physiological and psychosocial factors need to be considered as possible contributors. Many different medications are used, but agents that potentiate dopamine release and/or delay dopamine reuptake appear to be more effective in helping patients who exhibit apathy (Roth, Flashman, & McAllister, 2007). While using amantadine, modafinil, methylphenidate, or any other agents in this category, one should watch for increased confusion and aggressiveness, sleep disturbances, vivid hallucinations, or psychotic symptoms. To help patients who have a moderate degree of apathy and memory impairment, some have suggested use of electronics such as pagers (Wilson et al., 2001) or mobile phones (Wade & Troy, 2001) to automatically remind the patient to recall and initiate various tasks. Such approaches are *always preferable* to using medications if they can be successfully implemented in reducing the undesirable symptoms in patients.

Despite significant progress already made in our understanding the role of psychotropic medications and other agents in TBI population, there is still some scientific uncertainty and clinical disagreement among the experts. No single psychopharmacological agent will become accepted by all experts (Chew & Zafonte, 2009). What is usually agreed is that it is crucial to address the psychopharmacological issues. Of course, the rehabilitation team should consider nonpharmacological approaches, environmental changes, and interdisciplinary training programs such as nonviolent crisis intervention, neuropsychological testing, and behavioral modification for the behavioral management of TBI patients. However, there are times when such efforts alone may not be sufficient.

COPING WITH SPINAL CORD INJURY

Spinal cord injury (SCI) results in a sudden, abrupt, devastating loss of multiple body functions. The incidence of SCI in the United States is 12,000 new cases per year, and the prevalence is 273,000 persons with a range of 238,000 to 332,000 persons in the United States (National Spinal Cord Injury Statistical Center, 2013). Although SCI often results from direct trauma to the spinal cord, it may also result from degenerative or congenital disease. Predictors of adjustment to SCI include premorbid personality, premorbid employment, ability to drive a car, previous interests, work values, and age. SCI tends to fall in a bimodal distribution, with individuals in the younger age group involved in sports injuries, motor vehicle accidents, gunshot wounds, and war injuries, whereas individuals in an older group over 40 years of age are involved in work accidents, construction accidents, home accidents, and motor vehicle accidents. Both groups require psychiatric treatment to address the unique psychological problems of their age group. Younger persons may not have completed their education or prepared for an occupation. Some of them may have an impulsive personality that correlates with involvement in risky behaviors such as diving in unprotected waters, motorcycle accidents, drag racing, trampoline use, or gang warfare. Younger persons may feel cheated out of entering a sexual experience, marriage, and children. The mourning period for SCI is acute within the first 6 months after onset, but it may last for a lifetime. The severity of disability is not the only or even the most significant predictor of adjustment.

The use of hope in treating persons with SCI has been found to be more effective than an appraisal of threat to well-being (Kennedy, Evans, & Sandhu, 2009). Hope has to be tempered by a realistic appraisal of a person's functional capacities and chance of physical restoration. Kennedy et al. (2003) and King and Kennedy (1999) demonstrated that changing a person's negative appraisals of SCI led to a reduction of depression and anxiety. A meta-analysis of 10 studies with 424 subjects concluded that cognitive behavior therapy (CBT) has a significant short-term effect on adjustment of adults with SCI (Dorstyn, Mathias, & Denson, 2011). The effectiveness of CBT was also evaluated in nine studies using both randomized controls and nonrandomized control studies (Mehta, Orenczuk, & Hanssen, 2011). CBT was found to be a useful approach for reducing depression, anxiety, and coping problems.

Other treatment approaches include group therapy (Duchnick, Letsch, & Curtiss, 2009), individual psychotherapy, and social supports. Hospital ecology is very important in helping patients to use wheelchairs and other assistive devices. Community reintegration, especially among persons who are aging and require more social services, should begin in a rehabilitation hospital where psychologists and psychiatrists prepare a person for the inevitable hardship of adaptation to living in the community (Charlifue & Gerhart, 2004; Scelza et al., 2007).

DISCHARGE PHASE

As the active phase of rehabilitation continues, the rehabilitation team begins to consider various disposition choices. What was expected to be the original discharge plan does not seem possible at times, and the alternative disposition options may be disappointing to the patient and/or family. This moment may become another occasion when the patient's emotional ability to cope can be significantly challenged. It is not unusual to see patients or their family blame staff or others for a less than desirable outcome. In some cases, the discussion of the appropriate length of stay in a rehabilitation hospital can become heated on the part of all involved. Making the patient "eligible" to receive inpatient rehabilitation is becoming more challenging. Patients and their families, as well as staff, may feel disappointed when there is any perception that a patient had to be discharged prior to optimal accomplishment of active rehabilitation. This disappointment can frequently arise when a patient needs to go to a skilled nursing facility rather than to extend participation in active inpatient rehabilitation. Most patients are not aware of the recent progress being made in some skilled nursing facilities in terms of what they can offer by way of rehabilitation programs. Most patients and their families need to be educated that transferring patients to a skilled nursing facility is primarily a way to continue the rehabilitation process, and they should not necessarily see such disposition as a failure, poor outcome, or being "punished" for not working hard. Experienced staff can appreciate the reality of such situations and do their best to provide optimal post-discharge support for patients and their families.

Prior to discharge, the issues related to the cause of the injury need to be revisited and a plan devised to prevent the recurrence of such events. For example, the patient should be advised to avoid alcohol and other substances that can increase the risk of reinjury. If the patient's injury resulted from being assaulted, one should make sure the patient is no longer at risk for assault during rehabilitation or after discharge. The changing roles for family members and significant others need to be clearly discussed to ease the adjustment after discharge. We should support the family during the rehabilitation but at the same time, if needed, the families should be referred for their own outpatient counseling in the community. If all the support for the patients and their family is coming from the inpatient rehabilitation team, it is disruptive to have this support abruptly discontinued after the patient is discharged from the program. It is a certainty that the injury will have caused many changes for the patient and family. While patient mays understand such changes, they should be reminded that some of the definitions of who they are remain the same. For example, if patients have had a stroke or an amputation, regardless of loss of ability or limb they are still sons, daughters, sisters, brothers, or parents, as before. They should be reminded that they have *not* lost their position and identity as such. In fact, some patients and their families experience that their relationships have become even more meaningful. When patients return to the community, additional adaptations may be required. The most frequent and disturbing challenges for these patients are feelings of hopelessness and humiliation. Persons around the patient should be aware of such emotional struggles and reassure the patient. Knowing of such vulnerabilities in patients may help family and friends to adjust their interactions accordingly. We should address any improper conduct by patients—specifically, hostile or inappropriate sexually oriented comments and/or behavior. Although their neurological impairments can usually create sympathy for patients, hostility or sexual inappropriateness can cause significant anger and discomfort among families and friends. Patients with moderate cognitive or other neurological deficits have less trouble getting back to the community compared with patients who mainly tend to exhibit behavioral problems. The psychiatric team also monitors the interaction between patients and their relatives, and, if needed, will address any possible expected "role-changes." Needless to say, issues related to abuse of alcohol or other substances including smoking, lack of activity, improper feeding, and weight gain should be addressed along with post-discharge psychiatric care and advice regarding the safety of the patient (i.e., driving, operating heavy machinery, etc.).Finally, since patients and their families have received support from the staff at the time that they were emotionally most vulnerable, they may have established strong close therapeutic relationships with team members. Ideally, one should plan for sufficient time for them to be able to say goodbye prior to discharge.

PEDIATRIC REHABILITATION—SPECIAL CONSIDERATIONS

While most infants, young children, and adolescents require rehabilitation for conditions similar to those of adults, there are special considerations relevant to a pediatric population. Central nervous system disorders, physical injuries, and infections are the most frequent. Other diagnoses include chromosomal abnormalities, prematurity, cerebral palsy, congenital or genetic disorders, neonatal abstinence syndrome, muscular dystrophy, sickle cell anemia, and juvenile arthritis. Children are expected to acquire new abilities as they age; when that evolution is interrupted or prevented by a medical condition, the injustice is experienced with particular difficulty. Because parents are responsible for their child's care, it is essential that they receive education and be active participants in their child's rehabilitation. Within the context of family-centered care (Lucas, 2010), the child's development, school, and peers are a focus of attention for assessment and treatment planning. The pediatric psychiatrist functions in complex roles as a consultant in addressing both medical and psychosocial factors that affect the patient, as well as in a liaison capacity collaborating with the rehabilitation team (Shaw & Demaso, 2006; American Academy of Child and Adolescent Psychiatry Work Group on Quality Issues, 2009).

ADMISSION TO THE REHABILITATION HOSPITAL

Ideally, the pediatric psychiatrist should be involved in deciding if a patient is appropriate for admission to an inpatient rehabilitation hospital. Considerations include if the patient is judged to be suitable for a pediatric unit where infants, young children, and their families may be at physical risk or significantly uncomfortable (e.g., a brain injured patient who is dangerously aggressive and/or manifesting disinhibited sexual behaviors). If an older adolescent is deemed to be more appropriate for an adult unit because of such concerns—or because the patient is a parent himself/herself or because of the family's preference—pediatric consultation and resources to support adult unit staff should be available. The pediatric contribution may be, for example, education about adolescent development, involvement of the patient in child life activities with pediatric patients, tutoring, and planning for reintegration to school. Professional caregivers in acute hospitals do not always recognize the limitations of rehabilitation hospitals' resources to provide complex medical evaluation, treatment with potential risks, and/or behavioral control. Psychiatric inpatient units may be unable to offer necessary medical or rehabilitation care. Therefore, it is preferable to stabilize the patient in an acute care hospital until he or she can safely and appropriately begin rehabilitation.

DEVELOPMENT

The pediatric psychiatrist incorporates a developmentally based perspective into a biopsychosocial approach when evaluating and caring for both children and their families. A child's capacity to have insight into his deficits is determined by the developmental abilities attained prior to the medical condition, as well as the condition and its treatments. Young children and many adolescents are unable to imagine the impact of their medical condition on their lives. Visible or invisible abnormalities can affect adolescents' body image and self esteem (Orr, et al., 1989). Dependence on others is particularly difficult for adolescents and their parents, who are already struggling with the challenges of individuation and separation.

In addition to the regression commonly seen in hospitalized patients of all ages, children with central nervous system disorders manifest particularly frequent developmental changes that can reflect either recovery or a contrast to premorbid skills (e.g., as the child's ability to communicate progresses, the severity of his cognitive deficits becomes increasingly apparent). Improvements in physical, cognitive, and emotional acquisitions often have different trajectories (e.g., gait becomes normal, long-term memory is regained while short-term memory deficits persist, immature behaviors increase). Such discrepancies can lead patients and their families to be confused about the child's recovery, and create difficulty in establishing appropriate expectations and goals.

CONSULTATION

The pediatric psychiatrist plays an essential role in the very frequent need to differentiate whether a patient's medical condition, behaviors, or mood are of organic and/or psychological etiology(ies) (e.g., whether an irritable toddler is hypoglycemic or experiencing separation anxiety from an absent parent). Comprehensive evaluation of the precipitating medical event and past history often reveals problems and strengths that affect strategy for rehabilitation; for instance, it helps to know that the child with traumatic brain injury has a history of attention deficit disorder so that the threshold is lower to treat with a stimulant, or that the patient is an athlete familiar with rigorous rehabilitation. The psychiatrist's contributions may include differing degrees of involvement in individual psychotherapy, family psychotherapy, psychotropic medication management, and behavioral management. The choice of which type of participation is appropriate depends on the patient's abilities and needs as he/she improves or does not improve over time. Although every patient and his/her family might theoretically benefit from a psychiatrist's involvement, priorities need be established because of time constraints, the patient's and family's availability on the unit, and their receptiveness to contact with a psychiatrist. An appropriate member of the medical or rehabilitation staff should discuss the reason(s) for the psychiatry consult with the patient and parents, as would occur if other consultations were considered indicated (e.g., by a cardiologist or neurologist). It may be helpful to review the team's belief in the value of support to a child and family when medical conditions are so significant that they require inpatient hospitalization, describe the psychiatrist as an active member of the rehabilitation team, and explain how the psychiatrist's role includes recommending strategies to minimize or avoid the need for medication. When resistance is encountered, the psychiatrist still has opportunities to develop an alliance with the child and parents through informal encounters, as well as to continue to work with the team members.

There is often pressure for the psychiatrist to "fix" a behavior, anxiety, or depression, particularly if those symptoms interfere with compliance (e.g., in rehabilitation therapy, taking medication, eating, or drinking). The question, "Can't he or won't he?" is key, and may focus the need for additional medical evaluation, medication, psychotherapy, and/or behavioral interventions. Patients with traumatic brain injuries are especially challenging (Warschausky, Kewman, D., & Kay, 1999). When staff describe that the patient is "behavioral," the psychiatrist can help them to explore the reasons for the behavior(s) that warrant being addressed.

The psychiatrist's medical and psychiatric background enables him or her to observe and educate patients and their families. Decisions regarding the content, amount of detail, and timing of discussions should be titrated to their cognitive abilities, tolerance, preference, and needs. Staff and families should take care to avoid talking about certain content in the patient's presence, even if that patient is considered to be incapable of understanding.

PSYCHOTROPIC MEDICATION

Psychotropic medication should be initiated judiciously, particularly in patients with central nervous system disorders and in young children, employing the adage of "go low, go slow" and considering potential drug–drug interactions. Although many medications have not been approved by the Food and Drug Administration for children under 18 years old, clinical experience may justify their use—particularly in an inpatient setting where the patient can be closely monitored. Patients transferred from acute hospital settings frequently have disrupted sleep, and the success of sleep hygiene and behavioral strategies in any hospital setting is limited. Given the importance of sleep, the threshold to treat with sleep aid medication(s) should be low. Depending on the sleep pattern, medical condition, other medications, and the patient's age, options may include diphenhydramine, melatonin, trazodone, a short-acting benzodiazepine, zolpidem, and gabapentin. Side effects of daytime sedation or cognitive impairment are rare, and usually can be resolved by adjusting the timing and/or dosage of the medication(s). A short-acting benzodiazepine may be indicated when anxiety is significant or related to a rehabilitation therapy, with the hope of treating for a brief period and later transitioning to a long-acting preparation if necessary. What appears to be "depression" often resolves as the medical condition improves, endurance increases, and the patient's abilities improve (e.g., to walk, feed himself/herself, be more independent). It is important to observe the patient's interactions in various settings (e.g., with parents, siblings, peers, in rehabilitation therapies), which may heighten or diminish concerns regarding "depression" and guide appropriate treatment(s). Symptoms of inattention, impulsivity, and overactivity in patients with CNS disorders are very similar to those of ADD and ADHD, and often respond to stimulants. A stimulant may also be efficacious to target apathy and fatigue. A mood stabilizer may benefit patients with aggression or mood lability. Neuroleptics in children/adolescents should be reserved for significant, already observed or potentially dangerous behavior and alarming psychotic symptoms. Prescription of a chemical restraint is preferable to physical restraints; such an approach is particularly relevant in a rehabilitation hospital population because of the frequency of physical injuries and central nervous system disorders.

THE PATIENT'S FAMILY

The patient's family is an invaluable resource and should be included as an active member of the rehabilitation team. Parents have unique expertise in their child's personality, strengths, and weaknesses. They may be the only individuals who provide continuity from the onset of the patient's medical problems, and spend more time with the child than staff can. Their instincts and interpretations are frequently insightful. Patients often manifest progress sooner or more readily with family than with staff (e.g., begin to talk, are more willing to eat). It is important to educate parents about their child's medical and rehabilitation issues, remind them of their past competence dealing with behavior problems, and help them to set appropriate limits even though their child is ill.

Regardless of the cause of a child's medical condition, parents often feel a sense of guilt for not having protected their child and/or project blame onto others, including professional caregivers. In addition to attending to their child's rehabilitation and medical needs, some parents are obliged to learn complicated medical care, which may inflict discomfort or pain (e.g., when their child has a tracheotomy or requires injections). Parents may feel that their ability to nurture or be "in charge" has been lost (e.g., when an infant is unable to feed, or an adolescent "won't listen"). Many parents have stayed with their child for up to 24 hours per day at the acute care hospital, may continue to do so at the rehabilitation hospital, and are exhausted. They have little time and energy to attend to the patient's siblings, a spouse, work, financial concerns, or themselves. Because there is a paucity of inpatient rehabilitation facilities for children, the distance from home may be an additional stressor. Although parents are grateful for aid from the community (e.g., providing meals, raising money through benefits), such offerings usually disappear over time. Parents' coping abilities are significantly challenged and are affected by their past experiences and emotional stability (Beresin, 1990). While providing support, it is important for professionals to respect boundaries and to facilitate referring parents to a primary care physician, individual psychotherapist, and/or couples therapist when indicated. Separated, divorced, or foster parents may present additional challenges. Ideally, information regarding custody should be obtained by the time the patient is admitted to the hospital. When tensions arise between parents, they should be helped to move to an environment where the child is not present and be reminded to focus on what is in the child's best interest.

Siblings are almost invariably affected by the patient's medical crisis, the loss of the patient as a companion, parents' absence and tensions, and/or being cared for by a variety of different people. They are often overwhelmed by questions or rumors about the patient. Even older siblings can experience jealousy because of the attention the hospitalized child is receiving. Manifestations of siblings' frequently unaddressed distress can include sleep disturbance, anxiety, depression, somatic symptoms, "acting out," altered relationships with peers, and/or deterioration in academic performance.

LIAISON

The pediatric psychiatrist's interactions with staff, the patient, and the patient's family can be mutually beneficial to all involved and enhance understanding from each individual's perspective. Observing the patient during rehabilitation therapies is a rich source of information about the patient and helps staff to feel respected and supported. In an inpatient rehabilitation facility, the rehabilitation team functions as an essential entity in which multidisciplinary expertise and communication enhance care. Recommendations to the patient and family may be more readily accepted when they come from the team rather than from individual professionals. When preparing the patient for reentry into the community, it is helpful to discuss potential responses the patient and family may encounter from others (e.g., to the patient's being in a wheelchair, or if the patient's face is disfigured by burns). Behavior plans to improve motivation and/or compliance are most successful when developed with the patient, family, and staff, followed by ongoing adjustments and education. In comparison to staff who work with adults, pediatric staff are less experienced and often uncomfortable dealing with sexual issues (e.g., managing a brain injured patient who has sexualized behaviors, discussing sexuality and reproduction with a spinal cord injured patient). Fortunately, deaths on a pediatric rehabilitation unit are uncommon, but when they happen they evoke complex feelings among the staff, including profound sadness, guilt, anger, and identification with the patient's parent(s). Ethical concerns are not infrequent and evoke both professional and personal responses (Deaton, 1996).

A psychologist may function as a psychotherapist, be involved in behavioral management, and/or perform formal neuropsychological or psychological evaluations. Although most patients' cognition is evaluated by a speech therapist, patients who have brain injuries or other brain disorders also benefit from neuropsychological testing (Crowley & White-Waters, 2010). Elucidation of the patient's cognitive strengths and weaknesses provides a more precise understanding of his needs during hospitalization, as well as when he returns to school. Once such a baseline is established, serial evaluations over time may help to differentiate between premorbid versus acquired abnormalities and to document changes.

The child life specialist provides activities and fun to patients and siblings, while assessing their play and responses. The role may include helping patients deal with medical or surgical procedures or preparing them for surgery or radiation. Ongoing communication with the pediatric psychiatrist enriches both professionals' understandings of a patient's emotional state, social abilities, and behavior.

The social worker's role typically includes working primarily with parents, exploring and facilitating resources in the community, and communicating with social services agencies or courts. When the medical condition (e.g., failure to thrive without a medical cause, nonaccidental trauma, a gunshot injury) or parents' behavior during the hospitalization raise concerns, a decision to file a report for suspected abuse or neglect needs to be considered. Since social service agencies may lack extensive experience with children who have medical conditions, offering education and guidance is beneficial.

The case manager and the team are confronted with pressures from insurance companies to discharge the patient when he or she is not meeting the insurance's criteria of making functional gains in rehabilitation. Insurance benefits for care in the home are precise and limited; therefore, a parent may be obliged to stop working, which sometimes results in losing the family's medical insurance. Parents have difficulty dealing with an adolescent's insistence on going home. Young children may cope better at home, but outpatient rehabilitation resources that have experience with young children are often limited. The pediatric psychiatrist can offer a more global perspective, establish appropriate priorities, and support staff and families as they contend with systems limitations.

SCHOOL

As the team is assessing the patient's physical and/or cognitive needs, the pediatric psychiatrist provides input regarding the child's ability to cope with the psychosocial challenges he/she is likely to encounter. Considerations include when tutoring should begin in the hospital, if the school system is able to provide adequate resources, whether a day program or residential school should be pursued, and how soon the child may be ready to return to school.

If speech, educational, and/or neuropsychological testing reveals that a patient with previously high intellectual abilities has become "average" since a central nervous system injury, the child is at risk for not meeting the school system's criteria for services, being considered "lazy," and developing psychological as well as academic problems. Under such and all circumstances, parents should be educated to identify and advocate for their children's needs (Savage, Pearson, McDonald, Potoczny-Gray, & Marchese, 2001).

CHALLENGES AFTER DISCHARGE FROM THE HOSPITAL

Most pediatric patients who require inpatient rehabilitation have not had major health problems that affect their functioning prior to acquiring the medical condition for which they were admitted to an acute care hospital. Many children are capable of remarkable resilience and make rapid gains in rehabilitation. However, as patients improve, they and their families are confronted with the contrast between their previous lives and current limitations, uncertain prognoses for eventual recovery, and the many challenges they face in the near and distant future (Augutis, Levi, Asplund, & Berg-Kelly, 2007). Interactions with peers are often very difficult; past relationships may be lost. The medical condition may prohibit the patient's ability to engage in activities or be in certain settings (e.g., because of a contraindication to play contact sports after a brain injury, the inability to access a friend's home in a wheelchair). The frequent need that the patient be supervised by a parent can be a "mixed message" that complicates regaining age-appropriate independence. Parents' time, energy, and finances are stressed by responsibilities to care for the child at home, be involved in rehabilitation and medical appointments, and maintain employment (Brooke, Kahn, Osberg, & Rowe, 1996). Siblings may have difficulties adjusting to the changes in their interactions and relationship with the patient as well as their parents having less time and emotional availability.

Discussions during hospitalization to identify concerns, needs, strategies, and resources may alleviate some of these burdens and stressors. Outpatient psychotherapy to include the patient and family provides a forum in which to process their experiences, identify preexisting and current family strife, address psychodynamics, offer support at a critical time, and facilitate the patient's and family's coping. The recommendation to begin with family psychotherapy may help reduce the stigma for the hospitalized patient and allow time to assess each family member's needs, including if the patient is unable or unwilling to participate in individual psychotherapy. The inpatient pediatric psychiatrist has had the opportunity and privilege to "live" with the patient and his family for an unusually long time and during a period of crisis. Especially when outpatient mental health caregivers do not have extensive experience with medically ill children, the pediatric psychiatrist's communication at the time of discharge and availability for future conversations are greatly valued and, most importantly, enhance the patient's and family's care.

SUMMARY

Almost all rehabilitation patients have an emotional response to their injuries. Some patients going through the rehabilitation process may also have pre-existing and chronic psychiatric symptoms, such that their emotional responses to their injuries may be secondary to their premorbid psychiatric disorders. Occasionally, pre-existing psychiatric disorders are actually a *cause* of the physical injury that will inevitably further change them emotionally, socially, financially, vocationally, and in many other ways. In most cases, these changes are not just episodic but will affect the patient and the family for a long time, often for the rest of their lives. The role of the psychiatric team in a rehabilitation hospital is to help patients and staff to optimize the rehabilitation process while trying to assist with reactive and underlying emotional distresses.

The physiatrist leads the rehabilitation team, which consists of professionals who have different skills in helping patients who are in need of physical, cognitive, emotional, recreational, and social rehabilitation. Physiatrists are physicians who specialize in physical medicine and rehabilitation, a subspecialty of medicine that focuses on the diagnosis and treatment of musculoskeletal injury and pain, and neuromuscular disorders, and the rehabilitation of patients with severe impairments resulting from traumatic brain injury, spinal cord injury, stroke, and other disabling events.

Many patients and their families are not well acquainted with the rehabilitation process and with what to expect as an outcome. Some patients may minimize their problems while others may be overly vigilant and unnecessarily focus too much on the possibility of a poor outcome. While most infants, young children, and adolescents require rehabilitation for conditions similar to those of adults, there are special considerations relevant to the pediatric population. It is crucial that the psychiatric team working in a rehabilitation setting becomes intimately familiar with each patient's short-term and long-term goals and resolves the patient's emotional responses that may interfere with accomplishing the team's plan of care. The rehabilitation team expects the psychiatrist and the psychologist to use their expertise to clarify whether a patient cannot or will not fully cooperate, and why.

Each patient's coping process begins by recognizing the overwhelming devastation and loss of function, which in most instances happens within a blink of an eye. Initially the focus is on survival and acute medical treatments, but once the patient is admitted to a rehabilitation facility the significance of the injury or illness may begin to be more apparent to the patient and the family. The psychiatric team will try to assist the patient to adapt and try to achieve the best possible outcome by considering cognitive, behavioral, social, spiritual, environmental, recreational, psychotherapeutic, and psychopharmacological approaches, as appropriate.

As the active phase of rehabilitation continues, the rehabilitation team begins to anticipate a patient's upcoming discharge and various disposition choices. What was expected to be the original discharge plan may not seem possible at times, and the alternative disposition options may be disappointing to the patient and/or the family. This disappointment can frequently arise when a patient needs to go to a skilled nursing facility. Patients and/or their families are often not aware of the recent progress being made in such facilities, in terms of what they can offer by way of their rehabilitation programs. Community reintegration, especially among patients who are aging and require social services, should begin in a rehabilitation hospital to prepare the patient for the inevitable hardship of adapting to daily life in the community.

Prior to discharge, issues related to abuse of alcohol or other substances, as well as post-discharge psychiatric care, need to be addressed and advice given about the safety of the patient to self and others. Also, the cause of the injury needs to be revisited and a plan devised to prevent the recurrence of such events. The changing roles for family members and significant others need to be clearly discussed to ease the adjustment after discharge. Finally, since patients and their families have received support from the staff at a time that they were emotionally vulnerable, they may have established strong and close therapeutic relationships with the team members. Ideally, one should plan sufficient time for them to be able to say goodbye prior to discharge.

CLINICAL PEARLS

- When the patient and the family are no longer worried about the survival of the patient and begin to evaluate the patient's overall impairment, the stage of comparison with their previous lives begins.

- Misperceptions, partially due to wishful thinking and partly due to the wrong rehabilitation information given, can be minimized by requesting a consultation from a competent PM&R specialist to evaluate the patient in the acute hospital prior to the admission to a rehabilitation facility.

- Some patients are unable or unwilling to accept the intensity of their rehabilitation and we need to modify their treatment plan accordingly. In such cases more rehabilitation does not necessarily result in a better outcome and may have an "adverse effect."

- A patient who is in denial will find it difficult to continue to use denial as a defense mechanism when confronted repeatedly while working with the rehabilitation team; this may lead to refusal of the rehabilitation program, a problem that can be evaluated by a psychiatric consultant.

- Adaptation requires a patient to separate his concept of disability from his concept of himself.

- Clinicians must focus on the positive assets of the person rather than functional limitations imposed by disability (Wright, 1960).

- One task of psychiatry and psychology is to help a person with physical disability to incorporate a change in body image with a patient's former picture of him or herself.

- Devaluation of a person with disability is counteracted by focus on a patient's abilities, moral values, and contributions to community.

- Risk factors for patients who may leave against medical advice include those with traumatic brain injury who are 24–35 years old, and/or a history of intentional injury, alcohol abuse, or substance abuse.

- Patients with schizophrenia need to be cautiously observed for apprehensive reactions and avoidance behaviors during therapeutic contacts that encroach on what has been personal space.

- The staff working in a rehabilitation hospital may, with or without being fully aware of it, experience a range of emotional responses, including disappointment, sadness, frustration, and anger.

- At times the staff is confronted by patients who do not wish to improve and who resist any fair treatment plan or discharge dispositions.

- The rehabilitation team expects the psychiatrist and the psychologist to use their expertise to clarify whether the patient cannot or will not fully cooperate and why.

- Burn survivors may be visited by a SOAR volunteer.

- Quality of life includes acceptance by family and friends of the individual's impairments, integration in a community's social and work life that may include volunteer and part-time paid work, a safe environment tailored to the individual's optimal level of independence, and adaptation of the individual to the impairments.

- Individuals with an acquired brain injury are more vulnerable to psychiatric disorders for many years after injury (Bradbury et al., 2008).

- The individual must integrate the former self with the self that now exists post–TBI. The patient needs to understand that only some aspects of self may have changed, not all aspects.

- There is often a fallacious presumption that individuals with brain injury are unable to process the conceptual changes necessary for growth and adjustment. Therefore, treatment has focused on concrete and specific changes in behavior.

- Most individuals with mild traumatic brain injury and postconcussive symptoms recover within six months; however, 10%–20% of patients have persistent symptoms of headache, dizziness, fatigue, loss of memory, loss of concentration, noise intolerance, anxiety, confusion, and depression (Glenn, 2008).

- Most patients and their families need to be educated that transferring patients to a skilled nursing facility is mainly to continue the rehabilitation process.

DISCLOSURE STATEMENTS

Dr. Cahen, Dr. Goldberg, Dr. Herman, and Dr. Karamouz have no conflicts to disclose with respect to their contributions to this chapter.

REFERENCES

Alviar, M. J., Hale, T., & Dunoca, M. (2011). Pharmacologic interventions for treating phantom limb pain, *Cochrane Database of Systematic Reviews, 12*, CD006380

American Academy of Child and Adolescent Psychiatry Work Group on Quality Issues. (2009). Practice parameter for the psychiatric assessment and management of physically ill children and adolescents. *Journal of the American Academy of Child & Adolescent Psychiatry, 48*(2), 213–233.

American Academy of Pediatrics. (2000). Reducing the number of deaths and injuries from residential fires. *Pediatrics, 105*, 1355–1358.

American Burns Association. (2000). *Fact Sheet: Incidence of Treatment in the U. S.* Chicago: American Burns Association.

Arseniou, S., Arvaniti, A., & Samakouri, M. (2011). Post-stroke depression: recognition and treatment interventions. *Psychiatrike 22*(3), 240–248

Augutis, M., Levi, R., Asplund, K., & Berg-Kelly, K. (2007). Psychosocial aspects of traumatic spinal cord injury with onset during adolescence: a qualitative study. *Journal of Spinal Cord Medicine, 30*(Suppl 1), S55-S64.

Bellamy, C. J., Kane-Gill, S. L., Falcione, B. A., & Seybert, A. L. (2009). Neuroleptic malignant syndrome in traumatic brain injury patients treated with haloperidol. *Journal of Trauma, 66*(3), 954–958.

Beresin, E. V. (1990). The difficult parent. In M. S. Jellinek & D. B. Herzog (Eds.), *Massachusetts General Hospital Psychiatric Aspects of General Hospital Pediatrics* (pp. 67–75). Chicago: Year Book Medical Publishers, Inc.

Bradbury, C. L., Christensen, B. K., Lau, M. A., Ruttan, L. A., Arundine, A. L., & Green, R. E. (2008). The efficacy of cognitive behavior therapy in the treatment of emotional distress after acquired brain injury.

Archives of Physical Medicine and Rehabilitation, 89(12 Supplement), S61–S68.

Brooke, M. M., Patterson, D. R., Questad, K. A., Cardenas, D., & Farrel-Roberts, L. (1992). The treatment of agitation during initial hospitalization after traumatic brain injury, *Archives of Physical Medicine and Rehabilitation, 73*, 917–921.

Brooke, M., Kahn, P., Osberg, J. S., & Rowe, K. (1996). Pediatric trauma: impact on work and family finances. *Pediatrics, 98*(5), 890–897.

Browne, G., Byrne, C., Brown, B., Pennock, M., Streiner, D., Roberts, R., et al. (1985). Psychosocial adjustment of burn survivors. *Burns, 12*(1), 28–35.

Bruns, J. Jr., & Hauser, W. A. (2003). The epidemiology of traumatic brain injury: A review. *Epilepsia, 44*(Supplement)10, 2–10.

Campbell Burton, C. A., Holmes, J., Murray, J., Gillespie, D., Lightbody, C. E., Watkins, C. L., & Knapp, P. (2011). Interventions for treating anxiety after stroke. *Cochrane Database of Systematic Reviews, 12*, CD008860.

Cantor, J. B., Ashman, T. A., Schwartz, M. E., Gordan, W. A., Hibbard, M. R., Brown M., et al. (2005). The role of self discrepancy theory in understanding post traumatic brain injury affective disorders: A pilot study. *Journal of Head Trauma Rehabilitation, 20*(6), 527–543.

Charlifue, S., & Gerhart, K. (2004). Community integration in spinal cord injury of long duration. *NeuroRehabilitation, 19*(2), 91–101.

Chew, E., & Zafonte, R. D. (2009). Pharmacological management of neurobehavioral disorders following traumatic brain injury-a state-of-the-art review. *Journal of Rehabilitation Research & Development, 46*(6), 851–879.

Chollet, F., Tardy, J., Albucher, J. F., Thalamas, C., Berard, E., Lamy, C., et al. (2011). Fluoxetine for motor recovery after acute ischaemic stroke (FLAME): a randomized placebo-controlled trial. *Lancet Neurology, 10*(2), 123–130.

Coronado, V. G., Thomas, K. E., Sattin, R. W., & Johnson, R. L. (2005). The CDC traumatic brain injury surveillance system. *Journal of Head Trauma Rehabilitation, 20*(5), 215–228.

Corrigan, J. D. (1989). Development of a scale for assessment of agitation following traumatic brain injury. *Journal of Clinical and Experimental Neuropsychology, 9*(11), 261–277.

Cramer, S. C. (2011). Listening to fluoxetine: a hot message from the, F. L.AME trial of post stroke motor recovery, *International Journal of Stroke, 6*(4), 315–316.

Crowley, J. A., & White-Waters, K. (2010). Psychological assessment in pediatric rehabilitation. In M. A. Alexander & D. J. Matthews (Eds.), *Pediatric rehabilitation: principles and practice* (4th ed., pp. 21–52). New York: Demos Medical Publishing, LLC.

Deaton, A. V. (1996). Ethical issues in pediatric rehabilitation: exploring an uneven terrain. *Rehabilitation Psychology, 41*(1), 3–52.

Dejong, G., Tian, W., Smout, R. J., Horn, S. D., Putman, K., Smith, P., et al. (2009). Use of rehabilitation and other health care services by patients with joint replacement after discharge from skilled nursing and inpatient rehabilitation facilities, *Archives of Physical Medicine and Rehabilitation, 90*, 1297–1305.

Dembo, T. A., Leviton, G. L., & Wright, B. A. (1956). Adjustment to misfortune: A problem of social-psychological rehabilitation. *Artificial Limbs, 3*(2), 4–62.

Desai, A., Nierenberg, D. W., & Duhaime, A. C. (2010). Akathisia after mild traumatic head injury. *Journal of Neurosurgery: Pediatrics, 5*(5), 460–464.

Dewar, B. V., & Gracey, F. (2007). "Am not was": cognitive behavioural therapy for adjustment and identity change following herpes simplex encephalitis. *Neuropsychological Rehabilitation, 17*(4/5), 602–620.

Difede, J., Ptacek, J. T., & Roberts, J. (2002). Acute stress disorder after burn injury: A predictor of posttraumatic stress disorder? *Psychosomatic Medicine, 64*, 826–834.

Dikman, S. S., Bombardier, C. H., Machamer, J. E., Fann, J. R., & Tamkin, N. R. (2004). Natural history of depression in traumatic brain injury. *Archives of Physical Medicine and Rehabilitation, 85*, 1457–1464.

Dorstyn, D., Mathias, J., & Denson, L. (2011). Efficacy of cognitive behavior for the management of psychological outcomes following spinal cord injury: a meta-analysis. *Journal of Health Psychology, 16*(2), 374–391.

Douglas, I., Smeeth, L., & Irvine, D. (2011). The use of antidepressants and the risk of haemorrhagic stroke: a nested case control study. *British Journal of Clinical Pharmacology, 71*(1), 116–120.

Duchnick, J. J., Letsch, E. A., & Curtiss, G. (2009). Coping effectiveness training during acute rehabilitation of spinal cord injury/dysfunction: A randomized clinical trial. *Rehabilitation Psychology, 54*(2), 123–132.

Edwards, R. R., Magyar-Russell, G., Thombs, B., Smith M.T., Holavanahalli R.K., Patterson D.R., et al. (2007). Acute pain at discharge from hospitalization is a prospective predictor of long term suicidal ideation after burn injury. *Archives of Physical Medicine and Rehabilitation, 88*, S36–S42.

Ehde, D., Patterson, D. R., Wiechman, S. A., & Wilson, L. G. (2000). Post traumatic stress symptoms and distress one year after burn injury. *Journal of Burn Care & Rehabilitation, 21*, 105–111.

Elovic, E. P., Lansang, R., Li, Y., & Ricker, J. H. (2003). The use of atypical antipsychotics in traumatic brain injury. *Journal of Head Trauma Rehabilitation, 18*, 177–195.

Esselman, P. C., Askay, S. W., Carrougher, G. J., Lezotte, D. C., Holavanahalli, R. K., Magyar-Russell, G., et al. (2007). Barriers to return to work after burn injuries. *Archives of Physical Medicine and Rehabilitation, 88*, S50–S56.

Estraneo, A., Moretta, P., Loreto, V., Lanzillo, B., Santoro, L., & Trojano, L. (2010). Late recovery after traumatic, anoxic, or hemorrhagic long-lasting vegetative state. *Neurology, 75*(3), 239–245.

Fauerbach, J. A., Heinberg, L. J., Lawrence, J. W., Munster, A. M., Palombo, D. A., Richter, D., et al. (2000). Effect of early body image dissatisfaction on subsequent psychological and physical adjustment after disfiguring injury. *Psychosomatic Medicine, 62*(4), 576–582.

Fauerbach, J. A., Lawrence, J. W., Fogel, J., Richter, L., Magyar-Russell, G., McKibben, J. B., et al. (2009). Approach avoidance coping conflict in a sample of burn patients at risk for post traumatic stress disorder. *Depression and Anxiety, 26*(9), 838–850.

Fukunishi, I. (1999). Relationship of cosmetic disfigurement to the severity of posttraumatic stress disorder in burn injury or digital amputation. *Psychotherapy and Psychosomatics, 68*, 82–86.

Giacino, J. T., Whyte, J., Bagiella, E., Kalmar, K., Childs, N., Khademi, A., et al. (2012). Placebo-controlled trial of amantadine for severe traumatic brain injury. *New England Journal of Medicine, 366*, 819–826.

Glenn, M. B. (2010). Sudden cardiac death and stroke with the use of antipsychotic medications: implications for clinicians treating individuals with traumatic injury. *Journal of Head Trauma Rehabilitation, 25*(1), 68–70.

Glenn, M. B. (2008). Post concussion disorders. Chapter 138 in W. Frontera & J. Silver (Eds.), *Essentials of rehabilitation medicine.* Philadelphia: Hanley & Belfus.

Glenn, M. B., O'Neil-Pirozzi, T., Goldstein, R., Burke, D., & Jacob, L. (2001). Depression amongst outpatients with traumatic brain injury. *Brain Injury, 15*(9), 811–818.

Goldberg, R. T. (2003). Psychotherapy. In E. Leskowitz (Ed.). *Complementary and alternative medicine in rehabilitation* (pp.139–148). St. Louis: Churchill Livingstone Elsevier Science.

Goldberg, R. T. (1981). *The making of Franklin D. Roosevelt: triumph over disability.* Cambridge, MA: ABT Books.

Gritzer, G. and Arluke, A. (1985). *The making of rehabilitation: a political economy of medical specialization, 1890–1980.* Berkeley: University of California Press.

Halldorsson, J. G., Flekkoy, K. M., Arnkelsson, G. B., Tomasson, K., Magnadottir, H. B., & Arnarson, E. K. (2012). The scope of early traumatic brain injury as a long-term health concern in two nationwide samples: Prevalence and prognosis factors. *Brain Injury, 26*, 1–13.

Herndon, D. N., & Tompkins, R. G. (2004). Support of the metabolic response to burn injury. *Lancet, 363*, 1895–1902.

Hoffman, A. N., Cheng, J. P., Zafonte, R. D., & Kline, A. E. (2008). Administration of haloperidol and risperidone after neurobehavioral testing hinders the recovery of traumatic brain injury-induced deficits. *Life Sciences, 83*(17-18), 602–607.

Horgan, O., & MacLachlan, M. (2004). Psychosocial adjustment to lower limb amputation: A review. *Disability and Rehabilitation, 26*(14-15), 837–850.

Ilfed, B. M. (2001). Contentious peripheral nerve blocks: a review of published evidence. *Anesthesia & Analgesia, 113*(4), 904–925.

Jamora, C. W., Young, A., & Ruff, R. M. (2012). Comparison of subjective cognitive complaints with neuropsychological tests in individual with mild vs. more severe traumatic brain injuries. *Brain Injury, 26*(1), 36–47

Jones, C., Harvey, A. G., & Berwin, C. R. (2005). Traumatic brain injury, dissociation, and posttraumatic stress disorder in road traffic accident survivors. *Journal of Traumatic Stress, 18*(3), 181–191.

Jorge, R. E., Acion, L., Moser, D., Adams, H. P. Jr, & Robinson, R. G. (2010). Escitalopram and enhancement of cognitive recovery following stroke. *Archives of General Psychiatry, 67*(2), 187–196.

Judd, D. P., & Wilson, S. L. (2005). Psychotherapy with brain injury survivors: An investigation of the challenges encountered by clinicians and their modifications to therapeutic practice. *Brain Injury, 19*(6), 437–449.

Kadyan, V., Mysiw, W. J., Bogner, J. A., Corrigan, J. D., Fugate, L. P., & Clinchot, D. M. (2004). Gender differences in agitation after traumatic brain injury. *American Journal of Medical Rehabilitation, 83*(10), 747–752.

Kennedy, P., Evans, M., & Sandhu, N. (2009). Psychological adjustment to spinal cord injury: the contribution of coping, hope and cognitive appraisals. *Journal of Psychological Health Medicine, 14*(1), 17–33.

Kennedy, P., Duff, J., Evans, M., & Beedie, A. (2003). Coping effectiveness training reduces depression and anxiety following traumatic spinal cord injuries. *British Journal of Clinical Psychology, 42*(Pt 1), 41–52.

Kim, H., Colantonio, A., Bayley, M., & Dawson, D. (2011). Discharge against medical advice after traumatic brain injury: is intentional injury a predictor? *The Journal of Trauma: Injury, Infection, and Critical Care, 71*(5), 1219–1225.

King, C., & Kennedy, P. (1999). Coping effectiveness training for people with spinal cord injury: preliminary results of a controlled trial. *British Journal of Clinical Psychology, 38*(Pt1), 5–14.

Kline, A. E., Massucci, J. L., Zafonte, R. D., Dixon, C. E., DeFeon, J. R., Rogers, E. H. (2007). Differential effects of single versus multiple administrations of haloperidol and risperidone on functional outcome after experimental brain trauma. *Critical Care Medicine, 35*(3), 919–924.

Kline, A. E., Hoffman, A. N., Cheng, J. P., Zafonte, R. D., & Massucci, J. L. (2008). Chronic administration of antipsychotics impede behavioral recovery after experimental traumatic brain injury *Neuroscience Letters, 448*(3), 263–267.

Klein, M. B., Lezotte, D. C., Heltshe, S., Fauerbach J., Holavanahalli R.K., Rivara F.P., et al. (2011). Functional and psychosocial outcomes of older adults after burn injury: results from a multicenter data base of severe burn injury. *Journal of Burn Care Research, 32*(1), 66–78.

Kurosawa, S., Hashimoto, E., Ukai, W., Toki, S., Saito, S., & Saito, T. (2007). Olanzapine potentiates neuronal survival and neural stem cells differentiation: regulation of endoplasmic reticulum stress response proteins. *Journal of Neural Transmission, 114*, 1121–1128.

Kvigney, K., & Kirkevold, M. (2003). Living with body strangeness: Women's experiences of their changing and unpredictable body following stroke. *Quality Health Research, 13*(9), 1291–1310.

Larrabee, G. L. (1997). Neuropsychological outcome, post concussive symptoms, and forensic considerations in mild closed head trauma. *Seminar in Clinical Neuropsychiatry, 2*(3), 196–206.

Lefebvre, H., Cloutier, G., & Levert, M. J. (2008). Perspectives of survivors of traumatic brain injury and their caregivers on long term social integration. *Brain Injury, 22*(7-8), 535–543.

Lewis, L. (1991). A framework for developing a psychotherapy treatment plan with brain injured patients. *Journal of Head Trauma Rehabilitation, 6*, 22–29.

Lindesay, J. E. (1985). Multiple pain complaints in amputees. *Journal of the Royal Society of Medicine, 78*(6), 452–458.

Lombardi, F. (2008). Pharmacological treatment of neurobehavioral sequelae of traumatic brain injury. *European Journal of Anaesthesiology (Suppl) 42*, 131–136.

Løvstad, M., Frøslie, K. F., Giacino, J. T., Skandsen, T., Anke, A., & Schanke, A. K. (2010). *Journal of Head Trauma Rehabilitation, 25*(5), 349–356.

Luauté, J., Maucort-Boulch, D., Tell, L., Quelard, F., Sarraf, T., Iwaz, J., et al. (2010). Long-term outcomes of chronic minimally conscious and vegetative states. *Neurology, 75*(3), 246–252.

Lucas, L. R. (2010). Psychosocial aspects of pediatric rehabilitation. In M. A. Alexander & D. J. Matthews (Eds.), *Pediatric rehabilitation: principles and practice* (4th ed., pp. 493–500). New York: Demos Medical Publishing, LLC.

McCarthy, M. J., Powers, L. E., & Lyons, K. S. (2011). Post stroke depression: Social workers' role in addressing an under-recognized psychological problem for couples who have experienced stroke. *Health & Social Work, 36*(2), 139–148.

McNamee, S., Howe, L., Nakase-Richardson, R., & Peterson, M. (2012). NCS treatment of disorders of consciousness in the Veterans Health Administration polytrauma centers. *Journal of Head Trauma Rehabilitation, 27*(4), 244–252.

Mehta, S., Orenczuk S., Hanssen, K. T., Aubut, J.A., Hitzig, S.L., Legassic, M., et al. (2011). An evidenced based review of the effectiveness of cognitive behavioral therapy for psychosocial issues post- spinal cord injury. *Rehabilitation Psychology, 56*(1), 15–25.

Michals, M.L., Crismon, M.L., Roberts, S., Childs, A. (1993). Clozapine response and adverse effects in nine brain-injured patients. *Journal of Clinical Psychopharmacology, 13*(3), 198–203.

Mikami, K. Jorge, R. E., Adams, H. P., Davis, P. H., Leira, E. C., Jang, M. & Robinson, R. G. (2011). Effect of antidepressants on the course of disability following stroke. *American Journal of Geriatric Psychiatry, 19*(12), 1007–1015.

Mittenberg, W., & Strauman, S. (2000). Diagnosis of mild head injury and the post concussion syndrome. *Journal of Head Trauma and Rehabilitation, 15*(2), 783–791.

Mooney, G., & Speed, J. (2001). The association between mild traumatic brain injury and psychiatric conditions. *Brain Injury, 15*(10), 865–877.

National Spinal Cord Injury Statistical Center (2013), *Spinal Cord Injury Facts and Figures at a Glance*, Feb. 2013.

Nakase-Richardson, R., Whyte, J., Giacino, J. T., Pavawalla, S., Barnett, S. D., Yablon, S. A., et al. (2012). Longitudinal outcome of patients with disordered consciousness in the NIDRR TBI Model Systems Programs. *Journal of Neurotrauma, 29*(1), 59–65.

Nochi, M. (1998). Loss of self in the narratives of people with traumatic brain injuries: A qualitative analysis. *Social Science and Medicine, 46*(7), 869–878.

Oshinsky, D. M. (2005). *Polio: an American story*. New York, Oxford University Press.

O'Toole, D. M., Goldberg, R. T., & Ryan, B. (1985). Functional changes in vascular amputee patients: Evaluation by Barthel Index, Pulses Profile, and Escrow Scale. *Archives of Physical Medicine and Rehabilitation, 66*, 492–495.

Orr, D. A., Resnikoff, M., & Smith, G. M. (1989). Body image, self esteem, and depression in burn injured adolescents and young adults. *Journal of Burn Care Rehabilitation, 10*(5), 454–461.

Patterson, D. R., Placek, J. T., Cromes, F., Fauerbach, J. A., & Engrav, L. (2000). Describing and predicting distress and satisfaction with life for burn survivors. *Journal of Burn Care Rehabilitation, 21*(6), 490–498.

Paus, T. (2001). Primate anterior cingulate cortex: where motor control, drive and cognition interface. *Nature Reviews: Neuroscience, 2*, 417–424.

Ramasubbu, R. (2011). Therapy for prevention of post-stroke depression. *Expert Opinion on Pharmacotherapy*, 2011 Oct. *12*(4), 2177–2187.

Rapoport, M. J., McCullagh, S., Streiner, D., & Feinstein, A. (2003). The clinical significance of major depression following mild traumatic brain injury, *Psychosomatics, 44*(1), 31–37.

Raskin, S. A. (1997). The relationship between sexual abuse and mild traumatic brain injury. *Brain Injury, 11*(8), 587–603.

Reid, L. D., Jia, H. Feng, H., Cameon, R., Wang, X., Tueth, M., & Wu, S. S. (2011). Selective serotonin reuptake inhibitor treatment and depression are associated with post-stroke mortality. *Annals of Pharmacotherapy, 45*(7-8), 888–897.

Reid, L. D., Jia, H. Feng, H. Cameon, R. Wang, X. & Tueth, M. (2010). Does pre-stroke depression impact post-stroke depression treatment? *American Journal of Geriatric Psychiatry, 18*(7), 624–633.

Ropper, A. (2011). Brain injuries from blasts. *New England Journal of Medicine, 364*, 2156–2157.

Roth, R. M., Flashman, L. A., & McAllister, T. W. (2007). Apathy and its treatment. *Currrent Treatment Options in Neurology, 9*(5), 363–370.

Rothgangel, A. S., Braun, S. M., Beurskens, A. J., Setz, R. J., & Wade, D. T. (2011). The clinical aspects of mirror therapy in rehabilitation: A systematic review of the literature. *International Journal of Rehabilitation Research 34*(1), 1–13.

Rusk, H. A. (1972). *A World to Care for: Autobiography of Howard A. Rusk*. New York: Random House.

Savage, R. C., Pearson, S., McDonald, H., Potoczny-Gray, A., & Marchese, N. (2001). After hospital: working with schools and families to support the long term needs of children with brain injuries. *NeuroRehabilitation, 16*(1), 49–58.

Scelza, W. M., Kirshblum, S. C., Wuermser, L. A., Ho, C. H., Priebe, M. M., Chiodo, A. E. (2007). Spinal cord injury medicine. Community reintegration after spinal cord injury. *Archives of Physical Medicine and Rehabilitation, 88*(Suppl 1), S71–S75.

Schneider, J. (2010). Burn rehabilitation. In W. R. Frontera & J. A. Delisa (Eds.), *Delisa's physical medicine and rehabilitation: principles and practices* (5th ed., Volume II, pp. 1125–1150). Philadelphia: Lippincott Williams & Wilkins.

Seel, R. T., Sherer, M., Whyte, J., Katz, D. I., Giacino, J. T., Rosenbaum, A. M., et al. (2010). Assessment scales for disorders of consciousness: evidence-based recommendations for clinical practice and research. *Archives of Physical Medicine and Rehabilitation, 91*(12), 1795–1813.

Shahin, H., Gopinath, S. P., & Robertson, C. S. (2010). Influence of alcohol on early Glasgow Coma Scale in head injured patients. *Journal of Trauma, 69*(5), 1176–1181.

Shaw, R. J., & Demaso, D. R. (2006). *Clinical manual of pediatric psychosomatic medicine: mental health consultation with physically ill children and their families*. Washington, DC: American Psychiatric Publishing, Inc.

Silver, J. M., Hales, R. E., & Yudofsky, S. C. (2002). *Neuropsychiatric aspects of traumatic brain injury, neuropsychiatry and clinical neuroscience* (4th edition). Arlington, VA: American Psychiatric Publishing.

Skidmore, F. M., Drago, V., Foster, P. S., & Helman, K. M. (2009). Bilateral restless legs affecting a phantom limb treated with dopamine agonist. *Journal of Neurology, Neurosurgery & Psychiatry, 80*(5), 569–570.

Tharwani, H. M., Yerramsetty, P., Mannelli, P., Patkar, A., & Masand, P. (2007). Recent advances in poststroke depression. *Current Psychiatry Reports, 9*(3), 225–231.

Van Loey, N. E., Maas, C. J., Faber, A. W., Taal, L.A., (2003). Predictors of chronic post traumatic stress symptoms following burn injury: results of a longitudinal study. *Journal of Traumatic Stress, 16*, 361–369.

Wade, T. K., & Troy, J. C. (2001). Mobile phone as a new memory aid: a preliminary investigation using case studies. *Brain Injury, 15*(4), 305–320.

Wall, G. C., & Heyneman, C. A. (1999). Calcitonin in phantom pain. *Annals of Pharmacotherapy, 33*(4), 499–501.

Warschausky, S., Kewman, D., & Kay, J. (1999). Empirically supported psychological and behavioral therapies in pediatric rehabilitation of, T. B. I. *Journal of Head Trauma Rehabilitation, 14*(4), 373–383.

Weeks, D. L., Greer, C. L., Bray, B. S., Schwartz, C. R., & White, J. R. Jr. (2011). Association of antidepressant medication therapy with inpatient rehabilitation outcomes for stroke, traumatic brain injury, or traumatic spinal cord injury. *Archives of Physical Medicine and Rehabilitation, 92*(5), 683–695.

Weeks, S. R., Anderson-Barnes, V. C. & Tsao, J. W. (2010). Phantom limb pain: theories and therapies. *The Neurologist, 16*(5), 277–286.

Whitehouse, A. M. (1994). Applications of cognitive behavior. *Psychotherapy: An International Quarterly, 8*(2), 141–160.

Wiechman, S. A., Ptacek, J. T., Patterson, D. R., Gibran, N. S., Engrav, L. E., & Heimbach, D. M. (2001). Rates, trends, and severity of depression after burn injuries. *Journal of Burn Care & Rehabilitation, 22*, 417–424.

Wilson, B. A., Emslie, H. C., Quirk, K., & Evans, J. J. (2001). Reducing everyday memory and planning problems by means of paging system: a randomized control crossover study. *Journal of Neurology, Neurosurgery, and Psychiatry, 70*(4), 477–482.

World Health Organization. (1980). *International Classification of Impairments, Disabilities, and Handicaps*. Geneva: World Health Organization.

World Health Organization. (1997). *International Classification of Impairments, Activities, and Participation*. Geneva: World Health Organization.

Wright, B. A. (1960). *Physical disability: a psychological approach*. New York: Harper.

Writer, B. W., & Schillerstrom, J. E. (2009). Psychopharmacological treatment for cognitive impairment in survivors of traumatic brain injury: a critical review. *Journal of Neuropsychiatry and Clinical Neuroscience, 21*(4), 362–370.

PART III

PHARMACOLOGIC AND OTHER SOMATIC TREATMENTS

21.

PSYCHOPHARMACOLOGY IN THE MEDICAL PATIENT

Thomas Markham Brown, Alan Stoudemire, Barry S. Fogel, and Michael G. Moran

INTRODUCTION

The decision to use psychotropic agents in patients with combined medical and psychiatric illness requires careful risk/benefit assessment for a number of reasons. Psychotropic drugs can interact with underlying medical illness causing serious complications, as when tricyclic antidepressants exacerbate heart block in patients with cardiovascular disease. Metabolic abnormalities associated with physical illness can increase the chances of drug toxicity because of altered pharmacokinetics, as when lithium is used in patients with renal insufficiency. Since medical patients are likely to be taking other nonpsychotropic medications, the chance of a clinically significant drug interaction is increased. Finally, elderly medically ill patients are at higher risk for adverse central nervous system (CNS) effects because they have greater sensitivity to psychotropic agents. This chapter gives an overview of the basic psychopharmacologic principles that should be considered in selecting and using psychotropic agents in the medically ill. Individual specialty chapters in this volume discuss psychopharmacologic considerations in greater detail for specific patient populations.

CYCLIC ANTIDEPRESSANTS

CARDIOVASCULAR COMPLICATIONS

In this chapter, the abbreviation "CyADs" refers to unicyclic, bicyclic, tricyclic, tetracyclic, SSRIs, and new antidepressants, except the monoamine oxidase inhibitors. TCAs refer to tricyclic antidepressants only. The use of tricyclic antidepressants (TCAs) by psychiatrists has declined substantially in the past two decades (Luca et al., 2013). This decline is due in part to the improved safety profile of the newer psychotropics. The prescription of TCAs by nonpsychiatrists, however, remains robust. As many as 20% or more of geriatric patients may receive a TCA over the course of a year in some settings (Martinsson et al., 2012). Often the use of a TCA is in low dosage and for nonpsychiatric problems such as neuropathic pain. But even while the target population of TCA prescription evolves, basic issues of safety and management remain. Table 21.1 summarizes the side effect profiles of currently available CyADs.

Table 21.2 summarizes the more common drug interactions for TCAs (Billup, Delate, & Dugan, 2009; Dasgupta, 2008; Forget, Polain de Waroux, Wallemacq, & Gala, 2008).

Conduction Effects

TCAs such as imipramine and amitriptyline have quinidine-like effects on the electrocardiogram (ECG); they can increase the P-R interval, QRS duration, and QTc time, and can cause T wave flattening. Clinically significant lengthening of the P-R, QRS, and QT intervals may imply excessive plasma levels. Direct relationships have been demonstrated between TCA serum concentrations and slowing of intracardiac conduction under steady state conditions. The clinical implication of this relationship is that monitoring of TCA serum levels may be helpful in preventing clinically significant cardiac conduction delays in vulnerable patients.

Because of their quinidine-like effects, the TCAs have antiarrhythmic properties by inhibiting fast sodium channels and thus prolonging the refractory period of the action potential of the cardiac conduction system. When TCAs were used in depressed patients with cardiovascular disease, they were noted to suppress PVCs (Bigger, Giardina, Perel, Kantor, & Glassman, 1977). More recent data, however, suggest that chronic use of TCAs might increase cardiac morbidity and mortality, since when antiarrhythmic drugs (including those with quinidine-like properties) were used prophylactically to prevent post-MI arrhythmias, patients receiving prophylactic antiarrhythmic therapy actually had more cardiovascular complications than did control groups (Hamer et al., 2011).

Clinically relevant deleterious effects on conduction time at therapeutic dosage levels of TCAs are observed almost exclusively in patients with preexisting, usually advanced, conduction problems such as atrioventricular (AV) nodal block. Even in patients with first-degree block, quinidine-like actions of tricyclics at therapeutic doses usually are minor and need not necessarily impede treatment if this is the only evidence of cardiac disease. For example, Roose and colleagues compared 150 depressed patients with normal ECGs and 41 depressed patients with first-degree AV and/or bundle-branch block treated for depression with imipramine or nortriptyline. The likelihood of second-degree AV block developing during treatment was greater in patients who had preexisting bundle-branch block (defined as a QRS interval greater than

Table 21.1 SIDE EFFECT PROFILES OF THE CYAD*

MEDICATION	EFFECT ON SEROTONIN REUPTAKE	EFFECT ON NOREPINEPHRINE REUPTAKE	SEDATING EFFECT	ANTI-CHOLINERGIC EFFECT	ORTHOSTATIC EFFECT	DOSE RANGE (MG)[†]
Amitriptyline‡	++++	++	++++	++++	++++	75–300
Imipramine	++++	++	+++	+++	++++	75–300
Nortriptyline	+++	+++	++	++	+	50–150
Protriptyline	+++	++++	+	+++	+	10–60
Trazodone	+++	+	+++	+	++	200–600
Desipramine	+++	++++	+	+	++	75–300
Amoxapine	++	+++	++	++	++	75–600
Maprotiline	+	++	++	+	++	150–200
Doxepin	+++	++	+++	++	++	75–300
Trimipramine	+	+	++	++	++	50–300
Fluoxetine	++++	–	–	–	–	20–60
Sertraline	++++	–	–	–	–	50–200
Bupropion	–	–	–	+	–	150–450
Mirtazapine	–	–	+++	++	+	15–45
Nefazodone	++++	++	++	–	++	200–600
Venlafaxine	+++	++++	–	–	–	75–225
Paroxetine	++++	–	+	+	–	10–40
Citalopram	++++	–	–	–	–	20–40

* Relative potencies (some ratings are approximated) based partly on affinities for brain receptors in competitive binding studies; – none; + slight or indeterminate; ++ moderate; +++ marked; ++++ pronounced.

† Dose ranges are for treatment of major depression in healthy young adults. Lower doses may be appropriate for other therapeutic uses, and for use in the elderly and medically ill.

‡ Available in injectable form.

0.11 seconds) than it was in patients with normal pretreatment ECGs (9% versus 0.7%). However, more than 90% of patients with preexisting conduction disease did not develop second-degree heart block (Roose et al., 1987a).

Certain types of heart block present particularly high risks with TCAs. In patients with preexisting bundle-branch block (especially those with second-degree heart block), dissociative (third-degree) AV heart block may develop. If type 1 antiarrhythmic medications (quinidine, disopyramide, procainamide) are concurrently administered with tricyclics, additive prolongation on cardiac conduction are possible (Levenson, 1985). It is now suspected, but not proven, that TCAs might increase cardiac morbidity and mortality in depressed post-MI patients (Roose & Miyazaki, 2005). Certain calcium channel blockers may prolong AV conduction and could, at least theoretically, interact with TCAs in this regard. Diltiazem and verapamil both may slow AV conduction; nifedipine, in contrast, generally does not affect AV conduction, and this calcium channel blocker may be preferred if TCA/calcium channel blocker combination therapy was being considered in a patient with cardiac conduction disease.

Right and left bundle-branch blocks may be seen as a part of underlying cardiovascular disease but are not in themselves a contraindication for TCA treatment. When treating patients with these cardiac conduction defects, the psychiatrist and cardiologist should jointly establish a schedule for monitoring cardiac effects when TCA treatment is pursued. In almost all cases, the SSRIs and newer antidepressants now represent the drugs of choice in patients with cardiovascular disease.

Prolonged QT Syndromes and TCAs

One of the quinidine-like effects of TCAs on the electrocardiogram can be prolongation of the QT interval. This involves inhibition of the human ether-a-go-go (hERG) channel by TCAs. The hERG channel is a potassium channel critical in repolarizing cardiac myocytes. Inhibition of

Table 21.2 SELECTED DRUG INTERACTIONS WITH TRICYCLIC ANTIDEPRESSANTS

MEDICATIONS	INTERACTIVE EFFECT
Type 1A Antiarrhythmics (quinidine, procainamide)	May prolong cardiac conduction time
Phenothiazines	May prolong QT interval and raise TCA levels
Reserpine Guanethidine Clonidine	May decrease antihypertensive effect
Prazosin and other a-adrenergic blocking agents	Potentiate hypotensive effect
Parenteral	May cause slight increases in blood pressure
Sympathomimetic pressor amines (e.g., epinephrine)	
Disulfiram Methylphenidate Cimetidine Valproate Duloxetine Fluoxetine Paroxetine	Raise TCA levels
Oral contraceptives Ethanol Barbiturates Phenytoin St John's wort	May lower TCA levels
Dextromethorphan	Intoxication may occur with 2D6 inhibitors such as amitriptyline
Anticholinergic agents Cyclobenzaprine	TCA may potentiate side effects
Carbamazepine	Additive cardiotoxicity possible Lowers tricyclic levels
Propafenone (Type 1C antiarrhythmic)	May elevate tricyclic levels
SSRI Duloxetine Methylene blue St John's wort	May precipitate serotonin syndrome when combined with TCA

this channel prolongs the QT interval (Dennis, Nassal, Deschenes, Thomas, & Ficker, 2011). Significant prolongation may be associated with an increased risk of ventricular tachycardia and ventricular fibrillation, particularly in patients with congenital or acquired heart disease. Some patients have prolonged QT intervals that are genetic in origin. The QT interval ordinarily varies with heart rate, so that guidelines for TCAs used are best based on the corrected QT interval (QT_c), which is defined as the actual QT interval divided by the square root of the R-R interval. The upper limit of normal for the QT_c is usually quoted as 0.42 seconds for men and 0.43 seconds for women. The TCAs (and, in our opinion, the SSRI citalopram) should now be avoided in such high-risk patients.

Despite the safety of TCAs in the vast majority of patients without preexisting cardiac disease, malignant ventricular arrhythmias rarely have been reported as a complication of TCA treatment. Two groups of patients at risk are patients with the congenital long QT syndrome and patients who develop undue QT interval prolongation during antidepressant treatment (Flugelman, Tal, & Pollack, 1985).

The first group is identified by a pretreatment ECG. The second group is identified by a follow-up ECG on TCA treatment. While follow-up ECGs clearly are indicated in patients with significant baseline abnormalities, it is not clear which patients with normal baseline ECGs and no cardiac history need follow-up ECGs to screen for drug-induced QT prolongation. At present, we advise follow-up ECGs in patients with borderline elevated QT_c intervals at baseline and in patients with a family history of sudden cardiac death, as well as those with definite cardiac histories. A QT_c of 0.44 seconds is regarded by some cardiologists as an acceptable upper limit of QT prolongation (Schwartz & Wolf, 1978; Kallergis, Goudis, Simantirakis, Kochiadakis, & Vardas, 2012). We would recommend, however, the setting of a criterion for each individual case in consultation with a cardiologist.

Therefore, in evaluating cardiac patients with depression, particularly patients with a history of cardiac arrhythmias, special attention should be given to considering whether or not a quinidine-like effect would aggravate heart block or increase vulnerability to ventricular tachycardia/ventricular fibrillation. However, the cardiotoxic effects of tricyclics in inducing life-threatening arrhythmias have been documented primarily in overdose situations. Fortunately, the availability of new generation antidepressants without quinidine-like properties has made treatment of depression in cardiovascular patients much less problematic.

Wolff-Parkinson-White Syndrome and TCAs

Depressed patients with the Wolff-Parkinson-White (WPW) syndrome require special consideration if a clinician is considering the use of TCA antidepressants. WPW syndrome is characterized by the presence of a short P-R interval and widened QRS complex, associated with paroxysmal tachycardia. The condition is caused by an accessory pathway between the atrium and ventricle that allows atrial impulses to activate the ventricular tissue prematurely, short-circuiting the normal AV conduction system. Arrhythmias associated with WPW syndrome have been described as deriving from "circus movement"—that is, a reentrant tachycardia usually based on ventriculoatrial retrograde conduction over the accessory pathway and anterograde conduction through the AV node. Electrocardiographic findings reveal a prolonged QRS duration, a shortened P-R interval, and a delta wave (slowing of the upstroke component of the QRS complex).

In some patients with WPW syndrome, atrial flutter-fibrillation may occur. If quinidine-like drugs such as the TCAs are administered, the atrial rate may slow during atrial fibrillation-flutter to the extent that anterograde conduction via the anomalous accessory pathway will predominate, sometimes leading to ventricular tachycardia or ventricular fibrillation (O'Connell & Bernard, 2012; Sellers et al., 1977).

Patients with WPW syndrome who have a short (less than 0.27 second) refractory period are at higher risk for life-threatening ventricular tachycardia if they develop atrial fibrillation (O'Connell & Bernard, 2012; Wellens & Durrer, 1974). Patients with a short refractory period have been identified by a special cardiology procedure known as the *procainamide infusion test* in which patients with WPW are monitored with an ECG during an intravenous infusion of procainamide (a type 1A quinidine-like antiarrhythmic; see Schreibman, McPherson, Rosenfeld, Batsford, & Lampert, 2004). If the delta wave does not dissipate and the QRS duration shortens during this infusion, this indicates the presence of a short refractory period and vulnerability to atrial fibrillation (Vieweg et al., 1988; Wellens et al., 1982). All patients with WPW syndrome should be evaluated by a cardiologist prior to treatment with a TCA to assess if a quinidine effect would put them at high risk for arrhythmias. SSRIs and drugs free of quinidine-like properties would clearly be drugs of choice in these patients.

Congestive Heart Failure and TCAs

TCAs are relatively safe in the majority of patients with adequately treated cardiac heart failure unless the patient has symptomatic orthostatic hypotension or markedly impaired cardiac ejection fraction. In elderly patients (mean age 70) with evidence of preexisting left ventricular dysfunction, imipramine (mean daily dose 223 mg/day, mean plasma level 338 ng/ml) had little to no effect on cardiac ejection fraction as measured by first-pass radionuclide angiography (Glassman, Johnson, & Giardina, 1983). Nortriptyline also does not significantly affect ejection fraction in patients with stable congestive heart failure and may be less likely than imipramine to induce orthostatic hypotension (Roose, Glassman, & Giardina, 1986). Nortriptyline would thus be a reasonable first-choice TCA in a patient with stable congestive heart failure. The use of bupropion, fluoxetine, sertraline, venlafaxine, and other relatively new antidepressants in patients with cardiovascular disease is discussed later, since

these newer drugs are almost always preferred in patients with heart disease.

Orthostatic Hypotension and TCAs

The cardiovascular effect of TCAs most often leading to discontinuation of treatment is orthostatic hypotension. Orthostatic hypotension is defined as a fall in systolic blood pressure of 20 mmHg or more, and in diastolic blood pressure of 10 mmHg or more, measured 3 minutes after a person stands up from a supine position. Because many patients with orthostatic hypotension lack subjective symptoms of orthostasis, the clinician should assess for this when there exists a risk, such as with prescription of a TCA (Lanier, Mote, & Clay, 2011).

Antidepressant use travels with an increased risk of having a hip fracture among elderly patients (Oderda, Young, Asche, & Pepper, 2012). Orthostatic hypotension is an important factor in this increased risk. Elderly patients treated with TCAs have a 60% increase in the risk of hip fracture as compared to matched controls, with the highest risk period for falls being the first 90 days in treatment (Ray, Griffin, & Malcolm, 1991). In a study by Glassman and associates, almost half of the study patients had to discontinue the drug because of orthostatic hypotension (Glassman, Bigger, & Giardina, 1979). Impairment of left ventricular function with or without hypotension is a significant risk factor for the development of tricyclic-induced orthostatic hypotension (Glassman, Johnson, & Giardina, 1986). Bundle-branch block may be another risk factor for orthostatic hypotension during treatment (Roose, Glassman, & Giardina, 1986). Glassman, Bigger, and Giardina (1979) reported no consistent relationship between the daily dose of plasma level of imipramine and subsequent development of orthostatic hypotension. A similar lack of predictive correlation between plasma levels and subsequent orthostatic hypotension has also been observed with nortriptyline (Smith, Chojnacki, & Hu, 1980). One reason for the difficulty in correlating plasma levels with orthostatic hypotension may be the activity of P-glycoprotein (Pgp). Pgp is a cellular protein found lining the brain, heart, and intestines that regulates the flux of various compounds across the plasma membrane. TCAs, including amitriptyline and nortriptyline, are substrates of Pgp. Pgp would tend to extrude TCAs from its target organs. However, innate variations in Pgp activity, as well as inhibitors of Pgp, can cause TCAs to accumulate. This may enhance fall risk without being strictly linked to plasma level (Roberts, Joyce, Mulder, & Begg, 2002).

A recent report compared falls in depressed nursing home patients treated with TCAs versus SSRIs. While depressed patients had a higher rate of falls than nondepressed patients, there was no significant difference in falls between patients treated with SSRIs and TCAs. The risk of having a hip fracture among TCAs as a class is essentially the same as for the SSRIs as a class (Oderda et al., 2012). Thus, it appears that depression itself confers a risk of falling, possibly because of psychomotor retardation or dehydration causing syncope. In patients with preexisting CHF, TCAs still cause dramatically more hypotension than SSRIs do, SSRIs having almost no effect on blood pressure (Thapa et al., 1998).

Bupropion has minimal effect on the cardiovascular system and does not cause orthostatic hypotension (Roose et al., 1987b; Thase et al., 2008); it may even raise blood pressure. Fluoxetine, sertraline, paroxetine, and other SSRIs appear to have little to no clinically significant effect on blood pressure. Venlafaxine, at higher dose ranges (i.e., >225 millgrams per day) can raise blood pressure. Duloxetine and reboxetine can also elevate blood pressure (D. Taylor, 2008). No consistent trend on blood pressure has as yet been observed with mirtazapine, although in some patients it does cause a small decrease in supine blood pressure.

ANTICHOLINERGIC EFFECTS AND TCAS

Particularly in elderly patients, highly anticholinergic drugs are relatively poorly tolerated with common complications being constipation and delirium. In men with benign prostatic hypertrophy, urinary retention may be a major problem, sometimes even necessitating surgical correction before TCAs could be tolerated. In patients with diabetic gastroparesis, the anticholinergic side effects of TCAs exacerbate problems with delayed gastric motility. Precipitation of narrow-angle glaucoma "crises" may occur, although patients with narrow-angle glaucoma can be safely treated with TCAs if they have first been treated ophthalmologically. Open-angle glaucoma, which is much more common than the narrow-angle type, is not exacerbated by the anticholinergic effects of TCAs. And for those patients with narrow-angle glaucoma who have had laser iridotomy, anticholinergic agents are also relatively safe (Kato, Yoshida, Suzuki, Murase, & Gotoh, 2005; Lieberman & Stoudemire, 1987).

In patients prone to the anticholinergic side effects, drugs with lesser anticholinergic effects should be chosen. Drugs of choice among the older TCA agents are desipramine or nortriptyline. The newer agents—bupropion, sertraline, fluoxetine, and venlafaxine—have almost no anticholinergic effects. Paroxetine has distinct anticholinergic properties that can become clinically significant. Citalopram and escitalopram have almost no anticholinergic effects (Chew et al., 2008). While the use of trazodone does not appear to produce anticholinergic effects, it may rarely cause priapism or bladder outlet obstruction, and it frequently is excessively sedating in therapeutic doses (300–600 mg/day). Trazodone at therapeutic dose ranges also tends to cause orthostatic hypotension in elderly patients (Poon & Braun, 2005)

TCA EFFECTS IN PATIENTS WITH RENAL FAILURE

Psychiatric illness is seen in perhaps 5% to 20% of patients undergoing hemodialysis. Many of these patients are being treated for psychiatric disease. In the case of the tricyclic antidepressants, some of these patients may be receiving treatment for conditions related to their renal problem, such as diabetic neuropathy (Fraile et al., 2009). Clinicians have long noted that patients with renal failure and those on dialysis appear to be more sensitive to the side effects of TCAs, although the reasons for this phenomenon are not entirely clear (Levy, 1987). Hemodialysis does remove TCAs (Unterecker et al., 2012). However, hydroxylated tricyclic metabolites, which have been found to be markedly elevated in renal failure and dialysis patients, may be involved in producing side-effects (Dawling et al., 1982; Lieberman et al., 1985). Although the hydroxylated metabolites of tricyclics are higher in patients with renal disease as compared to normal control patients, serum levels of the parent tricyclic compounds (amitriptyline and nortriptyline) are generally only slightly higher in dialysis patients compared to control subjects after oral doses (Lieberman et al., 1985). Hence, although there are no data suggesting the need for routine measurement of the hydroxylated metabolites of TCAs in patients with chronic renal failure or those on dialysis, the likelihood that these metabolites contribute to side effect hypersensitivity argues for more conservative titration of doses in this patient population. Levels of fluoxetine have been studied in dialysis and renal failure patients and seem to be stable at the usual doses. The SSRIs have supplanted TCAs in renal failure patients for the management of depression.

DOSAGE AND PLASMA LEVELS OF TCAS

An essential principle for the safe use of any TCA in elderly and medically ill patients is careful titration of dosage. Starting doses of traditional tricyclic drugs such as imipramine, desipramine, and nortriptyline should be low (10 mg or 25 mg) in patients with proneness to or preexisting orthostatic hypotension or with other predictable vulnerabilities to side effects of TCAs. Doses may be increased every 2 to 4 days as tolerated. Assessment for expected side effects (e.g., hypotension or cardiac arrhythmia) should be carried out after each dosage increase. Peak plasma levels for most tricyclic antidepressants are reached 2 to 4 hours after oral ingestion. Because of the long half-life of most of the standard antidepressants, the dose may be given once daily in the evening, which can facilitate both sleep induction and compliance.

Obtaining a baseline electrocardiogram is strongly recommended. The serum tricyclic level has often been used to help determine whether or not a patient is on a therapeutic dose. Functional measures of effect, such as the QTc, can help to determine whether or not the same dose is potentially toxic. Just as the dose of a drug does not always translate into a predictable serum level, the serum level is in turn only a rough gauge of the drug's concentration within important target tissues, such as the heart. In other words, TCA dose is not as significant a measure of risk as serum TCA level, and the serum TCA level is not always as accurate an indicator of risk as a functional measure (Rodriguez de la Torre et al., 2001). Because widening of the QTc may be asymptomatic until it is frankly dangerous, a baseline ECG is needed.

PREDOMINATELY "SEROTONERGIC" ANTIDEPRESSANTS (SSRIS)

Fluoxetine

Fluoxetine, the classic serotonin reuptake blocker, has very little affinity for muscarinic, histaminic, dopaminergic, serotonergic (5-HT$_1$ or 5-HT$_2$), and a$_1$- or a$_2$-noradrenergic receptors in vitro (Stark, Fuller, & Wong, 1985). Its low affinity for other neurotransmitter systems probably accounts for its very low incidence of anticholinergic, antihistaminic, sedative, and hypotensive effects. In most of the early studies, the side effects that have been most frequently reported are anxiety, insomnia, anorexia, and nausea (Feighner et al., 1988). Anxiety, nervousness, and insomnia, which may affect 10%–15% of fluoxetine-treated patients, may represent a form of akathisia, a side effect that can limit treatment even if benzodiazepines or beta blockers are coadministered to attenuate it (Koliscak et al., 2009). Panic disorder patients are extremely sensitive to SSRIs and usually tolerate starting doses 50%–70% lower than starting doses for depression (e.g., 5 mg liquid fluoxetine).

Although fluoxetine causes insomnia in some patients, a substantial number of patients (10%–20%) experience drowsiness or sedation, especially in the early phases of treatment, which usually will decrease over time (Feighner & Cohn, 1985). The same observation is true for other SSRIs. The sedation may be continuous, or most pronounced in the late afternoon, a pattern also seen with monoamine oxidase inhibitors (MAOIs).

Fluoxetine is benign in respect to the heart. In a comprehensive study of the effects of fluoxetine on cardiac conduction, Fisch (1985) examined a total of 1506 ECGs from 753 patients treated with amitriptyline (54), doxepin (56), imipramine (165), fluoxetine (312), and placebo (166). No appreciable changes in the ECG were seen with the use of fluoxetine. This observation is confirmed by fluoxetine's lack of cardiotoxicity in overdose.

Accumulating sporadic case reports, however, reveal some cardiac side effects of fluoxetine although cause-and-effect relationships are difficult to assess because of the anecdotal nature of these observations. Case reports of bradycardia (with syncope) and of atrial fibrillation associated with fluoxetine have been published (Buff et al., 1991; Ellison, Milofsky, & Ely, 1990; Feder, 1991). The SSRIs in general are relatively benign, even in patients with significant degrees of cardiovascular illness. Exceptions do exist.

Two important exceptions to the idea that fluoxetine is benign with respect to the heart are the serotonin syndrome and drug–drug interactions. The serotonin syndrome is a catastrophic drug side effect discussed elsewhere. Fluoxetine can contribute to the development of the serotonin syndrome, including its occasionally fatal cardiovascular consequences. The potential pharmacokinetic drug–drug interactions of risk to the heart include some deliberate combinations with fluoxetine. For example, fluoxetine inhibits Pgp, a pump located in the plasma membrane the function of which is to move compounds from within the cell to the outside. Many drugs are substrates of Pgp and some drugs, such as fluoxetine, inhibit it (Argov, Kashi, Peer, & Margalit, 2009).

Fluoxetine has been reported to prolong the half-life of diazepam and reduce its clearance, resulting in higher plasma concentrations of diazepam and a reduction in the rate of formation of the active metabolite N-desmethyldiazepam. However, there is no evidence that this effect has any major clinical significance as judged by performance on tests of psychomotor abilities (Lemberger et al., 1988). A few other agents have been studied specifically for pharmacokinetic interactions with fluoxetine; no effect on plasma half-life has been observed for chlorothiazide or tolbutamide (Lemberger et al., 1985).

When fluoxetine is coadministered with other drugs that are highly protein-bound, displacement effects may occur that result in more unbound bioactive drug being available. Such effects are possible with warfarin and digitoxin (but much less so with digoxin). There is no strong evidence that such effects are large enough to require dosage adjustment of either warfarin, digitoxin, or fluoxetine in such situations when they are coadministered with each other. However, rechecking prothrombin times or drug levels after instituting fluoxetine is a reasonable precaution. Table 21.3 summarizes clinically significant drug interactions with the SSRIs including fluoxetine (Andrade, Sandarsh, Chethan, & Nagesh, 2010; Binkhorst et al., 2013; Gex-Fabry, Balant-Gorgia, & Balant, 2003; Go, Golightly, Barber, & Barron, 2010; Henderson, Yue, Bergquist, Gerden, & Arlett, 2002; Hersh, Pinto, & Moore, 2007; Hill & Lee, 2013; Mir et al., 2012; Nelson & Philbrick, 2012; Ng & Cameron, 2010; Rolan, 2012; Saruwatari et al., 2012; Spina et al., 2002; Teles, Fukuda, & Feder, 2012).

Fluoxetine's metabolism does appear to be affected by cirrhosis, since, in relatively stable alcoholic cirrhosis, the elimination of fluoxetine is substantially reduced. The mean half-life of fluoxetine was 6.6 days in middle-aged patients with cirrhosis compared to 2.2 days in age-matched volunteer controls. Formation of fluoxetine's principal metabolite, norfluoxetine, was delayed (Schenker et al., 1988). These data are compatible with previous studies in which other low-clearance drugs metabolized predominantly by demethylation have shown impaired elimination in liver disease (Secor & Schenker, 1987; Williams & Mamelok, 1980). It has been recommended that the doses of fluoxetine be reduced by as much as 50% in patients with liver disease, which can be accomplished practically by giving the drug on an every-other-day (or Monday-Wednesday-Friday) schedule. Because the half-life may be even more prolonged in patients with unstable or decompensating liver disease, even lower doses may need to be given. Even under normal circumstances in healthy patients, the elimination half-life of fluoxetine is 2 to 3 days, and that of norfluoxetine is 7 to 9 days. However, there is a great deal of individual variation. Furthermore, chronic high-dose therapy of 80 mg/day has been associated with half-lives of 8 days for fluoxetine and 19 days for norfluoxetine (Pato & Murphy, 1991). Thus, less-than-daily dosage is rational, and frequently necessary, particularly in

Table 21.3 SELECTED DRUG INTERACTIONS WITH SELECTIVE SEROTONIN REUPTAKE INHIBITORS

DRUG	INTERACTIVE EFFECT
FLUVOXAMINE	
Propranolol	Five-time increase in propranolol levels
Warfarin	Increase in warfarin concentrations by 60%; increased prothrombin time
Theophylline	Increase in theophylline levels by factor of three
Carbamazepine	Conflicting reports: increase in carbamazepine levels as well as stable carbamazepine levels reported when fluvoxamine added
Amitriptyline	Increase in tricyclic antidepressant serum levels
Clomipramine	No increase in demethylated metabolites of clomipramine
Atenolol	Some decrease in clinical effect of atenolol
Bromazepam	Increase in bromazepam levels
Imipramine	Increase in imipramine levels
Desipramine	Slight increase in desipramine levels when fluvoxamine added to patients with stable serum levels of desipramine
Lorazepam	No effect
Clozapine	Increase in clozapine levels
FLUOXETINE	
Imipramine	Increase in imipramine levels
Desipramine	Increase in desipramine levels
Nortriptyline	Increase in nortriptyline levels
Haloperidol	Increase in haloperidol levels
Olanzapine	Increase in olanzapine levels
Risperidone	Increase in risperidone levels
Perphenazine	Increase in perphenazine levels
Diazepam	Increase in diazepam levels
Alprazolam	Increase in alprazolam levels
Carbamazepine	Increase in both carbamazepine and carbamazepine 10,11-epoxide levels
Warfarin	No effect on half-life of warfarin or the prothrombin time
Pimozide	Bradycardia when fluoxetine was added; delirium also reported, probably caused by increased pimozide levels
Cyclosporine	No effect of fluoxetine on cyclosporine levels (variable)
Valproic acid	Increase in valproic acid serum levels

DRUG	INTERACTIVE EFFECT
Clozapine	Increase in clozapine levels
Phenytoin	Possible increase in phenytoin levels
Metoprolol	Bradycardia when fluoxetine was added
Digitoxin	Fluoxetine may displace digitoxin from binding sites
Protease inhibitors	Tend to increase serum fluoxetine levels
PAROXETINE	
Cimetidine	Increase in paroxetine levels by 50%
Phenobarbital	Decrease in paroxetine levels by 25%
Carbamazepine, valproate, and phenytoin	No effect on carbamazepine serum levels when paroxetine coadministered with these anticonvulsants
Phenytoin and carbamazepine	Possible decrease in paroxetine levels
Molindone	Increase in extrapyramidal side effects
Olanzapine	Increase in olanzapine levels
Risperidone	Increase in risperidone levels
Drugs metabolized via CyP450-2D6 (includes tricyclics)	Increase in serum levels of almost all CyP450-2D6 metabolized drugs
Fosamprenavir/ ritonavir	May lower serum paroxetine levels by more than 50%
Warfarin	May significantly increase bleeding tendency
Fexofenadine	Paroxetine delays fexofenadine elimination by 50%
SERTRALINE	
Tolbutamide	Decrease in tolbutamide levels
Warfarin	Increased prothrombin time
Atenolol	No effect on atenolol level
Drugs metabolized by CyP450-2D6	Slight increase in serum levels
Olanzapine	Increase in olanzapine levels
Risperidone	Increase in risperidone levels
Tricyclics (including desipramine)	Slight elevation of tricyclic antidepressant levels
Ritonavir	May raise serum sertraline levels
Efavirenz, nevirapine,	Each may lower serum sertraline levels ritonavir

(continued)

Table 21.3 CONTINUED

DRUG	INTERACTIVE EFFECT
CITALOPRAM & **ESCITALOPRAM**	
Metoprolol	Doubled levels of metoprolol
Cimetidine	Elevated levels of citalopram
Imipramine	50% increase in desipramine metabolite levels
Omeprazole*	Possible increase in citalopram levels
OTHER	
Tramadol	Can lose analgesic activity when 2D6 inhibition by SSRI prevents formation of analgesic metabolite. Parent compound can still precipitate serotonin syndrome when combined with an SSRI.
Codeine	Can lose analgesic activity when 2D6 inhibition by SSRI prevents formation of analgesic metabolite.
Tamoxifen	Inhibition of 2D6 by SSRIs can reduce formation of active metabolite endoxifen, and reduce efficacy of tamoxifen
NSAIDS,	In patients at risk of gastrointestinal bleeding, the ability of SSRIS
Aspirin, other Anti-platelet agents	to promote bleeding may heighten the risk of bleeding with other agents
St John's wort Triptans Methylene blue Linezolid	Risks serotonin syndrome when combined with an SSRI
Ondansetron	SSRIs can reduce antiemetic effect of ondansetron in some cancer patients receiving highly emetogenic therapy

* Omeprazole is a potent inhibitor of Cy450-C19

Adapted and updated from Stoudemire & Moran, 1998. Used with permission.

See also

elderly patients. The availability of fluoxetine in liquid form has rendered more dosing flexibility for patients needing lower daily doses.

It is now well established that fluoxetine, as well as SSRIs—particularly paroxetine—may increase the serum levels of tricyclics and trazodone, and if fluoxetine or paroxetine is added to the drug regimen of a patient with an established tricyclic level, abrupt elevation in tricyclic levels may result and cause tricyclic toxicity. Tricyclic overdoses in patients taking fluoxetine can lead to very prolonged elevation of tricyclic levels (Rosenstein, Takeshita, & Nelson, 1991). Fluoxetine primarily inhibits the CyP450-2D6 and CyP450-3A4 systems (Cavanaugh, 1990) and may elevate plasma levels of any medication that is demethylated, hydroxylated, dealkylated, or sulfoxidated—which would include most psychotropics, but not lithium (Fabre, Scharf, & Itil, 1991). Carbamazepine levels are known to rise significantly with coadministration of fluoxetine, with a 27% increase in the area under the concentration-time curve when 20 mg of fluoxetine was added to stable carbamazepine doses in a volunteer sample (Grimsley et al., 1991).

The syndrome of inappropriate secretion of antidiuretic hormone (SIADH) has been reported as a side effect of fluoxetine, particularly in the elderly (Cohen, Mahelsky, & Adler, 1990; Hwang & Magraw, 1989; Vishwanath et al., 1991). SIADH has also been observed occasionally and unpredictably with tricyclics, neuroleptics, and with essentially every SSRI.

Sertraline

Sertraline is an SSRI antidepressant with marked similarities to fluoxetine. As compared to fluoxetine, however, pharmacokinetic differences exist in that its elimination half-life is approximately 24 hours and steady state levels are reached more rapidly than with fluoxetine. The drug has selective effects on serotonin reuptake similar to those of fluoxetine, and thus has minimal effects on pulse rate and blood pressure and minimal or no anticholinergic effects. There do not appear to be clinically significant effects on cardiac conduction, at least in patients with normal pretreatment ECGs. There is some evidence that sertraline can cause sinus bradycardia in some patients (Fisch, 1991). Its cardiovascular side effect profile is as benign as that of fluoxetine, and data from its use in medically healthy adults suggest a very safe cardiac profile, although the risks of such events as the serotonin syndrome and unintended cardiac toxicity mediated through such pharmacokinetic mechanisms as P-glycoprotein inhibition also apply to sertraline (Kapoor et al., 2013).

Sertraline, like fluoxetine, theoretically may increase the prothrombin time by competing with warfarin for protein binding sites, leaving more unbound bioactive warfarin available; such effects are believed to be of minor clinical significance (Wilner et al., 1991). The modest increase seen in the prothrombin time with sertraline is likely not clinically significant (Apseloff et al., 1997). Sertraline also has been shown to have no clinically significant effect on the plasma concentration or renal clearance of digoxin (Forster et al., 1991). Sertraline has been reported to very rarely cause reversible elevations in aspartate aminotransferase (AST), alanine aminotransferase (ALT), and alkaline phosphatase levels (Cohn et al., 1991). Sertraline interacts minimally with the cytochrome P450-2D6 system in the liver and is less likely than fluoxetine and paroxetine to affect serum levels of the other medications. Its major route of metabolism is likely CyP450-3A.

Paroxetine

Paroxetine is another potent and selective inhibitor of neuronal reuptake of serotonin. It has a mean terminal elimination half-life of 24 hours. Like fluoxetine and sertraline, it does not appear to have clinically significant effects on the ECG. In doses of 30 mg to 40 mg/day, it also does not appear to alter heart rate or blood pressure. Paroxetine, of all the SSRIs, is the most potent inhibitor of CyP450-2D6.

Maximal plasma concentrations of paroxetine tend to increase with deteriorating renal function, but elimination half-life is prolonged only for patients with severe renal impairment. In patients with hepatic disease there is some evidence of reduced clearance, and patients in this population should be started on doses in the lower end of the therapeutic range. In vitro, paroxetine has more anticholinergic properties than other SSRIs, but this effect is usually of minimal clinical importance other than the side effect of dry mouth. This anticholinergic effect is likely to be detrimental to patients with Alzheimer's disease.

Fluvoxamine

The potent SSRI primarily marketed for obsessive convulsive disorder, fluvoxamine, is complicated most often by nausea, insomnia, sedation, anorexia, and agitation. The agitation leads to discontinuation of fluvoxamine therapy in as many as 6% of patients (Brown & Stoudemire, 1998). Hepatic impairment reduces the clearance of fluvoxamine, and renal impairment may do the same (DeVane & Gill, 1997). The risk of toxicity in special populations, such as patients with cardiovascular disease, is essentially the same for fluvoxamine as for other serotonergic antidepressants.

Fluvoxamine is metabolized in part through the P450-3A4 system, making it unsafe to combine this agent with astemizole. Fluvoxamine raises serum levels of alprazolam, carbamazepine, clozapine, diazepam, methadone, propranolol, theophylline, tricyclic antidepressants, and warfarin. The unanticipated rise in serum warfarin levels could theoretically result in hemorrhagic stroke. Benfield and Ward have reported that the introduction of fluvoxamine to a standing warfarin regimen can increase total serum warfarin levels by 60% with subsequent elevation of prothrombin time (PT) (Benfield & Ward, 1986). The same problem has been encountered with fluoxetine (Sansone & Sansone, 2009). In both cases, displacement of warfarin from binding sites on albumin may have contributed to the elevation in total serum warfarin levels (Stoudemire & Moran, 1998). When initiating fluvoxamine therapy in a patient who takes warfarin, the PT should be monitored until fluvoxamine is established and the patient stabilizes. Serum levels of atenolol and digoxin are unaffected (Brown & Stoudemire, 1998).

Citalopram

The SSRI citalopram was introduced in the United States in late 1998 (Medical Letter, 1998). Its average half-life is 35 hours, which is prolonged in patients with liver disease and in the elderly. It has minimal effects on cholinergic, histaminic, gamma-aminobutyric acid (GABA), dopamine, or norepinephrine receptors—thus a very low side effect profile. Usual dose ranges are 20–40 mg once daily. It has minimal binding to serum proteins and is very unlikely to displace other drugs from their binding sites. Citalopram is metabolized primarily by CyP450 isoenzymes 3A4 and 2C19. Drug interactions of clinical significance are summarized in Table 21.3 (Andrade, Sandarsh, Chethan, & Nagesh, 2010; Binkhorst et al., 2013; Gex-Fabry, Balant-Gorgia, & Balant, 2003; Go, Golightly, Barber, & Barron, 2010; Henderson, Yue, Bergquist, Gerden, & Arlett, 2002; Hersh, Pinto, & Moore, 2007; Hill & Lee, 2013; Mir et al., 2012; Nelson & Philbrick, 2012; Ng & Cameron, 2010; Rolan, 2012; Saruwatari et al., 2012; Spina et al., 2002; Teles, Fukuda, & Feder, 2012). CyP450-3A4 inhibitors such as ketoconazole and erythromycin will likely elevate this SSRI's serum levels, since CyP450-3A4 is involved in the initial step of citalopram's metabolism. Cimetidine will elevate citalopram levels. Citalopram will raise the level of the beta-blocker metoprolol and possibly other beta blockers as well. Citalopram can raise the levels of desipramine by 50%. Its effect on CyP450-2D6 is minimal. No clinically significant interactions have been noted with digoxin, lithium, warfarin, or carbamazepine. Omeprazole, which inhibits CyP450-2C19, might elevate citalopram levels.

The United States Food and Drug Administration (FDA) has determined that citalopram in doses greater than 40 milligrams daily may prolong the QT interval (Castro et al., 2013). Certainly one would want to obtain a baseline electrocardiogram prior to starting citalopram. Identifying patients at risk for symptomatic QT prolongation is also possible.

Escitalopram

The bioavailability of oral escitalopram is about 80%. The drug is 50%–60% bound by serum proteins. It is metabolized through CyP450-3A4 and 2C9. Its elimination half-life ranges from about 27–32 hours. This is roughly doubled in the elderly. Significant liver disease slows the metabolism of escitalopram, and the dosage should be halved.

Escitalopram may be more likely than citalopram to prolong the QT interval (Castro et al., 2013).

SSRIS AND SEROVASCULAR FUNCTION

A rare but important issue with SSRI therapy in general is the potential effect of altering the manner in which platelets handle serotonin, with alterations in their tendency to form clots. Concern about this has led some blood banks to decline blood donated by persons taking SSRIs (Reikvam et al., 2012). The SSRIs all block the serotonin-reuptake pump of platelets. Platelets release serotonin to dilate intact blood vessels, while causing vessels with damaged endothelium to contract and form platelet plugs that lodge in the damaged and contracting vessel. Basic science and large epidemiologic studies have found no consistent clinical impact of SSRIs on serovascular function (Maschino et al., 2012; Reikvam et al., 2012). Yet in some cases, it appears that SSRIs may significantly impair the ability of platelets to aggregate. This may rarely result in abnormal bleeding manifested by petechia or ecchymosis. Upper gastrointestinal bleeding is the likeliest injury in such cases (Hreinsson, Kalaitzakis, Gudmundsson, & Björnsson, 2013). More severe examples of platelet dysfunction, such as melena, are quite rare. Fluoxetine-induced abnormalities of platelet function are among the best described. These appear to be dose-dependent abnormalities, occurring most often when the dose of fluoxetine exceeds 20 mg per day (Alderman, Moritz, & Ben-Tovim, 1992). Interestingly, bleeding times return to normal 3–4 days after fluoxetine is discontinued, indicating that the primary effect on platelets is fluoxetine itself, since its principal metabolite, norfluoxetine, has a half-life of 10–14 days.

A final serovascular issue of great physiological importance, but of unmeasured epidemiologic significance, is the effect of blocking serotonin reuptake in the vasculature among patients with endothelial disease or abnormal responses to serotonin. Early reports of unexpected deaths among medically ill patients receiving fluoxetine sparked interest in the mechanisms by which cardiac disease might be aggravated by SSRI therapy (Spier & Frontera, 1991). It has been found that patients with angina, both typical and atypical, experience not the normal vasodilatory response to serotonin but rather vasoconstriction (Fricchione et al., 1993; McFadden et al., 1991). Patients with endothelial disease, including that induced by atherosclerosis, diabetes, and hyperlipidemia, have a similarly abnormal response to serotonin (Golino et al., 1991; Sikorski et al., 1993; Luscher et al., 1993). Again, in the aggregate there is no contraindication to the use of SSRIs among patients with cardiovascular disease. Overall, the SSRIs appear to benefit such patients (Paraskevaidis, Palios, Parissis, Filippatos, & Anastasiou-Nana, 2012).

One way to understand the potential risks of SSRIs and yet their overall safety for patients with a variety of cardiovascular diseases is to include the serovascular effects of depression in the discussion. The platelet of the depressed patient is hyperaggregable. The endothelial function of the depressed patient is also abnormal, and promotes vascular events ranging from atherosclerosis to myocardial ischemia (Pizzi et al., 2012). The initial and primarily pharmacologic effects of SSRIs, such as a transient elevation of serum serotonin, may aggravate the pathophysiology of the depressed platelet and endothelium. But with recovery from depression, platelet and endothelial physiology become more normal and the risk of a cardiovascular side effect declines.

SEROTONIN-NORADRENALINE REUPTAKE INHIBITORS (SNRIS)

Duloxetine

Duloxetine inhibits the reuptake of both serotonin and noradrenaline. This is sometimes referred to as a "balanced" reuptake inhibition. Duloxetine has good oral bioavailability, although with a slight reduction in uptake with food. The elimination half-life ranges from 8 to 17 hours. The drug is over 90% bound to serum proteins. Elimination is mainly via the kidneys (70%), but also in part through the gut (20%). Use of duloxetine is contraindicated in patients with liver or kidney impairment. Duloxetine is a substrate of CyP450-1A2 and 2D6, and tends to inhibit 2D6. Duloxetine tends to inhibit the metabolism of warfarin but less so than paroxetine, venlafaxine, or fluoxetine (Teles, Fukuda, & Feder, 2012).

Side effects with duloxetine tend to be mild and include primarily gastrointestinal complaints and sleep disturbances. More serious side effects, ranging from extrapyramidal side effects to the serotonin syndrome, may rarely occur (Karakaş Uğurlu, Onen, Bayındırlı, & Caykölü, 2013). Cardiovascular side effects with duloxetine are also rare (Xue, Strombom, Turnbull, Zhu, & Seeger, 2012). Overdose with duloxetine is rarely life-threatening (Darracq, Clark, Qian, & Cantrell, 2013).

Venlafaxine

Venlafaxine inhibits the reuptake of both serotonin and norepinephrine in a manner similar to that of most TCAs. It is five times as active at blocking the reuptake of serotonin as it is at blocking the reuptake of norepinephrine. Side effects are largely dose dependent, and the most commonly reported include sedation (up to 14%), dizziness (12%), initial anxiety (up to 12%), and increased blood pressure (Brown & Stoudemire, 1998).

Cardiovascular side effects attributable to venlafaxine alone are rare (McElroy, Keck, & Friedman, 1995). However, venlafaxine does have a dose-dependent effect on blood pressure. A sustained elevation of diastolic blood pressure greater than 10 mmHg, which is greater than the pretreatment baseline and exceeds 90 mmHg, is seen in 5% of patients taking over 200 mg/day of venlafaxine. This percentage rises to 13% when the total daily dosage exceeds 300 mg. Pharmacodynamic interactions may heighten the risk of cardiovascular side effects. An extreme example of this is the serotonin syndrome precipitated by venlafaxine (Gitlin, 1997). Overdosage of venlafaxine can lead to the serotonin syndrome complicated by left heart failure. The mechanism of the left heart failure is unclear (Batista et al., 2013).

Neither venlafaxine nor its active major metabolite, O-desmethylvenlafaxine, has significant activity at a-adrenergic, D-dopaminergic, histaminergic, muscarinic, or m-opioid receptors (Beliles & Stoudemire, 1998). Venlafaxine is bound minimally at approximately 25% to serum proteins. It has a balanced metabolism through both cytochromes P450-2D6 and 3A4. Its elimination half-life is considerably extended in both hepatic and renal impairment. Severe hepatic impairment may increase the elimination half-life by almost 200% (Stoudemire, 1996). Doses of venlafaxine in patients with hepatic or renal failure should be adjusted conservatively, as the half-life of the drug is prolonged in both categories of patients. Cimetidine raises the levels of venlafaxine but not its psychoactive primary metabolite O-desmethylvenlafaxine. This occurs because venlafaxine's "first pass" metabolism is inhibited by cimetidine, but O-desmethylvenlafaxine serum levels do not appear affected to any clinically significant degree. A long-acting controlled-release capsule form of this drug is now available.

Desvenlafaxine

Desvenlafaxine, or O-desmethylvenlafaxine, is a synthetic formulation of the major metabolite of venlafaxine. Because the majority of the actions of venlafaxine come from the activity of its major metabolite, desvenlafaxine, the benefits and risks of the two agents is very similar. The oral bioavailability of desvenlafaxine is about 80%. The drug is roughly 30% bound to serum proteins. It is metabolized mainly through hepatic conjugation, with a lesser role played by oxidation via CyP450-3A4. The elimination half-life is 10–11 hours, although this may be markedly prolonged in hepatic or renal failure. Almost half of the drug is excreted in the urine unchanged, while another 25% is renally excreted as metabolites.

Milnacipran

The bioavailability of oral milnacipran approaches 90%. The elimination half-life is 6–8 hours. Milnacipran is 13% bound to serum proteins. The drug undergoes hepatic metabolism. Milnacipran is a comparatively weak inhibitor of cytochromes P450 when compared to other antidepressants (Miguel & Albuquerque, 2011). Over 90% is excreted in the urine, and just over 50% is excreted as unchanged milnacipran (Li, Chin, Wangsa, & Ho, 2012). In moderate to severe renal failure, the dosage must be reduced (Nagler, Webster, Vanholder, & Zoccali, 2012).

A case exists of hypertension, tachycardia, and cardiomyopathy associated with milnacipran use. It was thought that the cardiomyopathy resulted from a hyperadrenergic state due to milnacipran use (Forman, Sutej, & Jackson, 2011). While this may be a uniquely bad outcome, it underscores the potential of milnacipran and agents like it to cause overstimulation of catecholamine and indoleamine systems. The serotonin syndrome, an example of indoleamine overactivity, has also been reported for milnacipran (Levine, Truitt, & O'Connor, 2011). Milnacipran is not available in the United States.

BUPROPION

Bupropion, active through dopaminergic neurotransmission, possibly by blockade of presynaptic dopamine reuptake, is a unique antidepressant different from the SSRIs and TCAs. Bupropion has a half-life of approximately 10 hours. A longer-acting form of bupropion is available, and its usefulness as part of smoking cessation programs is now well established. The drug has some structural similarities to amphetamine and to diethylpropion, a sympathomimetic agent. Although bupropion has an activating effect that can be beneficial in some patients, it can induce agitation or provoke psychosis (Kumar et al., 2011). The properties of bupropion of greatest interest to psychiatrists working with medical patients are its lack of cardiovascular toxicity and its association with seizures. Bupropion is metabolized primarily through CyP450-2B6.

Cardiovascular Disease and Bupropion

As noted briefly earlier, bupropion has an excellent side effect profile (Roose et al., 1991b). It has minimal anticholinergic properties and minimal effects on histamine and a_1- and a_2-adrenergic receptors. Its relative lack of sedative, anticholinergic, antihistaminic, and anti-a-adrenergic effects would make it particularly attractive for medically ill patients if its efficacy were conclusively demonstrated to be equal to that of more established agents.

Bupropion can prolong the QRS and QT intervals. This is the result of inhibition of inwardly-rectifying potassium currents, a relatively frequent source of drug-induced QT prolongation (Caillier et al., 2012). Yet, early studies demonstrated that bupropion had little clinically significant effect on blood pressure, heart rate, or the ECG, and that it was not associated with orthostatic hypotension. Bupropion-treated patients have nevertheless rarely reported symptoms of syncope, dizziness, and fainting. Occasional patients develop hypertension on bupropion.

Few studies have specifically focused on patients with concurrent advanced cardiovascular disease. Large epidemiologic studies report a relatively low rate of sudden cardiac death or arrhythmias among patients taking bupropion, even when compared to other safe antidepressants (Leonard, Bilker, Newcomb, Kimmel, & Hennessy, 2011). Roose and associates (1987b) compared the cardiovascular effects of bupropion to imipramine in a small series of depressed patients with congestive heart failure. In a randomized, double-blind, crossover trial, 10 depressed patients with left ventricular failure received bupropion (mean dose 445 mg/day) versus imipramine (mean dose 197 mg/day). Neither bupropion nor imipramine adversely affected ejection fraction or other indices of left ventricular function. Half of the patients treated with imipramine, however, developed severe orthostatic hypotension. Bupropion, in contrast, was well tolerated and did not cause orthostatic hypotension. Bupropion had no effect on the ECG.

A report (Roose et al., 1991b) on 36 depressed patients with cardiac disease confirmed bupropion's general safety in cardiac patients, indicating that (1) pulse rate was not changed; (2) supine blood pressure sometimes was elevated; (3) orthostatic hypotension was observed in only 1 of 36 study patients; (4) no significant effects were observed on cardiac conduction, nor were higher degrees of AV block induced in patients with preexisting bundle-branch block; (5) preexisting ventricular arrhythmias were not exacerbated; and (6) no effect was observed on ejection fraction in patients with impaired left ventricular function. In two patients, however, the drug had to be discontinued because of exacerbation of baseline hypertension.

Seizures and Bupropion

Seizures may occur in 0.35% to 0.44% of patients taking bupropion. This risk rises with the dose used, but the association with serum levels is weak enough that obtaining a bupropion serum level does not help stratify the risk. It may be that recreational abuse of bupropion by intranasal insufflation ("snorting") may increase the risk of having a seizure (Kim & Steinhart, 2010). This well-known concern with bupropion and seizures has decreased in general populations with the availability of its longer-acting form due to smoother serum levels and less "peaking" effect in the CNS. The drug should still not be used without anticonvulsant prophylaxis in patients with known risk factors for seizures.

Theoretically, bupropion might be relatively contraindicated in the treatment of depression in alcoholics because of their increased risk of seizures (as a result of head trauma, withdrawal, etc.). Furthermore, bupropion undergoes a first-pass effect influenced by alcoholic liver disease that can alter both pharmacokinetics and dose-response relationships. Although prolongation in the half-life of bupropion metabolites in patients with a history of alcoholism may be only minimal, the drug should be used with lower initial doses and carefully titrated, if it is used at all, in alcoholic patients (DeVane et al., 1990). Similar concerns exist for other high-risk patients in psychiatry, including patients with anorexia nervosa and malnourished patients.

NEFAZODONE

Nefazodone is unique among antidepressants in that its therapeutic action appears to involve both inhibition of serotonin reuptake and antagonism of $5HT_2$ receptors. Clinically significant fatigue, dizziness, blurred vision, and lightheadedness are attributed to nefazodone. These may be related to the tendency of nefazodone to lower systolic blood pressure slightly (Beliles & Stoudemire, 1998). As a single agent, nefazodone appears to have little effect on the EKG (Beliles & Stoudemire, 1998).

Nefazodone is metabolized primarily through CyP450 3A4, however, and may inhibit the metabolism of astemizole and interact with other drugs metabolized by this isoenzyme.

One of the major metabolites of nefazodone is the serotonin agonist and anxiogenic compound metachlorophenylpiperazine (mCPP), which is metabolized by CyP450-2D6. If an inhibitor of P450-2D6, like paroxetine, is discontinued and nefazodone added (before CyP450-2D6 activity recovers), high levels of mCPP will continue to circulate and cause severe anxiety. When switching from a long-acting SSRI (like fluoxetine) to nefazodone, a washout period should be allowed for the SSRI consistent with the SSRI's half-life. Activation of $5HT_{2c}$ receptors by mCPP may cause anxiety and akathisia (Brown & Stoudemire, 1998).

Hepatotoxicity is the most worrisome side effect usually attributed to nefazodone. By 2005, the FDA had received 55 reports of hepatic failure due to nefazodone, 20 of which resulted in death. This is a rate of about 1 case of hepatic failure per 250,000 to 300,000 patients. A reactive metabolite is thought to be responsible for the liver injury (Kalgutkar et al., 2005). Because of the infrequency of this catastrophic side-effect, predicting who is at risk is difficult. The product carries a black box warning for hepatic failure.

MIRTAZAPINE

While usually not formally classified as an SSRI, mirtazapine appears to have limited effects on the cardiovascular system and is relatively safe in overdose. However, over 50% of patients taking mirtazapine experience significant dose-dependent sedation. Increased appetite and weight gain also complicate mirtazapine therapy (Nelson, 1997; Watanabe et al., 2010). Although catastrophic side effects such as the serotonin syndrome can occur with mirtazapine, in general the drug is safe even in overdose (Waring, Good, & Bateman, 2007).

Mirtazapine has a unique mechanism of action. Mirtazapine antagonizes presynaptic a_2-adrenoreceptors, which "disinhibits" (facilitates) the release of central norepinephrine. Norepinephrine stimulates a_1-adrenoreceptors located on central serotonin neurons, which then causes the release of serotonin. Mirtazapine also blocks central $5HT_2$ and $5HT_3$ serotonin receptors, as well as central histamine H_1 receptors (deBoer, 1996). Blockade of central histamine receptors likely accounts for the sedating effect of mirtazapine. The net effect of mirtazapine's complex pharmacologic profile on the cardiovascular system is more difficult to predict. However, at this time mirtazapine alone appears to have little effect on the EKG.

Mirtazapine is 85% bound to plasma proteins. It undergoes extensive metabolism involving cytochromes P450-1A2, 2D6, and 3A4. It is not a potent inhibitor of any of these three isoenzymes (Delbressine & Vos, 1997). The manufacturer notes that hepatic impairment may reduce the clearance of mirtazapine by 30%, while renal impairment may reduce the clearance of mirtazapine by 30% to 50%.

NEUROLEPTICS

The major classes of "standard," or "traditional," or "typical" neuroleptics include phenothiazines (such as chlorpromazine, trifluoperazine, perphenazine, fluphenazine, and thioridazine), butyrophenones (such as haloperidol), thioxanthenes (such as thiothixene), dihydroindolones (such as molidone), and dibenzoxazepines (such as loxapine).

All neuroleptics are well absorbed from the gastrointestinal tract. Hypoacidity (as in antacid therapy) and increased gastric emptying may result in increased absorption, whereas increased gastric acidity and delayed gastric emptying will result in decreased absorption, although such effects are of doubtful clinical significance. Neuroleptics are highly lipophilic and highly protein-bound. Thus, as with cyclic antidepressants, dialysis is not useful in overdose. Neuroleptics are metabolized primarily via hepatic oxidation pathways. Portal hypertension or congestive failure can decrease first-pass metabolism and increase the activity of these drugs.

Common drug interactions with neuroleptics are listed in Table 21.4 (Laplane et al., 1992).

Neuroleptics may be broadly classified into three major categories: traditional "low-potency" agents such as chlorpromazine and thioridazine, traditional "high-potency" agents such as haloperidol and fluphenazine, and "atypical" agents such as clozapine, olanzapine, risperidone, and quetiapine. Differences among these agents are outlined below (Nordstrom et al., 1998).

Despite the vast improvement in side effects that the atypical agents have brought, the risks of the major neuropsychiatric side effects of antipsychotic medications, such as the neuroleptic malignant syndrome (NMS), likely remains with all available agents including the atypicals (Trayer & Fidler, 1998). For example, NMS has been reported with clozapine and with olanzapine (Apple & Haur, 1999). Both caution and optimism are warranted in this regard with the atypical agents.

The appropriate use of neuroleptics in the medically ill and geriatric populations requires considerable knowledge and care on the part of the physician. In addition to their use in psychiatric patients who have concurrent medical illnesses and in medically ill patients with secondary psychiatric symptoms, neuroleptics are widely used in geriatric patients to control such symptoms as agitation, wandering, behavioral dyscontrol, and confusion. In fact, neuroleptics at one time were the third most utilized class of drugs in nursing homes in the United States (Phillipson et al., 1990). The rate of use of these agents among the elderly in nursing homes remains high. A study of over 1.4 million nursing home residents across the country revealed that 22% were prescribed an antipsychotic. The most commonly prescribed were the atypical agents risperidone, quetiapine and olanzapine (Briesacher et al., 2013). In a similar though smaller study of residents in veterans' nursing homes, 26% of residents were prescribed an antipsychotic agent. However, only 60% had an evidence-based reason for receiving such medication (Gellad et al., 2012). The extensive use of these drugs in a group of patients who are especially susceptible to their untoward side effects calls for careful attention to treatment strategies and risk/benefit assessments. The availability of antipsychotics with minimal extrapyramidal side effects such as olanzapine, and especially quetiapine, has significantly changed the risk/benefit profile of using neuroleptics in the medically ill.

Other serious medical events have been linked to initiation of an antipsychotic. A worrisome pronouncement was made by the FDA in 2005 that the use of atypical antipsychotics among elderly patients was associated with a 1.6-fold to 1.7-fold increase in all-cause mortality (US Food and Drug Administration, 2005). Across 17 placebo-controlled studies, with a modal duration of 10 weeks, 4.5% of patients with psychosis attributed to dementia died versus 2.6% of

Table 21.4 REPORTED DRUG INTERACTIONS WITH NEUROLEPTICS

MEDICATION	INTERACTIVE EFFECT
Type 1A Antiarrhythmics	Chlorpromazine/thioridazine may prolong cardiac conduction
Tricyclics	
Beta blockers	
Chloramphenicol	
Disulfiram	Disulfiram can cause extrapyramidal symptoms and increases risk of EPS with neuroleptics
Fluoxetine	
Paroxetine	May increase neuroleptic levels
MAOIs	
Other SSRIs	
Acetaminophen	
Valproic acid/valproate	
Buspirone	
Barbiturates / Rifampin	Lower neuroleptic levels through induction of hepatic enzymes
Griseofulvin	
Phenylbutazone	
Carbamazepine	
Fluvoxamine	Raises clozapine levels
Rifampin	Lowers clozapine levels
Gel-type antacids	May interfere with neuroleptic absorption
Enflurane	Potentiate hypotensive effects of neuroleptics
Isoflurane	
Prazosin	Increase hypotensive effect
ACE inhibitors (captopril, enalapril)	
Narcotics	May increase sedative effects of neuroleptics
Tricyclics	
Barbiturates	
Iproniazid	May cause encephalopathy and hepatotoxicity when used with neuroleptics
Guanethidine Clonidine	Neuroleptics may decrease blood pressure control

such patients receiving a placebo. Cause of death varied, but tended to be the result of a cardiac event or pneumonia. These findings inspired a host of further studies intended to clarify these risks.

In a review of randomized trials and meta-analyses, Pratt and colleagues found that there was a 20%–30% increased rate of death among elderly patients prescribed an atypical antipsychotic, or 1 additional death per 100 patients. This compared favorably with the use of typical antipsychotics, which yielded between 2 and 7 additional deaths per 100 patients when compared to the use of atypical agents (Pratt, Roughead, Salter, & Ryan, 2012). Subsequent analysis of the FDA data revealed that for patients over 65 years old, whether demented or not, taking an antipsychotic was associated with a roughly twofold increase in the risk of pneumonia. The risk appeared greatest within the first week of starting antipsychotic therapy. Agents associated with pneumonia also seem to prolong the course of pneumonia, strengthening a causal link. Among typical antipsychotics, phenothiazines such as chlorpromazine may carry a greater risk of being followed by pneumonia than do butyrophenones such as haloperidol, although haloperidol does elevate the risk of pneumonia. Among atypical antipsychotics, clozapine, olanzapine, and risperidone carry a distinct risk. Yang and colleagues found among patients treated for bipolar disorder that certain combinations of agents carried a markedly increased risk of pneumonia. The combination of olanzapine with carbamazepine carried an adjusted risk ratio of 11.88 in their study. Clozapine combined with valproic acid carried an adjusted risk ratio for pneumonia of 4.80. Of note, Yang and colleagues found that carbamazepine and valproic acid, when used alone, did not increase the risk of developing pneumonia (Trifirò, 2011; Yang et al., 2013). Why antipsychotic agents may increase the risk of pneumonia is unclear. Sedation due to antihistaminic effects, inhibition of secretions through anticholinergic effects, and impairments of swallowing due to extrapyramidal side effects may all contribute to an increased risk of pneumonia. It is possible that immunomodulatory effects of psychotropics may be involved. For example, lithium appears frankly protective against pneumonia (Yang et al., 2013). Lithium has been found to inhibit the activities of several DNA viruses (Ren et al., 2011). Perhaps an as yet unrecognized property of antipsychotic agents undermines the pulmonary immune response.

Use of antipsychotic agents by elderly patients is also associated with an increased risk of having a cerebrovascular event. This risk is elevated within the first 30 days of taking such a medication, and may persist for as long as 2 years. Atypical antipsychotics, when compared to no use of an antipsychotic agent, may increase the risk of having a cerebrovascular event 2 to 3 times. However, the risk of having an event serious enough to warrant hospitalization is not increased (Pratt et al., 2012). This concern was raised initially by data generated by trials of risperidone and olanzapine among elderly demented patients with behavioral problems. There appeared to be an increased rate of cerebrovascular events with these agents, mainly risperidone. However, subsequent analysis of this data did not confirm a clear association between the use of either agent and having a cerebrovascular accident. Furthermore, the relative risk with risperidone compared with olanzapine may have been due to the greater inclusion of patients with histories of cerebrovascular events in the risperidone group (Herrmann et al., 2005). Subsequent studies have at times found an increased risk of having a cerebrovascular event, including stroke, among elderly patients receiving atypical antipsychotics, and sometimes not (Mittal, Kurup, Williamson, Muralee, & Tampi, 2011). The risk of having a cerebrovascular event when taking an atypical versus a typical is at times regarded as equal (Kales et al., 2007). However, in a large retrospective study of elderly patients with dementia prescribed psychotropics, Finkel and colleagues found that the risk of having a cerebrovascular event was roughly twice that with haloperidol compared to that with risperidone, olanzapine, or quetiapine. Furthermore, benzodiazepines conferred a risk of having a cerebrovascular event equal to that of haloperidol, or twice that of the atypical antipsychotics (Finkel et al., 2005). Why elderly demented patients may have an enhanced risk of having cerebrovascular events after initiating treatment with an antipsychotic is not clear. Alpha-adrenergic blockade leading to hypotension and subsequent cerebrovascular events is often cited. However, this is just one pharmacologic mechanism that may be responsible. In some cases, remote effects on the heart such as arrhythmia may be responsible. An interaction between the physiology of the agitated, demented patient and the pharmacology of the medication also cannot be excluded. The clinician should of course consider the use of an antipsychotic only when clearly indicated, begin at a low dose, and monitor closely for side effects.

There is some debate about the risk of having a myocardial infarction while taking an antipsychotic (Brauer et al., 2011). Patients receiving atypical antipsychotics may have a 50% greater risk of nonfatal myocardial infarction than patients taking typical antipsychotics. On the other hand, those patients taking a typical antipsychotic are at greater risk of death overall compared to those receiving an atypical antipsychotic (Vasilyeva et al., 2013). There may be distinct groups at relatively greater risk of a myocardial infarction or a related event. For example, initiation of an antipsychotic among demented patients taking cholinesterase inhibitors may carry a time-limited increase in the risk of having a myocardial infarction. Pariente and colleagues found that among thousands of such patients, the risk of having a myocardial infarction was increased 1.78-fold over the first 30 days, 1.67-fold from day 31 to day 60, and 1.37-fold from day 61 to day 90 (Pariente et al., 2012). Patients receiving an antipsychotic with a propensity to cause significant arrhythmias, such as thioridazine or droperidol, have a secondary increased risk of myocardial infarction (Pacher et al., 2004). Those at risk for orthostatic hypotension may experience greater hypotension with an antipsychotic, and a myocardial infarction may result (Gugger, 2011). Among patients with a recent acute coronary event, use of a phenothiazine antipsychotic increased the adjusted odds ratio of sudden cardiac death 10.9-fold compared to those not receiving a psychotropic. Use of a butyrophenone was associated with an adjusted odds ratio of 6.74 for having sudden cardiac death. Use of any antipsychotic in the setting of an acute coronary event led to an adjusted odds ratio of suffering sudden cardiac death of 3.44, while the odds ratio fell to 1.30 if the antipsychotic was an atypical agent (Honkola et al., 2012). The dose of antipsychotic is also, in general, linearly associated with the risk of sudden cardiac death (Ray et al., 2001). While interest in this issue increases, the clinician should cautiously consider the individual patient's risk of having a vascular event and weigh the potential risks of starting any antipsychotic against its potential benefits.

Antipsychotic agents also elevate the risk of having a hip fracture among the elderly. Leipzig and colleagues found that the use of a typical antipsychotic increased the risk of having a fall among the elderly 1.4-fold to 1.7-fold (Leipzig et al., 1999). This is significant, as 20%–30% of falls among the elderly result in a hip fracture. Furthermore, the typical agents may carry a 50% greater risk of hip fracture than the atypical antipsychotics (Ordera et al., 2012; Pratt et al., 2012). A variety of factors may affect the risk of having a hip fracture while taking an antipsychotic. These include falls due to hypotension, sedation, or Parkinsonism, low vitamin D levels, and the possibility of hyperprolactinemia causing bone loss (Kishimoto, De Hert, Carlson, Manu, & Correll, 2012). Besides medication, psychosis itself appears to convey an increased risk of increased bone loss (Partti et al., 2010). Weaving antipsychotic therapy into an elderly patient's medication regimen necessitates identifying risk factors for falls and then anticipating and managing these with the patient. A serum vitamin D level helps determine the need for replacement. Proper footwear should be encouraged. Exercise is essential as well. A baseline measure of blood pressure to assess for orthostasis is important, and minimization of psychotropics when possible can help (Moncada, 2011).

We recommend adhering to the following principles in the use of neuroleptics in the medically ill:

1. Whenever possible, identify and treat the underlying illness rather than treating superficial symptoms. For example, treat the etiology of a patient's delirium or cognitive impairment instead of merely controlling secondary symptoms of agitation or hallucinations. This is especially important, since, in the medically ill, neuroleptics can produce improvement in overt psychiatric symptoms while the underlying medical etiology of the symptoms progresses.

2. Avoid polypharmacy that is not scientifically based on the results of randomized, controlled, clinical trials and be cognizant of the potential for drug interactions and of pharmacokinetic and pharmacodynamic reasons for increased risks of adverse effects. For example, decreased albumin in malnourished patients implies the increased bioavailability of free fractions of protein-bound drugs and therefore more potent effects per milligram dosage (more unbound drug is available to act on receptor sites).

3. Identify specific target symptoms and carefully evaluate the treatment response objectively. Whereas agitation and behavioral symptoms may respond promptly, symptoms such as hallucinations and delusions may require weeks to respond.

4. Use the minimum effective dosage. High neuroleptic dosages are associated with increased side effects and do not necessarily increase antipsychotic efficacy (Kane, 1990). Even when higher doses give somewhat better control of positive psychotic symptoms, the patient's overall function may be worse because of extrapyramidal side effects of typical neuroleptics such as bradykinesia, apathy, akathisia, or rigidity. When treating geriatric patients, starting doses as low as 0.5 to 1 mg of risperidone, for example, are often quite sufficient.

LOW-POTENCY "TYPICAL" OR TRADITIONAL NEUROLEPTICS

Low-potency typical neuroleptics such as chlorpromazine and thioridazine have a side effect profile that includes a-adrenergic receptor blockage resulting in a risk of orthostatic hypotension, histaminic blockage resulting in sedation, and anticholinergic effects that can cause dry mouth, constipation, blurred vision, urinary retention, and sinus tachycardia.

In the elderly, the central anticholinergic actions of these medications are especially prone to cause memory deficits and place the patient at increased risk for central anticholinergic toxicity and delirium. In particular, patients with Alzheimer's disease are more susceptible to these deleterious side effects.

In addition, the low-potency typical neuroleptics are more likely to be associated with miscellaneous dermatologic and systemic side effects such as photosensitivity and cholestatic jaundice. Neuroleptic-induced cholestatic jaundice is almost always benign and is thought to be an allergic response, since it is frequently accompanied by rash, fever, and eosinophilia (Lader, 1989).

At higher doses (600–800 mg/day), thioridazine carries a small risk of pigmentary retinopathy; doses over 800 mg/day are contraindicated because of an unacceptable risk of this side effect. It is also the neuroleptic most likely to be associated with male sexual dysfunction (e.g., retrograde ejaculation, erectile dysfunction).

Low-potency phenothiazines such as chlorpromazine are also more likely to have quinidine-like side effects on myocardial conduction. This may result in P-R and QT interval prolongation and in flattening of the T wave on the ECG. These effects rarely are clinically significant unless the patient is also receiving a type 1 antiarrhythmic or has a preexisting heart block or prolonged QT syndrome (Stoudemire, Moran, & Fogel, 1991). Thioridazine appears to have the most pronounced quinidine-like effects of the neuroleptics and should not be used in patients with heart block (Wenzel-Seifert, Wittmann, M., & Haen, 2011).

Although all neuroleptics can lower the seizure threshold, the low-potency phenothiazine chlorpromazine is more strongly associated with seizures and should be avoided in epileptics and patients at high risk for seizures. Hematologic side effects such as agranulocytosis, transient leukopenia, and thrombocytopenia can occur with any neuroleptic but seem to have a higher incidence with the low-potency typical neuroleptics as compared to the high-potency typical agents (Balon & Berchou, 1986).

Reversible endocrinologic side effects of all typical neuroleptics include gynecomastia, amenorrhea, and galactorrhea due to stimulation of prolactin secretion.

In general, because of their propensity to cause orthostatic hypotension and sedation, low-potency typical neuroleptics should be avoided in patients with acute medical illness. This is especially true in delirious patients, in whom monitoring the sensorium is of critical importance, and in patients with cardiovascular or cerebrovascular disease, in whom an episode of hypotension could have catastrophic effects.

The use of low-potency agents in patients with chronic and stable medical illness is reasonable in the special situation in which a very small dose of a low-potency agent (e.g., 10–25 mg of thioridazine) gives dramatic relief of target symptoms. At very low dosages, the hypotensive, sedative, and anticholinergic effects of low-potency agents may be minimal or easily tolerated. If low doses of low-potency agents do not control symptoms, switching to a high-potency agent may be safer than raising the dose of the low-potency agent. New drugs like quetiapine and olanzapine will likely supplant the use of the older low-potency and higher potency "typical" neuroleptics in the geriatric population, especially if parenteral forms of these drugs become available.

HIGH-POTENCY TYPICAL NEUROLEPTICS

High-potency typical neuroleptics, with haloperidol as the prototypic agent, are less likely to induce orthostatic hypotension and sedation but are more likely to be associated with extrapyramidal side effects (EPS). Acute EPS syndromes include acute dystonias, parkinsonian symptoms, bradykinesia, akathisia, and the "rabbit syndrome"—an unusual rhythmic perioral tremor. In addition, high-potency typical neuroleptics are more commonly associated with neuroleptic-induced catatonia and neuroleptic malignant syndrome.

Acute Dystonias

The risk for acute dystonia is greatest in young men. Children constitute another high-risk group for dystonia and for EPS in general (Pringsheim et al., 2011). Dystonia may be manifested by torticollis, retrocollis, tongue protrusion, opisthotonos, facial grimacing, or an oculogyric crisis, which occurs in approximately 2.5% of patients receiving typical neuroleptics (Lader, 1989). Laryngospasm is a rarer form of acute dystonia, but may also result from antipsychotics or other agents, such as antiemetics, that work by blocking the dopamine D2 receptor (Derinoz & Caglar, 2013). The symptoms usually respond to 25–50 mg of diphenhydramine or 1–2 mg of benztropine intramuscularly or intravenously, followed by oral doses of diphenhydramine 25–50 mg three times daily or benztropine 1–2 mg three times daily. Trihexyphenidyl also is effective. If patients are unable to tolerate anticholinergic agents, amantadine, a weak dopamine agonist with very mild anticholinergic effects, can be used instead; 50–100 mg orally twice a day is the usual dose (Prigsheim et al., 2011; Stoudemire & Fogel, 1995).

Parkinsonian Symptoms

Parkinsonian side effects are particularly prevalent and problematic in elderly patients and can limit the use of typical high-potency neuroleptics in this population. Neuroleptic-induced parkinsonism can be clinically indistinguishable from idiopathic Parkinson's disease with masked facies, bradykinesia, rigidity, pill-rolling tremor that is greater at rest, and festinating gait.

However, parkinsonian side effects from typical neuroleptics comprise a continuum and functionally significant bradykinesia, rigidity, or gait disturbance can occur without a prominent tremor or the typical "cogwheeling" on examination of the limbs. The finding of rigidity in the neck and cogwheeling in the forearm and wrist muscles are useful confirmatory signs on physical examination when a partial parkinsonian syndrome is suspected. The occurrence of an incomplete parkinsonian syndrome should trigger the same management approach as a full syndrome, if the symptoms and signs are associated with either subjective distress or impairment in daily activities. Management strategies include reducing the dosage of neuroleptic, switching to a lower potency neuroleptic, prescribing concurrent antiparkinsonian agents, or switching to an atypical antipsychotic such as quetiapine.

The choice of antiparkinsonian drugs should depend on the specific EPS as well as medical risk factors. Anticholinergic drugs, such as trihexyphenidyl and benztropine, are rapidly effective for tremor and dystonia and can be given preventively but cause a full range of peripheral and central anticholinergic side effects. Patients with constipation, urinary retention, or vulnerability to confusion may tolerate them poorly. Amantadine, a dopamine agonist with mild anticholinergic effects, has fewer physical side effects although it can occasionally cause hallucinations, confusion, and other mental symptoms. It may be more effective for rigidity and akinesia than the anticholinergics. It is not available parenterally. Finally, severe and disabling drug-induced parkinsonism can be treated with major dopamine agonist drugs such as levodopa-carbidopa or bromocriptine. Because of the risk of mental side effects of these drugs, they would generally be used only if motor disability outweighed mental disability. Neuroleptics can also unmask subclinical idiopathic Parkinson's disease, and, even if antipsychotics are discontinued, up to 11% of patients may show persistent symptoms (Sakauye, 1990). Symptoms that persist after 6 months to a year after withdrawal of the antipsychotic likely represent idiopathic Parkinson's disease (Lim et al., 2013). With the atypical antipsychotics, the frequency of EPS is much lower—especially with quetiapine. Among elderly patients with dementia, the risk of EPS with quetiapine rivals that of risperidone and olanzapine when equivalent doses are used. Being male in the population carries a twofold greater risk of EPS with these atypical antipsychotics (Marras et al., 2012).

Akathisia

Akathisia (literally, "unable to remain seated") is an intense, unpleasant, subjective sense of inner restlessness and associated motor restlessness. The most common estimates of the prevalence in patients treated with typical neuroleptics range from about 5% to 20% (Bakker, de Groot, van Os, & van Harten, 2011). Unlike neuroleptic-induced parkinsonian symptoms, akathisia typically does not respond well to antiparkinsonian therapy but may respond to beta-adrenergic blockade. Beyond neuroleptic dose reduction, when feasible, propranolol 30–120 mg/day in divided doses may be effective in most patients, although concerns regarding hypotension and bradycardia in the medically ill may limit this option (Prigsheim et al., 2011). It is important to exclude other organic etiologies of the anxiety states such as hypoxia, drug withdrawal states, and metabolic abnormalities.

ATYPICAL NEUROLEPTICS

Aripiprazole

Aripiprazole's oral bioavailability is nearly 90%. There also exists an intramuscular version. Serum protein binding is 99%. The elimination half-life of aripiprazole is about 75 hours, and that of its active metabolite dehydroaripiprazole is 94 hours. Among slow metabolizers through CyP450-2D6, the elimination half-life of aripiprazole may double. About 55% of a dose of aripiprazole is eliminated in the feces and 25% in the urine. Aripiprazole appears to be well tolerated among those with renal or hepatic impairment (Mallikaarjun et al., 2008).

Among the main advantages claimed for aripiprazole when compared to other atypical antipsychotics is a reduced tendency to weight gain and an associated reduction in the risk of developing the metabolic syndrome (Khanna et al., 2013). The main limitation of aripiprazole is usually dose-related EPS, which is more common among children and adolescents than adults. The rate of EPS with aripiprazole appears to be more than that of most other atypical antipsychotics, but less than that of risperidone and of haloperidol (De Fazio et al., 2010; Rummel-Kluge et al., 2012).

Asenapine

Asenapine is among the newest of the atypical antipsychotics. The bioavailability of asenapine is less than 2% if swallowed, but rises to 35% when given sublingually. It is 95% bound to serum proteins. Its elimination half-life is about 24 hours. About 50% of a dose is excreted in the urine and 40% in the feces. Inducers of CyP1A2 may speed the elimination of asenapine (Minassian & Young, 2010). Side effects include somnolence in 24%, significant weight gain in nearly 20%, akathisia in 2%, and other EPS in 5% (McIntyre, 2011).

Iloperidone

Iloperidone is another of the newest atypical antipsychotics. It appears to be well absorbed. Iloperidone is metabolized through CyP4502D6 and 3A4 and has two active metabolites. The elimination half-life of iloperidone ranges from 18 hours among rapid 2D6 metabolizers to 33 hours among slow 2D6 metabolizers. Protein binding is about 95%. Metabolism occurs through CyP450-2D6 and 3A4. The drug is mainly excreted in the urine. However, it can be safely used in patients with impaired renal function. Patients with impaired hepatic function may require a dose adjustment or discontinuation (Citrome, 2011). Dose-dependent orthostatic hypotension obligates the clinician to a slow upward titration. Other important side effects are weight gain, tachycardia, somnolence, and QT prolongation similar to that of ziprasidone (Arif & Mitchell, 2011). Extrapyramidal symptoms, including akathisia, occur in about 2% of patients. In registration trial studies, use of iloperidone when CyP450-2D6 and 3A4 were simultaneously inhibited prolonged the QTc by an average of 19 milliseconds (Novartis 2013).

Lurasidone

Lurasidone is among the newest of the atypical antipsychotics. It has a low oral bioavailability of about 10% to 20%. Serum protein binding is 99%. Lurasidone is metabolized mainly through CyP450-3A4, and produces an active metabolite. The elimination half-life of lurasidone is 18 hours, while that of its active metabolite is 8 to 10 hours. No dosage adjustment is needed in either renal or hepatic impairment. Lurasidone is complicated by dose-dependent EPS that may be seen in as many as 10% of patients, and akathisia in as many as 20% (Yasui-Furukori, 2012). There appears to be no significant effects on weight, lipids or the QTc with lurasidone (Kantrowitz et al., 2012).

Risperidone

Table 21.5 contrasts the differences between typical and atypical neuroleptics. Risperidone in low doses embraces many of the benefits of the atypical antipsychotics. It is effective against negative symptoms of chronic psychosis and has a

Table 21.5 DIFFERENCES BETWEEN TRADITIONAL (TYPICAL) AND ATYPICAL NEUROLEPTICS

Traditional Neuroleptics	Atypical neuroleptics
Are associated with a high incidence of EPS (extrapyramidal symptoms)	Are associated with a low incidence of EPS
May cause tardive dyskinesia	May not cause tardive dyskinesia
Increase serum prolactin levels	Show minimal or no increase in serum prolactin levels
Treat mainly positive symptoms of psychosis (such as hallucinations), but not negative ones (such as social withdrawal)	Treat both positive and negative symptoms of psychosis
Cause catalepsy in animals	Do not cause catalepsy in animals

low rate of development of tardive dyskinesia. Quality of life during risperidone therapy appears demonstrably better than with typical antipsychotics such as haloperidol, and comparable to that of the other atypical agents. Quality of life is generally defined to incorporate measures of benefit, tolerability, and patient satisfaction (Bobes et al., 2007; Chouinard & Albright, 1997).

Neuropsychiatric side effects of risperidone include dose-dependent sedation (20% to over 40%), sleep disturbances (15%–30%), and impairments of memory and concentration (15% to over 20%) (Peuskens, 1995). Rarely, mania has been reported with risperidone (Diaz, 1996). In one suicide attempt, 240 mg of risperidone was ingested, with minimal side effects; the most significant abnormalities were cardiovascular with QRS and QT_c prolongation (K Brown et al., 1993). The risk of cardiovascular complications during therapy with usual doses of risperidone, however, appears to be low (Casey, 1997a).

With a daily dosage of under 4 mg/day of risperidone, the incidence of extrapyramidal side effects (EPS) is relatively low. However, when the daily dosage of risperidone is increased to between 4 mg/day and 8 mg/day, then the rate at which EPS emerge begins to resemble that of traditional neuroleptics, especially in elderly patients (Miller et al 2008; Owens, 1994). Reports of risperidone-induced neuroleptic malignant syndrome also exist (Arslankoylu et al., 2011; Dave, 1995; Singer, Richards, & Boland, 1995; Tarsy, 1996). The elderly and patients with renal and hepatic disease are at risk for reduced clearance of risperidone, as well as of its active metabolite 9-hydroxy-risperidone. Accumulation of these agents is associated with increased problems with EPS (Heykants et al., 1994).

Risperidone appears to exert its antipsychotic action through the potent blockade of both central serotonin $5HT_2$ and dopamine D_2 receptors (Kapur, Zipursky, & Remington, 1999). The $5HT_2$ antagonism is more potent than the D_2 antagonism, but after the daily dosage reaches 4 mg to 8 mg, the clinical effect of the greater potency for $5HT_2$ receptors is lost. Also of importance is the disinhibition of dopamine release from central dopamine neurons by risperidone. Presynaptic $5HT_2$ receptors located on central dopamine neurons inhibit the release of dopamine; blockage of these receptors by risperidone probably leads to increased release of dopamine. This may be a mechanism through which risperidone in low doses limits the emergence of EPS (Kapur & Remington, 1996). Blockade of $5HT_2$ receptors does not appear to be directly antipsychotic.

Risperidone is 90% bound to serum proteins. 9-Hydroxy-risperidone is 77% bound to serum proteins. The metabolism of risperidone is accomplished largely through cytochrome P450-2D6 (DeVane, 1996). Patients who are genetically poor metabolizers through this isoenzyme and patients receiving other medications that inhibit the activity of this isoenzyme may increase serum risperidone levels. Such effects may have reduced clinical consequences because the active metabolite of risperidone, 9-hydroxy-risperidone, has a pharmacologic and therapeutic profile very similar to that of the parent compound (Grant & Fitton, 1994; Keegan, 1994). Risperidone is associated with EPS, even in low doses, in children and in the elderly (Prigsheim et al., 2011).

Paliperidone

The bioavailability of oral paliperidone is 28%. Only about 30% of paliperidone is metabolized. This occurs mainly through CyP4502D6, and to a lesser extent through 3A4. The elimination half-life is 23 hours. The drug is 74% bound to serum proteins. Mild to moderate liver disease does not significantly affect the elimination of paliperidone. 59% of a dose of paliperidone is excreted as unchanged drug in the urine. However, because paliperidone is excreted in part by active transport in the renal tubules, impairment of renal function does slow the elimination of paliperidone (Marino, English, Caballero, & Harrington, 2012; Vermeir et al., 2008). For patients whose creatinine clearance (CrCl) is between 50 and 80 mL/min, the clearance of paliperidone falls by 32%. When the CrCl is between 30 and 50 mL/min, the clearance falls by 64%, and for those patients whose CrCl is below 30 mL/min the clearance of paliperidone falls by 71% (Janssen, 2012). The elimination half-life among elderly patients is 25 hours (Snoeck et al., 1995). For the elderly and those with renal disease, a reduction in dose is reasonable. Because Invega is prepared as a time-released product stored within a rigid capsule, patients with intestinal strictures should not take Invega.

Paliperidone treatment is limited by many of the same side-effects that limit treatment with risperidone. Extrapyramidal symptoms (EPS) that occur more often than with placebo include hypertonia, dystonia and akathisia. In a study comparing the safety and efficacy of paliperidone and quetiapine, EPS rates were higher with paliperidone, including akathisia (10% versus 3%), hypertonia (5% versus 1%), and drooling (6% versus 0%) (Vieta et al., 2010). Several cases of NMS have been attributed to paliperidone (Özdemir et al., 2012).

The usually modest QT-prolonging effects of risperidone are mainly due to paliperidone (Suzuki et al., 2012). Rodent and in vitro human data reveal that paliperidone prolongs the QT interval by inhibiting the hERG channel (Vigneault et al., 2011). Fortunately, the QTc prolongation of paliperidone is 4 milliseconds or less. Rarely is *torsades de pointes* a risk with paliperidone (Wenzel-Seifert et al., 2011). On the other hand, mild tachycardia is seen among 10% to 20% of patients receiving paliperidone. This does not usually have a significant effect on overall cardiac function (Marino et al., 2012).

Olanzapine

Olanzapine is an atypical neuroleptic both in terms of its pharmacologic activity as well as its efficacy for both positive and negative symptoms of chronic psychoses. Olanzapine is metabolized by the CyP450-1A2 isoenzyme and multiple others. Its use as an antipsychotic for the medically ill and delirious patients appears promising. This is because of the relatively mild side effect profile, as well as olanzapine's potential for use in patients with Parkinson's disease who become psychotic on otherwise therapeutic doses of dopaminergic agents. Especially promising is the very low rate of tardive dyskinesia with olanzapine. It has been estimated that the risk of developing tardive dyskinesia during olanzapine therapy may be about 1% per year, which is essentially the rate at which never-medicated psychotic patients develop tardive dyskinesia (Tollefson et al., 1997a, 1997b).

The side effect profile of olanzapine is characterized by a reduced risk of extrapyramidal side effects (EPS), although sedation and dizziness occur in 10%–20% of patients (Beasley et al., 1996; Lilly Research Laboratories, 1996). Olanzapine shares risperidone's relative freedom from direct cardiovascular toxicity and has significantly fewer EPS than risperidone (Casey, 1997a). In first-episode schizophrenia, olanzapine is associated with akathisia in about 10%, Parkinsonism in 6%, and very rarely dyskinesias and dystonia (Haddad et al., 2012). This is due to the slightly different pharmacodynamic activity of olanzapine (Kapur, Zipursky, & Remington, 1999).

As with other atypical neuroleptics, olanzapine potently antagonizes both the central $5HT_2$ serotonin receptor as well as the central D_2 dopamine receptor, with much greater affinity for the $5HT_2$ receptor than the D_2 receptor. However, olanzapine also binds to muscarinic cholinergic receptors, histamine H_1 receptors, and a_1-adrenergic receptors with a predictable but mild side effect profile.

Alcohol can increase olanzapine uptake from the gut. Cimetidine may increase serum olanzapine levels, probably through effects on multiple enzyme systems.

Olanzapine has been associated with significant weight gain (average about 2.3 kg) after 4–6 months of treatment and sometimes marked increases in serum triglycerides (Osser et al., 1998). Olanzapine has also been associated with the onset of diabetes (possibly type II due to weight gain) as well as exacerbation of preexisting diabetes. Like clozapine, olanzapine can cause sialorrhea (Perkins & McClure, 1998). At least one case of priapism has been reported with olanzapine (Deirmenjian et al., 1998).

Quetiapine

Quetiapine, a dibenzothiazepine, is another of the new atypical neuroleptics. It is characterized by having only rare EPS, although two anecdotal cases of the neuroleptic malignant syndrome have been ascribed to quetiapine. Dizziness, somnolence, and agitation each affect about 10% of patients (Small et al., 1997; Zeneca, 2013). Because of the development of cataracts in dogs ingesting doses of quetiapine, the manufacturer now recommends slit lamp examinations before initiating therapy with quetiapine and every 6 months thereafter (Zeneca, 2013).

Quetiapine is like the other typical antipsychotics in that it is a more potent antagonist of serotonin $5HT_2$ receptors than of dopamine D_2 receptors; however, quetiapine also potently antagonizes, in descending order of potency, histamine H_1 receptors, a_1-andrenergic receptors, and a_2-adrenergic receptors (Casey, 1997b). H_1 antagonism accounts for quetiapine's tendency to cause somnolence, while a_1-adrenergic blockade can produce some orthostatic hypotension.

The elimination half-life of quetiapine is about 6 hours. This drug is 83% bound to serum proteins but does not appear to alter warfarin pharmacokinetics. Quetiapine is metabolized to inactive metabolites through cytochrome P450-3A4.

Inhibitors of this isoenzyme, which include erythromycin, itraconazole, fluconazole, and ketoconazole, will slow the elimination of quetiapine and subsequently raise its serum levels. Phenytoin and thioridazine both reduce the serum quetiapine level. Quetiapine slightly raises serum lorazepam levels. Cimetidine, fluoxetine, haloperidol, imipramine, lithium, risperidone, and warfarin appear not to have pharmacokinetic interactions with quetiapine. Alcohol, antihistamines, and benzodiazepines are among the many drugs that have synergistic sedative effects with quetiapine.

Quetiapine may antagonize the action of dopamine agonists used in the treatment of Parkinson's disease (Zeneca, 2013), although reports suggest that it causes the least EPS in Parkinson's disease patients with the exception of clozapine. Early reports from some neurologists hail quetiapine as the new "drug of choice" for Parkinson's disease psychosis, with claims that quetiapine has minimal EPS in therapeutic doses even in Parkinson's disease. More research is needed to confirm this initial enthusiasm for quetiapine in Parkinson's disease patients.

Clozapine

Because of the risk of agranulocytosis, if clozapine is used the physician must access the distribution system for clozapine through the Sandoz Pharmaceuticals Corporation to ensure that weekly monitoring of serum white blood cell (WBC) levels occurs. Parameters for use of clozapine are outlined in Box 21.1 (Novartis, 1997) but may change.

***Box 21.1* PARAMETERS FOR CLOZAPINE USE**

Check white blood cell (WBC) and automated neutrophil count (ANC) prior to initiating treatment. If WBC >3500/mm³ and ANC >2000/mm³, and there is no prior history of a myeloproliferative disorder, including due to clozapine use, then treatment may begin.

During treatment, if cell counts remain as above then:

(a) for the first six months, check cell counts weekly;

(b) for the second six months, check cell counts every two weeks;

(c) after the first year, check cell counts monthly; and,

(d) after cessation of treatment, check white cell count after one month.

During treatment, clozapine use and monitoring changes as follows:

(a) for WBC counts between 3000 and 3500, or ANC between 1500 and 2000, check cell counts twice weekly;

(b) for WBC counts between 2000 and 3000, or ANC between 1000 and 1500, clozapine treatment is stopped until the abnormal finding has resolved; and,

(c) for WBC count <2000, or ANC <1000, clozapine treatment is permanently suspended.

Many of clozapine's side effects are predictable and result from its antihistaminic, anticholinergic, and antiadrenergic activity. In one multicenter study, the most frequent adverse side effects were sedation (21%), tachycardia (17%), constipation (16%), dizziness (14%), hypotension (13%), and hypersalivation (13%) (Kane et al., 1988). Although tremor, akathisia, and rigidity have been reported with clozapine treatment, these are uncommon (approximately 5%) and generally mild. Moreover, the drug does not appear to be associated with masked facies, acute dystonic reactions, and parkinsonian gait abnormalities.

Clozapine lowers the seizure threshold, with the incidence of seizures increasing with dosage: 1% at dosages below 300 mg/day, 2.7% at dosages of 300–599 mg/day, and 4.4% at higher dosages of 600–900 mg/day. The risk of seizures with clozapine is cumulative over time, reaching 10% at 3.8 years of treatment (DeVinsky, Honigfeld, & Patin, 1991). Clozapine is contraindicated in patients with myeloproliferative disorders or granulocytopenia and should not be used with other medications known to have myelosuppressive effects (e.g., carbamazepine).

If clozapine is needed in a patient with epilepsy, the patient should be switched to an anticonvulsant other than carbamazepine. To minimize the risk of seizures, anticonvulsant levels should be monitored frequently during initiation of clozapine and kept at the higher end of the therapeutic range. Some authors favor concurrent use of an anticonvulsant such as phenytoin or valproate if clozapine doses in excess of 500 mg are utilized, even in nonepileptic patients (Baldessarini & Frankenberg, 1991).

It is recommended that clozapine treatment be instituted at low dosages (12.5 mg–25 mg) in elderly patients because of its potential to induce marked sedation and hypotension. In elderly patients a starting dose of 12.5 mg twice daily is recommended. The typical therapeutic range for schizophrenia in physically healthy patients is 300–500 mg/day, with a maximum of 900 mg/day. Dosing should be on a twice or three times daily schedule (Lieberman, Kane, & Johns, 1989).

Fever up to 103°F may occur when starting clozapine and may persist with fluctuation for 4–6 weeks. Fever should be managed supportively with acetaminophen and is not in itself a reason to discontinue the drug. However, care should be taken to ensure that patients are adequately hydrated and to reassess patients frequently for symptoms suggesting an infectious cause for the fever or the possible emergence of NMS.

Friedman and Lannon reported on the successful treatment with clozapine of psychotic symptoms in six patients with Parkinson's disease. In patients who exhibited psychotic symptoms such as auditory hallucinations and paranoia, and who ranged in age from 52 to 78 years, they found that clozapine improved psychiatric symptoms without worsening motor manifestations of Parkinson's disease such as rigidity and gait disturbance. In two patients, parkinsonian symptoms actually improved. They noted that the likely explanation is that clozapine has relatively low affinity for striatal dopamine receptors. Its affinity for the D_2 receptor in the caudate nucleus is only 1/50 that of haloperidol and 1/10 that of chlorpromazine. The patients in this case series did not develop agranulocytosis, and the major side effect encountered was hypersalivation, which can be treated with clonidine. Psychotic symptoms were controlled with relatively low doses ranging from 25 or 50 mg/day up to 275 mg/day (Friedman & Lannon, 1989). Another original case report (Roberts, Dean, & Stoudemire, 1989) showed similar symptomatic improvement in hallucinosis and paranoia in a 64-year-old woman with Parkinson's disease. When treated with clozapine 25 mg by mouth every 4 hours, not only did mental symptoms improve but the patient's parkinsonian symptoms improved to the point at which specific parkinsonian pharmacotherapy (carbidopa, levodopa, and trihexyphenidyl) could be discontinued. These reports have been confirmed by several other papers (Bernardi & DelZampa, 1990; Kahn et al., 1991; Pfeiffer et al., 1990).

Due to clozapine's orthostatic effects, psychotic PD patients may need as little as 12.5 mg clozapine a day, and blood pressure should be monitored as the dose is raised.

Granulocyte colony–stimulating factor (G-CSF) has proven effective in reversing many cases of clozapine-induced neutropenia. In one case in which clozapine was the only effective and available antipsychotic for a young man with severe clozapine-induced neutropenia, coadministration of clozapine with G-CSF led to a prompt normalization of the patient's white blood cell count (Sperner-Unterweger et al., 1998).

Clozapine can have a profound effect on gut motility. The anticholinergic and antiserotonergic effects of clozapine are likely involved. Effects can range from constipation to severe ileus leading to necrosis and bowel perforation, and even death. When colonic dilatation develops in the absence of mechanical obstruction, the condition is called *Ogilvie's syndrome*. The triad of colonic dilatation of greater than 6 centimeters, inflammation of the colon, and septic shock is referred to as *toxic megacolon* (Alam, Fricchione, Guimaraes, & Zukerberg, 2009). Palmer and colleagues found that among 102 patients who developed life-threatening gastrointestinal hypomotility with clozapine, 28 died. Risk factors included recent initiation of clozapine, higher doses and serum levels of clozapine, concomitant use of other anticholinergic agents, and intercurrent illness (Palmer, McLean, Ellis, & Harrison-Woolrych, 2008). There is no specific medication used to manage clozapine's effects on the gut (Chukhin et al., 2013). Instead, management of clozapine's effects on the gut begin with the preparations to begin treatment. Patients with preexisting bowel problems, including those caused by other medications, would ideally have good control of these problems prior to starting treatment with clozapine. Since patients may not report bowel complaints spontaneously, especially those patients with prominent negative symptoms of psychosis, regular inquiries into bowel function must be made. When problems with bowel function do arise, they should be managed aggressively and monitored closely.

Ziprasidone

The bioavailability of oral ziprasidone is 60% or less; this is greatly enhanced by taking the medication with food. In some patients the bioavailability nearly doubles with food. The type of food appears to have little impact on the improvement in bioavailability (Miceli, Glue, Alderman, & Wilner, 2007). Its elimination half-life is 2–7 hours. Serum protein binding is 99%. Ziprasidone is extensively metabolized by the liver, although less than a third of this metabolism is through cytochromes P450, specifically 3A4 and to a lesser extent 1A2. The bulk of hepatic metabolism of ziprasidone is accomplished by aldehyde oxidase.

Compared to agents such as risperidone and perphenazine, patients on ziprasidone discontinue the medication because of EPS relatively infrequently (Miller et al., 2008). But ziprasidone is also generally considered less effective an antipsychotic than olanzapine or risperidone (Stip et al., 2011). Ziprasidone also has the greatest QT prolongation among available atypical antipsychotics (Wenzel-Seifert et al., 2011). The significance of this QT prolongation is debated, with some authors claiming that the nature and extent of ziprasidone's QT prolongation is clinically insignificant (Correll et al., 2011).

INJECTABLE DEPOT ATYPICAL ANTIPSYCHOTIC AGENTS

Injectable, long-acting, or depot forms of atypical antipsychotics exist for aripiprazole, olanzapine, paliperidone, and risperidone. These agents have the potential to improve the consistency of medication use. One of the main limitations of the agents is the persistence in the systemic circulation after side effects develop. For example, the offending agent in neuroleptic malignant syndrome or an allergic reaction is much easier to stop when given orally than when given as a depot agent, due to the protracted action of the depot agent.

Depot aripiprazole is marketed as Abilify Maintena. This agent is given as a monthly injection of 300 or 400 mg of long-acting aripiprazole. Side effects of depot aripiprazole include insomnia that may develop in 8% to 10% of patients, anxiety in 6% to 8%, akathisia in 6%, tremor in 2% to 6%, and weight gain in 7% to 10%. An important aspect of the large, 52-week registration study performed by Kane and colleagues was the initial 4-week to 12-week period of stabilization on oral aripiprazole. This period allowed an assessment of whether a patient would have a hypersensitivity reaction to aripiprazole (Kane et al., 2012).

A depot form of risperidone was the first atypical antipsychotic made available as a depot agent. It is marketed as Risperdal Consta. It is recommended that patients who may receive this agent begin with oral risperidone for 2 weeks prior to initiating depot risperidone, and for 3 weeks after beginning depot risperidone. This agent is given every 2 weeks in doses of 12.5 mg, 25 mg, 37.5 mg, or 50 mg. The formulation of Risperdal Consta causes less than 1% of the drug to be released immediately into the systemic circulation. The bulk of the release occurs around week 3, and is maintained between weeks 4 and 6. After four such injections, a steady state is achieved that lasts for 4–6 weeks after the last injection. The main reason for discontinuing depot risperidone is the emergence or worsening of movement disorders. Insomnia and anxiety are the most common side effects of treatment. Perhaps 15% of patients will develop or experience worsening of parkinsonism, and 15% of patients will have the same concern with regard to another form of EPS (Singh & O'Connor, 2009).

Depot paliperidone, currently marketed as Invega Sustenna, is a monthly injection that utilizes an induction protocol. Peak plasma levels are usually achieved on day 13, and the elimination half-life ranges from 25 to 50 days. The initial injection is a 234mg injection given on day 1. The next injection is a 156mg dose given on day 8. Injections thereafter are monthly. The monthly dose typically ranges from 39–234 milligrams based on such factors as weight, benefit, and side effects. Weight gain and elevations of prolactin are the most common concerns (Bishara, 2010). In general, side effects are the same as for oral paliperidone.

Olanzapine has been formulated for depot injection. It was introduced in 2010 as Zyprexa Relprevv. Recommended doses for acute schizophrenia are 210 or 300 mg every 2 weeks, or 405 mg monthly. For maintenance treatment of schizophrenia, the recommended doses are 150 or 300 mg every 2 weeks, or 405 mg monthly (Lindenmayer, 2010). The elimination half-life of this agent is 30 days. Steady state is achieved in 12 weeks. Typically, supplementation with oral olanzapine is not needed. An important complication of depot olanzapine treatment is a postinjection delirium sedation syndrome (PDSS). PDSS occurs in 0.07% of injections, and typically within 1 to 3 hours of receiving the injection. It resembles an overdose of olanzapine, and is characterized by sedation grading into somnolence, dizziness, confusion, and dysarthria. Cardiovascular function normally is preserved (Di Lorenzo & Brogli, 2010). PDSS is thought to result when there is a partial injection of the agent directly into the vascular space. Serum levels then may quickly rise above the expected range of 5 to 73 ng/ml. Levels approaching 600 ng/ml have been observed. The serum level usually resolves without a specific intervention within 24 to 72 hours (McDonnell et al., 2010). PDSS is thus generally a self-limiting side effect for which support but no specific intervention is needed (Duran-Sindreu et al., 2013). Experience with oral olanzapine overdoses indicates that severe central nervous system depression with tachycardia, orthostatic hypotension, hyperthermia, miosis, and respiratory depression requiring ventilation is possible (Tse, Warner, & Waring, 2008). Patients should wait in their injection clinic for 3 hours after each injection.

BENZODIAZEPINES

Benzodiazepines are commonly used in medically ill patients as anxiolytics, muscle relaxants, anticonvulsants, and hypnotics, and for sedation for procedures. The medically ill and elderly, however, are at increased risk for adverse side effects from these medications. There is also evidence that, in addition to pharmacokinetic changes related to aging, the elderly may be intrinsically more sensitive to both positive and negative clinical effects of the benzodiazepines (Greenblatt, Harmatz, & Shader, 1991). Benzodiazepine use may increase the risk of delirium among medically ill patients (Pisani, Murphy, Araujo, & Van Ness, 2010). Along with anticholinergic agents, benzodiazepines are among the agents most likely to impair cognitive functions such as short-term memory (Chavant, Favrelière, Lafay-Chebassier, Plazanet, & Pérault-Pochat, 2011). However, it is unclear as yet to what degree benzodiazepine use is a marker for patients at risk of developing delirium and to what degree their use actually precipitates delirium (Tse et al., 2012). A further potential complication of benzodiazepine use is their tendency to lower extracellular levels of neurotrophic factors (Tamaji et al., 2012). Reduction in the brain levels of brain-derived neurotrophic factor (BDNF) is a marker for neurodegeneration across disease states (Diniz & Teixeira, 2011). This may be one mechanism, besides sedation, by which benzodiazepines increase the risk of cognitive disorders such as delirium. Despite these risks, benzodiazepines, along with anticholinergic agents, are among the agents most commonly prescribed to elderly patients with mild cognitive impairment. Over 30% of such patients in the community are prescribed a benzodiazepine (Weston, Weinstein, Barton, & Yaffe, 2010).

Hypnotics, both the benzodiazepine and the nonbenzodiazepine, are associated with an increased risk of various types of morbidity as well as mortality. One controversial but persistent finding is an association between hypnotic use and an increased risk of cancer (Kao et al., 2012; Kripke, 2008). The risk of developing cancer is increased an average of 1.35-fold (95% CI: 1.18 to 1.55). This effect appears to be dose dependent and occurs across a surprising array of agents (Kripke, Langer, & Kline, 2012). Zopiclone, zolpidem, and ramelteon were found to be clastogenic in rodents during preliminary studies. These agents are associated with an increased risk of nonmelonoma skin cancers (Stebbing et al., 2005). Some authors caution that controlling carefully for other health risk factors can reduce the apparent size of the effect of hypnotics on overall mortality and some cancers, although it does not eliminate it (Hartz & Ross, 2012). The link between GABA-A–active agents and cancer may be related to GABA's role in modifying the behavior of stem cells (Young & Bordey, 2009). Other authors caution that the epidemiological association between the use of certain hypnotics and cancer does not prove causality (Phillips, 2012). Nonetheless, the association between hypnotic use and increased morbidity and mortality may be an argument for the use of behavior and lifestyle-modifying techniques for some patients with insomnia.

As a class, benzodiazepines share more similarities than differences in their intrinsic pharmacologic activity, which is mediated via the benzodiazepine receptor (increasing GABA-ergic tone), and side effect profile. There are, however, considerable differences in the pharmacokinetics of the various benzodiazepines. Thus, the knowledge of an individual benzodiazepine's pharmacokinetic profile may be more important, especially in the medically ill and the elderly, than the somewhat arbitrary distinctions between anxiolytic and hypnotic indications. Pharmacokinetic distinctions are especially significant because there is no convincing evidence that one benzodiazepine is clinically more effective than any other, and no evidence that benzodiazepines marketed as hypnotics for the treatment of insomnia are more effective for sleep than those marked as anxiolytics, and vice versa.

METABOLIC ROUTE AND ELIMINATION HALF-LIFE

Pharmacokinetic considerations in the use of benzodiazepines include the route of metabolism and biotransformation, elimination half-life, and relative lipophilicity. Most benzodiazepines, including diazepam, chlordiazepoxide, alprazolam, flurazepam, triazolam, and midazolam, undergo primary biotransformation in the liver via microsomal oxidative pathways. Thus, for these medications, drugs that inhibit hepatic microsomal enzymes, such as alcohol, isoniazid, and cimetidine, will increase plasma concentrations and elimination half-lives. Conversely, drugs that induce microsomal enzymes, such as estrogen, methylxanthines, rifampin, and cigarette smoking, will decrease the concentrations of these benzodiazepines. An example of the clinical significance of this latter observation is the fact that theophylline preparations and benzodiazepines are frequently used together in intensive care settings. If the theophylline were discontinued in a patient who was concurrently receiving a benzodiazepine, the patient would theoretically be at risk for a rise in the plasma concentration of the benzodiazepine that could result in a diminished level of consciousness and a degree of respiratory depression (Bonfiglio & Dasta, 1991). Since hepatic biotransformation is impaired by advanced age and hepatic disease, such as hepatitis and cirrhosis, benzodiazepines that are eliminated by hepatic oxidation should either be avoided or be given at reduced dosages and at increased time intervals. Drug interactions with benzodiazepines are listed in Table 21.6 (Barnes, Gerst, Smith, Terrell, & Mullins, 2006; Leach, Mohanraj, & Borland, 2012; Oliver, Keen, Rowse, & Mathers, 2001; Park & Jung, 2010; Stoudemire, Moran, & Fogel, 1991).

The parent compounds of benzodiazepines that are eliminated via oxidative metabolism typically are transformed into active metabolites that may be long-lived. For example, diazepam, chlordiazepoxide, clorazepate, and prazepam are metabolized to their common active metabolite, desmethyldiazepam, which has a half-life in excess of 50 hours in young, healthy patients and up to 175 hours in elderly or medically ill patients (Barbee & McLaulin, 1990). Similarly, the benzodiazepine hypnotics flurazepam and quazepam share the active metabolite desalkylflurazepam, which has an elimination half-life of 48 to 120 hours (Greenblatt, 1991). Two triazolobenzodiazepines that are metabolized by oxidative pathways but do not have significantly active metabolites are triazolam and alprazolam, with elimination half-lives of 3–5 hours and 12–15 hours, respectively.

Three available benzodiazepines are metabolized primarily in conjugation with glucuronic acid: lorazepam, oxazepam, and temazepam. These drugs, therefore, are less likely to accumulate in the elderly and in patients who have hepatic disease. For example, for a patient who presented with symptoms of alcohol withdrawal and had an unknown liver function status, lorazepam or oxazepam would be preferable to chlordiazepoxide. Lorazepam is also one of the only

Table 21.6 DRUG INTERACTIONS WITH BENZODIAZEPINES AND PSYCHOSTIMULANTS

MEDICATION	INTERACTIVE EFFECT
Benzodiazepines	
Cimetidine	May elevate serum levels of benzodiazepines
Disulfiram	Metabolized predominantly by oxidation
Ethanol	
Isoniazid	
Estrogens	Tend to lower benzodiazepine levels
Cigarettes	
Methylxanthine derivatives	
Rifampin	
Opiates	
Propylene glycol	Vehicle used for some intravenous preparations; can accumulate and cause toxicity; monitor osmolar gap
Olanzapine	May synergistically cause hypotension
Opiates	Synergistic sedation; may cause respiratory sedation
Psychostimulants	
Guanethidine	Decreased antihypertensive effect
Vasopressors	Increased pressor effect
Oral anticoagulants	Increased prothrombin time
Anticonvulsants	Increased levels of phenobarbital, primidone, phenytoin
	Stimulants may undermine efficacy of anticonvulsants
Tricyclics	Increased blood levels of TCA
	May precipitate mania, hyperadrenergic state, or hyperserotonergic state
MAOIs	Hypertension
	May precipitate mania, hyperadrenergic state, or hyperserotonergic state
SSRIs	Increased risk of serotonin syndrome
P-glycoprotein inhibitors	May increase brain concentrations of methylphenidate, but not of amphetamine or modafinil

two benzodiazepines (along with midazolam) that is reliably absorbed intramuscularly, should the patient be unable to take oral medications.

When drugs that inhibit the CyP450-3A enzyme are used (e.g., nefazodone), many benzodiazepines such as alprazolam will have increased serum levels.

Clonazepam, technically marketed as an anticonvulsant, has an elimination half-life of 30–40 hours. Its biotransformation is primarily by reduction of the 7-nitro group to the 4-amino derivative. This metabolite is acetylated, hydroxylated, and glucuronidated. Cy450-3A may play some role in the drug's reduction and oxidation. Clonazepam will be discussed in more detail in several other parts of this chapter.

TRIAZOLAM

Triazolam, an ultra-short-acting triazolobenzodiazepine marketed as a hypnotic, has been associated with reports of confusion, delirium, anterograde amnesia, and rebound insomnia and rebound anxiety. Bixler et al. (1991) examined 18 poor sleepers placed in three parallel groups treated with 0.5 mg of triazolam, 30 mg of temazepam, or placebo. Immediate recall was similar in all three groups; however, delayed recall was more impaired in the triazolam-treated patients. In addition, five of the six triazolam-treated subjects reported episodes of next-day memory impairment. Greenblatt et al. (1991) evaluated the sensitivity to triazolam in the elderly via a double-blind crossover study of 26 healthy, young (mean age 30 years) and 21 healthy, elderly (mean age 69 years) patients. Impaired psychomotor performance and memory, and increased psychomotor sedation were found in the elderly subjects. The authors recommend reducing the average dose of triazolam in the elderly by 50%, suggesting that clinical efficacy of 0.125 mg in the elderly is equivalent to 0.25 mg in healthy, young patients. We do not recommend the use of triazolam in the elderly or any other population.

It has also been suggested that triazolam may have a lower therapeutic index than other benzodiazepines, which, as a class, have a relatively high therapeutic index. A case report of coma with an overdose of only 0.5 mg has been described, whereas other benzodiazepines require approximately 100 times the clinical dose for serious overdose (Kales, 1990). Inhibition of Cyp450 3A4 or pf P-glycoprotein can increase serum levels of triazolam. Because many drugs and some foods, such as grapefruit juice, are potent inhibitors of both of these proteins, the risk of unintended increases in serum triazolam levels is significant (Bailey, Malcolm, Arnold, & Spence, 1998).

If a short-acting soporific drug is needed, the nonbenzodiazepine soporific zolpidem is likely somewhat more preferable, but it has been reported to have some of the side effects of triazolam with less frequency. We still tend to prefer the intermediate-acting benzodiazepine temazepam, which is metabolized by glucuronide conjugation and has an elimination half-life of about 12 hours.

Clonazepam

As noted, clonazepam has a half-life of 30–40 hours. Since it may take longer than 1 week to achieve steady state, elderly patients may be at increased risk for progressive oversedation, ataxia, and psychomotor slowing (Stoudemire, Fogel, & Gulley, 1991). The pharmacodynamic profile of clonazepam may provide a gradual physiologic "self-taper." For example, Patterson (1988) described successful detoxification in ten alprazolam-dependent patients, substituting clonazepam for alprazolam on a milligram-for-milligram equivalent basis and then discontinuing the clonazepam. Clinical experience indicates that clonazepam is one of the least sedating benzodiazepines. It is an excellent benzodiazepine for the treatment of panic disorder (Nardi et al., 2013).

Quazepam

Quazepam is a highly lipophilic benzodiazepine approved by the FDA for use as a sedative-hypnotic agent. It is rapidly absorbed and reaches peak plasma concentration 1.5 hours after ingestion of an oral dose. Quazepam is extensively metabolized in the liver, with an elimination half-life of 41 hours, although, as noted above, it is metabolized to the same long half-life metabolite as flurazepam, desalkylflurazepam (Kales, 1990). Recommended dosage is 15 mg orally for young adults and 7.5 mg orally for elderly patients. Its long elimination half-life diminishes the risk of rebound insomnia and withdrawal symptoms, at the expense of increased risk of accumulation and daytime sedation. Since it is more slowly absorbed and may cost slightly more than flurazepam, it seems to offer no particular advantages over already established hypnotics for regular use (Medical Letter, 1990). For occasional use, the relative selectivity of the parent compound and its 2-oxo metabolite for BZ1 benzodiazepine receptors may be relevant. Specifically, it may cause relatively less cognitive and motor side effects than flurazepam after a single dose. However, even this potential advantage is not well established. Inducers of Pgp and of Cyp450 3A4, such as St. John's wort, can lower serum quazepam levels (Izzo & Ernst, 2009).

Estazolam

Estazolam, like triazolam, is a triazolobenzodiazepine derivative with sedative-hypnotic efficacy. It is rapidly absorbed, with a mean time to maximum plasma concentration of less than 2 hours, and its half-life is approximately 14 hours (Gustavson & Carrigan, 1990), which is similar to that of temazepam. Estazolam is metabolized via microsomal oxidation and has no significant active metabolites. CyP450 3A4 is the primary responsible hepatic enzyme (Miura, Otani, & Ohkubo, 2005). The usual daily dose is 1–2 mg (clinical trials have found 2 mg of estazolam comparable to 30 mg of flurazepam; see Cohn et al., 1991; Scharf et al., 1990). Although it is clinically efficacious, there have been concerns that estazolam may share the increased toxicity and increased risk of withdrawal-rebound syndromes with the other triazolobenzodiazepines, triazolam and alprazolam.

Midazolam

Midazolam is primarily used as a parenteral preanesthetic in induction of general anesthesia and for sedation before short diagnostic procedures such as endoscopy. It can be administered intramuscularly or intravenously. However, its sedating and anxiolytic action, its remarkably short onset and duration of action, and the option of parenteral use suggest potential usefulness for psychiatric patients. This notion has been bolstered by case reports in the psychiatric literature of its efficacy in the management of acutely agitated and psychotic patients (Bond, Mandos, & Kurtz, 1989; Mendoza et al., 1987).

Midazolam is highly lipophilic at physiologic pH and, unlike most benzodiazepines, is rapidly and well absorbed intramuscularly (Matson & Thurlow, 1988). It has a very rapid onset of CNS effects, with sedation occurring within 5–15 minutes after intramuscular injection (3–5 minutes after intravenous administration) and reaching its peak within 30–60 minutes. Midazolam is rapidly displaced from benzodiazepine receptors and has a short duration of action of approximately 2 hours, with a range of 1–6 hours (Bond, Mandos, & Kurtz, 1989). Its biologic half-life is only 1.3 to 2.2 hours (Beck, Salom, & Holzer, 1983). Midazolam undergoes extensive biotransformation to its major pharmacologically active metabolite, 1-hydroxy-methylmidazolam, by way of microsomal oxidation. Critically ill patients, including infants and children, may experience a higher serum level of midazolam for any given dose due to illness-related decreases in CyP450 3A4 activity (Ince et al., 2012). Drug–drug interactions mediated through CyP450 3A4 and related 3A isoenzymes can have a profound effect on midazolam serum levels (Lichtenbelt et al., 2010). The problem of illness and drug–drug interactions can be an acutely important issue for midazolam use, since it is often given to very ill patients receiving multiple medications (see Box 21.2).

There is also evidence that there are significant age-related differences in the clearance of midazolam with decreased clearance in elderly patients, especially elderly men (Holazo, Winkler, & Patel, 1988). Lower initial doses are therefore recommended in patients older than 60 years. Although the drug is generally well tolerated, like other benzodiazepines, respiratory depression (including apnea) has been associated with its intravenous use. In addition, there have been case reports of hypotension (Matson & Thurlow, 1988), disinhibition of aggressive behavior (Bobo & Miwa, 1988), transient paranoia and agitation (Burnakis & Berman, 1989), and delirium, especially in the elderly. Advancing age and use of an opiate are each associated with an increased risk of acute confusion in the presence of midazolam (Colombo et al., 2012). This may be due in part to midazolam's well-described respiratory sedation, which may be greater among the elderly (Fredman et al., 1999; Huang, Chen, Yang, & Liu, 2012).

Midazolam may induce anterograde amnestic episodes, primarily when it is used intravenously during medical procedures. Retrograde amnesia is not usually achieved. But essentially all patients given midazolam will have anterograde amnesia if sufficient midazolam is given. In one study, 5 mg given intravenously appeared sufficient to produce anterograde amnesia in all patients (Bulach et al., 2005).

Midazolam is approximately three to four times as potent per milligram as diazepam, and initial intramuscular dosage is 0.07–0.08 mg/kg, with the average dosage in a healthy adult being 5 mg and lower dosages recommended in elderly or debilitated patients. Dosage guidelines in the psychiatric setting are not established. On occasion, midazolam may assist in the management of aggressive behavior. Bond, Mandos, and Kurtz (1989) reported three cases of use of midazolam in the treatment of mentally retarded patients with acute and refractory aggressivity and violence, using 5–10 mg of midazolam administered intramuscularly. The patients (a 14-year-old girl, a 17-year-old boy, and a 26-year-old man) showed rapid improvement in aggressive behavior. Mendoza et al. (1987) reported three patients with acute psychotic states with hyperarousal who responded favorably when treated with lower dosages of midazolam in a psychiatric emergency room setting. The patients included a 17-year-old boy, a 38-year-old man, and a 34-year-old woman. The authors noted the onset of sedation in these patients to occur within 6 to 8 minutes, with sedation lasting approximately 90 minutes after an intramuscular dose of 2.5–3 mg. More recent and larger studies paint a less optimistic picture. One randomized study of 301 patients compared midazolam 15 mg intramuscular injection for agitation in psychotic patients against an intramuscular combination of haloperidol 10 mg and promethazine 50 mg. Being asleep or tranquil at 20 minutes was the primary outcome measure. The two regimens were equally effective in achieving this. However, 6% more of the midazolam group had a second episode of aggression. There was one episode of respiratory

depression in the midazolam group, and none in the other (TREC Collaborative Group, 2003). A large, randomized, double-blind study involving 150 patients compared olanzapine, ziprasidone, haloperidol plus midazolam, haloperidol plus promethazine, or haloperidol alone in the management of acute agitation. After 12 hours, only the group randomized to receive haloperidol plus midazolam had high levels of agitation. They also had the most side effects (Baldaçara, Sanches, Cordeiro, & Jackoswski, 2011).

RELATIVE LIPOPHILICITY

In addition to metabolic fate and elimination half-life, the relative lipid solubility of a benzodiazepine is also important to consider. More highly lipophilic drugs, such as diazepam and midazolam, cross the blood–brain barrier quickly but also may be distributed more widely in the peripheral tissues. Diazepam is highly lipophilic and has a rapid onset of action when given intravenously, whereas lorazepam is relatively less lipophilic with less rapid onset of clinical activity when given intravenously (Greenblatt, 1991). When single doses of highly lipophilic drugs are given, redistribution rather than elimination determines the duration of clinical effect.

Elimination half-lives vary widely among individual benzodiazepines. Short half-life benzodiazepines are less likely to accumulate with repetitive dosing, since they reach steady state more rapidly (steady state is more than 90% achieved after approximately four times the elimination half-life; see Greenblatt, 1991). The ultra-short-acting benzodiazepines such as triazolam carry the risk of interdose anxiety, rebound anxiety, and insomnia.

One aspect of the clinical importance of the distinction between long and short half-life benzodiazepines is the propensity of long half-life medications to accumulate in the elderly and increase the risk of falling. In a large retrospective epidemiologic study, Ray, Griffin, and Downey (1989) examined the relative risk for hip fracture in patients age 65 and older who had suffered a hip fracture and had filled a prescription for benzodiazepines within the past 30 days, utilizing computerized pharmacy records available via the Saskatchewan, Canada, universal healthcare plan. These investigators found that current users of long half-life benzodiazepines (diazepam, chlordiazepoxide, flurazepam, clorazepate) had a 70% greater risk of hip fracture than did patients on no psychotropic medications. There was no increased risk in current users of short half-life benzodiazepines (alprazolam, lorazepam, oxazepam, triazolam, bromazepam) (Ray, Griffin, & Downey, 1989). Mortality rises significantly within the first few months after a hip fracture and gradually declines over several years (Yoon, Park, et al., 2011). In one 12-month study of over 500 elderly patients, the withdrawal of psychotropics, including benzodiazepines, led to an 8-fold reduction in the number of falls. In light of the significant and well established morbidity and mortality associated with hip fracture in the elderly (Kelsey & Hoffman, 1987), the clinician should minimize or avoid the use of long half-life benzodiazepines in elderly fragile patients because the prolonged elimination of these benzodiazepines leads to accumulation with daytime drowsiness or ataxia.

FINAL CONSIDERATIONS IN BENZODIAZEPINE USE

All benzodiazepines can lead to tolerance and psychological and physiological dependence. Risk factors for dependency include increased duration of treatment, utilization of higher doses, and a previous history of alcoholism. Physical dependence can occur within as short a time as 2–3 weeks, and often does occur within 4 months at two to five times the therapeutic dose. In addition, benzodiazepine discontinuation syndromes can include reemergence of symptoms that were targeted by treatment. Withdrawal symptoms in tolerant patients include rebound anxiety or insomnia, and major symptoms such as psychosis and seizures (Salzman, 1991).

Despite the high therapeutic index of benzodiazepines in healthy patients, their use should be considered carefully in medically ill patients. In addition to pharmacodynamic alterations and increased drug interactions, the medically ill may be particularly at risk for sedation, especially if benzodiazepines are used concurrently with other CNS depressants such as barbiturate anticonvulsants or narcotics. In addition, it is well established that benzodiazepines reduce the ventilatory response to hypoxia. In chronically hypercapnic patients who have lost their hypercapnic respiratory drive, the suppression of hypoxic drive may result in respiratory suppression. Therefore, baseline arterial blood gases should be obtained in patients with pulmonary disease, and the use of benzodiazepines should be avoided if pCO_2 is elevated (Stoudemire & Fogel, 1995). In addition, benzodiazepines are contraindicated in sleep apnea and may exacerbate symptoms in patients with undiagnosed sleep apnea syndromes (Mendelson, 1987). Agents such as zolpidem and triazolam may be used in sleep apnea cautiously, and only when the risk of respiratory depression is judged to be low (Aurora et al., 2012).

A final caveat regarding the use of benzodiazepines in the elderly and medically ill is that the clinician should give a high priority to the exclusion of underlying treatable pathophysiology before symptomatic treatment of anxiety and insomnia is undertaken. Insomnia, the most common reason for benzodiazepine prescriptions, can be due to underlying medical problems such as restless legs syndrome, the disturbed sleep/wake cycle of delirium or dementia, paroxysmal nocturnal dyspnea, or due to primary psychiatric syndromes such as major depression (Buysse, 2013; Moran & Stoudemire, 1992).

NONBENZODIAZEPINE ANXIOLYTICS AND HYPNOTICS

BUSPIRONE

Buspirone is a nonbenzodiazepine anxiolytic that is free from the side effect of respiratory depression and also lacks withdrawal symptoms on discontinuation (Apter & Allen, 1999). Buspirone's mean elimination half-life is 2 to 3 hours, although its metabolites may have elimination half-lives of 6 to 8 hours (Jann, 1988). While buspirone has significant anxiolytic activity, it is devoid of anticonvulsant, muscle relaxant, and sedative-hypnotic activity. There are no synergistic or additive effects between buspirone and alcohol or other sedative-hypnotics.

The pharmacokinetics of the drug have been studied in patients with impaired liver and kidney function. In patients with hepatic cirrhosis, after a single 20mg dose, the elimination half-life was 6.21 versus 1.79 hours in patients with cirrhosis compared to 4.19 versus 0.53 hours in healthy subjects (Dalhoff et al., 1987; Goa & Ward, 1986). In patients with impaired renal function, including some who were completely anuric, buspirone clearance decreased between 33% and 50%, with no correlation between the severity of renal impairment and buspirone clearance (Gammans, Mayol, & Labudde, 1986). Hence, small reductions in buspirone dosage are likely to be needed in patients with hepatic and renal disease, although the reported prolongation of elimination half-lives by liver or kidney failure is likely to represent an effect of smaller magnitude than normal interindividual differences in optimal dosage. Side effects are not generally more frequent or severe among patients with renal or hepatic impairment (Barbhaiya et al., 1994). No clinically significant prolongation of buspirone pharmacokinetics in elderly patients has been observed (Gammans et al., 1989). However, the pharmacokinetics are highly variable in the general population, implying a need to individualize dosage.

Drug Interactions

Buspirone does not induce or inhibit hepatic mixed oxidase enzymatic functions (Molitor et al., 1985). Buspirone is metabolized through Cyp450 3A4. Inhibitors of CyP450 3A4 can increase serum buspirone levels. Grapefruit juice, a potent inhibitor of CyP450 3A4, can elevate serum buspirone levels fourfold (Lilja, Kivistö, Backman, Lamberg, & Neuvonen, 1998). Similarly, inducers of Cyp450 3A4 such as rifampin can lower serum buspirone levels (Finch, Chrisman, Baciewicz, & Self, 2002). The ability of buspirone to displace phenytoin, warfarin, propranolol, and digoxin from protein binding has been studied in vitro (Gammans et al., 1985), and interaction with these drugs does not appear to be clinically significant. Buspirone also appears free from interaction with antihistamines, bronchodilators, H_2 histamine receptor blockers, oral contraceptives, nonsteroidal antiinflammatory drugs, benzodiazepine hypnotics, digitalis preparations, and oral hypoglycemics (Domantay & Napoliello, 1989; Levine & Napoliello, 1988). Pharmacokinetic interactions between buspirone and TCAs have not been found (Gammans, Mayol, & Labudde, 1986). However, buspirone has been observed to increase serum haloperidol concentrations (Sussman, 1987). Elevations in blood pressure have been observed in patients taking buspirone and MAOIs (Knapp, 1987), leading to the manufacturer's recommendations against this combination. There may be some slight prolongation in the metabolism of diazepam when it is used concurrently with buspirone, although this is of doubtful clinical significance (Meltzer & Fleming, 1982).

Some slight increase in sedation may occur if buspirone is used concurrently with diazepam (Gershon, 1982). Some anecdotal reports claim verapamil and diltiazem (calcium channel blockers) may elevate buspirone serum levels.

Buspirone is generally regarded as an agent with only mild side effects. Yet, buspirone may contribute to development of the serotonin syndrome. This may sometimes occur unexpectedly, as when buspirone is combined with linezolid (Morrison & Rowe, 2012). Linezolid is an antibiotic that reversibly inhibits monoamine oxidase, which creates the potential to amplify the serotonergic effects of medications such as buspirone (Taylor, Wilson, & Estes, 2006). Buspirone is sometimes used to induce therapeutic hypothermia. Its combination with meperidone is considered an effective regimen for induction of hypothermia (Sessler, 2009). However, meperidone combined with serotonergic agents is also capable of precipitating the serotonin syndrome (Gillman, 2005).

Buspirone and Pulmonary Disease

Buspirone is of value in patients with pulmonary disease. Animal studies suggest that buspirone may serve either as a partial respiratory stimulant or as an agent that improves alveolar oxygen diffusion (Garner et al., 1989; Meyer, Hetem, Fick, Mitchell, & Fuller, 2010). In an open study of 82 patients, buspirone was used safely for reduction of anxiety in patients with chronic lung disease. No problems developed from using buspirone together with bronchodilators such as theophylline and terbutaline (Brenes, 2003; Kiev & Domantay, 1988).

Buspirone and Other Conditions

Many case reports and studies indicate clinical efficacy for buspirone in a variety of conditions other than anxiety disorders. Buspirone has been used to treat autism (Brahm, Fast, & Brown, 2008; Realmuto, August, & Garfinkel, 1989), for the suppression of neuroleptic-induced akathisia (D'Mello, McNeil, & Harris, 1989), as an augmenting agent in antidepressant treatment (Robinson et al., 1989), and for ADHD in children. Antidepressant-induced bruxism is often effectively treated with buspirone (Albayrak & Ekinci, 2011). Buspirone can counteract SSRI-induced sexual dysfunction in some patients. It does not, however, appear to increase libido (Moll & Brown, 2011). Buspirone can help reduce anxiety and agitation in brain-injured patients and in patients with dementia (Colenda, 1988; Levine, 1988; Loane & Politis, 2012; Tiller, Dakis, & Shaw, 1988). Typically, relatively low doses are needed for this antiagitation effect (5–10 mg tid). Buspirone also may be helpful in smoking cessation (Carrão, Moreira, & Fuchs, 2007; Gawin, Compton, & Byck, 1989) and in luteal phase dysphoric disorder (Rickels, Freeman, & Sondheimer, 1989; Yatham, Barr, & Dinan, 1989). Current studies are investigating high doses of buspirone for the treatment of tardive dyskinesia. In this role, buspirone may help both by stimulating normal dopamine activity in the brain

and by offering neuroprotection (Lauterbach et al., 2010). Buspirone may also help treat functional dyspepsia, as it relaxes the fundus (Tack, Janssen, Masaoka, Farré R, & Van Oudenhove, 2012).

Stimulant Effect of Buspirone

Although buspirone has an anxiolytic effect that is maximal in 4 to 6 weeks, some patients experience early stimulation or agitation from the drug. The authors have seen several of these reactions in patients with diagnoses ranging from panic disorder to depression to mental retardation. The reaction is dose dependent and can be treated by discontinuing buspirone until the agitation or insomnia resolves, then restarting the drug at a lower dose. A reasonable approach to starting buspirone in "panicky" or neurologically impaired patients is to start no higher than 2.5 mg three times daily and warn the patient or caretaker about possible early and transient agitation. Since buspirone has a weak antidepressant effect at higher doses (30–90 mg/day), it may precipitate hypomania or mania. In some cases, the agitation represents akathisia caused by buspirone (Patterson, 1988). Akathisia related to serotonergic agents appears to be a separate entity from the anxiety or "jitteriness" that agents such as buspirone sometimes cause (Sinclair et al., 2009). However, drug-induced akathisia also tends to be dose dependent. Many patients who might develop these side effects with buspirone may tolerate the drug with a gradual upward taper. In some cases, however, it may be necessary to abandon treatment with buspirone.

MELATONIN

Melatonin spares psychomotor performance, unlike agents such as zaleplon, zopiclone and temazepam (Paul, Gray, Kenny, & Pigeau, 2003). Melatonin easily crosses the blood–brain barrier and stimulates endogenous receptors, promoting sleep. Melatonin indirectly also promotes the release of GABA and inhibits the release of glutamate (Banach, Gurdziel, Jędrych, & Borowicz, 2011). Melatonin lacks known toxicity in acute settings. It is not a mutagen in the Ames test (Anisimov, 2003). Endogenous melatonin is metabolized through CyP450 1A (Rifkind, 2006). Oral melatonin doses of 0.1–0.3 mg achieve serum levels that are similar to those normally seen at night. Sleep latency is reduced, and sleep duration is prolonged (Dollins, Zhdanova, Wurtman, Lynch, & Deng, 1994). Because of its relative benignity, as well as its potent antioxidant effects, melatonin use has been recommended for a variety of disorders including Alzheimer's disease, myocardial infarction, and diabetes (Korkmaz et al., 2012; Sánchez-Barceló et al., 2010). Doses of melatonin higher than 0.3 mg can cause protracted elevations of serum melatonin, and hence persistent daytime sedation. In some cases, while melatonin reduces the time it takes to fall asleep it does not prolong sleep, and patients wind up sleeping the same total amount of time and waking up earlier (Gringras et al., 2012).

RAMELTEON

The bioavailability of oral ramelteon is about 2%. Its elimination half-life is 1–3 hours, and that of its active metabolite is 2–5 hours. Over 80% of the drug is excreted as metabolites in the urine. Metabolism is primarily through CyP450s 1A2 and 2C19, with a small contribution from 3A4 (Obach & Ryder, 2010). Ramelteon is an agonist at melatonin MT1 and MT2 receptors. Although its active metabolite has some affinity for the serotonin 5HT2b receptor, there is no significant activity at other receptors including the GABA-A receptor. Significantly less impairment of cognition and of psychomotor performance is expected with ramelteon compared to those agents active through the GABA-A receptor (Mets et al., 2011). Ramelteon does not have significant withdrawal effects or lead to rebound insomnia on discontinuation. There are no significant effects on respiration among patients with pulmonary problems placed on ramelteon (Greenberg & Goss, 2009). Somnolence is the most common side effect with ramelteon and may affect 5% of patients (Kohsaka et al., 2011).

ESZOPICLONE

Eszopiclone is the s-enantiomer of zopiclone, a nonbenzodiazepine agent that is an allosteric modulator of the GABA-A channel. Its elimination half-life is 6 hours. The drug is 50% to 60% protein-bound. Over 75% is eliminated in the urine as metabolites; less than 10% is recovered in the urine as the parent compound. Eszopiclone is metabolized through CyP450 3A4. Inhibitors of CyP450 3A4, as well as advancing age and liver disease prolongs the elimination half-life (Greenblatt & Zammit, 2012). While sedation and dizziness do occur in a minority of patients, dose-dependent dysgeusia is the most common adverse event. Between 20% and 60% of patients prescribed eszopiclone will experience dysgeusia (Uchimura, Kamijo, & Takase, 2012). There is an elevated risk ratio of 1.4 for developing an infection during treatment with zopiclone or eszopiclone. These are usually mild. The reasons for this association are unclear (Joya, Kripke, Loving, Dawson, & Kline, 2009).

ZALEPLON

The bioavailability of oral zaleplon is about 30% (Drover, 2004). The elimination half-life of zaleplon is an hour. About 70% of the drug is excreted in the urine as metabolites and 17% in the feces as metabolites. Almost no unchanged drug is found in the urine. Zaleplon has a weaker association with mortality and cancer than do zolpidem and temazepam, based on the available data (Kripke et al., 2012). Overdose with zaleplon may cause ataxia, confusion, hallucinations, tachycardia, and vomiting, but these are not typically life threatening (Forrester, 2006). An advantage of zaleplon is that its very short elimination half-life helps minimize cognitive impairment the next day (Lieberman, 2007).

ZOLPIDEM

Among the agents used for insomnia, zolpidem has a relatively strong association with falls and fractures. Among 1,508 patients with fractures and insomnia, Kang and colleagues noted a relative risk of 1.72 (95% CI: 1.37 to 2.16) of having a fracture among patients taking zolpidem. The relative risk among patients taking a benzodiazepine was 1.00 (Kang et al., 2012). Zolpidem overdose has the same general presentation as overdose with zaleplon, although zolpidem is more likely to cause side effects requiring medical attention (Forrester, 2006). Zolpidem appears to be safe for patients with stable mild to moderate chronic obstructive pulmonary disease and for patients with treated sleep apnea (Estivill et al., 2003). Zolpidem is available both as an immediate-release agent and as an extended-release agent. The extended-release formulation permits 60% of the active agent to be taken up immediately, while the remaining 40% is released slowly. This reduces peak serum concentrations and extends the duration of action by 3 hours. Two important differences between the indications of immediate-release and sustained-release zolpidem are that the latter is indicated for sleep maintenance, not just sleep promotion, and also can be used chronically (Lieberman, 2007).

Zolpidem use has also been linked to cancer. The hazard ratio for oral cancer among patients taking more than 300 mg of zolpidem in a year was reported by Kao and colleagues (2012) to be 2.36 (95% CI: 1.57 to 3.56).

ZOPICLONE

The bioavailability of oral zopiclone is generally 70%–80%. The elimination half-life normally ranges from 3.5–6.5 hours. Plasma protein binding ranges from 45%–80% (Drover, 2004; Fernandez, Martin, Gimenez, & Farinotti, 1995). Potent inducers of CyP450 3A4, such as carbamazepine, phenytoin and rifampicin, speed the elimination and reduce the effects of zopiclone (Villikka, Kivistö Lamberg, Kantola, & Neuvonen, 1997). Zopiclone resembles zolpidem in being relatively safe for patients with pulmonary disease. Neither agent significantly impairs respiratory drive when used in recommended dosages (Estivill et al., 2003).

As discussed for eszopiclone, there is an increased risk of infection with zopiclone (Joya et al., 2009).

LITHIUM CARBONATE

EFFECT ON RENAL FUNCTION

Lithium is one of the older psychotropic agents still in use. Its benefits in managing mania remain the gold standard of treatment for bipolar disorder. And the robust neurotrophic effects of lithium continue to inspire research into its potential for other diseases, such as Alzheimer's disease (Diniz, Machado-Vieira, & Forlenza, 2013). Lithium has been used clinically for centuries. Moving into the 1900s, lithium was often used as a sedative or a treatment for gout. In the 1940s it was recommended as a "salt substitute" for patients with cardiovascular disease. This use of lithium led to marked toxicity in a vulnerable population, and by 1949 the drug was banned as too toxic for clinical use (Maletzky & Shore, 1978). That very year, however, Cade began publishing his studies of lithium in mania. Cade's thoughtful assessment of lithium's potential in the management of "psychotic excitement," including comments about the toxicity of lithium, inspired its reintroduction for clinical use (Cade, 1949). With the introduction of anticonvulsants for use in bipolar disorder, and more recently the atypical antipsychotics, use of lithium has been replaced or deferred in many patients. But lithium, with all of its potential benefits and side effects, remains an important therapeutic tool and frequent source of medical concern.

The primary metabolic consideration in the use of lithium in medically ill patients is renal function. Lithium is excreted by the kidney, and rates of excretion are affected by age and creatinine clearance. Before starting lithium, all patients require a routine assessment of renal function via measurement of serum electrolytes, blood urea nitrogen (BUN), and creatinine, along with a standard urinalysis. In patients with known or suspected kidney disease, a 24-hour urine collection to determine baseline creatinine clearance should also be obtained. Lithium excretion is primarily determined by glomerular filtration rate (GFR) and proximal reabsorption. Lithium is filtered freely at the glomerulus; then, approximately 55% of filtered lithium is reabsorbed in the proximal tubule (DePaulo, 1984) and a further 15% is reabsorbed in the descending loop. Sodium depletion increases the reabsorbed fraction of both sodium and lithium ions up to 95%, therefore decreasing clearance of lithium. Thiazide diuretics that act primarily at the distal tubule enhance proximal reabsorption of lithium because they deplete sodium, leading to enhanced proximal reabsorption of sodium and lithium. Loop diuretics such as furosemide appear to have less effect on lithium clearance, although they can deplete sodium as well. Potassium-sparing diuretics such as spironolactone and triamterene also may reduce lithium clearance, although they have been less well studied than other diuretics. Lithium toxicity has been reported with nonthiazide diuretics, however, such as indapamide (Hanna, Lobao, & Stewart, 1990).

Medications such as acetazolamide, theophylline, and aminophylline, which act as diuretics by inhibiting proximal tubular reabsorption, increase lithium excretion moderately and may therefore decrease serum levels. Nonsteroidal antiinflammatory drugs including indomethacin, ibuprofen, phenylbutazone, and piroxicam decrease renal lithium clearance and increase lithium levels (Ragheb, 1990; Rogers, 1985). Aspirin and sulindac, however, apparently have no effect on lithium clearance.

Patients on thiazide diuretics usually need approximately 50% less lithium to attain therapeutic levels, but there is considerable interindividual variation. Patients on diuretics should be dosed slowly, and lithium levels should be monitored at least twice a week during the initiation of therapy. Frequent monitoring of levels should be resumed for a few weeks after any change in diuretic dosage or in diet. Patients on diuretics

and their families deserve especially detailed warnings about the early signs of lithium intoxication; commercially available bracelets with imprinted medical warnings are appropriate for some patients. A report showed that furosemide (a loop diuretic) does not increase serum lithium as much as the distal tubular diuretic hydrochlorothiazide (Crabtree et al., 1991).

Lithium is dialyzable. Therefore, lithium should be given to patients after dialysis, with the usual dose being 300–600 mg by mouth. The dose need not be repeated until after the next dialysis. Serum levels of lithium should be taken several hours after dialysis, since plasma levels may actually rise in the postdialysis period when reequilibration with tissue stores occurs (Bennett, Muther, & Parker, 1980). The dialyzability of lithium can be exploited to rapidly reduce lithium levels in life-threatening cases of lithium toxicity. In cases of lithium intoxication, intermittent hemodialysis can also quickly reduce serum lithium levels. Once again, the problem of rebound in serum levels of lithium after discontinuation of hemodialysis requires ongoing monitoring for days, as lithium moves from intracellular compartments to the extracellular space (Sood & Richardson, 2007).

In virtually all patients on lithium there is some loss of the kidney's ability to concentrate the urine. This develops within 4 to 8 weeks of starting treatment with lithium. Occasionally, this leads to symptomatic polyuria and a diagnosis of nephrogenic diabetes insipidus (NDI). Even when these do not occur, a careful history reveals more frequent urination and larger urine volumes in most patients on lithium. The mechanism of these changes is a direct toxic effect of lithium on the loop of Henle and the distal tubule mediated by interference with the translocation and function of aquaporin-2. The effect is dose related. Usually, stopping lithium allows the renal defect to resolve. However, full recovery can take months or years. In 20% of patients with lithium-induced NDI the condition is permanent and resistant to arginine vasopressin (Bedford et al., 2008). Polyuria may disrupt work or sleep routines and can aggravate incontinence in patients with impaired bladder control. This problem can be partially mitigated by once-daily dosing of lithium.

Because of its potential acute toxicity, as well as its relentless effects on renal function, routine monitoring of renal function during lithium treatment is recommended. During the first 6 months of lithium therapy, renal function should be checked every 2–3 months. In a stable patient receiving chronic lithium therapy, renal function can be checked every 6 months to a year (Jefferson, 2010). Elevations in serum creatinine and reductions in the GFR are indications of possible lithium-induced renal injury. The GFR can be estimated from the serum creatinine. If the GFR falls below 60 mL/minute, as may occur in as many as 1 of 4 patients on lithium therapy for a year, consultation with a nephrologist is advised (Severus & Bauer, 2013). On average, it takes 20 years of lithium treatment to produce end-stage renal disease (Presne et al., 2003). Thyroid function tests should also be obtained. The TSH level, measured at quarterly intervals, is an excellent screen for lithium-induced hypothyroidism in its early asymptomatic stages. Serum electrolyte levels, calcium levels, and thyroid function studies should also be obtained. A baseline ECG is recommended prior to starting lithium treatment. When to repeat the ECG is largely a clinical decision. Finally, a pregnancy test should be obtained prior to starting lithium, since lithium is a teratogen. When to repeat this test is also a clinical decision.

When lithium-induced polyuria threatens to limit lithium treatment, there are several options open. One option is to shift lithium's contact with the kidney away from the collecting ducts. The treatment of choice in this case is the potassium-sparing diuretic amiloride (Oliveira et al., 2010). Amiloride binds to the epithelial sodium channel in the renal collecting duct and diverts lithium and its effects away from this portion of the kidney. Amiloride may help with this side effect in doses ranging from 5–20 mg per day (Bedford et al., 2008; Kosten & Forrest, 1986). In refractory cases, 50 mg/day of hydrochlorothiazide could be added. With or without adjunctive thiazide therapy, amiloride can increase lithium levels, potentially leading to lithium toxicity if levels are not monitored and dosage adjusted. If amiloride is used alone, hyperkalemia is a risk; electrolytes should be rechecked a few times after starting the drug. If amiloride is used with hydrochlorothiazide, lithium dosage must be reduced.

Thiazide diuretics may also be employed, with suitable precautions, to enhance lithium reabsorption at the proximal tubule, thereby protecting the more distal nephron from high lithium concentrations (Forrest, Cohen, & Torretti, 1974; Lippman, Wagemaker, & Tuker, 1981; MacNeil, Hanson-Nortey, & Paschalis, 1975; Mukhopadhyay, Gokulkrishnan, & Mohanaruban, 2001). The total lithium dose is reduced by as much as 50% if this strategy is used.

Angiotensin converting enzyme (ACE) inhibitors used in the treatment of hypertension have been reported to have a pharmacokinetic interaction with lithium. This may be due to ACE inhibitors–induced lithium retention (Baldwin & Safferman, 1990; Roughead, Kalisch, Barratt, & Gilbert, 2010). If the two classes of drugs are used together, lithium levels must be monitored closely (Douste-Blazy et al., 1986) for elevations of lithium levels. Similar problems have been reported with most ACE inhibitors, including enalapril, captopril, and lisinopril.

As a cation, lithium competes with other cations at various sites, including calcium, magnesium, potassium, and sodium. A host of ECG changes and cardiac effects can occur during lithium treatment. Among the changes that occur are QT prolongation and changes in the ST segment and T wave. These changes may result from a cumulative effect of lithium on cardiac tissues, and in intoxication (Kayrak et al., 2010). A normal serum lithium level does not mean that there is no potential for cardiotoxicity. Sinus node dysfunction and sinoatrial node block have been described, as well as rare episodes of ventricular irritability, even at therapeutic levels (Mitchell & MacKenzie, 1982). The most common cardiac abnormality associated with lithium in therapeutic doses is sinoatrial node dysfunction; aggravation of ventricular arrhythmias and heart block have been very rarely reported (Horgan et al., 1973; Jaffe, 1977; Tangedahl & Gau, 1972; Tilkian et al., 1976). In contrast, antiarrhythmic effects of lithium have also been described (Leonard et al., 2011; Levenson et al., 1986;

Polumbo et al., 1973). Clinically significant cardiovascular side effects of lithium, however, are sufficiently rare that they are seldom relevant to drug choice even in patients with cardiovascular disease. Electrocardiograms made before and after initiation of lithium therapy are an appropriate precaution for patients with asymptomatic abnormalities of cardiac conduction or repolarization. In patients with symptomatic arrhythmias, appropriate monitoring during initiation of lithium therapy should be worked out in collaboration with a cardiologist. Rarely, lithium may cause hypercalcemia by inducing parathyroid adenomas and elevated PTH levels, which can lead to EKG abnormalities and arrhythmias (Wolf et al., 1998). Lithium-induced thyroid dysfunction is another potential cause of arrhythmias.

Hypothyroidism and goiter are two common complications of lithium therapy. Although as many as 50% of patients may develop one or both of these abnormalities, clinically significant thyroid disease likely occurs much less frequently. Hypothyroidism may occur within the first few months of lithium treatment, but on average it takes about 18 months to develop. At-risk groups include women, those over 50 years old, patients who are positive for thyroid autoantibodies, and those with a family history of thyroid disease (Kibirige, Luzinda, & Ssekitoleko, 2013). Hyperthyroidism may also result from lithium therapy, but it is rare. Perhaps 1%–2% of patients chronically receiving lithium will develop hyperthyroidism (Bocchetta et al., 2007). In patients with known hypothyroidism, lithium is safe provided adequate thyroid replacement is given. Patients with Hashimoto's disease may have fluctuating thyroid levels; when they are treated with lithium, fluctuations may increase because lithium can cause increases or decreases in thyroid antibody levels. Obtaining TSH and free thyroxine levels is advisable whenever there is an unexplained change in physical or mental status in a patient with Hashimoto's disease who is taking lithium (Lazarus, 1986).

Both elderly patients and patients with brain disease are particularly susceptible to developing mild cognitive dysfunction, delirium, and tremor, even at therapeutic lithium levels (Babinsky & Levene, 2012; Stoudemire & Moran, 1998). Dosage aiming for the lower end of the therapeutic range is therefore recommended for elderly individuals and others susceptible to the neurologic side effects of lithium (Delva & Hawken, 2001). Maintenance doses of lithium for elderly patients usually are about 50% of the maintenance doses required in younger individuals. When lithium is used to potentiate tricyclics in elderly patients with unipolar depression, doses may be even smaller. At times, doses as small as 150 mg/day may yield therapeutic effects, with much less likelihood of CNS toxicity than with full antimanic dosage (Kushnir, 1986). If cognitive problems develop with lithium in elderly patients, valproate or an atypical antipsychotic such as risperidone may be considered as alternative agents. A syndrome of irreversible lithium-effectuated neurotoxicity, referred to as "SILENT," may develop. SILENT is characterized by persistent evidence of neurologic injury 2 months after discontinuation of lithium. SILENT may develop at any age. A characteristic feature of SILENT is the presence of cerebellar or brainstem findings. It is thought that injury to myelin may be involved in the pathophysiology of this side effect (Adityanjee, Munshi, & Thampy, 2005; Khanna & Sethi, 1993).

Lithium can be a risk factor for complications during electroconvulsive therapy (ECT). Lithium can prolong neuromuscular blockade induced by succinylcholine or pancuronium (Blackwell & Schmidt, 1984). Inhibition of acetylcholinesterases by lithium may explain this drug–drug interaction (Petraglio et al., 2008). If possible, lithium therapy should be discontinued during ECT treatment and prior to elective surgery. The aggravation of post-ECT confusion and amnesia by lithium in some patients is another reason to discontinue lithium during ECT (Naguib & Koorn, 2002). If lithium must be given during a course of ECT, the serum lithium level should be maintained at the lower end of therapeutic (Thirthalli, Harish, & Gangadhar, 2011).

LITHIUM IN CHRONIC RENAL FAILURE

Although lithium is not recommended in the presence of acute renal failure, there is no evidence that it is necessarily contraindicated in chronic renal failure (CRF) (DasGupta & Jefferson, 1990). In one study of patients with CRF continued on lithium, there is a trend toward a gradual decline in estimated GFR over 60 months compared to no decline in estimated GFR among patients with CRF whose lithium treatment was discontinued (Rej, Abitbol, Looper, & Segal, 2013). Thus, CRF is not an absolute contraindication to lithium therapy but must be weighed against the possible therapeutic advantages of continuing lithium versus stopping lithium. Lithium doses should be adjusted downward to accommodate decreases in creatinine clearance (Chiu, Shen, Chen, & Lu, 2007; Csernansky & Hollister, 1985). Since it is not known if lithium accelerates the progression of certain types of renal disease, close monitoring is indicated in patients with chronic renal disease (such as semiannual creatine clearance determination or quarterly BUN/creatinine levels). Alternative mood-stabilizing agents such as carbamazepine, valproate, and atypical antipsychotics should be considered if not contraindicated for other reasons. The use of lithium in hemodialysis appears to be both safe and effective if lithium doses are reduced to the range of 300–600 mg and if lithium doses are given after hemodialysis (Bjarnason et al., 2006; Lippman, Manshadi, & Gultekin, 1984; Port, Kroll, & Rosenzweig, 1979; Stoudemire & Fogel, 1995).

Since renal transplantation has become a relatively common procedure, clinicians increasingly will encounter renal transplant patients requiring lithium therapy for bipolar disorder or for mood disorders secondary to corticosteroids. Experience with the use of lithium in transplant recipients remains quite limited, but there are a few reports of its successful implementation (Blazer, Petric, & Wilson, 1976; Koecheler et al., 1986). Koecheler et al. recommended more conservative use of lithium in patients receiving cadaveric transplants, because their renal function is more unstable than in those with living related donor transplants. Cyclosporine can elevate lithium levels by decreasing lithium excretion, so lithium doses may need to be adjusted downward in patients receiving this drug (DasGupta & Jefferson, 1990; Dieperink et al., 1987; Vareesangthip et al., 2004; Vincent, Weimar, & Schalekamp, 1987). Close monitoring of lithium levels is essential given that the transplant's function may be unstable for weeks following transplantation. In animal models and in patients, the combination of lithium with cyclosporine can be synergistically nephrotoxic (Tariq, Morais, Sobki, Al Sulaiman, & Al Khader, 2000).

DRUG INTERACTIONS

Table 21.7 summarizes clinically significant drug interactions with lithium (Adan-Manes, Novalbos, López-Rodríguez, Ayuso-Mateos, & Abad-Santos, 2006; Beijnen, Bais, & tenBokkelHuinink, 1994; Dick, Towler, Whiting, & Forrester, 1992; Gardner & Lynd, 1998; Ma, Shiah, Chang, Kao, & Lee, 2012; Preskorn, 2007; Shirley, Walter, & Noormohamed, 2002; Su, Chang, & Hwang, 2007; Torre, Menon, & Power, 2009; Türck, Heinzel, & Luik, 2000.). Concurrent use of a tetracycline for lithium-induced acne may slightly lower lithium levels, but the effect is of no real clinical significance (Frankhauser et al., 1988).

Movement disorders, including cerebellar and extrapyramidal, may develop during lithium treatment (Lloyd, Perkins, & Schwartz, 2010). When this occurs, the clinician should suspect lithium toxicity (Reed, Wise, & Timmerman, 1989). At other times, a pharmacodynamic drug–drug interaction may be responsible (Bondon-Guitton et al., 2011). Choreoathetosis is a striking example of such a drug interaction with lithium. Choreoathetosis has been observed in one case when lithium was combined with verapamil (Helmuth et al., 1989). Other involuntary movements have been reported with the combined use of verapamil and lithium (Price & Giannini, 1986).

LITHIUM, DIABETES, AND THE METABOLIC SYNDROME.

The role of lithium in producing the metabolic syndrome or diabetes is unclear. Some studies suggest a greater risk of having the metabolic syndrome among bipolar patients treated with lithium versus those treated with carbamazepine, valproic acid, or antipsychotics (Ezzaher et al., 2011). There is evidence to suggest that, at least in some patients, lithium can decrease glucose tolerance (DasGupta & Jefferson, 1990). However, increased glucose tolerance also has been reported as a lithium effect (Vendsborg, 1979). Confounding these studies is the fact that mania and psychosis both impair pancreatic beta-cell function, which in turn promotes insulin resistance (Shiloah et al., 2003). Although glucose tolerance curves may be affected by lithium in some patients, there is no strong evidence that this is a clinically significant effect in the vast majority of patients nor is there evidence to suggest the need for routine glucose monitoring in patients treated with lithium other than diabetic patients with unstable control of

Table 21.7 DRUG INTERACTIONS WITH LITHIUM

MEDICATION	INTERACTIVE EFFECT
Thiazide diuretics	Raise lithium levels
Spironolactone	
Triamterene	
Enalapril	
Nonsteroidal antiinflammatory drugs (e.g., indomethacin, ibuprofen, meloxicam, phenylbutazone, piroxicam)	
Telmisartan	
Valsartan	
Cyclosporin	
Acetazolamide	Lower lithium levels
Theophylline	
Aminophylline	
Caffeine	
Theophylline	
Cisplatin	
Calcium channel blockers	May either raise or lower lithium levels, effects not clear; verapamil may cause bradycardia when used with lithium
Metronidazole	May increase lithium levels; may increase chances of nephrotoxicity
Tetracycline	Minor elevation of lithium levels
Antipsychotics	Pharmacodynamically increase the risk of neuroleptic malignant syndrome during lithium treatment
Serotonergic agents (e.g., SSRIs, MAOIs, venlafaxine, triptans)	Pharmacodynamically increases risk of serotonin syndrome during lithium treatment

blood glucose, who would undoubtedly be monitored closely anyway (DasGupta & Jefferson, 1990). Weight gain caused by lithium may be a factor to consider. As many as 30% of patients on chronic lithium therapy will gain 4 to 10 kilograms (Grandjean & Aubry, 2009).

LITHIUM AND EPILEPSY

Lithium administration is associated with EEG changes. Especially in overdose, lithium may induce seizures. Since nonconvulsive status epilepticus (NCSE) is one type of seizure that can occur in lithium intoxication, monitoring of the serum lithium level and making use of the EEG when patients on lithium develop altered mentation are very important (Yip & Yeung, 2007). Note that NCSE may be caused by lithium even when the serum lithium level is therapeutic

(Bellesi, Passamonti, Silvestrini, Bartolini, & Provinciali, 2006). However, lithium is not contraindicated for patients with epilepsy. A series of bipolar patients treated with lithium suggested that lithium may be benign in patients with epilepsy (Shukla, Mukherjec, & Decina, 1988). In an open study of eight patients, lithium levels were maintained in the 0.6 to 1.1 mEq/liter range, and concurrent anticonvulsants were limited to phenytoin and phenobarbital (no patients were on carbamazepine, sodium valproate, or clonazepam). Lithium prevented the recurrence of affective episodes without increasing seizure frequency in patients with incompletely controlled seizures and did not induce any seizures in well-controlled patients.

Although lithium should not be dismissed because of an undue concern about aggravation of seizures, the mood-stabilizing anticonvulsants carbamazepine and sodium valproate are natural alternatives for patients with concurrent bipolar disorder and epilepsy. When lithium and anticonvulsants are given simultaneously, pharmacodynamic interactions may lead to CNS side effects at lithium levels within the therapeutic range (Fogel, 1988), so the upper end of the therapeutic range of lithium levels usually should be avoided. A classic example of this would be cerebellar ataxias at therapeutic doses of phenytoin combined with lithium (Manto, 2012).

While lithium is problematic in many medically ill and elderly patients, the availability of valproate and of some atypical antipsychotics as antimanic agents has provided excellent alternative drugs for this patient population.

ANTICONVULSANTS AS PSYCHOTROPICS

As noted, in the last several years anticonvulsants have entered the mainstream of psychopharmacologic practice. Carbamazepine (Tegretol), valproate (Depakote, Depakene), and lamotrigine (Lamictal) and topiramate (Topamax) all have been widely employed for psychiatric indications. Anticonvulsants have found a particularly important place as alternatives or adjuncts to lithium in the treatment of bipolar disorder (Goodwin & Jamison, 1990; Pope et al., 1991; Prien & Gelenberg, 1989).

CARBAMAZEPINE

Issues to be considered when prescribing carbamazepine to medically ill patients include hematologic toxicity, hepatic toxicity, quinidine-like effects on cardiac conduction, antidiuretic actions, enzyme induction leading to drug interactions, clinical interpretation of carbamazepine blood levels, and management of carbamazepine overdose. Drug interactions are summarized in Table 21.8 (Bauler et al., 2012; Brzaković et al., 2012; Chrościńska-Krawczyk et al., 2011; Contin et al., 2002; Glue et al., 1997; May et al., 2007; Sockalingam et al., 2013; Spina, Pisani, & Perucca, 1996; Strack, Leckband, & Meyer, 2009; Yamamoto et al., 2012).

Table 21.8 SELECTED DRUG INTERACTIONS WITH CARBAMAZEPINE

MEDICATION	INTERACTIVE EFFECT
Erythromycin	May raise carbamazepine to toxic levels and precipitate heart block
Antiarrhythmics	May have additive effects on cardiac conduction time
Fluoxetine	May raise carbamazepine levels to toxic levels
Cimetidine	
Diltiazem	
Verapamil	
Acetazolamide	
Grapefruit juice	
Danazol	
Metronidazole	
Propoxyphene	
Nefazodone	
Quinidine	Serum levels lowered by carbamazepine
Carbamazepine	
Felbamate	
Lamotrigine	
Phenytoin	
Pregabalin	
Topiramate	
Valproate	
Warfarin	
Fluindione	
Tricyclic antidepressants	
Neuroleptics	
Propranolol	
Cyclosporine	
Boceprevir	
Telaprevir	
Theophylline	
Phenobarbital	Decreases serum levels of carbamazepine and increases concentrations of carbamazepine's epoxide metabolite
Phenytoin	Decreases levels of carbamazepine; phenytoin levels decrease when used with carbamazepine
Warfarin	Carbamazepine causes increased metabolism of anticoagulants due to hepatic enzyme induction
Oral contraceptives	Carbamazepine reduces efficacy; loss of contraceptive effect possible
Caffeine	Reduces anticonvulsant efficacy of carbamazepine and other anticonvulsants

One of the more important pharmacokinetic actions of carbamazepine is the induction of its own metabolism, as well as many other drugs metabolized through hepatic cytochromes P450. This effect typically takes 10 to 14 days to become maximal. At this time the serum level of carbamazepine should be checked, as it may become subtherapeutic. The same is true for many other medications coadministered with carbamazepine. P-glycoprotein does not appear to be affected by carbamazepine (Magnusson, Dahl, Cederberg, Karlsson, & Sandström, 2008). See also below.

A particularly common and relevant interaction for medical-psychiatric practices is the interaction of carbamazepine with the calcium channel blockers diltiazem and verapamil. These two drugs, but not nifedipine, raise carbamazepine levels substantially, frequently producing toxicity such as ataxia if carbamazepine dosage is not lowered (Bahls, Ozuna, & Ritchie, 1991; Wijdicks, Arendt, & Bazzell, 2004). Carbamazepine is now available in long-acting preparations.

HEMATOLOGIC TOXICITY

When carbamazepine was first introduced in the United States, the manufacturer recommended frequent blood counts because of concerns about the development of agranulocytosis. However, as evidence accumulated that these potentially fatal side effects were rare and idiosyncratic, this recommendation has been modified by major national clinical neurological associations. Present practice regarding monitoring for hematologic interactions is based on the idea that there are two different hematologic reactions to carbamazepine.

One reaction is a predictable and often transient drop in both red and white blood cell counts; the other is a rare and idiosyncratic failure of the bone marrow that can occur at any unpredictable time after initiation of therapy. Leukopenia occurs in 7% to 12% of treated patients. Leukopenia apparently is unrelated to aplastic anemia, which occurs in approximately 1 in 575,000 treated patients per year (Seetharam & Pellock, 1991). Among psychotropics, carbamazepine is second only to clozapine in causing severe blood dyscrasias (Stübner et al., 2004).

When patients have preexisting anemia or neutropenia, the predictable drop in red and white blood cell counts induced by carbamazepine occurs at a lower baseline. However, there is no evidence that patients with preexisting blood disorders are at greater risk in general for the life-threatening complications of aplastic anemia and agranulocytosis. Therefore, preexisting cytopenias are relative but not necessarily absolute contraindications to carbamazepine. The authors recommend that hematologic consultation be obtained prior to initiating carbamazepine in any patient with a baseline hemoglobin below 12 g/dl or a white blood cell count below 4000/mm^3. The consultant should be asked both for an individualized assessment of risk and for specific guidelines for monitoring and drug discontinuation if carbamazepine is begun.

Caution should be used when combining carbamazepine with other drugs known to cause severe blood dyscrasias, such as agranulocytosis. Ticlopidine, spironolactone, and antithyroid drugs are among the many agents that can affect blood cell production (Ibáñez, Vidal, Ballarín, & Laporte, 2005). It is tempting to consider combining carbamazepine with agents that increase blood cell counts. For example, lithium is known to increase serum white cell counts, in part through enhanced release and action of granulocyte colony-stimulating factor (G-CSF) (Focosi, Azzarà, Kast, Carulli, & Petrini, 2009). Patients receiving combined therapy with lithium and carbamazepine may be at somewhat less risk for a lowering of the white cell count because of lithium's mild stimulatory effects on white cell production (Brewerton, 1986; Vieweg et al., 1986–87). However, leukopenia has been reported with combined therapy (Sheehan & Shelley, 1990).

HEPATIC TOXICITY

In general, carbamazepine should be avoided, or only cautiously introduced, to children and to patients with preexisting liver disease, alcohol abuse or dependence, or patients with chronic acetaminophen use (Ferrajolo et al., 2010; Sedky, Nazir, Joshi, Kaur, & Lippmann, 2012). This is because, as in the case of hematologic toxicity, hepatic toxicity from carbamazepine comes in two kinds: frequent, predictable, and benign; and rare, idiosyncratic, and life threatening (Dreifuss & Langer, 1987). The relatively benign form of toxicity, seen in no more than 5% of patients (Jeavons, 1983), consists of mild asymptomatic elevations of AST and ALT, usually to less than twice the upper limit of their normal values. The life-threatening toxicity is acute hepatic necrosis with liver failure, occurring in less than 1 in 10,000 treated patients. Only 21 cases of this severe hepatic toxicity were reported in the first 20 years of carbamazepine's clinical use (Jeavons, 1983). Severe hepatic toxicity occurs unpredictably, usually within the first month of therapy but occasionally after several months of uneventful treatment. All patients should be advised to report for an examination and tests of liver enzymes should they develop anorexia, nausea, vomiting, or upper abdominal pain. Elevations of AST and ALT to less than twice the upper limit of normal would not necessitate discontinuation of the drug. Greater elevations would trigger either drug discontinuation or consultation with a gastroenterologist or a specialist in liver diseases.

In regard to monitoring liver enzymes, it should be noted that the gamma-glutamyl transpeptidase (GGT) level can be markedly elevated by carbamazepine, as well as by other anticonvulsants, in the absence of clinical symptoms of liver disease (Jeavons, 1983). An isolated elevation of GGT, even to high levels, would indicate consultation with a gastroenterologist but not necessarily discontinuation of the drug. A full panel of liver function tests, including a prothrombin time, should be taken into account when evaluating the significance of an elevated GGT level.

Prescription of carbamazepine to patients with preexisting liver disease has two risks (Sedky et al., 2012). The first is that any hepatic reaction to carbamazepine will occur on a lower baseline of liver function, so that a mild reaction could become symptomatic. The second is that carbamazepine will be metabolized more slowly, since its primary route of metabolism is hepatic. For this reason, significant liver disease is a relative contraindication to carbamazepine. Consultation with an internist should be obtained before prescribing carbamazepine to a patient with significant liver disease. In patients such as alcoholics who are at risk for liver disease that is not necessarily apparent on routine screening liver function tests, carbamazepine should be started more slowly than usual, with frequent determinations of liver enzymes, prothrombin time, and carbamazepine levels during the initiation of therapy.

EFFECTS ON CARDIAC CONDUCTION

Carbamazepine is similar in chemical structure to the TCAs and has similar effects on the heart, with the potential for slowing conduction through the AV node and suppressing ventricular automaticity (Benassi et al., 1987). It does not, however, apparently affect the QRS complex or QT interval at normal heart rates (Kenneback et al., 1991). Symptomatic heart block has been reported when carbamazepine has been given to patients with known or suspected preexisting cardiac disease (Beerman & Edhag, 1978), and cardiac rhythm disturbances are a feature of severe carbamazepine overdose. Therefore, pretreatment ECGs are warranted prior to carbamazepine therapy. If the ECG shows more severe block than first-degree AV block, right bundle-branch block, left anterior hemiblock, or asymptomatic Mobitz type I (Wenckebach-type) block, carbamazepine should not be prescribed on an outpatient basis unless the patient has been cleared first by a cardiologist (Jankovic & Dostik, 2012). In patients with benign, asymptomatic forms of heart block, a posttreatment ECG should be obtained to rule out aggravation of the heart block by carbamazepine. Valproate would be an excellent alternative drug for bipolar patients with cardiac disease.

ANTIDIURETIC ACTIONS OF CARBAMAZEPINE

Carbamazepine has an antidiuretic action and is associated both with clinically significant hyponatremia and with mild, asymptomatic reductions in serum sodium (Letmaier et al., 2012). The effect is thought to be via a direct action on the renal tubules. Patients with other factors predisposing to hyponatremia, including advanced age, diuretic use, and congestive heart failure, are especially at risk. They should have electrolyte determinations weekly during the first month of carbamazepine therapy, with additional determinations done if there is any change in mental or physical status or if there are significant changes in carbamazepine dosage or in their other medications.

As suggestions for practical management of carbamazepine-induced hyponatremia, the authors offer the following recommendations.

1. If the sodium level drops below 125 mEq/liter on carbamazepine, the drug should be discontinued.

2. If the sodium level drops to between 125 and 130 mEq/liter, and carbamazepine appears clinically useful, other drugs that may aggravate hyponatremia (such as thiazide diuretics) should be discontinued if possible. If the sodium level still remains below 130 mEq/liter, carbamazepine should be discontinued.

3. If the sodium level is between 130 and 135 mEq/liter, discontinuation of carbamazepine is not necessary but electrolytes should be followed weekly for 1 month to assure stability of the level. Serum sodium should be rechecked immediately if mental status changes.

4. An evaluation for SIADH should be carried out if the sodium level remains below 130 mEq/liter after carbamazepine discontinuation and is not otherwise explained (e.g., by congestive heart failure).

5. Discontinuation of long-term carbamazepine, when indicated by a low sodium level, should be gradual to avoid withdrawal phenomena such as cholinergic rebound or seizures.

6. When carbamazepine is being used for the indication of seizures, an alternate anticonvulsant less likely to cause hyponatremia should be initiated prior to tapering carbamazepine (e.g., phenytoin or valproate).

ENZYME INDUCTION LEADING TO DRUG–DRUG INTERACTIONS

Carbamazepine is known to be a potent inducer of the cytochrome P450 system. As such, it influences the metabolism of all drugs that rely on this system for their metabolism. One well-known consequence of enzyme induction is that it decreases its own serum level with increased dosages and induces its own metabolism; hence the need to gradually build up carbamazepine dosage over the first few weeks of treatment to maintain a steady blood level. Two other consequences are clinically significant. The first is that the blood levels of some drugs may drop if carbamazepine is added to the patient's medication regimen. This has been reported for benzodiazepines, with potentially clinically significant withdrawal when carbamazepine is added to a steady dosage of alprazolam, midazolam, triazolam, and other benzodiazepines (Arana et al., 1988; Yuan, Flockhart, & Balian, 1999). A similar concern exists for antipsychotics combined with carbamazepine, including aripiprazole, clozapine, haloperidol, quetiapine, risperidone, ziprasidone, and other agents metabolized through such cytochromes P450 as 3A4 (Arana et al., 1986; Besag & Berry, 2006; Strack, Leckband, & Meyer, 2009). Valproate levels for a given dose decrease when carbamazepine is given concurrently (Ieiri

et al., 1990); a similar effect has been reported on imipramine levels in children (Brown et al., 1990). Concurrent use of valproate with carbamazepine also increases the levels of the toxic epoxide metabolite of carbamazepine. Serum moclobemide levels are similarly reduced by carbamazepine (Rakic, Miljkovic, Todorovic, Timotijevic, & Pokrajac, 2009).

Carbamazepine may induce the metabolism and undermine the efficacy of agents used to treat HIV and AIDS. Serum levels of agents such as efavirenz and nevirapine may be lowered by coadministration of carbamazepine (Birbeck et al., 2012). Data on such interactions is limited, which means the clinician must proceed with caution when combining carbamazepine with antiviral agents.

The second effect is that drug metabolites not ordinarily clinically significant might be present in larger quantities as a result of carbamazepine-induced induction of metabolic enzymes. Hydroxymetabolites of desipramine have been reported to cause EKG changes in a patient concurrently treated with carbamazepine and desipramine, despite a desipramine level in the therapeutic range (Baldessarini et al., 1988; see discussion in TCA section of this chapter).

A practical implication of these observations with carbamazepine is that blood levels of drugs metabolized by the liver should be determined promptly if unexpected toxicity or lack of therapeutic effect occurs in the context of concurrent carbamazepine therapy. Furthermore, toxicity in the presence of apparently therapeutic blood levels is possible on the basis of unusually great concentrations of unmeasured metabolites. Specifically, medically ill patients on combined carbamazepine and tricyclic therapy should have posttreatment ECGs even if tricyclic blood levels appear normal.

CLINICAL INTERPRETATION OF CARBAMAZEPINE BLOOD LEVELS

Carbamazepine blood levels are published for the use of carbamazepine in the treatment of epilepsy. Typical normal ranges are 8–12 ng/ml for single-drug therapy and 4–8 ng/ml for combined therapy with other anticonvulsants. However, when carbamazepine is used as a psychotropic, or when it is used together with other medications in medically ill patients, the interpretation of levels is subject to several caveats. First, since carbamazepine is heavily protein-bound, free carbamazepine levels, on which both therapeutic and toxic effects depend, can vary if other drugs displace carbamazepine from its protein binding sites. This has been reported for agents as ubiquitous as aspirin. Second, pharmacodynamic interactions can induce neurotoxicity of carbamazepine at therapeutic blood levels when the drug is given in conjunction with other psychotropics (Fogel, 1988). This has been reported for coadministration with haloperidol and with lithium, although such reports have all but disappeared from the literature. The neurotoxicity of combined carbamazepine–lithium therapy has been shown to be additive rather than synergistic (McGinness, Kishimoto, & Hollister, 1990). Third, the level of carbamazepine needed for maximum psychotropic effect may be greater than the level optimal for seizure control.

Finally, usually unmeasured metabolites, such as carbamazepine 10,11-epoxide, can contribute to both therapeutic and toxic effects. While the ratio of the parent compound to the epoxide is fairly predictable among medically well persons, it may vary in the medically ill, particularly in the setting of liver disease or polypharmacy. As noted earlier, the combination of carbamazepine with valproate can produce toxic levels of carbamazepine 10,11-epoxide (Rambeck et al., 1990). A similar effect is seen when probenecid or a barbiturate is combined with carbamazepine (Kim, Oh, Park, & Park, 2005). In general, coadministered medications, younger age, larger doses of carbamazepine, and timing of carbamazepine doses may all influence the extent to which the epoxide is formed (Lanchote et al., 1995). For all these reasons, scrupulous and frequent clinical monitoring clinical reassessments must supplement blood levels in evaluating carbamazepine effect. Serum free carbamazepine and 10,11-epoxide levels can be obtained to supplement clinical observations.

MANAGEMENT OF CARBAMAZEPINE OVERDOSE

Because carbamazepine has been increasingly prescribed both as an anticonvulsant and psychotropic, the incidence of carbamazepine overdose has been increasing. The problems of carbamazepine overdose include coma, seizures, hypotension, and cardiac arrhythmia. The general approach to supportive management is similar to that used for TCA overdose. In treating carbamazepine overdose, vigorous use of activated charcoal and laxatives is helpful because the absorption of carbamazepine is quite slow, and much may remain in the intestine at the time the patient presents for emergency treatment. In cases of severe carbamazepine intoxication, hemodialysis can reduce serum carbamazepine levels (Ozhasenekler, Gökhan, Güloğlu, Orak, & Ustündağ, 2012). Hemodialysis can remove both carbamazepine and its 10,11-epoxide metabolite (Harder, Heung, Vilay, Mueller, & Segal, 2011). The phenomenon of prolonged absorption can lead to a recurrence of coma following apparent recovery as a result of the eventual absorption of drug remaining in the intestine (Fisher & Cysyk, 1988; Sethna et al., 1989). For this reason, patients with serious carbamazepine overdose should be observed in the hospital for a full 24 hours following the return of consciousness.

VALPROATE

Depakene is valproic acid, and Depakote is divalproex sodium, which is a stable compound of sodium valproate and valproic acid formed by the neutralizing effects of sodium hydroxide. Hence, sodium valproate causes fewer gastrointestinal side effects and is much better tolerated than valproic acid.

Issues to be considered when prescribing valproate to medically ill patients include (1) gastrointestinal side effects, (2) hepatic toxicity, (3) effects on coagulation, (4) drug interactions, (5) clinical interpretation of blood levels, and (6) management of overdose.

GASTROINTESTINAL TOXICITY

In comparative studies of anticonvulsant side effects, the most prominent and troublesome side effect of valproate has been nausea, often accompanied by vomiting. Medically ill patients, particularly those with diseases predisposing to nausea, may be at increased risk. Since valproate is much less likely to cause gastrointestinal upset than valproic acid, more frequent dosing, preferably after meals, is almost always better tolerated than larger doses taken fewer times per day. Occasional patients will be better on valproic acid syrup or Depakote "sprinkles," a pediatric preparation designed to be sprinkled on food. However, regardless of the preparation used, some patients simply will be unable to tolerate the drug. As noted earlier, we rarely have gastrointestinal problems with Depakote if it is taken on a full stomach. Elevated amylase levels may occur with valproic acid.

HEPATIC TOXICITY

Shortly after valproic acid was first introduced, there were several deaths from acute hepatic necrosis, and, as of 1988, approximately 100 fatalities had been reported from valproate-induced liver failure (Scheffner et al., 1988). These and subsequent cases inspired much research into the link between valproic acid use and liver injury (Neyns, Hoorens, & Stupp, 2008). These deaths also led to considerable caution in the use of the drug. As experiences have accumulated, however, it appears that hepatic necrosis is a major risk only for children under 2 years, particularly those given multiple-drug therapy for epilepsy.

Overall, the risk of severe liver injury with valproic acid is low (Gerstner et al., 2008). The incidence of hepatic necrosis in adults receiving valproate is well under 1 in 10,000 (Eadie, Hooper, & Dickinson, 1988) and may be as low as 1 in 50,000, with 95% of reported cases developing symptoms within the first 6 months of therapy (Scheffner et al., 1988). Given this very infrequent occurrence of life-threatening hepatic toxicity, routine long-term monitoring of liver function tests does not seem necessary unless patients have some form of liver disease or a history of liver disease. Periodic liver function tests for the first 6 months are a reasonable precaution but, as noted above, are not recommended as routine for all patients. All patients should be warned of the early signs of liver disease and be told to report immediately for repeat testing of liver function should those signs develop during valproate therapy. L-carnitine has been used successfully to manage some cases of hepatotoxicity due to valproic acid (Chan, Tse, & Lau, 2007). Hemodialysis is also effective in removing ammonia in hepatic encephalopathy (Thanacoody, 2009).

A much more common (although benign) hepatic effect of valproate is an increase in the serum ammonia level. A twofold increase in serum ammonia levels may be seen in the majority of patients starting treatment with valproic acid. In the vast majority of cases this is an asymptomatic change in liver function (Chicharro, de Marinis, & Kanner, 2007). This elevation in serum ammonia may, however, be of concern in individuals with preexisting liver disease, especially those in whom there is a history of hepatic encephalopathy. Significant liver disease is a relative contraindication to valproate therapy, and close monitoring of both liver enzymes and serum ammonia would be an appropriate precaution with alcoholic patients suspected to have subclinical cirrhosis of the liver. Other risk factors for clinically significant hyperammonemia during valproic acid therapy include doses of greater than 20 mg/kg/day and coadministration of either carbamazepine or topiramate (Yamamoto, Inoue, Matsuda, Takahashi, & Kagawa, 2012). Consultation with a gastroenterologist would be advisable before starting valproate in a patient with known liver or pancreatic disease.

Valproic acid may also cause pancreatitis. Pancreatitis is not dependent on the dose of valproic acid and often occurs when serum valproic acid levels are in the normal range. This is also not a toxicity that tends to develop upon initiation of treatment. Many patients have been tolerating valproic acid for years before they develop pancreatitis (Werlin & Fish, 2006). Fortunately this is an infrequent side effect of valproic acid therapy (Barreto, Tiong, & Williams, 2011).

EFFECTS ON COAGULATION

Valproate therapy can increase the prothrombin time, decrease fibrinogen levels, and reduce the platelet count. These findings, one or more of which may occur in as many as one-third of patients receiving valproate (Rochel & Ehrenthal, 1983), rarely lead to clinically significant bleeding. Children may be particularly susceptible to valproate-induced coagulopathy (Koenig et al., 2008). Among children, the risk of having a clinically significant valproate-induced coagulopathy is estimated to be 4% for those on chronic valproic acid therapy (Gerstner et al., 2006). Valproate-treated patients should have a full coagulation panel including a platelet count, bleeding time, prothrombin time, and partial thromboplastin time prior to undergoing surgery or dental work, and patients with preexisting anticoagulant therapy or bleeding diatheses require especially close monitoring during initiation of valproate therapy.

Valproic acid may also displace warfarin from serum protein binding sites. When valproic acid is initiated after a therapeutic dose of warfarin has been established, it is possible that a rise in free serum warfarin levels may lead to significant bleeding (Yoon, Giraldo, & Wijdicks, 2011).

DRUG INTERACTIONS

In contrast to carbamazepine, which is an enzyme inducer, valproate inhibits liver enzymes that metabolize other drugs (Perucca, 2006). Therefore, it can prolong the half-life of other drugs with mainly hepatic metabolism. This effect has been documented for diazepam and the tricyclics, which have a prolonged half-life in the presence of valproate. In general, the coadministration of long-acting benzodiazepines with valproate may be problematic, both because of the prolongation of benzodiazepine metabolism and because of additive sedation and ataxia. If a benzodiazepine must be given to a patient on valproate, lorazepam is a good choice since it is not likely to interact significantly. The full range of drugs that might have altered metabolism in the presence of valproate is not known, so the possibility of drug accumulation should be considered with other drugs that rely primarily on hepatic metabolism.

Interactions of valproate with other anticonvulsants have been studied extensively and are well established (Bourgeois, 1988). Carbamazepine, phenytoin, and phenobarbital all can lower valproate levels (May & Rambeck, 1985; Perucca, 2006). In contrast, valproate increases levels of phenobarbital by inhibiting its metabolism (Redenbaugh et al., 1980) and raises the free fraction of phenytoin by displacing the drug from protein binding sites. This phenomenon can lead to phenytoin toxicity at apparently "therapeutic" phenytoin levels (Bruno et al., 1980).

Of even greater interest to psychiatrists who might be using valproate together with carbamazepine for treatment-refractory mania is the observation that valproate raises the concentration of the carbamazepine 10,11-epoxide metabolite (Pisani et al., 1986). This metabolite, not usually measured, has additive toxicity with its parent drug carbamazepine (Bourgeois & Wad, 1984). Thus, when valproate is given concurrently, carbamazepine can produce toxicity at apparently therapeutic levels because of an increased level of the 10,11-epoxide carbamazepine metabolite.

Aspirin in usual antipyretic doses can raise both total and free valproate levels because of both metabolic enzyme inhibition and displacement of valproate from protein binding sites. Significant toxicity can result (Goulden et al., 1987). Therefore, alternate agents such as acetaminophen would be preferable for treating fever or minor pain in patients on valproate. A opiate-induced fatality has been reported when a child was given hydrocodone in addition to clarithromycin and valproic acid (Madadi et al., 2010). While clarithromycin likely was responsible for the majority of the opiate's accumulation, valproic acid may have contributed.

Pharmacodynamic interactions have been reported between valproate and neuroleptics, with the development of an encephalopathic syndrome with diffuse EEG slowing (Van Sweden & Van Moffaert, 1985) or increased parkinsonism (Puzynski & Klosiewicz, 1984). Valproate toxicity also has been reported to develop when erythromycin was given to a patient on valproate, leading to abrupt elevations in valproate levels (Redington, Wells, & Petito, 1992). A summary of established drug interactions with valproate is listed in Tables 21.9 and 21.10 (Blackford, Enlow, & Reed, 2013; Cervera et al., 2012; Coulter et al., 2013; De Dios, Fudio, & Lorenzo. 2011; de Jong et al., 2007; Diaz et al., 2008; Gu & Huang, 2009; Haslemo, Olsen, Lunde, & Molden, 2012; Lee, Lee, & Heo, 2002; Lin et al.,

Table 21.9 SELECTED DRUG INTERACTIONS WITH VALPROIC ACID/VALPROATE

MEDICATION	INTERACTIVE EFFECT
Benzodiazepines	Sedative effects and serum levels of benzodiazepines increased by valproate (except lorazepam)
Carbamazepine Phenytoin Phenobarbital	Lower levels of valproate
Phenobarbital	Phenobarbital levels increased by valproate
Phenytoin	Bioavailable phenytoin and carbamazepine increased
Carbamazepine	by valproate by displacing these drugs from their serum protein binding sites
10,11-epoxide metabolite	This metabolite's levels of CBZ increased by valproate of carbamazepine
Tricyclic antidepressants (TCAs)	TCA levels increased by valproate
Chlorpromazine Cimetidine Salicylates Guanfacine	Increased levels of valproate
Anticoagulants (warfarin)	Increased prothrombin times (valproate also inhibits secondary phase of platelet aggregation)

2008; Luszczki, Sawicka, Kozinska, Borowicz, & Czuczwar, 2007; Kim, Hwang, Jeon, & Do, 2012; Michaelis, Ha, Doerr, & Cinatl, 2008; Perucca, 2006; Pisani, 1992; Sandson, Marcucci, Bourke, & Smith-Lamacchia, 2006; Stewart, Nesmith, & Mattox, 2012; Taha, Hammond, & Sheth, 2013; Unterecker, Burger, Hohage, Deckert, & Pfuhlmann, 2013; Unterecker, Reif, et al., 2013; Yoon & Kim, 2013).

More recently, the effect of valproic acid on medications intended for HIV and other infections have been explored. Valproic acid may raise serum levels of agents such as lopinavir and zidovudine but not atazanavir, ritonavir, or efavirenz (Birbeck et al., 2012). On the other hand, meropenem lowers serum valproic acid levels and can result in therapeutic failure of the anticonvulsant. Seizures may result (Coves-Orts et al., 2005). This appears to be a class effect of the carbopenems on valproic acid (Mancl & Gidal, 2009). This pharmacokinetic interaction may be exacerbated by the tendency of penicillins to antagonize the GABA-A receptor. Valproic acid also appears to potentiate the replication of human cytomegalovirus, while undermining the antiviral effects of cidofovir, foscarnet, and ganciclovir (Michaelis, Ha, Doerr, & Cinatl, 2008).

While adverse drug interactions abound with valproic acid, there is also evidence that it may be helpful in settings

Table 21.10 EFFECTS OF VALPROATE ON ANTICONVULSANTS AND OTHER DRUGS: POTENTIALLY IMPORTANT INTERACTIONS

DRUG ADMINISTERED WITH DIVALPROEX SODIUM	INTERACTION
Amitriptyline	Adding valproate to amitriptyline can lead to a marked elevation of serum amitriptyline and nortriptyline levels
Antiviral agents	In vitro valproate inhibits the activity of cidofovir, foscarnet, and ganciclovir against human cytomegalovirus
Aspirin	Can displace valproate from protein binding sites and increase serum free valproate levels several-fold
Carbapenem	Serum levels of valproic acid decreased by 90%
Carbamazepine and	Serum levels of carbamazepine decreased by 17%.
10,11-epoxide of CBZ	Levels of carbamazepine-10,11-epoxide increased by 45% in patients with epilepsy taking valproate and carbamazepine
Cimetidine	Slows the elimination of valproate, and increases serum valproate levels
Cisplatin	Valproate may enhance sensitivity of tumor cells to cisplatin
Clonazepam	Concomitant use with valproic acid may induce absence status in patients with a history of absence-type seizures.
Clozapine	Valproate significantly lowers serum clozapine levels.
Diazepam	Valproate displaced diazepam from plasma albumin-binding sites and inhibited its metabolism. Coadministration of valproate 1500 mg/day to healthy volunteers increased the free fraction of diazepam (10 mg) by 90%; diazepam plasma clearance decreased by 25% and volume of distribution by 20%. Elimination half-life of diazepam did not change.
Doxepin	Valproate can double serum levels of doxepin plus N-doxepin
Ethosuximide	Valproate inhibited ethosuximide metabolism. Administration of a single 500 mg dose of ethosuximide with valproate (800-1600 mg/day) to healthy volunteers increased ethosuximide elimination half-life by 25% and decreased its total clearance by 15%. Serum levels of both drugs should be monitored in patients receiving valproate and ethosuximide, especially with other anticonvulsants.
Ertapenem	May decrease serum valproate concentrations

(continued)

Table 21.10 CONTINUED

DRUG ADMINISTERED WITH DIVALPROEX SODIUM	INTERACTION
Felbamate	Can increase serum valproate levels
Furosemide	Appears pharmacodynamically to enhance the anticonvulsant activity of valproate; significance uncertain
Imatinib	Valproate may restore sensitivity to imatinib in patients with certain tumors
Irinotecan	Serum levels of the active irinotecan metabolite SN-38 may be significantly lowered in the presence of valproate
Isoniazid	Can elevate serum valproate concentrations to toxic levels; valproate may also slow elimination of isoniazid
Lamotrigine	Coadministration of valproate to healthy volunteers increased lamotrigine elimination half-life from 26 to 70 hours. The dose of lamotrigine should be reduced when coadministered with valproate
Lorazepam	Valproate can slow elimination of lorazepam and cause stupor or coma
Meropenem	As is true for other carbapenems, may rapidly lower serum valproate concentrations
Olanzapine	Valproate can significantly lower serum olanzapine levels
Phenobarbital	Valproate inhibited phenobarbital metabolism, resulting in a 50% increase in phenobarbital half-life and a 30% decrease in plasma clearance. The fraction of phenobarbital dose excreted unchanged increased by 50%. There is evidence for severe central nervous system depression, with or without significant elevations of barbiturate or valproate serum concentrations. All patients receiving concomitant barbiturate therapy should be monitored closely for neurologic toxicity.
Primidone	Primidone is metabolized to a barbiturate and may be involved in a similar interaction with valproate.
Phenytoin	Valproate displaced phenytoin from its plasma albumin-binding sites and inhibited its hepatic metabolism. Coadministration of valproate 400 mg twice a day with phenytoin 250 mg to healthy volunteers increased the free fraction of phenytoin by 60%; total plasma clearance and apparent volume of distribution increased by 30%. Both the clearance and the apparent volume of distribution of free phenytoin were reduced by 25%. In patients with epilepsy, breakthrough seizures have occurred with the combination of valproate and phenytoin.

DRUG ADMINISTERED WITH DIVALPROEX SODIUM	INTERACTION
Quetiapine	Valproate may occasionally increase serum quetiapine levels significantly
Rocuronium	Valproate reduces efficacy of rocuronium, possibly through enhanced elimination of rocuronium
Rufinamide	Serum rufinamide levels may rise significantly as the serum level of valproate rises
Temsirolimus	Valproate reduces the maximum tolerated dose of temsirolimus, with mucositis being the dose-limiting toxicity
Tolbutamide	In vitro, the unbound fraction of tolbutamide was increased from 20% to 50% when added to plasma samples from patients treated with valproate. The clinical relevance of this displacement is unknown.
Topiramate	Topiramate may increase risk of hyperammonemia with valproic acid.
Warfarin	The potential exists for valproate to displace warfarin from its plasma albumin-binding sites. The therapeutic relevance of this displacement is unknown; coagulation tests should be monitored if divalproex sodium is initiated in patients taking anticoagulants.
Venlafaxine	Combining valproate with venlafaxine does not affect serum venlafaxine levels, but can significantly elevate serum levels of O-desmethylvenlafaxine
Zidovudine	In HIV-positive patients, the clearance of zidovudine 100 mg every 8 hours decreased by 38% after administration of valproate 250 or 500 mg every 8 hours; zidovudine half-life was unaffected.

Reprinted from Stoudemire & Moran, 1998. Used with permission.

other than the neurologic and psychiatric. For example, valproic acid may offer synergistic pharmacodynamic effects when combined with cytarabine for the treatment of pediatric acute myeloid leukemia. In this case, the ability of valproic acid to inhibit histone deacetylase may be of value (Xie et al., 2010). Similar benefits have been reported for the same disease when valproic acid is added to clofarabine or to gemtuzumab (ten Cate et al., 2007; Xie et al., 2012). Such off-label potential benefits require caution when being considered for use, as valproic acid continues to have its usual toxicities. However, if obliged to choose between one anticonvulsant and another in the management of a child with acute myeloid leukemia, this data may provide an argument for choosing valproic acid.

CLINICAL INTERPRETATION OF BLOOD LEVELS

Therapeutic blood levels for valproate in the treatment of epilepsy usually are reported as 50–125 ng/ml. The work of Bowden, McElroy, Keck, and others suggests that effective blood levels for bipolar disorder are similar and that little clinical effect is seen with blood levels less than 50 ng/ml (Gyulai et al., 2003). Toxic effects begin to occur with levels greater than 100 ng/ml, so the therapeutic index is quite low. Because of individual variations in metabolism of valproate, blood levels should be obtained routinely during upward titration of valproate dosage to assure that the blood level is indeed adequate and to avoid toxicity. Considering the relationship between blood levels and toxicity, it should be noted that toxicity may develop at apparently therapeutic levels when the patient is on multiple drugs, whereas levels above the usual therapeutic range may be tolerated in the context of single-drug therapy.

MANAGEMENT OF VALPROATE OVERDOSE

Because valproate is not toxic to the heart, patients receiving aggressive support have tolerated massive valproate overdoses, including ingestions of greater than 50 gm (Grynnerup et al., 2012). Current recommendations for managing valproate overdose focuses on supportive therapy; although gastric lavage might be considered early in an overdose, it is unlikely to be of much help later in an overdose because absorption of valproate is fairly rapid. Similar arguments hold for activated charcoal (Vannaprasaht, Tiamkao, Sirivongs, & Piyavhatkul, 2009). Hemodialysis is effective in clearing ammonia in cases of hyperammonemic encephalopathy. Coma caused by valproate overdose might be reversible by naloxone because of the latter's effects on GABA receptors (Alberto et al., 1989). Given the low toxicity of naloxone and its empiric use in overdoses of unknown agents, it is an appropriate consideration as adjunctive therapy even when a patient is known to have taken valproate rather than a narcotic (Manoguerra et al., 2008).

LAMOTRIGINE

Lamotrigine at one time inspired great interest for use in bipolar disorder, but in recent years its limitations have become more apparent. Though the drug clearly has value in the management of depression in bipolar disorder, it is not regarded as an effective first-line agent for mania. It is often used, however, as maintenance therapy in bipolar disorder (Tränkner, Sander, & Schönknecht, 2013). Lamotrigine is not recommended as monotherapy in bipolar disorder (Bowden & Singh, 2012).

Lamotrigine causes dizziness in 25% of patients, diplopia (21%), ataxia (16%), blurred vision (11%), somnolence (7%), exacerbation of seizures (3%–4%), and depression or psychosis (in less than 1% of patients). Lamotrigine can cause dose-dependent myoclonic jerks. These have been observed primarily in patients with idiopathic generalized epilepsy

(Crespel et al., 2005). Abrupt withdrawal of lamotrigine may cause a rebound increase in seizure frequency. In the extreme, status epilepticus may occur with secondary rhabdomyolysis and multisystem organ failure (Pellock, 1994; Schmidt & Kramer, 1994; Wang-Tilz et al., 2005). Perhaps the best known of lamotrigine's side effects is the risk of developing a rash. Perhaps 8% of adults receiving lamotrigine will develop a rash. This is usually a benign maculopapular rash that develops within the first 4 months of treatment. About 0.1% of patients develop a serious rash, such as Stevens-Johnson syndrome. Among children and adolescents, the risk of rashes appears to be higher. In one study of 102 such patients, 23 developed a rash within the first 7 weeks of treatment with lamotrigine. One of these cases was of the Stevens-Johnson syndrome (Tak et al., 2012). A black box warning for lamotrigine exists for rashes in children. Other risk factors for a lamotrigine-induced rash include coadministration of valproic acid, rapid upward titration of the medication, and higher doses of the medication.

The metabolism of lamotrigine is induced by acetaminophen, carbamazepine, and phenytoin. Valproic acid raises the serum lamotrigine level. Lamotrigine may pharmacodynamically increase the activity of L-dopa in the treatment of parkinsonism (Meldrum, 1994; Patsalos & Duncan, 1993). Lamotrigine appears to be a substrate of Pgp (Lovrić et al., 2012), and its distribution may be affected by other drugs acting on or though Pgp. Lamotrigine is also a substrate for organic cation transporter 1 (OCT1), which, like Pgp, lines the blood–brain barrier. Inhibitors of OCT1, such as quetiapine, may concentrate lamotrigine in target organs (Dickens et al., 2012).

EPILEPSY AND MENTAL ILLNESS

Diseases of the central nervous system are not only a reason to prescribe psychotropics, but issues that may confound their safe use, as well as side effects in some cases of psychotropic medications. Perhaps nowhere else in psychopharmacology is a side effect more striking—and often less obvious in its etiology—than a seizure. This is problematic for psychiatrists, because anticonvulsants are very often used as mood stabilizers, and various psychotropics may alter the seizure threshold. Excellent reviews exist that detail individual agents and their side effects (Cavanna, Ali, Rickards, & McCorry, 2010; Mula & Monaco, 2009). However, it is useful to have a general concept of the potential problems. There may be three ways in which anticonvulsants alter affect, behavior or cognition, and movement. First, an anticonvulsant's pharmacologic actions may affect some aspect of mentation. An obvious example would be sedation and subsequently impaired cognition, with agents that stimulate the GABA-A receptor. Second, anticonvulsants may interact with seizure disorders in complex ways that secondarily affect mood, behavior, or thought. Finally, if the brain has underlying structural or functional abnormalities manifesting as a seizure disorder, anticonvulsants may generate side effects or further impairments of brain function that present as disturbances of mood, behavior, or cognition.

MOOD DISTURBANCES

Depression is intimately linked to epilepsy. The rate of major depressive disorder among patients with epilepsy may approach 20% (Jones et al., 2005). Having depression is a risk factor for more severe or treatment-refractory epilepsy (Kanner, 2011). Patients with epilepsy are five times more likely than the general population to commit suicide. Among patients with complex partial seizures or temporal lobe epilepsy, this rate may soar to as high as 25 times that of the general population (Kalinin, 2007). Reasons for this may include frontal lobe hypometabolism, folate deficiency, and abnormalities of hippocampal structure and function (Beydoun, Shroff, Beydoun, & Zonderman, 2010; Bromfield et al., 1992; Pineda, Shin, Sankar, & Mazarati, 2010). Decreased levels of neurotrophins such as brain-derived neurotrophic factor may also foster the evolution of both epilepsy and mood disorders (LaFrance, Leaver, Stopa, Papandonatos, & Blum, 2010). Anticonvulsants may affect these rates both positively and negatively. Being seizure-free over a year, for example, is associated with a reduced risk of suicide (Ridsdale, Charlton, Ashworth, Richardson, & Gulliford, 2011). And, of course, anticonvulsants are routinely used in the management of bipolar disorder.

In 1999, Ketter and colleagues proposed the existence of two mechanisms by which anticonvulsants may affect mood, psychomotor activity, and cognition. The first mechanism was stimulation of GABA receptors, which would tend to be "sedating." The second mechanism was interference with glutamatergic activity at NMDA receptors, which would be "activating." Sedating agents were hypothesized to have antimanic potential, while the activating agents would potentially have an antidepressant effect (Ketter, Post, & Theodore, 1999). Some authors rightly argue that the simplicity of Ketter's hypothesis risks failing to explain the actions of complex agents (Roberts et al., 2005). Yet, research supports the idea that NMDA receptor antagonists such as ketamine may exert an antidepressant action (Autry et al., 2011). The role of GABA activity in the modulation of mood is also increasingly appreciated (Möhler, 2012). Interestingly, rapid cessation of anticonvulsants, and the mood and anxiety symptoms that may accompany their withdrawal, are also suggestive of a pharmacological basis of mood effects for anticonvulsants (Ketter et al., 1994).

The FDA issued a warning in 2008 that anticonvulsants may increase the risk of suicide (US Food and Drug Administration, 2008). This finding was based on registration trial studies of 11 anticonvulsants. Patorno and coauthors found that patients taking gabapentin, lamotrigine, oxcarbazepine, and tiagabine, when compared to those taking topiramate, had an increased risk of suicide or related behaviors (Patorno et al., 2010). Limiting these studies is the short duration and the fact that the time shortly after the diagnosis of epilepsy is known to be a time of increased risk for suicide. Arana and colleagues used a database of over 5 million patients, followed on average for 6 years, and found that the use of an anticonvulsant prescribed for epilepsy did not increase the risk of suicide (Arana, Wentworth, Ayuso-Mateos, & Arellano, 2010). Gibbons and colleagues found that the anticonvulsants assessed by the FDA also did not increase the risk of suicide among patients receiving anticonvulsants for bipolar disorder (Gibbons, Hur, Brown, & Mann, 2009). In a study of veterans over the age of 66 years old, VanCott and coauthors (2010) also noted no increase in the risk of suicide. This does not mean that compelling cases of apparent anticonvulsant-induced suicidality do not exist, and that attention to the mental health of persons prescribed anticonvulsants should not be monitored (Mago, Huege, Ahuja, & Kunkel, 2006). In general, though, it does appear that while having a mood disorder, whether as a consequence of epilepsy or independent of epilepsy, increases the risk of suicide, while being prescribed an anticonvulsant does not (Machado et al., 2011).

In treating the patient with epilepsy and depressed mood, several principles should be considered. First, the goal of anticonvulsant therapy should be freedom from seizures. In pursuing this goal, the gradual upward titration of the fewest possible agents appears to be the safest from the standpoint of avoiding psychiatric side effects. The time after initial diagnosis of epilepsy and in the initiation of treatment appears to be the period of greatest risk for suicidal thoughts and behaviors, so attention to the patient's mood and functioning is important. Anticonvulsant side effects that may increase the risk of depression or a change in mentation, such as a drop in serum folate or hyponatremia, should be considered. Finally, if depression does emerge, treating the patient with an antidepressant should be considered. Emerging data suggest that treating depressive states may actually improve the management of epilepsy. There may be many reasons for this. For example, a depressed patient may not comply as reliably with anticonvulsant therapy as a euthymic patient. Also, selective serotonin reuptake inhibitors (SSRIs) may increase the seizure threshold in epilepsy (Kondziella & Asztely, 2009). However, SSRIs may also occasionally cause hyponatremia, as may carbamazepine. Caution is warranted when combining these agents (Jackson & Turkington, 2005). Some agents may lower the seizure threshold, such as bupropion, and may not be suitable as first-line therapies.

DISTURBANCES OF THOUGHT

Anticonvulsants may occasionally provoke psychosis. This may occur in 1%–2% of patients with epilepsy. Gibbs was among the first to connect the treatment of epilepsy with the appearance of psychosis. He reported on the occasional development of psychosis among patients treated for temporal lobe epilepsy (Gibbs, 1951). Ethosuximide is an example of an established agent that continues to be recognized as a cause of psychiatric disturbances (Chien, 2011). For example, in a study of 105 patients taking ethosuximide, psychosis was seen in 3 subjects (Fischer, Korskjaer, & Pedersen, 1965). Landolt observed that psychosis may develop when seizure control is achieved through medication, and in 1953 called this "forced normalization" (Mula & Monaco et al., 2009). Trimble and Reynolds suspected that this resulted from pharmacologic actions associated with over-rapid normalization of the electroencephalogram (Trimble & Reynolds, 1976). Tellenbach broadened the relationship between epilepsy and psychosis—with seizures alternating with psychosis during seizure-free periods—by introducing the concept of "alternative psychosis" (Tellenbach, 1965). Tellenbach's formulation eliminated the need for a normalized EEG as part of the etiology of the psychosis, and hinted at the underlying seizure disorder as participating in what appeared to be a drug side effect. The concept of forced normalization is no longer widely accepted. The rate at which seizures are suppressed is simply not related to the risk of psychosis (Youroukos, Lazopoulou, Michelakou, & Karagianni, 2003). Inhibition of glutamatergic NMDA receptors, either directly or indirectly, as through inhibition of voltage-gated sodium channels, is a more current and useful way of conceptualizing the ability of some anticonvulsants to cause psychosis (Farber, Jiang, X. P., Heinkel, C., & Nemmers, 2002). However, despite decades of research the mechanism of ethosuximide's action—and thus its method of inducing psychosis, mania, and depression—are not known (Greenhill, Morgan, Massey, Woodhall, & Jones, 2012). It should be noted that psychosis with ethosuximide is not common, nor are changes in mentation necessarily more or less common with other anticonvulsants (Glauser et al., 2010).

In general, psychosis with anticonvulsants is rare. It appears to occur most often with temporal lobe epilepsy (Nadkarni et al., 2007). Starting with monotherapy and gradually increasing the dose of an anticonvulsant to the lowest effective dose may help avoid the development of drug-induced psychosis (Mula & Monaco et al., 2009). Difficulty with one anticonvulsant does not necessarily mean that another agent will also cause disturbances of thought, mood, or behavior. If psychosis develops, the clinician must determine whether another disorder such as depression or schizophrenia is also present. Among the disorders that must be considered is postictal confusion, which may result from medication ineffectiveness or noncompliance. At times an antipsychotic may be needed to manage anticonvulsant-induced psychosis. In such cases, agents known to lower the seizure threshold—such as clozapine, haloperidol, and chlorpromazine—should be avoided.

MOVEMENT DISORDERS

A postural tremor is one of the more common findings among patients receiving treatment for epilepsy. Valproic acid and carbamazepine, followed by phenytoin, are the most common offending agents (Zadikoff et al., 2007). When cerebellar dysfunction is the cause, phenytoin is among the most serious offenders. Phenytoin intoxication typically presents with cerebellar findings, including the pancerebellar syndrome (Luef, Chemelli, Birbamer, Aichner, & Bauer, 1994). In their seminal studies of phenytoin for epilepsy, Merritt and Putnam (1938) noted that about 15% of their patients developed cerebellar findings. These findings generally resolve as the free serum concentration of phenytoin falls to normal therapeutic limits. However, as many as 30% of patients receiving chronic phenytoin develop cerebellar atrophy. Duration of treatment appears to be the most important variable (De Marcos, Ghizoni, Kobayashi, Li, &

Cendes, 2003; Ney, Lantos, Barr, & Schaul, 1994). Typically patients present with the pancerebellar syndrome, including hypotonia, ataxia, nystagmus, and dysarthria. Radiography often reveals diffuse cerebellar atrophy. It does appear that acute phenytoin intoxication may also rarely cause cerebellar atrophy and the pancerebellar syndrome (Alioğlu, Sari, Velioğlu, & Oumlzmenoğlu, 2000). In the acute case, immediate discontinuation of phenytoin usually permits complete resolution of symptoms. This is more likely in the absence of cerebellar atrophy. The latter does not always respond to drug cessation, in which case symptoms may persist. The cause of this atrophy remains unknown.

Benzodiazepines may also cause cerebellar findings, including the pancerebellar syndrome. As is true for phenytoin, this occurs in intoxication. Though no longer routinely employed in the treatment of epilepsy, benzodiazepines are still often used to manage seizures, including those of alcohol withdrawal and status epilepticus (Nair, Kalita, & Misra, 2011). When a benzodiazepine is used for alcohol withdrawal, it is crucial to distinguish between the cerebellar findings of Wernicke's encephalopathy and the cerebellar findings that may be caused by the benzodiazepine. This distinction requires a good physical and mental status examination prior to starting treatment with the benzodiazepine. The role of thiamine in preventing the emergence or worsening of Wernicke's encephalopathy has been reviewed elsewhere and should be familiar to all clinicians (Thomson et al., 2002). Benzodiazepines do not cause cerebellar atrophy to the extent seen with phenytoin. But concern about neurodegeneration with benzodiazepines is not new (Poser, Poser, Roscher, & Argyrakis, 1983). Benzodiazepines may inhibit neurogenesis through stimulation of GABA-A receptors and may promote apoptosis through activation of peripheral benzodiazepine receptors (Jordà et al., 2005; Yamaguchi & Mori, 2005). This may be another set of reasons to use caution when considering chronic use of benzodiazepines.

SSRIs are also recognized as an important potential cause of EPS due to antidopaminergic effects. SSRI-induced EPS may consist of parkinsonism, akathisia, dyskinesias, or dystonias. Although EPS may be seen in less than 5% of patients, it must be anticipated as a potential source of worsening among susceptible patients (Stoudemire & Moran, 1998). Such patients include the elderly with subclinical Parkinson's disease. Paroxetine (because of its anticholinergic properties), and sertraline (because it potentiates brain dopaminergic transmission) may be relatively less likely to cause this side effect. Duloxetine frequently has been implicated in cases of SSRI-related EPS. However, EPS may develop with any of the currently available antidepressants. This is not a dose-dependent side effect and can develop at any time during antidepressant treatment (Madhusoodanan, Alexeenko, Sanders, & Brenner, 2010).

Anticonvulsants may at times cause or worsen EPS. This is an important problem, as anticonvulsants are often combined with antipsychotics in the management of bipolar disorder and because after cerebellar dysfunction, EPS may be the most common movement disorder caused by anticonvulsants. In a study of 201 patients with epilepsy receiving a wide variety of agents, Zadikoff and colleagues found that 9, or 4.5%, had EPS (Zadikoff et al., 2007). Valproic acid is likely the worst offender. Jamora and colleagues (2007) found 6 patients among 266 treated with valproic acid who developed parkinsonism. Valproic acid is also implicated in the development of parkinsonism coupled with cognitive decline. In a series of 364 patients, Ristić and colleagues (2006) observed reversible Parkinsonism with cognitive decline in 5. Fortunately this drug-induced syndrome, as well as simple EPS, reverses when valproic acid is stopped. Striking features of this syndrome include cerebrocortical atrophy that reverses upon discontinuation of valproic acid, a normal electroencephalogram, and a normal ammonia level (Evans, Shinar, & Yaari, 2011; Guerrini, Belmonte, Canapicchi, Casalini, & Perucca, 1998). Although EPS and EPS with cognitive impairment may arise shortly after initiation of treatment with valproic acid, in some cases patients tolerate the medication with good result for years and then develop these reversible side effects (Masmoudi, Gras-Champel, Masson, & Andréjak, 2006).

Ethosuximide may worsen the resting tremor of patients with Parkinson's disease and patients with neuroleptic-induced Parkinsonism (Pourcher, Gomez-Mancilla, & Bédard, 1992). A similar result can be seen with levetiracetam (Lyons et al., 2006). Other agents reported to cause or worsen extrapyramidal symptoms include carbamazepine, gabapentin, lamotrigine, phenytoin, vigabatrin, and zonisamide (Ertan et al., 2006; Raju, Walker, & Lee, 2007; Santens, Claeys, Vonck, & Boon, 2007; Zadikoff et al., 2007). Dystonias and tics are reported as rare side effects of a variety of anticonvulsants. These rarer examples of anticonvulsant-induced extrapyramidal dysfunction remind the clinician of the need to be vigilant when prescribing psychoactive medications, especially to patients whose brain structure or function may not be normal. In such cases a cautious reduction in the dose of the suspected offending agent is important. Another anticonvulsant can be substituted with equal benefit and less side effects in many cases.

Gabapentin may occasionally cause reversible myoclonus (Ege et al., 2008). This is more likely when toxic levels are reached, as may occur in renal disease (Zhang, Glenn, Bell, & O'Donovan, 2005). Other agents, including pregabalin and topiramate, may also rarely cause myoclonus (Healy, Ingle, G. T., & Brown, 2009; Miller, Prost, Bookstaver, & Gaines, 2010).

ACUTE CONFUSIONAL STATES

There are many ways in which anticonvulsants can provoke acute confusion. Valproic acid for example, commonly elevates serum ammonia levels. Serum ammonia levels may on average double after starting valproic acid. In most cases the rise in serum ammonia is not accompanied by changes in mentation (Chicharro et al., 2007). Yet, on occasion valproic acid causes hyperammonemic encephalopathy. This can be an acute and devastating example of an anticonvulsant-induced alteration in mentation. Treatments include lactulose, carnitine, and hemodialysis, and stopping valproic acid (Lheureux & Hanson, 2009; Thanacoody, 2009).

When a patient with a psychiatric disorder that may be treated with an anticonvulsant, (such as bipolar disorder) also has a seizure disorder, the anticonvulsant may worsen the seizure disorder. Table 21.11 lists the reported adverse effects of anticonvulsants on seizure disorders (Chiron & Dulac, 2011; Genton & McMenamin, 1998; Mantoan & Walker, 2011; Sazgar & Bourgeois, 2005). If a patient appears to be at risk for worsening of a seizure disorder, consultation with a neurologist should precede institution of the anticonvulsant if possible. Note that the cause of seizure worsening by anticonvulsants may be the result of either anticonvulsant withdrawal when tolerance has developed, anticonvulsant intoxication, or an adverse effect of an anticonvulsant on particular neurons at therapeutic drug levels (Perucca et al., 1998; Perruca, 2006). When any of these causes can be managed, then the patient may be able to remain on the anticonvulsant without harm.

MONOAMINE OXIDASE INHIBITORS

Despite the introduction of many new psychotropics, MAOIs remain an important alternative for several conditions, including atypical or tricyclic-refractory depression, panic disorder/agoraphobia, social phobia, and for some patients with obsessive compulsive disorder and posttraumatic stress disorder. Some patients have strikingly positive therapeutic responses to MAOIs with poor response to all other available medications. When such patients have a significant concurrent medical illness, situations arise in which risks and benefits must be balanced, and clinical strategies must be employed to contain risks that are not completely avoidable. This section deals with several such issues, including (1) general anesthesia for patients on MAOIs, (2) drug interactions, (3) dietary precautions, and (4) management of medically important side effects.

Before discussing these issues, we review some important differences among the MAOIs most commonly prescribed in the United States: phenelzine (Nardil), tranylcypromine (Parnate), and selegiline (Eldepryl) and selegiline transdermal system (Emsam). Phenelzine, tranylcypromine, and transdermal selegiline are FDA approved for psychiatric indications. Oral selegiline is approved for the treatment of Parkinson's disease but can be an effective antidepressant when used at higher doses sufficient to produce nonselective (MAO$_A$ plus MAO$_B$ isoenzyme) MAO inhibition (Mann et al., 1989). Moclobemide, a selective reversible MAO$_A$ inhibitor with less chance of tyramine reactions, is not currently available in the United States (available in Canada). It is also important to note the MAOI isocarboxazide is also available in the US market. Linezolid (Zyvox) is marketed as an antibiotic, but it too is an MAOI. Linezolid reversibly and competitively inhibits MAO$_A$.

The first main difference among the three drugs is that phenelzine and tranylcypromine are nonselective MAOIs (inhibiting both MAO$_A$ and MAO$_B$), whereas selegiline is a selective inhibitor of MAO$_B$ at doses up to approximately 20 mg/day. When selegiline is used at this lower,

Table 21.11 SEIZURE DISORDERS AND POTENTIAL WORSENING BY ANTICONVULSANTS

DRUG	SEIZURE DISORDER	EFFECT OF ADDING DRUG
Barbiturates	Absence	Aggravation
		Worsen Dravet syndrome
Benzodiazepines	Lennox-Gastaut syndrome	Serial tonic seizures
Carbamazepine	Benign "Rolandic" epilepsy	Drop attacks
	Childhood absence	Increases in absences
	Juvenile myoclonus epilepsy	Increases episodes of myoclonus
	Progressive myoclonus epilepsy	Increases episodes of myoclonus
		Worsens Dravet syndrome
	Absence	Aggravation
Gabapentin	Absence (any type)	Increases in absences
Lamotrigine	Severe myoclonic epilepsy	Aggravation
		Worsens Dravet syndrome
Oxcarbazepine	Juvenile myoclonus epilepsy	Increases episodes of myoclonus
Idiopathic generalized epilepsy		Increase in absences and myoclonus
Phenobarbital (large doses)	Childhood absence	Increases in absence
Phenytoin	Childhood absence	No efficacy; aggravation
	Other generalized epilepsies	No efficacy; aggravation
	Progressive myoclonus epilepsy	Long-term aggravation
	Juvenile myoclonus epilepsy	Increases episodes of myoclonus
Pregabalin	Juvenile myoclonus epilepsy	Increases episodes of myoclonus
Tiagabine	Nonconvulsive status epilepticus	Aggravation
	Juvenile myoclonus epilepsy	Increases episodes of myoclonus
Vigabatrin	Childhood absence	Increases in absences
	Juvenile myoclonus epilepsy	Increases episodes of myoclonus
	Myoclonic epilepsy	Increases in episodes of myoclonus

antiparkinson dose, no dietary restrictions or drug interaction precautions are necessary. At higher doses, although precautions may be necessary, tyramine sensitivity may be less than with tranylcypromine at a comparable dose (Bieck & Antonin, 1989; Wimbiscus, Kostenko, & Malone, 2010). When used as a transdermal patch, 6 mg per day is effective for the treatment of depression. Note that the bioavailability of transdermal selegiline is about 75%, versus 4% to 5% for oral selegiline (Wimbiscus et al., 2010). While some authors suggest that no dosage adjustment is required for selegiline in the presence of hepatic or renal impairment, or other factors routinely considered such as age, others note that this may not be true for all patients. For example, Nagler and colleagues (2012) argue for a dosage reduction if selegiline is given to patients with stage 3–5 chronic kidney disease.

Moclobemide is the reversible inhibitor of MAO_A. Its main potential advantage in the medically ill is that it typically does not cause weight gain like the classic $MAO_{A/B}$ inhibitors. It is also much less likely to cause tyramine reactions at normal dose levels than nonselective $MAO_{A/B}$ inhibitors such as phenelzine. Since MAO_A is responsible for the degradation of both serotonin and noradrenaline, it is at least of theoretical concern when a patient with severe endothelial disease such as hypertension is started on an inhibitor of MAO_A. Such patients may be at risk for the development of catecholaminergic or serotonergic toxicity if the MAO_A inhibitor is coadministered with a noradrenergic or serotonergic agent, such as a stimulating decongestant or an SSRI.

Moclobemide causes some dose-related excessive stimulation in roughly 3% of patients leading to agitation or insomnia; more severe side effects are rare. Seizures may occur in about 1.5% of patients; these are primarily patients who have preexisting seizure disorders. Severe hypertensive reactions have been noted, usually in conjunction with tyramine ingestion, in about 0.2% of patients, but tyramine reactions are much less likely than those from combined $MAO_{A/B}$ inhibitors. Hepatotoxicity is rare but may first manifest as an encephalopathy (Brown & Stoudemire, 1998). Cardiovascular side effects are rare and consist primarily of tachycardia. Occasional reports appear of ECG abnormalities, without a consistent pattern (Chen & Ruch, 1993).

The possibility of inducing the serotonin syndrome during treatment with moclobemide is important to consider for two reasons. First, it underscores a predictable pathophysiologic reaction to moclobemide for some patients. Second, although rare, the serotonin syndrome is occasionally fatal.

Drug interactions are potentially an important cause of toxicity with moclobemide. The most obvious are noted above, such as the ingestion of a stimulant, (e.g., phenylpropanolamine) with moclobemide; other important pharmacodynamic interactions include the coingestion of opiates such as morphine or dextropropoxyphene with moclobemide. In such cases, excessive stimulation of the central nervous system may occur. Cimetidine may prolong the normal 1-hour to 3-hour half-life of moclobemide by 100% (Callingham, 1993).

GENERAL GUIDELINES FOR ANESTHETIC MANAGEMENT OF PATIENTS ON MAO INHIBITORS

Patients taking MAOIs may safely have surgery, with some medication-specific cautions. Isocarboxazide, phenelzine, and tranylcypromine irreversibly inhibit monoamine oxidases. Because of this, normal monoamine oxidase activity typically takes weeks to regenerate, well after these MAOIs have been eliminated from the body. If an MAOI must be stopped prior to an operation or any other major procedure, or even a medication change, the clinician should assume the presence of residual monoamine oxidase inhibition for 2 weeks after discontinuation of the MAOI (Fiedorowicz & Swartz, 2004). Since untreated depression warrants as much caution as most potential drug side effects and interactions, discontinuation of an MAOI is not a routine recommendation prior to surgery.

1. Meperidine is absolutely contraindicated for postoperative analgesia in patients on MAOIs. Its use in such patients can produce hypertension, hyperthermia, and death. The problem is relatively specific to meperidine. Dextromethorphan, tramadol, and possibly fentanyl have been associated with deaths in combination with MAOIs. This is likely due to a hyperserotonergic state, such as the serotonin syndrome. Morphine and its analogues, such as codeine, have long been given without complications to patients on MAOIs (Gillman, 2005). Nonetheless, because of potential interactions, initial dosage of narcotic analgesics should be conservative. The availability of potent NSAIDs such as ketorolac, with analgesic potencies approaching that of narcotics, is an option for patients on MAO inhibitors.

2. Because it has an indirect sympathomimetic effect, curare should be avoided in MAOI-treated patients (Anonymous, 2003; Stack, Rogers, & Linter, 1988). If succinylcholine is given to a patient on phenelzine, monitoring of neuromuscular function and adequacy of respiration must be particularly careful because phenelzine can reduce pseudocholinesterase levels in some patients (Bodley, Halwax, & Potts, 1969).

3. If hypotension develops intraoperatively, initial correction should be attempted through volume expansion. If this is inadequate, then direct sympathomimetics such as norepinephrine are the preferred therapy. The clinician should bear in mind that the pressor response to the sympathomimetic may be amplified by residual MAOI activity (Dawson, Earnshaw, & Graham, 1995). Indirect-acting sympathomimetics such as metaraminol should be avoided, because they can produce hypertensive crises (Janowsky & Janowsky, 1985).

4. Previously, because of concerns about blood pressure stability, it was recommended that patients receiving prolonged anesthesia for major surgery should be monitored with an indwelling arterial catheter (Sides, 1987; Wong, 1986). While drug–drug interactions do require careful monitoring, it appears that use of either moclobemide or tranylcypromine is safe before surgery, that patients taking these agents have fewer episodes of intraoperative hypotension than patients not taking MAOIs, and that they have the same rate of bradycardia, tachycardia, and hypertension as do patients not taking MAOIs (van Haelst et al., 2012).

5. If significant hypertension develops during surgery, it can be managed with intravenous phentolamine or nitroprusside (Tuncel & Ram, 2003).

6. Because of the potential for various drug interactions, particular care must be taken to assure that all staff caring for surgical patients are aware of the patient's MAOI therapy and its implications. Prescribing or drug administration errors sometimes take place in the course of a patient's journey from operating room to recovery room to intensive care to surgical floor. At each point along the way, MAOI-related safety issues should be reinforced. As a practical precaution, a sticker stating that the patient is "allergic to Demerol (meperidine)" can be placed on the patient's chart.

DRUG INTERACTIONS WITH MAO INHIBITORS

The MAOIs are associated with a wide range of drug interactions, many of which are displayed in Table 21.12 (Barkhuizen, Petzer, & Petzer, 2013; Brown &Stoudemire, 1998; Huang & Gortney, 2006). These can be grouped into three general classes: interactions with indirect-acting sympathomimetics; interactions with serotonin drugs; and pharmacodynamic potentiation of other drugs' CNS side effects.

Selegiline is metabolized to its metabolites by CyP4502B6, 2A6, and 3A4 (Benetton et al., 2007). However, it does not appear to alter the disposition of drugs metabolized through cytochromes P450, including alprazolam, olanzapine, and risperidone (Azzaro, Ziemniak, Kemper, Campbell, & VanDenBerg, 2007). Moclobemide is a substrate of CyP450 2C19, and inhibits the activity of this enzyme and of 1A2 and 2D6. Little is known about the influence of tranylcypromine, phenelzine, or isocarboxazide on hepatic drug metabolism. Some data suggest that (like moclobemide) phenelzine and tranylcypromine may inhibit their own metabolism (Polasek et al., 2006).

When an indirect-acting sympathomimetic agent is given, excessive amounts of catecholamines can be released, leading to a hypertensive crisis. Indirect-acting sympathomimetics include cocaine, amphetamines, methylphenidate, ephedrine, pseudo-ephedrine, and phenylpropanolamine. As a practical point, the most frequent occasion for such reactions is patients' use of over-the-counter (OTC) cold remedies that include a sympathomimetic decongestant. The problem is complicated by the fact that many OTC drugs have multiple formulations with similar sounding names, some of which are safe and others of which are not.

Although not strictly sympathomimetics, L-dopa and carbidopa-levodopa (Sinemet) can also produce hypertensive reactions in combination with MAOIs. Direct-acting

Table 21.12 REPORTED DRUG INTERACTIONS WITH MONOAMINE OXIDASE INHIBITORS

MEDICATION	INTERACTIVE EFFECT
Meperidine	Fatal reaction
L-dopa	Elevation of blood pressure
Methyldopa, dopamine	
Buspirone, guanethidine	
Cyclic antidepressants	
Cyclobenzaprine	
Direct-acting sympathomimetics	Elevation of blood pressure
Epinephrine	
Norepinephrine	
Isoproterenol	
Methoxamine	
Indirect-acting sympathomimetics	Severe hypertension
Cocaine; amphetamines	
Tyramine	
Methylphenidate	
Phenethylamine;	
Metaraminol	
Ephedrine;	
Phenylpropanolamine	
Direct- and indirect-acting sympathomimetics	Extreme hypertension
Pseudoephedrine	
Metaraminol	
Phenylephrine	
Serotonergic agents	"Serotonin syndrome" (ataxia, nystagmus, confusion, fever, tremor)
SSRIs	
Tryptophan	
Sumatriptan	
Zolmitriptan	
Caffeine	Mild increase in blood pressure
Theophylline	
Aminophylline	
Hypoglycemic agents	Lowers blood glucose further
Anticoagulants	Prolonged PT
Succinylcholine	Phenelzine prolongs action
Diuretics	Increased hypotensive effect
Propranolol	
Prazosin	
Calcium channel blockers	
Other monoamine oxidase inhibitors	

MEDICATION	INTERACTIVE EFFECT
Nonselective	
Caffeine	
Linezolid	
Phenformin	
MAO-A	
Beta blockers	
Oxprenolol	
Pindolol	
Propranolol	
Local Anesthetics	
Dibucaine	
Lidocaine	
Prilocaine	
Procainamide	
Procaine	
Tetracaine	
Pentamidine	
MAO-B	
Antidepressants	
Amitriptyline	
Desipramine	
Doxepin	
Imipramine	
Antipsychotics	
Chlorpromazine	

antiparkinson drugs such as bromocriptine would presumably be safer if a patient with Parkinson's disease required MAOI therapy at antidepressant doses. The use of selegiline in antiparkinson doses of 10 mg/day is, of course, compatible with L-dopa or carbidopa-levodopa.

Direct-acting sympathomimetics can be used if necessary—for example, as bronchodilators for the treatment of asthma. Inhalers are safer than systemic drugs. Furthermore, a challenge with the inhaled drug, with blood pressure determination before and after, provides even greater security that a particular drug is safe in the face of MAOI therapy.

The second major type of drug interaction with MAOIs concerns their combination with serotonin drugs such as the SSRIs or buspirone. The interaction with meperidine may have a similar mechanism, since meperidine blocks serotonin reuptake (Guo et al., 2009).

Clinical symptoms of the "serotonin syndrome" include myoclonus, ataxia, fever, and confusion. Neuromuscular symptoms range from tremor to lead-pipe rigidity. Neurologic examination shows hyperreflexia, sometimes with clonus; nystagmus; altered mental status; and, frequently, rigidity. Blood pressure may be either normal or elevated, but hypertension, when it occurs, usually is not extreme. Fever usually is present, and at times there is hyperthermia. However, profuse sweating, so common in neuroleptic malignant syndrome, is not part of the serotonin syndrome. The syndrome is best prevented by avoiding the addition of serotonin drugs when patients are on MAO inhibitors. Furthermore, MAO inhibitors should be avoided for at least 5 weeks following discontinuation of fluoxetine because of the very long half-life of the latter drug and its active metabolite, norfluoxetine. If the safety of an MAOI is in question in a patient who has recently taken fluoxetine, a fluoxetine blood level should be obtained. Detectable levels of fluoxetine or norfluoxetine are a contraindication to starting MAO inhibitors. It is not known, but very unlikely, that a shorter SSRI "washout" period would be safe for short-acting SSRIs like sertraline.

Treatment begins with instituting supportive measures and discontinuing the drugs that promote the syndrome. Specific therapy has been reported anecdotally with a number of drugs with serotonin-blocking effects, including chlorpromazine and cyproheptadine (Gillman, 2005, see also Chapter 23).

The third type of drug interaction concerns pharmacodynamic potentiation of other drugs' CNS effects. For example, MAOIs potentiate the anticholinergic effects of atropine (Janowsky & Janowsky, 1985). Central nervous system depressant effects of narcotics, benzodiazepines, and barbiturates can be greater in patients taking MAOIs, as can sedative side effects of nonsteroidal antiinflammatory drugs. The mechanism of these pharmacodynamic interactions is not well understood, but their prevalence argues for particular conservatism in dosage of anticholinergics and CNS depressant drugs in MAOI-treated patients.

MAO INHIBITORS AND FOOD INTERACTIONS

The interaction of MAO inhibitors with tyramine-containing foods remains the primary deterrent to their wider use by psychiatrists, and may be a major reason for their nonuse by nonpsychiatric physicians. Moreover, burdensome dietary restrictions often are a reason that patients are reluctant to take MAOIs even when they are clinically helpful. Patients with concurrent medical diseases such as diabetes or renal failure that impose additional dietary restrictions may be particularly reluctant to restrict their diets further. For the otherwise healthy patient, the MAOIs impose only modest dietary restrictions. Box 21.3 outlines the amount of cheese—in particular cheddar cheese, which is typically rich in tyramine—that would be too much. Note that the amount of tyramine required to precipitate a pressor response, defined as a rise in the systolic blood pressure by 30 mmHg, is 2–3 times greater in the fed state compared to the fasting state (EMSAM, 2005; Wimbiscus et al., 2010).

Box 21.3 THE CHEESE REACTION: HOW MUCH IS TOO MUCH?

To Raise the Systolic Blood Pressure by 30 mmHg:

(1) a person not taking an MAOI would need to consume, when fasting, 500 mg of tyramine, or 2 pounds of cheddar cheese consumed in 30 minutes;

(2) for a patient on a 6 mg selegiline patch, again, 2 pounds of cheddar cheese;

(3) for a patient on tranylcypromine, 10 mg of tyramine if fasting, or 25 mg if taken with food, or about an ounce of cheddar cheese.

However, many patients' and physicians' problems with MAOI diets are both unnecessary and avoidable. Cheese, the food most often implicated in hypertensive reactions, varies enormously in its tyramine content. Cream cheese and cottage cheese are free from tyramine. The tyramine content of cheddar cheeses in a large sample varied from 0 to 1.4 mg/g of cheese—an astonishing number when one considers that the average threshold for 30 mmHg blood pressure elevation with tranylcypromine is only 10 mg of tyramine (EMSAM, 2005). Patients therefore should be told that the lack of a hypertensive reaction on one occasion does not imply that a particular aged cheese is safe. And, in general, one should assume that a cheese is aged if there is any uncertainty.

In the past, psychiatrists frequently confronted hospital diets or published recommendations that advocated stringent food restrictions for MAO inhibitors that are not supported by a critical review of the literature. Since spontaneous hypertensive reactions do occur with MAOIs, multiple reports of a particular food–drug interaction, along with chemical analyses or challenge studies, are needed to establish conclusively that a particular food is risky. We recommend explaining these issues to patients, encouraging them to be extremely scrupulous about high-risk foods, and less concerned about foods less definitely associated with hypertensive reactions. The list of foods that should absolutely be avoided is fairly short. Box 21.4 lists these (Gardner et al., 1996).

MANAGEMENT OF SIDE EFFECTS

Side effects of traditional A and B enzyme MAOIs that are particularly problematic in medically ill patients include orthostatic hypotension, hypertensive episodes, weight gain, and insomnia. An additional but infrequent side effect is potentiation of insulin-induced hypoglycemia by MAOIs in diabetic patients (Bodnar, Starr, & Halter, 2011; Cooper & Ashcroft, 1966; McIntyre, Soczynska, Konarski, & Kennedy, 2006). Active management of these side effects can enable patients who benefit from MAOI therapy to continue the treatment.

Orthostatic hypotension may occur with any of the MAOIs. Its initial management involves making sure the patient is safe and, for example, knows to stand slowly and be cautious of falling, and also clarifying whether the MAOI is indeed responsible. Orthostatic hypotension is approached initially by reducing or eliminating diuretics, vasodilators, and other medications that may lower blood pressure. Adequate hydration is assured, and salt intake is liberalized if it has been restricted. If these measures are insufficient, administration of fludrocortisone (Florinef) 0.1 mg/day may be helpful, at least for the short term (Simonson, 1964). Fludrocortisone should be used with caution in patients with congestive heart failure (Stumpf & Mitrzyk, 1994). In some cases it may be necessary to discontinue the MAOI.

Episodes of hypertension, whether spontaneous or attributable to food–drug or drug–drug interactions, pose particular risks in patients with cerebral vascular disease and cardiovascular disease, and in patients on anticoagulants. In these patients especially we recommend training patients to recognize the early signs of a hypertensive reaction, such as headache and flushing, and to carry with them an oral hypotensive medication. Patients are asked to seek medical attention urgently should they develop an episode, but immediate use of an oral hypotensive agent relieves some of the risk and discomfort they would otherwise face before getting medical attention. Among the first-line agents is oral nifedipine. The initial recommended dose is 20 mg. The medication should be swallowed, not bitten or otherwise taken sublingually, in order to avoid uncontrolled hypotension (van den Born et al., 2011). If symptoms do not resolve within 15 minutes for nifedipine, a second dose can be taken while the patient is in transit to an emergency room.

Insomnia is a common side effect of MAOIs that can be particularly problematic for patients with other medical conditions, such as arthritic pain, that keep them awake at night. In such patients the first step in managing insomnia is to identify and optimally treat medical problems that can interfere with sleep. If this is insufficient, options include a short-acting benzodiazepine at bedtime or trazodone 25–50 mg every four hours (Jacobsen, 1990). At times the atypical antipsychotics in low dose, such as quetiapine 50 mg at bedtime, can help if standard options fail to treat MAOI-related insomnia (Sokolski & Brown, 2006).

Weight gain in patients on MAOIs is particularly a problem for those with diabetes or hyperlipidemia. In such patients, tranylcypromine usually is the MAOI of choice because it is less likely to cause weight gain than phenelzine. If available, moclobemide might be the best choice in such a situation. If a patient must be switched to tranylcypromine from another MAOI, there must be a 2-week drug-free interval to avoid a hypertensive reaction. If weight gain persists on tranylcypromine, caloric restriction and exercise can be advised, but these prescriptions often are not successful.

Autonomic side effects such as urinary retention and impotence may be more likely in patients with preexisting autonomic problems, such as those with diabetes. It is rational to attempt management of these side effects with bethanechol, a cholinergic agonist drug that does not cross the blood–brain barrier. Initial dosage should be conservative—5 mg three or four times daily; the dose can be increased if tolerated and helpful. The main side effect is nausea.

Finally, the possibility that MAOIs may influence patients' response to insulin leads us to recommend that when insulin-dependent diabetics are started on MAOIs, blood sugar should be checked with a glucometer four times a day over the first 72 hours of treatment and for a similar period after each dosage increase.

PSYCHOSTIMULANTS

Psychostimulants offer some patients distinct advantages over traditional antidepressants. Unlike CyADs, psychostimulants produce an improvement in mood that, if it occurs, is rapid, usually within the first 24 to 48 hours of treatment. In addition, the psychostimulants are relatively well tolerated even in most older, medically ill patients. Patients with recent myocardial infarctions, congestive heart failure, or ventricular arrhythmias, and patients who were taking an MAOI within the last 2 weeks, are at risk for complications with psychostimulants (Berlim & Turecki, 2007). However, the possibilities of rebound depression after cessation of the drugs, habituation, abuse, and precipitation of paranoid reactions argue against routine usage of psychostimulants to treat major depression except in patients whose medical illness contraindicates use of standard antidepressants. Drug interactions with psychostimulants are listed in Table 21.9. Commonly used psychostimulants and their usual daily doses include methylphenidate (10–60 mg/day, usually divided in twice-daily doses), dextroamphetamine (10–40 mg/day divided in twice-daily doses), atomoxetine (40–120 mg/day divided in twice-daily doses), and pramipexole (0.25 to 1 mg three times daily).

Bupropion, with its CNS stimulant properties, might be considered as a long-term antidepressant for patients who respond well to dextroamphetamine or methylphenidate. Psychostimulants, however, remain valuable and essential treatment modalities for psychiatrists working with the medically ill.

Although little debate continues as to the short-term efficacy of psychostimulants in the treatment of depression among the medically ill, the use of methylphenidate among patients with a variety of neurological injuries has helped to clarify how methylphenidate and dextroamphetamine work and how they may be most effectively employed. Galynker et al. (1997) studied the effects of methylphenidate on negative symptoms (typically including social withdrawal, flattened affect, anhedonia), other measures of depression, and cognition. Negative symptoms and cognition both improved, whereas other measures of depression did not. This is consistent with many other studies in which methylphenidate and dextroamphetamine have been shown to improve psychomotor performance. In the severely ill patient, such as poststroke patients, linking the use of psychostimulants to rehabilitation such as physical therapy can have a synergistically beneficial effect (Delbari, Salman-Roghani, & Lokk, 2011; Max, Richards, & Hamdan-Allen, 1995; Van Dyck et al., 1997; Walker-Batson et al., 1995; Whyte et al., 1997). Psychostimulants can both hasten stroke therapy and improve the outcome (Grade et al., 1998).

Masand, Pickett, and Murray (1991) performed a retrospective, uncontrolled review of 4740 consecutive hospital consultations in patients with secondary depression (i.e., the onset of the depression coincided with or came after their medical illness). Of the 198 patients treated with psychostimulants (primarily dextroamphetamine), 82% experienced some improvement and 70% were retrospectively rated as markedly improved. Side effects encountered included confusion and agitation (4 patients), hypomania (3 patients), paranoid delusions (3 patients), elevated blood pressure and sinus tachycardia (3 patients each), and 1 case of atrial fibrillation. In another retrospective chart review study of 29 patients by Rosenberg, Ahmed, and Hurwitz (1991), although moderate or marked improvement was seen in 55% of the patients, significant side effects were noted in 28%, including agitation, tachycardia, and visual hallucinations. The presence of delirium predicted nonresponse.

Masand, Murray, and Pickett (1991) noted improvement in 82% of 17 poststroke patients studied retrospectively with equal efficacy with dextroamphetamine and methylphenidate. Improvement typically was rapid, usually within the first 2 days of treatment. Lingam and associates (1988) retrospectively studied the records of 25 patients with poststroke depression who were treated with methylphenidate at dosages of at least 20 mg/day for 5 consecutive days. These authors found "complete" recovery from depression in 52% of the patients. In a prospective study of another medically ill population, depressed cancer patients, Fernandez et al. (1987) treated 30 patients (7 men and 23 women) at an initial dose of 10 mg of methylphenidate three times daily, with 23 showing marked or moderate improvement. This study included 11 patients who were treated for 1 year at low doses of 5–10 mg/day without evidence of tolerance or abuse. One patient with dementia became more agitated and confused on the psychostimulant.

A subgroup of medically ill patients who may not fare well under psychostimulant treatment includes those infected with HIV or with hepatitis C virus. Studies with methamphetamine indicate that this particular amphetamine may both undermine the immune response to these viruses and enhance the neurotoxicity of HIV (Cadet & Krasnova, 2007; Ferris, Mactutus, & Booze, 2008; Ye et al., 2008). This finding may not apply to all viruses nor even to all psychostimulants. For example, methamphetamine appears to inhibit the replication of the influenza A virus (Chen, Wu, & Chen, 2012).

Although use of psychostimulants in the treatment of primary depression in physically healthy patients remains controversial, their use in medically ill patients—at least for short periods—is well accepted. It is important to remember, however, that there is no formal FDA approval for using these medicines as antidepressants.

The two most commonly used psychostimulants are methylphenidate and dextroamphetamine.

Dextroamphetamine is approximately twice as potent as methylphenidate, with typical therapeutic dosages of 10–20 mg/day for dextroamphetamine versus 20–40 mg/day for methylphenidate (Jenike, 1985). Higher doses may safely be used as need indicates (Berlim & Turecki, 2007). Dextroamphetamine excretion is influenced by urinary pH, and when urine is acidic, dextroamphetamine is excreted more rapidly and largely unchanged in the urine (Thus, ascorbic acid or cranberry juice could be used in the ambulatory treatment of mild dextroamphetamine toxicity.). Its plasma half-life is approximately 12 hours (Chiarello & Cole, 1987) as opposed to the 2-hour average half-life of methylphenidate, which is quickly metabolized by the liver to ritalinic acid, a metabolite with little CNS activity (Goff, 1986). Long-acting forms of dextroamphetamine and methylphenidate are available.

Adderall is a new stimulant approved for the treatment of attention deficit disorder with hyperactivity and for narcolepsy. It is a combination of mixed salts of amphetamine product consisting of dextroamphetamine sulfate, dextroamphetamine saccharate, amphetamine sulfate, and amphetamine aspartate. To our knowledge, it has not yet been used for depression in the medically ill.

In general, the psychostimulants are safe for short-term use. Occasional reports of important side effects encourage vigilance in monitoring patients' responses. Rarely, a switch into mania may be provoked by a psychostimulant (Parker & Brotchie, 2010). Among children taking psychostimulants for attention deficit hyperactivity disorder, over 90% of cases of psychostimulant-induced mania or psychosis occur in children with no history of either. Hallucinations are often visual or tactile (Mosholder, Gelperin, Hammad, Phelan, & Johann-Liang, 2009). Pramipexole has been associated with hypersexuality and impulse-control disorders such as pathological gambling among patients taking the medication for Parkinson's disease (Weintraub et al., 2010). For those patients with psychostimulant intoxication as the cause of their altered mentation, discontinuation of the offending agent and supportive care are usually sufficient. In those few patients in whom a diathesis has been activated—for example, those patients whose latent bipolar disorder is unmasked by a psychostimulant—more prolonged management may be required. In some cases, despite significant side effects it is not possible to eliminate some form of stimulant altogether. An example is Parkinson's disease, in which dopamine agonist therapy is often complicated by psychiatric side effects. In these cases, cautious selection of another agent to control side effects may be needed. Dose reductions of the psychostimulant, as well as lower potency antipsychotics such as clozapine and quetiapine, have been used with success in such cases (Georgiev et al., 2010; Rotondo, Bosco, Plastino, Consoli, & Bosco, 2010).

CLINICAL PEARLS

- Because many patients with orthostatic hypotension lack subjective symptoms of orthostasis, the clinician should assess postural signs when the mechanism of a drug predicts risk, such as with prescription of a TCA (Lanier et al., 2011).

- Antidepressant use travels with an increased risk of having a hip fracture among elderly patients, both for TCAs and SSRIs (Oderda et al., 2012).

- Citalopram will raise the level of the beta blocker metoprolol and possibly other beta blockers as well. No clinically significant interactions have been noted with digoxin, lithium, warfarin, or carbamazepine. Omeprazole, which inhibits CyP450-2C19, might elevate citalopram levels.

- The half-life of escitalopram is roughly doubled in the elderly. Significant liver disease slows the metabolism of escitalopram, and the dosage should be halved.

- Both citalopram and escitalopram can prolong the QT interval.

- We recommend adhering to the following principles in the use of neuroleptics in the medically ill:

  - Whenever possible, identify and treat the underlying illness rather than treating superficial symptoms. For example, treat the etiology of a patient's delirium or cognitive impairment instead of merely controlling secondary symptoms of agitation or hallucinations.
  - Avoid polypharmacy that is not scientifically based on the results of randomized, controlled, clinical trials and be cognizant of the potential for drug interactions and of pharmacokinetic and pharmacodynamic reasons for increased risks of adverse effects. For example, decreased albumin in malnourished patients implies the increased bioavailability of free fractions of protein-bound drugs and therefore more potent effects per milligram dosage (more unbound drug is available to act on receptor sites).
  - Identify specific target symptoms and carefully evaluate the treatment response objectively. Whereas agitation and behavioral symptoms may respond promptly,

symptoms such as hallucinations and delusions may require weeks to respond.
  - Use the minimum effective dosage.

- Lurasidone is complicated by dose-dependent EPS that may be seen in as many as 10% of patients, and akathisia in as many as 20% (Yasui-Furukori, 2012).

- Because Invega paliperidone is prepared as a time-released product stored within a rigid capsule, patients with intestinal strictures should not take it.

- Physical dependence to benzodiazepines can occur within as short a time as 2–3 weeks, and often does occur within 4 months, at 2–5 times the therapeutic dose.

- Buspirone may also help treat functional dyspepsia, as it relaxes the fundus (Tack et al., 2012).

- Pharmacokinetic distinctions are especially significant because there is no convincing evidence that one benzodiazepine is clinically more effective than any other, and no evidence that benzodiazepines marketed as hypnotics for the treatment of insomnia are more effective for sleep than those marked as anxiolytics, and vice versa.

- An important complication of depot olanzapine treatment is a postinjection delirium sedation syndrome (PDSS). PDSS occurs in 0.07% of injections and typically within 1 to 3 hours of receiving the injection. It resembles an overdose of olanzapine and is characterized by sedation grading into somnolence, dizziness, confusion, and dysarthria.

- At each point along the way, MAOI-related safety issues should be reinforced. As a practical precaution, a sticker stating that the patient is "allergic to Demerol (meperidine)" can be placed on the patient's chart.

DISCLOSURES

Dr. Brown has no potential conflicts to disclose.

Dr. Fogel is Chief Scientific Officer of Synchroneuron Inc., Managing Director of Anal-Gesic LLC, and Executive Vice President of PointRight Inc. He is the sole inventor or lead inventor on several pharmaceutical patents. In his opinion these affiliations do not entail any conflict of interest with regard to the editing of this book or his personal contributions to it. He has no other potential conflicts, direct or indirect, financial or otherwise, to disclose in connection with the editing of this book or his personal contributions to it.

REFERENCES

Adan-Manes, J., Novalbos, J., López-Rodríguez, R., Ayuso-Mateos, J. L., & Abad-Santos, F. (2006). Lithium and venlafaxine interaction: a case of serotonin syndrome. *Journal of Clinical Pharmacy and Therapeutics, 31*, 397–400.

Adityanjee, Munshi, K. R., & Thampy A. (2005). The syndrome of irreversible lithium–effectuated neurotoxicity. *Clinical Neuropharmacology, 28*, 38–49

Alam, H. B., Fricchione, G. L., Guimaraes, A. S., & Zukerberg, L. R. (2009). Case records of the Massachusetts General Hospital. Case 31-2009. A 26-year-old man with abdominal distention and shock. *New England Journal of Medicine, 361*, 1487–1496.

Albayrak, Y., & Ekinci, O. (2011). Duloxetine-induced nocturnal bruxism resolved by buspirone: case report. *Clinical Neuropharmacology, 34*, 137–138.

Alberto, G., Erickson, T., Popiel, R., et al. (1989). Central nervous system manifestations of a valproic acid overdose responsive to naloxone. *Annals of Emergency Medicine, 18*, 889–891.

Alderman, C. P., Moritz, C. K., & Ben-Tovim, D. I. (1992). Abnormal platelet aggregation associated with fluoxetine therapy. *Annals of Pharmacotherapy, 26*, 1517–1519.

Alioğlu, Z., Sari, A., Velioğlu, S. K., & Oumlzmenoğlu, M. (2000). Cerebellar atrophy following acute phenytoin intoxication. *Journal of Neuroradiology, 27*, 52–55.

American Psychiatric Association (1994). *Diagnostic and Statistical Manual of Mental Disorders.* (4th ed.), Washington, D.C.: American Psychiatric Association.

Andrade, C., Sandarsh, S., Chethan, K. B., & Nagesh, K. S. (2010). Serotonin reuptake inhibitor antidepressants and abnormal bleeding: a review for clinicians and a reconsideration of mechanisms. *Journal of Clinical Psychiatry, 71*, 1565–1575.

Anisimov, V. N. (2003). Effects of exogenous melatonin—a review. *Toxicologic Pathology, 31*, 589–603.

Anonymous: Phaeochromocytoma unmasked by drug therapy. Prescrire Int 12(67):181–182.

Apple, J. E., & Van Haver, G. (1999). Neuroleptic malignant syndrome associated with olanzapine therapy (Letter). *Psychosomatics, 40*, 1–2.

Apseloff, G., Wilner, K. D., Gerber, N., & Tremaine, L. M. (1997). Effect of sertraline on protein binding of warfarin. *Clinical Pharmacokinetics, 32*(Suppl 1), 37–42.

Apter, J. T., & Allen, L. A. (1999). Buspirone: future directions. *Journal of Clinical Psychopharmacology, 19*, 86–93.

Arana, A., Wentworth, C. E., Ayuso-Mateos, J. L., & Arellano, F. M. (2010). Suicide-related events in patients treated with antiepileptic drugs. *New England Journal of Medicine, 363*, 542–551.

Arana, G. W., Epstein, S., Molloy, M., et al. (1988). Carbamazepine-induced reduction of plasma alprazolam concentrations: a clinical case report. *Journal of Clinical Psychiatry, 49*, 448–449.

Arana, G. W., Goff, D. C., Friedman, H., Ornsteen, M., Greenblatt, D. J., Black, B., & Shader, R. I. (1986). Does carbamazepine-induced reduction of plasma haloperidol levels worsen psychotic symptoms? *American Journal of Psychiatry, 143*, 650–651.

Argov, M., Kashi, R., Peer, D., & Margalit R. (2009). Treatment of resistant human colon cancer xenografts by a fluoxetine-doxorubicin combination enhances therapeutic responses comparable to an aggressive bevacizumab regimen. *Cancer Letters, 274*, 118–125.

Arif, S. A., & Mitchell, M. M. (2011). Iloperidone: A new drug for the treatment of schizophrenia. *American Journal of Health-System Pharmacy, 68*, 301–308.

Arslankoylu, A. E., Kutuk, M. O., Okuyaz, C., & Toros F. (2011). Neuroleptic malignant syndrome due to risperidone misdiagnosed as status epilepticus. *Pediatric Reports, 3*, e19.

Ashton, M. G., Ball, S. G., Thomas, T. H., et al. (1977). Water intoxication associated with carbamazepine treatment. *British Medical Journal, 1*, 1134–1135.

Aurora, R. N., Chowdhuri, S., Ramar, K., Bista, S. R., Casey, K. R., Lamm, C. I., et al. (2012). The treatment of central sleep apnea syndromes in adults: practice parameters with an evidence-based literature review and meta-analyses. *Sleep, 35*, 17–40.

Autry, A. E., Adachi, M., Nosyreva, E., Na, E. S., Los, M. F., Cheng, P. F., et al. (2011). NMDA receptor blockade at rest triggers rapid behavioural antidepressant responses. *Nature, 475*(7354), 91–95.

Azzaro, A. J., Ziemniak, J., Kemper, E., Campbell, B. J., & VanDenBerg, C. (2007). Selegiline transdermal system: an examination of the potential for CYP450-dependent pharmacokinetic interactions with 3 psychotropic medications. *Journal of Clinical Pharmacology, 47*, 146–158.

Babinsky, E., & Levene RS. (2012). Multisystem atrophy made worse by lithium treatment in a hospice patient: a case report. *American Journal of Hospital Palliative Care, 29*, 570–573.

Bahls, F. H., Ozuna, J., & Ritchie, D. E. (1991). Interactions between calcium channel blockers and the anticonvulsants carbamazepine and phenytoin. *Neurology, 41*, 740–742.

Bailey, D. G., Malcolm, J., Arnold, O., & Spence, J. D. Grapefruit juice-drug interactions. *British Journal of Clinical Pharmacology*, (1998). 46, 101–110.

Bakker, P. R., de Groot, I. W., van Os, J., & van Harten, P. N. (2011). Long-stay psychiatric patients: a prospective study revealing persistent antipsychotic-induced movement disorder. *PLoS One, 6*, e25588

Baldaçara, L., Sanches, M., Cordeiro, D. C., & Jackoswski A. P. (2011). Rapid tranquilization for agitated patients in emergency psychiatric rooms: a randomized trial of olanzapine, ziprasidone, haloperidol plus promethazine, haloperidol plus midazolam and haloperidol alone. *Revista Brasileira de Psiquiatria, 33*, 30–39.

Baldessarini, R. J., & Frankenburg, F. R. (1991). Clozapine: a novel antipsychotic agent. *New England Journal of Medicine, 324*, 746–754.

Baldessarini, R. J., Teicher, M. H., Cassidy, J. W., & Stein, M. H. (1988). Anticonvulsant cotreatment may increase toxic metabolites of antidepressants and other psychotropic drugs (letter). *Journal of Clinical Psychopharmacology, 8*, 381–382.

Baldwin, C., & Safferman, A. (1990). A case of lisinopril-induced lithium toxicity. DICP, *Annals of Pharmacotherapy, 24*, 946–947.

Balon, R., & Berchou, R. (1986). Hematologic side effects of psychotropic drugs. *Psychosomatics, 27*, 119–127.

Banach, M., Gurdziel, E., Jędrych, M., & Borowicz, K. K. (2011). Melatonin in experimental seizures and epilepsy. *Pharmacological Reports, 63*, 1–11.

Barbee, J. G., & McLaulin, J. B. (1990). Anxiety disorders: diagnosis and pharmacotherapy in the elderly. *Psychiatric Annals, 20*, 439–445.

Barbhaiya, R. H., Shukla, U. A., Pfeffer, M., Pittman, K. A., Shrotriya, R., Laroudie, C., & Gammans, R. E. (1994). Disposition kinetics of buspirone in patients with renal or hepatic impairment after administration of single and multiple doses. *European Journal of Clinical Pharmacology, 46*, 41–47

Barkhuizen, M., Petzer, A., & Petzer, J. P. (2013). The inhibition of monoamine oxidase by phenformin and pentamidine. *Drug Research (Stuttgart)*, e-pub ahead of print

Barnes, B. J., Gerst, C., Smith, J. R., Terrell, A. R., & Mullins, M. E. (2006). Osmol gap as a surrogate marker for serum propylene glycol concentrations in patients receiving lorazepam for sedation. *Pharmacotherapy, 26*, 23–33.

Barreto, S. G., Tiong, L., & Williams, R. (2011). Drug-induced acute pancreatitis in a cohort of 328 patients. A single-centre experience from Australia. *Journal of Oncology Practice, 12*, 581–585.

Batista, M., Dugernier, T., Simon, M., Haufroid, V., Capron, A., Fonseca, S., et al. (2013). The spectrum of acute heart failure after venlafaxine overdose. *Clinical Toxicology, 51*, 92–95.

Bauler, S., Janoly-Dumenil, A., Sancho, P. O., Fromager, F., Gouraud, A., Rioufol, C., et al. (2012). Effect of carbamazepine on fluindione's anticoagulant activity: a case report. *Therapie, 67*, 488–489.

Beasley, C. M., Tollefson, G., Tran, P., Satterlee, W., Sanger, T., & Hamilton, S. (1996). Olanzapine versus placebo and haloperidol: acute phase results of the North American double-blind olanzapine trial. *Neuropsychopharmacology, 14*, 111–123.

Beck, H., Salom, M., & Holzer, J. (1983). Midazolam dosage studies in institutionalized geriatric patients. *British Journal of Pharmacology, 16*, 1335–1375.

Bedford, J. J., Weggery, S., Ellis, G., McDonald, F. J., Joyce, P. R., Leader, J. P., & Walker R. J. (2008). Lithium-induced nephrogenic diabetes insipidus: renal effects of amiloride. *Clinical Journal of the American Society of Nephrology, 3*, 1324–1331.

Beerman, B., & Edhag, O. (1978). Depressive effects of carbamazepine on idioventricular rhythm in man. *British Medical Journal, 2*, 171–172.

Beijnen, J. H., Bais, E. M., ten Bokkel Huinink, W.W. (1994). Lithium pharmacokinetics during cisplatin-based chemotherapy: a case report. *Cancer Chemotherapy and Pharmacology, 33*, 523–526.

Beliles, K., & Stoudemire, A. (1998). Psychopharmacologic treatment of depression in the medically ill. *Psychosomatics, 39*(Suppl), S1–S19.

Bellesi, M., Passamonti, L., Silvestrini, M., Bartolini, M., & Provinciali L. (2006). Non-convulsive status epilepticus during lithium treatment at therapeutic doses. *Neurological Sciences, 26*, 444–446.

Benassi, E., Bo, G. P., Cocito, L., Maffini, M., & Loeb, C. (1987). Carbamazepine and cardiac conduction disturbances. *Annals of Neurology, 22*, 280–281.

Benetton, S. A., Fang, C., Yang, Y. O., Alok, R., Year, M., Lin, C. C., & Yeh L. T. (2007). P450 phenotyping of the metabolism of selegiline to desmethylselegiline and methamphetamine. *Drug Metababolism and Pharmacokinetics, 22*, 78–87.

Benfield, P., & Ward, A. (1986). Fluvoxamine. A review of its pharmacodynamic and pharmacokinetic properties, and therapeutic efficacy in depressive illness. *Drugs, 32*, 313–334.

Bennett, W. M., Muther, R. S., & Parker, R. A. (1980). Drug therapy in renal failure: dosing guidelines for adults: Part II. Sedatives, hypnotics, and tranquilizers; cardiovascular, antihypertensive, and diuretic agents; miscellaneous agents. *Annals of Internal Medicine, 93*, 286–325.

Berlim, M. T., & Turecki, M. G. (2007). Using psychostimulants for treating residual symptoms in major depression. *Journal of Psychiatry & Neuroscience, 32*, 304.

Bernardi, F., & DelZampa, M. (1990). Clozapine in idiopathic Parkinson's disease. *Neurology, 40*, 1151.

Besag, F. M., & Berry, D. (2006). Interactions between antiepileptic and antipsychotic drugs. *Drug Safety, 29*, 95–118.

Beydoun, A., Uthman, B. M., & Sackellares, J. C. (1995). Gabapentin: pharmacokinetics, efficacy and safety. *Clinical Neuropharmacology, 18*, 469–481.

Beydoun, M. A., Shroff, M. R., Beydoun, H. A., & Zonderman, A. B. (2010). Serum folate, vitamin B-12, and homocysteine and their association with depressive symptoms among U.S. adults. *Psychosomatic Medicine, 72*, 862–873.

Bieck, P. R., & Antonin, K. H. (1989). Tyramine potentiation during treatment with MAO inhibitors: brofaromine and moclobemide vs. irreversible inhibitors. *Journal of Neural Transmission, 28*(suppl), 21–31.

Bigger, J. T., Giardina EGV, Perel, J. M., Kantor, S. J., & Glassman, A. H. (1977). Cardiac antiarrhythmic effect of imipramine hydrochloride. *New England Journal of Medicine, 296*, 206–208.

Billups, S. J., Delate, T., & Dugan, D. (2009). Evaluation of risk factors for elevated tricyclic antidepressant plasma concentrations. *Pharmacoepidemiology and Drug Safety, 18*, 253–257.

Binkhorst, L., Mathijssen, R. H., van Herk-Sukel, M. P., Bannink, M., Jager, A., Wiemer, E. A., & van Gelder, T. (2013). Unjustified prescribing of CYP2D6 inhibiting SSRIs in women treated with tamoxifen. *Breast Cancer Research and Treatment, 139*, 923–929.

Birbeck, G. L., French, J. A., Perucca, E., Simpson, D. M., Fraimow, H., George, J. M., et al. (2012). Quality Standards Subcommittee of the American Academy of Neurology; Ad Hoc Task Force of the Commission on Therapeutic Strategies of the International League Against Epilepsy: Evidence-based guideline: Antiepileptic drug selection for people with HIV/AIDS. Report of the Quality Standards Subcommittee of the American Academy of Neurology and the Ad Hoc Task Force of the Commission on Therapeutic Strategies of the International League Against Epilepsy. *Neurology, 78*, 139–145.

Bishara, D. (2010). Once-monthly paliperidone injection for the treatment of schizophrenia. *Neuropsychiatric Disease and Treatment, 6*, 561–572

Bixler, E. O., Kales, A., Manfredi, R. L., Vgontzas, A. N., Tyson, K. L., & Kales, J. D. (1991). Next-day memory impairment with triazolam use. *Lancet, 337*, 827–831.

Bjarnason, N. H., Munkner, R., Kampmann, J. P., Tornoe, C. W., Ladefoged, S., & Dalhoff, K. (2006). Optimizing lithium dosing in hemodialysis. *Therapeutic Drug Monitoring, 28*, 262–266.

Blackford, M. G., Do, S. T., Enlow, T. C., & Reed, M. D. (2013). Valproic acid and topiramate induced hyperammonemic encephalopathy in a patient with normal serum carnitine. *Journal of Pediatric Pharmacology and Therapeutics, 18*, 128–136.

Blackwell, B., & Schmidt, G. L. (1984). Drug interactions in psychopharmacology. *Psychiatric Clinics of North America, 7*, 625–637.

Blazer, D. G., Petrie, W. M., & Wilson, W. P. (1976). Affective psychoses following renal transplant. *Diseases of the Nervous System, 37*, 663–667.

Bobes, J., Garcia-Portilla, M. P., Bascaran, M. T., Saiz, P. A., & Bousoño M. (2007). Quality of life in schizophrenic patients. *Dialogues in Clinical Neuroscience, 9*, 215–226

Bobo, B. L., & Miwa, L. J. (1988). Midazolam disinhibition reaction. *Drug Intelligence & Clinical Pharmacy, 22*, 725.

Bocchetta, A., Cocco, F., Velluzzi, F., Del-Zompo, M., Mariotti, S., & Loviselli A. (2007). Fifteen-year follow-up of thyroid function in lithium patients. *Journal of Endocrinological Investigation, 30*, 363–366.

Bodley, R. P., Halwax, K., & Potts, L. (1969). Low serum cholinesterase levels complicating treatment with phenelzine. *British Medical Journal, 3*, 510–512.

Bodnar, T., Starr, K., & Halter, J. B. (2011). Linezolid-associated hypoglycemia in a 64-year-old man with type 2 diabetes. *American Journal of Geriatric Pharmacotherapy, 9*, 88–92

Bond, W. S., Mandos, L. A., & Kurtz, M. B. (1989). Midazolam for aggressivity and violence in three mentally retarded patients. *American Journal of Psychiatry, 146*, 925–926.

Bondon-Guitton, E., Perez-Lloret, S., Bagheri, H., Brefel, C., Rascol, O., & Montastruc, J. L. (2011). Drug-induced Parkinsonism: a review of 17 years' experience in a regional pharmacovigilance center in France. *Movement Disorders, 26*, 2226–2231.

Bonfiglio, M. F., & Dasta, J. F. (1991). Clinical significance of the benzodiazepine-theophylline interaction. *Pharmacotherapy, 11*, 85–87.

Bourgeois, B. F. D., & Wad, N. (1984). Individual and combined antiepileptic and neurotoxic activity of carbamazepine and carbamazepine-10, 11-epoxide in mice. *Journal of Pharmacological and Experimental Therapeutics, 231*, 411–415.

Bourgeois, B. F. D. (1988). Pharmacologic interactions between valproate and other drugs. *American Journal of Medicine, 84*(suppl 1A), 29–33.

Bowden, C. L., Nemeroff, C. B., & Potter, W. Z. (1991). *Practical clinical guidelines for the management of bipolar disorder. Monograph on Treatment.* Chicago: Abbott Laboratories.

Bowden, C. L., & Singh V. (2012). Lamotrigine (Lamictal IR) for the treatment of bipolar disorder. *Expert Opinion in Pharmacotherapy, 13*, 2565–2571.

Brahm, N. C., Fast, G. A., & Brown, R. C. (2008). Buspirone for autistic disorder in a woman with an intellectual disability. *Annals of Pharmacotherapy, 42*, 131–137.

Brenes, G. A. (2003). Anxiety and chronic obstructive pulmonary disease: prevalence, impact, and treatment. *Psychosomatic Medicine, 65*, 963–970

Brewerton, T. D. (1986). Lithium counteracts carbamazepine-induced leukopenia while increasing its therapeutic effect. *Biological Psychiatry, 21*, 677–685.

Briesacher, B. A., Tjia, J., Field, T., Peterson, D., & Gurwitz, J. H. (2013). Antipsychotic use among nursing home residents. *Journal of the American Medical Association, 309*, 440–442

Bromfield, E. B., Altshuler, L., Leiderman, D. B., Balish, M., Ketter, T. A., Devinsky, O., et al. (1992). Cerebral metabolism and depression in patients with complex partial seizures. *Archives of Neurology, 49*, 617–623.

Brown, C. S., Wells, B. G., Cold, J. A., Froemming, J. H., Self, T. H., & Jabbour, J. T. (1990). Possible influence of carbamazepine on plasma imipramine concentrations in children with attention deficit hyperactivity disorder. *Journal of Clinical Psychopharmacology, 10*, 359–362.

Brown, K., Levy, H., Brenner, C., Leffler, S., & Hamburg, E. L. (1993). Overdose of risperidone. *Annals of Emergency Medicine*, 22, 1908–1910.

Brown, T. C. K., & Cass, N. M. (1979). Beware—the use of MAO inhibitors is increasing again. *Anaesthesia and Intensive Care*, 7, 65–68.

Brown, T. M., & Stoudemire, A. (1998). Antidepressants. In Brown, T. M., & Stoudemire, A., eds., *Psychiatric side effects of prescription and over-the-counter medications* (pp. 53–82). Washington, D.C.: American Psychiatric Press.

Bruno, J., Gallo, J. M., Lee, C. S., et al. (1980). Interactions of valproic acid with phenytoin. *Neurology*, 30, 1233–1236.

Brzaković, B. B., Vezmar Kovačević, S. D., Vučićević, K. M., Miljković, B. R., Martinović Z. J., Pokrajac, M. V., & Prostran, M. Š. (2012). Impact of age, weight and concomitant treatment on lamotrigine pharmacokinetics. *Journal of Clinical Pharmacy and Therapeutics*, 37, 693–697.

Buff, D. D., Brenner, R., Kirtane, S. S., & Gilboa, R. (1991). Dysrhythmia associated with fluoxetine treatment in an elderly patient with cardiac disease. *Journal of Clinical Psychiatry*, 52, 174–176.

Bulach, R., Myles, P. S., & Russnak, M. (2005). Double-blind randomized controlled trial to determine extent of amnesia with midazolam given immediately before general anaesthesia. *British Journal of Anaesthesia*, 94, 300–305.

Burnakis, T. G., & Berman, D. E. (1989). Hostility and hallucinations as a consequence of midazolam administration. *Drug Intelligence & Clinical Pharmacy*, 23, 671–672.

Buysse, D. J. (2013). Insomnia. *Journal of the American Medical Association*, 309, 706–716.

Cade, J. F. J. (1949). Lithium salts in the treatment of psychotic excitement. *Medical Journal of Australia*, 11, 349–351.

Cadet, J. L., & Krasnova, I. N. (2007). Interactions of HIV and methamphetamine: cellular and molecular mechanisms of toxicity potentiation. *Neurotoxicity Research*, 12, 181–204.

Caillier, B., Pilote, S., Castonguay, A., Patoine, D., Ménard-Desrosiers, V., Vigneault, P., et al. (2012). QRS widening and QT prolongation under bupropion: a unique cardiac electrophysiological profile. *Fundamental & Clinical Pharmacology*, 26, 599–608.

Callingham, B. A. (1993). Drug interactions with reversible monoamine oxidase-A inhibitors. *Clinical Neuropharmacology*, 16(Suppl 2), 42–50.

CAPS (Cardiac Arrhythmic Pilot Study Investigators) (1988). Effects of encainide, flecainide, imipramine and moricizine on ventricular arrhythmias during the year after acute myocardial infarction. *American Journal of Cardiology*, 61, 501–509.

Carrão, J. L., Moreira, L. B., & Fuchs, F. D. (2007). The efficacy of the combination of sertraline with buspirone for smoking cessation. A randomized clinical trial in nondepressed smokers. *European Archives of Psychiatry and Clinical Neuroscience*, 257, 383–388

Casey, D. E. (1997a). How antipsychotic drug pharmacology relates to side effects. *Journal of Clinical Psychiatry, Monograph Series*, 15, 30–33.

Casey, D. E. (1997b). The relationship of pharmacology to side effects. *Journal of Clinical Psychiatry*, 59(Suppl 10), 55–62.

Castro, V. M., Clements, C. C., Murphy, S. N., Gainer, V. S., Fava, M., Weilburg, J. B., et al. (2013). QT interval and antidepressant use: a cross sectional study of electronic health records. *British Medical Journal*, 29, 346:f288.

Cavanaugh, S von A. (1990). Drug-drug interactions of fluoxetine with tricyclics. *Psychosomatics*, 31, 273–276.

Cavanna, A. E., Ali, F., Rickards, H. E., & McCorry D. (2010). Behavioral and cognitive effects of anti-epileptic drugs. *Discovery Medicine*, 9, 138–144

Cervera, E., Candelaria, M., López-Navarro, O., Labardini, J., Gonzalez-Fierro, A., Taja-Chayeb, L., et al. (2012). Epigenetic therapy with hydralazine and magnesium valproate reverses imatinib resistance in patients with chronic myeloid leukemia. *Clinical Lymphoma Myeloma and Leukemia*, 12, 207–212.

Chan, Y. C., Tse, M. L., & Lau, F. L. (2007). Two cases of valproic acid poisoning treated with L-carnitine. *Human & Experimental Toxicology*, 26, 967–969.

Chavant, F., Favrelière, S., Lafay-Chebassier, C., Plazanet, C., & Pérault-Pochat, M. C. (2011). Memory disorders associated with consumption of drugs: updating through a case/noncase study in the French PharmacoVigilance Database. *British Journal of Clinical Pharmacology*, 72, 898–904

Chen, D. T., & Ruch, R. (1993). Safety of moclobemide in clinical use. *Clinical Neuropharmacology*, 16(Suppl 2), S63–S68.

Chen, Y. H., Wu, K. L., & Chen, C. H. (2012). Methamphetamine reduces human influenza A virus replication. *PLoS One*, 7(11), e48335

Chew, M. L., Mulsant, B. H., Pollock, B. G., Lehman, M. E., Greenspan, A., Mahmoud, R. A., et al. (2008). Anticholinergic activity of 107 medications commonly used by older adults. *Journal of the American Geriatrics Society*, 56, 1333–1341.

Chiarello, R. J., & Cole, J. O. (1987). The use of psychostimulants in general psychiatry. *Archives of General Psychiatry*, 44, 286–295.

Chicharro, A. V., de Marinis, A. J., & Kanner, A. M. (2007). The measurement of ammonia blood levels in patients taking valproic acid: looking for problems where they do not exist? *Epilepsy & Behavior*, 11, 361–366

Chien J. (2011). Ethosuximide-induced mania in a 10-year-old boy. *Epilepsy & Behavior*, 21, 483–485

Chiron, C., & Dulac, O. (2011). The pharmacologic treatment of Dravet syndrome. *Epilepsia*, 52(Suppl 2), 72–75.

Chiu, C. C., Shen, W. W., Chen, K. P., & Lu, M. L. (2007). Application of the Cockcroft-Gault method to estimate lithium dosage requirement. *Psychiatry and Clinical Neurosciences*, 61, 269–274.

Chouinard, G., & Albright, P. S. (1997). Economic and health state utility determinations for schizophrenic patients treated with risperidone or haloperidol. *Journal of Clinical Psychopharmacology*, 17, 298–307.

Chouinard, G. (1987). Clonazepam in acute and maintenance treatment of bipolar affective disorder. *Journal of Clinical Psychiatry*, 48(Suppl), 29–37.

Chrościńska-Krawczyk, M., Jargiełło-Baszak, M., Wałek, M., Tylus, B., & Czuczwar, S. J. (2011). Caffeine and the anticonvulsant potency of antiepileptic drugs: experimental and clinical data. *Pharmacological Reports*, 63, 12–18

Chukhin, E., Takala, P., Hakko, H., Raidma, M., Putkonen, H., Räsänen, P., et al. (2013). In a randomized placebo-controlled add-on study orlistat significantly reduced clozapine-induced constipation. *International Clinical Psychopharmacology*, 28, 67–70.

Citrome, L. (2010). Iloperidone: chemistry, pharmacodynamics, pharmacokinetics and metabolism, clinical efficacy, safety and tolerability, regulatory affairs, and an opinion. *Expert Opinion on Drug Metabolism & Toxicology*, 6, 1551–1564.

Cohen, B. J., Mahelsky, M., & Adler, L. (1990). More cases of SIADH with fluoxetine (letter). *American Journal of Psychiatry*, 147, 948–949.

Cohn, J. B., Wilcox, C. S., Bremner, J., & Ettinger, M. (1991). Hypnotic efficacy of estazolam compared with flurazepam in outpatients with insomnia. *Journal of Clinical Pharmacology*, 31, 747–750.

Colenda, C. C. (1988). Buspirone in treatment of agitated demented patient. *Lancet*, 1, 1169.

Colombo, R., Corona, A., Praga, F., Minari, C., Giannotti, C., et al. (2012). A reorientation strategy for reducing delirium in the critically ill. Results of an interventional study. *Minerva Anestesiologica*, 78, 1026–1033.

Contin, M., Riva, R., Albani, F., Avoni, P., & Baruzzi, A. (2002). Topiramate therapeutic monitoring in patients with epilepsy: effect of concomitant antiepileptic drugs. *Therapeutic Drug Monitoring*, 24, 332–337.

Cooper, A. J., & Ashcroft, G. (1966). Potentiation of insulin hypoglycemia by MAOI antidepressant drugs. *Lancet*, 1, 407–409.

Correll, C. U., Lops, J. D., Figen, V., Malhotra, A. K., Kane, J. M., & Manu P. (2011). QT interval duration and dispersion in children and adolescents treated with ziprasidone. *Journal of Clinical Psychiatry*, 72, 854–860.

Coulter, D. W., Walko, C., Patel, J., Moats-Staats, B. M., McFadden, A., Smith, S. V., et al. (2013). Valproic acid reduces the tolerability of temsirolimus in children and adolescents with solid tumors. *Anticancer Drugs, 24,* 415–421.

Coves-Orts, F. J., Borrás-Blasco, J., Navarro-Ruiz, A., Murcia-López, A., & Palacios-Ortega, F. (2005). Acute seizures due to a probable interaction between valproic acid and meropenem. *Annals of Pharmacotherapy, 39,* 533–537.

Crabtree, B. L., Mack, J. E., Johnson, C. D., & Amyx, B. C. (1991). Comparison of the effects of hydrochlorothiazide and furosemide on lithium disposition. *American Journal of Psychiatry, 148,* 1060–1063

Crespel, A., Genton, P., Berramdane, M., Coubes, P., Monicard, C., Baldy-Moulinier, M., & Gelisse, P. (2005). Lamotrigine associated with exacerbation or de novo myoclonus in idiopathic generalized epilepsies. *Neurology, 65,* 762–764.

Csernansky, J. G., & Hollister, L. E. (1985). Using lithium in patients with cardiac and renal disease. *Hospital Formulary, 20,* 726–735.

D'Mello, D. A., McNeil, J. A., & Harris, W. (1989). Buspirone suppression of neuroleptic-induced akathisia: multiple case reports. *Journal of Clinical Psychopharmacology, 9,* 151–152.

Dalhoff, K., Poulsen, H. E., Garred, P., Placchi, M., Gammans, R. E., Mayol, R. F., & Pfeffer, M. (1987). Buspirone pharmacokinetics in patients with cirrhosis. *British Journal of Clinical Pharmacology, 24,* 547–550.

Darracq, M. A., Clark, A., Qian, L., & Cantrell, F. L. (2013). A retrospective review of isolated duloxetine-exposure cases. *Clinical Toxicology, 51,* 106–110.

Dasgupta, A. (2008). Herbal supplements and therapeutic drug monitoring: focus on digoxin immunoassays and interactions with St. John's wort. *Therapeutic Drug Monitoring, 30,* 212–217.

DasGupta, K., & Jefferson, J. W. (1990). The use of lithium in the medically ill. *General Hospital Psychiatry, 12,* 83–97.

Dave, M. (1995). Two cases of risperidone-induced neuroleptic malignant syndrome (letter), *American Journal of Psychiatry, 152,* 1233–1234.

Dawling, S., Crome, P., & Braithwaite, R. A. (1980). Pharmacokinetics of a single oral dose of nortriptyline in depressed elderly hospital patients and young healthy volunteers. *Clinical Pharmacokinetics, 5,* 394–401.

Dawling, S., Crome, P., Heyer, E. J., & Lewis, R. R. (1981). Nortriptyline therapy in elderly patients: dosage prediction from plasma concentration at 24 hours after a single 50 mg dose. *British Journal of Psychiatry, 139,* 413–416.

Dawling, S., Lynn, K., Rosser, R., & Braithwaite, R. (1982). Nortriptyline metabolism in chronic renal failure: metabolite elimination. *Clinical Pharmacology and Therapeutics, 32,* 322–329.

Dawson, J. K., Earnshaw, S. M., & Graham, C. S. (1995). Dangerous monoamine oxidase inhibitor interactions are still occurring in the 1990s. *Journal of Accident & Emergency Medicine, 12,* 49–51.

De Dios, C., Fudio, S., & Lorenzo, A. (2011). Reversible Parkinsonism and cognitive decline due to a possible interaction of valproic acid and quetiapine. *Journal of Clinical Pharmacy and Therapeutics, 36,* 430–432.

De Fazio, P., Girardi, P., Maina, G., Mauri, M. C., Mauri, M., Monteleone, P., et al. (2010). Aripiprazole in acute mania and long-term treatment of bipolar disorder: a critical review by an Italian working group. *Clinical Drug Investigation, 30,* 827–841.

de Jong, F. A., van der Bol, J. M., Mathijssen, R. H., Loos, W. J., Mathôt, R. A., Kitzen, J. J., et al. (2007). Irinotecan chemotherapy during valproic acid treatment: pharmacokinetic interaction and hepatotoxicity. *Cancer Biology & Therapy, 6,* 1368–1374.

De Marcos, F. A., Ghizoni, E., Kobayashi, E., Li, L. M., & Cendes, F. (2003). Cerebellar volume and long-term use of phenytoin. *Seizure, 12,* 312–315.

deBoer, T. (1996). The pharmacologic profile of mirtazapine. *Journal of Clinical Psychiatry, 57*(Suppl 4), 19–25.

Deirmenjian, J. M., Erhart, S. M., Wirshing, D. A., Spellberg, B. J., & Wirshing, W. C. (1998). Olanzapine-induced reversible priapism: a case report. *Journal of Clinical Psychopharmacology, 18,* 351–352.

Delbari, A., Salman-Roghani, R., & Lokk, J. (2011). Effect of methylphenidate and/or levodopa combined with physiotherapy on mood and cognition after stroke: a randomized, double-blind, placebo-controlled trial. *European Neurology, 66,* 7–13

Delbressine, L. P., & Vos, R. M. (1997). The clinical relevance of preclinical data: mirtazapine, a model compound. *Journal of Clinical Psychopharmacology, 17*(Suppl. 2), 29S–33S.

Delva, N. J., & Hawken, E. R. (2001). Preventing lithium intoxication. Guide for physicians. *Canadian Family Physician, 47,* 1595–1600.

Dennis, A. T., Nassal, D., Deschenes, I., Thomas, D., & Ficker, E. (2011). Antidepressant-induced ubiquitination and degradation of the cardiac potassium channel hERG. *Journal of Biological Chemistry, 286,* 34413–3442.5

DePaulo, J. R., Jr. (1984). Lithium. *Psychiatric Clinics of North America, 7,* 587–599.

Derinoz, O., & Caglar, A. A. (2013). Drug-induced movement disorders in children at paediatric emergency department: "dystonia." *Emergency Medicine Journal, 30,* 130–133

DeVane, C. L., & Gill, H. S. (1997). Clinical pharmacokinetics of fluvoxamine: applications to dosage regimen design. *Journal of Clinical Psychiatry, 58*(Suppl. 5), 7–14.

DeVane, C. L. (1996). Drug interactions and antipsychotic therapy. *Pharmacotherapy, 16*(1 Pt 2), 15S–20S.

DeVane, C. L., Laizure, S. C., Stewart, J. T., et al. (1990). Disposition of bupropion in healthy volunteers and subjects with alcoholic liver disease. *Journal of Clinical Psychopharmacology, 10,* 328–332.

Devinsky, O., Honigfeld, G., & Patin, J. (1991). Clozapine-related seizures. *Neurology, 41,* 369–371.

Di Lorenzo, R., & Brogli A. (2010). Profile of olanzapine long-acting injection for the maintenance treatment of adult patients with schizophrenia. *Neuropsychiatric Disease and Treatment, 6,* 573–581.

Diaz, F. J., Santoro, V., Spina, E., Cogollo, M., Rivera, T. E., Botts, S., & de Leon, J. (2008). Estimating the size of the effects of co-medications on plasma clozapine concentrations using a model that controls for clozapine doses and confounding variables. *Pharmacopsychiatry, 41,* 81–91.

Diaz, S. F. (1996). Mania associated with risperidone (letter). *Journal of Clinical Psychiatry, 57,* 41–42.

Dick, A. D., Towler, H. M., Whiting, P., & Forrester, J. V. (1992). The use of lithium clearance studies in the early detection of cyclosporin A (CsA) nephrotoxicity: a protocol of renal function assessment with CsA therapy. *Current Eye Research, 11*(Suppl), 215–218.

Dickens, D., Owen, A., Alfirevic, A., Giannoudis, A., Davies, A., Weksler, B., et al. (2012). Lamotrigine is a substrate for OCT1 in brain endothelial cells. *Biochemical Pharmacology, 183,* 805–814.

Dieperink, H., Leyssac, P. P., Kemp, E., Starklint, H., Frandsen, N. E., Tvede, N., et al. (1987). Nephrotoxicity of cyclosporin A in humans: effects on glomerular filtration and tubular reabsorption rates. *European Journal of Clinical Investigation, 17,* 493–496.

Diniz, B. S., Machado-Vieira, R., & Forlenza, O. V. (2013). Lithium and neuroprotection: translational evidence and implications for the treatment of neuropsychiatric disorders. *Neuropsychiatric Disease and Treatment, 9,* 493–500

Diniz, B. S., & Teixeira, A. L. (2011). Brain-derived neurotrophic factor and Alzheimer's disease: physiopathology and beyond. *Neuromolecular Medicine, 13,* 217–222.

Dollins, A. B., Zhdanova, I. V., Wurtman, R. J., Lynch, H. J., & Deng, M. H. (1994). Effect of inducing nocturnal serum melatonin concentrations in daytime on sleep, mood, body temperature, and performance. *Proceedings of the National Academy of Sciences USA, 91,* 1824–1828.

Domantay, A. G., & Napoliello, M. J. (1989). Buspirone for elderly anxious patients: a review of clinical studies. *Family Practice Recertification, 11*(9), 17–23.

Douste-Blazy, P., Rostin, M., Livarek, B., Tordjman, E., Montastruc, J. L., & Galinier, F. (1986). Angiotensin converting enzyme inhibitors and lithium treatment. *Lancet, 1*(8495), 1448.

Dreifuss, F. E., & Langer, D. H. (1987). Hepatic considerations in the use of antiepileptic drugs. *Epilepsia, 28*(suppl 2):523–529.

Drover, D. R. (2004). Comparative pharmacokinetics and pharmacodynamics of short-acting hypnosedatives: zaleplon, zolpidem and zopiclone. *Clinical Pharmacokinetics, 43,* 227–238.

Duran-Sindreu, S. F., Grasa-Bello, E., Corripio-Collado, I., Sauras-Quetcuti, R. B., Keymer-Gausset, A., Roldán-Bejarano, A., et al. (2013). Síndrome post-inyección por olanzapina de liberación retardada: Breve revisión a propósito de un caso. *Actas Espanas de Psiquiatria, 41*(1), 60–62.

Eadie, M. J., Hooper, W. D., & Dickinson, R. G. (1988). Valproate associated hepatotoxicity and its biochemical mechanisms. *Medical Toxicology and Adverse Drug Experience, 3*, 85–106.

Ege, F., Koçak, Y., Titiz, A. P., Ozturk, S. M., Oztürk, S., & Ozbakir S. (2008). Gabapentin-Induced myoclonus: case report (letter). *Movement Disorders, 23*, 1947–1948.

El-Ganzouri, A. R., Ivankovich, A. D., Braverman, B., & McCarthy, R. (1985). Monoamine oxidase inhibitors: should they be discontinued preoperatively? *Anesthesia and Analgesia, 64*, 592–596.

Ellison, J. M., Milofsky, J. E., & Ely, E. (1990). Fluoxetine-induced bradycardia and syncope in two patients. *Journal of Clinical Psychiatry, 51*, 385–386.

EMSAM, Selegiline Transdermal System. NDA 21,336/21,708. Psychopharmacologic Drugs Advisory Committee. October 26, 2005. http://www.fda.gov/ohrms/dockets/ac/05/briefing/2005-4186b2_01_01_somerset-emsam.pdf, accessed 30 April 2013.

Ertan, S., Ulu, M. O., Hanimoglu, H., Tanriverdi, T., Kafadar, A. M., Acar, Z. U., & Kiziltan G. (2006). Phenytoin-induced parkinsonism. *Singapore Medical Journal, 47*, 981–983

Estivill, E., Bové A, García-Borreguero, D., Gibert, J., Paniagua, J., Pin, G., et al; members of the Consensus Group. (2003). Consensus on drug treatment, definition and diagnosis for insomnia. *Clinical Drug Investigation, 23*, 351–385.

Evans, M. D., Shinar, R., & Yaari, R. (2011). Reversible dementia and gait disturbance after prolonged use of valproic acid. *Seizure, 20*, 509–511

Ezzaher, A., Haj, M. D., Mechri, A., Neffati, F., Douki, W., Gaha, L., & Najjar MF. (2011). Metabolic syndrome in Tunisian bipolar I patients. *African Health Sciences, 11*, 414–420.

Fabre, L. F., Scharf, M. B., & Itil, T. M. (1991). Comparative efficacy and safety of nortriptyline and fluoxetine in the treatment of major depression: a clinical study. *Journal of Clinical Psychiatry, 52*(suppl):62–67.

Farber, N. B., Jiang, X. P., Heinkel, C., & Nemmers, B. (2002). Antiepileptic drugs and agents that inhibit voltage-gated sodium channels prevent NMDA antagonist neurotoxicity. *Molecular Psychiatry, 7*, 726–733.

Feder, R. (1991). Bradycardia and syncope induced by fluoxetine (letter). *Journal of Clinical Psychiatry, 52*, 139.

Feighner, J. P., & Cohn, J. B. (1985). Double-blind comparative trials of fluoxetine and doxepin in geriatric patients with major depressive disorder. *Journal of Clinical Psychiatry, 46*, 20–25.

Feighner, J. P., Boyer, W. F., Meredith, C. H., & Hendrickson, G. (1988). An overview of fluoxetine in geriatric depression. *British Journal of Psychiatry, 153*, 105–108.

Fernandez, C., Martin, C., Gimenez, F., & Farinotti R. (1995). Clinical pharmacokinetics of zopiclone. *Clinical Pharmacokinetics, 29*, 431–441

Fernandez, F., Adams, F., Holmes, V. F., Levy, J. K., & Neidhart, M. (1987). Methylphenidate for depressive disorders in cancer patients. An alternative to standard antidepressants. *Psychosomatics, 28*, 455–461.

Ferrajolo, C., Capuano, A., Verhamme, K. M., Schuemie, M., Rossi, F., Stricker, B. H., & Sturkenboom, M. C. (2010). Drug-induced hepatic injury in children: a case/non-case study of suspected adverse drug reactions in VigiBase. *British Journal of Clinical Pharmacology, 70*, 721–728

Ferris, M. J., Mactutus, C. F., & Booze, R. M. (2008). Neurotoxic profiles of HIV, psychostimulant drugs of abuse, and their concerted effect on the brain: current status of dopamine system vulnerability in NeuroAIDS. *Neuroscience and Biobehavioral Reviews, 32*, 883–909.

Fiedorowicz, J. G., & Swartz, K. L. (2004). The role of monoamine oxidase inhibitors in current psychiatric practice. *Journal of Psychiatric Practice, 10*, 239–248.

Finch, C. K., Chrisman, C. R., Baciewicz, A. M., & Self, T. H. (2002). Rifampin and rifabutin drug interactions: an update. *Archives of Internal Medicine, 162*, 985–992.

Finkel, S., Kozma, C., Long, S., Greenspan, A., Mahmoud, R., Baser, O., & Engelhart L. (2005). Risperidone treatment in elderly patients with dementia: relative risk of cerebrovascular events versus other antipsychotics. *International Psychogeriatrics, 17*, 617–629.

Fisch, C. (1985). Effect of fluoxetine on the electrocardiogram. *Journal of Clinical Psychiatry, 46*, 42–44.

Fisch, C. (1991). Effects of sertraline on the ECG in non-elderly and elderly patients with major depression (abstract). *Biological Psychiatry, 29*, 353S–354S.

Fischer, M., Korskjaer, G., & Pedersen, E. (1965). Psychotic episodes in Zarondan treatment. Effects and side-effects in 105 patients. *Epilepsia, 6*, 325–334.

Fisher, R. S., & Cysyk, B. (1988). A fatal overdose of carbamazepine: case report and review of literature. *Journal of Toxicology and Clinical Toxicology, 26*, 477–486.

Flugelman, M. Y., Tal, A., & Pollack, S. (1985). Psychotropic drugs and long, Q. T.syndromes: case reports. *Journal of Clinical Psychiatry, 46*, 290–291.

Focosi, D., Azzarà, A., Kast, R. E., Carulli, G., & Petrini M. (2009). Lithium and hematology: established and proposed uses. *Journal of Leukocyte Biology, 85*, 20–28

Fogel, B. S. (1988). Combining anticonvulsants with conventional psychopharmacologic agents. In S. L. McElroy & H. G. Pope (Eds.), *Use of anticonvulsants in psychiatry: recent advances* (pp. 77–94). Clifton, NJ: Oxford Health Care.

Forget, P., le Polain de Waroux, B., Wallemacq, P., & Gala, J. L. (2008). Life-threatening dextromethorphan intoxication associated with interaction with amitriptyline in a poor CYP2D6 metabolizer: a single case re-exposure study. *Journal of Pain and Symptom Management, 36*, 92–96.

Forman, M. B., Sutej, P. G., & Jackson, E. K. (2011). Hypertension, tachycardia, and reversible cardiomyopathy temporally associated with milnacipran use. *Texas Heart Institute Journal, 38*, 714–718.

Forrest, J. N., Cohen, A. D., & Torretti, K. (1974). On the mechanism of lithium-induced diabetes insipidus in man and rate. *Journal of Clinical Investigation, 53*, 1115–1123.

Forster, P. L., Dewland, P. M., Muirhead, D., et al. (1991). The effects of sertraline on plasma concentration and renal clearance of digoxin (abstract). *Biological Psychiatry, 29*, 3555.

Fraile, P., Garcia-Cosmes, P., Garcia, T., Corbacho, L., Alvarez, M., & Tabernero, J. M. (2009). Hypotension, as consequence of the interaction between tacrolimus and mirtazapine, in a patient with renal transplant. *Nephrology, Dialysis, Transplantation, 24*, 1999–2001.

Frankhauser, M. P., Lindon, J. L., Connolly, B., & Healey, W. J. (1988). Evaluation of lithium-tetracycline interaction. *Clinical Pharmacology, 7*, 314–317.

Fredman, B., Lahav, M., Zohar, E., Golod, M., Paruta, I., & Jedeikin, R. (1999). The effect of midazolam premedication on mental and psychomotor recovery in geriatric patients undergoing brief surgical procedures. *Anesthesia and Analgesia, 89*, 1161–1166.

Fricchione, G. L., Woznicki, R. M., Klesmer, J., & Vlay, S. C. (1993). Vasoconstrictive effects and SSRIs (letter). *Journal of Clinical Psychiatry, 54*, 71–72.

Friedman, J. H., & Lannon, M. C. (1989). Clozapine in the treatment of psychosis in Parkinson's disease. *Neurology, 39*, 1219–1221.

Galynker, I., Ieronimo, C., Miner, C., Rosenblum, J., Vilkas, N., & Rosenthal, R. (1997). Methylphenidate treatment of negative symptoms in patients with dementia. *Journal of Neuropsychiatry and Clinical Neurosciences, 9*, 231–239.

Gammans, R. E., Bullen, W. W., Briner, L., et al. (1985). The effects of buspirone binding of digoxin, propranolol and warfarin to human plasma. *Federation Proceedings, 44*, 1123.

Gammans, R. E., Mayol, R. F., & Labudde, J. A. (1986). Metabolism and dispositions of buspirone. *American Journal of Medicine, 80*, 41–51.

Gammans, R. E., Westrick, M. L., Shea, J. P., Mayol, R. F., & LaBudde, J. A. (1989). Pharmacokinetics of buspirone in elderly subjects. *Journal of Clinical Pharmacology, 29*, 72–78.

Gardner, D. M., & Lynd, L. D. (1998). Sumatriptan contraindications and the serotonin syndrome. *Annals of Pharmacotherapy, 32,* 33–38.

Gardner, D. M., Shulman, K. I., Walker, S. E., & Tailor SA. (1996). The making of a user friendly MAOI diet. *Journal of Clinical Psychiatry, 57,* 99–104.

Garner, S. J., Eldridge, F. L., Wagner, P. G., & Dowell, R. T. (1989). Buspirone, an anxiolytic drug that stimulates respiration. *American Review of Respiratory Disease, 139,* 946–950.

Gawin, F., Compton, M., Byck, R. (1989). Buspirone reduces smoking. *Archives of General Psychiatry, 46,* 288–289.

Gellad, W. F., Aspinall, S. L., Handler, S. M., Stone, R. A., Castle, N., Semla, T. P., et al. (2012). Use of antipsychotics among older residents in VA nursing homes. *Medical Care, 50,* 954–960.

Genton, P., & McMenamin, J. (1998). Aggravation of seizures by antiepileptic drugs: what to do in clinical practice. *Epilepsia, 39*(Suppl. 3), S26–S29.

Genton, P., & McMenamin, J. (1998). Aggravation of seizures by antiepileptic drugs: what to do in clinical practice. *Epilepsia, 39*(Suppl 3), S26–S29. Used with permission.

Georgiev, D., Danieli, A., Ocepek, L., Novak, D., Zupancic-Kriznar, N., Trost, M., & Pirtosek Z. (2010). Othello syndrome in patients with Parkinson's disease. *Psychiatria Danubia, 22,* 94–98.

Gershon, S. (1982). Drug interactions in controlled clinical trials. *Journal of Clinical Psychiatry, 43,* 95–98.

Gerstner, T., Bell, N., & König S. (2008). Oral valproic acid for epilepsy—long-term experience in therapy and side effects. *Expert Opinion on Pharmacotherapy, 9,* 285–292

Gerstner, T., Teich, M., Bell, N., Longin, E., Dempfle, C. E., Brand, J., & König S. (2006). Valproate-associated coagulopathies are frequent and variable in children. *Epilepsia, 47,* 1136–1143.

Gex-Fabry, M., Balant-Gorgia, A. E., & Balant, L. P. (2003). Therapeutic drug monitoring of olanzapine: the combined effect of age, gender, smoking, and comedication. *Therapeutic Drug Monitoring, 25,* 46–53

Gibbons, R. D., Hur, K., Brown, C. H., & Mann, J. J. (2009). Relationship between antiepileptic drugs and suicide attempts in patients with bipolar disorder. *Archives of General Psychiatry, 66,* 1354–1360.

Gibbs, F. A. (1951). Ictal and non-ictal psychiatric disorders in temporal lobe epilepsy. *Journal of Nervous and Mental Disease, 113,* 522–528.

Gillman, P. K. (2005). Monoamine oxidase inhibitors, opioid analgesics and serotonin toxicity. *British Journal of Anaesthesia, 95,* 434–441

Gitlin, M. J. (1997). Venlafaxine, monoamine oxidase inhibitors, and the serotonin syndrome (letter). *Journal of Clinical Psychopharmacology, 17,* 66–67.

Glassman, A. H., Bigger, J. T., & Giardina, E. V. (1979). Clinical characteristics of imipramine-induced orthostatic hypotension. *Lancet, l,* 468–472.

Glassman, A. H., Johnson, L. L., & Giardina E. V. A. (1983). The use of imipramine in depressed patients with congestive heart failure. *Journal of the American Medical Association, 250,* 1977–2001.

Glauser, T. A., Cnaan, A., Shinnar, S., Hirtz, D. G., Dlugos, D., Masur, D., et al; Childhood Absence Epilepsy Study Group. (2010). Ethosuximide, valproic acid, and lamotrigine in childhood absence epilepsy. *New England Journal of Medicine, 362,* 790–799

Glue, P., Banfield, C. R., Perhach, J. L., Mather, G. G., Racha, J. K., & Levy, R. H. (1997). Pharmacokinetic interactions with felbamate. In vitro-in vivo correlation. *Clinical Pharmacokinetics, 33,* 214–224

Go, A. C., Golightly, L. K., Barber, G. R., & Barron, M. A. (2010). Linezolid interaction with serotonin reuptake inhibitors: report of two cases and incidence assessment. *Drug Metabolism and Drug Interactions, 25,* 41–47.

Goa, K. L., & Ward, A. (1986). Buspirone: a preliminary review of its pharmacologic properties and therapeutic efficacy an axiolytic. *Drugs, 32,* 114–129.

Goff, D. C. (1986). The stimulant challenge test in depression. *Journal of Clinical Psychiatry, 47,* 538–543.

Golino, P., Piscione, F., Willerson, J. T., Cappelli-Bigazzi, M., Focaccio, A., Villari, B., et al. (1991). Divergent effects of serotonin on coronary–artery dimensions and blood flow in patients with coronary atherosclerosis and control patients. *New England Journal of Medicine, 324,* 641–648.

Goodwin, F. K., & Jamison, K. R. (1990). *Manic-depressive illness.* New York: Oxford University Press.

Goulden, K. J., Dooley, J. M., Camfield, P. R., & Fraser, A. D. (1987). Clinical valproate toxicity induced by acetylsalicyclic acid. *Neurology, 37,* 1392–1394.

Grade, C., Redford, B., Chrostowski, J., Toussaint, L., & Blackwell, B. (1998). Methylphenidate in early post-stroke recovery: a double-blind, placebo-controlled study. *Archives of Physical Medicine and Rehabilitation, 79,* 1047–1050.

Grandjean, E. M., & Aubry, J. M. (2009). Lithium: updated human knowledge using an evidence-based approach: part III. clinical safety. *CNS Drugs, 23,* 397–418.

Grant, S., & Fitton, A. (1994). Risperidone. A review of its pharmacology and therapeutic potential in the treatment of schizophrenia. *Drugs, 48,* 253–273.

Greenberg, J., & Goss, J. B. (2009). Therapies for insomnia and comorbid chronic obstructive pulmonary disease with a focus on ramelteon (rozerem). *Pharmacy & Therapeutics, 34,* 502–508.

Greenblatt, D. J. (1991). Benzodiazepine hypnotics: sorting out the pharmacokinetic facts. *Journal of Clinical Psychiatry, 52*(9 Suppl):4–10.

Greenblatt, D. J., Harmatz, J. S., & Shader, R. I. (1991). Clinical pharmacokinetics of anxiolytics and hypnotics in the elderly. Part I. *Clinical Pharmacokinetics, 21,* 165–177.

Greenblatt, D. J., Harmatz, J. S., Shapiro, L., Engelhardt, N., Gouthro, T. A., & Shader, R. I. (1991). Sensitivity to triazolam in the elderly. *New England Journal of Medicine, 324,* 1691–1698.

Greenblatt, D. J., & Zammit, G. K. (2012). Pharmacokinetic evaluation of eszopiclone: clinical and therapeutic implications. *Expert Opinion on Drug Metabolism & Toxicology, 8,* 1609–1618.

Greenhill, S. D., Morgan, N. H., Massey, P. V., Woodhall, G. L., & Jones, R. S. (2012). Ethosuximide modifies network excitability in the rat entorhinal cortex via an increase in GABA release. *Neuropharmacology, 62,* 807–814.

Greenwald, B. S., Marin, D. B., & Silverman, S. M. (1986). Serotoninergic treatment of screaming and banging in dementia. *Lancet, 2,* 1464–1465.

Grimsley, S. R., Jann, M. W., Carter, J. G., D'Mello, A. P., & D'Souza, M. J. (1991). Increased carbamazepine plasma concentrations after fluoxetine coadministration. *Clinical Pharmacology & Therapeutics, 50,* 10–15.

Gringras, P., Gamble, C., Jones, A. P., Wiggs, L., Williamson, P. R., Sutcliffe, A., et al; MENDS Study Group. (2012). Melatonin for sleep problems in children with neurodevelopmental disorders: randomised double masked placebo controlled trial. *British Medical Journal, 345,* e6664.

Gu, J., & Huang, Y. (2009). Effect of concomitant administration of meropenem and valproic acid in an elderly Chinese patient. *American Journal of Geriatric Pharmacotherapy, 7,* 26–33.

Guerrini, R., Belmonte, A., Canapicchi, R., Casalini, C., & Perucca, E. (1998). Reversible pseudoatrophy of the brain and mental deterioration associated with valproate treatment. *Epilepsia, 39,* 27–32.

Gugger, J. J. (2011). Antipsychotic pharmacotherapy and orthostatic hypotension: identification and management. *CNS Drugs, 25,* 659–671.

Guo, S. L., Wu, T. J., Liu, C. C., Ng, C. C., Chien, C. C., & Sun, H. L. (2009). Meperidine-induced serotonin syndrome in a susceptible patient. *British Journal of Anaesthesia, 103,* 369–370.

Gustavson, L. E., & Carrigan, P. J. (1990). The clinical pharmacokinetics of single doses of estazolam. *American Journal of Medicine, 88*(Suppl 3A), 2S–5S.

Gyulai, L., Bowden, C. L., McElroy, S. L., Calabrese, J. R., Petty, F., Swann, A. C., et al. (2003). Maintenance efficacy of divalproex in the prevention of bipolar depression. *Neuropsychopharmacology, 28,* 1374–1382.

Haddad, P. M., Das, A., Keyhani, S., & Chaudhry, I. B. (2012). Antipsychotic drugs and extrapyramidal side effects in first episode psychosis: a systematic review of head-head comparisons. *Journal of Psychopharmacology, 26*(5 Suppl), 5–26.

Hamer, M., David Batty, G., Seldenrijk, A., & Kivimaki M. (2011). Antidepressant medication use and future risk of cardiovascular disease: the Scottish Health Survey. *European Heart Journal, 32*, 437–442.

Hanna, M. E., Lobao, C. B., & Stewart, J. T. (1990). Severe lithium toxicity associated with indapamide therapy (letter). *Journal of Clinical Psychopharmacology, 10*, 379.

Harder, J. L., Heung, M., Vilay, A. M., Mueller, B. A., & Segal, J. H. (2011). Carbamazepine and the active epoxide metabolite are effectively cleared by hemodialysis followed by continuous venovenous hemodialysis in an acute overdose. *Hemodialysis International, 15*, 412–415.

Hartz, A., & Ross, J. J. (2012). Cohort study of the association of hypnotic use with mortality in postmenopausal women. *British Medical Journal, 2*(5), pii: e001413.

Haslemo, T., Olsen, K., Lunde, H., & Molden, E. (2012). Valproic acid significantly lowers serum concentrations of olanzapine—an interaction effect comparable with smoking. *Therapeutic Drug Monitoring, 34*, 512–517.

Healy, D. G., Ingle, G. T., & Brown, P. (2009). Pregabalin- and gabapentin-associated myoclonus in a patient with chronic renal failure. *Movement Disorders, 24*, 2028–2029.

Helmuth, D., Ljaljevic, Z., Ramirez, L., & Meltzer, H. Y. (1989). Choreoathetosis induced by verapamil and lithium treatment. *Journal of Clinical Psychopharmacology, 9*, 454–455.

Henderson, L., Yue, Q. Y., Bergquist, C., Gerden, B., & Arlett, P. (2002). St John's wort (Hypericumperforatum): drug interactions and clinical outcomes. *British Journal of Clinical Pharmacology, 54*, 349–356.

Hersh, E. V., Pinto, A., & Moore, P. A. (2007). Adverse drug interactions involving common prescription and over-the-counter analgesic agents. *Clinical Therapeutics, 29*(Suppl), 2477–2497.

Heykants, J., Huang, M. L., Mannens, G., Meuldermans, W., Snoeck, E., Van Beijsterveldt, L., et al. (1994). The pharmacokinetics of risperidone in humans: a summary. *Journal of Clinical Psychiatry, 55*(Suppl. 5), 13–17.

Hill, L., & Lee, K. C. (2013). Pharmacotherapy considerations in patients with HIV and psychiatric disorders: focus on antidepressants and antipsychotics. *Annals of Pharmacotherapy, 47*, 75–89.

Holazo, A. A., Winkler, M. B., & Patel, I. H. (1988). Effects of age, gender and oral contraceptives on intramuscular midazolam pharmacokinetics. *Journal of Clinical Pharmacology, 28*, 104–105.

Honkola, J., Hookana, E., Malinen, S., Kaikkonen, K. S., Junttila, M. J., Isohanni, M., et al. (2012). Psychotropic medications and the risk of sudden cardiac death during an acute coronary event. *European Heart Journal, 33*, 745–751

Horgan, J. H., Proctor, J. D., Velandia, J., & Wasserman, A. J. (1973). Antiarrhythmic effect of lithium. *Archives Internationales de Pharmacodynamie et de Therapie, 206*, 105–112.

Hreinsson, J. P., Kalaitzakis, E., Gudmundsson, S., & Björnsson, E. S. (2013). Upper gastrointestinal bleeding: incidence, etiology and outcomes in a population-based setting. *Scandinavian Journal of Gastroenterology, 48*, 439–447

Huang, V., & Gortney, J. S. (2006). Risk of serotonin syndrome with concomitant administration of linezolid and serotonin agonists. *Pharmacotherapy, 26*, 1784–1793.

Huang, Z., Chen, Y. S., Yang, Z. L., & Liu, J. Y. (2012). Dexmedetomidine versus midazolam for the sedation of patients with non-invasive ventilation failure. *Internal Medicine, 51*, 2299–2305.

Hwang, A. S., & Magraw, R. M. (1989). Syndrome of inappropriate secretion of antidiuretic hormone due to fluoxetine (letter). *American Journal of Psychiatry, 146*, 399.

Ibáñez, L., Vidal, X., Ballarín, E., & Laporte J. R. (2005). Population-based drug-induced agranulocytosis. *Archives of Internal Medicine, 165*, 869–874.

Ieiri, I., Higuchi, S., Hirata, K., Yamada, H., & Aoyama, T. (1990). Analysis of the factors influencing anti-epileptic drug concentrations—valproic acid. *Journal of Clinical Pharmacology and Therapeutics, 15*, 351–363.

Ince, I., de Wildt, S. N., Peeters, M. Y., Murry, D. J., Tibboel, D., Danhof, M., & Knibbe, C. A. (2012). Critical illness is a major determinant of midazolam clearance in children aged 1 month to 17 years. *Therapeutic Drug Monitoring, 34*, 381–389.

Izzo, A. A., & Ernst, E. (2009). Interactions between herbal medicines and prescribed drugs: an updated systematic review. *Drugs, 69*, 1777–1798.

Jackson, M. J., & Turkington, D. (2005). Depression and anxiety in epilepsy. *Journal of Neurology, Neurosurgery, and Psychiatry, 76*(Suppl 1), i45–47.

Jacobsen, F. M. (1990). Low-dose trazodone as a hypnotic in patients treated with MAOIs and other psychotropics: a pilot study. *Journal of Clinical Psychiatry, 51*, 298–302.

Jaffe, C. M. (1977). First-degree atrioventricular block during lithium carbonate treatment. *American Journal of Psychiatry, 134*, 88–89.

Jamora, D., Lim, S. H., Pan, A., Tan, L., & Tan, E. K. (2007). Valproate-induced Parkinsonism in epilepsy patients. *Movement Disorders, 22*, 130–133.

Jankovic, S. M., & Dostic M. (2012). Choice of antiepileptic drugs for the elderly: possible drug interactions and adverse effects. *Expert Opinion on Drug Metabolism & Toxicology, 8*, 81–91.

Jann, M. W. (1988). Buspirone: an update on a unique anxiolytic agent. *Pharmacotherapy, 8*, 100–116.

Janowsky, D. S. (1988). *Journal of Clinical Psychopharmacology, 8*, 450.

Janowsky, E. C., & Janowsky, D. S. (1985). What precautions should be taken if a patient on an MAOI is scheduled to undergo anesthesia? *Journal of Clinical Psychopharmacology, 5*, 128–129.

Janssen Pharmaceuticals, Inc. (2012). InvegaR (extended-release paliperidone): product information. Titusville, New Jersey. http://www.invega.com/prescribing-information, last accessed 24 July 2014

Jeavons, P. M. (1983). Hepatoxicity in antiepileptic drugs. In J. Oxley, D. Janz, & H. Meinardi (Eds.), *Chronic toxicity of antiepileptic drugs* (pp. 1–46). New York: Raven Press.

Jefferson, J. W. (2010). A clinician's guide to monitoring kidney function in lithium-treated patients. *Journal of Clinical Psychiatry, 71*, 1153–1157.

Jenike, M. A. (1985). *Handbook of geriatric psychopharmacology* (pp. 73–87). Littleton, MA: PSG Publishing.

Jones, J. E., Hermann, B. P., Barry, J. J., Gilliam, F., Kanner, A. M., & Meador K. J. (2005). Clinical assessment of Axis I psychiatric morbidity in chronic epilepsy: a multicenter investigation. *Journal of Neuropsychiatry and Clinical Neurosciences, 17*, 172–179.

Jordà, E. G., Jiménez, A., Verdaguer, E., Canudas, A. M., Folch, J., Sureda, F. X., et al. (2005). Evidence in favour of a role for peripheral-type benzodiazepine receptor ligands in amplification of neuronal apoptosis. *Apoptosis, 10*(1), 91–104.

Joya, F. L., Kripke, D. F., Loving, R. T., Dawson, A., & Kline, L. E. (2009). Meta-analyses of hypnotics and infections: eszopiclone, ramelteon, zaleplon, and zolpidem. *Journal of Clinical Sleep Medicine, 5*, 377–383.

Kahn, N., Freeman, A., Juncos, J. L., Manning, D., & Watts, R. L. (1991). Clozapine is beneficial for psychosis in Parkinson's disease. *Neurology, 41*, 1699–1700.

Kales, A. (1990). Quazepam: hypnotic efficacy and side effects. *Pharmacotherapy, 10*, 1–12.

Kales, H. C., Valenstein, M., Kim, H. M., McCarthy, J. F., Ganoczy, D., Cunningham, F., & Blow, F. C. (2007). Mortality risk in patients with dementia treated with antipsychotics versus other psychiatric medications. *American Journal of Psychiatry, 164*, 1568–1576.

Kalgutkar, A. S., Vaz, A. D., Lame, M. E., Henne, K. R., Soglia, J., Zhao, S. X., et al. (2005). Bioactivation of the nontricyclic antidepressant nefazodone to a reactive quinone-imine species in human liver microsomes and recombinant cytochrome P450 3A4. *Drug Metabolism and Disposition, 33*, 243–253.

Kalinin, V. V. (2007). Suicidality and antiepileptic drugs: is there a link? *Drug Safety, 30*, 123–142.

Kallergis, E. M., Goudis, C. A., Simantirakis, E. N., Kochiadakis, G. E., & Vardas, P. E. (2012). Mechanisms, risk factors, and management of acquired long QT syndrome: a comprehensive review. *Scientific World Journal, 2012*, 212178.

Kane, J., Honigfeld, G., Singer J., et al. (1988). Clozapine for the treatment resistant schizophrenic. *Archives of General Psychiatry, 45*, 789–796.

Kane, J. M. (1990). Psychopharmacologic treatment issues. *Psychiatric Medicine, 8*, 111–112.

Kane, J. M., Sanchez, R., Perry, P. P., Jin, N., Johnson, B. R., Forbes, R. A., et al. (2012). Aripiprazole intramuscular depot as maintenance treatment in patients with schizophrenia: a 52-week, multicenter, randomized, double-blind, placebo-controlled study. *Journal of Clinical Psychiatry, 73*, 617–624.

Kang, D. Y., Park, S., Rhee, C. W., Kim, Y. J., Choi, N. K., Lee, J., & Park, B. J. (2012). Zolpidem use and risk of fracture in elderly insomnia patients. *Journal of Preventive Medicine and Public Health, 45*, 219–226.

Kanner, A. M. (2011). Is depression a risk factor of worse response to therapy in epilepsy? *Epilepsy Currents, 11*, 50–51.

Kantrowitz, J. T., & Citrome, L. (2012). Lurasidone for schizophrenia: what's different? *Expert Review of Neurotherapeutics, 12*, 265–273.

Kao, C. H., Sun, L. M., Liang, J. A., Chang, S. N., Sung, F. C., & Muo, C. H. (2012). Relationship of zolpidem and cancer risk: a Taiwanese population-based cohort study. *Mayo Clinic Proceedings, 87*, 430–436.

Kapoor, A., Iqbal, M., Petropoulos, S., Ho, H. L., Gibb, W., & Matthews, S. G. (2013). Effects of sertraline and fluoxetine on p-glycoprotein at barrier sites: in vivo and in vitro approaches. *PLoS One, 8*(2), e56525.

Kapur, S., Zipursky, R. B., & Remington, G. C. (1999). Clinical and theoretical implications of 5-HT2 and D2 receptor occupancy of clozapine, risperidone, and olanzapine in schizophrenia. *American Journal of Psychiatry, 156*, 286–293.

Karakaş Uğurlu, G., Onen, S., Bayındırlı, D., & Cayköylü, A. (2013) Acute dystonia after using single dose duloxetine: case report. *Psychiatry Investigation*, 2013 Mar; *10*(1), 95–7.

Kato, K., Yoshida, K., Suzuki, K., Murase, T., & Gotoh, M. (2005). Managing patients with an overactive bladder and glaucoma: a questionnaire survey of Japanese urologists on the use of anticholinergics. *BJU International, 95*, 98–101.

Kayrak, M., Ari, H., Duman, C., Gul, E. E., Ak, A., & Atalay, H. (2010). Lithium intoxication causing, S. T.segment elevation and wandering atrial rhythms in an elderly patient. *Cardiology Journal, 17*, 404–407.

Keegan D (1994). Risperidone: neurochemical, pharmacologic and clinical properties of a new antipsychotic drug. *Canadian Journal of Psychiatry, 39*, S46–S52.

Kelsey, J. L., & Hoffman, S. (1987). Risk factors for hip fracture. *New England Journal of Medicine, 316*, 404–406.

Kenneback, G., Bergfeldt, L., Vallin, H., et al. (1991). Electrophysiologic effects and clinical hazards of carbamazepine treatment for neurologic disorders in patients with abnormalities of the cardiac conduction system. *American Heart Journal, 121*, 1421–1429.

Ketter, T. A., Malow, B. A., Flamini, R., White, S. R., Post, R. M., & Theodore, W. H. (1994). Anticonvulsant withdrawal- emergent psychopathology. *Neurology, 44*, 55–61.

Ketter, T. A., Post, R. M., & Theodore, W. H. (1999). Positive and negative psychiatric effects of antiepileptic drugs in patients with seizure disorders. *Neurology, 53*(5 Suppl 2):S53–S67.

Khanna, P., Komossa, K., Rummel-Kluge, C., Hunger, H., Schwarz, S., El-Sayeh, H. G., & Leucht S. (2013). Aripiprazole versus other atypical antipsychotics for schizophrenia. *Cochrane Database of Systematic Reviews, 2*, CD006569.

Kibirige, D., Luzinda, K., & Ssekitoleko, R. (2013). Spectrum of lithium induced thyroid abnormalities: a current perspective. *Thyroid Research, 6*, 3.

Kiev, A., & Domantay, A. G. (1988). A study of buspirone coprescribed with bronchodilators in 82 anxious ambulatory patients. *Journal of Asthma, 25*, 281–284.

Kim, D., & Steinhart, B. (2010). Seizures induced by recreational abuse of bupropion tablets via nasal insufflation. *Canadian Journal of Emergency Medical Care, 12*, 158–161.

Kim, K. A., Oh, S. O., Park, P. W., & Park, J. Y. (2005). Effect of probenecid on the pharmacokinetics of carbamazepine in healthy subjects. *European Journal of Clinical Pharmacology, 61*, 275–280.

Kim, M. H., Hwang, J. W., Jeon, Y. T., & Do, S. H. (2012). Effects of valproic acid and magnesium sulphate on rocuronium requirement in patients undergoing craniotomy for cerebrovascular surgery. *British Journal of Anaesthesia, 109*, 407–412.

Kishimoto, T., De Hert, M., Carlson, H. E., Manu, P., & Correll, C. U. (2012). Osteoporosis and fracture risk in people with schizophrenia. *Current Opinion in Psychiatry, 25*, 415–429.

Knapp, J. E. (1987). Monoamine oxidase inhibitor interaction information. Medical update. Evansville, IN: Mead Johnson.

Koecheler, J. A., Canafax, D. M., Simmons, R. L., & Najarian, J. S. (1986). Lithium dosing in renal allograft recipients with changing renal function. *Drug Intelligence & Clinical Pharmacy, 20*, 623–624.

Koenig, S., Gerstner, T., Keller, A., Teich, M., Longin, E., & Dempfle, C. E. (2008). High incidence of vaproate–induced coagulation disorders in children receiving valproic acid: a prospective study. *Blood Coagulation & Fibrinolysis, 19*, 375–382.

Koliscak, L. P., & Makela, E. H. (2009). Selective serotonin reuptake inhibitor-induced akathisia. *Journal of the American Pharmacist Association, 49*, e28–36

Kondziella, D., Asztely, F. (2009). Don't be afraid to treat depression in patients with epilepsy! *Acta Neurolica Scandinavica, 119*, 75–80.

Korkmaz, A., Ma, S., Topal, T., Rosales-Corral, S., Tan, D. X., & Reiter, R. J. (2012). Glucose: a vital toxin and potential utility of melatonin in protecting against the diabetic state. *Molecular and Cellular Endocrinology, 349*, 128–137.

Kosten, T. N., & Forrest, J. N. (1986). Treatment of severe lithium-induced polyuria with amiloride. *American Journal of Psychiatry, 143*, 1563–1568.

Kripke, D. F., Langer, R. D., & Kline, L. E. (2012). Hypnotics' association with mortality or cancer: a matched cohort study. *British Medical Journal, Open 2*(1), e000850.

Kripke, D. F. (2008). Possibility that certain hypnotics might cause cancer in skin. *Journal of Sleep Research, 17*, 245–250.

Kumar, S., Kodela, S., Detweiler, J. G., Kim, K. Y., Detweiler, M. B. (2011). Bupropion-induced psychosis: folklore or a fact? A systematic review of the literature. *General Hospital Psychiatry, 33*, 612–617.

Kushnir, S. L. (1986). Lithium antidepressant combinations in treatment of depressed, physically ill geriatric patients. *American Journal of Psychiatry, 143*, 378–379.

Lader, M. (1989). Clinical pharmacology of antipsychotic drugs. *Journal of International Medical Research, 17*, 16–16.

LaFrance, W. C. Jr., Leaver, K., Stopa, E. G., Papandonatos, G. D., & Blum, A. S. (2010). Decreased serum BDNF levels in patients with epileptic and psychogenic nonepileptic seizures. *Neurology, 75*, 1285–1291.

Lanchote, V. L., Bonato, P. S., Campos, G. M., & Rodrigues, I. (1995). Factors influencing plasma concentrations of carbamazepine and carbamazepine-10,11-epoxide in epileptic children and adults. *Therapeutic Drug Monitoring, 17*, 47–52.

Lanier, J. B., Mote, M. B., Clay, E. C. (2011). Evaluation and management of orthostatic hypotension. *American Family Physician, 84*, 527–536.

Laplane, D., Attal, N., Sauron, B., de Billy, A., & Dubois, B. (1992). Lesions of basal ganglia due to disulfiram neurotoxicity. *Journal of Neurology, Neurosurgery, and Psychiatry, 55*, 925–929.

Lauterbach, E. C., Victoroff, J., Coburn, K. L., Shillcutt, S. D., Doonan, S. M., & Mendez, M. F. (2010). Psychopharmacological neuroprotection in neurodegenerative disease: assessing the preclinical data. *Journal of Neuropsychiatry and Clinical Neurosciences, 22*, 8–18.

Lazarus, J. H. (1986). *Endocrine and metabolic effects of lithium* (pp. 99–117). New York: Plenum.

Leach, J. P., Mohanraj, R., & Borland, W. (2012). Alcohol and drugs in epilepsy: pathophysiology, presentation, possibilities, and prevention. *Epilepsia, 53*(Suppl 4), 48–57.

Lee, S. A., Lee, J. K., & Heo, K. (2002). Coma probably induced by lorazepam-valproate interaction. *Seizure, 11*, 124–125.

Leipzig, R. M., Cumming, R. G., & Tinetti, M. E. (1999). Drugs and falls in older people: a systematic review and meta-analysis: I. Psychotropic drugs. *Journal of the American Geriatrics Society, 47*, 30–39.

Lemberger, L., Bergstrom, R. F., Wolen, R. L., Farid, N. A., Enas, G. G., & Aronoff, G. R. (1985). Fluoxetine: clinical pharmacology and physiologic disposition. *Journal of Clinical Psychiatry, 46,* 14–19.

Lemberger, L., Rowe, H., Bosomworth, J. C., Tenbarge, J. B., & Bergstrom, R. F. (1988). The effect of fluoxetine on the pharmacokinetics and psychomotor responses of diazepam. *Clinical Pharmacology & Therapeutics, 43,* 412–419.

Leonard, C. E., Bilker, W. B., Newcomb, C., Kimmel, S. E., & Hennessy, S. (2011). Antidepressants and the risk of sudden cardiac death and ventricular arrhythmia. *Pharmacoepidemiology and Drug Safety, 20,* 903–913.

Letmaier, M., Painold, A., Holl, A. K., Vergin, H., Engel, R., Konstantinidis, A., et al. (2012). Hyponatraemia during psychopharmacological treatment: results of a drug surveillance programme. *International Journal of Neuropsychopharmacology, 15,* 739–748.

Levenson, J. L. (1985). Neuroleptic malignant syndrome. *American Journal of Psychiatry, 142,* 1137–1145.

Levenson, J. L., Mishra, A., Bavernfeind, R. A., & Rea, R. F. (1986). Lithium treatment of mania in a patient with recurrent ventricular tachycardia. *Psychosomatics, 27,* 594–596.

Levine, A. (1988). Buspirone and agitation in head injury. *Brain Injury, 2,* 165–167.

Levine, M., Truitt, C. A., & O'Connor, A. D. (2011). Cardiotoxicity and serotonin syndrome complicating a milnacipran overdose. *Journal of Medical Toxicology, 7,* 312–316.

Levine, S., & Napoliello, M. J. (1988). A study of buspirone coprescribed with histamine H2-receptor antagonists in anxious outpatients. *International Clinical Psychopharmacology, 3,* 83–86.

Levy, N. B. (1987). Chronic renal disease, dialysis, and transplantation. In A. Stoudemire & B. S. Fogel (Eds.), *Principles of medical psychiatry* (Chap 27, pp. 583–594). Orlando, FL: Grune & Stratton.

Lheureux, P. E., & Hantson, P. (2009). Carnitine in the treatment of valproic acid-induced toxicity. *Clinical Toxicology (Philadelphia), 47,* 101–111.

Li, F., Chin, C., Wangsa, J., & Ho, J. (2012). Excretion and metabolism of milnacipran in humans after oral administration of milnacipran hydrochloride. *Drug Metabolism and Disposition, 40,* 1723–1735.

Lichtenbelt, B. J., Olofsen, E., Dahan, A., van Kleef, J. W., Struys, M. M., & Vuyk, J. (2010). Propofol reduces the distribution and clearance of midazolam. *Anesthesia and Analgesia, 110,* 1597–1606.

Lieberman, E., & Stoudemire, A. (1987). The use of tricyclic antidepressants in patients with glaucoma. *Psychosomatics, 28,* 145–148.

Lieberman, J. A., Cooper, T. B., Suckow, R. F., Steinberg, H., Borenstein, M., Brenner, R., & Kane, J. M. (1985). Tricyclic antidepressant and metabolite levels in chronic renal failure. *Clinical Pharmacology & Therapeutics, 37,* 301–307.

Lieberman, J. A., Kane, J. M., & Johns, C. A. (1989). Clozapine: guidelines for clinical management. *Journal of Clinical Psychiatry, 50,* 329–338.

Lieberman, J. A. (2007). Update on the safety considerations in the management of insomnia with hypnotics: incorporating modified-release formulations into primary care. *Primary Care Companion to the Journal of Clinical Psychiatry, 9,* 25–31.

Lilja, J. J., Kivistö, K. T., Backman, J. T., Lamberg, T. S., & Neuvonen, P. J. (1998). Grapefruit juice substantially increases plasma concentrations of buspirone. *Clinical Pharmacology & Therapeutics, 64,* 655–660

Lilly Research Laboratories. (1996). Data on file: Zyprexa™ (olanzapine). Indianapolis, IN: Eli Lilly Industries, Inc. http://pi.lilly.com/us/zyprexa-pi.pdf, last accessed 25 July 2014.

Lim, T. T., Ahmed, A., Itin, I., Gostkowski, M., Rudolph, J., Cooper, S., & Fernandez, H. H. (2013). Is 6 months of neuroleptic withdrawal sufficient to distinguish drug-induced parkinsonism from Parkinson's disease? *International Journal of Neuroscience, 123,* 170–174.

Lin, C. T., Lai, H. C., Lee, H. Y., Lin, W. H., Chang, C. C., Chu, T. Y., et al. (2008). Valproic acid resensitizes cisplatin-resistant ovarian cancer cells. *Cancer Science, 99,* 1218–1226.

Lindenmayer, J. P. (2010). Long-acting injectable antipsychotics: focus on olanzapine pamoate. *Neuropsychiatric Disease and Treatment, 6,* 261–267.

Lingam, V. R., Lazarus, L. W., Groves, L., et al. (1988). Methylphenidate in treating post-stroke depression. *Journal of Clinical Psychiatry, 49,* 151–153.

Lippman, S., Wagemaker, H., & Tuker D. (1981). A practice approach to management of lithium concurrent with hyponatremia, diuretic therapy, and/or chronic renal failure. *Journal of Clinical Psychiatry, 42,* 304–306.

Lippman, S. B., Manshadi, M. S., & Gultekin, A. (1984). Lithium in a patient with renal failure on hemodialysis. *Journal of Clinical Psychiatry, 45,* 444.

Lloyd, R. B., Perkins, R. E., & Schwartz, A. C. (2010). Choreoathetosis in the setting of lithium toxicity. *Psychosomatics, 51,* 529–531.

Loane, C., & Politis, M. (2012). Buspirone: what is it all about? *Brain Research, 1461,* 111–118

Lovrić, M., Božina, N., Hajnšek, S., Kuzman, M. R., Sporiš, D., Lalić, Z., et al. (2012). Association between lamotrigine concentrations and ABCB1 polymorphisms in patients with epilepsy. *Therapeutic Drug Monitoring, 34,* 518–525.

Luca, M., Prossimo, G., Messina, V., Luca, A., Romeo, S., & Calandra, C. (2013). Epidemiology and treatment of mood disorders in a day hospital setting from 1996 to 2007: an Italian study. *Neuropsychiatric Disease and Treatment, 9,* 169–176.

Luef, G., Chemelli, A., Birbamer, G., Aichner, F., & Bauer, G. (1994). Phenytoin overdosage and cerebellar atrophy in epileptic patients: clinical and MRI findings. *European Neurology, 34*(Suppl 1), 79–81.

Luscher, T. F., Tanner, F. C., Tschudi, M. R., & Noll, G. (1993). Endothelial dysfunction in coronary artery disease. *Annual Review of Medicine, 44,* 395–418.

Luszczki, J. J., Sawicka, K. M., Kozinska, J., Borowicz, K. K., & Czuczwar, S. J. (2007). Furosemide potentiates the anticonvulsant action of valproate in the mouse maximal electroshock seizure model. *Epilepsy Research, 76,* 66–72.

Lyons KE, Pahwa R. (2006) Efficacy and tolerability of levetiracetam in Parkinson disease patients with levodopa-induced dyskinesia. *Clinical Neuropharmacology, 29,* 148–153.

Ma, C. C., Shiah, I. S., Chang, S. W., Kao, Y. C., & Lee, W. K. (2012). Telmisartan-induced lithium intoxication in a patient with schizoaffective disorder (letter). *Psychiatry and Clinical Research, 66,* 165–166.

Machado, R. A., Espinosa, A. G., Melendrez, D., González, Y. R., García, V. F., & Rodríguez, Y. Q. (2011). Suicidal risk and suicide attempts in people treated with antiepileptic drugs for epilepsy. *Seizure, 20,* 280–284.

MacNeil, S., Hanson-Nortey, E., & Paschalis, C. (1975). Diuretics during lithium therapy. *Lancet, 1,* 1925–1926.

Madadi, P., Hildebrandt, D., Gong, I. Y., Schwarz, U. I., Ciszkowski, C., Ross, C. J., et al. (2010). Fatal hydrocodone overdose in a child: pharmacogenetics and drug interactions. *Pediatrics, 126,* e986–989.

Madhusoodanan, S., Alexeenko, L., Sanders, R., & Brenner, R. (2010). Extrapyramidal symptoms associated with antidepressants—a review of the literature and an analysis of spontaneous reports. *Annals of Clinical Psychiatry, 22,* 148–156.

Magnusson, M. O., Dahl, M. L., Cederberg, J., Karlsson, M. O., & Sandström, R. (2008). Pharmacodynamics of carbamazepine-mediated induction of CYP3A4, CYP1A2, and Pgp as assessed by probe substrates midazolam, caffeine, and digoxin. *Clinical Pharmacology & Therapeutics, 84,* 52–62.

Mago, R., Huege, S., Ahuja, N., & Kunkel, E. J. (2006). Zonisamide-induced suicidal ideation. *Psychosomatics, 47,* 68–69.

Maletzky, B. M., & Shore, J. H. (1978). Lithium treatment for psychiatric disorders. *Western Journal of Medicine, 128,* 488–498.

Mallikaarjun, S., Shoaf, S. E., Boulton, D. W., & Bramer, S. L. (2008). Effects of hepatic or renal impairment on the pharmacokinetics of aripiprazole. *Clinical Pharmacokinetics, 47,* 533–542.

Mancl, E. E., & Gidal, B. E. (2009). The effect of carbapenem antibiotics on plasma concentrations of valproic acid. *Annals of Pharmacotherapy, 43,* 2082–2087.

Mann, J. J., Aaron, S. F., Wilner, P. J., et al. (1989). A controlled study of the antidepressant efficacy and side effects of (-)deprenyl: a selective monoamine oxidase inhibitor. *Archives of General Psychiatry, 46*, 45–50.

Manoguerra, A. S., Erdman, A. R., Woolf, A. D., Chyka, P. A., Caravati, E. M., Scharman, E. J., et al. (2008). American Association of Poison Control Centers: Valproic acid poisoning: an evidence-based consensus guideline for out-of-hospital management. *Clinical Toxicology (Philadelphia), 46*, 661–676.

Manto, M. (2012). Toxic agents causing cerebellar ataxias. *Handbook of Clinical Neurology, 103*, 201–213.

Mantoan, L., & Walker, M. (2011). Treatment options in juvenile myoclonic epilepsy. *Current Treatment Options in Neurology, 13*, 355–370.

Marino, J., English, C., Caballero, J., & Harrington, C. (2012). The role of paliperidone extended release for the treatment of bipolar disorder. *Neuropsychiatric Disease and Treatment, 8*, 181–189.

Marras, C., Herrmann, N., Anderson, G. M., Fischer, H. D., Wang, X., & Rochon, P. A. (2012). Atypical antipsychotic use and parkinsonism in dementia: effects of drug, dose, and sex. *American Journal of Geriatric Pharmacotherapy, 10*, 381–389.

Masand, P., Murray, G. B., & Pickett, P. (1991). Psychostimulants in post-stroke depression. *Journal of Neuropsychiatry, 3*, 23–27.

Masand, P., Pickett, P., & Murray, G. B. (1991). Psychostimulants for secondary depression in medical illness. *Psychosomatics, 32*, 203–208.

Maschino, F., Hurault-Delarue, C., Chebbane, L., Fabry, V., Montastruc, J. L., & Bagheri, H. (2012). French Association of Regional Pharmacovigilance Centers: Bleeding adverse drug reactions (ADRs) in patients exposed to antiplatelet plus serotonin reuptake inhibitor drugs: analysis of the French Spontaneous Reporting Database for a controversial ADR. *European Journal of Clinical Pharmacology, 68*, 1557–1560.

Masmoudi, K., Gras-Champel, V., Masson, H., & Andréjak, M. (2006). Parkinsonism and/or cognitive impairment with valproic acid therapy: a report of ten cases. *Pharmacopsychiatry, 39*, 9–12.

Matson, A. M., & Thurlow, A. C. (1988). Hypotension and neurological sequelae following intramuscular midazolam (letter). *Anaesthesia, 43*, 896.

Max, J. E., Richards, L., Hamdan-Allen, G. (1995). Case study: antimanic effectiveness of dextroamphetamine in a brain-injured adolescent. *Journal of the American Academy of Child and Adolescent Psychiatry, 34*, 472–476.

May, T., & Rambeck, R. (1985). Serum concentrations of valproic acid: influence of dose and comedication. *Therapeutic Drug Monitoring, 7*, 387–390.

May, T. W., Rambeck, B., Neb, R., & Jürgens, U. (2007). Serum concentrations of pregabalin in patients with epilepsy: the influence of dose, age, and comedication. *Therapeutic Drug Monitoring, 29*, 789–794.

McDonnell, D. P., Detke, H. C., Bergstrom, R. F., Kothare, P., Johnson, J., Stickelmeyer, M., et al. (2010). Post-injection delirium/sedation syndrome in patients with schizophrenia treated with olanzapine long-acting injection, II: investigations of mechanism. *BMC Psychiatry, 10*, 45.

McElroy, S. L., Keck, P. E. Jr, Friedman, L. M. (1995). Minimizing and managing antidepressant side effects. *Journal of Clinical Psychiatry, 56*(Suppl 2), 49–55.

McElroy, S. L., Keck, P. E., Pope, H. G., & Hudson, J. I. (1989). Valproate in psychiatric disorders: literature review and clinical guidelines. *Journal of Clinical Psychiatry, 50*(suppl), 23–29.

McFadden, E. P., Clarke, J. G., Davies, G. J., Kaski, J. C., Haider, A. W., & Maseri, A. (1991). Effect of intracoronary serotonin on coronary vessels in patients with stable angina and patients with variant angina. *New England Journal of Medicine, 324*, 648–654.

McGinness, J., Kishimoto, A., & Hollister, L. E. (1990). Avoiding neurotoxicity with lithium-carbamazepine combinations. *Psychopharmacology Bulletin, 26*, 181–184.

McIntyre, R. S., Soczynska, J. K., Konarski, J. Z., & Kennedy, S. H. (2006). The effect of antidepressants on glucose homeostasis and insulin sensitivity: synthesis and mechanisms. *Expert Opinion on Drug Safety, 5*, 157–168.

McIntyre, R. S. (2011). Asenapine: a review of acute and extension phase data in bipolar disorder. CNS Neurosci Ther 17, 645–648.

Medical Letter. (1998). Citalopram for depression. *Medical Letter, 40*, 113–114.

Meldrum, B. S. (1994). The role of glutamate in epilepsy and other CNS disorders. *Neurology, 44*(Suppl. 8), S14–S32.

Meltzer, H. Y., & Fleming, R. (1982). Effect of buspirone on prolactin and growth hormone secretion in laboratory rodents and man. *Journal of Clinical Psychiatry, 43*, 76–79.

Mendelson, W. B. (1987). Pharmacotherapy of insomnia. *Psychiatric Clinics of North America, 10*, 555–563.

Mendoza, R., Djenderedjian, A. H., Adams, J., & Ananth, J. (1987). Midazolam in acute psychotic patients with hyperarousal. *Journal of Clinical Psychiatry, 48*, 291–292.

Merritt, H. H., & Putnam, T. J. (1938). Sodium diphenyl hydantoinate in the treatment of convulsive disorders. *Journal of the American Medical Association, 111*, 1068–1073.

Mets, M. A., de Vries, J. M., de Senerpont Domis, L. M., Volkerts, E. R., Olivier, B., & Verster, J. C. (2011). Next–day effects of ramelteon (8 mg), zopiclone (7.5 mg), and placebo on highway driving performance, memory functioning, psychomotor performance, and mood in healthy adult subjects. *Sleep, 34*, 1327–1334.

Meyer, L. C., Hetem, R. S., Fick, L. G., Mitchell, D., & Fuller A. (2010). Effects of serotonin agonists and doxapram on respiratory depression and hypoxemia in etorphine-immobilized impala (*Aepyceros melampus*). *Journal of Wildlife Diseases, 46*, 514–524.

Miceli, J. J., Glue, P., Alderman, J., & Wilner, K. (2007). The effect of food on the absorption of oral ziprasidone. *Psychopharmacology Bulletin, 40*, 58–68.

Michaelis, M., Ha, T. A., Doerr, H. W., & Cinatl, J. Jr. (2008). Valproic acid interferes with antiviral treatment in human cytomegalovirus-infected endothelial cells. *Cardiovascular Research, 77*, 544–550.

Michaelis, M., Ha, T.A., Doerr H. W., & Cinatl, J. Jr. (2008). Valproic acid interferes with antiviral treatment in human cytomegalovirus-infected endothelial cells. *Cardiovascular Research, 77*, 544–550.

Miguel, C., & Albuquerque, E. (2011). Drug interaction in psycho-oncology: antidepressants and antineoplastics. *Pharmacology, 88*, 333–339.

Miller, A. D., Prost, V. M., Bookstaver, P. B., & Gaines, K. J. (2010). Topiramate-induced myoclonus and psychosis during migraine prophylaxis. *American Journal of Health-System Pharmacy, 67*, 1178–1180.

Miller, D. D., Caroff, S. N., Davis, S. M., Rosenheck, R. A., McEvoy, J. P., Saltz, B. L., et al.; Clinical Antipsychotic Trials of Intervention Effectiveness (CATIE). Investigators. (2008). Extrapyramidal side-effects of antipsychotics in a randomised trial. *British Journal of Psychiatry, 193*, 279–288.

Minassian, A., & Young, J. W. (2010). Evaluation of the clinical efficacy of asenapine in schizophrenia. *Expert Opinion on Pharmacotherapy, 11*, 2107–2115.

Mir, O., Durand, J. P., Boudou-Rouquette, P., Giroux, J., Coriat, R., Cessot, A., et al. (2012). Interaction between serotonin reuptake inhibitors, 5-HT3 antagonists, and NK1 antagonists in cancer patients receiving highly emetogenic chemotherapy: a case-control study. *Supportive Care in Cancer, 20*, 2235–2239.

Mitchell, J. E., & MacKenzie, T. B. (1982). Cardiac effects of lithium therapy in man: a review. *Journal of Clinical Psychiatry, 43*, 47–51.

Mittal, V., Kurup, L., Williamson, D., Muralee, S., & Tampi, R. R. (2011). Risk of cerebrovascular adverse events and death in elderly patients with dementia when treated with antipsychotic medications: a literature review of evidence. *American Journal of Alzheimer's Disease and Other Dementias, 26*, 10–28.

Miura, M., Otani, K., & Ohkubo, T. (2005). Identification of human cytochrome P450 enzymes involved in the formation of 4-hydroxyestazolam from estazolam. *Xenobiotica, 35*, 455–465.

Möhler, H. (2012). The GABA system in anxiety and depression and its therapeutic potential. *Neuropharmacology, 62*, 42–53.

Molitor, J. A., Gammans, R. E., Carroll, C. M., et al. (1985). Effect of buspirone on mixed function oxidase in rats. *Federation Proceedings, 44,* 1257.

Moll, J. L., & Brown, C. S. (2011). The use of monoamine pharmacological agents in the treatment of sexual dysfunction: evidence in the literature. J Sex Med 8, 956–970

Moncada, L. V. (2011). Management of falls in older persons: a prescription for prevention. *American Family Physician, 84,* 1267–1276.

Moran, M. G., & Stoudemire, A. (1992). Sleep disorders in the medically ill patient. *Journal of Clinical Psychiatry, 53*(6, Suppl), 29–36.

Morrison, E. K., & Rowe, A. S. (2012). Probable drug-drug interaction leading to serotonin syndrome in a patient treated with concomitant buspirone and linezolid in the setting of therapeutic hypothermia. *Journal of Clinical Pharmacy and Therapeutics, 37,* 610–613

Mosholder, A. D., Gelperin, K., Hammad, T. A., Phelan, K., & Johann-Liang, R. (2009). Hallucinations and other psychotic symptoms associated with the use of attention-deficit/hyperactivity disorder drugs in children. *Pediatrics, 123,* 611–616.

Mukhopadhyay, D., Gokulkrishnan, L., & Mohanaruban, K. (2001). Lithium-induced nephrogenic diabetes insipidus in older people. *Age and Ageing, 30,* 347–350.

Mula, M., & Monaco, F. (2009). Antiepileptic drugs and psychopathology of epilepsy: an update. *Epileptic Disorders, 11,* 1–9.

Nadkarni, S., Arnedo, V., & Devinsky, O. (2007). Psychosis in epilepsy patients. *Epilepsia, 48*(Suppl 9), 17–19.

Nagler, E. V., Webster, A. C., Vanholder, R., & Zoccali, C. (2012). Antidepressants for depression in stage 3-5 chronic kidney disease: a systematic review of pharmacokinetics, efficacy and safety with recommendations by European Renal Best Practice (ERBP). *Nephrology, Dialysis, Transplantation, 27,* 3736–3745.

Naguib, M., & Koorn, R. (2002). Interactions between psychotropics, anaesthetics and electroconvulsive therapy: implications for drug choice and patient management. *CNS Drugs, 16,* 229–247.

Nair, P. P., Kalita, J., & Misra, U. K. (2011). Status epilepticus: why, what, and how. *Journal of Postgraduate Medicine, 57,* 242–252.

Nardi, A. E., Machado, S., Almada, L. F., Paes, F., Silva, A. C., Marques, R. J., et al. (2013). Clonazepam for the treatment of panic disorder. *Current Drug Targets, 14,* 353–364.

Nelson, E. M., & Philbrick, A. M. (2012). Avoiding serotonin syndrome: the nature of the interaction between tramadol and selective serotonin reuptake inhibitors. *Annals of Pharmacotherapy, 46,* 1712–1716.

Nelson, J. C. (1997). Safety and tolerability of the new antidepressants. *Journal of Clinical Psychiatry, 58*(Suppl. 6):26–31.

Ney, G. C., Lantos, G., Barr, W. B., & Schaul, N. (1994). Cerebellar atrophy in patients with long-term phenytoin exposure and epilepsy. *Archives of Neurology, 51,* 767–771.

Neyns, B., Hoorens, A., & Stupp, R. (2008). Valproic acid related idiosyncratic drug induced hepatotoxicity in a glioblastoma patient treated with temozolomide. *Acta Neurologica Belgica, 108,* 131–134.

Ng, B. K., & Cameron, A. J. (2010). The role of methylene blue in serotonin syndrome: a systematic review. *Psychosomatics, 51,* 194–200.

Nordstrom, A. L., Nyberg, S., Olsson, H., & Farde, L. (1998). Positron emission tomography finding of a high striatal D2 receptor occupancy in olanzapine-treated patients. *Archives of General Psychiatry, 55,* 283–284.

Novartis. (1997). Clozaril® (clozapine): prescribing information. Sandoz Pharmaceuticals Corporation, East Hanover, New Jersey.

Novartis. (2013). FANAPT (iloperidone): prescribing information. East Hanover, NJ. Novartis Pharmaceuticals Corp; January 2013.

O'Connell, M., & Bernard, A. (2012). A serious cause of panic attack. *Case Reports in Emergency Medicine, 2012,* 393275.

Obach, R. S., & Ryder, T. F. (2010). Metabolism of ramelteon in human liver microsomes and correlation with the effect of fluvoxamine on ramelteon pharmacokinetics. *Drug Metabolism and Disposition, 38,* 1381–1391.

Oderda, L. H., Young, J. R., Asche, C. V., & Pepper, G. A. (2012). Psychotropic-related hip fractures: meta-analysis of first-generation and second-generation antidepressant and antipsychotic drugs. *Annals of Pharmacotherapy, 46,* 917–928.

Oliveira, J. L., Silva Júnior, G. B., Abreu, K. L., Rocha Nde, A., Franco, L. F., Araújo, S. M., & Daher Ede, F. (2010). Lithium nephrotoxicity. *Revista da Associacao Medica Brasileira, 56,* 600–606.

Oliver, P., Keen, J., Rowse, G., & Mathers, N. (2001). Deaths from drugs of abuse in Sheffield, 1998: the role of prescribed medication. *British Journal of General Practice, 51,* 394–396

Osser, D. N., Naharian, D., Berman, I., et al. (1998). Olanapine increases weight and triglyceride levels. Abstract #NR688, American Psychiatric Association Annual Meeting, Toronto.

Owens, D. G. (1994). Extrapyramidal side effects and tolerability of risperidone: a review. *Journal of Clinical Psychiatry, 55*(5, Suppl.), 29–35.

Özdemir, A., Aksoy-Poyraz, C., & Kılıç-Yener E. (2012). Possible paliperidone-induced neuroleptic malignant syndrome: a case report. *Journal of Neuropsychiatry and Clinical Neurosciences, 24,* E22–23.

Ozhasenekler, A., Gökhan, S., Güloğlu, C., Orak, M., & Üstündağ, M. (2012). Benefit of hemodialysis in carbamazepine intoxications with neurological complications. *European Review for Medical and Pharmacological Sciences, 16*(Suppl 1), 43–47.

Pacher, P., & Kecskemeti, V. (2004). Cardiovascular side effects of new antidepressants and antipsychotics: new drugs, old concerns? *Current Pharmaceutical Design, 10*(20), 2463–2475.

Palmer, S. E., McLean, R. M., Ellis, P. M., & Harrison-Woolrych, M. (2008). Life-threatening clozapine-induced gastrointestinal hypomotility: an analysis of 102 cases. *Journal of Clinical Psychiatry, 69,* 759–768.

Paraskevaidis, I., Palios, J., Parissis, J., Filippatos, G., & Anastasiou-Nana, M. (2012). Treating depression in coronary artery disease and chronic heart failure: what's new in using selective serotonin re-uptake inhibitors? *Cardiovascular & Hematological Agents in Medical Chemistry, 10,* 109–115.

Pariente, A., Fourrier-Réglat, A., Ducruet, T., Farrington, P., Béland, S. G., Dartigues, J. F., et al. (2012). Antipsychotic use and myocardial infarction in older patients with treated dementia. *Archives of Internal Medicine, 172,* 648–653.

Park, Y. M., Jung, Y. K. (2010). Manic switch and serotonin syndrome induced by augmentation of paroxetine with methylphenidate in a patient with major depression (letter). *Progress in Neuropsychopharmacology and Biological Psychiatry, 34*(4), 719–720.

Parker, G., & Brotchie, H. (2010). Do the old psychostimulant drugs have a role in managing treatment-resistant depression? *Acta Psychiatrica Scandinavica, 121,* 308–314.

Partti, K., Heliövaara, M., Impivaara, O., Perälä J, Saarni, S. I., Lönnqvist, J., & Suvisaari, J. M. (2010). Skeletal status in psychotic disorders: a population-based study. *Psychosomatic Medicine, 72,* 933–940.

Pato, M. T., & Murphy, D. L. (1991). Sustained plasma concentrations of fluoxetine and/or norfluoxetine four and eight weeks after fluoxetine discontinuation. *Journal of Clinical Psychopharmacology, 11,* 224–225.

Patorno, E., Bohn, R. L., Wahl, P. M., Avorn, J., Patrick, A. R., Liu, J., & Schneeweiss, S. (2010). Anticonvulsant medications and the risk of suicide, attempted suicide, or violent death. *Journal of the American Medical Association, 303,* 1401–1409.

Patsalos, P. N., & Duncan, J. D. (1993). Antiepileptic drugs. A review of clinically significant drug interactions. *Drug Safety, 9,* 156–184.

Patterson, J. F. (1988). Alprazolam dependency: use of clonazepam for withdrawal. *Southern Medical Journal, 8,* 830–836.

Patterson, J. F. (1988). Akathisia associated with buspirone. *Journal of Clinical Psychopharmacology, 8,* 296–297.

Paul, M. A., Gray, G., Kenny, G., & Pigeau, R. A. (2003). Impact of melatonin, zaleplon, zopiclone, and temazepam on psychomotor performance. *Aviation, Space, and Environmental Medicine, 74,* 1263–1270.

Pellock, J. M. (1994). The clinical efficacy of lamotrigine as an antiepileptic drug. *Neurology, 44*(Suppl. 8), S29–S35.

Perkins, D. O., & McCLure, R. K. (1998). Hypersalivation coincident with olanzapine treatment. *American Journal of Psychiatry, 7,* 993–994.

Perucca, E., Gram, L., Avanzini, G., & Dulac, O. (1998). Antiepileptic drugs as a cause of worsening seizures. *Epilepsia, 39*, 5–17.

Perucca, E. (2006). Clinically relevant drug interactions with antiepileptic drugs. *British Journal of Clinical Pharmacology, 61*, 246–255.

Perucca, E. (2006). Clinically relevant drug interactions with antiepileptic drugs. *British Journal of Clinical Pharmacology, 61*, 246–255.

Petraglio, G., Bartolini, M., Branduardi, D., Andrisano, V., Recanatini, M., Gervasio, F. L., et al. (2008). The role of Li+, Na+, and K+ in the ligand binding inside the human acetylcholinesterase gorge. *Proteins, 70*, 779–785.

Peuskens, J. (1995). Risperidone in the treatment of patients with chronic schizophrenia: a multi-national, multi-centre, double-blind, parallel group study versus haloperidol. *British Journal of Psychiatry, 166*, 712–726.

Pfeiffer, R. F., Kang, J., Granber, B., Hofman, R., & Wilson, J. (1990). Clozapine for psychosis in parkinsonian patients with dopaminomimetic psychosis. *Movement Disorders, 5*, 239–242.

Phillipson, M., Moranville, J. T., Jeste, D. V., & Harris, M. J. (1990). Antipsychotics. *Clinics in Geriatric Medicine, 6*, 411–422.

Pineda, E., Shin, D., Sankar, R., & Mazarati, A. M. (2010). Comorbidity between epilepsy and depression: experimental evidence for the involvement of serotonergic, glucocorticoid, and neuroinflammatory mechanisms. *Epilepsia, 51*(Suppl 3), 110–114.

Pinner, E., & Rich, C. (1988). Effects of trazodone on aggressive behavior in seven patients with organic mental disorders. *American Journal of Psychiatry, 145*, 1295–1296.

Pisani, F. (1992). Influence of co-medication on the metabolism of valproate. *Pharmaceutisch Weekblad. Scientific Edition, 14*, 108–113.

Pisani, M. A., Murphy, T. E., Araujo, K. L. B., & Van Ness, P. H. (2010). Factors associated with persistent delirium following ICU admission in an older medical patient population. *Journal of Critical Care, 25*, 540.e1–540.e7.

Pisani, F., Fazio A., Orteri G., Ruello, C., Gitto, C., Russo, F., & Perucca, E. (1986). Sodium valproate and valpromide: Differential interactions with carbamazepine in epileptic patients. *Epilepsia, 27*, 548–552.

Pizzi, C., Santarella, L., Costa, M. G., Manfrini, O., Flacco, M. E., Capasso, L., et al. (2012). Pathophysiological mechanisms linking depression and atherosclerosis: an overview. *Journal of Biological Regulators and Homeostatic Agents, 26*, 775–782.

Polasek, T. M., Elliot, D. J., Somogyi, A. A., Gillam, E. M., Lewis, B. C., & Miners, J. O. (2006). An evaluation of potential mechanism-based inactivation of human drug metabolizing cytochromes P450 by monoamine oxidase inhibitors, including isoniazid. *British Journal of Clinical Pharmacology, 61*, 570–584.

Polumbo, R. A., Branzi, A., Schroeder, J. S., & Harrison, D. C. (1973). The antiarrhythmic effect of lithium chloride for experimental ouabain-induced arrhythmias. *Proceedings of the Society for Experimental Biology and Medicine, 142*, 1200–1204.

Poon, I. O., & Braun, U. (2005). High prevalence of orthostatic hypotension and its correlation with potentially causative medications among elderly veterans. *Journal of Clinical Pharmacy and Therapeutics, 30*, 173–178.

Pope, H. G., McElroy, S. L., Keck, P. E., & Hudson, J. I. (1991). Valproate in the treatment of acute mania. A placebo-controlled study. *Archives of General Psychiatry, 48*, 62–68.

Port, F. K., Kroll, P. D., & Rozenzweig, J. (1979). Lithium therapy during maintenance hemodialysis. *Psychosomatics, 20*, 130–131.

Poser, W., Poser, S., Roscher, D., & Argyrakis, A. (1983). Do benzodiazepines cause cerebral atrophy (letter)? *Lancet, 1*(8326 Pt 1), 715.

Pourcher, E., Gomez-Mancilla, B., & Bédard, P. J. (1992). Ethosuximide and tremor in Parkinson's disease: a pilot study. *Movement Disorders, 7*, 132–136.

Pratt, N., Roughead, E. E., Salter, A., & Ryan, P. (2012). Choice of observational study design impacts on measurement of antipsychotic risks in the elderly: a systematic review. *BMC Medical Research Methodology, 12*, 72.

Preskorn, S. H. (2007). Neuroleptic malignant syndrome resulting from a complex drug-drug interaction: "I don't see 'em!" *Journal of Psychiatric Practice, 13*, 328–333.

Presne, C., Fakhouri, F., Noël, L. H., Stengel, B., Even, C., Kreis, H., et al. (2003). Lithium-induced nephropathy: Rate of progression and prognostic factors. *Kidney International, 64*, 585–592.

Price, W., & Giannini, R. J. (1986). Neurotoxicity caused by lithium verapamil synergism. *Journal of Clinical Pharmacology, 26*, 717–719.

Prien, R. F., & Gelenberg, A. J. (1989). Alternatives to lithium for preventive treatment of bipolar disorder. *American Journal of Psychiatry, 146*, 840–848.

Puzynski, S., & Klosiewicz, I. (1984). Valproic acid amide in the treatment of affective and schizoaffective disorders. *Journal of Affective Disorders, 6*, 115–121.

Ragheb, M. (1990). The clinical significance of lithium-nonsteroidal and inflammatory drug interactions. *Journal of Clinical Psychopharmacology, 10*, 350–354.

Raju, P. M., Walker, R. W., & Lee, M. A. (2007). Dyskinesia induced by gabapentin in idiopathic Parkinson's disease. *Movement Disorders, 22*, 288–289.

Rakic, I. A., Miljkovic, B., Todorovic, D., Timotijevic, I., & Pokrajac, M. (2009). Moclobemide monotherapy vs. combined therapy with valproic acid or carbamazepine in depressive patients: a pharmacokinetic interaction study. *British Journal of Clinical Pharmacology, 67*, 199–208.

Rambeck, B., Salke-Treumann, A., May, T., & Boenigk, H. E. (1990). Valproic acid-induced carbamazepine-10,11-epoxide toxicity in children and adolescents. *European Neurology, 30*, 79–83.

Ratey, J. J., Sovner, R., Mikkelsen, E., & Chmielinski, H. E. (1989). Buspirone therapy for maladaptive behavior and anxiety in developmentally disabled person. *Journal of Clinical Psychiatry, 50*, 382–384.

Ray, W. A., Griffin, M. R., & Downey, M. (1989). Benzodiazepines of long and short life elimination and the risk of hip fracture. *Journal of the American Medical Association, 262*, 3303–3307.

Ray, W. A., Griffin, M. R., & Malcolm, E. (1991). Cyclic antidepressants and the risk of hip fracture. *Archives of Internal Medicine, 151*, 754–756.

Ray, W. A., Meredith, S., Thapa, P. B., Meador, K. G., Hall, K., & Murray, K. T. (2001). Antipsychotics and the risk of sudden cardiac death. *Archives of General Psychiatry, 58*, 1161–1167.

Realmuto, G. M., August, G. J., & Garfinkel, B. D. (1989). Clinical effect of buspirone in autistic children. *Journal of Clinical Psychopharmacology, 9*, 122–125.

Redenbaugh, J. E., Sato, S., Penry, J. K., Dreifuss, F. E., & Kupferberg, H. J. (1980). Sodium valproate: pharmacokinetics and effectiveness in treating intractable seizures. *Neurology, 30*, 1–6.

Redington, K., Wells, C., & Petito, F. (1992). Erythromycin and valproate interaction (letter). *Annals of Internal Medicine, 116*, 877–878.

Reed, S. M., Wise, M. G., & Timmerman, I. (1989). Choreoathetosis: a sign of lithium toxicity. *Journal of Neuropsychiatry, 1*, 57–60.

Reikvam, A. G., Hustad, S., Reikvam, H., Apelseth, T. O., Nepstad, I., & Hervig, T. A. (2012). The effects of selective serotonin reuptake inhibitors on platelet function in whole blood and platelet concentrates. *Platelets, 23*, 299–308.

Rej, S., Abitbol, R., Looper, K., & Segal, M. (2013). Chronic renal failure in lithium-using geriatric patients: effects of lithium continuation versus discontinuation-a 60-month retrospective study. *International Journal of Geriatric Psychiatry, 28*, 450–453.

Ren, X., Meng, F., Yin, J., Li, G., Li, X., Wang, C., & Herrler, G. (2011). Action mechanisms of lithium chloride on cell infection by transmissible gastroenteritis coronavirus. *PLoS One, 6*, e18669.

Rickels, K., Freeman, F., & Sondheimer, S. (1989). Buspirone in treatment of premenstrual syndrome. *Lancet, 1*, 777.

Ridsdale, L., Charlton, J., Ashworth, M., Richardson, M. P., & Gulliford, M. C. (2011). Epilepsy mortality and risk factors for death in epilepsy: a population-based study. *British Journal of General Practice, 61*, e271–e278.

Rifkind, A. B. (2006). CYP1A in TCDD toxicity and in physiology-with particular reference to CYP dependent arachidonic acid metabolism and other endogenous substrates. *Drug Metabolism Reviews, 38*, 291–335.

Ristić, A. J., Vojvodić, N., Janković, S., Sindelić, A., & Sokić, D. (2006). The frequency of reversible Parkinsonism and cognitive decline associated with valproate treatment: a study of 364 patients with different types of epilepsy. *Epilepsia*, *47*, 2183–2185.

Rizack, M. A., & Hillman, C. D. (1989). Tyramine table. In, M. A. Rizack & C. D. Hillman (Eds.), *The medical letter handbook of adverse drug interactions* (p. 143). New York: The Medical Letter.

Roberts, G. M., Majoie, H. J., Leenen, L. A., Bootsma, H. P., Kessels, A. G., Aldenkamp, A. P., & Leonard, B. E. (2005). Ketter's hypothesis of the mood effects of antiepileptic drugs coupled to the mechanism of action of topiramate and levetiracetam. *Epilepsy & Behavior*, *6*, 366–372

Roberts, H. E., Dean, R. C., & Stoudemire, A. (1989). Clozapine treatment of psychosis in Parkinson's disease. *Journal of Neuropsychiatry*, and Clin Neurosciences, 1, 190–192.

Roberts, R. L., Joyce, P. R., Mulder, R. T., Begg, E. J., & Kennedy, M. A. (2002). A common P-glycoprotein polymorphism is associated with nortriptyline-induced postural hypotension in patients treated for major depression. *Pharmacogenomics Journal*, *2*, 191–196.

Robinson, D. S., Alms, D. R., Shrotiya, R. C., Messina, M., & Wickramaratne, P. (1989). Serotonergic anxiolytics and treatment of depression. *Psychopathology*, *22*(suppl.1), 27–36.

Rochel, M., & Ehrenthal, W. (1983). Hematological side effects of valproic acid. In J. Oxley, D. Janz, & H. Meinardi (Eds.), *Chronic toxicity of antiepileptic drugs* (Chap 8, pp. 101–104). New York: Raven Press.

Rodriguez de la Torre, B., Dreher, J., Malevany, I., Bagli, M., Kolbinger, M., Omran, H., et al. (2001). Serum levels and cardiovascular effects of tricyclic antidepressants and selective serotonin reuptake inhibitors in depressed patients. *Therapeutic Drug Monitoring*, *23*, 435–440.

Rogers, M. P. (1985). Rheumatoid arthritis: psychiatric aspects and use of psychotropics. *Psychosomatics*, *26*, 915–925.

Rolan, P. E. (2012). Drug interactions with triptans: which are clinically significant? *CNS Drugs*, *26*, 949–957.

Roose, S. P., Dalack, G. W., Glassman, A. H., et al. (1991b). Cardiovascular effects of bupropion in depressed patients with heart disease. *American Journal of Psychiatry*, *148*, 512–516.

Roose, S. P., Glassman, A. H., & Giardina, E. G. V. (1986). Nortriptyline in depressed patients with left ventricular impairment. *Journal of the American Medical Association*, *256*, 3253–3257.

Roose, S. P., Glassman, A. H., Giardina, E. G., et al. (1987b). Cardiovascular effects of imipramine and bupropion in depressed patients with congestive heart failure. *Journal of Clinical Psychopharmacology*, *7*, 247–251.

Roose, S. P., Glassman, A. H., Giardina, E. G. V., et al. (1987a). Tricyclic antidepressants in depressed patients with cardiac conduction disease. *Archives of General Psychiatry*, *44*, 273–275.

Roose, S. P., & Miyazaki, M. (2005). Pharmacologic treatment of depression in patients with heart disease. *Psychosomatic Medicine*, *67*(Suppl 1), S54–S57.

Rosenberg, P. B., Ahmed, I., & Hurwitz, S. (1991). Methylphenidate in depressed medically ill patients. *Journal of Clinical Psychiatry*, *52*, 263–267.

Rosenstein, D. R., Takeshita, J., & Nelson, J. C. (1991). Fluoxetine-induced elevation and prolongation of tricyclic levels in overdose (letter to the editor). *American Journal of Psychiatry*, *148*, 807.

Rotondo, A., Bosco, D., Plastino, M., Consoli, A., & Bosco, F. (2010). Clozapine for medication-related pathological gambling in Parkinson disease. *Movement Disorders*, *25*, 1994–1995.

Roughead, E. E., Kalisch, L. M., Barratt, J. D., & Gilbert, A. L. (2010). Prevalence of potentially hazardous drug interactions amongst Australian veterans. *British Journal of Clinical Pharmacology*, *70*, 252–257.

Rummel-Kluge, C., Komossa, K., Schwarz, S., Hunger, H., Schmid, F., Kissling, W., et al. (2012). Second-generation antipsychotic drugs and extrapyramidal side effects: a systematic review and meta-analysis of head-to-head comparisons. *Schizophrenia Bulletin*, *38*, 167–177.

Sakauye, K. (1990). Psychotic disorders: guidelines and problems with antipsychotropic medications in the elderly. *Psychiatric Annals*, *20*, 456–465.

Salzman, C. (1987). Treatment of agitation in the elderly. In H. Y. Meltzer (Ed.), *Psychopharmacology, a generation of progress* (Chap 120, pp. 1167–1176). New York: Raven Press.

Sánchez–Barceló, E. J., Mediavilla, M. D., Tan, D. X., & Reiter, R. J. (2010). Clinical uses of melatonin: evaluation of human trials. *Current Medicinal Chemistry*, *17*, 2070–2095.

Sandson, N. B., Marcucci, C., Bourke, D. L., & Smith-Lamacchia, R. (2006). An interaction between aspirin and valproate: the relevance of plasma protein displacement drug-drug interactions. *American Journal of Psychiatry*, *163*, 1891–1896.

Sansone, R. A., & Sansone, L. A. (2009). Warfarin and antidepressants: happiness without hemorrhaging. *Psychiatry (Edgmont)*, *6*, 24–29.

Santens, P., Claeys, I., Vonck, K., & Boon, P. (2006). Parkinsonism due to lamotrigine. *Movement Disorders*, *21*, 2269–2270.

Saruwatari, J., Yasui-Furukori, N., Niioka, T., Akamine, Y., Takashima, A., Kaneko, S., & Uno, T. (2012). Different effects of the selective serotonin reuptake inhibitors fluvoxamine, paroxetine, and sertraline on the pharmacokinetics of fexofenadine in healthy volunteers. *Journal of Clinical Psychopharmacology*, *32*, 195–199.

Sazgar, M., & Bourgeois, B. F. (2005). Aggravation of epilepsy by antiepileptic drugs. *Pediatric Neurology*, *33*, 227–234.

Scharf, M. B., Roth, P. B., Dominguez, R. A., & Ware, J. C. (1990). Estazolam and flurazepam: a multicenter, placebo-controlled comparative study in outpatients with insomnia. *Journal of Clinical Pharmacology*, *30*, 461–467.

Scheffner, D., Konig, S., Rauterberg-Rutland, I., Kochen, W., Hofmann, W. J., & Unkelbach, S. (1988). Fatal liver failure in 16 children with valproate therapy. *Epilepsia*, *29*, 520–542.

Schenker, S., Bergstrom, R. F., Wolen, R. I., et al. (1988). Fluoxetine disposition and elimination in cirrhosis. *Clinical Pharmacology & Therapeutics*, *44*, 353–359.

Schizophrenia Letter. (September 1996). FDA panel recommends sertindole for approval. *Psychiatric Times*, *13* (Suppl), pp. 1 and 3.

Schmidt, D., & Kramer, G. (1994). The new anticonvulsant drugs: implications for avoidance of adverse effects. *Drug Safety*, *11*, 422–431.

Schreibman, D. S., McPherson, C. A., Rosenfeld, L. E., Batsford, W. P., & Lampert, R. (2004). Usefulness of procainamide challenge for electrophysiologic arrhythmia risk stratification. *American Journal of Cardiology*, *94*, 1435–1438.

Schwartz, P., & Wolf, S. (1978). QT interval prolongation as predictor of sudden death in patients with myocardial infarction. *Circulation*, *57*, 1074–1077.

Secor, J. W., & Schenker, S. (1987). Drug metabolism in patients with liver disease. *Advances in Internal Medicine*, *32*, 379–406.

Sedky, K., Nazir, R., Joshi, A., Kaur, G., & Lippmann, S. (2012). Which psychotropic medications induce hepatotoxicity? *General Hospital Psychiatry*, *34*, 53–61.

Seetharam, M. N., & Pellock, J. M. (1991). Risk-benefit assessment of carbamazepine in children. *Drug Safety*, *6*, 148–158.

Sellers, T. D. Jr., Campbell, R. W. F., Bashore, T. M., & Gallagher, J. J. (1977). Effects of procainamide and quinidine sulfate in the Wolff-Parkinson-White syndrome. *Circulation*, *55*, 15–22.

Sessler, D. I. (2009). Defeating normal thermoregulatory defenses: induction of therapeutic hypothermia. *Stroke*, *40*, e614–e621.

Sethna, M., Solomon, G., Cedarbaum, J., & Kutt, H. (1989). Successful treatment of massive carbamazepine overdose. *Epilepsia*, *30*, 71–73.

Severus, E., & Bauer, M. (2013). Managing the risk of lithium-induced nephropathy in the long-term treatment of patients with recurrent affective disorders. BMC Med 11, 34

Sheehan, J. D., & Shelley, R. D. (1990). Leucopenia secondary to carbamazepine despite concurrent lithium treatment. *British Journal of Psychiatry*, *157*, 911–912.

Shiloah, E., Witz, S., Abramovitch, Y., Cohen, O., Buchs, A., Ramot, Y., et al. (2003). Effect of acute psychotic stress in nondiabetic subjects on beta-cell function and insulin sensitivity. *Diabetes Care*, *26*, 1462–1467.

Shirley, D. G., Walter, S. J., & Noormohamed, F. H. (2002). Natriuretic effect of caffeine: assessment of segmental sodium reabsorption in humans. *Clinical Science (London)*, *103*, 461–466.

Shukla, S., Mukherjee, S., & Decina, P. (1988). Lithium in the treatment of bipolar disorders associated with epilepsy: an open study. *Journal of Clinical Psychopharmacology, 8*, 201–204.

Sides, C. A. (1987). Hypertension during anesthesia with monoamine oxidase inhibitors. *Anesthesia, 42*, 633–635.

Sikorski, B. W., James, G. M., Glance, S. D., Hodgson, W. C., & King, R. G. (1993). Effect of endothelium on diabetes-induced changes in constrictor responses mediated by 5-hydroxytryptamine in rat aorta. *Journal of Cardiovascular Pharmacology, 22*, 423–430.

Simonson, M. (1964). Controlling MAO inhibitor hypotension. *American Journal of Psychiatry, 120*, 1118–1119.

Sinclair, L. I., Christmas, D. M., Hood, S. D., Potokar, J. P., Robertson, A., Isaac, A., et al. (2009). Antidepressant-induced jitteriness/anxiety syndrome: systematic review. *British Journal of Psychiatry, 194*, 483–490.

Singer, S., Richards, C., & Boland, R. D. (1995). Two cases of risperidone-induced neuroleptic malignant syndrome (letter). *American Journal of Psychiatry, 152*, 1234.

Singh, D., & O'Connor, D. W. (2009). Efficacy and safety of risperidone long-acting injection in elderly people with schizophrenia. *Clinical Interventions in Aging, 4*, 351–355.

Small, J. G., Hirsch, S. R., Arvanitis, L. A., Miller, B. G., & Link, C. G. (1997). Quetiapine in patients with schizophrenia: a high-and-low double-blind comparison with placebo. *Archives of General Psychiatry, 54*, 549–557.

Smith, R. C., Chojnacki, M., Hu, R., & Mann, E. (1980). Cardiovascular effecs of therapeutic doses of tricyclic antidepressants: importance of blood level monitoring. *Journal of Clinical Psychiatry, 41*(12 Pt 2), 57–63.

Snoeck, E., Van Peer, A., Sack, M., Horton, M., Mannens, G., Woestenborghs, R., et al. (1995). Influence of age, renal and liver impairment on the pharmacokinetics of risperidone in man. *Psychopharmacology (Berlin), 122*, 223–229.

Sockalingam, S., Tseng, A., Giguere, P., & Wong, D. (2013). Psychiatric treatment considerations with direct acting antivirals in hepatitis C. *BMC Gastroenterology, 13*, 86.

Sood, M. M., & Richardson, R. (2007). Negative anion gap and elevated osmolar gap due to lithium overdose. *Canadian Medical Association Journal, 176*, 921–923

Sperner-Unterweger, B., Czepek, I., Gaggl, S., Geissler, D., Spiel, G., & Fleischhacker W. W. (1998). Treatment of severe clozapine-induced neutropenia with granulocyte colony-stimulating factor (G-CSF). Remission despite continuous treatment with clozapine. *British Journal of Psychiatry, 172*, 82–84.

Spier, S. A., & Frontera, M. A. (1991). Unexpected deaths in depressed medical inpatients treated with fluoxetine. *Journal of Clinical Psychiatry, 52*, 377–382.

Spina, E., Avenoso, A., Scordo, M. G., Ancione, M., Madia, A., Gatti, G., & Perucca, E. (2002). Inhibition of risperidone metabolism by fluoxetine in patients with schizophrenia: a clinically relevant pharmacokinetic drug interaction. *Journal of Clinical Psychopharmacology, 22*, 419–423.

Spina, E., Pisani, F., & Perucca, E. (1996). Clinically significant pharmacokinetic drug interactions with carbamazepine. An update. *Clinical Pharmacokinetics, 31*, 198–214.

Stack, C. G., Rogers, P., & Linter, S. P. K. (1988). Monoamine oxidase inhibitors and anaesthesia. *British Journal of Anaesthesia, 60*, 222–227.

Stark, P., Fuller, R. W., & Wong, D. T. (1985). The pharmacologic profile of fluoxetine. *Journal of Clinical Psychiatry, 46*, 7–13.

Stebbing, J., Waters, L., Davies, L., Mandalia, S., Nelson, M., Gazzard, B., & Bower, M. (2005). Incidence of cancer in individuals receiving chronic zopiclone or eszopiclone requires prospective study. *Journal of Clinical Oncology, 23*, 8134–8136.

Stewart, J. T., Nesmith, M. W., Mattox, K. M. (2012). A case of valproate toxicity related to isoniazid. *Journal of Clinical Psychopharmacology, 32*, 840–841.

Stip, E., Zhornitsky, S., Moteshafi, H., Létourneau, G., Stikarovska, I., Potvin, S., & Tourjman, V. (2011). Ziprasidone for psychotic disorders: a meta-analysis and systematic review of the relationship between pharmacokinetics, pharmacodynamics, and clinical profile. *Clinical Therapeutics, 33*, 1853–1867.

Stoudemire, A., & Clayton, L. (1989). Successful use of clozapine in a patient with a history of neuroleptic malignant syndrome. *Journal of Neuropsychiatry, 1*, 303–305.

Stoudemire, A., & Fogel, B. S. (1995). Psychopharmacology in the medical patient: an update. In A Stoudemire & BS Fogel (Eds.), *Medical psychiatric practice* (Vol. 3, Chap. 2, pp. 79–149). Washington, DC: American Psychiatric Press.

Stoudemire, A., & Moran, M. G. (1998). Psychopharmacology in the medically ill patient. In A. F. Schatzberg & C. B. Nemeroff (Eds.), *Textbook of psychopharmacology* (2nd ed., Chap. 45, pp. 931–959). Washington, DC: American Psychiatric Press.

Stoudemire, A. (1996). New antidepressant drugs and the treatment of depression in the medically ill patient. *Psychiatric Clinics of North America, 19*, 495–514.

Stoudemire, A., Fogel, B. S., & Gulley, L. R. (1991). Psychopharmacology in the medically ill: an update. In A. Stoudemire & B. S. Fogel (Eds.), *Medical psychiatric practice* (Vol. I, Chap. 2, pp. 29–97). Washington, DC: American Psychiatric Press.

Stoudemire, A., Hill, C. D., Lewison, B., et al. (1998). Lithium intolerance in a medical-psychiatric population. *General Hospital Psychiatry, 20*, 85–90.

Stoudemire, A., Moran, M. G., & Fogel, B. S. (1991). Psychotropic drug use in the medically ill: Part II. *Psychosomatics, 32*, 34–46.

Stoudemire, A., Moran, M. G. (1998). Psychopharmacology in the medically ill patient. In A. Schatzbert & C. Nemeroff (Eds.), *Textbook of psychopharmacology* (2nd edition, pp. 931–960). Washington, DC: American Psychiatric Press.

Strack, D. K., Leckband, S. G., & Meyer, J. M. (2009). Antipsychotic prescribing practices following withdrawal of concomitant carbamazepine. *Journal of Psychiatric Practice, 15*, 442–448.

Stübner, S., Grohmann, R., Engel, R., Bandelow, B., Ludwig, W. D., Wagner, G., et al. (2004). Blood dyscrasias induced by psychotropic drugs. *Pharmacopsychiatry, 37*(Suppl 1), S70–S78.

Stumpf, J. L., & Mitrzyk, B. (1994). Management of orthostatic hypotension. *American Journal of Hospital Pharmacy, 51*, 648–660.

Su, Y. P., Chang C. J., & Hwang, T. J. (2007). Lithium intoxication after valsartan treatment (letter). *Psychiatry and Clinical Research, 61*, 204.

Sussman, N. (1987). Treatment of anxiety with buspirone. *Psychiatric Annals, 17*, 114–117.

Suzuki, Y., Fukui, N., Watanabe, J., Ono, S., Sugai, T., Tsuneyama, N., et al. (2012). QT prolongation of the antipsychotic risperidone is predominantly related to its 9-hydroxy metabolite paliperidone. *Human Psychopharmacology, 27*, 39–42.

Tack, J., Janssen, P., Masaoka, T., Farré R., & Van Oudenhove, L. (2012). Efficacy of buspirone, a fundus-relaxing drug, in patients with functional dyspepsia. *Clinical Gastroenterology and Hepatology, 10*, 1239–1245.

Taha, F. A., Hammond, D. N., & Sheth, R. D. (2013). Seizures from valproate-carbapenem interaction. *Pediatric Neurology, 49*, 279–281.

Tak, H. J., Ahn, J. H., Kim, K. W., Kim, Y., Choi, S. W., Lee, K. Y., et al. (2012). Rash in psychiatric and nonpsychiatric adolescent patients receiving lamotrigine in Korea: a retrospective cohort study. *Psychiatry Investigation, 9*, 174–179.

Tamaji, A., Iwamoto, K., Kawamura, Y., Takahashi, M., Ebe, K., Kawano, N., et al. (2012). Differential effects of diazepam, tandospirone, and paroxetine on plasma brain-derived neurotrophic factor level under mental stress. *Human Psychopharmacology, 27*, 329–333.

Tangedahl, T. N., & Gau, G. T. (1972). Myocardial irritability associated with lithium carbonate therapy. *New England Journal of Medicine, 287*, 867–869.

Tariq, M., Morais, C., Sobki, S., Al Sulaiman, M., & Al Khader, A. (2000). Effect of lithium on cyclosporin induced nephrotoxicity in rats. Ren Fail 22, 545–560.

Tarsy, D. (1996). Risperidone and neuroleptic malignant syndrome (letter). *Journal of the American Medical Association, 275*, 446.

Taylor, D. (2008). Antidepressant drugs and cardiovascular pathology: a clinical overview of effectiveness and safety. *Acta Psychiatrica Scandinavica*, 118, 434–442.

Taylor, J. J., Wilson, J. W., & Estes, L. L. (2006). Linezolid and serotonergic drug interactions: a retrospective survey. *Clinical Infectious Diseases*, 43, 180–187.

Teles, J. S., Fukuda, E. Y., & Feder, D. (2012). Warfarin: pharmacological profile and drug interactions with antidepressants. *Einstein (Sao Paulo)*, 10, 110–115.

Tellenbach, H. (1965). Epilepsie als Anfallsleiden und als Psychose. Ueber alternative Psychoser paranoiden Prägung bei "forcierter Normalisierung" (Landolt) des Elektroencephalogramms Epileptischer. *Nervenarzt*, 36, 190–202.

ten Cate, B., Samplonius, D. F., Bijma, T., de Leij, L. F., Helfrich, W., & Bremer, E. (2007). The histone deacetylase inhibitor valproic acid potently augments gemtuzumab ozogamicin-induced apoptosis in acute myeloid leukemic cells. *Leukemia*, 21, 248–252.

Thanacoody, R. H. (2009). Extracorporeal elimination in acute valproic acid poisoning. *Clinical Toxicology (Philadelphia)*, 47, 609–616.

Thapa, P. B., Gideon, P., Cost, T. W., Milam, A. B., & Ray, W. A. (1998). Antidepressants and the risk of falls among nursing home residents. *New England Journal of Medicine*, 339, 875–882.

Thase, M. E., Haight, B. R., Johnson, M. C., Hunt, T., Krishen, A., Fleck, R. J., & Modell, J. G. (2008). A randomized, double-blind, placebo-controlled study of the effect of sustained-release bupropion on blood pressure in individuals with mild untreated hypertension. *Journal of Clinical Psychopharmacology*, 28, 302–307.

Thirthalli, J., Harish, T., & Gangadhar, B. N. (2011). A prospective comparative study of interaction between lithium and modified electroconvulsive therapy. *World Journal of Biological Psychiatry*, 12, 149–155.

Thomson, A. D., Cook, C. C., Touquet, R., Henry, J. A.; Royal College of Physicians, London. (2002). The Royal College of Physicians report on alcohol: guidelines for managing Wernicke's encephalopathy in the accident and emergency department. *Alcohol and Alcoholism*, 37, 513–521.

Tilkian, J. G., Schroeder, J. S., Cao, J., et al. (1976). Effect of lithium on cardiovascular performance. A report on extended ambulatory monitoring and exercise testing before and during lithium. *American Journal of Cardiology*, 38, 701–798.

Tiller, J. W. G., Dakis, J. A., & Shaw, J. M. (1988). Short-term buspirone treatment in disinhibition with dementia. *Lancet*, 2, 510.

Tollefson, G. D., Beasley, C. M., Tamura, R. N., Tran, P. V., & Potvin, J. H. (1997a). Blind, controlled, long-term study of the comparative incidence of treatment-emergent tardive dyskinesia with olanzapine or haloperidol, *American Journal of Psychiatry*, 154, 1248–1254.

Tollefson, G. D., Beasley, C. M., Tran, P. V., Street, J. S., Krueger, J. A., Tamura, R. N., et al. (1997b). Olanzapine versus haloperidol in the treatment of schizophrenia and schizoaffective and schizophreniform disorders: results of an international collaborative trial. *American Journal of Psychiatry*, 154, 457–465.

Torre, L. E., Menon, R., & Power, B. M. (2009). Prolonged serotonin toxicity with proserotonergic drugs in the intensive care unit. *Critical Care and Resuscitation*, 11, 272–275.

Tränkner, A., Sander, C., & Schönknecht, P. (2013). A critical review of the recent literature and selected therapy guidelines since 2006 on the use of lamotrigine in bipolar disorder. *Neuropsychiatric Disease and Treatment*, 9, 101–111.

Trayer, J. S., & Fidler, D. C. (1998). Neuroleptic malignant syndrome related to the use of clozapine (letter). *Journal of the American Osteopathic Association*, 98, 168–169.

TREC Collaborative Group. (2003). Rapid tranquillisation for agitated patients in emergency psychiatric rooms: a randomised trial of midazolam versus haloperidol plus promethazine. *British Medical Journal*, 327(7417), 708–713.

Trifirò, G. (2011). Antipsychotic drug use and community-acquired pneumonia. *Current Infectious Disease Reports*, 13, 262–268.

Trimble, M. R., & Reynolds, E. H. (1976). Anticonvulsant drugs and mental symptoms: a review. *Psychological Medicine*, 6(2), 169–178.

Tse, G. H., Warner, M. H., & Waring, W. S. (2008). Prolonged toxicity after massive olanzapine overdose: two cases with confirmatory laboratory data. *Journal of Toxicological Sciences*, 33, 363–365.

Tse, L., Schwarz SKW, Bowering, J. B., Moore, R. L., Burns, K. D., Richford, C. M., et al. (2012). Pharmacological risk factors for delirium after cardiac surgery: a review. *Current Neuropharmacology*, 10(3), 181–196.

Tuncel, M., & Ram, V. C. (2003). Hypertensive emergencies. Etiology and management. *American Journal of Cardiovascular Drugs*, 3, 21–31.

Türck, D., Heinzel, G., & Luik, G. (2000). Steady-state pharmacokinetics of lithium in healthy volunteers receiving concomitant meloxicam. *British Journal of Clinical Pharmacology*, 50, 197–204.

U.S. Food and Drug Administration. (2008). FDA alerts health care providers to risk of suicidal thoughts and behavior with antiepileptic medications. Retrieved from http://www.fda.gov/Drugs/DrugSafety/PostmarketDrugSafetyInformationforPatientsandProviders/ucm100200.htm., last accessed 25 July 2014.

U.S. Food and Drug Administration (2005). Public Health Advisory: Deaths with antipsychotics in elderly patients with behavioral disturbances. Silver Spring, MD: U.S. Food and Drug Administration; 11 April 2005. Retrieved from http://www.fda.gov/drugs/drugsafety/postmarketdrugsafetyinformationforpatientsandproviders/drugsafetyinformationforheathcareprofessionals/publichealthadvisories/ucm053171.htm, last accessed 25 July 2014.

Uchimura, N., Kamijo, A., & Takase, T. (2012). Effects of eszopiclone on safety, subjective measures of efficacy, and quality of life in elderly and nonelderly Japanese patients with chronic insomnia, both with and without comorbid psychiatric disorders: a 24-week, randomized, double-blind study. *Annals of General Psychiatry*, 11, 15.

Unterecker, S., Burger, R., Hohage, A., Deckert, J., & Pfuhlmann, B. (2013). Interaction of valproic acid and amitriptyline: analysis of therapeutic drug monitoring data under naturalistic conditions. *Journal of Clinical Psychopharmacology*, 33, 561–564.

Unterecker, S., Müller, P., Jacob, C., Riederer, P., & Pfuhlmann, B. (2012). Therapeutic drug monitoring of antidepressants in haemodialysis patients. *Clinical Drug Investigation*, 32, 539–545.

Unterecker, S., Reif, A., Hempel, S., Proft, F., Riederer, P., Deckert, J., & Pfuhlmann, B. (2013). Interaction of valproic acid and the antidepressant drugs doxepin and venlafaxine: analysis of therapeutic drug monitoring data under naturalistic conditions. *International Clinical Psychopharmacology*.

US Gabapentin Study Group No. 5 (1993). Gabapentin as add-on therapy in refractory partial epilepsy: a double-blind, placebo-controlled, parallel-group study. *Neurology*, 43, 2292–2298.

van den Born, B. J., Beutler, J. J., Gaillard, C. A., de Gooijer, A., van den Meiracker, A. H., & Kroon, A. A. (2011). Dutch guideline for the management of hypertensive crisis—2010 revision. *The Netherlands Journal of Medicine*, 69, 248–255.

Van Dyck, C. H., McMahon, T. J., Rosen, M. I., et al. (1997). Sustained-release methylphenidate for cognitive impairment in HIV-1-infected drug abusers: a pilot study. *Journal of Neuropsychiatry and Clinical Neurosciences*, 9, 29–36.

van Haelst, I. M., van Klei, W. A., Doodeman, H. J., Kalkman, C. J., Egberts, T. C.; MAOI Study Group. (2012). Antidepressive treatment with monoamine oxidase inhibitors and the occurrence of intraoperative hemodynamic events: a retrospective observational cohort study. *Journal of Clinical Psychiatry*, 73, 1103–1109.

Van Sweden, B., & Van Moffaert, M. (1985). Valproate as psychotropic agent. *Acta Psychiatrica Scandinavica*, 72, 315–317.

VanCott, A. C., Cramer, J. A., Copeland, L. A., Zeber, J. E., Steinman, M. A., Dersh, J. J., et al. (2010). Suicide-related behaviors in older patients with new anti-epileptic drug use: data from the VA hospital system. *BMC Medicine*, 8, 4.

Vannaprasaht, S., Tiamkao, S., Sirivongs, D., & Piyavhatkul, N. (2009). Acute valproic acid overdose: enhance elimination with multiple-doses activated charcoal. *Journal of the Medical Association of Thailand*, 92, 1113–1115.

Vareesangthip, K., Hanlakorn, P., Suwannaton, L., Larpkitkachorn, R., Chuawattana, D., Pidetcha, P., & Ong-Aj-Yooth, L. (2004).

Erythrocyte sodium lithium countertransport in renal transplant recipients with mycophenolate mofetil and low-dose cyclosporine. *Transplantation Proceedings, 36*, 3032–3035.

Vasilyeva, I., Biscontri, R. G., Enns, M. W., Metge, C. J., & Alessi-Severini, S. (2013). Adverse events in elderly users of antipsychotic pharmacotherapy in the province of Manitoba: a retrospective cohort study. *Journal of Clinical Psychopharmacology, 33*, 24–30.

Vendsborg, P. B. (1979). Lithium and glucose tolerance in manic-melancholic patients. *Acta Psychiatrica Scandinavica, 59*, 306–316.

Vermeir, M., Naessens, I., Remmerie, B., Mannens, G., Hendrickx, J., Sterkens, P., et al. (2008). Absorption, metabolism, and excretion of paliperidone, a new monoaminergic antagonist, in humans. *Drug Metabolism and Disposition, 36*, 769–779.

Vieta, E., Nuamah, I. F., Lim, P., Yuen, E. C., Palumbo, J. M., Hough, D. W., & Berwaerts, J. (2010). A randomized, placebo-and active-controlled study of paliperidone extended release for the treatment of acute manic and mixed episodes of bipolar I disorder. *Bipolar Disorders, 12*, 230–243.

Vieweg, W. V., Hillard, J. R., Hoffman, M. A., David, J. J., Spradlin, W. W. (1988). Depression and the Wolf-Parkinson-White syndrome. *Psychosomatics, 29*, 113–116.

Vieweg, W. V. R., & Godleski, L. S. (1988). Carbamazepine and hyponatremia. *American Journal of Psychiatry, 145*, 1323–1324.

Vieweg, V., Glick, J. L., Herring, S., Kerler, R., Godleski, L. S., Barber, J., et al. (1987). Absence of carbamazepine-induced hyponatremia among patients also given lithium. *American Journal of Psychiatry, 144*, 943–947.

Vieweg, W. V. R., Yank, G. R., Row, W. T., et al. (1986–87). Increase in white blood cell count and serum sodium level following the addition of lithium to carbamazepine treatment among three chronically psychotic male patients with disturbed affective states. *Psychiatric Quarterly, 58*, 213–217.

Vigneault, P., Kaddar, N., Bourgault, S., Caillier, B., Pilote, S., Patoine, D., et al. (2011). Prolongation of cardiac ventricular repolarization under paliperidone: how and how much? *Journal of Cardiovascular Pharmacology, 57*, 690–695.

Villikka, K., Kivistö KT, Lamberg, T. S., Kantola, T., & Neuvonen, P. J. (1997). Concentrations and effects of zopiclone are greatly reduced by rifampicin. *British Journal of Clinical Pharmacology, 43*, 471–474.

Vincent, H. H., Weimar, W., & Schalekamp, M. A. D. H. (1987). Effect of cyclosporine in fractional excretion of lithium and potassium in kidney transplant recipients. *Kidney International, 31*, 1048.

Vishwanath, B. M., Navalgund, A. A., Cusano, W., Navalgund, K. A. (1991). Fluoxetine as a cause of SIADH (letter); *American Journal of Psychiatry, 148*, 542–543.

Walker-Batson, D., Smith, P., Curtis, S., Unwin, H., & Greenlee, R. (1995). Amphetamine paired with physical therapy accelerates motor recovery after stroke. Further evidence. *Stroke, 26*, 2254–2259.

Wang-Tilz, Y., Tilz, C., Wang, B., Pauli, E., Koebnick, C., & Stefan, H. (2005). Changes of seizures activity during rapid withdrawal of lamotrigine. *European Journal of Neurology, 12*, 280–288.

Waring, W. S., Good, A. M., & Bateman, D. N. (2007). Lack of significant toxicity after mirtazapine overdose: a five-year review of cases admitted to a regional toxicology unit. *Clinical Toxicology (Philadelphia), 45*, 45–50.

Watanabe, N., Omori, I. M., Nakagawa, A., Cipriani, A., Barbui, C., McGuire, H., et al; MANGA (Meta-Analysis of New Generation Antidepressants). Study Group. (2010). Safety reporting and adverse-event profile of mirtazapine described in randomized controlled trials in comparison with other classes of antidepressants in the acute-phase treatment of adults with depression: systematic review and meta-analysis. *CNS Drugs, 24*, 35–53.

Weintraub, D., Koester, J., Potenza, M. N., Siderowf, A. D., Stacy, M., Voon, V., et al. (2010). Impulse control disorders in Parkinson disease: a cross-sectional study of 3090 patients. *Archives of Neurology, 67*, 589–595.

Wellens, H. J., & Durrer, D. (1974). Wolff-Parkinson-White syndrome and atrial fibrillation: relation between refractory period of accessory pathway and ventricular rate during atrial fibrillation. *American Journal of Cardiology, 34*, 777–782.

Wellens, H. J., Braat, S., Brugada, P., Gorgels, A. P., & Bär, F. W. (1982). Use of procainamide in patients with the Wolff-Parkinson-White syndrome to disclose a short refractory period of the accessory pathway. *American Journal of Cardiology, 50*, 1087–1089.

Wenzel-Seifert, K., Wittmann, M., & Haen, E. (2011). QTc prolongation by psychotropic drugs and the risk of Torsade de Pointes. *Deutsches Ärzteblatt International, 108*, 687–693.

Werlin, S. L., & Fish, D. L. (2006). The spectrum of valproic acid-associated pancreatitis. *Pediatrics, 118*, 1660–1663.

Weston, A. L., Weinstein, A. M., Barton, C., & Yaffe, K. (2010). Potentially inappropriate medication use in older adults with mild cognitive impairment. *Journals of Gerontology Series A: Biological Sciences and Medical Sciences, 65*, 318–321.

Whyte, J., Hart, T., Schuster, K., Fleming, M., Polansky, M., & Coslett, H. B. (1997). Effects of methylphenidate on attentional function after traumatic brain injury. A randomized, placebo-controlled trial. *American Journal of Physical & Medical Rehabilitation, 76*, 440–450.

Wijdicks, E. F., Arendt, C., & Bazzell, M. C. (2004). Postoperative ophthalmoplegia and ataxia due to carbamazepine toxicity facilitated by diltiazem (letter). *Journal of Neuroophthalmology, 24*, 95.

Williams, R. L., & Mamelok, R. D. (1980). Hepatic disease and drug pharmacokinetics. *Clinical Pharmacokinetics, 5*, 528–547.

Wilner, K. D., Lazar, J. D., Apseloff, G., et al. (1991). The effects of sertraline on the pharmacodynamics of warfarin in health volunteers (abstract). *Biological Psychiatry, 29*, 3545.

Wimbiscus, M., Kostenko, O., & Malone, D. (2010). MAO inhibitors: risks, benefits, and lore. *Cleveland Clinic Journal of Medicine, 77*, 859–882.

Wolf, M. E., Moffat, M., Ranade, V., Somberg, J. C., Lehrer, E., Mosnaim, A. D. (1998). Lithium, hypercalcemia, and arrhythmia. *Journal of Clinical Psychopharmacology, 18*, 420–423.

Wong, K. C. (1986). Preoperative discontinuation of monoamine oxidase inhibitor therapy: An old wives tale? *Seminars in Anesthesia, 5*, 145–148.

Xie, C., Edwards, H., Lograsso, S. B., Buck, S. A., Matherly, L. H., Taub, J. W., & Ge, Y. (2012). Valproic acid synergistically enhances the cytotoxicity of clofarabine in pediatric acute myeloid leukemia cells. *Pediatric Blood & Cancer, 59*, 1245–1251.

Xie, C., Edwards, H., Xu, X., Zhou, H., Buck, S. A., Stout, M. L., Yu, Q., et al. (2010). Mechanisms of synergistic antileukemic interactions between valproic acid and cytarabine in pediatric acute myeloid leukemia. *Clinical Cancer Research, 16*, 5499–5510.

Xue, F., Strombom, I., Turnbull, B., Zhu, S., & Seeger, J. (2012). Treatment with duloxetine in adults and the incidence of cardiovascular events. *Journal of Clinical Psychopharmacology, 32*, 23–30.

Yamaguchi, M., & Mori, K. (2005). Critical period for sensory experience-dependent survival of newly generated granule cells in the adult mouse olfactory bulb. *Proceedings of the National Academy of Sciences USA, 102*, 9697–9702.

Yamamoto, Y., Inoue, Y., Matsuda, K., Takahashi, Y., & Kagawa, Y. (2012). Influence of concomitant antiepileptic drugs on plasma lamotrigine concentration in adult Japanese epilepsy patients. *Biological & Pharmaceutical Bulletin, 35*, 487–493.

Yamamoto, Y., Takahashi, Y., Suzuki, E., Mishima, N., Inoue, K., Itoh, K., et al. (2012). Risk factors for hyperammonemia associated with valproic acid therapy in adult epilepsy patients. *Epilepsy Research, 101*, 202–209.

Yang, S. Y., Liao, Y. T., Liu, H. C., Chen, W. J., Chen, C. C., & Kuo, C. J. (2013). Antipsychotic drugs, mood stabilizers, and risk of pneumonia in bipolar disorder: a nationwide case-control study. *Journal of Clinical Psychiatry, 74*, e79–86.

Yasui-Furukori, N. (2012). Update on the development of lurasidone as a treatment for patients with acute schizophrenia. *Drug Design, Development and Therapy, 6*, 107–115.

Yatham, L. N., Barr, S., & Dinan, T. G. (1989). Serotonin receptors, buspirone, and premenstrual syndrome. *Lancet, 1*, 1447–1448.

Ye, L., Peng, J. S., Wang, X., Wang, Y. J., Luo, G. X., & Ho, W. Z. (2008). Methamphetamine enhances Hepatitis C virus replication in human hepatocytes. *Journal of Viral Hepatitis, 15*, 261–270.

Yip, K. K., & Yeung, W. T. (2007). Lithium overdose causing non-convulsive status epilepticus—the importance of lithium levels and the electroencephalography in diagnosis. *Hong Kong Medical Journal, 13*, 471–474.

Yoon H., & Kim, D. H. (2013). Unusual drug reaction between valproate sodium and meropenem. *International Journal of Clinical Pharmacology, 35*, 316–318.

Yoon, H. K., Park, C., Jang, S., Jang, S., Lee, Y. K., & Ha, Y. C. (2011). Incidence and mortality following hip fracture in Korea. *Journal of Korean Medical Science, 26*, 1087–1092.

Yoon, H. W., Giraldo, E. A., & Wijdicks, E. F. (2011). Valproic acid and warfarin: an underrecognized drug interaction. *Neurocritical Care, 15*, 182–185.

Young, R. C., Alexopolous, G. S., Shamoian, C. A., et al. (1985). Plasma 10-hydroxy-nortriptyline and ECG changes in elderly depressed patients. *American Journal of Psychiatry, 142*, 866–868.

Young, S. Z., & Bordey, A. (2009). GABA's control of stem and cancer cell proliferation in adult neural and peripheral niches. *Physiology (Bethesda), 24*, 171–185.

Youroukos, S., Lazopoulou, D., Michelakou, D., & Karagianni, J. (2003). Acute psychosis associated with levetiracetam. *Epileptic Disorders, 5*, 117–119.

Yuan, R., Flockhart, D. A., & Balian, J. D. (1999). Pharmacokinetic and pharmacodynamic consequences of metabolism-based drug interactions with alprazolam, midazolam, and triazolam. *Journal of Clinical Pharmacology, 39*, 1109–1125.

Zadikoff, C., Munhoz, R. P., Asante, A. N., Politzer, N., Wennberg, R., Carlen, P., & Lang, A. (2007). Movement disorders in patients taking anticonvulsants. *Journal of Neurology, Neurosurgery, and Psychiatry, 78*, 147–151.

Zeneca Pharmaceuticals. (2013). Seroquel* (quetiapine fumarate): product information. Zeneca, Inc., Wilmington, Delaware. Retrieved from http://www1.astrazeneca-us.com/pi/seroquel.pdf.

Zhang, C., Glenn, D. G., Bell, W. L., & O'Donovan, C. A. (2005). Gabapentin-induced myoclonus in end-stage renal disease. *Epilepsia, 46*, 156–158.

22.

PHARMACOKINETICS OF PSYCHOTROPIC DRUGS IN THE CONTEXT OF GENERAL MEDICAL ILLNESS

Cynthia A. Gutierrez and Barry S. Fogel

INTRODUCTION

Pharmacokinetics provides details of the relationship between the dose of drug administered and the alterations in drug concentration in the body over time (Varghese, Roberts, & Lipman, 2010). In patients with general medical illness, the pharmacokinetic parameters of many psychotropic agents can be altered, at times drastically. Chronic disease states, acute medical problems, surgery and other procedures, and concomitant nonpsychotropic medications all play a role. In addition to the influence of impaired hepatic or renal function, other factors relevant to pharmacokinetics include changes in protein binding and altered gastrointestinal function such as delayed gastric emptying or altered gastrointestinal transit time. Alternate nonenteral routes of administration and specialized oral formulations can have special relevance in the context of diseases that interfere with swallowing or gastrointestinal function. Changes in drug levels due to pharmacokinetic factors can lead to toxicity or to lack of efficacy, and the influence of psychotropic drugs on the pharmacokinetics of general medical drugs can cause toxicity or lack of efficacy of those medications. Therapeutic drug monitoring—and sometimes pharmacogenetic testing—can reduce risk in many cases, while in others the best risk mitigation strategy is to use a different drug or different dose. General advice such as "start low and go slow" is naïve and in some cases actually is counterproductive; when mental and behavioral symptoms are the greatest and most immediate threat to patients' function and well-being, it is far better to make the right choice of psychotropic drug and dosage as soon as possible.

Pharmacokinetics specifically deals with all of the steps between the administration of a dosage form and the elimination of the drug from the body (Shargel, Wu-Pong, & Yu, 2005). This includes the delivery of the drug to its ultimate site of action—the brain in the case of psychotropic drugs. Pharmacodynamics characterizes the relationship between the drug concentration at the site of action and the drug's clinical effects, both therapeutic and adverse. In other words, pharmacokinetics is what the body does to the drug, and pharmacodynamics is what the drug does to the body. The relevant steps in pharmacokinetics are summarized by the acronym ADME: Absorption, Distribution, Metabolism, and Excretion. These processes are sequential at the molecular level, but at the gross level they are simultaneous; one process can influence another, as when the action of a drug on the intestine influences the absorption of drugs still present there.

PHARMACOKINETICS VERSUS PHARMACODYNAMICS

Brain effects do not correspond directly to the blood concentrations of a drug for several reasons. First, the level of the drug in the blood can differ greatly from the level of the drug in the central nervous system (CNS) because of the blood–brain barrier. The difference in concentrations can be as great as two orders of magnitude; it is related to the lipophilicity of the drug, whether its entry into the brain is facilitated by its interaction with a transporter, and whether the drug is actively transported into or out of the cerebrospinal fluid (CSF). Second, the drug's mechanism of action may not require that the drug be continuously present; it may, for example, induce RNA transcription leading to the synthesis of a protein that will persist for hours or days. And third, the changes in neuronal function initially produced by the drug can cause secondary changes in the same neurons or connected neurons that produce clinically relevant effects. For example, if a drug blocks a neuron's dopamine receptors that neuron will synthesize additional receptors; also, activity in related glutamatergic neurons will increase. This in turn may have effects on the targets of those neurons' axons.

THE PHARMACOKINETIC CURVE

The pharmacokinetic (PK) curve, or time-concentration curve, is a plot showing time since drug administration on the x-axis and the drug's blood concentration (typically its plasma level) on the y-axis. It is illustrated in Figure 22.1. Three essential parameters of the PK curve, which do not totally define it but are critical to the drug's clinical effects, are the *maximum concentration attained* (Cmax), the *time needed to reach the maximum concentration* (Tmax), and the total *area under the PK curve* (AUC) (Shargel, Wu-Pong, & Yu, 2005). The AUC is based on extrapolation of the PK curve to infinity from the last actual measurement of concentration (Shargel,

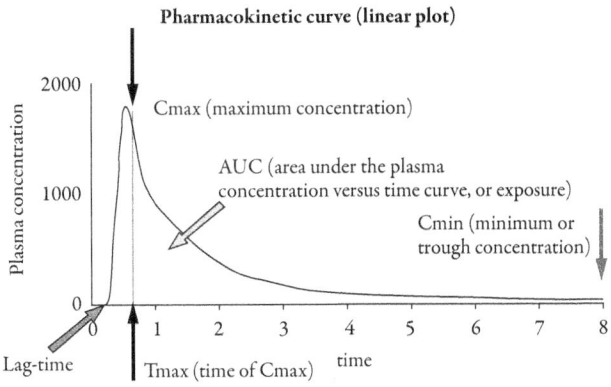

Pharmacokinetic curve (linear plot)

Figure 22.1 The Pharmacokinetic Curve.

Wu-Pong, & Yu, 2005). The definitions of some common PK terms including the parameters of the PK curve are shown in Table 22.1.

PHARMACOKINETICS AND GENERIC SUBSTITUTION

When generic equivalents of previously approved drugs receive regulatory approval they are required to be *bioequivalent*. This is defined as having a Cmax and an AUC whose 95% confidence limits in a clinical population lie between 80% and 125% of the (mean) Cmax and AUC of the originally approved drug (Center for Drug Evaluation and Research, 2003). Note that formulations that are bioequivalent are not necessarily identical in their pharmacokinetic properties, because (1) the Tmax and exact shape of the PK curve are not required to be equivalent; (2) the confidence limits of the new formulation's PK parameters can vary with the subject population tested; and (3) the excipients in the new formulation need not be the same as in the original one, and in some patients the excipients could have a biological effect—for example, if the patient was allergic to one of them. Of the noted reasons, the population-specificity of the PK curve is most relevant to medical psychiatrists. The similarity of two formulations of the same drug might be less in patients with abnormal gastrointestinal function, or in patients who are taking several other drugs with physiological actions that influence the absorption of the drug of interest. In addition, any specific patient can be an outlier in whom the ratios of Cmax and AUC lie outside the 80%–125% range.

These considerations do not rule out the substitution of generic for brand name drugs or of one generic drug for another; they only imply that the optimal dosage of two different formulations might not be the same for a specific patient, and that a specific patient might experience a different response—either therapeutic benefits, adverse effects, or both—with one formulation of a drug versus another. It is thus useful to know when a pharmacy substitutes one maker's formulation for another, particularly for drugs in which precise dosage is clinically important. If clinicians are aware of

Table 22.1 TERMINOLOGY IN PHARMACOKINETICS

PARAMETER (SYMBOL)	DESCRIPTION	TYPICAL UNITS
Dose (D)	Amount of drug administered	mg
Dosing interval (τ)	Time between drug dose administrations	hours
Maximum concentration (Cmax)	Peak plasma concentration of a drug after administration	mg/L, µg/ml
Tmax	Time to reach Cmax	hours
Minimum concentration (Cmin)	Lowest (trough) concentration that a drug reaches before the next dose is administered.	mg/L, µg/ml
Volume of distribution (Vd)	Apparent volume in which a drug is distributed (i.e., the parameter relating drug concentration to drug amount in the body)	liters
Concentration (C)	Amount of drug in a given volume of fluid, usually plasma	mg/L, ng/ml, µg/ml
Elimination half-life ($T_{1/2}$)	Time required for the concentration of the drug to reach half of its original value	hours
Elimination rate constant (k_e)	Rate at which a drug is removed from the body	hours^{-1}
Infusion rate (k_i)	Rate of infusion required to balance elimination	mg/hour, ml/hour
Area under the curve (AUC)	Integral of the concentration-time curve (after a single dose or in steady state)	(mg/L) * hours
Clearance (CL)	Volume of plasma cleared of the drug per unit time	L/hour
Bioavailability (F)	Systemically available fraction of a drug	percentage ≤100%

DeVane, 1990.

the potential for a difference in effects or tolerability, they will be quick to recognize it and respond accordingly. This is especially important for drugs with a narrow therapeutic index or a small range between concentrations required for therapeutic effect and those that cause toxicity.

There have been instances where change to generic formulations initially deemed bioequivalent by the FDA have resulted in decreased efficacy and/or increased toxicity. Phenytoin, carbamazepine, clozapine, and bupropion have each had reports of these issues with generic formulations (Hartley, Aleksandrowicz, Ng, McLain, Bowmer, et al., 1990; Jumao-as, Bella, Craig, Lowe, & Dasheiff, 1989; Chen, Allen Oxley, & Richens, 1982; Oles, Penry, Smith, Anderson, Dean, et al., 1992; Lam, Ereshefsky, Toney, & Gonzales, 2001; Kluznik, Walbek, Farnsworth, & Melstrom, 2001; Woodcock, Khan, & Yu, 2012). In the instance of the bupropion product, specifically the 300mg tablet, reports of decreased effectiveness led to further pharmacokinetic studies and subsequent withdrawal from the market (Woodcock, Khan, & Yu, 2012).

ABSORPTION

Absorption is both the rate and extent to which a drug leaves its administration site, passes through biological barriers, and reaches the systemic circulation (Buxton & Benet, 2011; Bauer, 2011). Absorption of a medication is dependent on many factors, including the surface area of the site(s) of absorption, blood flow to the site(s), the dissolution of the drug in body fluids (which often is pH-dependent), and the presence and functioning of active or passive transporters. Clinical focus typically is on *bioavailability*, the fraction of the dose administered that eventually reaches the circulation. (Note, however, that equal bioavailability of two versions of the same drug does not imply therapeutic equivalence, as the two versions can differ in the peak blood level they produce—Cmax—and in how rapidly a therapeutic threshold is reached—both factors of obvious therapeutic relevance.) Bioavailability is conventionally abbreviated by an upper case F.

For medications administered intravenously, F equals 1. For intramuscular medications, absorption can be erratic as the drug must pass one or more biological membranes to enter the systemic circulation. For patients with poor peripheral perfusion, as with shock, absorption after intramuscular administration may be delayed or incomplete. For enterally administered medications, bioavailability usually is less than 1 because absorption is often incomplete, and because drugs absorbed in the intestine are subject to metabolism prior to reaching the systemic circulation—the "first pass" effect. Most first-pass metabolism takes place in the liver, but for some drugs there is a significant contribution from metabolic enzymes in the intestinal mucosa. In addition to the absolute value of F, the *variability of F between patients* is a potentially important distinction between drugs. For example, when metabolism of a drug by CYP3A4 in the intestinal mucosa lowers a drug's bioavailability, patients with low activity of this enzyme will absorb more drug. It is known that CYP3A4 activity is highly variable in the general population, and hence that F for that drug will be highly variable as well. A few points related to drug absorption are useful in choosing drug oral drug formulations:

1. Solutions and suspensions are most rapidly absorbed; enteric-coated tablets are least rapidly absorbed; capsules are more rapidly absorbed than standard tablets. When a rapid onset of action is sought from a single oral dose of a medication, a solution or suspension is the ideal form when it is available and the patient will accept it.

2. Prodrugs—agents that become therapeutically active only after they are metabolized—usually are lipophilic compounds with high bioavailability; many have rapid absorption. Many prodrugs offer the additional benefit of avoiding a high Cmax of the active metabolite(s); this mitigates Cmax-related side effects and in some cases reduces the liability of the drug for abuse via intravenous injection. Slowly activated prodrugs can make once-a-day administration feasible for drugs that in their active form would require dosing several times a day for optimal effectiveness. Prodrugs usually are not suitable when a rapid onset of action is required because their activation rather than their absorption controls the rate of onset of therapeutic action, making rapid onset of action dependent upon rapid metabolism.

3. Extended-release or enteric-coated formulations should be avoided when a patient has diarrhea or another condition involving increased intestinal motility. In the latter situation, the pill may have passed into the colon or even have been eliminated before it is fully absorbed.

4. Delayed gastric emptying and/or decreased intestinal motility, caused either by disease or by anticholinergic drugs or opiates, can have variable and in some cases unpredictable effects on the absorption of psychotropic drugs. For most psychotropic drugs the bulk of absorption takes place in the proximal ileum (DeVane, 1990), and changes in gastrointestinal motility will alter the time after ingestion at which the drug reaches the absorptive site. Overall bioavailability can change, and in virtually all cases the PK curve will have different parameters with consequences for therapeutic efficacy or side effects.

5. For many psychotropic drugs, absorption will differ when the drug is taken with food versus in the fasting state. Food effects are measurable more often than they are clinically relevant, but they do matter for some drugs, as noted below. Effects can go in either direction. Because food slows gastric emptying and intestinal transit time, it can increase the absorption of drugs when the latter depends on time in contact with a particular area of the small intestine. For the same reason it can increase the time to peak concentration of the drug. On the other hand, if there are saturable transporters involved in intestinal absorption of the drug, substances in the food eaten can compete with the drug for spots on those

transporters and thereby reduce absorption. The bioavailability of ziprasidone *doubles* when it is taken with or just after a high-calorie meal as opposed to in the fasting state (Lincoln. Stewart, & Preskorn, 2010). Similarly, the antipsychotic lurasidone's AUC doubles, and Cmax increases threefold, when administered in the fed state and should be given with at least 350 calories for maximal absorption (Lurasidone Product Information, 2013). On the other hand, acamprosate, a drug used to suppress craving in recovering alcoholics, is 20%–30% less well absorbed if taken with food (Saivin, Hulot, Chabac, Potgieter, Durbin, et al., 1998), probably because of competition for amino acid Saivin transporters in the small intestine. Complicating matters further, the peak concentration nonetheless can be higher when acamprosate is taken with food. Medical conditions and their treatments often influence food intake, but there is little literature on food effects on psychotropic drug pharmacokinetics.

Patients receiving *intermittent* tube feedings can be dosed with drugs in either the fed or the fasting state. Those receiving *continuous* tube feedings are always in the fed state and therefore may require adjustment of dosage of drugs for which there is a significant food effect. Phenytoin pharmacokinetics especially are altered in the presence of tube feedings, with serum concentrations three to four times lower when given during continuous tube feedings, and should be administered at least 2 hours before and 2 hours after tube feedings (Bauer, 1982).

6. In addition to hepatic metabolism, the first-pass effect also includes active transport of drug from the portal circulation back into the intestinal lumen and metabolism of the drug by enzymes in the intestinal wall. Of these, CYP3A4 (see the discussion of the cytochrome p450 enzymes below) is particularly important because (1) it is the CYP enzyme most prevalent in intestinal cells, (2) it is involved in the metabolism of several commonly prescribed psychotropic drugs, and (3) it can be induced or inhibited by several common general medical drugs. Active transport of drugs from intestinal mucosal cells back to the intestinal lumen is mediated by P-glycoprotein (Pgp). This mechanism has clinically relevant magnitude for the antipsychotic drugs risperidone and paliperidone; when Pgp is inhibited by the calcium channel blocker verapamil, absorption of the drugs increases significantly (Nakagami, Yasui-Furukori, Saito, Tateishi, & Kaneo, 2005). The pharmacodynamic consequences are even greater than the pharmacokinetic effects, because Pgp is also present at the blood–brain barrier, and its inhibition increases the proportion of drug in the plasma that reaches the brain. Likewise, when Pgp activity is increased in the presence of a Pgp inducer, less substrate is able to reach the CNS. Other psychotropic drugs for which Pgp is important in controlling absorption (and distribution to the CNS) are the antidepressants amitriptyline, nortriptyline, doxepin, citalopram, paroxetine, sertraline, and venlafaxine; the anticonvulsants carbamazepine and topiramate; and the antipsychotics chlorpromazine, quetiapine, and olanzapine (Levine, 2012). Other common inhibitors of Pgp are cardiovascular drugs amiodarone, captopril, carvedilol, diltiazem, felodipine, and ranolazine, and the anti-infectives azithromycin, clarithromycin, erythromycin, itraconazole, and ketoconazole (U.S. Food and Drug Administration, 2011). Certain psychotropics including venlafaxine (though not desvenlafaxine) (Bachmeier, Beaulieu-Abdelahad, Ganey, Mullan, & Levin, 2011), and, to a lesser extent, nefazodone and trazodone, can induce Pgp, leading to a decrease in bioavailability and clinical efficacy of substrates such as protease inhibitors (Levine, 2012). Table 22.2 summarizes drugs that have been involved in clinically significant interactions through Pgp, are associated with strong warnings, or have recommendations for specific interventions, including several other drugs of medical-psychiatric interest.

7. When the first-pass effect leads to very low bioavailability or highly variable bioavailability (which can be a worse problem clinically), nonenteral options should be considered if they are available. These include intravenous, intramuscular, or subcutaneous injections; transdermal delivery systems; sublingual tablets; intranasal and inhaled preparations; and rectal suppositories—the latter effective because the lower rectal veins drain in to the systemic rather than the portal circulation.

DISTRIBUTION

Drug distribution refers to the disposition of drug from the plasma to various tissues of the body, including body fat, internal organs, and the brain. Once a drug has entered the systemic circulation, it is distributed to the interstitial and intracellular fluids (Buxton & Benet, 2011). Distribution immediately after drug administration is dependent on cardiac output, regional blood flow, and tissue volume. Initially, the drug is rapidly distributed to well-perfused organs including the heart, brain, kidneys, and liver. During the second phase, drug is distributed to and reaches equilibrium with other tissues such as muscle, skin, and adipose tissue, at a much slower rate (minutes to hours). Tissue distribution is dependent on lipophilicity and pH, but most significantly on the compound's ability to bind with plasma proteins and macromolecules (Buxton & Benet, 2011).

PROTEIN BINDING

In the context of pharmacokinetics, protein binding refers to the binding of drugs to *plasma* proteins, rather than to cellular proteins in the tissues that are the targets of drug action. Protein binding impacts the ability of drug to reach the desired target, as only unbound drug may cross tissue to the site of action, and only free, unbound drug is in equilibrium across membranes. Bound drug cannot cross the blood–brain barrier, nor can it be metabolized by the liver or excreted by a normal kidney. In general, acidic drugs bind to

Table 22.2 POTENTIALLY SIGNIFICANT INTERACTIONS WITH PSYCHOTROPIC AGENTS VIA ALTERATIONS IN Pgp ACTIVITY

Pgp SUBSTRATES	Pgp INHIBITORS (POTENTIALLY INCREASE CNS LEVEL OF SUBSTRATE)	Pgp INDUCERS (POTENTIALLY DECREASE CNS LEVEL OF SUBSTRATE)
Antidepressants Amitriptyline Citalopram Clomipramine Desipramine Imipramine Nortriptyline Paroxetine Sertraline Venlafaxine *Antiepileptic agents* Carbamazepine Phenytoin *Antipsychotic agents* Aripiprazole Clozapine Haloperidol Olanzapine Paliperidone Quetiapine Risperidone *Analgesics* Fentanyl Methadone Morphine	*Cardiovascular drugs* Amiodarone Atorvastatin Captopril Carvedilol Diltiazem Dronedarone *Felodipine* Lomitapide Lovastatin Nicardepine Nifedapine Propafenone Quinidine Ranolazine Spironolactone Ticagrelor Verapamil *Anti-infective agents* Atazanovir Bocepavir Clarithromycin Erythromycin Etravirine Fluconazole Itraconazole Ketoconazole Nelfinavir Quinine Ritonavir Saquinavir Telaprevir Telithromycin *Antidepressants* Fluoxetine Fluvoxamine Paroxetine *Antiepileptic agents* Ezogabine *Antineoplastics* Lapatinib *Proton Pump Inhibitors* Omeprazole Pantoprazole *Immunosuppressants* Cyclosporine *Other* Colchicine Conivaptan Grapefruit juice Mirabegron	*Antiepileptic agents* Carbamazepine Phenobarbital Phenytoin *Antidepressants* Venlafaxine St. John's wort *Antiinfectives* Rifampin *Antineoplastics* Doxorubicin *Other* Dexamethasone

albumin while basic molecules bind to alpha-1 glycoprotein (also known as alpha 1 acid glycoprotein, AAG, or orosomucoid, OSM). There is clinically relevant genetic variation in the binding properties of AAG in the general population. The extent of binding to other plasma proteins is much less, and not likely clinically relevant. Protein binding is a saturable, nonlinear process, with the amount bound dependent on drug concentration, affinity for protein binding sites, and the number of binding sites present. With most drugs within their usual therapeutic ranges the extent of protein binding as indicated by the free fraction is relatively constant (Buxton & Benet, 2011).

The degree of protein binding exhibited by a drug is expressed quantitatively as the free fraction—the concentration of free drug divided by the total concentration (free + bound). Binding of drugs to albumin or AAG is nonspecific, and, because the number of binding sites is limited, it is possible for the free fraction of a drug to increase if the patient is taking other drugs that bind to the same protein. At equilibrium the percentage of binding will not affect the free concentration of the drug. Nonetheless, there can be a transient change in the free concentration following the addition of a second drug that competes for the first for binding on the same protein. This can be relevant in drugs with slow elimination and a low therapeutic index. In malnourished patients with low serum protein concentrations, the binding sites for drugs will be saturated at lower concentrations, and clinical effects related to competition of drugs at protein binding sites may be greater.

Disease processes can alter the concentrations of albumin and AAG and thereby increase or decrease protein binding. Hypoalbuminemia, typically due to malnutrition, hepatic dysfunction, or proteinuria, can increase the free fraction of acidic drugs. The free fraction of basic drugs such as chlorpromazine can be decreased under conditions that increase AAG levels; these include inflammatory states due to infection, autoimmune disease, cancer, or myocardial infarction. Animal models suggest that even physiological stress without disease can elevate AAG levels. Cigarette smoking can elevate AAG levels; the clinical significance of this fact is uncertain. The basal concentration of AAG is much lower than that of albumin; however, in inflammatory states it can increase to a multiple of baseline (Dasgupta, 2007). In patients receiving the antipsychotic clozapine, plasma concentrations can be significantly elevated to toxic levels in the presence of severe inflammation and infection although signs of toxicity may not be present. This may be attributed to elevations of AAG, as the drug is highly bound to AAG (Espnes. Heimdal, & Spigset, 2012).

Changes in the free fraction (as opposed to the level of free drug) typically do not affect drug efficacy or toxicity at equilibrium, because the concentration of free drug is unchanged. Note, however, that, laboratory assays of drug levels typically measure total drug concentration. When therapeutic drug monitoring is utilized and dosing targets a particular range of blood levels, a change in free fraction can be problematic because published therapeutic ranges presume a typical free fraction (Schmidt, Gonzalez, & Derendorf, 2010; Dasgupta, 2007). Within an individual patient, a change in measured blood levels between two points in time can be due to a change

in protein binding rather than a change in free concentration; such a change should not be misinterpreted as a reason to change dosage or to suspect the drug is not being taken as prescribed. The free drug level should be monitored in this situation if therapeutic drug monitoring is clinically required. When highly protein-bound drugs are initiated in situations where decreased protein binding is likely to occur, as with hepatic cirrhosis or the nephrotic syndrome, the starting dose should be lower than usual. If lack of efficacy suggests the dose should be increased, monitoring of free drug levels—if available—will reduce the risk of toxicity (Israili & Dayton, 2001).

The above issues of protein binding and drug levels are clinically significant only for drugs that are highly protein bound, namely, with a free fraction <20% (Table 22.3). The mood-stabilizing antiepileptic drugs carbamazepine and valproate both are in this category. For these drugs, measurement of free drug levels is preferable when it is available—especially when a patient has risk factors for decreased protein binding such as low serum albumin and/or concomitant drugs that compete for albumin binding sites.

The total volume of distribution of a drug is a function of both body mass and body composition; obese patients can, for lipophilic compounds, have a significantly higher volume of distribution than those of normal weight, especially with highly lipophilic drugs (Hanley, Abernethy, & Greenblatt, 2010). They therefore can require higher doses for efficacy than patients with normal body weight. The need for a dosage adjustment, and how much dosage should be changed, is specific to the drug and its indication. Linear adjustment via mg/kg dosing is not generally appropriate because body *composition* is different in severely obese patients. In morbid obesity, 20%–40% of weight increase is attributable to an increase in lean body mass (De Baerdemaeker, Mortier, & Struys, 2004). The clinical relevance of obesity to pharmacokinetics is complex because obesity can affect drug metabolism as well as drug distribution, and it is often associated with inflammatory states that increase AAG levels, thereby increasing the protein binding of basic drugs. Appropriate adjustments for dosing for obesity will depend on the distribution and metabolism of the specific drug and whether the drug is intended for short-term or longer-term use. Before equilibrium is reached, a patient with a large volume of distribution can require larger than usual doses for an adequate therapeutic effect; after equilibrium is reached, the need for a dosage adjustment will depend more on whether the drug's metabolism was affected by a medical complication of obesity.

Finally, distribution of a drug across the blood–brain barrier is obviously relevant to its therapeutic effect; however, differences in such distribution rarely manifest as differences in blood concentrations because the brain contributes relatively little to the overall volume of distribution. Pgp, mentioned above in connection with its role in drug absorption, has special relevance to distribution across the blood–brain barrier; some drugs are actively transported from brain endothelial cells back into the bloodstream. Inhibitors of Pgp, therefore, will therefore increase the relative brain concentration of a drug that it actively transports. Inducers of Pgp will reduce the relative brain concentration of such a drug. The effect of Pgp at

Table 22.3 PSYCHOTROPIC MEDICATIONS THAT ARE HIGHLY PROTEIN-BOUND

DRUG	DEGREE OF PROTEIN BINDING
Antidepressants	
Bupropion	84%
Citalopram	80%
Doxepin	80%
Duloxetine	90%
Fluoxetine	95%
Fluvoxamine	80%
Mirtazapine	85%
Nefazodone	99%
Paroxetine	95%
Sertraline	98%
Selegiline	90%
Trazodone	95%
Vilazodone	99%
Antiepileptic Drugs	
Carbamazepine	90%
Phenytoin	95%
Tiagabine	96%
Valproic acid	90%
Antipsychotic Agents	
Aripiprazole	99%
Asenapine	95%
Chlorpromazine	97%
Clozapine	97%*
Fluphenazine	99%
Haloperidol	90%
Iloperidone	95%
Lurasidone	99%
Olanzapine	93%
Quetiapine	83%
Risperidone	90%
Ziprasidone	94%
Autonomic Agents	
Propranolol	90%
Analgesics	
Fentanyl	86%
Methadone	90%
Buprenorphine	95%

Most of the listed drugs are primarily bound to albumin. Those with significant binding to AAG are indicated with an asterisk. PK issues related to protein binding of albumin-bound drugs usually arise because of low serum albumin, typically due to liver disease, malnutrition or proteinuria. PK issues related to protein binding of AAG-bound drugs usually arise because of an increase in AAG with infection and with inflammatory or autoimmune disease.

the blood–brain barrier can be large and clinically important (Lin & Yamazaki, 2003). Drugs with clinically significant Pgp transport at the blood–brain barrier include the antidepressants fluvoxamine, citalopram and escitalopram, venlafaxine and desvenlafaxine; and the antipsychotic drugs haloperidol, risperidone, and paliperidone. The pharmacokinetic and pharmacodynamic effects of Pgp will go in the same direction; when induction of Pgp decreases a drug's blood level by decreasing its net intestinal absorption, it will also decrease the drug's brain

level by increasing the drug's transport across the blood–brain barrier from brain to blood. For some drugs, the difference in the brain:blood ratio can be more clinically important than the difference in blood level. Four general medical drugs known to be potent inhibitors of Pgp are erythromycin, ketoconazole, quinidine, and verapamil (Wang, Ruan, Taylor, Donovan, Markowitz, et al., 2004; Linnet & Ejsing, 2007). A frequently updated source of data on PK properties of drugs, including their interactions with transporters like Pgp, can be found on the Internet at www.drugbank.ca. The website provides PK information as well as supportive references.

ELIMINATION

METABOLISM

Most psychotropic drugs are lipophilic; this property facilitates their crossing the blood–brain barrier. Psychotropic drugs that are not lipophilic either are effective despite relatively low brain levels or have their access to the brain facilitated by transporters. In their unaltered form, lipophilic compounds are poorly excreted by the kidneys because they will be reabsorbed into the systemic circulation in the renal tubules. To terminate drug action and to allow for elimination from the body, drugs are transformed by metabolism to more polar, hydrophilic compounds. Hydrophilic metabolites usually are inactive, but some have useful therapeutic activity and have even been developed as drugs in their own right— for example, 9-hydroxyrisperidone (paliperidone).

Prodrugs are pharmaceuticals that are biologically inactive until they are metabolized; one or more of the metabolites has the desired therapeutic effect. Prodrugs are developed to address poor bioavailability and/or other pharmacokinetic challenges. Medical psychiatrists should be aware when a patient has a medical condition that can interfere with the metabolism of a prodrug into its active metabolite(s).

Biotransformation reactions can be classified as Phase I (oxidative) or Phase II (conjugative). Phase I oxidative reactions usually involve an enzyme of CYP (aka cytochrome P450) system. Phase II conjugation reactions, which bind the drug to be eliminated with a polar moiety such as glucuronic acid, a sulfate group, or glutathione, often involve the uridine 5-diphosphate glucuronosyltransferase (UGT) enzymatic system. The liver is the most important site of action of both the CYP and the UGT enzymes, though both classes of enzymes are found in the gut wall and to a lesser extent in other tissues.

Typically, drugs undergo Phase I metabolism followed by Phase II metabolism (Sandson, Armstrong, & Cozza, 2005). For most psychotropic drugs, Phase I metabolism is most important for terminating the drug's action; even for prodrugs that initially are activated by Phase I metabolism, subsequent Phase I metabolism of the active metabolite yields an inactive molecule. Changes in Phase II metabolism have particular clinical significance when the drug or active metabolite does not undergo Phase I metabolism (or when its Phase I metabolism is impaired). In this situation, an active molecule can accumulate to potentially toxic levels.

Cytochrome P450 enzymes, a family of heme-containing proteins, are so named because when they are in the reduced state and complexed with carbon monoxide, they are a red pigment with maximum absorption of light at a wavelength of 450 nm. The enzymes are officially designated by the initials CYP followed by an Arabic numeral, a capital letter, and another numeral to indicate the family, subfamily, and specific isoform of the enzyme. Their function is catalysis of oxidative reactions, most often the insertion of an oxygen atom into an organic compound, such as replacing a hydrogen atom with a hydroxyl group. Standard nomenclature is to refer to a CYP enzyme in a standard font and its associated gene in italics; for example, *CYP3A4* denotes the gene encoding the enzyme CYP3A4. Six enzymes are most important in the oxidation of CNS drugs: CYP1A2, 2C9, 2C19, 2D6, 2E1 and 3A4. Among these, 2D6 and 3A4 have the highest concentration in the human body. CYP2B6 and CYP2C8, while less important overall, still have a role in clinically significant interactions with common drugs.

Exogenous substances including foods, drugs, and environmental toxins can induce or inhibit the CYP enzymes. CYP *induction* usually entails increased synthesis of the enzyme beginning with increased mRNA transcription, although some CYP inducers raise CYP enzyme levels by inhibiting degradation of the enzyme. These mechanisms imply that the induction of a CYP enzyme will take hours, and maximal induction can take several days to weeks. In contrast to induction, *activation* of a CYP enzyme entails a direct interaction between a substance and the enzyme that increases the enzyme's catalytic activity with its intended substrate. Activation is an immediate process rather than a delayed one. Though it is frequently observed in vitro, activation is an uncommon cause of clinical drug interactions. CYP *inhibition* usually involves interaction of the substance with the enzyme rather than the substance influencing the synthesis and degradation of the enzyme. An inhibitor of a CYP enzyme can be a substrate, but not necessarily. Inhibitors can be reversible or irreversible, competitive or noncompetitive. Clinically relevant drug interactions involving CYP enzymes can be understood better if the specific mechanisms of the involved drugs' effect on the CYP enzymes in question are known (Hollenberg, 2002).

Most of the well-recognized, clinically significant drug interactions involving psychotropic drugs are related to Phase I oxidative metabolism of the drugs by the CYP system. Clinically significant interactions related to Phase II metabolism or to the action of membrane transporters like Pgp are less common. Because of the wider occurrence of clinically significant interactions related to Phase I metabolism, most studies of genetic variation in psychotropic drug metabolism have focused on genetic variability in the CYP system.

PHARMACOGENETICS

With respect to a particular CYP enzyme, individuals can be classified as *extensive metabolizers* (EM)—the usual or "wild-type" situation—or as poor (PM), intermediate (IM), or ultrarapid (UM) metabolizers. For some enzymes and substrates, UM status requires induction by exposure to the substrate. Patients with PM status have two defective copies of the gene for the CYP enzyme of interest, and therefore will metabolize the drug through an alternate pathway. Patients with IM status usually have one normal gene and one defective gene, so that the pathway using that CYP enzyme continues to be used but others become more relevant. Inhibition of a CYP enzyme can have a more profound clinical effect in IM patients, while having no effect at all in PM patients who don't use the enzyme in metabolizing the drug in question.

Particular ethnic groups are known to have a relatively high prevalence of non–wild type CYPs. Variability is especially well known and clinically important for CYP2D6, where 5%–10% of Caucasians are PM, 50% of Asians are IM, many Africans are IM, and UM status is common among those of Middle Eastern or North African descent (Cavallari & Lam, 2011).

The impact on the metabolism of a specific drug of a specific CYP variation will depend on whether the drug is primarily, substantially, or secondarily metabolized by that CYP enzyme. When a drug is primarily metabolized by a CYP enzyme—call it CYPx—no other CYP enzyme is involved in metabolizing the drug under usual conditions. In this situation of absent or diminished enzyme activity, CYPx will significantly raise the drug concentration because alternative metabolic pathways will be substantially less efficient. When the drug is substantially metabolized by CYPx, that enzyme will account for the metabolism of more than 50% of the drug under usual conditions. If another CYP enzyme, CYPy, accounts for the rest, diminished activity of enzyme CYPx will lead to a larger role for CYPy. The level of activity of CYPy will then determine whether the blood level of the drug is elevated. In that situation, diminished activity of enzyme B will become clinically relevant. When a drug is partially metabolized by CYPx—namely, when CYPx accounts for less than 50% of its metabolism under usual conditions—an *isolated* decrease in the activity of CYPx will not increase the drug level significantly, but a decrease in the activity of CYPx can be clinically important if there also is decreased activity of the CYPs that usually dominate the drug's metabolism. If the activity of CYPx is markedly *increased,* it doesn't matter whether that CYP is primarily, substantially, or partially involved. It will take over most of the metabolism of the drug, and the blood level will be lower than usual for a given dose. For this reason the ultrarapid phenotype for a CYP enzyme has broad clinical implications, because it can affect blood levels of drugs for which that enzyme is not usually the main metabolic route.

The following discussion of the CYP enzymes and drug interactions is introductory and heuristic; the reader is encouraged to consult standard references on potential drug interactions before starting any new drug. We will focus especially on situations where a single CYP enzyme is primary for a particular drug, as those situations offer good examples of the underlying principles.

INDICATIONS FOR PHARMACOGENETIC TESTING

The indications for pharmacogenetic testing are evolving with the increasing availability and decreasing cost of profiling patients' genetics of drug metabolism. Patients interested in gaining maximal control of their pharmacologic fate can already get pharmacogenetic profiles without a physician's order from several consumer-oriented clinical laboratories. Testing should be considered when patients have a strong personal or family history of unusual reactions to drugs that suggest PM or UM status, or when the patient belongs to an ethnic group known to have a high frequency of non-EM status for a CYP enzyme important in metabolizing a drug under consideration for use in treatment. An increased likelihood of PM status is especially relevant in when a drug to be prescribed has a low therapeutic index and/or when the patient will be on other drugs that can cause severe interactions in patients with PM or IM status.

From the practical viewpoint, CYP genotyping is widely available and the sample for analysis can be obtained by swabbing the patient's cheek—no blood draw is required. Laboratories will test for individual CYP enzymes or perform a panel of four, where the enzymes are known to affect the metabolism of many psychotropic drugs and to have a significant frequency of PM and or UM alleles in the general population, and where genotype and phenotype have an established association. These enzymes are CYP1A2, 2C9, 2C19, and 2D6. CYP3A4 has very wide variability in enzyme activity in the general population, and it has many single nucleotide polymorphisms. However, the genotype–phenotype associations are not sufficiently well established to infer the enzyme's metabolic activity from the genotype. For this reason, CYP3A4 is not included in pharmacogenetic testing even though interactions involving CYP3A4 are very common.

For many psychotropic drugs, the rate of metabolism is linear over a broad range of dosing (first order kinetics). For these drugs, clearance of the drug at therapeutic dosage can be inferred from clearance of the drug at a "microdose"—a dose small enough that significant adverse effects would be unlikely even in a patient with unusual sensitivity to the drug. The feasibility of assessing patients' profiles of CYP activity through assaying blood levels after microdosing of typical substrates for each of the CYP isozymes has been demonstrated in research contexts, but for both practical and regulatory reasons it is not clinically used. However, measuring the blood level of one specific drug of interest after a small test dose could be a rational clinical strategy when one plans to use a drug with widely variable pharmacokinetics and many potential interactions in a vulnerable patient with clinical conditions or on other drugs that could alter the activity of the relevant CYP enzyme(s) (Madakasira & Khazanie, 1985).

CYP ENZYMES ESPECIALLY RELEVANT TO PSYCHOTROPIC DRUG METABOLISM

Several CYP enzymes are especially relevant to the metabolism of commonly prescribed psychotropic drugs; there are some facts about each that are well established and of particular interest to medical psychiatrists.

CYP1A2

CYP1A2 is the primary route of metabolism for the antipsychotic drugs clozapine and olanzapine, for the SSRI fluvoxamine, for the stimulants caffeine and theophylline, for the adrenergic agents propranolol and tizanidine, and for the analgesic (and potentially hepatotoxic) drug acetaminophen. It has a substantial role in the metabolism of the antidepressants duloxetine, clomipramine, and imipramine, and the antipsychotic drug chlorpromazine. It is induced by cigarette smoking and by insulin, modafinil, and omeprazole among other drugs, and (at least in theory) by eating large quantities of cruciferous vegetables such as broccoli and cauliflower. It is strongly inhibited by fluvoxamine, ciprofloxacin, and several other fluoroquinolones, and potentially by herbal teas made from chamomile, dandelions, peppermint, or cannabis. It is worth noting that smoked cannabis, like smoked tobacco, *induces* CYP1A2 (Grant, Atkinson, Gouaux, & Wilsey, 2012).

Of particular concern to medical psychiatrists is the effect of alterations in CYP1A2 activity on concentrations of drugs such as clozapine and olanzapine, and of *discontinuing* agents that induce CYP1A2. General medical illness, and especially hospitalization, frequently is associated with smoking cessation, dietary changes, and/or discontinuation of drugs because they are deemed undesirable or unnecessary in the current medical context. When smoking cessation is initiated, drugs like clozapine and olanzapine can require dosage reductions of 30%–40% to maintain the prior blood level of the drug (Haslemo, Eikeseth, & Tanum, 2006). The effect of smoking to induce CYP1A2 can be maximal on as few as seven cigarettes a day, so even light smokers are vulnerable to the interaction (Lowe & Ackman, 2010).

There is substantial variability of CYP1A2 activity in the general population on a genetic basis; patients can be PM, IM, EM, or inducible UM, who develop ultra-rapid metabolism when exposed to a CYP1A2 inducer. The majority of patients of pure Japanese descent will have the UM phenotype; it is also very common in patients of sub-Saharan African background. While UM status is less common among patients of northern European background, it is common enough that it should be considered when a patient with such background fails to respond as expected to a conventional dose of a drug primarily metabolized by CYP1A2 (Mrazek, 2010).

CYP2C9

CYP2C9 is the primary metabolic enzyme for the SSRI fluoxetine and for the anesthetic (and potential antidepressant) ketamine. It is also the predominant metabolic enzyme for most of the nonsteroidal antiinflammatory drugs (NSAIDs), for the antiepileptic drug (AED) phenytoin, for several commonly prescribed oral hypoglycemic drugs, for the PDE5 inhibitor sildenafil and for the anticoagulant warfarin. It is strongly inhibited by valproate (Gunes, Bilir, Zengil, Babaoglu, Bozkurt, et al., 2007), by the antifungal drugs miconazole and fluconazole, by amentoflavone, a constituent of *Ginkgo biloba* and of St. John's wort (Kimura, Ito, Ohnishi, & Hatano, 2010), and by cannabis (Yamaori,

Koeda, Kushihara, Hada, Yamamoto, et al., 2012). The effect of valproate, one of the most common treatments for bipolar disorder, is of special interest to medical psychiatrists since it implies that patients treated for bipolar disorder with valproate can develop severe hypoglycemia on typical doses of oral hypoglycemic drugs, and can develop unexpectedly severe side effects from typical doses of NSAIDs or sildenafil. Whether the effect of *Ginkgo biloba* or St. John's wort on CYP2C9 will be clinically significant will depend on the dosage and on the amentoflavone content of the specific preparation consumed. Commercial preparations of these herbal remedies are standardized for their concentrations of ginkgosides and of hypericin, respectively, and not for their concentrations of amentoflavones; this introduces another element of uncertainty. Cannabis use should be taken into account when considering CYP2C9 substrates, especially in light of increasing legalization for both medical and recreational use. There are relatively few inducers of CYP2C9; the anti-TB drug rifampicin is the best known.

There is significant genetically based variability of the CYP2C9 phenotype in the general population. Of patients of European descent approximately 10% will be poor metabolizers. However, some ethnic groups have a particularly high prevalence of non-EM phenotypes. For example, over one-third of patients with Ashkenazi Jewish background have either an IM or PM phenotype (Scott, Edelmann, Kornreich, Erazo, & Desnick, 2007). Patients of Asian or African descent are unlikely to have non-EM phenotypes.

CYP 2C19

CYP2C19 is the predominant enzyme in the metabolism of the SSRIs citalopram and escitalopram, of the TCAs amitriptyline and clomipramine, and of the benzodiazepine diazepam and its active metabolite nordiazepam (Andersson, Cederberg, Edvardsson, Heggelund, & Lundborg, 1990). It has a substantial role in the metabolism of the TCAs doxepin, imipramine, and nortriptyline (Morinobu, Tanaka, Kawakatsu, Totsuka, Koyama, et al., 1997); the SSRI sertraline; and the MAO-A inhibitor moclobemide, as well as in the metabolism of the older AEDs phenytoin, primidone, and phenobarbital. It is induced by the AED carbamazepine, by the oral contraceptive norethisterone, by the corticosteroid prednisone, and by the anti-TB drug rifampicin, among others. It is strongly inhibited by fluvoxamine and fluoxetine (Jeppesen, Gram, Vistisen, Loft, Poulsen, et al., 1996).

Approximately 2% of patients of Northern European descent are PM for 2C19; 26% have the IM phenotype for 2C19. Among Chinese patients, however, only 25% of patients will have EM phenotypes, while 50% will have the IM phenotype and 25% will have the PM phenotype. Over 25% of patients of African descent will have PM phenotypes for 2C19. Four percent of the Northern European population have UM phenotypes and another 9% have a lesser degree of increased 2C19 activity. The UM phenotype is rare in Chinese patients. (Desta, Zhao, Shin, & Flockhart, 2002).

CYP2C19 is of special medical-psychiatric interest for several reasons. Prednisone is widely prescribed for a range of inflammatory and autoimmune conditions, many of which have depression as a psychiatric complication or comorbidity. If such patients are treated for their depression with citalopram or escitalopram, the drug may have less efficacy than expected because it will be more rapidly metabolized. Initiation of prednisone in a patient on long-term treatment with diazepam may reduce levels of diazepam and its active metabolite nordiazepam, leading to a rebound of anxiety. Citalopram is very widely prescribed as an antidepressant and is generally viewed as having low toxicity, but it can cause dose-dependent QT prolongation. QT prolongation could be clinically significant in patients with the PM phenotype treated with typical doses of this drug. Many oral contraceptive drugs contain norethisterone. Such contraceptives can make citalopram or escitalopram less efficacious at their usual doses by accelerating their metabolism.

CYP2D6

CYP2D6, the second most prevalent drug-metabolizing enzyme in the human body, is involved in the metabolism of hundreds of drugs. It is the primary enzyme involved in the metabolism of the SSRI antidepressants fluoxetine and paroxetine; the SNRI venlafaxine; the TCAs desipramine, doxepin, and nortriptyline; the first-generation antipsychotic drugs chlorpromazine, haloperidol, perphenazine, and thioridazine (von Bahr, Movin, Nordin, Lidén, Hammarlund-Udenaes, et al., 1991); and the second-generation antipsychotic drug risperidone (Spina, Avenoso, & Facciola, 2001). It is substantial in the metabolism of several other antidepressants and of the second-generation antipsychotic drugs aripiprazole and olanzapine. It is important (primary or substantial) in the metabolism of the opioids codeine, hydrocodone, oxycodone, and tramadol. Both codeine and tramadol are prodrugs requiring metabolism for activation; thus, patients with the PM phenotype for 2D6 may get poor pain relief from codeine or tramadol, while those with the UM phenotype may get a more rapid onset of effect, with greater abuse liability. CYP2D6 has a substantial role in the metabolism of most of the beta blockers, the amphetamines and atomoxetine, and the cholinesterase inhibitor donepezil.

CYP2D6 is induced by dexamethasone and by rifampin. It is strongly inhibited by the antidepressants fluoxetine, paroxetine, and bupropion; by quinidine; and by the antiretroviral agent ritonavir. The effect of quinidine to inhibit CYP2D6 is exploited to increase dextromethorphan concentrations in the fixed-dose combination of quinidine and dextromethorphan, which is indicated for treating pseudobulbar affect.

CYP2D6 shows clinically important genetic variability. Five to ten percent of Caucasian patients and more than 10% of those with sub-Saharan African background have the PM phenotype. About half of the Asian population have the IM phenotype. And, a significant number of patients of North African or Middle Eastern background have the UM phenotype.

The involvement of CYP2D6 in the metabolism of opiate analgesics is of particular medical-psychiatric interest because pain and depression are associated, and it is common for patients to receive both an opiate and an antidepressant. Fluoxetine, paroxetine, and bupropion can each prolong the effect of the commonly prescribed opiates oxycodone and hydrocodone, while interfering with the efficacy of codeine or tramadol.

CYP3A4

CYP3A4 is the most prevalent of all of the CYP enzymes. It is found in large quantities in the intestine as well as in the liver, and it is involved in the metabolism of hundreds of drugs. For psychotropic drugs, CYP3A4 typically is not the exclusive route of metabolism. When CYP3A4 is not the exclusive route of Phase I metabolism, the lack of CYP3A4 activity or its inhibition becomes clinically significant when the other CYP enzyme(s) involved also have diminished or absent activity.

Psychotropic drugs that are substrates for CYP3A4 include the tertiary amine TCAs; the SSRIs citalopram and escitalopram, norfluoxetine, and sertraline; the SNRI venlafaxine; trazodone and nefazodone; buspirone; several of the antipsychotic drugs including risperidone, iloperidone, haloperidol, aripiprazole, and ziprasidone; opiates including buprenorphine, codeine, fentanyl, and methadone; several of the benzodiazepines including alprazolam (Greenblatt, Wright, von Moltke, Harmatz, Ehrenberg, et al., 1998); the hypnotic "Z" drugs zolpidem, zaleplon, and eszopiclone; and the PDE5 inhibitors sildenafil and tadalafil. CYP3A4 is also involved in androgen and estrogen metabolism. Inducers of particular medical-psychiatric interest include the AEDs carbamazepine, oxcarbazepine, phenytoin, and phenobarbital; modafinil; glucocorticoids including prednisone; and the herbal remedy St. John's wort. Strong inhibitors include the antidepressant drug nefazodone, several of the antiretroviral drugs, the macrolide antibiotics clarithromycin and telithromycin, and the antifungal drugs ketoconazole and itraconazole. Several other agents of medical-psychiatric interest are inhibitors of lesser or unknown strength. These include grapefruit juice, the SSRIs fluoxetine (and its metabolite norfluoxetine) and fluvoxamine, and the herbal remedies valerian, milk thistle, and *Ginkgo biloba*.

CYP3A4 activity varies widely in the general population, but the phenotypic variability is not readily assessed by pharmacogenetic testing.

Of particular interest to medical psychiatrists is the role of CYP3A4 in the metabolism of commonly prescribed hypnotic drugs, antianxiety drugs, and opiate analgesics, as medical patients often receive these in conjunction with drugs than can induce or inhibit its activity. Inhibition of CYP3A4 by grapefruit juice (Lilja, Kivisto, Backman, Lamberg, & Neuvonen, 1998) and induction of CYP3A4 by St. John's wort have caused serious adverse events in well-documented cases.

CYP2E1

CYP2E1 metabolizes ethyl alcohol and several of the anesthetic drugs. While it typically has less of a role in ethanol metabolism compared to alcohol dehydrogenase, it is induced by chronic alcohol use, thereby making alcoholics more rapid metabolizers of alcohol.

DRUG METABOLISM AND SELECTION OF PSYCHOTROPIC DRUGS

The medical psychiatrist has an opportunity to prevent adverse drug interactions related to drug metabolism in three general clinical situations:

1. The patient is taking one or more psychotropic drugs chronically, then develops an acute medical illness—or an exacerbation or relapse of a chronic medical condition—that necessitates starting a general medical drug that interacts with one of the continuing psychotropic drugs. In this case, preventive strategies include prospective adjustment of the psychotropic drug dose and/or the general medical drug dose, monitoring clinical presentation, therapeutic drug monitoring, and/or switching to a noninteracting alternative within the same therapeutic class.

2. The patient is being treated for one or more general medical conditions and then develops a mental disorder or other condition requiring treatment with a psychotropic drug. In addition to the strategies for the first case, here the medical psychiatrist may have the option of prescribing or recommending a psychotropic drug within the relevant therapeutic class that is less likely to cause a clinically significant drug interaction. For example, it is generally wise to avoid initiating fluoxetine in patients with multiple general medical conditions because of its strongly inhibitory effect on CYP2D6 and other inhibitory actions on CYP2C19 and CYP3A4.

3. Hospitalization or other consequences of acute general medical illness implies cessation of smoking or discontinuation of nonprescribed drugs or supplements that have affected drug metabolism. Discontinuation of agents that induce or inhibit the metabolism of the patient's general medical or psychotropic drugs will alter the levels of those drugs, often with clinically significant consequences. Prevention is based on anticipating the effects and estimating their magnitude. If the expected effect is large, doses should be adjusted. If it is relatively small, closer clinical monitoring, potentially with checking drug levels, may suffice.

EXCRETION

Drugs and metabolites are removed from the body through excretion. The kidney is the primary organ for excretion of psychotropic medications, although there may be unabsorbed drug or metabolites secreted into the bile or directly into the intestinal tract that are excreted in the feces. Less clinically relevant, drugs may be excreted in sweat, saliva, tears, and breast milk. Renal excretion involves glomerular filtration, active tubular secretion, and passive tubular reabsorption.

Table 22.4 RELEVANT CYTOCHROME P450 DRUG INTERACTIONS

ENZYME	SUBSTRATE	INDUCER	INHIBITOR
CYP1A2	*Antidepressants* Fluvoxamine Clomipramine Duloxetine Imipramine *Antipsychotics* Clozapine Haloperidol Olanzapine Chlorpromazine *Stimulants* Caffeine *Autonomic Agents* Propranolol Tizanidine *Analgesics* Acetaminophen Naproxen	*Smoking* Cruciferous vegetables Insulin Modafinil Omeprazole	*Fluvoxamine Ciprofloxacin* Cimetidine Amiodarone Interferon
CYP2C9	*Antidepressants* Fluoxetine *Antiepileptic Drugs* Phenytoin *Analgesics* Diclofenac Ibuprofen Meloxicam Piroxicam Naproxen *Other* Ketamine	Rifampin Secobarbital	*Fluconazole* *Amiodarone* *Valproic acid and derivatives* *Fluvoxamine* *Isoniazid* *Ginkgo biloba* *St. John's wort*
2C19	*Antidepressants* Amitriptyline Citalopram Clomipramine Imipramine Moclobemide *Antiepileptic drugs* Diazepam Phenytoin Primidone *Autonomic agents* Propranolol *Analgesics* Indomethacin Carisoprodol	*Carbamazepine* *Norethindrone* *Prednisone* *Rifampicin*	*Omeprazole* Chloramphenicol Cimetidine Felbamate Fluoxetine Fluvoxamine Indomethacin Ketoconazole Modafinil Oxcarbazepine Probenicid Ticlopidine Topiramate
CYP2D6	*Antidepressants* Amitriptyline Clomipramine Desipramine Duloxetine Fluoxetine Fluvoxamine Imipramine Nortriptyline Paroxetine Venlafaxine	Dexamethasone Rifampin	*Bupropion* *Fluoxetine* *Paroxetine* *Quinidine* Cinacalcet Duloxetine Sertraline Terbinafine Amiodarone Cimetidine

(continued)

Table 22.4 (CONTINUED)

ENZYME	SUBSTRATE	INDUCER	INHIBITOR
	Antipsychotics Aripiprazole Chlorpromazine Haloperidol Iloperidone Perphenazine Risperidone Thioridazine		
	Stimulants Atomoxetine Amphetamine		
	Autonomic agents Clonidine Propranolol		
	Analgesics Codeine * Oxycodone Tramadol* Lidocaine		
	Cognitive enhancers Donepezil		
CYP2E1	Acetaminophen	Ethanol Isoniazid	Disulfiram
CYP3A4	*Antidepressants* Citalopram Escitalopram Levomilnacipran Nefazodone Sertraline Venlafaxine Trazodone	*Carbamazepine* Oxcarbazepine Phenytoin Phenobarbital Modafinil Prednisone Rifampin St. John's wort	*Nefazodone* *Indinavir* *Nelfinavir* *Ritonavir* *Clarithromycin* *Itraconazole* *Ketoconazole* Erythromycin Telithromycin Verapamil Diltiazem Fluvoxamine Norfluoxetine Grapefruit juice
	Anxiolytics Alprazolam Diazepam Midazolam Triazolam Buspirone		
	Hypnotics Zolpidem Zaleplon Eszopiclone		
	Antipsychotics Aripiprazole Haloperidol Iloperidone Lurasidone Risperidone Ziprasidone		
	Antiepileptic drugs Carbamazepine		
	Stimulants Modafinil Armodafinil		
	Analgesics Buprenorphine Codeine Fentanyl Methadone		

Potent inhibitors and inducers are indicated in bold italics.

*activation required for clinical activity.

Glomerular filtration controls the amount of drug entering the tubular lumen. As noted above, only unbound drug is filtered except in cases of proteinuria. Active tubular secretion occurs via transporters in the proximal renal tubule and can add drug to the tubular fluid. Reabsorption occurs mainly in the distal tubule via nonionic passive diffusion, though some active reabsorption by transporters also occurs.

Pgp transporters, discussed above in connection with intestinal absorption and in affecting relative brain concentrations, are also located in the proximal tubules of the kidney, where they actively excrete certain drugs. Inhibition of Pgp at the proximal tubule can also lead to reduced clearance of those drugs. Thus induction of Pgp transporters in the kidney can reduce a drug's effect, while Pgp inhibition can increase it—but this will be the case only if the form of drug excreted by the kidney is active. Paliperidone, for example, is excreted in active form. Note that Pgp activity always reduces the effect of a CNS drug, if it matters at all, by reducing the drug's absorption from the intestine, by increasing its elimination via the kidney, and by removing drug from the CSF and thereby reducing the ratio of brain concentration to plasma concentration.

CLEARANCE

Clearance (Cl) describes the body's ability to remove drug from the plasma; it is often used as a synonym for renal clearance, although other organs are often involved. It is expressed in units of ml/minute. It is affected by body weight and surface area, protein binding, blood flow to the liver and kidneys, extraction ratio, renal function, hepatic function, and cardiac output. Clearance is useful in determining the dosing rate to maintain a steady-state concentration within a therapeutic window. When a drug has first-order kinetics, the elimination of it is proportional to its concentration. This is the case for most drugs for which renal excretion is the primary route of elimination. When it has zero-order kinetics, there is a fixed amount of drug that can be eliminated per unit time. Zero-order kinetics are most often encountered when the drug is eliminated via a metabolic process that is saturated (i.e., maximal) at usual concentrations of the drug. The antiepileptic phenytoin, while following first-order kinetics at low doses, changes to zero-order when the dose is increased and maximum velocity of metabolism (Vmax) is reached (Richens, 1979). Of great importance to safe driving, the clearance via hepatic metabolism of ethyl alcohol has zero-order kinetics.

VOLUME OF DISTRIBUTION

Volume of distribution (Vd) relates the total amount of drug in the body at steady state to its plasma concentration. It is the volume of plasma that would be needed to yield the steady-state plasma concentration actually observed, if the entire body consisted only of plasma rather than an assortment of tissues with different affinities for the drug. A highly lipophilic drug can have a relatively large Vd because much of the drug will be absorbed by body fat. High protein binding is another factor that can raise the Vd. Loading doses often are employed when

initiating treatment with drugs that have a high Vd. Once the body is loaded with the drug, a steady-state concentration can be obtained with a lower daily dose of the drug, since only the drug that is free in the plasma can be eliminated.

ELIMINATION HALF-LIFE

Elimination half-life describes the rate of drug removal from the body. Specifically, $T_{1/2}$ is the time required for the plasma concentration (Cp) to decrease by 50%. Half-life is dependent on both clearance and volume of distribution:

$$T_{1/2} = 0.693 \times VD/CL$$

Elimination half-life is useful in predicting the time to achieve steady state with regular dosing. *Steady state* describes the point where daily drug elimination equals the bioavailable daily dose of the drug. Conventionally, the time to steady state is estimated as 5 times $T_{1/2}$. Three half-lives after a drug is initiated or a dosage is changed its plasma concentration, Cp is at nearly 88% of the predicted steady-state concentration (Css); after 5 half-lives, Cp is at nearly 97% of Css. The value of $T_{1/2}$ can be used to determine a maximum interval between doses of a drug compatible with maintaining Cp above a therapeutic threshold. For example, if a drug has a minimum plasma concentration of 100 ng/ml for therapeutic efficacy, its $T_{1/2}$ is 12 hours and its Cmax after an oral dose is 300 ng/ml the drug must be given twice daily, as the elimination half-life of 12 hours implies that Cp would be subtherapeutic 24 hours after a single dose.

THERAPEUTIC DRUG MONITORING

Therapeutic drug monitoring (TDM) is defined as the management of a patient's medication regimen based on the measured concentration of the drug in blood, plasma, serum, or another body fluid (Dasgupta, 2007). For drugs with a wide range between the concentration required for pharmacologic activity and toxicity—that is, drugs with a high *therapeutic index*—TDM is not routinely performed. For drugs with a low therapeutic index and a well-established therapeutic range—for example, lithium—the use of TDM is a standard of practice.

The measurement of drug levels in plasma, serum, or other body fluids has clinical utility in several situations where TDM is not the standard of practice. These situations arise often in medical psychiatry. They comprise the following:

1. A patient fails to respond to a prescription for a typical therapeutic dosage of a medication and does not have side effects typical for that medication. In this situation a low level of the drug in the blood can suggest an individual difference in ADME, implying that the typical dosage will be inadequate for that particular patient. Alternatively, the patient might not be taking the medication as prescribed.

2. A patient develops typical adverse effects of an excessive dose of a medication while under a prescription for a typical therapeutic dosage of a medication. In this situation a

high level of the drug in the blood can suggest an individual difference in ADME, implying that the typical dosage will be excessive for that particular patient. Alternatively, the patient might be taking more of the medication than is prescribed.

3. A patient has a history of poor adherence to prescriptions, or there is some other reason to believe that adherence to a prescription will be an issue. Checking a blood level after several scheduled doses can establish whether the patient is taking the medication. A patient's knowledge that the blood level will be checked can, in some cases, motivate the patient to be more adherent.

4. A patient has a known reason for having PK for a given drug differing from the general population. This could be having a genotype associated with poor metabolism or ultrarapid metabolism of the drug, having liver or kidney disease, being morbidly obese, or taking other medications that induce or inhibit the metabolism of the drug in question. In this situation a prospective dosage adjustment typically will be made based on an estimate of the patient's PK profile for the drug. Checking the blood level after one or several doses of the drug can inform a more accurate and patient-specific dosage adjustment.

5. A patient is taking a drug that does not have first-order kinetics and its therapeutic index is sufficiently low that there is a danger of toxicity during initial dosing adjustments.

Most psychotropic drugs follow first-order kinetics, in which the steady-state concentration of the drug is proportional to the total dose (Bauer, 2011). Exceptions are important, because when drugs do not have first-order kinetics small increments of dosage can produce large increases in blood levels, or, alternatively, large increments in dosage produce small increases in blood levels. Two antiepileptic drugs offer classic examples. In the case of phenytoin there is a maximum amount of drug that can be metabolized per day. If, for example, a dosage of 300 mg per day saturated the metabolic enzymes, a dosage of 350 mg per day might double the blood level of the drug. In the case of carbamazepine, the drug induces CYP3A4—the enzyme that is the principal enzyme in its own metabolism. When a patient is initiating therapy with carbamazepine, increases in dosage can be necessary just to maintain a constant blood level. Non–first-order kinetics are an especially relevant concern when a standard dosage increment (e.g., one pill per day) can alter a patient's blood level from a subtherapeutic to a toxic one, or when autoinduction of metabolism can lead to a loss of the drug's therapeutic effect.

PLASMA OR SERUM, TOTAL OR FREE CONCENTRATIONS

When physicians order "blood levels" of a drug, the clinical laboratory typically makes the decision about whether serum or plasma will be assayed for the drug. The difference between serum and plasma is the presence of clotting factors (proteins) in the latter

and the presence of substances released by clotting in the former. For drugs that are highly protein bound, the total concentration of drug can be greater in plasma than serum although the free drug concentration is the same in both. Therapeutic ranges for total drug concentration, therefore, can differ between serum and plasma. When feasible, measurement of the free drug concentration is the most reliable basis for TDM. When free drug levels are not available, protein binding effects should be considered in the interpretation of serum or plasma levels.

PK CONSIDERATIONS FOR SPECIFIC PSYCHOTROPIC DRUGS

For each psychotropic drug there are several PK considerations that together can help the medical psychiatrist anticipate issues that might necessitate dosage adjustments or even contraindicate the drug in particular patients. They are:

1. Hepatic metabolism
   a. Is it necessary to activate the drug?
   b. Is it necessary to inactivate the drug?
   c. Are there active metabolites, and, if so, do they require further hepatic metabolism to inactivate them?
   d. Are there active metabolites that can accumulate and cause toxicity?
   e. What enzymes are involved, and which are primary?
   f. Does the drug induce or inhibit its own metabolism?
   g. Is the drug's metabolism affected by drugs commonly prescribed together with it?

2. Renal elimination
   a. Is elimination by the kidney necessary to terminate action of the drug?
   b. Are there toxic metabolites that must be eliminated by the kidney?
   c. Is elimination of the drug and its metabolites dependent only on glomerular filtration, or is there a significant role for renal tubular function?
   d. To what extent is the drug eliminated by hemodialysis?

3. Protein binding
   a. Is the drug highly protein bound?
   b. Is the drug bound to albumin, AAG, or both?
   c. Is there significant binding to any other proteins?
   d. Is the difference between serum and plasma levels big enough to impact TDM?

4. Interindividual variability
   a. Is there large variability in the PK of the drug in the general population?
   b. Are there known associations with age, gender, race, or ethnicity of the patient?
   c. Are there well-established genetic issues affecting the drug's PK?

5. Nonlinear kinetics
   a. Does the drug have nonlinear kinetics over some part of its usual dosage range?
   b. Is the effect to increase or decrease the increase in blood concentration for a given dosage increase?

6. Nutritional issues
    a. Is there a measurable food effect on drug absorption?
    b. Is it clinically relevant?
    c. How does malnutrition affect the drug's PK?
    d. How does obesity affect the drug's PK?
    e. How does obesity surgery affect the drug's PK?

7. Clinical significance of blood levels
    a. Is there a well-defined therapeutic range ("therapeutic window")?
    b. Is there a minimum threshold level for therapeutic effect?
    c. Is there a maximum threshold above which significant toxicity is common?
    d. Is TDM the standard of practice for utilizing the drug?

8. Dosing-related issues
    a. How long does it take for the drug to reach steady state?
    b. What is the elimination half-life?

ALTERNATE ORAL FORMULATIONS AND ALTERNATE ROUTES OF ADMINISTRATION

Alternate oral formulations comprise alternatives to standard tablets and capsules. Each alternative is associated with specific properties of interest to medical psychiatrists.

1. *Liquids—solutions and suspensions.* Liquids are more suitable for patients who have difficulty swallowing solids but not liquids, or who are unwilling to swallow pills for emotional reasons. These may be preferred after gastric bypass surgery, as absorption of liquid preparations is more predictable postprocedure than tablets or capsules. They also can be administered via a nasogastric tube or gastrostomy.

2. *Orally disintegrating tablets (ODTs)*—tablets that disintegrate while still in the mouth, with the active ingredient dissolving in the patient's saliva. Though there may be some absorption in the buccal and pharyngeal regions, their absorption takes place primarily in the gastrointestinal tract. Their primary benefit is ease of administration. Typically there is no difference in Tmax or Cmax between ODTs and standard tablets, and the quantitative effect on bioavailability is not clinically significant.

3. *Sublingual tablets.* These have rapid onset of action and high bioavailability, since first-pass metabolism is bypassed as the buccal and pharyngeal regions drain to the superior vena cava rather than to the portal vein. They require a measure of patient cooperation to keep the tablet under the tongue rather than swallow it. For this reason they are unsuitable for cognitively impaired patients.

4. *Controlled-release or extended-release (ER) tablets or capsules.* One specific form is the gastric retentive (GR) tablet. GR tablets, when taken with food, remain in the stomach for several hours and slowly release the active ingredient into the gastric fluid. GR tablets must be taken with food to have optimal pharmacokinetics. Thus they work best with cooperative patients who eat regular meals. CR and ER tablets are helpful to individuals who are susceptible to adverse effects when the drug is at Cmax, as these tend to produce lower peak concentrations compared to standard formulations. CR and ER formulations can be suitable for less frequent dosing, which can improve treatment adherence. A special situation of note is the patient with cognitive impairment living in the community who can receive one supervised medication dose per day.

5. *Enteric-coated tablets*—tablets coated with a material impervious to stomach acid but soluble in the less acidic environment of the intestine. These are more tolerable to patients prone to dyspepsia, but their absorption can be adversely impacted by shortened intestine or a gastrointestinal hypermotility.

Non-oral routes of administration for psychotropic drugs similarly have properties with special medical-psychiatric interest. They have the common feature of increased bioavailability because they do not require intestinal absorption and they do not undergo first-pass metabolism.

1. *Injections*—intravenous (IV), intramuscular (IM), or subcutaneous (SC). Injections avoid treatment adherence issues—although not compliance issues in patients who are resistant to care in general or injections in particular.
    a. IV administration allows for 100% bioavailability, and when given as a bolus Tmax is instantaneous with a corresponding relatively high Cmax. This can be desirable in patients in severe distress, but can also produce severe adverse effects. Administering medications as an intravenous push runs the risk of the patient experiencing an anaphylactic reaction. Additionally, if an adverse event occurs, administration is already complete and cannot be terminated early. Intravenous infusion likewise results in 100% availability but allows for greater control of absorption rate by adjusting rate of the drip. The issue of respiratory depression is particularly salient with IV antianxiety drugs, antiepileptic drugs, and analgesics; these can interact with other CNS depressants and cause a life-threatening situation. In general, IV psychotropic drugs with respiratory depressant effects should not be given without anesthesiology backup. IV access can be difficult in patients who have scarred veins because of frequent prior IV access (e.g., patients receiving cancer chemotherapy) or IV drug abusers.
    b. IM injections have a slower onset of action and lower Cmax than IV injections. The onset of action can be especially slow in patients with poorly perfused muscle because of peripheral vascular disease, heart failure, or shock. They are also associated with an increase in serum CPK levels. While serum CPK is no longer used to diagnose myocardial infarction, it is used in the

diagnosis of neuroleptic malignant syndrome. A moderate elevation of CPK should be interpreted with caution when a patient with suspected neuroleptic malignant syndrome has recently received an IM injection of an antipsychotic drug—or any other drug. IM injections can be problematic in severely malnourished or cachectic patients with markedly decreased muscle bulk. In these patients the trauma to muscle can be clinically significant, while blood levels can rise more rapidly than in patients with normal muscle bulk.

c. SC injections are seldom used to administer psychotropic drugs.

d. Although not approved for intravenous use, haloperidol given IV for delirium can be effective. However, there is a higher risk of QTc prolongation and *torsades de pointes* with IV administration compared with oral. The FDA issued a safety alert in September 2007 detailing this information. The alert recommends ECG monitoring, should haloperidol be given IV (Food and Drug Administration, 2007). The antiemetic droperidol is sometimes provided in lieu of haloperidol, but it also carries the risk of QTc prolongation and *torsades de pointes*, with the FDA issuing a black box warning for the risk of sudden cardiac death in 2001 (Gan, 2004). Other parenteral antipsychotics are designed to be given as intramuscular injections and should not be given IV.

e. Benzodiazepines—specifically lorazepam, diazepam, and midazolam—may be administered IV. Because of increased lipophilicity compared to lorazepam, diazepam and midazolam more easily cross the blood–brain barrier and thus have a much more rapid onset of action.

2. *Depot intramuscular injections*, also known as long-acting injectable (LAI) formulations, mitigate problems of medication nonadherence in outpatients. However, once a depot injection has been given it is not feasible to remove it, so if a patient has an adverse reaction to the medication it may last a long time. When depot injections of antipsychotic drugs cause adverse neurological effects, these can persist for weeks or months. Depot injections of narcotic antagonists can complicate analgesic therapy if the patient develops a painful medical condition, has severe trauma, or requires major surgery while the drug is still on board. In general, depot injections are not a good choice for patients with multiple medical comorbidities.

   The pharmacokinetics of LAI antipsychotic drugs exhibit the "flip-flop" phenomenon, where the drug's half-life is determined by its absorption rate rather than by its elimination (Ereshefsky et al., 1983). Flip-flop kinetics occur when a drug's elimination rate is substantially shorter than the rate of absorption. The PK curve of haloperidol, a typical LAI antipsychotic drug, is shown in Figure 22.2. When a change in metabolism occurs, the plasma concentration changes but the terminal elimination half-life does not.

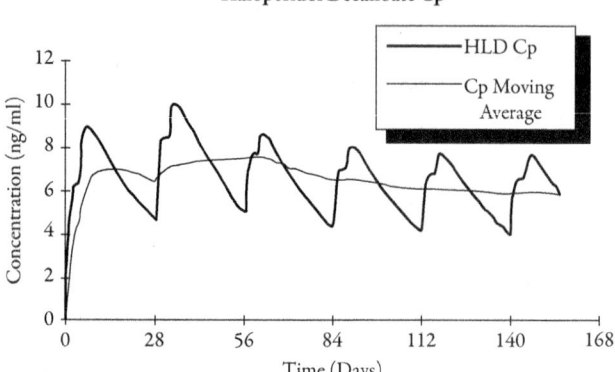

Figure 22.2 Pharmacokinetic Curve of Haloperidol Decanoate.

While medical psychiatrists would be unlikely to start an LAI antipsychotic drug in a person with an unstable medical condition, they are likely to encounter patients already receiving LAI antipsychotic drug therapy who need to start a general medical drug that might interact with the antipsychotic drug already on board. While the new drug likely won't affect absorption, it can effect distribution, metabolism, and excretion of the antipsychotic agent. For example, a patient on an LAI formulation of paliperidone might develop sedation or dystonia if started on cyclosporine, a potent inhibitor of Pgp. Or, a patient with schizoaffective disorder in remission on LAI olanzapine might experience an exacerbation of symptoms after the initiation of insulin for new-onset Type II diabetes, because insulin can induce CYP1A2.

3. *Rectal gels and suppositories*. Rectal administration may be considered if oral or parenteral routes are not viable options. However, absorption following rectal administration is erratic and often incomplete. Bioavailability is affected by drug placement: absorption in the lower rectal region bypasses first pass metabolism, while medication absorbed in the upper region passes through the portal vein. In general, 50% of drug absorbed rectally will bypass first-pass metabolism. These formulations have a limited role in the administration of psychotropic drugs. One exception is the use of rectal diazepam for the treatment of status epilepticus or delirium tremens in patients in which IV access is difficult to establish. In fact, diazepam is more rapidly absorbed as a rectal solution than either oral or IM administration, although rectal suppository results in decreased bioavailability and slower rate of absorption (Moolenaar, Bakker, Visser, & Huizinga, 1980). Diazepam is also commercially available as a rectal gel, which has 90% bioavailability with Tmax at 1.5 hours (Diastat Product Information).

4. *Transdermal patches*. Transdermal administration allows for a drug to be delivered into the systemic circulation via the skin. Transdermal patches are the most common formulation. Depending on the product, drug may be released immediately or over a prolonged period of time. Most formulations deliver drug at a constant rate

(zero-order process), providing a stable plateau plasma concentration. Transdermal administration bypasses first-pass metabolism and thereby increases bioavailability. Transdermal patches are more convenient than taking oral medication several times a day, when the pharmacokinetic properties of oral formulations would require it. Transdermal patches obviously avoid direct gastrointestinal irritation, and in some cases the lack of direct gastrointestinal effect reduces systemic toxicity. This is the case with the transdermal MAO inhibitor selegiline, which does not cause the food–drug interactions ("cheese effect") that limit the use of oral MAO inhibitors in treating depression. Finally, transdermal preparations do not produce high peak concentrations of drug that can be associated with adverse effects.

Transdermal delivery systems are available for an increasing number of psychotropic drugs. At this time there are transdermal delivery systems available for (1) selegiline, an MAO-B inhibitor antidepressant; (2) clonidine, an alpha-2 agonist used in treating tics and ADHD; (3) methylphenidate, a stimulant used in treating ADHD; (4) the opiate analgesics buprenorphine and fentanyl; (5) the cholinesterase inhibitors donepezil and rivastigmine; (6) nicotine, used for aid in smoking cessation; and (7) the sex hormones estradiol and testosterone. At this time there is no transdermal antipsychotic drug available.

Medical psychiatric patients for various reasons require individualization of drug dosage, and in some cases the optimal dose of a transdermally delivered drug can be less than the dose in the smallest marketed skin patch. In this situation, cutting of the patch often is considered—but this approach is not appropriate for transdermal systems based on a reservoir of drug rather than drug homogeneously embedded within a matrix. If a reservoir-based patch is cut, the entire dose of the drug can leak out at once. Successful transdermal therapy requires adequate blood flow to the skin and adequate adhesion of the patch to the skin. Patches should be applied to dry, hairless, and well-perfused skin for this reason. Absorption is variable in cachectic patients.

5. *Nasal sprays.* Because the nasal mucosa is highly vascularized, drugs administered by the intranasal route are rapidly absorbed into the systemic circulation; thus the nasal route is an alternative to injections when a rapid onset of action is required. These preparations have the same advantages as sublingual preparations; the nasal mucosa is well-perfused. Nasal disease is the primary limitation to their use. Nasal sprays can be problematic when the drug has a low therapeutic index and the patient is cognitively impaired or has a drug abuse liability. "Puffs" of a nasal spray can be large or small, and when a patient takes multiple puffs the resulting drug level may be toxic.

6. *Intranasal solutions.* While no solution of a psychotropic drug has been FDA approved for intranasal administration, it is feasible to administer solutions by the intranasal route if the volume of drug required is 1–2 ml or less.

When a solution is given this way the PK curve is similar to that produced by IV injection. Intranasal administration has been of particular interest in the treatment of narcotic overdose with naloxone and in the treatment of benzodiazepine overdose with flumazenil.

Off-label intranasal administration of solutions designed for injection might be contemplated if rapid onset of action is important and venous access is difficult. However, the very rapid onset of action with intranasal administration makes necessary the same precautions regarding cardiac, respiratory, and neurological side effects that are taken with intravenous administration.

Psychotropic drug administration by the intranasal route is entirely off-label. Notwithstanding, there is a community of interest in intranasal drug therapy including family members of opiate addicts and of children with intractable seizures. Intranasal benzodiazepines can abort status epilepticus as well as intravenous or rectal benzodiazepines (Holsti, Dudley, Schunk, Adelgais, Greenberg, et al., 2010), and intranasal naloxone can be life-saving in cases of opiate overdose (Robertson, Hendey, Stroh, & Shalit, 2009). Flumazenil, the benzodiazepine antagonist, might also be given by this route for emergency treatment of benzodiazepine overdose (Heard, Creighton, & Lerman, 2009).

7. *Aerosols for inhalation.* These offer a virtually instantaneous onset of action without requiring intravenous access. They lead to a high Cmax, which can be either helpful or harmful according to the circumstances. Inhaled products are rapidly absorbed if they reach the lower airways, which have a larger total surface area than the small intestine. This requires optimization of particle size to 1–4 microns in diameter; larger particles can be deposited in the large airways, and smaller ones can be exhaled prior to absorption (Rabinowitz, Lloyd, Munzar, Myers, Cross, et al., 2006).

The first-generation, mid-potency drug loxapine is available in an inhaled formulation (Lesem, Tran-Johnson, Riesenberg, Feifel, Allen, et al., 2011). The drug is rapidly absorbed into the systemic circulation with a Tmax of 2 minutes, unlike oral and intramuscular, which offers an average Tmax of 2 hours and 1 hour respectively (Spyker, Munzar, & Cassella, 2010).

AVAILABILITY OF ALTERNATE FORMULATIONS

Many psychotropic drugs come in alternate formulations that are FDA-approved. Others are at times administered off-label by routes other than the ones for which they are marketed. For example, capsules are emptied and dissolved in water to make a solution, or a drug designed for IM injection is given intravenously. These improvised approaches to drug delivery can have unwanted consequences when their implications for pharmacokinetics are not appreciated. When a solution intended for IM use is given IV, the Cmax will be higher and the Tmax will be shorter. This can potentially increase side effects dependent on Cmax such as cardiac arrhythmias or respiratory depression. On the other hand, the short Tmax makes intensive monitoring and emergency backup more practical. A CR tablet can be turned into an immediate-release product; doing the same for a GR tablet will destroy the physical properties that enable its retention in the stomach.

Availability (in the United States) of alternate formulations of psychotropic drugs is shown in Table 22.5. Drugs not ordinarily classed as psychiatric drugs are included if they are widely prescribed for psychiatric conditions; propranolol for symptoms of anxiety disorders is an example. The table includes only those alternate formulations that are FDA approved for some indication. Formulations made by compounding pharmacies or available in the United States only via personal importation are not included.

IMPACT OF ORGAN SYSTEM DISEASES ON PHARMACOKINETICS

KIDNEY DISEASE

Compounds with a high fraction of drug excreted unchanged remain active until they are eliminated by the kidney, so decreased renal function will affect their therapeutic action and their toxicity more than it will for drugs that are inactivated by hepatic metabolism or by conjugation with a hydrophilic moiety. Relevant examples are lithium, gabapentin, topiramate, and paliperidone.

Of drugs dependent on renal excretion for termination of their activity, lithium is considered the most problematic

Table 22.5 AVAILABLE FORMULATIONS OF PSYCHOTROPIC MEDICATIONS

MEDICATION	FORMULATION
Antidepressants	
Selective Serotonin Reuptake Inhibitors	
Citalopram	Tablet, oral solution
Escitalopram	Tablet, oral solution
Fluoxetine	Tablet, capsule, oral solution, weekly tablet
Fluvoxamine	Tablet, extended release capsule
Paroxetine	Tablet, controlled release tablet, oral suspension
Sertraline	Tablet, oral solution
Dual Reuptake Inhibitors	
Bupropion	Immediate release tablet, sustained release tablet, extended release tablet
Duloxetine	Delayed release capsule
Venlafaxine	Tablet, extended release tablet, extended release capsule
Desvenlafaxine	Extended release tablet
Levomilnacipran	Extended release capsule
Novel Mechanism Agents	
Mirtazapine	Tablet, oral disintegrating tablet
Nefazodone	Tablet
Trazodone	Tablet
Vilazodone	Tablet
Tricyclic Antidepressants	
Amitriptyline	Tablet
Clomipramine	Capsule
Desipramine	Tablet
Doxepin	Capsule, oral solution
Imipramine	Tablet, capsule
Nortriptyline	Capsule, oral solution
Monoamine Oxidase Inhibitors	
Isocarboxazid	Tablet
Phenelzine	Tablet
Selegiline	Transdermal patch

(continued)

Table 22.5 (CONTINUED)

MEDICATION	FORMULATION
Antipsychotics	
First Generation Agents	
Haloperidol	Tablet, oral solution, long-acting decanoate, short-acting IM solution
Fluphenazine	Tablet, oral elixir, long-acting decanoate, short-acting IM solution
Chlorpromazine	Oral tablet, injectable solution
Perphenazine	Tablet
Loxapine	Capsule, oral inhaler
Second Generation Agents	
Risperidone	Tablet, oral disintegrating tablet, oral solution, long-acting injectable suspension
Quetiapine	Tablet, extended release tablet
Olanzapine	Tablet, oral disintegrating tablet, long-acting injectable suspension, short-acting IM solution
Ziprasidone	Capsule, short-acting IM solution
Aripiprazole	Tablet, oral disintegrating tablet, oral solution, short-acting IM solution, long-acting injectable suspension
Paliperidone	Extended release tablet, long-acting injectable suspension
Iloperidone	Tablet
Asenapine	Sublingual tablet
Lurasidone	Tablet
Clozapine	Tablet, oral disintegrating tablet
Anxiolytics	
Buspirone	Tablet
Alprazolam	Tablet, oral disintegrating tablet, extended release tablet, oral solution
Chlordiazepoxide	Capsule
Clonazepam	Tablet, oral disintegrating tablet
Diazepam	Tablet, oral solution, injection solution, rectal gel
Lorazepam	Tablet, oral solution, injection solution
Oxazepam	Capsule
Clorazepate	Tablet, extended release tablet
Midazolam	Oral solution, oral syrup, injection solution
Sedative Hypnotics	
Estazolam	Tablet
Flurazepam	Capsule
Quazepam	Tablet
Temazepam	Capsule
Triazolam	Tablet
Eszopiclone	Tablet
Zaleplon	Capsule
Zolpidem	Tablet, extended release tablet, sublingual tablet, oral spray
Ramelteon	Tablet
Autonomic Agents	
Propranolol	Tablet, extended release capsule, oral solution, intravenous solution
Clonidine	Tablet, extended release tablet, transdermal patch
Guanfacine	Tablet, extended release tablet
Dexmedetomidine	Intravenous solution

(*continued*)

Table 22.5 (CONTINUED)

MEDICATION	FORMULATION
Antiepileptics and Lithium	
Valproic acid and derivatives	Capsule, delayed release capsule, delayed release tablet, extended release tablet, oral liquid, intravenous solution
Carbamazepine	Tablet, chewable tablet, extended release tablet, extended release capsule, oral suspension
Oxcarbazepine	Tablet, extended release tablet, oral suspension
Lamotrigine	Tablet, extended release tablet, chewable tablet, oral disintegrating tablet
Levetiracetam	Tablet, extended release tablet, oral solution, intravenous solution
Tiagabine	Tablet
Gabapentin	Tablet, capsule, oral solution
Topiramate	Tablet, capsule, extended release capsule
Lithium	Tablet, extended release tablet, capsule, oral solution, oral syrup
Stimulants	
Dexedrine	Tablet, extended release capsule, oral solution
Dextroamphetamine/Amphetamine	Tablet, extended release capsule
Methylphenidate	Tablet, extended release tablet, chewable tablet, extended release capsule, oral solution, oral suspension, transdermal patch
Lisdexamfetamine	Capsule
Atomoxetine	Capsule
Modafinil	Tablet
Armodafinil	Tablet
Cognition Enhancing Drugs	
Donepazil	Tablet, oral disintegrating tablet, transdermal patch
Rivastigmine	Capsule, oral solution, transdermal patch
Galantamine	Tablet, extended release capsule, oral solution
Memantine	Tablet, extended release capsule, oral solution
Drugs Used to Treat Addiction	
Naltrexone	Tablet, long-acting injection
Acamprosate	Delayed release tablet, enteric coated tablet
Buprenorphine/Naltrexone	Sublingual tablet, sublingual film
Varenicline	Tablet
Nicotine Replacement	Gum, lozenge, transdermal patch, oral inhaler, nasal spray

due to its narrow therapeutic index and significant risk of severe toxicity. The renal clearance of lithium is proportional to creatinine clearance down to a creatinine clearance of 30 ml/minute. Below this point, tubular reabsorption of lithium has a larger role, so the clearance of lithium decreases more rapidly than creatinine clearance. An essential point is that lithium is reabsorbed in the proximal tubules in proportion to sodium reabsorption, so lithium reabsorption is increased when aldosterone is increased, when patients are on thiazide diuretics, or when the patient has another clinical condition (e.g., heart failure) or is taking another drug associated with sodium retention. Hypokalemia can be an indicator of such conditions and should be a trigger for closer monitoring of lithium levels, slower titration of lithium dosage, and usually a lower ultimate dose of the drug. The complexity of giving lithium to patients with medical comorbidities has led many psychiatrists to avoid lithium in favor of other mood stabilizing agents, but this is not necessarily wise. Many patients with bipolar disorder attain a full remission on lithium but have only partial remissions on alternative agents. Furthermore, a full response to lithium makes neuroleptic drugs unnecessary; patients thus avoid the significant metabolic side effects of the latter drugs. Finally, there is some suggestion from recent research that consistent use of lithium can have a neuroprotective effect, preventing the loss of executive cognitive function that frequently complicates the long-term course of bipolar disorder (Diniz, Machado-Vieira, & Forlenza, 2013).

HEMODIALYSIS

Factors that affect drug removal by hemodialysis include water solubility, volume of distribution, molecule size, and degree of protein binding. Lipophilic or otherwise poorly soluble molecules are not dialyzed. When a drug has a high Vd, its concentration will change less with dialysis than one with a small Vd. Additionally, only free, unbound molecules can cross the dialysis membrane, so drugs with extensive protein binding will be less completely removed during the procedure. Information regarding psychotropic medications, renal impairment, and dialysis can be found in Table 22.6.

LIVER DISEASE

The liver is the primary site of drug metabolism, and thus the primary site of drug inactivation. The usual routes of inactivation of psychotropic drugs are oxidative reactions and conjugation with hydrophilic moieties; often the former are followed by the latter. Liver disease can alter any combination of pharmacokinetic parameters including bioavailability, the ratio of drug to metabolites, and conjugation of drug and/or metabolites as a prerequisite for renal excretion. For drugs metabolized by the liver, the typical effect of liver disease is an increase in drug level for a given oral dose—due to diminished

Table 22.6 DOSAGE ADJUSTMENTS OF SELECT PSYCHOTROPIC MEDICATIONS IN RENAL IMPAIRMENT

MEDICATION	RECOMMENDED DOSAGE ADJUSTMENT IN MILD TO MODERATE RENAL IMPAIRMENT (CRCL 30–50 ML/MIN)	RECOMMENDED DOSAGE ADJUSTMENT IN SIGNIFICANT RENAL IMPAIRMENT (CRCL 10–30 ML/MIN)	REMOVAL BY DIALYSIS
Antidepressants			
Selective Serotonin Reuptake Inhibitors			
Citalopram	None	None	None
Escitalopram	None	None	None
Fluoxetine	None	None	None
Fluvoxamine	None	None	None
Paroxetine	None	10–40 mg/day	None
Sertraline	None	None	Minimal
Dual Reuptake Inhibitors			
Bupropion	None	Reduce dose and/or frequency	Avoid with dialysis
Duloxetine	Initiate at 30 mg daily	Avoid use	No data
Venlafaxine	Decrease dose by 25%	Decrease dose by 50%	Minimal Decrease dose by 50%
Desvenlafaxine	Maximum 50 mg/day	50 mg every other day	None
Levomilnacipran	Maximum 80 mg/day	Maximum 40 mg/day	None *not recommended with ESRD (CrCl <15 ml/min)
Novel Mechanism Agents			
Mirtazapine	None	Reduced clearance, titrate slowly	No data
Nefazodone	None	None	None
Trazodone	None	None	No data
Vilazodone	None	None	No data
Tricyclic Antidepressants			
Amitriptyline	None	None	None
Clomipramine	None	None	None
Desipramine	None	None	None
Doxepin	None	None	None
Imipramine	None	None	None
Nortriptyline	None	None	None

(continued)

Table 22.6 (CONTINUED)

MEDICATION	RECOMMENDED DOSAGE ADJUSTMENT IN MILD TO MODERATE RENAL IMPAIRMENT (CRCL 30–50 ML/MIN)	RECOMMENDED DOSAGE ADJUSTMENT IN SIGNIFICANT RENAL IMPAIRMENT (CRCL 10–30 ML/MIN)	REMOVAL BY DIALYSIS
Monoamine Oxidase Inhibitors			
Isocarboxazid	None	None	No data
Phenelzine	None	None	No data
Selegiline	None	Caution	No data
Antipsychotics			
First Generation Agents			
Haloperidol	None	None	No data
Fluphenazine	None	None	No data
Chlorpromazine	None	None	None
Perphenazine	None	None	None
Loxapine	None	None	No data
Second Generation Agents			
Risperidone	None	Initial dose 0.5 mg bid, increase by 0.5 mg bid increments as needed	No data
Quetiapine	None	None	No data
Olanzapine	None	None	None
Ziprasidone	None	None	None
Aripiprazole	None	None	None
Paliperidone	Maximum dose 6 mg/day	Maximum dose 3 mg/day	No data
Iloperidone	None	None	No data
Asenapine	None	None	No data
Lurasidone	Starting dose 20 mg/day, maximum dose 80 mg/day	Starting dose 20 mg/day, maximum dose 80 mg/day	No data
Clozapine	None	None	No data
Anxiolytics			
Buspirone	None	None	None, use not recommended
Alprazolam	None	None	None
Chlordiazepoxide	None		None Decrease dose by 50%
Clonazepam	None	None	None
Diazepam	None	None	None
Lorazepam	None	None *caution with IV prolonged use—risk of propylene glycol toxicity	None
Oxazepam	None	None	None
Clorazepate	None	None	None
Midazolam	None	<10 ml/min—Decrease dose by 50%	None

(*continued*)

Table 22.6 (CONTINUED)

MEDICATION	RECOMMENDED DOSAGE ADJUSTMENT IN MILD TO MODERATE RENAL IMPAIRMENT (CRCL 30–50 ML/MIN)	RECOMMENDED DOSAGE ADJUSTMENT IN SIGNIFICANT RENAL IMPAIRMENT (CRCL 10–30 ML/MIN)	REMOVAL BY DIALYSIS
Sedative Hypnotics			
Estazolam	None	None	No data
Flurazepam	None	None	None
Quazepam	None	None	None
Temazepam	None	None	None
Triazolam	None	None	None
Eszopiclone	None	None	No data
Zaleplon	None	None	None
Zolpidem	None	None	None
Ramelteon	None	None	None
Autonomic Agents			
Propranolol	None	None	None
Clonidine	None	Consider lower initial dose	None
Guanfacine	None	Consider lower initial dose	None
Antiepileptics and Lithium			
Valproic acid and derivatives	None	None	None
Carbamazepine	None	None	None
Oxcarbazepine	None	None	No data
Lamotrigine	None	None	No data
Levetiracetam	250–750 mg q12h	250–500 mg q12h	Dialyzable; XR use not recommended; IR: 500–1000 mg daily, then 250–500 mg after hemodialysis
Gabapentin	400 mg tid	300 mg q12h to q2h4	Dialyzable; 100–300 mg daily, then 125–350 mg after hemodialysis
Topiramate	Reduce dose by 50%	Reduce dose by 75%	30% dialyzable; supplemental dose may be needed
Lithium	Reduce dose by 25%–50%	Reduce dose by 50%–75%	50%–100% dialyzable; dose after dialysis
Stimulants			
Dexedrine	No data	No data	No data
Dextroamphetamine/Amphetamine	No data	No data	No data
Methylphenidate	No data	No data	No data
Lisdexamfetamine	No data	No data	No data
Atomoxetine	None	None	No data
Modafinil	None	No data	No data
Armodafinil	None	No data	No data
Cognition Enhancing Drugs			
Donepazil	None	None	No data
Rivastigmine	None	None	No data
Galantamine	Maximum 16 mg/day	Maximum 16 mg/day	Do not use
Memantine	None	Maximum 5 mg bid	Do not use

(*continued*)

Table 22.6 (CONTINUED)

MEDICATION	RECOMMENDED DOSAGE ADJUSTMENT IN MILD TO MODERATE RENAL IMPAIRMENT (CRCL 30–50 ML/MIN)	RECOMMENDED DOSAGE ADJUSTMENT IN SIGNIFICANT RENAL IMPAIRMENT (CRCL 10–30 ML/MIN)	REMOVAL BY DIALYSIS
Drugs Used to Treat Addiction			
Naltrexone	None	No data	None
Acamprosate	333 mg tid	Do not use	Do not use
Buprenorphine/Naltrexone	None	Use with caution	None
Varenicline	None	Maximum 0.5 mg bid	Dialyzable. Maximum 0.5 mg daily
Nicotine Replacement	None	None	No data

hepatic inactivation, and potentially also to portal-systemic shunting that reduces first-pass metabolism. However, the relationship of liver disease to drug action has potential complexities. Impaired venous drainage of the intestines due to portal hypertension can reduce the intestinal absorption of drugs. Laxatives given to mitigate hepatic encephalopathy can decrease intestinal transit time and reduce drug absorption. Ascites and edema associated with advanced liver disease increase volume of distribution, which can initially reduce drug levels for a given oral dose but that will slow the elimination of the drug from the body. Decreased levels of serum proteins can increase the biologically active free fraction of drugs that are extensively protein bound. Furthermore, when the compound administered is a prodrug that requires metabolism for activation, liver disease can be associated with decreased levels of active metabolites and thus a decrease in therapeutic effect (Verbeck, 2008).

Another concern is that the *metabolic* activity of the liver is not directly measured by typical laboratory tests. "Liver enzymes" such as ALT and AST measure leakage of enzymes from damaged hepatocytes, and increased bilirubin levels reflect impaired biliary excretion (in the absence of hemolysis). Decreased albumin levels or increased clotting times typically reflect decreased hepatic protein synthesis. None of these phenomena have a consistent proportionality to changes in drug metabolism.

Because of these complexities, specific precautions in drug administration related to hepatic dysfunction have been arrived at largely through clinical experience and are based on Child Pugh scores. Child Pugh is based on factors including international normalized ratio, albumin levels, and bilirubin, as well as degree of ascites and encephalopathy (Child & Turcotte, 1964; Pugh, Murray-Lyon, Dawson, Pietroni, & Williams, 1973). Scores are used to assess prognosis in those with liver disease. Therapeutic drug monitoring may be required—especially with narrow therapeutic index medications such as tricyclic antidepressants—to minimize risk of significant toxicity. Psychotropic drugs that require significant dosage adjustment in patients with hepatic dysfunction can be found in Table 22.7.

HEART DISEASE

Medical psychiatrists' concerns about cardiovascular disease often have focused on cardiac rhythm; many psychotropic drugs affect the QT interval or potentially exacerbate conduction blocks; this issue is discussed in depth on cardiology chapter. However, both acute and chronic heart disease can have *pharmacokinetic* effects as well. Acute myocardial infarction or myocarditis can lead to increased levels of AAG, which will increase protein binding of basic drugs and lead to overestimation of the free drug concentration when the laboratory measures total concentration. The increase in protein binding can also slow the rate of renal clearance of the drug by increasing the volume of distribution. Heart failure can influence all four pharmacokinetic processes. Slowing of gastric motility can increase drug absorption, while decreased splanchnic blood flow can decrease it. Edema can increase volume of distribution. Hepatic congestion can lead to decreased drug metabolism. Decreased renal blood flow can imply decreased renal clearance, and clearance can be reduced further by sodium retention for drugs like lithium that are reabsorbed in the proximal tubules. The net effect will be greater with more severe heart failure, but the direction of effect, its magnitude, and its clinical relevance will depend on the drug—with, as always, drugs with a low therapeutic index being of greatest concern (Rodighiero, 1989). The drugs of greatest concern in patients with heart disease include tricyclic antidepressants and lithium, which not only have pharmacokinetic changes in patients with heart disease for the aforementioned reasons but also are known to have cardiotoxic effects (Roose, 1983; Roose, Glassman, & Dalack, 1989; Tilkian, Schroeder, Kao, & Hultgren, 1976).

RESPIRATORY DISEASE

Respiratory failure can influence the elimination of some drugs via metabolic acidosis. Decreased free fraction of basic drugs can occur (du Suich, McLean, Lalka, Erill, & Gibaldi, 1978), likely related to changes in alpha 1 glycoprotein concentrations. Further, decreased renal perfusion can impact elimination of drugs cleared by the kidney. Theoretically,

Table 22.7 DOSAGE ADJUSTMENTS OF PSYCHOTROPIC MEDICATIONS IN HEPATIC IMPAIRMENT

DRUG	RECOMMENDED DOSAGE ADJUSTMENT IN MILD HEPATIC IMPAIRMENT (CHILD-PUGH SCORE A)	RECOMMENDED DOSAGE ADJUSTMENT IN MODERATE HEPATIC IMPAIRMENT (CHILD-PUGH SCORE B)	RECOMMENDED DOSAGE ADJUSTMENT IN SEVERE HEPATIC IMPAIRMENT (CHILD-PUGH SCORE C)
Antidepressants			
Selective Serotonin Reuptake Inhibitors			
Citalopram	Maximum 20 mg/day	Maximum 20 mg/day	Maximum 20 mg/day
Escitalopram	10 mg/day	10 mg/day	10 mg/day
Fluoxetine	Use lower dose or extend dosing interval	Use lower dose or extend dosing interval	Reduce dose by 50%
Fluvoxamine		Reduce dose, titrate slowly	Reduce dose, titrate slowly
Paroxetine			Initiate at 10 mg/day, maximum daily dose 40 mg/day
Sertraline	Use lower dose or extend dosing interval	Use lower dose or extend dosing interval	Use lower dose or extend dosing interval
Dual Reuptake Inhibitors			
Bupropion	Use lower dose or extend dosing interval	Use lower dose or extend dosing interval	Immediate Release: maximum 75 mg/day Sustained Release: maximum 100 mg/day or 150 mg every other day Extended Release: 150 mg every other day
Duloxetine	Use not recommended	Use not recommended	Use not recommended
Venlafaxine		Reduce dose by 50%	Reduce dose by 50%
Desvenlafaxine	Maximum daily dose 100 mg	Maximum daily dose 100 mg	Maximum daily dose 100 mg
Tricyclic Antidepressants	Use with caution	Use with caution	Use with caution
Antipsychotics			
First Generation Agents			
Chlorpromazine			Avoid use
Second Generation Agents			
Risperidone			Initial dose 0.5 g mg bid, increase gradually
Quetiapine		Initial dose 25–50 mg, increase by 25–50 mg increments	Initial dose 25–50 mg, increase by 25–50 mg increments
Iloperidone	Use not recommended	Use not recommended	Use not recommended
Asenapine			Use not recommended
Lurasidone		Initial dose 20 mg daily, maximum daily dose 80 mg	Initial dose 20 mg daily, maximum daily dose 40 mg
Anxiolytics			
Buspirone			Use not recommended
Alprazolam		Reduce dose by 50%	Use not recommended
Chlordiazepoxide	Use not recommended	Use not recommended	Use not recommended
Diazepam	Reduce dose by 50%	Reduce dose by 50%	Reduce dose by 50%
Sedative Hypnotics			
Flurazepam	15 mg hs	15 mg hs	15 mg hs
Triazolam		Reduce dose	Avoid use
Eszopiclone			Initial dose 1 mg hs, maximum dose 2 mg hs

(continued)

Table 22.7 (CONTINUED)

DRUG	RECOMMENDED DOSAGE ADJUSTMENT IN MILD HEPATIC IMPAIRMENT (CHILD-PUGH SCORE A)	RECOMMENDED DOSAGE ADJUSTMENT IN MODERATE HEPATIC IMPAIRMENT (CHILD-PUGH SCORE B)	RECOMMENDED DOSAGE ADJUSTMENT IN SEVERE HEPATIC IMPAIRMENT (CHILD-PUGH SCORE C)
Zaleplon	Maximum 5 mg hs	Maximum 5 mg hs	Use not recommended
Zolpidem	Maximum 5 mg hs	Maximum 5 mg hs	Maximum 5 mg hs
Ramelteon			Avoid use
Antiepileptics and Lithium			
Valproic acid and derivatives	Avoid use	Avoid use	Avoid use
Carbamazepine			Avoid use
Oxcarbazepine			Avoid use
Lamotrigine		Decrease dose by 25%	Decrease dose by 50%
Stimulants			
Atomoxetine		Decrease dose by 50%	Decrease dose by 75%
Modafinil		Decrease dose by 50%	Decrease dose by 50%
Armodafinil		Decrease dose by 50%	Decrease dose by 50%
Cognition Enhancing Drugs			
Donepezil			
Rivastigmine	Maximum 4.6 mg/24 hour patch	Maximum 4.6 mg/24 hour patch	Avoid use
Galantamine		Maximum 16 mg/day	Avoid use
Drugs Used to Treat Addiction			
Naltrexone			Use with caution

hypoxia can lead to decreased biotransformation of drugs with decreased hepatic extraction ratios, thus decreasing rates of elimination (Taburet, Tollier, & Richard, 1990). In mild to moderate hypercapnia, an initial stress response leads to increased cardiac output and pulmonary pressure; however, as severity increases, cardiac output and vascular resistance decreases (Devlin, 2014). Mechanical ventilation and subsequent decreases in both cardiac output and hepatic blood flow can lead to increased plasma concentrations of drugs with high hepatic extraction ratios (Taburet, Tollier, & Richard, 1990), including certain antidepressants and antipsychotics such as amitriptyline and chlorpromazine, as well as propranolol. The benzodiazepine midazolam displays an extended elimination half-life when administered to those on mechanical ventilation (Byatt, Lewis, Dawling, & Cochrane, 1984).

INFECTIOUS AND INFLAMMATORY DISEASES

Infection and inflammatory processes can significantly impact both drug distribution to site of action as well as drug metabolism (Aitken, Richardson, & Morgan, 2006). Inflammation—as seen with acute infection, cancer, or chronic inflammatory disease such as rheumatoid arthritis—can lead to decreased expression of metabolic enzymes, including CYP enzymes, and drug transporters via proinflammatory cytokines including IL-6. Decreased metabolic enzyme activity is seen in both the liver and the gut (Xu, Wang, Sun, Chen, & Wei, 2006).

Increased plasma concentrations of drug can occur, along with toxicity. Decreased Pgp expression leads to greater penetration into the CNS for psychoactive drugs, increasing the risk for serious toxicity. Alternatively, use of targeted therapeutic proteins such as antitumor necrosis factor alpha or monoclonal antibody targeting IL-6 to treat chronic inflammatory diseases can cause an upregulation in metabolic enzymes and transporters, leading to increased clearance and decreased exposure to therapeutic medications and, ultimately, decreased therapeutic effect (Morgan, 2009). Alterations in pharmacokinetics of existing medications should be taken into account when therapy is initiated.

Infectious and inflammatory diseases can cause an increase in synthesis and release of acute phase proteins, including C-reactive protein and AAG (Morgan, 2009). Increased concentrations of AAG protein can lead to decreased free fractions of highly bound medications, including clozapine (as described above), and the synthetic opioid methadone (Kapur, Hutson, Chibber, Luk, & Selby, 2011).

MORBID OBESITY AND GASTRIC BYPASS SURGERY

As noted above, morbid obesity has complex effects on the pharmacokinetics of many medications, and predictions for dosing adjustments can be difficult to make. Alterations in Vd are dependent on protein binding, tissue blood flow, and physiochemical properties of the drug itself (Hanley, Abernethy, & Greenblatt, 2010). Obesity has little impact on albumin concentrations, but data, though mixed, suggest AAG concentrations can be elevated in obese persons and result in a lower free fraction of drug (Ghobadi, Johnson, Aarabi, Almond, Allabi, et al., 2011; Hanley, Abernethy, & Greenblatt, 2010). Tissue perfusion may be reduced in individuals who are obese, and cardiac output can be altered (Hanley, Abernethy, & Greenblatt, 2010). Stroke volume may be increased as well as heart rate, leading to greater cardiac output (Ghobadi, Johnson, Aarabi, Almond, Allabi, et al., 2011). Drugs that are highly lipophilic, such as diazepam or trazodone, have a much larger Vd in obese individuals and can accumulate in adipose tissue. Alterations in efficiency of drug metabolism have also been noted in obesity. Certain enzymes of the cytochrome P450 system display altered metabolic activity in obesity; activity of CYP3A4 can be decreased 10%–40%, while activity at CYP2E1 can be substantially increased, ranging from 10%–140% (Ghobadi, Johnson, Aarabi, Almond, Allabi, et al., 2011; Kotlyar & Carson, 1999). Alterations in other CYP enzymes have not been fully elucidated. (Kotlyar & Carson, 1999). Hepatic clearance can be increased, as seen with diazepam; likewise, GFR may be increased in obesity. Because obese individuals can have an increase in lean muscle mass as well as increased adipose tissue, estimating GFR can be complicated; using an adjusted body weight that falls between ideal body weight and actual body weight may be more accurate. If significant changes in Vd occur, while clearance remains constant or is altered less dramatically, $T_{1/2}$ can be greatly increased, as is seen with carbamazepine (Emery, Fisher, Chien, Kharasch, Dellinger, et al., 2003).

As the obesity epidemic in the United States has progressed, surgical treatment for obesity—typically with gastric bypass—has become much more common. Gastric bypass surgery reduces the absorptive surface of the intestine, usually decreasing drug absorption. Beneficial effects of weight loss on cardiac, hepatic, and/or renal function usually will decrease steady-state drug levels. Weight loss reduces volume of distribution. Initially postprocedure, absorption of oral tablets and capsules, either immediate release or extended release products, can be unpredictable and lead to exacerbation of illness. Use of oral liquids, crushed immediate release tablets, or alternate routes of administration may be preferred when available. (Hamad, Helsel, Perel, Kozak, McShea, et al., 2012). Delayed-release and extended-release products may be not absorbed completely, which can lead to clinical decompensation as seen with the antidepressant duloxetine, which is available as only a delayed-release capsule (Roerig, Steffen, Zimmerman, Mitchell, Crosby, et al., 2013). Whenever possible, immediate-release preparations should be provided. Drugs that require food for absorption, such as the antipsychotics ziprasidone and lurasidone, will have absorption rates of one-third to one-half of that when provided with a large calorie meal (Lincoln, Stewart, & Preskorn, 2010; Lurasidone Product Information, 2013), and alternate agents should be considered. Patients should be monitored carefully for worsening of symptoms postprocedure because of changes in drug absorption. Those who undergo gastric bypass may also experience changes in absorption of alcohol, with higher Cmax and shorter Tmax, leading to increased clinical effects (Maluenda, Cendes, De Aretxabala, Poniachik, Salvo, et al., 2010; Klockhoff, Naslund, & Jones, 2002).

Nutritional deficiencies are frequently seen after gastric bypass, with some of the most common being decreased levels of thiamine, folate, B_1, zinc, iron, copper, calcium, and fat-soluble vitamins A, D, E, and K. Problems such as Wernicke's encephalopathy and peripheral neuropathy can develop if deficiencies are not corrected (Bloomberg, Fleishman, Nalle, Herron, & Kini, 2005). Further, B_{12} and folate deficiencies are associated with depression (Tiemeier, van Tuijl, Hofman, Meijer, Kiliaan, et al., 2002; Alpert & Fava, 1997). Nearly 50% of those who have undergone gastric bypass develop unrecognized nutritional deficits (John & Hoegrel, 2009), and it is imperative that these be considered when evaluating patients.

CLINICAL PEARLS

- Brain effects do not correspond directly to the blood concentrations of a drug because:
  - The level of the drug in the blood can differ greatly from the level of the drug in the CNS because of the blood–brain barrier due to the lipophilicity of the drug; whether there is interaction with a transporter; and whether the drug is actively transported into or out of the CSF.
  - The drug's mechanism of action may not require that the drug be continuously present; it may, for example, induce RNA transcription, leading to the synthesis of a protein that will persist for hours or days.
  - The changes in neuronal function initially produced by the drug can cause secondary changes in the same neurons or connected neurons that produce clinically relevant effects. For example, if a drug blocks a neuron's dopamine receptors, that neuron will synthesize additional receptors; also, activity in related glutamatergic neurons will increase.
- Clinical focus typically is on *bioavailability*, the fraction of the dose administered that eventually reaches the circulation. (Note, however, that equal bioavailability of two versions of the same drug does not imply therapeutic equivalence, as the two versions can differ in the peak blood level they produce—Cmax—and in how rapidly a therapeutic threshold is reached.)
- Elimination half-life is useful in predicting the time to achieve steady state with regular dosing.
- CYP3A4 has very wide variability in enzyme activity in the general population, and it has many single nucleotide polymorphisms. However, the genotype–phenotype associations are not sufficiently well established to infer the enzyme's metabolic activity from the genotype. For this reason, CYP3A4 is not included in pharmacogenetic testing even though interactions involving CYP3A4 are very common.

- Sublingual tablets have rapid onset of action and high bioavailability, since first-pass metabolism is bypassed as the buccal and pharyngeal regions drain to the superior vena cava rather than to the portal vein. They require a measure of patient cooperation to keep the tablet under the tongue rather than swallow it. For this reason they are unsuitable for cognitively impaired patients.

- For many psychotropic drugs, absorption will differ when the drug is taken with food versus in the fasting state. Food effects are measurable more often than they are clinically relevant, but they do matter for some drugs, as has been noted. Effects can go in either direction.

- Nearly 50% of those who have undergone gastric bypass develop unrecognized nutritional deficits (John & Hoegrel, 2009), and it is imperative that these be considered when evaluating patients who have undergone this procedure.

DISCLOSURE STATEMENTS

Dr. Gutierrez has no conflicts of interest, direct or indirect, to disclose.

Dr. Fogel is Chief Scientific Officer of Synchroneuron Inc., Managing Director of Anal-Gesic LLC, and Executive Vice President of PointRight Inc. He is the sole inventor or lead inventor on several pharmaceutical patents. In his opinion these affiliations do not entail any conflict of interest with regard to the editing of this book or his personal contributions to it. He has no other potential conflicts, direct or indirect, financial or otherwise, to disclose in connection with the editing of this book or his personal contributions to it.

REFERENCES

Aitken, A. E., Richardson, T. A., & Morgan, E. T. (2006). Regulation of drug-metabolizing enzymes and transporters in inflammation. *Annual Review of Pharmacology and Toxicology, 46,* 123–149.

Alpert, J. E., & Fava, M. (1997). Nutrition and depression: the role of folate. *Nutrition Reviews, 55,* 145–149.

Andersson, T., Cederberg, C., Edvardsson, G., Heggelund, A., & Lundborg, P. (1990). Effect of omeprazole treatment on diazepam plasma levels in slow versus normal rapid metabolizers of omeprazole. *Clinical Pharmacology and Therapeutics, 47,* 79–85.

Bachmeier, C. J., Beaulieu-Abdelahad, D., Ganey, N. J., Mullan, M. J., & Levin, G. M. (2011). Induction of drug efflux protein expression by venlafaxine but not desvenlafaxine. *Biopharmaceutics & Drug Disposition, 32*(4), 233–244.

Bauer, L. A. (2014). Chapter 5. Clinical Pharmacokinetics and Pharmacodynamics. In DiPiro, J. T., Talbert, R. L., Yee, G. C., Matzke, G. R., Wells, B. G., Posey, L. (Eds.), Pharmacotherapy: A Pathophysiologic Approach, 9e. Retrieved July 27, 2014 from http://accesspharmacy.mhmedical.com/content.aspx?bookid=689&Sectionid=48811430.rt.

Bauer, L. A. (1982). Interference of oral phenytoin absorption by continuous nasogastric feedings. *Neurology, 32,* 570–572.

Bloomberg, R. D., Fleishman, A., Nalle, J. E., Herron, D. M., & Kini, S. (2005). Nutritional deficiencies following bariatric surgery: what have we learned? [review] *Obesity Surgery, 15,* 145–154.

Buxton, I. O., & Benet, L. Z. (2011). Chapter 2. Pharmacokinetics: The Dynamics of Drug Absorption, Distribution, Metabolism, and Elimination. In Brunton, L. L., Chabner, B. A., Knollmann, B. C. (Eds.), Goodman & Gilman's The Pharmacological Basis of Therapeutics, 12e. Retrieved July 27, 2014 from http://accesspharmacy.mhmedical.com/content.aspx?bookid=374&Sectionid=41266207.

Byatt, C. M., Lewis, L. D., Dawling, S., & Cochrane, G. M. (1984). Accumulation of midazolam after repeated dosage in patients receiving mechanical ventilation in an intensive care unit. *British Medical Journal, 289,* 799–800.

Cavallari, L. H., & Lam, Y. W. (2014). eChapter 6. Pharmacogenetics. In DiPiro, J. T., Talbert, R. L., Yee, G. C., Matzke, G. R., Wells, B. G., Posey, L. (Eds.), Pharmacotherapy: A Pathophysiologic Approach, 9e. Retrieved July 27, 2014 from http://accesspharmacy.mhmedical.com/content.aspx?bookid=689&Sectionid=48811431.

Center for Drug Evaluation and Research. (2003). *Guidance for industry: bioavailability and bioequivalence studies for orally administered drug products—general considerations.* Washington, DC: United States Food and Drug Administration.

Chen, S. S., Allen, J., Oxley, J., & Richens, A. (1982). Comparative bioavailability of phenytoin from generic formulations in the United Kingdom. *Epilepsia, 23,* 149–152.

Child, C. G., & Turcotte, J. G. (1964). Surgery and portal hypertension. In C. G. Child (Ed.), *The liver and portal hypertension.* (pp. 50–64). Philadelphia: Saunders.

Dasgupta, A. (2007). Usefulness of monitoring free (unbound) concentrations of therapeutic drugs in patient management. *International Journal of Clinical Chemistry, 377,* 1–13.

De Baerdemaeker, L., Mortier, E. P., & Struys, M. (2004). Pharmacokinetics in obese patients. *Continuing Education in Anaesthesia, Critical Care, & Pain, 4,* 152–155.

DeVane, C. L. (1990). Principles of pharmacokinetics. In, C. L. DeVane (Ed.), *Fundamentals of monitoring psychoactive drug therapy* (pp. 27–49). Baltimore, MD: Williams & Wilkins.

Desta, Z., Zhao, X., Shin, J. G., & Flockhart, D. A. (2002). Clinical significance of the cytochrome P450 2C19 genetic polymorphism. *Clinical Pharmacokinetics, 41*(12), 913–958.

Devlin, J. W. (2014). Chapter 37. Acid–Base Disorders. In DiPiro, J. T., Talbert, R. L., Yee, G. C., Matzke, G. R., Wells, B. G., Posey, L. (Eds.), Pharmacotherapy: A Pathophysiologic Approach, 9e. Retrieved September 13, 2013 from http://accesspharmacy.mhmedical.com/content.aspx?bookid=689&Sectionid=45310486.

Diniz, B. S., Machado-Vieira, R., & Forlenza, O. V. (2013). Lithium and neuroprotection: translational evidence and implications for the treatment of neuropsychiatric disorders. *Neuropsychiatric Disease and Treatment, 9,* 493–500.

Du Suich, P., McLean, A. J., Lalka, D., Erill, S., & Gibaldi M. (1978). Pulmonary disease and pharmacokinetics. *Clinical Pharmacokinetics, 3,* 257–266.

Emery, M. G., Fisher, J. M., Chien, J. Y., Kharasch, E. D., Dellinger, E. P., Kowdley, K. V., et al. (2003). CYP2E1 activity before and after weight loss in morbidly obese subjects with nonalcoholic fatty liver disease. *Hepatology, 38,* 428–35.

Ereshefsky, L., Saklad, S. R., Jann, M. W., Richards, A. L., & Davis, C. M. (1983). Pharmacokinetics of fluphenazine decanoate by high performance liquid chromatography. *Drug Intelligence Clinical Pharmacology, 17,* 436–437.

Espnes, K. A., Heimdal, K. O., & Spigset O. (2012). A puzzling case of increased serum clozapine levels in a patient with inflammation and infection. *Therapeutic Drug Monitoring, 34,* 489–492.

Gaedigk, A., Bradford, L. D., Marcucci, K. A., & Leeder, J. S. (2002). Unique CYP2D6 activity distribution and genotype-phenotype discordance in black Americans. *Clinical Pharmacology and Therapeutics, 72,* 76–89.

Gan, T. J. (2004). "Black Box" warning on droperidol: a report of the FDA convened expert panel. *Anesthesia and Analgesia, 98,* 1809.

Ghobadi, C., Johnson, T. N., Aarabi, M., Almond, L. M., Allabi, A. C., Rowland-Yeo, K., et al. (2011). Application of a systems approach to the bottom-up assessment of pharmacokinetics in obese patients: expected variations in clearance. *Clinical Pharmacokinetics, 50*, 809–822.

Grant, I., Atkinson, J. H., Gouaux, B., & Wilsey, B. (2012). Medical marijuana: clearing away the smoke. *Open Neurology Journal, 6*, 18–25.

Greenblatt, D. J., Wright, C. E., von Moltke, L. L., Harmatz, J. S., Ehrenberg, B. L., Harrel, L. M., et al. (1998). Ketoconazole inhibition of triazolam and alprazolam clearance: differential kinetic and dynamic consequences. *Clinical Pharmacology and Therapeutics, 64*, 237–247.

Gunes, A., Bilir, E., Zengil, H., Babaoglu, M. O., Bozkurt, A., & Yasar, U. (2007). Inhibitory effect of valproic acid on cytochrome P450 2C9 activity in epilepsy patients. *Basic & Clinical Pharmacology & Toxicology, 100*(6), 383–386.

Hamad, G. G., Helsel, J. C., Perel, J. M., Kozak, G. M., McShea, M. C., Hughes, C., et al. (2012). The effect of gastric bypass on the pharmacokinetics of serotonin reuptake inhibitors. *American Journal of Psychiatry, 169*, 256–263.

Hanley, M. J., Abernethy, D. R., & Greenblatt, D. J. (2010). Effect of obesity on the pharmacokinetics of drugs in humans. *Clinical Pharmacokinetics, 49*, 71–87.

Hartley, R., Aleksandrowicz, J., Ng, P. C., McLain, B., Bowmer, C. J., & Forsythe, W. I. (1990). Breakthrough seizures with generic carbamazepine: a consequence of poorer bioavailability. *British Journal of Clinical Practice, 44*, 270–227.

Haslemo, T., Eikeseth, P. H., & Tanum, L. (2006). The effect of variable cigarette consumption on the interaction with clozapine and olanzapine. *European Journal of Clinical Pharmacology, 62*, 1049–1053.

Heard, C., Creighton, P., & Lerman, J. (2009). Intranasal flumazenil and naloxone to reverse over-sedation in a child undergoing dental restorations. *Paediatric Anaesthesia, 19*, 795–797.

Hellriegel, E. T., Bjornsson, T. D., & Hauck, W. W. (1996). Interpatient variability in bioavailability is related to the extent of absorption: implications for bioavailability and bioequivalence studies. *Clinical Pharmacology and Therapeutics, 60*, 601–607.

Hollenberg, P. F. (2002). Characteristics and common properties of inhibitors, inducers and activators of CYP enzymes. *Drug Metabolism Reviews, 34*, 17–35.

Holsti, M., Dudley, N., Schunk, J., Adelgais, K., Greenberg, R., Olsen, C., et al. (2010). Intranasal midazolam vs rectal diazepam for the home treatment of acute seizures in pediatric patients with epilepsy. *Archives of Pediatric & Adolescent Medicine, 164*, 747–753.

Israili, Z. H., & Dayton, P. G. (2001). Human alpha-1-glycoprotein and its interactions with drugs. *Drug Metabolism Reviews, 33*, 61–235.

Jeppesen, U., Gram, L. F., Vistisen, K., Loft, S., Poulsen, H. E., & Brøsen, K. (1996). Dose-dependent inhibition of CYP1A2, CYP2C19 and CYP2D6 by citalopram, fluoxetine, fluvoxamine and paroxetine. *European Journal of Clinical Pharmacology, 51*, 73–78.

John, S., & Hoegerl, C. (2009). Nutritional deficiencies after gastric bypass surgery. *Journal of the American Osteopathic Association, 109*, 601–604.

Jumao-as, A., Bella, I., Craig, B., Lowe, J., & Dasheiff, R. M. (1989). Comparison of steady-state blood levels of two carbamazepine formulations. *Epilepsia, 30*, 67–70.

Kapur, B. M., Hutson, J. R., Chibber, T., Luk, A., & Selby, P. (2011). Methadone: a review of drug-drug and pathophysiological interactions. *Critical Reviews in Clinical Laboratory Sciences, 48*, 171–195.

Kimura, Y., Ito, H., Ohnishi, R., & Hatano, T. (2010). Inhibitory effects of polyphenols on human cytochrome p450 3A4 and 2C9 activity. *Food and Chemical Toxicology, 48*, 429–435.

Klockhoff, H., Naslund, I., & Jones A. W. (2002). Faster absorption of ethanol and higher peak concentration in women after gastric bypass surgery. *British Journal of Clinical Pharmacology, 54*, 587–591.

Kluznik, J. C., Walbek, N. H., Farnsworth, M. G., & Melstrom, K. (2001). Clinical effects of a randomized switch of patients from Clozaril to generic clozapine. *Journal of Clinical Psychiatry, 62*(suppl 5), 14–18.

Kotlyar, M., & Carson, S. W. (1999). Effects of obesity on the cytochrome p450 system. *Int J Clinical Pharmacology and Therapeutics, 37*, 8–19.

Lam, Y. W., Ereshefsky, L., Toney, G. B., & Gonzales, C. (2001). Branded versus generic clozapine: bioavailability comparison and interchangeability issues. *Journal of Clinical Psychiatry, 62*(suppl 5), 18–22.

Lesem, M. D., Tran-Johnson, T. K., Riesenberg, R. A., Feifel, D., Allen, M. H., Fishman, R., et al. (2011). Rapid acute treatment of agitation in individuals with schizophrenia: multicentre, randomised, placebo controlled study of inhaled loxapine. *British Journal of Psychiatry, 198*, 51–58.

Levine, G. M. (2012). P-glycoprotein: why this drug transporter may be clinically important. *Current Psychiatry, 11*, 38–40.

Lilja, J. J., Kivisto, K. T., Backman, J. T., Lamberg, T. S., & Neuvonen, P. J. (1998). Grapefruit juice substantially increases plasma concentrations of buspirone. *Clinical Pharmacology and Therapeutics, 64*, 655–660.

Lin, J. H., & Yamazaki, M. (2003). Role of P-glycoprotein in pharmacokinetics—clinical implications. *Clinical Pharmacokinetics, 42*, 59–98.

Lincoln, J., Stewart, M. E., & Preskorn, S. H. (2010). How sequential studies inform drug development: evaluating the effect of food intake on optimal bioavailability of ziprasidone. *Journal of Psychiatric Practice, 16*, 103–114.

Linnet, K., & Ejsing, T. B. (2008). A review on the impact of P-glycoprotein on the penetration of drugs into the brain. Focus on psychotropic drugs. *Journal of the European College of Neuropsychopharmacology, 18*, 157–169.

Lowe, E. J., & Ackman, M. L. (2010). Impact of tobacco smoking cessation on stable clozapine or olanzapine treatment. *Annals of Pharmacotherapy, 44*, 727–732.

Lurasidone (Latuda). (2013). *Product information*. Fort Lee, New Jersey: Sunovian. Accessed November 24, 2013 at http://www.google.com/url?sa=t&rct=j&q=&esrc=s&source=web&cd=1&ved=0CC8QFjAA&url=http%3A%2F%2Fwww.latuda.com%2FLatudaPrescribingInformation.pdf&ei=-rjVU5WUHMGC8QGV5YGYAQ&usg=AFQjCNH01TNyYsBUFNHXmkeYUltV0h9_mA

Madakasira, S., & Khazanie, P. G. (1985). Reliability of amitriptyline dose prediction based on single-dose plasma levels. *Clinical Pharmacology and Therapeutics, 37*, 145–149.

Maluenda, F., Cendes, A., De Aretxabala, X., Poniachik, J., Salvo, K., Delgado, I., et al. (2010). Alcohol absorption modification after a laparoscopic sleeve gastrectomy due to obesity. *Obesity Surgery, 20*, 744–748.

Moolenaar, F., Bakker, S., Visser, J., & Huizinga, T. (1980). Biopharmaceutics of rectal administration of drugs in man IX. Comparative biopharmaceutics of diazepam after single rectal, oral, intramuscular and intravenous administration in man. *International Journal of Pharmaceutics, 5*, 127–137.

Morgan, E. T. (2009). Impact of infectious and inflammatory disease on cytochrome P450-mediated drug metabolism and pharmacokinetics. *Nature, 85*, 434–438.

Morinobu, S., Tanaka, T., Kawakatsu, S., Totsuka, S., Koyama, E., Chiba, K., et al. (1997). Effects of genetic defects in the CYP2C19 gene on the N-demethylation of imipramine, and clinical outcome of imipramine therapy. *Psychiatry and Clinical Neuroscience, 51*, 253–257.

Mrazek, D. A. (2010). *Psychiatric pharmacogenomics*. New York: Oxford University Press.

Nakagami, T., Yasui-Furukori, N., Saito, M., Tateishi, T., & Kaneo S. (2005). Effect of verapamil on pharmacokinetics and pharmacodynamics of risperidone: in vivo evidence of involvement of P-glycoprotein in risperidone disposition. *Clinical Pharmacology and Therapeutics, 78*, 43–51.

Oles, K. S., Penry, J. K., Smith, L. D., Anderson, R. L., Dean, J. C., & Riela, A. R. (1992). Therapeutic bioequivalency study of brand name versus generic carbamazepine. *Neurology, 42*, 1147–1153.

P-glycoprotein drug interactions. (2013). *Pharmacist's Letter, 29*, PL Detail-Document #291008.

Pugh, R. N., Murray-Lyon, I. M., Dawson, J. L., Pietroni, M. C., & Williams, R. (1973). Transection of the oesophagus for bleeding oesophageal varices. *British Journal of Surgery, 60*, 646–649.

Rabinowitz, J. D., Lloyd, P. M., Munzar, P., Myers, D. J., Cross, S., Damani, R., et al. (2006). Ultrafast absorption of amorphous pure drug aerosols via deep lung inhalation. *Journal of Pharmaceutical Sciences, 95,* 2438–2451.

Richens, A. (1979). Clinical pharmacokinetics of phenytoin. *Clinical Pharmacokinetics, 4,* 153–169.

Robertson, T. M., Hendey, G. W., Stroh, G., & Shalit, M. (2009). Intranasal naloxone is a viable alternative to intravenous naloxone for prehospital narcotic overdose. *Prehospital Emergency Care, 13,* 512–515.

Rodighiero, V. (1989). Effects of cardiovascular disease on pharmacokinetics. *Cardiovascular Drugs and Therapy, 3,* 711–730.

Roerig, J. L., Steffen, K. J., Zimmerman, C., Mitchell, J. E., Crosby, R. D., & Cao, L. (2013). A comparison of duloxetine plasma levels in postbariatric surgery patients versus matched nonsurgical control subjects. *Journal of Clinical Psychopharmacology, 33,* 479–484.

Roose, J. C. (1983). Cardiac effects of antidepressant drugs: A comparison of the tricyclic antidepressants and fluvoxamine. *British Journal of Clinical Practice, 15*(Suppl 3), 439S–445S.

Roose, S. P., Glassman, A. H., & Dalack, G. W. (1989). Depression, heart disease, and tricyclic antidepressants. *Journal of Clinical Psychiatry, 50*(Suppl), 12–16.

Saivin, S., Hulot, T., Chabac, S., Potgieter, A., Durbin, P., & Houin, G. (1998). Clinical pharmacokinetics of acamprosate. *Clinical Pharmacokinetics, 35,* 331–345.

Sandson, N. B., Armstrong, S. C., & Cozza, K. L. (2005). An overview of psychotropic drug-drug interactions. *Psychosomatics, 46,* 464–494.

Schmidt, S., Gonzalez, D., & Derendorf, H. (2010). Significance of protein binding in pharmacokinetics and pharmacodynamics. *Journal of Pharmceutical Sciences, 99,* 1107–1122.

Scott, S. A., Edelmann, L., Kornreich, R., Erazo, M., & Desnick, R. J. (2007). CYP2C9, CYP2C19 and CYP2D6 allele frequencies in the Ashkenazi Jewish population. *Pharmacogenomics, 8*(7), 721–730.

Shargel, L., Wu-Pong, S., & Yu, A. B. C. (2005). Introduction to biopharmaceutics and pharmacokinetics. In *Applied Biopharmaceutics and Pharmacokinetics* (5th ed., pp. 1–20). New York: McGraw-Hill.

Spina, E., Avenoso, A., Facciola, G., Scordo, M. G., Ancione, M., & Madia, A. (2001). Plasma concentrations of risperidone and 9-hydroxyrisperidone during combined treatment with paroxetine. *Therapeutic Drug Monitoring, 23,* 223–227.

Spyker, D. A., Munzar, P., & Cassella, J. V. (2010). Pharmacokinetics of loxapine following inhalation of a thermally generated aerosol in healthy volunteers. *Journal of Clinical Pharmacology, 50,* 169–179.

Taburet, A. M., Tollier, C., & Richard, C. (1990). The effect of respiratory disorders on clinical pharmacokinetic variables. *Clinical Pharmacokinetics, 19,* 462–490.

Tiemeier, H., van Tuijl, R., Hofman, A., Meijer, J., Kiliaan, A. J., & Breteler, M. M. (2002). Vitamin B12, folate, and homocysteine in depression: The Rotterdam study. *American Journal of Psychiatry, 159,* 2099–2101.

Tilkian, A. G., Schroeder, J. S., Kao J, Hultgren H. (1976). Effect of lithium on cardiovascular performance: report on extended ambulatory monitoring and exercise testing before and during lithium therapy. *American Journal of Cardiology, 38,* 701–708.

U.S. Food and Drug Administration. (2011). *Drug development and drug interactions: Table of substrates, inhibitors and inducers.* Retrieved from http://www.fda.gov/drugs/developmentapprovalprocess/development resources/druginteractionslabeling/ucm093664.htm#inhibitors. Accessed October 23, 2013.

U.S. Food and Drug Administration. (2007). *Information for health care professionals: Haloperidol.* Retrieved from http://www.fda.gov/drugs/drugsafety/postmarketdrugsafetyinformationforpatient-sandproviders/drugsafetyinformationforheathcareprofessionals/ucm085203.htm. Accessed September 13, 2013.

Varghese, J. M., Roberts, J. A., & Lipman, J. (2010). Pharmacokinetics and pharmacodynamics in critically ill patients. *Current Opinion in Anaesthesiology, 23,* 472–478.

Verbeck, R. K. (2008). Pharmacokinetics and dosage adjustments in patients with hepatic dysfunction. *European Journal of Clinical Pharmacology, 64,* 1147–1161.

von Bahr, C., Movin, G., Nordin, C., Lidén, A., Hammarlund-Udenaes, M., Hedberg, A., et al. (1991). Plasma levels of thioridazine and metabolites are influenced by the debrisoquin phenotype. *Clinical Pharmacology and Therapeutics, 49,* 234–240.

Wang, J. S., Ruan, Y., Taylor, R. M., Donovan, J. L., Markowitz, J. S., & DeVane, C. L. (2004). The brain entry of risperidone and 9-hydroxyrisperidone is greatly limited by P-glycoprotein. *International Journal of Neuropsychopharmacology, 7,* 415–419.

Wellbutrin'. (2008). *Oral tablets, bupropion hydrochloride oral tablets.* Greenville, NC: GlaxoSmithKline. Accessed June 15, 2013 at https://www.gsksource.com/WELLBUTRIN-TABLETS-PI-MG.PDF

Woodcock, J., Khan, M., & Yu, L. X. (2012). Withdrawal of generic budeprion for nonbioequivalence. *New England Journal of Medicine, 367,* 2463–2465.

Xu, D. X., Wang, J. P., Sun, M. F., Chen, Y. H., & Wei, W. (2006). Lipopolysaccharide downregulates the expressions of intestinal pregnane X receptor and cytochrome P450 3a11. *European Journal of Pharmacology, 536,* 162–170.

Yamaori, S., Koeda, K., Kushihara, M., Hada, Y., Yamamoto, I., & Watanabe, K. (2012). Comparison in the in vitro inhibitory effects of major phytocannabinoids and polycyclic aromatic hydrocarbons contained in marijuana smoke on cytochrome P450 2C9 activity. *Drug Metabolism and Pharmacokinetics, 27,* 294–300.

23.

MEDICALLY SIGNIFICANT SIDE EFFECTS
OF PSYCHOTROPIC DRUGS

Thomas Markham Brown

INTRODUCTION

Among the side effects associated with the drug treatment of mental disorders are some that threaten life, impair function, or exacerbate the symptoms of one or more of the patient's illnesses. Such side effects represent legal as well as clinical risks. While some clinicians fail to recognize or respond to them, others deny their patients optimal psychopharmacological treatment because of excessive concern about them. This chapter reviews the clinical features, epidemiology, course, and treatment of the most important medical side effects of commonly prescribed psychiatric drug treatments. All but one of them are related to individuals' responses to the intrinsic pharmacodynamic actions of the drug prescribed; the one exception is Stevens-Johnson syndrome, which is an idiosyncratic allergic reaction.

The side effects described all can occur at dosages of the drugs within the usual therapeutic range, but all are more frequent and more severe at excessive doses. In many general psychiatric settings, intentional overdoses due to drug abuse or self-destructive intent are salient concerns. By contrast, in general medical settings overdoses are most likely to occur because of drug interactions or genetic variations in drug metabolism, or because of medication errors by patients or caregivers. Mitigating risk of severe adverse events involves systematic consideration of drug interactions, pharmacodynamics, potential medication errors, and barriers to treatment adherence such as cognitive impairment.

The side effects discussed in this chapter are (1) serotonin syndrome, (2) neuroleptic malignant syndrome and neuroleptic-induced catatonia, (3) central anticholinergic syndrome, (4) Stevens-Johnson syndrome and related skin rashes, (5) blood pressure changes (hypertension and orthostatic hypotension), (6) cardiac arrhythmias including heart block and ventricular tachycardia, and (7) metabolic syndrome.

SEROTONIN SYNDROME

CLINICAL FEATURES

The serotonin syndrome (SS) is an infrequent but potentially life-threatening side effect of serotonergic medications. The incidence is estimated by some to be less than one in 10,000 among patients taking serotonergic antidepressants (Mackay, Dunn, & Mann, 1999). However, in a retrospective study of fluoxetine overdoses, Borys and colleagues (1992) found that 5 of 67 adults who ingested fluoxetine alone developed tremor. This suggests the possibility that some cases of SS are overlooked. SS itself is a constellation of symptoms and signs involving the gut, the cardiovascular system, and the central nervous system. The symptom profile is similar to that associated with paroxysmal release of excessive serotonin in the carcinoid syndrome. Gastric distress, autonomic instability that may include hypertension and cardiac ischemia, delirium, and hyperreflexia with clonus are typical features. In contrast to the situation in the carcinoid syndrome, systemic levels of serotonin and its metabolites usually are normal—thus laboratory measures of serotonin or of its metabolites are of little use in making the diagnosis, which remains a clinical one.

Serotonin was first isolated and characterized in 1948 (Rapport, Green, & Page, 1948). The earliest descriptions of what may have been the SS appeared in the literature several years later when the mental, gastric, and autonomic changes of the carcinoid syndrome were linked to excessive serotonin (Bean & Funk, 1956–1957). In 1991, Sternbach proposed an operationalized pathophysiology of SS, as well as criteria for its diagnosis (Sternbach, 1991). This work inspired greater interest in and recognition of the disorder. Sternbach's criteria are still often cited in making the diagnosis, although other methods such as Hunter's criteria are increasingly used because of their improved sensitivity and specificity (Isbister, Buckley, & Whyte, 2007). Box 23.1 outlines one version of the Hunter criteria for SS (Altman & Jahangiri, 2010).

Obviously, these criteria are sensitive but nonspecific; many patients with delirium have one or more of these signs, and many may be on selective serotonin reuptake inhibitors (SSRIs) for treatment of depression or anxiety comorbid with or secondary to their primary medical problems. Many patients with delirium may have hyperreflexia and a few beats of clonus; what is distinctive about SS is the prominent and sustained clonus disproportionate to other signs of encephalopathy. The concurrence of gastrointestinal symptoms helps with the diagnosis, but the most useful point is a history of simultaneous onset of the CNS, autonomic, and GI symptoms in relation to a change in medications with serotonergic effects, or a change in medications that interact with a serotonergic medication to increase its level or its effect.

WHO IS AT RISK?

SS is caused by increased activity of neurons stimulated by serotonin. Thus drugs or medical conditions that increase serotonin release, drugs that impair the neuronal reuptake or systemic clearance of serotonin, and drugs that directly stimulate serotonin receptors all can contribute. Moreover, the neuromodulator nitric oxide shuts off serotonin release, so agents that reduce nitric oxide levels may indirectly increase serotonergic activity. The onset of SS usually is provoked by a change in one or more of these three factors.

Circumstances and substances that increase serotonin release include the following: acute stress, trauma, surgery, hypoxia, hypoglycemia, alcohol, opiates, cocaine, MDMA, amphetamines and other sympathomimetic agents, lithium, and the nutritional supplement 5-hydroxytryptophan (5-HTP), which is the immediate precursor of serotonin.

Drugs directly stimulating serotonin receptors include: triptans, buspirone, lithium, and LSD.

Drugs inhibiting neuronal reuptake of serotonin include SSRIs, selective noradrenaline reuptake inhibitors (SNRIs), tricyclic antidepressants (TCAs), monoamine oxidase inhibitors (MAOIs) and linezolid.

Drugs that inhibit nitric oxide (NO) synthesis include paroxetine, fluoxetine, and methylene blue (Ng & Cameron, 2010). It is thought that the former two SSRIs may carry increased risk of SS because of their dual effect on NO synthase and on serotonin reuptake.

SS is more common in smokers. Diabetes and hypertension are both associated with increased risk of the condition.

Patients undergoing acute medical illness, surgery, or trauma are overall at increased risk of SS because acute stress causes serotonin release.

TREATMENT

Treatment of SS involves removing potentially offending agents (to the extent medically feasible) and providing supportive care. More specific treatment options involve either augmenting endogenous serotonergic regulatory processes or blocking serotonin receptors with a drug. The magnitude of treatment response will depend on syndrome severity. Mild cases of SS will resolve within 72 hours of discontinuing the offending drug. Severe cases of SS may involve dehydration, hyperthermia, and rhabdomyolysis similar to that seen in neuroleptic malignant syndrome (see below). In such cases intensive care is needed, which may include neuromuscular paralysis and assisted ventilation (Brubacher, Hoffman, & Lurin, 1996; Zand, Hoffman, & Nyman, 2010; Ables & Nagubilli, 2010).

Endogenous regulation of serotonin release can be enhanced by administering nitroglycerin. This will stimulate the synthesis and release of nitric oxide and thus shut off serotonin release. Case series report its rapid effectiveness in severe and refractory cases of SS; the theoretical argument for its use is solid, but evidence from controlled trials is lacking (Brown, 2004). The authors suggest that nitroglycerin be considered in severe SS where the symptoms are a threat to the patient's life and health, and in cases of SS that show no improvement in the first 24 hours after discontinuation of offending medications and provision of symptomatic treatment with benzodiazepines and/or cyproheptadine. A necessary caution is to avoid nitroglycerin in a patient who has recently taken a PDE5 inhibitor, particularly the long-acting PDE5 inhibitor tadalafil (Cialis). Because of the frequent occurrence of sexual dysfunction as an SSRI side effect, it is not uncommon to find patients on a combination of SSRIs and PDE5 inhibitors.

Other drug treatments of SS include drugs that block serotonin receptors. Cyproheptadine, an antihistamine that blocks all types of serotonin receptors, has a relatively benign side-effect profile, with sedation being the most common reaction; however, it also has anticholinergic effects that can be problematic in some medically fragile patients. It is formulated as 4mg tablets; treatment can start with one or two tablets, and this dose of 4 mg or 8 mg of cyproheptadine may be repeated every 1 to 4 hours until symptoms of SS are resolved. Other reported treatments include benzodiazepines, ondansetron (a 5HT3 blocker), chlorpromazine, and olanzapine (which blocks 5HT2 receptors). Benzodiazepines are most helpful for agitation and hyperreflexia but may not be effective for the full syndrome. Chlorpromazine can be helpful for agitation and the GI symptoms but may exacerbate tremors and autonomic disturbances, and it has substantial anticholinergic effects. Ondansetron is highly effective for nausea and vomiting, but its relatively selective inhibition of 5HT3 receptors may actually disinhibit serotonin release in some brain regions. Similar considerations apply to olanzapine, with its relatively selective 5HT2 blocking action. Benzodiazepines, often the first choice for managing

SS, help with GI symptoms and agitation but can exacerbate neuromuscular symptoms and may disinhibit serotonin release by some neuronal populations (TM Brown, Skop, & Mareth, 1996; Brown, 2004; Brubacher et al., 1996; Jones & Story, 2005; Ables & Nagubilli, 2010; Zand et al., 2010). Because of these considerations, the authors recommend the use of benzodiazepines for mild cases with predominant agitation and hyperreflexia, cyproheptadine for mild to moderate cases with a combination of GI and CNS symptoms, and consideration of nitrates for severe cases. Ondansetron would be a good alternative when nausea and vomiting are the predominant symptoms. Hypotension, hypertension, and hyperthermia, when they occur, should be treated symptomatically. The authors do not recommend the use of neuroleptics to treat SS.

Restarting a serotonergic medication in a patient who has experienced SS can be safe. This is particularly true when one or more of the additional causal factors is no longer present. For example, if a patient developed SS while on the combination of an SSRI and an opiate, it might be safe to restart the SSRI if the patient no longer requires opiate analgesics. In this case, a note would be made to discontinue the SSRI if in the future the patient faced surgery or developed a painful condition for which opiates would be needed. If the patient was taking fluoxetine or citalopram when he or she developed SS, switching to citalopram, escitalopram, or sertraline would be reasonable because these agents do not inhibit nitric oxide synthase, thereby removing a factor that can contribute to the syndrome (Brown, 2004). In cases in which no manageable precipitating factor or drug can be identified as contributing to development of SS other than a serotonergic agent apart from fluoxetine or paroxetine, it would be prudent to avoid SSRIs and SNRIs for treating the patient's depression in the future. Several treatment options would remain, including bupropion, the TCA desipramine (which has the least serotonergic effect of the TCAs), and the nonpharmacologic somatic treatments ECT and rTMS.

NEUROLEPTIC MALIGNANT SYNDROME

The neuroleptic malignant syndrome, or NMS, may have been first described in 1959 by Walker, who reported a case of what appeared to be tetanus in a 19-year-old man given trifluoperazine—fever and profound parkinsonian rigidity that was partially relieved by trihexyphenidyl (Walker, 1959). Credit for identifying the disorder is usually, however, given to Delay and colleagues for their description in 1960 of "akinetic hypertonic syndrome," renamed *neuroleptic malignant syndrome* in 1968 by Delay and Deniker (Delay, Pichot Lempiere, Blissalde, & Peigne, 1960; Delay & Deniker, 1968). In 1986, the first case of NMS due to an atypical antipsychotic—in this case clozapine—was reported. This dashed hope that clozapine, with its greatly reduced propensity to cause extrapyramidal symptoms (EPS), would not cause NMS (Pope, Cole, Choras, & Fulwiler, 1986).

Levenson in 1985 proposed a set of major and minor criteria for diagnosing NMS (see Box 23.2). The condition would

---

Box 23.2 LEVENSON'S CRITERIA FOR NMS

Major Criteria
  fever
  rigidity
  elevated serum creatinine kinase

Minor Criteria
  tachycardia
  hypertension *or* hypotension
  altered mentation
  diaphoresis
  leukocytosis

---

be diagnosed if a patient had three or more major criteria, or two of the major criteria and four of the minor criteria (Levenson, 1985). Other criterion sets, including one proposed by the American Psychiatric Association, see fever and rigidity as essential to the diagnosis and add dysphagia, incontinence, mutism, and tremor to the minor criteria. The APA criteria require both severe rigidity and fever (rather than accepting just one of the two if there is an elevated creatine kinase); only two minor criteria must be present (American Psychiatric Association, 2000).

NMS occurs in approximately one in 500 patients treated with neuroleptics, though the incidence may be higher in particular vulnerable populations. In a retrospective study of 224,372 patients with psychiatric disorders, Nielsen and colleagues (2012) identified 83, or 0.04%, as having had NMS. Among 672 acutely manic men given antipsychotics, three (0.45%) who received haloperidol developed NMS (Sarkar, Natarajan, & Gode, 2009). Its importance is related to its mortality, which may exceed 10%, making it one of the most life-threatening adverse effects encountered in psychiatric drug therapy.

There is little disagreement about the clinical diagnosis of NMS when all of the characteristic features are present; diagnostic confusion arises when one of the typical features is obscured. For example, muscular rigidity is less severe if the offending drug is clozapine and may be absent if the patient suffered damage to the cerebellum as a consequence of severe and prolonged hyperthermia (Trollor, Chen, & Sachdev, 2009; Brown, 1999; Lee et al., 1989).

The combination of fever, rigidity, and altered mental status can be seen in several other conditions as described in Table 23.1. These include tetanus, (Walker, 1959) serotonin syndrome, malignant hyperthermia, neuroleptic-induced catatonia, and the central anticholinergic syndrome (Fink, 2011; O'Brien & Young, 1989). Differentiation of NMS from these conditions is based on the differences in the constellation of symptoms, association of the disorder with the initiation of neuroleptic therapy, a change in dosage, or initiation of a drug that interacts with a preexisting neuroleptic to raise its level or enhance its dopamine-blocking effects. As with serotonin syndrome, clinicians who have seen several cases of NMS often can recognize a distinctive overall pattern of history, symptoms, and signs.

CONDITION	HYPERTHERMIA	NEUROMUSCULAR	MENTAL STATUS	LABORATORY
NMS	Usual; often>104° F	Rigidity is usual; typically severe and tremulous	Cognition usually impaired; mutism common	Creatine kinase (CK) usually high, often extremely; myoglobinuria in severe cases
Tetanus	Fever in most cases but not usually over 104° F	Muscle spasms but not tremulous rigidity typical of neuroleptic-induced EPS	Confusion is sometimes present	Positive culture for *Clostridium tetani*
Serotonin syndrome	Inconsistently present	Hyperreflexia and clonus but not rigidity; sometimes tremor	Confusion is sometimes present	No specific finding; mild but not severe elevation of CK in some cases
Malignant catatonia	Often present but not essential	Catatonia ("waxy flexibility"); not severe rigidity; no tremor	Usually confused, often mute	No specific finding; CK may be mildly elevated
Malignant hyperthermia	Fever over 104° F	Rigidity usual but not necessarily extreme; not tremulous	Often confused but not necessarily	CK elevated, sometimes extremely; myoglobinuria in severe cases
Heat stroke	Fever is usual	Not rigid	Sometimes confused	No specific findings

WHO IS AT RISK?

NMS occurs in patients who have impaired dopamine transmission but not in all such patients, so other factors are involved. It can be precipitated not only by neuroleptics but also by other drugs that block dopamine receptors—for example, metoclopramide (Supariwala, Kant, & Jean, 2011)—or by drugs that deplete dopamine, such as tetrabenazine or reserpine (Guay, 2010). NMS may also be precipitated by the abrupt withdrawal of levodopa in a patient with Parkinson's disease (Gibb & Griffith, 1986).

Cautious use of other agents (such as statins) that can cause muscle injury is important, since such agents can markedly worsen the course of NMS even though there is no evidence that they cause it (Cooper & Jones, 2009). Some agents of abuse, such as ecstasy and methamphetamine, may also increase the risk of muscle injury and organ failure and of subsequent NMS (Matsusue et al., 2011; Russell, Riazi, Kraeva, Steel, & Hawryluck, 2012). Tantalizing associations between NMS and anesthetic agent–induced malignant hyperthermia have been identified, but after decades of research these entities appear pathophysiologically distinct (Matsusue et al., 2009; Wagner, Fink, & Stephenson, 2004).

NMS develops shortly after initiating a neuroleptic (or other dopamine blocking drug) or increasing its dose. Almost all cases begin within a month of starting neuroleptic therapy, increasing the dose, or adding a second drug that interacts with the first either to raise its blood level or to augment its effect on CNS dopamine receptors. Symptoms tend to evolve over 24–72 hours (Adnet, Lestavel, & Krivosic-Horber, 2000). Young men are the highest risk demographic. Clinical conditions associated with increased risk include agitation, dehydration, alcoholism, alcohol withdrawal, fever, structural brain injury, hyponatremia, iron deficiency, infection, and concomitant lithium therapy. Increased dopamine blockade increases risk: higher neuroleptic dosage, higher potency drugs, and intramuscular administration all carry a higher risk of NMS (O'Brien & Young, 1989). Atypical (second generation) neuroleptics carry less risk than typical (first generation) neuroleptics. Notwithstanding, numerous cases of NMS due to atypical neuroleptics have been reported. Among 20 patients between the ages of 11 and 18 years treated with atypical antipsychotic agents who suffered a total of 23 episodes of NMS, Nehut and colleagues found that the average time to onset of symptoms was 8.7 + 16.2 days (Neuhut, Lindenmayer, & Silva, 2009). Another risk factor for developing NMS is rechallenge with a neuroleptic drug in a patient who has had NMS in the past.

The symptoms of NMS are due to the combination of direct effects of dopamine blockade (or dopamine deficiency) and compensatory increases in the activity of other neurotransmitters due to the dopamine blockade. Activity of both monoamine neurotransmitters and glutamate is increased. It is worth noting that several of the conditions that increase the risk of NMS involve increased activity in sympathetic and glutamatergic systems. The pathophysiology of NMS is outlined in Figure 23.1 (Brown, 2001).

TREATMENT

NMS is always an emergency requiring hospitalization and in most cases intensive care. Treatment of NMS begins with discontinuing all potentially offending agents, including both antipsychotic drugs and other antidopamine agents such as metoclopramide. Supportive therapy is begun to manage fever, autonomic instability, and dehydration, as well as electrolyte abnormalities if these are present. Specific therapy for NMS is

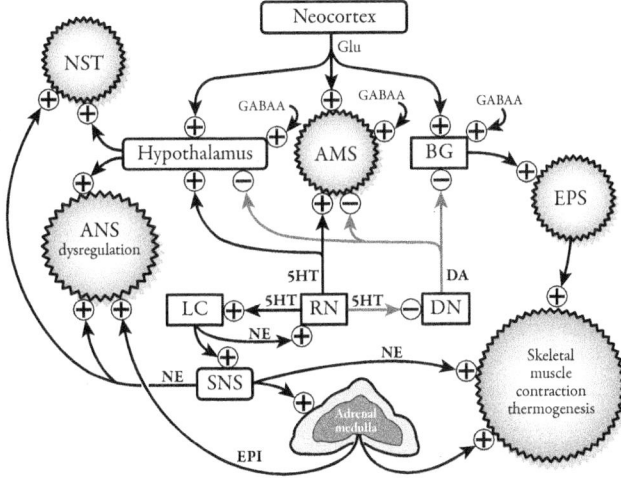

Figure 23.1 Actions of various neurotransmitters on brain structures and functions and their relationship to neuroleptic malignant syndrome (NMS). Abbreviations: + = stimulates release of neurotransmitter; − = inhibits release of neurotransmitter; AMS = altered mental status; ANS = autonomic nervous system; BG = basal ganglia; DA = dopamine; EPI = epinephrine; EPS = extrapyramidal side effects; GABA = gamma-aminobutyric acid; GABAA = GABAA receptor; GLU = glutamate; 5HT = serotonin; LC = locus coeruleus; NE = norepinephrine; NST = nonshivering thermogenesis; RN = raphe nuclei; SN = substantia nigra; SNS = sympathetic nervous system.

initiated with a dopamine agonist and a neuromuscular blocking agent that treats rigidity. The dopamine agonist most often utilized is bromocriptine; the dose is 5 mg by mouth or nasogastric tube every 6–8 hours. The usual neuromuscular blocking agent is dantrolene 50 mg IV every 6 hours. Rosenberg and Green (1989) observed that five patients with NMS who received only supportive treatments began to improve after an average of 6.8 days, while 15 patients who received bromocriptine began improving after an average of one day. Ten patients who received dantrolene began improving after an average of 1.7 days. Full resolution of symptoms took on average 15 days with supportive care only, compared with 9 days for bromocriptine and 10 days for dantrolene (Rosenberg & Green, 1989). Clinical experience over the subsequent two decades has corroborated their initial study. The authors recommend treating NMS with a dopamine agonist and dantrolene, maintaining the patient on dantrolene until muscular rigidity is completely resolved and the creatine kinase is normal, and continuing the dopamine agonist for 10 days beyond that point. Acceptable alternatives to bromocriptine are pramipexole, amantadine, and levodopa; the authors prefer bromocriptine because of the more extensive reported experience with that agent.

Patients in whom the distinction between NMS and catatonia is unclear can be challenged with intravenous lorazepam. This agent will often reverse catatonia but will not reverse the symptoms of NMS (Casamassima et al., 2010).

Laboratory tests that should be done as soon as NMS is seriously suspected include serum CK, a complete blood count, serum electrolytes, calcium, magnesium, iron, liver enzymes, and urine myoglobin. Liver enzymes should be retested after the patient has been on dantrolene for several days, as a small percentage of patients receiving dantrolene develop drug-induced hepatitis. Significant myoglobinuria implies a need for nephrology consultation and, potentially, hemodialysis. Shalev and colleagues reported that myoglobinuria and

renal failure were strongly predictive of mortality in NMS, with 50% of patients dying who had these findings (Shalev, Hermesh &, Munitz, 1989). Early and aggressive treatment of acute renal failure, for example with hemodialysis or hemofiltration, can restore renal function and prevent death in NMS (Sanai et al., 2006). As noted above, all but the mildest case of NMS warrants intensive care until hyperthermia and rigidity are resolved.

PREVENTION OF RECURRENCE

Many patients who develop NMS may subsequently need drug treatment for psychotic disorders. To minimize the risk of recurrence, high-potency neuroleptics should be avoided; most clinicians would opt for a second-generation neuroleptic or clozapine.

The patient who requires maintenance treatment for psychosis, but who has had an episode of NMS, requires some thought in order to manage the risk of recurrence of NMS. Authors who have studied this problem suggest that going from a high-potency antipsychotic to a different high-potency antipsychotic yields a much higher risk of recurrence than moving to an agent of lower potency with respect to dopamine D2 blockade (Mendhekar, Jiloha, Mehndiratta, & War, 2002; Shalev et al., 1989). Atypical antipsychotics may have a lower risk of causing severe NMS. The atypical antipsychotics as a class have a lower mortality (perhaps 3%) than the typical antipsychotics, estimated at 16% by Trollor and colleagues (2012). Among atypical antipsychotics, aripiprazole—despite its status as a partial agonist at the dopamine D2 receptor—does not appear to have a reduced risk of causing NMS (Patel & Brunetti, 2010).

Prophylaxis against NMS, as might theoretically be achieved by combining a dopamine agonist with an antipsychotic, is not an established intervention. Because withdrawal of dopamine agonists has caused NMS, their routine use is not necessarily benign (Man, 2011).

Certainly, addressing predisposing factors is crucial and may include reassessing the need for an antipsychotic. A patient with psychotic depression may do as well, for example, with electroconvulsive therapy. A non-antipsychotic mood stabilizer may help a patient with bipolar disorder.

Hospitalization of a patient with a history of NMS who requires resumption of an antipsychotic is also reasonable, to ensure that if NMS recurs it can be managed quickly.

CENTRAL ANTICHOLINERGIC SYNDROME

CLINICAL FEATURES

The central anticholinergic syndrome (CAS) is well described. This is due partly to the large number of agents that interfere with the central and peripheral actions of acetylcholine, acting primarily at muscarinic receptors. Atropine and hyoscine are classic offenders (Frampton & Spinks, 2005). In CAS, patients typically present with a combination of central and peripheral findings. In addition to confusion and agitation, the patient may have weakness, ataxia, dilated and poorly-reactive pupils with blurred vision, tachycardia, dry mucous membranes, hyperthermia, a flushed appearance, urinary retention, and constipation (Hall, Feinsilver, & Holt, 1981; Mintzer & Burns, 2000). Stupor, seizures, and coma may develop in severe cases. CAS may be fatal. A brief saying that describes the anticholinergic state is "hot as a hare, red as a beet, dry as a bone, blind as a bat, and mad as a hatter" (Ramjan, Williams, Isbister, & Elliott, 2007). Table 23.2 outlines some central and peripheral features of atropine intoxication (Brown, 1998).

The electroencephalogram (EEG) in CAS is essentially the same as that in delirium. Serum anticholinergic activity is one measure of the total serum anticholinergic medication burden but does not correlate well with the EEG (Thomas et al., 2008). While serum anticholinergic activity does identify agents that pose a risk of anticholinergic toxicity, it does not correlate reliably with clinically significant adverse events (Nishtala et al., 2009). There is no specific laboratory study that identifies CAS. However, in cases of hyperthermia and confusion some consideration should be given to infection and other processes that may also have these findings. See under Neuroleptic Malignant Syndrome, Table 23.1, for a selection of differential diagnoses.

WHO IS AT RISK?

Many drugs have anticholinergic activity. These include agents well known for such activity as well as agents that one might not expect to have any anticholinergic activity. Table 23.3 lists a few of these agents. Of note, some agents reported as having detectable serum anticholinergic activity may have such activity only at doses beyond those normally used. These include diazepam, digoxin, furosemide, metformin, and phenytoin (Chew et al., 2008; Gjerden, Bramness, & Slørdal, 2009; Mintzer & Burns, 2000). Cimetidine is a drug sometimes implicated in cases of CAS, but it is unclear if this is due to innate muscarinic anticholinergic activity, pharmacokinetic effects on more potent anticholinergic drugs, or a combination of these (Nishtala et al., 2009). Sometimes the causal agent in CAS is a surprise: Speich and Haller (1994) reported a clear case of CAS due to mefloquine. And in many cases, no one drug may be the cause of CAS; rather, a combination of drugs may be responsible.

The risk of CAS is often a matter of age complicated by the degree of muscarinic anticholinergic activity to which the patient is exposed. The very young and the very old are especially sensitive to anticholinergic agents (Garza, Osterhoudt, & Rutstein, 2000). Slow metabolizers—whether due to genotype, pharmacokinetic drug–drug interactions, or renal or liver disease—are also at risk. General anesthesia is another setting in which CAS may develop (Link, Papadopoulos, Dopjans, Guggenmoos-Holzmann, & Eyrich, 1997). Because many of these risks are common, including polypharmacy and being elderly, several groups have approached the task of identifying agents that pose significant central and peripheral anticholinergic risk. These include the American Geriatric Society's (AGS) Beers Criteria, as well as the Anticholinergic Risk Scale.

The Beers Criteria comprise a set of drugs that the AGS recommends be avoided among elderly patients (American Geriatrics Society, 2012). The AGS refers to the medications on the Beers list as "potentially inappropriate" for geriatric patients, although the medications pose risks as well for the very young, and for any age group when given in larger doses

Table 23.2 CENTRAL AND PERIPHERAL FEATURES OF ATROPINE INTOXICATION

ATROPINE DOSE (MILLIGRAMS)	CENTRAL EFFECTS	PERIPHERAL EFFECTS
0.5	Mild effects on arousal.	*Cardiac:* mild slowing *Pupillary:* minimal *Gut:* slight dryness of mouth
1.0	Increased effects on arousal. Some short-term memory impairment.	*Cardiac:* slight tachycardia *Pupillary:* dilatation *Gut:* increased oral dryness
2.0	Worsening of above effects.	*Cardiac:* marked tachycardia *Pupillary:* dilatation now complicated by impaired accommodation (blurred vision) *Gut:* marked oral dryness
5.0	Restlessness and fatigue. Onset of confusion and agitation. Visual hallucinations may occur.	*Cardiac:* marked tachycardia *Pupillary:* worsening of above *Gut:* swallowing difficult; constipation *Other:* urinary retention, skin dry
10	Delirium may progress to seizures, coma and death.	*Cardiac:* tachycardia may be complicated by reduced cardiac output *Pupillary:* pupils maximally dilated; paralysis of accommodation *Gut:* skin red, hot, dry

Table 23.3 ANTICHOLINERGIC RATING
SCALE: SELECTED AGENTS

1 POINT	2 POINTS	3 POINTS
carbidopa-levodopa	amantadine	amitriptyline
haloperidol	baclofen	atropine
paroxetine	cimetidine	benztropine
quetiapine	clozapine	cyproheptadine
ranitidine	cyclobenzaprine	diphenhydramine
risperidone	olanzapine	fluphenazine
trazodone	pseudoephedrine	hydroxyzine
ziprasidone		hyoscyamine
		imipramine
		perphenazine
		promethazine
		thioridazine
		tizanidine

or in combination. The AGS posts their list of potentially inappropriate medications on the Internet (see http://www.dcri.org/trial-participation/the-beers-list/). While the medications on the Beers list are regarded as risky based on their anticholinergic activity, it is possible for a medication to be potently anticholinergic and yet have poor central penetration. Glycopyrrolate is a valuable medication precisely when such effects are needed, as in managing bradycardia during electroconvulsive therapy. Such medications have reduced risk of causing CAS. This fact has led other groups to establish rating systems for anticholinergic activity based upon their combined peripheral and central risks. The Anticholinergic Risk Scale (ARS) is the product of one such effort.

The ARS rates a drug's risk of causing such central effects as cognitive impairment and delirium on a 0- to 3-point rating scale. A score of 0 would indicate no such risk. A score of 3 indicates marked risk of central anticholinergic side effects. A drug rated as a 3 would have a 70% chance of causing two or more anticholinergic side effects in a geriatric patient. The sum of each individual medication's score can be added to create a number that reflects the total anticholinergic burden for a given medication regimen. Table 23.3 lists some of the agents studied for inclusion in the ARS (Rudolph, Salow, Angelini, & McGlinchey, 2008).

The serum anticholinergic activity (SAA) assay is referenced in studies of anticholinergic drug effects. Tune and Coyle developed this laboratory assay in 1980 using competitive inhibition of the potent muscarinic agonist, tritiated quinuclidinyl benzilate (Tune & Coyle, 1980). When nonstandard solutions are assessed, such as the serum of patients taking multiple anticholinergic agents, confounding pharmacokinetic actions and patient-specific variables can undermine the utility of the assay (Carnahan, Lund, Perry, &

Pollock, 2002). Further limitations of this assay in clinical work include its inconsistent association with anticholinergic side effects, including central (Kersten et al., 2013). Some authors have, however, found the SAA assay useful in describing the risk of anticholinergic agents for large cohorts of patients (Pasina et al., 2013). This may represent a combination of endogenous and medication-specific effects, which may be valuable in itself even if it does not specifically reflect the anticholinergic risk of medications alone.

TREATMENT

Stopping offending agents as tolerated is the first step in managing CAS. As mentioned above, serum anticholinergic assays are not routinely helpful, nor are they usually immediately available. An EEG can be helpful in the hospital setting, but in an emergency the diagnosis is more likely to be made by clinical examination and history (Frampton & Spinks, 2005). Because CAS can be a lethal process, urgent attention to management of symptoms is crucial. Cooling blankets, antipyretics, and intravenous fluids can limit the effects of hyperthermia. Diazepam has been used to treat agitation and, on occasion, seizures. However, since the mid-19th century and the work of Thomas Fraser, the antidote to atropinism has been physostigmine (Proudfoot, 2006). Table 23.4 outlines an algorithm for management of CAS.

Physostigmine is a reversible anticholinersterase that crosses the blood–brain barrier. It has been used to treat CAS as well as to treat sedation after anesthesia, in which significant anticholinergic activity may occur (Frampton & Spinks, 2005; Panagopoulou, Tzimas, Arampatzis, Aroni, & Papadopoulos, 2011). The elimination $t_{1/2}$ of physostigmine appears to be under 20 minutes, although its anticholinesterase activity may average 80–90 minutes (Asthana et al., 1995). In a 6-week-old child with CAS, Kulka and colleagues (2004) used physostigmine 0.04 milligrams per kilogram intravenously. These authors administered two doses of physostigmine and noted full recovery within 24 hours. In adults, 2 mg may be pushed intravenously (Speich & Haller, 1994). The amount given should be titrated to effect, although caution is required to avoid overshooting the mark. Atropine can be used in cases of physostigmine intoxication. Nausea and vomiting are the most common side effects of physostigmine. These can be avoided by pushing the drug at a rate of 1 mg per minute or slower (Jastak, 1985). Some clinicians hesitate to use physostigmine because of concerns about seizures and arrhythmias. However, these side effects are more common when physostigmine is used in the absence of anticholinergic toxicity (Frascogna, 2007; Suchard, 2003).

Similarly, pyridostigmine, a reversible anticholinesterase that crosses the blood–brain barrier, has also been used to treat CAS. Its relatively long elimination $t_{1/2}$ of 1–2 hours, prolonged duration of action (roughly 6 hours), and availability for intravenous administration can make it more useful than other anticholinesterases in managing CAS (Aquilonius & Hartvig, 1986). It should be noted that the central penetration of pyridostigmine is limited, even in overdose (Almog et al., 1991). This means that confusion and hallucinations

Table 23.4 ALGORITHM FOR MANAGEMENT OF CAS

PRESENTATION	INTERVENTION
(1) CAS identified	(1) Patient should be transported to a hospital if not already in one, given the possibility that mild CAS may be the first evidence of more severe impending deterioration.
(2) Check ABCs	(2) *Place in darkened, quiet room.* This reduces agitation. *Gather data.* Measure oxygen saturation, and consider obtaining an arterial blood gas. Also obtain serum glucose level, electrolytes, and complete blood count. Consider serum CK level if patient is agitated. Obtain urine drug screen. Electrocardiogram for arrhythmias and ischemia. Chest x-ray. Consider neuroimaging, especially if evidence of trauma is present.
(3) Initiate treatment	(3) Establish intravenous access. Thiamine 200 mg IV every eight hours. Activated charcoal for gut decontamination. Cooling blankets or antipyretics for hyperthermia. Benzodiazepines for agitation. Consider physostigmine for severe intoxication. Urinary catheter for urinary retention.

in some patients may not respond significantly to pyridostigmine. Furthermore, contraindications to pyridostigmine tend to reflect its peripheral benefits. Contraindications to pyridostigmine are related to its parasympathetic effects: enhanced insulin secretion among diabetics, patients with functional or structural bowel dysfunction, patients with cardiac arrhythmias or conduction disturbances who may not tolerate parasympathetic effects, and so on (Hall et al., 1981). However, when used cautiously and as an antidote to CAS, pyridostigmine is generally safe. Pyridostigmine is given orally in doses of 0.1 milligram per kilogram.

REBOUND PSYCHOSIS

CLINICAL FEATURES

While antipsychotics treat psychosis, their abrupt discontinuation can provoke psychosis. This is called *rebound psychosis* or *supersensitivity psychosis*. Many examples exist of patients whose antipsychotic therapy was stopped, only to be follow by the swift emergence of psychosis, agitation, confusion, and movement disorders (Jacob, Ash, & Craighead, 2012). The

issue is, in large part, one of central adaptation to dopamine D2 receptor blockade. This fact is strikingly demonstrated when a potent D2 antagonist not given for mental illness, such as metoclopramide or domperidone, is abruptly stopped and frank psychosis ensues (Lu, Pan, Teng, Su, & Shen, 2002; Roy-Desruisseaux et al., 2011). The unexpected emergence of psychosis or confusion, or of an extrapyramidal movement disorder (or both) upon discontinuation of a D2 antagonist should lead the clinician to consider a withdrawal encephalopathy. In cases in which the patient has a history of mental illness for which a neuroleptic was prescribed, the clinician may need to distinguish between a drug side effect and the underlying mental illness.

Rebound psychosis differs from relapse into the initial psychotic state in being a relatively swift development after medication discontinuation. Rebound psychosis must be distinguished from frank withdrawal effects that may also occur with some antipsychotics. Shiovitz and colleagues (1996) studied this during a study of 28 patients with schizophrenia placed on clozapine for a month. The medication was abruptly discontinued after the single study month. Within 1 week after discontinuation of clozapine, one patient had developed frank psychosis requiring urgent hospitalization. Four patients experienced moderately severe withdrawal characterized by agitation, nausea, and vomiting. Only 11 patients had no evidence of withdrawal (Shiovitz et al., 1996). This study nicely illustrated key points in differentiating rebound psychosis from withdrawal. In withdrawal, one often sees the triad of a constellation of systemic findings, accompanied by a nonspecific change in mental status described generally as "agitation," and dyskinesias (Lambert, 2007). In the case of rebound psychosis, distinct symptoms of psychosis developed in the absence of systemic findings and dyskinesias. Table 23.5 outlines some distinguishing features of rebound psychosis (Miller, 2009).

WHO IS AT RISK?

As is true for drugs in general, individual antipsychotics have their own propensities for causing rebound psychosis. For example, some authors speculate that aripiprazole may be less likely to cause rebound psychosis (Tadokoro et al., 2011). Furthermore, the more anticholinergic an agent the less likely rebound psychosis may happen with abrupt discontinuation of that agent. Interestingly, patients who do not respond to antipsychotics may be less likely to suffer rebound psychosis when the medications are discontinued (Miller, 2009). Time on medication appears to be a reliably important risk factor for rebound psychosis: the longer the duration of treatment, the greater the potential risk. Older age, longer duration of illness, more psychotic symptoms, and a tendency not to tolerate minor life stressors may each increase the likelihood of rebound psychosis (Fallon & Dursun, 2011). Treatment-emergent movement disorders may also signal a risk of rebound psychosis. In the CATIE study, the presence of antipsychotic-induced movement disorders appeared to herald susceptibility both to rebound psychosis and to tardive dyskinesia. Both of these side effects are thought to be due to a "supersensitive" dopamine D2 receptor (Chouinard & Chouinard, 2008).

Table 23.5 DISTINGUISHING FEATURES OF REBOUND PSYCHOSIS

	REBOUND	WITHDRAWAL	RELAPSE
Time to occurrence after medication discontinuation	Typically days	Typically days	Gradual accumulation of cases over 1–2 years
Systemic findings	May or may not be seen	Usually present, and often accompanied by dyskinesias	Usually absent
Mental status changes	Typical psychosis	Non-specific with agitation or confusion	Typical psychosis
Effect of resuming discontinued medication	Gradual improvement	Swift resolution of systemic and mental status findings	Gradual improvement
Effect of not resuming medication	Gradual improvement may occur over weeks, but is not assured, and may be less likely with less anticholinergic agents	Gradual improvement occurs over weeks	No improvement without intervention

TREATMENT

Management of rebound psychosis begins with its anticipation. If a medication must be stopped, a gradual tapering and simultaneous initiation of another antipsychotic can help. Occasionally patients may experience rebound psychosis despite the clinician's best effort to make slow, tolerable changes. Hospitalization may, in such cases, be inevitable. For patients whose rebound psychosis is linked to noncompliance with treatment, depot antipsychotics may be helpful.

GABA-A ANTAGONISTS

CLINICAL FEATURES

A worrisome feature of some drugs is their antagonism of GABA-A receptors. This is most often recognized with antibiotics. Reuling and Cramer (1947) reported that intrathecal penicillin causes convulsions. The neurotoxicity of the beta-lactams, including the penicillins and cephalosporins, has subsequently become well established. Perhaps 1% or more of patients prescribed a beta-lactam will have a seizure. Sicker patients are at greater, and sometimes substantial, risk (Miller, Ball, Bookstaver, & Dornblaser, 2011). Among beta-lactam antibiotics, imipenem-cilastatin has the most worrisome record. In a study of 82 children with systemic cancer who received 143 courses of imipenem-cilastatin, 3 children suffered convulsions (Karadeniz, Oğuz, Canter, & Serdaroğlu, 2000). Among 200 patients with severe pneumonia who received imipenem-cilastatin, 11 had seizures. In the same study, in a separate group of 202 patients who received ciprofloxacin, only 3 had seizures (Fink et al., 1994). Benzylpenicillin and cefazolin are other beta-lactam antibiotics with a relatively high risk of neurotoxicity (Schliamser, Cars, & Norrby, 1991). This contrasts with other beta-lactams. For example, in a study of 4,872 patients who received meropenem and who represented a variety of ages and illnesses, the incidence of seizures due to meropenem was estimated to be 0.08% (Norrby & Gildon, 1999).

The central role of GABA-A receptor antagonism in producing the observed side effects helps the clinician to recognize the symptoms. Patients may experience a host of findings ranging from anxiety and hallucinations to myoclonus and disorientation, and even seizures. New-onset generalized status epilepticus has been reported with penicillins (Fernández-Torre, Santos-Sánchez, & Pelayo, 2010).

WHO IS AT RISK?

Patients who may be at increased risk of seizures with GABA-A antagonists include those with impairments of the blood–brain barrier—as can be caused for example by meningitis or structural brain lesions—as well as the elderly, those with lower body weight, and patients with renal impairment (Hoffman, Trimble, & Brophy, 2009). Renal function looms large as a risk factor. In a study of 1,951 patients who received doses of imipenem-cilastatin adjusted for renal function, only 4 developed seizures. Interestingly, even in this study the four who had seizures received inappropriately high doses of imipenem-cilastatin for their renal function (Pestotnik, Classen, Evans, Stevens, & Burke, 1993).

Other agents may facilitate the development of seizures among patients taking beta-lactams. For example, furosemide may cause hyponatremia, which increases the risk of seizures and antagonize GABA-A receptors (Korpi & Luddens, 1997). Withdrawal from alcohol, barbiturates, or benzodiazepines may also increase the risk of seizures with a GABA-A receptor antagonist.

TREATMENT

If GABA-A antagonism is thought to be present and symptomatic, an electroencephalogram can help to document the problem. A benzodiazepine can also provide insight into the pathophysiology of the process, as well as provide relief (Grill & Maganti, 2008).

While benzodiazepines are effective in managing beta-lactam–induced neurotoxicity, other anticonvulsants may not be. Serum valproic acid levels may be lowered by some beta-lactams, making this approach difficult and potentially confusing (Miller et al., 2011). Simply being on an anticonvulsant does not ensure protection against beta-lactam–induced neurotoxicity (Anzellotti et al., 2011). However, phenytoin has proved helpful in cases of beta-lactam-induced convulsions (Job & Dretler, 1990).

THE METABOLIC SYNDROME

CLINICAL FEATURES

Perhaps one in three or four persons worldwide meets criteria for the metabolic syndrome (MS) (Nieman, Brock, Butterworth, Utter, & Nieman, 2002). The MS is a constellation of findings that stems in large part from peripheral insulin resistance and that indicate an increased risk of cardiovascular disease (Reaven, 2006). In addition to peripheral insulin resistance, visceral adiposity appears to be another essential component, while atherogenic dyslipidemia and endothelial dysfunction round out the usual constellation of findings (Huang, 2009). The MS is of great concern to psychiatrists; it travels with many of the more worrisome features of mental illness, such as obesity and excess mortality, largely associated with cardiovascular disease and increasingly cancer. The MS is also a concern to psychiatrists because mental illness, and even chronic stress, is strongly associated with the development of insulin resistance and its consequences. Police officers who become depressed, for example, have a risk of developing the MS that increases with the degree of job stress and of depression (Hartley et al., 2012). While many medications provoke weight gain and thereby lead to insulin resistance, it is thought that atypical antipsychotics as a class may directly cause insulin resistance and thus contribute to the development of the MS (de Hert, Schreurs, Vancampfort, & Van Winkel, 2009). Why this may be so is as yet unclear (Stahl, Mignon, & Meyer, 2009). What is clear is that attention to the essential features of the MS, and some sense of what factors may affect their appearance and resolution, is an important element in the practice of modern psychopharmacology.

Several organizations have established criteria for the diagnosis of the MS. The American Heart Association with the National Heart, Lung, and Blood Institute (AHA/NHLBI) is among these, and their criteria are outlined in Box 23.3 below (Grundy et al., 2005). Using the AHA/NHLBI criteria, any three of the five findings is sufficient to make the diagnosis. Patients with chronic and severe mental illness develop the metabolic syndrome roughly two to three times more often than the general population (Toalson, Ahmed, Hardy, & Kabinoff, 2004). Frank diabetes is significantly more common among drug-naïve patients with schizophrenia than among healthy controls (Verma, Subramaniam, Liew, & Poon, 2009). Excess mortality among patients with severe mental illness is two to three times that of the general population. This translates into 13–30 years less life for the patient with severe mental illness, with the majority of the mortality stemming from cardiovascular events (de Hert et al., 2011). Recognizing and managing the MS is thus an urgent priority for the mentally ill.

With these criteria in mind, the clinician is able to look for evidence of the MS. The next step is identifying who may be

Box 23.3 AHA/NHLBI GUIDELINES FOR THE CLINICAL DIAGNOSIS OF THE METABOLIC SYNDROME

Measure Cut-off Values

Waist circumference > 102 cm (>40 inches) in men
  or
  > 88 cm (>35 inches) in women
Elevated > 150 mg/dL (1.7 mmol/L) triglycerides
  or
On drug treatment for elevated triglycerides
Reduced HDL-C < 40 mg/dL (1.03 mmol/L) in men
  or
  < 50 mg/dL (1.3 mmol/L) in women
  or
On drug treatment for reduced HDL-C
Elevated blood pressure >130 mmHg systolic blood pressure
  or
  > 85 mmHg diastolic blood pressure
  or
On antihypertensive drug treatment in a patient with a history of hypertension
Elevated fasting >100 mg/dL glucose
  or
On drug treatment for elevated glucose

at risk. Intriguingly, mental illness itself appears to be a risk factor for development of the MS.

WHO IS AT RISK?

The relationship between mental illness and insulin resistance is complex. Walter Cannon and colleagues described "emotional glycosuria," in which distressed patients transiently excreted glucose in their urine (Cannon, Shohl, & Wright, 1911). Kooy in 1919 reviewed the impact of emotions on the urinary excretion of glucose. He noted that while this "emotional" or "nervous" glycosuria sometimes deteriorated into frank diabetes, it did not always do so (Kooy, 1919). Kasanin noted in 1926 that "It seems safe to conclude that in psychogenic stupors one frequently encounters a decreased carbohydrate tolerance" (Kasanin, 1926). Depression, mania, and psychosis may each provoke an acute decline in insulin sensitivity. This may be seen in roughly a third or more of patients with severe mental illness (Freeman, 1946). More recent studies have found similarly large numbers of untreated mentally ill patients expressing insulin resistance, even in such disorders as posttraumatic stress disorder (de Hert et al., 2009; Weiss et al., 2011). Insulin resistance in mental illness clearly predates both modern psychopharmacology and the obesity epidemic. This raises the question: why might there be insulin resistance in mental illness?

One link between insulin resistance and mental illness may be neuroprotection (Wada, Yokoo, Yanagita, & Kobayashi, 2005). The brain operates on the brink of energetic failure. A constant supply of the substrates of aerobic metabolism, including glucose and oxygen, is required by the brain and helps to explain why brain activity accounts for 20% of the body's resting caloric expenses (Heiss, 2011). During periods of starvation or stress, a state sometimes called "fasting diabetes" develops: this is a state of adaptive insulin resistance in which glucose is diverted away from the periphery and toward the brain and a few other obligate consumers of glucose (Stannard & Johnson, 2004). Neel (1962) formulated the "thrifty gene hypothesis"—the idea that under stress, an inducible state of insulin resistance might be adaptive. Since then, the neuroprotective and neurotrophic roles of insulin have become clearer, indicating that the value of "fasting diabetes" or adaptive peripheral insulin resistance rests not solely in the diversion of glucose to the brain, but in the delivery of additional insulin to the brain as well (Jolivalt et al., 2008). Insulin coma therapy crudely but effectively capitalized on the potential benefits of enhancing insulin delivery to the brain (Sakel, 1938). And yet, as Neel and others have emphasized, a tendency to peripheral insulin resistance, no matter what the basis, may produce disease (Neel, 1962; Stannard & Johnson, 2004). The metabolic syndrome is one such disease state.

As a syndrome, there are several pathways to the MS and to insulin resistance in particular. Severe stress or mental illness are just two such pathways. Box 23.4 outlines some factors and conditions known to be associated with the MS. Many of these risk factors are commonly seen among patients with major mental illness (Chatterjee et al., 2010; Cornier et al., 2008; Hruz, 2011; Saad, 2009; Smith, Ju, Saha, Racette, & Fisher, 2004; Vardeny et al., 2011).

Box 23.4 FACTORS AND ASSOCIATED CONDITIONS THAT INCREASE THE RISK OF HAVING THE METABOLIC SYNDROME

Diseases
 hyperlipidemia
 hypotestosteronemia
 mental illness
 nonalcoholic fatty liver disease
 non–insulin-dependent diabetes mellitus
 obstructive sleep apnea
 polycystic ovarian disease

Medications
 antiretrovirals (mainly protease inhibitors, some nucleoside
  reverse transcriptase inhibitors)
 beta-blockers
 corticosteroids
 potassium-wasting diuretics
 agents that promote weight gain
 levodopa-carbidopa

Behavioral
 diets rich in refined carbohydrates, sugar, or fat
 physical inactivity
 obesity
 tobacco smoking

TREATMENT

Management of the MS begins with recognition of its antecedents. This may include making dietary changes, increasing physical activity, and assessing the potential roles on insulin sensitivity of coexisting diseases and their treatments. Baseline and regularly repeated measures of weight, waist circumference, blood pressure fasting glucose, and fasting lipid profiles are recommended (Newcomer, 2007). The American Diabetes Association and the American Psychiatric Association jointly developed recommendations for patients starting on treatment with atypical antipsychotics. The recommendations included baseline assessments of personal and family history, weight or body mass index (BMI), waist circumference, blood pressure, fasting plasma glucose, and a fasting lipid profile. The greatest emphasis was placed on tracking weight or BMI, with less frequent reassessment of the other items of interest. (American Diabetes Association et al., 2004) Of note, these consensus recommendations included checking weight or BMI every 4 weeks for the first 3 months. This underscores the fact that one's risk of having the MS may evolve quickly. Table 23.6 further outlines measures that may be useful in deciding whether a patient is at risk for the MS (Hadaegh et al., 2009; Kaur, Adams-Huet, Smith, & Jialal, 2013; Reaven, 2006).

The World Health Organization recommends intervening when BMI exceeds 27 in a person with evidence of obesity-related disease such as diabetes, or 30 in a person without acute evidence of obesity-related illness (McIntyre et al., 2012). If a medication is promoting weight gain or some other aspect of the MS, consideration should be given to a trial of an agent less likely to cause such side effects. Medication may also offer some relief from weight gain and its metabolic consequences. Among the agents added to atypical antipsychotics for management of weight gain, metformin is the best studied and most promising. Several large studies have concluded that this agent is beneficial as add-on treatment for antipsychotic-induced weight gain (Fiedorowicz et al., 2012). Metformin appears to be most effective when given early in the treatment of drug-naïve or first-episode adult patients. It is less effective for children and adolescents. Metformin's benefits include not just a reduction in weight gain but also improvement in insulin sensitivity (Smith, 2012). Doses of metformin tend to range from 1000 to 1500 milligrams a day. However, metformin is not the only option nor is it the most effective for every patient (Baptista et al., 2007).

Among the other options for antipsychotic-induced weight gain are orlistat, histamine H2 receptor antagonists, topiramate, amantadine, and various other agents with less substantiated utility. Orlistat is indicated for the management of obesity. It is a gastrointestinal lipase inhibitor. Orlistat 120 mg three times a day is generally safe and effective for weight loss and improves insulin sensitivity. Mild gastrointestinal distress, and very rarely severe liver injury, are important side effects (Ioannides-Demos, Piccenna, & McNeil, 2011).

It is not clear why H2 receptor antagonists such as nizatidine or famotidine may be helpful, but it is possible that peripheral suppression of cholecystokinin activity is helpful.

FACTOR	MEASURE	LIMITATIONS
Fasting insulin level	An elevated serum level suggests insulin resistance	Not every clinic has this study available.
Fasting glucose	A normal level is <100 mg/dL	Elevations may reflect a late stage of insulin resistance
HgbA1C	Normal values are 4% to 5.6%	Elevations may reflect a late stage of insulin resistance.
Triglyceride/HDL (fasting)	A ratio <3 suggests low risk for the MS, while a ratio >6 indicates a >50% risk of having the MS.	The "poor man's" insulin sensitivity assay. Lipoprotein lipase is under the control of insulin, and affected by insulin resistance. An independent disorder of lipid metabolism, or treatment for a lipid disorder, may skew results and reduce the value of this ratio as a measure of insulin sensitivity.
Waist circumference	Men: > 40 inches Women: > 35 inches	Increases the likelihood of metabolic syndrome, but overall contribution is only about 25%.
Body mass index	> 25: overweight > 30: obese > 40: morbid obesity	Highly correlated with waist circumference and obesity, with same limitation as for waist circumference
White cell count	Elevations are a well-established feature of the MS.	An elevated white cell count is very nonspecific.

Benefits with these agents are not as consistent as with metformin (Fiedorowicz et al., 2012). Topiramate 250 mg daily has been effective for some patients (Ko, Joe, Jung, & Kim, 2005). The FDA has approved Qysmia for weight reduction. This is a combination of low-dose phentermine and controlled-release topiramate (Garvey et al., 2012). Concerns about cardiovascular and pulmonary toxicity with phentermine are somewhat assuaged by the low-dose use in Qysmia as well as toxicity studies for the combination agent. Topiramate has well described unwanted cognitive effects. These are dose-dependent. However, because the serum levels achieved by a single dose of topiramate may vary by a factor of over 50 times among individuals, it is difficult to predict the impact of a single dose (Cirulli et al., 2012). Amantadine 200 mg daily when added to olanzapine separates from placebo in reducing weight gain (Hoffmann, Case, & Jacobson, 2012).

An inquiry should also be made into sleep quality and characteristics. If obstructive sleep apnea suggests itself in the patient's history, a sleep study should be considered to make a definitive diagnosis (Rajagopalan, 2011). For some patients, bariatric surgery may be significantly helpful in treating obesity and, as a result, the MS (Giugliano, Ceriello, & Esposito, 2008; Madan, Orth, Ternovits, & Tichansky, 2006).

DERMATOLOGICAL REACTIONS

CLINICAL FEATURES

The skin holds a special distinction among drug side effects as being the site of some of the drug reactions that are the most visible, violent, and difficult to diagnose. Among these reactions are the Stevens Johnson syndrome (SJS), drug rash with eosinophilia and systemic symptoms (DRESS) syndrome,

and toxic epidermal necrolysis (TEN). Acute hypersensitivity reactions may be difficult to anticipate. The clinician should, however, be aware of a few important points.

Many drugs can cause rashes: among the most common offenders are aromatic anticonvulsants; other psychotropics are less frequent offenders. The aromatic anticonvulsants include carbamazepine, lamotrigine, phenobarbital, phenytoin, and trileptal. Their metabolism rarely yields arene oxides, which are often implicated in the anticonvulsant hypersensitivity syndrome (AHS). AHS may also be an immune-mediated (or allergic) response. As many as 8% of all persons exposed to medications will develop some form of cutaneous side effect. Perhaps 3% of all patients prescribed carbamazepine will develop a drug eruption (Elias, Madhusoodanan, Pudukkadan, & Antony, 2006). In one retrospective study of patients started in lamotrigine, 13% developed a nonserious rash of some kind (Ginsberg, 2006). Most of these rashes are benign. A rash that spreads widely, is intensely pruritic, involves the mucous membranes of the eye or mouth, or has other systemic findings such as fever or lymphadenopathy, should raise alarm and lead to treatment of the rash and discontinuation of any medication suspected of causing it. Leukocytosis, especially with eosinophilia, and elevation of hepatic enzymes are also indicative of a more severe systemic reaction. But devastating hypersenstivity reactions to anticonvulsants, or AHS, are rare. First described in 1950 by Chaiken and colleagues, AHS typically occurs with older anticonvulsants such as carbamazepine, phenobarbital, phenytoin—but, as noted, it may occur with lamotrigine. Because of the relatively high incidence of seizures in the first decade of life, children may present relatively frequently with AHS (Chaiken, Goldberg, & Segal, 1950; Scaparrotta et al., 2011). The clinician must be concerned when an extensive rash develops that is complicated by fever, eosinophilia, lymphadenopathy, nephritis, or hepatitis (Cacoub et al., 2011).

WHO IS AT RISK?

As noted, those prescribed anticonvulsants are at relatively higher risk of developing a fulminant drug eruption. These include children, patients with epilepsy, patients receiving radiation therapy for brain tumors, and patients with psychiatric illnesses who are prescribed anticonvulsants mainly as mood stabilizers (Metro, Pino, Pellegrini, Sacerdoti, & Fabi, 2007). Those newly started on anticonvulsants are at higher risk of developing an AHS, which tends to develop within the first few weeks of treatment. Intriguingly, a genetic link exists. Among certain groups of Asians, including Han Chinese, carbamazepine-induced SJS and TENS occur relatively frequently among carriers of the HLA-B*1502 allele (Zhang et al., 2011). Lamotrigine-induced SJS or other adverse cutaneous reactions are currently not associated with the HLA-B*1502 allele among the Han Chinese (Shi et al., 2011) The HLA-B*1502 allele does not predict risk of AHS or maculopapular eruptions among persons of Asian descent. Among patients of European ancestry, the HLA-A*3101 allele is found in 2%–5%. This allele appears to confer some risk of developing SJS or TENS as well as milder adverse cutaneous reactions, such as maculopapular eruptions, when carbamazepine is prescribed (McCormack et al., 2011). It is not yet known how these alleles are associated with the risk of severe drug eruptions. Yet the connections are sufficiently sturdy that the risk of SJS and TENS among carriers of the HLA-B* 1502 allele is now advertised in a black box warning in package inserts for carbamazepine (Novartis, 2011).

The involvement of the immune system in severe drug-induced skin reactions such as SJS and TENS is clear. This relationship may be unmasked or underscored when there are other challenges to the immune system. An example of this is the suspected relationship between infection with certain human herpes viruses (HHV) and drug-induced hypersensitivity reactions. It is thought that infection with Epstein Barr virus, cytomegalovirus, HHV-6, and HHV-7 may increase the risk of a drug hypersensitivity reaction (Shiohara, Inaoka, & Kano, 2006). Typically a drug eruption precipitates reactivation of a latent HHV infection (Aihara et al., 2001). However, the reverse has also been observed (Calligaris et al., 2009; Saida et al., 2010). Because post-herpetic neuralgia may be treated with carbamazepine, the potential for a synergistic stimulation of the immune system against autoantigens may be significant in such cases (Garcia, Ferro, Carvalho, da Rocha, & de Souza, 2010).

TREATMENT

When a rash develops and might be caused by a medication, the patient and the clinician are faced with the question of which medication may be the offending agent and whether it should be stopped. The rash is usually exanthemous and starts within a week or so of beginning the causative agent. Certainly when large areas of skin as well as the mouth are involved in a rash, if the skin begins to break down, or in the presence of systemic findings such as fever or lymphadenopathy, it is important to consider stopping the medication. Oral antihistamines and topical steroids may be helpful in minor cases, whether or not the offending agent is stopped. Usually, the rash subsides over a few weeks after discontinuation of the responsible medication (Rawlin, 2011).

The treatment of a severe dermatologic reaction due to a medication begins with stopping the offending agent. Identifying the offending agent can at times be difficult, and a systematic approach to identifying the likeliest agent, agents, or circumstances is crucial. When an agent must be withdrawn abruptly, issues such as withdrawal and the ongoing need to treat other illnesses must be considered. Corticosteroids are routinely provided. Symptomatic measures may at times include life support but usually include intravenous fluids, pain medications, and ocular care. Improvement in skin manifestations and eosinophilia is often prompt with these interventions. However, in some cases substantial or full resolution may take months (Pereira de Silva, Piquioni, Kochen, & Saidon, 2011). Infection, neoplasia, other immune reactions, and other drugs are typically in the differential for a suspected drug-induced rash. Certainly when one aromatic anticonvulsant has caused an AHS, it is reasonable to avoid treatment with another aromatic anticonvulsant. Seitz and colleagues (2006) warned that TCAs are structurally similar to carbamazepine and may lead to a recurrence of a drug-induced hypersensitivity reaction among sensitive patients. Their rough data suggested that a third of patients with a history of AHS will have a recurrence when administered a structurally similar anticonvulsant or TCA.

In some cases it may be possible to pursue treatment with an agent that has caused a rash. For example, if a patient develops a rash during lamotrigine treatment, and if arene oxides are indeed the cause, it may be possible to limit their production by hepatic cytochromes P450 by increasing the dose slowly and perhaps to a lower final dosage (Naveen et al., 2012). Because a visible, pruritic rash may be a late development in what proves to be a severe systemic drug reaction, the clinician should be cautious in rechallenging a patient (Lonati et al., 2012).

HYPONATREMIA

CLINICAL FEATURES

Hyponatremia is generally defined as a serum sodium concentration less than 134–136 milliequivalents per deciliter (mEq/L). It is the most common electrolyte disturbance among hospitalized patients and may occur in as many as 15%–30%. The brain is particularly susceptible to edema and injury in hyponatremia, but overrapid correction of hyponatremia is also perilous. Hyponatremia may cause acute confusion, obtundation, and seizures. It may also cause more subtle problems. For example, motor and gait disturbances due to hyponatremia can reduce quality of life and increase the risk of falls. When the serum sodium falls below 115 mEq/L, the clinician may observe an altered sensorium in over 50% of patients, seizures in over 20%, nausea and vomiting in 5%, disturbances of gait and falls in 4%, dysarthia in 2%, and coma in another 2% (Douglas, 2006). Once discovered, hyponatremia requires clinical action. Box 23.5 outlines a clinical approach to hyponatremia (Chubb, 2009; Esposito, Piotti, Bianzina, Malul, & Dal Canton, 2011; Josiassen et al., 2012; Vaidya, Ho, & Freda, 2010).

A host of medications and conditions can cause, or encourage the development, of hyponatremia. Box 23.6 outlines the general categories of these agents and treatments.

WHO IS AT RISK?

Many factors increase the risk of developing hyponatremia. Being female, advancing age, commonly used medications such as thiazide diruetics and SSRIs, a variety of common medical problems including hypothyroidism, and a history of having hyponatremia are among the risk factors for developing it (Musham, Jarathi, & Pedraza, 2010). The syndrome of inappropriate antidiuretic hormone (SIADH) activity is the most common cause of hyponatremia (Hannon & Thompson, 2010). Patients with SIADH cannot dilute their urine despite hypoosmolar serum. Among medications, the SSRIs appear to be a common precipitant of SIADH.

Certainly SSRI-induced SIADH is not common: perhaps a few cases per thousand occur. And yet the SSRIs are prescribed so widely that the problem has become well known. Typically, SSRI-induced SIADH develops within 2 to 4 weeks of initiating treatment. Dosage does not appear to be a risk factor. But hyponatremia may develop 3 months or more after starting treatment with an SSRI (Liu et al., 1996; Madhusoodanan

et al., 2002), Fisher and colleagues (2002) found that the vast majority of patients with symptomatic hyponatremia due to citalopram were at least 70 years old and that three in four were women. It appears that the SSRIs increase the expression of aquaporin 2 in the inner medullary collecting duct of the kidney (Moyses, Nakandakari, & Magaldi, 2008). This enhances the renal response to ADH and leads to hyponatremia.

It is sometimes argued that other classes of antidepressant may pose less risk of hyponatremia and studies have found that the risk of hyponatremia with mirtazapine and venlafaxine was significantly less than with SSRIs (Jung, Jun, Kim, & Bahk, 2011). However, case reports of hyponatremia have been linked to essentially every class of antidepressant. Roxanas and colleagues reported in a prospective study that 10 of 58 patients over 65 years old started on venlafaxine developed hyponatremia within weeks (Roxanas, Hibbert, & Field, 2007).

Antipsychotics can also cause hyponatremia, and this is typically due to SIADH (Kohen, Voelker, & Manu, 2008). This risk may be just as great for antipsychotics as for antidepressants, but the risk may be overlooked in the presence of other agents with better known risk, such as SSRIs (Mannesse et al., 2010). Indeed, the combination of typical or atypical antipsychotics with other psychotropics known to cause SIADH, such as SSRIs, may compound the risk of developing hyponatremia (Vucicevic, Degoricija, Alfirevic, & Vukicevic-Badouin, 2007). The profile of the patient at risk for developing hyponatremia during antipsychotic therapy may differ from that of patients receiving antidepressants. Meulendijks and colleagues (2010) found that the majority of patients reported to have antipsychotic-induced hyponatremia were middle-aged men. Among the severely mentally ill, the possibility of psychogenic polydipsia must also be considered, as the incidence of psychogenic polydipsia in that group ranges from 6%–20% (Dudeja, McCormick, & Dudeja, 2010). Distinguishing psychogenic polydipsia from drug-induced SIADH is important. Table 23.7 outlines some important differences (Dundas, Harris, & Narasimhan, 2007).

Anticonvulsants are another well-known cause of hyponatremia. In a prospective study involving oxcarbazepine, 25% of patients developed hyponatremia after starting the drug, and in a third of these patients the serum sodium level fell to less than 128 mEq/L. Higher doses, and use in combination with other drugs capable of causing hyponatremia, increased the risk (Lin et al., 2010). Many other anticonvulsants have been linked to hyponatremia, with reports ranging from the frequent (for carbamazepine, phenytoin, and valproic acid) to the rare for agents such as pregabalin (Beers, van Puijenbroek, Bartelink, van der Linden, & Jansen, 2010; Blum, Simsolo, & Tatour, 2009).

There are several mechanisms by which medications may produce the syndrome of inappropriate antidiuretic hormone (SIADH) or some other form of hyponatremia. These include both central and peripheral actions (Esposito et al., 2011). Centrally, psychotropics may alter the regulation of sodium and water. In humans, hyponatremia may develop rapidly as a result (Karim, Jawairia, Rahman, Balsam, & Rubinstein, 2011). Agents that inhibit serotonin reuptake or promote serotonin release tend to cause rats to retain water and reduce their appetite for sodium. The net result is a centrally-mediated hypoosmolar hyponatremia (de Magalhães-Nunes et al., 2007). A direct effect on renal sodium and water handling may also be exerted by medications. For example, SSRIs such as fluoxetine may increase water reabsorption specifically within the kidney by increasing the number of aquaporin receptors in the inner medullary collecting duct (Moyses et al., 2008). Given the multitude of central and peripheral effects that medications may have on sodium and water handling, the clinician is obliged to be attentive to the possibility of iatrogenic hyponatremia.

TREATMENT

Correction of hyponatremia involves identifying modifiable risk factors and causes, clarifying the type of hyponatremia, and determining how recently the hyponatremia has developed. It is of course important to exclude pseudohyponatremia, in which the serum sodium concentration is low, but the serum osmolarity is normal, as may occur in hypertriglyceridemia or hyperproteinemia. Pseudohyponatremia may develop in conditions such as acute pancreatitis or myelomas (Douglas, 2006). Once pseudohyponatremia is excluded, and reversible causes of hyponatremia have been identified, and their reversal initiated, the clinician should move quickly to correcting the serum sodium level. The pacing of sodium replacement depends heavily upon the duration of the hyponatremia. As noted above, if hyponatremia has persisted beyond 48 hours, its correction should be gradual in order to avoid such injuries as central demyelination. Hyponatremia developing in less than 48 hours has not typically been accompanied by substantial movements of cellular sodium and can be treated more aggressively.

The replacement of serum sodium is designed to take place at a rate that will not produce significant osmotic changes with neurons, and with a goal of minimizing such neurological consequences of hyponatremia as seizures. A hypertonic saline solution of 3%, given at a rate of 1–2 mL/kg/hour, is often combined with a loop diuretic to enhance free water elimination. A fast rate may be used if seizures or other signs of neurologic deterioration are present. The serum sodium level should not rise faster than 2 mEq/L/hour. In the first 24 hours, the total rise should not be more than 12 mEq/L. The goal is a serum sodium level of 118 mEq/L and an asymptomatic patient. Once these are achieved, the rate of correction can be slowed further, with a goal of 125 mEq/L. In euvolemic and hypervolemic hyponatremia, fluid restriction

Table 23.7 DISTINGUISHING FEATURES OF PSYCHOGENIC POLYDIPSIA AND SIADH

FACTOR	PSYCHOGENIC POLYDIPSIA	SIADH
Urine osmolality	Low, and sometimes profoundly low. <100 mOsm/L	Not low given serum osmolality: >100 mOsm/L
Urine sodium levels	Low: <10 meq/L	Not low: >40 meq/L
ADH levels	Low or very low	Elevated
Plasma osmolality	Low	Low
Fluid intake	Increased	May be normal

may be useful (Douglas, 2006). In SIADH, restricting fluid intake to 800–1200 milliliters of water a day is the first-line treatment (Sherlock & Thompson, 2010).

In cases of chronic, asymptomatic hyponatremia, medications may be of use. Demeclocycline is an antagonist of vasopressin that reduces the urine concentration. It works in about 60% of patients by causing diabetes insipidus. Demeclocycline can cause nephrotoxicity, but this is usually reversible with discontinuation of the drug. A newer class of medication is that of the vasopressin type 2 receptor antagonist, or *vaptans* (Sherlock & Thompson, 2010). These relatively new agents are not widely used as yet, in part because of their newness and in part due to cost.

For the patient with medication-induced SIADH who requires treatment of a disorder such as depression, for which the recommended treatments caused SIADH, the clinician must decide with the patient how to manage both the medication-induced SIADH as well as the disorder for which the offending medication was prescribed. In some cases a different medication or treatment may be sufficient. Electroconvulsive therapy may substitute for an SSRI in a depressed patient. A patient with epilepsy may fare better with some anticonvulsant other than carbamazepine. For the patient who is obliged to continue treatment with a medication that lowers his or her serum sodium, options may include careful fluid restriction or a trial of a vaptan or demeclocycline. Careful monitoring of serum sodium is essential in such cases. In addition, the patient must be taught to recognize the signs and symptoms of hyponatremia such as subtle changes in gait, an increase in clumsiness, or worsening memory (van der Lubbe, Thompson, Zietse, & Hoorn, 2009). The patient must also know the consequences of such signs and symptoms and how to respond—for example, no driving if gait or memory worsens and a trip to see the clinician for testing of the serum sodium.

CLINICAL PEARLS

- On serotonin syndrome: Many patients with delirium may have hyperreflexia and a few beats of clonus; what is distinctive about SS is the prominent and sustained clonus disproportionate to other signs of encephalopathy. The concurrence of gastrointestinal symptoms helps with the diagnosis, but the most useful point is a history of simultaneous onset of the CNS, autonomic, and GI symptoms in relation to a change in medications with serotonergic effects or a change in medications that interact with a serotonergic medication to increase its level or its effect.

- Drugs directly stimulating serotonin receptors include triptans, buspirone, lithium, and LSD.

- Drugs inhibiting neuronal reuptake of serotonin include SSRIs, SNRIs, TCAs, MAOIs, and linezolid.

- Drugs that inhibit nitric oxide synthesis include paroxetine, fluoxetine, and methylene blue. It is thought that the former two SSRIs may carry increased risk of SS

because of their dual effect on NO synthase and on serotonin reuptake.

- SS is more common in smokers. Diabetes and hypertension are both associated with increased risk of the condition.

- Young men are the highest risk demographic for neuroleptic malignant syndrome.

- Clinical conditions associated with increased risk for NMS include agitation, dehydration, alcoholism, alcohol withdrawal, fever, structural brain injury, hyponatremia, iron deficiency, infection, and concomitant lithium therapy.

- Increased dopamine blockade increases risk: higher neuroleptic dosage, higher potency drugs, and intramuscular administration all carry a higher risk of NMS.

- Atypical (second generation) neuroleptics carry less risk than typical (first generation) neuroleptics. Notwithstanding, numerous cases of NMS due to atypical neuroleptics have been reported

DISCLOSURE STATEMENT

Dr. Brown has no financial or other disclosures to report.

REFERENCES

Ables, A. Z., & Nagubilli, R. (2010). Prevention, recognition, and management of serotonin syndrome. *American Family Physician, 81*, 1139–1142.

Adnet, P., Lestavel, P., & Krivosic-Horber, R. (2000). Neuroleptic malignant syndrome. *British Journal of Anaesthesia, 85*, 129–135.

Aihara, M., Sugita, Y., Takahashi, S., Nagatani, T., Arata, S., Takeuchi, K., & Ikezawa, Z. (2001). Anticonvulsant hypersensitivity syndrome associated with reactivation of cytomegalovirus. *British Journal of Dermatology, 144*, 1231–1234.

Almog, S., Winkler, E., Amitai, Y., Dani, S., Shefi, M., Tirosh, M., & Shemer, J. (1991). Acute pyridostigmine overdose: a report of nine cases. *Israeli Journal of Medical Science, 27*, 659–663.

Altman, C. S., & Jahangiri, M. F. (2010). Serotonin syndrome in the perioperative period. *Anesthesia and Analgesia, 110*, 526–528.

American Psychiatric Association. (2000). Diagnostic and Statistical Manual, Fourth Edition, Revised, 2000.

Anzellotti, F., Ricciardi, L., Monaco, D., Ciccocioppo, F., Borrelli, I., Zhuzhuni, H., & Onofrj, M. (2011). Cefixime-induced nonconvulsive status epilepticus. *Neurological Sciences, 33*, 325–329.

Aquilonius, S. M., & Hartvig, P. (1986). Clinical pharmacokinetics of cholinesterase inhibitors. *Clinical Pharmacokinetics, 11*, 236–249.

American Diabetes Association; American Psychiatric Association; American Association of Clinical Endocrinologists; North American Association for the Study of Obesity. (2004). Consensus development conference on antipsychotic drugs and obesity and diabetes. *Diabetes Care, 27*, 596–601.

American Geriatrics Society (2012). 2012 Beers Criteria Update Expert Panel: American Geriatrics Society updated Beers Criteria for potentially inappropriate medication use in older adults. *Journal of the American Geriatrics Society, 60*(4), 616–631.

Asthana, S., Greig, N. H., Hegedus, L., Holloway, H. H., Raffaele, K. C., Schapiro, M. B., & Soncrant, T. T. (1995). Clinical pharmacokinetics of physostigmine in patients with Alzheimer's disease. *Clinical Pharmacology and Therapeutics, 58*, 299–309.

Baptista, T., Rangel, N., Fernández, V., Carrizo, E., El Fakih, Y., Uzcátegui, E., et al. (2007). Metformin as an adjunctive treatment to control body weight and metabolic dysfunction during olanzapine administration: a multicentric, double-blind, placebo-controlled trial. *Schizophrenia Research, 93*, 99–108.

Bean, W. B., & Funk, D. (1956–1957). The vasculocardiac syndrome of metastatic carcinoid. *Transactions of the American Clinical and Climatological Association, 68*, 111–125.

Beers, E., van Puijenbroek, E. P., Bartelink, I. H., van der Linden, C. M., & Jansen, P. A. (2010). Syndrome of inappropriate antidiuretic hormone secretion (SIADH) or hyponatraemia associated with valproic Acid: four case reports from the Netherlands and a case/non-case analysis of vigibase. *Drug Safety, 33*, 47–55.

Blum, A., Simsolo, C., & Tatour, I. (2009). Hyponatremia and confusion caused by pregabalin. *Israeli Medical Association Journal, 11*, 699–700.

Borys, D. J., Setzer, S. C., Ling, L. J., Reisdorf, J. J., Day, L. C., & Krenzelok, E. P. (1999). Acute fluoxetine overdose: a report of 234 cases. *American Journal of Emergency Medicine*, (1992). 10, 115–120.

Brown, T. M. (1999). Clozapine, neuroleptic malignant syndrome, and pancerebellar syndrome. *Psychosomatics, 40*, 518–520.

Brown, T. M. (2004). Nitroglycerin in the treatment of the serotonin syndrome (letter). *American Journal of Emergency Medicine, 22*, 510.

Brown, T. M. (2001). Substance-induced delirium and related encephalopathies. In S. Yudofsky, et al. (Eds.), *Treatment of psychiatric disorders* (3rd Edition, pp. 413–479). Washington, DC, American Psychiatric Press.

Brown, T. M., Skop, B. P., & Mareth, T. R. (1996). Pathophysiology and management of the serotonin syndrome. *Annals of Pharmacotherapy, 30*, 527–533.

Brubacher, J. R., Hoffman, R. S., & Lurin, M. J. (1996). Serotonin syndrome from venlafaxine-tranylcypromine interaction. *Veterinary and Human Toxicology, 38*, 358–361.

Cacoub, P., Musette, P., Descamps, V., Meyer, O., Speirs, C., Finzi, L., & Roujeau, J. C. (2011). The DRESS syndrome: a literature review. *American Journal of Medicine, 124*, 588–597.

Calligaris, L., Stocco, G., De Iudicibus, S., Marino, S., Decorti, G., Barbi, E., et al. (2009). Carbamazepine hypersensitivity syndrome triggered by a human herpes virus reactivation in a genetically predisposed patient. *International Archives of Allergy and Immunology, 149*, 173–177.

Cannon, W. B., Shohl, A. T., & Wright, W. S. (1911). Emotional glycosuria. *American Journal of Physiology, 29*, 280–287.

Carnahan, R. M., Lund, B. C., Perry, P. J., & Pollock, B. G. (2002). A critical appraisal of the utility of the serum anticholinergic activity assay in research and clinical practice. *Psychopharmacology Bulletin, 36*, 24–39.

Casamassima, F., Lattanzi, L., Perlis, R. H., Litta, A., Fui, E., Bonuccelli, U., et al. (2010). Neuroleptic malignant syndrome: further lessons from a case report. *Psychosomatics, 51*, 349–354.

Chaiken, B. H., Goldberg, B. I., & Segal, J. P. (1950). Dilantin sensitivity—report of a case of hepatitis with jaundice, pyrexia and exfoliative dermatitis. *New England Journal of Medicine, 242*, 897–898.

Chatterjee, R., Yeh, H. C., Shafi, T., Selvin, E., Anderson, C., Pankow, J. S., et al. (2010). Serum and dietary potassium and risk of incident type 2 diabetes mellitus: The Atherosclerosis Risk in Communities (ARIC) study. *Archives of Internal Medicine, 170*, 1745–1751.

Chew, M. L., Mulsant, B. H., Pollock, B. G., Lehman, M. E., Greenspan, A., Mahmoud, R. A., et al. (2008). Anticholinergic activity of 107 medications commonly used by older adults. *Journal of the American Geriatrics Society, 56*, 1333–1341.

Chouinard, G., & Chouinard, V. A. (2008). Atypical antipsychotics: CATIE study, drug-induced movement disorder and resulting iatrogenic psychiatric-like symptoms, supersensitivity rebound psychosis and withdrawal discontinuation syndromes. *Psychotherapy and Psychosomatics, 77*, 69–77.

Chubb, S. A. (2009). Hyponatremia treatment guidelines 2007: expert panel recommendations. *Clinical Biochemist Reviews, 30*, 35–38.

Cirulli, E. T., Urban, T. J., Marino, S. E., Linney, K. N., Birnbaum, A. K., Depondt, C., et al. (2012). Genetic and environmental correlates of topiramate-induced cognitive impairment. *Epilepsia, 53*, e5–e8.

Cooper, J. M., Jones, A. L. (2009). Neuroleptic malignant syndrome or a statin drug reaction? A case report. *Clinical Neuropharmacology, 32*, 348–349.

Cornier, M. A., Dabelea, D., Hernandez, T. L., Lindstrom, R. C., Steig, A. J., Stob, N. R., et al. (2008). The metabolic syndrome. *Endocrine Reviews, 29*, 777–822.

de Hert, M., Correll, C. U., Bobes, J., Cetkovich-Bakmas, M., Cohen, D., Asai, I., et al. (2011). Physical illness in patients with severe mental disorders. I. Prevalence, impact of medications and disparities in health care. *World Psychiatry, 10*, 52–77.

de Hert, M., Schreurs, V., Vancampfort, D., & Van Winkel, R. (2009). Metabolic syndrome in people with schizophrenia: a review. World Psychiatry 8, 15–22.

de Magalhães-Nunes, A. P., Badauê-Passos, D. Jr., Ventura, R. R., Guedes Dda, S. Jr., Araújo, J. P., Granadeiro, P. C., et al. (2007). Sertraline, a selective serotonin reuptake inhibitor, affects thirst, salt appetite and plasma levels of oxytocin and vasopressin in rats. *Experimental Physiology, 92*, 913–922.

Delay, J., & Deniker, P. (1968). Drug-induced extrapyramidal syndromes. In P. Vinken & G. W. Bruyn (Eds.), *Handbook of clinical neurology:* Diseases of the Basal Ganglia (Volume 6, pp. 248–266). Amsterdam, North Holland Publishing Company.

Delay, J., Pichot, P., Lempiere, T., Blissalde, B., & Peigne, F. (1960). Un neuroleptique majeur non phenothiazinique et non réserpinique, l'halopéridol, dans le traitement des psychoses. *Annales Médico-psychologiques, Revue Psychiatrique, 18*, 145–152.

Douglas, I. (2006). Hyponatremia: why it matters, how it presents, how we can manage it. *Cleveland Clinic Journal of Medicine, 73*(Suppl 3), S4–S12.

Dudeja, S. J., McCormick, M., & Dudeja, R. K. (2010). Olanzapine induced hyponatraemia (letter). *Ulster Medical Journal, 79*, 104–105.

Dundas, B., Harris, M., & Narasimhan, M. (2007). Psychogenic polydipsia review: etiology, differential, and treatment. *Curr Psychiatry Rep, 9*, 236–241.

Elias, A., Madhusoodanan, S., Pudukkadan, D., & Antony, J. T. (2006). Angioedema and maculopapular eruptions associated with carbamazepine administration. *CNS Spectrum, 206*(11), 352–354.

Esposito, P., Piotti, G., Bianzina, S., Malul, Y., & Dal Canton, A. (2011). The syndrome of inappropriate antidiuresis: pathophysiology, clinical management and new therapeutic options. *Nephron. Clinical Practice, 119*, c62–c73.

Fallon, P., & Dursun, S. M. (2011). A naturalistic controlled study of relapsing schizophrenic patients with tardive dyskinesia and supersensitivity psychosis. *Journal of Psychopharmacology, 25*, 755–762.

Fernández-Torre, J. L., Santos-Sánchez, C., & Pelayo, A. L. (2010). De novo generalised non-convulsive status epilepticus triggered by piperacillin/tazobactam. *Seizure, 19*, 529–530.

Fiedorowicz, J. G., Miller, D. D., Bishop, J. R., Calarge, C. A., Ellingrod, V. L., & Haynes, W. G. (2012). Systematic review and meta-analysis of pharmacological interventions for weight gain from antipsychotics and mood stabilizers. *Current Psychiatry Reviews, 8*, 25–36.

Fink, M. (2011). Catatonia from its creation to DSM-V: Considerations for ICD. *Indian Journal of Psychiatry, 53*, 214–217.

Fink, M. P., Snydman, D. R., Niederman, M. S., Leeper, K. V. Jr., Johnson, R. H., Heard, S. O., et al. (1994). Treatment of severe pneumonia in hospitalized patients: results of a multicenter, randomized, double-blind trial comparing intravenous ciprofloxacin with imipenem-cilastatin. The Severe Pneumonia Study Group. *Antimicrobial Agents and Chemotherapy, 38*, 547–557.

Fisher, A., Davis, M., Croft-Baker, J., Purcell, P., & McLean, A. (2002). Citalopram-induced severe hyponatremia with coma and seizure. Case report with literature and spontaneous report review. *Adverse Drug Reactions and Toxicological Reviews, 21*, 179–187.

Frampton, A., & Spinks, J. (2005). Hyperthermia associated with central anticholinergic syndrome caused by a transdermal hyoscine patch in a child with cerebral palsy. *Emergency Medicine Journal, 22*, 678–679.

Frascogna, N. (2007). Physostigmine: is there a role for this antidote in pediatric poisonings? *Current Opinion in Pediatrics, 19*, 201–205.

Freeman, H. (1946). Resistance to insulin in mentally disturbed soldiers. *Archives of Neurology & Psychiatry, 56*, 74–78.

Garcia, J. B., Ferro, L. S., Carvalho, A. B., da Rocha, R. M., & de Souza, L. M. (2010). Severe carbamazepine-induced cutaneous reaction in the treatment of post-herpetic neuralgia. Case report. *Revista Brasileira Anestesiologia, 60*, 429–437.

Garza, M. B., Osterhoudt, K. C., & Rutstein, R. (2000). Central anticholinergic syndrome from orphenadrine in a 3 year old. *Pediatric Emergency Care, 16*, 97–98.

Garvey, W. T., Ryan, D. H., Look, M., Gadde, K. M., Allison, D. B., Peterson, C. A., et al. (2012). Two-year sustained weight loss and metabolic benefits with controlled-release phentermine/topiramate in obese and overweight adults (SEQUEL): a randomized, placebo-controlled, phase 3 extension study. *American Journal of Clinical Nutrition, 95*, 297–308.

Gibb, W. R., & Griffith, D. N. (1986). Levodopa withdrawal syndrome identical to neuroleptic malignant syndrome. *Journal of Postgraduate Medicine, 62*, 59–60.

Ginsberg, L. D. (2006). Efficacy and safety of lamotrigine for adults with bipolar disorder in a private practice setting. *CNS Spectrum, 11*, 376–382.

Giugliano, D., Ceriello, A., & Esposito, K. (2008). Are there specific treatments for the metabolic syndrome? *American Journal of Clinical Nutrition, 87*, 8–11.

Gjerden, P., Bramness, J. G., & Slørdal, L. (2009). The use and potential abuse of anticholinergic antiparkinson drugs in Norway: a pharmacoepidemiological study. *British Journal of Clinical Pharmacology, 67*, 228–233.

Grill, M. F., & Maganti, R. (2008). Cephalosporin-induced neurotoxicity: clinical manifestations, potential pathogenic mechanisms, and the role of electroencephalographic monitoring. *Annals of Pharmacotherapy, 42*, 1843–1850.

Grundy, S. M., Cleeman, J. I., Daniels, S. R., Donato, K. A., Eckel, R. H., Franklin, B. A., et al. (2005). American Heart Association; National Heart, Lung, and Blood Institute: Diagnosis and management of the metabolic syndrome: an American Heart Association/National Heart, Lung, and Blood Institute Scientific Statement. *Circulation, 112*, 2735–2752.

Guay, D. R. (2010). Tetrabenazine, a monoamine-depleting drug used in the treatment of hyperkinetic movement disorders. *American Journal of Geriatric Pharmacotherapy, 8*, 331–373.

Hadaegh, F., Khalili, D., Ghasemi, A., Tohidi, M., Sheikholeslami, F., & Azizi, F. (2009). Triglyceride/HDL-cholesterol ratio is an independent predictor for coronary heart disease in a population of Iranian men. *Nutrition, Metabolism, and Cardiovascular Diseases, 19*, 401–408.

Hall, R. C. W., Feinsilver, D. L., & Holt, R. E. (1981). Anticholinergic psychosis: differential diagnosis and management. *Psychosomatics, 22*, 581–587.

Hannon, M. J., & Thompson, C. J. (2010). The syndrome of inappropriate antidiuretic hormone: prevalence, causes and consequences. *European Journal of Endocrinology, 162*(Suppl 1), S5–S12.

Hartley, T. A., Knox, S. S., Fekedulegn, D., Barbosa-Leiker, C., Violanti, J. M., Andrew, M. E., & Burchfiel, C. M. (2012). Association between depressive symptoms and metabolic syndrome in police officers: results from two cross-sectional studies. *Journal of Environmental and Public Health 2012*, 861219.

Heiss, W. D. (2011). The ischemic penumbra: correlates in imaging and implications for treatment of ischemic stroke. The Johann Jacob Wepfer award 2011. *Cerebrovascular Disease, 32*, 307–320.

Hoffman, J., Trimble, J., & Brophy, G. M. (2009). Safety of imipenem/cilastatin in neurocritical care patients. *Neurocritical Care, 10*, 403–407.

Hoffmann, V. P., Case, M., & Jacobson, J. G. (2012). Assessment of treatment algorithms including amantadine, metformin, and zonisamide for the prevention of weight gain with olanzapine: a randomized controlled open-label study. *Journal of Clinical Psychiatry, 73*, 216–223.

Hruz, P. W. (2011). Molecular mechanisms for insulin resistance in treated, H. I.V-infection. Best Practice & Research. *Clinical Endocrinology and Metabolism, 25*, 459–468.

Huang, P. L. (2009). A comprehensive definition for metabolic syndrome. *Disease Model Mechanisms, 2*, 231–237.

Ioannides-Demos, L. L., Piccenna, L., & McNeil, J. J. (2011). Pharmacotherapies for obesity: past, current, and future therapies. *Journal of Obesity, 2011*, 179674.

Isbister, G. K., Buckley, N. A., & Whyte, I. M. (2007). Serotonin toxicity: a practical approach to diagnosis and treatment. *Medical Journal of Australia, 187*, 361–365.

Jacob, M. K., Ash, P., & Craighead, W. E. (2012). Adolescent female with withdrawal psychosis following abrupt termination of ziprasidone. *Eur Child Adolesc Psychiatry, 21*, 165–168.

Jastak, J. T. (1985). Physostigmine: an antidote for excessive central nervous system depression or paradoxical rage reactions resulting from intravenous diazepam. *Anesthesia Progress, 32*, 87–92.

Job, M. L., & Dretler, R. H. (1990). Seizure activity with imipenem therapy: incidence and risk factors. *DICP, 24*, 467–469.

Jolivalt, C. G., Lee, C. A., Beiswenger, K. K., Smith, J. L., Orlov, M., Torrance, M. A., & Masliah, E. (2008). Defective insulin signaling pathway and increased glycogen synthase kinase-3 activity in the brain of diabetic mice: parallels with Alzheimer's disease and correction by insulin. *Journal of Neuroscience Research, 86*, 3265–3274.

Jones, D., & Story, D. A. (2005). Serotonin syndrome and the anaesthetist. *Anaesthesia and Intensive Care, 33*, 181–187.

Josiassen, R. C., Filmyer, D. M., Geboy, A. G., Martin, D. M., Curtis, J. L., Shaughnessy, R. A., et al. (2012). Psychomotor deficits associated with hyponatremia: a retrospective analysis. *Clinical Neuropsychology, 26*, 74–87.

Jung, Y. E., Jun, T. Y., Kim, K. S., & Bahk, W. M. (2011). Hyponatremia associated with selective serotonin reuptake inhibitors, mirtazapine, and venlafaxine in Korean patients with major depressive disorder. *International Journal of Clinical Pharmacology and Therapeutics, 49*, 437–443.

Karadeniz, C., Oğuz, A., Canter, B., & Serdaroğlu, A. (2000). Incidence of seizures in pediatric cancer patients treated with imipenem/cilastatin. *Pediatric Hematology and Oncology, 17*, 585–590.

Karim, M. R., Jawairia, M., Rahman, S., Balsam, L., & Rubinstein, S. (2011). Cocaine-associated acute severe hyponatremia. *Clinical Nephrology, 75*(Suppl 1), 11–15.

Kasanin, J. (1926). The blood sugar curve in mental disease. *Archives of Neurology & Psychiatry, 16*, 414–419.

Kaur, H., Adams-Huet, B., Smith, G., & Jialal, I. (2013). Increased neutrophil count in nascent metabolic syndrome. *Metabolic Syndrome and Related Disorders, 11*, 128–131.

Kersten, H., Molden, E., Tolo, I. K., Skovlund, E., Engedal, K., & Wyller, T. B. (2013). Cognitive effects of reducing anticholinergic drug burden in a frail elderly population: a randomized controlled trial. *Journal of Gerontology. Series A, Biological Sciences and Medical Sciences, 68*, 271–278.

Ko, Y. H., Joe, S. H., Jung, I. K., & Kim, S. H. (2005). Topiramate as an adjuvant treatment with atypical antipsychotics in schizophrenic patients experiencing weight gain. *Clinical Neuropharmacology, 28*, 169–175.

Kohen, I., Voelker, S., & Manu, P. (2008). Antipsychotic-induced hyponatremia: case report and literature review. *American Journal of Therapeutics, 15*, 492–494.

Kooy, F. H. (1919). Hyperglycaemia in mental disorders. *Brain, 42*, 214–290.

Korpi, E. R., & Lüddens, H., (1997). Furosemide interactions with brain, GABAA receptors. *British Journal of Pharmacology, 120*, 741–748.

Kulka, P. J., Toker, H., Heim, J., Joist, A., & Jakschik, J. (2004). Suspected central anticholinergic syndrome in a 6-week-old infant. *Anesthesia and Analgesia, 99*, 1376–1378.

Lambert, T. J. (2007). Switching antipsychotic therapy: what to expect and clinical strategies for improving therapeutic outcomes. *Clin Psychiatry. 68*(Suppl 6), 10–13.

Lee, S., Merriam, A., Kim, T. S., Liebling, M., Dickson, D. W., & Moore, G. R. (1989). Cerebellar degeneration in neuroleptic malignant syndrome: neuropathologic findings and review of the literature concerning heat-related nervous system injury. *Journal of Neurology, Neurosurgery, & Psychiatry, 52*, 387–391.

Levenson, J. L. (1985). Neuroleptic malignant syndrome. *Am J Psychiatry, 142*, 1137–1145.

Lin, C. H., Lu, C. H., Wang, F. J., Tsai, M. H., Chang, W. N., Tsai, N. W., et al. (2010). Risk factors of oxcarbazepine-induced hyponatremia in patients with epilepsy. *Clinical Neuropharmacology, 33*, 293–296.

Link, J., Papadopoulos, G., Dopjans, D., Guggenmoos-Holzmann, I., & Eyrich, K. (1997). Distinct central anticholinergic syndrome following general anaesthesia. *European Journal of Anaesthesiology, 14*, 15–23.

Liu, B. A., Mittmann, N., Knowles, S. R., Shear, N. H. (1996). Hyponatremia and the syndrome of inappropriate secretion of antidiuretic hormone associated with the use of selective serotonin reuptake inhibitors: a review of spontaneous reports. *Canadian Medical Association Journal, 155*, 519–527.

Lonati, D., Zancan, A., Giampreti, A., Sparpaglione, D., Locatelli, C. A., & Manzo, L. (2012). An insidious skin rash without itch. *Clinical Toxicology (Philadelphia), 50*, 149–150.

Lu, M. L., Pan, J. J., Teng, H. W., Su, K. P., & Shen, W. W. (2002). Metoclopramide-induced supersensitivity psychosis. *Annals of Pharmacotherapy, 36*, 1387–1390.

Mackay, F. J., Dunn, N. R., & Mann, R. D. (1999). Antidepressants and the serotonin syndrome in general practice. *British Journal of General Practice, 49*, 871–874.

Madan, A. K., Orth, W., Ternovits, C. A., Tichansky, D. S. (2006). Metabolic syndrome: yet another co-morbidity gastric bypass helps cure. *Surgery for Obesity and Related Diseases, 2*, 48–51.

Madhusoodanan, S., Bogunovic, O. J., Moise, D., Brenner, R., Markowitz, S., & Sotelo, J. (2002). Hyponatremia associated with psychotropic medications. A review of the literature and spontaneous reports. *Adverse Drug Reactions and Toxicological Reviews, 21*, 17–29.

Man, S. P. (2011). An uncommon adverse effect of levodopa withdrawal in a patient taking antipsychotic medication: neuroleptic malignant-like syndrome. *Hong Kong Medical Journal, 17*, 74–76.

Mannesse, C. K., van Puijenbroek, E. P., Jansen, P. A., van Marum, R. J., Souverein, P. C., & Egberts, T. C. (2010). Hyponatraemia as an adverse drug reaction of antipsychotic drugs: a case-control study in VigiBase. *Drug Safety, 33*, 569–578.

Matsusue, A., Hara, K., Kageura, M., Kashiwagi, M., Lu, W., Ishigami, A., et al. (2009). Genetic analysis of ryanodine receptor 1 gene and carnitine palmitoyltransferase II gene: an autopsy case of neuroleptic malignant syndrome related to vegetamin. *Journal of Legal Medicine (Tokyo), 11*(Suppl 1), S570–S572.

Matsusue, A., Hara, K., Kashiwagi, M., Kageura, M., Sugimura, T., & Kubo, S. (2011). Genetic analysis of the rhabdomyolysis-associated genes in forensic autopsy cases of methamphetamine abusers. *Journal of Legal Medicine (Tokyo), 13*, 7–11.

McCormack, M., Alfirevic, A., Bourgeois, S., Farrell, J. J., Kasperavičiūtė D, Carrington, M., et al. (2011). HLA-A*3101 and carbamazepine-induced hypersensitivity reactions in Europeans. *New England Journal of Medicine, 364*, 1134–1143.

McIntyre, R. S., Rosenbluth, M., Ramasubbu, R., Bond, D. J., Taylor, V. H., Beaulieu, S., Schaffer A; Canadian Network for Mood and Anxiety Treatments (CANMAT) Task Force. (2012). Managing medical and psychiatric comorbidity in individuals with major depressive disorder and bipolar disorder. *Annals of Clinical Psychiatry, 24*, 163–169.

Mendhekar, D. N., Jiloha, R. C., Mehndiratta, M. M., & War, L. (2002). Challenge with atypical antipsychotic drugs in risperidone induced neuroleptic malignant syndrome: a case report. *Indian Journal of Psychiatry, 44*, 387–390.

Metro, G., Pino, S., Pellegrini, D., Sacerdoti, G., & Fabi, A. (2007). Brain radiotherapy during treatment with anticonvulsant therapy as a trigger for toxic epidermal necrolysis. *Anticancer Research, 27*, 1167–1169.

Meulendijks, D., Mannesse, C. K., Jansen, P. A., van Marum, R. J., & Egberts, T. C. (2010). Antipsychotic-induced hyponatraemia: a systematic review of the published evidence. *Drug Safety, 33*, 101–114.

Miller, A. D., Ball, A. M., Bookstaver, P. B., Dornblaser, E. K., & Bennett, C. L. (2011). Epileptogenic potential of carbapenem agents: mechanism of action, seizure rates, and clinical considerations. *Pharmacotherapy, 31*, 408–423.

Miller, R. (2009). Mechanisms of action of antipsychotic drugs of different classes, refractoriness to therapeutic effects of classical neuroleptics, and individual variation in sensitivity to their actions: Part II. *Current Neuropharmacology, 7*, 315–330.

Mintzer, J., & Burns, A. (2000). Anticholinergic side-effects of drugs in elderly people. *Journal of the Royal Society of Medicine, 93*, 457–462.

Moyses, Z. P., Nakandakari, F. K., & Magaldi, A. J. (2008). Fluoxetine effect on kidney water reabsorption. *Nephrology, Dialysis, Transplantation, 23*, 1173–1178.

Musham, C. K., Jarathi, A., & Pedraza, G. (2010). A rare case of fatal hyponatremia due to a combination of psychotropic polypharmacy and hypothyroidism. *Primary Care Companion. Journal of Clinical Psychiatry, 12*(4), PCC.09100897.

Naveen, K. N., Ravindra, M. S., Pai, V. V., Rai, V., Athanikar, S. B., & Girish, M. (2012). Lamotrigine induced DRESS syndrome. *Indian J Pharmacol, 44*, 798–800.

Neel, J. V. (1962). Diabetes mellitus: a "thrifty" genotype rendered detrimental by "progress"? *American Journal of Human Genetics, 14*, 353–362.

Neuhut, R., Lindenmayer, J. P., & Silva, R. (2009). Neuroleptic malignant syndrome in children and adolescents on atypical antipsychotic medication: a review. *Journal of Child and Adolescent Psychopharmacology, 19*, 415–422.

Newcomer, J. W. (2007). Metabolic syndrome and mental illness. *American Journal of Managed Care, 13*(7 Suppl), S170–S177.

Ng, B. K., & Cameron, A. J. (2010). The role of methylene blue in serotonin syndrome: a systematic review. *Psychosomatics, 51*, 194–200.

Nielsen, R. E., Wallenstein Jensen, S. O., & Nielsen, J. (2012). Neuroleptic malignant syndrome-an 11-year longitudinal case–control study. *Canadian Journal of Psychiatry, 57*, 512–518.

Nieman, D. C., Brock, D. W., Butterworth, D., Utter, A. C., & Nieman, C. C. (2002). Reducing diet and/or exercise training decreases the lipid and lipoprotein risk factors of moderately obese women. *Journal of the American College of Nutrition, 21*, 344–350.

Nishtala, R. A., McLachlan, A. J., Bell, J. S., Kelly, P. J., & Chen, T. F. (2009). Anticholinergic activity of commonly prescribed medications and neuropsychiatric adverse events in older people. *Journal of Clinical Pharmacology, 49*, 1176–1184.

Norrby, S. R., & Gildon, K. M. (1999). Safety profile of meropenem: a review of nearly 5,000 patients treated with meropenem. *Scandinavian Journal of Infectious Diseases, 31*, 3–10.

Novartis: Tegretol^R (carbamazepine). (2011). prescribing information. East Hanover, New Jersey, http://www.pharma.us.novartis.com/product/pi/pdf/tegretol.pdfSar

O'Brien, R. A., & Young, G. B. (1989). Neuroleptic malignant syndrome: a review. *Canadian Family Physician, 35*, 1119–1122.

Panagopoulou, V., Tzimas, P., Arampatzis, P., Aroni, F., & Papadopoulos, G. (2011). The effects of physostigmine on recovery from general anesthesia in elderly patients. *Minerva Anestesiologica, 77*, 401–407.

Pasina, L., Djade, C. D., Lucca, U., Nobili, A., Tettamanti, M., Franchi, C., et al. (2013). Association of anticholinergic burden with cognitive and functional status in a cohort of hospitalized elderly: comparison of the anticholinergic cognitive burden scale and anticholinergic risk scale: results from the REPOSI study. *Drugs and Aging, 30*, 103–112.

Patel, M. K., & Brunetti, L. (2010). Neuroleptic malignant syndrome secondary to aripiprazole initiation in a clozapine-intolerant patient. *American Journal of Health-System Pharmacy, 67*, 1254–1259.

Pereira de Silva, N., Piquioni, P., Kochen, S., & Saidon, P. (2011). Risk factors associated with, D. R. ESS syndrome produced by aromatic and non-aromatic antipiletic drugs. *European Journal of Clinical Pharmacology, 67*, 463–470.

Pestotnik, S. L., Classen, D. C., Evans, R. S., Stevens, L. E., & Burke, J. P. (1993). Prospective surveillance of imipenem/cilastatin use and associated seizures using a hospital information system. *Annals of Pharmacotherapy*, *27*, 497–501.

Pope, H. G. Jr, Cole, J. O., Choras, P. T., & Fulwiler, C. E. (1986). Apparent neuroleptic malignant syndrome with clozapine and lithium. *Journal of Nervous and Mental Disease*, *174*, 493–495.

Proudfoot, A. (2006). The early toxicology of physostigmine: a tale of beans, great men and egos. *Toxicological Reviews*, *25*, 99–138.

Rajagopalan, N. (2011). Obstructive sleep apnea: not just a sleep disorder. *Journal of Postgraduate Medicine*, *57*, 168–175.

Ramjan, K. A., Williams, A. J., Isbister, G. K., & Elliott, E. J. (2007). "Red as a beet and blind as a bat." Anticholinergic delirium in adolescents: lessons for the paediatrician. *Journal of Paediatrics and Child Health*, *43*, 779–780.

Rapport, M. M., Green, A. A., & Page, I. H. (1948). Serum vasoconstriction (serotonin), IV: isolation and characterization. *Journal of Biological Chemistry*, *176*, 1243–1251.

Rawlin, M. (2011). Exanthems and drug reactions. *Australian Family Physician*, *40*, 486–489.

Reaven, G. M. (2006). The metabolic syndrome: is this diagnosis necessary? *American Journal of Clinical Nutrition*, *83*, 1237–1247.

Reuling, J., & Cramer, C. (1947). Intrathecal penicillin. *JAMA*, *134*, 16–18.

Rosenberg, M. R., & Green, M. (1989). Neuroleptic malignant syndrome. Review of response to therapy. *Archives of Internal Medicine*, *149*, 1927–1931.

Roxanas, M., Hibbert, E., & Field, M. (2007). Venlafaxine hyponatraemia: incidence, mechanism and management. *Australian & New Zealand Journal of Psychiatry*, *41*, 411–418.

Roy-Desruisseaux, J., Landry, J., Bocti, C., Tessier, D., Hottin, P., & Trudel, J. F. (2011). Domperidone-induced tardive dyskinesia and withdrawal psychosis in an elderly woman with dementia. *Annals of Pharmacotherapy*, *45*, e51.

Rudolph, J. L., Salow, M. J., Angelini, M. C., & McGlinchey, R. E. (2008). The anticholinergic risk scale and anticholinergic adverse effects in older persons. *Archives of Internal Medicine*, *168*, 508–513.

Russell, T., Riazi, S., Kraeva,., Steel, A. C., & Hawryluck, L. A. (2012). Ecstacy-induced delayed rhabdomyolysis and neuroleptic malignant syndrome in a patient with a novel variant in the ryanodine receptor type 1 gene. *Anaesthesia*, *67*, 1021–1024.

Saad, F. (2009). The role of testosterone in type 2 diabetes and metabolic syndrome in men. *Arquivos Brasileiros de Endocrinologia & Metabologia*, *53*, 901–907.

Saida, S., Yoshida, A., Tanaka, R., & Abe, J. Hamahata, K., Okumura, M., & Momoi, T. (2010). A case of drug-induced hypersensitivity syndrome-like symptoms following HHV-6 encephalopathy. *Allergology International*, *59*, 83–86.

Sakel, M. (1938). Insulin therapy in the future of psychiatry. *Canadian Medical Association Journal*, *39*, 178–179.

Sanai, T., Matsui, R., Hirano, T., Torichigai, S., Yotsueda, H., Higashi, H., et al. (2006). Successful treatment of six patients with neuroleptic malignant syndrome associated with myoglobulinemic acute renal failure. *Renal Failure*, *28*, 51–55.

Sarkar, P., Natarajan, C., & Gode, N., (2009). Prevalence of neuroleptic malignant syndrome in 672 consecutive male in-patients. *Indian Journal of Psychiatry*, *51*, 202–205.

Scaparrotta, A., Verrotti, A., Consilvio, N. P., Cingolani, A., Di Pillo, S., Di Gioacchino, M., et al. (2011). Pathogenesis and clinical approaches to anticonvulsant hypersensitivity syndrome: current state of knowledge. *International Journal of Immunopathology and Pharmacology*, *24*, 277–284.

Schliamser, S. E., Cars, O., & Norrby, S. R. (1991). Neurotoxicity of beta-lactam antibiotics: predisposing factors and pathogenesis. *Journal of Antimicrobial Chemotherapy*, *27*, 405–425.

Seitz, C. S., Pfeuffer, P., Raith, P., Bröcker, E. B., & Trautmann, A. (2006). Anticonvulsant hypersensitivity syndrome: cross-reactivity with tricyclic antidepressant agents. *Annals of Allergy, Asthma and Immunology*, *97*, 698–702.

Shalev, A., Hermesh, H., & Munitz, H. (1989). Mortality from neuroleptic malignant syndrome. *Journal of Clinical Psychiatry*, *50*, 18–25.

Sherlock, M., Thompson, C. J. (2010). The syndrome of inappropriate antidiuretic hormone: current and future management options. *European Journal of Endocrinology*, *162*(Suppl 1), S13–S18.

Shi, Y. W., Min, F. L., Liu, X. R., Zan, L. X., Gao, M. M., Yu, M. J., & Liao, W. P. (2011). Hla-B alleles and lamotrigine-induced cutaneous adverse drug reactions in the Han Chinese population. *Basic Clinical Pharmacology & Toxicology*, *109*, 42–46.

Shiohara, T., Inaoka, M., & Kano, Y. (2006). Drug-induced hypersensitivity syndrome (DIHS): a reaction induced by a complex interplay among herpesviruses and antiviral and antidrug immune responses. *Allergology International*, *55*, 1–8.

Shiovitz, T. M., Welke, T. L., Tigel, P. D., Anand, R., Hartman, R. D., Sramek, J. J., et al. (1996). Cholinergic rebound and rapid onset psychosis following abrupt clozapine withdrawal. *Schizophrenia Bulletin*, *22*, 591–595.

Smith, J. L., Ju, J. S., Saha, B. M., Racette, B. A., & Fisher, J. S. (2004). Levodopa with carbidopa diminishes glycogen concentration, glycogen synthase activity, and insulin-stimulated glucose transport in rat skeletal muscle. *Journal of Applied Physiology*, *97*, 2339–2346.

Smith, R. C. (2012). Metformin as a treatment for antipsychotic drug side effects: special focus on women with schizophrenia. *American Journal of Psychiatry*, *169*, 774–776.

Speich, R., & Haller, A. (1994). Central anticholinergic syndrome with the antimalarial drug mefloquine. *New England Journal of Medicine*, *331*, 57–58.

Stahl, S. M., Mignon, L., & Meyer, J. M. (2009). Which comes first: atypical antipsychotic treatment or cardiometabolic risk? *Acta Psychiatrica Scandinavica*, *119*, 171–179.

Stannard, S. R., & Johnson, N. A. (2004). Insulin resistance and elevated triglyceride in muscle: more important for survival than "thrifty" genes? *Journal of Physiology*, *554*(Pt 3), 595–607.

Sternbach, H. (1991). The serotonin syndrome. *American Journal of Psychiatry*, *148*, 705–713.

Suchard, J. R. (2003). Assessing physostigmine's contraindication in cyclic antidepressant ingestions. *Journal of Emergency Medicine*, *25*, 185–191.

Supariwala, A., Kant, G., & Jean, R. E. (2011). Neuroleptic malignant syndrome with metoclopramide overdose coexisting with *Clostridium difficile* diarrhea. *Intensive Care Medicine*, *37*, 1706–1708.

Tadokoro, S., Okamura, N., Sekine, Y., Kanahara, N., Hashimoto, K., & Iyo, M. (2011). *Schizophrenia Bulletin*, *38*, 1012–1020.

Toalson, P., Ahmed, S., Hardy, T., & Kabinoff, G. (2004). The Metabolic Syndrome in Patients With Severe Mental Illnesses. *Primary Care Companion. Journal of Clinical Psychiatry*, *6*, 152–158.

Thomas, C., Hestermann, U., Kopitz, J., Plaschke, K., Oster, P., Driessen, M., et al. (2008). Serum anticholinergic activity and cerebral cholinergic dysfunction: an, E. E.G study in frail elderly with and without delirium. *BMC Neuroscience*, *9*, 86.

Trollor, J. N., Chen, X., Chitty, K., & Sachdev, P. S. (2012). Comparison of neuroleptic malignant syndrome induced by first- and second-generation antipsychotics. *British Journal of Psychiatry*, *201*, 52–56.

Trollor, J. N., Chen, X., & Sachdev, P. S. (2009). Neuroleptic malignant syndrome associated with atypical antipsychotic drugs. *CNS Drugs*, *23*, 477–492.

Tune, L., & Coyle, J. T. (1980). Serum levels of anticholinergic drugs in treatment of acute extrapyramidal side effects. *Archives of General Psychiatry*, *37*, 293–297.

Vaidya, C., Ho, W., & Freda, B. J. (2010). Management of hyponatremia: providing treatment and avoiding harm. *Cleveland Clinic Journal of Medicine*, *77*, 715–726.

Vardeny, O., Uno, H., Braunwald, E., Rouleau, J. L., Gersh, B., Maggioni, A. P., et al. (2011). Prevention of Events with an, A.C.E Inhibitor (PEACE) Investigators: Opposing effects of β blockers and angiotensin-converting enzyme inhibitors on development of new-onset diabetes mellitus in patients with stable coronary artery disease. *American Journal of Cardiology*, *107*, 1705–1709.

van der Lubbe, N., Thompson, C. J., Zietse, R., & Hoorn, E. J. (2009). The clinical challenge of SIADH—three cases. *NDT Plus, 2*(Suppl_3), iii20–iii24.

Verma, S. K., Subramaniam, M., Liew, A., & Poon, L. Y. (2009). Metabolic risk factors in drug-naive patients with first-episode psychosis. *Journal of Clinical Psychiatry, 70,* 997–1000.

Vucicevic, Z., Degoricija, V., Alfirevic, Z., & Vukicevic-Badouin, D. (2007). Fatal hyponatremia and other metabolic disturbances associated with psychotropic drug polypharmacy. *International Journal of Clinical Pharmacology and Therapeutics, 45,* 289–292.

Wada, A., Yokoo, H., Yanagita, T., & Kobayashi, H. (2005). New twist on neuronal insulin receptor signaling in health, disease, and therapeutics. *Journal of Pharmacological Sciences, 99,* 128–143.

Wagner, R., Fink, R. H., & Stephenson, D. G. (2004). Effects of chlorpromazine on excitation-contraction coupling events in fast-twitch skeletal muscle fibres of the rat. *British Journal of Pharmacology, 141,* 624–633.

Walker, M. F. C. (1959). Simulation of tetanus by trifluperazine overdosage. *Canadian Medical Association Journal, 81,* 109–110.

Weiss, T., Skelton, K., Phifer, J., Jovanovic, T., Gillespie, C. F., Smith, A., et al. (2011). Posttraumatic stress disorder is a risk factor for metabolic syndrome in an impoverished urban population. *General Hospital Psychiatry, 33,* 135–142.

Zand, L., Hoffman, S. J., & Nyman, M. A. (2010). 74-year-old woman with new-onset myoclonus. *Mayo Clinic Proceedings, 85,* 955–958.

Zhang, Y., Wang, J., Zhao, L. M., Peng, W., Shen, G. Q., Xue, L., et al. (2011). Strong association between, H. L.A-B*1502 and carbamazepine-induced Stevens-Johnson syndrome and toxic epidermal necrolysis in mainland Han Chinese patients. *European Journal of Clinical Pharmacology, 67,* 885–887.

24.

NEUROSTIMULATION: ECT, VNS, ʀTMS AND DBS

Lawrence Park

INTRODUCTION

Somatic therapies have played a prominent role in the history of psychiatric therapeutics. The term *somatic therapies* refers to a wide range of treatment modalities that utilize treatment interventions based in biological mechanisms. While it could be argued that pharmacological treatment is a form of somatic therapy, the term is typically used to distinguish biologically based therapies from pharmacological treatments. At the present time, pharmacological treatments serve as the mainstay of psychiatric therapeutics, but somatically based interventions are gaining in prominence and in the future may commonly be utilized in clinical settings.

Somatic treatments proliferated in the late 1800s and early 1900s as the foundations of modern neurology and psychiatry were being developed. During this period of time, the biological substrates of mental phenomena were just beginning to be understood, and a paucity of effective treatments existed (Shorter, 1997). Prior to the advent of modern psychopharmacology (i.e., generally considered to have started with the synthesis of chlorpromazine in 1954), a variety of somatic treatments were developed. Many treatments, such as hydrotherapy—the immersion of patients into hot water—had little scientific evidence to support their safety and effectiveness. Other interventions were based on a rudimentary understanding of the biological basis of psychiatric conditions and demonstrated marginal effectiveness and/or significant adverse events. For instance, Julius Wagner von Jauregg (an Austrian psychiatrist) investigated the use of pyrotherapy, the use of febrile illness to treat psychiatric conditions. Targeting dementia paralytica (dementia related to neurosyphilis), he injected patients with live malaria parasites from infected individuals. While the ensuing fevers from malaria were purported to be quite effective for eradicating treponema pallidum and treating tertiary syphilis, the patient was then left with another pernicious, and incurable, condition (malaria). For his work, von Jauregg was awarded the Nobel Prize for medicine in 1927. Another somatic treatment developed in this era was the use of insulin coma therapy. Manfred Sakel (a Polish psychiatrist) developed the technique of administering insulin to psychiatric patients (primarily for psychotic symptoms) in order to induce hypoglycemic coma (Sakel, 1958). Again, while beneficial outcomes were reported, the potential

complications of intentionally induced sustained hypoglycemia were significant. A final example of a somatic treatment during this era is the development of ablative surgical procedures for psychiatric symptoms. Colloquially referred to as "psychosurgery," anatomical targets of ablation, such as the frontal lobe, were proposed based on empirical experience of an individual who had sustained accidental brain injury (i.e., John Gage) and the resulting effects. As in the previous examples, proponents of ablative procedures, such as frontal lobotomy or lobectomy, reported positive outcomes on psychiatric target symptoms, but rigorous studies have never been conducted and significant and permanent neuropsychiatric complications are known to occur.

Recently, somatic treatments have focused on a number of neurostimulation techniques for the treatment of neurological and psychiatric indications. Neurostimulation techniques currently being investigated or used in clinical practice include electroconvulsive therapy (ECT), vagus nerve stimulation (VNS), repetitive transcranial magnetic stimulation (rTMS) and deep brain stimulation (DBS).

While the development of modern neurostimulation techniques rests on the previous crude somatic techniques described, it is important to recognize important distinctions between the two eras. First, current neurostimulation techniques are based on a more sophisticated understanding of the biological substrates of psychiatric illness (e.g., neurofunctional imaging of anatomical correlates, brain mechanisms of learning through long-term potentiation). As a result, interventions are designed with much more precision and therefore may maximize therapeutic effects and minimize associated side effects. Second, clinical investigations in the current era are conducted with much greater scientific rigor than in the past. As a result, a greater degree of certainty about safety and effectiveness can generally be gained from the current body of scientific data.

Based on greater insights into the biological mechanisms underlying neuropsychiatric disease, there has been a proliferation of modern somatically based technologies, including neurostimulation interventions utilizing various forms of stimulation (Rosa & Lisanby, 2012). In addition to neurostimulation using electrical and/or electromagnetic stimulation, a host of other modalities of intervention are being investigated. These interventions include light box therapy (for seasonal affective disorder; Terman et al., 1989), focal electrically administered seizure therapy (Spellman, Peterchev, & Lisanby, 2009), magnetic seizure therapy (Lisanby, Schlaepfer, Fisch, & Sackeim, 2001), low intensity pulsed ultrasound (Tyler et al., 2008), near infrared light therapy (Hamblin & Demidova, 2006), low field magnetic stimulation (Rohan et al., 2004) and optogenetic stimulation (in animals; see Yizhar et al., 2011). Each varies in the type of energy utilized and in the methods of application. Moreover, while each of these technologies is at a different stage of development, none have been approved or cleared for use by the FDA. These treatments remain investigational, and in the clinical setting they would only be encountered in patients participating in clinical trials studying their use.

This chapter will focus on neurostimulation treatments that have been approved or cleared for neurological and/or psychiatric indications. These treatments include well-established treatments such as ECT, which has a long history of use, as well as more recently developed interventions such as VNS, rTMS and DBS. These technologies are being used or investigated to treat a growing number of neuropsychiatric conditions such as seizure disorder, Parkinson's disease, essential tremor, dystonia, catatonia, obsessive compulsive disorder, and depression, and are currently being studied for numerous other diseases. We will examine the historical development and theoretical foundation of each treatment, the indications for use, potential associated adverse events, typical clinical management, and settings where these treatments may be encountered in the care of the medical patient.

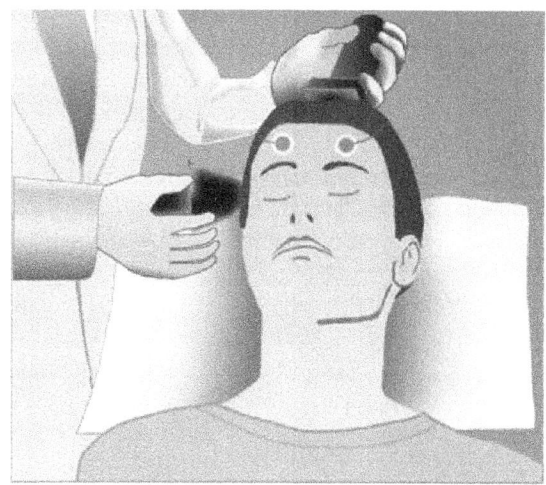

Figure 24.1 Electroconvulsive therapy (ECT)

ECT

Considered by many to be one of the most effective treatments for depression, ECT is also one of the oldest treatments still used for psychiatric conditions. The application of electricity to the scalp with the intention of causing a seizure was first conducted by two Italian physicians, Cerletti and Bini, in 1938 (Bini, 1995). Since that time, ECT has had a varied history with periods of significant use and relative disuse. In the 1940s and 1950s, given the relative lack of effective pharmacotherapy and used in association with psychosurgical techniques, ECT was used quite widely. At this time, ECT was administered without modern medical and anesthetic management. In the 1960s through the 1980s— pharmacotherapy became more effective, while there was increasing public concern about coercive treatment and the stigmatization of mentally ill people. In this context the usage of ECT waned, even for the treatment of patient populations in which it is remarkably effective. From the 1990s through the present, with the development of modern anesthesia (general anesthesia, muscle relaxation, cardiovascular and pulmonary management), modifications in the ECT technique, and increasing concern about treatment-resistant disease, ECT has once again become an important option in the treatment algorithm of severe, treatment-resistant depression.

Currently, ECT is used to treat depression (both unipolar and bipolar) and catatonia, as well as other conditions

such as psychotic depression, mania, and schizophrenia (U.S. Department of Health and Human Services, 1999). While a significant amount of research has been conducted on ECT for various indications, recent systematic reviews and meta-analyses of the literature support effectiveness only for depression, and only in the acute period within the first month after the course of treatment (Greenhalgh, Knight, Hind, Beverley, & Walters, 2005). For depression, ECT is generally considered after failure of multiple antidepressant trials and/or deterioration of the patient's psychiatric or medical condition creating a need for a rapid, definitive response (i.e., acutely suicidal, medically unstable; American Psychiatric Association, 2001). Because of the lack of other effective treatments, and the high mortality rate associated with treatment-resistant catatonia, in the clinical setting ECT is considered in treatment resistant catatonia (i.e., refractory to adequate trials—at least 2 mg parenteral lorazepam or equivalent—of benzodiazepine; Bush et al., 1996) as an off-label treatment.

Of all the treatment modalities discussed in this chapter, ECT is the most likely treatment intervention to be encountered in clinical practice. Treatment-resistant depression has been a growing concern (Rush et al., 2006) and individuals who have adequately responded to multiple antidepressant medication trials and suffer from severe symptomatology may be encountered in both the outpatient and inpatient setting. The catatonic syndrome, though uncommon, should be anticipated in the general hospital setting, given that the etiology may be medical, neurological, or psychiatric in nature, and the presentation may masquerade as a variety of related conditions. The typical course of ECT consists of 6–12 treatments, administered 2–3 times per week. Catatonic symptoms may be more persistent and may require longer courses of treatment. As previously noted, the effectiveness of ECT has been demonstrated in the acute period; symptom relapse after a successful course of ECT is a clinical concern. Clinical practice strategies that are intended to decrease the relapse rate include continuation pharmacotherapy using post-ECT administration of antidepressants, such as nortriptyline and lithium carbonate (Sackeim et al., 2001), or maintenance ECT (a tapered course of periodic administration after a full course of ECT, e.g., once/week, once/month, etc.) (Kellner et al., 2006).

ECT is associated with considerable medical and psychiatric risks. Adverse events of ECT are presented in Table 24.1.

Medical risks of ECT include acute cardiovascular adverse events (such as hypertension, hypotension, arrhythmias, ischemia, embolic or hemorrhagic strokes), pulmonary complications (such as aspiration pneumonia or prolonged apnea), prolonged or tardive seizures, physical trauma (including bodily/dental/oral/ocular injury, skin burns), pain/discomfort/nausea, adverse reaction to anesthesia, and death. Psychiatric risks of ECT treatment include induction of mania, post-ECT cognitive disorientation, anterograde memory impairment, and retrograde autobiographical memory impairment.

Developments in medical and anesthetic management have significantly improved the safety profile of the procedure. This includes the use of general anesthesia to render the patient unconscious during the procedure, neuromuscular blocking agents to prevent tonic clonic muscle activity, and cardiovascular/pulmonary management as well as ECG, EEG, and ventilatory monitoring. Of note, depolarizing muscle blockers such as succinylcholine are considered the first-line agents for muscle relaxation. Contraindications to the use of succinylcholine include inherited cholinesterase inhibitor deficiency that may result in prolonged recovery time, or neuromuscular conditions or other states of muscular inactivity that may predispose the patient to excess potassium release from muscle tissue during the procedure. A complete history and physical should be conducted prior to ECT—including past medical and family history for adverse reactions to general anesthesia or neuromuscular blocking agents—in order to assess the occurrence of past adverse events. The information gained in the initial evaluation may aid in the optimal selection of medications to be used during the procedure.

Overall, the use of general anesthesia and neuromuscular blockers have greatly reduced the discomfort and amount of physical trauma (i.e., fractures and soft tissue trauma) associated with ECT. Appropriate cardiovascular and pulmonary monitoring and management have also significantly decreased the medical risks of ECT.

Management of other risks of ECT include EEG monitoring during the procedure to assess for prolonged or tardive seizures. In the event of prolonged seizure activity, ready access to antiepileptic agents should be available. The use of bite blocks during the procedure prevents significant dental/oral trauma. Proper skin preparation, the use of conductivity gel and snug electrode placement minimize the occurrence of skin burns. Pain, discomfort, and nausea are treated symptomatically.

As with any procedure utilizing general anesthesia, a rare but potential adverse event is death. Estimates of the mortality rate associated with ECT are 1 per 10,000 patients or 1 per 80,000 treatments (American Psychiatric Association, 2001). This rate is similar to that of general anesthesia use associated with minor elective surgical procedures.

Psychiatric adverse events associated with ECT include inadvertent induction of mania, post-procedure disorientation and confusion, and anterograde and retrograde memory impairment. Induction of mania is a rare but documented possibility of ECT treatment. The occurrence of mania may indicate an underlying bipolar diathesis. If hypomania or mania occurs during a treatment course, ECT is often discontinued and, if needed, appropriate mood-stabilizing pharmacotherapy can be initiated. Post-procedure disorientation and confusion are commonly seen and typically resolve in the minutes to hours after treatment administration.

Perhaps the most concerning adverse events associated with ECT deal with memory impairment. It is generally accepted that ECT results in memory deficits in different domains, namely anterograde memory (i.e., recent memory or the creation new memories) and retrograde personal memory (i.e., memory for past autobiographical information). For both types of memory, impairment is greatest just after treatment. Studies suggest that anterograde memory deficits resolve within days to weeks of the cessation of treatment (Semkovska & McLoughlin, 2010). Studies examining retrograde autobiographical memory demonstrate that while there may be improvement over time, complete resolution of memory deficits has not been observed as far out as 6 months posttreatment (Fraser, O'Carroll, & Meier, 2008).

Selection of stimulation parameters may aid in the minimization of memory impairment. Greater memory impairment has been associated with sine wave stimulation, bilateral and unilateral dominant hemisphere electrode placement, increased frequency of treatment (i.e., 3/week vs. 2/week) and increasing doses of energy (for bilateral electrode placement only). In order to optimize the positive effects of ECT and minimize memory adverse events, the current standard for administering ECT is to use unilateral nondominant hemisphere placement, high energy dose (>3 times seizure threshold; seizure threshold determined by stimulus titration at the onset of treatment), and brief pulse (1–1.5 msec) waveform. Recent studies have examined the use of ultrabrief pulse stimulus (0.3 msec), which demonstrates some promise with regard to significantly decreasing memory adverse events (though this may occur at the expense of lost efficacy; see Sienaert, Vansteelandt, Demyttenaere, & Peuskens, 2010).

Because of the possibility of significant adverse events and past reports of coercive or inadequate informed consent procedures, an approved written informed consent process, with complete discussion of all the benefits and risks of treatment, should be undertaken prior to initiating any course of ECT.

A thorough psychiatric and medical evaluation is essential to ensure the safety of ECT. In addition to the treating psychiatrist, the initial workup should be conducted with the involvement of an appropriate anesthesia provider. A routine initial evaluation typically includes complete medical and psychiatric history, physical examination, laboratory tests (CBC, chemistries, UA), chest x-ray, and ECG. Preexisting medical conditions may warrant further consultation and workup (Park, Weiss, & Welch, 2004). While there are no absolute contraindications to ECT, several conditions deserve further attention before considering a course of ECT. Patients with coronary artery disease, recent myocardial ischemia/infarction, hypertension, vascular aneurysms, and cardiac arrhythmias often require cardiac consultation, further pre-ECT

Table 24.1 ADVERSE EVENTS ASSOCIATED WITH ECT AND POTENTIAL MITIGATING FACTORS

SYSTEM	ADVERSE EVENT	POTENTIAL MITIGATING FACTORS
Cardiovascular	Hypertension, hypotension, arrhythmias, ischemia, embolic or hemorrhagic strokes Frequency: BP changes common, CV uncommon, stroke rare. Severity: mild–severe	• Pre-ECT assessment (e.g., BP, EKG, echocardiogram, holter, neuroimaging, neurovascular studies) • Appropriate procedure monitoring (e.g., BP and rate control, anticoagulation for patients with atrial fibrillation) • Appropriate clinical management
Pulmonary	Apnea, aspiration Frequency: rare Severity: high	• Pre-ECT assessment (e.g., chest x-ray, pulmonary function tests) • Appropriate procedure monitoring • Appropriate clinical management
Neurological	Prolonged or tardive seizures Frequency: uncommon Severity: moderate-severe	• Pre-ECT neurological evaluation • EEG monitoring • Availability of seizure treatment during procedure
Physical	Fractures, soft tissue injury, dental fractures, dislocations, oral lacerations, prosthetic damage, corneal abrasions, burns at electrode site Frequency: uncommon Severity: mild–severe	• Pre-ECT dental assessment • Removal of prostheses • Use of general anesthetic agents and neuromuscular blocking agents • Use of mouth protection (bite blocks) • Skin preparation and electrode contact • Use of conductivity gel
Anesthesia-related	Adverse reaction or prolonged reaction to anesthetic agents, neuromuscular blocking agents Frequency: rare Severity: severe	• Pre-ECT assessment (medical, family history) • Appropriate procedure monitoring • Appropriate clinical management
Death	Resulting from other pathophysiological processes Frequency: rare Severity: severe	• Appropriate workup and management of specific medical and psychiatric risks
Pain/ discomfort/ nausea	Frequency: common Severity: mild–moderate	• Use of analgesic/antiemetic medications
Psychiatric		
Induction of mania	Frequency: uncommon Severity: moderate–severe	• Cessation of treatment • Administration of mood stabilizers
Cognition	Disorientation generally occurs posttreatment, but typically resolves minutes after completion of treatment. Frequency: common Severity: mild	• Use of square wave, direct current, brief pulse waveform stimulus (not sine wave) • Use of unilateral nondominant electrode placement • Use of ultra-brief pulse (0.3 msec) stimulus • Frequency of treatment no greater than twice weekly during a course of ECT
Memory	Anterograde memory impairment—appears to resolve within 3 months posttreatment. Retrograde autobiographical memory impairment—data out to 6 months do not demonstrate full resolution of impairment. Frequency: common Severity: mild–severe	• Exclusive use of square wave, direct current, brief pulse waveform stimulus • Use of unilateral nondominant electrode placement • Frequency of treatment no greater than twice weekly during a course of ECT • Use of ultra-brief pulse (0.3 msec) stimulus

Adapted from http://www.fda.gov/downloads/AdvisoryCommittees/CommitteesMeetingMaterials/MedicalDevices/MedicalDevicesAdvisoryCommittee/ NeurologicalDevicesPanel/UCM240933.pdf.

evaluation, and special observation and management (if ECT is pursued). In particular, individuals with cardiac valve disease (e.g., aortic stenosis) may require cardiac outflow studies and correction of the underlying structural anomaly prior to initiating ECT. Other conditions that warrant additional evaluation and management include pregnancy, space-occupying intracranial lesions, cerebral aneurysms, neurovascular malformations, and recent TIAs/strokes.

Some medications may have potentially problematic interactions with ECT and should be tapered or discontinued prior to treatment. Tricyclic antidepressant medications and MAO inhibitors may increase the risk of cardiac arrhythmias; therefore, they should be discontinued and/or cardiac status should be closely monitored. Lithium has been associated with increased confusion when used during a course of ECT; theophylline may increase the length of seizures. These medications are usually tapered during a course of treatment. Anticonvulsant agents (including benzodiazepines) increase the seizure threshold and therefore may interfere with seizure induction during the procedure. If adequate seizures are not being achieved, tapering or discontinuation of these agents may be indicated.

VNS

VNS involves the electrical stimulation of the left vagus nerve with the intention of affecting the functioning of limbic and higher cortical structures. VNS was initially explored as a potential treatment modality because of its role in the autonomic nervous system and direct connections to brainstem structures. It was theorized that because fibers from the vagus nerve synapse in the nucleus tractus solitarius (NTS), stimulation of the vagus nerve would affect NTS neurons, and from there could exert an ascending influence on other brain structures related to mood (George et al., 2000). Stimulation is targeted at the left vagus nerve because the majority of nerve fibers (80%) are ascending afferent fibers (in contract to the largely efferent right vagus nerve). Early investigations noted changes in cortical EEG (McLean, 1990) and anticonvulsant effects of VNS in animals (Zabara, 1992).

Based on these findings, VNS has been studied for seizure disorders and psychiatric disorders. In 1997, VNS was approved for adjunctive therapy in reducing the frequency of refractory partial-onset seizures in individuals 12 years of age and older. In 2005, VNS was approved for the long-term treatment of chronic or recurrent depression in adults who have not had an adequate response to four or more adequate antidepressant trials. For the one-third of patients who will suffer from medication refractory seizures, and who do not want or are not candidates for surgical resection, VNS may be a viable treatment alternative (Milby, Halpern, & Baltuch, 2008). VNS was also approved for treatment-resistant depression in 2005. The pivotal trial upon which approval was based (Rush et al., 2005) did not demonstrate a significant difference between active and sham groups at 10 weeks, though a post-hoc comparison of treatment-resistant depression patients receiving VNS and treatment as usual showed significant results favoring the VNS group (Rush & Siefert, 2009). Measures of depression improved over several months, with the investigators inferring that the maximal effect of VNS for depression occurs 6-12 months after implantation of the unit. Treatment response can increase over time when VNS is used for epilepsy as well. For example, Kuba et al. (2009), reporting a series of epilepsy patients who received VNS for 5 years or more, noted that one year after implantation of the unit 44.4% of patients were assessed as responders to treatment, while after two years 58.7% of patients were judged as responders. Given the potential delay in symptom improvement, VNS should not be viewed as an appropriate treatment for acute depression. In the treatment of chronic treatment-refractory depression the benefit of VNS *may* justify the expense and risk of adverse events, but it should be kept in mind that only a minority of patients treated will experience a remission of depression with VNS, and some will not improve as well. A retrospective study of Medicare beneficiaries with treatment resistant depression (TRD) (Feldman et al., 2013) suggests that there may be long-term economic benefits of VNS treatment on a population basis even if the benefit is not predictable for individual patients. They found that average medical costs per patient year *post-implantation* for Medicare beneficiaries with TRD receiving TNS were substantially lower than the costs for beneficiaries with TRD receiving other treatments.

The VNS device consists of an implanted pulse generator (IPG) and an electrode that attaches to the left vagus nerve. The IPG is surgically implanted into the left chest wall, either subcutaneously or in a pocket in the pectoral muscle, and the electrode is attached to the left vagus nerve, and then a connection is made with the IPG. In addition, the system also includes an external programming device that links to the IPG with a programming wand and a wristwatch style magnet that can be used to reset the microprocessor. After surgical implantation and an adequate time for healing, the treating physician may activate the device and program the settings. Typical stimulation parameters are presented in Table 24.2. Note that the VNS is active intermittently; the percentage of the time the unit is active is an important determinant both of side effects and of battery life.

Adverse events associated with the implantation and operation of a VNS unit include incisional pain, neck pain, dysphagia, nausea, paresthesias, increased cough, dyspnea, laryngismus, pharyngitis, voice alteration (hoarseness), and

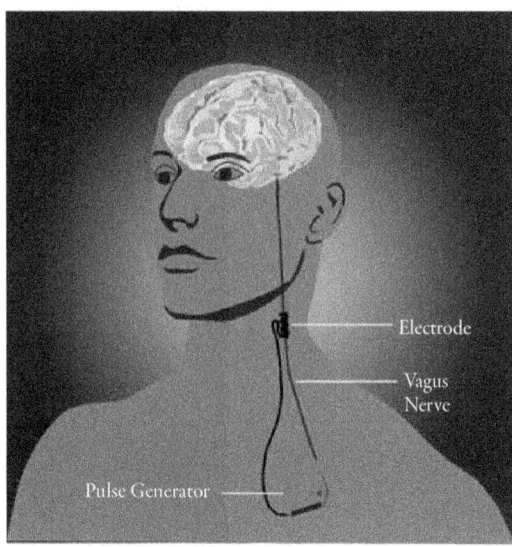

Electrode

Vagus Nerve

Pulse Generator

Figure 24.2 Vagus nerve stimulation (VNS)

Table 24.2 TYPICAL VNS STIMULATION PARAMETERS

PARAMETER	RANGE
Output current	0–3.5 mA
Frequency	1–30 Hz
Pulse width	130–1000 μsec
Duty cycle	
• Stimulation ON	≤60 sec
• Stimulation OFF	0.2–180 min

From Labiner & Ahern, 2007.

cardiac events (bradycardia, tachycardia, palpitations, postural hypotension, and syncope). Of these, the most common are hoarseness, coughing and dyspnea, neck pain, and dysphagia. These complications occur during the active stimulation phase and are generally uncomfortable but not severe. If patients do not acclimate to these effects over time, the frequency and intensity of the stimulus, or the percentage of time the stimulator is active, may be reduced to decrease their occurrence or severity. Bradycardia, hypotension, and syncope when they occur are typically seen during the active stimulation phase and are thought to be due to increased vagal tone. While quite concerning and potentially severe, cardiac complications are not commonly seen with VNS treatment. If they do occur, they are often successfully managed by decreasing or suspending stimulation.

Appropriate preimplantation workup includes a comprehensive medical and psychiatric evaluation involving psychiatrist, anesthesiologist, and neurosurgeon (Fahy, 2010). VNS placement is contraindicated in patients with a bilateral or left cervical vagotomy, and cardiac arrhythmias are a relative contraindication. VNS can cause or exacerbate bradycardia and rarely can induce asystole requiring resuscitation. It can exacerbate obstructive sleep apnea (OSA), or precipitate the onset of OSA in patients not previously affected. Patients with chronic lung disease may experience a worsening of dyspnea when the vagus nerve is stimulated. Postoperative arrhythmia will not necessarily be detected by a day of Holter monitoring conducted when the patient is asymptomatic; when a patient develops episodic faintness, syncope or palpitations following VNS an effort should be made to obtain an ECG when the patient is symptomatic. Patients with implanted VNS units should not receive diathermy treatments either utilizing short-wave or microwave radiation or therapeutic ultrasound. Magnetic resonance imaging (MRI) of the body, transcutaneous electrical nerve stimulation (TENS), defibrillation, and extracorporeal shockwave lithotripsy all have the potential to damage the VNS unit (Cyberonics, 2007). At the time of writing, VNS has been approved as adjunctive therapy for reducing seizure frequency in patients at least 12 years old with partial seizures refractory to antiepileptic medications, and as adjunctive long-term therapy for chronic or recurrent depression that has not had an adequate response to four or more adequate antidepressant treatments. Clinicians working in hospital settings are more likely to encounter patients with vagus nerve stimulators for the epilepsy indication than for the depression indication. While depression and epilepsy are the only approved indications for VNS, clinicians have published case series of its use in other conditions of interest to medical psychiatrists, notably fibromyalgia (Lange et al., 2011) and anxiety disorders (George et al., 2008).

Clinical situations that can arise in the management of VNS devices include battery depletion and device malfunction. Depending on the parameters of the VNS – amplitude and frequency of stimulation, and the percentage of the time the unit is activated – expected battery life ranges from less than one year to more than 10 years. In addition to battery depletion, another common device malfunction is lead breakage, which can be due to trauma to the chest or neck, or to growth in the case of adolescents treated for epilepsy with VNS. In both cases, stimulation can terminate abruptly and this can result in a precipitous exacerbation of symptoms. The nature of device malfunction usually can be established by externally querying the device with its remote control. Surgical revision would be required to replace or repair the defective components.

VNS is not compatible with full body MRI. MRI should not be performed with a body coil in transmit mode (this may result in heating of the VNS lead). Compatibility of VNS with brain MRI has been demonstrated with the stimulator in the off mode (i.e., current = 0 mA) with a transmit-and-receive type of head coil and a static magnetic field strength of 2 Tesla or less.[1] Finally, although several case reports have been published recently, the safety of administering ECT in patients with VNS has not been firmly established.

rTMS

Repetitive transcranial magnetic stimulation is a noninvasive brain stimulation technology that utilizes the principle of electromagnetic induction to subject the brain to an alternating electrical current by externally applying an alternating magnetic field. This technology is based on Ampère and Faraday's (Liao, Dourmashkin & Belcher, 2004) finding that passing a wire through a magnetic field generates an electric current—in other words, "a changing magnetic field can general electrical current in nearby wires, nerves or muscles" (George, 2010). The basic rTMS system consists of an external wire coil through which an alternating electrical current is passed. A fluctuating magnetic field is created around the coil, which induces an alternating electric current in underlying neuronal tissue. This current by altering the electrical environment of neurons influences theirfiring properties (Wassermann & Zimmermann, 2012). The magnetic fields penetrate tissues and are not subject to the electrical resistance of bone and soft tissues that limits the use of external

---

1. IPG output = 0 mA, transmit and receive head coil only, static magnetic field strength ≤ 2 T, specific absorption rate (SAR) < 1.3 W/kg for 70 kg patient, time-varying intensity of < 10 T/sec.

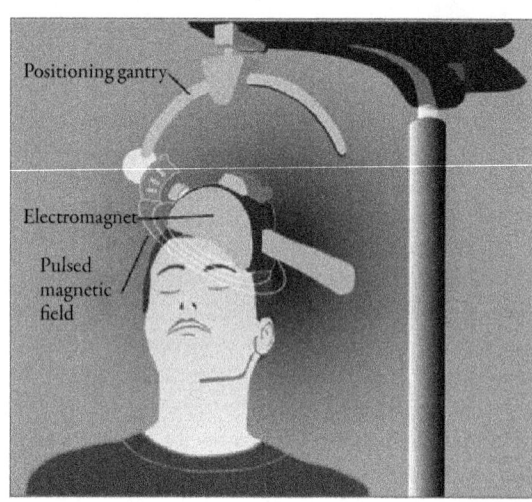

Positioning gantry

Electromagnet

Pulsed magnetic field

Figure 24.3 Repetitive transcranial megnetic stimulation (rTMS)

Table 24.3 MAXIMUM SAFE DURATION (IN SECONDS) OF SINGLE TRAINS OF RTMS

FREQ (HZ)	INTENSITY (% MT)				
	90	100	110	120	130
1	>1800	>1800	>1800	>360	>50
5	>10	>10	>10	>10	>10
10	>5	>5	>5	4.2	2.9
20	2.05	2.05	1.6	1.0	0.55
25	1.28	1.28	0.84	0.4	0.24

From Rossi et al., 2009, p. 2023.

electrical stimulation (though, however, transcranial direct current stimulation with low current is feasible and is under exploration as a therapy for depression and other conditions). Through the use of shaped coils, the magnetic flux may be focused on specific cortical anatomical targets. While magnetic stimulation utilizing different characteristics has been investigated (i.e., single pulse vs. repetitive, alternating vs. direct current), repetitive stimulation—rTMS, utilizing alternating current—has received the most attention. rTMS devices have been investigated in a number of different conditions. However, they are approved for only one condition, which is major depression. In 2008, an rTMS device was cleared for the treatment of major depressive disorder in adult patients who have failed to achieve satisfactory improvement from one prior antidepressant medication at or above the minimal effective dose and duration in the current episode.[2] The pivotal randomized controlled trial demonstrated a p-value of 0.057 for the prespecified primary effectiveness endpoint (difference between active and sham baseline to 4-week endpoint change on the Montgomery-Asberg Depression Rating Scale; see O'Reardon et al., 2007). Based on the evidence available, rTMS was cleared by the FDA for use in individuals with major depression who had failed one prior antidepressant trial.

While rTMS has not been cleared or approved for other indications, current investigations are examining its use for various conditions including schizophrenic hallucinations, PTSD, obsessive compulsive disorder, Parkinson's disease, Alzheimer's disease, neurorehabilitation, migraine headache, chronic pain, and tinnitus (Wassermann & Zimmermann, 2012).

The system includes a wrapped wire coil, a console (including energy source), and a patient chair. Coils are of various shapes (a common shape is "figure 8") to create an optimal magnetic field (Marangell, Martinez, Jurdi, & Zboyan, 2007). For depression, stimulation is localized over the left dorsolateral prefrontal cortex. Certain parameters are then set for the treatment, such as frequency of pulses, and intensity (as a percentage of motor threshold-MT, train duration, and total

2. www.accessdata.fda.gov/cdrh_docs/pdf8/K083538.pdf

number of pulses). Maximum safe stimulation criteria have been established, originally published by Wassermann (1998) and later updated by Rossi et al. (2009; see Table 24.3). rTMS is generally conducted in the outpatient setting, with a typical course of treatment comprising one-hour stimulation sessions five days a week for 4 to 6 weeks. Potential adverse events include seizures, induction of mania, pain over the stimulation site, headache, visual changes, dental pain, facial numbness or twitching, temporary or permanent hearing loss, and, in children and adolescents, neurocardiogenic syncope. The risk of a seizure can be minimized by adherence to safe stimulation criteria. EEG monitoring and appropriate antiepileptic management should be available in the event that seizures occur in the course of treatment. Induction of hypomania or mania is also a rare complication of rTMS, and should be managed by cessation of rTMS treatments and/or appropriate mood stabilizing interventions. Given the loudness of the rTMS device and the potential for permanent hearing loss, earplugs should be worn at all times by all patients and treaters. If rTMS is off-label for a child or adolescent the patient's blood pressure and pulse should be monitored because of the risk of neurocardiogenic syncope. Overall, however, the incidence of serious adverse events with rTMS is very low and the treatment should be regarded as relatively safe, as compared with ECT, multi-drug regimens and other treatment options for treatment-refractory depression. Contraindications to rTMS include any metal in the head (except in the oral cavity), increased intracranial pressure, cardiac pacemakers, implanted neurostimulators, medication pumps, and intracardiac lines. Other conditions that may preclude rTMS treatment or require additional monitoring and management include significant cardiac disease, pregnancy, history of bipolar disorder, stroke, brain lesions, suicide attempts, and personal or family history of seizure disorders.

DEEP BRAIN STIMULATION

Deep brain stimulation (DBS) is an invasive brain stimulation technique which involves direct electrical stimulation of cortical and subcortical brain structures through the precisely-localized implantation of an electrode into deep

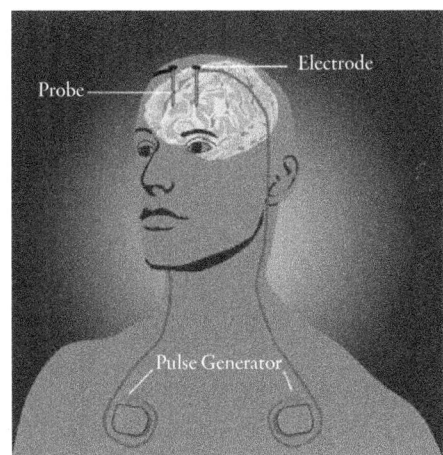

Figure 24.4 Deep brain stimulation (DBS)

brain structures. Electrodes are connected via a lead wire to neurostimulator pulse generators implanted under the skin in the chest wall. Like the implanted VNS device, the DBS system includes external programming devices for use by the physician and by the patient that control the implanted device via a radio frequency connection. External radio frequency stimulation can induce sufficient current in the implanted device to recharge its battery.

Perhaps more than any of the other neurostimulation techniques, DBS is rooted in a structural theory of brain function, and, while not an ablative procedure, is founded on the experience of past ablative neurosurgical procedures (Goodman & Insel, 2009). DBS was initially attempted by Heath in 1963 (Heath, 1963). Based on the understanding of motor circuitry in the brain involving cortical-thalamo-striatal-cortical circuits, treatments for movement disorders using DBS were developed. Theoretical advances in understanding were paralleled by technological advances in stereotactic neurosurgery, which provided the ability to precisely and accurately localize electrode placement in specific brain structures. While movement disorders were the initial indications of DBS research, DBS targeting limbic structures emerged as a new somatic treatment for severe primary mental disorders. The application of DBS to primary mental disorders has been informed by emerging neuroanatomy-based models of their pathophysiology. DBS is currently approved for several indications, including Parkinson's disease, essential tremor, dystonia, and obsessive compulsive disorder (OCD). Dystonia and OCD were approved by the FDA under a Humanitarian Device Exemption, which allows for a maximum annual number of patients treated of 4,000. In clinical practice, given the increased use and experience of DBS for movement disorders, patients with implanted DBS devices are most likely to be encountered by medical psychiatrists when they consult to neurology services. On occasion medical psychiatrists are asked to do pre-implantation assessments of candidates for DBS. Table 24.4 outlines the indications and anatomical targets.

In addition, DBS is currently being investigated at various locations for a number of other disorders. These disorders include major depression, epilepsy, Tourette

syndrome, headache, other chronic pain, eating disorders, and posttraumatic coma, (Perlmutter & Mink, 2006; Pluza, Perazza & Golub, 2011), PTSD, substance abuse, and Alzheimer's disease. Studies examining DBS for major depression have targeted locations such as subgenual cingulate white matter (Brodmann area 25; see Mayberg et al., 2005) and the ventral capsule/ventral striatum (Malone et al., 2009). Typical stimulation parameter ranges are presented in Table 24.5.

Table 24.4 CURRENTLY APPROVED DBS INDICATIONS

DISEASE	INDICATION	ANATOMICAL TARGET
Parkinson's Disease	Adjunctive therapy in reducing some of the symptoms of advanced, levodopa-responsive Parkinson's disease that are not adequately controlled with medication.	Bilateral stimulation of GPi or STN
Essential Tremor	Suppression of tremor in the upper extremity in patients who are diagnosed with essential tremor or parkinsonian tremor not adequately controlled by medications and where the tremor constitutes a significant functional disability.	Unilateral thalamic stimulation
Dystonia	Chronic, intractable (drug refractory) primary dystonia, hemidystonia, generalized and segmental dystonia, hemidystonia, and cervical dystonia (torticollis), for individuals 7 years of age or older.	Unilateral or bilateral stimulation of the GPi or STN
OCD	Chronic, severe, treatment-resistant OCD in adult patients who have failed at least 3 SSRIs.	Bilateral anterior limb of the internal capsule

From www.fda.gov.

Table 24.5 TYPICAL DBS STIMULATION PARAMETERS

PARAMETER	RANGE
Output current	0–2.25 mA
Frequency	<185 Hz
Amplitude	<3.5 V
Pulse width	<210 μsec
Charge density	30 μC/cm²/phase
Duty cycle	
• Stimulation ON	≤60 sec
• Stimulation OFF	0.3–180 min

From Kuncel & Grill, 2004.

The most serious adverse events associated with DBS are related to the surgical implantation of the stimulating apparatus; these include intracranial hemorrhage, stroke, seizures, cerebrospinal fluid (CSF) leaks, infections, allergic reactions, neurological symptoms, cardiovascular/pulmonary complications, incisional pain, and headaches. Intracranial hemorrhage occurs in approximately 2% of patients (Follett et al., 2010). The mortality rate for the procedure has been estimated at approximately 1%. While DBS implantation is relatively benign compared with other neurosurgical procedures, it represents a significant risk in the context of neuropsychiatric disorders and their standard non-surgical treatments.

In order to minimize surgery-related risks, a full preoperative medical evaluation should be conducted prior to DBS implantation. In addition to the usual anesthesia-related risks, bleeding disorders and cerebrovascular disease are especially relevant. Potential neuropsychiatric symptoms associated with deep brain stimulation itself (as opposed to device implantation) include confusion, depression or hypomania, suicidal ideation, agitation/irritability, cognitive/behavioral changes, speech disturbance. Specific symptoms are encountered with specific electrode placement sites. Neuropsychiatric symptoms sometimes can be mitigated or eliminated by adjusting stimulation parameters.

Device malfunction such as electrode migration, lead breakage, battery depletion or other malfunction of the implanted pulse generator usually requires surgical revision and/or replacement of the implanted device components.

As with all permanently implanted metallic devices, diathermy (including shortwave diathermy, microwave diathermy, and therapeutic ultrasound diathermy) is contraindicated with DBS devices because heating of the device components can occur and lead to severe injury or death. Undergoing MRI with an implanted DBS system may pose a safety risk; the possibility of safely performing an MRI procedure in a specific patient depends on the device, the specific image to be obtained, and the details of the MRI machine. There have been reports of serious injury and death in individuals with implanted DBS devices undergoing MRIs due to heating and/or movement of the implanted pulse generator, the electrodes or the leads that connect them (Rezai et al., 2004). The FDA has adopted a classification of "MR Safe", "MR Unsafe" and "MR Conditional" to describe safety in the MR environment for those with implanted devices.[3] Some manufacturers have conducted safety testing and provided this information in the approved labeling of the device. Provided the device-specific conditions set forth in the approved labeling are followed, there is a reasonable assurance that MR imaging can be performed safely. Finally, the safety of administering ECT in patients with DBS has not been established.

After electroconvulsive therapy (ECT), DBS is the second most common neurostimulation modality currently in clinical use. However, because of its invasiveness, and the limited evidence of efficacy for conditions other than movement disorders, it is not the first-line treatment for any condition.

Medical psychiatrists consulting to neurological services will encounter patients receiving DBS for movement disorders (Parkinson's disease, essential tremor, and dystonia). Often, consultation will be requested regarding management of symptoms that could either be adverse effects of DBS or symptoms of one of the psychiatric conditions commonly associated with the movement disorder (e.g., major depression with Parkinson's disease). If neuropsychiatric symptoms have arisen or worsened following a recent adjustment of device stimulation parameters, an attempt should be made to readjust stimulation initiating or changing psychopharmacologic treatment of the symptoms. In some cases the adjustment of stimulation parameters willworsen motor symptoms at the same time as it helps neuropsychiatric symptoms – a situation similar to the one that arises when levodopa is reduced in a patient with Parkinson's disease because of levodopa-induced mental status changes. An appropriate response is to assess and quantify the distress and functional impairment associated with the motor symptoms and the neuropsychiatric symptoms with different choices of stimulation parameters. This will inform a decision, which often involves a dialogue among the neurologist, the medical psychiatrist, and the patient. Finally, when a patient with a DBS devices has a sudden exacerbation of primary symptoms, the device should be interrogated via its remote controller to ensure that it is functioning properly. Abrupt device malfunction (or battery depletion) could be responsible for occurrences of sudden and severe rebound symptomatology.

SUMMARY

ECT is a standard treatment for refractory depression and DBS a standard treatment for certain severe movement disorders. With the development of newer technologies various forms of neurostimulation are finding broader application in neurology and psychiatry, and it is likely that some will emerge as standard treatments, competing with or complementing drug therapies. Each neurostimulation procedure and device is associated with specific adverse events with which the medical psychiatrist should be familiar.

CLINICAL PEARLS

Currently available neurostimulation techniques arebased on a more sophisticated understanding of the biological substrates of psychiatric illness than ECT, the historical option for treatment of psychiatric disorders with neurostimulation. Recent neurostimulation techniques have been designed with more precise targets and, with the exception of DBS, are safer than ECT. The level of evidence currently required to establish the safety and effectiveness of treatments for particular indications is much higher than what was required in the past.

A host of non-pharmacologic somatic therapies for mental disorders are under investigation or in off-label clinical use, including transcranial direct current stimulation (tDCS), light therapy (for seasonal affective disorder and delayed

---

3. http://www.fda.gov/MedicalDevices/DeviceRegulationandGuidance/GuidanceDocuments/ucm107705.htm

sleep phase, focal electrically administered seizure therapy (FEAST), magnetic seizure therapy (MST), focused ultrasound (FUS), near infrared light therapy (NILT), low field magnetic stimulation (LFMS), and optogenetic stimulation.

Because of the lack of other effective treatments and the high mortality rate associated with treatment-resistant catatonia, ECT is generally considered if catatonia is refractory to adequate trials or benzodiazepines (at least 2 mg parenteral lorazepam or equivalent) or if symptom relapse is experienced despite maximal benzodiazepine treatment.

Catatonic symptoms may be more persistent and may require longer courses of ECT treatment than major depression without catatonia.

With ECT, anterograde memory impairment appears to resolve within 3 months posttreatment. Retrograde autobiographical memory impairment for up to 6 months prior to the date of the first treatment does not fully resolve. Techniques to minimize memory impairment with ECT include exclusive use of square wave, direct current, brief pulse waveform stimulus; use of unilateral nondominant electrode placement; frequency of treatment no greater than twice weekly during a course of ECT; and the use of ultra-brief pulse (0.3 msec) stimulus.

In 2005, VNS was approved for the long-term treatment of chronic or recurrent depression in adults who have not had an adequate response to four or more adequate antidepressant trials. However, the pivotal trial upon which the approval was based showed only a 15% response rate in the active group at 12 weeks, not statistically significant when compared to 10% response rate in a control group receiving sham VNS. The rate of improvement was substantially higher after 6 to 12 months of treatment, implying that when VNS is utilized for treatment-refractory depression the patient and psychiatrist should by slow to decide whether treatment was efficacious. Further, VNS appears more suitable for truly chronic rather than relapsing-remitting depression.

For depression, rTMS is localized over the left dorsolateral prefrontal cortex.

Potential adverse events associated with rTMS include seizures, induction of mania, local pain, headache, visual changes, dental pain, facial numbness or twitching, and temporary or permanent hearing loss due to barotrauma from the very loud noise produced by the device. Neurocardiogenic syncope can occur in children and adolescents. The most concerning risk of rTMS is the rare possibility of seizures, which can be minimized by adherence to the safe stimulation criteria.

DBS is currently approved for Parkinson's disease, essential tremor, dystonia, and OCD. Dystonia and OCD are approved by the FDA as a Humanitarian Device Exemption, which allows for a maximum annual number of patients treated of 4,000.

Patients receiving DBS for movement disorders can develop new or worsened neuropsychiatric symptoms shortly after stimulation parameters have been adjusted. In this situation re-adjustment of stimulation parameters usually should precede new or altered pharmacologic treatment. When optimal treatment of motor symptoms entails an increase in neuropsychiatric symptoms, the distress and functional impairment from the movement disorder should be weighed against the distress and functional impairment from the neuropsychiatric symptoms, much as is done when adjusting dosage of levodopa in advanced Parkinson's disease with neuropsychiatric comorbidity.

DISCLOSURE STATEMENT

Dr. Park has no conflicts to disclose. He is a full-time employee of the U.S. Food and Drug Administration.

The mention of commercial products, their sources, or their use in connection with material reported herein is not to be construed as either an actual or implied endorsement of such products by the Department of Health and Human Services.

The material in this chapter was written by Dr. Park in his capacity as an employee of the Federal Government. It is therefore in the public domain and it may be reproduced freely without permission.

REFERENCES

American Psychiatric Association. (2001). *The practice of electroconvulsive therapy: recommendations for treatment, training and privileging—a task force report* (2nd ed.). Washington, DC: American Psychiatric Press.

Bini, L. (1995). Professor Bini's notes on the first electro-shock experiment. *Convulsive Therapy, 11*(4), 260–261.

Bush, G., Fink, M., Petrides, G., Dowling, F., & Francis, A. (1996). Catatonia: II—treatment with lorazepam and electroconvulsive therapy, *Acta Psychiatrica Scandinavia, 93*, 137–143.

Cyberonics (2007). *Brief Summary of Safety Information for the VNS Therapy™ System [Epilepsy and Depression Indications].* Houston, TX: Cyberonics, Inc.

Fahy, B. G. (2010). Intraoperative and perioperative complications with a vagus nerve stimulation device. *Journal of Clinical Anesthesia, 22,* 213–222.

Feldman, R. L., Dunner, D. L., Muller, J. S., & Stone, D. A. (2013). Medicare patient experience with vagus nerve stimulation for treatment-resistant depression. *Journal of Medical Economics, 16*(1), 62–74.

Follett, K. A., Weaver, F. M., Stern, M., Hur, K., Harris, C. L., Luo, P. et al. (2010). Pallidal versus subthalamic deep brain stimulation for Parkinson's disease. *New England Journal of Medicine, 362,* 2077–2091.

Fraser, L. M., O'Carroll, R. E., & Ebmeier, K. P. (2008). The effect of electroconvulsive therapy on autobiographical memory: a systematic review. *Journal of ECT, 24,* 10–17.

George, M. S. (2010). Transcranial magnetic stimulation for the treatment of depression. *Expert Review of Neurotherapeutics, 10*(11), 1761–1772.

George, M. S., Sackeim, H. A., Rush, A. J., Marangell, L. B., Nahas, Z., Husain, M. M., et al. (2000). Vagus nerve stimulation: A new tool for brain research and therapy. *Biological Psychiatry, 47,* 287–295.

George, M. S., Ward, H. E., Ninan, P. T., Pollack, M., Nahas, Z., Anderson, B., et al. (2008). A pilot study of vagus nerve stimulation (VNS) for treatment-resistant anxiety disorders. *Brain Stimulation, 1,* 112–121.

Greenhalgh, J., Knight, C., Hind, D., Beverley, C., & Walters, S. (2005). Clinical and cost-effectiveness of electroconvulsive therapy for depressive illness, schizophrenia, catatonia and mania: systematic reviews and economic modeling studies. *Health Technology Assessment, 9*(9), 1–170.

Goodman, W. K., & Insel, T. (2009). Deep brain stimulation in psychiatry: Concentrating on the road ahead. *Biological Psychiatry, 65,* 263–266.

Hamblin, M. R., & Demidova, T. N. (2006). Mechanisms of low level light therapy Proc. SPIE 6140, doi:10.1117/12.646294; http://dx.doi.org/10.1117/12.646294

Heath, R. G. (1963). Electrical self-stimulation of the brain in man. *American Journal of Psychiatry, 120*, 571–577.

Kellner, C. H., Knapp, R. G., Petrides, G., Rummans, T. A., Husain, M. M., Rasmussen, K., et al. (2006). Continuation electroconvulsive therapy vs pharmacotherapy for relapse prevention in major depression: a multi-site study from the consortium for research in electroconvulsive therapy (CORE). *Archives of General Psychiatry, 63*,1337–1344.

Kuba, R., Brázdil, M., Kalina, M., Procházka, T., Hovorka, J., Nezádal, T., et al. (2009). Vagus nerve stimulation: longitudinal follow-up of patients treated for 5 years. *Seizure, 18*(4), 269–274.

Kuncel, A. M., & Grill, W. M. (2004). Selection of stimulus parameters for deep brain stimulation. *Clinical Neurophysiology, 115*, 2431–41.

Labiner, D. M., & Ahern, G. L. (2007). Vagus nerve stimulation therapy in depression and epilepsy: therapeutic parameter settings. *Acta Neurologica Scandnavica, 115*, 23–33.

Lange, G., Janal, M. N., Maniker, A., FitzGibbons, J., Fobler, M., Cook, D., & Natelson, B. H. (2011). Safety and efficacy of vagus nerve stimulation in Fibromyalgia: A Phase I/II proof of concept trial. *Pain Medicine, 12*(9), 1406–1413.

Liao, S. B., & Dourmashkin, P., & Belcher J. (2004). *Introduction to Electricity and Magnetism.* Boston, Pearson Custom Publishing.

Lisanby, S. H., Schlaepfer, T. E., Fisch, H. U., Sackeim, H. A. (2001). Magnetic seizure therapy of major depression. *Archives of General Psychiatry, 58*(3), 303–305.

Malone, D. A., Dougherty, D. D., Rezai, A. R., Carpenter, L. L., Friehs, G. M., Eskandar, E. N., et al. (2009). Deep brain stimulation of the ventral capsule/ventral striatum for treatment-resistant depression. *Biological Psychiatry, 65*, 267–275.

Marangell, L. B., Martinez, M. Jurdi, R. A., & Zboyan, H. (2007). Neurostimulation therapies in depression: a review of new modalities. *Acta Psychiatrica Scandinavia, 116*, 174–181.

Mayberg, H. S., Lozano, A. M., Voon V., McNeely, H. E., Seminowicz, D., Hamani, C., et al. (2005). Deep brain stimulation for treatment-resistant depression. *Neuron, 45*, 651–660.

McLean, P. D. (1990). *The triune brain in evolution: Role in paleocerebral functions.* New York: Plenum Press.

Milby, A. H., Halpern, C. H., & Baltuch, G. H. (2008). Vagus nerve stimulation for epilepsy and depression. *Neurotherapeutics, 5*, 75–85.

O'Reardon, J. P., Solvason, H. B., Janicak, P. G., Sampson, S., Isenberg, K. E., Nahas, Z., et al. (2007). Efficacy and safety of transcranial magnetic stimulation in the acute treatment of major depression: a multisite randomized controlled trial. *Biological Psychiatry, 62*, 1208–1216.

Park, L., Weiss, A. P., & Welch, C. A. (2004). Electroconvulsvie therapy. In T. A. Stern & J. Herman (Eds.). *Massachusetts General Hospital psychiatry update and board preparation* (2nd edition). New York: McGraw-Hill.

Perlmutter, J. S., & Mink, J. W. (2006). Deep brain stimulation. *Annual Review of Neuroscience, 29*, 229–257.

Pluza, R. M., Perazza, G. D., & Bolub, R. M. (2011). Deep brain stimulation. *Journal of the American Medical Association, 305*(7), 732.

Rezai, A. R., Phillips, M., Baker, K. B., Sharan, A. D., Nyenhuis, J., et al. (2004). Neurostimulation system used for deep brain stimulation (DBS), MR safety issues and implications of failing to follow safety recommendations. *Investigative Radiology, 39*, 300–303.

Rohan, M., Parow, A., Stoll, A. L., Demopulos, C., Friedman, S., Dager, S., et al. (2004). Low-field magnetic stimulation in bipolar depression using an, M.R.I-based stimulator. *American Journal of Psychiatry, 161*, 93–98.

Rosa, M. A., & Lisanby, S. H. (2012). Somatic treatments for mood disorders. *Neuropsychopharmacology Reviews, 27*, 102–116.

Rush, A. J., Marangell, L. B., Sackeim, H. A., George, M. S., Brannan, S. K., Davis, S. M., et al. (2005). Vagus nerve stimulation for treatment-resistant depression: a randomized, controlled acute phase trial. *Biological Psychiatry, 58*, 347–354.

Rush, A. J., Siefert, S. E. (2009). Clinical issues in considering vagus nerve stimulation for treatment-resistant depression. *Experimental Neurology, 219*, 36–43.

Rush, A. J., Trivedi, M. L., Wisniewski, S. R., Nierenberg, A. A., Stewart, J. W., Warden, D., et al. (2006). Acute and longer-term outcomes in depressed outpatients requiring one or several treatment steps: A STAR*D report. *American Journal of Psychiatry, 163*, 1905–1917.

Rossi, S., Hallett, M., Rossini, P. M., Pascual-Leone, A.; Safety of TMS Consensus Group. (2009). Safety, ethical considerations, and application guidelines for the use of transcranial magnetic stimulation in clinical practice and research. *Clinical Neurophysiology, 120*, 2008–2039.

Sackeim, H. A., Haskett, R. F., Mulsant, B. H., Thase, M. E., Mann, J. J., Pettinati, H. M., et al. (2001). Continuation pharmacotherapy in the prevention of relapse following electroconvulsive therapy: a randomized controlled trial. *Journal of the American Medical Association, 285*(10), 1299–1307.

Sakel, M. (1958). *Schizophrenia.* New York: Philosophical Library.

Semkovska, M., & McLoughlin, D. M. (2010). Objective cognitive performance associated with electroconvulsive therapy for depression: A systematic review and meta-analysis. *Biological Psychiatry, 68*, 568–577.

Shorter E. (1997). *A history of psychiatry: From the age of the asylum to the era of Prozac.* New York: John Wiley and Sons.

Sienaert, P., Vansteelandt, K., Demyttenaere, K., & Peuskens J. (2010). Randomized comparison of ultra-brief bifrontal and unilateral electroconvulsive therapy for major depression: cognitive side effects. *Journal of Affective Disorders, 122*, 60–67.

Spellman, T., Peterchev, A. V., & Lisanby, S. H. (2009). Focal electrically administered seizure therapy: a novel form of ECT illustrates the roles of current directionality, polarity and electrode configuration in seizure induction. *Neuropsychopharmacology, 34*, 2002–2010.

Terman, M., Terman, J. S., Quitkin, F. M., McGrath, P. J., Stewart, J. W., Rafferty, B. et al. (1989). Light therapy for seasonal affective disorder: a review of efficacy. *Neuropsychopharmacology, 2*(1), 1–22.

Tyler, W. J., Tufail, Y., Finsterwald, M., Tauchmann, M. L., Olson, E. J., Majestic, C. (2008). Remote excitation of neuronal circuits using low-intensity, low-frequency ultrasound. *PLoS One, 3*(10), e3511.

U.S. Department of Health and Human Services. (1999). *Mental Health: A Report of the Surgeon General.* Rockville, MD: Substance Abuse and Mental Health Services Administration / Center for Mental Health Services; National Institutes of Health / National Institute of Mental Health.

Wassermann, E. M. (1998). Risk and safety of repetitive transcranial magnetic stimulation: report and suggested guidelines from the International Workshop on the Safety of Repetitive Transcranial Magnetic Stimulation, June 5–7, 1996. *Electroencephalography and Clinical Neurophysiology, 108*, 1–16.

Wassermann, E. M., & Zimmermann, T. (2012). Transcranial magnetic brain stimulation: Therapeutic promises and scientific gaps. *Pharmacology and Therapeutics, 133*, 98–107.

Yizhar, O., Fenno, L. E., Davidson, T. J., Mogri, M., & Deisseroth, K. (2011). Optogenetics in neural systems. *Neuron, 71*, 9–34.

Zabara, J. (1992). Inhibition of experimental seizures in canines by repetitive vagal stimulation. *Epilepsia, 33*, 1005–1012.

25.

ACUTE PAIN MANAGEMENT AND PSYCHOPHARMACOLOGY IN THE MEDICALLY ILL

Robert J. Boland, Monique V. Yohanan, and Richard J. Goldberg

The greatest evil is physical pain.   SAINT AUGUSTINE

INTRODUCTION

Pain is the most common reason a patient presents to a doctor. It is a common symptom in many types of trauma and disease. In a US National Health Survey, it was found that within the 3 months before the survey 29% of adult respondents had experienced lower back pain, 17% had had a severe headache, 15% had experienced neck pain, and 5% had experienced facial or jaw pain (Sondik, Madans, & Gentleman, 2011). The cost of pain in treatment, disability, and lost time at work is immeasurable.

Alleviating pain is one of our most fundamental roles. At times, this can be complex and frustrating. Often, however, through understanding some fundamental principles of pain management, even the inexperienced clinician gives some relief to the suffering patient.

Pain serves an important signaling function in the organism and often leads to recognition of an underlying disease that can be remedied. However, pain remains hard to describe and quantify. Of more concern is that it is often inadequately treated.

BARRIERS TO ADEQUATE PAIN MANAGEMENT

Historically, the undertreatment of pain has been an all too frequent reality. Well into the modern medical era, there have remained many barriers to adequate pain management. These barriers include cultural attitudes about pain as an inevitable part of the human condition, fear of analgesic misuse, fear of disciplinary action against those who prescribe such analgesics, and inadequate medical training in pain management. Some patient groups have been found to be at higher risk for inadequate pain control, including members of minority ethnicities, women, children, older patients, people with cognitive impairments, and those with a psychiatric diagnosis (Moskovitz et al., 2011; Groenewald, Rabbitts, Schroeder, & Harrison, 2012).

Although these problems have continued into the present, there has been a gradual shift in attitudes about a patient's right to adequate treatment. Although fear of legal prosecution sometimes is cited by physicians as a rationale for not providing prescriptions for opioid medications, it generally is accepted that appropriate pain management is an obligation of the doctor–patient relationship (Hall & Boswell, 2009). This obligation may be gaining some ground socially, ethically, and even legally as a fundamental human right (Brennan, Carr, & Cousins, 2007).

ASSESSMENT OF PAIN

One of the most common reasons for inadequate pain management is a discrepancy between the patient and physician assessment. Adequate assessment of pain usually follows the same basic principles as assessment of other medical problems. A history is taken in an attempt to classify the type and cause of pain. While this categorization has an important role in pain assessment, for most patients pain is not an isolated problem but an experience that may be affected by and impact medical, psychiatric, social, and spiritual concerns. Optimal pain management begins with an assessment that considers all these domains.

Usually we attempt to differentiate whether pain is acute or chronic. Acute pain is not only brief, it is also usually associated with clear injury or disease. Acute pain has biological purpose; it alerts the patient to injury or disease. It is commonly associated with activation of the sympathetic nervous system manifest as tachycardia, tachypnea, and diaphoresis, and, as such, elicits an empathetic response and tends to be easier for healthcare providers to recognize. Acute pain levels may change dramatically over a short period. An example of acute pain is postsurgical pain, in which the pain is reasonably well correlated to the degree of injury. While chronic pain may begin with an acute insult, it persists beyond a temporal association with the factors that initiated it and long past the point of any biological purpose.

In addition to determining the time course of the pain, it is also is common in assessment to distinguish between nociceptive and neuropathic pain. Nociceptive pain occurs when the nerves appropriately sense and respond to tissue damage. It is worse with stress or pressure and tends to respond to treatment with opioids and antiinflammatory agents. Patients may use words such as sharp, dull, aching, or throbbing when asked to describe this type pain. While radiation may be present, it is less common, and when it is noted it often does not follow a distinct nerve distribution.

Neuropathic pain reflects an abnormal functioning of the central or peripheral nervous system, which may be triggered by a direct nerve injury or systemic illness. Severe pain may occur with trivial stimuli, such as a light touch or a breeze on a patient's skin. Opiates are less helpful in alleviating neuropathic pain, and when they are used they tend to require higher doses to provide adequate analgesia. Patients may describe the pain as electric or burning. Radiation is common and tends to follow a typical nerve distribution.

The experience of pain in a particular patient may not always fit neatly into these categories. Patients may have acute surgical pain but a complicated postoperative course that ultimately leads to a chronic pain syndrome. Despite the limitations of the acute/chronic, nociceptive/neuropathic framework, it may be a useful starting point in developing a management approach.

In addition to categorizing pain in terms of its time course and mechanism, a common next step is to rate pain intensity. Since many patients will have more than one area of pain at any given time, rating pain is usually preceded by a determination of the total number of pain problems (and where they are located), and then describing and rating each. Various instruments are available to assess pain, including visual analog and numeric scales. Despite the limitations of numeric scales, they are commonly used and practical for bedside assessment. They are easily administered, require no special forms, and can be used to track changes over time (Hawker, Mian, Kendzerska, & French, 2011). Typically, the person administering the scale asks the patient to rate his/her pain intensity from 1 to 10, 1 being no pain and 10 being the worst pain imaginable. In addition to asking the patient to provide a number to rate his/her current pain level, it also can be helpful to ask, "What number would you like it to be?" Once this assessment has been performed, a common starting dose for patients who are opiate-naïve would be 5–10 mg of oral morphine equivalent every 4 hours. The lower dose range should be considered for patients who are older and who have renal or hepatic insufficiency, which may affect drug metabolism and effective half-life.

In addition to assessing the experience of pain itself, a thorough evaluation also should include an investigation for the presence of other associated non-pain symptoms that may be present. These include but are not limited to physical symptoms, such as dyspnea and nausea, and also an evaluation for psychiatric comorbidities or complications. Determining the degree to which a patient is suffering is essential. Suffering has been described as "a state of severe distress associated with events that threaten the intactness of the person" (Cassel, 1982). While suffering may be difficult to quantify, it has a significant impact on quality of life. If it is not addressed, it is unlikely that even the most thoughtfully chosen pain regimen will provide adequate palliation.

PAIN FROM A PSYCHIATRIC PERSPECTIVE

The various editions of the American Psychiatric Association's *Diagnostic and Statistical Manual* contain diagnoses related to pain; however, these all apply to chronic pain and continue to wrestle with the problem of whether pain can be subdivided into subtypes that are "primarily psychological" and "primarily medical." In the fifth edition of the manual, the work group responsible for this disorder recommended that these distinctions be dropped and the category of *Pain Disorder* be subsumed into a new, more general somatoform disorder (currently referred to as *Somatic Symptom Disorder*). Many individuals currently diagnosed with Pain Disorder would fit into this category, whereas for others, psychological factors affecting other medical conditions or an adjustment disorder would be more appropriate.

In clinical practice, the majority of pain patients—particularly acute pain patients—will not have a somatoform disorder. However, even short-term pain symptoms can predispose a patient to other psychiatric disorders, particularly depressive and anxiety disorders. In addition, even in the absence of a formal psychiatric disorder it should be remembered that all pain is, in part, a psychological phenomenon (Lavand'homme, 2011). The Institute of Medicine underscored this point in its description of the nature of pain: "The experience of pain is more than a simple sensory process. It is a complex perception that involves higher levels of the central nervous system, emotional status, and higher order mental processes" (Osterweis, 1988).

PHARMACOLOGIC TREATMENT FOR PAIN

While nonpharmacologic approaches may have an important role in acute pain management (and are addressed later in this chapter), most patients treated for acute pain will be medicated. The choice of analgesic therapy is based on the type and severity of pain, individual patient concerns and preferences, and knowledge of the clinical pharmacology of the drug prescribed, including its half-life and common drug–drug interactions. Attention to all these factors increases the likelihood of providing successful analgesia at any stage of treatment.

There are some instances of acute pain when correcting the underlying problem will immediately resolve severe pain symptoms. For example, while a patient with an acute hip dislocation may present with excruciating pain that warrants opiate medication prior to definitive therapy, when reduction is performed it may lead to immediate resolution of pain. This speaks to the idea of pattern matching. Appropriate pharmacological treatment of pain provides medication that addresses both the severity and likely time course of the pain condition.

Medication choice also will depend on patient-specific factors. If the patient has a previous history of using pain medication, the response to specific agents may be useful in guiding current therapy. The presence of renal and/or hepatic impairment will impact the choice of agent. If a patient has more than one symptom—for example, back pain and debilitating cough—a regimen that includes an opioid could reasonably be expected to palliate both symptoms.

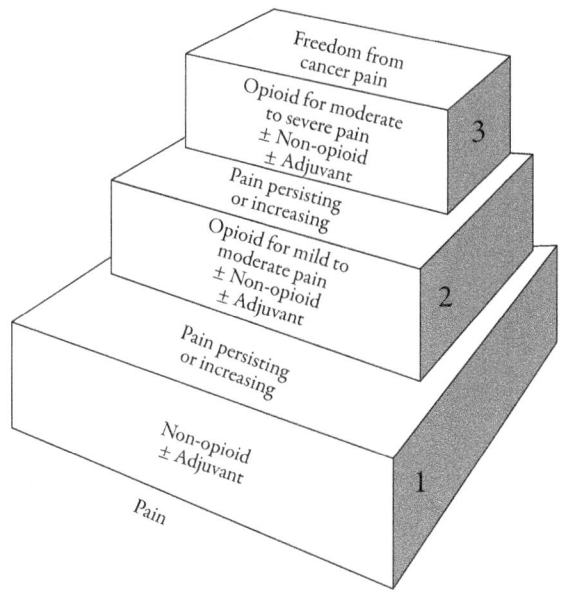

Figure 25.1. WHO Pain Ladder The World Health Organization (WHO) analgesic ladder for the management of cancer pain (reproduced with permission from WHO).

Although regimens should be individualized, general guiding principles are available. The World Health Organization (WHO) ladder (Ventafridda, Saita, Ripamonti, & De Conno, 1985) provides a step-wise approach for the treatment of cancer pain, which also may provide guidance for the management of noncancer pain (Figure 25.1). Step 1 addresses the management of mild to moderate pain and advises the use of non-opioid agents (e.g., nonsteroidal antiinflammatory drugs or paracetamol). Adjuvant agents may be used at any of the steps and include (but are not limited to) antidepressants, anticonvulsants, steroids, muscle relaxants, and behavioral therapy. When pain persists or increases, Step 2 suggests continuing the non-opioid drug and adding a low potency opioid (e.g., codeine). For pain that persists or increases despite this regimen, Step 3 recommends more potent opioids (e.g., morphine) as first-line therapy.

Minimizing polypharmacy is a preferred treatment strategy. This is in part because single agents may be more carefully titrated and have more predictable side effect profiles. In addition, the benefits of adding adjuvant medications, such as antidepressants, should be weighed against the potential for drug–drug interactions. The use of codeine illustrates this concern. The analgesic effect of codeine is dependent on conversion to an active metabolite by the CYP 450 2D6 substrate (Eissing, Lippert, & Willmann, 2012). Approximately 7% of the population lacks the 2D6 enzyme and are not benefited by this medication. The enzyme can also be blocked by many commonly prescribed medications, such as selective serotonin reuptake inhibitors (SSRIs) (Sindrup & Brosen, 1995) like paroxetine and fluoxetine that significantly inhibit the 2D6 enzyme.

EFFECTIVE USE OF OPIOIDS IN ACUTE PAIN

For patients with severe, acute pain, morphine represents the standard opioid against which all others are usually compared.

Unlike some other agents, including the NSAIDs, acetaminophen and the mixed agonist-antagonist analgesics, morphine has no ceiling effect.

Short-acting and long-acting opioid formulations are available, and each class has particular benefits and limitations in the treatment of acute pain. Short-acting opioid formulations with a quick onset of action may be of particular benefit in achieving immediate analgesia, and doses may be easily adjusted to address fluctuating pain levels. Opioids with longer half-lives, such as sustained-release morphine and methadone, may have a role for the patient whose acute pain has been stabilized on short-acting opioids and is likely to remain severe and continuous for several days or longer. The slow-release mechanism may result in fewer peak-and-trough fluctuations and therefore may cause fewer side effects such as nausea and vomiting (Walsh, 1984). Their delayed onset of action and lack of ability to be precisely titrated should be considered if they are used in treating a patient with acute pain.

DOSE AND FREQUENCY

The most common cause of inadequate acute pain management is the underuse of opioid analgesics. In fact, many doctors prescribe less than half the effective analgesic dose for their patients with pain (Marks et al., 2009). In addition to doses that are inadequate, opioids often are prescribed at time intervals that extend beyond the effective half-life of the drug. The use of suboptimal doses and excessive time between dose intervals may result from physician orders, nursing administration, or patient bias. Some patients attempt to endure pain and earn the respect of the nurses and doctors as "good" patients. When patients start to complain of severe pain before their next dose is "due," they often are thought of as "addicted" or excessively preoccupied with medication. In fact, such patients may only be expressing the fact that their pain has reemerged because their dose time has gone beyond the effective duration of the opioid. Table 25.1 lists usual dose ranges for commonly prescribed opioids and their average duration of action.

The consultant dealing with a pain patient who continues to complain despite "usually adequate treatment" should first look at the dose and frequency of analgesic delivered. Ask patients what level of relief they get within the first hour after their dose. If relief during that time is inadequate, the dose is too low. If pain relief is complete but reemerges before the next dose, the duration between doses is too long. It is essential to look directly at the drug administration record, not at orders or progress notes, to confirm what has actually been given to the patient and on what schedule. Opioids should be given on a schedule corresponding to their analgesic half-life (see Table 25.1).

Pain symptom palliation always should take into account the balance between opioid analgesic benefit and the suffering that common opioid side effects may cause. Many symptoms, such as nausea, constipation, respiratory suppression, and delirium, may be avoided or minimized, and strategies are discussed later in this chapter.

Table 25.1 OPIOIDS AND RELATED COMPOUNDS TYPICALLY USED FOR ANALGESIA

DRUG	USUAL PO DOSE (MG)	USUAL PARENTERAL DOSE (MG)	DOSING INTERVAL (HRS)	APPROXIMATE ORAL EQUIVALENT TO 30 MG ORAL MORPHINE (MG)	APPROXIMATE IV EQUIVALENT TO 10 MG IV MORPHINE (MG)	COMMENTS
Morphine and Related Compounds						
Morphine	30	3–6	3–4	–	–	
Sustained release	90–120	–	8–12	60		
Hydromorphone	6	1.5	3–4	3–4	1.3–2	
Oxymorphone	10–20	3–5	4–6	0.5–1	1	
Codeine and related compounds						
Codeine	60	3–5	3–4	180–300	100	Little benefit in doses beyond 60 mg, as higher doses may lead to agitation and dysphoria
Dihydrocodeine	16–32	–	3–4	120–150		Only available in combination with aspirin and caffeine
Hydrocodone	5	–	3–4	60		Only available in combination with acetaminophen, aspirin or ibuprofen
Oxycodone	5–30	–	3–4	12–15	10	Also available in combination with acetaminophen or aspirin.
Extended release	10–60		12			Extended release dose varies depending on tolerance.
Synthetic Opioids and Related Compounds						
Meperidine	Not recommended	100	3–4	250	80	Not recommended. Can be psychotoxic.
Fentanyl transdermal	(transdermal: 25 ug/h)		72	0.2		Immediate release available but primarily used for anesthesia
Methadone	20	4–6	8–12	2–10	2–10	Long half-life.
Levorphanol	4	2	6–8	4–8	2	
Tramadol	50		3–4	300		Is a mu receptor agonist, however is not an opioid.

FIXED VERSUS AS-NEEDED DOSE SCHEDULES

When acute pain has been diagnosed, physicians must consider whether analgesics should be prescribed on an as-needed or fixed-dose schedule. Severe, continuous pain is better treated on a fixed schedule. A routine schedule not only increases the likelihood of effective analgesia, but also will tend to minimize some of the common adverse effects associated with shifting blood levels, including nausea and respiratory depression (Lo Presti, Roscetti, Muriess, & Mammucari, 2010).

A schedule based on the half-life of the opioid prevents reemergence of pain before the next dose, but even well-intentioned efforts to provide as-needed medication based on half-life may provide insufficient analgesia, as drug metabolism and duration of benefit may vary among individual patients. The dose required to treat reemergent pain resulting from an as-needed or PRN (Latin: *pro re nata* literally, "from the thing born"; figuratively, "as the need arises") schedule often is larger than would be required to prevent it using a fixed schedule. Giving patients medications on a PRN basis places them in a dependent position. The requirement that they must ask staff for each dose of pain medication can be humiliating for the patient and can be negatively interpreted by care providers as an excessive preoccupation with receiving medication. In patients who do have a propensity for drug seeking, this type of regimen may reinforce this negative behavior. Patients who have cognitive impairments or fluctuating levels of alertness may have difficulty being able to ask for medication.

Another challenge to the PRN approach is in the management of nighttime pain. Lack of sleep creates a vicious cycle of increased pain, which causes more lack of sleep, and diminished sleep efficiency tends to lower the pain threshold. Strategies to address this problem include administering opioids before bedtime in patients whose sleep is being interrupted by pain or who awaken in the morning with excessive reemergent pain. Alternatively, the use of long-acting medications may be associated with improved sleep, although these formulations should be used with caution in older patients and those with renal insufficiency. Conversely, if a patient is sleeping well and is not awakening with increased perception of pain and its consequent anxiety, there is no need to schedule analgesic doses during the patient's sleep time.

An alternative opioid scheduling method is known as "reverse PRN." This method involves offering the medication to the patient on a scheduled basis, allowing the patient to accept, refuse, or delay the dose. This reverse PRN method ensures that the medication is made available and offered, but also helps the patient maintain some autonomy and control over titrating the dose.

Although standing dose regimens may be more appropriate for persistent, acute pain, there are circumstances in which PRN regimens are preferred. Patients with hepatic or renal impairment may not be optimal candidates for fixed dosing. There also are circumstances where pain is not continuous and can be predicted. If a patient is undergoing debridement of a decubitus ulcer, it is reasonable to provide short-acting premedication in anticipation of this event. When a fixed-dose pain regimen is ordered, it is common practice to write an accompanying order for PRN medication to provide breakthrough pain coverage. Generally, the appropriate PRN dose should be related to the total daily morphine equivalent of the standing dose medication. Frequent reassessments of the amount of PRN medication being accessed may be useful in guiding dose adjustments and optimizing pain management.

CHOICE OF ROUTE OF ADMINISTRATION

There are multiple routes available for opiate administration that may be appropriate in providing acute pain management. These vary in terms of onset, intensity, and duration of analgesic effect; ease of dispensing; availability; and cost. Conversion between forms is discussed later in this chapter.

ORAL

Oral analgesic administration offers simplicity and economy, avoids the discomforts and potential complications of repeated injections, makes the patient less dependent on others for care, and may obviate the need for hospitalization in some cases. Dosage forms include tablets, capsules, and liquids. Pure opiate and combination (opioid/NSAID or paracetamol) forms are available. Oral medications are available in short-acting, immediate-release, and long-acting release formulations. As discussed earlier in this chapter, short-acting opioid formulations with a quick onset of action are more likely to give immediate analgesia and are more easily adjusted than longer acting medications. Opioids with longer-half lives and extended release medications may have a role in acute pain after stabilization has been achieved with short-acting medications, if the pain is likely to remain severe and continuous for several days or longer.

Oral analgesics often are used in patients with dysphagia and/or feeding tubes. In these circumstances, the medications are crushed and mixed with food or liquid to allow for easier swallowing or feeding tube administration. Many long-acting pain formulations (e.g., morphine sulfate controlled release, oxycodone controlled release), should not be crushed, as this results in a bolus dose of the medication. Morphine sulfate extended release capsules, as well as liquid formulations of morphine and methadone, are available and may be used in these circumstances.

SUBLINGUAL

Sublingual administration may be a useful route when swallowing is impaired. Sublingual opioids are directly absorbed into the systemic circulation. The high opioid concentration of commonly available formulations (e.g., morphine sulfate concentrate), allows for immediate analgesia in patients with limited or absent ability to swallow even small amounts of liquid medication.

RECTAL

Substances absorbed by the rectal route provide another option when a patient cannot tolerate oral medication. Suppository forms of many opioids are commercially available. Alternately, many oral tablet formulations can be administered rectally when coated with glycerin gel.

INTRAVENOUS

Intravenous (IV) opioid administration remains the most rapid and effective means of delivering opioids to the systemic circulation (Miner, Moore, Gray, Skinner, & Biros, 2008). Most commonly, an IV dose is given at regular intervals. Proper use of this method requires understanding the pharmacokinetics of a drug to ensure that the blood level does not go below the minimum effective concentration. This can be particularly difficult when the drug is given on an "as needed" basis.

Continuous IV administration can be a very efficient way to provide pain relief for patients whose pain management requirements are anticipated to last for several days or weeks. To provide continuously effective pain relief, the blood level of the drug must always be kept above the minimally effective concentration. Since this can be particularly difficult at the beginning of continuous therapy, as a drug requires four to five half-lives to achieve steady-state concentration, a loading dose is recommended before starting continuous infusion.

PATIENT-CONTROLLED ANALGESIA

Patient-controlled analgesia (PCA) may be administered through the IV or subcutaneous routes. It has gained widespread use in several areas of acute pain management. Computerized programmable pumps allow bolus doses of opioid to be administered by the patient. This may be coupled with a background basal infusion of opioid. Bolus dose limits, "lock-out" intervals, and a maximum total hourly dose all are programmable by medical staff (Karci et al., 2003). Patients who are confused are not good candidates for this method of drug administration. In addition, patients with a drug addiction history may be unable to self-limit their utilization. Despite these limitations, for many patients PCA is a reasonable option that provides immediate pain relief while optimizing autonomy.

SUBCUTANEOUS

We know surprisingly little about the pharmacokinetics of subcutaneous (SC) opioids. For morphine, the blood levels achieved with SC administration are probably comparable to IV administration. Due to local irritant effects, the dose of opiate that may be administered via the SC route tends to be smaller than what is possible through the IV and intramuscular routes. Other limitations to subcutaneous administration include more difficult administration and erratic absorption in patients with severe cachexia.

INTRAMUSCULAR

Intramuscular (IM) administration of opioids, although a popular route, has significant limitations. Opioids given through this route are less predictably absorbed. IM injections are painful, and patients can alternate between toxicity and undertreatment. This method of administration should generally be reserved for unusual cases in which no other method of administration is feasible.

SPINAL ADMINISTRATION

Opioid analgesics may also be given through the spinal route, for example, epidurally (Marret, Remy, Bonnet, & Postoperative Pain Forum Group, 2007). Preoperative and perioperative use of epidural analgesia can significantly reduce the need for postoperative analgesia. Its use should be reserved for patients who have failed good trials of opioid medication by other routes.

TRANSDERMAL

The first transdermal opioid was the fentanyl citrate patch. The route of administration is often preferred by patients, and some side effects (such as nausea and constipation) may be less commonly seen than with oral opioids (Tassinari et al., 2009). Limitations include expense and erratic absorption in patients with severe cachexia.

SPECIFIC OPIOID MEDICATIONS

COMBINATION AGENTS

There are multiple available agents that combine a non-opioid drug (typically acetaminophen or NSAIDs) with an opioid agent (e.g., codeine, hydrocodone, or oxycodone; see Gaskell, Derry, Moore, & McQuay, 2009). These combination agents have many attractive features. They are inexpensive, readily obtainable, and maximize patient autonomy. There are, however, some limitations to their use. Acetaminophen combinations are limited by the drug's toxic effects. NSAID-containing combinations also carry with them the potential for gastrointestinal irritation and hemorrhage. The side effects of NSAIDs and acetaminophen are discussed in further detail later in this chapter.

CODEINE

Codeine is a pro-drug converted to its active metabolite, morphine, by the CYP450 2D6. It is an opioid agonist that produces analgesia, sedation, and antitussive effects. It is usually dispensed in an oral form (tablet or liquid) and is often compounded with other agents (e.g., acetaminophen, guaifenesin) depending on the desired effect. Its half-life generally ranges from 2–4 hours, and dosing may need to be adjusted in the presence of renal impairment. As noted above, approximately 7% of the general population lacks the enzyme necessary to convert this medication to its active metabolite (Sindrup & Brosen, 1995), and medications that inhibit the P450 2D6 enzyme can inhibit this conversion. In this circumstance the constipating effects of the medication still are present, but the patient may receive little to no analgesic benefit.

PROPOXYPHENE

Propoxyphene exerted its analgesic effect by binding various opioid receptors. It is metabolized in the liver by the CYP 450 3A4 enzyme, and also acts as an inhibitor of the 3A4 and 2D6. It was available in a tablet form both alone and in a combination form (with napsylate/acetaminophen). While the half-life of propoxyphene is 6–12 hours, the half-life of its active metabolite, norpropoxyphene, is 30–36 hours (Inturrisi et al., 1982). Black box warnings have called attention to numerous reports of overdose when this drug is taken alone or in combination with alcohol or other central nervous system depressants and also have cautioned against concomitant use with other CYP3A4 inhibitors (e.g., protease inhibitors, macrolide antibiotics, azole antifungals), as this may increase propoxyphene levels. There are numerous drug–drug interactions and associated side effects, including potential cardiac toxicity (Barkin, Barkin, & Barkin, 2006). As a result of concerns about increasing the risk of arrhythmias, the US Food and Drug Administration (FDA) announced a safety review in July of 2009, and in November of 2010 recommended against further use of the pain reliever (FDA, 2010), and it has been withdrawn from the US market. The European Medicines Agency decided on a phased withdrawal of propoxyphene from the European market in June of 2009.

MORPHINE

Morphine is metabolized by the liver and gastrointestinal tract by the CYP 450 enzyme. It is available in multiple forms include short-acting and long-acting tablets, liquid, a concentrated solution that may be administered sublingually, suppositories, and formulations that may be administered by the SC, IM, or IV routes. It undergoes significant first-pass metabolism (Wiffen & McQuay, 2007). Monitoring may include a baseline creatinine as well as assessment of respiratory function, particularly with epidural or intrathecal use. Black box warnings also stress concerns regarding abuse potential.

OXYCODONE

Oxycodone undergoes extensive liver metabolism by CYP450 3A4, although there is some 2D6 metabolism as well; an active metabolite is formed. It is available in short-acting and long-acting tablet forms, and a concentrated liquid that may be administered sublingually (Gaskell et al., 2009). Oxycodone seems to have a side-effect, safety, and efficacy profile similar to morphine. It may be a reasonable therapeutic option for patients unable to tolerate other opiates or who have special considerations such as renal insufficiency (Rischitelli & Karbowicz, 2002).

HYDROMORPHONE

Hydromorphone is metabolized by the liver (CYP450) and the upper gastrointestinal tract (1A3, 2B7), and some providers prefer it to morphine in patients with renal insufficiency. It is available in oral tablet, liquid, and suppository forms. It also may be administered via the SC, IM, and IV routes (Quigley, 2002). It is a reasonable choice for patients who need a more potent opioid option than morphine, but this same property also is responsible for its primary limitations. Its black box warning emphasizes its high potential for abuse and respiratory depression.

MEPERIDINE

Meperidine is a phenylpiperidine analgesic with CNS effects similar to those of morphine. Hypertension, excitation, delirium, hyperpyrexia, convulsions, respiratory depression, and death have been reported with meperidine monotherapy in relation to the accumulation of the metabolite normeperidine with a longer half-life and renal excretion, particularly in settings of longer use and renal insufficiency.

Meperidine is particularly contraindicated for concomitant administration with monoamine oxidase inhibitors (MAOIs), which may exacerbate this general cerebrotoxic effect. Although the mechanism of this interaction is not clear, it appears to be a central serotonin effect analogous to a "serotonin syndrome" (Latta, Ginsberg, & Barkin, 2002).

METHADONE

Methadone is metabolized by the liver, primarily via CYP 450 2B6, but also with minor effects by the 2C10, 2D6, and 34A enzymes. Chronic administration may lead to the drug inducing its own metabolism. It is available in multiple forms, including tablet and liquid, and may also be administered via the SC, IM, and IV routes. It is excreted in both the feces and urine and has a wildly variable half-life ranging from 8–60 hours. It tends to accumulate in the liver and other tissues and is slowly released from these sites. Its black box warning suggests that its use should be limited to practitioners who well understand its pharmacokinetics, and then only in patients for whom the potential analgesic benefits outweigh its significant risks. Its risk of inducing respiratory depression may last longer than its peak analgesic effects (Fainsinger, Schoeller, & Bruera, 1993).

FENTANYL

Fentanyl is available in transdermal and transmucosal (film, lozenge, tablet) formulations and also may be administered via the IM and IV routes. It is metabolized by the liver via the CYP450 3A4 substrate. Its half-life varies depending on formulation; the IM half-life is up to 4 hours, lozenge up to 7 hours, and transdermal up to 17 hours (the transdermal half-life may be prolonged due to continued absorption from drug deposition in the skin). Its most common use is for chronic moderate to severe pain. Transmucosal forms may only be prescribed by oncologists and pain specialists (Fine, Narayana, & Passik, 2010).

Conversions Among Opioids

There are several situations where improper opioid conversion leads to psychiatric consultation. These include (1) increasing or decreasing analgesic requirements (e.g., the need to switch from morphine to hydromorphone due to pain severity or renal insufficiency); (2) the need to change the type of medication provided based on the venue of care (e.g., converting IV medications used in the inpatient setting to oral formulations on discharge); or (3) the need for a different medication based on a change in the patient's medical condition (e.g., new inability to swallow).

When calculating conversions between opioid formulations, or to sort out the total opioid dose in situations where many analgesics have been used, it is helpful to convert all analgesics to a standard reference. This conversion among opioids is facilitated by converting all drugs to oral morphine equivalents (see Table 25.1). From a methodological viewpoint, the information for this table comes primarily from pain relief studies in cancer patients, whose acute pain needs and analgesia metabolism may be different from those of noncancer patients. In addition, the time-effect curves for studying various doses of analgesia generally result from single-dose experiments. Single-dose studies neglect the kinetic changes that take place following repeated dosing, especially with opioids such as methadone that have long half-lives. Finally, the conversion information presented in Table 25.1 does not acknowledge the probable differences in pain relief associated with age, sex, race, or quality of pain (Kaiko, Wallenstein, Rogers, & Houde, 1982).

A commonly used strategy is to calculate the 24-hour equivalent of the old drug (including both the amount of fixed-dose and PRN opiate being dispensed) and then use this calculation to determine the 24-hour equivalent of new drug (or new route of administration). Then the dosing interval of the new drug (based on its half-life) is divided into this 24-hour period to determine the appropriate dose. It is important to keep in mind cross-tolerance when converting a patient from one opioid regimen to another. For some patients, tolerance to one formulation may result in a decreased response to a new, structurally similar formulation. However, for other patients cross-tolerance is incomplete or paradoxical, and it is possible that a 1:1 conversion based on the daily morphine equivalent will deliver too high an effective dose. Predicting what an individual patient's response will be is, at best, an imprecise endeavor. One way to address this concern is to begin with a standing dose that is less than the calculated 24-hour morphine equivalent, and also provide PRN coverage. The dosage of the new opioid may then be titrated up or down based on the patient's response to the standing dose, as well as on PRN usage.

DEVELOPMENT OF TOLERANCE

In addition to complicating opioid conversion, the development of tolerance has other implications in acute pain management. Tolerance must be differentiated from loss of pain control due to new or advancing disease, inadequate dose, or inadequate duration. The tolerant patient is the one who notices a shortened duration of analgesic effect and an eventual decrease in pain relief. The rate of development of tolerance varies, but any patient who is exposed to continuous doses of opioids may develop tolerance; this may occur in as few as 5–7 days. It is often necessary to increase the dose in order to obtain the same pain relief, and even substantial tolerance can usually be surmounted and adequate analgesia restored by giving a higher dose. Unfortunately, staff may become anxious about continuing opioids for a long period and attempt to decrease the dose just at the time when the patient has developed tolerance and an increase in analgesic medication is called for. The consultant must explain this phenomenon and should anticipate some resistance to the recommendation to increase opioids for a "problem" patient just at the time when the staff expected a solution that included tapering opioids.

Tolerance also may be considered in relation to adverse dose-limiting effects of opioids, including respiratory and CNS depressant effects. While side effects will be discussed at greater length later in this chapter, in general they most commonly have a temporal relationship to shifts in serum opiate levels and tend to resolve once a steady state level is reached. Tolerance to the constipating effects of opioids is a notable exception to this general rule; constipation may persist even when opiate levels are at steady state.

FEAR OF THE ADDICTED PATIENT

A major concern among physicians and other healthcare workers is the fear of creating an addicted patient. There have been only a few studies examining this question, and most of the existing studies examine the use of long-term opioids for chronic pain. The studies are difficult to compare given their different definitions and methodologies, and the reported risks vary widely, ranging from 0% to 7.7% in cancer patients and 0% to as high as 50% in patients with chronic nonmalignant pain; the most rigorous of the studies for nonmalignant pain reported rates around 25% (Hojsted & Sjogren, 2007). In most of these studies, patients with an addiction history were not excluded, and the lengths of treatment were much longer than that seen with acute pain treatment. Taken as a whole, it would appear that iatrogenic addiction is unlikely but not impossible, and patients who are to receive more than a few days of opioid treatment should be evaluated for possible addictive behaviors. Such an evaluation should include an assessment of the patient's initial reaction to opioids; it has been suggested that patients who became addicted to opioid treatment experienced more euphoria when first taking the drug (Bieber et al., 2008).

TREATMENT OF ACUTE PAIN IN OPIOID ADDICTS

In situations involving acute pain treatment in the opioid addict, it is often helpful to keep the management of the addiction separate from the management of the pain. For example, the patient's underlying opioid addiction can be managed with methadone. Most street addicts can be adequately managed on an oral dose of methadone between 20 and 40 mg/day. With methadone used for maintenance of the underlying addiction, the pain can then be treated as a separate issue, using a different opioid at doses 50% greater than normal.

OPIOID WITHDRAWAL

If opioids are taken on a regular basis, physical dependence develops. It generally occurs in patients taking oral opioids for more than 3 to 4 weeks and, along with tolerance, is a characteristic feature of the opioids. Physical dependence on opioids is best defined as a condition that is associated with withdrawal symptoms after an abrupt discontinuation or significant decrease in dosage. The emergence of withdrawal symptoms occurs more rapidly and more intensely with the use of drugs with shorter half-lives. Withdrawal symptoms are best described as a noradrenergic and cholinergic hyperactivity state and include abdominal pain, diarrhea, muscle aching, yawning, rhinorrhea, and lacrimation. Opioid withdrawal (or abstinence) symptoms may create an acute management problem and occur on a predictable and observable basis. Significant objective symptoms—but not subjective anxiety or drug craving alone—warrant attention with increased opioid coverage.

There are several options available for discontinuing opioids in patients who have become physically dependent on them. One possibility is slow weaning from the specific opioid to minimize the development of withdrawal symptoms. Bedtime doses should be decreased last in order to minimize sleep disruption. For morphine, a 10% to 25% decrease each day is reasonable. The main drawbacks are the need to tolerate some withdrawal symptoms and the extension of drug use over time, especially when the process is initiated on the day the patient is otherwise medically ready to leave the hospital. Clonidine may allow for the rapid withdrawal of opiates.

OPIOID SIDE EFFECTS

PREVENTION AND TREATMENT OF OPIOID-INDUCED RESPIRATORY DEPRESSION

Like many of the side effects of opioids, respiratory depression tends to be associated with fluctuating opiate levels and tends to resolve once levels stabilize. There are important caveats to consider. The risk of respiratory depression may be greater with the concomitant administration of some medications, such as benzodiazepines. In addition, there may be patient specific factors, such as a history of emphysema, which may limit respiratory reserve. In patients who are older or who have renal or hepatic impairment, the functional half-life may be prolonged. A related concern is the phenomenon of dose stacking. This is most common when a long-acting medication, particularly one with a widely variable half-life, is dosed at an interval shorter than the drug's half-life. This can lead to

an accumulation of opioid and may precipitate acute respiratory depression. Finally, the respiratory depressant effects of opiates may persist beyond their analgesic effects, even in the absence of dose stacking (Dahan et al., 2004).

PREVENTION AND TREATMENT OF OPIOID-INDUCED GASTROINTESTINAL SIDE EFFECTS

Nausea and vomiting are among the most common side effects associated with opiate administration. There are a variety of mechanisms that may be at play, including anticipatory nausea prior to medical treatments (especially in cancer patients), medication-related histamine release (e.g., morphine), and shifts in dopamine levels prior to reaching a stable opiate dose. Premedication and/or treatment of frank nausea and vomiting should include careful assessment as to the most likely contributing factors and the choice of an agent whose pharmacology is appropriate to the situation at hand. In contrast to other opioid side effects, constipation tends to persist even when stable opiate doses are achieved. Constipation can be uncomfortable and disturbing to patients and can lead to severe cramping pain or even functional ileus or obstruction (Brock et al., 2012).

PSYCHOTOXICITY

Psychiatric consultation may be requested when the patient develops some behavioral disturbance and the question is raised whether it represents a reaction to opioids. All opioids have some psychotoxic potential, with more specific problems associated with meperidine, pentazocine, and nalbuphine. Opioids produce analgesia, drowsiness, changes in mood, and mental clouding, although analgesia should occur without loss of consciousness. For a given degree of analgesia, the mental clouding produced by therapeutic doses of morphine is considerably less pronounced and of a different character than that produced by alcohol or barbiturates. Morphine and its related analgesics rarely produce the garrulous, jocular, and emotionally labile behavior seen with alcohol or barbiturate intoxication. As the dose is increased, the subjective effects, including pain relief, become more pronounced. Moreover, in some individuals the euphoric effects become greater (Lawlor, 2002). For many patients these side effects are most pronounced during dose adjustments, which often abate or resolve once steady state levels are achieved.

OPIOID ALLERGIES

Idiosyncratic reactions to morphine and related opioids, such as nausea, vomiting, and dizziness, often are described by patients as an "allergy" to opioids. Actually, true allergic phenomena to opioids are uncommon and usually are manifested by urticaria, skin rashes, and dermatitis. More severe anaphylactoid reactions are rare. When severe pain requires opioids in an opioid-allergic patient, there are several options available. Obviously, a non-opioid analgesic should be considered, recognizing the hematologic and gastric risks associated with high-dose aspirin and nonsteroidal agents. No research data are available describing the degree of cross-reactivity of allergic responses within the family of opioid opioids. If one needs to use an opioid analgesic, an allergic reaction to one opioid does not necessarily imply an allergy to a chemically related congener. As there are other families of opioid analgesics, an alternative would be to use an opioid from a different family.

Non-Opioid Analgesics and Augmenting Agents

Non-opioid analgesics as potentiators of opioid analgesics, both alone and in combination, have been used for more than two decades. Despite this common practice there have been relatively few controlled studies of their effectiveness. They may have a particular role in situations where it is important for the patient to have a lower opioid dose (or to avoid opioids altogether) because of respiratory suppression, nausea, constipation, sedation, or other side effects.

NSAIDS

Nonsteroidal antiinflammatory drugs (NSAIDs), of which aspirin in the salicylate family is best known (see Table 25.2), control pain via the inhibition of prostaglandin synthetase function and thus prevent the formation of prostaglandin E_2. Most painful conditions are associated with some inflammation, which will at least in part be remediated by NSAIDs. These drugs have a role in treating a variety of painful conditions including arthritic pain, postoperative pain, dysmenorrhea, headaches, and metastatic bone pain. Ketorolac tromethamine is available in IM and oral forms and may be a useful alternative to opioids in postoperative patients for whom opioids are contraindicated. NSAIDs are not associated with the development of dependence, although discontinuation syndromes such as rebound headache may occur (Rapoport et al., 1996).

Table 25.2 ANALGESIC DURATION (WITH ORAL DOSING)

ANALGESIC	DURATION OF ACTION (hr)
Morphine	2.5–7
Meperidine	2–4
Methadone	4–7 (longer with chronic use)
Hydromorphone	4–6
Pentazocine	3–4
Codeine	4–7
Propoxyphene	4–7
Oxycodone	3–5
Tramadol	4–6

NSAIDs include the following drug families with the following representative members: salicylates (aspirin), pyrroles (indomethacin and sulindac), propionic acids (ibuprofen and naproxen), and oxicams (piroxicam). The pyrroles, propionic acids, and oxicams differ from aspirin primarily with respect to their higher analgesic potential and better patient tolerance (see Table 25.2) The non-aspirin salicylates differ primarily in their pharmacokinetics and duration of analgesic action, with their side effects and toxicities being essentially the same. Adverse effects that need to be taken into account and that may influence dosing include diminished platelet function, renal and hepatic insufficiency, and fluid retention (Dieppe, Bartlett, Davey, Doyal, & Ebrahim, 2004). Although CNS side effects including nervousness, anxiety, insomnia, and drowsiness are possible, these are less commonly reported. The gastrointestinal side effects, especially hemorrhage, are of particular concern. Although it is common practice to prescribe proton pump inhibitors in an attempt to limit this risk, the protective effect may be limited in some patients (Stillman & Stillman, 2007).

The risk of gastrointestinal hemorrhage with NSAIDs was one of the factors that drove the development of cyclooxygenase-2 (COX-2) inhibitors. COX2 inhibitors decrease inflammation and pain by selectively inhibition of the cyclooxygenase-2 and reduction of prostaglandin synthesis, and as such it was thought that they would have a decreased risk of peptic ulceration and gastrointestinal hemorrhage as compared with traditional NSAIDs. Although earlier reports did suggest that the drugs had improved side effect profiles, later data suggested that with chronic use the gastrointestinal benefits are not as apparent. In addition, the rates of other NSAID-related side effects, such as renal failure, were no better than with other NSAIDs. Of most concern, however, was the realization that COX-2 inhibitors lack some of the platelet-inhibiting properties of nonspecific NSAIDs and may have an increased risk for heart attack, thrombosis, and stroke (Bunimov & Laneuville, 2008). In 2004, rofecoxib (Vioxx) was voluntarily withdrawn from the market due to an increased risk of cardiovascular and cerebrovascular events. Valdecoxib (Bextra) was withdrawn from the market in 2005. Evidence to date has not suggested the same vascular risks with celecoxib; however, it includes a black box warning regarding the potential of these risks along with its gastrointestinal risks.

ACETAMINOPHEN

Para-aminophenol (acetaminophen) is the most widely used pharmaceutical analgesic and antipyretic agent in the United States and the world. It has similar analgesic potency to the NSAIDs. It is metabolized by the liver via CYP450 1A2 and 2E1 substrates, but its analgesic mechanism of action is not entirely understood. It is commonly used alone for mild pain relief, and in combination with various opiates for moderate pain. It is limited by its toxic effect on the liver, and a maximum dose of 4 grams/day is generally accepted. Its use is cautioned in patients with chronic alcohol use and/or hepatic impairment.

STEROIDS

Steroids are important analgesic adjuncts for acute pain syndromes associated with metastatic bone disease, epidural cord compression, headache due to increased intracranial pressure, and tumor infiltration of brachial and lumbar plexuses or other peripheral nerves. Steroids are thought to provide analgesia via their peripheral antiinflammatory effects and their central effects on neurotransmitters, and may be of particular benefit preceding and during radiation therapy for conditions ranging from epidural cord compression to nerve infiltration. They may also have the additional benefits of producing increased appetite, weight gain, and improved mood. Intra-articular steroid injections are a common treatment for managing degenerative joint disease.

Care must be taken when steroids are administered with NSAIDs because of the increased risk of gastrointestinal side effects (ulcers and gastrointestinal bleeding).

STIMULANTS

Stimulants represent another class of analgesic adjuvant most useful in patients with coexisting sedation, loss of alertness, or depressive symptoms. Dextroamphetamine has been shown to augment morphine analgesia while offsetting its sedative effects, without significantly changing vital signs. Amphetamine coprescribing is not common practice for several reasons—some of which, including suppression of sleep and appetite, may be exaggerated. Keeping these concerns in mind, many prescribers use lower doses of stimulants when treating patients who are older or medically frail, particularly those with coexisting heart disease.

In addition to the amphetamines, caffeine also may have analgesic benefit. Caffeine may act as a sympathomimetic and can potentiate the action of opiates and NSAIDs. It is not clear whether this effect is long-term or short-term (Palmer, Graham, Williams, & Day, 2010).

ANTIDEPRESSANTS

The analgesic effects of tricyclic antidepressants (TCAs) is well known and may represent the most common use of these drugs in the United States. While amitriptyline is the most commonly used antidepressant for pain treatment, other TCAs such as nortriptyline (a metabolite of amitriptyline) and doxepin may have fewer anticholinergic side effects. The analgesic effects of antidepressants possibly are mediated centrally by enhancing the transmission in monoamine pathways, which exert a regulatory effect in the brain. Norepinephrine release and beta receptor affinity varies between TCAs, which may account for some of the differences in analgesic effect among agents in this class (Saarto & Wiffen, 2007).

Although the serotonin transmitter is intimately involved in pain modulation, SSRIs have generally been reported to be less effective as analgesics than the TCAs. There have been some promising studies; however, they are limited and focus on the treatment of chronic neuropathies. It appears that combined effects on norepinephrine, as well as serotonin, are important for an analgesic effect; hence the increased efficacy of TCAs over SSRIs. With that in mind, investigators have looked at newer dual-acting agents such as the serotonin-norepinephrine reuptake inhibitors (SNRIs), which, theoretically, should have the benefits of the TCAs without the side effect profile. Venlafaxine appears to have an effect on pain similar to that of TCAs; however, there are only limited data to support this (Amr & Yousef, 2010). The SNRI duloxetine has been successfully used for a number of pain disorders, including diabetic peripheral neuropathic pain and fibromyalgia pain (Perahia, Pritchett, Desaiah, & Raskin, 2006), and is currently approved by the FDA for both conditions. Its effectiveness in more acute forms of pain is not well known.

It should be remembered, however, that anxiety and depression can significantly affect the emotional expression of pain, and both can cause an amplification of existing pain symptoms. In such cases, antidepressant treatment of any class can be dramatically helpful to the patient.

ANTICONVULSANTS

Anticonvulsants are also frequently used for pain; however again, most of the data is for the treatment of painful neuropathies. They may act by suppressing neuronal firing in damaged neurons. The FDA has approved many of these agents for pain management, including carbamazepine for trigeminal neuralgia and gabapentin for postherpetic neuralgia. There is good evidence to support the use of carbamazepine, gabapentin, and pregabalin for pain treatment (although primarily for chronic diabetic neuropathy) and there is preliminary evidence for lamotrigine (Vinik, 2005).

When used for pain, anticonvulsants are generally started slowly and gradually increased in dose to minimize side effects. Common side effects include dizziness, ataxia, drowsiness, blurred vision, and gastrointestinal irritation. Specific organ toxicities can present a problem: carbamazepine can cause bone marrow suppression, sodium valproate can cause liver toxicity, and both drugs require blood monitoring. Valproic acid and topiramate have not shown consistent efficacy for pain treatment, and phenytoin may cause a peripheral neuropathy (Wiffen et al., 2005).

LOCALLY ACTING AGENTS

Locally acting agents, such as lidocaine and 2-chlorprocaine, are used for peripheral neuropathies. These agents are generally used topically (Lin et al., 2008); other routes of administration, including intranasal, have been described. Capsaicin, another locally acting agent, can be applied topically as a cream to painful areas. It is an alkaloid irritant derived from chili peppers, which appears to work by depleting substance P. It has been shown to be useful for a number of syndromes including diabetic neuropathy, osteoarthritis, postherpetic neuralgia, and psoriasis (Zhang & Po, 1994).

NEUROLEPTICS

Although there are occasional analgesic reports of antipsychotics being used as co-analgesics, the primary use of phenothiazines in terminal cancer patients remains antiemetic or anxiolytic in conjunction with morphine (Seidel et al., 2008).

BENZODIAZEPINES

Benzodiazepines do not appear to have a significant role in the treatment of acute pain. They may modify the affective experience of pain and ameliorate some of the affective elements of nonpain symptoms such as nausea. Adjunctive use benzodiazepines with opiates may increase respiratory depressant effects. They may have some utility as muscle relaxants, which can be beneficial in addressing some types of acute musculoskeletal pain such as neck pain (Malanga et al., 2009).

TRAMADOL

Tramadol hydrochloride is a centrally acting analgesic. Tramadol is indicated for moderate to moderately severe pain, in a manner analogous to low-potency opioids. Although marketed as a "non-opioid analgesic" it acts as a weak mu-receptor agonist. It is also a weak norepinephrine and serotonin reuptake inhibitor and may act through this mechanism as well. The most common side effect associated with tramadol is nausea, and while it is generally considered to have fewer respiratory and gastrointestinal effects than traditional opioids, there are multiple adverse effects including lethargy, agitation, respiratory depression, and coma, which are possible with overdose. Patients with a history of seizures and those taking antidepressants, antipsychotics, or MAOIs appear to be at relatively higher risk for seizures with tramadol. Tramadol levels are raised by drugs that inhibit the cytochrome P-450 2D6 isoenzyme, such as paroxetine. Although initially described as "less abusable" than opioids, physical dependence and withdrawal syndromes have been described (Duhmke, Cornblath, & Hollingshead, 2004).

MIXED OPIOID AGONIST-ANTAGONIST DRUGS

The mixed opioid agonist-antagonist drugs have moderate to strong analgesic activity. The group consists of a number of drugs, including pentazocine, buprenorphine, and nalbuphine. All of the members of this group cause respiratory depression and can lead to physical dependence with prolonged use, and to an opioid withdrawal syndrome (Heel, Brogden, Speight, & Avery, 1978); therefore, these drugs should be tapered gradually after chronic use. Overall, the mixed agonist-antagonist group is likely to be used as an analgesic adjunct to anesthesia for relatively short-term pain problems.

CANNABINOIDS

Cannabinoids appear to have some analgesic effect. This effect is probably mediated by non-opioid receptors, which may argue for an adjunctive role in pain management. Some investigators have suggested that the cannabinergic neurotransmitter system serves to modulate pain sensitivity. Whether other cannabinoids such as dronabinol (an oral synthetic cannabinoid) offer similar benefits with fewer ill effects is a matter worthy of investigation. Dronabinol has the obvious advantage of being legally available throughout the United States; it is used for nausea and as an appetite stimulant. There is limited available evidence in the medical literature regarding whether it is effective as an analgesic (Kraft et al., 2008).

ALTERNATIVE AND COMPLEMENTARY TREATMENTS

A number of alternative treatments, such as Therapeutic Touch, Reiki Healing, herbal remedies, dietary changes, or nutritional supplements have all been used for the treatment of pain, and, anecdotally, many individuals have attested to the relief provided by one or another approaches. However, the few studies that have rigorously investigated these treatments have largely been either negative or too flawed to be convincing.

An exception to this may be acupuncture. Most studies investigating acupuncture also suffer from methodological difficulties; however, there is some convincing evidence for the efficacy of acupuncture in the treatment of dental pain, and preliminary data for lower back pain, headache, and fibromyalgia (Sierpina & Frenkel, 2005).

USE OF PLACEBOS

Placebo (Latin: "I shall please") is a term that evokes emotion in both healthcare givers and recipients. A placebo is an inert substance, given in any form, and without inherent pharmacologic property, which may have a desired effect on a given disorder by virtue of the environment in which it is taken, the psychological state of the recipient, and the specific neurophysiological processes of the recipient. Unfortunately, there remains significant misunderstanding within the medical community regarding placebos and their purpose (Goldberg, Leigh, & Quinlan, 1979). Up to 30%–40% of patients are placebo responders, which may explain why occasionally clinicians will administer placebo pills or injections when they are skeptical of a patient's report of pain. Attempting to deceive a patient is unethical, and a positive response to placebo does not prove that the pain was merely "in the patient's head." It is more likely that the pain is a very real phenomenon, probably mediated by the release of endogenous substances such as endorphins.

When placebo use is encountered or contemplated, the physician should ask, "What is happening in this treatment system?" Typical answers include the following: inadequate opioid medication is being used; the personality style of the patient has promoted the staff to become unduly suspicious; and/or the patient and staff are caught in ongoing interpersonal conflict. The only appropriate clinical role for placebos is in research protocols conducted with proper informed consent.

BEHAVIORAL TREATMENTS

Behavioral treatments are primarily used for chronic pain, with an emphasis on helping patients cope with the pain and minimize functional impairment. However, some behavioral strategies can be useful in the acute pain setting as well. Psychoeducation is crucial: patients should be instructed in the proper use of pain medication, particularly the importance of attempting to request pain medication (or use their PCA) at the emergence of pain and not wait until the pain has become unbearable. Similarly, patients should be reassured about their fears of becoming an addict should they use opioids.

Other behavioral techniques may be useful as well. Hypnosis has been shown useful in altering patient's perceptions; in a typical treatment a patient will receive the suggestion that his or her pain is another sensation, such as a sense of warmth. One advantage of hypnosis is that, with practice, patients can learn to hypnotize themselves. Relaxation training can be useful for a variety of pain conditions, particularly those in which tension plays a role, such as tension headaches. Biofeedback can reduce muscle contractions, which can also aid tension headaches. Cognitive therapy has been very useful in treating pain behavior and the conscious thoughts that influence such behavior; however, this is mainly used for chronic pain management.

CLINICAL PEARLS

- In addition to asking the patient to provide a number to rate his/her current pain level, it also can be helpful to ask, "What number would you like it to be?"

- In addition to assessing the experience of pain itself, a thorough evaluation also should include an investigation for the presence of other associated nonpain symptoms that may be present.

- If suffering is not addressed, it is unlikely that even the most thoughtfully chosen pain regimen will provide adequate palliation.

- Minimizing polypharmacy is a preferred treatment strategy.

- Opioids often are prescribed at time intervals that extend beyond the effective half-life of the drug.

- A routine schedule not only increases the likelihood of effective analgesia, but also will tend to minimize some of the common adverse effects associated with shifting blood levels, including nausea and respiratory depression (Lo Presti et al., 2010).

- The dose required to treat reemergent pain resulting from an as-needed or PRN schedule often is larger than would be required to prevent it using a fixed schedule.

- An alternative opioid scheduling method, "reverse PRN," involves offering the medication to the patient on a scheduled basis and allowing the patient to accept, refuse, or delay the dose.

- Morphine sulfate controlled release tablets and oxycodone controlled release tablets should not be crushed for use in feeding tubes, as this results in a bolus dose of the medication. Morphine sulfate extended-release capsules or liquid formulations of morphine and methadone are alternatives.

- The tolerant patient notices a shortened duration of analgesic effect and an eventual decrease in pain relief. The rate of development of tolerance varies, but any patient who is exposed to continuous doses of opioids may develop tolerance; this may occur in as few as 5–7 days.

- The emergence of withdrawal symptoms occurs more rapidly and more intensely with the use of drugs with shorter half-lives.

- If one needs to use an opioid analgesic, an allergic reaction to one opioid does not necessarily imply an allergy to chemically related congeners.

- Although CNS side effects from NSAIDs are possible, including nervousness, anxiety, insomnia, and drowsiness, these are less commonly reported.

DISCLOSURE STATEMENTS

Dr. Boland has no conflicts to disclose.

Dr. Yohanan works for MCG, a Hearst company that creates treatment guidelines.

Dr. Goldberg has no conflicts to disclose.

REFERENCES

Amr, Y. M., & Yousef, A. A. (2010). Evaluation of efficacy of the perioperative administration of venlafaxine or gabapentin on acute and chronic postmastectomy pain. *The Clinical Journal of Pain, 26*(5), 381–385.

Barkin, R. L., Barkin, S. J., & Barkin, D. S. (2006). Propoxyphene (dextropropoxyphene): A critical review of a weak opioid analgesic that should remain in antiquity. *American Journal of Therapeutics, 13*(6), 534–542.

Bieber, C. M., Fernandez, K., Borsook, D., Brennan, M. J., Butler, S. F., Jamison, R. N., et al. (2008). Retrospective accounts of initial subjective effects of opioids in patients treated for pain who do or do not develop opioid addiction: A pilot case-control study. *Experimental and Clinical Psychopharmacology, 16*(5), 429–434.

Brennan, F., Carr, D. B., & Cousins, M. (2007). Pain management: A fundamental human right. *Anesthesia and Analgesia, 105*(1), 205–221.

Brock, C., Olesen, S. S., Olesen, A. E., Frøkjaer, J. B., Andresen, T., & Drewes, A. M. (2012). Opioid-induced bowel dysfunction: pathophysiology and management. *Drugs, 72*(14), 1847–1865.

Bunimov, N., & Laneuville, O. (2008). Cyclooxygenase inhibitors: Instrumental drugs to understand cardiovascular homeostasis and arterial thrombosis. *Cardiovascular & Hematological Disorders Drug Targets, 8*(4), 268–277.

Cassel, E. J. (1982). The nature of suffering and the goals of medicine. *The New England Journal of Medicine, 306*(11), 639–645.

Dahan, A., Romberg, R., Teppema, L., Sarton, E., Bijl, H., & Olofsen, E. (2004). Simultaneous measurement and integrated analysis of analgesia and respiration after an intravenous morphine infusion. *Anesthesiology, 101*(5), 1201–1209.

Dieppe, P., Bartlett, C., Davey, P., Doyal, L., & Ebrahim, S. (2004). Balancing benefits and harms: The example of non-steroidal anti-inflammatory drugs. *BMJ (Clinical Research Ed.), 329*(7456), 31–34.

Duhmke, R. M., Cornblath, D. D., & Hollingshead, J. R. (2004). Tramadol for neuropathic pain. *Cochrane Database of Systematic Reviews (Online), (2)*(2), CD003726.

Eissing, T., Lippert, J., & Willmann, S. (2012). Pharmacogenomics of codeine, morphine, and morphine-6-glucuronide: model-based analysis of the influence of CYP2D6 activity, UGT2B7 activity, renal impairment, and CYP3A4 inhibition. *Molecular Diagnosis & Therapy, 16*(1), 43–53.

Fainsinger, R., Schoeller, T., & Bruera, E. (1993). Methadone in the management of cancer pain: A review. *Pain, 52*(2), 137–147.

FDA (2010). FDA Drug Safety Communication: FDA recommends against the continued use of propoxyphene. Available at http://www.fda.gov/Drugs/DrugSafety/ucm234338.htm.

Fine, P. G., Narayana, A., & Passik, S. D. (2010). Treatment of breakthrough pain with fentanyl buccal tablet in opioid-tolerant patients with chronic pain: Appropriate patient selection and management. *Pain Medicine (Malden, Mass.), 11*(7), 1024–1036.

Gaskell, H., Derry, S., Moore, R. A., & McQuay, H. J. (2009). Single dose oral oxycodone and oxycodone plus paracetamol (acetaminophen) for acute postoperative pain in adults. *Cochrane Database of Systematic Reviews (Online), (3)*(3), CD002763.

Goldberg, R. J., Leigh, H., & Quinlan, D. (1979). The current status of placebo in hospital practice. *General Hospital Psychiatry, 1*(3), 196–201.

Groenewald, C. B., Rabbitts, J. A., Schroeder, D. R., & Harrison, T. E. (2012). Prevalence of moderate-severe pain in hospitalized children. *Paediatric Anaesthesia, 22*(7), 661–668.

Hall, J. K, & Boswell, M. V. (2009). Ethics, law, and pain management as a patient right. *Pain Physician, 12*(3), 499–506.

Hawker, G. A., Mian, S., Kendzerska, T., & French, M. (2011). Measures of adult pain: Visual Analog Scale for Pain (VAS Pain), Numeric Rating Scale for Pain (NRS Pain), McGill Pain Questionnaire (MPQ), Short-Form McGill Pain Questionnaire (SF-MPQ), Chronic Pain Grade Scale (CPGS), Short Form-36 Bodily Pain Scale (SF-36 BPS), and Measure of Intermittent and Constant Osteoarthritis Pain (ICOAP). *Arthritis Care Research (Hoboken), Suppl 11*, S240–S252.

Heel, R. C., Brogden, R. N., Speight, T. M., & Avery, G. S. (1978). Butorphanol: A review of its pharmacological properties and therapeutic efficacy. *Drugs, 16*(6), 473–505.

Hojsted, J., & Sjogren, P. (2007). Addiction to opioids in chronic pain patients: A literature review. *European Journal of Pain (London, England), 11*(5), 490–518.

Inturrisi, C. E., Colburn, W. A., Verebey, K., Dayton, H. E., Woody, G. E., & O'Brien, C. P. (1982). Propoxyphene and norpropoxyphene kinetics after single and repeated doses of propoxyphene. *Clinical Pharmacology and Therapeutics, 31*(2), 157–167.

Kaiko, R. F., Wallenstein, S. L., Rogers, A. G., & Houde, R. W. (1982). Sources of variation in morphine analgesia in cancer patients with chronic pain. *NIDA Research Monograph, 41*, 294–300.

Karci, A., Tasdogen, A., Erkin, Y., Sahinoz, B., Kara, H., & Elar, Z. (2003). Evaluation of quality in patient-controlled analgesia provided by an acute pain service. *European Surgical Research. Europaische Chirurgische Forschung. Recherches Chirurgicales Europeennes, 35*(4), 363–371.

Kraft, B., Frickey, N. A., Kaufmann, R. M., Reif, M., Frey, R., Gustorff, B., et al. (2008). Lack of analgesia by oral standardized cannabis extract on acute inflammatory pain and hyperalgesia in volunteers. *Anesthesiology, 109*(1), 101–110.

Latta, K. S., Ginsberg, B., & Barkin, R. L. (2002). Meperidine: A critical review. *American Journal of Therapeutics, 9*(1), 53–68.

Lavand'homme, P. (2011). The progression from acute to chronic pain. *Current Opinion in Anaesthesiology, 24*(5), 545–550.

Lawlor, P. G. (2002). The panorama of opioid-related cognitive dysfunction in patients with cancer: A critical literature appraisal. *Cancer, 94*(6), 1836–1853.

Lin, P. L., Fan, S. Z., Huang, C. H., Huang, H. H., Tsai, M. C., Lin, C. J., et al. (2008). Analgesic effect of lidocaine patch 5% in the treatment of acute herpes zoster: A double-blind and vehicle-controlled study. *Regional Anesthesia and Pain Medicine, 33*(4), 320–325.

Lo Presti, C., Roscetti, A., Muriess, D., & Mammucari, M. (2010). Time to pain relief after immediate-release morphine in episodic pain: The TIME study. *Clinical Drug Investigation, 30*(Suppl 2), 49–55.

Malanga, G. A., Ruoff, G. E., Weil, A. J., Altman, C. A., Xie, F., & Borenstein, D. G. (2009). Cyclobenzaprine ER for muscle spasm associated with low back and neck pain: Two randomized, double-blind, placebo-controlled studies of identical design. *Current Medical Research and Opinion, 25*(5), 1179–1196.

Marks, D. M., Shah, M. J., Patkar, A. A., Masand, P. S., Park, G. Y., & Pae, C. U. (2009). Serotonin-norepinephrine reuptake inhibitors for pain control: Premise and promise. *Current Neuropharmacology, 7*(4), 331–336.

Marret, E., Remy, C., Bonnet, F., & Postoperative Pain Forum Group. (2007). Meta-analysis of epidural analgesia versus parenteral opioid analgesia after colorectal surgery. *The British Journal of Surgery, 94*(6), 665–673.

Miner, J. R., Moore, J., Gray, R. O., Skinner, L., & Biros, M. H. (2008). Oral versus intravenous opioid dosing for the initial treatment of acute musculoskeletal pain in the emergency department. *Academic Emergency Medicine: Official Journal of the Society for Academic Emergency Medicine, 15*(12), 1234–1240.

Moskovitz BL, Benson CJ, Patel AA, Chow W, Mody SH, McCarberg BH, Kim MS. (2011). Analgesic treatment for moderate-to-severe acute pain in the United States: patients' perspectives in the Physicians Partnering Against Pain (P3) survey. *Journal of Opioid Management, 7*(4), 277–286.

Osterweis, M. (1988). Perceptions not yet matched by research. *Journal of Palliative Care, 4*(1–2), 78–80.

Oxycodone pectinate (proladone) and other opiate suppositories. (1979). *Drug and Therapeutics Bulletin, 17*(6), 21–22.

Palmer, H., Graham, G., Williams, K., & Day, R. (2010). A risk-benefit assessment of paracetamol (acetaminophen) combined with caffeine. *Pain Medicine (Malden, Mass.), 11*(6), 951–965.

Perahia, D. G., Pritchett, Y. L., Desaiah, D., & Raskin, J. (2006). Efficacy of duloxetine in painful symptoms: An analgesic or antidepressant effect? *International Clinical Psychopharmacology, 21*(6), 311–317.

Quigley, C. (2002). Hydromorphone for acute and chronic pain. *Cochrane Database of Systematic Reviews (Online), (1)*(1), CD003447.

Rapoport, A., Stang, P., Gutterman, D. L., Cady, R., Markley, H., Weeks, R., et al. (1996). Analgesic rebound headache in clinical practice: Data from a physician survey. *Headache, 36*(1), 14–19.

Rischitelli, D. G., & Karbowicz, S. H. (2002). Safety and efficacy of controlled-release oxycodone: A systematic literature review. *Pharmacotherapy, 22*(7), 898–904.

Saarto, T., & Wiffen, P. J. (2007). Antidepressants for neuropathic pain. *Cochrane Database of Systematic Reviews (Online), (4)*(4), CD005454.

Seidel, S., Aigner, M., Ossege, M., Pernicka, E., Wildner, B., & Sycha, T. (2008). Antipsychotics for acute and chronic pain in adults. *Cochrane Database of Systematic Reviews (Online), (4)*(4), CD004844.

Sierpina, V. S., Frenkel, M. A. (2005). Acupuncture: a clinical review. *Southern Medical Journal, 98*, 330–337.

Sindrup, S. H., & Brosen, K. (1995). The pharmacogenetics of codeine hypoalgesia. *Pharmacogenetics, 5*(6), 335–346.

Sondik, E. J., Madans, J. H., & Gentleman, J. F. (2011). Summary health statistics for U.S. adults: National health interview survey. *National Center for Health Statistics, 256*(10).

Stillman, M. J., & Stillman, M. T. (2007). Choosing nonselective NSAIDs and selective COX-2 inhibitors in the elderly. A clinical use pathway. *Geriatrics, 62*(2), 26–34.

Tassinari, D., Sartori, S., Tamburini, E., Scarpi, E., Tombesi, P., Santelmo, C., et al. (2009). Transdermal fentanyl as a front-line approach to moderate-severe pain: A meta-analysis of randomized clinical trials. *Journal of Palliative Care, 25*(3), 172–180.

Ventafridda, V., Saita, L., Ripamonti, C., & De Conno, F. (1985). WHO guidelines for the use of analgesics in cancer pain. *International Journal of Tissue Reactions, 7*(1), 93–96.

Vinik, A. (2005). Clinical Review: Use of antiepileptic drugs in the treatment of chronic painful diabetic neuropathy. *The Journal of Clinical Endocrinology and Metabolism, 90*(8), 4936–4945.

Walsh, T. D. (1984). Oral morphine in chronic cancer pain. *Pain, 18*(1), 1–11.

Wiffen, P., Collins, S., McQuay, H., Carroll, D., Jadad, A., & Moore, A. (2005). Anticonvulsant drugs for acute and chronic pain. *Cochrane Database of Systematic Reviews (Online), (3)*(3), CD001133.

Wiffen, P. J., & McQuay, H. J. (2007). Oral morphine for cancer pain. *Cochrane Database of Systematic Reviews (Online), (4)*(4), CD003868.

Zhang, W. Y., & Li Wan Po, A. (1994). The effectiveness of topically applied capsaicin. A meta-analysis. *European Journal of Clinical Pharmacology, 46*(6), 517–522.

26.

PHARMACOLOGIC AND OTHER SOMATIC TREATMENTS OF NAUSEA AND VOMITING

Danielle N. Ko and Eva H. Chittenden

INTRODUCTION

Nausea and vomiting are common complaints in the general population. In one study 3% of people had nausea once a week, while 2% reported vomiting more than once a month (Talley, Zinsmeister, Schleck, & Melton, 1992). These symptoms are frequent causes of presentation to outpatient clinics (Britt & Fahridin, 2007; Frese, Klauss, Herrmann, & Sandholzer, 2011) as well as highly prevalent in the inpatient population. In patients with advanced cancer, nausea and vomiting are estimated to affect between 40%–70% of patients (Borison & Wang, 1953). Nausea is a common side effect of many medications.

Systematic and effective treatment of these often very distressing symptoms requires knowledge of the physiological mechanisms and potential treatments for nausea and vomiting. In some patients mental states significantly contribute to or exacerbate the experience of these symptoms. While the relationship between one's emotional state and gastrointestinal (GI) function has been the subject of medical discussion for centuries, (Van Oudenhove, Vandenberghe, Demyttenaere, & Tack, 2010), the details of these interactions remain an unresolved question. We hope to elucidate known contributions of the central nervous system to nausea and vomiting.

PATHOPHYSIOLOGY

The pathophysiology of nausea and vomiting involves both central nervous system (CNS) and peripheral mechanisms. The brainstem, specifically the medulla, is an important anatomic area for nausea and vomiting with two separate areas involved, the chemoreceptor trigger zone (CTZ) and the vomiting center (VC).

The CTZ is located in the area postrema in the floor of the fourth ventricle, a site with an ineffective or absent blood-brain barrier. The CTZ, despite its location in the CNS, can sample blood for endogenous or exogenous toxins. Electrolyte imbalances such as hypercalcemia and hyponatremia, liver or kidney failure with their associated endogenous toxins, and exogenous toxins such as medications (including chemotherapy agents) and chemicals found in spoiled food can all activate the CTZ. The CTZ then sends signals to the vomiting center (VC).

The VC is anatomically more diffuse and includes the nucleus of the tractus solitarius and the reticular formation of the medulla. The VC is stimulated via multiple pathways (described below) and, once activated, controls the physical act of vomiting by coordinating parasympathetic and motor efferent activity (Krakauer, et al., 2005; Mannix, 2005; Quigley, Hasler, & Parkman, 2001).

The relationship of nausea to vomiting is unclear but is hypothesized to be a quantitative one: nausea without vomiting occurs when the VC is not sufficiently stimulated to trigger the vomiting reflex. Vomiting without preceding nausea is less common and even less understood.

EMETOGENIC PATHWAYS

The Vomiting Center (VC), the final common pathway in vomiting, is triggered via four pathways:

1. The chemoreceptor trigger zone (CTZ), which is stimulated by various endogenous and exogenous chemicals in the bloodstream.

2. Afferent neural pathways from the GI tract. These include the vagus nerve, the splanchnic nerves, sympathetic ganglia, and the glossopharyngeal nerves. The vagus nerve is stimulated by mechanoreceptors in the GI tract that sense stretch or distension and by chemoreceptors that sense mucosal irritation or damage, usually through the secretion of serotonin by the GI mucosa. Conditions that cause stretch or distension include diabetic gastroparesis, slowed motility from opioids, bowel obstruction, and constipation. Conditions that cause mucosal irritation include infections such as candidiasis or viral/bacterial gastroenteritis, ulcers due to *H. pylori* infection or nonsteroidal antiinflammatory agents, alcoholic gastritis, and mucositis from chemotherapy. The vagus nerve sends signals directly to the VC.

3. Afferent neural pathways from the viscera and serosa of the thorax and abdomen. Signals originate in mechanoreceptors and chemoreceptors in all of

the viscera and serosa of the head and neck, thorax, abdomen, and pelvis. As in the GI tract, the mechano-receptors and chemoreceptors of the pharynx, heart, liver, and kidneys, communicate primarily through the vagus nerve. The vagus nerve (and to a lesser extent the splanchnic and sympathetic nerves) send nausea-inducing signals to the VC when organ capsules are stretched (e.g., hepatitis, liver metastases, or pyelonephritis) or when hollow organs, ducts or tubes are stretched (e.g., in cholelithiasis, choledocolithiasis, nephrolithiasis, or ectopic pregnancy.) The vagus nerve also sends nausea-inducing signals when serosal linings—the pleura, peritoneum or pericardium—are stretched.

4. Afferent neural pathways from CNS sites outside the medulla, including the vestibular system, the diencephalon, and the cerebral cortex. The vestibular system is activated by motion in susceptible individuals (i.e., motion sickness) and in conditions such as benign positional vertigo, labyrinthitis, and Meniere's disease. Rarely, the vestibular system may be sensitized by opioids, which can then cause nausea and vomiting through this pathway. Although the mechanism remains unclear, one hypothesis is that nausea is mediated by the mu receptors on the vestibular epithelium (Porreca & Ossipov, 2009). The vestibular system sends signals to the VC and perhaps also to the CTZ.

Increased intracranial pressure and mass effect from traumatic brain injury, hemorrhage, edema, or CNS infection can cause nausea and vomiting. Migraine headaches are often associated with nausea. The pathways involved are not fully understood.

It has been postulated that the relationship between gastrointestinal function and one's emotional/psychological state can be partially explained by the fact that CNS control of the gut is primarily located in the limbic system (anatomically comprised of the hypothalamus, amygdala, medial thalamus and anterior cingulate cortex), the same area responsible for one's emotions (Jones, Dilley, Drossman, & Crowell, 2006). In addition, serotonin is an important neurotransmitter in both the GI tract and CNS system.

The cerebral cortex may provide inhibitory input to the VC, much as it provides inhibitory input to nociceptive neurons in the spinal cord and brainstem, although the mechanisms are poorly understood. The rationale behind this thinking is based on the limited data suggesting that nonpharmacological interventions such as cognitive behavioral therapy and hypnosis decrease chemotherapy-related nausea and vomiting (Lotfi-Jam, Carey, Jefford, Schofield, Charleson, & Aranda, 2008).

Nausea is often accompanied by strong emotional as well as cognitive components (Muth, Stern, Thayer, Koch, 1996). The cerebral regions responsible for processing nausea in humans are not well elucidated, but it has been hypothesized that it is likely to include areas that are responsible for conscious awareness of internal body states, including the insular and dorsal anterior cingulate cortices (Napadow et al., 2013).

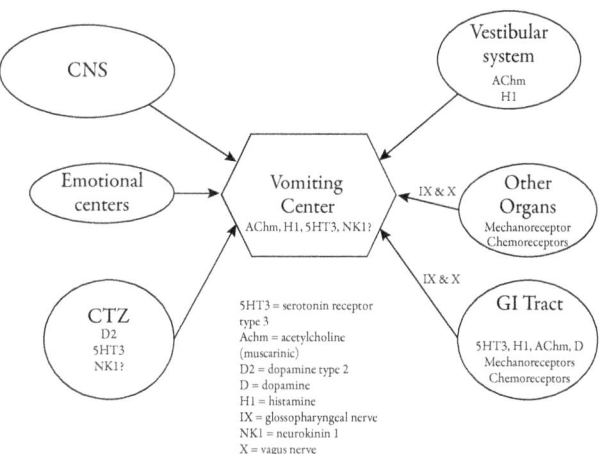

Figure 26.1 Pharmacologically relevant neuralpathways and neurotransmitters.

NEUROTRANSMITTERS AND RECEPTORS INVOLVED IN NAUSEA AND VOMITING

Figure 26.1 summarizes the neural pathways and neurotransmitters thought to be important in nausea and vomiting. The most important receptor in the CTZ is the dopamine type 2 (D2) receptor; the primary receptors in the VC are muscarinic cholinergic (AChm) and histamine (H1) receptors. Serotonin type 3 (5HT3) receptors are also present in both sites and serotonin type 2 (5HT2) receptors in the VC. Substance P is found in high concentrations in the CTZ and VC and binds to neurokinin 1 (NK1) receptors; a role for substance P in nausea and vomiting has been postulated. H1 and AChm receptors mediate nausea in the vestibular apparatus.

In the GI tract there are many receptors involved in nausea and vomiting, including serotonin, acetylcholine, histamine, and dopamine. 5HT3 receptors on vagal or glossopharyngeal afferents are stimulated by release of serotonin from enterochromaffin cells in the GI tract. Release of serotonin can occur with mucosal irritation from drugs, radiotherapy, or bacterial endotoxins. Dopamine is also thought to be an important neurotransmitter in the regulation of gastrointestinal function. While there are many subtypes of dopamine receptors throughout the GI tract, the mechanisms through which dopamine acts on the gut remain elusive. Outside the GI tract there are acetylcholine and histamine type 1 receptors on viscera and serosal surfaces (Mannix, 2005; Hernandez et al., 1987; Li, 2009; Krakauer et al., 2005; Mannix, 2005; Naylor & Inall, 1994).

ETIOLOGY

Table 26.1 is a comprehensive list of possible causes of nausea and vomiting. Acute causes usually are infectious, inflammatory or iatrogenic. Chronic nausea and vomiting have a wide differential diagnosis.

Table 26.1 DIFFERENTIAL DIAGNOSES OF NAUSEA AND VOMITING

GASTROINTESTINAL

General	*Obstruction*	*Functional*
Appendicitis	Adhesions	Chronic idiopathic nausea
Cholecystitis/cholangitis	Constipation (severe)	Cyclical vomiting
Hepatitis	Esophageal disorders	Functional vomiting
Inflammatory bowel disease	Intussusception	
Pancreatitis	Malignancy	
Peritonitis	Pyloric stenosis	
	Strangulated hernia	
Chronic intestinal pseudo-obstruction	Volvulus	
Gastroparesis		
Irritable bowel		
Peptic ulcer disease		
Non-ulcer dyspepsia		
Liver failure		

Infectious	*Metabolic/Endocrine*	*Medications/Toxins*
Acute otitis media (in children)	Adrenal disorders	Medications, including
Bacteria (e.g., shigella, salmonella, staphylococcal, cholera)	Diabetic ketoacidosis	Antiarrhythmics including digoxin
	Electrolyte imbalance e.g.,	Antibiotics
Pneumonia	hypercalcemia, hyponatremia	Anticonvulsants
Spontaneous bacterial peritonitis	Paraneoplastic syndromes	Chemotherpeutics
Urinary tract infection/pyelonephritis	Pregnancy	NSAIDS
Viruses (e.g., adenovirus, Norwalk, rotavirus)		Opiates
		Radiation therapy

(AGA, 2001; Hall & Driscoll, 2005; Mannix, 2005; Murtagh, 2011; Scorza, Williams, Phillips, & Shaw, 2007; Talley, 2007)

GASTROINTESTINAL CAUSES

Differential diagnosis of nausea and vomiting begins with a full exploration of the patient's history of other gastrointestinal symptoms. Presence or absence of abdominal pain, diarrhea or constipation, passing of flatus, fever, and jaundice should help in differentiating between the general gastrointestinal causes.

The sudden onset of severe abdominal pain radiating to the back associated with nausea and vomiting suggests acute pancreatitis. Conditions such as gastroesophageal reflux disease, irritable bowel syndrome, and peptic ulcer disease all can cause nausea and vomiting, but these rarely are the patient's chief complaint.

Bowel obstructions may present as acute, chronic, or acute on chronic, depending on the underlying cause, and are often associated with severe abdominal pain as well as inability to pass flatus/stool. Feculent vomitus is typical of ileal or colonic obstruction.

INFECTIOUS CAUSES

Infectious causes tend to present acutely and are usually self-limiting. Severe cases can lead to dehydration and electrolyte disturbances that must be corrected.

METABOLIC/ENDOCRINE CAUSES

Pregnancy, with nausea and vomiting occurring in more than 50% of cases, must be considered in any woman of childbearing age. *Hyperemesis gravidarum*, which occurs in less than 1% of pregnancies, is a severe form of pregnancy-related nausea and vomiting that can cause severe dehydration and electrolyte disturbance. Nausea and vomiting are present in the majority of cases of diabetic ketoacidosis and in Addisonian crisis.

MEDICATIONS/TOXINS

Almost any medication can cause nausea and/or vomiting. Symptoms tend to occur soon after starting a medication. In cases of chemotherapy there can be anticipatory nausea/vomiting. Delayed vomiting after chemotherapy, by definition, will occur at least one day post-chemotherapy. Digoxin toxicity, a medical emergency, often is associated with visual changes, mental status changes, and/or symptoms or signs of cardiac arrhythmia. Ethanol intoxication and withdrawal both are common causes of nausea and vomiting, as are opioid intoxication and withdrawal. Withdrawal of alcohol and opioids are associated with other typical physical and behavioral withdrawal symptoms.

CNS CAUSES

Patients with CNS causes of nausea and vomiting usually present with additional neurological symptoms and signs. Vertigo may be present if the labyrinth is involved. A classic presentation of migraine is one-sided headache, photophobia, nausea, and vomiting. Nausea and vomiting associated with severe gait disturbance points to cerebellar hemorrhage. Nausea and vomiting may also occur in seizure disorders. The rare presence of ictal vomiting usually indicates involvement of the nondominant insular cortex, but by itself it is not definitive in localizing the hemisphere in which the seizure arises. Nausea and vomiting are also associated with severe pain and with the eye pain of acute glaucoma.

MYOCARDIAL INFARCTION

Nausea is a common presenting symptom of myocardial infarction, occurring in 60%–70% of all infarcts. While nausea and vomiting were previously thought to be more common in inferior myocardial infarctions (Culic, Miric, & Eterovic, 2001), newer data assert that nausea is just as common in anterior MIs (Fuller, Alemu, Harper, & Feldman, 2009). Nausea may be associated with infarct size rather than location (Herlihy, McIvor, Cummings, Siu, & Alikahn, 1987; Quigley et al., 2001).

POSTOPERATIVE NAUSEA

Postoperative nausea and vomiting is estimated to complicate the post-operative period in approximately one third of patients undergoing general anaesthesia (Quinn, Brown, Wallace, & Asbury, 1994). Risk factors include younger age, female sex, use of certain inhalational agents such as nitrous oxide, longer duration of surgery and anaesthesia, and type of surgery (e.g., gynecological and middle ear surgery). Prophylactic treatment with ondansetron has been shown to be only mildly more effective and to cause more side effects when compared to symptomatic treatment. Prophylactic treatment is not considered to be cost efficient (Tramer, Phillips, Reynolds, McQuay, & Moore, 1999; AGA, 2001; Britt & Fahridin, 2007; Hall & Driscoll, 2005; Metz & Hebbard, 2007; Murtagh, 2011).

CHRONIC UNEXPLAINED NAUSEA AND VOMITING DISORDERS

There are patients who have chronic nausea and/or vomiting that remain undiagnosed after extensive diagnostic workup. Previously, patients with unexplained chronic nausea and vomiting were labeled as having "psychogenic" vomiting, namely, vomiting secondary to an emotional disorder (Hill, 1968). In one study 53% of patients met criteria for conversion disorder and 36% met criteria for depression (Muraoka, Mine, Matsumoto, Nakai, & Nakagawa, 1990). In a study that included controls with explained nausea and vomiting (unlike the Muraoka study), there was no difference in rates of psychiatric disease in patients with unexplained versus diagnosed conditions (Olden & Crowell, 2005). While there is clearly an overlap, the relationship between chronic gastrointestinal and psychiatric symptoms remains unclear (Talley, 2007). The pathophysiology of functional disorders is multi-factorial, with biological, psychological, and social factors influencing the presence and severity of disease, as well as presentation for medical care. Three types of functional vomiting disorders have been described as part of the Rome III classification of functional gastroduodenal and

bowel disorder: cyclical vomiting syndrome (CVS), chronic idiopathic nausea (CIN), and functional vomiting (FV) (Tack et al., 2006).

Cyclical vomiting syndrome (CVS), well described in children and more rare in adults, is a disorder in which the patient has stereotypical and severe episodes of nausea and vomiting lasting up to a week that occur three or more times per year. In between episodes, the patient is free of gastrointestinal symptoms. Diffuse abdominal pain is often present. In up to 25% of patients, there is a family or personal history of migraine headaches. A subset of these patients may have accelerated gastric emptying (Pasricha et al., 2011). While it can relieve nausea and vomiting, cannabis can also cause CVS. In such cases, complete cessation of cannabis use can lead to resolution of the cyclical vomiting disorder (Talley, 2007).

Anxiety and depression occur in about 60% of patients with CVS, a subset of which has panic attacks. Tricyclic antidepressants (TCAs), beginning with low-dose amitriptyline, have been used as an effective treatment—a treatment that would be efficacious for migraine as well as anxiety/depression. Clinicians called attention to chronic cannabis or opioid use and undiagnosed more serious psychiatric illness as possible causes of the vomiting syndrome in the 15% of non-responders to TCAs (Hejazi & McCallum, 2011). Use of acute migraine therapies, such as the triptan medications, can be effective during an acute attack. Beta-blockers, and the newer antiepileptic medications, such as levetiracetam, can be effective in preventing or decreasing the severity of vomiting episodes. In women with cyclical vomiting related to menstruation, the oral contraceptive pill can prevent episodes (Talley, 2007).

Chronic idiopathic nausea (CIN) is recurrent and unexplained nausea without vomiting that occurs at least once a week. It must be differentiated from non-ulcer dyspepsia, which usually occurs in relation to meals, and is associated with abdominal discomfort. It must also be differentiated from gastroesophageal reflux disease, which can rarely present as nausea in the absence of heartburn. Although promotility agents such as metocolopramide or antiemetics can be tried, there are no good treatments for chronic idiopathic nausea to date. Long-term use of metoclopramide is not recommended due to the possibility of developing extrapyramidal side effects (Talley, 2007).

Functional vomiting is defined as one or more episodes of vomiting weekly in the absence of an eating disorder, regurgitation, major psychiatric illness, chronic cannabinoid use, or any other organic etiology (Talley, 2007). There are limited treatments for functional vomiting. Tricyclic antidepressants have been anecdotally successful in the absence of depression. Antiemetics are marginally useful (Talley, 2007).

In a six-center study of patients with gastroparesis and more than 12 weeks of symptoms, the 106 (25%) patients with normal gastric emptying and chronic nausea did not differ in gastrointestinal symptoms, demographic characteristics, or depression from those without delayed gastric emptying. Only 12% of these patients were described by the stand alone criteria of functional vomiting or chronic idiopathic nausea. The majority in both groups qualified for the diagnosis of irritable bowel syndrome or chronic dyspepsia. The physiology remains unclear for these patients who do not differ in symptoms from those with gastroparesis (Pasricha et al., 2011).

PSYCHIATRIC CAUSES

Several psychiatric diagnoses should be considered when investigating unexplained chronic nausea and vomiting. These include not only depression and conversion disorder but also anxiety and panic disorder.

Nausea can be a somatic symptom of depression. In one study examining the relationship between somatic symptoms and depression, 13% of those suffering from major depressive disorder reported at least moderate levels of nausea and vomiting. Nonetheless, nausea was much less prevalent than fatigue, "feeling weak," headache, and other pain complaints. In fact, nausea was ranked 28th of the 28 somatic symptoms studied (Vaccarino, Sills, Evans, & Kalali, 2008). Morning nausea is seen in melancholia, the form of depression in which symptoms are often worse in the morning.

Patients with panic disorder most commonly present with a constellation of symptoms called the "cardiorespiratory subtype," in which dyspnea or chest pain are predominant. The next most common symptom cluster, called the "mixed somatic subtype," includes nausea, sweating, trembling, chills/hot flashes, and dizziness (Meuret et al., 2006). Generalized anxiety disorder can also feature nausea and, less commonly, vomiting. In anorexia nervosa and bulimia nervosa, patients can self-induce vomiting either by taking emetogenic drugs, by gagging themselves, or by gorging on food to the point of distending the stomach sufficiently to trigger vomiting. Some patients with these disorders train themselves to vomit without exogenous stimulation. Other psychiatric diagnoses that the clinician should include in the differential include factitious disorder and malingering, in which patients may self-administer emetogenic drugs like ipecac.

Conditioned or anticipatory nausea and vomiting is seen after multiple treatments of emetic chemotherapy; the patient is triggered by the thought of the chemotherapy, the location of treatment, the smells or sights associated with previous treatment, or the memory of the last food eaten before treatment. Reminders after treatment is over may evoke a similar response. This natural evolution of nausea, as a result of medical treatment, offers evidence of how conditioned nausea and vomiting can evolve in other settings in which the provocation for nausea and vomiting is not as obvious.

ASSESSMENT

The probable cause of nausea and vomiting usually is evident after a thorough history and physical examination, especially in acute cases. When the probable cause is viral gastroenteritis, laboratory tests are needed only in moderate to severe cases for detecting electrolyte abnormalities and assessing dehydration. When other causes are suspected, imaging studies and laboratory tests are directed to confirm and assess the suspected underlying cause. Nausea and vomiting in immunocompromised or frail elderly patients can be difficult to diagnose from history and examination alone and usually require an extensive diagnostic workup.

HISTORY

Nausea and vomiting are two distinct entities, and therefore each one should be assessed independently. Vomiting should also be distinguished from other symptoms such as retching, regurgitation, and rumination (see Box 26.1). The nature of the vomitus should be elicited. Coffeeground emesis is indicative of upper GI bleeding, whereas feculent vomiting suggests distal small bowel obstruction. The timeframe of symptoms should be established early as the differential diagnosis for acute (less than one month) and chronic nausea and/or vomiting are very different. Triggers as well as timing in relation to food intake may also provide helpful clues. A systems review must be performed to identify any accompanying symptoms, including neurological symptoms (e.g., vertigo, difficulty walking, and headache) or symptoms suggestive of infection. The patient should also be asked about prescriptions (e.g., digoxin, antibiotics) and any over-the-counter medications/supplements. In acute cases, a history of contact with other ill persons, recent travel, and recent food intake should be elicited. In chronic cases, questions that screen for depression, anxiety, and eating disorders (e.g., self-image, binge eating, and self-induced vomiting) should be used. Symptom diaries can also be kept. Such logs can help patients feel some sense of control and ownership of the problem. They can help healthcare providers by highlighting any patterns to symptoms, as well as helping both patients and clinicians track response to treatments. A number of assessment tools have been developed for nausea and vomiting, especially in the context of chemotherapy related nausea and vomiting,

---

Box 26.1 **DEFINITIONS**

Nausea is the unpleasant subjective sensation of needing to vomit.

Vomiting or emesis is the forceful expulsion of upper gastrointestinal contents through the mouth.

Retching involves the same physical act of vomiting but against a closed glottis.

Regurgitation, which is the effortless return of contents to the mouth without diaphragmatic contraction, should be distinguished from vomiting.

Rumination is the repeated regurgitation of undigested pleasant tasting food from the stomach back up into the mouth. It is likely a learned reflex response, not a conscious action.

which can aid in monitoring the frequency, severity, and duration of symptoms (Wood, Chapman, & Eilers, 2011; Rhodes &, McDaniel, 1999).

EXAMINATION

The physical examination should focus on the following:

1. Signs of dehydration including hypotension, orthostatic changes, tachycardia, decreased tissue turgor and dry mucous membranes.

2. Abdominal examination including observing for jaundice (involvement of the liver, bile duct, pancreas), abdominal distention that may indicate obstruction and hernias; palpating for focal or rebound tenderness or guarding, masses, or hepatomegaly; and rectal examination. Auscultation should focus on the presence or absence of bowel sounds (ileus) as well as the quality and frequency of bowel sounds (increased, high-pitched bowel sounds suggest obstruction). Presence of a succussion splash indicates gastric outlet obstruction.

3. Neurological examination. Any cranial nerve abnormality or gait disturbance suggests a brainstem lesion; cognitive mental status abnormalities suggest cortical disease. The optic disc should be examined for papilledema (raised intracranial pressure). Nystagmus indicates dysfunction of the vestibular system.

4. Signs of eating disorders (parotid gland enlargement, loss of tooth enamel, and lanugo), depression, and anxiety.

INVESTIGATIONS

Typical laboratory tests and imaging studies for patients presenting with nausea and vomiting are listed in Table 26.2.
In more severe or prolonged episodes of vomiting, elevated hemoglobin level and hematocrit may be seen secondary to volume contraction, while hypochloremia is seen following large losses of HCl with vomiting, often resulting in a hypochloremic metabolic alkalosis.

Further testing will be guided by clinical suspicion and may include serum drug levels (e.g., digoxin toxicity), gastroscopy (proximal lesions), small bowel follow-through (for lesions up to the terminal ileum), abdominal ultrasounds (for liver, gallbladder or pancreatic disease), computed tomography (CT) with oral and IV contrast, and CT or MRI of the brain (intracranial lesions).

(AGA, 2001; Metz & Hebbard, 2007; Murtagh, 2011; Scorza, et al., 2007)

MANAGEMENT

Initially, management should be directed toward stabilizing the patient via methods including rehydration and correction of any electrolyte abnormalities. Empiric treatment should also be instigated early in an attempt to provide some

Table 26.2 INITIAL TESTS

TEST	REASON
Laboratory tests	
Complete blood count	Increased white cell count if infection is suspected. Anemia would warrant further investigation for causes such as malignancy in chronic cases.
Electrolytes	To assess electrolyte abnormalities in more serious cases of nausea and vomiting e.g., hypokalemia, alkalosis
Liver enzymes/ Pancreatic enzymes	When liver or pancreatic disease is suspected
Calcium	Hypercalcemia
Blood glucose, urinary and blood ketones	If suspect diabetic ketoacidosis and in all patients with known diabetes
bHCG	Any woman of childbearing age
TSH	Patients with symptoms and signs of thyroid toxicity
Albumin	Cases of chronic vomiting to assess nutritional status
Urinary microscopy and culture	For suspected cases of UTI, pyelonephritis
Stool microscopy	Where there is associated diarrhea looking for bacterial or parasitic

symptomatic relief. When possible, the underlying cause should be corrected. Cases requiring hospital admission include moderate to severe dehydration (especially in the elderly), possible bowel obstruction, increased intracranial pressure, acute myocardial infarction, and other gastrointestinal and neurological emergencies.

NONPHARMACOLOGIC TREATMENTS

Simple measures such as avoiding noxious stimuli (e.g., strong odors) and eating food frequently and in small amounts can be helpful. For more chronic cases, such as chemotherapy related nausea and vomiting, a number of nonpharmacological techniques can be considered. Relaxation techniques including biofeedback, self-hypnosis, progressive muscle relaxation, cognitive distraction, guided imagery, and systematic desensitization can be helpful particularly for patients with anticipatory nausea and vomiting and for those with prominent anxiety around chemotherapy. While many patients find these techniques effective, there have been few controlled clinical trials. In an uncontrolled study of self-hypnosis for chemotherapy-related nausea and vomiting in 16 cancer patients, all had complete remission of anticipatory symptoms and major decreases in post-chemotherapy nausea and vomiting (Marchioro et al., 2000). However, there have been no controlled studies reported, and clinicians' experiences have been mixed. Patients' varying hypnotic susceptibility may account for much of the variability in response. There have been positive controlled studies of progressive muscle relaxation, with or without guided imagery, for chemotherapy-induced nausea and vomiting (Lyles, Burish, Krozely, & Oldham, 1982; Molassiotis, Yung, Yam, Chan, & Mok, 2002; Morrow & Morrell, 1982). The reported studies have shown decreases in incidence and duration of anxiety, nausea and vomiting during chemotherapy (Arakawa, 1997; Lyles, et al., 1982). The evidence for guided imagery alone is less effective than guided imagery combined with other techniques such as music therapy or progressive muscle relaxation (Yoo, Ahn, Kim, Kim, & Han, 2005). Both cognitive distraction and systematic densensitization are supported by more robust studies, with both techniques shown to significantly decrease both anticipatory nausea and vomiting as well as decrease post-chemotherapy symptoms (Hoffman, 1982; Vasterling, Jenkins, Tope, & Burish, 1993). Apart from greater relaxation, other potential benefits include decreased feelings of helplessness and an enhanced sense of control. Acupressure and acupuncture increasingly are being accepted by mainstream medicine as potentially useful for controlling nausea and vomiting in pregnancy, postoperative and chemotherapy-related contexts (NIH Consensus Conference, 1998). Studies systematically reviewing the efficacy of the wrist acupuncture point P6 have been generally positive, though virtually all have methodological limitations (Arsenault, et al., 2002; A. Lee & Done, 2004; E. J. Lee & Frazier, 2011).

In conclusion, all of the above treatments have some empirical support but none have become the standard of care. In practice, local availability of practitioners skilled in administering the treatment and patient preference are likely to determine the prescription for nonpharmacologic treatment.

PHARMACOLOGIC TREATMENTS

Over–the-Counter Medications/Supplements

Ginger (*Zingiber officinale*) is often advocated as beneficial for nausea and vomiting. A meta-analysis demonstrated that a fixed dose at least 1 g of ginger is more effective than placebo for the prevention of postoperative nausea and vomiting. Studies also suggest efficacy in pregnancy, but the evidence is inconsistent (Ernst & Pittler, 2000; Dennehy, 2011). Vitamin B_6 is also thought to be helpful, but again, it is not supported by high-level evidence.

Prescription Medications

Antiemetic medications are appropriate when a cause is identified but treatment of the underlying condition is impossible or does not provide adequate or timely relief. There are several steps involved in choosing an effective antiemetic. First, one must decide on the likely cause; then, the relevant emetogenic pathway(s) as well as major relevant neurotransmitters. Table 26.3 is a summary of representative antiemetics from each class of medication, the receptors and sites at which they act, the dosages used, and the main side effects.

D2 ANTAGONISTS

Haloperidol is the most potent antagonist of the D2 receptor at the CTZ. Small doses are often very effective. Prochlorperazine is a less potent D2 antagonist. Olanzapine, an atypical antipsychotic, has been effective for nausea even with highly emetic chemotherapy (Navari, Nagy, & Gray, 2013).

Metoclopramide is a prokinetic with potent activity in the GI tract to antagonize D2 and stimulate 5HT4 receptors. Acetylcholine is released by the stimulated

Table 26.3 REPRESENTATIVE ANTIEMETICS, THEIR RECEPTORS, AND INDICATIONS

MEDICATION	RECEPTOR ANTAGONIZED/ SITE OF ACTION	PRIMARY INDICATIONS	USUAL DOSAGES AND ROUTES	MAJOR SIDE-EFFECTS/ NOTES
Dopamine Antagonists				
Haloperidol	D2 in CTZ	Medication-induced nausea Chemical/metabolic causes of N and V	0.5–1 mg oral, subcutaneous, IV every 8 hours	Extrapyramidal reactions Caution re: prolonged QT, especially with IV route
Prochlorperazine	D2 in CTZ	Medication-induced nausea Chemical/metabolic causes of N and V	5–10 mg oral every 8 hours; 25 mg rectally twice a day	Extrapyramidal reactions
Metoclopramide	D2 in CTZ and GIT 5HT4 in GIT	Gastric stasis, ileus	10–20 mg oral, subcutaneous, iv, every 6 hours	Extrapyramidal reactions Caution re: prolonged QTc in higher doses or prolonged use

5HT4 receptors, which reverses gastroparesis in the upper GI tract. There is also some antidopaminergic action at the CTZ. Metoclopramide can be used in partial bowel obstruction, but should not be given if the patient has colic as this will likely exacerbate abdominal pain in an obstructed patient.

All of the D2-blocking medications can acutely produce the side effect of akathisia. With chronic use, they can cause tardive dyskinesia. In fact, there is a black box warning specifically concerning tardive dyskinesia risk with long-term use of metoclopramide.

ANTIHISTAMINES/ANTICHOLINERGIC MEDICATIONS

Scopolamine, meclizine, and dramamine are used classically for the nausea of motion sickness or as augmentation for nausea related to the distension of viscera.

SEROTONIN (5HT3) RECEPTOR ANTAGONISTS

Serotonin receptor antagonists are thought to be most effective through their effects in the GI tract. Emetogenic chemotherapies such as cisplatin induce serotonin release from enterochromaffin cells in the GI mucosa; the serotonin stimulates local vagal afferents that send messages to the VC. Although there are serotonin (5HT3) receptors in the CTZ and VC, the serotonin receptor antagonists are not thought to be effective at these sites.

CORTICOSTEROIDS

Corticosteroids have antiemetic effects, which can be potent in certain settings. The mechanisms of action are poorly understood but are likely multiple. Through their antiinflammatory effects, they are thought to decrease output from peripheral mechanoreceptors. Examples of nausea caused by swelling would include nausea from intracranial mass or hemorrhage, stretch of the liver capsule from metastases, hepatocellular carcinoma, or acute hepatitis. Corticosteroids can be given either intravenously or orally if the patient is not actively vomiting. The irritant effects of these medications on the stomach tend to occur with chronic use only and can be prevented with H2-blockers or proton pump inhibitors. These effects on the stomach do not commonly cause symptoms, but rather they can increase the chances of nonsymptomatic gastric bleeding from ulcers. Corticosteroids can help nausea at low or high doses. It is often prudent to start at low doses (e.g., 2 mg of dexamethasone) and increase the doses as needed given the acute side effect profile of insomnia and dysphoria or euphoria. The long-term side effects of hypertension, elevated sugars or diabetes, infection, and decreased bone density are less relevant when using these medications for acute nausea. When using long-term, it is usually in the setting of terminal disease, such as metastatic cancer, where these long-term side effects are no longer relevant.

NEUROKININ-1 ANTAGONISTS

Aprepitant is one neurokinin-1 antagonist used for chemotherapy induced vomiting with highly emetic drugs. It also has an indication for post-operative nausea and vomiting.

BENZODIAZEPINES

While benzodiazepines have no antiemetic properties at any of the nausea pathways described earlier in the chapter, they can be very useful in reducing the anxiety associated with nausea and in treating anticipatory nausea from chemotherapy and other triggers. One must be mindful of their sedating properties, especially in patients who have not used them before and especially when used in conjunction with other sedating antiemetics (e.g., D2 antagonists) or opioids. Patients with end-stage cancer often have nausea, anxiety, and pain. In this setting it is often more useful to use a dopamine antagonist such as haloperidol with opioids, as haloperidol is less sedating, helps with anxiety, and has more potent antiemetic properties than benzodiazepines (depending on the etiology of the nausea, of course).

CANNABINOIDS

Synthetic cannabinoid analogues may not be as effective as cannabis. Cannabinoids working at a distinct receptor have benefit for chemotherapy induced vomiting resistant to other antiemetics. Common side effects of somnolence, disturbances in thinking, psychotic symptoms, and dizziness may limit benefit (AGA, 2001; Arsenault, et al., 2002; Mannix, 2005; Murtagh, 2011; Naylor & Inall, 1994; Quigley, et al., 2001; Scorza, et al., 2007).

REFRACTORY NAUSEA AND VOMITING

If nausea and vomiting are significant, it is important to schedule medications around the clock, rather than as needed. If nausea and vomiting continue despite targeted antiemetics, reassess for missed diagnoses including contributing psychological factors. If using more than one antiemetic, use medications with different mechanisms of action while bearing in mind the suspected cause of the nausea and vomiting and the medications' side effects. Choosing an appropriate route of administration is important. Avoid the oral route in severely nauseated patients and use other routes such as IV, subcutaneous, rectal, sublingual, or topical.

SUMMARY

Many psychotropic drugs are antiemetic; they may be used to treat psychiatric syndromes at the same time as they act against nausea and vomiting—antipsychotics by virtue of dopamine blockade, benzodiazepines by suppressing conditioning, or antidepressants when depression or chronic anxiety is a major perpetuating cause. The nausea-producing serotoninergic side effects of serotonin reuptake inhibitors may be prevented with the antidote of ondansetron or similar 5HT3 antagonist. Olanzapine is mood stabilizing and has been shown effective for chemotherapy related emesis. The contributions of substance abuse and withdrawal to nausea—via alcohol, cannabis, and opiates—should be noted. Alleviation of motion-related nausea by antihistamines or benzodiazepines as well as the use of tricyclic antidepressants for the nausea of migraines and functional vomiting can be considered. Alleviation of anxiety by nonpharmacological modes can prevent the cascade of nausea when arousal is an element of conditioned nausea and vomiting.

CLINICAL PEARLS

- Ethanol intoxication and withdrawal both are common causes of nausea and vomiting, as are opioid intoxication and withdrawal

- During an acute attack of the functional disorder of cyclic vomiting, acute migraine therapies, such as the triptan medications, can be effective. In addition to low dose tricyclic antidepressants, beta-blockers, and the newer antiepileptic medications, such as levetiracetam, can be effective in preventing or decreasing the severity of vomiting episodes. In women with cyclical vomiting related to menstruation, the oral contraceptive pill can prevent episodes (Tulley NJ, 2007).

- Olanzapine, an atypical antipsychotic, has been effective for nausea even with highly emetic chemotherapy (Navari, 2013).

- Those patients with chronic nausea and vomiting with gastroparesis are not easily distinguished in their course and characteristics from those that do not have gastroparesis.

- Many psychotropic drugs are antiemetic; they may be used to treat psychiatric syndromes at the same time as they act against nausea and vomiting: antipsychotics by virtue of dopamine blockade, benzodiazepines by suppressing conditioning, antidepressants when depression is a major perpetuating cause.

- The nausea-producing serotoninergic side effects of serotonin reuptake inhibitors may be prevented with the antidote of ondansetron or similar 5HT3 antagonist. Olanzapine has been shown effective for chemotherapy related emesis.

- Alleviation of anxiety by non-pharmacological anti-anxiety techniques can prevent the cascade of nausea when arousal is an element of conditioned nausea and vomiting.

DISCLOSURE STATEMENTS

Dr. Ko has no conflicts of interest to disclose.
Dr. Chittenden has no conflicts of interest to disclose.

REFERENCES

AGA. (2001). American Gastroenterological Association medical position statement: nausea and vomiting. *Gastroenterology, 120*(1), 261–263.

Arakawa, S. (1997). Relaxation to reduce nausea, vomiting, and anxiety induced by chemotherapy in Japanese patients. *Cancer Nursing, 20*(5), 342–349.

Arsenault, M. Y., Lane, C. A., MacKinnon, C. J., Bartellas, E., Cargill, Y. M., Klein, M. C., et al. (2002). The management of nausea and vomiting of pregnancy. *Journal of Obstetrics & Gynaecolology, Canada, 24*(10), 817–831; quiz 832–813.

Borison, H. L., & Wang, S. C. (1953). Physiology and pharmacology of vomiting. *Pharmacology Reviews, 5*(2), 193–230.

Britt, H., & Fahridin, S. (2007). Presentations of nausea and vomiting. *Australian Family Physician, 36*(9), 682–683.

Culic, V., Miric, D., & Eterovic, D. (2001). Correlation between symptomatology and site of acute myocardial infarction. *International Journal of Cardiology, 77*(2–3), 163–168.

Dennehy, C. (2011). Omega-3 fatty acids and ginger in maternal health: pharmacology, efficacy, and safety. *Journal of Midwifery & Women's Health, 56*, 584–590, updates data on ginger; refs 35–44.

Ernst, E., & Pittler, M. H. (2000). Efficacy of ginger for nausea and vomiting: a systematic review of randomized clinical trials. *British Journal of Anaesthesia, 84*(3), 367–371.

Frese, T., Klauss, S., Herrmann, K., & Sandholzer, K. (2011). Nausea and Vomiting as the Reasons for Encounter. *Journal of Clinical Medicine Research, 3*(1).

Fuller, E. E., Alemu, R., Harper, J. F., & Feldman, M. (2009). Relation of nausea and vomiting in acute myocardial infarction to location of infarct. *American Journal of Cardiology, 104*(12), 1638–1640

Hernandez, D. E., Mason, G. A., Walker, C. H., & Valenzuela, J. E. (1987). Dopamine receptors in human gastrointestinal mucosa. *Life Sciences, 41*(25), 2717–2723.

Hall, J., & Driscoll, P. (2005). Nausea, vomiting and fever. *Emergency Medeicine Journal, 22*(3), 200–204.

Hejazi, R. A., & McCallum, R. W. (2011). Review article: cyclic vomiting syndrome in adults—rediscovering and redefining an old entity. *Alimentary Pharmacology & Therapeutics, 34*, 263–273.

Herlihy, T., McIvor, M. E., Cummings, C. C., Siu, C. O., & Alikahn, M. (1987). Nausea and vomiting during acute myocardial infarction and its relation to infarct size and location. *American Journal of Cardiology, 60*(1), 20–22.

Hill, O. W. (1968). Psychogenic vomiting. *Gut, 9*(3), 348–352.

Hoffman, M. L. (1982). Hypnotic desensitization for the management of anticipatory emesis in chemotherapy. *American Journal of Clinical Hypnosis, 25*(2–3), 173–176.

Jones, M. P., Dilley, J. B., Drossman, D., & Crowell, M. D. (2006). Brain-gut connections in functional GI disorders: anatomic and physiologic relationships. *Neurogastroenterology and Motility, 18*(2), 91–103.

Krakauer, E. L., Zhu, A. X., Bounds, B. C., Sahani, D., McDonald, K. R., & Brachtel, E. F. (2005). Case records of the Massachusetts General Hospital. Weekly clinicopathological exercises. Case 6-2005. A 58-year-old man with esophageal cancer and nausea, vomiting, and intractable hiccups. *New England Journal of Medicine, 352*(8), 817–825.

Lee, A., & Done, M. L. (2004). Stimulation of the wrist acupuncture point P6 for preventing postoperative nausea and vomiting. *Cochrane Database of Systematic Reviews*(3), CD003281.

Lee, E. J., & Frazier, S. K. (2011). The Efficacy of Acupressure for Symptom Management: A Systematic Review. *Journal of Pain Symptom Management, 42*(4), 589–603.

Lotfi-Jam, K., Carey, M., Jefford, M., Schofield, P., Charleson, C., & Aranda, S. (2008). Nonpharmacologic strategies for managing common chemotherapy adverse effects: a systematic review. *Journal of clinical oncology, 26*(34), 5618–5629.

Lyles, J. N., Burish, T. G., Krozely, M. G., & Oldham, R. K. (1982). Efficacy of relaxation training and guided imagery in reducing the aversiveness of cancer chemotherapy. *Journal of Consulting Clinical Psychology, 50*(4), 509–524.

Mannix, K. (2005). *Palliation of Nausea and Vomiting* (3rd ed.). Oxford, England: Oxford University Press.

Marchioro, G., Azzarello, G., Viviani, F., Barbato, F., Pavanetto, M., Rosetti, F., et al. (2000). Hypnosis in the treatment of anticipatory nausea and vomiting in patients receiving cancer chemotherapy. *Oncology, 59*(2), 100–104.

Metz, A., & Hebbard, G. (2007). Nausea and vomiting in adults—a diagnostic approach. *Australian Family Physician, 36*(9), 688–692.

Meuret, A. E., White, K. S., Ritz, T., Roth, W. T., Hofmann, S. G., & Brown, T. A. (2006). Panic attack symptom dimensions and their relationship to illness characteristics in panic disorder. *Journal of Psychiatric Research, 40*(6), 520–527.

Molassiotis, A., Yung, H. P., Yam, B. M., Chan, F. Y., & Mok, T. S. (2002). The effectiveness of progressive muscle relaxation training in managing chemotherapy-induced nausea and vomiting in Chinese breast cancer patients: a randomised controlled trial. *Supportive Care in Cancer, 10*(3), 237–246.

Morrow, G. R., & Morrell, C. (1982). Behavioral treatment for the anticipatory nausea and vomiting induced by cancer chemotherapy. *New England Journal of Medicine, 307*(24), 1476–1480.

Muraoka, M., Mine, K., Matsumoto, K., Nakai, Y., & Nakagawa, T. (1990). Psychogenic vomiting: the relation between patterns of vomiting and psychiatric diagnoses. *Gut, 31*(5), 526–528.

Murtagh, J. (2011). *John Murtagh's General Practice* (5th ed.). New York: McGraw Hill Medical Publishing.

Muth, E. R., Stern, R. M., Thayer, J. F., & Koch, K. L. (1996). Assessment of the multiple dimensions of nausea: the Nausea Profile (NP). *Journal of Psychosomatic Research, May;40*(5), 511–520.

Napadow, V., Sheehan, J. D., Kim, J., Lacount, L. T., Park, K., Kaptchuk, T. J., et al. (2013). The brain circuitry underlying the temporal evolution of nausea in humans. *Cerebral Cortex, 23*(4), 806–813.

Navari, R. M., Nagy, C. K., & Gray, S. E. (2013). The use of olanzapine versus metoclopramide for the treatment of breakthrough chemotherapy-induced nausea and vomiting in patients receiving highly emetogenic chemotherapy. *Supportive Care in Cancer, Jun;21*(6), 1655–1663.

Naylor, R. J., & Inall, F. C. (1994). The physiology and pharmacology of postoperative nausea and vomiting. *Anaesthesia, 49 Suppl,* 2–5.

NIH Consensus Conference. (1998). Acupuncture. *Journal of the American Medical Association, 280*(17), 1518–1524.

(1992). Psychogenic vomiting—a disorder of gastrointestinal motility? *Lancet, 339*(8788), 279.

Olden, K., & Crowell, M. D. (2005). Chronic nausea: New insights and approach to treatment. *Current Treatment Options in Gastroenterology, 8*(4), 305–310.

Pasricha, P. J., Colin, R., Yates, K., Hasler, W. L., Abell, T. L., Unalp-Arida, A., et al. (2011). Characteristics of patients with chronic unexplained nausea and vomiting and normal gastric emptying. *Clinical Gastroenterology and Hepatology, 9*(7), 567–576.

Porreca, F., & Ossipov, M. H. (2009). Nausea and vomiting side effects with opioid analgesics during treatment of chronic pain: mechanisms, implications, and management options. *Pain Medicine, May-Jun;10*(4), 654–662.

Quigley, E. M., Hasler, W. L., & Parkman, H. P. (2001). AGA technical review on nausea and vomiting. *Gastroenterology, 120*(1), 263–286.

Quinn, A. C., Brown, J. H., Wallace, P. G., & Asbury, A. J. (1994). Studies in postoperative sequelae. Nausea and vomiting—still a problem. *Anaesthesia, 49*(1), 62–65.

Rhodes, V. A. & McDaniel, R. W. (1999). The Index of nausea, vomiting and retching: a new format of the Index of Nausea and Vomiting. *Oncology Nursing Forum, 26*(5), 889–894.

Scorza, K., Williams, A., Phillips, J. D., & Shaw, J. (2007). Evaluation of nausea and vomiting. *American Family Physician, 76*(1), 76–84.

Tack, J., Talley, N. J., Camilleri, M., Holtmann, G., Hu, P., Maladelada, J-R., et al. (2006). Functional gastroduodenal disorders. *Gastroenterology, 130,* 1466–1479.

Talley, N. J. (2007). Functional nausea and vomiting. *Australian Family Physician, 36*(9), 694–697.

Talley, N. J., Zinsmeister, A. R., Schleck, C. D., & Melton, L. J. 3rd (1992). Dyspepsia and dyspepsia subgroups: a population-based study. *Gastroenterology, 102*(4 Pt 1), 1259–1268.

Tramer, M. R., Phillips, C., Reynolds, D. J., McQuay, H. J., & Moore, R. A. (1999). Cost-effectiveness of ondansetron for post-operative nausea and vomiting. *Anaesthesia, 54,* 226–234.

Vaccarino, A. L., Sills, T. L., Evans, K. R., & Kalali, A. H. (2008). Prevalence and association of somatic symptoms in patients with major depressive disorder. *Journal of Affective Disorders, 110*(3), 270–276.

Van Oudenhove, L., Vandenberghe, J., Demyttenaere, K., & Tack, J. (2010). Psychosocial factors, psychiatric illness and functional gastrointestinal disorders: a historical perspective. *Digestion, 82*(4), 201–210.

Vasterling, J., Jenkins, R. A., Tope, D. M., & Burish, T. G. (1993). Cognitive distraction and relaxation training for the control of side effects due to cancer chemotherapy. *Journal of Behavioral Medicine, 16*(1), 65–80.

Wood, J. M, Chapman, K., & Eilers, J. (2011). Tools for assessing nausea, vomiting, and retching. *Cancer Nursing, 34*(1), E14–34.

Yoo, H. J., Ahn, S. H., Kim, S. B., Kim, W. K., & Han, O. S. (2005). Efficacy of progressive muscle relaxation training and guided imagery in reducing chemotherapy side effects in patients with breast cancer and in improving their quality of life. *Supportive Care in Cancer, 13*(10), 826–833.

27.

PHARMACOLOGIC AND OTHER SOMATIC TREATMENTS OF DYSPNEA

Pedro E. Pérez-Cruz and Eva H. Chittenden

INTRODUCTION

The American Thoracic Society defines dyspnea as "a subjective experience of breathing discomfort that consists of qualitatively distinct sensations that vary in intensity" (Parshall et al., 2012) and is not necessarily associated with hypoxia or hypercarbia. Patients with dyspnea experience associated distress, functional impairment and decreased quality of life. Dyspnea has been recognized as a strong and independent predictor of mortality (Parshall et al., 2012). Physiologic, psychological, social and cultural factors influence the perception of dyspnea. The *perception* of dyspnea refers to the unique manner in which a particular individual experiences breathlessness and it consists of three distinct dimensions: a sensory dimension (i.e., the intensity of the symptom), an affective dimension (i.e., how unpleasant the symptom is), and a functional dimension (i.e., the impact or burden of the symptom). While the goal of the clinician is to resolve the underlying cause of the derangement, this is often not possible and leads to situations of chronic dyspnea in many patients with cardiopulmonary disease. Understanding the underlying pathophysiologic and emotional factors that impact dyspnea will help the clinician choose targeted interventions for these patients when the underlying cause cannot be cured or further treated. This chapter will review symptomatic treatments of dyspnea that decrease the sense of breathlessness and improve the patient's quality of life.

The reported prevalence of dyspnea in oncologic patients varies from 21% to 90% depending on the stage of cancer (Thomas & von Gunten, 2002). The prevalence of dyspnea in patients with cancer increases as patients approach death. In the National Hospice study, 70% of cancer patients reported dyspnea at least once during their last 6 weeks of life (Reuben & Mor, 1986). In patients with lung cancer dyspnea is the most distressing symptom, with a prevalence between 55% and 90% (Xue & Abernethy, 2010). Dyspnea is also a frequent symptom in the palliative care population. In a retrospective English study of patients referred to palliative care services, 31% of the patients had dyspnea at the time of referral (Potter, Hami, Bryan, & Quigley, 2003).

With a prevalence between 72.5% and 94%, dyspnea is the most common and distressing symptom in chronic obstructive pulmonary disease (COPD) patients (Pauwels, Buist, Calverley, Jenkins, & Hurd, 2001). It is also a predictor of all-cause mortality in COPD patients with stable disease (Esteban et al., 2008). Dyspnea is frequent in patients with congestive heart failure (CHF), and its prevalence increases before death. In the SUPPORT study 35% of patients with CHF had dyspnea 3 to 6 months before death, and this increased to over 60% during the last 3 days of life (Stuart, 2007).

PHYSIOLOGY OF THE RESPIRATORY CONTROL SYSTEM

The respiratory control system functions to maintain ventilatory homeostasis. Clusters of neurons in the medulla oblongata of the brainstem (the respiratory complex) send messages to the respiratory muscles to breathe. This structure is responsible for spontaneous breathing and the automatic adjustments to ventilation that maintain oxygenation and acid–base balance. It triggers contraction of the various muscle groups involved in breathing, increasing or decreasing the number and types of muscles activated. Under normal conditions breathing is an automatic phenomenon—patients do not need to think about inspiration or expiring air from the lungs—and functional adjustments are unconsciously regulated. Nevertheless, automatic breathing can be overridden by voluntary action: the motor cortex can stimulate respiratory muscles directly via the pyramidal motor system, bypassing the respiratory complex (American Thoracic Society, 1999).

There are several inputs to the medullary respiratory complex:

Chemoreceptors: Both peripheral and central chemoreceptors sense levels of oxygen and carbon dioxide in blood and send signals to the respiratory complex, which adjusts breathing as necessary to maintain oxygenation and acid–base balance. The peripheral chemoreceptors are located in the carotid and aortic bodies and are responsive to changes in the partial pressure of oxygen and, to a lesser extent, to variations in the partial pressure of carbon dioxide. The carotid bodies are innervated by the glossopharyngeal nerve and the aortic bodies by the vagus nerve; these nerves convey the information to the respiratory complex. Central chemoreceptors are located in the medulla oblongata and primarily sense carbon dioxide levels in the cerebrospinal fluid. Under normal conditions, the respiratory drive is mainly regulated by the partial pressure of carbon dioxide in the cerebrospinal fluid sensed at the central level. In certain circumstances during central nervous system depression (e.g., under the effect of anesthesia or when a patient has hypercarbia), the central chemoreceptors are inhibited and their ability to trigger normal ventilation is decreased. Unlike central chemoreceptors, peripheral chemoreceptors are not inhibited during central nervous system depression. In these situations, the respiratory drive is maintained by the partial pressure of oxygen sensed in the carotid and aortic bodies.

Vagal receptors: The upper airways have vagal receptors that are stimulated by cold air. There are stretch receptors in the smooth muscle of the larger airways that are activated by CO2 and inhaled furosamide (which can help the sensation of dyspnea). In the parenchyma of the lungs, there are pulmonary irritant receptors that react to chemical irritants such as cigarette smoke, to inflammatory mediators, and to fluid and inflammation in the lung parenchyma. Finally, there are C-fibre receptors that are in close proximity to either the pulmonary or bronchial circulation. At this point, there is no definitive evidence that stimulation of these receptors causes dyspnea.

Chest wall receptors: Mechanoreceptors in the joints, tendons and muscles of the chest wall send afferent signals to the respiratory complex.

Neural pathways from receptors to the brain: This wealth of information from the chemoreceptors in the medulla and bloodstream, vagal receptors in the airways and lung parenchyma, and mechanoreceptors in the chest wall provides continuous feedback to the respiratory complex in the medulla, which sends signals to the thalamus and up to the cortex. Neuroimaging studies of dyspnea show stimulation of specific areas of the brain cortex, including the anterior right insula, the cerebellar vermis, the amygdala, and the cingulated cortex. In response to these sensory inputs, the medullary respiratory complex (or the motor cortex when breathing is under conscious control) sends efferent commands to the ventilatory muscles.

Corollary motor discharge: When a motor command is sent to the respiratory muscles, a copy of this command, called corollary motor discharge, is relayed to the sensory cortex (with an "expected" response from the respiratory muscles). The motor response of the respiratory muscles will trigger a sensory input that will be also relayed to the sensory cortex, which represents the "actual" motor response. The corollary motor discharge ("expected" response) and the actual motor response received by the sensory cortex will be compared allowing the sensory cortex to detect discrepancy between these two sources of information. This mechanism could

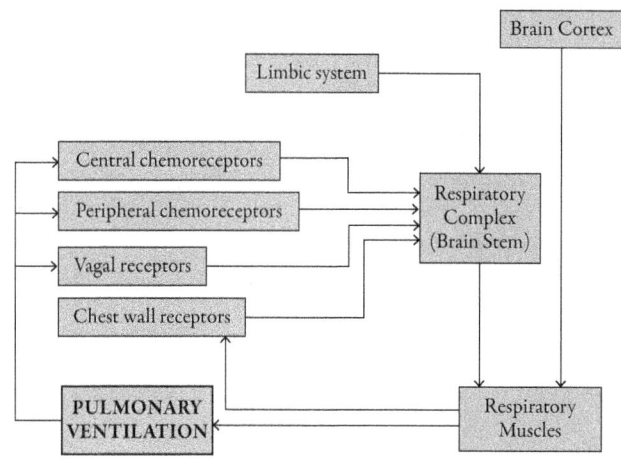

Figure 27.1 A schematic diagram of the structures involved in the control and regulation of breathing. Adapted from Duffin & Phillipson, 2010.

explain the conscious awareness of the effort of breathing that is described by some patients experiencing dyspnea (Nishino, 2011; Schwartzstein & Adams, 2010).

Figure 27.1 describes the pathways involved in the regulation of breathing. The respiratory complex triggers the involuntary activation of different respiratory muscle groups involved in breathing. The brain cortex can voluntarily activate the respiratory muscles. Changes in oxygenation, acid-base balance, lung function, and muscle effort will be communicated to the respiratory complex via a variety of receptors. Emotions, through limbic connections, influence the perception and functioning of the respiratory complex (De Peuter et al., 2004; Duffin & Phillipson, 2010; Evans, Shea, & Saykin, 1999).

PATHOPHYSIOLOGY OF DYSPNEA

Dyspnea is a complex symptom and its mechanisms are not completely understood. Hypercarbia and hypoxia can induce dyspnea in normal subjects, but in individual patients the sensation of breathlessness correlates poorly with the degree of the abnormality (Burki & Lee, 2010). Dyspnea associated with blood gas abnormalities results from increased respiratory motor activity mediated by chemoreceptor activation (American Thoracic Society, 1999), and it could also result from a direct dyspneogenic effect, independent of the ventilatory motor output (Burki & Lee, 2010). This sensation is not due to the resulting increased respiratory muscle activity as quadriplegic people experience dyspnea with hypercarbia. Studies of the hypoxic respiratory drive, in which pCO2 and ventilation are kept constant, show that PO2 has to drop below 6.7 kPa before subjects experience a sharp increase in dyspnea. The mechanism by which vagal afferents from the airways and lungs and the mechanoreceptors from the chest wall cause dyspnea is not known.

The corollary motor discharge from the respiratory center is thought to be key to the generation of the sensation of dyspnea. Others theorize that dyspnea results from a mismatch between respiratory drive and sensory inputs. Dyspnea is experienced when the respiratory complex sends greater than usual stimulus to the respiratory muscles but the sensors convey data implying insufficient ventilation, insufficient muscle contraction, or insufficient movement of air. In other words, there are more signals going out from the respiratory complex but not enough good news coming back from the chest wall mechanoreceptors, central and peripheral chemoreceptors, and vagal airway and pulmonary interoception.

Researchers hypothesize that dyspnea has an affective component in addition to the sensory dimension already discussed. In severe dyspnea, the insular cortex and anterior cingulated gyrus, both part of the limbic system, are activated in functional imaging studies. These areas are postulated to process the distress caused by the sensation of dyspnea, and they may also process the distress caused by physical pain. This evidence correlates well with what we know clinically, that the experience of dyspnea is often accompanied by anxiety and fear. Patients with chronic lung disease who suffer from dyspnea often exhibit anxiety and/or depressive symptoms (Gift & Cahill, 1990).

The association between dyspnea and psychological symptoms is well described in both healthy individuals and in populations with lung disease (Dales, Spitzer, Schechter, & Suissa, 1989; Neuman et al., 2006). Healthy and asthmatic patients with a personality characterized by high negative emotionality (anxiety and highly irritable) report more dyspnea than those with low negative emotionality, regardless of their pulmonary function (Bogaerts et al., 2005). Likewise, dyspnea in patients with stable asthma is explained by both the degree of airway obstruction and patient's emotional status (Martinez-Moragon, Perpina, Belloch, de Diego, & Martinez-Frances, 2003).

The degree of dyspnea experienced in populations of patients and in individuals does not correlate well with air-flow limitation or exercise performance. (De Peuter et al., 2004). Emotional and cognitive factors, as well as the ability to use adaptive techniques, such as distraction, influence the perception of dyspnea. For example, individuals experiencing dyspnea who are able to shift their attention to external stimuli have decreased sense of breathlessness (Thornby, Haas, & Axen, 1995). Likewise, patients with COPD who listen to music while on a rehabilitation program improve their performance compared to patients who do not listen to music (Bauldoff, Hoffman, Zullo, & Sciurba, 2002). Studies have also shown that situational or emotional cues associated with a particular symptom can trigger the symptom even in the absence of the physiological trigger (Rietveld, Everaerd, & Vanbeest, 1999). Negative emotions have been shown to be associated with decreased accuracy in dyspnea perception (De Peuter et al., 2004).

Dyspnea appears to involve qualitatively different sensations. Healthy subjects and patients describe three sensations: (1) "air hunger" or an "urge to breathe"; (2) an "increased work" of breathing; and (3) "chest tightness." Dyspnea that is due to acute hypercarbia or acute severe hypoxia and that is mediated by the peripheral and central chemoreceptors is often described as "air hunger," or an "urge or need to breathe." This description of dyspnea is also observed in the context of exercise-induced dyspnea, especially if ventilatory response is constrained (Parshall et al., 2012). It is related to a conscious awareness of inadequate respiratory motor complex output in relation to the afferent information sensed via corollary discharge (Mahler et al., 1996; Nishino, 2011; Parshall et al., 2012). Dyspnea that is due to either muscle weakness or an increased mechanical load causes an increased sense of respiratory effort, often described as increased work or effort to breathe. Both types of dyspnea, air hunger and increased work of breathing, are associated with increased respiratory drive. A third description of dyspnea is "chest tightness." This phrase is often used by asthmatics and is thought to be associated with bronchoconstriction. It has been suggested that chest tightness arises from stimulation of pulmonary receptors and not from and increased sense of effort (Nishino, 2011; Parshall et al., 2012). Thus, probing about the quality of the dyspnea can guide the clinician in diagnosing the underlying pathophysiologic mechanism, but it is important to keep an open mind because these mechanisms may overlap in complex patients.

ETIOLOGIES

The differential diagnosis of dyspnea is large and includes respiratory, cardiovascular, hematologic, neuromuscular, and psychiatric disorders. Identifying the underlying cause or causes and the likely pathophysiologic mechanisms will help in devising an appropriate treatment plan. Uncommon etiologies, such as chronic pulmonary microemboli and myasthenia gravis, should be ruled out before attributing dyspnea exclusively to a psychiatric cause. Etiologies of dypsnea are listed in Table 27.1.

The clinical history, physical examination, and appropriate testing will aid in determining the most likely system involved and the underlying etiology. There may be more than one process involved especially for patients with chronic dyspnea or for those with an acute exacerbation of chronic dyspnea. Emotional and cognitive factors influence the perception and the functional impact of dyspnea even when there is no primary or secondary mental disorder.

We will flesh out the psychiatric causes of dyspnea a bit more given these causes of dyspnea are less well understood and are often a diagnosis of exclusion after cardiopulmonary and hematologic disorders have been ruled out. Panic disorder, in which panic attacks are associated with concerns about recurrence and often lead to agoraphobia and high use of medical resources, often presents with somatic symptoms, including dyspnea and chest pain, along with a feeling of anxiety and impending doom. In a study of 55 primary care patients presenting with panic disorder, 39% had cardiac symptoms, such as chest pain, dypsnea, and tachycardia (W. Katon, 1984). In fact, a "respiratory subtype" of panic disorder has been described (Abrams, Rassovsky, & Kushner, 2006). Somatic symptoms such as headaches, lightheadedness and epigastric discomfort are often associated with panic disorder as well.

Table 27.1 ETIOLOGIES OF DYSPNEA

SYSTEM	SUBTYPE	MAJOR DISEASES
Respiratory	Airways Disease	Asthma, Chronic obstructive pulmonary diseases, Upper airway obstruction
	Parenchymal lung disease	Pneumonia, Interstitial lung disease, Adult respiratory distress syndrome, Lung cancer
	Pulmonary vascular disease	Pulmonary embolism, primary pulmonary hypertension, chronic pulmonary microemboli
	Pleural Disease	Pleural effusion, Pneumothorax
	Neuromuscular and chest wall diseases	Polymyositis, Myasthenia gravis, Guillain-Barre, kyphoscoliosis
Cardiovascular		Left-sided heart failure, mitral stenosis, pericardial tamponade
Psychiatric		Anxiety, panic attacks, somatization disorder
Other		Anemia

Dyspnea can occur in other mental disorders with a high level of somatization, including somatization disorder, social anxiety disorder, and stimulant abuse (W. Katon, Ries, & Kleinman, 1984; Kroenke & Rosmalen, 2006).

PSYCHIATRIC COMORBIDITIES IN PATIENTS WITH CARDIOPULMONARY DISEASE

Patients with asthma have a higher prevalence of panic disorder and panic attacks than the general population (Hasler et al., 2005). According to one literature review, patients with asthma have a frequency of panic attacks ranging between 6.5% and 24% (W. J. Katon, Richardson, Lozano, & McCauley, 2004). Patients with COPD have a higher prevalence of generalized anxiety disorder (10%–15.8%) and panic disorder (32%–37%) compared to the general population (3.6%–5.1% and 3.4% respectively) (Periyakoil, Skultety, & Sheikh, 2005). Depression is also common in patients with COPD (Chavannes et al., 2005). In patients with CHF dyspnea is associated with fatigue, perception of poor health, and depression. Dyspnea and depression are associated in patients with asthma, cancer, and in mechanically ventilated patients (Ramasamy et al., 2006).

ASSESSMENT

The goal of the clinical assessment is to characterize the magnitude and impact of the symptom and identify possible etiologies. Two major groups of patients must be recognized: those with no prior history of dyspnea, for whom we need to identify the cause of the symptom; and those with a known cardiovascular, respiratory, or muscular disease with worsening dyspnea, for whom we need to distinguish if the cause of the symptom is a new problem or worsening of the underlying disease (Parshall et al., 2012).

We would like to highlight again that as dyspnea is a symptom, it can only be perceived by the person experiencing it. In fact, the correct assessment of dyspnea depends on self report. Therefore, it is important for clinicians to distinguish dyspnea from the clinical signs that health care providers use as evidence of respiratory dysfunction such as increased respiratory rate, use of accessory breathing muscles and intercostal retraction (Parshall et al., 2012).

Dyspnea scales have been developed to standardize the magnitude or impact of the symptom. A large number and variety of tools have been developed to assess dyspnea but each tool measures specific domains. Recent reviews have recognized three different types of measures (Parshall et al., 2012): scales that assess the sensory-perceptual experience of the patient by measuring what breathing feels like to the patient (e.g.; modified Borg scale; Borg, 1982); scales that assess the affective stress by measuring associated distress and the impact/burden of the symptom, focusing on the functional ability of the patient (e.g., Medical Research Council—MRC scale; Fletcher, Elmes, Fairbairn, & Wood, 1959).

In patients with dyspnea, the history, past medical history, and physical examination are the most important components of the diagnostic evaluation.

The history should be directed at identifying the quality of dyspnea, associated symptoms, triggers or alleviating factors, and comorbidities.

A thorough past medical and social history will provide us with essential information about risk factors for dyspnea and for particular etiologies. The presence or absence of specific symptoms will orient us to a possible cause. For instance, dyspnea associated with cough, sputum, hemoptysis, or wheezing, may suggest a respiratory cause, although congestive heart failure can also present with cough and wheezing. The presence of stridor will point to central airway obstruction. The combination of dyspnea on exertion, orthopnea, and lower extremity edema suggests heart failure. Dyspnea associated with generalized muscle weakness raises the possibility of neuromuscular disease. If the physical examination is normal and additional workup is negative, one could consider a primary psychiatric condition, such as anxiety or depression. It is important to keep in mind that a patient may have multiple causes of dyspnea, especially if there is an acute worsening of chronic dyspnea.

A complete physical examination will help confirm or modify the initial hypothesis. Findings such as hyperinflation, dullness to lung percussion, rales, rhonchi, or wheezing will suggest pulmonary etiologies. A severe chest deformity or generalized muscle atrophy will lead us to think of problems with the respiratory pump. The presence of a third heart sound on cardiac auscultation, crackles in the lungs, and bilateral swelling of the lower extremities would point to heart failure. The presence of pale mucosa with tachycardia should make us think of anemia. Commonly used tests in the workup of dyspnea are listed in Table 27.2.

SYMPTOMATIC TREATMENT

The treatment of dyspnea should focus on the underlying cause and its complications. Interventions to treat the etiology will reduce the intensity of the dyspnea and increase the patient's comfort. Table 27.3 describes common reversible etiologies that cause dyspnea in terminal patients and their main treatments. Interventions should be focused on treating the

Table 27.2 INITIAL STUDIES TO EVALUATE DYSPNEA

TESTS	RATIONALE
Lab Tests	
Arterial and mixed venous blood gases	Assess oxygenation and acid-base status
CBC	Detect anemia and infection
Electrolytes and renal function	Estimate anion gap and assess kidney function
Sputum analysis and culture	Identify infectious etiology
Pleural fluid analysis and cultures	Identify cause of pleural effusion and infection
Pulmonary Function Tests	
Spirometry and lung volumes	Differentiate obstructive from restrictive lung disease
CO Diffusion	Assess alveolar diffusion
Cardiopulmonary exercise testing	Differentiate pulmonary, cardiovascular and musculoskeletal causes of dyspnea.
Imaging Techniques	
Chest X-ray	Assess multiple etiologies
Chest CT scan/ PE CT scan	Assess multiple etiologies and/ or detect PE
Cardiac Evaluation	
EKG	Detect arrhythmias or ischemia
Echocardiogram	Assess heart structure and function

Table 27.3 COMMON REVERSIBLE ETIOLOGIES AND TREATMENTS IN PATIENTS WITH DYSPNEA

UNDERLYING CAUSE	INTERVENTIONS
Pleural effusion	Drainage if significant, consider pleural catheter if indicated
Airway obstruction by tumor	Steroids, radiation therapy, stents
Carcinomatous lymphangitis	Steroids
COPD exacerbation	Bronchodilators, steroids, oxygen, antibiotics, non-invasive ventilatory support
Pulmonary embolism	Anticoagulation
Pneumonia	Antibiotics
Ascites	Paracentesis
Congestive Heart Failure	Diuretics, digoxin, betablockers, ACE inhibitors
Anemia	Transfusions of packed RBC

Adapted from Del Fabbro, Dalal, & Bruera, 2006.

breathlessness itself when the underlying disease cannot be effectively treated. Unfortunately, there are no completely satisfactory treatments for the various forms of dyspnea (Lanken et al., 2008). Treatment should focus on both the physical and psychological components of dyspnea. In this section we will describe the available nonpharmacologic and pharmacologic interventions for the symptomatic treatment of dyspnea.

NONPHARMACOLOGIC INTERVENTIONS

Nonpharmacologic interventions tend to be inexpensive and underutilized. A recent review published in the Cochrane database analyzed the effectiveness of these interventions (Bausewein, Booth, Gysels, & Higginson, 2008). In brief, the available and effective interventions include the following:

Fans: Hand-held fans that deliver cool air to the face have been shown to decrease dyspnea both in patients with COPD and in normal volunteers (American Thoracic Society, 1999). This intervention is effective for any severity of dyspnea at any stage of disease (Booth, Moffat, Burkin, Galbraith, & Bausewein, 2011). The mechanism of action may be related to stimulation of trigeminal receptors in the face.

Positioning: Leaning forward while standing or sitting improves the efficiency of accessory muscles. This position improves diaphragmatic function, especially in hyperinflated lungs as seen in emphysema and chronic severe asthma (American Thoracic Society, 1999; Booth et al., 2011). It is useful mainly for patients with dyspnea at rest. Other beneficial positions include lying on one's side in a semi-recumbent position or leaning forward into a stack of pillows (Booth et al., 2011).

Energy conservation interventions: Slowing one's gait can reduce physical effort and decrease the sense of breathlessness at any stage of illness. It is important to encourage patients to pace themselves and use available energy for the most important tasks. Energy conservation techniques can promote a sense of control and well-being.

Walking aids: Walking aids, such as canes or walkers, can reduce exertional breathlessness and increase walking distance (Probst et al., 2004). They may decrease dyspnea by prompting the patient to lean forward while walking.

Exercise training and rehabilitation programs: Pulmonary rehabilitation programs improve exercise capacity, health related quality of life and dyspnea in patients with COPD (Ries et al., 2007). Patients with chronic progressive lung disorders should be encouraged to participate early on in their illness, as these programs are less effective at advanced stages of disease. In fact, they are not indicated in patients with end-stage disease. Further, pulmonary rehabilitation prior to the terminal phase of an illness can be helpful in alleviating anxiety at the end of life (Booth et al., 2011; Lanken et al., 2008). Mechanisms for improvement may include increased aerobic capacity, a smaller increase in lactate levels during exercise, knowledge and use of relaxation techniques, increased mechanical efficiency (longer stride length), improvement of self-esteem (with an associated reduction in anxiety and depression) and desensitization to the sensation of dyspnea during exertion (American Thoracic Society, 1999).

Anxiety reduction interventions: These approaches, which include education and psychotherapeutic interventions, are postulated to work by modifying the central perception of breathlessness. Educating the patient about his or her disease and teaching and encouraging coping strategies can help patients feel a greater sense of control, which in turn, may improve their experience of breathlessness (Ben-Aharon, Gafter-Gvili, Paul, Leibovici, & Stemmer, 2008; Schwartzstein & Adams, 2010). Cognitive-behavioral approaches to modify the affective response have been shown to modify the intensity of the symptom. Sharing experiences with others in support groups and psychotherapy decreases patients' emotional distress and improves dyspnea in chronic lung disease (Ries et al., 2007; Schwartzstein & Adams, 2010). These interventions are more appropriate at earlier stages of disease, as they require motivation and active participation on the part of the patient.

Noninvasive positive pressure ventilation: The use of non-invasive ventilation can allow respiratory muscles to rest in patients with increased ventilatory demand due to increased respiratory muscle use. This intervention might reduce the need for intubation, the length of hospitalization, mortality, and dyspnea in patients with COPD exacerbations (Del Fabbro et al., 2006). It might also have a role in patients with acute CHF decompensation and in patients with amyotrophic lateral sclerosis. Unfortunately, these types of masks, which must fit tightly, can be highly uncomfortable and many patients cannot tolerate them. Clinicians must assess and discuss the burdens and benefits of this intervention, particularly at the end of life.

Other proven interventions include the use of specific breathing techniques such as diaphragmatic or pursed lip breathing, neuromuscular electrical stimulation to improve respiratory muscle weakness, use of music as an attention-diverting strategy, and acupuncture and acupressure.

PHARMACOLOGIC INTERVENTIONS

Oxygen therapy: There are both medical and symptomatic indications for chronic oxygen therapy. Medical indications include oxygen for any patient who is hypoxemic. Chronic hypoxemia can lead to the sequelae of pulmonary hypertension. In COPD patients who are severely hypoxemic, oxygen therapy prolongs survival and improves symptoms. In patients with chronic hypoxemia from other causes (e.g., interstitial lung disease, neuromuscular disease), oxygen therapy is indicated only for symptomatic relief. It does not modify patient survival. Side effects of oxygen therapy that should be taken into consideration when prescribing it include airway damage due to the direct effect of oxygen reactive species on the respiratory mucosa, and carbon dioxide retention, due to decreased lung ventilation induced by the abolition of the hypoxemic respiratory stimulus by increased blood oxygen levels. The role of oxygen therapy in non-hypoxemic patients is less clear. A recent randomized controlled trial compared the effect of oxygen versus room air (administered by nasal cannula) in relieving dyspnea in non-hypoxemic patients with advanced disease. The study demonstrated that oxygen is no better than room air (Abernethy et al., 2010). Both groups of patients had improved dyspnea at the end of the one-week study, supporting the idea that air movement near the face may improve the sensation of breathlessness.

Opioids: This family of drugs is the most effective for the treatment of dyspnea. They stimulate opioid receptors not only in the CNS, but also peripherally and in the lungs in particular. Opioids relieve dyspnea and improve exercise capacity in patients with COPD (Thomas & von Gunten, 2002). A systematic review of the use of opioids in patients with terminal disease from cancer, congestive heart failure, or COPD supports the use of oral and parenteral opioids for palliation of dyspnea (Jennings, Davies, Higgins, Gibbs, & Broadley, 2002). This same review did not show improvement of breathlessness when opioids were administered via inhalation. Side effects from opioids should be continuously assessed. The doses of opioids needed to treat dyspnea tend to be lower than those required for pain and do not affect respiratory rate or oxygen saturation if used appropriately (Thomas & von Gunten, 2002). In general, one should start with the lowest dose and titrate up cautiously. One would start with short-acting oral opioids and add in a long-acting opioid (such as long acting morphine) only if the patient was using more than the equivalent dose of the long-acting opioid in a 24-hour period. When starting a long acting opioid, it is good practice to continue the short acting opioid as needed for breakthrough dyspnea. Opioid starting doses for patients with chronic lung disease are described in Table 27.4. In patients with concurrent pain already on opioids, you can increase the opioids by about 25%. All of the various opioids relieve dyspnea equally. In general, patients quickly develop tolerance to the sedating effects of opioids if started slowly and titrated carefully, and clinicians need not be fearful of causing significant sedation or respiratory depression. On the other hand, patients rarely develop tolerance —or the need for increasing doses to obtain the same anti-dyspnea effect—to

Table 27.4 OPIOID DOSING IN PATIENTS WITH CHRONIC LUNG DISEASE

OPIOID	STARTING ORAL DOSE (SHORT-ACTING)	*STARTING ORAL DOSE (LONG-ACTING)	STARTING IV DOSE
Morphine	5–10 mg po q4 hours prn dyspnea	Long-acting morphine (e.g., MS Contin) 15 mg po q12 hours	1–2 mg IV q4 hours prn dyspnea
Oxycodone	5–10 mg po q4 hours prn dypsnea	Long-acting oxycodone (e.g., OxyContin) 10 mg po q12 hours	No IV formulation
Hydromorphone	1–2 mg po q4 hours prn dyspnea	No long acting formulation on the market currently	0.1–0.2 mg IV q3 hours prn dysnpea

*Only start long-acting if the patient is taking more than the equivalent dose of short-acting in a 24-hour period.

the anti-dypsnea effects of opioids. Most often, the need for increasing doses would signify a worsening of the underlying disease process. All patients on opioids develop physiologic dependence on opioids such that they will experience withdrawal symptoms if the medications are stopped suddenly.

Anxiolytics: In a systematic review of interventions for alleviating cancer-related dyspnea, only one study was identified that assessed the effect of benzodiazepines. In this study, the addition of a benzodiazepine to an opioid eased the sense of breathlessness compared to the opioid alone, without additional adverse effects (Ben-Aharon et al., 2008). However, there is no evidence to support the routine use of benzodiazepines in the management of dyspnea (Del Fabbro et al., 2006). Still, they may have a role in patients with significant anxiety related to their dyspnea. The clinician should monitor side effects closely and start the medications in sequence, not in parallel. One can also consider low-dose neuroleptics (e.g., quetiapine or olanzapine) or an SSRI for the chronic anxiety component related to the dyspnea. Given the high incidence of confusion or delirium in elderly patients or patients with chronic illness receiving benzodiazepines, as well as the potent sedation caused by the combination of opioids and benzodiazepines, many palliative care clinicians choose to use neuroleptics for anxiety related to dyspnea.

SUMMARY

Dyspnea is a common symptom in patients with cancer, cardiopulmonary disease and neuromuscular conditions that affect respiratory muscles. Anxiety often accompanies the dyspnea. While gaps in our knowledge remain, dyspnea is thought to represent a mismatch between the central respiratory motor command and incoming afferent information from sensory receptors. The perception of dyspnea is highly influenced by emotions. The history and physical examination and the judicious use of laboratory and functional tests will help identify the possible etiologies and underlying mechanisms of dyspnea. Treatment should be focused first and whenever possible on the underlying cause of the dyspnea and on the symptom itself when disease-modifying interventions are ineffective or have become burdensome. Opioids and other interventions, pharmacologic and non-pharmacologic, can be implemented effectively for the symptomatic treatment

of dyspnea. The challenge is to combine the tools of medicine and psychiatry to affect the emotional dimension.

CLINICAL PEARLS

- The *perception* of dyspnea refers to the unique manner in which a particular individual experiences breathlessness and it consists of three distinct dimensions: a sensory dimension, i.e., the intensity of the symptom; an affective dimension, i.e., how unpleasant the symptom is; and a functional dimension, i.e., the impact or burden of the symptom.

- Dyspnea in patients with stable asthma is explained by both the degree of airway obstruction and patient's emotional status (Martinez-Moragon, Perpina, Belloch, de Diego, & Martinez-Frances, 2003).

- In severe dyspnea, the insular cortex and anterior cingulated gyrus, both part of the limbic system, are activated in functional imaging studies. This evidence correlates well with what we know clinically, that the experience of dyspnea is often accompanied by anxiety and fear.

- Individuals experiencing dyspnea who are able to shift their attention to external stimuli have decreased sense of breathlessness (Thornby, Haas, & Axen, 1995). Likewise, patients with COPD who listen to music while on a rehabilitation program improve their performance compared to patients who do not listen to music (Bauldoff, Hoffman, Zullo, & Sciurba, 2002).

- Negative emotions have been shown to be associated with decreased accuracy in dyspnea perception (De Peuter et al., 2004).

- Both types of dyspnea, "air hunger" and "increased work of breathing" are associated with increased respiratory drive. A third description of dyspnea is "chest tightness." This phrase is often used by asthmatics and is thought to be associated with bronchoconstriction

- Hand-held fans that deliver cool air to the face have been shown to decrease dyspnea both in patients with COPD and in normal volunteers (American Thoracic Society, 1999). This intervention is effective for any severity of dyspnea at any stage of disease (Booth, Moffat, Burkin, Galbraith, & Bausewein, 2011).

- For dypsnea at rest, leaning forward while standing or sitting improves the efficiency of accessory muscles.

- Walking aids, such as canes or walkers, can reduce exertional breathlessness and increase walking distance (Probst et al., 2004).

- Cognitive-behavioral approaches to modify the affective response have been shown to modify the intensity of dyspnea. Sharing experiences with others in support groups and psychotherapy decreases patients' emotional distress and improves dyspnea in chronic lung disease (Ries et al., 2007; Schwartzstein & Adams, 2010).

- The role of oxygen therapy in non-hypoxemic patients is less clear. A recent randomized controlled trial compared the effect of oxygen versus room air (administered by nasal cannula) in relieving dyspnea in non-hypoxemic patients with advanced disease. The study demonstrated that oxygen is no better than room air (Abernethy et al., 2010).

- Opioids relieve dyspnea and improve exercise capacity in patients with COPD (Thomas & von Gunten, 2002).

DISCLOSURE STATEMENTS

Dr. Pérez-Cruz has no conflicts of interest to disclose.

Dr. Chittenden has no conflicts of interest to disclose.

REFERENCES

Abernethy, A. P., McDonald, C. F., Frith, P. A., Clark, K., Herndon, J. E., 2nd, Marcello, J., et al. (2010). Effect of palliative oxygen versus room air in relief of breathlessness in patients with refractory dyspnoea: a double-blind, randomised controlled trial. *Lancet*, *376*(9743), 784–793.

Abrams, K., Rassovsky, Y., & Kushner, M. G. (2006). Evidence for respiratory and nonrespiratory subtypes in panic disorder. *Depression and Anxiety*, *23*(8), 474–481.

American Thoracic Society. (1999). Dyspnea. Mechanisms, assessment, and management: a consensus statement. *American Journal of Respiriratory and Critical Care Medicine*, *159*(1), 321–340.

Bauldoff, G. S., Hoffman, L. A., Zullo, T. G., & Sciurba, F. C. (2002). Exercise maintenance following pulmonary rehabilitation: effect of distractive stimuli. *Chest*, *122*(3), 948–954.

Bausewein, C., Booth, S., Gysels, M., & Higginson, I. (2008). Non-pharmacological interventions for breathlessness in advanced stages of malignant and non-malignant diseases. *Cochrane Database of Systematic Reviews*, (2), CD005623.

Ben-Aharon, I., Gafter-Gvili, A., Paul, M., Leibovici, L., & Stemmer, S. M. (2008). Interventions for alleviating cancer-related dyspnea: a systematic review. *Journal of Clinical Oncology*, *26*(14), 2396–2404.

Bogaerts, K., Notebaert, K., Van Diest, I., Devriese, S., De Peuter, S., & Van den Bergh, O. (2005). Accuracy of respiratory symptom perception in different affective contexts. *Journal of Psychosomatic Research*, *58*(6), 537–543.

Booth, S., Moffat, C., Burkin, J., Galbraith, S., & Bausewein, C. (2011). Nonpharmacological interventions for breathlessness. *Current Opinion in Supportive and Palliative Care*, *5*(2), 77–86.

Borg, G. A. (1982). Psychophysical bases of perceived exertion. *Medicine & Science in Sports & Exercise*, *14*(5), 377–381.

Burki, N. K., & Lee, L. Y. (2010). Mechanisms of dyspnea. *Chest*, *138*(5), 1196–1201.

Chavannes, N. H., Huibers, M. J., Schermer, T. R., Hendriks, A., van Weel, C., Wouters, E. F., & van Schayck, C. P. (2005). Associations of depressive symptoms with gender, body mass index and dyspnea in primary care COPD patients. *Family Practice*, *22*(6), 604–607.

Dales, R. E., Spitzer, W. O., Schechter, M. T., & Suissa, S. (1989). The influence of psychological status on respiratory symptom reporting. *American Review of Respiratory Disease*, *139*(6), 1459–1463.

De Peuter, S., Van Diest, I., Lemaigre, V., Verleden, G., Demedts, M., & Van den Bergh, O. (2004). Dyspnea: the role of psychological processes. *Clinical Psychology Reviews*, *24*(5), 557–581.

Del Fabbro, E., Dalal, S., & Bruera, E. (2006). Symptom control in palliative care—Part III: dyspnea and delirium. *Journal of Palliative Medicine*, *9*(2), 422–436.

Duffin, J., & Phillipson, E. A. (2010). Hypoventilation and Hyperventilation Syndromes. In J. F. Murray & R. J. Mason (Eds.), *Murray and Nadel's textbook of respiratory medicine* (5th ed., pp. 1859–1880). Philadelphia, PA: Saunders/Elsevier.

Esteban, C., Quintana, J. M., Aburto, M., Moraza, J., Egurrola, M., Espana, P. P., . . . Capelastegui, A. (2008). Predictors of mortality in patients with stable COPD. *Journal of General Internal Medicine*, *23*(11), 1829–1834.

Evans, K. C., Shea, S. A., & Saykin, A. J. (1999). Functional MRI localisation of central nervous system regions associated with volitional inspiration in humans. *Journal of Physiology*, *520 Pt 2*, 383–392.

Fletcher, C. M., Elmes, P. C., Fairbairn, A. S., & Wood, C. H. (1959). The significance of respiratory symptoms and the diagnosis of chronic bronchitis in a working population. *British Medical Journal*, *2*(5147), 257–266.

Gift, A. G., & Cahill, C. A. (1990). Psychophysiologic aspects of dyspnea in chronic obstructive pulmonary disease: a pilot study. *Heart Lung*, *19*(3), 252–257.

Hasler, G., Gergen, P. J., Kleinbaum, D. G., Ajdacic, V., Gamma, A., Eich, D., . . . Angst, J. (2005). Asthma and panic in young adults: a 20-year prospective community study. *American Journal of Respiratory and Critical Care Medicine*, *171*(11), 1224–1230.

Jennings, A. L., Davies, A. N., Higgins, J. P., Gibbs, J. S., & Broadley, K. E. (2002). A systematic review of the use of opioids in the management of dyspnoea. *Thorax*, *57*(11), 939–944.

Katon, W. (1984). Panic disorder and somatization. Review of 55 cases. *American Journal of Medicine*, *77*(1), 101–106.

Katon, W., Ries, R. K., & Kleinman, A. (1984). The prevalence of somatization in primary care. *Comprehensive Psychiatry*, *25*(2), 208–215.

Katon, W. J., Richardson, L., Lozano, P., & McCauley, E. (2004). The relationship of asthma and anxiety disorders. *Psychosomatic Medicine*, *66*(3), 349–355.

Kroenke, K., & Rosmalen, J. G. (2006). Symptoms, syndromes, and the value of psychiatric diagnostics in patients who have functional somatic disorders. *Medical Clinics of North America*, *90*(4), 603–626.

Lanken, P. N., Terry, P. B., Delisser, H. M., Fahy, B. F., Hansen-Flaschen, J., Heffner, J. E., et al. (2008). An official American Thoracic Society clinical policy statement: palliative care for patients with respiratory diseases and critical illnesses. *American Journal of Respiratory and Critical Care Medicine*, *177*(8), 912–927.

Mahler, D. A., Harver, A., Lentine, T., Scott, J. A., Beck, K., & Schwartzstein, R. M. (1996). Descriptors of breathlessness in cardiorespiratory diseases. *American Journal of Respiratory and Critical Care Medicine*, *154*(5), 1357–1363.

Martinez-Moragon, E., Perpina, M., Belloch, A., de Diego, A., & Martinez-Frances, M. (2003). Determinants of dyspnea in patients with different grades of stable asthma. *Journal of Asthma*, *40*(4), 375–382.

Neuman, A., Gunnbjornsdottir, M., Tunsater, A., Nystrom, L., Franklin, K. A., Norrman, E., & Janson, C. (2006). Dyspnea in relation to symptoms of anxiety and depression: A prospective population study. *Respiratory Medicine, 100*(10), 1843–1849.

Nishino, T. (2011). Dyspnoea: underlying mechanisms and treatment. *British Journal of Anaesthesia, 106*(4), 463–474.

Parshall, M. B., Schwartzstein, R. M., Adams, L., Banzett, R. B., Manning, H. L., Bourbeau, J., et al; American Thoracic Society Committee on Dyspnea. (2012). An official American Thoracic Society statement: update on the mechanisms, assessment, and management of dyspnea. *American Journal of Respiratory and Critical Care Medicine, 185*(4), 435–452.

Pauwels, R. A., Buist, A. S., Calverley, P. M., Jenkins, C. R., & Hurd, S. S. (2001). Global strategy for the diagnosis, management, and prevention of chronic obstructive pulmonary disease. NHLBI/WHO Global Initiative for Chronic Obstructive Lung Disease (GOLD) Workshop summary. *American Journal of Respiratory and Critical Care Medicine, 163*(5), 1256–1276.

Periyakoil, V. S., Skultety, K., & Sheikh, J. (2005). Panic, anxiety, and chronic dyspnea. *Journal of Palliative Medicine, 8*(2), 453–459.

Potter, J., Hami, F., Bryan, T., & Quigley, C. (2003). Symptoms in 400 patients referred to palliative care services: prevalence and patterns. *Palliative Medicine, 17*(4), 310–314.

Probst, V. S., Troosters, T., Coosemans, I., Spruit, M. A., Pitta Fde, O., Decramer, M., & Gosselink, R. (2004). Mechanisms of improvement in exercise capacity using a rollator in patients with COPD. *Chest, 126*(4), 1102–1107.

Ramasamy, R., Hildebrandt, T., O'Hea, E., Patel, M., Clemow, L., Freudenberger, R., & Skotzko, C. (2006). Psychological and social factors that correlate with dyspnea in heart failure. *Psychosomatics, 47*(5), 430–434.

Reuben, D. B., & Mor, V. (1986). Dyspnea in terminally ill cancer patients. *Chest, 89*(2), 234–236.

Ries, A. L., Bauldoff, G. S., Carlin, B. W., Casaburi, R., Emery, C. F., Mahler, D. A., et al. (2007). Pulmonary Rehabilitation: Joint ACCP/AACVPR Evidence-Based Clinical Practice Guidelines. *Chest, 131*(5 Suppl), 4S–42S.

Rietveld, S., Everaerd, W., & Vanbeest, I. (1999). Can biased symptom perception explain false-alarm choking sensations? *Psychological Medicine, 29*(1), 121–126.

Schwartzstein, R. M., & Adams, L. (2010). Dyspnea. In J. F. Murray & R. J. Mason (Eds.), *Murray and Nadel's textbook of respiratory medicine* (5th ed., Vol. 1, pp. 613–627). Philadelphia, PA: Saunders/Elsevier.

Stuart, B. (2007). Palliative care and hospice in advanced heart failure. *Journal of Palliative Medicine, 10*(1), 210–228.

Thomas, J. R., & von Gunten, C. F. (2002). Clinical management of dyspnoea. *Lancet Oncology, 3*(4), 223–228.

Thornby, M. A., Haas, F., & Axen, K. (1995). Effect of distractive auditory stimuli on exercise tolerance in patients with COPD. *Chest, 107*(5), 1213–1217.

Xue, D., & Abernethy, A. P. (2010). Management of dyspnea in advanced lung cancer: recent data and emerging concepts. *Current Opinion in Supportive and Palliative Care, 4*(2), 85–91.

28.

THERAPEUTIC NUTRIENTS, HERBS, AND HORMONES

Patricia L. Gerbarg and Richard P. Brown

Editors' Preface

The editors think that Gerbarg and Brown's chapter on nutrients, herbs, and hormones in medical psychiatry warrants a special preface. In their chapter the authors present a thoughtful assessment of the current status of alternative, integrative, and less conventional nonprescription treatments for mental and behavioral symptoms. They present the scientific evidence related to the efficacy and safety of the most widely used nutrients, herbs, and nonprescription hormones, and describe how they use them in their own specialized integrative psychopharmacologic practice. Many of the treatments in this chapter are not yet considered to be part of standard psychiatric practice. Consequently, many medical psychiatrists are not cognizant of their potential benefits and do not know how to integrate these therapies into their practices. Virtually all psychiatrists treating patients with general medical illness will encounter individuals presenting for consultation who are already using these complementary and alternative treatments, or will have patients or family members asking whether such treatments might be helpful. When a patient presents for consultation already taking a nutrient, herb, or nonprescription hormone that is working well for its target symptoms and not causing adverse effects, if the clinician counsels discontinuation because he or she does not personally favor the treatment it will potentially worsen the clinical outcome. On the other hand, many patients who take such treatments on their own are unaware of potential interactions with prescription drugs and with general medical diseases and, as a result, take risks of which they are not aware.

Most of the treatments described in this chapter are not classified as pharmaceuticals by the US Food and Drug Administration; all are legal nonprescription supplements sold without claims of efficacy for any specific disease; some are prescription medications used by conventional psychiatrists in Europe. For some of the agents discussed here, the evidence from controlled clinical trials is similar in amount and quality to the evidence used to support a prescription drug's marketing approval. For others the evidence is less, and the support for use of the agent is based on a combination of open or pilot studies, personal and anecdotal clinical experience, preclinical data, and

the putative mechanism of action. Inquiring whether patients are using alternative therapies is essential, and, when they are, the medical psychiatrist must check an appropriate database for interactions of the agents being used with the patient's diseases and prescription drugs. It is also recommended, if feasible, to check each agent to determine whether the manufacturer is known to make a product of reliable potency and purity. Recommending alternative treatments is an optional part of medical psychiatric practice.

Medical-psychiatric patients are potentially attracted to nonprescription alternative treatments for several reasons: (1) they may believe that they are safer; (2) they may have a philosophical preference for "natural" treatments; (3) they may have had relevant personal or vicarious experience, either positive with alternative treatments and/or negative with conventional prescribed drug therapies; (4) many patients are unable to tolerate side effects from prescription medications; (5) complementary and alternative treatments may be less expensive and insurance companies often refuse to cover phsyician recommended prescription medications; (6) taking supplements without a doctor's prescription may give the patient a greater sense of control over his/her treatment in a context of general medical illness that always entails some loss of control over one's life; and (7) taking an agent to treat symptoms, with no psychiatric diagnosis (documentation of the diagnosis is necessary for a prescription medication) avoids potential stigma, keeps psychiatric content out of the medical record, and protects the patient from being identified as having a psychiatric disorder that could jeopardize their career if it became known, for example commercial pilots who are subject to drug testing and active duty military personnel. Medical psychiatrists frequently encounter patients who are open to herbal and nutritional therapies at a time when they would not accept a psychotropic drug prescription. The most common reason for consulting specialists in integrative psychopharmacology is that many, if not all, categories of conventional prescription treatments have been tried and failed. In such cases the physician must decide between telling the patient there is nothing left to offer relief or broadening the treatment options by integrating low risk, less conventional approaches.

In counseling a patient to begin an alternative treatment—or even to continue one the patient has already started—the psychiatrist assumes clinical and legal responsibility. The clinician should share with the patient what is known about the risks and benefits of the agent(s) involved and how they might interact with the patient's diseases and other treatments, and why the patient might do better with the alternative treatment than a conventional prescription psychotropic. This discussion should be documented in the record. Finally, the patient's treatment choice and response to treatment should be documented in the medical record.

INTRODUCTION

Medical patients suffer from the psychological effects of their medical conditions, the direct and indirect stressors of their illnesses, and the medications and procedures used to treat these conditions. Therapeutic nutrients and herbs have an emerging role in ameliorating neuropsychiatric and physical symptoms in medical patients. Synthetic psychotropic medications used to treat anxiety, insomnia, depression, and cognitive impairment can add to the burden of side effects in medical patients who may be more susceptible to adverse reactions and medication interactions. Furthermore, prescription anxiolytics, sedative hypnotics, and analgesics have the potential for habituation, addiction, overdose, and withdrawal symptoms. In general, herbs and nutrients have far fewer side effects and far less addiction potential. Rather than taking an encyclopedic approach, this chapter focuses on clinically useful treatments, their mechanisms of action, and the evidence for safety and efficacy. The safety of most herbs during pregnancy and breastfeeding has not been adequately studied. Herb–drug interactions and the use of herbs to counteract medication side effects are covered in the last sections of this chapter. Summaries of dose ranges, side effects, and drug interactions, are provided in Tables 28.1, 28.2 and 28.3.

Many herbs and nutrients have been considered to be part of complementary and alternative medicine (CAM). Advances in neurophysiology, molecular biology, and genomics have created a deeper understanding of the mechanisms of action and the potential benefits of treatments that were previously considered outside the purview of conventional medicine. Integrative medicine and integrative psychiatry are emerging fields that cultivate integrative approaches using herbs, nutrients, neurohormones, mind–body practices, and mainstream medical treatments.

GENERAL ISSUES IN THE PURSUIT OF QUALITY

STANDARDIZATION OF SUPPLEMENTS

Considerable progress has occurred in the standardization of botanical extracts based on the concentration of marker compounds believed to be essential for therapeutic activity and/or to be unique to the species. High-pressure liquid chromatography (HLPC) can be employed to measure the presence and concentration of marker compounds, and for most herbs this is sufficient. However, for certain rare and more expensive herbs, adulteration may still occur by "spiking" the product with marker chemicals. Usually the reporting of one or two marker compounds is adequate, but the testing of more marker compounds or comparison of the complete HPLC profiles would be preferable for more complex herbs. The ultimate test of an extract is proven efficacy in a good quality controlled trial, published in a peer-reviewed journal.

Most supplements are stable enough that their quality is not significantly affected by differences in processing. In this chapter, complex products whose quality is more affected by differences in cultivation and extraction procedures—for example, *Ginkgo biloba, Hypericum perforatum* (St. John's wort) and *Rhodiola rosea* (Arctic root)—will be identified. The relative amounts of active compounds in herbs are affected by the soil, climate, time of harvest, and age of the plant at the time of harvest. The composition of plant extracts depends upon the method of drying and extraction. Some compounds are soluble in water, others in alcohol. Procedures for extraction of certain herbs, such as *R. rosea*, use either water or alcohol or both. Volatile compounds can be lost if subjected to excessively high temperature during processing. Extracts are sold to companies that encapsulate and market products under various brand names. Companies may change the source of raw product as the cost and availability of plant extracts change. Product labels rarely state the source of extracts. *Ginkgo biloba* is one exception. Many products containing *Ginkgo biloba* identify their content as, for example, EGb 761 or Kira, which are both known to be reliable, potent extracts based on numerous scientific studies in which they were used. For other complex herbs, additional investigation is needed to identify products containing high-quality extracts. For example, the Swedish Herbal Institute has a long history of producing high-quality products with demonstrated efficacy in research studies. In determining the appropriate dosage, it is important to note not only the milligrams of the marker compounds but also the percentage of those marker compounds. For example, 150 mg of an *R. rosea* product containing 4% of marker compounds called *rosavins* is more potent than a brand containing 3% rosavins. The authors have provided lists of high-quality products in previous publications (Brown, Gerbarg, & Muskin, 2009; Brown & Gerbarg, 2011). Proprietary preparations do not always reveal the exact amount of each component. Companies may consider secrecy to be a business necessity; however, prescribing a product without knowing its exact contents is problematic for clinicians.

Improved verification of the authenticity and quality of herbal products is evolving with new technologies. Ideally, in the future herbs may be identified by genomic analysis, the concentration of key constituents assessed at each stage of production, and supplement brands systematically tested for purity and efficacy.

REGULATORY ISSUES

Each country has its own regulatory processes. Within the US Food and Drug Administration (FDA) the Center for Food Safety and Applied Nutrition monitors the safety of dietary supplements and the accuracy of labels and inserts. The US Federal Trade Commission requires and oversees truthfulness in product advertising (www.ftc.gov).

RELIABLE SOURCES FOR INFORMATION ABOUT QUALITY AND SAFETY OF SUPPLEMENTS

Information on the safety of specific supplements is available at the FDA website: www.fda.gov/Food/Dietary Supplements/Alerts. The "Alerts and Advisories" section of the National Center for Complementary and Alternative medicine (NCCAM) posts information about problematic supplements at www.nccam.nih.gov/news/alerts. The National Institute of Health National Library of Medicine maintains the *Dietary Supplement Labels Database* containing information about the ingredients in over 2,000 brands of supplements on their website, www.dietarysupplements.nlm.nih.gov/dietary.

In Germany, the German *Commission E* closely regulates the quality of phytomedicines and publishes highly respected monographs that are available at http://cms.herbalgram.org/commissione/index.html.

The American Herbal Pharmacopoeia (AHP) maintains authentic botanical reference materials to insure the identity and quality of medicinal plants. These are used by academic institutions, researchers, supplement manufacturers, and those who evaluate products, such as ConsumerLab. The AHP publishes scholarly qualitative and therapeutic monographs and books on herb safety (see http://www.herbal-ahp.org/order_online.htm).

The American Botanical Council (ABC) is an independent, nonprofit research and education organization that provides reliable information about herbs for consumers, healthcare practitioners, researchers, industry, and the media. The ABC publications are peer reviewed and include periodicals, books, monographs, safety reviews, continuing education materials, and searchable online databases. *Herbalgram*, the quarterly journal of the ABC, publishes extensive articles on the history of phytomedicines, modern uses, and current issues that affect cultivation and quality. *HerbClips* reviews current research studies and books. The ABC website is accessible at http://abc.herbalgram.org/site/PageServer.

The *Natural Medicines Comprehensive Database* (NMCD) covers a great deal of information, even on obscure herbs, with yearly updates. The drawbacks are that it cites articles that mention side effects even if based on weak or nonvalidated evidence. Most of the information is accurate, but some is not. Consequently, the long lists of potential side effects may include nonvalidated items, speculations based on information from in vitro or animal studies, or equivocal cases. The burden is on the reader to check the original citations to determine the degree of validity and clinical relevance of the information (Jellin, 2010).

ConsumerLab.com is one of the best nongovernmental resources for up-to-date, detailed, practical information on most of the supplements encountered in clinical practice. Companies pay a fee to ConsumerLab to analyze and report on the contents and quality of their products. Clinicians and consumers pay a modest annual fee for access to reports that cover thousands of brands. ConsumerLab purchases products from stores, not directly from the manufacturer, and sends them to independent laboratories for HPLC assessment of marker compounds and other constituents that play a role in therapeutic action. Products are tested for lead and other contaminants as appropriate. A passing score is given to products that meet US Pharmacopoeia standards for tablet disintegration, fulfill FDA labeling requirements, contain 100% of the label claims for content, do not exceed legal levels for lead contamination, and meet other product-specific quality indices.

Herbal Contraindications and Drug Interactions by Francis Brinker is an excellent resource providing precise explanations on the sources of information, limitations and contradictions in the literature, and the complexity of the available evidence (Brinker, 2010). The publisher posts free updates at www.eclecticherb.com/emp.

Herbs, Nutrients and Yoga in Mental Health Care by Richard P. Brown, Patricia Gerbarg, and Philip Muskin is a practical clinician's guide that includes sources of quality products, recommended dosages, how to combine standard, complementary, and alternative treatments, and case illustrations (Brown, Gerbarg, & Muskin, 2009).

REPORTING SIDE EFFECTS AND ADVERSE REACTIONS

As with prescription medications, adverse reactions to phytomedicines and nutritional supplements are underreported. Side effects can be reported to MedWatch by phone (1-888-463-6332) or through the FDA website at www.fda.gov/safety/MedWatch/How   ToReport/ucm053074.htms. For reporting serious adverse reactions, healthcare providers may call the MedWatch hotline at 1-800-FDA-1088.

LIABILITY ISSUES

Individuals who request CAM treatments are entitled to the same quality of diagnostic evaluation as those who seek conventional treatments. Malpractice experts note that the following categories of malpractice could be applied to CAM: misdiagnosis, failure to treat, failure of informed consent, fraud and misrepresentation, abandonment, vicarious liability, and breach of privacy and confidentiality (Cohen & Schouten, 2007). In general, the approach to liability issues—and to all categories of liability in integrative mental healthcare using nutrients and herbs—are similar to those for standard practices. The issue of failure to treat raises several potential scenarios worth noting:

1. The risk of liability is less if scientific evidence supports the safety and efficacy of a CAM treatment. In cases in

which a patient does not tolerate or respond to conventional treatments and whose condition could be treated effectively with a reasonably safe CAM therapy, one could argue that it would be negligent not to inform the patient of the CAM treatment and offer the option to try it.

2. If scientific evidence indicates that a particular CAM treatment is ineffective or is likely to cause harm, then the practitioner should try to dissuade the patient.

3. If the evidence for safety or efficacy of a CAM treatment is equivocal, then the patient should be informed of all known potential risks as well as the quality of the evidence both in favor and against the treatment. If the patient chooses to try the treatment after this discussion (and the discussion has been documented in the chart), then the practitioner should monitor the patient during the trial for benefits and side effects and should intervene if any adverse reactions occur.

4. If the patient has a condition that could be easily or rapidly cured by standard treatment, and if the use of CAM delays effective treatment such that the patient suffers harm or illness progresses, this could be considered malpractice, negligence, or substandard care.

The same principles that govern informed consent in conventional treatments can be applied to CAM. Each state has specific regulations governing the practice of CAM. The U.S. Federation of State Medical Boards (FSMB) has approved model guidelines for the use of CAM therapies in medical practice (Federation of State Medical Boards, 2007; see http://www.fsmb.org/pdf/2002_grpol_complementary_alternative_therapies.pdf). The FSMB recommends that the physician conduct an appropriate medical history, physical examination, and review of patient medical records before offering any recommendation for treatment. The FSMB Guidelines note that

"The evaluation shall include, but not be limited to, conventional methods of diagnosis and may include other methods of diagnosis as long as the methodology utilized for diagnosis is based upon the same standards of safety and reliability as conventional methods, and shall be documented in the patient's medical record. The medical record shall also document:

- what medical options have been discussed, offered or tried, and if so, to what effect, or a statement as to whether or not certain options have been refused by the patient or guardian; that proper referral has been offered for appropriate treatment;

- that the risks and benefits of the use of the recommended treatment to the extent known have been appropriately discussed with the patient or guardian;

- that the physician has determined the extent to which the treatment could interfere with any other recommended or ongoing treatment."

In their discussion of liability issues Brown, Gerberg, and Muskin include an example of a note for documentation of the decision-making process that leads to the use of a CAM treatment (Brown, Gerberg, & Muskin, 2009).

ANXIETY DISORDERS AND INSOMNIA

NUTRIENTS FOR ANXIETY DISORDERS AND INSOMNIA

Evaluating the nutritional status of medical patients is part of standard practice. Nutritional deficiencies develop in association with poor diet, chronic illness, loss of appetite, aging, dementia, chemotherapy, malabsorption, gastrointestinal problems, and substance abuse.

Gamma-aminobutyric Acid

Gamma-aminobutyric acid (GABA), the major central nervous system inhibitory neurotransmitter, is involved in cardiovascular regulation, pituitary function, immunity, fertilization, and renal function. Many foods contain small amounts of GABA, and fermented food products may contain high levels. Natural GABA produced by fermentation is widely used as a functional food supplement in Japan.

The effects on EEG of 100 mg of GABA produced by natural fermentation (pharma-GABA) were compared to 200 mg L-theanine and placebo in a double blind placebo controlled (DBPC) crossover study of 13 healthy adults. Alpha waves are associated with relaxed, effortless alertness. Beta waves occur in highly stressful situations and during difficulty with mental concentration. GABA intake resulted in a significantly greater increase in alpha and decrease in beta compared to both L-theanine and placebo control (Abdou et al., 2006). The high alpha/beta ratio indicates a state of arousal with relaxation or relaxed concentration. Low levels of salivary immunoglobulin-A (IgA) found in highly anxious individuals drop further in stressful situations. In a double blind randomized placebo controlled (DBRCT) study, 8 adults with acrophobia (fear of heights) walked across a suspension bridge 300 meters long and 54 meters above the ground. In the placebo group, IgA levels (a marker of stress and immune response) dropped substantially halfway across and at the end of the bridge. In comparison, in subjects given 100 mg GABA (pharma-GABA), IgA levels dropped only slightly midway and rose above baseline by the end of the bridge (Abdou et al., 2006).

Pregabalin is a synthetic structural analogue of GABA approved by the FDA for treatment of neuropathic pain and partial-onset seizures. It is being considered for approval as an adjunctive treatment for generalized anxiety disorder (GAD). Several randomized controlled trials (RCTs) confirm that pregabalin is comparable to lorazepam (Ativan), alprazolam (Xanax), and venlafaxine (Effexor) for moderate to severe GAD. Pregabalin is generally safe and well tolerated. Side effects include dizziness, somnolence, cognitive interference, incoordination, headache, and some potential for dependence. The onset of anxiolytic effects requires 1 week of daily treatment (Bandelow, Wedekind, & Leon, 2007). In clinical practice, the authors (PLG and RPB) use pregabalin only when first-line treatments have failed. Starting doses of 50 mg three times daily are titrated upward as tolerated.

L-lysine and L-arginine

Lysine is an essential limiting amino acid in wheat-based diets. In a 3-month DBRCT in poor Syrian families whose diet is based on wheat, lysine fortification of wheat resulted in improvements in anxiety and stress response (Smriga, Ghosh, Mouneimne, Pellett, & Scrimshaw, 2004). L-lysine combined with L-arginine may affect neurotransmitters involved in stress and anxiety. Acting as a partial serotonin receptor 4 (5-HT4) antagonist, L-lysine was found to reduce serum cortisol and brain–gut responses to stress. A study of men with high trait anxiety based on the Stait-Trait Anxiety Inventory found that L-lysine/L-arginine improved the ability to handle induced stress more than placebo (Jezova, Makatsori, Smriga, Morinaga, & Duncko, 2005). A double blind randomized placebo controlled (DBRPC) study found that after one week of L-lysine (2.64 g/day) plus L-arginine (2.64 g/day), healthy Japanese men had lower basal salivary cortisol levels and reduction in state anxiety (Smriga et al., 2007). Lysine supplementation may reduce anxiety in people with lysine-deficient diets. The combination of L-lysine and L-arginine may be useful in treating anxiety.

Magnesium in Combination Products

Although research has not shown magnesium monotherapy to be anxiolytic, a few studies of multivitamins containing magnesium show some positive effects. A multivitamin with calcium, magnesium, and zinc reduced anxiety in healthy young men in a 28-day DBRPC study (Carroll, Ring, Suter, & Willemsen, 2000). Another 1-month study of 200 mg magnesium plus 50 mg vitamin B_6 reduced premenstrual anxiety in a DBR crossover study (De Souza, Walker, Robinson, & Bolland, 2000). Without further study, however, anxiolytic effects in healthy normal subjects should not be extrapolated to those with anxiety disorders. In clinical practice, the authors (PLG and RPB) find 600–800 mg of magnesium to be beneficial for some anxious patients.

Omega-3 Fatty Acids

Although few studies have used omega-3 fatty acids (n-3 FAs) for anxiety disorders, evidence suggests that they may be beneficial, particularly in patients with low levels. Omega-3 FAs were approximately 30% lower in the red cell membranes of untreated patients with social anxiety disorder and showed a significant inverse correlation with social anxiety ratings (Green et al., 2006). In a 3-month DBRPC study of substance abusers with presumed poor dietary habits, 13 were given 3 gm of omega-3 polyunsaturated fatty acids (n-3 PUFAS; in this case, eicosapentaenoic acid, EPA + docosahexaenoic acid, DHA) versus 11 given placebo. Compared to the placebo group, those given n-3 PUFAS had significant progressive decline in anxiety scores over 6 months (Buydens-Branchey & Branchey, 2006). One DBRPC crossover trial of EPA alone in patients with obsessive compulsive disorder on serotonin reuptake inhibitors (SSRIs) found no effect on anxiety (Fux, Benjamin, & Nemets, 2004). It is possible that a combination of EPA + DHA might have been more effective than EPA alone. The testing of n-3 FA levels is not done routinely, but it is available. In light of the general health benefits and minimal side effects, n-3 FAs are worth trying in patients with anxiety disorders, particularly if nutrition has been compromised.

HERBAL TREATMENTS FOR ANXIETY DISORDERS

Traditional research has focused on isolating single active components from plants—for example, aspirin (salicylic acid) from white willow (*Salix alba*) or digitoxin from foxglove (*Digitalis purpurea*). However, many plant extracts contain tens or hundreds of bioactive compounds that often have synergistic and polyvalent effects (Sarris, Panossian, Schweitzer, Stough, & Scholey, 2011). *Synergy* implies that the sum of multiple compounds exerting one main biological effect is greater than the effect of any one alone. *Polyvalence* indicates that multiple biological actions contribute to an overall effect. This occurs when numerous constituents have varying physiological effects or when one constituent exerts multiple effects. Furthermore, one compound may influence the absorption, distribution, metabolism, or excretion of other components.

The mechanisms of action of phytomedicines include binding to neurotransmitters and receptors, effects on synthesis of neurotransmitters or the enzymes that metabolize them, stimulation or inhibition of CNS activities, modulation of neuroendocrine systems, neuroprotection (for example, against free radicals, oxidative stress, toxins, or hypoxia), enhancement of energy production and cellular repair, and support for neurogenesis. Sarris and colleagues (2011) use the term *herbomics* to mean the use of proteomic, genomic, and other "omic" technologies in herbal research. For example, in an animal model, after 8 weeks of daily doses St. John's wort extract (*Hypericum perforatum*) showed regulation of 66 genes compared with imipramine regulation of 74 genes. St. John's wort (SJW) and imipramine had 6 transcripts in common that were related to synaptic and energy metabolism (Wong et al., 2004).

A systematic review of clinical studies found strong evidence for herbal supplements containing passionflower (*Passiflora incarnata*) or kava (*Piper methysticum*) and insufficient evidence for SJW in the treatment of anxiety (Lakhan & Vieira, 2010). A subsequent review of psychopharmacological and clinical studies (Sarris et al., 2011) used the following defined levels of evidence:

A—meta-analysis or replicated RCTs with positive results;

B—one unreplicated RCT or studies with mixed but mainly positive results; or

C—one or more clinical trials with poor methodology or mixed evidence from clinical trials.

The level of clinical evidence for effects on anxiety was rated A for kava; and B for chamomile (*Matricaria recutita*), passionflower, and Arctic root or roseroot (*Rhodiola rosea*). Preclinical in vitro and animal studies indicate that anxiolytic phytomedicines commonly affect the GABA system by reducing CNS stimulation and quieting the overactivity of the amygdala that occurs in posttraumatic stress disorder (PTSD) and other anxiety disorders. Anxiolytic herbs that inhibit two enzymes known to metabolize GABA were tested in rat brain homogenates. Extracts of lemon balm (*Melissa officinalis*) showed the strongest inhibition of GABA transaminase; extracts of chamomile (*Matricicaria recutita*) and hops (*Humulus lupulus*) significantly inhibited glutamate acid decarboxylase (Awad et al., 2007).

Matricaria recutita (Chamomile)

Chamomile grows in Europe, Asia, North America, and Australia. The aromatic flowers are used to make tea. Active constituents include terpine bisabolol, farnesene, chamazulene, flavonoids (including apigenin, quescetin, patuletin, and luteolin) and coumarin. Traditional uses are for stomach ache and irritable bowel syndrome, and as a gentle sleep aid, mild laxative, antiinflammatory, and bactericidal. An 8-week RCT of moderately anxious GAD patients given 220–1100 mg/day of standardized chamomile extract found significant improvement on Hamilton Anxiety scores versus placebo (Amsterdam et al., 2009). Apigenin, a component of chamomile with high affinity for benzodiazepine GABA receptors, modulates monoamine neurotransmission and neuroendocrine activity but exerts minimal sedative or muscle-relaxant effects. Chamomile can trigger allergic reactions in people who have ragweed allergy. In one case a 70-year-old patient on warfarin experienced increased internal bleeding when she drank chamomile tea (Segal & Pilote, 2006).

Ginkgo biloba (Ginkgo)

An extract of ginkgo (EGb 761, Willmar Schwabe Pharmaceutical Co., Germany), distributed in the United States by Nature's Way as Ginkgold, reduced anxiety in two studies. A DBRPC study of 170 adults (aged 18–70 years) with GAD or adjustment disorder with anxious mood were given 480 mg/day EGb761, 240 mg/day EGb761, or placebo for 4 weeks. Hamilton Anxiety Rating scores decreased significantly (p = .0003) and (p = .003) in the higher and lower doses respectively compared to placebo (Woelk, Arnoldt,

Kieser, & Hoerr, 2007). European studies of ginkgo have tended to show more favorable results than American studies. This may be due to the use of better quality standardized ginkgo extracts in Europe. American researchers are becoming more aware of the importance of testing the best quality products in research studies. Whether the positive effects on anxiety seen with EGb761 would be the same with other ginkgo preparations remains to be proven. Ginkgo will be discussed in greater detail in the section titled Herbs for Treatment of Cognitive Dysfunction.

Piper methysticum (Kava)

Kava (extracted from *Piper methysticum*), a traditional social ceremonial drink in Pacific Islands, contains alpha-pyrones (kavalactones) which have been shown to block sodium and calcium channels, reduce excitatory neurotransmitter release, enhance ligand binding to GABA type A receptors, reversibly inhibit monoamine oxidase B, inhibit cyclogenase, and reduce reuptake of dopamine and noradrenaline. Kava has shown modest benefits in eight short-term RCTs of mild anxiety. In a 6-week double-blind, randomized, placebo-controlled trial in patients with generalized anxiety disorder (n = 75), Sarris and colleagues (2013a, 2013b) studied the effects of neurotransmitter polymorphisms on response to Kava. Subjects given 120/140 mg kavalactones per day had significant reductions in anxiety compared to placebo. GABA transporter polymorphisms rs2601126 and rs2697153 were associated with HAMA reduction in response to kava.

Since 1998, reports of hepatotoxicity, including liver failure requiring transplantation, led the FDA to issue a *Letter to Health Care Professionals* and a consumer advisory warning of potential liver injury (Kraft et al., 2001; US Food and Drug Administration, 2002). Ship's records left by Captain Cook from the 1800s describe kava intoxication in natives and seamen (Singh & Blumenthal, 1996). Among Maori in Australia, long-term kava users have developed facial swelling, scaly rash, increased patellar reflexes, dyspnea, low albumin levels, increased GGTPase, decreased white blood cell and platelet counts, hematuria, and tall P waves on ECGs consistent with pulmonary hypertension (Mathews et al., 1988). Side effects include gastrointestinal symptoms, allergic reactions, headache, and light sensitivity. Less common side effects are restlessness, drowsiness, lack of energy, and tremor. Investigations of adverse reactions implicate the use of incorrect plant parts or species, acetonic or ethanolic extraction, and poor storage resulting in hepatotoxic mold (Teschke, Qiu, & Lebot, 2011). Recent short-term studies using high quality standardized Kava report minimal side effects. Taking kava with alcohol, sedatives, or muscle relaxants can induce coma (Almeida & Grimsley, 1996). Extracts of kava and kava lactones inhibit P450 enzymes (see Herb–Drug Interactions) involved in the metabolism of many pharmaceuticals (Mathews, Etheridge, & Black, 2002; Gurley et al., 2005). Considering the risks of intoxication, abuse, dependency, medication interactions, and, rarely, severe adverse reactions, the authors do not recommend prescribing kava until more compelling data on safety and efficacy become available and until a consistently high quality of manufacturing and reliable batch testing are established.

Melissa officinalis (Lemon Balm)

In a DBRPC crossover study of *Melissa officinalis* using a 20-minute laboratory-induced psychological stressor, 20 healthy subjects were given single doses of 600 mg, 1000 mg, or 1600 mg of lemon balm or placebo. The 600 mg dose significantly improved self-ratings of calmness (Kennedy et al., 2003). Lemon balm may be helpful for mild anxiety, but in some cases it may work best in combination with other anxiolytic supplements.

Passiflora incarnate (Passionflower)

Passionflower (*Passiflora incarnata*) contains a dihydroflavone, chrysin, which binds to benzodiazepine receptors. Effects mediated via modulation of the GABA system include affinity for GABAA and GABAB receptors and effects on GABA uptake (Appel et al., 2011). In a DBRPC trial, 36 patients with a *DSM-IV* (American Psychiatric Association, 1994) GAD and Hamilton Anxiety Scale scores ≥14 were given passionflower extract 45 drops/day plus a placebo tablet, or oxazepam 30 mg/day plus placebo drops for 4 weeks. Although the oxazepam effect was more rapid, passionflower was as effective in reducing anxiety and showed a trend toward less impairment in job performance (Akhondzadeh et al., 2001). A study of presurgical anxiety (n = 60) showed that patients given passionflower had significantly greater reductions in anxiety compared with those given placebo (Movafegh, Alizadeh, Hajimohamadi, Esfehani, & Nejatfar, 2008). Larger controlled trials are needed to validate these findings. Side effects are usually mild and may include dizziness, confusion, incoordination, altered consciousness, and inflammation. This herb should not be used during pregnancy because it may cause uterine contractions. In practice, the authors begin with one or two pills 2–4 times a day as needed with gradual increase.

Melissa officinalis (Lemon Balm) and Valeriana officinalis (Valerian)

A combination of lemon balm and valerian in three doses (600 mg, 1200 mg, 1800 mg) was given to 24 healthy volunteers in a DBRPC crossover trial using a 20-minute laboratory-induced psychological stressor (Kennedy, Little, & Scholey 2004). Mood and anxiety were evaluated at baseline and at 1, 3, and 6 hours. The 600mg dose significantly reduced anxiety ratings, while the 1800mg dose somewhat increased anxiety ratings. Within a therapeutic window, the combination of *M. officinalis* and *V. officinalis* may reduce anxiety under stress. In a large uncontrolled multicenter study, a valerian/lemon balm product (Euvegal forte) was tested in 918 children under the age of 12 years with restlessness and dyssomnia (Muller & Klement, 2006). Substantial improvement occurred in 80.9% of the children with dyssomnia and 70.4% of those with restlessness. The tolerability of Euvegal forte was

evaluated as "good" or "very good" by 96.7% of the patients. No herb-related adverse events occurred.

Valeriana officinalis (Valerian) and Piper methysticum (Kava)

A DBRPC internet-based study of kava and valerian reported no significant differences between kava and placebo for anxiety or between valerian and placebo for sleep disturbance (Jacobs, Bent, Tice, Blackwell, & Cummings, 2005). Subject selection was based on State-Trait Anxiety Inventory subtest and on self-report of "a problem going to sleep or staying asleep over the past 2 weeks" rather than on standard diagnostic criteria. The negative results may have been due to selection of a heterogeneous population, comorbid conditions, inadequate doses of herbs, or other limitations of Internet surveys.

Butterbur (Ze 185: Petasites hybridus or Petasites officinalis), Valerian, Passionflower, Lemon Balm

In a 2-week RCT, 182 patients with somatoform disorders were randomized to three groups: (1) Ze 185, a combination of butterbur, valerian, passionflower and lemon balm; (2) valerian, passionflower, and lemon balm; (3) and placebo. Those on the 4-herb combination had greater improvements in anxiety and depression compared to the 3-herb combination. Both the 4-herb and the 3-herb outperformed placebo. Although there were nine complaints including dry mouth, headache, constipation, or drowsiness, no serious side effects occurred (Melzer, Schrader, Brattstrom, Schellenberg, & Saller, 2009).

Another RCT of 60 patients with migraine found that Petadolex—a preparation of butterbur containing 25 mg per capsule, given as two capsules twice a day for 12 weeks—significantly reduced the frequency of migraines compared to placebo (Grossmann & Schmidramsl, 2000). Butterbur extract was well tolerated with no significant side effects.

Rhodiola, Artic Root, Roseroot, Rosewort, Golden Root

Rhodiola rosea and several of its 18 related subspecies, including *R. kiriolowi, R. crenulata, R. imbricata,* and *R. sacra,* have been studied for adaptogenic properties. Plant adaptogens are metabolic regulators that enable organisms to resist many forms of stress (e.g., physical, mental, psychological, chemical, radiological, toxic, oxidative, hypoxic, and carcinogenic). The evidence has been reviewed that *R.rosea* alone and in combination with other adaptogens significantly improves mental and physical performance under stress (Brown, Gerbarg, & Muskin, 2009; Brown, Gerbarg, & Ramazanov, 2002; Panossian, 2013; Panossian & Wagner 2005). Psychoactive constituents of root extracts from *R. rosea,* phenolic compounds, structurally related to catecholamines, are involved in sympathetic nervous system (SNS) activation during stress response. Salidroside extracted from *R. rosea* protected PC 12 cells (derived from rat adrenal medulla pheochromocytoma) from glutamate toxicity—excitatory neurotransmitter whose damaging effects on emotion regulatory systems have been studied in PTSD (Cao, Du, & Wang, 2006). Studies have shown that *R. rosea* increases the capacity of muscle and nerve cells to maintain production of the high energy molecules adenosine triphosphate (ATP) and creatine phosphate (CP), needed to sustain cellular activities and repair mechanisms (Kurkin & Zapesochnaya, 1986b). In a pilot study (Bystritsky, Kerwin, & Feusner, 2008) 10 patients from the UCLA Anxiety Disorders Program between the ages of 34 and 55 with *DSM-IV* diagnosis of GAD, given a total daily dose of 340 mg *R. rosea* (Rhodax) for 10 weeks, showed significant decreases in mean Hamilton Anxiety Rating Scale scores at endpoint (t = 3.27, p = 0.01). Adverse events were generally mild or moderate, the most common being dizziness and dry mouth. These preliminary findings warrant further exploration. While the authors sometimes find moderate doses of *R. rosea* beneficial in anxiety disorders, its stimulative effects may initially increase agitation in sensitive individuals. Nevertheless, in clinical practices the authors note that over time it can increase stress resiliency and reduce symptoms of PTSD. Panossian and colleagues (Panossian, 2013; Panossian, Hamm, Wikman, & Effert, 2014) continue to explore the molecular and genomic bases for these actions: See Figure 28.1, *Hypothetical Neuroendocrine Mechanism of Stress Protection by Adaptogens* and Figure 28.2, *Hypothetical Molecular Mechanisms by which Adaptogens Activate Stress Response G-protein Coupled Receptors (GPCR) Pathways*. *R. rosea* will be discussed in greater detail under Herbs for Treatment of Cognitive Dysfunction.

Hypericum perforatum (St. John's Wort)

Extracts from the flowers and leaves of St. John's wort (*Hypericum perforatum*) are best known for their antidepressant effects. Case reports and some open-label studies of patients with generalized anxiety disorder suggesting response to SJW have appeared in the literature, but controlled studies have not been supportive (Kobak, Taylor, Warner, et al., 2005; Kobak, Taylor, Bystritsky, et al., 2005). In clinical practice with anxious patients, the authors prefer to use SJW brand Kira rather than Perika (Nature's Way) because it is less stimulating and therefore less likely to exacerbate anxiety and agitation. However, Perika may be more helpful in activating patients who have a sluggish depression (e.g., apathy or psychomotor retardation). Side effects and dosage will be discussed in the section on Herbs for Treatment of Mood Disorders.

Camellia sinensis (Green Tea, Theanine)

Green tea, made from leaves of *Camillia sinensis*, has been used for centuries for its calming and medicinal effects. Three to four cups of green tea contain 60–160 mg of theanine (5-N-ethylglutamine or γ-glutamylethylamide), an amino acid found in green tea that may reduce anxiety under conditions of stress. In animal studies, theanine perfusion into the brain increased dopamine release and possibly inhibited excitatory neurotransmission (Yamada, Terashima, Okubo, Juneja, & Yokogoshi, 2005). Small studies in humans have

shown mixed results. One DBRPC theanine study in 16 healthy volunteers showed some evidence of a mild relaxing effect under resting conditions, but not during experimentally induced anxiety (Lu et al., 2004). Another DBRPC study of 12 healthy subjects given a mental arithmetic task as a stressor found that those given L-theanine had reduced heart rate and attenuation of SNS activation (Kimura, Ozeki, Juneja, & Ohira, 2007). In clinical practice, the authors (RPB and PLG) find that theanine can be helpful in mild to moderate anxiety, particularly in patients who are highly sensitive to side effects of other agents. It has minimal and usually no side effects when given in a starting dose of 200 mg 1–3 times a day up to a maximum of 6 times a day. In brain damaged patients, large doses may cause paradoxical overactivation. Green tea and theanine have numerous health benefits, including antioxidant and antiproliferative activity. Decaffeinated green tea and capsules work well for anxious or agitated patients.

Valeriana officinalis (Valerian)

Studies in mice show that valerenic acid and vulerenos, two of the active constituents of valerian (*Valeriana officinalis*) extract, bind to GABAA receptors (Benke et al., 2009). Reviews of studies using Valerian for sleep show inconsistent or weak results (Bent, Padula, Moore, Patterson, & Mehling, 2006; Fernandez-San-Martin et al., 2010; Krystal & Ressler, 2001), possibly due to differences in product quality, methods of extraction, doses, and patient populations. Valerian's anxiolytic activity has been attributed to GABAA receptor effects. Also the effect of valerian improves over time and maximal benefit may take 2 weeks. One advantage of valerian over other sedative/hypnotics is that there have been no cases of habituation or abuse and only one case of possible withdrawal symptoms. Valerian should be avoided in pregnancy. Valerian is more effective when combined with other herbs, but isolated cases of adverse reactions in combination with benzodiazepines have been reported.

NEUROHORMONES FOR ANXIETY AND INSOMNIA

7-KETO DHEA (3-ACETYL-7-OXO-DEHYDROEPI-ANDROSTERONE) FOR PTSD

To date there is no specific pharmacological treatment for dissociative disorder in PTSD. In a small case series five women with severe chronic PTSD due to extreme childhood abuse, who were treated with 50–75 mg/day of a metabolite of dehydroepiandrosterone (DHEA) known as *7-keto DHEA*), experienced rapid, substantial improvement in dissociative symptoms, emotional numbing, avoidance, irritability, energy, mood, memory, concentration, cognitive function, libido, anxiety, and insomnia (Sageman & Brown, 2006). The patients had not responded previously to many years of psychotherapy and pharmacotherapy. No adverse side effects were reported. Previous studies have linked DHEA cortisol-lowering effects in PTSD with improvements in memory, cognition, and mood (Rasmusson et al., 2004). Unlike DHEA, 7-keto DHEA is not converted to testosterone or estrogen. Consequently, 7-keto DHEA is less likely to cause acne, baldness, hirsutism, prostatic changes, or increased estrogenicity. Chronic treatment-resistant PTSD in patients with serum DHEA and DHEAS levels in the lower 50% of normal may benefit from 7-keto DHEA. Side effects are minimal. Agitation may occur in some patients and there is an increased risk of mania in bipolar patients.

MELATONIN FOR INSOMNIA

Melatonin (N-acetyl-5-methoxytryptamine), a hormone secreted by the pineal gland, affects sleep circadian rhythms. Generally safe and easy to use, melatonin does not disturb sleep architecture nor lead to habituation. DBRPC trials show that melatonin improves sleep, reduces sleep onset latency (Kayumov, Brown, Jindal, Buttoo, & Shapiro, 2001), and restores sleep efficiency (Zhdanova et al., 2001). It is also effective in treating insomnia in dementia and Parkinson's (Dowling et al., 2005), "sundowning" (Cohen-Mansfield, Garfinkel, & Lipson, 2000), and rapid eye movement behavior disorder (RBD) (Pandi-Perumal, Zisapel, Srinivasan, & Cardinali, 2005). RBD, a chronic progressive parasomnia, occurs in neurodegenerative disorders and in Parkinson's patients treated with dopamine agonists and levodopa. In RBD the motor paralysis that normally occurs during rapid eye movement (REM) sleep is lost, such that patients may act out dreams, thrashing and kicking, hurting themselves or their partners. Stimulants, tricyclic antidepressants (TCAs), and SSRIs can trigger RBD (Schenck, Bundlie, Ettinger, & Mahowald, 1986), although this is more likely in patients with neurodegenerative diseases. Clonazepam or carbamazepine, the standard treatments for RBD, can exacerbate cognitive dysfunction or cause ataxia (increasing the risk of falls). Side effects rarely occur with melatonin, even at 9–12 mg h.s., the doses necessary to treat RBD (Kunz & Bes, 1997; Paparrigopoulos, 2005). In a DBRPC study of elderly melatonin-deficient insomniacs, 2 mg sustained-release melatonin given for 1 week improved sleep maintenance, while 2 mg fast-release melatonin improved sleep initiation with no adverse effects (Haimov et al., 1995). A review of 14 RCTs found that melatonin reduced sleep onset latency in people with delayed sleep phase syndrome (DSPS) more effectively than in those with a diagnosis of insomnia (Buscemi et al., 2005). The distinction between DSPS and insomnia accounted for much of the heterogeneity in previous studies. Melatonin has a low incidence of adverse events (headaches, drowsiness, dizziness, and nausea) with no difference between melatonin and placebo in any study. Furthermore, melatonin has strong antioxidant protective effects in the dopamine system.

MOOD DISORDERS

NUTRIENTS FOR MOOD DISORDERS

B Vitamins, Folic Acid, L-methylfolate

The most important vitamins for mental health, the B vitamins (including folic acid) are essential for the functioning of nerve cells and are the most likely to be depleted due to poor nutrition, malabsorption, rapid utilization, aging, chronic illness, diabetes, cancer, smoking, alcohol use, environmental stress, or the use of medications such as mood stabilizers, L-dopa, statins, oral antidiabetic drugs, and chemotherapy.

Dietary *folate* and *folic acid* (supplemental form) must be converted into *L-methylfolate* for use in numerous metabolic pathways, including the synthesis of neurotransmitters. The final step in this conversion depends upon methyltetrahydroxyfolate reductase (MTHFR), which is also required for production of methionine from homocysteine (see Figure 28.1 Methylation Cycle, Folate Cycle). Polymorphisms of the MTHFR gene affect the capacity of MTHFR to convert homocysteine to methionine, or methylene-tetrahydrofolate to L-methylfolate (see Box 28.1). For an in-depth discussion of the relationship between folate, other B vitamins,

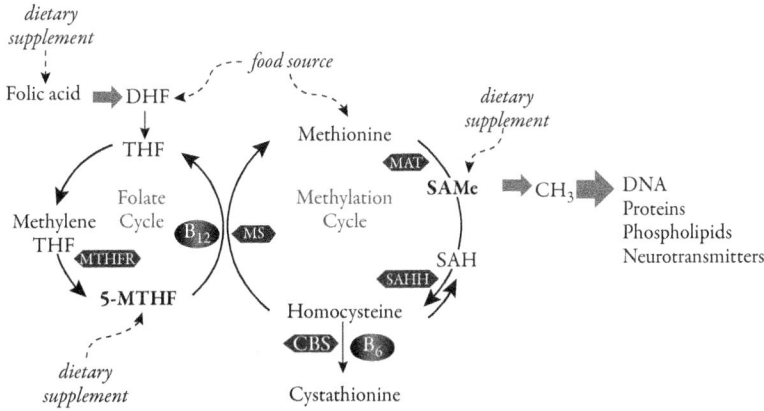

Figure 28.1 Methylation Cycle, Folate Cycle, SAMe, and B Vitamins. Key: Relationship between folate, vitamin B_{12} and methylation. Abbreviations: DHF, dihydrofolate; THF, tetrahydrofolate; 5-MTHF, 5-methyltetrahydrofolate; SAMe, S-adenosylmethionine; SAH, S-adenosylhomocysteine; MTHFR, methyltetrahydrofolate reductase; MS, methionine synthase; MAT, methionine adenosyltransferase; SAHH, S-adenosylhomocysteine hydrolase. Reproduced with permission of Dr. Teodoro Bottiglieri, adapted from *Psychiatric Clinics of North America*, 2013, 36(1):3.

homocysteine, and depression, see the scholarly discussions by Papakostos and Bottiglieri (Papakostos et al., 2005; Bottiglieri, 2013). A mutation on the MTHFR gene at the 677 base position—due to a substitution of a cytosine base (C) by a thymine (T), a C→T polymorphism—results in a less active form of the enzyme. The normal genotype C/C has 100% MTHFR activity. However, MTHRF activity declines to 71% with C/T and 34% with T/T genotypes. The consequences of a C/T or T/T polymorphism are increased homocysteine and reduced folate concentrations. About 40%–50% of the population has C/T mutation, while 10%–12% has T/T genotype. In addition, S-adenosylmethionine (SAMe) production may decline. Consequently, the reduction in SAMe and the metabolism of folate, along with the increase in homocysteine, may contribute to depression, poor response to antidepressants, and progression of other illnesses such as cardiovascular disease. Supplementation with L-methylfolate may be more effective than folic acid in patients with polymorphisms, because it bypasses the final MTHFR conversion step. L-methylfolate is well absorbed and readily crosses the blood–brain barrier. For example, in a DBRPC study of 123 patients with major depression or schizophrenia, 33% had low or borderline folate levels. Among the low-folate patients on standard psychotropic medication, the addition of 15 mg/day methylfolate resulted in significantly greater improvements compared to placebo (Procter, 1991). Studies suggest that L-methylfolate 15 mg/day is useful in the treatment of SSRI-resistant depression. Two DBR parallel sequential trials in adults with major depression (total n = 223) found 2 weeks of 15 mg/day L-methylfolate augmentation of SSRI to be safe, well tolerated, and significantly better in improving response rates and reducing scores on Hamilton Depression Scale compared with SSRI augmentation with placebo or 7.5 mg/day L-methylfolate (Papakostas et al., 2012). Testing of MTHFR polymorphisms is becoming more widely used to identify patients who would be more likely to benefit. Deplin, a prescription form of L-methylfolate is available. However, most insurance companies do not cover the costs. Consumers can obtain the supplement online from established commercial brands less expensively.

In depressed patients and in the elderly, low levels of B_{12} (cyanocobalamin) and folate have been associated with disorders of mood, memory, and cognition (Bottiglieri, 1996; Crellin, Bottiglieri, & Reynolds, 1993). Proton pump inhibitors interfere with B_{12} absorption. If there is reason to think that a patient may have impaired B_{12} absorption, for example, due to loss of intrinsic factor with aging or the use of a proton pump inhibitor (e.g., cimetidine, ranitidine, omeprazole, esomeprazole, famotidine), then sublingual B_{12} should be administered. Testing for serum methylmalonic acid provides a more accurate indicator of intracellular B_{12} than serum B_{12} levels.

Studies of B vitamins and folic acid as solo treatments for depression show mixed results. Methylfolate and B vitamins are generally quite safe and low in side effects. Allergic reactions may occur. B Vitamins and folic acid stimulate endothelial proliferation and may accelerate occlusion of cardiac stents, but only in men whose baseline homocysteine level is less than 15 mM/L (Lange et al., 2004). Poor gastric absorption of B_{12} may contribute to B_{12} deficiency, nonresponse to supplementation, and mixed results in clinical studies. Therefore, the use of sublingual B_{12} tablets may be more effective.

Vitamin D_3

Vitamin D_3 (cholecalciferol) is critical for normal brain development. Evidence from preclinical studies suggests that vitamin D can affect neurotransmitters, calcium homeostasis, hypothalamic-pituitary-adrenal (HPA) axis function, inflammatory markers, and nerve growth factor. Population studies indicate an association between low vitamin D levels and depression, Alzheimer's disease (AD), Parkinson's disease, and cognitive decline. Vitamin D deficiency occurs at serum levels below 20 ng/ml 25-hydroxyvitamin D [25(OH)D]; insufficiency occurs below 30 ng/ml; and optimal levels are between 30–80 ng/ml. Although small clinical trials showed improvement in symptoms of depression with vitamin D, large population studies have yielded mixed results. A cross-sectional study of 12,594 adults in a primary care clinic revealed that individuals with a prior history of depression showed a significant correlation between high vitamin D levels and reduced risk of depression, whereas those with no prior history of depression did not (Hoang et al., 2011). Reduction of light exposure during winter months results in a decrease in production of vitamin D. The relationship between sun exposure, vitamin D levels, and seasonal affective disorder has been explored in several small randomized studies with mixed results (Bell et al., 1992).

In a study of 104 adolescents presenting for treatment for serious acute symptoms of mental illness, 34% had vitamin D deficiency and 38% insufficiency. Vitamin D deficiency was strongly associated with psychotic features (Gracious, Finucane, Freidman-Campbell, Messing, & Parkhurst, 2012).

Administration of vitamin D to all depressed patients is not justifiable based on current evidence. However, it is appropriate to check 25(OH)D levels in those at risk for deficiency due to prior history of depression, age above 65 years, adolescents with severe mental illness, lack of regular outdoor activity, and residence in northern latitudes with reduced sun exposure. Documented vitamin D deficiency can be treated acutely with high-dose vitamin D_3 (cholecalciferol) until serum levels reach normal, followed by a maintenance dose of 2000 to 6,000 IU/day.

S-adenosyl-L-methionine, Adometionine, SAMe

SAMe (S-adenosyl-L-methionine or S-adenosylmethionine), a first-line mainstream antidepressant and antiarthritic in many European countries, is still viewed as an alternative treatment in the United States. The FDA approved its use as an over-the-counter nutraceutical in 1998. The US Department of Health and Human Services Agency for Healthcare Research and Quality published an evidence report (Agency for Healthcare Research and Quality, 2007) concluding that SAMe was equivalent to standard pharmacotherapy for treatment of

Box 28.1 NEUROPROTECTIVE EFFECTS OF SAME, FOLATE, AND VITAMIN B$_{12}$

AD is associated with decreased plasma folate and increased plasma homocysteine . Substantial evidence associates increased serum homocysteine with AD (Coppede, 2010) and low brain SAMe levels with AD. Folate deficiency leads to a decline in SAMe with decreased DNA methylation and increased DNA breakage during aging and AD (See Figure 28.3). The reduction in folate and SAMe potentiates AD risk factors—increased neurotoxicity from elevated homocysteine, presenilin-1 (PS-1) over-expression, reduced use of glutathione, and increased beta-amyloid deposition. The C677T polymorphism of MTHFR uses folate to regenerate methionine from homocysteine. Condensation of ATP and methionine produce SAMe. Therefore, insufficiency of tetrahydrofolate leads to accumulation of homocysteine and decreased production of SAMe as methionine becomes less available.

In human neuronal cells folate and B$_{12}$ deprivation were associated with reduced production of SAMe and methylation of the promoter of the preselin-1 (*PSEN1*) gene, resulting in increased production of preselin-1 and amyloid precursor protein. This epigenetic modification in the *PSEN1* gene would result in increased beta-amyloid (Aβ) peptide production. Furthermore, addition of SAMe to human neuroblastoma cell cultures led to downregulation of PSEN1 expression and a decrease in Aβ peptide production (Coppede, 2010). The MTHFR C677T polymorphism is an apolipoprotein E4-dependent risk factor for AD: as SAMe decreases, S-adenosylhomocysteine increases, further inhibiting methylation (Bottiglieri, 2013).

Cognitive impairment and increased aggression were found in mice lacking murine ApoE and mice expressing human E4 when fed a diet deficient in folic acid and vitamin E with iron-induced oxidative stress. Supplementation with SAMe attenuated these adverse effects. Furthermore, supplementation with SAMe improved cognitive performance in mice 9 to 12 months of age that were lacking murine ApoE and expressing human E2, E3, or E4 alleles. SAMe also indirectly contributed to acetylcholine synthesis (Chan, Tchantchou, Rogers, & Shea, 2009).

SAMe reduced impairments in primates and facilitated recovery from vascular lesions in motor and dorsolateral prefrontal cortex. In rats SAMe substantially decreased free radical production, increased glutathione, glutathione peroxidase, and transferase, and improved cholinergic function and learning. SAMe significantly improved survival when given within 24 hours of ischemia or hemorrhagic stroke (Monaco et al., 1996). In patients with traumatic brain injury (TBI), 1 month of SAMe decreased mean postconcussion symptom scores by 77% compared to 49% in a placebo group. Symptoms of headache, vertigo, depressed mood, cognitive slowing, slow thought, speech, and decreased concentration improved (Bacci Ballerini, Lopez Anguera, Alcaraz, & Hernandez Reyes, 1983).

through the condensation of methionine and ATP, a reaction catalyzed by methionine methyltransferase (MAT) (see Figure 28.3). SAMe donates methyl groups for production of DNA, proteins, phospholipids, neurotransmitters (serotonin, norepinephrine, and dopamine), and other cellular components. These methylation reactions are catalyzed by methyltransferase enzymes and require vitamin B$_{12}$ and folate as cofactors. SAMe also contributes sulfate groups for synthesis of the major endogenous antioxidant, glutathione (Bottiglieri, 2002, 2013). B$_{12}$ 1000 mcg/day, folic acid 400–800 mcg/day, and B$_6$ 50–100 mg/day can be effective for augmentation of SAMe and other antidepressants.

SAMe was shown to be safe and effective for the treatment of major depression in 16 open trials, 13 DBRPC studies, and 19 DBRCTs in comparison to standard antidepressants. See reviews of SAMe metabolism research (Brown, Gerbarg, & Bottiglieri, 2000; Bottiglieri, 2013) and clinical applications (Brown, Gerbarg, & Muskin, 2009).

A 12-week double-blind, randomized, placebo controlled trial of S-adenosylmethionine (SAMe) versus escitalopram in 189 outpatients with major depressive disorder (MDD) was reported as a failed trial by Mischoulon and colleagues (2014). No significant differences were found in response rates: 36% for SAMe, 34% for escitalopram, and 30% for placebo. Remission rates suggested that both SAMe and escitalopram had more robust effects compared to placebo: 28% for SAMe, 28% for escitalopram, and 17% for placebo. Placebo response rates ≥ 30% are correlated with lower risk ratio of response to antidepressants versus placebo (Iovieno and Papakostas, 2012). Studies with placebo response rates ≥ 30%, as seen in this study, reported worse performance of drug versus placebo (Rutherford and Roose, 2013). Furthermore, the sample size was only 2/3 of the number for which the study was powered.

Bias was introduced in the discussion of the study results. Mischoulon and colleagues wrote that the sample was large enough to provide a "conclusive statement about the efficacy of SAMe as a monotherapy for MDD" and that "SAMe may be better suited as an augmentation therapy than as a monotherapy." They made no such statement about escitalopram, though it performed no better than SAMe. A critique of this study noted, "The manner in which researchers discuss study results impacts clinical practice and can be particularly damaging in the case of less well known or less conventional treatments" and suggested that the causes for the failure of both treatments to produce higher response rates than placebo are "more likely be found in problems with the patient selection process and the heterogeneity within patient groups with respect to genomic and metabolic biomarkers. At the very least, until the true causes of invalidity are identified, such studies should not be used to create unwarranted doubt about the efficacy of highly beneficial treatments such as SAMe." (Gerbarg, Muskin, Bottiglieri, & Brown, 2014).

As a natural metabolite, SAMe is very low in side effects compared with synthetic antidepressants and it has a more rapid onset of action. There are credible reports of adverse interactions with other medications. In fact, SAMe protects the liver and bone marrow from toxic effects of other

depression and osteoarthritis. SAMe was also found to be more effective than placebo in reducing bilirubin and pruritis in intrahepatic cholestasis and cholestasis of pregnancy.

An essential molecule in hundreds of biochemical reactions within the cells of all organisms, SAMe is produced medications (Brown, Gerbarg, & Muskin, 2009). The most common side effect of SAMe is nausea. This can usually be relieved by eating a light snack before taking SAMe, using ginger capsules or tea, or by reducing the SAMe dose. Loose bowels, flatulence, and abdominal pain can occur. Occasionally patients complain of headache. In rare cases patients with palpitations have complained of an increase in irregular heartbeats when given SAMe, although it is generally well tolerated by individuals with cardiovascular disease. However, if it exacerbates symptoms it should be discontinued. The most serious potential side effect is the potential to induce mania in bipolar I patients.

As an activating antidepressant, SAMe helps energize patients whose depression is characterized by low energy, tiredness, low motivation, and hypersomnia. It absorbs best when taken at least 20–30 minutes before breakfast and lunch on an empty stomach or 2 hours after a meal. If taken late in the day, it may interfere with sleep. For patients whose depression includes anxiety and agitation, it may be necessary to use an anxiolytic during the first few weeks to counteract the stimulative effects of SAMe and to avoid exacerbating anxiety (as also occurs with stimulating antidepressants such as SSRIs). However, within 2–3 weeks, as the antidepressant action is established, it is usually possible to taper off of anxiolytics. SAMe does not cause sexual side effects, sedation, weight gain, or cognitive interference. In patients who have medication sensitivities, significant anxiety, gastrointestinal problems, or serious medical conditions, one can start with a test dose of 200 mg SAMe 20 minutes before breakfast for a few days. If this is well tolerated, it can be increased to 400 mg 20 minutes before breakfast for 3–7 days. The rate of increase in SAMe doses depends on clinical assessment of the patient. For elderly, frail, or unstable patients, more time may be needed before each increase. If the patient reports side effects, then more time may be allowed before the next increase. In general, the dose for mild depression is 400–600 mg/day; moderate depression 600–1200 mg/day; severe depression 1200–1600 mg/day; and very severe, treatment-resistant depression 1600–2400 mg/day.

Clinical Applications and Practical Considerations

SAMe has unique benefits in treating depression in patients with arthritis, fibromyalgia, liver disease, or HIV/AIDS. It should also be seriously considered for patients who take medications that may impair liver function, for example, statins and/or prescription antidepressants. SAMe has no adverse hepatic effects and it protects against liver damage from prescription medications (Torta et al., 1988).

Cost is a major drawback for SAMe because it is not yet covered by medical insurance in many countries. Prices vary from $20 to $60 for a package of 20 of the 400mg tablets. Patients can comparison shop (for quality brands) or get pharmaceutical grade SAMe online (Brown, Gerbarg, & Muskin, 2009). Unfortunately, at higher doses many people cannot afford the expense of SAMe. However, since SAMe combines well with all other antidepressants, it is possible to combine a smaller dose of SAMe with a reduced dose of a prescription antidepressant. This approach reduces side effects of the prescription antidepressant and reduces the cost of SAMe.

SAMe to Augment Antidepressants

There are few pharmacological agents for treatment resistant depression and overall outcomes are poor. Results from the US National Institute of Mental Health's (NIMH) STAR*D (Sequenced Treatment Alternatives to Relieve Depression) programme indicate that after the failure of two treatment trials, the chances of remission decrease significantly (Shelton, Osuntokun, Heinloth, & Corya, 2010).

The neuronal effects of SAMe overlap those of TCAs with additional dopamine stimulating effects, but SAMe has fewer side effects. Three controlled studies have shown that SAMe enhances the action of TCAs (Brown, Gerbarg, & Bottiglieri, 2000). One DBRPC trail (n = 350) demonstrated that SAMe accelerated the response to imipramine (Berlanga, Ortega-Soto, Ontiveros, & Senties, 1992). SAMe has been shown to enhance the effectiveness of prescription antidepressants and hasten onset of action. In an open trial at Massachusetts General Hospital, 30 depressed nonresponders to either SSRIs or venlafaxine were administered SAMe (800–1600 mg/day). SAMe augmentation showed a response rate of 50% and a remission rate of 43% (Alpert et al., 2004).

Further controlled trials for treatment resistant depression are warranted. A meta-analysis of European-licensed therapies in patients with MDD and inadequate response to antidepressant monotherapy identified 7 RCTs that met criteria for analysis. This meta-analysis concluded that the likelihood of response was significantly greater with SAMe augmentation versus placebo or lithium (Turner, Kantaria, & Young, 2014).

The addition of SAMe caused no adverse reactions in 500 patients on benzodiazepines, 60 on monoamine oxidase inhibitors (MAOIs), 45 on anticonvulsants, and 18 alcoholics on antidepressants or anticonvulsants. Moreover, SAMe reversed or prevented liver toxicity, reducing the elevated levels of gamma-glutamyl-transpeptidase (GGT) in all patients taking MAOIs, anticonvulsants, or antidepressants (Torta et al., 1988). SAMe is the only antidepressant that has been studied in combination with MAO inhibitors with good results and no adverse reactions. In addition to its antidepressant effects, SAMe has numerous long-term health benefits in a wide range of serious medical conditions.

SAMe for Treatment of Depression, Arthritis, and Fibromyalgia

Depression and arthritis are often comorbid and are exacerbated by chronic progressive pain, disrupted sleep, aging, debilitation, and side effects from antiinflammatory and pain medications. Twelve studies in more than 20,000 adults have shown that SAMe provides analgesic and antiinflammatory effects equal to nonsteroidal antiinflammatories in osteoarthritis, but causes fewer side effects. Six studies reported that SAMe improved both depression and pain in patients with fibromyalgia at doses equivalent to 800 mg/day with no side effects (Grassetto & Varatto, 1994; Ianiello et al.,

1994; Tavoni, Vitali, Bombardieri, & Pasero, 1987; Tavoni, Jeracitano, & Cirigliano, 1998).

SAMe for Treatment of Depression and Liver Disease

Patients with liver diseases often have comorbid depression that may be primary, secondary to the hepatic dysfunction, or due to medications (e.g., interferon). Moreover, psychotropic medications (particularly SSRIs) can cause elevations of liver function tests (LFTs) or exacerbate preexisting liver dysfunction. Alcohol abuse depletes the liver of SAMe and causes oxidative stress that contributes to tissue damage. Numerous studies have demonstrated that SAMe improves liver function and reverses biochemical markers (abnormal LFTs) in patients with cirrhosis or hepatitis due to alcohol, drugs, toxins, infections, or gallstones, including during pregnancy (Frezza, Centini, Cammareri, Le Grazie, & Di Padova, 1990; Friedel, Goa, & Benfield, 1989; Lieber, 1999; Mato et al., 1999; Milkiewicz et al., 1999). In a 2-year DBRPC study of alcohol-induced liver cirrhosis (Childs Class A and B cases) SAMe 1200 mg/day increased survival and delayed liver transplants (Mato et al., 1999). Many cases of undiagnosed hepatitis are discovered when LFTs rise in patients taking SSRIs for depression. Discontinuation of the prescription antidepressant and initiation of SAMe usually restores LFTs to normal range. Treatment of mildly elevated LFTs usually requires SAMe 800 mg in the morning (except in bipolar patients). In bipolar patients Ease-2 or Ease-Plus (CraneHerb)—Chinese herbal preparations containing bupleurum—may be used. Hepatoprotection by *Bupleurum kaoi* includes antiinflammatory and antifibrotic effects, enhanced glutathione production, and liver cell regeneration (Yen, Weng, Liu, Chai, & Lin, 2005). LFT increases greater than three times normal respond better to SAMe 1200–1600 mg/day enhanced with polyenylphosphatidylcholine. SAMe is depleted during the conversion of phosphatidyl ethanolamine to phosphatidylcholine. Taking polyenylphosphatidylcholine replenishes phosphatidylcholine supplies, preventing depletion of SAMe. As SAMe reserves increase, more glutathione is produced to counteract oxidative damage to the liver (Aleynik & Lieber, 2003; Lieber, 2001, 2005). In patients with serious underlying liver disease with documented fibrosis, adding B vitamins (including B_6) and alpha-lipoic acid can enhance response. If LFT elevations persist, betaine (trimethylglycine) can augment the response to SAMe by elevating glutathione (antioxidant), protecting the liver from chemical damage, and improving liver function (Barak, Beckenhauer, & Tuma, 1996; Kharbanda et al., 2005).

In a 24-week DBRPC trial, 37 outpatients with alcoholic liver disease were administered either SAMe 400 mg three times daily or placebo. No significant differences were found in LFTs or fibrosis in liver biopsies for the entire group. However, in the cases with less severe fibrosis, SAMe was more beneficial than placebo (Medici et al., 2011), but vitamin B_6 levels were subnormal. The negative results could be attributed to the severity of fibrosis, short duration of treatment compared with other studies, presence of subnormal B_6 levels, and/or the absence of supplemental support for the SAMe treatment. In cases of significant hepatic fibrosis, it is necessary to augment SAMe with polyenolphosphatidylcholine, L-methylfolate, B_{12}, B_6, and sometimes herbal formulas containing bupleurum. Without the necessary cofactors and maintenance of SAMe supplies, the treatment is not as effective.

SAMe for Treatment of Depression and Parkinson's Disease

Carbidopa is a common treatment for Parkinson's disease, a degenerative disorder characterized by difficulty initiating movements, dyskinesias, stiffness, tremor, rigidity, mask-like facies (loss of facial expression), and unsteady gait. It often leads to social withdrawal and the loss of all spontaneous activity and communication. L-dopa treatment further reduces the already depleted brain stores of SAMe in patients with Parkinson's, exacerbating the depression which is highly resistant to treatment with standard antidepressants. In a double blind crossover study of 21 patients with Parkinson's disease, depression improved significantly in 8 of the patients given SAMe 1200 mg/day (Carrieri, Indaco, & Gentile, 1990). Depression also improved in 11 out of 13 subjects in an open series of Parkinson's patients given SAMe 1600–4000 mg/day (Di Rocco, Rogers, Brown, Werner, & Bottiglieri, 2000). At these doses, neurological symptoms such as dyskinesia and poor balance also improved in some cases. A Phase II 12-week DBRPC study compared SAMe 1200–2400 mg versus escitalopram (Lexapro) 10–20 mg in the treatment of depression associated with Parkinson's disease. Both SAMe and escitalopram significantly reduced depression (HAMD) scores with greater improvements on escitalopram. However, SAMe significantly improved motor symptoms compared to no change on escitalopram (Varanese, Birnbaum, Rossi, & Di Rocco, 2011).

SAMe for Treatment of Depression and HIV/AIDS

Depression occurs in about 30%–50% of HIV+ patients and is associated with low immune response, disease progression, and diminished quality of life. SAMe deficiency has been found in HIV-infected patients. An open 8-week study of 20 patients with HIV and major depression, given SAMe 400 mg twice a day with folic acid (800 mcg/day) and B_{12} (1000 mcg/day), showed significant improvement in depression by week four (Shippy, Mendez, Jones, Cergnul, & Karpiak, 2004).

Perinatal Depression

Clinical studies show the safety and efficacy of SAMe for improving liver function in the treatment of cholestasis due to gallstones of pregnancy (Frezza et al., 1990; Friedel, Goa, & Benfield, 1989; Lieber, 1999; Mato et al., 1999; Milkiewicz et al., 1999). No adverse effects on infant development have been identified. The normal level of SAMe in the spinal fluid of infants is 3 to 7 times higher than that of adults (Surtees & Hyland, 1990). Studies of children with inborn errors of metabolism affecting methyl transfer pathways found that SAMe deficiency in the cerebrospinal fluid of children was associated with demyelination and that treatment with SAMe was associated with remyelination (Surtees, Leonard, & Austin, 1991); therefore, it is unlikely that the administration of therapeutic doses of SAMe to mothers experiencing perinatal depression would be harmful during pregnancy or breastfeeding (Brown, Gerbarg, & Muskin, 2009). Longer follow-up studies including neuropsychological testing of children would provide further assurance of safety during pregnancy.

SAMe for Treatment of Depression in Children

There are no published controlled studies on the safety and efficacy of SAMe in children. However, SAMe has been used successfully to treat depression in children and adolescents in clinical practice. Three cases were reported including two sisters, aged 8 and 11, and one boy, aged 16. Both parents of the girls had strong family histories of depression and credited SAMe with providing full relief of their own depressions. They did not want to expose their children to side effects from prescription medications. The girls had developed severe major depression including crying, withdrawal, sadness, and preoccupation with themes of death. The 11-year-old was started on 200 mg/day SAMe. When her dose was increased to 600 mg/day, her depression rapidly and completely remitted with no side effects. Her 8-year-old sister's depression also remitted on 200 mg SAMe twice a day (Schaller, Thomas, & Bazzan, 2004).

Quality and Potency of SAMe Brands

SAMe rapidly oxidizes when exposed to air. It is stabilized in the form of a salt. Tablets are enterically coated to resist degradation by gastric enzymes. The quality of the SAMe and the quality of the tablet are critical for maintaining potency over time. If the manufacturing is flawed, tablets lose most of their potency while sitting on shelves. Unfortunately, some companies are producing low-grade SAMe and selling it at bargain prices. Not only do these products lack efficacy, they can also cause more side effects. Patients should be advised to purchase only products of proven quality and those in which each tablet is protected within its own foil blister pack. SAMe should *not* be refrigerated because tablets can be damaged by condensation of water within the blister packs. Also, tablets should not be cut because the enteric coating would be disrupted.

Omega-3-Fatty Acids for Depression and Bipolar Disorder

Omega-3 fatty acids (n-3FAs), particularly eicosapentaenoic acid (EPA) and docosahexaenoic acid (DHA) help maintain cell membrane fluidity. EPA and DHA also reduce production of inflammatory eicosanoids and the release of proinflammatory cytokines. Data suggest that the substitution of omega-6FAs for n-3FAs in cell membranes is associated with unipolar and bipolar depression (Hirashima et al., 2004). The loss of membrane fluidity affecting membrane proteins

(enzymes, receptors, ion channels) may impair neurotransmission. Increased eicosanoids and proinflammatory cytokines may also be contributory. Omega-3 FA deficiency has been associated with increased depression and risk of suicide (McNamara et al., 2007; Sublette, Hibbeln, Galfalvy, Oquendo, & Mann, 2006), and n-3FA supplementation has been found to reduce depression and suicidality (Hallahan, Hibbeln, Davis, & Garland, 2007). For a clinical review of n-3FAs see Mischoulon and Freeman (2013). However, a meta-analysis of 13 RCTs, detecting heterogeneity and publication bias, concluded that although the balance of omega-3 to omega-6 fatty acids may be involved in the pathogenesis of depression, there was little evidence of significant benefit from n-3FAs in the treatment of major depressive disorder (Bloch & Hannestad, 2012).

Perinatal Depression

Omega 3-FAs are crucial for brain development in utero and after birth, particularly arachidonic acid (AA) and DHA. The recommended intake of DHA during pregnancy is 200–300 mg/day. During the first 6 months of life, a ratio of 4:10 n-6FA:n-3FAs is advised (Rombaldi Bernardi, de Souza Escobar, Ferreira, & Pelufo Silveira, 2012). Omega3 FAs are generally considered to be safe during pregnancy and breastfeeding, although an upper dose limit has not been established. Many prenatal vitamins and infant formulas contain n-3 FAs. In their review of n-FAs, Mischoulon and Freedman (2013) found that DBRCTs in pregnant and postpartum women yielded mixed results. They concluded that n-3FAs could help to alleviate perinatal depression in a ratio of 2:1 EPA:DHA as an alternative or adjunctive to standard treatment. Lin and colleagues (2012) observed that 5 meta-analyses concluded that n-3 FAs had antidepressant effects in patients with major depressive disorder based on *DSM* criteria, but that evidence did not support mood improvement in symptomatic individuals with unconfirmed diagnoses. They critiqued a meta-analysis that included studies that reported no benefits from n-FAs, in which the subjects were not evaluated for major depressive disorder with rigorous measures such as the HAMD.

Omega-3 Fatty Acids and Bipolar Disorder

Depressive symptoms in bipolar disorder respond better to adjunctive treatment with a combination of EPA and DHA using total daily doses ranging from 1–9 gm (Frangou, Lewis, & McCrone, 2006; Osher, Bersudsky, & Belmaker, 2005; Stoll et al., 1999). Although there have been some reports of n-3FAs triggering manic symptoms, this did not occur in the studies by Frangou, Osher, or Stoll. Anecdotally, some cases show marked improvement in both manic and depressive symptoms enabling reduction of prescription medication doses. In a meta-analysis of n-3FAs for bipolar disorder, Sarris and colleagues found a significant effect on bipolar depression and a nonspecific effect for mania (Sarris, Mischoulon, & Schweitzer, 2012).

Geriatric Depression

Depression in the elderly is often overlooked, and depletion of n-3FAs has been associated with depression. An 8-week

DBRPC parallel group study of 46 elderly (65–95 years) depressed women in a nursing home found that 2.5g/day of n-3FA (EPA:DHA of 2:1) significantly improved scores on the Geriatric Depression Scale and lowered the ratio of AA to EPA in whole blood and red cell membranes (Rizzo et al., 2012).

Side Effects and Dosages

The most common side effects of n-3FAs are gastrointestinal: nausea, heartburn, stomach pain, belching, bloating, or diarrhea. These are more likely to occur at doses above 6 g/day. The FDA has approved prescription forms of fish oil, Omacor and Lovaza, for treatment of hypertriglyceridemia (Medical Letter, 2006). Each 900mg capsule contains 465 mg EPA and 375 mg DHA. Nonprescription high-quality refined fish oil in concentrated liquid form has a light, non-fishy taste and is less likely to cause gastrointestinal side effects. Because n-3FAs reduce platelet aggregation, patients on anticoagulants should be monitored more closely when taking n-3FAs. It is best to refrigerate fish oil products to prevent them from turning rancid.

5-Hydroxy-L-Tryptophan (5-HTP)

The rationale for using the amino acid, 5-hydroxy-L-tryptophan (5-HTP) for depression is based on its role as the precursor for synthesis of serotonin. 5-HTP replaced L-tryptophan, which was taken off the market in 1989 after a contaminated product from a single manufacturer was linked to eosinophilia malignant syndrome. Since then, studies of 5-HTP have found no evidence of toxicity (Das, Bagchi, Bagchi, & Preuss, 2004). The efficacy of 5-HTP in depression has been reviewed (Das et al., 2004; Turner, Loftis, & Blackwell, 2006). Out of 27 studies 11 were DBRPC. Of the 11 DBRPC studies, 7 reported that 5-HTP performed better than placebo, but only 5 of those showed statistical significance. Several studies have shown that the addition of 5-HTP to prescription antidepressants such as nialamide, chlomipramine, and nomifensine significantly improved antidepressant response. The average dosage of 5-HTP in adults is 200–300 mg/day given in divided doses. Overall, studies suggest that 5-HTP may have limited benefit for depression with some support for its use as an augmentation. Common side effects include nausea, vomiting, and diarrhea. Less frequent side effects include headache and insomnia. Although rodent studies have shown that doses above 100 mg/kg/day induce serotonin syndrome, no cases of serotonin syndrome have been reported in humans using 5-HTP alone or in combination with SSRIs. Studies combining 5-HTP with MAOIs report no adverse effects. The use of a peripheral decarboxylase inhibitor such as carbidopa may increase the level of 5-HTP in serum 14-fold (Gijsman et al., 2002).

N-Acetylcysteine for Bipolar Disorder

N-acetylcysteine (NAC) is a precursor for synthesis of the antioxidant glutathione. In animal studies oral administration of NAC over time increased peripheral glutathione levels and reduced markers of oxidative stress. Increased oxidative stress and disturbed glutathione metabolism have been associated with bipolar disorder and depression. In a 6-month DBRPC study of 75 patients with bipolar disorder, the addition of NAC 2g/day to the usual treatment regimen resulted in significant improvements on measures of depression, mania, quality of life, and social and occupational functioning compared to placebo. Response took 8–12 weeks with no significant side effects (Berk, Copolov, Dean, et al., 2008b).

Psychotropic medications, particularly antipsychotics, can damage fibers in the striatum leading to tremors, stiffness, or abnormal movements. In animal studies NAC protected rat striatum from oxidative stress and lipid peroxidation due to an antipsychotic medication, haloperidol (Haldol). This raises the possibility that NAC could protect patients from some of the adverse effects of treatment with antipsychotic medications. NAC has also been used to treat acetaminophen overdose and to reduce the risk of respiratory infections and flu. Because NAC is safe, well tolerated, and has additional health benefits, it is a useful complementary treatment. A positive response usually takes 8–12 weeks using daily doses of 2400–3600 mg/day.

HERBS FOR TREATMENT OF MOOD DISORDERS

Hypericum perforatum (St. John's Wort)

Meta-analyses of RCTs of St. John's wort for mild to moderate depression show significant benefits compared to placebo, effects comparable to imipramine and SSRIs, and far fewer side effects than synthetic antidepressants but slower onset of action (3–6 weeks imipramine vs. 6–12 weeks SJW) (Linde et al., 1996; Rahimi, Nikfar, & Abdollahi, 2009; Sarris et al., 2011, 2013). See section titled Herb–Drug Interactions.

Rigorous research has shown more consistent results in studies using adequate doses of better quality standardized pharmaceutical grade SJW extracts, such as Kira (LI 160) 600 mg three times daily (Vorbach, Arnoldt, & Hubner, 1997) or Remotiv (ZE 117) 500 mg/day (Schrader, 2000) for mild to moderate depression and Ws5570 900-1800 mg/day for moderate to severe depression (Szegedi, Kohnen, Dienel, & Kieser, 2005). Treating severe depression with SJW requires higher doses (1800 mg/day) for longer periods of time (6–12 weeks). At higher doses SJW has side effects that are milder but similar to SSRIs, including nausea, heartburn, loose stools, sexual dysfunction, bruxism (teeth clenching), and restless leg syndrome. SJW can augment response to antidepressants such as tricyclics, buproprion, venlafaxine, and SAMe, but it should not be combined with MAOIs. Combining SJW with other serotonergic antidepressants may increase the risk of serotonin syndrome. SJW can induce mania in bipolar patients. A review of data from 35 DBRCTs found that dropout and adverse effects rates in patients receiving SJW extracts were similar to placebo. However, medically ill patients probably have higher rates of adverse reactions than patients selected for depression studies, which usually exclude serious medical illness and patients on medication. Phototoxic rash occurs in less than 1% of people taking SJW 900 mg/day or more. SJW should be discontinued 2 or 3 weeks prior to surgery because it can affect heart rate and blood pressure during anesthesia. SJW has been found to interfere with absorption and metabolism of numerous medications in humans. See the section on Herb–Drug Interactions for discussion of clinically significant effects that are probably due to induction of cytochrome P450 3A4 and 1A2 enzymes as well as intestinal wall P-glycoprotein (Knuppel & Linde, 2004; Russo, Scicchitano, Whalley, Mazzitello, Ciriaco, Esposito, et al., 2014). Nevertheless, in some settings SJW is particularly beneficial, for example, in mild depression with wintertime seasonal affective disorder (Cott & Fugh-Berman, 1998; Hansgen, Vesper, & Ploch, 1994; Wheatley, 1999) and in somatoform disorder (Volz, Murck, Kasper, & Moller, 2002). The authors (PLG and RPB) usually do not recommend SJW as a first-line solo treatment for depression unless the patient has a history of good response to low dose SSRI (e.g., 5mg/day fluoxetine) but complains of intolerable side effects such as weight gain or sexual dysfunction. Because there is such variability in the quality of SJW products, selecting brands that are standardized (0.3%–0.5% hyperforin) and that have proven efficacy based on their use in clinical trials is advised.

Rhodiola rosea (Roseroot, Arctic Root, Golden Root)

Although *Rhodiola rosea* has mainly been used for fatigue, cognitive disorders, memory, and performance under stress (see below), it can alleviate depression, increase transport of tryptophan and 5-HT (serotonin) into the brain, and support cellular energy transport. In the first study of *R. rosea* as a treatment for for depression, 128 patients with mixed types of depression were given 150 mg three times daily of *R. rosea* or placebo. Two-thirds of those on *R. rosea* improved significantly (Brichenko & Skorokhodova, 1987). Although this study did not fulfill modern methodological standards, it suggested positive effects. More recently, a standardized extract (SHR-5 from Swedish Herbal Institute) of *R. rosea* rhizomes was used in a DBRPC study of 89 adults between 18 and 70 years of age who met *DSM-IV* criteria for mild to moderate depression (HAMD scores 12–31). Subjects were randomly assigned to three groups. Group A received moderate doses of SHR-5 (340 mg/day); Group B received SHR-5 680 mg/day; and Group C received placebo. At the end of six weeks, mean HAMD scores dropped significantly in Groups A and B but not in Group C. No serious side effects were reported in any group (Darbinyan et al., 2007).

The authors routinely use *R. rosea* as augmentation in treating depression because it increases mental and physical energy, which are often low. It also improves mood and stress tolerance. Prescription antidepressants may alleviate negative mood states but often fall short of producing positive mood. Many patients anecdotally report that addition of *R. rosea* engenders a sense of well-being with increased motivation to get out of bed and do things. In the authors' clinical experience, patients with asthenia (mental and physical fatigue)

respond well to *R. rosea*. For a discussion of mechanisms of action, see the section titled Herbs for Treatment of Cognitive Dysfunction.

Rhodiola rosea for Depression in Menopause

Although it has not been formally studied in menopausal women for depression, fatigue, and memory decline, the authors (PLG and RPB) find that *R. rosea* restores energy, mental clarity, and sense of joyfulness. For further discussion, see subsections on Herbal Treatments for Cognitive Dysfunction and Herbs for Female Sexual Function.

Rhodiola rosea Side Effects and Dosage

R. rosea has an energizing or mildly stimulating effect but is usually emotionally calming. Unlike prescription stimulants (e.g., amphetamines) this adaptogen does not cause addiction, habituation, or withdrawal symptoms. Individuals who are sensitive to stimulants such as caffeine may initially feel more anxious, agitated, jittery, or "wired." Patients should reduce their intake of caffeine when using this herb, because the stimulative effects can be additive. For those who are sensitive it is possible to give a fraction of the usual dose and then increase gradually as tolerated. Starting doses of 100–150 mg in the morning on the first 2 days for mild to moderate depression can be increased by one capsule every 3–7 days to a maximum of 600 mg/day. As an adjunctive treatment for depression, *R. rosea* is usually effective in doses of 200–400 mg/day. As a solo treatment, higher doses up to 750 mg/day are sometimes needed. Above 900 mg/day, mild effects on blood coagulation may occur with increased bruising. *R. rosea* should be given with caution and with close monitoring to patients taking anticoagulants. Physicians should question patients who use sports drinks, which can contain 1000 mg or more of *R. rosea* often in combination with caffeine. This may increase the risk of adverse effects such as tachycardia, particularly in athletes who may consume more than one bottle of such drinks to enhance sports performance. There is no evidence that increasing the dose of *R. rosea* above 900 mg/day provides greater benefits, and it may entail increased risks. *R. rosea* should be taken in the early part of the day to avoid interference with sleep. Some people report vivid dreams (not nightmares) during the first 2 weeks. Occasionally, the herb may cause mild nausea. This can usually be managed by taking two ginger capsules 20 minutes before ingesting *R. rosea* or by drinking ginger tea. For discussion of potential hormonal and anticarcinogenic effects, see the section on Adaptogens and Herbs with Adaptogenic Properties for Menopause and Herb–Drug Interactions.

Quality and Potency of Rhodiola rosea

R. rosea is one of the complex herbs whose quality can be affected by the factors described in the section on Standardization of Supplements. Among the dozens of medicinal compounds in *R. rosea* root extracts, salidrosides and rosavins have been identified as active components and used as marker compounds, although no one has yet identified which combinations of the numerous antioxidants and other bioactive constituents are responsible for its many effects. Also, it may be subject to the addition of marker compounds to products that have been adulterated with less expensive herbs. The marker compounds alone do not account for all of the medicinal effects; therefore, it is important to use only those brands that have been proven to be clinically effective or that have been tested for at least 6 marker compounds.

Eleutherococcus senticosus or *Acanthopanax senticosus* (Siberian Ginseng)

Extracts from the fruit and seeds of *Eleutherococcus senticosus* were studied in the USSR for mental disorders. In their reviews, Panossian and Wikman found that the methodologies in most of the Soviet studies between 1950 and 1980 do not meet current standards. Nevertheless, the improvements reported in depression, bipolar disorder, schizophrenia, addictions, and alcoholic hallucinosis would be intriguing pathways for future research (Panossian & Wikman, 2009; Panossian, 2013). In a more recent study, *E. senticosus* 750 mg three times daily augmentation of lithium resulted in response and remission rates that were comparable to augmentation of lithium with fluoxetine 20 mg/day in a 6-week DBRCT of 79 Chinese adolescents with bipolar disorder. Furthermore, side effects and switching to mania were far less with *E. senticosus* than with fluoxetine (Weng, 2007).

Crocus sativus (Saffron)

Concentrated extracts of the stamen and petals of saffron were tested in two RCTs and found to significantly improve depression compared to placebo (Akhondzadeh et al., 2005; Moshiri et al., 2006). In three additional RCTs, the effects of *C. sativus* on HAMD scores were equivalent to the effects of imipramine and fluoxetine (Akhondzadeh Basti, et al., 2007; Moshiri, Noorbala, et al., 2007; Noorbala, Akhondzadeh, Tahmacebi-Pour, & Jamshidi, 2005). The occurrence of side effects including anxiety, tachycardia, nausea, dyspepsia, and appetite changes was not statistically significant compared to placebo. All of the studies thus far have been conducted by one group of researchers. Trials at other centers would help validate these encouraging findings. Evidence from one RCT suggested that saffron can reduce carbohydrate craving and help with weight loss (Gout, Bourges, & Paineau-Dubreuil, 2010). For a clinical review see Modabbernia and Akhondzadeh (2013).

Curcuma longa (Curcumin from Tumeric)

Curcuminoids from the spice, turmeric, piperine, the alkaloid that gives black pepper its taste, is used to enhance the absorption of nutrients.

A randomized double-blind placebo-controlled 8-week trial of curcumin 500 mg twice daily showed that curcumin was more effective than placebo in improving scores on the Inventory of Depressive Symptomatology ad the Spielberger State-Traint Anxiety inventory. Greater benefits were found in patients with atypical depression (Lopresti et al., 2014).

In a double-blind study, 11 adults with MDD were randomized to receive stanhdard antidepressants or standard antidepressants augmented with curcuminoids-piperine compbination 1000/10 mg/day). Reductions in BDI-II and MADS were significantly greater in the group given curcuminoids versus control (p < 0.001) (Panahi et al., 2014).

Curumen is very low in side effects, may be better absorbed in combination with piperine, and could serve as a useful add-on to standard antidepressants.

COGNITIVE FUNCTION

Disorders of cognition and memory develop from processes in which the damage to neurons compromises function and exceeds the capacity for repair. Nutrients and herbs that are neuroprotective and that support brain functions, energy production, cellular repair, and neuroplasticity will be reviewed. *Neural fatigue* or *neurasthenia* refers to a condition in which the patient experiences excess mental fatigue after a shorter than normal period of cognitive activity (resulting in reduced work capacity), increased perception of effort, and reduced endurance for sustained mental activity. It is more likely to occur under stress and/or following brain injury of any kind. Adaptogens have been shown to be particularly beneficial in patients with symptoms of neurasthenia or neural fatigue, which include a subjective sense of mental fatigue, reduced efficiency for mental tasks, and decreased work productivity (usually occurring with mental exertion), often with headache or malaise. The term *synaptic fatigue* attributes mental fatigue to depletion of presynaptic neurotransmitters, but more recently central fatigue has been linked to activation of microglia and/or increased cytokines and chemokines in the brain, implicating dysfunction in the ascending arousal system; pathways connecting basal ganglia, thalamus, limbic system, and higher cortical centers; sleep executive control areas; reward areas; and the suprachiasmatic nucleus. (Harrington, 2012).

PATHOPHYSIOLOGICAL TARGETS FOR INTEGRATIVE TREATMENTS

Nutrients and phytomedicines target mediators of the stress response, energy metabolism, neuroprotection, cellular repair, neuroplasticity, and the neuroendocrine system.

The membrane hypothesis of aging proposes that oxidative damage to cellular membranes leads to loss of permeability, increased intracellular density, accumulation of cross-linked proteins and lipofuscin (waste products), breaks in DNA, slowing of RNA synthesis, and decreased protein turnover and repair. Free radical damage to mitochondria compromises the ability of the cell to maintain sufficient energy production to sustain normal functions and to fuel cellular repair systems. Substances that have antioxidant properties or that increase production of antioxidants are candidates for prevention and treatment of age-associated cognitive and memory

Table 28.1 ANXIETY DISORDERS AND INSOMNIA IN THE MEDICAL PATIENT

	CONDITIONS/ SYMPTOMS	DOSE RANGES	SIDE EFFECTS*	DRUG INTERACTIONS	COMMENTS
NUTRIENTS					
Gamma amino-butyric acid GABA	Anxiety, stress phobias	100 mg/d	Minimal		
Magnesium	Anxiety Premenstrual syndrome	200–400 mg/d			Most studies are in combination with vitamins + minerals
Omega-3-fatty acids	Anxiety	2–4 gm/d	Belching, loose stools		EPA:DHA ratio 2:1
HERBS					
Butterbur *Petasites hybridus*	Migraines, allergic rhinitis	100 mg 2–4 times/d	Minimal	Poor quality brands may interact with CYP3A4 substrates	Use in combination with lemon balm, passion flower, valerian.
Chamomile *Matricaria recutita*	Minimal sedative Generalized Anxiety Disorder	200–1000 mg/d	Ragweed family—allergic reactions		Avoid during pregnancy
Ginkgo *Ginkgo biloba*	Anxiety depression dementia	240–280 mg/d	Minimal: headache	Anticoagulants**	Discontinue 2 weeks prior to surgery
Kava *Piper methysticum*	Anxiety, insomnia	100 mg standardized extract (70 mg kavalactones) t.i.d.	Gastrointestinal distress, allergic rash, photosensitivity, headache, Occasional: ↓ energy, drowsiness, tremor, restlessness, dystonia, hepatitis, liver failure.	↓ effects of levodopa	Avoid during pregnancy Toxicity may occur at doses > 240 mg kavalactones/d
Lemon balm *Melissa officianalis*	Anxiety, insomnia	(400–600 mg/d depending on preparation)	No serious side effects		Mild anxiolytic
Passionflower *Passiflora incarnate*	Anxiety, insomnia	500–1000 mg 2–4/d	Minimal		Mild anxiolytic

Supplement	Indication	Dose	Side Effects	Drug Interactions	Cautions/Contraindications
Rhodiola Arctic Root *Rhodiola rosea*	PTSD Combat stress	50–900 mg/d	Agitation, insomnia, anxiety, headache Rare: palpitations, chest pain	Doses > 750 mg/d may ↓ platelet aggregation	Can trigger mania in Bipolar disorder
St. John's wort *Hypericum perforatum*	Depression mild–mod	300–600 mg t.i.d.	Nausea, heartburn, loose bowels, jitteriness, insomnia, fatigue, bruxism, phototoxic rash, mania in bipolar.	Induces CYP 3A4, and P-glycoprotein: ↓ digoxin, warfarin, indivir, cyclosporine, theophylline, birth control pills, anesthetics, and others.	Discontinue 2 weeks prior to surgery. Avoid during pregnancy. Evidence for use in depression is weak.
Theanine Green tea *Camellia sinensis*	Mild anxiety	200 mg 1–3x/d	Minimal	Anticoagulants	Monitor if given with anticoagulants
Valerian *Valeriana officianalis*	Sleep	450–900 mg h.s.	Occasional gastrointestinal distress, headaches, minimal hangover on high doses > 600 mg.		Avoid during pregnancy. Contraindication: hepatic disease
NEUROHORMONES					
7-keto DHEA	PTSD dissociative symptoms	25–200 mg/d	Bipolar patients may become agitated, irritable, anxious.		Contraindication: Estrogen sensitive or prostate cancer patients.
Melatonin	Sleep	1–12 mg h.s.	Occasional agitation, abdominal cramps, fatigue, dizziness, headache, vivid dreams.		Contraindication: pregnancy

*In addition to the listed side effects, rare side effects can occur. Most supplements have not been tested for safety during pregnancy and breastfeeding. Patients taking anticoagulants and those with high blood pressure, diabetes, hepatic disease, or any chronic or serious medical condition may be at increased risk for side effects and therefore require closer monitoring. Herbal side effects are more frequent with lower quality products which may contain contaminants or adulterants.

**No cases of bleeding have been reported with products containing pharmaceutical grade *Ginkgo biloba*, such as EGb761.

Key: PTSD, Posttraumatic stress disorder; EPA, eicosapentanoic acid; DHA, dicosahexaenoic acid; hs, bedtime; b.i.d., twice a day; t.i.d., three times a day; gm, grams; mg, milligrams; mcg, microgram; ↓, decreases decline as well as cerebrovascular and neurodegenerative diseases (Aliev, Palacios, & Obrenovich, 2011).

Mitochondrial energy enhancers support production of molecules such as ATP, necessary for energy transport within cells.

The *calcium hypothesis* of neuronal aging has been modified in tandem with increasing information about the role of subtle age-related changes in Ca^{2+} in mitochondrial dysfunction (Toescu & Verkhratsky, 2007). According to the *membrane hypothesis* (Long & Pekala, 1996; Zs-Nagy, 1997), reactive oxygen species damage cell membranes and organelles through lipid peroxidation that contributes to neurodegenerative disorders such as Alzheimer's (AD) and Parkinson's disease (PD).

Endothelial damage due to arteriosclerosis and free radicals leads to hypoperfusion in cerebrovascular diseases such as multi-infarct dementia and ischemic stroke. Cerebral vasodilators and antioxidants can be used to prevent or ameliorate perfusion-related problems. Membrane fluidity, which is essential for neurotransmission, enables receptors to fold and unfold for optimal opening and closing of membrane ion channels. Oxidative damage and loss of membrane n-3FAs contribute to increased membrane rigidity. Evidence suggests that sustained inflammation may also be a factor in neurodegenerative disorders such as AD and PD.

The *cholinergic hypothesis* attributes a significant role in the pathophysiology of AD to loss of cholinergic neurons resulting in synaptic changes in cerebral cortex, hippocampus, and other brain areas involved in cognitive functions (Arciniegas, 2001).

Neuroplasticity, involving changes in synaptic connectivity and neurogenesis depends on brain-derived neurotrophic factor (BDNF). BDNF and its receptor, tropomyosin receptor–related kinase B, modulate numerous neuroprotective functions. Long-term potentiation, a form of neuroplasticity, is based on increased interneuronal connectivity. N-methyl-D-aspartate (NMDA) excitatory amino acid receptors modulated by BDNF are involved in rapid connectivity changes such as long-term potentiation.

Mediators of stress response include neuropeptide Y, nitric oxide, membrane bound G-protein receptors, heat shock proteins, and others, and will be discussed in the section on Mediators of the Stress Response.

VITAMINS AND NUTRIENTS FOR COGNITIVE FUNCTION

Vitamins and trace elements are essential for energy production, brain development, cognitive function, neuroprotection, and recovery from damage (Bourre, 2006; Brown, Gerbarg, & Muskin, 2009; Brown & Gerbarg, 2011). Limited evidence suggests that a combination of Vitamins C and E may reduce the incidence of AD (Zandi et al., 2004). Synthetic vitamin E (d-alpha tocopherol) is no longer recommended for prevention of cognitive decline because a prospective study of 35,533 healthy men followed for 7 to 12 years found that the absolute increase in risk of prostate cancer per 1000 person-years was 1.6 for synthetic vitamin E (400 IU/d of all rac-α-tocopheryl acetate), 0.8 for selenium, and 0.4 for a combination of the two (Klein et al., 2011). Suboptimal vitamin D levels may be

a risk factor for cognitive decline and AD (Eyles, Burne, & McGrath, 2012; Annweiler et al., 2012). Stronger evidence supports the combined use of B vitamins, folic acid, S-adenosylmethionine, and n-3FAs in disorders of cognition, including age-related cognitive decline, dementia, AD, stroke, and traumatic brain injury.

B Vitamins, Folic Acid, S-adenosylmethionine (SAMe)

Methylation (donation of methyl groups) pathways, dependent on B vitamins and folate cofactors, are essential for synthesis of proteins, neurotransmitters, antioxidants, and other cellular components used to maintain function, membrane integrity, and repair of DNA and RNA (Bottiglieri, 1996, 2013; Hassing, Wahlin, Winblad, & Backman, 1999). SAMe, the body's most active donator of methyl groups, participates in more than 200 different biochemical reactions in humans, including three central metabolic pathways: transmethylation (donation of methyl groups, CH_3); transsulfuration (donation of sulfur); and transaminopropylation (donation of aminopropyl moieties; see Figure 28.3). Foods supply part of the body's need for SAMe, the remainder being generated by de novo synthesis from methionine and ATP—primarily in the liver, which produces 3 gms/day. SAMe levels are easily increased by oral supplementation.

Vitamin and Nutrient Formulas

Three studies using a vitamin/nutrient formula (NF) containing folic acid 400 mcg, B_{12} 6 mcg, vitamin E alpha-tocopherol 30 IU, S-adenosylmethionine 400 mg, N-acetylcysteine 600 mg, and acetyl-L-carnitine 500 mg found positive effects on cognitive function. A DBRPC study of 115 community-dwelling adults aged 22–73 years without dementia found that after 2 weeks, the test scores of subjects taking NF improved significantly on the California Verbal Learning Test II (CLVT) and the Trail-making Test compared with those on placebo. This was followed by a 3-month open-label extension during which those taking NF showed additional improvement. During a 3-month discontinuation of NF, test measures reverted to baseline. Resumption of NF restored improvements (Chan et al., 2010). A 12-month open label study of the same NF given to 14 community-dwelling adults with early-stage AD rated mild to moderate on the Dementia Rating Scale (DRS) found that within 6 months, total performance on DRS improved significantly by about 30% (p < .02) with improvements maintained at 12 months (Chan, Paskavitz, Remington, Rasmussen, & Shea, 2008). Another DBRPC study of NF in 12 institutionalized patients with moderate to late-stage AD showed that those given the NF had clinically significant delay in decline on DRS and on the Clock Drawing Test (CLOX 1 and 2) over a period of 9 months compared to those given placebo (Remington, Chan, Paskavitz, & Shea, 2009). These small studies are promising but should be interpreted with some caution pending validation by large studies done by other research groups. Given recent controversy regarding increased risk of prostate cancer in men taking vitamin E, the vitamin/nutrient formula may need to be modified. The composition of vitamin/nutrient/herbal formulas (VNHF) could include constituents that target as many as possible of the relevant pathophysiological mechanisms described above to optimize synergistic effects.

B Vitamins and Antioxidants

Combining B vitamins with antioxidants may be more effective than either alone. However, there may be differences in the absorption and activity of natural vitamins compared to synthetic. For example, natural folate is absorbed less than synthetic. The authors prefer to use a product called Bio-Strath containing natural vitamins produced by yeast cultivated with vitamin enriched nutrients. In a 3-month DBRPC trial, Bio-Strath (B vitamin + antioxidants) at double the usual adult dose was given to 75 patients aged 55–85 years with mild dementia. The placebo group deteriorated while the Bio-Strath group showed improvement in short-term memory with physical and emotional benefits at 3 months (Pelka & Leuchtgens, 1995). For geriatric patients with neurodegenerative disorders and cognitive decline, studies suggest a dose of 2 tablets three times a day or 1 tablespoon twice a day of the liquid preparation. In healthy adults, 3 tablets twice a day or 1 teaspoon three times daily is usually sufficient. Alternatively, patients can be treated with folic acid 400–800 mcg/day, B_{12} 500 mcg/day (preferably sublingual), and B_6 in the range of 25 mg/day. Considering the importance of B vitamins for cognitive function and the low incidence of side effects, the authors use them in the treatment of patients with brain injury, dementia, and many other conditions affecting brain function. Sublingual B_{12} is better absorbed than oral capsules, particularly in patients with impaired gastrointestinal absorption. Serum methylmalonic acid is a more accurate measure of intracellular B_{12} than serum B_{12}.

In some studies folic acid, B_{12}, and B_6 have been found to lower homocysteine levels. A review of the literature found the evidence on the homocysteine-lowering effect of folic acid and B vitamin therapy in coronary artery restenosis to be contradictory (van Hattum, Doevendans, & Moll, 2007). In a 7-month DBRPC study of 205 patients following balloon angioplasty, among those treated with folic acid and B vitamins the rate of restenosis in subjects without stents was 10.3% versus placebo 41.9% (p <0.001); in subjects with stents it was 20.6% versus 29.9% (p = 0.32) respectively (Schnyder et al., 2001). A 6-month DBRPC study of coronary stent replacement in 636 patients found that reduction in restenosis was associated with the lowering of homocysteine by folic acid and B vitamins, the greatest reductions occurring in women and men with baseline homocysteine levels above 15 μM/L. However, an 8% increase in the rate of restenosis was found only in men (not in women) with baseline homocysteine levels less than 15 μM/L, who were given folic acid with B_{12} and B_6 supplementation (Lange et al., 2004). No study reported a significant difference in cardiovascular events in patients treated with folic acid versus placebo. There does not appear to be any increased risk of vascular occlusion in individuals who take folic acid and B vitamins and who do not have cardiac stents.

Omega-3 Fatty Acids (n-3FAs)

Polyunsaturated fatty acids (PUFAs), including the n-3FAs, DHA, EPA, and AA are necessary to maintain cell membrane function and the production of molecules involved in inflammatory modulation (Bourre, 2005). It is preferable to take a 1000mg/day blend of EPA and DHA in a 2:1 ratio. For mechanisms of action, dosages, and side effects, see the section on Omega-3 Fatty Acids for Depression and Bipolar Disorder.

Low levels of n-3FAs have been found in patients with dementia and AD. In an 8-year prospective study of 1,200 elderly subjects, those with low serum DHA had a 67% greater chance of developing AD than those with high DHA (Kyle & Arterburn, 1998). A 5-year prospective study of 210 healthy men aged 70–89 years found that those who ate fish equivalent to EPA/DHA 400 mg/day had slower cognitive decline than those who did not (van Gelder, Tijhuis, Kalmijn, & Kromhout, 2007). Another study of 2251 older adults found less decline in verbal ability in those with higher serum levels of EPA/DHA, especially in those with high blood pressure and high lipid levels (Beydoun, Kaufman, Satia, Rosamond, & Folsom, 2007).

DHA supplementation improved neurological symptoms in Alzheimer's patients (Nidecker, 1997). In a DBRPC study of 174 very mildly impaired Alzheimer's disease patients, 600 mg EPA slowed cognitive decline over a 6-month period (Freund-Levi et al., 2006). More studies are needed to confirm the neuroprotective effects of antioxidants and n-3FAs in patients with neurodegenerative conditions. Patients unwilling to eat fish regularly can be encouraged to take fish oil or flax oil capsules. In general, fish oils are preferable because only a fraction of the linolenic acid in flax oil gets converted into DHA. Credible evidence suggests that PUFAs enhance cognitive development and protect against neurodegeneration. While increasing dietary unsaturated nonhydrogenated fats may lower the risk of AD, large amounts of saturated trans fats increase the risk of AD (Morris et al., 2003).

Phosphatidylserine

Phosphatidylserine (Pdt Ser) is a naturally occurring phospholipid thought to contribute to nerve cell membrane fluidity. DBRPC studies of bovine-derived Ptd Ser (containing high amounts of DHA) showing modest memory improvements in age-associated memory decline have been reported with bovine Ptd Ser. However, the risk of acquiring prions, an infectious agent composed of misfolded protein from animals with Mad Cow disease, has not been assessed. At this time we advise limiting the use of Ptd Ser to products derived from fish, soy beans, or cows raised in New Zealand and Australia where surveillance for prion-related diseases is carefully regulated. Ptd Ser may be safer when derived from cow blood as opposed to neural tissues or organs where prions accumulate. Although studies of soy-derived Ptd Ser are limited, it appears to be of some benefit. Ptd Ser is often combined with other nutrients such as ginkgo (McDaniel, Maier, & Einstein, 2003). In clinical practice, soy-derived Ptd Ser may be a useful complementary treatment for age-associated

Table 28.2 MOOD DISORDERS IN THE MEDICAL PATIENT

	CONDITIONS/SYMPTOMS	DOSE RANGES	SIDE EFFECTS*	DRUG INTERACTIONS	COMMENTS
NUTRIENTS					
B vitamins	Depression Energy	B_{12} 1,000 mcg	Rare: activation		
Cholecalciferol Vitamin D3	Depression	2,000–6,000 IU/d			Use in vitamin D deficient patients
Folic acid L-methylfolate	Depression Depression	400 mcg/d 7.5–15 mg/d			8% ↑ risk occlusion cardiac stents men with baseline homocysteine < 15 mM/L** Use L-methylfolate for MTHFR polymorphisms
5-hydroxytryptophan 5-HTP	Depression	200–300 mg/d	Headache, insomnia, nausea, vomiting, diarrhea		
Inositol	Depression	12–20 g	Gas, loose bowels, mania		Caution: Bipolar
Choline	Mania	2,000–7,200 mg	Excess doses: depression		
N-acetylcysteine (NAC)	Bipolar depression and mania	2,400–3,600 mg/d	Rare: heartburn when taken on empty stomach		Response may take 8–12 weeks
Omega-3-fatty acids	Depression Bipolar depression	1–9 gm/day	Belching, loose stools, nausea, abdominal pain	Anticoagulants –monitor	EPA:DHA 2:1
S-adenosyl-L-methionine (SAMe)	Depression mild to severe Arthritis, fibromyalgia, liver disease Liver diseases Parkinson's depression	400–1,600mg/d 800–1,200 mg/d 800–1,200 mg/d 1,600–4,800 mg/d	Nausea, loose bowels, activation, anxiety, headache, occasional palpitations	None Use to augment other antidepressants	Can trigger mania in Bipolar
HERBS					
Eleuthero, Acanthopanax Eleutherococcus senticosus	Augmentation in depression and bipolar	750 mg t.i.d.	Minimal		
Rhodiola Arctic Root Rhodiola rosea	Depression, fatigue, amotivation Augment other antidepressants	50–900 mg/d	Agitation, insomnia, anxiety, headache. Rarely: palpitations, chest pain	Doses > 750 mg/d may affect platelet aggregation and ↑ bruising	Caution in Bipolar
Saffron Crocus sativa	Depression	88.25 mg 2–4 caps/d	Minimal Anticoagulants		Optimized saffron
St. John's wort Hypericum perforatum	Depression mild–moderate Seasonal affective disorder Somatoform	300–600 mg t.i.d.	Nausea, heartburn, loose bowels, jitteriness, insomnia, fatigue, bruxism, phototoxic rash, mania in bipolar patients, restless leg syndrome.	Induces CYP 3A4 and P-glycoprotein: ↓ digoxin, warfarin, indivir, cyclosporine, theophylline, birth control pills, anaesthetics and other medications. Serotonin syndrome	Discontinue 2 weeks prior to surgery. Avoid during pregnancy.

* In addition to the listed side effects, rare side effects can occur. Most supplements have not been tested for safety during pregnancy and breastfeeding. Patients taking anticoagulants and those with high blood pressure, diabetes, hepatic disease, or any chronic or serious medical condition may be at increased risk for side effects and therefore require closer monitoring. Herbal side effects are more frequent with lower quality products which may contain contaminants or adulterants.

** Folate + B_{12} + B_6 reduce the rate of cardiac stent restenosis in women and in men with baseline homocysteine level >15 mM/L.

Table Key: b.i.d., twice a day; t.i.d., three times a day; gm, grams; mg, milligrams; mcg, microgram; IU, International Units; ↑, increases; ↓, decreases; <, less than; >, more than memory decline but not for more severe memory disorders. A marine source of PtS with omega-3 long chain polyunsaturated fatty acids attached to its backbone, PS-DHA, was used in a 15-week DBRPC study of 157 nondemented elderly persons with memory complaints. Those who received PS-DHA (300 mg PS/day) showed significant improvements in immediate verbal recall. Those with higher baseline cognitive status had additional improvements in delayed verbal recall, learning abilities, and time to copy figures (Vakhapova, Richter, Cohen, Herzog, & Korczyn, 2011).

Mitochondrial Energy Production and Antioxidant Protection

Substances that support mitochondrial ATP-producing electron transport help maintain adequate energy supplies for cellular function, production of antioxidants, cellular repair, and neurogenesis.

Acetyl-L-Carnitine and Propionyl-L-Carnitine

Derivatives of carnitine, an essential nutrient, improve mitochondrial function and reduce oxidative damage. Acetyl-L-carnitine (ALC) facilitates acetyl coenzyme A uptake into mitochondria during fatty acid oxidation and increases energy production via the oxidative phosphorylation chain (Pettegrew, Levine, & McClure, 2000; Abdul Muneer, Alikunju, Szlachetka, & Haorah, 2011). Malaguarrera (2012) reviewed preclinical and clinical studies of ALC, PLC, and other carnitines. Positive effects of ALC were reported in diabetic, antiretroviral, and chemotherapy-induced neuropathies, insulin resistance, hypertension, Peyronie's disease, coronary artery disease, hepatic encephalopathy, sperm motility, and fibromyalgia. In animal models, ALC was neuroprotective and enhanced recovery from stroke (Lolic, Fiskum, & Rosenthal, 1997). In a study of oxidative toxicity using 4-hydroxy-2-nonenal, ALC plus alpha-lipoic acid (see below) protected rat cortical neurons from protein oxidation, lipid peroxidation, antioxidant depletion, and apoptosis (Abdul & Butterfield, 2007). ALC protected neurons from ethanol-induced oxidative injury in animal brain tissue slices (Rump et al., 2010). In an in vitro study of human brain endothelial cells, ALC stabilized superoxide dismutase (antioxidant preventing mitochondrial membrane damage) and protected the blood–brain barrier, brain vascular tone, and vasodilation (Haorah, Floreani, Knipe, & Persidsky, 2011). ALC may be more effective in delaying age-related deterioration of mitochondria when combined with alpha-lipoic acid, CoQ10, and essential fatty acids (Di Donato et al., 1986; Lolic, Fiskum, & Rosenthal, 1997). Alcar showed modest slowing of the development of AD in subjects 60 years of age or younger (Brooks, Yesavage, Carta, & Bravi, 1998). In a DBPC study of 12 elderly subjects with cerebral vascular disease, alcar improved reaction time, memory, and cognitive performance (Arrigo, Casale, Buonocore, & Ciano, 1990). Alcar 1500 mg administered intravenuosly increased regional cerebral blood flow in 8 out of 10 men with cerebral ischemia (Rosadini, Marenco, Nobili, Novellone, & Rodriguez, 1990). Although studies of ALC in AD are weak, it may have a role in prevention

or in augmentation of cholinesterase inhibitors in mild AD (Bianchetti, Rozzini, & Trabucchi, 2003). In patients with TBI and cerebrovascular disease, the authors find that ALC 1500 mg twice daily often improves energy and cognitive function within 2 weeks. ALC is low-risk and has few side effects. Rarely, it may trigger mania in bipolar patients.

Alpha-Lipoic Acid

Alpha-lipoic acid (ALA), a metabolic antioxidant, has been used as a prescription drug in Europe for treatment of cardiac autonomic problems related to diabetic neuropathy as well as other consequences of diabetes. Neuroprotective effects have been described in cerebral ischemia/reperfusion animal models, excitotoxic amino acid brain injury, mitochondrial dysfunction, diabetic neuropathy, inborn errors of metabolism, and other causes of acute or chronic damage to nerve tissue including excess levels of iron, copper, or other metals (Packer & Colman, 1999). ALA and CoQ-10 may be helpful in poststroke recovery and ischemic heart disease. ALA generates large amounts of glutathione in animal brain models (similar to SAMe). For patients who cannot afford SAMe, ALA in combination with vinpocetine (cerebral vasodilator) can be helpful when ischemia is a major factor and in other brain injuries. The authors find an ALA dose of 300 mg three times daily to be useful in TBI.

Coenzyme Q-10 (Idebenone)

Coenzyme Q10 (CoQ10, idebenone) enhances ATP-producing mitochondrial electron transport (Gillis, Benefield, & McTavish, 1994; Matsumoto et al., 1998). CoQ10 variants which enhance both cellular energy production and antioxidant defense are of interest for prevention and treatment of neurodegenerative, cerebrovascular, and cardiovascular diseases. In clinical practice the authors find that sluggish, psychomotor-retarded patients respond well to idebenone, which improves alertness. For individuals who become overstimulated by prescription cholinesterase inhibitors (e.g., donepezil, Aricept), idebenone serves as a less stimulating alternative. Combined with other supplements, it is particularly useful in cerebrovascular disease (e.g., multi-infarct dementia) and disorders of mitochondrial function (e.g., Friedreich's Ataxia) (Brown & Gerbarg, 2011). Ubiquinol, a reduced form of CoQ10, is an effective antioxidant protecting membranes from peroxidation. Muscle biopsies from patients with myopathies (e.g., myofiber atrophy and muscular dystrophy) showed significant positive correlations between CoQ10 and ubiquinone concentrations versus the percentage of myofibrils containing mitochondrial aggregates (Miles et al., 2005). The authors find ubiquinol to be beneficial in treating statin-induced myopathy.

Creatine

Creatine enhances cellular energy production in brain injury, muscular dystrophy, and other mitochondrial cytopathies (Brown & Gerbarg, 2011). Phosphorylated creatine provides a phosphate group in the conversion of ADP to ATP. In an open-label RCT pilot study, 39 children with TBI were

Table 28.3 COGNITIVE DISORDERS IN THE MEDICAL PATIENT

NUTRIENTS	CONDITIONS/SYMPTOMS	DOSE RANGES	SIDE EFFECTS*	DRUG INTERACTIONS	COMMENTS
Acetyl-L-carnitine ALCAR	TBI, AD, CVA, CVD, Alzheimers, fatigue, energy, alertness	500 mg b.i.d. starting dose Up to maximum dose 1,500 mg b.i.d.	Mild gastric upset, heartburn.	None	May slow progression of AD Take with food.
Alpha-lipoic acid	CVD, TBI, ischemia	300 mg t.i.d			
(Apoaequorin Synthetic jelly fish protein)	TBI, memory	10–40 mg/day	Headache, drowsiness, allergic reactions	Unknown	One RCT (n = 218)
B-vitamins	TBI, stroke, dementia, cognitive decline Neurodegenerative disorders, energy	B$_{12}$ 1,000 mcg	Rare: activation		
Centrophenoxine (Meclophenoxate)	TBI, Alzheimers Memory, alertness, focus	250 mg b.i.d starting dose Up to maximum dose 1,000 mg b.i.d.	Minimal, gastric upset, heartburn	When combined with other cholinergic agents: headache, muscle tension, insomnia, irritability, agitation, facial tics	
Citicholine CDP-Choline	CVD, TBI, acute ischemic stroke, ischemia, multi-infarct dementia	1,000–7,200 mg/d	Occasional: agitation Excess doses: depression		
Coenzyme Q10 Ubiquinol	CVD, TBI, Alzheimers, Neurodegenerative disease	270–900 mg/d	None		Less stimulating alternative to cholinesterase inhibitors
Creatine	TBI, memory, cognition, focus	0.4 gm/kg/d 5000 mg q.i.d for 5 days, then 5000 mg b.i.d.	Minimal		One study positive effects in children
Folic acid L-methylfolate	Depression, memory, cognition Depression, memory, cognition	400 mcg/d 7.5–15 mg/d			8% ↑ risk occlusion of cardiac stents in men with baseline homocysteine level < 15 mM/L**
L-Deprenyl	CVD, TBI, Alzheimers, Parkinsons's, cognitive, memory, preventive	2.5–5 mg/d	Minimal	None	<10 mg/d has no significant MAOI effect
Omega-3-fatty acids	Alzheimer's, neurodegeneration	2,000–3,000 mg/d	Belching, loose stools, nausea, abdominal pain	Anticoagulants: monitor	EFA:DHA ratio 2:1
Phosphatidyl serine	AAMI	Loading dose 300 mg/d for 1 month, Then 100 mg/d	Minimal	None	

Name	Uses	Dose	Side Effects	Comments
Picamilon	TBI, CVA, CVD, ischemia, Parkinsons, toxic brain lesions	50 mg b.i.d. up to 100 mg t.i.d.	High dose: postural hypotension	In CVD improves alertness, confusion, anxiety, depression
Pyrrolodones Racetams aniracetam, piracetam, pramiracetam	Poststroke aphasia, dyslexia Med-related cognitive impairment	aniracetam 750 mg b.i.d.	Minimal. Rarely: anxiety, insomnia, agitation, irritability, headache	Safe in children
S-adenosyl-L-methionine (SAMe)	Alzheimer's, Parkinson's TBI Depression Arthritis, liver diseases	400–4,000 mg/d in divided doses 400–1,600 mg/d 1,200–1,600 mg/d	Nausea, loose bowels, activation, anxiety, headache, occasional palpitations	Combines well and augments all classes of antidepressants tested. Give with L-dopa to reverse depletion of SAMe
HERBS				
Eleuthero, Acanthopanax *Eleutherococcus senticosus*	Fatigue, alertness	750 mg t.i.d.	Uncommon: diarrhea, dizziness, insomnia, headache, hypertension, irregular or rapid heart beat	Interferes with some digoxin tests, but does not lower digoxin levels / Combine with R. rosea and other adaptogens
Galantamine *Galanthus nivalis*	Alzheimers, TBI, CVD	8–32 mg/d	Mild nausea, GI upset	
Ginkgo biloba	Neuropsychiatric symptoms in AAMI, MCI, CVD, VAD, Alzheimers. Attention, memory. Peripheral vascular disease, claudication. Vascular related vertigo and tinnitus.	60–120 mg b.i.d.	Minimal, headache, gastrointestinal upset, nausea, ↓ platelet aggregation. Rare agitation, allergic reactions. Reported cases of bleeding not confirmed by recent reviews**	Monitor with anticoagulants and antiplatelet drugs** Anesthetics / Combine with acetylcholinesterase inhibitors for better effect in dementia. Discontinue 2 weeks prior to surgery.
Ginseng *Panax ginseng*	Dementia, cognitive function, alertness, focus, neurasthenia	300–800 mg/d	Activation, gastrointestinal, anxiety, insomnia, tachycardia, ↓ platelet aggregation, diarrhea. Hormonal: vaginal bleeding, swollen breasts. Excess doses: headache, vomiting, nervousness. Doses > 3 gm/d may have toxic effects: ↑ blood pressure, agitation, confusion	Anticoagulants, steroids, MAOIs / For CVA, TBI: better combined with adaptogens. Caution: Bipolar, hypertension. Contraindication: hormone sensitive cancers.
Huperzine	Alzheimers, AAMI, TBI, vascular dementia	200–400 mcg/d	Minimal	
Maca *Lepidium myenii*	Neural fatigue, memory, hearing, energy	Approximately 750 mg t.i.d. (dose depends on preparation)	Occasional: overactivation, jitteriness, insomnia, headache	Human studies are needed. Contraindication: hormone sensitive cancers.

(continued)

Table 28.3 (CONTINUED)

	CONDITIONS/SYMPTOMS	DOSE RANGES	SIDE EFFECTS*	DRUG INTERACTIONS	COMMENTS
Rhodiola Arctic Root *Rhodiola rosea*	TBI, post CNS infection (e.g., Neuro-Lyme), post stroke, dementia for cognitive recovery and memory	50–900 mg/d	Occasional: Agitation, insomnia, anxiety, headache Rare: palpitations, chest pain	Doses >750 mg/d may ↓ platelet aggregation. Additive effects with other stimulants (eg. caffeine)	Caution in Bipolar: may benefit depression but may exacerbate mania
Saffron	Mild–moderate Alzheimers, cognition, ↓ agitation	88.25 mg 2–4 caps/d	Minimal	Anticoagulants	Optimized saffron
Schizandra *Schizandra chinensis*	Concentration, energy, agitation	110–200 mg/d	Heartburn, acid indigestion, stomach pain, allergic rashes		Emotional calming
St. John's wort *Hypericum perforatum*	Depression mild–moderate	300–600 mg t.i.d.	Nausea, heartburn, loose bowels, jitteriness, insomnia, fatigue, bruxism, phototoxic rash, mania in bipolar.	Induces CYP 3A4, and P-glycoprotein: ↓ digoxin, warfarin, indivir, cyclosporine, birth control pills, anesthetics, theophyline, and others.	Discontinue 2 weeks prior to surgery. Avoid during pregnancy.
Vinpocetine Snowdrop *Vinca minor*	CVA, CVD, ischemia	10 mg t.i.d.	Mild indigestion, nausea, dizziness, anxiety, facial flushing, insomnia, headache, drowsiness and dry mouth	Monitor closely with agents that ↓ platelet aggregation	
NEUROHORMONES					
Dehydro-epiandrosterone DHEA	Cognitive, memory	25–100 mg/d	Mild insomnia, irritability. Bipolar patients may become agitated, irritable, or anxious.	Steroids	Pharmaceutical grade is best. Benefits patients with low or low normal baseline DHEA levels. Contraindications: Estrogen sensitive or prostate cancer
Melatonin	Sleep, 'sundowning'	1–12 mg h.s.	Occasional agitation, abdominal cramps, fatigue, dizziness, headache, vivid dreams.		Avoid during pregnancy

* In addition to the listed side effects, rare side effects can occur. Most supplements have not been tested for safety during pregnancy or breastfeeding. Patients taking anticoagulants and those with high blood pressure, diabetes, hepatic disease, or any chronic or serious medical condition may be at increased risk for side effects and therefore require closer monitoring. Herbal side effects are more frequent with lower quality products which may contain contaminants or adulturants.

** Folate + B$_{12}$+ B$_6$ may increase the rate of cardiac stent restenosis in in men only with baseline homocysteine level <15 mM/L.

*** Recent trials with pharmaceutical grade *Ginkgo biloba*, EGb761 do not confirm earlier reports of bleeding (Diamond, 2013).

Table Key: AAMI, Age Associated Memory Impairment; CVD, cerebrovascular disease; CVA, cerebrovascular accident; MCI, minimal cognitive impairment; TBI, traumatic brain injury; VAD, vascular dementia; h.s., bedtime; b.i.d., twice a day; t.i.d., three times a day; g, grams; mg, milligrams; mcg, microgram; ↓, decreases; ↑, increases; <, less than; >, more than.

randomized to standard treatment alone versus standard treatment plus creatine for 6 months. The duration of posttraumatic amnesia, intubation, and ICU stay were reduced in children treated with 0.4 g/kg/day creatine. Those given creatine showed significant improvement in headaches, dizziness, and fatigue compared with the standard treatment only group (Sakellaris et al., 2008). The authors note that creatine can ameliorate neural fatigue, dizziness, and headaches in TBI patients.

Cholinergic Enhancing Treatments

Cholinergic deficits underlie the main symptoms of AD. Treatments that enhance cholinergic transmission—by protecting cholinergic neurons, increasing availability of choline (precursor of acetyl choline), or reducing breakdown of acetyl choline (ACh)—improve cognitive function and delay deterioration in some studies of cerebrovascular accidents, AD, and other dementias and brain disorders (Akhondzadeh, Gerberg, & Brown, 2013). Plant-derived alkaloid extracts that act as acetyl cholinesterase inhibitors (AChEI) are discussed in Herbal Treatments for Cognitive Dysfunction.

Citicholine (CDP-choline, Cch)

Cytidine 5'-diphosphocholine (CDP-choline), a phospholipid cholinergic precursor used to treat stroke, dementia, and brain injury (Alvarez et al., 1999) is well absorbed, crosses the blood–brain barrier, and breaks down into choline and cytidine (a ribonucleoside). Acetyl coenzyme A and choline form the neurotransmitter acetyl choline. Choline is incorporated into cell membrane phospholipids, improves mitochondrial metabolism, increases ATP levels and synthesis of phospholipids, reduces glutamate release, and raises levels of norepinephrine, dopamine, and 5HT. In animal models it alleviates cerebral hypoxia and protects against ischemia, edema, and neuronal death in the cerebral cortex, forebrain, and hippocampus (Baskaya, Dogan, Rao, & Dempsey, 2000; Hurtado et al., 2005; Rao, Hatcher, & Dempsey, 1999). In rat brain injury and aging models, CDP-choline improved memory and cognitive performance and potentiated neuroplasticity (Dixon, Ma, & Marion, 1997).

A 6-week study of 214 patients with acute middle cerebral artery ischemic stroke found that those given CDP-choline within the first 24 hours showed significantly less enlargement in lesion volume on repeat MRI 12 weeks after the stroke (Mitka, 2002). Meta-analysis of controlled trials of CDP-choline by the Cochrane Stroke Review Group concluded that there is some evidence that CDP-choline has positive effects on memory and behavior in the short to medium term in cerebral disorders in the elderly (Fioravanti & Yanagi, 2005). It may be necessary to start CDP-choline within 24 hours of stroke onset for benefits to occur (Parnetti, Mignini, Tomassoni, Traini, & Amenta, 2007). In a review of 4 trials with a total of 1,472 patients, oral CDP-choline improved recovery when started within 24 hours of the onset of stroke symptoms. Maintenance on CDP-choline in first-stroke patients for 6 months prevented cognitive decline and improved temporal orientation, attention, and executive functions (Alvarez-Sabin & Roman, 2011). A review of eight studies (including three DBRPC trials) of TBI found evidence of acute and long-term benefits (Arenth, Russell, Ricker, H., & Zafonte, 2011). Davalos and colleagues (2012) conducted a 6-week multicenter DBRPC of CDP-choline 2000 mg/day in patients (n = 2,298) with moderate to severe acute ischemic stroke. Unlike previous studies, patients given CDP-choline did not have better outcomes than the placebo group. A subgroup analysis revealed better outcomes with CDP-choline in patients above 70 years old, those with moderate stroke severity, and those who were not being given a fibrinolytic (Davalos et al., 2012). A review of choline in mental and behavioral disorders by Akhondzadeh and colleagues pointed out that the multicenter study by Davelos used a dose of 2000 mg/day CDP-choline, which could have been subtherapeutic in comparison to findings from previous studies that doses greater than 2000 mg/day had greater efficacy (Akhondzadeh, Gerberg, & Brown, 2013). Moreover, the duration (6 weeks) was short considering that benefits are generally seen 9–12 weeks after the initiation of treatment. A comprehensive review of drug surveillance studies in over 4,000 acute ischemic stroke patients concluded that CDP-choline was associated with better outcomes than standard treatment alone (Cho & Kim, 2009; Leon-Jimenez et al., 2010). CDP-choline is safe with virtually no side effects.

Cerebral Vasodilators

Picamilon

Picamilon, a cerebral vasodilator, is composed of GABA and Vitamin B_3 (niacin). Vasodilation through reduction of smooth muscle tone in the walls of cerebral blood vessels increases cerebral blood flow (Mirzoian, Gan'shina, Kosoi, Aleksandrin, & Aleksandrin, 1989). Picamilon has both a mild tranquilizing action that can reduce aggressive behavior and a mild stimulative action that can improve alertness and cognitive function. Picamilon readily crosses the blood–brain barrier (Dorofeev & Kholodov 1991) and has low toxicity in animal experiments (median lethal oral dose >10 g/kg of body weight). Large open clinical trials in 16 medical centers in Russia, using picamilon 20-50 mg 2 to 3 times a day in treatments ranging from 2 weeks to 3 months, showed the best results in patients with organic brain syndromes due to head trauma, cerebral atherosclerosis, and toxic brain lesions (Kruglikova, 1997). Controlled trials are warranted. In clinical practice the authors find picamilon to be beneficial in patients with cerebral vascular impairment, particularly with decreased alertness, confusion, anxiety, and depression as the following case illustrates.

CASE STUDY: 80 YEAR-OLD WOMAN WITH CEREBRAL INSUFFICIENCY RESPONDS TO CEREBRAL VASODILATOR

An active 80-year-old, Joyce managed her home, balanced the checkbook, and drove herself to the grocery store, church, and volunteer activities. Her mild bipolar disorder was well controlled with quetiapine 50 mg h.s. until she required surgery for hernia repair. After awakening from anesthesia, Joyce was in a confusional state that persisted for 4 weeks after leaving the hospital. Her family took shifts caring for her, as she tended to sit for hours doing nothing unless prompted. Usually outspoken, her responses dwindled to a few barely audible words. Based on an fMRI showing reduced perfusion and the possibility that surgical anesthesia had further compromised cerebral circulation, she was treated with a cerebral vasodilator, picamilon 100 mg twice daily. Two days into treatment she began to improve. At follow-up three 3 weeks later Joyce was talkative, oriented, and reengaged in her previous activities. Nine months later, the patient's family brought her for re-evaluation of recurrent symptoms of confusion, reduced activity and paucity of speech. Joyce had stopped taking picamilon four weeks earlier when her supply ran out. Once she resumed taking the cerebral vasodilator, all of these symptoms remitted within two weeks.

Apoaequorin (Aequorea Victoria)

Apoaequorin is a calcium binding protein first isolated from jellyfish (*Aequorea victoria*). Potassium calcium channels in smooth muscle and endothelial cells are involved in regulation of vascular tone. Vascular dysfunction during ischemia reperfusion is associated with modulations of potassium and calcium. A company that marketings apoaequorin conducted a 90-day DBRPC study in 218 adults aged 40 to 91 years with self-reported memory issues. Compared to placebo, subjects given apoaequorin showed significant improvements on tests of recall performance, executive functioning, memory, delayed recall, and verbal learning. The study reported no adverse events and good tolerability (Underwood, Sivesind, Gabourie, & Lerner, 2011). Peer-reviewed studies by research groups are needed to evaluate apoaequorin as a potential treatment for cognitive and memory decline. However, in light of the low risks, clinicians could offer patients the option of a 3-month to 6-month trial in doses of 10, 20, or 40 mg/day.

HERBAL TREATMENTS FOR COGNITIVE DYSFUNCTION

Medicinal plants contain bioactive substances in the roots, leaves, flowers, and fruit. Unlike most synthetic drugs with one target of action, the presence of numerous medicinal compounds within one herb results in multiple effects. While the active constituents have been identified in some herbs, in others they have not. Moreover, the synergistic effects of constituents can be more powerful than any one alone. See the excellent review by Howes and Perry on the mechanisms of action and the use of phytochemicals in prevention and treatment of dementia (Howes & Perry, 2011). In vitro and animal studies are shedding light on physiological and genetic aspects of herbal medicines. For example, the cognitive enhancing effects observed with galantamine and huperzine may be due to potentiation of cholinergic and NMDA activity (Narahashi, Moriguchi, Zhao, Marszalec, & Yeh, 2004).

Huperzia serrata (Huperzine-A)

Huperzine-A, an alkaloid derived from Chinese club moss (Huperzia serrata) is a strong, selective, reversible AChEI

with neuroprotective properties including protection against hydrogen peroxide free radicals, B-amyloid protein formation, glutamate, and ischemia (Zhao et al., 2011). It protects mitochondria, reduces oxidative stress, and upregulates nerve growth factor. Huperzine-A is rapidly absorbed, readily penetrates the blood–brain barrier, and has a relatively long duration of AChE inhibitory action. In animal and primate studies it improves learning and memory (Tang, 1996). Three DBRCTs with more than 450 people and one open trial done in China showed significant benefits in AD. Four trials in vascular dementia and AD, using huperzine-A in combination with other medicines, nicergoline (a nootropic antiinflammatory that upregulates neurotrophic factors in glial cells), and estrogen compounds or mental training, showed favorable outcomes. In a DBRPC study of 78 patients with mild to moderate vascular dementia (VaD), those given Huperzine A 0.1 mg twice daily significantly improved in scores on the Mini Mental Status Exam (MMSE), clinical dementia rating, and activities of daily living after 12 weeks (p < .01) No significant adverse events occurred (Xu et al., 2011). A 16-week DBRPC study of 210 individuals with mild-to-moderate AD reported cognitive enhancement only at doses above 0.4 mg/day at week 16 (Rafii et al., 2011). Other trials showed positive outcomes in vascular dementia, TBI, age-associate memory decline, and schizophrenia (Akhondzadeh & Abbasi, 2006; Wang, Yan, & Tang, 2006). Huperzine-A is well tolerated with few side effects and minimal peripheral cholinergic effects.

Galanthus nivalis (Snowdrop) Galantamine

An alkaloid extract of snowdrop (*Galanthus nivalis*) was used in folk medicines of Russia and Eastern Europe to preserve memory as people aged. Galantamine, FDA-approved for treatment of AD, is an allosteric modulator of nicotinic receptors and a weak inhibitor of acetylcholinesterase (Raskind, Peskind, Wessel, & Yuan, 2000). In an open–label study, 280 AD patients included in the Swedish Alzheimer Treatment Study were given galantamine starting with 8 mg/day and gradually increasing to 16 mg/day at 4 weeks and then 24 mg/day as tolerated. After 3 years, subjects had mean increases of 2.6 points on the MMSE and 5.6 points in Alzheimer's Disease Assessment Scale-Cognitive (ADAS-cog) (Wallin, Wattmo, & Minthon 2011). Many patients do not tolerate the gastrointestinal disturbances caused by prescription galantamine or donepezil. In the author's (RPB) clinical experience, the herbal extract of *Galanthus nivalis* combined with *R. rosea* can be as effective as galantamine and more tolerable.

Vinpocetine from Vinca minor (the Lesser Periwinkle)

Vinpocetine (ethyl apovincaminate), is a semisynthetic ethyl ester of an alkaloid extract from leaves of the lesser periwinkle (*Vinca minor*). As a cerebrovascular vasodilator, it has been used for treatment of cerebrovascular disorders. Studies show neuroprotectant and anticonvulsant activity through inhibition of calcium/

calmodulin–dependent cyclic guanosine monophosphate-phosphodiesterase, enhancing intracellular cyclic guanosine monophosphate levels in vascular smooth muscle, reducing resistance of cerebral blood vessels, and increasing blood flow without significantly affecting blood pressure or peripheral vascular resistance (Patyar, Prakash, Modi, & Medhi, 2011). Vinpocetine inhibits the molecular cascade caused by the rise of intracellular calcium and selectively inhibits voltage-sensitive sodiaum channels, reducing excess extracellular calcium associated with ischemia/reperfusion, edema, and glutamate toxicity (Brown & Gerberg, 2011; Patyar et al., 2011). It scavenges hydroxyl radicals, inhibits IKB kinase complex, inhibits platelet aggregation, and increases erythrocyte deformability, reducing blood viscosity and further enhancing blood flow. Stimulation of locus ceruleus neurons may enhance alertness, concentration and information processing. In a DBRPC study of 43 stroke patients, transcranial Doppler and near infrared spectroscopy showed that vinpocetine improved cerebral perfusion in the peristroke area (Bönöczk et al., 2002). PET scans of 13 stroke patients showed improved peristroke cerebral glucose kinetics and blood flow (Szilagyi et al., 2005). In a 1-year study of 61 children with hypoxic ischemic encephalopathy due to intracranial birth trauma, vinpocetine reduced seizures, intracranial hypertension, and psychomotor sequelae (Dutov et al., 1991). Mild side effects include indigestion, nausea, dizziness, anxiety, facial flushing, insomnia, headache, drowsiness, and dry mouth. Patients taking other blood thinners concurrently should be closely monitored. The average dose is 10 mg three times a day. The authors find vinpocetine to be most helpful in cases with evidence of blood flow abnormalities on brain imaging studies.

Adaptogens: *Rhodiola rosea, Schizandra chinensis, Eleutherococcus senticosus, Panax ginseng, Lepidium peruvianum Chacon*

An adaptogen is a plant that increases resistance against multiple stressors (biological, chemical, or physical), normalizes physiological parameters, and does not disturb normal body functions more than necessary to improve resistance (Brekhman & Dardymov, 1969). Adaptogens contain bioactive compounds that function as metabolic regulators. In reviewing the effects of adaptogens on the central nervous system, Panossian and Wagner (2005) suggest that extracts from adaptogenic herbs have synergistic effects on stress response. *R. rosea* qualified as an adaptogen because it protected every organism tested, from snails to humans, against physical and mental stress including fatigue, heat, cold, toxins, chemotherapy cytotoxicity, heavy metals, ischemia, hypoxia, and radiation (Panossian & Wagner, 2005; Brown, 2002; Brown & Gerberg, 2004).

Panossian, Wikman, Wagner, and colleagues have been testing hypotheses regarding the mechanisms by which adaptogens exert numerous effects, including improving stress resilience, energy, mood, cognitive function, attention, memory, physical performance, and others (Panossian, 2013; Panossian & Wikman, 2009; Panossian, Wikman, Kaur, & Asea, 2012). They propose that adaptogens support homeostasis and regulation of the HPA axis via mediators of the stress response. Furthermore, they propose that adaptogens modulate gene expression of key mediators of stress-induced transduction pathways (Panossian et al., 2013). A full discussion of these hypotheses and their evidence base is beyond the scope of this chapter. Here we briefly outline the hypotheses and refer to the works of Panossian and colleagues for the details.

MEDIATORS OF THE STRESS RESPONSE

Molecular Chaperones, Heat Shock Proteins

Heat shock proteins (HSP70) protect cellular proteins from free radicals and enable the repair of damaged proteins, the disposal of defective proteins, and the inhibition of cell death. ADAPT- 232 (a fixed combination of *R. rosea, E. senticosus,* and *S. chinensis*) and salidroside (an active constituent of *R. rosea*) were found to increase serum levels of HSP70 in mice under stress and the expression and release of HSP70 from human neuroglial cells in vitro (See Figure 29.2).

Neuropeptide Y

During stress response, neuropeptide Y (NPY) is released from sympathetic nerves. Peripherally, it potentiates the stress response. Centrally NPY inhibits SNS activity and has an anxiolytic effect. NPY can promote ATP formation, inhibit NO synthesis (relieving the suppression of ATP formation by NO), reduce elevated protein kinases, affect modulators of immune response that control DNA transcription, and modulate the release of neuropeptides from the hypothalamus (See Figure 28.2). ADAPT-232 and salidroside have been shown to increase expression and release of NPY from human glioblastoma cells in culture. Panossian and colleagues hypothesize that, analogous to the strengthening effects of regular physical exercise, adaptogens act as mild stressors that increase stress tolerance and adaptation by stimulating the release of stress mediators HSP70 and NPY (Panossian et al., 2012; Panossian, 2014).

MODULATION OF GENE EXPRESSION

Genomic studies show that in combination, *R. rosea, E. senticosus,* and *S. chinensis* upregulate and downregulate a total of 2,188 genes in human neuroglial cells T98G. One active constituent, salidroside, alters expression of more than 700 genes. Among the genes affected by these adaptogens are those that encode cell membrane bound G-protein coupled receptors, including $5\text{-}HT_3$ receptors involved in the release of neurotransmitters and neurohormones (Panossian et al., 2013). Adaptogens also target SERPIN1, the gene encoding neuroserpin, which is involved in growth of axons, development of synapses, and synaptic plasticity (Panossian, 2013). Further studies in human neuroglial cells found that extract of Rhodiola upregulated 336 genes and down-regulated 295. Downstream effects of these genes are associated with cardiovascular (72 genes), metabolic (63 genes), gastrointestinal (163 genes), neurological (95 genes), endocrine (60 genes),

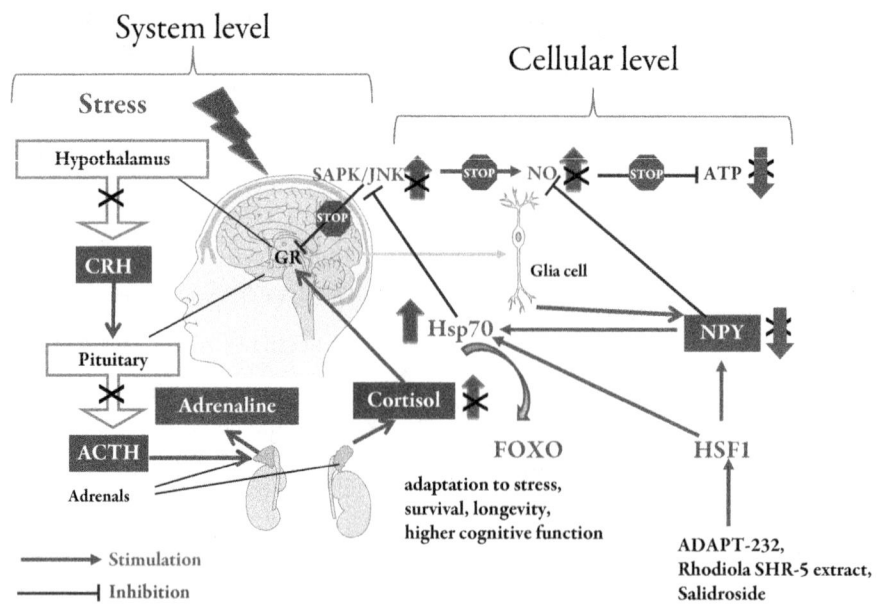

Figure 28.2 Hypothetical Mechanisms of Stress Protection by Adaptogens: Rhodiola SHR-5 extract, salidroside, and ADAPT-232. Reproduced with permission of Dr. Alexander Panossian (Panossian, 2013). Key: Stress induces hypothalamic release of corticotropin releasing hormone (CRH) followed by pituitary release of adrenocorticotropic releasing hormone (ACTH), which simulates release of adrenal hormones and Neuropeptide Y (NPY) to mobilize energy resources and cope with the stress. Feedback regulation of overreaction is initiated by cortisol release from adrenal cortex. Cortisol binds to glucocorticoid receptors (GR) in the brain, stopping further release of brain neurohormones and reducing the stress induced increase of cortisol down to baseline (pre-stress) levels. Although brief and mild stress (eustress or challenge) is essential to life, severe stress (distress or overload) is associated with extensive generation of oxygen free radicals, including nitric oxide (NO), which inhibit adenosine triphosphate (ATP) formation. Stress-activated protein kinases (SAPK/JNK/MAPK) inhibit GR, blocking this feedback downregulation such that serum cortisol remains high in fatigue, depression, and other stress-related conditions. Adaptogens normalize stress-induced elevated levels of cortisol and other extracellular and intracellular mediators of stress response, including elevated NO, SAPK (via upregulation of NPY expression), heat shock factor (HSF-1) and heat shock proteins (Hsp70), which inhibit SAPK. Consequently, NO generation is reduced and ATP production is no longer suppressed. Intracellularly Hsp70 enhances antiapoptotic mechanisms and protects proteins against mitochondria generated oxygen-containing radicals, including NO and superoxide anion. Hsp70 acts as an endogenous danger signal and has a vital role in immune stimulation. NPY is crucial in the HPA axis function and energy balance maintenance. Both NPY and Hsp70 are involved in enhancement of cellular adaptation to stress, survival, longevity and cognitive function. Hsp70 inhibits foxhead O transcription factor (FOXO), playing an important role in adaptation to stress and longevity. These pathways contribute to adaptogenic effects, such as antifatigue, improved attention and enhanced cognitive function. cognitivecognitive function.

behavioral (50 genes), and psychological disorders (62 genes) (Panossian, et al., 2014).

Rhodiola, Golden Root, Arctic Root, or Roseroot (*Rhodiola rosea*)

Although many of the 19 species in the Rhodiola genus are used as traditional medicines in Europe and Asia, *Rhodiola rosea* has been the most intensely studied. Starting in the 1950s under the Ministry of Defense of the former Soviet Union, 30 years of unpublished systematic research was kept in classified documents while the strategic use of *R. rosea* and other adaptogenic herbs to enhance physical, cognitive, and psychological functions was explored in military personnel, cosmonauts, Olympic athletes, scientists, and students (Baranov, 1994; Brown, Gerbarg, & Ramazanov, 2002; Brown & Gerbarg, 2004; Brown, Gerbarg, & Muskin, 2009; Stancheva, Mosharrof, & Petkov, 1986; Panossian, 2013). A formula called ADAPT, containing *Rhodiola rosea, Eleutherococcus senticosus*, and *Schizandra chinensis* was developed and tested the most extensively. Most of these studies were written as government reports, not for publication. However, current research is confirming many of the findings. Since the 1960s the Russian Pharmacopoeia has described the approved medicinal uses of root extracts of *R. rosea*. Soviet researchers observed therapeutic effects in posttraumatic and vascular brain lesions, especially in early post-injury stages. Rhodiola species

contain many antioxidant compounds and mitochondrial enhancers found to maintain higher levels of ATP and creatine phosphate (CP) in brain, muscle, liver, and blood (Furmanowa, Skopinska-Rozewska, Rogala, & Malgorzata, 1998; Kurkin & Zapesochnaya, 1986a). In animal studies *R. rosea* was shown to increase brain norepinephrine, DA, and 5-HT and stimulate nicotinic cholinergic systems (Petkov et al., 1986; Stancheva & Mosharrof, 1987). *R. rosea* increases blood–brain barrier permeability to DA and 5-HT precursors, consistent with activation of the cerebral cortex and limbic systems. Extracts also reversed the blockage of acetylcholine in pathways ascending from limbic system to cortex that are involved in memory. Two flavonoid glycosides (gossypetin-7-O-l-rhamnopyranoside and rhodio-flavonoside) from the alcohol extract of *R. rosea* (5 g/L) were found to cause 58 ± 15% and 38 ± 4% AChE inhibition respectively and may account in part for cognitive and memory-enhancing properties (Hill-House, Ming, French, & Towers, 2004).

In healthy individuals, *R. rosea* enhances intellectual work capacity, abstract thinking, accuracy on tedious tasks, and reaction time (Shevtsov et al., 2003; Spasov, Mandrikov, & Mironova, 2000). For example, a DBRPC study of 60 first-year college students under stress found that those given low-dose *R. rosea* (100 mg/day) had significant improvement in mental fatigue, psychomotor function, overall well-being, physical work capacity, and heart rate (Spasov, Wikman, Mandrikov, Mironova, & Neumoin, 2000). The ADAPT formula, now labeled ADAPT-232 (Swedish Herbal Institute) was recently tested in a DBRPC single-dose effect study in 40 healthy but psychologically stressed, tired women aged 20–68 years. Compared to the placebo group, within 2 hours of consuming 270 mg ADAPT-232 subjects gained significant improvements in attention, speed, and accuracy during stressful cognitive tasks (Aslanyan et al., 2010). *R. rosea* has no reported adverse interactions with drugs. However, caffeine and other stimulants can have additive effects. In older Soviet studies, *R. rosea* was reported to exacerbate a condition in patients described as "volatile or euphoric" (Saratikov & Krasnov, 1987). These were probably patients with bipolar disorder and there may be some risk of inducing mania in bipolar patients, as can occur with antidepressants and stimulants. However, in the authors' (PLG and RPB) experience, *R. rosea* can be quite helpful for depression and for patients on mood stabilizers whose mood swings are primarily the depressed type with occasional mild hypomanic symptoms.

In patients with brain injury, *R. rosea* has a mild cognitive stimulant effect while it is also emotionally calming. Doses and precautions are the same as described in the section titled Herbs for Treatment of Mood Disorders. Highly anxious patients may not tolerate higher doses, because the activating effects sometimes exacerbate anxiety. *R. rosea* is best absorbed when ingested 20 minutes before breakfast and/or lunch when the stomach is empty, starting with 150 mg/day and increasing by 150 mg every 3–7 days. If tolerated, the entire dose can be given in the morning to increase compliance. In some cases the single morning dose has a better effect. Elderly, medically ill, or anxious patients should start by taking one-fourth to one-half of a capsule (37–75 mg) per day dissolved in tea or juice and increased slowly. Response takes 1–12 weeks.

Since *R. rosea* is known to have a mild effect on platelet aggregation at high doses, patients should be advised to watch for signs of increased bruising, especially at doses above 750 mg/day. Patients on coumadin or other medications that affect platelet aggregation or clotting factors should have their International Normalized Ratio (INR) checked (following each increase in *R. rosea* dose) and their coumadin doses adjusted accordingly (see section on Herb–Drug Interactions).

The authors find *R. rosea* to be effective in a variety of conditions: disorders of memory, cognition, and fatigue; enhancement of physical endurance, cognitive performance, memory, and energy in healthy individuals and in those with a wide range of disorders including age-related cognitive decline, poststroke, TBI, and cognitive impairment due to medical illness (e.g., cancer, HIV, or other chronic conditions); reduction of medication side effects; and recovery from central nervous system infections such as neuro-Lyme disease. Augmentation of *R. rosea* with *Eleutherococcus senticosus, Schizandra chinensis, Panax ginseng, Ginkgo biloba, Withania somnifera* (ashwaganda), and/or piracetam can further increase the beneficial effects on memory and cognition. Patients often report improved energy, mental clarity, and memory. Energy usually improves within the first week. Improvements in cognitive function and memory may take 1–12 weeks. Some individuals experience a decline in effectiveness after 3 to 12 months. In such cases a dose increase or a 2-week "holiday" off of the herb may restore efficacy. Alternatively, using a well-tested, quality brand may increase and sustain the benefits longer. This adaptogen can be used intermittently, prior to and during times of increased stress, or continuously for chronic conditions. For example, *R. rosea* could be started 2 or 3 weeks before examinations to reduce stress and improve academic performance.

Schizandra chinensis (Schizandra or Schisandra)

Schizandra chinensis is a Chinese medicinal herb (Bei Wu Wei Zi or Chosen-Gomishi) used to improve concentration, energy, and physical endurance. Bioactive components (lignans), including schizandrin and gomisan A, are polyphenolic. Extracts of the schizandra fruit showed significant AChE inhibition (Hung et al., 2007) as well as antidepressant, antiinflammatory, and hepatoprotective effects. The emotional calming effect of *S. chinensis* counterbalances the stimulating effect of *R. rosea* in patients who tend to become anxious. The pharmacology and clinical research on schizandra has been reviewed (Panossian & Wikman, 2008).

Eleutherococcus senticosus or *Acanthopanax senticosus* (Siberian Ginseng or Eleuthero)

Eleutherococcus senticosus is often called *Acanthopanax senticosus*, Oriental ginseng, or Siberian ginseng, though it is not in the ginseng family. A thorny shrub that grows in Siberia and northern China, it has a long history of use in Russia, China, Korea, and Japan as an adaptogen to enhance nonspecific resistance to stress and fatigue. Animal studies of bioactive compounds from *E. senticosus*, including eleutherosides and isoflaxidin, demonstrated reduced fatigue and improved recovery of natural killer cell activity and corticosterone levels following stress induced by swimming in mice. *E. senticosus*, used as an antiinflammatory in rheumatic diseases in oriental medicine, was found to downregulate inflammatory inducible nitric oxide synthase (iNOS) expression (Jung et al., 2007). Extracts have been used by athletes to enhance physical strength and endurance. While human studies of *E. senticosus* monotherapy are limited, it has been shown to contribute to the anti-fatigue and mental stimulatory effects of adaptogen combination formulas, particularly ADAPT-232 (Panossian & Wagner, 2005). Adverse events have been reported with intravenous administration but not with oral ingestions (Weng et al., 2007).

Panax ginseng (Korean or Asian Ginseng) and *Panax quinquefolius* (American Ginseng)

Ginsengs contain numerous bioactive compounds. *Panax ginseng* increases nitric oxide production in endothelial cells, which is essential for blood flow and oxygen delivery. *Panax ginseng* (400 mg/day) significantly improved abstract thinking and reaction time compared to placebo in a DBRPC

8-week study of healthy volunteers (age >40 years). However, there was no effect on memory or concentration (Sorensen & Sonne, 1996). *Panax ginseng* 100 mg also significantly improved reaction time, accuracy, calmness, and working memory in a DBRPC crossover study of 32 healthy adults aged 18–40 years (Reay, Scholey, & Kennedy, 2010). In a 12-week RCT of 97 Alzheimer disease patients, improvements were reported in cognitive function and MMSE (Lee, Chu, et al., 2008). However, literature reviews find methodological limitations in ginseng studies, a lack of convincing evidence, and a need for better quality studies (Geng et al., 2010).

A DBRPC trial in 32 healthy young adults found significant acute improvements in working memory in subjects given a single dose of 100, 200, and 400 mg American ginseng, *P. quinquefolius* (Cereboost, standardized to 10.65% ginsenosides) compared to those given placebo (Scholey et al., 2010). Of note, American ginseng (preparation HT100) significantly improved verbal memory and reduced extrapyramidal symptoms in a 4-week DBRPC study of 64 schizophrenic patients (Chen & Hui, 2012). American ginseng is less activating than *Panax ginseng*. The concentration of active ginsenosides in *P. ginseng* preparations can vary considerably.

In clinical practice, ginseng augments the activating effects of other agents, improving alertness, mental focus, energy, and cognitive function. One of the authors (RPB) attains better results by combining *P. ginseng*, American ginseng, and *E. senticosus* when treating cognitive dysfunction due to stroke, trauma, or vascular disease.

Lepidium myenii Walpers, Lepidium peruvianum Chacon (Maca)

Maca is a Peruvian adaptogenic herb that grows at high altitudes in the Andes. The Peruvian species has been referred to as *Lepidium myenii*, but the Peruvian government and universities chose to recognize its official name as *Lepidium peruvianum Chacon*. Its many active components include alkaloids, polyunsaturated acids, and their amides, and plant sterols. Maca is used as a nutritional supplement to improve alertness, mental focus, and physical resilience. Although it is mainly used to enhance sexual function and fertility, the roots have other medicinal properties. *L. peruvianum* is considered to be a nonhormonal phytomedicine that has the properties of an adaptogen. The key active constituents have not been identified. Among the 13 phenotypes of *L. peruvianum*, each has its own color and variation in the balance of active constituents. A review of maca studies discussed the following findings (Gonzales, 2012).

The black variety of maca shows positive effects on learning and memory in animal models. Black maca reduced human brain malondialdehyde levels (marker of oxidative stress) and decreased acetylcholinesterase levels in ovariectomized mice. Toxic effects have not been reported if the herb is boiled before consumption. It is neither teratogenic nor carcinogenic. The authors (PLG and RPB) find maca to be a useful adjunctive treatment for neural fatigue.

Ginkgo biloba (Ginkgo) from Leaves of the Maidenhair Tree

Leaf extracts of *Ginkgo biloba* contain flavones associated with antioxidant effects and terpene lactones responsible for anti–platelet activating factor. The EEG profile associated with ginkgo is indicative of cognitive activation with increased alpha and low-beta frequencies as well as decreased slow theta and delta, a pattern typical of cognitive activators (such as donepezil) and stimulants. A review of 22 controlled ginkgo studies in cerebrovascular disease, memory impairment, cognitive impairment, AD, multi-infarct dementia, subarachnoid hemorrhage, aging, hypoxia, and vestibular disorder, and in healthy volunteers, found evidence for clinically meaningful (though subtle) improvements (Diamond et al., 2000; Diamond & Bailey, 2013). In a DBRPC 52-week study of 236 Alzheimer's patients, *G. biloba* (EGB 761) 120 mg/day improved cognitive performance in patients with mild to moderate cognitive impairment and slowed deterioration in patients with severe impairment. A DBRPC 22-week trial of 400 patients with mild to moderate dementia given 240 mg/day EGB 761 documented that the ginkgo group had better cognitive outcome compared to placebo (Napryeyenko, Borzenko, & Gindem-Np Study Group, 2007). Although 120 mg twice daily of ginkgo (EGb761) failed to prevent dementia in the DBRPC Ginkgo Evaluation of Memory study of over 3,000 subjects followed for an average of 6.1 years (DeKosky et al., 2008), issues of compliance and diagnostic heterogeneity limit conclusions. Other DBRPC studies indicate that gingko may be particularly beneficial for neuropsychiatric and behavioral symptoms in dementia, especially when combined with 10 mg/day donepezil (Bachinskaya, Hoerr, & Ihl, 2011; Ihl, 2012; Ihl et al., 2012). A comprehensive review of EGb761 by Diamond and Bailey (2013) noted that the largest proportion of cognitive effects in RCTs are in fluid intelligence, selective attention, short-term and long-term verbal and visual memory, and executive functions. They also reviewed RCTs showing EGB761 to be beneficial for multiple sclerosis and anxiety disorders (Diamond & Bailey, 2013). EGb761 is standardized to contain 24% ginkgo-flavone glycosides and 6% terpenoids with numerous other active constituents, which may account for its effects on cerebrovascular tone, neurotransmitter and receptor activity, glucose metabolism, and electrical activity.

The authors' clinical experience suggests that ginkgo is best used to augment centrophenoxine and racetams (see below) in patients with TBI because its effects alone are mild. Side effects are rare with occasional nausea, headache, or rash. Cases of bleeding in patients with poor quality ginkgo, and usually with concurrent antiplatelet or anticoagulant medications, have been reported. High quality pharmaceutical grade ginkgo such as EGb761 has not been shown to affect bleeding time and does not potentiate anticoagulant drugs (Weinmann, Roll, Schwarzbach, Vauth, & Willich, 2010). Nevertheless, the current recommendations in the medical literature are that ginkgo not be given with warfarin and that it be discontinued 2 weeks prior to surgery.

Labiatae Family: *Melissa officinalis* (Lemon Balm), *Salvia officianalis* (Sage) and *Salvia lavandulaefolia* (Spanish Sage)

Modabbernia and Akhondzadeh (2013) recently reviewed the use of Labiatae phytomedicines in mental health. Preliminary small RCTs suggest that lemon balm and sage may enhance cognition and reduce agitation in patients with dementia (Akhondzadeh & Abbasi, 2006; Akhondzadeh et al., 2003). In 4-week DBRPC trial in 71 severely demented patients, *M. officianalis* aromatherapy decreased agitation and withdrawal and improved activities of daily living. A DBRPC trial in 18 healthy volunteers found that a 300 mg/day dose improved math processing speed while maintaining accuracy. Furthermore, at 600 mg/day lemon balm reduced effects of stress and improved calmness (Kennedy, Little, & Scholey, 2004). Side effects are insignificant. The authors find that 800 mg lemon balm helps reduce agitation in patients with dementia.

A DBRPC crossover study in 24 healthy undergraduates (ages 18–37) found that those given 50 μl Spanish sage had significant improvements in speed of memory, alertness, calmness, and contentedness compared to those on placebo. Spanish sage (*S. lavandulaefolia*) was used instead of sage (*S. officianalis*) because it contains the same bioactive compounds as *S. officianalis* but has a lower concentration of thujone, a terpenoid ketone that can be toxic in high doses (Tildesley et al., 2005). Side effects and drug interactions of sage and Spanish sage are minimal. In the authors' experience with dementia, 50 drops of 1.5% tincture of Spanish sage improves memory and alertness while ameliorating agitation. The cognitive effects of these herbs warrant further study.

Croccus sativus (Saffron)

Preclinical and clinical evidence on the benefits of saffron have been reviewed (Modabbernia & Akhondzadeh, 2013). It may exert AChEI effects, antagonize glutamatergic activity at NMDA receptors, and inhibit aggregation and deposition of amyloid β. In a 16-week DBRPC trial of 46 patients with probable mild to moderate AD, those treated with saffron 15 mg twice daily (extracted from stigmas of saffron) improved significantly on tests of cognitive function and had markedly reduced agitation compared to placebo (Akhondzadeh, Sabet, et al., 2010). A DBRPC Phase II 22-week trial (n = 54) found saffron 15 mg b.i.d. to be as effective as donepezil 10 mg/day in community dwelling adults over the age of 55 years with mild-to-moderate Alzheimer's disease (Akhondzadeh, Shafiee Sabet, et al., 2010).

NOOTROPICS—CENTROPHENOXINE (MECLOFENOXATE, LUCIDRIL), L-DEPRENYL (SELEGILINE), PYRROLIDINONES (RACETAMS)

Nootropics are manufactured cognitive enhancing and neuroprotective agents that have been extensively studied and prescribed in Europe, but are not well known in the United States. Froestl and colleagues recently proposed a nootropic classification system with 19 categories based on mechanisms of action—for example, interactions with receptors, enzymes, ion channels, nerve growth factors, reuptake transporters, antioxidants, metal chelators, and monoclonal antibodies interacting with amyloid-B and tau (Froestl, Muhs, & Pfeifer, 2012). They have reviewed the interactions of nootropics with enzymes, receptors, (Froestl, Muhs, & Pfeifer, 2013) and other targets (Froestl, Pfeifer, & Muhs, 2012). Evidence suggests that nootropics improve antioxidant status, membrane fluidity, mitochondrial function, neurotransmitter levels, mRNA protein synthesis, cerebral blood flow, neuroplasticity, and long-term potentiation (Brown, Gerbarg, & Muskin, 2009).

Pyrrolidinones (Racetams): Piracetam, Aniracetam, Pramiracetam

The modest neuroprotective effects of piracetam can be potentiated by CDP-choline, idebenone, vinpocetine, centrophenoxine, and deprenyl. Oxiracetam, aniracetam, and pramiracetam produce somewhat stronger effects than piracetam (Brown, Gerbarg, & Muskin, 2009). Large DBPC studies indicate that racetams improve symptoms in dyslexia and augment the benefits of speech therapy in poststroke aphasia (De Deyn, Reuck, Deberdt, Vlietinck, & Orgogozo, 1997). One PET scan study demonstrated improved task-related blood flow in left hemisphere speech areas (Kessler, Thiel, Karbe, & Heiss, 2000). In postconcussion syndrome, piracetam may reduce symptoms (especially vertigo and headache) and accelerate recovery with EEG normalization. In patients with dyslexia and aphasia, ginkgo improved attention and perception and augmented piracetam in cognitive retraining (Deberdt, 1994; Enderby, Broeckx, Hospers, Schildermans, & Deberdt, 1994).

In a DBRPC study of cognitive impairment and ischemic stroke following coronary artery bypass surgery, 98 patients were randomized to either placebo or piracetam IV (150 mg/kg/day; 300 mg/kg on the day of surgery) starting 1 day before surgery to 6 days after surgery and then 12 mg/day orally for up to 6 weeks. Patients given piracetam showed significant improvement in cognitive function compared to placebo (Szalma et al., 2006).

Racetams are very low in side effects. The authors (PLG and RPB) use aniracetam 750 mg twice daily to improve cognitive function in adults and children with learning disabilities, dyslexia, stuttering, anticonvulsant-induced cognitive impairment, bipolar disorder, unipolar depressives on antidepressants, and chronic fatigue syndrome. For the treatment of children, pramiracetam is less activating and more calming than aniracetam.

L-Deprenyl (Eldepryl, Selegiline, Emsam, Jumex)

Although L-deprenyl is a prescription MAOI antidepressant in the United States, most physicians are not aware of its neuroprotective effects. In low doses (<10 mg/day) it does not act as an MAO-A inhibitor and does not require a low tyramine diet. Preclinical evidence suggests that selegiline enhances mesencephalic drive regulation and resiliency under stress; increases release of BDNF, catecholamines, and 5HT, (most markedly in the hippocampus; see Knoll 2000, 2003); improves dopamine function and cognitive function; and exerts neuroprotective effects (particularly in catecholaminergic and cholinergic neurons) including protection against glutamate excitotoxicity (Ebadi et al., 2006). In ultra-low doses (2.5–5.0 mg/d) L-deprenyl may be modestly beneficial in treatment of TBI, AAMD, neurodegenerative or vascular cognitive impairment, AD, or a family history of dementia. As an enhancer regulator, L-deprenyl was associated with increased activity levels in enhancer-sensitive neurons that are associated with delay in age-related neurodegenerative changes, and it significantly increased longevity in 6 different animal species (Denes, Szilagyi, Gal, Bori, & Nagy, 2006). Further study on neuroprotection is needed.

Centrophenoxine (Meclofenoxate, Lucidril)

Dimethyl-aminoethanol (DMAE) is the precursor to phosphatidyl-DMAE, an avid scavenger of OH-radicals in cell membranes. Centrophenoxine (CPH) is an ester of DMAE and p-chlorophenoxyacetic acid, a synthetic form of a plant growth hormone (Nandy, 1978). CPH elevates levels of brain acetyl choline (ACh) and has antioxidant properties. CPH delivers DMAE rapidly to the brain where it is incorporated into nerve cell membranes as phosphatidyl-DMAE thereby providing antioxidant protective effects (Zs-Nagy, Dajko, Uray, & Zs-Nagy, 1994). In animal models of ischemia and in aged rats, CPH reduced cognitive deficits (Liao, Wang, & Tang, 2004). CPH increased activity of catalase, superoxide dismutase, glutathione reductase, and glutathione, as well as diminishing lipid peroxidation (Bhalla & Nehru, 2005). Significantly increased psychomotor and behavioral performance was observed in patients treated with centrophenoxine compared to placebo in an 8-week DBRPC trial in patients with moderate dementia (Pek, Fulop, & Zs-Nagy, 1989). In a 3-month DBRPC study 62 geriatric patients with mild to moderate AD, a preparation of CPH, vitamins, and nutrients (Antagonic Stress) was associated with significant improvements in memory, cognitive function, and behavior compared to nicergoline (Schneider et al., 1994). Nootropics may be more effective when combined with vitamins, minerals, and other nootropics (Fischer, Schmidt, & Wustmann, 1984).

HORMONES FOR COGNITIVE DYSFUNCTION
Dehydroepiandrosterone (DHEA)

Clinical studies of memory and cognitive enhancement with DHEA, produced primarily in the adrenal glands and secondarily in the ovaries and testes, show mixed results. In a 3-month study of normal older men, DHEA showed no impact on cognition or well-being (van Niekerk, Huppert, & Herbert, 2001). Patients whose DHEA is low for age, menopausal women who have had ovariectomies and adrenalectomies (Gurnell & Chatterjee, 2001), and debilitated geriatric patients are more likely to respond to DHEA with improvements in energy, memory, mood, and weight maintenance. Side effects, including insomnia and irritability, are usually mild. Slight increases in estrogen, potential interactions with steroids, and effects on prostate are concerns. Serial prostate-specific antigen testing is advisable. Patients with a history of prostate cancer or other hormone-sensitive cancers should not be given DHEA. Pharmaceutical grade DHEA is preferable in doses sufficient to restore physiologic levels, usually 25–50 mg/day.

Melatonin

Melatonin, a methoxyindole neurohormone secreted primarily by the pineal gland, diffuses readily through membranes and enters cell organelles. Best known for its role in sleep and circadian rhythms, melatonin is also a robust neuroprotectant that avidly scavenges reactive oxygen species including reactive hydroxyl radicals, carbonate radicals, and reactive nitrogen species (Srinivasan, Pandi-Perumal, Cardinali, Poeggeler, & Hardeland, 2006). In addition, melatonin prevents excitation-dependent generation of free radicals, reduces lipid peroxidation, upregulates antioxidant enzymes, and potentiates other antioxidants. Melatonin levels decline with aging and in neurodegenerative conditions. Beneficial effects of melatonin in AD and PD may involve antioxidant protection of mitochondrial membranes and DNA, enhanced glutathione production and regeneration, improved electron transport capacity, and anti–amyloid-β and antifibrillogenic effects. In elderly patients, early AD, and mild cognitive impairment (MCI), small studies found that melatonin improved sleep, mood, memory, and sundowning, and possibly slowed progression of cognitive decline. In a DBPC study of 20 patients with AD, those given melatonin 3 mg at bedtime showed significantly greater improvements on ADAS cognitive and noncognitive behavioral scores compared to the placebo group, but no significant differences were found on MMSE (Asayama et al., 2003). A review of melatonin studies in patients with MCI included 5 DBRPC trials and 1 open-label retrospective study, and all concurred in finding that evening treatment with melatonin significantly improved sleep quality and cognitive performance (Cardinali, Furio, & Brusco, 2010). Studies with additional measures also showed better mood. Larger studies are needed to evaluate long-term benefits of melatonin on disease progression in AD. In elderly patients, including those with AD and PD, melatonin in doses of 3–9 mg at bedtime can help to improve sleep, mood, memory, and sundowning. It probably slows progression of cognitive decline in MCI and, possibly, early AD. Melatonin may have a role in long-term prevention of neurodegeneration, particularly if begun by age 45.

MENOPAUSE, ANDROPAUSE, AND SEXUAL FUNCTION

PHYTOESTROGENS AND OTHER HERBS FOR FEMALE MENOPAUSE

Recent reviews pertaining to the safety and efficacy of phytoestrogens for menopausal symptoms, bone loss, and breast cancer highlight difficulties interpreting research studies and the complexities of clinical decision making (Bedell, Nachtigall, & Naftolin, 2012; Lagari & Levis, 2012; Leclercq & Jacquot, 2012). Interest in alternatives to hormone replacement therapy (HRT) has been growing, particularly in light of long-term studies showing increased risk of breast and uterine cancer among women taking HRT. Evidence of risk versus benefit is insufficient to justify the use of HRT to prevent osteoporosis, cardiovascular disease, or dementia. Although dietary supplements and herbs are widely used for relief of menopausal symptoms, more research is needed to confirm their benefits and safety.

Phytoestrogens

Phytoestrogens are plant-derived selective estrogen receptor modulators (SERMs) with structural similarities to estradiol. They bind to estrogen receptors and may act as estrogen agonists or antagonists depending on the specific tissue, the presence of other SERMs, and their ability to recruit coactivator or corepressor complexes (Bedell, Nachtigall, & Naftolin, 2012). Current research on SERMs aims to reduce menopausal symptoms and the risk of bone fractures and cardiovascular disease without increasing the risk of breast, uterine, or ovarian cancer (Blizzard, 2008). An ideal SERM would exert agonistic effects on estrogen receptors in bone, the cardiovascular system, and the central nervous system, but have anti-estrogenic or no effects on healthy breast and endometrial tissues (Hendrix & McNeeley, 2001). Tamoxifen, the first SERM used to reduce breast cancer risk, increased risks of endometrial cancer and blood clots (Cuzick et al., 2013). Other synthetic SERMs (e.g., ralozafen and bazedoxifene) have shown mixed results and side effects such as headache, arthralgias, hot flashes, and back pain (Gatti, Rossini, Sblendorio, & Lello, 2013; Kawate & Takayanagi, 2011). Research is needed on the potential role of plant-derived SERMs in treating menopausal symptoms and reducing risks of osteoporosis, cardiovascular disease, and breast cancer.

Plants containing phystoestrogens—for example, soy (*Glycine max*), red clover (*Trifolium pratense*), and hops (*Humulus lupulus*)—have been widely used and studied. Soy constituents include phytoestrogen isoflavones, diadzein, and genistein, as well as the precursor to mammalian lignans. Although the mechanisms of action are not entirely known, soy isoflavones show selective weak binding to estrogen receptors, preferentially estrogen receptor B. Mildly estrogenic isoflavones in red clover, similar to those in soy, also bind to human estrogen receptors (Booth et al., 2006). Extracts from red clover and hops upregulate progesterone receptor mRNA, interact with transcription factors (NF-KappaB), and possess antioxidant activity (Overk et al., 2005). Hops, traditionally used to brew beer, binds to estrogen receptors in vitro but does not stimulate uterine growth in ovariectomized rats (Beckham, 1995; Fackleman, 1998). In vitro studies indicate that one constituent, 8-prenylnaringenin, has high estrogenic activity and binding to estrogen receptors A and B (Milligan et al., 2000). Hops may have mild additive effects with other sedative agents.

Epidemiologic data and animal studies suggest that the health benefits of soy (lowering cholesterol and cancer prevention) are best obtained from whole soy (i.e., whole food) rather than from isolated isoflavones. A review of 22 RCTs by the American Heart Association Nutrition Committee concluded that isolated soy protein with isoflavones, compared with milk or other proteins, decreased LDL cholesterol concentrations on average approximately 3%—a small change relative to the large amount of soy protein (averaging 50 g/day) tested. There were no significant effects on HDL cholesterol, triglycerides, lipoprotein, or blood pressure. Furthermore, in 19 studies of soy isoflavones, the average effect on LDL cholesterol and other lipid risk factors was nil.

Isoflavones exert estrogenic and anti-estrogenic effects, both stimulating and inhibiting growth in breast cancer cells in vitro. The net effect has been no change in the risks of breast, endometrial, or other cancers. A meta-analysis of soy studies identified a small reduction in breast cancer risk associated with the use of whole soy but not high-dose isoflavone supplements (Trock, Hilakivi-Clarke, & Clarke, 2006). A prospective study of 15,555 women aged 50–69 concluded that high intake of isoflavones had no significant relationship to breast cancer risk (Keinan-Boker, van Der Schouw, Grobbee, & Peeters, 2004).

The efficacy and safety of soy isoflavones for preventing or treating cancer of the breast, endometrium, and prostate are not established. No evidence from clinical trials points to increased risk of cancer. The use of isoflavone supplements in food or pills is not recommended. Earlier research indicating that soy protein has important favorable effects compared to other proteins has not been confirmed. The benefits of many soy products may be attributed partly to the high content of polyunsaturated fats, fiber, vitamins, and minerals, and low content of saturated fat (Sacks et al., 2006).

Animal studies suggest that red clover isoflavones decrease bone loss induced by ovariectomy, probably by reducing the rate of bone turnover via inhibition of bone resorption (Occhiuto et al., 2007). Most clinical studies show lack of effectiveness of isoflavones derived from soy or red clover in preventing menopause-related bone loss. However, three meta-analyses of RCTs in menopausal women found evidence that ingesting soy isoflavones for 6 months significantly but moderately improved bone marrow density in the lumbar spine but not in total hip, femoral neck, and trochanter. The supplements were associated with significant reductions in urine deoxypyridinoline (a bone resorption marker) but not serum alkaline phosphatase or osteocalcin (Taku, Melby, Nishi, Omori, & Kurzer, 2011). Further studies are needed to assess the magnitude of these effects and potential interactions between isoflavones and anti-osteoporosis drugs. In a

DBRPC study of women aged 45–60 years within 5 years of menopause, with baseline bone marrow density T score >− 2.0, daily intake of 200 mg isoflavone tablets for 2 years did not prevent bone loss or menopausal symptoms (Levis et al., 2011). However, interpretation of this study should be cautious because it included women who were up to 5 years postmenopausal. Isoflavones in soy foods and red clover may have a modest positive effect on plasma lipid concentrations, bone mass density, and cognitive function.

The evidence for the therapeutic value of phytoestrogens in perimenopause is mixed with more positive results in recent studies. Stronger evidence supports the use of isoflavones for management of vasomotor symptoms (Molla, Hidalgo-Mora, & Soteras, 2011). For example, In a 12-week DBRPC study of 84 postmenopausal women, those given 30 mg/day synthetic genistein experienced a 51% decrease in the number and duration of hot flushes versus a 27% decrease in the placebo group (p = 0.026). There were no differences between groups in follicle stimulating hormone (FSH), 17-β-estradiol, endometrial thickness, or adverse events (Evans, Elliott, Sharma, Berman, & Guthrie, 2011). Assessment of risks and benefits of phytoestrogens in women with breast cancer and breast cancer survivors remains controversial. Recent studies have not found an increase in the risk of breast cancer or endometrial hyperplasia. However, trials specifically designed to detect cancer are needed. Lignans do not seem to increase risk of blood clots. Most studies suggest minimal health risks with phytoestrogens (Bedell, Nachtigall, & Naftolin, 2012). Including whole soy in the diet of postmenopausal women may be beneficial, but the optimal dose range remains unknown. Women could be informed that although there is some evidence of efficacy, it is not conclusive. While there is no evidence of harm, long-term safety studies in humans have not been done.

Recent assessments of previous reviews of hundreds of phytoestrogen studies find inconsistencies that could be attributed to several important factors.

1. Patient selection: The inclusion of women who are more than 1 year postmenopause, whose menopausal symptoms would wane naturally over time, reduces the likelihood of positive results.

2. Targets of measurements: Although it is easier to measure changes in frequency of hot flushes rather than severity, the latter is a better indicator of efficacy.

3. Increased consumption of phytoestrogens and exposure to endocrine disruptors: Longer term studies may be affected by the increasing consumption of phystoestrogens such as soy in commercial products and the exposure to estrogenic substances in products such as cosmetics, food containers, and meat from animals given hormones (Guerrero-Bosagna & Skinner, 2012).

4. Polymorphisms: Genetic polymorphisms of enzymes involved in metabolism of phytoestrogens play a role in the individual and ethnic differences that occur in digestion, absorption, and dose requirements for efficacy.

5. Gastrointestinal microflora: Soybean isoflavones are hydrolyzed to aglycone, diadzein, and genistein by intestinal enzymes and further metabolized to other compounds such as equol. The estrogen-agonist potency of equol is much higher than diadzein. Women who lack the intestinal microflora needed to convert daidzein to equol are called "nonproducers." Equol production can be affected by diet, antibiotics, and illness. Consequently, women who are nonproducers of equol would have less response to the ingestion of isoflavones (Bedell, Nachtigall, & Naftolin, 2012). The differentiation of women's capacities for equol production may be relevant for interpretation of study results and for adjusting either isoflavone dosages and/or correcting factors that may influence microflora.

Based on more recent research, Bedell and colleagues are more optimistic about phytoestrogens, particularly isoflavones, lignans, and coumestoms for treatment of vasomotor symptoms, vaginal atrophy, insomnia, and osteoporosis. They concluded that phytoestrogens reduce the intensity of hot flushes and that some combinations reduce the frequency. Their review indicates that phystoestrogens can reduce vaginal atrophy, improve sleep, cognition, and possibly bone health, primarily in the spine (Bedell, Nachtigall, & Naftolin, 2012). Leclercq and colleagues note that phytoestrogens can induce epigenetic change in genes involved in estrogen receptor regulation, for example, DNA methylation and histone acetylation/methylation. Their investigations in breast cancer cell lines incubated with genistein and daidzen documented effects on DNA hypermethylation and the restoration of the expression of BRCA1 and BRCA2 oncosupressor gene expression. They support a quest for specific estrogen receptor ligands to treat endocrine-disrupting diseases, including breast cancer (Leclercq & Jacquot, 2012).

Data from large RCTs suggest that SSRIs and SNRIs are promising treatments for perimenopausal vasomotor and mood symptoms. However, SSRIs (e.g., fluoxetine, paroxetine) inhibit CYP2D6 and can interfere with the clinical benefit of anticancer drugs such as tamoxifen. While estrogen receptor modulators (e.g., raloxifene and bazedoxifene) may reduce vulvovaginal atrophy, vasomotor symptoms, and the risk of osteoporosis, they impart an increased risk of venous thrombosis, stroke, or blood clots in the legs, lungs, or eyes. Other side effects of raloxifene are vasodilation (hot flushes), affecting about 10%–25% of users, and leg cramps, affecting about 7% (Wooltorton, 2006). The long-term safety (beyond 3 years) of SERMs regarding cancer and cardiovascular risks has not yet been established (Levine, 2011). Women who object to raloxifene and bazedoxifene, find them intolerable, or cannot afford the costs may consider herbal or nutritional therapy after being fully informed of the risks and limitations of the evidence of safety and efficacy.

Black Cohosh (Cimicifuga racemosa or Actaea racemosa)

Black cohosh has been used for over 60 years in Europe for its ability to decrease hot flushes by reducing the level of luteinizing hormone (LH). Studies show no binding to estrogen receptors in vitro, no clinical estrogenic effect, no carcinogenicity, and no more side effects than placebo at usual dosages. In fact, black cohosh augmented the antiproliferative activity of tamoxifen in vitro (Fackleman, 1998; Foster, 1999; Lieberman, 1998). Although stimulation of some uterine growth in ovariectomized rats had been reported, in a multinational study of 400 postmenopausal women given 40 mg/day black cohosh (*Cimicifuga racemosa* BNO 1055) for 52 weeks, there were no cases of endometrial hyperplasia. The number and intensity of hot flushes was markedly reduced and the herb was well tolerated (Raus, Brucker, Gorkow, & Wuttke, 2006). Several controlled studies, including one DBRPC study, showed efficacy equivalent to estrogen replacement therapy (Foster, 1999; Lieberman, 1998).

Studies of black cohosh have yielded inconsistent results. For example, a DBRPC 12-week study assigned 62 postmenopausal women to *Cimicifuga racemosa* extract (CR BNO 1055), the equivalent of 40 mg/day of the raw herb; conjugated estrogens (0.6 mg/day); or placebo. Women in the groups receiving conjugated estrogens or black cohosh extract had better sleep quality and fewer menopausal symptoms than those taking placebo. Both CR BNO 1055 and conjugated estrogens increased vaginal superficial cells; CR BNO 1055 had no effect on endometrial thickness, which was significantly increased by conjugated estrogens (Wuttke, Seidlova-Wuttke, & Gorkow, 2003). In contrast, a one-year DBRPC study of 351 women (ages 45–55 years) found no difference between frequency or intensity of vasomotor symptoms in those given a different herbal preparation of 160 mg/day black cohosh (Pure World, Inc. *Cimicifuga racemosa*; 2.5% triterpine glycosides; 70% ethanol extract) versus placebo (Newton et al., 2006). This study was limited to women in late menopausal transition or postmenopause. Although this study concluded that black cohosh is unlikely to have an important role in the treatment of vasomotor symptoms, the findings may not be generalizable because in late menopause hot flushes usually subside within a year, the length of the study.

Differences in the outcomes of DBRPCs may be due to differences in herbal preparations, patient selection criteria, length of study, and symptom measurements. Levels of bioactive compounds can be significantly affected by extraction procedures. A major problem in assessing this research is that studies using proprietary components may not reveal the process that makes their product "special." This leaves open the question of whether the difference in outcomes of studies using BNO 1055 versus other brands could be due to significant differences in the quality and efficacy of the products or to other factors. Nonetheless, given the excellent safety profile of black cohosh, it could be recommended for relief of menopausal symptoms in women who do not want or do not respond well to conventional treatments such as SSRIs, SNRIs, or synthetic SERMs. Compared to synthetic SERMs, black cohosh reduces menopausal symptoms without stimulating uterine estrogen receptors, has fewer side effects, and provides additional health benefits.

Dong Quai (Angelica sinensis)

Dong quai has been used in traditional Chinese medicine in tonics for thousands of years. Now it is added to many combination products. Evidence of estrogenicity includes strong binding to estrogen receptors in vitro, stimulation of uterine growth in ovariectomized rats, and induction of progesterone secretion (Belford-Courtney, 1993). The water-soluble extract regulates uterine contractions, while the essential oil relaxes uterine muscles. One DBRPC trial of dong quai as a monotherapy found no benefits for menopause (Hirata et al., 1997). The use of dong quai for perimenopausal symptoms, especially in women with breast cancer may entail some risks due to estrogen agonist effects. Considering the lack of evidence for effectiveness and the well-documented risks, the use of dong quai is not recommended.

Vitex (Vitex agnus castus)

Vitex from chaste tree berry, often used to relieve symptoms in premenstrual syndrome, modulates prolactin secretion and binds to dopamine receptors. Vitex slightly binds to estrogen receptors in vitro and modestly stimulates uterine growth in ovariectomized rats. Although vitex has not been studied in menopause, anecdotal reports suggest beneficial effects for hot flushes, fluid retention, and weight gain. It has been used to treat hyperprolactinemia (Wuttke, Jarry, Christoffel, Spengler, & Seidlova-Wuttke, 2003). One of the authors (RPB) finds vitex to effectively counteract elevations in prolactin levels induced by antipsychotic medications without interfering with antipsychotic effects. Vitex has been shown to be safe in studies lasting up to 18 months. Infrequent side effects include gastrointestinal upset, headache, diarrhea, nausea, itching, urticaria, rash, acne, insomnia, weight gain, and irregular menstrual bleeding. It may be unsafe during pregnancy.

ADAPTOGENS AND HERBS WITH ADAPTOGENIC PROPERTIES FOR MENOPAUSE

Rhodiola, Arctic Root, Golden Root, Roseroot (*Rhodiola Rosea*)

Rhodiola rosea has been used for centuries in Russia, Asia, Eastern Europe, and Scandinavia to enhance fertility and sexual function in people living at high altitudes, where it grows naturally in cold climates. The authors (PLG) found evidence for the use of *R. rosea* in an epic poem dating back to Bronze Age Greece (Brown & Gerbarg, 2004).

In an open study of 40 women with primary and secondary amenorrhea given *R. rosea* extract 100 mg twice daily, normal menstrual cycles were restored and uterine length increased to normal size in 25 women. Of these, 11 became pregnant (Gerasimova, 1970). Dr. Patricia Eagon at the University of Pittsburgh discovered that *R. rosea* showed strong estrogen receptor binding in vitro, but it did not activate estrogen receptors, elevate circulating estradiol levels, nor increase uterine size in ovariectomized rats (Eagon et al., 2003). These findings indicate that *R. rosea* could also be considered to contain selective estrogen receptor modulator(s). Of note, Eagon also found that when ovariectomized rats given estrogen implants (which elevate circulating estradiol to levels above normal) were fed *R. rosea*, the excess estradiol levels decreased toward normal. This is an example of the normalizing effect of adaptogens. The discrepancy between the lack of estrogenicity in the Eagon study versus Gerasimova's observations is most likely due to differences in the method of preparation and/or route of administration. Gerasimova administered the herb intraperitoneally. Dr. Eagon fed the animals a proprietary *Rhodiola rosea* product, Rosavin (Ameriden International) that is used in humans. Digestion and metabolism of the orally ingested herb alters the properties of constituents. Other differences were in the source of the herb (wild-grown versus cultivated) and extraction procedures. Evidence suggests that *R. rosea* may exert anticarcinogenic as well as hepatoprotective effects (see section on Adaptogens in Cancer Treatment).

In clinical practice, the authors (PLG and RPB) find that *R. rosea* can reduce vaginal dryness and improve libido in many cases. It is be particularly beneficial in menopausal women for symptoms of fatigue, forgetfulness, cognitive dysfunction, and depressed mood.

Many women who delay childbirth encounter problems with infertility. The onset of menopause can range from the mid 30s to the late 50s and is generally not predictable. It may be possible for women who delay childbearing past the age of 35 to use *R. rosea,* maca, and vitex to prolong fertility and possibly delay the onset of menopause. Given a choice, some women would opt to start *R. rosea* by age 35 to possibly maintain fertility if they find it necessary to delay childbearing.

Studies show that *R. rosea* enhances cognitive function (see section on Adaptogens for Cognitive Dysfunction). Although no specific studies have been done on perimenopausal women, the authors (PLG and RPB) have found in more than 100 cases that it is particularly helpful in improving memory, mental clarity, cognitive speed, energy, and mood in women before, during, and after menopause. These clinical observations should be extended through research on the mechanisms of action and clinical applications of *R. rosea* in treating perimenopausal decline in memory and cognitive functions, as well as other hormone-related conditions.

Ginkgo biloba and *Panax ginseng* (Ginkgo and Asian Ginseng)

Trials of *G. biloba* for fatigue and cognitive decline in menopause have had mixed results. In a 6-week DBRPC study of *G. biloba* in postmenopausal women, those in Stage +1 (mean age 55) performed better than those in Stage +2 (mean age 61) at baseline on tests of memory and cognitive function. After 6 weeks, in the ginkgo group the only clear benefit was greater mental flexibility among Stage +2 women (Elsabagh, Hartley, & File, 2005). In a 12-week DBRPC study, 57 postmenopausal women (aged 51–66 years) were given *G. biloba* 120 mg plus *P. ginseng* 200 mg or placebo. No significant effects were found

on mood, menopausal symptoms, attention, or memory (Hartley, Elsabagh, & File, 2004).

Lepidium peruvianum Chacon, formerly *Lepidium meyenii* (Maca)

In the Andean region of Peru, people living in the mountains traditionally use maca to enhance fertility in humans and in livestock, particularly at high altitudes (see section on Herbs for Female Sexual Function). A systematic review found four RCTs showing positive benefits for menopausal symptoms. Due to the small sample size and mixed quality of methodologies, no firm conclusions were drawn (Lee, Shin, Yang, Lim, & Ernst, 2011). Estrogenic effects are a contraindication for use in women with fibroids, breast cancer, or endometriosis. Effects on long-term cancer risk are unknown.

Hypericum perforatum (St. John's Wort)

St. John's wort 900 mg/day given to 111 menopausal women in a 12-week open series significantly improved self-esteem, self-image, irritability, anxiety, and depression. Improvements not reaching statistical significance were observed in psychosomatic symptoms (insomnia, headache, and palpitations), vasomotor symptoms (sweating, flushing, and dizziness), and sexual desire (Grube, Walper, & Wheatley, 1999). In clinical practice, the authors find SJW to be mildly helpful in menopause, but the risk of drug interactions and phototoxicity may outweigh the benefits.

Linum usitatissimum (Flaxseed) and *Triticum aestivum* or *vulgaris* (Wheat germ)

Flaxseed and wheat germ have been used to relieve hot flushes and night sweats. A DBRPC trial comparing flaxseed to wheat germ in menopausal women found them equally helpful in relieving hot flushes, but neither improved bone mineral density or lipid profile (Dodin et al., 2005). Flaxseed is rich in lignans which have weak estrogenic and weak anti-estrogenic effects. Lignans and their metabolites increase serum estrogens by stimulating synthesis of sex hormone binding globulin (SHBG), which reduces clearance of circulating estrogens. Lignans also bind to estrogen receptors, act as SERMs, and theoretically could impede tumor genesis (Bedell, Nachtigall, & Naftolin, 2012).

HORMONAL TREATMENTS FOR FEMALE MENOPAUSE

Dehydroepiandrosterone (DHEA), dehydroepiandrosterone sulfate (DHEAS) and 7-keto DHEA

The authors have found that patients whose DHEA and/or DHEAS levels are low normal or below normal for age (particularly menopausal women) often respond to treatment with DHEA 25–75 mg/day with enhanced mood, cognitive function, memory, energy, and sexual function (see discussion of DHEA in the sections Hormones for Treatment of Cognitive Dysfunction, Menopause, Andropause, and Sexual Function). A starting daily morning dose of DHEA 25 mg and a maintenance dose of 50 mg each morning are generally sufficient for menopausal symptoms. Side effects are usually minimal and include activation, anxiety, agitation, and occasionally seborrhea. DHEA, DHEAS, and total and free testosterone levels should be checked before treatment. If testosterone is low, DHEA may modestly increase levels enough to alleviate cognitive and sexual dysfunction but not enough to correct androgen deficiency states. However, treatment with testosterone resulting in higher testosterone levels may increase long-term risk of breast cancer. Therefore, in comparison to treatment with testosterone DHEA may provide a more modest but safer elevation of testosterone into the low normal range, enhancing DHEAS and sexual function. Because there are no clear data on DHEA and long-term risk of breast cancer, DHEA is relatively contraindicated in women with a personal or family history of breast cancer. In such cases 7-keto DHEA would be preferable, as it does not convert to testosterone, estrogen, or progesterone.

Intravaginal DHEA is a promising treatment for sexual function (Tan, Bradshaw, & Carr, 2012). In a 12-week DBRPC Phase II trial, 216 postmenopausal women were randomized to four groups. Each group was instructed to insert at bedtime a different concentration of DHEA: 0 mg, 3.25 mg, 6.5 mg, or 13 mg. Sexual function showed significant time-dependent and dose-dependent improvements in desire, arousal/sensation, arousal/lubrication, orgasm, and dryness during intercourse. The doses of DHEA were low enough that serum steroids stayed within normal postmenopausal range. Unlike estrogens, which only affect superficial epithelial cells, the DHEA transforms into androgens and/or estrogens locally and appears to affect cells in all three layers of the vagina (epithelium, lamina propria, and muscularis) (Labrie et al., 2009). Long-term trials are needed to verify safety.

INTEGRATIVE APPROACH FOR MENOPAUSE-RELATED DISORDERS

Evaluating patients who might benefit from integrative treatments begins with obtaining the personal and family history regarding menstruation, menopause, cancer, and cancer risk factors to identify contraindications for hormonal, phytoestrogen, or other herbal treatments. Target symptoms of concern to the patient may include hot flushes, vaginal dryness, dyspareunia, sexual dysfunction, insomnia, cognitive impairment, memory decline, fatigue, low energy, or mood changes. If the history reveals insomnia, daytime fatigue, snoring, gaps in breathing, leg movements at night, or uncomfortable leg sensations relieved by walking, a sleep evaluation (often followed by polysomnography) is indicated to rule out sleep apnea and restless leg syndrome. Appropriate laboratory testing of hormone levels includes FSH, LH, estrogens, progesterone, DHEA, DHEAS, free testosterone, total testosterone, thyroid functions, and possibly prolactin.

In addition to dietary improvements, exercise, sleep hygiene, and stress reduction, the following integrative treatments can be considered for specific target symptoms. Each treatment can be added to the others sequentially for stronger synergistic effects.

1. Hot flushes: black cohosh.

2. Vaginal dryness, dyspareunia: intravaginal DHEA as an alternative to estrogen cream, DHEA, *R. rosea*.

3. Hot flushes with cognitive/memory impairment and low energy: black cohosh plus *R. rosea*.

4. Primarily complaints of cognition/memory decline: *R. rosea* and/or DHEA or 7-keto DHEA (in women with low DHEA or DHEAS).

5. Low energy, fatigue: *R. rosea*.

6. Sexual dysfunction:
   a. low libido: maca, *R. rosea, P. ginseng*, marapuama, DHEA, 7-keto DHEA
   b. problems of arousal, sensation or orgasm: *R. rosea*, maca, *P. ginseng*, L-arginine, DHEA, 7-keto DHEA

7. Mood changes or depression: DHEA, 7-keto DHEA, *R. rosea*.

8. Pervasive complaints (hot flushes, cognitive, memory, low energy, sexual dysfunction) in women with low DHEA or DHEAS (lower quartile or subnormal), a trial of DHEA or 7-keto DHEA with cognitive enhancers is often helpful.

FEMALE SEXUAL ENHANCEMENT

Sexual function in women can be affected by psychological or physical stressors, age-related hormonal changes, relationship issues, medical illnesses, or medications. In many cultures potions from plants and animal parts have been used for centuries as aphrodisiacs. Scientific evidence for improvement in sexual function using herbs and nutrients is limited. Nevertheless, products promising sexual enhancement are sold widely. Possible mechanisms of action include vasodilation, improved circulation, antiinflammatory, antioxidant, hormonal, stimulant, and mood enhancement (Rowland & Tai, 2003). This discussion is limited to sexual enhancers for which there is some research evidence, frequent consumer use, and/or positive clinical experience. Herbs and nutrients can be helpful adjuncts to standard treatments including psychotherapy, pharmacotherapy, couples counseling, sex therapy, and life style changes to improve physical fitness and to reduce stress, fatigue, and substance abuse.

Herbs for Female Sexual Function

Panax ginseng (Asian or Korean Ginseng)

In a DBRPC trial, 32 postmenopausal women aged 40–60 years who had no menses for 1 year were given 1 g Korean red ginseng three times daily or placebo. Twenty-eight out of 32 reported improved sexual arousal with ginseng compared to placebo. Two cases of vaginal bleeding were reported (Oh et al., 2010). Infrequent side effects include insomnia, amenorrhea, pruritus, headache, and vertigo. Human studies suggest that ginseng does not affect platelet aggregation. Because ginseng may have hypoglycemic effects, insulin-dependent patients may require dose reductions when taking ginseng (Natural Medicines Database, 2010, pp. 780–781).

Lepidium peruvianum Chacon, Lepidium myenii (Maca)

Maca is a Peruvian adaptogen used to improve energy, sexual function, fertility at high altitudes, stress tolerance, nutritional status, and menopausal symptoms; it contains sterols, glucosinolates, and alkaloid components. Increased FSH, estrogen, and testosterone levels were noted in female rats given doses far in excess of those used clinically (Quiros & Cardenas, 1997; Chacon, 1997). These effects have not been found to occur in humans using clinical doses. An aqueous extract of yellow maca increased litter size in female mice and increased uterine weight in ovariectomized rodents, evidence of estrogenic effects (Ruiz-Luna et al., 2005). These findings cannot be extrapolated to humans without further clinical trials. Excess doses may cause over-activation or breast tenderness. Maca should not be used in patients with fibroids, estrogen receptor–related cancer risk, family history of breast cancer, or endometriosis. No behavioral toxicity has been reported in human or animal studies. However, the authors find that maca may precipitate agitation or mania in bipolar patients. Therefore, it should be used cautiously and in lower doses in cases of bipolar disorder. In clinical practice, the authors (RPB and PLG) find that monotherapy with a good quality brand of maca at doses between 3000 and 6000 mg/day can help many men and women improve libido, arousal, sensation, and orgasm. The effects may be mild, moderate, or strong. Maca can be useful in treating sexual dysfunction due to medical illness or medications (SSRI, SNRI, or antipsychotics). In a DBRCT in subjects (intent-to-treat n = 16) with SSRI-induced sexual dysfunction, 3.0 g/day of maca significantly improved libido (p < 0.05) on the Arizona Sexual Scale and the Massachusetts General Hospital Function Questionnaire (Dording et al., 2008). The benefits can be augmented with *R. rosea, P. ginseng*, and occasionally *Epimidium sagitatum* (see below).

Ptychopetalium olacoides or Uncinatum guyanna (Muira puama or Marapuama)

Marapuama, from the rain forests of Brazil, is used as an aphrodisiac, nerve tonic, and antiarthritic (Mowrey, 1996). An open trial in 202 healthy women complaining of low sex drive found that after 1 month of taking marapuama combined with *G. biloba* 65% reported improvements in libido, intercourse, sexual satisfaction, intensity of orgasm, and other measures (Waynberg & Brewer, 2000). Mechanisms of action, side effects, and drug interactions have not been studied. Controlled studies with objective measures are needed.

Crocus sativus (Saffron)

The ability of saffron to reverse SSRI-induced sexual dysfunction was evaluated in a DBRPC study of 38 women (ages 18–45 years) with major depressive disorder who had responded to fluoxetine 40 mg/day with at least 50% improvement in depression. All of the women continued fluoxetine 40 mg/day. Those who were also given saffron 15 mg twice daily had significantly greater improvements in sexual arousal on the Female Sexual Function Inventory, lubrication, and reduction in pain with intercourse. The reduction in pain may be attributed to antinociceptive effects of saffron (Kashani et al., 2012).

Nutrients and Combination Formulas for Female Sexual Function

L-Arginine (2-amino-5-guanidinopentanoic acid)

L-arginine is the precursor to nitric oxide (NO), which is involved in vasodilation of genitalia during sexual arousal. Arginine in combination products has been used to enhance sexual dysfunction in women. A multi-herb supplement, ArginMax comes in two gender-specific forms. Arginmax for Women contains L-arginine, *P. ginseng, G. biloba*, damiana leaf (*Turnera diffusa*), multiple B-vitamins, folic acid, vitamins A, C, and E, calcium, iron, and zinc. Damiana is considered safe in medicinal doses, but excess amounts may have adverse effects.

In a 4-week DBRPC study of 77 women, 73.5% of the subjects taking ArginMax reported improvements in their sex lives, including improved desire, vaginal lubrication, frequency of intercourse and orgasm, and clitoral sensation, versus 37.2% of those on placebo. ArginMax had no significant side effects (Ito, Trant, & Polan, 2001). In a 4-week DBRPC trial, ArginMax for Women was studied in 108 women (aged 22–73 years) who had reported lack of sexual desire. Among the premenopausal subjects, those taking ArginMax reported significant improvements in sexual desire, frequency of intercourse, and satisfaction with sex life compared with the placebo group. Perimenopausal women reported improvements in frequency of intercourse, less vaginal dryness, and greater satisfaction with their sexual relationships compared with the placebo group. Postmenopausal women showed an increased level of sexual desire (51%) compared with placebo (8%). Anecdotally, the authors find ArginMax to be beneficial for sexual dysfunction secondary to medical illness or medications. This study highlights two important issues. First, the effects of herbal treatments can vary with hormonal status. Second, combinations of synergistic herbs and other nutrients can be more effective than monotherapies.

In vitro studies of ArginMax have not shown estrogenic activity (Ito, Polan, Whipple, & Trant, 2006). Infrequent side effects included abdominal pain, bloating, gout, allergic response, or exacerbation of airway inflammation in asthma (Jellin et al., 2010). There have been no long-term toxicity studies. The balance of L-arginine and lysine affects replication of herpes virus. In practice, the authors (RPB and PLG) have seen outbreaks of oral-buccal herpes in patients who take L-arginine or ArginMax. This can be prevented or treated by the addition of lysine tablets and/or lip balm.

Hormones for Female Sexual Function

Dehydroepiandrosterone (DHEA) for Sexual Arousal

A double-blind randomized crossover study of 16 postmenopausal sexually active women showed that a single oral dose of 300 mg DHEA taken 60 minutes before viewing an erotic video increased subjective ratings of physical (p < 0.036) and mental (p < 0.016) arousal compared to placebo (Hackbert & Heiman, 2002). The possible risks of intermittent use of relatively high-dose DHEA for sexual enhancement compared with the risks of testosterone or other treatments has not been studied.

Integrative Approach to Sexual Dysfunction in Women

1. History and physical examination.

2. Rule out medical conditions that could affect sexual function. Also, evaluate for iatrogenic factors such as medications that may impair libido, arousal, and/or orgasm, such as birth control pills or other hormonal products, antidepressants (particularly SSRIs, venlafaxine), antipsychotics, blood pressure medications, and over-the-counter preparations.

3. Evaluate psychological, emotional, and relationship factors contributing to sexual dysfunction.

4. Obtain the following laboratory studies: DHEA, DHEAS, free testosterone, total testosterone, and prolactin. DHEA or DHEAS levels in the lower quartile may be worth treating in patients with sexual dysfunction or depression. Increased levels of prolactin—not uncommon in patients taking antipsychotics or SSRIs—are often missed.

5. If stress or lack of sleep are significant causative factors, then advise life style changes and mind-body practices such as yoga breathing, yoga postures, meditation, and exercise.

6. For lack of libido in women, try maca, *R. rosea*, Herbal-vX (*Muira puama* + ginkgo), or DHEA.

7. For problems with arousal or orgasm, suggest ArginMax, maca, *R. rosea*, DHEA or 7-keto-DHEA. These treatments can be layered for combined effects.

MALE SEXUAL FUNCTION AND ANDROPAUSE

Physical or psychological stress, anxiety, depression, fatigue, poor nutrition, substance abuse, low hormone levels, environmental toxins, alcohol abuse, medical conditions (e.g., benign prostatic hypertrophy, hypertension, and vascular disease), and medications such as nonthiazide diuretics, benzodiazepines, antidepressants (particularly SSRIs and venlafaxine) can adversely affect sexual function in men. Although low libido, disorders of arousal, premature ejaculation, and inability to climax can occur at any age, these problems tend to worsen after age 45 during andropause when changes in hormone levels and prostatic enlargement are occurring.

While standard treatments for sexual performance (e.g., phosphodiesterase-5 inhibitors) can be helpful in many cases, conventional treatments for loss of libido are more limited. Herbs and nutrients for treatment of sexual dysfunction will be discussed first, followed by treatments for benign prostatic hypertrophy.

Erectile Dysfunction

Erectile dysfunction (ED) is the most frequent among male sexual function disorders. Although 60%–70% of men respond to phosphodiesterase-5 inhibitors such as sildenafil with improved erectile function, many cannot tolerate side effects such as headache, gastrointestinal upset, and nasal congestion. Rare side effects include anterior ischemic optic neuropathy and deafness. Serious risks with this class of drugs involve interactions with nitrates, pulmonary hypertension, rarely anterior ischemic optic neuropathy, and deafness, especially with long-acting phosphodiesterase-5 inhibitors such as tadalafil (Cialis).

Herbs for Male Sexual Function

Panax ginseng (Asian or Korean ginseng)

Panax ginseng is a sexual stimulant often found in herbal preparations. It has been shown to increase nitric oxide synthesis, sperm count, testicular weight, testosterone level, and mating counts in animal studies (Kang, Kim, Schini, & Kim, 1995). *P. ginseng* 300 mg/day improved sexual performance more than placebo in a 3-month controlled study of 60 men (Choi, Seong, & Rha, 1995). In an 8-week DBRPC study 143 men with ED were given 1000 mg twice daily *P. ginseng*). Among the 86 completers, the ginseng extract significantly improved libido, erectile function, and orgasmic function compared to placebo. Insignificant changes in testosterone levels were found in the ginseng group. Levels of FSH, LH, prolactin, and estradiol did not change significantly (Kim et al., 2009). There have been anecdotal reports of hypersexual behavior induced by ginseng. Further studies are needed.

Ginkgo biloba (Ginkgo)

Ginkgo increases blood flow to the brain and genitalia. In an open 6-month nonblinded study of 50 men with ED with antidepressant-induced sexual dysfunction, ginkgo (EGb761) was reported to improve erectile function (Sohn & Sikora, 1991). These studies suffered from poor methodology. Furthermore, studies of treatments for sexual dysfunction tend to have high rates of placebo response. An 8-week DBRPC study (n=37) of antidepressant-induced sexual dysfunction found no difference between *G. biloba* and placebo (Kang, Lee, Kim, & Cho, 2002). Limited evidence supports benefits of ginkgo monotherapy for mild symptoms of impotence in middle-aged men, but not for problems with libido or orgasm, when given alone.

Maca (Lepidium myenii)

Peruvians living at high altitudes where maca (*Lepidium myenii*) grows have used it for centuries to enhance sexual function and fertility. In reviewing maca research, Gonzales noted that, in rodent studies, black maca increased testosterone levels and spermatogenesis, prevented high-altitude spermatogenic disruption, and improved sexual performance in normal rats and in those with erectile dysfunction (Gonzales, 2012). One small study (n = 9) of normal men found that 4 months of taking maca resulted in increased seminal volume, sperm count, and sperm motility. Serum hormone levels were not changed by maca. Larger studies are needed to confirm long-term safety and efficacy (Gonzales et al., 2001). In a 12-week DBRPC trial of two different maca doses (1500 mg or 3000 mg/day), among the 57 men taking maca 40% reported significant improvements in self-perception of sexual desire at week 8 and 42.2% at week 12 compared to 0.0% in the placebo group. Nine men who were treated with maca in this study were selected for additional testing, which showed no increases in serum testosterone, LH, FSH, prolactin, or estradiol, and no change in ratings for depression (or anxiety. A weakness in this study was that the assessment of sexual desire was based on one question only with a scale of 0–5 (Gonzales et al., 2002). It would be worthwhile to replicate these findings using additional validated assessments of desire. No major side effects have been reported in human or animal studies. Excess doses may cause overactivation. Prostate cancer may be a contraindication to the use of maca.

Ptychopetalium olacoides or *Ptychopetalium unicatum* (*Muira Puama or Marpuama*) and *Ptychopetali lignum* (*Muira Puama Wood*)

Extracts from the bark and roots of small trees in the Amazon rainforest, *Ptychopetalium olacoides* or *Ptychopetalium unicatum,* are used to make an aphrodisiac called "muira puama."

In an open study of 262 men complaining of lack of sexual desire and impotence who were treated with muira puama 1500 mg/day for 2 weeks, 62% reported enhanced libido and 51% reported better erections (Waynberg, 1990). Controlled studies with objective measures are needed to confirm these findings. The authors (RPB and PLG) observe that some patients report significant improvement in sexual desire and satisfaction with muira puama, whereas most have no response. Side effects tend to be mild.

Pinus maritime (*French Maritime Pine Bark, Pycnogenol*)

A standardized extract of *Pinus maritime* called "pycnogenol" inhibits cyclo-oxygenase and reduces prostaglandin production and inflammation. When combined with the substrate L-arginine, pycnogenol increases production of NO by nitric oxide synthase, relaxing the cavernous smooth muscle that is necessary for penile erection. A 3-month open study of men with ED compared L-arginine (1.7 g/day) with L-arginine (1.7 g/day) plus pycnogenol (40 mg twice daily for 2 months, then 40 mg three times daily for the third month). Of the men given the combination, 92.5% reported normal erections (Stanislavov & Nikolova, 2003). The lack of placebo control or objective documentation of erectile function limits the import of this study. Pycnogenol showed no mutagenicity,

teratogenicity, effects on fertility, or other adverse effects in dogs given 150 mg/kg. Among 2,000 patients, a 1.5% incidence of minor side effects was reported including gastrointestinal disturbance, dizziness, nausea, and headache (Rohdewald, 2002). Evidence suggests that pycnogenol may impart long-term health benefits, including antioxidant, anti-inflammatory, antihypertensive, and cognitive enhancement.

Combination Formulas for Male Sexual Function

Arginine and ArginMax for Men

ArginMax for Men contains L-arginine, *P. ginseng*, ginkgo, and 13 vitamins and minerals. L-Arginine is a precursor to nitric oxide (NO). The NO signaling pathway affects specific sexual dysfunctions. In a small DBRPC study of 50 men with ED, L-arginine monotherapy resulted in 9/29 responders versus 2/17 on placebo. All nine responders had reduced NO excretion or production at baseline (Chen et al., 1999). A 2-week DBRPC crossover study of 45 men with ED compared a combination of L-arginine glutamate 6 gm/day plus yohimbine 6 mg/day; yohimbine 6 mg/day alone; and placebo taken 1–2 hours prior to sexual intercourse. At the end of each treatment period, erectile function domain scores for L-arginine plus yohimbine, yohimbine alone, and placebo were 17.2+/−7.17, 15.4+/−6.49 and 14.1+/−6.56, respectively. The difference between L-arginine plus yohimbine versus placebo reached statistical significance (p = 0.006). Stratification according to baseline scores above 14 indicated that patients with mild to moderate ED had better erectile function domain responses to both treatments compared to placebo (Lebret, Herve, Gorny, Worcel, & Botto, 2002).

Prelox is a proprietary blend containing 720 mg total of L-arginine HCl, aspartic acid, pycnogenol, and 50 mg of *Epimedium sagittatum* extract standardized to 60.0% (30 mg) icariin. *E. sagittatum* is used in traditional Chinese medicine to prolong male sexual response. A DBRPC study of 50 men with mild to moderate ED found that those given Prelox more than doubled the mean number of intercourse events and significantly increased testosterone levels. Systolic and diastolic blood pressure both declined. No adverse effects were observed. The onset of action required 1–9 days (Stanislova, Nikolova, & Rohdewald, 2008). In a 6-month DBRPC study of 124 men ages 30–50 years with moderate ED and normal baseline testosterone levels, Prelox significantly improved ED and testosterone levels compared to placebo (Ledda, Belcaro, Cesarone, Dugall, & Schonlau, 2010). For a discussion of side effects see Nutrients and Combination Formulas for Female Sexual Function. In most studies and in clinical practice, L-arginine is effective when combined with other herbs.

Yohimbine (*Pausinystalia yohimbe or Corynanthe johimbe*)

Yohimbine, extracted from the bark of a tropical African tree (*P. yohimbe*), contains an alkaloid chemically similar to reserpine. Yohimbine inhibits adrenergic receptors that innervate the genitals. A meta-analysis of seven well-done DBPC studies surmised that 15–43 mg/day yohimbine alleviated ED more effectively than placebo in 40% of men with sexual dysfunction (Ernst & Pittler, 1998). Higher quality prescription yohimbine is preferable in 5.4 mg pills, with a usual dose of 18–42 mg/day. Over-the-counter products account for 98% of reported side effects and these often contain only negligible amounts of yohimbine (Betz, White, & der Marderosian, 1995). Some patients, for example the elderly, are unable to tolerate yohimbine side effects such as anxiety, nausea, dizziness, chills, sweating, headache, insomnia, and, at higher doses, increased blood pressure. Yohimbine can exacerbate symptoms in patients with anxiety, panic, obsessive compulsive disorder, or posttraumatic stress disorder.

Epimidium sagittatum (Horny Goat Weed)

Epimidium sagittatum contains the phystoestrogens icariin, genistein, and daidzein. Icariin inhibits phosphodiesterase-5 and enhances cGMP in cells of cavernous smooth muscle. It is used in traditional Chinese medicine to prolong male sexual response. In vitro and animal studies of icariin and of herbal products containing *E. sagittatum* show no serious adverse effects and stronger phosphodiesterase inhibition than sildenafil (Ning et al., 2006). However, human safety and efficacy trials are needed. The authors use *E. sagittatum* occasionally to augment other herbs.

Hormones for Male Sexual Function

Dehydroepiandrosterone (DHEA)

Serum DHEA-S levels were found to be inversely correlated with the prevalence of ED in the Massachusetts Male Aging Study (Feldman, Goldstein, Hatzichristou, Krane, & McKinlay, 1994). In 40 men with serum DHEA-S levels below 1.5 μmol/L, a 24-week DBRPC study revealed that the men given DHEA 50 mg/day achieved significantly greater improvements in erectile function, orgasmic function, sexual desire, and intercourse satisfaction than those given placebo (Reiter et al., 2001).

Nutrients for Male Sexual Function

Acetyl-L-carnitine (ALC) and propionyl-L-carnitine (PLC)

In a DBRPC study of 96 men after bilateral nerve-sparing retropubic prostatectomy, ALC significantly augmented sildenafil in alleviating ED in comparison to men given sildenafil monotherapy or placebo. ALC plus sildenafil resulted in significantly greater improvements in ED, sexual intercourse satisfaction, orgasm, and general sexual well-being (Cavallini, Modenini, Vitali, & Koverech, 2005). In a 6-month DBRPC study of 120 men aged 60–74 years, those who received testosterone undecanoate 160 mg/day plus ALC 2 g/day plus PLC 2 g/day had significantly more improvement in erectile function score, depression melancholia scale score, and fatigue than those given testosterone plus placebo. Carnitines had more effect on erectile function score than testosterone alone. Unlike testosterone supplementation, carnitines do not increase prostate volume (Cavallini, Caracciolo, Vitali,

Modenini, & Biagiotti, 2004). Evidence suggests that carnitines can enhance the response to sildenafil.

Prostatic Enlargement and Sexual Dysfunction

Pygeum (Pygeum africanum), Saw Palmetto (Serenoa repens), and Stinging Nettle Root (Urtica dioica)

Prostatic enlargement is a common factor in sexual dysfunction in middle and late life. Free testosterone declines, and the prostate is stimulated by increasing levels of estradiol, prolactin, SHBG, and dihydrotestosterone. Reducing the size of an enlarged prostate sometimes improves sexual function. Treatments for benign prostatic hypertrophy (BPH) include finasteride, alpha-adrenergic blockers (terazosin, doxazosin, or tamsulosin), and surgery. Surgical procedures are expensive and may exacerbate sexual dysfunction. Alpha adrenergic blockers can cause tiredness, dizziness, depression, headache, abnormal ejaculation, and rhinitis (Medical Letter, 1997). Reduction of BPH has been reported for three herbs: saw palmetto (*Serenoa repens*), pygeum (*Pygeum africanum*), and stinging nettle root (*Urtica dioica*). Recent studies and systematic reviews of saw palmetto find no evidence to support its use for sexual dysfunction related to BPH (Barry et al., 2011; Tacklind, Macdonald, Rutks, Stanke, & Wilt, 2012).

Pygeum Bark (Pygeum africanum) and Stinging Nettle (Urtica dioica)

Production of extracts from the fragile African pygeum tree may not be ecologically sustainable. Pygeum bark extract increases prostate secretions and inhibits prostate cell growth and aromatase, which reduces the estrogen/testosterone ratio. It also reduces prolactin, inflammation, cholesterol, and the uptake of testosterone in the prostate (Bassi et al., 1987). Pygeum has been shown to significantly improve lower urinary tract symptoms (LUTS) without side effects in DBRPC trials (Barlet et al., 1990), but only one small open study supports its use for sexual activity in older men (Carani et al., 1991). Several DBRPC studies indicate that stinging nettle root alone and in combination with other plant extracts improves LUTS without adverse effects in men with BPH. However, effects on sexual function have not been adequately studied. Reduction in LUTS and prostatic volume have been attributed to blockage of prostate cell growth receptors and 5-alpha-reductase, inhibition of aromatase and SHBG binding, and antiinflammatory activity (Lichius & Muth, 1997; Sokeland & Albrecht, 1997). These benefits were demonstrated at a dose of 300 mg/day (Safarinejad, 2005). In a 60-week DBRPC of 140 elderly outpatients, a combination of 160 mg WS1473 saw palmetto and 120 mg WS1031 stinging nettle (PRO 160/120) was as effective as tamsulosin (alpha1-adrenoceptor antagonist) for LUTS caused by BPH (Engelmann, Walther, Bondarenko, Funk, & Schlafke, 2006).

HERB–DRUG INTERACTIONS

Concerns about herb–drug interactions (HDIs) prevent many clinicians from offering patients the full range of treatment options. Phytomedicines can either interfere with or enhance the benefits of synthetic drugs such as psychotropics, anticoagulants, or chemotherapy agents. Among the herbs discussed in this chapter, only a few pose clinically significant risks of HDIs. Assessing the likelihood of HDIs and methods to minimize or obviate risks will be highlighted before addressing specific herbs. Understanding these issues will enable clinicians to take advantage of the therapeutic contribution of phytomedicines while avoiding adverse effects.

PHARMACOKINETIC AND PHARMACODYNAMIC INTERACTIONS

The two main aspects of pharmacokinetic interactions that can affect medication serum levels are the induction or inhibition of cytochrome P450 (CYP) isozymes and p-glycoproteins. Pharmacodynamic interactions include risks of increased CNS side effects (e.g., serotonin syndrome), hepatotoxicity, or bleeding. Additive effects such as excess sedation or activation can occur in the absence of pharmacokinetic or pharmacodynamic interactions. In a systematic review of 21 whole herb extracts (not isolated constituents) with human-level evidence regarding HDIs, Kennedy and Seely (2010) acknowledge the limitations of the information about potential HDIs. When isolated, the concentration of a constituent far exceeds that which occurs in the whole herb extract. This review made several important points.

1. Many herb–drug combinations that had preclinical evidence of drug interaction in vitro and in animal studies showed no evidence of interaction in humans.

2. For most of the herbs that had evidence of drug interaction in preclinical studies, the actual effect on serum levels of medications is quite small and of no clinical significance.

3. Caution is most needed when combining herbs with drugs that have a narrow therapeutic window such as warfarin or digoxin.

4. The effects of whole herbs or whole herbal extracts are often different from those of single isolated constituents.

5. The impact of a botanical extract on the CYP450 metabolism of one drug does not necessarily generalize to other drugs that are processed by the same isoenzyme because they may have different binding affinities. The affinity of the botanical extract could be stronger for one drug but weaker for another.

6. The interaction of herbs with many anesthetics and antidepressants requires further study.

The impact of a botanical extract on CYP450 metabolism from in vitro and in vivo animal studies is often not seen in human studies and may merely indicate a need for additional information. For example, not only phytomedicinals but also common fruits and vegetables consumed in our daily diet inhibit or induce CYP450 isozymes in vitro but have no significant HDIs in humans. The gastrointestinal digestion, absorption, and metabolism of herbal constituents alter their properties and, therefore, their effects in living organisms as opposed to tissue cultures. Potential risks can be minimized by systematic monitoring for efficacy, side effects, and serum levels of medications that have a low therapeutic index (a small margin of safety between therapeutic and toxic effects or between therapeutic and subtherapeutic benefits) and meaningful serum levels. Herbs that have demonstrated, verified, serious HDIs in humans should not be used in combination with those specific medications. For extensive reviews showing the level of the evidence on HDIs, including whether the study is based on in vitro, in vivo, animal, or human trials, see Kennedy and Seely (2010). In his highly recommended book, *Herbal Contraindications and Drug Interactions*, Francis Brinker not only provides extensive details on HDIs and the evidence sources but also differentiates herbal effects on each of three phases of metabolism: Phase I, CYP450 system of isozymes; Phase II, conjugating enzymes; and phase III, transporter proteins (Brinker, 2010).

Phytomedicines can potentially enhance the effectiveness of chemotherapy agents and reduce chemotoxic effects. Studies of human tumors in animals with metabolizing enzyme systems similar to humans would clarify when to use and when to avoid herbals in patients undergoing cancer treatments. To date most cancer-related studies have been done in cell cultures or in rodents whose enzyme systems differ too much from human systems to permit extrapolation of results. However, clinical studies are appearing that will take into account the digestive and metabolic factors as well as tissue-specific and tumor-specific effects. Overall, the available evidence indicates potential for highly significant benefits of phytomedicinals in cancer treatment.

Actea racemosa (Black Cohosh)

Human studies of black cohosh demonstrate no impact on CYP3A4, CYP1A2, CYP2E1, or digoxin pharmacokinetics. At doses above therapeutic level, there was weak, insignificant inhibition of CYP2D6. In vitro studies of estrogen-responsive breast cancer cells showed that black cohosh enhanced the antiproliferative activity of tamoxifen (Kennedy & Seely, 2010).

Curcuma longa or *Curcuma domestica* (Curcumin)

No adverse interactions with drugs have been reported. In vitro and animal studies indicate that curcumin at high doses (over 15 gms/day) can inhibit platelet aggregation. Curcumin extract reduced or enhanced antitumor effects of chemotherapy agents and reduced hepatotoxic and cardiotoxic effects in vitro and in animal studies, depending on the type of cancer (Brinker, 2010).

Angelica sinensis (Dong Quai)

In vitro and animal studies found that water and ethanol extracts of dong quai increased activity of CYP2D6 and

CYP3A subfamily. Dong quai is not recommended for patients taking chemotherapy medications such as tamoxifen, temsirolimus, and other drugs metabolized by these enzymes (Yap, Kuo, Lee, Chui, & Chan, 2010). Individual case reports showed that concurrent use of dong quai with warfarin increased prothrombin time and INR (Brinker, 2010). Theoretically, antiplatelet/anticoagulant effects of dong quai could increase the risk of bleeding in patients on anticoagulants. The clinical use of dong quai is not recommended.

Camellia sinensis (Green Tea)

A supplement containing decaffeinated green tea had no effect on CYP3A4 or CYP2D6. A study using drug probes found no impact on CYP2D6, 1A2, or 2C9. A 20% increase in buspirone area under the curve (AUC), indicating some inhibition of CYP3A4, was deemed not to be clinically significant (Kennedy & Seely, 2010).

Eleuthero, Siberian Ginseng (Eleutherococcus senticosus, Acanthopanax)

Preliminary evidence from in vitro and animal studies of *E. senticosus* suggested possible inhibition of P450 enzymes 1A2, 2C9, 2D6, and 3A4. However, human studies of *E. senticosus* show no impact on any of these isozymes and no evidence of effects on digoxin levels (Kennedy & Seely, 2010). Mild hypoglycemic effects indicate a need to monitor serum blood sugar of insulin dependent diabetics and adjust the dosage of antidiabetic medications as needed.

Zingiber officinale (Ginger)

Although ginger has exhibited antiinflammatory and antiplatelet activity, it did not alter clotting states or warfarin pharmacokinetics at doses of 3.6 gms/day for one week or 100 mg/kg for 4 days in human trials (Kennedy & Seely, 2010). Rare cases of increased bleeding have been reported in patients on long-term phenprocoumon.

Ginkgo biloba (Ginkgo)

In reviewing studies of ginkgo, Diamond and Bailey (2013) pointed out that flavones, ginkolides A and B, and bilobalide are thought to be involved in antioxidant, metabolic, neurotransmitter, and regulatory actions. Ginkolides inhibit platelet anti-activating factor. Although ginkgo has been shown to reduce blood viscosity and to thereby increase perfusion in elderly patients and in peripheral artery disease, it has not shown significant effects on platelet aggregation, fibrinogen, partial thromboplastin time, or prothrombin time. Case reports of increased bleeding include patients on warfarin, aspirin, nonsteroidal antiinflammatories, and other drugs. Attribution of bleeding to ginkgo is unsubstantiated in most cases. Reviews of RCTs and case reports did not find changes in objective measures of coagulation (Diamond & Bailey, 2013). Induction of

CYP3A2 by higher than therapeutic doses occurred in an animal study. Diamond and Bailey (2013) concluded that in therapeutic doses (80 to 720 mg/day in divided doses), standardized high quality ginkgo extracts are generally safe but may entail synergistic effects when administered with anticoagulants such as warfarin or aspirin (Diamond & Bailey, 2013).

Panax ginseng (Asian or Korean Ginseng)

Human studies had shown no impact of *P. ginseng* on probe substrates of CYP2D6, CYP3A4, CYP2E1 or CYP1A2. The herb also had no effect of serum levels of warfarin (Kennedy & Seely, 2010). However, in a more recent study, 12 healthy adults were given an oral dose of midazolam 8 mg (a CYP3A substrate) and fexofenadine 120 mg (probe for P-gp function) before and after taking *P. ginseng* 500 mg twice daily (Vitamar Laboratories, 5% ginsenocides from whole root powder) for 28 days. Pharmacokinetic calculations comparing before and after midazolam serum levels found reductions in AUC of 0.66 (0.55–0.78), half-life of 0.71 (0.53–0.90), and maximum concentration of 0.74 (0.56–0.93). No change occurred in fexofenadine pharmacokinetics (Malati et al., 2012). As a CYP3A probe, the metabolism of midazolam can vary significantly depending on CYP3A polymorphisms (Elens et al., 2013).

Panax quinquefolius (American Ginseng)

American ginseng extract (1 g q8 hrs for 14 days) had no effect on the pharmacokinetics of indinavir (800 mg q8 hrs for 3 days) (Andrade et al., 2008). Two weeks of American ginseng extract 200 mg twice daily did not alter zidovudine pharmacokinetics, but it did reduce oxidative stress markers (Lee, Wise, et al., 2008). However, in a 4-week DBRPC study, 20 healthy subjects were given warfarin 5 mg/day for 3 consecutive days during weeks 1 and 4. After the first week they received either American ginseng 1.0 g/day or placebo for 3 weeks. The peak INR, peak plasma warfarin level, and warfarin AUC significantly decreased after 2 weeks of ginseng administration, indicating that American ginseng can reduce the anticoagulant effect of warfarin (Yuan et al., 2004).

Piper methysticum (Kava)

In vitro studies of the effects of kava extract and kava lactones on human liver microsomes found significant inhibition of P450 enzymes (CYP1A2, 2C9, 2C19, 2D6, 3A4, and 4A9/11) (Mathews, Etheridge, & Black, 2002) and CYP2E1 (Gurley et al., 2005) involved in the metabolism of many pharmaceuticals. Taking kava with alcohol, sedatives, or muscle relaxants can induce coma (Almeida & Grimsley, 1996). Hepatotoxic effects have been reported, particularly when kava is consumed by individuals who regularly drink alcohol.

Rhodiola, Arctic Root, Rose Root (*Rhodiola rosea*)

An in vitro study found that 95% ethanol extracts from *R. rosea* plants grown in different areas of Norway showed inhibition of CYP3A4 and P-glycoprotein (P-gp) in cell cultures (Hellum et al., 2010). There was no correlation between the concentrations of the six marker constituents (which were presumed to be active) with these inhibitory effects. The component(s) responsible for in vitro inhibition of CYP3A4 and P-gp have not been identified. However, as with other herbs, CYP3A4 inhibitory activity in vitro did not translate to CYP3A4 inhibitory activity in vivo or in humans. In a rat study, *R. rosea* (SHR-5) was given with either warfarin (CYP450 test substrate) or theophylline (CYP1A2 substrate). No significant effects on drug pharmacokinetics were found and there were no significant changes in the anticoagulant activity of warfarin (Panossian, Hovhannisyan, Abrahamyan, Gabrielyan, & Wikman, 2009). The authors (RPB and PLG) have used *R. rosea* in patients taking many different medications without adverse effects (Brown, Gerbarg, Muskin 2009). One author (RPB) treated one patient on warfarin with *R. rosea* 150 mg/day and another on warfarin with *R. rosea* 300 mg/day. There was no change in INR in either case. Without information from in vivo and human studies, it cannot be assumed that *R. rosea* would interact adversely with medications. Nevertheless, the checking of serum levels (eg. digoxin) and INR (eg. warfarin) would minimize any potential risks.

Serenoa repens (Saw Palmetto)

Two studies indicate that saw palmetto does not affect CYP3A4, CYP1A2, CYP2D6, or CYP2E1 activity (Kennedy & Seely, 2010). A study of 10 adults given saw palmetto for 2 weeks found no increase in coagulation time or platelet function. One case of intraoperative hemorrhage in association with saw palmetto use was reported. In vitro studies of saw palmetto extracts show inhibition of tamsulosin binding to alpha$_1$-adrenoceptors. Saw palmetto alpha$_1$-adrenoceptors antagonism was less than for prazosin in human trials (Brinker, 2010). Until more studies are completed, discontinuation of saw palmetto 2 weeks prior to surgery is advised. Given the lack of clinical effect in the most recent studies and reviews, it is hard to justify the use of saw palmetto (Tacklind et al., 2012).

Schizandra chinensis and Schisandra sphenanthera (Schisandra)

In vitro studies show that schisandra inhibits CYP3A4 enzymes. However, schisandra induces the same enzymes in in vivo animal studies. Molecular changes that occur through digestion of herbals can alter their effects on CYP450 enzymes. In animal models schisandra reduced warfarin levels, but this has not been demonstrated in human subjects. Until more is known, INR should be monitored in patients taking anticoagulants who are given schisandra. In rat studies multiple dosing of *Schisandra chinensis* alcoholic extract (1.5 g × kg (−1), qd × 7d) significantly induced CYP2E1, inhibited CYP2D2, and had no effect on CYP2C6, CYP3A1/2, CYP1A2 or (Wang, Hu, Sheng, & Li, 2011). In China *Schisandra sphenanthera* is commonly used with tacrolimus, an immunosuppressant that reduces organ rejection in transplant patients. Compared to treatments with tacrolimus alone, liver transplant patients given both tacrolimus and schisandra showed markedly increased serum concentrations of tacrolimus, improved liver function, and reduced incidence of tacrolimus-associated side effects of diarrhea and agitation (Jiang, Wang, Xu, & Kong, 2010).

Hypericum perforatum (St. John's Wort)

St. John's wort extracts induce cytochrome P450 isozymes including CYP3A4, 2C19, 2C9, and 1A2, as well as intestinal wall p-glycoprotein (P-gp) transporter. Case reports and human studies indicate SJW can interfere with absorption, metabolism, and clinical effectiveness of numerous medications including digoxin, warfarin, phenprocoumon, HIV protease inhibitors, reverse transcriptase inhibitors, indinavir, irinotecan, theophylline, cyclosporine, alprazolam, amitriptyline, clonazapine, dextromethorphan, simvastatin, tacrolimus, and oral contraceptives (Knuppel & Linde, 2004; Van Strater & Bogers, 2012). SJW constituents hypericin, hyperforin, and flavones are used for standardization. The hypericin content is associated with antidepressant effects and hyperforin is associated with CYP3A4 induction. An excellent review of SJW by Sarris noted that studies using high-dose hyperforin extracts >10 mg/day induced CYP3A4, whereas those containing low-dose hyperforin <4 mg/day showed no significant effects on CYP3A4 (Sarris, 2013). However, low-dose hyperforin extracts are not clinically effective. SJW should be discontinued 2–3 weeks prior to surgery because it can affect heart rate and blood pressure during anesthesia.

Valeriana officianalis (Valerian)

Two studies evaluating valerian did not find any effects on CYP1A2, CYP2E1, CYP2D6, or CYP3A4/5 activity (Kennedy & Seely, 2010). However, in 12 healthy subjects the maximum concentration of alprazolam (CYP3A4 substrate) at baseline was significantly increased after 14 days of taking 1000 mg nightly of valerian extract (1.1% valerenic acids), a dose that is greater than the usual clinical dose (Donovan et al., 2004). In a study of 12 adults taking 375 mg/day for 28 days of a valerian root extract that did not contain valerenic acids, there was no effect on metabolism of the CYP3A4 substrate midazolam (Brinker, 2010). The absence of the active compound, valerenic acid, limits the clinical usefulness of this study. This illustrates the point that differences in the content of extracts and variations in affinities among substrates of the same isozymes can yield different effects. Based on animal studies, valerian could potentiate the action of sedative drugs, possibly by additive effects.

Vitex agnes-castus (Vitex, Chaste Tree)

In fluorogenic in vitro assays a vitex preparation did not affect CYP1A1 or CYP2C9, but it impacted CYP2C19 and CYP3A4 (Ho, Singh, Holloway, & Crankshaw, 2011). No HDIs involving vitex in humans have been reported, although caution is recommended when used with dopamine agonists, hormone replacement therapy, and possibly birth control pills. A systematic review of adverse events based on data from clinical trials, postmarketing surveillance studies, surveys, spontaneous reporting, manufacturers, and herbalist organizations reported no drug interactions (Daniele, Thompson Coon, Pittler, & Ernst, 2005).

SUMMARY

Many physicians are reluctant to recommend or condone the use of herbal medicines because they lack familiarity with the benefits, the potential side effects, and the simple methods to minimize risks. In contrast, most physicians become comfortable prescribing medications that are known to have more frequent and more severe drug interactions and side effects. Although the number of phytomedicines may seem daunting at first, in reality only a handful of them would have a significant impact in most clinical practices. Knowledge of just a few of the most useful herbs, how to monitor for benefits and side effects, and where to obtain reliable brands, would enable the physician to responsibly integrate phytomedicines with standard treatments to optimize patient outcomes (Brown, Gerbarg, & Muskin, 2009).

COUNTERACTING MEDICATION SIDE EFFECTS WITH NUTRIENTS AND HERBS

Intolerance of medication side effects is a major cause of noncompliance. When dose reduction or switching medications is ineffective, herbs, nutrients, and hormones can be used either to substitute for the offending medication or to counteract side effects of medications that cannot be discontinued. Although only a few natural medicines have been studied as antidotes to side effects, in clinical practice, the authors find the following treatments to be useful in preventing or reversing medication-induced side effects. Dosage guidelines are included for some supplements. Where there is no specific dose recommended, the practitioner should start by following the instructions on the product label and increase gradually while monitoring for symptom relief and side effects.

ASTHENIA, FATIGUE, SOMNOLENCE

Many drugs cause fatigue or somnolence, particularly psychotropics, antihypertensives, antihistamines, opiates, beta blockers, tamsulosin, and chemotherapy treatments. If it is not possible to change the medication, the following treatments can be combined to increase daytime energy (mental and physical) without causing addiction: *R. rosea* (300–750 mg/day), *E. senticosus* (500 mg b.i.d.), and *P. ginseng* (300 mg or more/day). If this combination is not effective enough, maca (3–4 × 750 mg tablets b.i.d.) may be added. ADAPT-232 (2–4 tablets/day) contains *R. rosea, E. senticosus,* and *S. chinensis.*

CACHEXIA IN CANCER PATIENTS ON CHEMOTHERAPY OR RADIATION THERAPY

Cancer cachexia is characterized by anorexia, weight loss, muscle wasting, weakness, fatigue, and changes in metabolism of carbohydrates, lipids, and proteins. Oxidative stress and systemic inflammation are considered to be contributory factors.

Bio-Strath

Bio-Strath, a traditional Swiss herbal preparation derived from brewer's yeast grown on a bed rich in medicinal alpine herbs, contains a high concentration of B Vitamins and antioxidants. A DBRPC stratified trial in 177 cancer patients undergoing radiation therapy found that those who were administered Bio-Strath showed improved energy, appetite, weight gain, and red blood cell counts compared with placebo. Bio-Strath did not affect tumor growth or the antitumor effect of radiotherapy (Schwarzenbach & Brunner, 1996).

L-Carnitine

A review of L-carnitine found evidence that it can reduce chronic inflammation and oxidative stress in cancer patients. Cancer patients are at risk for carnitine deficiency due to reduced food intake, increased metabolic demands, and interference by chemotherapy drugs with carnitine absorption, synthesis, and excretion. Studies of carnitine (4 g/day) in cancer patients find improvement in fatigue, mood, sleep, and appetite, with an increase in lean body mass (Silverio, Laviano, Rossi Fanelli, & Seelaender, 2011). A review of L-carnitine reported evidence that it helps reduce the side effects of radiochemotherapy (Kahn, 2004). Animal studies demonstrate protection against radiation-induced germ cell apoptosis and reduced damage to brain, retina, cochlea, and kidneys. L-carnitine has been used to prevent cardiotoxicity from chemotherapy.

Rhodiola rosea

A nonblinded 28-week RCT in 58 patients with advanced nonsmall-cell lung cancer showed that those who were given 10 intravenous 30-hour ATP infusions at 2- to 4-week intervals had statistically significant improvements in weight, serum albumin, muscle strength, energy and fatigue (p <0.0001), and quality of life. Side effects included chest heaviness (Agteresch, Dagnelie, van der Gaast, Stijnen, & Wilson, 2000). While this treatment was effective, it has limited practicality because of the need for intravenous infusion. However, since *R. rosea* can be easily given by mouth it would be worthwhile to study this as a simpler way to increase ATP (Panossian, 2013), particularly because it has already been found to improve muscle strength, energy, and fatigue in animal studies, normal subjects, and patients with other illnesses.

NAUSEA AND VOMITING

Nausea and vomiting sometimes respond to ginger tea or ginger capsules taken 40 minutes prior to medication. A small container of candied ginger can be carried easily for sudden episodes of nausea. Nausea can also be relieved using acupressure bands applied to acupressure points at the wrist. Amrit Kalash (two complex Ayurvedic herbal formulas) can be used for severe nausea, fatigue, and other side effects of chemotherapy.

HEPATIC DYSFUNCTION

Many medications can cause hepatitis as indicated by elevations in liver enzymes. See the section titled Nutrients for Mood Disorders for a discussion of the hepatoprotection by SAMe, polyenolphosphatidyl serine, and bupleurum.

CONSTIPATION, HEMORRHOIDS, AND VARICOSE VEINS

Constipation caused by medications often responds to triphala 2–4 capsules/day (an Ayurvedic herbal preparation) (Munshi et al., 2011) or magnesium 600–800 mg/day (Guerrera, Volpe, & Mao, 2009). Patients who become constipated on medications (e.g., opioids) may engage in constipation-prolonged forceful valsalva during defecation, which can exacerbate hemorrhoids. Herbs that strengthen the walls of blood vessels and help to heal and prevent hemorrhoids and varicose veins include *Ruscus aculeatus* (butchers broom; CircuCaps) and *Aesculus hippocastanum* (horse chestnut extract). These vasotonic herbs also reduce capillary filtration rate and edema in chronic venous insufficiency (MacKay, 2001). In addition, butcher's broom has antiinflammatory properties and inhibits macromolecular permeability and elastase. Meta-analysis of 20 clinical trials of Cyclo 3 Fort (root extract of the *Ruscus aculeatus* 150 mg, hesperidin methyl chalcone 150 mg, and ascorbic acid 100 mg)—including 20 placebo controlled, randomized double blind studies and 5 randomized studies against a comparator drug— found strong evidence of efficacy in the treatment of chronic venous insufficiency (Boyle, Diehm, & Robertson, 2003). Horse chestnut exhibits vasotonic, vascular protective, antiinflammatory, and free-radical scavenging properties. In vitro studies demonstrated inhibition of the enzymes elastase and hyaluronidase. These herbs are safe and generally well tolerated. Isolated adverse effects of horse chestnut have been reported in one patient on anticoagulant medication with angiomyolipoma and in one anorexic patient with renal insufficiency.

NERVOUS SYSTEM

Extrapyramidal Symptoms

Controlled studies of herbs and nutrients in psychotic disorders are limited. However, considering the devastating effects of psychotic disorders, the severity of antipsychotic medication side effects (e.g., weight gain, diabetes, cardiovascular disease, sedation, fatigue, extrapyramidal symptoms, and tardive dyskinesia) and the low side-effect risk with herbs and nutrients, a lower threshold of evidence is reasonable in offering complementary treatments. Oxidative stress causing damage to neurotransmitter systems, particularly dopaminergic nerves in striatal tissues, has been implicated in the pathogenesis of the following psychotropic medication side effects:

1. Extrapyramidal symptoms: dystonias (muscle spasms), oculogyric crises (spasm of muscles controlling eye movements), pseudoparkinsonism (muscle rigidity, tremor, bradykinesia, mask-like facies), akinesia (difficulty initiating movement), akathisia (motor restlessness), restless legs, bruxism (jaw clenching), and blepherospasm (eyelid spasms).

2. Tardive dyskinesia (TD): involuntary movements of the tongue, jaw, trunk, or extremities may be choreiform (rapid, jerky, discontinuous) or athetoid (slow, sinuous, continuous).

Reduced levels of antioxidant defense enzymes in schizophrenic patients, oxidative damage, toxins, and inflammatory processes may contribute to the development of schizophrenia and medication side effects (Sivrioglu, Kirli, Sipahioglu, Gursoy, & Sarandol, 2007). The incidence and severity of side effects could be ameliorated by substances with known neuroprotective, cognitive enhancing, antioxidant, and antiinflammatory actions in patients taking antipsychotic medications.

Ginkgo Biloba

Ginkgo increases circulating and membrane PUFAs (particularly eicosapentanoic acid) and protects against oxidative stress in vivo (Drieu et al., 2000). Reducing oxidative damage to neurons by increasing PUFAs could help alleviate adverse effects of antipsychotic medications. Ginkgo may protect against the neural damage associated with antipsychotics and extrapyramidal symptoms. For example, a 12-week DBRPC trial in patients with treatment-resistant schizophrenia compared (n = 56) ginkgo 360 mg/day plus haloperidol 0.25 mg/kg/day with (n = 53) placebo plus haloperidol 0.25 mg/kg/day; 57% of the ginkgo group were rated as responders versus 38% of the placebo group. The ginkgo group showed a lower incidence of extrapyramidal symptoms and greater improvement in positive symptoms of schizophrenia such as delusions, hallucinations, disorganized speech, grossly disorganized or catatonic behavior, and in negative symptoms such as flattening of affect, alogia (restriction in the fluency and productivity of thought and speech), and avolition (restriction in goal-directed behavior) (Zhang et al., 2001). Similarly, in an 8-week DBRCT of schizophrenic patients those given olanzapine with gingko (EGb) augmentation (n = 15) had a significant reduction on the Positive Syndrome Scale (PANSS) versus those given olanzapine alone (n = 14).

The group taking gingko had significantly greater reductions in superoxide dismutase and catalase, indicating reduced oxidative stress (Atmaca, Tezcan, Kuloglu, Ustundag, & Kirtas, 2005).

B Vitamins

Pyridoxine (vitamin B_6) may reduce side effects of antipsychotic medications. In a 4-week DBPCR trial in 15 schizophrenic and schizo-affective patients with TD, B6 400 mg/day markedly reduced TD symptoms (Lerner et al., 2001). A 5-day DBRPC study of 20 schizophrenic and schizo-affective patients with neuroleptic-induced akathisia found B6 600 mg b.i.d. improved the subjective sense of restlessness, distress and global ratings significantly more than placebo (Lerner, Bergman, Statsenko, & Miodownik, 2004). In another DBRPC trail, 60 schizophrenia and schizoaffective inpatients with neuroleptic-induced akathisia were randomized to receive vitamin B_6 1200 mg/day, mianserin 15 mg/day (tricyclic noradrenergic and specific serotonergic antidepressant), or placebo for 5 days. Compared with the placebo group, the vitamin B_6-treated and mianserin-treated patients had a significant improvement in subjective distress and Clinical Global Impression subscales, but not in the objective subscale. A reduction of at least 2 points on the Barnes Akathisia Rating Scale global subscale was noted in the vitamin B_6 group (13/23, 56%) and in the mianserin groups (13/20, 65%) compared to only one patient in the placebo group (Miodownik et al., 2006). High doses of B_6 with low doses of mianserin may be a useful addition to current treatments of neuroleptic-induced akathisia.

Combination Supplement—Omega-3 FA, Vitamin E, and Vitamin C

In an open study, 17 schizophrenic patients being treated with haloperidol were given a 1000 mg capsule of n-3 FAs (180 mg EPA + 120 mg DHA) twice daily, vitamin E 400 IU twice daily and vitamin C 1000 mg/day for 4 months. At the end of the study, scores were significantly lower compared to baseline on the Brief Psychiatric Rating Scale, Scale for the Assessment of Negative Symptoms, Simpson Angus Scale, and Barnes Akathisia Rating Scale. In addition, superoxide dismutase levels were significantly lower at the end of study, but gluthatione peroxidase, malondialdehyde, vitamin E and C levels were not (Sivrioglu et al., 2007).

N-acetylcysteine

N-acetylcysteine scavenges for free radicals and increases intracellular glutathione, the primary neuroprotective antioxidant in the brain. Studies of animals given haloperidol 1.5 mg/kg/day for 21 days showed significant elevations in striatal superoxide (free radicals) and lipid peroxidation (free radical damage to membranes) compared with animals not given haloperidol. Next, both groups of animals were given N-acetylcysteine (NAC) for 21 days in 3 different doses: 50 mg/day, 500 mg/day, and 1500 mg/day. All three doses of NAC prevented the haloperidol-induced increase in superoxide (free radical) levels. The 1500 mg/day dose of NAC prevented haloperidol-induced increase in lipid peroxidation and improved the glutathione/reduced glutathione ratio. In animals not pretreated with haloperidol, 50 mg/day and 500 mg/day NAC reduced oxidative stress markers, but 1500 mg/day increased levels of superoxide, decreased lipid peroxidation, and increased consumption of reduced glutathione (Harvey, Joubert, du Preez, & Berk, 2007). Doses up to 1800 mg twice daily are being used in human studies. Excessive doses of NAC may promote oxidative processes. Caution is advised in the use of high-dose intravenous NAC. The use of NAC in addiction, compulsive and grooming disorders, schizophrenia, and bipolar disorder has been reviewed (Dean, Giorlando, & Berk 2011).

In a 6-month DBRPC study of 140 patients with schizophrenia, NAC 1000 mg twice daily reduced symptoms of akathisia and improved Clinical Global Impression (effect size = 0.40) compared to placebo (Berk, Copolov, Dean, et al., 2008a). In appropriate doses, NAC may reduce prevent or reduce medication-induced damage to striatal tissues and the ensuing side effects. NAC is available in 600 mg tablets in the United States. Two 600mg tablets twice a day would have about the same effect as the doses used in clinical trials.

Dehydroepiandrosterone (DHEA)

In a 12-week DBRPC study of chronic schizophrenic patients (n = 40), DHEA (up to 150 mg/day) reduced negative symptoms, extrapyramidal symptoms, akathisia, and glucose levels better than placebo (Strous et al., 2007). The reduction in negative symptoms and medication side effects may be attributable to potentiation of NMDA-receptor activity, suppression of GABA inhibition, and enhancement of frontal dopamine release.

Melatonin

Melatonin (10 mg/day sustained release) alleviated symptoms of TD in 17 out of 22 patients with schizophrenia (mean duration of 25 years) in a 6-week DBPC crossover study. Scores on the Abnormal Involuntary Movement Scale decreased 3 points in seven patients on melatonin versus one patient on placebo (Shamir et al., 2001).

Restless Leg Syndrome

Restless leg syndrome is characterized by abnormal uncomfortable sensations and/or movements of the legs, usually worse at night or at rest and often relieved by walking around. Antipsychotics and antidepressants, particularly SSRIs, can cause restless leg syndrome with secondary loss of sleep. A combination of lemon balm, passion flower, and valerian can be helpful.

Cognition, Memory, and Word Finding

Patients often complain of cognitive impairment, decreased memory, and/or word-finding problems related to medication. Many of the treatments described in the section titled Cognitive Function can help to counteract cognitive and memory dysfunction due to medication side effects, including the following: *R.rosea* 450–750 mg/day; ADAPT-232 2–4 tablets/day; Aniracetam 750 mg twice daily; and Huperzine-A 200–400 mg twice daily. Artichoke extract may be of benefit in cognitive impairment secondary to chronic use of benzodiazepines, based on animal studies.

In a DBRCT of schizophrenic inpatients (n = 42) with elevated homocysteine (increased oxidative stress), those who were given a daily vitamin combination (folic acid 2 mg, B_{12} 400 mcg, B_6 25 mg) showed significantly greater reduction in homocysteine levels and PANSS scores and improved cognitive function compared to the placebo group (Levine et al., 2006).

Insomnia

Medication-induced insomnia can respond to Melatonin 3–9 mg hs. Melatonin reduces sleep onset latency; extended release melatonin maintains sleep. Chronic schizophrenic patients have shown blunted nocturnal melatonin levels. A DBRPC study in schizophrenic outpatients (n = 40) demonstrated that in patients receiving haloperidol 10-15 mg/day, melatonin 3 mg hs improved sleep measures and quality of life in comparison to placebo (Kumar, Andrade, Bhakta, & Singh, 2007).

CARDIOVASCULAR SYSTEM

Pedal Edema

Antipsychotics, mood stabilizers (such as valproate and lithium carbonate), SSRIs, and other medications can cause pedal edema (swelling of the feet and ankles due to leakage of fluid from veins into tissues. (See section on constipation, hemorrhoids, and venous insufficiency.) By strengthening the veins, butcher's broom (Sanhelios CircuCaps 900 mg/d) and horse chestnut extract (Natures Way Standardized Extract 1 tablet b.i.d.) can reduce pedal edema.

MUSCULOSKELETAL SYSTEM

In a university department of cardiology clinic, more than 30% of patients taking statins reported myopathy, myalgia, or myositis (Riphagen, van der Veer, Muskiet, & DeJongste, 2012). Statin myotoxicity has been linked to impairment of mitochondrial functions, such as electron transport, and depletion of CoQ10. Preliminary studies of CoQ10 supplementation to relieve statin-induced myalgia and muscle weakness have yielded inconsistent results. Patients on maintenance statin treatment should have CoQ10 levels monitored. If the levels are low, or if the patient develops symptoms of muscle pain or weakness, then supplemental CoQ10 (preferably ubiquinol, a reduced form of CoQ10) is indicated. The ongoing *Co-Enzyme Q10 in Statin Myopathy* study intends to determine the effects of CoQ10 on pain intensity in patients with statin-induced myalgia who are being treated for hypercholesterolemia (Parker et al., 2013).

HEMATOLOGICAL DISORDERS, IMMUNE DEFENSE, CHEMOTHERAPY TOXICITY

Erythrocytes

Medication-induced decreases in red blood cell count with a hematocrit >32 can be reversed with *R. rosea, E. senticosus,* and/or shark liver oil. Toxicity from contaminants and gastrointestinal disturbances with low-quality shark liver oil products has been reported. Therefore, the authors recommend only high-quality shark oil products such as Immunofin 2–6 capsules/day (Lane Labs) or shark liver oil (Life Extension Foundation) (Brown et al., 2009).

Leukocytes

Medication-induced decreases in white cells with a total count >3500 and a neutrophil count >1500, can be reversed using shark liver oil (2–6 capsules/day Immunofin,) *E. senticosus* 500 mg b.i.d., Astragalus, and/or lithium 600 mg/day or more (Brown et al., 2009).

Platelets

Medication-induced decreases in platelets, when the count is >80,000 and without bruising or bleeding, can sometimes be treated with shark liver oil (Immunofin) 2–6 capsules/day. The platelet count should be monitored to avoid supranormal levels (Brown et al., 2009).

If erythrocyte, leukocyte, or platelet counts drop below the minimal levels mentioned above, then the offending medication should be discontinued and the natural treatments continued until cell counts return to normal. If cell counts continue to decline or fail to improve, a hematologist should be consulted.

ADAPTOGENS IN CANCER TREATMENT REDUCE CHEMOTOXIC EFFECTS ON BONE MARROW AND LIVER

Chemotherapy drugs often damage stem cells in the liver and bone marrow, resulting in increased susceptibility to infections and other medical problems. When blood cell counts fall too low, chemotherapy may be interrupted.

Rhodiola rosea extracts demonstrated antitumor and antimetastatic activity in studies of human cancers transplanted into mice (Lewis lung carcinoma, Ehrlich's sarcoma, Pliss lymphosarcoma, NK/Ly tumor, and melanoma B16). Moreover, *R. rosea* protected liver and bone marrow cells from chemotoxic effects of adriamycin and cyclophosphamide, while at the same time enhancing the effectiveness of the chemotherapy in destroying cancer cells and reducing metastases (Dement'eva & Iaremenko, 1987; Razina, Zueva, Amosova, & Krylova, 2000; Udintsev, Krylova, & Fomina, 1992; Udintsev & Schakhov, 1989, 1990, 1991).

In 12 patients with superficial bladder carcinoma, *R. rosea* improved urothelial tissue, leukocyte integrines, and T-cell immunity with a trend toward reduction in frequency of relapse (Bocharova et al., 1995). A 95% ethanol extract of

R. rosea stems exhibited cytotoxic activity against prostate cancer cells (Ming et al., 2005).

Studies in rodents with transplants of human cancers (Lewis lung sarcoma, Pliss lymphosarcoma, Ehrlich's sarcoma, NKY/LY tumor, and melanoma B16) given adriamycin or cyclophosphamide found that the addition of *R. rosea* did not interfere with the actions of the chemotherapy agents. In fact, the *R. rosea* increased the effectiveness of the chemotherapy drugs, reduced metastases, and protected the liver and bone marrow stem cells from toxic effects of the chemotherapy. *R. rosea* is administered to cancer patients in the former Soviet Union. RCTs are needed to confirm safety and efficacy. Since fatigue is the most common complaint among cancer patients and since *R. rosea* is so beneficial for fatigue, trials would be helpful in cancer treatment and recovery.

The inaccessibility of *R. rosea* cancer research (much of which is published in foreign language journals) combined with reluctance to use herbal preparations in cancer patients and lack of funding to study adaptogens has prevented oncologists from discovering the potential benefits of *R. rosea* and other adaptogenic herbs.

Adaptogen Combination Treatments

In a study of 28 women with stage III–IV ovarian cancer treated with cisplatin and cyclophosphamide, subjects who took AdMax 270 mg/day (combination of extracts from roots of *Leuzea carthamoides, R. rosea, E. senticosus,* and fruits of *S. chinensis*) for 4 weeks following chemotherapy showed increases in T cell subclasses (CD3, CD4, CD5, and CD8), IgG and IgM compared with those who did not (Kormosh, Laktionov, & Antoshechkina, 2006).

Ashwagandha (Withania somnifera)
Ashwagandha is an adaptogenic herb known in Indian medicine for its antistress, antiinflammatory, antioxidant, analgesic, antidepressant, and immunomodulatory effects. An in vitro and in vivo study of selective tumor inhibition by an ashwagandha leaf extract found that one of the constituents, withanone, activated p53, a gene responsible for tumor cell apoptosis. The herbal extract selectively killed various human tumor cells but not normal human cells (Widodo et al., 2007). However, because ashwaganda has estrogenic properties, further studies are needed regarding long-term safety in women.

Amrit Kalash
Amrit Kalash, a proprietary Ayurvedic formula containing many herbs including ashwagandha, enhanced immune function and protected against free radical damage and toxic effects of chemotherapy in animal and cell culture studies. Amrit Nectar tablets (MA-7, containing 38 herbs) showed antioxidant activity and protected against toxicity from adriamycin and cisplatin (Dwivedi, Natarajan, & Matthees, 2005). It is reported to improve energy, well being, sleep, appetite, vomiting, diarrhea, and tolerance of cancer treatment without interfering with chemotherapy agents. Additional RCTs are needed to confirm safety and efficacy for cancer patients. In clinical practice the authors find that patients who take Amrit Kalash during a course of chemotherapy report improved energy, digestion, and sense of well-being, as well as little or no hair loss.

RESPIRATORY INFECTIONS

Certain medications (e.g., modafinil) increase the occurrence of upper respiratory infections. Herbs and vitamins for stimulating immune defense include sambucol (concentrated extract of elderberries) and astragalus, reishi, shiitake, and maitake mushrooms. Red mangrove (*Rhizophora mangle*) bark extract from Fiji (Nature's Nurse, Respigard) is used to increase resistance to respiratory infection and to accelerate recovery. Traditional Polynesian medicine uses red mangrove for its astringent, antiseptic, hemostatic, antifungal, and anti-ulcerogenic properties (de Armas, Sarracent, Marrero, Fernandez, & Branford-White, 2005; Marrero et al., 2006). Based on in vitro and in vivo studies, *Andrographis paniculata* (king of bitters), an Asian phytomedicinal, manifests anticancer, antiinflammatory, and immunomodulatory action, and possibly reduction of autoimmune responses (Denzler , Waters, Jacobs, Rochon, & Langland, 2010; Iruretagoyena et al., 2005; Yang et al., 2010).

SUMMARY

Phytomedicines, nutrients, and neurohormones have the potential to relieve psychological and physical symptoms in medical patients. The growing reliance on synthetic medications has brought unintended consequences: side effects, serious adverse reactions, drug interactions, high costs of development passed on to consumers, substance abuse, and withdrawal symptoms. In addition, the manufacturing of synthetic drugs creates environmental pollutants, and the disposal of nonbiodegradable medications contributes to toxic water pollution. In comparison, herbs and nutrients have far fewer side effects, less addiction potential, and lower costs.

Biodiversity in medicinal plants and their innumerable related species is an untapped resource for the future development of medical treatments. Once the bioactive constituents are identified in a plant part, it is possible to alter the relative concentrations of therapeutic compounds by cross-breeding and by changing the composition of nutrients in the soil and water. Such methods mimic some of the forces of natural evolution and, therefore, are less likely to produce harmful new compounds with unexpected effects as compared to artificial synthetic processes or genetic insertions. Genomic analysis is expanding our understanding of speciation and the subtle genetic differences that may determine therapeutic effectiveness. Furthermore, phytomedicines are a natural, renewable resource that can help farming communities flourish.

CLINICAL PEARLS

- Considerable progress has been made in the standardization of botanical extracts based on the concentration of marker compounds believed to be essential for therapeutic activity and/or to be unique to the species.

- The ultimate test of an extract is proven efficacy in a good quality controlled trial published in a peer-reviewed journal.

- Safety of most herbs during pregnancy and breastfeeding has not been adequately studied.

- Certain complex products are more affected by differences in cultivation and extraction procedures; for example *Ginkgo biloba, Hypericum perforatum* (St. John's wort) and *Rhodiola rosea* (Arctic root).

- Product labels rarely state the source of extracts; *Ginkgo biloba* is one exception.

- In determining dosage, take note not only of the milligrams of the marker compounds but also of the percentage of the same marker compounds.

- ConsumerLab.com is one of the best nongovernmental resources for up-to-date, detailed, practical information on most of the supplements encountered in clinical practice.

- Natural GABA, produced by fermentation, is widely used as a functional food supplement in Japan

- Herbs and nutritional supplements have a role in treatment of anxiety, mood, cognitive function, menopause, andropause, and sexual function.

- Kava and kava lactones carry risk of intoxication, abuse, dependency, medication interactions, and rarely severe adverse reactions (e.g., liver injury). Only high quality Kava should be considered for clinical use.

- Supplementation with l-methylfolate may be more effective than folic acid in patients with polymorphisms because it bypasses the final MTHFR conversion step.

- The quality of S-adenosyl-L-methionine (SAMe) and the quality of the tablet are critical for maintaining potency over time.

- In herb–drug interactions, pharmacodynamic interactions include risks of increased CNS side effects (e.g., serotonin syndrome), hepatotoxicity, or bleeding Pharmacokinetic concerns entail effects on the P450 cytochrome system.

ACKNOWLEDGMENTS

We wish to thank Dr. Teodoro Bottiglieri and Dr. Alexander Panossian for their support in the preparation of this chapter.

DISCLOSURE STATEMENTS

Dr. Richard P. Brown holds a patent for the use of 3-acetyl-7-oxo-dehydroepi-androsterone (7-Keto DHEA) in the treatments of PTSD and dissociative disorders. He has no other conflicts of interest.

Dr. Patricia L. Gerbarg is married to Dr. Richard P. Brown who holds a pantent on the use of 3-acetyl-7-oxo-dehydroepi-androsterone (7-Keto DHEA) in the treatments of PTSD and dissociative disorders. She has no other conflicts of interest.

REFERENCES

Abdou, A. M., Higashiguchi, S., Horie, K., Kim, M., Hatta, H., & Yokogoshi, H. (2006). Relaxation and immunity enhancement effects of gamma-aminobutyric acid (GABA) administration in humans. *Biofactors, 26*(3), 201–208.

Abdul, H. M., & Butterfield, D. A. (2007). Involvement of PI3K/PKG/ERK1/2 signaling pathways in cortical neurons to trigger protection by cotreatment of acetyl-L-carnitine and alpha-lipoic acid against HNE-mediated oxidative stress and neurotoxicity: implications for Alzheimer's disease. *Free Radical Biology and Medicine, 42*(3), 371–384.

Abdul Muneer, P. M., Alikunju, S., Szlachetka, A. M., & Haorah, J. (2011). Methamphetamine inhibits the glucose uptake by human neurons and astrocytes: stabilization by acetyl-L-carnitine. *PLoS One, 6*(4), e19258.

Agency for Healthcare Research and Quality (AHRQ). (2007). *S-adenosyl-L-metionine for treatment of depression, osteoarthritis, and liver disease.* Retrieved October 8, 2007 from http://www.ahrq.gov/clinic/epcsums/samesum.htm.

Agteresch, H. J., Dagnelie, P. C., van der Gaast, A., Stijnen, T., & Wilson, J. H. (2000). Randomized clinical trial of adenosine 5'-triphosphate in patients with advanced non-small-cell lung cancer. *Journal of the National Cancer Institute, 92*(4), 321–328.

Akhondzadeh Basti, A., Moshiri, E., Noorbala, A. A., Jamshidi, A. H., Abbasi, S. H., & Akhondzadeh, S. (2007). Comparison of petal of Crocus sativus L. and fluoxetine in the treatment of depressed outpatients: a pilot double-blind randomized trial. *Progress in Neuropsychopharmacology and Biological Psychiatry, 31*(2), 439–442.

Akhondzadeh S., Gerbarg, P. L., & Brown, R. P. (2013). Nutrients for prevention and treatment of mental health disorders *Psychiatric Clinics of North America, March, 3*(61):25–36.

Akhondzadeh, S., & Abbasi, S. H. (2006). Herbal medicine in the treatment of Alzheimer's disease. [Review]. *American Journal of Alzheimer's Disease and Other Dementias, 21*(2), 113–118.

Akhondzadeh, S., Naghavi, H. R., Vazirian, M., Shayeganpour, A., Rashidi, H., & Khani, M. (2001). Passionflower in the treatment of generalized anxiety: a pilot double-blind randomized controlled trial with oxazepam. *Journal of Clinical Pharmacy and Therapeutics, 26*(5), 363–367.

Akhondzadeh, S., Noroozian, M., Mohammadi, M., Ohadinia, S., Jamshidi, A. H., & Khani, M. (2003). Melissa officinalis extract in the treatment of patients with mild to moderate Alzheimer's disease: a double blind, randomised, placebo controlled trial. *Journal of Neurology, Neurosurgry, and Psychiatry, 74*(7), 863–866.

Akhondzadeh, S., Sabet, M. S., Harirchian, M. H., Togha, M., Cheraghmakani, H., Razeghi, S., et al. (2010). Saffron in the treatment of patients with mild to moderate Alzheimer's disease: a 16-week, randomized and placebo-controlled trial. *Journal of Clinical Pharmacy and Therapeutics, 35*(5), 581–588.

Akhondzadeh, S., Shafiee Sabet, M., Harirchian, M. H., Togha, M., Cheraghmakani, H., Razeghi, S., et al. (2010). A 22-week, multicenter, randomized, double-blind controlled trial of Crocus sativus in the treatment of mild-to-moderate Alzheimer's disease. *Psychopharmacology (Berl), 207*(4), 637–643.

Akhondzadeh, S., Tahmacebi-Pour, N., Noorbala, A. A., Amini, H., Fallah-Pour, H., Jamshidi, A. H., & Khani, M. (2005). Crocus sativus L. in the treatment of mild to moderate depression: a double-blind, randomized and placebo-controlled trial. *Phytotherapy Research, 19*(2), 148–151.

Aleynik, S. I., & Lieber, C. S. (2003). Polyenylphosphatidylcholine corrects the alcohol-induced hepatic oxidative stress by restoring s-adenosylmethionine. *Alcohol Alcoholism, 38*(3), 208–212.

Aliev, G., Li, Y., Palacios, H. H., & Obrenovich, M. E. (2011). Oxidative stress induced mitochondrial DNA deletion as a hallmark for the drug development in the context of the cerebrovascular diseases. *Recent Patents on Cardiovascular Drug Discovery, 6*(3), 222–241.

Almeida, J. C., & Grimsley, E. W. (1996). Coma from the health food store: interaction between kava and alprazolam. *Annals of Internal Medicine, 125*(11), 940–941.

Alpert, J. E., Papakostas, G., Mischoulon, D., Worthington, J. J., 3rd, Petersen, T., Mahal, Y., et al. (2004). S-adenosyl-L-methionine (SAMe) as an adjunct for resistant major depressive disorder: an open trial following partial or nonresponse to selective serotonin reuptake inhibitors or venlafaxine. *Journal of Clinical Psychopharmacology, 24*(6), 661–664.

Alvarez-Sabin, J., & Roman, G. C. (2011). Citicoline in vascular cognitive impairment and vascular dementia after stroke. *Stroke, 42*(1 Suppl), S40–S43.

Alvarez, X. A., Mouzo, R., Pichel, V., Perez, P., Laredo, M., Fernandez-Novoa, L., et al. (1999). Double-blind placebo-controlled study with citicoline in APOE genotyped Alzheimer's disease patients. Effects on cognitive performance, brain bioelectrical activity and cerebral perfusion. *Methods and Findings in Experimental and Clinical Pharmacology, 21*(9), 633–644.

American Psychiatric Association. (1994). *Diagnostic and statistical manual* (4th ed.). Washington, D. C.: American Psychiatric Press.

Amsterdam, J. D., Li, Y., Soeller, I., Rockwell, K., Mao, J. J., & Shults, J. (2009). A randomized, double-blind, placebo-controlled trial of oral Matricaria recutita (chamomile) extract therapy for generalized anxiety disorder. *Journal of Clinical Psychopharmacology, 29*(4), 378–382.

Andrade, A. S., Hendrix, C., Parsons, T. L., Caballero, B., Yuan, C. S., Flexner, C. W., et al. (2008). Pharmacokinetic and metabolic effects of American ginseng (Panax quinquefolius) in healthy volunteers receiving the HIV protease inhibitor indinavir. *BMC Complementary and Alternative Medicine, 8*, 50.

Annweiler, C., Rolland, Y., Schott, A. M., Blain, H., Vellas, B., Herrmann, F. R., & Beauchet, O. (2012). Higher vitamin D dietary intake is associated with lower risk of Alzheimer's disease: A 7-year follow-up. *Journals of Gerontology. Series A Biological Sciences and Medical Sciences.*

Appel, K., Rose, T., Fiebich, B., Kammler, T., Hoffmann, C., & Weiss, G. (2011). Modulation of the gamma-aminobutyric acid (GABA) system by Passiflora incarnata L. *Phytotherapy Research, 25*(6), 838–843.

Arciniegas, D. B. (2001). Traumatic brain injury and cognitive impairment: the cholinergic hypothesis. *Neuropsychiatry Reviews*, 17–20.

Arenth, P. M., Russell, K. C., Ricker, J. H., & Zafonte, R. D. (2011). CDP-choline as a biological supplement during neurorecovery: a focused review. *PM & R, 3*(6 Suppl 1), S123–S131.

Arrigo, A., Casale, R., Buonocore, M., & Ciano, C. (1990). Effects of acetyl-L-carnitine on reaction times in patients with cerebrovascular insufficiency. *International Journal of Clinical Pharmacology Research, 10*(1–2), 133–137.

Asayama, K., Yamadera, H., Ito, T., Suzuki, H., Kudo, Y., & Endo, S. (2003). Double blind study of melatonin effects on the sleep-wake rhythm, cognitive and non-cognitive functions in Alzheimer type dementia. *Journal of Nippon Medical School, 70*(4), 334–341.

Aslanyan, G., Amroyan, E., Gabrielyan, E., Nylander, M., Wikman, G., & Panossian, A. (2010). Double-blind, placebo-controlled, randomised study of single dose effects of ADAPT-232 on cognitive functions. *Phytomedicine, 17*(7), 494–499.

Atmaca, M., Tezcan, E., Kuloglu, M., Ustundag, B., & Kirtas, O. (2005). The effect of extract of ginkgo biloba addition to olanzapine on therapeutic effect and antioxidant enzyme levels in patients with schizophrenia. *Psychiatry and Clinical Neuroscience, 59*(6), 652–656.

Awad, R., Levac, D., Cybulska, P., Merali, Z., Trudeau, V. L., & Arnason, J. T. (2007). Effects of traditionally used anxiolytic botanicals on enzymes of the gamma-aminobutyric acid (GABA) system. *Canadian Journal of Physiology and Pharmacology, 85*(9), 933–942.

Bacci Ballerini, F., Lopez Anguera, A., Alcaraz, P., & Hernandez Reyes, N. (1983). Treatment of postconcussion syndrome with S-adenosylmethionine. *Medicina Clinica, 80*(4), 161–164.

Bachinskaya, N., Hoerr, R., & Ihl, R. (2011). Alleviating neuropsychiatric symptoms in dementia: the effects of Ginkgo biloba extract EGb 761. Findings from a randomized controlled trial. *Neuropsychiatric Disease and Treatment, 7*, 209–215.

Bandelow, B., Wedekind, D., & Leon, T. (2007). Pregabalin for the treatment of generalized anxiety disorder: a novel pharmacologic intervention. [Review]. *Expert Review of Neurotherapeutics, 7*(7), 769–781.

Barak, A. J., Beckenhauer, H. C., & Tuma, D. J. (1996). Betaine effects on hepatic methionine metabolism elicited by short-term ethanol feeding. *Alcohol, 13*(5), 483–486.

Baranov, V. B. (Ed.). (1994). *Experimental trials of herbal adaptogen effect on the quality of operation activity, mental and professional work capacity. Contract 93-11-615 Stage 2 Phase I.* Moscow: Russian Federation Ministry of Health Institute of Medical and Biological Problems (IMBP).

Barlet, A., Albrecht, J., Aubert, A., Fischer, M., Grof, F., Grothuesmann, H. G., et al. (1990). [Efficacy of Pygeum africanum extract in the medical therapy of urination disorders due to benign prostatic hyperplasia: evaluation of objective and subjective parameters. A placebo-controlled double-blind multicenter study]. *Wien Klin Wochenschr, 102*(22), 667–673.

Barry, M. J., Meleth, S., Lee, J. Y., Kreder, K. J., Avins, A. L., Nickel, J. C., et al. (2011). Effect of increasing doses of saw palmetto extract on lower urinary tract symptoms: a randomized trial. *Journal of the American Medical Association, 306*(12), 1344–1351.

Baskaya, M. K., Dogan, A., Rao, A. M., & Dempsey, R. J. (2000). Neuroprotective effects of citicoline on brain edema and blood-brain barrier breakdown after traumatic brain injury. *Journal of Neurosurgery, 92*(3), 448–452.

Bassi, P., Artibani. W., De Luca, V., Zattoni, F., Lembo, A. (1987). [Standardized extract of Pygeum africanum in the treatment of benign prostatic hypertrophy. Controlled clinical study versus placebo]. *Minerva Urologica e Nefrologica, 39*(1), 45–50. [Italian]

Beckham, N. (1995). Phyto-oestrogens and compounds that affect oestrogen metabolism, part II. *Australian Journal of Medical Herbalism, 7*(2), 27–33.

Bedell, S., Nachtigall, M., & Naftolin, F. (2014). The pros and cons of plant estrogens for menopause. *Journal of Steroid Biochemistry and Molecular Biology, 139*, 225–236.

Belford-Courtney, R. (1993). Comparison of Chinese and Western users of Angelica sinensis. *Australian Journal of Medical Herbalisms, 5*(4), 87–91.

Bell, I. R., Edman, J. S., Morrow, F. D., Marby, D. W., Perrone, G., Kayne, H. L., et al. (1992). Brief communication. Vitamin B1, B2, and B6 augmentation of tricyclic antidepressant treatment in geriatric depression with cognitive dysfunction. *Journal of the American College of Nutrition, 11*(2), 159–163.

Benke, D., Barberis, A., Kopp, S., Altmann, K. H., Schubiger, M., Vogt, K. E., et al. (2008). GABA A receptors as in vivo substrate for the anxiolytic action of valerenic acid, a major constituent of valerian root extracts. *Neuropharmacology, 56*(1), 174–81.

Bent, S., Padula, A., Moore, D., Patterson, M., & Mehling, W. (2006). Valerian for sleep: a systematic review and meta-analysis. *American Journal of Medicine, 119*(12), 1005–1012.

Berk, M., Copolov, D., Dean, O., Lu, K., Jeavons, S., Schapkaitz, I., et al. (2008a). N-acetyl cysteine as a glutathione precursor for schizophrenia—a double-blind, randomized, placebo-controlled trial. *Biological Psychiatry, 64*(5), 361–368.

Berk, M., Copolov, D. L., Dean, O., Lu, K., Jeavons, S., Schapkaitz, I., et al. (2008b). N-acetyl cysteine for depressive symptoms in bipolar disorder—a double-blind randomized placebo-controlled trial. *Biological Psychiatry, 64*(6), 468–475.

Berlanga, C., Ortega-Soto, H. A., Ontiveros, M., & Senties, H. (1992). Efficacy of S-adenosyl-L-methionine in speeding the onset of action of imipramine. *Psychiatry Research, 44*(3), 257–262.

Betz, J. M., White, K. D., & der Marderosian, A. H. (1995). Gas chromatographic determination of yohimbine in commercial yohimbe products. *Journal of AOAC International, 78*(5), 1189–1194.

Beydoun, M. A., Kaufman, J. S., Satia, J. A., Rosamond, W., & Folsom, A. R. (2007). Plasma n-3 fatty acids and the risk of cognitive decline in older adults: the Atherosclerosis Risk in Communities Study. *American Journal of Clinical Nutrition, 85*(4), 1103–1111.

Bhalla, P., & Nehru, B. (2005). Modulatory effects of centrophenoxine on different regions of ageing rat brain. *Experimental Gerontology, 40*(10), 801–806.

Bianchetti, A., Rozzini, R., & Trabucchi, M. (2003). Effects of acetyl-L-carnitine in Alzheimer's disease patients unresponsive to acetylcholinesterase inhibitors. *Current Medical Research and Opinion, 19*(4), 350–353.

Blizzard, T. A. (2008). Selective estrogen receptor modulator medicinal chemistry at Merck. *A review. Current Topics in Medicinal Chemistry, 8*(9), 792–812.

Bloch, M. H., & Hannestad, J. (2012). Omega-3 fatty acids for the treatment of depression: systematic review and meta-analysis. *Molecular Psychiatry, 17*(12), 1272–82.

Federation of State Medical Board. (2007). *Model guidelines for physician use of complementary and alternative therapies in medical practice.* Retrieved from www.fsmb.org/pdf/2002_grpol_Complementary_Alternative_Terapies.pdf.

Bocharova, O. A., Matveev, B. P., Baryshnikov, A. I. u., Figurin, K. M., Serebriakova, R. V., & Bodrova, N. B. (1995). The effect of a Rhodiola rosea extract on the incidence of recurrences of a superficial bladder cancer (experimental clinical research). *Urologiia I Nefrologiia, (2)*, 46–47.

Bönöczk, P., Gulyas, B., Adam-Vizi, V., Nemes, A., Karpati, E., Kiss, B., et al. (2000). Role of sodium channel inhibition in neuroprotection: effect of vinpocetine. *Brain Research Bulletin, 53*(3), 245–254.

Booth, N. L., Overk, C. R., Yao, P., Burdette, J. E., Nikolic, D., Chen, S. N., et al. (2006). The chemical and biologic profile of a red clover (Trifoliumpratense L.) phase II clinical extract. *Journal of Alternative and Complementary Medicine, 12*(2), 133–139.

Bottiglieri, T. (1996). Folate, vitamin B12, and neuropsychiatric disorders. *Nutrition Reviews, 54*(12), 382–390.

Bottiglieri, T. (2002). S-Adenosyl-L-methionine (SAMe): from the bench to the bedside--molecular basis of a pleiotrophic molecule. *American Journal of Clinical Nutrition, 76*(5), 1151S–1157S.

Bottiglieri, T. (2013). Folate, vitamin B12, and S-adenosylmethionine. *Psychiatric Clinics of North America, 36*(1), 1–13.

Bourre, J. M. (2005). Dietary omega-3 Fatty acids and psychiatry: mood, behaviour, stress, depression, dementia and aging. *Journal of Nutrition, Health & Aging, 9*(1), 31–38.

Bourre, J. M. (2006). Effects of nutrients (in food) on the structure and function of the nervous system: update on dietary requirements for brain. Part 1: micronutrients. *Journal of Nutrition, Health & Aging, 10*(5), 377–385.

Boyle, P., Diehm, C., & Robertson, C. (2003). Meta-analysis of clinical trials of Cyclo 3 Fort in the treatment of chronic venous insufficiency. *Journal of the International Union of Angiology, 22*(3), 250–262.

Brekhman, I. I., & Dardymov, I. V. (1969). New substances of plant origin which increase non-specific resistance. *Annual Review of Pharmacology, 9*, 419–430.

Brichenko, V. S., & Skorokhodova, T. F. (1987). Herbal adaptogens in rehabilitation of patients with depression. *Clinical and organisational aspects of early manifestations of nervous and mental diseases* (p. 15). Altajskoe Knižnoe Izd: Barnaul.

Brinker, F. (2010). *Herbal contraindications and drug interactions plus herbal adjuncts with medicines* (4th ed.). Sandy, Oregon: Eclectic Medical Publications.

Brooks, J. O., 3rd, Yesavage, J. A., Carta, A., & Bravi, D. (1998). Acetyl L-carnitine slows decline in younger patients with Alzheimer's disease: a reanalysis of a double-blind, placebo-controlled study using the trilinear approach. *International Psychogeriatrics, 10*(2), 193–203.

Brown, R. P., & Gerbarg, P. L. (2004). *The rhodiola revolution: Transform your health with the herbal breakthrough of the 21st century.* Emmaus, PA: Rodale.

Brown, R. P. & Gerbarg, P. L. (2011). Complementary and integrative treatments in brain injury. In J. M. Silver, T. W. McAllister, S. C. Yudofsky (Eds.), *Textbook of traumatic brain injury* (2nd ed., pp. 599–622). Washington, DC: American Psychiatric Press, Inc.

Brown, R. P., Gerbarg, P. L., & Bottiglieri, T. (2000). S-Adenosylmethionine (SAMe) in the clincial practice of psychiatry, neurology, and internal medicine. *Clinical Practice of Alternative Medicine, 1*(4), 230–241.

Brown, R. P., Gerbarg, P. L., & Muskin, P. R. (2009). *How to use herbs, nutrients and yoga in mental health care.* New York: W. W. Norton.

Brown, R. P., Gerbarg, P. L., & Ramazanov, Z. (2002). A phythomedical review of rhodiola rosea. *Herbalgram, 56*, 40–62.

Buscemi, N., Vandermeer, B., Hooton, N., Pandya, R., Tjosvold, L., Hartling, L., et al. (2005). The efficacy and safety of exogenous melatonin for primary sleep disorders. A meta-analysis. *Journal of General Internal Medicine, 20*(12), 1151–1158.

Buydens-Branchey, L., & Branchey, M. (2006). n-3 polyunsaturated fatty acids decrease anxiety feelings in a population of substance abusers. *Journal of Clinical Psychopharmacology, 26*(6), 661–665.

Bystritsky, A., Kerwin, L., & Feusner, J. D. (2008). A pilot study of Rhodiola rosea (Rhodax) for generalized anxiety disorder (GAD). *Journal of Alternative and Complementary Medicine, 14*(2), 175–180.

Cao, L. L., Du, G. H., & Wang, M. W. (2006). The effect of salidroside on cell damage induced by glutamate and intracellular free calcium in PC12 cells. *Journal of Asian Natural Products Research, 8*(1–2), 159–165.

Carani, C., Salvioli, V., Scuteri, A., Borelli, A., Baldini, A., Granata, A. R., & Marrama, P. (1991). [Urological and sexual evaluation of treatment of benign prostatic disease using Pygeum africanum at high doses]. *Archivio italiano di urologia, nefrologia, andrologia : organo ufficiale dell'Associazione per la ricerca in urologia = Urological, nephrological, and andrological sciences, 63*(3), 341–345.

Cardinali, D. P., Furio, A. M., & Brusco, L. I. (2010). Clinical aspects of melatonin intervention in Alzheimer's disease progression. *Current Neuropharmacology, 8*(3), 218–227.

Carrieri, P. B., Indaco, A., & Gentile, S. (1990). S-Adenosylmethionine treatment of depression in patients with Parkinson's disease: a double-blind crossover study versus placebo. *Current Theraputic Research, 48*, 154–160.

Carroll, D., Ring, C., Suter, M., & Willemsen, G. (2000). The effects of an oral multivitamin combination with calcium, magnesium, and zinc on psychological well-being in healthy young male volunteers: a double-blind placebo-controlled trial. *Psychopharmacology (Berl), 150*(2), 220–225.

Cavallini, G., Caracciolo, S., Vitali, G., Modenini, F., & Biagiotti, G. (2004). Carnitine versus androgen administration in the treatment of sexual dysfunction, depressed mood, and fatigue associated with male aging. *Urology, 63*(4), 641–646.

Cavallini, G., Modenini, F., Vitali, G., & Koverech, A. (2005). Acetyl-L-carnitine plus propionyl-L-carnitine improve efficacy of sildenafil in treatment of erectile dysfunction after bilateral nerve-sparing radical retropubic prostatectomy. *Urology, 66*(5), 1080–1085.

Chacon, G. A. (1997). *La importancia de Lepidium peruvianum Chacon ("Maca") en la alimentacion y salud humano y animal 2,000 anos antes y despues de cristo y en el siglo XXI.* Unpublished dissertation. Lima, Peru: Universidad Nacional Mayor de San Marcos.

Chan, A., Paskavitz, J., Remington, R., Rasmussen, S., & Shea, T. B. (2008). Efficacy of a vitamin/nutriceutical formulation for early-stage Alzheimer's disease: a 1-year, open-label pilot study with an 16-month caregiver extension. *American Journal of Alzheimer's Disease and Other Dementias, 23*(6), 571–585.

Chan, A., Remington, R., Kotyla, E., Lepore, A., Zemianek, J., & Shea, T. B. (2010). A vitamin/nutriceutical formulation improves memory and cognitive performance in community-dwelling adults without dementia. *Journal of Nutrition, Health & Aging, 14*(3), 224–230.

Chan, A., Tchantchou, F., Rogers, E. J., & Shea, T. B. (2009). Dietary deficiency increases presenilin expression, gamma-secretase activity, and Abeta levels: potentiation by ApoE genotype and alleviation by S-adenosyl methionine. *Journal of Neurochemistry, 110*(3), 831–836.

Chen, E. Y., & Hui, C. L. (2012). HT1001, A proprietary North American ginseng extract, improves working memory in schizophrenia: A double-blind, placebo-controlled study. *Phytotherapy Research, 26*(8), 1166–1172.

Chen, J., Wollman, Y., Chernichovsky, T., Iaina, A., Sofer, M., & Matzkin, H. (1999). Effect of oral administration of high-dose nitric oxide donor L- arginine in men with organic erectile dysfunction: results of a double- blind, randomized, placebo-controlled study. *British Journal of Urology International, 83*(3), 269–273.

Cho, H. J., & Kim, Y. J. (2009). Efficacy and safety of oral citicoline in acute ischemic stroke: drug surveillance study in 4,191 cases. *Methods and Findings in Experimental and Clinical Pharmacology, 31*(3), 171–176.

Choi, H. K., Seong, D. H., & Rha, K. H. (1995). Clinical efficacy of Korean red ginseng for erectile dysfunction. *International Journal of Impotence Research, 7*(3), 181–186.

Cohen-Mansfield, J., Garfinkel, D., & Lipson, S. (2000). Melatonin for treatment of sundowning in elderly persons with dementia—a preliminary study. *Archives of Gerontology and Geriatrics, 31*, 65–76.

Cohen, M. H., & Schouten, R. (2007). Legal, regulatory, and ethical issues. In J. Lake, & D. Spiegel (Eds.), *Complementary and alternative treatments in mental health care* (pp. 21–33). Washington, DC: American Psychiatric Publishing, Inc.

Coppede, F. (2010). One-carbon metabolism and Alzheimer's disease: focus on epigenetics. *Current Genomics, 11*(4), 246–260.

Cott, J. M., & Fugh-Berman, A. (1998). Is St. John's wort (Hypericum perforatum) an effective antidepressant? *Journal of Nervous and Mental Disease, 186*(8), 500–501.

Crellin, R., Bottiglieri, T., & Reynolds, E. H. (1993). Folates and psychiatric disorders. Clinical potential. *Drugs, 45*(5), 623–636.

Cuzick, J., Sestak, I., Bonanni, B., Costantino, J. P., Cummings, S., DeCensi, A., et al. (2013). Selective oestrogen receptor modulators in prevention of breast cancer: an updated meta-analysis of individual participant data. *Lancet, 25, 381*(9880), 1827–1834.

Daniele, C., Thompson Coon, J., Pittler, M. H., & Ernst, E. (2005). Vitex agnus castus: a systematic review of adverse events. *Drug Safety, 28*(4), 319–332.

Darbinyan, V., Aslanyan, G., Amroyan, E., Gabrielyan, E., Malmstrom, C., & Panossian, A. (2007). Clinical trial of Rhodiola rosea L. extract SHR-5 in the treatment of mild to moderate depression. *Nordic Journal of Psychiatry, 61*(5), 343–348.

Das, Y. T., Bagchi, M., Bagchi, D., & Preuss, H. G. (2004). Safety of 5-hydroxy-L-tryptophan. *Toxicology Letters, 150*(1), 111–122.

Davalos, A., Alvarez-Sabin, J., Castillo, J., Diez-Tejedor, E., Ferro, J., Martinez-Vila, E., et al. (2012). Citicoline in the treatment of acute ischaemic stroke: an international, randomised, multicentre, placebo-controlled study (ICTUS trial). *Lancet, 380*(9839), 349–357.

de Armas, E., Sarracent, Y., Marrero, E., Fernandez, O., & Branford-White, C. (2005). Efficacy of Rhizophora mangle aqueous bark extract (RMABE) in the treatment of aphthous ulcers: a pilot study. *Current Medical Research and Opinion, 21*(11), 1711–1715.

De Deyn, P. P., Reuck, J. D., Deberdt, W., Vlietinck, R., & Orgogozo, J. M. (1997). Treatment of acute ischemic stroke with piracetam.

Members of the Piracetam in Acute Stroke Study (PASS) Group. *Stroke, 28*(12), 2347–2352.

De Souza, M. C., Walker, A. F., Robinson, P. A., & Bolland, K. (2000). A synergistic effect of a daily supplement for 1 month of 200 mg magnesium plus 50 mg vitamin B6 for the relief of anxiety-related premenstrual symptoms: a randomized, double-blind, crossover study. *Journal of Women's Health & Gender Based Medicine, 9*(2), 131–139.

Dean, O., Giorlando, F., & Berk, M. (2011). N-acetylcysteine in psychiatry: current therapeutic evidence and potential mechanisms of action. *Journal of Psychiatry & Neroscience, 36*(2), 78–86.

Deberdt, W. (1994). Interaction between psychological and pharmacological treatment in cognitive impairment. *Life Sciences, 55*(25–26), 2057–2066.

DeKosky, S. T., Williamson, J. D., Fitzpatrick, A. L., Kronmal, R. A., Ives, D. G., Saxton, J. A., et al. (2008). Ginkgo biloba for prevention of dementia: a randomized controlled trial. *Journal of the American Medical Association, 300*(19), 2253–2262.

Dement'eva, L. A., & Iaremenko, K. V. (1987). [Effect of a Rhodiola extract on the tumor process in an experiment]. *Voprosy Onkologii, 33*(7), 57–60.

Denes, L., Szilagyi, G., Gal, A., Bori, Z., & Nagy, Z. (2006). Cytoprotective effect of two synthetic enhancer substances, (-)-BPAP and (-)-deprenyl, on human brain capillary endothelial cells and rat PC12 cells. *Life Sciences, 79*(11), 1034–1039.

Denzler, K. L., Waters, R., Jacobs, B. L., Rochon, Y., & Langland, J. O. (2010). Regulation of inflammatory gene expression in PBMCs by immunostimulatory botanicals. *PLoS One, 5*(9), e12561.

Di Donato, S., Frerman, F. E., Rimoldi, M., Rinaldo, P., Taroni, F., & Wiesmann, U. N. (1986). Systemic carnitine deficiency due to lack of electron transfer flavoprotein:ubiquinone oxidoreductase. *Neurology, 36*(7), 957–963.

Di Rocco, A., Rogers, J. D., Brown, R., Werner, P., & Bottiglieri, T. (2000). S-adenosyl-l-methionine improves depression in patients with Parkinson's disease in an open label clinical trial. *Journal of the Movement Disorder Society, 15*(6), 1225–1229.

Diamond, B. J., Bailey, M. R. (2013). Ginkgo biloba: indications, mechanisms, and safety. *Psychiatric Clinics of North America, 36*(1), 73–84.

Diamond, B. J., Shiflett, S. C., Feiwel, N., Matheis, R. J., Noskin, O., Richards, J. A., & Schoenberger, N. E. (2000). Ginkgo biloba extract: mechanisms and clinical indications. *Archives of Physical Medicine and Rehabilitation, 81*(5), 668–678.

Dixon, C. E., Ma, X., &Marion, D. W. (1997). Effects of CDP-choline treatment on neurobehavioral deficits after TBI and on hippocampal and neocortical acetylcholine release. *Journal of Neurotrauma, 14*(3), 161–169.

Dodin, S., Lemay, A., Jacques, H., Legare, F., Forest, J. C., & Masse, B. (2005). The effects of flaxseed dietary supplement on lipid profile, bone mineral density, and symptoms in menopausal women: a randomized, double-blind, wheat germ placebo-controlled clinical trial. *Journal of Clinical Endocrinology and Metabolism, 90*(3), 1390–1397.

Donovan, J. L., DeVane, C. L., Chavin, K. D., Wang, J. S., Gibson, B. B., Gefroh, H. A., & Markowitz, J. S. (2004). Multiple night-time doses of valerian (Valeriana officinalis) had minimal effects on CYP3A4 activity and no effect on CYP2D6 activity in healthy volunteers. *Drug Metabolism and Disposition, 32*(12), 1333–1336.

Dording, C. M., Fisher, L., Papakostas, G., Farabaugh, A., Sonawalla, S., Fava, M., & Mischoulon, D. (2008). A double-blind, randomized, pilot dose-finding study of maca root (*L. meyenii*) for the management of SSRI-induced sexual dysfunction. *CNS Neuroscience & Therapeutics, 14*(3), 182–191.

Dorofeev, B. F., & Kholodov, L. E. (1991). [Pikamilon pharmacokinetics in animals]. *Farmakologiia I Toksikologiia, 54*(2), 66–69.

Dowling, G. A., Mastick, J., Colling, E., Carter, J. H., Singer, C. M., & Aminoff, M. J. (2005). Melatonin for sleep disturbances in Parkinson's disease. *Sleep Medicine, 6*(5), 459–466.

Drieu, K., Vranckx, R., Benassayad, C., Haourigi, M., Hassid, J., Yoa, R. G., et al. (2000). Effect of the extract of Ginkgo biloba (EGb 761) on the circulating and cellular profiles of polyunsaturated fatty acids: correlation with the anti-oxidant properties of the extract.

Prostaglandins, Leukotrienes, and Essential Fatty Acids, 63(5), 293–300.

Dutov, A. A., Gal'tvanitsa, G. A., Volkova, V. A., Sukhanova, O. N., Lavrishcheva, T. G., & Petrov, A. P. (1991). [Cavinton in the prevention of the convulsive syndrome in children after birth injury]. *Zhurnal Nevropatologii I Psikhiatrii Imeni S.S. Korsakova, 91*(8), 21–22.

Dwivedi, C., Natarajan, K., & Matthees, D. P. (2005). Chemopreventive effects of dietary flaxseed oil on colon tumor development. *Nutrition and Cancer, 51*(1), 52–58.

Eagon, P. K., Elm, M. S., Gerberg, P. L., Brown, R. P., Check J. J., Diorio, G. J., & Houghton, F. Jr. (2004). Evaluation of the medicinal botanical rhodiola rosea for estrogenicity [Abstract #2878]. *Proceedings of the American Association for Cancer Research, 2004*(1), 663.

Ebadi, M., Brown-Borg, H., Ren, J., Sharma, S., Shavali, S., El ReFaey, H., & Carlson, E. C. (2006). Therapeutic efficacy of selegiline in neurodegenerative disorders and neurological diseases. *Current Drug Targets, 7*(11), 1513–1529.

Elens, L., Nieuweboer, A., Clarke, S. J., Charles, K. A., de Graan, A. J., Haufroid, V., et al. (2013). CYP3A4 intron 6 C>T SNP (CYP3A4*22) encodes lower CYP3A4 activity in cancer patients, as measured with probes midazolam and erythromycin. *Pharmacogenomics, 14*(2), 137–149.

Elsabagh, S., Hartley, D. E., & File, S. E. (2005). Limited cognitive benefits in Stage +2 postmenopausal women after 6 weeks of treatment with Ginkgo biloba. *Journal of Psychopharmacology, 19*(2), 173–181.

Enderby, P., Broeckx, J., Hospers, W., Schildermans, F., & Deberdt, W. (1994). Effect of piracetam on recovery and rehabilitation after stroke: a double-blind, placebo-controlled study. *Clinical Neuropharmacology, 17*(4), 320–331.

Engelmann, U., Walther, C., Bondarenko, B., Funk, P., & Schlafke, S. (2006). Efficacy and safety of a combination of sabal and urtica extract in lower urinary tract symptoms. A randomized, double-blind study versus tamsulosin. *Arzneimittel-Forschung, 56*(3), 222–229.

Ernst, E., & Pittler, M. H. (1998). Yohimbine for erectile dysfunction: a systematic review and meta- analysis of randomized clinical trials. *Journal of Urology, 159*(2), 433–436.

Evans, M., Elliott, J. G., Sharma, P., Berman, R., & Guthrie, N. (2011). The effect of synthetic genistein on menopause symptom management in healthy postmenopausal women: a multi-center, randomized, placebo-controlled study. *Maturitas, 68*(2), 189–196.

Eyles, D. W., Burne, T. H., & McGrath, J. J. (2012). Vitamin D, effects on brain development, adult brain function and the links between low levels of vitamin D and neuropsychiatric disease. *Frontiers in Neuroendocrinology, 34*(1), 47–64.

Fackleman, K. (1998). Medicine for menopause. *Science News, 153*, 392–393.

Federation of State Medical Boards. (2007). *Model guidelines for physician use of complementary and alternative therapies in medical practice.* Retrieved from www.fsmb.org/pdf/2002_grpol_Complementary_ Alternative_Terapies.pdf.

Feldman, H. A., Goldstein, I., Hatzichristou, D. G., Krane, R. J., & McKinlay, J. B. (1994). Impotence and its medical and psychosocial correlates: results of the Massachusetts Male Aging Study. *Journal of Urology, 151*(1), 54–61.

Fernandez-San-Martin, M. I., Masa-Font, R., Palacios-Soler, L., Sancho-Gomez, P., Calbo-Caldentey, C., & Flores-Mateo, G. (2010). Effectiveness of valerian on insomnia: a meta-analysis of randomized placebo-controlled trials [meta-analysis]. *Sleep Medicine, 11*(6), 505–511.

Fioravanti, M., & Yanagi, M. (2005). Cytidinediphosphocholine (CDP-choline) for cognitive and behavioural disturbances associated with chronic cerebral disorders in the elderly. *Cochrane Database of Systematic Reviews, (2),* CD000269.

Fischer, H. D., Schmidt, J., & Wustmann, C. (1984). On some mechanisms of antihypoxic actions of nootropic drugs. *Biomedica Biochimica Acta, 43*(4), 541–543.

Foster, S. (1999). Black cohosh *cimicifugae racemosa*: a literature review. *Herbalgram, 45*, 36–49.

Frangou, S., Lewis, M., & McCrone, P. (2006). Efficacy of ethyl-eicosapentaenoic acid in bipolar depression: randomised double-blind placebo-controlled study. *British Journal of Psychiatry, 188*, 46–50.

Freund-Levi, Y., Eriksdotter-Jonhagen, M., Cederholm, T., Basun, H., Faxen-Irving, G., Garlind, A., et al. (2006). Omega-3 fatty acid treatment in 174 patients with mild to moderate Alzheimer disease: OmegAD study: a randomized double-blind trial. *Archives of Neurology, 63*(10), 1402–1408.

Frezza, M., Centini, G., Cammareri, G., Le Grazie, C., & Di Padova, C. (1990). S-adenosylmethionine for the treatment of intrahepatic cholestasis of pregnancy. Results of a controlled clinical trial. *Hepatogastroenterology, 37*(Suppl 2), 122–125.

Friedel, H. A., Goa, K. L., & Benfield, P. (1989). S-adenosyl-L-methionine. A review of its pharmacological properties and therapeutic potential in liver dysfunction and affective disorders in relation to its physiological role in cell metabolism. *Drugs, 38*(3), 389–416.

Froestl, W., Muhs, A., & Pfeifer, A. (2012). Cognitive enhancers (nootropics). Part 1: drugs interacting with receptors. *Journal of Alzheimer's Disease, 32*(4), 793–887.

Froestl, W., Muhs, A., & Pfeifer, A. (2013). Cognitive enhancers (nootropics). Part 2: drugs interacting with enzymes. *Journal of Alzheimer's Disease, 33*(3), 547–658.

Froestl, W., Pfeifer, A., & Muhs, A. (2012). Cognitive Enhancers (Nootropics). Part 3: Drugs Interacting with Targets other than Receptors or Enzymes. Disease-modifying Drugs. *Journal of Alzheimer's Disease, 34*(1), 1–114.

Furmanowa, M., Skopinska-Rozewska, E., Rogala, E., & Malgorzata, H. (1998). Rhodiola rosea in vitro culture—phytochemical analysis and antioxidant action. *Acta Societis Botanicorum Poloniae, 76*(1), 69–73.

Fux, M., Benjamin, J., & Nemets, B. (2004). A placebo-controlled cross-over trial of adjunctive EPA in OCD. *Journal of Psychiatric Research, 38*(3), 323–325.

Gatti, D., Rossini, M., Sblendorio, I., & Lello, S. (2013). Pharmacokinetic evaluation of bazedoxifene for the treatment of osteoporosis. *Expert Opinion on Drug Metabolism & Toxicology, 9*(7), 883–892.

Geng, J., Dong, J., Ni, H., Lee, M. S., Wu, T., Jiang, K., et al. (2010). Ginseng for cognition. *Cochrane Database of Systematic Reviews, (12),* CD007769.

Gerasimova, H. D. (1970). Effect of Rhodiola rosea extract on ovarian functional activity. *Proceedings of Scientific Conference on Endocrinology and Gynecology,* 46–48.

Gerberg, P. L. & Brown, R. P. (2013). Phytomedicines for Prevention and Treatment of Mental Health Disorders. In Complementary and Integrative Therapies for Psychiatric Disorders, Edited by P. R. Muskin, P. L. Gerberg, and R. P. Brown. *Psychiatric Clinics of North America, 36*(1), 37–47.

Gerberg, P. L., Muskin, P. R., Bottiglieri, T., Brown, R. P. (2014). Failed studies should not be used to malign good treatments. Letter to the editor. *Journal of Clinical Psychiatry, 75*(11), e1328.

Gijsman, H. J., van Gerven, J. M., de Kam, M. L., Schoemaker, R. C., Pieters, M. S., Weemaes, M., et al. (2002). Placebo-controlled comparison of three dose-regimens of 5-hydroxytryptophan challenge test in healthy volunteers. *Journal of Clinical Psychopharmacology, 22*(2), 183–189.

Gillis, J. C., Benefield, P., & McTavish, D. (1994). Idebenone. A review of its pharmacodynamic and pharmacokinetic properties, and therapeutic use in age-related cognitive disorders. *Drugs & Aging, 5*(2), 133–152.

Gonzales, G. F. (2012). Ethnobiology and ethnopharmacology of lepidium meyenii (Maca), a plant from the Peruvian Highlands. *Evidence-Based Complementary and Alternative Medicine, 2012*, 193496.

Gonzales, G. F., Cordova, A., Gonzales, C., Chung, A., Vega, K., & Villena, A. (2001). Lepidium meyenii (Maca) improved semen parameters in adult men. *Asian Journal of Andrology, 3*(4), 301–303.

Gonzales, G. F., Cordova, A., Vega, K., Chung, A., Villena, A., Gonez, C., & Castillo, S. (2002). Effect of Lepidium meyenii (MACA) on sexual desire and its absent relationship with serum testosterone levels in adult healthy men. *Andrologia, 34*(6), 367–372.

Gout, B., Bourges, C., & Paineau-Dubreuil, S. (2010). Satiereal, a Crocus sativus L extract, reduces snacking and increases satiety in a randomized placebo-controlled study of mildly overweight, healthy women. *Nutrition Research, 30*(5), 305–313.

Gracious, B. L., Finucane, T. L., Freidman-Campbell, M., Messing, S., & Parkhurst, M. M. (2012). Vitamin D deficiency and psychotic features in mentally ill adolescents: A cross-sectional study. *BMC Psychiatry, 12*(1), 38.

Grassetto, M., & Varatto, A. (1994). Primary Fibromyalgia is responsive to S-adenosyl-L-methionine. *Current Theraputic Research, 55,* 797–806.

Green, P., Hermesh, H., Monselise, A., Marom, S., Presburger, G., & Weizman, A. (2006). Red cell membrane omega-3 fatty acids are decreased in nondepressed patients with social anxiety disorder. *Journal of the European College of Neuropsychopharmacology, 16*(2), 107–113.

Grossmann, M., & Schmidramsl, H. (2000). An extract of Petasitis hybridus is effective in the prophylaxis of migraine. *International Journal of Clinical Pharmacology and Therapeutics, 38*(9), 430–435.

Grube, B., Walper, A., & Wheatley, D. (1999). St. John's Wort extract efficacy for menopausal symptoms of psychological origin. *Advance in Therapy, 16*(4), 177–186.

Guerrera, M. P., Volpe, S. L., & Mao, J. J. (2009). Therapeutic uses of magnesium. [Review]. *American Family Physician, 80*(2), 157–162.

Guerrero-Bosagna, C. M., & Skinner, M. K. (2014). Environmental epigenetics and phytoestrogen/phytochemical exposures. *Journal of Steroid Biochemistry and Molecular Biology, 139,* 270–276.

Gurley, B. J., Gardner, S. F., Hubbard, M. A., Williams, D. K., Gentry, W. B., Khan, I. A., & Shah, A. (2005). In vivo effects of goldenseal, kava kava, black cohosh, and valerian on human cytochrome P450 1A2, 2D6, 2E1, and 3A4/5 phenotypes. *Clinical Pharmacology and Therapeutics, 77*(5), 415–426.

Gurnell, E. M., & Chatterjee, V. K. (2001). Dehydroepiandrosterone replacement therapy. *European Journal of Endocrinology, 145*(2), 103–106.

Hackbert, L., & Heiman, J. R. (2002). Acute dehydroepiandrosterone (DHEA) effects on sexual arousal in postmenopausal women. *Journal of Women's Health & Gender Based Medicine, 11*(2), 155–162.

Haimov, I., Lavie, P., Laudon, M., Herer, P., Vigder, C., & Zisapel, N. (1995). Melatonin replacement therapy of elderly insomniacs. *Sleep, 18*(7), 598–603.

Hallahan, B., Hibbeln, J. R., Davis, J. M., & Garland, M. R. (2007). Omega-3 fatty acid supplementation in patients with recurrent self-harm. Single-centre double-blind randomised controlled trial. *British Journal of Psychiatry, 190,* 118–122.

Hansgen, K. D., Vesper, J., & Ploch, M. (1994). Multicenter double-blind study examining the antidepressant effectiveness of the hypericum extract LI 160. *Journal of Geriatric Psychiatry and Neurology, 7*(Suppl 1), S15–S18.

Haorah, J., Floreani, N. A., Knipe, B., & Persidsky, Y. (2011). Stabilization of superoxide dismutase by acetyl-l-carnitine in human brain endothelium during alcohol exposure: novel protective approach. *Free Radical Biology and Medicine, 51*(8), 1601–1609.

Harrington, M. E. (2012). Neurobiological studies of fatigue. *Progress in Neurobiology, 99*(2), 93–105.

Hartley, D. E., Elsabagh, S., & File, S. E. (2004). Gincosan (a combination of Ginkgo biloba and Panax ginseng): the effects on mood and cognition of 6 and 12 weeks' treatment in post-menopausal women. *Nutritional Neuroscience, 7*(5–6), 325–333.

Harvey, B. H., Joubert, C., du Preez, J. L., & Berk, M. (2007). Effect of chronic n-acetyl cysteine administration on oxidative status in the presence and absence of induced oxidative stress in rat striatum. *Neurochemical Research, 33*(3), 508–517.

Hassing, L., Wahlin, A., Winblad, B., & Backman, L. (1999). Further evidence on the effects of vitamin B12 and folate levels on episodic memory functioning: a population-based study of healthy very old adults. *Biological Psychiatry, 45*(11), 1472–1480.

Hellum, B. H., Tosse, A., Hoybakk, K., Thomsen, M., Rohloff, J., & Georg Nilsen, O. (2010). Potent in vitro inhibition of CYP3A4 and P-glycoprotein by Rhodiola rosea. *Planta Medica, 76*(4), 331–338.

Hendrix, S. L., & McNeeley, S. G. (2001). Effect of selective estrogen receptor modulators on reproductive tissues other than endometrium. *Annals of the New York Academy of Sciences, 949,* 243–250.

Hill-House, B. J., Ming, D. S., French, C. J., & Towers, N. G. H. (2004). Acetylcholine esterase inhibitors in rhodiolarosea. *Pharmaceutical Biology, 42*(1), 68–72.

Hirashima, F., Parow, A. M., Stoll, A. L., Demopulos, C. M., Damico, K. E., Rohan, M. L., et al. (2004). Omega-3 fatty acid treatment and T(2) whole brain relaxation times in bipolar disorder. *American Journal of Psychiatry, 161*(10), 1922–1924.

Hirata, J. D., Swiersz, L. M., Zell, B., Small, R., & Ettinger, B. (1997). Does dong quai have estrogenic effects in postmenopausal women? A double-blind placebo controlled trial. *Fertility and Sterility, 68,* 981–986.

Ho, S. H., Singh, M., Holloway, A. C., & Crankshaw, D. J. (2011). The effects of commercial preparations of herbal supplements commonly used by women on the biotransformation of fluorogenic substrates by human cytochromes P450. *Phytotherapy Research, 25*(7), 983–989.

Hoang, M. T., Defina, L. F., Willis, B. L., Leonard, D. S., Weiner, M. F., & Brown, E. S. (2011). Association between low serum 25-hydroxyvitamin D and depression in a large sample of healthy adults: the CooperCenter longitudinal study. *Mayo Clinic Proceedings, 86*(11), 1050–1055.

Howes, M. J., & Perry, E. (2011). The role of phytochemicals in the treatment and prevention of dementia. *Drugs & Aging, 28*(6), 439–468.

Hung, T. M., Na, M., Min, B. S., Ngoc, T. M., Lee, I., Zhang, X., & Bae, K. (2007). Acetylcholinesterase inhibitory effect of lignans isolated from Schizandra chinensis. *Archives of Pharmacal Research, 30*(6), 685–690.

Hurtado, O., Moro, M. A., Cardenas, A., Sanchez, V., Fernandez-Tome, P., Leza, J. C., et al. (2005). Neuroprotection afforded by prior citicoline administration in experimental brain ischemia: effects on glutamate transport. *Neurobiology of Disease, 18*(2), 336–345.

Ianiello, A., Ostuni, P. A., Sfriso, P., Menenghetti, L., Zennaro, A., & Silvan Todesco, S. (1994). S-adenosyl-L-methionine in Sjogren's Syndrome and fibromyalgia. *Current Theraputic Research, 55,* 699–705.

Ihl, R. (2012). Gingko biloba extract EGb 761(R): clinical data in dementia. [Review]. *International Psychogeriatrics, 24*(Suppl 1), S35–40.

Ihl, R., Tribanek, M., Bachinskaya, N., & Group, G. S. (2012). Efficacy and tolerability of a once daily formulation of *Ginkgo biloba* extract EGb 761(R) in Alzheimer's disease and vascular dementia: results from a randomised controlled trial. *Pharmacopsychiatry, 45*(2), 41–46.

Iovieno, N. & Papakostas, G. I. (2012). Correlation between different levels of placebo response rate and clinical outcome in major depressive disorder: a meta-analysis. *Journal of Clinical Psychiatry, 73*(10), 1300–1306.

Iruretagoyena, M. I., Tobar, J. A., Gonzalez, P. A., Sepulveda, S. E., Figueroa, C. A., Burgos, R. A., et al. (2005). Andrographolide interferes with T cell activation and reduces experimental autoimmune encephalomyelitis in the mouse. *Journal of Pharmacology and Experimental Therapeutics, 312*(1), 366–372.

Ito, T. Y., Polan, M. L., Whipple, B., & Trant, A. S. (2006). The enhancement of female sexual function with ArginMax, a nutritional supplement, among women differing in menopausal status. *Journal of Sex and Marital Therapy, 32*(5), 369–378.

Ito, T. Y., Trant, A. S., & Polan, M. L. (2001). A double-blind placebo-controlled study of ArginMax, a nutritional supplement for enhancement of female sexual function. *Journal of Sex and Marital Therapy, 27*(5), 541–549.

Jacobs, B. P., Bent, S., Tice, J. A., Blackwell, T., & Cummings, S. R. (2005). An internet-based randomized, placebo-controlled trial of kava and valerian for anxiety and insomnia. *Medicine (Baltimore)*, 84(4), 197–207.

Jellin, J. M., (Ed.); Therapeutic Research Faculty. (2010). *Pharmacist's letter/prescriber's letter natural medicines comprehensive database.* (12th ed.). Stockton, CA: Pharmacist's Letter.

Jezova, D., A. Makatsori, M. Smriga, Y. Morinaga, & Duncko, R. (2005). Subchronic treatment with amino acid mixture of L-lysine and L-arginine modifies neuroendocrine activation during psychosocial stress in subjects with high trait anxiety. *Nutritional Neuroscience*, 8(3), 155–160.

Jiang, W., Wang, X., Xu, X., & Kong, L. (2010). Effect of Schisandra sphenanthera extract on the concentration of tacrolimus in the blood of liver transplant patients. *International Journal of Clinical Pharmacology and Therapeutics*, 48(3), 224–229.

Jung, C. H., Jung, H., Shin, Y. C., Park, J. H., Jun, C. Y., Kim, H. M., et al. (2007). Eleutherococcus senticosus extract attenuates LPS-induced iNOS expression through the inhibition of Akt and JNK pathways in murine macrophage. *Journal of Ethnopharmacology*, 113(1), 183–187.

Kahn, E. (Ed.). (2004). *"Ha" breathe "Ou ka Leo O ka Pu" the voice of the shell sounds.* Hawaii: Zen Care.

Kang, B. J., Lee, S. J., Kim, M. D., & Cho, M. J. (2002). A placebo-controlled, double-blind trial of Ginkgo biloba for antidepressant-induced sexual dysfunction. *Human Psychopharmacology*, 17(6), 279–284.

Kang, S. Y., Kim, S. H., Schini, V. B., & Kim, N. D. (1995). Dietary ginsenosides improve endothelium-dependent relaxation in the thoracic aorta of hypercholesterolemic rabbit. *General Pharmacology*, 26(3), 483–487.

Kashani, L., Raisi, F., Saroukhani, S., Sohrabi, H., Modabbernia, A., Nasehi, A. A., et al. (2012). Saffron for treatment of fluoxetine-induced sexual dysfunction in women: randomized double-blind placebo-controlled study. *Human Psychopharmacology*, 28(1), 54–60.

Kawate, H., & Takayanagi, R. (2011). Efficacy and safety of bazedoxifene for postmenopausal osteoporosis. *Clinical Interventions in Aging*, 6, 151–60.

Kayumov, L., Brown, G., Jindal, R., Buttoo, K., & Shapiro, C. M. (2001). A randomized, double-blind, placebo-controlled crossover study of the effect of exogenous melatonin on delayed sleep phase syndrome. *Psychosomatic Medicine*, 63(1), 40–48.

Keinan-Boker, L., van Der Schouw, Y. T., Grobbee, D. E., & Peeters, P. H. (2004). Dietary phytoestrogens and breast cancer risk. *American Journal of Clinical Nutrition*, 79(2), 282–288.

Kennedy, D. A., & Seely, D. (2010). Clinically based evidence of drug-herb interactions: a systematic review. [Review]. *Expert Opinion on Drug Safety*, 9(1), 79–124.

Kennedy, D. O., Little, W., & Scholey, A. B. (2004). Attenuation of laboratory-induced stress in humans after acute administration of *Melissa officinalis* (lemon balm). *Psychosomatic Medicine*, 66(4), 607–613.

Kennedy, D. O., Wake, G., Savelev, S., Tildesley, N. T., Perry, E. K., Wesnes, K. A., & Scholey, A. B. (2003). Modulation of mood and cognitive performance following acute administration of single doses of *Melissa officinalis* (lemon balm) with human CNS nicotinic and muscarinic receptor-binding properties. *Neuropsychopharmacology*, 28(10), 1871–1881.

Kessler, J., Thiel, A., Karbe, H., & Heiss, W. D. (2000). Piracetam improves activated blood flow and facilitates rehabilitation of post-stroke aphasic patients. *Stroke*, 31(9), 2112–2116.

Kharbanda, K. K., Rogers, D. D. 2nd, Mailliard, M. E., Siford, G. L., Barak, A. J., Beckenhauer, H. C., et al. (2005). A comparison of the effects of betaine and S-adenosylmethionine on ethanol-induced changes in methionine metabolism and steatosis in rat hepatocytes. *Journal of Nutrition*, 135(3), 519–524.

Kim, T. H., Jeon, S. H., Hahn, E. J., Paek, K. Y., Park, J. K., Youn, N. Y., & Lee, H. L. (2009). Effects of tissue-cultured mountain ginseng (Panax ginseng CA Meyer) extract on male patients with erectile dysfunction. *Asian Journal of Andrology*, 11(3), 356–361.

Kimura, K., Ozeki, M., Juneja, L. R., & Ohira, H. (2007). L-Theanine reduces psychological and physiological stress responses. *Biological Psychology*, 74(1), 39–45.

Klein, E. A., Thompson, I. M., Jr., Tangen, C. M., Crowley, J. J., Lucia, M. S., Goodman, P. J., et al. (2011). Vitamin E and the risk of prostate cancer: the Selenium and Vitamin E Cancer Prevention Trial (SELECT). *Journal of the American Medical Association*, 306(14), 1549–1556.

Knoll, J. (2000). (-)Deprenyl (Selegiline): past, present and future. *Neurobiology*, 8(2), 179–199.

Knoll, J. (2003). Enhancer regulation/endogenous and synthetic enhancer compounds: a neurochemical concept of the innate and acquired drives. *Neurochemical Research*, 28(8), 1275–1297.

Knuppel, L., & Linde, K. (2004). Adverse effects of St. John's wort: a systematic review. *Journal of Clinical Psychiatry*, 65(11), 1470–1479.

Kobak, K. A., Taylor, L. V., Bystritsky, A., Kohlenberg, C. J., Greist, J. H., Tucker, P., et al. (2005). St John's wort versus placebo in obsessive-compulsive disorder: results from a double-blind study. *International Clinical Psychopharmacology*, 20(6), 299–304.

Kobak, K. A., Taylor, L. V., Warner, G., & Futterer, R. (2005). St. John's wort versus placebo in social phobia: results from a placebo-controlled pilot study. *Journal of Clinical Psychopharmacology*, 25(1), 51–58.

Kormosh, N., Laktionov, K., & Antoshechkina, M. (2006). Effect of a combination of extract from several plants on cell-mediated and humoral immunity of patients with advanced ovarian cancer. *Phytotherapy Research*, 20(5), 424–425.

Kraft, M., Spahn, T. W., Menzel, J., Senninger, N., Dietl, K. H., Herbst, H., et al. (2001). [Fulminant liver failure after administration of the herbal antidepressant Kava-Kava]. *Deutsche Medizinische Wochenschrift*, 126(36), 970–972.

Kruglikova, R. P. (1997). How and why picamilon works. *Life Extension*, (Jul), 34–38.

Krystal. A. D., & Ressler, I. (2001). The use of valerian in neuropsychiatry. *CNS Spectrums*, 6(10), 841–847.

Kumar, P. N. S., Andrade, C., Bhakta, S. G., & Singh, N. M. (2007). Melatonin in schizophrenic outpatients with insomnia: a double-blind, placebo-controlled study. *Journal of Clinical Psychiatry*, 68, 237–241.

Kunz, D., & Bes, F. (1997). Melatonin effects in a patient with severe REM sleep behavior disorder: case report and theoretical considerations. *Neuropsychobiology*, 36(4), 211–214.

Kurkin, V. A., & Zapesochnaya, G. G. (1986a). Chemical composition and pharmacological properties of *Rhodiola rosea*. *Chemical and Pharmaceutical Journal (Moscow)*, 20(10), 1231–1244.

Kurkin, V. A., & Zapesochnaya, G. G. (1986b). Khimicheskiy sostav i farmakologicheskiye svoystva rasteniy roda Rhodiola. Obzor. (Chemical composition and pharmacological properties of *Rhodiola rosea*). *Khim-Farm Zh (Chemical and Pharmaceutical Journal Moscow)*, 20(10), 1231–1244.

Kyle, D. J., & Arterburn, L. M. (1998). Single cell oil sources of docosahexaenoic acid: clinical studies. *World Review of Nutrition and Dietetics*, 83, 116–131.

Labrie, F., Archer, D., Bouchard, C., Fortier, M., Cusan, L., Gomez, J. L., et al. (2009). Serum steroid levels during 12-week intravaginal dehydroepiandrosterone administration. *Menopause*, 16(5), 897–906.

Lagari, V. S., & Levis, S. (2012). Phytoestrogens for menopausal bone loss and climacteric symptoms. *Journal of Steroid Biochemistry and Molecular Biology*, 139, 294–301.

Lakhan, S. E., & Vieira, K. F. (2010). Nutritional and herbal supplements for anxiety and anxiety-related disorders: a systematic review. *Nutrition Journal*, 9, 42.

Lange, H., Suryapranata, H., De Luca, G., Borner, C., Dille, J., Kallmayer, K., et al. (2004). Folate therapy and in-stent restenosis after coronary stenting. *New England Journal of Medicine*, 350(26), 2673–2681.

Lebret, T., Herve, J. M., Gorny, P., Worcel, M., & Botto, H. (2002). Efficacy and safety of a novel combination of L-arginine glutamate and yohimbine hydrochloride: a new oral therapy for erectile dysfunction. *European Urology*, 41(6), 608–613; discussion 613.

Leclercq, G., & Jacquot, Y. (2014). Interactions of isoflavones and other plant derived estrogens with estrogen receptors for prevention and treatment of breast cancer—considerations concerning related efficacy and safety. *Journal of Steroid Biochemistry and Molecular Biology, 139*, 237–244.

Ledda, A., Belcaro, G., Cesarone, M. R., Dugall, M., & Schonlau, F. (2010). Investigation of a complex plant extract for mild to moderate erectile dysfunction in a randomized, double-blind, placebo-controlled, parallel-arm study. *BJU International, 106*(7), 1030–1033.

Lee, L. S., Wise, S. D., Chan, C., Parsons, T. L., Flexner, C., & Lietman, P. S. (2008). Possible differential induction of phase 2 enzyme and antioxidant pathways by american ginseng, *Panax quinquefolius*. *Journal of Clinical Pharmacology, 48*(5), 599–609.

Lee, M. S., Shin, B. C., Yang, E. J., Lim, H. J., & Ernst, E. (2011). Maca (*Lepidium meyenii*) for treatment of menopausal symptoms: A systematic review. *Maturitas, 70*(3), 227–233.

Lee, S. T., Chu, K., Sim, J. Y., Heo, J. H., & Kim, M. (2008). *Panax ginseng* enhances cognitive performance in Alzheimer disease. *Alzheimer Disease and Associated Disorders, 22*(3), 222–226.

Leon-Jimenez, C., Chiquete, E., Cantu, C., Miramontes-Saldana, M. J., Andrade-Ramos, M. A., & Ruiz-Sandoval, J. L. (2010). Citicoline for acute ischemic stroke in Mexican hospitals: a retrospective postmarketing analysis. *Methods and Findings in Experimental and Clinical Pharmacology, 32*(5), 325–330.

Lerner, V., Bergman, J., Statsenko, N., & Miodownik, C. (2004). Vitamin B6 treatment in acute neuroleptic-induced akathisia: a randomized, double-blind, placebo-controlled study. *Journal of Clinical Psychiatry, 65*(11), 1550–1554.

Lerner, V., Miodownik, C., Kaptsan, A., Cohen, H., Matar, M., Loewenthal, U., & Kotler, M. (2001). Vitamin B(6) in the treatment of tardive dyskinesia: a double-blind, placebo-controlled, crossover study. *American Journal of Psychiatry, 158*(9), 1511–1514.

Levine, J., Stahl, Z., Sela, B. A., Ruderman, V., Shumaico, O., Babushkin, I., et al. (2006). Homocysteine-reducing strategies improve symptoms in chronic schizophrenic patients with hyperhomocysteinemia. *Biological Psychiatry, 60*(3), 265–269.

Levine, J. P. (2011). Treating menopausal symptoms with a tissue-selective estrogen complex. Gender Medicine, 8(2), 57–68.

Levis, S., Strickman-Stein, N., Ganjei-Azar, P., Xu, P., Doerge, D. R., & Krischer, J. (2011). Soy isoflavones in the prevention of menopausal bone loss and menopausal symptoms: a randomized, double-blind trial. *Archives of Internal Medicine, 171*(15), 1363–1369.

Liao, Y., Wang, R., & Tang, X. C. (2004). Centrophenoxine improves chronic cerebral ischemia induced cognitive deficit and neuronal degeneration in rats. *Acta Pharmacologica Sinica, 25*(12), 1590–1596.

Lichius, J. J., & Muth, C. (1997). The inhibiting effects of Urtica dioica root extracts on experimentally induced prostatic hyperplasia in the mouse. *Planta Medica, 63*(4), 307–310.

Lieber, C. S. (1999). Role of S-adenosyl-L-methionine in the treatment of liver diseases. *Journal of Hepatology, 30*(6), 1155–1159.

Lieber, C. S. (2001). Liver diseases by alcohol and hepatitis C: early detection and new insights in pathogenesis lead to improved treatment. *American Journal of Addictions, 10*(Suppl), 29–50.

Lieber, C. S. (2005). Pathogenesis and treatment of alcoholic liver disease: progress over the last 50 years. *Rocz Roczniki Akademii Medycznej w Bialymstoku, 50*, 7–20.

Lieberman, S. (1998). A review of the effectiveness of Cimicifuga racemosa (black cohosh) for the symptoms of menopause. *Journal of Women's Health, 7*(5), 525–529.

Lin, P. Y., Mischoulon, D., Freeman, M. P., Matsuoka, Y., Hibbeln, J., Belmaker, R. H., & Su, K. P. (2012). Are omega-3 fatty acids antidepressants or just mood-improving agents? The effect depends upon diagnosis, supplement preparation, and severity of depression. *Molecular Psychiatry, 17*(12), 1161–1163; author reply 1163–1167.

Linde, K., Ramirez, G., Mulrow, C. D., Pauls, A., Weidenhammer, W., & Melchart, D. (1996). St John's wort for depression—an overview and meta-analysis of randomised clinical trials. *British Medical Journal, 313*(7052), 253–258.

Lolic, M. M., Fiskum, G., & Rosenthal, R. E. (1997). Neuroprotective effects of acetyl-L-carnitine after stroke in rats. *Annals of Emergency Medicine, 29*(6), 758–765.

Long, S. D., & Pekala, P. H. (1996). Regulation of GLUT4 gene expression by arachidonic acid. Evidence for multiple pathways, one of which requires oxidation to prostaglandin E2. *Journal of Biological Chemistry, 271*(2), 1138–1144.

Lopresti, A. L., Maes, M., Maker, G. L., Hood, S. D., Drummond, P. D. (2014). Curcumin for the treatment of major depression: A randomised, double-blind, placebo controlled study. *Journal of Affecctive Disorders, 167*, 368–375.

Lu, K., Gray, M. A., Oliver, C., Liley, D. T., Harrison, B. J., Bartholomeusz, C. F., et al. (2004). The acute effects of L-theanine in comparison with alprazolam on anticipatory anxiety in humans. *Human Psychopharmacology, 19*(7), 457–465.

MacKay, D. (2001). Hemorrhoids and varicose veins: a review of treatment options. [Review]. *Alternative Medicine Review, 6*(2), 126–140.

Malaguarnera, M. (2012). Carnitine derivatives: clinical usefulness. *Current Opinion in Gastroenterology, 28*(2), 166–176.

Malati, C. Y., Robertson, S. M., Hunt, J. D., Chairez, C., Alfaro, R. M., Kovacs, J. A., & Penzak, S. R. (2012). Influence of *Panax ginseng* on cytochrome P450 (CYP)3A and P-glycoprotein (P-gp) activity in healthy participants. *Journal of Clinical Pharmacology, 52*(6), 932–939.

Marrero, E., Sanchez, J., de Armas, E., Escobar, A., Melchor, G., Abad, M. J., et al. (2006). COX-2 and sPLA2 inhibitory activity of aqueous extract and polyphenols of *Rhizophora mangle* (red mangrove). *Fitoterapia, 77*(4), 313–315.

Mathews, J. D., Riley, M. D., Fejo, L., Munoz, E., Milns, N. R., Gardner, I. D., et al. (1988). Effects of the heavy usage of kava on physical health: summary of a pilot survey in an aboriginal community. *Medical Journal of Australia, 148*(11), 548–555.

Mathews, J. M., Etheridge, A. S., & Black, S. R. (2002). Inhibition of human cytochrome P450 activities by kava extract and kavalactones. *Drug Metabolism and Disposition, 30*(11), 1153–1157.

Mato, J. M., Camara, J., Fernandez de Paz, J., Caballeria, L., Coll, S., Caballero, A., et al. (1999). S-adenosylmethionine in alcoholic liver cirrhosis: a randomized, placebo-controlled, double-blind, multicenter clinical trial. *Journal of Hepatology, 30*(6), 1081–1089.

Matsumoto, S., Mori, N., Tsuchihashi, N., Ogata, T., Lin, Y., Yokoyama, H., & Ishida, S. (1998). Enhancement of nitroxide-reducing activity in rats after chronic administration of vitamin E, vitamin C, and idebenone examined by an in vivo electron spin resonance technique. *Magnetic Resonance in Medicine, 40*(2), 330–333.

McDaniel, M. A., Maier, S. F., & Einstein, G. O. (2003). "Brain-specific" nutrients: a memory cure? *Nutrition, 19*(11–12), 957–975.

McNamara, R. K., Hahn, C. G., Jandacek, R., Rider, T., Tso, P., Stanford, K. E., & Richtand, N. M. (2007). Selective deficits in the omega-3 fatty acid docosahexaenoic acid in the postmortem orbitofrontal cortex of patients with major depressive disorder. *Biological Psychiatry, 62*(1), 17–24.

Medical Letter, The. (2006). Fish oil supplements. *Medical Letter on Drugs and Therapeutics, 48*(1239), 59–60.

Medical Letter, The. (1997). Tamsulosin for benign prostatic hyperplasia. *Medical Letter on Drugs and Therapeutics, 39*(1011), 96.

Medici, V., Virata, M. C., Peerson, J. M., Stabler, S. P., French, S. W., Gregory, J. F. 3rd, et al. (2011). S-adenosyl-L-methionine treatment for alcoholic liver disease: a double-blinded, randomized, placebo-controlled trial. *Alcoholism, Clinical and Experimental Research, 35*(11), 1960–1965.

Melzer, J., Schrader, E., Brattstrom, A., Schellenberg, R., & Saller, R. (2009). Fixed herbal drug combination with and without butterbur (Ze 185) for the treatment of patients with somatoform disorders: randomized, placebo-controlled pharmaco-clinical trial. *Phytotherapy Research, 23*(9), 1303–1308.

Miles, L., Miles, M. V., Tang, P. H., Horn, P. S., Wong, B. L., DeGrauw, T. J., et al. (2005). Muscle coenzyme Q: a potential test for mitochondrial activity and redox status. *Pediatric Neurology, 32*(5), 318–324.

Milkiewicz, P., Mills, C. O., Roma, M. G., Ahmed-Choudhury, J., Elias, E., & Coleman, R. (1999). Tauroursodeoxycholate and

S-adenosyl-L-methionine exert an additive ameliorating effect on taurolithocholate-induced cholestasis: a study in isolated rat hepatocyte couplets. *Hepatology, 29*(2), 471–476.

Milligan, S. R., Kalita, J. C., Pocock, V., Van De Kauter, V., Stevens, J. F., Deinzer, M. L., et al. (2000). The endocrine activities of 8-prenylnaringenin and related hop (Humulus lupulus L.) flavonoids. *Journal of Clinical Endocrinology and Metabolism, 85*(12), 4912–4915.

Ming, D. S., Hillhouse, B. J., Guns, E. S., Eberding, A., Xie, S., Vimalanathan, S., & Towers, G. H. (2005). Bioactive compounds from *Rhodiola rosea* (Crassulaceae). *Phytotherapy Research, 19*(9), 740–743.

Miodownik, C., Lerner, V., Statsenko, N., Dwolatzky, T., Nemets, B., Berzak, E., & Bergman, J. (2006). Vitamin B6 versus mianserin and placebo in acute neuroleptic-induced akathisia: a randomized, double-blind, controlled study. *Clinical Neuropharmacology, 29*(2), 68–72.

Mirzoian, R. S., Gan'shina, T. S., Kosoi, M. I., Aleksandrin, V. V., & Aleksandrin, P. N. (1989). [Effect of pikamilon on the cortical blood supply and microcirculation in the pial arteriole system]. *Biulleten' Eksperimental' Noi Biologii I Meditsiny, 107*(5), 581–582.

Mischoulon, D., & Freeman, M. P. (2013). Omega-3 fatty acids in psychiatry. *Psychiatric Clinics of North America, 36*(1), 15–23.

Mischoulon, D., Price, L.,H., Carpenter, L. L., Tyrka, A. R., Papakostas, G. I., Baer, L., et al. (2014). A double-blind randomized, placebo-controlled clinical trial of S-adenosylmethionine (SAMe) versus escitalopram in major depressive disorder. *Journal of Clinical Psychiatry, 75*(4), 370–376.

Mitka, M. (2002). News about neuroprotectants for the treatment of stroke. *Journal of the American Medical Association, 287*(10), 1253–1254.

Modabbernia, A., & Akhondzadeh, S. (2013). Saffron, passionflower, valerian and sage for mental health. *Psychiatric Clinics of North America, 36*(1), 85–91.

Molla, M. D., Hidalgo-Mora, J. J., & Soteras, M. G. (2011). Phytotherapy as alternative to hormone replacement therapy. *Frontiers Bioscience (Scholar Edition), 3*, 191–204.

Monaco, P., Pastore, L., Rizzo, S., Avarello, S., Collone, A., & Gasparro, S. (1996). Safety and tolerability of adometionine (ADE) SD for inpatients with stroke: a pilot randomized, double-blind, placebo controlled study [abstract] presented at the Third World Stroke Conference and Fifth European Stroke Conference, Sept. 1–5, 1996, Munich, Germany.

Morris, M. C., Evans, D. A., Bienias, J. L., Tangney, C. C., Bennett, D. A., Aggarwal, N., et al. (2003). Dietary fats and the risk of incident Alzheimer disease. *Archives of Neurology, 60*(2), 194–200.

Moshiri, E., Basti, A. A., Noorbala, A. A., Jamshidi, A. H., Hesameddin Abbasi, S., & Akhondzadeh, S. (2006). *Crocus sativus L.* (petal) in the treatment of mild-to-moderate depression: a double-blind, randomized and placebo-controlled trial. *Phytomedicine, 13*(9–10), 607–611.

Movafegh, A., Alizadeh, R., Hajimohamadi, F., Esfehani, F., & Nejatfar, M. (2008). Preoperative oral *Passiflora incarnata* reduces anxiety in ambulatory surgery patients: a double-blind, placebo-controlled study. *Anesthesia and Analgesia, 106*(6), 1728–1732.

Mowrey, D. B. (1996). *Muira-Puama (Liriosma ovata), in herbal tonic therapies.* Avenel, NJ: Wings Books.

Muller, S. F., & Klement, S. (2006). A combination of valerian and lemon balm is effective in the treatment of restlessness and dyssomnia in children. *Phytomedicine, 13*(6), 383–387.

Munshi, R., Bhalerao, S., Rathi, P., Kuber, V. V., Nipanikar, S. U., & Kadbhane, K. P. (2011). An open-label, prospective clinical study to evaluate the efficacy and safety of TLPL/AY/01/2008 in the management of functional constipation. *Journal of Ayurveda and Integrative Medicine, 2*(3), 144–152.

Nandy, K. (1978). Centrophenoxine: effects on aging mammalian brain. *Journal of the American Geriatrics Society, 26*(2), 74–81.

Napryeyenko, O., Borzenko, I., & Gindem-Np Study Group. (2007). Ginkgo biloba special extract in dementia with neuropsychiatric features. A randomised, placebo-controlled, double-blind clinical trial. *Arzneimittel-Forschung, 57*(1), 4–11.

Narahashi, T., Moriguchi, S., Zhao, X., Marszalec, W., & Yeh, J. Z. (2004). Mechanisms of action of cognitive enhancers on neuroreceptors. *Biological & Pharmaceutical Bulletin, 27*(11), 1701–1706.

Newton, K. M., Reed, S. D., LaCroix, A. Z., Grothaus, L. C., Ehrlich, K., & Guiltinan, J. (2006). Treatment of vasomotor symptoms of menopause with black cohosh, multibotanicals, soy, hormone therapy, or placebo: a randomized trial. *Annals of Internal Medicine, 145*(12), 869–879.

Nidecker, A. (1997). Probing genes, drugs, and fatty acids in dementia. *Clinical Psychiatry News, 4.*

Ning, H., Xin, Z. C., Lin, G., Banie, L., Lue, T. F., & Lin, C. S. (2006). Effects of icariin on phosphodiesterase-5 activity in vitro and cyclic guanosine monophosphate level in cavernous smooth muscle cells. *Urology, 68*(6), 1350–1354.

Noorbala, A. A., Akhondzadeh, S., Tahmacebi-Pour, N., & Jamshidi, A. H. (2005). Hydro-alcoholic extract of *Crocus sativus L.* versus fluoxetine in the treatment of mild to moderate depression: a double-blind, randomized pilot trial. *Journal of Ethnopharmacology, 97*(2), 281–284.

Occhiuto, F., Pasquale, R. D., Guglielmo, G., Palumbo, D. R., Zangla, G., Samperi, S., et al. (2007). Effects of phytoestrogenic isoflavones from red clover (*Trifolium pratense L.*) on experimental osteoporosis. *Phytotherapy Research, 21*(2), 130–134.

Oh, K. J., Chae, M. J., Lee, H. S., Hong, H. D., & Park, K. (2010). Effects of Korean red ginseng on sexual arousal in menopausal women: placebo-controlled, double-blind crossover clinical study. *Journal of Sexual Medicine, 7(4 Pt 1),* 1469–1477.

Osher, Y., Bersudsky, Y., & Belmaker, R. H. (2005). Omega-3 eicosapentaenoic acid in bipolar depression: report of a small open-label study. *Journal of Clinical Psychiatry, 66*(6), 726–729.

Overk, C. R., Yao, P., Chadwick, L. R., Nikolic, D., Sun, Y., Cuendet, M. A., et al. (2005). Comparison of the in vitro estrogenic activities of compounds from hops (*Humulus lupulus*) and red clover (*Trifolium pratense*). *Journal of Agricultural and Food Chemistry, 53*(16), 6246–6253.

Packer, L., & Colman, C. (1999). *The antioxidant miracle.* New York: Wiley.

Panahi, Y., Badeli, R., Karami, N., & Sahebkar, A. (1914). Investigation of the efficacy of adjunctive therapy with bioavailability-boosted curcuminoids in major depressive disorder. *Phythotherapy Research, 28,* [in press].

Pandi-Perumal, S. R., Zisapel, N., Srinivasan, V., & Cardinali, D. P. (2005). Melatonin and sleep in aging population. *Experimental Gerontology, 40*(12), 911–925.

Panossian, A. (2013). Adaptogens in mental and behavioural disorders. *Psychiatric Clinics of North America, 36*(1), 49–64.

Panossian, A., Hamm, R., Wikman, G., & Efferth, T. (2013). Synergy and antagonism of active constituents of ADAPT-232 on transcriptional level of metabolic regulation in isolated neuroglia cells *Frontiers in Neuroendocrinology, 7*(16), 1–17.

Panossian, A., Hamm, R., Wikman, G., & Efferth, T. (2014). Mechanisms of action of Rhodiola, salidroside, tyrosol and triandrin in isolated neuroglial cells: An interactive pathway analysis of the downstream effects using RNA microarray data. *Phytomedicine, 21,* 1325–1348.

Panossian, A., Hovhannisyan, A., Abrahamyan, H., Gabrielyan, E., & Wikman, G. (2009). Pharmacokinetic and pharmacodynamic study of interaction of *Rhodiola rosea* SHR-5 extract with warfarin and theophylline in rats. *Phytotherapy Research, 23*(3), 351–357.

Panossian, A., & Wagner, H. (2005). Stimulating effect of adaptogens: an overview with particular reference to their efficacy following single dose administration. *Phytotherapy Research, 19*(10), 819–838.

Panossian, A., & Wikman, G. (2008). Pharmacology of Schisandra chinensis Bail.: an overview of Russian research and uses in medicine. *Journal of Ethnopharmacology, 118*(2), 183–212.

Panossian, A., & Wikman, G. (2009). Evidence-based efficacy of adaptogens in fatigue, and molecular mechanisms related to their stress-protective activity. [Review]. *Current Clinical Pharmacology*, *4*(3), 198–219.

Panossian, A., Wikman, G., Kaur, P., & Asea, A. (2012). Adaptogens stimulate neuropeptide y and hsp72 expression and release in neuroglia cells. *Frontiers in Neuroscience*, *6*, 6.

Papakostas, G. I., Petersen, T., Lebowitz, B. D., Mischoulon, D., Ryan, J. L., Nierenberg, A. A., et al. (2005). The relationship between serum folate, vitamin B12, and homocysteine levels in major depressive disorder and the timing of improvement with fluoxetine. *International Journal of Neuropsychopharmacology*, *8*(4), 523–528.

Papakostas, G. I., Shelton, R. C., Zajecka, J. M., Etemad, B., Rickels, K., Clain, A., et al. (2012). l-Methylfolate as adjunctive therapy for SSRI-resistant major depression: Results of two randomized, double-blind, parallel-sequential trials. *American Journal of Psychiatry*, *169*(12), 1267–1274.

Paparrigopoulos, T. J. (2005). REM sleep behaviour disorder: clinical profiles and pathophysiology. *International Review of Psychiatry*, *17*(4), 293–300.

Parker, B. A., Gregory, S., M., Lorson, L., Polk, D., White, C. M., & Thompson, P. D. (2013). A randomized trial of coenzyme Q10 in patients with statin myopathy: Rationale and study design. *Journal of Clinical Lipidology*, *7*(3), 187–93.

Parnetti, L., Mignini, F., Tomassoni, D., Traini, E., & Amenta, F. (2007). Cholinergic precursors in the treatment of cognitive impairment of vascular origin: Ineffective approaches or need for re-evaluation? *Journal of the Neurological Sciences*, *257*(1–2), 264–269.

Patyar, S., Prakash, A., Modi, M., & Medhi, B. (2011). Role of vinpocetine in cerebrovascular diseases. [Review]. *Pharmacological Reports*, *63*(3), 618–628.

Pek, G., Fulop, T., & Zs-Nagy, I. (1989). Gerontopsychological studies using NAI ("Nurnberger Alters-Inventar") on patients with organic psychosyndrome (DSM III, Category 1) treated with centrophenoxine in a double blind, comparative, randomized clinical trial. *Archives of Gerontology and Geriatrics*, *9*(1), 17–30.

Pelka, R. B., & Leuchtgens, H. (1995). Pre-Alzheimer study: action of a herbal yeast preparation (Bio-Strath) in a randomised double-blind trial. *Ars Medici*, *85*, 1–5.

Petkov, V. D., Yonkov, D., Mosharoff, A., Kambourova, T., Alova, L., Petkov, V. V., & Todorov, I. (1986). Effects of alcohol aqueous extract from Rhodiola rosea L. roots on learning and memory. *Acta Physiologica et Pharmacologica Bulgarica*, *12*(1), 3–16.

Pettegrew, J. W., Levine, J., & McClure, R. J. (2000). Acetyl-L-carnitine physical-chemical, metabolic, and therapeutic properties: relevance for its mode of action in Alzheimer's disease and geriatric depression. *Molecular Psychiatry*, *5*(6), 616–632.

Procter, A. (1991). Enhancement of recovery from psychiatric illness by methylfolate. *British Journal of Psychiatry*, *159*, 271–272.

Quiros, C. F., & Cardenas, R. A. (1997). *Maca (Lepidium meyenii Walp)* (Vol. 21). Rome, Italy: Institute of Plant Genetics and Crop Plant Research, Gatersleben/ International Plant Resources Institute.

Rafii, M. S., Walsh, S., Little, J. T., Behan, K., Reynolds, B., Ward, C., et al. (2011). A phase II trial of huperzine A in mild to moderate Alzheimer disease. *Neurology*, *76*(16), 1389–1394.

Rahimi, R., Nikfar, S., & Abdollahi, M. (2009). Efficacy and tolerability of *Hypericum perforatum* in major depressive disorder in comparison with selective serotonin reuptake inhibitors: a meta-analysis. *Progress in Neuropsychopharmacology and Biological Psychiatry*, *33*(1), 118–127.

Rao, A. M., Hatcher, J. F., & Dempsey, R. J. (1999). CDP-choline: neuroprotection in transient forebrain ischemia of gerbils. *Journal of Neuroscience Research*, *58*(5), 697–705.

Raskind, M. A., Peskind, E. R., Wessel, T., & Yuan, W. (2000). Galantamine in AD: A 6-month randomized, placebo-controlled trial with a 6-month extension. The Galantamine USA-1 Study Group. *Neurology*, *54*(12), 2261–2268.

Rasmusson, A. M., Vasek, J., Lipschitz, D. S., Vojvoda, D., Mustone, M. E., Shi, Q., et al. (2004). An increased capacity for adrenal DHEA release is associated with decreased avoidance and negative mood symptoms in women with PTSD. *Neuropsychopharmacology*, *29*(8), 1546–1557.

Raus, K., Brucker, C., Gorkow, C., & Wuttke, W. (2006). First-time proof of endometrial safety of the special black cohosh extract (*Actaea* or *Cimicifuga racemosa* extract) CR BNO 1055. *Menopause*, *13*(4), 678–691.

Razina, T. G., Zueva, E. P., Amosova, E. N., & Krylova, S. G. (2000). [Medicinal plant preparations used as adjuvant therapeutics in experimental oncology]. *Eksperimental'naia I Klinicheskaia Farmakologiia*, *63*(5), 59–61.

Reay, J. L., Scholey, A. B., & Kennedy, D. O. (2010). Panax ginseng (G115) improves aspects of working memory performance and subjective ratings of calmness in healthy young adults. *Human Psychopharmacology*, *25*(6), 462–471.

Reiter, W. J., Schatzl, G., Mark, I., Zeiner, A., Pycha, A., & Marberger, M. (2001). Dehydroepiandrosterone in the treatment of erectile dysfunction in patients with different organic etiologies. *Urological Research*, *29*(4), 278–281.

Remington, R., Chan, A., Paskavitz, J., & Shea, T. B. (2009). Efficacy of a vitamin/nutriceutical formulation for moderate-stage to later-stage Alzheimer's disease: a placebo-controlled pilot study. *American Journal of Alzheimer's Disease and Other Dementias*, *24*(1), 27–33.

Riphagen, I. J., van der Veer, E., Muskiet, F. A, & DeJongste, M. J. (2012). Myopathy during statin therapy in the daily practice of an outpatient cardiology clinic: prevalence, predictors and relation with vitamin D. *Current Medical Research and Opinion*, *28*(7), 1247–1252.

Rizzo, A. M., Corsetto, P. A., Montorfano, G., Opizzi, A., Faliva, M., Giacosa, A., et al. (2012). Comparison between the AA/EPA ratio in depressed and nondepressed elderly females: omega-3 fatty acid supplementation correlates with improved symptoms but does not change immunological parameters. *Nutrition Journal*, *11*, 82.

Rohdewald, P. (2002). A review of the French maritime pine bark extract (Pycnogenol), a herbal medication with a diverse clinical pharmacology. *International Journal of Clinical Pharmacology and Therapeutics*, *40*(4), 158–168.

Rombaldi Bernardi, J., de Souza Escobar, R., Ferreira, C. F., & Pelufo Silveira, P. (2012). Fetal and neonatal levels of omega-3: effects on neurodevelopment, nutrition, and growth. *Scientific World Journal*, *2012*, ID 202473. Retrieved from: http://www.hindawi.com/journals/tswj/2012/202473.

Rosadini, G., Marenco, S., Nobili, F., Novellone, G., & Rodriguez, G. (1990). Acute effects of acetyl-L-carnitine on regional cerebral blood flow in patients with brain ischaemia. *International Journal of Clinical Pharmacology Research*, *10*(1–2), 123–128.

Rowland, D. L., & Tai, W. (2003). A review of plant-derived and herbal approaches to the treatment of sexual dysfunctions. *Journal of Sex and Marital Therapy*, *29*(3), 185–205.

Ruiz-Luna, A. C., Salazar, S., Aspajo, N. J., Rubio, J., Gasco, M., & Gonzales, G. F. (2005). Lepidium meyenii (Maca) increases litter size in normal adult female mice. *Reproductive Biology and Endocrinology*, *3*, 16.

Rump, T. J., Abdul Muneer, P. M., Szlachetka, A. M., Lamb, A., Haorei, C., Alikunju, S., et al. (2010). Acetyl-L-carnitine protects neuronal function from alcohol-induced oxidative damage in the brain. *Free Radical Biology and Medicine*, *49*(10), 1494–1504.

Rutherford, B. R. & Roose, S. P. (2013). A model of placebo response in antidepressant clinical trials. *American Journal of Psychiatry*, *170*(7), 723–733.

Sacks, F. M., Lichtenstein, A., Van Horn, L., Harris, W., Kris-Etherton, P., Winston, M., & American Heart Association Nutrition Committee. (2006). Soy protein, isoflavones, and cardiovascular health: an American Heart Association Science Advisory for professionals from the Nutrition Committee. *Circulation*, *113*(7), 1034–1044.

Safarinejad, M. R. (2005). Urtica dioica for treatment of benign prostatic hyperplasia: a prospective, randomized, double-blind, placebo-controlled, crossover study. *Journal of Herbal Pharmacotherapy, 5*(4), 1–11.

Sageman, S., & Brown, R. P. (2006). 3-acetyl-7-oxo-dehydroepiandrosterone for healing treatment-resistant posttraumatic stress disorder in women: 5 case reports. *Journal of Clinical Psychiatry, 67*(3), 493–496.

Sakellaris, G., Nasis, G., Kotsiou, M., Tamiolaki, M., Charissis, G., & Evangeliou, A. (2008). Prevention of traumatic headache, dizziness and fatigue with creatine administration. A pilot study. *Acta Paediatrica, 97*(1), 31–4.

Saratikov, A.S., & Krasnov, E.A. (1987). Clinical studies of Rhodiola. In A. S. Saratikov, & E. A. Krasnov (Eds.), *Rhodiola rosea is a valuable medicinal plant. (Golden root)*. Tomsk, Russia: Tomsk State University Press.

Sarris, J. (2013). St. John's wort for the treatment of psychiatric disorders. *Psychiatric Clinics of North America, 36*(1), 65–72.

Sarris, J., Mischoulon, D., & Schweitzer, I. (2012). Omega-3 for bipolar disorder: meta-analyses of use in mania and bipolar depression. *Journal of Clinical Psychiatry, 73*(1), 81–86.

Sarris, J., Panossian, A., Schweitzer, I., Stough, C., & Scholey, A. (2011). Herbal medicine for depression, anxiety and insomnia: a review of psychopharmacology and clinical evidence. *Journal of the European College of Neuropsychopharmacology, 21*(12), 841–860.

Sarris, J., Stough, C., Bousman, C. A., Wahid, Z. T., Murray, G., Teschke, R. et al. (2013a). Kava in the treatment of generalized anxiety disorder. A double-blind, randomized, placebo-controlled study. *Journal of Clinical Psychopharmacology, 33*(5), 1–6.

Sarris, J., Stough, C., Teschke, R., Wahid, Z. T., Bousman, C. A., Murray, G., et al. (2013b). Kava for the treatment of generalized anxiety disorder RCT: analysis of adverse reactions, liver function, addiction, and sexual effects. *Phytotherapy Research, 27*(11), 1723–1728.

Schaller, J. L., Thomas, J., & Bazzan, A. J. (2004). SAMe use in children and adolescents. [Case Reports Letter]. *European Child & Adolescent Psychiatry, 13*(5), 332–334.

Schenck, C. H., Bundlie, S. R., Ettinger, M. G., & Mahowald, M. W. (1986). Chronic behavioral disorders of human REM sleep: a new category of parasomnia. *Sleep, 9*(2), 293–308.

Schneider, F., Popa, R., Mihalas, G., Stefaniga, P., Mihalas, I. G., Maties, R., & Mateescu, R. (1994). Superiority of antagonic-stress composition versus nicergoline in gerontopsychiatry. *Annals of the New York Academy of Sciences, 717*, 332–42.

Schnyder, G., Roffi, M., Pin, R., Flammer, Y., Lange, H., Eberli, F. R., et al. (2001). Decreased rate of coronary restenosis after lowering of plasma homocysteine levels. *New England Journal of Medicine, 345*(22), 1593–1600.

Scholey, A., Ossoukhova, A., Owen, L., Ibarra, A., Pipingas, A., He, K., et al. (2010). Effects of American ginseng (*Panax quinquefolius*) on neurocognitive function: an acute, randomised, double-blind, placebo-controlled, crossover study. *Psychopharmacology (Berl), 212*(3), 345–356.

Schrader, E. (2000). Equivalence of St John's wort extract (Ze 117) and fluoxetine: a randomized, controlled study in mild-moderate depression. *International Clinical Psychopharmacology, 15*(2), 61–68.

Schwarzenbach, F. H., & Brunner, K. W. (1996). Effects of a herbal yeast preparation in convalescent patients. *Schweizerische Zeitschrift Ganzheits Medizin*, 226–273.

Segal, R., & Pilote, L. (2006). Warfarin interaction with *Matricaria chamomilla*. [Case Reports Letter]. *Centre for Advanced Materials Joining, 174*(9), 1281–1282.

Shamir, E., Barak, Y., Shalman, I., Laudon, M., Zisapel, N., Tarrasch, R., et al. (2001). Melatonin treatment for tardive dyskinesia: a double-blind, placebo- controlled, crossover study. *Archives of General Psychiatry, 58*(11), 1049–1052.

Shelton, R. C., Osuntokun, O., Heinloth, A. N., & Corya, S. A. (2010). Therapeutic options for treatment-resistant depression. *Central Nervous Sysytem Drugs, 24*(2), 131–161.

Shevtsov, V. A., Zholus, B. I., Shervarly, V. I., Vol'skij, V. B., Korovin, Y. P., Khristich, M. P., et al. (2003). A randomized trial of two different doses of a SHR-5 *Rhodiola rosea* extract versus placebo

and control of capacity for mental work. *Phytomedicine, 10*(2–3), 95–105.

Shippy, R. A., Mendez, D., Jones, K., Cergnul, I., & Karpiak, S. E. (2004). S-adenosylmethionine (SAM-e) for the treatment of depression in people living with HIV/AIDS. *BMC Psychiatry, 4*, 38.

Silverio, R., Laviano, A., Rossi Fanelli, F., & Seelaender, M. (2011). l-carnitine and cancer cachexia: Clinical and experimental aspects. *Journal of Cachexia, Sarcopenia and Muscle, 2*(1), 37–44.

Singh, Y. N., & Blumenthal, M. (1996). Kava: an overview. *Herbalgram, Special Review, 39*, 33–55.

Sivrioglu, E. Y., Kirli, S., Sipahioglu, D., Gursoy, B., & Sarandol, E. (2007). The impact of omega-3 fatty acids, vitamins E and C supplementation on treatment outcome and side effects in schizophrenia patients treated with haloperidol: an open-label pilot study. *Progress in Neuropsychopharmacology and Biological Psychiatry, 31*(7), 1493–1499.

Smriga, M., T. Ando, M. Akutsu, Y. Furukawa, K. Miwa, & Morinaga, Y. (2007). Oral treatment with L-lysine and L-arginine reduces anxiety and basal cortisol levels in healthy humans. *Biomedical Research, 28*(2), 85–90.

Smriga, M., Ghosh, S., Mouneimne, Y., Pellett, P. L., & Scrimshaw, N. S. (2004). Lysine fortification reduces anxiety and lessens stress in family members in economically weak communities in Northwest Syria. *Proceedings of the National Academy of Sciences of the United States of America, 101*(22), 8285–8288.

Sohn, M., & Sikora, R. (1991). *Ginkgo biloba* extract in the therapy of erectile dysfunction. *Journal of Sex Education Therapy, 17*, 53–61.

Sokeland, J., & Albrecht, J. (1997). [Combination of Sabal and Urtica extract vs. finasteride in benign prostatic hyperplasia (Aiken stages I to II). Comparison of therapeutic effectiveness in a one year double-blind study]. *Urologe A, 36*(4), 327–333.

Sorensen, H., & Sonne, J. (1996). A double-masked study of the effects of ginseng on cognitive functions. *Current Therapeutic Research, 57*(12), 959–968.

Spasov, A. A., Mandrikov, V. B., & Mironova, I. A. (2000). The effect of the preparation rodakson on the psychophysiological and physical adaptation of students to an academic load. *Eksperimental'naia I Klinicheskaia Farmakologiia, 63*(1), 76–78.

Spasov, A. A., Wikman, G. K., Mandrikov, V. B., Mironova, I. A., & Neumoin, V. V. (2000). A double-blind, placebo-controlled pilot study of the stimulating and adaptogenic effect of Rhodiola rosea SHR-5 extract on the fatigue of students caused by stress during an examination period with a repeated low-dose regimen. *Phytomedicine, 7*(2), 85–89.

Srinivasan, V., Pandi-Perumal, S., Cardinali, D., Poeggeler, B., & Hardeland, R. (2006). Melatonin in Alzheimer's disease and other neurodegenerative disorders. *Behavioral and Brain Function, 2*(1), 15.

Stancheva, S., Mosharrof, A., & Petkov, V. (1986). *Effect of Rhodiola rosea L. extract on the brain level of monoamines in rat. [abstract No. 34P]*. Lublin, Poland: Ninth Congress of the Polish Pharmacological Society.

Stancheva, S. L., & Mosharrof, A. (1987). Effect of the extract of *Rhodiola rosea L.* on the content of the brain biogenic monoamines. *Medecine Physiologie Comptes rendus de l'Academie bulgare des Sciences, 40*(6), 85–87.

Stanislavov, R., & Nikolova, V. (2003). Treatment of erectile dysfunction with pycnogenol and L-arginine. *Journal of Sex and Marital Therapy, 29*(3), 207–213.

Stanislavov, R., Nikolova, V., Rohdewald, P. (2008). Improvement of erectile function with Prelox: a randomized, double-blind, placebo-controlled, crossover trial. *International Journal of Impotence Research, 20*(2), 173–180.

Stoll, A. L., Severus, W. E., Freeman, M. P., et al. (1999). Omega 3 fatty acids in bipolar disorder. *Archives of General Psychiatry, 56*, 407–412.

Strous, R. D., Stryjer, R., Maayan, R., Gal, G., Viglin, D., Katz, E., et al. (2007). Analysis of clinical symptomatology, extrapyramidal symptoms and neurocognitive dysfunction following dehydroepiandrosterone (DHEA) administration in olanzapine treated schizophrenia patients: a randomized, double-blind placebo controlled trial. *Psychoneuroendocrinology, 32*(2), 96–105.

Sublette, M. E., Hibbeln, J. R., Galfalvy, H., Oquendo, M. A., & Mann, J. J. (2006). Omega-3 polyunsaturated essential fatty acid status as a predictor of future suicide risk. *American Journal of Psychiatry, 163*(6), 1100–1102.

Surtees, R., & Hyland, K. (1990). Cerebrospinal fluid concentrations of S-adenosylmethionine, methionine, and 5-methyltetrahydrofolate in a reference population: cerebrospinal fluid S-adenosylmethionine declines with age in humans. *Biochemistry Medicine and Metabolic Biology, 44*(2), 192–199.

Surtees, R., Leonard, J., & Austin, S. (1991). Association of demyelination with deficiency of cerebrospinal fluid S-adenosylmethioninein inborn errors of methyl-transfer pathway. *Lancet, 338*(8782-8783), 1550–1554.

Szalma, I., Kiss, A., Kardos, L., Horvath, G., Nyitrai, E., Tordai, Z., & Csiba, L. (2006). Piracetam prevents cognitive decline in coronary artery bypass: a randomized trial versus placebo. *Annals of Thoracic Surgery, 82*(4), 1430–1435.

Szegedi, A., Kohnen, R., Dienel, A., & Kieser, M. (2005). Acute treatment of moderate to severe depression with hypericum extract WS 5570 (St John's wort): randomised controlled double blind non-inferiority trial versus paroxetine. *British Medical Journal, 330*(7490), 503.

Szilagyi, G., Nagy, Z., Balkay, L., Boros, I., Emri, M., Lehel, S., et al. (2005). Effects of vinpocetine on the redistribution of cerebral blood flow and glucose metabolism in chronic ischemic stroke patients: a PET study. *Journal of the Neurological Sciences, 229–230,* 275–284.

Tacklind, J., Macdonald, R., Rutks, I., Stanke, J. U., & Wilt, T. J. (2012). Serenoa repens for benign prostatic hyperplasia. *Cochrane Database of Systematic Reviews, 12,* CD001423.

Taku, K., Melby, M. K., Nishi, N., Omori, T., & Kurzer, M. S. (2011). Soy isoflavones for osteoporosis: An evidence-based approach. *Maturitas, 70*(4), 333–338.

Tan, O., Bradshaw, K., & Carr, B. R. (2012). Management of vulvovaginal atrophy-related sexual dysfunction in postmenopausal women: an up-to-date review. *Menopause, 19*(1), 109–117.

Tang, X. C. (1996). Huperzine A (shuangyiping): a promising drug for Alzheimer's disease. *Acta Pharmacologica Sinica, 17*(6), 481–484.

Tavoni, A., Jeracitano, G., & Cirigliano, G. (1998). Evaluation of S-adenosylmethionine in secondary fibromyalgia: a double- blind study. [letter]. *Clinical and Experimental Rheumatology, 16*(1), 106–107.

Tavoni, A., Vitali, C., Bombardieri, S., & Pasero, G. (1987). Evaluation of S-adenosylmethionine in primary fibromyalgia. A double-blind crossover study. *American Journal of Medicine, 83*(5A), 107–110.

Teschke, R., Qiu, S. X., & Lebot, V. (2011). Herbal hepatotoxicity by kava: update on pipermethystine, flavokavain B, and mould hepatotoxins as primarily assumed culprits. [Review]. *Digestive and Liver Disease, 43*(9), 676–681.

Tildesley, N. T., Kennedy, D. O., Perry, E. K., Ballard, C. G., Wesnes, K. A., & Scholey, A. B. (2005). Positive modulation of mood and cognitive performance following administration of acute doses of *Salvia lavandulaefolia* essential oil to healthy young volunteers. *Physiology & Behavior, 83*(5), 699–709.

Toescu, E. C., & Verkhratsky, A. (2007). The importance of being subtle: small changes in calcium homeostasis control cognitive decline in normal aging. [Review]. *Aging Cell, 6*(3), 267–273.

Torta, R., Zanalda, F., Rocca, P., & Ravizza, L. (1988). Inhibitory activity of S-adenosyl-L-methionine on serum gamma-glutamyl-transpeptidase increase induced by psychodrugs and anticonvulsants. *Current Therapeutic Research, 44,* 144–159.

Trock, B. J., Hilakivi-Clarke, L., & Clarke, R. (2006). Meta-analysis of soy intake and breast cancer risk. *Journal of the National Cancer Institute, 98*(7), 459–471.

Turner, E. H., Loftis, J. M., & Blackwell, A. D. (2006). Serotonin a la carte: supplementation with the serotonin precursor 5-hydroxytryptophan. *Pharmacology & Therapeutics, 109*(3), 325–338.

Turner, P., Kantaria, R., & Young, A. H. (2014). A systematic review and meta-analysis of the evidence base for add-on treatment for patients with major depressive disorder who have not responded to antidepressant treatment: a European perspective. *Journal of Psychopharmacology, 28*(2), 85–98.

Udintsev, S. N., Krylova, S. G., & Fomina, T. I. (1992). The enhancement of the efficacy of adriamycin by using hepatoprotectors of plant origin in metastases of Ehrlich's adenocarcinoma to the liver in mice. *Voprosy Onkologii, 38*(10), 1217–1222.

Udintsev, S. N., & Schakhov, V. P. (1991). Decrease of cyclophosphamide haematotoxicity by Rhodiola rosea root extract in mice with Ehrlich and Lewis transplantable tumors. [letter]. *European Journal of Cancer, 27*(9), 1182.

Udintsev, S. N., & Shakhov, V. P. (1989). Decrease in the growth rate of Ehrlich's tumor and Pliss' lymphosarcoma with partial hepatectomy. *Voprosy Onkologii, 35*(9), 1072–1075.

Udintsev, S. N., & Shakhov, V. P. (1990). Changes in clonogenic properties of bone marrow and transplantable mice tumor cells during combined use of cyclophosphane and biological response modifiers of adaptogenic origin. *Eksperimental'naia Onkologiia, 12*(6), 55–56.

Underwood, M., Sivesind, P. A., Gabourie, T. A., & Lerner, K. C. (2011). *The effects of the calcium binding protein apoaequorin on memory and cognitive functioning in adults.* (July, pp. 1–8). Madison, Wisconson: Quincy Bioscience.

U S Food and Drug Administration. (2002, Nov. 25, 2011). *Consumer advisory: kava-containing dietary supplements may be associated with severe liver injury.* Retrieved from http://www.cdc.gov/mmwr/preview/mmwrhtml/mm5147a1.htm.

Vakhapova, V., Richter, Y., Cohen, T., Herzog, Y., & Korczyn, A. D. (2011). Safety of phosphatidylserine containing omega-3 fatty acids in non-demented elderly: a double-blind placebo-controlled trial followed by an open-label extension. *BMC Neurology, 11,* 79.

van Gelder, B. M., Tijhuis, M., Kalmijn, S., & Kromhout, D. (2007). Fish consumption, n-3 fatty acids, and subsequent 5-y cognitive decline in elderly men: the Zutphen Elderly Study. *American Journal of Clinical Nutrition, 85*(4), 1142–1147.

van Hattum, E. S., Doevendans, P. A., & Moll, F. L. (2007). Does folate therapy reduce the risk of coronary restenosis? *Netherlands Heart Journal, 15*(1), 12–15.

van Niekerk, J. K., Huppert, F. A., & Herbert, J. (2001). Salivary cortisol and DHEA: association with measures of cognition and well-being in normal older men, and effects of three months of DHEA supplementation. *Psychoneuroendocrinology, 26*(6), 591–612.

Van Strater, A. C., & Bogers, J. P. (2012). Interaction of St John's wort (Hypericum perforatum) with clozapine. [Case Reports]. *International Clinical Psychopharmacology, 27*(2), 121–124.

Varanese, S., Birnbaum, Z., Rossi, R., & Di Rocco, A. (2011). Treatment of advanced Parkinson's disease. *Parkinson's Disease, 2010,* 480260.

Volz, H. P., Murck, H., Kasper, S., & Moller, H. J. (2002). St John's wort extract (LI 160) in somatoform disorders: results of a placebo-controlled trial. *Psychopharmacology (Berlin), 164*(3), 294–300.

Vorbach, E. U., Arnoldt, K. H., & Hubner, W. D. (1997). Efficacy and tolerability of St. John's wort extract LI 160 versus imipramine in patients with severe depressive episodes according to ICD- 10. *Pharmacopsychiatry, 30*(Suppl 2), 81–85.

Wallin, A. K., Wattmo, C., & Minthon, L. (2011). Galantamine treatment in Alzheimer's disease: response and long-term outcome in a routine clinical setting. *Neuropsychiatric Disease and Treatment, 7,* 565–576.

Wang, B. L., Hu, J. P., Sheng, L., & Li, Y. (2011). [Effects of *Schisandra chinensis* (Wuweizi) constituents on the activity of hepatic microsomal CYP450 isozymes in rats detected by using a cocktail probe substrates method]. *Yao Xue Xue Bao, 46*(8), 922–927.

Wang, R., Yan, H., & Tang, X. C. (2006). Progress in studies of huperzine A, a natural cholinesterase inhibitor from Chinese herbal medicine. *Acta Pharmacologica Sinica, 27*(1), 1–26.

Waynberg, J. (1990). *Aphrodesiacs: contribution to the clinical validation of traditional use of Ptychopetalum guyanna:* Presentation at the First International Congress on Ethnopharmacology. Strasbourg, France, June 5–9.

Waynberg, J., & Brewer, S. (2000). Effects of Herbal vX on libido and sexual activity in premenopausal and postmenopausal women. *Advance in Therapy, 17*(5), 255–262.

Weinmann, S., Roll, S., Schwarzbach, C., Vauth, C., & Willich, S. N. (2010). Effects of *Ginkgo biloba* in dementia: systematic review and meta-analysis. *BMC Geriatrics, 10,* 14.

Weng, S., Tang, J., Wang, G. et al. (2007). Comparison of the addition of Siberian Ginseng (*Acanthopanax senticosus*) versus fluoxetine to lithium for the treatment of bipolar disorder in adolescents: a randomized, double-blind trial. *Current Therapeutic Research, Clinical and Experimental, 68*(4), 280–290.

Wheatley, D. (1999). Hypericum in seasonal affective disorder (SAD). *Current Medical Research and Opinion, 15*(1), 33–37.

Widodo, N., Kaur, K., Shrestha, B. G., Takagi, Y., Ishii, T., Wadhwa, R., & Kaul, S. C. (2007). Selective killing of cancer cells by leaf extract of Ashwagandha: identification of a tumor-inhibitory factor and the first molecular insights to its effect. *Clinical Cancer Research, 13*(7), 2298–2306.

Woelk, H., Arnoldt, K. H., Kieser, M., & Hoerr, R. (2007). *Ginkgo biloba* special extract EGb 761 in generalized anxiety disorder and adjustment disorder with anxious mood: a randomized, double-blind, placebo-controlled trial. *Journal of Psychiatric Research, 41*(6), 472–480.

Wong, M. L., O'Kirwan, F., Hannestad, J. P., Irizarry, K. J., Elashoff, D., & Licinio, J. (2004). St John's wort and imipramine-induced gene expression profiles identify cellular functions relevant to antidepressant action and novel pharmacogenetic candidates for the phenotype of antidepressant treatment response. *Molecular Psychiatry, 9*(3), 237–251.

Wooltorton, E. (2006). Osteoporosis treatment: raloxifene (Evista) and stroke mortality. *Centre for Advanced Materials Joining, 175*(2), 147.

Wuttke, W., Jarry, H., Christoffel, V., Spengler, B., & Seidlova-Wuttke, D. (2003). Chaste tree (Vitex agnus-castus)—pharmacology and clinical indications. *Phytomedicine, 10*(4), 348–357.

Wuttke, W., Seidlova-Wuttke, D., & Gorkow, C. (2003). The Cimicifuga preparation BNO 1055 vs. conjugated estrogens in a double-blind placebo-controlled study: effects on menopause symptoms and bone markers. *Maturitas, 44*(Suppl 1), S67–77.

Xu, F., Hongbin, H., Yan, J., Chen, H., He, Q., Xu, W., et al. (2011). Greatly improved neuroprotective efficiency of citicoline by stereotactic delivery in treatment of ischemic injury. *Drug Delivery, 18*(7), 461–467.

Yamada, T., Terashima, T., Okubo, T., Juneja, L. R., & Yokogoshi, H. (2005). Effects of theanine, r-glutamylethylamide, on neurotransmitter release and its relationship with glutamic acid neurotransmission. *Nutritional Neuroscience, 8*(4), 219–226.

Yang, S., Evens, A. M., Prachand, S., Singh, A. T., Bhalla, S., David, K., & Gordon, L. I. (2010). Mitochondrial-mediated apoptosis in lymphoma cells by the diterpenoid lactone andrographolide, the active component of *Andrographis paniculata. Clinical Cancer Research, 16*(19), 4755–4768.

Yap, K. Y., Kuo, E. Y., Lee, J. J., Chui, W. K., & Chan, A. (2010). An onco-informatics database for anticancer drug interactions with complementary and alternative medicines used in cancer treatment and supportive care: an overview of the OncoRx project. *Support Care Cancer, 18*(7), 883–891.

Yen, M. H., Weng, T. C., Liu, S. Y., Chai, C. Y., & Lin, C. C. (2005). The hepatoprotective effect of Bupleurum kaoi, an endemic plant to Taiwan, against dimethylnitrosamine-induced hepatic fibrosis in rats. *Biological & Pharmaceutical Bulletin, 28*(3), 442–448.

Yuan, C. S., Wei, G., Dey, L., Karrison, T., Nahlik, L., Maleckar, S., et al. (2004). Brief communication: American ginseng reduces warfarin's effect in healthy patients: a randomized, controlled trial. *Annals of Internal Medicine, 141*(1), 23–27.

Zandi, P. P., Anthony, J. C., Khachaturian, A. S., Stone, S. V., Gustafson, D., Tschanz, J. T., et al. (2004). Reduced risk of Alzheimer disease in users of antioxidant vitamin supplements: the Cache County Study. *Archives of Neurology, 61*(1), 82–88.

Zhang, X. Y., Zhou, D. F., Zhang, P. Y., Wu, G. Y., Su, J. M., Cao, L. Y. (2001). A double-blind, placebo-controlled trial of extract of Ginkgo biloba added to haloperidol in treatment-resistant patients with schizophrenia. *Journal of Clinical Psychiatry, 62*(11), 878–883.

Zhao, Y., Dou, J., Luo, J., Li, W., Chan, H. H., Cui, W., et al. (2011). Neuroprotection against excitotoxic and ischemic insults by bis(12)-hupyridone, a novel anti-acetylcholinesterase dimer, possibly via acting on multiple targets. *Brain Research, 1421,* 100–109.

Zhdanova, I. V., Wurtman, R. J., Regan, M. M., Taylor, J. A., Shi, J. P., & Leclair, O. U. (2001). Melatonin treatment for age-related insomnia. *Journal of Clinical Endocrinology and Metabolism, 86*(10), 4727–4730.

Zs-Nagy, I. (1997). The membrane hypothesis of aging: its relevance to recent progress in genetic research. *Journal Molecular Medicine, 75*(10), 703–714.

Zs-Nagy, K., Dajko, G., Uray, I., & Zs-Nagy, I. (1994). Comparative studies on the free radical scavenger properties of two nootropic drugs, CPH and BCE-001. *Annals of the New York Academy of Sciences, 717,* 115–121.

PART IV

MAJOR SYMPTOMS AND SYNDROMES

29.

GRIEF, COMPLICATED GRIEF, AND BEREAVEMENT-RELATED DEPRESSION

Alana Iglewicz and Sidney Zisook

INTRODUCTION

Grief is a universal mammalian experience. Generally, grief is considered to be self-limited, adaptive, and outside the general domain of psychiatric concerns. However, there are times when grieving persons can and should be referred for mental health care, such as when the death of a loved one also triggers a major depressive disorder, a prolonged stress or trauma reaction, or when healing does not occur spontaneously—a condition called "complicated grief." In those circumstances grief can be associated with important general medical and mental health consequences (Ajdacic-Gross et al., 2008; M. K. Shear et al., 2011; Stroebe, Stroebe, & Abakoumkin, 2005; Zisook & Shear, 2009). This chapter will cover the clinical features of "normal" grief, the complex relationship between grief and depression (where does one end and the other begin?), the clinical features of complicated grief (CG), and evidence-based interventions for bereavement-related depression and CG.

TERMINOLOGY

Since terms used to describe emotions and behaviors following the death of a loved one are imprecise and used idiosyncratically by clinicians and experts alike, it is useful to review contemporary definitions of key terms. *Grief* may be defined as the constellation of feelings, cognitions, behaviors, and changes in function associated with loss of any kind. This definition applies to the medically ill population, as many medically ill individuals are grieving numerous losses including their loss of health, function, and independence; and to individuals undergoing any number of other losses, such as divorce, financial security, employment, and home. Alternatively, *bereavement*, the state of having lost a loved one or someone close specifically through death, is sometimes used to connote grief after the death of a loved one (Stroebe, Hansson, Stroebe, & Schut, 2001). For the purposes of the rest of this chapter, *grief* and *bereavement* will be used interchangeably. Another term that sometimes is used to refer to grief reactions is *mourning*. We define mourning as the social, cultural, and behavioral rituals of grief, while Shear et al. define mourning as the psychosocial process by which one transitions from acute to integrated grief (M. K. Shear et al., 2011).

ACUTE, INTEGRATED, AND COMPLICATED GRIEF

Grief can be further subcategorized as *acute grief*, the initial painful response, and *integrated grief*, the ongoing, attenuated adaptation to the death of a loved one. *Complicated grief*, sometimes called prolonged, traumatic, or unresolved grief, refers to *acute* grief that remains intense and persistent without transitioning into integrated grief.

ACUTE GRIEF

Grief is conceptualized as a universal, natural, adaptive, and instinctual reaction to the loss of a loved one. The *acute* manifestations of grief can span the full gamut of intensity from barely noticeable discomfort and dysfunction to among the most painful, distressing, and debilitating experiences of a person's life. In acute grief there may be disbelief and difficulty comprehending the finality of the loss. Acute grief is a preoccupying experience in which feelings of yearning and longing for the deceased are accompanied by pangs of intense emotions, often experienced as unfamiliar and difficult to control. The bereaved person is consumed with thoughts and memories of the deceased and relatively uninterested in other people and usual life occupations. However, even when the predominant features are pain and loss, pleasant and positive emotions also occur. The bereaved person may experience enjoyment in recalling happy times and sharing amusing anecdotes, warmth in recalling closeness, pride in honoring the deceased, relief from the burden, and joy in being alive (Bonanno, Moskowitz, Papa, & Folkman, 2005). Typically, intense emotions come in waves, the so-called *pangs* of grief, which gradually become less frequent and intense. While there is no accepted time frame for grief to last, the current consensus is that the most painful features at least begin to abate by about 6 months. By then, wounds begin to heal, and the bereaved person finds his or her way back to a fulfilling life. The reality and meaning of the death are assimilated, and the bereaved are able to engage once again in pleasurable and satisfying relationships and activities (Zisook & Shear, 2009).

INTEGRATED GRIEF

Normally, acute grief instinctively transitions to *integrated grief* within several months. As the permanence of the loss is comprehended, acute grief resolves, and memories of the deceased are integrated into the ongoing psychological life of the bereaved. Engagement in constructive daily occupations is reestablished, and the person is able to fully resume old roles and functions as well as develop new ones that may be necessary for ongoing life. Thoughts and memories of the deceased remain accessible but are no longer preoccupying. After such integration there is diminished intensity of sadness and retreat of preoccupying thoughts. Integrated grief may be life-long and often continues to evolve over time (M. K. Shear, 2010). Notably, symptoms of acute grief can recur transiently, oftentimes during anniversaries, holidays, stresses, special occasions, and other losses.

COMPLICATED GRIEF

Complicated grief is a recognizable syndrome of prolonged, intense grief that occurs when acute grief does not transition to integrated grief by 6 months (Zisook, Simon et al., 2010). Time moves on, but healing does not. It is not always clear why the natural healing process of grief is impeded in any given individual, but several risk factors have been identified. For example, CG has been found more often after suicide or when the deceased is a "soul-mate" (Jordan, 2008; M. K. Shear et al., 2011). Past and current major depressive disorder also is associated with increased risk for CG. Sometimes, the resolution of grief is impeded by maladaptive attitudes and behaviors such as intense blame of self or others, fear of being overwhelmed by the intensity of grief, persistent avoidance of reminders of the deceased, the prospect of life without the deceased, or a disinclination to engage in activities that were shared with the deceased (Boelen, van den Bout, & van den Hout, 2006; K. Shear et al., 2007). On occasion, practical and/or interpersonal problems may complicate the adjustment process and delay the healing of grief. Persistent avoidance of reminders of the loss is another major impediment to adjustment. When resolution of acute grief is blocked, the resulting complicated grief can persist for years, decades, or even a lifetime, with prolonged suffering and failure to find avenues for constructive activities in a world without the deceased.

Approximately 10% of bereaved individuals may experience CG (Middleton, Raphael, Burnett, & Martinek, 1998; H. G. Prigerson et al., 2009). A recent large population-based study of older adults in the Netherlands indicates a CG prevalence of 4.8% of the general older adult population, 7% of the general 75–85-year-old population, and 25.4% of the older grieving population (Newson, Boelen, Hek, Hofman, & Tiemeier, 2011). CG is observed across various ethnic groups in the United States (Cruz et al., 2007; Goldsmith, Morrison, Vanderwerker, & Prigerson, 2008) and cultures throughout the world (Bonanno, Papa, Lalande, Zhang, & Noll, 2005; Ghaffari-Nejad, Ahmadi-Mousavi, Gandomkar, & Reihani-Kermani, 2007; Kersting et al., 2007; Langner & Maercker, 2005; Momartin, Silove, Manicavasagar, & Steel,

2004; Morina, Rudari, Bleichhardt, & Prigerson, 2010; H. Prigerson et al., 2002; Schaal, Elbert, & Neuner, 2009).

Box 29.1 provides a brief screening questionnaire for CG. The clinical symptoms of CG include persistent difficulty accepting the death, preoccupation with thoughts and images of the deceased, recurrent pangs of intense grief, avoidance of reminders of the loss, anger, guilt, and difficulty adjusting to life without the deceased (H. G. Prigerson et al., 1995; M. K. Shear, 2010). Excessive proximity-seeking is common, and in its most extreme form can manifest as wishes to die or suicidal behavior with the belief that life has no purpose or meaning without the deceased. Additionally, individuals with CG often experience ruminating thoughts about the circumstances around the death (M. K. Shear et al., 2011). Without treatment, CG tends to persist indefinitely.

Although CG often is comorbid with major depressive disorder (MDD)—either as a risk and/or as a consequence—it is important to differentiate between the two conditions, as treatments and prognosis vary (M. K. Shear et al., 2011). A key difference is that the core features of CG—longing, pining, preoccupation, and avoidance—are not characteristic features of MDD. The core features of MDD (persistent and pervasive sadness, anhedonia, and low self esteem) are not characteristic features of CG. Table 29.1 summarizes phenomenological and clinical distinctions between CG and MDD. CG also shares many features with posttraumatic stress disorder (PTSD) and often co-occurs with PTSD, but they can be differentiated by several key distinguishing features (M. K. Shear et al., 2011). The predominant trauma in CG is loss-related, while the major trauma in PTSD is threat-related. The characteristic affects of CG (longing and yearning) are not the same as the predominant affect of PTSD (fear).

CG is associated with functional impairment in multiple modalities, including daily activities (Monk, Houck, & Shear, 2006), socializing (Boelen & Prigerson, 2007; Melhem, Moritz, Walker, Shear, & Brent, 2007), work (Lannen, Wolfe, Prigerson, Onelov, & Kreicbergs, 2008; H. G. Prigerson et al., 1997), and relationships (Monk, Houck, & Shear, 2006). Additionally, individuals with CG have increased rates of

---

Box 29.1 **BRIEF GRIEF QUESTIONNAIRE: A SCREENING TOOL FOR COMPLICATED GRIEF**

Rate as: 0 = Not at all, 1 = Somewhat, 2 = A lot
Screen positive: Scores ≥4

1. How much trouble are you having accepting the death?

2. How much does grief interfere with your life?

3. Are you having troublesome or preoccupying images or thoughts of _____?

4. Are there things you used to do when _____ was alive that you don't feel comfortable doing anymore, that you avoid?

5. How much are you feeling cut off or distant from other people since _____ died?

(Shear et al., Psychiatric Service, 2006).

Table 29.1 PHENOMENOLOGICAL DIFFERENCES BETWEEN COMPLICATED GRIEF AND DEPRESSION (ZISOOK ET AL, JCP 2010)

	COMPLICATED GRIEF	MAJOR DEPRESSIVE DISORDER
Mood/Sadness	Pangs of emotion triggered by reminders of the loss	Pervasive
Anhedonia	Related to missing loved one	Pervasive
Suicidal Ideation	If present, focused on joining the deceased loved one	Frequent, focused on not being worthy of living
Preoccupying Thoughts	Of the deceased; guilt and self blame focused on the deceased	Of low self esteem and related to a sense of guilt or shame
Avoidance	Avoidance of activities, situations and people because of the death	General withdrawal from activities and people
Intrusive Images	Prominent—of the deceased	Not prominent
Yearning and Longing	Frequent—for the deceased	Not typically seen

psychiatric comorbidity (Newson, Boelen, Hek, Hofman, & Tiemeier, 2011; Simon et al., 2007), worsening symptoms of other psychiatric illnesses (M. K. Shear et al., 2011), and insomnia (Hardison, Neimeyer, & Lichstein, 2005). Importantly, CG is associated with increased suicidal ideation and behavior across various age groups (Latham & Prigerson, 2004; Mitchell, Kim, Prigerson, & Mortimer, 2005; H. G. Prigerson et al., 1999; Szanto, Prigerson, Houck, Ehrenpreis, & Reynolds, 1997; Szanto et al., 2006).

In addition, CG negatively affects individuals' physical health outcomes (Lichtenthal, Cruess, & Prigerson, 2004; M. Stroebe et al., 2007). CG is associated with increased tobacco and alcohol use (Zisook, Shuchter, & Lyons, 1987). In their study of bereaved widows and widowers, H. G. Prigerson et al. (1997) found that CG predicted numerous negative health changes. Individuals with CG had increased rates of cancer, cardiac disease, and hypertension. Moreover, widows and widowers with CG had significantly higher rates of the flu, headaches, and cardiac issues around the anniversary of the death of their spouse than did bereaved spouses without CG. Gender differences exist in these health outcomes. Widowers with CG tend to have worse health outcomes than do widows (Chen et al., 1999). Despite their increased risk for developing health problems, individuals with CG underutilize health services (H. Prigerson et al., 2001). Overall, untreated CG results in suffering, impairment, and poor health outcomes.

TREATMENT OF COMPLICATED GRIEF

Considering that grief is a normal, adaptive response to loss, noncomplicated grief that is not comorbid with depression does not warrant any intervention in most circumstances. When support, reassurance, and information generally provided by family, friends, and sometimes clergy, is not available or sufficient, bereavement support groups may help fill the gap (Lieberman & Videkasherman, 1986; Marmar, Horowitz, Weiss, Wilner, & Kaltreider, 1988). Support groups can be particularly helpful after traumatic losses such as the death of a child, a death after suicide, or deaths from other "unnatural" causes. While we do not mean to imply that acute grief is a pathological condition, certain individuals find that their desire to explore and make sense of their grief motivates them to initiate a productive exploratory or supportive therapy.

Uncomplicated acute and integrated grief generally do not require formal interventions—but CG does. Without treatment, CG symptoms follow an unrelenting course. The effectiveness and role of pharmacologic management of CG is not yet established. An open pilot study (Pasternak et al., 1991) and a randomized controlled trial (Reynolds et al., 1999) of bereavement-related major depression in patients—many of whom also had symptoms of CG—demonstrated little response in grief symptoms to nortriptyline. Another small, open trial of sustained-release bupropion for recently bereaved individuals with bereavement-related depression was associated with an improvement in both grief and depressive symptoms (Zisook, Shuchter, Pedrelli, Sable, & Deaciuc, 2001), but CG was not targeted in this study. However, a small case series of participants with CG suggested that escitalopram may be an effective treatment for CG (Simon, Thompson, Pollack, & Shear, 2007), and another study indicated that the response of individuals with CG to two forms of psychotherapy improved with concurrent escitalopram treatment (Simon et al., 2008). In light of these findings suggesting a potential role for pharmacological interventions for CG, a large multisite randomized controlled trial exploring the efficacy of citalopram for the treatment of CG is currently in progress (http://clinicaltrials.gov/ct2/show/NCT01179568).

A recent meta-analysis of studies assessing psychotherapeutic strategies for the prevention and treatment of CG was not able to confirm the effectiveness of preventive interventions, but it did show that certain psychotherapy interventions are effective. Moreover, benefits increase over time (Wittouck, Van Autreve, De Jaegere, Portzky, & van Heeringen, 2011). Studies substantiate the use of cognitive behavioral therapy (Boelen & Prigerson, 2007; Wagner, Knaevelsrud, & Maercker, 2006), time-limited interpretive group therapy (Piper, McCallum, Joyce, Rosie, & Ogrodniczuk, 2001; Piper, Ogrodniczuk, Joyce, Weideman, & Rosie, 2007; Saindon et al., 2014), and complicated grief therapy (K. Shear, Frank, Houck, & Reynolds, 2005).

Complicated grief therapy (CGT) was developed specifically for persons with complicated grief. The basic principle underlying CGT is that acute grief will progress instinctively to integrated grief if the complications of the grief are addressed and the natural mourning process is supported. Integrating treatment strategies from cognitive behavioral, interpersonal, exposure, motivational, and gestalt therapies, CGT focuses both (1) on the *loss* (e.g., through imaginal revisiting exercises, in vivo exposure, imaginal conversations, actual revisiting of painful places and activities, review of pictures, etc.) and (2) on *life* without the deceased (e.g., through goal-setting exercises, planning for holidays and special occasions, and working on interpersonal difficulties). Significant others are educated, supported, and asked to participate in treatment both during certain sessions and between sessions. Pilot (M. K. Shear et al., 2001) and two randomized controlled trials funded by the National Institute of Mental Health (NIMH) (Shear, Frank, Houck, & Reynolds, 2005; Simon et al., 2008) support the robust efficacy of CGT for the treatment of CG.

BEREAVEMENT-RELATED DEPRESSION AND THE BEREAVEMENT EXCLUSION

MDD is a heterogeneous group of disorders that often, but not invariably, is triggered by stressful life events. Bereavement bears a special relationship to MDD, as it is simultaneously one of the most virulent precipitants of major depressive episodes (MDE) while also being the only life event that might have, according to *DSM-III* and *IV* conventions, negated the diagnosis of MDD. Thus, when an MDE was ostensibly triggered by other losses—such as divorce, terminal illness, unemployment, homelessness, or new onset disability—if full symptomatic criteria weree met for >2 weeks, the diagnosis of MDE was made. Not so for depression that occurred in the context of the death of a loved one based on the *DSM-III* and *IV*. In this singular instance, unless the depression was particularly severe or prolonged (described in more detail below), a V-code (no mental illness) of "bereavement" was given rather than a clinical diagnosis of MDE. Of note, this diagnostic distinction afforded depression following bereavement, the so called "bereavement exclusion," is not provided by the *International Diagnostic Classification of Diseases*–10. Based on the literature subsequently reviewed in this chapter, the bereavement exclusion was removed from the *DSM-5*. The removal of the bereavement exclusion was one of the most heavily debated changes in the *DSM-5*. Because of the unique status afforded to bereavement there remains great confusion in the United States and in other countries that use the *DSM* for diagnosis about when and how to diagnose and treat depression occurring in the context of the death of a loved one. The rest of this chapter will attempt to clarify those uncertainties.

History of the Bereavement Exclusion in *DSM III* and *IV*

Diagnosing MDE in the aftermath of the death of a loved one is complicated by the fact that bereavement was an exclusion criterion for depression in the *DSM-IV-TR*. According to *DSM-IV-TR*, if the depressive symptoms begin within 2 months of the death of a loved one and do not continue beyond these 2 months, then the diagnosis of depression should not be made. Several exceptions existed, including if the symptoms were associated with marked functional impairment or if one or more of the following "conditional" features were present: suicidal ideation, morbid preoccupation with worthlessness, psychotic symptoms, and/or profound psychomotor retardation.

The bereavement exclusion criteria were first introduced in the *DSM III*, mainly based on the pivotal work of Clayton et al. (Clayton, Desmarai, & Winokur, 1968; Clayton, 1990; Clayton & Darvish, 1979) who showed a high rate of major depressive syndromes in recently bereaved individuals. These depressive syndromes were relatively mild, differed from clinical depression in several aspects, and often resolved over time without treatment. Notably, there are no such exclusion criteria in the International Diagnostic Classification of Diseases.

Research Indicating a Reconsideration of the Validity of the Bereavement Exclusion and Changes in the *DSM-5*

Several comprehensive reviews (Iglewicz, Seay, Vigeant, et al., 2013; Iglewicz, Seay, Zetumer, & Zisook, 2013; Zisook, Corruble, Duan, et al., 2012; Zisook & Kendler, 2007; Zisook, Shear, & Kendler, 2007) and data from subsequent studies focusing on the validity of the bereavement exclusion for the diagnosis of MDD suggested that it was time to eliminate the bereavement exclusion (Brent, Melhem, Donohoe, & Walker, 2009; Corruble, Chouinard, Letierce, Gorwood, & Chouinard, 2009; Corruble, Falissard, & Gorwood, 2011; Corruble, Gorwood, & Chouinard, 2010; Karam et al., 2009; Kendler, Myers, & Zisook, 2008; Kessing, Bukh, Bock, Vinberg, & Gether, 2010; Wakefield, Schmitz, First, & Horwitz, 2007).

First, in a secondary analysis of the National Comorbidity Study, Wakefield and colleagues (2007) compared MDD after bereavement to depressive syndromes occurring after other stressful life events. They found that MDD after bereavement was far more similar than different to MDD after other life events. Although the investigators did not conclude that the data support removal of the bereavement exclusion, other experts have debated these conclusions (Kendler & Zisook, 2009; Pies & Zisook, 2010; Wakefield, Schmitz, First, & Horwitz, 2009).

In another secondary analysis of a large community-based study, Kendler, Myers, and Zisook (2008) also compared individuals with bereavement-related depression to those with MDD related to other stressful life events and found that bereavement-related depressions were strikingly similar to non-bereavement, stress-related depressions in most demographic risk factors, familiality, past histories of MDD, personality characteristics, comorbidity, symptom patterns, intensity, impairment, and course. The investigators concluded that there was no rational reason to single out bereavement as the lone disqualifying life event for the diagnosis of MDD. Thus, they recommended removing the bereavement exclusion from future editions of the *DSM*. Similar results were found in population-based studies in Lebanon (Karam et al., 2009), in US children who lost parents to suicide, accident, or sudden natural death (Brent, Melhem, Donohoe, & Walker, 2009), and in studies of clinical populations in Denmark (Kessing, Bukh, Bock, Vinberg, & Gether, 2010) and France (Corruble, Chouinard, Letierce, Gorwood, & Chouinard, 2009; Corruble, Falissard, & Gorwood, 2011; Corruble, Gorwood, & Chouinard, 2010). In the latter series of studies, participants who were not given the diagnosis of MDE on the basis of clinicians' understanding of *DSM-IV* criteria were found to have more severe symptoms of depression than were MDE controls without bereavement, and they responded at least as well to antidepressant medications. In addition, many individuals who should have been excluded based on *DSM-IV* criteria were not, suggesting that the bereavement exclusion is not being used as intended and may lead to more confusion than clarity of diagnosis (Corruble, 2013; Corruble, Chouinard, Letierce, Gorwood, & Chouinard, 2009; Corruble, Falissard, & Gorwood, 2011). These studies made a strong argument that bereavement-related depression is more similar than not to other, nonbereavement-related instances of MDD, laid the foundation for the American Psychiatric Association's *DSM-5* Mood Disorders Taskforce proposal to eliminate the bereavement exclusion from *DSM-5* (M. K. Shear et al., 2011; http://www.dsm5.org/proposedrevision/Pages/DepressiveDisorders.aspx), and ultimately set the stage for the removal of the bereavement exclusion from the *DSM-5*. The respective changes in the *DSM*-5 regarding diagnostic criteria for a major depressive disorder denote that depressive syndromes occurring in the context of bereavement should be taken as seriously as depressive symptoms occurring in any other context.

DISTINGUISHING BETWEEN GRIEF AND DEPRESSION

Diagnosing MDD in the context of acute grief can challenge even the most experienced clinicians. Several features of "normal" grief and depression overlap. Mood changes, anhedonia, guilt, sleep disturbance, and, at times, suicidal ideation may be present in both conditions (Lamb, Pies, & Zisook, 2010; Pies, 2009; Zisook, Reynolds et al., 2010). Yet, the quality of these symptoms differs between grief and depression (Lamb, Pies, &

Zisook, 2010; Zisook, Reynolds, et al., 2010). These qualitative differences are thus key aspects of differential diagnosis. Although sadness is present in both grief and depression, the sadness typically is pervasive in depression, whereas with grief the sadness comes in waves and is intermixed with pleasant emotions and memories. Similarly, the anhedonia in depression is omnipresent, whereas the anhedonia in grief is tied specifically to longing for the deceased. Depression-related guilt is often associated with feelings of worthlessness. Meanwhile, grief-related guilt characteristically centers on thoughts of letting the deceased loved one down (i.e., not doing enough for them while they were alive, the "could haves" and "should haves"). In the absence of co-occurring MDD, grieving individuals are rarely suicidal. However, when thoughts of dying are present in bereaved individuals they tend to be focused on a longing for reunion with the deceased. In contrast, suicidal ideation in depressed individuals often relates to feelings of worthlessness and not deserving to live (Zisook & Shear, 2009). Even the perception of time can be used to distinguish between grief and depression. Grieving individuals often understand that grief is limited and life will improve over time. But, depressed individuals can experience time as slowed or frozen and their depression as inexhaustible (Lamb, Pies, & Zisook, 2010).

Table 29.2 compares the distinguishing phenomenology of grief and depression. Yet, even when one is cognizant of the distinguishing qualitative features, determining whether an independent MDE is present in an acutely bereaved individual can be perplexing. It is important for the clinician to remember that the timing of the onset of symptoms is just one of many features to consider. Even more important are severity and pervasiveness of symptoms and their effects on functioning. When in doubt, past and family histories can be helpful. It is useful for clinicians to remember that the death of a loved one may trigger **BOTH** acute grief **AND** the onset or worsening of an MDE; grief and depression often occur simultaneously. Subsequently, the decision regarding whether a bereaved person is "just grieving" or also has a co-occurring MDE should not be reduced to an either/or conundrum. Recognizing the possibility of MDD in the context of bereavement is not meant to "medicalize" grief; rather, it is meant to facilitate accurate diagnosis and appropriate treatment for those bereaved individuals suffering from an episode of major depression.

Table 29.2 QUALITATIVE PHENOMENOLOGICAL DIFFERENCES BETWEEN GRIEF AND DEPRESSION

	GRIEF	MAJOR DEPRESSIVE DISORDER
Mood/Sadness	Comes in waves and mixed with happy emotions, especially when recounting pleasant memories of the deceased loved one	Pervasive
Anhedonia	Related to longing for the deceased loved one	Pervasive
Suicidal Ideation	Connected with longing for reunion with the deceased loved one	Connected with feelings of not deserving to live
Guilt	Focused on letting the deceased loved one down	Focused on self loathing and worthlessness
Functional Impairment	Intermittent, typically lasts days to weeks	Pervasive, often lasts weeks to months

CONCURRENT GRIEF AND DEPRESSION

Bereavement is a stressor that places vulnerable individuals at higher risk for developing a clinically significant MDE (Umberson, Wortman, & Kessler, 1992). A systematic review of risk factors for MDE in older adults indicates that recent bereavement is a stronger predictor of the development of MDE than are prior episodes of depression, female gender, disability, and sleep disturbance (odds ratio of 3.3 compared to 2.3, 1.4, 2.5, and 2.6 respectively; see Cole & Dendukuri, 2003). Approximately 20% of bereaved adults (Zisook, Paulus, Shuchter, & Judd, 1997; Zisook & Shuchter, 1993) and children (D. Brent, Melhem, Donohoe, & Walker, 2009; D. A. Brent, Peters, & Weller, 1994; Melhem, Walker, Moritz, & Brent, 2008) may experience a comorbid MDE. Although the rates of MDE decrease over time after the loss, the best predictor of MDE 13 months after the loss of a loved one is MDE at 2 months after the loss, even more so than other risk factors such as a family history of MDD, lack of treatment, and the deceased having died by suicide (Zisook, Paulus, Shuchter, & Judd, 1997). When grief and depression occur together, the grief is more protracted and severe than grief without depression. For example, bereaved widows who develop MDE within 2 months of their loss have more difficult physical and emotional experiences with grief than do bereaved widows without comorbid depression (Zisook & Shuchter, 1993). Since bereavement is a universal stressor that places certain individuals at higher risk for depression and concurrent grief, and depression is associated with worse physical and psychological outcomes than grief alone, it is imperative that we recognize and treat depression in grieving individuals.

TREATMENT OF BEREAVEMENT-RELATED DEPRESSION

The two key questions are (1) when to treat and (2) how to treat. Regarding the first, decisions likely should be made just as in depressions triggered by other stressful life circumstances. The diagnosis of MDD is not enough to warrant active treatment, as many episodes are short-lived and may remit without formal interventions (Posternak et al., 2006). As in other, nonbereavement instances of MDD, the decision rests on the severity, intensity, and pervasiveness of symptoms; past history of MDD; previous outcomes to treatment; comorbidities; safety; and patient preferences. Sometimes the best initial treatment combines support, education, and watchful waiting; but if symptoms worsen, persist, or interfere with functioning, more active treatment should be considered. For someone with a past history of severe or life-threatening MDD who is not currently on maintenance treatment, the clinician might strongly consider reinstituting treatment even before symptoms emerge when there is either an impending or recent death of a loved one.

The second question, how to treat, also bears resemblance to optimizing treatment options for any bereavement or non-bereavement related depressions. At present there is a paucity of data confirming the effectiveness of psychotherapy for either preventing or treating MDD associated with bereavement. Yet, there is no reason to suspect that psychotherapy should not be as effective, either alone or in combination with medications, as it is in other, nonbereavement-related instances of MDD. On the other hand, there are at least eight studies documenting the effectiveness of antidepressant medications for bereavement-related depression (Corruble, Falissard, & Gorwood, 2011; Hensley, Slonimski, Uhlenhuth, & Clayton, 2009; Jacobs, Nelson, & Zisook, 1987; Kessing, Bukh, Bock, Vinberg, & Gether, 2010; Pasternak et al., 1991; Reynolds et al., 1999; Zisook, Shuchter, Pedrelli, Sable, & Deaciuc, 2001). The authors favor following American Psychiatric Association Treatment Guidelines (American Psychiatric Association, 2010), which suggest either psychotherapy or medications for relatively mild depressions depending on past responses, availability, costs, and patient preferences. For more severe depressions, medications play a more predominant role, but combinations of psychotherapy and medications are the treatments of choice for very severe or complicated MDD or when a single approach has not been sufficient. The key is to not dismiss treating depression when grief is present, falsely rationalizing that depression is "understandable." Rather, in light of the profound physical and psychological burden of concurrent grief and depression, the depression should be recognized and treated with the same compassion and diligence utilized when treating depression associated with other life stressors (Ganadjian & Zisook, 2009; Zisook, Reynolds et al., 2010).

SUMMARY

Bereavement is a severe psychosocial stressor which often triggers a grief response that, albeit painful and distressing, is self-limiting, becomes integrated into the ongoing fabric of one's being, and does not require professional attention. However, in vulnerable individuals the grief process can become derailed, impeding healing and leading to the syndrome of CG. In addition, bereavement may trigger MDD in vulnerable individuals whether or not CG occurs. Each of these untoward adverse consequences of bereavement is fraught with diagnostic challenges, is often missed in clinical populations, and may lead to ongoing suffering and morbidity. When accurately diagnosed, both CG and MDD associated with bereavement respond to targeted treatments that can profoundly improve the quality of life of certain grieving individuals, oftentimes making the difference between a life of ongoing suffering and disability and a life filled with meaning and satisfaction. Studies of CG and bereavement-related depression are in their infancy, but as these conditions become better known, understood, and legitimized as appropriate targets for scientific study, future investigations will no doubt lead to more refined diagnostic strategies and treatment guidelines.

CLINICAL PEARLS

- Up to 10% may have complicated grief.

- Maladaptive attitudes and behaviors that impede resolution of grief include the following: intense blame of self or others, fear of being overwhelmed by the intensity of grief, persistent avoidance of reminders of the deceased, the prospect of life without the deceased, or a disinclination to engage in activities that were shared with the deceased.

- Death by suicide or death of soul mate are additional risk factors for complicated grief.

- The core features of complicated grief—longing, pining, preoccupation and avoidance—are not characteristic features of major depressive disorder.

- Complicated grief often co-occurs with PTSD, but the predominant affect of complicated grief is longing and yearning rather than fear.

- It is useful for clinicians to remember that the death of a loved one may trigger **BOTH** acute grief **AND** the onset or worsening of a major depressive episode.

- A meaningful minority of bereaved adults and children will experience a clinically meaningful and persistent major depressive episode in the wake of their loss.

- The best predictor of a major depressive episode 13 months after the loss of a loved one is a major depressive episode at 2 months after the loss.

- For someone with a past history of severe or life-threatening major depressive disorder who is not currently on maintenance treatment, the clinician might strongly consider reinstituting treatment (psychotherapy and/or medication) even before symptoms emerge when there is either an impending or recent death of a loved one.

DISCLOSURE STATEMENTS

Dr. Iglewicz has no potential conflicts, direct or indirect, financial or otherwise, to disclose in connection with the chapter submitted.

Dr. Zisook has no conflicts of interest or relationships with industry to disclose.

REFERENCES

Ajdacic-Gross, V., Ring, M., Gadola, E., Lauber, C., Bopp, M., Gutzwiller, F., et al. (2008). Suicide after bereavement: an overlooked problem. *Psychological Medicine*, 38(5), 673–676.

American Psychiatric Association. (2010). Practice Guideline for the Treatment of Patients with Major Depressive Disorder. *American Journal of Psychiatry*, 167(Oct. Suppl.), 1–118.

Boelen, P. A., & Prigerson, H. G. (2007). The influence of symptoms of prolonged grief disorder, depression, and anxiety on quality of life among bereaved adults. *European Archives of Psychiatry and Clinical Neuroscience*, 257(8), 444–452.

Boelen, P. A., van den Bout, J., & van den Hout, M. A. (2006). Negative cognitions and avoidance in emotional problems after bereavement: A prospective study. *Behaviour Research and Therapy*, 44(11), 1657–1672.

Bonanno, G. A., Moskowitz, J. T., Papa, A., & Folkman, S. (2005). Resilience to loss in bereaved spouses, bereaved parents, and bereaved gay men. *Journal of Personality and Social Psychology*, 88(5), 827–843.

Bonanno, G. A., Papa, A., Lalande, K., Zhang, N. P., & Noll, J. G. (2005). Grief processing and deliberate grief avoidance: A prospective comparison of bereaved spouses and parents in the United States and the People's Republic of China. *Journal of Consulting and Clinical Psychology*, 73(1), 86–98.

Brent, D., Melhem, N., Donohoe, M. B., & Walker, M. (2009). The incidence and course of depression in bereaved youth 21 months after the loss of a parent to suicide, accident, or sudden natural death. *American Journal of Psychiatry*, 166(7), 786–794.

Brent, D. A., Peters, M. J., & Weller, E. (1994). Resolved—several weeks of depressive symptoms after exposure to a friends suicide is major depressive disorder. *Journal of the American Academy of Child and Adolescent Psychiatry*, 33(4), 582–587.

Chen, J. H., Bierhals, A. J., Prigerson, H. G., Kasl, S. V., Mazure, C. M., & Jacobs, S. (1999). Gender differences in the effects of bereavement-related psychological distress in health outcomes. *Psychological Medicine*, 29(2), 367–380.

Clayton, P., Desmarai, L., & Winokur, G. (1968). A Study of Normal Bereavement. *American Journal of Psychiatry*, 125(2), 168–178.

Clayton, P. J. (1990). Bereavement and depression. *Journal of Clinical Psychiatry*, 51, 34–38.

Clayton, P. J., & Darvish, H. S. (1979). Course of depressive symptoms following the stress of bereavement. In Barrett, J. E., R. M. Rose and G. L. Klerman (Eds.), *Stress and Mental Disorder* (pp. 121–136). New York: Raven Press.

Cole, M. G., & Dendukuri, N. (2003). Risk factors for depression among elderly community subjects: A systematic review and meta-analysis. *American Journal of Psychiatry*, 160(6), 1147–1156.

Corruble, E. (2013). The discriminant validity of DSM-IV bereavement exclusion for the diagnosis of major depression: results of naturalistic real-world studies in France. *Psychiatry Annual*, 43(6), 272–275.

Corruble, E., Chouinard, V.-A., Letierce, A., Gorwood, P. A. P. A., & Chouinard, G. (2009). Is DSM-IV bereavement exclusion for major depressive episode relevant to severity and pattern of symptoms? A case-control, cross-sectional study. *Journal of Clinical Psychiatry*, 70(8), 1091–1097.

Corruble, E., Falissard, B., & Gorwood, P. (2011). Is DSM-IV bereavement exclusion for major depression relevant to treatment response? A case-control, prospective study. *Journal of Clinical Psychiatry*, 72(7), 898–902.

Corruble, E., Gorwood, P. A. P. M., & Chouinard, G. (2010). Dr. Corruble and colleagues reply. *Journal of Clinical Psychiatry*, 71(3), 360–360.

Cruz, M., Scott, J., Houck, P., Reynolds, C. F., III, Frank, E., & Shear, M. K. (2007). Clinical presentation and treatment outcome of African Americans with complicated grief. *Psychiatric Services*, 58(5), 700–702.

Ganadjian, K., & Zisook, S. (2009). Bereavement. In R. E. Ingram (Ed.), *The encyclopedia of depression* (pp. 70–73). New York: Spinger Publishing Company.

Ghaffari-Nejad, A., Ahmadi-Mousavi, M., Gandomkar, M., & Reihani-Kermani, H. (2007). The prevalence of complicated grief among Bam earthquake survivors in Iran. *Archives of Iranian Medicine*, 10(4), 525–528.

Goldsmith, B., Morrison, R. S., Vanderwerker, L. C., & Prigerson, H. G. (2008). Elevated rates of prolonged grief disorder in African Americans. *Death Studies*, 32(4), 352–365.

Hardison, H. G., Neimeyer, R. A., & Lichstein, K. L. (2005). Insomnia and complicated grief symptoms in bereaved college students. *Behavioral sleep medicine*, 3(2), 99–111.

Hensley, P. L., Slonimski, C. K., Uhlenhuth, E. H., & Clayton, P. J. (2009). Escitalopram: An open-label study of bereavement-related depression and grief. *Journal of Affective Disorders*, 113(1–2), 142–149.

Iglewicz, A., Seay, K., Vigeant, S., Jouhal, S. K., & Zisook, S. (2013). The bereavement exclusion: the truth between pathology and politics. *Psychiatry Annual*, 43(6), 261–266.

Iglewicz, A., Seay, K., Zetumer, S. D., & Zisook, S. (2013). The removal of the bereavement exclusion in the DSM-5: exploring the evidence. *Current Psychiatry Reports*, 15(11), 413.

Jacobs, S. C., Nelson, J. C., & Zisook, S. (1987). Treating depressions of bereavement with antidepressants—a pilot-study. *Psychiatric Clinics of North America*, 10(3), 501–510.

Jordan, J. R. (2008). Bereavement after suicide. *Psychiatric Annals*, 38(10), 679–685.

Karam, E. G., Tabet, C. C., Alam, D., Shamseddeen, W., Chatila, Y., Mneimneh, Z., et al. (2009). Bereavement related and non-bereavement related depressions: A comparative field study. *Journal of Affective Disorders*, 112(1–3), 102–110.

Kendler, K. S., Myers, J., & Zisook, S. (2008). Does bereavement-related major depression differ from major depression associated with other stressful life events? *American Journal of Psychiatry*, 165(11), 1449–1455.

Kendler, K. S., & Zisook, S. (2009). The importance of the main effect even within an interaction model: Elimination vs. expansion of the bereavement exclusion in the diagnostic criteria for depression reply. *American Journal of Psychiatry*, 166(4), 492–493.

Kersting, A., Kroker, K., Steinhard, J., Luedorff, K., Wesselmann, U., Ohrmann, P., et al. (2007). Complicated grief after traumatic loss—A 14-month follow up study. *European Archives of Psychiatry and Clinical Neuroscience*, 257(8), 437–443.

Kessing, L. V., Bukh, J. D., Bock, C., Vinberg, M., & Gether, U. (2010). Does bereavement-related first episode depression differ from other kinds of first depressions? *Social Psychiatry and Psychiatric Epidemiology*, 45(8), 801–808.

Lamb, K., Pies, R., & Zisook, S. (2010). The bereavement exclusion for the diagnosis of major depression: To be, or not to be. *Psychiatry (Edgmont)*, 7(7), 19–25.

Langner, R., & Maercker, A. (2005). Complicated grief as a stress response disorder: evaluating diagnostic criteria in a German sample. *Journal of Psychosomatic Research*, 58(3), 235–242.

Lannen, P. K., Wolfe, J., Prigerson, H. G., Onelov, E., & Kreicbergs, U. C. (2008). Unresolved grief in a national sample of bereaved parents: Impaired mental and physical health 4 to 9 years later. *Journal of Clinical Oncology*, 26(36), 5870–5876.

Latham, A. E., & Prigerson, H. G. (2004). Suicidality and bereavement: Complicated grief as psychiatric disorder presenting greatest risk for suicidality. *Suicide and Life-Threatening Behavior*, 34(4), 350–362.

Lichtenthal, W. G., Cruess, D. G., & Prigerson, H. G. (2004). A case for establishing complicated grief as a distinct mental disorder in DSM-V. *Clinical Psychology Review*, 24(6), 637–662.

Lieberman, M. A., & Videkasherman, L. (1986). The impact of self-help groups on the mental-health of widows and widowers. *American Journal of Orthopsychiatry*, 56(3), 435–449.

Marmar, C. R., Horowitz, M. J., Weiss, D. S., Wilner, N. R., & Kaltreider, N. B. (1988). A controlled trial of brief psychotherapy and mutual-help group treatment of conjugal bereavement. *American Journal of Psychiatry*, 145(2), 203–209.

Melhem, N. M., Moritz, G., Walker, M., Shear, M. K., & Brent, D. (2007). Phenomenology and correlates of complicated grief in children and adolescents. *Journal of the American Academy of Child and Adolescent Psychiatry*, 46(4), 493–499.

Melhem, N. M., Walker, M., Moritz, G., & Brent, D. A. (2008). Antecedents and sequelae of sudden parental death in offspring and surviving caregivers. *Archives of Pediatrics & Adolescent Medicine*, 162(5), 403–410.

Middleton, W., Raphael, B., Burnett, P., & Martinek, N. (1998). A longitudinal study comparing bereavement phenomena in recently bereaved spouses, adult children and parents. *Australian and New Zealand Journal of Psychiatry*, 32(2), 235–241.

Mitchell, A. M., Kim, Y., Prigerson, H. G., & Mortimer, M. K. (2005). Complicated grief and suicidal ideation in adult survivors of suicide. *Suicide and Life-Threatening Behavior*, 35(5), 498–506.

Momartin, S., Silove, D., Manicavasagar, V., & Steel, Z. (2004). Complicated grief in Bosnian refugees: Associations with posttraumatic stress disorder and depression. *Comprehensive Psychiatry*, 45(6), 475–482.

Monk, T. H., Houck, P. R., & Shear, M. K. (2006). The daily life of complicated grief patients—What gets missed, what gets added? *Death Studies*, 30(1), 77–85.

Morina, N., Rudari, V., Bleichhardt, G., & Prigerson, H. G. (2010). Prolonged grief disorder, depression, and posttraumatic stress disorder among bereaved Kosovar civilian war survivors: a preliminary investigation. *International Journal of Social Psychiatry*, 56(3), 288–297.

Newson, R. S., Boelen, P. A., Hek, K., Hofman, A., & Tiemeier, H. (2011). The prevalence and characteristics of complicated grief in older adults. *Journal of Affective Disorders*, 132(1–2), 231–238.

Pasternak, R. E., Reynolds, C. F., Schlernitzauer, M., Hoch, C. C., Buysse, D. J., Houck, P. R., et al. (1991). Acute open-trial nortriptyline therapy of bereavement-related depression in late life. *Journal of Clinical Psychiatry*, 52(7), 307–310.

Pies R, & Zisook S. (2010). Grief and depression redux: response to Dr. Frances's "compromise". *Psychiatric Times*. http://www.psychiatrictimes.com/dsm-5/content/article/10168/1679026

Pies, R. W. (2009). Pseudoresistant bipolar depression. *Journal of Clinical Psychiatry*, 70(10), 1476–1477.

Piper, W. E., McCallum, M., Joyce, A. S., Rosie, J. S., & Ogrodniczuk, J. S. (2001). Patient personality and time-limited group psychotherapy for complicated grief. *International Journal of Group Psychotherapy*, 51(4), 525–552.

Piper, W. E., Ogrodniczuk, J. S., Joyce, A. S., Weideman, R., & Rosie, J. S. (2007). Group composition and group therapy for complicated grief. *Journal of Consulting and Clinical Psychology*, 75(1), 116–125.

Posternak, M. A., Solomon, D. A., Leon, A. C., Mueller, T. I., Shea, M. T., Endicott, J., et al. (2006). The naturalistic course of unipolar major depression in the absence of somatic therapy. *Journal of Nervous and Mental Disease*, 194(5), 324–329.

Prigerson, H., Ahmed, I., Silverman, G. K., Saxena, A. K., Maciejewski, P. K., Jacobs, S. C., et al. (2002). Rates and risks of complicated grief among psychiatric clinic patients in Karachi, Pakistan. *Death Studies*, 26(10), 781–792.

Prigerson, H., Silverman, G., Jacobs, S., Maciejewski, P., Kasl, S., & Rosenheck, R. (2001). Traumatic grief, disability and the underutilization of health services: a preliminary look. *Prim Psychiatry*(8), 61–69.

Prigerson, H. G., Bierhals, A. J., Kasl, S. V., Reynolds, C. F., Shear, M. K., Day, N., et al. (1997). Traumatic grief as a risk factor for mental and physical morbidity. *American Journal of Psychiatry*, 154(5), 616–623.

Prigerson, H. G., Bridge, J., Maciejewski, P. K., Beery, L. C., Rosenheck, R. A., Jacobs, S. C., et al. (1999). Influence of traumatic grief on suicidal ideation among young adults. *American Journal of Psychiatry*, 156(12), 1994–1995.

Prigerson, H. G., Horowitz, M. J., Jacobs, S. C., Parkes, C. M., Aslan, M., Goodkin, K., et al. (2009). Prolonged grief disorder: Psychometric validation of criteria proposed for DSM-V and ICD-11. *Plos Medicine*, 6(8).

Prigerson, H. G., Maciejewski, P. K., Reynolds, C. F., Bierhals, A. J., Newsom, J. T., Fasiczka, A., et al. (1995). Inventory of complicated grief: A scale to measure maladaptive symptoms of loss. *Psychiatry Research*, 59(1–2), 65–79.

Reynolds, C. F., Miller, M. D., Pasternak, R. E., Frank, E., Perel, J. M., Cornes, C., et al. (1999). Treatment of bereavement-related major depressive episodes in later life: A controlled study of acute and continuation treatment with nortriptyline and interpersonal psychotherapy. *American Journal of Psychiatry*, 156(2), 202–208.

Saindon, C., et al. (2014). Restorative retelling for violent loss: an open clinical trial. *Death studies*, 38(4).

Schaal, S., Elbert, T., & Neuner, F. (2009). Prolonged grief disorder and depression in widows due to the Rwandan genocide. *Omega–Journal of Death and Dying*, 59(3), 203–219.

Shear, K., Frank, E., Houck, P. R., & Reynolds, C. F. (2005). Treatment of complicated grief—A randomized controlled trial. *Journal of the American Medical Association*, 293(21), 2601–2608.

Shear, K., Monk, T., Houck, P., Melhem, N., Frank, E., Reynolds, C., et al. (2007). An attachment-based model of complicated grief including the role of avoidance. *European Archives of Psychiatry and Clinical Neuroscience*, 257(8), 453–461.

Shear, M. K. (2010). Exploring the role of experiential avoidance from the perspective of attachment theory and the dual process model. *Omega–Journal of Death and Dying, 61*(4), 357–369.

Shear, M. K., Frank, E., Foa, E., Cherry, C., Reynolds, C. F., Vander Bilt, J., et al. (2001). Traumatic grief treatment: A pilot study. *American Journal of Psychiatry, 158*(9), 1506–1508.

Shear, M. K., Simon, N., Wall, M., Zisook, S., Neimeyer, R., Duan, N., et al. (2011). Complicated grief and related bereavement issues for DSM-5. *Depression and Anxiety, 28*(2), 103–117.

Simon, N. M., Shear, K. M., Thompson, E. H., Zalta, A. K., Perlman, C., Reynolds, C. F., et al. (2007). The prevalence and correlates of psychiatric comorbidity in individuals with complicated grief. *Comprehensive Psychiatry, 48*(5), 395–399.

Simon, N. M., Shear, M. K., Fagiolini, A., Frank, E., Zalta, A., Thompson, E. H., et al. (2008). Impact of concurrent naturalistic pharmacotherapy on psychotherapy of complicated grief. *Psychiatry Research, 159*(1–2), 31–36. http://clinicaltrials.gov/ct2/show/NCT01244295?term=complicated+grief+treatment&rank=1

Simon, N. M., Thompson, E. H., Pollack, M. H., & Shear, M. K. (2007). Complicated grief: A case series using Escitalopram. *American Journal of Psychiatry, 164*(11), 1760–1761.

Stroebe, M., Boelen, P. A., van den Hout, M., Stroebe, W., Salemink, E., & van den Bout, J. (2007). Ruminative coping as avoidance—A reinterpretation of its function in adjustment to bereavement. *European Archives of Psychiatry and Clinical Neuroscience, 257*(8), 462–472.

Stroebe, M., Hansson, R., Stroebe, W., & Schut, H. (2001). *Handbook of bereavement research: consequences, coping and care.* Washington, DC: American Psychological Association.

Stroebe, M., Stroebe, W., & Abakoumkin, G. (2005). The broken heart: Suicidal ideation in bereavement. *American Journal of Psychiatry, 162*(11), 2178–U2173.

Szanto, K., Prigerson, H., Houck, P., Ehrenpreis, L., & Reynolds, C. F. (1997). Suicidal ideation in elderly bereaved: The role of complicated grief. *Suicide and Life-Threatening Behavior, 27*(2), 194–207.

Szanto, K., Shear, M. K., Houck, P. R., Reynolds, C. F., Frank, E., Caroff, K., et al. (2006). Indirect self-destructive behavior and overt suicidality in patients with complicated grief. *Journal of Clinical Psychiatry, 67*(2), 233–239.

Umberson, D., Wortman, C. B., & Kessler, R. C. (1992). Widowhood and depression—Explaining long-term gender differences in vulnerability. *Journal of Health and Social Behavior, 33*(1), 10–24.

Wagner, B., Knaevelsrud, C., & Maercker, A. (2006). Internet-based cognitive-behavioral therapy for complicated grief: A randomized controlled trial. *Death Studies, 30*(5), 429–453.

Wakefield, J. C., Schmitz, M. F., First, M. B., & Horwitz, A. V. (2007). Extending the bereavement exclusion for major depression to other losses—Evidence from the National Comorbidity Survey. *Archives of General Psychiatry, 64*(4), 433–440.

Wakefield, J. C., Schmitz, M. F., First, M. B., & Horwitz, A. V. (2009). The importance of the main effect even within an interaction model: Elimination vs. expansion of the bereavement exclusion in the diagnostic criteria for depression. *American Journal of Psychiatry, 166*(4), 491–492.

Wittouck, C., Van Autreve, S., De Jaegere, E., Portzky, G., & van Heeringen, K. (2011). The prevention and treatment of complicated grief: A meta-analysis. *Clinical Psychology Review, 31*(1), 69–78.

Zisook, S., Corruble, E., Duan, N., Iglewicz, A., Karam, E. G., Lanouette, N., et al. (2012). The bereavement exclusion and DSM-5. *Depress Anxiety, 29*(5), 425–443.

Zisook S, Reynolds CF, Pies R, & et al. (2010). Bereavement, complicated grief, and DSM, part 1: depression. *Journal of Clinical Psychiatry, 71*, 955–956.

Zisook, S., & Kendler, K. S. (2007). Is bereavement-related depression different than non-bereavement-related depression? *Psychological Medicine, 37*(6), 779–794.

Zisook, S., Paulus, M., Shuchter, S. R., & Judd, L. L. (1997). The many faces of depression following spousal bereavement. *Journal of Affective Disorders, 45*(1–2), 85–94.

Zisook, S., Reynolds, C. F., III, Pies, R., Simon, N., Lebowitz, B., Madowitz, J., et al. (2010). Bereavement, complicated grief, and DSM, Part 1: Depression. *Journal of Clinical Psychiatry, 71*(7), 955–956.

Zisook, S., & Shear, K. (2009). Grief and bereavement: What psychiatrists need to know. *World Psychiatry, 8*(2), 67–74.

Zisook, S., Shear, K., & Kendler, K. S. (2007). Validity of the bereavement exclusion criterion for the diagnosis of major depressive episode. *World Psychiatry, 6*(2), 38–43.

Zisook, S., & Shuchter, S. R. (1993). Uncomplicated bereavement. *Journal of Clinical Psychiatry, 54*(10), 365–372.

Zisook, S., Shuchter, S. R., & Lyons, L. E. (1987). Predictors of psychological reactions during the early stages of widowhood. *Psychiatric Clinics of North America, 10*(3), 355–368.

Zisook, S., Shuchter, S. R., Pedrelli, P., Sable, J., & Deaciuc, S. C. (2001). Bupropion sustained release for bereavement: Results of an open trial. *Journal of Clinical Psychiatry, 62*(4), 227–230.

Zisook, S., Simon, N. M., Reynolds, C. F., III, Pies, R., Lebowitz, B., Young, I. T., et al. (2010). Bereavement, complicated grief, and DSM, Part 2: Complicated grief. *Journal of Clinical Psychiatry, 71*(8), 1097–1098.

30.

ACUTE AND CHRONIC REACTIONS TO TRAUMA

T. H. Eric Bui, M. Alexandra Kredlow, Meredith E. Charney, Mary C. Zeng, and Naomi M. Simon

INTRODUCTION

Psychological reactions to trauma have been vividly described since antiquity (Birmes et al., 2010). According to Plutarch (1920), in his biography of famous lives, general and Roman consul Caius Marius (157–86 BC), when presented with a reminder of one of his dreaded enemies, was gripped with an "overpowering thought of a new war, of fresh struggles, of terrors known by experience to be dreadful" and descended "into a state of dreadful despair, and was prey to nightly terrors and harassing dreams." Although described since antiquity, these psychological responses had not been viewed under a pathological lens until the first descriptions of "traumatic neuroses" in the 19th century (Oppenheim, 1889). Finally, it was in the aftermath of the Vietnam War that trauma-related psychological disturbances truly became an independent field of research.

Exposure to a traumatic event may lead to the development of a variety of reactions ranging from relatively mild (causing minor disruptions in the individual's life) to severe and debilitating. It is worth highlighting that most traumatized people will develop some level of psychological stress responses which are generally brief and short lived. In some, however, symptoms do not spontaneously remit and instead become clinically significant, persistent, and impairing.

Reactions to trauma exposure have thus been defined according to their time frame: immediate or peritraumatic reactions, lasting minutes to hours; acute stress disorder (ASD), which lasts between 2 days and 1 month; and post-traumatic stress disorder (PTSD), when symptoms persist for more than a month. PTSD can also occur after a symptom-free period of up to several years. However, by definition, delayed-onset PTSD refers to cases in which symptoms occur at least 6 months after the trauma. Although other psychiatric conditions such as depression might also result from traumatization, in this chapter we will review the different types of psychopathological reactions specific to trauma.

TRAUMA AND TRAUMATIC EVENTS

DEFINITIONS

Trauma, which derives from the Greek word τραῦμα, meaning *wound*, has been medically defined for centuries as "an injury (as a wound) to living tissue caused by an extrinsic agent" (Merriam-Webster, 1995). It was not until 1889, however, that this word was applied to the field that was yet to be known as mental health, by Oppenheim (1889) in his clinical descriptions of "traumatic neuroses" in victims of railroad accidents. From then on, the term *trauma* endorsed both a physical and a psychological signification.

A traumatic event has been commonly described as presenting three characteristics: (1) it happens suddenly and unexpectedly, (2) it threatens the individual's physical integrity, and (3) it does not belong in the normal range of events experienced during life. These three specific features differentiate it from other distressing events such as grief, medical disease, or romantic breakups. Furthermore, Terr suggested that psychological trauma, regardless of its being sudden or not, should be defined based on whether the traumatic events are repeated or not (Terr, 1991). According to her, type I traumas are time-limited single traumatic events (accident, disaster, etc.), and type II concern long-standing or repeated exposure to traumatic events that can be without the element of surprise (abuse, torture, combat situation, etc.).

While in the fourth edition of the *Diagnostic and Statistical Manual of Mental Disorders* (*DSM-IV*) traumatic events were defined as "events that involve actual or threatened death or serious injury, or a threat to the physical integrity of oneself or others" (criterion A1) accompanied by a feeling of "intense fear, helplessness, or horror" (criterion A2), the fifth edition (*DSM-5*) has dropped the required subjective reaction (A2) to the trauma (APA, 2013). Traumatic events include direct exposure (i.e., being a victim), witnessing a traumatic event, or learning that it occurred to someone close. The new definition also includes extreme and repeated exposure to trauma details (as experienced by first responders), but excludes exposure through the media unless it is work-related.

Of note, while the stressor criteria of the *DSM-III-R* (APA, 1983) necessitated that the traumatic event be "outside the range of normal human experience," this is no longer the case in either the *DSM-IV-TR* or the *DSM-5*. Thus, while the *DSM-III-R* excluded life-threatening illness as a stressor qualifying for criterion A of the PTSD diagnosis, the *DSM-IV-TR* and *DSM-5* include it as a potential traumatic event.

This subsequently paved the way for an increasing number of studies on the traumatizing effects of medical illnesses, such as cancer. Thus, potential cancer-related traumatic events could be receiving the diagnosis, fear of the surgery and chemotherapy, or detecting a lump (Mehnert & Koch, 2007). This is important as it suggests that clinicians should be aware that giving a diagnosis of cancer may results in PTSD, which may in turn result in poorer psychological and physical outcome. Further, death may also be considered an A1 qualifying event.

EPIDEMIOLOGY

Estimates of the lifetime prevalence of exposure to a traumatic event range from 39% to 74% for the United States and Canada (Kessler, Sonnega, Bromet, Hughes, & Nelson, 1995; Norris, 1992; Resnick, Kilpatrick, Dansky, Saunders, & Best, 1993); some other developed countries (e.g., Netherlands and New Zealand) fall within that range but some studies suggest a lower rate for others (Hepp et al., 2006; Perkonigg, Kessler, Storz, & Wittchen, 2000; Vaiva et al., 2008). Variances might be accounted for by confounders such as age, gender, or type of events (Breslau, 2001). Additionally, discrepancies might result from differences in measurement methods and the way traumatic events have been defined (Solomon & Davidson, 1997).

Although research on the prevalence of medical illness-related traumatic events is scarce, some studies reported that a substantial amount of life threatening illness patients met *DSM-IV* PTSD criterion A, as is typical in 41%–54% of breast cancer patients (Mehnert & Koch, 2007; Palmer, Kagee, Coyne, & DeMichele, 2004).

PERITRAUMATIC REACTIONS

When confronted with a traumatic event, individuals often develop immediate reactions of distress. Reactions experienced during and immediately after trauma are called *peritraumatic* and recent developments have identified certain trauma-specific peritraumatic reactions (distress defined in a specific way) and dissociation as robust predictors of the development of chronic and debilitating PTSD (Brewin, Andrews, & Valentine, 2000; Ozer, Best, Lipsey, & Weiss, 2003). While peritraumatic dissociation has been studied for a significant period of time, peritraumatic distress has only become the focus of attention lately.

Peritraumatic distress was proposed as a measure of the intensity of *DSM-IV* PTSD criterion A2 (Brunet et al., 2001)—the feeling of "fear, helplessness and horror" experienced by an individual during or immediately after exposure to a traumatizing event. Furthermore, this dimension also includes such phenomena as "feeling ashamed of one's emotional reactions" or "having difficulty controlling one's bowel and bladder." The Peritraumatic Distress Inventory (PDI) was introduced in 2001 as a measure of peritraumatic distress criterion A2 (Brunet et al., 2001) and evaluates feelings of helplessness, sadness, guilt, shame, frustration, fright, horror, passing out, worry for others, loss of bowel and bladder control, physical reactions, and thoughts of dying. The self-report PDI includes 13 Likert-type items scored from 0–4 ("not at all true" to "extremely true") with a total score ranging from 0 to 52 (Table 30.1). To date, no cut-off has been reported

Table 30.1 PERITRAUMATIC DISTRESS INVENTORY

Please check the boxes corresponding to the best to what you felt during and immediately after the event. If the phrase doesn't apply to how you experienced the event, check the box *"not true at all."*

HOW MUCH IS EACH OF THE FOLLOWING STATEMENTS TRUE OF YOU?	NOT AT ALL TRUE				EXTREMELY TRUE
1. I felt helpless to do more	0	1	2	3	4
2. I felt sadness and grief	0	1	2	3	4
3. I felt frustrated or angry I could not do more	0	1	2	3	4
4. I felt afraid for my safety	0	1	2	3	4
5. I felt guilt that more was not done	0	1	2	3	4
6. I felt ashamed of my emotional reactions	0	1	2	3	4
7. I felt worried about the safety of others	0	1	2	3	4
8. I had the feeling I was about to lose control of my emotions	0	1	2	3	4
9. I had difficulty controlling my bowel and bladder	0	1	2	3	4
10. I was horrified by what happened	0	1	2	3	4
11. I had physical reactions like sweating, shaking, and pounding heart	0	1	2	3	4
12. I felt I might pass out	0	1	2	3	4
13. I thought I might die	0	1	2	3	4

(Brunet et al., 2001)

in the literature. Peritraumatic distress might be considered to be a predictor of PTSD because psychological (Brewin & Holmes, 2003) and neurobiological (Cahill, Prins, Weber, & McGaugh, 1994) models of PTSD both emphasize perceived life threat as a key component in the development of this disorder. In line with this, a number of prospective studies reported that individuals experiencing increased levels of peritraumatic distress were also at risk for PTSD symptoms (Allenou et al., 2010; Bui, Brunet, et al., 2010; Bui, Joubert, et al., 2010). On a conceptual level, PTSD is a fear-based disorder and patients do not really *develop* this disorder per se, but rather still present clinical symptoms of distress and dysfunction 1 month after the trauma. In this sense, *peritraumatic distress* would be more accurately described as a risk factor for the continuation of clinically significant symptoms 1 month after the trauma. In other words, the more "frightened" the individual is during the trauma, the more likely he is to still be frightened 1 month later.

Peritraumatic dissociation refers to alterations in an individual's experience of time, place and person during or shortly after exposure to a traumatic event. The 10-item Peritraumatic Dissociative Experiences Questionnaire has been proposed as a measure of peritraumatic dissociation (Marmar et al., 2007; Tichenor, Marmar, Weiss, Metzler, & Ronfeldt, 1996) and includes items measuring blanking out, a feeling that one is on autopilot, time distortion ("slow motion"), depersonalization (feeling of watching oneself act while having no control over the situation), derealization (feeling of strangeness and unreality of the external world), confusion, amnesia, and reduced awareness.

Dissociative reactions to an extreme stress factor were previously conceptualized as adaptive, viewed as a way to remove oneself from experiencing feelings that are too intense (van der Hart, van Ochten, van Son, Steele, & Lensvelt-Mulders, 2008). Contrary to this belief, empirical studies have recently found that dissociation did not prevent the development of psychopathology and was in fact a risk factor for PTSD (Ozer et al., 2003). These findings are in line with an older theory according to which dissociative reactions reflect a failure in coping and other adaptive psychological mechanisms (Janet, 1909).

Besides these two trauma-specific immediate reactions, traumatized individuals may also develop immediate nonspecific reactions, such as somatic functional symptoms or they might experience aggravation of a preexisting psychiatric condition.

One possible cause of the discrepancy between the prevalence of trauma exposure and the prevalence of PTSD might lie in an interindividual variability of what people experience as traumatizing. Based on data from the National Comorbidity Survey (Kessler et al., 1995), Table 30.2 presents the lifetime prevalence of different trauma types and the probability that a particular trauma type, once selected as the basis for the assessment of PTSD, will be associated with PTSD.

The issue of whether exposure to an event has to be accompanied by a negative subjective reaction (such as fear) to be qualified as "traumatic" has been an ongoing source of discussion. Including negative immediate reactions in the definition of a traumatic event and the diagnostic criteria for PTSD suggests that the trauma is a subjective experience and that it

Table 30.2 LIFETIME PREVALENCE OF TRAUMA AND PROBABILITY TO DEVELOP PTSD BASED ON THE NATIONAL COMORBID SURVEY

| | LIFETIME PREVALENCE OF TRAUMA % (SE) | | PROBABILITY OF PTSD* % (SE) | |
Traumatic Event	Men (n = 2812)	Women (n = 3065)	Men (n = 2812)	Women (n = 3065)
Rape	0.7% (0.2)	9.2% (0.8)	65.0% (15.6)	45.9% (5.9)
Molestation	2.8% (0.5)	12.3% (1.0)	12.2% (5.3)	26.5% (4.0)
Physical attack	11.1% (1.0)	6.9% (0.9)	1.8% (0.9)	21.3% (7.3)
Combat	6.4% (0.9)	0% (n/a)	38.8% (9.9)	n/a
Shock	11.4% (1.1)	12.4% (1.1)	4.4% (1.4)	10.4% (2.0)
Threat with weapon	19% (1.3)	6.8% (0.6)	1.9% (0.8)	32.6% (7.8)
Accident	25% (1.2)	13.8% (1.1)	6.3% (1.8)	8.8% (4.3)
Natural disaster with fire	18.9% (1.4)	15.2% (1.2)	3.7% (1.8)	5.4% (3.8)
Witness	35.6% (2.0)	14.5% (0.7)	6.4% (1.2)	7.5% (1.7)
Neglect	2.1% (0.4)	3.4% (0.5)	23.9% (10.3)	19.7% (7.7)
Physical abuse	3.2% (0.4)	4.8% (0.6)	22.3% (5.2)	48.5% (9.5)
Other qualifying trauma	2.2% (0.5)	2.7% (0.4)	12.7% (4.8)	33.4% (8.0)
Any trauma	60.7% (1.9)	51.2% (1.9)	8.1% (1.0)	20.4% (1.5)

* The probability that a particular trauma type, once selected as the basis for the assessment of PTSD, will be associated with PTSD.

is this subjective negative experience of an event that results in PTSD. Excluding this requirement suggests that only the objective events, in themselves, can result in PTSD. In other words, the question is whether it is the actual event that produces the symptoms.

However, the retention of the negative subjective experience of the stressor (criterion A2) in the current revision of the *DSM* has been the focus of much recent debate, as it has been suggested to confound the stressor and its reaction (Friedman, Resick, Bryant, & Brewin, 2011; Karam et al., 2010). This resulted in the removal of the requirement for a negative subjective experience of the stressor from the PTSD criteria in the current *DSM-5*.

ACUTE STRESS DISORDER

CLINICAL FEATURES

Acute stress disorder, which is a clinical entity occurring in a limited timeframe after trauma exposure, was introduced in the *DSM-IV* in order to differentiate between PTSD, a chronic condition, and short-lived, self-limited, distressing, and impairing reactions to trauma (Koopman, Classen, Cardeña, & Spiegel, 1995). Patients with ASD are individuals at risk for a diagnosis of PTSD one month later (Spiegel, Koopman, Cardeña, & Classen, 1996).

According to the *DSM-5* criteria, ASD may occur when an individual is exposed to a traumatic event through direct exposure (i.e., being a victim) to a life-threatening event, witnessing it, or learning that it occurred to someone close. Clinical presentation is characterized by a cluster of anxiety and dissociative symptoms. In *DSM-IV-TR*, the requisite criteria for diagnosis comprise at least three dissociative symptoms (such as numbing, detachment, reduction in awareness of one's surroundings, derealization, depersonalization, dissociative amnesia), one reexperiencing symptom (such as recurrent images, thoughts, nightmares, or flashback episodes, or distress when confronted with reminders of the traumatic event), avoidance of reminders, and hyperarousal. This is no longer the case in *DSM-V*. The main diagnostic criterion now requires meeting 9 of 14 symptoms, without any particular cluster. Furthermore, like all psychiatric disorder diagnoses, marked distress or impairment is also required. The differences between ASD and PTSD lie in the presence of dissociative symptoms among the symptoms of ASD and the different timeframes: ASD occurs between 3 days and 4 weeks following the traumatic event (Criteria G), while symptoms lasting over 1 month point to a diagnosis of PTSD.

EPIDEMIOLOGY

Across different studies, prevalence rates of ASD in trauma exposed individuals range from 7% to 59% (Bryant, Creamer, O'Donnell, Silove, & McFarlane, 2008; Elklit & Christiansen, 2010) with a mean prevalence of 17.4% (Bryant, 2011). Although one study (Mehnert & Koch, 2007) reported

a relatively low prevalence rate for cancer-related ASD (2.4%), the majority of the literature found rates ranging from 28%–35% (Kangas, Henry, & Bryant, 2005; McGarvey et al., 1998; Pedersen & Zachariae, 2010).

RELATIONSHIP OF ASD TO PTSD

Given that ASD was introduced in order to identify individuals at risk for PTSD and shares similarities with PTSD, studies reported that ASD symptoms significantly predicted the occurrence of PTSD symptoms (Bui, Tremblay, et al., 2010; McKibben, Bresnick, Wiechman Askay, & Fauerbach, 2008; Yasan, Guzel, Tamam, & Ozkan, 2009). It has been consistently found, however, that the majority of persons who experience early posttraumatic symptoms adjust in the following weeks or months (Blanchard et al., 1996; Hamanaka et al., 2006). Furthermore, recent developments have found that ASD symptoms fail to adequately identify people who will later suffer from PTSD. More precisely, a recent systematic review of the literature on 22 published longitudinal studies reported that while ASD's positive predictive power was reasonable, its sensitivity (proportion of people meeting ASD criteria who eventually develop PTSD) was poor (20%–72%), suggesting that most trauma survivors who subsequently develop PTSD do not meet full criteria for ASD (Bryant, 2011).

In conclusion, ASD should be considered as an entity that captures a significant level of distress and impairment and identifies individuals who might require clinical attention. Nonetheless, ASD symptoms or subsyndromal ASD (i.e., symptoms of reexperiencing, arousal, and avoidance, but without dissociation) might still be indicative of a possible subsequent PTSD diagnosis (Bryant, 2011).

ASSESSMENT

The Stanford Acute Stress Reaction Questionnaire (Cardena, Koopman, Classen, Waelde, & Spiegel, 2000), a self-report questionnaire composed of 30 items rated from 0–5 (Box 30.1), has been developed to evaluate ASD symptoms. The Acute Stress Disorder Interview (Bryant, Harvey, Dang, & Sackville, 1998), a 19-item dichotomously scored interview, has been developed to identify individuals suffering from ASD. Both instruments have shown sound psychometric properties and can be used in clinical settings (Bryant, et al., 1998; Cardena, et al., 2000). Because clinician-administered interviews are usually time consuming, self-report measures are preferred for screening purposes.

POSTTRAUMATIC STRESS DISORDER

CLINICAL FEATURES

Consistent with the ASD diagnostic criteria, the *DSM-5* requires for PTSD diagnosis that the individual be subject to a traumatic event (direct exposure, witnessing it, or learning that it occurred to someone close; criterion A). Again,

Box 30.1 STANFORD ACUTE STRESS REACTION QUESTIONNAIRE

Stanford Acute Stress Reaction Questionnaire

Recall the stressful events that occurred in your life during the PAST MONTH.

Briefly describe the one event that was the most disturbing on the lines below:
How disturbing was this event to you? (Please mark one):

Not at all disturbing _____
Somewhat disturbing _____
Moderately disturbing _____
Very disturbing _____
Extremely disturbing _____

Below is a list of experiences people sometimes have during and after a stressful event. Please read each item carefully and decide how well it describes your experience since the stressful event described above. Refer to this event in answering the items that mention "the stressful event." Use the 0–5 point scale shown below and circle the number that best describes your experience. (0 = not experienced, 1 = very rarely experienced, 2 = rarely experienced, 3 = sometimes experienced, 4 = often experienced, 5 = very often experienced)

1. I had difficulty falling or staying asleep.
2. I felt restless.
3. I felt a sense of timelessness.
4. I was slow to respond.
5. I tried to avoid feelings about the stressful event.
6. I had repeated distressing dreams of the stressful event.
7. I felt extremely upset if exposed to events that reminded me of an aspect of the stressful event.
8. I would jump in surprise at the least thing.
9. The stressful event made it difficult for me to perform work or other things I needed to do.
10. I did not have the usual sense of who I am.
11. I tried to avoid activities that reminded me of the stressful event.
12. I felt hypervigilant or "on edge".
13. I experienced myself as though I were a stranger.
14. I tried to avoid conversations about the stressful event.
15. I had a bodily reaction when exposed to reminders of the stressful event.
16. I had problems remembering important details about the stressful event.
17. I tried to avoid thoughts about the stressful event.
18. Things I saw looked different to me from how I know they really looked.
19. I had repeated and unwanted memories of the stressful event.
20. I felt distant from my own emotions.
21. I felt irritable or had outbursts of anger.
22. I avoided contact with people who reminded me of the stressful event.
23. I would suddenly act or feel as if the stressful event was happening again.
24. My mind went blank.
25. I had amnesia for large periods of the stressful event.
26. The stressful event caused problems in my relationships with other people.
27. I had difficulty concentrating.
28. I felt estranged or detached from other people.
29. I had a vivid sense that the stressful event was happening all over again.
30. I tried to stay away from places that reminded me of the stressful event.

On how many days did you experience any of the above symptoms of distress? (Please mark one):
No days _____
One day _____
Two days _____
Three days _____
Four days _____
Five or more days _____

From Stanford Center on Stress and Health website: http://stresshealthcenter.stanford.edu/research/measures.html

life-threatening situations are diverse. Contrary to some earlier concepts of nosology, the life-threatening situation that is the basis of PTSD does not need to be outside the range of normal human experience.

The diagnosis is further defined in criteria B–E as necessitating the presence of symptoms in the four clusters of intrusion, avoidance, alterations in mood and cognition, and alterations in arousal and reactivity. In particular, the following symptoms related to the traumatic event are additionally required for diagnosis:

Criterion B—one or more intrusion symptoms (recurrent, distressing memories or dreams; dissociative experiences such as flashbacks; intense or prolonged psychological distress; and marked physiological reactions);

Criterion C—one or both avoidance symptoms (efforts to avoid distressing memories, thoughts, or feelings; and efforts to avoid external reminders);

Criterion D—two or more negative alterations in cognitions and mood (including dissociative amnesia, exaggerated negative beliefs about the self, diminished interest, feelings of detachment, and inability to experience positive emotions); and

Criterion E—two or more alterations in arousal and reactivity (including irritable or self-destructive behavior, hypervigiliance, exaggerated startle response, difficulty with sleep, and difficulty with concentration).

The duration of the disturbance due to criteria B–E symptoms must last for at least 1 month (criterion F), must cause significant functional impairment (criterion G), and must not be attributable to the effects of a substance or better explained by another medical or psychiatric condition (criterion H).

In contrast to ASD, dissociative symptoms are not included in the diagnostic criteria for PTSD in the *DSM-5*. They are, instead, utilized as a specifier for a PTSD diagnosis. Therefore, if an individual who meets the criteria for PTSD also experiences the symptoms of either depersonalization ("persistent or recurrent experiences of feeling detached from, and as if one were an outside observer of, one's mental processes or body") or derealization ("persistent or recurrent experiences of unreality of surroundings"), that individual is diagnosed with PTSD with dissociative symptoms. The *DSM-5* also includes a specifier for delayed-onset PTSD, which is described as "with delayed expression" if the interval between the traumatic event and the onset of symptoms is more than 6 months; these cases are rare, and patients usually present with some subsyndromal distress prior to developing full-blown PTSD. Clinically significant distress and impairment in the context of a subthreshold PTSD might warrant clinical attention.

Of note, the criteria listed for PTSD above apply to individuals over the age of six years. For children six years and younger, the *DSM-5* has outlined separate but similar diagnostic criteria in an effort to improve the recognition of this disorder in young children.

EPIDEMIOLOGY

Although lifetime prevalence rates reported in Europe are somewhat lower—for example, 1.9% in six European countries (Alonso et al., 2004b)—it is estimated that 6.8%–9.2% of people in North America have suffered from PTSD over the course of their lifetime (Breslau, Davis, Andreski, & Peterson, 1991; Kessler et al., 2005; Kessler, et al., 1995). Twelve-month prevalence rates have been shown to range from 3.5%–4.9%

in North America (Kessler, Chiu, Demler, Merikangas, & Walters, 2005; Kilpatrick et al., 2003; Norris, 1992; Resnick, et al., 1993), again contrasting with somewhat lower reported rates in Europe (Alonso, et al., 2004b; Darves-Bornoz et al., 2008; Hepp, et al., 2006; Perkonigg, et al., 2000; Vaiva, et al., 2008; van Zelst, de Beurs, Beekman, Deeg, & van Dyck, 2003).

Rates of PTSD or PTSD symptoms ranging from 5%–63% have been reported among intensive care unit survivors, depending on the assessment methods and the populations (Jackson et al., 2007), with an estimated prevalence ranging from 19%–22% (Davydow, Gifford, Desai, Needham, & Bienvenu, 2008). Prevalence rates of PTSD for those with cancer reported in the literature are also divergent, ranging from 0% to 32% (Matsuoka et al., 2002; Naidich & Motta, 2000). However, a recent large epidemiogical study reported that significant PTSD symptoms were present in 20.1% and 14.3% of Danish breast cancer survivors, 3 and 15 months after surgery, respectively (O'Connor, Christensen, Jensen, Moller, & Zachariae, 2011).

Posttraumatic stress disorder is a distressing and debilitating condition at the individual level, and it represents a significant burden to society because of its prevalence (Kessler, 2000). In addition to being a risk factor for other psychiatric conditions, such as substance abuse or depression, PTSD also leads to an increased likelihood of divorce, unemployment, academic failure, and early pregnancy. In terms of work days lost, PTSD is among the most impairing conditions ahead of even a number of somatic illnesses, such as heart disease (Alonso et al., 2004a).

A number of studies have investigated risk factors for PTSD. Pretraumatic risk factors included female gender (Breslau et al., 1991; Brewin et al., 2000; Yehuda, 2004), low education, previous trauma, history of childhood adversity, and prior personal or familial psychiatric history (Brewin et al., 2000; Ozer et al., 2003). Lack of social support is a strong posttraumatic risk factor for PTSD (Ozer et al., 2003). Severe peritraumatic distress is a predictor of PTSD (Brewin et al., 2000; Ozer et al., 2003). Finally, the type of trauma also influences the likelihood of developing PTSD; interpersonal trauma and sexual assault in particular have been shown to more frequently result in PTSD than non-interpersonal trauma such as natural disaster (Adler et al., 2008; Rose, Bisson, Churchill, & Wessely, 2002). In the community, it is estimated that one in five victims of assaultive violence develops PTSD compared to 6% of victims of other injury (Rose et al., 2002).

Because of their high rates of exposure to trauma, prevalence rates of PTSD are high in veterans. It is estimated that 12%–13% of veterans returning from the Gulf and Afghanistan wars suffered from PTSD (Seal, Bertenthal, Miner, Sen, & Marmar, 2007; Board on Population Health and Public Health Practice at the National Academies of Science, 2008). Furthermore, among veterans this disorder tends to become chronic—9% of Vietnam veterans still suffered from symptoms of PTSD in 1990 (Dohrenwend et al., 2006). Recently, it has been reported that among National Guard members preparing for deployment to Iraq, those previously deployed in Afghanistan (Operation Enduring Freedom) or Iraq (Operation Iraqi Freedom) were more than 3 times more likely to screen positive for PTSD (Kline et al., 2010).

Table 30.3 COMMONLY USED INSTRUMENTS FOR ASSESSING POSTTRAUMATIC STRESS DISORDER IN MEDICAL PATIENTS

INSTRUMENT	ABBREVIATION	METHOD OF ADMINISTRATION	# ITEMS	ADVANTAGES	LIMITATIONS	COMMENTS	TIME REQUIREMENT
Structured Clinical Interview for the *DSM–IV*	SCID–I	Interviewer–rated	21	Comprehensive assessment tool; Flexibility in administration	Dichotomous rating; focus on "worst event" experienced; lengthy; recommended for only trained clinicians	Can use only the PTSD module; Anxiety disorders, mood disorders, and substance use disorders modules recommended	2–10 minutes for PTSD module, 20 mins—several hours for the entire instrument
Clinician Administered PTSD Scale	CAPS	Interviewer–rated	30	Separate ratings for frequency and intensity; Flexibility in administration	Needs training; Time-consuming	Shorten by only assessing 17 core symptoms; Child Adolescent Version CAPS–CA	30 mins—1 hour
PTSD Symptom Scale Interview	PSS–I	Interviewer–rated	17	Can be administered by trained paraprofessionals	Measures symptoms over past 2 weeks rather than 1 month	Recommended for use with sexual assault survivors; Child Adolescent Version CPSS	20 mins
Structured Interview for PTSD	SI–PTSD	Interviewer–rated	27	Can be administered by trained paraprofessionals		Also assesses survival and behavioral guilt	10–30 mins
Anxiety Disorders Interview Schedule–PTSD	ADIS–PTSD	Interviewer–rated		Yields both dichotomous and continuous information	Mixed results in reliability and validity studies; recommended for only trained interviewers	Module of ADIS–IV	
Short Post–Traumatic Stress Disorder Rating Interview	SPRINT	Interviewer–rated	8	Used for screening	Not diagnostic	Sensitive to change	3 min
PTSD–Interview	PTSD–I	Interviewer–rated / Self–report		Yields both dichotomous and continuous information		Patients are given a copy of the scale to read along with interviewer	
Impact of Event Scale—Revised	IES–R	Self–report	22	Short; Widely used, enabling comparisons	Does not closely match *DSM–IV* criteria	Widely used	10 mins
Mississippi Scale for Combat–Related PTSD	M–PTSD	Self–report	35	Well validated for combat–related PTSD	Correspond to *DSM–III* criteria	Recommended for use with combat–related PTSD	10–15 mins
Keane PTSD Scale of the MMPI–2	MMPI–2, PK	Self–report	46		Dichotomous rating	Recommended for use with veterans	15 mins
Posttraumatic Stress Diagnostic Scale	PDS	Self–report	49	Yields both dichotomous and continuous information			10–15 mins
PTSD Checklist	PCL	Self–report	17	Closely match *DSM–IV* criteria	Does not provide diagnosis	Civilian Version (PCL–C), Military Version (PCL–M) and Specific Version (PCL–S)	5–10 mins
Los Angeles Symptom Checklist	LASC	Self–report	43	Yields both dichotomous and continuous information		Also assesses general psychological distress	15 mins
Distressing Events Questionnaire	DEQ	Self–report	35	Yields both dichotomous and continuous information	Does not assess criterion A1	Also assesses guilt, anger, and grief	5–7 mins

DIFFERENTIAL DIAGNOSES

The time elapsed since the trauma is the main point to consider when determining the difference between PTSD and ASD, although ASD also comprises dissociative symptom that are not included in the syndrome of PTSD except as a specifier. Generally, ASD occurs within the first month after trauma exposure, while PTSD is diagnosed beyond that.

Patients with anxiety disorders (panic disorder, general anxiety disorder, social anxiety disorder, etc) also may experience a certain level of hyperarousal and avoidant behaviors; however, both the trauma exposure and the reexperiencing of symptoms are missing from their clinical presentation. Depressive disorders may be triggered by a stressful experience and can also include concentration difficulties, insomnia, social withdrawal or detachment, and anhedonia, but they do not include trauma reexperiencing or trauma-related avoidance. Finally, an adjustment disorder can also occur after exposure to a stressor. However, in that condition either the stressor is not extreme or life threatening (e.g., divorce or job loss) and/or the reaction to it is not severe enough to meet criteria for PTSD. Furthermore, according to criterion C for adjustment disorder, meeting the criteria for any other mental disorder preempts a diagnosis of adjustment disorder.

COMORBIDITIES

PTSD commonly co-occurs with other psychiatric disorders, such as other anxiety disorders, affective disorders (depression, dysthymia, bipolar disorder), and substance use disorders (Kessler et al., 1995). Typically, PTSD precedes the development of the comorbid condition (Kessler et al., 1995; Perkonigg et al., 2000), although PTSD can occur before, after, or concurrently with any other mental disorder. As noted, preexisting psychiatric conditions serve as risk factors for PTSD in the face of trauma exposure. Regarding comorbidity of PTSD and other conditions, it may be important to address PTSD first in order to adequately treat the comorbid problem. A recent study of women treated for comorbid PTSD and substance dependence showed that a reduction in

---

Box 30.2 PRIMARY CARE PTSD SCREEN

In your life, have you ever had any experience that was so frightening, horrible, or upsetting that, in the past month, you . . .

1. Have had nightmares about it or thought about it when you did not want to?
   YES NO

2. Tried hard not to think about it or went out of your way to avoid situations that reminded you of it?
   YES NO

3. Were constantly on guard, watchful, or easily startled?
   YES NO

4. Felt numb or detached from others, activities, or your surroundings?
   YES NO

PTSD symptoms with specific PTSD treatment was associated with a reduction in substance use. In contrast, reduction in substance use did not necessarily reduce PTSD symptoms in this study (Hien et al., 2010).

PTSD is also comorbid with physical conditions. A recent study reported that even after adjusting for sociodemographics and comorbid psychiatric disorders, PTSD was significantly associated with an increased likelihood of suffering from a physical disorder in the past year, including neurological, vascular, gastrointestinal, metabolic, as well as auto-immune, bone, and joint conditions (Sareen, Cox, Clara, & Asmundson, 2005). Thus, chronic PTSD and chronic medical conditions can influence one another adversely. Medical conditions that are painful or life-threatening can increase arousal and thereby aggravate PTSD symptoms. At the same time patients with PTSD may have problems with medical treatment adherence, may have unhealthy behavior, and may show adverse physiologic effects of their chronic stress (Shemesh et al., 2001). There is evidence that PTSD is accompanied by dysregulation in the hypothalamic-pituitary-adrenal axis, associated with low cortisol levels frequently found in PTSD patients (Meewisse, Reitsma, de Vries, Gersons, & Olff, 2007). Further, recent data also suggest that patients with PTSD may exhibit immune modifications including increased circulating inflammatory markers, reactivity to antigen skin tests, and lower natural killer cell activity or total T lymphocyte counts (Pace & Heim, 2011).

ASSESSMENT

A range of both lengthy interviewer-based and brief self-rated instruments have been developed to assess or screen for PTSD (Pratt, Brief, & Keane, 2006). Although exhaustive description of all available instruments is beyond the score of the present chapter, Table 30.3 reports those most commonly used in clinical practice, along with their usefulness and the time needed to administer them. Of note, the gold standard to assess PTSD is not the SCID, but the clinician-administered PTSD scale (Blake et al., 1995), which usually takes up to one hour to be administered. A number of the self-report scales, such as the Impact of Event Scale–Revised and the Posttraumatic Stress Diagnostic Scale have been used as screening instruments in medical settings with consistently strong results (Davydow, et al., 2008). Recently, a 4-item screening instrument has been developed for use in primary care (Box 30.2). Endorsing three items (yes/no) yields a sensitivity of 0.77 with a specificity of 0.85 for detecting PTSD (Prins et al., 2004).

TREATMENTS AND PREVENTION

PRINCIPLES OF ACUTE STRESS DISORDER TREATMENT AND POSTTRAUMATIC STRESS DISORDER PREVENTION

It is worth highlighting that many individuals will experience a range of psychological and somatic stress response symptoms in the wake of trauma such as hyperarousal, anxiety,

	AUTHOR, YEAR	RESULTS
Brief Psychotherapy		
Cognitive Behavioral Therapy (CBT)	Bryant, 1998a	Brief (5 sessions) CBT within 2 weeks > Supportive counseling in preventing PTSD
	Bryant, 1999	Brief (5 sessions) PE or PE + Anxiety mgmt > Supportive counseling in preventing PTSD
	Bryant, 2003	Brief (5 sessions) CBT > Supportive Counseling in preventing PTSD
	Bryant, 2008a	Brief (5 sessions) ET > CT > No Tx in preventing PTSD
	Resnick, 2007	Video intervention reduces PTSD vs. standard care
Self–Help (SH)	Scholes, 2007	no group differences between SH and no Tx
	Turpin, 2005	no group differences in PTSD between SH and no Tx
Structured Writing Therapy (SWT)	van Emmerik, 2008	Efficacy of SWT was comparable to CBT
	Bugg, 2009	No differences between writing and self help (information only) groups
Memory Structured Intervention (MSI)	Gidron, 2007	No differences between MSI and supportive listening
Pharmacotherapy		
Propranolol	Pitman, 2002	Significant improvement post–acute stress
	Stein, 2007	No difference from placebo (gabapentin or propanolol)
	Reist, 2001	Recall of arousing story was reduced
	Vaiva, 2003	PTSD rate and symptoms lower in the propanolol group
Cortisol	Schelling, 2004	Hydrocortisone administered during cardiac surgery reduced chronic stress symptom scores
	Aerni, 2004	Low–dose cortisol for 1 month reduces the cardinal symptoms of PTSD
Morphine	Bryant et al. (2008c)	Patients with PTSD received significantly less morphine than those who did not develop PTSD
	Holbrook et al. (2010)	Wounded, morphine shortly after the injury reduced development of PTSD

From 2010 VA/DOD *Clinical Practice Guidelines for Management of Post–Traumatic Stress.*

and emotional distress. These may not show enough severity or impairment to meet ASD criteria; when they do not, they usually do not require professional intervention and the symptoms generally resolve spontaneously. Requiring acutely traumatized individuals to "debrief" in a group setting, termed *critical incident debriefing*, may actually increase rates of PTSD and related distress through interference with individuals' spontaneous coping mechanisms (Adler et al., 2008; Rose et al., 2002; van Emmerik, Kamphuis, Hulsbosch, & Emmelkamp, 2002). While those who seek professional assistance following a traumatic event and those who display the syndrome of ASD should always be offered care, it is not advisable to require or urge all individuals exposed to a trauma to talk about the trauma in detail, to participate in groups, or to receive services from a mental health professional. It is enough to ensure that trauma survivors have access to information about the usual course and reactions to trauma, to focus on basic medical and safety needs and to facilitate access to social supports (Zohar, Sonnino, Juven-Wetzler, & Cohen, 2009).

Because of the short timeframe in which ASD occurs and its potential role in predicting PTSD, naturally studies investigating its treatment somewhat overlap with those aiming to prevent PTSD (Table 30.4). Available research indicates that effective treatment techniques exist for treating ASD in trauma-exposed populations including sexual and nonsexual assault survivors, motor vehicle accident survivors, and survivors of industrial accidents. In particular, brief trauma-focused cognitive behavioral therapy has been shown to be effective in treating ASD and preventing development of PTSD (Roberts, Kitchiner, Kenardy, & Bisson, 2010). However, the administration of psychological interventions requires trained therapists. Unfortunately, there remains insufficient availability of professionals trained to administer these types of treatments, particularly in medical settings.

Another potential approach to treatment of ASD and prevention of PTSD could be a pharmacological one (Friedman, 2010), which is often more readily available across treatment settings; unfortunately, to date no data support the efficacy of any pharmacological agent for this indication. Limited and mixed evidence suggest that propranolol (McGhee et al., 2009; Pitman et al., 2002; Vaiva et al., 2003), hydrocortisone (Schelling et al., 2004), and morphine (Holbrook, Galarneau, Dye, Quinn, & Dougherty, 2010) might be potential candidates for further investigations. In addition, studies are under way using selective serotonin reuptake inhibitors (SSRIs) for this indication (Zohar et al., 2009), although data from children suffering from burns and ASD symptoms did not demonstrate greater benefit from imipramine or fluoxetine than from placebo (Robert et al., 2008). Finally, although trauma patients usually present with acute signs of anxiety and benzodiazepines are well known for their efficient and rapid action on these symptoms, including insomnia, their benefit in trauma patients is much less clear. Recent studies found that not only do benzodiazepines not seem to prevent the development of PTSD, they might actually even increase the risk for this condition (Davydow, et al., 2008; Gelpin, Bonne, Peri, Brandes, & Shalev, 1996; Mellman, Bustamante, David, & Fins, 2002). This may in part be due to interference with natural resolution of fear responses to trauma that occur with time (i.e., extinction learning). Animal data have also suggested that early benzodiazepine administration after a stressor may interfere with successful responses to stress exposures later on, potentially via effects on the HPA axis (Matar, Zohar, Kaplan, & Cohen, 2009). In other words, while no strong data support the use of any medication in the early aftermath after trauma exposure, clinicians should at least avoid using benzodiazepines during that period.

PRINCIPLES OF POSTTRAUMATIC STRESS DISORDER TREATMENT

Two primary types of treatments are available for PTSD: psychological interventions and pharmacotherapy. Psychotherapeutic techniques that have yielded the most consistent findings in PTSD are different forms of cognitive–behavioral therapies (CBT). CBT adapted to PTSD usually includes elements of exposure therapy, and, to date, results from over 30 randomized controlled trials (RCT) provide evidence for the use of individual CBT as a first-line treatment in PTSD (Orsillo, Raja, & Hammond, 2002). Two types of CBT with strong randomized controlled data supporting safety and efficacy in the treatment of PTSD are *Prolonged Exposure (PE) Therapy* (Foa et al., 2005; Schnurr et al., 2007) *and Cognitive Processing (CP) Therapy* (Monson et al., 2006; Resick et al., 2008; Resick, Nishith, Weaver, Astin, & Feuer, 2002). There is no evidence supporting differential efficacy for PE compared to CPT for PTSD to date, although there may be individual patient or clinician preferences (Resick et al., 2002). PE focuses on repeated imaginal exposure to the traumatic event as well as repeated in vivo exposure to safe situations that are currently avoided as they trigger traumatic reminders. These exposures promote extinction learning and resolution of symptoms. CPT focuses predominantly on cognitive interventions including challenging and modifying dysfunctional beliefs related to the trauma (e.g., lack of safety, difficulty trusting others), but also includes exposure via writing about the trauma.

Another technique found to be effective in PTSD is eye movement desensitization and reprocessing (EMDR). Although EMDR integrates elements of psychodynamic, cognitive behavioral, cognitive, interpersonal, systems, and body-oriented therapies (Seiffge-Krenke & Klessinger, 2000), it possesses a unique feature of bilateral brain stimulation (e.g., eye movements). This therapy follows an eight-phase structure and aims to allow patients to develop more adaptive coping mechanisms by processing distressing memories and reducing their influence. It has been suggested that EMDR makes use of a dual attention awareness to allow the patient to alternate between the traumatic memories and the safety of the present moment. A body of literature found that this therapy is effective in the treatment of PTSD (Amoyal et al., 2011; Orsillo et al., 2002); this suggests that it may be considered a first-line psychological treatment (Bisson et al., 2007). However, there is evidence that the eye movements may be an unnecessary part of the treatment and that the treatment effect is a result of the exposure component (P. R. Davidson & Parker, 2001). Although group CBT and stress management seem to be effective in PTSD, the effect has been reported to be weaker than individual CBT and EMDR, which prevents their use as first-line treatments (Bisson et al., 2007). Please see Table 30.5 for a comparison of EMDR, cognitive-based therapies, and exposure-based therapies. Other psychotherapeutic interventions such as couple and family therapy, psychodynamic therapy, hypnosis, creative therapy, etc., have also been proposed; however, to date, strong empirical support for their efficacy in PTSD is still lacking (Bisson, et al., 2007). A detailed review of available data supporting the different psychotherapy treatment approaches is available in the recent VA/DoD Clinical Practice Guidelines for the Management of Posttraumatic Stress (Department of Veterans Affairs & Department of Defense, 2010).

Table 30.5 ELEMENTS OF PSYCHOTHERAPEUTIC APPROACHES VALIDATED FOR POSTTRAUMATIC STRESS DISORDER

CORE COMPONENTS	ADDITIONAL POSSIBLE COMPONENTS
Exposure–based therapies	
In–vivo, imaginal, and narrative exposure to the traumatic event	Cognitive restructuring
	Relaxation techniques
	Self–montoring of anxiety
Cognitive–based therapies	
Cognitive restructuring (challenging automatic or acquired beliefs connected to the traumatic event)	Relaxation techniques
	Discussion/narration of the traumatic event
Eye Movement Desensitization and Reprocessing (EMDR)	
Alternating eye–movements or attention to tones, tapping, or other stimuli	Imaginal and/or narrative exposure to the traumatic event
	Cognitive restructuring
	Relaxation techniques
	Self–montoring of anxiety

First-line pharmacological treatment of PTSD focuses on SSRIs, with some support for comparable efficacy of serotonin norepinephrine reuptake inhibitors such as venlafaxine (J. Davidson et al., 2006). Although recent research suggests that SSRIs might not be as effective as previously thought (Orsillo et al., 2002; van Emmerik et al., 2002) and that chronic combat-related PTSD may be somewhat less responsive, there is strong empirical evidence suggesting that SSRIs should be the preferred first-line medication for PTSD based on results from a number of well-conducted random controlled trials. To date, two agents have been approved by the Food and Drug Administration for the treatment of PTSD: sertraline and paroxetine. SSRIs are well tolerated and may also be useful to treat comorbid depression; however, because of a possible initial increase in anxiety symptoms, they should be initiated more slowly than in depression. Other medications that have been studied as monotherapy in the treatment of PTSD include other antidepressants, anticonvulsants, antipsychotics, and antihypertensive drugs. While evidence supporting their use as first-line treatments is limited by the lack of large randomized controlled trials, several antidepressants including mirtazapine, nefazodone, amitriptyline, imipramine and phenelzine might be considered as second-line choices for monotherapy (Department of Veterans Affairs & Department of Defense, 2010).

Although atypical antipsychotics such as risperidone and olanzapine have not been shown to be effective in monotherapy on PTSD symptoms, some evidence suggests that their use as adjunctive may be beneficial on associated symptoms of psychosis (Department of Veterans Affairs & Department of Defense, 2010). No large randomized studies support the efficacy of benzodiazepines for PTSD. While they may be useful as adjunctive agents in limited cases, those with PTSD are at heightened risk for substance abuse and dependence. In addition, benzodiazepines may interfere with CBT efficacy, potentially even more so when used on an as needed basis. Some data support the use of alternative agents for insomnia and nightmares in patients with PTSD. These include the alpha blocker prazosin and newer sleep agents such as eszopiclone (Pollack et al., 2011; Taylor et al., 2008). Again, an excellent review of evidence for pharmacotherapy approaches beyond the scope of this chapter is available in the recent VA/DoD *Clinical Practice Guidelines for the* Management *of Post-traumatic Stress* (Department of Veterans Affairs & Department of Defense, 2010).

FUTURE AND CONTROVERSIES

The fifth revision of the *DSM* includes a number of changes in the formulation of the diagnostic criteria for acute and chronic reactions to trauma. ASD and PTSD no longer belong to the anxiety disorder spectrum, but to a new class of trauma and stressor-related disorders. The requirement for a subjective negative response to the stressor (*DSM–IV–TR* criterion A2, "intense fear, helplessness, horror") has been suppressed in both ASD and PTSD. Finally, in the *DSM–V,* ASD symptoms are no longer organized in four symptom clusters but are now grouped into one single criterion. PTSD symptoms are now reclassified into four clusters (reexperiencing, avoidance, alterations in cognition and mood, hyperarousal) instead of three. Future studies will determine whether these changes in symptoms criteria will result in changes in prevalence rates, and yield significant clinical implications.

SUMMARY

In recent years research has blossomed in understanding the underlying risk factors, phenomenology and biology, prevention and early intervention, and treatment for ASD and PTSD. However, more data are needed to guide the optimal identification of trauma-exposed individuals at risk and to provide optimal prevention and intervention strategies. Perhaps the greatest advances have been in the development of exposure based psychotherapies, which can be considered first line for ASD and PTSD. Although many more practitioners are now aware of these treatments, additional dissemination of these evidence based psychotherapies is needed to increase availability. Further, the avoidance and stigma associated with PTSD can interfere with patients seeking or continuing with treatment, suggesting it is important for practitioners to screen for and educate about PTSD amongst trauma exposed individuals. First-line pharmacotherapy for PTSD is an antidepressant drug, but not all patients respond. PTSD is a heterogeneous condition associated with high rates of psychiatric, substance, and medical comorbidities that should be assessed and may require targeted treatment. More research is needed to develop novel pharmacotherapies and increase the evidence base for commonly employed pharmacotherapeutic approaches to PTSD. With many basic science and clinical research studies ongoing and increasing attention to the field, it is hopeful that growing scientific knowledge will lead to improved prevention and better outcomes in the coming years.

CLINICAL PEARLS

- Peritraumatic reactions are those experienced during and immediately after trauma. Certain trauma-specific peritraumatic reactions—distress and dissociation—are robust predictors of the development of chronic and debilitating PTSD (Brewin et al., 2000; Ozer et al., 2003). In other words, the more "frightened" the individual is during the trauma, the more likely he is to still be frightened 1 month later.

- The majority of persons who experience early post-traumatic symptoms adjust in the following weeks or months (Blanchard et al., 1996; Hamanaka et al., 2006).

- Most trauma survivors who subsequently develop PTSD do not meet full criteria for ASD (R. A. Bryant, 2011).

- Risk factors for PTSD included female gender (Breslau et al., 1991; Brewin et al., 2000; Yehuda, 2004), low education, previous trauma, history of childhood adversity, and prior personal or familial psychiatric history (Brewin et al., 2000; Ozer et al., 2003), lack of social support (Ozer et al., 2003), severe peritraumatic distress (Brewin et al., 2000; Ozer et al., 2003), and, finally, interpersonal trauma and sexual assault (Adler et al., 2008; Rose et al., 2002).

- In the community, it is estimated that one of five victims of assaultive violence develops PTSD compared to 6% of victims of other injury (Rose et al., 2002).

- Among National Guard members preparing for deployment to Iraq, those previously deployed in Afghanistan (Operation Enduring Freedom) or Iraq (Operation Iraqi Freedom) were more than 3 times more likely to screen positive for PTSD (Kline et al., 2010).

- Patients with other anxiety disorders (panic disorder, general anxiety disorder, social anxiety disorder, etc) also may experience a certain level of hyperarousal and avoidant behaviors; however, both the trauma exposure and the reexperiencing symptoms are missing from their clinical presentation.

- A recent study of women treated for comorbid PTSD and substance dependence showed that a reduction in PTSD symptoms with specific PTSD treatment was associated with a reduction in substance use. In contrast, in this study, reduction in substance use did not necessarily reduce PTSD symptoms (Hien et al., 2010).

- Medical conditions that are painful or life-threatening can increase arousal and thereby aggravate PTSD symptoms.

- Requiring acutely traumatized individuals to "debrief" in a group setting, termed *critical incident debriefing,* may actually increase rates of PTSD and related distress through interference with individuals' spontaneous coping mechanisms (Adler et al., 2008; Rose et al., 2002; van Emmerik et al., 2002).

- It is not advisable to require or urge all individuals exposed to a trauma to talk about the trauma in detail, to participate in groups, or to receive services from a mental health professional. It is enough to ensure that trauma survivors have access to information about the usual course and reactions to trauma, to focus on basic medical and safety needs and to facilitate access to social supports (Zohar et al., 2009).

- Brief trauma-focused cognitive behavioral therapy has been shown to be effective in treating ASD and preventing development of PTSD (Roberts et al., 2010).

- Benzodiazepines do not seem to prevent the development of PTSD, but they might actually even increase the risk for this condition.

- Strong empirical evidence suggests that SSRIs should be the preferred first-line medication for PTSD based on results from a number of well-conducted random controlled trials.

DISCLOSURE STATEMENTS

Dr. Bui does not have any conflict of interest to disclose.

Dr. Charney does not have any conflict of interest to disclose.

Ms. Kredlow does not have any conflict of interest to disclose.

Dr. Simon receives grant support from NIH, DOD, AFSP, ACS, Highland Street Foundation, Forest Laboratories, Inc. She receives financial compensation from the MGH Psychiatry Academy. Her spouse receives equity from Elan, Dandreon, G–Zero, Gatekeeper.

Dr. Zeng does not have any conflict of interest to disclose.

REFERENCES

Adler, A. B., Litz, B. T., Castro, C. A., Suvak, M., Thomas, J. L., Burrell, L., et al. (2008). A group randomized trial of critical incident stress debriefing provided to U.S. peacekeepers. *Journal of Traumatic Stress, 21*(3), 253–263.

Allenou, C., Olliac, B., Bourdet-Loubere, S., Brunet, A., David, A. C., Claudet, I., et al. (2010). Symptoms of traumatic stress in mothers of children victims of a motor vehicle accident. *Depression and Anxiety, 27*(7), 652–657.

Alonso, J., Angermeyer, M. C., Bernert, S., Bruffaerts, R., Brugha, T. S., Bryson, H., et al. (2004a). Disability and quality of life impact of mental disorders in Europe: results from the European study of the epidemiology of mental disorders (ESEMeD) project. *Acta Psychiatrica Scandinavica, Supplementum,* (420), 38–46.

Alonso, J., Angermeyer, M. C., Bernert, S., Bruffaerts, R., Brugha, T. S., Bryson, H., et al. (2004b). Prevalence of mental disorders in Europe: results from the European Study of the Epidemiology of Mental Disorders (ESEMeD) project. *Acta Psychiatrica Scandinavica, Supplementum,* (420), 21–27.

Amoyal, N. R., Mason, S. T., Gould, N. F., Corry, N., Mahfouz, S., Barkey, A., & Fauerbach, J. A. (2011). Measuring coping behavior in patients with major burn injuries: a psychometric evaluation of the BCOPE. *Journal of Burn Care & Research, 32*(3), 392–398.

APA. (1983). *Diagnostic and statistical manual of mental disorders, DSM-III.* (3rd ed., Rev.). Washington, DC: American Psychiatric Publishing.

APA. (2000). *Diagnostic and statistical manual of mental disorders, DSM-IV-TR.* (4th ed. Rev.). Washington, DC: American Psychiatric Publishing.

APA. (2013). *Diagnostic and statistical manual of mental disorders, DSM5.* (5th ed.). Washington, DC: American Psychiatric Publishing.

Birmes, P., Bui, E., Klein, K., Billard, J., Schmitt, L., Allenou, C., et al. (2010). Psychotraumatology in antiquity. *Stress & Health, 26*(1), 21–31.

Bisson, J. I., Ehlers, A., Matthews, R., Pilling, S., Richards, D., & Turner, S. (2007). Psychological treatments for chronic post-traumatic stress disorder. Systematic review and meta-analysis. *British Journal of Psychiatry, 190,* 97–104.

Blake, D. D., Weathers, F. W., Nagy, L. M., Kaloupek, D. G., Gusman, F. D., Charney, D. S., & Keane, T. M. (1995). The development of a Clinician-Administered PTSD Scale. *Journal of Traumatic Stress, 8*(1), 75–90.

Blanchard, E. B., Hickling, E. J., Barton, K. A., Taylor, A. E., Loos, W. R., & Jones-Alexander, J. (1996). One-year prospective follow-up of motor vehicle accident victims. *Behaviour Research and Therapy, 34*(10), 775–786.

Board on Population Health and Public Health Practice at the National Academies of Science. (2008). *Committee on Gulf War and health: Updated literature review of depleted uranium, institute of medicine.* Retrieved from http://www.nap.edu/catalog.php?record id=12183.

Breslau, N. (2001). The epidemiology of posttraumatic stress disorder: what is the extent of the problem? *Journal of Clinical Psychiatry, 62*(Suppl 17), 16–22.

Breslau, N., Davis, G. C., Andreski, P., & Peterson, E. (1991). Traumatic events and posttraumatic stress disorder in an urban population of young adults. *Archives of General Psychiatry, 48*(3), 216–222.

Brewin, C. R., Andrews, B., & Valentine, J. D. (2000). Meta-analysis of risk factors for posttraumatic stress disorder in trauma-exposed adults. *Journal of Consulting and Clinical Psychology, 68*(5), 748–766.

Brewin, C. R., & Holmes, E. A. (2003). Psychological theories of post-traumatic stress disorder. *Clinical Psychology Review, 23*(3), 339–376.

Brunet, A., Weiss, D. S., Metzler, T. J., Best, S. R., Neylan, T. C., Rogers, C., et al. (2001). The Peritraumatic Distress Inventory: a proposed measure of PTSD criterion A2. *American Journal of Psychiatry, 158*(9), 1480–1485.

Bryant, R. A. (2011). Acute stress disorder as a predictor of posttraumatic stress disorder: a systematic review. *Journal of Clinical Psychiatry, 72*(2), 233–239.

Bryant, R. A., Creamer, M., O'Donnell, M. L., Silove, D., & McFarlane, A. C. (2008). A multisite study of the capacity of acute stress disorder diagnosis to predict posttraumatic stress disorder. *Journal of Clinical Psychiatry, 69*(6), 923–929.

Bryant, R. A., Harvey, A. G., Dang, S. T., & Sackville, T. (1998). Assessing acute stress disorder: Psychometric properties of a structured clinical interview. *Psychological Assessment, 10*(3), 215–220.

Bui, E., Brunet, A., Allenou, C., Camassel, C., Raynaud, J. P., Claudet, I., et al. (2010). Peritraumatic reactions and posttraumatic stress symptoms in school-aged children victims of road traffic accident. *General Hospital Psychiatry, 32*(3), 330–333.

Bui, E., Joubert, S., Manetti, A., Camassel, C., Charpentier, S., Ribereau-Gayon, R., et al. (2010). Peritraumatic distress predicts posttraumatic stress symptoms in older people. *International Journal of Geriatric Psychiatry, 25*(12), 1306–1307.

Bui, E., Tremblay, L., Brunet, A., Rodgers, R., Jehel, L., Very, E., et al. (2010). Course of posttraumatic stress symptoms over the 5 years following an industrial disaster: a structural equation modeling study. *Journal of Traumatic Stress, 23*(6), 759–766.

Cahill, L., Prins, B., Weber, M., & McGaugh, J. L. (1994). Beta-adrenergic activation and memory for emotional events. *Nature, 371*(6499), 702–704.

Cardena, E., Koopman, C., Classen, C., Waelde, L. C., & Spiegel, D. (2000). Psychometric properties of the Stanford Acute Stress Reaction Questionnaire (SASRQ): a valid and reliable measure of acute stress. *Journal of Traumatic Stress, 13*(4), 719–734.

Darves-Bornoz, J. M., Alonso, J., de Girolamo, G., de Graaf, R., Haro, J. M., Kovess-Masfety, V., et al. (2008). Main traumatic events in Europe: PTSD in the European study of the epidemiology of mental disorders survey. *Journal of Traumatic Stress, 21*(5), 455–462.

Davidson, J., Rothbaum, B. O., Tucker, P., Asnis, G., Benattia, I., & Musgnung, J. J. (2006). Venlafaxine extended release in posttraumatic stress disorder: a sertraline- and placebo-controlled study. *Journal of Clinical Psychopharmacology, 26*(3), 259–267.

Davidson, P. R., & Parker, K. C. (2001). Eye movement desensitization and reprocessing (EMDR): a meta-analysis. [Meta-Analysis Research Support, Non-U.S. Gov't]. *Journal of Consulting and Clinical Psychology, 69*(2), 305–316.

Davydow, D. S., Gifford, J. M., Desai, S. V., Needham, D. M., & Bienvenu, O. J. (2008). Posttraumatic stress disorder in general intensive care unit survivors: a systematic review. *General Hospital Psychiatry, 30*(5), 421–434.

Department of Veterans Affairs, & Department of Defense. (2010). *VA/DOD clinical practice guideline for management of post-traumatic stress.* Retrieved from http://www.healthquality.va.gov/Post Traumatic Stress Disorder PTSD.asp.

Dohrenwend, B. P., Turner, J. B., Turse, N. A., Adams, B. G., Koenen, K. C., & Marshall, R. (2006). The psychological risks of Vietnam for U.S. veterans: a revisit with new data and methods. *Science, 313*(5789), 979–982.

Elklit, A., & Christiansen, D. M. (2010). ASD and PTSD in rape victims. *Journal of Interpersonal Violence, 25*(8), 1470–1488.

Foa, E. B., Hembree, E. A., Cahill, S. P., Rauch, S. A., Riggs, D. S., Feeny, N. C., & Yadin, E. (2005). Randomized trial of prolonged exposure for posttraumatic stress disorder with and without cognitive restructuring: outcome at academic and community clinics. [Randomized Controlled Trial Research Support, N.I.H., Extramural]. *Journal of Consulting and Clinical Psychology, 73*(5), 953–964.

Friedman, M. J. (2010). Prevention of psychiatric problems among military personnel and their spouses. *New England Journal of Medicine, 362*(2), 168–170.

Friedman, M. J., Resick, P. A., Bryant, R. A., & Brewin, C. R. (2011). Considering PTSD for DSM-5. *Depression and Anxiety, 28*(9), 750–769.

Gelpin, E., Bonne, O., Peri, T., Brandes, D., & Shalev, A. Y. (1996). Treatment of recent trauma survivors with benzodiazepines: a prospective study. *Journal of Clinical Psychiatry, 57*(9), 390–394.

Hamanaka, S., Asukai, N., Kamijo, Y., Hatta, K., Kishimoto, J., & Miyaoka, H. (2006). Acute stress disorder and posttraumatic stress disorder symptoms among patients severely injured in motor vehicle accidents in Japan. *General Hospital Psychiatry, 28*(3), 234–241.

Hepp, U., Gamma, A., Milos, G., Eich, D., Ajdacic-Gross, V., Rossler, W., et al. (2006). Prevalence of exposure to potentially traumatic events and PTSD. The Zurich Cohort Study. *European Archives of Psychiatry and Clinical Neuroscience, 256*(3), 151–158.

Hien, D. A., Jiang, H., Campbell, A. N. C., Hu, M.-C., Miele, G. M., Cohen, L. R., et al. (2010). Do Treatment Improvements in PTSD Severity Affect Substance Use Outcomes? A Secondary Analysis From a Randomized Clinical Trial in NIDA's Clinical Trials Network. *American Journal of Psychiatry, 167*(1), 95–101.

Holbrook, T. L., Galarneau, M. R., Dye, J. L., Quinn, K., & Dougherty, A. L. (2010). Morphine use after combat injury in Iraq and post-traumatic stress disorder. *New England Journal of Medicine, 362*(2), 110–117.

Jackson, J., Hart, R., Gordon, S., Hopkins, R., Girard, T., & Ely, E. W. (2007). Post-traumatic stress disorder and post-traumatic stress symptoms following critical illness in medical intensive care unit patients: assessing the magnitude of the problem. *Critical Care, 11*(1), R27.

Janet, P. (1909). Problèmes psychologiques de l'émotion. *Revue Neurologique, 17,* 1551–1687.

Kangas, M., Henry, J. L., & Bryant, R. A. (2005). The relationship between acute stress disorder and posttraumatic stress disorder following cancer. *Journal of Consulting and Clinical Psychology, 73*(2), 360–364.

Karam, E. G., Andrews, G., Bromet, E., Petukhova, M., Ruscio, A. M., Salamoun, M., et al. (2010). The role of criterion A2 in the DSM-IV diagnosis of posttraumatic stress disorder. *Biological Psychiatry, 68*(5), 465–473.

Kessler, R. C. (2000). Posttraumatic stress disorder: the burden to the individual and to society. *Journal of Clinical Psychiatry, 61*(Suppl 5), 4–12; discussion 13–14.

Kessler, R. C., Berglund, P., Demler, O., Jin, R., Merikangas, K. R., & Walters, E. E. (2005). Lifetime prevalence and age-of-onset distributions of DSM-IV disorders in the National Comorbidity Survey Replication. *Archives of General Psychiatry, 62*(6), 593–602.

Kessler, R. C., Chiu, W. T., Demler, O., Merikangas, K. R., & Walters, E. E. (2005). Prevalence, severity, and comorbidity of 12-month DSM-IV disorders in the National Comorbidity Survey Replication. *Archives of General Psychiatry, 62*(6), 617–627.

Kessler, R. C., Sonnega, A., Bromet, E., Hughes, M., & Nelson, C. B. (1995). Posttraumatic stress disorder in the National Comorbidity Survey. *Archives of General Psychiatry, 52*(12), 1048–1060.

Kilpatrick, D. G., Ruggiero, K. J., Acierno, R., Saunders, B. E., Resnick, H. S., & Best, C. L. (2003). Violence and risk of PTSD, major depression, substance abuse/dependence, and comorbidity: results from the National Survey of Adolescents. *Journal of Consulting and Clinical Psychology, 71*(4), 692–700.

Kline, A., Falca-Dodson, M., Sussner, B., Ciccone, D. S., Chandler, H., Callahan, L., & Losonczy, M. (2010). Effects of Repeated Deployment to Iraq and Afghanistan on the Health of New Jersey Army National Guard Troops: Implications for Military Readiness. *American Journal of Public Health, 100*(2), 276–283.

Koopman, C., Classen, C., Cardeña, E., & Spiegel, D. (1995). When disaster strikes, acute stress disorder may follow. *Journal of Traumatic Stress, 8*(1), 29–46.

Marmar, C. R., Metzler, T. J., Otte, C., McCaslin, S., Inslicht, S., & Henn Haase, C. (2007). The peritraumatic dissociative experiences questionnaire: An international perspective. In J. P. Wilson & C. So-kum Tang (Eds.), *Cross-cultural assessment of psychological trauma and PTSD* (pp. 197–217). New York: Springer US.

Matar, M. A., Zohar, J., Kaplan, Z., & Cohen, H. (2009). Alprazolam treatment immediately after stress exposure interferes with the normal HPA-stress response and increases vulnerability to subsequent stress in an animal model of PTSD. *European Neuropsychopharmacology, 19*(4), 283–295.

Matsuoka, Y., Nakano, T., Inagaki, M., Sugawara, Y., Akechi, T., Imoto, S., et al. (2002). Cancer-related intrusive thoughts as an indicator of poor psychological adjustment at 3 or more years after breast surgery: A preliminary study. *Breast Cancer Research and Treatment, 76*(2), 117–124.

McGarvey, E. L., Canterbury, R. J., Koopman, C., Clavet, G. J., Cohen, R., Largay, K., & Spiegel, D. (1998). Acute stress disorder following diagnosis of cancer. *International Journal of Rehabilitation and Health, 4*(1), 1–15.

McGhee, L. L., Maani, C. V., Garza, T. H., Desocio, P. A., Gaylord, K. M., & Black, I. H. (2009). The effect of propranolol on posttraumatic stress disorder in burned service members. *Journal of Burn Care & Research, 30*(1), 92–97.

McKibben, J. B., Bresnick, M. G., Wiechman Askay, S. A., & Fauerbach, J. A. (2008). Acute stress disorder and posttraumatic stress disorder: a prospective study of prevalence, course, and predictors in a sample with major burn injuries. *Journal of Burn Care & Research, 29*(1), 22–35.

Meewisse, M. L., Reitsma, J. B., de Vries, G. J., Gersons, B. P., & Olff, M. (2007). Cortisol and post-traumatic stress disorder in adults: systematic review and meta-analysis. [Meta-Analysis Review]. *The British Journal of Psychiatry, 191,* 387–392.

Mehnert, A., & Koch, U. (2007). Prevalence of acute and post-traumatic stress disorder and comorbid mental disorders in breast cancer patients during primary cancer care: a prospective study. *Psycho-Oncology, 16*(3), 181–188.

Mellman, T. A., Bustamante, V., David, D., & Fins, A. I. (2002). Hypnotic medication in the aftermath of trauma. *Journal of Clinical Psychiatry, 63*(12), 1183–1184.

Merriam-Webster. (1995). trauma (n.d.).

Monson, C. M., Schnurr, P. P., Resick, P. A., Friedman, M. J., Young-Xu, Y., & Stevens, S. P. (2006). Cognitive processing therapy for veterans with military-related posttraumatic stress disorder. [Randomized Controlled Trial]. *Journal of Consulting and Clinical Psychology, 74*(5), 898–907.

Naidich, J. B., & Motta, R. W. (2000). PTSD-related symptoms in women with breast cancer. *Journal of Psychotherapy in Independent Practice, 1*(1), 35–54.

Norris, F. H. (1992). Epidemiology of trauma: frequency and impact of different potentially traumatic events on different demographic groups. *Journal of Consulting and Clinical Psychology, 60*(3), 409–418.

O'Connor, M., Christensen, S., Jensen, A. B., Moller, S., & Zachariae, R. (2011). How traumatic is breast cancer? Post-traumatic stress symptoms (PTSS) and risk factors for severe PTSS at 3 and 15 months after surgery in a nationwide cohort of Danish women treated for primary breast cancer. *British Journal of Cancer, 104*(3), 419–426.

Oppenheim, H. (1889). *Die traumatischen Neurosen.* Berlin: Kessinger Publishing.

Orsillo, S. M., Raja, S., & Hammond, C. (2002). Gender issues in PTSD with comorbid mental health disorders. In R. Kimerling, P. Ouimette & J. Wolfe (Eds.), *Gender and PTSD* (pp. 207–231). New York: The Guilford Press.

Ozer, E. J., Best, S. R., Lipsey, T. L., & Weiss, D. S. (2003). Predictors of posttraumatic stress disorder and symptoms in adults: a meta-analysis. *Psychological Bulletin, 129*(1), 52–73.

Pace, T. W., & Heim, C. M. (2011). A short review on the psychoneuroimmunology of posttraumatic stress disorder: from risk factors to medical comorbidities. [Review]. *Brain, Behavior, and Immunity*, *25*(1), 6–13.

Palmer, S. C., Kagee, A., Coyne, J. C., & DeMichele, A. (2004). Experience of trauma, distress, and posttraumatic stress disorder among breast cancer patients. *Psychosomatic Medicine, 66*(2), 258–264.

Pedersen, A. F., & Zachariae, R. (2010). Cancer, acute stress disorder, and repressive coping. *Scandinavian Journal of Psychology, 51*(1), 84–91.

Perkonigg, A., Kessler, R. C., Storz, S., & Wittchen, H. U. (2000). Traumatic events and post-traumatic stress disorder in the community: prevalence, risk factors and comorbidity. *Acta Psychiatrica Scandinavica, 101*(1), 46–59.

Pitman, R. K., Sanders, K. M., Zusman, R. M., Healy, A. R., Cheema, F., Lasko, N. B., et al. (2002). Pilot study of secondary prevention of posttraumatic stress disorder with propranolol. *Biological Psychiatry, 51*(2), 189–192.

Plutarch. (1920). *Plutarch's Lives* (Vol. 9). London: William Heinemann.

Pollack, M. H., Hoge, E. A., Worthington, J. J., Moshier, S. J., Wechsler, R. S., Brandes, M., & Simon, N. M. (2011). Eszopiclone for the treatment of posttraumatic stress disorder and associated insomnia: a randomized, double-blind, placebo-controlled trial. *Journal of Clinical Psychiatry, 72*(7), 892–897.

Pratt, E. M., Brief, D. J., & Keane, T. M. (2006). Recent advances in psychological assessment of adults with posttraumatic stress disorder. In V. M. Follette & J. I. Ruzek (Eds.), *Cognitive-behavioral therapies for trauma* (2nd ed., pp. 34–61). New York: Guilford Press.

Prins, A., Ouimette, P., Kimerling, R., Camerond, R. P., Hugelshofer, D. S., Shaw-Hegwer, J., et al. (2004). The primary care PTSD screen (PC-PTSD): development and operating characteristics. *Primary Care Psychiatry, 9*(1), 9–14.

Resick, P. A., Galovski, T. E., O'Brien Uhlmansiek, M., Scher, C. D., Clum, G. A., & Young-Xu, Y. (2008). A randomized clinical trial to dismantle components of cognitive processing therapy for posttraumatic stress disorder in female victims of interpersonal violence. [Comparative Study Randomized Controlled Trial Research Support, N.I.H., Extramural]. *Journal of Consulting and Clinical Psychology, 76*(2), 243–258.

Resick, P. A., Nishith, P., Weaver, T. L., Astin, M. C., & Feuer, C. A. (2002). A comparison of cognitive-processing therapy with prolonged exposure and a waiting condition for the treatment of chronic posttraumatic stress disorder in female rape victims. [Clinical Trial Comparative Study Randomized Controlled Trial Research Support, U.S. Gov't, P.H.S.]. *Journal of Consulting and Clinical Psychology, 70*(4), 867–879.

Resnick, H. S., Kilpatrick, D. G., Dansky, B. S., Saunders, B. E., & Best, C. L. (1993). Prevalence of civilian trauma and posttraumatic stress disorder in a representative national sample of women. *Journal of Consulting and Clinical Psychology, 61*(6), 984–991.

Robert, R., Tcheung, W. J., Rosenberg, L., Rosenberg, M., Mitchell, C., Villarreal, C., et al. (2008). Treating thermally injured children suffering symptoms of acute stress with imipramine and fluoxetine: a randomized, double-blind study. *Burns, 34*(7), 919–928.

Roberts, N. P., Kitchiner, N. J., Kenardy, J., & Bisson, J. I. (2010). Early psychological interventions to treat acute traumatic stress symptoms. *Cochrane Database of Systematic Reviews, 3*, CD007944.

Rose, S., Bisson, J., Churchill, R., & Wessely, S. (2002). Psychological debriefing for preventing post traumatic stress disorder (PTSD). *Cochrane Database of Systematic Reviews,* (2), CD000560.

Sareen, J., Cox, B. J., Clara, I., & Asmundson, G. J. G. (2005). The relationship between anxiety disorders and physical disorders in the U.S. National Comorbidity Survey. *Depression and Anxiety, 21*(4), 193–202.

Schelling, G., Kilger, E., Roozendaal, B., de Quervain, D. J., Briegel, J., Dagge, A., et al. (2004). Stress doses of hydrocortisone, traumatic memories, and symptoms of posttraumatic stress disorder in patients after cardiac surgery: a randomized study. *Biological Psychiatry, 55*(6), 627–633.

Schnurr, P. P., Friedman, M. J., Engel, C. C., Foa, E. B., Shea, M. T., Chow, B. K., et al. (2007). Cognitive behavioral therapy for posttraumatic stress disorder in women: a randomized controlled trial. [Comparative Study Multicenter Study Randomized Controlled Trial Research Support, U.S. Gov't, Non-P.H.S.]. *Journal of the American Medical Association, 297*(8), 820–830.

Seal, K. H., Bertenthal, D., Miner, C. R., Sen, S., & Marmar, C. (2007). Bringing the war back home: mental health disorders among 103,788 US veterans returning from Iraq and Afghanistan seen at Department of Veterans Affairs facilities. *Archives of Internal Medicine, 167*(5), 476–482.

Seiffge-Krenke, I., & Klessinger, N. (2000). Long-term effects of avoidant coping on adolescents' depressive symptoms. *Journal of Youth and Adolescence, 29*(6), 617–630.

Shemesh, E., Rudnick, A., Kaluski, E., Milovanov, O., Salah, A., Alon, D., et al. (2001). A prospective study of posttraumatic stress symptoms and nonadherence in survivors of a myocardial infarction (MI). *General Hospital Psychiatry, 23*(4), 215–222.

Solomon, S. D., & Davidson, J. R. (1997). Trauma: prevalence, impairment, service use, and cost. *Journal of Clinical Psychiatry, 58*(Suppl 9), 5–11.

Spiegel, D., Koopman, C., Cardeña, E., & Classen, C. (1996). Dissociative symptoms in the diagnosis of acute stress disorder. Handbook of dissociation: Theoretical, empirical, and clinical perspectives. In L. K. Michelson & W. J. Ray (Eds.), *Handbook of dissociation: Theoretical, empirical, and clinical perspectives* (pp. 367–380). New York: Plenum Press.

Taylor, F. B., Martin, P., Thompson, C., Williams, J., Mellman, T. A., Gross, C., et al. (2008). Prazosin effects on objective sleep measures and clinical symptoms in civilian trauma posttraumatic stress disorder: a placebo-controlled study. *Biological Psychiatry, 63*(6), 629–632.

Terr, L. C. (1991). Childhood traumas: an outline and overview. *American Journal of Psychiatry, 148*(1), 10–20.

Tichenor, V., Marmar, C. R., Weiss, D. S., Metzler, T. J., & Ronfeldt, H. M. (1996). The relationship of peritraumatic dissociation and posttraumatic stress: findings in female Vietnam theater veterans. *Journal of Consulting and Clinical Psychology, 64*(5), 1054–1059.

Vaiva, G., Ducrocq, F., Jezequel, K., Averland, B., Lestavel, P., Brunet, A., & Marmar, C. R. (2003). Immediate treatment with propranolol decreases posttraumatic stress disorder two months after trauma. *Biological Psychiatry, 54*(9), 947–949.

Vaiva, G., Jehel, L., Cottencin, O., Ducrocq, F., Duchet, C., Omnes, C., et al. (2008). [Prevalence of trauma-related disorders in the French WHO study: Santé mentale en population générale (SMPG)]. *Encephale, 34*(6), 577–583.

van der Hart, O., van Ochten, J. M., van Son, M. J., Steele, K., & Lensvelt-Mulders, G. (2008). Relations among peritraumatic dissociation and posttraumatic stress: a critical review. *Journal of Trauma & Dissociation, 9*(4), 481–505.

van Emmerik, A. A., Kamphuis, J. H., Hulsbosch, A. M., & Emmelkamp, P. M. (2002). Single session debriefing after psychological trauma: a meta-analysis. *Lancet, 360*(9335), 766–771.

van Zelst, W. H., de Beurs, E., Beekman, A. T., Deeg, D. J., & van Dyck, R. (2003). Prevalence and risk factors of posttraumatic stress disorder in older adults. *Psychotherapy & Psychosomatics, 72*(6), 333–342.

Yasan, A., Guzel, A., Tamam, Y., & Ozkan, M. (2009). Predictive factors for acute stress disorder and posttraumatic stress disorder after motor vehicle accidents. *Psychopathology, 42*(4), 236–241.

Yehuda, R. (2004). Risk and resilience in posttraumatic stress disorder. *Journal of Clinical Psychiatry, 65* (Suppl 1), 29–36.

Zohar, J., Sonnino, R., Juven-Wetzler, A., & Cohen, H. (2009). Can posttraumatic stress disorder be prevented? *CNS Spectrums, 14*(1 Suppl 1), 44–51.

31.

ANXIETY IN THE MEDICALLY ILL

Richard J. Goldberg and Donna B. Greenberg

INTRODUCTION

The anxiety that accompanies medical illness contributes greatly to each patient's functional impairment (Marcus et al., 1997). Recognition and reduction of excessive anxiety facilitates the ability to cope. This chapter presents an approach to the evaluation and treatment of anxiety in medical patients that includes both biological and psychological dimensions and requires full medical and psychiatric consideration. First, we review medication-induced or substance-induced symptoms and notable underlying medical bases for anxiety. Once these possibilities have been considered, a clinician draws on the patient's personal and psychiatric history to determine whether anxiety is part of an underlying psychiatric disorder, such as panic disorder, mood disorder, or personality disorder. Simultaneously, the clinician assesses the anxiety as a reactive psychological adjustment response.

MEDICAL DISORDERS THAT PRESENT AS ANXIETY

Medical disorders can produce anxiety directly or indirectly. Some medical disorders have specific effects on neurotransmitter systems that stimulate anxiety, such as hyperthyroidism (Hall, 1983; MacCrimmon et al., 1979); others have specific effects on neuroanatomic sites associated directly with the production of anxiety, for example, tumors of the temporal lobe (Dietch, 1984). Other medical disorders produce anxiety through autonomic arousal, which the patient interprets as a psychological state. Medical disorders that can present with anxiety as a prominent symptom are listed in Box 31.1.

TOXIC AND WITHDRAWAL EFFECTS OF DRUGS

The toxic and withdrawal effects of drugs are a common cause of anxiety in medical patients See Box 31.2. If there is any doubt about what drugs the patient has been taking, a toxicology screen should be ordered. Such screening is especially useful when the patient is suspected of surreptitious drug use. Review of the patient's medication list should also pay attention to what drugs have been stopped.

Caffeine

Caffeine is one of the most widely used psychotropic drugs in the United States and one which causes anxiety; it is found in many beverages and drug combinations (Abelson & Fishburne, 1976). The approximate amount of caffeine in a cup of coffee is 150 mg; tea generally has about 50–100 mg per cup; cola drinks have about 40–50 mg/12 oz.; and a small chocolate bar has about 15–25 mg. Caffeine-containing medications (as it is usually combined with aspirin or acetaminophen) have about 32 mg of caffeine per tablet. Consumption of these medications is associated with an increase in sleep difficulties (Brown et al., 1995). Although sensitivity varies, symptoms of caffeinism may occur at doses of only 200 mg (Victor, Lubetsky, & Greden, 1981). Patients with generalized anxiety disorder are abnormally sensitive to caffeine for both subjective and physiologic arousal measures (Bruce et al., 1992). Caffeine increases norepinephrine levels in the plasma and urine (Robertson et al., 1978), inhibits phosphodiesterase breakdown of cyclic adenosine monophosphate in the central nervous system (CNS), and sensitizes central catecholamine receptors, particularly for dopamine (Waldeck, 1975). Caffeine can precipitate an actual panic attack in patients with panic disorder (Charney, Heninger, & Jatlow, 1985). In chronic users, caffeine abstinence should also be considered as a possible source of intermittent anxiety (White et al., 1980). After ceasing consumption, people who have consumed even low or moderate amounts of caffeine (mean amounts of 235 mg/day, which is equivalent to 2.5 cups of coffee) may have withdrawal syndromes such as moderate to severe headache, fatigue, or psychic distress (Silverman et al., 1992). Since caffeine is like other psychoactive drugs with the development of dependence and withdrawal syndrome (Strain et al., 1994), patients should be advised to taper off caffeine gradually rather than stop abruptly.

Energy drinks have moderate to relatively high levels and concentrations of caffeine (2.5–35.7 mg per oz) compared to other caffeinated beverages such as a 12oz. cola or 6oz. cup of coffee (see Box 31.3). Energy shots are low volume (1–2oz.) and have an even higher concentration of caffeine than other energy drinks. Also, hot beverages like coffee are usually drunk more slowly than cold energy drinks, so in the latter case larger quantities of caffeine can be consumed in short order. Energy drinks have also been linked to drinking high

Box 31.1 MEDICAL CONDITIONS ASSOCIATED WITH ANXIETY SYMPTOMS

Cardiovascular Conditions

Angina pectoris
Arrhythmias
Congestive heart failure
Hypovolemia
Myocardial infarction
Valvular disease

Endocrine Conditions

Carcinoid syndrome
Hyperadrenalism
Hypercalcemia
Hyperthyroidism
Hypocalcemia
Hypothyroidism
Pheochromocytoma

Metabolic Conditions

Hyperkalemia
Hyperthermia
Hypoglycemia
Hyponatremia
Hypoxia
Porphyria

Neurologic Conditions

Akathisia
Encephalopathy
Mass lesion
Postconcussion syndrome
Seizure disorder
Vertigo

Peptic Ulcer Disease

Respiratory Conditions

Asthma
Chronic obstructive pulmonary disease
Pneumothorax
Pulmonary edema
Pulmonary embolism

Immunologic Conditions

Anaphylaxis
Systemic lupus erythematosus

Box 31.2 DRUGS THAT CAUSE ANXIETY

Stimulants

Amphetamines
Aminophylline
Caffeine
Cocaine
Methylphenidate
Theophylline

Sympathomimetics

Ephedrine
Epinephrine
Phentermine
Phenylpropanolamine
Pseudoephedrine

Drug Withdrawal

Benzodiazepines
Narcotics
Barbiturates
Sedatives
Alcohol

Anticholinergics

Trihexyphenidyl
Benztropine
Diphenhydramine
Oxybutynin
Propantheline
Meperidine
Tricyclics
Pilocarpine (including ocular)

Dopaminergics

Amantadine
Bromocriptine
L-dopa
Carbidopa-leuodopa
Metoclopramide
Neuroleptics
Pergolide

Miscellaneous

Baclofen
Cycloserine
Hallucinogens
Indomethacin
Anabolic steroids
Captopril
Disopyramide
Dronabinol
Estrogens
Fluoroquinolone antibiotics
Metrizamide

volumes of alcohol per drinking session, with more injudicious consequences (Arria & O'Brien, 2011). The American Academy of Pediatrics recommends that adolescents should not have more than 100 mg of caffeine each day, and adults should limit caffeine to 500 mg per day. Older patients may be

Metronidazole
Procaine derivatives
Progestins
Sumatriptan and other triptans

Other

SSRIs (may be confused with akathisia)
   Interferon

more sensitive to caffeine (Brown & Stoudemire, 1998; Torpy & Livingston, 2013; American Academy of Pediatrics, 2011).

Cocaine, Methamphetamine and Marijuana

Symptoms of anxiety, irritability, tremulousness, fatigue, or depression may appear soon after the initial euphoriant effects of cocaine (Resnick, Kestenbaum, & Schwartz, 1976; Abramowicz, 1986). Cocaine has been reported to induce

---

Box 31.3 CAFFEINE CONTENT OF BEVERAGES AND OTHER PRODUCTS

Energy Drinks and Caffeine Content (mg)
  5-hour Energy 207
  Amp, 16 oz. 143
  BAWLS guarana 16 oz. 100
  Full throttle, 16 oz. 197
  Monster, 16 oz. 160
  No Fear, 16 oz. 174
  NOS, 16 oz. 260
  Red Bull, 16 oz. 152
  Rip it 16 oz. 200
  Rockstar, 16 oz. 160
  SPIKE Shooter 286

Sodas and Caffeine Content (mg)
  Coca Cola 20 oz. bottle 58
  Dr. Pepper 20 oz. bottle 70
  Mountain Dew 20 oz. bottle 90
  Pepsi, 20 oz. bottle 63
  Pepsi MAX 20 oz. bottle 115
  Vault 20 oz. bottle 118

Other
  Arizona Iced Tea, green 16 oz. 15
  Black tea (brwed) 8 oz. 55
  Coffee (brewed) 16 oz. 170
  Excedrin Extra Strength 2 pills 130
  Hot chocolate 8 oz. 9
  NoDoz Maimum Strength 1 pill 200
  StayAlert gum 1 piece 100
  Vivarin 1 pill 200

*Average values; individual brands may vary.
Source: Center for Military Psychiatry and Neuroscience at the Walter Reed Army Institute of Research 2012 (more info on www.jama.com)
From Torpy & Livingston,2013)

---

panic attacks in susceptible individuals and actually to precipitate panic disorder, which continues autonomously even after the cocaine use is discontinued (Aronson & Craig, 1986). Detectable amounts of cocaine are found in the urine or plasma only for a few hours after use, although one of the metabolites, benzoylecgonine, can be detected in a urine sample for as long as 48 hours after use and longer after chronic use (Preston et al., 2002). Abuse of methamphetamine, which has a half-life of 12 hours (longer than cocaine), can present with anxiety in the setting of intoxication or withdrawal. In withdrawal, the depression may be more prolonged and worse than that of cocaine withdrawal (Winslow, Voorhees, & Pehl, 2007) Among marijuana users anxiety is prominent with panic reactions noted most often in naïve users (Green et al., 2003). Tolerance to the intoxicating effects of marijuana can develop, and anxiety, insomnia, appetite disturbance, and depression can occur upon withdrawal (Budeny & Hughes, 2006; Maldonado et al., 2011).

Alcohol and Sedative Withdrawal

Since many hospitalized medical patients have unhealthy alcohol use (Moore, 1985; Saltz et al., 2005), alcohol withdrawal (Lerner & Fallon, 1985) is a frequent etiology for agitation and anxiety in this population. Minor abstinence syndrome, which has its modal onset about 24 hours after cessation of drinking, presents with anxiety, tremulousness (the shakes), and insomnia. The major concern is whether such symptoms are the harbinger of alcohol withdrawal delirium (delirium tremens), which has a modal onset 72 hours following cessation or significant reduction of drinking but can also occur as early as 24 hours or up to 7 days later. In major abstinence, anxiety and tremulousness are accompanied by symptoms of autonomic arousal, and should be considered a serious medical problem that requires supervised medical management (Sellers & Kalant, 1976). The classic signs and symptoms of sedative withdrawal can be masked by the concurrent use of other medications. For example, mydriasis may be absent if the patient is on narcotics, and tachycardia may be masked by beta-blockers. Because of the association of Wernicke-Korsakoff syndrome with alcohol use (Reuler, Girard, & Cooney, 1985), such patients should always be given thiamine.

Opiate Withdrawal

Narcotic abstinence is always accompanied by anxiety. Iatrogenic withdrawal (and recurrent pain) may occur when patients are changed from parenteral to oral narcotics without consideration of differences in oral/parenteral potency ratios.

Neuroleptics and Other Dopamine Blockers

Akathisia, an extrapyramidal side effect of typical neuroleptics, mimics anxiety. Patients may be aware of inability to keep their legs still and their desire to move. They may rock from foot to foot, and may have insomnia. Signs of akathisia range from occasional fidgety movements to walking on the spot. In the outpatient setting patients may get up from their chair as they describe anxiety and insomnia and pace around the room (Barnes, 2003). Typical antipsychotics as well as prochlorperazine and other dopamine receptor blockers like metoclopramide can cause akathisia. Risperidone, ziprasidone, and aripiprazole have a higher risk of akathisia than the atypical antipsychotics olanzapine, or quetiapine (Kumar & Sachdev, 2009). Patients with bipolar disorder and depression are more prone to akathisia than those with schizophrenia. Akathisia with aripiprazole in schizophrenic patients occurred in 12.5% as compared to 24% with haloperidol (Kane et al., 2010). Among schizophrenic patients in a large study (the Clinical Antipsychotic Trials of Intervention Effectiveness Schizophrenia Trial), a moderate dose of perphenazine produced comparable rates of akathisia to ziprasidone, risperidone, and olanzapine (Caroff, Hurford, Lybrand, & Campbell, 2011).

Akathisia may be treated by lowering the neuroleptic dose of the offending drug or by a switch to an atypical agent with less potential for akathisia. While other extrapyramidal side effects like acute dystonia and parkinsonism respond to anticholinergic drugs, it is not clear that they are helpful for akathisia. Benzodiazepines such as lorazepam 0.5 mg three times daily or clonazepam 0.5 mg once daily offer another treatment option (Fleischhacker, Roth, & Kane, 1990; Wells et al., 1991; Rathbone & Soares-Weiser, 2006). Propranolol 40–80 mg twice daily has been effective. Mirtazapine 15 mg each day may also be effective (Poyurovsky, 2010).

Antidepressants

Akathisia-like jitteriness is a common side effect of fluoxetine and other specific serotonin reuptake inhibitors (SSRI) (Lipinski et al., 1989) characterized by motor restlessness and anxiety that is indistinguishable from neuroleptic-induced anxiety. The side effect appears to be similar to the jitteriness associated with tricyclic antidepressants (TCAs) (Nierenberg & Cole, 1991; Pohl et al., 1988). Such jitteriness (including increased anxiety and insomnia) can occur even at low doses. A review of anti-depressant induced jitteriness/anxiety syndrome did not find robust evidence of a different incidence between tricyclics and SSRIs. This jitteriness syndrome is sometimes thought to be distinct from the akathisia typical of neuroleptics. Common treatment strategies are slower titration of antidepressants and the addition of benzodiazepines (Sinclair et al., 2009).

Agitation, insomnia, and tremor are also among the most common side effects of bupropion (Bryant, Guernsey, & Ingrim, 1983; Gardner, 1983). Tolerance usually develops with continuation of treatment. As with neuroleptic-induced akathisia, beta-adrenergic blockers or benzodiazepines may be helpful in reducing or abolishing the symptoms, although dose reduction is often necessary.

Other Drugs

Alpha-adrenergic stimulants such as pseudoephedrine are often included in over-the-counter decongestants. These agents are closely related to amphetamines and can produce symptoms of anxiety, restlessness, irritability, and insomnia (Weiner, 1980).

Bronchodilators, which chemically resemble the catecholamines (such as isoproterenol and albuterol), have peripheral effects that include increased heart rate and blood pressure that contribute to feelings of anxiety. Systemic effects, reported even with metered-dose inhalers (Harris, 1985), include symptoms of anxiety, restlessness, nervousness, tremor, irritability, insomnia, and emotional lability.

Theophylline, a methylxanthine related chemically to caffeine, is capable of producing powerful cardiovascular effects with tachycardia, along with nervousness and anxiety states (Jacobs, Senior, & Kessler, 1976).

Nifedipine and verapamil have been reported to produce neuropsychiatric symptoms that include anxiety, tremulousness, jitteriness, and sleep disturbance (Bela & Raftery, 1980; Mueller & Chahine, 1981; Rinkenberger et al., 1980; Singh, Ellrodt, & Peter, 1978).

Other drugs reported to produce anxiety as a side effect include amphetamines and similar anorexic agents, antihistamines, cycloserine, and indomethacin (Abramowicz, 1989).

OTHER MEDICAL DISORDERS

Hypoglycemia

Diabetes has a high rate of comorbid depression and anxiety disorder; however, anxiety symptoms must be evaluated with consideration of hypoglycemia. Hypoglycemia provokes adrenergic or catecholamine-mediated symptoms that may include anxiety, tachycardia, diaphoresis, tremor, weakness, hunger, irritability, and palpitations. Patients taking insulin, glinides, metformin, or sulfonuria are most at risk. Patients can be educated to be alert to glucose readings below 70 mg/dL. This threshold allows for inaccurate readings and comes before symptoms develop. Patients need not always treat themselves with glucose at this reading but should avoid exercise or driving until the glucose is higher. Older patients and patients who have recurrent hypoglycemia are less likely to have the sympathetic symptoms and are more at risk of becoming confused without the forewarning of anxiety (Seaquist et al., 2013). Hypoglycemia is discussed further in Chapter 6.

Complex Partial Seizures

Anxiety is the most common ictal emotion associated with temporal lobe epilepsy (Weil, 1959). Simple partial seizures from a mesial temporal structural lesion can mimic panic disorder (Young et al., 1995). The phenomenology of panic attacks and temporal lobe epilepsy can be difficult to distinguish, especially when the electroencephalogram (EEG) does not support the diagnosis of temporal lobe epilepsy. McNamara and Fogel (1990) reported five cases of patients with panic attacks with associated paroxysmal emotional, autonomic, or psychosensory symptoms. The EEG findings, although compatible with interictal temporal lobe epilepsy, were nonspecific. However, the cases responded well to anticonvulsant therapy. The likelihood of complex partial seizures is increased if the patient has a history of head injury, febrile convulsions in childhood, birth trauma, or encephalitis, or a personal or family history of seizures.

The characteristic abnormality in temporal lobe seizures is the anterior temporal spike focus; however, in the waking state at least one half of patients have normal EEGs (Gibbs & Gibbs, 1952). A sleep record does increase the percentage of abnormal EEGs in epileptic patients, although the measure of false negatives remains about 30% to 40%. The value of nasopharyngeal and sphenoidal leads is uncertain, although the use of continuous ambulatory EEG monitoring (Kristensen & Sendrup, 1978; Lieb et al., 1976; McNamara & Fogel, 1990; Zijlmans et al., 2008) can increase the diagnostic yield (see Chapter 43). Because of the high incidence of false-negatives, the EEG is not a definitive test, and the diagnosis of temporal lobe seizure disorder often must be made on clinical grounds and tested by an empiric trial of anticonvulsants.

Angina Pectoris

Angina may present as anxiety with episodes of dyspnea and palpitations accompanied by only mild chest discomfort. When such episodes are precipitated by exercise or emotional stress, angina should be suspected and cardiac evaluation considered, especially in patients over 40 years of age or those with a cardiac history. However, when such evaluations are done, panic disorder is found to be a common cause of chest pain in patients with negative cardiac test results (Katon, 1990).

Cardiac Arrhythmias

Because cardiac arrhythmias may produce symptoms mistaken for anxiety, pulse regularity should always be checked during an episode of anxiety. For instance, paroxysmal supraventricular tachycardia may be misdiagnosed as panic disorder (McCrank, Schurmans, & Lefkoe, 1998). If the diagnosis of recurrent arrhythmias is suspected, ambulatory monitoring may be helpful. For those patients with arrhythmias, a host of medical conditions that are also associated with anxiety symptoms need to be considered, such as hyperthyroidism, caffeinism, and nicotine abuse (Lynch et al., 1977). Implantable defibrillators have been reported to cause PTSD after repeated discharges. (Habibovic, van den Broek, Alings, van der Voort, & Denollet, 2012; Hamner et al., 1999).

Mitral Valve Prolapse

Both patients with panic disorder and patients with mitral valve prolapse complain of chest pain, dyspnea, fatigue, dizziness, and a fainting sensation. About half of patients with mitral valve prolapse at one time or another complain of palpitations, but continuous cardiac monitoring of such patients often reveals no relationship between the complaint of palpitations and any form of cardiac rhythm disturbance (Devereux et al., 1976; Shear et al., 1984). Studies looking for an association between the two syndromes have provided inconsistent results over the last 40 years, and more recent studies have not found an association (Filho et al., 2008, 2011).

Recurrent Pulmonary Emboli

Recurrent pulmonary emboli can present as repeated episodes of acute anxiety associated with hyperventilation and dyspnea (Ferrer, 1968). The most common symptoms of pulmonary embolus in patients who did not have preexisting cardiopulmonary disease (as noted in the Prospective Investigation of Pulmonary Embolism Diagnosis II) were dyspnea at rest or with exertion, pleuritic pain, cough, more than two-pillow orthopnea, calf or thigh pain/swelling, and wheezing. Tachypnea and tachycardia were the most common signs (Stein et al., 2007).

Arterial blood gases may reveal decreased partial pressure of oxygen during an episode but not always, and the confirmatory tests most in use are the computerized tomography pulmonary angiography (CT-PA), ventilation-perfusion lung scan and D-dimer. This diagnosis should be considered in those patients who have some predisposition, such as immobilization, surgery within the last 3 months, stroke, paresis, paralysis, central venous instrumentation within the last 3 months, cancer, chronic heart disease, autoimmune diseases, and history of venous thromboembolism (Thompson & Hales, 2014).

Heart Failure and Pulmonary Edema

Insomnia and anxiety may be early signs of heart failure, as patients find their sleep disrupted, must sit up or sleep with pillows due to orthopnea, and have paroxysmal nocturnal dyspnea.

Hyperthyroidism

Hyperthyroidism usually presents with symptoms of nervousness, palpitations, diaphoresis, heat intolerance, and diarrhea. Signs include tachycardia, tremor, weight loss, and hot, moist skin. The contribution of hyperthyroidism to anxiety, along with its diagnosis and treatment, are discussed in Chapters 6 and 55.

Pheochromocytoma

Pheochromocytoma is a rare tumor of the adrenal medulla or sympathetic ganglia (paragangliomas) which can secrete catecholamines (norepinephrine, epinephrine, or dopamine) (Hodin, 2014). The output of catecholamines may be episodic or continuous, producing acute or chronic symptoms of anxiety that are often accompanied by headache, sweating, and flushing (Lishman, 1987). Although anxiety symptoms may be prominent, panic attacks are not always seen (Starkman et al., 1985). Episodes of palpitations and anxiety may be subtle, and the classic signs of flushing and headache may be absent (Hodin, 2014). Hypertension is usually present during acute episodes, and 60% to 80% of patients have sustained hypertension. Urinary and plasma catecholamines and fractionated metanephrine and normetanephrine are assessed for diagnosis. Plasma free metanephrine levels and fractionated metanephrine levels in the urine are most sensitive to exclude the tumor (Pacak et al., 2005). The diagnosis is pursued in the setting of resistant hypertension, hyperadrenergic episodes, an incidental adrenal tumor on imaging, cardiomyopathy in a young person, and family history of a predisposing syndrome. Familial syndromes are multiple endocrine neoplasia type 2, von Hippel-Lindau syndrome, neurofibromatosis type 1, and familial paraganglioma. Further details of the evaluation can be found in Chapter 6.

Hyperventilation Syndrome

Hyperventilation syndrome (HVS), like panic disorder, is a syndrome that harks back to descriptions of nineteenth century soldiers with an irritable heart and predates the current definition of panic disorder. It was estimated to have a prevalence of 10% in a general medical clinic years ago (Rice, 1950), and 5% in a neurology clinic practice (Pincus & Tucker, 1985). Anxiety is a cardinal symptom along with a variety of other medical symptoms, including faintness, visual disturbances, nausea, vertigo, headache, palpitations, dyspnea, diaphoresis, and paresthesias. Patients may or may not be aware that they are hyperventilating, and repeated sighing is often a visible sign. The diagnosis of HVS can be made on the basis of the patient's response to overbreathing (breathing by mouth for up to 3 minutes or until dizzy). If the symptoms in question are entirely reproduced, without an alternative explanation by physical examination, medical history, or laboratory tests, the diagnosis can be established.

Hyperventilation syndrome probably represents a form of panic disorder in most cases, and patients may qualify for both syndromes (Cowley & Roy-Byrne, 1987). Hyperventilation leads to excessive elimination of carbon dioxide, acute respiratory alkalosis, and cerebral arterial constriction. In 240 seconds of overbreathing, cerebral blood flow can be reduced by 40% (Plum & Posner, 1972), causing EEG slowing (Gotoh, Meyer, & Takagi, 1965). Muscular tension is heightened by a decreased ionization of calcium associated with the increase in pH (Neill & Hattenhauer, 1975). Hyperventilation also causes increased coronary artery resistance and can cause chest discomfort that is difficult to distinguish from angina pectoris (Evans & Lum, 1977), along with nonspecific downward depression of the ST segment and T wave flattening (Christensen, 1946). Unlike ischemic ST changes, those caused by hyperventilation usually appear early during exercise and tend to disappear as exercise continues (McHenry et al., 1970).

Postconcussion Syndrome

Cerebral concussion is classically regarded as a disorder that produces no irreversible anatomic lesions. Clinically, concussion results in an instantaneous diminution of function or loss of consciousness followed by rapid and complete recovery. The episode may be surrounded by a sphere of amnesia, with about one-tenth of the total as retrograde amnesia (Parkinson, 1977). Mild head trauma (1-minute to 2-minute loss of consciousness without external signs of trauma) has been reported to lead to an increase in catecholamines lasting for about 4 months (Wortsman et al., 1980). Initially patients complain of feeling fuzzy or slowed down, unable to sleep, tired, headachey or dizzy with visual problems. They feel anxious, irritable or depressed (Silver, 2014). For most patients, the symptoms abate after a few weeks to a few months A fraction of patients have persistent symptoms for more than a few months after a concussion associated with pre- trauma conditions like substance abuse and mood disorder and social factors: lack of social support or anticipated litigation and compensation (Silver, 2014).

There has been controversy about whether postconcussive syndrome is a long-term consequence of mild traumatic brain injury. A study of the prospective course of postconcussion syndrome found that mild traumatic brain injury did not predict postconcussive syndrome among those who entered a Level 1 trauma unit after mild traumatic brain injury. A pre-injury depressive or anxiety disorder and acute posttraumatic stress were early markers of postconcussive syndrome regardless of brain injury (Meares, Shores, Taylor, Batchelor, & Bryant, 2011) Anxiety in patients was endorsed by 16% at 5 days and 29% at 106 days, along with the symptoms of headache, dizziness, irritability, impairment of memory and concentration, fatigue, noise intolerance, depression, mood swings, insomnia, and malaise.

Psychiatric aspects of head trauma are discussed in Chapter 45.

Nonspecific Medical Causes

Many medical disorders may be associated with a broad array of psychiatric symptoms, including anxiety as a nonspecific reaction to delirium, although not as a prominent feature. Such disorders include Cushing's syndrome (Lishman, 1987), hyponatremia (Gehi et al., 1981), renal failure (Marshall, 1979), hypoparathyroidism (Denko & Kaelbling, 1962), and other electrolyte imbalances (Webb & Gehi, 1981). Hypomagnesemia (Hall & Joffe, 1973) in particular may be associated with hypocalcemia, and the drop of ionized calcium with hyperventilation may be accentuated by symptoms of tetany. The diagnostic workup for a physiologic cause of anxiety must be guided by the clinical review of systems and a complete survey of current and recently discontinued drugs and medications, and known concurrent medical conditions. In an otherwise healthy patient with significant sustained anxiety, thyroid screening alone might be sufficient. At the other end of the spectrum (e.g., new-onset sustained anxiety in the elderly), a comprehensive metabolic and neurologic assessment is needed.

CONCURRENT PSYCHIATRIC DISORDERS IN MEDICAL PATIENTS

The second step in evaluating the presentation of anxiety in a medical or surgical patient is to evaluate for the possibility of underlying psychiatric disorder, exploring past history and family history. Anxiety disorder is the most common psychiatric diagnosis with a lifetime prevalence of 29% (Kessler et al., 2005). In primary care as many as 20 percent of patients have at least one anxiety disorder with a range of 6–9% for post-traumatic stress disorder, panic disorder, social anxiety disorder, and generalized anxiety disorder (Kroenke et al., 2007). Higher rates are seen in selected subgroups such as those with Parkinson's disease (Stein et al., 1990), chest pain patients with normal coronary angiograms (Beitman et al., 1991), irritable bowel syndrome (Lydiard et al., 1993) and high utilizers of medical care (Katon et al., 1990).

Panic disorder is associated with an array of somatic symptoms and fear of symptoms, leading to more evaluation by doctors (Barsky et al., 1999; Rudaz et al., 2010). In primary care, the most common panic disorder symptoms are cardiac, neurological, and gastrointestinal (Katon, 1986). In addition, vestibular and respiratory clusters of symptoms help to define which specialist will subsequently be seeing the patient (Sansone & Sansone, 2009). Palpitations, shortness of breath, choking, chest pain, and numbness, have defined a cardio-respiratory type associated with fear of dying. A second constellation includes sweating, trembling, nausea, hot flashes, and dizziness. The thoughts that accompany panic attacks, a cognitive constellation: a feeling of unreality, fear of going crazy, and fear of losing control serve as clues to the diagnosis of panic disorder (Meuret et al., 2006).

Anxiety is often a significant component of a mood disorder. Anxiety disorders may predate a secondary depression or panic attacks may present at the onset of a clinical depression. In fact, anxiety disorder and depression are often seen together in patients coming to primary care physicians with first complaints (McLaughlin, et al., 2006; Toft et al., 2005). Anxious depression has a more chronic course of illness, an increased incidence of suicidal thoughts, and greater occupational impairment among patients with depressive disorder (Rao & Zisook, 2009). Patients with comorbid major depressive disorder and panic disorder before and after treatment with SSRIs have poorer quality of life and more impairment of function than patients with major depressive disorder alone (IsHak et al., 2014).

Those with anxiety and depression have more somatic symptoms without an identified medical cause; the more the symptoms the more likely the patient has anxiety and depression (Kroenke et al., 1994; Katon et al., 2007). Those patients preoccupied with somatic symptoms much of the time for at least 6 months such that they are distressed or have significant disruption of functioning as well as excessive and disproportionate thoughts, feelings, and behaviors around the symptoms are diagnosed as having somatic symptom disorder (APA, 2013). Those with persistent anxiety about illness who constantly check for illness or avoid doctors but have no somatic symptoms carry the diagnosis of illness anxiety disorder. What had been called hypochondriasis is now subsumed under somatic symptom disorder if both anxiety and somatic symptoms are present (APA, 2013; Warwick & Salkovskis, 1990).

For those with somatic symptom disorder the contribution of anxiety disorder and anxious depression should be considered seriously and treated as part of management (Croicu et al., 2014). Substance abuse should be tracked and its contribution considered in the differential diagnosis.

In addition to clinical evaluation of anxiety and depressive disorders, the Patient Health Questionnaire-9 (PHQ 9) and the Generalized Anxiety Disorder Questionnaire 7 (GAD 7) (Kroenke et al., 2007, 2010; Spitzer et al., 2006) have been useful self-report questionnaires. The Somatic Symptom Scale-8 measures somatic symptom burden and its severity and can be used to follow patients (Barsky, 2014; Gierk et al., 2014). Other aspects of management of illness behavior are discussed in Chapter 37.

Patients with anxiety disorders often come to attention in the medical setting because of their claustrophobia, which prevents magnetic resonance imaging, or because they have phobias of having blood drawn. They may not be able to take the elevator to the doctor's office or acquiesce to radiation treatment. Patients may be especially anxious when trapped by traction in the orthopedic setting. These patients often have great anticipatory anxiety and are likely to focus on catastrophic events 6 months down the line when the physician is speaking to them about a treatment plan for the current week. Conditioned anxiety can be seen after multiple treatments of chemotherapy or dressing changes and can be triggered when patients approach the hospital or other territory that reminds them of past treatment.

Anxiety has both positive and negative symptoms; the positive symptoms of panic attacks and sympathetic arousal are more visible in the medical setting than the negative symptoms of avoidance, non-compliance, and indecision. Patients avoid the settings of past anxiety attacks and challenges that may arouse anxiety; therefore, they may avoid coming to medical appointments. The ways that anxiety has restricted the lives of patients, the way that they do not move into the social sphere or try new things may not be as obvious to the clinician or to the patient unless the clinician considers the negative symptoms of anxiety in a fuller evaluation.

A full psychiatric evaluation may also recognize that anxiety presents in the setting of psychotic disorder, borderline personality disorder (Nisenson et al., 1998) or cognitive impairment, and incipient dementia.

PSYCHOSOCIAL ISSUES AND ANXIETY IN MEDICAL PATIENTS

No evaluation of the anxious medical patient is complete without an inquiry into the psychosocial dimension of the patient's experience. The psychosocial dimension encompasses the intrapsychic meanings that patients attach to experiences and their behaviorally conditioned responses. Although physicians often assume that the distress associated with illness is accounted for by the physical morbidity, a significant component of the distress associated with cancer, for example, relates to psychosocial adjustment (Goldberg & Cullen, 1985). It is often therapeutic to help the patient identify emotional problem areas that are being transformed into symptoms and to help contain the anxiety by putting it into words. The following sections discuss four major areas worth reviewing in terms of understanding potential psychological sources of anxiety.

ALIENATION

Social support plays an important role in maintaining mental and physical health. Anxiety over separation, loss, abandonment, and isolation can be even more important than fear associated with the disease itself. The physician should identify the patient's major social supports and assess their involvement. Whenever possible, the physician should meet with patient and key supports together to observe their interaction and to facilitate better sharing and communication. The patient's intrapsychic concern about abandonment is sometimes best dealt with by a concrete intervention, such as arranging homemaker or visiting nurse assistance.

As disease progresses, patients may become anxious because of a growing sense of distance from the physician. Patients nearing the end of an intensive treatment program are noted to experience an increase in anxiety rather than a sense of relief (Mastrovito, 1972; Peck & Boland, 1977), fearing that the detachment will jeopardize their survival. Maintenance of a regular contact and communication of concern are valuable positive interventions, although to the action-oriented physician such visits may seem like doing very little.

LOSS OF CONTROL

For many patients, the loss of control inherent in illness may be the crucial factor underlying anxiety symptoms. The consultant must be creative in identifying areas in which the patient can exercise some control without jeopardizing medical treatment. Intellectual mastery is another means of reasserting control for some patients. Sharing information in a way appropriate to the patient's personality style should therefore be considered an important means of reducing anxiety, although physicians often worry that patients may become more upset by hearing about their diagnosis (Goldberg, 1983).

PHYSICAL DAMAGE

Threatened or real loss of bodily integrity or a body part can trigger profound anxiety, along with insomnia, anorexia, and difficulty in concentrating. Patients who view themselves as less than whole may withdraw from relationships because of anxiety over rejection. Before surgery, patients can become panicked and feel they have a poor chance of survival (Bard & Sutherland, 1977). It is always important to explore what patients have heard from others about the procedure they are awaiting because misconceptions can arise from stories about a friend or relative who did poorly in a similar situation or information gleaned from chat rooms. Preoperative review of potential misconceptions may even decrease certain surgical complications (Egbert et al., 1964).

With anxious patients who ask, "Am I going to be all right?", there is a tendency to reassure prematurely rather than to explore difficult feelings. Furthermore, some preoperative anxiety can be helpful, since it stimulates realistic planning. Patients who are extraordinarily calm may be masking fears that place them at higher risk for not coping with later inevitable events (Sutherland et al., 1977).

DEATH

The issue of dying may or may not be brought up directly by the patient; it may emerge instead through some related symptoms of anxiety. As long as patients with life-threatening illness function adaptively, elements of denial play an important role in continued function (Dimsdale & Hackett, 1982). The natural course of progressive illness, however, usually challenges the patient to slowly adjust denial mechanisms to the emerging medical reality (Weisman, 1979). Recurrence of disease often erodes initial optimism and creates a situation in which the patient for the first time deals with issues of dying. Signs of physician willingness to engage the patient on these issues are important in allaying fears, which otherwise would remain unexpressed. Dealing in some way with their own sense of mortality probably is important for clinicians to be effective in dealing with patients' anxiety about death. See Chapters 81 and 84 on end of life issues for children and adults.

PHARMACOLOGICAL MANAGEMENT

BENZODIAZEPINES

The best indication for using benzodiazepines is for relief when a time-limited cause of anxiety can be identified, as in the case of the patient awaiting a cardiac catheterization. Benzodiazepines are also helpful in treating primary anxiety disorders, and adjunctively for patients with physiologic/endogenous anxiety syndromes (see Chapter 21). They are particularly helpful when they mitigate the suffering of acute medical management. Alternatives to benzodiazepines are sought for chronic anxiety because patients may become tolerant and dependent to these medications, and those with a history of substance abuse may add benzodiazepines to alcohol or narcotics.

Pharmacokinetics

All the benzodiazepines are well absorbed orally and reach peak blood levels after a single oral dose in times varying from 1 to 6 hours. The differences in time to reach peak plasma level largely reflect differences in gastrointestinal absorption. As metabolites reach a steady state, however, initial differences related to absorption and distribution disappear and differences related to metabolism become prominent. Chlordiazepoxide (Greenblatt et al., 1974) and diazepam (Greenblatt & Koch-Weser, 1976) are poorly and unpredictably absorbed from intramuscular (IM) sites, whereas lorazepam and midazolam have the distinct property of prompt and reliable IM absorption (Greenblatt et al., 1982). The metabolic fate of various benzodiazepines may be simplified by appreciating that they fall into two classes—long acting and short acting (see Table 31.1).

Drug accumulation, with potential impairment of cognitive and motor performance, is a special risk to be kept in mind with long-acting agents, especially for older patients and those with liver impairment (Greenblatt et al., 1980; Greenblatt, Miller, & Shader, 1987). Despite the long half-lives and accumulation of active substances, chronic use of these drugs usually does not lead to oversedation. The sedative and anti-anxiety effects of benzodiazepines appear to be distinct, and the CNS seems to adapt to the nonspecific sedative effects as a steady state is reached (Johnson & Chernik, 1982). However, there is an age-related increase in the sensitivity of elderly individuals to the central depressant effects of long-acting benzodiazepines (Pomara et al., 1985).

Drug Interactions

Benzodiazepines have relatively few significant adverse drug interactions. Their major drug interaction, augmentation of other CNS depressants, can be controlled by adjusting dosage downward. An extensive discussion of benzodiazepines can be found in Chapters 21, 22, and 23.

Side Effects

The most common adverse effects of the benzodiazepines involve CNS depression: muscle weakness, ataxia, dysarthria, vertigo, somnolence, and confusion. These side effects can be a major problem, especially for the medically ill patient who may be weak from prolonged bed rest or already impaired by other CNS illness. Older patients are especially susceptible to psychomotor impairment and falls (Ray, Griffin, & Downey, 1989; Tinetti, Speechley, & Ginter, 1988). There is always the risk that treating anxiety secondary to depression may not only mask the depression but actually exacerbate it.

There is some question whether or not benzodiazepines may stimulate some people (Hall & Joffe, 1972) or release hostility and rage reactions (Karch, 1979). Such instances are infrequent (Dietch & Jennings, 1988). Disinhibition seems most common in patients with preexisting personality disorders, substance abuse, or underlying organic brain disorders. However, benzodiazepines can produce or increase depressive symptomatology (Greenblatt & Shader, 1974; Ryan et al., 1968).

Van der Kropf (1979) first reported finding depersonalization, anxiety, and paranoia in subjects with chronic insomnia treated with triazolam. Benzodiazepines impair memory function in two ways. The first is an acute anterograde amnestic effect, usually after intravenous use. However, this effect is also reported with therapeutic oral doses of the high-potency and short half-life benzodiazepines such as triazolam, especially if taken with alcohol (Healey et al., 1983; Scharf et al., 1984; Shader et al., 1986; Wolkowitz et al., 1987). The second type of memory impairment involves recall during chronic use. Because benzodiazepines interfere with memory consolidation, users, especially the elderly (Nikaido et al., 1987), may have impaired long-term recall (Angus & Romney, 1984; Lucki, Rickels, & Geller, 1986).

Large doses of benzodiazepines produce only minor changes in cardiovascular function even in patients with underlying cardiac disease (Rao et al., 1973). In patients without pulmonary disease, changes in tidal volume and response to elevated pCO_2 are barely detectable (Lakshminarayan et al., 1976). In a single-blind study, diazepam actually improved the breathlessness of patients with chronic airflow obstruction associated with emphysema (Mitchells-Heggs et al., 1980).

The respiratory depressant effects of benzodiazepines appear to be most marked in patients with carbon dioxide retention. Benzodiazepines should not be given to patients with clinically significant pulmonary disease who might be retaining carbon dioxide before measuring arterial blood gases. Anxious carbon dioxide retainers may be treated with buspirone or low-dose neuroleptics, which do not alter respiratory drive. Intravenous benzodiazepines given concurrently with parenteral narcotics produce significant respiratory depression of a greater degree than is found with opiates alone, especially in patients with some pulmonary impairment (Cohen, Finn, & Steen, 1969).

Toxicity and Dependence

Benzodiazepines are relatively nonlethal in overdose. In the medical literature there have been fewer than a dozen reported suicides by diazepam ingestion alone (Finkel, McCloskey, & Goodman, 1979). However, benzodiazepines are often used in combination with other sedative drugs and ethanol in fatal overdoses.

Overall, the risks of overuse, dependence, and addiction are low considering the widespread use of benzodiazepines (Rifkin et al., 1989; Uhlenhuth et al., 1988; O'Brien. 2005). However, abuse can occur in high-risk patients for chemical dependency and abuse when benzodiazepines are used regularly for at least several months. The potential for addiction is greater for alcoholic patients (Ciraulo, Sands, & Shader, 1988).

Withdrawal

Symptoms of benzodiazepine withdrawal may include anxiety, insomnia, dizziness, headache, anorexia, hypotension, hyperthermia, neuromuscular irritability, tinnitus, blurred vision, shakiness, and psychosis. Higher doses taken over longer durations create a greater risk of moderate to severe withdrawal (Hollister, Motzenbecker, & Degnan, 1961). There are reports of abstinence phenomena beginning at 5–7 days and lasting 2–4 weeks after cessation of usual therapeutic

Table 31.1 PHARMACOKINETIC SUMMARY COMPARISON OF BENZODIAZEPINES

DRUG GIVEN	PEAK PLASMA LEVEL (HOURS)	MEAN (RANGE) ELIMINATION HALF-LIFE (HOURS)[†]	ACTIVE METABOLITES	MEAN (RANGE) ELIMINATION HALF-LIFE (HOURS)	APPROXIMATE DOSE EQUIVALENT (MG)[‡]
Alprazolam (Xanax)	1–2	11(6–16)	Alphahydroxyalprazolam	6	0.5
Chlordiazepoxide (Librium)	0.5–4	10(5–30)	Desmethylchlordiazepoxide	(24–96)	10
			Demoxepam	(14–95)	
			Desmethyldiazepam	73(30–100)	
			Oxazepam	7(5–15)	
Clonazepam (Klonopin)	1–4	23(18–50)	None		0.25
Clorazepate (Tranxene)	1–2	*	Desmethyldiazepam	73(30–100)	7.5
			Oxazepam	7(5–15)	
Diazepam (Valium)	1–2	43(20–70)	Desmethyldiazepam	73(30–100)	5
			Oxazepam	7(5–15)	
Estazolam (ProSom)	2	14(10–24)	2 metabolites with low concentrations and potencies	10–14	1.0
Flurazepam (Dalmane)	0.5–2	*	N-desalkylflurazepam	74(36–120)	5
Lorazepam (Ativan)	1–2 PO	14(10–25)	None		1.0
	(20 min IM)	14			
Midazolam	5 min IV	68 min	None		For sedation 1–2 mg IV up to 0.15 mg/kg
Oxazepam (Serax)	2	7(5–15)	None		15
Prazepam (Centrax)	6	*	Desmethyldiazepam	73(30–100)	
			Oxazepam	7(5–15)	
Quazepam (Doral)	1–3	39	2-oxoquazepam	39	
			N-desalkylflurazepam	74(36–120)	
Temazepam (Restoril)	1–1.5	13(8–20)	None		15
Triazolam (Halcion)	1–2	2	None		0.25
	(0.25 sl)	3(1.5–5.5)			

[†]Drugs marked with (*) are prodrugs; all CNS effects are due to their active metabolites.

[‡]Dose equivalence compared to 1.0 mg lorazepam; e.g., 1.0 mg lorazepam-5 mg diazepam.

doses of diazepam (Busto et al., 1986; Pevnick, Jasinski, & Haertzen, 1978; Winokur et al., 1980). There are also reports of seizures occurring in association with the discontinuation of moderate doses of lorazepam (de la Fuenta et al., 1980) and triazolam (Tien & Gujavarty, 1985). One advantage of long-acting benzodiazepines such as clonazepam is that they tend to self-taper if discontinued. Although abrupt discontinuation of long-acting benzodiazepines is usually not dangerous, it can lead to a persistent state of heightened anxiety. The short-acting benzodiazepines are associated with a greater prevalence and severity of withdrawal reactions, because their plasma concentrations decline more rapidly following discontinuation. Withdrawal symptoms can be minimized by slow tapering rather than abruptly discontinuing the drug.

During withdrawal, autonomic symptoms can be relieved by a beta-adrenergic blocker (Abernethy, Greenblatt, & Shader, 1981) and possibly by carbamazepine as well (Malcolm et al., 1989; Ries et al., 1989). It should be kept in mind that withdrawal symptoms from alprazolam and triazolam may not be fully covered by other benzodiazepines (Schneider, Syapin, &

Table 31.2 COMPARISON OF BENZODIAZEPINES AND
BUSPIRONE

	BENZODIAZEPINES	BUSPIRONE
Anxiolytic effect	1	1
Psychomotor impairment	1	2
Cognitive impairment	1	2
Sedation	1	2
Addiction potential	1	2
Sedative augmentation	1	2
Respiratory depression	1	2
Withdrawal	1	2
Muscle relaxation	1	2
Anticonvulsant	1	2

Pawluczyk, 1987; Zipursky, Baker, & Zimmer, 1985). In these cases, substitution with clonazepam is an effective alternative (Albeck, 1987; Patterson, 1988). Benzodiazepine withdrawal may take months to accomplish. We recommend approximately a 10% dose reduction per week for patients who have been treated with these drugs for 12 months or longer.

Clonazepam

Clonazepam has achieved widespread use for the treatment of anxiety. Originally introduced in the United States for the treatment of specific seizure disorders, it has also found application for the treatment of myoclonus, restless leg syndrome, akathisia, bipolar disorder, acute mania, and neuroleptic-induced somnambulism. Clonazepam is mainly metabolized in the liver by nitro reduction, which may be slightly impaired by cimetidine, but does not appear to be affected by age (Greenblatt et al., 1985). Clonazepam's half-life is approximately 24 hours. Compared to alprazolam, which has a half-life of 10–12 hours, there is less likelihood of symptom rebound (such as symptoms associated with a missed dose) or interdose rebound. While many clinicians now prefer to cross alprazolam patients over to clonazepam to facilitate withdrawal, one study found that gradual reduction of alprazolam worked just as well (Schweizer et al., 1990). The long-hour half-life of clonazepam does not mitigate against the possibility of significant withdrawal symptoms (including delirium and psychosis) if the medication is suddenly stopped (Freeman, 1997). Like any other benzodiazepine, clonazepam effectively reduces a wide variety of anxiety symptoms. Daily doses of about 1.0–2.0 mg/day are generally effective for the treatment of panic disorder (Rosenbaum et al., 1997), with increased rates of somnolence and ataxia at daily doses of 3.0 mg/day. Higher doses have been associated with depression, dizziness, fatigue, and irritability as adverse effects similar to other benzodiazepines.

BUSPIRONE

Buspirone is a nonbenzodiazepine anxiolytic that has an anxiolytic effect without the sedative or cognitive side effects associated with the benzodiazepines. Its mechanism of action is thought to involve its function as a partial agonist at the serotonin 1A receptor (Eison & Eison, 1984; Eison & Temple, 1986).

Table 31.1 summarizes the pertinent clinical issues involving buspirone, in comparison with benzodiazepines. Buspirone does not have acute effects. In fact, it usually takes at least 7 to 10 days (and often 4 weeks) to have an effect. Therefore, it is best used for patients with chronic generalized anxiety.

Aside from generalized anxiety disorder itself for which buspirone is approved by the Federal Drug Administration, medical patients with chronic symptoms related to autonomic arousal may benefit from buspirone. These groups include, for example, patients with irritable bowel syndrome, asthma, and chronic obstructive pulmonary disease (COPD) with anxiety-related dyspnea. Patients whose symptoms are increased by anxiety, such as those with epilepsy, may benefit from anxiety reduction with buspirone.

There are, in addition, several niches for buspirone that emerge from its clinical profile. Because buspirone does not augment other sedative drug effects, it may be particularly helpful for those anxious patients who are prone to misuse or who are taking concomitant sedatives. For example, buspirone has helped reduce anxiety in anxious drug users with AIDS (Batki, 1990). Buspirone does not impair respiratory drive as the benzodiazepines do, and in fact may be somewhat of a respiratory stimulant (Garner et al., 1989; Rapoport & Mendelson, 1989). Therefore, it is safe to treat anxious carbon dioxide–retaining patients with buspirone, whereas it would not be safe to do so with a benzodiazepine. Buspirone also does not augment the sedative potential of other CNS sedatives. Therefore, anxious patients on other sedatives (such as anticonvulsants, antihistamines, and narcotic analgesics) may be able to benefit from anxiolytic treatment without the additive sedative effects associated with the benzodiazepines. Unlike the benzodiazepines, buspirone lacks muscle relaxant, anticonvulsant, and hypnotic activities; it does not block the withdrawal syndrome associated with CNS sedatives (Schweizer & Rickels, 1986).

Pharmacokinetics

Buspirone is rapidly and completely absorbed from the gastrointestinal tract, with extensive first-pass hepatic metabolism. Taking the drug with food appears to decrease its rate of absorption and its first-pass metabolism, making more of the drug available. Peak plasma level is reached in about 1 hour. Average elimination half-life is 2.5 hours. About 65% is eliminated by the kidneys, mostly in a metabolized form, and 35% undergoes fecal elimination. There have not been any adverse reports about liver or renal impairment on drug effects.

Side Effects

The major side effects include dizziness, headache, and nervousness. Buspirone is not sedative, which is one of its primary advantages (Cohn & Wilcox, 1986; Newton et al., 1986). In fact, buspirone causes no more drowsiness than placebo and does not impair psychomotor performance skills, such as driving. There have been no deaths reported as a result of buspirone overdose in more than 375 cases. Major sequelae of overdose have included nausea and vomiting, dizziness, drowsiness, and miosis. No withdrawal syndrome has been reported following the abrupt discontinuation of its use.

Buspirone has no abuse potential (Griffith, Jasinski, & Mc-Kinney, 1986), lacking euphoric properties and actually having some dysphoric properties with repeated excessive use and higher dose. This property, coupled with the fact that it does not potentiate the sedative effects of alcohol (or other CNS sedatives), seems to make buspirone a good drug for the treatment of anxiety in chemically dependent or abuse patients (Kastenholz & Crismon, 1984; Meyer, 1986).

Drug Interactions

There are few reports of drug interactions in humans; use of buspirone with monoamine oxidase inhibitors is considered contraindicated because of potential hypertensive reactions or serotonin syndrome. The calcium channel inhibitors verapamil and diltiazem may increase buspirone levels (Lamberg et al., 1998).

Clinical Use

Buspirone has been demonstrated to have clinical anxiolytic efficacy comparable to that of the benzodiazepines (Cohn et al., 1986; Rickels et al., 1982; Schuckit, 1984). However, a dose of 5 mg three times daily often is inadequate. More patients show a response to 10 mg three times daily but some cannot start this high without developing tinnitus, light-headedness, or aggravation of anxiety. From 10 mg, dosage should be raised by 10mg/day increments every 7 to 10 days as needed up to a maximum of 60 mg/day. Since the anxiolytic effects of buspirone may take several weeks to occur, the patient may become prematurely discouraged about the potential effectiveness of this medication. An additional issue, the significance of which is yet to be determined, is that some patients who have been on benzodiazepines appear not to report comparable anxiolytic benefit from buspirone (Schweizer, Rickels, & Lucki, 1986). However, buspirone may be helpful in concurrent use with benzodiazepines in treating panic disorder and helping prevent relapse after withdrawal of benzodiazepines.

Buspirone also appears to have a clinically relevant antiaggression effect and can suppress disinhibition which may be helpful in populations with different types of brain damage, including the episodic hyperarousal that accompanies head injury (Levine, 1988), mental retardation (Ratey et al., 1989), dementia (Colenda, 1988), and attention deficit disorder (Balon, 1990). In these patients, a lower initial dose (no more than 5 mg three times daily) is recommended because some patients with brain damage can show an agitation response at a higher initial dose.

BETA-ADRENERGIC BLOCKING AGENTS

Autonomic symptoms associated with anxiety (such as palpitations and tremulousness) are mediated by beta-adrenergic sympathetic activity. Beta-adrenergic blocking agents, such as propranolol which has highly lipophilic properties to cross the blood-brain barrier, have been demonstrated to antagonize both the somatic (Granville-Grossman & Turner, 1966; Tyrer & Lader, 1974) and the emotional (Kathol et al., 1980) symptoms of anxiety.

It has been suggested that propranolol has a unique role for patients with acute situational distress, such as public performance anxiety, in which the psychomotor intellectual impairment produced by benzodiazepines is not desirable. Forty milligrams of propranolol given 90 minutes before performance was shown to have a positive effect in decreasing performance anxiety in a group of musicians (James et al., 1978).

Evaluation of the effectiveness of beta-blockers in anxiety has become more complex with the recognition that these agents (especially propranolol) enter the CNS and can produce direct neurologic and behavioral effects. Although weakness and depression are the most common neuropsychiatric symptoms associated with propranolol, patients may also have insomnia, vivid nightmares, hypnogogic hallucinations, or toxic psychosis, even at relatively low doses (Fraser & Carr, 1976; Gershon et al., 1979). Such mental changes tend to reverse within 48 hours after discontinuation of propranolol. Nadolol and atenolol are beta-blockers that do not cross the blood-brain barrier to any significant clinical extent but also seem to improve some components of anxiety. It may be that the central effects are exerted by some kind of neurohumoral feedback to the CNS rather than by a direct action. Finally, pindolol (with intrinsic sympathomimetic activity) and labetalol (with alpha$_1$-blocking activity) are beta-blockers that do not tend to lower pulse rate. However, their antianxiety effects remain relatively unproven. Pindolol has been studied as an augmenting agent for SSRIs (Whale, Terao, Cowen, Freemantle, & Geddes, 2010).

Issues in Prescribing

Propranolol is almost completely absorbed following oral administration. It undergoes extensive first-pass metabolism in the liver, and variation in this component results in as much as 20-fold variability in plasma concentration among individuals on comparable doses. The half-life is initially about 3 hours, which may increase to 4 hours during chronic use. It is 90%–95% bound to plasma protein, which also may contribute to its variabilities in plasma concentrations. Propranolol is almost completely metabolized in the liver before urinary excretion. Nadolol is poorly absorbed from the gastrointestinal tract (Dreyfuss et al., 1979) and is excreted largely by the kidney in unchanged form (Frishman, 1981). The elimination half-life is 14–24 hours, which increases dramatically in patients with renal dysfunction. Contraindications to the use of beta-blockers include bradycardia and atrioventricular block. Beta blockers may be used in patients with heart failure or may exacerbate heart failure depending on the context; so its use should be worked out with physicians managing the heart condition. In patients with angina, the cessation of chronic beta blockade may worsen chest pain. Because of their effects on bronchial smooth muscle, beta-blockers are relatively contraindicated in patients with bronchospastic disease or COPD. They should be used cautiously in diabetics because they can mask clinical signs of hypoglycemia and interfere with glycogenolysis during hypoglycemia.

Beta-receptor blockade has little effect on the normal heart at rest, although there is some decrease in heart rate, cardiac output, and blood pressure. During exercise and anxiety, however, sympathetic responses may be significantly blocked. Maximum exercise tolerance may therefore be decreased in otherwise normal patients.

ANTIDEPRESSANTS

Antidepressants treat not only depression but also the anxiety symptoms that accompany depression, as well as primary anxiety disorders such as panic disorder, generalized anxiety disorder, obsessive-compulsive disorder, and PTSD, probably on the basis of serotonergic augmentation. For many years, the tricyclic antidepressants (TCAs) and monoamine oxidase inhibitors were recommended for the treatment of panic attacks (Klein, 1982; Pohl, Berchou, & Rainey, 1982; Sheehan, Ballenger, & Jacobsen, 1980; Zitrin, Klein, & Woerner, 1978). Both groups of drugs were also effective in patients with mixed anxiety and depression (Paykel et al., 1982; Rickels et al., 1974), especially in so-called *atypical depressions*, which were characterized by high levels of anxiety (Robinson et al., 1973). It was also noted that TCAs were effective in the treatment of some patients with chronic anxiety alone (Lipman et al., 1981, Kahn et al., 1986). In a double blind placebo controlled study (even eliminating patients with panic-phobic syndromes) of the treatment of anxiety with imipramine, chlordiazepoxide, or placebo, the antianxiety effects of imipramine were superior to those of the others by the second treatment week and became clearly more significant thereafter, independent of baseline levels of depression and anxiety (Kahn et al., 1986).

SSRIs have a similar efficacy as tricyclics for generalized anxiety disorder. Paroxetine, citalopram, escitalopram, and the serotonin-noradrenaline reuptake inhibitor venlafaxine extended-release have proved their effectiveness (Fricchione, 2004). Our practice is to start with very low doses and increase the dosage slowly. Benzodiazepines can be a useful adjunct in the first weeks of adjusting to the antidepressant. For patients who are more problematic, it is helpful to know that benzodiazepine-antidepressant treatment with SSRIs have been shown to be effective, and fewer patients did not complete the studies (Furukawa, Streiner, & Young, 2002).

NEUROLEPTICS

There are certain situations in which neuroleptics can be effectively used to treat anxiety, especially for short periods of time so the risk of tardive dyskinesia is much less of an issue (Rickels, 1983; Fann, Lake, & Majors, 1974). These situations include acute anxiety in patients with carbon dioxide retention, in whom suppression of the hypoxic respiratory drive by benzodiazepines should be avoided, anxiety that represents an incipient psychotic disorganization (as in some borderline personality–disordered patients under stress), schizophrenia, anxiety syndromes due to medical causes with disorganized cognition or behavior (as in the severely anxious patient with racing thoughts precipitated by steroids), and anxiety in the context of significant delirium. Some of the more sedative typical neuroleptics, such as thioridazine and perphenazine, are more anxiolytic than high-potency agents such as haloperidol. Atypical antipsychotics are similarly more sedating. However, no neuroleptic maintains a Food and Drug Administration indication for treating anxiety alone. We have grown to prefer olanzapine and quetiapine for use in the medically ill because of lower rates of akathisia and extrapyramidal symptoms (EPS). It makes sense to monitor postural signs and anticholinergic side effects when atypical agents are used acutely. In studies of off-label uses of atypical antipsychotics, quetiapine has shown benefit for generalized anxiety disorder, and risperidone for obsessive-compulsive disorder. The side effects in non-elderly adults are weight gain (particularly for olanzapine), fatigue, sedation, akathisia (for aripiprazole) and EPS (Maher et al., 2011).

ANTIHISTAMINES

Antihistamines such as hydroxyzine and diphenhydramine are sometimes prescribed to treat anxiety. They have no specific anxiolytic properties (Rickels et al., 1970), although patients may feel less anxious on them because of their sedative effects. There is little rationale to support their use; they have a number of unwanted side effects such as anticholinergic properties, especially if used in repeated doses. However, review of limited studies with hydroxyzine has found it more effective for generalized anxiety disorder than placebo, and more sedating (Guaiana, Barbui, & Cipriani, 2010). Diphenhydramine is less effective than benzodiazepines for sleep induction (Rickels et al., 1983). The only situation involving anxiety in which antihistamines might have a special use would be when anxiety is the accompaniment of an allergic response for which their antihistaminic properties are of primary value.

GABAPENTIN AND PREGABALIN

Both gabapentin and pregabalin are anticonvulsants that may reduce anxiety although their most recognized indication is treatment of neuropathic pain and fibromyalgia (Wiffen et al., 2013). They selectively bind at alpha2-delta subunit of presynaptic voltage-dependent calcium channels. While the drugs are analogues of GABA, they do not act at GABA receptors.

In patients with generalized anxiety disorder, pregabalin reduces anxiety relatively rapidly, usually in less than a week. It affects both somatic and cognitive symptoms of anxiety. Its acute side effects are somnolence, dizziness. (Frampton, 2014) For treatment of generalized anxiety disorder it has been approved in Europe. Although it has not been compared directly to serotonin reuptake inhibitors, pregabalin has been used for augmentation (Rickels et al., 2012) and also to facilitate taper of long-term benzodiazepines (Hadley, Mandel, & Schweitzer, 2012; Frampton, 2014).

Pregabalin can also reduce preoperative anxiety, postoperative pain, and prevent chronic post-surgical pain, nausea, and vomiting. At doses of 150–450 mg per day it has helped to prevent relapse of alcohol dependence (Guglielmo et al., 2012).

Gabapentin has reduced anxiety symptoms in the medical setting, for instance, for breast cancer survivors who may also benefit from its effect on hot flashes (Lavigne et al., 2012). It treats preoperative anxiety and postoperative nausea and vomiting (Guttuso, 2014) as well as social anxiety disorder (Blanco et al., 2013; Pande, 1999) and alcohol dependence (Mason et al., 2014). Common side effects are dizziness, ataxia, somnolence, and occasionally peripheral edema.

Both these agents are metabolized by the kidney, and dose reduction is warranted in those with renal impairment. These medications should be tapered over a week or more.

SELF-REGULATION METHODS

It is now well established that most patients can be taught techniques that induce relaxation. These techniques should be considered appropriate for generalized anxiety, for desensitization therapy in specific anxiety-producing situations, and for reduction of medical symptoms sustained by chronic stress.

MUSCLE RELAXATION THERAPIES

Learning to specifically sense and control muscle tension is a widely utilized and effective method for anxiety reduction. The Jacobson method of progressive relaxation depends on systematically tensing and relaxing muscle groups starting with the feet and eventually involving the entire body (Jacobson, 1938). Of course, it is important to discuss the intent of the procedure with the patient beforehand and to elicit any specific questions, misconceptions, or concerns the patient might have. A comfortable and quiet setting without interruptions is important. Although tape-recorded or printed instructions can be used, the initial session with the physician can be an important factor in establishing a positive alliance for future work.

ELECTROMYOGRAPHIC BIOFEEDBACK

The Jacobson method was devised to induce relaxation by heightening awareness of muscle tension. Electromyographic (EMG) biofeedback goes one step further by providing the person with precise information about the electrical potentials of selected muscle groups. In EMG biofeedback treatment of anxiety, the frontalis muscle is usually selected for monitoring because the frontalis EMG activity level is regarded as an index of overall physiologic arousal. Patients learn to reduce muscle tension, but the benefit is related to the importance of muscle tension as a symptom of anxiety. A review of studies of biofeedback for chronic anxiety suggested that multimodal treatment using EMG with EEG feedback or with thermal feedback may be most effective (Schoenberg & David, 2014).

MEDITATION TECHNIQUES AND THE RELAXATION RESPONSE

Meditation has been shown to produce a physiologic state of restful alertness that is different from sleeping or waking (Wallace, 1970). Physiologic findings during meditation are generally opposite to those encountered in an anxiety patient. After reviewing a range of meditative practices, Benson concluded that within the apparent multiplicity of practices common features reside that could serve as the basis for a nonsectarian form of practice capable of inducing a state he called the *relaxation response* (Benson, Beary, & Carol, 1974). The technique for eliciting the relaxation response consists of four basic elements:

1. A *mental device.* There needs to be some constant stimulus—for example, a sound, a word (such as "one"), or a phrase repeated silently or audibly. Fixed gazing at an object is a suitable alternative. The purpose of this procedure is to focus attention away from the continuous flow of sensory distractions and intellectual preoccupations.

2. *A passive attitude.* During the aural or visual practice, distracting thoughts are to be disregarded. One should not be concerned with performance standards. When lapses are recognized, the practitioner should patiently return to the mental device without self-criticism or concern about success or failure.

3. *Decreased muscle tone.* The subject should be in a comfortable position to minimize any muscular strain or tension.

4. *A quiet environment.* A suitable room should be chosen with decreased stimuli and where there is no concern about unexpected interruptions. Most techniques instruct the practitioner to close the eyes.

The relaxation response has achieved wide recognition and has emerged as a technique to manage anxiety and a wide array of stress-related disorders (Chang, Dusek, & Benson, 2011; Goldberg, 1982a, b; Nakao et al., 2001). Chapter 17 discusses the concepts of mind-body medicine that have evolved from this recognition, and Chapter 16 discusses the use of hypnosis for anxiety and procedural phobias.

BEHAVIORAL TECHNIQUES USED WITH ANXIETY DISORDER PATIENTS AND THE MEDICALLY ILL

Cognitive behavioral treatment is an effective evidence-based treatment for anxiety in the medical setting. It can be used as an adjunct to medication but becomes even more important in cases in which the patient is hesitant to take medication or when medication alone is not enough or is completely contraindicated. It is typically both structured and time-limited form of treatment. Cognitive behavioral treatments for patients with anxiety disorders as well as the anxiety-provoking challenges of medical illness are discussed in Chapter 14. For the very ill, the challenge may be to tailor the structured treatment so that it is available on the same day as other medical visits or via telephone or video-conference. The skills to reduce chronic anxiety may be modified to offer additional strategies for patients to cope with the realistic adverse events that may be most likely (Greer et al., 2012).

One area in which behavioral techniques have proven successful is in the management of blood and injury phobias. Blood phobias are unique in that, unlike other phobias, they do not result in the typical sympathetic arousal, tachycardia, dyspnea, and paresthesias. Rather, blood phobias usually result in an initial rise in heart rate that is often quickly followed by vasovagal bradycardia, decrease in blood pressure, and eventually syncope. It is estimated that approximately 3.1% of the normal population experience severe blood phobia (Agras, Sylvester, & Oliveau, 1969). Such a phobia can represent a severe threat if it results in avoidance of life-saving medical procedures such as insulin injections, surgery, and blood transfusions.

A variety of behavioral treatments for blood and injury phobia have been elaborated. Of all these treatments, the most frequently reported have been in vivo exposure to needles and blood (Leitenberg et al., 1970) and exposure to films of venipuncture, surgery, and injury in an emergency room (Marks et al., 1977). However, a variety of other behavioral treatments, such as systematic desensitization (Cohn, Kron, & Brady, 1976), controlled breathing and modeling (Moore, Geffken, & Royal, 1995), implosion (Ollendick & Gruen, 1972), an applied tension procedure (Ost, Sterner, & Fellenius, 1989) and relaxation techniques (Ost et al., 1984), have been used with varying degrees of success. Another area in which behavioral techniques such as progressive relaxation and biofeedback have been shown to be beneficial has been with patients who suffer from asthma and chronic obstructive pulmonary disease (COPD) (Gift, Moore, & Seeken, 1992; Hock et al., 1978). Dyspnea often leads the patient to become more anxious, which results in increased muscle tension and increased need for oxygen. As this happens, dyspnea becomes magnified and a vicious cycle of increasing muscle tension, anxiety, and dyspnea ensues. Biofeedback (Acosta, 1988; Hannich et al., 2004) hypnosis (Treggiari-Venzi, Suter, De Tonnac, & Romand, 2000), coaching (especially by a familiar nurse), verbal reassurance, distraction, and music have also been used to address the anxiety associated with weaning from a ventilator. See Chapter 27 on dyspnea.

Finally, the relaxation response has reduced stress and psychophysiologic reactivity in postmyocardial infarction patients (Gatchel, Gaffney, & Smith, 1986). It reduces pre-operative anxiety in ambulatory surgery patients (Domar, Noe, & Benson, 1987) and reduces anxiety and esophageal acid exposure in patients with gastroesophageal reflux disease (McDonald-Haile et al., 1999).

While we mentioned specifically CBT and mind-body medicine, all psychotherapeutic modalities (Part II) considered in this book including individual and group psychotherapy, family therapy and parent guidance, and attention to spiritual issues deepen the approach to this complex symptom.

CLINICAL PEARLS

- The approach to evaluation of anxiety in the medical setting requires a synthetic medical and psychiatric assessment including review of medications and recreational substances that have been started or stopped and medical disorders that present with anxiety. The history should allow assessment of psychiatric diagnoses as well as the psychological challenge of the patient's predicament.

- Alienation (fear of separation and abandonment), loss of control, threat to body integrity, and fear of death are themes to be explored.

- Energy drinks have moderate to relatively high levels and concentrations of caffeine (2.5–35.7 mg per oz.) compared to other caffeinated beverages such as a 12oz. cola or a 6oz. cup of coffee.

- Abuse of methamphetamine, which has a half-life of 12 hours (longer than cocaine) can present with anxiety in the setting of intoxication or withdrawal. In withdrawal, the depression may be more prolonged and worse than that of cocaine withdrawal (Winslow, Voorhees, & Pehl, 2007).

- The most common symptoms of pulmonary embolus in patients who did not have preexisting cardiopulmonary disease (noted in the Prospective Investigation of Pulmonary Embolism Diagnosis II) were dyspnea at rest or with exertion, pleuritic pain, cough, more than two-pillow orthopnea, calf or thigh pain/swelling, and wheezing. Tachypnea and tachycardia were the most common signs (Stein et al., 2007).

- In order to avoid episodes of hypoglycemia, diabetic patients can be educated to be alert to glucose readings below 70 mg/dL (Seaquist et al., 2013).

- Among schizophrenic patients in a large study (CATIE), a moderate dose of perphenazine produced comparable rates of akathisia to ziprasidone, risperidone, and olanzapine (Caroff et al., 2011).

- In addition to benzodiazepines and propranolol, mirtazapine 15 mg each day may also be effective for treatment of akathisia (Poyurovsky, 2010).

- Anxious depression has a more chronic course of illness, an increased incidence of suicidal thoughts, and greater occupational impairment (Rao & Zisook, 2009).

- The Somatic Symptom Scale-8 measures somatic symptom burden and its severity and can be used to follow patients (Barsky, 2014; Gierk et al., 2014).

- The ways that anxiety has restricted the lives of patients, the way that they do not move into the social sphere or try new things may not be as obvious to the clinician or to the patient unless the clinician considers the negative symptoms of anxiety (avoidance) in a fuller evaluation.

DISCLOSURE STATEMENTS

Dr. Goldberg had no conflicts related to his contribution to this chapter.

Dr. Greenberg has no conflicts of interest to disclose.

REFERENCES

Abelson, H. I., & Fishburne, P. M. (1976). *Nonmedical use of psychoactive substances: 1975–1976.* Princeton, NJ: Response Analysis Corporation.

Abernethy, D. R., Greenblatt, D. J., & Shader, R. I. (1981). Treatment of diazepam withdrawal syndrome with propranolol. *Annals of Internal Medicine, 94,* 354–355.

Abramowicz, M. (1986). Crack. *Medical Letter on Drugs and Therapeutics, 28,* 69–70.

Abramowicz, M. (1989). Drugs that cause psychiatric symptoms. *Medical Letter on Drugs and Therapeutics, 31,* 113–118.

Agras, S., Silvester, D., & Oliveau, D. (1969). Epidemiology of common fears and phobias. *Comprehensive Psychiatry, 10,* 151–156.

Albeck, J. H. (1987). Withdrawal and detoxification from benzodiazepine dependence: A potential role for clonazepam. *Journal of Clinical Psychiatry, 48,* 10S.

American Academy of Pediatrics. (2011). Clinical report—sports drinks and energy drinks for children and adolescents: Are they appropriate? Retrieved from Pediatrics.aappublications.org/content/early/2011/05/25/peds.2011-0965.

American Psychiatric Association. (2013). *Diagnostic and statistical manual of mental disorders. 5th edition.* Washington, D.C., American Psychiatric Association.

Angus, W. R., & Romney, D. M. (1984). The effect of diazepam on patients' memory. *Journal of Clinical Psychopharmacology, 4,* 203–206.

Aronson, T. A., & Craig, T. J. (1986). Cocaine precipitation of panic disorder. *American Journal of Psychiatry, 143,* 643–645.

Arria, A. M., & O'Brien, M. C. (2011). The "High" risk of energy drinks. *Journal of the American Medical Association, 305,* 600–601.

Balon, R. (1990). Buspirone for attention deficit hyperactivity disorder? *Journal of Clinical Psychopharmacology, 10,* 77.

Bard, M., & Sutherland, A. M. (1977). *Adaptation to radical mastectomy. The psychological impact of cancer* (Ch. 3, pp. 55–71). New York: American Cancer Society.

Barnes, T. R. (2003). The Barnes Akathisia Rating Scale-revisited. *Journal of Psychopharmacology, 17*(4), 365–370.

Barsky, A. J. (2014). Assessing somatic symptoms in clinical practice. *Journal of the American Medical Association Internal Medicine, 174,* 407–408.

Barsky, A. J., Delamater, B. A., & Orav, J. E. (1999). Panic disorder patients and their medical care. *Psychosomatics, 40*(1), 50–56.

Batki, S. L. (1990). Buspirone in drug users with AIDS or AIDS-related complex. *Journal of Clinical Psychopharmacology, 10,* 111S–115S.

Beitman, B. D., Kushner, M. G., Basha, I., et al. (1991). Follow-up status of patients with angiographically normal coronary arteries and panic disorder. *Journal of the American Medical Association, 265,* 1545–1549.

Bela, S. V., & Raftery, E. F. (1980). The role of verapamil in chronic stable angina: A controlled study with computerized multistage treadmill exercise. *Lancet, 1,* 841–844.

Benson, H., Beary, J. F., & Carol, M. P. (1974). The relaxation response. *Psychiatry, 37,* 37–46.

Blanco, C., Bragdon, L. B., Schneier, F. R., & Liebowitz, M. R. (2013). The evidence-based pharmacotherapy of social anxiety disorder. *International Journal of Neuropsychopharmacology, 16,* 235–249.

Bodkin, J. A. & Teicher, M. H. (1989). Fluoxetine may antagonize the anxiolytic action of buspirone. *Journal of Clinical Psychopharmacology, 9,* 150.

Brown, S. L., Salive, M. E., Pahor, M., et al. (1995). Occult caffeine as a source of sleep problems in an older population. *Journal of the American Geriatrics Society, 43,* 860–864.

Bruce, M., Scott, N., Shine, P., et al. (1992). Anxiogenic effects of caffeine in patients with anxiety disorder. *Archives of General Psychiatry, 49,* 867–869.

Brown, T. M., & Stoudemire, A. (1998). *Psychiatric side effects of prescription and over-the-counter medications.* Washington, D.C.: American Psychiatric Press.

Bryant, S. G., Guernsey, G. B., & Ingrim, N. B. (1983). Review of bupropion. *Clinical Pharmacy, 2,* 525–537.

Budney, A. J., & Hughes, J. R. (2006). The dannabis withdrawal syndrome. *Current Opinion in Psychiatry, 19,* 233–238.

Busto, U., Sillers, E. M., Naranjo, C. A., et al. (1986).Withdrawal reaction after long-term therapeutic use of benzodiazepine. *New England Journal of Medicine, 315,* 854–859.

Caroff, S. N., Hurford, I., Lybrand, J., & Campbell, E. C. (2011). Movement disorders induced by antipsychotic drugs: implications of the CATIE schizophrenia trial. *Neurologic Clinics, 29,* 127–128.

Chang, B. H., Dusek, J. A., & Benson, H. (2011). Psychobiological changes from relaxation response elicitation; long-term practitioners vs. novices. *Psychosomatics, 52,* 550–559.

Charney, D. S., Heninger, G. R., & Jatlow, P. I. (1985). Increased anxiogenic effects of caffeine in panic disorders. *Archives of General Psychiatry, 423,* 233–243.

Christensen, B. (1946). Studies on hyperventilation: II. Electrocardiographic changes in normal man during voluntary hyperventilation. *Journal of Clinical Investigation, 24,* 880.

Ciraulo, D. A., Sands, B. F., & Shader, R. I. (1988). Critical review of liability for benzodiazepines: Abuse among alcoholics. *American Journal of Psychiatry, 145,* 1501–1506.

Cohen, R. B., Finn, H., & Steen, S. M. (1969). Effect of diazepam and meperidine, alone and in combination, on the respiratory response to carbon dioxide. *Anesthesia and Analgesia, 48,* 353–355.

Cohn, C. K., Kron, R. A., & Brady, J. P. (1976). A case study of blood-illness-injury phobia treated behaviorally. *Journal of Nervous and Mental Disease, 162,* 65–68.

Cohn, J. B., Bowden, C. L., Fisher, J. G., et al. (1986). Double-blind comparison of buspirone and clorazepate in anxious outpatients. *American Journal of Medicine, 80*(Suppl 3B), 10–16.

Cohn, J. B. & Wilcox, C. S. (1986). Low-sedation potential of buspirone compared with alprazolam and lorazepam in the treatment of anxious patients: A double-blind study. *Journal of Clinical Psychiatry, 47,* 409–412.

Colenda, C. C. (1988). Buspirone in treatment of agitated demented patient. *Lancet, 1,* 169.

Cowley, D. S., & Roy-Byrne, P. P. (1987). Hyperventilation and panic disorder. *American Journal of Medicine, 83,* 929–937.

Croicu, C., Chwastiak, L., & Katon, W. (2014). Approach to the patient with multiple somatic symptoms. *Medical Clinics of North America, 98,* 1079–1095.

de la Fuenta, J. R., Rosenbaum, A. H., Martin, H. R., et al. (1980). Lorazepam-related withdrawal seizures. *Mayo Clinic Proceedings, 55,* 190–192.

Denko, J. D., & Kaelbling, R. (1962). The psychiatric aspects of hypoparathyroidism. *Acta Psychiatrica Scandinavica, 38*(suppl 164), 61–70.

Devereux, R. B., Perloff, J. K., Reichek, N., et al. (1976). Mitral valve prolapse. *Circulation, 54,* 7–14.

Dietch, J. T. (1984). Cerebral tumor presenting with panic attacks. *Psychosomatics, 25,* 861–863.

Dietch, J. T., & Jennings, R. K. (1988). Aggressive dyscontrol in patients treated with benzodiazepines. *Journal of Clinical Psychiatry, 49,* 184–188.

Dimsdale, J. E., & Hackett, T. P. (1982). Effect of denial on cardiac health and psychological assessment. *American Journal of Psychiatry, 139,* 1477–1480.

Domar, A. D., Noe, J. M., & Benson, H. (1987). The preoperative use of the relaxation response with ambulatory surgery patients. *Journal of Human Stress, 13,* 101–107.

Dreyfuss, J., Griffith, D. L., Singhvi, S. M., et al. (1979). Pharmacokinetics of nadolol, a beta-receptor antagonist: Administration of therapeutic single and multiple-dosage regimens to hypertensive patients. *Journal of Clinical Pharmacology, 19,* 712–720.

Egbert, L. D., Battit, G. E., Welch, C. E., et al. (1964). Reduction of post-operative pain by encouragement and instruction of patients: A study of doctor-patient rapport. *New England Journal of Medicine, 270,* 825–827.

Eison, A. S., & Temple, D. L. Jr. (1986). Buspirone: Review of its pharmacology and current perspectives on its mechanism of action. *American Journal of Medicine, 80*(Suppl 3B), 1–9.

Eison, M. S., & Eison, A. S. (1984). Buspirone as a midbrain modulator: Anxiolysis unrelated to traditional benzodiazepine mechanisms. *Drug Development Research, 4,* 109–119.

Epstein, S. A., Kay, G., Clauw, D., Heaton, R., Klein, D., Krupp, L., et al. (1999). Psychiatric disorders in patients with fibromyalgia. *Psychosomatics, 40,* 57–63.

Evans, D. W., & Lum, L. C. (1977). Hyperventilation: An important cause of pseudoangina. *Lancet, 1,* 155–157.

Fann, W. E., Lake, R. C., & Majors, L. F. (1974). Thioridazine in neurotic, anxious, and depressed patients. *Psychosomatics, 15,* 117–121.

Ferrer, M. (1968). Mistaken psychiatric referral of occult serious cardiovascular disease. *Archives of General Psychiatry, 18,* 112–113.

Filho, A. S., Maciel, B. C., Martin-Santos, R., Romano, M. M. D., & Crippa, J. A. (2008). Does the association between mitral valve prolapse and panic disorder really exist? *Primary Care Companion J Clinical Pyschiatry, 10,* 38–47.

Filho, A. S., Maciel, B. C., Romano, M. M., Lascala, T. F., Trzesniak, C., Freitas-Ferrari, M. C., et al. (2011). Mitral valve prolapse and anxiety disorders. *British Journal Psychiatry, 199,* 247–248.

Finkel, B. S., McCloskey, K. L., & Goodman, L. S. (1979). Diazepam and drug-associated deaths. *Journal of the American Medical Association, 242,* 429–434.

Fleischhacker, W. W., Roth, S. D., & Kane, J. M. (1990). The pharmacologic treatment of neuroleptic-induced akathisia. *Journal of Clinical Psychopharmacology, 10,* 12–21.

Frampton, J. E. (2014). Pregabalin: A review of its use in adults with generalized anxiety disorder. *CNS Drugs, 28,* 835–854.

Fraser, H. S., & Carr, A. C. (1976). Propranolol psychosis. *British Journal of Psychiatry, 129,* 508–509.

Freeman, S. (1997). The realities of clonazepam discontinuation. *Psychiatric Services, 48,* 881–882.

Fricchione, G. (2004). Generalized anxiety disorder. *New England Journal of Medicine, 351,* 675–682.

Furukawa, T. A., Streiner, D. L., & Young, L. T. (2002). Antidepressant and benzodiazepine for major depression. *Cochrane Database Systematic Review, 1,* CD001026.

Gardner, E. A. (1983). Long-term preventive care in depression: The use of bupropion in patients intolerant of other antidepressants. *Journal of Clinical Psychiatry, 44,* 157–162.

Garner, S. J., Eldridge, F. L., Wagner, P. G., et al. (1989). Buspirone, an anxiolytic drug that stimulates respiration. *American Review of Respiratory Disease, 139,* 946–950.

Gatchel, R. J., Gaffney, F. A., & Smith, J. E. (1986). Comparative efficacy of behavioral stress management versus propranolol in reducing psychophysiological reactivity in post-myocardial infarction patients. *Journal of Behavioral Medicine, 9,* 503–513.

Gehi, M. M., Rosenthal, R. H., Fizette, N. B., et al. (1981). Psychiatric manifestations of hyponatremia. *Psychosomatics, 22,* 739–743.

Gershon, E. S., Goldstein, R. E., Moss, A. J., et al. (1979). Psychosis with ordinary doses of propranolol. *Annals of Internal Medicine, 90,* 938–940.

Gibbs, F. A., & Gibbs, E. C. (1952). *Atlas of electroencephalography* (Vol. 2). Cambridge, MA: Addison-Wesley.

Gierk, B., Kohlmann, S., Kroenke, K., Spangenberg, L., Zenger, M., et al. (2014) The Somatic Symptom Scale-8 (SSS-8) A brief measure of somatic symptom burden. *Journal of American Medical Association Internal Medicine 174,* 399–407.

Gift, A. G., Moore, T., & Seeken, K. (1992). Relaxation to reduce dyspnea and anxiety in COPD patients. *Nursing Research, 41*(4), 242–246.

Goldberg, R. J. (1982a). *Anxiety: A guide to biobehavioral diagnosis and therapy for physicians and mental health clinicians.* New York: Free Press.

Goldberg, R. J. (1982b). Anxiety reduction by self-regulation: Theory, practice and evaluation. *Annals of Internal Medicine, 96,* 483–487.

Goldberg, R. J. (1983). Personality types and personality disorders. In H. Leigh (Ed.), *Psychiatry in the practice of medicine* (Ch. 4, pp. 37–56). Menlo Park: Addison-Wesley.

Goldberg, R. J., & Cullen, L. O. (1985). Factors important to psychosocial adjustment to cancer: A review of the evidence. *Social Science & Medicine, 20,* 803–807.

Goldberg, R. J., Morris, P., Christian, F., et al. (1990). Panic disorder in cardiac outpatients. *Psychosomatics, 31,* 168–173.

Gotoh, F., Meyer, J. S., & Takagi, Y. (1965). Cerebral effects of hyperventilation in man. *Archives of Neurology, 12,* 10.

Granville-Grossman, K. L., & Turner, P. (1966). The effect of propranolol on anxiety. *Lancet, 1,* 788–790.

Green, B., Kavanagh, D., Young, R. (2003). Being stoned: a review of self-reported cannabis effects. *Drug and Alcohol Review, 22,* 453–460.

Greenblatt, D. J., Allen, M. D., Harmatz, M. J., et al. (1980). Diazepam disposition determinants. *Clinical Pharmacology and Therapeutics, 27,* 301–312.

Greenblatt, D. J., Divoll, M., Harmatz, J. S., et al. (1982). Pharmacokinetic comparison of sublingual lorazepam with intravenous, intramuscular and oral lorazepam. *Journal of Pharmaceutical Sciences, 71,* 248–252.

Greenblatt, D. J., & Koch-Weser, J. (1976). Intramuscular injection of drugs. *New England Journal of Medicine, 295,* 542–546.

Greenblatt, D. J., & Shader, R. I. (1974). *Benzodiazepines in clinical practice.* New York: Raven Press.

Greenblatt, D. J., Shader, R. I., Koch-Weser, J., et al. (1974). Slow absorption of intramuscular chlordiazepoxide. *New England Journal of Medicine, 291,* 1116–1118.

Greenblatt, D. J., Abernethy, D. R., Locniskar, A., et al. (1985). Age, sex, and nitrazepam kinetics: relation to antipyrine disposition. *Clinical Pharmacology and Therapeutics, 38,* 697–703.

Greenblatt, D. J., Miller, L. G., & Shader, R. I. (1987). Clonazepam pharmacokinetics, brain uptake, and receptor interactions. *Journal of Clinical Psychiatry, 48,* 2–9.

Greer, J. A., Traeger, L., Bemis, H., Solis, J. Hendriksen, E. S., & Park, E. R. (2012). A pilot randomized controlled trial of brief cognitive-behavioral therapy for anxiety in patients with terminal cancer. *The Oncologist, 17*, 1337–1345.

Griffith, J. D., Jasinski, D. R., & McKinney, G. R. (1986). Investigation of the abuse liability of buspirone in alcohol-dependent patients. *American Journal of Medicine, 80*(Suppl 3B), 30–35.

Guiana, G., Barbui, C., & Cipriani, A. (2010). Hydroxyzine for generalised anxiety disorder. *Cochrane Database Systematic Review, 8*, CD006815.

Guttuso, T., Jr. (2014). Gabapentin's anti-nausea and anti-emetic effects: A review. *Experimental Brain Research, 232*, 2535–2539.

Habibovic, M., van den Broek, K. C., Alings, M., van der Voort, P. H., & Denollet, J. (2012). Posttraumatic stress 18 months following cardioverter defibrillator implantation: shocks, anxiety, and personality. *Health Psychology, 31*, 186–193.

Hadley, S. J., Mandel, F. S., & Schweizer, E. (2012). Switching rom long-term benzodiazepine therapy to pregabalin in patients with generalized anxiety disorder; a double-blind, placebo-controlled trial. *Journal of Psychopharmacology (Oxf), 26*, 461–470.

Hall, R. C. (1983). Psychiatric effects on thyroid hormone disturbance. *Psychosomatics, 24*, 18.

Hall, R. C., & Joffe, J. R. (1972). Aberrant response to diazepam: A new syndrome. *American Journal of Psychiatry, 126P*, 738–742.

Hall, R. C., & Joffe, J. R. (1973). Hypomagnesemia: Physical and psychiatric symptoms. *Journal of the American Medical Association, 224*, 1749–1751.

Hamner, M., Hunt, N., Gee, J., Garrell, R., & Monroe, R. (1999). PTSD and automatic implantable cardioverter defibrillators. *Psychosomatics, 40*, 82–85.

Hannich, H. J., Hartmann, U., Lehmann, C. H., Grundling, M., Pavlovic, D., & Reinhardt, F. (2004). Biofeedback as a supportive method in weaning long-term ventilated critically ill patients. *Medical Hypotheses, 63*, 21–25.

Harris, M. C. (1985). The use and abuse of pocket nebulizers in the treatment of asthma. *Postgraduate Medicine, 23*, 170–173.

Healey, M., Pickens, R., Meisch, R., et al. (1983). Effects of clorazepate, diazepam, lorazepam, and placebo on human memory. *Journal of Clinical Psychiatry, 44*, 436–439.

Hock, R. A., Rodgers, C. H., Redd, C., et al. (1978). Medical-psychological interventions in male asthmatic children: An evaluation of psychological change. *Psychosomatic Medicine, 40*, 210–215.

Hodin, R., Lubitz, C., Phitayakorn, R., & Stephen, A. (2014). Diagnosis and management of pheochromocytoma. *Current Problems in Surgery, 51*, 151–187.

Hollister, L. E., Motzenbecker, F. P., & Degnan, R. O. (1961). Withdrawal reactions from chlordiazepoxide (Librium). *Psychopharmacologia, 2*, 63–68.

IsHak, W. W., Mirocha, J., Christensen, S., Wu, F., Kwock, R., Behjat, J., et al. (2014). Patient-reported outcomes of quality of life, functioning, and depressive symptom severity in major depressive disorder comorbid with panic disorder before and after ssri treatment in the star*d trial. *Depression and Anxiety, 8*, 707–716.

Jacobs, M. A., Senior, R. M., & Kessler, G. (1976). Clinical experience with theophylline: Relationship between dosage, serum concentration, and toxicity. *Journal of the American Medical Association, 235*, 1983–1986.

Jacobson, E. (1938). *Progressive relaxation* (2nd ed.). Chicago: University of Chicago Press.

James, I. M., Pearson, R. M., Griffith, D. N., et al. (1978). Reducing the somatic manifestations of anxiety by beta-blockage: A study of stage fright. *Journal of Psychosomatic Research, 22*, 327–337.

Johnson, L. C., & Chernik, D. A. (1982). Sedative-hypnotics and human performance. *Psychopharmacology, 76*, 101–113.

Kahn, R. J., McNair, D. M., Lipman, R. S., et al. (1986). Imipramine and chlordiazepoxide in depressive and anxiety disorders: II. Efficacy in anxious outpatients. *Archives of General Psychiatry, 43*, 79–85.

Kane, J. M., Barnes, T. R., Correll, C. U., Sachs, G., Buckley, P., Eudicone, J., et al. (2010). Evaluation of akathisia in patients with schizophrenia, schizoaffective disorder, or bipolar I disorder: a post hoc analysis of pooled data from short- and long-term aripiprazole trials. *Journal of Psychopharmacology, 24*, 1019–1029.

Karajgi, B., Rifkin, A., Doddi, S., et al. (1990). The prevalence of anxiety disorders in patients with chronic obstructive pulmonary disease. *American Journal of Psychiatry, 147*, 200–201.

Karch, F. E. (1979). Rage reaction associated with clorazepate dipotassium. *Annals of Internal Medicine, 91*, 61–62.

Kastenholz, K. V., & Crismon, M. L. (1984). Buspirone, a novel nonbenzodiazepine anxiolytic. *Clinical Pharmacology, 3*, 600–607.

Kathol, R. G., Noyes, R. Jr., Slymen, D. J., et al. (1980). Propranolol in chronic anxiety disorders. A controlled study. *Archives of General Psychiatry, 37*, 1361–1365.

Katon, W. (1986). Panic disorder: epidemiology, diagnosis, and treatment in primary care. *Journal of Clinical Psychiatry, 47*, 21–30.

Katon, W. J. (1990). Chest pain, cardiac disease, and panic disorder. *Journal of Clinical Psychiatry, 51*, 17–30.

Katon, W., Lin, E. H., Kroenke, K., et al. (2007). The association of depression and anxiety with medical symptom burden in patients with chronic medical illness. *General Hospital Psychiatry, 29*, 147–155.Katon, W., VonKorff, M., Lin, E., et al. (1990). Distressed high utilizers of medical care. DSM-III-R diagnoses and treatment needs. *General Hospital Psychiatry, 12*, 355–362.

Kessler, R. C., Berglund, P., Demier, O., Jin, R., Merkangas, K. R., & Walters, E. E. (2005). Lifetime prevalence and age-of-onset distributions of DSM-IV disorders in the National Comorbidity Survey Replication. *Archives General Psychiatry, 62*, 593–602.

Klein, D. F. (1982). Medication in the treatment of panic attacks and phobic states. *Psychopharmacology Bulletin, 18*, 85–90.

Koch-Weser, J., & Frishman, W. H. (1981). b-Adrenergic antagonists: New drugs and new indications. *New England Journal of Medicine, 305*, 500–505.

Kristensen, O., & Sendrup, E. H. (1978). Sphenoidal electrodes. *Acta Neurologica Scandinavica, 58*, 157–166.

Kroenke, K., Spitzer, R. L., Williams, J. B., et al. (1994). Physical symptoms in primary care: predictors of psychiatric disorders and functional impairment. *Archives Family Medicine, 3*, 774–779.

Kroenke, K., Spitzer, R. L., Williams, J. B., & Lowe, B. (2010). The Patient Health Questionnaire somatic, anxiety, and depressive symptom scales: a systematic review. *General Hospital Psychiatry, 32*, 345–359.

Kroenke, K., Spitzer, R. L., Williams, J. B., Monahan, P. O., & Lowe, B. (2007). Anxiety disorders in primary care: Prevalence, impairment, comorbidity, and detection. *Annals Internal Medicine, 146*, 317–325.

Kumar, R., & Sachdev, P. S. (2009). Akathisia and second generation antipsychotic drugs. *Current Opinion in Psychiatry, 2*, 293–299.

Lakshminarayan, M. D., Sahn, S. A., Hudson, L. D., et al. (1976). Effect of diazepam on ventilatory responses. *Clinical Pharmacology and Therapeutics, 20*, 178–183.

Lamberg, T. S., Kivisto, K. T., & Neuvonen, P. J. (1998). Effects of verapamil and diltiazem on the pharmacokinetics of buspirone. *Clinical Pharmacology and Therapeutics, 63*, 640–645.

Leitenberg, H., Wincze, J. P., Butz, R. A., et al. (1970). Comparison of the effects of instructions and reinforcement in the treatment of a neurotic avoidance response: A single case experiment. *Journal of Behavior Therapy and Experimental Psychiatry, 1*, 53–58.

Lerner, W. D., & Fallon, H. J. (1985). The alcohol withdrawal syndrome. *New England Journal of Medicine, 313*, 951–952.

Levine, A. M. (1988). Buspirone and agitation in head injury. *Brain Injury, 2*, 165–167.

Lieb, J. P., Walsh, G. O. Babb, T. L., et al. (1976). A comparison of EEG seizure patterns recorded with surface and depth electrodes in patients with temporal lobe epilepsy. *Epilepsia, 17*, 137–160.

Lipinski, J. F., Mallya, G., Zimmerman, P., et al. (1989). Fluoxetine-induced akathisia: Clinical and theoretical implications. *Journal of Clinical Psychiatry, 50*, 339–342.

Lipman, R. S., Covi, L., Downing, R. W., et al. (1981). Pharmacotherapy of anxiety and depression. *Psychopharmacology Bulletin, 17*, 91–103.

Linzer, M., Varia, I., Pontinen, M., et al. (1992). Medically unexplained syncope: relationship to psychiatric illness. *American Journal of Medicine, 92*, 18S–25S.

Lishman, W. A. (1987). Endocrine disorders and metabolic disorders. In *Organic psychiatry* (Ch. 11, pp. 428–485). London: Blackwell.

Lucki, I., Rickels, K., & Geller, A. M. (1986). Chronic use of benzodiazepines and psychomotor and cognitive test performance. *Psychopharmacology, 89*, S55.

Lydiard, R. B., Fossey, M. D., Marsh, W., et al. (1993). Prevalence of psychiatric disorders in patients with irritable bowel syndrome. *Psychosomatics, 34*, 229–234.

Lynch, J. J., Paskewitz, D. A., Gimbel, K. S., et al. (1977). Psychological aspects of cardiac arrhythmia. *American Heart Journal, 93*, 645–657.

MacCrimmon, D. J., Wallace, J. E., Goldberg, W. M., et al. (1979). Emotional disturbance and cognitive deficits in hyperthyroidism. *Psychosomatic Medicine, 41*, 331–340.

Maldonado, R., Berrendero, F., Ozaita, A., & Robledo, P. (2011). Neurochemical basis of cannabis addiction. *Neuroscience, 181*, 11–17.

Malcolm, R., Ballenger, J. C., Sturgis, E. T., et al. (1989). Double-blind controlled trial comparing carbamazepine to oxazepam treatment of alcohol withdrawal. *American Journal of Psychiatry, 146*, 617–621.

Maher, A. R., Maglione, M., Bagley, S., Suttorp, M., Hu, J-H., Ewing, B., et al. (2011) Efficacy and comparative effectiveness of atypical antipsychotic medications for off-label uses in adults. *Journal of American Medical Association, 306*, 1359–1369.

Marcus, S. C., Olfson, M., Pincus, H. A., et al. (1997). Self-reported anxiety, general medical conditions, and disability bed days. *American Journal of Psychiatry, 154*, 1766–1768.

Marks, I. M., Hallam, R. S., Connolly, J., et al. (1977). *Nursing in behavioral psychotherapy: An advanced role for nurses.* London: Royal College of Nursing.

Marshall, J. R. (1979). Neuropsychiatric aspects of renal failure. *Journal of Clinical Psychiatry, 40*, 81–85.

Mason, B. J., Quello, S., Goodell, V., Shadan, F., Kyle, M., & Begovic, A. (2014). Gabapentin treatment for alcohol dependence: A randomized clinical trial. *JAMA Internal Medicine, 174*, 70–77.

Mastrovito, R. C. (1972). Symposium: Emotional considerations in cancer and stroke. *New York State Journal of Medicine, 72*, 2874–2877.

McDonald-Haile, J., Bradley, L. A., Bailey, M. A., et al. (1994). Relaxation training reduces symptom reports and acid exposure in patients with gastroesophageal reflux disease. *Gastroenterology, 107*(1), 61–67.

McHenry, P. L., Cogan, O. J., Elliott, W. C., et al. (1970). False-positive ECG response to exercise secondary to hyperventilation: Cineangiographic correlation. *American Heart Journal, 79*, 683–687.

McCrank, E., Schurmans, K., & Lefcoe, D. (1998). Paroxysmal supraventricular tachycardia misdiagnosed as panic disorder. *Archives Internal Medicine, 158*, 297.

McLaughlin, T. P., Khandker, R. K., Kruzikas, D. T., et al. (2006). Overlap of anxiety and depression in a managed care population: prevalence and association with resource utilization. *Journal of Clinical Psychiatry, 67*, 1187–1193.

McNamara, M. E., & Fogel, B. S. (1990). Anticonvulsant-responsive panic attacks with temporal lobe EEG abnormalities. *Journal of Neuropsychiatry and Clinical Neurosciences, 2*, 193–196.

Meares, S., Shores, E. A., Taylor, A. J., Batchelor, J., & Bryant, R. A. (2011). The prospective course of postconcussion syndrome: the role of mild traumatic brain injury *Neuropsychology, 25*, 454–465.

Meuret, A. E., White, K. S., Ritz, T., Roth, W. T., Hofmann, S. G., & Brown, T. A. (2006). Panic attack symptom dimensions and their relationship to illness characteristics in panic disorder. *Journal of Psychiatric Research, 40*, 520–527.

Meyer, R. E. (1986). Anxiolytics and the alcoholic patient. *Journal of Studies on Alcohol, 47*, 269–273.

Mitchells-Heggs, P., Murphy, K., Minty, K., et al. (1980). Diazepam in the treatment of dyspnea in the "pink puffer" syndrome. *Quarterly Journal of Medicine, 49*, 19–20.

Moore, K. E., Geffken, G. R., & Royal, G. P. (1995). Behavioral intervention to reduce child distress during self-injection. *Clinical Pediatrics, 34*(10), 530–534.

Moore, R. A. (1985).The prevalence of alcoholism in medical and surgical patients. In M. A. Schuckit, & A. E. Slaby (Eds.), *Alcohol patterns and problems* (Ch. 8, pp. 247–265). New Brunswick, NJ: Rutgers University Press.

Mueller, H. S. & Chahine, R. A. (1981). Interim report of multicenter double-blind placebo-controlled studies of nifedipine in chronic stable angina. *American Journal of Medicine 71*, 645–657.

Nakao, M., Fricchione, G., Myers, P., Zuttermeister, P. C., Baim, M., Mandle, C. L., et al. (2001). Anxiety is a good indicator for somatic symptom reduction through behavioral medicine intervention in a mind/body medicine clinic. *Psychotherapy and Psychosomatics, 70*, 50–57.

Neill, W. A., & Hattenhauer, M. (1975). Impairment of myocardial O_2 supply due to hyperventilation. *Circulation, 52*, 854–858.

Newton, R. E., Marunycz, J. D., Alderdice, M. T., et al. (1986). Review of the side-effect profile of buspirone. *American Journal of Medicine, 80*(Suppl 3B), 17–21.

Nierenberg, A., & Cole, J. O. (1991). Antidepressant adverse drug reactions. *Journal of Clinical Psychiatry, 52*, 40–47.

Nikaido, A. M., Ellinwood, E. H., Heatherly, D., et al. (1987). Differential, C. N.S effects of diazepam in elderly adults. *Pharmacology, Biochemistry, and Behavior, 27*, 273–281.

Nisenson, L. G., Pepper, C. M., Schwenk, T. L., et al. (1998). The nature and prevalence of anxiety disorders in primary care. *General Hospital Psychiatry, 20*, 11–28.

O'Brien, C. P. (2005). Benzodiazepine use, abuse, and dependence. *Journal Clinical Psychiatry, 66* Suppl 2, 28–33.

Olfson, M., Fireman, B., Weissman, M. M., et al. (1997). Mental disorders and disability among patients in a primary care group practice. *American Journal of Psychiatry, 154*, 1734–1740.

Ollendick, T. H., & Gruen, G. E. (1972). Treatment of a bodily injury phobia with implosive therapy. *Journal of Consulting and Clinical Psychology, 38*, 389–393.

Ost, L. G., Lindahl, I. L., Sterner, U., et al. (1984). Exposure in vivo vs. applied relaxation in the treatment of blood phobia. *Behavior Research and Therapy, 22*, 205–216.

Ost, L. G., Sterner, U., & Fellenius, J. (1989). Applied tension, applied relaxation and the combination in treatment of blood phobia. *Behavior Research and Therapy, 27*, 109–121.

Pacak, K., Eisenhofer, G., Ahlman, H., et al. (2005). Pheochromocytoma: recommendations for clinical practice from the First International Symposium. *Nature Clinical Practice Endocrinology and Metabolim, 88*, 2656–2666.

Pande, A. C., Davidson, R. T., Jefferson, J. W., Janney, C. A., et al. (1999). Treatment of social phobia with gabapentin: a placebo controlled study. *Journal of Clinical Psychopharmacology 19*, 341–348.

Paradis, C. M., Friedman, S., Lazar, R. M., et al. (1993). Anxiety disorders in a neuromuscular clinic. *American Journal of Psychiatry, 150*, 1102–1104.

Parkinson, D. (1977). Concussion. *Mayo Clinic Proceedings, 52*, 492–496.

Patterson, J. (1988). Alprazolam dependency: Use of clonazepam for withdrawal. *Southern Medical Journal, 81*, 830–831.

Paykel, E. S., Rowman, P. R., Parker, R. R., et al. (1982). Response to phenelzine and amitriptyline in subtypes of outpatient depression. *Archives of General Psychiatry, 39*, 041–1049.

Peck, A., & Boland, J. (1977). Emotional reactions to radiation treatment. *Cancer, 40*, 184–184.

Perna, G. et al. (1997). Asthma and panic attacks. *Biological Psychiatry, 42*, 625–630.

Pevnick, J. S., Jasinski, D. R., & Haertzen, C. A. (1978). Abrupt withdrawal from therapeutically administered diazepam. *Archives of General Psychiatry, 35*, 995–998.

Pincus, J. H., & Tucker, G. J. (1985). *Behavioral neurology* (3rd ed.). New York: Oxford University Press.

Plum, F., & Posner, J. B. (1972). Diagnosis of stupor and coma (2nd ed.). *Contemporary neurology series*. Philadelphia: FA Davis.

Pohl, R., Berchou, R., & Rainey, J. M. (1982). Tricyclic antidepressants and monoamine oxidase inhibitors in the treatment of agoraphobia. *Journal of Clinical Psychopharmacology, 2*, 399–407.

Pohl, R., Yeragani, V. K., Balon, R., et al. (1988). The jitteriness syndrome in panic disorder patients treated with antidepressants. *Journal of Clinical Psychiatry, 49*, 100–104.

Pollack, M. H., Kradin, R., Otto, M. W., et al. (1996). Prevalence of panic in patients referred for pulmonary function testing at a major medical center. *American Journal of Psychiatry, 153*, 110–113.

Pomara, N., Stanley, B., Block, R., et al. (1985). Increased sensitivity of the elderly to the central depressant effects of diazepam. *Journal of Clinical Psychiatry, 46*, 185–187.

Popkin, M. K., Callies, A. L., Lentz, R. D., et al. (1988). Prevalence of major depression, simple phobia and other psychiatric disorders in patients with long-standing type I diabetes mellitus. *Archives of General Psychiatry, 45*, 54–68.

Poyurovsky, M. (2010). Acute antipsychotic-induced akathisia revisited. *British Journal of Psychiatry, 196*, 89–91.

Preston, K. L., Epstein, D. H., Cone, E. J., et al. (2002). Urinary elimination of cocaine metabolites in chronic cocaine users during cessation. *Journal of Analytical Toxicology, 26*, 93.

Rao, S., Sherbaniuk, R. W., Prasad, K., et al. (1973). Cardiopulmonary effects of diazepam. *Clinical Pharmacology and Therapeutics, 14*, 182–189.

Rao, S., & Zisook, S. (2009) Anxious depression: Clinical features and treatment. *Current Psychiatry Reports, 11*, 429–436.

Rapoport, D. M., & Mendelson, W. H. (1989). Buspirone: A new respiratory stimulant [abstract]. *American Review of Respiratory Disease, 139*, A625.

Rathbone, J., & Soares-Weiser, K. (2006). Anticholinergics for neuroleptic-induced acute akathisia. *Cochrane Database Systematic Reviews. 4*, CD003727.

Ratey, J. J., Sovner, R., Mikkelsen, E., et al. (1989). Buspirone therapy for maladaptive behavior and anxiety in developmentally disabled persons. *Journal of Clinical Psychiatry, 509*, 382–384.

Ray, W. A., Griffin, M. R., & Downey, W. (1989). Benzodiazepines of long and short elimination half-life and the risk of hip fracture. *Journal of the American Medical Association, 262*, 3303–3307.

Resnick, R. B., Kestenbaum, R. S., & Schwartz, L. K. (1976). Acute systemic effects of cocaine in man: A controlled study by intranasal and intravenous routes. *Science, 195*, 96–698.

Reuler, J. B., Girard, D. E., & Cooney, T. G. (1985). Wernicke's encephalopathy. *New England Journal of Medicine, 312*, 1035–1039.

Rice, R. L. (1950). Symptom patterns of the hyperventilation syndrome. *American Journal of Medicine, 8*, 691–700.

Rickels, K. (1983). Nonbenzodiazepine anxiolytics: Clinical usefulness. *Journal of Clinical Psychiatry, 44*(11 sec 2), 38–43.

Rickels, K., Csanalosi, I., Chung, H. R., et al. (1974). Amitriptyline in anxious-depressed outpatinets: A controlled study. *American Journal of Psychiatry, 131*, 25–30.

Rickels, K., Gordon, P. E., Zamostein, B. B., et al. (1970). Hydroxyzine and chlordiazepoxide in anxious neurotic outpatients: A collaborative controlled study. *Comprehensive Psychiatry, 11*, 457–474.

Rickels, K., Morris, R. J., Newman, H., et al. (1983). Diphenhydramine in insomniac family practice patients: A double-blind study. *Journal of Clinical Pharmacology, 23*, 235–242.

Rickels, K., Shiovitz, T. M., Ramey, T. S., et al. (2012). Adjunctive therapy with pregabalin in generalized anxiety disorder patients with partial response to SSRI or SNRI treatment. *International Clinical Psychopharmacology, 27*, 142–150.

Rickels, K., Weisman, K., Norstad, N., et al. (1982). Buspirone and diazepam in anxiety: A controlled study. *Journal of Clinical Psychiatry, 43*(12, sec 2), 81–86.

Ries, R. K., Roy-Byrne, P. P., Ward, N. G., et al. (1989). Carbamazepine treatment for benzodiazepine withdrawal. *American Journal of Psychiatry, 146*, 536–537.

Rifkin, A., Doddi, S., Karajgi, B., et al. (1989). Benzodiazepine use and abuse by patients at outpatient clinics. *American Journal of Psychiatry, 146*, 1331–1332.

Rinkenberger, R. L., Psystowsky, E. N., Heger, J. J., et al. (1980). Effect of intravenous and chronic oral verapamil administration in patients with supraventricular arrhythmias. *Circulation, 62*, 996–1010.

Robertson, D., Frolich, J. C., Carr, R. K., et al. (1978). Effects of caffeine on plasma renin activity, catecholamines and blood pressure. *New England Journal of Medicine, 298*, 181–186.

Robinson, D. S., Nies, A., Ravaris, C. L., et al. (1973). The monoamine oxidase inhibitor, phenelzine, in the treatment of depressive-anxiety states: A controlled clinical trial. *Archives of General Psychiatry, 29*, 407–413.

Rosenbaum, J. F., Moroz, G., & Bowden, C. L. (1997). Clonazepam in the treatment of panic disorder with or without agoraphobia: a dose-response study of efficacy, safety, and discontinuance. *Journal of Clinical Psychopharmacology, 17*, 390–400.

Rudaz, M., Craske, M. G., Becker, E. S., Ledermann, T., & Margraf, J. (2010). Health anxiety and fear of fear in panic disorder and agoraphobia vs. Social phobia: a prospective longitudnal study. *Depression & Anxiety, 27*, 404–411.

Ryan, H. F., Merrill, F. B., Scott, G. E., et al. (1968). Increase in suicidal thoughts and tendencies: Association with diazepam therapy. *Journal of the American Medical Association, 203*, 1137–1139.

Saltz, R., Freedner, N., Palfai, T. P., Horton, N. J., & Samet, J. H. (2005). The severity of unhealthy alcohol use in hospitalized medical patients. *Journal of General Internal Medicine, 21*, 381–385.

Sansone, R. A., & Sanson, L. A. (2009). Panic disorder subtypes: deceptive somatic impersonatorsl. *Psychiatry, 7*, 33–37.

Scharf, M. B., Khosla, N., Brocker, N., et al. (1984). Differential amnestic properties of short and long-acting benzodiazepines. *Journal of Clinical Psychiatry, 45*, 51–53.

Schneider, L. S., Syapin, P. J., & Pawluczyk, S. (1987). Seizures following triazolam withdrawal despite benzodiazepine treatment. *Journal of Clinical Psychiatry, 48*, 418–419.

Schuckit, M. A. (1984). Clinical studies of buspirone. *Psychopathology, 17*(Suppl 3), 61–68.

Schweizer, E., & Rickels, K. (1986). Failure of buspirone to manage benzodiazepine withdrawal. *American Journal of Psychiatry, 143*, 1590–1592.

Schweizer, E., Rickels, K., & Lucki, I. (1986). Resistance to the antianxiety effect of buspirone in patients with a history of benzodiazepine use. *New England Journal of Medicine, 314*, 719–720.

Schweizer, E., Rickels, K., Case, W. G., et al. (1990). Long-term therapeutic use of benzodiazepine: II effects of gradual taper. *Archives of General Psychiatry, 47*, 908–915.

Seaquist, E. R., Anderson, J., Childs, B., Cryer, P., et al. (2013). Hypoglycemia and diabetes: a report of a workgroup of the American Diabetes Association and The Endocrine Society. *Journal of Clinical Endocrinology and Metabolism, 98*, 1845–1859.

Sellers, E. M., & Kalant, H. (1976). Alcohol intoxication and withdrawal. *New England Journal of Medicine, 294*, 757–762.

Shader, R. I., Dreyfuss, D., Gerrein, J. R., et al. (1986). Sedative effects and impaired learning and recall following single oral doses of lorazepam. *Clinical Pharmacology and Therapeutics, 39*, 526–529.

Sheehan, D. V., Ballenger, J., & Jacobsen, G. (1980). Treatment of endogenous anxiety with phobic, hysterical and hypochondriacal symptoms. *Archives of General Psychiatry, 37*, 51–59.

Silver, J. M. (2014). Neuropsychiatry of persistent symptoms after concussion. *Psychiatric Clinics of North America 37*, 91–102.

Silverman, K., Evans, S. M., Strain, E. C., et al. (1992). Withdrawal syndrome after the double-blind cessation of caffeine consumption. *New England Journal of Medicine, 327*, 1109–1114.

Sinclair, L. I., Christmas, D. M., Hood, S. D., Potokar, J. P., et al. (2009). Antidepressant-induced jitteriness/anxiety syndrome: systematic review. *British Journal of Psychiatry, 194*, 83–490.

Singh, B. N., Ellrodt, G., & Peter, C. T. (1978). Verapamil: A review of its pharmacological properties and therapeutic use. *Drugs, 15*, 169–197.

Spitzer, R. L., Kroenke, K., Williams, J. B., et al. (2006). A brief measure for assessing generalized anxiety disorder: the GAD-7. *Archives Internal Medicine, 146*, 317–325.

Starkman, M. N., Zelnik, T. C., Nesse, R. M., et al. (1985). Anxiety in patients with pheochromocytomas. *Archives of Internal Medicine, 145,* 248–252.

Stein, M. B., Heuser, I. J., Juncos, J. L., et al. (1990). Anxiety disorders in patients with Parkinson's disease. *American Journal of Psychiatry, 147,* 217–220.

Stein, P. D., Beemath, A., Matta, F., et al. (2007). Clinical characteristics of patients with acute pulmonary embolism: data from PIOPED II. *American Journal of Medicine, 120,* 71.

Strain, E. C., Mumford, G. K., Silverman, K., et al. (1994). Caffeine dependence syndrome. Evidence from case histories and experimental evaluations. *Journal of the American Medical Association, 272,* 1043–1048.

Sutherland, A. M., Orbach, C. E., Duk, R. B., et al. (1977). Adaptation to the dry colostomy; preliminary report and summary of findings. In the *psychological impact of cancer* (pp. 1–16). New York: American Cancer Society.

Thompson, B. T. & Hales, C. A. (2014). Diagnosis of acute pulmonary embolism and overview of acute pulmonary embolism. In: Basow, D. S. (ed) UpToDate.

Tien, A. Y., & Gujavarty, K. S. (1985). Seizure following withdrawal from triazolam [letter to the editor]. *American Journal of Psychiatry, 142,* 1516–1517.

Tinetti, M. E., Speechley, M., & Ginter, S. F. (1988). Risk factors for falls among elderly persons living in the community. *New England Journal of Medicine, 319,* 1701–1707.

Toft, T., Fink, P., Oernboel, E., et al. (2005). Mental disorders in primary care: prevalence and co-morbidity among disorders. Results from the functional illness in primary care (FIP) study. *Psychological Medicine 35,* 1175–1184.

Torpy, J. M., & Livingston, E. H. (2013). Energy drinks. *Journal of the American Medical Association, 309*(3), 297.

Treggiari-Venzi, M. M., Suter, P. M., De Tonnac, N., & Romand, J. A. (2000). Successful use of hypnosis as an adjunctive therapy for weaning from mechanical ventilation. *Anesthesiology, 92,* 890–892.

Tyrer, P. J., & Lader, M. H. (1974). Response to propranolol and diazepam in somatic anxiety. *British Medical Journal, 2,* 14–16.

Uhlenhuth, E. H., DeWit, H., Balter, M. B., et al. (1988). Risks and benefits of long-term benzodiazepine use. *Journal of Clinical Psychopharmacology, 8,* 161–167.

Van der Kropf, C. (1979). Reactions to triazolam. *Lancet, 2,* 26.

Victor, B. S., Lubetsky, M., & Greden, J. F. (1981). Somatic manifestations of caffeinism. *Journal of Clinical Psychiatry, 42,* 185–188.

Waldeck, B. (1975). Effect of caffeine on locomotor activity in central catecholamine mechanisms: A study with special reference to drug interaction. *Acta Pharmacologica et Toxicologica, 36,* 9–23.

Wallace, R. K. (1970). Physiological effects of transcendental meditation. *Science, 167,* 1751–1754.

Warwick, H. M., & Salkovskis, P. M. (1990). Hypochondriasis. *Behavior Research and Therapy, 28,* 105–117.

Webb, W. L., & Gehi, M. (1981). Electrolyte and fluid imbalance: Neuropsychiatric manifestations. *Psychosomatics, 22,* 199–203.

Weil, A. A. (1959). Ictal emotions occurring in temporal lobe dysfunction. *Archives of Neurology, 1,* 87–97.

Weiner, N. (1980). Norephedrine, ephedrine, and sympathomimetic amines. In A. G. Goodman, L. S. Goodman, & A. Gilman (Eds.), *Pharmacological basis of therapeutics* (p. 163). New York: Macmillan.

Weisman, A. (1979). *Coping with cancer.* New York: McGraw-Hill.

Wells, B. G., Cold, J. A., Marken, P. A., et al. (1991). A placebo-controlled trial of Nadolol in the treatment of neuroleptic-induced akathisia. *Journal of Clinical Psychiatry, 52,* 255–260.

Whale, R., Terao, T., Cowen, P., Freemantle, N., & Geddes, J. (2010). Pindolol augmentation of serotonin reuptake inhibitors for the treatment of depressive disorder. A systemic review. *Journal of Psychopharmacology, 24,* 513–520.

White, B. C., Lincoln, C. A., Pearce, N. W., et al. (1980). Anxiety and muscle tension as consequences of caffeine withdrawal. *Science, 209,* 1547–1548.

Wiffen, P. J., Derry, S., Moore, R. A., Aldington, D., Cole, P., Rice, A. S., et al. (2013) Antiepileptic drugs for neuropathic pain and fibromyalgia—an overview of Cochrane reviews. *Cochrane Database Syst Rev, 11,* CD010567.

Winokur, A., Rickels, K., Greenblatt, D. J., et al. (1980). Withdrawal reaction from long-term low-dosage administration of diazepam. *Archives of General Psychiatry, 37,* 101–105.

Winslow, B. R., Voorhees, K. I., & Pehl, K. A. (2007). Methamphetamine abuse. *American Family Physician, 76,* 1169–1176.

Wolkowitz, O. M., Weingartner, H., Thompson, K., et al. (1987). Diazepam-induced amnesia: A neuropharmacological model of an "organic amnestic syndrome." *American Journal of Psychiatry, 144,* 25–29.

Wortsman, J., Burns, G., Van Beek, A. L., et al. (1980). Hyperadrenergic state after trauma to the neuroaxis. *Journal of the American Medical Association, 243,* 1459–1460.

Yingling, K. W., Wulsin, L. R., Arnold, L. M., et al. (1993). Estimated prevalences of panic disorder and depression among consecutive patients seen in an emergency department with acute chest pain. *Journal of General Internal Medicine, 8,* 231–235.

Young, G. B., Chandarana, P. C., Blume, W. T., McLachlan, R. S., Munoz, D. G., Girin, J. P. (1995). Mesial temporal lobe seizures presenting as anxiety disorders. *Journal of Neuropsychiatry & Clinical Neurosciences, 7,* 352–357.

Zijlmans, M., Huiskamp, G. M., van Huffelen, A. C., Spetgens, W. P., & Leijten, F. S. (2008). Detection of temproal lobe spikes: Comparing nasopharyngeal, cheek and anterior temporal electrodes to simultaneous subdural recordings. *Clinical Neurophysiology, 119,* 1771–1777.

Zipursky, R. B., Baker, R. W., & Zimmer, B. (1985). Alprazolam withdrawal delirium unresponsibe to diazepam: Case report. *Journal of Clinical Psychiatry, 46,* 344–345.

Zitrin, C. M., Klein, D. F., Woerner, M. G. (1978). Behavior therapy, supportive psychotherapy, imipramine and phobias. *Archives of General Psychiatry, 35,* 307–316.

32.

EATING DISORDERS

Megan Moore Brennan, Caitlin M. Nevins, and Jennifer J. Thomas

INTRODUCTION

Eating disorders (EDs) are common, especially among young women. EDs are serious illnesses associated with significant medical and psychiatric morbidity. Particularly when chronic and severe, EDs have relatively high mortality rates when compared with other psychiatric disorders. Because of the ego-syntonic nature of many EDs, patients often first present in the medical sector due to the unwanted and unintended physical consequences. Frequently patients are embarrassed about the underlying behaviors causing their physical problems and are therefore reluctant to report disordered eating. For these reasons, it is crucial that clinicians be knowledgeable about EDs and know when to suspect that one is present. Early identification and treatment can help prevent the associated morbidity and mortality.

DIAGNOSIS

In 2013, the *Diagnostic and Statistical Manual of Mental Disorders fourth edition text revision (DSM-IV-TR)* was updated to the *fifth edition (DSM-5)*. The Eating Disorders Work Group made several revisions to enhance the clinical utility of ED diagnoses in *DSM-5*. The primary *DSM-5* changes included combining feeding disorders and EDs into a single chapter; broadening and clarifying the criteria for anorexia nervosa (AN) and bulimia nervosa (BN); adding binge eating disorder (BED) as a formal diagnosis; and re-classifying feeding disorder of infancy or early childhood as avoidant/restrictive food intake disorder (ARFID). Moreover, *DSM-5* separated the single *DSM-IV* residual category of eating disorder not otherwise specified (EDNOS) into two separate residual categories of other specified feeding or eating disorder (OSFED) and unspecified feeding or eating disorder (UFED). OSFED comprises a list of five example presentations, whereas UFED is reserved for cases in which a clinically significant ED is present but the clinician does not have sufficient information to characterize the presentation (e.g., in an emergency room setting) (see below). In this chapter, we will focus mainly on AN, BN and BED because their phenomenology and treatment is currently better understood, and clinicians treating adults are most likely to encounter patients with these diagnoses. See Table 32.1 for descriptions of each ED diagnosis.

The hallmark of AN is low body weight for sex and age. To meet criteria for AN, individuals must either express an intense fear of becoming fat or exhibit behaviors that interfere with weight restoration; and exhibit a lack of recognition of the possible health consequences of low weight. *DSM-5* no longer requires cessation of menstruation for 3 months (American Psychiatric Association, 2013). Low body weight is considered a body mass index (BMI) < 18.5 for adults, or a BMI < 5th percentile for sex and age using growth charts for children and adolescents (American Psychiatric Association, 2013).

In contrast to those with AN, individuals with BN are normal weight, overweight, or obese. BN is characterized by a pattern of binge eating followed by compensatory behaviors to make up for calories consumed, occurring at least once weekly for at least 3 months. Compensatory behavior may comprise purging (i.e., self-induced vomiting, laxative or diuretic misuse) or non-purging (i.e., fasting, excessive exercise) symptoms. Similar to AN, the self-image of individuals with BN is dominated by their weight and shape. *DSM-5* differentiates subtypes of AN (restricting and binge-eating/purging type), such that an individual who meets criteria for both disorders would be diagnosed as AN binge-eating/purging type (American Psychiatric Association, 2013).

BED is characterized by frequent episodes of binge eating, but does not feature the compensatory behaviors that characterize BN. To meet diagnostic criteria, binge episodes must be associated with at least 3 of 5 key physical and psychological characteristics (e.g., eating rapidly or when not hungry; feeling disgusted or guilty after bingeing). To distinguish binge eating from simple overeating, binges are defined as consuming a large amount of food in a short period of time while concurrently feeling out of control (i.e., unable to stop eating) (American Psychiatric Publishing, 2013).

OSFED, previously referred as EDNOS, comprises five non-exhaustive example presentations: atypical anorexia nervosa (anorexic features without low weight), subthreshold BN (bingeing and purging less than once per week or for fewer than 3 months), subthreshold BED (binge eating less than once per week or for fewer than 3 months), purging disorder (regular purging in the absence of binge eating), and night eating syndrome (characterized by nocturnal eating episodes after awakening from sleep, or consuming a large proportion of daily calories after the evening meal). Although many *DSM-5* changes aimed to reduce the large number of patients

Table 32.1 EATING DISORDERS

EATING DISORDER	DESCRIPTION
Anorexia Nervosa	Low body weight for sex and age accompanied by an intense fear of becoming fat and/or persistent behaviors that interfere with gaining weight; and lack of recognition of the possible health consequences of low weight. Subtypes are based on whether low weight is maintained by pure restriction or by bingeing and/or purging.
Bulimia Nervosa	Binge eating followed by compensatory behaviors to make up for calories consumed, occurring at least once weekly for at least 3 months. Self-image is dominated by weight and shape. Individuals with BN can be normal weight, overweight, or obese.
Binge Eating Disorder	Frequent episodes of binge eating that are not followed by compensatory behaviors. During binges individuals feel out of control. Afterward, they may feel embarrassed, disgusted with themselves, depressed, and/or guilty. Patients can be normal weight, overweight, or obese.
Other Specified Feeding or Eating Disorder	This group comprises eating disturbances that cause clinical impairment but do not meet diagnostic criteria for AN, BN, BED, or ARFID. Specific examples include partial syndromes of either AN or BN, as well as other forms of ED such as repeatedly purging in the absence of binge eating, or night eating syndrome.

falling into this residual category, available data suggest that a substantial minority of cases will still receive an OSFED or UFED diagnosis (Thomas et al., under review).

EPIDEMIOLOGY

Although epidemiological data on EDs are limited, findings from the National Comorbidity Survey Replication (NCS-R) provide estimates (Hudson, Hiripi, Pope, & Kessler, 2007). Lifetime prevalence estimates for women and men are 0.9% and 0.3% for AN, 1.5% and 0.5% for BN, and 3.5% and 2.0% for BED, respectively (Hudson et al., 2007). These are likely underestimates, given that individuals with disordered eating may be reluctant to report behaviors and also because the NCS-R did not include operational definitions, OSFED examples or new *DSM-5* presentations such as ARFID.

Also according to NCS-R data, only a minority of individuals with EDs seek mental health treatment. In this representative study, only 50%–63% of those with lifetime EDs had ever sought treatment for emotional problems, and less than 50% had ever sought treatment specifically for EDs. For those patients with 12-month histories of ED, only 15.6% of those with BN and 28.5% of those with BED reported seeking treatment for emotional problems in the preceding 12 months.

The most common site of treatment in the NCS-R study was the medical sector (e.g., primary care). In medical settings patients rarely present with a chief complaint of disordered eating (e.g., restricting food, purging, using laxatives); rather, most present with nonspecific physical or emotional complaints. For example, patients with AN may report lightheadedness or constipation; patients with BN may present with acid reflux or other gastrointestinal problems; and patients with BED may present with obesity or depression. In our clinical experience, it is sometimes only after months of frustrating and seemingly treatment-resistant physical symptoms that suspicion of an ED develops.

At times a patient is relieved when a clinician ascertains a covert ED. In turn, the patient may become forthcoming with information and motivated to accept treatment. This is satisfying for both patient and clinician. However, when a patient continues to deny there is an eating problem and refuses recommended treatments, the clinician may feel frustrated, exhausted, and unsure how to proceed—especially when behaviors have potentially dangerous medical consequences. Although difficult for all involved, this is a crucial time to strengthen the patient–clinician alliance and motivate the patient toward ED treatment.

COMORBIDITY

EDs are typically comorbid with other psychiatric disorders. Traits common to AN and BN include perfectionism and dysphoric mood. Other traits presage the specific ED symptoms that an individual may ultimately adopt. For example, obsessive compulsive traits contribute to restrictive eating patterns, whereas borderline personality traits promote impulsive eating patterns such as binge eating and self-induced vomiting (Sansone & Sansone, 2010). Similarly, high constraint, constricted affect, and asceticism are often associated with AN, whereas high impulsivity and sensation-seeking are associated with BN (Kaye, 2008). Impulse control disorders have been associated with both normal-weight and obese presentations of BED (Keel, Holm-Denoma, & Crosby, 2011).

The majority of individuals with EDs in the NCS-R also had a lifetime history of another psychiatric disorder. Anxiety, mood, and substance use disorders are highly comorbid with EDs. Rates of lifetime anxiety disorders among patients with EDs range from 54%–83% (Kaye, 2007). Patients with AN who binge and purge have higher rates of substance use disorders than patients with restricting-type AN (Root et al., 2010). Higher comorbidity is typically associated with worse overall ED outcome.

Personality disorders are also common among patients with EDs, but available data raise questions about the reliability of personality disorder diagnoses at initial consultation, when erratic or isolative behaviors may be secondary to nutritional compromise. For example, one study demonstrated that at 5-year follow-up from initial inpatient treatment, 43% of ED patients had a diagnosable personality disorder compared to 78% during the inpatient baseline (Vrabel, Ro, Martinsen, Hoffart, & Rosenvinge, 2010). Additionally, a 5-year naturalistic study of patients with BN and EDNOS found that the presence of comorbid personality disorders did not significantly alter time to remission or relapse (Grilo et al., 2007), suggesting that ED outcomes may be independent of personality pathology. These more recent studies provide optimism that patients with comorbid eating and personality disorders can and do improve.

Lastly, but importantly, suicidality is common among individuals with ED. AN has among the highest mortality rates of any psychiatric disorder, with the majority of deaths attributable to malnutrition-related medical complications and suicide (Harris & Barraclough, 1998; Papadopoulos, Ekbom, Brandt, & Ekselius, 2009). Despite a higher mortality rate related to completed suicides in patients with AN, a higher percentage of patients with BN make suicide attempts: 3%–20% in AN and 25%–35% in BN (Franko & Keel, 2006). A combination of traits including low self-directedness, reward dependence, and impulsivity may increase the risk of making suicide attempts in individuals with BN (Forcano et al., 2009). Additionally, literature suggests that a switch from restrictive-type AN to binge-purge type increases risk of suicidal behavior (Foulon et al., 2007). A review of suicidality among patients with EDs identified purging behaviors, depression, substance abuse, and a history of childhood physical or sexual abuse as correlates of suicidality (Franko & Keel, 2006).

COURSE OF ILLNESS

Research on ED course and outcomes is limited, and outcomes vary substantially depending on study duration and level of care.

ANOREXIA NERVOSA

Compared to BN and BED, adult AN tends to be more diagnostically stable over time and follow a more chronic course with overall worse outcomes (Fichter & Quadflieg, 2007). Studies demonstrate that even when remission from AN is achieved, patients persistently have higher anxious, depressive, and obsessive symptoms compared to controls (Wagner et al., 2006). Follow-up studies of AN range from 2.5 years (Clausen, 2008) to 18 years (Wentz, Gillber, Anckarsater, Gillberg, & Rastam, 2006). One 12-year course and outcome study of inpatients with AN reported global outcome scores with 27.5% having a good outcome, 25.3% an intermediate outcome, 39.6% a poor outcome, and 7.7% deceased (Fichter, Quadflieg, & Hedlund, 2006). In this study a poor outcome

was defined as never achieving normal weight. Impulsivity, baseline symptom severity, and chronicity predicted a worse 12-year outcome. Given that the point of entry for this study was an inpatient unit, a selection bias likely makes the outcomes appear graver than for the broader AN population. Follow-up studies with less severely ill populations demonstrate more optimistic outcome data, for example, remission rates of 76% at 5 years and 82% at 8 years. In a recent review of outcomes in AN, mortality rates ranged from zero to 8% across studies with a cumulative mortality rate of 2.8% (9 deaths in 318 cases who were followed for an average of 11 years; see Keel et al., 2010). Another study reviewed 177 cases and found crude mortality rates of 4% (Crow et al., 2009).

BULIMIA NERVOSA

Overall, outcomes for individuals with BN are better than for AN. Remission rates in shorter duration studies are close to 30% and increase to 70% at 10-year follow-up (Keel et al., 2010). Similar to studies of AN, outcome studies for BN range from a few months to 20 years (Keel et al., 2010), and, as length of time to follow-up increases, so do response and remission rates. That said, studies demonstrate that similar to AN, even when remission is achieved patients persistently have psychopathology and altered serotonin function (Wagner et al., 2006, Kaye et al., 1998). In a recent review of outcomes in BN, mortality rates ranged from zero to 2% across studies with a cumulative mortality rate of 0.4% (2 deaths in 459 cases who were followed for an average of 7 years) (Keel & Brown, 2010). Another study of 906 patients with BN reported a crude mortality rate of 3.9% over 8–25 years (Crow et al., 2009).

BINGE EATING DISORDER

Because it is a more recently defined disorder, outcomes for BED are not as well studied as those for AN and BN. Available data suggest that, although individuals with BED may relapse after first remission, many are able to achieve lasting remission over time. One longitudinal study of 104 patients with BED, recruited from college campuses, demonstrated high rates of relapse for individuals with BED within the first 6 months after remission (Agras, Crow, Mitchell, Halmi & Bryson, 2009). However, the same study also demonstrated that that 82% of individuals with BED had remitted after 4 years compared with just 47% of the BN group and 57% of the AN group (Agras et al., 2009). At a 12-year follow-up another study reported a 67% remission rate for 68 female patients with BED who were first recruited during inpatient treatment (Fichter et al., 2008).

IDENTIFICATION AND DIAGNOSIS

Often long before ED patients are willing to accept treatment, they seek substitute treatment for care for the unintended—and often distressing and dangerous—physical consequences (Ogg, Millar, Pusztai, & Thom, 1997). Many patients with ED, particularly AN and BN, present with medical complaints that are atypical or more severe than would be expected given their demographics and otherwise healthy status. For example, a high-school girl may present with hair loss, early satiety, and constipation; or an undergraduate male may present with a 20-pound weight gain over 1 year, insomnia, and heartburn. While hypothyroidism in the former case and numerous medical conditions in the latter should be considered on the differential diagnosis, EDs are common in otherwise healthy youth and should be investigated before embarking on extensive and costly medical tests. Indeed, if the patient exhibits signs and symptoms clearly consistent with an ED, and in the absence of any atypical medical or neurological symptoms, there is no need to exhaust all possible alternative medical explanations before intervening (Mehler & Andersen, 2010). There are very few case reports of serious illness masquerading as an ED, for example, a right frontal brain tumor presenting as AN (Houy, Debono, Dechelotte, & Thibaut, 2007). These cases typically have unusual manifestations (e.g., neurological symptoms) that distinguish them from typical EDs and cue the physician to investigate further.

Many patients do not report ED behaviors to health professionals unless directly queried about eating and weight concerns (Becker, Thomas, Franko, & Herzog, 2005). This is rarely due to any specific gain in lying or deceiving clinicians; usually it is out of embarrassment, fear the clinician will not understand, or a reluctance to give up valued behaviors. However maladaptive and destructive the behaviors appear to the outside observer, they likely serve crucial functions for patients (e.g., providing a sense of control, regulating emotions). Although the patient's illness and life may appear out of control and would seem improved with less disordered eating, paradoxically, patients often feel their lives are *only* in control with the ED and believe that their lives will spiral further out of control or feel intolerable without the behaviors.

SCREENING PATIENTS FOR EATING DISORDERS IN GENERAL MEDICAL SETTINGS

The SCOFF questionnaire is a brief, 5-item screening tool that is easy to administer in clinical settings (Morgan, Reid, & Lacey, 1999; see Table 32.2). It is similar in format to the CAGE questions used to screen for alcohol abuse (Ewing, 1984). It is rapid, sensitive, and requires no special training to use. Validity was initially tested in a group of patients with known AN or BN and a group of controls with no known EDs. With a threshold of two or more positive answers raising concern for a probable ED, there was 100% sensitivity and 87.5% specificity for AN and BN, and 87.5% specificity for controls. The false positive rate was just 12.5%, a reasonable trade-off for the high sensitivity.

In a follow-up study of 341 women ages 18–50 within general practice (Luck et al., 2002), the SCOFF questionnaire detected all cases of AN and BN (4 total) and nearly all cases of EDNOS (7 of 9). One of the EDNOS cases was missed due

Table 32.2 SCOFF QUESTIONS

S	1. Do you make yourself *Sick* because you feel uncomfortably full?
C	2. Do you worry you have lost *Control* over how much you eat?
O	3. Have you recently lost more than *One* stone (about 15 pounds) in a 3-month period?
F	4. Do you believe yourself to be *Fat* when others say you are too thin?
F	5. Would you say that *Food* dominates your life?
Scoring	One point for every "yes"; a score of ≥2 indicates a likely case of AN or BN

From Morgan, Reid, & Lacey, 1999.

to patient nondisclosure. There is some evidence that disclosure increases when patients answer the SCOFF questions privately in written format before their appointments (Perry et al., 2002). The sensitivity was 84.6%, specificity 89.6%, and there were 34 false positives.

One SCOFF feasibility study demonstrated that although clinicians found the screening tool easy to use they did not know what to do with positive results, rarely recorded the results in medical notes, and infrequently offered treatment (Johnston, Fornal, Cabrini, & Kendrick, 2007). The study suggests that screening should be augmented by a standard protocol for triaging patients with likely EDs. Also important to note, the SCOFF was specifically designed to screen for AN and BN, so its sensitivity and specificity for other *DSM-5* ED presentations (e.g., BED, OSFED) remains unknown.

Once suspicion is raised for a possible ED, the next step is to clarify the specific diagnosis. There is significant overlap in symptoms and behaviors among patients with AN and BN; there is less overlap between AN and BED. Patients with restricting type anorexia, who do not engage in bingeing or inappropriate compensatory behaviors (e.g., self-induced vomiting, laxative use), are more easily distinguished from patients with BN. To meet criteria for AN, patients must be significantly underweight (BMI < 18.5 in adults). Moreover, fear of gaining weight or becoming fat is thought to be a central feature and driving force in perpetuating the illness. Interestingly, there is a subset of patients with *DSM-5* AN who do not explicitly endorse fear of fatness but nonetheless exhibit behaviors that interfere with weight restoration. Such patients are especially common in culturally non-Western and youth populations (Becker, Thomas, & Pike, 2009). These patients are characterized as *non–fat phobic AN*, and it is unclear how they may differ from patients with classic AN in terms of diagnosis, treatment, and outcomes (Becker et al., 2009).

Patients with bingeing and purging present more of a diagnostic challenge. Regular bingeing and compensatory behaviors are a core and highly distressing feature of BN, and one or both are also present in the AN binge-eating/purge subtype. The key distinction is that AN patients are significantly underweight, whereas BN patients are normal weight or overweight. In some ways, AN is an illness marked by over-control of behaviors and BN by out-of-control behaviors.

In the evaluation of BED, it is important to distinguish simple overeating from a bona fide ED. Although patients who overeat may be unhappy about it, patients with BED engage in discrete, episodic binges during which they eat large amounts of food, feel out of control, and are highly distressed.

EVALUATION OF PATIENTS WITH EATING DISORDERS

In the initial evaluation of ED patients, it is important to assess current psychiatric and medical issues and to determine their acuity.

PSYCHIATRIC ASSESSMENT

Psychiatric assessments should explore ED symptoms as well as any co-occurring mental illnesses and safety concerns.

Beginning with assessment of the ED, it is critical to investigate daily food consumption in detail. This can vary from complete food and water refusal to bingeing on upwards of 10,000 kilocalories several times per day. A direct and specific, yet empathic, approach will maximize information gathering.

During the initial evaluation we suggest asking patients specifically what they ate and drank for all meals and snacks on the day prior to evaluation. This circumvents vague answers and also exposes distorted perceptions of food. With less targeted questions about what is typically eaten, patients may respond with vague answers such as "three pretty good meals." When asked what these meals comprise it would not be uncommon to discover that "three pretty good meals" is actually a half a cup of cereal with skim milk and a large coffee for breakfast, two cups of lettuce with nonfat dressing for lunch, and one cup of stir-fried vegetables for dinner. As the day reported may not represent most days, it is helpful to ask whether food intake varies from day to day. If it does, ask the patient to describe a highest and lowest intake day. Individuals with BN may respond well to queries about the differences in food consumption on binge days (during which eating restraint is relaxed) versus nonbinge days (when eating is typically more restrictive).

If patients are willing, it is often helpful to have them keep a food diary where they write down everything eaten immediately following consumption. Then, at follow-up appointments, the food diary can be scanned briefly rather than using a lot of time drawing out the information on interview. Characterizing the predominant pattern of eating sheds light on diagnosis—a restrictive eating pattern with no objective

binges is consistent with AN (restricting type); frequent bingeing and compensatory behaviors is consistent with BN (or AN binge eating/purging type); and regular eating, overeating, or grazing with frequent episodes of bingeing is consistent with BED.

In addition to assessing food intake, behaviors used to maintain weight or compensate for specific eating episodes should be evaluated. This is crucial, especially since these behaviors contribute to much of the morbidity associated with EDs. Compensatory behaviors include vomiting (either self-induced or with emetics), laxatives, diuretics, fasting, and excessive exercise. Compensatory behaviors are a core feature of BN, as well as the AN binge-eating/purging subtype. When purging becomes frequent, medical morbidity increases significantly. It can be helpful to ask in a way that decreases shame, for example, "Some patients who are struggling with controlling their eating and weight induce vomiting or use laxatives. Have you found yourself doing this?" If patients endorse purging it is important to assess the frequency and method. A review of systems and physical exam will be important to identify the presence of purging-related medical complications.

Regarding excessive exercise, a common compensatory behavior to control weight, try to evaluate the quality and quantity of exercise per day and week. Although the definition of recommended and excessive exercise varies, anything more than the 30 minutes of moderate to high-intensity physical activity recommended by the US Surgeon General should be carefully explored. Excessive exercise may also be defined as compulsively exercising even when injured or sick, or exercising more than what coaches or physicians recommend. Patients with EDs are known to underreport the extent of their physical activity (Bratland et al., 2010). Patients trying to hide their ED also may exercise covertly in their daily routines (e.g., walking everywhere instead of driving, standing at times it would be more socially appropriate to sit), so it is helpful to specifically ask how much of their day is spent active (i.e., not sitting down).

While disordered eating behaviors are immediately salient, cognitive and emotional aspects of the illness are intimately related with the behaviors but may go unnoticed if not explored. Simply asking patients how distressed or preoccupied they are by thoughts about food and weight can suggest their level of impairment. Some patients are so consumed by their illness that 95% of their mental time and activities are spent thinking about or acting out behaviors related to the illness. This leaves little time for other activities, and it is common for patients to forgo their usual activities and pleasures to engage in ED behaviors. The 16-item Clinical Impairment Assessment (Fairburn & Bohn, 2008) is an easy-to-administer inventory of the myriad life domains that may be impaired by a patient's ED.

For all patients with ED, regardless of the type, it is equally important to assess for comorbid psychiatric illness and patient safety (i.e., self-injurious behavior, suicidality, and homicidality). As mentioned previously, EDs are highly comorbid with mood, anxiety, personality, and substance use disorders. Therefore, it is important to screen for any concurrent depressive and anxiety disorders, and in particular, alcohol/drug use and safety concerns (dangerousness to self or others).

Some patients may not be ready to accept ED treatment; however, they may accept treatment for comorbid mood or anxiety problems. In general, severity of distress level, depression, anxiety, self-injurious behavior, and suicidal thoughts will determine how rapidly patients need to be referred for further psychiatric evaluation. Any patients who are moderately to severely distressed, depressed or anxious, or who have histories of self-injury or suicide attempts should be referred rapidly to psychiatry (within a few weeks) and have frequent follow-up with the treating clinician as well as instructions for what to do if symptoms worsen (e.g., call the medical clinic or go to the emergency room) until the referral to psychiatry is completed. Patients with severe distress, depression, or recent or current self-injurious or suicidal thoughts and behaviors should be referred for emergent evaluation (either same-day or emergency room).

MEDICAL ASSESSMENT

Medical assessment of ED patients is crucial given high rates of medical morbidity associated with malnutrition and disordered eating behaviors. Routine examination with a comprehensive history, review of systems, weight, height, vital signs, and physical exam is likely to identify ED signs and symptoms as well as related medical complications. Information gathered in the history, physical, and laboratory evaluations will determine medical acuity.

The review of systems is an important part of the general medical assessment of patients with EDs. Given the often severe and widespread physical ramifications of ED, there may be pertinent positives and negatives in nearly all systems. Table 32.3 outlines symptoms commonly elicited on review of systems.

When evaluating the ED it is also helpful to assess how rapidly weight is changing. Barring other uncommon factors accountable for weight change, rapid weight gain or loss typically indicates a severe degree of behaviors such as restricting, bingeing, purging, or excessive exercising. Although some patients avoid weighing themselves, others obsessively weigh themselves—sometimes several times per day. Begin by asking patients if they know their weight and if it has changed in the past few months or weeks. It is also helpful to know patients' lifetime highest and lowest weights to get a sense of how severe the illness has been in the past and how their current status compares. While these conversations can yield important information, obtaining a current, accurate, objective weight is necessary to determine acuity and identify possible underreporting of symptoms.

Recording weight and height allows for calculation of body mass index (BMI), an important factor in diagnostic assessment and treatment planning. BMI can be calculated by hand (i.e., weight in kilograms divided by height [in meters] squared) or through an online calculator or mobile app. For adults, BMI < 18.5 kg/mg^2 is underweight (and possibly consistent with a diagnosis of AN), BMI > 18.5 kg/mg^2 but < 25.0 kg/mg^2 is healthy weight, and BMI >= 25.0 kg/mg^2 is overweight. For children and adolescents, BMI < 5th percentile for age and height is underweight, BMI > 5th percentile but < 85th percentile is healthy weight, and BMI >=85th percentile is overweight. Of note, patients with AN or who are underweight should be weighed in a hospital gown to prevent patients putting weights and other heavy objects in pockets and orifices to falsely elevate weight. Additionally, patients may "water load" (drink excessive amounts of water) prior to

Table 32.3 PERTINENT FINDINGS ON REVIEW OF SYSTEMS IN PATIENTS WITH EATING DISORDERS

SYSTEM	SYMPTOMS	ASSOCIATED EATING DISORDER BEHAVIOR
General	High, low, or dramatic change in weight	Restricting, bingeing and/or purging
	Lethargy	Restricting/starvation
HEENT	Dental cavities, halitosis, throat pain	Purging
GI	Altered appetite, early fullness, constipation, bloating	Starvation/restricting
	Heartburn	Purging
	Diarrhea, rectal prolapse	Laxative abuse
Gyn	Irregular menses or amenorrhea	Low body fat and/or low weight, stress
MSK	Joint pain, stress fractures, muscle/tendon injuries	Excessive exercise
	Bone fractures	Osteoporosis from prolonged restriction/starvation
Endocrine	Cold sensitivity, brittle/thinning hair	Restricting/starvation
Neuro	Lightheadedness, fainting	Food/fluid restriction, low weight/starvation, excessive exercise
	Numbness, tingling	Starvation (vitamin deficiencies)

Key: HEENT–head, eyes, ears, nose, throat. GI–Gastrointestinal. Gyn–gynecological. MSK–musculoskeletal. Neuro–neurological.

Table 32.4 COMMON SIGNS ON PHYSICAL EXAM

EATING DISORDER	PHYSICAL SIGNS
Anorexia Nervosa	• Sinus bradycardia, hypotension, orthostatic hypotension, and hypothermia • Cachexia • Parotid and submandibular gland swelling (if purging) • Brittle and thinning head hair and presence of lanugo • Acrocyanosis • Breast atrophy • Diminished bowel sounds
Bulimia Nervosa	• Hypotension and tachycardia • Bilateral parotid gland swelling • Erosion of enamel on the lingual surface of teeth • Periodontal disease and dental carries • Russell's sign (scarring and abrasions on the knuckles of the dominant hand from repeated self-induced vomiting) • Pedal edema (protein malnourishment)
Binge Eating Disorder	• Obesity • Hypertension

the weigh-in to falsely increase weight. Checking urine specific gravity can help rule out water loading.

For many patients, being weighed is highly distressing. It is therefore a difficult procedure for clinicians who are working diligently to decrease patients' distress, not increase it. Instead of forgoing the weighing procedure entirely or engaging in lengthy struggles with patients, we suggest taking an empathic but firm approach with patients. The following statement may be used: "I realize getting weighed may be difficult for you. In order for me to provide you with good and safe care, I will have to weigh you at each visit. It is likely to be more difficult in the beginning and get easier with time. Let's go ahead and get it out of the way for today's visit." The majority of patients, however reluctant, typically agree to be weighed.

Although the physical signs common to EDs are nonspecific, patterns or combinations of physical signs can help identify an ED and support diagnosis. Table 32.4 outlines some of the physical signs common to EDs.

Attention to vital signs is important for all ED patients, but particularly for those who are significantly underweight or with severe bingeing, purging, or hyper-exercise. Sinus bradycardia, low blood pressure, orthostatic hypotension, and hypothermia are ominous signs of starvation and typically indications for inpatient hospitalization on a medical unit to begin weight restoration and nutrition repletion. In a study of medical findings in community-dwelling patients with AN, 41.3% had bradycardia, 16.1% hypotension, and 22.4% had hypothermia (Miller et al., 2005). In normal-weight patients with BN, changes in heart rate and blood pressure, particularly hypotension and tachycardia, may indicate presence of rapid fluid shifts and dehydration from bingeing and purging as well as more concerning behaviors such as ipecac use, which is known to cause cardiomyopathy (Rashid, 2006; Schneider et al., 1996).

Medical Assessment in Anorexia Nervosa

Physical signs common to patients with AN are related to food restriction, malnutrition, and bingeing/purging if those behaviors are present. On physical exam, cachexia, parotid and submandibular gland swelling (if purging type), brittle and thinning head hair, lanugo, acrocyanosis, and breast atrophy are typical. Assessment of the cardiovascular system on physical exam typically reveals sinus bradycardia. There may be signs associated with mitral valve prolapse, which occurs related to reduced left ventricular mass (Cooke & Chambers, 1995). Echocardiograms of patients with AN often demonstrate atrophic myocardium and low cardiac output (Casiero, 2006). In very underweight patients (e.g. BMI less than or equal to 13.5 kg/mg^2), pericardial effusion may be present. It is most often asymptomatic but in rare cases may require pericardiocentesis to prevent tamponade (Docx et al., 2010; Polli et al., 2006). Electrocardiogram may demonstrate prolongation of the QTc and PR intervals, first-degree heart block, and ST-T wave abnormalities. Most cardiac abnormalities improve with careful nutritional rehabilitation.

Evaluation of the gastrointestinal system in patients with AN may reveal diminished bowel sounds consistent with inactivity and slowed metabolism. Although rare, there have been several reports of patients with AN having massive gastric dilatation following binges (Barada et al., 2006; Mathevon, Rougier, Ducher, Pic, Garcier, & Schmidt, 2004), as well as gastric rupture and death (Sinicina, Pankratz, Büttner, & Mall, 2005). Patients with common complaints of early fullness, nausea, and bloating are often referred to gastroenterology to rule out organic pathology. Gastric and bowel studies, in the absence of organic pathology, are often positive for delayed emptying (Zipfel et al., 2006, Hultson & Wald, 1990; Benini et al., 2004) and increased whole bowel and colonic transit time (Waldholtz & Andersen, 1990). Studies demonstrate that nutritional rehabilitation improves gastrointestinal dysfunction (Rigaud et al., 1988).

Muskuloskeletal problems are common to patients with AN, particularly in those with a chronic and severe course and who engage in hyper-exercise. Long-standing starvation can lead to early osteoporosis and fractures, and hyper-exercise often leads to overuse injuries. In younger patients, starvation may lead to deficits in bone mass accrual and arrested skeletal growth (Misra, 2008; Lacey, Crisp, Hart, & Kirkwood, 1979).

Lab abnormalities in AN patients typically reflect changes associated with starvation, as well as with purging (if present). One study demonstrated that among 214 community-dwelling patients with AN, 38.6% had anemia, 34.4% leucopenia, 19.7% hyponatremia, 19.7% hypokalemia, and 12.2% elevated alanine aminotransferase concentration (Miller et al., 2005).

Medical Assessment in Bulimia Nervosa

Compared to patients with AN, patients with BN have fewer physical findings associated with starvation and more medical morbidity related to bingeing and especially to compensatory behaviors. Some patients have a normal physical exam; however, as disease severity increases there are typically physical signs that may include bilateral parotid gland swelling, erosion of enamel on the lingual surface of teeth, periodontal disease, dental caries, and pedal edema (protein malnourishment). Russell's sign (scarring and abrasions on the knuckles of the dominant hand from repeated self-induced vomiting) is more common in the beginning of the illness as individuals with chronic BN can typically induce vomiting at will.

The cardiovascular system of patients with BN may be affected by both malnourishment and bingeing and purging behaviors, which can lead to fluid shifts and electrolyte abnormalities that destabilize the electrical activity of the heart. Electrocardiograms may demonstrate QTc prolongation (Takimoto et al., 2004; Contaldo, Di Paolo, Mazzacano, Di Biase, & Giumetti, 1990), increased PR interval, hypokalemia-related widened QRS complex, and *torsade de pointes* (Suri, Poist, Hager, & Gross, 1999), as well as increased supraventricular and ventricular ectopic rhythms and arrythmias (Takimoto, Yoshiuchi, Kumano, & Kuboki, 2006).

In BN, bingeing and purging behaviors are the main cause of gastrointestinal complications. Recurrent vomiting exposes the esophagus to acidic gastric contents potentially leading to esophagitis, esophageal ulcers, strictures, vascular tears (Mallory-Weiss tear), and even rupture. Esophagitis is a risk factor for esophageal cancer, and cases have been reported in otherwise healthy women with BN (Navab, Avunduk, Gang, & Frankel, 1996). Lowered esophageal sphincter tone from recurrent vomiting often leads to gastroesophageal reflux disease. Although uncommon, bingeing can lead to acute gastric dilatation, sometimes with fatal outcomes (Pandey, Maqbool, & Jayachandran, 2009; Bravender & Story, 2007; Gyurkovics et al., 2006).

Patients who purge with stimulant laxatives often develop complications of the colon and rectum. Chronic use of laxatives can lead to a vicious cycle of decreased colonic tone, chronic constipation, and further dependence on laxatives to move fecal matter. Rectal prolapse has also been associated with laxative abuse (Malik, Stratton, & Sweeney, 1997).

Similar to patients with AN, patients with BN are often referred to gastroenterology for evaluation of common complaints (e.g., dyspepsia, nausea, bloating) and may have delayed gastric emptying and slowed motility (Kamal et al., 1991) in the absence of primary gastrointestinal pathology.

Patients with severe BN may develop lower extremity edema from two processes, either protein malnutrition or abrupt cessation of purging behaviors, which leads to unopposed high aldosterone levels and salt retention (Mehler & Andersen, 2004). The latter scenario can be a vicious cycle as patients then try to solve the edema by taking more diuretics and laxatives.

Dental problems are nearly universal in patients who engage in purging by vomiting, and enamel erosions can be seen after just 6 months (Altshuler, Dechow, Waller, & Hardy, 1990). The American Dental Association currently recommends that patients not brush their teeth immediately after vomiting but rather rinse with baking soda, which helps to neutralize the destructive effects of the stomach acid (http://www.mouthhealthy.org/en/az-topics/e/eating-disorders).

Laboratory findings in patients with BN are variable depending on nutrition status, frequency of bingeing and purging, and methods of purging. Hypokalemia, hypochloremia, hyperphosphatemia, and metabolic alkalosis are common, especially in underweight patients with BN who frequently induce vomiting (Rushing, Jones, & Carney, 2003). Patients who primarily abuse laxatives may present with metabolic acidosis due to alkaline fluid loss from the bowels (Mitchell, Hatsukami, & Pyle, 1987), and patients using multiple purging methods may have mixed acid-base findings making it difficult to diagnose the purging method by lab results. BN patients with severe hypokalemia and hypovolemia often need aggressive fluid repletion in order to correct the hypokalemia; as volume status improves the metabolic alkalosis corrects and inactivates the rennin-angiotensin axis (Mehler & Andersen, 2004).

Serum amylase is commonly elevated in patients who regularly vomit; however, only the salivary fractionate has been shown to be useful in differentiating patients with elevated amylase due to purging behaviors (Walsh, Wong, Pesce, Hadigan, & Bodourian, 1990). In the majority of patients, extent of amylase elevation is correlated with frequency of vomiting (Kinzl, Biebl, & Herold, 1993). Salivary amylase can be a sensitive laboratory test for detecting surreptitious vomiting.

Patients with suppressed TSH in the absence of primary thyroid disorder may be abusing thyroid hormone in an effort to lose weight (Kaplan, 1998).

Medical Assessment in Binge Eating Disorder

BED is associated with a range of physical problems different from patients with AN and BN. The physical exam of BED patients is typically remarkable for obesity. Related more to obesity than to BED, patients commonly have hypertension, gall bladder disease, musculoskeletal problems, and obstructive sleep apnea. Laboratory tests often demonstrate presence of metabolic syndromes including diabetes and dyslipidemia. Interestingly, a recent study suggested that individuals with BED have a higher risk of metabolic syndrome over and above the risk conferred by obesity alone (Hudson et al., 2010).

In addition to a comprehensive history and physical, Table 32.5 (adapted from the American Psychiatric Association practice guideline for EDs) outlines laboratory and diagnostic tests to obtain as part of the initial evaluation.

TREATMENT

The goals of care for all EDs are similar and include establishing regular eating patterns, nutritional rehabilitation, and restoration of a healthy weight range; treating the emotional, cognitive, and behavioral aspects of the disorder as well as any psychiatric comorbidities; and providing regular medical surveillance and treatment.

For patients with severe illness, an interdisciplinary team composed of a primary care physician, therapist, psychiatrist, and dietitian—preferably with some or all members having experience in treating EDs—is ideal. For less complicated patients, other combinations can sufficiently comprise a team. For example, a therapist experienced with ED, along with a primary care physician, can adequately treat patients with milder forms of illness. Patients who lack significant psychiatric comorbidities do not necessarily need a psychiatrist. Indeed, BN is the only ED that has an FDA-approved medication (fluoxetine), and primary care physicians are often comfortable prescribing this. It is helpful to assess at the outset, and periodically through treatment, patients' particular needs and clinicians' level of comfort treating patients with EDs, in order to readjust as indicated.

Medical, psychological, and pharmacological treatments for each ED are reviewed below. Table 32.6 outlines current psychological treatments for EDs.

ANOREXIA NERVOSA

The initial treatment focus for patients with AN is nutritional rehabilitation and weight restoration. The importance of weight restoration is underscored in recent studies, with the most significant predictor of weight maintenance following intensive treatment for AN being higher BMI at discharge

Table 32.5 RECOMMENDED LABORATORY AND DIAGNOSTIC TESTS

PATIENT INDICATION	LABORATORY TESTS	DIAGNOSTIC STUDIES
All patients	Serum electrolytes, blood urea nitrogen, creatinine, TSH, CBC with differential, erythrocyte sedimentation rate, aspartate aminotransferase, alanine aminotransferase, alkaline phosphatase, urinalysis	
Malnourished and severely symptomatic patients	Complement component 3a, serum calcium, magnesium, phosphorus, ferritin, 24-hour urine for creatinine clearance	Electrocardiogram
Amenorrheic >6 months		Dual-energy X-ray absorptiometry, serum estradiol in female patients
Suspected substance use	Toxicology screen	
Suspected surreptitious vomiting	Serum amylase (fractionated for salivary gland isoenzyme)	
Persistent amenorrhea but normal weight	Serum luteinizing hormone, follicle-stimulating hormone, B-human chorionic gonadotropin, prolactin	
Significant cognitive deficits, neurological soft signs, unremitting course or other atypical features		Brain magnetic resonance imaging, computed tomography
Suspected GI bleeding		Stool guaiac
Suspected laxative abuse	Stool or urine for bisacodyl, emodin, aloe-emodin, rhein*	
Obesity	Cholesterol (total, HDL, LDL), triglycerides, fasting glucose	

Adapted from American Psychiatric Association, 2006.

*Rhein, emodin, and aloe-emodin are common ingredients and active metabolites found in laxatives.

Table 32.6 SUMMARY OF PSYCHOLOGICAL TREATMENTS FOR EDS

DIAGNOSIS	TREATMENT	SUMMARY	EVIDENCE OF EFFICACY IN AT LEAST 2 RCTS
Anorexia Nervosa	Family Based Treatment	Parents restore patient's weight by taking charge of refeeding their child, exploring how the illness affects family dynamics, and working to support patient's ability to make proper food choices.	Yes
	Cognitive Behavioral Therapy	Educates patients about how thoughts and behaviors maintain AN. Patients normalize their eating while concurrently challenging and reducing thoughts and behaviors that maintain AN.	Yes
	Specialist Supportive Clinical Management	Interventions are similar to CBT, but with a broader focus on supportive therapy techniques such as active listening, validation, and praise.	Yes
	Cognitive Remediation Therapy	Patients identify and examine how rigid and narrow thought patterns maintain AN behaviors. In-session exercises promote cognitive flexibility and big-picture thinking.	No
	Uniting Couples in the Treatment of Anorexia Nervosa	Educates patients and their partners about AN and teaches couples how to deal with interpersonal issues that arise from AN symptoms.	No
	Emotion Acceptance Behavior Therapy	Educates patients about how AN is used for emotion avoidance and helps patients return to regular life activities.	No
	Exposure and Response Prevention	Assists patients in developing a hierarchy of fear foods and then systematically incorporates these foods while refraining from avoidance behaviors.	No
Bulimia Nervosa	Cognitive Behavior Therapy	Patients learn how thoughts and behaviors maintain BN. Patients normalize their eating while concurrently challenging and reducing thoughts and behaviors that maintain BN. Patients also identify and reduce triggers for binge eating such as dietary restriction, poor body image, and mood intolerance.	Yes
	Family Based Treatment	Enlists parents in helping patients refrain from bingeing and purging, exploring how the illness affects family dynamics, and working to support the patient's ability to make proper food choices.	Yes
	Interpersonal Psychotherapy	Identifies interpersonal difficulties that are influencing BN behaviors. Patients focus on one of four interpersonal issues during therapy including interpersonal deficits, interpersonal role disputes, role transitions, and grief.	Yes
	Dialectical Behavioral Therapy	Focuses on emotion regulation, distress tolerance, interpersonal effectiveness, and mindfulness.	No
	Integrative Cognitive Affective Therapy	Identifies how self-directed behaviors (i.e., dieting or purging) are used to cope with perceived discrepancies between the actual and ideal self.	No

(continued)

Table 32.6 (CONTINUED)

DIAGNOSIS	TREATMENT	SUMMARY	EVIDENCE OF EFFICACY IN AT LEAST 2 RCTS
Binge Eating Disorder	Cognitive Behavioral Therapy	Normalizes eating behaviors and decreases maladaptive thoughts about weight and shape. Emphasizes healthy dietary restraint with patients who are overweight.	Yes
	Interpersonal Psychotherapy	Identifies interpersonal difficulties that are influencing BED behaviors. Patients focus on one of four interpersonal issues during therapy including interpersonal deficits, interpersonal role disputes, role transitions, and grief.	Yes
	Behavioral Weight Loss Treatment	Regulates eating patterns and promotes healthy dietary restraint to facilitate modest weight loss and reduce obesity-related risks to mental and physical health.	Yes

and slower rate of weight loss following discharge (Kaplan et al., 2009). More specifically, lower rates of weight loss over the first 28 days postdischarge predicted better weight maintenance at 6 and 12 months (Kaplan et al., 2009). Additionally, many of the medical complications improve or entirely reverse with weight restoration.

For the most acute patients, inpatient medical and/or psychiatric hospitalization is necessary. Psychiatric units vary considerably in their capacity to manage medically ill patients; inpatient medical admission is indicated if BMI is very low or if any of the following are present: significant bradycardia (<40bpm), hypothermia, significant or symptomatic orthostatic hypotension, hypokalemia or electrolyte disarray, signs of organ failure, or any acute medical complications (e.g., hematemesis).

Given the risks associated with refeeding syndrome—a potentially life-threatening syndrome involving large fluid and electrolyte shifts associated with introducing nutrition to the severely malnourished—refeeding severely underweight patients (i.e., BMI < 16.0 kg/m², Mehler et al., 2010) is done in a medically monitored setting. Refeeding syndrome is associated with hypophosphatemia, hypomagnesemia, hypokalemia, congestive heart failure, edema, delirium, coma, and even death (Gunarathne, McKay, Pillans, McKinlay, & Crockett, 2010). It can be prevented by gradually introducing nutrition and closely monitoring electrolytes, volume status, and vital organ function. In general, nutrition starts very slowly to make sure organ systems demonstrate capacity to withstand the stress of reintroducing nutrition. During acute starvation, AN patients typically have a suppressed resting metabolic rate even when accounting for their low weight. Therefore, during refeeding patients' metabolic rates increase substantially and they often require a very high daily caloric intake to gain weight, for example, as much as 100 kcal/kg per day. Consulting dieticians with experience refeeding severely malnourished patients is essential for safe and effective treatment. Patients can be transitioned to other levels of care once they reach reasonable medical stability. "Medical stability" is somewhat vague, but in general it is when patients are no longer at risk of refeeding syndrome, demonstrate stable

vital organ function, and have achieved steady weight gain. This is a critical transition period, and, without ongoing intensive treatment, patients tend to relapse rapidly.

Patients with AN are generally hospitalized on inpatient psychiatry units for any of the following combinations of criteria: underweight or rapidly changing weight but not yet significantly medically compromised, moderate to severe ED behaviors (e.g., bingeing and purging multiple times per day, severe restriction), moderate to severe comorbid psychiatric illness (e.g., major depression), self-injurious behavior and/or suicidality (intensifying or active thoughts, developing intentions or plans to act on thoughts). In our experience, insurance companies will generally approve inpatient treatment when patients meet any of the above criteria. For patients who are on the borderline of these criteria, lower levels of care such as residential or intensive outpatient programs may be covered. If physicians come up against resistance from insurance companies, it is helpful to emphasize that patients are failing the current level of treatment and, therefore, no less intensive option exists.

Given high rates of relapse following inpatient treatment for refeeding, a range of treatment options between the inpatient and outpatient setting have developed in recent years including residential (Delinsky et al., 2010), day hospital, and intensive outpatient treatments.

Psychological Treatments for Anorexia Nervosa

Family-Based Treatment

The psychosocial treatment modality for AN with the greatest empirical support is a three-phase manualized family-based treatment (FBT) designed for the outpatient care of adolescent patients (Lock, le Grange, Agras, & Dare, 2001). In phase one, the patient's parents are encouraged to correct the patient's malnutrition by planning and implementing a nutritious, calorie-dense meal plan. The therapist supports the parents in their efforts by absolving them of blame for the etiology of the illness and helping them encourage their child to eat adequately during an in-session family meal. After steady weight gain has been established, food choices are gradually returned to the patient during phase two, and the family is encouraged to explore the ways in which AN has affected familial dynamics. In the final phase, when the patient has reached a stable weight, therapy focuses on enhancing the patient's autonomy and orchestrating a smooth return to normal adolescent development. Elements of FBT have been adapted for delivery in separate but simultaneous parents-only and patient-only sessions (Eisler, Simic, Russell, & Dare, 2007), and in a multifamily group format (Zucker, Marcus, & Bulik, 2006). The professionally moderated website http://www.maudsleyparents.org/ is a helpful resource for parents who would like to learn more about FBT through articles, videos, and interactive online discussion.

In comparison to individual therapy, FBT has produced greater improvements in body weight and ED psychopathology at 1-year (Lock et. al., 2010) and 5-year (Eisler et al., 1997) follow-up—especially among young patients with a short duration of illness (Eisler et al., 1997). However, data suggest that FBT is less effective with non-intact versus intact families (Lock, Agras, Bryson, & Kraemer, 2005) and highly critical versus less critical parents (Eisler et al., 2007). Furthermore, FBT's lack of applicability to older patients (trials typically don't include young adults who are over 18) highlights the ongoing need for novel therapy development.

Cognitive Behavioral Therapy

The most recent version of cognitive behavioral therapy (CBT) for AN (Fairburn, 2008) provides psychoeducation on the consequences of starvation, encourages the patient to consider the long-term advantages of achieving a healthy body weight, and addresses the patient's overvaluation of shape and weight by reducing body checking and avoidance behaviors. In contrast to the parental control of meal planning in FBT, in CBT patients are encouraged to make their own food choices as long as they eat three meals and two-three snacks per day. The therapist facilitates weight gain by helping the patient to design behavioral experiments in which the patient purposefully breaks dietary rules in order to evaluate whether feared consequences—such as instantaneous obesity or never-ending anxiety—actually occur.

Although CBT is the gold standard treatment for adult BN, its evidence base in AN is mixed. CBT was superior to the nutrition counseling alone in a post-hospitalization relapse prevention trial for AN (Pike, Walsh, Vitousek, Wilson, & Bauer, 2003) but no better than specialist supportive clinical management or interpersonal psychotherapy in a randomized outpatient trial (McIntosh et al., 2005). Moreover, in a placebo-controlled medication trial in which all patients received CBT, approximately half of patients in both groups either relapsed or dropped out within 1 year (Walsh et al., 2006). Challenges to implementing CBT for AN include the ego-syntonicity of the illness and the cognitive rigidity of underweight patients. CBT has also been critiqued for its potentially inadequate involvement of significant others (Bulik, Baucom, Kirby, & Pisetsky, 2011) and its preferential focus on cognitive rather than behavioral strategies despite both being components of the treatment (Steinglass et al., 2010).

Novel Therapies for AN

Catalyzed in part by a 2003 request for applications by the National Institute of Mental Health, several novel therapies for AN have recently been developed, including specialist supportive clinical management, cognitive remediation therapy, uniting couples in the treatment of anorexia nervosa, emotion acceptance behavior therapy, and exposure and response prevention. Although the evidence base is still somewhat limited, clinicians may wish to draw upon techniques from these novel therapies when working with adult patients who have not responded favorably to first-line therapies.

Specialist Supportive Clinical Management (SSCM)

SSCM was originally developed as a comparison therapy for a trial examining the efficacy of CBT versus IPT for adult AN (McIntosh et al., 2005), but the surprising finding that SSCM was comparable to CBT and superior to IPT in promoting weight gain sparked independent clinical interest in SSCM. Although SSCM utilizes some interventions that overlap with CBT (e.g., psychoeducation, self-monitoring), its overarching focus on supportive therapy techniques such as active listening, validation, praise, reassurance, and therapist self-disclosure (McIntosh et al., 2006) suggests that nonspecific therapeutic interventions may have promise in the treatment of AN.

COGNITIVE REMEDIATION THERAPY (CRT) Rather than addressing the content of distorted AN cognitions directly, CRT addresses the hallmark rigidity that characterizes cognitive processing in AN. CRT is a 3-session (Lopez, Roberts, Tchanturia, & Treasure, 2008) to 10-session (Tchanturia, Davies, & Campbell, 2007) adjunctive treatment to standard care and includes a neuropsychological battery designed to identify deficits in set-shifting and central coherence, feedback on how neuropsychological deficits impact both eating and noneating-related life domains, and exercises designed to increase cognitive flexibility. Although CRT has yet to be tested in a randomized controlled trial, several case studies and patient series suggest that CRT is acceptable to patients and is associated with improvements in set-shifting abilities (Davies & Tchanturia, 2005; Lopez et al., 2008; Tchanturia, Whitney, & Treasure, 2006; Tchanturia et al., 2007). Because it directly targets maladaptive thinking styles, CRT is designed to augment rather than replace therapies that focus on normalizing eating and restoring weight.

UNITING COUPLES IN THE TREATMENT OF ANOREXIA NERVOSA (UCAN) The success of family therapy with adolescent AN has inspired the recent application of couples therapy to adult AN (Bulik, Baucom, Kirby, & Pisetsky, 2011). UCAN provides the AN patient and his or her partner with psychoeducation on illness and recovery, teaches the couple effective communication skills, addresses interpersonal conflicts that arise from AN symptoms (e.g., secrecy, restricting, purging), and facilitates the development of a relapse prevention plan (Bulik et al., 2011). A controlled trial testing the efficacy of UCAN is still underway, http://www.med.unc.edu/psych/eatingdisorders/patient-care-1/clinical-trials/ucan-uniting-couples-in-the-treatment-of-anorexia-nervosa.

EMOTION ACCEPTANCE BEHAVIOR THERAPY (EABT) Individuals with AN endorse high levels of emotional avoidance (Wildes, Ringham, & Marcus, 2010). Therefore, Wildes and Marcus (2011) developed EABT in order educate patients about the role of AN symptoms in facilitating emotion avoidance, to encourage greater awareness of emotions, and to facilitate a return to valued (albeit anxiety-provoking) life activities. In an uncontrolled case series of five patients, three showed modest weight gain, highlighting the potential promise of conducting larger-scale trials of EABT.

Exposure and Response Prevention (ERP)

Based on the overlap between eating and anxiety disorders, Steinglass and colleagues (2010) have developed an ERP intervention in which AN patients are repeatedly exposed to specific fear foods (e.g., pizza) and prevented from engaging in safety or avoidance behaviors (e.g., blotting with a napkin, looking away while eating). In a small, randomized controlled trial, AN patients who received ERP consumed more calories at a posttreatment test meal in comparison to those who received treatment as usual without ERP (Steinglass et al., 2007).

Pharmacological Interventions for AN

Psychotropic medication has a relatively limited role in the treatment of acute AN. The main "pharmacological" intervention is nutrition. To date, there are no FDA-approved medications for the treatment of AN, though numerous medications in nearly all psychotropic classes have been studied. The evidence base is significantly limited, as there are few randomized controlled trials (RCTs) and most studies are not blinded or are case reports or series. Among controlled trials, results are mixed but mostly negative. Outcomes are typically rate of weight gain during the acute treatment phase, maintaining stability once weight is restored, and the cognitive and behavioral aspects of the disorder. Few medications are significantly effective when patients are underweight, even when nutritional supplements are taken (Barbarich et al., 2004).

Given the typically undesirable weight gain associated with olanzapine in other patient populations, it has been studied as a weight-promoting agent in patients with AN. One RCT involved a 10-week flexible dose trial where 34 patients were randomized to olanzapine plus hospital day treatment or placebo plus hospital day treatment (Bissada, Tasca, Barber, & Bradwejn, 2008). The dose range was 2.5 mg to 10 mg per day with a mean dose of 6.61 mg per day. Although differences were not large between the control and placebo group, patients randomized to olanzapine did demonstrate more rapid weight gain, reached target BMI sooner, and had a greater decrease in obsessive thoughts. Underscoring the difficulty in conducting large studies in patients with AN, over half the patients approached refused to participate. Other small, controlled trials have

demonstrated potential benefit of low-dose olanzapine (2.5–5 mg) in reducing psychopathological aspects of AN and promoting weight stability (Brambilla et al., 2007, Mondraty et al., 2005). Given that olanzapine can prolong QTc, and patients with AN are prone to QTc prolongation, patients should have an electrocardiogram to ensure that the baseline QTc is less than 450 msec. Additionally, hypomagnesemia and hypokalemia contribute to the risk of cardiac arrhythmias. Because patients with AN frequently have electrolyte disturbances, magnesium and potassium should be monitored closely.

Although an earlier, smaller RCT demonstrated some preliminary evidence that fluoxetine may improve outcomes following inpatient treatment for weight restoration (Kaye et al., 2001), a later, larger RCT with improved completion rates was negative. The latter study sought to evaluate whether fluoxetine promotes maintenance of recovery in weight- restored anorexic patients; fluoxetine did not demonstrate any significant benefit compared to placebo (Walsh et al., 2006). All patients in this study received outpatient individual cognitive behavioral therapy for the duration of the 1-year study.

Despite the lackluster results of medications in trials and lack of FDA-approved psychopharmacological treatments, when patients are significantly underweight and psychopathological symptoms are severe, as long as there are no significant contraindications we support a trial of low-dose olanzapine during the acute recovery to promote weight gain and reduce psychopathological symptoms. Of note: although there is no empirical evidence to guide treatment duration with olanzapine, given the known long-term morbidity associated with its use we caution against long-term treatment. Additionally, as previously stated, QTc, potassium, and magnesium must be carefully monitored during treatment with olanzapine to minimize the risk of cardiac arrhythmias. Similarly, we support a trial of fluoxetine up to 60 mg daily to treat psychopathological symptoms and promote weight maintenance during the acute and long-term recovery.

BULIMIA NERVOSA

Psychological Treatments for Bulimia Nervosa

Cognitive Behavioral Therapy–Enhanced

CBT is the gold standard for the treatment of adult BN. More specifically, cognitive behavioral therapy–enhanced (CBT-E; Fairburn, 2008) is an updated and enhanced version of the original form of CBT for BN (Fairburn et al., 1993). CBT-E is a 4-stage individualized treatment that focuses on creating a personalized formulation for each patient. Throughout therapy, the therapist works with the patient to identify binge triggers and address negative body image and rigid dieting behaviors. CBT-E emphasizes self-monitoring, which allows the patient to pay attention to his or her behaviors and urges in real time. This self-monitoring may also highlight the frequent use of body checking and avoidance, a result of the patient's overvaluation of weight and shape. Throughout treatment the therapist may encourage the patient to complete behavioral experiments that challenge the rigid food rules often present in EDs. For example, a patient may believe that eating refined carbohydrates will cause rapid weight gain. This patient would be asked to weigh herself one day, eat the feared food, and then weigh herself again the next day. CBT-E also encourages patients to problem-solve for themselves and to replace binge episodes with healthy, pleasurable activities such as knitting, going for a walk, or socializing with others. While there is a set structure to CBT-E, it has the added advantage of being personalized to the unique maintaining mechanisms of each patient's ED. Specifically, the therapist can implement specific interventions designed to address perfectionism, core self-esteem, mood intolerance, and/or interpersonal difficulties if desired. However, these added modules have not been shown to improve treatment outcomes when added to standard CBT-E (Fairburn et al., 2009). Toward the end of treatment the focus shifts to relapse prevention and the importance of maintaining the positive skills previously set in place. Treatment goals and strategies are reassessed at each stage depending on the efficacy of the prior stage (Fairburn, 2008).

In a randomized controlled study, CBT-E produced positive results when compared to an 8-week treatment delay; patients receiving CBT-E showed substantial symptom reduction at the end of treatment, and roughly half of patients exhibited ED features within one standard deviation of community norms (Fairburn et al., 2009). Even more strikingly, in a randomized controlled trial comparing CBT-E to psychoanalytic psychotherapy for BN, 42% of patients in CBT-E but just 6% of patients in psychoanalytic therapy had stopped bingeing and purging after 5 months of treatment (Poulsen et al., 2014). At 2 years, BN remission rates were nearly half (44%) for CBT-E but just 15% for psychoanalytic therapy, suggesting that CBT-E should be considered the first-line treatment for adults with BN.

Interpersonal Psychotherapy

Although approximately half of individuals with BN respond positively to CBT, the corollary is that the other half will remain symptomatic at the end of treatment, highlighting the need for alternative modalities. Interpersonal psychotherapy (IPT) for BN is a short-term supportive therapy that focuses on the interpersonal difficulties that serve as a backdrop to ED symptoms (Agras et al., 2000). More specifically, patients select one of four possible interpersonal problems on which to focus the therapy: interpersonal deficits, interpersonal role disputes, role transitions, or grief (Grilo & Mitchell, 2010). A randomized trial comparing IPT to CBT provides support for the potential efficacy of IPT for treating BN. CBT was superior to IPT at end of treatment in promoting recovery (defined as having no binge or purge behaviors in the previous 28 days Agras et al., 2000); however, no significant difference was observed between CBT and IPT at the 1-year follow-up (Agras et al., 2000). Thus IPT shows promise for BN, although it may not work as quickly as CBT, and more evidence is needed to better understand its efficacy.

Novel Treatments

Nearly half (47.3%) of individuals with BN are not recovered at the completion of CBT-E (Fairburn et al., 2009). For that reason, several novel psychosocial treatments are under study including dialectical behavioral therapy, family based treatment, and integrative cognitive affective therapy.

Dialectical Behavioral Therapy (DBT)

DBT was originally developed for the treatment of borderline personality disorder and has since been adapted to fit other populations, giving it the added benefit of being transdiagnostic across ED diagnoses. The main treatment foci of DBT are emotion regulation, distress tolerance, interpersonal effectiveness, and mindfulness (Chen & Safer, 2010). In a study examining the effectiveness of DBT for patients with borderline personality disorder and either AN or BN, participants in both categories demonstrated a benefit from DBT at follow-up. Specifically, AN participants showed a significant weight increase, and BN participants showed a reduction in binge frequency (Kroger et al., 2010). However, the low remission rates and lack of change in ED psychopathology demonstrated a need for further research. Another DBT treatment called *appetite-focused DBT* (DBT-AF) is in the early phases of testing (Hill, Craighead, Safer, 2010). This therapy is a combination of appetite awareness training and DBT and combines awareness of internal appetite cues with awareness of emotional state. At the conclusion of a treatment development study, DBT-AF participants reported fewer BN symptoms than participants in the delayed treatment control group (Hill et al., 2010). Given the impulsive nature of BN, it may be beneficial to collect more evidence on both forms of DBT.

Family Based Treatment (FBT)

FBT has shown previous success for adolescent AN (Lock et al., 2010) and may also be a viable option for the treatment of adolescent BN. In a randomized controlled comparison of FBT and supportive therapy, FBT demonstrated an advantage over supportive therapy in the reduction of core bulimic symptoms at end of treatment and follow-up. Furthermore, compared to supportive therapy, FBT appears to achieve therapeutic results at a more rapid rate (le Grange, Crosby, Rathouz, & Leventhal, 2007).

Integrative Cognitive Affective Therapy (ICAT)

ICAT targets BN by exploring the relationship between self-discrepancies (i.e., differences between actual and ideal self) and self-directed coping mechanisms (Wonderlich et al., 2008). For example, patients with BN may use self-directed behaviors (i.e., dieting, purging, over-exercising) as an attempt to distract from or minimize self-discrepancies. In an assessment-only study comparing individuals with BN and a non-ED control group, BN participants showed higher levels of self-discrepancy. Higher levels of self-discrepancy were also associated with more negative self-directed styles in both the BN and control groups (Wonderlich et al., 2008). The first randomized controlled trial comparing ICAT to CBT-E—the current gold-standard treatment for BN—identified no differences in treatment outcome (Wonderlich et al., 2013), highlighting the potential promise of ICAT as a novel treatment modality.

Pharmacological Therapies for BN

Similar to AN, psychosocial therapies are the main and most effective treatments for BN. However, different from AN, some medications have demonstrated consistent efficacy in reducing the psychopathological and behavioral symptoms of BN. The best studied medication (and also the only one with an FDA approval for treatment of BN) is fluoxetine (60 mg daily). It has been shown in reasonably sized RCTs to reduce the frequency of bingeing and purging behaviors and to improve depression, pathological attitudes about eating, and carbohydrate craving ("Fluoxetine in the Treatment", 1992; Goldbloom & Olmsted, 1993; Goldstein, Wilson, Thompson, Potvin, & Rampey, 1995). Studies demonstrate efficacy of fluoxetine as an adjunctive treatment to psychotherapy (Goldbloom & Olmsted, 1997), particularly if patients are responding poorly to psychotherapy alone (Walsh et al., 2000). Additionally, fluoxetine has been shown to improve long-term outcomes and decrease likelihood of relapse (Romano, Halmi, Sarkar, Koke, & Lee, 2002). Other selective serotonin reuptake inhibitors (SSRIs), including sertraline and citalopram, have demonstrated efficacy in trials, suggesting that SSRIs as a class are likely moderately effective in reducing symptoms of BN (Sloan, Mizes, Helbok, & Muck, 2004; Milano, Petrella, Sabatino, & Capasso, 2004; Leombruni et al., 2006). Similar to the SSRIs, several tricyclic antidepressants have been studied and found to be effective in patients with BN, but they are quite limited by unpleasant side effect profiles and rarely used as first-line treatment (Pope, Hudson, & Jonas, 1983).

Although the SSRIs have been studied the most, other medications demonstrate effectiveness in reducing symptoms of BN. Several RCTs have demonstrated that topiramate (50–400 mg daily) is effective in reducing behaviors and psychopathological features of BN (Hoopes et al., 2003; Hedges et al., 2003; Nickel et al., C). Given the role of endogenous opiates in regulating food ingestion, the opiate antagonist naltrexone has been studied in one small RCT and several non-blinded, non–placebo controlled studies (Marrazzi, Bacon, Kinzie, & Luby, 1995; Maremmani, Castrogiovanni, P., & Deltito, 1996). It is effective in reducing bingeing and purging behaviors; however, risks and benefits in patients with preexisting liver disease should be weighed carefully given the risk of hepatic toxicity.

Bupropion carries a relative contraindication for use in patients with BN due to increased seizure risk. A study of immediate-release bupropion in patients with active bingeing and purging found bupropion to be effective in reducing behaviors; however, 4 of 55 subjects had grand mal seizures (Horne et al., 1998), a rate of seizures much higher than the general population. Three of those four were taking 375 mg immediate-release bupropion daily. Although it is established that the immediate-release formulation and peak concentration is associated with increased risk of seizure, no follow-up studies of sustained-release or extended-release formulations have been done in patients with BN. For patients with serious comorbid depression and prior failed trials of other antidepressants, weighing of all risks and benefits may favor a trial of slow-release formulations of bupropion despite this early study of immediate-release bupropion and the relative contraindication.

BINGE EATING DISORDER

Psychological Treatments for Binge Eating Disorder

Cognitive Behavioral Therapy

Several therapies have been studied for the treatment of BED, with CBT having the most support to date. Similar to CBT for BN, CBT for BED addresses the mechanisms that maintain disordered eating (Fairburn, 2008). CBT for BED focuses on establishing normalized eating behaviors and editing maladaptive thoughts surrounding weight and shape. An added advantage of CBT for BED is that it can be delivered in therapist-led or self-help versions. Self-led therapy involves limited or no interaction with a clinician. Instead, the individual guides his or her own treatment, usually based on a manual such as *Overcoming Binge Eating* (Fairburn, 2013). Self-led treatment has the benefit of being cost effective and widely disseminable to nonspecialty treatment settings (Grilo & Mitchel, 2010).

In recent studies CBT has shown promising results for the treatment of BED. When compared to treatment as usual, CBTgsh (guided self-help, in which patients read *Overcoming Binge Eating* and met with a therapist for eight 20-minute sessions over a 12-week period) led to greater abstinence from binge episodes and an improvement in restraint, eating, weight and shape concerns, depression, and social adjustment (Striegel-Moore et al., 2010). CBTgsh has also shown to be more effective than behavioral weight loss treatment (BWLT) for patients who do not rapidly respond to treatment. In this case, rapid response is defined as a 65% or greater reduction in binge symptoms by the fourth week of treatment (Masheb & Grilo, 2007). Nonrapid responders showed a greater reduction in binge episodes after receiving CBTgsh. While this research supports the use of CBTgsh, future research should aim to compare the efficacy of self-help methods verses therapist-led CBT (Sysko & Walsh, 2008). CBT (whether self-led or therapist-led) should currently be considered the first-line treatment for BED.

Interpersonal Psychotherapy

Interpersonal psychotherapy (IPT) has shown comparable results to CBT for the treatment of BED (Wilson et al., 2010). Similar to IPT for BN, IPT for BED examines interpersonal functioning and its relationship to disordered eating. When compared to CBTgsh and BWLT, IPT and CBTgsh showed greater remission than BWLT (Wilson et al., 2010). Results suggest that, while CBT is still the best option for the treatment of BED, IPT may be beneficial for BED patients who simultaneously endorse low self-esteem and high ED psychopathology (Wilson et al., 2010).

Behavioral Weight Loss Treatment

Many individuals with BED are obese, putting their physical as well as mental health at risk (Grilo et al., 2005). Although

CBT is highly effective in reducing binge eating among individuals with BED, its impact on body weight is negligible. Behavioral Weight Loss Treatment (BWLT) addresses both binge eating and weight-loss simultaneously by focusing on regulating eating patterns in conjunction with healthy dietary restriction (Grilo et al., 2005). In a study comparing BWLT to CBT, both treatments showed significant improvement from baseline to end of treatment, yet BWLT resulted in a faster and larger reductions in BMI than CBT (Munsch et al., 2007). However, it is important to note that two-year follow-up results show that patients who undergo BWLT actually tend to gain the weight back, bringing into question the long-term efficacy of this therapy (Wilson, Wilfley, Agras, & Bryson, 2010). While BWLT does put an important emphasis on healthy weight control, CBT appears to have an advantage for reducing the binge eating episodes that comprise the core psychopathology of BED (Grilo & Masheb, 2005; Munsch et al., 2007; Wilson et al., 2010).

Pharmacological Interventions

Given successful trials with SSRIs in reducing symptoms of BN, numerous studies of SSRIs in BED have followed suit. Small to moderate sized, short-term (6–24 weeks) RCTs of fluoxetine, citalopram, sertraline, fluvoxamine, and escitalopram have demonstrated that SSRIs as a class may be effective in reducing bingeing frequency, weight, and psychopathological features of the illness (Arnold et al., 2002; McElroy et al., 2003; Guerdjikova et al., 2008; Leombruni et al., 2008). Although sometimes significant when compared to placebo, the amount of weight loss is modest at best and generally unsatisfactory to patients and clinicians. In several placebo-controlled RCTs, topiramate has established efficacy in reducing symptoms of BED (McElroy et al., 2003, 2004, 2007). Atomoxetine, a norepinephrine reuptake inhibitor, was studied in a small 10-week flexible-dose placebo-controlled trial, was found to be effective in reducing symptoms of BED, and was well tolerated (McElroy, 2007).

Although in several RCTs sibutramine demonstrated efficacy in treating BED in obese patients (Willfley et al., 2008; Milano et al., 2005; Appolinario et al., 2003), it was recently withdrawn from the United States market due to increased cardiovascular events and strokes (James et al., 2010).

OTHER SPECIFIED FEEDING OR EATING DISORDER

Given that a substantial minority of individuals with eating disorders will remain in the residual category (i.e., OSFED or UFED) even after DSM-5 changes (e.g., Thomas et al., under review), findings from randomized controlled trials based on strict DSM diagnoses may not generalize to all patients seen in clinical practice. Fortunately, CBT-E was designed to be transdiagnostic—that is, flexibly based on a patient's individualized formulation rather than a specific ED profile (Fairburn et al., 2009). For example, patients with atypical AN may benefit from CBT-E targeted toward AN-like symptoms, and patients with subthreshold BN or purging disorder may benefit from CBT-E targeted toward BN-like symptoms. Fortunately, many studies to date have shown the efficacy of disorder-specific therapies for patients with subthreshold classification, and CBT has been the most widely studied therapy in this regard. For example, in a CBT study that included both strict and lenient weight criteria for AN, no significant difference was found between the two subgroups on either symptom severity or therapy outcome (McIntosh et al., 2005). These results were further supported in a long-term efficacy study of CBT for AN and subthreshold AN (s-AN) (Ricca et al., 2010). In this study s-AN participants met all DSM-IV diagnostic criteria for AN excluding amenorrhea and underweight. AN and s-AN did not show significant differences on clinical measures at baseline, end of treatment, or follow-up, with both groups demonstrating weight gain and a reduction in ED psychopathology (Ricca et al., 2010). Similarly, in a study using both BN and EDNOS participants, all participants regardless of disorder criterion benefited from CBTgsh for the reduction of binge-eating symptoms (Schmidt et al., 2007).

PATIENTS WHO ARE RELUCTANT TO ACCEPT TREATMENT

It is always frustrating when patients are very ill but still refuse treatment. This is common among patients with ED. In general, when medical and psychiatric problems are not emergent patients reserve the right to refuse treatment. For example, a treatment team may recommend inpatient hospitalization for a young woman with AN who has not made any progress after 3 months in outpatient treatment. However, if she is maintaining a BMI of 17.5 kg/m^2, has no laboratory abnormalities, and demonstrates cardiovascular stability, she reserves the right to refuse treatment. Mental hygiene laws in most states do not support involuntary treatment in nonemergent situations.

In these situations efforts are best focused on building treatment alliance, clarifying thresholds for increasing the level of care, and enhancing motivation for change. Taking the above situation as an example, we would recommend first stabilizing the treatment alliance by expressing both an empathic understanding of the patient's position and your specific concerns regarding her health and reasons for recommending more intensive treatment. Clearly outline for the patient the requirements to maintain a minimum level of safe care, as well as what is necessary to remain in treatment. Enlist the patient in this problem-solving exercise to increase her sense of ownership and control in treatment. Make the requirements explicit with the patient; it can be helpful to co-create a written contract that the patient and team members co-sign. For this particular patient example, the clinician might require the patient to have weekly visits for weight check-in, laboratory evaluation, and vital signs. It would be reasonable to require inpatient treatment should any of these become unstable (e.g., BMI < 16.0 kg/m^2, laboratory abnormalities, altered vital signs) and to require increased level of care should the patient make no progress (weight gain) with another 4 weeks of outpatient treatment. If patients repeatedly fail to follow through, this may be grounds for termination from treatment—although we recommend first consulting with your particular clinic or hospital supervisors given medico-legal issues surrounding termination.

MOTIVATIONAL ENHANCEMENT THERAPY

ED patients are often ambivalent about recovery, which can lead to treatment attrition and relapse. Motivational enhancement therapy (MET) addresses the discrepancy between the patient's motivators and life goals and his or her ED. Although the format is similar to the motivational interviewing originally developed to help patients with substance abuse, the content is specific to the symptoms of ED. Therapy can be applied prior to formal, change-oriented treatment or as an adjunctive or stand-alone treatment. In contrast to CBT and IPT, MET is nondirective, allowing the patient to make his or her own arguments for symptom change. Patients are asked to identify personal goals for the future, such as going to college or having children, and then to critically evaluate how their ED either supports or obstructs these aspirations. Other common interventions include identifying the pros and cons of valued ED symptoms, imagining one's life free from ED, and identifying core life values (e.g., honesty, companionship, spirituality). In a randomized controlled trial comparing MET to treatment as usual, MET patients appeared to show longer-term motivation and engagement in treatment (Dean Touyz, Rieger, & Thornton, 2008). Furthermore, in a two-phase trial study treatment outcomes did not differ whether the patients received MET or CBT in the first phase (Katzman et al., 2010). To date most MET studies have been short or uncontrolled, but, given its attempt to address the ego-syntonic nature of ED, MET appears to be a promising treatment approach.

INVOLUNTARY TREATMENT

Involuntary hospitalization usually occurs when there are emergent psychiatric or medical problems. Psychiatrically this is when patients are suicidal, homicidal, actively engaging in severe self-harm behavior, or suffering severe comorbid illness such as depression, mania, or psychosis. For example, a patient with BN who gains 20 pounds, develops suicidal thoughts, and buys a bottle of acetaminophen with the intention to overdose would be hospitalized involuntarily on a psychiatric unit.

Medically, patients may be hospitalized and treated against their will when two conditions are met: (1) when emergent medical conditions related to the ED arise, and (2) when patients fail to demonstrate adequate decision-making capacity. In these situations clinicians must make a determination of whether the patient maintains decision-making capacity to refuse treatment, similar to any other situation in medicine when patients refuse treatment. An example would be a young woman with AN with a BMI of 14.0 kg/m^2, heart rate of 40 beats per minute, low potassium, and complete food and water refusal. She refuses to be hospitalized for refeeding despite a thorough explanation of the risks of refusing treatment because she believes she is fat and does not believe the cardiac risks actually apply to her. She is both in an emergent medical situation and fails to demonstrate adequate decision-making capacity. She would be hospitalized and treated despite her preference to leave against advice.

A full discussion of decision-making capacity is beyond the scope of this chapter. This clinical dilemma is not an uncommon challenge when treating patients with severe EDs and acute AN in particular. Often patients are able to recite verbatim the risks of refusing treatment, yet are unable to appreciate how these risks apply to themselves (i.e., they are in denial of their ill status); their thought styles are overly rigid, and they display poor reasoning skills. In situations where a patient fails to demonstrate decision-making capacity in an emergent situation, treatment is generally instituted while ongoing efforts are made to restore the patient's decision-making capacity. In rare situations a legal guardian may be appointed to help make treatment decisions.

Needless to say, it is difficult for both patients and clinicians when involuntary hospitalization occurs. Clinicians face the dilemma of delicately balancing patients' rights, the treatment alliance, and medical and psychiatric safety. On the one hand, unless there is an associated grave risk of not being hospitalized the long-term utility of involuntary hospitalizations is unclear and may alienate patients from treatment. On the other hand, a study of inpatients with EDs found that nearly half of the patients who felt they did not need inpatient treatment at the time of admission had acknowledged that they indeed did need inpatient treatment at 2-week follow-up (Guarda et al., 2007) suggesting that once in treatment (and perhaps feeling better) they able to accept the help they need.

SUMMARY

In summary, EDs are common psychiatric illnesses that are associated with substantial medical and psychiatric morbidity. As most patients with ED first present in the medical setting, medical clinicians are uniquely poised to make the first diagnosis of a previously covert ED. Patients with EDs often require multidisciplinary teams composed of a medical clinician, therapist, and sometimes a dietitian and/or psychiatrist. With treatment, most patients achieve significant improvement and many fully remit. Although treatment can be challenging for both patients and clinicians, it can be rewarding as well. Increasingly there are empirically supported psychosocial and pharmacologic treatments for EDs. Although nutritional stabilization and psychosocial therapies remain mainstays of treatment, some pharmacological interventions, particularly fluoxetine in BN, have demonstrated efficacy. The main supported treatments currently are FBT for AN; CBT and fluoxetine for BN; and CBT (including a guided self-help format) for BED. Research into promising novel therapies is needed and is ongoing.

CLINICAL PEARLS

- Early identification and treatment can help prevent the associated morbidity and mortality of eating disorders.

- Patients with eating disorders present most often in medical settings, but rarely with a chief complaint of disordered eating (e.g., restricting food, purging, using laxatives). Rather, they present with nonspecific physical or emotional complaints. For example, patients with AN may report lightheadedness or constipation; patients with BN may present with acid reflux or other gastrointestinal complaints; and patients with BED may present with obesity or depression.

- Traits common to AN and BN include perfectionism and dysphoric mood.

- Anxiety, mood, and substance use disorders are highly comorbid with EDs. AN has among the highest mortality rates of any psychiatric disorder, with the majority of deaths attributable to medical complications related to severe malnutrition and suicide (Harris & Barraclough, 1998; Papadopoulous et al., 2009).

- A higher percentage of patients with BN make suicide attempts: 3%–20% in AN and 25%–35% in BN.

- Overall, outcomes for individuals with BN are better than for AN.

- Many patients with ED, particularly AN and BN, present with medical complaints that are atypical or more severe than would be expected given their demographics and otherwise healthy status.

- Interestingly, there is a subset of patients who meet all the criteria for AN except for not endorsing fear of weight gain. Such patients are especially common in culturally non-Western and youth populations (Becker et al., 2009).

- During the initial evaluation we suggest asking patients specifically what they ate and drank for all meals and snacks on the day prior to evaluation.

- It can be helpful to ask in a way that decreases shame; for example, "Some patients who are struggling with controlling their eating and weight induce vomiting or use laxatives. Have you found yourself doing this?"

- To assess exercise, it is helpful to specifically ask how much of the day is spent active (e.g., not sitting down).

- For an empathic but firm approach, the following statement may be used to ease the anguish about getting weighed: "I realize getting weighed may be difficult for you. In order for me to provide you with good and safe care, I will have to weigh you at each visit. It is likely to be more difficult in the beginning and get easier with time. Let's go ahead and get it out of the way for today's visit."

- The American Dental Association (ADA) currently recommends that patients not brush their teeth immediately after vomiting but rather rinse with baking soda, which helps to neutralize the destructive effects of the stomach acid (http://www.mouthhealthy.org/en/az-topics/e/eating-disorders).

- Approximately 30% of ED patients do not meet full criteria for AN, BN, or BED, and will fall into the residual category of Other Specified Feeding or Eating Disorder (Thomas et al., under review).

DISCLOSURES

Dr. Brennan and Ms. Nevins have no conflicts of interest to disclose. Dr. Thomas receives royalties from Hazelden and Harvard Health Publications for the sale of her book, *Almost Anorexic: Is My (Or My Loved One's) Relationship with Food a Problem?*.

REFERENCES

Eating Disorders. (n.d.). In *HealthMouth*. Retrieved August 25, 2014, from http://www.mouthhealthy.org/en/az-topics/e/eating-disorders

Agras, W. S., Walsh, T., Fairburn, C. G., Wilson, G. T., & Kraemer, H. C. (2000). A multicenter comparison of cognitive-behavioral therapy and interpersonal psychotherapy for bulimia nervosa. *Archives of General Psychiatry, 57,* 459–466.

Agras, W. S., Crow, S., Mitchell J. E., Halmi K. A., Bryson S. (2009). A 4-year prospective study of eating disorder NOS compared with full eating disorder syndromes. *International Journal of Eating Disorders, 42,* 565–570.

Altshuler, B. D., Dechow, P. C., Waller, D. A., Hardy, B. W. (1990). An investigation of the oral pathologies occurring in bulimia nervosa. *International Journal of Eating Disorders, 9,* 191.

American Psychiatric Association. (2006). Treatment of patients with eating disorders, 3rd edition. *American Journal of Psychiatry, 163*(7 suppl), 4–54.

American Psychiatric Association. (2000). *Diagnostic and statistical manual of mental disorders* (Revised 4th ed.). Washington, DC: Author.

American Psychiatric Association. (2013). Diagnostic and statistical manual of mental disorders (5th ed.). Arlington, VA: American Psychiatric Publishing.

Appolinario, J. C., Bacaltchuk, J., Sichieri, R., Claudino, A. M., Godoy-Matos, A., Morgan, C., et al. (2003). A randomized, double-blind, placebo-controlled study of sibutramine in the treatment of binge eating disorder. *Archives of General Psychiatry, 60,* 1109–1116.

Arnold, J. M., McElroy, S. L., Hudson, J. I., Welge, J. A., Bennett, A. J., & Keck, P. E. (2002). A placebo-controlled, randomized trial of fluoxetine in the treatment of binge-eating disorder. *Journal of Clinical Psychology, 63,* 1028–1033.

Barada, K. A., Azar, C. R., Al-Kutoubi, A. O., Harb, R. S., Hazimeh, Y. M., Abbas, J. S., et al. (2006). Massive gastric dilatation after a single binge in an anorectic woman. *International Journal of Eating Disorders, 39,* 166–169.

Becker, A. E., Thomas, J. J., Franko, D. L., & Herzog, D. B. (2005). Disclosure patterns of eating and weight concerns to clinicians, educational professionals, family and peers. *International Journal of Eating Disorders, 38,* 18–23.

Becker, A. E., Thomas, J. J., & Pike, K. M. (2009). Should non-fat phobic anorexia nervosa be included in DSM-V? *International Journal of Eating Disorders, 42,* 620–635.

Barbarich, N. C., McConaha, C. W., Halmi, K. A., Gendall, K., Sunday, S. R., Gaskill, J., et al. (2004). Use of nutritional supplements to increase the efficacy of fluoxetine in the treatment of anorexia nervosa. *International Journal of Eating Disorders, 35*, 10–15.

Benini, L., Todesco, T., Dalle Grave, R., Deiorio, F., Salandini, L., & Vantini, I. (2004). Gastric emptying in patients with restricting and binge/purging subtypes of anorexia nervosa. *American Journal of Gastroenterology, 99*(8), 1448–1454.

Bissada, H., Tasca, G. A., Barber, A. M., & Bradwejn, J. (2008). Olanzapine in the treatment of low body weight and obsessive thinking in women with anorexia nervosa: a randomized, double-blind, placebo-controlled trial. *American Journal of Psychiatry, 165*, 1281–1288.

Brambilla, F., Garcia, C. S., Fassino, S., Daga, G. A., Favaro, A., Santonastaso, P., et al. (2007). Olanzapine therapy in anorexia nervosa: psychobiological effects. *International Clinical Psychopharmacology, 22*, 197–204.

Bratland, Sanda S., Sundgot-Borgen, J., Ro, O., Rosenvinge, J. H., Hoffart, A., & Martinsen, E. W. (2010). "I'm not physically active—I only go for walks": physical activity in patients with longstanding eating disorders. *International Journal of Eating Disorders, 43*, 88–92.

Bravender, T., & Story, L. (2007). Massive binge eating, gastric dilation and unsuccessful purging in a young woman with bulimia nervosa. *Journal of Adolescent Health, 41*, 516–518.

Bulik, C. M., Baucom, D. H., Kirby, J. S., & Pisetsky, E. (2011). Uniting couples (in the treatment of) anorexia nervosa (UCAN). *The International Journal of Eating Disorders, 44*, 19–28.

Bulimia Nervosa Collaborative Study Group. (1992). Fluoxetine in the treatment of bulimia nervosa. A multicenter, placebo-conrolled, double-blind trial. *Archives of General Psychiatry, 49*, 139–147.

Casiero, D., & Frishman, W. H. (2006). Cardiovascular complications of eating disorders. *Cardiology in Review, 14*, 227–231.

Chen, E. Y., & Safer, D. L. (2010). Dialectical behavior therapy for bulimia nervosa and binge-eating disorder. In C. Grilo & J. Mitchell (Eds.), *The treatment of eating disorders: a clinical handbook* (pp. 294–316). New York: Guilford.

Clausen, L. (2008). Time to remission for eating disorder patients: A 2(1/2)-year follow-up study of outcome and predictors. *Nordic Journal of Psychiatry, 62*, 151–159.

Department of Psychiatry. (n.d.) *Cognitive Behavior Therapy and Eating Disorders (Fairburn, 2008)*. Retrieved from http://www.psychiatry.ox.ac.uk/research/researchunits/credo/cbt_and_eating_disorders.

Contaldo, F., Di Paolo, M. R., Mazzacano, C., Di Biase, G., & Giumetti, D. (1990). Hypopotassemia and prolongation of the QT interval in a patient with severe malnutrition caused by bulimia and post-prandial vomiting. *Recenti Progressi in Medicina, 81*, 266–268.

Cooke, R. A., & Chambers, J. B. (1995). Anorexia nervosa and the heart. *British Journal of Hospital Medicine, 54*, 313–317.

Crow, S. J., Peterson, C. B., Swanson, S. A., Raymond, N. C., Eckert, E. D., & Mitchell, J. E. (2009). Increased mortality in bulimia nervosa and other eating disorders. *The American Journal of Psychiatry, 166*, 1342–1346.

Davies, H., & Tchanturia, K. (2005). Cognitive remediation therapy as an intervention for acute anorexia nervosa: a case report. *European Eating Disorders Review, 13*, 311–316.

Delinsky S. S., St. Germain S. A., Thomas J. J., Craigen, K. E., Fagley, W. H., Weigel, T. J., et al. (2010). Naturalistic study of course, effectiveness, and predictors of outcome among female adolescents in residential treatment for eating disorders. *Eating Weight Disorders, 15*, e127–e135.

Dean, H. Y., Touyz, S. W., Rieger, E., & Thornton, C. E. (2008). Group motivational enhancement therapy as an adjunct to inpatient treatment for eating disorders: A preliminary study. *European Eating Disorders Review: The Journal of the Eating Disorders Association, 16*, 256–267.

Docx, M. K., Gewillig, M., Simons, A., Vandenberghe, P., Weyler, J., Ramet, J., & Mertens, L. (2010). Pericardial effusions in adolescent girls with anorexia nervosa: clinical course and risk factors. *Eating Disorders, 18*, 218–225.

Eisler, I., Dare, C., Russell, G. F., Szmukler, G., le Grange, D., & Dodge, E. (1997). Family and individual therapy in anorexia nervosa. A 5-year follow-up. *Archives of General Psychiatry, 54*, 1025–30.

Eisler, I., Simic, M., Russell, G., & Dare, C. (2007). A randomized controlled treatment trial of two forms of family therapy in adolescent anorexia nervosa: a five-year follow-up. *Journal of Child Psychology and Psychiatry, 48*, 552–560.

Ewing, J. A. (1984). Detecting alcoholism: The CAGE questionnaire. *The Journal of the American Medical Association, 252*, 1905–1907.

Fairburn, C. G. (2013). *Overcoming Binge Eating: The Proven Program to Learn why You Binge and how You Can Stop*. Guilford Press.

Fairburn, C. G., Jones, R., Peveler, R. C., Hope, R. A., & O'Connor, M. (1993). Psychotherapy and bulimia nervosa: longer-term effects of interpersonal psychotherapy, behavior therapy, and cognitive behavior therapy. *Archives of General Psychiatry, 50*, 419–428.

Fairburn, C. G., & Bohn, K. (2008). Appendix III: The Clinical Impairment Assessment Questionnaire (CIA). In C. Fairburn (Ed.), *Cognitive Behavior Therapy and Eating Disorders* (pp. 315–317). New York: Guilford.

Fairburn, C. G. (2008). *Cognitive behavior therapy and eating disorders*. New York: Guilford Press.

Fairburn, C. G., Cooper, Z., Doll, H. A., O'Connor, M. E., Bohn, K., Hawker, D. M., et al. (2009). Transdiagnostic cognitive-behavioral therapy for patients with eating disorders: A two-site trial with 60-week follow-up. *The American Journal of Psychiatry, 166*, 311–319.

Fichter, M. M., Quadflieg, N., & Hedlund, S. (2008). Long-term course of binge eating disorder and bulimia nervosa: relevance for nosology and diagnostic criteria, *International Journal of Eating Disorders, 41*, 577–586.

Fichter, M. M., & Quadflieg, N. (2007). Long-term stability of eating disorder diagnoses. *International Journal of Eating Disorders, 40*(Suppl), S61–S66.

Fichter, M. M., Quadflieg, N., & Hedlund, S. (2006). Twelve-year course and outcome predictors of anorexia nervosa, *International Journal of Eating Disorders, 39*, 87–100.

Fluoxetine in the treatment of bulimia nervosa. A multicenter, placebo-controlled, double-blind trial. Fluoxetine Bulimia Nervosa Collaborative Study Group, (1992), *Archives of General Psychiatry, 49*(2), 139–147.

Forcano, L., Fernández-Aranda, F., Álvarez-Moya, E., Bulik, C., Granero, R., Gratacòs, M., & . . . Estivill, X. (2009). Suicide attempts in bulimia nervosa: Personality and psychopathological correlates. *European Psychiatry, 24*(2), 91–97. doi:10.1016/j.eurpsy.2008.10.002

Foulon, C., Guelfi J. D., Kipman, A., Ades, J., Romo, L., Houdeyer, K., et al. (2007). Switching to the bingeing/purging subtype of anorexia nervosa is frequently associated with suicidal attempts. *European Psychiatry, 22*(8), 513–519.

Franko, D. L., & Keel, P. K. (2006). Suicidality in eating disorders: occurrence, correlates, and clinical implications. *Clinical Psychology Review, 26*, 769–782.

Goldbloom, D. S., & Olmsted, M. P. (1993). Pharmacotherapy of bulimia nervosa with fluoxetine: assessment of clinically significant attitudinal change. *American Journal of Psychiatry, 150*, 770–774.

Goldstein, D. J., Wilson, M. G., Thompson, V. L., Potvin, J. H., & Rampey, A. H. Jr. (1995). Long-term fluoxetine treatment of bulimia nervosa. Fluoxetine Nervosa Research Group. *British Journal of Psychiatry, 166*, 660–666.

Grilo, C. M., & Masheb, R. M. (2005). A randomized controlled comparison of guided self-help cognitive behavioral therapy and behavioral weight loss for binge eating disorder. *Behaviour Research and Therapy, 43*, 1509–1525.

Grilo, C. M., & Mitchell, J. E. (2010). *The treatment of eating disorders: a clinical handbook*. New York: Guilford.

Grilo, C. M., Pagano, M. E., Skodol, A. E., Sanislow, C. A., McGlashan, T. H., Gunderson, J. G., & Stout, R. L. (2007). Natural course of bulimia nervosa and of eating disorder not otherwise specified: 5-year prospective study of remissions, relapses, and the effects of personality disorder psychopathology. *The Journal of clinical psychiatry, 68*(5), 738.

Guarda, A., Pinto, A., Coughlin, J., Hussain, S., Haug, N., & Heinberg, L. (2007). Perceived coercion and change in perceived need for admission in patients hospitalized for eating disorders. *The American Journal of Psychiatry, 164*(1), 108–114.

Guerdjikova, A. I., McElroy, S. L., Kotwal, R., Welge, J. A., Nelson, E., Lake, K., et al. (2008). High-dose escitalopram in the treatment of binge-eating disorder with obesity: a placebo-controlled monotherapy trial. *Human Psychopharmacology, 23*, 1–11.

Gunarathne, T., McKay, R., Pillans, L., McKinlay, A., & Crockett, P. (2010). Refeeding syndrome in a patient with anorexia nervosa. *British Medical Journal, 340*, c56.

Gyurkovics, E., Tihanyi, B., Szijarto, A., Kaliszky, P., Temesi, V., Hedvig, S. A., & Kupcsuli, P. (2006). Fatal outcome from extreme acute gastric dilation after an eating binge. *International Journal of Eating Disorders, 39*, 602–605.

Harris, E. C., & Barraclough, B. (1998). Excess mortality of mental disorder. *British Journal of Psychiatry, 173*, 11–53.

Hedges, D. W., Reimherr, F. W., Hoopes, S. P., Rosenthal, N. R., Kamin, M., Karm, R., & Capece, J. A. (2003). Treatment of bulimia nervosa with topiramate in a randomized, double-blind, placebo-controlled trial, part 2: improvement in psychiatric measures. *Journal of Clinical Psychology, 64*, 1449–1454.

Hill, D. M., Craighead, L. W., & Safer, D. L. (2010). Appetite-focused dialectical behavior therapy for the treatment of binge eating with purging: A preliminary trial. *The International Journal of Eating Disorders, 44*(3), 249–261.

Hoopes, S. P., Reimherr, F. W., Hedges, D. W., Rosenthal, N. R., Kamin, M., Karm, R., et al. (2003). Treatment of bulimia nervosa with topiramate in a randomized, double-blind, placebo-controlled trial, part 1: improvement in binge and purge measures. *Journal of Clinical Psychology, 64*, 1335–1341.

Houy, E., Debono, B., Dechelotte, P., & Thibaut, F. (2007). Anorexia nervosa associated with right frontal brain lesion. *International Journal of Eating Disorders, 40*(8), 758–761.

Horne, R. L., Ferguson, J. M., Pope, H. G. Jr., Hudson, J. I., Lineberry, C. G., Ascher, J., & Cato, A. (1998). Treatment of bulimia with bupropion: a multicenter controlled trial. *Journal of Clinical Psychology, 49*, 262–266.

Hudson, J. L., Lalonde, J. K., Coit, C. E., Tsuang, M. T., McElroy, S. L., Crow, S. J., et al. (2010). Longitudinal study of the diagnosis of components of the metabolic syndrome in individuals with binge-eating disorder. *The American Journal of Clinical Nutrition, 91*, 1568–1573.

Hudson, J. I., Hiripi, E., Pope, H. G., & Kessler, R. C. (2007). The prevalence and correlates of eating disorders in the national comorbidity survey replication, *Biological Psychiatry, 61*, 348–358.

Hudson, J. I., McElroy, S. L., & Raymond, N. C. (1998). Fluvoxamine treatment of binge eating disorder: a multicenter, placebo-controlled double-blind trial. *American Journal of Psychiatry, 155*, 1756–1762.

Hultson, W. R., & Wald, A. (1990). Gastric emptying in patients with bulimia nervosa and anorexia nervosa. *The American Journal of Gastrenterology, 85*, 41–46.

James, W. P., Caterson, I. D., Coutinho, W., Finer, N., Van Gaal, L. F., Maggioni, A. P., et al. (2010). Effect of sibutramine on cardiovascular outcomes in overweight and obese subjects. *The New England Journal of Medicine, 363*, 905–917.

Kaplan, R. (1998). Thyroxine abuse. *Australia and New Zealand Journal of Pyschiatry, 32*(3), 464–465.

Johnston, O., Fornal, G., Cabrini, S., & Kendrick, T. (2007). Feasibility and acceptability of screening for eating disorders in primary care. *Family Practice, 24*, 511–517.

Kamal, N., Chami, T., Andersen, A. Rosell, F A., Schuster, M. M., & Whitehead, W. E. (1991). Delayed gastrointestinal transit times in anorexia nervosa and bulimia nervosa. *Gastroenterology, 101*, 1320–1324.

Kaplan, A. S., Walsh, B. T., Olmsted, M., Attia, E., Carter, J. C., Devlin, M. J., et al. (2009). The slippery slope: prediction of successful weight maintenance in anorexia nervosa. *Psychological Medicine, 39*, 1037–1045.

Katzman, M., Bara-Carril, N., Rabe-Hesketh, S., Schmidt, U., Troop, N., & Treasure, J. (2010). A randomized controlled two-stage trial in the treatment of bulimia nervosa, comparing CBT versus motivational enhancement in Phase 1 followed by group versus individual CBT in Phase 2. *Psychosomatic Medicine, 72*(7), 656–663. doi:10.1097/PSY.0b013e3181ec5373

Kaye, W. H., Greeno, C. G., Moss, H., Fernstrom, J., Ferstrom, M., Lilenfeld, L. R., et al. (1998). Alterations in serotonin activity and psychiatric symptoms after recovery from bulimia nervosa. *Archives of General Psychiatry, 55*, 927–935.

Kaye, W. (2008). Neurobiology of anorexia and bulimia nervosa. *Physiology & Behavior 94*, 121–135.

Kaye, W. H., Nagata, T., Weltzin, T. E., Hsu, L. K., Sokol, M. S., McConaha, C., et al. (2001). Double-blind placebo-controlled administration of fluoxetine in restricting- and restricting-purging-type anorexia nervosa. *Biological Psychology, 49*, 644–652.

Keel, P. K., Gravener, J. A., Joiner, T. E. Jr., & Haedt, A. A. (2010). Twenty-year follow-up of bulimia nervosa and related eating disorders not otherwise specified, *The International Journal of Eating Disorders, 43*, 492–497.

Keel P. K., Holm-Denoma J. M., & Crosby, R. (2011). Clinical significance and distinctiveness of purging disorder and binge eating disorder. *The International Journal of Eating Disorders, 44*(4), 311–316.

Keel, P. K., & Brown, T. A. (2010). Update on course and outcome in eating disorders, *International Journal of Eating Disorders, 43*, 195–204.

Kinzl, J., Biebl, W., & Herold, M. (1993). Significance of vomiting for hyperamylasemia and sialadenosis in patients with eating disorders. *The International Journal of Eating Disorders, 13*, 117–124.

Kroger, C., Schweiger, U., Sipos, V., Kliem, S., Arnold, R., Schunert, T., & Reinecker, H. (2010). Dialectical behaviour therapy and an added cognitive behavioural treatment module for eating disorders in women with borderline personality disorder and anorexia nervosa or bulimia nervosa who failed to respond to previous treatments. an open trial with a 15-month follow-up. *Journal of Behavior Therapy and Experimental Psychiatry, 41*, 381–388.

Lacey, J. H., Crisp, A. H., Hart, G., & Kirkwood, B. A. (1979). Weight and skeletal maturation—a study of radiological and chronological age in an anorexia nervosa population. *Postgraduate Medical Journal, 55*(644), 381–385.

le Grange, D., Crosby, R. D., Rathouz, P. J., & Leventhal, B. L. (2007). A randomized controlled comparison of family-based treatment and supportive psychotherapy for adolescent bulimia nervosa. *Archives of General Psychiatry, 64*, 1049–1056.

Leombruni, P., Piero, A., Lavagnino, L., Brustolin, A., Campisi, S., & Fassino, S. (2008). A randomized, double-blind trial comparing sertraline and fluoxetine 6-month treatment in obese patients with binge eating disorder. *Progress in Neuro-Psychopharmacology and Biological Psychiatry, 32*, 1599–1605.

Leombruni, P., Amianto, F., Delsedime, N., Gramaglia, C., Abbbate-Daga, G., & Fassino, S. (2006). Citalopram versus fluoxetine for the treatment of patients with bulimia nervosa: a single-blind randomized controlled trial. *Advances in Therapy, 23*, 481–494.

Lock, J., le Grange, D., Agras, W. S., & Dare, C. (2001). *Treatment manual for anorexia nervosa: A family based approach.* New York: Guilford.

Lock, J., Agras, W. S., Bryson, S., & Kraemer, H. C. (2005). A comparison of short- and long-term family therapy for adolescent anorexia nervosa. *Journal of the American Academy of Child and Adolescent Psychiatry, 44*, 632–639.

Lock, J., Le Grange, D., Agras, W. S., Moye, A., Bryson, S. W., & Jo, B. (2010). Randomized clinical trial comparing family-based treatment with adolescent-focused individual therapy for adolescents with anorexia nervosa. *Archives of General Psychiatry, 67*, 1025–1032.

Lopez, C., Roberts, M. E., Tchanturia, K., & Treasure, J. (2008). Using neuropsychological feedback therapeutically in treatment for anorexia nervosa: Two illustrative case reports. *European Eating Disorders Review: The Journal of the Eating Disorders Association, 16*, 411–420.

Luck, A. J., Morgan, J. F., Reid, F., O'Brien, A., Brunton, J., Price, C., et al. (2002). The SCOFF questionnaire and clinical interview for eating disorders in general practice: comparative study. *British Medical Journal, 325,* 755–756.

Malik, M., Stratton, J., & Sweeney, W. B. (1997). Rectal prolapse associated with bulimia nervosa: report of seven cases. *Diseases of the Colon and Rectum, 40,* 1382–1385.

Maremmani, I., Marini, G., Castrogiovanni, P., & Deltito, J. (1996). The effectiveness of the combination fluoxetine-naltrexone in bulimia nervosa. *European Psychiatry, 11,* 322–324.

Marrazzi, M. A., Bacon, J. P., Kinzie, J., & Luby, E. D. (1995). Naltrexone use in the treatment of anorexia nervosa and bulimia nervosa. *International Clinical Psychopharmacology, 10,* 163–172.

Masheb, R. M., & Grilo, C. M. (2007). Rapid response predicts treatment outcomes in binge eating disorder: Implications for stepped care. *Journal of Consulting and Clinical Psychology, 75,* 639–644.

Mathevon, T., Rougier, C., Ducher, E., Pic, D., Garcier, J. M., & Schmidt, J. (2004). Acute abdominal dilatation, a serious complication in the case of anorexia nervosa. *Presse Medical Journal, 33,* 601–603.

McElroy, S. L., Guerdjikova, A., Kotwal, R., Welge, J. A., Nelson, E. B., Lake, K. A., et al. (2007). Atomoxetine in the treatment of binge-eating disorder: a randomized placebo-controlled trial. *Journal of Clinical Psychology, 68,* 390–398.

McElroy, S. L., Hudson, J. I., Capece, J. A., Beyers, K., Fisher, A. C., & Rosenthal, N. R. (2007). Topiramate for the treatment of binge eating disorder associated with obesity: a placebo-controlled study. *Biological Psychiatry, 61,* 1039–1048.

McElroy, S. L., Shapira, N. A., Arnold, L. M., Keck, P. E., Rosenthal, N. R., Wu, S. C., et al. (2004). Topiramate in the long-term treatment of binge-eating disorder associated with obesity. *Journal of Clinical Psychology, 65,* 1463–1469.

McElroy, S. L., Hudson, J. I., Malhotra, S., Welge, J. A., Nelson, E. B., & Keck, P. E. Jr. (2003). Citalopram in the treatment of binge-eating disorder: a placebo-controlled trial. *Journal of Clinical Psychology, 64,* 807–813.

McElroy, S. L., Arnold, L. M., Shapira, N. A., Keck, P. E., Rosenthal, N. R., Karim, M. R., et al. (2003). Topiramate in the treatment of binge eating disorder associated with obesity: a randomized, placebo controlled trial. *American Journal of Psychiatry, 160,* 255–261.

McIntosh, V. V., Jordan, J., Carter, F. A., Luty, S. E., McKenzie, J. M., Bulik, C. M., et al. (2005). Three psychotherapies for anorexia nervosa: A randomized, controlled trial. *The American Journal of Psychiatry, 162,* 741–747.

McIntosh, V. V., Jordan, J., Luty, S. E., Carter, F. A., McKenzie, J. M., Bulik, C. M., et al. (2006). Specialist supportive clinical management for anorexia nervosa. *The International Journal of Eating Disorders, 39,* 625–632.

Mehler, P. S., Winkelman, A. B., Andersen, D. M., & Gaudiani, J. L. (2010). Nutritional rehabilitation: practical guidelines for refeeding the anorectic patient. *Journal of Nutrition and Metabolism.*

Mehler, P. S., & Andersen, A. E. (2010). *Eating disorders: a guide to medical care and complications.* Baltimore: Johns Hopkins University Press.

Milano, W., Petrella, C., Casella, A., Capasso, A., Carrino, S., & Milano, L. (2005). Use of sibutramine, an inhibitor of the reuptake of serotonin and noradrenaline, in the treatment of binge eating disorder: a placebo-controlled study. *Advances in Therapy, 22,* 25–31.

Milano, W., Petrella, C., Sabatino, C., & Capasso, A. (2004). Treatment of bulimia nervosa with sertraline: a randomized controlled trial. *Advances in Therapy, 21,* 232–237.

Miller, K. K., Grinspoon, M. D., Ciampa, J., Hier, J., Herzog, D., & Klibanski, A. (2005). Medical findings in outpatients with anorexia nervosa. *Archives Internal Medicine, 165,* 561–566.

Misra, M. (2008). Long-term skeletal effects of eating disorders with onset in adolescence. *Annals of the New York Academy of Sciences, 1135,* 212–218.

Mitchell, J. E., Hatsukami, D., & Pyle, R. L. (1987). Metabolic acidosis as a marker for laxative abuse in patients with bulimia. *The International Journal of Eating Disorders, 6,* 557–560.

Mondraty, N., Birmingham, C. L., Touyz, S., Sundakov, V., Chapman, L., & Beumont, P. (2005). Randomized controlled trial of olanzapine

in the treatment of cognitions in anorexia nervosa. *Australasian Psychiatry, 13,* 72–75.

Mood Disorder News and Headlines. (n.d.). *Mood Disorder News and Headlines.* Retrieved February 15, 2011, from http://dsm–5.org

Morgan, J. F., Reid, F., & Lacey, H (1999). The SCOFF questionnaire: assessment of a new screening tool for eating disorders. *British Medical Journal, 319,* 1467–68.

Munsch, S., Biedert, E., Meyer, A., Michael, T., Schlup, B., Tuch, A., et al. (2007). A randomized comparison of cognitive behavioral therapy and behavioral weight loss treatment for overweight individuals with binge eating disorder. *The International Journal of Eating Disorders, 40,* 102–113.

Navab, F., Avunduk, C., Gang, D., & Frankel, K. (1996). Bulimia nervosa complicated by Barrett's esophagus and esophageal cancer. *Gastrointestinal Endoscopy, 44,* 492–494.

Nickel, C., Tritt, K., Muehlbacher, M., Pedrosa, Gil F., Mitterlehner, F. O., Kaplan, P., et al. (2005). Topiramate treatment in bulimia nervosa patients: a randomized, double-blind, placebo-controlled trial. *The International Journal of Eating Disorders, 38,* 295–300.

Ogg, E. C., Millar, H. R., Pusztai, E. E., & Thom, A. S. (1997). General practice consultation patterns preceding diagnosis of eating disorders. *The International Journal of Eating Disorders, 22,* 89–93.

Pandey, R., Maqbool, A., & Jayachandran, N. (2009). Medical Image. Massive gastric dilatation secondary to a binge episode in bulimia nervosa. *The New Zealand Medical Journal, 122*(1289), 85–86.

Papadopoulous, F. C., Ekbom, A., Brandt, L., & Ekselius, L. (2009). Excess mortality, causes of death and prognostic factors in anorexia nervosa. *British Journal of Psychiatry, 194,* 10–17.

Perry, L., Morgan, J., Reid, F., Brunton, J., O'Brien, A., Luck, A., & Lacey, H. (2002). Screening for syptoms of eating disorders: reliability of the SCOFF screening tool with written compared to oral delivery. *The International Journal of Eating Disorders, 32,* 466–472.

Pike, K. M., Walsh, T. B., Vitousek, K., Wilson, G. T., & Bauer, J. (2003). Cognitive behavior therapy in the posthospitalization treatment of anorexia nervosa. *American Journal of Psychiatry, 160,* 2046–2049.

Polli, N., Blengino, S., Moro, M., Zappulli, D., Scacchi, M., & Cavagnini, F. (2006). Pericardial effusion requiring pericardiocentesis in a girl with anorexia nervosa. *The International Journal of Eating Disorders, 39,* 609–611.

Pope, H. G., Hudson, J. I., & Jonas, J. M. (1983). Bulimia treated with imipramine: a pleacebo-controlled, double-blind study. *American Journal of Psychiatry, 140,* 554–558.

Poulsen, S., Lunn, S., Daniel, S. I., Folke, S., Mathiesen, B. B., Katznelson, H., & Fairburn, C. G. (2014). A randomized controlled trial of psychoanalytic psychotherapy or cognitive-behavioral therapy for bulimia nervosa. *American Journal of Psychiatry, 171,* 109–116.

Ricca, V., Castellini, G., Lo Sauro, C., Mannucci, E., Ravaldi, C., Rotella, F., et al. (2010). Cognitive-behavioral therapy for threshold and subthreshold anorexia nervosa: A three-year follow-up study. *Psychotherapy and Psychosomatics, 79,* 238–248.

Rashid, N. (2006). Medically unexplained myopathy due to ipecac abuse. *Psychosomatics, 47,* 167–169.

Rigaud, D., Bedig, G., Merrouche, M., Vulpillat, M., Bonfils, S., & Apfebaum, M. (1998). Delayed gastric emptying in anorexia nervosa is improved by completion of a renutrition program. *Digestive Diseases and Sciences, 33,* 919–925.

Romano, S. J., Halmi, K. A., Sarkar, N. P., Koke, S. C., & Lee, J. S. (2002). A placebo-controlled study of fluoxetine in continued treatment of bulimia nervosa after successful acute fluoxetine treatment. *American Journal of Psychiatry, 159,* 96–102.

Root, T. L., Pesetsky, E. M., Thornton, L., Lichtenstein, P., Pedersen, N. L., & Bulik, C. M. (2010). Patterns of co-morbidity of eating disorders and substance use in Swedish females, *Psychological Medicine, 40,* 105–115.

Rushing, J. M., Jones, L. E., & Carney, C. P. (2003). Bulimia *Nervosa: A Primary Care Review. Primary Care Companion. Journal of Clinical Psychology, 5,* 217–224.

Sansone, R. A., & Sansone, L. A. (2010). Personality disorders as risk factors for eating disorders: clinical implications. *Nutrition in Clinical Practice, 25,* 116–121.

Schmidt, U., Lee, S., Beecham, J., Perkins, S., Treasure, J., Yi, I., et al. (2007). A randomized controlled trial of family therapy and cognitive behavior therapy guided self-care for adolescents with bulimia nervosa and related disorders. *The American Journal of Psychiatry, 164*, 591–598.

Schneider, D. J., Perez, A., Knilamus, T. E., Daniels, S. R., Bove, K. E., & Bonnell, H. (1996). Clinical and pathologic aspects of cardiomyopathy from ipecac administration in muchausen's syndrome by proxy. *Pediatrics, 97*, 902–906.

Sinicina, I., Pankratz, H., Büttner, A., & Mall, G. (2005). Death due to neurogenic shock following gastric rupture in an anorexia nervosa patient. *Forensic Science International, 155*, 7–12.

Sloan, D. M., Mizes, J. S., Helbok, C., & Muck, R. (2004). Efficacy of sertraline for bulimia nervosa. *The International Journal of Eating Disorders, 36*, 48–54.

Steinglass, J. E., Sysko, R., Glasofer, D., Albano, A. M., Simpson, H. B., & Walsh, B. T. (2010). Rationale for the application of exposure and response prevention to the treatment of anorexia nervosa. *International Journal of Eating Disorders, 44*, 134–141.

Steinglass, J., Sysko, R., Schebendach, J., Broft, A., Strober, M., & Walsh, B. T. (2007). The application of exposure therapy and D-cycloserine to the treatment of anorexia nervosa: A preliminary trial. *Journal of Psychiatric Practice, 13*, 238–245.

Striegel-Moore, R. H., Wilson, G. T., DeBar, L., Perrin, N., Lynch, F., Rosselli, F., et al. (2010). Cognitive behavioral guided self-help for the treatment of recurrent binge eating. *Journal of Consulting and Clinical Psychology, 78*, 312–321.

Suri, R., Poist, E. S., Hager, W. D., & Gross, J. B. (1999). Unrecognized bulimia nervosa: a potential cause of perioperative cardiac dysrhythmias. *Canadian Journal of Anesthesia, 46*, 1048–1052.

Sysko, R., & Walsh, B. T. (2008). A critical evaluation of the efficacy of self-help interventions for the treatment of bulimia nervosa and binge-eating disorder. *The International Journal of Eating Disorders, 41*, 97–112.

Takimoto, Y., Yoshiuchi, K., Kumano, H., & Kuboki, T. (2006). Bulimia nervosa and abnormal cardiac repolarization. *Journal of Psychosomatic Research, 60*, 105–107.

Takimoto, Y., Yoshiuchi, K., Kumano, H., Yamanaka, G., Sasaki, T., Suematsu, H., et al. (2004). QT interval and QT dispersion in eating disorders. *Psychotherapy and Psychosomatics, 73*(5), 324–328.

Tchanturia, K., Davies, H., & Campbell, I. C. (2007). Cognitive remediation therapy for patients with anorexia nervosa: Preliminary findings. *Annals of General Psychiatry, 6*, 14.

Tchanturia, K., Whitney, J., & Treasure, J. (2006). Can cognitive exercises help treat anorexia nervosa? *Eating and Weight Disorders, 11*, e112–e116.

Thomas, J. J., Eddy, K. T., Murray, H. B., Tromp, M. D. P., Hartmann, A. S., Stone, M. T., Levendusky, P. G., Becker, A. E. (under review). Impact of revised DSM-5 criteria on the relative distribution, comparative psychopathology, and inter-rater reliability of eating disorder diagnoses in a residential treatment setting.

Thomas, J. J., Vartanian, L. R., & Brownell, K. D. (2009). The relationship between eating disorder not otherwise specified (EDNOS) and officially recognized eating disorders: Meta-analysis and implications for DSM. *Psychological Bulletin, 135*, 407–433.

Vrabel, K. R., Ro, O., Martinsen, E. W., Hoffart, A., & Rosenvinge, J. H. (2010). Five-year prospective study of personality disorders in adults with longstanding eating disorders. *The International Journal of Eating Disorders, 43*, 22–28.

Wagner, A., Barbarich-Marsteller, N. C., Frank, G. K., Bailer, U. F., Wonderlich, S. A., Crosby, R. D., et al. (2006). Personality traits after recovery from eating disorders: Do subtypes differ? *International Journal of Eating Disorders, 39*, 276–284.

Waldholtz, B. D., & Andersen, A. E. (1990). Gastrointestinal symptoms in anorexia nervosa. A prospective study. *Gastroenterology, 98*, 1415–1419.

Walsh, B. F., Wilson, G. T., Loeb, K. L., Devlin, M. J., Pike, K. M., Roose, S. P., et al. (1997). Medication and psychotherapy in the treatment of bulimia nervosa. *American Journal of Psychiatry, 154*, 523–531.

Walsh, B. T., Agras, W. S., Devlin, M. J., Fairburn, C. G., Wilson, G. T., Kahn, C., & Chally, M. K. (2000). Fluoxetine for bulimia nervosa following poor response to psychotherapy. *American Journal of Psychiatry, 157*, 1332–1334.

Walsh, B. T., Kaplan, A. S., Attia, E., Olmsted, M., Parides, M., Carter, J. C., et al. (2006). Fluoxetine after weight restoration in anorexia nervosa: a randomized controlled trial. *The Journal of the American Medical Association, 295*, 2605–2612.

Walsh, B. T., Wong, L. M., Pesce, M. A., Hadigan, C. M., & Bodourian, S. H. (1990). Hyperamylasemia in bulimia nervosa. *Journal of Clinical Psychiatry, 51*, 373–377.

Walsh. (n.d.). Report of the DSM-5 Eating Disorders Work Group | APA DSM-5. *Home | APA DSM-5*. Retrieved February 21, 2011, from http://www.dsm5.org/ProgressReports/Pages/0904 Report of the DSM–V EatingDisordersWorkGroup.aspx

Wentz, E., Gillber, I. C., Anckarsater, H., Gillberg, C., & Rastam, M. (2006). Adolescent-onset anorexia nervosa: 18 year outcome. *The British Journal of Psychiatry, 39*, 87–100.

Wildes, J. E., & Marcus, M. D. (2011). Development of emotion acceptance behavior therapy for anorexia nervosa: A case series. *The International Journal of Eating Disorders, 44*(5), 421–427.

Wildes, J. E., Ringham, R. M., & Marcus, M. D. (2010). Emotion avoidance in patients with anorexia nervosa: Initial test of a functional model. *International Journal of Eating Disorders, 43*, 398–404.

Willfley, D. E., Crow, S. J., Hudson, J. I., Mitchell, J. E., Berkowitz, R. I., Blakesley, V., & Walsh, B. T. (2008). Efficacy of sibutramine for the treatment of binge eating disorder: a randomized multicenter placebo-controlled double-blind study. *The American Journal of Psychiatry, 165*, 51–58.

Wilson, G. T., Wilfley, D. E., Agras, W. S., & Bryson, S. W. (2010). Psychological treatments of binge eating disorder. *Archives of General Psychiatry, 67*, 94–101.

Wonderlich, S. A., Engel, S. G., Peterson, C. B., Robinson, M. D., Crosby, R. D., Mitchell, J. E., et al. (2008). Examining the conceptual model of integrative cognitive-affective therapy for BN: Two assessment studies. *The International Journal of Eating Disorders, 41*, 748–754.

Wonderlich, S. A., Peterson, C. B., Crosby, R. D., Smith, T. L., Klein, M. H., Mitchell, J. E., & Crow, S. J. (2014). A randomized controlled comparison of integrative cognitive-affective therapy (ICAT) and enhanced cognitive-behavioral therapy (CBT-E) for bulimia nervosa. *Psychological Medicine, 44*, 543–553.

Zipfel, S., Sammet, I., Rapps, N., Herzog, W., Herpertz, S., & Martens, U. (2006). Gastrointestinal disturbances in eating disorders: clinical and neurobiological aspects. *Autonomic Neuroscience, 129*, 99–106.

Zucker, N. L., Marcus, M., & Bulik, C. (2006). A group parent-training program: A novel approach for eating disorder management. *Eating and Weight Disorders, 11*, 78–82.

33.

PRIMARY SLEEP DISORDERS IN MEDICAL AND NEUROLOGICAL PATIENTS

Amit Chopra and Jarrett W. Richardson

INTRODUCTION

The consulting psychiatrist may be called on to help manage variety of psychiatric issues that arise during hospitalization in a medical or surgical setting, including intensive care settings. Sleep disturbances and their consequences are amongst the most common reasons for consultation. Assessment of sleep is a critical component of the psychiatric evaluation in medically ill patients due to multi-factorial etiology of sleep complaints in this population. Comorbid psychiatric disorders, iatrogenic causes, or an undiagnosed primary sleep disorder associated with medical/neurological disorders may lead to sleep complaints in hospitalized patients. This chapter reviews the spectrum of the primary sleep disorders commonly encountered in medical, neurological and ICU patients. This chapter also covers the effects on sleep of medications and environmental factors in hospital settings.

PRIMARY SLEEP DISORDERS IN MEDICAL PATIENTS

ENDOCRINE DISORDERS

Hypothyroidism

Patients with hypothyroidism may present with excessive sleepiness and fatigue. Polysomnography changes in sleep in hypothyroid patients include decreased slow wave sleep (SWS), which tends to normalize after thyroid replacement. A higher incidence of obstructive sleep apnea (OSA) has been noted in patients with untreated hypothyroidism. Factors such as obesity, myopathy, and upper airway edema may contribute to increased incidence of OSA in patients with hypothyroidism.

Acromegaly

Acromegaly is characterized by hypersecretion of growth hormone, usually secondary to pituitary adenoma. Approximately 60%–80% of the patients with acromegaly complain of sleep apnea which is primarily obstructive in nature, although,

central apnea is noted in one-third of the patients. Orofacial anatomic abnormalities secondary to excess growth hormone secretion may lead to development of sleep apnea in patients with acromegaly. Sleep evaluation should be considered in patients with suspected apnea syndromes. Neurosurgical treatment of pituitary adenoma and medication treatments including bromocriptine and octreotide may improve sleep apnea. Patients with persistent apneic episodes despite surgical and medical treatments may benefit from positive airway pressure therapy.

Cushing Syndrome

Patients with Cushing syndrome have an excess of adrenocorticosteroid hormones. Sleep complaints, including insomnia and OSA, are common. Fat accumulation in the parapharyngeal area may play an important role in pathogenesis of OSA. Polysomnography findings include changes in sleep architecture, decreased sleep efficiency, increased sleep fragmentation, decreased slow wave sleep, decreased REM latency, and increased REM density.

Diabetes Mellitus

Type 2 diabetes is a major public health concern with high morbidity, mortality, and health-care costs. Increased prevalence of sleep problems including difficulty initiating sleep, difficulty maintaining sleep, excessive daytime drowsiness, and sleep-disordered breathing have been reported in patients with type 2 diabetes mellitus.

A growing number of epidemiologic studies, originating from various geographic regions and involving diverse study populations, have suggested the existence of an independent link between markers of severity of OSA and an increased risk of type 2 diabetes. Numerous studies have examined the effects of continuous positive airway pressure (CPAP) treatment on glucose metabolism both in diabetic and nondiabetic populations. There is accumulating evidence suggesting that metabolic abnormalities can be partially corrected by CPAP treatment, which supports the concept of a causal link between OSA and altered glucose control.

The pathophysiological mechanisms leading to alterations in glucose metabolism in OSA patients are likely to be multiple. High sympathetic nervous system activity, intermittent hypoxia, sleep fragmentation and sleep loss, dysregulation of the hypothalamic-pituitary axis, endothelial dysfunction, and alterations in cytokine and adipokine release have all been proposed as potential mechanisms for abnormal glucose metabolism in OSA patients.

Obesity

Obesity is a serious medical disorder resulting in increased risk of morbidity and mortality due to both acute and chronic medical conditions. Sleep disorders including sleep-disordered breathing (SDB), excessive daytime somnolence, night eating syndrome, and sleep-related eating disorders have been noted in obese patients.

Increased incidence of SDB, including OSA and obesity hypoventilation syndrome, has been noted in obese patients. For every 10 kg increment in weight, the risk for OSA increases by more than twofold, while an increase in the body mass index (BMI) by one standard deviation is associated with a fourfold increase in the prevalence of OSA. The possible etiological factors may include gender (OSA more common in obese males), anatomical and neuromuscular factors, and hormonal and genetic factors.

Obesity hypoventilation syndrome is defined as a combination of obesity, chronic daytime hypercapnia ($PaCO_2 > 45$ mm Hg), and a SDB in the absence of other known causes of hypercapnia. The prevalence of OHS in sleep apnea syndrome is 8%–10% when BMI is between 30–34 kg/m2 and 18%–25% when BMI is >40 kg/m2. Conversely, not all patients with OHS have sleep apnea syndrome. In approximately 90% of patients with OHS the SDB consists of OSA. The remaining 10% of patients with OHS have an apnea–hypopnea index less than 5. The pathophysiology of OHS results from complex interactions, among which are increased work of breathing related to obesity, abnormal load responsiveness, and repeated airway occlusion during sleep.

The most important therapy for OSA in obese patients is weight loss. Weight loss changes pharyngeal anatomy and decreases airway collapsibility by increasing the pharyngeal closing pressure. A longitudinal study with a 4-year polysomnogram follow-up showed that a 3% change in AHI was noted with each percent change in weight. In one controlled study, 23 obese patients were assigned to receive either dietary counseling or no intervention. Those who experienced weight loss of 10 kg or more had significant reduction in apnea index (AI), improvement in daytime sleepiness, and oxyhemoglobin saturation. The most impressive results of AHI improvement are derived from those morbidly obese patients who underwent bariatric surgery. One of the studies noted a 72% reduction in the mean AHI of 47 morbidly obese patients after 1 year of undergoing Roux-en-Y gastric surgery. However, at 7-year follow-up, 47% had regained considerable weight and were diagnosed with severe OSA. Alternative treatment options for OSA and OHS in obese patients include CPAP and bilevel positive airway pressure (BPAP) devices.

PULMONARY DISORDERS

More than 50% of the patients with COPD experience difficulty initiating and maintaining sleep. Sleep is interrupted in COPD patients due to production of secretions, coughing, and dyspnea related to airway constriction. Patients complain of multiple awakenings during night, daytime fatigue and somnolence. COPD is associated with nocturnal hypoxemia, especially during REM sleep, due to loss of muscle tone of the accessory muscles of respiration during REM sleep. Coexistence of obstructive sleep apnea (OSA) and COPD is termed *overlap syndrome,* and its prevalence has been estimated at 29% according to one study. Patients with overlap syndrome are at greater risk of prolonged oxygen desaturations at night as compared to those with OSA alone, and it appears to be associated with increased morbidity and mortality in these patients. Treatment of OSA with CPAP therapy has been associated with improved outcomes and decreased mortality in patients with overlap syndrome.

Patients with restrictive lung disorders and chest wall abnormalities (kyphoscoliosis) are at risk of sleep related hypoventilation/hypoxemia. Polysomnography findings include frequent arousals, increased wakefulness after sleep onset, and nocturnal hypoxemia. Other consequences of nocturnal hypoxemia include pulmonary hypertension, *cor pulmonale,* and neurocognitive dysfunction. These patients likely require BPAP for treatment of sleep-related hypoventilation/hypoxemia.

CARDIOVASCULAR DISORDERS

Consistent data suggest strong associations between sleep-disordered breathing and hypertension, coronary artery disease, congestive heart failure, and cardiac arrhythmias. Potential mechanisms of increased of cardiovascular events in patients with OSA include increased sympathetic activity during sleep, inflammation due to increased proinflammatory cytokines in OSA, hypercoagulability, endothelial dysfunction, oxidative stress, and insulin resistance.

OSA has been implicated as a cause of nocturnal ST depression and angina pectoris. Higher incidence of fatal and non-fatal cardiovascular events has been reported in patients with severe OSA. Nocturnal arrhythmias may contribute to higher night time prevalence of sudden death in patients with OSA. Early recognition and treatment of sleep-disordered breathing with positive airway pressure therapy in patients with cardiovascular disorders has been associated with improved morbidity and mortality.

Patients with congestive heart failure (CHF) may develop both OSA and central sleep apnea (CSA). CHF patients CSA may develop Cheyne Stokes respiration (CSR) with periodic crescendo-decrescendo breathing accompanied with apneas predominantly during NREM stages 1 and 2. The risk factors for CSA-CSR pattern include old age, male gender, $PaCO_2$ <38 mm Hg, atrial fibrillation, and left ventricular ejection fraction <40%. CHF patients with CSA-CSR pattern have a greater mortality risk as compared to those without CSR pattern. Therapy for CSA-CSR pattern begins with optimization of medical treatment of heart failure. Treatment with CPAP, adaptive servoventilation device, and supplemental O2 should be considered for CSA-CSR.

RENAL DISORDERS

Sleep apnea is prevalent in over 50% of the patients with chronic kidney disease (CKD) and end stage renal disease (ESRD). Factors including fluid overload and altered control of breathing have been proposed as causative factors for sleep apnea in ESRD patients.

Presence of untreated sleep apnea in CKD and ESRD patients may have detrimental effect on renal function as sleep apnea has been associated with nocturnal hypoxemia, increased systemic blood pressure, inflammatory cytokines, and increased sympathetic activity. In addition, sleep apnea can lead to disturbed night sleep, daytime sleepiness, and diminished quality of life in these patients. Use of positive airway pressure therapy, nocturnal hemodialysis, and renal transplant have been found to be effective in treatment of sleep apnea in CKD and ESRD.

Patients with CKD and ESRD also have increased prevalence (20%–80%) of restless legs syndrome and periodic limb movement disorder leading to sleep disruption. Increased periodic limb movement index may adversely affect sleep continuity and lead to cyclical apneas due to ventilatory instability. Periodic limb movement disorder has been shown to be better predictor of mortality than serum albumin and other parameters monitored in dialysis patients. Treatment with dopamine agonists and gabapentin (adjusted dose due to renal elimination) may be helpful in these patients. Iron supplementation and erythropoietin for correction of anemia may be considered as well.

GASTROINTESTINAL DISORDERS

Nocturnal gastroesophageal reflux disease (GERD) appears to be common in patients with OSA. In one study, approximately 50% of the episodes of GERD occurring in patients with OSA were related to apneas or hypopneas. Polysomnography findings in patients with GERD include repeated arousals followed by swallowing as represented by an increase in chin EMG activity. GERD episodes may be related to sleep-related laryngospasm which is characterized by sudden awakening accompanied with sensation of suffocation and apnea lasting from 5–45 seconds followed by stridor.

Therapy may involve elevating the head of the bed, pharmacotherapy (proton pump inhibitors), or antireflux surgery. CPAP therapy has been shown to decrease the frequency of nocturnal GERD symptoms both in patients with and without OSA. This antireflux activity may be attributed to elevation of intraesophageal pressure as well as to constriction of lower esophageal sphincter.

RHEUMATOLOGICAL DISORDERS

Arthritis is the leading cause of chronic illness in the United States.

Seventy-two percent of the adults aged 55 years and older with arthritis report sleep difficulties.

Sleep complaints and related daytime symptoms occur in 54%–70% of adult Rheumatoid arthritis (RA) patients, including difficulty falling asleep, poor quality sleep, non-restorative sleep, numerous awakenings during the night, early morning awakening, excessive daytime sleepiness, and fatigue. Sleep architecture—total sleep time, rapid eye movement (REM) sleep latency, non-REM (NREM) sleep stages, REM sleep, and number of sleep cycles—in RA patients is usually normal. NREM sleep latency is usually normal but may be prolonged during disease flare.

Improvement in sleep parameters, including an increase in SWS together with a decrease in REM sleep, correlated with a decrease in pain and morning stiffness; a decrease in wake stage was followed by a decrease in pain level and morning stiffness in RA. Associated primary sleep disorders, including sleep apnea and periodic leg movements of sleep can impair sleep. Sleep apnea affects 7.5%–30.8% in RA subjects and can result from temporomandibular joint destruction narrowing the posterior airspace or compromised position of the head and neck, limited mouth opening, and distorted anatomy with reduced upper airway tone. Depressive symptoms are present in 13%–20% of RA patients. Data from studies in RA patients suggest that pain exacerbates sleep complaints in RA patients and that both pain and sleep disturbances may contribute to depression.

Systemic lupus erythematosus (SLE) is associated with complaints of poor sleep quality, fatigue, pain, and depression. Polysomnographic findings associated with increased disease activity include reduced sleep efficiency, reduced delta sleep, sleep fragmentation, increased arousals, and alpha intrusions. Associated primary sleep disorders include sleep apnea, periodic leg movements of sleep, and narcolepsy with cataplexy. Pain, depression, and insomnia are common complaints associated with osteoarthritis. Polysomnography demonstrates increased Stage 1 NREM sleep, reduced Stage 2 NREM sleep, and increased sleep fragmentation.

Adequate treatment of arthritic pain, use of cognitive behavioral therapy for insomnia (CBT-I), and/or judicious use of hypnotic/sedative medications along with assessment of comorbid depressive symptoms should be considered for insomnia related to rheumatological disorders. Associated sleep disorders include sleep apnea, narcolepsy, and periodic limb movements of sleep; these should be adequately treated to improve outcomes.

CHRONIC FATIGUE AND FIBROMYALGIA SYNDROMES

Sleep disorders—including insomnia, restless legs syndrome, periodic leg movements of sleep, and sleep-disordered breathing—are common in chronic fatigue and fibromyalgia syndromes. PSG findings in fibromyalgia patients include poor sleep efficiency, slightly longer sleep latency with increased wakefulness in the first half of the night. In CFS, longer sleep latency (including REM sleep latency) with reduced REM sleep have been noted. Non-restorative sleep has been linked to alpha activity in

NREM sleep in fibromyalgia patients, although this may be a nonspecific finding and has not been correlated with symptom severity. Fibromyalgia patients have been shown to consistently demonstrate fewer sleep spindles during stage 2 of sleep.

PAIN SYNDROMES (ACUTE AND CHRONIC)

Sleep and pain appear to have bidirectional interaction as pain can lead to sleep interruption, and, conversely, poor sleep can magnify perception of pain intensity. Patients with acute post-operative pain demonstrate shortened and fragmented sleep reduced amount of slow wave and REM sleep as demonstrated in polysomnography studies. The sleep architecture tends to normalize after resolution of acute pain.

Patients with chronic pain often complain of insomnia and daytime somnolence and inactivity, which further exacerbate insomnia. Iatrogenic sleep disturbances due to medications, especially opiates, may further worsen symptoms of daytime drowsiness and fatigue. Patients on chronic opiate therapy, especially at higher doses, are at greater risk of development of central sleep apnea syndromes. Development of depression in patients with chronic pain may further lead to sleep disturbances.

Treatment of sleep disturbances in patients with pain syndromes involves adequate management of pain with judicious use of painkiller medications, adequate sleep hygiene, physical exercise, and treatment of comorbid psychiatric disorders such as depression. Patients with chronic pain refractory to pain medications should be considered for referral to chronic pain management programs. Use of medications such as benzodiazepines in patients on chronic opiate treatment is a concern due to risk of respiratory depression, worsening of sleep apnea syndromes, and increased daytime sedation. Nonmedication therapies such as CBT for insomnia may as well be considered in these patients.

MALIGNANCY

Cancer patients frequently report disturbed sleep and daytime fatigue as distressing symptoms; sleep disturbances may be prevalent in 40%–50% of cancer patients. Prevalence of sleep disturbance may be relatively higher in younger patients (54%), and it may be attributed to higher rates of anxiety and depression in younger patients. Pain, depression, and anxiety are among the common etiologic factors for sleep disturbances—although other factors, including delirium in the later stages of malignant illness, medications (steroids, bronchodilators, chemotherapeutic agents), and environmental factors in institutionalized patients may also be implicated. Adequate treatment of pain has been associated with increases in total sleep time and sleep quality in cancer patients. Recognition and treatment of depression and anxiety can be associated with improved sleep outcomes in cancer patients.

HIV/AIDS

Insomnia has been reported in 73% of the patients meeting criteria for HIV/AIDS and risk factors for insomnia include anxiety, depression, and cognitive impairment. Somatic symptoms associated with sleep disturbance in HIV/AIDS patients include night sweats, chills, headache, and diarrhea. Polysomnography studies show increased slow-wave sleep in patients with early asymptomatic HIV infection. These findings have been linked to release of cytokines (sleep inducing effect), which are also associated with fatigue and subjective sleepiness. Slow wave sleep has been reported to be decreased in patients with advanced AIDS.

Addressing sleep complaints in HIV/AIDS patients involves comprehensive assessment and treatment of factors such as aggressive management of CNS involvement (CNS metastases, delirium, AIDS-related complex), adequate management of pain, amelioration of medical symptoms (including cough, dyspnea, headaches and diarrhea), and adequate treatment of anxiety and depression. In addition, other measures including sleep hygiene, progressive muscle relaxation, biofeedback, and guided imagery may be helpful.

PRIMARY SLEEP DISORDERS IN NEUROLOGICAL PATIENTS

ALZHEIMER'S DEMENTIA

Sleep disorders in Alzheimer's dementia (AD) are frequently correlated with severity of disease progression. Sleep disorders may range from insomnia, hypersomnia, SDB, parasomnias, sleep-related movement disorders, and circadian rhythm sleep disorders. Polysomnography findings in AD patients include reduced sleep efficiency, reduced sleep time, reduction in spindles and K complexes, reduced REM sleep, and increased arousals. Sleep fragmentation is associated with insomnia, nocturnal wandering, daytime sleepiness and cognitive impairment. Degeneration of specific nuclei in the brain including cholinergic neurons in the nucleus basalis of Meynert, pedunculopontine nucleus, and laterodorsal tegmental nuclei may be implicated in decreased REM sleep in AD patients. Degeneration of suprachiasmatic nucleus is thought to be primarily responsible for circadian rhythm disorders in AD.

Nonpharmacological interventions for sleep disorders include behavioral, environmental, psychosocial management (CBT), and support and education for families have been associated with improved outcomes in AD patients. Treatable causes of sleep disruption including anxiety, depression, and sleep apnea should be addressed. Phototherapy may be helpful in AD patients with circadian rhythm disorders. Medications such as sedatives-hypnotics should be used cautiously due to risk of falls, cognitive impairment, and worsening of preexisting SDB. Medications may be used in AD patients with severe nocturnal agitation and agents such as trazodone and low dose antipsychotics can be considered for specific target symptoms. The use of these medications should be carefully and regularly reviewed due to potential drug-associated adverse effects.

PARKINSON'S DISEASE

Sleep complaints are common non-motor symptoms of Parkinson's disease and related syndromes with prevalence in 60%–90% of the patients. Sleep disorders can range from insomnia, sleep fragmentation, early morning awakenings, restless legs syndrome, REM sleep behavior disorder, excessive daytime drowsiness, and sleep attacks. Polysomnographic findings in PD patients include decreased total sleep time, poor sleep efficiency, reduced SWS, reduced REM sleep, and REM sleep without atonia. The etiology of sleep problems in PD is multifactorial including motor symptoms of PD (difficulty turning in bed, dyskinesias) interrupting sleep, comorbid psychiatric disorders (depression and anxiety), and medication effects. Sleep disturbance, depression, and lack of independence are the primary determinants of poor quality of life.

Improved sleep hygiene plays an important role in treatment of insomnia in PD patients. Use of dopaminergic agents to treat motor symptoms of PD is the mainstay of treatment. Preliminary evidence suggests that deep brain stimulation for treatment of advanced PD may improve sleep architecture, restless legs syndrome, and daytime sleepiness, although deep brain stimulation has no impact on REM sleep behavior disorder (RBD). Treatment of restless legs syndrome with dopamine agonists (pramipexole/ropinirole) should be considered, as L-dopa treatment may be associated with increased rates of augmentation as compared to dopamine agonists. RBD symptoms may respond to treatment with low-dose clonazepam and melatonin. Comorbid psychiatric disorders such as anxiety and depression should be adequately treated using medication and psychological therapies. Close monitoring of side effects of anti-parkinsonian medications including excessive daytime drowsiness and hallucinations is essential. Adjustment in medication dosages under the supervision of neurologists and use of low dose atypical antipsychotics (quetiapine, clozapine) may be effective in treatment of dopaminergic-induced hallucinations.

EPILEPSY

The interactions between sleep and epilepsy are complex and multidimensional. Sleep deprivation can activate epileptiform activity and interfere with seizure control whereas seizures can disrupt sleep, especially nocturnal epilepsy syndromes, and lead to excessive daytime drowsiness, as do anticonvulsant medications. NREM sleep has been associated with greater tendency for propagation of epileptiform discharges when compared to REM sleep due to excessive diffuse cortical synchronization. Polysomnography findings in epilepsy patients include increase in sleep latency, increase wake time after sleep onset, increased N1 and N2 sleep, and decreased slow wave and REM sleep.

Certain seizure disorders occur predominantly or exclusively during sleep and these may include nocturnal frontal lobe epilepsy (NFLE), benign rolandic epilepsy of childhood with centrotemporal spikes, and juvenile myoclonic epilepsy. Clinical features of sleep-related seizures include abrupt awakenings, abnormal motor activity (automatisms, focal or generalized tonic clonic movements, tongue biting), and urinary incontinence. Postictal confusion may be evident after nocturnal seizures. Abnormal sleep related behaviors such as parasomnias and pseudo-seizures need to be considered in differential diagnosis of nocturnal epilepsy syndromes.

Obstructive sleep apnea (OSA) may have detrimental effects on various aspects of epilepsy: seizure control, mood disorders, cognitive dysfunction, and quality of life. Higher prevalence (up to 30%) of OSA has been reported in drug-resistant epilepsy patients (Malow, Levy, Maturen, & Bowes, 2000), while older epilepsy patients with OSA have been found to show poor seizure control compared with age-matched epilepsy patients not affected by OSA (Chihorek, Abou-Khalil, & Malow, 2007). Continuous positive airway pressure treatment (CPAP) of patients with epilepsy and OSA was found to reduce EEG interictal epileptiform activity (Oliveira, Zamagni, Dolso, Bassetti, & Gigli, 2000) and improved seizure control after CPAP in epilepsy patients with coexisting OSA has also been reported. In a pilot study of patients with drug-resistant epilepsy plus OSA, randomized to receive therapeutic or sham continuous CPAP, seizures were reduced by 50% or more (compared with the baseline period) in 28% of the patients undergoing therapeutic CPAP versus 15% of those receiving sham CPAP (Malow, Foldvary-Schaefer, Vaughn, Selwa, Chervin, et al., 2008).

Several factors can contribute to insomnia in epilepsy patients. These include the fragmentation of sleep due to recurrent seizures; the effects of some antiepileptic drugs (AEDs) such as lamotrigine, felbamate and levetiracetam; and the effects of comorbid anxiety and depression. Sleep fragmentation is frequently reported in nocturnal frontal lobel epilepsy (NFLE) and also in temporal lobe epilepsy (TLE), in which the frequent association with depression may also play an important role in inducing insomnia. Epileptic patients with sleep disturbance, mainly those with insomnia, were reported to have quality of life scores lower than patients without sleep complaints (Piperidou, Karlovasitou, Triantafyllou, Terzoudi, Constantinidis, et al., 2008a; Piperidou, Karlovasitou, Triantafyllou, Dimitrakoudi, Terzoudi, et al., 2008b).

Epilepsy patients frequently experience excessive daytime sleepiness (EDS), a complaint of multifactorial origin. Factors associated with EDS in epilepsy patients include poor or insufficient sleep, nocturnal seizures, AEDs, depression, and sleep disorders such as OSA (Manni & Tartara, 2000).

STROKE

Patients with deep hemispheric lesions may present with increased yawning and hypersomnia, while patients with thalamic, subcortical, and pontine strokes are likely to suffer from insomnia. Comorbid depression may further contribute to sleep disturbances in stroke patients.

Higher prevalence of OSA (up to 60%) has been noted in patients with cerebrovascular events. OSA is the most common form of SDB in these patients, whereas CSA and Cheyne stokes breathing pattern may be present in 30%–40% of the patients. OSA is known to increase the risk of cerebrovascular disease, with obstructive apneas being associated with cerebral hypoperfusion. Other factors such as altered cerebral autoregulation, impaired endothelial function, and accelerated proinflammatory states may play a role as well.

Restless legs syndrome has been noted in patients with pontine, thalamic, basal ganglia and corona radiata infarcts. Pontine tegmental strokes can lead to RBD, where patients can act out violent dreams with evidence of REM sleep without atonia on polysomnography studies. Sleep disordered breathing and sleep–wake disturbances negatively affect short and long term stroke outcomes, length of hospitalization, and stroke recurrence risk.

CPAP therapy is the treatment of choice for obstructive sleep apnea (OSA) and this treatment has potential to reverse vascular risk in stroke patients. An adaptive servoventilation device should be considered for treatment of central sleep apnea syndromes. Hypnotics and sedative antidepressants may aggravate SDB and neurologic recovery and should be used with caution. Modafinil or activating antidepressants may be considered for management of hypersomnia. Poststroke sleep-related movement disorders can be treated with dopaminergic drugs (pramipexole/ropinirole); REM sleep behavior disorder can be treated with clonazepam or melatonin (Hermann & Bassetti, 2009).

TRAUMATIC BRAIN INJURY

Approximately 30%–70% of the patients with TBI experience sleep disturbances which often exacerbate TBI symptoms and impede both rehabilitation process and ability to return to work. Insomnia is one of the most common and well documented syndromes seen in patients with TBI. Risk factors associated with insomnia include mild TBI, higher levels of fatigue, depression, and pain. Insomnia not only represents a problem immediately following injury but also appears to persist for months and years after a TBI. Insomnia is often associated with daytime fatigue and drowsiness in TBI patients.

Higher incidence of other sleep disorders including OSA, periodic limb movements, and narcolepsy has been noted in TBI patients. Among circadian rhythm disorders, delayed sleep phase syndrome is the most common and is often misinterpreted as insomnia by patients and clinicians alike (Orff, Ayalon, & Drummond, 2009).

Cognitive behavioral therapy for insomnia (CBT-I) holds promise for treatment of insomnia in general but the use of this therapy is not extensively studied in these patients. Use of hypnotic medications should be carefully considered due to potential side effects including daytime drowsiness, dizziness or lightheadedness, and cognitive and psychomotor impairments, all of which are likely to be particularly detrimental for TBI patients. Treatment of delayed sleep phase syndrome in TBI patients can be considered with use of bright light therapy in the morning and use of low dose melatonin in the evening time. TBI patients with suspected SDB should undergo polysomnography evaluation and use of CPAP for treatment of OSA should be considered. Daytime hypersomnia may respond to use of modafinil or stimulant medications.

PRIMARY SLEEP DISORDERS IN CRITICALLY ILL PATIENTS (ICU SETTING)

Sleep disruption and deprivation with resultant daytime sleepiness are common phenomenon in ICU patients and are result of multitude of factors including acute illness, iatrogenic factors (medications, medical interventions), pain, environmental (sound and light exposure), and psychosocial factors. Polysomnography studies in ICU patients have shown prolonged sleep latency, decreased sleep efficiency, predominance of stage 1 and 2 NREM sleep, decreased or absent stage 3 NREM and REM sleep, and sleep fragmentation associated with frequent arousals. Those factors endorsed by patients to be most stressful in the ICU setting are the presence of endotracheal tubes, being injected with needles, experiencing pain, and being physically disturbed (Cochran & Ganong, 1989). According to nursing literature in the ICU setting, being restrained and experiencing loss of personal control have the most distressing effect on patients.

Parasomnias are common problems for patients with significant medical disorders. Of the injurious sleep-related behavior that occurs in hospitalized patients, REM sleep behavior disorder is the most common (85%) in the ICU, and night terrors and sleepwalking accounting for the remainder (Schenck & Mahowald, 1991). Parasomnias associated with ICU situations include (1) parasomnias originating in the ICU (e.g., stroke-induced); (2) admission to ICUs resulting from parasomnia-induced injuries; and (3) parasomnias in patients admitted to ICU for other medical problems. Parasomnias including REM sleep behavior disorder, night terrors, somnambulism, and confusional arousals in hospitalized patients, particularly those with known CNS disorders (dementia syndromes, Parkinson's disease, CVAs, and toxic/metabolic states), are important in the differential diagnosis of patients with nocturnal injurious behavior.

Changes in behavior and cognition have been associated with sleep deprivation in ICU patients and these include fatigue, mood changes, irritability, disorientation, short-term memory impairment, perceptual disturbances and visual hallucinations. Sleep deprivation has been considered as an important contributor to the development of ICU syndrome which is noted in up to 40% of the patients admitted to the ICU. Delirium with sleep–wake irregularities is integral to the ICU syndrome. The symptoms of ICU syndrome are rapid in onset and include disorientation, fluctuating levels of consciousness, delusions, hallucinations, and behavioral symptoms including aggression, lasting generally for 24–48 hours.

Daytime sleepiness and cognitive impairment associated with sleep disturbance can compromise the ability of ICU patients to engage in complex tasks such as respiratory muscle training, coughing, and deep breathing that are required to facilitate weaning from mechanical ventilation. Sleep disturbance in the ICU has been associated with increased morbidity and mortality, which is at least partly due to the impaired cellular function and immunity that results from sleep disturbance (Krachman, S'Alonzo, & Criner, 1995). Sleep disturbance in the ICU that persists after hospitalization has been associated with poor outcomes (Hurel, Loirat, Saulnier, Nicolas, & Brivet, 1997).

Interventions used in ICU settings to improve sleep and behavioral symptoms vary from supportive care to aggressive pharmacological management. These interventions may include providing psychological support, minimizing environmental noise and light exposure during night, optimizing pain treatment, avoidance of medications disrupting sleep architecture, orientation to day/night patterns, and judicious use of sedative/hypnotic medications. Medications including benzodiazepines and opiates may be associated with respiratory depression and worsening of SDB in patients, and therefore should be used carefully. Medical management of severely disrupted sleep/wake patterns may include aggressive pharmacologic overnight sedation with intravenous midazolam or propofol in the ICU, which has been shown to benefit sleep but not necessarily reduce anxiety or depression (Treggiari-Venzi, Borgeat, Fuchs-Buder, Gachoud, & Suter, 1996; Krachman, S'Alonzo, & Criner, 1995).

EFFECT OF MEDICATIONS

In addition to the effects of the primary illness, pain, environmental disturbances, and caregiver influences, many of the medications that are used to treat medically ill patients have significant effects on sleep. As a rule, any drug that crosses the blood–brain barrier is likely to have an effect on receptors that affect sleep. Sleep is known to be affected by the action of drugs on many receptors, as seen in Table 33.1 (Pascue, 1994). Essentially all centrally acting substances that have been studied have been found to have effects on sleep. Some agents affect primarily the circadian pacemaker

Table 33.1 RELATIONSHIP OF NEURO-TRANSMITTERS TO SLEEP

5HT	(agonist—normal activity helps with sleep maintenance, excessive 5HT activity leads to increased number of awakenings, more stage one and less stage REM sleep)
NE	(agonist—normal activity helps with sustained alertness, excessive NE activity leads to sleep disruption)
	(antagonist—leads to sedation)
DA	(agonist—excessive activity leads to increased wakefulness)
	(antagonist—leads to sedation)
Ach	(agonist—activity higher in REM than non-REM sleep, and increased in daytime arousal; excessive activity leads to excessive arousal)
	(antagonist—anticholinergic activity decreases REM-related phenomena)
H1	(antagonists—produce increased daytime drowsiness but little effect on Wake After Sleep Onset)
	(agonists—lead to increased wakefulness)
H2	(antagonists—little effect on daytime or sleep but have been reported to cause confusion)
H3	(regulates histamine release—agonist produces deeper sleep in rats)
	Adenosine (neuromodulator—inhibits release of Ach, NE, DA, 5HT, GABA)
	(antagonism by methylxanthines is excitatory)

system—arginine-vasopressin, GABA, melatonin, gastrin-releasing peptide, neuropeptide-Y, peptide histidine isoleucine, vasoactive intestinal peptide, glutamate, pancreatic polypeptide, and corticosteroids (Dawson & Armstrong, 1996).

Other substances and medications affect various sleep components such as initial sleep latency, number of awakenings, number of sleep stage shifts, percent stage one, percent stage two, percent REM sleep, REM sleep density, REM sleep latency, slow wave sleep, and the number of arousals or discontinuities in sleep as well as evidences of sleep interruptions manifest by alpha rhythm intrusion or K-complexes. Many medications have sedating effects during the daytime that adversely affect subjective or objective functioning, and drugs that disturb sleep may lead to similar daytime problems (Dietrich, 1997; Liborio & Terzano, 1996; Nicholson, Bradley, & Pascoe, 1994; Novak & Shapiro, 1997; Obermeyer & Benca, 1996). See Table 33.2 and chapters 30 and 31.

Very few drugs have a beneficial effect on sleep, and drugs may have different effects on normal subjects than on patients with an illness. Drugs generally decrease slow wave sleep and decrease REM sleep unless proven otherwise. The exceptions are few and seldom helpful enough to compensate for other adverse effects on sleep properties. Alcohol in healthy young adults, lithium, clonidine (a_2 agonist), some TCAs, and chlorpromazine have been reported in some limited situations to increase slow wave sleep. Reserpine, yohimbine (a_2 antagonist), physostigmine (cholinomimetic), and steroids under certain circumstances increase REM sleep. Some drugs that may initially increase a particular sleep component over time will decrease this stage of sleep if administration is continued. If the drug improves some underlying disorder with secondary improvement in sleep, only then is it likely to have long-term benefit.

Rather than assume that these various factors are too complex to be useful in the psychiatric care of the medically ill patient, the medical psychiatrist can learn the few basic groups of drugs that have demonstrated empirically significant effects on sleep, and use knowledge of sleep physiology to logically infer the effects of most other drugs on sleep. Another way to organize an understanding of effects of drugs on sleep is to group drugs according to their most likely adverse effects on sleep/wake behavior (Novak & Shapiro, 1997). Drugs most likely to cause insomnia are those that are CNS stimulants such as ephedrine, caffeine, anorectics, amphetamines, and methylphenidate. Drugs that disturb REM sleep may produce nightmares and other sleep disturbance (e.g., opioids, corticosteroids) that also commonly lead to increased wake after sleep onset, and increased number of awakenings.

Drugs that most commonly cause parasomnias include TCAs, which lead to an increased incidence of periodic limb movements (PLMS), and drugs that are most commonly associated with nightmares such as corticosteroids, certain antineoplastic agents, MAOIs, L-dopa, and certain antihypertensive agents (particularly a_2 antagonists, lipophilic beta blockers such as propranolol, and reserpine). Abrupt withdrawal from agents that suppress REM sleep can also produce nightmares. In particular, withdrawal from sedative/hypnotics, TCAs, MAOIs, and venlafaxine commonly

Table 33.2 EFFECTS OF MEDICATIONS ON SLEEP

SUBSTANCE	TST	#A	SL	%II	%SWS	% REM	REML	INSOMNIA	VIGILANCE	SEDATION	PARA
ACETYLCHOLINESTERASE INHIBITORS											
ALCOHOL											
Acute	1	–	–		1	–	1	6			1
Withdrawal	–	1	1		–	1	–	1	1		111
ANALGESICS											
Opioids											
Acute	6	1	–		–	–		6		1	1
Withdrawal	–	1	1	–	–						
Acetyl salicylic acid		1	1	1	–						
ANORECTICS								1			
ANTIBIOTIC											
Quinolones						–		1			
ANTICHOLINERGICS		–	–	1		–	1			6	6
ANTICONVULSANTS											
Carbamazepine	1						1			1	
Phenytoin	–		–								
Valproate	1									1	
ANTIDEPRESSANTS											
Bupropion								1		Nightmares and PLMs	
MAOI											
Acute	–					–	1				
Withdrawal					1	1	1				
Mirtazepine	–	–		1					–		
SSRI	6	6	6			–	1	6		6	
Trazodone	–	–		1			1			1	

(*continued*)

Table 33.2 (CONTINUED)

SUBSTANCE	TST	#A	SL	%II	%SWS	% REM	REML	INSOMNIA	VIGILANCE	SEDATION	PARA
Tricyclics											
Acute	1	–	6	1		–	–				
Withdrawal	–	1	1			1	1	1			
Venlafaxine	1	–	–	1							
ANTIHISTAMINES											
H1 agonists		11								1	
H1 antagonists		–									
ANTIHYPERTENSIVES											
2 agonist	1	1	1	1	–		1			1	Nightmares
1 antagonist	1									1	
ACE inhibitors											Nightmares
B-blocker											
Lipophilic		1				–			–		Nightmares
Ca channel agonist								1			
5HT2 agonist					1						
Methyldopa		–				1	–				Nightmares
ANTINEOPLASTIC											
Flutamide							1	1		1	Nightmares
Procarbazine		1								1	Nightmares
Interferons					1			–			
ANTIPARKINSONIAN											
L-dopa											
Acute	–	1			–	–		1			Nightmares
Chronic								1			
Amantadine	1	–						–			
Selegiline											

	SL	%II	%SWS	%REM	TST	#A	REML	
ANTIPSYCHOTICS								
Acute	1	–	–	1	1	–	1	
Withdrawal	–	1	1	–	–	1	1	
ANXIOLYTICS							1	
Buspirone								
BARBITURATES AND								
BENZODIAZEPINES	1	–	–	1	1	–	1	
Acute	–	1	1	–	1		1	
Withdrawal	–	1	1					
CAFFEINE	1	1	1	–	1	1		Nightmares
CORTICOSTEROIDS	1	1	1	–	–	1	1	
LITHIUM								
NICOTINE	–	–						
Acute	1	1					1	
Withdrawal	–	1	1	–	1	1	1	
STIMULANTS	1	–						
TETRAHYDROCANNABINOL	1	1	1		1		1	
Yohimbine								

(1) = that the drug is known to produce an increase in the sleep parameter or phenomenon; (–) = that the drug is known to produce a decrease in the sleep parameter or phenomenon; (6) = that the drug is known to produce variable effect on the sleep parameter or phenomenon; (blank) = indicates that there are no reliable data on the effect of this drug on sleep parameters; (11) or (111) = degree of the effect; (NO) = zero effect; TST = total sleep time; #A = number of arousals; SL = sleep latency; %II = percentage stage II sleep; %SWS = percent slow wave sleep; %REM = percent rapid eye movement sleep; REML = REM sleep latency.

produce REM sleep rebound and often nightmares, though withdrawal from other antidepressants can, less commonly, cause sleep disturbance.

Excessive daytime sleepiness is associated with drugs that cause sleep loss or sleep disruption as well as withdrawal from chronic CNS stimulants and direct effects of opioids, antihistamines, certain beta blockers, and many dopamine antagonists including antiemetics. Hypnotics such as flurazepam, with long half-lives or active metabolites that have long half-lives, commonly produce daytime "hangovers" and sedation.

Neuroleptics, commonly used in medical patients for psychosis, delirium, and behavior dyscontrol, may produce akathisia that may be manifest as disturbances in nocturnal sleep/wake behavior. Typical neuroleptics may worsen sleep by exacerbating an underlying restless legs syndrome and periodic movements in sleep. The differential diagnosis between these two phenomena is often difficult. Distinguishing features are that akathisia is not characteristically predominant in the evening and at bedtime as is the syndrome of restless legs. Restless legs are not commonly manifest in the morning or midday hours, except in advanced cases. The differential diagnosis is important because of significant differences in recommended treatment. Treatment for akathisia is reduction of the neuroleptic (or rarely an SSRI), introduction of anticholinergic agents, or low-dose propranolol. Appropriate treatment of restless legs syndrome is reduction of the exacerbating agent, the addition of dopaminergic agents or clonazepam, or, in severe cases, narcotics.

Another source of complexity in evaluating the sleep in medical patients is the increasingly common use of unregulated over-the-counter herbal preparations. Aside from the likelihood that these preparations may be contaminated with unknown substances (antiinflammatory agents, steroids, diuretics, antihistamines, tranquilizers, hormones, and heavy metals), there is more information becoming available about potential adverse effects of herbal preparations taken as sleep aids, daytime stimulants, or for other purposes. Table 33.3 indicates toxicity described from the use of herbal substances for sedative or stimulant purposes as abstracted from a review of the use of herbal medications among consultation populations (Crone & Wise, 1998).

HOSPITAL ENVIRONMENTAL FACTORS

Hospitalization is in itself anxiety provoking, with the presence of the significant illness that led to admission amplified by a strange environment and the attendant procedures, many of which are painful and require preparation that may be uncomfortable at least. In addition, care routines seldom conform to the patient's home schedule, and new nursing personnel appear at least three times a day. The cadre of laboratory workers, medical students, residents, fellows and attendings, and consulting services have a schedule of their own that keep days very active and often allow little time for rest and recuperation from the previous tests or procedures.

The hospital day usually begins very early, as the patient is awakened from (usually) a restless night's sleep in a strange room with a strange bed. The first experience in the morning is often a needle stick for blood work, an opportunity for a hurried bath, and preparations for tests that may include enemas and missed meals. The familiar bed partner's absence and changes in ambient noises and temperatures also contribute to unsettled sleep patterns and sleep depth, resulting in fragmented sleep and disturbed circadian rhythms. The many circadian, hormonal, and behavioral factors that contribute to stable state of well-being are disrupted, and there is seldom any exposure to ambient light of the right frequency, strength, and duration to reset the important internal sleep–wake cycle

Table 33.3 HERBAL MEDICATIONS WITH SLEEP/WAKE TOXICITY

HERBAL MEDICATIONS	TOXICITY
Preparations used as sedatives	
Broom (*Cystisus scoparius*)	vomiting, uterine contractions, bradycardia
Kava Kava (*Piper methysticum*)	dermatitis, hallucinations, shortness of breath
Passion flower (*Passiflora caerulea*)	seizures, hypotension, hallucinations
Valerian (*Valeriana officinalis*)	dystonic reactions, hepatotoxicity
Preparations with excessive stimulation and insomnia as side/toxic effects	
Echinacea (*Echinacea augustifolia* or E. purpurea)	central nervous system stimulant, dermatitis, anaphylaxis
Ginseng (*Panax ginseng*)	hypertension, mastalgia, agitation, anxiety, depression, insomnia
Golden seal (*Hydrastis canadensis*)	nausea and vomiting, central nervous system stimulant, paralysis/paresthesia, respiratory failure
Ma huang (*Ephedra sinica*)	mania/psychosis, hypertension, tachycardia
Yohimbine bark (*Pausinystalia yohimbine* or *Corynanthe yohimbe*)	hallucinogen/anxiety, hypertension/tachycardia, nausea/vomiting

pacemakers. Medications may be changed or administered at unfamiliar times, and any over-the-counter pain or sleeping medications that patients have been taking are often omitted.

In addition to these changes in the patient's experience, the staff working with the patient may be either sleep-deprived or functioning on a poorly organized shift-work schedule so that suboptimal emotional and intellectual functioning is the norm rather than the exception in many hospitals. In a setting where extra patience and sensitivity is needed by the patient, staff—particularly junior medical and nursing staff—are themselves anxious and under a great deal of pressure, something that patients often perceive and that adds to their own anxiety.

The minimal effect of all these factors is a tired patient who has some difficulty cooperating maximally with needed care and tests/procedures. Often the patient is also irritable or hypersensitive to perceived slowness of response to calls for help, and interpersonal conflicts with caregivers may arise over otherwise relatively insignificant issues. This phenomenon may lead to changes in the caregivers' approach to the patient, which escalates rather than diffuses things. By the time a psychiatry consult is called, psychological concerns may have been greatly amplified.

While sleep-related problems in the hospital have been noted for many years as being important, formal studies have only been done in recent decades. In the early 1980s the negative effects on sleep of noise in a children's hospital ward in Australia were described by Keipert (1985). Both the ambient and the peak noise levels on the ward were greater than those recommended for hospitals, and at times were even greater than those recommended for outdoor activities. Ward staff were most concerned about the noise of cleaning machines and the sound of crying infants. Noise of staff conversations and staff activity has been documented to be disturbing to patients (Cochran & Ganong, 1989).

Recommended changes in nursing practices include (1) efforts to reduce nighttime noise and unnecessary patient interaction; (2) attention to environmental noise in the form of cleaning machines; (3) decreasing noise of technologic monitoring devices; (4) minimizing staff conversation; (5) timing "morning chores" (such as very early morning baths) and morning laboratory interruptions (such as very early visits from the phlebotomy staff) to the sleep cycle of the patient; (6) attending to the need for reduced light at night; (7) optimal light exposure in the daytime; (8) some semblance of regularity of meals, plus exercise when at all possible; and (9) definite rest periods during the daytime without long periods of daytime sleep.

CLINICAL PEARLS

- Sleep apnea is common in hypothyroid patients and patients with acromegaly.

- There is accumulating evidence suggesting that metabolic abnormalities in diabetics can be partially corrected by CPAP treatment, which supports the concept of a causal link between OSA and altered glucose control.

- For every 10 kg increment in weight the risk for OSA increases by more than twofold.

- The most important therapy for OSA in obese patients is weight loss.

- More than 50% of the patients with COPD experience difficulty initiating and maintaining sleep.

- COPD is associated with nocturnal hypoxemia, especially during REM sleep, due to loss of muscle tone of the accessory muscles of respiration during REM sleep.

- Patients with restrictive lung disorders and chest wall abnormalities (kyphoscoliosis) are at risk of sleep-related hypoventilation/hypoxemia. Polysomnography findings include frequent arousals, increased wakefulness after sleep onset, and nocturnal hypoxemia. Other consequences of nocturnal hypoxemia include pulmonary hypertension, *cor pulmonale*, and neurocognitive dysfunction.

- Periodic limb movement disorder has been shown to be a better predictor of mortality than serum albumin and other parameters monitored in dialysis patients. Treatment with dopamine agonists and gabapentin (adjusted dose due to renal elimination) may be helpful.

- Phototherapy may be helpful in Alzheimer's disease patients with circadian rhythm disorders.

- Certain seizure disorders occur predominantly or exclusively during sleep: nocturnal frontal lobe epilepsy (NFLE), benign rolandic epilepsy of childhood with centrotemporal spikes, and juvenile myoclonic epilepsy.

- CPAP treating obstructive sleep apnea in patients with epilepsy has improved seizure control.

- Patients with deep hemispheric lesions may present with increased yawning and hypersomnia, while patients with thalamic, subcortical, and pontine strokes are likely to suffer from insomnia.

- Restless legs syndrome has been noted in patients with pontine, thalamic, basal ganglia, and corona radiata infarcts.

- Adaptive servoventilation devices should be considered for treatment of central sleep apnea syndromes in stroke patients.

- Insomnia is one of the most common and well documented syndromes seen in patients with traumatic brain injury.

- Among circadian rhythm disorders, delayed sleep phase syndrome is the most common in traumatic brain injury patients and is often misinterpreted as insomnia.

- Drugs generally decrease slow wave sleep and decrease REM sleep unless proven otherwise.

- Withdrawal from sedative/hypnotics, TCAs, MAOIs, and venlafaxine commonly produce REM sleep rebound and often nightmares.

- Akathisia is not characteristically predominant in the evening and at bedtime, as is the syndrome of restless legs.

- Among many changes in hospital that challenge sleep, medications may be changed or administered at unfamiliar times, and any over-the-counter pain or sleeping medications that patients have been taking are often omitted.

DISCLOSURE STATEMENTS

Dr. Chopra has no conflict of interest to disclose.

Dr. Richardson has no conflict of interest to disclose.

REFERENCES

Chihorek, A. M., Abou-Khalil, B., & Malow, B. A. (2007). Obstructive sleep apnea is associated with seizure occurrence in older adults with epilepsy. *Neurology, 69*, 1823–1827.

Cochran, J., & Ganong, L. H. (1989). A comparison of nurses' and patient's perceptions of intensive care unit stressors. *Journal of Advanced Nursing, 14*(12), 1038–1043.

Crone, C. C., & Wise, T. N. (1998). Use of herbal medicines among consultation-liason populations: a review of current information regarding risks, interactions and efficacy. *Psychosomatics, 39*(1), 3–13.

Dawson, D., & Armstrong, S. M. (1996). Chronobiotics: drugs that shift rhythm. *Pharmacology & Therapeutics, 69*(1), 15–36.

Dietrich, B. (1997). Polysomnography in drug development. *Journal of Clinical Pharmacology, 37*, 70S–78S.

Hermann, D. M., & Bassetti, C. L. (2009). Sleep-related breathing and sleep-wake disturbances in ischemic stroke. *Neurology, 73*(16), 1313–1322.

Hurel, D., Loirat, P., Saulnier, F., Nicolas, F., & Brivet, F. (1997). Quality of life six months after intensive care: results of a prospective multicenter study using a generic health status scale and a satisfaction scale. *Intensive Care Medicine, 23*(3), 331–337.

Keipert, J. A. (1985). The harmful effects of noise in a children's ward. *Australian Paediatric Journal, 21*(2), 101–113.

Krachman, S. L., S'Alonzo, G. E., & Criner, G. J. (1995). Sleep in the intensive care unit. *Chest, 107*(6), 1730–1720.

Liborio, P., & Terzano, M. G. (1996). Polysomnographic effects of hypnotic drugs: a review. *Psychopharmacology, 126*, 1–16.

Malow, B. A., Levy, K., Maturen, K., & Bowes, R. (2000). Obstructive sleep apnea is common in medically refractory epilepsy patients. *Neurology, 55*, 1002–1007.

Malow, B. A., Foldvary-Schaefer, N., Vaughn, B. V., Selwa, L. M., Chervin, R. D., Weatherwax, K. J., et al. (2008). Treating obstructive sleep apnea in adults with epilepsy. A randomized pilot study. *Neurology, 71*, 572–577.

Manni, R., & Tartara, A. (2000). Evaluation of sleepiness in epilepsy. *Clinical Neurophysiology, 111*(S2), 111–114.

Nicholson, A. H., Bradley, C. M., & Pascoe, P. A. (1994). Medications: effects on sleep and wakefulness. In M. H. Kryger, T. Roth, & W. C. Dement (Eds), *Principles and practice of sleep medicine* (2nd ed., pp. 364–372). Philadelphia: W.B. Saunders.

Novak, M., & Shapiro, C. M. (1997). Drug-induced sleep disturbances: focus on nonpsychotropic medications. *Drug Safety, 16*(2), 133–149.

Obermeyer, W. H., & Benca, R. M. (1996). Effects of drugs on sleep. *Neurologic Clinics, 14*(4), 827–840.

Oliveira, A. J., Zamagni, M., Dolso, P. Bassetti, M. A., & Gigli, G. L. (2000). Respiratory disorders during sleep in patients with epilepsy: effect of ventilatory therapy on EEG interictal epileptiform discharges. *Clinical Neurophysiology, 111*(S2), 141–145.

Orff, H. J., Ayalon, L., & Drummond, S. P. (2009). Traumatic brain injury and sleep disturbance: a review of current research. *Journal of Head Trauma Rehabilitation, 24*(3), 155–165.

Pascue, P. D. (1994). Drugs and the sleep-wakefulness continuum. *Pharmacology & Therapeutics, 61*, 227–236.

Piperidou, C., Karlovasitou, A., Triantafyllou, N., Terzoudi, A., Constantinidis, T., Vadikolias, K., et al. (2008a). Influence of sleep disturbance on quality of life of patients with epilepsy. *Seizure, 17*(7), 588–594.

Piperidou, C., Karlovasitou, A., Triantafyllou, N., Dimitrakoudi, E., Terzoudi, A., Mavraki, E., et al. (2008b). Association of demographic, clinical and treatment variables with quality of life of patients with epilepsy in Greece. *Quality of Life Research, 17*(7), 987–996.

Schenck, C. H., & Mahowald, M. W. (1991). Injurious sleep behavior disorders (parasomnias) affecting patients on intensive care units. *Intensive Care Medicine, 17*(4), 219–224.

Treggiari-Venzi, M., Borgeat, A., Fuchs-Buder, T., Gachoud, J. P., & Suter, P. M. (1996). Overnight sedation with midazolam or propofol in the ICU: effects on sleep quality, anxiety, and depression. *Intensive Care Medicine, 22*(11), 1186–1190.

MEDICAL AND PSYCHIATRIC ASPECTS OF CHRONIC FATIGUE SYNDROMES AND APATHY

Linda L. M. Worley and Donna B. Greenberg

INTRODUCTION

Of every five patients seeking medical care, one complains of fatigue; this accounts for more than 7 million office visits per year (Epstein, 1995). Frequently no treatable cause is found. Over 800 research articles reflect the scientific and medical community's vigorous efforts to uncover the etiology and cure for a spectrum of complaints characterized globally as chronic fatigue syndrome (CFS).

CFS denotes a syndrome of severe disabling physical and mental fatigue lasting at least 6 months that substantially impairs functioning, is exacerbated by minimal exertion, and is unexplained by a conventional biomedical diagnosis (Fukuda et al., 1994; Sharpe et al., 1997). It is typically accompanied by other symptoms such as myalgias, sleep disturbances, and mood disorders. There is a high prevalence of comorbid psychiatric illness (Katon et al., 1991; Manu, Matthews, & Lane, 1988) and comorbid fibromyalgia (Bombardier & Buchwald, 1996).

To date, an identifiable etiology for CFS has not been reproducible. Physicians have very few proven treatments to offer. Obviously, it is difficult to treat a syndrome of symptoms effectively if the etiology is unknown.

Patients become disillusioned and angry if they perceive that the authenticity of their suffering is questioned in light of repeated negative findings. Many patients become dissatisfied with their physicians and seek alternative, nontraditional, and nonscientific sources of care (Denz-Penhey & Murdoch, 1993; Murdoch, unpublished). This chapter is a guide for psychiatrists who are evaluating and managing chronically fatigued patients.

DESCRIPTION OF CHRONIC FATIGUE SYNDROME

Chronic fatigue syndrome is a clinically defined condition characterized by severe disabling fatigue and a combination of symptoms that prominently feature self-reported impairments in concentration and short-term memory, sleep disturbances, and musculoskeletal pain. The diagnosis of CFS can be made only after medical and psychiatric causes of chronic fatiguing illness have been excluded (Fukuda et al., 1994).

DIAGNOSTIC CRITERIA

The earliest three operationally qualified working definitions for chronic fatigue syndrome are the CDC version (Fukuda et al., 1994), the British version, and the Australian version (Bates et al., 1994; Wessely, 1995). The CDC version remains the most cited and the best validated although at least five others have been added (Brurberg et al. [2014]; Johnston et al. [2013]). These criteria were designed as a basis for research into CFS to insure uniformity in patient selection. The CDC criteria differ by requiring multiple minor signs and symptoms. The British criteria require a definite onset of the illness, and the Australian criteria require the presence of post-exertional fatigue (Bates et al., 1994).

The CDC guidelines describe the symptom of fatigue as "severe mental and physical exhaustion." It is not somnolence or lack of motivation and cannot be attributed to exertion or diagnosable disease (Fukuda et al., 1994).

Definitions for and clinical evaluation of prolonged fatigue and chronic fatigue according to the current CDC guidelines are as follows: prolonged fatigue is self-reported persistent fatigue lasting 1 month or longer; chronic fatigue is self-reported persistent or relapsing fatigue lasting 6 or more consecutive months. Figure 34.1 describes the evaluation and classification of unexplained chronic fatigue (Fukuda et al., 1994).

Prolonged or chronic fatigue mandates a thorough clinical evaluation to identify potentially treatable underlying or contributing conditions. CFS as defined by the CDC cannot be diagnosed without such an evaluation. This clinical evaluation should include the following:

1. A thorough history to evaluate the following:
   a. the medical and psychosocial circumstances at the onset of fatigue
   b. -past medical history (including history of thyroid disease, anemia, etc.)
   c. the presence or history of depressive or other psychiatric disorders
   d. any previous episodes of medically unexplained symptoms
   e. alcohol or other substance abuse
   f. current use of prescription and over-the-counter medications and/or food supplements.

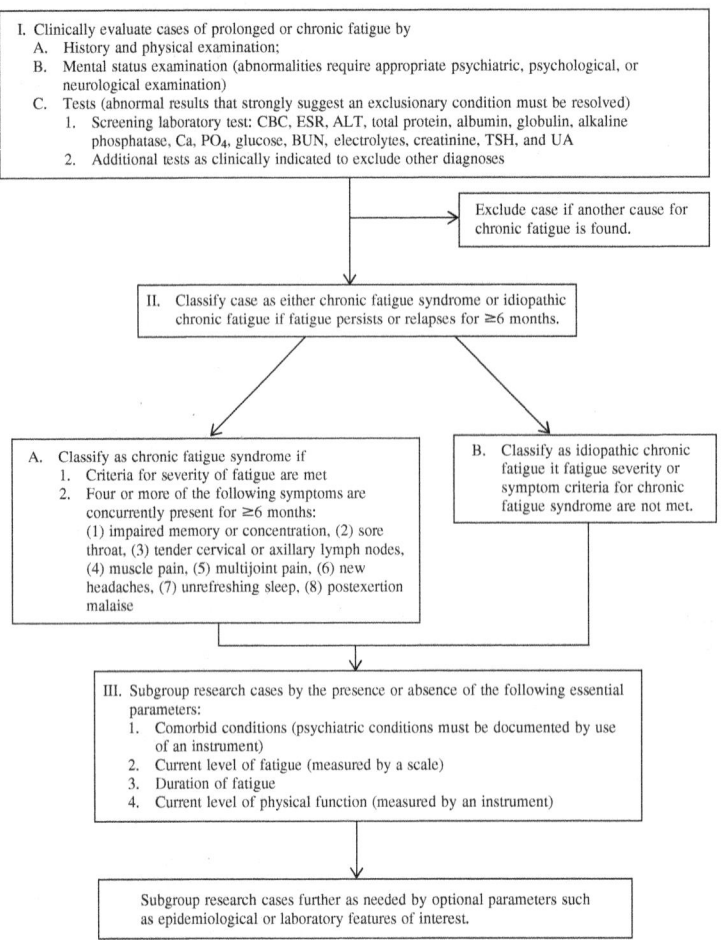

I. Clinically evaluate cases of prolonged or chronic fatigue by
  A. History and physical examination;
  B. Mental status examination (abnormalities require appropriate psychiatric, psychological, or neurological examination)
  C. Tests (abnormal results that strongly suggest an exclusionary condition must be resolved)
     1. Screening laboratory test: CBC, ESR, ALT, total protein, albumin, globulin, alkaline phosphatase, Ca, PO₄, glucose, BUN, electrolytes, creatinine, TSH, and UA
     2. Additional tests as clinically indicated to exclude other diagnoses

Exclude case if another cause for chronic fatigue is found.

II. Classify case as either chronic fatigue syndrome or idiopathic chronic fatigue if fatigue persists or relapses for ≥6 months.

A. Classify as chronic fatigue syndrome if
  1. Criteria for severity of fatigue are met
  2. Four or more of the following symptoms are concurrently present for ≥6 months:
     (1) impaired memory or concentration, (2) sore throat, (3) tender cervical or axillary lymph nodes, (4) muscle pain, (5) multijoint pain, (6) new headaches, (7) unrefreshing sleep, (8) postexertion malaise

B. Classify as idiopathic chronic fatigue if fatigue severity or symptom criteria for chronic fatigue syndrome are not met.

III. Subgroup research cases by the presence or absence of the following essential parameters:
  1. Comorbid conditions (psychiatric conditions must be documented by use of an instrument)
  2. Current level of fatigue (measured by a scale)
  3. Duration of fatigue
  4. Current level of physical function (measured by an instrument)

Subgroup research cases further as needed by optional parameters such as epidemiological or laboratory features of interest.

Figure 34.1 Evaluation and classification of unexplained chronic fatigue. ALT = alanine aminotransferase; BUN = blood urea nitrogen; CBC = complete blood counts; ESR = erythrocyte sedimentation rate; PO₄ = phosphorus; TSH = thyroid-stimulating hormone; UA = urinalysis. *Source:* Adapted from Fukada, Straus Hickie, et al. (1994). The chronic fatigue syndrome: a comprehensive approach to its definition and study. *Annals of Internal Medicine, 121,* 953–959. Used with permission.

2. A mental status examination should be performed, searching for abnormalities in mood, intellectual function, memory, and/or personality. Particular attention should be directed toward current symptoms of depression or anxiety, self-destructive thoughts, and observable signs such as psychomotor retardation. Evidence of a psychiatric or neurologic disorder requires an appropriate psychiatric, psychological, or neurologic evaluation.

3. A thorough physical examination.

4. A minimum battery of laboratory screening tests including complete blood count with leukocyte differential; erythrocyte sedimentation rate; serum levels of alanine aminotransferase, total protein, albumin, globulin, alkaline phosphatase, calcium, phosphorus, glucose, blood urea nitrogen, electrolytes, and creatinine; determination of thyroid-stimulating hormone (TSH); and urinalysis (Fukuda et al., 1994). Further tests should be judiciously included as warranted by suggestive findings in the comprehensive history and physical—for example, human immunodeficiency virus (HIV), Epstein-Barr Virus (EBV) viral capsid antigen immunoglobulin M (EBV VCA IgM) to consider acute mononucleosis -,

enzyme-linked immunosorbent assay (ELISA) and Western blot for *Borrelia burgdorferi*, treponemal (fluorescent treponemal antibody absorption [FTA-Abs]) or non-treponemal tests(VDRL or rapid plasma reagin [RPR] test for syphilis), sleep studies (polysomnography by a certified sleep laboratory), and reproductive/endocrine workup).

Conditions that potentially explain chronic fatigue symptoms include the following:

1. Any active medical condition that may explain the presence of chronic fatigue (Kroenke, 1989), such as untreated hypothyroidism, cancer, sleep apnea, narcolepsy, and iatrogenic conditions such as side effects of medication(s). Unfortunately, much of the research describing CFS patients has included samples of patients with these comorbid conditions.

2. Any previously diagnosed medical condition whose resolution has not been documented beyond reasonable clinical doubt and whose continued activity may explain the chronic fatiguing illness.

3. Any past or current diagnosis of a major depressive disorder with psychotic or melancholic features as well as bipolar mood disorder, schizophrenia of any subtype, delusional disorders of any subtype, dementias of any subtype, anorexia nervosa, or bulimia nervosa.

4. Alcohol or other substance abuse within 2 years of the onset of the chronic fatigue and any time thereafter.

5. Severe obesity as defined by a body mass index (body mass index = weight in kilograms/(height in meters)^2) >45.

Any unexplained physical examination finding or laboratory/ imaging test abnormality that suggests the presence of an exclusionary condition must be resolved before further classification.

Conditions that by definition do not adequately explain chronic fatigue or exclude them from the diagnosis of unexplained chronic fatigue include the following:

1. Any condition defined primarily by symptoms that cannot be confirmed by diagnostic laboratory tests, including fibromyalgia, anxiety disorders, somatic symptom disorders, nonpsychotic or nonmelancholic depression, "neurasthenia," and /or multiple chemical sensitivity syndrome.

2. Any condition under specific treatment sufficient to alleviate all symptoms related to that condition for which the adequacy of treatment has been documented. Such conditions include hypothyroidism for which the adequacy of replacement hormone has been verified by normal TSH levels or asthma in which the adequacy of treatment has been determined by pulmonary function and other testing.

3. Any condition, such as Lyme disease or syphilis, treated with definitive therapy prior to the development of chronic symptomatic sequelae.

4. Any isolated/unexplained physical examination finding or an abnormal laboratory or imaging test insufficient to confirm the existence of an exclusionary condition. For example, an elevated antinuclear antibody titer (ANA) without other laboratory or clinical evidence to support the diagnosis of a discrete connective tissue disorder.

Major Classification Categories

Clinically evaluated, unexplained cases of chronic fatigue can be separated into either the chronic fatigue syndrome or idiopathic chronic fatigue on the basis of the following criteria:

1. Clinically evaluated, unexplained, persistent, or relapsing chronic fatigue that
   a. is of new or definite onset (has not been lifelong); is not the result of ongoing exertion; is not substantially alleviated by rest
   b. results in substantial reduction in previous levels of occupational, educational, social, or personal activities

2. The concurrence of four or more of the following symptoms, all of which must have persisted or recurred during 6 or more consecutive months of illness and must not have predated the fatigue:
   c. self-reported impairment in short-term memory or concentration severe enough to cause substantial reduction in previous levels of occupational, educational, social, or personal activities
   d. sore throat
   e. tender cervical or axillary lymph nodes
   f. muscle pain, multi-joint pain without joint swelling or redness
   g. headaches of a new type, pattern, or severity
   h. unrefreshing sleep
   i. post-exertional malaise lasting more than 24 hours.

A case of idiopathic chronic fatigue is defined as clinically evaluated, unexplained chronic fatigue that fails to meet full, operationally defined criteria for the chronic fatigue syndrome. The reasons for failing to meet the criteria should be specified.

PREVALENCE

In the United States, 24% of the general adult population has had fatigue lasting 2 weeks or longer; 59% to 64% of these persons report that their fatigue has no medical cause (Price et al., 1992; Walker, Katon, & Jemelka, 1993). In one study, 24% of patients in primary care clinics reported having had prolonged fatigue for a month or more (Kroenke et al., 1988). In a community setting study, Buchwald et al. found a point prevalence of 98 to 267 per 100,000 for CFS and 2316 to 6321 per 100,000 for idiopathic chronic fatigue (Bombardier & Buchwald, 1996). More recent studies have reported prevalence rates of 0.24% to 2.6% (Vincent et al., 2012).

COMORBIDITY WITH OTHER CONDITIONS

Approximately 50% of patients meeting criteria for CFS have comorbid mood disorders. Another 25% have other psychiatric disorders such as anxiety disorders or somatic symptom disorders. The remaining 25%–33% of patients with CFS do not have an identifiable psychiatric diagnosis. The overlap between psychological disorders and CFS is not surprising. One of the most robust findings in psychiatric epidemiology is a positive correlation between the number of somatic symptoms and the risk of psychiatric disorder (Goldberg & Huxley, 1992; Simon & VonKorff, 1991). Similarly, the greater the number of pain symptoms, the greater risk of depression (Dworkin, VonKorff, & LeResche, 1990). Fatigue itself may be a feature which augments severity or presence of "caseness" in psychiatric diagnoses (Hickie, Hadzi-Pavlovic, & Ricci, 1997).

An interesting study, prospectively following nearly 3,000 patients without chronic fatigue or psychiatric disorder from age 36, showed that 7% had developed fatigue at age 43. Neuroticism and being female were risk factors for fatigue with or without psychiatric disorder. Of those who reported fatigue at age 43 (with a duration of more than 1 month or fatigue that was present for 12 months on at least 2 days each week), 45% had a comorbid psychiatric disorder. For those who had fatigue and a psychiatric disorder, predictors were family history of psychiatric illness and negative life events. Those with mild and moderate fatigue without psychiatric disorder had increased risk of psychiatric disorders at age 53. The predictors of fatigue without psychiatric disorder were excessive childhood energy reported by teachers at age 13 or being overweight as an adult. These distinct risk factors may suggest a path to a diagnosis of neurasthenia (Harvey et al., 2009).

In the *International Classification of Diseases* [Tenth Edition (ICD-10)] the psychiatric diagnosis of *neurasthenia* would identify almost all subjects with CDC-defined CFS (Farmer et al., 1995). The *DSM-IV* or *V* did not include neurasthenia as a diagnostic category (Sharpe, 1996; DSM-V, 2013). In an international study of mental illness in general health care Ustun and Sartorius (1995) report a 5.4% prevalence of neurasthenia, with two-thirds of those afflicted also having disorders of comorbid anxiety and depression. Merikangas has suggested that neurasthenia in adolescents may be a prodrome of bipolar disorder (Merikangas & Angst, 1994). In adults about one-fourth may have associated hypomanic symptoms (Gastpar & Kielholz, 1991).

Fibromyalgia is a syndrome with prominent muscle pain and specific trigger points (bilateral, above and below the diaphragm) that is often associated with fatigue, insomnia, and anxiety (see chapter 61). The presence of fibromyalgia does not preclude the diagnosis of CFS. Fibromyalgia is also associated with depression and irritable bowel syndrome. Low doses of sedating tricyclic antidepressants have been useful in treating this syndrome (Carrette, Bell & Reynolds, 1994). One theory of fibromyalgia is that symptoms result from a nonspecific sleep disorder, sometimes characterized by "intrusive" alpha waves into deeper levels of sleep; hence, tricyclic antidepressants may be treating a sleep disorder or a moderate mood disorder. Many psychiatrists regard fibromyalgia as somatized depression. Both CFS and fibromyalgia have been seen as conditions of central sensitization, with several top-down and bottom-up mechanisms contributing to the hyperresponsiveness of the CNS to a variety of inputs (Nijs et al., 2012; Clauw et al., 2011).

Vincent and colleagues reviewed the medical records of potential cases of CFS identified from 1998–2002 in the Rochester MN Epidemiology Project, a population-based database. Of those 482 patients who met criteria for CFS, the most common comorbid medical conditions were irritable bowel syndrome (46%), fibromyalgia (38%), and hypertension (30%). Insomnia occurred in 59%, depression in 70%, anxiety in 51%, somatoform disorder in 5%, and dysthymic disorder in 22%. The most common exclusionary conditions were obstructive sleep apnea (33%), restless legs syndrome (12%), and substance abuse (10%), all treatable conditions. Other exclusionary conditions were chronic obstructive pulmonary disease, heart failure, bipolar disorder, recent pregnancy, cancer within 5 years, dementia, rheumatoid arthritis, hepatitis B or C, stroke without full recovery, epilepsy, schizophrenia, Parkinson's disease, insulin-dependent diabetes, narcolepsy, depression with psychotic features, and systemic lupus erythematosus. In addition, there were a few cases of melancholic depression, eating disorder within 5 years, multiple sclerosis, cirrhosis, current chemotherapy, organ transplant, morbid obesity, and polymyalgia rheumatica. These serve as guides to diagnoses that should be part of a complete evaluation. They highlight the need to consider whether fatigue or other symptoms should be attributed to exclusionary or comorbid conditions. Careful attribution to the correct underlying condition will ensure disease-specific care.

ETIOLOGY OF CFS

The standardized criteria for CFS have been the basis of research and have defined the syndrome for the public mind, but unfortunately they define a very heterogeneous group of patients with a probable broad spectrum of triggers (Komaroff, 1997). Despite considerable research effort, no pathophysiologic mechanism has yet been established for CFS, and the symptoms remain largely unexplained (Sharpe, 1996; Taerk & Gnam, 1994). There are several hypotheses as to the etiology and pathology of CFS (Gonzalez, Cousins, & Doraiswamy, 1996).

HYPOTHALAMIC-PITUITARY-ADRENAL (HPA) AXIS/CNS ABNORMALITY

Demitrack et al. proposed that the biologic as well as behavioral features of CFS may be linked to an endocrine dysfunction of the HPA axis (Demitrack, 1994b). Dinan and associates reported a blunted serotonergic activation of the HPA axis in CFS (Dinan, 1997). The prominent fatigue associated with adrenal insufficiency has led several researchers to hypothesize that adrenal function is also impaired in patients with CFS (Poteliakhoff, 1981; Sharpe, 1996). Poteliakhoff (1981) showed that individuals with either chronic or acute fatigue had a clear reduction in diurnal levels of cortisol in comparison to nonfatigued controls. Demitrack studied the HPA axis of 30 patients with CFS compared to 72 healthy controls and reported a significant reduction in both plasma and urinary glucocorticoid levels, accompanied by an impairment in the stimulated activity of the axis for the patients with CFS (Demitrack, 1994a; 1997; Demitrack et al., 1991). There is evidence that some patients with CFS have both low levels of cortisol and an abnormal adrenal response to stress and exertion (Sharpe, 1996). Tak et al. (2011) did find evidence in a meta-analysis of 85 studies of statistically significant basal hypocortisolism in CFS subjects compared to controls but not in patients with fibromyalgia or irritable bowel syndrome.

This finding is by no means universal in this patient population. Evidence of hypocortisolism has also been associated with CFS in adolescents with normalization with treatment success (Nijhof, et al., 2014).

Low-dose hydrocortisone (i.e., 20–30 mg q8AM and 5 mg q2PM for 12 weeks) administered to CFS patients in a randomized, placebo-controlled, double-blind therapeutic trial, between 1992 and 1996 resulted in slight (not statistically significant), apparently mild but consistent improvement on a global wellness rating scale, compared to placebo-treated controls. Other self-reported rating scales did not reflect an improvement. Predictably, patients receiving hydrocortisone developed statistically significant adrenal suppression. The most frequent milder side effects of the steroid included insomnia, weight gain, and acne. The final conclusion from this study was that the slight improvement that might be attributable to hydrocortisone treatment was achieved at the expense of significant adrenal suppression precluding its practical use for CFS. Hydrocortisone itself, at these dose levels, has mood-elevating effects (McKenzie et al., 1998).

Of note, a variety of other stress-associated clinical syndromes also manifest disruptions in the integrity of the HPA axis, such as posttraumatic stress disorder (Yehuda et al., 1993) and athletes suffering from "overtraining syndrome" (Barron et al., 1985). How all of these clinical syndromes arrive at the common biochemical disturbance of reduced glucocorticoid output is unclear and may require an integrated, multidimensional model of disease pathogenesis (Demitrack, 1997).

Regardless of the specific hypothesis, the occurrence of neurologic (Komaroff & Buchwald, 1991), affective (Krupp et al., 1994), neuroendocrine (Demitrack et al., 1991), as well as cognitive (DeLuca et al., 1995) abnormalities suggest that the CFS disease process affects the brain (Bell, 1994). It remains to be conclusively shown whether the brain abnormalities are the cause, result, or mediator of the CFS patient's symptoms and how much brain involvement might influence the outcome or prognosis of CFS (Gonzalez et al., 1996).

PSYCHIATRY AND NEUROPSYCHIATRY

Another hypothesis focuses on CFS as a primary mood spectrum disorder, in particular, a type of chronic depression (Demitrack & Engleberg, 1994). Some authors have attempted to integrate the psychiatric and physiologic aspects of the illness (Taerk & Gnam, 1994; Taerk et al., 1987; Salit, 1985, 1987) and propose that CFS reflects the interplay between physical and psychological factors in psychologically vulnerable individuals with a depressive diathesis. They point to the biologic changes in both the hypothalamic-pituitary-adrenal axis and the immune system of individuals who have experienced early traumatic events or losses (Coe et al., 1992; Gunnar, 1992; Laudenslager, Dapitanio & Reite, 1985) and hypothesize a relationship between these changes and CFS (Taerk & Gnam, 1994). Figure 31.2 is the explanatory model for disease susceptibility applied to CFS (Taerk & Gnam, 1994).

It has been suggested that CFS and mood-related psychiatric disorders share a common origin in both neurobiologic and psychosocial dysfunction (Wessely, 1996). The risk of CFS is increased in patients with a history of depression. Rates of comorbid psychiatric syndromes are high—higher than would be expected if the medical dimension of CFS led to psychological consequences (Holgate et al., 2011).

Formal disorders of intellect and memory cannot be confirmed in CFS, despite the severity of the subjective complaints, but a disorder of sustained attention seems probable. Patients with CFS have scored lower on tests in which motor and cognitive processing speeds were a critical factor: tasks of reaction time and tasks of working memory (Christley et al., 2013). However, the cognitive status of patients with CFS did not differ from patients with a history of dysthymia or depression matched for age and intelligence quotient (Marshall et al., 1997). These neuropsychological findings are typical of those found in depressed patients.

Cerebral perfusion studies have shown decreased perfusion to the brain stem in CFS patients (Costa, Tannock, & Brostoff, 1995), although similar if not identical abnormalities have been noted in patients with depression (Sharpe,

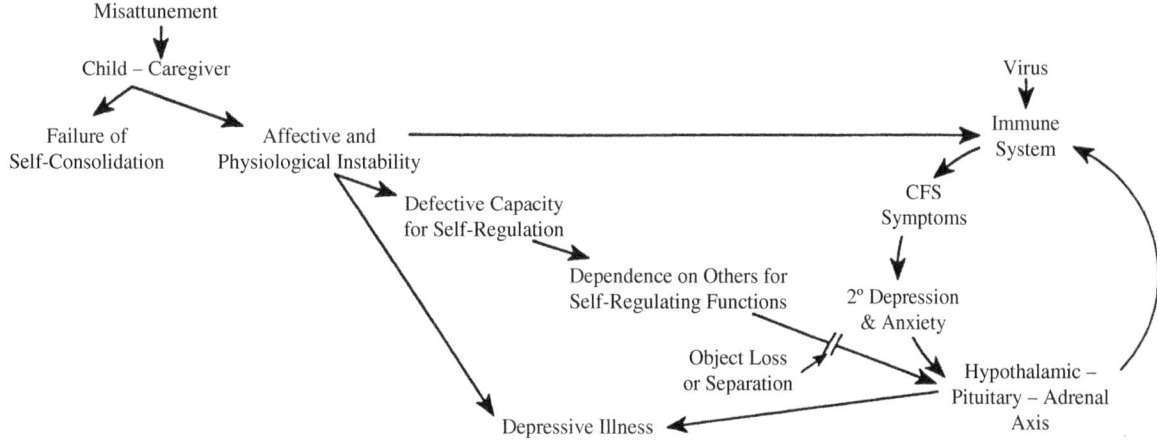

Figure 34.2 One explanatory model of chronic fatigue syndrome.

1996). These studies have not been replicated to our knowledge under controlled conditions with blinded raters of the diagnosis during scan assessment.

EEG spectral coherence data have been able to distinguish unmedicated patients who meet criteria for CFS from those depressed or healthy controls (Duffy et al., 2011). Review of other studies of central nervous system changes in CFS patients show abnormalities but no alterations in specific regions associated with CFS (Nater, Heim, & Raison, 2012).

SLEEP ABNORMALITIES

Unrefreshing sleep is an almost ubiquitous complaint of people suffering from CFS (Sharpe et al., 1992). Morriss reported that 87% of CFS patients surveyed experience sleep disorders such as poor sleep hygiene, restless legs syndrome, and more daytime sleepiness and napping than depressed patients or controls (Morriss, Wearden, & Battersby, 1997). As noted earlier, simple disruption of (deep) slow-wave sleep where alpha waves (associated with relaxed wakefulness with closed eyes) intrude into the sleep pattern is an observation in some with CFS (Morriss et al., 1993; Sharpe, 1996) and may lead to a sensation of low energy. This type of sleep pattern is seen in about one-third of patients with fibromyalgia. Some patients describe their sleep to feel as though they "skim just below the surface of sleep," feeling as if they are awake during sleep, and completely misjudging the duration before sleep onset and the total duration of sleep (Shapiro, Devins, & Hussain, 1993). As noted above, similar complaints of disrupted sleep are found in fibromyalgia (classically associated with nonrestorative sleep) and in symptomatic perimenopausal women, who report longer and more numerous arousals than nonperimenopausal women (Baker, Simpson, & Dawson, 1997). Although inefficient sleep could contribute to daytime fatigue, its etiologic role and specificity in CFS remain uncertain (Sharpe, 1996). Experimental sleep deprivation can reproduce both the symptoms and neuroendocrine profiles of CFS (Leese et al., 1996; Moldofsky & Scarisbrick, 1976). A study by Sharpley et al. (1997) found that patients with CFS had more abnormalities in sleep continuity than the control group but no significant difference in the actual time spent in individual sleep stages. CFS patients spent significantly longer in bed trying to sleep, reflecting an inefficient sleep pattern, but that did not appear to be a major cause of daytime fatigue. A study of sleep in monozygotic twins discordant for CFS found that the percentage of Stage 3 and REM sleep were greater among the CFS twins than their healthy twins, but no other differences in sleep architecture were noted. The study did not provide strong evidence for a major role of sleep architecture abnormality in CFS. (Bali et al., 2004).

AUTONOMIC NERVOUS SYSTEM DYSFUNCTION

It has been proposed that CFS is a variant (or "6th form") of neurocirculatory asthenia (van Waveren, 1996) and is due to a dysfunction of the autonomic nervous system, particularly the sympathetic system, with the predominant symptom being that of fatigue (Martinez-Martinez et al., 2014). (Theories and hypotheses for CFS are in no short supply; proof of their validity is).

Postural hypotension has been noted in patients with CFS (Bou-Holaigah et al., 1995; Van Cauwenbergh et al., 2014), but this may be a consequence of inactivity (Sharpe, 1996).

POSTINFECTIOUS ETIOLOGIES

Epidemiologic data do not confirm a link between CFS and the common infective agents encountered in everyday life. In a controlled prospective study of the outcome of over 1000 symptomatic infective episodes seen in British primary care patients, researchers were unable to demonstrate any link between clinical viral infection and subsequent chronic fatigue or CFS (Wessely, 1995). In contrast, a distinct fatigue syndrome that persisted for the 6-month duration of a single prospective longitudinal primary care study was identified following acute mononucleosis (glandular fever), aseptic meningitis, and hepatitis (White et al., 1995). This fatigue syndrome differed from that seen in CFS, as it was associated with hypersomnia in contrast to the insomnia generally seen in CFS (White et al., 1995).

Although CFS was at one time thought to be due to chronic EBV, attribution of chronic fatigue to EBV infection would now rest on the recognition of recent acute mononucleosis, typically acute pharyngitis, lymphadenopathy, and hepatospenomegaly. IgM to viral capsid antigen (VCA-IgM) titers may be elevated for 4–8 weeks. Elevated IgG antibodies may persist in some patients, so their presence does not indicate recent infection or symptomatic chronic infection. In adolescents with acute mononucleosis, baseline autonomic symptoms and days spent in bed since diagnosis, proxies of severity of illness, were the only significant predictors of those who met CFS criteria at 6 months. (Jason et al., 2014). An Australian prospective study of patients with EBV, Q fever, or epidemic polyarthritis (Ross River virus) found that 11% of 253 patients met criteria for CFS at the end of 6 months, and this was predicted also primarily by severity of illness (Hickie et al, 2006). This then could be a post-infectious pathway that could trigger CFS but not fully explain it Holgate, 2011). Coxiella burnetti, parvovirus B19, human herpesvirus-6, and enteroviruses have also been studied as triggers (Duffy, 2011).

Chronic Lyme disease due to infection by the spirochete *Borrelia burgdorferi* had also been linked to chronic fatigue in some cases (Ellenbogen, 1997), but it is extremely unlikely that fatigue would be the only sign of Lyme disease (Dawson & Sabin, 1993). The presence of neurologic findings or arthritic complaints of the knee, hip, or shoulders suggestive of the clinical characteristics of Lyme disease would be an indication for an ELISA test and a Western blot test for *Borrelia burgdorferi*. Typically, non-specific symptoms improve over 6 months following diagnosis and treatment.

Post-Lyme disease syndrome, a syndrome subjectively similar to CFS, was defined to describe documented cases of early or late Lyme disease treated with a generally accepted antibiotic treatment regimen with objective resolution or stabilization of objective manifestations of Lyme disease, who within 6 months of diagnosis then develop fatigue, widespread musculoskeletal pain, or complaints of cognitive difficulties. Patients were excluded if before the diagnosis of Lyme they had fibromyalgia, unexplained somatic complaints like fatigue or musculoskeletal symptoms or chronic fatigue syndrome. Patients with objective abnormalities on neuropsychologic testing that may explain the patient's complaints were also excluded (Wormser et al., 2006). Very few patients meet these criteria, and antibiotics have not shown benefit for persistent non-specific symptoms. In fact, chronic Lyme disease is now seen as a misnomer (Feder et al., 2007; Baker, 2008).

IMMUNE DYSFUNCTION

Another theory proposes that CFS is a persistent immune dysfunction initiated by some infectious process, such as an unknown virus (Zubieta et al., 1994). It is recognized that fatigue is a prominent symptom in HIV. Research has claimed alterations in immune functioning in some CSF patients, the most consistent finding reported within T-cell subsets (Buchwald & Komaroff, 1991). Unfortunately these abnormalities have not been placed in an epidemiologic context (Wessely, 1995), and the findings have not been consistently replicated. The possibility that any changes might be secondary to confounders such as neurohormonal variables, sleep disorder, or psychological distress has been insufficiently addressed. The presence of immunologic dysfunction has not been associated with clinical status or clinical outcome (Wessely, 1996).

MUSCLE DYSFUNCTION

There is no consistent evidence of a primary disorder of muscle in most studies, nor is there evidence of any change in muscle structure that could not be explained by the consequence of illness (Wessely, 1996).

SJÖGREN'S SYNDROME

Sjögren's syndrome (SS) is a rheumatologic disease of unknown etiology that is characterized by a classic triad of dryness of eyes and mouth accompanied by symptoms of joint inflammation. It is often associated with an enhanced immunologic reactivity (SS-B antibodies, presence of rheumatoid factor, elevated ESR, and occasional proteinuria reflective of interstitial nephritis). Diagnostic procedures such as the Schirmer test (measuring the quantity of tears secreted in 5 minutes to irritation from a filter paper strip placed under a lower eyelid moistening less than 5 mm/5 min), the ocular staining test, tear breakup time, tear lysozyme concentration, and slit-lamp examination are useful. Subjective manifestations of SS such as neurocognitive dysfunction and fatigue have been stressed by some observers. It has been suggested that SS may represent a common and frequently overlooked clinical subset of CFS (Calabrese, Davis, & Wilke, 1994).

CONFOUNDING VARIABLES TO RESEARCH

Unfortunately, most studies of CFS have suffered from methodologic shortcomings (Schluederberg et al., 1992; Sharpe, 1996). The principal shortcoming has been in patient selection. Most etiologic studies recruit their CFS patients from tertiary care clinics and self-help groups. Diagnostic criteria have been both modified capriciously and applied inconsistently (Schluederberg et al., 1992) in this often disabled population of patients, many of whom are completely confined to bed (Wessely, 1995). Numerous studies have reported abnormalities that could be a result of chronic inactivity, which is known to have profound effects on muscle function and chemistry, cardiac function, immune function, and psychological status (Wessely, 1995).

PROGNOSIS OF CFS

There is a paucity of information on the prognosis of patients with CFS (Salit, 1996), especially regarding the natural history of CFS in the community or primary care (Wessely, 1996). Studies in tertiary care settings give both guarded and pessimistic views. Salit recommends that patients with CFS be reassured about the generally positive outcome, stating that most individuals will improve over the first several years after diagnosis, but that the long term prognosis is unknown (Salit, 1996). He indicates that while many patients do improve, few report complete recovery at 2 to 3 years after diagnosis and only a minority of patients show significant deterioration over time. He adds that "CFS is not fatal, although some patients do commit suicide" (Salit, 1996). Komaroff reports that 12% of individuals with CFS return to normal health but half of these relapse. He found the typical course to be very difficult the first 6 months with a gradual improvement thereafter—either because of overall improvement or because patients adjusted their expectations (Komaroff, 1997).

In a small study of patients undergoing cognitive-behavioral therapy (Deale et al., 1997), poor outcome was associated with taking medical retirement or making a new claim for a disability-related benefit during treatment.

The majority of children who are diagnosed with CFS have been reported to recover (Joyce, Hotopf, & Wessely, 1997; Nijhof et al., 2013).

Overall, the greater fatigue severity, the more likely the prognosis will be worse (Vincent, 2012, Taylor et al., 2002; Jason et al., 2011). Consistent risk factors for poor prognosis include duration of disease, lifetime dysthymia (Clark et al., 1993), the strength of belief in a physical cause for symptoms, untreated psychological distress, and the use of avoidant coping strategies such as reducing activity and imposing dietary, social, and other restrictions (Wessely, 1996; Joyce et al., 1997).

EPIDEMIOLOGY

PREMORBID PERSONALITY CHARACTERISTICS

While the criteria define a syndrome with symptoms that may be alleviated, the underlying lifetime vulnerability of patients may be more relevant (Hickie et al., 1997). Baseline fatigue scores are a predictor of chronic fatigue in the general population. Severity and chronicity of fatigue fluctuates over time with intermittent fulfillment of the criteria for CFS. Stressors and constitution then interact with distress as an independent factor (Lawrie et al., 1997). Both research studies and clinical experience suggest that many persons with CFS have a tendency toward hard-driving, perfectionistic, or obsessive compulsive personalities and an overactive premorbid lifestyle (Fry & Martin, 1996; Sharpe, 1996). Loneliness is a predictor of chronic fatigue (Kellner, 1991). Studying a population in Georgia, Nater et al. (2010) found a greater prevalence of CFS patients had a personality disorder compared to well controls.

Many children attending specialist centers in the United Kingdom who have a diagnosis of CFS are described to be high achievers and often "have anxieties about their school performance, which cause them to work excessively hard to achieve at the limits of their ability" (Wessely, 1996; Lievesley, Rimes, & Chalder, 2014). In addition, psychological factors contribute to CFS in children including a complex family dynamic of involvement, high expectations, limited communication regarding emotional issues, and previous experience of illness (Wessely, 1996).

GENDER

Women with CFS are overrepresented in specialty clinics. The relative risk for women to develop CFS in community samples has been reported to be 1.3–1.7. The relative risk for women increases as the diagnostic criteria used for CFS become increasingly stringent (e.g., duration, percentage of time the patient was fatigued, presence of myalgias; see Wessely, 1995).

SOCIAL CLASS

There is no clear link to social class or occupational group; these associations relate to attendance at tertiary center clinics, not to prevalence in the general population (Wessely, 1996). There is no evidence that ethnic minorities are at less risk (Wessely, 1995).

DIFFERENTIAL DIAGNOSES

CANCER-RELATED FATIGUE

In order to study the syndromes of fatigue related to cancer, the syndrome has been defined as a distressing, persistent, and subjective sense of physical, emotional, and/or cognitive tiredness or exhaustion related to cancer or cancer treatment that is not proportional to recent activity and that interferes with usual functioning (Berger et al., 2010). Patients who have had chemotherapy experience a syndrome of fatigue following treatment that may be related in part to regulation of inflammation (Bower et al., 2011). Radiation treatment is also associated with a fatigue syndrome. Both are typically time-limited and related to intensity of treatment. This syndrome is often embedded with other side effects of treatment like menopausal symptoms, sleep dysfunction, depression or the presence of persistent tumor like lymphoma. In controlled studies stimulants have had mixed results. Methylphenidate led to positive results in one trial, and modafinil has been useful for more severe fatigue. Exercise programs have reduced cancer-related fatigue with effect sizes ranging from 0.18 to 0.37 in a meta-analysis (Cramp & Daniel, 2008). Energy conservation or activity management, teaching self-care or coping techniques, and education about fatigue have been helpful (Pachman et al., 2012; Goedendorp et al., 2009).

APATHY OR DIMINISHED MOTIVATION

Diminished motivation or apathy without dysphoria may present as chronic fatigue without defined somatic symptoms and may be more effectively reexamined with a neuropsychiatric differential diagnosis. Apathy is seen in dementia and is a common symptom in first episode psychosis cohort 10 years after illness debut. Its presence in psychotic patients relates to impaired functioning and poorer subjective quality of life (Evensen, Rossberg, & Barder, 2012).

Apathy is a condition of diminished motivation even in the presence of normal consciousness, attention, cognitive capacity and mood. Patients are able to initiate and sustain behavior, describe their plans, goals, and interests, and react emotionally to significant events and experiences; however, they do all of these things less often than normal patients. Goal-related aspects of overt behavior, thought content, and emotion are decreased. (Marin, 1990; Marin & Wilkosz, 2005).

When apathy worsens, the patient is seen as having abulia, poverty of behavior and speech output, lack of initiative, loss of emotional response, psychomotor slowing, and prolonged speech latency. Akinetic mutism is the total absence of these behaviors. In the differential diagnosis of these states is stupor with altered consciousness, catatonia with waxy flexibility, and clinical depression with depressed mood.

The core circuit for motivation is the anterior cingulum, nucleus accumbens, ventral pallidum, medial dorsal nucleus of the thalamus, and the ventral tegmental area. Frontal and diencephalic diseases are prominent in the etiology of these syndromes. Therefore, the exam should assess olfactory function, visual acuity, visual fields, frontal release signs, *gegenhalten*, and extrapyramidal motor signs.

Loss of incentive and a sense of overwhelming loss of control can lead to apathy as a psychological dimension. Demoralization and despair can be factors that diminish motivation. Major depressive disorder, delirium, and dementia may present with syndromes of apathy.

The severity of apathy may be measured with the Apathy Evaluation Scale, an 18-item list graded from 1–4 (Marin, Biedrzycki, & Firinciogullari, 1991). The items ask whether the interview supports these characteristics of the patient: interested in things, gets things done during the day, whether getting things started on his own is important to him, whether she is interested in new experiences, interested in learning new things, whether she puts little effort into anything or approaches life with intensity, sees a job through to the end, or spends time doing things that interest her. Does someone have to tell him what to do each day? Is he less concerned about problems than he should be? Does she have friends and get together with them? When something good happens, does he get excited? Does she have an accurate understanding of her problems? Is it true that getting things done during the day is important to him, that he has initiative and motivation?

Strategies for treatment of apathy include optimizing medical status, diagnosing other conditions like Parkinson's disease or hyperthyroidism, sometimes eliminating doses of psychotropics like SSRIs or dopamine antagonists and at other times treating depression or psychosis effectively (Brodaty & Burns, 2012). Specific drugs to increase motivation include dopamine agonist stimulants, and cholinesterase inhibitors (donepezil, galantamine, and rivastigmine). Pramipexole, amantadine, bromocriptine, selegiline, pergolide, l-dopa/carbidopa, and modafinil, may have a role as well as methylphenidate, dextroamphetamine, bupropion, protriptyline, and venlafaxine (Bowman, et al., 1997; Berman, et al., 2012).

TREATMENT OF CHRONIC FATIGUE SYNDROME

STEP 1: INITIAL PATIENT VISIT

Establish an understanding of the problem.

Help me understand what you are hoping that I can help with.

It is essential to carefully observe and listen to patients with complaints of CFS to understand what they are experiencing (Conn et al., 1978). Acknowledge and respond to their nonverbal cues and strong emotions (Ekman & Friesen, 1975) in order to fully appreciate the impact of their illness. This allows the physician to respond appropriately to any preconceived notions or lingering ill feelings that patients may harbor regarding previous experiences with health care providers who did not seem supportive in treating their illness. Listen carefully (taking notes if necessary) to learn exactly what it feels like to be in their shoes and how the illness has affected their life. Reflect back to the patient what they have reported (preferably in their own words), clarifying as necessary. For example,

Let me see if I understand. You've been so exhausted physically and mentally over the past 8 months that you lost the job you loved and are now afraid that your husband is sorry he married you. This has you feeling sad,

---

Box 34.1 CONDITIONS ASSOCIATED WITH APATHY, ABULIA, AND AKINETIC MUTISM

Neurological Disorders

Frontal Lobe

Frontotemporal dementia
Anterior cerebral infarction
Tumor
Hydrocephalus
Trauma

Right Hemisphere

Right middle cerebral artery infarction
Cerebral white matter disease
Ischemic white matter disease
Multiple sclerosis
Binswanger's encephalopathy
HIV

Basal Ganglia

Parkinson's disease
Huntington's disease
Progressive supranuclear palsy
Carbon monoxide poisoning
Diencephalon
Degenerative or infraction of thalamus
Wernicke-Korsakoff disease

Amygdala

Kluver-Bucy syndrome

Multifocal Disease

Alzheimer's disease (prefrontal cortex, parietal cortex and amygdala)

Medical Disorders

Apathetic hyperthyroidism
Hypothyroidism
Pseudohypoparathyroidism
Lyme disease
Chronic fatigue syndrome
Testosterone deficiency
Debilitating medical conditions, e.g. cancer, heart or renal failure

Drug-Induced

Neuroleptics, esp. typical
Selective serotonin reuptake inhibitors
Marijuana dependence
Amphetamine or cocaine withdrawal

Loss of Incentive or Perceived Control

Role change
Institutionalization

(adapted from Marin & Wikosz, 2003, Table 1)

desperate, and alone. You are coming to me to find out what has you so exhausted, and you want to feel better! What am I missing?

Sometimes patients will breathe a sigh of relief, feeling understood. There remains a high risk of disappointing the patient who wants a firm diagnosis and who comes with a great deal of distrust (Ax, Gregg, & Jones, 1997).

Formulate a diagnostic plan acceptable to the patient. Explain that there are numerous causes for fatigue and exhaustion and that it will be important to go through a comprehensive (1) history, followed by (2) a complete physical examination (including a careful neurological examination and a mental status examination) and finally, (3) perform selected laboratory testing as medically indicated. If the patient agrees with this plan, proceed with the evaluation. Teach throughout this diagnostic process, so that the patient is an active participant and understands the necessity of searching each area. This is very reassuring for the patient to understand that a serious physical etiology will be found if it exists.

1. Obtain a comprehensive history (Sharpe et al., 1997), including medical, psychiatric, and psychosocial issues. See Box 34.2.

2. Perform thorough physical and psychiatric examinations to rule out common causes of chronic fatigue (Epstein, 1995). See Box 34.3.

3. Recommended minimal laboratory testing (Fukuda et al., 1994): See Box 34.4.

Additional selected tests (i.e., HIV, VDRL, EBV, Lyme titer, ANA) are guided by an excellent medical evaluation. A conservative approach is prudent, basing each patient's diagnostic workup on suggestive findings and risk factors.

STEP 2: SCHEDULE REGULAR FOLLOW-UP PATIENT VISITS

Review Findings

Review the positive and negative findings from the history, physical examination, and laboratory testing, teaching how each finding relates to fatigue. Treat any underlying medical and/or psychiatric conditions appropriately. If no explanation is identified for the fatigue, patients may be reassured and educated about CFS:

> *You have an illness called "chronic fatigue syndrome." It is not an illness that leads to death. Despite a great deal of research, there is no single cause; many factors may contribute. There are no scientifically proven cures, but there are many claims for cure. You must be extremely cautious not to fall prey to particularly expensive treatment programs promising spectacular results.*
>
> *It will take a lot of work to fight this illness and I will continue to help you in this long uphill battle. What we do know is that strategies of strict inactivity make CFS*

---

much worse in the long run. The most useful treatments include maximizing your overall health (this allows your body to heal itself naturally), normalizing your sleep, and increasing your activity level extremely slowly within a structured cognitive behavioral therapy program for CFS.

It is important to observe the patient's reactions to this news (Salit, 1985), including nonverbal communications (Ekman & Friesen, 1975), and to inquire as to thoughts, feelings, questions, and concerns.

Plan Comprehensive Treatment Strategy

Design the treatment strategy tailored for each unique patient, maximizing overall positive health behaviors (Denz-Penhey & Murdoch, 1993).

1. Normalize sleep patterns (Shapiro et al., 1993). Review the sleep hygiene of the patient. Even small changes in activity make a difference. Ensure that the patient does not take daytime naps or have any unnecessary nocturnal interruptions of sleep. Consolidate sleep and restrict bedtime to improve sleep efficiency. Paradoxically, hypnotic drugs which may improve sleep may heighten daytime fatigue and create dependency problems such as with the benzodiazepines. Consider the possibility of a primary sleep disorder and investigate accordingly. Avoid caffeine, nicotine, or any other stimulating substance. Limit activities in the bedroom to sleep and intimacy. A sleep diary may be helpful.

2. Initiate cognitive behavioral therapy (CBT). There are at least 6 published cognitive behavior therapy randomized controlled trials noted in a Cochrane review 2008 (Price et al., 2008) and then in the review of clinical evidence (Reid, 2010) (Deale et al., 1997; Lloyd et al., 1993; Sharpe, et al., 1996; Prins et al., 2001; O'Dowd et al., 2006; Jason, 2007).

Sessions 1 to 3 involved engaging the patient(s) in therapy and offering a detailed treatment rationale. Presenting problems were assessed, and patients kept diaries in which they recorded hourly details of activity, rest, and fatigue.

At session 4 a schedule of planned, consistent, graded activity and rest was agreed upon. The initial targets were modest and small enough to be sustained despite fluctuations in symptoms. Rather than being symptom-dependent, activity and rest were divided into small, manageable portions spread throughout the day (for example, three 5-minute walks daily rather than a 45-minute walk once a week). Patients were encouraged to persevere with their targets and not to reduce them on a bad day or exceed them on a good day.

Once a structured schedule was established, activity was gradually increased and rest was reduced, step by step as tolerance developed. Therapist and patient agreed on specific daily targets covering a range of activities—for example, walking, reading, visiting friends, or gardening. A sleep routine was established—stopping daytime sleep, rising at a specific time each morning, reducing time in bed, and using stimulus control techniques for insomnia (Lacks, 1987).

Cognitive strategies were introduced at session 8 (while the graded activity program continued). Patients recorded any unhelpful or distressing thoughts and, in discussion and as homework, practiced generating alternatives (Beck et al., 1979). The unhelpful or distressing thoughts included fears about symptoms and treatment, perfectionism, self-criticism, guilt, and performance expectations.

In the final sessions, strategies for dealing with setbacks were rehearsed and patients drew up action plans to guide them through the coming months. The importance of maintaining the principles of therapy after discharge was reinforced.

CBT techniques directly confront the maladaptive cognitive and behavioral changes often associated with CFS that have lead to symptom perpetuation. Other related illnesses (anxiety, depression, chronic low back pain, rheumatoid arthritis, and atypical chest pain) have been successfully treated and managed with CBT (Wilson et al., 1994).

Successful CBT interventions for CFS involve several key elements including: goal setting (increased activity levels, increased social and pleasurable events); education about the illness; relaxation training; exposure to avoided activities; restructuring of potential cognitive errors involving misinterpretation of events or stimuli (i.e., fearing the worst, "I'm bound to relapse"); and the evaluation of possible social, family, or personal reinforcers of disability. Several attempts at utilizing CBT for CFS have not been effective; these attempts utilized a shorter duration of treatment with a different form of reintroduction of activity than described by Deale. Adolescents with chronic fatigue syndrome have been treated effectively with internet-based CBT (Nijhof et al., 2013).

3. Encourage physical rehabilitation and exercise (Wilson et al., 1994). Muscle performance (including endurance and recovery) is normal in patients with CFS. It is important to educate patients that exercise will not harm them, but will benefit their recovery when done very gradually. Initially, activity may exacerbate symptoms (initial worsening followed by improvement). In population studies, inactivity has been shown to be associated with more reports of fatigue and greater risk of depression. 4. Maximize balanced nutrition (Morris, 1993). Patients with CFS are advised to eat a varied (normal) diet selected from and within the basic food groups to ensure adequate nutrient intake to reach and maintain a healthy body weight.

4. Unproven diet therapies for patients with CFS include megavitamin/mineral supplements; royal jelly and other dietary supplements; and elimination, avoidance, and rotation diets. Claims that these therapies relieve CFS symptoms and promote recovery are anecdotal and have not been substantiated by clinical research. The yeast-avoidance and sugar-free diets, both promoted to combat *Candida albicans* overgrowth, are of no proven value in treating patients with CFS. Diet strategies that call for the avoidance of food additives, preservatives, sweeteners, and other ingredients are not supported by scientific evidence and are not practical for patients with CFS (Morris, 1993).

5. Maximize physical health through preventative medical and dental care. It is important that patients with CFS have annual medical examinations to rule out occult or new illnesses (Denz-Penhey & Murdoch, 1993) and abnormalities throughout the year are investigated and treated appropriately. It is also essential to maintain dentition in good repair.

6. Treat psychiatric illness and operantly decrease sick role behavior. Be vigilant for comorbid depression, anxiety, and somatoform disorders and treat them vigorously. Help patients to identify and appropriately express their emotions. Contained emotions such as anger are exhausting. Encourage patients to be direct about their needs and limitations rather than needing to maintain a "sick role" to avoid being overwhelmed by the expectations and requests of others. Accept and encourage patients to appropriately grieve for the losses they have experienced (both personal and professional) as a result of having CFS. Assist them to redefine meaningful,

realistic life/career goals and support their efforts to strive for them. Continue to elicit a detailed understanding of their lives, including overwhelming stressors, psychosocial and financial pressures, and lifelong patterns of behavior. Attempt to understand possible perpetuating factors (e.g., the role of the family in the patient's functioning).

7. Overcome facilitating factors. Individuals with CFS develop avoidance behavior toward activities perceived to worsen their fatigue. For example, many individuals exercise in spurts, overdoing it and suffering grave consequences. They then carefully avoid all levels of exercise, fearing the worst (Nijs et al., 2013). Figure 31.3 illustrates a cognitive model of the perpetuation of CFS (Fry & Martin, 1996).

8. Control symptoms. No available *somatic treatment* has been found to be consistently effective for CFS in controlled trials (Vercoulen et al., 1996). This leaves patients who suffer with CFS open to purveyors of folk remedies, unorthodox treatments, and exploitive practitioners and charlatans from a variety of health-related professions. Therefore, when patients find treatment programs that are particularly expensive and unproven, they should be advised to be particularly cautious.

The use of antidepressant medications (Wilson et al., 1994; Jorge, 1997), predominantly tricyclic agents, in patients with CFS has achieved widespread theoretical and clinical support despite a lack of controlled studies. In uncontrolled samples 70% to 80% of patients are said to have benefited (Jones & Straus, 1987; Manu et al., 1989). The rationale for the use of these medications includes their utility in primary depression with associated fatigue, sleep disturbances, and related disorders such as fibromyalgia; their site of action within the central nervous system; and the high rates of depression reported in CFS subjects. Clinical experience suggests that tricyclic antidepressants are often poorly tolerated in patients with CFS, even in low doses, due to their sedative and anticholinergic effects. In patients with fibromyalgia, tricyclic antidepressant agents such as nortriptyline have been evaluated in randomized, placebo-controlled studies and found to be effective in comparison to placebo and nonsteroidal antiinflammatory drugs (see Chapter 61).

Fluoxetine 20 mg per day was found to be ineffective in a randomized, double blind placebo controlled 8-week trial for treating CFS irrespective of whether depressive symptoms were present (Vercoulen et al., 1996). It should be noted here that fluoxetine is a drug developed, proved effective, and FDA approved for depression.

Controlled studies utilizing newer psychopharmacologic agents for the treatment of CFS are lacking although one trial of for neurasthenia suggested the power of treatment with CBT and then mirtazapine produced additive benefits. The timing of therapy and/or antidepressants may be important (Stubhaug et al., 2008). When treating comorbid depressive or anxiety disorders, antidepressants should be titrated and tailored to each patient. If insomnia is prominent, then more-sedating medications may be better tolerated. Non-sedating medications like bupropion or adjunctive agents like methylphenidate may be useful, especially since the patient will not be alarmed by sedation.

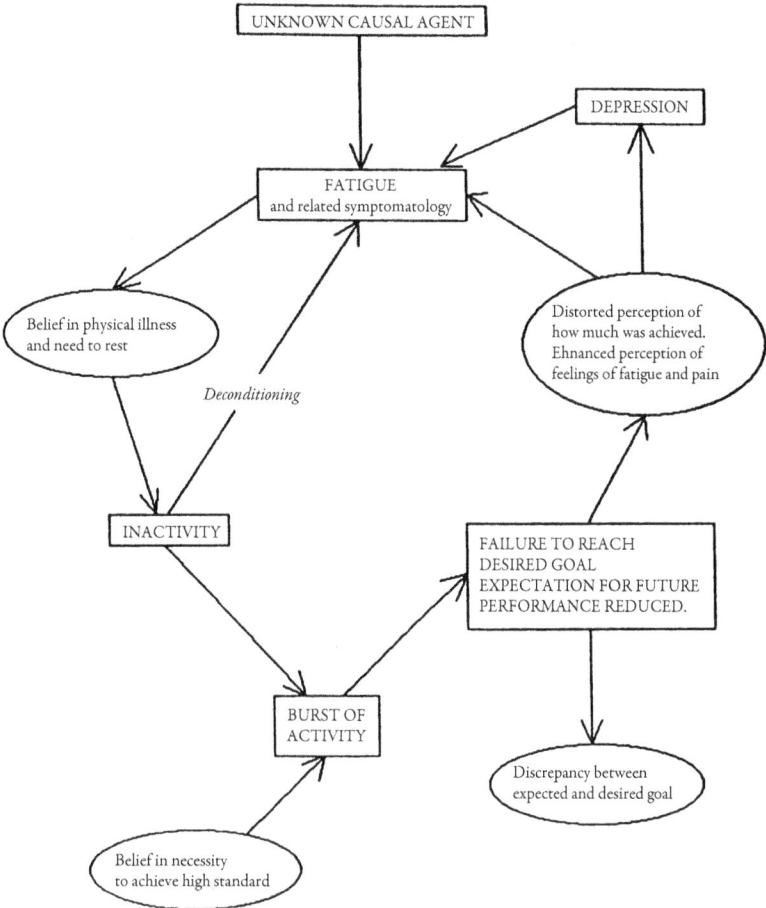

Figure 34.3 A cognitive model of chronic fatigue syndrome and the pathways that perpetuate it. From Fry & Martin, 1996.

Novel pharmacologic agents are available, but they are not yet proven to be clinically efficacious by reproducible double-blind randomized placebo-controlled trials. A recent review of the effect of treatments for CFS (Reid et al., 2011) concluded that the effectiveness of corticosteroids and intramuscular magnesium are unknown. Dietary supplements, evening primrose oil, oral nicotinamide adenine dinucleotide, homeopathy, and prolonged rest have not been studied in enough detail to draw conclusions. In one single randomized control study galantamine was no better than placebo. For gammaglobulin, two double blind placebo controlled trials were conducted utilizing intravenous gammaglobulin in adults with CFS. One study showed a significant improvement, but results were not replicated in the second study. A third study of 99 adults showed side effects but no benefit; therefore, gammaglobulin in the management of CFS cannot be recommended (Vollmer-Conna et al., 1997; Wilson et al., 1994).

Rintatolimod (trade name ampligen), known as PolyI; poly C12U, is an experimental immunomodulatory double-stranded RNA preparation thought to have both antiviral and immunomodulatory properties. When administered to CFS patients in a randomized multicenter placebo controlled double blind study for 24 weeks it was found to significantly improve global performance and perceived cognition (Strayer et al., 1994). Unfortunately, the patient group studied was atypical in that they were severely affected (many subjects were bedbound), and the magnitude of the therapeutic effect was small (Wilson et al., 1994). A double blind placebo controlled randomized clinical trial of this toll-like receptor 3 agonist and inducer of innate immune responses involved 234 subjects with long-standing debilitating CFS at 12 sites. The outcome of exercise tolerance was improved in the drug-treated group (Strayer et al., 2012); however, this orphan drug has not been approved.

9. Recognize countertransference. Recognize that it is normal to experience frustration and helplessness in treating patients with CFS. Be cautious not to base professional gratification on patient improvement. Patients often need unconditional empathy whether they are fatigued or energetic. Empathy, however, must be balanced with active efforts to mobilize these patients from sick and disability roles they may have adopted. In our present state of knowledge it is just as likely for clinicians to reinforce symptoms of CFS, including sick role behaviors, versus diminishing their severity.

CLINICAL PEARLS

- The risk of CFS is increased in patients with a history of depression. Rates of comorbid psychiatric syndromes are high—higher than would be expected if the medical dimension of CFS led to psychological consequences (Holgate et al., 2011).

- Overall, the greater fatigue severity the more likely that the prognosis is worse (Vincent, 2012; Taylor, 2002; Jason, 2011). Consistent risk factors for poor prognosis include duration of disease, lifetime dysthymia (Clark et al., 1993), the strength of belief in a physical cause for symptoms, untreated psychological distress, and the use of avoidant coping strategies such as reducing activity and imposing dietary, social, and other restrictions (Wessely, 1996; Joyce et al., 1997).

- Diminished motivation or apathy without dysphoria may present as chronic fatigue without defined somatic symptoms and may be more effectively reexamined with a neuropsychiatric differential diagnosis.

- Apathy is seen in dementia and is a common symptom in first episode psychosis cohort 10 years after illness debut.

- Strategies for treatment of apathy include optimizing medical status, diagnosing other conditions like Parkinson's disease or hyperthyroidism, eliminating doses of psychotropics like SSRIs, dopamine antagonists, and treating depression effectively. Specific medications to increase motivation through stimulants include dopamine agonist stimulants, and cholinesterase inhibitors (donepezil, galantamine, and rivastigmine). Pramipexole, amantadine, bromocriptine, selegiline, pergolide, l-dopa/carbidopa, modafinil, may have a role as well as methylphenidate, dextroamphetamine, bupropion, protriptyline, and venlafaxine.

- For the patient with chronic fatigue:

  (a) Acknowledge and respond to their nonverbal cues and strong emotions in order to appreciate fully the impact of their illness.
  (b) Review the positive and negative findings from the history, physical examination, and laboratory testing, teaching how each finding relates to fatigue.
  (c) Normalize sleep patterns.
  (d) Use the techniques of cognitive behavioral treatment.
  (e) Treat comorbid psychiatric disorders.
  (f) Decrease sick role behavior.
  (g) Add in physical therapy and graded exercise.
  (h) Recognize countertransference.

DISCLOSURE STATEMENTS

Dr. Worley has no conflicts to disclose. She is funded by the Veterans Health Administration, and the Vanderbilt School of Medicine Center for Professional Health.

Dr. Greenberg has no conflicts of interest to disclose.

REFERENCES

American Psychiatric Association (2013). *Diagnostic and Statistical Manual of Mental Disorders*. Washington, D.C. American Psychiatric Publishing, Inc.

Ax, S., Gregg, V., & Jones, D. (1997). Chronic fatigue syndrome: sufferers' evaluation of medical support. *Journal of the Royal Society of Medicine*, (90), 250–254.

Baker, A., Simpson, S., & Dawson, D. (1997). Sleep disruption and mood changes associated with menopause. *Journal of Psychosomatic Research*, 43(4), 359–369.

Baker, P. J. (2008). Perspectives on "Chronic Lyme Disease." *American Journal of Medicine*, 121, 562–564.

Bali, N., Buchwald, D. S., Schmidt, D., Goldberg, J., Ashton, S., & Armitage, R. (2004). Monozygotic twins discordant for chronic fatigue syndrome: objective measures of sleep. *Journal of Psychosomatic Research*, 56, 207–212.

Barron, J. L., Noakes, T. D., Levy, W., Smith, C., & Millar R. P. (1985). Hypothalamic dysfunction in overtrained athletes. *Journal of Endocrinology and Metabolism*, 60(4), 803–806.

Bates, D. W., Buchwald, D., Lee, J., Kith, P., Doolittle, T. H., & Umali, P. (1994). A comparison of case definitions of chronic fatigue syndrome. *Clinical Infectious Diseases*, 18(Suppl 1), S11–15.

Beck, A., Rush, A., Shaw, B., & Emery G. (Eds.). (1979). *Cognitive therapy of depression*. New York: Guilford Press.

Bell, D. S. (1994). Chronic fatigue syndrome update. Findings now point to CNS involvement. *Postgraduate Medicine*, 96(6), 73–76, 79–81.

Berger, A. M., Abernethy, A. P., Atkinson, A., Barsevick, A. M., Breitbart, W. S., & Cella, D. (2010). Cancer-related fatigue. *Journal of the National Comprehensive Cancer Network*, 8, 904–931.

Berman, K., Brodaty, H., Withall, A., & Seeber, K. (2012). Pharmacologic treatment of apathy in dementia. *American Journal of Geriatric Psychiatry*, 20, 104–122.

Bombardier, C. H., & Buchwald, D. (1996). Chronic fatigue, chronic fatigue syndrome, and fibromyalgia. Disability and health-care use. *Medical Care*, 34(9), 924–930.

Bou-Holaigah, I., Rowe, P. C., Kan, J., & Calkins, H. (1995). The relationship between neurally mediated hypotension and the chronic fatigue syndrome. *Journal of the American Medical Association*, 274(12), 961–967.

Bower, J. E., Ganz, P. A., Irwin, M. R., Kwan, L., Breen E. C., Cole, S. W. (2011). Inflammation and behavioral symptoms after breast cancer treatment: Do fatigue depression and sleep disturbance share a common underlying mechanism? *Journal of Clinical Oncology*, 29, 3517–3522.

Bowman, M. A., Kirk, J. K., Michielutte, R., & Preisser, J. S. (1997). Use of amantadine for chronic fatigue syndrome [letter]. *Archives of Internal Medicine*, 157(11), 1264–1265.

Brurberg, K. G., Fonhus, M. S., Larun, L., Flottorp, S., & Malterud, K. (2014). Case definitions for chronic fatigue syndrome/myalgic encephalomyelitis (CFS/ME): a systematic review. *British Medical Journal Open*, 4,e003973, 1–9.

Brodaty, H., & Burns, K. (2012). Nonpharmacological management of apathy in dementia: a systematic review. *American Journal of Geriatric Psychiatry*, 20, 549–564.

Buchwald, D., & Komaroff, A. (1991). Review of laboratory findings for patients with chronic fatigue syndrome. *Reviews of Infectious Diseases*, 13(Suppl 1), 12–18.

Calabrese, L. H., Davis, M. E., &Wilke, W. S. (1994). Chronic fatigue syndrome and a disorder resembling Sjogren's syndrome: preliminary report. *Clinical Infectious Diseases*, 18(Suppl 1), S28–31.

Carrette, S., Bell, M., & Reynolds, J. (1994). Comparison of amitriptyline, cyclobenzaprine, and placebo in the treatment of fibromyalgia: a randomized double blind clinical trial. *Arthritis and Rheumatism*, 37, 32–40.

Christley, Y., Duffy, T., Everall, I. P., & Martin, C. R. (2013). The neuropsychiatric and neuropsychological features of chronic fatigue syndrome; revisiting the enigma. *Current Psychiatry Reports*, 15(4), 353–362.

Clark, M., Sullivan, M., Katon, W., Russo, J. E., Fischl, M., Dobie, R. A., et al. (1993). Psychiatric and medical factors associated with disability in patients with dizziness. *Psychosomatics, 34*(5), 409–415.

Clauw, D. J., Arnold, L. M., & McCarberg, B. H. (2011). The science of fibromyalgia. *Mayo Clinic Proceedings, 86*, 907–911.

Coe, C., Lubach, G., Schneider, M., Dierschke, D. J., & Ershler, W. B. (1992). Early rearing conditions alter immune responses in the developing infant primate. *Pediatrics, 90*, 505–509.

Conn, H., Rakel, R., & Johnson, T. (Eds.) (1978). *Family practice.* Philadelphia: W.B. Saunders.

Costa, D. C., Tannock, C., & Brostoff, J. (1995). Brainstem perfusion is impaired in chronic fatigue syndrome [see comments]. *Journal of the Association of Physicians, 88*(11), 767–773.

Cramp, F., & Daniel, J. (2008). Exercise for the management of cancer-related fatigue in adults. *Cochrane Database of Systematic Reviews, 2*, CD006145.

Dawson, D., & Sabin, T. (Eds.) (1993). *Chronic fatigue syndrome.* Boston: Little, Brown.

Deale, A., Chalder, T., Marks, I., & Wessely, S. (1997). Cognitive behavior therapy for chronic fatigue syndrome: a randomized controlled trial. *American Journal of Psychiatry, 154*(3), 408–414.

DeLuca, J., Johnson, S. K., Beldowicz, D., & Natelson, B. H. (1995). Neuropsychological impairments in chronic fatigue syndrome, multiple sclerosis, and depression. *Journal of Neurology, Neurosurgery, and Psychiatry, 58*(1), 38–43.

Demitrack, M. (1994a). Neuroendocrine aspects of chronic fatigue syndrome: implications for diagnosis and research. In S. Straus (Ed.), *Chronic fatigue syndrome.* New York: Marcel Dekker.

Demitrack, M., Dale, J., Straus, S., Laue, L., Listwak, S. J., Kruesi, M. J., et al. (1991). Evidence for impaired activation of the hypothalamic-pituitary-adrenal axis in patients with chronic fatigue syndrome. *Journal of Endocrinology and Metabolism, 73*(6), 1224–1234.

Demitrack, M. A. (1994b). Chronic fatigue syndrome: a disease of the hypothalamic-pituitary-adrenal axis? [editorial]. *Annals of Medicine, 26*(1), 1–5.

Demitrack, M. A. (1997). Neuroendocrine correlates of chronic fatigue syndrome: a brief review. *Journal of Psychiatric Research, 31*(1), 69–82.

Demitrack, M. A., & Engleberg, N. C. (1994). Chronic fatigue syndrome. *Current Therapy in Endocrinology and Metabolism, 5*, 135–142.

Denz-Penhey, H., & Murdoch, J. (1993). Service delivery for people with chronic fatigue syndrome: a pilot action research study. *Family Practice, 10*(1), 14–18.

Dinan, T. G. (1997). Blunted serotonin-mediated activation of the hypothalamic-pituitary-adrenal axis in chronic fatigue syndrome. *Psychoneuroendocrinology, 22*(4), 261–267.

Duffy, F. H., McAnulty, G. B., McCreary, M. C., Cuchural, G. J., & Komaroff, A. L. (2011). EEG spectral coherence data distinguish chronic fatigue syndrome patients from healthy controls and depressed patients—a case control study. *BMC Neurology, 11*, 8294.

Dworkin, S., VonKorff, M., & LeResche, L. (1990). Multiple pains and psychiatric disturbance: an epidemiologic investigation. *Archives of General Psychiatry, 47*, 239–244.

Ekman, P., & Friesen, W. (1975). *Unmasking the face.* Englewood Cliffs, NJ: Prentice-Hall.

Ellenbogen, C. (1997). Lyme disease. Shift the paradigm. *Archives in Family Medicine, 6*(2), 191–195.

Epstein, K. (1995). The chronically fatigued patient. *Medical Clinics of North America, 79*(2), 315–327.

Evensen, J., Rossberg, J. I., & Barder, H. (2012). Apathy in first episode psychosis patients: a ten year longitudinal follow up study. *Schizophrenia Research, 136*, 19–24.

Farmer, A., Jones, I., Hillier, J., Llewelyn, M., Borysiewicz, L., & Smith, A. (1995). Neuraesthenia revisited: ICD-10 and, D. S.M-III-R psychiatric syndromes in chronic fatigue patients and comparison subjects. *British Journal of Psychiatry, 167*(4), 503–506.

Feder, H. M., Johnson, B. J. B., O'Connell, S. O., Shapiro E. D., Steere, A. C., Wormser, G. P., et al. (2007). A critical appraisal of "chronic Lyme disease." *New England Journal of Medicine, 357*, 1422–1430.

Fry, A. M., & Martin, M. (1996). Fatigue in the chronic fatigue syndrome: a cognitive phenomenon? *Journal of Psychosomatic Research, 41*(5), 415–426.

Fukuda, K., Straus, S. E., Hickie, I., Sharpe, M. C., Dobbins, J. G., & Komaroff, A. (1994). The chronic fatigue syndrome: a comprehensive approach to its definition and study. International Chronic Fatigue Syndrome Study Group [see comments]. *Annals of Internal Medicine, 121*(12), 953–959.

Gastpar, M. & Kielholz, P. (Eds.) (1991). *Problems in psychiatry in general practice.* Lewiston, NY: Hogrefe and Huber Publishers.

Goedendorp, M. M., Gielissen, M. F., Verhagen, C. A., & Bleijenberg, G. (2009). Psychosocial interventions for reducing fatigue during cancer treatment in adults. *Cochrane Database of Systematic Reviews, 1*, CD006953.

Goldberg, D., & Huxley, P. (1992). *Common mental disorders: A biosocial model.* London: Tavistock/Routledge.

Gonzalez, M. B., Cousins, J. C., & Doraiswamy, P. M. (1996). Neurobiology of chronic fatigue syndrome. *Progress in Neuro-Psychopharmacology & Biological Psychiatry, 20*(5), 749–759.

Gunnar, R. (1992). Reactivity of the hypothalamic-pituitary-adrenocortical system to stressors in normal infants and children. *Pediatrics, 90*, 491–497.

Harvey, S. B., Wessely, S., Kuh, D., & Hotopf, M. (2009). The relationship between fatigue and psychiatric disorders: Evidence for the concept of neurasthenia. *Journal of Psychosomatic Research, 6*, 445–454.

Hickie, I., Hadzi-Pavlovic, D., & Ricci, C. (1997). Editorial: Reviving the diagnosis of neurasthenia. *Psychological Medicine, 27*, 989–994.

Hickie, I., Davenport, T., Wakefield, D., Vollmer-Conna, U., Cameron, B., Vernon, S. D., et al. (2006). Post-infective and chronic fatigue syndromes precipitated by viral and non-viral pathogens: prospective cohort study. *British Medical Journal, 333*, 575–581.

Holgate, S. T., Komaroff, A. L., Mangan, D., & Wessely, S. (2011). Chronic fatigue syndrome: understanding a complex illness. *Nature Reviews. Neuroscience, 12*, 539–544.

Jason, L. A.T. (2007). Non-pharmacologic interventions for CFS: a randomized trial. *Journal of Clinical Psychological Medicine, 14*, 275–296.

Jason, L. A., Katz, B. Z., Shiraishi, Y., Mears, C. J., Im, Y., & Taylor, R. (2014). Predictors of post-infectious chronic fatigue syndrome in adolescents. *Health Psychology and Behavioral Medicine, 2*(1), 41–51.

Jason, L. A., Porter, N., Hunnell, J., Brown, A., Rademaker, A., & Richman, J. A. (2011). A natural history study of chronic fatigue syndrome. *Rehabilitation Psychology, 56*, 32–42.

Jones, J., & Straus, S. (1987). Chronic Epstein-Barr virus infection. *Annual Review of Medicine, 38*, 195–209.

Jorge, C. M. (1997). Chronic fatigue syndrome and depression: biological differentiation and treatment. *Psychiatric Annals, 27*(5), 365–371.

Johnston, S., Brenu, E. W., Staines, D. R., & Marshall-Gradisnik, S. (2013). The adoption of chronic fatigue syndrome/myalgic encephalomyelitis case definitions to assess prevalence: a systematic review. *Annals of Epidemiology, 23*, 371–376.

Joyce, J., Hotopf, M., & Wessely, S. (1997). The prognosis of chronic fatigue and chronic fatigue syndrome: a systematic review. *Journal of the Association of Physicians, 90*(3), 223–233.

Katon, W., Buchwald, D., Simon, G., Russo, J. E., & Mease, P. J. (1991). Psychiatric illness in patients with chronic fatigue and rheumatoid arthritis. *Journal of General Internal Medicine, 6*, 77.

Kellner, R. (1991). *Psychosomatic syndromes and somatic symptoms.* Washington, DC: American Psychiatric Press.

Komaroff, A. (1997). A 56-year-old woman with chronic fatigue syndrome. *Journal of the American Medical Association, 278*, 1179–1187.

Komaroff, A., & Buchwald, D. (1991). Symptoms and signs of chronic fatigue syndrome. *Reviews of Infectious Diseases, 13*(Suppl 1), S8–S11.

Kroenke, K. (1989). Chronic fatigue: frequency, causes, evaluation, and management. *Comprehensive Therapy, 15*, 3–7.

Kroenke, K., Wood, D. R., Mangelsdorff, A. D., Meier, N. J., & Powell, J. B. (1988). Chronic fatigue in primary care. Prevalence, patient characteristics and outcome. *Journal of the American Medical Association, 206,* 929–934.

Krupp, L., Sliwinski, M., Masur, D., Friedberg, F., & Coyle, P. K. (1994). Cognitive functioning and depression in patients with chronic fatigue syndrome and multiple sclerosis. *Archives of Neurology, 51,* 705–710.

Lacks, P. (1987). *Behavioral treatment of persistent insomnia.* New York: Pergamon Press.

Laudenslager, M., Dapitanio, J., & Reite, M. (1985). Possible effects of early separation experiences on subsequent immune function in adult macaque monkeys. *American Journal of Psychiatry, 142,* 862–866.

Lawrie, S., MacHale, S., Power, M., & Goodwin, G. M. (1997). Is the chronic fatigue syndrome best understood as a primary disturbance of sense of effort? *Psychological Medicine, 27,* 995–999.

Lievesley, K., Rimes, K. A., & Chalder, T. (2014). A review of the predisposing, precipitating and perpetuating factors in chronic fatigue syndrome in children and adolescents. *Clincal Psychology Reiew 24,* 233–248.

Leese, G., Chattington, P., Fraser, W., Vora, J., Edwards, R., & Williams, G. (1996). Short-term night-shift working mimics the pituitary-adrenocortical dysfunction in chronic fatigue syndrome. *Journal of Clinical Endocrinology and Metabolism, 81*(5), 1867–1870.

Lloyd, A., Hickie, I., Brockman, A., Hickie, C., Wilson, A., Dwyer, J., et al. (1993). Immunologic and psychologic therapy for patients with chronic fatigue syndrome: a double-blind, placebo-controlled trial. *American Journal of Medicine, 94,* 197–203.

Marin, R. S. (1990). Differential diagnosis and classification of apathy. *American Journal of Psychiatry, 147,* 22–30.

Marin, R. S., Biedrzycki, R. C., & Firinciogullari, S. (1991). Reliability and validity of the apathy evaluation scale. *Psychiatry Research, 38,* 143–162.

Marin, R. S., & Wilkosz, P. A. (2005). Disorders of diminished motivation. *Journal of Head Trauma Rehabilitation, 20,* 377–388.

Manu, P., Matthews, D., & Lane, T. (1988). The mental health of patients with a chief complaint of chronic fatigue. *Archives of Internal Medicine, 148,* 213.

Manu, P., Matthews, D., Lane, T., Tennen, H., Hesselbrock, V., Mendola, R., et al. (1989). Depression among patients with a primary complaint of chronic fatigue. *Journal of Affective Disorders, 17,* 165–172.

Marshall, P., Forstot, M., Callies, A., Peterson, P. K., & Schenck, C. H. (1997). Cognitive slowing and working memory difficulties in chronic fatigue syndrome. *Psychosomatic Medicine, (59),* 58–66.

Martinez-Martinez, L. A., Mora, T., Vargas, A., Fuentes-Iniestra, M., & Martinez-Lavin, M. (2014). Sympathetic nervous system dysfunction in fibromyalgia, chronic fatigue syndrome, irritable bowel syndrome, and interstitial cystitis: a review of case-control studies. *Journal of Clinical Rheumatology 20,* 146–150.

McKenzie, R., Fallon, A., Dale, J., Demitrack, M., Sharma, G., Deloria, M., et al. (1998). Low-dose hydrocortisone for treatment of chronic fatigue syndrome. *Journal of the American Medical Association, 280,* 1061–1066.

Merikangas, K., & Angst, J. (1994). Neurasthenia in a longitudinal cohort of young adults. *Psychological Medicine, 24,* 1013–1024.

Moldofsky, H., & Scarisbrick, P. (1976). Induction of neurasthenia musculoskeletal pain syndrome by selective sleep deprivations. *Psychosomatic Medicine, 38,* 35–44.

Morris, D. H. (1993). Unproven diet therapies in the treatment of the chronic fatigue syndrome. *Archives of Family Medicine, 2*(2), 181–186.

Morriss, R., Sharpe, M., Sharpley, A., Cowen, P. J., Hawton, K., & Morris, J. (1993). Abnormalities of sleep in patients with chronic fatigue syndrome. *British Medical Journal, 306*(6886), 1161–1164.

Morriss, R., Wearden, A., & Battersby, L. (1997). The relation of sleep difficulties to fatigue, mood and disability in chronic fatigue syndrome. *Journal of Psychosomatic Research, 42*(6), 597–605.

Nater, U. M., Heim, C. M., & Raison, C. (2012). Chronic fatigue syndrome. In T. E. Schlaepfer & C. B. Nemeroff (eds.), *Handbook of Clinical Neurology, vol 106 (3rd series) Neurobiology of Psychiatric Disorders,* Amsterdam: Elsevier B.V., 573–587.

Nater, U. M., Jones, J. F., Lin, J-M. S., Maloney, E., Reeves, W. C., & Heim, C. (2010). Personality features and personality disorders in chronic fatigue syndrome: a population-based study. *Psychotherapy and Psychosomatics, 79,* 312–318.

Nijhof, S. L., Priesterbach, L. P., Uiterwaal, C. S., Bleijenberg, G., Kimpen, J. L., & van de Putte, E. M. (2013). Internet-based therapy for adolescents with chronic fatigue syndrome: long-term follow-up. *Pediatrics, 131,e* 1788–1795.

Nijhof, S. L., Rutten, J. M., Uiterwaal, C. S., Bleijenberg, G., Kimpen, J. L., & van de Putte, E. M. (2014). The role of hypocortisolism in chronic fatigue syndrome. *Psychoneuroendocrinology, 42,* 199–206.

Nijs, J., Meeus, M., Van Oosterwijck, J., Ickmans, K., Moorkens, G., Hans, G. & DeClerck, L. S. (2012). In the mind or in the brain? Scientific evidence for central sensitization in chronic fatigue syndrome. *European Journal of Clinical Investigation, 42,* 203–212.

Nijs, J., Roussel, N., van Oosterwijck, J., De Kooning, M., Ickmans, K., Struyf, F., et al. (2013). Fear of movement and avoidance behavior toward physical activity in chronic-fatigue syndrome and fibromyalgia: state of the art and implications for clinical practice. *Clinical Rheumatology, 32,* 1121–1129.

O'Dowd, H., Gladwell, P., Rogers, C. A., Hollinghurst, S., & Gregory, A. (2006). Cognitive behavioral therapy in chronic fatigue syndrome: A randomized controlled trial of an outpatient group program. *Health Technology Assessment, 10,* iii–iv, ix–x, 1–121.

Pachman, D. R., Barton, D. L., Swetz, K. M., & Loprinzi, C. L. (2012). Troublesome symptoms in cancer survivors: fatigue, insomnia, neuropathy, and pain. *Journal of Clinical Oncology, 30,* 3687–3696.

Poteliakhoff, A. (1981). Adrenocortical activity and some clinical findings in acute and chronic fatigue. *Journal of Psychosomatic Research,* (25), 91–95.

Price, J., Mitchell, E., Tidy, E., & Hunot V. (2008). Cognitive behavior therapy for chronic fatigue syndrome in adults. In *The Cochrane Library* (Issue 2, 2010). Chichester, UK: John Wiley & Sons, Ltd.

Price, R. K., North, C. S., Wessely, S., & Fraser, V. J. (1992). Estimating the prevalence of chronic fatigue syndrome and associated symptoms in the community. *Public Health Reports, 107,* 514–522.

Prins, J. B., Bleijenberg, G., Bazelmans, E., Elving, L. D., de Boo, T. M., Severens, J. L., et al. (2001). Cognitive behavior therapy for chronic fatigue syndrome: a multicentre randomized controlled trial. *Lancet, 357,* 841–847.

Reid, S., Chalder, T., Cleare, A., Hotopf, M., & Wessely, S. (2011). Chronic fatigue syndrome. *Clinical Evidence, 05,* 1101–1156

Salit, I. E. (1985). Sporadic post infectious neuromyasthenia. Clinical and community studies. *Canadian Medical Association Journal, 133,* 659–663.

Salit, I. E. (1987). Chronic EBV infection (post-infectious neuromyasthenia). *Medical Clinics of North America, 10,* 1944–1950.

Salit, I. E. (1996). The chronic fatigue syndrome: a position paper. *Journal of Rheumatology, 23*(3), 540–544.

Schluederberg, A., Straus, S., Peterson, P., Blumenthal, S., Komaroff, A. L., Spring, S. B., et al. (1992). NIH Conference. Chronic fatigue syndrome research. Definition and medical outcome assessment. *Annals of Internal Medicine, 117*(4), 325–331.

Shapiro, C. M., Devins, G. M., & Hussain, M. R. (1993). ABC of sleep disorders. Sleep problems in patients with medical illness. *British Medical Journal, 306*(6891), 1532–1535.

Sharpe, M. (1996). Chronic fatigue syndrome. *Psychiatric Clinics of North America, 19*(3), 549–573.

Sharpe, M., Chalder, T., Palmer, I., & Wessely, S. (1997). Chronic fatigue syndrome. A practical guide to assessment and management. *General Hospital Psychiatry, 19*(3), 185–199.

Sharpe, M., Hawton, K., Seagroatt, V., & Pasvol, G. (1992). Follow up of patients presenting with fatigue to an infectious diseases clinic. *British Medical Journal, 305,* 147–152.

Sharpe, M., Hawton, K., Simkin, S. Surawy, C., Hackmann, A., Klimes, I., et al. (1996). Cognitive behavior therapy for the chronic fatigue syndrome: a randomized controlled trial. *British Medical Journal, 312,* 22–26.

Sharpley, A., Clements, A., Hawton, K., & Sharpe, M. (1997). Do patients with "pure" CFS (neurasthenia) have abnormal sleep? *Psychosomatic Medicine, 59*, 592–596.

Simon, G., & Von Korff, M. (1991). Somatization and psychiatric disorder in the NIMH Epidemiologic Catchment Area Study. *American Journal of Psychiatry, 148*, 1494–1500.

Strayer, D. R., Carter, W. A., Brodsky, I., Cheney, P., Peterson, D., Salvato, P., et al. (1994). A controlled clinical trial with a specifically configured RNA drug, poly(I).poly(C12U), in chronic fatigue syndrome. *Clinical Infectious Diseases, 18*(Suppl 1), S88–S95.

Strayer, D. R., Carter, W. A., Stouch, B. C. V., Steven, S. R., Bateman, L., Cimoch, P. J., et al. (2012). A double-blind, placebo-controlled, randomized, clinical trial of the TLR-3 agonist rintatolimod in severe cases of chronic fatigue syndrome. *PLoS One, 7*, e31334–e31319.

Streeten, D. H. (1998). The nature of chronic fatigue. (editorial/review). *Journal of the American Medical Association, 280*, 1094–1095.

Stubhaug, B., Lie, S. A., Ursin, H., & Eriksen, H. R. (2008). Cognitive-behavioural therapy v. mirtazapine for chronic fatigue and neurasthenia: randomised plaebo-controlled trial. *British Journal of Psychiatry, 192*, 217–223.

Taerk, G. & Gnam, W. (1994). A psychodynamic view of the chronic fatigue syndrome: the role of object relations in etiology and treatment. *General Hospital Psychiatry 16*, 319–325.

Taerk, G. S., Toner, B. B., Salit, I. E., Garkinkel, P. E., & Ozersky, S. (1987). Depression in patients with neuromyasthenia (benign myalgic encephalomyelitis). *International Journal of Psychiatry in Medicine, 17*, 49–56.

Tak, L. M., Cleare, A. J., Ormel, J., Manoharan, A., Kok, I. C., Wessely, S., et al. (2011). Meta-analysis and meta-regression of hypothalamic-pituitary adrenal axis activity in functional somatic disorders. *Biological Psychology, 87*, 183–194.

Taylor, R. R., Jason, L. A., & Curie, C. J. (2002). Prognosis of chronic fatigue in a community-based sample. *Psychosomatic Medicine, 64*, 319–327.

Ustun, T., & Sartorius, N. (Eds.) (1995). *Mental illness in general health care: An international study.* Chichester: John Wiley & Sons.

van Cauwenbergh, D., Nijs, J., Kos, D., van Weijnen, L., Struyf, F., & Meeus, M. (2014). Malfunctioning of the autonomic nervous system in patients with chronic fatigue syndrome: a systematic literature review. *European Journal of Clinical Investigation, 44*, 516–526.

vanWaveren, E. K. (1996). The rise and fall of the chronic fatigue syndrome as defined by Holmes et al. *Medical Hypotheses, 46*(2), 63–66.

Vercoulen, J. H., Hoofs, M. P., Bleijenberg, G., Swanink, C. M., Vreden, S. G., Fennis, J. F., et al. (1996). Randomised, double-blind, placebo-controlled study of fluoxetine in chronic fatigue syndrome. *Lancet, 347*(9005), 858–861.

Vincent, A., Brimmer, D. J., Whipple, M. O., Jones, J. F., Boneva, R., Lahr, B. D., et al. (2012). Prevalence, incidence, and classification of chronic fatigue syndrome in Olmsted County, Minnesota, as estimated using the Rochester Epidemiology Project. *Mayo Clinic Proceedings, 87*, 1145–1152.

Vollmer-Conna, U., Hickie, I., Hadzi-Pavlovic, D., Tymms, K., Wakefield, D., Dwyer, J., et al. (1997). Intravenous immunoglobulin is ineffective in the treatment of patients with chronic fatigue syndrome. *American Journal of Medicine, 103*, 38–43.

Walker, E. A., Katon, W. J., & Jemelka, R. P. (1993). Psychiatric disorders and medical care utilization among people in the general population who report fatigue. *Journal of General Internal Medicine, 8*, 436–440.

Wessely, S. (1995). The epidemiology of chronic fatigue syndrome. *Epidemiologic Review, 17*(1), 139–151.

Wessely, S. (1996). Chronic fatigue syndrome: summary of a report of a joint committee of the Royal Colleges of Physicians, Psychiatrists & General Practitioners. *Journal of Royal College of Physicians of London, 30*(6), 497–504.

White, P. D., Grover, S. A., Kangro, H. O., Thomas, J. M., Amess, J., & Clare, A. W. (1995). The validity and reliability of the fatigue syndrome that follows glandular fever. *Psychological Medicine, 25*(5), 917–924.

Wilson, A., Hickie, I., Lloyd, A., & Wakefield, D. (1994). The treatment of chronic fatigue syndrome: science and speculation. *American Journal of Medicine, 96*(6), 544–550.

Wormser, G.P., Dattwyler, R. J., Shapiro, E.D., Halperin, J. J., Steere, A.C., Klempner, M. S., et al. (2006). The clinical assessment, treatment and prevention of Lyme disease, human granulocytic anaplasmosis, and babesiosis: Clinical practice guidelines by the Infectious Diseases Society of America. *Clinical Infectious Diseases, 43*, 1089.

Yehuda, R., Southwick, S., Krystal, J., Bremner, D., Charney, D. S., & Mason, J. W. (1993). Enhanced suppression of cortisol following dexamethasone administration in posttraumatic stress disorder. *American Journal of Psychiatry, 150*(1), 83–86.

Zubieta, J., Englenberg, N., Yargic, I., Pande, A. C., & Demitrack, M. A. (1994). Seasonal symptom variation in patients with chronic fatigue: comparison with major mood disorders. *Journal of Psychiatric Research, 28*(1), 13–22.

35.

SEXUAL DYSFUNCTION

Barry S. Fogel and Donna B. Greenberg

INTRODUCTION

Patients may bring to the medical psychiatrist their concerns about sexual function, their preoccupations about sex, or the quality of the sexual relationship with a partner. On occasion, sexual issues will be identified in the course of medical psychiatric assessment for a nonsexual presenting problem such as chronic pain or depression. In either case the medical psychiatrist often is the only medical professional who engages the patient in a detailed exploration of sexual issues. Patients for whom the presenting issue is not sexual sometimes are reticent to talk about their sexuality. Reluctance to talk openly about the subject does not signify that it is unimportant to the patient; epidemiologic studies suggest that the minority of individuals with common forms of sexual dysfunction, such as erectile dysfunction or postmenopausal dyspareunia, will bring their problems to a physician's attention. A satisfying sexual life contributes to a patient's happiness and overall life satisfaction, and, when it is a life goal, not having one can affect a patient's self-confidence and self-esteem. Thus, even when discussion of sexual issues is not timely at the initial encounter with the patient, the topic should remain as an open item in the psychiatrist's mind—one to be explored in the future with the patient if the professional relationship continues. The association of sexual dysfunction with internal disease, especially in men, is another reason to explore sexual issues that are not spontaneously raised. Erectile dysfunction before age 60 is associated with a significant increase in the risk of myocardial infarction, even after controlling for hypertension, hypercholesterolemia, and smoking. Mainstream cardiologists have recommended that the new onset of erectile dysfunction in a younger man warrants an cardiogram and a stress test, and some have gone so far as to recommend CT scan assessment of coronary calcification in this situation even when the stress test is negative (Nehra et al., 2013; Miner et al., 2014). In addition to cardiovascular disease, testosterone deficiency is another prevalent condition that can present with erectile dysfunction—with or without loss of sexual interest.

A trusted physician explaining the connection between health-related behaviors and sexual function can be useful in motivating a patient to make valuable changes in lifestyle. A man's belief that changes in his diet or exercise habits will improve his sexual performance can be more effective than general knowledge about lifestyle and longevity, and the experience of improved sexual performance can be immediately reinforcing.

On a population level, better health is unequivocally correlated with more sexual activity and greater sexual satisfaction. For example, older heterosexual couples who engage in regular sexual intercourse have lower levels of depressive symptoms, better cardiovascular health, and a lower waist circumference than similarly aged couples that don't (Brody, 2010). More generally, individuals with good to excellent self-reported health are more likely to be sexually active than those with fair to poor self-reported health (Lindau & Gavrilova, 2010). Some patients will realize apparent physical and mental health benefits from an active sexual life while others enjoy good health without one. It is reasonable to assume that a younger patient who has never had a satisfying sexual life is likely to want one, and that an older patient who has previously had a satisfactory sexual life will feel a loss if sexual activity is no longer feasible, physically possible, or satisfying. Expectations of sexual behavior later in sexual life differ widely according to culture and according to age cohort. Regarding the latter effect, Beckman, Waern, Gustafson, and Skoog (2008) analyzed cross-sectional data from populations surveys in Gothenburg, Sweden, and found that between 1971 and 2000 the percentage of married men reporting sexual intercourse rose from 52% to 68%; for married women the percentage rose from 38% to 56%. The most dramatic increase was seen in rates of sexual intercourse among unmarried 70-year-old women, which rose to 12% in 2000 from less than 1% in 1971. Sexual life continues into very old age if health permits and a partner is available. An Australian study of men over 75 found that among men aged 75 to 79 years, 40% had been sexually active in the prior year; the percentage decreased with age to 11% for men aged 90–95 (Hyde et al., 2010). Longitudinal studies of aging suggest that some people remain sexually active past age 100 if a partner is available. However, many people regard it as normal to completely stop having sexual intercourse at some point in their later years, even if they live with a spouse or partner with whom they have been sexually active in the past (Lindau et al., 2007).

Interest in sex (a desire to be sexual) and sexual interest (a desire to have sex, whether in general or with a specific actual or fantasied partner) are not the same. A patient can wish to have sexual desire but not feel it. If the medical psychiatrist determines that a patient wishes to be sexual, this is sufficient reason to explore the issue further even if the patient has not been sexually active recently or has not recently experienced sexual desire. The medical psychiatrist can determine what aspects of the sexual experience are most related to the patient's satisfaction; this will influence the focus of treatment. For some patients having an orgasm is less important than physical closeness to or the satisfaction of a spouse or partner. For others, arousal without orgasm is an intensely unpleasant experience. The mechanical aspects of sex—physical arousal, erection or lubrication, and orgasm—often are the easiest ones to address. For each there is a reasonable base of evidence for differential diagnosis and for treatment. In the 15 years since the last edition of this volume was written, accurate diagnosis and effective treatment for mechanical aspects of sex have become more widely available, and information about almost any sexual topic has become easy to find on the Internet (though not always accurate). Notwithstanding, even now patients with addressable physical impediments to sexual satisfaction do not necessarily seek treatment for them, and this is true even when the patient's sexual issues cause them emotional distress or adversely affect the quality of their marital relationship.

While there is much written about the workup of sexual dysfunction, the authors find it useful to think about the sexuality of medical-psychiatric patients in a broader context.

This chapter offers a framework for conceptualizing sexual issues in patients with general medical illness. Detailed discussion of physiological aspects of male sexual function and dysfunction can be found in this book's chapters on urology and on spinal cord injury.

ANALYZING SEXUALITY IN MEDICAL PSYCHIATRIC PATIENTS

The following sequence of questions describes the scope of an ideal inquiry into the sexual issues of a medical-psychiatric patient. The actual questions the clinician will ask will depend on the reason for the consultation, the amount of time available, the setting of the interview, the patient's current mental status, and, importantly, the scope of the clinician's "license". The latter will be quite different when the medical psychiatrist is intervening in a crisis where a patient is resistant to medically necessary care versus when he or she is responding to a patient's personal request for help in coping with the emotional impact of a serious illness.

1. *Set the context.* Is the patient sexually active in any way— with a partner or solo? If not, does the patient wish to be? If there is a wish but no activity, what is the reason? When was the patient last sexually active and what was the sexual experience like at that time? If there is no wish to be sexually active, when did they last have such a wish? If the patient has a regular sexual relationship how frequently do they have sex? Who usually initiates the sexual encounter?

2. *Assess sexual interest.* If the patient does not wish to be sexual at all, what is the reason? Is it related to a specific

traumatic event? Is the lack of an interest in sex due to a belief of some kind? For example, does the patient who has no sexual partner feel undesirable to a potential partner because of their age, appearance, or health status? Does the patient feel masturbation is wrong or harmful? Or, does the patient simply not care about sexuality at this particular point in their life? Is there any distress or perplexity associated with the loss of interest in sex? If the patient does not wish to be sexual because the spouse or partner is not interested, why does the spouse or partner lack interest? What is the recent history of the couple's sexual relationship? Does the spouse or partner find the lack of a sexual relationship to be acceptable?

3. *Assess desire.* If the patient wishes to be sexual but feels no desire, is that loss of interest generalized or specific to the current spouse or partner? Desire can be viewed as a balance of impulse and inhibition. It can be assessed over days or over hours. General medical illness, medications, and emotional reactions to illness can affect either impulse, inhibition, or both. Fatigue reduces the impulse, while the irritability that comes with fatigue increases the power of environmental effects to inhibit desire. How would the patient describe the interplay of impulse and inhibition in their own experience? Can they offer examples where they noticed a lack of response to circumstances that they would expect to find arousing? Can they recall specific reasons why sexual activity didn't take place because something interfered? Does the patient have a problem with sleep or with sleepiness? Sleep disorders are common. Lack of sleep is associated with reduced desire, greater vulnerability of desire to inhibition by distraction or discomfort, and decreased physical arousal. Snoring, restless legs or a disturbing parasomnia can inhibit the arousal of the partner.

4. *Assess arousal.* If the patient or partner is a woman, does she experience emotional arousal? If so, is there associated lubrication or does the vagina remain dry? If the patient or partner is a man, does he have an erection? Is the erection persistent? Is it firm enough for penetration?

5. *Assess sexually related pain.* Does the patient have, anticipate having, or fear having some form of physical discomfort during sexual activity? In the medical psychiatric contexts sexually related discomfort encompasses much more than dyspareunia. Sexually related discomforts range broadly from dyspnea on exertion to muscle pain to neuropathic dysesthesia of the pelvis or thighs to postcoital migraine. These symptoms or avoidance of them not only can cause conscious avoidance of sex but can also inhibit the patient's desire. Eventually "yes but" becomes "not tonight" and then just "no".

6. *Assess orgasm, including its qualitative aspects.* Does the patient have orgasms, and if so, is it qualitatively the same as in times past? If the patient is a woman, has she ever had an orgasm? If so has she had one with intercourse? If she does not have orgasms does she come close to having one? Is the experience of arousal without orgasm pleasant or unpleasant? If the patient is a man and he does not now

have orgasms does he get close to having one? Is the experience of arousal without orgasm pleasant or unpleasant? If he has an orgasm does he ejaculate normally? Does he ejaculate earlier than he desires? And with how much stimulation? Does he have a sense of control over his ejaculation?

7. *Assess the patient's view of the spouse or partner's sexual function.*

8. *Assess satisfaction and frustration of the patient and partner, qualitatively and quantitatively.* How does the patient's sexual dysfunction affect the quality of the sexual relationship? How distressing does the patient find the sexual dysfunction? Does the patient find intimacy with their spouse or partner to be satisfying despite the sexual dysfunction? What is the spouse or partner's point of view on these matters?

9. *Explore consideration of sexual alternatives*: Is the patient willing to consider alternatives to their customary sexual repertoire before illness? For example, willingness to consider alternatives to vaginal intercourse varies greatly with patients' cultural background and openness to new experiences. Even with the greater permissiveness of mainstream culture in Western countries, many patients come from a cultural or religious background that restricts the acceptable forms of sexual expression. Patients with such issues vary in their acceptance of permission to experiment when the permission is given by a physician. The patient's personality is relevant as well; those patients with personalities that are high on the openness factor are more likely to accept alternative forms of sexual expression.

10. *Consider specialist referral.* Is the patient open to referral to a specialist in sexual medicine? Such a referral would be a second or third referral, following the referral to the medical psychiatrist, which in itself might have come through another medical specialist or through a nonphysician mental health professional. Accepting this referral, which is based on an explicitly sex-related reason, requires that a patient believes that the sexual issue is important enough to deserve an investment of time and resources, that there is some hope of a good outcome, and that the specialist is competent, trustworthy, and will maintain confidentiality. Furthermore, it may require the approval—or at least the nonopposition—of a spouse or significant other. A referral to a specialist in sexual medicine may be more acceptable to a patient if the medical psychiatrist takes sufficient time to explore relationship issues, interest in sex, openness to alternatives, and the relationships of these sexual issues to the patient's personal history and current physical and mental health problems. Through the process of exploration, the explicitly sexual issue can become part of the patient's personal problem list. With this motivation a specialty referral usually will be appreciated; without it the patient may not follow through.

SCREENING PATIENTS FOR SEXUAL DYSFUNCTION

Studies of sexual dysfunction in medical patients have led to the development of efficient screening questions for detecting the most common sexual issues. Questions can be asked in writing via questionnaires to be completed by the patient or asked orally by the physician as part of the overall history and examination. Questionnaires and self-rated instruments sometimes will elicit information about sexual concerns that would not come out in a face-to-face interview. When they are available and applicable, sexuality related rating scales specific to the patient's medical illness or condition can be more informative than general scales of sexual function and dysfunction.

INTERVIEW QUESTIONS SCREENING FOR SEXUAL DYSFUNCTION

The following short list of sexuality related questions was recommended by Shafer (2008) for inclusion in a general diagnostic interview. Questions can be reworded if this would make the interview more comfortable for the patient.

1. Are you active sexually? With men, women, or both?

2. In your sex life:
   a. is there anything you would like to change?
   b. have there been any changes recently?
   c. are you satisfied?

Additional screening questions have been suggested by Althof and colleagues (2013):
For both men and women:

1. Do you identify yourself as heterosexual, homosexual, or bisexual?

2. Are you satisfied with the level of your sexual desire or interest?

3. Are you satisfied with the frequency of lovemaking?

4. Do you experience pain during lovemaking?

5. Are you satisfied with the overall quality of your sexual life?

For men:

1. Are you satisfied with your ability to achieve and maintain an erection?

2. Do you frequently have difficulty ejaculating?

3. Do you frequently ejaculate too quickly without wanting to?

4. Have you noticed any changes to the shape of your penis?

For women:

1. During lovemaking do you have difficulty becoming mentally aroused?

2. During lovemaking do you have difficulty with genital lubrication (wetness)?

3. Do you have difficulty achieving orgasm when you want to?

QUESTIONNAIRES AND SELF-RATED INSTRUMENTS

Questionnaires for assessing sexual dysfunction can be either generic or problem-specific. Generic rating scales should be considered for use in medical-psychiatric settings where sexual dysfunction has a high prevalence and it is feasible to follow up any issues identified. Once a sexual issue has been identified, a problem-specific scale can be helpful in better characterizing it, gauging its severity, and assessing its response to treatment. Table 35.1 lists sexual dysfunction scales widely used in clinical research and increasingly in clinical practice.

An additional instrument, the Sexual Excitation/Sexual Inhibition Inventory for Women and Men (SESII-W/M; Milhausen, Graham, Sanders, Yarber, & Maitland, 2010), is a questionnaire comprising 30 four-point bidirectional ordinal items concerning what excites and what inhibits individuals' sexual desire. There are six domains: (1) inhibitory cognitions—for example, "Sometimes I have so many worries that I am unable to be aroused"; (2) relationship importance—for example, "I really need to trust a partner to be fully aroused"; (3) arousability—for example, "Just talking about sex is enough to put me in a sexual mood"; (4) partner characteristics and behaviors—for example, "If a partner surprises me by doing chores it sparks my sexual interest"; (5) setting—for example, "Having sex in a different setting than usual is a real turn on for me"; and (6) dyadic elements of the sexual interaction—for example, "It interferes with my arousal if there is not a balance of giving and receiving pleasure during sex". When counseling a patient with sexual dysfunction in the context of general medical illness, the clinician should help the patient and spouse or partner find practical strategies to increase excitement and decrease inhibition. Specific items on the SESII-W/M offer clues to these strategies, and the discussion of each other's answers to the questions on the instrument can help a couple communicate about issues related to sexual interest as opposed to performance.

INVOLVING THE SPOUSE OR PARTNER

When a patient is in an ongoing sexual relationship it is often—but not always—useful to involve the partner in addressing an issue of sexual dysfunction. The patient and the spouse or partner must agree to be seen together. If one and/or the other do not agree to this, the reason can be diagnostically informative. Whether the medical psychiatrist sees the couple or refers the couple to another professional for couples therapy or sex therapy will depend specifically on the medical psychiatrist's scope of expertise, expectations for the duration, and scope and focus for his/her future work with the patient. If the expectation is for time-limited or intermittent therapy with a practical focus on coping with a general medical illness it is usually a positive for the medical psychiatrist to see the couple personally. If the expectation is for long-term psychodynamic psychotherapy, a referral for the couple probably will be more compatible with the patient's future treatment.

When a patient is not in a sexual relationship but wants to be in one, and is deterred by fear of a sexual dysfunction (such as erectile dysfunction, premature ejaculation, or vaginismus), referral to a sex therapy clinic is an attractive option when it is feasible. Such clinics offer sex education, evidence-based cognitive behavioral therapy, physical treatment for vaginismus, and in some cases treatment involving a surrogate partner. A referral for sex therapy offers the patient access to the most effective available treatments, while avoiding the ethical and transference-related risks of the psychiatrist's getting overinvolved in a patient's sex life.

LOSS OF SEXUAL INTEREST (LOSS OF LIBIDO)

Patients of either sex can have the symptom of low libido, that is, the relative or complete absence of sexual fantasies or desire to engage in sexual activity. A patient may or may not be troubled by a loss of libido—in other words, patients without sexual interest may or may not retain an interest in sex. Loss of sexual interest is a common accompaniment of general medical illness and a side effect of numerous medications that affect the CNS, whether or not a CNS disease was their target. When evaluating a patient with this complaint, the medical psychiatrist should first determine if any of the following situations applies:

- The patient has some specific form of sexual dysfunction (e.g., ED or PE) and is not interested in sex because he or she does not wish to repeat an unhappy sexual experience.

- The patient's sexual function is intact, but the patient wishes to avoid physical symptoms, expecting or fearing that they will accompany or follow sexual activity.

- The patient has symptoms such as fatigue or pain that interfere with sexual arousal.

- The patient has a general loss of interest and pleasure in many activities, sex being one of them.

Each of these conditions implies a medical differential diagnosis, and in most cases there is some prospect for a return of sexual interest if the underlying medical condition is addressed or if an offending drug is discontinued. Most endocrine and neurological conditions that affect sexual interest also have other somatic and mental symptoms. Hypothyroidism, a relatively common endocrine disorder, causes a loss of libido that is reversed when the patient becomes euthyroid, though loss of libido would rarely be the *sole* symptom of the disorder at the time of presentation. A relatively specific loss of libido *can* be seen due to a deficiency of testosterone in men, or due to a deficiency of estrogen or testosterone in women (Yasui et al., 2012).

Table 35.1 SEXUAL DYSFUNCTION QUESTIONNAIRES

TEST	DESCRIPTION	REFERENCE
For Either Gender		
Arizona Sexual Experience Inventory (ASEX)	5-item questionnaire comprising six-point ordinal items; one week look-back period. Questions concern (1) sex drive; (2) ease of arousal; (3) erectile function for men, lubrication for women; (4) ease of reaching orgasm; (5) satisfaction with orgasms	McGahuey et al., 2000.
For Men		
Male Sexual Health Questionnaire (MSHQ)		Rosen et al., 2004
Sexual Health Inventory for Men (SHIM)	5-item screening form of IIEF. Also known as the IIEF-5.	Rosen et al., 1999; Vroege, 1999; Cappeliere & Rosen, 1999
International Index of Erectile Function (IIEF)	15-item questionnaire; 5- or 6-point ordinal items; five domains: erectile function, orgasmic function, sexual desire, intercourse satisfaction, overall satisfaction	Rosen et al., 1997; Rosen et al., 2002
Premature Ejaculation Diagnostic Tool (PEDT)	5-item questionnaire comprising 5-point ordinal items. Questions concern timing of ejaculation, sense of control, ejaculation with minimal stimulation, frustration with the problem, concern for partner's satisfaction	Symonds et al., 2007a; Symonds et al., 2007b; Abraham et al., 2008
Brief Sexual Function Inventory (BSFI)	11-item questionnaire; 5-point ordinal items. Five domains: sex drive, erection, ejaculation, perception of sexual problems, overall satisfaction	O'Leary et al., 1995
For Women		
Female Sexual Function Index (FSFI)	19-item questionnaire; 5-point ordinal items; 4-week look-back; six domains: desire, arousal, lubrication, orgasm, satisfaction, pain	Rosen et al., 2000
Female Sexual Distress Scale (FSDS)	12-item questionnaire; 5-point ordinal items rated on frequency; focus on distress, embarrassment, and other negative feelings related to sexual problems	Derogatis et al., 2002
Sexual Interest and Desire Inventory—Female (SIDI-F)	54-item interview based scale with 5-point ordinal items. Assesses four dimensions: evaluative, physiological, motivational, negative/aversive.	Clayton et al., 2006
Profile of Female Sexual Function (PFSF)	37-item questionnaire focused on HSDD, 6-point ordinal items measuring frequency. Seven domains: desire, arousal, orgasm, sexual pleasure, sexual concerns, sexual responsiveness, sexual self-image	Derogatis et al., 2004

MALE SEXUAL DYSFUNCTION

The most prevalent types of male sexual dysfunction in general medical settings are erectile dysfunction (ED), premature ejaculation (PE), loss of sexual interest, and ejaculatory dysfunction. All can usefully be viewed as conditions that are rarely purely "psychogenic" but almost always have emotional dimensions.

ERECTILE DYSFUNCTION

ED is defined as the inability of a man to maintain an erection sufficient to engage in intercourse. The prevalence of ED increases with age, mainly due to age-associated disease rather than to aging per se. ED in men under 60 especially raises the

suspicion of systemic disease, specifically cardiovascular or peripheral vascular disease, neuropathy, or endocrine disease. ED is seen in more than half of men with diabetes, and it can be the first symptom of the disease. A clearly new onset of ED in a man of any age should trigger a full medical reassessment, including an electrocardiogram and stress test, screening for glucose intolerance, and measurement of serum testosterone (Shamloul & Ghanem, 2013; Ghanem, Salonia, & Martin-Morales, 2013; Miner et al., 2014).

The medical causes of ED can be grouped into central (endocrine and neuropsychiatric), vascular and neurogenic. Under ordinary circumstances a man's erection begins with a central message of sexual arousal that is itself triggered by a sensory stimulus, a memory, or an association, sending a message through the autonomic nervous system to the penis. This triggers engorgement of the corpora cavernosa, a process involving the inflow of arterial blood and the blockage of venous outflow. ED is explained by altered function at one or more points along this pathway. The various diagnostic tests that have been developed for diagnosing the cause of ED all aim to establish or rule out dysfunction at specific points in the pathway. For example, a Doppler ultrasound study of penile blood flow after intracavernous injection of prostaglandin specifically assesses whether arterial flow to the penis is adequate and whether the venous outflow is blocked without excessive leakage.

Historically physicians have been concerned with distinguishing "organic" from "psychogenic" ED. Practice has been moving away from this dualism because most patients with persistent ED have one or more general medical conditions that contribute to it, and ED in patients due to known general medical problems can be better or worse according to the patient's mental state and situation. For this reason, the nocturnal penile tumescence (NPT) test is now seldom done, though medical psychiatrists will occasionally encounter the test. The NPT test uses an electrical strain gauge applied to the base and tip of the penis to determine the number of times and the degree to which the penis becomes rigid during sleep. The occurrence of multiple rigid erections during a night of sleep confirms that a complaint of ED is not due to peripheral neural or vascular factors. A lack of erections, or a lack of sufficient rigidity, suggests there are such neural or vascular factors contributing to the ED. The limitation of the NPT test is that a patient with normal erections during sleep can still have a nonpsychological reason for ED, for example, low testosterone. And a patient with impaired erections during sleep may have a significant emotional component to his ED in addition to the neural and/or vascular factors.

PDE5 Inhibitors

The advent of phophodiesterase-5 (PDE5) inhibitors radically changed the diagnosis of ED as well as its treatment. At this time, most men without gross urological or neurological pathology who present to a physician with ED will have a general medical assessment followed by a trial of a PDE5 inhibitor, unless they are taking nitrates for angina pectoris or the general medical workup reveals unstable cardiac disease. If the PDE5 inhibitor is effective the patient receives an ongoing prescription for one of them. If it is not, a further workup is done.

While this practice has made ED treatment much more widely available—and has thus encouraged men to recognize the problem and talk about it—it has two significant drawbacks. One is that important and treatable contributors to ED can be neglected if a PDE5 inhibitor works despite them. The second is that many men will try a PDE5 inhibitor as prescribed by their primary care physician or urologist, find that it doesn't work or has intolerable side effects, and then give up on restoring their sexual potency—much as some patients who appropriately receive an SSRI for depression from their primary care physician may abandon efforts to treat their depression if that SSRI is not tolerated or is ineffective at the dose at which it was prescribed. In many of these cases either a different PDE5 or a different dose will be tolerated and effective; in others, another intervention in place of or in addition to a PDE5 inhibitor will work.

There are four PDE5 inhibitors approved in the US for treatment of ED: sildenafil (Viagra), tadalfil (Cialis), vardenifil (Levitra) and avanafil (Stendra). They are equally efficacious for treating ED but differ in their pharmacokinetics and in their specificity for inhibition of PDE5. The latter may account for some of the differences in side effect profiles. Sildenafil, the first PDE5 inhibitor to be approved, will be the first to be available in a lower cost generic version.

Table 35.2 summarizes the differences between the four PDE5 inhibitors available in the United States. Note that of the four, vardenafil is the only one associated with QT prolongation. Vardenafil is not recommended in patients taking type 1A or type 3 antiarrhythmics or those who have a prolonged QT interval (Corona, Razzoli, Forti, & Maggi, 2008). All of the PDE5 inhibitors can cause headache, flushing, nasal or sinus congestion, or dyspepsia. While about one-third of men will develop one or more side effects from use of a PDE5 inhibitor, fewer than 10% will discontinue the medication because of one of these side effects—and that percentage is even lower with tadalafil and avanafil. Considerations in the

Table 35.2 COMPARISON OF APPROVED PDE5 INHIBITORS

DRUG	ONSET OF ACTION	COMMENTS
Avanafil	Tmax 30–45 minutes; half-life 5 hours.	Most specific for PDE5; most rapid onset. No food effect. More flushing and headache than others. Lowest reported rate of discontinuation for side effects in clinical trials.
Sildenafil	Tmax 1 hour; half-life 4 hours	Absorption delayed by high-fat meal. Least specific for PDE5; most reports of vision or hearing loss; more benign visual symptoms than others. First to go off-patent.
Tadalafil	Tmax 2 hours; half-life 17.5 hours	Approved for daily use. More myalgias than others. No food effect. Preferred by most men who have tried several.
Vardenafil	T max 1 hour: half-life 4 hours	Associated with QT prolongation. Absorption delayed by high-fat meal. More back pain than others.

(Yuan et al., 2013; Raheem & Kell, 2009).

choice of a PDE5 inhibitor for a specific patient were comprehensively reviewed by Corona et al. (2011).

All of the PDE5 inhibitors will cause hypotensive reactions when combined with nitrates; because these reactions can be of life-threatening severity the combination is absolutely contraindicated. The combination of a PDE5 inhibitor with an alpha-adrenergic blocker can cause hypotension as well, although the degree is variable and the combination is not contraindicated; in fact, the combination can have additive benefits in patients with lower urinary tract symptoms (LUTS) due to benign prostate disease. When using the two drugs together, the risk of symptomatic hypotension is minimized by choosing an alpha blocker such as tamulosin that is more specific for urinary tract alpha receptors, and by introducing the medicines one at a time with the second one started at a low dose and increased slowly.

Two very rare adverse effects of PDE5 inhibitors must be mentioned in the process of informed consent for their use (they are also likely to be mentioned by patients who are especially attuned to rare but serious potential side effects of medications). These are sudden loss of vision due to ischemic optic neuropathy and sudden loss of hearing due to ischemic cochlear damage. The risk of these adverse effects probably is less than one in 10,000 patients treated. The risk of either is greater at higher dosages; thus drug interactions due to CYP3A4 inhibition will increase the risk.

Nonarteritic anterior ischemic optic neuropathy (NAION) is a rare condition that can cause loss of visual acuity and even blindness. While numerous cases have been reported of NAION in men taking PDE5 inhibitors, the relationship of the drug to the eye disease is poorly understood. The overall incidence of NAION in adults over 50 is 2 to 10 per 100,000 per year. Thus, an extremely large sample would be needed to show the statistical significance of an increase in risk associated with a drug. Most patients who take PDE5 inhibitors have other risk factors of NAION, such as hypertension, nocturnal hypotension, smoking, sleep apnea, diabetes, hyperlipidemia, and/or prothrombotic factors. Notwithstanding, there are well-documented cases, most involving sildenafil, in which men developed sudden visual loss after talking a PDE5 inhibitor. The visual loss was resolved when the drug was stopped and recurred when the drug was restarted. There were other cases in which men lost vision in one eye coincident with taking a PDE5 inhibitor and lost vision in the other eye when rechallenged with the drug. The putative mechanism is hypotension in the branches of the posterior ciliary artery that supply the optic nerve head, possibly compounded by a loss of autoregulation of blood flow, endothelial dysfunction and choking off of the blood supply to the disc by ischemia-related edema. The last of these mechanisms can occur in men with small optic discs and a relatively small optic cup—so-called "discs at risk" (Danesh-Meyer & Levin, 2007). Patients should be warned about this potential issue and advised to stop their PDE5 inhibitor and consult an ophthalmologist immediately if they experience a sudden loss of visual acuity. Patients who have visible arterial disease in the optic fundi, small optic discs, and small optic cups should be warned that they are at particular risk for this side effect. If a patient with an elevated risk for

NAION wishes to try PDE5 therapy for ED and there are no other contraindications, low-dose daily tadalafil might be better than PRN sildenafil as it would avoid high peak levels of drug. However, there is no published evidence one way or the other.

Patients taking PDE5 inhibitors, especially sildenafil, can have benign visual symptoms such as altered color vision or increased glare sensitivity that do not alter or threaten to alter visual acuity and are completely unrelated to NAION. These are related to the effect of incidental PDE6 inhibition on retinal rods and cones. PDE6 is not found in the ophthalmic blood vessels (Laties & Sharlip, 2006). Among the four approved PDE5 inhibitors, avanafil is most specific for PDE5; a patient who develops troublesome though benign visual side effects on sildenafil might be switched to avanafil.

Sudden onset of sensorineural hearing impairment has been reported in association with PDE5 administration. Epidemiological evidence supports a potentially significant relationship to the use of sildenafil but not necessarily tadalafil or vardenafil. It is unclear if the mechanism of hearing loss is causally related: it could be due to local ischemia, to direct ototoxicity, or to eustachian tube obstruction with elevated middle ear pressure (McGwin, 2010). In a series of 18 men taking PDE5 inhibitors and monitored prospectively for hearing loss, four showed transient changes in auditory thresholds (Okuyucu, Guven, Akoglu, Uçar, & Dagli, 2009). However, the transient hearing loss observed by Okuyucu and colleagues is not necessarily due to the same mechanism as sudden and persistent hearing loss.

Among the PDE5 inhibitors, tadalafil is preferred by the majority of patients who have tried two or more. The preference has been attributed to the long half-life of the drug, which allows for greater spontaneity in the patient's sexual activity. Even so, some patients do not mind taking medication shortly before they anticipate having intercourse, and they may prefer avanafil or vardenafil because of their more rapid onset of action. In addition, a patient can have a side effect like headache, dyspepsia, or muscle pain with one PDE5 inhibitor and not with another.

All of the approved PDE5 inhibitors are metabolized by CYP3A4. Therefore, adjustment of the dosage of the PDE5 inhibitor often will be necessary if the patient is also taking another drug that induces or strongly inhibits CYP3A4. Patients suspected of having slow metabolism of CYP3A4 substrates because of their experience with other drugs should be started on lower than usual doses of PDE5 inhibitors.

In clinical use the PDE5 inhibitors raise issues homologous to those that arise with SSRI antidepressants: While the efficacy of the alternatives is the same in populations, individual patients can tolerate one better than another or can prefer one to another. Avanafil, the most PDE5-selective of the approved PDE5 inhibitors, may have the lowest incidence of adverse effects; in a recent Korean study fewer than 3% of men treated with avanafil over a 1-year period discontinued the drug because of side effects (Sanford, 2013). Dosage must be individualized and there are many potential drug interactions. A patient should be offered a trial of a different PDE5 inhibitor if they don't respond to the first one at the maximum tolerated approved dosage or if they have unpleasant (though not medically serious) side effects at the minimum efficacious dosage. Four attempts at intercourse with a specific PDE5 inhibitor and dose are sufficient to make a judgment about its efficacy.

A patient with ED and a low testosterone level (total T level <300 ng/mL) who does not responds to PDE5 inhibitor therapy may become a responder when testosterone supplementation is added (Shamloul et al., 2005). A patient with ED and chronic lower urinary tract symptoms (e.g., from chronic prostatitis or BPH) who does not respond to PDE5 inhibitors may become a responder when an alpha-adrenergic blocker is added. However, the combination is associated with the potential for symptomatic hypotension. Some patients with a partial but not satisfactory response to intermittent PDE5 therapy will respond to daily tadalafil, though the dosage required may be higher than the approved dosage of 5 mg per day. Daily tadalafil therapy is of particular interest in men with both ED and LUTS. LUTS can improve significantly with daily tadalafil, though tadalafil is not approved for this indication the improvement is of similar magnitude to that seen with alpha-adrenergic blockers (Park, Won, Sorsaburu, Rivera, & Lee, 2013).

Several other options are available for treatment of ED not responsive to PDE5 therapy. PDE5 inhibitors require sufficiently intact parasympathetic innervation of the penis. In cases of neuropathic or surgically related denervation of the penis, an intra-urethral pellet of prostaglandin E1 (PGE1; alprostadil) administered via an applicator may be efficacious, as the effect of PGE1 effect on the blood supply to the corpora cavernosa is independent of neural inputs to the blood vessels. Intracavernosal injections of alprostadil are even more efficacious in the same situation, though less preferred by most patients than the urethral suppositories because of the inconvenience of injection; in addition they can cause—albeit rarely—priapism or penile fibrosis (Costa & Potempa, 2012).

When ED is based on leakage from the veins of the corpora cavernosa an erection can be maintained by placing an elastic band around the base of the penis to block the outflow of blood. When arterial inflow is insufficient none of the above treatments can work; in this situation a penile prosthesis is the remaining option. There are both semirigid and inflatable prostheses; the choice is a matter of patient preference (Porst et al., 2013).

Thus, most cases of ED based on neural factors, vascular disease, and/or testosterone deficiency can be treated effectively. Optimal results in terms of a satisfying sexual life often require nonpharmacologic therapy in addition. Patients with significant general medical illness can have issues of depression, anxiety, or specific fears that affect their sexuality. Couple issues may contribute. Men with limited and largely disappointing sexual experience associated with ED can be in a self-defeating cycle in which they lack confidence and approach potential sexual relationships with anxiety that adversely affects their erectile function as well as their communication with their potential sexual partner. Cognitive behavioral therapy and group therapy can be helpful to such patients. Patients with disabilities that they fear will put off a potential partner might be appropriate candidates for sex therapy with a surrogate partner. In this case the patient would be referred to a well-reputed sex therapy clinic with an established surrogate program; less formal arrangements would be complicated by the potential for ethical and reputational issues.

PREMATURE EJACULATION

Premature ejaculation has been defined by the American Urological Association as ejaculation that occurs sooner than desired, either before or shortly after penetration, causing distress to one or both partners. A variety of alternative criteria have been proposed, some of which specify that ejaculation occurs within less than one minute or less than two minutes after penetration. However, the AUA definition is an inclusive one that is consistent with a patient-centered approach to the problem (Serefoglu & Saitz, 2012). The best established instrument for confirming a diagnosis of PE is the Premature Ejaculation Diagnostic Tool (PEDT; see Symonds et al., 2007; Althof & Symonds, 2007). The prevalence of PE in community studies has ranged widely, corresponding to the inclusiveness of the diagnostic criteria used. A recent study of almost 5,000 men using a criterion of PEDT ≥11 found a community prevalence of 16% (McMahon, Lee, Park, & Adaikan, 2012). Patients with PE usually do not seek treatment for it, and some younger men with the disorder will avoid sexual relationships or even intimacy with sexual potential because of embarrassment over the condition. Others present in infertility clinics, where a detailed history reveals that ejaculation prior to penetration has prevented fertilization.

PE can be either lifelong and consistent or acquired. Lifelong PE can persist for life if not treated; it represents a biological predisposition but is not due to medical disease. Acquired and subsequently persistent PE in a man with previously satisfactory ejaculatory function suggests either urological or endocrine disease, a drug side effect, or a psychological or relationship problem (Serefoglu & Saitz, 2012). Among psychological factors, anxiety related to the sexual relationship or the sexual act commonly contributes.

Treatment of lifelong PE should begin with sex education; treatment of acquired PE should begin with a medical-psychiatric evaluation. If the patient is in a marriage or other regular sexual relationship the spouse or partner usually should participate, although there are cases in which the patient wants to "own the problem" himself or in which working with the couple is otherwise complicated.

There are several efficacious pharmacological treatments, one of which is approved and available OTC. The approved treatment is a proprietary formulation of topical lidocaine—a eutectic lidocaine spray that the patient applies to the head and shaft of the penis about 10 minutes before intercourse. The lidocaine is formulated to penetrate the skin, providing sufficient reduction in sensation to increase the patient's time to orgasm. Systemic absorption is negligible, and there is not enough lidocaine transferred to impair the partner's sensation. The patient adjusts the number of sprays to the minimum necessary to attain a satisfactory post-penetration ejaculatory latency (McMahon, 2009; Promescent package insert).

Three off-label options are tramadol, SSRIs, and PDE5 inhibitors. Tramadol 25 mg taken shortly before intercourse can remarkably prolong intravaginal ejaculatory latency time (IELT); in one study IELT was extended by over 6 minutes (Salem et al., 2008). Tramadol has the potential to cause nausea, constipation, and sedation, as it does when used as an analgesic.

SSRIs taken daily at antidepressant doses will delay ejaculation, with a peak of effect after 1–2 weeks of treatment. A single dose of an SSRI taken 4–6 hours before intercourse can help, though less reliably than daily dosing. Loss of libido, ED, and orgasmic dysfunction are potential side effects in addition to the usual nonsexual side effects of SSRIs. Of greater concern to patients trying to conceive, SSRIs impair spermatogenesis and adversely affect semen quality (Safarinejad, 2008; Tanrikut, Feldman, Altemus, & Paduch, 2010; Koyuncu et al., 2011; Koyuncu, Serefoglu, Ozdemir, & Hellstrom, 2012; Alzahrani, 2012; Attia & Bakheet, 2013).

While PDE5 inhibitors don't prolong ejaculatory latency, they can help patients with PD in several ways. First, they address concomitant ED when it is present and, in any case, improve sexual confidence. Second, they reduce the refractory period following ejaculation, and patients who ejaculate prematurely with initial intercourse may have longer IELT on a second attempt a few minutes later. Third, they can mitigate ED that would otherwise be a side effect of topical lidocaine or SSRIs used to treat PE.

As with ED, combination of pharmacologic and nonpharmacologic therapy may be required for optimal outcome. However, it is worth noting that in men with lifelong PE pharmacologic therapies have larger effect sizes and more consistent results than psychotherapeutic and behavioral interventions. Psychotherapy and behavioral interventions have a more central role in acquired PE when the latter is not due to a new-onset endocrine or urological condition or a drug side effect.

ORGASMIC DYSFUNCTION

Orgasmic dysfunction can refer either to inhibited orgasm or to retrograde ejaculation; both conditions can be causes of male infertility. Retrograde ejaculation—semen discharge into the bladder rather than into the penile urethra, occurs when the internal urethral sphincter does not close during orgasm. Causes include prostate surgery and side effects of alpha-adrenergic blockers. Orgasm can be delayed by neuropathic sensory loss in the penis as well as by opiates; as noted above tramadol can profoundly affect time to ejaculation. Several classes of antidepressants can cause orgasmic dysfunction including SSRIs, SNRIs, MAOIs, and TCAs; among the latter clomipramine and amitriptyline are the worst as they have the greatest effects on serotonergic transmission. Anorgasmia due to these drugs sometimes can be reversed with PRN use of cyproheptadine, a serotonin antagonist. The dose is 4 mg 30–60 minutes before intercourse is planned; the main side effects are sedation and anticholinergic effects (which at worst can lead to ED). Yohimbine has also been used successful to reverse anorgasmia induced by antidepressants (Keller, Hamer, & Rosen, 1997); in contrast to cyproheptadine, it sometimes can improve arousal and erectile function.

While drugs with potent effects on serotonergic transmission can affect libido, arousal, and erection as well as orgasm, they often cause orgasmic dysfunction disproportionate to changes in other aspects of sexual function. A wide range of other drugs that cause orgasmic dysfunction usually do so more in proportion to other sexual side effects.

When a patient in a long-term sexual relationship newly develops orgasmic dysfunction not explained by a drug side effect, it is likely that there is a relationship issue. An effort should be made to assess the couple, either directly by the medical psychiatrist or through a referral. When the patient is the only willing participant in the treatment, the spouse or partner's role in the couple's dysfunction must be inferred and addressed indirectly.

Drugs with effects on adrenergic and serotonergic function are most frequently associated with orgasmic dysfunction. However, any of a broad range of drugs that have been associated with sexual dysfunction in general can cause orgasmic dysfunction in some patients. A list of common offenders is provided later in this chapter. Typically orgasmic dysfunction due to medications develops within weeks of starting the drug. Suspicion of inducing orgasmic dysfunction should thus fall mainly on drugs recently introduced or increased in dosage and on medications with blood levels or effects that might have increased recently because of interaction with another medication recently introduced, discontinued, or changed in dosage.

The literature on drug-induced orgasmic dysfunction has focused more on ejaculatory dysfunction in men than on impaired orgasm in women. If a woman newly develops inhibited orgasm after a change in medication regimen, this possibility should be considered, especially if the drug is relatively new to the market, notwithstanding the absence of published reports concerning female orgasmic dysfunction with the new medication.

LOSS OF LIBIDO

Loss of libido—decreased sexual interest, desire, and ease of sexual arousal—is a common accompaniment of chronic medical diseases, a typical symptom of depression, and a side effect of several commonly prescribed classes of drugs including the beta blockers and thiazide diuretics, as well as SSRIs and other agents affecting serotonergic neurotransmission. Specific diseases and drugs will be discussed later in this chapter.

A common intermediate factor linking chronic diseases with loss of libido—or accentuating the effect of chronic diseases on sexual function—is androgen deficiency (Traish, Miner, Morgentaler, & Zitzmann, 2011). Low testosterone causes a characteristic combination of symptoms including muscle wasting, abdominal obesity (sometimes with the metabolic syndrome), diminished vigor, and loss of libido. The testosterone level required for normal sexual function differs significantly among men (Finkelstein et al., 2013). When a man has a serum testosterone of <200 ng/mL, accepted practice is to give testosterone supplementation. When the testosterone level is borderline low—between 200 ng/mL and 300 ng/mL—*and* the patient has one or more characteristic symptoms of androgen deficiency, the patient should be given a trial of testosterone supplementation to bring the serum level to the middle of the normal range. If several weeks of supplementation to this level provides clear-cut symptomatic benefit, the treatment should be continued. Testosterone supplementation is given transdermally via a gel or a patch. A history of prostate cancer has until recently been regarded as a contraindication to testosterone therapy, and a survey of physicians suggested that fear of increasing prostate cancer risk was their greatest concern about testosterone replacement. However, no correlation has been demonstrated between testosterone levels and prostate cancer incidence in the general male population, and a multiple controlled trials of testosterone supplementation did not show a greater incidence of prostate cancer in men receiving testosterone than in those receiving placebo (Traish et al., 2011; Raynaud 2006; Shabsigh et al., 2004; Cui, Zong, Yan, & Zhang, 2014; Khera, Crawford, Morales, Salonia, & Morgentaler, 2014). Pastuszak et al. (2013) published a case series of men who had received radiation therapy for prostate cancer and subsequently received testosterone replacement therapy; none developed any recurrence of their cancer.

Morgentaler et al. (2011) have advanced the hypothesis that prostatic androgen receptors are saturated at a level of testosterone well below the threshold for symptomatic hypogonadism, so that men with prostate cancer and low testosterone levels who have not been castrated or treated with anti-androgens still have enough testosterone to saturate prostatic androgen receptors even though there are significant somatic symptoms of androgen deficiency. They infer that testosterone replacement to physiologic levels would not incrementally stimulate prostate growth, and thus that symptomatic testosterone deficiency could safely be treated in men with prostate cancer following cancer treatment that is appropriate for the size and stage of the cancer (Morgentaler et al., 2011). Notwithstanding, there remains some uncertainty on this point (Corona & Maggi, 2013). A conservative approach would be to monitor the patient for cancer recurrence for several months, then, if there were no evidence of recurrence and symptoms of hypogonadism were distressing, to replace testosterone to the physiological range. If the symptoms attributed to hypogonadism resolved and there were no increase in prostate-specific antigen or hemoglobin or change on the prostate examination, testosterone therapy would be continued. In most cases of sexual dysfunction encountered in medical psychiatric practice, testosterone deficiency is not the sole cause. However, correcting testosterone deficiency can be a necessary (though not usually sufficient) step to treat the dysfunction. For maximum diagnostic value, testosterone levels should be drawn in the morning. If results are borderline the test should be repeated, and free testosterone should be measured if the test is available.

FEMALE SEXUAL DYSFUNCTION

The most prevalent types of female sexual dysfunction are lack of sexual desire, impaired arousal, orgasmic dysfunction, dyspareunia (painful intercourse), and vaginismus (involuntary spasm of the vagina that prevents insertion of the penis into the vagina). The point prevalence of any sexual dysfunction in American women was 43% in a recent survey; however, only 12% of the women reporting sexual dysfunction reported being distressed by it. Most women with sexual dysfunction do not seek help for it. However, many more women will report sexual dysfunction to a physician if they are asked specifically about it. For example, in one gynecology outpatient clinic the frequency of spontaneous complaints of sexual dysfunction was 3%, but 19% of patients acknowledged a complaint if directly asked (Buster, 2013). A focus on changes in sexual interest (desire) is a useful point of departure for eliciting, diagnosing, and treating female sexual dysfunction. Often diminished desire and another sexual dysfunction will have the same cause, for example, diminished desire and orgasmic dysfunction due to an SSRI. And, if desire is strong, a patient will be motivated to address other sexual dysfunctions and relevant relationship and communication issues.

SEXUALLY RELATED PAIN: VAGINISMUS

Vaginismus is pain and spasm of the distal third of the vagina when penetration is attempted or, in severe cases, even contemplated. The spasm physically prevents vaginal intercourse; the condition is the most common reason for unconsummated marriages. Some women with vaginismus have a lifetime history of the condition, for example, always having been unable to use tampons during their menstrual periods. Others develop the condition suddenly after a history of successful vaginal intercourse. Acquired vaginismus can occur after sexual or emotional trauma, but many cases are unexplained. In milder cases suggestions by the patient's gynecologist are sufficient to resolve the problem. These include the following: (1) do Kegel exercises to build control of the pubococcygeal muscle; (2) use a generous amount of lubricant when intercourse is attempted; (3) use the female-superior position, as this gives the woman control over the rate of insertion; (4) attempt intercourse in a generally relaxed state in a pleasant environment; (5) practice the insertion of objects of progressively larger diameter into the vagina. The gynecologist can use (or provide) a graduated set of vaginal dilators; a cooperative spouse or sexual partner can use fingers to accomplish the same purpose. The medical psychiatrist can address the patient's fear and anxiety associated with either pharmacologic or nonpharmacologic treatment. Here too a cooperative spouse or partner sometimes can help.

The situation may arise where a woman with vaginismus has no partner and avoids romantic relationships because of concern they will lead to sex—a prospect that raises fears not only of pain but also embarrassment and possibly romantic abandonment. Treatment of such a patient by a sex therapy clinic that provides a surrogate partner might be considered when the option is available.

More severe cases of vaginismus may yield to progressive dilation of the vagina under anesthesia. If a patient's vaginismus does not resolve with these maneuvers it may respond to injections of botulinum toxin into the levator ani muscle

(Ferreira & Souza, 2012). Uncontrolled case series suggest a high response rate (Pacik, 2011).

SEXUALLY RELATED PAIN: DYSPAREUNIA

Dyspareunia is pain with vaginal intercourse. It can be secondary to any of a number of gynecologic conditions including infections, tumors, and endometriosis. However, the most common cause of dyspareunia that medical psychiatrists will encounter is postmenopausal vaginal and vulvar atrophy, a condition that affects as many as 45% of women later in life (North American Menopause Society, 2013). During and after the menopause, the deficiency of estrogen leads to thinning of the vaginal mucosa and a loss of secretions. In this condition, called *atrophic vaginitis* or *vulvovaginal atrophy*, the vaginal wall can be tender or simply can be dry and subject to irritation by the friction of intercourse. In addition to pain there can be a blood-tinged discharge following intercourse that a woman may find frightening. Pain with vaginal intercourse can lead to reduced sexual desire that in turn reduces the woman's motivation to address and resolve the dyspareunia. The treatment of atrophic vaginitis has been comprehensively reviewed by Tan and colleagues (2012).

Physicians treating postmenopausal dyspareunia tend to avoid systemic hormone replacement therapy (HRT) because of concerns about cancer risk and thromboembolic risk; they consider use of systemic HRT when there are other problems such as vasomotor symptoms and insomnia in addition to the vaginitis. When dyspareunia is the sole or main problem, the usual treatment is topical estrogen delivered as a cream (e.g., Premarin or Estrace cream), a vaginal tablet (e.g., Vagifem), or a ring-shaped pessary (e.g., Estring) (Archer, 2010; Castelo-Branco, Cancelo, Villero, Nohales, & Juliá, 2005). Topical estrogens are intended to be safe for long-term use without a concomitant progestin; the amount of estrogen absorbed systemically should be low enough that there is no thickening of the endometrium, no increased risk of endometrial cancer, Patients taking vaginal estrogen therapy that does not significantly raise estrogen blood levels appear to have no increased risk of breast cancer. However, the safety of vaginal estrogens for patients with estrogen receptor–positive breast cancer, including those taking aromatase inhibitors, is unknown (Ponzone et al., 2005).

While serum levels of estrogens in patients taking one of the commonly used vaginal estrogen preparations *usually* are well within the usual postmenopausal range, the systemic absorption and subsequent metabolism of estrogens from topical preparations is in fact variable, with some postmenopausal women having serum estrogen levels outside the normal postmenopausal range (Bhamra et al., 2011)—or suppression of their FSH levels—when taking the labeled dosage of estrogen cream or the now discontinued 25 μg dosage of the Vagifem estradiol tablet. Absorption of estrogens will depend in part on the condition of the vaginal mucosa. Once absorbed, estradiol is metabolized by CYP3A4, so whatever estradiol is systemically absorbed from the vagina will accumulate more if CYP3A4 is inhibited or if the patient is, for genetic reasons, a slow metabolizer of CYP3A4

substrates. Medically significant elevation of serum estrogen would be unusual but not completely impossible with the 10 μg Vagifem tablet or with Estring, which delivers approximately 7.5 μg/day of topical estradiol. In a safety study of 336 women sponsored by its manufacturer, the 10 μg Vagifem tablet (estradiol), taken once daily for 2 weeks and twice weekly thereafter, did not increase estradiol levels beyond the postmenopausal range or suppress FSH. Patients who took it showed no thickening of the endometrium on ultrasound examination or endometrial biopsy after 1 year of use (Chollet, 2011; Simon & Maamari, 2013).

A more conservative option for treating dyspareunia due to atrophic vaginitis is using a vaginal moisturizer on a regular basis (e.g., three times weekly). Many women first deal with postmenopausal dyspareunia by using a lubricant to facilitate intercourse. However, thrice-weekly use of a vaginal moisturizer is fundamentally more helpful for symptoms of vaginal atrophy than occasional use of a lubricant. It makes the vaginal wall thicker and more flexible as well as wetter, reducing itching, lowering vaginal pH, and, over several weeks, eventually providing as much relief from painful intercourse as vaginal estrogens for most (though not all) patients who take them (Bygdeman & Swahn, 1996). Replens and similar vaginal moisturizers use have ingredients similar to those used in sustained-release oral tablets; they might be thought of as "sustained release water" delivered to the dry vaginal surface.

A newly approved therapy for dyspareunia due to vulvar and vaginal atrophy is ospemifene, a selective estrogen receptor modulator (SERM). Given orally at a dose of 60 mg per day ospemifene restores the vaginal mucosa and relieves dyspareunia, without affecting the endometrium and thereby requiring concurrent progestin administration. It may have benefits for preventing osteoporosis like the SERM raloxifene, and preclinical studies suggest it might actually reduce breast cancer risk. As it was very recently approved, clinical experience and Phase 4 studies will be needed to delineate its place in the spectrum of treatment options (Soe, Wurz, Kao, & Degregorio, 2013).

There is some evidence that low doses of systemic testosterone (e.g., a 200 mg testosterone transdermal patch) can help atrophic vaginitis and restore sexual interest in postmenopausal women. Low-dose testosterone does not necessarily have unacceptable masculinizing effects (Davis et al., 2008; Braunstein et al., 2005), and it appears to be safe in this population (Shifren, Monz, Russo, Segreti, & Johannes, 2008). However, Endocrine Society guidelines do not at this time recommend androgens to menopausal symptoms (Wierman et al., 2006). Topical use of testosterone or DHEA may be an option for women who do not tolerate topical vaginal estrogens (Tan, Bradshaw, & Carr, 2012); research is ongoing.

Finally, some cases of discomfort with sexual intercourse are related to muscle pain that can be addressed by improving the tone of the pelvic muscles. This is done with the same Kegel exercises that are recommended for stress urinary incontinence, for vaginismus, and for preparation for pregnancy.

ORGASMIC DYSFUNCTION

In women orgasmic dysfunction refers to the lack of orgasm, delay of orgasm, or orgasms of markedly diminished intensity despite adequate stimulation and a high level of sexual arousal. Regarding the definition of "adequate stimulation," note that most women require stimulation of the clitoris to reach an orgasm. The indirect stimulation of the clitoris during vaginal intercourse is sufficient for some women to reach orgasm, but most will usually require some degree of direct clitoral stimulation. Anorgasmia, the complete lack of orgasms, can be either primary or secondary. Women with primary anorgasmia have never experienced an orgasm; those with secondary anorgasmia have experienced orgasm and subsequently lost the capacity to do so. The International Society for Sexual Medicine has recently published practice guidelines for evaluating and treating female orgasmic disorders (Laan, Rellini, & Barnes, 2013).

The clitoral complex includes the glans clitoris and clitoral bodies and bulbs; it is larger than the glans only and extends to the perineal body (Foldes & Buisson, 2009). While many people think of the clitoris as just the glans clitoris, stimulation of any part of the clitoral complex can bring about an orgasm. Pressure on and movement of the clitoris's root during vaginal penetration and subsequent perineal contraction may explain the sensitivity of the anterior vaginal wall. Systematic study has not confirmed the existence of "G Spot" in the vagina that has clitoris-like sensitivity to stimulation. When a woman reports inability to have an orgasm, the first step in evaluation is to confirm that direct and sustained stimulation of the clitoris has been tried either by the woman's spouse or partner or by the woman herself while masturbating. Individual differences in the ability to have an orgasm without direct clitoral stimulation relate both to differences in genital anatomy and differences in the central processing of genital stimuli.

Women who have never experienced orgasm usually can do so with masturbation; some women require the permission implicit in getting medical treatment to feel comfortable with self-stimulation. Overall, an educational approach is often successful, with referral to a sex therapy clinic the second step.

When a female patient who has previously experienced orgasm loses the ability there are several initial considerations:

1. Does the patient experience the same degree of sexual arousal as she did when she was orgasmic? If not, is there a lack of desire or a lack of arousal despite adequate desire?

2. Does the patient suffer pain or discomfort—or the fear of pain or discomfort—during intercourse?

3. Has there been a change in the partner's sexual technique, so that there has been a change in clitoral stimulation?

4. Does the patient almost but not quite reach orgasm? This is a common experience among patients who develop orgasmic dysfunction as a side effect of antidepressant medications that affect serotonergic transmission.

Sometimes changes in sexual technique can facilitate orgasm during intercourse. Alternatively, the patient's spouse or partner can bring her to orgasm with oral or manual stimulation and follow with vaginal intercourse. Good communication between the partners about sexual matters helps greatly; sometimes this can be facilitated by a single clinical visit by the couple in which the mechanics of intercourse are discussed in more detail than might be natural at home.

LOSS OF LIBIDO AND HYPOACTIVE SEXUAL DESIRE DISORDER

Women's sexual desire is highest when estradiol levels peak, at the time of ovulation. Estrogenic action increases vaginal blood flow and the release of vasoactive substances such as nitric oxide by endothelial cells, leading to vasodilatation and an increase of peripheral vibratory sensation. The postpartum period is a time of transition, and about half of women report less desire over 3 months after parturition. The majority of women (80%) resume sexual activity by 6 weeks after a baby is born. Another decline in desire occurs in the menopausal transition, the last phase before the final menses as estrogen is declining (Bitzer, Giraldi, & Pfaus, 2013). A persistent loss of sexual interest and desire that goes beyond normal changes with the menstrual cycle and life cycle, and that cause a woman significant distress and/or interpersonal difficulties may meet criteria for a diagnosis of Hypoactive Sexual Desire Disorder (HSDD). Given the wide variation in normal women's sexuality, the element of distress is critical diagnostically. It can be measured quantitatively, for example, with the Female Sexual Distress Inventory (Derogatis, Clayton, Lewis-D'Agostino, Wunderlich, & Fu, 2008) or the Sexual Interest and Desire Inventory-Female (Clayton et al., 2006).

Clinical depression can cause low sexual desire in both sexes (40% for women and 30% for men). A study characterizing sexual dysfunction in a group of depressed premenopausal women as they were about to participate in an antidepressant study, found that 18% had hypoactive sexual desire disorder, 3% sexual aversion disorder, 6% arousal disorder, and 8% orgasmic disorder. The more severe the depression, the more severe the sexual dysfunction (Fabre & Smith, 2012). Aversion to sex, when not a consequence of sexual trauma, often is a reflection of anxiety and is viewed by some as a phobic disorder rather than a sexual dysfunction. Both behavioral treatments and antidepressant treatment can help relieve it, with the usual warning that the most commonly prescribed antidepressants frequently cause a loss of libido—thus, ironically, replacing an aversion to sex with simple lack of interest. Alternatively, the patient might be treated with an antidepressant less associated with sexual side effects, such as mirtazapine, or bupropion. Vilazodone, a new SSRI with 5-HT1A partial agonist effects, might have a lower incidence of sexual dysfunction and the other SSRIs (Clayton, Kennedy, Edwards, Gallipoli, & Reed, 2013). Each has its own unique side effects of potential medical-psychiatric relevance, such as lowering of the seizure threshold with bupropion or sedation and weight gain with mirtazapine. Vilazodone is relatively new to the market, and its place in the spectrum of antidepressants is not yet established.

The psychological contribution to diminished sexual desire is complex, particularly for women. To make this point, Basson and colleagues (2010) note that depression is the major factor determining whether women with multiple sclerosis, renal failure, or diabetes have sexual dysfunction. Automatic negative thoughts during sexual activity are the strongest predictors of decreased desire. Patients' general medical symptoms show indirect effects via distraction or anxious thoughts about sexual failure. Patients' negative past experiences or beliefs that sex is bad or sinful may color current attitudes. Concerns about body image or low self-esteem related to illness or disability can reduce desire.

Conflicts that reduce libido may be intrapsychic or may be between the patient and her spouse or partner. Besides the interpersonal relationship, personal psychological factors of importance include self-image, comfort with being vulnerable, and ability to allow intimacy with another despite the risk of suffering grief if that person is lost. In other words, the anxious and avoidant attachment styles are problematic for sexuality. Basson and colleagues (2010) also note that many women engage in routine intercourse-focused sexual activity that lacks eroticism, pleasure, and intimacy. Distinguishing these psychological factors in order to define a group of women with an isolated ego-dystonic reduction in desire for intercourse—in other words, hypoactive sexual desire disorder (HSDD)—is a challenging requirement for research.

Testosterone influences social behavior, and social behavior affects testosterone levels. The basal level of testosterone remains fairly constant in men and women and may define a trait. In women with ovariectomy, testosterone drops precipitously compared to natural menopause. 200 mg transdermal testosterone patches have been used off-label in ovariectomized women and those with natural menopause to increase sexual desire and frequency of sex. Potential side effects include hair growth and acne, though these would be expected to be rare at dosages that simply restored testosterone to the range ordinarily seen in premenopausal women. Data support the safety of testosterone for postmenopausal women; there are insufficient data to comment on safety for premenopausal women (Shifren et al., 2008).

As of this writing no medication is approved for the treatment of HSDD in women, and the evidence in support of specific medications is limited. Given the relative lack of an evidence base to guide treatment decisions, effective pharmacological treatment of HSDD is likely to involve both psychological and pharmacological exploration in a context of a trusting therapeutic relationship, informed consent, and careful analysis of the subjective and objective effects of each drug that is tried. Bloemers et al. (2013) have suggested that different women have different causal mechanisms for an intrinsic sexual desire disorder. Some women have a relative insensitivity for sexual cues, while others are inhibited during sexual stimulation. Sublingual testosterone 0.5 mg increases the sensitivity of the brain to sexual cues with a delay in effect of about 4 hours; this might be effective preparation for the arousal-enhancing benefit from a PDE5 inhibitor, the actions of which are contingent on the presence of sexual desire. In addition, a 5HT1A receptor agonist timed for maximal effect during a woman's window of increased sensitivity to sexual cues might be helpful to reduce inhibition. Thus, the combination of testosterone and a PDE5 inhibitor may be effective for those with low sensitivity for sexual cues, while adding a 5HT1A receptor agonist medication to testosterone may work for women with sexual inhibitions (Poels et al., 2013; Van Rooij et al., 2013). The treatment of HSDD can be even more challenging in women with chronic general medical illness that are taking multiple medications for those conditions. A woman must really "want to want to" have sexual relations to succeed in the process. For this reason a more comprehensive medical-psychiatric assessment, including involvement of the patient's spouse or partner when feasible, should precede intervention more narrowly focused on the sexual issue. Conversely, it often makes sense to revisit issues of sexuality—including both the desire to be sexual and sexual desire—several visits into a course of treatment of a medical-psychiatric patient. If medical-psychiatric involvement continues over the long-term course of a chronic illness, issues of sexuality should be reopened from time to time. Such issues might only become relevant or only become addressable after more pressing issues like management of pain, treatment of depression, or coping with trauma or loss have been addressed.

Good communication between partners—whether explicit and verbal or implicit and nonverbal—is essential to a good long-term sexual relationship. Sex therapy and less specific communication skills training probably have equal efficacy for sexual dysfunction in couples with a stable relationship and previously satisfactory sex. Given that communication skills training has other benefits and may be less threatening to patients or their partners, it should be an early consideration. Most couples can understand that coping with general medical illness requires especially good communication, and that even a couple that has communicated adequately under normal circumstances might benefit from communication skills training to help them face the unusual challenges posed by illness.

Sexual behavior is inextricably intertwined with relationship issues, which is yet another reason to explore the sexual relationship when evaluating a patient with a chronic medical-psychiatric issue. In the acute medical situation, there are more pressing concerns, though occasionally a patient's concern about the impact of the general medical illness on future sexual life is a major contributor to depression or anxiety. Exploring a change in a couples' sexual relationship sometimes reveals information about the behavior or mood of the patient and the patient's spouse or partner. The discussion may be an opening to patients' misconceptions about general medical illness or to revelations about a dysfunctional caregiving relationship.

A history of sexual abuse does not always result in difficulty with orgasm nor can it be presumed to be the cause of dysfunction. Childhood experiences may, but do not necessarily, affect present attitudes. Among survivors of sexual abuse, low desire is the most common sexual symptom reported.

When the focus is sex with a spouse or partner, the spouse or partner should be involved in evaluation, and marital conflicts and/or communication difficulties should be addressed first. Behavioral sex therapy overlaps with couple therapy. An approach of graded increases in treatment, the PLISSIT model (Annon, 1976) begins with a physician providing **P**ermission, **L**imited **I**nformation, **S**pecific **S**uggestions, and ultimately more **I**ntensive **T**herapy and referral.

For women with primary anorgasmia, the International Society for Sexual Medicine recommends cognitive behavioral psychotherapies with an initial focus on directed masturbation training. This training—which has been delivered successfully in group, individual, couples, and self-directed reading contexts—involves graded exposure to genital stimulation and may include role playing an orgasmic response and the use of sexual fantasy with or without a vibrator (Heiman, 2002).

Sensate focus can be added to this treatment. This strategy for couples includes graded exposure from nonsexual to sexual focusing, building trust and communication, and relieving anxiety first before focusing on a goal of intercourse or orgasm. It improves attention to pleasurable sensual and sexual feelings without demanding the outcome of intercourse.

SPECIFIC MEDICAL CAUSES OF SEXUAL DYSFUNCTION

DEPRESSION

Major depression, a common and remarkably morbid condition, most often occurs as a primary mental disorder and is more prevalent in women than in men. The syndrome of major depression frequently complicates general medical conditions that involve pain and/or loss of function. Some chronic diseases cause depression disproportionately, which implies that a specific endocrine, neurological, biochemical, or immunological process is mediating the connection of the general medical disease with the mood disorder. Major depression in turn causes sexual dysfunction that usually resolves when the depression remits. Low sexual desire is a symptom reported by approximately 40% of women and 30% of men with major depression. Greater severity of depression is associated with greater sexual dysfunction. Thus, when a patient with general medical illness has diminished sexual interest, depression should be identified and treated if it is present. The decision whether to treat the depression and the sexual dysfunction sequentially versus simultaneously should take into account the patient's presenting complaints and whether actual or feared loss of sexual function is an important contributor to the patient's emotional distress. In the latter case fully evaluating other potential causes of sexual dysfunction is essential.

SEXUAL DYSFUNCTION IN SPECIFIC MEDICAL CONDITIONS

ENDOCRINE DISORDERS

Sexual dysfunction can be caused or exacerbated by excess or deficiency of any of several hormones, and restoration of normal hormone levels is a usually necessary and sometimes sufficient treatment for that dysfunction. There are nonetheless areas of ambiguity, particularly when hormonal abnormalities are "subclinical" apart from their hypothesized effects on sexual function.

Obviously, changes in the reproductive endocrine system can cause sexual dysfunction. Hyperprolactinemia reduces sexual interest and erectile function in men at levels greater than 35 ng/mL (735 IU/L), though many cases of hyperprolactinemia in men are caused by pituitary tumors that can have effects on other hormones, notably testosterone (Maggi, Buvat, Corona, Guay, & Torres, 2013). The endocrine environment of the immediate postpartum period (high prolactin and suddenly decreased estrogen and progesterone) is associated with low libido, as is the endocrine environment of the late perimenopause.

Thyroid disorders have remarkably specific patterns of associated sexual dysfunction. Carani et al. (2005) found that of 34 adult men with hyperthyroidism, 50% had premature ejaculation; other sexual dysfunctions were much less common. Of 14 men with hypothyroidism, 65% had orgasmic dysfunction (delayed ejaculation). The hypothyroid men had similarly high rates of loss of libido and ED, but only 7% had premature ejaculation.

The literature on male sexual dysfunction in acromegaly is mixed; it is unclear whether GH excess has a specific effect on sexual function. Low DHEA levels have been hypothesized to be related to various age-associated symptoms including sexual dysfunction. However, controlled trials have not shown improved male sexual function with DHEA supplementation (Maggi et al., 2013).

NEUROLOGICAL DISEASES

Neurological diseases can affect sexual function directly, via depression, via drug side effects, or via alterations in the couples' relationships due to caregiving burdens and changes in personality or behavior due to brain dysfunction. Three chronic neurological diseases have an especially high prevalence of sexual dysfunction: Multiple sclerosis, temporal lobe epilepsy, and Parkinson's disease.

In multiple sclerosis patients sexual dysfunction affects up to 50%–90% of men and 40%–85% of women. Both men and women with MS often have decreased libido. Men with MS may also have ED and/or ejaculatory dysfunction. Women may also have abnormal vaginal sensation, decreased vaginal lubrication, and orgasmic dysfunction. Sildenafil has been shown to alleviate MS-associated ED in a randomized controlled trial (Samkoff & Goodman, 2011).

Decreased libido is also seen in both men and women with temporal lobe epilepsy (TLE) (Sivaraaman & Mintzer, 2011). In men there may be hypogonadotropic hypogonadism, with a low testosterone level and an inappropriately low or low normal LH; these men also can have ED. In women there may be irregular menses and dysregulation of the cycle of LH and FSH. In both cases addressing the reproductive endocrine problem is necessary to normalize sexual function, but often it is not sufficient. For some patients with TLE hyposexuality is lifelong. Several of the older antiepileptic drugs (e.g., phenytoin and carbamazepine) reduce bioactive testosterone by increasing sex hormone binding globulin. Those drugs that induce CYP3A4 will reduce the blood level of a PDE5 inhibitor for a given dose and thereby diminish the efficacy of that dose.

Neuropathies that affect pelvic sensory and/or autonomic function are associated with sexual dysfunction, as might be expected. Considering ED in a variety of neurological diseases, those with upper motor neuron lesions are more likely to respond to PDE5 inhibitors than those with lower motor neuron involvement. Men with the latter problem but without vascular disease might require a local treatment such as intraurethral alprostadil to attain a satisfactory erection. When neuropathic sensory loss is the issue, changes in sexual technique to increase stimulation sometimes can resolve issues both with ED and with orgasmic dysfunction.

Parkinson's disease (PD) is not only associated with a prevalence of sexual dysfunction as high as 80% in some studies, but also is remarkable for the very wide range of types of sexual dysfunction it can cause. Patients with PD can display any combination of decreased libido, problems with arousal, diminished lubrication in women, sexually associated pain in men and in women, impaired or premature ejaculation, orgasmic dysfunction, dissatisfaction with the quality of sexual experience, and problems with communication about sexual matters. Nonetheless most patients with PD, especially those with young-onset disease, are interested in maintaining a sexual life, and many men with PD regard sexual dysfunction as the single most troublesome nonmotor manifestation of their illness. In addition, men with PD can become hypersexual on dopamine-agonist treatment of PD, leading to conflicts with their spouse or partner over the frequency of sexual activity and to sexually inappropriate behavior in cases where cognitive changes of PD impair insight and impulse control. Sexual dysfunction, like other nonmotor symptoms of PD, can precede motor symptoms or can be disproportionate to them. Several points can be distilled from the extensive literature on the subject: (1) Patients with PD should be asked about sexual and marital issues both during their initial evaluation and periodically after that, as the disease progresses. (2) If the patient has impaired cognition and/or impaired insight, their spouse or partner should be asked about sexual issues. (3) Evaluation of sexual dysfunction should include measurement of testosterone levels, as many men with PD will develop androgen deficiency. (4) Both male and female patients should be asked about sexually related pain and discomfort, the latter including muscle pain related to the motor symptoms of PD. (5) Patients should be screened for anxiety and depression. (6) In patients with motor fluctuations the relationship between sexual dysfunction and motor status should be explored. (7) Interviews with couples should include exploration of incompatible levels of interest, quality of communication about sexual matters, and ways in which physical changes associated with PD might turn off the desire of the spouse or partner. (8) Autonomic symptoms should be considered in planning treatment, including both orthostatic hypotension that can increase the risk of PDE5 inhibitors and incontinence associated with sexual activity. (9) Positive and negative effects of medications should be considered, with special attention to effects of antidepressants that are frequently prescribed to treat comorbid depression or anxiety.

Successful treatment of sexual dysfunction in PD usually requires the involvement of multiple specialties including neurology, psychiatry, and gynecology or urology. While the task is complex, it is worth pursuing both because sexuality matters greatly to many patients and because optimizing sexual function can aid in optimizing other aspects of the patient's treatment and in improving overall health-related quality of life.

END-STAGE RENAL DISEASE

Both men and women with end-stage renal disease (ESRD) suffer sexual dysfunction. The full spectrum of sexual function is affected from desire through orgasm; women with ESRD have lower desire, less arousal, worse lubrication, more orgasmic dysfunction, and a higher prevalence of dyspareunia (Kettas et al., 2008). The prevalence of sexual dysfunction is highest on patients receiving hemodialysis as compared with those treated with peritoneal dialysis or with renal transplantation. The underlying causes include anemia, endocrine disturbances, the disease(s) responsible for the renal failure (including diabetes and hypertension), side effects of medications, and depression (a condition highly prevalent in ESRD patients). Overall, approximately 50% of male pre-dialysis chronic kidney disease patients have ED, 80% of male patients on dialysis have ED, and 50% of women on dialysis have difficulties with arousal (Vecchio et al., 2010).

Sexual dysfunction in ESRD has been studied extensively, in part because there are many patients with ESRD of an age at which an active sexual life is a general expectation. Typically male sexual function is measured with the IIEF, and female sexual dysfunction is measured with the FSFI or the ASEX. Two consistent findings are that there is a strong correlation between depression and sexual dysfunction, and that sexual function is associated with a higher health-related quality of life and better self-rated physical health. Men on hemodialysis for ESRD have a higher divorce rate than those treated with transplantation or peritoneal dialysis. By contrast, most male transplant recipients who are in relationships are sexually active and satisfied with their relationship (Hegarty & Olsburgh, 2012).

While the relationships of sexual function, relationship satisfaction, self-rated health, and depression are all bidirectional, sexual dysfunction can be a productive focus for medical intervention when it is present and distressing to the patient. Efforts to resolve it can lead to more effective antidepressant treatment tailored to minimize sexual side effect, and can draw attention to suboptimally treated anemia or endocrine dysfunction. Meta-analysis of controlled clinical trials shows Class I evidence in support of the use of PDE5 for ED in men with ESRD. There also is evidence to support the benefit of oral zinc supplementation on testosterone levels, frequency of intercourse, and erectile function. In women with ESRD on hemodialysis sexual dysfunction is the rule. A recent cross-sectional study of women on hemodialysis in Europe and South America who completed the Female Sexual Function Inventory showed that 84% of 659 women had sexual dysfunction of some kind. Disorders of arousal, orgasm, and desire were the prevalent, but all aspects of sexual function were affected. Factors with independent contributions to the risk of sexual dysfunction were age, lower educational level, menopause, diabetes, low serum albumin, and the use of diuretics (Strippoli et al., 2012).

CARDIOVASCULAR DISEASES

ED in men should lead to a full assessment for coronary artery disease and cardiac risk factors, and to a cardiac stress test in patients who have a profile implying increased risk of heart disease. ED is a risk factor for myocardial infarction beyond the risk associated with the disorders that are common risk factors for both, such as diabetes, hypertension, hyperlipidemia, and smoking (Morano, 2003).

Patients with congestive heart failure (CHF) have a prevalence of sexual dysfunction of approximately 80%, and 30% are not sexually active at all (Alberti et al., 2013). Sexual dysfunction in patients with CHF can affect any part of the process from desire through orgasm. Sexual activity usually is safe for CHF patients of NYHA Class I or II; patients with more severe heart failure can experience exacerbation of symptoms with the exertion of sexual intercourse. Chronic therapy with a PDE5 inhibitor for the ED associated with CHF may actually improve the symptoms of CHF by reducing pulmonary hypertension and improving endothelial function. While PDE5 inhibitors are not approved for treatment of pulmonary hypertension associated with CHF, it would be logical to use daily tadalafil rather than intermittent PDE5 therapy for a man with CHF who was in a stable sexual relationship. Recently attention has been drawn to the high frequency of testosterone deficiency in patients with heart failure: 26% to 37% of men with heart failure have been found to be testosterone deficient (Naghi, Philip, DiLibero, Willix & Schwarz, 2011). Testosterone supplementation potentially could improve their overall clinical status (e.g., by reversing anabolic deficiency and/or increasing exercise tolerance) and not only their sexual function (Alberti et al., 2013).

Many patients, both men and women, who have had a myocardial infarction (MI) are fearful about returning to sexual activity, especially if they have not received specific guidance on this subject from their cardiologist. The majority of both men and women who have had a myocardial infarction are less sexually active than in the year before their MI (Lindau et al., 2012). The standard guidelines for care after an MI suggest that stable patients without complications can resume sexual activity with their usual partners in a week to 10 days (Anderson et al., 2007). The implication is that sexual activity with a new partner involves greater arousal and in some cases involves anxiety, both of which entail sympathetic activation that could increase the risk myocardial ischemia. Overall, the risk of

myocardial infarction and sudden cardiac death associated with sexual intercourse is low, even in patients with coronary disease. The heart's ability to tolerate sexual activity is related to the functional reserve—how much the heart rate, blood pressure, and oxygen consumption approach the peak response to exercise. Cardiac symptoms during sex rarely occur in patients who have tolerated exercise testing at a level of 6 METs (i.e., exercise involving oxygen consumption six times the basal level of 3.5 mL O_2 /kg/min). Sexual activity pre-orgasm typically requires 2–3 METs and orgasm requires 3–4 METs. For comparison, 3 METs is the energy expenditure for walking on level ground at 5 km/hour (Alberti et al., 2013).

For men, there is less physical exertion if the woman is positioned on top. The risk of MI is not increased by the use of PDE5 inhibitors (DeBusk, 2000; Cheitlin, 2005). A recent review and meta-analysis found that both life style modification and medications to improve cardiovascular risk factors are associated with a statistically significant improvement in the severity of erectile dysfunction (Gupta et al., 2011).

Several of the drugs used to prevent or treat cardiovascular diseases cause sexual dysfunction, ED in particular. Thiazide diuretics, beta blockers (with the exception of nebivolol), clofibrate, digoxin, amiodarone, and disopyramide all can cause ED. Beta blockers and statin drugs have been implicated in orgasmic dysfunction. Nitrates used to treat angina pectoris are an absolute contraindication to the use of PDE5 inhibitors because of the potential for the combination to cause life-threatening hypotension.

CHRONIC OBSTRUCTIVE PULMONARY DISEASE

COPD is not a contraindication to sexual activity. In fact, oxygenation tends to improve during sexual intercourse, which increases the rate and depth of respiration and improves the balance of ventilation and perfusion. Patients with exercise-induced bronchospasm may require premedication with an inhaler prior to intercourse.

SEXUAL SIDE EFFECTS OF MEDICATIONS

A wide range of medications can cause sexual side effects; a complete survey is beyond the scope of this chapter. However, some drugs very commonly encountered—or prescribed—by medical psychiatrists cause sexual side effects frequently enough to be a major factor in treatment adherence. Several classes of such drugs will be discussed here.

Drug-induced sexual dysfunction should be suspected when a patient's sexual function changes soon after the introduction of a new drug, the discontinuation of a drug, or a change in the dose of a drug. In medical-psychiatric settings patients usually are taking multiple drugs, with the potential for pharmacokinetic or pharmacodynamic drug interactions. For example, a drug that is not itself suspected of causing sexual dysfunction can precipitate it, if via a pharmacokinetic interaction it increases the blood level of a second drug that is associated with sexual side effects. Or, discontinuation of a drug that mitigates the sexual side effects of a second drug could cause sexual dysfunction: for example, the discontinuation of bupropion in a patient also on an SSRI could unmask sexual dysfunction caused by the latter drug.

ANTIHYPERTENSIVE DRUGS

Hypertension itself is associated with sexual dysfunctions including ED in men and loss of libido in both men and women. Effective treatment of hypertension improves sexual function as long as the treatment does not itself have sexual side effects. The sexual side effects of antihypertensive medications were comprehensively reviewed by Manolis and Doumas (2012). They concluded that thiazide diuretics and most beta blockers frequently have adverse effects on sexual function, whereas ARBs, ACE inhibitors, and calcium channel blockers were less likely to do so. In an earlier publications the same authors make the important point that when sexual dysfunction develops in a patient taking antihypertensive drugs it can be a warning sign of vascular disease needing a thorough investigation; sexual dysfunction developing on an antihypertensive medication is not necessarily due to that medication (Manolis & Doumas, 2008).

Pharmacological differences among the different beta blockers may explain their different propensity to cause sexual side effects. The lipophilic beta-blockers such as propranolol and metoprolol can cross the blood–brain barrier and affect libido by central mechanisms; hydrophilic drugs such as atenolol can cause ED but may be less likely to affect libido (Fogari et al., 1998, 2002). Drugs more selective for β_1 adrenergic receptors appear less likely to cause ED than nonselective beta blockers. Carvedilol (a nonselective beta blocker and an α_1 –adrenergic blocker that is moderately lipophilic) is a beta blocker that is especially likely to cause sexual dysfunction by multiple mechanisms (Cordero et al., 2010; Hackett, 2010; Baumhakel et al., 2011). Nebivolol, a lipophilic beta blocker that is β_1-selective and also enhances the release of endothelial nitric oxide, essentially does not cause ED. Male patients who have ED while taking another beta blocker can regain erectile function if switched to nebivolol. For example, Doumas et al. (2006) reported on a series of 29 patients with hypertension and ED at baseline who were treated with atenolol, bisoprolol, or metoprolol for 6 months and continued to have ED despite control of their hypertension; after a switch of beta blocker to nebivolol, erectile function improved in 20 (69%) and normalized completely in 11 (38%).

In women, beta blockers can affect libido, arousal, and the capacity for orgasm. Switching a patient from another beta blocker to nebivolol or an ARB has the potential to improve sexual function, both in men and in women. Alpha adrenergic blockers have the potential to cause sexual dysfunction though they do so far less often than beta blockers. There is a potential for causing symptomatic hypotension when combining alpha blockers with PDE5 inhibitors; this risk can be mitigated by low initial dosage and slow dosage change for the drug that is started second.

ANTIDEPRESSANT DRUGS

Sexual dysfunction can occur with SSRIs; many patients who initially have sexual side effects will improve after 2 weeks to 4 months on treatment. If a patient has persistent sexual side effects after 4 months—or if they cannot tolerate the sexual side effects at an earlier time—options are to change the dosage, change the drug, or add an adjunctive agent that may both improve sexual function and treat residual symptoms of depression. Dosage reduction alone should be considered only if the patient's depression is in remission; patients who are only partially improved are likely to get worse on a lower dose of the same drug. A switch to a different class of antidepressant would be preferred if the patient had an incomplete response to the SSRI (Baldwin, 2014). Options with a lower incidence of sexual side effects than SSRIs include mirtazapine and bupropion. Vilazodone *may* have a lower incidence of sexual side effects than the SSRIs, but the drug is relatively new, and clinical experience is still accumulating (Clayton et al., 2013; Wang, Han, & Lee, 2013). There have been no randomized studies comparing vilazodone with SSRIs; such studies would be needed to conclusively prove that vilazodone was superior with regard to sexual side effects. In the medical-psychiatric population, mirtazepine's frequent side effects of weight gain and sedation could be either a positive or a negative depending on the patient's nutritional status and sleep quality.

Augmentation of an SSRI with bupropion can potentially convert a partial remission of depression into a full remission. In addition, it can relieve sexual side effects of the SSRIs. PDE5 inhibitors may have the same effect. Used PRN they can be efficacious for antidepressant-associated ED (Fava & Rankin, 2002; Nurnberg et al., 2008). Shim and colleagues (2014) showed that daily use of the PDE5 inhibitor udenafil improved measures of depression, cognition, and somatization in men with erectile dysfunction, lower urinary tract symptoms and no concurrent psychiatric diagnosis. Tadalafil, the only PDE5 inhibitor currently approved in the United States for daily use, may show benefits for mood as well as erectile function when used in a dose as small as 5 mg every other day (Choi et al., 2014). The effect of a daily PDE5 inhibitor on female patients, whether taking SSRIs or otherwise, has not been systematically studied. In a *Cochrane* review of strategies to manage sexual dysfunction induced by SSRI antidepressant medication that looked at 23 trials for antidepressant-induced erectile dysfunction, the addition of sildenafil or tadalafil appeared to be an effective strategy for men. For women with antidepressant induced sexual function, the addition of bupropion at higher doses appears to be the most promising approach studied so far (Taylor et al., 2013).

As noted above, both TCAs and MAOIs can cause sexual dysfunction of various types. MAOIs are particularly associated with orgasmic dysfunction. TCAs' anticholinergic effects can contribute to sexual dysfunction; these are less with nortriptyline and desipramine. Mitigation of

TCAs' anticholinergic effects with low dose donepezil or with Huperzine A with cholinergic agents is an off-label option when a TCA is an especially efficacious antidepressant for a particular patient and anticholinergic effects—not limited to sexual dysfunction—make the therapy intolerable. Trazodone is unique among the antidepressants in its potential for causing priapism as a side effect.

ANTIPSYCHOTIC DRUGS

In first-episode patients with schizophrenia (Baggaley, 2008) the disease itself influences sexual dysfunction. However, all of the antipsychotic drugs are associated with sexual side effects. Among the antipsychotic drugs olanzapine, risperidone, haloperidol, clozapine, and thioridazine have been associated with higher rates of sexual dysfunction than quetiapine, ziprasidone, aripiprazole, and perphenazine (Serretti & Chiesa, 2011). If the prolactin level is high with an antipsychotic drug such as risperidone or olanzapine, then the particular antipsychotic might be changed to one with lesser effect on prolactin, since hyperprolactinemia alone can cause erectile dysfunction, amenorrhea, and galactorrhea (Seeman, 2013). Peripheral anticholinergic and alpha-adrenergic blocking actions of antipsychotics can also contribute to the sexual dysfunction.

OPIATE ANALGESICS

Opiate analgesics are associated with ED in men and diminished libido in both men and women. The problem appears to be a class effect, but some opiates are worse than others. For example, men on methadone maintenance have been noted to have a higher rate of erectile dysfunction than men on buprenorphine maintenance treatment (Hallinan et al., 2008). Individual patients might have more sexual dysfunction on one opiate than another, so a change in drug might be considered for patients who require long-term opiate therapy for chronic pain. Tramadol has a remarkable propensity to delay orgasm. This can be used therapeutically in the treatment of men with premature ejaculation; for other patients it can be a problem.

H2 BLOCKERS

The H2 blockers cimetidine and ranitidine have anti-androgenic effects that can cause ED or loss of libido. An alternative H2 blocker or a proton pump inhibitor should be substituted if these side effects develop.

OTHER DRUGS WITH ANTI-ANDROGENIC EFFECTS

Any drug with anti-adrenergic effects—whether intentional or incidental—can affect libido or male erectile function. Common examples are leuprolide, gosrelin, zoladex, finasteride, flutamide, ketoconazole, and spironolactone. In some cases alternate therapies may be available with lesser sexual side effects; when this is not feasible treatment of ED with a PDE5 inhibitor may be effective.

SEXUAL ISSUES IN CANCER SURVIVORS

Cancer and its treatment often have major effects on patients' sexuality, mediated by the patient's emotional reaction to a life-threating illness, changes in body image, pain and other distressing symptoms, and changes in the couple's relationship, as well as the effects of cancer treatments on the endocrine and nervous systems. When the cancer involves the urogenital system issues such as erectile dysfunction or pain on intercourse may contribute (Bober & Varela, 2012). Yet, it often is worth the effort for a patient to overcome the barriers to a satisfying sexual life despite his or her cancer; healthy sexuality is a powerful affirmation of physical and emotional survival.

Anti-estrogen treatment for breast cancer precipitates an abrupt menopause, with symptoms of atrophic vaginitis, loss of lubrication, dyspareunia, and loss of libido. These local symptoms are common when aromatase inhibitors are part of the oncologic treatment regimen (Baumgart et al., 2013). Women taking aromatase inhibitors tend to report global sexual problems, including not only dyspareunia but also reduced sexual desire, difficulty becoming sexually aroused, and problems with orgasm (Bradford, 2013). For many patients the principal problem is vaginal pain related to lack of lubrication but not fully resolved by lubricants. Short-term studies of low-dose topical hormonal treatments with vaginal estradiol or testosterone have shown promise but long term data are not available. Because the elevation of systemic estrogen levels by topical hormone therapy is negligible at the doses needed to relieve vaginal atrophy, such treatment is unlikely to increase the risk of cancer recurrence (Witherby et al., 2011; Kendall, Dowsett, Folkerd, & Smith, 2006).

With mastectomy and reconstruction, women who are satisfied with cosmetic results may still need to adjust to loss of breast and nipple sensation. Women who have had pelvic radiation may have complications of vaginal fibrosis, stenosis, and loss of lubrication. Colon cancer surgery can affect nerves important for erectile function in men and decrease vaginal function in women. Patients with ostomies must overcome social barriers to sexual contact, and patients who have had bone marrow transplants may have sexual dysfunction and fears about bacterial contagion in an immune deficiency state. Patients with head and neck surgery are sensitive about physical deformities that follow treatment; those who have tumors related to human papilloma virus may feel guilt about the effect of a sexually transmitted disease. Successful resolution of any of these cancer-related issues usually comes with some combination of individual and couples counseling, education, adjustment of sexual technique, and medical interventions. As an example of the latter, vaginal stenosis following radiation therapy can be addressed by the physical dilation of the vagina (Miles & Johnson, 2010).

Resolution of cancer-associated sexual dysfunction requires significant motivation on the part of the patient and his/her spouse or partner, and a commitment of time and energy. Thus illness-associated fatigue and apathy may be addressed, either sequentially or simultaneously, along with the more narrowly defined sexual issues; the expectations of the patient and the spouse or partner should be aligned.

Other things being equal, younger patients are more likely to regain sexual function after treatment for cancer. This may partly be due to differences in vigor, but differences in expectations also play a role. Young cancer patients usually expect to have an active sexual life. Older ones—with the age threshold differing by cultural background and family tradition—may see an episode of cancer as an indicator that their sexual life is over. This belief should be explored by the clinician; it is especially important to identify when the expectations of the patient and his/her spouse or partner are different in this regard.

SEXUAL DYSFUNCTION AFTER RADICAL PROSTATECTOMY

Sexual dysfunction affects the majority of men who have a radical prostatectomy (RP) for prostate cancer, although its incidence is lower with nerve-sparing procedures. It is noteworthy that medical centers differ significantly in their rates of sexual dysfunction following RP; a discussion of the risk of postoperative sexual dysfunction should be part of the informed consent discussion, and in the authors' opinion this should include comparison of local rates of postoperative sexual dysfunction with appropriate benchmarks. Depending on the extent of nerve damage during prostatectomy, postoperative erectile dysfunction might or might not respond to PDE5 inhibitors. If it does not, erectile function can be restored with one of the more invasive treatments described above. Identifying and intervening to restore sexual function relatively soon after surgery is associated with a better long-term outlook for recovery of sexual function. Moreover, early recovery of sexual function can help a man's emotional recovery from the trauma and loss associated with cancer and its treatment.

A specific problem common after RP is loss of urine during orgasm in an otherwise continent man. This problem improves with time in about half of those affected. The problem can be mitigated by emptying the bladder before intercourse, lying on the back or side during orgasm, and/or wearing a condom. Some men find Kegel exercises useful for this symptom. On occasion the symptom is so bothersome and persistent that surgical treatment is offered; it is usually successful. Other sexual complications seen after RP are shortening of the penis and orgasm without ejaculation.

Radiation therapy of prostate cancer reduces ejaculatory volume and can alter the experience of orgasm even when the capacity for orgasm is preserved. Anti-androgen treatment for prostate cancer can shorten the penis, cause testicular atrophy, and diminish desire, although these effects are variable (Higano, 2012). Most men on anti-androgen treatment continue to have sexual thoughts and erotic dreams, and many are able to continue sexual activity. When ED is present, PDE5 inhibitors may be effective despite the lack of androgens, although this too is variable.

Overall, the various and variable effects of prostate cancer treatment on sexual function call for especially good communication between a concerned physician, the patient, and the patient's spouse or partner. Depending on the center where the patient is treated, discussion and intervention concerning sexual issues can involve the oncologist, an urologist, a medical psychiatrist, and/or a specialist in sexual medicine. When a medical psychiatrist is involved—often for a nonsexual presenting complaint such as depression, anxiety, or chronic pain—they should ensure that sexual concerns are elicited and discussed, and that someone takes responsibility for following them up.

CANCER AND COUPLE RELATIONSHIPS

Cancer and its treatment take an emotional toll on the spouse or partner of the patient, and the spouse or partner's emotional issues often are compounded by problems in the couple's communication. The emotional impact on the spouse or partner can affect *their* sexual function, and communication problems impede their resolution. For example, partners of patients who had hematopoietic stem cell transplantation reported a high burden of depression and sexual problems long after the transplant took place (Bishop et al., 2007). In the setting of metastatic breast cancer, sexual problems were associated with depressive symptoms for both women and their partners; however, depressive symptoms were reduced by mutual constructive communication. Successful communication included mutual discussion of cancer-related issues, expression of feelings, understanding of views, and a feeling that the issue was resolved. In contrast to this successful pattern of communication, one often encounters the pattern of demand–withdrawal communication in which one partner wants to talk about issues related to cancer and the other partner does not, responding by withdrawing emotionally (Milbury & Badr, 2013). This communication pattern is associated with a less satisfactory sexual relationship, whether or not the cancer-related issues concern sexual dysfunction. At best, the crisis of cancer—or any other major or life-threatening illness—can be an occasion for a couple to have increased intimacy and communication, one that draws out expressions of the partners' concern, love, and commitment. The medical psychiatrist should be alert to opportunities to facilitate this constructive outcome.

SUMMARY

Regular, satisfying sexual activity improves a patient's health-related quality of life. For couples in which one member suffers functional impairments due to chronic disease, a happy sexual relationship can mitigate some of the stress of caregiving. Moreover, uncovering and addressing the causes of sexual dysfunction can lead to new and important diagnoses and can contribute positively to the patients overall care and its outcomes. In many chronic diseases sexual dysfunction affects more than half of patients at some point in their course. However, in any given clinical encounter with a general medical physician or even a medical psychiatrist, sexual concerns seldom are in the foreground. Active effort on a clinician's part, at a propitious time in the patient's course of treatment, usually is needed to open the dialogue; screening tests and rating scales can help focus the conversation. The yield is high and the effort is worth making.

CLINICAL PEARLS

- Even when discussion of sexual issues is not timely at the initial encounter, the topic should remain an open item in the psychiatrist's mind—one to be explored in the future with the patient if the professional relationship continues.

- A desire to be sexual and desire to have sex, whether in general or with a specific actual or fantasied partner are not the same. If the medical psychiatrist determines that a patient wishes to be sexual this is a sufficient reason to explore the issue further, even if the patient has not been sexually active recently and has not recently experienced sexual desire.

- Clearly new onset erectile dysfunction in a man of any age should trigger a full medical reassessment, including an electrocardiogram and stress test, screening for glucose intolerance, and measurement of serum testosterone. (Shamloul & Ghanem, 2013; Miner et al., 2014)

- A patient can have a side effect like headache, dyspepsia or muscle pain with one PDE5 inhibitor and not with another.

- A newly approved therapy for dyspareunia due to vulvar and vaginal atrophy is ospemifene, a selective estrogen receptor modulator (SERM). Given orally at a dose of 60 mg per day ospemifene restores the vaginal mucosa and relieves dyspareunia, without affecting the endometrium and thereby requiring concurrent progestin administration

- Thiazide diuretics and most beta blockers frequently have adverse effects on sexual function, whereas ARBs, ACE inhibitors, and calcium channel blockers were less likely to do so. (Manolis & Doumas, 2012).

- Three common neurological diseases—multiple sclerosis, Parkinson's disease, and temporal lobe epilepsy—are associated with a disproportionately high rate of sexual dysfunction.

DISCLOSURE STATEMENTS

Dr. Fogel is Chief Scientific Officer of Synchroneuron Inc., Managing Director of Anal-Gesic LLC, and Executive Vice President of PointRight Inc. He is the sole inventor or lead inventor on several pharmaceutical patents. In his opinion these affiliations do not entail any conflict of interest with regard to the editing of this book or his personal contributions to it. He has no other potential conflicts, direct or indirect, financial or otherwise, to disclose in connection with the editing of this book or his personal contributions to it.

Dr. Greenberg has no conflicts of interest to disclose.

REFERENCES

Abraham, L., Symonds, T., & Morris, M. F. (2008). Psychometric validation of a sexual quality of life questionnaire for use in men with premature ejaculation or erectile dysfunction. *Journal of Sexual Medicine, 5*, 595–601.

Alberti, L., Torlasco, C., Lauretta, L., Loffi, M., Maranta, F., Salonia, A., et al. (2013). Erectile function in heart failure patients: a critical reappraisal. *Andrology, 1*, 177–191.

Althof, S., & Symonds, T. (2007). Patient reported outcomes used in the assessment of premature ejaculation. In A. Seftel, & M. Resnick (Eds.), *Urologic clinics of North, America* (pp.581–589). New York: Elsevier.

Althof, S. E., Rosen, R. C., Perelman, M. A., & Rubio-Aurioles, E. (2013). Standard operating procedures for taking a sexual history. *Journal of Sexual Medicine, 10*, 26–35.

Alzahrani, H. A. S. (2012). Sister chromatid exchanges and sperm abnormalities produced by antidepressant drug fluoxetine in mouse treated in vivo. *European Review for Medical and Pharmacological Sciences, 16*, 2154–2161.

Anderson, J., Adams, C., Antman, E., Bridges, C., Califf, R., Casey, D. E. Jr., et al. (2007). ACC/AHA (2007) guidelines for the management of patients with unstable angina/non-ST-elevation myocardial infarction: a report of the American College of Cardiology/American Heart Association Task Force on Practice Guidelines: developed in collaboration with the American College of Emergency Physicians, Society for Academic Emergency Medicine, Society for Cardiovascular Angiography and Interventions, and Society of Thoracic Surgeons. *Journal of the American College of Cardiology, 50*, e1–e157.

Annon, J. (1976). *Behavioral Treatment of Sexual Problems: Brief Therapy*, vol. 1. New York, Harper & Row.

Archer, D. F. (2010). Efficacy and tolerability of local estrogen therapy for urogenital atrophy. *Menopause, 17*, 194–203.

Attia, S. M., & Bakheet, S. A. (2013). Citalopram at the recommended human doses after long-term treatment is genotoxic for male germ cell. *Food and Chemical Toxicology, 53*, 281–285.

Baggaley, M. (2008). Sexual dysfunction in schizophrenia: Focus on recent evidence. *Human Psychopharmacology, 23*, 201–209.

Baldwin, D. S. (2004). Sexual dysfunction associated with antidepressant drugs. *Expert Opinion on Drug Safety, 3*, 457–470.

Basson, R., Brotto, La, Petkau, A. J., & Labrie, F. (2010). Role of androgens in women's sexual dysfunction. *Menopause, 17*, 962–971.

Basson, R. (2010). Is it time to move on from "hypoactive sexual desire disorder?" *Menopause, 17*, 1097–1098.

Baumgart, J., Nilsson, K., Evers, A. S., et al. (2013). Sexual dysfunction in women on adjuvant endocrine therapy after breast cancer. *Menopause, 20*, 162–168.

Baumhakel, M., Schlimmer, N., Kratz, M., et al. (2011). Cardiovascular risk, drugs and erectile function—a systematic analysis. *International Journal of Clinical Practice, 65*, 289–298.

Beckman, N., Waern, M., Gustafson, D., & Skoog, I. (2008). Secular trends in self-reported sexual activity and satisfaction in Swedish 70 year olds: cross sectional survey of four populations, 1971–2001. *BMJ, 337*, a279.

Bhamra, R. K.1, Margolis, M. B., Liu, J. H., Hendy, C. H., Jenkins, R. G., & DiLiberti, C. E. (2011). A randomized, multiple-dose parallel study to compare the pharmacokinetic parameters of synthetic conjugated estrogens, A, administered as oral tablet or vaginal cream. *Menopause, 18*, 393–399.

Bishop, M. M., Beaumont, J. L., Hahn, E. A., Cella, D., Andrykowski, M. A., Brady, M. J., et al. (2007). Late effects of cancer and hematopoietic stem-cell transplantation on spouses or partners compared with survivors and survivor-matched controls. *Journal of Clinical Oncology, 25*, 1403–1411.

Bitzer, J., Giraldi, A., & Pfaus, J. (2013). Sexual desire and hypoactive sexual desire disorder in women. Introduction and overview. Standard operating procedure (SOP Part 1). *Journal of Sexual Medicine, 10*, 36–49.

Bloemers, J., van Rooij, K., Poels, S., Goldstein, I., Everaerd, W., Koppeschaar, H., et al. (2013). Toward personalized sexual medicine (part 1): Integrating the "dual control model" into differential drug treatments for hypoactive sexual desire disorder and female sexual arousal disorder. *Journal of Sexual Medicine, 10*, 791–809.

Bober, S. L., & Varela, V. S. (2012). Sexuality in adult cancer survivors: challenges and intervention. *Journal of Clinical Oncology, 30*, 3712–3719.

Bradford, A. (2013). Sexual outcomes of aromatase inhibitor therapy in women with breast cancer: time for intervention. *Menopause, 20*, 128–129.

Braunstein, G. D., Sundwall, D. A., Katz, M., Shifren, J. L., Buster, J. E., Simon, J. A., et al. (2005). Safety and efficacy of a testosterone patch for the treatment of hypoactive sexual desire disorder in surgically menopausal women; a randomized, placebo-controlled trial. *Archives of Internal Medicine, 165*, 1582–1589.

Brody, S. (2010). The relative health benefits of different sexual activities. *Journal of Sexual Medicine, 7*(4 Pt 1), 1336–1361.

Buster, J. E. (2013). Managing female sexual dysfunction. *Fertility and Sterility, 100*, 905–915.

Bygdeman, M., & Swahn, M. L. (1996). Replens versus dienoestriol cream in the symptomatic treatment of vaginal atrophy in postmenopausal women. *Maturitas, 23*, 259–263.

Carani, C., Isidori, A. M., Granata, A., Carosa, E., Maggi, M., et al. (2005). Multicenter study on the prevalence of sexual symptoms in male hypo- and hyperthyroid patients. *Journal of Clinical Endocrinology & Metabolism, 90*, 6472–6479.

Castelo-Branco, C., Cancelo, M. J., Villero, J., Nohales, F., & Juliá, M. D. (2005). Management of post-menopausal vaginal atrophy and atrophic vaginitis. *Maturitas, 52*, S46–S52.

Cheitlin, M. D. (2005). Sexual activity and cardiac risk. *American Journal of Cardiology, 96*(suppl), 24M–28M.

Choi, H., Kim, J.-H., Shim, J.-S., Park, J. Y., Kang, S. H., Moon, D. G., et al. (2014). Comparison of the efficacy and safety of 5-mg once-daily versus 5-mg alternate-day tadalafil in men with erectile dysfunction and lower urinary tract symptoms. *International Journal of Impotence Research*, epubdoi: 10.1038/ijir.2014.19

Chollet, J. A. (2011). Efficacy and safety of ultra-low-dose Vagifem. *Patient Preference and Adherence, 5*, 571–574.

Clayton, A. H., Segraves, R. T., Leiblum, S., Basson, R., Pyke, R., Cotton, D., et al. (2006). Reliability and validity of the Sexual Interest and Desire Inventory-Female (SIDI-F), a scale designed to measure severity of female hypoactive sexual desire disorder. *Journal of Sex and Marital Therapy, 32*, 115–135.

Clayton, A. H., Kennedy, S. H., Edwards, J. B., Gallipoli, S., & Reed, C. R. (2013). The effect of vilazodone on sexual function during the treatment of major depressive disorder. *Journal of Sexual Medicine, 10*, 2465–2476.

Cordero, A., Bertomeu-Martinez, Mazón, P., Fácila, L., Bertomeu-González, V., Conthe, P., et al. (2010). Erectile dysfunction in high-risk hypertensive patients treated with beta-blockade agents. *Cardiovascular Therapeutics, 28*, 15–22.

Corona, G., & Maggi, M. (2013). Re: Testosterone replacement therapy in the setting of prostate cancer treated with radiation. *European Urology, 63*(3), 583.

Corona, G., Razzoli, E., Forti, G., & Maggi, M.(2008). The use of phophodiesterase 5 inhibitors with concomitant medications. *Journal of Endocrinological Investigation, 31*, 799–808.

Corona, G., Mondaini, N., Ungar, A., Razzoli, E., Rossi, A., & Fusco, F. (2011). Phosphodiesterase type 5 (PDE5) inhibitors in erectile dysfunction: the proper drug for the proper patient. *Journal of Sexual Medicine, 8*, 3418–3432.

Costa, P., & Potempa, A. J. (2012). Intraurethral alprostadil for erectile dysfunction: a review of the literature. *Drugs, 72*, 2243–2254.

Cui, Y., Zong, H., Yan, H., & Zhang, Y. (2014). The effect of testosterone replacement therapy on prostate cancer: a systematic review and meta-analysis. *Prostate Cancer and Prostatic Disease*, 1–12.

Danesh-Meyer, H. V., & Levin, L. A. (2007). Erectile dysfunction drugs and risk of anterior ischaemic optic neuropathy: casual or causal association? *British Journal of Ophthalmology, 91*, 1551–1555.

Davis, S. R., Moreau, M., Kroll, R., Bouchard, C., Panay, N., Gass, M., et al. (2008). Testosterone for low libido in postmenopausal women not taking estrogen. *New England Journal of Medicine, 259*, 2005–2017.

DeBusk, R. F. (2000). Evaluating the cardiovascular tolerance for sex. *American Journal of Cardiology, 86*(suppl), 51F–56F.

Derogatis, L., Clayton, A., Lewis-D'Agostino, D. Wunderlich, G., & Fu, Y. (2008). Validation of the female sexual distress scale-revised for assessing distress in women with hypoactive sexual desire disorder. *Journal of Sexual Medicine, 5*, 357–364,

Derogatis, L. R., Rosen, R. C., Leiblum, S., Burnett, A., & Heiman, J. (2002). The female sexual distress scale (FSDS): initial validation of a standardized scale for assessment of sexually related personal distress in women. *Journal of Sex & Marital Therapy, 28*, 317–330.

Derogatis, L. R., Rust, J., Golombok, S., Bouchard, C., Nachtigall, L., Rodenberg, C., et al. (2004). Validation of the profile of female sexual function (PFSF) in surgically and naturally menopausal women. *Journal of Sex & Marital Therapy, 30*, 25–36.

Doumas, M., Tsakiris, A., Douma, S., Grigorakis, A., Papadopoulos, A., Hounta, A., et al. (2006). Beneficial effects of switching from beta-blockers to nebivolol on the erectile function of hypertensive patients. *Asian Journal of Andrology, 8*, 177–182.

Fabre, L. F., & Smith, L. C. (2012). The effect of major depression on sexual function in women. *Journal of Sexual Medicine, 9*, 231–239.

Fava, M., & Rankin, M. (2002). Sexual functioning and SSRIs. *Journal of Clinical Psychiatry, 63*(Suppl 5), 13–16.

Ferreira, J. R., & Souza, R. P. (2012). Botulinum toxin for vaginismus treatment. *Pharmacology, 89*, 256–259.

Finkelstein, J. S., Lee, H., Burnett-Bowie, S. M., Pallais, J. C., Yu, E. W., Borges, L., et al. (2013). Gonadal steroids and body composition, strength, and sexual function in men. *New England Journal of Medicine, 369*, 1011–1022.

Fogari, R., Preti, P., Derosa, G., Marasi, G., Zoppi, A., Rinaldi, A., et al. (2002). Effect of antihypertensive treatment with valsartan or atenolol on sexual activity and plasma testosterone in hypertensive men. *European Journal of Clinical Pharmacology, 28*, 177–180.

Fogari, R., Zoppi, A., Corradi, L, Mugellini, A., Poletti, L., & Lusardi, P. (1998). Sexual function in hypertensive males treated with lisinopril or atenolol: a cross-over study. *American Journal of Hypertension, 11*, 1244–1247.

Foldes, P., & Buisson, O. (2009). The clitoral complex: A dynamic sonographic study. *Journal of Sexual Medicine, 6*, 1223–1231.

Ghanem, H. M., Salonia, A., & Martin-Morales, A. (2013). SOP: Physical examination and laboratory testing for men with erectile dysfunction. *Journal of Sexual Medicine, 10*, 108–110.

Gupta, B. P., Murad, M. H., Clifton, M. M., Prokop, L., Nehra, A., & Kopecky, S. L. (2011). The effect of lifestyle modification and cardiovascular risk factor reduction on erectile dysfunction: A systematic review and meta-analysis. *Archives of Internal Medicine, 71*, 1797–1803.

Hackett, G. (2010). Hypertensive medication and erectile dysfunction. *Cardiovascular Therapeutics, 28*, 5–7.

Hallinan, R., Byrne, A., Agho, K., McMahon, C., Tynan, P., & Attia, J. (2008). Erectile dysfunction in men receiving methadone and buprenorphine maintenance treatment. *Journal of Sexual Medicine, 5*, 684–692.

Hegarty, P. K., & Olsburgh, J. (2012). Renal replacement and male sexuality. *Transplant Proceedings, 44*, 1804–1805.

Heiman, J. R. (2002). Psychologic treatments for female sexual dysfunction: Are they effective and do we need them? *Archives of Sexual Behavior, 31*, 445–450.

Higano, C. S. (2012). Sexuality and intimacy after definitive treatment and subsequent androgen deprivation therapy for prostate cancer. *Journal of Clinical Oncology, 30*, 3720–3725.

Hyde, Z., Flicker, L., Hankey, G. J., Almeida, O. P., McCaul, K. A., Chubb, S. A. P., & Yeap, B. B. (2010). Prevalence of sexual activity and associated factors in men aged 75 to 95 years: A cohort study. *Annals of Internal Medicine, 153*(11), 693–702.

Irwig, M. S. (2012). Depressive symptoms and suicidal thoughts among former users of finasteride with persistent sexual side effects. *Journal of Clinical Psychiatry, 73*, 1220–1223.

Keller, A. A., Hamer, R., & Rosen, R. C. (1997). Serotonin reuptake inhibitor-induced sexual dysfunction and its treatment: a large-scale retrospective study of 596 psychiatric outpatients. *Journal of Sex and Marital Therapy, 23*, 165–175.

Kendall, A., Dowsett, M., Folkerd, E., & Smith, I. (2006). Caution: Vaginal estradiol appears to be contraindicated in postmenopausal women on adjuvant aromatase inhibitors. *Annals of Oncology, 17*, 584–587.

Kettaş E, Cayan, F., Akbay, E., Kiykim, A., & Cayan, S. (2008). Sexual dysfunction and associated risk factors in women with end-stage renal disease. *Journal of Sexual Medicine, 5*, 872–877.

Khera, M., Crawford, D., Morales, A., Salonia, A., & Morgentaler, A. (2014). A new era of testosterone and prostate cancer: From physiology to clinical implications. *European Urology, 65*, 115–123.

Koyuncu, H., Serefoglu, E. C., Ozdemir, A. T., & Hellstrom, W. J. (2012). Deleterious effects of selective serotonin reuptake inhibitor treatment on semen parameters in patients with lifelong premature ejaculation. *International Journal of Impotence Research, 24*, 171–173.

Koyuncu, H., Serefoglu, E. C., Yencilek, E., Atalay, H., Akbas, N. B., & Sarıca, K. (2011). Escitalopram treatment for premature ejaculation has a negative effect on semen parameters. *International Journal of Impotence Research, 23*, 257–261.

Laan, E., Rellini, A. H., & Barnes, T. (2013). Standard operating procedures for female orgasmic disorder: consensus of the International Society for Sexual Medicine. *Journal of Sexual Medicine, 10*, 74–82.

Laties, A., & Sharlip, I. (2006). Ocular safety in patients using sildenafil citrate therapy for erectile dysfunction. *Journal of Sexual Medicine, 3*, 12–27.

Lindau, S. T., & Gavrilova, N (2010). Sex, health, and years of sexually active life gained due to good health: evidence from two US population based cross sectional surveys of ageing. *BMJ, 340*, c810.

Lindau, S. T., Scumm, L. P., Laumann, E. O., Levinson, W., O'Muircheartaigh, C. A., Waite, L. J., et al. (2007). A study of sexuality and health among older adults in the United States. *New England Journal of Medicine, 357*, 762–774.

Lindau, S. T., Abramsohn, E., & Gosch, K., Wroblewski, K., Spatz, E. S., Chan, P. S., et al. (2012). Patterns and loss of sexual activity in the year following hospitalization for acute myocardial infraction (a United States National Multisite Observational Study). *American Journal of Cardiology, 109*, 1439–1444.

Maggi, M., Buvat, J., Corona, G., Guay, A., & Torres, L. O. (2013). Hormonal causes of male sexual dysfunctions and their management (hyperprolactinemia, thyroid disorder, GH disorders, and DHEA). *Journal of Sexual Medicine, 10*, 661–677.

Manolis, A., & Doumas, M. (2008). Sexual dysfunction: the 'prima ballerina' of hypertension-related quality-of-life complications. *Journal of Hypertension, 26*, 2074–2084.

Manolis, A., & Doumas, M. (2012). Antihypertensive treatment and sexual dysfunction. *Current Hypertension Reports, 14*, 285–292.

McGahuey, C. A., Gelenberg, A. J., Laukes, C. A., Moreno, F. A., Delgado, P. L., McKnight, K. M., et al. (2000). The Arizona Sexual Experience Scale (ASEX): reliability and validity. *Journal of Sex and Marital Therapy, 20*, 25–40.

McGwin, G. (2010). Phosphodiesterase type 5 inhibitor use and hearing impairment. *Archives of Otolaryngology—Head & Neck Surgery, 136*, 488–492.

McMahon, C. G. (2009). Sexual dysfunction: anesthetic spray improves premature ejaculation. *Nature Reviews. Urology, 6*, 472–473.

McMahon, C. G., Lee, G., Park, J. K., & Adaikan, P. G. (2012). Premature ejaculation and erectile dysfunction prevalence and attitudes in the Asia-Pacific region. *Journal of Sexual Medicine, 9*, 454–465.

Milbury, K., & Badr, H. (2013). Sexual problems, communication patterns, and depressive symptoms in couples coping with metastatic breast cancer. *Psycho-oncology, 22*, 814–822.

Miles, T., & Johnson, N. (2010). Vaginal dilator therapy for women receiving pelvic radiotherapy. *Cochrane Database of Systematic Reviews, 9*, CD007291.

Milhausen, R. R., Graham, C. A., Sanders, S. A., Yarber, W. L., & Maitland, S. B. (2010). Validation of the sexual excitation/sexual inhibition inventory for women and men. *Archives of Sexual Behavior, 39*, 1091–1104.

Miner, M., Nehra, A., Jackson, G., Bhasin, S., Billups, K., Burnett, A. L., et al. (2014). All men with vasculogenic erectile dysfunction require a cardiovascular workup. *American Journal of Medicine, 127*, 174–182.

Morano, S. (2003). Pathophysiology of diabetic sexual dysfunction. *Journal of Endocrinological Investigation, 26*(3 Suppl), 65–69.

Morgentaler, A., Lipshultz, L. I., Bennett, R., Sweeney, M., Avila, D. Jr., & Khera, M. (2011). Testosterone therapy in men with untreated prostate cancer. *Journal of Urology, 185*, 1256–1261.

Naghi, J. J., Philip, K. J., DiLibero, D., Willix, R., & Schwarz, E., R. (2011). Testosterone therapy: treatment of metabolic disturbances in heart failure. *Journal of Cardiovascular Pharmacology and Therapeutics, 16*(1), 14–23.

Nehra, A., Jackson, G., Miner, M., Billups, K. L., Burnett, A. L., Buvat, J., et al. (2013). Diagnosis and treatment of erectile dysfunction for reduction of cardiovascular risk. *Journal of Urology, 189*(6), 2031–2038.

North American Menopause Society (2013). Management of symptomatic vulvovaginal atrophy: 2013 position statement of The North American Menopause Society. *Menopause, 20*, 888–902.

Nurnberg, H. G., Hensley, P. L., Heiman, Jr., Croft, H. A., Debattista, C., & Paine S. (2008). Sildenafil treatment of women with antidepressant-associated sexual dysfunction: A randomized controlled trial. *Journal of the American Medical Association, 300*, 395–404.

Okuyucu, S., Guven, O. E., Akoglu, E., Uçar, E., & Dagli, S. (2009) Effect of phosphodiesterase-5 inhibitor on hearing. *Journal of Laryngology and Otology, 123*, 718–722.

O'Leary, M. P., Fowler, F. J., Lenderking, W. R., Barber, B., Sagnier, P. P., Guess, H. A., et al. (1995). A brief male sexual function inventory for urology. *Urology, 46*, 697–706.

Pacik, P. T. (2011). Vaginismus: Review of current concepts and treatment using, Botox injections, bupivacaine injections, and progressive dilation with the patient under anesthesia. *Aesthetic Plastic Surgery, 35*, 1160–1164.

Park, H. J., Won, J. E., Sorsaburu, S., Rivera, P. D., & Lee, S. W. (2013). Urinary Tract Symptoms (LUTS) Secondary to Benign Prostatic Hyperplasia (BPH) and LUTS/BPH with erectile dysfunction in Asian men: A systematic review focusing on Tadalafil. *World Journal of Men's Health, 31*, 193–207.

Pastuszak, A. W., Pearlman, A. M., Godoy, G., Miles, B. J., Lipshultz, L. I., & Khera, M. (2013). Testosterone replacement therapy in the setting of prostate cancer treated with radiation. *International Journal of Impotence Research, 25*(1), 4–8.

Poels, S., Bloemers, J., van Rooij, K., Goldstein, I., Gerritsen, J., van Ham, D., et al. (2013). Toward personalized sexual medicine (part 2): Testosterone combined with a PDE5 inhibitor increases sexual satisfaction in women with HSDD and FSAD, and a low sensitive system for sexual cues. *Journal of Sexual Medicine, 10*, 810–823.

Ponzone, R., Biglia, N., Jacomuzzi, M. E., Maggiorotto, F., Mariani, L., & Sismondi, P. (2005). Vaginal oestrogen therapy after breast cancer: Is it safe? *European Journal of Cancer, 41*, 2673–2681.

Porst, H., Burnett, A., Brock, G., Ghanem, H., Giuliano, F., Glina, S., et al. (2013). ISSM Standards Committee for Sexual Medicine SOP conservative (medical and mechanical) treatment of erectile dysfunction. *Journal of Sexual Medicine, 10*, 130–171.

Raheem, A. A., & Kell, P. (2009). Patient preference and satisfaction in erectile dysfunction therapy: a comparison of the three phosphodiesterase-5 inhibitors sildenafil, vardenafil and tadalfil. *Patient Preference and Adherence, 3*, 99–104.

Raynaud, J. P. (2006). Prostate cancer risk in testosterone-treated men. *Steroid Biochemistry and Molecular Biology, 102*, 261–266.

Rosen, R. C., Brown, C., Heiman, J., Leiblum, S., Meston, C., Shabsigh, R., et al. (2000). The Female Sexual Function Inventory (FSFI): a multidimensional self-report instrument for the assessment of female sexual function. *Journal of Sex & Marital Therapy, 26,* 191–208.

Rosen, R. C., Cappelleri, J. C., & Gendrano, N. (2002). The International Index of Erectile Function (IIEF): A state-of-the-science review. *International Journal of Impotence Research, 14,* 226–244.

Rosen, R. C., Cappelleri, J. C., Smith, M. D., Lipsky, J., & Peña, B. M. (1999). Development and evaluation of an abridged, 5-item version of the International Index of Erectile Function (IIEF-5) as a diagnostic tool for erectile dysfunction. *International Journal of Impotence Research, 11,* 319–326.

Rosen, R. C., Catania, J., Pollack, L., Althof, S., O'Leary, M., & Seftel, A. D. (2004). Male Sexual Health Questionnaire (MSHQ): scale development and psychometric validation. *Urology, 64,* 777–782.

Rosen, R. C., Riley, A., Wagener, G., Osterloh, I. H., Kirkpatrick, J., & Mishra, A. (1997). The international index of erectile function (IIEF): A multidimensional scale for assessment of erectile dysfunction. *Urology, 49,* 822–830.

Safarinejad, M. R. (2008). Sperm DNA damage and semen quality impairment after treatment with selective serotonin reuptake inhibitors detected using semen analysis and sperm chromatin structure assay. *Journal of Urology, 180,* 2124–2128.

Salem, E. A., Wilson, S. K., Bissada, N. K., Delk, J. R., Hellstrom, W. J., Cleves, M. A. (2008). Tramadol, H. C. L has promise in on-demand use to treat premature ejaculation. *Journal of Sexual Medicine, 5,* 188–193.

Samkoff, L. M., & Goodman, A. D. (2011). Symptomatic management in multiple sclerosis. *Neurologic Clinics, 29,* 449–463.

Sanford, M. (2013). Avanafil: a review of its use in patients with erectile dysfunction. *Drugs and Aging, 30,* 853–862.

Seeman, M. V. (2013). Loss of libido in a woman with schizophrenia. *American Journal of Psychiatry, 170,* 471–475.

Serefoglu, E. C., & Saitz, T. R. (2012). New insights on premature ejaculation: a review of definition, classification, prevalence and treatment. *Asian Journal of Andrology, 14,* 822–829.

Serretti, A., & Chiesa, A. (2011). A meta-analysis of sexual dysfunction in psychiatric patients taking antipsychotics. *International Clinical Psychopharmacology, 26,* 130–140.

Shabsigh, R., Crawford, E. D., Nehra, A., & Slawin, K. M. (2009). Testosterone therapy in hypogonadal men and potential prostate cancer risk: a systematic review. *International Journal of Impotence Research, 21,* 9–23.

Shabsigh, R., Kaufman, J. M., Steidle, C., & Padma-Nathan, H. (2004). Randomized study of testosterone gel as adjunctive therapy to sildenafil in hypogonadal men with erectile dysfunction who do not reponsd to sildenafil alone. *Journal of Urology, 172,* 658–663.

Shafer, L. C. (2008). Sexual disorders and sexual dysfunction. In T. A. Stern, J. F. Rosenbaum, M. Fava, et al. (Eds.), *Massachusetts General Hospital comprehensive clinical psychiatry.* Philadelphia: Mosby Elsevier.

Shamloul, R., & Ghanem, H. (2013). Erectile dysfunction. *Lancet, 381*(9681), 153–165.

Shamloul, R., Ghanem, H., Fahmy, I., El-Meleigy, A., Ashoor, S., Elnashaar, A., et al. (2005). Testosterone therapy can enhance erectile function response to sildenafil in patients with PADAM: A pilot study. *Journal of Sexual Medicine, 2,* 559–564.

Shifren, J. L., Monz, B. U., Russo, P. A., Segreti, A., & Johannes, C. B. (2008). Sexual problems and distress in, United States women: prevalence and correlates. *Obstetrics and Gynecology, 112,* 970–978.

Shim, Y. S., Pae, C. U., Cho, K. J., Kim, S. V. V., Kim, J. C., & Koh, J. S. (2014). Effects of daily low-dose treatment with phosphodiesterase type 5 inhibitor on cognition, depression, somatization and erectile function in patients with erectile dysfunction: a double-blind, placebo-controlled study. *International Journal of Impotence Research, 2,* 76–80.

Simon, J. A., & Maamari, R. V. (2013). Ultra-low-dose estrogen tablets for the treatment of postmenopausal vaginal atrophy. *Climacteric, 16*(Suppl 1), 37–43.

Sivaraaman, K., & Mintzer, S. (2011). Hormonal consequences of epilepsy and its treatment in men. *Current Opinion in Endocrinology, Diabetes, and Obesity, 18,* 204–209.

Soe, L. H., Wurz, G. T., Kao, C. J., & Degregorio, M. W. (2013). Ospemifene for the treatment of dyspareunia associated with vulvar and vaginal atrophy: potential benefits in bone and breast. *International Journal of Women's Health, 5,* 605–611.

Strippoli, G. F., Collaborative Depression and Sexual Dysfunction (CDS) in Hemodialysis Working Group, Vecchio, M., Palmer, S., De Berardis, G., Craig, J., et al. (2012). Sexual dysfunction in women with ESRD requiring hemodialysis. *Clinical Journal of the American Society of Nephrology, 7*(6), 974–981.

Symonds, T., Perelman, M., Althof, S., Giuliano, F., Martin, M., May, K., et al. (2007a). Development and validation of a premature ejaculation diagnostic tool. *European Urology, 52,* 565–573.

Symonds, T., Perelman, M., Althof, S., Giuliano, F., Martin, M., Abraham, L., et al. (2007b). Further evidence of the reliability and validity of the premature ejaculation diagnostic tool. *International Journal of Impotence Research, 19,* 521–525.

Tan, O., Bradshaw, K., & Carr, B. R. (2012). Management of vulvovaginal atrophy-related sexual dysfunction in postmenopausal women: An up-to-date review. *Menopause, 9,* 109–117.

Tanrikut, C., Feldman, A. S., Altemus, M., & Paduch, D. A. (2010). Adverse effect of paroxetine on sperm. *Fertility and Sterility, 94*(3), 1021–1026.

Taylor, M. J., Rudkin, L., Bullemor-Day, P., Lubin, J., Chukwujekwu, C., & Hawton, K. (2013). Strategies for managing sexual dysfunction induced by antidepressant medication. *Cochrane Database of Systematic Reviews, 5*(1), 1361–6137.

Traish, A. M., Miner, M. M., Morgentaler, A., & Zitzmann, M. (2011). Testosterone deficiency. *American Journal of Medicine 124,* 578–587.

Van Rooij, K., Poels, S., Bloemers, J., Goldstein, I., Gerritsen, J., van Ham, D., et al. (2013). Toward personalized sexual medicine (part 3): Testosterone combined with a serotonin 1A receptor agonist increases sexual satisfaction in women with HSDD and FSAD, and dysfunctional activation of sexual inhibitory mechanism. *Journal of Sexual Medicine, 10,* 824–837.

Vecchio, M., Navaneethan, S. D., Johnson, D. W., Lucisano, G., Graziano, G., et al. (2010). Interventions for treating sexual dysfunction in patients with chronic kidney disease. *Cochrane Database Systematic Reviews,* 12:CD007747

Vroege, J. A. (1999). The sexual health inventory for men (IIEF-5). *International Journal of Impotence Research, 11,* 177.

Wang, C., Nieschlag, E., Swerdloff, R., Behre, H. M., Hellstrom, W. J., Gooren, L. J., et al. (2009). Investigation, treatment and monitoring of late-onset hypogonadism in males: ISA, ISSAM, EAU, EAA, and ASA recommendations. *European Urology, 55,* 121–130.

Wang, S. M., Han, C., & Lee, S. J. (2013). A review of current evidence for vilazodone in major depressive disorder. *International Journal of Psychiatry in Clinical Practices, 17,* 160–169.

Wierman, M. E., Basson, R., Davis, S. R., Khosla, S., Miller, K. K., Rosner, W., et al. (2006). Androgen therapy in women: an endocrine society clinical practice guideline. *Journal of Clinical Endocrinology and Metabolism, 91,* 3697–3710.

Witherby, S., Johnson, J., Demers, L., Mount, S., Littenberg, B., Maclean, C. D., et al. (2011). Topical testosterone for breast cancer patients with vaginal atrophy related to aromatase inhibitors: A phase I/II study. *Oncologist, 16,* 424–431.

Yasui, T., Matsui, S., Tani, A., Kunimi, K., Yamamoto, S., & Irahara, M. (2012). Androgen in postmenopausal women. *Journal of Medical Investigation,, 59,* 12–27.

Yuan, J., Zhang, R., Yang, Z., Lee, J., Liu, Y., Tian, J., et al. (2013). Comparative effectiveness and safety of oral phosphodiesterase type 5 inhibitors for erectile dysfunction: a systematic review and network meta-analysis. *European Urology, 63,* 902–912.

36.

CHRONIC PAIN

David Borsook

INTRODUCTION

Chronic pain is defined as pain lasting for more than three months. It has reached pandemic proportions in Western countries, affecting over 100 million people in the United States alone. The evidence base for therapies is very small relative to the size of the *problem*. For the therapies that are considered effective—essentially, only pharmaceutical medication, based on randomized trials—the outcomes are relatively poor, with around a 30% efficacy rate, where "efficacy" is essentially a 2-point improvement on a 10-point scale. Increasing recognition of the chronic pain pandemic and the lack of well-established therapies has led to increased research on both the pathophysiology and the treatment of the condition. New research is leading to a new conceptualization of chronic pain that is likely to improve future treatment outcomes.

COMMON DISORDERS—IMPORTANT INSIGHTS

If one evaluates the conditions that are most prevalent in chronic pain, there are those that may be categorized along the lines of disease-based chronic pain problems. While mechanistic approaches in defining chronic pain are clearly the way forward, common pain clinical syndromes are provided as examples of disease states because of the special features that they provide for conceptualizing the problems that we face in treating chronic pain.

OSTEOARTHRITIS—NOT JUST A PERIPHERAL PAIN PROBLEM

Osteoarthritis is a disease of joints that affects millions of individuals. Osteoarthritis has been considered a chronic nociceptive pain disorder that is characterized by pain due to inflammation, local tissue damage, and attempts at tissue repair (Sofat et al., 2011). Although it is considered a predominantly peripheral pain disorder, more recent data have suggested central processes are at play, including central sensitization (Gwilym et al., 2009). While pain may be mostly exacerbated by activity, the activity produces increased pain processing in the brain, leading to changes such as thalamic atrophy (Gwilym et al., 2010). The ongoing pain may also

produce changes in brain systems (Parks et al., 2011). Thus targeted therapies and anti-inflammatory drugs, including non-steroidals (NSAIDs), have been a mainstay of symptomatic treatment (Hinz & Brune, 2004); however, patients often do not get complete relief. Given that osteoarthritis is a disease predominantly affecting the elderly, under-treatment may be a major issue (Marcum et al., 2011). Until better disease-modifying agents become routine, pain will continue to be a major problem in this group of patients.

CANCER PAIN—FROM DISEASE TO TREATMENT-INDUCED PAIN

Aside from the disease of cancer's initiating pain through multiple mechanisms (inflammation, nerve entrapment, mass effect), treatment effects for cancer are the leading causes of chronic pain. All these, including radiotherapy, chemotherapy, and surgery, may result in a chronic neuropathic pain condition. Many of these treatment-induced syndromes, including chemotherapy-induced peripheral neuropathic pain, may be highly resistant to treatment. Of the chemotherapies that cause neuropathic pain, paclitaxel is perhaps the most noteworthy, but other chemotherapeutic drugs also produce the same problem (Loprinzi et al., 2011). Paclitaxel has been postulated to produce nerve damage through damage to mitochondria (Zheng et al., 2011). It should be noted that muscle pain is also a significant problem following chemotherapy—presumably because of similar damage to muscle fibers (Alvarez et al., 2011). Some agents have been thought useful in preventing pain related to chemotherapy-induced peripheral neuropathy (CIPN), including intravenous calcium and magnesium infusions and glutathione (Pachman et al., 2011); however, no benefit of intravenous calcium/magnesium to prevent oxaliplatin-induced sensory neurotoxicity was found in a recent placebo-controlled, double-blind study (Loprinzi et al., 2013). Unfortunately, there are few well-defined therapies for CIPN.

NEUROPATHIC PAIN—TRAUMATIC INDUCED NEUROPATHIES ARE EPIDEMIC

Neuropathic pain includes all pain—peripheral or central—that results from damage to pain pathways (Borsook, 2011). Many diseases produce neuropathic pain, such as diabetes, complex regional pain syndrome, degenerative spine disease, trigeminal neuralgia, and spinal cord compression, to name a few. A review on neuropathic pain and its mechanisms has been provided elsewhere (Costigan et al., 2009; Baron et al., 2010) . However, one neuropathic pain condition that follows surgery is the so-called surgically induced neuropathic pain (SNPP) that affects 15–50% of individuals undergoing surgery (Kehlet et al., 2006). Given that there are around 29 million surgeries in the United States each year, the prevalence is epidemic. Neuropathic pain results in spontaneous pain (burning, shooting) and evoked pain (allodynia, hyperalgesia, and hyperpathia). It is now clear that significant changes in brain function and structure occur as a result of ongoing neuropathic pain. Such changes affect not only sensory systems but also emotional and cognitive systems. As such, many comorbid features arise from the condition, including depression, anxiety, and addiction.

Pharmacological treatment with neuropathic pain is largely empirical, with a trial-and-error approach utilizing some drugs that have shown to be effective in clinical trials (e.g., gabapentinoids, duloxetine, and others). These drugs may be grouped into calcium channel modulators (e.g., gabapentin), membrane stabilizers (e.g., mexilitene, sodium channel-blocking activity of amitriptyline, lidocaine patch), gamma-amino-butyric acid (GABA) inhibitors (e.g., baclofen), n-methyl-D-Aspartate (NMDA) antagonists (e.g., ketamine), capsaicin, and opioids. Other treatment modalities including neuromodulatory (spinal cord stimulation) and behavioral (e.g., cognitive therapy, biofeedback), and unconventional approaches such as acupuncture have all been deployed in trying to treat chronic neuropathic pain. In controlled trials, efficacy of around 30% has usually been achieved. Evidence-based approaches have been issued by a number of groups (Dworkin et al., 2007).

VISCERAL PAIN—FROM IRRITABLE BOWEL SYNDROME TO PANCREATITIS

Visceral pain is among the most difficult to evaluate and control. Visceral pain syndromes include chronic pancreatitis, cystitis, testicular pain, and irritable bowel syndrome (IBS). Even phantom visceral pain conditions have been described (Puhse et al., 2010). IBS is considered a hypersensitivity disorder (Barbara et al., 2011). Visceral hypersensitivity is an increased perception of events occurring in the gastrointestinal tract. It is characterized by hyperalgesia, an enhanced response to painful stimuli, and allodynia, a painful response to an innocuous stimulus. Central brain changes (Price et al., 2009) and significant aberrant behavioral processes are associated with IBS (Elsenbruch, 2011). The condition is also associated with mucosal abnormalities (e.g., immune, neural, etc.). However, compared with somatic pain, the syndrome is far less well understood (Sengupta, 2009), and includes abnormal inhibitory modulation of pain. Significant changes are present in the central nervous system (CNS) in IBS patients (Seminowicz et al., 2010), and there is evidence of decreased brainstem inhibition of pain (Berman et al.,

2008). Other visceral pain conditions have no understood etiology or mechanism (e.g., functional bowel disorders and chronic pelvic pain). Chronic pancreatitis is among the most difficult pain conditions to manage (Drewes et al., 2008), and treatments have included radical surgical approaches (Schnelldorfer et al., 2007). Inflammation of the pancreas that may include alterations in cytokines, glial function, and immune changes may produce a chronic inflammation in the organ suggestive of an autoimmune etiology (Sanchez-Castanon et al., 2010). Like many chronic pain syndromes, it "reorganizes" the central nervous system (Dimcevski et al., 2007; Fregni et al., 2007). By whatever mechanism, visceral pain syndromes are made more complex and more resistant to treatments, perhaps in part by the frequently associated comorbid features of depression, anxiety, and cognitive alterations that are often observed to be present in these patients. Functional abdominal pain syndromes are even more complex (Sperber & Drossman, 2011).

Visceral analgesic therapies, including pharmacological ones, are suboptimal (Camilleri, 2010). The new 5-HT(4) agonists like prucalopride seem to have a safer cardiac profile, and other agents such as intestinal secretagogues (e.g., chloride channel activators and guanylate cyclase-C agonists) may provide useful approaches to the treatment of the disease (Camilleri, 2010). {table visceral analgesia}

MIGRAINE—COMMON AND FORGOTTEN

Migraine is considered by the World Health Organization (WHO) to be in the top 20 causes of disability worldwide (Buse et al., 2009) and affects patients during their formative and most productive periods of their lives, between age 25 and 55 (Lipton et al., 2001; Lipton et al., 2002). It frequently starts in childhood, particularly around puberty, and affects women more than men. It has significant effects on the brain (Antonaci et al., 2014). The major challenge in migraine is developing preventive treatments or disease-modifying treatments (Barbanti et al., 2011). Acute therapies for migraine work reasonably well (triptans, NSAIDs), and they work best if taken at the onset of the attack (Burstein et al., 2004). While some treatments for chronic migraine or chronic daily headache (more than 14 headache days per month) have shown efficacy in controlled trials (e.g., topiramate; Ferrari et al., 2011), and botulinum toxin (Diener et al., 2010), these effects are not very strong, and other medications continue to be used (valproate, β-blockers, and tricyclic antidepressants). The continued migraine attacks change the brain and may make the condition prone to transforming from acute episodic migraine to chronic daily headaches. Of note, medication overuse, particularly of triptans and opioids (Bigal & Lipton, 2009) may contribute to such transformation. Mechanisms for transformation by medication have been reviewed elsewhere and may include processes of amplification including central sensitization and descending facilitation (De Felice et al., 2011a). Reversal of this state may also be possible with opioid withdrawal.

BRAIN-DERIVED PAIN SYNDROMES

The following discussion reviews examples of two pain syndromes wherein pain becomes a manifestation of changes or drivers within the nervous system.

Depression and Pain

While depression may be a consequence of pain (Haley et al., 1985; Wilson et al., 2002), it is also true that depressed individuals with no history of pain or tissue damage are at increased risk for the development of neuropathic pain (Gureje et al., 2001; Breslau et al., 2003). As a reward-deficit state, chronic pain may reduce the capacity to suppress negative emotion and may contribute to the evolution of unipolar depression (Levesque et al., 2003). Numerous studies have indicated common changes in the prefrontal cortex (PFC) in depression and chronic pain, including a decrease in volume of gray matter (Drevets et al., 1998; Apkarian et al., 2004) and dysfunction in prefrontal cortical processing (Drevets, 2000; Apkarian et al., 2001). Structural changes in the cortex have been linked with functional changes in pain experience (Apkarian et al., 2004; Horton et al., 2004), and functional imaging of chronic pain patients indicates significant alterations of frontal lobe function (Casey et al., 2003). The role of brain-reward systems in depression, the idea that an altered brain-reward system may be the underlying brain mechanism of the loss of pleasure and interest experienced in major depressive disorder, has been reviewed elsewhere (Naranjo et al., 2001). Thus, the intriguing feature of pain evolving from depression is that it implies that depression causes an alteration in neural circuits that produces a generalized pain syndrome. This is not unique to depression, since patients who are opioid addicts may have similar changes in which their drug intake may alter their neural networks such that they are more sensitive to pain (experimentally and clinically).

Fibromyalgia

Fibromyalgia is a syndrome that has widespread pain, and it is now considered to have an origin in the brain (Clauw, 2009; Clauw et al., 2011). It is an under-diagnosed condition, principally because it does not have a precise definition or objective measure. Although criteria for definition of the disease have been defined, these are not specific. Aside from pain, other significant clinical manifestations are noted, including fatigue, non-restorative sleep, and cognitive dysfunction. Treatment of fibromyalgia is challenging. Pharmacological approaches include classical antidepressants, and serotonin and noradrenaline reuptake inhibitors, used in sub-antidepressant doses, seem to be the most effective.

PAIN MECHANISMS

Reviews for disease conditions and their mechanisms are noted elsewhere: neuropathic pain (Baron et al., 2010; Nickel et al., 2011); migraine (Goadsby et al., 2009; Akerman et al., 2011); osteoarthritis (Mease et al., 2011); complex regional pain syndrome (Bruehl, 2010); irritable bowel syndrome (Barbara et al., 2011; Zhou & Verne, 2011); fibromyalgia (Staud & Rodriguez, 2006); trigeminal neuralgia (Iwata et al., 2011); chronic pancreatitis (Vardanyan & Rilo, 2010); diabetic neuropathic pain (Calcutt & Backonja, 2007; Fischer & Waxman, 2010b); post-herpetic neuralgia (Fields et al., 1998); and central pain syndromes such as thalamic pain (Boivie et al., 1989; Kumar et al., 2009; etc.). Mechanistic approaches are currently a major focus, since therapies can be more logically targeted and developed. A number of important advances have occurred in the pain field in the past ten years. In the sections that follow, a brief overview of some of these is discussed.

GENETIC

Numerous candidate pain genes have been discovered (see Pain Genes Data Base (http://www.jbldesign.com/jmogil/enter.html)). Genetic association studies have identified approximately 20 genes that contain single nucleotide polymorphisms (SNPs) that may confer differences in response to acute and chronic pain (Muralidharan & Smith, 2011). Some SNPs associated with pain genes include the potassium channel alpha subunit *KCNS1* that is a prognostic indicator of chronic pain (Costigan et al., 2010). Others seem to regulate pain sensitivity and persistence, such as GTP cyclohydrolase (*GCH1*) (Tegeder et al., 2006). A haplotype of the *GCH1* gene was significantly associated with less pain following diskectomy for persistent radicular low-back pain (Tegeder et al., 2006). Such discoveries will contribute to significant changes in the way we evaluate and treat patients with chronic pain. Similarly, genetic variants in individual drug responses (pharmacogenomics) also have important contributions to make in the future evaluation and treatment of patients (Webster, 2008; Stamer et al., 2010).

MOLECULAR MECHANISMS

Perhaps the most interesting molecular candidate has been the discovery of the transient receptor potential (TRP) channel vanilloid receptor (TRPV1; Caterina et al., 1999). It is expressed predominantly in the peripheral nervous system and has been a target for drug development (Wong & Gavva, 2009). Mice lacking the receptor have impaired analgesia (Caterina et al., 2000). Six TRPs (TRPV1, TRPV2, TRPV3, TRPV4, TRPM8, and TRPA1) have subsequently been shown to express in primary afferent nociceptors (Levine & Alessandri-Haber, 2007). Loss-of-function mutations in another gene, the *Nav1.7* gene, underlie congenital indifference to pain (Goldberg et al., 2007), while a gain of function of the same gene is linked to erythromelalgia (Fischer & Waxman, 2010a). Such insights point to new opportunities to evolving new concepts in pain and its treatment. Other channelopathies (calcium) are associated with other painful diseases such as familial hemiplegic migraine (Barrett et al., 2008). Many other ion channels have been implicated in chronic pain (Raouf et al., 2010).

GENDER AND PAIN

Clear differences in pain are seen across gender. Women have lower thresholds to experimental pain and are more likely to seek treatment for their pain and have differences to analgesics (Fillingim & Ness, 2000; Craft et al., 2004). While the exact role of hormonal differences in altering acute and chronic pain responses between sexes is not completely understood, clearly, alterations in the hormonal milieu must change neurons and glia across central and peripheral nerve systems (Aloisi & Bonifazi, 2006). Gender differences in pain modulation have also been shown (Popescu et al., 2010).

PERIPHERAL AND CENTRAL SENSITIZATION

Sensitization refers to the process of increased responses to normal stimuli. It may involve the peripheral nerve (peripheral sensitization) or the central nervous system (central sensitization) (Woolf, 2007). In the latter, it has been defined as "prolonged but reversible increase in the excitability and synaptic efficacy of neurons" (Woolf, 2011). Centralization has been inferred across most chronic pain conditions. It is important that the concept be understood as alteration in responses to stimuli but it may also have innate effects on the spontaneous pain condition, including chronification of the disease. Examples of central sensitization include photophobia in migraine, and opioid-induced hyperalgesia (Bannister & Dickenson, 2010). Opioid-induced hyperalgesia has been validated in normal human volunteers receiving chronic morphine infusions; and improvements in paradoxical pain intensity upon discontinuation of opioid therapy have been noted in patients on longtime opioids imply the need for a multidisciplinary approach to chronic pain. Numerous processes may contribute to central sensitization, including genetic, catastrophizing, gender, etc.

ALTERATION IN ENDOGENOUS PAIN MODULATION IN CHRONIC PAIN

Pain modulatory systems include those well documented in the brainstem such as the periaqueductal gray, the cuneiform nucleus, and the raphe magnus (Gebhart, 2004; Mason, 2005; Ossipov et al., 2010). However, it is now well known that other, more rostral brain regions, including the frontal cortex, the cingulate and basal ganglia, may all be involved in the pain modulation. The understanding of pain modulation will have implications for which treatments may augment endogenous processes of pain modulation. The placebo response is one "output" through which these endogenous systems may participate in placebo-induced analgesia (placebo response) or increased pain (nocebo response) (Pollo & Benedetti, 2009). Different brain mechanisms such as expectation, anxiety, and reward are all involved, as well as a variety of learning phenomena (Benedetti et al., 2011). Neuroimaging studies in healthy subjects have contributed to our understanding of placebo responses (Bingel & Tracey, 2008; Bingel, 2010). In a variety of chronic pain conditions, these endogenous systems show diminished inhibition of pain (Staud, 2009) and indeed may show facilitation of pain as demonstrated in animal models

(Edelmayer et al., 2009), while enhanced descending modulation protects against chronic pain (Vera-Portocarrero et al., 2006; De Felice et al., 2011b). Thus, understanding abnormal processing of descending controls (which are affected by a variety of processes, including catastrophizing, medications, affect, and placebo response) and how we can best delay or enhance them would seem like an important addition to our clinical approach to patients (Vanegas & Schaible, 2004).

GLIA AND CHRONIC PAIN

Evidence for astrocytes and glia involvement in chronic pain has become a new force in understanding chronic pain and developing novel therapies for the condition (Austin & Moalem-Taylor, 2010; Gao & Ji, 2010; Gosselin et al., 2010). Perhaps one of the best insights into this issue is the presence of glial hyperactivity in a patient with chronic pain following amputation: positron-emission tomography (PET) imaging displayed increased binding of a specific ligand to glia in the contralateral thalamus (Banati et al., 2001).

EPIGENETIC MECHANISMS

Epigenetic changes affect processes that modify chromatin and subsequently change gene activity without altering the DNA sequence (Geranton, 2011). The importance of understanding epigenetic mechanisms is that they may be potential targets for disease modification.

CENTRALIZATION OF PAIN

The term *centralization of pain* refers to progressive changes in brain systems that result from peripheral nerve injury; for example, changes in brain systems that produce pain such as depression. Perhaps the best examples are the progressive changes seen in brain dysfunction in patients who have a trivial nerve injury and then have manifestations of spread of pain beyond the area (frequently involving the whole body), alterations in autonomic tone, alterations in parietal function (e.g., hemi-inattention), changes in cognition, and movement disorders. These occur in various combinations in complex regional pain syndrome (CRPS). Clearly, a simple injury has not only produced chronic pain, but has led to changes in neuronal circuitry that have now been shown in brain-imaging studies, and correlate with many of the behavior syndromes described above.

CHRONIC PAIN—A COMPLEX DISORDER

Clearly, chronic pain is a disease of the nervous system that encompasses sensory, emotional, cognitive, and other changes as a result of ongoing pain. In addition, comorbid features include a variety of defined conditions, including depression (Nicolson et al., 2009), anxiety (Gureje, 2008; Nicolson et al., 2009; Robinson et al., 2009), addiction (Bailey et al., 2010), or traumatic brain injury (Nampiaparampil, 2008; Robinson et al., 2009; Jain et al., 2011). Thus, treating a chronic pain patient is a complex problem demanding complex interventions that are, or should be, primarily "brain targeted" therapies. In the elderly, a group with increasing pain issues, other processes make the therapeutic approach more difficult, including cognitive decline (e.g., Alzheimer's disease) and decreased mobility. In a recent review of neurological conditions and chronic pain, significant numbers of patients across the spectrum of neurological disease had high rates of depression (Borsook, 2011). In addition, many primary psychiatric diseases have chronic pain as a manifestation of their disease (e.g., depression, addiction, post-traumatic stress disorder [PTSD] or altered pain processing [schizophrenia]). Thus multimodal approaches are required for complex disease interactions (Kirsh & Fishman, 2011).

Psychological Factors

Many psychological factors are processed in chronic pain and an individual's adjustment to chronic pain (Jensen et al., 2011). Among these, "catastrophizing" ranks the highest. Catastrophizing is a concept or term that relates to having a more intense pain experience and increased emotional distress; it is thus a negative cognitive-affective response to anticipated or actual pain (Quartana et al., 2009). It is a predictor for post-surgical chronic pain (Khan et al., 2011). Other psychological factors are important; for example, anxiety sensitivity is reportedly strongly associated with fearful appraisals of pain (Ocanez et al., 2010).

Reward-Aversion

Pain and pleasure are at opposite ends of a behavioral spectrum (Becerra et al., 2001). Thus, aversion (pain) may be considered opposite to reward (pain relief/analgesia) and indeed these two are postulated to utilize similar "reward-based" brain networks (Leknes & Tracey, 2008). Chronic pain may be considered a "reward-deficit state" (Elman et al., 2011). Pain-relief is a rewarding process (Leknes et al., 2011). Pain relief is a concept that incorporates not only pain intensity reduction, but also other emotional and cognitive components related to the condition, including pleasantness. Patients are thus in a state where life is less eventful and satisfying, and this may lead to significant comorbid features such as depression and suicide.

TREATMENTS

Treatment of chronic pain is a real challenge because there are no good treatments. Current approaches are many (some are listed below), and the overall issue is to balance efficacy and adverse effects. In the pharmacological domain this is more easily done, because we have data on drug side effects and can change drugs. For interventional therapies, some are reversible (e.g., spinal cord stimulators) and others (e.g., lesions) are not. In the following sections, information on the possible impact of particular treatment domains is provided. This is not a "how to" approach (which can be found in many texts on pain treatment) but rather an attempt to provide an overall sense of

current therapeutic approaches. The number needed to treat (NNT) before a 50% benefit is observed in a single patient is observed has provided a sense of treatment efficacy; while the number needed to harm (NNH) is the same approach related to measures of side effects (Selph et al., 2011).

PHARMACOTHERAPY

Cochrane Database (and Other) Summaries of Drug Treatments

Anticonvulsants

The gabapentinoids are among the most commonly used drugs for neuropathic pain. Pregabalin at doses of 300 mg, 450 mg, and 600 mg daily was effective in patients with post-herpetic neuralgia, painful diabetic neuropathy, central neuropathic pain, and fibromyalgia (19 studies, 7,003 participants). Pregabalin at 150 mg/d was generally ineffective (Moore et al., 2009). However, as noted in this review, "A minority of patients will have substantial benefit with pregabalin, and more will have moderate benefit. Many will have no or trivial benefit, or will discontinue because of adverse events." The NNH for minor harm for gabapentin accumulated in randomized clinical studies is reported to be 3.7, and the NNT is 2.9 for diabetic neuropathy and 3.9 for post-herpetic neuralgia (Wiffen et al., 2011). When NNTs were evaluated for other "anticonvulsants" and specific neuropathic pain conditions, the following was reported in the Cochrane Database: carbamazepine for trigeminal neuralgia is 2.5 vs. 3.2 for gabapentin; for diabetic neuropathy the NNTs are 2.3 for carbamazepine, 2.1 for phenytoin, and 3.8 for gabapentin. However, the NNH (minor harm) were 3.7, 3.5, and 3.2 for each of these drugs, respectively (Wiffen et al., 2010). As can be seen from these data sets, different drugs have different NNTs that relate to individual differences that determine response rates at a population level, but not for the individual being treated. Nevertheless, they provide one approach to a more rational choice of drug until better methods that are adaptable to the pressures of normal "clinic life" become available.

Antidepressants

Current evidence supports the use of tricyclic antidepressants (amitriptyline, nortriptyline, desipramine) in neuropathic pain, headaches, low back pain, fibromyalgia, and IBS. No evidence supports the use of SSRIs (fluoxetine, paroxetine, citalopram) in chronic pain (Verdu et al., 2008). More recent evidence has shown efficacy for the SNRIs (duloxetine, venlafaxine) across a spectrum of chronic pain (back pain, fibromyalgia, and osteoarthritis) (Dharmshaktu et al., 2011). NNTs for duloxetine (60mg/d but not 20mg/d) for diabetic neuropathy are 6 and for fibromyalgia are 8, but there were adverse effects.

Opioids

The evidence for chronic opioid use in chronic pain is controversial. A recent systematic review of randomized trials on the use of opioids for the treatment of chronic non-cancer pain reported that only tramadol is useful (fair) in osteoarthritis, with poor evidence for all other opioids and chronic pain conditions. Therefore, the use of opioids is mostly based on non-randomized studies. None of the trials went beyond 12 weeks. Because of the relatively few studies, important additional insights into tolerance, addiction, and other aspects of chronic opioid use are not easily evaluated (Kalso et al., 2004). Evidence was insufficient to determine if long-acting opioids as a class are more effective or associated with fewer side effects (harms) than short-acting opioids (Carson et al., 2011).

Lidocaine

In a Cochrane-based review of 31 trials that met the inclusion criteria, lidocaine and oral analogues were safe drugs in controlled clinical trials for neuropathic pain and were better than placebo, and as effective as other analgesics (Challapalli et al., 2005). Currently, there is insufficient evidence to recommend the topical lidocaine patch as a first-line agent in the treatment of post-herpetic neuralgia (PHN) with allodynia (Khaliq et al., 2007). However, when considering side effects, newer studies have indicated that a lidocaine patch is associated with comparable levels of analgesia in patients with PHN or diabetic peripheral neuropathy (DPN) but substantially fewer frequent adverse events than pregabalin (Baron et al., 2009).

Ketamine

This antagonist of the N-methyl-D-Aspartatic Acid (NMDA) receptor has been increasingly used in chronic pain. It has been administered intravenously and orally. Norketamine is the pharmacologically active metabolite believed to contribute to the analgesic effect of oral ketamine. It may be considered in resistant cases, and increasing dosing may have increased clinical efficacy (Borsook, 2009), although it is unclear how this is mediated, since the drug also has deleterious effects on neuronal populations.

High-dose Capsaicin

High dose (8%) capsaicin patches may be useful for neuropathic pain, although the evidence is not strongly supported.

Opioids

Initially used for cancer pain, opioids had been increasingly used for chronic pain (Przewlocki & Przewlocka, 2001), but their use still remains controversial (Katz & Benoit, 2005; Przewlocki & Przewlocka, 2001). Indeed, there is no evidence that they are effective for chronic pain conditions such as neuropathic pain (Carson et al., 2011). Their use seems justified under some circumstances, but risks of side effects like addiction and constipation need to be evaluated and managed. In recent years, there has been a move away from opioids, principally for three reasons—first, there is no good evidence for their efficacy in chronic pain; second, there are significant legal issues surrounding their use because of increased abuse of prescription opioids (Hernandez & Nelson, 2010), and third, because of increasing evidence that opioids alter brain systems (Upadhyay et al., 2010) in a way that may not be reversible. With respect to the latter, this may contribute to either more pain or resistance to other pharmacological treatments, as is observed in migraine (Bigal & Lipton, 2009; De Felice & Porreca, 2009).

Combination Pharmacological Treatments

The notion of combination pharmacological treatments' improving pain gained notoriety following a publication in the *New England Journal of Medicine*, on gabapentin and opioids' significantly improving pain (Gilron et al., 2005). Importantly, the combination provided better analgesia at lower doses than did independent use of each drug. While long-term data are not available, such studies are suggesting the potential to enhance treatments with fewer side effects. For example, more recent data have indicated that combination therapy with duloxetine and pregabalin; lidocaine patch and pregabalin; or gabapentin with imipramine, nortriptyline, or venlafaxine, may have had a potential benefit compared with monotherapy, but there was an increased risk of adverse events (see Selph et al., 2011). Clearly, additional clinical studies are warranted (Vorobeychik et al., 2011).

Other Treatments

Botulinum Toxin

Evidence-based data indicate that administration of botulinum toxin in several human conditions (*viz.*, chronic migraine) can alleviate refractory pain (Jabbari & Machado, 2011). However, further studies are clearly indicated to evaluate the potential use of the drug in post-operative pain and chronic neuropathic pain (Jeynes & Gauci, 2008).

Expert Consensus Reviews on Pharmacotherapy for Pain

Because of the overriding lack of evidence for many pharmacological agents, particularly comparing one agent against another, guidelines from task forces have tried to provide a rational approach to treatment of chronic pain, including chronic neuropathic pain. For example, the European Federation of Neurological Societies Task Force (EFNS) (Attal et al., 2010) summarized their results in the PubMed abstract:

> Drugs generally have similar efficacy in various conditions, except in trigeminal neuralgia, chronic radiculopathy and HIV neuropathy, with level A evidence in support of tricyclic antidepressants (TCA), pregabalin, gabapentin, tramadol and opioids (in various conditions), duloxetine, venlafaxine, topical lidocaine and capsaicin patches (in restricted conditions). Combination therapy appears useful for TCA-gabapentin and gabapentin-opioids (level A).

Another group, Special Interest Group on Neuropathic Pain (NEUPSIG), has evaluated drugs for chronic neuropathic pain and has put forward similar guidelines for pain management of this condition (Dworkin et al., 2010):

Tricyclic antidepressants, dual reuptake inhibitors of serotonin and norepinephrine, calcium channel alpha(2)-delta ligands (i.e., gabapentin and pregabalin), and topical lidocaine were recommended as first-line treatment options on the basis of the results of randomized clinical trials. Opioid analgesics and tramadol were recommended as second-line treatments.

Increasingly, it has become difficult to show efficacy of drugs vs. placebo in controlled trials for chronic pain as exemplified for lacosamide (Ziegler et al., 2010) or lamotrigine (Irizarry et al., 2009).

ACTIVITY-RELATED TREATMENTS

General fitness seems to confer benefits in chronic pain as well (Schaafsma et al., 2010). Similarly, appropriate physical therapy by individuals skilled in treating chronic pain (as opposed, for example, to treatment of acute orthopedic problems) can make a significant difference in chronic pain. The effects are not only related to muscle strengthening but seem to have changes on sensorimotor processing akin to the effects of prostheses in chronic pain that provide additional feedback in patients with amputations (Flor, 2003). The approach has to do with reorganizing the abnormalities producing chronic pain (Karl et al., 2001) by reconstituting cortical processes that these rehabilitation processes confer (see Giraux & Sirigu, 2003). Appropriate exercises specific to a pain problem (e.g., back pain, "frozen shoulder" pain) are easily implemented and may provide some of the best treatment outcomes. Proper clinical trials are needed to define this further (see Cherkin et al., 1998).

USE OF INTERVENTIONAL THERAPIES

Interventional therapies include injections of local anesthetics, steroids, intrathecal infusions of drugs, and neuroablation or stimulation (Shah et al., 2003; Markman & Philip, 2007; Bottger & Diehlmann, 2011). Repetitive nerve blocks as a monotherapeutic treatment are losing their importance in the therapy of chronic pain (Donner et al., 1998). Spinal cord stimulation is addressed above. There are no good outcome studies for any of these studies. However, in some cases, patients may receive benefit, and even if it is short-term, the provision of a respite may help them with accessing and getting involved in other therapies including increased activity (Abdelshafi et al., 2011). More aggressive approaches are used in cancer patients, including intrathecal administration of opioids, local anesthetics, or clonidine (Miguel, 2000). Obviously, invasive techniques may have some complications, but overall these seem to be relatively rare. What are clearly needed are outcome studies to define efficacy in a more rigorous manner.

PSYCHOLOGICAL/BEHAVIORAL THERAPIES

A recent Cochrane Database review reports on the efficacy of psychological therapies for chronic pain, based on a systematic review of randomized controlled trials (Eccleston et al., 2009). Of the behavioral methods studied, only cognitive-behavioral therapy (CBT) showed even small positive effects for pain, disability, and mood. Thus, there are insufficient data on quality or content of behavioral therapies to evaluate their influence on outcome. In a similar Cochrane Database evaluation of psychological treatments in children and adolescents, such treatments were noted to be effective in pain control for children with headache (Eccleston et al., 2009). Psychological treatments may also improve pain control for children with musculoskeletal and recurrent abdominal pain.

NEUROMODULATION

Epidural motor cortex stimulation (MCS) was first reported to be useful for the treatment of refractory neuropathic pain, although its mechanism of action remains poorly understood (Lazorthes et al., 2007). Subsequent use of transcranial magnetic stimulation (TMS) has also provided seemingly beneficial results for a number of pain conditions, including neuropathic pain (Schwenkreis et al., 2010) and fibromyalgia (Mhalla et al., 2011), visceral pain (Villanueva, 2011), and migraine (Lipton et al., 2010). The attractive feature of TMS is that it is non-invasive and may augment other treatments like pharmacotherapy (Antal & Paulus, 2011).

The European Federation of Neurological Societies (EFNS) task force guidelines on the use of neurostimulation for neuropathic pain state:

> Spinal cord stimulation (SCS) is efficacious in failed back surgery syndrome (FBSS) and complex regional pain syndrome (CRPS). Motor cortex stimulation (MCS) is efficacious in central post-stroke and facial pain at lower levels of efficacy. Deep brain stimulation (DBS) should only be performed in experienced centers. (Cruccu et al., 2007)

PAIN ETHICS

While the treatment of pain and access to treatment for pain should be considered a universal right (Lohman et al., 2010), the problem is that, by and large, treatments are relatively ineffective, and trial and error may help produce a best possible option. As noted by McGee and colleagues:

> Raising awareness about chronic pain, improving access and outcomes to quality pain care, and resolving public policy debates about the use of opioids in chronic pain populations are the first steps to ensuring a morally justifiable approach to chronic pain management in the 21st century. (McGee et al., 2011)

In approaching this, there several issues that can be addressed, including disparities in treatment across age and gender, access to pain, standards of care, prevention of discrimination, and the need to enhance studies that provide evidence-based outcomes to guide treatment. Doing better with the current armamentarium based on best practice seems like a reasonable measure to start with, while developments in these domains improve pain treatments. In a report from the Institute of Medicine (IOM), it is noted that:

> Pain is a major driver for visits to physicians, a major reason for taking medications, a major cause of disability, and a key factor in quality of life and productivity. Given the burden of pain in human lives, dollars, and social consequences, relieving pain should be a national priority. (Relieving Pain in America: A Blueprint for Transforming Prevention, Care, Education, and Research; http://www.iom.edu/Reports/2011/Relieving-Pain-in-America-A-Blueprint-for-Transforming-Prevention-Care-Education-Research.aspx)

By getting rid of treatments that do not benefit patients, by education about what is possible based on scientific evidence, we can provide a more honest approach to patients who suffer from chronic pain.

MISSING ELEMENTS AND INTEGRATED TREATMENTS

Pain treatment is at a crossroads. There needs to be a modification of our approaches that incorporate integrated approaches. This is different from the so-called multidisciplinary approaches where the patient "hops from one discipline to another." The approach needs to be patient-centric and treatments need to be measured according to the diagnosis. The best example is a recent paper on chronic back pain. It defines the contributions of additive therapies based on the level of the disease (Hill et al., 2011). By stratifying care into three therapeutic pathways according to the estimated risk of poor prognosis (defined in their study as persistent disability because of back pain), the authors improved clinical outcomes while remaining cost-effective.

For integrated treatments, there are numerous missing elements. While the mainstays of advanced pain treatments have been mostly procedural, there lately seems to be a major change in the way we approach pain treatment, based on the increasing demand for outcome studies on treatment efficacy. In order to improve our position, the following issues will need to be addressed:

1. Chronic pain needs to be understood as a disease of the CNS. Understanding reward-aversion processing and alterations in endogenous pain processing are critical.

2. Missing "elements" in pain treatment including neurology (Borsook, 2011) and psychiatry (Elman et al., 2011), which may provide additional approaches to patient evaluation and treatment. These two disciplines by and large do not involve themselves in pain.

3. Objective assays (biomarkers) for the diagnosis of pain and treatment (Borsook et al., 2011a, 2011b) or for segregating patient groups based on mechanism (Scholz et al., 2009) are needed.

4. Mechanism-based treatments should be the focus of therapy (Woolf, 2004).

5. Evidence-based management of chronic pain conditions is a critical need. Integrating science into the clinic will no doubt contribute to accelerating the development of improved treatment approaches.

CLINICAL PEARLS

- Chronic pain is defined as pain lasting for more than three months.

- Neuropathic pain includes all pain—peripheral or central—that results from damage to pain pathways (Borsook, 2011).

- Neuropathic pain results in spontaneous pain (burning, shooting) and evoked pain (allodynia, hyperalgesia, and hyperpathia).

- Changes in brain function and structure occur as a result of ongoing neuropathic pain.

- Irritable bowel syndrome (IBS) is a visceral hypersensitivity disorder (Barbara et al., 2011).

- Continued migraine attacks change the brain and may make the condition prone to transforming from acute episodic migraine to chronic daily headaches; medication overuse, particularly triptans and opioids, may contribute to such transformation.

- *Sensitization* refers to the process of increased responses to normal stimuli.

- Pain modulatory systems include those well documented in the brainstem and other more rostral brain regions, including the frontal cortex, the cingulate, and basal ganglia.

- Enhanced descending modulation protects against chronic pain; thus, understanding abnormal processing of descending controls is an important addition to the clinical approach.

- Centralization of pain implicates progressive changes in brain systems that occur as a result of peripheral nerve injury.

- Catastrophizing, the negative cognitive-affective response to anticipated or actual pain, is a prominent psychological factor contributing to the pain experience.

- In consideration of the reward-aversion pathways, pain relief incorporates not only pain reduction but improvements in emotional and cognitive components.

- No evidence supports the use of serotonin reuptake inhibitors in chronic pain (Verdu et al., 2008).

- Use of opioids in chronic pain is mostly based on non-randomized studies; none of the trials went beyond 12 weeks.

- Evidence was insufficient to determine if long-acting opioids as a class are more effective or associated with fewer side effects than short-acting opioids (Carson et al, 2011).

- There is increasing evidence that opioids alter brain systems that may not be reversible (Upadhyay et al., 2010).

- Combination therapy with duloxetine and pregabalin; lidocaine patch and pregabalin; or gabapentin with imipramine, nortriptyline, or venlafaxine may have a potential benefit compared to monotherapy (Selph et al., 2011).

- General fitness seems to confer benefits in chronic pain (Schaafsma et al., 2010).

DISCLOSURE STATEMENT

Dr. Borsook has no Conflicts related to this chapter.

REFERENCES

Abdelshafi, M. E., Yosry, M., Elmulla, A. F., Al-Shahawy, E. A., Adou Aly, M., & Eliewa, E. A. (2011). Relief of chronic shoulder pain: A comparative study of three approaches. *Middle East Journal of Anesthesiology, 21*, 83–92.

Akerman, S., Holland, P. R., & Goadsby, P. J. (2011). Diencephalic and brainstem mechanisms in migraine. *Nature Reviews in the Neurosciences, 12*, 570–584.

Aloisi, A. M., & Bonifazi, M. (2006). Sex hormones, central nervous system and pain. *Hormones & Behavior, 50*, 1–7.

Alvarez, P., Ferrari, L. F., & Levine, J. D. (2011). Muscle pain in models of chemotherapy-induced and alcohol-induced peripheral neuropathy. *Annals of Neurology, 70*, 101–109.

Antal, A., & Paulus, W. (2011). A case of refractory orofacial pain treated by transcranial direct current stimulation applied over hand motor area in combination with NMDA agonist drug intake. *Brain Stimulation, 4*, 117–121.

Antonaci, F., Voiticovschi-Iosob, C., Di Stefano, A. L., Galli, F., Ozge, A., Balottin, U. (2014). The evolution of headache from childhood to adulthood: a review of the literature. *Journal of Headache Pain*, Mar;18(15), 15. doi: 10.1186/1129-2377-15-15.

Apkarian, A. V., Sosa, Y., Sonty, S., et al. (2004). Chronic back pain is associated with decreased prefrontal and thalamic gray matter density. *Journal of Neuroscience, 24*, 104–105.

Apkarian, A. V., Thomas, P. S., Krauss, B. R., & Szeverenyi, N. M. (2001). Prefrontal cortical hyperactivity in patients with sympathetically mediated chronic pain. *Neuroscience Letters, 311*, 193–197.

Attal, N., Cruccu, G., Baron, R., et al. (2010). EFNS guidelines on the pharmacological treatment of neuropathic pain: 2010 revision. *European Journal of Neurology, 17*, e1113–e1188.

Austin, P. J., & Moalem-Taylor, G. (2010). The neuro-immune balance in neuropathic pain: Involvement of inflammatory immune cells, immune-like glial cells and cytokines. *Journal of Neuroimmunology, 229*, 26–50.

Bailey, J. A., Hurley, R. W., & Gold, M. S. (2010). Crossroads of pain and addiction. *Pain Medicine, 11*, 1803–1818.

Banati, R. B., Cagnin, A., Brooks, D. J., et al. (2001). Long-term trans-synaptic glial responses in the human thalamus after peripheral nerve injury. *Neuroreport, 12*, 3439–3442.

Bannister, K., & Dickenson, A. H. (2010). Opioid hyperalgesia. *Current Opinion in Supportive & Palliative Care, 4*, 1–5.

Barbanti, P., Aurilia, C., Egeo, G., & Fofi, L. (2011). Migraine prophylaxis: What is new and what do we need? *Neurological Sciences, 32*(Suppl 1), S111–S115.

Barbara, G., Cremon, C., De Giorgio, R., et al. (2011). Mechanisms underlying visceral hypersensitivity in irritable bowel syndrome. *Current Gastroenterology Reports, 13*, 308–315.

Baron, R., Binder, A., & Wasner, G. (2010). Neuropathic pain: Diagnosis, pathophysiological mechanisms, and treatment. *Lancet Neurology, 9*, 807–819.

Baron, R., Mayoral, V., Leijon, G., Binder, A., Steigerwald, I., & Serpell, M. (2009). Efficacy and safety of 5% lidocaine (lignocaine) medicated plaster in comparison with pregabalin in patients with postherpetic neuralgia and diabetic polyneuropathy: Interim analysis from an open-label, two-stage adaptive, randomized, controlled trial. *Clinical Drug Investigation, 29*, 231–241.

Barrett, C. F., van den Maagdenberg, A. M., Frants, R. R., & Ferrari, M. D. (2008). Familial hemiplegic migraine. *Advances in Genetics, 63*, 57–83.

Becerra, L., Breiter, H. C., Wise, R., Gonzalez, R. G., & Borsook, D. (2001). Reward circuitry activation by noxious thermal stimuli. *Neuron, 32*, 927–946.

Benedetti, F., Carlino, E., & Pollo, A. (2011). How placebos change the patient's brain. *Neuropsychopharmacology, 36*, 339–354.

Berman, S. M., Naliboff, B. D., Suyenobu, B., et al. (2008). Reduced brainstem inhibition during anticipated pelvic visceral pain correlates with enhanced brain response to the visceral stimulus in women with irritable bowel syndrome. *Journal of Neuroscience, 28*, 349–359.

Bigal, M. E., & Lipton, R. B. (2009). Overuse of acute migraine medications and migraine chronification. *Current Pain & Headache Reports, 13*, 301–307.

Bingel, U. (2010). [Mechanisms of endogenous pain modulation illustrated by placebo analgesia: Functional imaging findings]. *Schmerz, 24*, 122–129.

Bingel, U., & Tracey, I. (2008). Imaging CNS modulation of pain in humans. *Physiology (Bethesda), 23*, 371–380.

Boivie, J., Leijon, G., & Johansson, I. (1989). Central post-stroke pain—a study of the mechanisms through analyses of the sensory abnormalities. *Pain, 37*, 173–185.

Borsook, D. (2009). Ketamine and chronic pain—going the distance. *Pain, 145*, 271–272.

Borsook, D. (2011). Neurological diseases and pain. *Brain*.

Borsook, D., Becerra, L., & Hargreaves, R. (2011a). Biomarkers for chronic pain and analgesia. Part 2: How, where, and what to look for using functional imaging. *Discovery Medicine, 11*, 209–219.

Borsook, D., Becerra, L., & Hargreaves, R. (2011b). Biomarkers for chronic pain and analgesia. Part 1: The need, reality, challenges, and solutions. *Discovery Medicine, 11*, 197–207.

Bottger, E., & Diehlmann, K. (2011). Selected interventional methods for the treatment of chronic pain: Part 1: Peripheral nerve block and sympathetic block. *Anaesthesist, 60*, 479–491; quiz, 492.

Breslau, N., Lipton, R. B., Stewart, W. F., Schultz, L. R., & Welch, K. M. (2003). Comorbidity of migraine and depression: Investigating potential etiology and prognosis. *Neurology, 60*, 1308–1312.

Bruehl, S. (2010). An update on the pathophysiology of complex regional pain syndrome. *Anesthesiology, 113*, 713–725.

Burstein, R., Collins, B., & Jakubowski, M. (2004). Defeating migraine pain with triptans: A race against the development of cutaneous allodynia. *Annals of Neurology, 55*, 19–26.

Buse, D. C., Rupnow, M. F., & Lipton, R. B. (2009). Assessing and managing all aspects of migraine: Migraine attacks, migraine-related functional impairment, common comorbidities, and quality of life. *Mayo Clinic Proceedings, 84*, 422–435.

Calcutt, N. A., & Backonja, M. M. (2007). Pathogenesis of pain in peripheral diabetic neuropathy. *Current Diabetes Reports, 7*, 429–434.

Camilleri, M. (2010). Review article: New receptor targets for medical therapy in irritable bowel syndrome. *Alimentary Pharmacology & Therapeutics, 31*, 35–46.

Carson, S., Thakurta, S., Low, A., Smith, B., & Chou, R. (2011). Drug class review: long-acting opioid analgesics: Final Update 6 Report [Internet]. *Drug Class Reviews*. Portland (OR): Oregon Health & Science University.

Casey, K. L., Lorenz, J., & Minoshima, S. (2003). Insights into the pathophysiology of neuropathic pain through functional brain imaging. *Experimental Neurology, 184*(Suppl 1), S80–S88.

Caterina, M. J., Leffler, A., Malmberg, A. B., et al. (2000). Impaired nociception and pain sensation in mice lacking the capsaicin receptor. *Science, 288*, 306–313.

Caterina, M. J., Rosen, T. A., Tominaga, M., Brake, A. J., & Julius, D. (1999). A capsaicin-receptor homologue with a high threshold for noxious heat. *Nature, 398*, 436–441.

Challapalli, V., Tremont-Lukats, I. W., McNicol, E. D., Lau, J., & Carr, D. B. (2005). Systemic administration of local anesthetic agents to relieve neuropathic pain. *Cochrane Database of Systematic Reviews, 101*(6), 1738–49, CD003345.

Cherkin, D. C., Deyo, R. A., Battie, M., Street, J., & Barlow, W. (1998). A comparison of physical therapy, chiropractic manipulation, and provision of an educational booklet for the treatment of patients with low back pain. *New England Journal of Medicine, 339*, 1021–1029.

Clauw, D. J. (2009). Fibromyalgia: An overview. *American Journal of Medicine, 122*, S3–S13.

Clauw, D. J., Arnold, L. M., & McCarberg, B. H. (2011). The science of fibromyalgia. *Mayo Clinic Proceedings, 86*, 907–911.

Costigan, M., et al. (2010). Multiple chronic pain states are associated with a common amino acid-changing allele in KCNS1. *Brain, 133*, 2519–2527.

Costigan, M., Scholz, J., & Woolf, C. J. (2009). Neuropathic pain: A maladaptive response of the nervous system to damage. *Annual Reviews in the Neurosciences, 32*, 1–32.

Craft, R. M., Mogil, J. S., & Aloisi, A. M. (2004). Sex differences in pain and analgesia: The role of gonadal hormones. *European Journal of Pain, 8*, 397–411.

Cruccu, G., Aziz, T. Z., Garcia-Larrea, L., Hansson, P., Jensen, T. S., Lefaucheur, J. P., et al. (2007). EFNS guidelines on neurostimulation therapy for neuropathic pain. *European Journal of Neurology, 14*(9), 952–970.

De Felice, M., & Porreca, F. (2009). Opiate-induced persistent pro-nociceptive trigeminal neural adaptations: Potential relevance to opiate-induced medication overuse headache. *Cephalalgia, 29*, 1277–1284.

De Felice, M., Ossipov, M. H., & Porreca, F. (2011a). Persistent medication-induced neural adaptations, descending facilitation, and medication overuse headache. *Current Opinion in Neurology, 24*, 193–196.

De Felice, M., Sanoja, R., Wang, R., et al. (2011b). Engagement of descending inhibition from the rostral ventromedial medulla protects against chronic neuropathic pain. *Pain, 152*, 2701–2709.

Dharmshaktu, P., Tayal, V., & Kalra, B. S. (2011). Efficacy of antidepressants as analgesics: A review. *Journal of Clinical Pharmacology*, Jan;52(1), 6–17.

Diener, H. C., Dodick, D. W., Aurora, S. K., et al. (2010). Onabotulinumtoxin A for treatment of chronic migraine: Results from the double-blind, randomized, placebo-controlled phase of the PREEMPT 2 trial. *Cephalalgia, 30*, 804–814.

Dimcevski, G., Sami, S. A., Funch-Jensen, P., et al. (2007). Pain in chronic pancreatitis: The role of reorganization in the central nervous system. *Gastroenterology, 132*, 1546–1556.

Donner, B., Schnell, P., & Zenz, M. (1998). [Indications and limits of nerve block techniques]. *Zeitschrift für ärztliche Fortbildung und Qualität im Gesundheitswesen, 92*, 29–33.

Drevets, W. C. (2000). Functional anatomical abnormalities in limbic and prefrontal cortical structures in major depression. *Progress in Brain Research, 126*, 413–431.

Drevets, W. C., Ongur, D., & Price, J. L. (1998). Neuroimaging abnormalities in the subgenual prefrontal cortex: Implications for the pathophysiology of familial mood disorders. *Molecular Psychiatry, 3*, 220–226.

Drewes, A. M., Krarup, A. L., Detlefsen, S., Malmstrom, M. L., Dimcevski, G., & Funch-Jensen, P. (2008). Pain in chronic pancreatitis: The role of neuropathic pain mechanisms. *Gut, 57*, 1616–1627.

Dworkin, R. H., O'Connor, A. B., Audette, J., Baron, R., Gourlay, G. K., Haanpää, M. L., et al. (2010). Recommendations for the pharmacological management of neuropathic pain: An overview and literature update. *Mayo Clinic Proceedings, 85*, S3–S14.

Dworkin, R. H., O'Connor, A. B., Backonja, M., et al. (2007). Pharmacologic management of neuropathic pain: Evidence-based recommendations. *Pain, 132*, 237–251.

Eccleston, C., Williams, A. C., & Morley, S. (2009). Psychological therapies for the management of chronic pain (excluding headache) in adults. *Cochrane Database of Systematic Reviews, 11*: CD007407.

Edelmayer, R. M., Vanderah, T. W., Majuta, L., et al. (2009). Medullary pain facilitating neurons mediate allodynia in headache-related pain. *Annals of Neurology, 65*, 184–193.

Elman, I., Zubieta, J. K., & Borsook, D. (2011). The missing p in psychiatric training: Why it is important to teach pain to psychiatrists. *Archives of General Psychiatry, 68*, 12–20.

Elsenbruch, S. (2011). Abdominal pain in irritable bowel syndrome: A review of putative psychological, neural and neuro-immune mechanisms. *Brain, Behavior, & Immunity, 25*, 386–394.

Ferrari, A., Tiraferri, I., Neri, L., & Sternieri, E. (2011). Clinical pharmacology of topiramate in migraine prevention. *Expert Opinion on Drug Metabolism & Toxicology, 7*, 1169–1181.

Fields, H. L., Rowbotham, M., & Baron, R. (1998). Postherpetic neuralgia: Irritable nociceptors and deafferentation. *Neurobiology of Disease, 5*, 209–227.

Fillingim, R. B., & Ness, T. J. (2000). Sex-related hormonal influences on pain and analgesic responses. *Neuroscience & Biobehavioral Reviews, 24*, 485–501.

Fischer, T. Z., & Waxman, S. G. (2010a). Familial pain syndromes from mutations of the NaV1.7 sodium channel. *Annals of the New York Academy of Sciences, 1184*, 196–207.

Fischer, T. Z., & Waxman, S. G. (2010b). Neuropathic pain in diabetes—evidence for a central mechanism. *Nature Revue Neurologique (Paris), 6*, 462–466.

Flor, H. (2003). Remapping somatosensory cortex after injury. *Advances in Neurology, 93*, 195–204.

Fregni, F., Pascual-Leone, A., & Freedman, S. D. (2007). Pain in chronic pancreatitis: A salutogenic mechanism or a maladaptive brain response? *Pancreatology, 7*, 411–422.

Gao, Y. J., & Ji, R. R. (2010). Targeting astrocyte signaling for chronic pain. *Neurotherapeutics, 7*, 482–493.

Gebhart, G. F. (2004). Descending modulation of pain. *Neuroscience & Biobehavioral Reviews, 27*, 729–737.

Geranton, S. M. (2011). Targeting epigenetic mechanisms for pain relief. *Current Opinion in Pharmacology*, Feb;12(1), 35–41. doi: 10.1016/j.coph.2011.10.012.

Gilron, I., Bailey, J. M., Tu, D., Holden, R. R., Weaver, D. F., & Houlden, R. L. (2005). Morphine, gabapentin, or their combination for neuropathic pain. *New England Journal of Medicine, 352*, 1324–1334.

Giraux, P., & Sirigu, A. (2003). Illusory movements of the paralyzed limb restore motor cortex activity. *Neuroimage, 20*(Suppl 1), S107–S111.

Goadsby, P. J., Charbit, A. R., Andreou, A. P., Akerman, S., & Holland, P. R. (2009). Neurobiology of migraine. *Neuroscience, 161*, 327–341.

Goldberg, Y. P., et al. (2007). Loss-of-function mutations in the Nav1.7 gene underlie congenital indifference to pain in multiple human populations. *Clinical Genetics, 71*, 311–319.

Gosselin, R. D., Suter, M. R., Ji, R. R., & Decosterd, I. (2010). Glial cells and chronic pain. *Neuroscientist, 16*, 519–531.

Gureje, O. (2008). Comorbidity of pain and anxiety disorders. *Current Psychiatry Report, 10*, 318–322.

Gureje, O., Simon, G. E., & Von Korff, M. (2001). A cross-national study of the course of persistent pain in primary care. *Pain, 92*, 195–200.

Gwilym, S. E., Filippini, N., Douaud, G., Carr, A. J., & Tracey, I. (2010). Thalamic atrophy associated with painful osteoarthritis of the hip is reversible after arthroplasty: A longitudinal voxel-based morphometric study. *Arthritis & Rheumatism, 62,* 2930–2940.

Gwilym, S. E., Keltner, J. R., Warnaby, C. E., et al. (2009). Psychophysical and functional imaging evidence supporting the presence of central sensitization in a cohort of osteoarthritis patients. *Arthritis & Rheumatism, 61,* 1226–1234.

Haley, W. E., Turner, J. A., & Romano, J. M. (1985). Depression in chronic pain patients: Relation to pain, activity, and sex differences. *Pain, 23,* 337–343.

Hernandez, S. H., & Nelson, L. S. (2010). Prescription drug abuse: Insight into the epidemic. *Clinical Pharmacology & Therapeutics, 88,* 307–317.

Hill, J. C., Whitehurst, D. G., Lewis, M., et al. (2011). Comparison of stratified primary care management for low back pain with current best practice (STarT Back): A randomised controlled trial. *Lancet, 378,* 1560–1571.

Hinz, B., & Brune, K. (2004). Pain and osteoarthritis: New drugs and mechanisms. *Current Opinion in Rheumatology, 16,* 628–633.

Horton, J. E., Crawford, H. J., Harrington, G., & Downs, J. H., 3rd (2004). Increased anterior corpus callosum size associated positively with hypnotizability and the ability to control pain. *Brain, 127,* 1741–1747.

Irizarry, M. C., Webb, D. J., Ali, Z., et al. (2009). Predictors of placebo response in pooled lamotrigine neuropathic pain clinical trials. *Clinical Journal of Pain, 25,* 469–476.

Iwata, K., Imamura, Y., Honda, K., & Shinoda, M. (2011). Physiological mechanisms of neuropathic pain: The orofacial region. *International Review of Neurobiology, 97,* 227–250.

Jabbari, B., & Machado, D. (2011). Treatment of refractory pain with botulinum toxins—An evidence-based review. *Pain Medicine,* Nov;*12*(11), 1594–1606.

Jain, R., Jain, S., Raison, C. L., & Maletic, V. (2011). Painful diabetic neuropathy is more than pain alone: Examining the role of anxiety and depression as mediators and complicators. *Current Diabetes Reports, 11,* 275–284.

Jensen, M. P., Moore, M. R., Bockow, T. B., Ehde, D. M., & Engel, J. M. (2011). Psychosocial factors and adjustment to chronic pain in persons with physical disabilities: A systematic review. *Archives of Physical Medicine and Rehabilitation, 92*(1), 146–160.

Jeynes, L. C., & Gauci, C. A. (2008). Evidence for the use of botulinum toxin in the chronic pain setting—a review of the literature. *Pain Practice, 8,* 269–276.

Kalso, E., Edwards, J. E., Moore, R. A., & McQuay, H. J. (2004). Opioids in chronic non-cancer pain: Systematic review of efficacy and safety. *Pain, 112,* 372–380.

Karl, A., Birbaumer, N., Lutzenberger, W., Cohen, L. G., & Flor, H. (2001). Reorganization of motor and somatosensory cortex in upper extremity amputees with phantom limb pain. *Journal of Neuroscience, 21,* 3609–3618.

Katz, N., & Benoit, C. (2005). Opioids for neuropathic pain. *Current Pain & Headache Reports, 9,* 153–160.

Kehlet, H., Jensen, T. S., & Woolf, C. J. (2006). Persistent postsurgical pain: Risk factors and prevention. *Lancet, 367,* 1618–1625.

Khaliq, W., Alam, S., & Puri, N. (2007). Topical lidocaine for the treatment of postherpetic neuralgia. *Cochrane Database of Systematic Reviews,* 10:CD004846.

Khan, R. S., Ahmed, K., Blakeway, E., et al. (2011). Catastrophizing: A predictive factor for postoperative pain. *American Journal of Surgery, 201,* 122–131.

Kirsh, K. L., & Fishman, S. M. (2011). Multimodal approaches to optimize outcomes of chronic opioid therapy in the management of chronic pain. *Pain Medicine, 12*(Suppl 1), S1–S11.

Kumar, B., Kalita, J., Kumar, G., & Misra, U. K. (2009). Central poststroke pain: A review of pathophysiology and treatment. *Anesthesia & Analgesia, 108,* 1645–1657.

Lazorthes, Y., Sol, J. C., Fowo, S., Roux, F. E., & Verdie, J. C. (2007). Motor cortex stimulation for neuropathic pain. *Acta Neurochirurgica Supplement, 97,* 37–44.

Leknes, S., & Tracey, I. (2008). A common neurobiology for pain and pleasure. *Nature Reviews in the Neurosciences, 9,* 314–320.

Leknes, S., Lee, M., Berna, C., Andersson, J., & Tracey, I. (2011). Relief as a reward: Hedonic and neural responses to safety from pain. *PLoS One, 6,* e17870.

Levesque, J., Eugene, F., Joanette, Y., et al. (2003). Neural circuitry underlying voluntary suppression of sadness. *Biological Psychiatry, 53,* 502–510.

Levine, J. D., & Alessandri-Haber, N. (2007). TRP channels: Targets for the relief of pain. *Biochimica et Biophysica Acta, 1772,* 989–1003.

Lipton, R. B., Diamond, S., Reed, M., Diamond, M. L., & Stewart, W. F. (2001). Migraine diagnosis and treatment: Results from the American Migraine Study II. *Headache, 41,* 638–645.

Lipton, R. B., Dodick, D. W., Silberstein, S. D., et al. (2010). Single-pulse transcranial magnetic stimulation for acute treatment of migraine with aura: A randomised, double-blind, parallel-group, sham-controlled trial. *Lancet Neurology, 9,* 373–380.

Lipton, R. B., Scher, A. I., Kolodner, K., Liberman, J., Steiner, T. J., & Stewart, W. F. (2002). Migraine in the United States: Epidemiology and patterns of health care use. *Neurology, 58,* 885–894.

Lohman, D., Schleifer, R., & Amon, J. J. (2010). Access to pain treatment as a human right. *BioMed Central Medicine, 8,* 8.

Loprinzi, C. L., Qin, R., Shaker, R., et al. (2013). Phase III randomized, placebo (PL)-controlled, double-blind study of intravenous calcium/magnesium to prevent oxaliplatin-induced sensory neurotoxicity, N08CB: An alliance for clinical trials in oncology study. *Journal of Clinical Oncology,* ASCO Annual Meeting Proceedings 31:15 suppl (May 20 Supp), 3501.

Loprinzi, C. L., Reeves, B. N., Dakhil, S. R., et al. (2011). Natural history of paclitaxel-associated acute pain syndrome: Prospective cohort study NCCTG N08C1. *Journal of Clinical Oncology, 29,* 1472–1478.

Marcum, Z. A., Perera, S., Donohue, J. M., Boudreau, R. M., Newman, A. B., Ruby, C. M. et al. (2011). Analgesic use for knee and hip osteoarthritis in community-dwelling elders. *Pain Medicine,* Nov;*12*(11), 1628–1636.

Markman, J. D., & Philip, A. (2007). Interventional approaches to pain management. *Anesthesiology Clinics, 25,* 883–898, viii.

Mason, P. (2005). Ventromedial medulla: Pain modulation and beyond. *Journal of Comparative Neurology, 493,* 2–8.

McGee, S. J., Kaylor, B. D., Emmott, H., & Christopher, M. J. (2011). Defining chronic pain ethics. *Pain Medicine, 12,* 1376–1384.

Mease, P. J., Hanna, S., Frakes, E. P., & Altman, R. D. (2011). Pain mechanisms in osteoarthritis: Understanding the role of central pain and current approaches to its treatment. *Journal of Rheumatology, 38,* 1546–1551.

Mhalla, A., Baudic, S., Ciampi de Andrade, D., et al. (2011). Long-term maintenance of the analgesic effects of transcranial magnetic stimulation in fibromyalgia. *Pain, 152,* 1478–1485.

Miguel, R. (2000). Interventional treatment of cancer pain: The fourth step in the World Health Organization analgesic ladder? *Cancer Control, 7,* 149–156.

Moore, R. A., Straube, S., Wiffen, P. J., Derry, S., & McQuay, H. J. (2009). Pregabalin for acute and chronic pain in adults. *Cochrane Database of Systematic Reviews,* 3:CD007076.

Muralidharan, A., & Smith, M. T. (2011). Pain, analgesia and genetics. *Journal of Pharmacy & Pharmacology, 63,* 1387–1400.

Nampiaparampil, D. E. (2008). Prevalence of chronic pain after traumatic brain injury: A systematic review. *Journal of the American Medical Association, 300,* 711–719.

Naranjo, C. A., Tremblay, L. K., & Busto, U. E. (2001). The role of the brain reward system in depression. *Progress in Neuropsychopharmacology & Biological Psychiatry, 25,* 781–823.

Nickel, F. T., Seifert, F., Lanz, S., & Maihofner, C. (2011). Mechanisms of neuropathic pain. *European Neuropsychopharmacology,* Feb;*22*(2), 81–91.

Nicolson, S. E., Caplan, J. P., Williams, D. E., & Stern, T. A. (2009). Comorbid pain, depression, and anxiety: Multifaceted pathology allows for multifaceted treatment. *Harvard Review of Psychiatry, 17,* 407–420.

Ocanez, K. L., McHugh, R. K., & Otto, M. W. (2010). A meta-analytic review of the association between anxiety sensitivity and pain. *Journal of Depression & Anxiety, 27*, 760–767.

Ossipov, M. H., Dussor, G. O., & Porreca, F. (2010). Central modulation of pain. *Journal of Clinical Investigation, 120*, 3779–3787.

Pachman, D. R., Barton, D. L., Watson, J. C., & Loprinzi, C. L. (2011). Chemotherapy-induced peripheral neuropathy: Prevention and treatment. *Clinical Pharmacology & Therapeutics, 90*, 377–387.

Parks, E. L., Geha, P. Y., Baliki, M. N., Katz, J., Schnitzer, T. J., & Apkarian, A. V. (2011). Brain activity for chronic knee osteoarthritis: Dissociating evoked pain from spontaneous pain. *European Journal of Pain, 15*, 843, e841–814.

Pollo, A., & Benedetti, F. (2009). The placebo response: Neurobiological and clinical issues of neurological relevance. *Progress in Brain Research, 175*, 283–294.

Popescu, A., LeResche, L., Truelove, E. L., & Drangsholt, M. T. (2010). Gender differences in pain modulation by diffuse noxious inhibitory controls: A systematic review. *Pain, 150*, 309–318.

Price, D. D., Craggs, J. G., Zhou, Q., Verne, G. N., Perlstein, W. M., & Robinson, M. E. (2009). Widespread hyperalgesia in irritable bowel syndrome is dynamically maintained by tonic visceral impulse input and placebo/nocebo factors: Evidence from human psychophysics, animal models, and neuroimaging. *Neuroimage, 47*, 995–1001.

Przewlocki, R., & Przewlocka, B. (2001). Opioids in chronic pain. *European Journal of Pharmacology, 429*, 79–91.

Puhse, G., Wachsmuth, J. U., Kemper, S., Husstedt, I. W., Kliesch, S., & Evers, S. (2010). Phantom testis syndrome: Prevalence, phenomenology and putative mechanisms. *International Journal of Andrology, 33*, e216–e220.

Quartana, P. J., Campbell, C. M., & Edwards, R. R. (2009). Pain catastrophizing: A critical review. *Expert Review of Neurotherapeutics, 9*, 745–758.

Raouf, R., Quick, K., & Wood, J. N. (2010). Pain as a channelopathy. *Journal of Clinical Investigation, 120*, 3745–3752.

Robinson, M. J., Edwards, S. E., Iyengar, S., Bymaster, F., Clark, M., & Katon, W. (2009). Depression and pain. *Frontiers in Bioscience, 14*, 5031–5051.

Sanchez-Castanon, M., de las Heras-Castano, G., Lopez-& Hoyos, M. (2010). Autoimmune pancreatitis: An underdiagnosed autoimmune disease with clinical, imaging and serological features. *Autoimmunity Reviews, 9*, 237–240.

Schaafsma, F., Schonstein, E., Whelan, K. M., Ulvestad, E., Kenny, D. T., & Verbeek, J. H. (2010). Physical conditioning programs for improving work outcomes in workers with back pain. *Cochrane Database of Systematic Reviews, 1*:CD001822.

Schnelldorfer, T., Lewin, D. N., & Adams, D. B. (2007). Operative management of chronic pancreatitis: Long-term results in 372 patients. *Journal of the American College of Surgery, 204*, 1039–1045; discussion, 1045–1037.

Scholz, J., Mannion, R. J., Hord, D. E., et al. (2009). A novel tool for the assessment of pain: Validation in low back pain. *PLoS Medicine, 6*, e1000047.

Schwenkreis, P., Scherens, A., Ronnau, A. K., Hoffken, O., Tegenthoff, M., & Maier, C. (2010). Cortical disinhibition occurs in chronic neuropathic, but not in chronic nociceptive pain. *BioMed Central Neuroscience, 11*, 73.

Selph, S., Carson, S., Fu, R., Thakurta, S., Low, A., & McDonagh, M. (2011). Drug Class Review: Neuropathic Pain: Final Update 1 Report [Internet]. Portland (OR): Oregon Health & Science University.

Seminowicz, D. A., Labus, J. S., Bueller, J. A., et al. (2010). Regional gray matter density changes in brains of patients with irritable bowel syndrome. *Gastroenterology, 139*, 48–57 e42.

Sengupta, J. N. (2009). Visceral pain: The neurophysiological mechanism. *Handbook of Experimental Pharmacology, 194*, 31–74.

Shah, R. V., Ericksen, J. J., & Lacerte, M. (2003). Interventions in chronic pain management. 2. New frontiers: Invasive nonsurgical interventions. *Archives of Physical Medicine & Rehabilitation, 84*, S39–S44.

Sofat, N., Ejindu, V., & Kiely, P. (2011). What makes osteoarthritis painful? The evidence for local and central pain processing. *Rheumatology (Oxford)*, Dec;*50*(12), 2157–2165.

Sperber, A. D., & Drossman, D. A. (2011). Review article: The functional abdominal pain syndrome. *Alimentary Pharmacology & Therapeutics, 33*, 514–524.

Stamer, U. M., Zhang, L., & Stuber, F. (2010). Personalized therapy in pain management: Where do we stand? *Pharmacogenomics, 11*, 843–864.

Staud, R. (2009). Abnormal pain modulation in patients with spatially distributed chronic pain: Fibromyalgia. *Rheumatic Disease Clinics of North America, 35*, 263–274.

Staud, R., & Rodriguez, M. E. (2006). Mechanisms of disease: Pain in fibromyalgia syndrome. *Nature Clinical Practice Rheumatology, 2*, 90–98.

Tegeder, I., et al. (2006). GTP cyclohydrolase and tetrahydrobiopterin regulate pain sensitivity and persistence. *Nature Medicine, 12*, 1269–1277.

Upadhyay, J., Maleki, N., Potter, J., et al. (2010). Alterations in brain structure and functional connectivity in prescription opioid-dependent patients. *Brain, 133*, 2098–2114.

Vanegas, H., & Schaible, H. G. (2004). Descending control of persistent pain: Inhibitory or facilitatory? *Brain Research Reviews, 46*, 295–309.

Vardanyan, M., & Rilo, H. L. (2010). Pathogenesis of chronic pancreatitis-induced pain. *Discovery Medicine, 9*, 304–310.

Vera-Portocarrero, L. P., Xie, J. Y., Kowal, J., Ossipov, M. H., King, T., & Porreca, F. (2006). Descending facilitation from the rostral ventromedial medulla maintains visceral pain in rats with experimental pancreatitis. *Gastroenterology, 130*, 2155–2164.

Verdu, B., Decosterd, I., Buclin, T., Stiefel, F., & Berney, A. (2008). Antidepressants for the treatment of chronic pain. *Drugs, 68*, 2611–2632.

Villanueva, L. (2011). Repetitive transcranial magnetic stimulation (rTMS) as a tool for the treatment of chronic visceral pain. *European Journal of Pain, 15*, 1–2.

Vorobeychik, Y., Gordin, V., Mao, J., & Chen, L. (2011). Combination therapy for neuropathic pain: A review of current evidence. *Central Nervous System Drugs*, Dec 1;*25*(12), 1023–1034.

Webster, L. R. (2008). Pharmacogenetics in pain management: The clinical need. *Clinics in Laboratory Medicine, 28*, 569–579.

Wiffen, P. J., Collins, S., McQuay, H. J., Carroll, D., Jadad, A., & Moore, R. A. (2005). Anticonvulsant drugs for acute and chronic pain. *Cochrane Database of Systematic Reviews, 3*:CD001133.

Wiffen, P. J., McQuay, H. J., Edwards, J., & Moore, R. A. (2005). Withdrawn: Gabapentin for acute and chronic pain. *Cochrane Database of Systematic Reviews, 3*:CD005452.

Wilson, K. G., Eriksson, M. Y., D'Eon, J. L., Mikail, S. F., & Emery, P. C. (2002). Major depression and insomnia in chronic pain. *Clinical Journal of Pain, 18*, 77–83.

Wong, G. Y., & Gavva, N. R. (2009). Therapeutic potential of vanilloid receptor TRPV1 agonists and antagonists as analgesics: Recent advances and setbacks. *Brain Research Reviews, 60*, 267–277.

Woolf, C. J. (2004). Pain: Moving from symptom control toward mechanism-specific pharmacologic management. *Annals of Internal Medicine, 140*, 441–451.

Woolf, C. J. (2007). Central sensitization: Uncovering the relation between pain and plasticity. *Anesthesiology, 106*, 864–867.

Woolf, C. J. (2011). Central sensitization: Implications for the diagnosis and treatment of pain. *Pain, 152*, S2–S15.

Zheng, H., Xiao, W. H., & Bennett, G. J. (2011). Functional deficits in peripheral nerve mitochondria in rats with paclitaxel- and oxaliplatin-evoked painful peripheral neuropathy. *Experimental Neurology, 232*, 154–161.

Zhou, Q., & Verne, G. N. (2011). New insights into visceral hypersensitivity—clinical implications in IBS. *Nature Reviews Gastroenterology & Hepatology, 8*, 349–355.

Ziegler, D., Hidvegi, T., Gurieva, I., et al. (2010). Efficacy and safety of lacosamide in painful diabetic neuropathy. *Diabetes Care, 33*, 839–841.

37.

EXCESSIVE ILLNESS BEHAVIOR

James C. Hamilton, Krystal A. Hedge, and Marc D. Feldman

INTRODUCTION

This chapter concerns the clinically important problem of patients whose reports of medical illness, physical discomfort, and disability are greater than one would expect on the basis of objective measures of disease or injury. These patients generally experience poor health outcomes and poor quality of life, despite minimal evidence of actual disease or injury. In addition, these patients can cause an admixture of anger and anxiety among their medical doctors, who may doubt the authenticity of the patient's complaints, but fear that the patient has a genuine problem that they have somehow failed to uncover. When a mental health referral is made in these cases, it often comes after the patient's relationship with medical caregivers has become strained by insinuations that the patient's complaints are not legitimate. This dynamic creates a guarded attitude in the patient that puts the consulting psychiatrist or psychologist at a disadvantage right from the start.

The goal of this chapter is to help the psychiatrist or psychologist and other medical physicians to better understand the problem of excessive illness behavior, and to provide them with the tools they need to manage patients who present in this way.

A BIOPSYCHOSOCIAL VIEW OF EXCESSIVE ILLNESS BEHAVIOR

The biopsychosocial approach to modern medicine (Engel, 1977) highlights a crucial distinction between disease and injury on one hand, and illness on the other. Whereas *disease* and *injury* can be defined in fairly narrow biological terms, the concept of *illness* expands from these biological realities to include the psychological, interpersonal, social, and even economic and political dimensions of having a disease or injury. An illness comprises the thoughts, feelings, and actions that a disease or injury provokes, as well as the changes in social and occupational functioning that occur in response to a disease or injury. It is these psychosocial aspects of the illness experience, not the biomedical ones, that cause people to seek medical care. A patient with a broken bone does not visit a doctor to get the bone fixed *per se*, but rather to be relieved of psychological distress (e.g., pain) and to return to normal functioning. Fixing the bone is the way to achieve those ends.

The term "illness behavior" can be used to encompass the intra- and interpersonal reactions of a patient to a disease or injury (Mechanic, 1966; Schwartz et al., 1994). Ideally, illness behaviors serve the purpose of protecting a person with a disease or injury (e.g., "guarding" behavior), and promoting physical recovery (e.g., increased sleep and rest for patients with a cold or flu). Illnesses are communicated to others who help the patient recover (e.g., allowing them to miss school or work). In some cases, illness behavior becomes dysfunctional, no longer serving the goals of prevention or recovery (Pilowsky, 1978). Excessive illness behavior can actually impede recovery, worsen the underlying disease or injury, or cause additional iatrogenic medical problems. For example, among persons with chronic back pain, guarding against re-injury and reduced activity level, which are adaptive short-term reactions to acute injury, can impede recovery over the long term: lack of exercise will reduce muscle support of the spinal architecture, predisposing the patient to more pain problems, and it may also increase broader health risks related to obesity and hypertension (Gatchel, Peng, Peters, Fuchs, & Turk, 2007). Patients who repeatedly seek out diagnostic testing to explain poorly defined physical complaints are at risk for false-positive results and the inevitable cascade of further tests and interventions that can lead to genuine, but iatrogenic, medical problems (Kouyanou, Pither, & Wessely, 1997).

The point of this discussion of the biopsychosocial model is to raise awareness of the fact that psychosocial variables that distinguish illness from disease or injury operate in every medical patient. In some cases, the clinical picture is complicated by too little illness behavior and a neglectful social milieu. In others, illness behavior may be excessive. The convenient dichotomy between patients who are genuinely ill and those whose problems are "all in their heads" is false and unhelpful. Instead, it may be best to regard every case as a complex interplay of biological and psychosocial factors that combine to produce the patient's unique experience and expression of his or her illness. Therefore, we believe there is value in attending to the psychosocial influences on the illness experience for all patients, not just the "difficult" ones.

The primary obstacle to the effective management of cases with excessive illness behavior is the stigma that attends psychological explanations of illness experiences. If the medical culture changed to more routinely consider the full spectrum of factors that affect the illness experience, we could vastly decrease that stigma and clear the way for effective biopsychosocial case management.

DEFINING AND CHARACTERIZING EXCESSIVE ILLNESS BEHAVIOR

THE LANDSCAPE OF EXCESSIVE ILLNESS BEHAVIOR

Psychiatric training related to excessive illness behavior has traditionally been limited to discussions of disorders in the *Diagnostic and Statistical Manual of Mental Disorders* (DSM) for which excessive illness behavior is a central diagnostic criterion. These disorders include the somatoform disorders and factitious disorders. Beyond these official DSM diagnoses, there are a number of other clinical presentations in which excessive illness behavior is an important feature, and mental health consultants should be aware of them.

Somatoform Disorders

The somatoform disorders (SFD) in the DSM include six specific disorders: *Hypochondriasis, Conversion disorder, Somatization disorder, Pain disorder, Undifferentiated somatoform disorder,* and *Somatoform disorder not otherwise specified* (American Psychiatric Association, 2000). Each of these disorders is characterized by excessive illness behavior. For each disorder, the patient is presumed to believe that he or she has a medical problem and is unaware of psychosocial influences on their illness experiences or behaviors. That is to say, the illness behavior is regarded as an expression of unconscious or implicit psychological processes.

Generally speaking, this category of diagnoses has been a failure (Creed, 2006; Levenson, 2011). The disorders lack affirmative psychological signs or symptoms, and are instead fundamentally diagnoses of exclusion (i.e., excluding a physical explanation): they cannot be verified without considerable medical information (Voigt et al., 2010). These disorder categories have also been criticized as overly restrictive, excluding persons with clinically significant, persistent excessive illness behavior and attendant distress and disability (Escobar, Waitzkin, Silver, Gara, & Holman, 1998). Unlike most other DSM diagnoses that rely on self-reports, it is doubtful that patients are either able or willing to accurately describe their medical complaints as "excessive." Consequently, the somatoform disorders have been omitted from most of the major self-report-based epidemiological studies of mental illness (Simon & VonKorff, 1991; Swartz, Landerman, Blazer, & George, 1989). Smaller-scale studies have addressed these disorders individually, but few have made comparisons among them.

The DSM-5 (DSM, 5th edition) includes major revisions to this category. The most sensible of these proposals are to: (a) distinguish health anxiety issues that are the hallmark of hypochondriasis, from disease conviction issues; and (b) combine the remaining somatoform disorders into a single category (with the exception of *Conversion disorder*, which is renamed but otherwise unchanged). In addition, the new criteria include previously uncategorized cases of persistent and disabling excessive illness behavior for which an official diagnosis would be appropriate and helpful to the patient.

Factitious Disorder

Factitious disorder (FD) is characterized by conscious and intentional medical deception. Patients with FD may exaggerate, lie about, simulate, or actually induce disease or injury. They do so primarily for the purpose of enacting or occupying the sick role: to be regarded as sick by friends, family, and medical professionals; to receive medical assessment and treatment, often including hospitalization; and to receive the signs of love, concern, and nurturance that are typically afforded to the seriously ill (American Psychiatric Association Task Force on DSM-IV, 2000).

Since the inclusion of SFD and FD in the DSM-III (DSM, 3rd ed.), these two types of disorders have been segregated into completely different chapters, despite the fact that both types of disorders are fundamentally problems of excessive illness behavior. The distinction is based on the persistent belief that patients with SFD are not consciously and intentionally producing their excessive illness behavior, whereas patients with FD are believed to consciously and intentionally feign or induce illness. For reasons that are more historical than empirical, the DSM's authors chose to require affirmative evidence of intentional feigning or self-injury for the diagnosis of FD. In practice, such evidence is only available in the most audacious cases, in which patients enact medical deceptions, creating the possibility that the patient can be "caught in the act." In the absence of tangible physical evidence of medical deception, the DSM presumes that excessive illness behavior is driven by unconscious processes, and therefore should be diagnosed as an SFD. This somewhat arbitrary nuance of the DSM criteria has cast FD as a rare, severe, and intractable disorder (Feldman, Hamilton, & Deemer, 2001). In doing this, it has also de-emphasized important motivational processes that may promote excessive illness behavior, in favor of cognitive explanations.

Malingering

Malingering is similar to FD in that its primary clinical feature is conscious and intentional medical deception. The key distinction is that, in malingering, the reason for the medical deception is to secure a tangible or instrumental benefit of some sort (e.g., a financial settlement, prescription drugs, disability income). Because these motivations do not distinguish malingerers from common criminals who commit fraud to secure benefits they are not otherwise entitled to, the DSM does not classify malingering as a psychiatric disorder, though neuropsychological testing can be valuable in the detection of malingering in forensic cases (Hamilton, Feldman, & Cunnien, 2008).

Functional Somatic Syndromes (FSS)

The medical literature describes several medical syndromes—functional somatic syndromes (FSS)—that are characterized by subjective medical complaints and a moderate to high degree of personal distress, but not by any hallmark finding of disease or injury. The patient's distress may stem from the functional impairments associated with their symptoms, the uncertainty of not knowing exactly what is wrong with them, or the inability to obtain symptom relief. The FSS conditions include chronic fatigue syndrome, irritable bowel syndrome (IBS), fibromyalgia, and environmental intolerance (previously called "multiple chemical sensitivities"). These conditions have in common a clinical presentation that is predominated by subjective complaints (e.g., fatigue, gastrointestinal discomfort, pain) and a lack of reliable physical markers that distinguish them from the unaffected population.

Heated controversy surrounds these conditions, and the controversies exemplify the core issues addressed in the preceding section on the biopsychosocial model. Patient advocacy groups insist that these conditions are genuine physical diseases and vehemently oppose suggestions that psychological factors influence the sufferers' illness experiences or illness behavior. These reactions are perfectly predictable responses in the context of a society that views medical problems as more authentic, important, legitimate, and reimbursable than psychological problems. In this way, their reactions also show how far away society is from fully realizing a biopsychosocial view of health and illness.

Medically Unexplained Symptoms

The vast majority of empirical evidence about excessive illness behavior comes from studies of patients or community members whose illness behavior is excessive but may not meet the strict DSM criteria for an SFD or FD, or whose symptoms do not match one of the FSS. In addition to "medically unexplained symptoms" (MUS), these studies may refer to excessive illness behavior as "unexplained medical complaints" or "functional somatic symptoms," or they may focus on patients who are frequent clinic visitors or "high utilizers" of healthcare services. Also included in this category are studies that focus on subclinical levels of excessive illness behavior that do not meet DSM criteria for a somatoform disorder but meet various provisional or research criteria (Escobar et al., 1998; Kroenke et al., 1997). It is safe to say that the majority of our scientifically based knowledge of excessive illness behavior comes from studies falling into this category.

THE EPIDEMIOLOGY AND ETIOLOGY OF EXCESSIVE ILLNESS BEHAVIOR

PREVALENCE

Numerous studies suggest that roughly 20–30% of primary care *visits* are associated with patient complaints that are not clearly linked to an identifiable disease or injury. In some sub-specialties, this figure may be as high as 50–80% (Nimnuan, Hotopf, & Wessely, 2001). These astronomical figures come mostly from chart review studies and may be inflated by reports of benign and self-limiting complaints with no particular psychological significance (Swanson, Hamilton, & Feldman, 2010). Physician surveys, which have both advantages and disadvantages, typically set the rate much lower, at around 10% (Swanson et al., 2010). More to the point is the prevalence of patients who present with persistent or multiple unexplained medical complaints. Studies of primary care patients set the prevalence rate between 0.3% (Smith, McGorm, Weller, Burton, & Sharpe, 2009) and 20% (Escobar et al., 1998; Steinbrecher, Koerber, Frieser, & Hiller, 2011), and the rate may be higher in specialty care. Rates for FSS are usually lower, around 7–10% (Aggarwal, McBeth, Zakrzewska, Lunt, & Macfarlane, 2006). Rates for the somatoform disorders are intermediate, at approximately 15–20% for any somatoform disorder (de Waal, Arnold, Eekhof, & van Hemert, 2004); however, the majority of these cases receive a diagnosis of "undifferentiated somatoform disorder" or "somatoform disorder NOS" (Faravelli et al., 1997; Fink, Hansen, & Oxhoj, 2004). In general, healthcare contacts for unexplained medical problems appear to be clustered in patients who use a disproportionate amount of health services. In a startling study, Fink (1992) found that 56 "persistent somatizers" accounted for 3% of the annual non-psychiatric health care visits made in the entire nation of Denmark.

DEMOGRAPHICS

Given the wide landscape of excessive illness behavior, summarizing the demographics of patients with excessive illness behavior might seem like a daunting task. Actually, it is not. With only very minor exceptions, the demographic features of patients with SD, FD, FSS, and general MUS are highly similar. First, these cases are overwhelmingly female. Second, in all these settings, the prevalence is greatest among patients around 30 to 45 years of age. In studies of European populations, there is a consistent finding of high rates among the less well-educated, the unemployed, unmarried persons, and members of racial and ethnic minority groups. Similar findings are reported for American samples, but the results are less consistent.

PSYCHIATRIC COMORBIDITY AND FUNCTIONAL IMPAIRMENT

Patients with persistent excessive illness behavior lead difficult lives. There is a very high comorbidity between excessive illness behavior problems and anxiety and depression (Henningsen, Zimmermann, & Sattel, 2003; Schur et al., 2007; Steinbrecher et al., 2011). The functional status of patients with excessive illness behavior is also generally poor, with the worst functioning in those with comorbid anxiety and depression (de Waal et al., 2004; Dirkzwager & Verhaak, 2007). Interestingly, studies of specific FSS suggest that the distress and functional impairment associated with unexplained symptoms are as bad as, or worse than, what is observed in patients with comparable confirmed disease; e.g., epilepsy and psychogenic non-epileptic seizures (Krumholz & Hopp, 2006) or irritable bowel syndrome and inflammatory bowel diseases (Pace et al., 2003; Reuber & Elger, 2003).

COURSE

Findings related to the persistence of excessive illness behavior are generally consistent in showing that 20–50% of patients continue to have difficulty a year or more after baseline assessment. A study of multi-somatoform disorder found that unexplained symptoms persisted for five years in 21% of patients (Jackson & Kroenke, 2008). Lieb and colleagues (2002) found that somatoform disorder persisted in 48% of patients after one year. Persistence of non-epileptic events was reported to be 71% after four years, with a poorer prognosis for cases with accompanying non-neurological unexplained symptoms (Reuber & Elger, 2003). It appears that the persistence of excessive illness behavior, and deterioration, are likeliest among patients with more physical complaints and greater psychiatric comorbidity at baseline (olde Hartman et al., 2009).

COSTS

In addition to the personal costs to patients of excessive illness behavior, this problem places an enormous financial burden on the healthcare system (Barsky, Ettner, Horsky, & Bates, 2001; Barsky, Orav, & Bates, 2005). A recent study by Barsky and colleagues suggests that in the United States alone, the annual costs of direct medical care related to somatization may exceed $250 billion (Barsky et al., 2005).

CAUSES

Research has consistently found that excessive illness behavior is highly comorbid with anxiety and depression, particularly depression, and associated with high levels of negative affectivity and the basic personality trait of neuroticism (Watson & Pennebaker, 1989). From these findings, a group of theories has emerged that suggest that excessive illness behavior is a product of some combination of heightened autonomic arousal, hypervigilance toward bodily cues, and a tendency toward negative and exaggerated interpretation of these physical experiences (Barsky, Goodson, Lane, & Cleary, 1988; Brown, 2004; Deary, Chalder, & Sharpe, 2007; Looper & Kirmayer, 2002). More recent research suggests that the relationship between neuroticism and somatic complaints may be more due to a bias toward experiencing distress, rather than to heightened attention to bodily sensations (Marcus, Gurley, Marchi, & Bauer, 2007). This view is in harmony with the idea that excessive illness behavior is a dissociative phenomenon (Brown, Brunt, Poliakoff, & Lloyd, 2010). The majority of interventions for excessive illness behavior are based on these cognitive or information-processing models.

Emotion-regulation models view excessive illness behavior as an indirect expression of psychological distress that patients are not able to express directly (Gottlieb, 2003; Waller & Scheidt, 2006). The term "alexithymia" is used to describe a dispositional deficit in the processing of emotional experiences. Studies linking alexithymia to excessive illness behavior have produced mixed results. A review of the literature found that one aspect of alexithymia, difficulty identifying emotions, was consistently associated with symptom reporting—not necessarily unexplained symptoms (De Gucht & Heiser, 2003). However, subsequent studies suggest that alexythmia does not prospectively predict the emergence of new somatic symptoms (De Gucht, Fischler, & Heiser, 2004; Kooiman, Bolk, Rooijmans, & Trijsburg, 2004), and some studies that control for the effects of other variables, such as negative affect, anxiety, and depression, fail to show a unique relationship of alexithymia to symptom reporting (Bewley, Murphy, Mallows, & Baker, 2005; De Gucht et al., 2004). Using a language-analysis coding system to operationalize deficits in emotion processing, Lane and colleagues found evidence that low levels of emotional awareness predict the level and nature of physical symptom reporting, and that these effects are independent of negative affectivity, anxiety, and depression (Lane, Carmichael, & Reis, 2011; Subic-Wrana, Bruder, Thomas, Lane, & Kohle, 2005).

Motivational or functional explanations of excessive illness behavior suggest that illness behavior leads to psychosocial benefits that serve to perpetuate it (Hotopf, 2004). The benefits of the sick role were formally described by Parsons (1951), and referred to in psychoanalytic writing as "secondary gains" (Fishbain, Rosomoff, Cutler, & Rosomoff, 1995). They include tangible benefits such as legal settlements, worker's compensation awards, Social Security Disability income, relief from military service or unpleasant jobs, and prescriptions for medications that can be used for recreational purposes or sold for profit. The benefits of illness behavior may also include predominantly psychological ones, such as avoidance of conflict, or securing care, nurturance, and forbearance from friends and loved ones. The existence of these psychological benefits is affirmed by the DSM-IV-TR (DSM-IV Text Revision), which lists them as the defining motivation of the illness behavior observed in FD.

Relatively little modern research has been done on the specific psychological benefits of illness behavior, or the individual characteristics that predispose some people to be so strongly drawn to them. Hamilton and Janata (1997) suggested that for persons with poor self-esteem or identity problems, the sick role may be a vehicle for securing a sense of uniqueness or importance, and it appears that certain features of the sick role may have desirable self-presentational effects (Hamilton, Deemer, & Janata, 2003). More recently, a well-replicated relation between MUS and *insecure attachment* (Taylor, Marshall, Mann, & Goldberg, 2011) has led to the development of an interpersonal theory of illness behavior (Noyes, Stuart, & Watson, 2008). According to this view, persons with attachment insecurity are reinforced by the care and nurturance that the sick role elicits in others, and are drawn into patterns of excessive illness behavior. This theory is certainly consistent with the clinical evidence that links FD to borderline and narcissistic personality types (Ehlers & Plassmann, 1994).

SUMMARY

Excessive illness behavior is common in all medical settings, and exacts substantial personal costs from patients and their care providers, at a substantial cost to healthcare delivery systems. Despite a wide array of outward presentations and diagnostic labels, cases of excessive illness behavior share a core pattern of demographic features, psychiatric comorbidities, and psychosocial impairments. The psychosocial mechanisms that underlie excessive illness behavior are not well understood, and research in this area has reflected the aforementioned bias in the DSM that casts excessive illness behavior in terms of faulty information-processing rather than as functionally related to sick-role benefits or other reinforcers.

MANAGEMENT OF EXCESSIVE ILLNESS BEHAVIOR

There are two ways mental health professionals might contribute to the management of cases with excessive illness behavior. The first is by helping primary medical care providers and allied health professionals, who are usually the first to encounter these cases. The second is through direct care of patients with excessive illness behavior.

EDUCATION AND CONSULTATION

Providers who encounter a patient with excessive illness behavior may initially view the case as a challenge. When all efforts to diagnose and treat the patient's problems fail, the provider may passively dismiss the patient's concerns by providing reassurance and acquiescing to requests for assessments and treatments that the provider views as unnecessary but harmless. Alternatively, the provider may confront the patient by suggesting that his or her problems are "psychological" and suggest that the patient seek the help of a mental health professional. Still other providers may simply pass the patients along to other doctors, with whom the process will probably be repeated. None of these strategies advances the care of the patient. Medical providers should be encouraged to think about illness behavior from the biopsychosocial perspective outlined above. Specifically, they should be helped to view physical disease or injury and illness behavior as two interdependent influences on the patient's health-related quality of life, and taught the basic clinical skills necessary to assess and manage psychosocial influences on illness behavior.

Communication

It is frequently assumed that patients with excessive illness behavior insist on strictly physical interpretations of their problems. However, important research by Salmon and colleagues contradicts the belief that patients demand somatic interpretations and interventions (Salmon, Humphris, Ring, Davies, & Dowrick, 2006, 2007). Instead, it appears that patients often broach psychosocial issues during medical visits, and that focus on somatic issues is reduced when physicians are responsive to those disclosures. Ironically, it appears that physician interactions with patients with medically unexplained complaints are especially lacking in the type of patient-centered communication that facilitates discussion of psychological issues (Epstein et al., 2006). Another study showed that patients with unexplained complaints were generally willing to accept a strategy of watchful waiting, but this acceptance was dependent on good communication between physicians and patients (van Bokhoven et al., 2009). Thus, the available research suggests unnecessary somatic interventions can be avoided if primary care physicians are able to effectively communicate with their patients about psychological distress and other psychosocial issues.

Identifying and Correcting Factual Errors

So what should physicians be encouraged to talk about? Important research by Leventhal and others on illness representations suggests that patients develop ideas about their diseases and injuries that include its name, symptoms, cause, course, and treatability/controllability (Leventhal, Leventhal, & Contrada, 1998). Frequently, patients' excessive illness behavior can be attributed to providers' failure to assess the accuracy of patients' information about these dimensions and to provide accurate corrective feedback. For example, in some cases, excessive health service use can occur because patients mistakenly believe that symptom flare-ups reflect a dangerous progression of their disease, when this is not necessarily the case. Physician colleagues should be advised to ask patients about these crucial dimensions of their illness representations, correct misconceptions, provide accurate information, and help patients cope with the fact that sometimes their questions do not have clear answers. Substantive conversations like these provide the foundation for meaningful reassurance about the patient's physical health.

Discussing the Role of Psychological Factors

Among the more important issues to openly discuss with a patient is the possible role of psychosocial factors that impact the illness experience. The key to an effective discussion of psychological factors is to clearly and directly reassure the patient that acknowledging the role of psychological factors is not tantamount to declaring that the patient does not have a legitimate medical problem. The focus should be on the role that stress and distress can play in the development of disease and in shaping reactions to disease. Physicians can be advised to call upon their knowledge of the effects of stress on the hypothalamic-pituitary-adrenal (HPA) axis to explain to patients, in biological terms, how stress and physical health can be intertwined. In addition, physicians can explain to patients how pain experiences are affected both by basic interpretation of pain sensations and by emotional centers of the brain that are responsible for the experience of pain distress. In either model, a case can be made for why understanding and managing the patient's stress and distress are important in a comprehensive approach to maximizing the patient's health-related quality of life.

Maintaining Standards of Care

The care of patients with excessive illness behavior can be compromised by departures from standard clinical practice. In the early phases of care for these patients, the greatest risk is succumbing to patients' persistent complaints by over-treating them. When suspicions arise about the authenticity of the complaints, the opposite error can occur: doing less than is indicated. This pattern is most clearly apparent in cases of FD. As educators or consultants, mental health professionals can caution physicians about this pattern and urge them to make medical decisions based on medical data. Elsewhere we have likened this approach to a pilot flying in bad weather: pilots are encouraged to follow procedures and trust their instruments (Hamilton & Feldman, 2011). Physicians should be encouraged to do likewise: to do no more and no fewer tests and interventions than they would for patients with less dramatic illness behavior.

An interesting lesson from the literature on FD is that more medical errors are made *before* the possibility of FD is raised than after. This is because suspicions about excessive illness behavior and about a major influence of psychological factors in a case cause physicians to avoid departures from standard care. We believe heightened attention to psychological factors can have the same positive results in the management of all cases along the spectrum of excessive illness behavior.

Finding and Disrupting Adventitious Reinforcement

There are benefits that accompany the sick role; that is, illness behavior is often reinforced. This is true regardless of whether a patient intentionally seeks reinforcement or reinforcement occurs by accident. Unpleasant work is put off, demanding spouses and bosses temporarily relent, time is available for pleasure reading, and friends send fruit baskets. The kind attention of physicians and the palliative treatments they provide can also be reinforcing. These reinforcing consequences of illness behavior cannot be avoided entirely. However, excessive illness behavior can be reduced by paying attention to, and controlling, the contingent relationships between illness behaviors and reinforcers. For example, physicians sometimes react to patients with excessive illness behavior by putting them off, seeing them only when their complaints are urgent or alarming. This approach unintentionally reinforces the report of increasingly more urgent and alarming symptoms. Such cases might be better handled by scheduling regular appointments in order to break the contingent relationship between health crises and physician attention. This approach to managing pain-contingent care and attention is a standard part of cognitive-behavioral pain-management programs (Turk, 1999).

A Focus on Functioning

Another important theme in the care of patients with excessive illness behavior is an emphasis on the patients' social and occupational functioning over symptom reduction. Whereas patients believe that their medical problems cause or require limitations in their functioning, it is probably more often true that reduced activity and engagement exacerbate the patients' experience of their medical problems. Often patients hold beliefs that a decrease in normal daily activities is an important part of physical recuperation or preventing a worsening of their condition (Sullivan & Stanish, 2003). Physicians should take the time to explore these beliefs and provide accurate information about the relationship of activities to the medical condition, and when appropriate, to explain the physical and psychological benefits of gradually increasing their activity and engagement. The patient can be reminded that, ultimately, the problem is not their physical symptoms, but rather the effects the symptoms have on the quality of their lives. This perspective supports the usefulness of working directly on improved functioning and overall quality of life as a primary clinical goal.

Reattribution Therapy

There have been several attempts to create systematic physician-delivered interventions for excessive illness behavior. Reattribution therapy is among the better known and most systematically researched of these interventions. In reattribution therapy, physicians are taught to provide psycho-education and cognitive restructuring to their patients, with the goal of encouraging less alarming and disabling attributions for patients' physical experiences (Edwards, Stern, Clarke, Ivbijaro, & Kasney, 2010); or, in other words, to have patients "see their symptoms in a different way" (Goldberg, Gask, & O'Dowd, 1989, p. 690).

This model comprises three main stages. In the first stage, the physician aims to ensure that the patient feels understood, which is achieved through a thorough examination and history-taking, including social history. The second stage consists of "broadening the agenda beyond physical symptoms" (Edwards et al., 2010, p. 212). Goldberg, Gask, and O'Dowd (1989) suggest the physician achieve this goal by (a) summarizing the findings from the first stage; (b) empathically validating the patient's experience of symptoms and distress; and (c) suggesting other meanings or explanations of their distress and symptoms. The goal of the final stage is to address psychological factors that emerged in the first stage and normalize the relationship between psychosocial stressors and physical symptoms. This step involves drawing a direct connection between the patient's pain or physical complaints and potential psychological etiology. While Goldberg, Gask, and O'Dowd (1989) suggest a number of specific approaches to presenting this link, at the most fundamental level, each approach focuses on normalizing the connection between physical symptoms and psychosocial stressors. They describe the process as a negotiation in which the physician finds a model of the link that is acceptable to the patient, but that allows him or her to move past an exclusive focus on physical causes and somatic interventions (see also Morriss et al., 2006).

Research on reattribution therapy has generally shown that physicians find the approach acceptable, and that they report feeling better able to manage patients presenting with unexplained medical complaints (Morriss et al., 2006). Also, there is evidence that the approach does increase communication about psychosocial issues between doctors and their patients (Morriss et al., 2010) and that it improves patient knowledge and satisfaction (Morriss et al., 2007). However, Morriss et al. (2010) report that 30% of their patients did not provide any psychosocial information, despite direct prompts from physicians. Qualitative analysis indicated patients failed to disclose emotional issues for fear their physician would not consider the possible physical underpinnings of their presenting problem.

There are mixed findings regarding the efficacy of this approach for reducing symptom reports and decreasing distress and disability (Morriss et al., 2006). A study conducted in Spain, with 39 physicians seeing 152 patients with unexplained medical symptoms, demonstrated significant improvement in general physical health, vitality, social functioning, and mental health (Aiarzaguena et al., 2007). There is little evidence that the approach reduces excessive illness behavior, and several studies show no effects, or even less improvement than treatment as usual, for more severe cases of excessive illness behavior (Morriss et al., 2007; Toft et al., 2010).

Consultation Letters

Another approach to the management of patients with excessive illness behavior is a one-time consultation between the patient and a mental health professional, followed by a consultation letter to the referring physician. The consultation ideally provides definitive information about the role of psychological factors in the patient's case, assures that medical risks in such cases are statistically low, and provides guidance on the management of the case (e.g., avoiding excessive assessments and treatments: scheduling frequent, regular appointments). Hoedeman and colleagues (2010) recently published a Cochrane review of the literature on consultation letters. Few studies met the rigorous inclusion criteria; however, the available evidence suggests that this simple intervention results in reduced medical expenditures and improved physical functioning in patients with medically unexplained symptoms.

DIRECT INTERVENTIONS

For cases in which the patient accepts a mental health referral, there are several effective approaches to therapy and case management. It should be noted that many of the same problems that arise in physician-delivered interventions also apply to the direct treatment of these patients by mental health professionals, particularly the issue of effective and empathic communication.

Cognitive-Behavioral Therapy

Cognitive-behavioral therapy (CBT) is perhaps the most well-researched treatment approach for patients with excessive illness behavior (Witthöft & Hiller, 2010). This approach includes "identifying and restricting automatic, dysfunctional thoughts that may compound, perpetuate, or worsen somatic symptoms" (Huang & McCarron, 2011, p. 30). There are several published models of excessive illness behavior that provide the conceptual basis for this application of CBT, and these models are generally consistent with one another (Brown, 2004; Deary et al., 2007; Looper & Kirmayer, 2002). Addressing the effectiveness of extant treatments for excessive illness behavior problems, Kroenke (2007) described CBT as "the one treatment for which there seems to be convincing evidence" (p. 885).

Kroenke and Swindle (2000) conducted a meta-analysis of 31 studies on the effects of CBT for somatization and functional syndromes. Twenty of 28 (71%) studies revealed significant improvement in physical symptoms, but fewer studies reported improved functional status (47%) or decreased psychological distress (38%). Results indicated that treatment outcome did not differ as a function of the frequency, duration, or mode (e.g., group versus individual therapy) of the CBT approach. However, as few as five sessions were found to be effective in treating somatization and functional syndromes, and outcomes were maintained for up to 12 months in nearly all studies. In a subsequent review of randomized controlled trials, Kroenke (2007) found that CBT produced better outcomes than treatment with antidepressants, psychiatric consultation letters, brief primary care interventions, and non-CBT psychotherapy. CBT was effective in treating somatoform disorder and subclinical levels of excessive illness behavior on at least one outcome variable in 11 of 13 studies. Results were inconclusive with regard to conversion disorder, and functional somatic syndromes and chronic symptoms (e.g., back pain) were not included in this meta-analysis.

Martin, Rauh, Fichter, and Rief (2007) conducted a study on the efficacy of a single three- to four-hour session of group CBT intervention with 104 primary care patients diagnosed with an SFD. They report a decrease in the number of medical visits in the CBT group compared to a control group. Medication usage and the number of sick days taken also decreased in the CBT group. However, the CBT group did not experience a significant decrease in the number of somatoform symptoms. Overall, it appears one session of CBT can have a beneficial effect on certain aspects of excessive illness behavior, especially the number of doctor visits and symptom severity. Escobar et al. (2007) found similar results regarding the effectiveness of brief CBT (ten sessions), with 60% of primary care patients who received CBT reporting relief from medically unexplained and depressive symptoms. However, benefit from the treatment was not sustained over time.

Heijmans et al. (2011) noted that studies examining CBT-based interventions have used varying and diverse combinations of basic CBT components. The lack of consistency across studies (which is expected at this stage of development) raises questions about which components are most effective in reducing the various expressions of excessive illness behavior.

Psychodynamic Treatment Approaches

Psychodynamic psychotherapy has also been used to treat excessive illness behavior. This treatment approach targets unconscious processes, defense mechanisms, and attachment styles (Abbass, Campbell, Magee, & Tarzwell, 2009; Nickel, Ademmer, & Egle, 2010). At its core, "psychodynamically oriented theory holds that negative or dysfunctional attachment and experiences cause a high vulnerability toward stress as well as forming a basis for the therapists' intervention" (Nickel et al., 2010, p. 225). Edwards, et al. (2010) noted this approach to have small to medium effects in empirical studies.

In a study using a pre-post design with a short-term dynamic psychotherapy approach, Abbass et al. (2009) compared rates of emergency room visits for patients with a provisional diagnosis of somatization, anxiety, or pain in the absence of a known acute cause. Results indicated emergency room visits decreased by 69% following the intervention. In addition, patients who were treated with short-term psychodynamic psychotherapy also had decreased scores on the Brief Symptom Inventory (BSI), indicating a decrease in somatic symptoms.

While some research may show improvement after treatment utilizing a psychodynamic approach, the accessibility of this approach serves as a major barrier in its implementation (Edwards et al., 2010). Psychodynamic interventions require significantly more training to be implemented than other approaches, such as CBT. Time-intensive training programs are required to fully understand and competently administer this intervention, which may not be practical for primary care physicians. Thus, the applicability of this approach will be limited if patients with excessive illness behavior refuse any treatment beyond standard medical care (e.g., psychotherapy).

Medication

The use of medication, especially antidepressants, was cited by 23 of 30 published papers as an important component in the management of excessive illness behavior (Heijmans et al., 2011). The effectiveness of this approach appears to be at least partially the result of a reduction of symptoms of depression or anxiety disorders that are frequently observed in patients with excessive illness behavior. One study found comorbid mood disorders in over 80% of a sample of outpatients with unexplained chronic pain (Aguera, Failde, Cervilla, Diaz-Fernandez, & Mico, 2010), which indicates that the use of antidepressant medications may be especially helpful in the management of excessive illness behavior in the large proportion of individuals with comorbid disorders. In a review of treatments for medically unexplained symptoms, Edwards et al. (2010) noted antidepressants might also reduce pain severity. A meta-analysis indicated improvement through the use of antidepressant medications in 69% of patients with unexplained symptoms or symptom syndromes on at least one outcome measure (O'Malley et al., 1999). Han et al. (2008) conducted a study in which they compared the effects of fluoxetine and sertraline on 32 outpatients with undifferentiated somatoform disorder. The study design included a randomized, 12-week trial of the medication. A decrease in subjective ratings on the Patient Health Questionnaire (PHQ), indicating an improvement in somatic symptoms, was reported. In addition, patients reported improvement in depressive symptoms as measured on the Beck Depression Inventory (BDI). There was no statistically significant difference between the sertraline and fluoxetine groups on the outcome variables. While it may appear that the improvement in somatic symptoms was a byproduct of improvement in depression and/or anxiety symptoms, individuals with Axis I disorders that may explain somatic symptoms were excluded from the study. In general, medication used to address anxiety and/or depression appears to be effective in the management of these issues.

GENERAL TREATMENT GUIDELINES

In response to the disorganized nature of the literature on treatments for excessive illness behavior, Heijmans et al. (2011) performed a qualitative analysis of articles that contained clinical guidance on the treatment and management of these cases. Their review revealed four common themes: (a) creating a "safe therapeutic environment" (p. 3); (b) implementing generic interventions; (c) implementing specific interventions; and (d) taking a multicomponent approach. The authors suggest that empathy, demonstrating a willingness to help the patient, and clear, direct communication provide the basis of a safe doctor–patient relationship. Generic treatment interventions include motivational interviewing techniques, explanation of symptoms, reassurance, and regularly scheduled appointments. Specific interventions included cognitive approaches, pharmacotherapy (especially antidepressants), activating therapy (e.g., exercise, creative writing), and complementary and alternative medicine. Finally, effective treatment appears to require the strategic use of several of these treatment approaches. It is important to note that these recommendations derived from themes that emerged from the literature that was reviewed, but they have not been subjected to empirical tests. However, similar ideas emerged in a previous edition of this book (see Box 37.1).

A collaborative care model was also noted to be an effective approach in the management of excessive illness behavior (Edwards et al., 2010). This approach was typically described as collaboration among a number of healthcare professionals from a variety of fields (e.g., primary care physician, social worker, mental health practitioner). These teams work closely with patients, and often their families, to "define problems and jointly develop treatment goals and actions" (Edwards et al., 2010, p. 215). It is recommended that these collaborative efforts take place in a medical healthcare setting to maximize the patients' response to mental health involvement, as many patients may reject freestanding mental health treatment. This approach, which is widely used and highly effective in the management of chronic pain, may be particularly useful in the management of excessive illness behavior, as there is a high prevalence of comorbid mood disorders among these patients (Aguera et al., 2010).

PREVENTION AND EARLY INTERVENTION

In more severe or chronic cases of excessive illness behavior, the patient may become so entrenched in the sick role that it is difficult for him or her to relinquish it. Such patients may have encountered doubts and questions about the legitimacy of their health problems, or been told that their illnesses are "all in your head." Patients in this situation may be highly resistant to any psychological interpretation of, or interventions for, their suffering. The literature that we have reviewed on treatments for excessive illness behavior collectively suggests that many patients with mild excessive illness behavior problems are amenable to treatment. However, those with more severe or chronic problems (e.g., factitious disorder) often are not. Thus, prevention, or early intervention, may be

particularly important in addressing the problems of excessive illness behavior.

In recent years, there has been increased attention paid to excessive illness behavior in children (Campo & Fritz, 2001; Eminson, 2007; Kashikar-Zuck, 2006; Schulte & Petermann, 2011). The rates of excessive illness behavior problems in pediatric settings appear to be similar to those observed in adult primary care settings (Schulte & Petermann, 2011). Although there is a paucity of studies that directly address the question of whether patterns of excessive illness behavior that emerge in childhood continue on into adulthood, several lines of thinking support this possibility (Mulvaney, Lambert, Garber, & Walker, 2006). If so, interventions for children and families in which excessive illness behavior is observed by pediatricians or educators may be a particularly important strategy for reducing the overall burden of excessive illness behavior.

SUMMARY

There are several conclusions that can safely be drawn from the literature on managing excessive illness behavior. The first is that patients prefer to be helped by their primary care physicians rather than mental health professionals, but primary care physicians do not seem to be particularly effective in managing these patients. The second is that interventions provided by trained mental health professionals appear to be effective, but patients are disinclined to avail themselves of this type of care. For both primary care interventions and mental health interventions, emphasis has been placed on effective doctor–patient communication, and on presenting patients with explanations for their illness experiences that integrate the role of psychosocial factors. However, it appears that this is precisely the point at which attempts to help patients with excessive illness behavior fail. That is, it appears that we have yet to develop an effective way of raising the issue of psychosocial influences that does not undermine patients' trust in their doctors or cause patients to fear that their medical care is being neglected. Within a culturally accepted belief system that portrays biological and psychological causes of human suffering as mutually exclusive explanations, such fears are inevitable.

Excessive illness behavior is a pervasive problem in nearly all medical settings. Left unaddressed, it erodes the quality of patients' lives, and places them at risk for iatrogenic disease or injury, which further degrades their quality of life. In a time when rising medical costs constitute a developing national crisis in the United States, we can ill afford to spend millions of dollars on unnecessary assessments and treatments for these patients.

The literature on the conceptualization and management of excessive illness behavior shows relatively close agreement on the role of faulty information-processing in the promotion and perpetuation of excessive illness behavior. Less attention has been paid to functional or motivational influences on excessive illness behavior, and, with the exception of comprehensive pain management programs, attention to these factors has been conspicuously poor in discussions of intervention. Nevertheless, CBT interventions designed primarily to reshape the way patients think about their physical symptoms appear to have meaningful effects on healthcare use and health-related quality of life for the patients who are willing to accept a mental health referral. However, patient acceptance of such referrals, and of the possible role of psychosocial factors in their experience of their illness, appears to be the pivotal problem in the management of these cases.

We believe that more careful and specific attention must be paid to the details of how psychosocial conceptualizations can be presented to patients in ways they will accept. A good place to start would be to call on the growing body of research that links psychological stress and distress to metabolic and immune functions through the activation of the HPA axis. In addition, we can call upon emerging evidence that there is considerable overlap in neural systems that respond to physical threats and those that respond to social and emotional threats. Both of these lines of research provide a compelling way of connecting psychological factors to physical experiences in ways that do not undermine the authenticity or legitimacy of the patient's illness experience. Patients will not believe a "story" about the role of psychosocial influences on their illness experiences that care providers do not themselves believe. The available evidence does not simply support the believability of the story of how psychological processes may affect physical ones, and vice versa; it supports the basic truth of the story.

Ultimately, patients' acceptance of the role of psychosocial factors in physical illness and wellness will require a more widespread acceptance of the biopsychosocial model and its practical implementation in primary care. Until attention to patients' social and psychological functioning becomes a routine part of medical evaluations, the belief will persist, both among patients and doctors, that medical complaints derive either from genuine disease or illness or from psychological causes in a mutually exclusive manner. Patients will continue to view inquiry into their psychosocial functioning as a rare event, and as a frightening sign that their complaints are not regarded by their doctors as genuine.

The integration of the biopsychosocial model into primary care can be advanced through several means. These include greater emphasis on mental health training in general medical education and more training in the process of building and maintaining effective doctor–patient relationships. The cause can also be advanced by the promotion of collaborative and integrative care models in which mental health professionals become routinely involved in patient assessment and care (Gallo et al., 2004).

CLINICAL PEARLS

- Patients with excessive illness behavior are those whose reports of medical illness, physical discomfort, and disability are greater than one would expect on the basis of objective measures of disease or injury. These patients generally experience poor health outcomes and poor quality

of life and can cause an admixture of anger and anxiety among their medical doctors.

- The concept of illness expands from these biological realities to include psychological, interpersonal, social, and even economic and political dimensions of having a disease or injury.

- The demographic features of patients with SD, FD, FSS, and general MUS are highly similar. These cases are overwhelmingly female, with the prevalence greatest among patients around 30 to 45 years of age.

- Excessive illness behavior problems and anxiety and depression are highly comorbid (Henningsen, Zimmermann, & Sattel, 2003; Schur et al., 2007; Steinbrecher et al., 2011). The functional status of these patients is generally poor, with the worst functioning in those with comorbid anxiety and depression (de Waal et al., 2004; Dirkzwager & Verhaak, 2007).

- Illness behavior leads to psychosocial benefits that serve to perpetuate it (Hotopf, 2004).

- Persons with attachment insecurity are reinforced by the care and nurturance that the sick role elicits in others and are drawn into patterns of excessive illness behavior.

GUIDELINES OF MANAGEMENT

- Communication: Patients with unexplained complaints are generally willing to accept a strategy of watchful waiting, but this acceptance depends on good communication between physicians and patients (van Bokhoven et al., 2009).

- Ask patients about crucial dimensions of their patients' illness representations, correct their misconceptions, provide accurate information, and help them cope with the fact that sometimes the questions do not have clear answers.

- Educate patients about the role that stress and distress can play in the development of disease and in shaping their reactions to disease.

- The care of patients with excessive illness behavior can be compromised by departures from standard clinical practice.

- Excessive illness behavior can be reduced by paying attention to, and controlling, the contingent relationships between illness behaviors and reinforcers.

- Emphasize the patients' social and occupational functioning over symptom reduction.

- Focus on normalizing the connection between physical symptoms and psychosocial stressors: The physician negotiates with the patient a link that is acceptable to the patient, but allows the patient to move past an exclusive focus on physical causes and somatic interventions (see Morriss et al., 2006).

- Goldberg, Gask, and O'Dowd (1989) suggest the physician (a) summarize the findings from the first stage; (b) empathically validate the patient's experience of symptoms and distress; and (c) suggest other meanings or explanations of distress and symptoms.

- A meta-analysis indicated improvement through the use of antidepressant medications in 69% of patients with unexplained symptoms or symptom syndromes on at least one outcome measure (O'Malley et al., 1999).

- Empathy demonstrates a willingness to help the patient, and clear, direct communication provides the basis of a safe doctor–patient relationship.

- Generic treatment interventions include motivational interviewing techniques, explanation of symptoms, reassurance, and regularly scheduled appointments. Specific interventions included cognitive approaches, pharmacotherapy (especially antidepressants), activating therapy (e.g., exercise, creative writing), and complementary and alternative medicine.

- Finally, effective treatment appears to require the strategic use of several of these treatment approaches.

DISCLOSURE STATEMENTS

Dr. Hamilton has no conflicts of interest that might affect the objectivity of his scholarly contributions to this chapter.

Ms. Hedge has no conflicts of interest that might affect the objectivity of his scholarly contributions to this chapter

Dr. Feldman has no conflicts of interest that might affect the objectivity of his scholarly contributions to this chapter

REFERENCES

Abbass, A., Campbell, S., Magee, K., & Tarzwell, R. (2009). Intensive short-term dynamic psychotherapy to reduce rates of emergency department return visits for patients with medically unexplained symptoms: preliminary evidence from a pre-post intervention study. *Canadian Journal of Emergency Medicine, 11*(6), 529–534.

Aggarwal, V. R., McBeth, J., Zakrzewska, J. M., Lunt, M., & Macfarlane, G. J. (2006). The epidemiology of chronic syndromes that are frequently unexplained: do they have common associated factors? *International Journal of Epidemiology, 35*(2), 468–476.

Aguera, L., Failde, I., Cervilla, J. A., Diaz-Fernandez, P., & Mico, J. A. (2010). Medically unexplained pain complaints are associated with underlying unrecognized mood disorders in primary care. *BioMed Central Family Practice, 11*, 17.

Aiarzaguena, J. M., Grandes, G., Gaminde, I., Salazar, A., Sanchez, A., & Arino, J. (2007). A randomized controlled clinical trial of a psychosocial and communication intervention carried out by GPs for patients with medically unexplained symptoms. *Psychological Medicine, 37*(2), 283–294.

American Psychiatric Association & American Psychiatric Association. Task Force on DSM-IV. (2000). *Diagnostic and statistical manual of mental disorders: DSM-IV-TR* (4th ed.). Washington, DC: American Psychiatric Association.

American Psychiatric Association (2000). *Diagnostic criteria from DSM-IV-TR.* Washington, DC: American Psychiatric Association.

Barsky, A. J., Goodson, J., Lane, R., & Cleary, P. (1988). The amplification of somatic symptoms. *Psychosomatic Medicine, 50*(5), 510–519.

Barsky, A. J., Orav, E. J., & Bates, D. W. (2005). Somatization increases medical utilization and costs independent of psychiatric and medical comorbidity. *Archives of General Psychiatry, 62*(8), 903–910.

Barsky, A., Ettner, S., Horsky, J., & Bates, D. (2001). Resource utilization of patients with hypochondriacal health anxiety and somatization. *Medical Care, 39*(7), 705–715.

Bewley, J., Murphy, P. N., Mallows, J., & Baker, G. A. (2005). Does alexithymia differentiate between patients with nonepileptic seizures, patients with epilepsy and nonpatient controls. *Epilepsy & Behavior, 7*, 1165–1173.

Brown, R. J. (2004). Psychological mechanisms of medically unexplained symptoms: An Integrative conceptual model. *Psychological Bulletin, 130*(5), 793.

Brown, R. J., Brunt, N., Poliakoff, E., & Lloyd, D. M. (2010). Illusory touch and tactile perception in somatoform dissociators. *Journal of Psychosomatic Research, 69*(3), 241–248.

Campo, J. V., & Fritz, G. (2001). A management model for pediatric somatization. [Literature review.] *Psychosomatics: Journal of Consultation Liaison Psychiatry, 42*(6), 467–476.

Creed, F. (2006). Can DSM-V facilitate productive research into the somatoform disorders? *Journal of Psychosomatic Research, 60*(4), 331–334.

De Gucht, V., & Heiser, W. (2003). Alexithymia and somatisation. A quantitative review of the literature. *Journal of Psychosomatic Research, 54*(5), 425–434.

De Gucht, V., Fischler, B., & Heiser, W. (2004). Personality and affect as determinants of medically unexplained symptoms in primary care: A follow-up study. *Journal of Psychosomatic Research, 56*(3), 279–285.

de Waal, M. W., Arnold, I. A., Eekhof, J. A., & van Hemert, A. M. (2004). Somatoform disorders in general practice: prevalence, functional impairment and comorbidity with anxiety and depressive disorders. *British Journal of Psychiatry, 184*, 470–476.

Deary, V., Chalder, T., & Sharpe, M. (2007). The cognitive behavioural model of medically unexplained symptoms: a theoretical and empirical review. *Clinical Psychology Review, 27*(7), 781–797.

Dirkzwager, A. J., & Verhaak, P. F. (2007). Patients with persistent medically unexplained symptoms in general practice: characteristics and quality of care. *BCM Family Practice, 8*, 33.

Edwards, T. M., Stern, A., Clarke, D. D., Ivbijaro, G., & Kasney, L. M. (2010). The treatment of patients with medically unexplained symptoms in primary care: A review of the literature. *Mental Health in Family Medicine, 7*, 209–221.

Ehlers, W., & Plassmann, R. (1994). Diagnosis of narcissistic self-esteem regulation in patients with factitious illness (Munchausen syndrome). *Psychotherapy & Psychosomatics, 62*(1–2), 69–77.

Eminson, D. M. (2007). Medically unexplained symptoms in children and adolescents. *Clinical Psychology Review, 27*(7), 855–871.

Engel, G. L. (1977). The need for a new medical model: a challenge for biomedicine. *Science, 196*(4286), 129–136.

Epstein, R. M., Shields, C. G., Meldrum, S. C., Fiscella, K., Carroll, J., Carney, P. A., et al. (2006). Physicians' responses to patients' medically unexplained symptoms. [Empirical study quantitative study.] *Psychosomatic Medicine, 68*(2), 269–276.

Escobar, J. I., Gara, M. A., Diaz-Martinez, A. M., Interian, A., Warman, M., Allen, L. A., et al. (2007). Effectiveness of a time-limited cognitive behavior therapy type intervention among primary care patients with medically unexplained symptoms. *Annals of Family Medicine, 5*(4), 328–335.

Escobar, J. I., Waitzkin, H., Silver, R. C., Gara, M., & Holman, A. (1998). Abridged somatization: a study in primary care. *Psychosomatic Medicine, 60*(4), 466–472.

Faravelli, C., Salvatori, S., Galassi, F., Aiazzi, L., Drei, C., & Cabras, P. (1997). Epidemiology of somatoform disorders: a community survey in Florence. *Social Psychiatry & Psychiatric Epidemiology, 32*(1), 24–29.

Feldman, M. D., Hamilton, J. C., & Deemer, H. N. (2001). Factitious disorder. In K. A. Phillips (Ed.), *Somatoform and factitious disorders.* (pp. 129–166). Washington, DC: American Psychiatric Association.

Fink, P. (1992). The use of hospitalizations by persistent somatizing patients. *Psychological Medicine, 22*(1), 173–180.

Fink, P., Hansen, M. S., & Oxhoj, M. L. (2004). The prevalence of somatoform disorders among internal medical inpatients. *Journal of Psychosomatic Research, 56*(4), 413–418.

Fishbain, D. A., Rosomoff, H. L., Cutler, R. B., & Rosomoff, R. S. (1995). Secondary gain concept: A review of the scientific evidence. [Literature review.] *The Clinical Journal of Pain, 11*(1), 6–21.

Folks, D. G., Feldman, M. D., & Ford, C. V. (2000). Somatoform disorders, factitious disorders, and malingering. In A. Stoudemire, B. S. Fogel, D. B. Greenberg (Eds.), *Psychiatric Care of the Medical Patient, 2nd ed* (pp. 459–475). New York, Oxford University Press.

Gallo, J. J., Zubritsky, C., Maxwell, J., Nazar, M., Bogner, H. R., Quijano, L. M., et al. (2004). Primary care clinicians evaluate integrated and referral models of behavioral health care for older adults: results from a multisite effectiveness trial (PRISM-e). *Annals of Family Medicine, 2*(4), 305–309.

Gatchel, R. J., Peng, Y. B., Peters, M. L., Fuchs, P. N., & Turk, D. C. (2007). The biopsychosocial approach to chronic pain: scientific advances and future directions. *Psychological Bulletin, 133*(4), 581–624.

Goldberg, D., Gask, L., & O'Dowd, T. (1989). The treatment of somatization: teaching techniques of reattribution. *Journal of Psychosomatic Research, 33*(6), 689–695.

Gottlieb, R. M. (2003). Psychosomatic medicine: the divergent legacies of Freud and Janet. *Journal of the American Psychoanalytic Association, 51*(3), 857–881.

Hamilton, J. C., & Feldman, M. D. (2011). Munchausen syndrome. *Medscape Reference.* Retrieved from http://emedicine.medscape.com/article/295127-overview.

Hamilton, J. C., & Janata, J. W. (1997). Dying to be ill: The role of self-enhancement motives in the spectrum of factitious disorders. *Journal of Social and Clinical Psychology, 16*(2), 178–199.

Hamilton, J. C., Deemer, H. N., & Janata, J. W. (2003). Feeling bad but looking good: Sick role features that lead to favorable interpersonal judgments. *Journal of Social and Clinical Psychology, 22*, 253–274.

Hamilton, J. C., Feldman, M. D., & Cunnien, A. J. (2008). Factitious disorder in medical and psychiatric practices. In R. Rogers (Ed.), *Clinical assessment of malingering and deception* (3rd ed., pp. 128–144). New York: Guilford Press.

Han, C., Pae, C. U., Lee, B. H., Ko, Y. H., Masand, P. S., Patkar, A. A., et al. (2008). Fluoxetine versus sertraline in the treatment of patients with undifferentiated somatoform disorder: a randomized, open-label, 12-week, parallel-group trial. *Progress in Neuropsychopharmacology & Biological Psychiatry, 32*(2), 437–444.

Heijmans, M., Olde Hartman, T. C., van Weel-Baumgarten, E., Dowrick, C., Lucassen, P. L., & van Weel, C. (2011). Experts' opinions on the management of medically unexplained symptoms in primary care. A qualitative analysis of narrative reviews and scientific editorials. *Family Practice, 28*(4), 444–455.

Henningsen, P., Zimmermann, T., & Sattel, H. (2003). Medically unexplained physical symptoms, anxiety, and depression: a meta-analytic review. *Psychosomatic Medicine, 65*(4), 528–533.

Hoedeman, R., Blankenstein, A. H., van der Feltz-Cornelis, C. M., Krol, B., Stewart, R., & Groothoff, J. W. (2010). Consultation letters for medically unexplained physical symptoms in primary care. *Cochrane Database of Systematic Reviews,* (12), CD006524.

Hotopf, M. (2004). Preventing somatization. *Psychological Medicine: A Journal of Research in Psychiatry and the Allied Sciences, 34*(2), 195–198.

Huang, H., & McCarron, R. M. (2011). Medically unexplained physical symptoms: Evidence-based interventions. *Current Psychiatry, 10*(7), 17–20, 30–31.

Jackson, J. L., & Kroenke, K. (2008). Prevalence, impact, and prognosis of multisomatoform disorder in primary care: a 5-year follow-up study. *Psychosomatic Medicine, 70*(4), 430–434.

Kashikar-Zuck, S. (2006). Treatment of children with unexplained chronic pain. *The Lancet, 367*(9508), 380–382.

Kooiman, C. G., Bolk, J. H., Rooijmans, H. G., & Trijsburg, R. W. (2004). Alexithymia does not predict the persistence of medically unexplained physical symptoms. *Psychosomatic Medicine, 66*(2), 224–232.

Kouyanou, K., Pither, C. E., & Wessely, S. (1997). Iatrogenic factors and chronic pain. *Psychosomatic Medicine, 59*(6), 597–604.

Kroenke, K. (2007). Efficacy of treatment for somatoform disorders: a review of randomized controlled trials. *Psychosomatic Medicine, 69*(9), 881–888.

Kroenke, K., & Swindle, R. (2000). Cognitive-behavioral therapy for somatization and symptom syndromes: a critical review of controlled clinical trials. *Psychotherapy & Psychosomatics, 69*(4), 205–215.

Kroenke, K., Spitzer, R. L., deGruy, F. V., III, Hahn, S. R., Linzer, M., Williams, J. B., et al. (1997). Multisomatoform disorder: An alternative to undifferentiated somatoform disorder for the somatizing patient in primary care. *Archives of General Psychiatry, 54*, 352–358.

Krumholz, A., & Hopp, J. (2006). Psychogenic (nonepileptic) seizures. *Seminars in Neurology, 26*(3), 341–350.

Lane, R. D., Carmichael, C., & Reis, H. T. (2011). Differentiation in the momentary rating of somatic symptoms covaries with trait emotional awareness in patients at risk for sudden cardiac death. *Psychosomatic Medicine, 73*(2), 185–192.

Levenson, J. L. (2011). The somatoform disorders: Six characters in search of an author. *Psychiatric Clinics of North America, 34*(3), 515–524.

Leventhal, H., Leventhal, E. A., & Contrada, R. J. (1998). Self-regulation, health, and behavior: A perceptual-cognitive approach. *Psychology & Health, 13*(4), 717–733.

Lieb, R., Zimmermann, P., Friis, R. H., Hofler, M., Tholen, S., & Wittchen, H. U. (2002). The natural course of DSM-IV somatoform disorders and syndromes among adolescents and young adults: a prospective-longitudinal community study. *European Psychiatry, 17*(6), 321–331.

Looper, K. J., & Kirmayer, L. J. (2002). Behavioral medicine approaches to somatoform disorders. *Journal of Consulting and Clinical Psychology, 70*(3), 810–827.

Marcus, D. K., Gurley, J. R., Marchi, M. M., & Bauer, C. (2007). Cognitive and perceptual variables in hypochondriasis and health anxiety: A systematic review. [Literature review systematic review.] *Clinical Psychology Review, 27*(2), 127–139.

Martin, A., Rauh, E., Fichter, M., & Rief, W. (2007). A one-session treatment for patients suffering from medically unexplained symptoms in primary care: a randomized clinical trial. *Psychosomatics, 48*(4), 294–303.

Mechanic, D. (1966). Response factors in illness: The study of illness behavior. *Social Psychology, 1*(1), 11–20.

Morriss, R., Dowrick, C., Salmon, P., Peters, S., Dunn, G., Rogers, A., et al. (2007). Cluster randomised controlled trial of training practices in reattribution for medically unexplained symptoms. *British Journal of Psychiatry, 191*, 536–542.

Morriss, R., Dowrick, C., Salmon, P., Peters, S., Rogers, A., Dunn, G., et al. (2006). Turning theory into practice: rationale, feasibility and external validity of an exploratory randomized controlled trial of training family practitioners in reattribution to manage patients with medically unexplained symptoms (the MUST). *General Hospital Psychiatry, 28*(4), 343–351.

Morriss, R., Gask, L., Dowrick, C., Dunn, G., Peters, S., Ring, A., et al. (2010). Randomized trial of reattribution on psychosocial talk between doctors and patients with medically unexplained symptoms. *Psychological Medicine, 40*(2), 325–333.

Mulvaney, S., Lambert, E. W., Garber, J., & Walker, L. S. (2006). Trajectories of symptoms and impairment for pediatric patients with functional abdominal pain: a 5-year longitudinal study. *Journal of the American Academy of Child & Adolescent Psychiatry, 45*(6), 737–744.

Nickel, R., Ademmer, K., & Egle, U. T. (2010). Manualized psychodynamic-interactional group therapy for the treatment of somatoform pain disorders. *Bulletin of the Menninger Clinic, 74*(3), 219–237.

Nimnuan, C., Hotopf, M., & Wessely, S. (2001). Medically unexplained symptoms: an epidemiological study in seven specialities. *Journal of Psychosomatic Research, 51*(1), 361–367.

Noyes, R., Jr., Stuart, S. P., & Watson, D. B. (2008). A reconceptualization of the somatoform disorders. *Psychosomatics, 49*(1), 14–22.

O'Malley, P. G., Jackson, J. L., Santoro, J., Tomkins, G., Balden, E., & Kroenke, K. (1999). Antidepressant therapy for unexplained symptoms and symptom syndromes. *Journal of Family Practice, 48*(12), 980–990.

olde Hartman, T. C., Borghuis, M. S., Lucassen, P. L., van de Laar, F. A., Speckens, A. E., & van Weel, C. (2009). Medically unexplained symptoms, somatisation disorder and hypochondriasis: course and prognosis. A systematic review. *Journal of Psychosomatic Research, 66*(5), 363–377.

Pace, F., Molteni, P., Bollani, S., Sarzi-Puttini, P., Stockbrugger, R., Bianchi Porro, G., et al. (2003). Inflammatory bowel disease versus irritable bowel syndrome: a hospital-based, case-control study of disease impact on quality of life. *Scandinavian Journal of Gastroenterology, 38*(10), 1031–1038.

Parsons, T. (1951). *The social system.* New York: Free Press.

Pilowsky, I. (1978). A general classification of abnormal illness behaviours. *British Journal of Medical Psychology, 51*(2), 131–137. doi:10.1111/j.20448341.1978.tb02457.x

Reuber, M., & Elger, C. (2003). Psychogenic nonepileptic seizures: Review and update. *Epilepsy & Behavior, 4*, 11.

Salmon, P., Humphris, G. M., Ring, A., Davies, J. C., & Dowrick, C. F. (2006). Why do primary care physicians propose medical care to patients with medically unexplained symptoms? A new method of sequence analysis to test theories of patient pressure. [Empirical Study Quantitative Study.] *Psychosomatic Medicine, 68*(4), 570–577.

Salmon, P., Humphris, G. M., Ring, A., Davies, J. C., & Dowrick, C. F. (2007). Primary care consultations about medically unexplained symptoms: Patient presentations and doctor responses that influence the probability of somatic intervention. [Empirical Study Quantitative Study.] *Psychosomatic Medicine, 69*(6), 571–577.

Schulte, I. E., & Petermann, F. (2011). Somatoform disorders: 30 years of debate about criteria! What about children and adolescents? [Literature review.] *Journal of Psychosomatic Research, 70*(3), 218–228.

Schur, E. A., Afari, N., Furberg, H., Olarte, M., Goldberg, J., Sullivan, P. F., et al. (2007). Feeling bad in more ways than one: comorbidity patterns of medically unexplained and psychiatric conditions. *Journal of General Internal Medicine, 22*(6), 818–821.

Schwartz, S. M., Gramling, S. E., & Mancini, T. (1994). The influence of life stress, personality, and illness history on illness behavior. *Journal of Behavior Therapy and Experimental Psychiatry, 25*(2), 135–142.

Simon, G. E., & VonKorff, M. (1991). Somatization and psychiatric disorder in the NIMH Epidemiologic Catchment Area study. *American Journal of Psychiatry, 148*(11), 1494–1500.

Smith, B. J., McGorm, K. J., Weller, D., Burton, C., & Sharpe, M. (2009). The identification in primary care of patients who have been repeatedly referred to hospital for medically unexplained symptoms: a pilot study. *Journal of Psychosomatic Research, 67*(3), 207–211.

Steinbrecher, N., Koerber, S., Frieser, D., & Hiller, W. (2011). The prevalence of medically unexplained symptoms in primary care. *Psychosomatics, 52*(3), 263–271.

Subic-Wrana, C., Bruder, S., Thomas, W., Lane, R. D., & Kohle, K. (2005). Emotional awareness deficits in inpatients of a psychosomatic ward: a comparison of two different measures of alexithymia. *Psychosomatic Medicine, 67*(3), 483–489.

Sullivan, M. J., & Stanish, W. D. (2003). Psychologically based occupational rehabilitation: the Pain-Disability Prevention Program. *Clinical Journal of Pain, 19*(2), 97–104.

Swanson, L. M., Hamilton, J. C., & Feldman, M. D. (2010). Physician-based estimates of medically unexplained symptoms: a comparison of four case definitions. *Family Practice, 27*(5), 487–493.

Swartz, M., Landerman, R., Blazer, D., & George, L. (1989). Somatization symptoms in the community: a rural/urban comparison. *Psychosomatics, 30*(1), 44–53.

Taylor, R. E., Marshall, T., Mann, A., & Goldberg, D. P. (2011). Insecure attachment and frequent attendance in primary care: a longitudinal cohort study of medically unexplained symptom presentations in ten UK general practices. *Psychological Medicine*, 1–10.

Toft, T., Rosendal, M., Ornbol, E., Olesen, F., Frostholm, L., & Fink, P. (2010). Training general practitioners in the treatment of functional somatic symptoms: effects on patient health in a cluster-randomised controlled trial (the Functional Illness in Primary Care study). *Psychotherapy & Psychosomatics, 79*(4), 227–237.

Turk, D. C. (1999). The role of psychological factors in chronic pain. *Acta Anaesthesiologica Scandinavica, 43*(9), 885–888.

van Bokhoven, M. A., Koch, H., van der Weijden, T., Grol, R. P. T. M., Kester, A. D., Rinkens, P. E. L. M., et al. (2009). Influence of watchful waiting on satisfaction and anxiety among patients seeking care for unexplained complaints. [Empirical Study Quantitative Study.] *Annals of Family Medicine, 7*(2), 112–120.

Voigt, K., Nagel, A., Meyer, B., Langs, G., Braukhaus, C., & Lowe, B. (2010). Towards positive diagnostic criteria: a systematic review of somatoform disorder diagnoses and suggestions for future classification. *Journal of Psychosomatic Research, 68*(5), 403–414.

Waller, E., & Scheidt, C. E. (2006). Somatoform disorders as disorders of affect regulation: a development perspective. *International Review of Psychiatry, 18*(1), 13–24.

Watson, D., & Pennebaker, J. (1989). Health complaints, stress, and distress: Exploring the central role of negative affectivity. *Psychological Review, 96*(2), 234–254.

Witthoft, M., & Hiller, W. (2010). Psychological approaches to origins and treatments of somatoform disorders. *Annual Review of Clinical Psychology, 6*, 257–283.

38.

TREATMENT OF ADDICTIONS AND RELATED DISORDERS

Robert Swift

INTRODUCTION

Patients with addictive disorders present a special challenge to clinicians who treat in medical settings. On average, addictive disorders, including smoking, are involved in the cases of more than one-third of patients presenting to general hospitals (Smothers & Yahr, 2005) and in similar numbers of patients in ambulatory settings. In public settings and Veterans Affairs (VA) medical centers, this figure is likely to be higher. Almost a third of all patients treated in emergency departments and about half of severely injured trauma patients screen positive for alcohol problems. The addictive disorder may be etiologically related to presenting medical or surgical problems, and it complicates the medical and surgical treatment of other illnesses.

THE NEUROBIOLOGY OF ADDICTIONS

Current thinking about addictive disorders posits that addiction is a chronic, relapsing condition with a multifactorial etiology that includes genetic, neurobiological, psychological, and environmental components (Koob & Volkow, 2010). In this regard, addictive disorders are similar to other medical illness (e.g., asthma, hyperlipidemia, and type 2 diabetes) and psychiatric illnesses (e.g., bipolar disorder, schizophrenia), for which there are complex genetic, biological, and psychosocial causes for the syndrome and for which the optimal treatment combines both biological and psychosocial treatments (McLellan, Lewis, O'Brien, & Kleber, 2000).

Drugs, alcohol, and compulsive behaviors such as gambling share common neurochemical substrates that produce acutely rewarding effects, relief of distress, and long-term neuroadaptations that can ultimately lead to addiction (Koob & Volkow, 2010). Although it is unclear precisely how these neural systems lead to dependence, it is thought that drugs of abuse and alcohol initially enhance reward mechanisms (Robinson & Berridge, 1993; Wise & Bozarth, 1987). Over time, continued use engenders a state of withdrawal, dysphoria, and distress, called *allostasis* (Koob & Le Moal, 2001) that is relieved only by continued drug and alcohol use. Individuals vary in their sensitivity to drug reward and susceptibility to allostasis; both environmental factors and genetic factors account for this variance, as well as gene by environment interactions.

Drug, alcohol, and behavioral rewards are, in part, mediated through activation of the mesolimbic dopamine pathway. The mesolimbic pathway and related limbic circuits, including the amygdala, hippocampus, and medial prefrontal cortex, are part of the motivational system that regulates responses to natural reinforcers, such as food and beverages, sex, and social interaction (Volkow et al., 2007). Activation of dopamine neurons in the ventral tegmental area of the midbrain increases dopamine release in the nucleus accumbens (also called the ventral striatum) and other areas of the limbic forebrain, such as the amygdala and prefrontal cortex. Dopamine is associated with reward and an increased salience for the stimulus. It is thought that repeated activation of this motivation-reward system sensitizes the system, resulting in increased craving in response to stimuli associated with substance use and compulsion with the development of craving (Nestler, 2001). Some drugs, like cocaine and stimulants, activate the mesolimbic pathway directly. Other drugs, like nicotine, cannabinoids, and alcohol, activate the pathway indirectly. Alcohol, morphine, and addictive behaviors like gambling also enhance endogenous opioid pathways that innervate the ventral tegmental area and the nucleus accumbens, producing a net effect of increasing dopamine release.

Most drug and alcohol dependence is associated with an unpleasant and distressing withdrawal syndrome that appears upon cessation of drug use; avoidance of withdrawal is an important factor in maintaining drug use. The withdrawal from most substances has two phases: an acute, intense withdrawal beginning within hours after the cessation of drug or alcohol use, lasting several days to a few weeks; and a chronic or protracted and more indolent withdrawal that can last from weeks to months. The duration and intensity of acute and chronic withdrawal symptoms depend on the pharmacokinetics and pharmacodynamics of the drug, the amount and duration of drug use, and individual differences in vulnerability to experiencing withdrawal. Withdrawal occurs because of adaptive changes in the nervous system in response to chronic drug or alcohol use. Typically, withdrawal symptoms are behaviorally opposite to the drug effects. Thus, sedative drugs like alcohol or benzodiazepines produce a withdrawal characterized by excitation; stimulant drugs like cocaine or amphetamines produce a withdrawal characterized by lethargy.

Chronic alcohol and drug use also activates the stress response system, resulting in abnormalities in corticotrophin releasing factor (CRF), neuropeptide Y (NPY), and other neurotransmitters involved in stress response, and inducing a neural state of chronic stress (Koob, 2008). The inability to tolerate this internal stress and/or external stressors can precipitate drug use or compulsive behaviors (Elman et al., 2012). Long after acute withdrawal symptoms have abated, abstinent drug and alcohol dependent individuals continue to experience the protracted, distressing state of allostasis, characterized by increased anxiety, dysphoria, difficulty coping with stress, and just not feeling "right." Because this allostasis can be relieved by the alcohol or drugs, it is a powerful inducer of relapse.

ADDICTION TREATMENTS ARE EFFECTIVE

A large body of research confirms that treatment for alcohol and drug addiction can be effective, both in reducing consumption of the substance and in reducing the medical, psychological, and social consequences of addiction (National Institute of Drug Abuse [NIDA], 2012). With proper diagnosis, intervention, and treatment, abstinence rates of 50–90% or significant reductions in substance use can be achieved on a long-term basis in recovery from drug and alcohol addiction. Although complete abstinence is the ideal for treatment, reduction in quantity and frequency of substance use can still result in *harm reduction*. Controlled research studies have demonstrated that treatment of addictive disorders is also cost-effective (Holder et al., 1991; Hoffmann et al., 1993; the Substance Abuse and Mental Health Service Administration [SAMHSA], 2009) in terms of reducing subsequent medical and psychiatric treatment utilization. The evidence for the effectiveness and cost effectiveness of addiction treatment has led to laws requiring parity for insurance coverage and equal access to treatment for addictive disorders.

Despite the high prevalence of psychoactive substance use among patients and its demonstrated morbidity and social costs, many clinicians are ill prepared to identify substance dependence and abuse and to treat these conditions. The sources of these deficiencies include poor training in the identification and treatment of substance use and dependence; a lack of knowledge of treatment resources; lack of confidence in treatment efficacy; and negative attitudes toward alcohol and substance abusers as patients (Geller et al., 1989; Holden, 1985; Samet et al., 1996). Effective treatment of substance abuse and dependence requires knowledge about therapies for the acute management of intoxicated patients or patients undergoing withdrawal, and knowledge about options for long-term treatment and rehabilitation. This chapter provides basic information on the etiology of addictive disorders, procedures for screening and diagnosis, and evidence-based treatment of these disorders in medical patients.

CRITERIA FOR THE DIAGNOSIS OF ADDICTION

The description of addictive disorders is complicated by ambiguity in the words used to describe psychoactive substance use. Words such as *tolerance, dependence, withdrawal, abuse,* and *addiction* are often confused. *Tolerance* is a pharmacological concept describing the need for a larger dose of a drug to achieve the same effect after repeated drug use. *Withdrawal* describes a physiological state that follows cessation or reduction in amount of the drug used. *Dependence* refers to both a condition in which a drug-specific withdrawal state follows cessation or reduction in drug dose (pharmacological dependence) and also to continued drug use despite adverse consequences. *Addiction* describes a repertoire of pathological behaviors that serve to maintain drug use (e.g., compulsive use, loss of control over drug use). The concept of "addictive disorders" is also complicated by basic questions of whether use of psychoactive substances constitutes a medical or a "moral" condition. In addressing these issues, organizations such as the World Health Organization (WHO) and the American Psychiatric Association (APA) consider problem-causing use of psychoactive substances to be a "medical disorder" with defined diagnostic criteria. This definition does not rule out the role of personal responsibility for seeking and complying with treatment, and does not legally excuse patients for crime or damages to others that are a consequence of alcohol and substance use.

The latest published edition of the *Diagnostic and Statistical Manual of Mental Disorders* (DSM-5) of the American Psychiatric Association (APA, 2013) classifies the acute and chronic effects of psychoactive substances under two major categories: *Substance use disorders* (SUD) and *Substance-induced disorders.* There is now one substance use disorder, which combines the concepts of *Substance dependence and abuse* and describes behavioral symptoms and maladaptive behaviors resulting from the acute or chronic effects of the drug. These include repeated use with negative consequences, in hazardous situations, despite interpersonal issues, for longer or in larger quantities than intended, causing neglect of other important activities, and despite known continuing adverse consequences on health; tolerance, withdrawal syndromes, cravings, unsuccessful desire and/or attempts to cut down drug use; and long periods taken to obtain drugs or recover from the effect.

Fewer than two positive criteria are indicative of no SUD diagnosis. If two to three criteria are positive, this is indicative of a substance use disorder of mild severity. Four or five positive criteria are indicative of and SUD of moderate severity. Six or more positive criteria indicate a severe substance use disorder.

Substance-induced disorders describe the direct effects of the drug on the central nervous system (CNS). These include *Substance intoxication, Substance withdrawal, Substance-induced psychotic disorder, Substance-induced mood disorder, Substance-induced anxiety, Substance-induced sleep disorder, Substance-induced persisting dementia (and amnestic) disorders,* and *Substance-induced sexual dysfunction.*

There have been changes in the classification and criteria for diagnosis of addictive disorders. In DSM 5, the criteria are under the heading "Substance Use and Addictive Disorders." The change in diagnostic classification to eliminate the "abuse" category and instead to redefine "dependence" as mild, moderate, or severe, brings the DSM-5 more into concordance with the International Classification of Diseases (ICD-10) classification of the World Health Organization (WHO). The diagnostic criteria for the disorders remain identical, except that "craving" is added as a criterion, "committing illegal acts" is deleted as a criterion, and only two of 11 criteria are required for diagnosis instead of three of 11. Compulsive gambling is included as a non-pharmacological addiction.

Eleven distinct classes of psychoactive substances had been designated by the DSM-IV: alcohol; amphetamine or related substances; caffeine; cannabis; cocaine; hallucinogens; inhalants; opioids; nicotine; phencyclidine or related substances; sedatives, hypnotics, or anxiolytics. Each class is associated with both a primarily neurophysiological (organic) mental disorder and a substance use disorder. Under the category of *Substance use disorders*, ten of these classes (all but nicotine) are associated with abuse and dependence; dependence only is defined for nicotine. *Polysubstance dependence* is defined using three or more categories of substances. A category for *Other substance use disorders* includes use of anabolic steroids, nitrate inhalants, anticholinergic agents, and other psychoactive substances.

EVALUATING SUBSTANCE USE IN PATIENTS

Although some patients present with an addictive disorder or its sequelae as a chief complaint, many patients present with other medical or surgical problems and only later reveal an addictive disorder through physical or laboratory findings, or incidental discovery. Patients as well as their family members are reluctant to report the extent of their drug and alcohol use to physicians or other healthcare providers due to denial, guilt, and shame. Patients experiencing an altered mental status due to intoxication or withdrawal may be cognitively incapable of providing an accurate history. In situations where a patient is unable to give a history of substance use, it is important to obtain additional history from family or acquaintances of the patient. Such information should be obtained with the patient's knowledge and consent, if possible, but under emergency conditions this may not be possible. It is also important to examine pill bottles or other medications in the patient's possession.

The primary task of the physician or consulting psychiatrist evaluating a patient for problem substance use or addiction is to establish an effective therapeutic relationship with the patient. In the context of this relationship, the clinician should conduct a detailed alcohol and drug history, conduct a physical and mental status examination, order and interpret necessary laboratory tests, and call or meet with family or significant others to obtain additional information and promptly involve them in evaluation and treatment. While obtaining information about the patient's alcohol and drug use, most clinicians routinely ask "quantity" and "frequency" questions about psychoactive substances, such as "how much?" and "how often?" A more effective interview method focuses on whether the patient has experienced negative consequences from use of psychoactive substances, has poor control of use, or has received criticism from others about the substance use. The description of personal, social, familial, occupational, and physical consequences of alcohol and substance use is usually more useful for diagnosis than reporting the actual amount consumed—which may be under-reported. Several practical, efficient, well-validated, formalized interviews have been developed that discriminate problem alcohol use using these criteria. Two of the most reliable and commonly used screens, with sensitivity of 90–98%, are the ten-question Alcohol Use Disorders Identification Test (AUDIT) (see Box 38.1) and the 25-item *Michigan Alcohol Screening Test* (MAST). Both of these scales identify abnormal drinking through the amount and frequency of alcohol use and its social and behavioral consequences (Selzer, 1971; Saunders et al., 1993). Shortened versions of these tests, the three-item AUDIT-C and the ten-item Brief MAST have similar efficacy. Because of its brevity and high sensitivity in identifying alcohol problems, the AUDIT-C is used by several large healthcare systems, including the Department of Veterans Affairs (VA) to screen all primary care patients. Another widely used, simple, and highly sensitive test is the CAGE questionnaire (Ewing, 1984). This four-item test uses the letters *C, A, G, E* as a mnemonic for the questions about alcohol use (Box 38.4). An affirmative answer on more than one question is considered suspicious for alcohol abuse. A discussion of several alcoholism screens and their use in specialized medical populations can be found at the following reference (National Institute Alcohol Abuse and Alcoholism [NIAAA], 2005).

Although less documentation exists regarding the optimal interview for the assessment of the drug-abusing patient, the same considerations apply: it is more effective to ask about the behavioral consequences of drug abuse from the patient, family, and significant others than to ask questions about quantity and frequency of use. Other red flags in the patient history that should increase suspicion about psychoactive substance use include divorce, problems at work (frequent job changes, chronic tardiness, absenteeism, work-related injuries), injuries (falls, auto accidents, fights), arrests, driving while intoxicated, leisure activities involving drugs or alcohol, financial problems, and the usual physical stigmata such as unusually ruddy face and nose, spider angioma, "beer gut," estrogenic effects in men, hepatomegaly, evidence of head trauma, malnutrition, cerebellar signs, cognitive deficits, Wernicke's syndrome, and testicular atrophy. Having an alcohol- or drug-abusing biological parent or spouse or a concomitant psychiatric disorder increases the risk for problem substance use significantly.

THE PHYSICAL EXAMINATION

As noted above, the physical examination of the patient provides important information about the presence of substance abuse and its medical complications. Signs of repeated trauma, especially to the head, strongly suggest substance abuse (Skinner et al., 1984). Other physical stigmata of addictive disorders include track marks of intravenous drug abuse, a necrotic nasal septum from cocaine abuse, peripheral

Box 38.1 ALCOHOL USE DISORDERS IDENTIFICATION TEST (AUDIT)

The Alcohol Use Disorders Identification Test: Interview Version

Read questions as written. Record answers carefully. Begin the AUDIT by saying "Now I am going to ask you some questions about your use of alcoholic beverages during this past year." Explain what is meant by "alcoholic beverages" by using local examples of beer, wine, vodka, etc. Code answers in terms of "standard drinks". Place the correct answer number in the box at the right.

1. How often do you have a drink containing alcohol?

   (0) Never [Skip to Qs 9-10]
   (1) Monthly or less
   (2) 2 to 4 times a month
   (3) 2 to 3 times a week
   (4) 4 or more times a week

2. How many drinks containing alcohol do you have on a typical day when you are drinking?

   (0) 1 or 2
   (1) 3 or 4
   (2) 5 or 6
   (3) 7, 8, or 9
   (4) 10 or more

3. How often do you have six or more drinks on one occasion?

   (0) Never
   (1) Less than monthly
   (2) Monthly
   (3) Weekly
   (4) Daily or almost daily

   Skip to Questions 9 and 10 if Total Score for Questions 2 and 3 = 0

4. How often during the last year have you found that you were not able to stop drinking once you had started?

   (0) Never
   (1) Less than monthly
   (2) Monthly
   (3) Weekly
   (4) Daily or almost daily

5. How often during the last year have you failed to do what was normally expected from you because of drinking?

   (0) Never
   (1) Less than monthly
   (2) Monthly
   (3) Weekly
   (4) Daily or almost daily

6. How often during the last year have you needed a first drink in the morning to get yourself going after a heavy drinking session?

   (0) Never
   (1) Less than monthly
   (2) Monthly
   (3) Weekly
   (4) Daily or almost daily

7. How often during the last year have you had a feeling of guilt or remorse after drinking?

   (0) Never
   (1) Less than monthly
   (2) Monthly
   (3) Weekly
   (4) Daily or almost daily

8. How often during the last year have you been unable to remember what happened the night before because you had been drinking?

   (0) Never
   (1) Less than monthly
   (2) Monthly
   (3) Weekly
   (4) Daily or almost daily

9. Have you or someone else been injured as a result of your drinking?

   (0)   No
   (2)   Yes, but not in the last year
   (4)   Yes, during the last year

10. Has a relative or friend or a doctor or another health worker been concerned about your drinking or suggested you cut down?

    (0)   No
    (2)   Yes, but not in the last year
    (4)   Yes, during the last year

Record total of specific items here

If total is greater than recommended cut-off, consult User's Manual.

The AUDIT can detect alcohol problems experienced in the last year. A total score of 8 or more on the AUDIT generally indicates harmful or hazardous drinking and requires further evaluation. Questions 1–8 = 0, 1, 2, 3, or 4 points. Questions 9 and 10 are scored 0, 2, or 4 only.

The AUDIT-C (Alcohol Use Disorders Identification Test—Consumption) consists of the first three questions of the audit only. The Audit-C is scored on a scale of 0 to 12 (a score of 0 reflects no alcohol use). A score of 3 or more in older adults is considered positive and suggests the need for further evaluation.

Source: From AUDIT: The Alcohol Use Disorders Identification Test. Guidelines for Use in Primary Care (2nd ed.). Geneva: World Health Organization. Available at: http://whqlibdoc.who.int/hq/2001/who_msd_msb_01.6a.pdf.

neuropathy from solvent inhalation, signs of liver disease from alcoholism and needle-acquired hepatitis B or hepatitis C, and signs and symptoms of acquired immunodeficiency syndrome (AIDS) or HIV-related illnesses (Stein, 1990). Wernicke's syndrome, also known as Wernicke's encephalopathy, consists of evidence of sixth nerve palsy, ataxia, nystagmus, language dysfunction, and confusion. Wernike's syndrome frequently coexists with Korsakoff syndrome, and is a substance-induced persisting amnestic disorder characterized by anterograde amnesia, confabulation, and other cognitive deficits.

MENTAL STATUS EXAMINATION

Each patient should receive a mental status examination to assess them for cognitive, neurological, or psychiatric impairments. Psychiatric disorders such as mood disorders, anxiety disorders, and personality disorders commonly coexist with alcohol and substance use (Grant et al., 2004; Regier et al., 1990). Cognitive mental status testing should be particularly detailed, because alcohol and drug abusers may have significant deficits in memory, concentration, and abstract reasoning, yet at the same time pass simple bedside tests of orientation, calculation, and immediate memory. The Mini-Mental Status Examination (MMSE) is useful for basic initial bedside testing (Crum et al., 1993). Formal neuropsychological testing is useful for detecting subtle deficits in attention, cognition, and performance and can better identify the type and localization of cerebral dysfunction (Berg, Franzen, & Wedding, 1987). Its expense limits its practical utility, and the expense involved must be justified by the value of the clinical information to be derived from the results.

LABORATORY SCREENING

Abnormal results on laboratory testing provide an important adjunct for confirming the diagnosis of substance abuse, but are not entirely reliable or specific. Few tests can

---

Box 38.3 EFFECTIVE INTERVENTIONS IN LONG-TERM TREATMENT OF ADDICTIONS

Psychotherapy—individual, group, and family
Pharmacotherapy
Changes in residence or living situation
Changes in work situation
Changes in friendships

Box 38.4 CLINICAL INSTITUTE WITHDRAWAL ASSESSMENT FOR ALCOHOL—REVISED (CIWA–AR)

Each of the following ten items is evaluated, scored on a 0 to 7 scale, where 0 is normal and 7 is severe, and the item scores are totaled. A total score of 10 or greater is indicative of mild withdrawal, greater than 24 is indicative of a moderate to severe withdrawal state.

1. **Nausea and vomiting.** Ask "Do you feel sick to your stomach? Have you vomited?" Observation.

2. **Tremor,** arms extended and fingers spread apart. Observation.

3. **Paroxysmal sweats.** Observation.

4. **Anxiety.** Ask "Do you feel nervous?" Observation.

5. **Agitation.** Observation.

6. **Tactile disturbances.** Ask "Have you any itching, pins-and-needles sensations, burning, numbness, or do you feel 'bugs' crawling on or under your skin?" Observation.

7. **Auditory disturbances.** Ask "Are you more aware of sounds around you? Are they harsh? Do they frighten you? Are you hearing anything that is disturbing to you? Are you hearing things you know are not there?" Observation.

8. **Visual disturbances.** Ask "Does the light appear to be too bright? Is its color different? Does it hurt your eyes? Are you seeing anything that is disturbing to you? Are you seeing things you know are not there?" Observation.

9. **Headache,** fullness in head. Ask "Does your head feel different? Does it feel like there is a band around your head?" Do not rate for dizziness or lightheadedness. Otherwise, rate severity

10. **Orientation** and clouding of sensorium.

(Sullivan et al., 1989)

---

determine how much of a substance was used and exactly when the usage occurred (Miller et al., 1990). In heavy users of alcohol, laboratory tests such as mean corpuscular volume (MCV), and liver function tests such as aspartate aminotransferase (AST) and gamma glutamyl transferase (GGT) may be abnormal in a high percentage of patients. Elevated GGT levels are as sensitive as screening questionnaires, such as the CAGE, in detecting heavy alcohol use (Litten et al., 1995; Beresford et al., 1990). However, medical illnesses, such as liver disease and nutritional deficiencies, may produce similar abnormal results. Several other biochemical tests have been proposed to "detect" or at least raise suspicion for alcohol use, including carbohydrate-deficient glycoproteins (especially transferrin), high-density lipoprotein (HDL) cholesterol, fatty acid ethyl-esters, and ethyl glucuronide (Salaspuro, 1995; Takase et al., 1985). The carbohydrate-deficient transferrin (CDT) test is based on the observation that alcohol inhibits the addition of sialic acid to glycoproteins, such as serum transferrin. Percent CDT has been found to be effective in discriminating heavy drinking (Litten et al., 1995). Ethylglucuronide, present in the urine, is formed by the condensation of glucuronic acid and ethanol. Because it persists in the body substantially longer than alcohol, it can detect even moderate drinking up to 72 hours after alcohol consumption. Fatty acid ethyl esters are condensations between fatty acids and ethanol. They are extremely long lasting and can be measured in hair samples, meconium, or other body tissues.

TOXICOLOGICAL SCREENING

Serum and urine toxicology screens have an important role in the assessment and treatment of patients with substance use disorders. Advances in testing technology have made drug testing widely available and reduced the per sample costs of testing. However, it is important that such testing be properly conducted and that the results be interpreted with great expertise. As with all laboratory tests, both false-positive and false-negative results may be obtained; and the test result may be affected by methods of sample collection and the accuracy of the laboratory (Hansen, Caudhill, & Boone, 1985). Most initial drug testing uses immunoassay methods to detect drugs or their metabolites in a body fluid, most commonly urine. Tests for five to ten different drugs are typically combined in a "panel." To minimize collection errors, samples should be obtained under direct but discreet observation. Optimally, informed consent should be obtained for all drug testing. Sometimes such screening is required by court order. Samples of both serum and urine should be obtained, as substances may be differentially distributed in body fluids. When drug testing is legally mandated, positive results must be confirmed by an alternate method, and for negative tests, validity verification testing must be conducted to identify possible tampering. For example, use of sympathomimetic agents to treat asthma may yield a positive urine test for amphetamines. A positive test suggests past use of a psychoactive substance but may not indicate the extent of the use, when it occurred, or whether there was behavioral impairment because of the use. The analysis of drugs in hair clippings can be used to detect substance use over long time periods, but this has little applicability to the immediate clinical situation. Details of laboratory testing in drug users and in psychiatric patients are discussed in several published reviews (Hawks & Chiang, 1986; Schwartz, 1988; Swift, Griffiths, & Camara, 1991).

THE TREATMENT OF ADDICTIVE DISORDERS

GENERAL CONSIDERATIONS

Addiction treatment may be defined as "medical, psychological, and social interventions to reduce or eliminate the harmful effects of psychoactive substances (drugs and alcohol) on the individual, and on others in society." Treatment usually consists of several components:

Intervention: Initiation of treatment and/or referral

Detoxification: Removal of alcohol or drug from the body and the treatment of withdrawal

Rehabilitation: Medical, psychological, and social measures to help the person avoid the use of psychoactive substances in the future

Aftercare: Processes to assist them in maintaining a sober or drug-free state.

Treatment ranges from very low-cost, less intensive methods (e.g., brief advice to stop drinking or drug use and self-help programs such as Alcoholics Anonymous), to higher cost, more intensive methods (e.g., inpatient detoxification and residential rehabilitation programs) (Holder et al., 1991). Different treatment settings may have different philosophical orientations, ranging from the medical and biological to the spiritual and religious. Intervention includes the ability to identify patients with alcohol and drug disorders, to stratify patients diagnostically, and to triage patients to the most appropriate treatment level, such as brief initial interventions, counseling, and outpatient versus hospital detoxification. The treatment plan should be practical, economical, and based on well-established scientific principles. The American Society of Addiction Medicine (ASAM) has developed guidelines that match the severity of the addiction to the intensity of the treatment (ASAM, 2001). For patients with moderate to severe addictions, the goals of treatment usually include detoxification and the establishment of a drug- or alcohol-free state. If total abstinence is not realistically obtainable, a significant reduction in harmful drug or alcohol use may be of some benefit as a start toward achieving total abstinence. For patients with problem use without addiction, the goal should be a reduction in harmful drug or alcohol use and the associated pathological behaviors. The objectives of detoxification include: (1) establishment of a drug- or alcohol-free state, (2) relief of distress and discomfort due to intoxication or withdrawal, (3) stabilization of comorbid medical conditions, and (4) preparation and education for and referral to aftercare treatment or rehabilitation (Kosten & O'Connor, 2003). The objectives for longer-term treatment or rehabilitation are depicted in Box 38.5 and include: (1) maintenance of the alcohol- or drug-free state, and (2) psychological, family, and vocational interventions to ensure compliance. Dramatic changes in living situation, work situation, or friendships may be necessary to decrease drug availability and to reduce peer pressure to use drugs. Halfway houses, therapeutic communities, and other residential treatment situations are useful in this regard. Ongoing, sometimes lifelong, individual and group psychotherapy can be useful for understanding the role of the drug in the individual's life, to stabilize the family system, to improve their self-esteem, to provide alternative methods of relieving psychosocial distress, and to reinforce the need for abstinence. Treatment of underlying psychiatric or medical illness may markedly reduce the psychiatric and physical morbidity and mortality associated with illicit drugs and abuse of alcohol (e.g., anxiety, depression, accidents, burns). Self-help groups, such as Alcoholics Anonymous (AA), Narcotics Anonymous (NA), Rational Recovery (RR), Secular Organization for Sobriety, and Al-Anon (for family members) provide treatment, education, emotional support, and hope to substance users and their families (Emrick, 1987).

Many patients presenting for treatment are part of a dysfunctional family. Sometimes the family dysfunction and substance or alcohol use are multigenerational and due to genetic and/or sociocultural factors. It is important for the clinician to be aware of dysfunctional family dynamics and any substance abuse, denial, defensiveness, and hostility present in family members. Family members need education, emotional and social support, and empathic confrontation of their possible role in maintaining denial and rescuing and facilitating the problem drinker or addict, a behavior pattern referred to as "co-dependency." Organizations such as Al-Anon and Alateen also may provide meaningful education and support for spouses and family members. It is important to involve the family in the patient's treatment as much as possible, and to recommend treatment for other family members, when appropriate.

Currently, the mainstay of addiction treatment in the United States has been psychosocial treatment. In spite of the evidence for a biological etiology of addictive disorders, clinicians and patients have been slow to adopt biologically based treatments. Some of the reasons for the reluctance to use evidence-based pharmacotherapies as adjunctive treatments include clinicians' lack of knowledge about the neurobiology of addiction, lack of knowledge about the effectiveness of medications, the increased cost of adding medications to treatment, and a paucity of prescribers (Thomas et al., 2003). Moreover, some clinicians and patients are uncomfortable in treating a drug problem with another drug. However, the evidence for the effectiveness of adjunctive pharmacotherapy in addiction treatment, along with the increased number of agents available, is gradually increasing the use of adjunctive medications by clinicians and their patients.

ALCOHOL

Alcohol dependence (AD) afflicts more than 12% of the U.S. population over the course of their lifetime, and causes serious morbidity and mortality, increased healthcare costs, and lost productivity (Hasin et al., 2007). *Alcoholism* is defined as a "repetitive, but inconsistent and sometimes unpredictable loss of control of drinking which produces symptoms of serious dysfunction or disability" (Clark, 1981). Alcohol-related problems were found in approximately 40% of U.S. general hospital admissions; and of those positive for alcohol problems, only 24% were referred to treatment (Smothers et al., 2004). In an American Medical Association (AMA)–sponsored poll of physicians, 71% felt they were either not competent enough or were too ambivalent to treat alcoholic patients correctly (Kennedy, 1985).

In the past decade, several methods have been developed to help general medical physicians and surgeons successfully identify and intervene with alcoholic patients (Samet et al., 1996). "The Physician's Guide to Helping Patients with Alcohol Problems," published by the National Institute on Alcohol Abuse and Alcoholism (NIAAA), presents several useful brief intervention methods (NIAAA, 1995). NIAAA defines "at risk" drinking (that is, at risk for adverse consequences) as more than 14 drinks per week or four drinks per occasion for men, and more than seven drinks per week or three drinks per occasion for women.

Brief interventions can consist of one or more sessions in the physician's office, during which education about substance use and dependence is provided and a plan for cutting down or eliminating substance use is negotiated. The patient and physician together should develop a contract, preferably written, defining the treatment and intervention plan. A formal means of assessment of effectiveness and follow-up should be part of the plan. Motivational interviewing, a technique that identifies and motivates patients to utilize their own treatment resources, is effective in engaging patients in treatment and reducing use of addictive substances (Miller & Rollnick, 1991; Miller, Benefield, & Tonigan, 1993). Meta-analyses of multiple studies of brief interventions in primary care settings found modest, but significant reductions in drinking (Bertholet et al., 2005; Moyer et al., 2002).

TREATMENT OF ALCOHOL INTOXICATION AND WITHDRAWAL

The treatment of alcohol intoxication consists of supporting vital physiological functions, maintaining metabolic homeostasis, and preventing behavioral problems. Patients using alcohol should *always* be medicated with thiamine and other B-vitamin supplements before being fed or receiving glucose to prevent the development of "Wernicke-Korsakoff syndrome," to use the classic terminology for the disorder. This frequently underdiagnosed condition is characterized by ocular disturbances (nystagmus and sixth nerve ophthalmoplegia), ataxia, and mental status changes, although many patients will not have the full triad of signs at any one time. The etiology is thiamine deficiency. Its presence should be considered a medical emergency, as delay in treatment diminishes chances of its reversibility. Because alcoholics may not absorb oral thiamine from the gastrointestinal (GI) tract, patients should receive high oral thiamine doses of 300–500 mg daily or receive 50–100 mg intramuscular thiamine daily for three days to ensure proper dosing (Thomson, 2000). In patients with florid neurological symptoms or signs, saving minutes may be critical, and thiamine should be administered intravenously at 100 mg three times per day. Magnesium and other electrolyte levels should be obtained and deficits corrected. Low magnesium and abnormal electrolytes may intensify withdrawal and predispose to seizures (Mennecier et al., 2008).

Physical dependence on alcohol and the alcohol withdrawal syndrome are due to compensatory central nervous system (CNS) changes in response to a chronically administered depressant substance (ethanol). The withdrawal syndrome results from increased rebound neuronal activity in the central and peripheral nervous systems following the cessation of chronic alcohol intake. The acute actions of alcohol include facilitation of inhibitory GABAergic neurotransmission and inhibition of excitatory glutamate neurotransmission.(Hunt, 1983) With repeated and chronic alcohol administration, the brain adapts to downregulate the inhibitory gamma aminobutyric acid (GABA) receptors and upregulate the excitatory glutamate receptors, producing an excitatory state that balances the sedative effects of alcohol (Tsai, et al., 1995). When the alcohol-dependent person stops drinking abruptly, the sedative alcohol is no longer present and the person experiences a state of generalized CNS excitation, typically anxiety, tremors, insomnia, and in severe cases, seizures and hallucinations (*delirium tremens*, or DTs) (Swift, 1999). It has been suggested that withdrawal symptoms intensify and become more protracted as withdrawal episodes grow in number, a phenomenon called "kindling" (Heilig et al., 2010). Although most individuals experience mild anxiety, tremulousness, and insomnia, approximately 5–10% of alcohol-dependent individuals undergoing detoxification will develop complicated withdrawal characterized by alcohol withdrawal DTs or withdrawal seizures (Mennecier et al., 2008). Predictors of withdrawal delirium include structural brain lesions, hypokalemia, and thrombocytopenia; predictors of a withdrawal seizure are a previous seizure or structural brain lesion (Eyer et al., 2011). Alcohol-dependent patients are also at risk for other serious medical complications, including pneumonia and other infections, myocardial infarction, cardiac arrhythmias, electrolyte disturbances, and serious physiological derangements, including hypertension, tachycardia, tremors, agitation, and insomnia (McIntosh, 1982). The basic physiological mechanisms of delirium are discussed in Chapter 41.

The clinician should be aware that signs and symptoms of withdrawal can obscure an underlying illness. For example, fever and change in mental status associated with withdrawal may coexist with pneumonia, head injury, or an infection of the CNS, and require neuroimaging and/or lumbar puncture for diagnosis. Treatment of the alcohol withdrawal syndrome includes correction of physiological abnormalities, hydration, nutritional support, and pharmacological therapy for the increased activity of the nervous system (Sellers & Kalant, 1976). The American Society of Addiction Medicine has developed formal guidelines for management of alcohol withdrawal (Mayo-Smith, 1997; Mee-Lee, 2001).

PHARMACOLOGICAL TREATMENT OF ALCOHOL WITHDRAWAL

It has long been known that re-administration of CNS-depressant substances markedly attenuates the signs and symptoms of withdrawal and greatly decreases medical morbidity and mortality. Historically, many pharmacological agents have been used to reduce the signs and symptoms of the withdrawal syndrome, including: chloral derivatives (e.g., chloral hydrate), paraldehyde, barbiturates, antihistamines, neuroleptics, antidepressants, beta-adrenergic blocking agents, and benzodiazepines (Golbert et al., 1967; Palestine & Alatorre, 1976; Sellers et al., 1980). Indeed, almost any CNS-depressant substance may be effective (Liskow & Goodwin, 1987; Litten & Allen, 1991).

Benzodiazepines

Benzodiazepine derivatives are the treatment of choice for alcohol withdrawal (Table 38.1), and their efficacy is well established by double-blind controlled studies (Ozdemir et al., 1994). Benzodiazepines bind to a distinct binding site on the GABA receptor-chloride ion channel complex and facilitate the inhibitory action of GABA on neurons (Johnston, 1996). Benzodiazepines are superior to other agents because of their low toxicity and anticonvulsant effects. Benzodiazepine use is optimal when the dose is titrated according to a withdrawal severity scale such as the Clinical Institute Withdrawal Assessment of Alcohol revised (CIWA-Ar) Scale (Sullivan et al., 1989; Saitz et al., 1994), reproduced in Box 38.4. Several methods have been described for titrating medication dosage to symptoms. The "symptom-triggered method" appears to have utility in many patients (Sellers et al., 1983). Its advantages include the avoidance of both under-medication and over-medication. Long half-life benzodiazepines (e.g., 10 mg diazepam intravenous [IV] or orally [PO], or 50–100 mg chlordiazepoxide PO) or short half-life benzodiazepines (e.g., lorazepam 1.0 mg PO, IV, or intramuscular [IM], or oxazepam 30 mg PO), are dosed every hour until the patient is sedated, develops nystagmus, or has a significant decrease in withdrawal signs and symptoms as shown by a withdrawal scale score, such as a CIWA-Ar score of less than 8. Those treated with long half-life medication may require no additional medication for their detoxification. Those receiving shorter half-life benzodiazepines will require continued dosing for three to five days. Withdrawal signs and symptoms of most patients treated with effective doses of sedatives are reduced within several hours. Occasionally, patients do require additional doses of medication after several days, to suppress re-emergent symptoms. During the period of benzodiazepine treatment, patients must be closely observed to avoid under-medication or over-medication. Patients with respiratory disease, cardiovascular disease, or hepatic disease must be monitored closely, and short half-life benzodiazepines that are glucuronidated (lorazepam or oxazepam) are preferred (D'Onofrio et al., 1999).

Two other medications used to treat alcohol withdrawal include barbiturates and clomethiazole. Barbiturates, like benzodiazepines, potentiate the action of GABA at the GABA-receptor chloride channel complex. However, barbiturates differ from benzodiazepines in binding to a different site and more strongly potentiating the effects of GABA. This

Table 38.1 PHARMACOLOGICAL THERAPIES FOR ALCOHOL WITHDRAWAL AND PREVENTION OF RELAPSE

TREATMENT PHASE AND DRUG CLASS	EXAMPLES	EFFECTS
ALCOHOL WITHDRAWAL:		
Benzodiazepines	Chlordiazepoxide*	Decreased severity of withdrawal; stabilization of vital signs: prevention of seizures and delirium tremens (alcohol withdrawal delirium)
	Diazepam*	
	Oxazepam*	
	Lorazepam and others†	
Beta-blockers	Atenolol	Improvement in vital signs; reduction in craving
	Propranolol	Propranolol has more CNS penetration due to lipophilicity
Alpha-agonists	Clonidine	Decreased withdrawal symptoms
Anti-epileptics	Carbamazepine	Decreased severity of withdrawal; prevention of seizures (may cause ataxia, hyponatremia, or elevate liver function tests [LFTs]).
PREVENTION OF RELAPSE:		
Alcohol sensitizers	Disulfiram*	Decreased alcohol use among those who relapse
		Associated with severe toxicity when alcohol ingested
Opioid antagonists	Naltrexone*	Increased abstinence, decreased no. of drinking days
Homotaurine derivatives	Acamprosate*	Increased abstinence
Anti-epileptics	Topiramate	Decreased drinking

*The drug has a Food and Drug Administration–approved indication for this use in the United States.

Adapted from O'Connor, P. G., & Shottenfeld, R. S. (1998). Patients with alcohol problems. *New England Journal of Medicine, 338*(9), 597.

increased potency of barbiturates increases their sedation and narrows the therapeutic window between effectiveness in suppressing alcohol withdrawal symptoms and toxicity. Nevertheless, long half-life barbiturates like phenobarbital are sometimes used to treat alcohol withdrawal and are preferred by some clinicians to treat more complicated, severe withdrawal (Mayo-Smith et al., 2004). Clomethiazole is a sedative and anticonvulsant medication used in Europe for the treatment of alcohol withdrawal. Clomethiazole potentiates GABA by acting as a positive allosteric modulator at the barbiturate-binding site at the GABA-receptor chloride channel complex.

Other Agents Used for Alcohol Withdrawal

Several other non-benzodiazepine GABA-ergic compounds have been used off-label and in research studies to treat alcohol withdrawal and have been found to be effective. These include: baclofen, a GABA-B receptor agonist; and the anti-epileptic medications carbamazepine, gabapentin, pregabalin, tiagabine, topiramate, and valproic acid (Leggio et al., 2008). Beta-adrenergic blocking drugs such as propranolol and atenolol have been exclusively used as primary agents in the treatment of alcohol withdrawal (Sellers & Kalant, 1976). However, beta-blockers are most effective in reduction of peripheral autonomic signs of withdrawal, and less so for central nervous system signs such as withdrawal delirium or seizures. Beta-blockers are particularly useful for controlling tachycardia and hypertension for patients with coronary artery disease. These agents should be considered as adjuncts in withdrawal regimens and usually are not needed if benzodiazepines are used in adequate doses.

Since most medications used to treat alcohol withdrawal are anti-epileptic, single seizures may be managed with an increase in medication and do not require another anti-epileptic medication. For patients with multiple seizures during withdrawal, or with a chronic seizure disorder, the addition of an anti-epileptic medication such as phenytoin may be indicated. Given that many alcoholics are noncompliant with treatment, the erratic use of anti-epileptics on an outpatient basis may actually worsen a seizure problem (Hillbom & Hjelm-Jager, 1984). Neuroleptics, such as risperidone or quetiapine, are specifically indicated for the treatment of hallucinosis and paranoid symptoms, but are not primary agents for withdrawal.

NONPHARMACOLOGICAL TREATMENT METHODS

Recently, the widespread use of pharmacological agents in the detoxification from alcohol has been called into question.

Some alcohol-treatment facilities provide "social setting detoxification," a non-drug method. This procedure relies on the extensive use of peer and group support and usually occurs in non-medical settings. This method seems effective in reducing withdrawal signs and symptoms, without an increased incidence of medical complications. Yet Shaw et al. (1981) claimed that even within a medical setting, most patients respond to "supportive care" and do not require pharmacological intervention. In a double-blind study comparing parenteral diazepam treatment with placebo, over half the patients receiving a placebo injection responded with a marked attenuation of withdrawal symptoms within five hours (Sellers et al., 1983).

In summary, although some alcohol-dependent individuals may be detoxified without the use of sedatives or other psychotropic drugs, medication-assisted detoxification smooths the withdrawal symptoms, causes less distress to patients, decreases the chances of seizures and hallucinations, and is a more humane approach.

OUTPATIENT VERSUS INPATIENT ALCOHOL DETOXIFICATION

Successful alcohol detoxification can be performed in day-treatment and outpatient settings at lower cost and with less disruption to the patient and family than hospital-based treatment (Abbott et al., 1995). Patients should be observed on a daily basis, and medications for withdrawal prescribed in small amounts, according to the severity of withdrawal signs and symptoms. Whitfield et al. (1978) reported large numbers of patients who were successfully detoxified from alcohol in an outpatient setting without the use of psychotropic drugs, although high-risk patients were excluded from this study.

Although few data exist for clinicians to predict which alcohol-dependent patients are candidates for outpatient detoxification, those with a stable living situation, history of mild withdrawal, and lack of medical and psychiatric problems are likely to be the best candidates. A history of DTs or seizures, the presence of medical disorders (such as diabetes, trauma, or pain), or surgical or psychiatric disorders increases the need for closer medical supervision and indicates that detoxification should be performed in an inpatient setting.

During and after detoxification, many alcoholic patients will appear to suffer from major depression and anxiety disorders. Some of these mood disorders are directly related to alcohol and will gradually resolve within two to four weeks after detoxification. Major depressive symptoms persisting beyond this time should be considered for treatment with antidepressants or electroconvulsive therapy (ECT). Patients previously known to have recurrent mood disorders should be treated immediately after detoxification if mood symptoms are severe. Non-dependence-producing anxiolytics such as buspirone or selective serotonin-reuptake inhibitor (SSRI) antidepressants may be excellent anxiolytics for patients with persistent anxiety disorders.

REHABILITATION AND AFTERCARE

The goals of rehabilitation and aftercare include maintaining a state of abstinence from alcohol and establishing psychological, family, and social interventions that serve to maintain this recovery. These goals may be best achieved through the patient's participation in a comprehensive treatment program, beginning after discharge from the acute-care setting. Nevertheless, there are aspects of the long-term treatment that should be initiated during an acute hospital stay.

There are several effective, evidence-based behavioral treatments for alcohol dependence. These include motivational interviewing (MI), cognitive-behavioral therapy (CBT), Twelve Step (AA) facilitation, supportive counseling, marital/family therapy, community reinforcement, and case-management (Miller et al., 2003). Patients with a history of recurrent relapses or who are homeless may benefit from residential treatment in a sober setting. Self-help organizations such as Alcoholics Anonymous (AA) or Rational Recovery (RR) are independent groups composed of alcoholics at various stages of recovery that help individuals maintain total abstinence from alcohol and other addictive substances through group and individual interactions. Self-help programs benefit many patients, but there is a paucity of objective outcome data on the actual long-term efficacy of such groups (Emrick, 1974, 1987). Most detoxification and rehabilitation programs encourage liberal attendance at self-help meetings. General hospitals often are used as meeting sites by local AA groups, and medical and surgical inpatients may easily attend these meetings.

MEDICATIONS TO REDUCE ALCOHOL CONSUMPTION

Four medications are currently approved for the treatment of alcohol dependence in the United States: disulfiram, oral naltrexone, extended-release (injectable) naltrexone, and acamprosate. Several other medications, including topiramate, are used off-label, or are only approved abroad. Federal agencies, including the National Institute on Alcohol Abuse and Alcoholism (NIAAA) and the Center for Substance Abuse Treatment (CSAT), recommend consideration of the approved pharmacotherapies in the treatment of all patients (NIAAA, 2007; CSAT, 2009). Unfortunately, there have been few comparative effectiveness studies of the several approved medications to match patients with the optimal medication.

DISULFIRAM

Disulfiram (e.g., Antabuse) is an inhibitor of the enzyme acetaldehyde dehydrogenase, and is used as an adjunctive treatment in selected alcoholics. If alcohol is consumed in the presence of disulfiram, the toxic metabolite acetaldehyde accumulates, producing tachycardia, flushing of skin, dyspnea, nausea, and vomiting. This unpleasant reaction provides a powerful deterrent to the consumption of alcohol (Chick et al., 1992, Brewer, 1993). Disulfiram is most effective when its administration is supervised by medical personnel or by a partner or significant other (Krampe & Ehrenreich, 2010). Patients started on disulfiram must be informed about the dangers of even small amounts of alcohol. Alcohol present in foods, cosmetics, mouthwashes, and over-the-counter medications may produce a disulfiram reaction. A usual dose of disulfiram is 250–500 mg, once daily. Disulfiram may interact with other medications, notably anticoagulants and phenytoin. It is contraindicated for patients with liver disease and psychosis.

ORAL NALTREXONE

Controlled clinical trials with the opioid-antagonist naltrexone show effects on reducing alcohol consumption in alcohol-dependent patients. Two different systemic reviews of literature and meta-analyses of published randomized, controlled clinical trials assessing oral naltrexone in alcohol dependence, found that naltrexone reduced the relapse rate to heavy drinking significantly, but with a small effect size. There was a non-significant trend in reduction of the abstinence rate (Bouza et al., 2004; Srisurapanont & Jarusuraisin, 2005). The large American multisite COMBINE Study, involving 1,380 alcohol-dependent patients, found naltrexone, compared to placebo, to produce small but significant reductions in relapses to heavy drinking in patients receiving a medically oriented behavioral intervention (Anton et al., 2006).

Naltrexone is believed to reduce alcohol consumption by reducing the pleasurable and positive reinforcing properties of alcohol. Both social drinkers and alcoholics receiving naltrexone and alcohol report less positive reinforcement and more intensely sedative effects of alcohol. Naltrexone also reduces craving for alcohol in response to alcohol cues. Predictors of a positive response to naltrexone include a high level of craving, a positive family history of alcoholism (Rubio et al., 2005), and possessing a specific genetic polymorphism (Asn40Asp) in the μ opioid receptor gene (Oslin et al., 2003).

The usual oral naltrexone dose is 50 mg per day, although doses of 25–100 mg per day have been reported to be effective. Naltrexone should be used only in the context of a comprehensive alcoholism-treatment program, which includes counseling and other psychosocial therapies (O'Malley, 1992). The most common side effects include anxiety, sedation, and nausea, in approximately 10% of patients. High doses of naltrexone (300 mg per day) have been associated with hepatotoxicity; however, hepatic toxicity is rarely observed at a 50 mg per day dose of naltrexone. It is recommended that liver function be monitored prior to naltrexone treatment and periodically thereafter. Patients with hepatitis or severe liver disease should receive naltrexone only with close monitoring.

Nalmefene is a μ-opioid antagonist that is similar to naltrexone. It currently is approved for the reversal of acute opioid intoxication and overdose in the United States, but is approved for the treatment of alcoholism in Europe. Studies in alcohol-dependent patients using a targeted approach of taking nalmefene during periods of high risk for drinking find decreased drinking and increased abstinence in those receiving the medication (Soyka & Rosner, 2010).

EXTENDED-RELEASE NALTREXONE

Because the effectiveness of naltrexone depends upon medication adherence, a sustained release, once-monthly injectable formulation of naltrexone was developed. A sustained-released naltrexone preparation, marketed as Vivitrol', was Food and Drug Administration (FDA) approved for the treatment of alcohol dependence in 2004. A six-month, multicenter, randomized, controlled trial of placebo and two doses of sustained-release naltrexone in 627 actively drinking alcohol-dependent adults showed a significant dose-dependent decrease in the rate of heavy drinking (26% at the highest dose) compared with placebo (Garbutt et al., 2005). The most common adverse events associated with extended-release naltrexone are injection site tenderness, nausea (which affected 33%), headache, and fatigue. Occasionally abscesses occur at the injection site and have engendered an FDA warning letter. In addition to improved adherence, sustained-release naltrexone may produce less hepatotoxicity than oral naltrexone, as the injected, sustained-release drug does not undergo first-pass metabolism in the liver.

ACAMPROSATE

Acamprosate (calcium acetylhomotaurine) is a structural analogue of taurine, a brain amino acid with unknown function. Its mechanism of action is not completely understood but most likely involves modulation of the metabotropic glutamate receptor, which is upregulated in chronic alcoholism (Littleton, 1995). Acamprosate has been shown to reduce alcohol consumption in several animal models of alcoholism (Nalpas et al., 1990). In several European clinical trials involving alcoholic human subjects, acamprosate reduced craving for alcohol, reduced relapse drinking, and had minimal side effects (Lhuintre et al., 1990; Sass et al., 1996). Meta-analyses that compare acamprosate statistically across several studies have supported the efficacy of acamprosate in improving rates of abstinence and increasing time to first drink, although with small effect sizes (Bouza et al., 2004). Interestingly, the efficacy of acamprosate appears primarily in clinical trials conducted in Europe; two American trials, a six-month multi-site study (Mason et al., 2006) and the COMBINE Study (Anton et al., 2006) failed to find similar efficacy. The reasons for the differences in effectiveness of acamprosate between European and American studies are unclear. Researchers have suggested that differences in terms of severity of alcoholism, typologies of patients, and the use of inpatient detoxification in Europe account for the discrepant outcomes.

TOPIRAMATE

The anti-epileptic medication topiramate, although not approved by the FDA for the treatment of alcohol dependence, is endorsed as an effective alcoholism treatment medication by NIAAA in its "Clinicians Guide" (NIAAA, 1997). In a 12-week, randomized, controlled trial in 150 patients with alcohol dependence receiving medication-adherence therapy, topiramate treatment significantly decreased the numbers of drinks per day, drinks per drinking day, and drinking days, and increased the number of days of abstinence, compared to placebo (Johnson et al., 2003). A subsequent U.S. multi-site trial (Johnson et al., 2007) demonstrated the efficacy of a 300 mg daily dose of topiramate to reduce heavy drinking and to improve quality of life. An advantage of topiramate is that it does not require patients be detoxified prior to starting the medication. Topiramate causes a number of dose-dependent neurological and cognitive side-effects and must be titrated slowly over several weeks.

SEROTONERGIC MEDICATIONS

Studies show that almost 25% of alcoholics are treated with antidepressants, whether or not they are diagnosed with major depression. SSRIs, such as fluoxetine and sertraline, which augment serotonergic function, also appear to reduce alcohol consumption in animals and non-depressed humans (Naranjo et al., 1990). Several human studies on non-depressed heavy drinkers found SSRIs to reduce overall alcohol consumption by some 15–20%. Patients receiving SSRIs report decreased desire and liking for alcohol. Other studies of patients with greater alcohol-dependency, however, have yielded less impressive results. A double-blind study comparing fluoxetine and placebo treatment in non-depressed alcoholics receiving psychotherapy found no difference in drinking between groups (Kranzler et al., 1995). However, when alcoholics were subtyped into early onset, high-psychopathology (Type B) and late onset, less psychopathology (Type A), the Type B alcoholics drank more with sertraline. Similar results were found in a study of sertraline in non-depressed alcoholics, in which the Type A alcoholics drank less (Pettinati et al., 2000).

In alcoholics with comorbid major depressive disorders, antidepressants may improve both drinking and depression. In a double-blind, placebo-controlled antidepressant trial with imipramine in alcoholics with major depression or dysthymia, those treated with the antidepressant reported improved mood and decreased drinking (McGrath et al., 1996). A trial of fluoxetine in 12 depressed, suicidal alcoholics showed decreased depression and alcohol consumption, compared to pretreatment (Cornelius et al., 1997). A recent study of depressed alcoholics found that the combination of sertraline plus naltrexone reduced their drinking and improved depression (Pettinati et al., 2010). The results of these antidepressant studies indicated that depressed alcoholics may have improved mood and sometimes lessened drinking (Nunes and Levin, 2004), but that antidepressants should not be used in non-depressed drinkers.

AMPHETAMINES AND SIMILARLY ACTING SYMPATHOMIMETIC AMINES

The amphetamines are a group of drugs structurally related to the catecholamine neurotransmitters norepinephrine, epinephrine, and dopamine. Amphetamines release catecholamines from nerve endings and act as catecholamine agonists at receptors in the peripheral autonomic and central nervous systems. Intoxication with stimulants such as amphetamines, methylphenidate, or other sympathomimetics produces a clinical picture of sympathetic and behavioral hyperactivity (Dietz, 1981). Chronic amphetamine users progressively increase drug doses for periods of several days to weeks, followed by a period of abstinence. An "amphetamine psychosis" with manifestations of agitation, paranoia, delusions, and hallucinosis, mimicking paranoid schizophrenia, may follow chronic high-dose use of these drugs (Ellinwood, 1969). Neuroimaging studies find that chronic users show dysregulation of corticolimbic connections. This results in chronic users' experiencing poor executive functioning, impulsivity, and deficits in information processing (Aron & Paulus, 2007).

Antipsychotic medication such as haloperidol, risperidone, or olanzepine can be used in the treatment of stimulant psychoses; however, such patients frequently require psychiatric hospitalization. Severe hypertension is seen in overdose and may be treated with alpha-adrenergic blockers such as phentolamine. The patient's cardiovascular status (EKG) also may need monitoring. A paranoid psychosis symptomatically similar to schizophrenia may occur with chronic use and persist following cessation of stimulant use. A withdrawal syndrome characterized by marked dysphoria, fatigue, and restlessness may occur. Stimulant users may suffer also from underlying psychiatric disorders such as mood disorders and attention deficit disorders (ADD). Thus, all patients should receive a comprehensive psychiatric evaluation both before and after the acute intoxication or psychosis.

The current treatment of stimulant dependence is predominantly psychosocially based (Lee and Rawson, 2008). No definitive pharmacologically based treatments that can address the underlying neurobiology of amphetamine dependence exist. There are ongoing clinical trials of modafinil, topiramate, and other medications that have been shown to be effective for other substances. One small, single-site trial using D-amphetamine as a substitution treatment for methamphetamine found reductions in methamphetamine use and better retention than placebo (Longo et al., 2010).

BARBITURATES AND OTHER SEDATIVE HYPNOTICS AND ANXIOLYTICS

Sedative medications are a major source of adverse drug interactions and drug emergencies, including overdose (Gottschalk et al., 1979). Sedatives are used clinically for their anxiolytic and hypnotic effects and to induce anesthesia and conscious sedation for medical procedures. Medications in this group include barbiturates, benzodiazepines, chloral derivatives, ethchlorvynol, gamma hydroxybutyrate (GBH), glutethimide, meprobamate, and methaqualone. Patients may obtain these medications illicitly from the street or from physicians who, wittingly or unwittingly, may be contributing to abuse or dependence. Certain sedatives, such as methaqualone, GBH, and flunitrazepam, are not FDA approved and therefore are not marketed in the United States, yet they are widely available on the illicit market. Potent sedative agents like GBH are sometimes administered to unsuspecting individuals for nefarious purposes, such as date rape.

Medications in this group, like the benzodiazepines, derive their pharmacological activity by affecting the chloride channel-GABA receptor complex in the brain (Seeman, 1972). Specific binding sites exist for benzodiazepines, barbiturates, and other drugs, which, when occupied by such a drug, increase hyperpolarization (and inhibition) of neurons (Costa & Guidotti, 1979; Schulz & MacDonald, 1981; Skolnick et al., 1981). Since alcohol also has inhibitory effects at the GABA-A receptor, alcohol and sedatives can interact to significantly enhance sedation. Chronic use of sedative medications causes the brain receptors to adapt to the sedative medication by becoming less sensitive to inhibition and producing tolerance.

As with alcohol treatment, treatment of the sedative abuser occurs in four stages: intervention, detoxification, long-term rehabilitation, and aftercare. The withdrawal syndrome that follows cessation of sedative drug use may be severe, including seizures, cardiac arrhythmias, and death. The need for detoxification depends on the duration and amount of sedative drug abuse, which can be estimated by means of a pentobarbital challenge test (Wesson & Smith, 1977; Wikler, 1968). In this protocol, pentobarbital 200 mg is administered orally and the patient observed one hour later. The patient's condition after the test dose will range from no effect to sleep. If the patient develops drowsiness or nystagmus on a 200 mg dose, the patient is not barbiturate-dependent. If 200 mg lacks effect, the dose should be repeated hourly until nystagmus or drowsiness develops. The total dosage administered at this endpoint approximates the patient's daily barbiturate habit and may be used as a starting point for detoxification. The barbiturate dose should be tapered over ten days, with approximately a 10% reduction each day. Alternatively, the patient can be given a loading dose of a long-acting benzodiazepine such as diazepam or clonazepam, and this medication tapered over seven to ten days (Patterson, 1990).

An alternative treatment increasingly used for sedative detoxification is carbamazepine (Klein et al., 1986). The medication is administered until blood levels are in the range for effective anticonvulsant activity, maintained for up to two weeks, and then tapered and discontinued. Carbamazepine may affect a class of endogenous benzodiazepine receptors known as "peripheral" benzodiazepine receptors, although the brain is rich in these receptor sites.

Following detoxification, the patient should be engaged in long-term individualized treatment, which may include residential drug-free programs, outpatient counseling, or self-help groups such as AA or Narcotics Anonymous (NA).

CAFFEINE

Caffeine, and the related methylxanthines theophylline and theobromine, are ubiquitous drugs in modern society. These agents occur in coffee, tea, cola, and other carbonated drinks, and are consumed by more than 80% of the population (Dews, 1982). Caffeine is present in chocolate, and in many prescribed and over-the-counter medications, including stimulants (NoDoz), appetite suppressants (Dexatrim), analgesics (Anacin, Excedrin, APC tablets), and cold and sinus preparations (Dristan, Contac). CNS effects of caffeine include psychomotor stimulation, increased attention and concentration, suppression of the need for sleep, and unpleasant insomnia. Even at low or moderate doses, caffeine can exacerbate symptoms of anxiety disorders, precipitate panic attacks, and may increase requirements for neuroleptic or sedative medications (Charney et al., 1985). At high doses and in sensitive individuals, methylxanthines may produce tolerance and behavioral symptoms of tremor, insomnia, jitteriness, and agitation. Moderate to heavy users experience a withdrawal syndrome, characterized by lethargy, hypersomnia, irritability, and severe, continuous headache (which may persist for as long as a week), beginning within 24 hours of cessation of use. Clinically significant caffeine withdrawal symptoms are commonly observed in even low to moderate users of caffeine (Hughes et al., 1991) and may occur with reduced caffeine intake occurring during a medical or psychiatric hospitalization. The signs and symptoms of caffeine intoxication or caffeine withdrawal may complicate medical or psychiatric treatment by increasing patient distress and by leading to an unnecessary evaluation for other disorders.

Methylxanthines produce physiological effects through actions at the cellular level. They produce cardiac stimulation, diuresis, bronchodilation, and CNS stimulation through several mechanisms. They inhibit the enzyme cyclic adenosine monophosphate (AMP) phosphodiesterase and increase intracellular levels of this second messenger, thereby augmenting the action of many hormones and neurotransmitters, such as norepinephrine. They also have a directly inhibitory effect on adenosine receptors and may have other neurotransmitter effects as well.

Treatment of caffeine dependence relies on gradually decreasing consumption of caffeine-containing foods, medications, and beverages over a period of usually four to six weeks. Beverages such as coffee or cola may be substituted by their decaffeinated forms. Often, patients are unaware of the extent of their caffeine consumption and of the caffeine content of consumables. They require education about the caffeine content of these substances. Withdrawal symptoms such as headache and lethargy may be treated with caffeine taper or symptomatically with analgesics, such as nonsteroidal anti-inflammatory drugs (NSAIDs) or acetaminophen, which are of variable help.

COCAINE

The use of cocaine in the United States has undergone a dramatic increase in the last three decades. The prevalence of cocaine use peaked in the mid-1980s and has slowly declined since. Based on the 1996 National Survey of Drug Abuse, over 20 million Americans tried cocaine at least once, and 2.6 million used it during the preceding year. During the mid-1970s, the pattern of cocaine use changed from intranasal "snorting" of cocaine powder to smoking or intravenous injection of the more potent cocaine "freebase." Freebase cocaine is now widely available in a product called "crack," which is extremely potent, very cheap, and easily distributed. Crack is self-administered by smoking, usually by adding a small piece to a burning cigarette and inhaling the vapor. Because crack is so inexpensive and freely available, it has greatly increased the pool of cocaine users, particularly among the poor. For example, the babies of "crack mothers" and the addiction of their mothers are major public health problems for almost all cities, and even in small towns. The tragic effects of crack on the fetus and newborns are similar to the effects of cocaine and are described below.

Cocaine has major physiological and behavioral effects (Gawin & Ellinwood, 1988):

1. It is a local anesthetic of high potency, the only naturally occurring local anesthetic. It blocks the initiation and propagation of nerve impulses by affecting the sodium conductance of nerve cell membranes (Seeman, 1972).

2. It is a potent sympathomimetic agent that potentiates the actions of catecholamines in the autonomic nervous system, producing tachycardia and hypertension. It is a potent vasoconstrictor.

3. Cocaine is a potent stimulant of the central nervous system, potentiating the action of central catecholamine neurotransmitters, norepinephrine and dopamine. Its effects include increased arousal, euphoria, a sense of creativity, expansiveness, excitement, and motor activation. At high doses, the effects may progress to agitation, irritability, apprehension, and paranoia. Cocaine easily mimics the symptoms of mania.

Cocaine intoxication produces elation, euphoria, excitement, pressured speech, restlessness, stereotyped movements, and bruxism. Physiological signs of sympathetic stimulation are present, including tachycardia, mydriasis, and sweating. With chronic use, paranoia, suspiciousness, and frank psychotic symptoms may occur over time, even after withdrawal. Overdose of cocaine produces cardiac arrhythmias, hyperpyrexia, hyperreflexia, and seizures, which may progress to coma, respiratory arrest, and death. Propranolol and

haloperidol administration have anecdotally been reported to be useful in overdose (Rappolt, Gay, & Inaba, 1977). Cocaine also has major deleterious effects on pregnancy, producing low-birth-weight infants, *abruptio placentae*, and behavioral abnormalities in the newborn (Chasnoff et al., 1985).

The plasma half-life of cocaine following oral, nasal, or intravenous administration is approximately one to two hours, which correlates with its behavioral effects (Van Dyke et al., 1978). With the decline in plasma levels, most users experience a period of dysphoria or "crash," which often leads to additional cocaine use within a short period. The dysphoria of the "crash" is intensified and prolonged following repeated use.

COCAINE TREATMENT

The optimal treatment of the chronic cocaine user is still not established; perhaps no "optimal" treatment yet exists. While cessation of cocaine use is not followed by a physiological withdrawal syndrome of the magnitude of that seen with opioids or alcohol, the dysphoria, depression, and drug craving that follow chronic cocaine use are often intense and make abstinence difficult. Psychotherapies, group therapy, and behavior modification are all somewhat useful in maintaining abstinence (Rounsaville et al., 1985). An innovative, behaviorally oriented treatment program using payment vouchers to provide positive reinforcement for cocaine abstinence has shown considerable success in reducing cocaine use in research settings (Higgins et al., 1994; Higgins, 1996). Patients are essentially "paid" not to use cocaine.

Self-help groups such as Narcotics Anonymous (NA) may be useful both as a primary treatment modality for cocaine dependence and as an adjunct to other treatment. For recidivists, long-term residential drug-free programs, including therapeutic communities, may be efficacious for some patients, depending on their motivation and capability to change.

Various pharmacological agents have been proposed as adjunctive treatments. Several reports suggest antidepressant agents such as imipramine, desipramine, lithium, or trazodone can reduce cocaine craving and usage in some patients (Gawin & Kleber, 1984; Tennant & Rawson, 1983). The doses of medication used were similar to those used for antidepressant therapy. Carbamazepine was initially reported as a useful adjunct for treatment (Halikas et al., 1991) but was shown not to be effective in a placebo-controlled clinical trial. The dopamine-2 receptor agonists bromocriptine, methylphenidate, and amantadine have all been reported to be "somewhat useful" in cocaine treatment and may block cocaine craving (Dackis & Gold, 1985), but they are by no means universally effective, and what efficacy they possess is usually measured over relatively short periods of follow-up (6–12 months at most).

Dopamine-1 and dopamine-3 receptor agonists and antagonists reduce cocaine self-administration in animals and are being tested in human cocaine users. However, in spite of considerable research, no pharmacological agent has been proven effective in cocaine treatment (Meyer, 1992). Cocaine use is a complex problem involving multiple social and cultural variables, and expecting an unlikely "biological" cure is naïve.

Certain psychiatric disorders such as depression and ADD may be common in cocaine users. Recognition and effective treatment of these underlying disorders might add to the likelihood that the patient will stop using cocaine. Many cocaine users also use alcohol or other drugs, particularly sedatives and heroin, and will require treatment for these substances as well. The use of naltrexone in opiate dependence is discussed later.

CANNABIS

Cannabis sativa, also called marijuana or hemp, is a plant indigenous to India but now grown worldwide. The leaves, flowers, and seeds of the plant contain many biologically active compounds, the most important of which are the lipophilic cannabinoids, especially delta 9-tetrahydrocannabinol (THC) and cannabidiol. The plant is also grown as a legal cash crop for hemp fiber. Cannabinoids have behavioral effects because they mimic the action of naturally occurring lipid-signaling molecules anandamide and 2-arachidonylglycerol (2-AG) at brain cannabinoid receptors, a G-protein linked receptor (Mackie, 2008). The biologically active substances are administered by smoking or ingesting dried plant parts (marijuana, bhang, ganga), the resin from the plant (hashish), or extracts of the resin (THC or hash oil). After inhalation or ingestion, THC rapidly enters the CNS. It has biphasic elimination with a short initial half-life (1–2 hours) reflecting redistribution, and a second half-life of days to weeks. THC is hydroxylated and excreted in bile and urine.

Cannabis intoxication is characterized by tachycardia, muscle relaxation, euphoria, and a sense of well-being. Time-sense is altered and emotional lability, particularly inappropriate laughter, may be seen. Performance on psychomotor tasks, including driving, is impaired (Klonoff, 1974; Fletcher et al., 1996). Occasionally, with high doses of the drug, depersonalization, paranoia, and anxiety reactions occur. Although tolerance to the effects of cannabis occurs with chronic use, cessation of use does not usually produce significant withdrawal phenomena; but some report anxiety, insomnia, appetite disturbance, and depression (Budney & Hughes, 2006). Chronic use of cannabis has been associated with an apathetic amotivational state, and even feminization effects in men, which usually improve upon discontinuation of the drug (Gersten, 1980). Marijuana has antiemetic and analgesic effects; it stimulates appetite in wasting illness, such as AIDS and cancer; and reduces intraocular pressure in glaucoma. Delta 9-THC is now available by prescription for the medical treatment of these conditions. As of the date of publication, marijuana use is legal in Colorado and Washington, and "medical marijuana" is available legally by physician prescription in several states, although the federal government has challenged its distribution in this manner (Annas, 1997).

TREATMENT

Treatment of cannabis dependence is similar to treatment of other drug dependencies. As part of the initial assessment, all patients should undergo complete psychiatric and medical examinations. Short-term goals should focus on reducing or stopping cannabis use and interventions to ensure compliance. Inpatient treatment may be necessary to achieve an abstinent state. Since many patients with cannabis dependence are adolescents or young adults, involvement of the family in assessment and treatment is important.

Long-term treatment should involve addictive disorder specialists to implement behavioral and psychological interventions to maintain an abstinent state. Often, a change in social situation is necessary to decrease drug availability and reduce peer pressure. Individual and group psychotherapy may be useful for understanding the role of the drug in the individual's life, improving self-esteem, and providing alternate methods of relieving psychosocial distress. Self-help groups can provide group and individual support and are most effective when patients are matched with an appropriate peer group. There is interest in using dronabinol (pharmaceutical THC) as a potential substitution treatment in cannabis dependence. Dronabinol has been shown to block some of the intoxicating effects of marijuana and to reduce cannabis withdrawal symptoms. Other medications, including the alpha2 agonist lofexidine and lithium, are currently being studied as potential treatments.

INHALANTS

Inhalants are dangerous volatile organic compounds that are used for their psychotropic effects. Substances in this class include organic solvents, such as gasoline, toluene, ethyl ether, fluorocarbons, and volatile nitrates, including nitrous oxide and butyl nitrate. Inhalants are ubiquitous and readily available in most households and places of employment. At low doses, inhalants produce mood changes and ataxia; at high doses they may produce dissociative states and hallucinosis. Dangers of organic solvent use include suffocation and organ damage, especially hepatotoxicity and neurotoxicity in the central and peripheral nervous systems (Watson, 1982). Cardiac arrhythmias and sudden death may occur. Inhaled nitrates may produce hypotension and methemoglobinemia.

The typical user of inhalants is a male teenager. According to the National Household Survey on Drug Abuse, 9.1% of 12–17-year-olds and 12.8% of 18–25-year-olds have tried an inhalant at least once.

Optimal treatment of the inhalant user is not well established. Since most users are adolescents, treatment, as with other disorders in this category, must involve the family. Long-term residential treatment may be helpful for heavy users. Inhalants are perhaps the most lethal form of substance abuse, other than drunk driving.

NICOTINE

Nicotine is an alkaloid drug present in the leaves of the tobacco plant, *Nicotiana tabacum*. Native Americans have used the plant for centuries in ceremonies, rituals, and as a medicinal herb. Since its discovery by Europeans, tobacco use has spread worldwide, and today nicotine is the most prevalent psychoactive drug in use. Over 60 million persons in the United States (29% of the population) are daily users of cigarettes, with another 10 million using another form of tobacco. Since the publication of the U.S. Surgeon General's *Report on Smoking and Health* in 1964, there has been a gradual decline in the percentage of Americans who smoke. Most of this decline has occurred among men. The number of young women who smoke has increased, as has the prevalence of lung cancer among women. The use of other tobacco products such as smokeless tobacco has also increased. The morbidity and mortality resulting from use of nicotine are extensive and include an increase in cardiovascular and respiratory disease and in cancers, particularly of the lung and oropharynx. Many of the deleterious effects of tobacco are not due to nicotine, but to toxic and carcinogenic compounds present in tobacco extract or smoke. The morbidity and mortality associated with this legal drug of addiction dwarf the human misery caused by all other drugs combined. Society's tolerance of this lethal agent is one of the great paradoxes of history.

To maximize the absorption of nicotine, tobacco products are usually smoked as pipe tobacco, cigars, or cigarettes, or instilled intranasally or intraorally as snuff and chewing tobacco, or "smokeless tobacco." Following absorption from the lungs or buccal mucosa, nicotine levels peak rapidly and then decline, with a half-life of 30–60 minutes.

Nicotine has several effects on the peripheral autonomic and central nervous systems. It is an agonist at "nicotinic" cholinergic receptor sites and stimulates autonomic ganglia in the parasympathetic and sympathetic nervous systems, producing salivation, increased gastric motility and acid secretion, and increased catecholamine release. In the CNS, nicotine acts as a mild psychomotor stimulant, producing increased alertness, increased attention and concentration, and appetite suppression. The fact that tobacco use can prevent weight gain makes the drug attractive, particularly to young women who as adolescents are most susceptible to peer pressures associated with body weight and the "sophistication" attached to smoking and other tobacco use.

Repeated use of nicotine produces tolerance and dependence. The degree of dependence is considerable, as over 70% of dependent individuals relapse within one year of stopping use. Cessation of nicotine use in dependent individuals is followed by a withdrawal syndrome characterized by increased irritability, decreased attention and concentration, and an intense craving for and preoccupation with nicotine. Frequently, appetite and food consumption increase, and a significant weight gain occurs. Withdrawal symptoms may begin within several hours of cessation of use or reduction in dosage, and typically last about a week. Craving and weight gain may persist for weeks or even months, however.

The treatment of nicotine dependence should follow the principles of treatment common to all psychoactive substances. Short-term goals should consist of the reduction or cessation of tobacco use. Few patients are able to reduce tobacco use on their own, and a supportive, encouraging relationship with a physician and/or the use of a smoking-cessation group program are usually necessary to ensure success (Greene, Goldberg, & Ockene, 1988). The most successful treatment of nicotine dependence occurs with interventions that combine pharmacological (nicotine replacement or bupropion) and behavioral therapies (Hughes, Goldstein, & Hurt et al., 1999). According to the clinical practice guidelines review (U.S. Dept. of Health & Human Services [USDHHS], 2000), all nicotine-dependent patients should be offered some form of pharmacotherapy unless medical conditions contraindicate it. The treatment of nicotine dependence is discussed in great detail in Chapter 53.

OPIOIDS

Opioid addiction is a significant sociological and medical problem worldwide, with an estimated U.S. opioid addict population of greater than 700,000. These patients are frequent users of medical and surgical services because of the propensity for overdose and the multiple medical sequelae of intravenous drug use and its associated lifestyle. Over the past decade, there has been an increasing trend away from intravenous heroin to high-potency oral opioids (e.g., oxycodone), as users have become aware of the risks of HIV infection associated with intravenous injection.

Opiate drugs produce euphoria, decreases in stress and anxiety, and analgesia because they bind to neuronal opioid receptors and mimic the action of the endogenous opioid peptide neurotransmitters: enkephalin, endorphin, and dynorphin. Recent evidence suggests that there are at least three distinct types of opioid receptors, which are designated by the Greek letters *mu, delta,* and *kappa.* The closely related nociceptin/orphanin receptor is also stimulated by opioid peptides and certain opiate medications (New & Wong, 2003). Most of the opioid medications used clinically and most of those abused have their predominant effects on mu opioid receptors. With regular use of a mu opioid agonist, mu opioid receptors downregulate and other neuronal systems adapt, so that chronic opiate users develop tolerance and dependence. Then, cessation of opiate use results in an unpleasant withdrawal syndrome Jaffe & Martin (1985).

Opiate overdose is a life-threatening emergency that should be suspected in any patient presenting with coma and respiratory suppression. While miotic pupils are usually present, they are nondiagnostic and may not appear with ingestion of mixed agonist-antagonist opioids. Other effects of intoxication include hypotension, seizures, and pulmonary edema. Treatment of suspected overdose includes emergency support of respiration and cardiovascular functions. Parenteral administration of the opioid antagonist naloxone 0.4–0.8 mg or of nalmefene is of both diagnostic and therapeutic value (Martin, 1976). While opioid antagonists will rapidly reverse the effects of opioids, including coma and respiratory suppression, they do not reverse CNS depression caused by other drugs, such as alcohol or sedative-hypnotics. Opioid antagonists will precipitate withdrawal in any patient who is dependent on opioids— sometimes causing a patient whose life was just saved to be "less than grateful."

OPIOID WITHDRAWAL

The opioid withdrawal syndrome is characterized by sympathetic hyperactivity, anxiety, agitation, pain, and intense craving for opioids. Although not life-threatening, the symptoms are extremely distressing and often lead to reinstitution of opioid use. Reduction of withdrawal signs and symptoms is usually accomplished through slow taper of opiates (usually methadone) or the use of alpha-2 agonist agents, such as clonidine or lofexidine. Alpha-2 agonists act at presynaptic noradrenergic neurons in the locus coeruleus, block the activation of central norepinephrine systems in the brain that occurs during opioid withdrawal, and ameliorate the agitation and anxiety of withdrawal (Aghajanian, 1976; Gold, Redmond, & Kleber, 1979). The time course of withdrawal depends on the pharmacokinetics of the opiate drug that causes the dependence. Withdrawal from short half-life drugs, such as heroin or oxycodone, begins within hours of stopping drug use and usually lasts for five to seven days. Withdrawal from long half-life opioids, such as methadone, begins 24–48 hours after stopping drug use and can last from 10–14 days. Two scales that are helpful for clinicians to assess the intensity of opioid withdrawal symptoms over time are the Subjective Opiate Withdrawal Scale (SOWS) and the Objective Opioid Withdrawal Scale (OOWS) (see Boxes 38.5 and 38.6).

TREATMENT OF OPIOID ADDICTION

Nonpharmacological and behavioral modalities are quite efficacious in the treatment of the opioid abuser. Programs may differ in their lengths of stay, their intensity, and their theoretical orientation. Long-term residential treatment may be most useful

---

Box 38.5 THE SUBJECTIVE OPIATE WITHDRAWAL SCALE (SOWS)

Time:

Date ....   Time ....

PLEASE SCORE EACH OF THE 16 ITEMS BELOW ACCORDING TO HOW YOU FEEL NOW (CIRCLE ONE NUMBER)

	SYMPTOM	NOT AT ALL	A LITTLE	MODERATELY	QUITE A BIT	EXTREMELY
1	I feel anxious	0	1	2	3	4
2	I feel like yawning	0	1	2	3	4
3	I am perspiring	0	1	2	3	4
4	My eyes are teary	0	1	2	3	4
5	My nose is running	0	1	2	3	4
6	I have goosebumps	0	1	2	3	4
7	I am shaking	0	1	2	3	4
8	I have hot flushes	0	1	2	3	4
9	I have cold flushes	0	1	2	3	4
10	My bones and muscles ache	0	1	2	3	4
11	I feel restless	0	1	2	3	4
12	I feel nauseous	0	1	2	3	4
13	I feel like vomiting	0	1	2	3	4
14	My muscles twitch	0	1	2	3	4
15	I have stomach cramps	0	1	2	3	4
16	I feel like using now	0	1	2	3	4

Total score range, 0–64.
Source: From Handelsman et al., 1987.
Score 1 to 10 = Mild withdrawal; Score 11 to 20 = Moderate withdrawal; Score ≥ 21 = Severe withdrawal.

Box 38.6 THE OBJECTIVE OPIOID WITHDRAWAL SCALE (OOWS)

DATE ....   TIME ....

OBSERVE THE PATIENT DURING A 5 *MINUTE OBSERVATION PERIOD* THEN INDICATE A SCORE FOR EACH OF THE OPIOID WITHDRAWAL SIGNS LISTED BELOW (ITEMS 1–13). ADD THE SCORES FOR EACH ITEM TO OBTAIN THE TOTAL SCORE

	SIGN	MEASURES		SCORE
1	Yawning	0 = no yawns	1 = ≥ 1 yawn	
2	Rhinorrhoea	0 = < 3 sniffs	1 = ≥ 3 sniffs	
3	Piloerection (observe arm)	0 = absent	1 = present	
4	Perspiration	0 = absent	1 = present	
5	Lacrimation	0 = absent	1 = present	
6	Tremor (hands)	0 = absent	1 = present	
7	Mydriasis	0 = absent	1 = ≥ 3mm	
8	Hot and cold flushes	0 = absent	1 = shivering / huddling for warmth	
9	Restlessness	0 = absent	1 = frequent shifts of position	
10	Vomiting	0 = absent	1 = present	
11	Muscle twitches	0 = absent	1 = present	
12	Abdominal cramps	0 = absent	1 = Holding stomach	
13	Anxiety	0 = absent	1 = mild to severe	
	TOTAL SCORE			

Total score range 0–13.
Source: From Handelsman et al., 1987.

---

for the chronic opioid abuser who requires a change in lifestyle, with vocational and psychological rehabilitation. Attending Narcotics Anonymous is helpful for motivated patients.

Opioid Substitution

The concept of opioid substitution is to provide patients with a medically monitored opiate substitute to maintain opioid dependence, thereby preventing withdrawal and increasing tolerance to diminish the effects of illicit opiates. In this harm-reduction paradigm, patients remain opioid dependent, but typically stop the use of illicit opioids. Two medications are FDA approved for substitution: methadone and buprenorphine. All of these medications are best used in the setting of a structured, maintenance treatment program, which includes monitored medication-administration; periodic, random urine toxicological screening to assess compliance; and intensive psychological, medical and vocational services.

Methadone Maintenance

Methadone is a synthetic opiate, which is orally active, possesses a long duration of action, produces minimal sedation or "high," and has few side effects at therapeutic doses.

Methadone was first shown to be an effective treatment in an open-label study of 22 patients in New York City (Dole & Nyswander, 1965) and is now used worldwide. Over the past 40 years, studies consistently have shown methadone maintenance to be effective in the treatment of addicts who are dependent on heroin and other opiates (Senay, 1985; O'Brien, 2008). A meta-analysis of studies comparing methadone maintenance to placebo or drug-free treatment found methadone maintenance to be significantly better than non-pharmacological therapy in reducing heroin use and improving program retention (Mattick et al., 2003). In addition, methadone maintenance has been shown to reduce opiate-related mortality and morbidity, reduce HIV transmission, decrease criminal activity, and increase employment (Vocci et al. 2005). A longitudinal study that compared more than 100 representative methadone maintenance programs found that the most effective programs provided intensive psychosocial and medical services and flexibility in methadone dosing, and allowed higher doses of methadone, in excess of 80 mg per day (D'Aunno & Pollack, 2002).

Methadone treatment is integrated with a comprehensive psychosocial treatment program. Methadone is dissolved in a flavored liquid and is administered to patients daily, under observation. Daily doses usually range from 20 mg per day to over 100 mg per day. (Long-standing program participants are allowed to "take home" some doses of methadone under a contingency contract that permits take-home doses as long as treatment compliance is maintained.) Counseling sessions are held weekly with a counselor trained and certified in addiction treatment. Medical care, employment counseling, and other rehabilitative services are provided on a regular basis. Urine toxicological screening is performed randomly and periodically to assess compliance with treatment. Higher doses are shown to be generally associated with better treatment retention.

Buprenorphine

In 2002, the FDA approved sublingual buprenorphine tablets (Subutex®) and buprenorphine/naloxone tablets (Suboxone®) for the management of opiate dependence (Ling et al., 1994; Vocci et al., 2005). In 2012, the sublingual tablets were phased out in favor of dissolving strips, which are less subject to diversion for illicit sales. Buprenorphine is a partial mu- and kappa-agonist opiate that was used medically as an analgesic. Importantly, the drug's agonist properties predominate at lower doses, and antagonist properties predominate at higher doses. These properties have led to its increasing use as an adjunctive substitution and maintenance treatment for opioid dependence. A randomized trial comparing buprenorphine maintenance to methadone maintenance for 16 weeks in 164 newly treated opiate users showed similar reductions in illicit drug use and similar retention in treatment (Strain et al., 1994). A six-month study comparing methadone maintenance with a approach to buprenorphine found identical rates of treatment retention (Kakko et al., 1997). Possible advantages of buprenorphine compared to methadone include a less intense withdrawal upon discontinuation and less potential for abuse, as agonist effects diminish at higher doses.

Federal law now permits individual physicians who are certified in buprenorphine and possess a special license from the Drug Enforcement Administration (DEA) to prescribe buprenorphine and buprenorphine/naloxone to up to 100 opioid-dependent patients who are also receiving psychosocial treatment. In the setting of a structured treatment program, daily buprenorphine dosing has been shown to be an effective maintenance treatment. Medication doses usually range from 4 mg per day to up to 16 mg per day, administered sublingually, since the medication is not effective orally.

In spite of the demonstrated evidence of effectiveness of maintenance treatment with methadone and buprenorphine, the concept of opioid substitution therapy remains extremely controversial. Indeed, opioid substitution therapies are among the most highly regulated treatments, and must follow strict guidelines described in the Code of Federal Regulations (CFR 42, section 8).

Naltrexone

Another pharmacological adjunctive treatment for the treatment of opioid dependence is antagonist therapy with naltrexone. Naltrexone is an opioid antagonist at mu-, kappa-, and delta-opioid receptors. When taken regularly, an oral daily dose of 50 mg naltrexone completely blocks the euphoric, analgesic, and sedative properties of opiates (Resnick et al., 1980). Patients receiving naltrexone first must be completely detoxified from opiates, or risk experiencing opioid withdrawal. In spite of its potential, studies with oral naltrexone as an adjunctive treatment have shown high treatment dropout and poor medication compliance, particularly in poorly motivated individuals with poor social supports (Capone et al., 1986). Naltrexone was most effective in highly motivated individuals, such as impaired professionals and parolees (Kleber and Kosten, 1984).

To address poor medication adherence with oral naltrexone, several sustained-release, injectable forms of naltrexone have been developed. Sixty detoxified opioid-dependent patients receiving once-monthly injections of a sustained-release naltrexone preparation in conjunction with twice-weekly counseling, showed dose-dependent reductions in illicit drug use and improvements in treatment retention (Comer, et al., 2006). A 24-week double-blind placebo-controlled multi-site study of extended-release naltrexone in 250 opioid-dependent patients conducted in Russia found significantly reduced relapse, reduce opioid craving, and improved study retention in the naltrexone group (Krupitsky et al., 2011). Based on these findings, the extended-release naltrexone preparation (Vivitrol®) initially marketed for the treatment of alcohol dependence, was FDA approved for opioid dependence treatment in 2011. The preparation, containing 380 mg of naltrexone, is injected monthly and causes blockade of opioid receptors for approximately 30 days. A potential concern for opioid-addicted patients treated with sustained-release naltrexone is the possibility of an overdose if opioids are used after treatment with naltrexone stops, due to loss of opioid tolerance.

HALLUCINOGENS AND PHENCYCLIDINE

Drugs used for their hallucinogenic or psychotomimetic effects include psychedelics such as lysergic acid diethylamide (LSD), mescaline, psilocybin ("mushrooms"), and dimethyltryptamine; hallucinogenic amphetamines such as methylenedioxyamphetamine (MDA) and methylenedioxymethamphetamine (MDMA, or Ecstasy [XTC]); phencyclidine (PCP, or "angel dust"), ketamine, and similarly acting arylcyclohexylamines; and anticholinergics, such as scopolamine. All cause a state of intoxication characterized by hallucinosis, mood lability, and delusional states. The mechanism of action of hallucinogens is not well understood and varies according to the drug. Hallucinogens of the LSD and amphetamine class are thought to act on dopaminergic and/or serotonergic brain systems (Abraham et al., 1996). Hallucinogens related to PCP and ketamine act at the n-methyl-d-aspartate (NMDA) glutamate receptor. Anticholinergics act at muscarinic cholinergic receptors. The rate of current use of hallucinogens in the American population has been stable at 0.6% in 1996. However, among youth ages 12–17, the rate nearly doubled in two years (1.1% in 1994 to 2.0% in 1996).

PCP intoxication has several definitive features (Young et al., 1987). Patients often present with impulsive violence, either directed at themselves or at others. Eye signs, including vertical and horizontal nystagmus, are often present. Myoclonus and ataxia are frequent. Autonomic instability, with hypertension and tachycardia, is common. Ketamine, used clinically as a dissociative anesthetic in pediatric surgery, has become increasingly popular as a party drug ("Special K") to induce hallucinosis and euphoria, and to perpetrate date rape.

The differential diagnosis of hallucinogen- or PCP-induced psychosis includes schizophrenia, bipolar mood disorder, delusional disorder, neurophysiological mental disorders such as encephalitis and brain tumor, and other toxic ingestions. Psychoses, including those that are drug-induced, may produce an analgesic state, and the clinician needs to be aware of any coexisting medical problems, such as injuries, head trauma, or an acute abdomen that may be painless.

Treatment of the psychotic state includes supportive measures to prevent patients from harming themselves or others, maintaining their cardiovascular and respiratory functions, and urgent amelioration of agitation and psychotic symptoms. Often agitation and psychosis respond to decreased sensory stimulation and verbal reassurance; still, patients usually require sedation with benzodiazepines or high-potency neuroleptics. Lorazepam 1–2 mg PO or IV every 1–2 hours as needed, or diazepam 5–10 mg PO every 2–4 hours as needed, can be given to calm and sedate them. For PCP, the acute symptoms of intoxication and withdrawal are diminished or reversed by intramuscular haloperidol 5–10 mg or oral risperidone every 1–6 hours as needed for behavioral control. Lorazepam 1–2 mg IV or diazepam 5–10 mg PO every 1–6 hours can also be given as needed. Severe tachycardia and hypertension, if present, can be treated with antihypertensives.

Most cases of hallucinogen intoxication are short-lived (lasting several hours) and resolve without incident; however, occasionally, prolonged drug-induced psychoses may occur. This is particularly common with use of PCP, which may produce a prolonged psychosis lasting from two days to a week (Walker et al., 1981). In addition, it is believed that hallucinogenic drug use may precipitate psychotic illnesses in certain individuals predisposed to the development of such disorders (Bowers & Swigar, 1983). If psychosis persists beyond two weeks after hallucinogen ingestion, it should be regarded as another primary psychiatric illness and treated accordingly, with a concurrent addiction program. Following detoxification, the patient should be engaged in long-term treatment, which may include residential drug-free programs, outpatient counseling, and self-help groups.

ANABOLIC STEROIDS

The use of anabolic steroids and performance-enhancing drugs, once predominantly a problem in weightlifters and body builders, has become an increasingly prevalent problem in professional and amateur athletes, and is common among adolescents and young adults. A recent study found 6.5% of adolescent boys and 1.9% of adolescent girls reported using anabolic steroids without a doctor's prescription (DuRant et al., 1993). A survey of high school students found that 2.5% and 1.8% of twelfth-grade boys used anabolic steroids in 2005 and 2011, respectively (Johnston et al., 2012). The use of anabolic steroids is often associated with the use of other substances, including cocaine, alcohol, injectable drugs, marijuana, and cigarettes.

Medical complications of anabolic steroid use include liver disease and altered lipid metabolism, leading to myocardial infarction and stroke. There is a significant effect on endocrine hormones in both males and females, altering growth and sexual development (Daly et al., 2003). Women can develop masculinizing features, including baldness, and men can develop enlarged breasts and smaller testicles. Abscesses and HIV infection have been associated with shared needle use in steroid injectors. Psychiatric symptoms associated with anabolic steroid use include severe depression, psychotic (paranoid) symptoms, aggressive behavior, homicidal impulses, euphoria, irritability, anxiety, and hyperactivity (Pope & Katz, 1988). While most of these symptoms will gradually abate with drug discontinuation, depression, fatigue, decreased sex drive, insomnia, anorexia, and dissatisfaction with body image may continue. Users are usually completely naïve about or deny the medical hazards of anabolic steroid use.

The treatment of anabolic steroid dependence should be within the same general model of other addictions, with due consideration to the high likelihood of dependency on other drugs, particularly in adolescents. Psychiatric management of drug-induced mood and paranoid syndromes is necessary. Issues regarding dysmorphic body image are often present in certain athletes and body builders and should be considered in their psychotherapy.

CLINICAL PEARLS

- It is thought that drugs of abuse and alcohol initially enhance reward mechanisms (Robinson & Berridge, 1993; Wise & Bozarth, 1987). Over time, continued use engenders a state of withdrawal, dysphoria, and distress, called *allostasis* (Koob & Le Moal, 2001), that is relieved only by continued drug and alcohol use.

- Dopamine is associated with reward and an increased salience for the stimulus; it is thought that repeated activation of this motivation-reward system sensitizes the system, resulting in increased craving in response to stimuli associated with substance use and compulsion with the development of craving (Nestler, 2001).

- The withdrawal from most substances has two phases: an acute, intense withdrawal beginning within hours after the cessation of drug or alcohol use, lasting from several days to a few weeks; and a chronic or protracted and more indolent withdrawal that can last weeks or months.

- Although complete abstinence is the ideal for treatment, reduction in quantity and frequency of substance use can still result in *harm reduction.*

- Rather than asking how much or how often a person uses, a more effective interview method focuses on whether the patient has experienced negative consequences from use of psychoactive substances, has poor control of use, or has received criticism from others about the substance use.

- Cognitive mental status testing should be particularly detailed, because alcohol and drug abusers may have significant deficits in memory, concentration, and abstract reasoning, yet at the same time pass simple bedside tests of orientation, calculation, and immediate memory.

- Percent carbohydrate-deficient transferrin (CDT) has been found to be effective in discriminating heavy drinking (Litten et al., 1995).

- A false positive in drug testing: use of sympathomimetic agents to treat asthma may yield a positive urine test for amphetamines.

- NIAAA defines "at risk" drinking (that is, at risk for adverse consequences) as more than 14 drinks per week or four drinks per occasion for men, and more than seven drinks per week or three drinks per occasion for women.

- Predictors of withdrawal delirium include structural brain lesions, hypokalemia, and thrombocytopenia; predictors of a withdrawal seizure are a previous seizure or structural brain lesion (Eyer et al., 2011).

- During and after detoxification, many alcoholic patients will appear to suffer from major depression and anxiety disorders. Some of these mood disorders are directly related to alcohol and will gradually resolve within two to four weeks after detoxification.

- Predictors of a positive response to naltrexone include a high level of craving, a positive family history of alcoholism (Rubio et al., 2005), and possessing a specific genetic polymorphism (Asn40Asp) in the μ opioid receptor gene (Oslin et al., 2003).

- Antidepressants in depressed alcoholics may improve their mood and sometimes their drinking (Nunes and Levin, 2004), but antidepressants should not be used in non-depressed drinkers.

- Chronic amphetamine users progressively increase their drug doses for periods of several days to weeks, followed by a period of abstinence.

- Chronic use of cannabis has been associated with an apathetic amotivational state, and even feminization effects in men, which usually improve upon discontinuation of the drug (Gersten, 1980).

- In 2012, sublingual buprenorphine tablets (Subutex®) and buprenorphine/naloxone tablets (Suboxone®) for the management of opiate dependence were phased out in favor of dissolving strips, which are less subject to diversion.

DISCLOSURE STATEMENT

Dr. Swift has received research funding and consultation fees from Farmaceutico CT. He is an advisory board member for D&A Pharma and has received consultant fees from this company. He has been a speaker for Lundbeck and received travel reimbursement and fees.

REFERENCES

Abbott, P. J., Quinn, D., & Knox, L. (1995). Ambulatory medical detoxification from alcohol. *American Journal of Drug & Alcohol Abuse, 21*(4), 549–563.

Abraham, H. D., Aldridge, A. M., & Gogia, P. (1996). The psychopharmacology of hallucinogens. *Neuropsychopharmacology, 14*(4), 285–298.

Aghajanian, G. K. (1976). Tolerance of locus ceruleus neurons to morphine and inhibition of withdrawal response by clonidine. *Nature, 276,* 186–188.

American Psychiatric Association (1995a). *Diagnostic and Statistical Manual of Mental Disorders* (4th ed.). Washington, DC: American Psychiatric Association Press.

American Psychiatric Association (1995b). *Diagnostic and Statistical Manual of Mental Disorders* (4th ed.), Primary Care Version. Washington, DC: American Psychiatric Association Press.

Annas, G. J. (1997). Reefer madness—The federal response to California's medical marijuana law. *New England Journal of Medicine, 337*(6), 435–439.

Anton, R. F., O'Malley, S. S., Ciraulo, D. A., Cisler, R. A., Couper, D., Donovan, D. M., et al. (2006). Combined pharmacotherapies and behavioral interventions for alcohol dependence: the COMBINE study: a randomized controlled trial. *Journal of the American Medical Association, 295,* 2003–2017.

Aron, J. L., & Paulus, M. P. (2007). Location, location: using functional magnetic resonance imaging to pinpoint brain differences relevant to stimulant use. *Addiction, 102*(suppl 1), 33–43.

Beresford, T. P., Blow, K. C., Hill, E., et al. (1990). Clinical practice: Comparison of CAGE questionnaire and computer assisted laboratory profiles in screening for covert alcoholism. *Lancet, 336,* 482–485.

Berg, R., Franzen, M., & Wedding, D. (1987). *Screening for brain impairment.* New York: Springer-Verlag.

Bertholet, N., Daeppen, J. B., Wietlisbach, V., Fleming, M., et al. (2005). Reduction of alcohol consumption by brief alcohol intervention in primary care: Systematic review and meta-analysis. *Archives of Internal Medicine, 165*(9), 986–995.

Bouza, C., Angeles, M., Munoz, A., & Amate, J. M. (2004). Efficacy and safety of naltrexone and acamprosate in the treatment of alcohol dependence: a systematic review. *Addiction, 99,* 811–828.

Bowers, M. B., & Swigar, M. E. (1983). Vulnerability to psychosis associated with hallucinogen use. *Psychiatry Research, 9,* 91–97.

Brewer, C. (1993). Recent developments in disulfiram treatment. *Alcohol & Alcoholism, 28,* 383–395.

Budney, A. J., & Hughes, J. R. (2006). The cannabis withdrawal syndrome. *Current Opinion in Psychiatry, 19,* 233–238.

Capone, T., Brahen, L., Condren, R., Kordal, N., Melchionda, R., & Peterson, M. (1986). Retention and outcome in a narcotic antagonist treatment program. *Journal of Clinical Psychology, 42,* 825–833.

Comer, S. D., Sullivan, M. A., Yu, E., Rothenberg, J. L., Kelber, H. D., Kampman, K., et al. (2006). Injectable, sustained-release naltrexone for the treatment of opioid dependence: a randomized, placebo-controlled trial. *Archives General Psychiatry, 63,* 210–218.

Charney, D. S., Henninger, G. R., & Jatlow, P. I. (1985). Increased anxiogenic effects of caffeine in panic disorders. *Archives of General Psychiatry, 42,* 233–243.

Charney, D. S., Sternberg, D. E., Kleber, H. D., et al. (1981). Clinical use of clonidine in abrupt withdrawal from methadone. *Archives of General Psychiatry, 38,* 1273–1278.

Chasnoff, I. J., Burns, W. J., Schnoll, S. H., et al. (1985). Cocaine use in pregnancy. *New England Journal of Medicine, 313*, 666–669.

Chick, J., Gough, K., Falkowski, W. (1992). Disulfiram treatment of alcoholism. *British Journal of Psychiatry, 161*, 84–89.

Clark, W. D. (1981). Alcoholism: Blocks to diagnosis and treatment. *American Journal of Medicine, 71*, 275–285.

Cornelius, J. R., Salloum, I. M., Ehler, J. G., et al. (1997). Fluoxetine in depressed alcoholics: A double-blind placebo-controlled trial. *Archives of General Psychiatry, 54*, 700–705.

Costa, E., & Guidotti, A. (1979). Molecular mechanisms in the receptor action of benzodiazepines. *Annual Review of Pharmacology & Toxicology, 19*, 531–545.

Crum, R. M., Anthony, J. C., Bassett, S. S., et al. (1993). Population-based norms for the Mini-Mental State Examination by age and educational level. *Journal of the American Medical Association, 269*(18), 2386–2391.

Daly, R. C., Su T. P., Schmidt, P. J., Pagliaro, M., Pickar, D., & Rubinow, D. R. (2003). Neuroendocrine and behavioral effects of high-dose anabolic steroid administration in male normal volunteers. *Psychoneuroendocrinology, 28*, 317–331.

D'Aunno, T., & Pollack, H. A. (2002). Changes in methadone treatment practices: Results from a national panel study, 1988–2000. *JAMA, 288*, 850–856.

D'Onofrio, G, Rathlev, N. K., Ulrich, A. S., et al. (1999). Lorazepam for the prevention of recurrent seizures related to alcohol. *New England Journal of Medicine, 340*, 915–919.

Dackis, C. A., & Gold, M. (1985). Bromocriptine as treatment of cocaine abuse. *Lancet, 1*, 151.

Dews, P. B. (1982). Caffeine. *Annual Review of Nutrition, 2*, 323–341.

Dietz, A. J. (1981). Amphetamine-like reactions to phenylpropanolamine. *Journal of the American Medical Association, 245*, 601–602.

Dole, V. P., & Nyswander, M. (1965). A medical treatment for diacetylmorphine (heroin) addiction: Clinical trial with methadone hydrochloride. *Journal of the American Medical Association, 193*, 646–650.

DuRant, R. H., Rickert, V. I., Ashworth, C. S., et al. (1993). The use of multiple drugs among adolescents who use anabolic steroids. *New England Journal of Medicine, 328*, 922–926.

Ellinwood, E. H. (1969). Amphetamine psychosis: A multidimensional process. *Seminars in Psychiatry, 1*, 208–226.

Elman, I., Becerra, L., Tschibelu, E., Yamamoto, R., George, E., & Borsook, D. (2012). Yohimbine-induced amygdala activation in pathological gamblers: A pilot study. *PLoS One, 7*(2), e31118.

Emrick, C. (1974). A review of psychologically oriented treatment of alcoholism. *Quarterly Journal of Studies on Alcohol, 38*, 1004–1031.

Emrick, C. D. (1987). Alcoholics Anonymous: Affiliation processes and effectiveness as treatment. *Alcoholism, 11*, 416–423.

Ewing, J. A. (1984). Detecting alcoholism: The CAGE questionaire-questionnaire. *Journal of the American Medical Association, 252*, 1905–1907.

Eyer, F., Schuster, T., Felgenhauer, N., Pfab, R., Strubel, T., Saugel, B., Zilker, T., et al. (2011). Risk assessment of moderate to severe alcohol withdrawal—Predictors for seizures and delirium tremens in the course of withdrawal. *Alcohol and Alcoholism, 46*(4), 427–433.

Fletcher, J. M., Page, J. B., Francis, D. J., et al. (1996). Cognitive correlates of long-term cannabis use in Costa Rican men. *Archives of General Psychiatry, 53*, 1051–1057.

Garbutt, J. C., Kranzler, H. R., O'Malley, S. S., Gastfriend, D. R., Pettinati, H. M., Silverman, B. L., Loewy, J. W., Ehrich, E. W.; Vivitrex Study Group (2005). Efficacy and tolerability of long-acting injectable naltrexone for alcohol dependence: a randomized controlled trial. *Journal of the American Medical Association, 293*, 1617–1625.

Gawin, F. H., & Ellinwood, E. H. Jr. (1988). Cocaine and other stimulants. Actions, abuse and treatment. *New England Journal of Medicine, 318*(18), 1173–1182.

Gawin, F. H., & Kleber, H. D. (1984). Cocaine abuse treatment: Open trial with desiprimine and lithium carbonate. *Archives of General Psychiatry, 41*, 903–909.

Geller, G., Levine, D. M., Mamom, J. A., et al. (1989). Knowledge, attitudes and reported practices of medical students and house staff regarding the diagnosis and treatment of alcoholism. *Journal of the American Medical Association, 261*(21), 3115–3120.

Gersten, S. P. (1980). Long-term adverse effects of brief marijuana usage. *Journal of Clinical Psychiatry, 41*(2), 60.

Golbert, T. M., Sanz, C. J., Rose, H. D., et al. (1967). Comparative evaluation of treatments of alcohol withdrawal syndromes. *Journal of the American Medical Association, 201*, 113–116.

Gold, M. S., Redmond, D. E. Jr, & Kleber, H. D. (1979). Noradrenergic hyperactivity in opiate withdrawal supressed by clonidine. *American Journal of Psychiatry, 136*, 100–102.

Gottschalk, L., McGuire, F., Heiser, J., et al. (1979). Drug abuse deaths in nine cities: A survey report. NIDA Research Monograph, No 29. Washington, DC: U.S. Government Printing Office.

Grant, B. F., Stinson, F. S., Dawson, D. A., Chou, S. P., Dufour, M. C., Compton, W., Pickering, R. P., Kaplan, K., et al. (2004). Prevalence and co-occurrence of substance use disorders and independent mood and anxiety disorders: Results from the National Epidemiologic Survey on Alcohol and Related Conditions. Copyright 2004 American Medical Association. All Rights Reserved. *Archives of General Psychiatry, 61*(8), 807–816.

Greene, H. L., Goldberg, R., & Ockene, J. K. (1988). Cigarette smoking: The physician's role in cessation and maintenance. *Journal of General Internal Medicine, 3*, 75–87.

Halikas, J. A., Crosby, R. D., Carlson, G. A., et al. (1991). Cocaine reduction in unmotivated crack users using carbamazepine versus placebo in a short-term, double-blind crossover design. *Clinical Pharmacology & Therapeutics, 50*(1), 81–95.

Handelsman, L., Cochrane, K. J., Aronson, M. J., Ness, R. A., Rubenstein, K. J., & Kanof, P. D. (1987). Two new rating scales for opiate withdrawal. *American Journal of Drug & Alcohol Abuse, 13*, 293–308.

Hansen, H. J., Caudhill, S. P., & Boone, D. J. (1985). Crisis in drug testing: Results of the CDC blind study. *Journal of the American Medical Association, 253*, 2382–2387.

Hasin, D. S., Stinson, F. S., Ogburn, E., & Grant, B. F. (2007). Prevalence, correlates, disability, and comorbidity of DSM-IV alcohol abuse and dependence in the United States: Results from the National Epidemiologic Survey on Alcohol and Related Conditions. *Archives of General Psychiatry, 64*(7), 830–842.

Hawks, R. L., & Chiang, C. N. (1986). Urine testing for drugs of abuse. *NIDA Research Monograph 73.* Washington, D.C.: Department of Health and Human Services.

Heilig, M., Egli, M., Crabbe, J. C., & Becker, H. C. (2010). Acute withdrawal, protracted abstinence and negative affect in alcoholism: Are they linked? *Addiction Biology, 15*(2), 169–184.

Higgins, S. T. (1996). Some potential contributions of reinforcement and consumer-demand theory to reducing cocaine use. *Addictive Behaviors, 21*, 803–816.

Higgins, S. T., Budney, A. J., & Bickel, W. K. (1994). Applying behavioral concepts and principles to the treatment of cocaine dependence. *Drug & Alcohol Dependency, 34*(2), 87–97.

Hillbom, M. E., & Hjelm-Jager, M. (1984). Should alcohol withdrawal seizures be treated with anti-epileptic drugs? *Acta Neurologica Scandinavica, 69*, 39–42.

Hoffmann, N. G., DeHart, S. S., & Fulkerson, J. A. (1993). Medical care utilization as a function of recovery status following chemical addictions treatment. *Journal of Addictive Diseases, 12*, 97–108.

Holden, C. (1985). The neglected disease in medical education. *Science, 229*, 741–742.

Holder, H., Longabaugh, R., Miller, W. R., et al. (1991). The cost effectiveness of alcoholism treatment: An approximation. *Journal of Studies on Alcohol, 52*(6), 517–540.

Hughes, J. R., Goldstein, M. G., Hurt, R. D., et al. (1999). Recent advances in the pharmacotherapy of smoking. *Journal of the American Medical Association, 281*, 72–76.

Hughes, J. R., Higgins, S. T., Bickel, W. K., et al. (1991). Caffeine self-administration, withdrawal and adverse effects among coffee drinkers. *Archives of General Psychiatry, 48*(7), 611–617.

Hunt, W. A. (1983). The effect of ethanol on GABAergic transmission. *Neuroscience & Biobehavioral Reviews, 7*, 87–95.

Jaffe, J. H., & Martin, W. R. (1985). Opioid analgesics and antagonists. In A. C. Gilman, L. S. Goodman, T. W. Rall, et al. (Eds.), *The Pharmacological Basis of Therapeutics* (7th ed.). New York: Macmillan.

Johnson, B. A., Ait-Daoud, N., Bowden, C. L., DiClemente, C. C., Roache, J. D., Lawson, K., Javors, M. A., & Ma, J. Z. (2003). Oral topiramte for treatment of alcohol dependence: a randomised controlled trial. *Lancet, 17*;361(9370), 1677–1685.

Johnson, B. A., Rosenthal, N., Capece, J. A., Wiegand, F., Mao, L., Beyers, K., et al. (2007). Topiramate for treating alcohol dependence: a randomized controlled trial. *Journal American Medical Association, 298*, 1641–1651.

Johnston, G. A. R. (1996). GABA$_A$ receptor pharmacology. *Pharmacology and Therapeutics, 69*(3), 173–198.

Johnston, L. D., O'Malley, P. M., Bachman, J. G., & Schulenberg, J. E. (2012). Monitoring the future: National survey results on drug use, 1975–2011: Volume II, College students and adults ages 19–50. Ann Arbor, MI: Institute for Social Research, The University of Michigan. Available at: Http://www.monitoringthefuture.org//pubs/monographs/mtf-vol2_2011.pdf

Kakko, J., Gronbladh, L., Svanborg, K. D., von Wachenfeldt, J., Ruck C., Rawlings, B., Nilsson, L. H., & Heilig, M. (1997). A stepped care strategy using buprenorphine and methadone versus conventional methadone maintenance in heroin dependence: a randomized controlled trial. *American Journal of Psychiatry, 164*, 797–803.

Kennedy, W. (1985). Chemical dependency: A treatable disease. *Ohio State Medical Journal, 71*, 77–79.

Klein, E., Uhde, T., & Post, R. M. (1986). Preliminary evidence for the utility of carbamazepine in alprazolam withdrawal. *American Journal of Psychiatry, 143*(2), 235–236.

Kleber, H. D., & Kosten, T. R. (1984). Naltrexone induction: psychologic and pharmacologic strategies. *Journal of Clinical Psychiatry, 45*, 29–38.

Klonoff, H. (1974). Marijuana and driving in real-life situations. *Science, 186*, 317–324.

Koob, G. F. (2008). A role for brain stress systems in addiction. *Neuron, 10, 59*(1), 11–34.

Koob, G. F., & Le Moal, M. (2001). Drug addiction, dysregulation of reward, and allostasis. *Neuropsychopharmacology, 24*(2), 97–129.

Koob, G. F., & Volkow, N. D. (2010). Neurocircuitry of addiction. *Neuropsychopharmacology, 35*(1), 217–238.

Kosten, T. R., & Kleber, H. D. (1988). Differential diagnosis of psychiatric comorbidity in substance abusers. *Journal of Substance Abuse Treatment, 5*, 201–206.

Kosten, T. R., & O'Connor, P. G. (2003). Management of drug and alcohol withdrawal. *New England Journal of Medicine, 348*(18), 1786–1795.

Krampe, H., & Ehrenreich, H. (2010). Supervised disulfiram as adjunct to psychotherapy in alcoholism treatment. *Current Pharmaceutical Design, 16*, 2076–2090.

Kranzler, H., Burleson, J. A., Korner, P., et al. (1995). Placebo-controlled trial of fluoxetine as an adjunct to relapse prevention in alcoholics. *American Journal of Psychiatry, 152*, 391–397.

Krupitsky, E., Nunes, E. V., Ling, W., Illeperuma, A., Gastfriend, D. R., & Silverman, B. L. (2011). Injectable extended-release naltrexone for opioid dependence: A double-blind, placebo-controlled, multicentre randomised trial. *The Lancet*, Volume, *377*(9776), 1506–1513.

Lee, N. K., & Rawson RA. (2008). A systematic review of cognitive and behavioural therapies for methamphetamine dependence. *Drug & Alcohol Review, 27*(3), 309–317.

Leggio, L., Kenna, G. A., & Swift, R. M. (2008). New developments for the pharmacological treatment of alcohol withdrawal syndrome. A focus on non-benzodiazepine GABAergic medications. *Progress in Neuro-Psychopharmacology and Biological Psychiatry, 32*, 1106–1117.

Lhuintre, J. P., Moore, N., Tran, G., et al. (1990). Acamprosate appears to decrease alcohol intake in weaned alcoholics. *Alcohol & Alcoholism, 25*, 613–622.

Ling, W., Rawson, R. A., & Compton, P. A. (1994). Substitution pharmacotherapies for opioid addiction: From methadone to LAAM and buprenorphine. *Journal of Psychoactive Drugs, 26*, 119–128.

Littleton, J. (1995). Acamprosate in acohol dependence: how does it work? *Addiction, 90*, 1179–1188.

Liskow, B. I., & Goodwin, D. W. (1987). Pharmacological treatment of alcohol intoxication, withdrawal and dependence: A critical review. *Journal of Studies on Alcohol, 48*, 356–370.

Litten, R. Z., & Allen, J. P. (1991). Pharmacotherapies for alcoholism: Promising agents and clinical issues. *Alcoholism: Clinical & Experimental Research, 15*(4), 620–633.

Litten, R. Z., Allen, J. P., & Fertig, J. B. (1995). Gamma-glutamyltranspeptidase and carbohydrate deficient transferrin: Alternative measures of excessive alcohol consumption. *Alcoholism: Clinical & Experimental Research, 19*(6), 1541–1546.

Longo, M., Wickes, W., Smout, M., Harrison, S., Cahill, S., & White, J. M. (2010). Randomized controlled trial of dexamphetamine maintenance for the treatment of methamphetamine dependence. *Addiction, 105*(1), 146–154.

Mackie, K. (2008). Cannabinoid receptors: where they are and what they do. *Journal of Neuroendocrinology, Suppl 1*, 10–14.

Martin, W. R. (1976). Naloxone. *Annals of Internal Medicine, 85*, 765–768.

Mason, B. J., Goodman, A. M., Chabac, S., & Lehert, P. (2006). Effect of oral acamprosate on abstinence in patients with alcohol dependence in a double-blind, placebo-controlled trial: the role of patients motivation. *Journal of Psychiatric Research, 40*, 383–393.

Mason, B. J., Kocsis, J. H., Ritvo, E. C., et al. (1996). A double-blind, placebo-controlled trial of desipramine for primary alcohol dependence stratified on the presence or absence of major depression [(see comments)]. *Journal of the American Medical Association, 275*, 761–767.

Mattick, R. P., Breen, C., Kimber, J., & Davoli, M. (2003). Methadone maintenance therapy versus no opioid replacement therapy for opioid dependence. *Cochrane Database Systematic Review, 3*, CD002209.

Mayo-Smith, M. F. (1997). Pharmacological management of alcohol withdrawal. A meta-analysis and evidence-based practice guideline. (1997). American Society of Addiction Medicine working group on pharmacological management of alcohol withdrawal. *Journal of the American Medical Association, 278*, 144.

Mayo-Smith, M. F., Beecher, L. H., Fischer, T. L., et al. (2004). Working group on the management of alcohol withdrawal delirium, practice guidelines committee, American Society of Addiction Medicine. Management of alcohol withdrawal delirium. An evidence-based practice guideline. *Archives of Internal Medicine, 164*, 1405–1412.

McGrath, P. J., Nunes, E. V., Stewart, J. W., et al. (1996). Imipramine treatment of alcoholics with major depression: A placebo controlled clinical trial. *Archives of General Psychiatry, 53*, 232–240.

McIntosh, I. (1982). Alcohol-related disabilities in general hospital patients: A critical assessment of the evidence. *International Journal of Addiction, 17*, 609–639.

McLellan, A. T., Lewis, D. C., O'Brien, C. P., & Kleber, H. D. (2000). Drug dependence, a chronic medical illness: implications for treatment, insurance, and outcome evaluation. *Journal of the American Medical Association, 284*, 1689–1695.

Mee-Lee, D. (Ed.) (2001). *ASAM Patient Placement Criteria for the Treatment of Substance-Related Disorders, Second Edition—Revised*. Mee-Lee, D (Editor-in-Chief): April, 2001.

Mennecier, D., Thomas, M., Arvers, P., Corberand, D., Sinayoko, L., Bonnefoy, S., Harnois, F., Thiolet, C., et al. (2008). Factors predictive of complicated or severe alcohol withdrawal in alcohol dependent inpatients. *Gastroenterologie Clinique et Biologique, 32*, 792–7.

Meyer, R. E. (1992). New pharmacotherapies for cocaine dependence . . . revisited. *Archives of General Psychiatry, 49*, 900–904.

Miller, N. S., Giannin, A. J., Gold, M. S., Philomena, J. A. (1990). Drug testing: Medical, legal, and ethical issues. *Journal of Substance Abuse Treatment, 7*(4), 239–244.

Miller, W., et al., (2003). What works? A summary of treatment outcome research. In R. Hester and & W. Miller (Eds.), *Handbook of alcoholism treatment approaches: Effective alternatives* (3rd ed.) (pp. 13–63). Boston: Allyn & Bacon.

Miller, W. R., & Rollnick, S. (1991). *Motivational interviewing. Preparing people to change addictive behavior*. New York: Guilford Press.

Miller, W. R., Benefield, R. G., & Tonigan, J. S. (1993). Enhancing motivation for change in problem drinking: A controlled comparison of two therapist styles. *Journal of Consulting and Clinical Psychology*ol, *61*, 455–461.

Moyer, A., Finney, J. W., Swearingen, C. E., & Vergun P. (2002). Brief interventions for alcohol problems: a meta-analytic review of controlled investigations in treatment-seeking and non-treatment-seeking populations. *Addiction, 97*, 279.

Nalpas, B., Dabadie, H., Parot, P., et al. (1990). Acamprosate: From pharmacology to therapeutics. *Encephale, 16*, 175–179.

Naranjo, C. A., Kadlac, K. E., Sanhueza, P., et al. (1990). Fluoxetine differentially alters alcohol intake and other consumatory behaviors in problem drinkers. *Clinical Pharmacology & Therapeutics, 47*, 490–498.

National Consensus Development Panel on Effective Medical Treatment of Opiate Addiction (1998). Effective medical treatment of opiate addiction. *Journal of the American Medical Association, 280*, 1936–1943.

Nestler, E. J. (2001). Molecular neurobiology of addiction. *American Journal on Addictions, 10*, 201–217.

New, D. C., & Wong, Y. H. (2003). The ORL1 receptor: molecular pharmacology and signalling mechanisms. *Neurosignals, 11*(4), 197–212.

NIAAA (1995). The physician's guide to helping patients with alcohol problems. NIH Publication No. 95–3769. (revised 1997).

NIAAA (2005). Alcohol Alert, 65: Screening for alcohol use and alcohol-related problems. Available at: http://pubs.niaaa.nih.gov/publications/aa65/AA65.pdf

NIDA (2012). National Institute on Drug Abuse. Principles of drug addiction treatment: A research-based guide (3third edition). NIH Pub Number: 12–4180. Available at: http://www.drugabuse.gov/publications/principles-drug-addiction-treatment

Nunes, E. V., & Levin, F. R. (2004). Treatment of depression in patients with alcohol or other drug dependence: a meta-analysis. *Journal of the American Medical Association, 291*, 1887.

O'Brien, C. P. (2008). A 50-year-old woman addicted to heroin: review of treatment of heroin addiction. *Journal of the American Medical Association, 300*, 314–321.

O'Malley, S. S. (1992). Integration of opioid antagonists and psychosocial therapy in the treatment of narcotic and alcohol dependence. *Journal of Clinical Psychology, 56*(Suppl 7), 30–38.

Oslin, D. W., Berrettini, W., Kranzler, H. R., Pettinati, H., Gelernter, J., Volpicelli, J. R., & O'Brien, C. P. (2003). A functional polymorphism of the mu-opioid receptor gene is associated with naltrexone response in alcohol-dependent patients. *Neuropsychopharmacology, 28*, 1546–1552.

Ozdemir, V., Bremner, K. E., & Naranjo, C. A. (1994). Treatment of alcohol withdrawal syndrome. *Annals of Medicine, 26*(2), 101–105.

Palestine, M. L., & Alatorre, E. (1976). Control of acute alcoholic withdrawal symptoms: A comparative study of haloperidol and chlordiazepoxide. *Current Therapeutic Research, 20*, 289–299.

Patterson, J. F. (1990). Withdrawal from alprazolam using clonazepam: Clinical observations. *Journal of Clinical Psychiatry, 51*(5) (Suppl), 47–49.

Pettinati, H. M., Oslin, D. W., Kampman, K. M., Dundon, W. D., Xie, H., Gallis, T. L., et al. (2010). A double-blind, placebo-controlled trial combining sertraline and naltrexone for treating co-occurring depression and alcohol dependence. *American Journal of Psychiatry, 167*, 668–675.

Pettinati, H. M., Volpicelli, J. R., Kranzler, H. R., Luck, G., Rukstalis, M. R., & Cnaan, A. (2000). Sertraline treatment for alcohol dependence: interactive effects of medication and alcoholic subtype. *Alcohol Clinical & Experimental Research, 24*, 1041–1049.

Pope, H. G., & Katz, D. A. (1988). Affective and psychotic symptoms associated with anabolic steroid use. *American Journal of Psychiatry, 145*, 487–490.

Rappolt, R. T., Gay, G. R., & Inaba, D. (1977). Propranolol: A specific antagonist to cocaine. *Clinical Toxicology, 10*, 265–271.

Regier, D. A., Farmer, M. E., Rae, D. S., Locke, B. Z., Keith, S. J., Judd, L. L., Goodwin, F. K., et al. (1990). Comorbidity of mental disorders with alcohol and other drug abuse: Results from the Epidemiologic Catchment Area (ECA) study. *Journal of the American Medical Association, 264*(19), 2511–2518.

Resnick, R. B., Schuyten-Resnick, E., & Washton, A. M. (1980). Assessment of narcotic antagonists in the treatment of opioid dependence. *Annual Review of Pharmacology & Toxicology, 20*, 463–474.

Robinson, T. E., & Berridge KC. (1993). The neural basis of drug craving: an incentive-sensitization theory of addiction. *Brain Research: Brain Research Reviews, 18*(3), 247–291.

Rounsaville, B. J., Gawin, F. H., & Kleber, H. D. (1985). Interpersonal psychotherapy adapted for ambulatory cocaine users. *American Journal of Drug & Alcohol Abuse, 11*, 171.

Rubio, G., Ponce, G., Rodriguez-Jimenez, R., Jimenez-Arriero, M. A., Hoenicka, J., & Palomo, T. (2005). Clinical predictors of response to naltrexone in alcoholic patients: who benefits most from treatment with naltrexone? *Alcohol and Alcoholism, 40*, 227–233.

Saitz, R., Mayo-Smith, M. F., Roberts, M. S., et al. (1994). Individualized treatment for alcohol withdrawal: A randomized double-blind clinical trial. *Journal of the American Medical Association, 272*, 519–523.

Salaspuro, M. (1995). Biological markers of alcohol consumption. In B. Tabakoff and & P. L. Hoffman (Eds.), *Biological aspects of alcoholism* (pp. 123–162). Seattle, WA: Hogref & Huber.

Samet, J. H., Rollnick, S., & Barnes, H. (1996). Beyond CAGE. A brief clinical approach after detection of substance abuse. *Archives of Internal Medicine, 156*, 2287–2293.

SAMHSA (2009). Cost offset of treatment services. Available at: http://www.samhsa.gov/grants/CSAT-GPRA/general/SAIS_GPRA_CostOffsetSubstanceAbuse.pdf

Sass, H., Soyka, M., Mann, K., et al. (1996). Relapse prevention by acamprosate: Results from a placebo-controlled study on alcohol dependence. *Archives of General Psychiatry, 53*, 673–680.

Saunders, J. B., Aasland O. G., Babor, T. F., de la Fuente, J. R., & Grant, M. (1993). Development of the Alcohol Use Disorders Identification Test (AUDIT): WHO Collaborative project on early detection of persons with harmful alcohol consumption II. *Addiction, 88*, 791–804.

Schulz, D. W., & Macdonald, R. L. (1981). Barbiturate enhancement of GABA-mediated inhibition and activation of chloride channel conductance: Correlation with anticonvulsant and anesthetic actions. *Brain Research, 209*, 177–188.

Schwartz, R. H. (1988). Urine testing in the detection of drugs of abuse. *Archives of Internal Medicine, 148*, 2407–2412.

Seeman, P. (1972). Membrane effects of anesthetics and tranquilizers. *Pharmocology Review, 24*, 583–655.

Sellers, E. M., & Kalant, H. (1976). Drug therapy: Alcohol intoxication and withdrawal. *New England Journal of Medicine, 294*, 757–762.

Sellers, E. M., Cooper, S. D., Zilm, D. H., et al. (1980). Lithium treatment during alcoholic withdrawal. *Clinical Pharmacology & Therapeutics, 20*, 199–206.

Sellers, E. M., Naranjo, C. A., Harrison, M., et al. (1983). Diazepam loading: Simplified treatment for alcohol withdrawal. *Clinical Pharmacology & Therapeutics, 6*, 822–826.

Selzer, M. L. (1971). The Michigan Alcoholism Screening Test: The quest for a new diagnostic instrument. *American Journal of Psychiatry, 127*, 1653–1658.

Senay, E. C. (1985). Methadone maintenance treatment. *International Journal of Addiction, 20*, 803–821.

Shaw, J. M., Kolesar, G. S., Sellers, E. M., et al. (1981). Development of optimal treatment tactics for alcohol withdrawal: Assessment and effectiveness of supportive care. *Journal of Clinical Psychopharmacology, 1*, 382–387.

Skinner, H. A., Holt, S., Schuller, R., et al. (1984). Identification of alcohol abuse using laboratory tests and a history of trauma. *Annals of Internal Medicine, 101*, 847–851.

Skolnick, P., Moncada, V., Barker J., et al. (1981). Pentobarbital: Dual action to increase brain benzodiazepine affinity. *Science, 211*, 1448–1450.

Smothers, B. A., & Yahr, H. T. (2005). Alcohol use disorder and illicit drug use in admissions to general hospitals in the United States. *American Journal of Addiction, 14*(3), 256–267

Smothers, B. A., Yahr, H. T., & Ruhl, C. E. (2004). Detection of alcohol use disorders in general hospital admissions in the United States. *Archives of Internal Medicine, 164*(7), 749–756.

Soyka, M., & Rösner, S. (2010). Nalmefene for treatment of alcohol dependence. *Expert Opinion on Investigational Drugs, 19*(11), 1451–1459.

Srisurapanont, M., & Jarusuraisin, N. (2005). Naltrexone for the treatment of alcoholism: a meta-analysis of randomized controlled trials. *International Journal of Neuropsychopharmacology, 8,* 267–280.

Stein, M. (1990). Medical consequences of intravenous drug abuse. *Journal of General Internal Medicine, 5,* 249–257.

Strain, E. C., Stitzer M. L., Liebson, I. A., & Bigelow, G. E. (1994). Buprenorphine versus methadone in the treatment of opioid-dependent cocaine users. *Psychopharmacology, 116,* 401–406.

Sullivan, J. T., Sykora, K., Schneiderman, J., Naranjo, C. A., & Sellers, E. M. (1989). Assessment of alcohol withdrawal: The revised clinical institute withdrawal assessment for alcohol scale (CIWA-Ar). *British Journal of Addiction, 84*(11), 1353.

Swift, R. M. (1999). Drug therapy for alcohol dependence. *New England Journal of Medicine, 340,* 1482–1490.

Swift, R. M., Griffiths, W., & Camara, P. (1991). Special technical considerations in laboratory testing for illicit drugs. In A. Stoudemire & B. S. Fogel (Eds.), *Medical psychiatric practice* (Vol. 1). Washington, DC: American Psychiatric Association Press.

Takase, S., Takada, A., Tsutsumi, M., et al. (1985). Biochemical markers of chronic alcoholism. *Alcohol, 2,* 405–410.

Tennant, F. S., & Rawson, R. A. (1983). Cocaine and amphetamine dependence treated with desipramine. In L. Harris (Ed.), *Problems of drug dependence* (pp. 351–355), NIDA Monograph Series 43. Rockville, MD: National Institute of Drug Abuse.

Thomas, C., Wallack, S., Swift, R., Bishop, C., McCarty, D., & Simoni-Wastila L. (2003). Research to practice: Adoption of naltrexone in alcoholism treatment. *Journal of Substance Abuse Treatment, 24*(1), 1–11.

Thomson, A. D. (2000). Mechanisms of vitamin deficiency in chronic alcohol misusers and the development of the Wernike-Korsakoff syndrome. *Alcohol and Alcoholism, 35*(Suppl 1), 2–7.

Tsai, G., Gastfriend, D. R., & Coyle, J. T. (1995). The glutamatergic basis of human alcoholism. *American Journal of Psychiatry, 152,* 332–40.

Van Dyke, C., Jatlow, P., Ungerer, J., et al. (1978). Oral cocaine: Plasma concentration and central effects. *Science, 200,* 211–213.

Vocci, F. J., Acri, J., & Elkashef, A. (2005). Medication development for addictive disorders: the state of the science. *American Journal Psychiatry, 162,* 1432–1440.

Volkow, N. D., Fowler, J. S., Wang, G. J., Swanson, J. M., & Telang, F. (2007). Dopamine in drug abuse and addiction: Results of imaging studies and treatment implications. *Archives of Neurology, 64*(11), 1575–1579.

Walker, S., Yesavage, J. A., & Tinklenberg, J. R. (1981). Acute phencyclidine (PCP) intoxication. Quantitative urine levels and clinical management. *American Journal of Psychiatry, 138,* 674–675.

Watson, J. M. (1982). Solvent abuse: Presentation and clinical diagnosis. *Human Toxicology, 1,* 249–256.

Wesson, D. R., & Smith, D. E. (1977). A new method for the treatment of barbiturate dependence. *Journal of the American Medical Association, 231,* 294–295.

Whitfield, C. L., Thompson, G., Lamb, A., et al. (1978). Detoxification of 1024 alcoholic patients without psychoactive drugs. *Journal of the American Medical Association, 239,* 1409–1410.

Wikler, A. (1968). Diagnosis and treatment of drug dependence of the barbiturate type. *American Journal of Psychiatry, 125,* 758–765.

Wise, R., & Bozarth, M. (1987). A psychomotor stimulant theory of addiction. *Psychology Review, 94,* 469–492.

Young, T., Lawson, G. W., & Gacocn, C. B. (1987). Clinical aspects of phencyclidine (PCP). *International Journal of Addiction, 22,* 1–15.

EVALUATING AND MANAGING SUICIDE RISK AND VIOLENCE RISK IN THE MEDICAL SETTING

Phillip M. Kleespies, Douglas H. Hughes, Sarah R. Weintraub, and Ashley S. Hart

INTRODUCTION

In the medical setting, the management of the suicidal or aggressive patient differs in a number of ways from the management of such patients in a psychiatric unit or facility. In a psychiatric unit or hospital, suicidal and aggressive behavior is relatively commonplace, and there are clear levels of observation and guidelines for management. In the medical setting, however, the patients are physically ill, and the staff is focused on their acute medical problems as well as on any potential medical emergencies that might occur. The suicidal or aggressive patient is unusual or atypical, and the staff is not necessarily well trained to manage emotional and behavioral crises or emergencies. This problem is often exacerbated during nights and weekends when the staffing volume tends to be lower than on day shifts during the week.

On a psychiatric unit, there is great emphasis on sensitivity to the patient's emotional needs and reactions. The relationship or alliance with the patient is viewed as crucial. On the other hand, as Kelly, Mufson, and Rogers (1999) have noted, medical units currently use multidisciplinary treatment teams that are organized by specialty, and it is not uncommon to have two or three specialty teams consulting on the same patient. Contacts with the patient are often brief and concerned with specific medical issues, and, at times, it is hard to know who has the primary relationship with the patient and who is in charge. Especially with patients who have serious mental illness, such circumstances may not foster a strong working alliance.

Psychiatric units put a priority on providing a safe physical environment. They are scrutinized for objects or structural features that patients might use in attempts to harm themselves or others. On the other hand, medical wards often have many pieces of equipment in the patient's room that could be wielded as weapons. Some treatments can even offer the patient a means for self-harm, as, for example, with the dialysis patient who could remove an arteriovenous shunt and bleed to death.

Psychiatric units typically have graduated levels of observation and containment that can be tailored to the estimated risk level of the individual patient. As Kelly and colleagues (Kelly et al., 1999) have pointed out, however, options are more limited in a medical setting where the approach to managing aggressive and suicidal behavior is done on an "all or nothing" basis; that is, either restraints and/or constant observation by a "sitter," or management that is no different from that for any other medical patient.

In a medical setting, it is critical that medical practitioners have a strong knowledge base about suicidal or aggressive behavior. More specifically, it is important for staff to recognize that behavioral risk can emerge from at least two sources: (1) from a patient who has a known mental illness but is being treated for a medical condition; and (2) from a patient who has no known mental illness but has a medical illness with an associated risk for suicide or violence.

In this chapter, we attempt to provide a knowledge base for the evaluation and management of suicidal and aggressive behavior, as well as a discussion of how to proceed with evaluating and managing such behavioral crises or emergencies in a medical setting. The chapter is divided into two major components: (1) the evaluation and management of suicide risk in a medical setting; and (2) the evaluation and management of violence risk in a medical setting. Under the first heading, we discuss:

(a) medical illness as an independent risk factor for suicide;

(b) specific medical illnesses with an associated risk of suicide;

(c) a framework for evaluating the acute risk of suicide; and

(d) the management of acute risk of suicide in a medical setting.

Under the second heading, we discuss:

(a) medical illness and the risk of violence;

(b) specific medical illnesses with an associated risk of violence;

(c) a framework for evaluating the acute risk of violence; and

(d) the management of acute risk of violence in a medical setting.

THE EVALUATION AND MANAGEMENT OF SUICIDE RISK IN A MEDICAL SETTING

MEDICAL ILLNESS AS AN INDEPENDENT RISK FACTOR FOR SUICIDE

As reported in detail by Clark and Horton-Deutsch (1992), community-based psychological autopsy studies have consistently found that over 90% of suicides (per official coroner reports) had a mental or emotional disorder. Less well known is the estimate that between 34% and 43% of those who ended their lives by suicide had a medical illness at the time of death (MacKenzie & Popkin, 1990; Whitlock, 1986), and that physical health problems were thought to contribute to suicide in 62% of a sample of elderly suicide victims (Harwood, Hawton, Hope, Harriss, & Jacoby, 2006).

Although mental illness seems more prevalent than physical illness among suicides, the findings above have led to further investigation of whether physical illness might have an independent association with suicide and suicidal behavior, an issue that is clearly significant for those who must assess suicide risk in a medical setting. Using data from a national comorbidity study of late adolescents and adults (ages 15–54), Goodwin, Marusic, and Hoven (2003) examined associations between a self-report checklist of medical illnesses and a question about lifetime suicide attempts. They found significantly increased odds of a suicide attempt with physical illness, even after controlling for demographic characteristics and mental disorders. They also found a linear, dose–response association between the total number of physical illnesses and the likelihood of a suicide attempt. In addition, Ruzicka, Choi, and Sadkowsky (2005), following the introduction of multiple-cause-of-death coding in Australia, reviewed all completed suicides over a five-year period (1997–2001) and compared them with deaths by accident. Their findings confirmed the significant relationship of suicide with mental health problems, but they also indicated that certain physical diseases (most notably HIV and cancer) were significantly associated with suicide. In general, mental disorders were more prevalent than physical illnesses among suicide victims under age 60, while physical illnesses were more prevalent than mental disorders among the suicide victims age 60 and over.

Finally, Waern et al. (2002) and Conwell et al. (2009) did case-control studies to examine the association of suicide with medical illness and psychiatric illness. In both studies, the authors examined samples of individuals who had committed suicide ($n = 85$ and $n = 86$, respectively) with matched living-community samples. In the study by Waern et al. (2002), the data for the suicide group were gathered from interviews with next-of-kin and by record review, while the data for the community sample were gathered directly by interview with control-group participants. In the study by Conwell et al. (2009), the data for both groups were gathered from interviews with next-of-kin and by record review.

The results in both studies supported previous findings of an association between psychiatric illness and suicide, and they also both found that physical illness was a significant, independent risk factor for suicide in the elderly. In the study by Conwell et al., it was also found that perception of deteriorating health status and functional impairment were significant risk factors, with functional impairment being the more robust predictor of suicide.

The findings above, of course, do not necessarily indicate a direct relationship between physical illness and suicidal behavior. As Ruzicka et al. (2005) have noted, the suicide risk associated with certain physical illnesses could be mediated by secondary mood or affective symptoms; or, as suggested by Conwell et al. (2009), perceived health status or functional impairment might also mediate risk. Nonetheless, the emerging data seem to suggest that certain physical illnesses (and particularly the burden of multiple concurrent physical illnesses in the elderly) warrant inclusion as risk factors for suicide.

Pertinent to this conclusion, it is noteworthy that in Oregon, assisted suicide for the terminally ill is legal under the Oregon Death with Dignity Act (ODDA). Of those people who have used the ODDA, 80.8% have had cancer. Under the ODDA, physicians are required to refer patients for psychiatric or psychological evaluation if their judgement is considered to be impaired by virtue of a mental disorder; yet, only 7.5% of patients using the Act have been referred (Oregon Public Health Services, 2011). These data suggest that most of these individuals with a terminal illness either did not have a mental disorder, or, if some proportion of them did, it did not seem to significantly impair their decision-making capacity for choosing an assisted death.

SPECIFIC MEDICAL ILLNESSES WITH AN ASSOCIATED RISK OF SUICIDE

There are a great many medical illnesses and conditions, and most of them, as single diseases or injuries, have no known associated risk of suicide (Harris & Barraclough, 1994). There is evidence, however, that a few specific illnesses or conditions are associated with an elevated risk (see Table 39.1 for a listing of illnesses or conditions and the factors that may lead to increased risk within each illness or condition). In terms of risk and specific illnesses, the evidence presented below is based, primarily, on large register linkage studies and meta-analytic reviews. If a particular illness or condition is not mentioned, it does not mean that there is no suicide risk associated with it, but only that we did not detect any large, trustworthy studies that would support its inclusion here.

HIV/AIDS

HIV/AIDS has long been associated with increased risk of suicide. In their frequently cited review of studies from 1966–1992, Harris and Barraclough (1994) found that the relative risk of suicide for men with HIV was seven times

Table 39.1 MEDICAL ILLNESSES/CONDITIONS AND INCREASED RISK OF SUICIDE

ILLNESS/CONDITION[*]	INCREASED RISK	SELECTED REFERENCES
HIV/AIDS	With progression of disease	Lu et al. (2006) Keiser et al. (2010)
Cancer	First 1–2 months post-hospital discharge First year after diagnosis	Lin, Wu, & Lee (2009) Ahn et al. (2010)
End-Stage Renal Disease	Age > 60 for dialysis patients First 16 months after transplant	Kurella et al. (2005) Ojo et al. (2000)
Epilepsy	Female gender Chronic epilepsy Comorbid depression	Christensen et al. (2007) Mainio et al. (2007)
Stroke	Age < 50 First 5 years after stroke History of prior stroke Pre-stroke depression	Teasdale & Engberg (2001a) Forsstrom et al. (2010)
Traumatic Brain Injury	Cerebral contusions or intracranial hemorrhage	Teasdale & Engberg (2001b) Harrison-Felix et al. (2009)
Multiple Sclerosis	First year after diagnosis Male and age < 40 Comorbid depression	Bronnum-Hansen et al. (2005) Fredrikson et al. (2003) Beiske et al. (2008)
Huntington's Disease	Anticipation of diagnosis Predictive test result Stage 2–decrease in independent functioning Comorbid depression	Larsson et al. (2006) Almqvist et al. (1999) Lipe et al. (1993)
Spinal Cord Injury	2–5 years post-injury Post-injury despondency Experiences of helplessness and feelings of shame	Soden et al. (2000) Charlfue & Gerhardt (1991)

[*]This listing of medical illnesses and conditions with associated suicide risk is not intended as an exhaustive list of medical illnesses and conditions with an associated suicide risk.

higher than the rate for men in the general population. With the introduction in 1996 of improved treatments such as highly active antiretroviral therapy (HAART), however, the level of risk may have been modified.

A review of the literature on the impact of HAART on suicide risk suggests that the evidence is mixed, with recent register linkage studies and meta-analytic reviews linking HAART to both an increase (Lu et al. 2006; Krentz, Kliewer, & Gill, 2005) and a decrease (Keiser et al., 2010; Komiti et al., 2001; Rice, Smith, & Delpech, 2010) in the incidence of suicide. Researchers who found a decrease in incidence linked this reduced suicide risk to "HAART-related improvements in disease status" (Keiser et al., 2010, p. 4). Those who found an increase in incidence attributed it in part to the difficult side effects of lifelong treatment with HAART, including mood disorders and other conditions, that impair quality of life (Carrico et al., 2007).

As Komiti et al. (2001) have noted, the psychological impact of improved medical treatments may be complex. For example, it is possible that cultural differences could account for the mixed findings. Indeed, the findings cited involve participants in Great Britain, Switzerland, Australia, Canada, and Taiwan, where differences in availability of and approach to health care, as well as community attitudes about HIV/AIDS, might affect the impact of new medical treatments on suicide risk.

The heightened incidence of suicide among people living with HIV/AIDS, of course, has also been linked to stigma, discrimination, and social isolation, as well as to mental health problems, including anxiety, depression, and substance abuse (Komiti et al., 2001; Mahajan et al., 2008). In the study by Keiser et al. (2010), the results of a survey of the infectious-disease staff involved with the care of the study patients who committed suicide suggested that, in the staff's opinion, the most common reason for the patients' suicides was the progression of the HIV infection followed by psychosocial problems. This finding suggests that clinicians may need to exercise greater caution about suicide in the HIV/AIDS population as the disease progresses.

Although the causes may be multiple, it is clear that the evidence converges on the conclusion that HIV/AIDS continues to be a risk factor for suicide, although the risk may be diminished since the introduction of treatments such as HAART.

Cancer

Large cohort studies linking national cancer and death registries for the past several decades have revealed significantly higher suicide rates among cancer patients than in the general population (Ahn et al., 2010; Kleespies, Hough, & Romeo, 2009). In the United States, for example, the incidence of suicide among more than 3.5 million patients diagnosed with cancer between 1973 and 2002 was nearly twice the rate in the general U.S. population (Standardized Mortality Ratio [SMR] = 1.88; Misono, Weiss, Fann, Redman, & Yueh, 2008). Similar to gender differences in suicide in the general U.S. population, the frequency of completed suicides for female cancer patients has been found to be one-fifth that of males, with a hazard ratio of 6.2 for male suicide relative to female suicide (Kendal, 2007).

Research has also pointed to an association between cancer-related suicide and age at diagnosis. In a case-control study of suicide risk associated with medical illness among New Jersey residents age 65 and older, cancer was the only medical condition that remained associated with suicide in adjusted analyses that accounted for psychiatric illness and the risk of dying within a year (Miller, Mogun, Azrael, Hempstead, & Solomon, 2008). In addition, Misono and colleagues (2008) documented higher rates of suicide with increasing age at cancer diagnosis among men. An examination of suicide rates by age at cancer diagnosis revealed that the highest SMR of 2.51 occurred for male and female patients in the uppermost age bracket of 85 years and older.

Two periods of heightened risk of committing suicide have been identified for cancer patients—one being shortly after discharge from the hospital. Lin, Wu, and Lee (2009) examined suicides occurring within three months of hospital discharge among cancer patients in Taiwan during the period of 2002–2004. Almost half (46.3%) of the post-discharge suicides occurred within 14 days, and approximately 60% of suicides occurred within the first month after discharge. The mean interval from discharge to suicide was 39.7 days.

The second period of elevated cancer-related suicide risk was the year following diagnosis. Ahn et al. (2010) and Robinson, Renshaw, Okello, Moller, and Davies (2009) reported a downward trend in relative risk of suicide with increasing time since cancer diagnosis, with the greatest risk occurring in the first year after diagnosis for both men and women (SMRs = 2.42 and 1.44, respectively). An increased risk of suicide within one year post-diagnosis has been repeatedly documented for prostate cancer patients. Among men in the United States diagnosed with prostate cancer from 1979–2004, the risk of suicide was elevated during the first year (SMR = 1.4), and especially during the first three months after diagnosis (SMR = 1.9; Fang et al., 2010).

Evidence indicates that poor prognosis and cancer stage at diagnosis confer additional risk of suicide. In a study by Dormer and colleagues (2008), specific types of cancer were grouped according to prognosis (i.e., five-year relative survival rates), and the very high SMR of 12.07 occurred for the poor-prognosis group in the first three months after diagnosis. Similarly, Robinson et al. (2009) found that cancers with high fatality carried a higher risk of suicide in both men (SMR = 2.67) and women (SMR = 2.17) compared to cancers with low fatality. Several studies have also found that suicide risk is related to cancer stage at diagnosis. Rates of suicide have been noted to be higher for patients in the United States with advanced disease at diagnosis (Misono et al., 2008). For example, data indicate that risk of suicide is elevated for metastatic disease at diagnosis (Kendal, 2007), particularly for prostate cancer (Fang et al., 2010). Kendal (2007) also found that cancer-directed surgery that could not be carried out (for head and neck cancers), high-grade tumors, and treatment contraindications all were associated with elevated suicide risk. Examining suicide rates across various types of cancer, Robinson and colleagues (2009) reported a strong effect of advanced stage of disease in women.

These findings suggest that varying rates of suicide across cancer sites may be explained at least in part by variations in associated survival rates. However, it is notable that even when the likelihood of survival is high, cancer is still associated with increased suicide risk relative to the general population (Christensen, Yousaf, Engholm, & Storm, 2006).

End-Stage Renal Disease

As Levy (2000) has pointed out, there are many stresses and losses associated with end-stage renal disease (ESRD) and with renal dialysis. Functional limitations typically lead to a loss of employment, a loss of income, and potentially a loss of one's role in the family. There can be a loss of sexual function and a fear of death, as the patient must rely on a life-sustaining treatment. With hemodialysis, patients become dependent on the dialysis machine and the dialysis staff. The routine of being dialyzed several times a week can become tedious. Continuous ambulatory peritoneal dialysis (CAPD), which can be performed at home, can reduce feelings of dependency, but the patient must observe the scrupulous antiseptic technique that is needed to avoid infections. Regardless of the dialysis technique, the individual needs to adhere to a low-phosphate, low-potassium, low-sodium, and restricted fluid intake diet. These stressors can make the patient more vulnerable to demoralization and possibly depression. Under such conditions, it is not surprising that suicide risk may be increased.

Bostwick and Cohen (2009), however, have contended that, by current standards, the suicide rate for ESRD patients may have been somewhat inflated in years past. They base their argument on the fact that ethical thought about the rights of patients to refuse life-sustaining medical treatment (LSMT) has markedly shifted over the past 30–35 years in the direction of respecting the autonomous choices of the patient. Thus, in the more paternalistic healthcare system of the past, an ESRD patient's refusal of, or request to discontinue, renal dialysis may have been more likely to be viewed as a suicidal act; while in the current U.S. healthcare system, competent patients are seen as having the right to refuse any LSMT, renal dialysis included, that they find invasive and not in keeping with personal control of their body. Death under such circumstances is typically not considered a suicide.

Be that as it may, there nonetheless appears to be a moderately elevated rate of suicide among ESRD patients in the United States. In a large study, a total of 465,563 patients who initiated dialysis between 1995 and 2000 and were registered in the United States Renal Data System (USRDS) were linked to the ESRD Death Notification Form register (Kurella, Kimmel, Young, & Chertow, 2005). The ESRD Death Notification Form makes a distinction between those who decide to withdraw from dialysis before death, and those who commit suicide. Having made this distinction, the investigators nonetheless found a suicide incidence ratio of 1.84, indicating that the ESRD patients had a suicide rate that was 84% higher than the rate for the general population, even after accounting for demographic differences.

The rates of suicide among renal dialysis patients in the study by Kurella et al. (2005) tended to increase with age, with those 60 and over having the highest rates. There appears to be a somewhat different picture, however, with renal disease patients who have received a kidney transplant. Ojo et al. (2000) took a sample of 86,502 kidney transplant patients who were registered with the United Network for Organ Sharing or with USRDS between 1988 and 1997, and linked them with cause-of-death information from a transplant recipient follow-up form and with the ESRD Death Notification Form. They found an elevated rate of suicide for transplant patients (15.7 per 100,000 persons a year) relative to the general population rate (9 per 100,000 persons a year). Interestingly, 35% of the suicides occurred in the first 12 months after the transplant, and 16 months was the median time from transplantation to suicide. The mean age of the sample was 39 years, suggesting a higher risk of suicide at a younger age for transplant patients relative to the dialysis patients in the Kurella et al. study. The reason(s) for this apparent age difference are as yet undetermined.

Epilepsy

Increased rates of depression and suicidality among patients with epilepsy are well documented. In one study, a history of major depression was found to be almost two times as common in patients with seizures compared to those without seizures, and a history of a suicide attempt was five times as common (Hesdorffer, Hauser, Olafsson, Ludvigsson, & Kjartansson, 2006). In one meta-analysis, suicide was found to be the cause of death for up to 13.5% of all patients with epilepsy (Pompili, Girardi, & Tatarelli, 2006).

Recent population-based studies have explored the heightened risk of suicide among patients with epilepsy,

pointing out the role of comorbid psychiatric disease, seizure status and disease progression, and demographic variables in moderating suicide risk (e.g., Christensen, Vestergaard, Mortensen, Sidenius, & Agerbo, 2007; Mainio, Alamaki, Karvonen, Hakko, Sarkioja, & Rasanen, 2007). Christensen et al. (2007) found that patients with epilepsy had a risk of suicide that was three times higher than matched controls. They also found that the relationship among epilepsy, psychiatric diagnosis, and suicide was stronger in women compared to men.

Using another population-based sample, in northern Finland, Mainio et al. (2007) examined suicide among multiple populations (n = 1877) from 1988 to 2002. They found that the percentage of previous suicide attempts among suicide victims with epilepsy was double that of people without epilepsy. In general, suicide victims with epilepsy were older, were more likely to have suffered from depression, and were more often female. It should be noted that it is unusual to find a population in which women have more suicides than men. The factors that may contribute to such a finding with epilepsy patients have not yet been investigated. Disease status also influenced risk of suicide, with a heightened risk of suicide occurring among patients with chronic epilepsy.

Another line of research has explored the relationship between anti-epileptic drug use (AEDS) and the heightened risk of suicide among epilepsy patients (Bell & Sander, 2009). Research findings gathered by pharmaceutical companies, which used placebo-controlled trials of 11 different AEDs, determined that the odds ratio for suicidal ideation or behavior was significantly increased among patients taking AEDs for epilepsy, but not among patients taking AEDS for psychiatric or other medical problems. A recent, large, case control study in Great Britain, however, found a significant relationship between AEDs and suicide-related events when AEDs were used with patients with depression (Arana, Wentworth, Ayuso-Mateos, & Arellano, 2010). Which patients (i.e., those with epilepsy or those with psychiatric disorders) have an associated risk of suicidality when using AEDs has therefore not been settled. Nonetheless, the clinician should be aware that the U.S. Food and Drug Administration (FDA) issued a warning about AEDs and suicidality in 2008 (US FDA, 2008).

Stroke

Patients with stroke have also been shown to have an increased risk of suicide. Teasdale and Engberg (2001a) identified 114,098 stroke patients discharged alive from the hospital between 1979 and 1993 and screened this cohort in Denmark's national death register over the same time period. The suicide rate was nearly doubled for stroke patients, with SMRs of 1.88 and 1.78 for men and women, respectively. Suicide risk was greatest for patients under 50 years of age (SMR = 2.85) and was smallest for patients 80 years of age or older (SMR = 1.3). The rate of suicide was also greater for patients with a shorter duration of hospitalization (i.e., less than two weeks versus more than three months; SMR = 2.32). Survival analysis indicated that the risk for suicide is greatest up to five years after a stroke.

Data indicate that depression and a history of prior stroke are risk factors for suicide following stroke. Pre-stroke depression more than doubled the risk of suicide relative to an absence of lifetime depression (Forsström, Hakko, Nordström, Räsänen, & Mainio, 2010).

Traumatic Brain Injury

Several studies have found a heightened risk of psychiatric disorders (notably major depression, panic disorder, obsessive-compulsive disorder, substance abuse) and an increased risk of suicidal ideation and suicide attempts in patients with traumatic brain injury (TBI) (e.g., Silver, Kramer, Greenwald, & Weissman, 2001; Simpson & Tate, 2002). Teasdale and Engberg (2001b) conducted a seminal study in Denmark focusing on TBI and risk of completed suicide. These investigators selected patients on a national register of hospital admissions from 1979 to 1993 for three types of traumatic brain injuries: concussion ($n = 126,114$), cranial fracture ($n = 7560$), and cerebral contusion or traumatic intracranial hemorrhage ($n = 11,766$). They then linked these lists of patients to a national register of deaths for the same period. Relative to the general population, the incidence of completed suicide was increased for all three groups with SMRs stratified by sex and age that equaled 3.0, 2.7, and 4.1, respectively. Using regression analyses for proportional hazards, patients with more serious brain injuries such as cerebral contusions or intracranial hemorrhages were found to have significantly greater risk of suicide than patients with concussions and cranial fractures,. It is worthy of note, however, that even patients with no more than a concussion or a cranial fracture had an increased risk for suicide.

In a more recent U.S.-based study of mortality after traumatic brain injury, Harrison-Felix et al. (2009) have presented evidence supportive of an increased risk of suicide in TBI patients. These investigators linked all patients admitted to a rehabilitation hospital over a 40-year span ($n = 1,678$) to the Social Security Administration's Death Index. They found that TBI patients in their sample had an estimated average life expectancy reduction of four years overall and were three times more likely to commit suicide than people in the general population of similar age, sex, and race.

The causes of the increased risk of suicide in patients with TBI are likely to be complex and may include cognitive, psychosocial, emotional, and neurobiological changes. In the clinical setting, it is important to remain aware of the risk, particularly among those with a more serious TBI.

Multiple Sclerosis

Multiple sclerosis (MS) is a chronic disease of the central nervous system that involves cognitive, motor, and sensory impairments. MS often leads to problems of living (e.g., financial difficulties, disruption in family life), in addition to significant emotional distress, including anxiety and depression (Gay et al., 2010). According to meta-analyses conducted in the 1990s (e.g., Harris & Barraclough, 1994, Stenager & Stenager, 1992), patients with MS appeared to have a suicide rate that was twice that of the general population. This finding has been confirmed in more recent record-linkage studies in Denmark and Sweden.

In Denmark, for example, Bronnum-Hansen, Stenager, Stenager, and Koch-Henriksen (2005) linked the Danish Multiple Sclerosis Registry, consisting of more than 10,000 patients, and Cause of Death Registry over the period from 1953 to 1996. They found that the SMR for suicide indicated that the risk for patients with MS was more than twice that for the general population (SMR = 2.12). The increased risk was particularly high in the first year after diagnosis (SMR = 3.15), but it also remained elevated for more than 20 years after diagnosis.

In Sweden, investigators linked all 12,284 cases of MS in the Swedish Hospital Inpatient Register during the period from 1969–1996 with the Swedish Cause of Death Register (Fredrikson, Cheng, Jiang, & Wasserman, 2003). Suicide risk of patients with MS was again found to be more than twice that of the general population (SMR = 2.3). As in the Danish study, suicide risk was particularly high in the first year after diagnosis. In this study, however, a gender difference was noted; the elevation in risk seemed to be greatest in young men (below age 40), while the risk for women was greatest for those between ages 30 and 59.

Studies have repeatedly found high rates of depression in patients with MS, with lifetime prevalence estimated in the range of 40–60% (e.g., Beiske, Svennson, Sandanger et al., 2008). Depression in MS patients often goes unrecognized and untreated (McGuigan & Hutchinson, 2006). Given that it is the mental disorder most frequently found among those who complete suicide, it seems critical that practitioners detect and treat symptoms of depression in these patients, particularly in the year following diagnosis. It should be noted, however, that not all suicides among individuals with MS occur in the context of a depressive episode. Other factors (e.g., decreased quality of life, decreased ability to participate in meaningful activity, loss of self-determination and control) may also be implicated (Williams et al., 2005).

Huntington's Disease

Research has revealed an elevated risk of suicide in relation to Huntington's disease (HD), a hereditary and progressive neurodegenerative disorder (see review in Kleespies, Hough, & Romeo, 2009). Additional studies have supported this linkage. Baliko, Csala, and Czopf (2004) found that, in the period from 1920–1997, suicide accounted for 10% of deaths among 96 Hungarian families with HD and occurred at a higher rate than in the general population of Hungary.

Studies have examined the psychosocial impact of gaining knowledge about one's genetic status as a result of predictive testing for HD. In a worldwide study of 4,527 HD test participants, Almqvist, Bloch, Brinkman, Craufurd, and Hayden (1999) found that the majority of individuals (84%) who experienced an adverse event—suicide, suicide attempt, or psychiatric hospitalization—had received a predictive testing result indicating increased risk of HD. Most individuals in the increased-risk group (62%) experienced an adverse event within the first year after receiving the result, and most (65%) were symptomatic at the time of the event.

Data also point to an elevated risk of suicide during the period leading up to predictive testing for HD among individuals at risk for the disease (Robins Wahlin et al., 2000; Larsson, Luszcz, Bui, and Robins Wahlin, 2006). The findings are consistent with previous work indicating that the two critical periods of elevated risk for suicide in HD are just before a formal diagnosis is received, and in Stage 2 of the disease, when independent functioning diminishes (see Kleespies et al., 2009).

A few studies have identified factors associated with increased risk of suicide in HD. A retrospective case-controlled study of instances of suicide in HD revealed that, among a variety of clinical and social variables, having no children was the most important risk factor and had an odds ratio of 13.6 (Lipe, Schultz, & Bird, 1993). In the study by Almqvist and colleagues (1999), both employment status and psychiatric history within the five years leading up to testing were significantly related to the frequency of an adverse event following predictive testing for HD; and age, gender, and marital status did not influence the likelihood of an event. Furthermore, in a recent prospective study of patients with prodromal HD, Fiedorowicz, Mills, Ruggle, Langbehn, and Paulsen (2011) found that a history of suicide attempts and the presence of depression were strongly predictive of suicidal behavior in these patients versus a control group.

Spinal Cord Injury or Disorder

Spinal cord injury or disorder (SCI/D) can cause complications and dysfunction in several organ systems leading to decreased survival or longevity. SCI/D patients often die from secondary illnesses such as pneumonia, septicemia, pulmonary emboli, or stroke. Over the past three or four decades, however, improvements in early care and in rehabilitation have led to an increased life expectancy that approaches 70% of normal for those with complete quadriplegia and 86% of normal for those with complete paraplegia. Yet, during this same time period, a study in Australia found that the death rate by suicide had reportedly trebled from an SMR of 2.5 before 1980 to an SMR of 8.7 since 1980 (Soden et al., 2000). The reasons for this increase are undetermined but may involve psychosocial issues that affect the quality of life and the mental health of SCI/D patients.

A recent register-linkage study in Norway that combined deaths by suicide and accidental poisoning (Hagen,

Lie, Rekand, Gilhus, & Gronning, 2010; SMR = 5.79) has confirmed findings in previous studies of an elevated rate of suicide for patients with traumatic spinal cord injury. Some have hypothesized that the elevated rate may, in part, be a function of heightened rates of mood disorder and substance abuse disorder in the SCI/D population. It is not uncommon for alcohol or drug intoxication to be involved in accidents that result in spinal cord injuries. Moreover, suicide attempts by individuals who are depressed and/or abusing alcohol or drugs can lead to spinal cord injuries. With regard to the latter, estimates of spinal cord injuries that result from suicide attempts have been modest; that is, in the range of 1.6–6.8% (see, e.g., Stanford, Soden, Bartrop, Mikk, & Taylor, 2007). Stanford et al. found that approximately 8% of the SCI/D patients in their study who had sustained their SCI/D in a prior suicide attempt eventually committed suicide. Relative to rates of suicide for the general population, this finding suggests that these patients constitute a high-risk group.

Suicide risk among patients with SCI/D tends to be greatest in the first two to five years after the injury (Soden et al., 2000). In a study of 5,200 individuals with SCI/D covering a 30-year period, Charlifue and Gerhart (1991) found that, of those who died by suicide, 50% did so within three years of SCI/D onset, and 76% did so within four years. Factors that distinguished suicides from matched non-suicidal people with SCI/D included (1) post-injury despondency, (2) experiences of helplessness and feelings of shame, and (3) pre-injury family fragmentation.

A FRAMEWORK FOR EVALUATING PATIENTS AT RISK FOR SUICIDE

A frequently used framework for evaluating patients at high risk for suicide has been described by Rudd, Joiner, and Rajab (2001). In this framework, the clinician examines the patient for predisposing or distal risk factors, acute or proximal risk factors, and protective factors. Distal risk factors form the background from which suicidal behavior can emerge. They contribute to what makes an individual vulnerable when proximal risk factors occur. Proximal risk factors, on the other hand, tend to be precipitating events that are closer in time to the occurrence of the behavior. In most circumstances, they are not sufficient to fully explain the occurrence, but, in combination with a significant set of distal risk factors, they can interact to create the conditions needed for these behaviors to occur. Protective factors are conditions or characteristics that, if present, may attenuate the risk of life-threatening behaviors, but, if absent or diminished, may make such behaviors more likely. Research on protective factors has unfortunately been under-developed.

The degree of risk for suicide can be estimated, ranging from minimal to severe, by weighing these three types of factors. An individual at minimal risk for life-threatening behavior might have no known distal risk factors or proximal risk factors and multiple protective factors. Someone at moderate risk, however, might have some distal and proximal risk factors, and some protective factors that are beginning to weaken. Those at serious or severe risk might have multiple distal and proximal risk factors and essentially lack protective factors.

In the section that follows, we will use this framework in presenting factors to consider in a mental health or psychiatric evaluation of suicide risk. Those who work in a medical setting should, of course, also consider the risk factors related to medical illness (as presented above) in any effort to weigh the level of risk in the medically ill.

EVALUATING FOR THE ACUTE RISK OF SUICIDE

In this subsection, some of the major risk and protective factors for suicide that have empirical support in the research literature are presented. Given space limitations, it is not an exhaustive review.

Distal Risk Factors

Demographic Factors

By age group, the elderly (ages 75–84) have typically had the highest rate of suicide in America. Although the annual incidence of suicide for the elderly remains high, the suicide rate for the middle-aged (ages 45–54) has exceeded that of the elderly since 2006. The most recent national statistics indicate that, in 2010, the incidence of suicide for the middle aged (ages 45–54) was 19.6/100,000/year versus 15.7/100,000/year for the elderly (U.S.A. Suicide: 2010 Official Final Data, 2012). Youth suicide (ages 15–24 and 25–34) rose through the 1980s and early 1990s, then seemed to peak in the mid-90s, decline, and plateau. In terms of gender, men are approximately four times more likely than women to complete suicide, while women are approximately three times more likely than men to engage in non-fatal suicidal behavior. By race or ethnicity, whites typically have a suicide rate that is two to three times higher than that of African-Americans, and white males account for approximately 70% of all suicides in the United States. Socioeconomic status is not a strong predictor of suicide.

Serious Mental Illness

Literature reviews have summarized findings from a number of psychological autopsy studies indicating that over 90% of adults and adolescents who commit suicide have a history of a psychiatric disorder (Kleespies & Dettmer, 2000; Miller & Emanuele, 2009; Sullivan & Bongar, 2009). Mental illness is clearly a distal risk factor for suicide. Some mental illnesses can be both distal and proximal risk factors, such as when there is an acute exacerbation of depression in a patient with a history of chronic or recurrent depression. The literature reviews noted above have identified affective disorders, alcohol abuse, and schizophrenia as diagnoses most commonly found among those who commit suicide. It is estimated that 80–85% of adults who commit suicide have one of these diagnoses in their history, and many have comorbid conditions. Combat-related post-traumatic stress disorder (PTSD), bipolar II disorder, and borderline personality disorder have also been found to have an elevated risk

of suicide (Bullman & Kang, 1994; Rihmer & Kiss, 2002; Duberstein & Witte, 2009).

Family-Related Factors

There is considerable evidence of a familial and probably a genetic contribution to the risk of suicide (Brent, Bridge, Johnson, & Connolly, 1996; Mann & Arango, 1999; Moscicki, 1997: Roy, Nielsen, Rylander, & Sarchiapone, 2000). A genetic contribution may be indirect, in that some of the psychiatric disorders associated with a heightened risk of suicide (e.g., major depression and schizophrenia) have been found to have a genetic loading in their etiology. On the other hand, evidence in studies with monozygotic and dizygotic twin pairs and in adoption studies supports the hypothesis that, after controlling for psychopathology (including depression), there may be an independent genetic loading for suicidal behavior (Roy et al., 2000). Moreover, a now-classic study of the Old Order Amish of Lancaster County in Pennsylvania (Egeland & Sussex, 1985) found that certain family pedigrees had a heavy loading for affective disorders and suicide, while other family pedigrees had a heavy loading only for affective disorders but not for suicide. The investigators concluded that their findings indicated that there is an increased risk of suicide for patients with a diagnosis of major affective disorder and a strong family history of suicide.

Although there may be a genetic contribution to some suicides, most investigators continue to agree that suicide is typically a multi-determined act with psychological, social, and biological factors involved. Thus, families of suicidal individuals have been found to exhibit poor communication and problem-solving skills (McLean & Taylor, 1994). Moreover, it is possible that, in some cases, suicidal behavior may be a learned strategy for communicating with family members or coping with difficult situations. With adolescents, poor parent–child communication and negative family interactions have been identified as risk factors (King, Segal, Naylor, & Evans, 1993).

Proximal Risk Factors

Acute Risk Factors Within High-Risk Diagnoses

Most patients with high-risk diagnoses do not commit suicide. The question then becomes what acute risk factors within these diagnoses might differentiate those who are at high risk for suicide.

Fawcett et al. (1987), in a multi-site prospective study, identified several symptoms that heighten the risk of suicide for those with an affective disorder. They include severe anhedonia, global insomnia, severe anxiety (and/or panic), obsessive-compulsive features, and active alcohol abuse. Whether the patient is reporting suicidal ideation or not, the clinician would do well to exercise caution when the patient is depressed and presents with some or all of these symptoms. Among individuals with schizophrenia, prospective studies have found suicide risk is most associated with feelings of hopelessness, depression, obsessive-compulsive features, paranoid ideation, and subjective distress (Cohen, Test, & Brown, 1990; Peuskens et al., 1997). Risk is greatest for male schizophrenic patients under age 40, particularly when these patients are not acutely psychotic, have a heightened awareness of the debilitating effects of their illness, and become depressed.

Among individuals with alcohol use disorder, retrospective studies examining risk factors for suicide have suggested that comorbid depression and the recent loss of a significant relationship are acute risk factors (Murphy, 1992). Suicide among patients with alcohol problems is generally more likely in mid-life and following a prolonged history of alcohol abuse and dependence. It is most likely to occur during an active phase of drinking. Increased risk of suicidal behavior and/or suicide has also been reported among inhalant users (Howard et al., 2010), heroin users (Darke & Ross, 2002), and cocaine users (Marzuk et al., 1992). Little is known about factors associated with the use of these substances that may increase risk. Borges, Walters, and Kessler (2000) found that the major risk of suicidal behavior was linked to the current use of these substances rather than to a history of use or abuse. They also found that polysubstance use was more important than a particular, single substance in predicting first suicide attempts.

Hopelessness

Hopelessness has been defined as a state of negative expectancies about the future (Weishaar & Beck, 1992). As a construct and a risk factor for suicide, it has been most intensively studied by Aaron Beck and his colleagues. In Beck's studies, hopelessness has been found to be more strongly related to suicidal intent than depression for both suicide ideators and suicide attempters. In a study of depressed and non-depressed schizophrenic patients, it was found that even non-depressed patients who had high levels of hopelessness had high levels of suicidal intent. In prospective studies, hopelessness has been strongly supported as a risk factor for completed suicide (see, e.g., Beck, Brown, Berchick, Stewart, & Steer, 1990; Fawcett et al., 1987). Hopelessness may be a factor to consider with patients who are suffering from serious medical illness or multiple medical illnesses or who have been given bad news about prognosis.

Protective Factors

As mentioned earlier, protective factors, when present, attenuate risk and increase resilience. When one is assessing risk, they are important parts of the equation used to determine the level or degree of risk. Although the research on protective factors is less developed than research on risk factors, several factors have received some empirical support.

Family Relationships

Positive family relationships appear to offer significant protection against suicidal ideation and behavior. Being married or in a committed relationship and having children under age 18 living in the home have been found to reduce suicide risk (Lester, 1987; Fawcett et al., 1987). With adolescents in particular, family connectedness and cohesion have been found to be strong protective factors that lower the risk of suicidal

ideation and behavior (Resnick et al., 1997; Rubenstein, Heeren, Housman, Rubin, & Stechler, 1989).

Social Support Outside of the Family

Friendships have been found to be protective for both adults and adolescents. Also, there is some evidence that religious commitment or membership in a church or temple reduces the risk of suicide (Stack, 1994). While having a few close friends is important for adults, acceptance and integration into a social group or a sense of connectedness to school have been found to be protective against suicide in adolescents (Resnick et al., 1997; Rubenstein et al., 1989).

Reasons for Living

It seems intuitive that having a sense of purpose and meaning in life would be protective against suicide. Linehan, Goodstein, Nielsen, and Chiles (1983) developed a scale to assess reasons for living (e.g., responsibility toward family and children, moral objections to suicide, fears of social disapproval, and pain involved in suicide). Subsequent studies have supported the assertion that such reasons for living or beliefs differentiate individuals with and without suicidal ideation and serve as protective factors against suicidal behavior in adolescents and adults (Gutierrez et al., 2002; Jobes & Mann, 1999). Other studies have identified additional protective factors such as hopefulness, spiritual well-being, and employment (Stack, 2000).

MANAGING THE ACUTE RISK OF SUICIDE

Both the inpatient medical setting and the outpatient medical setting present challenges for managing suicide risk. In this regard, it can be helpful for the clinician to think not only in terms of distal and proximal risk factors, but also in terms of static and dynamic risk factors. Often, proximal risk factors are dynamic and changeable. If the clinician can intervene to improve dynamic risk factors and/or strengthen protective factors, he or she may lessen the risk level.

In the Medical Inpatient Setting

Physicians generally under-treat emotional or mental conditions in the medically ill. Yet, there is evidence from a Swedish study (Rutz, von Knorring, & Walinder, 1989) that educating physicians about the diagnosis and treatment of affective disorders can lead to a significant improvement in the identification and treatment of depression and to an apparent reduction in the suicide rate. Having a staff that is informed and aware that certain medical conditions have an elevated risk for suicide and that psychiatric patients with particular diagnoses can be at heightened risk is an excellent starting point for managing suicide risk in the inpatient and outpatient medical setting. Awareness can be heightened by in-service presentations from the psychiatry or mental health service. Beyond awareness, however, it is important to ask patients how they are coping emotionally with their medical problems. If a patient has been given bad news, for example, a subsequent inquiry might include asking whether he or she is feeling discouraged, depressed, hopeless, or like giving up. Questions about thoughts of ending his or her life might follow.

If these inquiries reveal that the patient is having difficulty coping or has thoughts of wanting to end his or her life, a consultation with the psychiatry consultation/liaison (c/l) team should be initiated. The psychiatry c/l team will assess the patient's emotional and mental condition, including his or her level of suicide risk. If the patient were to be considered at imminent risk (i.e., might harm him- or herself in next few minutes, hours, or days), a "sitter" might be assigned to be with the patient at all times until the crisis has passed. The sitter, of course, would notify staff if the patient were to make efforts to actively harm him- or herself or if he or she were to attempt to leave the hospital. If the patient made active efforts at self-harm or elopement, leather restraints might be necessary to prevent self-destructive efforts. Sedating medication to calm an agitated patient can also be helpful. Staff need to be aware, however, that antidepressant medication can take weeks to have an effect on mood and will not provide any rapid relief for a patient during a short hospital stay.

Unfortunately, as noted earlier in this chapter, the patient who is not considered at imminent or acute risk in a medical setting is typically treated like any other medical patient. The psychiatry c/l team may continue to follow the patient with daily contacts or contacts every several days, but there are rarely other levels of observation for moderate levels of risk. Management is therefore dependent on the staff's continuing to stay in contact with the patient about his or her emotional state and remaining aware of any signs of deterioration and increased risk.

In the Medical Outpatient Setting

Numerous studies have found that a high percentage of patients who committed suicide had not necessarily visited an outpatient mental health provider prior to their death, but had visited their physician. Conwell (1997), for example, found that an average of 62% of a sample of elderly people who committed suicide saw a primary care provider within 30 days of death, and an average of 35.5% had done so within a week of death. Studies such as these led Murphy (1986) to refer to the physician's office as "the primary suicide prevention center" (p. 171).

As in the inpatient medical setting, having physicians and a staff in the outpatient setting who are aware and informed that certain medical conditions have an elevated risk for suicide and that psychiatric patients with particular diagnoses can be at heightened risk is crucial in terms of managing suicide risk. Questions about how the patient is coping with his or her illness and about any wishes to "give up or die" should be part of routine questioning during an outpatient visit. If a patient reports significant emotional distress, a referral for psychiatric or mental health follow-up can be made. If suicidal thoughts or intentions are reported, the patient can be seen more immediately by psychiatry or

mental health in the emergency department. There, it will be the mental health clinician's responsibility to determine whether the patient's risk is at a level that can be managed on an outpatient basis or whether psychiatric hospitalization is necessary.

The current clinical standard of care for patients who are at mild or moderate suicide risk is mental health outpatient follow-up with a plan outlining what the patient can do to maintain safety in the event that his or her risk increases. So, as Stanley and Brown (2011) have suggested, the clinician and the patient can collaborate on identifying warning signs of increasing risk and then identify coping strategies that the patient might employ to take his or her mind off of troubling situations. The plan might next involve identifying people whom the patient might contact because they might provide distraction. If these efforts fail, the patient might identify people whom he or she might trust to tell about the risk, or professionals and agencies that could be contacted if the risk seems significant.

In terms of therapy, there is evidence from several randomized controlled trials that cognitive-behavioral approaches that make suicidality the central focus of the therapy sessions can be effective in reducing suicidal behavior (Rudd, Joiner, Trotter, Williams, & Cordero, 2009). Cognitive-behavioral approaches emphasize the identifying and correcting of cognitive distortions about self and others, learning emotion-regulation skills, learning problem-solving skills, and learning interpersonal relationship skills. If risk nonetheless begins to increase, the mental health clinician has options that include: (1) increasing the frequency of visits or having interim telephone contacts; (2) arranging for 24-hour availability or coverage; (3) reevaluating the treatment plan, including the medication regimen; and (4) evaluating the patient for hospitalization. Hospitalization is typically necessary when the risk has become severe, when it is not possible to establish or reestablish a firm treatment alliance, when crisis intervention techniques fail, and when the patient continues to have intent to commit suicide in the immediate future (Comstock, 1992). Although there is no evidence that hospitalization ultimately prevents suicide, it does provide a safer environment during a period of heightened risk. Typically, one or two hours with a patient who maintains imminent suicidal intent are sufficient to persuade clinicians to hospitalize them, either on a voluntary basis (if the patient is cooperative) or, if necessary, on an involuntary temporary commitment.

Clinical experience indicates there are times when involuntary hospitalization can damage the patient–clinician relationship. This damage can often be repaired once the patient has become more emotionally stable. It may also be possible to lessen the risk of such damage if the patient has been informed early in the treatment relationship that there are limits to confidentiality and that, if the patient is considered to be at imminent risk of seriously harming himself or herself or others, the clinician is ethically and legally obligated to break confidentiality to protect the patient or others who may be at risk from the patient.

THE EVALUATION AND MANAGEMENT OF VIOLENCE RISK IN A MEDICAL SETTING

MEDICAL ILLNESS AND RISK FOR VIOLENCE

There has been little systematic investigation of whether medical illness in general might be an independent risk factor for violence. There has been relatively strong interest, however, in the neurobiological bases of aggression and violence and in the associations of certain neurological conditions with risk for violence. Thus, considerable research has converged on the importance of brain circuitry involving activation of the limbic system (e.g., hippocampus and amygdala), and the regulating influence of the frontal lobes and particularly the prefrontal cortex (PFC) in aggressive behavior (Denson, 2011). This circuitry involves the interaction of the so-called phylogenetically older, reflexive parts of the brain that we share with other animals, and the newer parts of the brain that are unique to humans and that help them function more reflectively.

It should also be noted that the neurotransmitter serotonin has been found to facilitate the functioning of PFC regions, and depletion of serotonin has been associated with violent and impulsive acts. On the other hand, the selective serotonin-reuptake inhibitors (or SSRIs) that are typically prescribed for depression have been found to reduce impulsive aggression in personality-disordered subjects (Coccaro & Kavoussi, 1997). As a result, there has also been great interest in the role of serotonin in the functioning of the brain circuitry mentioned above.

In terms of neurological conditions associated with violence, a prospective study of patients with traumatic brain injury (TBI) found that aggressive or violent behavior was significantly more frequent among patients with TBI than among a comparable group of patients with traumatic injury that did not involve the brain (Tateno, Jorge, & Robinson, 2003). More specifically, and consistent with previously cited research, such behavior was associated with injuries to the frontal lobes and/or the prefrontal cortex as well as with depression, substance abuse, and impaired social functioning. The authors concluded that aggression following TBI was associated with multiple biological and psychosocial factors including the presence of frontal lobe impairment. Also, in a retrospective study known as the Vietnam Head Injury Study (VHIS) (Grafman et al., 1996), veterans with lesions limited to the frontal lobes were found to show more aggressive and violent behaviors than veterans with non-frontal head injuries and controls without head injury. Moreover, there have been multiple neuropsychological and neuroimaging studies (as reviewed by Bowser & Price, 2001) pointing to a strong association between increased aggression and impaired prefrontal cortical activity in TBI patients relative to control subjects.

Several primary progressive dementing disorders also affect the frontal lobes (White, Krengel, & Thompson, 2009). These disorders include Pick's disease and fronto-temporal dementia. The primary presentation of these diseases typically involves a loss of behavioral control. These patients become irritable and unable to inhibit aggressive acts that they were able to inhibit premorbidly. In a study contrasting patients with fronto-temporal dementia with patients with Alzheimer's dementia, Miller, Darby, Benson, Cummings, and Miller (1997) found that patients with fronto-temporal dementia were significantly more likely to have exhibited antisocial behaviors such as assault, indecent exposure, and shoplifting than were Alzheimer's patients. In similar fashion, an increased risk of aggression or violence has been found with other neurological conditions such as cerebrovascular disease (multi-infarct dementia) and multiple sclerosis when there are lesions or demyelination involving the frontal lobes.

Findings such as those above comparing fronto-temporal dementia patients and Alzheimer's patients do not necessarily imply that those with Alzheimer's dementia are free of aggressive or violent behaviors. O'Leary, Jyringi, and Sedler (2005) evaluated 198 elderly patients with dementia related to Alzheimer's disease. They found that compared to elderly patients without dementia, those with dementia had displayed significantly higher levels of physical aggression against their partners. Twenty-five percent of Alzheimer's patients had engaged in physical aggression against their caregivers in the past year, and 33% had engaged in an act of physical aggression against any individual in the past two weeks. Dementia severity affected the frequency of aggressive acts, with acts of physical aggression more likely to occur in later than in earlier stages of the disease process. Physical aggression was related to agitation and most often included hitting, throwing, and grabbing.

Psychotic symptoms in Alzheimer's patients may also lead to aggression. In their review of research, Shub, Ball, Abbas, Gottumukkala, and Kunik (2010) found that eight out of nine studies (including both cross-sectional and longitudinal studies) showed a significant association between psychosis and aggression. For example, in a study of 771 patients with Alzheimer's disease, Mizrahi et al. (2006) found delusions to be significantly associated with overt aggression and agitation. Likewise, in their study of 194 dementia patients, Petrov et al. (2007) found that psychosis was significantly related to agitation, irritability, hallucinations, and anxiety. Treatment studies, however, have had more mixed results, and Shub et al. (2010) have noted that there is a need for prospective studies to confirm a stronger causal link between psychosis and aggression in dementia patients.

Huntington's chorea, the rare autosomal dominant genetic disease with increased suicide risk, is another neurological disorder that is associated with a heightened risk of violence. Huntington's patients seem to have difficulty inhibiting impulsive behavior. As noted by White et al. (2009), there is a great deal of evidence of antisocial behavior among Huntington's disease patients, including physical assaults and child abuse. There is controversy, however, about the degree to which these aggressive behaviors are a function of the neuropathology of the disease and/or the social effects of being in a family that must live with the specter of such a debilitating and incurable condition.

Of course, there are various metabolic disturbances that can cause delirium, the acute brain syndrome that can also lead to agitation and violence. The delirious patient is typically disoriented and confused and may experience perceptual distortions or frank hallucinations. Delirium is typically reversible, so the initial efforts are focused on determining the cause and treating it before there is more serious damage. The immediate management of the delirious patient is behavioral and environmental and is aimed at keeping the patient and others safe, while not obscuring the clinical presentation.

EVALUATING FOR THE ACUTE RISK OF VIOLENCE

In this subsection, we propose that the clinician use the same process of weighing distal risk factors, proximal risk factors, and protective factors as proposed earlier for the evaluation of suicide risk, but apply it to the evaluation of violence risk (Kleespies & Hill, 2011). Of course, those who work in a medical setting should also consider the medical illnesses with associated risk of violence (as noted above) in any effort to weigh the level of risk. If time is available, there are several decision-support tools that can be utilized in assessing for risk of violence. These tools are not psychological tests, but were constructed in the framework known as "structured professional judgement." The items included in these instruments were typically expert-generated. Several of them that have good reliability and predictive validity are the *Historical-Clinical-Risk Management–20* (HCR-20; Webster, Douglas, Eaves, & Hart, 1997), the *Structured Assessment of Violence Risk in Youth* (SAVRY; Borum, Bartel, & Forth, 2006), and the *Spousal Assault Risk Assessment Guide* (SARA; Kropp, Hart, Webster, & Eaves, 2008).

Distal Risk Factors

Demographic Factors
It is well known that adolescents and young adults have higher rates of violence, but, as noted in the section on specific medical illnesses and associated violence, elderly patients who suffer from dementia also have an increased rate of violence. It is also well known that, in the general population, men are far more likely to be violent than women (U.S. Bureau of Justice Statistics, 2010). Women with acute mental illness, however, have been found to be as likely as men with acute mental illness to become violent; but men with mental illness remain more likely to engage in more serious forms of violence (Monahan et al., 2001). Race or ethnicity has not been found to be a strong predictor of violence when socioeconomic level is controlled. Lower socioeconomic level itself, however, has been associated with increased risk (Swanson, Holzer, Ganju, & Jono, 1990).

Serious Mental Illness
Although having a major mental illness is a risk factor for violence, it is important to note that most violence in our society is not committed by the mentally ill (Fazel & Grann, 2006). We need to be careful not to "demonize" the mentally ill as extremely violent. As is the case with risk for suicide, however, certain mental illnesses are both distal and proximal risk

factors for violence. These include schizophrenia, schizoaffective disorder, bipolar disorder, and major depression (McNiel, Gregory, Lam, Binder, & Sullivan, 2003). In addition, military veterans with PTSD, and especially those with a history of war zone violence (Hiley-Young, Blake, Abueg, Rozynko, & Gusman, 1995), have been found to be at increased risk.

Personality disorders that are marked by impulsivity and poor behavioral control (e.g., antisocial personality disorder and borderline personality disorder) have also been associated with violent behavior. In adolescents, conduct disorders as well as attention-deficit and hyperactivity disorders (ADHD) are at elevated risk of violence (Saterfield & Schell, 1997).

Historical and Dispositional Factors
It is widely known that the best predictor of future violence is a history of violent behavior. The risk level of future violence increases, however, when there has been an early onset of violent and aggressive behavior in the person's life. If children have engaged in violent acts or delinquent behavior before age 12, they are more likely to engage in violent and criminal activities over the course of their lifespan (Tolan & Thomas, 1995). In general, the greater the number of violent acts, the greater the likelihood of future violence (Borum, 2000).

Childhood maltreatment, physical abuse, and exposure to violence between parents increases the risk of perpetration of violence in adulthood (Ehrensaft et al., 2003). Such experiences are thought to model, reward, or reinforce the use and display of violence.

There is a constellation of affective, interpersonal, and behavioral characteristics, referred to as *psychopathy*, that has been found to be a clear risk factor for violence (see, e.g., Forth, Hart, & Hare, 1990). "Psychopathy" is said to refer to characteristics that include "egocentricity; impulsivity; irresponsibility; shallow emotions; lack of empathy, guilt, or remorse; [and] manipulativeness" (Hare, 1998; p. 188). Hare (1991) developed a 20-item measure of the concept entitled the *Hare Psychopathy Checklist—Revised* (or *PCL-R*). The PCL-R has been found to be a good predictor of violence in diverse populations, including schizophrenic and personality disordered individuals (Harris, Rice, & Quinsey, 1993). Psychopathy is considered a static risk factor since treatment has not been effective in making substantial changes in psychopathic individuals.

Proximal Risk Factors

Acute Mental Illness and Substance Abuse
McNiel et al. (2003) have noted that schizophrenic patients are most at risk for violence when they are having a psychotic episode, and bipolar patients are most at risk when they are having a manic episode. In a hospital setting, manic patients often exhibit behavior that requires limit setting, but it is important to remember that manic patients often react with aggression to efforts at containment and limit-setting.

Active substance use significantly increases the risk of violence when it co-occurs in persons with serious mental illness. Swanson (1994), for example, studied mental illness, substance abuse, and community violence in a sample of

10,000 people. He found that mental disorder alone was twice as likely to be present in violent individuals as in those who were non-violent. He also found that substance abuse alone and in combination with comorbid mental illness was five times as likely to be present in the violent as opposed to the non-violent group.

Clinical Symptoms as Proximal Risk Factors

McNiel (1998, 2009) has noted that certain clinical symptoms can be used to estimate short-term risk for violence. McNiel and Binder (1994) studied a sample of decompensating patients at the time of admission to a psychiatric unit. They found that symptoms described as hostile-suspiciousness, agitation-excitement, and disturbed thinking (unusual thought content/hallucinations) were associated with aggressive behavior in the first hours or days after admission. In a similar vein, Link and Steuve (1994) identified a delusional state that they referred to as *threat/control override*. The term refers to a delusional state in which the person feels personally threatened to the point that he or she feels justified in overriding self-control to eliminate the threat. Beliefs such as these have been found to predict violent behavior by male patients (Teasdale, Silver, & Monahan, 2006). Finally, an acute risk of violence has been found with *command hallucinations*; that is, a *voice* telling the patient to harm or kill someone else. The risk is heightened further if the command is consistent with a delusional belief (e.g., a patient who hears a voice telling him to attack a supervisor whom he believes is a member of a devil-worshipping cult) (Monahan et al., 2001).

Situational or Contextual Factors

Family members of patients with major mental illness and violent behavior are at high risk. Straznickas, McNiel, and Binder (1993) evaluated 113 acute psychiatric patients admitted after a violent event. They found that 56% of the patients had assaulted a family member. Moreover, it has long been known that mothers who live with adult children who have schizophrenia have an increased risk of violent victimization (Estroff, Swanson, Lachiotte, Swartz, & Bolduc, 1998).

Despite the fact that we do not have good empirical evidence on female-to-male violence (Riggs, Caulfield, & Fair, 2009), Resnick, Acierno, Holmes, Dammeyer, & Kilpatrick (2000) have noted that female victims of rape, who fear being harmed again or who have feelings of anger and fear, have been known to express homicidal thoughts. These researchers recommend that their feelings of anger and fear be validated and that their risk of retaliating with violence be assessed.

Although there is little empirical evidence linking weapon availability and risk for violence in individual cases, it is clear that most homicides in the United States are by firearm (U.S. Department of Justice Statistics, 2010). Moreover, higher rates of gun-related violence have been reported in locales with greater access to guns (Kaplan & Gelig, 1998). It seems reasonable to assume that those who have ready access to weapons, if they become violent, are at greater risk of engaging in more serious forms of violence.

Protective Factors

Research on protective factors for risk of violence is even less developed than that for risk of suicide. There has been an effort to examine treatments that might reduce violence risk (Monahan & Applebaum, 1999), but there has been little emphasis on "personal strengths, resources, and protective or 'buffer' factors" (Hart, 2001, p. 21). Good personal and family support and involvement in a treatment or support program have been viewed as protective factors (Estroff & Zimmer, 1994). Some studies have noted factors that are, in essence, the reverse of known risk factors and therefore might reduce risk. For example, it has been reported that non-abusive men were less likely to have experienced violence during childhood, to have attitudes tolerant of spouse abuse, or to engage in impulsive behaviors (Hanson, Cadsy, Harris, & LaLonde, 1997). Clearly, however, further research on protective factors is needed and might improve the specificity of who is less likely to engage in violence.

MANAGING THE ACUTE RISK OF VIOLENCE

As with managing suicide risk, there are differences in how patients who are at risk for violence can be managed in the inpatient medical setting versus the outpatient medical setting.

In the Medical Inpatient Setting

In providing medical treatment for a patient who, by virtue of his or her medical condition or by virtue of a preexisting mental illness, poses a possible risk of violence, treatment providers would benefit from an awareness of certain verbal and behavioral signs of potential loss of control. Aggressive verbal statements or threats should be taken seriously. Clinical experience, however, has informed us that observing certain behavioral signs can also be important. These include: (1) psychomotor restlessness such as pacing, fidgeting, clenching fists, startle response, grinding teeth, or inability to sit or lie down; (2) affective and facial changes which may reflect either hostility, fear, or paranoia; and (3) the tone and loudness of the patient's speech.

If a patient seems hostile, agitated, or tense, initial empathic comments about his or her apparent distress should allow the staff member to observe how the patient responds. If he or she is able to verbalize what the issue(s) may be, it might be possible to de-escalate a potential crisis by discussing an immediate problem and finding an acceptable solution. It may also be the beginning of a working alliance. If the patient is not responsive to verbal efforts to reduce tension, however, a consultation with the psychiatry consult/liaison team should be initiated. As in cases of suicide risk, the psychiatry team will assess the patient's emotional and mental condition, including his or her level of risk for violence. If the level of immediate risk is considered mild or moderate, the psychiatry team might recommend the initiation of, or the addition of, a psychotropic medication to calm the patient. A sitter might be assigned if needed or helpful, and psychiatry could continue to follow the patient on a daily basis, as needed, until the crisis is resolved and the patient is in better behavioral control.

If these efforts at intervention fail, however, and the patient continues to escalate or is at risk of losing behavioral control, there is typically a psychiatric emergency code team that can be called. At times, such a "show of force" (which includes members from the facility police or security service) helps the patient realize that, in the interests of the safety of others, there are limits to what behavior can be tolerated. If the patient continues to be agitated and is in marginal control, he or she can be offered medication. For short-term control of agitation and potentially violent behavior, benzodiazepines and anti-psychotics have been the medications of choice. Although benzodiazepines have sometimes been reported to increase aggressive behavior, it is a relatively rare phenomenon, and, far more typically, they have a sedating effect. If a patient is already prescribed an antipsychotic medication, more of the same can be offered. Otherwise, haloperidol (i.e., Haldol) 5 mg by mouth or intramuscularly, as well as a benzodiazepine such as lorazepam (i.e., Ativan) 1 to 2 mg by mouth or intramuscularly, is customary for an initial trial. Individually, these medications are both sedating within 30 minutes. When both of these medications are administered sequentially to a patient, the sedative effects are significantly augmented. So for female, young, and elderly patients, administering haloperidol or lorazepam as a single sedating agent may be sufficient. Alternatively, a clinician could also administer lower doses of each agent—for example, haloperidol 2 mg and lorazepam 0.5 to 1.0 mg—to achieve a comfortable sedative effect. For a robust adult male patient, doses may range from haloperidol 5 to 10 mg and lorazepam 1 to 2 mg to achieve a calming effect. Clinicians should be careful when administering sedating medication to patients who may have recently ingested or injected medications that have depressing central nervous system properties. The above dosages can be repeated in 30 to 60 minutes if the patient's agitation persists. Benztropine (i.e., Cogentin) is sometimes added as a prophylactic against dystonias and extrapyramidal side effects. Cardiac irregularities or changes in heart rhythm can also be a rare side effect of haloperidol.

Haldoperidol and lorazepam are medications that have the advantage of being readily available and familiar to emergency psychiatry personnel. The risk of extrapyramidal side effects decreases dramatically after age 40, so the use of an atypical antipsychotic or of benztropine prophylaxis is indicated only for younger patients. It is recommended that patients with liver disease be given lorazepam or oxazepam as the benzodiazepines of choice because they metabolize quickly and are eliminated by the kidneys (Saitz, Ciraulo, Shader, & Ciraulo, 2003). It is noteworthy that benzodiazepines such as lorazepam tend to be less effective for those who have developed a tolerance for them. Since both benzodiazepines and alcohol work on the same neural receptors, a tolerance can develop through excessive use of the medication or through excessive use of alcohol.

One of the most serious and life-threatening side effects of rapid administration of a neuroleptic medication is neuroleptic malignant syndrome (NMS). It is an uncommon disorder, with an incidence of less than 1.0%, but it can be fatal. The signs of NMS include fever, muscle rigidity, autonomic instability, and an elevated white blood cell count and creatine kinase level. Treatment involves discontinuation of all neuroleptic medication. Acute admission to an intensive care unit (ICU) is recommended for full life-supportive measures. Should a patient have a history of NMS, employing lorazepam and the avoidance of acute administration of a neuroleptic may be wise.

Studies have found that beta-blockers help diminish aggressive behavior, particularly in patients with dementia, brain injuries, and mental retardation. The anti-aggressive effects of beta-blockers, however, usually occur four to eight weeks after the effective dose is reached, and they are not particularly helpful under emergency conditions. Lithium is the medication most likely to control aggression in the long run, but, again, it is not useful in circumstances that call for rapid action to reduce acute behavioral risk. Patients must be carefully educated about the potential side effects of any medication employed, and clinicians should try to select a medication with a side-effect profile compatible with a patient's lifestyle to increase the likelihood of compliance.

If the patient will not voluntarily accept medication and/or continues to be agitated and threatening, or actually loses control, it may be necessary to consider more restrictive measures as a humane response to a situation that could otherwise lead to serious injury. Of course, patients have a legal and ethical right to refuse care. There are, however, exceptions to this rule, including patients who lack competency and/or patients who are at acute risk to harm themselves or others. The clinician in these life-threatening situations needs to employ and document the least restrictive but effective means available to help the patient regain composure. In the process, the clinician needs to be cognizant of state laws regarding the use of physical restraints and forced medication. Restraints, in most states but not all, are seen as less restrictive than forced medications. It is also difficult and potentially dangerous to administer intramuscular injections to an aggressive and unrestrained patient. A patient who has met criteria for physical restraints, however, does not necessarily or automatically meet criteria for forced medication. If the patient is still at demonstrable risk for harm to self or others while in restraints, the clinician may then force medication.

The physical restraint of an aggressive or agitated patient involves some risk to both patient and staff and should not be undertaken unless there is no good alternative. While some patients are cooperative with the restraint procedure, many are not. A sufficient number of staff is needed to manage a resistant patient; that is, one trained person to control each limb and one to protect and control the head. A sixth person should be available to coordinate the procedure and talk with the patient. Vital signs and agitation may increase for the first few minutes after a patient is placed in restraints. The positioning of the patient should be given some consideration, particularly for those who have been traumatized by violence or abuse in the past. Most patients are restrained in the face-up position, but those who have experienced sexual trauma may become more agitated by being placed in such a vulnerable position. For these patients, restraint while lying on their side may be preferred.

After a patient is restrained, a staff member needs to sit with the patient to monitor his or her emotional and physical condition. Legal requirements and hospital policies can vary by state and by whether the patient is an adult or under 18 years of age; however, guidelines generally require that leather restraints be checked every 15 minutes to ensure that there is no interference with circulation. Unless it is unsafe to do so, each limb is to be removed from restraint for exercise once per hour. Restraint and the establishment of control have a calming effect on some patients. Others, however, may continue to be agitated or become more agitated. In such cases, and as noted above, it may be necessary to use medication to ease the patient's distress and help him or her to regain self-control. Restraints should be maintained for the minimum time necessary for this process to occur.

It is important for clinicians to be aware that coercing a patient to take medications ("If you don't take any medication, we will have to hospitalize you") is not ethical and could constitute an inappropriate use of involuntary medication. In an emergency situation, the clinician needs to apprise his or her patient of the consequences of their noncompliance, but the line between patient education and coercion can get blurred. If a physically restrained patient requires involuntary medication, it is important to continue to try to elicit his or her cooperation and select the least invasive and traumatic means to administer medication. Thus, the clinician should offer oral medications over injections. If the patient refuses oral medication, asking in which arm the patient would want the injection still provides him or her with some choice. Informing the patient that he or she will get an injection if they do not cooperate and take oral medication, depending on the tone of voice and manner of the clinician, could be perceived as crossing the line from patient education and voluntary medication into coercion and involuntary medication.

While oral and intramuscular medications are common in emergency situations, intravenous medications are not common. Intravenous administration of sedating medication has a rapid onset, which can approximate general anesthesia with all its inherent risks for respiratory and cardiac complications. There are exceptions, particularly in intensive care units when intravenous lines are already established and the patient's vital signs are already being electronically monitored by experienced critical care personal who are equipped to deal with any adverse respiratory or cardiac sequelae.

Of course, in circumstances where physical restraints and forced medication are utilized, it is crucial for clinicians to document the facts in the chart, and his or her rationale in a risk-benefit note. This documentation should include clinical examples that clearly demonstrate how less-invasive techniques, including physical restraints, failed to contain the patient's behavior, and why involuntary medication was required.

In the Medical Outpatient Setting

If a medical outpatient makes threats or exhibits threatening behavior to staff, a psychiatric emergency code team can be called, as one might do in the inpatient setting. If the patient, however, makes comments or threats that indicate that he or she may be at serious risk to harm others in the community, the patient should be escorted to the hospital emergency department (ED) for evaluation by the mental health clinician on duty. If the patient were to refuse to go to the ED, the code team could be called to assess whether the patient should be escorted to the ED involuntarily for evaluation in a safer setting.

Depending on the estimated level of risk, Monahan (1993) has suggested three types of intervention for managing the patient at risk to others: (1) intensifying treatment; (2) hardening the target; and (3) incapacitation of the patient. If the patient is evaluated and does not appear to pose an imminent risk of violence, it may be possible to initiate follow-up mental health treatment, or intensify an ongoing treatment, as a way of managing risk in the community. Thus, the patient could be scheduled for therapy sessions that are more frequent than usual. He or she could have telephone safety checks, be asked to enter a more structured outpatient or partial hospitalization program, or be asked to enter a substance abuse treatment program (if needed). Medication that might reduce agitation or modulate mood could be considered or increased. A plan for 24-hour emergency coverage should also be developed, and there should be frequent reassessments of the level of risk. The focus of therapy sessions should be on developing strategies to reduce the likelihood of violence: for example, increasing insight, anger-management techniques, increasing frustration tolerance, improving affect regulation, and so forth.

If the patient were to elope from the medical setting without a plan for managing risk, it might be necessary to warn any intended victims and complete a temporary involuntary commitment form so that the local or state police might locate the patient and bring him or her to an emergency room for further evaluation. Warning the intended victim has become known as "hardening the target." In the case of the intended victim, this makes it possible for him or her to take protective measures. After the Tarasoff case in California, warning the intended victim became known to clinicians as the "duty to warn" (*Tarasoff* v. *Regents of University of California*, 1974). The California court, however, reviewed the case two years later and revised its opinion to what has now become known as the "duty to protect" (*Tarasoff* v. *Regents of University of California*, 1976). In effect, the Court's revised opinion was that therapists do have a duty to protect the intended victim or victims of their patients, and there are several ways to do so. Warning the individual in question may be one way, but it is not the only way or, depending on circumstances, necessarily the best way.

Borum (2009) has noted that warning the intended victim can be frightening to the individual and should be reserved for times when other interventions have been rejected by the patient or are not feasible. If a warning is given, his advice is that the clinician be careful in reviewing the nature and seriousness of the threat, and then work with the individual to find sources of assistance and develop protective measures.

If a patient is evaluated and is considered to be a serious threat to others, it may be necessary to incapacitate the patient. Incapacitating the patient means utilizing measures that directly decrease the person's ability to act out in a violent manner. These measures can include involuntary hospitalization, the administration of sedating medication against the wishes of the patient, and physical restraints or seclusion. These are obviously very intrusive interventions and should be used only in situations where the danger of serious harm is great and less restrictive means have failed or are likely to be ineffective. As noted above in the discussion of restraints, the use of these means is typically regulated by law and institutional or agency policy. Their use is sometimes necessary to avoid a worse alternative (i.e., serious harm or death of an intended victim). They are not a solution to the longer-term risk of violence, but prevent immediate harm. They may also allow for a diagnostic evaluation and the initiation of treatment that may have longer lasting benefit.

SUMMARY

In the medical setting, the clinician must weigh the possible contributions of both mental illness and medical illness when assessing and managing the risk of suicide or the risk of violence. It is also important to note that the vulnerability to becoming suicidal and the vulnerability to becoming violent may not be entirely independent. Research has indicated that those who had a history of violence were at increased risk of suicidal behavior, and that rates of lifetime aggression and impulsivity were significantly greater in suicide attempters than in those who had never attempted suicide (Mann, Waternaux, Haas, & Malone, 1999). Thus, when evaluating a patient for risk of violence, the clinician may be well advised to also consider the possibility of risk of suicide, and vice versa.

Finally, in evaluating a patient for risk of suicide or risk of violence, the importance of practicing good risk-management practices should not go unnoted. First and foremost, good risk management includes documentation and consultation. Documentation should focus on statements that reflect that a risk–benefit analysis was done in arriving at a rationale for case decisions; while seeking the consultation of a colleague is one of the better ways to meet the community standard for working with a high-risk patient.

CLINICAL PEARLS

- Physical illness is a significant, independent risk factor for suicide in the elderly. In the study by Conwell et al. (2010) it was also found that perception of deteriorating health status and functional impairment were significant risk factors, with functional impairment being the more robust predictor of suicide.

- There is considerable evidence of a familial and a probable genetic contribution to the risk of suicide (Brent, Bridge, Johnson, & Connolly, 1996; Mann & Arango, 1999; Moscicki, 1997: Roy, Nielsen, Rylander, & Sarchiapone, 2000). Most investigators, however, continue to agree that suicide is a multi-determined act, with psychological, social, and biological factors involved.

- For male schizophrenic patients under age 40, the risk of suicide is higher when these patients are not acutely psychotic, have a heightened awareness of the debilitating effects of their illness, and become depressed.

- Suicide among patients with alcohol problems is generally more likely in mid-life and following a prolonged history of alcohol abuse and dependence. It is most likely to occur during an active phase of drinking.

- In prospective studies, hopelessness has been strongly supported as a risk factor for completed suicide (see, e.g., Beck, Brown, Berchick, Stewart, & Steer, 1990; Fawcett et al., 1987).

- The best predictor of future violence is a history of violent behavior. The risk level of future violence is increased, however, when there has been an early onset of violent and aggressive behavior in the person's life.

- Schizophrenic patients are most at risk for violence when they are having a psychotic episode, and bipolar patients are most at risk when they are having a manic episode.

- Certain behavioral signs can also be important signs of impending violent behavior: (1) psychomotor restlessness such as pacing, fidgeting, clenching fists, startle response, grinding teeth, or inability to sit or lie down; (2) affective and facial changes that may reflect either hostility, fear, or paranoia; and (3) the tone and loudness of the patient's speech.

- A patient who has met criteria for physical restraints does not necessarily or automatically meet criteria for forced medication.

- Coercing a patient to take medications ("If you don't take any medication, we will have to hospitalize you") is not ethical and could constitute an inappropriate use of involuntary medication.

- Depending on the estimated level of risk of violence, Monahan (1993) has suggested three types of intervention for managing the patient at risk to others: (1) intensifying treatment; (2) "hardening the target" (warning/protecting an identified victim); and (3) incapacitation of the patient.

- Those who had a history of violence were at increased risk of suicidal behavior, and rates of lifetime aggression and impulsivity were significantly greater in suicide attempters than in those who had never attempted suicide (Mann, Waternaux, Haas, & Malone, 1999).

DISCLOSURE STATEMENTS

Dr. Kleespies, Dr. Hughes, Dr. Weintraub, and Dr. Hart do not have any conflicts of interest to disclose.

REFERENCES

Ahn, E., Shin, D., Cho, S., Park, S., Won, Y., & Yun, Y. (2010). Suicide rates and risk factors among Korean cancer patients, 1993-2005. *Cancer Epidemiology, Biomarkers & Prevention, 19,* 2097-2105.

Almqvist, E. W., Bloch, M., Brinkman, R., Craufurd, D., & Hayden, M. R. (1999). A worldwide assessment of the frequency of suicide, suicide attempts, or psychiatric hospitalization after predictive testing for Huntington disease. *American Journal of Human Genetics, 64,* 1293-1304.

Arana, A., Wentworth, C., Ayuso-Mateos, J., & Arellano, F. (2010). Suicide-related events in patients treated with antiepileptic drugs. *The New England Journal of Medicine, 363,* 542-551.

Baliko, L., Csala, B., & Czopf, J. (2004). Suicide in Hungarian Huntington's disease patients. *Neuroepidemiology, 23,* 258-260.

Beck, A., Brown, G., Berchick, R., Stewart, B., & Steer, R. (1990). Relationship between hopelessness and ultimate suicide: A replication with psychiatric outpatients. *American Journal of Psychiatry, 147,* 190-195.

Beiske, A.G., Svensson, E., Sandanger, I., et al. (2008). Depression and anxiety amongst multiple sclerosis patients. *European Journal of Neurology, 15*(3), 239-245.

Bell, G. S., & Sander, J. W. (2009). Suicide and epilepsy. *Current Opinions in Neurology, 22,* 174-178.

Borum, R. (2000). Assessing violence risk among youth. *Journal of Clinical Psychology, 56,* 1263-1288.

Borum, R. (2009). Children and adolescents at risk of violence. In P. Kleespies (Ed.), *Behavioral emergencies: An evidence-based resource for evaluating and managing risk of suicide, violence, and victimization* (pp. 147-163). Washington, DC: APA Books.

Borum, R., Bartel, P., & Forth, A. (2006). *Structured assessment of violence risk in youth: Professional manual.* Lutz, FL: Psychological Assessment Resources.

Bostwick, J., & Cohen, L. (2009). Differentiating suicide from life-ending acts and end- of-life decisions: A model based on chronic kidney disease and dialysis. *Psychosomatics, 50,* 1-7.

Bowser, M., & Price, B. (2001). Neuropsychiatry of frontal lobe dysfunction in violent and criminal behavior: A critical review. *Journal of Neurology, Neurosurgery, & Psychiatry, 71,* 720-726.

Brent, D., Bridge, J., Johnson, B., & Connolly, J. (1996). Suicidal behavior runs in families: A controlled family study of adolescent suicide victims. *Archives of General Psychiatry, 41,* 888-891.

Bronnum-Hansen, H., Stenager, E., Stenager, E. N., et al. (2005). Suicide among Danes with multiple sclerosis. *Journal of Neurology, Neurosurgery, & Psychiatry, 76,* 1457-1459.

Bullman, T., & Kang, H. (1994). Posttraumatic stress disorder and the risk of traumatic deaths among Vietnam veterans. *The Journal of Nervous and Mental Disease, 182,* 604-610.

Carrico, A. W., Johnson, M. O., Morin, S. F., et al. (2007). Correlates of suicidal ideation among HIV-positive persons. *AIDS, 21,* 1199-1203.

Charlifue, S., & Gerhart, K. (1991). Behavioral and demographic predictors of suicide after traumatic spinal cord injury. *Archives of Physical Medicine & Rehabilitation, 72,* 488-492.

Christensen, J., Vestergaard, M., Mortensen, P. B., Sidenius, P., & Agerbo, E. (2007). Epilepsy and risk of suicide: A population-based case-control study. *Lancet Neurology, 6*(8), 693-698.

Christensen, M.-L. M., Yousaf, U., Engholm, G., & Storm, H. H. (2006). Increased suicide risk among Danish women with non-melanoma skin cancer, 1971-1999. *European Journal of Cancer Prevention, 15,* 266-268.

Clark, D., & Horton-Deutsch, S. (1992). Assessment *in absentia:* The value of the psychological autopsy method for studying antecedents of suicide and predicting future suicides. In R. Maris, A. Berman, J. Maltsberger, & R. Yufit (Eds.), *Assessment and prediction of suicide* (pp. 144-182). New York: The Guilford Press.

Coccaro, E., & Kavoussi, R. (1997). Fluoxetine and impulsive aggressive behavior in personality-disordered subjects. *Archives of General Psychiatry, 54,* 1081-1088.

Cohen, L., Test, M., & Brown, R. (1990). Suicide and schizophrenia: Data from a prospective community study. *American Journal of Psychiatry, 147,* 602-607.

Comstock, B. (1992). Decision to hospitalize and alternatives to hospitalization. In B. Bongar (Ed.), *Suicide: Guidelines for assessment, management, and treatment.* (pp. 204-217). New York: Oxford University Press.

Conwell, Y. (1997). Management of suicidal behavior in the elderly. *The Psychiatric Clinics of North America, 20,* 667-683.

Conwell, Y., Duberstein, P., Hirsch, J., Conner, K., Eberly, S., & Caine, E. (2010). Health status and suicide in the second half of life. *International Journal of Geriatric Psychiatry, 25,* 371-379.

Darke, S., & Ross, J. (2002). Suicide among heroin users: Rates, risk factors, and methods. *Addiction, 97,* 1383-1394.

Denson, T. (2011). A social neuroscience perspective on the neurobiological bases of aggression. In P. Shaver & M. Mikulincer (Eds.), *Human aggression and violence: Causes, manifestations, and consequences* (pp. 105-120). Washington, DC: APA Books.

Dormer, N. R. C., McCaul, K. A., & Kristjanson, L. J. (2008). Risk of suicide in cancer patients in Western Australia, 1981-2002. *Medical Journal of Australia, 188,* 140-143.

Duberstein, P., & Witte, T. (2009). Suicide risk in personality disorders: An argument for a public health perspective. In P. Kleespies (Ed.), *Behavioral emergencies: An evidence-based resource for evaluating and managing risk of suicide, violence, and victimization* (pp. 257-286). Washington, DC: APA Books.

Egeland, J., & Sussex, J. (1985). Suicide and family loading for affective disorders. *Journal of the American Medical Association, 254,* 915-918.

Ehrensaft, M., Cohen, P., Brown, J., Smailes, E., Chen, H., & Johnson, J. (2003). Intergenerational transmission of partner violence: A 20-year prospective study. *Journal of Consulting & Clinical Psychology, 71,* 741-753.

Estroff, S., & Zimmer, C. (1994). Social networks, social support, and violence among persons with severe, persistent mental illness. In J. Monahan & H. Steadman (Eds.), *Violence and mental disorder: Developments in risk assessment* (pp. 259-295). Chicago: University of Chicago Press.

Estroff, S., Swanson, J., Lachiotte, W., Swartz, M., & Bolduc, M. (1998). Risk reconsidered: Targets of violence in the social networks of people with serious psychiatric disorders. *Social Psychiatry & Psychiatric Epidemiology, 33,* S95-S101.

Fang, F., Keating, N. L., Mucci, L. A., et al. (2010). Immediate risk of suicide and cardiovascular death after a prostate cancer diagnosis: Cohort study in the United States. *Journal of the National Cancer Institute, 102,* 307-314.

Fawcett, J., Scheftner, W., Clark, D., Hedeker, D., Gibbons, R., & Coryell, W. (1987). Clinical predictors of suicide in patients with major affective disorder. *American Journal of Psychiatry, 144,* 1189-1194.

Fazel, S., & Grann, M. (2006). The population impact of severe mental illness on violent crime. *Hospital & Community Psychiatry, 163,* 1397-1403.

Fiedorowicz, J., Mills, J., Ruggle, A., Langbehn, D., & Paulsen, J. (2011). Suicidal behavior in prodromal Huntington disease. *Neurodegenerative Disease, 8,* 483-490.

Forsström, E., Hakko, H., Nordström, T., Räsänen, P., & Mainio, A. (2010). Suicide in patients with stroke: A population-based study of suicide victims through the years 1988-2007 in Northern Finland. *Journal of Neuropsychiatry & Clinical Neurosciences, 22,* 182-187.

Forth, A., Hart, S., & Hare. R. (1990). Assessment of psychopathy in male young offenders. *Psychological Assessment: A Journal of Consulting & Clinical Psychology, 2,* 342-344.

Fredrikson, S., Cheng, Q., Jiang, G., & Wasserman, D. (2003). Elevated suicide risk among patients with multiple sclerosis in Sweden. *Neuroepidemiology, 22,* 146–152.

Gay, M., Vrignaud, P., Garitte, C., & Meunier, C. (2010). Predictors of depression in multiple sclerosis patients. *Acta Neurologica Scandinavica, 121,* 161–170.

Goodwin, R., Marusic, A., & Hoven, C. (2003). Suicide attempts in the United States: The role of physical illness. *Social Science & Medicine, 56,* 1783–1788.

Grafman, J., Schwab, K., Warden, D., Pridgen, A., Brown, H., & Salazar, A. (1996). Frontal lobe injuries, violence, and aggression: A report of the Vietnam Head Injury Study. *Neurology, 46,* 1231–1238.

Gutierrez, P., Osman, A., Barios, F., Kopper, B., Baker, M., & Haraburda, C. (2002). Development of the Reasons for Living Inventory for young adults. *Journal of Clinical Psychology, 58,* 339–357.

Hagen, E. M., Lie, S. A., Rekand, T., Gilhus, N., & Gronning, M. (2010). *Journal of Neurology, Neurosurgery, & Psychiatry, 81,* 368–373.

Hanson, R., Cadsy, O., Harris, A., & LaLonde, C. (1997). Correlates of battering among 997 men: Family history, adjustment, and attitudinal differences. *Violence & Victims, 12,* 191–208.

Hare, R. (1991). *Manual for the Hare Psychopathy Checklist—Revised.* Toronto: Multi-Health Systems.

Hare, R. (1998). Psychopaths and their nature: Implications for the mental health and criminal justice systems. In T. Milton, E. Simonsen, M. Birkett-Smith, & R. Davis (Eds.), *Psychopathy: Antisocial, criminal, and violent behavior* (pp. 188–223). New York: Guilford Press.

Harris, E., & Barraclough, B. (1994). Suicide as an outcome for medical disorders. *Medicine Baltimore, 73,* 281–296.

Harris, G., Rice, M., & Quinsey, V. (1993). Violent recidivism of mentally disordered offenders: The development of a statistical prediction instrument. *Criminal Justice & Behavior, 20,* 315–335.

Harrison-Felix, C., Whiteneck, G., Jha, A., DeVivo, M., Hammond, F., & Hart, D. (2009). Mortality over four decades after traumatic brain injury rehabilitation: A retrospective cohort study. *Archives of Physical & Medical Rehabilitation, 90,* 1506–1513.

Hart, S. (2001). Assessing and managing violence risk. In K. Douglas, C. Webster, S. Hart, D. Eaves, & J. Ogloff (Eds.), *HCR-20: Violence risk management companion guide* (pp. 13–25). Burnaby, British Columbia: Mental Health, Law, and Policy Institute, Simon Fraser University.

Harwood, D., Hawton, K., Hope, T., Harriss, L., & Jacoby, R. (2006). Life problems and physical illness as risk factors for suicide in older people: A descriptive and case-control study. *Psychological Medicine, 36,* 1265–1274.

Hesdorffer, D. C., Hauser, W. A., Olafsson, E., Ludvigsson, P., & Kjartansson, O. (2006). Depression and suicide attempt as risk factors for incident unprovoked seizures. *Annals of Neurology, 59,* 35–41.

Hiley-Young, B., Blake, D., Abueg, F., Rozynko, V., & Gusman, F. (1995). War zone violence in Vietnam: An examination of premilitary, military, and postmilitary factors in PTSD inpatients. *Journal of Traumatic Stress, 8,* 125–141.

Howard, M., Perron, B., Sacco, P., Ilgen, M., Vaughn, M., Garland, E., & Freedentahl, S. (2010). Suicide ideation and attempts among inhalant users: Results from the National Epidemiologic Survey on alcohol and related conditions. *Suicide and Life-PPThreatening Behavior, 40,* 276–286.

Jobes, D., & Mann, R. (1999). Reasons for living versus reasons for dying: Examining the internal debate of suicide. *Suicide & Life-Threatening Behavior, 29,* 97–104.

Kaplan, M., & Gelig, O. (1998). Firearm suicides and homicide in the United States: Regional variations and patterns of gun ownership. *Social Science & Medicine, 46,* 1227–1233.

Keiser, O., Spoerri, A., Brinkhof, M. W. G., et al. (2010). Suicide in HIV-infected individuals and the general population in Switzerland, 1988–2008. *American Journal of Psychiatry, 167*(2), 1–8.

Kelly, M., Mufson, M., & Rogers, M. (1999). Medical settings and suicide. In D. Jacobs (Ed.), *The Harvard Medical School guide to suicide assessment & intervention* (pp. 491–519). San Francisco: Jossey-Bass Publishers.

Kendal, W. S. (2007). Suicide and cancer: A gender-comparative study. *Annals of Oncology, 18,* 381–387.

King, C., Segal, H., Naylor, M., & Evans, T. (1993). Family functioning and suicidal behavior in adolescent inpatients with mood disorders. *Journal of the American Academy of Child & Adolescent Psychiatry, 32,* 1198–1206.

Kleespies, P. M., Hough, S., & Romeo, A. M. (2009). Suicide risk in people with medical and terminal illness. In P. M. Kleespies (Ed.), *Behavioral emergencies: An evidence-based resource for evaluating and managing risk of suicide, violence, and victimization* (pp. 103–121). Washington, DC: American Psychological Association.

Kleespies, P., & Dettmer, E. (2000). An evidence-based approach to evaluating and managing suicidal emergencies. *Journal of Clinical Psychology, 56,* 1109–1130.

Kleespies, P., & Hill, J. (2011). Behavioral emergencies and crises. In D. Barlow (Ed.), *The Oxford handbook of clinical psychology* (pp. 739–761). New York: Oxford University Press.

Komiti, A., Judd, F., Grech, P., et al. (2001). Suicidal behavior in people with HIV/AIDS: A review. *Australian & New Zealand Journal of Psychiatry, 35,* 747–757.

Krentz, H., Kliewer, G., & Gill, M. (2005). Changing mortality rates and causes of death for HIV-infected individuals living in Southern Alberta, Canada, from 1984 to 2003. *HIV Medicine, 6,* 99–106.

Kropp, P.R., Hart, S., Webster, C., & Eaves, D. (2008). *Manual for the Spousal Assault Risk Assessment guide.* Vancouver, British Columbia: Proactive Resolutions.

Kurella, M., Kimmel, P., Young, B., & Chertow, G. (2005). Suicide in the United States End-Stage Renal Disease Program. *Journal of the American Society of Nephrology, 16,* 774–781.

Larsson, M. U., Luszcz, M. A., Bui, T.-H., & Robins Wahlin, T.-B. (2006). Depression and suicidal ideation after predictive testing for Huntington's disease: A two-year follow-up study. *Journal of Genetic Counseling, 15,* 361–374.

Lester, D. (1987). Benefits of marriage for reducing risk of violent death from suicide and homicide for white and non-white persons: Generalizing Gove's findings. *Psychological Reports, 61,* 198.

Levy, N. (2000). Psychiatric considerations in the primary medical care of the patient with renal failure. *Advances in Renal Replacement Therapy, 7,* 231–238.

Lin, H.-C., Wu, C.-H., & Lee, H.-C. (2009). Risk factors for suicide following hospital discharge among cancer patients. *Psycho-Oncology, 18,* 1038–1044.

Linehan, M., Goodstein, J., Nielsen, S., & Chiles, J. (1983). Reasons for staying alive when you are thinking of killing yourself: The Reasons for Living Inventory. *Journal of Clinical & Consulting Psychology, 51,* 276–286.

Lipe, H., Schultz, A., & Bird, T. D. (1993). Risk factors for suicide in Huntington's disease: A retrospective case-controlled study. *American Journal of Medical Genetics, 48,* 231–233.

Lu, T., Chang, H., Chen, L., Chu, M., Ou, N., & Jen, I. (2006). Changes in causes of death and associated conditions among persons with HIV/AIDS after the introduction of highly active antiretroviral therapy in Taiwan. *Journal of the Formosan Medical Association, 105,* 604–609.

Mackenzie, P., & Popkin, M. (1990). Medical illness and suicide. In S. Blumenthal & D. Kupfer (Eds.), *Suicide over the life cycle: Risk factors, assessment, and treatment of suicidal patients* (pp. 205–232). Washington, DC: American Psychiatric Press.

Mahajan, A. P., Sayles, J. N., Patel, V. A., et al. (2008). Stigma in the HIV/AIDS epidemic: A review of the literature and recommendations for the way forwards. *AIDS, 22*(Suppl 2), S67–S79.

Mainio, A., Alamaki, K., Karvonen, K., Hakko, H., Sarkioja, T., & Rasanen, P. (2007). Depression and suicide in epileptic victims: A population-based study of suicide victims during the years 1988–2002 in northern Finland. *Epilepsy & Behavior, 11,* 389–393.

Mann, J., & Arango, V. (1999). The neurobiology of suicidal behavior. In D. Jacobs (Ed.), *The Harvard Medical School guide to suicide assessment and intervention.* San Francisco: Jossey-Bass Publishers.

Mann, J., Waternaux, C., Haas, G., & Malone, K. (1999). Toward a clinical model of suicidal behavior in psychiatric patients. *American Journal of Psychiatry, 156*, 181–188.

Marzuk, P., Tardiff, K., Leon, A., Stajic, M., Morgan, E., & Mann, J. (1992). Prevalence of cocaine use among residents of New York City who committed suicide during a one-year period. *American Journal of Psychiatry, 149*, 371–375.

McGuigan, C., & Hutchinson, M. (2006). Unrecognised symptoms of depression in a community-based population with multiple sclerosis. *Journal of Neurology, 252*, 219–223.

McLean, P., & Taylor, S. (1994). Family therapy for suicidal people. *Death Studies, 18*, 409–426.

McNiel, D. (1998). Empirically based clinical evaluation and management of the potentially violent patient. In Kleespies, P. (Ed.), *Emergencies in mental health practice: Evaluation and management* (pp. 95–116). New York: Guilford Press.

McNiel, D. (2009). Assessment and management of acute risk of violence in adult patients. In P. Kleespies (Ed.), *Behavioral emergencies: An evidence-based resource for evaluating and managing risk of suicide, violence, and victimization* (pp. 125–145). Washington, DC: APA Books.

McNiel, D., Gregory, A., Lam, J., Binder, R., & Sullivan, G. (2003). Utility of decision support tools for assessing acute risk of violence. *Journal of Consulting & Clinical Psychology, 71*, 945–953.

Miller, B., Darby, A., Benson, D., Cummings, J., & Miller, M. (1997). Aggressive, socially disruptive, and antisocial behaviour associated with fronto-temporal dementia. *British Journal of Psychiatry, 170*, 150–155.

Miller, M., Mogun, H., Azrael, D., Hempstead, K., & Solomon, D. H. (2008). Cancer and the risk of suicide in older Americans. *Journal of Clinical Oncology, 26*, 4720–4724.

Misono, S., Weiss, N. S., Fann, J. R., Redman, M., & Yueh, B. (2008). Incidence of suicide in persons with cancer. *Journal of Clinical Oncology, 26*, 4731–4738.

Mizrahi, R., Starkstein, S. E., Jorge R., & Robinson, R. G. (2006). Phenomenology and clinical correlates of delusions in Alzheimer disease. *American Journal of Geriatric Psychiatry, 14*, 573–581.

Monahan, J. (1993). Limiting therapist exposure to *Tarasoff* liability: Guidelines for risk containment. *American Psychologist, 48*, 242–250.

Monahan, J., & Applebaum, P. (1999). Reducing violence risk: Diagnostically based clues from the MacArthur Violence Risk Assessment Study. In S. Hodgins (Ed.), *Violence among the mentally ill: Effective treatments and management strategies* (pp. 19–34). Boston: Kluwer Academic Publishers.

Monahan, J., Steadman, H., Silver. E., et al. (2001). *Rethinking risk assessment: The MacArthur Study of mental disorder and violence.* New York: Oxford University Press.

Moscicki, E. (1997). Identification of suicide risk factors using epidemiologic studies, *Psychiatric Clinics of North America, 20*, 499–517.

Murphy, G. (1986). The physician's role in suicide prevention. In A. Roy (Ed.), *Suicide* (pp. 171–179). Baltimore, MD: Williams & Wilkins.

Murphy, G. (1992). *Suicide in alcoholism.* New York: Oxford University Press.

O'Leary, D. O., Jyringi, D., & Sedler, M. (2005). Childhood conduct problems, stages of Alzheimer's disease, and physical aggression against caregivers. *International Journal of Geriatric Psychiatry, 20*, 401–405.

Ojo, A., Hanson, J., Wolfe, R., Leichtman, A., Agodoa, L., & Port, F. (2000). Long-term survival in renal transplant recipients with graft function. *Kidney International, 57*, 307–313.

Oregon Public Health Services (2011). Thirteenth annual report on Oregon's Death with Dignity Act. Retrieved August 11, 2011, from http://public.health.oregon.gov/ProviderPartnerResources/EvaluationResearch/DeathwithDignityAct/Pages/index.aspx.

Petrov, M., Hurt, C., Collins, D., et al. (2007). Clustering of behavioural and psychological symptoms in dementia: A European Alzheimer's Disease Consortium (EADC) study. *Acta Clinica Belgica, 62*, 426–432.

Peuskins, J., DeHert, M., Cosyns, P., Pieters, G., Theys, P., & Vermotte, R. (1997). Suicide in young schizophrenic patients during and after inpatient treatment. *International Journal of Mental Health, 25*, 39–44.

Pompili, M., Girardi, P., & Tatarelli, R. (2006). Death from suicide versus mortality from epilepsy in the epilepsies: A meta-analysis. *Epilepsy & Behavior, 9*, 641–648.

Resnick, M., Bearman, P., Blum, R., et al. (1997). Protecting adolescents from harm: Findings from the National Longitudinal Study on Adolescent Health. *Journal of the American Medical Association, 278*, 823–832.

Rihmer, Z., & Kiss, K. (2002). Bipolar disorders and suicidal behavior. *Bipolar Disorder, 4* (Suppl 1), 21–25.

Rice, B., Smith, R., & Delpech, V. (2010). HIV infection and suicide in the era of HAART in England, Wales, and Northern Ireland. *AIDS, 24*, 1795–1797.

Riggs, D., Caulfield, M., & Fair, K. (2009). Risk for intimate partner violence: Factors associated with perpetration and victimization. In P. Kleespies (Ed.), *Behavioral emergencies: An evidence-based resource for evaluating and managing risk of suicide, violence, and victimization* (pp. 189–208). Washington, DC: APA Books.

Robins Wahlin, T.-B., Bäckman, L., Lundin, A., Haegermark, A., Winblad, B., & Anvret, M. (2000). High suicidal ideation in persons testing for Huntington's disease. *Acta Neurologica Scandinavica, 102*, 150–161.

Robinson, D., Renshaw, C., Okello, C., Møller, H., & Davies, E. A. (2009). Suicide in cancer patients in South East England from 1996 to 2005: A population-based study. *British Journal of Cancer, 101*, 198–201.

Roy, A., Nielsen, D., Rylander, G., & Sarchiapone, M. (2000). The genetics of suicidal behavior. In K. Hawton & K. van Heeringen (Eds.), *The international handbook of suicide and attempted suicide* (pp. 209–221). New York: J. W. Wiley & Sons.

Rubenstein, J., Heeren, T., Housman, T., Rubin, C., & Stechler, G. (1989). Suicidal behavior in "normal" adolescents: Risk and protective factors. *American Journal of Orthopsychiatry, 59*, 59–7–1.

Rudd, M. D., Joiner, T., & Rajab, M. H. (2001). *Treating suicidal behavior: An effective, time-limited approach.* New York: Guilford Press.

Rudd, M. D., Joiner, T., Trotter, D., Williams, B., & Cordero, L. (2009). The psychosocial treatment of suicidal behavior: A critique of what we know (and don't know). In P. Kleespies (Ed.), *Behavioral emergencies: An evidence-based resource for evaluating and managing risk of suicide, violence, and victimization* (pp. 339–350). Washington, DC: APA Books.

Rutz, W., von Knorring, L., & Walinder, J. (1989). Frequency of suicide on Gotland after systematic postgraduate education of general practitioners. *Acta Psychiatrica Scandinavica, 80*, 151–154.

Ruzicka, L., Choi, C., & Sadkowsky, K. (2005). Medical disorders of suicides in Australia: Analysis using a multiple-cause-of-death approach. *Social Science & Medicine, 61*, 333–341.

Saitz, R., Ciraulo, D., Shader, R., & Ciraulo, A. (2003). Treatment of alcohol withdrawal. In R. Shader (Ed.), *Manual of psychiatric therapeutics* (3rd ed., pp. 127–168). Philadelphia, PA: Lippincott, Williams, & Wilkins.

Saterfield, J. & Schelll, A. (1997). A prospective study of hyperactive boys with conduct problems and normal boys: Adolescent and adult criminality. *Journal of the American Academy of Child & Adolescent Psychiatry. 36*, 1726–1735.

Shub, D., Ball, V., Abbas, A. A., Gottumukkala, A., & Kunik, M. E. (2010). The link between psychosis and aggression in persons with dementia: A systematic review. *Psychiatric Quarterly, 81*, 97–110.

Silver, J., Kramer, R., Greenwald, S., & Weissman, M. (2001). The association between head injuries and psychiatric disorders: The findings of the New Haven NIMH Epidemiological Catchment Area Study. *Brain Injury, 15*, 935–945.

Simpson, G., & Tate, R. (2002). Suicidality after traumatic brain injury: Demographic, injury, and clinical correlates. *Psychological Medicine, 32*, 687–697.

Soden, R., Walsh, J., Middleton, J., Craven, M., Rutkowski, S., & Yeo, J. (2000). Causes of death after spinal cord injury. *Spinal Cord, 38,* 604–610.

Stack, S. (1994). Marriage, family, religion, and suicide. In R. Maris, A. Berman, J. Maltsberger, & R. Yufit (Eds.), *Assessment and prediction of suicide* (pp. 540–552). New York: Guilford Press.

Stack, S. (2000). Work and the economy. In R. Maris, A. Berman, & M. Silverman (Eds.), *Comprehensive textbook of suicidology* (pp. 193–221). New York: Guilford Press.

Stanford, R., Soden, R., Bartrop, R., Mikk, M., & Taylor, T. (2007). Spinal cord and related injuries after attempted suicide: Psychiatric diagnosis and long-term follow-up. *Spinal Cord, 45,* 437–443.

Stanley, B., & Brown, G. (2011). Safety planning intervention: A brief intervention to mitigate suicide risk. *Cognitive & Behavioral Practice,* doi: 10.1016/j.cbpra.2011.01.001

Stenager, E. N., & Stenager, E. (1992). Suicide and patients with neurologic diseases. *Archives of Neurology, 49,* 1296–1303.

Straznickas, K., McNiel, D., & Binder, R. (1993). Violence toward family caregivers by mentally ill relatives. *Hospital & Community Psychiatry, 44,* 385–387.

Swanson, J., Holzer, C., Ganju, V., & Joni, R. (1990). Violence and psychiatric disorder in the community. Evidence from the Epidemiologic Catchment Area surveys. *Hospital & Community Psychiatry, 41,* 761–770.

Tarasoff v. Regents of University of California (1974). S29 P. 2d 553, 118 Cal Rptr. 129.

Tarasoff v. *Regents of University of California* (1976). 17 Cal. 3d 425, 551 P. 2d 334, 131 Cal Rptr, 14.

Tateno, A., Jorge, R., & Robinson, R. (2003). Clinical correlates of aggressive behavior after traumatic brain injury. *The Journal of Neuropsychiatry & Clinical Neurosciences, 15,* 155–160.

Teasdale, T., & Engberg, A. (2001a). Suicide after stroke: A population study. *Journal of Epidemiology & Community Health, 55,* 863–866.

Teasdale, T., & Engberg, A. (2001b). Suicide after traumatic brain injury: A population study. *Journal of Neurology, Neurosurgery, & Psychiatry, 71,* 436–440.

Teasdale, B., Silver, E., & Monahan, J. (2006). Gender, threat/control override delusions and violence. *Law and Human Behavior, 30,* 649–658.

Tolan, P., & Thomas, P. (1995). The implications of age of onset for delinquency risk: II. Longitudinal data. *Journal of Abnormal Child Psychology, 23,* 157–181.

U.S. Bureau of Justice Statistics (2008). Retrieved September 14, 2010, from http://bjs.ojp.usdoj.gov/content/homicide/gender.cfm.

U.S.A. Suicide: 2010 Official Final Data (2012). Retrieved on November 26, 2012, from http://www.suicidology.org/web/guest/stats-and-tools/fact-sheets.

Waern, M., Rubenowitz, E., Runeson, B., Skoog, I., Wilhelmson, K., & Allebeck, P. (2002). Burden of illness and suicide in elderly people: Case-control study. *British Medical Journal, 324,* 1355–1358.

Webster, C., Douglas, K., Eaves, D., & Hart, S. (1997). *HCR-20: Assessing risk for violence (Version 2).* Burnaby, British Columbia: Mental Health, Law, and Policy Institute, Simon Fraser University.

Weishaar, M., & Beck, A. (1992). Clinical and cognitive predictors of suicide. In R. Maris, A. Berman, J. Maltsberger, & R. Yufit (Eds.), *Assessment and prediction of suicide* (pp. 467–483). New York: Guilford Publications.

White, R., Krengel, M., & Thompson, T. (2009). Common neurological disorders associated with psychological-behavioral problems. In P. Kleespies (Ed.), *Behavioral emergencies: An evidence-based resource for evaluating and managing risk of suicide, violence, and victimization* (pp. 289–309). Washington, DC: APA Books.

Whitlock, F. (1986). Suicide and physical illness. In A. Roy (Ed.): *Suicide* (pp. 151–170). Baltimore: Lippincott Williams & Wilkens.

Williams, R., Turner, A., Hatzakis, M. Jr., Bowen, J., Rodriquez, A., & Haselkorn, J. (2005). Prevalence and correlates of depression among veterans with multiple sclerosis. *Neurology, 64,* 75–80.

40.

PERSONALITY DISORDERS IN THE MEDICAL SETTING

Barry S. Fogel

INTRODUCTION

Medical psychiatrists have long been interested in the impact of personality disorders and personality traits on physician–patient relationships, patients' behavior in general medical settings, and patients' adherence to medical treatment recommendations. Fifty years ago, Ralph Kahana and Grete Bibring (1964), psychoanalysts who consulted in a general hospital, described prototypes of different personality styles (e.g., hysterical and compulsive) and suggested how treatment instructions could be adapted to the patient's personality to promote treatment adherence. Their classic article illustrated the fundamental principle of customizing the details of treatment to respect individual differences in personality.

This chapter offers a contemporary perspective on the medical-psychiatric implications of personality issues. It takes account of the current context of medical-psychiatric practice. Specifically:

1. Accepted diagnostic practice combines categorical and dimensional views of personality pathology;

2. Questionnaire-based personality tests are ubiquitous;

3. Epidemiological studies have established the very high prevalence of personality disorders in several of the most common medical-psychiatric conditions;

4. Specific pharmacological and non-pharmacological therapies for borderline personality disorder are supported by high-level evidence;

5. Nonspecific effects of medical treatment—e.g., positive and negative placebo effects—are receiving renewed scientific interest;

6. Subjective and functional outcomes of medical care, including patient satisfaction, are regularly measured and utilized by healthcare systems; and

7. Boundary issues and obligations of physicians to their patients, always important ethical concerns, have become conspicuous legal issues as well.

ALTERNATE WAYS TO DESCRIBE PERSONALITY

Personality traits and personality disorders can be described in various ways that have different uses and different limitations. The clinical context suggests the perspectives on personality that are likely to be the most useful. The medical psychiatrist can make a valuable contribution to a case by choosing the best perspective to apply to the presenting problem. Diagnostic nomenclature will follow from the choice of perspective. Alternative perspectives comprise the following: *categorical, dimensional, mechanistic, typological,* and *based on analysis of defenses.*

CATEGORICAL PERSPECTIVE

In the categorical perspective, a patient is assigned or not assigned to a diagnostic category, such as *Borderline Personality Disorder.* This binary decision is based on whether the patient meets a sufficient number of criteria related to his or her history, behavior, and mental status. Maladaptive personality traits not meeting a sufficient number of criteria for a particular personality disorder can still be conceptualized categorically by describing them as "sub-syndromal" for the personality disorder(s) for which they almost meet criteria.

Advantages of the categorical perspective for medical-psychiatric usage include:

- Wide recognition of certain categorical diagnoses within the medical profession, even outside of psychiatry, including such diagnoses as borderline personality and antisocial personality (psychopathy). Using these diagnoses, a consulting psychiatrist can communicate a great deal in a few words.

- Extensive epidemiological literature on comorbidity of specific personality disorders with specific Axis I conditions and specific general medical disorders.

- Evidence that Axis II comorbidity—expressed in categorical terms—can help predict prognosis and treatment outcome of Axis I conditions, as well as the occurrence of specific salient outcomes like suicide attempts or violence against others.

- Evidence for efficacy of specific pharmacological and non-pharmacological treatments for symptoms of borderline personality disorder, a condition relatively common in the general medical population, and one that is especially likely to disrupt medical treatment or worsen its outcome.

The primary drawback of a categorical diagnosis of personality disorders in the medical-psychiatric context is the lack of reliability and stability of categorical diagnoses made in the face of acute illness on Axis I and/or Axis III. Trauma, pain, loss, and emotional reactions to them, like depression and anxiety, can transiently worsen maladaptive personality traits and/or evoke conspicuous misbehavior, pushing a patient "over the line" to meet categorical diagnostic criteria. This problem can be mitigated by making categorical personality disorder diagnoses based on assessment when a patient is not acutely ill and by utilizing collateral data on the patient's premorbid personality and behavior.

DIMENSIONAL PERSPECTIVE

In the dimensional perspective, a patient is described according to a set of personality dimensions that are applicable to normal people as well as to patients with personality pathology. A patient can be diagnosed as having a personality disorder or problematic personality traits when a statistically abnormal pattern of personality dimensions is combined with emotional distress and/or functional impairment. The five-factor dimensional description of personality promoted by Paul Costa and Robert McCrae (McCrae & Costa, 2010) is probably the most widely known dimensional scheme. The five factors are Extraversion-Introversion, Neuroticism, Openness, Conscientiousness, and Agreeableness. Advantages of the dimensional approach include:

- Stability of personality dimensions over decades of life, without flipping across binary categorical boundaries, even in the face of anxiety or depression and stressful life events. When a patient shows a major change in a personality dimension, the clinician should suspect brain disease, drug effects, or extraordinary circumstances.

- Applicability to improving physicians' understanding of individual differences among their patients, including the majority who do not have any personality disorder diagnosis.

- Face validity of the personality factors, which can be easily understood by patients as well as healthcare professionals, and which are not in themselves associated with stigma.

- Free online resources for assessment and for patient education.

The five-factor characterization of personality can help the medical psychiatrist match patients with treatments and with treatment providers. A patient with above-average scores on extraversion and openness is more likely to do well in a patient support group than one with below-average scores on those dimensions. Knowing a patient is low on the conscientiousness and agreeableness dimensions might guide a clinician to refer the patient to a competent medical specialist who is patient and tolerant, rather than another who is highly rated but arrogant and very busy. The best medical advice can be ineffective if it is not followed.

The principal drawback of the dimensional perspective is that it is not categorical, so it does not easily fit into clinical diagnostic practices and the conventions of coding and reimbursement. Furthermore, evidence on comorbidity, prognosis, and treatment outcomes is usually not organized dimensionally. Knowledge of a dimensional personality profile complements knowledge of a personality disorder diagnosis or its absence, but it does not substitute for it.

MECHANISTIC PERSPECTIVE

The mechanistic perspective on personality is a variant of the dimensional perspective that emphasizes underlying relationships of personality traits to neurochemical or neuroanatomical systems. A widely known mechanistic perspective on personality is the one expounded by Robert Cloninger and his colleagues (Cloninger et al., 1993). It identifies four temperamental dimensions: novelty seeking, harm avoidance, reward dependence, and persistence; and three characterological dimensions: self-directedness, cooperativeness, and self-transcendence. In Cloninger's theory, the four fundamental dimensions of temperament are based on individual differences in neurotransmission and the function of brain circuits. Novelty seeking is associated with dopamine, harm avoidance with serotonin, and reward dependence with norepinephrine. Persistence is associated with the functioning of the frontal executive systems. The seven dimensions of personality described by Cloninger are measured by a 240-item self-rated questionnaire comprising true-false items, the Temperament and Character Inventory (TCI) (Cloninger, 1994).

A particular value of the mechanistic approach is that it enables the linkage of neuropsychiatric conditions with personality change. Three examples illustrate the point:

1. Novelty seeking is related to low dopamine. A patient with Parkinson's disease (PD) progressively loses dopaminergic function, so might be expected to show an increase in impulsive behavior to the extent his or her motor function permitted it. In fact, patients with PD can develop sexual impulsivity, compulsive gambling, and other impulse-control disorders when treatment of the motor disorder enables them to act on their impulses. Another example is the association of major depression with harm avoidance.

2. Patients with major depression can show an increase in harm avoidance that reverts to normal when the patient's depression is successfully treated. This makes sense if the patients' major depression is linked to disruption of serotonergic transmission and is relieved by treatment with a selective serotonin reuptake inhibitor (SSRI).

3. Persistence (effective goal-directedness) is associated with good functioning of frontal executive systems. Patients with early frontotemporal dementia can display a personality change manifested by failing to follow through on plans, keep their word, and honor obligations.

The characterological dimensions of Cloninger's system have neuroanatomical correlates demonstrable on quantitative brain imaging, but there is a less developed understanding of their relationships to specific brain circuits and transmitters than there is for the temperamental dimensions. All three dimensions are positively correlated with better physical and mental health and with better ability to cope with adversity (resilience). Knowing these dimensions can help a clinician assess a patients' vulnerability to developing mental disorders in the face of illness or trauma, and the personal assets they might have to help cope with their current adversity.

TYPOLOGICAL PERSPECTIVE

Typological approaches are hybrids of the dimensional and categorical approaches to personality. They focus more on normal variations than on personality pathology, although extreme examples of personality types can qualify for personality disorder diagnoses. Two useful typological approaches are the Myers-Briggs Type Indicator (MBTI) and the typology of attachment styles.

The Myers-Briggs Type Indicator (MBTI) characterizes individuals into one of 16 types, based on four preferences in their cognitive and emotional processes: Extroversion (E)/Introversion (I), Sensation (S)/Intuition (N), Thinking (T)/Feeling (F), and Perceiving (P)/Judging (J) (Myers, 1998). Individuals' preferences on these four dichotomies can be more or less strong. For example, a person might be characterized as INTP if he or she were introverted, experienced the world more intuitively than through direct sensory experience, usually reached conclusions through reasoning rather than emotionally, and were relatively slow to make final judgments about experiences and issues. Scores on the MBTI are used to classify individuals into one of the 16 types. The MBTI comprises 93 binary items. There are also abbreviated and expanded versions, as well as options for confidential online administration. An extensive literature has related psychological type as measured by the MBTI to occupations, social roles, intimate relationships, and typical interpersonal conflicts. An example of how the MBTI relates to occupations is the correlation of psychological type and the choice of medical specialty by physicians: A physician of type INTP is 2.75 times more likely to become a neurologist and 0.44 times less likely to become an OB/GYN than would be expected from the distribution of medical specialists.

The typological view has been utilized extensively in organizational psychology and in marital therapy. It deserves consideration as an aid to understanding how physician–patient relationships can go wrong, and in judging whether a change in physician or some form of advice to the physician and/or patient is a practicable way to resolve a problem.

For example, consider the physician–patient relationship when the physician's type is INTP and the patient's type is ESFJ. The physician might quickly make a correct diagnosis and communicate it in a matter-of-fact way to the patient, while not taking the time to build rapport and warm feelings with the patient, and not doing a visibly meticulous examination. The patient, whose judgments are driven by feelings and immediate sensations, may reject or deny the diagnosis, not because it is incorrect, but because of the mismatch of the physician and the patient's personality style.

Another example is suggested by a recent report that the risk tolerance of surgeons is correlated with their personality type (Contessa et al., 2013). Greater risk tolerance is associated with higher scores on scales of extraversion, thinking, and perceiving. If there is a choice of similarly qualified surgeons, one might attempt to align the risk tolerance of the patient with that of the surgeon when making a referral.

Another typological perspective—limited in its scope but clinically useful—is expressed in the classification of attachment styles based on the attachment theory of the psychoanalyst John Bowlby (Bowlby, 1988), and further developed by numerous other psychodynamically-oriented psychologists and psychiatrists. Individuals are described with respect to dimensions of their close relationships: Are they avoided? Is their importance minimized? Are their attachments insecure? Both interview-based and questionnaire-based scales are available for assessing attachment styles (Ravitz et al., 2010). Moreover, detailed behavioral profiles of the four main attachment styles enable medical psychiatrists to characterize most patients from clinical information they would routinely collect (Maunder & Hunter, 2009). Because attachment styles are coherent (Hunter & Maunder, 2001) and strongly correlated with illness behavior, the characterization of a patient has predictive value. Some specific, simple and accessible self-report scales include the Relationship Scales Questionnaire (RSQ) (Bartholomew & Horowitz, 1991) and its four-item brief version, the Relationship Questionnaire (RQ); and the Experiences in Close Relationships Scale–Revised (ECR-R). The RSQ comprises 20 bidirectional (Likert) 7-point items; e.g., the patient is asked to rate how much the statement "I find it difficult to depend on other people" does or does not apply to him or her. Based on their responses to these questions, patients' attachment style can be characterized as *secure* (positive view of self and other), *anxious/preoccupied* (negative view of self, positive view of other), *avoidant/fearful* (negative view of self and other), or *dismissive* (positive view of self, negative view of other). The ECR focuses on romantic relationships and comprises 36 7-point Likert-type ordinal items (Fraley et al., 2000; Brennan et al., 1998).

Relationship style is remarkably stable over time. Relationship style predicts patients' relationships with their physicians, other professionals, their caregivers, and their intimates, thus affecting their ability to successfully navigate the healthcare system, get the care they need, adhere to their treatment, modify health-related behaviors, and cope with their symptoms and impairments. Several examples from recent research reports illustrate the value of the attachment style perspective:

1. Avoidant attachment style was linked to a higher incidence of post-traumatic stress disorder (PTSD) following operative birth (Ayers et al., 2014);

2. Avoidant attachment style was associated with a higher incidence of unsafe sexual encounters in gay men (Starks & Parsons, 2014);

3. Women in primary care with anxious attachment had more unsafe sexual encounters; women with avoidant attachment were more likely to be smokers (Ahrens et al., 2012);

4. In chronic pain patients, insecure attachment styles were associated with more pain intensity, pain-related behavior, pain-related disability, depressive symptoms, and a greater perception of a negative spousal responses (Forsythe et al., 2012);

5. In an oncology practice, insecurely attached patients were less likely to trust their oncologist or be satisfied with care one year after their cancer diagnosis (Hillen et al., 2014). More generally, avoidant and dismissive styles are associated with less trust in physicians and poorer adherence to treatment, while anxious/insecure attachment is associated with more psychosomatic complaints and greater utilization of healthcare resources.

Even without the results of questionnaires, medical psychiatrists can assess patients' attachment styles from their explicit responses and their behavior during the diagnostic interview. Patients' attachment styles can be kept in mind when planning treatment and aid in setting realistic expectations for patient behavior and treatment outcome with the patient, family caregivers, and medical colleagues.

PERSPECTIVE BASED ON ANALYSIS OF DEFENSES

One of the gifts of psychoanalysis to general psychiatry is the conceptualization and description of defense mechanisms—ways in which people cope with psychological stress using characteristic patterns of perceiving, thinking, and acting. These mechanisms also have been termed "involuntary coping mechanisms" by George Vaillant, who has done extensive longitudinal studies of defense mechanism and their lifetime implications (Vaillant, 2011). Defenses have six characteristics:

1. They mitigate the distressing effects of both emotion and cognitive dissonance;

2. They are unconscious (i.e., involuntary);

3. They are discrete from one another;

4. They are dynamic and reversible;

5. They can be adaptive and even creative as well as pathological; and

6. They are invisible to the user but not to observers (Vaillant, 1977).

Defenses have been organized into a hierarchy of four groups:

1. *Psychotic*, including delusional projection, psychotic denial, and psychotic distortion;

2. *Immature*, including acting out, dissociation, passive aggression, and non-psychotic projection;

3. *Intermediate (neurotic)*, including displacement, isolation, and repression; and

4. *Mature*, including humor, altruism, sublimation, and suppression.

Patients' defensive styles can be assessed using the Defense Styles Questionnaire (DSQ) (Bond, 1986). The questionnaire comes in various versions, with 88, 60, or 40 ordinal items. Scoring yields an overall assessment of defensive functioning. Defenses can be expressed in terms of three factors or placed into a seven-level hierarchy. The three factors are *image distorting, affect regulating,* and *adaptive.* The seven levels are *action, major image distortion, disavowal, minor image distortion, neurotic, obsessional,* and *adaptive.* Clinicians can appraise patients' defensive styles without questionnaires making use of their clinical observations and both the verbal and nonverbal responses of patients' to their questions during a diagnostic interview. The description and classification of the defensive styles utilized in the interpretation of questionnaires is applicable to interpretation of data from the medical record and clinical encounters.

Defense mechanisms have been associated with patients' symptoms and with medical outcomes across a broad range of medical conditions: patients with neurotic defenses have more symptoms, sick or well, than those with adaptive defenses (Hyphantis et al., 2013). Supportive psychotherapeutic interventions for medical-psychiatric patients—regardless of their severity of general medical illness—aim to identify, bolster, and mobilize patients' adaptive defenses and diminish the use of lower-level defenses by psychotherapeutic, behavioral, environmental, and/or pharmacological means.

Even patients with healthy personalities might utilize lower-level defense mechanisms when suffering from illness, trauma, loss, or other severe stress. The resulting adaptive failure can lead to a medical-psychiatric consultation. A perspective based on the analysis of defenses can be helpful to medical psychiatrists in conceiving their short-term psychotherapeutic work with such patients. The clinician aims to identify adaptive defenses that worked for the patient in the past, to discover why the patient is not using them or why they are not currently effective, and to get the patient to "move up" the hierarchy of defenses. This might involve pointing out alternatives and encouraging their use, or addressing impediments to the use of previously effective defenses. As an example of the latter tactic, note that many of the adaptive defenses have substantial cognitive demands. If a patient with cognitively intense adaptive defenses is given a benzodiazepine that impairs his or her cognition, it can actually cause an increase in anxiety due to the loss of an effective defense mechanism. Stopping the anti-anxiety drug could actually reduce anxiety in this situation. Similarly, when a patient has adaptive defenses that require substantial mental energy and the latter has been reduced by general medical illness, giving a stimulant might reduce anxiety by helping the patient mobilize his or her adaptive defenses. In other patients with a different defensive style, benzodiazepines might relieve anxiety and stimulants might worsen it.

TIPS ON CATEGORICAL DIAGNOSIS

It is assumed that the reader is familiar with the *Diagnostic and Statistical Manual of Mental Disorders* (DSM) classification of personality disorders and with the ways in which patients with particular personality disorders are likely to show problematic behavior in medical settings. When the presence of a personality disorder or maladaptive personality trait impedes medical treatment, the specific personality diagnosis is relevant to the selection of a management strategy, but a current (re)assessment of the patient's defensive style and quality of interpersonal relationships is also necessary. This assessment is most important for individuals with narcissistic, histrionic, dependent, and passive-aggressive traits, who can have relatively more or less mature defenses and more or less unstable interpersonal relations. For example, histrionic or "hysterical" patients with relatively good impulse control and a more mature defensive structure require different management from less mature, impulsive histrionic patients with borderline features.

Antisocial personalities, diagnosed on the basis of history, always should be presumed to have "psychotic" or "immature" defenses, even if they appear to be functioning at a higher level on a single cross-sectional assessment.

The formal diagnosis of *Borderline Personality Disorder* (BPD) by DSM criteria is less important for medical-psychiatric management than identification of the patient as one with a poor quality of interpersonal relationships and a tendency to use the defenses of splitting and projective identification. Patients with a history of childhood sexual abuse, factitious illness, or multiple suicide attempts are highly likely to have a borderline personality organization.

Patients with *passive-aggressive* and *dependent* personalities can have either more mature or less mature defensive structures and object relations. More primitive passive-aggressive patients might passively attempt to sabotage medical treatment as an expression of rage against the physician, who serves as a transference figure. By contrast, the passive-aggressive patient with higher-level defenses primarily might have conflicts over control and autonomy, or might be identifying with a passive-aggressive parent. Management should be in accord with the patient's defensive style and specific emotional conflicts.

Schizoid and *avoidant personalities* may be difficult to distinguish on a single cross-sectional assessment. Both, however, fear closeness and may fear being controlled by others.

The enforced intimacy of medical settings and the attendant loss of control lead to anxiety, which is expressed according to the patient's defensive style.

Narcissistic personalities can have either a low or a high level of functioning. More severely impaired individuals might display demanding, manipulative, exploitative, entitled, and/or dishonest behavior that disrupts medical treatment and engenders angry reactions from their caregivers. Better-functioning narcissistic personalities might be less dramatically "entitled" but might reveal an excessive vulnerability to criticism, disappointment, and feelings of shame or embarrassment. They might overvalue particular physical or mental attributes and have an unusually difficult time adjusting to the limitations of a chronic illness. The physician, if not devalued, might be idealized to the point of discomfort. Physicians can find themselves rapidly idealized and then equally rapidly devalued.

SPECIAL ISSUES IN OLDER PATIENTS

As problematic as categorical personality disorder diagnosis can be in general medical patients, it can be even more difficult in older medical patients, because neither diagnostic criteria nor their application are age-neutral. The criminal behavior that is required for a diagnosis of antisocial personality is less prevalent during old age, as are the identity disturbances typical of borderline personality in young adults. Yet personality traits are relatively stable with age, suggesting that personality disorders do not disappear altogether but change their form according to the patient's life stage. Antisocial personalities might give up crime and turn to alcoholism and hypochondriasis, and borderline personalities can develop stable social and occupational functioning but fail to form close personal relationships. The focus of patients' concerns and conflicts shifts with life stage: narcissistic individuals might inflate their past accomplishments or the talent of their grandchildren; borderline personalities might apply splitting and projective identification to their caregivers and to their children instead of to their parents, spouses, or partners.

Age-specific events can evoke symptoms of personality disorder. Such situations include bereavement, institutionalization, forced intimacy with caretakers, and cognitive changes, particularly those of early dementia. Personality disorders thus can emerge during old age, especially in individuals who had sub-syndromal traits earlier in life.

Because categorical personality disorder diagnoses can help with prognosis, treatment planning and communicating with other clinicians it is worth the effort to attempt a categorical personality diagnosis in an older patient with evident maladaptive personality traits This exercise can be aided by: (1) obtaining information on the patient's earlier adaptation, especially from reliable informants or old records; (2) considering traits and defensive style and de-emphasizing whether formal criteria are met; and (3) considering the possibility that disordered personality can emerge during old age as a function of changed life circumstances or alterations in brain function (Sadavoy & Fogel, 1992).

PRESENTATION OF PERSONALITY DISORDERS IN GENERAL MEDICAL SETTINGS

In general medical settings, patients with personality disorders are brought to the attention of the psychiatrist because:

1. They display angry, manipulative, self-destructive behavior, violent behavior, or make threats to harm themselves or others;

2. They adhere poorly to treatment recommendations or show unexpectedly poor treatment outcomes;

3. They develop somatic complaints in excess of diagnosable general medical conditions;

4. They develop severe anxiety or depression;

5. They show signs of an Axis I condition requiring treatment in its own right (e.g., substance abuse, PTSD, or psychosis);

6. Their treatment for an Axis I condition by their primary care physician or other principal physician is not successful;

7. They abuse or misuse prescribed medications;

8. They evoke frustration and anger in their family members or other informal caregivers;

9. They evoke negative or inappropriate emotional reactions in clinicians, or evoke conflict between clinicians caring for them;

10. They initiate or induce legal actions, either civil or criminal.

Most medical-psychiatric involvement with patients with personality disorders is reactive to one of the above situations. Prospective identification and preventive intervention with patients with personality disorders is an appealing alternative when a medical psychiatrist operates as a liaison to a service treating a clinical population with a high prevalence of Axis II comorbidity, such as patients with chronic pain, patients with addictions, or patients with somatoform disorders. The author's view is that when patients are diagnosed with a major chronic general medical disease, their personalities should be assessed, whether formally or informally, and the results of the assessment should be used to adapt the treatment to the patient. If the patient has borderline personality disorder (BPD), he or she should be offered evidence-based treatment to mitigate the symptoms of BPD, since improvement in the BPD will necessarily improve coping with the general medical illness; and the best time for therapeutic intervention is when the patient is both motivated by a momentous diagnosis and not so physically sick that psychiatric treatment is either irrelevant or intolerable.

Incorporating an understanding of *normal variations* of personality into treatment planning and patient management should be part of a medical psychiatrist's usual practice. When the medical psychiatrist will be involved in the long-term management of a patient with a chronic or relapsing-remitting general medical condition, it is useful both to assess the patient for Axis II disorders and to characterize the patient's personality qualitatively from one or more of the different perspectives described above. Self-rated questionnaires are useful, but even without using specific questionnaires, the conceptual schemes that underlie them can be employed to organize the clinician's observations into descriptors that can be used to approach the literature and to communicate with colleagues.

AXIS I AND AXIS II COMORBIDITY

The large literature on the comorbidity of Axis I and Axis II will not be reviewed here. I will confine myself to several general observations that are well supported by empirical evidence and have special applicability in the medical-psychiatric setting.

1. *Avoidant personality* overlaps greatly with *social anxiety disorder* (social phobia). Both conditions can interfere with patients' relationships with healthcare providers and thus with medical treatment adherence. Social anxiety disorder, more than avoidant personality alone, has evidence-based and frequently effective pharmacological and cognitive-behavioral treatments. When a patient with social anxiety disorder is diagnosed with a chronic general medical illness, or is at high risk for developing one, intervention to treat the social anxiety prepares the patient to have a better course of treatment for his or her medical problem.

2. *Schizotypy* is a continuum from schizotypal traits to schizotypal personality to schizophrenia (Nelson et al., 2013). Schizotypal personality is a risk factor for developing schizophrenia, and patients with severe schizotypal personality have a very high risk of developing schizophrenia (Barrantes-Vidal et al., 2013). On brain imaging, patients with schizotypal personality and patients with schizophrenia share abnormalities in the temporal lobe, but schizotypal personality disorder patients without schizophrenia lack the relative atrophy of the frontal lobes seen in the latter disorder (Fervaha & Remington, 2013). With stronger frontal systems functioning, they are able to compensate better for their temporal dysfunction and thus prevent the emergence of full-blown psychosis. Schizotypal personality thus reflects a balance between a tendency toward psychosis and inhibitory mechanisms. Stress, general medical illness, traumatic brain injury, and/or the effects of alcohol or drugs can upset this balance, leading to the onset of overt psychosis. When providing comprehensive medical care to a patient with schizotypal personality disorder, great attention should be paid to brain health—discouraging alcohol and drug use, assessing potential central nervous system (CNS) side effects of drugs used for general medical conditions, etc.

3. *Obsessive-compulsive personality* overlaps with *obsessive-compulsive disorder* (OCD). The latter condition has evidence-based and often effective pharmacological and

cognitive-behavioral treatment. Some compulsive rituals cause medical harm; others interfere with patients' treatment for general medical conditions. These situations argue for the importance of treating OCD even when the patient's distress from his or her compulsions is not severe.

4. Patients who present with *major depression* often have a comorbid personality disorder. The effectiveness of treatment for major depression is lower when there is a comorbid personality disorder. Furthermore, depression can increase the severity of personality disorder symptoms or move a patient across the line into personality disorder from sub-syndromal status. Patients with major depression and comorbid personality disorder require especially conscientious treatment of the major depression that takes the distinctive interpersonal and defensive style of the patient into account.

5. Patients with *substance abuse* frequently have personality disorders—with antisocial and borderline personality disorder (BPD) especially common (Skodol et al., 1999). Patients with antisocial personality should be treated with appropriate mistrust and with precautions to avoid violent or criminal acting-out. Patients with borderline personality may benefit from non-pharmacological treatment of their BPD after they are abstinent from their substances of abuse.

6. Patients with BPD have a high rate of comorbid somatoform disorders, and the prevalence of BPD is high in patients with chronic pain and patients with medically unexplained symptoms or other forms of excessive illness behavior. When a patient presents with a new diagnosis of a somatoform disorder, the diagnosis of BPD should be considered.

7. In considering Axis I comorbidity in patients with BPD, the "80% rule" is useful: Over 80% of patients with BPD have a lifetime history of an anxiety disorder, over 80% have a lifetime history of a mood disorder, and slightly fewer than 80% have a lifetime history of a substance use disorder.

8. Adolescents and adults with *attention-deficit hyperactivity disorder* (ADHD) may display angry, impulsive, and uncooperative behavior in the hospital environment because of the combination of overstimulation and enforced passivity. Such patients' behavior can remove remarkably when they are given stimulants, and even some patients with comorbid BPD will show behavioral improvement. However, stimulants can precipitate psychotic symptoms in BPD patients, and it is difficult to predict which ones will have this reaction. A conservative approach would be to use stimulants in patients with comorbid ADHD and BPD in acute medical-psychiatric contexts only when prior treatment with stimulants has been an unequivocal success. Even greater caution applies to the use of stimulants in patients with comorbid ADHD and schizotypal personality. When ADHD occurs without either of these comorbidities, stimulants usually help hospitalized patients' agitation and inattention. The author's impression from decades of consultations is that when patients hospitalized for acute medical illness become agitated, ADHD is relatively neglected in the differential diagnosis, and stimulants are neglected as a therapeutic option. A childhood history of ADHD or learning disability and the absence of delirium should prompt consideration of the diagnosis; if ADHD is present, the clinician should consider whether there is a psychiatric or general medical comorbidity that would contraindicate the use of stimulants.

AXIS II COMORBIDITY WITH GENERAL MEDICAL CONDITIONS

The study of the comorbidity of personality disorders with general medical illness is confounded by the relationship of personality with patterns of help-seeking and interaction with clinicians and institutions. For example, patients with BPD would be more likely to seek treatment for a general medical condition in an emergency room because of the intensity of the distress they might feel when ill and their inability to tolerate waiting for an outpatient appointment. A patient with avoidant personality might avoid seeking treatment for a medical condition until its symptoms became intolerable. Studying the comorbidity of general medical illness and personality disorder in population-based surveys has other shortcomings—an avoidant person with serious general medical illness might not respond to a telephone survey or home visit by a surveyor; neither might a person with significant paranoid traits. Hospitals, clinics, and physicians' offices are full of patients with personality disorders that rarely are diagnosed by non-psychiatric physicians. Specific medical populations with a high proportion of patients with personality disorders include: patients with chronic pain, patients with somatoform disorders, patients with sexually transmitted diseases, patients with self-inflicted injuries, patients injured in violent altercations, patients seeking disability status, and patients with eating disorders. Systematic screening for personality disorders and characterization of personality traits is clinically warranted in these populations, even if patients do not present in a way that demands immediate psychiatric attention.

Experienced primary care physicians with long-term patient relationships often have a good grasp of their patients' personality traits and characteristic responses to stressful life events. However, they are unlikely to make personality disorder diagnoses, even in situations in which a psychiatrist could make them. Missed diagnoses of personality disorders most often are missed opportunities to make a potentially helpful referral or modification of treatment strategy. However, in some cases, missed Axis II diagnoses are dangerous. Not recognizing that a patient has an antisocial personality, a physician might be manipulated into prescribing controlled substances that are then illegally diverted (e.g., resold). Or, not giving in to inappropriate demands for controlled substances, the physician might be physically threatened or attacked. Not recognizing that a patient has a borderline personality, a physician might be seduced into a boundary violation, or give in to the patient's pressure to do unnecessary tests or procedures. In multi-specialty practices, non-psychiatric physicians should be encouraged to get psychiatric consultation routinely when an unfamiliar patient begins pushing for procedures or treatments despite the physician's reluctance—including prescription of controlled substances—or asks for a physician's help in documenting disability status that is not supported by objective signs.

PROBLEM-ORIENTED MEDICAL-PSYCHIATRIC CONSULTATION

Medical psychiatrists often are consulted by general medical physicians to assess patients with problematic behavior in a hospital or clinic or in the physician–patient relationship. Many of the patients involved in such difficult situations have personality disorders or personality trait disturbances. A practical approach to problem-focused consultations might consider these points in the initial assessment:

1. What is the patient's view of the problem? Is there a legitimate, practically resolvable issue? Is there a misunderstanding between the patient and the medical staff that needs clarification? The patient might have a valid concern, even if he or she expresses the concern in a way that is self-defeating or impinges on others.

2. Are there practical, negotiable issues compounded by emotional issues and interpersonal conflicts? If the practical concerns could be separated from the emotional and interpersonal ones, could they be resolved?

3. Is there evidence of an Axis I diagnosis? In particular, is there a treatable Axis I diagnosis that is more directly linked to the immediate problem than is the patient's personality? For example, non-adherence to general medical treatment by a patient with avoidant personality might be explained by social phobia or agoraphobia. Treating the phobia could improve their medical treatment adherence without requiring a change in the underlying personality.

4. Is the patient under the influence of prescribed medications, alcohol, or illicit drugs, or withdrawing from such substances? Patients with Cluster B personality disorders—antisocial, borderline, histrionic, or narcissistic—are more likely than patients in general to use and to abuse psychoactive substances. The proximate cause of a behavioral problem in a patient with a Cluster B personality disorder might be a manageable substance-related problem.

5. What is the patient's perception of the physician–patient relationship and of the patient's role in the treatment? Malalignment of expectations of the patient for the physician and the physician for the patient can cause trouble in any circumstance, though the troubles are worse when one of the discordant parties has a personality disorder.

6. Is the immediate problem provoked by inappropriate or inflexible behavior by a physician, nurse, or other health-care provider? Tactless or inept limit-setting can bring out the worst in a patient with a borderline personality.

7. Has a medical disorder or medication side-effect been overlooked or misdiagnosed? Just because personality disorders can impair physician–patient communication, patients with personality disorders are more likely to get incorrect diagnoses, have under-treated or over-treated symptoms, or have unrecognized medication side effects. At the same time, patients with personality disorders can express emotional distress as physical symptoms disproportionate to the medical illness, and insist that a diagnosis has been missed or that medication side effects have been neglected. At best, a medical-psychiatric consultant can assess these issues with eyes unclouded by countertransference or the effects of an already-difficult physician–patient relationship.

When information from the interview, collateral sources, healthcare providers, and the medical record is synthesized, a tentative personality diagnosis might be possible, as well as a concise statement of the behavioral problem needing resolution. Specific strategies can be employed to address behavioral problems according to the patient's personality type, while concurrent Axis I and general medical problems receive appropriate pharmacological or psychotherapeutic attention, or both.

MANAGEMENT STRATEGY

Management strategy for patients with personality disorders in general medical settings comprises tactical responses to short-term problem situations; longer-term approaches to preventing crises, disruptions of medical treatment, and non-adherence to treatment for chronic conditions; and, where feasible, interventions to decrease the distress and impairments caused by the personality disorder itself in areas beyond their participation in general medical treatment. The strategy is based on a personality diagnosis that includes a categorical diagnosis of a specific personality disorder, if one is justified. Tactics for short-term problems with behavior, treatment adherence, or physician–patient relationships are selected with consideration of current defensive functioning. Longer-term considerations in treatment planning may include consideration of personality dimensions, attachment style, and psychological type.

When approaching acute behavioral problems in general medical settings that are potentially related to the patient's personality, the medical psychiatrist gathers data from the patient interview, medical records, and collateral sources and synthesizes them to make a tentative personality diagnosis that comprises an assignment of an Axis II diagnosis if appropriate, and an assessment of current defensive operations and the quality of the patient's interpersonal relations. Axis I and

Axis III disorders that contribute to the behavioral problem also are diagnosed, and their treatment is initiated or modified as appropriate. In this connection substance abuse, CNS side effects of prescribed medications, and brain diseases with frequent neuropsychiatric complications deserve special attention. The psychiatrist then develops a management strategy to reduce the interference of the patient's maladaptive personality traits and less mature defenses with his or her medical treatment.

Specific tactics for handling short-term problem situations are part of the tradition of consultation-liaison psychiatry. While evidence to support them is largely anecdotal, they are widely taught, and the author, among others, has found them useful. Several will be described here.

When the medical psychiatrist has an ongoing relationship with a subspecialty clinic, it may be feasible to prospectively identify patients with personality disorders or evident trait disturbances and act preemptively to prevent non-adherence or disruptive behavior. Identification of candidates for preventive action can be done informally, or a clinic can include some self-rated instruments in its intake process. While the latter step is unusual at this time, it would seem rational for a clinic that treats chronic diseases with a very high prevalence of psychiatric comorbidity.

However a patient with a personality disorder is identified, the Axis II condition should be dealt with like any other comorbid condition—psychiatric or medical—that can affect the outcome of the primary illness being treated. For example, a management strategy for a patient under the care of a rheumatologist with newly diagnosed systemic lupus erythematosus (SLE) and a BPD might include referral of the patient for a course of dialectical behavioral therapy or transference-focused therapy for BPD, and a trial of a mood-stabilizing antiepileptic drug if the patient has prominent affective instability. This might be combined with an informal conference with the members of the rheumatologist's practice team alerting them to the borderline patient's potential for splitting, and suggesting that they develop an explicit written plan of treatment that could be accessed by any physician who might be providing coverage for the patient after hours or on a weekend or holiday.

TACTICS FOR PATIENTS WITH IMMATURE DEFENSES

When managing a patient with less mature defenses, the physician must not assume *a priori* a trusting relationship or the patient's capacity to be consistent. Consistency and appropriateness must be provided by the physician, who must not be unduly moved by pleas, demands, manipulations, or threats, or be personally affronted by the patient's mistrust (Dawson, 1988).

Because patients with less mature defenses may react dramatically to disappointment, it is all-important to clarify treatment expectations. The patient's view of his or her implicit therapeutic contract with their physician(s) should be explored and the goals and limits of the patient's medical treatment made clear at the outset. Conflicts can be minimized by frequently reorienting the patient, the significant others, and healthcare providers toward a basic and circumscribed treatment contract. Whenever possible, this implicit contract should be restated in the patient's own words. Management tactics useful for patients with immature defenses involve giving the patient a sense of control, simplifying the treatment plan, being consistent, taking the "one-down" position, limit-setting, avoiding or limiting hospitalization, and anti-splitting maneuvers.

GIVING THE PATIENT A SENSE OF CONTROL

Giving the patient a sense of control is maximizing the appropriate influence the patient has over the treatment situation. Maximizing patient autonomy while remaining consistent—or almost consistent—with evidence-based practice is a widely accepted principle in the United States, though perhaps patient autonomy receives less weight in some other countries with national health systems in which the patient is not viewed as a customer. Notwithstanding, given the time constraints and customary procedures of busy practices, physicians often tell patients what a plan of treatment will be, rather than ask them for their preferences. Patients with mature defenses usually will speak up and negotiate with a physician if the recommendation does not work for them; those with immature defenses are more likely to respond maladaptively, for example by getting angry, breaking off the treatment relationship, not showing up for appointments, or not taking medications as prescribed. These problems can be reduced by inviting patients to express their preferences before settling on the details of treatment; for example, a schedule of outpatient visits, a prescription of medication, or the hospital discharge date. Incorporating patient preferences sometimes requires deviation from usual procedures and sometimes requires the physician to advocate within a hospital, clinic, or health system on behalf of the patient. This can make sense when the alternative is worse; the physician should bear in mind that a treatment plan that perfectly follows evidence-based practice guidelines or the policies of the hospital or health plan is of little value if the patient does not accept it. For risk management purposes the reasoning for making an exception should be documented, and comment on the patient's personality or behavioral issues is sometimes necessary to support the physician's decision.

SIMPLIFYING THE TREATMENT PLAN

Following a medical treatment plan almost always involves behavior change on the patient's part. Intentional, consistent, and adaptive behavior can be difficult for any patient: consider the success rate with attempts at smoking cessation, weight loss, or increasing exercise! It is an even greater challenge for patients with immature defenses who are less able to manage anxiety and frustration and who might have deficits in executive control systems. The physician in charge of coordinating a patient's care—*and there should be one*—should determine the top short-term priorities for behavior change (including treatment adherence) and limit what is asked of the patient at one time. This can mean delaying attention to a known medical problem until other problems are under control. Here, too, the reason for deviation from ideal practice should be documented.

BEING CONSISTENT

Being consistent means minimizing changes in the treatment plan, the healthcare providers involved, and the language in which information is conveyed, thereby reducing opportunities for confusion or misunderstanding. It is facilitated by giving the patient some control and simplifying the plan. Instructions should be written, and patients should be asked to restate them in their own words. When several healthcare providers are involved, one of them must "get the license" to coordinate the plans and recommendations of all. When patients have multiple comorbid conditions, it might be unrealistic for the primary care physician to be the team captain. In the author's experience, the best coordinator usually is the specialist treating the condition currently most critical to the patient's outcome: for example, the oncologist for a patient being treated for cancer, the cardiologist for a patient with a recent myocardial infarction, or the medical psychiatrist for a patient with melancholia and suicidal ideation.

Communication by email has can either be an aid or an impediment to being consistent. If patients email different physicians and other healthcare providers separately, they can accumulate inconsistent or even contradictory written advice. If all email communication goes through a common secure portal, designed so that all involved healthcare providers can see all of the messages, it can be a powerful tool for aligning everyone's advice and for identifying differences of opinion so they can be promptly resolved. Many health systems offer such patient portals. For a portal to work to promote consistency, everyone involved has to agree to use it and to not have side communications with the patient, and the patient has to agree that information will be shared among all of their providers.

TAKING THE "ONE-DOWN" POSITION

Taking the "one-down" position means realistically recognizing one's limitations in affecting another person's behavior, and approaching the patient with genuine and appropriate humility. It includes "allowing" some degree of pathological behavior to go unchallenged if it is not immediately or severely harmful to the patient. This approach—more an attitude than a tactic—forestalls many potential control struggles with personality-disordered patients. Taking the one-down position implies yielding control in some areas of contention between physician and patient; the empowerment of the patient helps alleviate any feelings of helplessness and vulnerability that can lead to rage reactions and defensive aggression. Distinguishing between appropriate humility and yielding to a patient's threats and manipulation is sometimes difficult, however. Consultation with a colleague can help clinically and is also a useful risk management strategy in high-stakes situations.

Taking the one-down position also includes setting appropriately modest expectations regarding all treatments, both psychiatric and medical. Treatment with psychotropic drugs in particular should be preceded by a "universal disclaimer"—the physician's statement that, while any drug prescription will be supported by evidence, such evidence will only show that a given drug is better than a placebo or better than an alternative, and not that it will work for everyone. They should also note that individuals have different sensitivity to adverse effects and that dosage might need to be individualized. A careful personal and family history of relevant drug responses should be taken, and where applicable, pharmacogenomic testing, therapeutic drug monitoring, or scheduled email follow-up with questionnaires about symptoms and side effects should be considered.

LIMIT SETTING

Limit setting is the trump card—to be played if a patient is seriously impeding treatment or is endangering someone. For outpatients, typical circumstances for limit setting are diversion of prescription drugs, verbal abuse of the office staff, or threats of violence. For inpatients, limit setting is an appropriate response to such behavior as deliberately pulling out intravenous lines, smoking in a room with oxygen, or screaming all night in a room full of sick patients, when such behavior is not an expression of delirium or psychosis.

In the inpatient case, all involved healthcare providers are told of the problem and decide together what limits will be set. The patient is told without anger which behaviors are unacceptable "*in this hospital*" (or in this clinic or other setting of practice). If limits are set angrily, the patient responds more to the anger than to the limit. Reference to "in this [setting of practice]" restricts the control struggle to one setting rather than to the whole world. In the outpatient case, the patient is told that the physician will not continue to treat the patient (or prescribe medication, or continue certifying disability, or whatever) if the behavior continues. Appropriate alternative sources of care would be discussed with the patient to forestall accusations of abandonment.

In the variation called "sympathetic limit setting," the physician acknowledges that there is something that could understandably provoke the patient's behavior, *but* that the behavior is nonetheless unacceptable in the current setting of care.

In the inpatient case, whether limits are set with or without an expression of sympathy, the patient is told that termination of the current treatment arrangement is inevitable if the unacceptable behavior continues. The patient will either be discharged from the hospital with a referral for some kind for follow-up, or, if involuntary psychiatric treatment is indicated because of a risk to self or others, a request for temporary certification is completed, and the patient is transferred an appropriate psychiatric facility. If the patient is too medically unstable for such a referral, control of violent or potentially self-injurious behavior is maintained with antipsychotic drugs, special observation, and/or physical restraints until the patient's physical condition permits either transfer to a secure psychiatric facility or discharge to the community with a referral for follow-up. The referral usually will be to an organized care setting such as a community mental health center that has the staff and resources to provide continuous coverage and to respond to a psychiatric emergency.

The clinician's countertransference is a common—if not the most common—impediment to effective limit setting. Limit setting with obvious anger is one expression of countertransference; another is a failure to set limits either because of the clinician's fear of the patient's anger or the clinician's defense against his or her own unconscious anger.

Another reason why clinicians fail to set necessary limits is fear of litigation or a complaint to a professional licensing board; increasingly, the expression of "consumer dissatisfaction" or a complaint to a hospital or health plan is a concern. Complaints to licensing boards can be challenging for clinicians, because clinicians do not necessarily have the protection of legal due process, and an articulate but malignant individual can paint a convincing though distorted picture of the clinician's actions (Gutheil, 2005). Furthermore, applications for medical staff appointments frequently ask whether a physician has been the subject of patient complaints, even if those complaints have not been substantiated. Notwithstanding, the failure to set appropriate limits will inevitably make matters worse. Good clinical practice as well as risk management call for setting the necessary limits while thoroughly documenting the situation, consulting with colleagues to validate one's reasoning and assess one's countertransference, and providing a reasonable referral if the patient is to be dismissed from one's practice.

AVOIDING OR LIMITING HOSPITALIZATION

Hospitalization itself can aggravate regressive behavior in borderline patients. It may be difficult to get a borderline patient out of a helpless, dependent position once he or she is in it. The environment of the hospital can evokes immature defenses, either by increasing anxiety or by providing powerful transference figures (physicians and nurses) or situations that evoke imagery of past traumatic events. For this reason, both hospitalizations and their length should be limited, even when it means ignoring patients' threats or demands aimed at initiating or prolonging a stay in hospital. Strict criteria of medical necessity should be applied when making the decision to hospitalize a borderline patient. The goals of medical hospitalizations should be limited to carrying out the procedures and treatments that can be done only in hospital, and the goals of psychiatric hospitalizations usually should be limited to containing a patient when there is a high short-term risk of violent or self-injurious behavior, or making a diagnosis and initiating treatment of an Axis I disorder when this would not be feasible on an outpatient basis. To assess immediate suicide risk, the clinician can supplement clinical judgment with a widely recognized rating scale like the Columbia Suicide Severity Rating Scale (C-SSRS): If the scale score is low, it makes the clinician's judgment more defensible if the patient acts out self-destructively; if the scale score is high, it helps support the legal or financial case for continued hospitalization. An exception to this general rule is the planned admission of a patient with BPD to a specialized medium-to-long-term inpatient treatment program. Such an admission might be part of a long-term strategy for managing a patient with BPD and a comorbid chronic medical illness, but it would not be a response to an acute behavioral crisis in a general medical setting.

ANTI-SPLITTING MANEUVERS

The "splitting defense," typically employed by borderline and lower-functioning narcissistic personalities, divides the important people in the patient's world into "good guys" and "bad guys"—the former loved and idealized, the latter hated and devalued. Patients' splitting behavior can induce among physicians and staff intense differences in attitude and feeling toward the patient, so that care providers split into two factions with strongly held and opposing views regarding the patient's diagnosis or treatment. Issues frequently disputed include pain management, the need for and choice of psychotropic or analgesic medication, the validity of the patient's physical complaints, and the limits that should be set on the patient's behavior.

Splitting of care providers can arise in three ways. First, the patient may manipulate some caretakers into a particular viewpoint, whereas others, unaffected by the manipulation, disagree and might view the patient negatively as "manipulative." Second, caretakers might have differing reactions to the patient's behavior. Some might respond with sympathy and protectiveness, whereas others respond with anger and annoyance. Third, the patient might have different transferences to different care providers, leading to quite different behavior with each of them in the absence of any conscious intent to manipulate or create chaos.

The consequences of splitting can include inconsistent care, inappropriate medication, and burdensome emotional demands on care providers. Clinical outcomes can be affected, not only for the patient doing the splitting, but also for others cared for by the same clinicians.

The basic "anti-splitting" maneuver is the network meeting. All physicians and staff involved in the patient's care are brought together, whether in person, by conference call, or via an online meeting. The medical psychiatrist identifies the problem of splitting and initially encourages ventilation of feelings and disagreements. The psychiatrist then points out that these feelings and disagreements are induced by the patient's behavior and that they provide valuable information about the patient. The psychiatrist then explains that the patient must be treated with the utmost consistency. A rational treatment plan must be agreed on and carried out, regardless of the patient's varying reactions to different care providers and despite any attempts made at manipulation. The psychiatrist works with the staff to develop a consensus on an appropriate care plan, and this plan is written down. The psychiatrist or other physician with a "license" to coordinate the patient's care then informs the patient of the meeting and reviews the key points of the care plan with the patient. It is sometimes appropriate for patients with relatively higher functioning to be invited to join the meeting at the end and hear the consensus directly.

Meetings of involved physicians and staff might be required periodically if the patient's length of stay in the hospital is relatively long, or if the patient is receiving ongoing outpatient care from multiple specialties or disciplines.

The most common error during network meetings held to combat splitting is the failure to include an important stakeholder. When this error occurs, those who have attended the meeting and those who have not can wind up on opposite sides of a split. If several physicians are involved regularly in the patient's care, all must be present. In inpatient settings, if nurses on day and evening shifts are split, both shifts must be represented at the meeting.

Splitting in outpatient settings can occur when patients with borderline personality organization see multiple physicians for different medical problems. They seek opinions from each physician, often asking one to comment on the opinions or care given by another, and attending carefully to any differences or discrepancies among physicians' opinions. Perceptions of a lack of consensus can lead to noncompliance or to the patient's devaluing one physician while idealizing another.

Outpatient anti-splitting maneuvers are similar to inpatient ones, with three salient differences:

1. It is less clear than in the inpatient setting who has authority to call a meeting with a reasonable expectation that others will participate, since there is no one with the formal authority of an inpatient attending physician. The medical psychiatrist leading the meeting will need time and effort to line up the participants, often calling on either the primary care physician or a respected specialist for help.

2. Electronic communication by conference call or web conferencing usually will be necessary to include all relevant stakeholders.

3. If there is a friend or family member loved and trusted by the patient, who is higher functioning than the patient, it usually makes sense to include him or her, subject as always to the patient's consent.

When anti-splitting maneuvers are implemented, borderline patients can become anxious or enraged. Some will defect from treatment. Others remain in treatment but might require short-term antipsychotic drug therapy to contain the anxiety that emerges when the splitting defense is effectively confronted. Despite these problems, anti-splitting maneuvers probably are safer for the patient than ignoring the problem, because persistent splitting can induce errors in physicians' or other providers' judgments that lead to a poor clinical outcome.

COMBINING TACTICS FOR LESS MATURE DEFENSES

For patients with less mature defenses, begin by clarifying expectations, being consistent, giving them a sense of control,

and taking the "one-down" position. Even if there is a past history of inappropriate behavior in the medical setting, there usually is no need to set limits until the patient acts or threatens to act destructively. Then limit setting can be done—sympathetically in the case of borderline and antisocial patients, and matter-of-factly with paranoid and schizotypal patients. Sympathetic limit setting should not be used with paranoid, avoidant, and schizotypal patients because sympathy can arouse further anxiety by implying closeness. If sympathetic limit setting is ineffective with a borderline or antisocial patient, one should proceed with matter-of-fact limit setting. Limits framed so they save face for the patient often are embraced gratefully by patients with more primitive narcissistic personalities. When splitting of healthcare providers occurs, anti-splitting maneuvers should be instituted.

TACTICS FOR PATIENTS WITH MORE MATURE DEFENSES

Tactics for patients with more mature defenses and better-quality interpersonal relationships presuppose a reasonable degree of trust and consistency; they attempt to use these patients' personality styles and personal issues as leverage to help them comply with prescribed therapeutic interventions. Tactics for these personalities include use of strategic reframing statements and personal leverage.

REFRAMING

"Reframing" is the tactic of presenting medical instructions in language that is most consistent with the patient's characteristic coping style. For example, after presenting a plan of treatment to a narcissistic patient, one might say, "Many patients would have difficulty with these instructions. Only a highly motivated and competent person could really follow this regimen as it was intended." The medical need for treatment adherence and its associated behavior change is expressed in language appealing to the patient's sense of specialness. A compulsive patient might be asked to carry out an instruction because "it will save you time and money." In this case, adherence to the treatment plan would be linked to the patient's concern with efficiency.

Reframing statements might emphasize illness as an occasion for personal growth, or the mastery of illness as a route to greater independence. These types of statements are particularly appealing to individuals with more mature defenses who have sympathy for the ideas of humanistic psychology and the concept of the physician and patient as peers. Reframing statements preferably use the patient's own language and focus on the patient's individual concerns. The process of creating reframing statements is similar to that used when developing hypnotic suggestions and self-hypnotic routines and can be combined with formal trance procedures by clinicians with sufficient expertise in hypnosis. Applications of self-induced trance in medical settings are described by Spiegel and Spiegel (1978).

PARADOXICAL INTENTION

"Paradoxical intention" includes tactics such as predicting a patient will fail at a proposed treatment or asking him or her to continue the problem behavior with even greater vigor. This somewhat controversial technique has worked with passive-aggressive patients who have an unconscious investment in proving the physician wrong or demonstrating their inability to comply with recommendations. It also can be applied with dependent personalities who fear they will lose their relationship with their physician if they improve, and because they fear the loss of the relationship more than they fear the continuation of their symptoms or disability.

For example, a passive-aggressive patient being treated as an outpatient for depression might be asked at each appointment "How badly did things go?" or the physician might conspicuously focus on questions concerning medication side effects. The patient could then prove the physician wrong by reporting only improvement or denying side effects. A patient disabled by a somatoform disorder who had a dependent personality might be given a detailed plan for a gradual return to normal activity and be told that it would be difficult to carry it out and that he or she probably could do it only by having weekly visits with the psychiatrist for support. Even then, if he or she did succeed, it would be largely due to perseverance in the face of a challenging situation. The medical psychiatrist would see him or her, however, only if he or she complied with the rehabilitative activities. A dependent patient lacking in self-confidence would thus be offered a situation in which he or she would get all the credit if they succeeded but no blame if treatment failed. The patient is also offered the opportunity to depend on the psychiatrist for support because of participation in rehabilitation rather than because of complaints or signs of psychopathology.

Paradoxical intention should be avoided with borderline personalities and other patients with immature defenses. Lacking a sense of humor and not crediting the physician's goodwill, they can be offended by the psychiatrist's well-intentioned manipulation and respond with self-destructive or hostile acting out.

PERSONAL LEVERAGE

Using personal leverage means motivating the patient with poor self-esteem by relating medically therapeutic behavior to an important personal relationship. The source of leverage can be a long-term primary care physician, a nurse, a consultant, a family member, or a member of the clergy. Personal leverage can involve suggestions, direct orders, recommendations, reassurance, or handwritten instructions. Typical statements are as follows: (1) "As your personal physician I recommend this treatment"; (2) "Dr. X, the top cardiologist in New York, thinks this is the best option"; (3) "For the sake of your children, now is the time to move to an assisted living facility."

In some cases, having a personally influential person talk to the patient about the medical treatment or personal problems is most helpful. For instance, a spouse might be invited by the doctor to help explain a procedure to the patient, assuming that the spouse has previously been shown to be positively influential toward the patient's overall health.

Personal leverage is particularly relevant when there is a well-defined decision to be made or behavior to be changed, when the patient has a stable and positive relationship with someone who can be an ally in the treatment, and when a more rational, cognitive approach did not work or, based on the patient's history, would be unlikely to work. The technique is not suitable for borderline patients with unstable relationships, and the clinician should take care to avoid the appearance of condescension. Personal leverage usually is not effective with compulsive patients, who tend to mistrust personal appeals and are much more comfortable with a rational, factually oriented approach.

Appeals to religious or philosophical beliefs, expectations of one's family or one's community, and other transpersonal concerns are variants of personal leverage that can be extraordinarily effective if the clinician has sufficient understanding of the patient's cultural milieu and belief system. This topic is discussed further in this book's chapter on spirituality.

COMBINING TACTICS FOR MORE MATURE DEFENSES

For patients with more mature defenses, the psychiatric interview determines the personal issue underlying the patient's noncompliance or emotional difficulty. The physician then attempts to describe the proposed treatment in a way that addresses the personal issue. Typical concerns are associated with different personality disorders, traits, types, and attachment styles. Typical concerns can help guide an interview that aims to arrive at a specific, shared conception of the patient's current personal issue.

For patients who avoid intimacy, whether they are avoidant, schizoid, schizotypal, paranoid, or simply have an avoidant or dismissive attachment style, it is useful for the physician to adopt a neutral, predictable, matter-of-fact manner with the patient. In inpatient settings, where other healthcare providers are involved with the patient, the medical psychiatrist might recommend that they do the same. In the author's experience, nurses and house officers with less clinical experience are most likely to display unwanted warmth and sympathy to such patients. Adopting a cooler style with these patients helps avert the anxiety evoked when they experience intimacy. Reducing anxiety can diminish the expression of immature defenses against that anxiety.

TRAITS AND TREATMENT: TEACHABLE TIPS

Medical psychiatrists are consulted by their general medical colleagues to solve problems; less often a psychiatrist attached to a specialty service can help institute screening for mental disorders—including personality disorders—and actively intervene to prevent acute behavioral problems and to improve medical outcomes and health-related quality of life. A third contribution medical psychiatrists can make to general medical care is raising their colleagues' awareness of mental and behavioral issues in their practices. This can take place in formal rounds and conferences, but informal interactions in hospitals and clinics probably have more impact.

Physicians of all specialties are interested in their patients' adherence to prescribed treatment, their satisfaction with care, and their clinical outcomes, and in not being the target of complaints and lawsuits. Medical psychiatrists can relate their informal advice to these shared objectives.

In this connection, personality traits and types, as captured by the five factors and by the classification of attachment styles, are teachable concepts with an obvious applicability to clinical practice. The idea of linking traits with treatment can be conveyed in brief bits of advice. For example:

1. "This patient really doesn't like intimacy. Don't be too warm with him—if he wants more information about his kind of cancer, refer him to the American Cancer Society website."

2. "This woman is very conventional and not very open to new ideas, but she'll trust you if there are no surprises. If you follow the practice guidelines, she'll follow your prescription, but don't give her anything off-label—it will make her nervous."

3. "This guy is very neurotic and complains all the time. But, if he comes in with a complaint you've never heard before, take it very seriously."

4. "This lady is very disagreeable, to be sure, and her son is even worse. Document everything you do; if anybody's going to see a lawyer if something goes wrong, she and her son are the ones."

USE OF PSYCHOTROPIC MEDICATIONS

Patients with personality disorders frequently are treated with psychotropic drugs. Even so, there is no medication approved for the treatment of any specific personality disorder. Moreover, a meta-analysis of adult patient preferences indicates that patients in general prefer psychological therapy over drug therapy by a wide margin (McHugh et al., 2013). To treat personality disorders with medications is an off-label adventure. Drugs are given to patients with personality disorders either: (1) to treat a concurrent Axis I disorder such as major depression or generalized anxiety; (2) to treat symptoms such as transient psychotic phenomena; or (3) to treat specific personality traits such as negative and unstable affect in BPD or cognitive and perceptual distortions in BPD or schizotypal personality disorder.

Regardless of the purpose for which psychotropic medication is given, some general principles are applicable:

1. The details of how a prescription is given to the patient will affect not only the likelihood the medication will be taken as prescribed, but also the how the patient will respond if there is an adverse reaction to it. The patient's personality should be considered when deciding how to ask him or her to report any side effects. Compulsive patients might be asked to send a the physician a daily email reporting the side effects they experience, since some are expected in every case, and their pattern should be observed to determine whether they are a reason to modify the treatment. Schizoid and paranoid patients might simply be asked to read the package insert and let the physician know if they have any questions—the physician avoiding an interaction that might seem too warm or giving the impression that potential negatives are being glossed over.

2. Medications can have personal meanings to patients with personality disorders that go beyond their pharmacological effects. For some patients with primitive personalities, a familiar medication is an anchoring point in a chaotic world, and they will resist changing it even if there are problems with its efficacy or its side effects. For other patients, the use of an as-needed anxiolytic or analgesic is a psychological defense mechanism that they greatly fear losing, even though they are not physiologically dependent on the medication and do not necessarily misuse it.

3. Since patients with personality disorders have problems in living and associated emotional symptoms which will continue even when their Axis I condition is effectively treated, it is important to identify the specific symptoms that are the target of psychotropic drug therapy. The symptoms should be regularly measured with a rating scale. This approach helps align the expectations of the patient and the physician.

4. Patients with unstable lives due to low-level personality disorders and patients with the personality trait of carelessness (low conscientiousness) should be given prescriptions that are as simple as possible. If feasible, medication regimens should be tailored to reduce the requirement for the patient's effort and consistency. Specifically, the following should be considered: (a) choosing regimens for all of the patient's psychiatric and general medical conditions so that medication is taken just once a day, with some flexibility in the time at which it is taken; (b) reducing the number of discrete medications by using combination formulations; and (c) using long-acting formulations like depot antipsychotic drugs or transdermal patches.

5. When patients with borderline or antisocial personalities are given prescriptions for controlled substances, precautions should be taken reduce the risk of abuse or diversion—even if the patient does not have a history of drug abuse. Potential precautions include non-refillable prescriptions, random drug testing and written treatment contracts. The latter should make clear that medications must be filled at one specific pharmacy, that there will be no emergency refills or extra medication if doses are lost, that the patient will not get prescriptions for the same or similar medication from another physician, and that the penalty for violating the rules will be termination of the relationship and a referral for drug abuse treatment.

6. Benzodiazepines should not be prescribed to borderline personalities or other patients with poor behavioral inhibition. However, when a patient with BPD, or a history of dramatic acting out without the full syndrome of BPD, comes into treatment already on chronic benzodiazepine treatment, the psychiatrist should withdraw benzodiazepine treatment very slowly, alert to the potential for exacerbation of behavioral problems by drug withdrawal effects. If the patient has been taking short-acting benzodiazepines regularly, whether on a schedule or as needed, rebound anxiety can create a vicious cycle that mimics addictive behavior. Switching to a long-acting benzodiazepine and withdrawing the latter slowly may help.

TREATING AXIS I DISORDERS IN PATIENTS WITH PERSONALITY DISORDERS

While treatment outcomes for Axis I disorders can be worse when there is Axis II comorbidity, there is only one situation I am aware of in which a personality disorder is a potential contraindication to an otherwise efficacious treatment for an Axis I disorder: the treatment of ADHD with stimulants. Here there are concerns that stimulants will be abused or diverted by patients with comorbid antisocial personality disorder, and that they will precipitate psychosis in patients with borderline personality disorder. However, a large-population pharmaco-epidemiological study of ADHD treatment and criminality showed that treatment of ADHD, principally with methylphenidate, reduced criminal behavior by 32% in men and 41% in women, and that the effect was seen independently of whether there was a comorbid personality disorder diagnosis (Lichtenstein et al., 2012). A Medline search revealed no controlled study of stimulant treatment of ADHD with comorbid BPD, but it did turn up a report that open-label use of methylphenidate in adolescent girls with comorbid ADHD and BPD improved symptoms of both conditions without precipitating psychotic symptoms (Golubchik et al., 2008). A cautious conclusion is that ADHD comorbid with borderline or antisocial personality may be treated with stimulants *if* there are well-defined target symptoms and appropriate precautions are taken. In the case of patients with antisocial personality, atomoxetine or lisdexamfetamine would appear preferable to methylphenidate, dextroamphetamine, or Adderall, as the first two drugs are not suitable for abuse by the intravenous route. In the case of patients with BPD and ADHD, stimulants should be started gradually, with frequent visits during dosage titration and specific inquiry about any psychotic and pre-psychotic symptoms. Medical psychiatrists specifically may encounter patients with ADHD on Axis I, borderline or antisocial personality on Axis II, and a significant chronic medical condition on Axis III, in whom the inattention and disorganization due to ADHD prevent effective treatment of the general medical condition. In this situation, effective treatment of the ADHD can improve the outcome of the medical condition, supporting the idea of an ADHD treatment trial despite the complexity added by the comorbid personality disorder.

TREATING SHORT-TERM SYMPTOMS OF PERSONALITY DISORDERS

One of the main problem-focused interventions of medical psychiatrists is advising on pharmacological treatment of patients with personality disorders who display anger, hostility, agitation, and/or aggressive behavior that disrupts medical treatment. This can be accompanied by psychotic thinking or perceptions, particularly in the case of patients with borderline or schizotypal personalities. Evidence supports the use of antipsychotic drugs to manage these symptoms in the case of borderline and schizotypal personality; the doses required can be lower than typically used in treating schizophrenia, but this is not necessarily the case. Antipsychotic drug treatment for transient aggressive or psychotic symptoms in borderline or schizotypal patients should begin with testing the efficacy of a low dose before advancing to full antipsychotic dosage if necessary. With schizotypal and borderline personalities, antipsychotic drug treatment for these symptoms is therapeutic and supported by controlled studies of efficacy. In contrast, the use of antipsychotic drugs to manage angry and aggressive behavior in non-psychotic patients with decompensated narcissistic or antisocial personalities is better viewed as "chemical restraint." It may be warranted when necessary to permit essential medical treatment. When it is used, the duration of treatment should be limited to that needed to permit necessary medical care, and the necessity for antipsychotic drugs should be well documented. Nonetheless, given the overlap between the various Axis II disorders and the high comorbidity of Axis II and Axis I, there will be patients with personality disorders other than borderline or schizotypal who develop brief psychotic episodes or mood disorders with psychotic features. In those cases, there is a sound, evidence-based justification for antipsychotic drug therapy that goes beyond symptom management.

TREATING COMPONENT TRAITS OF PERSONALITY DISORDERS

The concept of treating specific traits associated with a personality disorder is best developed for BPD, where negative and unstable affect, impulsiveness/disinhibition, and aggressive/antagonistic behavior are consistent behavioral dispositions that are potential, measurable targets for treatment. A recent review of controlled trials of drug treatment for these traits in BPD (Ripoll, 2012) reached the following conclusions:

1. Olanzapine and aripiprazole (but not ziprasidone), in dosages lower than typically used for treating schizophrenia, have a moderate effect on traits of antagonism, negative affectivity, disinhibition, psychotic symptoms, and interpersonal dysfunction;

2. Antiepileptic drugs (AEDs) have shown moderate-to-large effects on the traits of antagonism, disinhibition, and negative affectivity. Specifically, valproate has shown benefits for antagonism and disinhibition, lamotrigine for disinhibition and negative affectivity, and topiramate for all of the above-mentioned traits.

3. The omega-3 fatty acid eicosapentanoic acid (EPA) has shown moderate-to-large effects on the traits of antagonism and negative affectivity.

An open-label trial of quetiapine showed a highly significant reduction in impulsiveness in patients with BPD, most of whom did not have psychotic symptoms (Villeneuve & Lemelin, 2005). On the other hand, a review of antipsychotic drugs in BPD that included first-generation neuroleptics concluded that the overall effect of antipsychotic drugs on global functioning was small (Ingenhoven & Duivenvoorden, 2011).

The challenge with the medical-psychiatric population is that all of the medications proved to be useful in treating BPD can in various ways exacerbate medical problems known to have a higher prevalence in individuals with BPD. BPD is associated with an increased prevalence of obesity and type 2 diabetes; the metabolic side effects of olanzapine in particular make these conditions worse. Cognitive impairment often is the dose-limiting side effect of topiramate, and the attentional and executive functions made worse by topiramate are frequently impaired in BPD prior to any drug treatment. Lamotrigine requires a lengthy dosage titration to minimize the risk of severe dermatological reactions; patients with BPD may have a particularly hard time complying with a prescription while waiting many weeks to see its benefit.

The author's conclusion is that BPD patients, particularly those with cardiovascular risk factors, should be prescribed omega-3 fatty acid supplementation unless the compliance burden of taking the supplements would diminish a specific patient's adherence to other, more essential, treatment. Antipsychotic drugs should not be given chronically for treatment of BPD as such, but if the patient has a psychotic disorder on Axis I, or their psychotic symptoms were significant enough to impair function or to interfere with necessary general medical treatment, the antipsychotic of choice would be aripiprazole if the patient was overweight, had glucose intolerance, cardiovascular risk factors, or a family history of diabetes or coronary artery disease. Olanzapine could be a first-line treatment in a patient who was underweight or normal weight without increased risk of a metabolic syndrome. Antiepileptic drugs cannot yet be seen as first-line treatment for BPD, but there would be good support for giving lamotrigine or valproate if the patient had comorbid bipolar disorder, and for trying topiramate if the patient had migraines and did not have significant cognitive impairment.

Psychotropic drugs have also been studied in randomized controlled trials as a treatment for schizotypal personality disorder. In this population, antipsychotic drugs have a moderate-to-large effect on anger, a moderate effect on cognitive-perceptual symptoms, and a small effect on global functioning. Mood-stabilizing AEDs were more efficacious overall, except for cognitive-perceptual symptoms, than the antipsychotic drugs, and antidepressants were of little benefit, even for patients with depressed mood (Ingenhoven et al., 2010).

Omega-3 fatty acid supplementation, EPA in particular, might be helpful in preventing the development of frank psychosis in patients with schizotypal personality. The evidence supporting this potential for EPA supplementation comes from a controlled study of omega-3 fatty acids at a dose of 1.2 g per day (700 mg EPA, 480 mg DHA) in preventing the development of a first episode of schizophreniform psychosis in patients aged 13–25 with sub-threshold psychotic symptoms (Amminger et al., 2010).

A conservative view would be that in patients with schizotypal personality, antipsychotic drugs should be reserved for those with cognitive-perceptual symptoms of near-psychotic proportions and those with intermittent psychotic symptoms or continuous low-level psychotic symptoms. As with BPD patients, schizotypal patients should be encouraged to take omega-3 fatty acid supplements, if adding the supplements will not unacceptably raise the burden of treatment compliance. If a schizotypal patient has cardiac risk factors, the case for doing this is even stronger.

Avoidant personality disorder overlaps significantly with the Axis I disorder of social anxiety disorder; treating the latter can alleviate symptoms of the former, including the avoidance of social situations and the morbid fear of rejection. The antidepressants sertraline, paroxetine, and venlafaxine are approved for social anxiety disorder; while not approved for this indication, monoamine oxidase inhibitors (MAOIs) have shown effectiveness in controlled trials (Dalrymple, 2012). MAOIs can help patients who do not respond adequately to SSRIs or serotonin-norepinephrine reuptake inhibitors (SNRIs) (Blanco et al., 2013). However, in the context of chronic medical disease, the use of MAOIs is fraught with risks of interactions with food and drugs. However, if patients are so avoidant that they do not show up for medical appointments, the option might be considered with appropriate risk management. While there is no controlled evidence to support its use for social avoidance *per se*, transdermal selegiline, an MAO-B selective MAO inhibitor—is an effective treatment of depression with particular efficacy for anxiety symptoms (Robinson et al., 2007). Unlike the approved oral formulations of MAOIs, transdermal selegiline does not require food restrictions, and it does not have pharmacokinetic interactions with drugs metabolized by the CYP450 system (Azzaro et al., 2007). It would a rational choice for an avoidant, anxious, depressed patient for whom first-line therapies had failed and social anxiety was compromising medical treatment.

PSYCHIATRIC LIAISON VERSUS PSYCHIATRIC PRINCIPAL CARE

Patients with less mature defenses and poor interpersonal relations are particularly likely to produce anger in the people who care for them; the consequence of their splitting defenses is the polarization of the caregivers. For these patients, psychiatric consultation rarely helps unless the reactions of attending physicians and nursing staff are addressed explicitly. Attention to the requester of the consultation, liaison work with nursing staff, and ongoing availability of the consultant are needed to forestall crises. Weekend and holiday coverage for the consultant must be arranged to promote maximum consistency of advice given to all involved.

When dealing with other healthcare providers, the consultant should permit ventilation of anger and disagreement and then emphasize that these reactions provide diagnostic information about the patient. The consultant should help them "cool down," so the basic principles of being consistent, giving a sense of control, and setting limits without anger can be emphasized. (Further details are offered in the earlier section in this chapter on preventing and managing staff splitting.)

Often, suggestion of a pharmacological intervention, such as recommending short-term antipsychotic drug treatment for the patient, permits a face-saving reappraisal of the patient by the staff. If the patient can be viewed as "stabilized" by an external agent, anger over the patient's past behavior can be rationalized. These pharmacological interventions must not be carried out solely for their effect on staff, but should be indicated by the patient's diagnosis and behavior.

Sometimes consultation, even with liaison and follow-up, is insufficient to contain the self-destructive, disruptive, or noncompliant behavior of the medically ill patient with a severe personality disorder. At other times, as with some pain patients, personality problems can prevent proper diagnosis and management in a purely medical setting. In these situations, principal care of the patient by the psychiatrist can facilitate resolution of the problem. When this arrangement is chosen, all orders are written by the psychiatrist, who sees the patient daily and uses medical specialists as consultants. At hospitals where there is a medical-psychiatric unit, an inpatient usually can be transferred there. Psychiatric primary care can greatly improve consistency of management because it puts the psychiatrist in the front-line position of deciding whether particular physical complaints need medical intervention or should be dealt with as somatic expression of a psychiatric disorder.

Psychiatric principal care is unsuitable if the medical problem is unstable; in such a case, concurrent care is better. Medical-psychiatric units may do better at containing the behavior of personality-disordered patients than they do at changing their maladaptive defenses; longer-stay, milieu-oriented units and outpatient therapy are more suited to promoting enduring behavioral change. Therefore, patients with severe personality disorders and active medical illness usually should be stabilized on a medical service or medical-psychiatric unit and then transferred to a conventional psychiatric unit if milieu-oriented inpatient treatment is still needed after medical stabilization.

Psychiatric principal care at times is suitable for long-term outpatient treatment. The patient's coping with the chronic illness and health care system can be used as a focus for psychotherapeutic exploration and behavioral change.

HEALTHCARE PROVIDERS' REACTIONS TO PATIENTS WITH PERSONALITY DISORDERS

Reactions to patients with personality disorders cover a wide range of possibilities, including hate, anger, desire to avoid or abandon the patient, personal attraction, overprotectiveness, and taking sides with the patient against family members or other healthcare professionals. The detection of countertransference reactions can be more difficult when they are defended against with reaction formation. For example, compulsive over-concern or excessive inclusiveness during a medical workup can be a defense against an unacceptable desire to avoid the patient.

Gallop and Wynn (1987), observing the reactions of nurses and psychiatry residents to hospitalized patients with severe personality disorders, noted that nurses were likely to be explicitly angry, rejecting, and devaluing of the patients. The psychiatry residents were likely to feel incompetent and powerless, and to develop conflicts with their supervisors.

Even the *label* of personality disorder has effects on countertransference. Including the term "personality disorder" in a case vignette of a patient with a major depression led to a lower rate of psychiatrists' recommendations for antidepressant drug treatment and to inferences that the patient was not motivated, or even seriously ill (Lewis & Appleby, 1988). (Patients with BPD don't like being called "borderline," either.)

In general psychiatric settings, a barrier to healthcare providers' recognizing their countertransference is defensiveness, sometimes related to a feeling that that countertransference is undesirable, avoidable, or simply embarrassing. In medical-psychiatric settings, the greatest barrier to a clear awareness of countertransference is the distraction of the patient's general medical care. On medical-psychiatric units, psychiatrists and nurses can lose sight of countertransference issues that would not escape their notice in a general psychiatric setting.

PERSONALITY DISORDERS IN LONG-TERM CARE

Elderly and/or disabled people living in nursing homes, assisted living facilities, or other long-term care facilities must contend with a loss of privacy and a loss of control, and unfortunately often with inappropriately familiar treatment by caregiving staff. Leaving the problematic situation is often difficult, because the facility is the person's home and not merely a temporary locus of healthcare. Patients with mature defenses and an agreeable personality can tolerate these problems, and might even enjoy the social environment of a long-term care facility (if it is a good one). Patients with immature defenses can decompensate and, in addition to feeling distress, they might resist care, verbally abuse caregivers, become physically agitated, make threats, and show other forms of disturbing behavior.

In these situations, a consistent, regular, supportive psychotherapeutic relationship can have a remarkably stabilizing effect on the patient's behavior. Indeed, many of these patients had supportive relationships with family members or primary care physicians prior to their move to a long-term care facility. The patient's move to a facility might have been triggered by the loss of supportive relationship. Or, the move to the facility might lead to a loss of a supportive relationship, as when the facility is inconvenient for a significant person to visit frequently.

Liaison interventions with the staff of long-term care facilities should focus on reducing the caregivers' level of affect and intimacy with the patient when it is clear that the patient is overwhelmed and the situation is becoming chaotic. Neuroleptic therapy, when considered because of acting-out behavior, should be kept to the low doses appropriate for treating personality disorders; full antipsychotic doses rarely are necessary and are associated with a high rate of disabling side effects. Second-generation antipsychotic drugs such as quetiapine or aripiprazole are preferable to first-generation agents or risperidone.

Age prejudice can lead to insensitivity to the distress of older patients with personality disorders; alternatively, over-solicitousness and excessive sympathy can lead to an under-utilization of appropriate confrontation and limit-setting. Psychiatrists must carefully examine their own attitudes toward aging and aged people as well as the attitudes of the caregivers seeking consultation. Caregivers' beliefs about old age should be explored; even experienced caregivers can have misconceptions they have not questioned, despite contradictory experience. For example, many clinicians believe that older patients are more hypochondriacal than younger ones. Actually, they simply suffer from more diseases, and when this is controlled for, they do not display more illness behavior or worse self-rated health (Costa & McCrae, 1985).

BOUNDARY ISSUES

Psychiatrists' training sensitizes them to boundary issues with their psychotherapy patients; even a first-year psychiatry resident would not offer a patient a ride home from the clinic or purchase an investment on a patient's recommendation. The physical examination of a psychotherapy patient is constrained by concern about the implications of touching the patient's body and the potential for mis-understanding of the psychiatrist's intentions. On the other hand, a patient receiving electroconvulsive therapy (ECT) would necessarily require a physical examination by the psychiatrist, as would one suspected of having the neuroleptic malignant syndrome. In medical psychiatry, boundary issues are subtler. For example, when excessive illness behavior is suspected, the physical examination of the patient can give the psychiatrist a deeper understanding of the patient's actual physical condition and can occasion-ally provide new diagnostic information for the patient's non-psychiatric physicians. Or, in palliative care situations, the touch of the psychiatrist can be comforting and healing. How much the medical psychiatrist physically touches the patient ideally should be a flexible decision, responsive to the clinical issue and the context of care. However, when the patient has a personality disorder—particularly BPD or a personality disorder with paranoid features—the risk that the patient will perceive a boundary violation can be so high that it outweighs the benefit of physical examination by the psychiatrist. Of course, if there is a medical emergency, the psychiatrist should do what is necessary, though even then a third party should be present if at all possible. In other situ-ations where there is a strong case for a physical examina-tion by the psychiatrist, consultation with a colleague—and documentation of the clinical reasoning—is recommended.

Similar issues arise when treating chronically disabled patients who cannot easily leave their homes but require psy-chiatric treatment. When the psychiatrist sees the patient in their home, there is a threshold that is literally crossed—but often quite appropriately. When the patient has—or is sus-pected of having—a severe personality disorder, the risk of a destructive interaction with the patient can be reduced by having a third party at hand when the psychiatrist visits the patient's home, whether a nurse, a paid caregiver, or a family member.

LEGAL CONCERNS

Patients with less mature defenses and personality disor-ders who have unstable interpersonal relations can rapidly turn against their physicians because of disappointment or disagreement. If there has been an error of judgment or an unexpectedly poor medical outcome, the patient might sue the physician or threaten litigation with manipulative intent. Lawyers, not understanding the dynamics of borderline per-sonality, might with good intentions pursue patient claims that are based more on near-psychotic transference reactions than on reality (Gutheil, 1985).

In general medical settings, psychiatrists frequently are called to consult when a physician–patient relationship has begun to deteriorate and a threat of a malpractice suit has been made. While psychiatric interventions with the patient and involved clinicians are made to "cool down" the situation, the physician threatened with litigation should be asked to obtain a second opinion on their care of the patient to date and the current plan of treatment, and to document thoroughly the reasons for the medical decisions made to date if they are not completely clear from the medical record. With the medical records and the second opinion in hand, the medical psychia-trist discusses past medical treatment and future plans with the physician at risk. Then, with a good understanding of the medical issues, the psychiatrist interviews the patient, with the aim of separating problems in the physician–patient relation-ship from issues about the medical treatment as such. After the interview, the psychiatrist usually will know whether the patient and the physician at risk can work out their differences with the psychiatrist's help. If not, the psychiatrist's task is to prepare both the patient and the physician at risk for a transi-tion of care that demonstrates compassion, empathy, and lack of defensiveness on the part of the physicians involved.

Occasionally, the psychiatrist has an opportunity for primary prevention of litigiousness against a general medi-cal physician. The opportunity presents if the psychiatrist knows that patient with a chronic illness has a borderline or low-level narcissistic personality and becomes aware that the patient is idealizing their principal physician. In this situation, the psychiatrist can advise the physician to gently disillusion the patient, repeatedly reminding him or her of the uncertainty of medical outcomes, the limitations of treatment, and the limitations of any physician facing chronic disease. The psychiatrist can prompt the physician to scrupulously document informed consent, to obtain second opinions whenever a suggested treatment has known adverse effects and there are reasonable alternatives, and in general to use the language of humble collaboration rather than of rescue. Specifically as regards consent, merely having the patient fill out a form that perfunctorily lists risks of a procedure or treatment is not sufficient. The physician should note specifically which risks were discussed orally, what other information was provided to the patient (e.g., video recordings or websites), and any specific questions the patient asked and how they were answered. It is admittedly burdensome to do all of this, and for most patients it is unnecessary. However, experience teaches us that the more extreme forms of idealization are no compliment to a physician—they are a warning that is best heeded.

CLINICAL PEARLS

- Different constructs of personality can be helpful to help the patient or caretakers to understand the patient. Besides DSM diagnoses, these constructs include attachment styles, Myers-Briggs types, Cloninger's dimensions of temperament and character, and analysis of defenses.

- Patients' different personality styles suggest that they will do better with physicians of certain personalities. The challenge is to make the best match.

- The medical psychiatrist's solution of a problem in a patient with personality disorder should consider:

  - the patient's view of the problem;

  - the practical, negotiable issues, which are compounded by emotional issues and interpersonal conflicts;

  - evidence of an Axis I diagnosis;

  - the influence of prescribed medications, alcohol, or illicit drugs, or withdrawal;

  - the patient's perception of the physician–patient relationship and of the patient's role in the treatment;

  - whether the immediate problem is provoked by inappropriate or inflexible behavior by a physician, nurse, or other healthcare provider;

  - whether a medical disorder or medication side-effect been overlooked or misdiagnosed.

- The physician in charge of coordinating a patient's care—and there should be one—should determine the top short-term priorities for behavior change (including treatment adherence) and limit what is asked of the patient at one time.

- In the setting of a patient with personality disorder, the need for consistency makes different email communication systems a problem. If all email communication goes through a common secure portal, designed so that all involved healthcare providers can see all of the messages, it can be a powerful tool for aligning everyone's advice and for identifying differences of opinion so they can be promptly resolved.

- Taking the "one-down" position means realistically recognizing one's limitations in affecting another person's behavior and approaching the patient with genuine and appropriate humility.

- Limit setting is the trump card—to be played if a patient is seriously impeding treatment or is endangering someone.

- For outpatients, typical circumstances for limit setting are diversion of prescription drugs, verbal abuse of the office staff, and threats of violence.

- Sympathetic limit setting should not be used with paranoid, avoidant, and schizotypal patients because sympathy can arouse further anxiety by implying closeness.

- Limits framed so they save face for the patient often are embraced gratefully by patients with more primitive narcissistic personalities.

- Reframing aligns the physician's directive with the patient's style. In the case of narcissism, the medical need for treatment adherence is expressed in language appealing to the patient's sense of specialness.

- Experience teaches us that the more extreme forms of idealization are no compliment to a physician—they are a warning that is best heeded.

DISCLOSURE STATEMENT

Dr. Fogel is Chief Scientific Officer of Synchroneuron Inc., Managing Director of Anal-Gesic LLC, and Executive Vice President of PointRight Inc. He is the sole inventor or lead inventor on several pharmaceutical patents. In his opinion, these affiliations do not entail any conflict of interest with regard to the editing of this book or his personal contributions to it. He has no other potential conflicts, direct or indirect, financial or otherwise, to disclose in connection with the editing of this book or his personal contributions to it.

REFERENCES

Ahrens, K. R., Ciechanowski, P., & Katon, W. (2012). Associations between adult attachment style and health risk behavior in an adult female primary care population. *Journal of Psychosomatic Research*, 72(5), published online: doi:10.1016/j.jpsychores.2012.02.002

Amminger, G. P., Schager, M. R., Papageorgiou, K., Klier, C. M., Cotton, S. M., Harrigan, S. M., et al. (2010). Long-chain omega-3 fatty acids for indicated prevention of psychotic disorders: A randomized placebo-controlled trial. *Archives of General Psychiatry*, 67, 146–154.

Ayers, S., Jessop, D., Pike, A., Parfitt, Y., & Ford, E. (2014). The role of adult attachment style, birth intervention and support in posttraumatic stress after childbirth: A prospective study. *Journal of Affective Disorders*, 155, 295–298.

Azzaro, A. J., Ziemniak, J., Kemper, E., Campbell, B. J., & VanDenBerg, C. (2007). Selegiline transdermal system: an examination of the potential for CYP450-dependent pharmacokinetic interactions with 3 psychotropic medications. *Journal of Clinical Pharmacology, 47*, 146–158.

Barrantes-Vidal, N., Gross, G. M., Sheinbaum, T., Mitjavila, M., Ballespí, S., & Kwapil, T. R. (2013). Positive and negative schizotypy are associated with prodromal and schizophrenia-spectrum symptoms. *Schizophrenia Research, 145*, 50–55.

Bartholomew, K., & Horowitz, L. M. (1991). Attachment styles among young adults: A test of a four-category model. *Journal of Personality & Social Psychology, 61*, 226–244.

Blanco, C., Bragdon, L. B., Schneier, F. R., & Liebowitz, M. R. (2013). The evidence-based pharmacotherapy of social anxiety disorder. *International Journal of Neuropsychopharmacology, 16*, 235–249.

Bond, M. (1986). Defense style questionnaire. In G. E. Vaillant (Ed.), *Empirical studies of ego mechanisms of defense* (pp. 146–152). Washington, DC: American Psychiatric Press.

Bowlby, J. (1988). *A secure base: Clinical applications of attachment theory.* London: Routledge.

Brennan, K. A., Clark, C. L., & Shaver, P. R. (1998). Self-report measurement of adult attachment: An integrative overview. In J. A., Simpson & W. S. Rholes (Eds.), *Attachment theory and close relationships* (pp. 46–76). New York: Guilford Press.

Cloninger, C. R. (1994). *The temperament and character inventory (TCI): A guide to its development and use.* St. Louis, MO: Center for Psychobiology of Personality, Washington University.

Cloninger, C. R., Svrakic, D. M., & Przybeck, T. R. (2013). A psychobiological model of temperament and character. *Archives of General Psychiatry, 50*, 970–975.

Contessa, J., Suarez, L., Kyriakides, T., & Nadzam, G. (2013). The influence of surgeon personality factors on risk tolerance: a pilot study. *Journal of Surgical Education, 70*, 806–812.

Costa, P. T., & McCrae, R. R. (1985). Hypochondriasis, neuroticism and aging: When are somatic complaints unfounded? *American Psychologist, 40*, 19–28.

Dalrymple, K. L. (2012). Issues and controversies surrounding the diagnosis and treatment of social anxiety disorder. *Expert Review of Neurotherapeutics, 12*, 993–1009.

Dawson, D. F. (1988). Treatment of the borderline patient: Relationship management. *Canadian Journal of Psychiatry, 33*, 370–374.

Fervaha, G., & Remington, G. (2013). Neuroimaging findings in schizotypal personality disorder: A systematic review. *Progress in Neuro-Pharmacology & Biological Psychiatry, 43*, 96–107.

Forsythe, L. P., Romano, J. M., Jensen, M. P., & and Thorn, B. E. (2012). Attachment style is associated with perceived spouse responses and pain-related outcomes. *Rehabilitation Psychology, 57*, 290–300.

Fraley, R. C., Waller, N. G., & Brennan, K. A. (2000). An item-response theory analysis of self-report measures of adult attachment. *Journal of Personality and Social Psychology, 78*, 350–365.

Gallop, R., & Wynn, F. (1987). The difficult inpatient: Identification and response by staff. *Canadian Journal of Psychiatry, 32*, 211–215.

Golubchik, P., Sever, J., Zalsman, G., & Weizman, A. (2008). Methylphenidate in the treatment of female adolescents with co-occurrence of attention deficit/hyperactivity disorder and borderline personality disorder: A preliminary open-label trial. *International Clinical Psychopharmacology, 23*, 228–231.

Gutheil, T. G. (1985). Medicolegal pitfalls in the treatment of borderline patients. *American Journal of Psychiatry, 142*, 9–14.

Gutheil, T. G. (2005). Boundaries, blackmail and double binds: A pattern observed in malpractice consultation. *Journal of the American Academy of Psychiatry & the Law, 33*, 476–481.

Hillen, M. A., deHaes, H. C., Stalpers, L. J., Klinkenbijl, J. H., Eddes, E. H., Verdam, M. G., et al. (2014). How attachment style and locus of control influence patients' trust in their oncologist. *Journal of Psychosomatic Research, 76*, 221–226.

Hunter, J. J., & Maunder, R. G. (2001). Using attachment theory to understand illness behavior. *General Hospital Psychiatry, 23*, 177–182.

Hyphantis, T., Goulia, P., & Carvalho, A. F. (2013). Personality traits, defense mechanisms and hostility features associated with somatic symptom severity in both health and disease. *Journal of Psychosomatic Research, 75*, 362–369.

Ingenhoven, T. J. M., & Duivenvoorden, H. J. (2011). Differential effectiveness of antipsychotics in borderline personality disorder: Meta-analyses of placebo-controlled, randomized clinical trials on symptomatic outcome domains. *Journal of Clinical Psychopharmacology, 31*, 489–496.

Ingenhoven, T. J. M., & Duivenvoorden, H. J. (2011). Differential effectiveness of antipsychotics in borderline personality disorder: Meta-analyses of placebo-controlled, randomized clinical trials on symptomatic outcome domains. *Journal of Clinical Psychopharmacology, 31*, 489–496.

Ingenhoven, T., Lafay, P., Rinne, T., Passchier, J., & Duivenvoorden, H. (2010). Effectiveness of pharmacotherapy for severe personality disorders: meta-analyses of randomized controlled trials. *Journal of Clinical Psychiatry, 71*, 14–25.

Kahana, R. J., & Bibring, G. L. (1964). Personality types in medical management. In N. E. Zinberg (Ed.), *Psychiatry and medical practice in a general hospital* (pp. 108–123). New York: International Universities Press.

Lewis, G., & Appleby, L. (1988). Personality disorder: The patients psychiatrists dislike. *British Journal of Psychiatry, 153*, 44–49.

Lichtenstein, P., Halldner, L., Zettergvist, J., Sjölander, A., Serlachius, E., Fazel, S., et al. (2012). Medication for attention-deficit hyperactivity disorder and criminality. *New England Journal of Medicine, 367*, 2006–2014.

Maunder, R. G., & Hunter, J. J. (2009). Assessing patterns of adult attachment in medical patients. *General Hospital Psychiatry, 31*, 123–130.

McCrae, R. R., & Costa, P. T. (2010). *NEO inventories: Professional manual.* Lutz, FL: Psychological Assessment Resources, Inc.

McHugh, R. K., Whitton, S. W., & Peckham, A. D. (2013). Patient preference for psychological vs. pharmacologic treatment of psychiatric disorders: A meta-analytic review. *Journal of Clinical Psychiatry, 74*, 595–602.

Myers, I. B. (1998). *Introduction to type.* Palo Alto, CA: Consulting Psychologists Press.

Myers, I. B., McCaulley, M. H., Quenk, N. L., & Hammer, A. L. (1998). *MBTI manual* (3rd ed.). Palo Alto, CA: Consulting Psychologists Press.

Nelson, M. T., Seal, M. L., Pantelis, C., & Philips, L. J. (2013). Evidence for a dimensional relationship between schizotypy and schizophrenia: A systematic review. *Neuroscience and Biobehavioral Reviews, 37*, 317–327.

Ravitz, P., Maunder, R., Hunter, J., Sthankiya, B., & Lancee, W. (2010). Adult attachment measures: A 25-year review. *Journal of Psychosomatic Research, 69*, 419–432.

Ripoll, L. H. (2012). Clinical psychopharmacology of borderline personality disorder: an update on the available evidence in light of the Diagnostic and Statistical Manual of Mental Disorders–5. *Current Opinion in Psychiatry, 25*, 52–58.

Robinson, D. S., Gilmor, M. L., Yang, Y., Moonsammy, G., Azzaro, A. J., Oren, D. A., et al. (2007). Treatment effects of selegiline transdermal system on symptoms of major depressive disorder: a meta-analysis of short-term, placebo-controlled, efficacy trials. *Psychopharmacology Bulletin, 40*, 15–28.

Sadavoy, J., & Fogel, B. (1992). Personality disorders in old age. In J. E. Birren, R. B. Sloan, & G. Cohen (Eds.), *Handbook of mental health and aging* (2nd ed.). Orlando, FL: Academic Press.

Skodol, A. E., Oldham, J. M., & Gallaher, P. E. (1999). Axis II comorbidity of substance use disorders among patients referred for treatment of personality disorders. *American Journal of Psychiatry, 156*, 733–738.

Spiegel, H., & Spiegel, D. (1978). *Trance and treatment.* New York: Basic Books.

Starks, T. J., & Parsons, J. T. (2014). Adult attachment among partnered gay men: Patterns and associations with sexual relationship quality. *Archives of Sexual Behavior, 43*, 107–117.

Vaillant, G. E. (1997). *Adaptation to life.* Boston, MA: Little Brown.

Vaillant, G. E. (2011). Involuntary coping mechanisms: A psychodynamic perspective. *Dialogues in Clinical Neuroscience, 13*, 366–370.

Villeneuve, E., & Lemelin, S. (2005). Open-label study of atypical neuroleptic quetiapine for treatment of borderline personality disorder: impulsivity as main target. *Journal of Clinical Psychiatry, 66*, 1298–1303.

PART V

NEUROPSYCHIATRIC DISORDERS

41.

DELIRIUM

NEUROBIOLOGY, CHARACTERISTICS, AND MANAGEMENT

José R. Maldonado

INTRODUCTION

Epidemiologically, delirium is likely the most common psychiatric syndrome found in the general hospital setting. Its occurrence parallels the severity of the underlying medical processes. Clinically, delirium presents as an acute or subacute organic mental syndrome characterized by disturbance of consciousness, global cognitive impairment, disorientation, perceptual disturbance, deficits in attention, changes in psychomotor activity, disordered sleep–wake cycles, and fluctuations in symptom severity, all representing a significant change over the patient's baseline level of cognitive and behavioral functioning. Etiologically, delirium is a neurobehavioral syndrome caused by the transient disruption of normal neuronal activity secondary to disturbances of systemic physiology. The phenotypes of delirium (i.e., hyperactive, hypoactive, mixed) are likely a function of which of the various neurotransmitter systems predominates, which can change due to progression of illness or the influence of environmental and/or pharmacological agents.

Hippocrates provided a clear description of the syndrome, but called it *phrenitis,* meaning an "acute inflammation of mind and body" (Lipowski, 1991). In fact, *phrenitis* literally means "inflammation of the mind or diaphragm" (Greek *phren* = mind, diaphragm; *itis* = inflammation) (Sakai, 1991; Frederiks, 2000). It was an ancient disease concept or descriptive notion that denoted a disease consisting of a combination of a mental disorder and fever (the term *phrenes* had a double meaning, indicating both a mental and a somatic domain), distinguishing phrenitis from conventional madness (Sakai, 1991; Frederiks, 2000).

The term *delirium* is reported to have been first used by the lay Roman writer Celsus (A.D. 1) (Adamis et al., 2007) and described in his compendium *De Medicina* as "a madness which is both acute and happens in a fever; the Greeks call it phrenitis" (Celsus, 1814, Chapter XVIII, p. 115). According to Celsus, a fever becomes a phrenitis "when the delirium begins to continue without interruption; or when the patient, though he still have his reason, yet forms to himself some vain images: it is perfect, when the mind gives itself up to these images" (Celsus, 1814). It was also Celsus who was the first to declare that "not all deliria were reversible, but in some cases, although the causes disappeared, patients continued

to be demented." *Delirium* is derived from the Latin roots *de* (meaning "away from"), *lira* (meaning "furrow in a field"), and *ium* (Latin for singular), and literally means "a going off the plowed track; a madness." Celsus described the various forms of delirium: "Now there are several kinds of it: for among phrenitic people some are merry, others sad; other grow outrageous, and do acts of violence.... Those, who are more violent in their actions, it is proper to bind, lest they should hurt either themselves or any other person." Despite Celsus's introduction of the term *delirium*, the syndrome continued to be referred to as "phrenitis."

In the second century A.D., Aretaeus classified diseases as "acute" or "chronic." Among the known mental disorders of the time, phrenitis and lethargy (*lethargus*) were the chief acute diseases, and both were believed to be caused by fever or poisons and thus reflecting brain disease (Lipowski, 1991). The ancient description of phrenitis typically involved restlessness, insomnia, and hallucinations, and appears consistent with our current understanding of *hyperactive delirium*. Conversely, lethargy, involving undue quietness and sleepiness, is more akin to what we now call *hypoactive delirium*.

It was not until the sixteenth century that we find the first description of delirium in the English medical literature, in the textbook *The Method of Physick* (Barrough, 1583). Barrough called it "frenesie" and described it involved the derangement of three main functions: imagination, cogitation, and memory; also featuring disturbed sleep.

Thomas Willis (1621–1675) described delirium as resulting from "fever, poisoning, hemorrhage, lack of sleep, and drunkenness" (Willis, 1672). According to Willis, its core features included "incongruous conceptions and confused thoughts," distorted visual perceptions, and disturbed behavior. Willis referred to phrenitis as "an inflammation of the whole sensitive soul and animal spirits" (Bynum, 2000).

It was not until the nineteenth century that the term *phrenitis* was replaced by the word "delirium," in part due to the efforts of Gerard van Swieten (1700–1772), Giovanni Battista Morgagni (1682–1771), and Philippe Pinel (1745–1826) (Byl & Szafran, 1996; Frederiks, 2000). After the works of these luminaries of medicine, the word *phrenitis* fell into disuse, replaced by the term *febrile delirium* (Berrios, 1981). In 1813, the British physician Thomas Sutton introduced the term *delirium tremens* to designate delirium caused by the withdrawal from "spirits, and in consequence of excess or habitual indulgence in them" (Sutton, 1813). In modern times, the term is exclusively applied to delirium resulting from alcohol withdrawal (2001). In the 1817 German treatise "The Dream and the Feverish Insanity" (*Der Traum und des fieberhafte Irreseyn*), Greiner first pioneered the term "clouding of consciousness" (*Verdunkelung des Bewusstseins*) to describe the pathophysiological abnormality responsible for delirium, and linking disordered consciousness to the phenomenon of delirium (Greiner, 1817). This relationship was further developed by Jackson, who viewed delirium as a clinical manifestation of disordered consciousness (Jackson, 1932). To Jackson, delirium represented a state of reduced consciousness that ranged from the "slightest confusion of thought to coma," and was due to some degree of "dissolution" of the topmost layer of the nervous centers and consequent release from inhibition of the evolutionarily lower centers.

Some of the most significant contributions in the field of delirium include the works of:

Engel and Romano (1959), who demonstrated that the behavioral and cognitive manifestations of delirium were a reflection of an underlying metabolic derangement, and demonstrated the relationship between reduction of brain metabolic rate and electroencephalogram (EEG) slowing;

Blass et al. (1981), who first proposed that impaired cerebral oxidative metabolism resulted in reduced synthesis of various neurotransmitters, particularly acetylcholine, leading to some of the characteristic deficits; and

Lipowski (1967, 1980, 1987), considered by many the contemporary father of the study of delirium, who, in his early seminal work, summarized the history of the field, highlighted the problem with nomenclature, characterized its clinical features, summarized known etiological factors, suggested diagnostic criteria and management, and influenced the course of delirium research for years.

Unfortunately, one of the factors contributing to confusion about delirium is that there are many other terms used by various medical disciplines to describe the same phenomenon: for example, "ICU (intensive care unit) psychosis," "sundowning," "acute confusional state," "toxic confusional state," "post-anesthetic excitement," "acute postoperative psychosis," "post-cardiotomy delirium," and "toxic-metabolic encephalopathy." The author personally prefers the term *acute brain failure*, as this term is compatible with multiple etiologies and settings, describes the acuteness of the onset, implies that the most important organ in the body, the brain, is failing, and this may be associated with significant cognitive decline, morbidity, and mortality.

EPIDEMIOLOGY OF DELIRIUM

Delirium's prevalence surpasses that of all other psychiatric syndromes in the general medical setting (Maldonado, 2008b; NICE, 2010). In fact, delirium has been reported to be one of the six most common preventable conditions in hospitalized elderly patients (Rothschild & Leape, 2000). Some specific medical conditions and surgical procedures are associated with a particularly high incidence of delirium during the postoperative period and among critical care unit patients (see Table 41.1). Terminally ill cancer patients, patients with moderate to severe traumatic brain injury, frail elders, and the critically ill are clinical populations generally recognized to have a high incidence of delirium over their course of illness, due to factors such as polypharmacy, comorbid medical conditions, and metabolic dysfunction.

A recent study at a large general hospital found that delirium had a point prevalence of one in every five inpatients, with some variation in certain medico-surgical units and populations (Ryan, et al. 2013). The frequency of delirium varies from 15% to 60% in hospitalized general medical and surgical patients (Smith & Dimsdale, 1989; Francis, Martin, & Kapoor, 1990; Levkoff et al., 1992; Schor et al., 1992; Williams-Russo, Urquhart, Sharrock, & Carlson, 1992; Pompei et al. 1994; Parikh & Chung, 1995; van der Mast & Roest, 1996; Elie, Cole, Primeau, & Bellavance, 1998; Bucht, Gustafson, & Sandburg, 1999; Fann Alfano, Roth-Roemer, Katon, & Syrjala, 2007; Aldemir Ozen, Kara, Sir, & Bac, 2001; Lepouse, Lautner, Liu, Gomis, & Leon, 2006; Siddiqi, House, & Holmes, 2006; Hala, 2007; Lundstrom et al., 2007; Maldonado, 2008b; Katznelson et al., 2009; Maldonado et al., 2009; Tognoni et al., 2011; Ryan et al., 2013). The rate of postoperative delirium has been reported to range from 10% to 74% (Dyer, Ashton, & Teasdale, 1995; Vaurio, Sands, Wang, Mullen, & Leung, 2006; Bruce, Ritchie, Blizard, Lai, & Raven, 2007; Maldonado et al., 2009; Wiesel, Klausner, Soffer & Zold, 2011). Studies have demonstrated that up to 87% of critically ill patients develop delirium during their ICU stay (Ely, Margolin, et al., 2001). Delirium is common among cancer patients (Adams, 1988; Weinrich & Sarna, 1994; Morita, Tei, Tsunoda, Inoue, & Chihara, 2001; Breitbart, Gibson, & Tremblay, 2002; Centeno, Sanz, & Bruera, 2004; Gaudreau, Gagnon, Harel, Tremblay, & Roy, 2005, Gaudreau, Gagnon, Roy, Harel & Tremblay, 2007).

Among the elderly, studies have found that between 14% and 24% of elderly patients are admitted to the hospital with delirium (Inouye, 1998). It is estimated that new cases arise in 6%–46% of hospitalized elderly patients (Inouye, 1993). In the emergency department, the prevalence in elderly patients is 9.6% (Elie et al., 2000). This data is consistent with more recent studies demonstrating that among those aged 85+ years, the prevalence of delirium is about 10%, rising up to 22% in populations with higher percentages of demented elders and as high as 70% for those in long-term care facilities (de Lange, Verhaak, & van der Meer, 2013).

The occurrence of delirium seems to be highest among the very sick. Various studies have repeatedly demonstrated that up to 87% of those critically ill develop delirium during their stay in critical care units (Ely, Margolin, et al., 2001).

MEDICAL POPULATIONS UNDER STUDY	PREVALENCE OF DELIRIUM (%)
General Medicine Wards	9–24% (Ritchie et al., 1996; Valdes et al., 2000; Maldonado, Dhami, & Wise, 2003; Gonzalez, de Pablo, et al., 2004; Speed et al., 2007)
HIV/AIDS	30%–40% (Fernandez, Levy, & Mansell, 1989; Uldall et al., 2000)
Medical-ICU	60%–80% (Ely et al., 2001)
Post-Stroke	13%–48% (McManus et al., 2007)
Surgery	
Postoperative Delirium	10%–74% (Vaurio et al., 2006; Wiesel, Klausner, et al., 2011)
General Surgical Wards	7%–52% (Dyer & Teasdale, 1995; Bucht, Gustafson, & Sandburgh, 1999)
Spine Surgery	12.5% (Kawaguchi et al., 2006)
Post-CABG	25%–32% (Nevin, Colchester, et al., 1989; Ebert & Herrmann 2001)
Post-Cardiotomy	50%–67% (Smith & Dimsdale, 1989; van der Mast & Roest, 1996; Maldonado et al., 2009)
Abdominal Aneurysm Repair	33% (Benoit et al., 2005)
Geriatrics	
Outpatient Minor (Cataract) Surgery	4.4% (Milstein et al., 2002)
At Time of Hospitalization	10%–15%
In Nursing Homes	15%–60%
Frail Elderly Patient	60% (Francis et al., 1990)
Elective Hip or Knee Replacement	25% (Gustafson, Berggren, et al., 1988; Marcantonio, Flacker, et al., 2000)
Bilateral Knee Replacement	41% (Williams-Russo et al., 1992)
Femoral Neck Fracture Repair	65% (Gustafson, Bucht, et al., 1988; Marcantonio et al., 2000)
Oncology	
General Prevalence	25%–40% (Weinrich & Sarna, 1994; Olofsson et al., 1996; Tuma & DeAngelis, 2000)
Palliative Care Units	26%–44% (Lawlor, Pereira, et al., 2000; Morita, Tei, et al., 2001; Lawlor, 2002; Centeno, Sanz, & Bruera, 2004)
Bone Marrow Transplantation	73% (Fann et al., 2007)
Advanced Cancer	Up to 85% (Lawlor et al., 2000)
Psychiatry	
Among Psychiatric Patients	14.6% (Ritchie et al., 1996)

In addition, delirium is common among cancer patients (Adams, 1988; Weinrich & Sarna, 1994; Morita et al., 2001; Breitbart et al., 2002; Centeno, Sanz, & Bruera, 2004; Gaudreau et al., 2005b). Among those with advanced cancer, delirium was diagnosed in 42% of patients on admission, while it developed in 45% of hospitalized cancer patients who were not delirious at the time of admission (Lawlor et al., 2000). Similar to patients in critical care units, terminal delirium occurs in up to 88% of patients dying of cancer (Lawlor et al., 2000).

The large variation of incidence and prevalence data reported by the various studies reflects differences in patient populations studied, the severity of their medical conditions, and the diagnostic criteria used.

IMPACT OF DELIRIUM

MORBIDITY AND MORTALITY RELATED TO DELIRIUM

Across many hospital settings (e.g., emergency department, general medical ward, postoperative, critical care units) and after controlling for multiple variables (e.g., demographics, age, gender, illness severity, and comorbid medical conditions), patients who develop delirium fare much worse than comparable nondelirious cohorts (Vasilevskis, Han, Hughes, Ely, 2012). A recent meta-analysis, including 16 studies ($n = 6410$) among critically ill patients, demonstrated that, despite modern advances, when compared to their nondelirious counterparts, hospitalized patients with delirium had higher mortality rates (odds ratio [OR]: 3.22; 95% confidence interval [CI]: 2.30–4.52); had longer lengths of stay in both the ICU (weighted mean difference [WMD]: 7.32 days; 95% CI: 4.63–10.01) and in the general hospital (WMD: 6.53 days; 95% CI: 3.03–10.03); spent more time on mechanical ventilation (WMD: 7.22; 95% CI: 5.15–9.29); experienced a higher rate (6X) of complications (e.g., acute respiratory extubation, removal of catheter, cardiac arrhythmia; OR: 6.5; 95% CI: 2.7–15.6); and were more likely to be discharged to skilled placement (OR: 2.59; 95% CI: 1.59–4.21) (Zhang, Pan, & Ni, 2013).

Delirious patients, when compared with patients suffering from the same medical problem who do not develop delirium as a complication, experience prolonged hospital stays—five to ten days longer on average (Francis, Martin, & Kapoor, 1990; O'Keeffe & Lavan, 1997; Ely, Gautam, et al. 2001; Maldonado, Dhami, & Wise, 2003; Ely, Shintani et al., 2004). Significantly more patients who develop delirium in the hospital ultimately require institutional post-acute care, such as placement in a skilled nursing facility (e.g., 16% for delirium patients versus 3% for those without delirium), even after controlling for illness severity, activities of daily living (ADL) status, prior cognitive impairment, and fever (Francis, Martin, & Kapoor, 1990; O'Keeffe & Lavan, 1997). Psychiatric hospital inpatients with delirium had hospital stays that were 62.1% longer than those of patients without delirium (Ritchie, Steiner, & Abrahamowicz, 1996).

Among critically ill patients there is an independent association between delirium present within 24 hours after admission to the critical care unit with an increased in-hospital mortality (i.e., 16.2% for delirious patients vs. 5.7% for nondelirious; van den Boogaard et al., 2010). Others have reported that patients who developed delirium in critical care units experience higher mortality, both at 90 days (11% vs. 3%; Pompei et al., 1994) and at 6 months (34% vs. 15%; Ely et al., 2004; (See http://jama.jamanetwork.com/article.aspx?articleid=198503)). A recent meta-analysis of clinical observational studies in critically ill patients revealed that, when compared with their nondelirious counterparts, delirious patients had higher mortality rate (OR: 3.22; 95% CI: 2.30–4.52); a higher rate of complications including removal of catheter, self-extubation, reintubation, acute respiratory distress syndrome, nosocomial pneumonia, cardiopulmonary edema, and cardiac arrhythmia (OR: 6.5; 95% CI: 2.7–15.6); longer length of stay in both the critical care unit (weighted mean difference [WMD]: 7.32 days; 95% CI: 4.63–10.01) and hospital (WMD: 6.53 days; 95% CI: 3.03–10.03); spent more time on mechanical ventilation (WMD: 7.22 days; 95% CI: 5.15–9.29); and were more likely to be discharged to skilled placement (OR: 2.59; 95% CI: 1.59–4.21) (Zhang et al., 2013).

Delirium's impact among the elderly is even greater. The mortality rate for elderly patients in acute care hospitals is much higher among those with delirium than those without delirium: 8% versus 1% in one study (Francis, Martin, & Kapoor, 1990). Among hospitalized, elderly, medically ill patients, incident delirium was associated with an excess stay after diagnosis of 7.78 days, even after controlling for covariates (McCusker, Cole, et al., 2003). Similarly, studies have demonstrated that delirium in the emergency department was an independent predictor of prolonged hospital length of stay (twice as long), compared to nondelirious patients, even after adjusting for confounding factors (Han et al., 2011). Furthermore, the number of days of delirium older patients experience while in the critical care unit is significantly associated with time to death within 1 year post-ICU admission, after controlling for age, severity of illness, comorbid conditions, psychoactive medication use, and baseline cognitive and functional status (hazard $p = 0.001$; hazard ratio, 1.10; 95% CI, 1.02–1.18); see Thoracic Society Journals, http://www.atsjournals.org/doi/abs/10.1164/rccm.200904-0537OC?url_ver=Z39.88-2003&rfr_id=ori:rid:crossref.org&rfr_dat=cr_pub%3dpubmed&#.VB9cea10wfg – Figure 2 Pisani, Kong, et al., 2009.

These bleak prognoses apply not only to severe cases; even patients with prevalent subsyndromal delirium (SSD) have been shown to experience longer acute-care hospital stay, increased post-discharge mortality, more symptoms of delirium, and a lower cognitive and functional level at follow-up than patients with no SSD (Cole, McCusker, Dendukuri, & Han, 2003). Among patients admitted to an intensive care unit, when comparing no delirium versus SSD, the mortality rate goes up from 2.4% to 10.6% ($p < 0.001$), ICU length of stay goes up from 2.5 to 5.2 days ($p < 0.001$), and the overall hospital length of stay goes up from 12.9 to 16.7 days ($p < 0.001$) (Ouimet, Kavanaugh, Gottfried, & Skrobik, 2007).

COGNITIVE AND BEHAVIORAL SEQUELAE

There appears to be a reciprocal relationship between delirium and cognitive decline, with evidence demonstrating that the presence of baseline cognitive deficits, including dementia, lowers the threshold to develop delirium (Inouye, 1998; Wahlund & Bjorlin, 1999; Litaker, Locala, Franco, Bronson, & Tannous, 2001; McNicoll et al., 2003; Benoit et al., 2005; Kalisvaart et al., 2006; Wacker, Nunes, Cabrita, & Forlenza, 2006; Smith, Attix, Weldon, Greene, & Monk, 2009; Franco, Valencia, et al., 2010; Tognoni et al., 2011). Data suggests that baseline dementia is the strongest risk factor for delirium among older patients (Elie et al., 1998; McCusker et al., 2003; McAvay et al., 2006; Inouye et al., 2007). On the other hand, the development of delirium appears to increase the risk of cognitive decline, including long-term cognitive impairment (LTCI) and dementia (Rockwood et al., 1999; Morandi et al., 2012). A number of pathways and mechanisms have been proposed, yet, despite of some suggestive evidence, none has been conclusively proven as causative (see Box 41.1).

Both clinical experience and research data suggests that many patients do not fully recover (cognitively) from delirium, particularly the elderly. The proportion of patients with residual cognitive impairment reported in various studies depends on the clinical population under study, the cause of the delirium (when it is known), and the threshold and criteria used for diagnosing. In fact, a substantial number of patients who survive delirium are left with post-delirium cognitive impairment (Wacker et al., 2006; Griffiths & Jones, 2007; Bickel, Gradinger, Kochs, & Forstl, 2008; Kat et al., 2008; Maldonado, 2008b; Fong et al., 2009; MacLullich, Beaglehole, Hall, & Meagher, 2009; Girard et al., 2010). Data demonstrates that, when compared to controls, patients diagnosed with delirium are much more likely to experience LTCI (Macdonald, 1999; Rockwood et al., 1999; Jackson, Gordon, Hart, Hopkins, & Ely, 2004; Gunther, Jackson, & Ely, 2007). A study of mechanically ventilated patients who experienced in-hospital delirium found that at 3-month and 12-month follow-ups, 79% and 71% of survivors had cognitive impairment, respectively, with 62% and 36% being severely impaired (Girard et al., 2010). These studies demonstrate that delirium duration was independently associated with long-term cognitive outcome (i.e., the longer the duration of delirium, the more significant the cognitive deficits). For example, an increase from 1 day of delirium to 5 days was independently associated with nearly a 5-point decline (i.e., a one-half standard deviation [SD] decline) in the cognitive battery mean score (95% CI, −9.2 to −0.1).In fact, more than 20 prospective studies (> 5,000 patients) during the last three decades demonstrate a significant association between delirium and long-term cognitive dysfunction (MacLullich et al., 2009; Witlox et al., 2010). The studies suggest that about 40% of patients with delirium develop some form of cognitive impairment when followed up from about 3 months to 5 years after an episode of delirium (Levkoff et al. 1992, McCusker, Cole, Dendukuri, Belzile, & Primeau, 2001; Jackson et al., 2004; Witlox et al., 2010). A comprehensive meta-analysis concluded that there is greater cognitive impairment among patients with delirium than matched controls; there is a higher incidence of dementia in patients with a history of delirium; and that one of three survivors of critical illness with delirium developed cognitive impairment (Jackson et al., 2004). A systematic search

---

Box 41.1 MECHANISMS MEDIATING DELIRIUM AND COGNITIVE IMPAIRMENT

1. A number of factors and mechanisms leading to delirium may also directly cause CNS damage and neuronal dysfunction, and thus mediate both the manifestations of delirium and long-term cognitive impairment, including:

    a) cytokine release and other neuroinflammatory mediators;

    b) decrease perfusion and oxygenation, leading to decreased cerebral oxidative metabolism;

    c) changes in blood–brain barrier permeability;

    d) hyper-catabolic states;

    e) water and electrolyte imbalances;

    f) excessive glucocorticoid levels and other HPA-axis dysfunctions;

    g) melatonin and sleep-wake cycle abnormalities

    h) genetic factors (e.g., some have described an association between APOE4 and prolonged delirium duration)

    i) Amyloid-β deposition (e.g., increased amyloid-β levels have been associated with subjective cognitive dysfunction in critical illness survivors)

2. Pharmacological agents used to treat the underlying causes of the delirium (e.g., steroids, calcineurin inhibitors, other immunosuppressants, dopamine) or the agents used to treat delirium (e.g., dopamine-blocking agents, benzodiazepines) may themselves lead to neuronal damage in a fragile brain.

3. Any of the mechanisms listed above may themselves lead to alterations in neurotransmitter concentration or receptor sensitivity, which itself may underlie the different symptoms and clinical presentations of delirium and/or long-term cognitive dysfunction. Thus, the same mechanisms that cause the substrate for delirium may mediate the cognitive impairments observed after the acute presentation of delirium has resolved.

4. It is possible that instead of causing cognitive deficits or dementia, delirium (and its underlying causes) only serves as a catabolic agent leading to an acceleration of normal, physiological, cerebral aging mechanisms leading to dementia.

5. It is also possible that an episode of delirium simply unmasks subtle cognitive deficits already present, although not yet identified.

of studies published between January 1981 and April 2010 found that delirium is associated with an increased risk of death compared with controls (38.0% vs. 27.5%); that patients who experienced delirium were at increased risk of institutionalization (33.4% vs. 10.7%); and that patients who experienced delirium were at increased risk of dementia (62.5% vs. 8.1%) (Witlox et al., 2010).

Some have postulated four possible putative mechanisms or explanations for the relationship between delirium and long-term cognitive impairment: (1) that delirium is a marker of chronic progressive pathology but unrelated to any progression; (2) that delirium is a consequence of acute brain damage, which is also responsible for a "single hit" or triggering of active processes causing LTCI; (3) that delirium itself is the cause of the LTCI; and/or (4) that pharmacological agents used for the treatment of delirium or other conditions are the cause of the LTCI associated with delirium (MacLullich et al., 2009).

There appears to be a "dose effect" of delirium on cognition, with a longer duration of delirium found to be associated with worse average performance on neuropsychological testing at 3 and 12 months follow-up ($p = 0.02$ and $p = 0.03$, respectively) even after adjusting for age, education, preexisting cognitive function, severity of illness, severe sepsis, and exposure to sedative medications in the critical care unit (Girard et al., 2010). An increase from 1 to 5 days of delirium was independently associated with a 7-point decline in the cognitive battery mean score at 12 months follow-up ($p = 0.03$) (Girard et al., 2010). Various factors may be associated with this dose effect: neuroinflammatory changes; changes in brain–blood barrier permeability; the effect of psychoactive medications; anemia, hypoxia, anoxia, and other low-perfusion states; or systemic organ failure (Maldonado, 2008a, 2013).

Yet, whatever the cause, there appears to be an association between longer duration of delirium and greater brain atrophy as measured by a larger ventricle-to-brain ratio at hospital discharge ($p = 0.03$) and at 3-month follow-up ($p = 0.05$) (Gunther et al., 2012). As expected, greater brain atrophy (higher ventricle-to-brain ratio) at 3 months was associated with worse cognitive performance (executive functioning and visual attention) at 12 months ($p = 0.04$) (Gunther et al., 2012). Others have found that the longer the duration of delirium, the greater the degree of white matter disruption in the genu of the corpus callosum and anterior limb of the internal capsule ($p = .01$), up to 3 months after hospital discharge (Morandi, Rogers, et al., 2012).

A prospective study followed older hospitalized delirious patients who suffered from prevalent or incident delirium detected during the first week of hospitalization for up to a year and found that 39%, 38.5%, and 48.9% of patients with dementia met delirium criteria at discharge, 6-month, and 12-month follow-ups, respectively, compared to 11.1%, 8.8%, and 14.8% of patients without dementia (McCusker, Cole, et al., 2003). However, cognitive improvement during hospitalization and long-term changes in the number of symptoms were remarkably similar in the two groups, with inattention, disorientation, and impaired memory being the most common symptoms.

Another study found that only 4% of delirious patients experienced full resolution of all symptoms of delirium before discharge from the hospital (Levkoff et al., 1992). In this case, after following this sample longitudinally, an additional 20.8% experienced resolution of symptoms by the third month after hospital discharge, with an additional 17.7% by the sixth month after discharge from the hospital. Among elderly hip surgery patients, delirium was a strong independent predictor of cognitive impairment and the occurrence of severe dependency in ADL. In fact, 38 months after discharge from the hospital, 53.8% of the surviving patients with postoperative delirium continued to experience cognitive impairment, compared to only 4.4% of the nondelirious subjects (Bickel et al., 2008). Similarly, a prospective, matched, controlled cohort study of elderly hip surgery patients demonstrated that the risk of dementia or mild cognitive impairment (MCI) over a 30-month follow-up was almost twice as high in patients with postoperative delirium as in those without (Kat et al., 2008).

A large systematic evidence review demonstrated that the proportion of persistent delirium in older hospital patients at discharge, 1, 3, and 6 months was 44.7%, 32.8%, 25.6%, and 21% respectively; one study reported a proportion of 41% at 12 months after discharge (Cole, Ciampi, Belzile, & Zhong, 2009) (see Figure 41.1). The data suggest that many older hospital patients do not recover from delirium and that the persistence of delirium is associated with adverse outcomes. In some of the studies, the long-term outcomes (mortality, nursing home placement, cognition, function) of patients with persistent delirium were consistently worse than the outcomes of patients who had recovered from delirium.

Furthermore, the data shows that SSD (associated with critical illness), in the absence of full-blown delirium, has also been found to result in long-term cognitive dysfunction 2 months to 6 years following critical illness (e.g., 46%–70% of patients showed signs of cognitive dysfunction at 1 year and 25% at 6 years) (Cole et al., 2003; Morandi, McCurley, et al., 2012).

On the other hand, the data suggests that among elderly patients there is a significant acceleration in the slope of cognitive decline in those with Alzheimer's disease (AD) following an episode of delirium (Fong et al., 2009). In fact, prospective data from hospitalized patients with AD (n = 263; median follow-up duration 3.2 years) found that after adjusting for dementia severity, comorbidity, and demographic characteristics, patients who had developed in-hospital delirium experienced greater cognitive deterioration in the year following hospitalization relative to patients who had not developed delirium (Gross et al., 2012). Cognitive deterioration following delirium in the year after hospitalization accelerated to twice the rate of patients who did not develop delirium. This rate of cognitive deterioration among delirious patients continued throughout a 5-year period following hospitalization (Gross et al., 2012). The Vantaa 85+ study (population-based cohort; n = 553 patients aged ≥85 years at baseline) followed examined individuals at 3, 5, 8, and 10 years after delirium and found that delirium increased the risk of incident dementia (OR 8.7, 95% CI, 2.1–3.5) and was associated with the loss of an additional 1 point per year in the Mini-Mental State

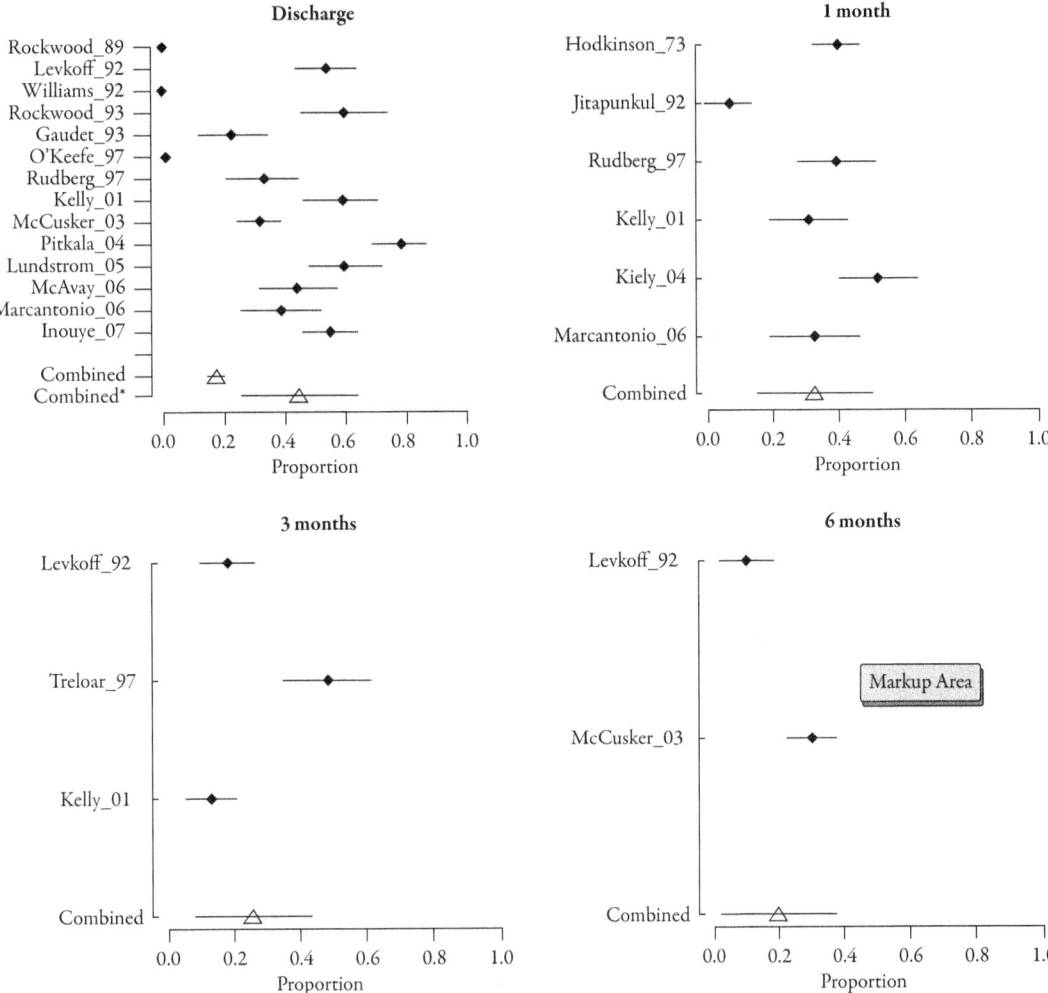

Figure 41.1 Individual and combined proportions (and 95% confidence intervals) for persistent delirium at discharge and one, three, and six months after enrollment. *Source:* (Cole, Ciampi et al., 2009)

Examination compared to those with no history of delirium (95% CI, 0.11–1.89) (Davis et al., 2012).

A prospective cohort study of 53 patients admitted for hip fracture surgery aged 75 years and older found that at the 3 months preoperative assessment, patients who had experienced postoperative delirium showed poorer performance on tests of global cognition and episodic memory, even after adjusting for age, gender, and baseline cognitive impairment (Basinski, Alfano, Katon, Syrjala, & Fann, 2010). No difference was found on tests of attention between patients with and without history of delirium after adjusting for relevant confounders. Another study of elderly patients (≥60) undergoing cardiac surgery (i.e., coronary-artery bypass grafting or valve replacement) found that at 6 months post-surgery, a higher percentage of patients with delirium than those without delirium had not returned to their preoperative baseline level of functioning (40% vs. 24%, $p = 0.01$), although that difference was not significant at 12 months (31% vs. 20%, $p = 0.055$) (Saczynski et al., 2012).

A different type of residual syndrome is post-traumatic stress disorder (PTSD) secondary to the dramatic and bizarre delusional and hallucinatory experiences that occur during a delirious state. The incidence of PTSD related to postoperative delirium has been shown to be related to the nature and level of the sedation and analgesia, degree of factual memory recall, incidence of delirium, and underlying prevalence of preexisting psychiatric morbidity (Blank & Perry, 1984; Bourgon, 1985; Stukas et al., 1999; Dew et al., 2001; Jones, Griffiths, Humphris, Skirrow, 2001; Breitbart et al., 2002; DiMartini, Dew, Kormos, McCurry, & Fontes, 2007; Griffiths & Jones, 2007; Roberts, Rickard, Rajbhandari, & Reynolds, 2007; O'Malley, Leonard, Meagher, & O'Keeffe, 2008; Basinski et al., 2010).

Finally, a number of factors associated with the medical setting may exacerbate the experience of hypnagogic hallucinations, such as medication use, physical restraints, and social isolation (Jones et al., 2001). Patients describe memories of these experiences as being very vivid, detailed, and frightening. A frightening "hallucinated" memory of a nurse trying to kill the patient or removing his organs, without a balancing memory of their medical condition and the care provided by the same nurse, is likely to contribute to the development of pseudo-memories with great emotional valence for that patient.

Studies have found that patients with delirium within the 4 weeks after myeloablative hematopoietic cell transplantation had significantly more distress and fatigue at 6 months ($P < .004$) and at 1 year ($P < .03$) and had worse symptoms of depression and post-traumatic stress at 1 year ($P < .03$), compared with patients without delirium (Basinski et al., 2010). Others have found that family members of delirious ICU patients can also develop PTSD. Both family caregivers (76%) and nurses (73%) have reported severe emotional distress related to a patient's delirium (Breitbart et al., 2002). In that study, family members were most distressed by patients' hyperactivity and functional impairment; nurses were most distressed by the severity of the patients' symptoms and by the presence of perceptual disturbances.

Data suggest that the impact of delirium on outcome may be changed by therapeutic interventions. (Please see the section on delirium management later in this chapter.)

THE COST OF DELIRIUM

The increased morbidity and extended hospital care associated with delirium have been associated with greater care costs (Inouye, 2000; Ely et al., 2004; Milbrandt et al., 2004). Delirious hospital inpatients require more nursing time per patient and have higher per-diem hospital costs, in addition to their increased lengths of stay (Siddiqi, Stockdale, Britton, & Holmes, 2007). The economic impact of delirium is substantial, rivaling the health care costs of falls and myocardial infarction (Hall et al., 1988; Rizzo, McAvay & Tinetti, 1996; Inouye, 2000).

A retrospective chart review of patients who received step-down critical care at a large university hospital showed that the 14% of the ICU population who developed delirium utilized 22% of total inpatient days (Maldonado, Dhami, & Wise, 2003). The treated group consisted of the patients for whom a psychosomatic medicine consult was obtained and the team implemented at least 80% of the recommended regimen (as detailed in the treatment section at the end of this chapter). The average number of days from symptomatic onset to resolution was 10.8 days for untreated patients and 6.3 days for treated patients. As a group, delirious patients were older (71.3 vs. 63.6 years), remained hospitalized longer (16.4 vs. 6.6 days), and had greater total costs per case ($63,900 vs. $30,800). Another study of ICU delirium demonstrated that even after adjusting for age, comorbidity, severity of illness, degree of organ dysfunction, nosocomial infection, hospital mortality, and other potential confounders, delirium was associated with 39% higher ICU and 31% higher hospital costs (Milbrandt et al., 2004). They also found that the severity and duration of delirium were associated with incremental greater care cost. Similarly, a study of hospitalized medically ill elderly patients the average cost per day was 2.5-fold greater in those with delirium, and the total excess cost attributable to delirium ranged from $16,303 to $64,421 per patient (Leslie, Marcantonio, Zhang, & Leo-Summers, 2008).

The total annual direct healthcare costs attributable to delirium in the United States might be as high as $152 billion (Leslie et al., 2008). These costs accrue after hospital discharge due to the greater need for long-term care or additional home health care, rehabilitation services, and informal caregiving. A recent study looking at costs over one year following an episode of delirium estimated that delirium is responsible for an additional cost of $60,000 to $64,000 per patient for the year following the index hospitalization (Leslie et al., 2008).

ETIOLOGY OF DELIRIUM

Many factors potentially contribute to the development of delirium (see Table 41.2). I use the mnemonic "End Acute Brain Failure," to help recall the 20 of the most clinically relevant risk factors. The reason to use this term is to convey to all members of the medical team the seriousness of delirium—indeed, during delirium, the brain is experiencing acute failure, with potentially disastrous consequences. Only some of the risk factors are discussed here; readers are referred to my comprehensive review of delirium risk factors for further details (Maldonado, 2008b). In general, risk factors can be grouped as *non-modifiable* and *potentially modifiable*.

NON-MODIFIABLE RISK FACTORS

Recognition of the non-modifiable factors can help identify patients at high risk for delirium in order to provide enhanced surveillance and implement preventive measures. (Table 41.3). Four important non-modifiable factors are older age, baseline cognitive impairment, severity of underlying medical illness, and preexisting mental disorders.

Age

Old age is likely to be a contributor due to a greater number of medical comorbidities and overall frailty. The aging process itself is associated with some degree of cognitive deficits and increased risk of dementia. Finally, aging is associated with age-related cerebral changes in stress-regulating neurotransmitter and intracellular signal transduction systems. Chronic neurodegeneration is accompanied by an inflammatory response characterized by a chronic, but selective, activation of central nervous system (CNS) microglial cells that are "primed" to produce exaggerated inflammatory responses to immunological challenges. This inflammation is assumed to contribute to disease progression through the production of inflammatory mediators, including cytokines and acute phase proteins (Cunningham, Wilcockson, Campion, Lunnon, & Perry, 2005,; Cunningham et al., 2009). Aging is also associated with decreased volume of acetylcholine (Ach)-producing cells and decreased cerebral oxidative metabolism. Thus, the decline in cognitive functioning associated with the normal aging process is aggravated by the presence of even mild hypoxia, which further inhibits ACh synthesis and its release.

Among elderly patients in the ICU, the probability of developing delirium increases by 2% per year of age for each year after age 65 (Figure 41.2) (Pandharipande et al., 2006). Many other studies confirm that older age is an independent

Table 41.2 DELIRIUM: PREDISPOSING AND PRECIPITATING RISK FACTORS—"END ACUTE BRAIN FAILURE"

RISK FACTOR	EXAMPLES
Electrolyte imbalance and dehydration	Electrolyte disturbances (e.g., hyperammonemia, hypercalcemia, hypo/hyperkalemia, hypomagnesemia, hypo/hypernatremia)
Neurological disorder and injury	All neurological disorders: e.g., CNS malignancies, abscesses, cerebrovascular accident (CVA), vasculitis, multiple sclerosis (MS), epilepsy, Parkinson's disease, normal pressure hydrocephalus (NPH), traumatic brain injury (TBI), diffuse axonal injury (DAI), limbic encephalitis (both non-paraneoplastic and paraneoplastic syndrome).
	Of the various forms of sensory impairment, only visual impairment has been shown to contribute to delirium. Visual impairment can increase the risk of delirium 3.5-fold.
Deficiencies (nutritional)	Nutritional deficiencies (e.g., malnutrition, low serum protein/albumin, low caloric intake, "failure to thrive"), malabsorption disorders (e.g., celiac disease), and hypovitaminosis; specifically deficiencies in cobalamine (B_{12}), folate (B_9), niacin (B_3; leading to pellagra), thiamine (B_1; leading to beriberi and Wernicke's disorder).
Age	Age [>65] and Gender [m>f]
Cognition	Baseline cognitive functioning, including dementia and other cognitive disorders and/or a past history of delirium have all been shown to increase the likelihood of delirium.
U-Tox (intoxication and withdrawal)	Substances of abuse—Acute illicit substance intoxication (e.g., cocaine, PCP, LSD, hallucinogens), as well as poisons, pesticides, solvents, and heavy metals (i.e., lead, manganese, mercury)—and substances withdrawal.
Trauma Toxins	Physical trauma and injury; heat stroke, hyperthermia, hypothermia, severe burns, including trauma of surgical procedures.
	Various toxins, including bio-toxins (animal poison); heavy metals (lead, manganese, mercury); insecticides; poisons; carbon dioxide; toxic effect of pharmacological agents (i.e., serotonin syndrome, neuroleptic malignant syndrome, anticholinergic states); blood levels (toxic levels of various therapeutic substances; e.g., lithium, VPA, carbamazepine, immunosuppressant agents).
Endocrine disturbance	Endocrinopathies such as hyper/hypo-adrenal corticoid; hyper/hypoglycemia; hyper/hypothyroidism.
Behavioral—psychiatric	Certain psychiatric diagnoses, including undue emotional distress; a history of alcohol and other substance abuse, as well as depression, schizophrenia, and bipolar disorder have been associated with a higher incidence of delirium.
Rx and other toxins	Several pharmacological agents have been identified, especially those with high anticholinergic activity, including prescribed agents (especially narcotics and GABA-ergic agents) and various OTC agents (especially anticholinergic substances; polypharmacy).
Anemia, anoxia, hypoxia, and low perfusion states	Any state that may contribute to decreased oxygenation (e.g., pulmonary or cardiac failure, hypotension, anemia, hypoperfusion, intraoperative complications, hypoxia, anoxia, carbon monoxide poisoning, shock).
Infectious	Pneumonia, urinary tract infections, sepsis, encephalitis, meningitis, HIV/AIDS.
Noxious stimuli (pain)	Data suggest that both pain and medications used for the treatment of pain have been associated with the development of delirium. Studies have demonstrated that the presence of postoperative pain is an independent predictor of delirium after surgery. On the other hand, the use of opioid agents has also been implicated in the development of delirium.
Failure (organ)	Organ and systemic failure; usually cardiac, hepatic, pulmonary, and renal failure.
APACHE score (severity of illness)	Evidence shows that the probability of transitioning to delirium increases dramatically for each additional point in the Acute Physiology and Chronic Health Evaluation (APACHE II) severity of illness score.
Intracranial processes	Stroke (especially non-dominant hemispheric); intracranial bleed; meningitis; encephalitis; neoplasms.
Light, sleep, and circadian rhythm	Sleep deprivation and insomnia, sleep disorders (e.g., obstructive sleep apnea) and disturbances/reversal in sleep-wake cycle.

(continued)

Table 41.2 (CONTINUED)

RISK FACTOR	EXAMPLES
Uremia and other metabolic disorders	Acidosis, alkalosis, hyperammonemia, hypersensitivity reactions; glucose, acid–base disturbances.
Restraints and any factors causing immobility	The use of restraints, including endotracheal tubes (ventilator), soft and leather restraints, intravenous lines, bladder catheters, and intermittent pneumatic leg-compression devices, casts, and traction devices all have been associated with an increased incidence of delirium.
Emergence delirium	Emergence from medication-induced sedation, coma, or paralysis; which may be associated with CNS depressant withdrawal, opioid withdrawal, REM-rebound, sleep deprivation.

risk factor among medically ill and surgical patients, with the increase in rate per year dependent on the specific context in which incidence is measured (Milstein, Pollack, Kleinman, & Barak, 2002; Khurana, Gambhir, & Kishore, 2011; Lee et al., 2011; Rudolph et al., 2011; Srinonprasert et al., 2011).

Baseline Cognitive Impairment

Baseline cognitive deficits, even those not rising to the level of dementia, significantly increase the risk of developing delirium. It is well established that individuals with compromised cognitive ability preoperatively (e.g., dementia) are at greater risk of delirium (Franco et al., 2010; Inouye, 1998; Litaker et al., 2001; McNicoll et al., 2003; Benoit et al., 2005). But recent evidence suggests that decrements in higher order cognitive functions, such as executive function (e.g., problem solving, processing speed, planning, complex sequencing, and reasoning), may also predict postoperative delirium in the absence of frank cognitive impairment (Rudolph et al.,

Table 41.3 DELIRIUM RISK FACTORS

MODIFIABLE FACTORS	NON-MODIFIABLE FACTORS
• Various pharmacological agents, especially GABA-ergic and opioid agents, and medications with anticholinergic effects • Prolonged and/or uninterrupted sedation • Immobility • Acute substance intoxication • Substance withdrawal states • Use of physical restraints • Water and electrolyte imbalances • Nutritional deficiencies • Metabolic disturbances and endocrinopathies (primarily deficiency or excess of cortisol) • Poor oxygenation states (e.g., hypo-perfusion, hypoxemia, anemia) • Disruption of the sleep-wake cycle • Uncontrolled pain • Emergence delirium	• Older age • Baseline cognitive impairment • Severity of underlying medical illness • Preexisting mental disorders

2006). A study of nondemented elderly patients undergoing elective orthopedic surgery demonstrated that subtle preoperative attention deficits, as tested by digit vigilance and reaction time testing, were closely associated with postoperative delirium (Lowery, & Ballard, 2007). In fact, these subtle changes predicted a 4-fold to 5-fold increased risk of postoperative delirium for subjects >1 SD above the sample means on these variables. Of note, in this study none of the previously identified risk factors for delirium was significantly associated with delirium (i.e., urea/creatinine ratio, visual impairment, blood pressure, sodium levels, hematocrit, bilirubin). Finally, a study of nearly 1,000 surgical patients found that preoperative executive dysfunction was associated with a greater incidence of postoperative delirium, independent of other risk factors (Smith et al., 2009). Furthermore, patients exhibiting both executive dysfunction and clinically significant levels of depression were at greatest risk for developing delirium postoperatively.

A study of elderly patients undergoing hip surgery found that preoperative Mini-Mental State Exam (MMSE) scores were an independent predictor of postoperative delirium (Kalisvaart et al., 2006). Similarly, a study of elderly subjects undergoing hip or knee replacement demonstrated that the presence of

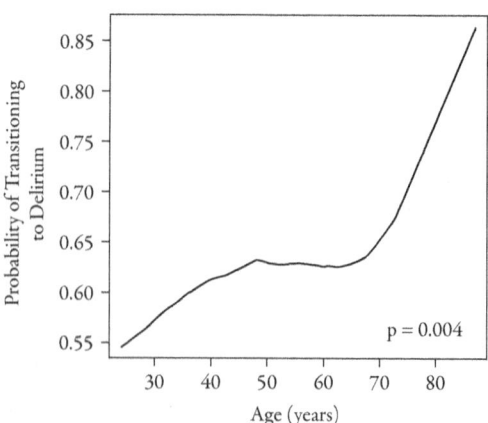

Figure 41.2 Age and the probability of transitioning to delirium. The most notable finding related to age was that probability of transitioning to delirium increased dramatically for each year of life after 65 years. Adjusted Odds Ratio –1.01 (1.00, 1.02) $p = 0.03$. *Abbreviations:* Y-axis = probability; X-axis = age in years. *Source:* (Pandharipande et al., 2006)

dementia increased the incidence of postoperative delirium from 32% to 100% (Wacker et al., 2006). Approximately 70% of elderly patients admitted to a specialized delirium ward had a preexisting cognitive disorder—either dementia or MCI (Wahlund & Bjorlin, 1999). A recent study of elderly patients undergoing urological surgery confirmed that age, baseline cognitive impairment, and previous history of delirium all were associated with a higher rate of postoperative delirium (Tognoni et al., 2011). The relationship between cognitive deficits and dementia seems to be reciprocal. So, while it is clear from the evidence presented above that the presence of baseline cognitive deficits, including dementia, lowers the threshold to develop delirium, data suggest that among elderly patients there is a significant acceleration in the slope of cognitive decline in patients with AD following an episode of delirium (Fong et al., 2009). This raises the question of whether prevention of delirium might ameliorate or delay cognitive decline in patients at risk, particularly those with AD.

Severity of Medical Illness

Studies have also shown that the severity of the patient's underlying medical problems has a significant effect on the development and progression of delirium (Ouimet et al., 2007; Girard et al., 2008; Maldonado, 2008b; Khan, Kahn, & Bourgeois, 2009; Pisani, Kong, et al., 2009; Maldonado, 2011; Srinonprasert et al., 2011; Ryan et al., 2013). A study of adult, mechanically ventilated ICU patients found that increased *severity of illness*, as measured by the modified Acute Physiology and Chronic Health Evaluation (APACHE II; a modified-APACHE II is reached by subtracting the Glasgow Coma Scale score from the usual calculation of the APACHE II total score) was associated with a greater probability of developing delirium (Pandharipande et al., 2006). The incremental risk increased with APACHE score until the latter reached 18 (see Figure 41.3), suggesting that for each additional point on the APACHE II scale, the probability of delirium increased by 6%. These findings were replicated in a

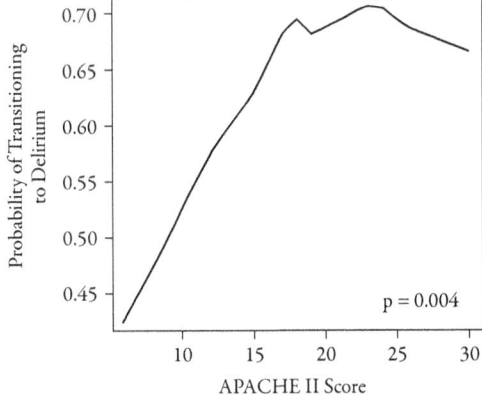

Figure 41.3 Severity of Illness and the Probability of Transitioning to Delirium. The probability of transitioning to delirium increased dramatically for each additional point in the Acute Physiology and Chronic Health Evaluation II (APACHE II) severity of illness score, until reaching a plateau APACHE score of 18. (Pandharipande et al., 2006)

study of elderly patients undergoing hip surgery (Kalisvaart et al., 2006) and another, of critically ill patients (Tsuruta et al., 2010), where APACHE II scores were identified as an independent predictor of delirium when controlling for the use of mechanical ventilation and length of ICU stay.

Preexisting Mental Disorders

A 1996 study retrospectively investigated incidence rates and risk factors for delirium among hospitalized psychiatric patients (Ritchie, Steiner, & Abrahamowicz, 1996). The overall incidence of delirium in the study sample was 15%. Patients with bipolar disorder had the highest incidence of delirium (36%). Only 48% of delirious patients were actually recognized as having delirium at the time it occurred. The hospital stays of patients with delirium were 62% longer than those without.

Delirious mania, also known as "Bell's mania," is defined as "a syndrome of acute onset of excitement, grandiosity, emotional lability, delusions and insomnia characteristic of mania, and the disorientation and altered consciousness characteristic of delirium. Almost all patients exhibit signs of catatonia" (Bell, 1849; Fink, 1999). The syndrome consists of a constellation of symptoms that can arise from both psychotic and affective psychiatric diseases, as well as from many medical diseases. It has been described as a subtype of the catatonia syndrome, having a rapid onset with signs of mania, delirium, and catatonia (Friedman, Mufson, Eisenberg, & Patel, 2003).

Among patients undergoing cardiac surgery—after adjustment for sex, older age, cross-clamp time, hemoglobin, and psychotropic drug use—major depression was significantly associated with delirium (OR = 3.86, 95% CI 1.42–10.52, $p = 0.001$) (Tully, Baker, Winefield, & Turnbull, 2010). A more recent study of cardiac surgery patients found that patients with a preoperative diagnosis of depression had an independently associated increased risk of developing postsurgical delirium (Kazmierski, Banys, Latek, Bourke, & Jaszewski, 2013). Thus, major depressive disorder has been associated with incident delirium after various types of surgical procedures, as well as among general hospital inpatients, independent of other risk factors (Schneider et al., 2002; Dasgupta & Dumbrell, 2006; Kazmierski et al., 2006; McAvay et al., 2007; Smith et al., 2009). A study of geriatric surgical subjects showed that patients with a greater number of preoperative depressive symptoms were more likely to develop postoperative delirium and experience a longer duration of postoperative delirium, even after adjusting for covariates (i.e., age, educational level, functional status, and preoperative alcohol use) (Leung, Sands, Mullen, Wang, & Vaurio, 2005).

Long-term benzodiazepine use is usually associated with the presence of an underlying psychiatric disorder (e.g., anxiety, depression, insomnia, alcohol abuse, benzodiazepine abuse), and thus it may be considered a marker of underlying psychiatric comorbidity. Studies have looked at the presence of postoperative delirium between long-term benzodiazepine users and nonusers and found that the incidence of delirium after orthopedic surgery in the elderly was significantly more frequent in long-term benzodiazepine users (26%) than in short-term users (13%)

(Kudoh, Takase, Takahira, & Takazawa, 2004). Benzodiazepines have been demonstrated to have a negative effect on memory (Lister, 1985; Ghoneim & Mewaldt, 1990; Ghoneim, Block, Ping, el-Zahaby, & Hinrichs, 1993), and it has been demonstrated that benzodiazepine use induces both nonamnestic and amnestic MCI (Tannenbaum, Paquette, Hilmer, Holroyd-Leduc, & Carnahan, 2012). Furthermore, chronic BZDP users had a significantly higher risk of cognitive decline in global cognitive and attention tests compared with non-BZDP users (Mura et al., 2013). It appears that even though there may be an improvement after BZDP discontinuation, there remains a significant impairment in most areas of cognition when compared to controls (Barker, Greenwood, Jackson, & Crowe, 2004, 2005).

As we discussed before, there is a relationship between dementia and development of delirium. New data suggest that the use of benzodiazepine is associated with an increased risk of Alzheimer's disease (adjusted OR 1.51, 95% CI, 1.36–1.69) (Billioti de Gage et al., 2014). Furthermore, the risk increases with cumulative exposure: 1.32 (1.01 to 1.74) for 3 to 6 months, and 1.84 (1.62 to 2.08) for more than 6 months (Billioti de Gage et al., 2014). Similarly, in a large nested-control study, after controlling for multiple variables (i.e., age, gender, education level, living alone, alcohol consumption, psychiatric history, and depressive symptomatology), the ongoing use of benzodiazepines was associated with a significantly increased risk of dementia (adjusted OR, 1.7; 95% CI, 1.2–2.4), while former use was associated with a significantly increased risk of dementia (adjusted OR, 2.3; 95% CI, 1.2–4.5) (Lagnaoui et al., 2002). Others have found similar results, with a marked increased incidence of dementia (OR = 3.50, 95% CI 1.57 to 7.79, $p = 0.002$) among those on long-term BZDP use (Gallacher et al., 2012). Finally, among subjects seeking acute treatment for alcohol withdrawal, 6.9% developed alcohol withdrawal delirium despite adequate treatment with benzodiazepine agents (Palmstierna, 2001). These findings raise the possibility that the use of benzodiazepines, when combined with other risk factors, may contribute or accelerate the rate of cognitive decline following delirium.

POTENTIALLY MODIFIABLE RISK FACTORS

Among the significant factors that are amenable to early intervention or prevention are electrolyte imbalances and nutritional deficiencies, metabolic disturbances and endocrinopathies, low oxygenation states, environmental factors disrupting the sleep-wake cycle and impeding adequate rest, pain and its treatment, the use of drugs with anticholinergic effects, substance intoxication and withdrawal states, the use of physical restraints, and the development of "emergence delirium" (i.e., an altered mental status occurring as a patient "emerges" from deep sedation or medication-induced coma).

Electrolyte Imbalances and Nutritional Deficiencies

Irrespective of the etiology, a water and electrolyte imbalance (primarily magnesium, phosphate, potassium, and chloride) provoking a hypo- or hyperosmolar state causes metabolic encephalopathy or delirium (Mattle, 1985; Schmickaly et al.,

1989; Wetterling, Kanitz, Veltrup, & Driessen, 1994; Aldemir et al., 2001; Lawlor, 2002; Sagawa, Akechi, et al., 2009; Caplan & Chang, 2010). The correction of these electrolyte disturbances has been shown to significantly shorten the duration of delirium (Koizumi, Shiraishi, Ofuku, & Suzuki, 1988). The relationship between nutritional deficiencies and delirium has long been documented, and it is the clearest in patients suffering from Wernicke's encephalopathy (B_1 or thiamine deficiency) (Hoes, 1979; Newman, Grocott, et al., 2001; Onishi, Sugimasa, Kawanishi, & Onose, 2005). In addition, vitamin B_6 and B_{12} deficiency have all been associated with delirium (Peters & Neumann, 1960; Hoes, 1979; Buchman, Mendelsson, et al., 1999; Lerner & Kanevsky, 2002). Some data suggest that vitamin B_{12} supplementation (in patients with documented deficiencies) reduced the duration of delirium in elderly demented subjects. And, others have found a relationship between low albumin levels and the development of delirium among elderly demented patients (Culp & Cacchione, 2008).

Metabolic Disturbances and Endocrinopathies

Metabolic disturbances and various endocrinopathies have been associated with the development of delirium, primarily deficiency or excess of cortisol (Thiele & Hohmann, 1961; Millerowa, 1966; McIntosh et al., 1985; Basavaraju & Phillips, 1989; Olsson, Astrom, Eriksson, & Forssell, 1989; Fassbender, Schmidt, Mossner, Daffertshofer, & Hennerici, 1994; O'Keeffe & Devlin, 1994; Johansson, Olsson, Carlberg, Karlsson, & Fagerlund, 1997; Olsson, 1999; Robertsson et al., 2001; Abildstrom, Christiansen, Sirsma, & Rasmussen, 2004; Nemoto, Kawanishi, Suzuki, Mizukami, & Asada, 2007; Weng, Chang, & Weng, 2008) or thyroid hormone (Vidal & Vidal, 1961; Goldfarb, Varma, & Roginsky, 1980; Nibuya, Suda, Mori, & Ishiguro, 2000; El-Kaissi, Kotowicz, Berk, & Wall, 2005), and either high or low blood glucose levels (Fishbain & Rotundo, 1988; Aldemir, Ozen, et al., 2001; Miller, 2008). There have been case reports of Cushing's disease caused by adrenocorticotropic hormone (ACTH)–producing pituitary adenomas, in patients who lacked the phenotypical signs of hypercortisolism (e.g., facial plethora, supraclavicular fat pads, buffalo hump, truncal obesity, and purple striae) and whose most prominent and distressing symptoms were severe myopathy and altered mental status (Tran & Elias, 2003). Similarly, there have been reports of hypoactive delirium as the primary presentation of a patient with tonsillar abscess and associated panhypopituitarism and secondary hyponatremia (Umekawa Yoshida, Sakane, & Kondo, 1996) and of a patient experiencing delirium secondary to serendipitously diagnosed hypocortisolemia, who presented none of the usual signs of adrenal insufficiency or endocrinopathy (Fang & Jaspan, 1989). Others have demonstrated that, among demented inpatients with no acute medical illness, there was a strong relationship between delirium and dexamethasone suppression test (DST) pathology, irrespective of age and the severity of dementia; suggesting the possibility that an impaired hypothalamus–pituitary–adrenal (HPA) system and a low delirium threshold may lead to delirium as a response to stress (Robertsson et al., 2001).

Low Oxygenation States

Poor oxygenation (i.e., hypoperfusion, hypoxemia, anemia) has long been associated with the development of delirium (Kinney, Duke, et al., 1970; Weissman et al., 1984; McGee, Veremakis, & Wilson, 1988; Fine, Anderson, Rothstein, Williams, & Gochuico, 1997; Maldonado, 2008a,b). Inadequate oxidative metabolism may be one of the underlying causes of the basic metabolic problems initiating the cascade that leads to the development of delirium; namely, inability to maintain ionic gradients, causing cortical spreading depression (i.e., spreading of a self-propagating wave of cellular depolarization in the cerebral cortex) (Moghaddam, Schenk, Stewart, & Hansen, 1987; Somjen et al., 1989, 1990; Iijima, Shimase, Iwao, & Sankawa, 1998; Shimizu-Sasamata, Bosque-Hamilton, Huang, Moskowitz, & Lo, 1998; Basarsky, Feighan, & MacVicar, 1999); abnormal neurotransmitter synthesis, metabolism, and release (Globus, Busto et al., 1988b, 1989, 1990; Busto et al., 1989; 1990; Globus, Wester, Busto, & Dietrich, 1992; Takagi, Ginsberg, et al., 1994; Busto, Dietrich, Globus, Alonso, & Dietrich, 1995; Busto, Dietrich, et al., 1997); and a failure to effectively eliminate neurotoxic byproducts (Busto, Globus, et al., 1989; Globus, Busto, et al., 1990; Globus, Alonso, et al., 1995).

Study findings correlate the development of delirium with findings suggestive of premorbid oxidative metabolism impairment. In a study of ICU patients, three measures of oxygenation (i.e., hemoglobin, hematocrit, and pulse oximetry) were worse in the patients who later developed delirium (Figure 41.4) (Seaman, Schillerstrom, Carroll, & Brown, 2006). Similarly, two measures of oxidative stress (sepsis, pneumonia) occurred more frequently among those diagnosed with delirium. Others have demonstrated that intraoperative cerebral oxygen desaturation (as measured by cerebral oximeter) is significantly associated with an increased risk of postoperative delirium and early cognitive decline and was associated with a nearly threefold increased risk of prolonged hospital stay after cardiac surgery (CABG) (Figure 41.5) (Slater et al., 2009). Finally, another large study of urgent cardiac surgery demonstrated that preoperative and intraoperative ScO_2 readings were lower in the group of patients who developed delirium. The binary logistic regression identified older age, lower MMSE, neurological or psychiatric disease, and lower preoperative ScO2 as independent predictors of postoperative delirium (Figure 41.6) (Schoen et al., 2011).

Sleep Disturbances

Sleep is another factor that seems to play a significant role in developing delirium in the ICU. Sleep deprivation has long been linked to the development of delirium (Lipowski, 1987) and psychosis (Berger, Vollmann, et al., 1997). Patients in the ICU experience severe alterations of sleep, with sleep loss, sleep fragmentation, and sleep–wake cycle disorganization. Continuous polysomnographic recordings have demonstrated that despite sedative practices, the average amount of sleep in ICU patients is limited (e.g., as short as 1 hour and 51 minutes

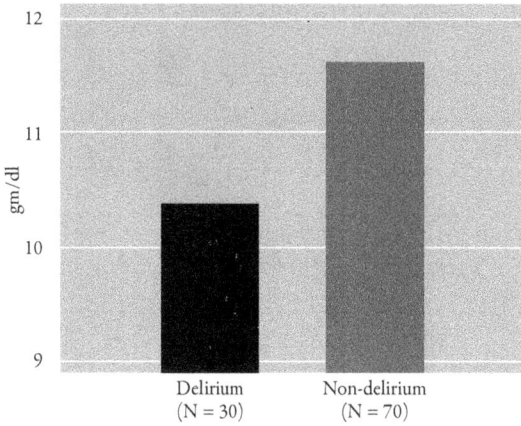

Note: p<0.004; Student's t-test with equal variances not assumed (Levene's test).

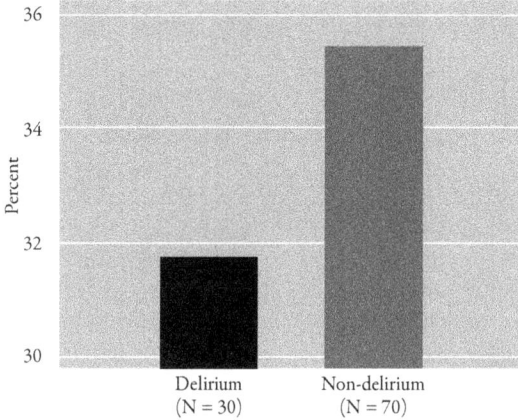

Note: p<0.006; Student's t-test with equal variances not assumed.

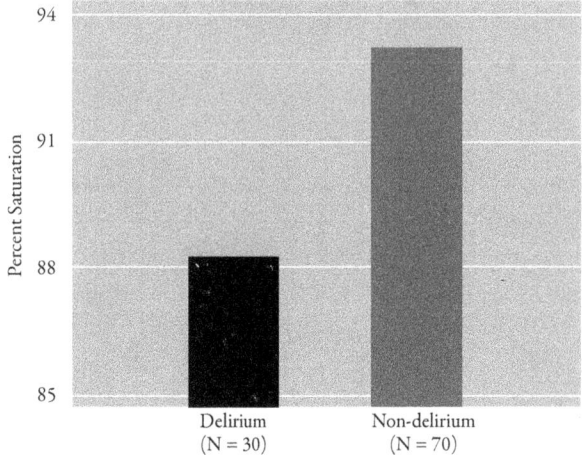

Note: p<0.006; Student's t-test with equal variances not assumed.

Figure 41.4 Oxidative Stress Hypothesis. Three measures of oxygenation (Hg, Hct, pulse ox.) were worse in the patients who later developed delirium.

per 24-hour period) (Aurell & Elmqvist, 1985). Sleep in ICU patients is characterized by prolonged sleep latencies, sleep fragmentation, decreased sleep efficiency, frequent arousals, a predominance of stage 1 and stage 2 non-rapid eye movement (REM) sleep, decreased or absent stage 3 and 4 non-REM sleep,

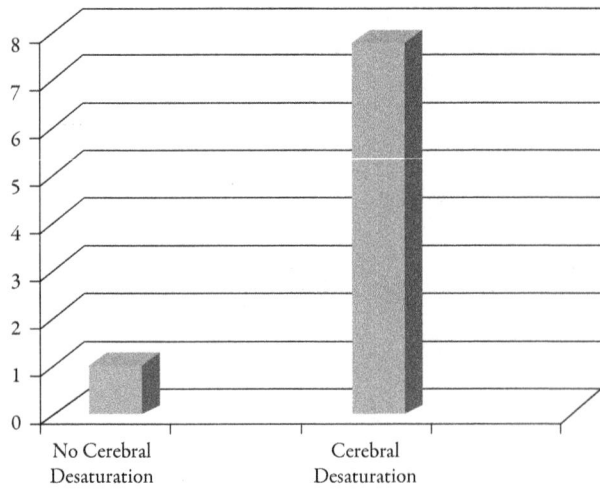

Figure 41.5 Cerebral Desaturation and Postoperative Delirium. Intraoperative cerebral O2 desaturation was a significant risk factor for postoperative delirium in CABG patients. (Slater et al., 2009)

and decreased or absent REM sleep (Weinhouse & Schwab, 2006; Drouot, Cabello, d'Ortho, & Brochard, 2008; Friese, 2008b).

There are many factors that may contribute to sleep debt in the hospital, and particularly in the ICU. These include frequent diagnostic and therapeutic interventions and procedures; anxiety, fear, pain, and underlying illness and disease severity; and environmental factors, such as around-the-clock medical care (e.g., suctioning, ventilator settings, blood draws, line

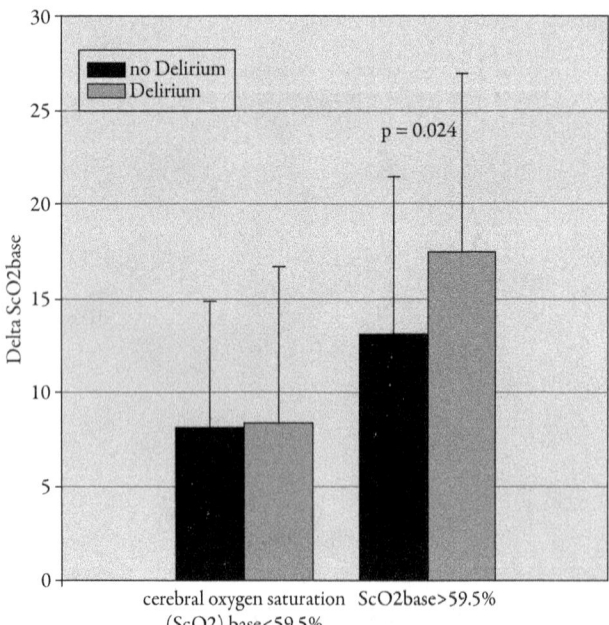

Figure 41.6 Preoperative and Intraoperative Cerebral O2 Saturation (ScO2) Values Influenced the Risk of Post-op Delirium Intraoperative changes in ScO2 in patients with or without delirium classified by normal or low preoperative ScO2. Delta ScO2base, difference between preoperative regional cerebral oxygen saturation with oxygen supplementation and minimal intraoperative regional cerebral oxygen saturation; ScO2base, regional cerebral oxygen saturation with supplemental oxygen. (Schoen et al., 2011)

changes/placement), noise, light, and discomfort (Weinhouse & Schwab 2006; Drouot et al., 2008; Friese, 2008b). Another large factor in sleep debt in ventilated patients is continuous sedation. In fact, studies have demonstrated that propofol and benzodiazepine agents (the primary agents used for continuous sedation) have a negative effect on sleep (e.g., severe alterations of sleep with sleep loss, ↓ REM sleep, loss of circadian rhythm, extreme sleep fragmentation, sleep–wake cycle disorganization) (Drouot et al., 2008; Matthews, 2011; Boyko, Ording, & Jennum, 2012; Hofhuis, Langevoort, Rommes, & Spronk, 2012; Kamdar, Needham, & Collop, 2012; McKinley et al., 2012; Nakos, 2012; Watson, Ceriana, & Fanfulla, 2012; Andersen, Boesen, & Olsen, 2013; Brummel & Girard, 2013; Gomez Sanz, 2013).

Pain Management

As in the case with sleep, both the experience of pain and some of the pharmacological agents used for the treatment of pain have been associated with the development of delirium. In fact, the presence of postoperative pain has been shown to be an independent predictor of postoperative delirium (Vaurio et al., 2006). There is also a direct relationship between levels of preoperative pain and the risk of developing postoperative delirium. Unfortunately, some opioid agents have also been implicated in the development of delirium (Fong, Sands, & Leung, 2006; Vella-Brincat & Macleod, 2007; Wang, Sands, Vaurio, Mullen, & Leung, 2007). In fact, opioid agents have been implicated in nearly 60% of the cases of delirium in patients with advanced cancer (Centeno, Sanz, & Bruera, 2004). Studies among cancer patients revealed significant associations between opioids and delirium (Gaudreau et al., 2007). The association remained significant after adjustment for corticosteroid, benzodiazepine, and antipsychotic exposure using generalized estimating equation regressions (OR of 1.37; $P = .0033$). Others have suggested that patients who used oral opioid analgesic agents as their sole means of postoperative pain control are at decreased risk of developing delirium compared to subjects using intravenous (IV) opioid-based, patient-controlled analgesia (PCA) (Vaurio et al., 2006; Wang et al., 2007).

Some opioid agents (e.g., meperidine) may have greater deliriogenic potential than others (Marcantonio et al., 1994; Morrison et al., 2003; Fong et al., 2006). Studies suggest that an opioid rotation to less deliriogenic agents like fentanyl or hydromorphone has been associated with improved pain management and lower delirium rating scores (Morita et al., 2005). The exact mechanism of delirium causation is unclear, but agent half-life, the presence of active metabolites, and anticholinergic potential have all been implicated in opioid-induced delirium (Slatkin & Rhiner, 2004). Some clinicians prefer the use of PCA, as the common wisdom is that patients usually "self-titrate" and end up receiving lower doses of medication, thus lowering delirium risk. This may be true in the cognitively intact individual; but in the cognitively impaired or already delirious patient, PCAs are contraindicated. The risk of a PCA apparatus for a patient who is already confused is that they may not know how to use it, what to do with the button. Essentially the question to answer is, is the patient cognitively intact and competent enough to use PCA appropriately? A simple rule: if the patient is experiencing any sign of confusion (e.g., disorientation, finger agnosia), do not use a PCA. This may be resumed when the patient's delirium resolves.

Medications

Besides opioid agents, a great number of *medications* have been associated with an increased risk of delirium (Table 41.4). Some have said that the highest incidence of medication-induced delirium has been observed in patients taking the greater number of agents (Inouye & Charpentier, 1996), agents with high *anticholinergic potential* (Tune, Carr, Cooper, Klug, & Golinger, 1993), and medications with significant psychoactive effects (Francis, Martin, & Kapoor, 1990; Olofsson, Weitzner, Valentine, Baile, & Meyers, 1996; Brauer, Morrison, Silberzweig, & Siu, 2000; Lawlor et al., 2000; Tuma & DeAngelis, 2000; Morita et al., 2001; Breitbart et al., 2002; Gaudreau & Gagnon, 2005). Among this latter group, opioids, corticosteroids, and benzodiazepines have been identified as major contributors to delirium in several studies (see Figure 41.7) (Gaudreau, Gagnon, et al., 2005b). In fact, narcotics, benzodiazepines, corticosteroids, and other psychoactive agents use have been associated with 3-fold to 11-fold increases in the prevalence of delirium (Morita et al., 2001; Morrison et al., 2003; Gaudreau & Gagnon, 2005; Gaudreau et al., 2005b, 2007; Fong et al., 2006; Pisani, Murphy, et al., 2009; van Munster et al., 2010).

There is significant evidence linking a medication's anticholinergic potential (as measured by serum anticholinergic activity) and their incidence of causing delirium (Tune, et al., 1981, 1993; Tune, Carr, Hoag, & Cooper, 1992; Golinger al., 1987; Milusheva et al., 1990; Inouye & Charpentier, 1996; Flacker et al., 1998; Tune & Egeli, 1999; Tune, 2000; Kojima, Terao, & Yoshimura, 1993; Meyer, Meyer, & Kressig, 2010). Several studies have identified some of these substances, and we have become increasingly aware of the importance of understanding the cumulative serum anticholinergic activity (Tune et al., 1981; Tune & Folstein 1986; Tune et al., 1992, 1993; Tune & Egeli, 1999; Tune, 2000) (see Table 41.5). Others have demonstrated that, among medical inpatients, exposure to anticholinergic agents is an independent risk factor for the development of delirium and is specifically associated with a subsequent increase in delirium symptom severity (Han et al., 2001).

Despite its apparent usefulness, there are limitations to the use of the serum anticholinergic activity (SAA) assay in clinical practice: (1) assays of standard drug solutions do not account for pharmacokinetic differences among drugs, which limits the interpretation of such measurements; (2) emerging evidence has suggested that anticholinergic medications may not be the only cause of elevated SAA (Carnahan, Lund et al., 2002). For example, naturally occurring SAAs have been described in the absence of exposure to known anticholinergic pharmacological agents; their etiology, although they are postulated to be related to the primary illness state (or aging process), and their clinical significance remain unknown (Flacker & Wei, 2001). Despite these limitations, elevated SAA has been consistently associated with cognitive

Table 41.4 COMMONLY USED MEDICINES THAT HAVE ANTICHOLINERGIC EFFECTS

ANTIHISTAMINES

Chlorpheniramine

Cyproheptadine

Dexchlorpheniramine

Diphenhydramine

Dimenhydrinate

Hydroxyzine

Meclizine

Promethazine

ANTIPARKINSONIAN

Benztropine

Biperiden

Levodopa

Trihexyphenidyl

CARDIOVASCULAR

Amiodarone

Beta-blockers

Captopril

Chlorthalidone

Digoxin

Diltiazem

Dipyridamole

Disopyramide

Dopamine

Ergotamine

Furosemide

Hydrochlorothiazide

Hydralazine

Isosorbide mononitrate

Lanoxin

Lidocaine

Methyldopa

Nifedipine

Procainamide

Quinidine

Triamterene

Warfarin

(continued)

Table 41.4 (CONTINUED)

CENTRAL NERVOUS SYSTEM

Barbiturates

Benzodiazepines

Carbamazepine

Chloral hydrate

Dextromethorphan

Heterocyclic antidepressants (esp. amitriptyline, clomipramine, doxepin, imipramine, trimipramine)

Lithium

Low-potency neuroleptics (esp. chlorpromazine, thioridazine)

Midazolam

Meprobamate

Monoamino oxidase inhibitors (MAOIs)

Phenytoin

Propofol

SGAs (some: clozapine, olanzapine)

SSRIs (some: paroxetine)

CORTICOSTEROIDS

Betamethasone

Cortisone

Dexamethasone

Hydrocortisone

Prednisolone

GASTROINTESTINAL

Atropine

Belladonna

Clinidum

Dicyclomine

Dimenhydrinate

Diphenoxylate

H2-antagonists (cimetidine, famotidine, nizatidine, ranitidine)

Hyoscyamine

Lomotil

Loperamide

Meclizine

Metoclopramide

Promethazine

Table 41.4 (CONTINUED)

Propantheline

Scopolamine

GENITOURINARY

Oxybutinin

IMMUNE ACTIVITY/IMMUNOSUPPRESSION

Azathioprine

Cyclosporine

Interleukin-2

Interferon

INFECTIOUS

Amphotericin-B

Ampicillin

Cefalothin

Cefamandole

Cefoxitin

Clindamycin

Cotrimazole

Cycloserine

Fluoroquinolones

Gentamicin

Itraconazole

Mefloquine

Piperacillin

Tobramycin

Vancomycin

MUSCLE RELAXANTS

Baclofen

Carisoprodol

Cyclobenzaprine

Metaxalone

Orphanedrine

Pancuronium

Tizanidine

ONCOLOGY

Asparaginase

Fluorouracil (5-FU)

Tamoxifen

(*continued*)

Table 41.4 (CONTINUED)

OTC

Cold/sinus preparations (antihistamines, pseudoephedrine)

Sleep aids (diphenhydramine, alcohol-containing elixirs)

Stay-awake preparations

PAIN MANAGEMENT

Codeine

Meperidine

NSAIDs (esp. indomethacin and COX2-inhibitors)

Oxycodone

Pentazocine

Propoxyphene

Tramadol

RESPIRATORY SYSTEM

Theophylline

Table 41.5 ANTICHOLINERGIC DRUG LEVELS IN 25 MEDICATIONS RANKED BY THE FREQUENCY OF THEIR PRESCRIPTION FOR ELDERLY PATIENTS

MEDICATION[†]	ANTICHOLINERGIC DRUG LEVEL § (NG/ML OF ATROPINE EQUIVALENTS)
1. Furosemide	0.22
2. Digoxin	0.25
3. Dyazide	0.08
4. Lanoxin	0.25
5. Hydrochlorothiazide	0.00
6. Propranolol	0.00
7. Salicylic acid	0.00
8. Dipyridamole	0.11
9. Theophylline anhydrous	0.44
10. Nitroglycerin	0.00
11. Insulin	0.00
12. Warfarin	0.12

†= At a 10^{-8} M concentration.

§ =Threshold for delirium = 0.80ng/ml.

Source: Tune et al., 1992

impairment and delirium in a number of research settings. In recent years, new data has renewed the concern regarding the relationship between anticholinergic agents and the neurocognitive disorders, including delirium and dementia. In fact, cumulative evidence has demonstrated a strong correlation between the use of anticholinergic agents and incident dementia (Lopez-Alvarez, Zea Sevilla et al. 2014, Gray, Anderson et al. 2015, Mate, Kerr et al. 2015) and an increased risk of hospitalization for confusion (Kalisch Ellett, Pratt et al. 2014).

Among the main offenders, GABA-ergic medications have been increasingly implicated in the development of delirium (Marcantonio et al., 1994; Meuret et al., 2000; Pain, Jeltsch, et al., 2000; Wang et al., 2000; Ely, Gautam, et al., 2001). Several studies have demonstrated a relationship between benzodiazepine use and delirium (Tune & Bylsma, 1991; Marcantonio et al., 1994; Ely, Gautam, et al., 2001; Kudoh et al., 2004). In fact, the benzodiazepine agent lorazepam has been found to be an independent risk factor for daily transition to delirium (see Figure 41.8) (Pandharipande et al., 2006). A recent study found that among ventilated burn patients, exposure to benzodiazepines was an independent risk factor for the development of delirium (P <.001) (Agarwal, et al., 2010). Similarly, the use of various general anesthetics has been associated to structural changes leading to disruption of blood–brain barrier (BBB) integrity (Forsberg et al., 2014). This will be discussed in further detail under the inflammatory hypothesis of delirium.

There are many mechanisms by which sedative agents, particularly GABA-ergic agents, mediate delirium. These may include interruption of physiological melatonin and sleep patterns, interference with central cholinergic transmission, disruption of thalamic gating, and acute and long-term

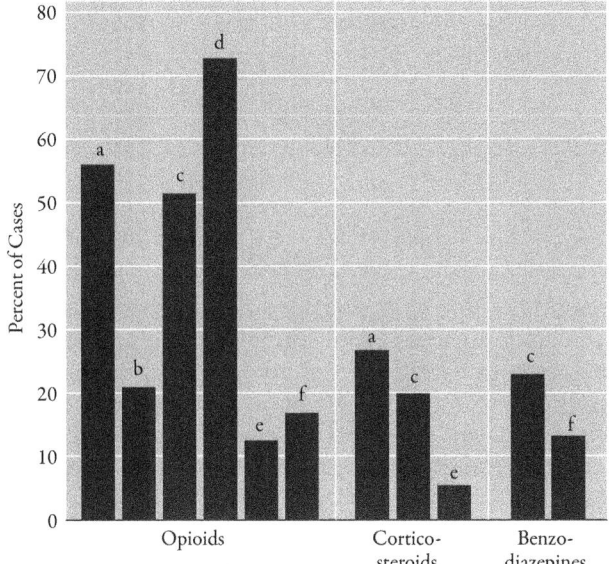

[a]Breitbart et al. 2002[26]
[b]Morita et al. 2001[29]
[c]Tuma and DeAngelis 2000[30]
[d]Lawlor et al. 2000[14]
[e]Olofsson et al. 1996[27]
[f]Francis et al. 1999[9]

Figure 41.7 Delirium Potentially Caused by Opioids, Corticosteroids, and Benzodiazepines in Six Case Series. (Gaudreau, Gagnon, et al., 2005b)

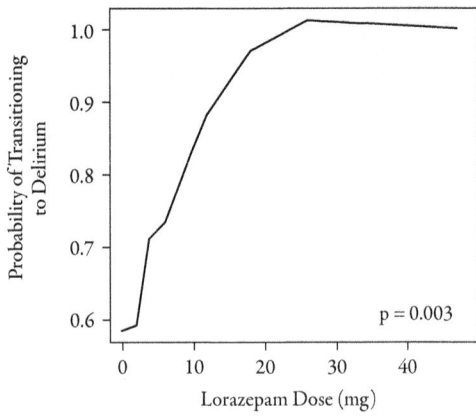

Figure 41.8 Lorazepam and the Probability of Transitioning to Delirium
The probability of transitioning to delirium increased with the dose of lorazepam administered in the previous 24 hours. This incremental risk was large at low doses and plateaued at around 20 mg/day.
Abbreviations: Y-axis = delirium risk; X-axis = lorazepam dose (in mg)   (Pandharipande et al., 2006)

cognitive disturb ances. Please see Box 41.2 for a comprehensive list of the 12 mechanisms by which sedative and analgesic agents mediate their deliriogenic effects. Similar to more classic anticholinergic agents, acute benzodiazepine use has been linked to agitation, confusion and delirium (Daman Willems and Dillon 1986, Short, Forrest et al. 1987, Miller and Gold 1991, O'Reilly and Smith 1991, Trewin, Lawrence et al. 1992, Lechin, van der Dijs et al. 1996, Hofmann 2013); and chronic use is linked to Alzheimer's disease (Billioti de Gage, Moride et al. 2014, Kmietowicz 2014, Yaffe and Boustani 2014).

Box 41.2 **SEDATIVE AND ANALGESIC AGENTS'
DELIRIOGENIC MECHANISMS:**

Sedative agents (mostly GABA-ergic) and opioids may contribute to the development of delirium by one of twelve possible mechanisms:

1. Acutely, benzodiazepines (BZDP) are associated with the development of psychomotor retardation, cognitive blunting, ataxia, poor balance, and decreased mobility, all known contributing factors for delirium (Sarasin, Ghoneim, & Block, 1996).

2. BZDP have been demonstrated to have a negative effect on memory (Lister, 1985; Ghoneim & Mewaldt, 1990; Ghoneim et al., 1993).

3. BZDP use induces both non-amnestic and amnestic mild cognitive impairment (Tannenbaum et al., 2012)

4. Chronic administration of BZDP induces a down-regulation of BZDP-receptors (Hutchinson, Smith, & Darlington, 1996), and a reduction in the number of these receptors seems to be correlated with cognitive decline (Shimohama, Taniguchi, Fujiwara, & Kameyama, 1988).

5. Long term BZDP use may induce a limitation in cognitive reserve capacity, which further reduces a person's ability to cope with early phase brain lesions by soliciting accessory neuronal networks (Stern, 2002).

6. New evidence suggests that BZDP use may be associated with an increased cumulative risk of dementia (Billioti de Gage et al., 2014).

7. BZDP use interferes with central cholinergic function muscarinic transmission at the level of the basal forebrain and hippocampus (i.e., causing a centrally mediated acetylcholine deficient state) (Schneck & Rupreht, 1989; Meuret, Backman, et al., 2000; Pain et al., 2000; Wang et al., 2000); furthermore, BZDP activate GABAA receptors, which inhibit glutamate effect on NMDA receptors, thus limiting Ach release (Cervetto & Taccola, 2008).

8. BZDP use interferes with physiological sleep patterns (e.g., ↓ slow wave sleep→ ↑REM latency→↓REM periods duration→REM deprivation) (Borbely, Mattmann, et al., 1985; Achermann & Borbely, 1987; Bastien, LeBlanc, Carrier, & Morin, 2003, Qureshi & Lee-Chiong, 2004; Mazza et al., 2014).

9. BZDP use disrupts the circadian rhythm of melatonin release (Olofsson et al., 2004).

10. Long-term use of BZDP increases compensatory up-regulation of N-methyl D-aspartate (NMDA) and kainate receptors and Ca^{2+} channels (Chaudieu, St-Pierre, Quirion, & Boksa, 1994; Heikkinen, Moykkynen, & Korpi, 2009); enhancing NMDA-induced neuronal damage (Zhu, Cottrell, & Kass, 1997).

11. BZDP use disrupts thalamic gating function (Gaudreau & Gagnon, 2005).

12. Long-term BZDP use may lead to CNS-depressant withdrawal syndromes, upon abrupt discontinuation.

Immobility

Immobility—due to disease conditions, physical restraints, or medical apparatus that effectively limits the patient's mobility (e.g., ET tube [ventilator], IV lines, bladder catheters, intermittent pneumatic leg-compression devices, casts, traction devices)— has been shown to increase the incidence of delirium (McCusker, Verdon, Caplan, Meldon, & Jacobs, 2002; Inouye et al., 2007). Some may include chemical restraints in this group. Data show that patients who are mobilized early (i.e., alerted and provided physical and occupational therapy) during the course of illness demonstrate greater return to independent functional status at hospital discharge (59% vs. 35%), spend less time in the ICU (2 vs. 4 days), and experience less delirium (33% vs. 57%) compared to a control cohort (Schweickert et al., 2009).

Both psychoactive medications and immobility may contribute to emergence delirium (ED) or emergence agitation (EA), a postoperative behavior that may occur upon awakening in patients exposed to general anesthesia (Bastron & Moyers, 1967; Gutstein, 1996; Haynes, 1999; Fong et al., 2006; Maldonado, 2008b) and that has been described in both children and adults (Albin, Bunegin, Massopust, & Jannetta, 1974; Lepouse, et al., 2006; Abu-Shahwan, 2008; Fronapfel, 2008; Hudek, 2009). Even though there is some suggestion that the incidence may be increased after the use of volatile (inhaled) anesthetic agents (Bajwa, Costi, & Cyna, 2010), many other agents commonly used for anesthesia and sedation in the ICU have been implicated (as already discussed above). All forms of conventional sedation may be associated with emergence delirium, although some are better than others. As a general rule, propofol is less deliriogenic than midazolam, but dexmedetomidine is less deliriogenic than both. The use of opioids as a sedative agent may be one of the main contributors of emergence delirium and should be avoided. The rule should be: Use sedative agents for sedation and narcotics for pain management, rather than the commonly practiced narcosedation. Another contributor to emergence delirium may be CNS depressants (e.g., narcotics, benzodiazepines, other GABA-ergic agents) when a patient has been exposed to these agents for a long period of time, and the primary team feels "it is time to extubate" so the patient is quickly taken off these agents rather than being carefully weaned off them. Being more mindful of this practice and its effects, and better planning, may significantly reduce delirium's occurrence.

NEUROPATHOGENESIS OF DELIRIUM

Many theories have been proposed to explain the etiology of delirium, but Engel and Romano explained it best:

> We thus arrive at the proposition that a derangement in functional metabolism underlies all instances of delirium and that this is reflected at the clinical level by the characteristic disturbance in cognitive functions.
>
> (Engel & Romano, 1959)

Thus we will start with the premise that delirium is a neurobehavioral syndrome caused by the transient disruption of normal neuronal activity secondary to systemic disturbances (Engel & Romano, 1959; Lipowski, 1992; Brown, 2000). Over the years, a number of theories have been proposed in an attempt to explain the processes leading to the development of delirium (Maldonado, 2008a). Most of these theories are complementary, rather than competing (see Figure 41.9). It is

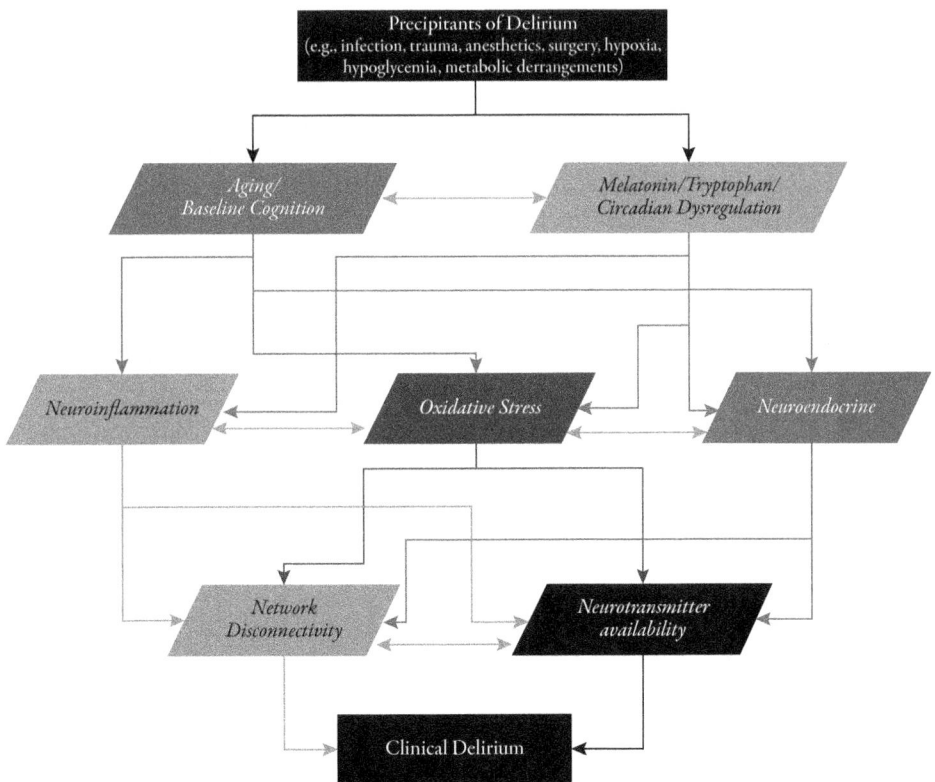

Figure 41.9 Neuropathogenesis of Delirium Schematics of the interrelationship of current theories on the pathophysiology of delirium and how they may relate to each other. Each proposed theory has focused on a specific mechanism or pathologic process (e.g., dopamine excess or acetylcholine deficiency theories), observational and experiential evidence (e.g., sleep deprivation, aging), or empirical data (e.g., specific pharmacological agents' association with post-operative delirium; intra-operative hypoxia). Most of these theories are complementary rather than competing, with many areas of intersection and reciprocal influence. In the end, it is unlikely that any one of these theories is fully capable of explaining the etiology or phenomenological manifestations of delirium, but rather that their interaction leads to the biochemical derangement and, ultimately, to the complex cognitive and behavioral changes characteristic of delirium. (Adapted from Maldonado, 2013).

likely that none of these theories by itself explains the phenomena of delirium, but rather that two or more of these, if not all, act together to lead to the biochemical derangement we know as delirium. Here we will highlight four of them. A detailed review of all has been published elsewhere (Maldonado, 2008a, 2013).

NEUROINFLAMMATORY HYPOTHESIS

The neuroinflammatory hypothesis suggests that acute peripheral inflammatory processes (e.g., infections, surgery, trauma) induce activation of brain parenchymal cells and expression of proinflammatory cytokines and inflammatory mediators in the central nervous system, which in turn induces neuronal and synaptic dysfunction that may serve as the substrate for the neurobehavioral and cognitive symptoms characteristic of delirium (Godbout et al., 2005, Dantzer,

O'Connor, Freund, Johnson, & Kelley, 2008; Cunningham et al., 2009; Godbout & Johnson, 2009; Cerejeira, Firmino, Vaz-Serra, & Mukaetova-Ladinska, 2010; Cunningham, 2011) (Figure 41.10). Previous studies have already demonstrated the brain's ability to monitor the presence of systemic inflammatory processes (e.g., outside the BBB) and the development of nonspecific physiological (e.g., fever, pain, malaise, fatigue, and anorexia) and behavioral adaptations (e.g., anhedonia, lethargy, social withdrawal, depressed mood, cognitive impairment) upon exposure to infection or inflammation collectively known as "sickness behavior."

According to the neuroinflammatory hypothesis, delirium represents the CNS manifestation of a systemic disease state that has crossed the blood–brain barrier (Maldonado, 2008b). Indeed, many of the circumstances associated with a high occurrence of delirium (e.g., infections, postoperative states) can also be associated with compromise of BBB

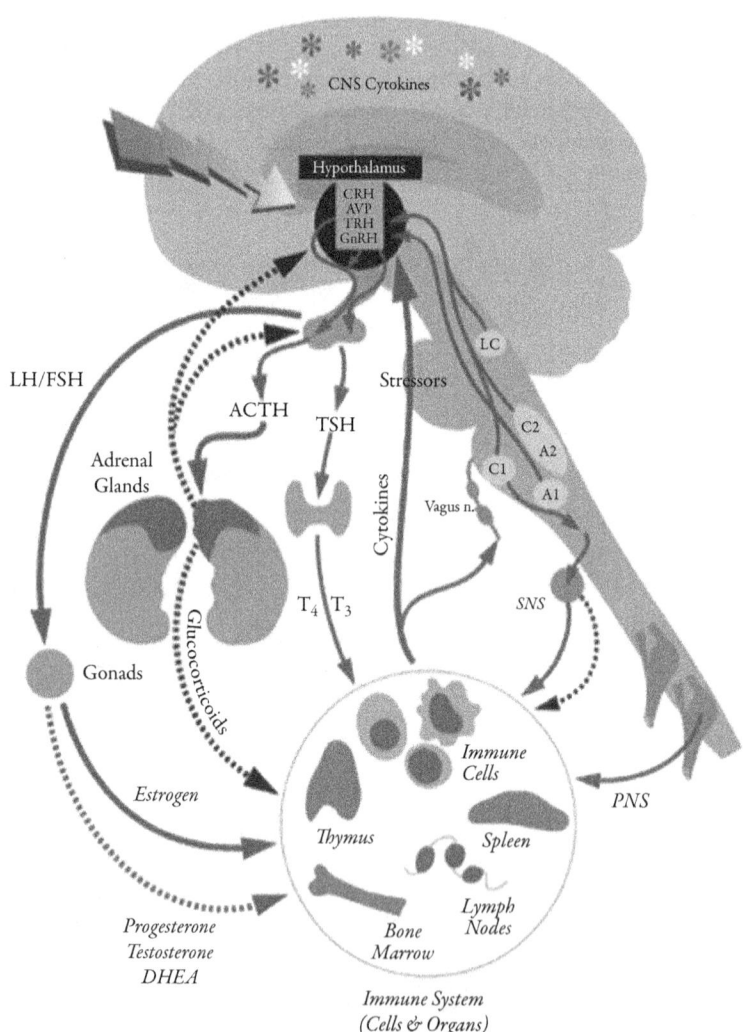

Figure 41.10 Schematic Illustration of Neural-Immune Interactions Immune signaling of the CNS via systemic routes and the vagus nerve (Vagus n.) and CNS regulation of immunity via the HPA, hypothalamic–pituitary-thyroid, and hypothalamic–pituitary–gonadal axes and the sympathetic nervous system (SNS) and parasympathetic nervous system (PNS). Cytokine expression within the CNS is represented by asterisks within the brain. Dotted lines represent negative regulatory pathways, and solid lines represent positive regulatory pathways. CRH: corticotrophin-releasing hormone; AVP: arginine vasopressin; TRH: thyrotropin-releasing hormone; GnRH: gonadotropin-releasing hormone; ACTH: adrenocorticotrophin hormone; TSH: thyroid-stimulating hormone; T4: thyroxine; T3: triio-dothyronine; LH: luteinizing hormone; FSH: follicle-stimulating hormone; LC: locus coeruleus; Al, Cl, A2, C2: brainstem adrenergic nuclei. (Marques-Deak, Cizza, & Sternberg, 2005)

integrity. It has been postulated that several illness processes (i.e., trauma, infections) and surgical procedures may introduce triggering factors leading to the activation of the inflammatory cascade: extensive tissue trauma, presence of foreign organisms or substances, elevated hormone levels, blood loss and anemia, blood transfusions, use of extracorporeal circulation, hypoxia, ischemia and reperfusion, formation of heparineprotamine complexes, and microemboli formation and migration (reviewed by Maldonado, 2008b, 2013). In addition, other factors associated with illness and surgery may directly lead to compromise of the BBB. For example, recent data suggests that the use of various general anesthetics (e.g., sevoflurane, isoflurane) can caused marked flattening of the surfaces of brain vascular endothelial cells along with disruption of BBB-associated tight junctions at cell margins, leading to holes in the vascular endothelial lining and increased BBB permeability, thus facilitating plasma influx into the brain interstitium (Forsberg et al., 2014). The frequency and magnitude of this effect increases with age, thus potentially serving as a mechanism to mediate postoperative delirium and its increased occurrence among elderly patients (Figure 41.11).

At least four pathways through which immune signals from the periphery are transduced to the brain have been proposed (Figure 41.12) (Dantzer et al., 2008). In the neural pathway, locally produced cytokines activate primary afferent nerves (e.g., vagus). In the humoral pathway, toll-like receptors on macrophage-like cells residing in the circumventricular organs and the choroid plexus respond to circulating pathogen-associated molecular patterns by producing proinflammatory cytokines, which enter the brain by diffusion. In the cytokine transporters pathway, proinflammatory cytokines overflowing in the systemic circulation can gain access to the brain through these saturable transport systems at the blood–brain barrier. The prostaglandin pathway involves

IL-1 receptors that are located on perivascular macrophages and endothelial cells of brain venules. Activation of these IL-1 receptors by circulating cytokines results in the local production of prostaglandin E2.

The neuroinflammatory hypothesis proposes that several conditions associated with delirium are characterized by activation of the inflammatory cascade with acute release of inflammatory mediators into the bloodstream (Cerejeira et al., 2010). CNS resident cells react to the presence of peripheral immune signals (cytokines and lipopolysaccharide [LPS]), leading to production of cytokines and other mediators in the brain, cell proliferation, and activation of the HPA axis (thus linking it with the neuroendocrine hypothesis, discussed next) through a complex system of interactions (Figure 41.13). These neuroinflammatory changes induce neuronal and synaptic dysfunction (i.e., affecting various neurotransmitter systems), leading to the neurobehavioral and cognitive symptoms characteristic of delirium.

Animal studies have shown that the administration of LPS induces sickness behavior, which requires activation of proinflammatory cytokine signaling in the brain (Dantzer et al. 1998; Dantzer, 2004). Microglia are the primary recipients of peripheral inflammatory signals that reach the brain (Figure 41.14) (Miller, Maletic, & Raison, 2009, Miller, Haroon, Raison, & Felger, 2013). Activated microglia, in turn, initiate an inflammatory cascade whereby release of relevant cytokines, chemokines, inflammatory mediators, reactive nitrogen species (RNS), and reactive oxygen species (ROS) induces mutual activation of astroglia, thereby amplifying inflammatory signals within the CNS. Cytokines, including IL-1, IL-6, and TNF-alpha, as well as IFN-alpha and IFN-gamma (from T cells), induce the enzyme indoleamine 2,3 dioxygenase (IDO), which breaks down tryptophan (TRP), the primary precursor of 5-HT, into quinolinic acid (QUIN), a

Proposed mechanism for link between post-surgical delirium, subsequent cognitive decline and eventual Alzheimer's disease

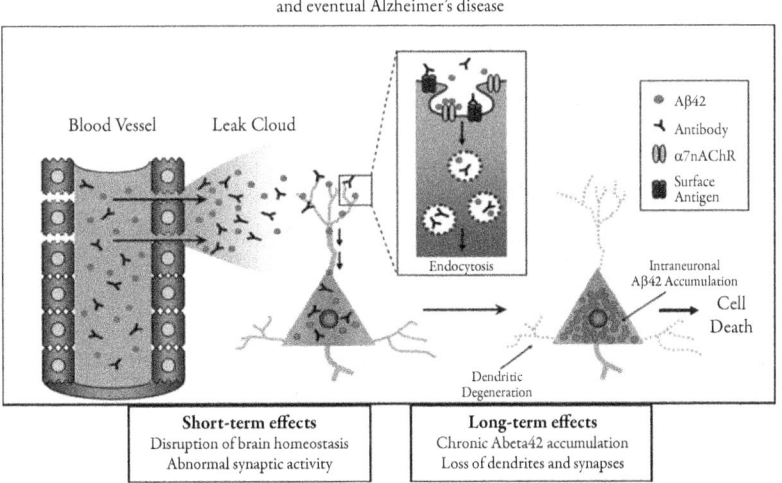

Figure 41.11 Exposure to anesthetics causes an immediate, short-term breakdown of BBB integrity. This leads to an influx of plasma components into the brain tissue that causes disruption of brain homeostasis and neuronal misfiring, all culminating into the array of symptoms that hallmark delirium. Failure to completely restore BBB integrity (most common in the elderly) may trigger long-term BBB breakdown, which can drive chronic plasma influx, more permanent disruption of brain homeostasis, and impairment of neuronal function. Chronic binding of bloodborne brain-reactive autoantibodies and soluble amyloid peptide (Abeta42) to neurons, and their internalization via endocytosis, are essential features of subsequent cognitive decline and early Alzheimer's disease pathology. (Forsberg et al., 2014)

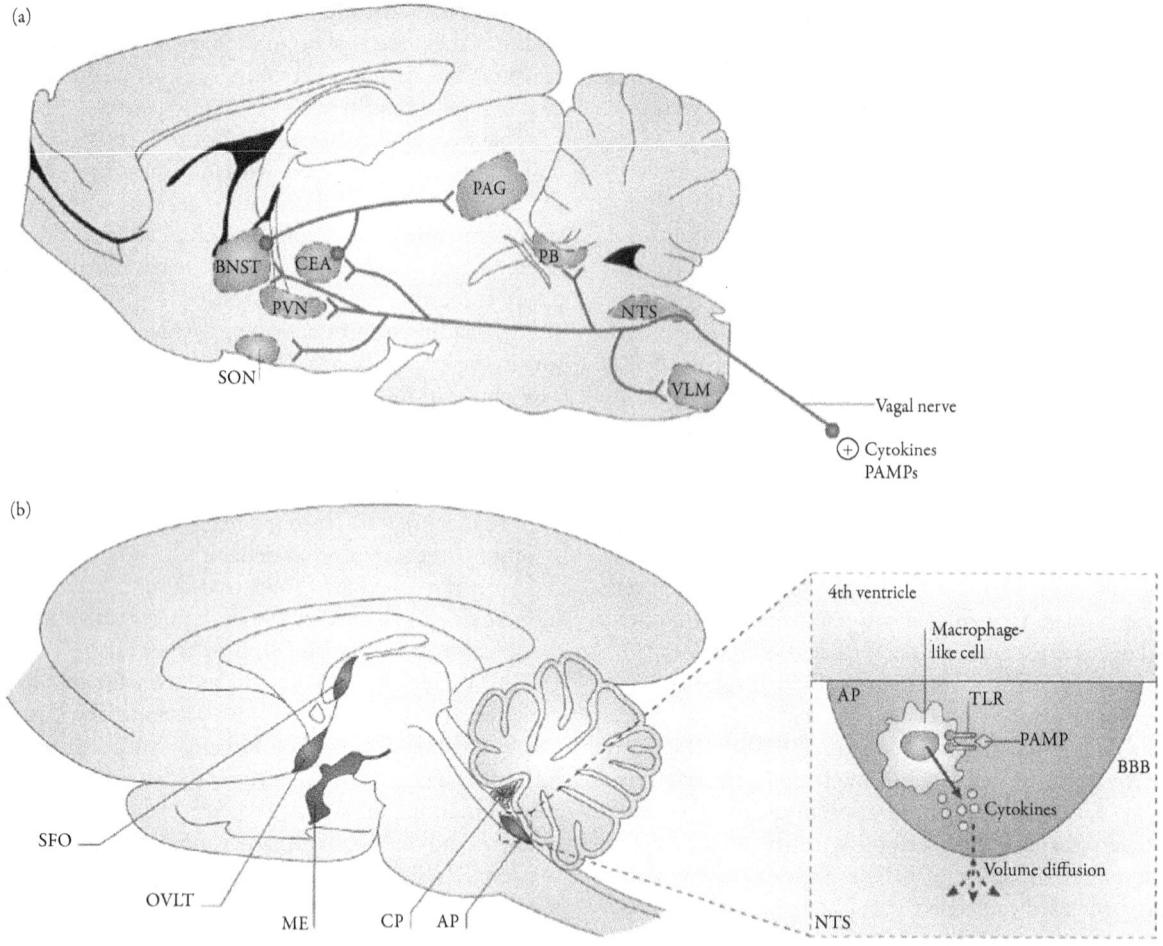

Figure 41.12 Pathways that Transduce Immune Signals from the Periphery to the Brain The brain and the immune system communicate through different pathways. (a) In the neural pathway, peripherally produced pathogen-associated molecular patterns (PAMPs) and cytokines activate primary afferent nerves (e.g., vagal nerve, trigeminal nerves). (b) The humoral pathway involves circulating PAMPs that reach the brain at the level of the choroid plexus (CP) and the circumventricular organs, where PAMPs induce the production and release of proinflammatory cytokines, likely reaching the brain by diffusion. (Dantzer et al., 2008)

potent NMDA agonist and stimulator of glutamate (GLU) release. Multiple astrocytic functions are compromised due to excessive exposure to cytokines, QUIN, and RNS/ROS, ultimately leading to downregulation of glutamate transporters, impaired glutamate reuptake, and increased glutamate release, as well as decreased production of neurotrophic factors. Of note, oligodendroglia are especially sensitive to the CNS inflammatory cascade and suffer damage due to overexposure to cytokines such as TNF-alpha, which has a direct toxic effect on these cells, potentially contributing to apoptosis and demyelination. The confluence of excessive astrocytic glutamate release, its inadequate reuptake by astrocytes and oligodendroglia, activation of NMDA receptors by QUIN, increased glutamate binding and activation of extrasynaptic NMDA receptors (accessible to glutamate released from glial elements and associated with inhibition of brain-derived neurotrophic factor [BDNF] expression), decline in neurotrophic support, and oxidative stress ultimately disrupt neural plasticity through excitotoxicity and apoptosis (Figure 41.15)

(Behan & Stone, 2000; Stone, Behan, Jones, Darlington, & Smith, 2001; Darlington et al., 2007, 2010; Stone, Forrest, & Darlington, 2012).

Human studies have confirmed these findings. A study of adult patients admitted to inpatient medicine wards showed that those who developed delirium had significantly elevated levels (i.e., above the detection limit) of IL-6 (53% versus 31%) and IL-8 (45% versus 22%), compared with patients who did not develop delirium, even after adjusting for infection, age, and cognitive impairment (de Rooij, van Munster, Korevaar, & Levi, 2007). This was the first study to show a relationship between peripherally measured cytokine levels and delirium as a symptom of sickness behavior in acutely admitted elderly. It also showed that cognitive function can be impaired by a systemic infection in patients with a neurodegenerative disorder such as Alzheimer's disease, and that this cognitive decline is preceded by raised serum levels of IL-1h. Furthermore, aging and neurodegenerative disorders exaggerate microglial responses following stimulation by

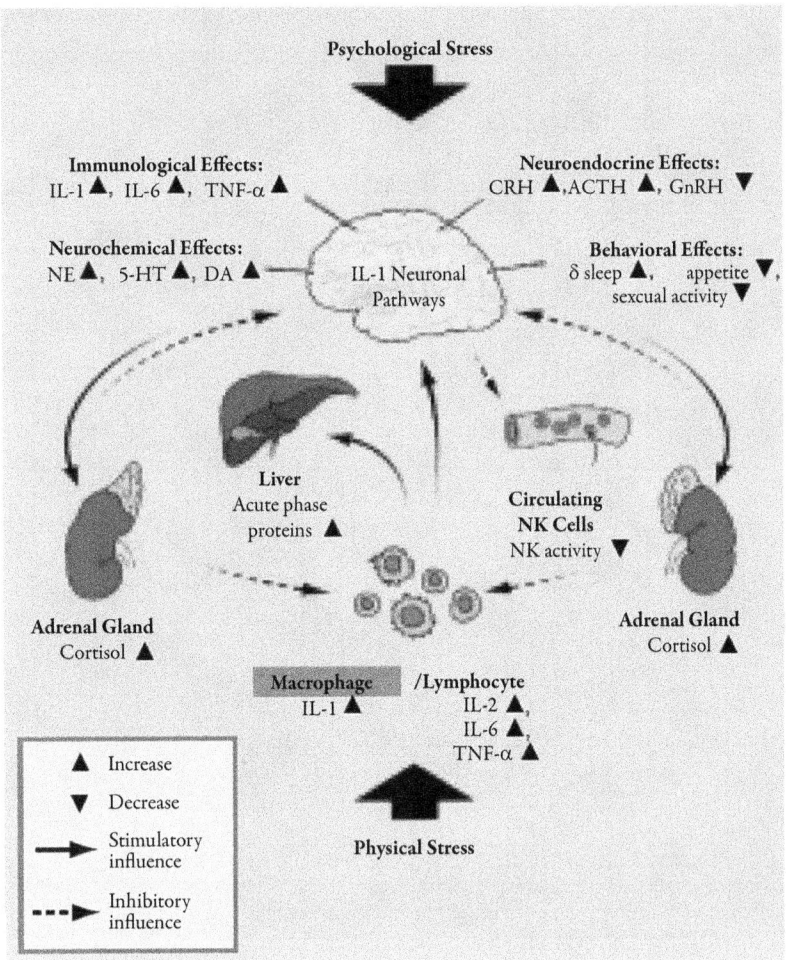

Figure 41.13 Interlukins and the Stress Response Both psychological stress (e.g., stress, depression) and physical stress (e.g., infection, trauma, surgery) can activate interleukin-1, which will trigger various phenomena both peripherally (e.g., cascade activation of other cytokines, induction of acute phase proteins) and centrally (e.g., various immunologic, neurochemical, neuroendocrine, and behavioral effects). Feedback mechanisms occur at several levels and include negative feedback exerted by cortisol. Abbreviations: IL = interleukin, TNF-α = tumor necrosis factor-α, CRH = corticotropinreleasing hormone, GnRH = gonadotropin-releasing hormone, NE = norepinephrine, 5-HT = serotonin, DA = dopamine, NK = natural killer. (Kronfol & Remick, 2000)

systemic immune stimuli such as peripheral inflammation and/or infection (as described in the neural aging hypothesis).

NEUROENDOCRINE HYPOTHESIS

The neuroendocrine hypothesis suggests excessive glucocorticoid (GC) levels may induce a vulnerable state in neurons. Glucocorticoids are hormones released during the stress response that are well known for their immunosuppressive and antiinflammatory properties; however, recent advances have uncovered situations wherein they have effects in the opposite direction (Sorrells, Caso, Munhoz, & Sapolsky, 2009). An extensive body of work has substantiated the idea that repeated or prolonged exposure to GCs has a deleterious impact on brain function, and has also provided evidence that GCs probably contribute to age-related decline in brain function (Goosens & Sapolsky, 2007). Others have

already demonstrated how stress (induced by illness processes, such as hypoxia/ischemia, hypoglycemia, or seizures) can lead to excess glucocorticoid release, which can exacerbate cell death by inhibiting glucose transport into cells (Figure 41.16 (Sapolsky & Pulsinelli, 1985; Sapolsky, 1990, 1996; Dinkel, Ogle, & Sapolsky, 2002). But there is growing evidence showing that GCs may have proinflammatory effects in the brain and can even enhance neuroinflammation at multiple levels in the pathway linking LPS exposure to inflammation (Figure 41.17) (Munhoz, Sorrells, Caso, Scavone, & Sapolsky, 2010; Schiepers, Wichers, & Maes, 2005). In addition, glucocorticoids can increase proinflammatory cell migration, cytokine production, and even transcription factor activity in the brain (Sorrells & Sapolsky, 2007). This can lead to a number of deleterious effects, including inhibition of glutamate reuptake in the synaptic cleft, inhibition of Ca+ efflux or sequestration, exacerbation of the breakdown of cytoskeletal proteins (i.e., tau), increase

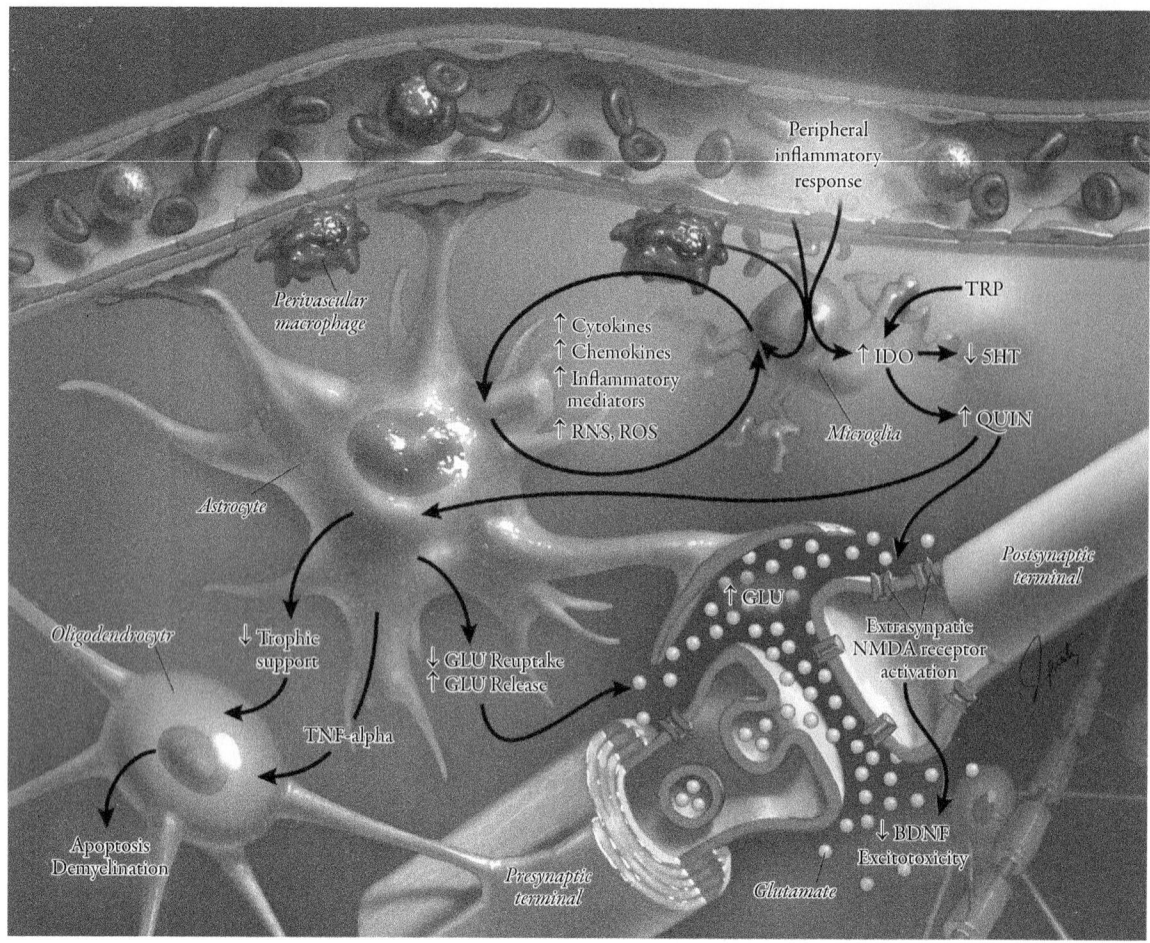

Figure 41.14 Effects of the CNS Inflammatory Cascade on Neural Plasticity. Microglia are the primary recipients of peripheral inflammatory signals that reach the brain. When activated, microglia initiate an inflammatory cascade (e.g., releasing cytokines, chemokines, inflammatory mediators, reactive nitrogen species, and reactive oxygen species) leading to the activation of astroglia, thus amplifying inflammatory signals within the CNS. Cytokines (e.g., IL-1, IL-6, and TNF-alpha, as well as IFN-alpha and IFN-gamma [from T cells]), induce the enzyme indoleamine 2,3 dioxygenase, affecting tryptophan metabolism and thus increasing quinolinic acid production, a potent NMDA agonist and stimulator of glutamate release. Eventually, there is astrocytic function compromise leading to downregulation of glutamate transporters, impaired glutamate reuptake, and increased glutamate release, as well as decreased production of neurotrophic factors. Oligodendroglia are especially sensitive to the CNS inflammatory cascade which leads to apoptosis and demyelination. The confluence of these factors leads to a decline in neurotrophic support, oxidative stress, and, ultimately, disruption of neural plasticity through excitotoxicity and apoptosis. Abbreviations: 5-HT, serotonin; BDNF, brain-derived neurotrophic factor; CNS, central nervous system; GLU, glutamate; IDO, indolamine 2,3 dioxygenase; IFN, interferon; IL, interleukin; NMDA, N-methyl-D-aspartate; QUIN, quinolinic acid; RNS, reactive nitrogen species; ROS, reactive oxygen species; TNF, tumor necrosis factor; TRP, tryptophan. (Miller, Maletic, & Raison, 2009)

in reactive oxygen species, decrease in activity of antioxidant enzymes, decreased release of inhibitory neurotransmitters (i.e., GABA), and decreased production of neurotrophins (i.e., BDNF).

Disturbances of the HPA system have also been found in several studies on delirium. Studies have found that patients experiencing postoperative delirium had an impaired stress-regulating system, with significantly elevated mean plasma cortisol levels compared to the preoperative baseline and nondelirious patients (McIntosh et al., 1985). Among delirious patients triggered by lower respiratory tract infection, 78% were found to be nonsuppressors on the DST compared to 14% of the patients without delirium (O'Keeffe & Devlin, 1994). Among non–medically ill demented patients, those who develop delirium exhibited significant differences between basal cortisol levels compared to demented, non-delirious patients (Robertsson et al., 2001). But, the most important finding of the study was a strong relationship between delirium and DST pathology irrespective of age and severity of dementia, with significant differences in post-DST cortisol levels between patients with different degrees of delirium: the greater the intensity of delirium, the greater the level of nonsuppression. Similarly, delirious patients after stroke exhibited significantly increased activation of the HPA system compared to those without acute confusion (Olsson et al., 1989; Olsson, Marklund, Gustafson, & Nasman, 1992; Fassbender et al., 1994; Johansson et al., 1997; Slowik et al., 2002).

The hippocampus is a major target for these effects, with its dense concentration of glucocorticoid receptors. The

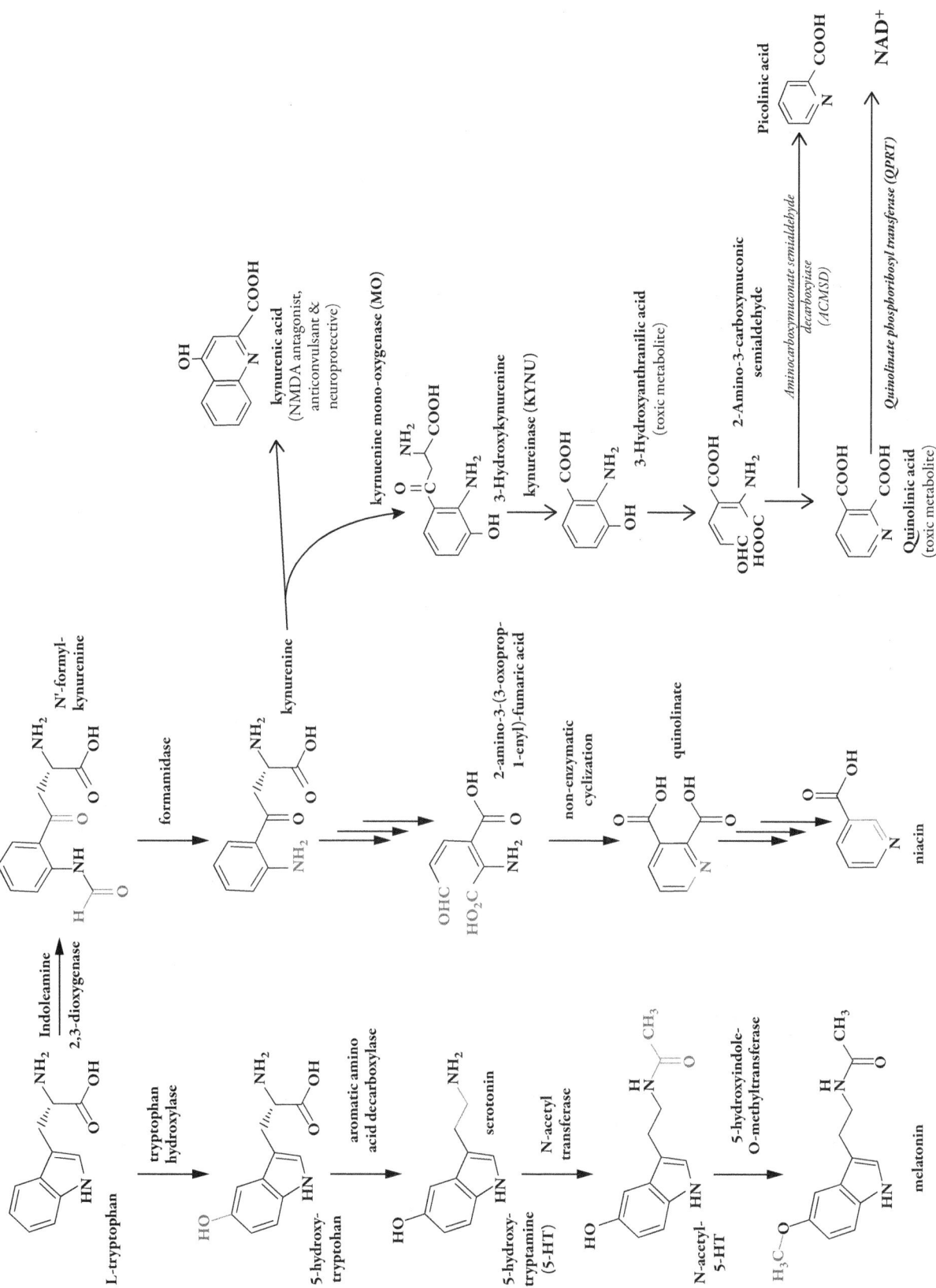

Figure 41.15 Metabolic Pattern of Tryptophan, Serotonin, Melatonin, Kynurenic and Quinolinic Acid. Evidence suggest that some proinflammatory cytokines can not only induce sickness behavior, but also enhance activity of the ubiquitous indoleamine 2,3 dioxygenase (IDO), leading to deficient tryptophan (TRP) levels, thus a reduction in 5HT and melatonin production, and a shift to the production of kynurenine (KYN) and other neurotoxic tryptophan-derived metabolites. (Maldonado 2013; modified from Darlington et al. 2010, and Stone, Forrest, & Darlington, 2012)

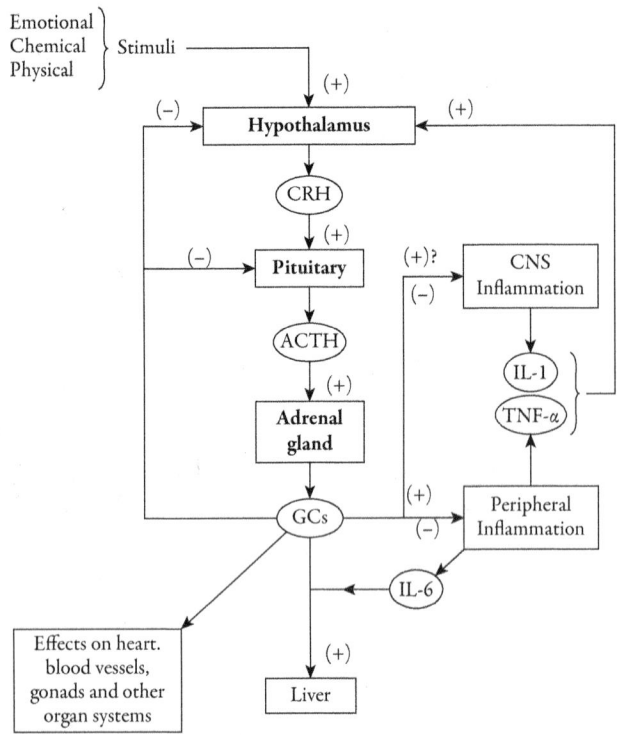

Figure 41.16 Neuroendocrine Circuits and the Effects of Inflammation. Various stressors can activate the HPA axis. The hypothalamus is stimulated to secrete CRH, which leads to ACTH secretion into the peripheral circulation. ACTH in turn triggers adrenal GC release and production. The CRH system is inhibited by GCs in a negative feedback loop. TNF-κ and IL-1 are produced from inflammatory sites and are potent activators of the HPA axis. IL-6 acts synergistically with GCs to stimulate the hepatic secretion of acute phase proteins. Although GCs are widely known for their anti-inflammatory actions, "(–)," more recently also proinflammatory effects have repeatedly been reported, "(+)?" Abbreviations: HPA = hypothalamic-pituitary-adrenal; CRH = corticotrophin-releasing hormone; ACTH = adrenocorticotrophic hormone; GCs = glucocorticoids; IL = interleukin; TNF = tumor necrosis factor; (+) = enhancing; (–) = suppressing. (Dinkel, Ogle, & Sapolsky, 2002)

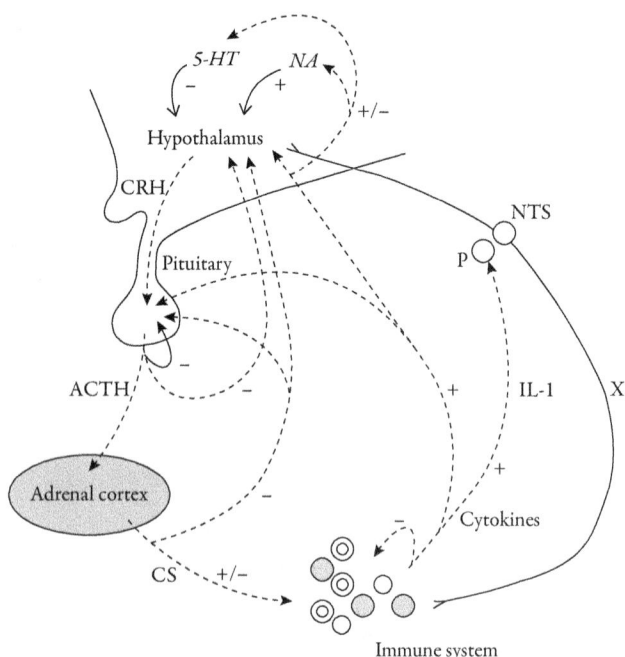

Figure 41.17 Inflammation, Neurotransmitters & the HPA Axis. The brain regulates the immune system, and the immune system modulates brain activity through various interactions. The hypothalamic–pituitary–adrenal (HPA) axis is the main route of immunoregulation, next to (para)sympathetic innervation of organs of the immune system. Immune cells secrete cytokines, which not only regulate the immune response but also act to block the actions of other humoral substances at different levels of the HPA axis (black bars). (Schiepers, Wichers, & Maes, 2005)

hippocampal–adrenal circuit may contribute to the amplification of deliriogenic factors. There is evidence that, relatively early during the metabolic stress leading to delirium, the hippocampus begins to malfunction. This may explain some of the memory dysfunction and errors in information processing, leading to the confabulations that are commonly seen in delirious patients. The loss of normal inhibition of adrenal steroidogenesis results in the continuous secretion of peak amounts of corticosteroids, leading to further mitochondrial dysfunction and apoptosis and further exacerbation of the catecholamine disturbances. A key abnormality related to cortisol excess in delirium seems to be abnormal "shut-off" of the HPA axis tested by the DST. In experimental models, the hippocampal formation is of prime importance for normal HPA axis shut-off (Olsson, 1999). In this brain area, a close interaction between neurotransmitters—notably ACH, 5HT, and NE—and glucocorticoid receptors is relevant for the development of delirium in elderly patients with stroke and neurodegenerative brain diseases.

OXIDATIVE STRESS HYPOTHESIS

The oxidative stress hypothesis proposes that decreased brain oxidative metabolism leads to abnormalities of various neurotransmitter systems, causing cerebral dysfunction and the behavioral symptoms of delirium. Thus, severe illness processes, combined with both decreased oxygen supply and/or increased oxygen demand, may lead to the same common end problem; namely, decreased oxygen availability to cerebral tissue. This has been the subject of an extensive review described elsewhere Figure 41.18 (Maldonado, 2013). In summary, hypoxia triggers diverse reconfigurations of widespread neuronal network at all levels of the nervous system (i.e., molecular, cellular, synaptic, neuronal, network): synaptic transmission is depressed through presynaptic mechanisms and excitatory/inhibitory alterations involving K+, Na+, and Ca2+ channels. Cerebral ischemia leads to a rapid depletion of energy stores, triggering a complex cascade of cellular events, including cellular depolarization and Ca2+ influx, resulting in excitotoxic cell death (see Figure 41.19).

Inadequate oxidative metabolism may be one of the causes of the problems observed in delirium; namely, inability to maintain ionic gradients causing "spreading depression"; abnormal neurotransmitter synthesis, metabolism and release; and a failure to effectively eliminate neurotoxic byproducts. Decreased oxygenation causes a failure in oxidative

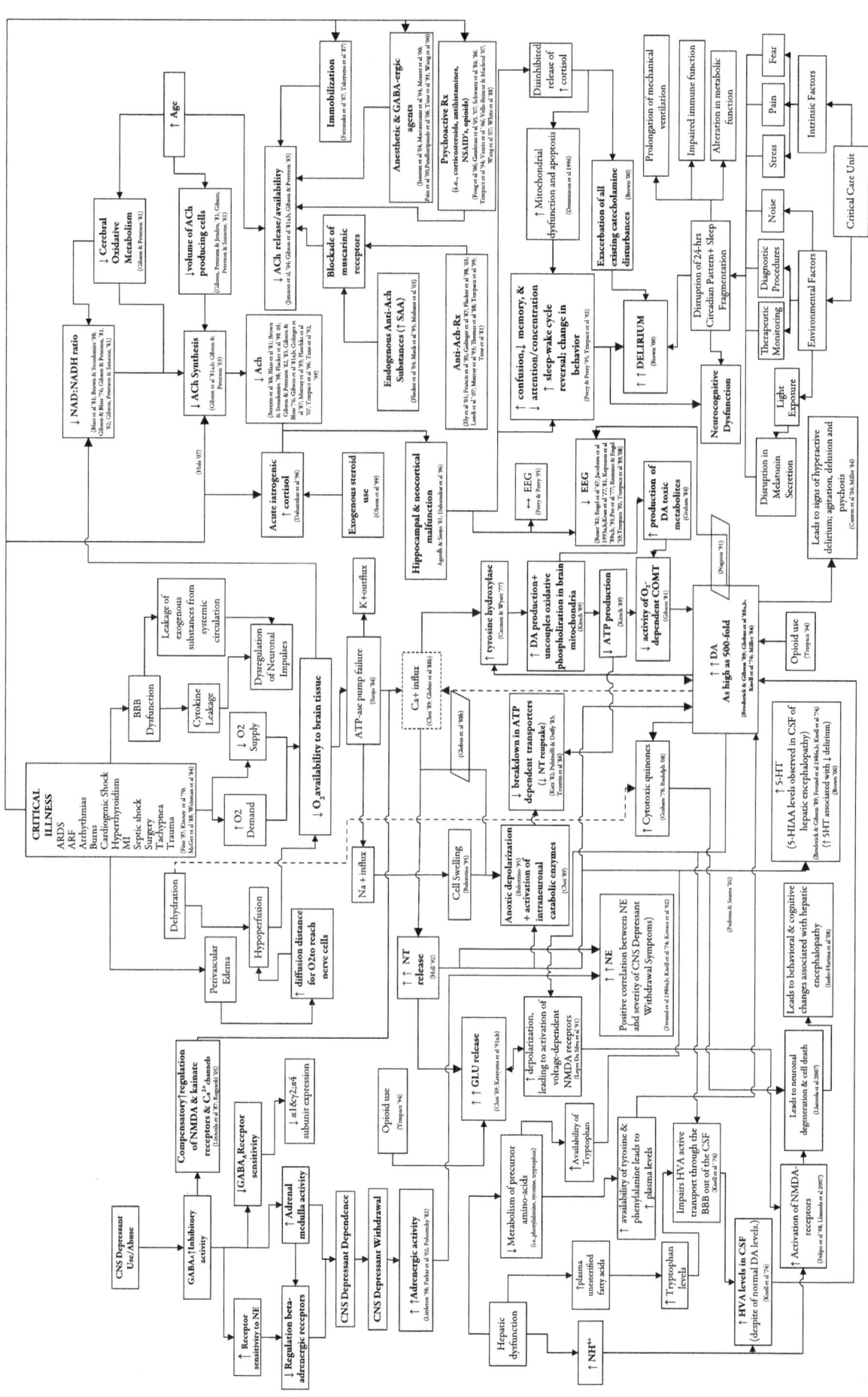

Figure 41.18 A Basic Pathoetiological Model of Delirium. This figure illustrates the theorized intersections between the oxidative stress hypothesis (OSH) and the neurotransmitter hypothesis (NTH) of delirium, demonstrating potential common biochemical outcomes, which may explain the complex cognitive and behavioral changes characteristic of delirium. The OSH proposes that a number of physiological processes (e.g., hypoxia, severe illness, infectious processes) may give rise to increased oxygen consumption and/or decreased oxygen availability, with associated increased energy expenditure and reduced cerebral oxidative metabolism, leading to cerebral dysfunction and associated cognitive and behavioral symptoms of delirium. The NTH was proposed after clinical observations that delirium occurred after the use of substances (e.g., medications, toxins) that alter neurotransmitter function or availability. The OSH intersects with the NTH as decreased oxygenation causes a failure in oxidative metabolism, leading to a failure of the ATP-ase pump system, which leads to an inability to maintain adequate ionic gradients, which in turn leads to significant electrolyte alterations (e.g., influx of Na+ and Ca2+; efflux of K+) and subsequent alterations (e.g., excess release or decreased availability) of several neurotransmitters (e.g., GLU, DA, Ach). (Maldonado 2008b, 2013).

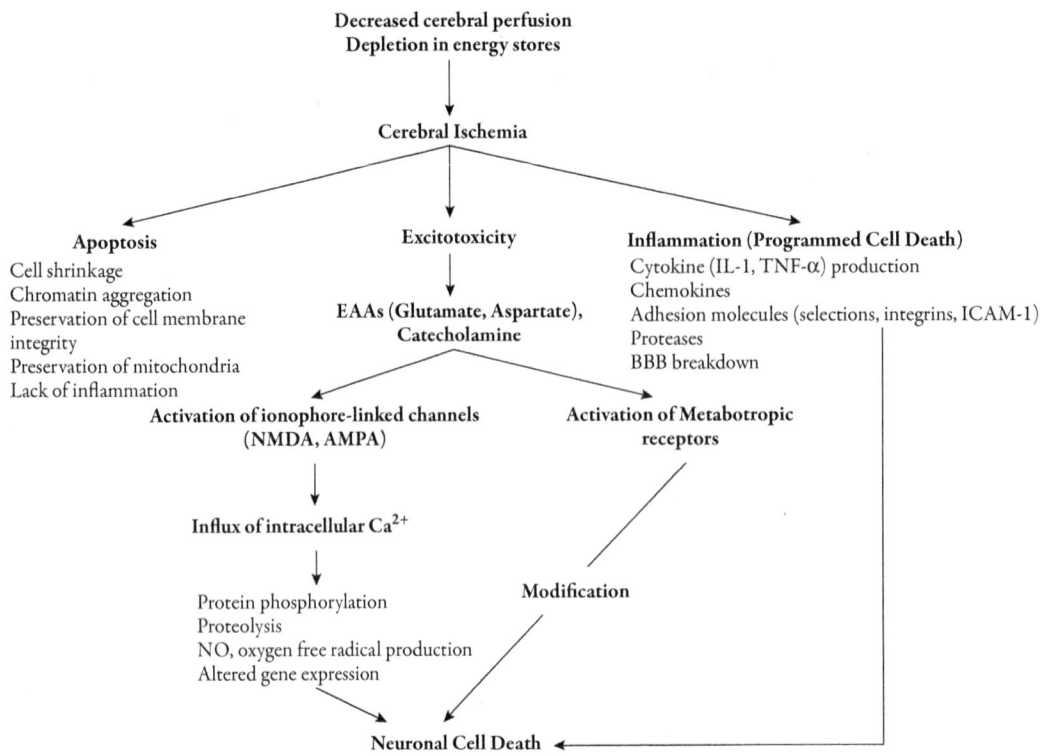

Decreased cerebral perfusion
Depletion in energy stores

↓

Cerebral Ischemia

Apoptosis
Cell shrinkage
Chromatin aggregation
Preservation of cell membrane integrity
Preservation of mitochondria
Lack of inflammation

Excitotoxicity

↓

EAAs (Glutamate, Aspartate), Catecholamine

Inflammation (Programmed Cell Death)
Cytokine (IL-1, TNF-α) production
Chemokines
Adhesion molecules (selections, integrins, ICAM-1)
Proteases
BBB breakdown

Activation of ionophore-linked channels (NMDA, AMPA)

Activation of Metabotropic receptors

↓

Influx of intracellular Ca²⁺

↓

Protein phosphorylation
Proteolysis
NO, oxygen free radical production
Altered gene expression

Modification

Neuronal Cell Death

Schematic diagram representing events leading to ischemic brain injury.
Harukuni & Bhardwaj, Neurol Clin 2006.

Figure 41.19 Mechanisms of Brain Injury after Global Cerebral Ischemia. During cerebral ischemia, excess glutamate exits into the extracellular compartment due to cellular depolarization, coupled with its impaired uptake, which results in increases in intracellular Ca2+. The cascade of events responsible for glutamate excitotoxicity includes three distinct processes: (1) induction, whereby extracellular glutamate efflux is transduced by receptors on the neuronal membrane to cause intracellular Ca2+ overload, which leads to lethal intracellular derangements; (2) amplification of the derangement, with an increase in intensity and involvement of other neurons; and (3) expression of cell death triggered by cytotoxic cascades. Excess release of Ca2+ and its intracellular influx is thought to be the primary trigger for a variety of complex, deleterious intracellular processes that result from activation of catabolic enzymes such as phospholipases (which lead to cell membrane breakdown, arachidonic acid, and free radical formation) and endonucleases (which lead to fragmentation of genomic DNA and energy failure due to mitochondrial dysfunction). (Harukuni & Bhardwaj, 2006)

metabolism, which leads to a failure of the Adenosine triphosphate (ATP)-ase pump system. When the pump fails, the ionic gradients cannot be maintained, leading to significant influxes of sodium (Na⁺) followed by calcium (Ca²⁺), while potassium (K⁺) moves out of the cell. Some have theorized that it is the excess inward flux of Ca²⁺ that precipitates the most significant neurobehavioral disturbances observed in delirious patients. The influx of Ca²⁺ during hypoxic conditions is associated with the dramatic release of several neurotransmitters, particularly glutamate (GLU) and dopamine (DA). Glutamate further potentiates its own release as GLU stimulates the influx of Ca²⁺, and it accumulates in the extracellular space as its reuptake and metabolism in glial cells is impeded by the ATP-ase pump failure. In addition, at least two factors facilitate dramatic increases in DA: first, the conversion of DA to norepinephrine (NE), which is oxygen dependent, is significantly decreased; second, the catechol-o-methyl transferase (COMT) enzymes, required for degradation of DA, get inhibited by toxic metabolites under hypoxic conditions, leading to even greater accumulation of DA (Graham, 1984). At the same time, serotonin (5HT) levels fall moderately in the cortex, increase in the striatum, and remain stable in the brainstem (Broderick & Gibson, 1989).

Hypoxia also leads to a reduced synthesis and release of acetylcholine, especially in the basal forebrain cholinergic centers. Indeed, cholinergic neurotransmission is particularly sensitive to metabolic insults, such as diminished availability of glucose and oxygen. ACh synthesis requires acetyl coenzyme A, which is a key intermediate linking the glycolytic pathway and the citric acid cycle. Thus, reduction in cerebral oxygen and glucose supply and deficiencies in enzyme cofactors such as thiamine may induce delirium by impairing ACh production.

There are definite data correlating poor oxygenation and cerebral dysfunction. Studies have demonstrated a strong correlation between intraoperative oxygen saturation and postoperative mental function (Rosenberg & Kehlet, 1993). Studies have demonstrated that delirium can be induced in healthy control subjects by dropping PaO₂ to 35 mmHg (Gibson & Peterson, 1981). A study of ICU patients demonstrated that three measures of oxygenation (i.e., hemoglobin level, hematocrit, pulse oximetry; see Figure 41.4) were worse in the patients who later developed delirium, and that clinical factors associated with greater oxidative stress (e.g., sepsis, pneumonia) occurred more frequently among those diagnosed with delirium (Seaman et al., 2006).

A recent study demonstrated that intraoperative cerebral oxygen desaturation was a significant risk factor for post-operative delirium in CABG patients (Figure 41.5) (Slater et al., 2009).

DIURNAL DYSREGULATION OR MELATONIN DYSREGULATION HYPOTHESIS

The diurnal dysregulation or melatonin dysregulation hypothesis suggests that the 24-hour internal "clock" (circadian pattern) is maintained by environmental factors, primarily light exposure, which affect melatonin secretion (BaHammam, 2006). Sleep deprivation may lead to the development of memory deficits (Walker & Stickgold, 2004). In fact, "chronic partial sleep deprivation" (i.e., sleeping limited to 4 hours per night, for 5 consecutive nights) has been shown to lead into cumulative impairment in attention, critical thinking, reaction time, and recall (Dinges, 2006). In turn, sleep deprivation (even just 36 consecutive hours) may lead to symptoms of emotional imbalance (i.e., short temper, mood swings, and excessive emotional response). Cumulative sleep debt can cause delirium in itself, and can aggravate or perpetuate delirium (Ito, Harada, Hayashida, Ishino, & Nakayama, 2006; Pandharipande & Ely, 2006). Similarly, others have found sleep deprivation to consistently precede onset of delirium in cardiac surgical patients (Sveinsson, 1975), and that ICU patients with sleep deprivation were significantly more likely to develop delirium than patients without sleep deprivation (Helton, Gordon, & Nunnery, 1980).

Melatonin plays important roles in multiple bodily functions (Reiter, 1991; Brzezinski, 1997; Verster, 2009). It has a chronobiotic effect (affecting aspects of biological time structure), sleep–wake cycle regulatory effects, and helps reset circadian rhythm disturbances. It has extensive antioxidant activity (with a particular role in the protection of nuclear and mitochondrial DNA), extensive anti-inflammatory activity, and some anti-nociceptive and analgesic effects; and data suggest that melatonin receptors appear to be important in mechanisms of learning and memory. Melatonin also inhibits the aggregation of the amyloid beta protein into neurotoxic micro-aggregates responsible for the neurofibrillary tangles characteristic of Alzheimer's disease, and it prevents the hyperphosphorylation of the tau protein. All of these factors may have potential implications regarding the development of delirium in the medically ill and postoperative patient.

In addition, current evidence suggests that acute and chronic sleep deprivation is associated with decreased proportions of natural killer cells, lower antibody titers following influenza-virus immunization, reduced lymphokine-activated killer activity, and reduced IL-2 production. Conversely, cytokines may play a role in normal sleep regulation by increasing non-REM sleep and decreasing REM sleep, and, during inflammatory events, an increase in cytokine levels may intensify their effects on sleep regulation. Moreover, sleep deprivation may alter endocrine and metabolic functions, altering the normal pattern of cortisol release and contributing to impairment of the regulation of glucocorticoid secretion via negative feedback mechanisms, insulin resistance, and glucose intolerance.

Several studies have demonstrated a relationship between melatonin secretion and delirium. A study of elderly patients after major abdominal surgery had their plasma melatonin levels measured preoperatively and every 2 hours during the postoperative period, and demonstrated that those who did not develop delirium did not have significant changes in plasma melatonin levels compared with preoperative values (Shigeta, Yasui, et al., 2001). Furthermore, patients who experienced postoperative delirium could be broken down into two groups: those who became delirious postoperatively, with an otherwise uncomplicated recovery; and those who developed postoperative complications such as pneumonia. Patients who went on to become delirious, but without other complications, demonstrated reduced plasma melatonin levels. Those delirious but with other complications had elevated plasma melatonin levels, similar to that seen in early sepsis (Mundigler et al., 2002). Similarly, a study of subjects undergoing thoracic esophagectomy demonstrated a significant correlation between ICU psychosis (i.e., delirium) and an irregular melatonin circadian rhythm (i.e., abnormally low serum levels of melatonin), measured every 6 hours during the first 4 postoperative days (P =.0001) (Miyazaki et al., 2003).

Of note, some have observed a relationship between the motoric delirium subtype and melatonin levels. A study of hospitalized elderly medical patients evaluated them daily using the Delerium Rating Scale (DRS) and conducted urinary measures of their 6-sulphatoxymelatonin (6-SMT), the chief metabolite of melatonin and a reliable proxy for serum melatonin (Matthews, Guerin, & Wang, 1991). The mean and standard deviation values of 6-SMT for each of the three motoric subtypes were calculated, and it was found that during periods of hyperactive delirium, subjects had decreased urinary 6-SMT levels compared with when they had recovered. Patients with hypoactive delirium had raised 6-SMT levels compared with when they had recovered, while those with the mixed form of delirium had no difference in urinary metabolite concentrations (Balan et al., 2003).

NEURONAL AGING HYPOTHESIS

Finally, the neuronal aging hypothesis suggests that elderly patients are at increased risk for developing delirium, based on the fact that aging is associated with age-related cerebral changes in stress-regulating neurotransmitter and intracellular signal transduction systems, and observations suggesting that chronic neurodegeneration is accompanied by an inflammatory response characterized by a chronic, but selective, activation of CNS microglial cells that are "primed" to produce exaggerated inflammatory responses to immunological challenges (Figure 41.20) (Cunningham et al., 2005, 2009). This inflammation is assumed to contribute to disease progression through the production of inflammatory mediators. Data suggest that the aging process is associated with a twofold to fourfold increase in baseline levels of circulating inflammatory mediators, including cytokines and acute phase proteins (Rosczyk, Sparkman, & Johnson, 2008). This may help explain why even minor surgical trauma was associated with increased IL-1b hippocampal expression in

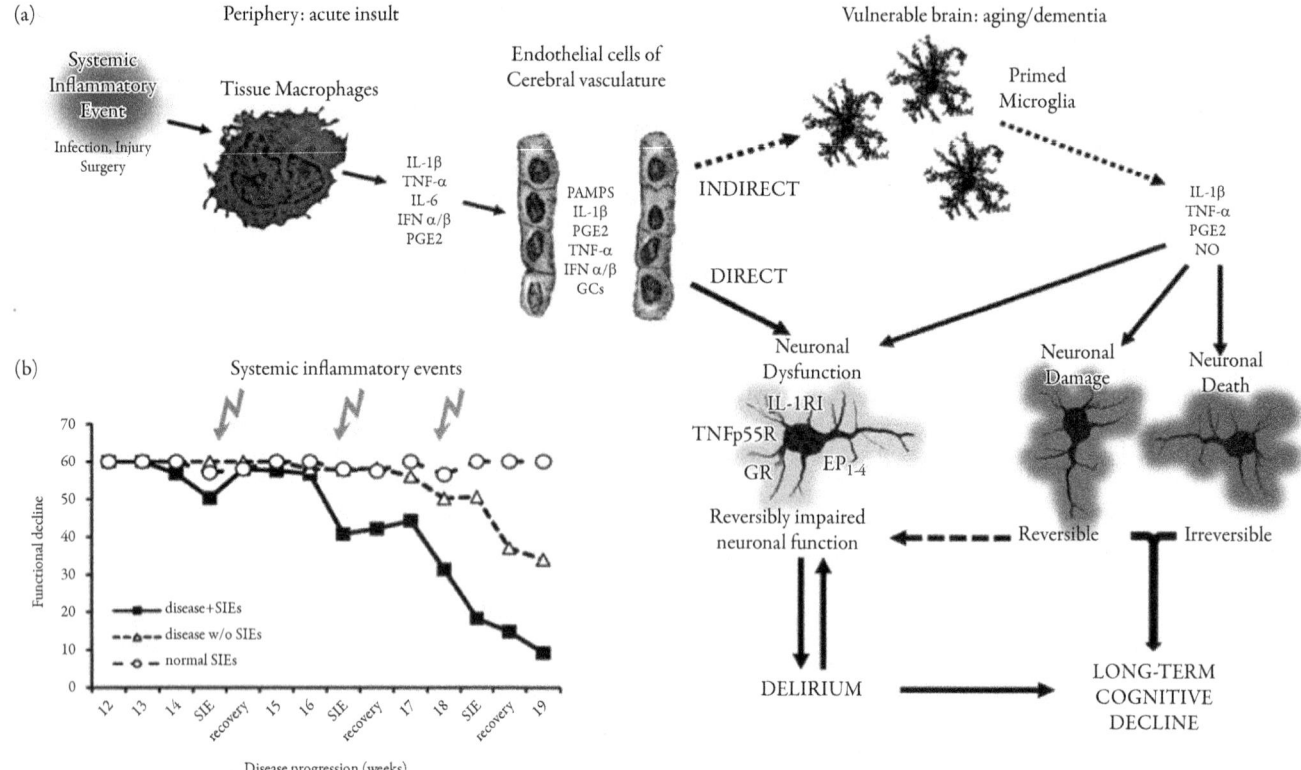

Figure 41.20 Effect of Inflammation on the Aging Brain. (a) Systemic inflammatory events trigger the release of inflammatory mediators by tissue macrophages and brain vascular endothelial cells. These mediators may affect neuronal function directly, or via the activation of microglial cells that have become primed by neurodegenerative disease or aging. Inflammatory mediators may cause reversible disruption of neuronal function, leading to various neurobehavioral syndromes including delirium. These mediators may also induce acute neuronal synaptic or dendritic damage that may be reversible and contribute to delirium, or may be irreversible and contribute to long-term cognitive decline. (b) Successive systemic inflammatory insults induce acute dysfunction, which is progressively less reversible each time, and also contribute to the progression of permanent disability. Abbreviations: IL-1RI, interleukin 1 receptor type I; TNFp55, TNFp55 receptor; GCs, glucocorticoids; GR, glucocorticoid receptor; NO, nitric oxide; EP1–4, prostaglandin receptors 1–4; PAMPs: pathogen-associated molecular patterns; IFNα/β, interferon α/β; SIEs, systemic inflammatory events.

animal studies. Aging is also associated with decreased volume of ACh-producing cells and decreased cerebral oxidative metabolism. Thus, the decline in cognitive functioning associated with the normal aging process is aggravated by the presence of even mild hypoxia, which further inhibits ACh synthesis and its release. As previously discussed, the probability of experiencing delirium rises with age. Of note, some have suggested that prostaglandins are responsible for the LPS-induced inhibition of sickness behaviors, either independent of cytokine activity or as complement (i.e., sensitizing certain targets to the effect of cytokines) (Teeling et al., 2007).

There has been some controversy about the contribution of apolipoprotein E and the development of postoperative cognitive dysfunction (POCD). To date, there have been nine published papers on the topic; four of them found that APOE-E4 genotype was not associated with POCD (Abildstrom et al., 2004; Tagarakis et al., 2007; van Munster, Korevaar, de Rooij, Levi, & Zwinderman, 2007; Bryson et al., 2011), while the other five suggested a positive relationship between POCD and APOE genotype (Adamis et al., 2007; Ely et al., 2007; Leung et al., 2007; Zhang et al., 2008; van Munster, Korevaar, Zwinderman, Leeflang, & de Rooij, 2009). (For a summary of all published studies see Table 41.6.) Of note, the only

published meta-analysis on the matter found a positive association between POCD and the APOE sigma4 allele.

In the end, any or all of the above theories lead to the same common result: changes in neurotransmitter concentration or receptor sensitivity (due to any of the mechanisms discussed by the previous hypotheses) mediate the different symptoms and clinical presentations of delirium. In general, the most commonly described neurotransmitter changes associated with delirium are excess release of norepinephrine (↑NE), dopamine (↑DA), and/or glutamate (↑GLU), and increased Ca+ channel activity (↑Ca+ Ch); reduced availability of acetylcholine (↓ Ach) and/or melatonin (↓MEL); and either a decreased and increased activity in serotonin (↓↑5HT), histamine (↓↑H1&2), and/or gamma-amino butyric acid (↓↑GABA), probably depending on the etiology or motoric presentation (see Table 41.7).

CLINICAL PRESENTATION OF DELIRIUM

Delirium is an acute or subacute organic mental syndrome characterized by disturbance in attention (often evidenced by a reduced ability to direct, focus, sustain, and shift attention) and awareness (with impaired orientation to the

Table 41.6 ASSOCIATION BETWEEN APOLIPOPROTEIN E GENOTYPE AND POSTOPERATIVE COGNITIVE DYSFUNCTION

STUDY(N = 10)	POPULATION	FINDINGS	P-VALUE
Abildstrom et al., 2004 Prospective, n = 967	Patients aged 40 yrs. and older undergoing non-cardiac surgery	• One week after surgery, the incidence of POCD was 11.7% in patients with the epsilon 4 allele and 9.9% in patients without the epsilon4 allele. • Conclusion: unable to show a significant association between apolipoprotein E genotype and POCD.	P = 0.41
Adamis et al., 2007 Prospective, n = 164	≥70 y/o hospitalized medically ill patients	• Recovery was significantly (P <.05) associated with lack of APOE 4 allele and higher initial interferon (IFN)-gamma. • A model incorporating gender, APOE epsilon4 status and IGF-I levels predicted recovery or not from delirium in 76.5% of cases, with a sensitivity 0.77 and specificity 0.75. • It further found a positive relationship between delirium with APOE genotype, IFN-gamma, and IGF-I, but not with IL-6, IL-1, TNF-alpha, and leukemia inhibitory factor.	p < 0.05
Leung et al., 2007 Prospective, n = 190	nested cohort study; patients aged ≥ 65 yr, scheduled to undergo major noncardiac surgery requiring anesthesia.	• The presence of one copy of the e4 allele was associated with an increased risk of early postoperative delirium (28.3% vs. 11.1%; P = 0.005). Even after adjusting for covariates, patients with one copy of the e4 allele were still more likely to have an increased risk of early postoperative delirium (OR, 3.64; 95% CI, 1.51–8.77) compared with those without the e4 allele.	P = 0.005
Tagarakis et al., 2007, n = 137	Elderly adults undergoing cardiac bypass surgery; excluded dementia	• Study confirmed the high incidence of cognitive decline and delirium after coronary surgery, but it does not support the role of the APOE-epsilon 4 allele in the occurrence of delirium.	NS
Van Munster et al., 2007 n = 415	Acutely admitted patients to the Department of Medicine of 65 yrs and over	The OR for carriers of an APOE epsilon 4-allele compared with patients without an APOE epsilon 4-allele for developing delirium was 1.17 (95% CI: 0.49–2.78) in the cognitively intact patients and 0.42 (95% CI: 0.14–1.30) in the cognitively impaired patients. No relation existed between the total number of APOE epsilon 4-alleles and the different delirium subtypes (P = 0.12).	P = 0.12
Ely et al., 2007 n = 53	Mechanically ventilated ICU patients	Using multivariable regression analysis to adjust for age, admission diagnosis of sepsis or acute respiratory distress syndrome or pneumonia, severity of illness, and duration of coma, the presence of APOE4 allele was the strongest predictor of delirium duration (OR, 7.32; 95% CI, 1.82–29.51, p =.005).	p = .005
Zhang et al., 2008 n = 196	Elderly patients (>60 yo) scheduled for major abdominal surgery requiring general anesthesia	The presence of the e4 allele and low level of education were both associated with an increased risk of EA (36.9% vs. 15.8%, P = 0.005; 30% vs. 14.3%, P = 0.01). After adjustment for covariates, the patients with the copy of the e4 allele were shown to have a greater likeliness of an increased risk of EA (OR: 4.32; 95% CI: 1.75–10.05).	P = 0.01
Van Munster et al., 2009 n = 656 + Meta-analysis	Medical department and orthopedic/traumatology department of university hospital from 2003 to 2007.	The OR for delirium adjusted for age, cognitive, and functional impairment of sigma4 carriers compared with non-sigma4 carriers was 1.7 (95% CI: 1.1–2.6). Four studies were added to the meta-analysis, which included 1,099 patients in total. The OR for delirium in the meta-analysis was 1.6 (95% CI: 0.9–2.7) of sigma4 carriers compared with non-sigma4 carriers. This study and meta-analysis suggest an association between delirium and the APOE sigma4 allele.	P = 0.04
Bryson et al., 2011 n = 88	Patients ≥60 yrs. of age undergoing open aortic repair.	Delirium predicted POCD at discharge (OR 2.86; 95% CIs 0.99 to 8.27) but not at three months. Apolipoprotein E-ε4 genotype was not associated with either delirium or POCD following adjustment for covariates.	p = 0.625

Table 41.7 THEORIZED NEUROCHEMICAL MECHANISMS ASSOCIATED WITH CONDITIONS LEADING TO DELIRIUM

DELIRIUM SOURCE	ACH	DA	GLU	GABA	5HT	NE	TRP	PHE	HIS	CYTOK	HPA AXIS	NMDA ACTIVITY	CHANGES IN RBF	EEG	MEL	INFLAM	CORT
Anoxia/hypoxia	↓	↑	↑	↑	↓	↓	⇕	↑	↑,↓	⇑	⇑	↑	⇑	↓	↓		↑
Aging	↓	↓	↓	↓	↓	↓	↓	↓	↓	⇑	⇑	↓	⇑	↓	↓	↑	↑
TBI	↑	↑	↑	↑	↑	↑	↑	↑	↓	⇑↑	↑	↑	↑	↓	↓	⇑	↑
CVA	↓	↑	↑	↑	↑	↑↓	↑	↑	↓	↑	↑	↑	⇑	↓	↓	⇑	↑
Hepatic failure (encephalopathy)	⇕	↓	↑	↑	↑	↑	↑	↑	↑	⇑	⇑	↑	⇑	↓	↓		↑
Sleep deprivation	↓	↓	⇑	↑	↓	↑	↓	↑	↑	↑	↑	↑	↑	↑	⇓	⇑	↑
Trauma, Sx, & Post-op	↓	↑	↑	↑	↓	↑	↓	↑	↑	↑	↑	↑	⇑	↑	↓	↑	↑
ETOH and CNS depressants withdrawal	↑	↑	↑	↓	↑	↑	↑	↑	↑	↑	⇑	↑	↓	↑	↓		↑
Infection/sepsis	↓	↑	↑	↑	↑	↑	↑	↓	↓	↑	⇑	⇑	⇑	↑	↓	↑	↑
Dehydration and electrolyte imbalance	⇕	↑	↑	⇑	↓	↑	?	?	↓	↑	↑	↑	↓	⇑	↓	⇑	↑
Medical illness	↓	↑	↑	↑	↓	↑	↓	↑	↑	↑	↑	↑	⇑	⇑	↓	⇑	↑

Legend & Abbreviations: ↑ = likely to be increased or activated; ↓ = likely to be decreased or slowed; ⇕ = no significant changes; ⇑ = probably a contributor, exact mechanism is unclear; (−) = likely not to be a contributing factor; CVA = cerebro-vascular accident; Sx = surgery; ETOH = alcohol; CNS-Dep = central nervous system depressant agent; ACH = acetylcholine; DA = dopamine; GLU = glutamate; GABA = gamma-amino butyric acid; 5HT = 5-hydroxytryptamine or serotonin; NE = norepinephrine; Trp = tryptophan; Phe = phenylalanine; His = histamine; Cytok = cyokines; HPA axis = hypothalamic-pituitary-adrenocortical axis; NMDA = N-methyl-D-aspartic acid; RBF = regional blood flow; EEG = electroencephalograph; Mel = melatonin; Inflam = inflammation; Cort = cortisol.

Source: Adapted from Maldonado, J. R. (2013). Neuropathogenesis of delirium: Review of current etiologic theories and common pathways. *American Journal of Geriatric Psychiatry, 21,* 1190–1222.

environment; Criterion A; APA, 1994). An additional disturbance is present in cognition (e.g., memory deficit, disorientation), language, visuospatial ability, or perception (e.g., hallucinations or delusions; Criterion C; APA, 1994). Often, the syndrome is accompanied by a disordered sleep–wake cycle, (e.g., sleep–wake cycle reversal, sundowning) and alterations in psychomotor activity (e.g., decreased or increased depending on the type of delirium; APA, 1994). By definition, these changes develop over a relatively short period of time (i.e., hours to days) and represent a change from baseline attention and awareness, and have a tendency to fluctuate in severity during the course of a day (e.g., waxing and waning; Criterion B; APA, 1994). Similarly, the presentation cannot be better explained by a preexisting psychiatric disorder (e.g., schizophrenia or dementia) and are deemed to be caused as a result of a primary medical disorder and/or its treatment, or mediated by psychoactive substances (e.g., acute use or intoxication, or substance withdrawal, as in delirium tremens; Criteria D & E; APA, 1994).

Some have suggested there are three core domains of delirium: *cognitive deficits* (characterized by attention and vigilance disturbances); *circadian rhythm dysregulation* (characterized by fragmentation of the sleep–wake cycle); and *higher cortical dysfunction* (characterized by semantic and comprehension deficits, executive dysfunction, and thought process disturbances) (Meagher et al., 2007). In fact, sleep–wake cycle disturbance, inattention, and language/thought process/comprehension abnormalities were the most frequent, consistent, and differentiating symptoms of delirium in medical/surgical populations (Trzepacz et al., 2001; Meagher et al., 2007; Franco, Trzepacz, Mejia, & Ochoa, 2009).

The clinical features of delirium include a prodromal phase, usually marked by restlessness, anxiety, irritability; and the experiencing of nightmares, transient hallucinations (often hypnagogic), and sleep disturbances, which usually develop over a period of several hours to days before the patient exhibits the full-blown syndrome. Often patients recover from a comatose or medication-induced state (e.g., midazolam or propofol infusion) in a confused and agitated state (i.e., emergence delirium).

Even though delirium was originally defined as a transient syndrome, "chronic" forms may be seen in patients experiencing protracted medical problems (e.g., chronic infections), those with concomitant psychiatric disorders (e.g., bipolar disease, psychosis), those with baseline cognitive impairment (e.g., delirium superimposed on dementia, traumatic brain injury [TBI]), and patients with combined delirium and CNS-depressant withdrawal (e.g., delirium tremens, opioid or benzodiazepine withdrawal) (see "Impact of Delirium" section). More commonly, patients exhibit a rapid and fluctuating course with symptoms varying rapidly over time, giving rise to the classic waxing and waning picture. Patients often experience the appearance or exacerbation of behavioral disturbances in the evening and at night, leading to the classic "sundowning" syndrome (Cardinali, Brusco, Liberczuk, & Furio, 2002). Whether this represents a function of biological circadian rhythm or results from decreased sensory input is unclear. The appearance of lucid intervals in the clinical course is an important observation and may even aid in the diagnosis of delirium.

As described above, global disturbance of cognition is a cardinal feature of delirium. All "main cognitive functions" (e.g., perception, thinking, memory) are impaired or abnormal to some extent. In addition, delirious patients have difficulty sustaining attention and responding to stimuli selectively. Usually, patients are easily distracted by their surrounding environment. Delirium may be better understood as a disorder of awareness, not arousal. Yet, arousal problems may be associated with the various presentations of delirium. For example, in the case of hypoactive delirium, the activating system may be hypoactive, in which case the patient would appear apathetic, somnolent, and quietly confused. In other patients, the brainstem's activating system may be hyperactive, in which case the patient is agitated and hypervigilant, exhibiting psychomotor hyperactivity and agitation, leading to the hyperactive type of delirium.

Often, the sleep–wake cycle is disturbed. This is not only symptomatic of delirium, but in itself may either cause or exacerbate the condition due to sleep deprivation. More commonly, patients exhibit sleep–awake cycle reversal: night sleep is usually shortened and fragmented; while daytime wakefulness is often reduced, presenting in the form of drowsiness and the tendency to nap or being difficult to arouse during the day.

Problems with orientation are likely to be associated with the patients' inability to adequately process incoming information and their impaired memory formation. In fact, delirious patients seem to experience a reduced ability to discriminate and integrate perceptions. This may include a reduced ability to relate incoming stimuli meaningfully to previously acquired knowledge. Thus, often patients have a difficult time telling apart perceptions, images, dreams, illusions, and hallucinations. This may be the reason why patients commonly report their experiences as happening "as if dreaming while still awake." Often patients experience emotional dysregulation or lability.

Delirious patients' memory is often impaired in most aspects (i.e., registration, retention, and recall). They may exhibit various degrees of both anterograde and retrograde amnesia, though their remote memory is often spared. Delirious patients often exhibit a disorganized and fragmented thinking pattern. The disturbances range from an inability to direct thoughts at will, to a complete inability to think coherently. This includes an inability to reason, solve problems, anticipate the consequences of actions, and grasp the meaning of abstract words. This disorganization of thinking, coupled with memory disturbance and misinterpretation of environmental stimuli, often leads to the development of delusional thinking (usually of paranoid nature) and confabulation.

DELIRIUM SUBTYPES

Historically, the first delirium subtypes have been based on behavioral and motoric characteristics (Liptzin & Levkoff, 1992). Factor analysis has confirmed the existence of at least two different clusters of symptoms: hyperalert/hyperactive features (e.g., agitation, hyperreactivity, aggressiveness, hallucinations, delusions); and the hypoalert/hypoactive features (e.g., decreased reactivity, motor and speech retardation, facial inexpressiveness) (Camus et al., 2000).

Subsequent studies have suggested that there are at least three types of delirium, based on their clinical (motoric) manifestations: hyperactive, hypoactive, and mixed (Meagher, O'Hanlon, O'Mahony, Casey, & Trzepacz, 2000; Meagher & Trzepacz, 2000). It is important to recognize that delirium seems to manifest differently in different populations under study (see Figure 41.21). For example, studies in the general adult medical population revealed that, among referrals to a consultation psychiatry service, the most common type appeared to the mixed type (46%), followed by the hyperactive (30%) and the hypoactive (24%) among those meeting *International Classification of Diseases–10* (ICD-10) (Box 41.3) criteria for delirium (Meagher et al., 2000). Yet, the numbers seem quite different when we look at the critically ill populations. Among medical ICU (MICU) patients, the most common type continues to be the mixed type (54.9%), but there is a significant reversal on the remaining types, with a much larger percentage of hypoactive (43.5%) than hyperactive (1.6%) types (Peterson et al., 2006). Meanwhile, among surgical ICU (SICU) patients, there is a significant reversal on the types of delirium found, with the most common form of delirium being the hypoactive type (64%), followed by the mixed type (27%), and only a minority of subjects exhibiting the purely hyperactive (9%) type (Pandharipande, Cotton et al., 2007). Finally, a study of elderly patients in the medicine wards found that the significant majority of subjects experienced the hypoactive subtype (65%), compared to the hyperactive (25%) or mixed (10%) subtypes (Khurana et al., 2011).

What is most significant about these findings is not only that hypoactive delirium is often missed or misdiagnosed (Liptzin & Levkoff, 1992), but that these patients experienced the worst prognosis (e.g., prolonged hospital stay, higher morbidity and mortality) (Kiely, Jones, Bergmann, & Marcantonio, 2007). Frequently these patients present with depressive-like symptoms (e.g., unawareness of the environment, lethargy, apathy, decreased level of alertness, psychomotor retardation, decreased speech production, and episodes of unresponsiveness or staring). Patients with hypoactive delirium often endorsed depressive symptoms, such as low mood (60%), worthlessness (68%), and frequent thoughts of death (52%) (Farrell & Ganzini, 1995). Studies have demonstrated that a large percentage of these patients are inappropriately diagnosed and treated as depressed. Hypoactive delirium is unrecognized (and therefore untreated or mismanaged) in 66%–84% of patients. In fact, studies have found that patients with hypoactive delirium demonstrated a seven-fold risk of under-recognition by nurses and that older, visually impaired, demented patients with hypoactive delirium were 20 times less likely to be recognized by nurses as having delirium (Inouye, Foreman, Mion, Katz, & Cooney, 2001). Our own experience at Stanford University Hospital, in parallel to that of others (Farrell & Ganzini, 1995; Kishi et al., 2007), found that 42% of the time when the psychiatry consultation service was called to treat a patient for "depression," the patient's correct diagnosis was hypoactive delirium (Maldonado, Dhami, & Wise, 2003). The same study found that nearly 80% of these patients had been inappropriately prescribed antidepressant medications.

To most physicians, the clearest and most recognizable form is the hyperactive type. Most clinicians agree that a confused, disoriented patient who does not have a preexisting psychiatric diagnosis, who suddenly becomes agitated, combative, and/or assaultive, is probably suffering from the hyperactive or "agitated type" of delirium. We use the term "mixed type" to describe the classic "waxing and waning" pattern, commonly seen in medically ill patients who appear

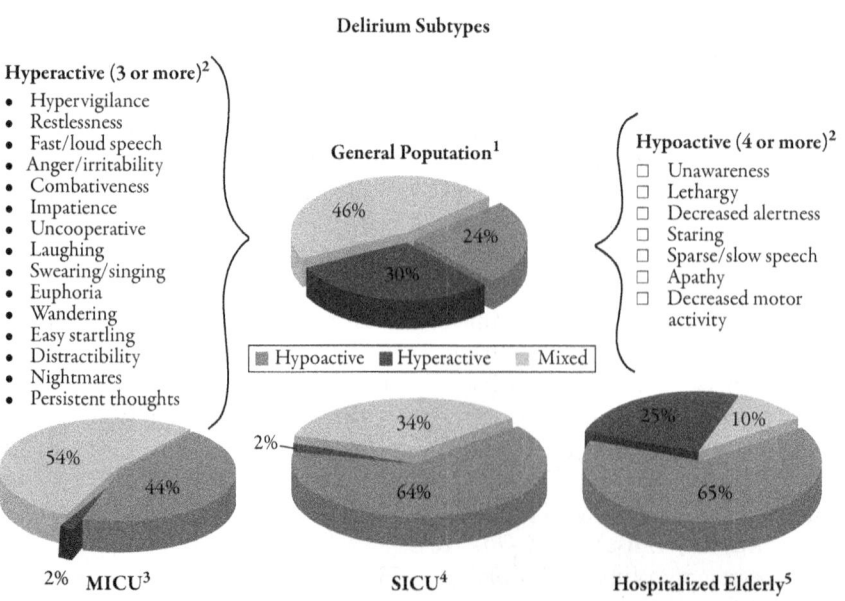

Figure 41.21 Motoric subtype of delirium depending on population under study.

Box 41.3 ICD-10 DIAGNOSTIC CRITERIA FOR DELIRIUM

For a definite diagnosis, delirium symptoms, mild or severe, should be present in each one of the following areas:

1. Impairment of consciousness and attention, on a continuum from clouding to coma (e.g., reduced ability to direct, focus, sustain, and shift attention);

2. Global disturbance of cognition (e.g., perceptual distortions, illusions and hallucinations—most often visual; impairment of abstract thinking and comprehension, with or without transient delusions, but typically with some degree of incoherence; impairment of immediate recall and of recent memory but with relatively intact remote memory; disorientation for time as well as, in more severe cases, for place and person);

3. Psychomotor disturbances (e.g., hypo- or hyperactivity and unpredictable shifts from one to the other; increased reaction time; increased or decreased flow of speech; enhanced startle reaction);

4. Disturbance of the sleep-wake cycle (e.g., insomnia or, in severe cases, total sleep loss or reversal of the sleep-wake cycle; daytime drowsiness; nocturnal worsening of symptoms; disturbing dreams or nightmares, which may continue as hallucinations after awakening);

5. Emotional disturbance (e.g. depression, anxiety or fear, irritability, euphoria, apathy, or wondering perplexity).

The onset is usually rapid, the course diurnally fluctuating, and the total duration of the condition less than six months. The above clinical picture is so characteristic that a fairly confident diagnosis of delirium can be made even if the underlying cause is not clearly established. In addition to a history of an underlying physical or brain disease, evidence of cerebral dysfunction (e.g., an abnormal electroencephalogram, usually but not invariably showing a slowing of the background activity) may be required if the diagnosis is in doubt.

---

agitated and combative at times, with alternating episodes of somnolence and hypoactivity.

In addition to motoric subtypes, researchers have recently described a new delirium presentation form: subsyndromal delirium (SSD). Different from the other three described above, this is not differentiated by motor type but by an incomplete presentation of diagnostic criteria, along with cognitive impairment. In one study, patients with SSD (defined as meeting ≥ 2 DSM-delirium criteria, but did not meet Confusion Assessment Method [CAM] diagnostic criteria for delirium) had outcomes similar to or worse than those with mild CAM-defined delirium (e.g., nursing home placement or death at 6 months: 27% vs. 0%) (Marcantonio, Ta, Duthie, & Resnick, 2002). Others have demonstrated that when the appropriate screening or diagnostic test is used to allow differentiation between no delirium, subsyndromal delirium, and clinical delirium (e.g., severity scale), patients with SSD in the general medical wards experienced longer acute care hospital stays, increased post-discharge mortality, more symptoms of delirium, and a lower cognitive and functional level at follow-up than patients with no SSD, even after adjusting for illness severity, baseline cognitive status, and severity of baseline functional status (Cole et al., 2003). In addition, patients with SSD had the same set of risk factors that predict the likelihood of developing DSM-defined delirium (e.g., older age, baseline dementia, and greater physiological severity of illness). A recent ICU study similarly concluded that patients with SSD (which defined SSD as patients who have <4 points on the Intensive Care Delirium Screening Checklist [ICDSC]) (Bergeron, Dubois, Dumont, Dial, & Skrobik, 2001) experienced greater mortality (10.6% vs. 2.4%; $P < 0.001$), longer ICU length of stay (5.2 days vs. 2.5 days; $P < 0.001$), and longer overall hospital stay (40.9 days vs. 31.7 days;

$P = 0.002$); conversely, patients with no delirium were more likely to be discharged home and less likely to need convalescence or long-term care than those with SSD (see Table 41.8) (Ouimet et al., 2007).

DIAGNOSING DELIRIUM

Several studies have demonstrated that hospital staff in general, and physicians in particular, are not good at identifying delirium. In fact, studies have demonstrated that delirium is misdiagnosed, detected late, or missed in over 50% of cases across the various healthcare settings (Kean & Ryan, 2008). Despite its high prevalence in critically ill patients, delirium remains unrecognized in as many as 66%–84% of patients experiencing this complication (Francis et al., 1990; Inouye, 1994; Rolfson, McElhaney, et al., 1999; Ely, Margolin et al., 2001; Inouye et al., 2001; Pisani, Redlich et al., 2003; Pisani, Inouye et al., 2003; Pandharipande et al., 2007; Steis & Fick, 2008; Swigart, Kishi, Thurber, Kathol, & Meller, 2008; Steis, Shaughnessy, & Gordon, 2012). Unfortunately, the associated mental status changes are often misattributed to dementia, depression, or just an expected occurrence of medical illness. Several studies have demonstrated a high rate (45%–66%) of missed diagnosis (i.e., either missed completely or misattributed to another disorder) of delirium by general medicine and surgical services (Farrell & Ganzini, 1995; Armstrong, Cozza, & Watanabe, 1997; Kishi et al., 2007). A recent study of an adult, acute hospital population found that only 63.6% of patients with delirium were recognized by nursing staff to be confused or delirious, whereas 43.6% had confusion documented in the medical case notes (Ryan et al., 2013). The authors concluded that "even if some

Table 41.8 SUBSYNDROMAL DELIRIUM AND CLINICAL OUTCOMES

	NO DELIRIUM (ND)	SUBSYNDROMAL (SD)	CLINICAL (CD)	*P* VALUE*
ICU Mortality	2.4%	10.6%	15.9%	*P* < 0.001
ICU LOS	2.5 d	5.2 d	10.8 d	*P* < 0.001
Hospital LOS	31.7 d	40.9 d	36.4 d	ND vs. SD, *P* = 0.002 ND vs. CD, *P* < 0.001 SD vs. CD, *P* = 0.137
Severity of illness (APACHE II)	12.9	16.7	18.6	ND vs. SD, *P* < 0.001 ND vs. CD, *P* < 0.001 SD vs. CD, *P* < 0.016

*Pair-wise comparison

Source: Ouimet et al., 2007

recognized, but undocumented, delirium cases occurred, these findings suggest that delirium is not a high diagnostic and therapeutic priority, despite its treatability and relevance to outcomes, especially for poorer prognosis in the elderly" (Ryan et al., 2013).

Factors contributing to the poor detection rate of delirium can be divided into three large components, which have significant interplay (Table 41.9):

1. *Patient factors* (e.g., older subjects, patients experiencing comorbid dementia, fluctuating course of presentation, presence of hypoactive features) (Liptzin & Levkoff, 1992; Inouye et al., 1993; Farrell & Ganzini, 1995; Inouye, 1999; Inouye et al., 2001; Pisani et al., 2003; Peterson et al., 2006; Kiely et al., 2007; Lowery et al., 2007; McAlpine et al., 2008; Meagher et al., 2008; Givens, Jones, & Inouye, 2009; Leonard et al., 2009; Collins, Blanchard, Tookman, & Sampson, 2010; Khurana et al., 2011; Srinonprasert et al., 2011; Morandi, McCurley, et al., 2012; Steis & Fick, 2012; Ryan et al., 2013);

2. *Clinician/practitioner factors* (e.g., lack of knowledge and training, lack of confidence, lack of suspicion, lack of time of the clinical staff, expectation that altered mental status

or delirium are a "normal occurrence" in certain medical settings, such as the ICU) (Wong, Chiu, & Chu, 2005; Wong, Holroyd-Leduc, et al., 2010; Adams, 1988; Inouye, 1991; Ely, Siegel, & Inouye 2001; Breitbart et al., 2002; Rabinowitz, 2002; Carnes, Howell, et al., 2003; Cole et al., 2003; Pisani et al., 2003; Dantzer, Capuron, et al., 2008; Steis & Fick, 2008; Davis & MacLullich, 2009; Khan et al., 2009; Collins et al., 2010; Boot, 2012; Steis et al., 2012); and

3. *Systems factors* (e.g., lack of consensus over the optimal assessment of delirium, location of care [worse in surgical than in medical settings], busy clinical settings [especially low nurse-to-patient ratio], inadequate application of "sedation holidays" in sedated-ventilated patients, and the rapid transfer of patients from one unit to another, which may decrease the proper documentation and diagnosis) (Inouye, 1991, 1998; Inouye, Schlesinger, & Lydon, 1999; Shinn & Maldonado, 2000; Inouye et al., 2001; Pisani, Redlich, McNicoll, Ely, & Inouye, 2003; (Pisani, Redlich et al. 2003) Siddiqi & House, 2006; Bickel et al., 2008; Davis & MacLullich, 2009; Collins et al., 2010; NICE, 2010; Wong et al., 2010; Boot, 2012; Brummel, Morandi, et al., 2012; Neto, Nassar, et al., 2012; Steis et al., 2012).

Table 41.9 FACTORS CONTRIBUTING TO THE POOR DETECTION RATE OF DELIRIUM

PATIENT FACTORS	CLINICIAN/PRACTITIONER FACTORS	SYSTEMS FACTORS
• Older subjects • Patients experiencing comorbid dementia • Fluctuating course of presentation • Presence of hypoactive features	• Lack of knowledge and training • Lack of confidence • Lack of suspicion • Lack of time of the clinical staff • Expectation that altered mental status or delirium are a "normal occurrence" in certain medical settings, such as the ICU	• Lack of consensus over the optimal assessment of delirium • Location of care (worse in surgical rather than medical settings) • Busy clinical settings (especially low nurse-to-patient ratio) • Inadequate application of sedation holidays in sedated-ventilated patients • The rapid transfer of patients from one unit to another, which may decrease the proper documentation and diagnosis

In order to accurately diagnose delirium, clinicians need to be vigilant and have a high level of suspicion, particularly in patient populations at higher risk, such as the elderly and those with the risk factors included in the mnemonic "end acute brain failure" (see Table 41.2).

To date, the diagnostic gold standard for delirium remains the *Diagnostic and Statistical Manual for Mental Disorders* (DSM). The previously published version was the Fourth Edition-Text Revised, published in 1994 (DSM-IV-TR; APA, 1994). A new DSM-5 (5th Edition) has changed the criteria slightly. The new DSM criteria change the diagnostic focus away from a "disturbance of consciousness" (DSM-IV) to a "disturbance in attention"—Criterion A. Criterion B relates to the acute or subacute onset of symptoms (to differentiate from more chronic cognitive deficits such as dementia; formerly Criterion C). New Criterion C refers to additional disturbances in cognition not better explained by another neurocognitive disorder (akin to former Criterion B in DSM-IV). New to DSM-5 is Criterion D, which stipulates that A and B "do not occur in the context of severely reduced level of arousal or coma." And, finally, Criterion E is identical to Criterion D in DSM-IV, which stipulates that there is physical evidence that can give an organic etiology for the syndrome. Notice that DSM-5 seems to have got rid of the presence of psychotic symptomatology (formerly Criterion B in DSM-IV) as part of the diagnostic criteria.

The *International Statistical Classification of Diseases and Related Health Problems* (ICD-10; see Box 41.3) provides its own diagnostic criteria (WHO, 1992, 2010). Yet, both criteria have at their core the same three cardinal features: disturbance of consciousness (i.e., reduced clarity of awareness of the environment, with reduced ability to focus, sustain, or shift attention); global disturbance of cognition (e.g., problem-solving impairment or memory impairment) and/ or perceptual disturbance (e.g., illusions or hallucinations); and an acute or subacute onset with a tendency to fluctuate (WHO, 2010; APA, 2013). These criteria are commonly used by medical personnel for the definite diagnosis of delirium. There are numerous clinically available instruments (see Box 41.4) developed to help medical providers screen for the presence of delirium. These instruments were designed to help nonpsychiatrists (e.g., nurses, internists, and research assistants) diagnose and follow the progression of delirium (Trzepacz, Baker, & Greenhouse, 1988; Marcantonio et al., 1994). All of these scales have been derived from, and validated against, expert psychiatric assessments using DSM or ICD diagnostic criteria. Some of these tools were designed and are better used for the purpose of screening for delirium (e.g., CAM, based on DSM-III-R, original sample size *n* = 56 [Inouye et al., 1990], CAM-ICU, based on CAM, original sample size *n* = 38 [Ely et al., 2001]). The CAM and CAM-ICU offer a binary result (i.e., delirium or no delirium), and there is no severity scale. Unfortunately, these tools have a high false-positive rate (as high as 10%); therefore, the team that developed the instrument recommends that all patients identified as delirious by screening instruments "have further evaluation to confirm the diagnosis" (Inouye et al., 1990; Liptzin & Levkoff, 1992). In fact, some have expressed

---

Box 41.4 OBJECTIVE MEASURES FOR THE DIAGNOSIS OF DELIRIUM

- DSM-IV-TR ("Gold Standard"; APA, 1994)
- Delirium Rating Scale (DRS) (Trzepacz, Baker, et al., 1988)
- Confusion Rating Scale (CRS) (Williams, Ward, et al., 1988)
- Confusion Assessment Method (CAM) (Inouye et al., 1990)
- Delirium Symptom Interview (DSI) (Albert et al., 1992)
- Delirium Assessment Scale (DAS) (O'Keeffe, 1994)
- Cognitive Test for Delirium (CTD) (Hart et al., 1996)
- NEECHAM Confusion Scale (Neelon & Champagne, 1996)
- Confusional State Evaluation (CSE) (Robertsson, Karlsson, et al., 1997)
- Memorial Delirium Assessment Scale (MDAS) (Breitbart et al., 1997)
- Delirium Severity Scale (DSS) (Bettin, Maletta, et al., 1998)
- Delirium Index (DI) (McCusker, Cole, et al., 1998)
- Delirium Rating Scale–Revised-98 (DRS-R-98) (Trzepacz et al., 2001)
- Intensive Care Delirium Screening Checklist (ICDSC) (Bergeron et al., 2001)
- Confusion Assessment Method for the Intensive Care unit (CAM-ICU) (Ely, Margolin, et al., 2001)
- Delirium Detection Score (DDS) (Otter, Martin, et al., 2005)
- Nursing Delirium Screening Scale (Nu-DESC) (Gaudreau et al., 2005a)
- Delirium Detection Tool–Provisional (DDT-pro) (Kean, Trzepacz, et al., 2010)
- *Diagnostic and Statistical Manual of Mental Disorders, 5th Edition* (DSM-5) ("New Gold Standard") (APA, 2013)

---

concerns regarding the generalizability of the CAM-ICU findings (Young & Arseven, 2010; Boot, 2012):

On closer scrutiny of the methodology of CAM-ICU studies, it is important to highlight some considerations when interpreting the data: (1) three of the studies examined were conducted by the tool's author who may have had a vested interest, and given that only 39% of the study population were intubated, it is difficult to conclude CAM-ICU's validity in intubated patients (van Eijk, van Marum, et al., 2009); (2) the study population sizes were relatively small, thus CAM-ICU adaptability into different healthcare organizations remains unclear (Page, Navarange, et al., 2009); (3) examination of the exclusion criteria (e.g., history of psychosis, learning disabilities, depression, dementia) of these studies raises questions to CAM-ICU transferability to these populations, especially as these conditions can have similar characteristics but very different treatment pathways; (4) studies have demonstrated although CAM-ICU has high validity in the non-intubated ICU patients, it seems to fail to detect milder, subtler symptoms of hypoactive delirium; (5) individuals with a history of mental illness (e.g., psychosis, learning disabilities, depression, dementia) were excluded, despite reports indicating delirium being of a medical cause (Boot, 2012, p.187))

In fact, a prospective study was used to assess the diagnostic validity of the CAM administered at the bedside by nurses in daily practice during a 5-month period to all patients ($n = 258$) consecutively admitted to an acute geriatric ward of a university hospital (Lemiengre, Nelis, et al., 2006). The CAM as administered by bedside nurses had a 66.7% sensitivity and a 90.7% specificity. The study suggested that bedside nurses had difficulties with the identification of elderly patients with delirium and that additional education about delirium is warranted, with special attention to guided training of bedside nurses in the use of an assessment strategy such as the CAM for the recognition of delirium symptoms.

A subsequent study compared the diagnostic accuracy of "delirium experts who diagnosed delirium in 75/181 subjects vs. the CAM-ICU as performed in 'routine practice'" (i.e., nonresearch setting, conducted by a nonresearch nurse), where delirium was diagnosed in 35 out of 181 cases. This yielded a sensitivity of 47% (95% CI = 35%–58%), specificity of 98% (95% CI = 93%–100%), positive predictive value of 95% (95% CI = 80%–99%), and negative predictive value of 72% (95% CI = 64%–79%). This suggested that the "specificity of the CAM-ICU as performed in routine, daily practice appears to be high but sensitivity low. The low sensitivity hampers early detection of delirium by the CAM-ICU" (Van Eijk et al., 2011).

Moreover, a recent systematic review and meta-analysis of studies on delirium in critically ill patients (i.e., intensive care units, surgical wards, emergency rooms) published between 1966 and 2011 (including 16 studies, $n = 1,523$; and covering five delirium screening tools) demonstrated that the CAM-ICU was the most specific bedside tool for the assessment of delirium in critically ill patients (Neto et al., 2012). Considering only the two most commonly used tools, the pooled sensitivities and specificities of the CAM-ICU for detection of delirium were 75.5% and 95.8%, compared to the ICDSC at 80.1% and 74.6%, respectively. All but one study was performed in a research setting, and that study suggested that, with routine use of the CAM-ICU, half of the patients with delirium were not detected. The authors concluded that "the low sensitivity of the CAM-ICU in routine, daily practice may limit its use as a screening test" (Neto et al., 2012).

Other scales have been designed to diagnose and assess the severity of a delirium episode. These include the Delirium Rating Scale (DRS), based on DSM-III, original sample size $n = 20$ (Trzepacz et al., 1988); the DRS-98, based on DSM-IV, original sample size $n = 68$ (Trzepacz, Mittal, et al., 2001); the Memorial Delirium Assessment Scale (MDAS), based on DSM-IV, original sample size $n = 68$ (Breitbart et al., 1997); and the Intensive Care Delirium Screening Checklist (ICDSC), based on DSM-IV, original sample size $n = 93$ (Bergeron et al., 2001), among others. (Please see Box 41.4 for a comprehensive list of delirium diagnostic tools.) A significant advantage of diagnostic tools that measure delirium

---

Box 41.5 PRIMITIVE REFLEXES

Primitive reflexes are clinical features that indicate brain dysfunction but that cannot be precisely localized or lateralized. When present, these signs suggest cortical disease, especially frontal cortex, resulting in disinhibition of usually extinguished or suppressed primitive reflexes. Their clinical significance is uncertain and is difficult to correlate with psychiatric illnesses and other behavior disorders, including delirium.

- *Glabellar Reflex*: With the examiner's fingers outside of patient's visual field, tap the glabellar region at a rate of one tap per second. A pathological response is either absence of blink, no habituation, or a shower of blinks. Normal response = blinking to the first few taps with rapid habituation.

- *Rooting Reflex*: Tested by stroking the corner of the patient's lips and drawing away. Pursing of the lips and movement of the lips or head toward the stroking is a positive response.

- *Snout Reflex*: Elicited by tapping the patient's upper lip with finger or percussion hammer causing the lips to purse and the mouth to pout.

- *Suck Reflex:* Tested by placing your knuckles between the patient's lips. A positive response would be puckering of the lips.

- *Grasp Reflex*: Elicited by stroking the patient's palm toward fingers or crosswise while the patient is distracted, causing the patient's hand to grasps the examiner's fingers.

- *Palmomental Reflex*: Test by scratching the base of the patient's thumb (noxious stimulus of thenar eminence). A positive response occurs when the ipsilateral lower lip and jaw move slightly downward, and does not extinguish with repeated stimulation.

- *Babinski Sign:* Downward (flexor response) movement of the great toe in response to plantar stimulation.

- *Adventitious Motor Overflow*: Seen as the examiner tests one hand for sequential finger movements, and the fingers of the other hand wiggle or tap. Also if there are choreiform movements.

- *Double Simultaneous Stimulation Discrimination*: Tested with the patient's eyes closed. The examiner simultaneously brushes a finger against one of the patient's cheeks and another finger against one of the patient's hands, asking the patient where he has been touched.

severity is that they provide clinicians a means to measure the severity of the episode and determine whether the condition seems to be worsening or improving (i.e., consecutive measures). A severity score is also useful in research studies, as particular interventions may not be able to fully prevent delirium but may lessen the severity of the episode. Finally, severity scales may provide the ability to diagnose subsyndromal delirium (i.e., patients presenting with mental status changes that do not rise to the level of full DSM or ICD diagnostic criteria). Clinical experience and accumulating research data seem to indicate that the presence of subsyndromal symptoms may have similarly negative effects in the patients who are experiencing them. A study of ICU patients demonstrated that patients experiencing subsyndromal delirium experienced significantly greater ICU mortality (10.6% vs. 2.4%), longer ICU stays (5.2 days vs. 2.5 days), and longer total hospital stays (40.9 days vs. 31.7 days) compared to patients experiencing similar medical illness but without delirium (Ouimet et al., 2007). As expected, these subsyndromal patients experienced less ICU mortality (10.6% vs. 15.9%), shorter ICU stays (5.2 days vs. 10.8 days), but longer total hospital stays (40.9 days vs. 36.4 days) compared to patients experiencing similar medical illness but with full clinical delirium (see Table 41.8).

In general, no delirium screening or assessment tool is expected to be perfect. Some have criticized the fact that even the two psychometrically valid scales most commonly used in the ICU (i.e., CAM-ICU, ICDSC) have detection ranges of delirium from 10% to >80%, in similar populations. It may very well be that vigilance and close clinical monitoring are more useful than any commonly used tool. In fact, some authors have reported that the CAM-ICU scoring may be affected by sedation, thus limiting its diagnostic accuracy (Kress, 2010). A study of "real-life" conditions (as opposed to a research setting) suggested that "the CAM-ICU in daily practice showed not quite as good test characteristics as presented in the original validation studies" (van Eijk et al., 2011). In fact, these authors found that "after stratification according to type of delirium, sensitivity of the CAM-ICU was lowest in the hypoactive subgroup (31%; 95% CI, 17%–48%); highest in the hyperactive delirious patients (100%; 95% CI, 56%–100%); and intermediate in the mixed-type patients (53%; 95% CI, 35%–74%); exhibiting particularly poor test characteristics in neurocritical care patients (sensitivity 17%; 95% CI, 1%–64%) (van Eijk et al., 2011). A recent study suggested that clinical assessments by critical care physicians may identify delirium more rapidly and more accurately than screening tool assessments (Bigatello et al., 2013).

It is unclear what the new DSM-5 diagnostic criteria will mean to the diagnostic accuracy of existing tools. It is likely that some of them may require revisions, yet all will need to be validated taking the new criteria into consideration. Nonetheless, it may be important for the clinician to be aware that the 2013 American College of Critical Care Medicine (ACCM)/Society of Critical Care Medicine (SCCM) clinical practice guidelines for pain, agitation, and delirium (PAD), based on available evidence, strongly recommend that critically ill patients be routinely monitored for delirium in the ICU using a validated tool. After their review of available delirium assessment tools, the 2013 PAD guideline group concluded that the Confusion Assessment Method for the ICU (CAM-ICU) and the Intensive Care Delirium Screening Checklist (ICDSC) are the ICU delirium screening tools with the strongest validity and reliability (Davidson, Harvey, Bemis-Dougherty, Smith, & Hopkins, 2013).

The most critical part of the assessment, given the characteristic waxing and waning of this syndrome, is to add to the clinical examination all available clinical information, including interview of the family members and caregivers, nursing and medical staff, and a thorough review of the chart for behaviors exhibited during the preceding 24 hours. Another potential clue of the presence of delirium may come from a thorough neurological examination. In our clinical experience, patients with delirium tend to exhibit a reemergence of primitive signs (see Box 41.5). This appears to be more consistent in cases of hypoactive delirium. The relationship between poor cognitive status and primitive reflexes has been described in patients suffering from HIV-related cognitive disorders (Tremont-Lukats, Teixeira, et al., 1999) and in cases of dementia (Paulson, 1977). One study described the presence of primitive reflexes in post-cardiotomy patients suffering from postoperative neuropsychiatric complications (Liu & Hsieh, 1993). A second study found that 55% of patients exhibiting at least two primitive reflexes and 80% of those exhibiting at least three primitive reflexes in the postoperative period developed delirium (Nicolson, Chabon, et al., 2011). Further studies are needed to determine whether an assessment for the presence of primitive reflexes may add to the diagnostic accuracy for delirium or at least assist in the characterization of delirium type, and whether such assessment has any prognostic value.

Some have advocated the use of the electroencephalogram (EEG) as a way to identify and diagnose delirium. Engel and Romano were the first to describe the relationship between delirium and the diffuse slowing and progressive disorganization of rhythm seen in the EEG (Engel, Webb, & Ferris, 1945) (Engel, Webb et al. 1945). The most common EEG findings in delirium include slowing of peak and average frequencies, and decreased alpha activity but increased theta and delta waves. Studies suggest that EEG changes correlate with the degree of cognitive deficit, but there does not appear to be a relationship between EEG patterns and delirium motoric type (Romano & Engel, 1944; Engel & Romano, 1959; Koponen, Partanen, et al., 1989; Koponen, Hurri, et al., 1989; Trzepacz, Sclabassi, & Van Thiel, 1989; Trzepacz, Leavitt, et al., 1992; Engel & Romano, 2004; Plaschke, Hill, et al., 2007). The clinical usefulness of EEG in the diagnosis of delirium may be constrained by its limited specificity (given that there are many conditions and medications that may affect the EEG) and the practicality of conducting the test (particularly in the case of agitated and combative patients). Still, the EEG can be useful in differentiating delirium from other psychiatric and neurological conditions such as catatonic states, seizure activity (e.g., nonconvulsive status), medication side effects (e.g., posterior reversible encephalopathy syndrome due to the use of calcineurin inhibitors), or the manifestations of the behavioral and psychological symptoms associated with dementia (BPSD). BPSD affects between 50% and 90% of patients suffering from dementia and is usually characterized by three main syndromes: agitation/aggression, psychosis, and an affective component. At times, apathy (as in the case of hypoactive delirium) or disinhibition (as in the case of hyperactive delirium) can be seen, particularly when there is frontal lobe involvement (Finkel, Costa e Silva, et al., 1996).

Finally, a 24-hour accelerometer-based activity monitor has been used to categorize the motoric behavior of patients with delirium. The continuous wavelet transform (CWT) provided by the instrument can then be used to characterize a delirium as hyperactive, hypoactive, or mixed (Godfrey, Conway, et al., 2009, 2010; Meagher, 2009). The technique has yet to find a clinical use, however.

MANAGEMENT OF DELIRIUM

ADEQUATE MEDICAL MANAGEMENT

The management of delirium has five main components (see Box 41.6):

1. Recognition of patients at risk (see Tables 41.1 and 41.2);

2. Implementation of prevention techniques (with pharmacological and nonpharmacological approaches), especially in populations identified to be at high risk;

3. Enhanced surveillance and screening;

Box 41.6 ALGORITHM FOR THE MANAGEMENT OF DELIRIUM

I. Recognition of patients at risk
   A. A particular patient's odds of developing delirium are associated with the interaction between the following conditions:
      i. Knowledge of a patient's characteristics.
      ii. Predisposing and precipitating medical risk factors (Table 41.4).
      iii. Modifiable and non-modifiable risk factors for that particular patient or patient population (Table 41.5).
      iv. Specific medical conditions and surgical procedures the patient is exposed to.
   B. Obtaining the patient's baseline level of cognitive functioning using information from accessory sources (e.g., Informant Questionnaire on Cognitive Decline in the Elderly [IQCODE]).
II. Implementation of prevention techniques
   A. A key focus should be placed on prevention strategies, particularly in "at risk" populations.
      i. Avoid all pharmacological agents with high deliriogenic potential or anticholinergic load, if possible.
      ii. Promote a non-pharmacological sleep protocol.
      iii. Early mobilization.
   B. For patients in the ICU, especially those on ventilation or IV sedation, consider:
      i. Sedating to a prescribed or target sedation level (e.g., RASS).
      ii. Consider using the sedative agent with lowest deliriogenic potential:
         • Dexmedetomidine use is associated with the lowest incidence of delirium.
         • Propofol use is a good second choice; followed by midazolam.
      iii. Reassess pain levels daily and titrate opioid agents to the lowest effective level required to maintain adequate analgesia.
         • Hydromorphone is preferred as baseline agent of choice for pain management.
         • Limit the use of fentanyl to rapid initiation of analgesia and as rescue agent.
         • Avoid the use of opioid agents for sedation or management of agitation or delirium.
      iv. Provide daily sedation holidays:
         • Interrupt sedative infusions daily until the patient is awake
         • Restart sedation, if needed, at the lowest effective dose
         • Reassess target sedation level (e.g., RASS).
III. Enhanced surveillance, screening and early detection
   A. Most important aspects of surveillance:
      i. Knowledge about the condition and presenting symptoms.
      ii. A high level of suspicion.
   B. Be vigilant for the development of delirium in high-risk groups:
      i. Use a standardized surveillance tools (e.g., DRS-R-98; MDAS; CAM)
      ii. Use psychiatric consultants (i.e., DSM-5/ICD-10 criteria)
      iii. Be particularly aware of the presence of hypoactive delirium and its different manifestations.
   C. Use psychiatric consultants to help with assessment and design of the treatment plan, if available.
   D. Train medical personnel at all levels.
IV. Treatment of all forms of delirium
   A. Identify and treat underlying medical causes.

(continued)

B. Treat or correct underlying medical problems and potential reversible factors.

C. Conduct an inventory of all pharmacological agents that have been administered to the patient.

    i. Discontinue any medication or agent known to cause delirium or to have high anticholinergic potential, if possible, or institute a suitable alternative.

D. Implement early mobilization techniques, to include ALL of the following components:

    i. Daily awakening protocols (sedation holiday), as described above.

    ii. Remove IV lines, bladder catheters, physical restraints, and any other immobilizing apparatuses as early as possible.

    iii. Initiate aggressive PT and OT as soon as it is medically safe to do.

        a. In bedridden patients, therapy may be limited to daily passive range of motion.

        b. Once medically stable, get the patient up and moving as early as possible.

    iv. Provide patients with any required sensory aids (i.e., eyeglasses, hearing aids).

    v. Promote as normal a circadian light rhythm as possible.

        a. Better if this can be achieved by environmental manipulations, such as light control (i.e., lights on and curtains open during the day; lights off at night) and noise control (i.e., provide ear plugs, turn off TVs, minimize night staff chatter).

        b. Provide as much natural light as possible during the daytime.

    vi. Provide adequate intellectual and environmental stimulation as early as possible.

E. Avoid using GABA-ergic agents to control agitation, if possible.

    • *Exception*: cases of CNS-depressant withdrawal (i.e., alcohol, benzodiazepines, barbiturates); or when more appropriate agents have failed and sedations are needed to prevent patient's harm.

F. Adequately assess and treat pain.

    i. Avoid the use of opioid agents for behavioral control of agitation.

    ii. Rotate opioid agents from morphine to hydromorphone or fentanyl.

G. For the treatment of delirium (all types), consider using:

    i. Acetylcholinesterase inhibitor (e.g., rivastigmine) for patients with a history of recurrent delirium or delirium superimposed on known cognitive deficits. Physostigmine, for known causes of anticholinergic delirium.

    ii. Melatonin (e.g., 3 mg q HS) or melatonin agonists (e.g., ramelteon 8 mg q HS) to promote a more natural sleep. If that is ineffective, consider trazodone (e.g., 25–100 mg q HS) or mirtazapine (e.g., 3.75–7.5 mg q HS).

    iii. Serotonin antagonist (e.g., ondansetron).

H. In case of *hyperactive delirium,* consider the use of the following agents:

    i. Dopamine antagonist agents (to address DA excess) (e.g., haloperidol, risperidone, quetiapine, aripiprazole).

        a. Moderate-dose haloperidol (e.g., <20 mg/24 hr in divided doses), is still considered the treatment of choice, if the patient's cardiac condition allows it.

        b. Before using haloperidol:

            • Obtain 12-lead ECG; measure QTc.

            • Check electrolytes; correct K+ and Mg+, if needed.

            • Carefully review the patient's medication list and identify any other agents with the ability to prolong QTc.

            • If possible, avoid other medications known to increase QTc and/or inhibitors of CPY3A4.

        c. When the use of haloperidol is contraindicated or not desirable, atypical antipsychotics should be considered:

            • There is better evidence for risperidone and quetiapine.

            • ii.Limited data for: olanzapine, aripiprazole, perospirone.

            • Avoid: clozapine, ziprasidone.

        d. Discontinue dopamine antagonist agents' use if QTc increases to >25% of baseline or >500 msec.

    ii. Alpha-2 agonist agents (to address the NE excess) (e.g., dexmedetomidine, clonidine, guanfacine)

        a. Consider changing primary sedative agents from GABA-ergic agents (e.g., propofol or midazolam) to an alpha-2 agent (e.g., dexmedetomidine), starting at 0.4 mcg/kg/hr, then titrate dose every 20 minutes to targeted RASS goal.

    iii. Anticonvulsant and other agents with glutamate antagonism or Ca+ Ch modulation (e.g., VPA, gabapentin, amantadine, memantine).

I. Consider the use of NMDA-receptor blocking agents, to minimize glutamate-induced neuronal injury (e.g., amantadine, memantine), particularly in cases of TBI and CVA.

J. G. In case of hypoactive delirium:

    i. Evidence suggests that DA antagonists may still have a place, given the excess DA theory.

        a. If haloperidol is used, recommended doses are in the very low range (i.e., 0.25–1.0 mg/24 hr). This is usually given as a single nighttime dose, just before sundown.

        b. If an atypical is preferred, consider an agent with low sedation (i.e., risperidone, aripiprazole).

    ii. In cases of extreme psychomotor retardation or catatonic features, in the absence of agitation or psychosis, consider the use of psychostimulant agents (e.g., methylphenidate, dextroamphetamine, modafinil) or conventional dopamine agonists (e.g., bromocriptine, amantadine, memantine).

(Modified from Maldonado, 2008a, 2009, 2011)

4. Treatment or correction of underlying medical problems and potentially reversible factors (e.g., correction of electrolyte imbalances, infection, end organ failure, sleep deprivation, pain, metabolic and endocrinological disturbances, substance or medication intoxication or withdrawal); and

5. Treatment of all forms of delirium (with pharmacological and nonpharmacological approaches).

We advocate an integrative approach that incorporates input and collaboration among all pertinent medical teams, including psychosomatic medicine, critical care, internal medicine, surgery, neurology, nursing, respiratory therapy, physical therapy, and occupational therapy teams, which we like to call the "CNS pharmacotherapy algorithm" (see Figure 41.22) (Maldonado, 2008a, 2011, 2014). The idea is to optimize patient comfort (i.e., adequate sedation), minimize pain (i.e., adequate analgesia), prevent or treat delirium, restore an adequate sleep–wake pattern, begin physical mobilization as early as possible, improve cognitive recovery, and return to baseline functional level as soon as medically possible. Others

have found psychiatric consultations to be superior to a multidisciplinary geriatric team approach in treating individuals with depression and delirium (Cole, Fenton, et al., 1991).

The recognition of patients at risk begins with knowledge of your patient's characteristics; an assessment of the predisposing and precipitating medical risk factors to which your patient is, or may be, exposed (Table 41.2); and being acquainted with the modifiable and nonmodifiable risk factors for that particular patient or patient population (Table 41.3). Finally, certain medical conditions and surgical procedures are more likely to be associated with the development of delirium than others. It is likely that a particular patient's odds of developing delirium are associated with the interactions among these conditions. These have been discussed in detail elsewhere (Maldonado, 2008a, 2014).

Prevention techniques have been found to be rather effective, especially when targeted to patients at high risk for developing delirium. There is a whole host of pharmacological and nonpharmacological techniques available. It is important that providers carefully consider the potential side effects versus the benefits associated with effective delirium prevention.

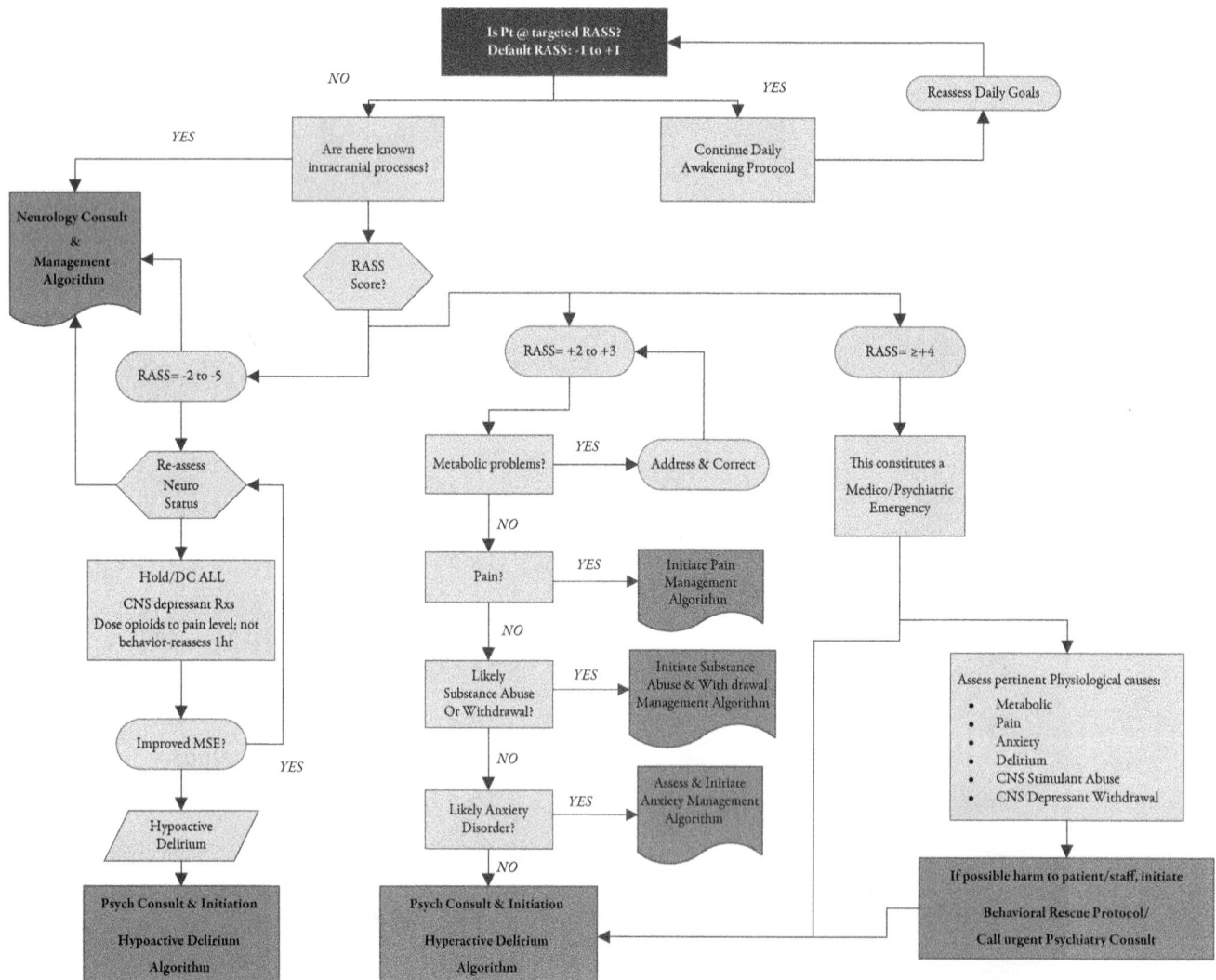

Figure 41.22 CNS Pharmacotherapy Model. (Adapted from Maldonado, 2008a, 2011, 2014)

The early recognition and prompt treatment of delirium is of utmost importance, not only because of issues of safety for patient and staff, but also because of the serious negative consequences of no treatment or delayed treatment. In fact, a recent study demonstrated that patients whose delirium treatment was delayed were more frequently mechanically ventilated (50.0% vs. 22.3%; $p = 0.012$), had more nosocomial infections (including pneumonia) ($p < 0.05$), and had a higher mortality rate ($p < 0.001$) (see Figure 41.23) than patients whose treatment was promptly started (Heymann et al., 2010). These data suggest that a delay in initiating delirium therapy may be associated with increased morbidity and mortality.

The most important aspects of adequate surveillance and early detection include knowledge about the condition and presenting symptoms (of all motor forms) and maintaining a high level of suspicion, especially in populations at risk. There are several surveillance tools and techniques (discussed earlier in this chapter) that can be used to efficiently screen subjects, especially those at greatest risk. Adequate training of medical personnel at all levels is paramount. Surveillance should be effectively implemented by all practitioners.

Once diagnosed, adequate management of delirium includes the following steps:

1. Management of the behavioral and psychiatric manifestations and symptoms to prevent the patient from self-harm or harming of others (e.g., use of tranquilizing agents to manage agitation);

2. Treatment or correction of underlying medical problems and potentially reversible factors (e.g., correction of electrolyte imbalances, infection, end organ failure, sleep deprivation, pain, metabolic and endocrinological disturbances, substance or medication intoxication or withdrawal); and

3. Correction of the neurochemical derangement (triggered by the underlying cause) which leads to the behavioral manifestations of delirium (see Table 41.7).

NONPHARMACOLOGICAL MANAGEMENT STRATEGIES

Nineteen studies have been published on nonpharmacological prevention strategy in the non-ICU environment (see Table 41.10). The original study suggesting that nonpharmacological approaches may be of use was a nonrandomized clinical trial, where hospitalized elderly patients were assessed for manifestations of delirium in response to the correction of environmental factors commonly associated with increased risk for delirium (Inouye et al., 1999). The multicomponent protocol consisted of simple techniques applied by the hospital staff, including reorientation, appropriate cognitive stimulation three times a day, the implementation of a nonpharmacological sleep protocol to help normalize patient's sleep–wake cycle, early mobilization after surgery or extubation, timely removal of catheters and restraints, correction of sensory deficiencies (i.e., by eyeglasses and hearing aids), and early correction of dehydration and electrolyte abnormalities. As a result of these environmental manipulations, they observed an astonishing 40% reduction in the risk of delirium (see Figure 41.24). This landmark work was preceded by two negative studies and followed by seven positive and five negative ones. Among the positive studies, there were three positive randomized clinical trials, and these are condensed in Table 41.11. They were all conducted among elderly orthopedic patients, and all found that the implementation of nonpharmacological multicomponent interventions led to a reduction in the occurrence of delirium and fewer medical complications in the intervention groups (Marcantonio, Flacker, 2001; Vidan, Serra, Moreno, Riquelme, & Ortiz, 2005; Lundstrom et al., 2007). Given the findings reported by others, a multicomponent approach has been developed that targets identified, treatable contributing factors and addresses them early on: the Hospital Elder Life Program (Inouye & Charpentier, 1996; Inouye, Bogardus, et al., 1999). This program involves the implementation, by an interdisciplinary team, of targeted interventions for known risk factors (i.e., cognitive impairment, sleep deprivation, immobility, dehydration, vision or hearing impairment) for cognitive decline in the elderly.

More recently, a meta-analysis of published studies has found that, although the multicomponent interventions appeared to be effective in preventing delirium among postoperative hip replacement patients, the intervention made no difference in a number of important secondary measures, including discharge location or post-discharge dependency, length of hospital stay ($p = 0.12$), or mortality rate ($p = 0.77$) between intervention and control groups (Holroyd-Leduc,

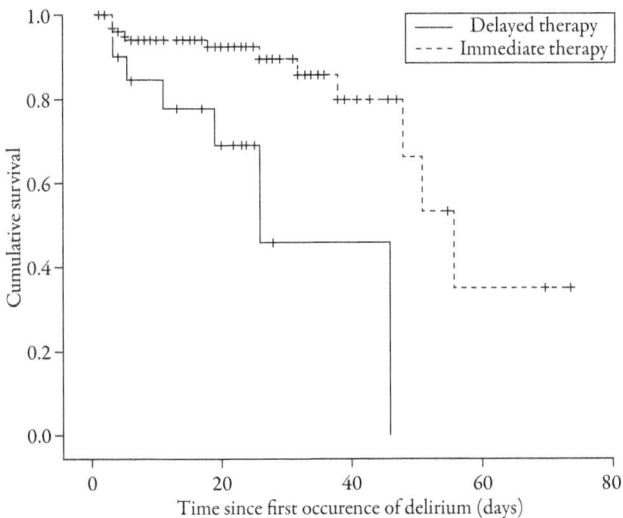

Figure 41.23 Survival Estimates for Delirious ICU Patients with Immediate or Delayed Delirium Treatment. Kaplan–Meier survival estimates for 184 ICU patients with delirium treated within 24 hours of diagnosis (immediate therapy group) and 20 patients in whom delirium treatment started > 24 hours after diagnosis (delayed therapy group); the delayed therapy group showed a lower probability of surviving until ICU discharge than the immediate therapy group (vertical markers show censorship points). There was a significantly higher risk of death in the delayed therapy group versus the immediate therapy group (log rank test, *P < 0.001*; Breslow test, *P = 0.013*). (Heymann et al., 2010)

Table 41.10 NONPHARMACOLOGICAL PREVENTION STRATEGY STUDIES IN THE NON-ICU ENVIRONMENT

STUDY (N = 19)	POPULATION	INTERVENTION	DELIRIUM DEFINITION	DELIRIUM INCIDENCE % CONTROL	DELIRIUM INCIDENCE % INTERVENTION	P VALUE
Schindler et al., 1989 RCT, $n = 33$	CABG	NP—peri-op Psych intervention vs. usual care	DSM-III	0 (0/17)	12.5 (2/16)	ns
Wanich et al., 1992 NRCT, $n = 235$	Gen IM elderly patients	NP—nursing intervention for elderly hospitalized patients vs. usual care	DSM-III	22 (22/100)	19 (26/135)	$p = 0.61$
Inouye et al., 1999 NRCT, $n = 852$	Gen IM elderly patients	NP—multi-component intervention vs. usual care	CAM	15 (64/426)	9.9 (42/426)	$p = 0.02$
Millisen et al., 2001 NRCT, $n = 120$	Traumatic hip Fx Sx repair	NP—multi-component vs. usual care	CAM	23.3 (14/60)	20 (12/60)	$p = 0.82$
Marcantonio et al., 2001 RCT, $n = 126$	Elderly pts. after Hip Fx Sx	NP—multi-component intervention vs. usual care	CAM	50 (32/64)	32 (20/62)	$p = 0.04$
Tabet et al., 2005 NRCT, $n = 250$	Gen IM elderly patients	NP—Staff education vs. usual care	Single assessment psychiatrist	19.5 (25/128)	9.8 (12/122)	$p = 0.034$
Wong et al., 2005 Pre- and post-eval	Traumatic hip Fx Sx repair	NP—multi-component vs. usual care	CAM	35.7 (10/28)	12.7 (9/71)	$p = 0.012$
Vidan et al., 2005 RCT, $n = 319$	Elderly pts. after Hip Fx Sx	NP—multi-component intervention vs. usual care	CAM	45.2 (70/155)	61.7 (100/164)	$p = 0.003$ For ≥1 major complications
Lundstrom et al., 2007 RCT, $n = 199$	Elderly pts. after Hip Fx Sx	NP—multi-component intervention vs. usual care	Organic Brain Syndrome Scale (OBSs)	75.3 (73/97)	54.9 (56/102)	$p = 0.003$
(Caplan & Harper, 2007) Pre–post eval, $n = 37$	Geriatric ward	NP—usual care vs. volunteer-mediated intervention (Inouye style)	CAM	38.1 (8/21)	6.3 (1/16)	$p = 0.032$
Taguchi et al., 2007 RCT, $n = 11$	Esophageal CA subjects	Normalization of their natural circadian rhythm by light therapy	NEECHAM scale	40 (2/5)	16 (1/6)	$P = 0.014$
Benedict, Hazelett, et al., 2009 NRCT, $n = 65$	Acute Care for Elders (ACE) units	NP—Delirium prevention protocol vs. usual care	Modified NEECHAM scale	[3.24]	[3.76]	$p = 0.368$
Schweickert et al., 2009 RCT, $n = 104$	MICU	Early exercise and mobilization (PT & OT) at daily sedation interruption vs. sedation interruption	CAM-ICU	Return to independence by D/H: 35% Delirium duration: 4 days	Return to independence by D/H: 59% Delirium duration: 2 days	$pp = 0.0202$

Study	Population	Intervention	Assessment tool	Pre-implementation incidence	Post-implementation incidence	p
Holroyd-Leduc et al., 2010 NRCT, $n = 134$	Traumatic hip Fx Sx repair	NP—multi-component delirium strategies	CAM	33 (23/70)	31 (20/64)	$p = 0.84$
Holroyd-Leduc et al., 2010 Meta-analysis, 3 studies ($n = 489$)		Comprehensive geriatric assessment and multi-component interventions targeted at precipitants of delirium	CAM (2) Organic Brain Syndrome Scale (1)			*The multicomponent interventions for the management of delirium had:* • *No effect on mortality (summary RR 1.08, 95% CI 0.81–1.44; p for heterogeneity = 0.77).* • *No effect on length of stay (summary weighted mean difference 3.25 days, 95% CI -2.85 to 9.34 days; p for heterogeneity =0.12)* • There was no impact on post-discharge dependency, function, or the need for institutional care.
Björkelund, Hommel, et al., 2010 NRCT, $n = 263$	Elderly hip Fx repair	NP—multi-component delirium strategies	OBS Scale	34 (45/132)	22 (29/131)	$p = 0.096$
Colombo et al., 2012; $n = 314$;	All patients admitted to mixed (med/surg) ICU over a year	NP—patients underwent both a reorientation strategy and environmental, acoustic, and visual stimulation. Study compared pts. in observation arm (control) vs. intervention arm	CAM-ICU	35.5 (60/170)	22 (31/144)	$p = 0.020$
Gagnon et al., 2012, randomized delirium prevention trial; $n = 1516$	Palliative care patients, in 2 cancer centers	NP—multi-component administered to patient and family education vs. usual care	Confusion rating scale (CRS)	43.9 (370/842)	49.1 (330/674)	$P = 0.045$
Martinez et al., 2012 $n = 287$	Older adults in gen medicine ward	Randomized to receive a multi-component management protocol, delivered by family members (144 patients) or standard management (143 patients).	CAM	13.3 (19/143)	5.6 (8kal/144)	$P = 0.027$

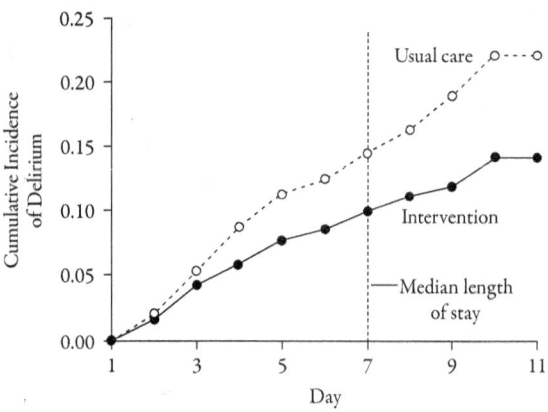

Figure 41.24 A MultiComponent Intervention to Prevent Delirium in Hospitalized Older Patients. (Inouye et al., 1999)

had no effect on the primary outcome, overall delirium incidence ($p = 0.66$); and, similarly, it had no effect on secondary outcomes of delirium severity, total delirious days, or duration of the first delirium episode (Gagnon, Allard, Gagnon, Merette, & Tardif, 2012).

Finally, a study examined the administration of nonprofessional, family-provided multicomponent intervention among high-risk elderly patients admitted to a medicine ward (Martinez, Tobar, Beddings, Vallejo, & Fuentes, 2012). The intervention consisted of educating family members about the clinical features and prognostic implications of delirium, plus the usual content of the traditional multicomponent intervention, but fully administered by family members. They found a significant reduction in the occurrence of delirium in the intervention group ($p = 0.027$). It is unclear why the multicomponent protocol yielded no results when implemented by the nursing staff in a "real world" scenario, but a possible explanation is that the average medicosurgical unit may not have the same nurse-to-patient ratio as research units, making the implementation of the protocol challenging. Therefore, an approach that combines the best of all available protocols and that takes into consideration available resources and limitations of each clinical setting may work best.

Of significance, a study of mechanically ventilated, critically ill patients used a combination of early physical and occupational therapy during periods of daily interruption of sedation to demonstrate a significantly greater return to independent functional status ($p = 0.02$), shorter duration of delirium ($p = 0.02$), and more ventilator-free days ($p = 0.05$) (Schweickert

Khandwala, & Sink, 2010). A separate study on the same population and by the same researcher, but this one conducted in a nonresearch environment, found that the intervention had no effect on the overall delirium rate ($p = 0.84$) and no significant difference on secondary measures (i.e., mean length of hospital stay), falls, or discharge to long-term care facilities (Holroyd-Leduc et al., 2010). Finally, a large study ($n = 1,516$) followed patients from admission to death at seven palliative care centers and compared usual care versus a nonpharmacological delirium-preventive intervention. The study found that the multicomponent preventive intervention

Table 41.11 SELECTED NONPHARMACOLOGICAL RCT-PREVENTION INTERVENTION STUDIES

STUDY AUTHORS; TYPE; SIZE	STUDY DETAILS	FINDINGS
Marcantonio et al., 2001 RCT, $n = 126$	Studied the effectiveness of proactive geriatric consultation compared to usual care in reducing delirium in patients 65 and older admitted emergently for surgical repair of hip fracture.	While there were not statistical differences between intervention and control groups regarding baseline measures and characteristics, the study found a reduction in the occurrence of delirium in the intervention group (32%) compared to usual care (50%) ($P = 0.04$). There was an even greater reduction in cases of "severe delirium," occurring in 12% of intervention patients and 29% of usual-care patients. Despite this reduction in delirium, length of stay did not significantly differ between intervention and usual care.
Vidan et al., 2005 RCT, $n = 319$	Studied patients were randomly assigned to daily multidisciplinary geriatric intervention or usual care during hospitalization in the acute phase of hip fracture.	The study showed that intervention subjects experienced shorter hospital stay (median length 16 vs. 18 days) ($P = 0.06$); lower in-hospital mortality (0.6% vs. 5.8%, $P = 0.03$) and lower rate of major medical complications (45.2% vs. 61.7%, $P = 0.003$). Overall, after adjustment for confounding variables, the geriatric intervention was associated with a 45% lower probability of death or major complications. More patients in the geriatric intervention group achieved a partial recovery at 3 months (57% vs. 44%, $P = 0.03$), but there were no difference between groups at 6 and 12 months assessments.
Lundström et al., 2007 RCT, $n = 199$	Studied randomly assigned elderly patients after femoral neck fracture repair to postoperative care in a specialized geriatric ward (i.e., staff education focusing on the assessment, prevention, and treatment of delirium and associated complications) or a conventional orthopedic ward.	Patients in the intervention group experience less postoperative delirium (54.9% vs. 75.3%, $p = 0.003$); those who did experience delirium did so for a shorter duration compared with controls (5.0 ± 7.1 days vs. 10.2 ± 13.3 days, $p = 0.009$). Patients in the intervention group suffered from fewer complications (e.g., decubitus ulcers, urinary tract infections, nutritional complications, sleeping problems, and falls) and shorter hospital stays (28.0 ± 17.9 days vs. 38.0 ± 40.6 days, $p = 0.028$).

et al., 2009). This is the first randomized, nonpharmacological intervention study shown to reduce ICU delirium. Others have found similar results (i.e., lower total amount benzodiazepine use, higher level of functional mobility, and reduction in delirium rates) by combining sedation reduction and early mobilization with physical rehabilitation (Needham & Korupolu, 2010). It is likely that the minimization of offending agents (e.g., sedatives), along with early mobility, may have something to do with the decreased rate of delirium among this cohort. Previously, I have suggested an approach that incorporates nonpharmacological and pharmacological approaches to the prevention and treatment of delirium, which is summarized in Box 41.6 but expanded elsewhere (Maldonado, 2008a, 2009, 2011). Given the significant adverse consequences of delirium, the primary goal should be prevention, particularly in populations at high risk. Key among them is minimizing the detrimental effects of prolonged and uninterrupted sedation. Therefore, we recommend that sedation be targeted to a predetermined goal using sedation scales such as the Richmond Agitation Sedation Scale (RASS; see Sessler, et al., 2002). As previously noted, daily awakening and sedation holidays are highly recommended. These will allow patients to awaken; then, if still needed, sedation should be restarted at the lowest needed level—again targeting a predetermined sedation level. Certain sedative agents are preferred to others, given pharmacological and pharmacodynamic qualities; and some appear to have less deliriogenic potential than others (Maldonado, van der Starre, Wysong, & Block, 2004; Pandharipande, Pun et al., 2007; Maldonado, 2008a, 2009, 2011; Riker et al., 2009). Therefore, dexmedetomidine may be the preferred choice when clinically indicated and tolerated, followed by propofol, and last by midazolam. Similarly, some analgesic agents may be better at preventing or controlling delirium. For example, despite its faster onset of action, fentanyl's clearance is much slower than hydromorphone; thus it tends to accumulate, and this may be problematic (see Figure 41.25). Therefore, we prefer the use of hydromorphone as the baseline agent of choice for pain management and sedation supplementation and limit the use of fentanyl for rapid initiation of analgesia and as a rescue agent.

More recently, a randomized study suggested that not using sedation, compared to the standard treatment with sedation and a daily wake-up trial, may further reduce the

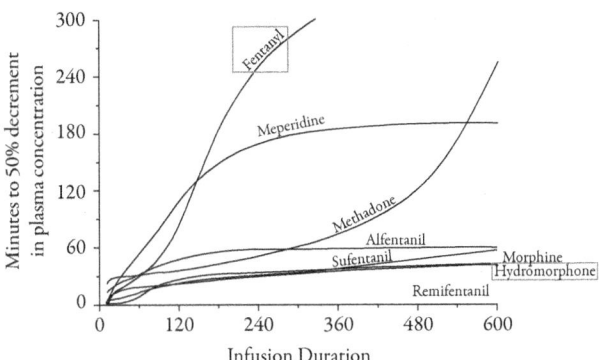

Figure 41.25 Minutes to 50% decrement in plasma concentration of commonly used opioid agents.

time patients require mechanical ventilation, shorten the length of the patient's stay in the intensive care unit, and decrease the overall hospital length of stay (Strom & Toft, 2011), thus providing further evidence that the use of sedative drugs should be reduced. Patients should be mobilized as early as possible, and individual patient sedative needs should be evaluated on a daily basis to minimize the untoward effects of these agents and optimize the care of each individual patient.

Given the high rate of underdiagnosed and missed cases, the routine use of assessment scales or diagnostic interviews by properly trained personnel will facilitate timely treatment and prevention of complications of delirium. Early involvement of a medical-psychiatric team is valuable for both prevention and early intervention. An active search for possible etiologies of delirium must first rule out the common causes of the syndrome (see Table 41.2). This must include a review of all medications and identification, and possible discontinuation of agents with high deliriogenic potential (see Table 41.4). Appropriate diagnostic tests and assays should be ordered and reviewed in a timely fashion and all abnormal findings addressed accordingly.

Conduct an inventory of all pharmacological agents that have been administered to the patient. Any medication or agent known to cause delirium (see Table 41.4) or to have high anticholinergic potential (see Table 41.5) should be discontinued if possible; if not, a suitable less anticholinergic alternative should be substituted.

Immobilizing lines and devices (e.g., chest tubes, IV lines, bladder catheters) should be removed as early as possible. Similarly, physical restraints should be avoided and eliminated as soon as it is safe to do. More importantly, early mobilization (e.g., daily interruption of sedation, minimization of restraint use, early physical and occupational therapy) has proven to be a key factor in minimizing delirium and improving the odds of returning to independent functioning upon discharge home (Schweickert et al., 2009).

Early correction of sensory deficits should be undertaken. That is, eyeglasses and hearing aids should be replaced or fitted (if the patient was not using them before the hospitalization) as soon as possible. This will allow patients to familiarize themselves with the environment and reorient themselves early on. It will also minimize the occurrence of misperceptions or misinterpretation of environmental cues and stimuli. Environmental isolation should be minimized if possible. Family members and loved ones should be encouraged to visit and provide a familiar and friendly environment, as well as provide appropriate orientation and stimulation to patients, especially those with baseline cognitive deficits. Dehydration and electrolyte abnormalities should be corrected as quickly and safely as possible. Malnutrition should be corrected, unless the patient is end-stage and their delirium is a pre-terminal phenomenon. In that situation, the decision to use a feeding tube, for example, would be a personal decision that different patients and families would make differently.

For intubated, sedated ICU patients, the approach must include judicious management of sedative and pain management agents in order to allow for early extubation, minimize time in bed, and limit the amount of potentially deliriogenic agents a patient is exposed to. Daily cessation of sedative protocols combined with daily spontaneous breathing trials and early mobilization (through physical and occupational therapy) have resulted in a significant decrease in the duration of mechanical ventilation, the length of stay in intensive care, and the number of days patients experienced acute brain dysfunction, compared with control groups (Kress, Pohlman, O'Connor, & Hall, 2000; Kress et al., 2003; Girard et al., 2008; Schweickert et al., 2009; Needham, Korupolu, et al., 2010).

Finally, environmental manipulations to normalize the sleep–wake cycle may be considered, from reducing noise levels and decreasing nighttime tests and procedures to increasing the amount of natural light during daytime hours. Early correction of sleep disturbance, preferably by nonpharmacological means, should be attempted.

Some have advocated the use of bright light therapy (similar to that used for the treatment of seasonal affective disorder) as an alternative to medication agents but despite the logic behind this approach, very little evidence for it exists. A small pilot study demonstrated that bright light therapy (5000 lux applied for 2 hours in the morning) led to a significant difference ($P = 0.014$) in the incidence of delirium (Taguchi, Yano, & Kido, 2007). Yet there were serious methodological problems with this study, including a very small sample, lack of blinding, and late initiation of the intervention (after extubation rather than immediately after surgery). A second, larger study ($n = 228$) conducted in a geriatric monitoring unit compared bright light therapy (2000–3000 lux; 6–10 pm daily) against placebo. The study found that among those randomized to bright light therapy, there were significant improvements in modified Barthel Index (MBI) scores, especially for the hyperactive and mixed delirium subtypes ($P < 0.05$); significant improvements on the DRS sleep–wake disturbance subscore, for all delirium subtypes; and improvements in the mean total sleep time (from 6.4 hours to 7.7) ($P < 0.05$) and length of first sleep bout (SB; 6.0 compared with 5.3 hours) ($P < 0.05$), with decreased mean number of SBs and awakenings when compared to those in the placebo group (Chong, Tan, Tay, Wong, & Ancoli-Israel, 2013).

The National Institute for Health and Clinical Excellence (NICE) provided a set of guidelines containing 13 specific recommendations for the prevention of delirium in elderly at-risk patients (O'Mahony, Murthy et al., 2011). They are mostly based on the correction of modifiable factors that may precipitate delirium, and the implementation of the multicomponent intervention package. The full version of these recommendations can be found at their website: http://guidance.nice.org.uk/CG103/Guidance/pdf/English. Similarly, the Society of Critical Care Medicine has developed pain, agitation, and delirium guidelines, promoted mobility to improve care of critically ill patients, and has developed tools to facilitate and rapidly implement the translation of guideline care recommendations into practice (Davidson et al., 2013).

PHARMACOLOGICAL MANAGEMENT STRATEGIES

It cannot be overstated that the "definitive treatment" of delirium is the accurate identification and treatment of its underlying cause(s). Nevertheless, pharmacological intervention with various psychoactive agents is often needed to help manage agitated patients and for the correction of the neurotransmitter derangements associated with delirium symptoms. Of note, no pharmacological agent has received Food and Drug Administration (FDA) approval for the treatment of delirium.

In an attempt to "first, do no harm," we should first identify all agents that may contribute to, exacerbate, or perpetuate delirium. Chief among these are anticholinergic substances and GABA-ergic agents (Box 41.2). As described above, all such agents (e.g., benzodiazepines, propofol) may cause or aggravate delirium and its behavioral manifestations (Marcantonio et al., 1994; Ely et al., 2001; Pandharipande, Shintani, et al., 2006). The use of benzodiazepines in the management of delirium should be limited to (a) patients experiencing delirium related to the withdrawal from a CNS-depressant agent (e.g., alcohol, barbiturates, benzodiazepines), or (b) when other more appropriate agents have failed and the level of agitation and need for behavioral control outweighs the potentially detrimental effects of benzodiazepines. Following the same principle, we should avoid the use of opioid agents for behavioral control of agitated patients and use these agents only for pain management, as opioids have been implicated in the development of delirium in many patient populations (Morrison et al., 2003; Centeno, Sanz, & Bruera, 2004; Morita et al., 2005; Fong et al., 2006; Vaurio et al., 2006; Gaudreau et al., 2007, Vella-Brincat & Macleod, 2007; Wang et al., 2007). A summary of a comprehensive delirium management algorithm can be found in Figure 41.26.

Pharmacological management strategies have mostly been limited to the use of antipsychotic agents, acetyl cholinesterase inhibitors, and sedative-hypnotic agents. In this section, I will address possible pharmacological interventions based on the neurotransmitter being targeted. In general, delirious patients have an excess of dopamine, norepinephrine, glutamate, and hyperactivity of calcium channels (Ca+ Ch); reduced levels of acetylcholine and melatonin; and variable levels of serotonin, histamine, and gamma-aminobutyric acid, depending on the type and cause of delirium. We will tailor the discussion regarding pharmacological prophylaxis and treatment based on these assumptions. Studies will be discussed in order of publication. In the only published set of guidelines for sedation management of critically ill adults, the Society of Critical Care Medicine recommended haloperidol as "the preferred agent for the treatment of delirium in critically ill patients" (Jacobi, Fraser, et al., 2002). Accordingly, haloperidol is used by about 78%–80% of intensivists as the standard pharmacological agent to manage delirium in the ICU, while novel agents, the second-generation antipsychotics, are gaining popularity for delirium management, are now being used by 35%–40% of ICU physicians (Patel, Gambrell, et al., 2009; MacSweeney, Barber, et al., 2010). A more recent

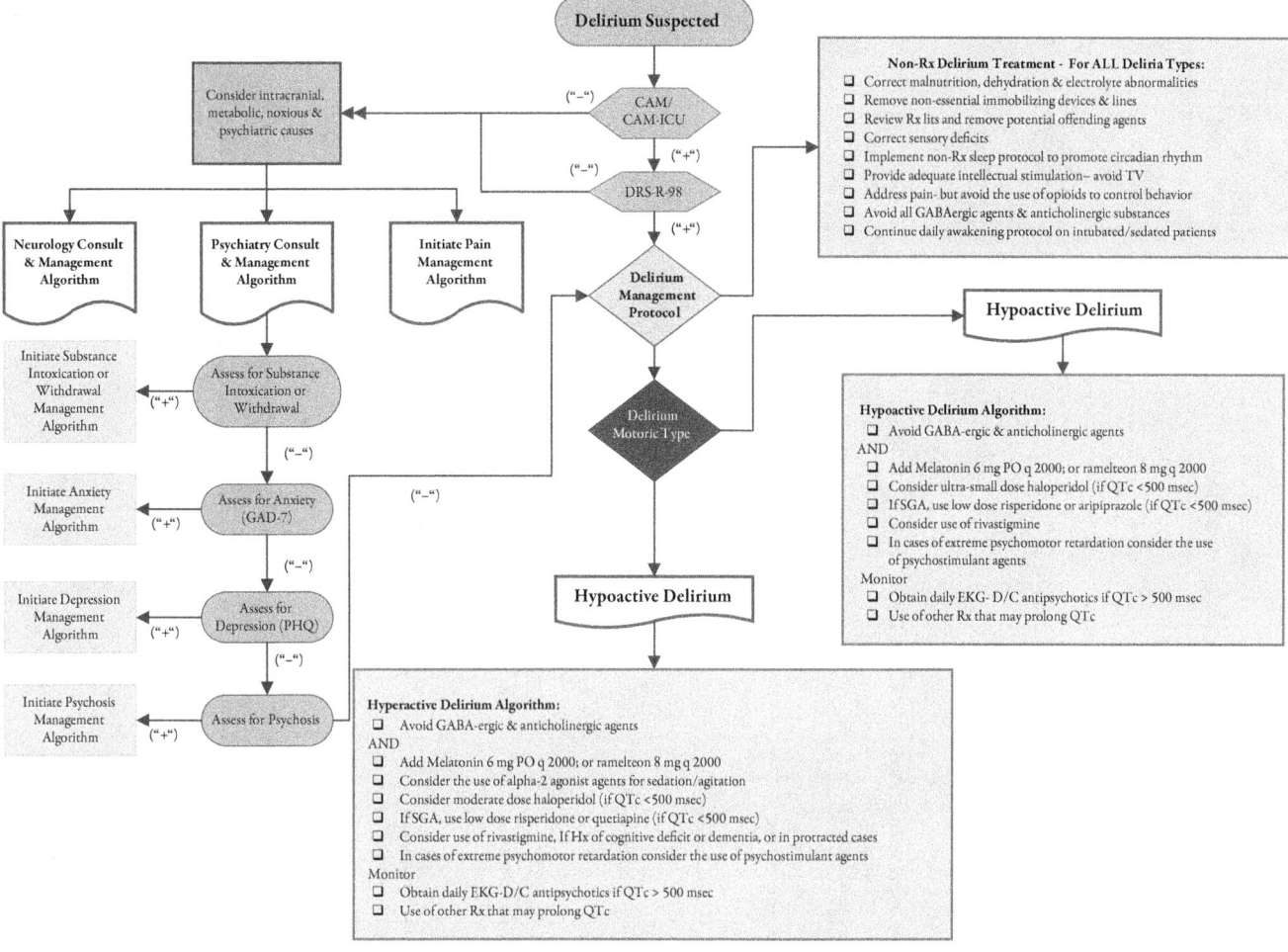

COMPREHENSIVE DELIRIUM ALGORITHM

Delirium Suspected

Consider intracranial, metabolic, noxious & psychiatric causes

CAM/ CAM-ICU

DRS-R-98

Non-Rx Delirium Treatment - For ALL Deliria Types:
- ☐ Correct malnutrition, dehydration & electrolyte abnormalities
- ☐ Remove non-essential immobilizing devices & lines
- ☐ Review Rx lits and remove potential offending agents
- ☐ Correct sensory deficits
- ☐ Implement non-Rx sleep protocol to promote circadian rhythm
- ☐ Provide adequate intellectual stimulation– avoid TV
- ☐ Address pain- but avoid the use of opioids to control behavior
- ☐ Avoid all GABAergic agents & anticholinergic substances
- ☐ Continue daily awakening protocol on intubated/sedated patients

Neurology Consult & Management Algorithm

Psychiatry Consult & Management Algorithm

Initiate Pain Management Algorithm

Delirium Management Protocol

Delirium Motoric Type

Hypoactive Delirium

Initiate Substance Intoxication or Withdrawal Management Algorithm

Assess for Substance Intoxication or Withdrawal

Hypoactive Delirium Algorithm:
- ☐ Avoid GABA-ergic & anticholinergic agents

AND
- ☐ Add Melatonin 6 mg PO q 2000; or ramelteon 8 mg q 2000
- ☐ Consider ultra-small dose haloperidol (if QTc <500 msec)
- ☐ If SGA, use low dose risperidone or aripiprazole (if QTc <500 msec)
- ☐ Consider use of rivastigmine
- ☐ In cases of extreme psychomotor retardation consider the use of psychostimulant agents

Monitor
- ☐ Obtain daily EKG- D/C antipsychotics if QTc > 500 msec
- ☐ Use of other Rx that may prolong QTc

Initiate Anxiety Management Algorithm

Assess for Anxiety (GAD-7)

Initiate Depression Management Algorithm

Assess for Depression (PHQ)

Hypoactive Delirium

Initiate Psychosis Management Algorithm

Assess for Psychosis

Hyperactive Delirium Algorithm:
- ☐ Avoid GABA-ergic & anticholinergic agents

AND
- ☐ Add Melatonin 6 mg PO q 2000; or ramelteon 8 mg q 2000
- ☐ Consider the use of alpha-2 agonist agents for sedation/agitation
- ☐ Consider moderate dose haloperidol (if QTc <500 msec)
- ☐ If SGA, use low dose risperidone or quetiapine (if QTc <500 msec)
- ☐ Consider use of rivastigmine, If Hx of cognitive deficit or dementia, or in protracted cases
- ☐ In cases of extreme psychomotor retardation consider the use of psychostimulant agents

Monitor
- ☐ Obtain daily EKG-D/C antipsychotics if QTc > 500 msec
- ☐ Use of other Rx that may prolong QTc

Figure 41.26 Comprehensive Delirium Algorithm. *Source:* (Maldonado, 2008a, 2011)

"post-publication perspective" of practice guidelines added no new information about pharmacological agents for the management of delirium in the ICU, but emphasized the benefits of early detection and patient mobilization. It is important to point out that soon after the publication of these perspectives a number of significant studies were published, all conclusively demonstrating the delirium-prophylactic benefits of antipsychotic agents in at-risk populations, which will be discussed in the next section.

Of note, no pharmacological agent has received FDA approval for the prevention of delirium.

Dopamine Excess

Dopamine Antagonists for Delirium Prevention

There are very few control studies on the efficacy of antipsychotic agents for the prevention of delirium, yet most studies suggest a positive effect (see Table 41.12). The first randomized controlled trial compared haloperidol to placebo in at-risk, elderly orthopedic patients (Kaneko, Jianhui, et al., 1999). The incidence of delirium was significantly lower in

the treatment group (10.5% vs. 32.5%; p <.05). Similarly, the intensity and duration of postoperative delirium were more severe and lasted longer in the control group.

The first double-blind, randomized, placebo control studies (DBRPCT) compared haloperidol to placebo, also in at-risk elderly orthopedic patients (Kalisvaart, de Jonghe, et al., 2005). Subjects received oral haloperidol 0.5 mg/d up to 72 hours preoperatively and then until the third postoperative day. The study found that prophylactic haloperidol use did not alter the incidence of postoperative delirium when compared with placebo (15.1 vs.16.5%; $p = ns$). Nevertheless, it did have a positive effect on the severity (the mean highest DRS-R-98 score ±SD was 14.4 ± 3.4 vs. 18.4 ± 4.3; P <.001) and duration (5.4 vs. 11.8 days; P <.001) of delirium and shortened the length of hospital stay (mean number of days in the hospital was 17.1±11.1 vs. 22.6 ± 16.7; *P <.001*).

Many additional studies have followed, all with positive findings. A study of patients undergoing cardiac surgery with cardiopulmonary bypass (CPB), randomly assigned to receive either 1 mg of risperidone or placebo sublingually as soon as they regained consciousness postoperatively,

Table 41.12 ANTIPSYCHOTIC AGENTS FOR PREVENTION OF DELIRIUM

STUDY (N = 9)	POPULATION	INTERVENTION	DELIRIUM DEFINITION	DELIRIUM INCIDENCE% CONTROL/INTERVENTION		P-VALUE
Kaneko et al., 1999; RPCT	GI surgery	Prophylaxis haloperidol vs. PBO IV postoperatively for 5 days	DSM-III-R	32.5	10.5	p < 0.05
Kalisvaart et al., 2005 DBRPCT, n = 430	Elderly hip-replacement Sx	PBO vs. haloperidol 1.5 mg/d started preop, continued for up to 3 days postop.	DSM-IV CAM DRS-R98	16.5 (36/216)	15.1 (32/212)	p = 0.91
Prakanrattana & Prapaitrakool, 2007 DBRPCT, n = 126	Cardiac Sx under CPB	PBO vs. sublingual risperidone immediately p-Sx	CAM	31.7 (20/63)	11.1 (7/63)	p = 0.009
Girard et al., 2010* DBRPCT, n = 101	Med/Surg ICU in mechanical ventilation	PBO vs. haloperidol vs. ziprasidone: days alive without delirium or coma; conducted in 6 tertiary medical centers.	CAM-ICU	12.5 [1.2–17.2] days 14.0 [6.0–18.0] days	15.0 [9.1–18.0] days	p = 0.66
Larsen et al. 2010 DBRPCT, n = 495	Elderly elective total joint-replacement	PBO vs. 5 mg of orally disintegrating olanzapine 1-dose pre- and 1-dose post-surgery	DSM-III-R	40.2 (82/204)	14.3 (28/196)	p < 0.001
Wang et al., 2012 DBRPCT, n = 457	Elderly, non-cardiac Sx	PBO vs. HAL (0.5 mg bolus, followed by cont infusion 0.1 mg/hr x 12hrs)	CAM	23.2	15.3	p = 0.031
van den Boogaard et al., 2013, 2013)DBRPCT, n = 476	ICU patients at "high risk"	PBO vs. HAL (1 mg/8 hr.) within 24 hrs. of admission to ICU	CAM-ICU	75	65	P = 0.01
Hirota & Kishi, 2013; Meta-analysis (RCTs), 6 studies, n = 1689	Various clinical settings	Meta-analysis of 6 studies (3 HAL, 1 olanzapine, 2 risperidone) using antipsychotic agent for delirium prophylaxis	Various tools	Sensitivity analysis showed that SGA were superior to PBO (NNT = 4; p < 0.0001), whereas HAL failed to show superiority to PBO		P < 0.00001
Teslyar et al., 2013; Meta-analysis (RCTs); 5 studies, n = 1491	Postoperative elderly patients	Medication administered included haloperidol (3), risperidone (1), and olanzapine (1).	Various tools	The pooled relative risk of the five studies resulted in a 50% reduction in the relative risk of delirium among those receiving antipsychotic medication compared with placebo.		P < 0.01

* Underpowered.

Abbreviations: RPCT=randomized placebo control trial; GI=gastrointestinal; PBO=placebo; DBRPCT=double blind randomized, placebo controlled trial; DSM=Diagnostic and Statistical Manual of Mental Disorders; CAM= Confusion Assessment Method; DRS=Delirium Rating Scale; Sx=surgery; CPB=cardio-pulmonary by-pass machine; ICU=intensive care unit. APA=antipsychotic agent; OLA=olanzapine; HAL=haloperidol; RIS=risperidone demonstrated a significantly lower incidence of postoperative delirium in the risperidone group (11.1% vs. 31.7%; *P = 0.009*) (Prakanrattana & Prapaitrakool, 2007). A study examined the effects of olanzapine pretreatment (5 mg Zydis formulation administered just preoperatively, and again 5 mg administered immediately after surgery upon awakening) to placebo in elderly subjects undergoing orthopedic joint-replacement surgery. The incidence of delirium in the intervention group was significantly lower in the study group compared to placebo (15% vs. 41%; *P < 0.0001*) (Larsen, 2007).

A large (*n* = 457; ages ≥65) postoperative delirium prevention study compared the efficacy and safety of low-dose IV-haloperidol (i.e., 0.5 mg intravenous bolus injection, followed by continuous infusion at a rate of 0.1 mg/hr for 12 hrs vs. placebo) vs. placebo in critically ill patients after noncardiac surgery. The study found the incidence of delirium during the first 7 days after surgery was 15.3% in the haloperidol group vs. 23.2% in the control group (*p* = .031). Other measures also appeared significantly improved: the mean time to onset of delirium and the mean number of delirium-free days were significantly longer (6.2 days [95% CI 5.9–6.4] vs. 5.7 days [95% CI 5.4–6.0]; *p* = .021; and 6.8 ± 0.5 days vs. 6.7 ± 0.8 days; *p* = .027, respectively); the median length of ICU stay was significantly shorter (21.3 hrs [95% CI, 20.3–22.2] vs. 23.0 hrs [95% CI, 20.9–25.1]; *p* = .024) in the haloperidol group than in the control group. There was no significant difference with regard to all-cause 28-day mortality between the two groups (0.9% [2/229] vs. 2.6% [6/228]; *p* = .175). No drug-related side effects were documented (Wang et al., 2012).

Finally, a study assessed the efficacy of haloperidol prophylaxis against delirium in "at risk" ICU patients (*n* = 177) (van den Boogaard, Schoonhoven, van Achterberg, van der Hoeven, & Pickkers, 2013). The results of the intervention were compared to a historical control group and a contemporary group that did not receive haloperidol prophylaxis, mainly due to noncompliance to the protocol, mostly during the implementation phase. The protocol consisted of low-dose haloperidol infusion (i.e., IV-haloperidol 1 mg/8 hr (or a lower dose, for patients ≥80 years), started as soon as patients were identified to be at increased risk, within the 24-hour period after ICU admission. All patients experiencing delirium received therapeutic doses of haloperidol according to the unit's customary protocol. Patient characteristics were comparable between the prevention and the control groups; with the exception of prophylactic haloperidol, as per study protocol. The intervention resulted in a lower delirium incidence (65% vs. 75%, *p* =.01), more delirium-free days (median, 20 days [interquartile range 8 to 27] vs. median 13 days [3 to 27], *p* =.003), fewer ICU readmissions (11% vs. 18%, *p* =.03), and less frequent unplanned removal of tubes/lines (12% vs., 19%, *p* =.02) in the intervention group compared to the control group. Beneficial effects of haloperidol appeared most pronounced in the patients with the highest risk for delirium. Haloperidol was stopped in 12 patients because of QTc-time prolongation (*n* = 9), renal failure (*n* = 1) or suspected neurological side-effects (*n* = 2). No other side effects

were reported, including *torsades de point* (TdP) (van den Boogaard et al., 2013).

Two meta-analyses of studies using dopamine antagonist agents for delirium prophylaxis found that pooled relative risk of published studies suggested a 50% reduction in the relative risk of delirium among those receiving antipsychotic medication compared with placebo (*p* <0.01). The studies suggest that perioperative use of prophylactic dopamine antagonist agents (both typical and second-generation antipsychotics), compared to placebo, may effectively reduce the overall risk of postoperative delirium, thereby potentially reducing mortality, disease burden, length of hospital stay, and associated healthcare costs (Hirota & Kishi, 2013; Teslyar, Stock, et al., 2013). A third meta-analysis, including all postoperative prevention strategies, found that both typical (3 RCTs; *n* = 965; RR = 0.71; 95% CI = 0.54–0.93) and atypical antipsychotics (3 RCTs; *n* = 627; RR = 0.36; 95% CI = 0.26–0.50) decreased delirium occurrence, compared to placebos (Zhang et al., 2013).

Dopamine Antagonists for Delirium Treatment

The literature has long recognized that intravenous neuroleptic agents are the recommended emergency treatment for agitated and mixed type delirium (Adams, Fernandez, & Andersson, 1986; Fernandez, Holmes, Adams, & Kavanaugh, 1988; Sanders, Murray, & Cassem, 1991; Ziehm, 1991; Riker, Fraser, & Cox, 1994; Inouye et al., 1999). Intravenous administration of haloperidol has always been thought superior to oral administration because the IV route has more reliable absorption, even in cases of systemic organ failure. Intravenous haloperidol use has the added advantage of requiring no patient cooperation, thus facilitating its use even in uncooperative and agitated patients. Studies suggest that the IV use of high-potency neuroleptic agents is associated with minimal effects on blood pressure, respiration, and heart rate (Ayd, 1978; Tesar, Murray, & Cassem, 1985; Adams, 1988; Sanders et al., 1991; Riker et al., 1994; Stern, 1994; Segatore & Adams, 2001). And, some have suggested that haloperidol has a lower incidence of extrapyramidal symptoms when administered IV versus orally (7.2% vs. 22.6%; *p* <0.01) (see Figure 41.27) (Sanders, Minnema, & Murray, 1989; Maldonado & Kang, 2003).

Intravenous haloperidol has been identified as the agent of choice for the management of delirious critically ill patients by a

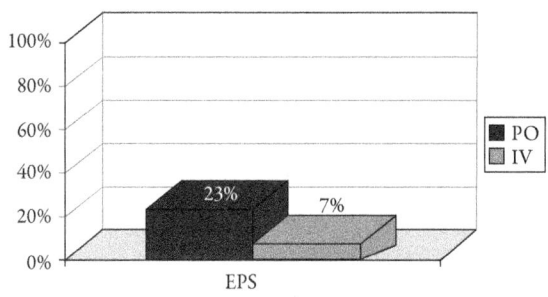

Figure 41.27 Haloperidol Route of Administration and Incidence of EPS. Rate of extrapyramidal symptoms and their association to mode of administration for haloperidol. (Maldonado, 2003)

number of national organizations, including Britain's National Institute for Health and Clinical Excellence (NICE, 2010) the American Psychiatric Association (APA, 1999, 2004) and the Society of Critical Care Medicine (Shapiro et al., 1995; Jacobi et al., 2002). Since then, a "best evidence topic in cardiac surgery" was written according to a structured protocol, addressing the issue of haloperidol safety for critically ill patients (Khasati, Thompson, & Dunning, 2004). Their search included 294 papers and concluded that haloperidol should be considered the first-line drug for agitated patients following cardiac surgery. Of note, in September of 2007, the FDA issued a "black-box" warning for the off-label clinical practice of using IV-haloperidol (FDA, 2007). It is important to remember that haloperidol has never been approved by the FDA for IV use.

Other antipsychotic agents have been studied for the treatment of delirium. Most of these include atypical or second-generation antipsychotic (SGA) agents. Because of the stigma and potential side effects associated with typical antipsychotics, SGAs have being been used at increasing rates over the last few years for the management of psychiatric and behavioral symptoms (e.g., agitation, psychosis, delirium) in medically ill patients. Large studies, particularly head-to-head comparisons between SGAs and more conventional agents (i.e., haloperidol), are lacking; therefore, most clinical practice is derived from case reports and open-label (OL) studies. Following are summaries of the only seven RCTs available; all others are summarized in Table 41.13.

The first study was a DBRCT that compared haloperidol (average. dose 1.4 mg/d) vs. chlorpromazine (average dose 36.0 mg/d) versus lorazepam (avg. dose 4.6 mg/d) among HIV/AIDS patients (Breitbart et al., 1996). Results showed that treatment with either haloperidol or chlorpromazine in relatively low doses resulted in significant improvement in the symptoms of delirium, while no improvement was found in the lorazepam group. Treatment with either neuroleptic was associated with an extremely low prevalence of extrapyramidal side effects; all patients receiving lorazepam, however, developed treatment-limiting adverse effects.

Table 41.13 DOPAMINE ANTAGONIST—ANTIPSYCHOTIC AGENTS AS TREATMENT OF DELIRIUM

STUDY(N = 32)	POPULATION	INTERVENTION	DELIRIUM DEFINITION/ MEASURE OF RESPONSE	RESULTS
Breitbart et al., 1996; DBRCT, *n* = 30	AIDS, medical patients	Haloperidol vs. chlorpromazine vs. lorazepam	DSM-IIIR/DRS	Tx either HAL or CPM resulted in significant improvement in the symptoms of delirium, while no improvement was found in the LOR group. Tx neuroleptic was associated with an extremely low prevalence of EPS, while all patients receiving LOR developed treatment-limiting adverse effects.
Sipahimalani & Masand, 1998; OL, *n* = 22	Med/Surg patients	Haloperidol vs. olanzapine	DRS	Improvement was similar in both groups (mean DRS +SD H = 11.1 ± 7.1; O = 10.3 ± 4.8; *P* = 0.760), with extrapyramidal symptoms found only in haloperidol patients. No side effects in olanzapine group.
Schwartz et al., 2000; Single-blind; *n* = 11	Med/Surg patients	Quetiapine vs. haloperidol— retrospective chart review	DRS	Effectiveness of ³50% in reducing DRS scores. When compared with haloperidol, there was no difference in onset of symptom resolution, duration of treatment, and overall clinical improvement.
Kim et al., 2001; OL, *n* = 20	Med/Surg patients	Olanzapine PO, variable dose	DSM-IV/DRS	50% decrease in Delirium Rating Scale scores (from pre of 20.0 ± 3.6, to post of 9.3 ± 4.6; *P* < 0.01). No side effects, including EPS.
Breitbart et al., 2002; OL, *n* = 79	Hospitalized cancer patients	Olanzapine PO, variable dose	DSM-IV/MDAS	Olanzapine was effective in treating 76% of delirium patients as evidenced by the MDAS; caused excessive sedation in 30% of patients.
Horikawa et al., 2003; OL, *n* = 10	Med/Surg patients	Risperidone PO	DSM-IV/DRS	At a low dose of 1.7 mg/d, on average, risperidone was effective in 80% of patients, and the effect appeared within a few days. Most commonly cited adverse effects included sleepiness (30%) and mild drug-induced Parkinsonism (10%).

(continued)

Table 41.13 (CONTINUED)

STUDY (*N* = 32)	POPULATION	INTERVENTION	DELIRIUM DEFINITION/ MEASURE OF RESPONSE	RESULTS
Sasaki et al., 2003; OL, *n* = 12	Med/Surg patients	Quetiapine PO, flexible doses	DSM-IV/DRS	100% of patients on quetiapine achieved resolution of delirium (mean on day 4.8 ± 3.5 days); no EPS reported.
Kim et al., 2003; OL, *n* = 12	Elderly medical inpatients	Quetiapine PO, flexible doses	DSM-IV/DRS	100% of patients on quetiapine achieved resolution of delirium by day 10 (mean on day 5.9 ± 2.2 days); no EPS reported. Delirium Rating Scale scores along with scores of the Mini-Mental State Examination and Clock Drawing Test continued to improve throughout the 3-month study period.
Liu et al., 2004; retrospective record review, *n* = 77	Med/Surg patients with hyperactive delirium	Risperidone (average dose 1.17±0.76 mg/d) vs. haloperidol (avg. dose 4.25±2.62 mg/d)	DSM-IV/various	Patients treated with haloperidol were younger than patients treated with risperidone ($P < 0.05$). The mean hyperactive syndrome scale score was higher in the haloperidol than that of the risperidone group. The authors found no significant difference in the efficacy or frequency of response rate between haloperidol and risperidone (100% vs. 95%; *p* = *ns*). Patients on risperidone experienced less EPS (7% vs. 69%).
Mittal et al., 2004; OL, *n* = 10	Patients admitted to Med-Surg unit	Risperidone, 0.5 mg PO BID, flexible PRNs	DSM-IV/DRS	Rapid resolution of delirium while receiving low dose risperidone (mean dose 0.75 mg/d); no EPS reported.
Parellada, Baeza, et al., 2004; OL	Prospective, multicenter, observational 7-day study	Risperidone PO	DSM-IV/ DRS PANSS-P MMSE	Risperidone was administered at the time of diagnosis, and treatment was maintained according to clinical response. Found a significant decrease in DRS scores in 90.6% of treated patients and significantly improved all symptoms measured by the scales from baseline to day 7 ($p < 0.0$); only 3% side effects.
Pae, Lee, et al., 2004 OL, *n* = 22	Med/Surg patients	Quetiapine PO	DRS-R9/ CGI8	DRS-R-98 and clinical global scores were significantly reduced by 57.3% and 55.1%, respectively. Quetiapine was effective and safe.
Han et al., 2004; DBRCT, *n* = 28	Med/Surg patients	Haloperidol vs. risperidone, 7 days medication trial	CAM/ DRS MDAS	Both groups showed significant improvement in baseline DRS and MDAS scores with either haloperidol (75%) or risperidone (42%) ($P < 0.05$). There was no significant difference in improvement of DRS ($p = 0.35$) or MDAS ($p = 0.51$) scores, comparing haloperidol with risperidone patients.
Hu et al., 2004; RPCT, *n* = 175	Med/Surg elderly patients	Haloperidol vs. olanzapine vs. placebo, 7 days medication trial	DRS/ CGI	All groups showed a decrease in DRS scores by 7th day, compared with baseline ($p < 0.01$). Decrease in DRS scores of treated patients at day 7 (OLA 72.2%; HAL 70.4%) differed significantly from DRS scores of PBO patients (29.7%; ($p < 0.01$), but not from each other ($p > 0.05$).

(*continued*)

Table 41.13 (CONTINUED)

STUDY (N = 32)	POPULATION	INTERVENTION	DELIRIUM DEFINITION/ MEASURE OF RESPONSE	RESULTS
Skrobik et al., 2004; OL-prospective RCT, n = 73	Critically ill Med/ Surg patients	Haloperidol (avg. 6.5 mg/d) vs. olanzapine (avg. 4.5 mg/d)	DIS	ICU Delirium Index Screening Checklist Scores were reduced in both groups, compared with baseline (p < 0.05), but there was no significant difference in DIS scores between active Tx groups ($p = 0.9$). EPS were found in 13% of haloperidol patients, but 0% in olanzapine group.
Toda et al., 2005; n = 10	Elderly inpatient general medicine	Risperidone, OL, 0.5 mg oral sol.; flexible titration, PRN	DSM-IV/ DRS	Resolution reported in 7 subjects (mean dose 0.92 ± 0.47 mg/d); 1 non-responder; side effects requiring Tx discontinuation reported in 2.
Lee et al., 2005; RCT, n = 40	Med/Surg patients	Amisulpride vs. quetiapine	DRS-R98/ CGI	After treatment, DRS-R-98 scores were significantly decreased from the baseline in both treatment groups ($P < 0.001$) without group difference. Both atypical antipsychotics were generally well tolerated.
Straker et al., 2006 OL, n = 14	Medically ill patients	Aripiprazole PO was used in a flexible dosing range, from 5 mg/day to 15 mg/day, titrated as clinically indicated	DSM-IV/ DRS-R98 CGI	50% of patients had improved significantly by day 5, as indicated by a 50% reduction in DRS-R-98 scores. 86% of patients had a 50% reduction in their DRS-R- 98 scores by end of treatment. Mean CGI Severity scores at the beginning of treatment were 5.2, with a mean CGI Improvement score after treatment of 2.1, indicating much improvement.
Takeuchi et al., 2007; OL, n = 38	Med/Surg patients	Perospirone, OL	DSM-IV/ DRS-R98	Perospirone was effective in 86.8% of patients, within several days (5.1 ± 4.9 days). The initial dose was 6.5 ± 3.7 mg/day and maximum dose of perospirone was 10.0 ± 5.3 mg/day. There were no serious adverse effects.
Maneeton, Maneeton, & Srisurapanont, 2007; OL, n = 17	Medically ill patients	Quetiapine, flexible dosing	CAM/DRS, CGI	88% subjects responded. Means (SDs) dose and duration (SD) of quetiapine treatment were 45.7 (28.7) mg/day and 6.5 (2.0) days, respectively. The DRS and CGI-S scores of days 2–7 were significantly lower than those of day 0 (p < 0. 001) for all comparisons. Only two subjects were shown to have mild tremor.
Reade et al., 2009; OL-RCT	Med/Surg ICU	Agitated delirium were randomized to receive an infusion of either haloperidol 0.5 to 2 mg/hour or dexmedetomidine 0.2 to 0.7 µg/kg/hr	ICDSC Time	DEX significantly shortened median time to extubation from 42.5 to 19.9 hours ($P = 0.016$); it significantly decreased ICU length of stay, from 6.5 to 1.5 days ($P = 0.004$); and of patients requiring ongoing sedation, it reduced the time propofol was required in half (79.5% vs. 41.2%; $P = 0.05$).
Devlin et al., 2010; DBRPCT, n = 36	MICU	PBO vs. quetiapine (50 mg BID) (multienter-3)	ICDSC	Tx w QUE was associated with: a shorter time to first resolution of delirium (*p =.001*), a reduced duration of delirium (*p =.006*), less agitation (*p =.02*), greater chance to be discharged home vs. long-term-care facility (*p =.06*), and lower requirement of as-needed haloperidol (*p =.05*).

(continued)

Table 41.13 (CONTINUED)

STUDY(*N* = 32)	POPULATION	INTERVENTION	DELIRIUM DEFINITION/ MEASURE OF RESPONSE	RESULTS
Girard et al., 2010; DBRPCT, *n* = 101	Mechanically ventilated Med/Surg ICU patients	PBO vs. HAL vs. Ziprasidone	CAM-ICU	Patients in the haloperidol group spent a similar number days alive without delirium or coma (14.0 [6.0 –18.0] days) as did those on ziprasidone (15.0 [9.1–18.0] days) and PBO groups (12.5 [1.2–17.2] days; *p* = 0.66).
Kim et al., 2010; SB-RCT, *n* = 32	Elderly, Med/Surg patients	Risperidone vs. olanzapine	DSM-IV/DRS-r-98	Significant within-group improvements in the DRS-R-98 scores over time were observed at every time point in both treatment groups. The response rates did not differ significantly between the two groups (risperidone group: 64.7%, olanzapine group: 73.3%); and there were no difference in the safety profiles and side effects between groups.
Tahir et al., 2010; DBRCT, *n* = 42	Med/Surg patients	Quetiapine vs. placebo	DSM-IV/DRS-r-98, CGI	Quetiapine has the potential to more quickly reduce the severity of non-cognitive aspects of delirium. The study was underpowered for treatment comparisons.
Grover et al., 2011; Prospective, single blind, *n* = 64	Med/Surg patients	Haloperidol (0.25 to 10 mg) vs. olanzapine (1.25 to 20 mg) vs. risperidone (0.25 to 4), flexible dosing	DSM-IV/DRS-r-98	Patient in all three groups experience a significant reduction in DRS-R98 severity scores and a significant improvement in MMSE scores over the period of 6 days; with no difference between the treatment groups. Rate of side effects was also similar.
Boettger et al., 2011; OL, *n* = 21	Med/Surg patients at Cancer Center	Aripiprazole, flexible dosing	DSM-IV/MDAS	The mean dosage of aripiprazole required was 18.3 mg (range of 5–30) daily at T3. Patients treated for delirium with aripiprazole experienced significant improvement and resolution of delirium, with MDAS scores declining from a mean of 18.0 at baseline (T1) to mean of 10.8 at T2 and a mean of 8.3 at T3. There was a 100% resolution of hypoactive delirium, compared to patients with hyperactive delirium (58.3%).
Hakim et al., 2012; PCRCT	Patients aged 65 yrs. or older who experienced subsyndromal delirium after on-pump cardiac surgery	Randomized using a computer-generated list to receive placebo (*n* = 50) or 0.5 mg risperidone (*n* = 51) every 12 hrs by mouth	ICDSC	Seven (13.7%) patients in the risperidone group experienced delirium vs. 17 (34%) in the placebo group (*p* = 0.031). Competing-risks regression analysis showed that failure to treat subsyndromal delirium with risperidone was an independent risk factor for delirium (*p* = 0.002). Two (3.9%) patients in the risperidone group experienced extrapyramidal manifestations versus one (2%) in the placebo group (*p* = 1.0).
Kishi et al., 2012; OL, *n* = 29	Adult delirious cancer patients	Risperidone given orally once per day (mean dosage, 1.4 ± 1.3 mg/day	DRS-R98	Entry DRS-R-98 score = 19.8 ± 6.8; 7-d follow-up score = 14.3 ± 7.8, results demonstrate DRS-R98 scores were improved in 79.3% of patients during the study period (*p* < 0.001); 38% achieved remission (i.e., DRS-R-98 ≤10).

(continued)

Table 41.13 (CONTINUED)

STUDY($N = 32$)	POPULATION	INTERVENTION	DELIRIUM DEFINITION/ MEASURE OF RESPONSE	RESULTS
Tagarakis et al., 2012; $n = 80$	Consecutive patients who developed post-op delirium after on-pump heart surgery	Ondansetron IV (8 mg) vs. haloperidol IV (5 mg); patients were evaluated before and 10 min after the injection	Self-developed rating scale: 0–4	Noted a statistically significant improvement in the test score rating after the administration of both ondansetron (from 3.1 to 1.2, percentage improvement 61.29%, $p < 0.01$) and haloperidol (from 3.1 to 1.3, ± percentage improvement 58.064%, $p < 0.01$).
Yoon et al., 2013; Observational study; $n = 80$	Patients with delirium at a tertiary level hospital	Assigned to receive either haloperidol ($n = 23$), risperidone ($n = 21$), olanzapine ($n = 18$), or quetiapine ($n = 18$)	Korean version of the Delirium Rating Scale–Revised-98 (DRS-K)	Haloperidol, risperidone, olanzapine, and quetiapine were equally efficacious and safe in the treatment of delirium. The treatment response rate was lower in patients over 75 years old than in patients under 75 years old, especially for olanzapine.
Maneeton et al., 2013; DBRCT, $n = 52$	Medically ill patients with delirium	25–100 mg/day of quetiapine ($n = 24$) or 0.5–2.0 mg/day of haloperidol ($n = 28$)	DRS-R-98 and total sleep time	Over the trial period, means (standard deviation) of the DRS-R-98 severity scores were not significantly different between the quetiapine and haloperidol groups (-22.9 [6.9] versus -21.7 [6.7]; $P = 0.59$). Concluding that low-dose quetiapine and haloperidol may be equally effective and safe for controlling delirium symptoms.

Abbreviations: RPCT=randomized placebo control trial; DBRPCT=double blind randomized, placebo controlled trial; OL=open label; trial; DSM=Diagnostic and Statistical Manual of Mental Disorders; CAM= Confusion Assessment Method; DRS=Delirium Rating Scale; MDAS=Memorial Delirium Assessment Scale; GI=gastrointestinal; PBO=placebo; Sx=surgery; CPB=cardio-pulmonary by-pass machine; ICU=intensive care unit. APA=antipsychotic agent; OLA=olanzapine; HAL=haloperidol; RIS=risperidone; AIDS=autoimmune deficiency syndrome; CPM=chlorpromazine; EPS= extra-pyramidal syndrome; LOR=lorazepam; PO= by mouth.

The second included a head-to-head comparison between haloperidol and an SGA (risperidone), demonstrating that delirium scores decreased significantly over the study period with no significant differences between groups (Han & Kim, 2004). An RPCT 7-day treatment trial compared haloperidol to olanzapine versus placebo among hospitalized elderly subjects, again showing no difference in the rate of improvement of delirium with either active agent, but significantly greater for each than placebo (olanzapine 72.2%; haloperidol 70.4%; placebo 29.7%; $p < 0.01$, against PBO) (Hu, Deng, & Yang, 2004). Another study compared enteral haloperidol (avg. dose 6.5 mg/d) versus olanzapine (avg. dose 4.5 mg/d) in the critical care setting (Skrobik, Bergeron, Dumont, & Gottfried, 2004). Results show that measures of delirium decreased over time in both groups, as did the administered dose of as-needed (PRN) benzodiazepines, with the degree of clinical improvement being similar in both treatment arms.

An RCT comparing the antipsychotics amisulpride versus quetiapine showed that after intervention, DRS-R-98 scores were significantly decreased from the baseline in both treatment groups ($P < 0.001$) without group difference, and that both SGAs were generally well tolerated (Lee, Won, et al., 2005). A study on the use of SGA involved the comparison of quetiapine (50 mg twice daily [BID]) versus placebo in medical ICU patients in three academic centers (Devlin, Roberts, et al., 2010). The study found that treatment with quetiapine was associated with a shorter time to first resolution of delirium (1.0 vs. 4.5 days; $p = .001$), a reduced duration of delirium (36 vs. 120 hrs.; $p = .006$), less agitation based on the Sedation-Agitation Scale score (6 vs. 36 hrs.; $p = .02$), greater chance to be discharged home versus long-term-care facility (89% vs. 56%; $p = .06$), and lower requirement of PRN haloperidol (3 vs. 4 days; $p = .05$).

The most recent published blinded RCT compared quetiapine (flexible dosing regimen of 25 to 175 mg per day, in divided doses) versus placebo among medico-surgical patients (Tahir et al., 2010). Results indicated the quetiapine group improved more rapidly, 82.7% faster (standard error [S.E.] 37.1%, $P = .026$) than the placebo group, in terms of the DRS-R-98 severity score; and 57.7% faster (S.E. 29.2%, $P = .048$) than the placebo group, in terms of the noncognitive subscale.

A Cochrane Database review compared haloperidol with risperidone, olanzapine, and placebo in the management of delirium and concluded that there was no significant difference between low-dose haloperidol (<3.0 mg per day) and the atypical antipsychotics olanzapine and risperidone (OR 0.63, $p = 0.25$); that low-dose haloperidol did not have a higher incidence of adverse effects than the atypical antipsychotics; and that low-dose haloperidol was effective in decreasing the intensity and duration of delirium in postoperative patients, compared with placebo (Lonergan, Britton, Luxenberg, & Wyller, 2007).

A subsequent meta-analysis on atypical antipsychotic agents for the treatment of delirium found that risperidone was the most thoroughly studied SGA for the management of delirium (Ozbolt, Paniagua, & Kaiser, 2008). Most studies found that risperidone was approximately 80%–85% effective in treating the behavioral disturbances of delirium at doses of 0.5–4.0 mg per day. On the other hand, olanzapine was approximately 70%–76% effective in treating the behavioral manifestations of delirium at doses of 2.5–11.6 mg per day. There were very few studies conducted using quetiapine; although available data suggest that it also appears to be a safe and effective alternative to high-potency antipsychotics. In the limited number of trials comparing SGAs to haloperidol, haloperidol consistently produced a higher rate (an additional 10%–13%) of extrapyramidal side effects.

Finally, there have been two case reports on the use of aripiprazole as an effective treatment of delirium (Alao & Moskowitz, 2006; Straker, Shapiro, & Muskin, 2006); and a retrospective case-matched study of aripiprazole vs. haloperidol that found an identical delirium resolution rate (76.2%) for both agents (Boettger, Friedlander, Breitbart, & Passik, 2011). In addition, there are two single case reports on the use of ziprasidone for the management of delirium (Leso & Schwartz, 2002; Young & Lujan, 2004) and one OL study (*n* = 38) on the use of perospirone, a recently developed atypical antipsychotic with potent serotonin 5-HT2 and dopamine D2 antagonist activity (Takeuchi et al., 2007).

A systematic literature review of 28 delirium treatment studies with antipsychotic agents concluded that:

1. Around 75% of delirious patients who receive short-term treatment with low-dose antipsychotics experience clinical response;

2. This response rate appears quite consistent across different patient groups and treatment settings;

3. Evidence does not indicate major differences in response rates between clinical subtypes of delirium; and

4. There are no significant differences in efficacy for haloperidol versus atypical agents (Meagher et al., 2013).

Regarding side-effect incidence, a meta-analysis of all randomized controlled trials in which SGAs have been compared with conventional drugs concluded that of the SGAs, only clozapine was associated with significantly fewer extrapyramidal symptoms (EPS ($p = 0.008$) and higher efficacy than low-potency conventional drugs. A reduced frequency of EPS was noted with olanzapine, which was of borderline significance ($p = 0.07$) (Leucht, Wahlbeck, Hamann, & Kissling, 2003). Another study analyzed the data on neuroleptics acquired in the German multicenter drug surveillance program database (Projekt "Arzneimittelsicherheit in der Psychiatrie") program from 1993 to 2000 and found that severe adverse drug reactions (ADRs) occurred in 1.1% of the patients (Bender, Grohmann, et al., 2004). In contrast to the results from controlled trials, atypical neuroleptics caused more severe ADRs than did typical neuroleptics. Overall, SGAs were found to be superior in EPS and urological ADRs, but when clozapine is excluded, typicals and SGAs have similar occurrence rates of severe ADRs. Other problems to consider when choosing an alternative agent include the fact that SGAs may be associated with weight gain, dyslipidemia, high blood pressure, and ultimately with cardiovascular disease, diabetes, and metabolic syndrome (Henderson, 2008). Therefore, when considering the use of SGAs, clinicians must consider these factors and weigh potential risks and benefits before prescribing these agents to a critically ill patient. Finally, there have been numerous reports attributing the onset of delirium to the use of SGAs (e.g., clozapine, olanzapine), probably due to their anticholinergic potential (Bender, Grohmann, et al., 2004). But these data are limited to small case reports (see Box 41.7).

Box 41.7 CASE REPORTS LINKING SGA TO DELIRIUM GENERATION

- Case reports implicating risperidone use in causing delirium:
  - Kato et al. (2005), *Psychosomatics*
  - Morikawa and Kishimoto (2002), *Canadian Journal of Psychology*
  - Tavcar and Dernovsek (1998), *Canadian Journal of Psychology*
  - Chen Chen and Cardasis (1996), *American Journal of Psychology*
- Case reports implicating quetiapine use in causing the delirium:
  - Sim, Brunet, and Conacher (2000), *Canadian Journal of Psychology* - Balit et al. (2003), *Annals of Emergency Medicine*
  - Miodownik et al. (2008), *Clinical Neuropharmacology*
- Case reports implicating olanzapine use in causing the delirium:
  - Robinson, Burk, & Raman (2003), *Journal of Postgraduate Medicine*
  - Steil (2003) *Der Nervenartzt*
  - Samuels and Fang (2004), *Journal of Clinical Psychology* - Morita et al. (2004) *Journal of Pain & Symptom Management*
  - Prommer (2005) *Journal of Pain & Symptom Management*
  - Tuglu, Erdogan, & Ebay (2005) *Journal of Korean Medicine*
  - Weizberg et al. (2006) *Clinical Toxicology*
  - Lim, Travino, & Tampi (2006), *Annals of Pharmacotherapy*

Please note that antipsychotic agents should only be used short-term for treating agitation in the cognitively impaired individual. Serious concerns have been raised about the stroke and mortality risk of atypical antipsychotics when administered long-term for the management of agitation in patients with dementia. The dementia antipsychotic withdrawal trial (DART-AD) found that at 12 months, the cumulative probability of survival was similar in the active group and the placebo group (70% versus 77%; $p = ns$) (Ballard, Hanney, et al., 2009). Yet, there was a reduction in survival of the patients who continued to receive antipsychotics (after 12 months) compared with those who received placebo (24-month survival 46% vs. 71%; 36-month survival 30% vs. 59%).

Regarding concerns for QTc prolongation, data from the FDA Division of CardioRenal Drug Products Consultation suggested that all antipsychotic agents lengthen the QTc to varying degrees. They based their conclusions on a study of antipsychotic agents in psychotic subjects with normal baseline ECGs who were titrated to the "highest tolerated dose" of one of six antipsychotic agents (see Table 41.14) (FDA, 2000; Huffman & Stern, 2003). It may be reasonable to assume the doses used may have been substantially lower than the doses used for the treatment of hyperactive delirium. We also need to consider the fact that when these agents are used for the management of delirium, patients often received parenteral formulations (when available) due to noncompliance, and they often experience a number of comorbid medical issues (Huffman & Stern, 2003). When antipsychotic agents are recommended, it is wise to review the patient's medication list and identify any other agents with the ability to prolong QTc. If possible, avoid other medications known to increase QTc and/or inhibitors of CPY3A4. Before and during the use of continuous antipsychotic management, you should obtain a 12-lead ECG, and measure QTc and electrolytes. All electrolyte abnormalities should be corrected (especially K+ and Mg+) and the QTc pattern monitored. Recommendations

Table 41.14 EFFECTS OF ORALLY ADMINISTERED ANTIPSYCHOTICS ON THE QTC INTERVAL[a]

DRUG	MEAN INCREASE IN QTC (MS)	% OF SUBJECTS WITH > 60 MS INCREASE IN QTC
Thioridazine	35.8	29
Ziprasidone	20.6	21
Quetiapine	14.5	11
Risperidone	10.0	4
Olanzapine	6.4	4
Haloperidol	4.7	4

Data from Huffman JC, Stern TA. (2003).QTc Prolongation and the use of antipsychotics: A case discussion. *Primary Care Companion to the Journal of Clinical Psychiatry,* 5(6), 278–81.

[a] Data adapted from the U.S. Food and Drug Administration's Center for Drug Evaluation and Research, Psychopharmacological Drugs Advisory Committee (FDA, 2000), adapted by Huffman & Stern, 2003.

are to discontinue antipsychotic use if QTc increases to >25% of baseline or >500 msec. Of note, studies suggest that haloperidol may have the lowest ratio of cardiac death among all dopamine-antagonist agents, both typical and atypical (Hatta, Takahashi, et al., 2001; Harrigan, Miceli, et al., 2004).

Our recommended schedule in the case of hyperactive states is to use antipsychotic agents (e.g., haloperidol, risperidone, quetiapine) at one of the following time schedules: "TID" (thrice daily) schedule (0600 hrs, 1000, 2000) or "QID" (four times a day) schedule (0600, 1000, 1600, 2200). The idea is to enhance behavioral control during the daytime and help promote better nighttime rest without causing oversedation. Therefore, daytime doses are significantly lower than the nighttime dose (e.g., a 20 mg/d haloperidol dose will be distributed as 5 mg IV q 0600, 1000, and 1600; plus 10 mg at 2200 hrs).

When treating hypoactive delirium, we recommend doses in the very low range (i.e., haloperidol and risperidone in the 0.25 to 1 mg/24 hr). Data available suggest that the dopamine excess observed in delirious subjects occurs in all cases, even hypoactive forms. The same data demonstrate that antipsychotic use helps prevent and treat all forms of deliria, including the hypoactive type. In these cases, it is usually given as a single nighttime dose, just before sundown. Given their hypoactive state, very sedating agents (e.g., quetiapine, olanzapine) are usually not recommended. In the experience of the author, aripiprazole may prove to be a particularly good choice for hypoactive cases (usually starting at doses as low as 1 mg at bedtime), probably due to its partial dopamine antagonist-agonist properties that may have positive effects on attention, concentration, and sleep–wake cycle reversal in delirium, and its minimal muscarinic and histaminic antagonist activity (thus minimizing adverse cognitive effects). Recent reports seem to support this clinical experience, confirming the usefulness of aripiprazole, particularly in hypoactive delirium (Alao & Moskowitz, 2006; Straker, Shapiro, & Muskin, 2006; Boettger & Breitbart, 2011). Aripiprazole had enjoyed the reputation of being the only SGA not to be associated with QTc-prolongation or TdP, confirmed by both clinical trials data and clinical experience (Gulisano, Cali, et al., 2011; Germano, Italiano, et al., 2014; Li, Luo, et al., 2014; Marder et al., 2003). Yet there are at least two case reports of aripiprazole-induced cardiac arrest due to TdP, when it was used as a single agent (Nelson & Leung, 2013). There is at least one case report of aripiprazole-associated QTc prolongation in a geriatric patient (Hategan & Bourgeois, 2014). Before this, all other cases of QTc prolongation had either been associated with concomitant use of another antipsychotic agent or occurred after an overdose (LoVecchio, Watts, & Winchell, 2005; Nelson & Leung, 2013).

Norepinephrine Excess

$α_2$-Adrenergic Receptors Agonists versus Conventional Sedative Agents: Effect on Delirium Prevention

There have been several randomized clinical trials looking at anesthetic practice and delirium prevention (see Table 41.15).

Table 41.15 A$_2$-ADRENERGIC RECEPTORS AGONISTS AND ALTERNATIVE SEDATIVE AGENTS VERSUS
CONVENTIONAL ANESTHETICS: EFFECT ON DELIRIUM PREVENTION AND TREATMENT

STUDY($N = 11$)	POPULATION	INTERVENTION	DELIRIUM DEFINITION	DELIRIUM INCIDENCE % CONTROL/INTERVENTION			P-VALUE
Berggren et al., 1987; RCT, $n = 57$	Femoral neck Fx repair	Epidural vs. halothane anesthesia	DSM-III	38% (11/29)	50% (14/28)		$P < 0.05$
Williams-Russo et al., 1992; RCT, $n = 60$	B knee replacement Sx	Continuous epidural bupivacaine + fentanyl vs. continuous IV fentanyl	DSM-III	44% (11/25)	38% (10/26)		$p = 0.69$
Aizawa et al., 2002; OL, $n = 42$	GI surgery	Usual care vs. BZD administration to promote sleep p-Sx	DSM-IV	35% (7/20)	5% (1/20)		$p = 0.023$
Maldonado et al., 2003, 2009; RCT, $n = 118$	Cardiac valve Sx	Post-op anesthesia w/ MID vs. PROP vs. DEX	DSM-IV DRS-R-98	Midazolam 50% (15/30)	Propofol 50% (15/30)	Dexmedeto-midine 3% (1/30)	$p < 0.001$
Pandharipande et al., 2007; DBRPCT, $n = 106$	Med/Surg ICU in mechanical ventilation	DEX vs. lorazepam (2 tertiary care centers); days alive w/o delirium or coma	CAM-ICU	3.0d	7.0d		$p = 0.01$
Reade et al., 2009; randomized, open-label, parallel groups pilot trial; $n = 20$	Tx-agitated ICU patients	IV haloperidol 0.5 to 2 mg/hour vs. dexmedetomidine 0.2 to 0.7 µg/kg/hr	ICDSC	42.2 hrs	20 hrs		$p = 0.016$
				Above numbers represent time to extubation; prolonged intubation attributed to delirium and agitation			
Riker et al., 2009; DBRPCT, $n = 375$	Med/Surg ICU in mechanical ventilation	Midazolam vs. DEX; trial conducted in 68 centers in 5 countries	CAM-ICU	76.6% (93/122)	54% (32/244)		$p<0.001$
Hudetz et al., 2009; DBRPCT, $n = 58$	Elective CABG or valve replacement/ repair w CPB	PBO vs. IV ketamine (0.5 mg/kg) bolus during the induction of anesthesia	Intensive Care Delirium Screening Checklist (ICDSC)	31% (9/29)	3% (1/29)		$p = 0.01$
Shehabi et al., 2009; DBRPCT, $n = 306$	Elderly patients after cardiac surgery	Morphine vs. DEX	CAM-ICU	15%	8.6%		$p =.088$
Rubino et al., 2010; DBRPCT, $n = 30$	Acute type-A aortic dissection repair	PBO vs. clonidine IV on delirium neurological outcome and respiratory function	Delirium Detection Score (DDS)→	1.8 ± 0.8	0.6 ± 0.7		$p = 0.001$
Jakob, Ruokonen, et al., 2012; RDBCT; $n = 498$	Adult ICU patients receiving mechanical ventilation	PROP vs. DEX	CAM-ICU	29% (71/247)	18% (45/251)		$p = 0.008$

Abbreviations: RCT=randomized control trial; RPCT=randomized placebo control trial; DBRPCT=double blind randomized, placebo controlled trial; OL=open label; trial; DSM=Diagnostic and Statistical Manual of Mental Disorders; CAM= Confusion Assessment Method; DRS=Delirium Rating Scale; MDAS=Memorial Delirium Assessment Scale; GI=gastrointestinal; PBO=placebo; Sx=surgery; CPB=cardio-pulmonary by-pass machine; ICU=intensive care unit. APA=antipsychotic agent; BZDP=benzodiazepine; DEX=dexmedetomidine; OLA=olanzapine; HAL=haloperidol; RIS=risperidone; AIDS=autoimmune deficiency syndrome; CPM=chlorpromazine; EPS= extra-pyramidal syndrome; LOR=lorazepam; PO= by mouth.

The earliest study examined epidural versus halothane anesthesia to assess postoperative delirium and found no difference between the two approaches (Berggren et al., 1987). A second study compared the effects of continuous epidural bupivacaine plus fentanyl versus continuous IV fentanyl anesthesia on postoperative delirium, and again found no differences between these approaches (Williams-Russo et al., 1992).

The majority of patients in the ICU, particularly those who are mechanically ventilated, receive some form of sedation to reduce their anxiety, encourage sleep, and increase tolerance of the critical care environment, including multiple IV lines, pain management, endotracheal tubes, and ventilators. Sedative and analgesic drugs are among the most commonly prescribed medications in the ICU (Farina, Levati, & Tognoni, 1981). As discussed, sedative agents (mostly GABA-ergic) and opioids may contribute to the development of delirium by one of six mechanisms: interfering with physiological sleep patterns; interfering with central cholinergic function; increasing compensatory upregulation of NMDA and kainite receptors and Ca^2+ channels; disrupting the circadian rhythm of melatonin release; disrupting thalamic gating function; and leading to CNS-depressant dependence and withdrawal. Therefore, sedating alternatives have been thought promising in decreasing medication/sedation-induced delirium.

The first study involving ketamine in delirium prevention was a DBRPCT involving children undergoing dental repair in sevoflurane-induced anesthesia (Abu-Shahwan & Chowdary, 2007). The study demonstrated a substantially lower incidence of emergence agitation in the ketamine group compared with placebo (16.6% vs. 34.2%), but no difference in time to meet recovery room discharge criteria between the two groups. A second study compared the effects of IV ketamine versus placebo on postoperative delirium in patients undergoing acute type-A aortic dissection repair, which found a significant reduction in the incidence of delirium in patients in the ketamine group (3% vs. 31%, $p = 0.01$) (Hudetz et al., 2009). Postoperative C-reactive protein concentration was also lower ($p <0.05$) in the ketamine-treated patients compared with the placebo-treated patients.

In an attempt to demonstrate that different sedative strategies may achieve delirium reduction, the author and his team (Maldonado, 2003) were the first to report on the use of the novel sedative agent dexmedetomidine (DEX) as an alternative to the use of benzodiazepines and related agents (e.g., midazolam [MID], propofol [PRO]) during the postoperative state (Maldonado, 2003; Maldonado et al., 2003, 2004). Post-cardiotomy patients were selected, given the high incidence of delirium in such patients (around 57%) nationwide (Ebert, Walzer, Huth, & Herrmann, 2001). We studied patients ($n = 118$) undergoing cardiac surgery (i.e., repair or replacement) with cardiopulmonary bypass (Maldonado et al., 2009). Intraoperative anesthesia for the surgical procedures was standardized for all subjects in all three studied groups. All procedures were performed via median sternotomy in conjunction with CPB and induction of moderate hypothermia. After successful weaning from CPB, patients were started on one of three randomly assigned, postoperative sedation regimens: DEX (loading dose: 0.4 µg/kg, followed by a maintenance drip of 0.2–0.7 µg/kg/hour), PRO drip (25–50 µg/kg/minute), or MID drip (0.5–2 mg/hour), all titrated to achieve a target sedation level (i.e., a Ramsay Sedation Score of 3 before extubation and 2 after extubation). Upon arrival at the ICU, a standardized protocol for postoperative care was implemented for all patients. Study results showed there were no significant preoperative or intraoperative differences between treatment groups (e.g., age, sex, American Society of Anesthesiology classification, bypass time, clamp time, or lowest temperature achieved) (see Table 41.16). The only real difference in management between groups was the type of postoperative sedation. Final results demonstrated an incidence of delirium of 3% for patients on DEX, compared to 50% for PRO and 50% for MID ($p <.01$). The absolute risk reduction in the incidence of delirium associated with using DEX was 47% (95% CI 28%–66%) corresponding to a number-to-treat of 2.1 patients (95% CI 1.5–3.6). Similarly, the number of delirious days was also significantly lower in the DEX group compared to PRO and MID (1% vs. 16% vs. 29%, respectively; $p <.001$).

Since then, two DBRPCT have confirmed the original findings and demonstrated the delirium-sparing effects of DEX. The first of these compared DEX with lorazepam (LOR) in the ICU on mechanical ventilation. The study found that DEX-treated patients had more delirium-free days (7 days vs. 3 days, $p =.01$), had a lower prevalence of coma ($p <0.001$), and spent more time within sedation goals ($p =.04$) than LOR-treated subjects (Pandharipande et al., 2007). Similarly, a second, much larger trial (i.e., 68 ICUs in five countries) compared the incidence of delirium among ICU-ventilated subjects sedated with either DEX or MID and found a lower delirium incidence (54% vs. 76.6%, $p <.001$), shorter intubation time (median time to extubation was 3.7 days DEX vs. 5.6 days MID; $p =.01$), and less tachycardia and hypertension in the DEX-treated group (Riker et al., 2009).

A study assessing the effects of different classes of sedative agents compared variable doses of morphine or dexmedetomidine, with open-label propofol titrated to effect (Shehabi et al., 2009). This study found that the incidence of delirium was comparable between morphine 22 (15.0%) and DEX 13 (8.6%) (95% CI: 0.256–1.099, $p =.088$). Yet DEX-managed patients spent 3 fewer days (2 vs. 5) delirious (95% CI: 1.09–6.67, $p =.0317$), were more likely to be extubated earlier (95% CI: 1.01–1.60, $p =.040$), experienced less systolic hypotension (23% *vs.* 38.1%, $p =.006$), and required less norepinephrine ($p < 0.001$), than morphine-treated patients.

Finally, a subsequent study assessed the role of clonidine IV (0.5 microg/kg bolus, followed by continuous infusion at 1–2 microg/kg/hr) versus placebo on delirium in post-cardiotomy patients and found no significant difference in the incidence of delirium between groups (33% vs. 40%, $p = 0.705$) (Rubino et al., 2010). Yet, delirium scores were significantly lower in patients treated with clonidine compared to placebo ($P = 0.001$), suggesting that the beneficial effects in delirium prevention previously seen with DEX may extend to all alpha-2 agonists (Rubino et al., 2010).

Despite evidence demonstrating that prophylactic use of DEX in reducing the incidence of delirium and plenty of clinical evidence that it is useful in the management of agitation related to hyperactive delirium, there is no study to

	DEXMEDE-TOMIDINE (N = 30)	PROPOFOL (N = 30)	MIDAZOLAM (N = 30)	OVERALL P-VALUE	DEX VS. PROPOFOL	DEX VS. MIDAZOLAM
Delirium						
Incidence of delirium (per protocol)	1/30 (3%)	15/30 (50%)	15/30 (50%)	<0.001	<0.001	<0.001
Incidence of delirium	4/40 (10%)	16/36 (44%)	17/40 (44%)	<0.001	0.001	0.002
Number of days delirious	2/216 (1%)	45/276 (16%)	75/259 (29%)	<0.001	<0.001	<0.001
Average length of delirium days)	2.0 ± 0	3.0 ± 3.1	5.4 ± 6.6	0.82	0.93	0.63
Time Variables						
ICU length of stay (days)	1.9 ±.9	3.0 ± 2.0	3.0 ± 3.0	0.11	0,14	0.14
Hospital length of stay (days)	7.1 ± 1.9	8.2 ± 3.8	8.9 ± 4.7	0.39	0.42	0.12
Intubation time (hours)	11.9 ± 4.5	11.1 ± 4.6	12.7 ± 8.5	0.64	0.91	0.34
PRN Medications						
Fentanyl (mcg)	320 ± 355	364 ± 320	1088 ± 832	<0.001	0.93	<0.001
Total Morphine equivalents (mg) P‡P	50.3 ± 38	51.6 ± 36	122.5 ± 84	<0.001	0.99	<0.001
Antiemetic use*	15/30 (50%)	17/30 (57%)	19/30 (63%)	0.58		
PRN Medications for the Management of Delirium**						
Lorazepam	1/30 (3%)	7/30 (23%)	6/30 (20%)	0.07	0.06	0.11
Haloperidol	0/30	3/30 (10%)	2/30 (7%)	0.23	0.07	0.15

† Percent of patients who developed delirium.

‡ Sum of average morphine equivalents (fentanyl, oxycodone, and hydrocodone) received in postoperative days 1–3.

* Number of patients who received dolasetron mesylate and/or promethazine HCl in postoperative day 1.

** Average amount over three days. None of these medications were given until a diagnosis of delirium was established.

Source: Maldonado, 2008a.

date confirming its potential in the treatment of delirium. A randomized, open-label trial of agitated delirium assigned subjects to receive an infusion of either haloperidol 0.5–2.0 mg/hour or dexmedetomidine 0.2–0.7 μg/kg/hr (Reade et al., 2009). Results found that DEX significantly shortened median time to extubation (from 42.5 to 19.9 hours; $P = 0.016$), significantly decreased ICU length of stay (from 6.5 to 1.5 days; $P = 0.004$), and, in patients requiring ongoing sedation, DEX cut in half the time propofol was needed (79.5% vs. 41.2%; $P = 0.05$). Finally, a recent meta-analysis including all postoperative prevention strategies found that DEX sedation was associated with less delirium compared to sedation produced by other drugs (2 RCTs with 415 patients, pooled RR = 0.39; 95% CI = 0.16–0.95) (Zhang et al., 2013).

The detailed proposed mechanisms for delirium reduction have been described elsewhere (Maldonado, 2008a). They can be summarized in six postulated theories: The first suggests that DEX has an intrinsic *delirium-sparing effects,* which may be explained by DEX's pharmacological characteristics. The second theory suggests that the reason patients had significantly less delirium in the DEX group was not because of its use per se, but because those patients were not exposed to other sedative agents with much greater delirium potential (e.g., GABA-ergic agents, such as propofol and midazolam, and lower doses of opioid agents). Third, data suggest that the neuroprotective effect of DEX is mediated by activation of the alpha2A adrenergic receptor subtype (Ma et al., 2004). Fourth, it is worth noticing that DEX has been shown to have significant neuroprotective effect, in vivo and in vitro, against glutamate-induced damage via an increased astrocyte expression of BDNF through an extracellular signal-regulated kinase-dependent pathway (Engelhard et al., 2003; Ma et al., 2004; Sato, Kimura, Nishikawa, Tobe, & Masaki, 2010; Degos et al., 2013). Fifth, it is also hypothesized that DEX increases the expression of active (autophosphorylated) focal adhesion kinase, a non-receptor tyrosine kinase playing a pivotal role in cellular plasticity and survival (Dahmani, Rouelle, Gressens, & Mantz, 2005). The sixth theory involves DEX's unique mechanism for inducing sleep. Data suggest that DEX induces a qualitatively similar pattern of c-Fos expression as seen during normal NREM sleep by acting on endogenous sleep pathways (i.e., a decrease in the locus ceruleus and tuberomammillary nucleus and an increase in the ventrolateral preoptic nucleus) (Nelson et al., 2003).

It is certainly possible that a combination of any or all of these six mechanisms work together, leading to the results obtained in the above-mentioned studies. It is this author's experience that all centrally acting α_2-adrenergic receptors agonists are to some extent useful in the management of hyperactive delirium. In fact, our team uses clonidine to help transition patients off IV-DEX with good success (see Table 41.17). We also use clonidine, orally and transdermally, for prevention of alcohol withdrawal, with excellent results. Another α_2-adrenergic receptor agonist worth considering is guanfacine. This agent is even more α_2 / α_1 selective and is available in oral dose form. This makes it an excellent alternative to DEX (which requires an IV drip and a monitored bed) and is less hypotensive than clonidine. Our team has been using this agent, as we have clonidine, both as adjunct treatment of hyperactive delirium and as a primary agent in the prevention and treatment of alcohol withdrawal.

Glutamate Excess

Glutamate Antagonists and Ca+ Channel Modulators for Delirium Management

A number of agents with antiglutamatergic and Ca+ channel blocking qualities are worth considering here: lamotrigine, amantadine, memantine, gabapentin, and valproic acid (VPA) (see Table 41.18).

Both amantadine and memantine have been recognized as having neuroprotective effects, probably mediated by their protection from glutamate-induced exocytosis (by blocking excessive N-methyl-D-aspartic acid receptors without disrupting physiological synaptic activity, thus preventing excessive calcium influx into neurons—believed to be the key early step in GLU-induced exocytosis); reducing the release of proinflammatory factors from activated microglia; inducing expression of neurotrophic factors, such as glial cell line–derived neurotrophic factor in astroglia; and limiting oxidative injury and dendritic degeneration induced by anticholinesterase neurotoxicity (Giacino & Whyte, 2003; Zaja-Milatovic, Gupta, Aschner, & Milatovic, 2009; Ossola et al., 2011; Kutzing, Luo, & Firestein, 2012). Thus, it makes sense to consider their use in various syndromes associated with excess glutamate and subsequent cognitive decline (e.g., traumatic brain injury, stroke, delirium). In fact, studies have demonstrated that memantine may be effective in reducing the damage induced by acute ischemia/reperfusion (Yigit et al., 2011), while amantadine has been shown to enhance cognitive recovery and minimize delirium after severe TBI in humans (Giacino et al., 2012).

A DBPCRT compared the use of gabapentin as an add-on agent in the treatment of postoperative pain (i.e., spine surgery under general anesthesia) to reduce the occurrence of postoperative delirium (Leung et al., 2006). Subjects received either placebo or gabapentin 900 mg administered orally one to two hours before surgery, and continued once a day for the first 3 postoperative days. Results demonstrated that gabapentin was superior to placebo in reducing delirium occurrence (0% vs. 42%, $p = 0.045$). Even though the study authors attributed this to gabapentin's opioid-sparing effect, they failed to consider gabapentin's true modes of action (i.e., modulation of voltage-sensitive Ca2+ channels, NMDA receptor antagonism, activation of spinal alpha-2 receptors, attenuation of Na+ dependent action potentials) as potential mediators of its deliriolytic effect.

Even though many of us routinely use VPA (either oral or IV) in the management of agitated delirious patients who either are not responsive or cannot tolerate conventional treatment, there is very little literature investigating the effectiveness of this practice. In fact, there are no RCT or even OL studies on the matter. The only published report on the effectiveness of VPA for delirium treatment comes from a report of six cases (Bourgeois, Koike, Simmons, Telles, & Egglestone,

Table 41.17 CENTRALLY ACTING A₂-ADRENERGIC RECEPTOR AGONISTS

DRUG	A₂/A₁ SELECTIVITY	DT ½	ET ½	PRODUCT AVAILABILITY	BIOAVAILABILITY	PROTEIN BINDING
Guanfacine	2,640	2.5 hr	17 hr	PO	~100%	70%
Dexmedetomidine	1,600	6 m	2 hr	IV	70–80%	94%
Medetomidine	1,200					
Clonidine	220	11 m	13 hr	PO TDS	100% PO 60% TDS	40%
Methyldopa		12 m	105 m	PO/IV	50%	<20%
Guanabenz		60 m	6 hr	PO	75%	90%

Abbreviations: dT1/2= time to onset; eT1/2= elimination half-life; PO=by mouth; IV=intravenous; TDS= transdermal delivery (patch).

DRUG	T ½	PRODUCT AVAILABILITY	BIO-AVAILABILITY	METABOLISM	PROTEIN BINDING	MECHANISM ACTION
Lamotrigine	25 hr	PO	~100%	Hepatic	55%	• Stabilizes neuronal membranes • Inhibits voltage-sensitive Na+ channels and/or Ca+ channels→ ↓ cortical GLU release • Calcium channel blockers • Excitatory amino acid antagonists
Amantadine	17 ± 4 hr	PO	86–90%	None Renal excretion	67%	• NMDA receptor antagonist • ↑ synthesis and release of dopamine
Memantine	60–80 hr	PO	100%	Mostly unchanged renal excretion	45%	• Noncompetitive NMDA receptor antagonist • Blocks the effects of excessive levels of GLU • Some Ca+ channel blockade • 5HT3 antagonist
Gabapentin	5–7 hr	PO	60%	None Renal excretion	<3%	• Voltage-gated Ca+ channel blockade → ↓ cortical GLU release • NMDA antagonism • Activation of spinal alpha2-adrenergic receptors • Attenuation of Na+ dependent action potential
VPA	9–16 hr	PO/IV	90%	Hepatic conjugation	90%	• GABA transaminase inhibitor → ↑ GABA • Inhibits voltage-sensitive Na+ channels→ ↓ cortical GLU release • ↓ release of the epileptogenic amino acid gamma-hydroxybutyric acid (GHB)

Abbreviations: T1/2=elimination half-life.

2005). The authors reported that "in all six cases, the use of VPA combined with conventional antidelirium medications resulted in improved control of behavioral symptoms without significant side effects." In all cases, standard psychotropic medication regimens commonly used for the management of delirium and/or nonspecific agitation in the general hospital setting (i.e., antipsychotics and/or benzodiazepines) had initially been tried with limited success, and in all cases the addition of VPA to the existing regimens resulted in improved clinical response. Daily doses ranged between 0.5 to 2.5 grams in divided doses, without significant side effects and with discernible therapeutic benefits.

Similarly, the Stanford's Psychosomatic Medicine Research Lab presented a larger case series (*n* = 16) equally demonstrating the usefulness and safety of VPA in the management of agitated/hyperactive delirium, as an add-on to ineffective response to conventional therapy (Sher, Lolak, Miller, & Maldonado, 2013). In this series, the dose ranged between 0.5 to 3.0 grams per day in divided doses. All subjects in this case series improved in their clinical status with eventual resolution of delirium. In the case of intubated patients,

addition of VPA frequently allowed prompt extubation, since agitation and related desaturation were better controlled. No significant side effects were identified in any of the subjects, with the exception of nonclinically significant decreases in the number of platelets in few subjects. Of note, as in the case of SGAs, there have been case reports on VPA-induced delirium. The availability of IV (Depacon) and elixir (Depakene, ideal for administration via feeding tube, if needed) forms allow administration in non-cooperative subjects, or those intubated and unable to take PO medication. The IV formulation even allows for loading to quickly establish therapeutic serum levels, then continuing for maintenance or converting to PO when medically indicated. Others have described the usefulness of VPA in the management of destructive and aggressive behavior associated with brain injury (Wroblewski, Joseph, Kupfer, & Kalliel, 1997) and dementia (Haas, Vincent, Holt, & Lippmann, 1997; Narayan & Nelson, 1997; Tariot, 1999; Porsteinsson, Tariot, et al., 2003; Sival, Duivenvoorden, et al., 2004). As in any patient receiving VPA, close monitoring of liver function tests, bilirubin, platelet count, and amylase are advisable, especially in the critically ill patient.

Cholinergic Deficit

Acetylcholinesterase Inhibitors for Delirium Prevention

Despite the logical premise behind the prophylactic use of acetylcholinesterase inhibitor agents, studies have not consistently demonstrated positive results (see Table 41.19). The first publication suggesting the promise of acetylcholinesterase inhibitors in delirium prevention comes from a study on the use of rivastigmine for delirium prevention among hospitalized elderly patients who had been chronically treated with rivastigmine for dementia (Dautzenberg, Mulder, Olde Rikkert, Wouters, & Loonen, 2004). A retrospective chart review showed that those on rivastigmine had a significantly lower incidence of delirium compared to subjects not treated (45.5% vs. 88.9%; p <0.05). Similarly, a prospective study of elderly subjects suffering from vascular dementia randomly placed patients on either rivastigmine (6 mg/d) or aspirin (100 mg/d) and followed them at regular intervals for 24 months (Moretti, Torre, Antonello, Cattaruzza, & Cazzato, 2004). The results suggested that those on rivastigmine had a substantially lower incidence of delirium compared to aspirin

(40% vs. 62%; p <0.001). Also of significance, when subjects developed delirium, the mean duration of delirium was shorter (mean duration 4 ± 1.71 days vs. 7.86 ± 2.73 days; p <0.01), and the use of benzodiazepine and neuroleptic agents for management of agitation was significantly less in the rivastigmine group (p <0.05). Furthermore, analysis of behavioral data (as measured by Behavioral Pathology in Alzheimer's Disease (BEHAVE-AD) scale), found that total scores in the rivastigmine group were significantly improved over baseline and at the end of the study (all p <0.001). Further sub-analysis of the BEHAVE-AD individual items indicated that rivastigmine provided benefits on all items of the scale, except for delusions, throughout the study.

Unfortunately, the only DBRCT of rivastigmine failed to demonstrate efficacy in the prevention of postoperative delirium. In a study in cardiac surgery patients comparing rivastigmine (1.5 mg/d for 3 days preoperatively) against placebo found no benefits of the active drug use (Gamberini et al., 2009).

Similarly, results have been negative with the use of donepezil. The first study was a DBRPCT involving elderly patients undergoing elective total joint replacement surgery

Table 41.19 ACETYLCHOLINESTERASE INHIBITORS IN DELIRIUM PREVENTION

STUDY(N = 7)	POPULATION	INTERVENTION	DELIRIUM DEFINITION	DELIRIUM INCIDENCE %		
				CONTROL	INTERVENTION	*P*-VALUE
Dautzenberg et al., 2004 OL, Retrospective review, n = 51	(P) ≥65y/o hospitalized demented patients	Patients who used rivastigmine chronically with a randomly selected subgroup of all patients not treated	Retrospective chart review of geriatric service consultations	88.9 (26/29)	45.5 (4/11)	P < 0.05
Moretti et al., 2004 RCT, n = 230	(P) ≥65y/o–o/p, w/ vasc dementia (24-month f/u)	Cardioaspirin vs. rivastigmine PO qD	CAM BEHAVE-AD	62 (71/115)	40 (46/115)	P < 0.001
Liptzin et al., 2005 DBRPCT n = 80	(P) Elderly elective total joint replacement	PBO vs. donepezil (14 days pre + 14 days post Sx)	DSM-IV	17.1 (7/41)	20.5 (8/39)	p = 0.69
Sampson et al., 2007 DBRPCT, n = 33	(P) Elderly elective hip replacement	PBO vs. donepezil 5 mg immediately p-Sx + 3 days	DSI	35.7 (5/14)	9.5 (2/19)	p = 0.08
Oldenbeuving et al., 2008 N = 26	(P) Delirium p CVA	Rivastigmine 3→ 12 mg/d; no PBO	DRS ≥ 12	In 16/17 (94%) delirium severity improved; mean decrease 14.8→8.5; mean duration: 6.7 days; no side effects		
Gamberini et al., 2009 DBRPCT, n = 120	(P) Cardiac Sx under CPB	PBO vs. PO rivastigmine 1.5[1] pre-op, until POD #6	CAM	30 (17/57)	32 (18/56)	p = 0.8
van Eijk et al., 2010 DBRPCT, n = 109	(Tx) >18 y/o in ICU	2 arms, both receiving haloperidol, trial PBO vs. rivastigmine	CAM-ICU	3d	5d	p = 0.06
				Above refers to delirium duration in days; trial halted due to mortality in rivastigmine (n = 12, 22%) was > than in placebo group (n = 4, 8%; p = 0.07)		

[1] Rivastigmine-treated patients who experienced delirium had a shorter duration, lower use of benzodiazepine and neuroleptic for management of agitation, and improvement in all behavioral aspects measured by the BEHAVE-AD.

(Liptzin, Laki, Garb, Fingeroth, & Krushell, 2005). Subjects in the active treatment group received donepezil or placebo for 14 days before surgery and 14 days afterward, and no significant differences between groups were found ($p = 0.69$). A second RCT also failed to demonstrate efficacy of donepezil (5 mg immediately postoperatively and every 24 hrs thereafter for the first 3 postoperative days) over placebo in preventing postoperative delirium after elective total hip replacement surgery in older people without preexisting dementia (9.5% donepezil vs. 35.7% PBO; $p = 0.08$) (Sampson et al., 2007). Even though this was a negative study, the trend was in the right direction (lower incidence of delirium; shorter length of stay [9.9 vs. 12.1 days; $p = 0.09$] and shorter delirium duration [1.5 vs. 1.8 days; $p = 0.83$]), and the study had Type-II errors (i.e., it was grossly underpowered).

The results of the acetylcholinesterase trials seem to suggest that these agents are either (a) just not good for delirium prevention; or (b) they need to be used for much longer periods of time (as in the case of Dautzenberg and Moretti's study); or (c) they need to be used at doses much higher than we currently use them in order to achieve acute clinical efficacy.

A note of warning: more recently a DBRPCT comparing rivastigmine to placebo was stopped after members of the data safety and monitoring board unblinded the results and performed an interim analysis, halting the study due to concerns about a higher mortality rate in the rivastigmine group ($p = 0.07$) (van Eijk et al., 2010). The authors failed to explain the mechanism by which rivastigmine use may have led to the higher mortality reported. It is difficult to interpret their report, as less than 25% of the sample had been studied, and the causes of death for those on the study drug were heterogeneous. It is clear that the study relied on a very fast rivastigmine titration (essentially doubling the dose every 3 days until reaching the goal of 6 mg BID by day 10). This could have contributed to untoward side effects, which could have potentially worsened underlying cardiovascular or metabolic processes. Unlike in other delirium studies, the population in this study was not homogeneous, as it involved patients with all types of disease in the ICU. As the authors reported, "we cannot exclude that the recorded difference in mortality is due to chance" (van Eijk et al., 2010, p.1835).

Acetylcholinesterase Inhibitors for Delirium Treatment

Addressing the theory that proposes that delirium is caused by a central cholinergic deficiency state, some researchers and clinicians have experimented with the use of acetylcholinesterase inhibitor agents. Most of the published data consist of small series of case reports associated with the use of rivastigmine in the treatment of delirium in older persons (Dautzenberg, Mulder, et al., 2004; van den Bliek & Maas, 2004)(van den Bliek and Maas 2004). There have been at least 19 papers, mostly case reports, suggesting that acetylcholinesterase inhibitor agents (e.g., donepezil, galantamine, physostigmine, rivastigmine) may be effective in the treatment of delirium (see Box 41.8).

Box 41.8 CASE REPORTS SUGGESTING A POSITIVE EFFECT OF ACETYLCHOLINESTERASE INHIBITORS IN THE TREATMENT OF DELIRIUM

- Burt, 2000
- Bruera, Strasser, et al., 2003
- Dautzenberg, et al., 2003, 2004
- Fisher et al., 2001
- Gleason, 2003
- Hasse & Rundshagen, 2007
- Hori, Tominaga, et al., 2003
- Kaufer, Catt, et al., 1998
- Kobayashi et al., 2004
- Logan & Stewart, 2007
- Moretti et al., 2004
- Palmer, 2004
- Rabinowitz, 2002
- Weizberg et al., 2006
- Wengel, Roccaforte, & Burke 1998
- Wengel, Burke, & Roccaforte, 1999

Physostigmine and Delirium

Acetylcholine deficiency has been postulated as one of the potential causes of delirium; whether this is caused by normal physiological causes (e.g., aging) or due to exogenous factors (e.g., use of anticholinergic substances). Thus, among the tools to treat delirium, particularly when it is presumed to be due to the ingestion of substances with anticholinergic potential, we should consider the potential use of physostigmine. Physostigmine, a short-acting acetylcholinesterase inhibitor, increases synaptic acetylcholine concentrations and can overcome the postsynaptic muscarinic receptor-blockade produced by anticholinergic agents. As a tertiary amine, it can pass freely into the CNS and reverse both central and peripheral anticholinergic effects.

Many reports have demonstrated its utility and safety in cases when delirium has been caused by medication overdose (whether accidental or intentional) (Stern, 1983); Lipowski, 1992; Beaver & Gavin, 1998; Richardson, Williams, & Carstairs, 2004; Eyer et al., 2011; Hail, Obafemi, & Kleinschmidt, 2013). Physostigmine has been successfully used to treat emergence delirium in both adults (Brown, Heller, & Barkin, 2004; Haase & Rundshagen, 2007) and pediatric patients (Funk, Hollnberger, & Geroldinger, 2008). It has been reported that physostigmine attenuates several withdrawal states, especially alcohol delirium and opiate and nitrous oxide withdrawal syndromes; and it may offer a protective mechanism against hypoxic damage of the brain (Powers, Decoskey, & Kahrilas, 1981; Ruprecht, Schneck, & Dworacek, 1989).

Despite many psychiatrists' concerns about physostigmine administration, its use as a diagnostic test appears to be rather safe. In a series of 39 adults treated with varying doses of physostigmine (range 0.5–2.0 mg), 56% of all cases experienced full reversal of delirium. Among the cases known to be antimuscarinic in etiology (e.g., overdose with a known substance) 100% of patients experience full reversal. In this sample, no patient experience dysrhythmias or signs of cholinergic excess, or required the administration of atropine. One (2.6%) in 39 patients experienced a brief convulsion, with no known adverse sequelae (Schneir et al., 2003). Similarly, others have reported that among 52 consecutive patients with suspected anticholinergic delirium, physostigmine controlled agitation and reversed delirium in 96% and 87% of cases, respectively (Burns, Linden Graudins, Brown, & Fletcher, 2000). Again, no significant side effects were reported.

Given its safety profile and effectiveness, physostigmine should be considered when a delirious patient's examination exhibits signs of a central anticholinergic state (e.g., confusion, sinus tachycardia, markedly dilated and fixed pupils, dry mouth, hypoactive bowels sounds, dry and flushed skin; see Box 41.9) and/or when it is known that the patient's altered mental status is due to the use of known anticholinergic substances (e.g., diphenhydramine). An initial physostigmine dose of 1–2 mg (0.5 mg in children) given intravenously over 3 to 5 minutes is the recommended dose. If the response is incomplete, additional doses of 0.5–1.0 mg every 5 minutes may be given until delirium resolves or there are signs of cholinergic excess (e.g., diaphoresis, salivation, vomiting, diarrhea). A prolonged PR interval (>200 ms) or QRS complex (>100 ms and not related to bundle branch block) interval on ECG are considered the only absolute contraindications for physostigmine use.

Melatonin and Sleep Deficit

Sleep deprivation is one of the major theories on the development of delirium, whether caused by medication effect, environmental factors, or patient characteristics. Many sedative and hypnotic agents may worsen sleep and thus are not recommended. As described in the prevention section, various sedative hypnotic agents are commonly used in the medical setting, but most of them have significant problems, including causing or worsening delirium, cognitive clouding, and respiratory depression.

Box 41.9 ANTICHOLINERGIC SIDE EFFECTS

Cognitive impairment
Delirium
Dilated and fixed pupils, blurred vision
Dry and flushed skin
Dry mouth
Fever
Hallucinations
Hypoactive bowels sounds, constipation, ileus
Sinus tachycardia
Urinary retention

Various sedative hypnotic agents are commonly used in the medical setting. Nevertheless, benzodiazepines and the benzodiazepine-receptor agonists (e.g., zolpidem) may cause or exacerbate delirium. Other sedating agents, such as antidepressants (e.g., trazodone, mirtazapine) and antipsychotics (e.g., olanzapine) have been used off-label to promote sleep, but these agents have not been tested in the critically ill population. Clinicians must also consider factors such as drug–drug interaction and medication half-lives when prescribing. For example, mirtazapine and trazodone may indeed promote night sleep, but their effects may last well into the next day, interfering with cognition, attention, and concentration. Sedative agents with high anticholinergic load, such as antihistaminic agents (e.g., diphenhydramine, hydroxyzine) or tricyclic antidepressants (e.g., amitriptyline) should be avoided, as they will aggravate delirium even if they are immediately effective in promoting sleep. Similarly, benzodiazepines should also be avoided if at all possible.

An alternative to these is the use of non-benzodiazepine agents, such as melatonin or melatonin agonists (i.e., ramelteon). Melatonin has been shown to play an important role in the regulation of circadian rhythm and maintenance of a physiological, well-regulated sleep-wake pattern (Brzezinski, 1997). Multiple studies have demonstrated a number of abnormalities linking melatonin and delirium, including (a) irregular patterns of melatonin circadian rhythm (Miyazaki et al., 2003; Olofsson, Alling, Lundberg, & Malmros, 2004); and (b) decreased melatonin secretion (Shigeta et al., 2001; Guo, Kuzumi, Charman, & Vuylsteke, 2002) and abnormalities in the 24-hour urinary excretion of 6-sulphatoxymelatonin (6-SMT); the chief metabolite of melatonin (Balan, Leibovitz, et al., 2003). (See Table 41.20 for publications on melatonin abnormalities in delirium.) It is also theorized that melatonin may have protective effects, at least in cases of global cerebral ischemia/reperfusion injury, which may have implications for delirium onset (Sun, Lin, et al., 2002; Zhang, Guo, et al., 2002; Cheung, 2003; Cervantes, Morali, et al., 2008). In fact, melatonin may have a number of beneficial physiological effects which may prove benefical in the management of medically ill, delirious patients (see Box 41.10).

Melatonin in Delirium Prevention

Several case reports have described the successful use of melatonin in preventing postoperative delirium (Hanania & Kitain, 2002). A small DBRPCT demonstrated that the use of melatonin (10 mg q HS) was associated with longer and better sleep quality ($p = 0.04$) (Bourne et al., 2008). A recent DBRPCT ($n = 222$) compared the effects of melatonin versus placebo among elderly patients undergoing hip arthroplasty under spinal anesthesia and found that those receiving melatonin showed a statistically significant decrease in the percentage of postoperative delirium (9.43% vs. 2.65%, $p = 0.003$) (Sultan, 2010). Similarly, a recent DBRPCT ($n = 145$) among tertiary-care medicine service elderly individuals demonstrated that the administration of low-dose (i.e., 0.5 mg) melatonin was associated with a lower risk of delirium (12.0% vs. 31.0%, $p = 0.014$), adjusted for dementia and other comorbidities (Al-Aama et al., 2011).

Table 41.20 DELIRIUM-ASSOCIATED MELATONIN ABNORMALITIES

STUDY	POPULATION	INTERVENTION	DELIRIUM DEFINITION	RESULTS
Shigeta et al., 2001 $N = 29$	Men and women undergoing laparotomy for digestive disease	None; observational	CAM	All patients without delirium showed nearly identical preoperative and postoperative melatonin secretion for 24 hours.
				Conclusions: Abnormal melatonin secretion may be involved in postoperative sleep disturbances, which triggered delirium in elderly patients.
Guo et al., 2002 $N = 12$	Males undergoing elective CABG with CPB	None; observational		Only three patients regained circadian secretion of cortisol.
				Conclusion: melatonin and cortisol secretion were disrupted during cardiac surgery with CPB and in the immediate postoperative period
Miyazaki et al., 2003 $N = 41$	s/p esophagectomy for CA	None; observational	CE	A significant correlation was seen between ICU psychosis and an irregular melatonin circadian rhythm ($P = .0001$).
Balan et al., 2003 $N = 31$	Patients who developed delirium during hospitalization	None; patients were divided into: hyperactive (7), hypoactive (10), mixed (14)	ICD-10 DRS	24-hr urinary excretion of 6-sulphatoxymelatonin (6-SMT)—the chief metabolite of melatonin.
				Among hyperactive patients, the levels of 6-SMT were lower during the acute delirium than after recovery ($p<0.001$). Among hypoactive patients, 6-SMT levels were higher during the acute delirium than after recovery ($p < 0.01$). No difference in mixed.
Yoshitaka, Egi, et al., 2013 $N = 40$	40 postoperative patients in intensive care unit	None; observational	CAM	There was no difference in preoperative melatonin concentration. The Δ melatonin concentration at 1-hr post-op was significantly lower in patients with delirium than in those without delirium ($P = .036$). After adjustment of relevant confounders, Δ melatonin concentration was independently associated with risk of delirium (OR, 0.50; $P = .047$).

Melatonin and Melatonin Agonists in Delirium Treatment

Several case reports have described the successful use of melatonin in treating severe postoperative delirium unresponsive to antipsychotics or benzodiazepines (Hanania & Kitain, 2002). As part of the Sultan (2010) DBRPCT noted above ($n = 222$), comparing the effects of melatonin versus placebo among elderly patients undergoing hip arthroplasty under spinal anesthesia, a number of subjects developed postoperative delirium and received postoperative melatonin for treatment ($n = 62$). It was found that 58% of subjects experienced delirium resolution after treatment administration (Sultan, 2010).

Box 41.10 MELATONIN PHYSIOLOGICAL EFFECTS

- Melatonin plays important roles in multiple bodily functions, which may have implications for the development of delirium in the medically ill:
    - Chronobiotic effect (affecting aspects of biological time structure)
    - Sleep–wake cycle regulatory effects
    - Helps reset circadian rhythm disturbances
    - Extensive antioxidant activity (with a particular role in the protection of nuclear and mitochondrial DNA)
    - Extensive antiinflammatory activity
    - Anti-nociceptive and analgesic effects
    - Melatonin receptors appear to be important in mechanisms of learning and memory
    - Inhibits the aggregation of the amyloid beta protein into neurotoxic microaggregates responsible for the neurofibrillary tangles characteristics of Alzheimer's disease, and it prevents the hyperphosphorylation of the tau protein.

Adapted from Maldonado (Maldonado, 2008a).

Darlington, L. G., C. M. Forrest, G. M. Mackay, R. A. Smith, A. J. Smith, N. Stoy and T. W. Stone (2010). "On the Biological Importance of the 3-hydroxyanthranilic Acid: Anthranilic Acid Ratio." *Int J Tryptophan Res* 3: 51–59.

Of note, a systematic literature search of all papers published on the use of melatonin for the treatment in dementia revealed a significant improvement in sundowning/agitated behavior (de Jonghe, Korevaar, van Munster, & de Rooij, 2010). This may be particularly important given the presence of circadian rhythm disturbances, like sundowning, in both dementia and delirium. Similarly, case reports have suggested the usefulness of ramelteon, a melatonin agonist, in the treatment of delirium (Kimura et al., 2011).

Similarly, there are two case reports of the successful use of ramelteon (a novel selective melatonin-receptor agonist) in the treatment of patients with delirium (Kimura et al., 2011; Furuya et al., 2012). (See Table 41.21 for a summary of published case reports and studies on the use of melatonin for the treatment of delirium.)

When it comes to sleep and delirium, the clinician must consider both risks and benefits of the intervention.

In general, lack of sleep may lead to delirium, especially in patients at high risk (e.g., the elderly; the seriously medically ill); thus, promoting sleep is paramount. The first step, as always, is prevention. Therefore, the implementation of nonpharmacological sleep protocols as described above is important. If the patient still has difficulty sleeping, the use of melatonin (or melatonin agonists) is probably the best first pharmacological option. When this is not enough, clinicians should consider the use of trazodone, followed by mirtazapine. If needed, zolpidem may be an acceptable choice. Compared to conventional benzodiazepine agents, zolpidem may have a lower deliriogenic potential. Certainly, some of the other delirium treatment alternatives already discussed above may be beneficial for sleep promotion, such as the use of nighttime gabapentin or VPA or the use of low-dose quetiapine. As a general rule, it is advisable to avoid the use of diphenhydramine due to its anticholinergic effects. Although

Table 41.21 MELATONIN AND ANALOG FOR DELIRIUM MANAGEMENT

STUDY $N = 7$	POPULATION	INTERVENTION	DELIRIUM DEFINITION	RESULTS
Bourne et al., 2008 $N = 24$ DBPCT	S/p tracheostomy to assist weaning from vent	Melatonin (MEL) 10 mg PO @ 2000	Bispectral index (BIS)	Melatonin use was associated with a 1-hour increase in nocturnal sleep ($P = 0.09$) and a decrease in BIS AUC indicating "better" sleep. Melatonin use was associated with increased nocturnal sleep efficiency.
Al-Aama, Brymer, et al., 2011 $N = 145$	Individuals aged ≥65 y/o admitted through the ED to a medical unit	Randomized to MEL 0.5 mg vs. PBO every night for 14 days or until discharge.	CAM	Melatonin was associated with a lower risk of delirium (12.0% vs. 31.0%, $p = 0.014$).
Sultan, 2010 $N = 300$	≥ 65 y/o scheduled for hip arthroplasty under spinal anesthesia	Randomized to: 1. PBO 2. Melatonin 5 mg 3. Midazolam 7.5 mg 4. Clonidine 100 μg	Abbreviated Mental Test (AMT)	The melatonin group showed a statistically significant decrease in the percentage of postoperative delirium to 9.43%. POD: PBO—32.7 %; MEL—9.4 % ($p = 0.003$); MID—44 and ($p = 0.245$) CLO—37.3 % ($p = 0.629$); Melatonin was successful in treating 58.06% of patients who suffered postoperative delirium.
de Jonghe et al., 2010 Review	Meta-analysis		Various	Nine papers, including RCTs ($n = 243$), and five case series ($n = 87$) were reviewed. Two of the RCTs found a significant improvement on sundowning/agitated behavior. All five case series found an improvement.
de Jonghe, van Munster, et al., 2011 $N = 452$	≥65 y/o admitted for surgical repair of hip fracture	Randomized to: PBO Melatonin 3 mg @ 2100	CAM	Ongoing
Kimura et al., 2011 $N = 3$ (case report)	Pts >59 y/o, medically ill	Open label; ramelteon 8 mg q HS	DSM-IV-TR MDAS-Jap	All three cases demonstrated significant improvement in delirium scores as measured by MDAS, with steady improvement over 7 days, ramelteon 8 mg at HS.
Furuya et al., 2012 $N = 5$ (case report)	Mostly demented, medically ill patients	Open label; ramelteon 8 mg	DSM-IV-TR	Authors reported the successful treatment of five cases of delirium within 1 day, after ramelteon 8 mg at HS.

Abbreviations: MEL=melatonin; BIS= Bispectral index (BIS) monitor.

low-dose doxepin is an excellent alternative for many adult patients, it is unclear if it would still have enough anticholinergic effect to make it wise avoid it. Certainly, the use of conventional benzodiazepine agents is discouraged due to their inherit deliriogenic effect.

SLEEP RESTORATION IN DELIRIUM TREATMENT

As described above, in delirium treatment we highly recommend starting with the implementation of nonpharmacological sleep protocols. If the patient still has difficulty sleeping, the use of melatonin (or melatonin agonists) is probably the best first pharmacological option (e.g., 3 mg PO q, 2000; for prophylaxis). Several case reports have described the successful use of melatonin (e.g., 1–36 mg HS PO, for treatment) and melatonin agonists in treating severe postoperative delirium that is unresponsive to antipsychotics or benzodiazepines (Sultan, 2010; Kimura et al., 2011; Furuya et al., 2012).

If that fails, clinicians should consider the use of non-benzodiazepine agents, such as trazodone or mirtazapine. If absolutely necessary, zolpidem may be an acceptable choice, but take into consideration the moderately high incidence of disordered sleep behaviors while on zolpidem and similar drugs. Given its short half-life and high sedation effect, low-dose quetiapine may also be an acceptable short-term solution, especially in patients experiencing sundowning.

OTHER AGENTS THAT HAVE SHOWN SOME PROMISE IN DELIRIUM MANAGEMENT

Some have theorized that an impaired serotonin metabolism may play a role in the development of delirium (Maldonado, 2008a,b). The original open-label study found that the antiemetic agent ondansetron, a selective serotonin 5-HT$_3$-type receptor antagonist, may be effective in the treatment of "hyperactive delirium" ($P = 0.001$) (Bayindir, Guden Akpinar, Sanisoglu, & Sagbas, 2001). More recently, there was a second study (DBRCT; $n = 80$) comparing ondansetron (8 mg IV) to haloperidol (5 mg IV) in the treatment of post-cardiotomy "delirium." The authors reported no significant baseline difference between the groups and similar clinical improvement, from delirious baseline, in both groups ($p < 0.01$). Unfortunately, this study did not use a standardized and validated delirium severity measure. The nonvalidated "scale" used by these researchers (different in each case) appeared to have been more a nonstandardized measure of agitation, rather than delirium. It is also not clear how the groups were randomly assessed, and it is difficult to make sense pharmacologically of the time for assessment, given very different pharmacokinetics of both agents (e.g., after IV administration, haloperidol's half-life is 10–20 hrs., vs. ondansetron's 5 hrs.; onset of action is also expected to be quite varied). Given the nature of these studies, and the fact it did not rely on the use of a validated diagnostic method, further, better designed studies are needed.

Finally, an open-label, prospective NRCT of patients undergoing cardiac surgery compared placebo versus statin administration for prevention of delirium in elderly patients (Katznelson et al., 2009). The authors remarked that statin administration has been shown to decrease morbidity and mortality after cardiac and major noncardiac surgery, and that animal and human studies have demonstrated the beneficial effect of statins in central neural system injury. Thus they theorized that the antithrombotic, antiinflammatory, and immunomodulatory properties of statins may be responsible for these protective effects, and that the same qualities may help protect against delirium. In fact, their study demonstrated that the administration of statins had a significant protective effect, reducing the odds of delirium by 46% among patients 60 years old and older. Of interest, these delirium-sparing effects did not manifest in patients younger than 60 years old.

DELIRIUM MANAGEMENT: SUMMARY

In summary, in order to prevent delirium, we recommend incorporating nonpharmacological and pharmacological approaches. Key among the possible interventions is the minimization of prolonged and uninterrupted sedation, by scheduling daily sedation holidays and titration of sedation to a targeted goal, assisted by the use of sedation scales. The choice of sedative and analgesic agents may also make a significant difference. It is important to be mindful of the additive effect that certain pharmacological agents may have, including sedative, deliriogenic, and anticholinergic potential. A good prevention strategy is the routine inspection of the patient's medication list, wise choice of agents (avoiding anticholinergic and benzodiazepine agents, if possible) and eliminating all unnecessary agents. Remember the rule: the greater the number of pharmacological agents the patient is exposed to, the greater the risk for delirium. The implementation of delirium surveillance methods (such as any of the widely available delirium detection tools) enables the early recognition of delirium, and sometimes the detection of subsyndromal forms of delirium, allowing for prompt action before a full-blown syndrome has developed. Early mobilization is paramount. As a rule, the more vertical and restriction-free a patient is, the lower the incidence of delirium. It is important to eliminate restrictive devices and to reduce or eliminate sedation and analgesia as soon as medically appropriate and safe, and to promote getting patients mobilized and out of bed as soon as possible. Once they are capable of leaving the bed, patients should be encouraged to eat all meals sitting at the bedside chair rather than in bed. The implementation of a multicomponent, nonpharmacological protocol (especially with training and involvement of family and friends) may make a big difference for many patients, their family, and hospital staff. When safe, family and staff should be encouraged to get the patient out of the unit and to see that the patient receives as much direct sunlight as possible. This will assist the process of normalizing the sleep–wake cycle naturally by manipulating the amount of ambient light. When this is not possible, consider the use of melatonin or a melatonin-agonist, as well as any of a whole host of nonpharmacological sleep-promoting interventions (e.g., avoid scheduling unnecessary blood draws and vital sign checks in the middle of the night [if the patient's medical condition allows it], minimize ambient noise and unnecessary light exposure, limit the amount of TV-watching after a certain time of day, and offer ear plugs and eye masks to enhance the patient's comfort). Melatonin and melatonin agonists may offer more benefit and fewer side effects than conventional sedative agents. The selective use of prophylactic antipsychotic agents should be considered, particularly in patients at high risk or those with a prior history of developing delirium in the medical environment. When delirium has already developed, the judicious use of dopamine antagonist agents seems to have the most evidence for a prompt recovery. When it comes to the use of acetylcholinesterase inhibitors, the data available seem to suggest that they work only in patients who have been on them long-term (i.e., for dementia). Thus their use may be considered in patients with moderate to severe cognitive impairment who suffer from multiple medical and chronic medical issues and who are expected to repeatedly return to the medical environment. Yet, data suggest that physostigmine is an underutilized therapeutic option we should consider in obvious cases of anticholinergic delirium.

SUMMARY

Delirium is a neurobehavioral syndrome caused by the transient disruption of normal neuronal activity secondary to systemic disturbances, and is the most common psychiatric syndrome found in the general hospital setting. In addition to causing distress to patients, families, and medical caregivers, the development of delirium has been associated with increased morbidity and mortality, increased cost of care, increased hospital-acquired complications, poor functional and cognitive recovery, decreased quality of life, prolonged hospital stays, and increased placement in specialized intermediate and long-term care facilities.

Clinical experience and research data suggest that once delirium has occurred, it is possible the patients may not return to their pre-delirium cognitive functional level. In fact, data suggests delirium the occurrence of delirium is associated with an increased risk of dementia, and acceleration in the rate of cognitive decline in those demented patients who develop delirium. Therefore, given increasing evidence that delirium is not always reversible, and given the potentially numerous negative sequelae associated with its development, physicians must do everything possible to prevent its occurrence.

The data also suggest that there may be a "dose-effect" for delirium, meaning that the longer a patient is delirious, the worse is the expected outcome. This is particularly true of hypoactive delirium, which unfortunately is the most commonly occurring type, particularly in the elderly. Therefore, clinicians are encouraged to implement as many prevention strategies as are available to them in order to improve patient outcome and prevent or minimize the occurrence of delirium, thus minimizing its morbidity.

Because delirium is common, it is important that physicians be mindful and implement surveillance and monitoring strategies to allow for early detection and the implementation of techniques that may shorten its duration. When delirium occurs, it is important to immediately correct the underlying contributing causes and use treatment strategies directed at preventing harm to the patient and others and to shorten the duration of the delirium episode, thus improving the odds of recovering baseline functional status.

The psychosomatic medicine specialist has much to contribute to the diagnosis, treatment, and study of delirium. In the author's experience, better results at implementing change, fostering psychiatric consultation, and greater involvement of our services come from getting involved in multidisciplinary quality-improvement projects that involve physicians, nurses, and ancillary staff in the process of recognition and treatment of delirious patients. Active participation in educational programs (e.g., continuing education, grand rounds, clinical case conferences) and development of a multidisciplinary task force charged with assessing the problem and developing an action plan are key to being recognized as an expert in the field, the one to go to for advice. At our institution, we developed a "CNS Pharmacotherapy Task-Force" that developed protocols for the ICU in sedation, pain management, neurological assessment, and delirium monitoring, prevention, and treatment. Its success has led to this model being replicated throughout the institution, with a greater recognition of delirium as a problem and of psychosomatic medicine specialists as the experts in the field. The author's team has implemented regular didactic sessions for nursing, regular rounding sessions in the MICU and SICU, and a monthly "psychiatric mortality and morbidity" review in the internal medicine program that has been invaluable in helping the medical staff change their perception and practice toward delirium, leading to greater joint participation between psychiatry and medico-surgical services.

CLINICAL PEARLS

- Four important non-modifiable factors for delirium are older age, baseline cognitive impairment, severity of underlying medical illness, and preexisting mental disorders.

- Among patients with preexisting mental disorders, patients with bipolar disorder had the highest incidence of delirium.

- Opioids, corticosteroids, and benzodiazepines are major contributors to delirium see Figure 41.7 (Gaudreau, Gagnon, et al., 2005b).

- A study of adult patients admitted to inpatient medicine wards showed that those who developed delirium had significantly elevated levels (i.e., above the detection limit) of IL-6 (53% versus 31%) and IL-8 (45% versus 22%), compared with patients who did not develop delirium, even after adjusting for infection, age, and cognitive impairment (de Rooij, van Munster, Korevaar, & Levi, 2007). This is the first study to show a relationship between peripherally measured cytokine levels and delirium as a symptom of sickness behavior in acutely admitted elderly.

- Three core domains of delirium are *cognitive deficits* (characterized by attention and vigilance disturbances), *circadian rhythm dysregulation* (characterized by fragmentation of the sleep–wake cycle), and *higher cortical dysfunction* (characterized by semantic and comprehension deficits, executive dysfunction, and thought-process disturbances) (Meagher et al., 2007).

- Hypoactive delirium is often missed or misdiagnosed as depression (Liptzin & Levkoff 1992), and these patients have experienced the worst prognosis (e.g., prolonged hospital stay, higher morbidity and mortality) (Kiely et al., 2007).

- The severity scales of delirium may provide an added benefit—the ability to diagnose subsyndromal delirium.

- In our clinical experience, patients with delirium tend to exhibit a reemergence of primitive signs (see Box 41.5).

- Although the EEG is nonspecific and difficult to obtain in agitated patients, it can be useful in differentiating delirium from other conditions such as catatonic states, seizure activity, somatoform disorders, and malingering.

DISCLOSURE STATEMENTS

Dr. Maldonado has no proprietary or commercial interest in any product mentioned or concept discussed in this chapter.

REFERENCES

Abildstrom, H., Christiansen, M., Siersma, V. D., & Rasmussen, L. S. (2004). Apolipoprotein E genotype and cognitive dysfunction after noncardiac surgery. *Anesthesiology, 101*(4), 855–861.

Abu-Shahwan, I. (2008). Effect of propofol on emergence behavior in children after sevoflurane general anesthesia. *Paediatric Anaesthesia, 18*(1), 55–59.

Abu-Shahwan, I., & Chowdary, K. (2007). Ketamine is effective in decreasing the incidence of emergence agitation in children undergoing dental repair under sevoflurane general anesthesia. *Paediatric Anaesthesia, 17*(9), 846–850.

Adamis, D., Treloar, A., Martin., F. C., Gregson, N., Hamilton, G., & Macdonald, A. J. (2007). APOE and cytokines as biological markers for recovery of prevalent delirium in elderly medical inpatients. *International Journal of Geriatric Psychiatry, 22*(7), 688–694.

Adams, F. (1988). Neuropsychiatric evaluation and treatment of delirium in cancer patients. *Adv Psychosomatic Medicine, 18*: 26–36.

Adams, F., Fernandez, F., & Andersson, B. (1986). Emergency pharmacotherapy of delirium in the critically ill cancer patient. *Psychosomatics, 27*(1 Suppl), 33–38.

Agarwal, V., O'Neill, P. J., Cotton, B. A., Pun, B. T., Haney, S., Thompson, J., et al. (2010). Prevalence and risk factors for development of delirium in burn intensive care unit patients. *Journal of Burn Care & Research, 31*(5), 706–715.

Al-Aama, T., Brymer, C., Gutmanis, I., Woolmore-Goodwin, S. M., Esbaugh, J., & Dasgupta, M. (2011). Melatonin decreases delirium in elderly patients: a randomized, placebo-controlled trial. *International Journal of Geriatric Psychiatry, 26*(7), 687–694.

Alao, A. O., & Moskowitz, L. (2006). Aripiprazole and delirium. *Annals of Clinical Psychiatry, 18*(4), 267–269.

Albin, M. S., Bunegin, L., Massopust Jr., L. C., & Jannetta, P. J. (1974). Ketamine-induced postanesthetic delirium attenuated by tetrahydroaminoacridine. *Experimental Neurology, 44*(1), 126–129.

Albert, M. S., Levkoff, S. E., Reilly, C., et al. (1992). The delirium symptom interview: an interview for the detection of delirium symptoms in hospitalized patients. *Journal of Geriatric Psychiatry & Neurology, 5*(1), 14–21.

Aldemir, M., Ozen, S., Kara, I. H., Sir, A., & Bac, B. (2001). Predisposing factors for delirium in the surgical intensive care unit. *Critical Care, 5*(5), 265–270.

Andersen, J. H., Boesen, H. C., & Olsen, K. S. (2013). Sleep in the intensive care unit measured by polysomnography. *Minerva Anestesiologica, 79*(7), 804–815.

APA (1994). *Diagnostic and Statistical Manual of Mental Disorders— 4th Edition.* Washington, DC: American Psychiatric Association.

APA (2013). *Diagnostic and Statistical Manual of Mental Disorders, 5th Edition.* Washington, DC: American Psychiatric Association.

APA (1999). Practice Guideline for the Treatment of Patients With Delirium. *American Psychiatric Association Steering Committee on Practice Guidelines.* P. Trzepacz, W. Breitbart, J. Franklin, et al., eds. Washington DC: American Psychiatric Association.

APA (2004). Guideline Watch: Practice Guideline for the Treatment of Patients With Delirium. *American Psychiatric Association Practice Guidelines.* I. A. Cook, ed. Washington DC: American Psychiatric Association.

Armstrong, S. C., Cozza, K. L., & Watanabe, K. S. (1997). The misdiagnosis of delirium. *Psychosomatics, 38*(5), 433–439.

Aurell, J., & Elmqvist, D. (1985). Sleep in the surgical intensive care unit: continuous polygraphic recording of sleep in nine patients receiving postoperative care. *British Medical Journal (Clinical Research Edition), 290*(6474), 1029–1032.

Ayd, F. J. Jr. (1978). Haloperidol: twenty years' clinical experience. *Journal of Clinical Psychiatry, 39*(11), 807–814.

BaHammam, A. (2006). Sleep in acute care units. *Sleep and Breathing, 10*(1), 6–15.

Bajwa, S. A., Costi, D., & Cyna, (2010). A comparison of emergence delirium scales following general anesthesia in children. *Paediatric Anaesthesia, 20*(8), 704–711.

Balan, S., Leibovitz, A., Zila, S. O., Ruth, M., Chana, W., Yassica, B., et al. (2003). The relation between the clinical subtypes of delirium and the urinary level of 6–SMT. *Journal of Neuropsychiatry & Clinical Neurosciences, 15*(3), 363–366.

Ballard, C., Hanney, M. L., Theodoulou, M., Douglas, S., McShane, R., Kossakowski, K., et al. (2009). The dementia antipsychotic withdrawal trial (DART-AD): long-term follow-up of a randomised placebo-controlled trial. *Lancet Neurology, 8*(2), 151–157.

Barker, M. J., Greenwood, K. M., Jackson, M., & Crowe, S. F. (2004). Persistence of cognitive effects after withdrawal from long–term benzodiazepine use: a meta–analysis. *Archives of Clinical Neuropsychology, 19*(3), 437–454.

Barker, M. J., Greenwood, K. M., Jackson, M., & Crowe, S. F. (2005). An evaluation of persisting cognitive effects after withdrawal from long-term benzodiazepine use. *Journal of the International Neuropsycholocy Society, 11*(3), 281–289.

Basarsky, T. A., Feighan, D., & MacVicar, B. A. (1999). Glutamate release through volume–activated channels during spreading depression. *Journal of Neuroscience, 19*(15), 6439–6445.

Basavaraju, N., & Phillips, S. L. (1989). Cortisol deficient state. A cause of reversible cognitive impairment and delirium in the elderly. *Journal of the American Geriatrics Society, 37*(1), 49–51.

Basinski, J. R., Alfano, C. M., Katon, W. J., Syrjala, K. L., & Fann, J. R. (2010). Impact of delirium on distress, health–related quality of life, and cognition 6 months and 1 year after hematopoietic cell transplant. *Biology of Blood and Bone Marrow Transplantation, 16*(6), 824–831.

Bastron, R. D., & Moyers, J. (1967). Emergence delirium. *Journal of the American Medical Association, 200*(10), 883.

Bayindir, O., Guden, M., Akpinar, B., Sanisoglu, I., & Sagbas, E. (2001). Ondansetron hydrochloride for the treatment of delirium after coronary artery surgery. *Journal of Thoracic and Cardiovascular Surgery, 121*(1), 176–177.

Beaver, K. M., & Gavin, T. J. (1998). Treatment of acute anticholinergic poisoning with physostigmine. *American Journal of Emergency Medicine, 16*(5), 505–507.

Behan, W. M., & Stone, T. W. (2000). Role of kynurenines in the neurotoxic actions of kainic acid. *British Journal of Pharmacol 129*(8), 1764–1770.

Bell, L. (1849). On a form of disease resembling some advanced stages of mania and fever, but so contradistinguished form ordinarily observed or described combination of symptoms as to render it probable that it may be an overlooked and hitherto unrecorded malady. *American Journal of Insanity, 6*, 97–127.

Benedict, L., Hazelett, S., Fleming, E., Ludwick, R., Anthony, M., Fosnight, S., et al. (2009). Prevention, detection and intervention with delirium in an acute care hospital: a feasibility study. *Int Journal of Older People Nurs, 4*(3), 194–202.

Bender, S., Grohmann, R., Engel, R. R., Degner, D., Dittmann-Balcar, A., & Ruther, E. (2004). Severe adverse drug reactions in psychiatric inpatients treated with neuroleptics. *Pharmacopsychiatry, 37*(Suppl 1): S46–53.

Benoit, A. G., Campbell, B. I., Tanner, J. R., et al. (2005). Risk factors and prevalence of perioperative cognitive dysfunction in abdominal aneurysm patients. *Journal of Vascular Surgery, 42*(5), 884–890.

Berger, M., Vollmann, J., Hohagen, F., Konig, A., Lohner, H., Voderholzer, U., & Riemann, D. (1997). Sleep deprivation combined with consecutive sleep phase advance as a fast–acting therapy in depression: an open pilot trial in medicated and unmedicated patients. *American Journal of Psychiatry, 154*(6), 870–872.

Bergeron, N., Dubois, M. J., Dumont, M., Dial, S., & Skrobik, Y. (2001). Intensive Care Delirium Screening Checklist: Evaluation of a new screening tool. *Intensive Care Medicine, 27*(5), 859–864.

Berggren, D., Gustafson, Y., Eriksson, B., Bucht, G., Hansson, L., Reiz, I. S., & Winblad, B. (1987). Postoperative confusion after anesthesia in elderly patients with femoral neck fractures. *Anesthesia and Analgesia, 66*(6), 497–504.

Berrios, G. E. (1981). Delirium and confusion in the 19th century: a conceptual history. *British Journal of Psychiatry 139*: 439–449.

Bettin, K. M., Maletta, G. J., Dysken, M. W., et al. (1998). Measuring delirium severity in older general hospital inpatients without dementia. The Delirium Severity Scale. *American Journal of Geriatric Psychiatry, 6*(4), 296–307.

Bickel, H., Gradinger R., Kochs, E., & Forstl, H. (2008). High risk of cognitive and functional decline after postoperative delirium. A three-year prospective study. *Dementia and Geriatric Cognitive Disorders, 26*(1), 26–31.

Billioti de Gage, S., Moride, Y., Ducruet, T., Kurth, T., Verdoux, H., Tournier, M., et al. (2014). Benzodiazepine use and risk of Alzheimer's disease: case-control study. *BMJ, 349*, g5205.

Bjorkelund, K. B., Hommel, A., Thorngren, K. G., Gustafson, L., Larsson, S., & Lundberg, D. (2010). Reducing delirium in elderly patients with hip fracture: a multi-factorial intervention study. *Acta Anaesthesiologica Scandinavica, 54*(6), 678–688.

Blank, K., & Perry, S. (1984). Relationship of psychological processes during delirium to outcome. *American Journal of Psychiatry, 141*(7), 843–847.

Blass, J., Gibson, G., Duffy, T., et al. (1981). Cholinergic dysfunction: a common denominator in metabolic encephalopathies. In: Pepeu, G., & Ladinsky, H. (Eds.) *Cholinergic Mechanisms* (pp. 921–928). New York: Plenum Publishing Corp.

Boettger, S., Friedlander, M., Breitbart, W., & Passik, S. (2011). Aripiprazole and haloperidol in the treatment of delirium. *The Australia and New Zealand Journal of Psychiatry, 45*(6), 477–482.

Boot, R. (2012). Delirium: a review of the nurses role in the intensive care unit. *Intensive and Critical Care Nursing, 28*(3), 185–189.

Borbely, A. A., Mattmann, P., Loepfe, M., Strauch, I., & Lehmann, D. (1985). Effect of benzodiazepine hypnotics on all-night sleep EEG spectra. *Human Neurobiology, 4*(3), 189–194.

Bourgeois, J. A., Koike, A. K., Simmons, J. E., Telles, S., & Eggleston, C. (2005). Adjunctive valproic acid for delirium and/or agitation on a consultation–liaison service: a report of six cases. *Journal of Neuropsychiatry & Clinical Neurosciences, 17*(2), 232–238.

Bourgon, L. (1985). Psychotic processes in delirium. *American Journal of Psychiatry, 142*(3), 392.

Bourne, R. S., Mills, G. H., & Minelli, C. (2008). Melatonin therapy to improve nocturnal sleep in critically ill patients: encouraging results from a small randomised controlled trial. *Critical Care, 12*(2), R52.

Boyko, Y., Ording, H., & Jennum, P. (2012). Sleep disturbances in critically ill patients in ICU: how much do we know? *Acta Anaesthesiologica Scandinavica, 56*(8), 950–958.

Brauer, C., Morrison, R. S., Silberzweig S. B., & Siu, A. L. (2000). The cause of delirium in patients with hip fracture. *Archives of Internal Medicine, 160*(12), 1856–1860.

Breitbart, W., Gibson, C., & Tremblay, A. (2002). The delirium experience: delirium recall and delirium–related distress in hospitalized patients with cancer, their spouses/caregivers, and their nurses. *Psychosomatics, 43*(3), 183–194.

Breitbart, W., Marotta, R., Platt, M. M., Weisman, Derevenco, M., Grau, C., et al. (1996). A H. double–blind trial of haloperidol, chlorpromazine, and lorazepam in the treatment of delirium in hospitalized AIDS patients. *American Journal of Psychiatry, 153*(2), 231–237.

Breitbart, W., Rosenfeld, B., Roth, A., Smith, M. J., Cohen, K., & Passik, S. (1997). The Memorial Delirium Assessment Scale. *Journal of Pain & Symptom Management, 13*(3), 128–137.

Broderick, P. A., & Gibson, G. E. (1989). Dopamine and serotonin in rat striatum during in vivo hypoxic–hypoxia. *Metabolic Brain Disease, 4*(2), 143–153.

Brown, D. V., Heller, F., & Barkin, R. (2004). Anticholinergic syndrome after anesthesia: a case report and review. *American Journal of Therapeutics, 11*(2), 144–153.

Brown, T. M. (2000). Basic mechanisms in the pathogenesis of delirium. In: F. B. Stoudemire, F. B., & Greenberg, A. (Eds.) *The Psychiatric Care of the Medical Patient* (pp. 571–580). New York: Oxford University Press.

Bruce, A. J., Ritchie, C. W., Blizard, R., Lai, R., & Raven, P. (2007). The incidence of delirium associated with orthopedic surgery: a meta–analytic review. *International Psychogeriatrics, 19*(2), 197–214.

Bruera, E., Strasser, F., Shen, L., et al. (2003). The effect of donepezil on sedation and other symptoms in patients receiving opioids for cancer pain: A pilot study. *Journal of Pain & Symptom Management, 26*(5), 1049–1054.

Brummel, N. E., & Girard, T. D. (2013). Preventing delirium in the intensive care unit. *Critical Care Clinics, 29*(1), 51–65.

Brummel, N. E., Morandi, A., & Vasilevskis, E. E. (2012). Intensive care unit delirium monitoring in Australia. *Critical Care Resusc, 14*(1), 89–90; author reply 91–82.

Bryson, G. L., Wyand, A., Wozny, D., Rees, L., Taljaard, M., & Nathan, H. (2011). A prospective cohort study evaluating associations among delirium, postoperative cognitive dysfunction, and apolipoprotein E genotype following open aortic repair. *Canadian Journal of Anaesthesia, 58*(3), 246–255.

Brzezinski, A. (1997). Melatonin in humans. *The New England Journal of Medicine, 336*(3), 186–195.

Buchman, N., Mendelsson, E., Lerner, V., & Kotler, M. (1999). Delirium associated with vitamin B12 deficiency after pneumonia. *Clinical Neuropharmacology, 22*(6), 356–358.

Bucht, G., Gustafson, Y., & Sandberg, O. (1999). Epidemiology of delirium. *Dementia & Geriatric Cognitive Disorders, 10*(5), 315–318.

Burns, M. J., Linden, C. H., Graudins, A., Brown, R. M., & Fletcher, K. E. (2000). A comparison of physostigmine and benzodiazepines for the treatment of anticholinergic poisoning. *Annals of Emergency Medicine, 35*(4), 374–381.

Burt, T. (2000). Donepezil and related cholinesterase inhibitors as mood and behavioral controlling agents. *Current Psychiatry Report, 2*(6), 473–478.

Busto, R., Dietrich, W. D., Globus, M. Y., Alonso, O., & Ginsberg, M. D. (1997). Extracellular release of serotonin following fluid–percussion brain injury in rats. *Journal of Neurotrauma, 14*(1), 35–42.

Busto, R., Globus, M. Y., Dietrich, W. D., Martinez, E., Valdes, I., & Ginsberg, M. D. (1989). Effect of mild hypothermia on ischemia-induced release of neurotransmitters and free fatty acids in rat brain. *Stroke, 20*(7), 904–910.

Byl, S., & Szafran, W. (1996). [Phrenitis in the Hippocratic Corpus: a philological and medical study]. *Vesalius, 2*(2), 98–105.

Bynum, B. (2000). Phrenitis: what's in a name? *Lancet, 356*(9245), 1936.

Camus, V., Burtin, B., Simeone, I., Schwed, P., Gonthier, R., & Dubos, G. (2000). Factor analysis supports the evidence of existing hyperactive and hypoactive subtypes of delirium. *International Journal of Geriatric Psychiatry, 15*(4), 313–316.

Caplan, J. P., & Chang, G. (2010). Refeeding syndrome as an iatrogenic cause of delirium: a retrospective pilot study. *Psychosomatics, 51*(5), 419–424.

Cardinali, D. P., Brusco, L. I., Liberczuk, C., & Furio, A. M. (2002). The use of melatonin in Alzheimer's disease. *Neuro Endocrinology Letters 23, Suppl 1*: 20–23.

Carnahan, R. M., Lund, B. C., Perry, P. J., & Pollock, B. G. (2002). A critical appraisal of the utility of the serum anticholinergic activity assay in research and clinical practice. *Psychopharmacology Bulletin, 36*(2), 24–39.

Carnes, M., Howell, T., Rosenberg, M., Francis, J., Hildebrand, C., & Knuppel, J. (2003). Physicians vary in approaches to the clinical management of delirium. *Journal of the American Geriatrics Society, 51*(2), 234–239.

Celsus, A. C. (1814). *Of Medicine.* Edinburgh: Edinburgh University Press.

Centeno, C., Sanz, A., & Bruera, E. (2004). Delirium in advanced cancer patients. *Palliative Medicine, 18*(3), 184–194.

Cerejeira, J., Firmino, H., Vaz-Serra, A., & Mukaetova-Ladinska, E. B. (2010). The neuroinflammatory hypothesis of delirium. *Acta Neuropathologica, 119*(6), 737–754.

Cervantes, M., Morali, G., & Letechipia-Vallejo, G. (2008). Melatonin and ischemia-reperfusion injury of the brain. *Journal of Pineal Research, 45*(1), 1–7.

Cheung, R. T. (2003). The utility of melatonin in reducing cerebral damage resulting from ischemia and reperfusion. *Journal of Pineal Research, 34*(3), 153–160.

Chong, M. S., Tan, K. T., Tay, L., Wong, Y. M., & Ancoli-Israel, S. (2013). Bright light therapy as part of a multicomponent management program improves sleep and functional outcomes in delirious older hospitalized adults. *Journal of Clinical Interventions in Aging, 8*, 565–572.

Cole, M. G., Fenton, F. R., Engelsmann, F., & Mansouri, I. (1991). Effectiveness of geriatric psychiatry consultation in an acute care hospital: a randomized clinical trial. *Jounal of the American Geriatrics Society, 39*(12), 1183–1188.

Cole, M., McCusker, J., Dendukuri, N., & Han, L. (2003). The prognostic significance of subsyndromal delirium in elderly medical inpatients. *Journal of the American Geriatrics Society, 51*(6), 754–760.

Cole, M. G., Ciampi, A., Belzile, E., & Zhong, L. (2009). Persistent delirium in older hospital patients: a systematic review of frequency and prognosis. *Age and Ageing, 38*(1), 19–26.

Collins, N., Blanchard, M. R., Tookman, A., & Sampson, E. L. (2010). Detection of delirium in the acute hospital. *Age Ageing, 39*(1), 131–135.

Culp, K. R., & Cacchione, P. Z. (2008). Nutritional status and delirium in long-term care elderly individuals. *Applied Nursing Research, 21*(2), 66–74.

Cunningham, C. (2011). Systemic inflammation and delirium: important co–factors in the progression of dementia. *Biochemical Society Transactions, 39*(4), 945–953.

Cunningham, C., Campion, S., Lunnon, K., Murray, C. L., Woods, J. F., Deacon, R. M., et al. (2009). Systemic inflammation induces acute behavioral and cognitive changes and accelerates neurodegenerative disease. *Biological Psychiatry, 65*(4), 304–312.

Cunningham, C., Wilcockson, D. C., Campion, S., Lunnon, K., & Perry, V. H. (2005). Central and systemic endotoxin challenges exacerbate the local inflammatory response and increase neuronal death during chronic neurodegeneration. *Journal of Neuroscience, 25*(40), 9275–9284.

Dahmani, S., Rouelle, D., Gressens, P., & Mantz, J. (2005). Effects of dexmedetomidine on hippocampal focal adhesion kinase tyrosine phosphorylation in physiologic and ischemic conditions. *Anesthesiology, 103*(5), 969–977.

Daman Willems, C. E., & Dillon, M. J. (1986). Confusion after admission to hospital in elderly patients using benzodiazepines. *British Medical Journal (Clinical Research Edition), 293*(6561), 1569.

Dantzer, R. (2004). Cytokine–induced sickness behaviour: a neuroimmune response to activation of innate immunity. *European Journal of Pharmacology, 500*(1–3), 399–411.

Dantzer, R., Bluthe, R. M., Laye, S., Bret-Dibat, J. L., Parnet, P., & Kelley, K. W. (1998). Cytokines and sickness behavior. *Ann N Y Acad Sci, 840*, 586–590.

Dantzer, R., Capuron, L., Irwin, M. R., Miller, A. H., Ollat, H., Perry, V. H., et al. (2008). Identification and treatment of symptoms associated with inflammation in medically ill patients. *Psychoneuroendocrinology, 33*(1), 18–29.

Darlington, L. G., Forrest, C. M., Mackay, G. M., Smith, R. A., Smith, A. J., Stoy, N., & Stone, T. W. (2010). On the biological importance of the 3-hydroxyanthranilic acid: anthranilic acid ratio. *International Journal of Tryptophan Research, 3*, 51–59.

Darlington, L. G., Mackay, G. M., Forrest, C. M., Stoy, N., George, C., & Stone, T. W. (2007). Altered kynurenine metabolism correlates with infarct volume in stroke. *Europpean Journal of Neuroscience, 26*(8), 2211–2221.

Dasgupta, M., & Dumbrell, A. C. (2006). Preoperative risk assessment for delirium after noncardiac surgery: a systematic review. *Journal of the American Geriatrics Society, 54*(10), 1578–1589.

Dautzenberg, P. L., Mulder, L. J., Olde Rikkert, M. G., Wouters, C. J., & Loonen, A J. (2004). Delirium in elderly hospitalised patients: Protective effects of chronic rivastigmine usage. *International Journal of Geriatric Psychiatry, 19*(7), 641–644.

Davidson, J. E., Harvey, M. A., Bemis-Dougherty, A., Smith, J. M., & Hopkins, R. O. (2013). Implementation of the Pain, Agitation, and Delirium Clinical Practice Guidelines and promoting patient mobility to prevent post–intensive care syndrome. *Critical Care Medicine, 41*(9 Suppl 1), S136–145.

Davis, D., & MacLullich, A. (2009). Understanding barriers to delirium care: a multicentre survey of knowledge and attitudes amongst UK junior doctors. *Age Ageing, 38*(5), 559–563.

Davis, D. H., Muniz Terrera, G., Keage, H., Rahkonen, T., Oinas, M., Matthews, F. E., et al. (2012). Delirium is a strong risk factor for dementia in the oldest-old: a population-based cohort study. *Brain, 135*(Pt 9), 2809–2816.

de Jonghe, A., Korevaar, J. C., van Munster, B. C., & de Rooij, S. E. (2010). Effectiveness of melatonin treatment on circadian rhythm disturbances in dementia. Are there implications for delirium? A systematic review. *International Journal of Geriatric Psychiatry 25*(12), 1201–1208.

de Jonghe, A., van Munster, B. C., van Oosten, H. E., Goslings, J. C., Kloen, P., van Rees, C., et al. (2011). The effects of melatonin versus placebo on delirium in hip fracture patients: study protocol of a randomised, placebo-controlled, double blind trial. *BMC Geriatrics, 11*(1), 34.

de Lange, E., Verhaak, P. F., & van der Meer, K. (2013). Prevalence, presentation and prognosis of delirium in older people in the population, at home and in long term care: a review. *International Journal of Geriatric Psychiatry, 28*(2), 127–134.

de Rooij, S. E., van Munster, B. C., Korevaar, J. C., & Levi, M. (2007). Cytokines and acute phase response in delirium. *Journal of Psychosomatic Research, 62*(5), 521–525.

Degos, V., Charpentier T. L., Chhor V., Brissaud O., Lebon S., Schwendimann L., et al. (2013). Neuroprotective effects of dexmedetomidine against glutamate agonist–induced neuronal cell death are related to increased astrocyte brain–derived neurotrophic factor expression. *Anesthesiology*, *118*(5), 1123–1132.

Devlin, J. W., Roberts, R. J., Fong, J. J., Skrobik, Y., Riker, R. R., Hill, N. S., et al. (2010). Efficacy and safety of quetiapine in critically ill patients with delirium: a prospective, multicenter, randomized, double-blind, placebo-controlled pilot study. *Critical Care Medicine*, *38*(2), 419–427.

Dew, M. A., Kormos, R. L., DiMartini, A. F., Switzer, G. E., Schulberg, H. C., Roth, L. H., & Griffith, B. P. (2001). Prevalence and risk of depression and anxiety–related disorders during the first three years after heart transplantation. *Psychosomatics*, *42*(4), 300–313.

DiMartini, A., Dew, M. A., Kormos, R., McCurry, K., & Fontes, P. (2007). Posttraumatic stress disorder caused by hallucinations and delusions experienced in delirium. *Psychosomatics*, *48*(5), 436–439.

Dinges, D. F. (2006). The state of sleep deprivation: From functional biology to functional consequences. *Sleep Medicine Reviews*, *10*(5), 303–305.

Drouot, X., Cabello, B., d'Ortho, M. P., & Brochard, L. (2008). Sleep in the intensive care unit. *Sleep Medicine Reviews*, *12*(5), 391–403.

Dyer, C. B., Ashton, C. M., & Teasdale, T. A. (1995). Postoperative delirium. A review of 80 primary data-collection studies. *Archives of Internal Medicine*, *155*(5), 461–465.

Ebert, A. D., Walzer, T. A., Huth, C., & Herrmann, M. (2001). Early neurobehavioral disorders after cardiac surgery: A comparative analysis of coronary artery bypass graft surgery and valve replacement. *Journal of Cardiothoracic & Vascular Anesthesia*, *15*(1), 15–19.

El-Kaissi, S., Kotowicz, M. A., Berk, M., & Wall, J. R. (2005). Acute delirium in the setting of primary hypothyroidism: the role of thyroid hormone replacement therapy. *Thyroid*, *15*(9), 1099–1101.

Elie, M., Cole, M. G., Primeau, F. J., & Bellavance, F. (1998). Delirium risk factors in elderly hospitalized patients. *Journal of General Internal Medicine*, *13*(3), 204–212.

Elie, M., Rousseau, F., Cole, M., Primeau, F., McCusker, J., & Bellavance, F. (2000). Prevalence and detection of delirium in elderly emergency department patients. *Canadian Medical Association Journal*, *163*(8), 977–981.

Ely, E. W., Gautam, S., Margolin, R., et al. (2001). The impact of delirium in the intensive care unit on hospital length of stay. *Intensive Care Medicine*, *27*(12), 1892–1900.

Ely, E. W., Girard T. D., Shintani A. K., Jackson J. C., Gordon S. M., Thomason J. W., et al. (2007). Apolipoprotein E4 polymorphism as a genetic predisposition to delirium in critically ill patients. *Critical Care Medicine*, *35*(1), 112–117.

Ely, E. W., Margolin, R., Francis, J., et al. (2001). Evaluation of delirium in critically ill patients: Validation of the Confusion Assessment Method for the Intensive Care Unit (CAM-ICU). *Critical Care Medicine*, *29*(7), 1370–1379.

Ely, E. W., Shintani, A., Truman, B., Speroff T., Gordon S. M., Harrell, F. E. Jr., et al. (2004). Delirium as a predictor of mortality in mechanically ventilated patients in the intensive care unit. *Journal of the American Medical Association*, *291*(14), 1753–1762.

Ely, E. W., Siegel, M. D., & Inouye, S. K. (2001). Delirium in the intensive care unit: an under-recognized syndrome of organ dysfunction. *Seminars Respiratory and Critical Care Medicine*, *22*(2), 115–126.

Engel, G. L., & Romano, J. (1959). Delirium, a syndrome of cerebral insufficiency. *Journal of Chronic Diseases*, *9*(3), 260–277.

Engel, G. L. & Romano, J. (2004). Delirium, a syndrome of cerebral insufficiency. 1959. *Journal of Neuropsychiatry Clinical Neuroscience*, *16*(4), 526–538.

Engel, G. L., Webb, J. P., & Ferris, E. B. (1945). Quantitative Electroencephalographic Studies of Anoxia in Humans; Comparison with Acute Alcoholic Intoxication and Hypoglycemia. *Journal of the Clinical Invest*, *24*(5), 691–697.

Engelhard, K., Werner, C., Eberspacher, E., Bachl, M., Blobner, M., Hildt, E., Pet, al. (2003). The effect of the alpha 2–agonist dexmedetomidine and the N-methyl–D–aspartate antagonist S(+)-ketamine on the expression of apoptosis–regulating proteins after incomplete cerebral ischemia and reperfusion in rats. *Anesthesia and Analgesia*, *96*(2), 524–531.

Eyer, F., Pfab, R., Felgenhauer, N., Strubel, T., Saugel, B., & Zilker, T. (2011). Clinical and analytical features of severe suicidal quetiapine overdoses––a retrospective cohort study. *Clinical Toxicology, (Phila)* *49*(9), 846–853.

Fang, V. S., & Jaspan, J. B. (1989). Delirium and neuromuscular symptoms in an elderly man with isolated corticotroph–deficiency syndrome completely reversed with glucocorticoid replacement. *Journal of Clinical Endocrinology and Metabolism*, *69*(5), 1073–1077.

Fann, J. R., Alfano, C. M., Roth-Roemer, S., Katon, W. J., & Syrjala, K. L. (2007). Impact of delirium on cognition, distress, and health-related quality of life after hematopoietic stem-cell transplantation. *Journal of Clinical Oncology*, *25*(10), 1223–1231.

Farina, M. L., Levati, A., & Tognoni, G. (1981). A multicenter study of ICU drug utilization. *Intensive Care Medicine*, *7*(3), 125–131.

Farrell, K. R., & Ganzini, L. (1995). Misdiagnosing delirium as depression in medically ill elderly patients. *Archives of Internal Medicine*, *155*(22), 2459–2464.

Fassbender, K., Schmidt, R., Mossner, R., Daffertshofer, M., & Hennerici, M. (1994). Pattern of activation of the hypothalamic–pituitary–adrenal axis in acute stroke. Relation to acute confusional state, extent of brain damage, and clinical outcome. *Stroke*, *25*(6), 1105–1108.

FDA (2000). Center for Drug Evaluation and research Psychopharmacological Drug Advisory Committee—Meeting transcript for the approval of ziprasidone. Retrieved 7/31/2011 from http://www.fda.gov/ohrms/dockets/ac/00/backgrd/3619b1b.pdf.

FDA (2007). Information for Healthcare Professionals: Haloperidol (marketed as Haldol, Haldol Decanoate and Haldol Lactate). Retrieved from www.fda.gov/cder/drug/InfoSheets/HCP/haloperidol.htm.

Fernandez, F., Holmes, V. F., Adams, F., & Kavanaugh, J. J. (1988). Treatment of severe, refractory agitation with a haloperidol drip. *Journal of Clinical Psychiatry*, *49*(6), 239–241.

Fernandez, F., Levy, J. K., & Mansell, P. W. (1989). Management of delirium in terminally ill AIDS patients. *International Journal of Psychiatry in Medicine*, *19*(2), 165–172.

Fine, A., Anderson, N. L., Rothstein, T. L., Williams, M. C., & Gochuico, B. R. (1997). Fas expression in pulmonary alveolar type II cells. *American Journal of Physiology*, *273*(1 Pt 1), L64–71.

Fink, M. (1999). Delirious mania. *Bipolar Disord 1*(1), 54–60.

Finkel, S. I., Costa e Silva, J., Cohen, G., Miller, S., & Sartorius, N. (1996). Behavioral and psychological signs and symptoms of dementia: a consensus statement on current knowledge and implications for research and treatment. *International Psychogeriatrics*, *8*(Suppl 3), 497–500.

Fishbain, D. A., & Rotundo, D. (1988). Frequency of hypoglycemic delirium in a psychiatric emergency service. *Psychosomatics*, *29*(3), 346–348.

Fisher, R. S., Bortz, J. J., Blum, D. E., Duncan, B., & Burke, H. (2001). A pilot study of donepezil for memory problems in epilepsy. *Epilepsy & Behavior*, *2*(4), 330–334.

Flacker, J. M., Cummings, V., Mach, J. R. Jr., Bettin, K., Kiely, D. K., & Wei, J. (1998). The association of serum anticholinergic activity with delirium in elderly medical patients. *American Journal of Geriatric Psychiatry*, *6*(1), 31–41.

Flacker, J. M., & Wei, J. Y. (2001). Endogenous anticholinergic substances may exist during acute illness in elderly medical patients. *Journals of Gerontology - Series A: Biological Sciences and Medical Sciences*, *56*(6), M353–355.

Fong, H. K., Sands, L. P., & Leung, J. M. (2006). The role of postoperative analgesia in delirium and cognitive decline in elderly patients: a systematic review. *Anesthesia and Analgesia*, *102*(4), 1255–1266.

Fong, T. G., Jones, R. N., Shi P., Marcantonio E. R., Yap L., Rudolph J. L., et al. (2009). Delirium accelerates cognitive decline in Alzheimer disease. *Neurology*, *72*(18), 1570–1575.

Francis, J., Martin, D., & Kapoor, W. N. (1990). A prospective study of delirium in hospitalized elderly. *Journal of the American Academy of Medicine*, *263*(8), 1097–1101.

Franco, J. G., Trzepacz, P. T., Mejia, M. A., & Ochoa, S. B. (2009). Factor analysis of the Colombian translation of the Delirium Rating Scale (DRS), Revised-98. *Psychosomatics*, *50*(3), 255–262.

Frederiks, J. A. (2000). Inflammation of the mind. On the 300th anniversary of Gerard van Swieten. *Journal of the History of the Neurosciences, 9*(3), 307–310.

Friedman, R. S., Mufson, M. J., Eisenberg, T. D., & Patel, M. R. (2003). Medically and psychiatrically ill: the challenge of delirious mania. *Harvard Review Psychiatry, 11*(2), 91–98.

Friese, R. S. (2008b). Sleep and recovery from critical illness and injury: a review of theory, current practice, and future directions. *Critical Care Medicine, 36*(3), 697–705.

Fronapfel, P. J. (2008). Prevention of emergence delirium. *Paediatric Anaesthesia, 18*(11), 1113–1114.

Funk, W., Hollnberger, H., & Geroldinger, J. (2008). Physostigmine and anaesthesia emergence delirium in preschool children: a randomized blinded trial. *European Journal of Anaesthesiology, 25*(1), 37–42.

Furuya, M., Miyaoka, T., Yasuda, H., Yamashita, S., Tanaka, I., Otsuka, S., Wake, R., & Horiguchi, J. (2012). Marked improvement in delirium with ramelteon: five case reports. *Psychogeriatrics, 12*(4), 259–262.

Gagnon, P., Allard P., Gagnon, B., Merette, C., & Tardif, F. (2012). Delirium prevention in terminal cancer: assessment of a multicomponent intervention. *Psychooncology, 21*(2), 187–194.

Gallacher, J., Elwood, P., Pickering, J., Bayer, A., Fish, M., & Ben-Shlomo, Y. (2012). Benzodiazepine use and risk of dementia: evidence from the Caerphilly Prospective Study (CaPS). *Journal of Epidemiology & Community Health, 66*(10), 869–873.

Gamberini, M., Bolliger, D., Lurati Buse, G. A., Burkhart, C. S., Grapow, M., Gagneux, A., et al. (2009). Rivastigmine for the prevention of postoperative delirium in elderly patients undergoing elective cardiac surgery—a randomized controlled trial. *Critical Care Medicine, 37*(5), 1762–1768.

Gaudreau, J. D., Gagnon, P., Harel, F., Tremblay, A., & Roy, M. A. (2005). Fast, systematic, and continuous delirium assessment in hospitalized patients: The Nursing Delirium Screening Scale. *Journal of Pain & Symptom Management, 29*(4), 368–375.

Gaudreau, J. D., Gagnon, P., Roy, M. A., Harel, F., & Tremblay, A. (2005). Association between psychoactive medications and delirium in hospitalized patients: a critical review. *Psychosomatics, 46*(4), 302–316.

Gaudreau, J. D., Gagnon, P., Roy, M. A., Harel, F., & Tremblay, A. (2007). Opioid medications and longitudinal risk of delirium in hospitalized cancer patients. *Cancer, 109*(11), 2365–2373.

Germano, E., Italiano, D., Lamberti, M., Guerriero, L., Privitera, C., D'Amico, G., et al. (2014). ECG parameters in children and adolescents treated with aripiprazole and risperidone. *Progress in Neuropsychopharmacology & Biological Psychiatry, 51*, 23–27.

Giacino, J. T., & Whyte, J. (2003). Amantadine to improve neurorecovery in traumatic brain injury–associated diffuse axonal injury: a pilot double–blind randomized trial. *Journal of Head Trauma Rehabilitation, 18*(1), 4–5; author reply 5–6.

Giacino, J. T., Whyte, J., Bagiella, E., Kalmar, K., Childs, N., Khademi, A., et al. (2012). Placebo–controlled trial of amantadine for severe traumatic brain injury. *New England Journal of Medicine, 366*(9), 819–826.

Gibson, G. E., & Peterson, C. (1981). Aging decreases oxidative metabolism and the release and synthesis of acetylcholine. *Journal of Neurochem, 37*(4), 978–984.

Girard, T. D., Jackson, J. C., Pandharipande, P. P., Pun, B. T., Thompson, J. L., Shintani, A. K., et al. Ely (2010). Delirium as a predictor of long–term cognitive impairment in survivors of critical illness. *Critical Care Medicine, 38*(7), 1513–1520.

Girard, T. D., Kress, J. P., Fuchs, B. D., Thomason, J. W., Schweickert, W. D., Pun, B. T., et al. (2008). Efficacy and safety of a paired sedation and ventilator weaning protocol for mechanically ventilated patients in intensive care (Awakening and Breathing Controlled trial), a randomised controlled trial. *Lancet 371*(9607), 126–134.

Givens, J. L., Jones, R. N., & Inouye, S. K. (2009). The overlap syndrome of depression and delirium in older hospitalized patients. *Journal of Amercian Geriatric Soceity, 57*(8), 1347–1353.

Gleason, O. C. (2003). Donepezil for postoperative delirium. *Psychosomatics, 44*(5), 437–438.

Globus, M. Y., Alonso, O., Dietrich, W. D., Busto, R., & Ginsberg, M. D. (1995). Glutamate release and free radical production following brain injury: effects of posttraumatic hypothermia. *J Neurochem 65*(4), 1704–1711.

Globus, M. Y., Busto, R., Dietrich, W. D., Martinez, E., Valdes, I., & Ginsberg, M. D. (1988b). Intra-ischemic extracellular release of dopamine and glutamate is associated with striatal vulnerability to ischemia. *Neurosci Lett 91*(1), 36–40.

Globus, M. Y., R. Busto, W. D. Dietrich, E. Martinez, I. Valdes and M. D. Ginsberg (1989). Direct evidence for acute and massive norepinephrine release in the hippocampus during transient ischemia. *J Cereb Blood Flow Metab 9*(6), 892–896.

Globus, M. Y., Busto, R., Martinez, E., Valdes, I., & Dietrich, W. D. (1990). Ischemia induces release of glutamate in regions spared from histopathologic damage in the rat. *Stroke, 21*(11 Suppl), III43–46.

Globus, M. Y., Wester, P, Busto, R., & Dietrich, W. D. (1992). Ischemia–induced extracellular release of serotonin plays a role in CA1 neuronal cell death in rats. *Stroke, 23*(11), 1595–1601.

Godbout, J. P., Chen, J., Abraham, J., Richwine, A. F., Berg, B. M., Kelley, K. W., & Johnson, R. W. (2005). Exaggerated neuroinflammation and sickness behavior in aged mice following activation of the peripheral innate immune system. *FASEB Journal, 19*(10), 1329–1331.

Godbout, J. P., & Johnson, R. W. (2009). Age and neuroinflammation: a lifetime of psychoneuroimmune consequences. *Immunolology and Allergy Clinics of North America, 29*(2), 321–337.

Godfrey, A., Conway, R., Leonard, M., Meagher, D., & Olaighin, G. M. (2009). A continuous wavelet transform and classification method for delirium motoric subtyping. *IEEE transactions on neural systems and rehabilitation engineering: a publication of the IEEE Engineering in Medicine and Biology Society, 17*(3), 298–307.

Godfrey, A., Conway, R., Leonard, M., Meagher, D., & Olaighin, G. M. (2010). Motion analysis in delirium: a discrete approach in determining physical activity for the purpose of delirium motoric subtyping. *Medical Engineering & Physics, 32*(2), 101–110.

Goldfarb, C. R., Varma, C., & Roginsky, M. S. (1980). Diagnosis in delirium: prompt confirmation of thyroid storm. *Clin Nucl Med, 5*(2), 66.

Golinger, R. C., Peet, T., & Tune, L. E. (1987). Association of elevated plasma anticholinergic activity with delirium in surgical patients. *American Journal of Psychiatry, 144*(9), 1218–1220.

Gomez Sanz, C. A. (2013). [Quality of sleep in patients hospitalized in an intensive care unit]. *Enferm Intensiva, 24*(1), 3–11.

Gonzalez, M., de Pablo, J., Fuente, E., Valdes, M., Peri, J. M., Nomdedeu, M., & Matrai, S. (2004). Instrument for detection of delirium in general hospitals: Adaptation of the confusion assessment method. *Psychosomatics, 45*(5), 426–431.

Goosens, K. A., & Sapolsky, R. M. (2007). Stress and glucocorticoid contributions to normal and pathological aging.

Graham, D. G. (1984). Catecholamine toxicity: a proposal for the molecular pathogenesis of manganese neurotoxicity and Parkinson's disease. *Neurotoxicology 5*(1), 83–95.

Gray, S. L., Anderson, M. L., Dublin, S., Hanlon, J. T., Hubbard, R., Walker, R., et al. (2015). Cumulative Use of Strong Anticholinergics and Incident Dementia: A Prospective Cohort Study. *JAMA Intern Med.*

Greiner, G. F. C. (1817). *Der Traum und das fieberhafte Irreseyn.* Germany, F. A. Brockhaus.

Griffiths, R. D., & Jones, C. (2007). Delirium, cognitive dysfunction and posttraumatic stress disorder. *Current Opinion in Anaesthesiology, 20*(2), 124–129.

Gross, A. L., Jones, R. N., Habtemariam, D. A., Fong, T. G., Tommet, D., Quach, L. et al. (2012). Delirium and long-term cognitive trajectory among persons with dementia. *Archives of Internal Medicine, 172*(17), 1324–1331.

Gulisano, M., Cali, P. V., Cavanna, A. E., Eddy, C., Rickards, H., & Rizzo, R. (2011). Cardiovascular safety of aripiprazole and pimozide in young patients with Tourette syndrome. *Journal of the Neurological Sciences, 32*(6), 1213–1217.

Gunther, M. L., Jackson, J. C., & Ely, E. W. (2007). The cognitive consequences of critical illness: practical recommendations for screening and assessment. *Critical Care Clinics, 23*(3), 491–506.

Gunther, M. L., Morandi, A., Krauskopf, E., Pandharipande, P., Girard, T. D., Jackson, J. C., et al. (2012). The association between brain volumes, delirium duration, and cognitive outcomes in intensive care unit survivors: the VISIONS cohort magnetic resonance imaging study*. *Critical Care Medicine, 40*(7), 2022–2032.

Gustafson, Y., Berggren, D., Brannstrom, B., Bucht, G., Norberg, A., Hansson, L. I., & Winblad, B. (1988). Acute confusional states in elderly patients treated for femoral neck fracture. *Journal of Amercian Geriatric Soceity, 36*(6), 525–530.

Gutstein, H. B. (1996). Potential physiologic mechanism for ketamine–induced emergence delirium. *Anesthesiology 84*(2), 474.

Haas, S., Vincent, K., Holt, J., & Lippmann, S. (1997). Divalproex: a possible treatment alternative for demented, elderly aggressive patients. *Annals of clinical psychiatry: official journal of the American Academy of Clinical Psychiatrists, 9*(3), 145–147.

Haase, U., & Rundshagen, I. (2007). [Pharmacotherapy—physostigmine administered postoperatively]. *Anästhesiologie, Intensivmedizin, Notfallmedizin, Schmerztherapie, 42*(3), 188–189.

Hail, S. L., Obafemi, A., & Kleinschmidt, K. C. (2013). Successful management of olanzapine-induced anticholinergic agitation and delirium with a continuous intravenous infusion of physostigmine in a pediatric patient. *Clinical Toxicology, (Phila) 51*(3), 162–166.

Hala, M. (2007). Pathophysiology of postoperative delirium: systemic inflammation as a response to surgical trauma causes diffuse microcirculatory impairment. *Medical Hypotheses, 68*(1), 194–196.

Hall, J. P., Heller, R. F., Dobson, A. J., Lloyd, D. M., Sanson-Fisher, R. W., & Leeder, S. R. (1988). A cost–effectiveness analysis of alternative strategies for the prevention of heart disease. *Medical Journal of Australia, 148*(6), 273–277.

Han, C. S., & Kim, Y. K. (2004). A double–blind trial of risperidone and haloperidol for the treatment of delirium. *Psychosomatics, 45*(4), 297–301.

Han, J. H., Eden, S., Shintani, A., Morandi, A., Schnelle, J., Dittus, R. S., et al. (2011). Delirium in older emergency department patients is an independent predictor of hospital length of stay. *Acadademic Emergency Medicine, 18*(5), 451–457.

Han, L., McCusker J., Cole, M., Abrahamowicz, M., Primeau, F., & Elie, M. (2001). Use of medications with anticholinergic effect predicts clinical severity of delirium symptoms in older medical inpatients. *Archives of Internal Medicine, 161*(8), 1099–1105.

Hanania, M., & Kitain, E. (2002). Melatonin for treatment and prevention of postoperative delirium. *Anesthesia and Analgesia, 94*(2), 338–339, table of contents.

Harrigan, E. P., Miceli, J. J., Anziano, R., Watsky, E., Reeves, K. R., Cutler, N. R., et al. (2004). A randomized evaluation of the effects of six antipsychotic agents on QTc, in the absence and presence of metabolic inhibition. *Journal of Clinical Psychopharmacology, 24*(1), 62–69.

Hart, R. P., Levenson, J. L., Sessler, C N., Best, A. M., Schwartz, S. M., & Rutherford, L. E. (1996). Validation of a cognitive test for delirium in medical ICU patients. *Psychosomatics, 37*(6), 533–546.

Hategan, A., & Bourgeois, J. A. (2014). Aripiprazole-associated QTc prolongation in a geriatric patient. *Journal of Clinical Psychopharmacology, 34*(6), 766–768.

Hatta, K., Takahashi, T., Nakamura, H., Yamashiro, H., Asukai, N., Matsuzaki, I., & Yonezawa, Y. (2001). The association between intravenous haloperidol and prolonged QT interval. *Journal of Clinical Psychopharmacology, 21*(3), 257–261.

Haynes, C. (1999). Emergence delirium: a literature review. *British Journal of Theatre Nursing, 9*(11), 502–503, 506–510.

Helton, M. C., Gordon, S. H., & Nunnery, S. L. (1980). The correlation between sleep deprivation and the intensive care unit syndrome. *Heart Lung Journal, 9*(3), 464–468.

Henderson, D. C. (2008). Managing weight gain and metabolic issues in patients treated with atypical antipsychotics. *Journal of Clinical Psychiatry, 69*(2), e04.

Hirota, T., & Kishi, T. (2013). Prophylactic antipsychotic use for postoperative delirium: a systematic review and meta–analysis. *Journal of Clinical Psychiatry, 74*(12), e1136–1144.

Hoes, M. J. (1979). The significance of the serum levels of vitamin B-1 and magnesium in delirium tremens and alcoholism. *Journal of Clinical Psychiatry, 40*(11), 476–479.

Hofhuis, J. G., Langevoort, G., Rommes, J. H., & Spronk, P. E. (2012). Sleep disturbances and sedation practices in the intensive care unit––a postal survey in the Netherlands. *Intensive and Critical Care Nursing, 28*(3), 141–149.

Hofmann, W. (2013). [Benzodiazepines in geriatrics]. *Z Gerontology Geriatric, 46*(8), 769–776; quiz 776.

Holroyd-Leduc, J. M., Abelseth, G. A., Khandwala, F., Silvius, J. L., Hogan, D. B., Schmaltz, H. N., et al. (2010). A pragmatic study exploring the prevention of delirium among hospitalized older hip fracture patients: Applying evidence to routine clinical practice using clinical decision support. *Implementation Science, 5*, 81.

Holroyd-Leduc, J. M., Khandwala, F., &. Sink, K. M (2010). How can delirium best be prevented and managed in older patients in hospital? *Canadian Medical Association Journal, 182*(5), 465–470.

Hori, K., Tominaga, I., Inada, T., Oda, T., Hirai, S., Hori, I., et al. (2003). Donepezil-responsive alcohol-related prolonged delirium. *Psychiatry & Clinical Neurosciences, 57*(6), 603–604.

Hu, H., Deng, W., & Yang, H. (2004). A prospective random control study comparison of olanzapine and haloperidol in senile delirium. *Chongging Medical Journal*, (8), 1234–1237.

Hudek, K. (2009). Emergence delirium: a nursing perspective. *AORN Journal, 89*(3), 509–516; quiz 517–509.

Hudetz, J. A., Patterson, K. M., Iqbal, Z., Gandhi, S. D., Byrne, A. J., Hudetz, A. G., et al. (2009). Ketamine attenuates delirium after cardiac surgery with cardiopulmonary bypass. *Journal of Cardiothoracic and Vascular Anethesia, 23*(5), 651–657.

Huffman, J. C., & Stern, T. A. (2003). QTc prolongation and the use of antipsychotics: A case discussion. *Primary Care Companion, Journal of Clinical Psychiatry, 5*(6), 278–281.

Iijima, T., Shimase, C., Iwao, Y., & Sankawa, H. (1998). Relationships between glutamate release, blood flow and spreading depression: real–time monitoring using an electroenzymatic dialysis electrode. *Neuroscience Research, 32*(3), 201–207.

Inouye, S., van Dyck, C., Alessi, C., Balkin, S., Siegal, A. P., & Horwitz, R. I. (1990). Clarifying confusion: The confusion assessment method. A new method for detection of delirium. *Annals of Internal Medicine, 113*(12), 941–948.

Inouye, S., Zhang, Y., Jones, R., Kiely, D. K., Yang, F., & Marcantonio, E. R. (2007). Risk factors for delirium at discharge: development and validation of a predictive model. *Archives of Internal Medicine, 167*(13), 1406–1413.

Inouye, S. K. (1991). The recognition of delirium. *Hospital Pract (Off Ed), 26*(4A), 61–62.

Inouye, S. K. (1993). Delirium in hospitalized elderly patients: recognition, evaluation, and management. *Connecticut Medicine, 57*(5), 309–315.

Inouye, S. K. (1994). The dilemma of delirium: clinical and research controversies regarding diagnosis and evaluation of delirium in hospitalized elderly medical patients. *Am J Med 97*(3), 278–288.

Inouye, S. K. (1998). Delirium in hospitalized older patients. *Clinics in Geriatric Medicine, 14*(4), 745–764.

Inouye, S. K. (1998). Delirium in hospitalized older patients: recognition and risk factors. *Journal of Geriatric Psychiatry and Neurology, 11*(3), 118–125; discussion 157–118.

Inouye, S. K. (1999). Predisposing and precipitating factors for delirium in hospitalized older patients. *Dementia and Geriatric Cognitive Disorders, 10*(5), 393–400.

Inouye, S. K. (2000). Prevention of delirium in hospitalized older patients: risk factors and targeted intervention strategies. *Annals of Medicine, 32*(4), 257–263.

Inouye, S. K., & Charpentier, P. A. (1996). Precipitating factors for delirium in hospitalized elderly persons. Predictive model and interrelationship with baseline vulnerability. *Journal of the American Medical Association, 275*(11), 852–857.

Inouye, S. K., Schlesinger, M. J., & Lydon, T. J. (1999). Delirium: a symptom of how hospital care is failing older persons and a window to improve quality of hospital care. *American Journal of Medicine, 106*(5), 565–573.

Inouye, S., Bogardus Jr., S., Charpentier, P., Leo-Summers, L., Acampora, D., Holford, T. R., & Cooney Jr., L. M. (1999). A multicomponent intervention to prevent delirium in hospitalized older patients. *New England Journal of Medicine, 340*(9), 669–676.

Inouye, S., Viscoli, C. M., Horwitz, R. I., Hurst, L. D., Tinetti, M. E. (1993). A predictive model for delirium in hospitalized elderly medical patients based on admission characteristics. *Annals of Internal Medicine, 119*(6), 474–481.

Inouye, S. K., Foreman, M. D., Mion, L. C., Katz, K. H., & Cooney, L. M. Jr. (2001). Nurses' recognition of delirium and its symptoms: comparison of nurse and researcher ratings. *Archives of Internal Medicine, 161*(20), 2467–2473.

Ito, H., Harada, D., Hayashida, K., Ishino, H., & Nakayama, K. (2006). [Psychiatry and sleep disorders––delirium]. *Seishin Shinkeigaku Zasshi, 108*(11), 1217–1221.

Jackson, J. C., Gordon, S. M., Hart, R. P., Hopkins, R. O., & Ely, E. W. (2004). The association between delirium and cognitive decline: a review of the empirical literature. *Neuropsychology Review, 14*(2), 87–98.

Jackson, J. H. (1932). *Selected writings of John Hughlings Jackson*. London: Hodder and Stoughton.

Jacobi, J., Fraser, G., Coursin, D., Riker, R. R., Fontaine, D., Wittbrodt, E. T., et al. (2002). Clinical practice guidelines for the sustained use of sedatives and analgesics in the critically ill adult. *Critical Care Medicine, 30*(1), 119–141.

Jakob, S. M., Ruokonen, E., Grounds, R. M., Sarapohja, T., Garratt, C., Pocock, S. J., et al., I. Dexmedetomidine for Long-Term Sedation (2012). Dexmedetomidine vs midazolam or propofol for sedation during prolonged mechanical ventilation: two randomized controlled trials. *JAMA, 307*(11), 1151–1160.

Johansson, A., Olsson, T., Carlberg, B., Karlsson, K., & Fagerlund, M. (1997). Hypercortisolism after stroke––partly cytokine-mediated? *Journal of the Neurological Sciences, 147*(1), 43–47.

Jones, C., Griffiths, R., Humphris, G., & Skirrow, P. M. (2001). Memory, delusions, and the development of acute posttraumatic stress disorder–related symptoms after intensive care. *Critical Care Medicine, 29*(3), 573–580.

Kalisch Ellett, L. M., Pratt, N. L., Ramsay, E. N., Barratt, J. D., & Roughead, E. E. (2014). Multiple anticholinergic medication use and risk of hospital admission for confusion or dementia. *Journal of American Geriatric Society, 62*(10), 1916–1922.

Kalisvaart, K., de Jonghe, J., Bogaards, M., Vreeswijk, R., Egberts, T. C., Burger, B. J., et al. (2005). Haloperidol prophylaxis for elderly hip-surgery patients at risk for delirium: a randomized placebo-controlled study. *Journal of American Geriatric Society, 53*(10), 1658–1666.

Kalisvaart, K., Vreeswijk, R., de Jonghe, J., van der Ploeg, T., van Gool, W. A., & Eikelenboom, P. (2006). Risk factors and prediction of postoperative delirium in elderly hip surgery patients: implementation and validation of a medical risk factor model. *Journal of the American Geriatrics Society, 54*(5), 817–822.

Kamdar, B. B., Needham, D. M., &. Collop, N. A. (2012). Sleep deprivation in critical illness: its role in physical and psychological recovery. *Journal of Intensive Care Medicine, 27*(2), 97–111.

Kat, M. G., Vreeswijk, R., de Jonghe, J. F., van der Ploeg, T., van Gool, W. A., Eikelenboom, P., & Kalisvaart, K. J. (2008). Long-term cognitive outcome of delirium in elderly hip surgery patients. A prospective matched controlled study over two and a half years. *Dementia and Geriatric Cognitive Disorders, 26*(1), 1–8.

Katznelson, R., Djaiani, G., Mitsakakis, N., Lindsay, T. F., Tait, G., Friedman, Z., et al. (2009). Delirium following vascular surgery: increased incidence with preoperative beta-blocker administration. *Canadian Journal of Anaesthesia, 56*(11), 793–801.

Kaufer, D. I., Catt, K. E., Lopez, O. L., & DeKosky, S. T. (1998). Dementia with Lewy bodies: Response of delirium-like features to donepezil. *Neurology, 51*(5), 1512.

Kawaguchi, Y., Kanamori, M., Ishihara, H., et al. (2006). Postoperative delirium in spine surgery. *Spine Journal, 6*(2), 164–169.

Kazmierski, J., Banys, A., Latek, J., Bourke, J., & Jaszewski, R. (2013). Cortisol levels and neuropsychiatric diagnosis as markers of postoperative delirium: a prospective cohort study. *Critical Care, 17*(2), R38.

Kazmierski, J., Kowman M., Banach M., Pawelczyk T., Okonski P., Iwaszkiewicz A., et al. (2006). Preoperative predictors of delirium after cardiac surgery: a preliminary study. *General Hospital Psychiatry, 28*(6), 536–538.

Kean, J., & Ryan, K. (2008). Delirium detection in clinical practice and research: critique of current tools and suggestions for future development. *Journal of Psychosomatic Research, 65*(3), 255–259.

Kean, J., Trzepacz, P. T., Murray, L. L., Abell, M., & Trexler, L. (2010). Initial validation of a brief provisional diagnostic scale for delirium. *Brain Injury, 24*(10), 1222–1230.

Khan, R. A., Kahn, D., & Bourgeois, J. A. (2009). Delirium: sifting through the confusion. *Current Psychiatry Reports, 11*(3), 226–234.

Khasati, N., Thompson, J., & Dunning, J. (2004). Is haloperidol or a benzodiazepine the safest treatment for acute psychosis in the critically ill patient? *Interactive Cardiovascular and Thoracic Surgery, 3*(2), 233–236.

Khurana, V., Gambhir, I. S., & Kishore, D. (2011). Evaluation of delirium in elderly: A hospital–based study. *Geriatrics & Gerontology International, 11*(4), 467–473.

Kiely, D. K., Jones, R. N., Bergmann, M. A., & Marcantonio, E. R. (2007). Association between psychomotor activity delirium subtypes and mortality among newly admitted post–acute facility patients. *Journals of Gerontology - Series A: Biological Sciences and Medical Sciences, 62*(2), 174–179.

Kimura, R., Mori K., Kumazaki, H., Yanagida, M., Taguchi, S., & Matsunaga, H. (2011). Treatment of delirium with ramelteon: initial experience in three patients. *General hospital psychiatry 33*(4), 407–409.

Kinney, J. M., Duke Jr., J. H., Long, C. L., & Gump, F. E. (1970). Tissue fuel and weight loss after injury. *Journal of Clinical Pathology, Suppl (R Coll Pathol), 4*, 65–72.

Kishi, Y., Kato, M., Okuyama, T., Hosaka, T., Mikami, K., Meller, W., et al. (2007). Delirium: patient characteristics that predict a missed diagnosis at psychiatric consultation. *General Hospital Psychiatry, 29*(5), 442–445.

Kmietowicz, Z. (2014). Benzodiazepines may be linked to Alzheimer's disease, study finds. *BMJ, 349*, g5555.

Kobayashi, K., Higashima, M., Mutou, K., et al. (2004). Severe delirium due to basal forebrain vascular lesion and efficacy of donepezil. *Progress in Neuropsychopharmacology & Biological Psychiatry, 28*(7), 1189–1194.

Koizumi, J., Shiraishi, H., Ofuku, K., & Suzuki, T. (1988). Duration of delirium shortened by the correction of electrolyte imbalance. *Japanese Journal of Psychiatry and Neurology, 42*(1), 81–88.

Kojima, H., Terao, T., & Yoshimura, R. (1993). Serotonin syndrome during clomipramine and lithium treatment. *American Journal of Psychiatry, 150*(12), 1897.

Koponen, H., Hurri, L., Stenback, U., Mattila, E., Soininen, H., & Riekkinen, P. J. (1989). Computed tomography findings in delirium. *Journal of Nervous and Mental Disease, 177*(4), 226–231.

Koponen, H., Partanen, J., Paakkonen, A., Mattila, E., & Riekkinen, P. J. (1989). EEG spectral analysis in delirium. *Journal of Neurology Neurosurgery Psychiatry, 52*(8), 980–985.

Kress, J. P. (2010). The complex interplay between delirium, sepsis and sedation. *Critical Care, 14*(3), 164.

Kress, J. P., Gehlbach, B., Lacy, M., Pliskin, N., Pohlman, A. S., & Hall, J. B. (2003). The long-term psychological effects of daily sedative interruption on critically ill patients. *American Journal of Respiratory and Critical Care Medicine, 168*(12), 1457–1461.

Kress, J. P., Pohlman, A. S., O'Connor, M. F., & Hall, J. B. (2000). Daily interruption of sedative infusions in critically ill patients undergoing mechanical ventilation. *New England Journal of Medicine, 342*(20), 1471–1477.

Kudoh, A., Takase, H., Takahira, Y., & Takazawa, T. (2004). Postoperative confusion increases in elderly long-term benzodiazepine users. *Anesthesia and Analgesia, 99*(6), 1674–1678, table of contents.

Kutzing, M. K., Luo, V., & Firestein, B. L. (2012). Protection from glutamate–induced excitotoxicity by memantine. *Annals of Biomedical Engineering, 40*(5), 1170–1181.

Lagnaoui, R., Begaud B., Moore N., Chaslerie A., Fourrier A., Letenneur L., et al. (2002). Benzodiazepine use and risk of dementia: a nested case-control study. *J Clin Epidemiol 55*(3), 314–318.

Lawlor, P. G. (2002). Delirium and dehydration: Some fluid for thought? *Supportive Care in Cancer, 10*(6), 445–454.

Lawlor, P. G., Gagnon, B., Mancini, I. L., et al. (2000). Occurence, causes, and outcome of delirium in patients with advanced cancer: A prospective study. *Archives of Internal Medicine, 160*(6), 786–794.

Lechin, F., van der Dijs, B., & Benaim, M. (1996). Benzodiazepines: tolerability in elderly patients. *Psychotheraphy Psychosomatics, 65*(4), 171–182.

Lee, K. U., Won, W. Y., Lee, H. K., Kweon, Y. S., Lee, C. T., Pae, C. U., & Bahk, W. M. (2005). Amisulpride versus quetiapine for the treatment of delirium: a randomized, open prospective study. *International Clinical Clinical Psychopharmacology, 20*(6), 311–314.

Lee, H. B., Mears, S. C., Rosenberg, P. B., Leoutsakos, J. M., Gottschalk, A., & Sieber, F. E. (2011). Predisposing factors for postoperative delirium after hip fracture repair in individuals with and without dementia. *Journal of the American Geriatrics Society, 59*(12), 2306–2313.

Lemiengre, J., Nelis, T., Joosten, E., Braes, T., Foreman, M., Gastmans, C., & Milisen, K. (2006). Detection of delirium by bedside nurses using the confusion assessment method. *Journal of American Geriatric Society, 54*(4), 685–689.

Leonard, M., Spiller, J., Keen, J., MacLullich, A., Kamholtz, B., & Meagher, D. (2009). Symptoms of depression and delirium assessed serially in palliative-care inpatients. *Psychosomatics, 50*(5), 506–514.

Lepouse, C., Lautner, C. A., Liu, L., Gomis, P., & Leon, A. (2006). Emergence delirium in adults in the post-anaesthesia care unit. *British Journal of Anaesthesia, 96*(6), 747–753.

Leslie, D. L., Marcantonio, E. R., Zhang, Y., Leo-Summers, L., & Inouye, S. K. (2008). One-year health care costs associated with delirium in the elderly population. *Archives of Internal Medicine, 168*(1), 27–32.

Leso, L., & Schwartz, T. L. (2002). Ziprasidone treatment of delirium. *Psychosomatics, 43*(1), 61–62.

Leucht, S., Wahlbeck, K., Hamann, J., & Kissling, W. (2003). New generation antipsychotics versus low-potency conventional antipsychotics: a systematic review and meta-analysis. *Lancet, 361*(9369), 1581–1589.

Leung, J. M., Sands, L. P., Mullen, E. A., Wang, Y., & Vaurio, L. (2005). Are preoperative depressive symptoms associated with postoperative delirium in geriatric surgical patients? *Journals of Gerontology - Series A: Biological Sciences and Medical Sciences, 60*(12), 1563–1568.

Leung, J. M., Sands, L. P., Rico, M., Petersen, K. L., Rowbotham, M. C., Dahl, J. B., et al. (2006). Pilot clinical trial of gabapentin to decrease postoperative delirium in older patients. *Neurology, 67*(7), 1251–1253.

Leung, J. M., Sands, L. P., Wang, Y., Poon, A., Kwok, P. Y., Kane, J. P., & Pullinger, C. R. (2007). Apolipoprotein E e4 allele increases the risk of early postoperative delirium in older patients undergoing noncardiac surgery. *Anesthesiology, 107*(3), 406–411.

Levkoff, S. E., Evans, D. A., Liptzin, B., Cleary, P. D., Lipsitz, L. A., Wetle, T. T., et al. (1992). Delirium. The occurence and persistence of symptoms among elderly hospitalized patients. *Archives of Internal Medicine, 152*(2), 334–340.

Li, H., Luo, J., Wang, C., Xie, S., Xu, X., Wang, X., et al. (2014). Efficacy and safety of aripiprazole in Chinese Han schizophrenia subjects: a randomized, double-blind, active parallel-controlled, multicenter clinical trial. *Schizophrenia Research, 157*(1–3), 112–119.

Lipowski, Z. J. (1967). Delirium, clouding of consciousness and confusion. *Journal of Nervous and Mental Disease, 145*(3), 227–255.

Lipowski, Z. J. (1980). Delirium updated. *Comprehensive Psychiatry, 21*(3), 190–196.

Lipowski, Z. J. (1987). Delirium (acute confusional states). *Journal of the American Medical Association, 258*(13), 1789–1792.

Lipowski, Z. J. (1991). Delirium: how its concept has developed. *International Psychogeriatrics, 3*(2), 115–120.

Lipowski, Z. J. (1992). Update on delirium. *Psychiatr Clin North Am 15*(2), 335–346.

Liptzin, B., Laki, A., Garb, J. L., Fingeroth, R., & Krushell, R. (2005). Donepezil in the prevention and treatment of post-surgical delirium. *American Journal of Geriatric Psychiatry, 13*(12), 1100–1106.

Liptzin, B., & Levkoff, S. E. (1992). An empirical study of delirium subtypes. *British Journal of Psychiatry, 161*: 843–845.

Litaker, D., Locala J., Franco, K., Bronson, D. L., & Tannous, Z. (2001). Preoperative risk factors for postoperative delirium. *General Hospital Psychiatry, 23*(2), 84–89.

Liu, C. Y., & Hsieh, J. C. (1993). [Post cardiopulmonary-bypass neuropsychiatric complications]. *Changgeng Yi Xue Za Zhi, 16*(1), 52–58.

Logan, C. J., & Stewart, J. T. (2007). Treatment of post-electroconvulsive therapy delirium and agitation with donepezil. *Journal of ECT, 23*(1), 28–29.

Lonergan, E., Britton, A. M., Luxenberg, J., & Wyller, T. (2007). Antipsychotics for delirium. *Cochrane Database System Reviews*(2), CD005594.

Lopez-Alvarez, J., Zea Sevilla, M. A., Aguera Ortiz, L., Fernandez Blazquez, M. A., Valenti Soler, M., & Martinez-Martin, P. (2014). Effect of anticholinergic drugs on cognitive impairment in the elderly. *Rev Psiquiatr Salud Ment*.

LoVecchio, F., Watts, D., & Winchell, J. (2005). One-year experience with aripiprazole exposures. *American Journal of Emergency Medicine, 23*(4), 585–586.

Lowery, D. P., Wesnes, K., & Ballard, C. G. (2007). Subtle attentional deficits in the absence of dementia are associated with an increased risk of post-operative delirium. *Dementia and Geriatric Cognitive Disorders, 23*(6), 390–394.

Lundstrom, M., Olofsson, B., Stenvall, M., Karlsson, S., Nyberg, L., Englund, U., et al. (2007). Postoperative delirium in old patients with femoral neck fracture: a randomized intervention study. *Aging Clinical and Experimental Research, 19*(3), 178–186.

Ma, D., Hossain M., Rajakumaraswamy, N., Arshad, M., Sanders, R. D., Franks, N. P., & Maze, M. (2004). Dexmedetomidine produces its neuroprotective effect via the alpha 2A–adrenoceptor subtype. *European Journal of Pharmacology, 502*(1–2), 87–97.

Macdonald, A. J. (1999). Can delirium be separated from dementia? *Dementia and Geriatric Cognitive Disorders, 10*(5), 386–388.

MacLullich, A. M., Beaglehole, A., Hall, R. J., & Meagher, D. J. (2009). Delirium and long-term cognitive impairment. *International Review of Psychiatry, 21*(1), 30–42.

Mac Sweeney, R., Barber, V., Page, V., Ely, E. W., Perkins, G. D., Young, J. D., et al. (2010). A national survey of the management of delirium in UK intensive care units. *QJM, 103*(4), 243–251.

Maldonado, J. (2009). Delirium risk factors and treatment algorithm. *Focus: The Journal of Lifelong Learning in Psychiatry*, VII (3), 336–342.

Maldonado, J. R. (2008). Delirium in the acute care setting: Characteristics, diagnosis and treatment. *Critical Care Clinics, 24*(4), 657–722.

Maldonado, J. R. (2008). Pathoetiological model of delirium: A comprehensive understanding of the neurobiology of delirium and an evidence-based approach to prevention and treatment. *Critical Care Clinics, 24*(4), 789–856.

Maldonado, J. R. (2011). Delirio. *Protocolos en Cuidado Critico*. S. Rodriguez-Villar. Madrid, Marban: pp. 636–645.

Maldonado, J. R. (2013). Neuropathogenesis of delirium: A review of current etiological theories and common pathways. *American Journal of Geriatric Psychiatry, 21*(12), 1190–1222.

Maldonado, J. R., Dhami, N., & Wise, L. (2003). Clinical implications of the recognition and management of delirium in general medical and surgical wards. *Psychosomatics, 44*(2), 157–158.

Maldonado, J., & Kang, H. (2003). Evidence of decreased incidence of extra-pyramidal symptoms with intravenous haloperidol. *Journal of Psychosomatic Research, 55*, 140–141.

Maldonado, J. R., van der Starre, P. J., Block, T., Wysong, A. (2003). Post-operative sedation and the incidence of delirium and cognitive deficits in cardiac surgery patients. *Anesthesiology, 99*, 465.

Maldonado, J. R., van der Starre, P., Wysong, A., & Block, T. (2004). Dexmedetomidine: Can it reduce the incidence of ICU delirium in postcardiotomy patients? *Psychosomatics, 45*(2), 173.

Maldonado J. R., Wysong, A., & van der Starre, P. J. (2003). The role of the novel anesthetic agent dexmedetomidine on reduction of the incidence of ICU delirium in postcardiotomy patients. *Journal of Psychosomatic Research, 55*(2), 150.

Maldonado, J. R., Wysong, A., van der Starre, P. J., Block, T., Miller, C., & Reitz, B. A. (2009). Dexmedetomidine and the reduction of postoperative delirium after cardiac surgery. *Psychosomatics, 50*(3), 206–217.

Marcantonio, E. R., Flacker, J. M., Wright, R. J., & Resnick, N. M. (2001). Reducing delirium after hip fracture: a randomized trial. *Journal of American Geriatric Society, 49*(5), 516–522.

Marcantonio, E., Ta, T., Duthie, E., & Resnick, N. M. (2002). Delirium severity and psychomotor types: their relationship with outcomes after hip fracture repair. *Journal of the American Geriatrics Society, 50*(5), 850–857.

Marcantonio, E. R., Juarez, G. Goldman, L., Mangione, C. M., Ludwig, L. E., Lind, L., et al. (1994). The relationship of postoperative delirium with psychoactive medications. *Journal of the American Medical Association, 272*(19), 1518–1522.

Marcantonio, E. R., Flacker, J. M., Michaels, M., & Resnick, N. M. (2000). Delirium is independently associated with poor functional recovery after hip fracture. *Journal of the American Geriatric Society, 48*(6), 618–624.

Marder, S. R., McQuade R. D., Stock E., Kaplita S., Marcus R., Safferman A. Z., et al. (2003). Aripiprazole in the treatment of schizophrenia: safety and tolerability in short–term, placebo–controlled trials. *Schizophrenia Research, 61*(2–3), 123–136.

Martinez, F. T., Tobar, C., Beddings, C. I., Vallejo, G., & Fuentes, P. (2012). Preventing delirium in an acute hospital using a non-pharmacological intervention. *Age and Ageing 41*(5), 629–634.

Mate, K. E., Kerr, K. P., Pond, D., Williams, E. J., Marley, J., Disler, P., et al. (2015). Impact of Multiple Low-Level Anticholinergic Medications on Anticholinergic Load of Community-Dwelling Elderly With and Without Dementia. *Drugs Aging.*

Matthews, C. D., Guerin, M. V., & Wang, X. (1991). Human plasma melatonin and urinary 6–sulphatoxy melatonin: studies in natural annual photoperiod and in extended darkness. *Clinical Endocrinology, 35*(1), 21–27.

Matthews, E. E. (2011). Sleep disturbances and fatigue in critically ill patients. *AACN Advanced Critical Care, 22*(3), 204–224.

Mattle, H. (1985). [Neurologic manifestations of osmolality disorders]. *Schweizerische medizinische Wochenschrift, 115*(26), 882–889.

McAlpine, J. N., Hodgson, E. J., Abramowitz, S., Richman, S. M., Su, Y., Kelly, M. G., et al. (2008). The incidence and risk factors associated with postoperative delirium in geriatric patients undergoing surgery for suspected gynecologic malignancies. *Gynecologic Oncology, 109*(2), 296–302.

McAvay, G. J., Van Ness, P. H., Bogardus, S. T. Jr., Zhang, Y., Leslie, D. L., Leo-Summers, L. S., & Inouye, S. K. (2006). Older adults discharged from the hospital with delirium: 1–year outcomes. *Journal of the American Geriatrics Society, 54*(8), 1245–1250.

McAvay, G. J., Van Ness, P. H., Bogardus, S. T. Jr., Zhang, Y., Leslie, D. L., Leo-Summers, L. S., & Inouye, S. K. (2007). Depressive symptoms and the risk of incident delirium in older hospitalized adults. *Journal of the American Geriatrics Society, 55*(5), 684–691.

McCusker, J., Cole, M., Bellavance, F., & Primeau, F. (1998). Reliability and validity of a new measure of severity of delirium. *International Psychogeriatrics, 10*(4), 421–433.

McCusker, J., Cole, M., Dendukuri, N., Belzile, E., & Primeau, F. (2001). Delirium in older medical inpatients and subsequent cognitive and functional status: a prospective study. *Canadian Medical Association Journal, 165*(5), 575–583.

McCusker, J., Cole, M., Dendukuri, N., Han, L., & Belzile, E. (2003). The course of delirium in older medical inpatients: a prospective study. *Journal of General Internal Medicine, 18*(9), 696–704.

McCusker, J., Cole, M. G., Dendukuri, N., & Belzile, E. (2003). Does delirium increase hospital stay? *Journal of American Geriatric Society, 51*(11), 1539–1546.

McCusker, J., Verdon, J., Caplan, G. A., Meldon, S. W., & Jacobs, P. (2002). Older persons in the emergency medical care system. *Journal of the American Geriatrics Society, 50*(12), 2103–2105.(McCusker, Cole et al. 2003)

McGee, W., Veremakis, C., & Wilson, G. L. (1988). Clinical importance of tissue oxygenation and use to the mixed venous blood gas. *Res Medica, 4*(2), 15–24.

McIntosh, T. K., Bush, H. L., Yeston, N. S., Grasberger, R., Palter, M., Aun, F., & Egdahl R. H. (1985). Beta-endorphin, cortisol and postoperative delirium: a preliminary report. *Psychoneuroendocrinology, 10*(3), 303–313.

McKinley, S., Aitken, L. M., Alison, J. A., King, M., Leslie, G., Burmeister, E., & Elliott, D. (2012). Sleep and other factors associated with mental health and psychological distress after intensive care for critical illness. *Intensive Care Medicine, 38*(4), 627–633.

McNicoll, L., Pisani, M. A., Zhang, Y., Ely, E. W., Siegel, M. D., & Inouye, S. K. (2003). Delirium in the intensive care unit: occurrence and clinical course in older patients. *Journal of the American Geriatrics Society, 51*(5), 591–598.

Meagher, D. (2009). Motor subtypes of delirium: past, present and future. *International Rreview of Psychiatry, 21*(1), 59–73.

Meagher, D. J., McLoughlin, L., Leonard, M., Hannon, N., Dunne, C., & O'Regan, N. (2013). What do we really know about the treatment of delirium with antipsychotics? ten key issues for delirium pharmacotherapy. *American Journal of Geriatric Psychiatry, 21*(12), 1223–1238.

Meagher, D. J., Moran, M., Raju, B., Gibbons, D., Donnelly, S., Saunders, J., & Trzepacz, P. T. (2007). Phenomenology of delirium. Assessment of 100 adult cases using standardised measures. *British Journal of Psychiatry 190*: 135–141.

Meagher, D. J., O'Hanlon, D., O'Mahony, E., Casey, P. R., & Trzepacz, P. T. (2000). Relationship between symptoms and motoric subtype of delirium. *Journal of Neuropsychiatry & Clinical Neurosciences, 12*(1), 51–56.

Meagher, D. J., & Trzepacz, P. T. (2000). Motoric subtypes of delirium. *Seminars in Clinical Neuropsychiatry, 5*(2), 75–85.

Meuret, P., Backman, S. B., Bonhomme, V., Plourde, G., & Fiset, P. (2000). Physostigmine reverses propofol-induced unconsciousness and attenuation of the auditory steady state response and bispectral index in human volunteers. *Anesthesiology, 93*(3), 708–717.

Meyer, O., Meyer, S., & Kressig, R. W. (2010). [Diagnosis of delirium]. *Therapeutische Umschau, 67*(2), 69–73.

Milbrandt, E. B., Deppen S., Harrison P. L., Shintani A. K., Speroff T., Stiles R. A., et al. (2004). Costs associated with delirium in mechanically ventilated patients. *Critical Care Medicine, 32*(4), 955–962.

Miller, M. O. (2008). Evaluation and management of delirium in hospitalized older patients. *American Family Physician, 78*(11), 1265–1270.

Miller, N. S., & Gold, M. S. (1991). Benzodiazepines: a major problem. Introduction. *Journal of Subst Abuse Treat, 8*(1–2), 3–7.

Miller, A. H., Haroon, E., Raison, C. L., & Felger, J. C. (2013). Cytokine targets in the brain: impact on neurotransmitters and neurocircuits. *Depression and Anxiety, 30*(4), 297–306.

Millerowa, D. (1966). [Delirium syndrome during corticoid therapy in a leukemic child]. *Pediatria Polska, 41*(1), 101–103.

McManus, J., Pathansali, R., Stewart, R., Macdonald, A., & Jackson, S. (2007). Delirium post-stroke. *Age & Ageing, 36*(6), 613–618.

Milstein, A., Pollack, A., Kleinman, G., & Barak, Y. (2002). Confusion/delirium following cataract surgery: An incidence study of 1-year duration. *International Psychogeriatrics, 14*(3), 301–306.

Milusheva, E., Sperlagh, B., Kiss, B., Szporny, L., Pasztor, E., Papasova, M., & Vizi, E. S. (1990). Inhibitory effect of hypoxic condition on acetylcholine release is partly due to the effect of adenosine released from the tissue. *Brain Research Bulletin, 24*(3), 369–373.

Miyazaki, T., Kuwano, H., Kato, H., Ando, H., Kimura, H., Inose, T., et al. (2003). Correlation between serum melatonin circadian rhythm and intensive care unit psychosis after thoracic esophagectomy. *Surgery, 133*(6), 662–668.

Moghaddam, B., Schenk, J. O., Stewart, W. B., & Hansen, A. J. (1987). Temporal relationship between neurotransmitter release and ion flux during spreading depression and anoxia. *Canadian Journal of Physiology and Pharmacology, 65*(5), 1105–1110.

Morandi, A., McCurley J., Vasilevskis E. E., Fick D. M., Bellelli G., Lee P., et al. (2012). Tools to detect delirium superimposed on dementia: a systematic review. *Journal of the American Geriatrics Society, 60*(11), 2005–2013.

Morandi, A., Pandharipande, P. P., Jackson, J. C., Bellelli, G., Trabucchi, M., & Ely, E. W. (2012). Understanding terminology of delirium and long-term cognitive impairment in critically ill patients. *Psychiatry and Clinical Neurosciences, 26*(3), 267–276.

Morandi, A., Rogers B. P., Gunther M. L., Merkle K., Pandharipande P., Girard T. D., et al. (2012). The relationship between delirium duration, white matter integrity, and cognitive impairment in intensive care unit survivors as determined by diffusion tensor imaging: the VISIONS prospective cohort magnetic resonance imaging study*. *Critical Care Medicine, 40*(7), 2182–2189.

Moretti, R., Torre, P., Antonello, R. M., Cattaruzza, T., & Cazzato, G. (2004). Cholinesterase inhibition as a possible therapy for delirium in vascular dementia: A controlled, open 24-month study of 246 patients. *American Journal of Alzheimer's Disease & Other Dementias, 19*(6), 333–339.

Morita, T., Takigawa, C., Onishi, H., Tajima, T., Tani, K., Matsubara, T., et al. (2005). Opioid rotation from morphine to fentanyl in delirious cancer patients: an open–label trial. *Journal of Pain and Symptom Management, 30*(1), 96–103.

Morita, T., Tei, Y., Tsunoda, J., Inoue, S., & Chihara, S. (2001). Underlying pathologies and their associations with clinical features in terminal delirium of cancer patients. *Journal of Pain & Symptom Management, 22*(6), 997–1006.

Morrison, R. S., Magaziner, J., Gilbert, M., Koval, K. J., McLaughlin, M. A., Orosz, G., et al. (2003). Relationship between pain and opioid analgesics on the development of delirium following hip fracture. *Journals of Gerontology - Series A: Biological Sciences and Medical Sciences, 58*(1), 76–81.

Mundigler, G., Delle-Karth G., Koreny M., Zehetgruber M., Steindl-Munda P., Marktl W., et al. (2002). Impaired circadian rhythm of melatonin secretion in sedated critically ill patients with severe sepsis. *Critical Care Medicine, 30*(3), 536–540.

Munhoz, C. D., Sorrells, S. F., Caso, J. R., Scavone, C., & Sapolsky, R. M. (2010). Glucocorticoids exacerbate lipopolysaccharide–induced signaling in the frontal cortex and hippocampus in a dose-dependent manner. *Journal of Neuroscience, 30*(41), 13690–13698.

Mura, T., Proust-Lima, C., Akbaraly, T., Amieva, H., Tzourio, C., Chevassus, H., et al. (2013). Chronic use of benzodiazepines and latent cognitive decline in the elderly: results from the Three–city study. *European Neuropsychopharmacology, 23*(3), 212–223.

Nakos, G. (2012). Sleep deprivation in ICU. *Minerva Anestesiologica, 78*(4), 395–396.

Narayan, M., & Nelson, J. C. (1997). Treatment of dementia with behavioral disturbance using divalproex or a combination of divalproex and a neuroleptic. *The Journal of Clinical Psychiatry, 58*(8), 351–354.

Needham, D. M., & Korupolu, R. (2010). Rehabilitation quality improvement in an intensive care unit setting: implementation of a quality improvement model. *Topics in Stroke Rehabilitation, 17*(4), 271–281.

Needham, D. M., Korupolu, R., Zanni, J. M., Pradhan, P., Colantuoni, E., Palmer, J. B., et al. (2010). Early physical medicine and rehabilitation for patients with acute respiratory failure: a quality improvement project. *Archives of Physical Medicine and Rehabilitation, 91*(4), 536–542.

Neelon, V. J., Champagne, M. T., Carlson, J. R., & Funk, S. G. (1996). The NEECHAM Confusion Scale: Construction, validation, and clinical testing. *Nursing Research, 45*(6), 324–330.

Nelson, L. E., Lu, J., Guo, T., Saper, C. B., Franks, N. P., & Maze, M. (2003). The alpha2–adrenoceptor agonist dexmedetomidine converges on an endogenous sleep–promoting pathway to exert its sedative effects. *Anesthesiology, 98*(2), 428–436.

Nelson, S., & Leung, J. G. (2013). Torsades de pointes after administration of low–dose aripiprazole. *Ann Pharmacother 47*(2), e11.

Nemoto, K., Kawanishi, Y., Suzuki, H., Mizukami, K., & Asada, T. (2007). Isolated adrenocorticotropic hormone deficiency presenting with delirium. *American Journal of Psychiatry, 164*(9), 1440.

Neto, A. S., Nassar Jr., A. P., Cardoso, S. O., Manetta, J. A., Pereira, V. G., Esposito, D. C., et al. (2012). Delirium screening in critically ill patients: a systematic review and meta-analysis. *Criticial Care Medicine, 40*(6), 1946–1951.

Nevin, M., Colchester, A. C., Adams, S., & Pepper, J. R. (1989). Prediction of neurological damage after cardiopulmonary bypass surgery. Use of the cerebral function analysing monitor. *Anaesthesia, 44*(9), 725–729.

Newman, M. F., Grocott, H. P., Mathew, J. P., White, W. D., Landolfo, K., Reves, J. G., et al. (2001). Report of the substudy assessing the impact of neurocognitive function on quality of life 5 years after cardiac surgery. *Stroke, 32*(12), 2874–2881.

Nibuya, M., Suda, S., Mori, K., & Ishiguro, T. (2000). Delirium with autoimmune thyroiditis induced by interferon alpha. *American Journal of Psychiatry, 157*(10), 1705–1706.

Nicolson, S. E., Chabon, B., Larsen, K. A., Kelly, S. E., Potter, A. W., & Stern, T. A. (2011). Primitive reflexes associated with delirium: a prospective trial. *Psychosomatics, 52*(6), 507–512.

NICE (2010). Delirium: Diagnosis, prevention and management. Manchester, United Kingdom: National Institute for Health and Clinical Excellence.

O'Keeffe, S. (1994). Rating the severity of delirium: The delirium assessment scale. *International Journal of Geriatric Psychiatry, 9*(7), 551–556.

O'Keeffe, S., & Lavan, J. (1997). The prognostic significance of delirium in older hospital patients. *Journal of the American Geriatrics Society, 45*(2), 174–178.

O'Keeffe, S. T., & Devlin, J. G. (1994). Delirium and the dexamethasone suppression test in the elderly. *Neuropsychobiology, 30*(4), 153–156.

O'Mahony, R., Murthy, L., Akunne, A., Young, J., & Guideline Development Group. (2011). Synopsis of the National Institute for Health and Clinical Excellence guideline for prevention of delirium. *Annals of Internal Medicine, 154*(11), 746–751.

O'Malley, G., Leonard, M., Meagher D., & O'Keeffe, S. T. (2008). The delirium experience: a review. *Journal of Psychosomatic Research, 65*(3), 223–228.

O'Reilly, R. L., & Smith, D. (1991). Benzodiazepines and Confusion in Medically Ill Alcoholics: Balancimg safety against toxicity. *Cancer Family Physician, 37*, 2609–2644.

Olofsson, S. M., Weitzner, M. A., Valentine, A. D., Baile, W. F., & Meyers, C. A. (1996). A retrospective study of the psychiatric management and outcome of delirium in the cancer patient. *Supportive Care in Cancer, 4*(5), 351–357.

Olsson, T. (1999). Activity in the hypothalamic–pituitary–adrenal axis and delirium. *Dementia and Geriatric Cognitive Disorders, 10*(5), 345–349.

Olsson, T., Astrom, M., Eriksson, S., & Forssell, A. (1989). Hypercortisolism revealed by the dexamethasone suppression test in patients [corrected] with acute ischemic stroke. *Stroke, 20*(12), 1685–1690.

Olsson, T., Marklund, N., Gustafson, Y., & Nasman, B. (1992). Abnormalities at different levels of the hypothalamic–pituitary–adrenocortical axis early after stroke. *Stroke, 23*(11), 1573–1576.

Onishi, H., Sugimasa, Y., Kawanishi, C., & Onose, M. (2005). Wernicke encephalopathy presented in the form of postoperative delirium in a patient with hepatocellular carcinoma and liver cirrhosis: a case report and review of the literature. *Palliative & Supportive Care, 3*(4), 337–340.

Ossola, B., Schendzielorz, N., Chen, S. H., Bird, G. S., Tuominen, R. K., Mannisto, P. T., & Hong, J. S. (2011). Amantadine protects dopamine neurons by a dual action: reducing activation of microglia and inducing expression of GNDF in astroglia. *Neuropharmacology, 61*(4), 574–582.

Otter, H., Martin, J., Basell, K., von Heymann, C., Hein, O. V., Bollert, P., et al. (2005). Validity and reliability of the DDS for severity of delirium in the ICU. *NeuroCritical Care, 2*(2), 150–158.

Ouimet, S., Kavanagh, B. P., Gottfried, S. B., & Skrobik, Y. (2007). Incidence, risk factors and consequences of ICU delirium. *Intensive Care Medicine, 33*(1), 66–73.

Ozbolt, L. B., Paniagua, M. A., & Kaiser, R. M. (2008). Atypical antipsychotics for the treatment of delirious elders. *Journal of the American Medical Directors Association, 9*(1), 18–28.

Pae, C. U., Lee, S. J., Lee, C. U., Lee, C., & Paik, I. H. (2004). A pilot trial of quetiapine for the treatment of patients with delirium. *Human Psychopharmacology, 19*(2), 125–127.

Page, V. J., Navarange, S., Gama, S., & McAuley, D. F. (2009). Routine delirium monitoring in a UK critical care unit. *Critical Care, 13*(1), R16.

Pain, L., Jeltsch, H., Lehmann, O., Lazarus, C., Laalou, F. Z., & Cassel, J. C. (2000). Central cholinergic depletion induced by 192 IgG–saporin alleviates the sedative effects of propofol in rats. *British Journal of Anaesthesia, 85*(6), 869–873.

Palmer, T. R. (2004). Donepezil in advanced dementia, or delirium? *Journal of the American Medical Directors Association, 5*(1), 67.

Palmstierna, T. (2001). A model for predicting alcohol withdrawal delirium. *Psychiatric Services,ices, 52*(6), 820–823.

Pandharipande, P., Cotton, B. A., Shintani, A., Thompson, J., Costabile, S., Truman, B., et al. (2007). Motoric subtypes of delirium in mechanically ventilated surgical and trauma intensive care unit patients. *Intensive Care Medicine, 33*(10), 1726–1731.

Pandharipande, P., & Ely, E. W. (2006). Sedative and analgesic medications: risk factors for delirium and sleep disturbances in the critically ill. *Critical Care Clinics, 22*(2), 313–327, vii.

Pandharipande, P. P., Pun, B. T., Herr, D. L., Maze, M., Girard, T. D., Miller, R. R., et al. (2007). Effect of sedation with dexmedetomidine vs lorazepam on acute brain dysfunction in mechanically ventilated patients: the MENDS randomized controlled trial. *Journal of the American Medical Association, 298*(22), 2644–2653.

Pandharipande, P., Shintani, A., Peterson, J., Pun, B. T., Wilkinson, G. R., Dittus, R. S., et al. (2006). Lorazepam is an independent risk factor for transitioning to delirium in intensive care unit patients. *Anesthesiology, 104*(1), 21–26.

Parellada, E., Baeza, I., de Pablo, J., & Martinez, G. (2004). Risperidone in the treatment of patients with delirium. *Journal of Clinical Psychiatry, 65*(3), 348–353.

Parikh, S. S., & Chung, F. (1995). Postoperative delirium in the elderly. *Anesthesia and Analgesia, 80*(6), 1223–1232.

Patel, R. P., Gambrell, M., Speroff, T., Scott, T. A., Pun, B. T., Okahashi, J., et al. (2009). Delirium and sedation in the intensive care unit: survey of behaviors and attitudes of 1384 healthcare professionals. *Critical Care Medicine, 37*(3), 825–832.

Paulson, G. W. (1977). The neurological examination in dementia. *Contemp Neurol Ser, 15*, 169–188.

Peters, U. H., & Neumann, H. (1960). [Vitamin B6 deficiency in delirium tremens]. *Arch Psychiatr Nervenkr Z Gesamte Neurol Psychiatr, 201*: 165–172.

Peterson, J. F., Pun, B. T., Dittus, R. S., Thomason, J. W., Jackson, J. C., Shintani, A. K., & Ely, E. W. (2006). Delirium and its motoric subtypes: a study of 614 critically ill patients. *Journal of the American Geriatrics Society, 54*(3), 479–484.

Pisani, M. A., Inouye, S. K., McNicoll, L., & Redlich, C. A. (2003). Screening for preexisting cognitive impairment in older intensive care unit patients: use of proxy assessment. *Journal of the American Geriatrics Society, 51*(5), 689–693.

Pisani, M. A., Kong, S. Y., Kasl, S. V., Murphy, T. E., Araujo, K. L., & Van Ness, P. H. (2009). Days of delirium are associated with 1-year mortality in an older intensive care unit population. *American Journal of Respiratory and Critical Care Medicine, 180*(11), 1092–1097.

Pisani, M. A., Murphy, T. E., Araujo, K. L., Slattum, P., Van Ness, P. H., & Inouye, S. K. (2009). Benzodiazepine and opioid use and the duration of intensive care unit delirium in an older population. *Critical Care Medicine, 37*(1), 177–183.

Pisani, M. A., Redlich C., McNicoll, L., Ely, E. W., & Inouye, S. K. (2003). Underrecognition of preexisting cognitive impairment by physicians in older ICU patients. *Chest, 124*(6), 2267–2274.

Plaschke, K., Hill, H., Engelhardt, R., Thomas, C., von Haken, R., Scholz, M., et al. (2007). EEG changes and serum anticholinergic activity measured in patients with delirium in the intensive care unit. *Anaesthesia, 62*(12), 1217–1223.

Pompei, P., Foreman, M., Rudberg, M. A., Inouye, S. K., Braund, V., & Cassel, C. K. (1994). Delirium in hospitalized older persons: outcomes and predictors. *Journal of the American Geriatrics Society, 42*(8), 809–815.

Porsteinsson, A. P., Tariot, P. N., Jakimovich, L. J., Kowalski, N., Holt, C., Erb, R., & Cox, C. (2003). Valproate therapy for agitation in dementia: open-label extension of a double-blind trial. *The American Journal of Geriatric Psychiatry: Official Journal of the American Association for Geriatric Psychiatry, 11*(4), 434–440.

Powers, J. S., Decoskey, D., & Kahrilas, P. J. (1981). Physostigmine for treatment of delirium tremens. *Journal of Clinical Pharmacology, 21*(1), 57–60.

Prakanrattana, U., & Prapaitrakool, S. (2007). Efficacy of risperidone for prevention of postoperative delirium in cardiac surgery. *Anaesth Intensive Care, 35*(5), 714–719.

Rabinowitz, T. (2002). Delirium: An important (but often unrecognized) clinical syndrome. *Current Psychiatry Report, 4*(3), 202–208.

Reiter, R. J. (1991). Pineal melatonin: cell biology of its synthesis and of its physiological interactions. *Endocrine Reviews, 12*(2), 151–180.

Richardson, W. H. 3rd, Williams, S. R., & Carstairs, S. D. (2004). A picturesque reversal of antimuscarinic delirium. *Journal of Emergency Medicine, 26*(4), 463.

Riker, R. R., Fraser, G. L., & Cox, P. M. (1994). Continuous infusion of haloperidol controls agitation in critically ill patients. *Critical Care Medicine, 22*(3), 433–440.

Riker, R. R., Shehabi, Y., Bokesch, P. M., Ceraso, D., Wisemandle, W., Koura, F., et al. (2009). Dexmedetomidine vs midazolam for sedation of critically ill patients: a randomized trial. *Journal of the American Medical Association, 301*(5), 489–499.

Ritchie, J., Steiner, W., & Abrahamowicz, M. (1996). Incidence of and risk factors for delirium among psychiatric inpatients. *Psychiatric Services, 47*(7), 727–730.

Rizzo, J. A., Baker, D. I., McAvay, G., & Tinetti, M. E. (1996). The cost-effectiveness of a multifactorial targeted prevention program for falls among community elderly persons. *Medical Care, 34*(9), 954–969.

Roberts, B. L., Rickard, C. M., Rajbhandari, D., & Reynolds, P. (2007). Factual memories of ICU: recall at two years post–discharge and comparison with delirium status during ICU admission––a multicentre cohort study. *Journal of Clinical Nursing, 16*(9), 1669–1677.

Robertsson, B., Karlsson, I., Styrud, E., & Gottfries, C. G. (1997). Confusional State Evaluation (CSE): an instrument for measuring severity of delirium in the elderly. *British Journal of Psychiatry, 170*, 565–570.

Robertsson, B., Blennow, K., Brane, G., Edman, A., Karlsson, I., Wallin, A., & Gottfries, C. G. (2001). Hyperactivity in the hypothalamic–pituitary–adrenal axis in demented patients with delirium. *International Clinical Psychopharmacology, 16*(1), 39–47.

Rockwood, K., Cosway, S., Carver, D., Jarrett, P., Stadnyk K., & Fisk, J. (1999). The risk of dementia and death after delirium. *Age and Ageing 28*(6), 551–556.

Rolfson, D. B., McElhaney, J. E., Jhangri, G. S., & Rockwood, K. (1999). Validity of the confusion assessment method in detecting postoperative delirium in the elderly. *International Psychogeriatrics, 11*(4), 431–438.

Romano, J., & Engel, G. (1944). Delirium. I. EEG data. *Archives of Neurological Psychiatry, 51*, 356–377.

Rosczyk, H. A., Sparkman, N. L., & Johnson, R. W. (2008). Neuroinflammation and cognitive function in aged mice following minor surgery. *Experimental Gerontology, 43*(9), 840–846.

Rosenberg, J., & Kehlet, H. (1993). Postoperative mental confusion—association with postoperative hypoxemia. *Surgery, 114*(1), 76–81.

Rothschild, J., & Leape, L. (2000). *The nature and extent of medical injury in older patients: executive summary.* Public Policy Institute, AARP, Washington, DC.

Rubino, A. S., Onorati, F., Caroleo, S., Galato, E., Nucera, S., Amantea, B., et al. (2010). Impact of clonidine administration on delirium and related respiratory weaning after surgical correction of acute type-A aortic dissection: results of a pilot study. *Interactive Cardiovascular and Thoracic Surgery, 10*(1), 58–62.

Rudolph, J. L., Harrington, M. B., Lucatorto, M. A., et al.; Veterans and Delirium Working Group. (2011). Validation of a medical record–based delirium risk assessment. *Journal of the American Geriatrics Society, 59 Suppl 2,* S289–294.

Rudolph, J. L., Jones, R. N., Grande, L. J., Milberg, W. P., King, E. G., Lipsitz, L. A., et al. (2006). Impaired executive function is associated with delirium after coronary artery bypass graft surgery. *Journal of the American Geriatrics Society, 54*(6), 937–941.

Rupreht, J., Schneck, H. J., & Dworacek, B. (1989). [Physostigmine–recent pharmacologic data and their significance for practical use]. *Anaesthesiology & Reanimation, 14*(4), 235–241.

Ryan, D. J., O'Regan, N. A., Caoimh, R. O., Clare, J., O'Connor, M., Leonard, M., et al. (2013). Delirium in an adult acute hospital population: predictors, prevalence and detection. *British Medical Journal, Open 3*(1).

Saczynski, J. S., Marcantonio, E. R., Quach, L., Fong, T. G., Gross, A., Inouye, S. K., & Jones, R. N. (2012). Cognitive trajectories after postoperative delirium. *New England Journal of Medicine, 367*(1), 30–39.

Sagawa, R., Akechi, T., Okuyama, T., Uchida, M., & Furukawa, T. A. (2009). Etiologies of delirium and their relationship to reversibility and motor subtype in cancer patients. *Jpn Journal of Clinical Oncology, 39*(3), 175–182.

Sakai, A. (1991). Phrenitis: inflammation of the mind and the body. *History of Psychiatry, 2*(6), 193–205.

Sampson, E. L., Raven, P. R., Ndhlovu, P. N., Vallance, A., Garlick, N., Watts, J., et al. (2007). A randomized, double–blind, placebo–controlled trial of donepezil hydrochloride (Aricept) for reducing the incidence of postoperative delirium after elective total hip replacement. *International Journal of Geriatric Psychiatry, 22*(4), 343–349.

Sanders, K. M., Minnema, M. A., & Murray, G. B. (1989). Low Incidence of Extrapyramidal Symptoms in Treatment of Delirium with Intravenous Haloperidol and Lorazepam in the Intensive Care Unit. *Journal of Intensive Care Medicine, 4*(5), 201–204.

Sanders, K. M., Murray, G. B., & Cassem, N. H. (1991). High–dose intravenous haloperidol for agitated delirium in a cardiac patient on intra-aortic balloon pump. *Journal of Clinical Psychopharmacology, 11*(2), 146–147.

Sapolsky, R. M. (1990). Glucocorticoids, hippocampal damage and the glutamatergic synapse. *Progress in Brain Research, 86,* 13–23.

Sapolsky, R. M. (1996). Stress, Glucocorticoids, and Damage to the Nervous System: The Current State of Confusion. *Stress, 1*(1), 1–19.

Sapolsky, R. M., & Pulsinelli, W. A. (1985). Glucocorticoids potentiate ischemic injury to neurons: therapeutic implications. *Science, 229*(4720), 1397–1400.

Sato, K., Kimura, T., Nishikawa, T., Tobe, Y., & Masaki, Y. (2010). Neuroprotective effects of a combination of dexmedetomidine and hypothermia after incomplete cerebral ischemia in rats. *Acta Anaesthesiologica Scandinavica, 54*(3), 377–382.

Schiepers, O. J., Wichers, M. C., & Maes, M. (2005). Cytokines and major depression. *Progress in Neuropsychopharmacology & Biological Psychiatry, 29*(2), 201–217.

Schmickaly, R., Nickel, B., Jarisch, M., Kursawe, H. K., Sachs, E., & Karson, A. (1989). [Electrolyte disorders, EEG changes and epileptic seizures in alcohol withdrawal delirium]. *Psychiatrie, Neurologie Und Medizinische Psychologie (Psychiatr Neurol Med Psychol (Leipz)), 41*(12), 722–729.

Schneider, F., H. Bohner, U. Habel, J. B. Salloum, A. Stierstorfer, T. C. Hummel, C. Miller, R. Friedrichs, E. E. Muller and W. Sandmann (2002). Risk factors for postoperative delirium in vascular surgery. *General Hospital Psychiatry, 24*(1), 28–34.

Schneir, A. B., Offerman, S. R., Ly, B. T., Davis, J. M., Baldwin, R. T., Williams, S. R., & Clark R. F. (2003). Complications of diagnostic physostigmine administration to emergency department patients. *Annals of Emergency Medicine, 42*(1), 14–19.

Schor, J. D., Levkoff, S. E., Lipsitz, L. A., Reilly, C. H., Cleary, P. D., Rowe, J. W., & Evans, D. A. (1992). Risk factors for delirium in hospitalized elderly. *Journal of the American Medical Association, 267*(6), 827–831.

Schweickert, W. D., Pohlman M. C., Pohlman A. S., Nigos C., Pawlik A. J., Esbrook C. L., et al. (2009). Early physical and occupational therapy in mechanically ventilated, critically ill patients: a randomised controlled trial. *Lancet, 373*(9678), 1874–1882.

Seaman, J. S., Schillerstrom, J., Carroll, D., & Brown, T. M. (2006). Impaired oxidative metabolism precipitates delirium: a study of 101 ICU patients. *Psychosomatics, 47*(1), 56–61.

Segatore, M., & Adams, D. (2001). Managing delirium and agitation in elderly hospitalized orthopaedic patients: Part 2—Interventions. *Orthopaedic Nursing, 20*(2), 61–73; quiz 73–65.

Sessler, C. N., Gosnell, M. S., Grap, M. J., et al. (2002). The Richmond Agitation-Sedation Scale: Validity and reliability in adult intensive care unit patients. *American Journal of Respiratory and Critical Care Medicine, 166*(10), 1338–1344. Available online at: http://www.ats-journals.org/doi/full/10.1164/rccm.2107138#.UxentT9dW5K

Shapiro, B. A., Warren, J., Egol, A. B., Greenbaum, D. M., Jacobi, J., Nasraway, S. A., et al. (1995). Practice parameters for intravenous analgesia and sedation for adult patients in the intensive care unit: an executive summary. Society of Critical Care Medicine. *Critical Care Medicine, 23*(9), 1596–1600.

Shehabi, Y., Grant, P., Wolfenden, H., Hammond, N., Bass, F., Campbell, M., & Chen, J. (2009). Prevalence of delirium with dexmedetomidine compared with morphine based therapy after cardiac surgery: a randomized controlled trial (DEXmedetomidine COmpared to Morphine–DEXCOM Study). *Anesthesiology, 111*(5), 1075–1084.

Sher, Y., Lolak, S., Miller, C., & Maldonado, J. (2013). Valproic Acid in Treatment of Delirium: Case Series and Literature Review. *American Delirium Society.* Indiannapolis, Indiana.

Shigeta, H., Yasui, A., Nimura, Y., Machida, N., Kageyama, M., Miura, M., et al. (2001). Postoperative delirium and melatonin levels in elderly patients. *American Journal of Surgery, 182*(5), 449–454.

Shimizu-Sasamata, M., Bosque-Hamilton, P., Huang, P. L., Moskowitz, M. A., & Lo, E. H. (1998). Attenuated neurotransmitter release and spreading depression-like depolarizations after focal ischemia in mutant mice with disrupted type I nitric oxide synthase gene. *Journal of Neuroscience, 18*(22), 9564–9571.

Shinn, J. A., & Maldonado, J. R. (2000). Performance improvement: increasing recognition and treatment of postoperative delirium. *Progress Cardiovascular Nursing, 15*(3), 114–115.

Short, T. G., Forrest, P., & Galletly, D. C. (1987). Paradoxical reactions to benzodiazepines—a genetically determined phenomenon? *Anaesth Intensive Care, 15*(3), 330–331.

Siddiqi, N., & House, A. (2006). Delirium: an update on diagnosis, treatment and prevention. *Clinical Medicine, 6*(6), 540–543.

Siddiqi, N., House, A. O., & Holmes, J. D. (2006). Occurrence and outcome of delirium in medical in–patients: a systematic literature review. *Age and Ageing, 35*(4), 350–364.

Siddiqi, N., Stockdale, R., Britton, A. M., & Holmes, J. (2007). Interventions for preventing delirium in hospitalised patients. *Cochrane Database Systems Review*(2), CD005563.

Sival, R. C., Duivenvoorden, H. J., Jansen, P. A., Haffmans, P. M., Duursma, S. A., & Eikelenboom, P. (2004). Sodium valproate in aggressive behaviour in dementia: a twelve-week open label follow-up study. *International Journal of Geriatric Psychiatry, 19*(4), 305–312.

Skrobik, Y. K., Bergeron, N., Dumont, M., & Gottfried, S. B. (2004). Olanzapine vs haloperidol: treating delirium in a critical care setting. *Intensive Care Medicine, 30*(3), 444–449.

Slatkin, N., & Rhiner, M. (2004). Treatment of opioid–induced delirium with acetylcholinesterase inhibitors: a case report. *Journal of Pain and Symptom Management, 27*(3), 268–273.

Slowik, A., Turaj, W., Pankiewicz, J., Dziedzic, T., Szermer, P., & Szczudlik, A. (2002). Hypercortisolemia in acute stroke is related to the inflammatory response. *Journal of the Neurological Sciences, 196*(1–2), 27–32.

Smith, P. J., Attix, D. K., Weldon, B. C., Greene, N. H., & Monk, T. G. (2009). Executive function and depression as independent risk factors for postoperative delirium. *Anesthesiology, 110*(4), 781–787.

Smith, L. W., & Dimsdale, J. E. (1989). Postcardiotomy delirium: Conclusions after 25 years? *American Journal of Psychiatry, 146*(4), 452–458.

Somjen, G. G., Aitken, P. G., Balestrino, M., Herreras, O., & Kawasaki, K. (1990). Spreading depression-like depolarization and selective vulnerability of neurons. A brief review. *Stroke, 21*(11 Suppl), III179–183.

Somjen, G. G., Aitken, P. G., Balestrino, M., Crain, B. J. Czeh, G., Kawasaki, K., et al. (1989). Extracellular ions, hypoxic irreversible loss of function and delayed postischemic neuron degeneration studied in vitro. *Acta Physiologica Scandinavica, Suppl 582*, 58.

Sorrells, S. F., Caso, J. R., Munhoz, C. D., & Sapolsky, R. M. (2009). The stressed CNS: when glucocorticoids aggravate inflammation. *Neuron, 64*(1), 33–39.

Sorrells, S. F., & Sapolsky, R. M. (2007). An inflammatory review of glucocorticoid actions in the CNS. *Brain, Behavior, & Immunity, 21*(3), 259–272.

Speed, G., Wynaden, D., McGowan, S., Hare, M., & Landsborough, I. (2007). Prevalence rate of delirium at two hospitals in Western Australia. *Australian Journal of Advanced Nursing, 25*(1), 38–43.

Srinonprasert, V., Pakdeewongse, S., Assanasen, J., Eiamjinnasuwat, W., Sirisuwat, A., Limmathuroskul, D., & Praditsuwan, R. (2011). Risk factors for developing delirium in older patients admitted to general medical wards. *Journal of the Medical Association of Thailand, 94 Suppl 1*: S99–104.

Steis, M. R., & Fick, D. M. (2008). Are nurses recognizing delirium? A systematic review. *Journal of Gerontological Nursing, 34*(9), 40–48.

Steis, M. R., Shaughnessy, M., & Gordon, S. M. (2012). Delirium: a very common problem you may not recognize. *J of Psychosocial Nursing and Mental Health Services, 50*(7), 17–20.

Stern, T. A. (1983). Continuous infusion of physostigmine in anticholinergic delirium: case report. *Journal of Clinical Psychiatry, 44*(12), 463–464.

Stern, T. A. (1994). Continuous infusion of haloperidol in agitated, critically ill patients. *Critical Care Medicine, 22*(3), 378–379.

Stone, T. W., Behan, W. M., Jones, P. A., Darlington, L. G., & Smith, R. A. (2001). The role of kynurenines in the production of neuronal death, and the neuroprotective effect of purines. *Journal of Alzheimers Disease, 3*(4), 355–366.

Strom, T., & Toft, P. (2011). Time to wake up the patients in the ICU: a crazy idea or common sense? *Minerva Anestesiologica, 77*(1), 59–63.

Stukas, A. A. Jr., Dew, M. A., Switzer, G. E., DiMartini, A., Kormos, R. L., & Griffith, B. P. (1999). PTSD in heart transplant recipients and their primary family caregivers. *Psychosomatics, 40*(3), 212–221.

Sultan, S. S. (2010). Assessment of role of perioperative melatonin in prevention and treatment of postoperative delirium after hip arthroplasty under spinal anesthesia in the elderly. *Saudi Journal of Anaesthesia, 4*(3), 169–173.

Sun, F. Y., Lin, X., Mao, L. Z., Ge, W. H., Zhang, L. M., Huang, Y. L., & Gu, J. (2002). Neuroprotection by melatonin against ischemic neuronal injury associated with modulation of DNA damage and repair in the rat following a transient cerebral ischemia. *Journal of Pineal Research, 33*(1), 48–56.

Sveinsson, I. S. (1975). Postoperative psychosis after heart surgery. *The Journal of Thoracic and Cardiovascular Surgery, 70*(4), 717–726.

Swigart, S. E., Kishi, Y., Thurber, S., Kathol, R. G., & Meller, W. H. (2008). Misdiagnosed delirium in patient referrals to a university–based hospital psychiatry department. *Psychosomatics, 49*(2), 104–108.

Tagarakis, G. I., Tsolaki-Tagaraki, F., Tsolaki, M., Diegeler, A., Tsilimingas, N. B., & Papassotiropoulos, A. (2007). The role of apolipoprotein E in cognitive decline and delirium after bypass heart operations. *American Journal of Alzheimer's Disease & Other Dementias, 22*(3), 223–228.

Taguchi, T., Yano, M., & Kido, Y. (2007). Influence of bright light therapy on postoperative patients: a pilot study. *Intensive and Critical Care Nursing, 23*(5), 289–297.

Tahir, T. A., Eeles, E., Karapareddy, V., Muthuvelu, P., Chapple, S., Phillips, B., et al. (2010). A randomized controlled trial of quetiapine versus placebo in the treatment of delirium. *Journal of Psychosomatic Research, 69*(5), 485–490.

Takagi, K., Ginsberg, M. D., Globus, M. Y., Martinez, E., & Busto, R. (1994). Effect of hyperthermia on glutamate release in ischemic penumbra after middle cerebral artery occlusion in rats. *American Journal of Physiology, 267*(5 Pt 2), H1770–1776.

Takeuchi, T., Furuta K., Hirasawa T., Masaki H., Yukizane T., Atsuta, H., & Nishikawa, T. (2007). Perospirone in the treatment of patients with delirium. *Psychiatry and Clinical Neurosciences, 61*(1), 67–70.

Tariot, P. N. (1999). Treatment of agitation in dementia. *The Journal of Clinical Psychiatry, 60*(Suppl 8), 11–20.

Teeling, J. L., Felton L. M., Deacon, R. M., Cunningham, C., Rawlins, J. N., & Perry, V. H. (2007). Sub-pyrogenic systemic inflammation impacts on brain and behavior, independent of cytokines. *Brain, Behavior, & Immunity, 21*(6), 836–850.

Tesar, G. E., Murray, G. B., & Cassem, N. H. (1985). Use of high–dose intravenous haloperidol in the treatment of agitated cardiac patients. *Journal of Clinical Psychopharmacology, 5*(6), 344–347.

Teslyar, P., Stock, V. M., Wilk, C. M., Camsari, U., Ehrenreich, M. J., & Himelhoch, S. (2013). Prophylaxis with antipsychotic medication reduces the risk of post-operative delirium in elderly patients: a meta-analysis. *Psychosomatics, 54*(2), 124–131.

Thiele, W., & Hohmann, H. (1961). [Corticoid treatment of delirium tremens]. *Nervenarzt, 32*, 405–408.

Tognoni, P., Simonato A., Robutti N., Pisani M., Cataldi A., Monacelli F., et al. (2011). Preoperative risk factors for postoperative delirium (POD) after urological surgery in the elderly. *Archives of Gerontology and Geriatrics, 52*(3), e166–169.

Tran, M., & Elias, A. N. (2003). Severe myopathy and psychosis in a patient with Cushing's disease macroadenoma. *Clinical Neurology and Neurosurgery, 106*(1), 1–4.

Tremont-Lukats, I. W., Teixeira, G. M., & Hernandez, D. E. (1999). Primitive reflexes in a case-control study of patients with advanced human immunodeficiency virus type 1. *Journal of Neurology, 246*(7), 540–543.

Trewin, V. F., Lawrence, C. J., & Veitch, G. B. (1992). An investigation of the association of benzodiazepines and other hypnotics with the incidence of falls in the elderly. *Journal of Clinical Pharmacology Therapy, 17*(2), 129–133.

Trzepacz, P. T., Baker, R. W., & Greenhouse, J. (1988). A symptom rating scale for delirium. *Psychiatry Research, 23*(1), 89–97.

Trzepacz, P. T., Sclabassi, R. J., & Van Thiel, D. H. (1989). Delirium: A subcortical phenomenon? *Journal of Neuropsychiatry Clinical Neuroscience, 1*(3), 283–290.

Trzepacz, P. T., Mittal, D., Torres, R., Kanary, K., Norton, J., & Jimerson, N. (2001). Validation of the Delirium Rating Scale–Revised-98: Comparison with the delirium rating scale and the cognitive test for delirium. *Journal of Neuropsychiatry & Clinical Neurosciences, 13*(2), 229–242.

Trzepacz, P. T., Leavitt, M. & Ciongoli, K. (1992). "An animal model for delirium." *Psychosomatics, 33*(4), 404–415.

Tsuruta, R., T. Nakahara, T. Miyauchi, S. Kutsuna, Y., Ogino, T., Yamamoto, T., et al. (2010). Prevalence and associated factors for delirium in critically ill patients at a Japanese intensive care unit. *General Hospital Psychiatry, 32*(6), 607–611.

Tully, P. J., Baker, R. A., Winefield, H. R., & Turnbull, D. A. (2010). Depression, anxiety disorders and Type D personality as risk factors for delirium after cardiac surgery. *Australia and New Zealand Journal of Psychiatry, 44*(11), 1005–1011.

Tuma, R., & DeAngelis, L. M. (2000). Altered mental status in patients with cancer. *Archives of Neurology, 57*(12), 1727–1731.

Tune, L. E. (2000). Serum anticholinergic activity levels and delirium in the elderly. *Seminars in Clinical Neuropsychiatry, 5*(2), 149–153.

Tune, L. E., & Bylsma, F. W. (1991). Benzodiazepine–induced and anticholinergic–induced delirium in the elderly. *International Psychogeriatrics, 3*(2), 397–408.

Tune, L., Carr, S., Hoag, E., & Cooper, T. (1992). Anticholinergic effects of drugs commonly prescribed for the elderly: potential means for assessing risk of delirium. *Amercian Journal of Psychiatry, 149*(10), 1393–1394.

Tune, L., Carr, S., Cooper, T., Klug, B., & Golinger, R. C. (1993). Association of anticholinergic activity of prescribed medications with postoperative delirium. *Journal of Neuropsychiatry & Clinical Neurosciences, 5*(2), 208–210.

Tune, L., & Folstein, M. F. (1986). Post–operative delirium. *Advances in Psychosomatic Medicine, 15,* 51–68.

Tune, L. E., Damlouji, N. F., Holland, A., Gardner, T. J., Folstein, M. F., & Coyle, J. T. (1981). Association of postoperative delirium with raised serum levels of anticholinergic drugs. *Lancet, 2*(8248), 651–653.

Tune, L. E., & Egeli, S. (1999). Acetylcholine and delirium. *Dementia and Geriatric Cognitive Disorders, 10*(5), 342–344.

Uldall, K. K., Ryan, R., Berghuis, J. P., & Harris, V. L. (2000). Association between delirium and death in AIDS patients. *AIDS Patient Care STDS, 14*(2), 95–100.

Umekawa, T., Yoshida, T., Sakane, N., & Kondo, M. (1996). A case of Sheehan's syndrome with delirium. *Psychiatry and Clinical Neurosciences, 50*(6), 327–330.

Valdes, M., de Pablo, J., Campos, R., et al. (2000). [Multinational European project and multicenter Spanish study of quality improvement of assistance on consultation-liaison psychiatry in general hospital: Clinical profile in Spain]. *Medicina Clinica (Barcelona), 115*(18), 690–694.

van den Bliek, B. M., & Maas, H. A. (2004). [Successful treatment of three elderly patients suffering from prolonged delirium using the cholinesterase inhibitor rivastigmine]. *Ned Tijdschr Geneeskd, 148*(43), 2149; author reply 2149.

van den Boogaard, M., Peters, S. A., van der Hoeven, J. G., Dagnelie, P. C., Leffers, P., Pickkers, P., & Schoonhoven, L. (2010). The impact of delirium on the prediction of in–hospital mortality in intensive care patients. *Critical Care, 14*(4), R146.

van der Mast, R. C., & Roest, F. H. (1996). Delirium after cardiac surgery: A critical review. *Journal of Psychosomatic Research, 41*(1), 13–30.

van Eijk, M. M., van Marum, R. J., Klijn, I. A., de Wit, N., Kesecioglu, J., & Slooter, A. J. (2009). Comparison of delirium assessment tools in a mixed intensive care unit. *Critical Care Medicine, 37*(6), 1881–1885.

van Eijk, M. van den Boogaard M., M., van Marum R. J., Benner P., Eikelenboom P., Honing M. L., et al. (2011). Routine use of the confusion assessment method for the intensive care unit: a multicenter study. *American Journal of Respiratory and Critical Care Medicine, 184*(3), 340–344.

van Munster, B. C., Bisschop P. H., Zwinderman A. H., Korevaar J. C., Endert E., Wiersinga W. J., et al. (2010). Cortisol, interleukins and S100B in delirium in the elderly. *Brain and Cognition, 74*(1), 18–23.

van Munster, B. C., Korevaar, J. C., de Rooij, S. E., Levi, M., & Zwinderman, A. H. (2007). The association between delirium and the apolipoprotein E epsilon4 allele in the elderly. *Psychiatric Genetics, 17*(5), 261–266.

van Munster, B. C., Korevaar, J. C., Zwinderman, A. H., Leeflang, M. M., & de Rooij, S. E. (2009). The association between delirium and the apolipoprotein E epsilon 4 allele: new study results and a meta–analysis. *American Journal of Geriatric Psychiatry, 17*(10), 856–862.

Vasilevskis, E. E., Han, J. H., Hughes, C. G., & Ely, E. W. (2012). Epidemiology and risk factors for delirium across hospital settings. *Best Pract Res Clin Anaesthesiol 26*(3), 277–287.

Vaurio, L. E., Sands, L. P., Wang, Y., Mullen, E. A., & Leung, J. M. (2006). Postoperative delirium: The importance of pain and pain management. *Anesthesia & Analgesia, 102*(4), 1267–1273.

Vella-Brincat, J., & Macleod, A. D. (2007). Adverse effects of opioids on the central nervous systems of palliative care patients. *Journal of Pain and Palliative Care Pharmacotherapy, 21*(1), 15–25.

Verster, G. C. (2009). Melatonin and its agonists, circadian rhythms and psychiatry. *African Journal of Psychiatry, 12*(1), 42–46.

Vidal, G., & Vidal, B. (1961). [Acute delirium after thyroidectomy]. *Toulouse Médical, 62,* 142–143.

Wacker, P., Nunes, P. V., Cabrita, H., & Forlenza, O. V. (2006). Post–operative delirium is associated with poor cognitive outcome and dementia. *Dementia and Geriatric Cognitive Disorders, 21*(4), 221–227.

Wahlund, L., & Bjorlin, G. A. (1999). Delirium in clinical practice: experiences from a specialized delirium ward. *Dementia and Geriatric Cognitive Disorders, 10*(5), 389–392.

Walker, M. P., & Stickgold, R. (2004). Sleep-dependent learning and memory consolidation. *Neuron 44*(1), 121–133.

Wang, W., Li, H. L., Wang, D. X., Zhu, X., Li, S. L., Yao, G. Q., et al. (2012). Haloperidol prophylaxis decreases delirium incidence in elderly patients after noncardiac surgery: a randomized controlled trial*. *Critical Care Medicine, 40*(3), 731–739.

Wang, Y., Sands, L. P., Vaurio, L., Mullen, E. A., & Leung, J. M. (2007). The effects of postoperative pain and its management on postoperative cognitive dysfunction. *American Journal of Geriatric Psychiatry, 15*(1), 50–59.

Watson, P. L., Ceriana, P., & Fanfulla, F. (2012). Delirium: is sleep important? *Best Practice & Research Clinical Anaesthesiology, 26*(3), 355–366.

Weinhouse, G. L., & Schwab, R. J. (2006). Sleep in the critically ill patient. *Sleep, 29*(5), 707–716.

Weinrich, S., & Sarna, L. (1994). Delirium in the older person with cancer. *Cancer, 74*(7 Suppl), 2079–2091.

Weissman, C., Kemper, M., Damask, M. C., Askanazi, J., Hyman, A. I., & Kinney, J. M. (1984). Effect of routine intensive care interactions on metabolic rate. *Chest, 86*(6), 815–818.

Weizberg, M., Su, M., Mazzola, J. L., Bird, S. B., Brush, D. E., & Boyer, E. W. (2006). Altered mental status from olanzapine overdose treated with physostigmine. *Clinical Toxicology (Philadelphia), 44*(3), 319–325.

Weng, Y. M., Chang, M. W., & Weng, C. S. (2008). Pituitary apoplexy associated with cortisol–induced hyperglycemia and acute delirium. *American Journal of Emergency Medicine, 26*(9), 1068 e1061–1063.

Wengel, S. P., Burke, W. J., & Roccaforte, W. H. (1999). Donepezil for postoperative delirium associated with Alzheimer's disease. *Journal of the American Geriatric Society, 47*(3), 379–380.

Wengel, S. P., Roccaforte, W. H., & Burke, W. J. (1998). Donepezil improves symptoms of delirium in dementia: Implications for future research. *Journal of Geriatric Psychiatry & Neurology, 11*(3), 159–161.

Wetterling, T., Kanitz, R. D., Veltrup, C., & Driessen, M. (1994). Clinical predictors of alcohol withdrawal delirium. *Alcoholism: Clinical and Experimental Research, 18*(5), 1100–1102.

WHO (1992). *The International Statistical Classification of Diseases and Related Health Problems (ICD-10): Classification of Mental and Behavioural Disorders.* Geneva: World Health Organization.

WHO (2010). *International Statistical Classification of Diseases and Related Health Problems* (ICD-10). Geneva: World Health Organization.

Wiesel, O., Klausner, J., Soffer, D., & Szold, O. (2011). [Postoperative delirium of the elderly patient—an iceberg?]. *Harefuah, 150*(3), 260–263, 303.

Williams, M. A., Ward, S. E., & Campbell, E. B. (1988). Confusion: Testing versus observation. *Journal of Gerontological Nursing, 14*(1), 25–30.

Williams-Russo, P., Urquhart, B. L., Sharrock, N. E., & Charlson, M. E. (1992). Postoperative delirium: Predictors and prognosis in elderly orthopedic patients. *Journal of the American Geriatric Society, 40*(8), 759–767.

Willis, T. (1672). *De Anima Brutorum.* London: Ric. Davis Oxford.

Witlox, J., Eurelings L. S., de Jonghe, J. F., Kalisvaart, K. J., Eikelenboom, P., & van Gool, W. A. (2010). Delirium in elderly patients and the risk of postdischarge mortality, institutionalization, and dementia: a meta-analysis. *Journal of the American Medical Association, 304*(4), 443–451.

Wong, C. P., Chiu, P. K., & Chu, L. W. (2005). Zopiclone withdrawal: an unusual cause of delirium in the elderly. *Age Ageing, 34*(5), 526–527.

Wong, C. L., Holroyd-Leduc, J., Simel, D. L., & Straus, S. E. (2010). Does this patient have delirium?: value of bedside instruments. *JAMA, 304*(7), 779–786.

Wroblewski, B. A., Joseph, A. B., Kupfer, J., & Kalliel, K. (1997). Effectiveness of valproic acid on destructive and aggressive behaviours in patients with acquired brain injury. *Brain Injury, 11*(1), 37–47.

Yaffe, K., & Boustani, M. (2014). Benzodiazepines and risk of Alzheimer's disease. *BMJ, 349,* g5312.

Yigit, U., Erdenoz, S., Uslu, U., Oba, E., Cumbul, A., Cagatay, H., et al. (2011). An immunohistochemical analysis of the neuroprotective effects of memantine, hyperbaric oxygen therapy, and brimonidine after acute ischemia reperfusion injury. *Molecular Vision, 17*, 1024–1033.

Yoshitaka, S., Egi, M., Morimatsu, H., Kanazawa, T., Toda, Y., & Morita, K. (2013). Perioperative plasma melatonin concentration in postoperative critically ill patients: its association with delirium. *Journal of Critical Care, 28*(3), 236–242.

Young, R. S., & Arseven, A. (2010). Diagnosing delirium. *JAMA, 304*(19), 2125–2126; author reply 2126–2127.

Young, C. C., & Lujan, E. (2004). Intravenous ziprasidone for treatment of delirium in the intensive care unit. *Anesthesiology, 101*(3), 794–795.

Zaja-Milatovic, S., Gupta, R. C., Aschner, M., & Milatovic, D. (2009). Protection of DFP–induced oxidative damage and neurodegeneration by antioxidants and NMDA receptor antagonist. *Toxicology and Applied Pharmacology, 240*(2), 124–131.

Zhang, J., Guo, J. D., Xing, S. H., Gu, S. L., & Dai, T. J. (2002). [The protective effects of melatonin on global cerebral ischemia-reperfusion injury in gerbils]. *Yao Xue Xue Bao, 37*(5), 329–333.

Zhang, F., Lewis, M., Yang, G., Iriondo-Perez, J., Zeng, Y., & Liu, J. (2008). Apolipoprotein E polymorphism, life stress and self–reported health among older adults. *Journal of Epidemiology & Community Health, 62*(4), e3.

Zhang, H., Y. Lu, M. Liu, Z. Zou, L. Wang, F. Y. Xu and X. Y. Shi (2013). Strategies for prevention of postoperative delirium: a systematic review and meta–analysis of randomized trials. *Critical Care, 17*(2), R47.

Zhang, Z., Pan, L., & Ni, H. (2013). Impact of delirium on clinical outcome in critically ill patients: a meta–analysis. *General Hospital Psychiatry, 35*(2), 105–111.

Ziehm, S. R. (1991). Intravenous haloperidol for tranquilization in critical care patients: a review and critique. *AACN Clinical Issues in Critical Care Nursing, 2*(4), 765–777.

42.

DEMENTIA: DIAGNOSIS AND TREATMENT

Scott McGinnis

INTRODUCTION

Dementia is a highly prevalent and ever-increasing cause of morbidity and mortality throughout the world. At present it is already one of the leading causes of years lost due to disability and healthcare expenditures in high-income countries; and with the rapidly growing older segments of the population developing dementia, the number of affected individuals will increase exponentially (*The Global Burden of Disease: 2004 Report*; Hebert, Scherr, Bienias, Bennett, & Evans, 2003). Dementia likewise stands ready to produce a significant public health challenge to the developing world, in which the number of affected individuals is rising most rapidly (Ferri et al., 2005). Medical practitioners in most disciplines encounter patients with dementia; it particularly behooves general practitioners, geriatricians, neurologists, psychiatrists, and psychologists to have a thorough understanding of its diagnosis and management.

Dementia is defined as a progressive impairment in cognition or behavior of sufficient severity to interfere with one's usual activities, and occurring in the absence of delirium. As such, it can present with a variety of different clinical manifestations and can be due to a variety of underlying brain conditions. Increasing knowledge about the phenotypes and pathophysiologies of neurodegenerative dementias, coupled with increasing availability of disease-specific biomarkers, has revolutionized diagnostic practice. Old practices of excluding reversible causes and lumping any remaining cases under the headings of "senile dementia" or "Alzheimer's disease" have given way to a process of proactively identifying specific clinical syndromes and attempting to determine neuropathology *in vivo*. The value of this new process is not purely academic, as identification of a specific condition carries both important prognostic and educational value for patients and caregivers and significant ramifications regarding strategies for symptomatic treatment. Identification of pathology *in vivo* also forms a critical component in the development and application of disease-modifying treatments for neurodegenerative dementia.

This chapter first reviews a general approach to diagnosis of dementia, focusing on the use of history and examination to localize cognitive dysfunction and to establish its time course and severity. A discussion of the differential diagnosis of dementia follows, including the epidemiology, genetics, clinical manifestations, diagnostic studies, clinical/pathological associations, and treatments for specific clinical syndromes. The chapter closes by presenting strategies for management of dementia cases in general.

APPROACH TO DIAGNOSIS: GENERAL PRINCIPLES

As with any neurological or psychiatric illness, a detailed history and examination provide the most important diagnostic information in the assessment of a patient with suspected cognitive impairment or dementia (see Chapters 1–4 of this volume). Goals of the history and examination include localizing the impairment to regions and/or large-scale networks in the brain, establishing the time course and severity of symptoms, reviewing potentially modifiable contributing medical and psychiatric factors, and reviewing pertinent aspects of the patient's developmental, social, and family histories.

LOCALIZATION OF COGNITIVE DYSFUNCTION

Important considerations when localizing cognitive dysfunction include determining whether a pattern of deficits is predominantly *cortical* or *subcortical*, determining whether deficits are focal, multifocal, or diffuse, and determining which large-scale networks in the brain are implicated. Cortical cognitive symptoms or signs reflect dysfunction in networks containing at least one node in a cortical zone, such as limbic, paralimbic, heteromodal, or unimodal association cortex (Marsel Mesulam, 2000). Examples of cortical deficits include, but are not limited to, amnesia, aphasia, alexia, apraxia, and agnosia. Cortical deficits may be *unimodal* (confined to processing in a single sensory/motor modality) or *transmodal* (involving multiple modalities), depending on whether dysfunction exists in unimodal or transmodal regions of the brain. Neurodegenerative illnesses with cortical pathology such as Alzheimer disease (AD) and dementia with Lewy bodies (DLB) are the most common causes of cortical dementia.

In contrast to cortical dementias, subcortical dementias present with a profile of slowed processing speed, impaired attention, apathy, mood symptoms, and motor symptoms (Albert, Feldman, & Willis, 1974). Subcortical dementias are associated with forgetfulness, but in contrast to the temporolimbic amnesia of a condition such as AD, memory difficulties are predominantly at levels of encoding and retrieving information, so recognition and cued memory are preserved. Subcortical dementias localize to subcortical white matter and/or deep gray structures. Examples of conditions producing subcortical dementia include vascular dementia (VaD), HIV-associated dementia, progressive supranuclear palsy (PSP), normal pressure hydrocephalus (NPH), and gliomatosis cerebri.[1]

Our understanding of the organization of large-scale networks in the brain has grown dramatically in recent years with the availability of new technologies, including functional connectivity magnetic resonance imaging (fcMRI) and diffusion tensor imaging (DTI; Yeo et al., 2011). For purposes of clinical care, it is useful to employ a simplified approach and categorize networks broadly by the cognitive functions they subserve. In this scheme, one can consider cognitive domains such as episodic memory, language, complex attention/executive functions, visuospatial functions, and behavioral regulation/social cognition. Language functions localize to the perisylvian networks in the dominant (usually left) hemisphere (Hickok & Poeppel, 2007). Visuospatial functions localize to two visual streams, a dorsal occipitoparietal stream important for localization of items in space and integration with one's own sense of body position, and a ventral occipitoparietal stream important for the identification of items (Ungerleider & Haxby, 1994). The domain of complex attention and executive functions, comprising numerous component processes, localizes predominantly to frontoparietal and frontal/subcortical networks in the brain (Cummings, 1993). Episodic memory localizes both to temporolimbic networks (important for encoding, retrieval, and storage), and frontal networks (important for encoding and retrieval) (Budson & Price, 2005). Behavioral regulation and social cognitive processes recruit networks predominantly involving paralimbic regions such as the orbitofrontal cortex, anterior cingulate cortex, and insula (Gleichgerrcht, Ibanez, Roca, Torralva, & Manes, 2010). In the case of each of these networks, connectivity exists between cortical nodes and other cortical nodes, cortical nodes and subcortical structures (striatum, thalamus), and between subcortical structures (Marsel Mesulam, 2000). Lesions at any point in the network can give rise to dysfunction, producing (in uncommon instances) cortical deficits from subcortical lesions.

Localization of cognitive symptoms to large-scale networks in the brain has particular value in the approach to dementia because neurodegenerative processes appear to target specific networks early in the course of the illness. Specific types of misfolded proteins accumulate with a limited range of possible distributions, starting focally and spreading along particular anatomical lines until there is diffuse involvement of the brain at the later stages of illness (Pievani, de Haan, Wu, Seeley, & Frisoni, 2011).[2] Additionally, circumscribed patterns

of atrophy in specific neurodegenerative syndromes correspond to regions of the brain that are highly structurally and functionally connected. These findings have given rise to the *network degeneration hypothesis*, which postulates that neurodegenerative processes target large-scale networks in the brain to produce characteristic progressions of neurodegeneration and clinical symptoms that depend on the pathology and networks targeted (Seeley, Crawford, Zhou, Miller, & Greicius, 2009). Further research is required to delineate the roles of misfolded proteins in the pathogenesis of specific diseases, the factors underlying network specificity, and the relationship between distribution of misfolded proteins and the distribution of neurodegeneration as marked by cell death and atrophy.

Despite enormous progress in recent years, there remain limitations to the approach of attempting to determine pathology in any given patient on the basis of history, examination, and structural neuroimaging alone. Such limitations arise from the following factors:

1. A single clinical syndrome or phenotype may be observed with different types of underlying pathology with varying probabilities, reflecting the fact that large-scale networks may be targeted by more than one type of disease process;

2. Clinical syndromes that share common underlying pathologies frequently overlap (e.g., a single patient may have features of multiple syndromes)[3];

3. Different neurodegenerative pathologies frequently coexist within the same individual, and with vascular pathology (Schneider, Arvanitakis, Bang, & Bennett, 2007); and

4. Very old age (90 years old or greater) increases not only the probability that AD pathology will be found in the non-demented, but also the probability that amnestic dementia will be found in the absence of AD pathology (Savva et al., 2009).

These limitations highlight the need to further develop *in vivo* biomarkers of pathology. Efforts at present are most advanced for AD, for which cerebrospinal fluid (CSF) analysis of β-amyloid, total tau (t-tau), and phosphorylated tau (p-tau) is already available for clinical use, and amyloid positron emission tomography (PET) imaging may become available in the near future.

TIME COURSE AND SEVERITY

The usual time course of a neurodegenerative dementia is one of insidious onset and gradual progression over months to

---

fused in sarcoma protein (FUS), and prion protein. See Table 42.3 and the text for specific clinical and pathological correlations.

3. Examples of overlapping clinical syndromes include those associated with AD pathology (amnestic AD, posterior cortical atrophy, logopenic primary progressive aphasia), those associated with Lewy body pathology (DLB and Parkinson disease dementia), and those associated with primary tau pathology (agrammatic primary progressive aphasia, behavioral-variant frontotemporal dementia, corticobasal syndrome, PSP syndrome).

---

1. See Chapters 46, 49, and 63 for detailed discussions of NPH, gliomas, and HIV-associated dementia, respectively.

2. Misfolded proteins in neurodegenerative dementia include (but are not limited to) β-amyloid, tau, α-synuclein, TAR DNA-binding protein 43 (TDP-43),

Table 42.1 DIFFERENTIAL DIAGNOSIS OF DEMENTIA

PROCESS	CONDITIONS
Vascular	Infarcts (strategic or disseminated)*, ischemia, CNS vasculitis, CAA, non-inflammatory vasculopathy, hyperviscosity states, subdural hematomas, venous sinus thrombosis, dural AVF
Infectious	Viral (HIV*, PML, HSV, others), bacterial (CNS Whipple, *Bartonella*, TB, neurosyphilis, Lyme), fungal, parasitic
Toxic	Alcohol, heavy metals, organic solvents, heroin
Autoimmune/inflammatory†	Multiple sclerosis, antibody-associated encephalitis (paraneoplastic or non-paraneoplastic), HE, other NAIM, neurosarcoidosis, Beçhet disease, celiac disease
Metabolic	Thyroid dysfunction, uremia, hepatic encephalopathy, vitamin deficiency (B_{12}, thiamine, niacin, vitamin E), porphyria
Iatrogenic	Medications, chemotherapy, radiation therapy
Neoplastic†	Primary CNS lymphoma, intravascular lymphoma, gliomatosis cerebri*, lymphomatoid granulomatosis, metastases
Structural	Hydrocephalus (obstructive or normal pressure)*, FTBSS
Genetic	Hereditary leukodystrophies, lysozomal disorders, mitochondrial encephalopathies
Psychiatric	Catatonia, psychosis, severe melancholic depression, somatoform disorders, malingering
Degenerative†	AD, PCA, FTD (bv-FTD, PPA-S, PPA-G, FTDP, FTD-ALS, CBS, PSP*), PPA-L, PDD, DLB, HD, prion diseases

Abbreviations: AVF = arteriovenous fistula; PML = progressive multifocal leukoencephalopathy; HSV = herpes simplex virus; TB = tuberculosis; FTBSS = frontotemporal brain sagging syndrome; FTDP = frontotemporal dementia with Parkinsonism; HD = Huntington disease. Please refer to chapter text for other abbreviations.

* Denotes conditions commonly associated with subcortical dementia.

† Denotes conditions associated with rapidly progressive dementia.

years. Atypical, rapid progression over days to weeks may occur in individuals with prion disease, autoimmune or inflammatory encephalitides, atypical forms of neurodegenerative conditions that usually progress more slowly, certain infections, or other rare causes of dementia (Table 42.1). Sudden onset of symptoms occurs most frequently with vascular conditions such as ischemic stroke or hemorrhage, although the absence of a sudden onset and/or stepwise progression does not exclude vascular disease as a primary or contributing factor. It is likewise important to note that, for any given neurodegenerative condition such as AD, there is considerable variability between individuals in terms of how quickly symptoms progress, as well as variability within the same individual in different stages of illness (Doody et al., 2010). A static time course or a course of fluctuating cognitive impairment without steady progression may occur in a variety of medical and psychiatric conditions[4] (Millan et al., 2012).

Numerous methods have been devised to rate the severity of cognitive dysfunction and dementia. A general distinction can be made between individuals with normal cognition for their age and education, those with cognitive dysfunction beyond what can be attributed to aging that nevertheless does not interfere with their usual activities, and those whose performance in usual activities has been disrupted by cognitive dysfunction. Individuals with impaired cognition that does not interfere with usual activities may be classified as having mild cognitive impairment (MCI), conceptualized as an intermediate stage between normal aging and dementia[5] (Petersen, 2004). Individuals with MCI are at an increased risk of progressing to a diagnosis of dementia when compared with cognitively normal individuals; the annual rate of progression in community-based populations has been estimated at 5–10%, the annual rate in specialty clinics at 10–15% (Petersen, 2011).

There are no strict guidelines that distinguish between mild, moderate, and severe dementia, although multiple schemes provide a conceptual framework for such classification. The Clinical Dementia Rating scale (CDR) is a widely used measure applicable to AD that relies on a semi-structured clinical interview and examination with a patient and reliable informant (Morris et al., 1997). Application of this scale generates ratings ranging from 0.5 (questionable

---

4. A thorough discussion of cognitive dysfunction associated with medical and psychiatric illness is beyond the scope of this chapter. Common mimics of dementia are discussed below in the section "Differential Diagnosis of Dementia." For review of the cognitive dysfunction associated with psychiatric illness, see Millan et al., 2012.

5. More specifically, standard criteria for MCI require a report of cognitive impairment by a patient (or caregiver) and evidence by history with or without exam that the individual is not normal for age, not demented, has sustained a decline in cognition, and has essentially normal functional activities. MCI may be further classified according to whether or not there is memory impairment (amnestic vs. non-amnestic) and whether a single domain or multiple domains of cognition have been affected (Petersen, 2004).

or very mild dementia), to 1 (mild dementia), 2 (moderate dementia) or 3 (severe dementia) for the domains of memory, orientation, judgement and problem solving, community affairs, home and hobbies, and personal care.[6] Various brief cognitive batteries including, but not limited to, the Montreal Cognitive Assessment (MoCA), the Mini-Mental State Exam (MMSE), the Kokmen Short Test of Mental Status, and the Addenbrooke's Cognitive Examination (ACE-R) are available to provide a longitudinal measure of global cognitive function and performance within selected sub-domains of cognition (Folstein, Folstein, & McHugh, 1975; Kokmen, Naessens, & Offord, 1987; Mioshi, Dawson, Mitchell, Arnold, & Hodges, 2006; Nasreddine et al., 2005). Each has its strengths and weaknesses; for example, the MoCA is relatively sensitive for attentional and executive dysfunction, whereas the ACE-R offers a more thorough examination of language and semantic processing. It is best to gain familiarity with a measure and to use it consistently so as to provide an index of change.

Increasing attention in research is being paid to the *preclinical* stage of neurodegenerative dementias, defined as the stage in which pathophysiological processes are active but have yet to produce clinically apparent symptoms. For AD, this stage may last for ten years or more prior to the onset of symptoms (Morris, 2005). Identification of neurodegenerative illness in the preclinical stage by definition requires the use of biomarkers of the pathophysiological process. At present, for AD, investigators have proposed models for the presence and progression of different biomarkers (Jack et al., 2010). Studies that will allow us to further refine these models and thus improve our ability to use biomarkers clinically are currently underway (Trojanowski et al., 2010).

DIFFERENTIAL DIAGNOSIS OF DEMENTIA

Table 42.1 lists causes of cognitive dysfunction and dementia categorized by the mechanism of illness: vascular, infectious, toxic, autoimmune/inflammatory, metabolic, iatrogenic, neoplastic, structural, genetic, psychiatric, and degenerative. A key question in formulating the differential diagnosis for a particular patient is whether or not the presentation suggests a relatively common condition such as AD, VaD, or cognitive dysfunction in the setting of general medical or psychiatric illness. Certain *red flags* that may suggest a less common cause of cognitive dysfunction include a non-amnestic cognitive profile, rapid progression of symptoms over days to weeks, or the early presence of additional

neurological symptoms such as pyramidal or extrapyramidal motor signs, myoclonus, cerebellar signs, apraxia, psychosis, autonomic dysfunction, rapid-eye-movement (REM) sleep behavior disorder, or seizures. Other red flags of note include young age (onset of symptoms before age 65, and especially before age 50), a family history suggestive of an autosomal dominant mode of inheritance, and prominent evidence of systemic medical or organ-specific illness not yet accounted for.

In a practice parameter for diagnosis of dementia, the Quality Standards Subcommittee of the American Academy of Neurology (AAN) recommended structural neuroimaging of the brain with computed tomography (CT) or magnetic resonance imaging (MRI), as well as routine screening for depression, vitamin B_{12} deficiency, and hypothyroidism as a part of one's routine evaluation (Knopman et al., 2001). Many practitioners also obtain additional laboratory measures such as comprehensive metabolic profile, complete blood count (CBC), and urinalysis. Table 42.2 lists selected additional labs and studies available for use in cases of diagnostic uncertainty.

The vast majority of late-onset dementias (onset of symptoms at age ≥ 65) are attributable to neurodegenerative pathology, vascular disease, or mixed degenerative/vascular pathology (Jellinger, Danielczyk, Fischer, & Gabriel, 1990; Schneider et al., 2007). Of the degenerative pathologies, AD is by far the most common in this age group, followed by Lewy body pathology. In the population of individuals with early-onset dementia (onset of symptoms between ages 45 and 65), AD and VaD continue to represent the most common etiologies, but a much higher proportion of cases are due to frontotemporal lobar degeneration (FTLD) pathology than in the population with late-onset dementia (Garre-Olmo et al., 2010; Picard, Pasquier, Martinaud, Hannequin, & Godefroy, 2011).

Table 42.3 summarizes the epidemiology, genetics, neuropsychology, imaging, and associated pathologies for selected neurodegenerative dementia phenotypes. One should note that nomenclature in the literature and in clinical practice has been inconsistent and rapidly evolving. This chapter groups the primary progressive aphasias (PPAs) together due to their common involvement of language, while noting that semantic PPA (PPA-S) and agrammatic PPA are also frequently classified as frontotemporal dementias (FTDs) due to their anatomical distributions and associations with FTLD pathology[7] (Josephs et al., 2011). PSP syndrome (PSPS) and corticobasal syndrome (CBS) are considered together as extrapyramidal syndromes frequently associated with FTLD-tau pathology.

---

6. From these ratings, a global dementia score and "sum of box scores" are derived. Examples of guiding criteria include the specification that patients with moderate dementia may appear well enough to be taken to functions outside of the home, are not able to function independently outside the home, perform only simple chores, have very restricted interests, and often require assistance in matters of dressing and personal hygiene. Individuals with severe dementia appear too ill to be taken to most functions outside of the home, require near-total assistance for functions within the home, and require much help with personal care.

7. FTLD pathology broadly comprises three specific subtypes based upon type of protein inclusion: FTLD-tau, FTLD-TDP, and FTLD-FUS. There are, at present, six subtypes of FTLD-tau (Pick, PSP, corticobasal degeneration, argyrophilic grain disease, multisystem tauopathy, diffuse neurofibrillary tangle with calcifications), four subtypes of FTLD-TDP (FTLD-TDP1-4), and three subtypes of FTLD-FUS (neuronal intermediate filament inclusion disease, basophilic inclusion body disease, atypical FTLD with ubiquitin-only immunoreactive changes). See Josephs et al., 2011, for review.

Table 42.2 ANCILLARY STUDIES IN THE DIAGNOSIS OF DEMENTIA

STUDY	INDICATIONS
Neuropsychological examination	Inadequate mental status examination; need for more detailed delineation of cognitive profile
Blood: RPR, HIV, Lyme Ab, other infection labs	Epidemiological setting for exposure; clinical evidence of infection[1]
Blood: ANA, ESR, CRP, anti-thyroid Abs, encephalitis Abs, other rheumatological labs	Suspicion for autoimmune/inflammatory causes of dementia[2]
Blood: thrombophilia labs, toxicology, copper/ceruloplasmin, homocysteine, MMA, vitamins, other metabolic labs	Suspicion for underlying condition
Blood: genetic tests for neurodegenerative conditions, CADASIL, leukodystrophies, lysozomal, mitochondrial disorders	Family history suggestive of autosomal dominant inheritance (if applicable); suspicion for underlying condition[3]
Urine: toxicology screen, copper, heavy metals, metabolic labs	Suspicion for toxic or metabolic condition[4]
CSF: cell counts, protein, glucose, infection labs, IgG synthesis/index, oligoclonal bands, paraneoplastic Abs, cytology/flow cytometry	Suspicion for autoimmune/inflammatory, infectious, neoplastic cause of dementia
CSF: β-amyloid, t-tau, p-tau, 14-3-3 protein	Suspicion for AD pathology or CJD
Imaging: CXR, CT C/A/P ± PET, mammography, echocardiography	Suspected systemic condition, including infection, inflammatory, neoplasm
Imaging: cerebral angiography (CT, MR, or conventional), CNIS, MR spectroscopy	Suspected vasculitis, vasculopathy, neoplasm
Imaging: brain FDG-PET or SPECT, PiB or AV-45 amyloid PET[5]	Biomarker evidence for AD vs. other degenerative dementias
DAT PET or SPECT, MIBG myocardial scintigraphy, polysomnography	Evidence for degenerative cause of Parkinsonism, DLB, sleep disorder
EEG, EMG/NCS, autonomic studies	Suspicion for seizures, HE/NAIM, CJD, neuropathy, MND, dysautonomia
Brain biopsy	Other studies non-diagnostic; note low sensitivity (~55–65%)[6]

Abbreviations: Ab = antibody; C/A/P = chest/abdomen/pelvis; CNIS = carotid noninvasive ultrasound; PiB = Pittsburgh Compound B; DAT = dopamine transporter. Please refer to chapter text for other abbreviations.

[1] Reviewed in McGinnis, S. M. (2011). Infectious causes of rapidly progressive dementia. *Seminars in Neurology, 31*(3), 266–285.

[2] Reviewed in Rosenbloom, M. H., Smith, S., Akdal, G., & Gleschwind, M. D. (2009). Immunologically mediated dementias. *Current Neurology & Neuroscience Reports, 9*(5), 359–367.

[3] Reviewed in Paulson, H. L., & Igo, I. (2011). Genetics of dementia. *Seminars in Neurology, 31*(5), 449–460.

[4] Reviewed in Ghosh, A. (2010). Endocrine, metabolic, nutritional, and toxic disorders leading to dementia. *Annals of the Indian Academy of Neurology, 13*, S63–S68.

[5] Not yet available for clinical use.

[6] Warren, J. D., Schott, J. M., Fox, N. C., Thom, M., Revesz, T., Holton, J. L., et al. (2005). Brain biopsy in dementia. *Brain 128*(9), 2016–2025; Josephson, S. A., Papanastassiou, A. M., Berger, M. S., Barbaro, N. M., McDermott, M. W., Hilton, J. F., et al. (2007). The diagnostic utility of brain biopsy procedures in patients with rapidly deteriorating neurological conditions or dementia. *Journal of Neurosurgery, 106*(1), 72–75.

ALZHEIMER DISEASE

Epidemiology and Genetics of Alzheimer Disease

AD is the most common cause of dementia, constituting approximately 50–70% of late-onset dementias and 20–40% of early-onset dementias diagnosed clinically (Garre-Olmo et al., 2010; Jellinger et al., 1990; Picard et al., 2011). Age is the primary risk factor for AD and for all-cause dementia; the incidences of AD and all-cause dementia increase exponentially after the age of 65 (Corrada, Brookmeyer, Paganini-Hill, Berlau, & Kawas, 2010; Jorm & Jolley, 1998). The current prevalence of AD in the United States is estimated to be 13% in individuals 65 and over, increasing to approximately 43% in individuals 85 and over (Thies & Bleiler, 2011). The estimated number of persons older than 65 with AD in the United States is projected to increase from approximately 5.1 million in 2010 to 13.2 million in 2050 (Hebert et al., 2003).

Approximately 94–99% of AD cases are late-onset (Bird, 2008). The average lifetime risk of AD in the general population is approximately 10–12% in a 75–80-year lifespan (Goldman et al., 2011). This risk at least doubles when one has a first-degree relative with AD. Although multiple candidate genes are under investigation, the only well-documented genetic association for late-onset AD is with the apolipoprotein E (*APOE*) gene, of which there are three isoforms: ε2, ε3, and ε4. Multiple studies have reported that approximately

Table 42.3 SELECTED NEURODEGENERATIVE DEMENTIA SYNDROMES

SYNDROME	ASSOCIATED PATHOLOGIES	EPIDEMIOLOGY	GENETICS	COGNITIVE PROFILE AND NEUROPSYCHIATRY	PATTERN OF ATROPHY	OTHER STUDIES
AD	AD >> others	Prevalence ~13% in people ≥ 65, ~43% in people ≥ 85[1]	APOE ε4 PSEN1 PSEN2 APP	↓↓ Memory; ↓ language, ↓ EF, ↓ VS; Depression, anxiety, apathy, irritability, agitation	Medial temporal, temporoparietal	FDG-PET, SPECT CSF β-amyloid, t-tau, p-tau
PCA	AD >> LB, CBD, others[2]	Age of onset usually 50s–early 60s[2]	Unknown	↓↓ VS, ↓ EF, ↓ language, ↓ memory; Depression, anxiety, VH	Parietal, occipital	FDG-PET, SPECT CSF β-amyloid, t-tau, p-tau
DLB	LB ± AD >> others	Prevalence ~0.7% in people ≥ 65[3]	SNCA	↓↓ VS, ↓↓ EF, ↓ memory; Depression, apathy, VH, delusions	Preservation of medial temporal volume vs. AD[4]	DAT-PET/SPECT, MIBG myocardial scintigraphy
PPA-G	tau > TDP, AD[5]	FTLD epidemiology*[5]	GRN	↓↓ Language (syntax, grammar), AOS; ± sx of bvFTD, CBS, PSP	Left posterior frontal, insula[6]	FDG-PET, SPECT
PPA-S	TDP >> tau, AD[5]	FTLD epidemiology[5]	Unknown	↓↓ Language (naming, comprehension); Behavioral rigidity	Left anterior temporal[6]	FDG-PET, SPECT
PPA-L	AD > TDP, tau[5]	Unknown	Unknown	↓↓ Language (word-finding, repeating phrases)	Left temporoparietal[6]	FDG-PET, SPECT CSF β-amyloid, t-tau, p-tau
bvFTD	tau ~ TDP >> FUS, others[7]	FTLD epidemiology[5]	MAPT GRN C9ORF72	↓ EF, ↓ decision making, ↓ social cog; Disinhibition, apathy, perseveration	Mesial frontal, orbitofrontal, anterior insula[7]	FDG-PET, SPECT

Abbreviations: EF = executive functions; VS = visuospatial functions; VH = visual hallucinations; LB = Lewy body pathology. Please refer to chapter text for other abbreviations.

* FTLD epidemiology: estimated prevalence of 3.5–15 cases per 100,000 for all syndromes associated with FTLD (bvFTD, PPA-S, PPA-G) in the age group 45–64.

[1] Thies, W., & Bleiler, L. (2011). 2011 Alzheimer's disease facts and figures. *Alzheimer's Dementia, 7*(2), 208–244.

[2] Crutch, S. J., Lehmann, M., Schott, J. M., Rabinovici, G. D., Rossor, M. N., & Fox, N. C. (2012). Posterior cortical atrophy. *Lancet Neurology, 11*(2), 170–178.

[3] McKeith, I., Mintzer, J., Aarsland, D., Burn, D., Chiu, H., Cohen-Mansfield, J., et al. (2004). Dementia with Lewy bodies. *Lancet Neurology, 3*(1), 19–28.

[4] Kantarci, K., Lowe, V. J., Boeve, B. F., Weigand, S. D., Senjem, M. L., Przybelski, S. A., et al. (2012). Multimodality imaging characteristics of dementia with Lewy bodies. *Neurobiology of Aging, 33*(9), 2091–2105.

[5] Grossman, M. (2010). Primary progressive aphasia: Clinicopathological correlations. *Nature Reviews Neurology, 6*(2), 88–97.

[6] Gorno-Tempini, M. L., Hillis, A. E., Weintraub, S., Kertesz, A., Mendez, M., Cappa, S. F., et al. (2011). Classification of primary progressive aphasia and its variants. *Neurology, 76*(11), 1006–1014.

[7] Piguet, O., Hornberger, M., Mioshi, E., & Hodges, J. R. (2011). Behavioural-variant frontotemporal dementia: Diagnosis, clinical staging, and management. *Lancet Neurology, 10*(2), 162–172.

50–70% of people with late-onset AD carry at least one ε4 allele, suggesting a two- to three-fold increase in risk of AD for *APOE* ε4 heterozygotes. However, these results may be biased by oversampling "younger-old" individuals, as other studies imply that the ε4 allele shifts the onset of AD towards an earlier age without altering one's overall lifetime risk (Khachaturian, Corcoran, Mayer, Zandi, & Breitner, 2004). Because of its lack of sensitivity and specificity, testing for *APOE* status is not recommended as part of a routine work-up for dementia or AD.

Approximately 60% of early-onset AD is familial (defined by the presence of two or more family members affected), and approximately 13% of cases appear to be inherited in an autosomal dominant fashion (suggested by ≥ three generations affected) (Campion et al., 1999). Familial autosomal dominant early-onset AD thus constitutes < 2% of all cases of AD (Bird, 2008). The three known gene associations for familial autosomal dominant early-onset AD involve the presenilin-1 gene on chromosome 14 (*PSEN1*), the amyloid precursor protein gene on chromosome 21 (*APP*), and the presenilin-2 gene on chromosome 1 (*PSEN2*). Mutations in *PSEN1* account for 20–70% of cases, mutations in APP for 10–15% of cases, and mutations in *PSEN2* are rare. Essentially all individuals with Down syndrome develop AD pathology after age 40, presumably because they have three copies of the *APP* gene. Experts recommend that testing for gene mutations associated with familial autosomal dominant early-onset AD be offered to individuals with early-onset AD and family history of dementia (or unknown family history), individuals with a family history suggestive of autosomal dominant dementia and at least one case of early-onset AD, and individuals with a relative who has a known gene mutation (Goldman et al., 2011). Referral to a genetic counselor is imperative for all individuals who desire testing, and recommended for those who are undecided and would like to discuss the issue further.

Strong medical or environmental risk factors for AD have yet to be established. There is some suggestion from epidemiological data that vascular risk factors increase one's risk for cognitive decline or AD, independent of stroke. Observational studies have demonstrated a correlation between hypertension in middle age (40–60 years of age) and cognitive impairment later in life (Whitmer, Sidney, Selby, Johnston, & Yaffe, 2005). Similarly, type 2 diabetes mellitus and obesity appear to independently increase one's risk of AD (Profenno, Porsteinsson, & Faraone, 2010). Although data regarding cholesterol levels and AD have been inconsistent, most studies involving individuals assessed in middle age have suggested that high blood levels of total cholesterol and/or low density lipoprotein (LDL) cholesterol confer increased risk of AD later in life (Shepardson, Shankar, & Selkoe, 2011). Some, but not all, studies concerning head trauma and risk of AD later in life have suggested an association, particularly in men and in individuals with a family history of dementia (Fleminger, Oliver, Lovestone, Rabe-Hesketh, & Giora, 2003).

Clinical Manifestations and Diagnosis of Alzheimer Disease

AD most commonly presents with insidious onset and gradual progression of difficulty with memory for recent events. Early impairments in language (usually difficulty finding words), executive functioning, and/or visuospatial functioning of varying severity are also frequently present. Although comportment and social demeanor are typically preserved until late in the course of the illness, neuropsychiatric features including mild apathy, social withdrawal, anxiety, and irritability are common early (Lyketsos et al., 2011). Insight into deficits is variable between patients, but at least somewhat reduced as a rule, and (as with other deficits) it worsens with the progression of the disease (McDaniel, Edland, & Heyman, 1995). Behavioral agitation is estimated to occur in approximately 80% of patients with AD, typically later in the disease course (Jost & Grossberg, 1996). Additional neurological manifestations such as seizures, myoclonus, and pyramidal or extrapyramidal motor signs usually do not occur until later stages of illness (Friedman, Honig, & Scarmeas, 2011; Portet, Scarmeas, Cosentino, Helzner, & Stern, 2009).

A clinical diagnosis of dementia due to probable AD is usually made by establishing a history of progressive cognitive impairment of sufficient severity to interfere with usual activities, with deficits in memory and at least one other cognitive domain apparent on examination, in the absence of other causative conditions (McKhann et al., 2011). Supportive features from mental status examination (MSE) or neuropsychological examination of a patient with mild dementia due to AD include impairments in episodic memory (encoding, retrieval, and storage), confrontation naming, semantic fluency, and, frequently, impairments on more challenging tests of complex attention/executive function and/or visuospatial function (see Chapter 3). Structural neuroimaging commonly reveals focal atrophy in the medial temporal and/or posterior temporoparietal regions, progressing to generalized atrophy with progression of disease and correlating with density of neurofibrillary tangles at autopsy (Figure 42.1) (Jack et al., 2004; Whitwell et al., 2008).

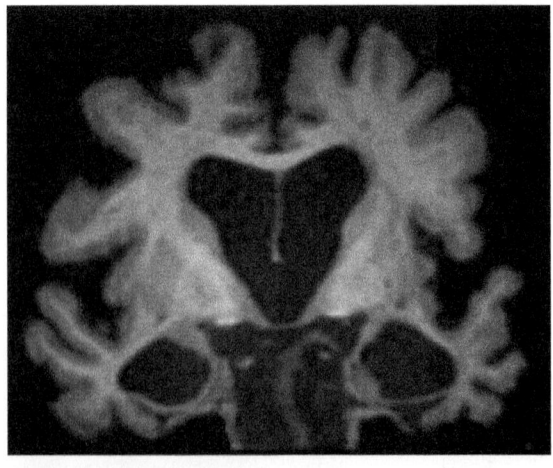

Figure 42.1 Coronal T1-weighted MRI of a patient with Alzheimer disease. This image demonstrates severe atrophy of the bilateral medial temporal cortices.

In uncommon instances, AD presents with symptoms other than memory impairment as the most prominent initial symptom. Examples include situations in which executive dysfunction, language, or visuospatial symptoms predominate. Cases of posterior cortical atrophy (PCA) and logopenic PPA due to AD pathology represent extreme versions of this situation, discussed in greater detail below. Even more rarely, AD pathology is uncovered to be the principal pathology in patients with the clinical syndromes of behavioral-variant FTD (bvFTD), PPA-S, or CBS (Alladi et al., 2007). Non-amnestic presentations appear to occur more frequently in the population with early-onset AD (Balasa et al., 2011; Koedam et al., 2010).

In cases of diagnostic ambiguity, biomarker evidence for AD can be obtained with 18-fluorodeoxyglucose positron emission tomography (FDG-PET), perfusion single-photon emission computed tomography (SPECT), or CSF analysis of β-amyloid 42, t-tau, and p-tau levels. FDG-PET or perfusion SPECT in AD reveals a characteristic pattern of hypometabolism or hypoperfusion in bilateral temporoparietal and posterior cingulate/precuneus cortex with variable involvement of the lobes and sparing of primary sensorimotor cortices. Elements of this pattern have yielded diagnostic sensitivities in the range of 86–94% and specificities ranging from 63–93% comparing AD with other degenerative dementias in studies with pathological confirmation of diagnosis (Devous, 2002; O'Brien, 2007).

The characteristic CSF profile of AD consists of a low level of β-amyloid 42 and elevated levels of t-tau and p-tau. CSF data from a cohort of 56 subjects with autopsy-confirmed AD and 52 age-matched controls revealed a diagnostic sensitivity of approximately 96% for low β-amyloid 42 levels (Shaw et al., 2009). Levels of t-tau had the greatest specificity (92%) in distinguishing AD from controls. Limited data comparing CSF biomarkers in AD compared to other neurodegenerative dementias with pathological confirmation suggest that combined use of β-amyloid 42 and p-tau levels yields a sensitivity of over 95% and a specificity of over 80% (Schoonenboom et al., 2012).

The availability of biomarker evidence of the AD pathophysiological process is one factor that prompted a revision of clinical diagnostic criteria for AD by the National Institute on Aging–Alzheimer's Association (NIA-AA) workgroups on diagnostic guidelines for Alzheimer's disease (Albert et al., 2011; McKhann et al., 2011). The new criteria allow for diagnosis of "probable AD dementia with evidence of the AD pathophysiological process" as well as "MCI due to AD." For each of these diagnoses, one must meet a set of core criteria for either probable AD dementia or MCI, and on top of that possess biomarkers of β-amyloid deposition and/or downstream neuronal degeneration or injury.[8] While not recommended for routine clinical use at this juncture, AD biomarker tests may be offered to patients for whom greater

diagnostic certainty sooner rather than later is likely to alter the plan of care.

Pathology and Pathophysiology of Alzheimer Disease

As with every neurodegenerative dementia, pathology represents the gold standard for the diagnosis of AD. Various criteria for the pathological diagnosis of AD have been proposed over the past several decades, each requiring a progression of extracellular fibrillar β-amyloid (senile plaques, and in particular a subset called neuritic plaques) and intracellular neurofibrillary tangles (NFTs) (Braak & Braak, 1991; Hyman et al., 2012; Hyman & Trojanowski, 1997; Khachaturian, 1985). Clinical and pathological studies have suggested that a clinical diagnosis of dementia due to AD predicts underlying AD pathology in approximately 85–95% of cases (Gearing et al., 1995; Jellinger et al., 1990; Mayeux et al., 1998; Schneider et al., 2007).

Despite the clearly established pathology of AD, questions remain about its fundamental etiology and pathophysiology. The amyloid hypothesis is based on evidence that accumulation of β-amyloid occurs as an upstream event preceding neurodegeneration, and the fact that the only gene mutations known to cause AD lead directly to overproduction of β-amyloid 42. Research has suggested that oligomeric forms of β-amyloid are toxic to synapses (Shankar et al., 2008) and that accumulation of β-amyloid directly or indirectly causes downstream events including inflammation, oxidative injury, tau hyperphosphorylation, and neuronal dysfunction and death (Hardy & Selkoe, 2002). It is possible that other mechanisms such as factors pertaining to neuronal energy metabolism, changes in intracellular and synaptic functions, and/or chronic neuroinflammatory response to an inciting injury occur upstream of or concomitantly with β-amyloid accumulation (Bero et al., 2011; Herrup, 2010; Pimplikar, Nixon, Robakis, Shen, & Tsai, 2010).

Compatible with a network-based model of neurodegeneration, amyloid deposition appears to target the default mode network—a network of brain regions including the medial temporal cortex, medial temporal cortex, temporoparietal cortex, and posterior cingulate/precuneus cortex (Buckner et al., 2005). Recent research has also suggested that once the cascade of tau hyperphosphorylation and NFT formation has been initiated, tau pathology spreads outward from entorhinal cortex along network lines via trans-synaptic mechanisms (Liu et al., 2012).

Treatment of Alzheimer Disease

Despite recent advances in our understanding of the pathophysiology of AD, disease-modifying therapies aimed at slowing or reversing the pathophysiological process have remained elusive. There are two types of symptomatic medications currently approved for use in dementia due to AD: cholinesterase inhibitors and memantine (Table 42.4).

In addition to the neuropathology of AD reviewed above, postmortem studies have revealed that the illness is associated with a significant loss of neurons in the basal forebrain—specifically

---

8. Current biomarkers of β-amyloid deposition include CSF β-amyloid 42 and PET amyloid imaging. Biomarkers of neuronal injury include CSF t-tau/p-tau, quantitative structural MRI measures, FDG-PET, SPECT, and other less well validated biomarkers (see Albert et al., 2011).

Table 42.4 SELECTED MEDICATIONS IN THE SYMPTOMATIC TREATMENT OF DEMENTIA

TYPE	INDICATIONS	EXAMPLES	STARTING DOSE	MAINTENANCE DOSE	COMMENTS
Cholinesterase inhibitors	AD, DLB/PDD, VaD*; cognition, mood, apathy, anxiety, psychosis	donepezil rivastigmine galantamine ER	5 mg QHS 1.5 mg BID† 8 mg QD	10 mg QHS 6 mg BID† 16–24 mg QD	Monitor GI s/e, sleep, HR, muscle cramps, fatigue
Memantine	AD, DLB/PDD*, VaD*, PPA*, bvFTD*; cognition, apathy*, agitation*	memantine	5 mg QD	10 mg BID	Monitor GI s/e, HA, dizziness, BP
SSRIs	mood*, anxiety*, irritability*, agitation*	sertraline citalopram	12.5 mg QD 5 mg QD	lowest effective (up to 200 mg QD) lowest effective (up to 40 mg QD)	Monitor QTc, GI s/e, HA, sleep, tremor, sexual s/e, fatigue, apathy
SNRIs	mood*, anxiety*	venlafaxine ER	37.5 mg QD	lowest effective (up to 225 mg QD)	Monitor GI s/e, HA, sleep, BP, diaphoresis
Bupropion	mood*, apathy*	bupropion SR	100 mg QD	lowest effective (up to 200 mg BID)	Monitor GI s/e, HA, sleep, tremor, anxiety
Mood stabilizers	mood lability*, agitation*	carbamazepine ER lamotrigine	100 mg BID 25 mg QD	lowest effective (up to 800 mg BID) lowest effective (up to 200 mg QD)	Monitor labs, GI s/e, HA, sleep, tremor, ataxia, fatigue, rash‡
Melatonin receptor agonists	insomnia*	melatonin ramelteon	3 mg QHS 8 mg QHS	lowest effective (up to 12 mg QHS) 8 mg QHS	Take within 30 minutes of bedtime
Stimulants	apathy*	methylphenidate	5 mg QD	lowest effective (up to 60 mg QD)	Monitor weight, sleep, anxiety, HR, BP
Atypical antipsychotics	aggressive agitation* (short term), psychosis,* insomnia*	quetiapine olanzapine aripiprazole	12.5 mg QHS 2.5 mg QHS 2 mg QD	lowest effective (up to 400 mg BID) lowest effective (up to 20 mg QHS) lowest effective (up to 30 mg QD)	Monitor QTc, weight, GI s/e, fatigue, extrapyramidal s/e§; note ↑ risk of stroke, mortality in older pts

Abbreviations: s/e = side effects; HR = heart rate; HA = headache; BP = blood pressure; QTc = QTc interval on electrocardiogram. Please refer to chapter text for additional abbreviations.

* Indicates off-label use and/or weaker evidence of efficacy.

† Also available in transdermal patch, which may reduce risk of GI s/e; starting dose 4.6 mg/24 hour, maintenance dose 9.5 mg/24 hour.

‡ Carbamazepine requires monitoring of CBC, BUN/creatinine, liver function tests, TSH, urinalysis; lamotrigine requires monitoring for Stevens-Johnson syndrome, and slow dose escalation (e.g., 25 mg QD × 2 weeks → 50 mg QD × 2 weeks → 100 mg QD × 1 week → 200 mg QD).

§ Patients with DLB or PDD may demonstrate severe sensitivity to neuroleptic medications. Only agents with low dopamine receptor antagonism (e.g., quetiapine, clozapine) should be used, and when used, used with caution.

the nucleus basalis of Meynert—that provide cholinergic projects to widespread areas of the cerebral cortex (Whitehouse et al., 1982). Cholinesterase inhibitors act by reducing the breakdown of acetylcholine, a neurotransmitter important for the modulation of attentional, memory, and sensory processing in the brain (Bentley, Driver, & Dolan, 2011). Studies have revealed modest but significant treatment effects of cholinesterase inhibitors vs. placebo in subjects with dementia due to AD on measures of cognition, behavior, and daily functioning (Raina et al., 2008). Response to treatment in any given individual is variable. More extensive data are available for mild to moderate dementia, but some studies suggest modest efficacy in severe dementia as well. Although selected subsets of patients with MCI may benefit, studies have not suggested that treatment with cholinesterase inhibitors delays progression to dementia in the population of individuals with MCI on the whole (Raschetti, Albanese, Vanacore, & Maggini, 2007).

Available data do not suggest clear superiority of any one of the three cholinesterase inhibitors currently in wide use (donepezil, galantamine, rivastigmine). The most common side effects associated with cholinesterase inhibitors include gastrointestinal (GI) side effects (diarrhea, nausea, vomiting, and loss of appetite), muscle cramps, insomnia, and fatigue. One should exercise caution in patients with significant bradycardia or heart block, history of ulcers or occult gastrointestinal bleeding, or severe obstructive pulmonary disease.

Memantine acts as a low to moderate affinity antagonist to glutamate NMDA (N-methyl-D-aspartate) receptors. Small beneficial effects on measures of cognition and behavior have been observed in treatment trials involving subjects with AD dementia, most apparent in moderate to severe disease (Smith, Wells, & Borrie, 2006). Combination therapy with both a cholinesterase inhibitor and memantine appears to provide benefit beyond treatment with just a cholinesterase inhibitor (Atri, Shaughnessy, Locascio, & Growdon, 2008). Potential side effects of memantine include dizziness, headache, GI side effects, hypertension, and confusion.

The Future of the Field: Disease-Modifying Therapies

Significant efforts to develop disease-modifying therapies for AD have been underway in recent years. Many strategies have centered on reducing β-amyloid formation, blocking its aggregation, or hastening its clearance from the brain. Other strategies have focused on inhibiting the phosphorylation and aggregation of tau, or on neuroprotection via reduction of oxidative stress, inflammation, or mitochondrial dysfunction.

Amyloid-based therapies have included inhibitors of the enzymes β-secretase and γ-secretase (responsible for cleaving the trans-membrane amyloid precursor protein into fragments of toxic β-amyloid) and active or passive immunization against β-amyloid. Thus far, there is good evidence from human and non-human studies that these agents do indeed lower levels of fibrillar β-amyloid in the brain, but completed studies to date have demonstrated either no or equivocal clinical efficacy (Citron, 2010; Rafii & Aisen, 2009). One hypothesis for why this has been the case is that studies to date have been conducted predominantly in subjects with mild to moderate dementia due to AD, stages in which the pathological burden is considerable and in which pathophysiological mechanisms downstream of β-amyloid accumulation may be less responsive to its reduction (Sperling, Jack, & Aisen, 2011). Multiple large-scale studies of amyloid-based therapies are ongoing at the time of this review, and additional studies are in the planning phases. Such studies are increasingly using biomarkers to establish the diagnosis of AD at the stages of MCI or preclinical illness.

POSTERIOR CORTICAL ATROPHY

The clinical syndrome of posterior cortical atrophy (PCA) involves insidious onset and gradual progression of visual deficits and/or apraxia, usually but not always associated with underlying AD pathology. Visual deficits include visuospatial impairments localizing to the dorsal (occipitoparietal) visual stream, visuoperceptual deficits localizing to the ventral (occipitotemporal) visual stream, and/or visual field cuts localizing to primary visual cortex. Accurate data regarding prevalence and incidence of PCA are currently lacking due to poor general awareness of the syndrome and a lack of consistent diagnostic criteria (Crutch et al., 2012). Most studies have suggested a younger average age of onset (50s to early 60s) for PCA compared to amnestic AD, in keeping with the hypothesis that non-amnestic presentations are more likely to occur as early-onset dementias.

Patients with PCA frequently present with problems navigating in space, reading, or carrying out arithmetic, although a subset may present to an ophthalmologist for evaluation regarding more basic elements of vision. Examination commonly reveals elements of the syndromes of Bálint (simultagnosia, optic ataxia, and oculomotor apraxia) and Gerstmann (agraphia, acalculia, left-right confusion, and finger agnosia[9]). Impairments in executive functions, language, and memory are variable early in the course of illness, but memory storage is frequently preserved. PCA patients commonly report visual hallucinations and/or positive perceptual phenomena, including color after-images, reverse size phenomena, perception of movement of static stimuli, and visual crowding (Crutch et al., 2012). Depression and anxiety are highly prevalent in this population, perhaps because insight into deficits tends to be more preserved than in amnestic AD (Mendez, Ghajarania, & Perryman, 2002). Structural neuroimaging with MRI in patients with PCA usually reveals atrophy in the bilateral parietal and occipital lobes that is apparent on gross inspection (Figure 42.2).

Limited clinical/pathological correlation series have suggested that AD pathology is found in approximately 80% of cases of PCA, with other associated pathologies including Lewy body pathology, corticobasal degeneration pathology, prion pathology, and subcortical gliosis each being found in 10% or fewer of cases (Crutch et al., 2012). Series involving

---

9. Finger agnosia, defined as an inability to distinguish, name, or recognize fingers, usually occurs in the setting of a more generalized disturbance in awareness of body parts and their orientation, also associated with disturbances in balance and/or dressing apraxia.

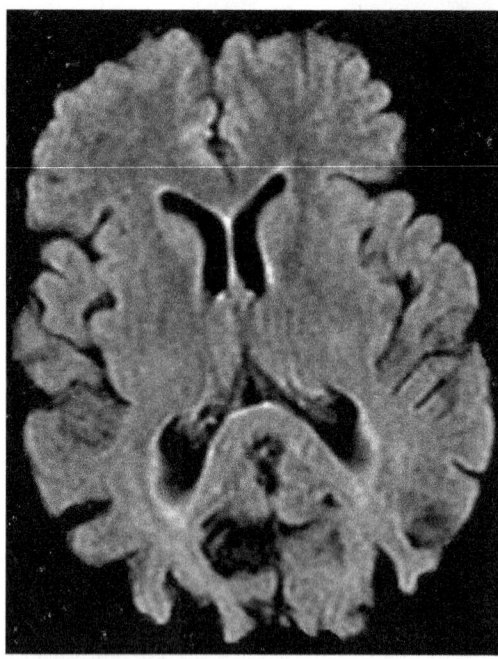

Figure 42.2 Axial FLAIR (fluid attenuated inversion recovery) MRI of a patient with posterior cortical atrophy. This image demonstrates severe atrophy of the posterior parietal and occipital cortices.

CSF analysis of AD biomarkers have revealed a profile suggestive of AD in a similar proportion of cases.

There are, at present, no medications with proven benefit for the visual and cognitive symptoms associated with PCA. Due to the pathological association between PCA and AD and information from case reports suggesting a potential benefit, many practitioners institute empirical trials of cholinesterase inhibitors for their patients. Treatment with antidepressant medications, anti-anxiety medications (Table 42.4), and/or symptomatic medications for Parkinsonism may provide benefit in appropriate circumstances. Occupational therapists and/or vision therapists can often provide strategies for modifying the home environment to optimize recognition of important objects or locations, along with other practical coping strategies and resources for the visually impaired.

DEMENTIA WITH LEWY BODIES AND PARKINSON DISEASE DEMENTIA

Dementias associated with Lewy body pathology—Parkinson disease dementia (PDD) and dementia with Lewy bodies (DLB)—are the second most common type of neurodegenerative dementia after AD (McKeith et al., 2004). Although epidemiological studies have been hindered by a lack of pathological criteria to distinguish between the two and (until recently) a lack of validated clinical diagnostic criteria for PDD, population-based clinical studies have estimated the prevalences of DLB and PDD to be 0.7% and 0.3%, respectively, in the population of individuals aged 65 and older. These estimates are in keeping with a prevalence of 10–15% for DLB in hospital-based autopsy series of dementia.

DLB and PDD frequently share clinical features and are distinguished somewhat arbitrarily by the timing of Parkinsonian symptoms relative to the onset of dementia; individuals with onset of dementia within one year of Parkinsonism are considered to have DLB. As no single individual symptom reliably distinguishes between DLB and PDD, and certain gene mutations have produced kindreds containing both disorders, experts have argued that they may exist along a spectrum of Lewy body disease with distribution of neurodegeneration determining phenotype (McKeith et al., 2004). The cognitive profile of both PDD and DLB usually involves early dysfunction in complex attention, executive functions, and visuospatial processing (Bradshaw, Saling, Anderson, Hopwood, & Brodtmann, 2006; Mosimann et al., 2004). Fluctuations in attention, alertness, or cognition of varying intensity and duration are considered to be a *core* feature of DLB (present in 50–75% of cases), but are also observed frequently in PDD (McKeith et al., 2005).[10] The other two core features of DLB are visual hallucinations that are often vivid, three-dimensional hallucinations of animate objects, and Parkinsonism, which is present in 25–50% of patients at diagnosis and develops in approximately 75% throughout the course of the illness. Visual hallucinations occur in an estimated 50% of patients with idiopathic Parkinson disease (Aarsland et al., 2007). Other neuropsychiatric symptoms common to both disorders include depression, anxiety, apathy, and delusions.

In comparison to the Parkinsonism of idiopathic PD, the Parkinsonism of DLB tends to be more bilaterally symmetrical and less responsive to treatment with levodopa (Molloy, McKeith, O'Brien, & Burn, 2005). Tremor is less common and less severe in DLB than in idiopathic PD, which is interesting in light of the fact that individuals with idiopathic PD and prominent early resting tremor are less likely to develop cognitive impairment than those with more prominent instability of posture and impaired gait (Burn et al., 2006). Additional features that may be present in both DLB and PDD (but that are more commonly present in DLB) include REM sleep behavior disorder, severe sensitivity to neuroleptic medications, and autonomic dysfunction. REM sleep behavior disorder manifests as vivid dreams without accompanying muscle atonia, leading to an individual's "acting out" dreams. REM sleep behavior disorder may precede other symptoms of DLB, PD, or multiple system atrophy (another α-synucleinopathy) by years or even decades (Iranzo et al., 2006). Autonomic dysfunction often produces orthostatic hypotension (with concomitant lightheadedness or syncope), urinary retention or incontinence, constipation, or impotence.

Structural neuroimaging demonstrating relative sparing of medial temporal lobe volume and/or thickness supports a diagnosis of DLB rather than AD in the correct clinical context, as does hypoperfusion or hypometabolism in the occipital and posterior temporoparietal cortices with sparing of the posterior cingulate/precuneus on perfusion SPECT or FDG-PET imaging (Kantarci et al., 2011). Dopamine

---

10. The third report of the DLB Consortium outlines clinical criteria for the diagnosis of "probable DLB" and "possible DLB" (McKeith et al., 2005).

transporter PET or SPECT and myocardial scintigraphy with 123-I-metaiodobenzylguanidine (MIBG) are approved imaging modalities with diagnostic utility for DLB and limited but increasing availability in the clinical setting (McKeith et al., 2007; Yoshita et al., 2006).

DLB and PDD are both associated with Lewy bodies—filamentous intraneuronal protein inclusions containing the protein α-synuclein, distributed throughout the central, peripheral, and autonomic nervous systems. Staging schemes have been proposed for both DLB (McKeith et al., 2005) and PD (Braak et al., 2003), based on the quantity and distribution of α-synuclein pathology in brainstem, subcortical, limbic, and neocortical brain regions. However, whether and to what degree the quantity and distribution of this pathology correlates with symptom type, severity, and progression in Lewy body disorders remains a matter of debate (Burke, Dauer, & Vonsattel, 2008; Jellinger, 2008). Synaptic dysfunction and/or cell loss may provide better correlates of clinical dysfunction. Most patients with DLB have some level of AD pathology, with burden of tangle pathology influencing the likelihood of Alzheimer-type manifestations.

Treatment of DLB and PDD centers on pharmacological and non-pharmacological management of cognitive, neuropsychiatric, motor, and autonomic symptoms. Multiple studies, including a randomized placebo-controlled study with rivastigmine, have suggested efficacy of cholinesterase inhibitors for treatment of cognition, and neuropsychiatric symptoms (McKeith et al., 2000; Samuel et al., 2000). One should be mindful of the potential for these medications to exacerbate postural hypotension, falls, and hypersalivation in patients with DLB. Fewer data are available regarding memantine, but some studies suggest benefits on global clinical status and behavioral symptoms in patients with mild to moderate DLB (Emre et al., 2010). Because of the potential for neuroleptic sensitivity, antipsychotic medications should be avoided in this patient population when possible. If psychotic symptoms are very intrusive and do not respond to cholinesterase inhibitors, memantine, or behavioral strategies, low doses of atypical antipsychotics with low dopamine receptor antagonism (e.g., quetiapine or clozapine) should be used with caution (see Table 42.4). Parkinsonian symptoms may be treated with carbidopa/levodopa monotherapy, starting at low doses and increasing gradually with monitoring for worsening psychotic symptoms in particular. Low-dose melatonin (3 mg at bedtime [QHS]) or clonazepam (0.25 mg QHS) may be effective for REM sleep behavior disorder. Fludricortisone and/or midodrine may be useful in the treatment of orthostatic hypotension. Modafinil has been studied on a limited basis for treatment of fatigue and daytime somnolence in PD, with some suggestion of benefit (Tyne, Taylor, Baker, & Steiger, 2010).

PRIMARY PROGRESSIVE APHASIA

Primary progressive aphasia (PPA) is a neurodegenerative syndrome characterized by early degeneration of left hemisphere perisylvian language networks. Capturing the specificity of early PPA for language, standard diagnostic criteria require that a patient present with a prominent isolated impairment of language, and that this impairment start insidiously, progress gradually, and account for all major limitations in activities of daily living for the initial phase of the illness (Mesulam, 2001).[11] Although PPAs may exist on a continuum in which various aspects of language such as word finding, object naming, syntax, or word comprehension may be more or less affected, most cases of PPA can be categorized in the early stages primarily as disorders of grammatical processing (PPA-G), semantic processing (PPA-S), or reduced verbal output with word-finding difficulties and frequently impaired repetition of sentences or phrases (logopenic PPA, or PPA-L) (Gorno-Tempini et al., 2011). There is a paucity of epidemiological data directly pertaining to PPA and its subtypes, but inference from the literature on FTLD and PPA-L suggests a prevalence on the order of 1–6 cases per 100,000, an annual incidence on the order of 0.4–1.4 cases per 100,000 person-years, and an average age of onset in the 50s or early 60s (Grossman, 2010; Mesulam, 2008).

PPA-G is characterized by effortful, non-fluent speech with impaired syntax and grammar. Apraxia of speech (AOS), a motor-based disorder of speech that produces speech sound errors, errors of stress assignment, and trial-and-error attempts to correct articulation, is frequently present (Josephs, Duffy, et al., 2006). Whereas comprehension of syntactically complex sentences is often impaired, comprehension of single words and knowledge of objects are typically preserved. Structural and functional imaging studies suggest that the left posterior frontal cortex (including premotor, supplementary motor area, and posterior inferior frontal areas) and insula degenerate early (Gorno-Tempini et al., 2004; Josephs, Duffy, et al., 2006). The majority of PPA-G cases examined pathologically have exhibited underlying FTLD-tau pathology, particularly when associated with AOS. Less frequently, PPA-G has been associated with underlying AD pathology or FTLD-TDP pathology (Grossman, 2010; Josephs, Duffy et al., 2006; M. Mesulam, 2008).

PPA-S is characterized by fluent, grammatical speech with dramatic early impairments in confrontation naming and understanding the meaning of single words. Examination frequently reveals additional features such as impaired reading or spelling of orthographically irregular words (i.e., surface dyslexia or dysgraphia), and impaired object knowledge (Gorno-Tempini et al., 2011). Neuropsychiatric features including obsessive-compulsive tendencies and behavioral disinhibition frequently follow language dysfunction (Seeley et al., 2005). Significant early atrophy and hypometabolism/hypoperfusion in PPA-S occurs in the anterior temporal lobes, usually ventral, lateral, and asymmetrical, left greater than right (Figure 42.3) (Gorno-Tempini et al., 2011). Patients with asymmetrical right greater than left early anterior temporal degeneration more frequently develop behavioral symptoms, topographical disorientation, or prosopagnosia prior to language impairment (Chan et al., 2009; Josephs,

11. See Mesulam, 2001; and Gorno-Tempini et al., 2011, for full diagnostic criteria.

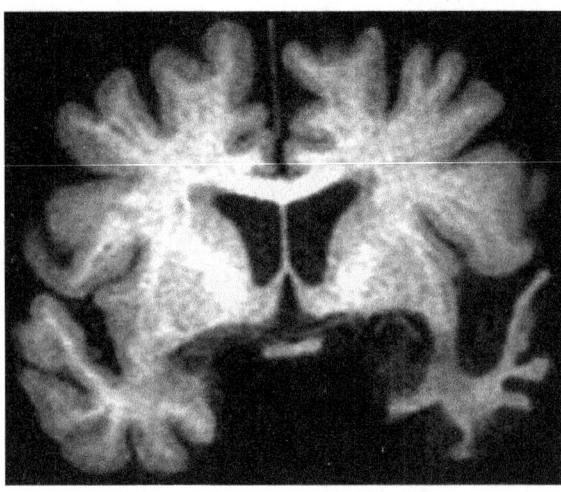

Figure 42.3 Coronal T1-weighted MRI of a patient with semantic primary progressive aphasia. This image demonstrates severe atrophy of the left anterior temporal lobe and insula.

Whitwell, et al., 2009). Neuropathological studies have suggested that the majority of PPA-S cases have underlying FLTD-TDP pathology (Grossman, 2010).

PPA-L is characterized by significant word-retrieval difficulties poor repetition of phrases and sentences, phonological errors in speech, but preserved grammar, motor output, and repetition and comprehension of single words (Gorno-Tempini et al., 2004). Imaging evidence consists of atrophy and/or hypoperfusion or hypometabolism in left posterior perisylvian temporal and parietal cortex (Gorno-Tempini et al., 2011). There are few clinical/pathological reports pertaining to logopenic PPA, but the data available suggest that a majority of cases exhibit underlying AD pathology (Grossman, 2010; M. Mesulam, 2008).

To date no medications have proven symptomatic benefit for PPA. Additional data are required to determine whether or not cholinesterase inhibitors and/or memantine may have benefit for subsets of patients (Boxer et al., 2009; Johnson et al., 2010; Kertesz et al., 2008). Speech and language therapy may provide patients and their families with compensatory strategies for coping with changes and optimizing language function.

BEHAVIORAL-VARIANT FRONTOTEMPORAL DEMENTIA

Unlike most other neurodegenerative dementias, the behavioral- variant of frontotemporal dementia (bvFTD) produces dramatic early changes in personality, comportment, and demeanor. Such changes frequently take the form of apathy, disinhibition, stereotyped or stimulus-bound behaviors, perseveration, mental rigidity, hoarding, loss of empathy, blunted affect, and changes in food preference, typically towards sweet foods. Insight into cognitive and behavioral changes is typically quite limited. Early diagnosis can be challenging because of the overlap between bvFTD and psychiatric disorders and because cognitive difficulties are usually overshadowed by behavioral changes. A subset of patients, usually male, who meet

behavioral criteria for a diagnosis of bvFTD but remain stable as opposed to progressing to incapacitating dementia may have developmental disorders on the spectrum of Asperger syndrome with decompensation in middle age related to altered life circumstances (Davies et al., 2006; Piguet, Hornberger, Mioshi, & Hodges, 2011). Documentation of clear impairment on neuropsychological measures of executive function, unambiguous progression, and abnormalities on structural or functional neuroimaging increase the likelihood of progressive, degenerative bvFTD[12] (Rascovsky et al., 2007).

The incidence of bvFTD is highest in the group of individuals with early-onset dementia (aged 45–64), although less common cases occur in the very young (20s-30s) or the very old. Epidemiological studies suggest a prevalence of 3.5–15 cases per 100,000 for all syndromes associated with FTLD (bvFTD, PPA-S, PPA-G) in the age group 45–64, of which approximately 60–80% of cases are bvFTD (Grossman et al., 2007; Knopman et al., 2005; Snowden, Neary, & Mann, 2007). Gene mutations account for about 10–20% of cases, with an autosomal dominant pattern of inheritance clear in about 10% (Piguet et al., 2011). Mutations in the genes encoding tau and progranulin (*MAPT* and *GRN*) account for the greatest proportion of genetic cases. Genetic counseling and screening for mutations in these genes may be offered to individuals with one or more first degree relatives with an illness in the FTD spectrum. A smaller proportion of genetic cases are due to mutations in the genes *C9ORF72, VCP, TARDBP*, or *CHMP2B*.

Performance on standard neuropsychological measures and on scales such as the MMSE may be largely preserved early, but selected tests of executive function, decision making, emotion detection, and theory of mind have utility (Torralva, Roca, Gleichgerrcht, Bekinschtein, & Manes, 2009). General neurological examination may reveal evidence of motor neuron disease (frontotemporal dementia with amyotrophic lateral sclerosis, or FTD-ALS), which occurs concomitantly with bvFTD in approximately 10% of cases. Parkinsonism and bvFTD may coexist in cases with underlying FTLD-tau pathology such as with *MAPT* mutations, CBD, or PSP, as well as familial cohorts with FTLD-TDP pathology due to mutations in *GRN* or *C9ORF72*. Structural imaging findings in bvFTD series are heterogeneous but most frequently reveal atrophy of the mesial frontal, orbitofrontal and anterior insula cortices (Figure 42.4) (Seeley et al., 2008). Similarly, perfusion SPECT and FDG-PET reveal a frontal distribution of hypoperfusion or hypometabolism (Kanda et al., 2008; Varma et al., 2002).

In the future, quantitative imaging techniques may be available for clinical application to predict pathological

---

12. International consensus criteria for a diagnosis of "possible" bvFTD require evidence of progressive deterioration in behavior and/or cognition plus three or more of the following: (1) early behavioral disinhibition; (2) early apathy or inertia; (3) early loss of sympathy or empathy; (4) early perseverative, stereotyped, or compulsive/ritualistic behavior; (5) hyperorality and dietary changes; (6) neuropsychological profile with executive function deficits. Certainty can be increased to "probable" bvFTD by presence of significant functional decline and imaging results consistent with bvFTD. Certainty can be increased to "definite" bvFTD with histopathological evidence of FTLD on post mortem examination or presence of a known pathogenic mutation.

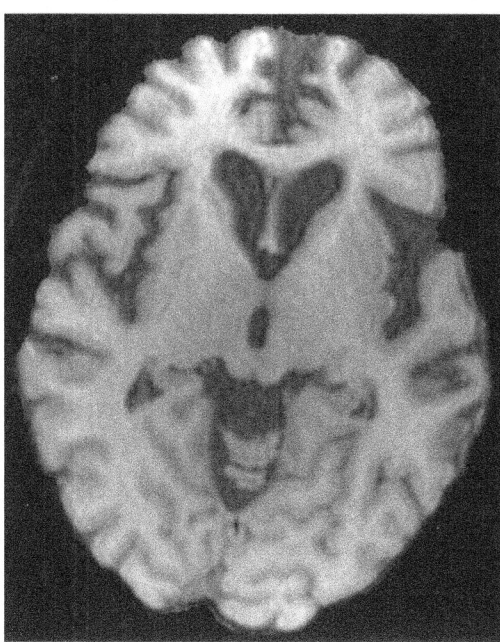

Figure 42.4 Axial T1-weighted MRI of a patient with behavioral-variant frontotemporal dementia. This image demonstrates atrophy of the frontal lobes bilaterally.

apraxia and extrapyramidal symptoms (rigidity, bradykinesia, tremor, dystonia) accompanied by signs of cortical involvement such as alien limb syndrome, cortical sensory loss, hemisensory neglect, visuospatial deficits, or myoclonus (Kouri, Whitwell, Josephs, Rademakers, & Dickson, 2011; Rebeiz, Kolodny, & Richardson, 1968). Other aspects of cognitive dysfunction including executive dysfunction, aphasia, and memory loss are highly variable but not uncommon (Murray et al., 2007; Wenning et al., 1998). PSPS characteristically involves severe early postural instability and falls, supranuclear gaze impairment that manifests with decreased saccade velocity or ophthalmoplegia, and an extrapyramidal syndrome with prominent axial rigidity (Steele, Richardson, & Olszewski, 1964; D. R. Williams & Lees, 2009). A majority of patients with PSPS develop a dementia syndrome with frontal and subcortical features such as disinhibition or impulsivity, apathy, social withdrawal, stimulus bound/imitative/utilization behavior, psychomotor slowing, executive dysfunction, and pseudobulbar affect (Golbe & Ohman-Strickland, 2007; Litvan, Mega, Cummings, & Fairbanks, 1996). As aforementioned, there can be substantial clinical overlap between the syndromes of CBS and PSPS in any given patient, as well as overlap with PPA-G and bvFTD (Kertesz, McMonagle, Blair, Davidson, & Munoz, 2005).

MRI in CBS characteristically reveals asymmetric atrophy of the perirolandic cortex and basal ganglia, whereas PSPS has been associated consistently with atrophy of the brainstem (particularly midbrain and superior cerebellar peduncle) and frontal white matter with lesser involvement of the frontal cortex (Boxer et al., 2006; Josephs et al., 2008). As with bvFTD, quantitative neuroimaging may help to determine underlying pathology in CBS and PSPS (Whitwell & Josephs, 2012). Although CBS is pathologically heterogeneous, focal atrophy of the posterior frontal cortex has been found to predict CBD (FTLD-tau) pathology, more widespread frontotemporal atrophy to predict FTLD-TAR DNA binding protein-43 (TDP) pathology, and more widespread temporoparietal atrophy to predict AD pathology (Whitwell et al., 2010). Unlike CBS, nearly all PSPS cases exhibit underlying FTLD-tau pathology, most commonly PSP pathology, less commonly CBD pathology (Josephs, Petersen, et al., 2006).

Pharmacological management of CBS and PSPS consists of symptomatic treatment of motor, cognitive, and mood dysfunction. One may do so in a manner analogous to that described for DLB and PDD above, noting that many CBS and PSPS patients will be less responsive to levodopa and cholinesterase inhibitors, and also less likely to demonstrate neuroleptic sensitivity. Disease-modifying therapies based on proposed pathophysiological mechanisms are being considered (Stamelou et al., 2010).

subtype in bvFTD and other syndromes associated with FTLD pathology (Whitwell & Josephs, 2012). This would be particularly useful for bvFTD, a pathologically heterogeneous syndrome associated with FTLD-tau or FTLD-TDP pathologies in 90–95% of cases (in roughly equal proportions) and FTLD-FUS and other pathologies in the remainder of cases. In addition to being associated with these protein inclusions, bvFTD is characterized pathologically by bilateral frontotemporal atrophy, neuronal loss, microvacuolation, and varying degrees of astrocytic gliosis.

Few treatment trials have been conducted to assess the efficacy of pharmacological interventions in bvFTD. Mostly anecdotal evidence suggests some benefit from selective serotonin reuptake inhibitors (SSRIs) for treating impulsivity, repetitive or obsessive-compulsive behaviors, and eating disorders (Mendez, 2009). Atypical antipsychotics may be used in low doses for significant agitation, aggression, or psychosis. Cholinesterase inhibitors do not appear to be effective. Memantine has shown some promise in limited studies; further investigation with placebo-controlled trials is required (Boxer et al., 2009). Caregiver education and support are indispensable in the management of bvFTD, as strategies for dealing with problematic behaviors are required and caregiver burden is very high compared to other types of dementia (Riedijk et al., 2006).

CORTICOBASAL SYNDROME AND PROGRESSIVE SUPRANUCLEAR PALSY

Corticobasal syndrome (CBS) and progressive supranuclear palsy syndrome (PSPS) are syndromes characterized by atypical parkinsonism with varying levels of cognitive impairment and dementia. The hallmarks of CBS are asymmetrical

VASCULAR COGNITIVE IMPAIRMENT AND DEMENTIA

Vascular cognitive impairment (VCI) is an umbrella term that encompasses patients with MCI due to cerebrovascular disease (also termed VCI-no dementia), vascular dementia

(VaD), and mixed vascular-degenerative dementia. VaD is the second most common form of dementia in developed countries after AD (Fratiglioni et al., 2000; Lobo et al., 2000); about a third of dementia cases show significant vascular pathology at autopsy, and the estimated prevalence of VCI in people over 65 is about 5% (Moorhouse & Rockwood, 2008). Challenges in the diagnosis of VaD are posed by its pathophysiological heterogeneity, lack of a consensus pathological gold standard, and frequent coexistence with neurodegenerative pathology. Diverse processes such as large-vessel cerebrovascular disease, small-vessel disease, chronic non-infarct ischemic changes, and hemorrhage are all associated with VaD. Although both correlation between the time course of stroke and cognitive dysfunction and neuroimaging evidence of vascular disease can provide useful evidence of VaD, the sensitivity of these features has been demonstrated to be suboptimal (Gold et al., 2002).

The nature and severity of cognitive dysfunction depend on the volume, quantity, and location of infarctions, ischemia, and atrophy referable to vascular disease. Deficits may be predominantly cortical or subcortical. The time course of progression may be gradual or stepwise. Single strategic infarcts in the thalamus, angular gyrus, caudate, globus pallidus, basal forebrain, or hippocampus may be sufficient to produce dementia, but many cases of VaD arise due to the cumulative effects of multifocal cortical or subcortical infarcts. Leukoaraiosis, a term for non-specific signal changes in the white matter detectable by CT or MRI, is associated with cognitive and functional decline, but as of yet without clear associations with particular cognitive domains (Moorhouse & Rockwood, 2008). Although executive dysfunction is not uncommon in VaD, and diffuse subcortical infarcts or ischemia may produce a syndrome of subcortical dementia with prominent executive impairment, clinical/pathological studies suggest that executive dysfunction is neither sensitive nor specific for VaD and should not be employed as a diagnostic marker (Reed et al., 2007).

Diagnosis of VCI and VaD requires a clinical judgement that vascular disease is contributing significantly to a patient's cognitive or behavioral dysfunction. Such judgement is most frequently based on: (1) history (including history of stroke and risk factors for stroke); (2) examination (including examination of blood pressure, heart rate, body mass index, waist circumference, examination of the cardiovascular system, and examination for focal neurological signs in addition to a detailed MSE); and (3) neuroimaging, bearing in mind the lack of pathognomonic neuroimaging features[13] and possible lack of correlation between infarct location and cognitive profile. Limitations in the current diagnostic criteria for VaD

most commonly used, the National Institute of Neurological Disorders and Stroke and Association Internationale pour la Recherché et l'Enseignement en Neurosciences (NINDS-AIREN) criteria, prompted the National Institute for Neurological Disorders and Stroke (NINDS) and the Canadian Stroke Network to recommend a comprehensive set of clinical and research standards for the description and study of VCI (Hachinski et al., 2006; Roman et al., 1993). These standards represent an important step in the direction of establishing a consensus diagnostic gold standard.

Treating modifiable risk factors for stroke such as hypertension, hypercholesterolemia, diabetes mellitus, smoking, and excessive alcohol intake is recommended in the treatment and prevention of VaD, although data demonstrating benefit with respect to primary and secondary prevention of stroke are more robust than data demonstrating direct benefits on cognition. Similarly, while antiplatelet therapy with aspirin, aspirin/dipyridamole, or clopidogrel offer benefit with respect to prevention of stroke in individuals at risk, no clinical trials have addressed the issue of efficacy for VaD (Williams, Spector, Orrell, & Rands, 2000). Randomized controlled trials of cholinesterase inhibitors and memantine over six months in mild to moderate VaD have suggested small benefits of uncertain clinical significance (Kavirajan & Schneider, 2007). Further studies are required to determine whether subgroups of patients might benefit.

RAPIDLY PROGRESSIVE DEMENTIAS

Rapidly progressive dementias (RPDs) involve progression of cognitive dysfunction sub-acutely over days, weeks, or several months as opposed to the progression over months to years usually witnessed with degenerative dementias. Rapid progression should prompt consideration of a differential diagnosis highlighting prion diseases, autoimmune/inflammatory encephalopathies, and unusual presentations of typically chronic neurodegenerative dementias.

Prion Diseases

Prion diseases account for the majority of cases of RPD (Geschwind, Shu, Haman, Sejvar, & Miller, 2008; Josephs, Ahlskog, et al., 2009). Human prion diseases include Creutzfeldt-Jakob disease (CJD), variant Creutzfeldt-Jakob disease (vCJD; "mad cow disease"), kuru, familial fatal insomnia, and Gerstmann-Sträussler-Scheinker syndrome (GSS). Prion diseases most frequently occur sporadically, but may also be transmitted genetically (due to autosomal dominant mutations in the prion protein gene), iatrogenically (via contaminated surgical instruments, tissue grafts, or use of cadaveric pituitary hormones), or, in cases of kuru or variant CJD, by ingestion of contaminated tissues. Sporadic CJD (sCJD) constitutes the most common form of human prion disease, with an incidence of approximately one case per million individuals per year worldwide (Ladogana et al., 2005).

Characteristic features of CJD, in addition to rapid cognitive decline, include focal higher cortical signs (such as apraxia, agnosia, or aphasia), akinetic mutism, myoclonus, pyramidal

---

13. In selected uncommon circumstances such as VCI/VaD due to cerebral autosomal dominant arteriopathy with subcortical infarcts and leukoencephalopathy (CADASIL) or cerebral amyloid angiopathy (CAA), MRI results have high sensitivity and specificity. CADASIL characteristically produces T2 hyperintensities in the temporal poles and external capsules. CAA characteristically produces multiple hemorrhages (apparent on gradient echo or susceptibility weighted MRI) restricted to lobar, cortical, or cortico-subcortical regions. See Knudsen et al. (2001), *Neurology 56*(4), 537–539; O'Sullivan et al. (2001), *Neurology 56*(5), 628–634.

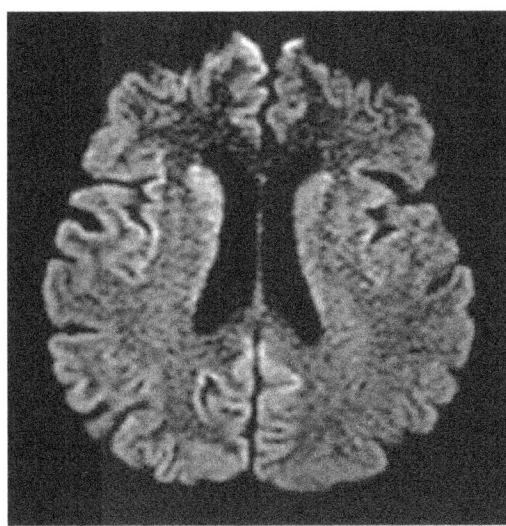

Figure 42.5 Diffusion-weighted MRI of a patient with Creutzfeldt-Jakob disease. This image demonstrates restricted diffusion diffusely along the cortical ribbon and in the basal ganglia.

or extrapyramidal signs, cerebellar signs, and visual dysfunction. The presence of restricted diffusion along the cortical ribbon and/or within deep gray structures (striatum and/or thalamus) is both sensitive and specific for CJD (Figure 42.5) (Vitali et al., 2011; Young et al., 2005). Diagnosis may be supported by the presence of periodic sharp wave complexes (PSWCs) on EEG and/or 14-3-3 protein in the CSF. Median survival is five months from onset of symptoms (Collins et al., 2006). Disease phenotype, including symptoms, signs, distribution of MRI signal abnormalities, EEG results, CSF results, and disease duration, is influenced considerably by the molecular subtype of illness (Parchi et al., 1999).[14]

Prion diseases have characteristic pathological features, including neuronal loss, glial proliferation, vacuoles in the neuropil (producing a "spongiform" appearance), and absence of inflammation (Prusiner, 1998). Pathophysiology involves the transformation of a normal cellular prion protein (PRPc) to a pathogenic isoform (PRPsc) via a three-dimensional conformational change. Pathogenic PRPsc spreads rapidly through the brain via trans-synaptic mechanisms. There are no treatments with established efficacy for prion diseases.

Autoimmune/Inflammatory Encephalopathies

Autoimmune or inflammatory causes of dementia merit consideration in the appropriate clinical setting, especially because they may respond to treatment more dramatically than other types of dementia such as neurodegenerative illness. The spectrum of autoimmune dementias is large; in some instances specific autoantibodies have been defined and pathogenic mechanisms relatively well delineated, while in others, disease mechanisms remain poorly defined and

the presence of autoimmunity is inferred on the basis of responsiveness to immunosuppression (Flanagan et al., 2010; Rosenbloom, Smith, Akdal, & Geschwind, 2009). Clinical features that should prompt consideration of an autoimmune cause of dementia include subacute onset and rapid progression of cognitive dysfunction, fluctuating course, coexisting organ-specific autoimmunity, evidence of inflammation in the CSF, or MRI suggestive of encephalitis.

Hashimoto encephalopathy (HE) and antibody-associated encephalitis (AAE) are two types of autoimmune illness particularly noteworthy in the context of RPD. HE is defined by cognitive dysfunction in the setting of high titers of anti-thyroid antibodies (anti-thyroid peroxidase, anti-thyroglobulin, or anti-microsomal antibodies), and absence of any other clear etiology for the cognitive dysfunction (Brain, Jellinek, & Ball, 1966; Chong, Rowland, & Utiger, 2003). The majority of individuals with HE have a fluctuating, relapsing, and remitting course; the minority, a subacute progressive course. Transient aphasia, tremor, seizures, gait ataxia, and hypersomnolence are frequently observed features, although the presentation is highly variable and numerous other signs and symptoms have been reported (Marshall & Doyle, 2006). Approximately 80% of cases exhibit elevated levels of total protein in the CSF; much fewer have elevated leukocytes, oligoclonal bands, or elevated IgG synthesis or index. Greater than 90% of reported cases have EEG abnormalities, most frequently consisting of generalized slowing, less frequently of focal slowing, epileptiform changes, or triphasic waves. MRI findings have consisted of normal or nonspecific findings in the majority of reported cases, although a few reported cases have demonstrated diffuse T2 hyperintensities in white matter.

The pathogenesis of HE remains unclear, as does the role, if any, anti-thyroid antibodies play in the encephalopathy. Limited pathological studies have most commonly revealed perivascular lymphocytic infiltrates in the brain parenchyma and/or leptomeninges, with or without gliosis. Similar clinical characteristics and pathology have been reported in encephalopathies in patients with other autoimmune diseases such as Sjögren syndrome and systemic lupus erythematosus, leading some authors to group these conditions under the rubric of nonvasculitic autoimmune inflammatory meningoencephalitis (NAIM) (Caselli, Boeve, Scheithauer, O'Duffy, & Hunder, 1999; Lyons, Caselli, & Parisi, 2008). Clinicians have most frequently treated HE and NAIM with high-dose intravenous corticosteroids as a first line of therapy (Castillo et al., 2006), additionally treating hypothyroidism and seizures as necessary. Alternative immunomodulatory treatments, including cyclophosphamide, azathioprine, methotrexate, intravenous immunoglobulin (IVIg), and plasmapheresis, have been employed with some success in cases where corticosteroids were not effective or were contraindicated (Marshall & Doyle, 2006).

Antibody-associated encephalitides (AAE) are encephalitides associated with antibodies reactive to neuronal antigens. Several such antibodies have been established, including (but not limited to) anti-Hu, anti-Ma2, anti-CV2, anti-VGKC, anti-amphiphysin, anti-Yo, anti-nCMAg, anti-Ma1, anti-Ri,

14. Subtypes, defined by the methionine-valine polymorphism at codon 129 of the prion protein and by the type of prion protein (type 1 or type 2): MM1 and MV1 ("classic"), VV2 ("ataxic"), MV2 ("kuru plaque"), MM2-cortical, MM2-thalamic, and VV1. MM1 and MV1 account for ~70% of cases and are characterized most frequently by cognitive deficits, myoclonus, ataxia, pyramidal signs, PSWCs on EEG, and 14-3-3 protein in CSF.

anti-GAD65, anti-NMDAR, and anti-neuropil antibodies. In many cases, AAE is paraneoplastic, either preceding or following the diagnosis of cancer by weeks, months, or rarely, one to several years. The most common neoplasms associated with paraneoplastic AAE include small-cell lung cancer, germ-cell tumors, thymoma, Hodgkin's lymphoma, and breast cancer (Gultekin et al., 2000). Age of onset of AAE ranges from childhood to older adulthood, depending in part upon the tumor and antibody associations involved.

AAE may occur as focal limbic encephalitis or be associated with more widespread involvement of the nervous system (i.e., brainstem, cerebellum, spinal cord). Limbic encephalitis frequently presents as a subacute amnestic syndrome with accompanying neuropsychiatric symptoms (depression, personality changes, anxiety, emotional lability) and seizures. More than 80% of these patients have an abnormality in the CSF, most frequently a mild elevation in protein with or without a mild pleocytosis (Daffner, Sherman, Gonzalez, & Hasserjian, 2008). Over 90% demonstrate abnormalities on EEG, including focal or generalized slowing and/or epileptiform activity. Only about 50–65% demonstrate MRI abnormalities of increased T2 signal in the medial temporal lobes and/or other limbic structures.

Comprehensive workup to evaluate for an underlying neoplasm is indicated in all cases of suspected or confirmed AAE. This workup may include CT scanning of the whole body, with and without contrast; PET scanning of the whole body; tests for tumor markers in the blood; mammography; and ultrasound studies. Aggressive treatment of an underlying neoplasm in conjunction with immunomodulatory therapies with IVIg, plasmapheresis, corticosteroids, or cytotoxic agents provides benefit to a subset of patients. Presence of antibodies reactive to cell membrane antigens (anti-VGKC, anti-NMDAR) may confer a more favorable prognosis than presence of antibodies reactive to intracellular antigens (Bataller et al., 2007).

COMMON DEMENTIA MIMICS

A fair proportion of individuals presenting for evaluation of cognitive changes turn out to have potentially reversible medical or psychiatric illness. Though not entirely specific, potential concern about symptoms by the patient exceeding that of loved ones is one predictive factor of non-progressive, non-degenerative illness. As noted above, one should screen for symptoms of depression, anxiety, and bipolar disease as a routine part of the cognitive assessment. Such symptoms may not be superficially apparent in patients who have cognitive dysfunction related to a maladaptive response to significant life stressors. This syndrome may exist on a spectrum with post-traumatic stress disorder. Characteristics include elements of dissociation and a cognitive profile suggestive of attentional/executive dysfunction, and poor memory encoding and retrieval.

This cognitive profile is common to other medical and psychiatric causes of cognitive dysfunction (Millan et al., 2012). Relatively common medical contributing factors include obstructive sleep apnea, history of chemotherapy, and chronic pain (Aloia, Arnedt, Davis, Riggs, & Byrd, 2004; Kannarkat, Lasher, & Schiff, 2007). Severe melancholic and/or psychotic depression in older individuals can cause dementia but be mistaken for neurodegenerative illness, especially when it is not responsive to antidepressant medications (Wagner, McClintock, Rosenquist, McCall, & Kahn, 2011). Electroconvulsive therapy may provide cognitive as well as mood benefits in such patients.

TREATMENT OF DEMENTIA

This section discusses treatment issues pertaining to dementia patients in general, specifically: (1) behavioral and lifestyle recommendations; (2) management of the neuropsychiatric symptoms of dementia; and (3) use of ancillary services and providers.

BEHAVIORAL AND LIFESTYLE RECOMMENDATIONS
Cognitive Performance and Quality of Life

In most cases, a diagnosis of dementia induces substantial fear and dread about what the future holds for patients and their families. Direct but compassionate communication by the provider about the diagnosis and what can and cannot be predicted is essential to address preconceived notions and to advocate for an active, safe lifestyle. Components of an active lifestyle that may provide psychological, physical, and even cognitive benefits include regular exercise, stimulating cognitive activities, social activities, and a healthy diet. In making lifestyle recommendations to patients and caregivers, it is important to remain aware that apathy and anxiety concerning reduced functionality are very frequent features of dementia that may lead to resistance to activities by the patient. Goals should therefore be realistic, adaptable, and always in keeping with a positive subjective experience for the patient.

Multiple studies have examined the effects of exercise on cognitive, behavioral, and psychiatric symptoms in dementia, with positive results. Exercise may improve physical functioning in patients with dementia and reduce problems related to agitation, wandering, and insomnia (Potter, Ellard, Rees, & Thorogood, 2011; Thune-Boyle, Iliffe, Cerga-Pashoja, Lowery, & Warner, 2011). A recent meta-analysis of studies pertaining to aerobic exercise and cognition suggested that exercise not only reduces risk of future MCI and dementia in healthy individuals, but it also improves cognitive scores and imaging biomarkers of cognition after 6 to 12 months in patients with MCI or dementia, compared with sedentary controls (Ahlskog, Geda, Graff-Radford, & Petersen, 2011).

As with exercise, accumulating evidence suggests that a healthy diet not only reduces risk for cardiovascular and cerebrovascular disease, but also may influence the risk and rate of progression of neurodegenerative pathology. Specifically, adherence to a "Mediterranean-type" diet appears to reduce the risk of cognitive impairment and dementia in healthy individuals, and it may slow cognitive decline in individuals diagnosed with MCI or AD (Solfrizzi et al., 2011). The Mediterranean diet emphasizes consumption of vegetables, fruits, unrefined whole-grain foods, and fish, while limiting foods containing trans-fat, cholesterol, added sugars, and salt.

Data from trials support the notion that activities that offer cognitive and social stimulation to patients with dementia are more likely to provide benefit than those that do not. Cognitive stimulation, an intervention usually presenting a range of activities aimed at general enhancement of cognitive and social functioning in a small-group setting, appears to consistently promote cognition, and possibly overall quality of life in patients with mild to moderate dementia (Buschert, Bokde, & Hampel, 2010; Woods, Aguirre, Spector, & Orrell, 2012). These data are consistent with studies in healthy older people suggesting that cognitively stimulating activities and social activity are associated with a lower risk of incipient dementia (James, Wilson, Barnes, & Bennett, 2011; Wilson et al., 2003).

Safety

The loss of independence inherently associated with dementia is one of the most challenging aspects of the condition for both patients and caregivers. Continued performance of routine activities within a patient's capabilities should be encouraged, as long as the safety of the patient or of others is not compromised. Driving is perhaps the most common example of an activity that poses substantial risk, usually not recognized by the patient. More than loss of memory, impairments in attention, executive functions, and visuospatial functions increase one's risk of accidents (Silva, Laks, & Engelhardt, 2009). An AAN practice parameter published in 2010 identified the following factors as predictive for unsafe driving: (1) dementia severity, including CDR global score of 1 or greater and/or MMSE of 24 or below; (2) self-reported situational avoidance or reduced driving mileage; (3) caregiver's rating of driving as "marginal" or "unsafe"; (4) a history of accidents or citations; and (5) impulsive or aggressive personality characteristics (Iverson et al., 2010). Individuals with dementia at low to moderate risk of accidents should be strongly encouraged to consider voluntary surrender of driving privileges or to undergo a professional driving evaluation. Noncompliant patients determined to be at high risk of accidents should be subject to intervention per applicable laws.

Examples of other potentially unsafe situations or activities include cooking without supervision when there is the potential to leave a stove or oven on, operating power tools or appliances during which a lapse in attention could cause significant bodily harm, and keeping firearms or other weapons in the house. Patients with dementia who have a propensity to wander but who do not require 24-hour supervision for other indications may benefit from wearing a monitor and/or from measures to prevent them from leaving the house unsupervised. Patient self-administration of medications should be monitored for errors, and assistance provided when necessary. Pill boxes with designated slots for different days and times may help reduce confusion about what medications should be taken when.

MANAGEMENT OF THE NEUROPSYCHIATRIC SYMPTOMS OF DEMENTIA

As reviewed above for specific dementia syndromes, neuropsychiatric symptoms of dementia (also termed "behavioral and psychological symptoms of dementia," or BPSD, in the literature) arise in nearly every dementia patient. Neuropsychiatric symptoms tend to cluster into syndromes of agitation, psychosis, or mood disorders, but these syndromes frequently coexist in the same patient (Ballard & Corbett, 2010). Pharmacological and non-pharmacological treatment strategies should be tailored to the type and severity of symptoms.

Depression, Anxiety, and Apathy

Despite the high prevalence of depression in dementia, relatively few randomized, controlled clinical trials have assessed the efficacy of the antidepressant medications most widely used in clinical practice. Those that have—for example, recent trials evaluating the efficacy of sertraline or mirtazapine for depressive symptoms in patients with AD—have not suggested benefit vs. placebo and have suggested a relatively high rate of side effects (Banerjee et al., 2011; Rosenberg et al., 2010). For this reason, consideration should be given to non-pharmacological treatments as a first line of therapy unless depression is severe. Non-pharmacological treatments may include cognitive stimulation, psychotherapy, exercise, occupational therapy with attention to environmental factors contributing to mood, and teaching caregivers behavioral management techniques (Brodaty, 2011). If not already started for enhancement of cognition, a cholinesterase inhibitor may also enhance mood, particularly in AD or Lewy body disorders (Ballard & Corbett, 2010). SSRIs may have greater efficacy for treatment of anxiety and irritability in dementia, although most data on the issue pertain to patients with more severe agitation and aggression (discussed below).

Most of the available evidence for pharmacological treatment of apathy in dementia comes from studies in which the primary endpoints involved other symptoms of dementia and measures of apathy were embedded in behavioral scales such as the Neuropsychiatric Inventory (Berman, Brodaty, Withall, & Seeher, 2012). From these studies, conducted largely in patients with AD, cholinesterase inhibitors demonstrated the clearest and most consistent benefits. Limited studies containing apathy measures that evaluated memantine or methylphenidate have likewise suggested benefit (Dolder, Davis, & McKinsey, 2010). Although available data do not suggest considerable benefit from antidepressant medications, those studied have not included the more "activating" antidepressants such as bupropion or serotonin-norepinephrine reuptake inhibitors (SNRIs). Dopamine agonists have been used off-label with some success for treating apathy related to other neurological conditions, such as stroke (Kohno et al., 2010), but have not been widely studied in dementia. Non-pharmacological treatments for apathy in dementia, including cognitive stimulation, cognitive-communication therapy, and multisensory stimulation, require further investigation (Roth, Flashman, & McAllister, 2007).

Insomnia

Disturbances of sleep are highly prevalent in dementia, and may be due to any number of factors, such as effects of the neurodegenerative process on neural mechanisms underlying the circadian rhythm, primary sleep disorders occurring concomitantly with the dementia, medical or psychiatric comorbidities, medication side effects, and environmental or behavioral factors. Accordingly, one's first step in managing insomnia in a patient with dementia should be to identify and treat the specific factors contributing to insomnia in that particular patient. Polysomnography may be useful to identify sleep disorders such as restless legs syndrome (RLS), periodic limb movements in sleep, REM sleep behavior disorder, and obstructive or central sleep apnea. Non-essential medications associated with insomnia, including cholinesterase inhibitors and anti-Parkinsonian medications, should be discontinued. Non-pharmacological therapies such as light therapy, daytime exercise, and behavioral interventions[15] should be employed prior to the use of medications.

There is no clear standard of care in the pharmacological treatment of insomnia in dementia. Of the available options, melatonin and the melatonin receptor agonist ramelteon have the lowest likelihood of adverse cognitive effects, although some studies have suggested limited efficacy (Serfaty, Kennell-Webb, Warner, Blizard, & Raven, 2002; Singer et al., 2003). Antihistamines should be avoided due to frequent side effects such as anticholinergic effects that can exacerbate cognitive impairment. Despite its widespread use, evidence for the efficacy of trazodone in insomnia is scant (Mendelson, 2005). Other options, including non-benzodiazepine hypnotics (zolpidem, zaleplon, eszopiclone) and atypical antipsychotics (e.g., quetiapine or olanzapine) should be used with caution and closely monitored for potential side effects. As a rule, the lowest possible effective dose should be sought over a time-limited trial, employing "as needed" rather than scheduled dosing.

Agitation and Aggression

Like insomnia, agitation and aggression occur in dementia with a multitude of possible underlying factors. Pharmacological treatment should be employed only as a last resort for patients with distressing symptoms of agitation or aggression that are unresponsive to non-pharmacological measures, unless there is imminent risk of harm to self or others. A recommended strategy is to first assess for infections, pain, constipation, or dehydration; to optimize treatment of visual and auditory impairment; and to address potential environmental triggers such as low light or extreme noise levels (Ballard & Corbett, 2010). Non-essential medications with the potential to cause or exacerbate confusion should be eliminated, as should a patient's access to alcohol. As recommended above, the patient's sleep cycle should be reinforced via adherence to a regular schedule with good sleep hygiene.

Where possible, situations that provoke anger or agitation should be identified and avoided. For example, if a certain mode of bathing or showering is not well tolerated, alternative modes should be explored, in particular those that foster a greater sense of relative autonomy in the patient. Rather than attempt to reason with a demented patient in situations of resistance or disagreement, a caregiver should distract or gently redirect the patient. Agitation frequently arises as a response to a perceived threat, so a calm demeanor and a predictable environment with cues that promote relaxation such as music and warm lighting may provide benefit. Patient stress may also be alleviated by routine exercise in moderation, "pet" therapy with animals, validation therapy, structured social interaction, other individualized meaningful activities, and aromatherapy with lavender oil or *Melissa officinalis* lemon balm (Ballard, O'Brien, Reichelt, & Perry, 2002).

When medications are required, atypical antipsychotics have the best evidence of benefit for short-term (up to 12 weeks) treatment of aggression (Ballard & Corbett, 2010). Potential adverse reactions include extrapyramidal symptoms, drowsiness, peripheral edema, stroke, acceleration in the rate of cognitive decline, and increase in mortality. Other types of medication, including memantine, carbamazepine, or SSRIs, have limited, but better evidence for treatment of non-aggressive agitation (Gauthier, Loft, & Cummings, 2008; Pollock et al., 2007; Tariot, Loy, Ryan, Porsteinsson, & Ismail, 2002). Benzodiazepines often exacerbate cognitive and motor difficulties and may cause frank confusion or paradoxical agitation.

USE OF ANCILLARY SERVICES AND PRACTITIONERS

As reviewed above, dementia poses a variety of different medical, psychological, and social challenges. A team-based approach to treatment offers the advantage of expertise in specialized areas of treatment. Such an approach works best when one physician is the point-person for the patient and his or her caregivers, coordinating the plan of care and facilitating communication between parties when necessary.

Education about a patient's illness, its expected sequelae, and common issues it raises frequently reduces stress in patients and their caregivers. Social workers with expertise in dementia, neuropsychiatry, and/or geriatric medicine can often provide information above and beyond that offered by the primary treating physician. They may also offer strategies for dealing with specific stressors or recurrent problematic situations, psychotherapy, guidance regarding financial and legal planning, and referral information for resources in the community. Information and support are also frequently available through nonprofit organizations such as the Alzheimer's Association,

---

15. Behavioral interventions include maintaining consistent bedtimes and rising times; following a relaxing bedtime routine; limiting daytime napping and time spent in bed; exposing the patient to bright light (preferably sunlight) in the day; keeping sleep areas dark, quiet, and temperate at night; avoiding caffeine, alcohol, and nicotine; establishing regular meal times; avoiding excessive fluid intake in the evening; emptying the bladder before bed; and treating musculoskeletal pain.

the Association for Frontotemporal Degeneration, the Lewy Body Dementia Association, and other disease-specific groups. Certain patients and caregivers, in particular those with uncommon or lesser-known conditions, often benefit from attending support groups, where people can discuss common experiences and strategies.

Symptom-specific rehabilitation provides a stimulus for attempting to maintain function and, when this is not possible, methods for compensation. Physical therapy (PT) and occupational therapy (OT) directly address changes in motor function, including loss of dexterity, difficulty completing skilled movements or tasks, and problems with balance and gait. Assessments and plans often include recommendations regarding exercise programs and guidance about when a walking-assistance device (e.g., a cane or walker) is indicated. Home safety evaluations, frequently conducted by OT, identify modifiable features of the home environment that increase a patient's risk for falls or other potential sources of harm. Speech and language therapy targets language and other aspects of cognition. Numerous studies have suggested therapeutic benefits and adaptive brain changes associated with cognitive intervention programs in MCI and mild to moderate dementia due to AD (Buschert et al., 2010).

As with any area of medicine, knowing one's own breadth of expertise and "comfort zone" in evaluating and treating specific problems is essential so that consultation with other providers will be obtained when necessary. In the case of dementia, specific consultations within medical, neurological, or psychiatric subspecialties may be sought, depending upon the circumstance. Geriatric psychopharmacologists can provide guidance with respect to the use of medications. Various types of individual and group psychotherapy are available for consideration and selection when appropriate.

Part of the art of dementia care consists of maintaining focus on the present while simultaneously addressing selected key matters of the future in advance. A patient's wishes pertaining to end-of-life care and surrogate medical and financial decision-making should be discussed while he or she has capacity to make decisions in these areas. Legal consultation with an elder law attorney may be appropriate. Longitudinal care of the dementia patient importantly requires longitudinal monitoring of caregiver resources and stress. When a need for increased supervision or services arises, options include home care, day programs, assisted living, and nursing home care. Selecting from among these options requires careful consideration of a patient's specific needs, desires, and resources (see Chapter 83).

SUMMARY

Dementia is a major source of morbidity and mortality worldwide. Most dementias are neurodegenerative, with age being the primary risk factor. Clinical evaluation of the patient presenting with change in cognition centers on determining the dysfunction of large-scale brain networks, establishing the time course and severity, and utilizing selected laboratory and imaging data to support one's hypothesis regarding underlying etiology. Familiarity with the key features of common causes of dementia such as AD and VaD assists in the process, as does familiarity with the salient features of less common causes including Lewy body disorders, PCA, FTD, PPA, common causes of rapidly progressive dementia, and medical and psychiatric illnesses that can cause or mimic dementia.

Symptomatic treatment of dementia includes behavioral and lifestyle modifications; optimization of factors that contribute to cognition, such as mood, anxiety, sleep, pain, and concomitant medical illness; attention to issues of safety and quality of life; and use of medications for symptomatic enhancement of cognition. Cholinesterase inhibitors and/or memantine may provide modest cognitive and behavioral benefit for patients with AD, Lewy body disorders, and possibly subgroups of patients with other types of dementia. Non-pharmacological strategies are generally preferred in the management of neuropsychiatric symptoms of dementia. When necessary and when potential benefits outweigh risks, SSRIs, other antidepressants, mood stabilizers, stimulants, and atypical antipsychotics may be useful. One should use such medications with close monitoring for side effects.

There are no disease-modifying therapies currently available for neurodegenerative dementias. Recent research has focused on the neurodegenerative process as targeting large-scale brain networks in a focal manner early in the course of illness and spreading along the lines of these networks as illnesses progress. The specific role of pathologically misfolded proteins, a feature common to the pathology of different neurodegenerative illnesses, remains unclear. Lack of efficacy of drugs targeting ß-amyloid in clinical trials for patients with dementia due to AD may be due to intervention at stages that are too advanced to provide benefit. Accordingly, efforts are underway to intervene at the stages of MCI or preclinical disease, using biomarkers to establish the diagnosis. As our understanding of neurodegenerative dementias continues to expand at an incredibly rapid rate, the future holds significant promise for more effective interventions.

CLINICAL PEARLS

- Old practices of excluding reversible causes and lumping remaining cases under the headings of "senile dementia" or "Alzheimer's disease" have given way to a process of proactively identifying specific clinical syndromes and attempting to determine neuropathology *in vivo*.

- When localizing cognitive dysfunction, determine whether a pattern of deficits is predominantly *cortical* or *subcortical*; determine whether deficits are focal, multifocal, or diffuse; and determine which large-scale networks in the brain are implicated.

- In contrast to cortical dementias, subcortical dementias present with a profile of slowed processing speed, impaired attention, apathy, mood symptoms, and motor symptoms

(Albert, Feldman, & Willis, 1974). Subcortical dementias are associated with forgetfulness, but memory difficulties are predominantly at levels of encoding and retrieving information so that recognition and cued memory are preserved.

- The domain of complex attention and executive functions localizes predominantly to frontoparietal and frontal/subcortical networks in the brain (Cummings, 1993). Episodic memory localizes both to temporolimbic networks (important for encoding, retrieval, and storage), and frontal networks (important for encoding and retrieval) (Budson & Price, 2005). Behavioral regulation and social cognitive processes recruit networks predominantly involving paralimbic regions such as the orbitofrontal cortex, anterior cingulate cortex, and insula (Gleichgerrcht, Ibanez, Roca, Torralva, & Manes, 2010).

- Specific types of misfolded proteins accumulate with a limited range of possible distributions, starting focally and spreading along particular anatomical lines until there is diffuse involvement of the brain at the later stages of illness.

- The *network degeneration hypothesis* postulates that neurodegenerative processes target large-scale networks in the brain to produce characteristic progressions of neurodegeneration and clinical symptoms that depend on the pathology and networks targeted (Seeley, Crawford, Zhou, Miller, & Greicius, 2009).

- There is a need to further develop *in vivo* biomarkers of pathology. Efforts now are most advanced for AD, for which CSF analysis of β-amyloid, total tau (t-tau), and phosphorylated tau (p-tau) are already available for clinical use, and amyloid PET imaging may become available in the near future.

- Certain *red flags* suggest a less common cause of cognitive dysfunction: a non-amnestic cognitive profile, rapid progression of symptoms over days to weeks, or the early presence of additional neurological symptoms such as pyramidal or extrapyramidal motor signs, myoclonus, cerebellar signs, apraxia, psychosis, autonomic dysfunction, REM sleep behavior disorder, or seizures. Other red flags include young age (onset of symptoms before age 65 and especially before age 50), a family history suggesting autosomal dominant mode of inheritance, and prominent evidence of systemic medical or organ-specific illness not yet accounted for.

- For a diagnosis of dementia, the Quality Standards Subcommittee of the American Academy of Neurology (AAN) recommended structural neuroimaging of the brain with CT or MRI, routine screening for depression, vitamin B_{12} deficiency, and hypothyroidism as part of a routine evaluation (Knopman et al., 2001). Many practitioners also obtain a comprehensive metabolic profile, CBC, and urinalysis (see Table 42.2).

- In the population of those with early-onset dementia (onset of symptoms between the ages of 45 and 65),

Alzheimer's disease and vascular dementia continue to be the most common etiologies, but a much higher proportion of cases is due to frontotemporal lobar degeneration (FTLD) pathology compared to the population with late-onset dementia (Garre-Olmo et al., 2010; Picard, Pasquier, Martinaud, Hannequin, & Godefroy, 2011).

- Experts recommend offering testing for gene mutations associated with familial, autosomal dominant, early-onset AD to individuals with early-onset AD and a family history of dementia (or unknown family history); individuals with a family history suggestive of autosomal dominant dementia and at least one case of early-onset AD, and individuals with a relative who has a known gene mutation (Goldman et al., 2011). Referral to a genetic counselor is imperative for all individuals who desire testing, and recommended for those who are undecided and would like to discuss the issue further.

- Although comportment and social demeanor are typically preserved until late in the course of AD, neuropsychiatric features such as mild apathy, social withdrawal, anxiety, and irritability are common early (Lyketsos et al., 2011).

- Available data do not suggest clear superiority of any one of the three cholinesterase inhibitors currently in wide use (donepezil, galantamine, rivastigmine).

- Limited data on CSF biomarkers in AD compared to other neurodegenerative dementias with pathological confirmation suggest that combined use of β-amyloid 42 and p-tau levels yields a sensitivity of over 95% and a specificity of over 80% (Schoonenboom et al., 2012).

- Combination therapy with both a cholinesterase inhibitor and memantine appears to provide benefit beyond treatment with just a cholinesterase inhibitor (Atri, Shaughnessy, Locascio, & Growdon, 2008). Potential side effects of memantine include dizziness, headache, GI side effects, hypertension, and confusion.

- Examination of patients with posterior cortical atrophy (PCA) commonly reveals elements of the syndromes of Bálint (simultagnosia, optic ataxia, and oculomotor apraxia) and Gerstmann (agraphia, acalculia, left-right confusion, and finger agnosia[16]). Impairments in executive functions, language, and memory are variable early in the course of illness, but memory storage is frequently preserved. PCA patients commonly report visual hallucinations and/or positive perceptual phenomena, including color after-images, reverse size phenomena, perception of movement of static stimuli, and visual crowding (Crutch et al., 2012). Treatment for depression, anxiety, and Parkinsonism may provide benefit in some cases.

---

16. Finger agnosia, defined as an inability to distinguish, name, or recognize fingers, usually occurs in the setting of a more generalized disturbance in awareness of body parts and their orientation, and is also associated with disturbances in balance and/or dressing apraxia.

- The cognitive profile of both PDD and DLB usually involves early dysfunction in complex attention, executive functions, and visuospatial processing (Bradshaw, Saling, Anderson, Hopwood, & Brodtmann, 2006; Mosimann et al., 2004). Fluctuations in attention, alertness, or cognition of varying intensity and duration are considered to be a *core* feature of DLB (present in 50–75% of cases), but are also observed frequently in PDD (McKeith et al., 2005).[17] The other two core features of DLB are visual hallucinations that are often vivid, three-dimensional hallucinations of animate objects, and parkinsonism.

- Additional features that may be present in both DLB and PDD (but that are more commonly present in DLB) include REM sleep behavior disorder, severe sensitivity to neuroleptic medications, and autonomic dysfunction.

- Unlike most other neurodegenerative dementias, the behavioral-variant of frontotemporal dementia (bvFTD) produces dramatic early changes in personality, comportment, and demeanor, in the form of apathy, disinhibition, stereotyped or stimulus-bound behaviors, perseveration, mental rigidity, hoarding, loss of empathy, blunted affect, and changes in food preference, typically towards sweet foods. The patient's insight into these cognitive and behavioral changes is typically quite limited.

- Hashimoto encephalopathy (HE) and antibody-associated encephalitis (AAE) are two types of autoimmune illness. HE is defined by cognitive dysfunction in the setting of high titers of anti-thyroid antibodies (anti-thyroid peroxidase, anti-thyroglobulin, or anti-microsomal antibodies), and absence of any other clear etiology for the cognitive dysfunction (Brain, Jellinek, & Ball, 1966; Chong, Rowland, & Utiger, 2003).

- The most common neoplasms associated with paraneoplastic AAE include small-cell lung cancer, germ-cell tumors, thymoma, Hodgkin lymphoma, and breast cancer (Gultekin et al., 2000).

DISCLOSURE STATEMENT

Dr. McGinnis has no conflicts to disclose.

REFERENCES

Aarsland, D., Bronnick, K., Ehrt, U., De Deyn, P. P., Tekin, S., Emre, M., et al. (2007). Neuropsychiatric symptoms in patients with Parkinson's disease and dementia: frequency, profile and associated care giver stress. *Journal of Neurology, Neurosurgery, & Psychiatry, 78*(1), 36–42.

Ahlskog, J. E., Geda, Y. E., Graff-Radford, N. R., & Petersen, R. C. (2011). Physical exercise as a preventive or disease-modifying treatment of dementia and brain aging. *Mayo Clinic Proceedings, 86*(9), 876–884.

Albert, M. L., Feldman, R. G., & Willis, A. L. (1974). The "subcortical dementia" of progressive supranuclear palsy. *Journal of Neurology, Neurosurgery, & Psychiatry, 37*(2), 121–130.

Albert, M. S., DeKosky, S. T., Dickson, D., Dubois, B., Feldman, H. H., Fox, N. C., et al. (2011). The diagnosis of mild cognitive impairment due to Alzheimer's disease: recommendations from the National Institute on Aging–Alzheimer's Association workgroups on diagnostic guidelines for Alzheimer's disease. *Alzheimer's Dementia, 7*(3), 270–279.

Alladi, S., Xuereb, J., Bak, T., Nestor, P., Knibb, J., Patterson, K., et al. (2007). Focal cortical presentations of Alzheimer's disease. *Brain, 130*(Pt 10), 2636–2645.

Aloia, M. S., Arnedt, J. T., Davis, J. D., Riggs, R. L., & Byrd, D. (2004). Neuropsychological sequelae of obstructive sleep apnea-hypopnea syndrome: a critical review. *Journal of the International Neuropsychological Society, 10*(5), 772–785.

Atri, A., Shaughnessy, L. W., Locascio, J. J., & Growdon, J. H. (2008). Long-term course and effectiveness of combination therapy in Alzheimer disease. *Alzheimer's Disease & Associated Disorders, 22*(3), 209–221.

Balasa, M., Gelpi, E., Antonell, A., Rey, M. J., Sanchez-Valle, R., Molinuevo, J. L., et al. (2011). Clinical features and APOE genotype of pathologically proven early-onset Alzheimer disease. *Neurology, 76*(20), 1720–1725.

Ballard, C. G., O'Brien, J. T., Reichelt, K., & Perry, E. K. (2002). Aromatherapy as a safe and effective treatment for the management of agitation in severe dementia: the results of a double-blind, placebo-controlled trial with Melissa. *Journal of Clinical Psychiatry, 63*(7), 553–558.

Ballard, C., & Corbett, A. (2010). Management of neuropsychiatric symptoms in people with dementia. *Central Nervous System Drugs, 24*(9), 729–739.

Banerjee, S., Hellier, J., Dewey, M., Romeo, R., Ballard, C., Baldwin, R., et al. (2011). Sertraline or mirtazapine for depression in dementia (HTA-SADD): a randomised, multicentre, double-blind, placebo-controlled trial. *Lancet, 378*(9789), 403–411.

Bataller, L., Kleopa, K. A., Wu, G. F., Rossi, J. E., Rosenfeld, M. R., & Dalmau, J. (2007). Autoimmune limbic encephalitis in 39 patients: immunophenotypes and outcomes. *Journal of Neurology, Neurosurgery, & Psychiatry, 78*(4), 381–385.

Bentley, P., Driver, J., & Dolan, R. J. (2011). Cholinergic modulation of cognition: insights from human pharmacological functional neuroimaging. *Progress in Neurobiology, 94*(4), 360–388.

Berman, K., Brodaty, H., Withall, A., & Seeher, K. (2012). Pharmacologic treatment of apathy in dementia. *American Journal of Geriatric Psychiatry, 20*(2), 104–122.

Bero, A. W., Yan, P., Roh, J. H., Cirrito, J. R., Stewart, F. R., Raichle, M. E., et al. (2011). Neuronal activity regulates the regional vulnerability to amyloid-beta deposition. *Nature Neuroscience, 14*(6), 750–756.

Bird, T. D. (2008). Genetic aspects of Alzheimer disease. *Genetics in Medicine, 10*(4), 231–239.

Boxer, A. L., Geschwind, M. D., Belfor, N., Gorno-Tempini, M. L., Schauer, G. F., Miller, B. L., et al. (2006). Patterns of brain atrophy that differentiate corticobasal degeneration syndrome from progressive supranuclear palsy. *Archives of Neurology, 63*(1), 81–86.

Boxer, A. L., Lipton, A. M., Womack, K., Merrilees, J., Neuhaus, J., Pavlic, D., et al. (2009). An open-label study of memantine treatment in 3 subtypes of frontotemporal lobar degeneration. *Alzheimer's Disease & Associated Disorders, 23*(3), 211–217.

Braak, H., & Braak, E. (1991). Neuropathological staging of Alzheimer-related changes. *Acta Neuropathologica, 82*(4), 239–259.

Braak, H., Del Tredici, K., Rub, U., de Vos, R. A., Jansen Steur, E. N., & Braak, E. (2003). Staging of brain pathology related to sporadic Parkinson's disease. *Neurobiology of Aging, 24*(2), 197–211.

---

17. The third report of the DLB Consortium outlines clinical criteria for the diagnosis of "probable DLB" and "possible DLB" (McKeith et al., 2005).

Bradshaw, J. M., Saling, M., Anderson, V., Hopwood, M., & Brodtmann, A. (2006). Higher cortical deficits influence attentional processing in dementia with Lewy bodies, relative to patients with dementia of the Alzheimer's type and controls. *Journal of Neurology, Neurosurgery, & Psychiatry*, 77(10), 1129–1135.

Brain, L., Jellinek, E. H., & Ball, K. (1966). Hashimoto's disease and encephalopathy. *Lancet*, 2(7462), 512–514.

Brodaty, H. (2011). Antidepressant treatment in Alzheimer's disease. *Lancet*, 378(9789), 375–376.

Buckner, R. L., Snyder, A. Z., Shannon, B. J., LaRossa, G., Sachs, R., Fotenos, A. F., et al. (2005). Molecular, structural, and functional characterization of Alzheimer's disease: evidence for a relationship between default activity, amyloid, and memory. *Journal of Neuroscience*, 25(34), 7709–7717.

Budson, A. E., & Price, B. H. (2005). Memory dysfunction. *New England Journal of Medicine*, 352(7), 692–699.

Burke, R. E., Dauer, W. T., & Vonsattel, J. P. (2008). A critical evaluation of the Braak staging scheme for Parkinson's disease. *Annals of Neurology*, 64(5), 485–491.

Burn, D. J., Rowan, E. N., Allan, L. M., Molloy, S., O'Brien, J. T., & McKeith, I. G. (2006). Motor subtype and cognitive decline in Parkinson's disease, Parkinson's disease with dementia, and dementia with Lewy bodies. *Journal of Neurology, Neurosurgery, & Psychiatry*, 77(5), 585–589.

Buschert, V., Bokde, A. L., & Hampel, H. (2010). Cognitive intervention in Alzheimer disease. *Nature Reviews Neurology*, 6(9), 508–517.

Campion, D., Dumanchin, C., Hannequin, D., Dubois, B., Belliard, S., Puel, M., et al. (1999). Early-onset autosomal dominant Alzheimer disease: prevalence, genetic heterogeneity, and mutation spectrum. *American Journal of Human Genetics*, 65(3), 664–670.

Caselli, R. J., Boeve, B. F., Scheithauer, B. W., O'Duffy, J. D., & Hunder, G. G. (1999). Nonvasculitic autoimmune inflammatory meningoencephalitis (NAIM): a reversible form of encephalopathy. *Neurology*, 53(7), 1579–1581.

Castillo, P., Woodruff, B., Caselli, R., Vernino, S., Lucchinetti, C., Swanson, J., et al. (2006). Steroid-responsive encephalopathy associated with autoimmune thyroiditis. *Archives of Neurology*, 63(2), 197–202.

Chan, D., Anderson, V., Pijnenburg, Y., Whitwell, J., Barnes, J., Scahill, R., et al. (2009). The clinical profile of right temporal lobe atrophy. *Brain*, 132(Pt 5), 1287–1298.

Chong, J. Y., Rowland, L. P., & Utiger, R. D. (2003). Hashimoto encephalopathy: syndrome or myth? *Archives of Neurology*, 60(2), 164–171.

Citron, M. (2010). Alzheimer's disease: strategies for disease modification. *Nature Reviews Drug Discovery*, 9(5), 387–398.

Collins, S. J., Sanchez-Juan, P., Masters, C. L., Klug, G. M., van Duijn, C., Poleggi, A., et al. (2006). Determinants of diagnostic investigation sensitivities across the clinical spectrum of sporadic Creutzfeldt-Jakob disease. *Brain*, 129(Pt 9), 2278–2287.

Corrada, M. M., Brookmeyer, R., Paganini-Hill, A., Berlau, D., & Kawas, C. H. (2010). Dementia incidence continues to increase with age in the oldest old: the 90+ study. *Annals of Neurology*, 67(1), 114–121.

Crutch, S. J., Lehmann, M., Schott, J. M., Rabinovici, G. D., Rossor, M. N., & Fox, N. C. (2012). Posterior cortical atrophy. *Lancet Neurology*, 11(2), 170–178.

Cummings, J. L. (1993). Frontal-subcortical circuits and human behavior. *Archives of Neurology*, 50(8), 873–880.

Daffner, K. R., Sherman, J. C., Gonzalez, R. G., & Hasserjian, R. P. (2008). Case records of the Massachusetts General Hospital. Case 35-2008. A 65-year-old man with confusion and memory loss. *New England Journal of Medicine*, 359(20), 2155–2164.

Davies, R. R., Kipps, C. M., Mitchell, J., Kril, J. J., Halliday, G. M., & Hodges, J. R. (2006). Progression in frontotemporal dementia: identifying a benign behavioral variant by magnetic resonance imaging. *Archives of Neurology*, 63(11), 1627–1631.

Devous, M. D., Sr. (2002). Functional brain imaging in the dementias: role in early detection, differential diagnosis, and longitudinal studies. *European Journal of Nuclear Medicine & Molecular Imaging*, 29(12), 1685–1696.

Dolder, C. R., Davis, L. N., & McKinsey, J. (2010). Use of psychostimulants in patients with dementia. *Annals of Pharmacotherapy*, 44(10), 1624–1632.

Doody, R. S., Pavlik, V., Massman, P., Rountree, S., Darby, E., & Chan, W. (2010). Predicting progression of Alzheimer's disease. *Alzheimer's Research & Therapy*, 2(1), 2.

Emre, M., Tsolaki, M., Bonuccelli, U., Destee, A., Tolosa, E., Kutzelnigg, A., et al. (2010). Memantine for patients with Parkinson's disease dementia or dementia with Lewy bodies: a randomised, double-blind, placebo-controlled trial. *Lancet Neurology*, 9(10), 969–977.

Ferri, C. P., Prince, M., Brayne, C., Brodaty, H., Fratiglioni, L., Ganguli, M., et al. (2005). Global prevalence of dementia: a Delphi consensus study. *Lancet*, 366(9503), 2112–2117.

Flanagan, E. P., McKeon, A., Lennon, V. A., Boeve, B. F., Trenerry, M. R., Tan, K. M., et al. (2010). Autoimmune dementia: clinical course and predictors of immunotherapy response. *Mayo Clinic Proceedings*, 85(10), 881–897.

Fleminger, S., Oliver, D. L., Lovestone, S., Rabe-Hesketh, S., & Giora, A. (2003). Head injury as a risk factor for Alzheimer's disease: the evidence 10 years on; a partial replication. *Journal of Neurology, Neurosurgery, & Psychiatry*, 74(7), 857–862.

Folstein, M. F., Folstein, S. E., & McHugh, P. R. (1975). "Mini-mental state": A practical method for grading the cognitive state of patients for the clinician. *Journal of Psychiatric Research*, 12(3), 189–198.

Fratiglioni, L., Launer, L. J., Andersen, K., Breteler, M. M., Copeland, J. R., Dartigues, J. F., et al. (2000). Incidence of dementia and major subtypes in Europe: A collaborative study of population-based cohorts. Neurologic Diseases in the Elderly Research Group. *Neurology*, 54(11 Suppl 5), S10–S15.

Friedman, D., Honig, L. S., & Scarmeas, N. (2011). Seizures and epilepsy in Alzheimer's disease. *Central Nervous System Neuroscience & Therapeutics*, 18(4), 285–294.

Garre-Olmo, J., Genis Batlle, D., del Mar Fernandez, M., Marquez Daniel, F., de Eugenio Huelamo, R., Casadevall, T., et al. (2010). Incidence and subtypes of early-onset dementia in a geographically defined general population. *Neurology*, 75(14), 1249–1255.

Gauthier, S., Loft, H., & Cummings, J. (2008). Improvement in behavioural symptoms in patients with moderate to severe Alzheimer's disease by memantine: a pooled data analysis. *International Journal of Geriatric Psychiatry*, 23(5), 537–545.

Gearing, M., Mirra, S. S., Hedreen, J. C., Sumi, S. M., Hansen, L. A., & Heyman, A. (1995). The Consortium to Establish a Registry for Alzheimer's Disease (CERAD). Part X: Neuropathology confirmation of the clinical diagnosis of Alzheimer's disease. *Neurology*, 45(3 Pt 1), 461–466.

Geschwind, M. D., Shu, H., Haman, A., Sejvar, J. J., & Miller, B. L. (2008). Rapidly progressive dementia. *Annals of Neurology*, 64(1), 97–108.

Ghosh, A. (2010). Endocrine, metabolic, nutritional, and toxic disorders leading to dementia. *Annals of the Indian Academy of Neurology*, 13, S63–S68.

Gleichgerrcht, E., Ibanez, A., Roca, M., Torralva, T., & Manes, F. (2010). Decision-making cognition in neurodegenerative diseases. *Nature Reviews Neurology*, 6(11), 611–623.

Golbe, L. I., & Ohman-Strickland, P. A. (2007). A clinical rating scale for progressive supranuclear palsy. *Brain*, 130(Pt 6), 1552–1565.

Gold, G., Bouras, C., Canuto, A., Bergallo, M. F., Herrmann, F. R., Hof, P. R., et al. (2002). Clinicopathological validation study of four sets of clinical criteria for vascular dementia. *American Journal of Psychiatry*, 159(1), 82–87.

Goldman, J. S., Hahn, S. E., Catania, J. W., LaRusse-Eckert, S., Butson, M. B., Rumbaugh, M., et al. (2011). Genetic counseling and testing for Alzheimer disease: joint practice guidelines of the American College of Medical Genetics and the National Society of Genetic Counselors. *Genetics in Medicine*, 13(6), 597–605.

Gorno-Tempini, M. L., Dronkers, N. F., Rankin, K. P., Ogar, J. M., Phengrasamy, L., Rosen, H. J., et al. (2004). Cognition and anatomy in three variants of primary progressive aphasia. *Annals of Neurology*, 55(3), 335–346.

Gorno-Tempini, M. L., Hillis, A. E., Weintraub, S., Kertesz, A., Mendez, M., Cappa, S. F., et al. (2011). Classification of primary progressive aphasia and its variants. *Neurology, 76*(11), 1006–1014.

Grossman, M. (2010). Primary progressive aphasia: clinicopathological correlations. *Nature Reviews Neurology, 6*(2), 88–97.

Grossman, M., Libon, D. J., Forman, M. S., Massimo, L., Wood, E., Moore, P., et al. (2007). Distinct antemortem profiles in patients with pathologically defined frontotemporal dementia. *Archives of Neurology, 64*(11), 1601–1609.

Gultekin, S. H., Rosenfeld, M. R., Voltz, R., Eichen, J., Posner, J. B., & Dalmau, J. (2000). Paraneoplastic limbic encephalitis: neurological symptoms, immunological findings and tumour association in 50 patients. *Brain, 123*(Pt 7), 1481–1494.

Hachinski, V., Iadecola, C., Petersen, R. C., Breteler, M. M., Nyenhuis, D. L., Black, S. E., et al. (2006). National Institute of Neurological Disorders and Stroke–Canadian Stroke Network vascular cognitive impairment harmonization standards. *Stroke, 37*(9), 2220–2241.

Hardy, J., & Selkoe, D. J. (2002). The amyloid hypothesis of Alzheimer's disease: progress and problems on the road to therapeutics. *Science, 297*(5580), 353–356.

Hebert, L. E., Scherr, P. A., Bienias, J. L., Bennett, D. A., & Evans, D. A. (2003). Alzheimer disease in the US population: prevalence estimates using the 2000 Census. *Archives of Neurology, 60*(8), 1119–1122.

Herrup, K. (2010). Reimagining Alzheimer's disease—an age-based hypothesis. *Journal of Neuroscience, 30*(50), 16755–16762.

Hickok, G., & Poeppel, D. (2007). The cortical organization of speech processing. *Nature Reviews Neuroscience, 8*(5), 393–402.

Hyman, B. T., & Trojanowski, J. Q. (1997). Consensus recommendations for the postmortem diagnosis of Alzheimer disease from the National Institute on Aging and the Reagan Institute Working Group on diagnostic criteria for the neuropathological assessment of Alzheimer disease. *Journal of Neuropathology & Experimental Neurology, 56*(10), 1095–1097.

Hyman, B. T., Phelps, C. H., Beach, T. G., Bigio, E. H., Cairns, N. J., Carrillo, M. C., et al. (2012). National Institute on Aging–Alzheimer's Association guidelines for the neuropathologic assessment of Alzheimer's disease. *Alzheimer's Dementia, 8*(1), 1–13.

Iranzo, A., Molinuevo, J. L., Santamaria, J., Serradell, M., Marti, M. J., Valldeoriola, F., et al. (2006). Rapid-eye-movement sleep behaviour disorder as an early marker for a neurodegenerative disorder: a descriptive study. *Lancet Neurology, 5*(7), 572–577.

Iverson, D. J., Gronseth, G. S., Reger, M. A., Classen, S., Dubinsky, R. M., & Rizzo, M. (2010). Practice parameter update: evaluation and management of driving risk in dementia: report of the Quality Standards Subcommittee of the American Academy of Neurology. *Neurology, 74*(16), 1316–1324.

Jack, C. R., Jr., Knopman, D. S., Jagust, W. J., Shaw, L. M., Aisen, P. S., Weiner, M. W., et al. (2010). Hypothetical model of dynamic biomarkers of the Alzheimer's pathological cascade. *Lancet Neurology, 9*(1), 119–128.

Jack, C. R., Jr., Shiung, M. M., Gunter, J. L., O'Brien, P. C., Weigand, S. D., Knopman, D. S., et al. (2004). Comparison of different MRI brain atrophy rate measures with clinical disease progression in AD. *Neurology, 62*(4), 591–600.

James, B. D., Wilson, R. S., Barnes, L. L., & Bennett, D. A. (2011). Late-life social activity and cognitive decline in old age. *Journal of the International Neuropsychological Society, 17*(6), 998–1005.

Jellinger, K. A. (2008). A critical reappraisal of current staging of Lewy-related pathology in human brain. *Acta Neuropathologica, 116*(1), 1–16.

Jellinger, K., Danielczyk, W., Fischer, P., & Gabriel, E. (1990). Clinicopathological analysis of dementia disorders in the elderly. *Journal of the Neurological Sciences, 95*(3), 239–258.

Johnson, N. A., Rademaker, A., Weintraub, S., Gitelman, D., Wienecke, C., & Mesulam, M. (2010). Pilot trial of memantine in primary progressive aphasia. *Alzheimer's Disease & Associated Disorders, 24*(3), 308.

Jorm, A. F., & Jolley, D. (1998). The incidence of dementia: a meta-analysis. *Neurology, 51*(3), 728–733.

Josephs, K. A., Ahlskog, J. E., Parisi, J. E., Boeve, B. F., Crum, B. A., Giannini, C., et al. (2009). Rapidly progressive neurodegenerative dementias. *Archives of Neurology, 66*(2), 201–207.

Josephs, K. A., Duffy, J. R., Strand, E. A., Whitwell, J. L., Layton, K. F., Parisi, J. E., et al. (2006). Clinicopathological and imaging correlates of progressive aphasia and apraxia of speech. *Brain, 129*(Pt 6), 1385–1398.

Josephs, K. A., Hodges, J. R., Snowden, J. S., Mackenzie, I. R., Neumann, M., Mann, D. M., et al. (2011). Neuropathological background of phenotypical variability in frontotemporal dementia. *Acta Neuropathologica, 122*(2), 137–153.

Josephs, K. A., Petersen, R. C., Knopman, D. S., Boeve, B. F., Whitwell, J. L., Duffy, J. R., et al. (2006). Clinicopathologic analysis of frontotemporal and corticobasal degenerations and PSP. *Neurology, 66*(1), 41–48.

Josephs, K. A., Whitwell, J. L., Dickson, D. W., Boeve, B. F., Knopman, D. S., Petersen, R. C., et al. (2008). Voxel-based morphometry in autopsy proven PSP and CBD. *Neurobiology of Aging, 29*(2), 280–289.

Josephs, K. A., Whitwell, J. L., Knopman, D. S., Boeve, B. F., Vemuri, P., Senjem, M. L., et al. (2009). Two distinct subtypes of right temporal variant frontotemporal dementia. *Neurology, 73*(18), 1443–1450.

Josephson, S. A., Papanastassiou, A. M., Berger, M. S., Barbaro, N. M., McDermott, M. W., Hilton, J. F., et al. (2007). The diagnostic utility of brain biopsy procedures in patients with rapidly deteriorating neurological conditions or dementia. *Journal of Neurosurgery, 106*(1), 72–75.

Jost, B. C., & Grossberg, G. T. (1996). The evolution of psychiatric symptoms in Alzheimer's disease: a natural history study. *Journal of the American Geriatric Society, 44*(9), 1078–1081.

Kanda, T., Ishii, K., Uemura, T., Miyamoto, N., Yoshikawa, T., Kono, A. K., et al. (2008). Comparison of grey matter and metabolic reductions in frontotemporal dementia using FDG-PET and voxel-based morphometric MR studies. *European Journal of Nuclear Medicine & Molecular Imaging, 35*(12), 2227–2234.

Kannarkat, G., Lasher, E. E., & Schiff, D. (2007). Neurologic complications of chemotherapy agents. *Current Opinion in Neurology, 20*(6), 719–725.

Kantarci, K., Lowe, V. J., Boeve, B. F., Weigand, S. D., Senjem, M. L., Przybelski, S. A., et al. (2012). Multimodality imaging characteristics of dementia with Lewy bodies. *Neurobiology of Aging, 33*(9), 2091–2105.

Kavirajan, H., & Schneider, L. S. (2007). Efficacy and adverse effects of cholinesterase inhibitors and memantine in vascular dementia: a meta-analysis of randomised controlled trials. *Lancet Neurology, 6*(9), 782–792.

Kertesz, A., McMonagle, P., Blair, M., Davidson, W., & Munoz, D. G. (2005). The evolution and pathology of frontotemporal dementia. *Brain, 128*(Pt 9), 1996–2005.

Kertesz, A., Morlog, D., Light, M., Blair, M., Davidson, W., Jesso, S., et al. (2008). Galantamine in frontotemporal dementia and primary progressive aphasia. *Dementia & Geriatric Cognitive Disorders, 25*(2), 178–185.

Khachaturian, A. S., Corcoran, C. D., Mayer, L. S., Zandi, P. P., & Breitner, J. C. (2004). Apolipoprotein E epsilon4 count affects age at onset of Alzheimer disease, but not lifetime susceptibility: The Cache County Study. *Archives of General Psychiatry, 61*(5), 518–524.

Khachaturian, Z. S. (1985). Diagnosis of Alzheimer's disease. *Archives of Neurology, 42*(11), 1097–1105.

Knopman, D. S., Boeve, B. F., Parisi, J. E., Dickson, D. W., Smith, G. E., Ivnik, R. J., et al. (2005). Antemortem diagnosis of frontotemporal lobar degeneration. *Annals of Neurology, 57*(4), 480–488.

Knopman, D. S., DeKosky, S. T., Cummings, J. L., Chui, H., Corey-Bloom, J., Relkin, N., et al. (2001). Practice parameter: diagnosis of dementia (an evidence-based review). Report of the Quality Standards Subcommittee of the American Academy of Neurology. *Neurology, 56*(9), 1143–1153.

Koedam, E. L., Lauffer, V., van der Vlies, A. E., van der Flier, W. M., Scheltens, P., & Pijnenburg, Y. A. (2010). Early-versus late-onset

Alzheimer's disease: more than age alone. *Journal of Alzheimer's Disease, 19*(4), 1401–1408.

Kohno, N., Abe, S., Toyoda, G., Oguro, H., Bokura, H., & Yamaguchi, S. (2010). Successful treatment of post-stroke apathy by the dopamine receptor agonist ropinirole. *Journal of Clinical Neuroscience, 17*(6), 804–806.

Kokmen, E., Naessens, J. M., & Offord, K. P. (1987). A short test of mental status: description and preliminary results. *Mayo Clinic Proceedings, 62*(4), 281–288.

Kouri, N., Whitwell, J. L., Josephs, K. A., Rademakers, R., & Dickson, D. W. (2011). Corticobasal degeneration: a pathologically distinct 4R tauopathy. *Nature Reviews Neurology, 7*(5), 263–272.

Ladogana, A., Puopolo, M., Croes, E. A., Budka, H., Jarius, C., Collins, S., et al. (2005). Mortality from Creutzfeldt-Jakob disease and related disorders in Europe, Australia, and Canada. *Neurology, 64*(9), 1586–1591.

Litvan, I., Mega, M. S., Cummings, J. L., & Fairbanks, L. (1996). Neuropsychiatric aspects of progressive supranuclear palsy. *Neurology, 47*(5), 1184–1189.

Liu, L., Drouet, V., Wu, J. W., Witter, M. P., Small, S. A., Clelland, C., et al. (2012). Trans-synaptic spread of tau pathology in vivo. *PLoS One, 7*(2), e31302.

Lobo, A., Launer, L. J., Fratiglioni, L., Andersen, K., Di Carlo, A., Breteler, M. M., et al. (2000). Prevalence of dementia and major subtypes in Europe: A collaborative study of population-based cohorts. Neurologic Diseases in the Elderly Research Group. *Neurology, 54*(11 Suppl 5), S4–S9.

Lyketsos, C. G., Carrillo, M. C., Ryan, J. M., Khachaturian, A. S., Trzepacz, P., Amatniek, J., et al. (2011). Neuropsychiatric symptoms in Alzheimer's disease. *Alzheimer's Dementia, 7*(5), 532–539.

Lyons, M. K., Caselli, R. J., & Parisi, J. E. (2008). Nonvasculitic autoimmune inflammatory meningoencephalitis as a cause of potentially reversible dementia: report of 4 cases. *Journal of Neurosurgery, 108*(5), 1024–1027.

Marshall, G. A., & Doyle, J. J. (2006). Long-term treatment of Hashimoto's encephalopathy. *Journal of Neuropsychiatry & Clinical Neurosciences, 18*(1), 14–20.

Mayeux, R., Saunders, A. M., Shea, S., Mirra, S., Evans, D., Roses, A. D., et al. (1998). Utility of the apolipoprotein E genotype in the diagnosis of Alzheimer's disease. Alzheimer's Disease Centers Consortium on Apolipoprotein E and Alzheimer's Disease. *New England Journal of Medicine, 338*(8), 506–511.

McDaniel, K. D., Edland, S. D., & Heyman, A. (1995). Relationship between level of insight and severity of dementia in Alzheimer disease. CERAD Clinical Investigators. Consortium to Establish a Registry for Alzheimer's Disease. *Alzheimer's Disease & Associated Disorders, 9*(2), 101–104.

McGinnis, S. M. (2011). Infectious causes of rapidly progressive dementia. *Seminars in Neurology, 31*(3), 266–285.

McKeith, I. G., Dickson, D. W., Lowe, J., Emre, M., O'Brien, J. T., Feldman, H., et al. (2005). Diagnosis and management of dementia with Lewy bodies: third report of the DLB Consortium. *Neurology, 65*(12), 1863–1872.

McKeith, I., Del Ser, T., Spano, P., Emre, M., Wesnes, K., Anand, R., et al. (2000). Efficacy of rivastigmine in dementia with Lewy bodies: a randomised, double-blind, placebo-controlled international study. *Lancet, 356*(9247), 2031–2036.

McKeith, I., Mintzer, J., Aarsland, D., Burn, D., Chiu, H., Cohen-Mansfield, J., et al. (2004). Dementia with Lewy bodies. *Lancet Neurology, 3*(1), 19–28.

McKeith, I., O'Brien, J., Walker, Z., Tatsch, K., Booij, J., Darcourt, J., et al. (2007). Sensitivity and specificity of dopamine transporter imaging with 123I-FP-CIT SPECT in dementia with Lewy bodies: a phase III, multicentre study. *Lancet Neurology, 6*(4), 305–313.

McKhann, G. M., Knopman, D. S., Chertkow, H., Hyman, B. T., Jack, C. R., Jr., Kawas, C. H., et al. (2011). The diagnosis of dementia due to Alzheimer's disease: recommendations from the National Institute on Aging-Alzheimer's Association workgroups on diagnostic guidelines for Alzheimer's disease. *Alzheimer's Dementia, 7*(3), 263–269.

Mendelson, W. B. (2005). A review of the evidence for the efficacy and safety of trazodone in insomnia. *Journal of Clinical Psychiatry, 66*(4), 469–476.

Mendez, M. F. (2009). Frontotemporal dementia: therapeutic interventions. *Frontiers of Neurology & Neuroscience, 24*, 168–178.

Mendez, M. F., Ghajarania, M., & Perryman, K. M. (2002). Posterior cortical atrophy: clinical characteristics and differences compared to Alzheimer's disease. *Dementia & Geriatric Cognitive Disorders, 14*(1), 33–40.

Mesulam, M. (2008). Primary progressive aphasia pathology. *Annals of Neurology, 63*(1), 124–125.

Mesulam, M. M. (2000). *Principles of behavioral and cognitive neurology* (2nd ed.). Oxford; New York: Oxford University Press.

Mesulam, M. M. (2001). Primary progressive aphasia. *Annals of Neurology, 49*(4), 425–432.

Millan, M. J., Agid, Y., Brune, M., Bullmore, E. T., Carter, C. S., Clayton, N. S., et al. (2012). Cognitive dysfunction in psychiatric disorders: characteristics, causes and the quest for improved therapy. *Nature Reviews Drug Discovery, 11*(2), 141–168.

Mioshi, E., Dawson, K., Mitchell, J., Arnold, R., & Hodges, J. R. (2006). The Addenbrooke's Cognitive Examination–Revised (ACE-R): a brief cognitive test battery for dementia screening. *International Journal of Geriatric Psychiatry, 21*(11), 1078–1085.

Molloy, S., McKeith, I. G., O'Brien, J. T., & Burn, D. J. (2005). The role of levodopa in the management of dementia with Lewy bodies. *Journal of Neurology, Neurosurgery, & Psychiatry, 76*(9), 1200–1203.

Moorhouse, P., & Rockwood, K. (2008). Vascular cognitive impairment: current concepts and clinical developments. *Lancet Neurology, 7*(3), 246–255.

Morris, J. C. (2005). Early-stage and preclinical Alzheimer disease. *Alzheimer's Disease & Associated Disorders, 19*(3), 163–165.

Morris, J. C., Ernesto, C., Schafer, K., Coats, M., Leon, S., Sano, M., et al. (1997). Clinical dementia rating training and reliability in multicenter studies: the Alzheimer's Disease Cooperative Study experience. *Neurology, 48*(6), 1508–1510.

Mosimann, U. P., Mather, G., Wesnes, K. A., O'Brien, J. T., Burn, D. J., & McKeith, I. G. (2004). Visual perception in Parkinson disease dementia and dementia with Lewy bodies. *Neurology, 63*(11), 2091–2096.

Murray, R., Neumann, M., Forman, M. S., Farmer, J., Massimo, L., Rice, A., et al. (2007). Cognitive and motor assessment in autopsy-proven corticobasal degeneration. *Neurology, 68*(16), 1274–1283.

Nasreddine, Z. S., Phillips, N. A., Bedirian, V., Charbonneau, S., Whitehead, V., Collin, I., et al. (2005). The Montreal Cognitive Assessment, MoCA: a brief screening tool for mild cognitive impairment. *Journal of the American Geriatric Society, 53*(4), 695–699.

O'Brien, J. T. (2007). Role of imaging techniques in the diagnosis of dementia. *British Journal of Radiology, 80* (Spec No 2), S71–S77.

Parchi, P., Giese, A., Capellari, S., Brown, P., Schulz-Schaeffer, W., Windl, O., et al. (1999). Classification of sporadic Creutzfeldt-Jakob disease based on molecular and phenotypic analysis of 300 subjects. *Annals of Neurology, 46*(2), 224–233.

Paulson, H. L., Igo, I. (2011). Genetics of dementia. *Seminars in Neurology, 31*(5), 449–460.

Petersen, R. C. (2004). Mild cognitive impairment as a diagnostic entity. *Journal of Internal Medicine, 256*(3), 183–194.

Petersen, R. C. (2011). Clinical practice. Mild cognitive impairment. *New England Journal of Medicine, 364*(23), 2227–2234.

Picard, C., Pasquier, F., Martinaud, O., Hannequin, D., & Godefroy, O. (2011). Early onset dementia: characteristics in a large cohort from academic memory clinics. *Alzheimer's Disease & Associated Disorders, 25*(3), 203–205.

Pievani, M., de Haan, W., Wu, T., Seeley, W. W., & Frisoni, G. B. (2011). Functional network disruption in the degenerative dementias. *Lancet Neurology, 10*(9), 829–843.

Piguet, O., Hornberger, M., Mioshi, E., & Hodges, J. R. (2011). Behavioural-variant frontotemporal dementia: diagnosis, clinical staging, and management. *Lancet Neurology, 10*(2), 162–172.

Pimplikar, S. W., Nixon, R. A., Robakis, N. K., Shen, J., & Tsai, L. H. (2010). Amyloid-independent mechanisms in Alzheimer's disease pathogenesis. *Journal of Neuroscience, 30*(45), 14946–14954.

Pollock, B. G., Mulsant, B. H., Rosen, J., Mazumdar, S., Blakesley, R. E., Houck, P. R., et al. (2007). A double-blind comparison of citalopram and risperidone for the treatment of behavioral and psychotic symptoms associated with dementia. *American Journal of Geriatric Psychiatry, 15*(11), 942–952.

Portet, F., Scarmeas, N., Cosentino, S., Helzner, E. P., & Stern, Y. (2009). Extrapyramidal signs before and after diagnosis of incident Alzheimer disease in a prospective population study. *Archives of Neurology, 66*(9), 1120–1126.

Potter, R., Ellard, D., Rees, K., & Thorogood, M. (2011). A systematic review of the effects of physical activity on physical functioning, quality of life and depression in older people with dementia. *International Journal of Geriatric Psychiatry, 26*(10), 1000–1011.

Profenno, L. A., Porsteinsson, A. P., & Faraone, S. V. (2010). Meta-analysis of Alzheimer's disease risk with obesity, diabetes, and related disorders. *Biological Psychiatry, 67*(6), 505–512.

Prusiner, S. B. (1998). Prions. *Proceedings of the National Academy of Sciences, USA, 95*(23), 13363–13383.

Rafii, M. S., & Aisen, P. S. (2009). Recent developments in Alzheimer's disease therapeutics. *BioMed Central Medicine, 7,* 7.

Raina, P., Santaguida, P., Ismaila, A., Patterson, C., Cowan, D., Levine, M., et al. (2008). Effectiveness of cholinesterase inhibitors and memantine for treating dementia: evidence review for a clinical practice guideline. *Annals of Internal Medicine, 148*(5), 379–397.

Raschetti, R., Albanese, E., Vanacore, N., & Maggini, M. (2007). Cholinesterase inhibitors in mild cognitive impairment: a systematic review of randomised trials. *PLoS Medicine, 4*(11), e338.

Rascovsky, K., Hodges, J. R., Kipps, C. M., Johnson, J. K., Seeley, W. W., Mendez, M. F., et al. (2007). Diagnostic criteria for the behavioral variant of frontotemporal dementia (bvFTD): current limitations and future directions. *Alzheimer's Disease & Associated Disorders, 21*(4), S14–S18.

Rebeiz, J. J., Kolodny, E. H., & Richardson, E. P., Jr. (1968). Corticodentatonigral degeneration with neuronal achromasia. *Archives of Neurology, 18*(1), 20–33.

Reed, B. R., Mungas, D. M., Kramer, J. H., Ellis, W., Vinters, H. V., Zarow, C., et al. (2007). Profiles of neuropsychological impairment in autopsy-defined Alzheimer's disease and cerebrovascular disease. *Brain, 130*(Pt 3), 731–739.

Riedijk, S. R., De Vugt, M. E., Duivenvoorden, H. J., Niermeijer, M. F., Van Swieten, J. C., Verhey, F. R., et al. (2006). Caregiver burden, health-related quality of life and coping in dementia caregivers: a comparison of frontotemporal dementia and Alzheimer's disease. *Dementia & Geriatric Cognitive Disorders, 22*(5–6), 405–412.

Roman, G. C., Tatemichi, T. K., Erkinjuntti, T., Cummings, J. L., Masdeu, J. C., Garcia, J. H., et al. (1993). Vascular dementia: diagnostic criteria for research studies. Report of the NINDS-AIREN International Workshop. *Neurology, 43*(2), 250–260.

Rosenberg, P. B., Drye, L. T., Martin, B. K., Frangakis, C., Mintzer, J. E., Weintraub, D., et al. (2010). Sertraline for the treatment of depression in Alzheimer disease. *American Journal of Geriatric Psychiatry, 18*(2), 136–145.

Rosenbloom, M. H., Smith, S., Akdal, G., & Geschwind, M. D. (2009). Immunologically mediated dementias. *Current Neurology & Neuroscience Reports, 9*(5), 359–367.

Roth, R. M., Flashman, L. A., & McAllister, T. W. (2007). Apathy and its treatment. *Current Treatment Options in Neurology, 9*(5), 363–370.

Samuel, W., Caligiuri, M., Galasko, D., Lacro, J., Marini, M., McClure, F. S., et al. (2000). Better cognitive and psychopathologic response to donepezil in patients prospectively diagnosed as dementia with Lewy bodies: a preliminary study. *International Journal of Geriatric Psychiatry, 15*(9), 794–802.

Savva, G. M., Wharton, S. B., Ince, P. G., Forster, G., Matthews, F. E., & Brayne, C. (2009). Age, neuropathology, and dementia. *New England Journal of Medicine, 360*(22), 2302–2309.

Schneider, J. A., Arvanitakis, Z., Bang, W., & Bennett, D. A. (2007). Mixed brain pathologies account for most dementia cases in community-dwelling older persons. *Neurology, 69*(24), 2197–2204.

Schoonenboom, N. S., Reesink, F. E., Verwey, N. A., Kester, M. I., Teunissen, C. E., van de Ven, P. M., et al. (2012). Cerebrospinal fluid markers for differential dementia diagnosis in a large memory clinic cohort. *Neurology, 78*(1), 47–54.

Seeley, W. W., Bauer, A. M., Miller, B. L., Gorno-Tempini, M. L., Kramer, J. H., Weiner, M., et al. (2005). The natural history of temporal variant frontotemporal dementia. *Neurology, 64*(8), 1384–1390.

Seeley, W. W., Crawford, R. K., Zhou, J., Miller, B. L., & Greicius, M. D. (2009). Neurodegenerative diseases target large-scale human brain networks. *Neuron, 62*(1), 42–52.

Seeley, W. W., Crawford, R., Rascovsky, K., Kramer, J. H., Weiner, M., Miller, B. L., et al. (2008). Frontal paralimbic network atrophy in very mild behavioral variant frontotemporal dementia. *Archives of Neurology, 65*(2), 249–255.

Serfaty, M., Kennell-Webb, S., Warner, J., Blizard, R., & Raven, P. (2002). Double blind randomised placebo controlled trial of low dose melatonin for sleep disorders in dementia. *International Journal of Geriatric Psychiatry, 17*(12), 1120–1127.

Shankar, G. M., Li, S., Mehta, T. H., Garcia-Munoz, A., Shepardson, N. E., Smith, I., et al. (2008). Amyloid-beta protein dimers isolated directly from Alzheimer's brains impair synaptic plasticity and memory. *Nature Medicine, 14*(8), 837–842.

Shaw, L. M., Vanderstichele, H., Knapik-Czajka, M., Clark, C. M., Aisen, P. S., Petersen, R. C., et al. (2009). Cerebrospinal fluid biomarker signature in Alzheimer's disease neuroimaging initiative subjects. *Annals of Neurology, 65*(4), 403–413.

Shepardson, N. E., Shankar, G. M., & Selkoe, D. J. (2011). Cholesterol level and statin use in Alzheimer disease: I. Review of epidemiological and preclinical studies. *Archives of Neurology, 68*(10), 1239–1244.

Silva, M. T., Laks, J., & Engelhardt, E. (2009). Neuropsychological tests and driving in dementia: a review of the recent literature. *Revista da Associação Médica Brasileira, 55*(4), 484–488.

Singer, C., Tractenberg, R. E., Kaye, J., Schafer, K., Gamst, A., Grundman, M., et al. (2003). A multicenter, placebo-controlled trial of melatonin for sleep disturbance in Alzheimer's disease. *Sleep, 26*(7), 893–901.

Smith, M., Wells, J., & Borrie, M. (2006). Treatment effect size of memantine therapy in Alzheimer disease and vascular dementia. *Alzheimer's Disease & Associated Disorders, 20*(3), 133–137.

Snowden, J., Neary, D., & Mann, D. (2007). Frontotemporal lobar degeneration: clinical and pathological relationships. *Acta Neuropathologica, 114*(1), 31–38.

Solfrizzi, V., Frisardi, V., Seripa, D., Logroscino, G., Imbimbo, B. P., D'Onofrio, G., et al. (2011). Mediterranean diet in predementia and dementia syndromes. *Current Alzheimer Research, 8*(5), 520–542.

Sperling, R. A., Jack, C. R., Jr., & Aisen, P. S. (2011). Testing the right target and right drug at the right stage. *Science Translational Medicine, 3*(111), 1–5.

Stamelou, M., de Silva, R., Arias-Carrion, O., Boura, E., Hollerhage, M., Oertel, W. H., et al. (2010). Rational therapeutic approaches to progressive supranuclear palsy. *Brain, 133*(Pt 6), 1578–1590.

Steele, J. C., Richardson, J. C., & Olszewski, J. (1964). Progressive supranuclear palsy: A heterogeneous degeneration involving the brain stem, basal ganglia and cerebellum with vertical gaze and pseudobulbar palsy, nuchal dystonia and dementia. *Archives of Neurology, 10,* 333–359.

Tariot, P. N., Loy, R., Ryan, J. M., Porsteinsson, A., & Ismail, S. (2002). Mood stabilizers in Alzheimer's disease: symptomatic and neuroprotective rationales. *Advanced Drug Delivery Reviews, 54*(12), 1567–1577.

Thies, W., & Bleiler, L. (2011). 2011 Alzheimer's disease facts and figures. *Alzheimer's Dementia, 7*(2), 208–244.

Thune-Boyle, I. C., Iliffe, S., Cerga-Pashoja, A., Lowery, D., & Warner, J. (2011). The effect of exercise on behavioral and psychological symptoms of dementia: towards a research agenda. *International Psychogeriatrics,* 1–12.

Torralva, T., Roca, M., Gleichgerrcht, E., Bekinschtein, T., & Manes, F. (2009). A neuropsychological battery to detect specific executive and social cognitive impairments in early frontotemporal dementia. *Brain, 132*(Pt 5), 1299–1309.

Trojanowski, J. Q., Vandeerstichele, H., Korecka, M., Clark, C. M., Aisen, P. S., Petersen, R. C., et al. (2010). Update on the biomarker core of the Alzheimer's Disease Neuroimaging Initiative subjects. *Alzheimer's Dementia, 6*(3), 230–238.

Tyne, H. L., Taylor, J., Baker, G. A., & Steiger, M. J. (2010). Modafinil for Parkinson's disease fatigue. *Journal of Neurology, 257*(3), 452–456.

Ungerleider, L. G., & Haxby, J. V. (1994). "What" and "where" in the human brain. *Current Opinion in Neurobiology, 4*(2), 157–165.

Varma, A. R., Adams, W., Lloyd, J. J., Carson, K. J., Snowden, J. S., Testa, H. J., et al. (2002). Diagnostic patterns of regional atrophy on MRI and regional cerebral blood flow change on SPECT in young onset patients with Alzheimer's disease, frontotemporal dementia and vascular dementia. *Acta Neurologica Scandinavica, 105*(4), 261–269.

Vitali, P., Maccagnano, E., Caverzasi, E., Henry, R. G., Haman, A., Torres-Chae, C., et al. (2011). Diffusion-weighted MRI hyperintensity patterns differentiate CJD from other rapid dementias. *Neurology, 76*(20), 1711–1719.

Wagner, G. S., McClintock, S. M., Rosenquist, P. B., McCall, W. V., & Kahn, D. A. (2011). Major depressive disorder with psychotic features may lead to misdiagnosis of dementia: a case report and review of the literature. *Journal of Psychiatric Practice, 17*(6), 432–438.

Warren, J. D., Schott, J. M., Fox, N. C., Thom, M., Revesz, T., Holton, J. L., et al. (2005). Brain biopsy in dementia. *Brain, 128*(9), 2016–2025.

Wenning, G. K., Litvan, I., Jankovic, J., Granata, R., Mangone, C. A., McKee, A., et al. (1998). Natural history and survival of 14 patients with corticobasal degeneration confirmed at postmortem examination. *Journal of Neurology, Neurosurgery, & Psychiatry, 64*(2), 184–189.

Whitehouse, P. J., Price, D. L., Struble, R. G., Clark, A. W., Coyle, J. T., & Delon, M. R. (1982). Alzheimer's disease and senile dementia: loss of neurons in the basal forebrain. *Science, 215*(4537), 1237–1239.

Whitmer, R. A., Sidney, S., Selby, J., Johnston, S. C., & Yaffe, K. (2005). Midlife cardiovascular risk factors and risk of dementia in late life. *Neurology, 64*(2), 277–281.

Whitwell, J. L., & Josephs, K. A. (2012). Neuroimaging in frontotemporal lobar degeneration-predicting molecular pathology. *Nature Reviews Neurology, 8*(3), 131–142.

Whitwell, J. L., Jack, C. R., Jr., Boeve, B. F., Parisi, J. E., Ahlskog, J. E., Drubach, D. A., et al. (2010). Imaging correlates of pathology in corticobasal syndrome. *Neurology, 75*(21), 1879–1887.

Whitwell, J. L., Josephs, K. A., Murray, M. E., Kantarci, K., Przybelski, S. A., Weigand, S. D., et al. (2008). MRI correlates of neurofibrillary tangle pathology at autopsy: a voxel-based morphometry study. *Neurology, 71*(10), 743–749.

WHO (2004). *The global burden of disease: 2004 report.* Geneva: World Health Organization.

Williams, D. R., & Lees, A. J. (2009). Progressive supranuclear palsy: clinicopathological concepts and diagnostic challenges. *Lancet Neurology, 8*(3), 270–279.

Williams, P. S., Spector, A., Orrell, M., & Rands, G. (2000). Aspirin for vascular dementia. *Cochrane Database of Systematic Reviews,* (2), CD001296.

Wilson, R. S., Bennett, D. A., Bienias, J. L., Mendes de Leon, C. F., Morris, M. C., & Evans, D. A. (2003). Cognitive activity and cognitive decline in a biracial community population. *Neurology, 61*(6), 812–816.

Woods, B., Aguirre, E., Spector, A. E., & Orrell, M. (2012). Cognitive stimulation to improve cognitive functioning in people with dementia. *Cochrane Database of Systematic Reviews, 2,* CD005562.

Yeo, B. T., Krienen, F. M., Sepulcre, J., Sabuncu, M. R., Lashkari, D., Hollinshead, M., et al. (2011). The organization of the human cerebral cortex estimated by intrinsic functional connectivity. *Journal of Neurophysiology, 106*(3), 1125–1165.

Yoshita, M., Taki, J., Yokoyama, K., Noguchi-Shinohara, M., Matsumoto, Y., Nakajima, K., et al. (2006). Value of 123I-MIBG radioactivity in the differential diagnosis of DLB from AD. *Neurology, 66*(12), 1850–1854.

Young, G. S., Geschwind, M. D., Fischbein, N. J., Martindale, J. L., Henry, R. G., Liu, S., et al. (2005). Diffusion-weighted and fluid-attenuated inversion recovery imaging in Creutzfeldt-Jakob disease: high sensitivity and specificity for diagnosis. *American Journal of Neuroradiology, 26*(6), 1551–1562.

43.

EPILEPSY AND SEIZURES

W. Curt LaFrance, Jr., and Andres M. Kanner

INTRODUCTION

When evaluating a patient with seizures, the first step is to establish whether the paroxysmal episodes are in fact epileptic seizures or physiological non-epileptic events or psychogenic non-epileptic seizures (Kaplan & Fisher, 2005; Schachter & LaFrance Jr., 2010). Indeed, one out of every four to five patients admitted to an epilepsy center with a diagnosis of treatment-resistant epilepsy (TRE) does not suffer from epilepsy. Several physiological non-epileptic events must be considered; such as sleep disorders, syncope, migraines, or transient ischemic attacks, as well as movement disorders. If the patient has epilepsy, it is essential to establish the type of epileptic syndrome and the type of seizures. As with any other neurological or psychiatric disorder, a detailed history of the paroxysmal events is of the essence.

The initial workup of the patient with seizures includes an electroencephalogram (EEG) with awake and asleep recordings and activation procedures, structural neuroimaging, and also an evaluation of the psychiatric comorbidities in epilepsy. If the routine EEG study coupled with the clinical history and neurological exam does not provide enough information to reach an adequate diagnosis, a prolonged (24–72-hour) EEG study can be considered, either as an ambulatory outpatient study or an inpatient one, preferably with video. Patients with focal epilepsy or refractory seizures should undergo pre-surgical evaluation (Fountain, Van Ness, Swain-Eng, Tonn, & Bever, 2010). A list of anti-seizure medications used for treatment of epilepsy and their pharmacological activity is found in Tables 43.1 and 43.2.

COMORBID DISORDERS IN EPILEPSY

Patients with epilepsy (PWE) have been found to be at higher risk of suffering from mood, anxiety, psychotic, and attention-deficit disorders and non-epileptic seizures (Benbadis, Agrawal, & Tatum IV, 2001; Benbadis & Hauser, 2000;; Bredkjaer, Mortensen, & Parnas, 1998; Brown et al., 2001; Currie, Heathfield, Henson, & Scott, 1971; Edeh & Toone, 1987; Ettinger et al., 2005; Jacoby, Baker, Steen, Potts, & Chadwick, 1996; Kessler et al., 1994; Kogeorgos, Fonagy, & Scott, 1982; McDermott et al., 1995; Mendez, Cummings, & Benson, 1986; O'Donoghue, Goodridge, Redhead, Sander, & Duncan, 1999; Onuma, Adachi, Ishida,

Katou, & Uesugi, 1995; Pariente, Lepine, & Lellouch, 1991; Perini et al., 1996; Regier et al., 1993; Roy-Byrne et al., 1999; Rutter et al., 1970; Schmitz & Wolf, 1995; Semrud-Clikeman & Wical, 1999; Walsh et al., 1986). (See Table 43.3.) The wide ranges of prevalence reflect the different patient populations surveyed and the different assessment techniques.

By the same token, there is evidence of a bidirectional relationship between some psychiatric disorders and epilepsy. Patients with a history of major depressive disorders or suicidality (independent of a major depressive disorder) have a four- to seven-fold greater risk of developing epilepsy (Forsgren & Nystrom, 1990; Hesdorffer, Hauser, Annegers, & Cascino, 2000; Hesdorffer, Hauser, Olafsson, Ludvigsson, & Kjartansson, 2006). Furthermore, children with a history of attention-deficit disorder of the inattentive type have a 3.7-fold higher risk of developing epilepsy (Hesdorffer et al., 2004). Further support of the bidirectional relationship model comes from a study of patients with chronic temporal lobe epilepsy (TLE), revealing progression of psychiatric comorbidity even after controlling for premorbid psychiatric history (Jones, Bell, et al., 2007). Jones et al. (Jones, Watson, et al., 2007) found that 45% of adolescents with new-onset epilepsy met criteria for an Axis I diagnosis according to the *Diagnostic and Statistical Manual of Mental Disorders IV Text Revision* (DSM-IV-TR) classification, while McAfee et al. reported that children with a psychiatric comorbid diagnosis were almost three times more likely to develop epilepsy than those without (McAfee et al., 2007). Clearly, the relationship between psychiatric disorders and epilepsy is complex and is not only the consequence of the epileptic disorder.

BIDIRECTIONAL RELATIONSHIP AND ANIMAL MODELS

Experimental animal data have supported the bidirectional relationship between epilepsy and depression. The assessment of "symptoms of depression" in rats (Sillaber, Holsboer, & Wotjak, 2009) has been carried out with two tests, among others: the quantification of saccharin in water (saccharin consumption test [SCT]), where a lower consumption is considered to be equivalent to anhedonia, as rats love this ingredient. The second test, known as the freezing swim test (FST), is based on the rats' dislike of swimming in water and their tendency to "freeze" when placed in a container of water. It consists of a measurement of immobility time when

**Table 43.1 CHOICE OF AEDS FOR SPECIFIC SEIZURE/
EPILEPSY TYPES**

EPILEPSY TYPE	FIRST LINE	SECOND LINE	THIRD LINE
Focal (Partial)	Carbamazepine Phenytoin Valproate Tiagabine Ethotoin Oxcarbazepine Primidone	Gabapentin Lamotrigine Topiramate Ezogabine Levetiracetam Zonisamide Lacosamide Pregabalin Oxcarbazepine	Phenobarbital Primidone Felbamate
Idiopathic Generalized:			
Absence	Ethosuximide Valproate Methsuximide	Methsuximide Clonazepam	
Myoclonic	Valproate Lamotrigine Topiramate Primidone	Clonazepam Levetiracetam	
Tonic-clonic	Valproate Phenytoin Carbamazepine Primidone Ethotoin	Lamotrigine Topiramate Levetiracetam	Phenobarbital Primidone
Symptomatic Generalized:			
	Valproate	Clonazepam Lamotrigine Topiramate Levetiracetam	Felbamate

Primidone: generalized *"grand mal"*, psychomotor, focal

Rufinamide/clobazam—adjunctive for treatment of seizures associated with Lennox-Gastaut syndrome

Idiopathic generalized epilepsy: Levetiracetam

placed in a container with water. A long period of immobility when placed in a water container is considered to be a symptom equivalent of "despair." Finally, separation of newly born rats from their dam has also been used as an animal model of depression. The assessment of "symptoms of anxiety" in rats is done by measuring the time spent in the open arms of the elevated plus maze, a behavioral experimental paradigm. A reduced time spent in the open arms is considered to be equivalent to symptoms of anxiety.

Epilepsy Facilitates the Development of Phenomena Equivalent to Depression in Animal Models

Using a common animal model of temporal lobe epilepsy (TLE), the lithium and pilocarpine-induced status epilepticus (SE) model with male Wistar rats, Mazarati et al. (Mazarati et al., 2008) demonstrated an increase in immobility time in the FST and decreased consumption of saccharin in the SCT in post-SE animals. This finding was associated with a decrease of serotonin (5-HT) concentrations and turnover in the hippocampus, and of 5-HT release from the hippocampus in response to raphe nuclei stimulation.

Depression Facilitates the Development of Epileptic Activity

Three studies have shown that early maternal separation (MS) of rats or cross-fostering at birth can accelerate the kindling process. In two of the three studies, male and female non-epileptic rats underwent MS on postnatal days 2–14 for 180 min/day or early handling (EH) and brief separation (15 min/day). At seven weeks of age, rats of both genders exposed to MS displayed significantly increased anxiety, as evidenced by reduced time spent in the open arms of the elevated plus maze compared with EH rats. In females, but not in males, fewer stimulations were required following MS than EH to reach the fully kindled state ($39.6 +/- 6.4$ vs. $67.1 +/- 9.4$; $p < 0.0001$) (Jones et al., 2009; Salzberg et al., 2007). Likewise, in the third study, cross-fostering was used as a model for early-life stress in seizure-prone (FAST) and seizure resistant (SLOW) rats. The animals underwent amygdala kindling (where repeated stimulation generated seizures), until six Class V seizures were recorded. An increased kindling rate was observed among all cross-fostered rats compared to non-fostered rats (Gilby et al., 2009).

Comorbidity of epilepsy and depressive and anxiety disorders has also been identified in other animal models. The genetically epilepsy-prone rat (GEPR) with its two strains, GEPR3 and GEPR9, is an animal model of epilepsy with comorbid behaviors equivalent to depressive symptomatology manifested by decreased sucrose consumption in the SCT and increased immobility time in the FST (Jobe, 2006). The GEPR harbors inborn defects in pre- and post-synaptic transmission of both serotonin (5-HT) and norepinephrine (NE), resulting from deficient arborization of noradrenergic and serotonergic neurons arising from the locus ceruleus and raphe nuclei (Jobe et al., 1994). Likewise, the Genetic Absence Epilepsy Rats from Strasbourg (GAERS) illustrate the existence of epilepsy semiology (or characteristics of the seizure) and comorbid symptoms equivalent to symptoms of depression and anxiety in an animal model of generalized epilepsy (Jones et al., 2008). One study of 47 GAERS and 73 control rats without epilepsy (CwoE) were subjected to behavioral measures of depression (Sucrose Preference Test [SPT]) and anxiety (Elevated Plus Maze [EPM]), and the Open Field Arena (OFA) at 7 and 13 weeks of age, ages prior to and after seizure onset. The GAERS exhibited significantly greater levels of behaviors equivalent to symptoms of depression and anxiety on these measures, including reduced consumption of sucrose solution in the SPT, shorter time in the open arms of the EPM, and reduced exploratory activity and less time spent in the inner area of the OFA. These differences were evident *preceding* and *following* the onset of epilepsy. Clearly, increased anxiety- and depressive-like behaviors in GAERS were not a consequence of seizures, but rather an expression of comorbid neurological and psychiatric-like conditions.

Table 43.2 ANTIEPILEPTIC DRUGS (AEDS)

DRUG	MECHANISM	METABOLISM	PROTEIN BINDING	HALF LIFE (HOURS)*	DOSE (P-PEDIATRIC; A-ADULT)
Phenobarbital	1, 2	Hepatic	50%	96	P: 2–5 mg/kg A: 90–120 mg
Phenytoin (Dilantin)	1	Hepatic	85–90%	12–36	P: 4–7 mg/kg A: 200–500 mg
Ethosuximide (Zarontin)	5	Hepatic	<5%	30–60	P: 15–40 mg/kg A: 500–2000 mg
Clonazepam (Klonopin)	1, 2	Hepatic	47%	18–50	P: 0.1–0.2 mg A: 2–6 mg
Carbamazepine (Tegretol)	1	Hepatic	65–90%	14–27	P: 5–20 mg/kg A: 600–1600 mg
Valproic acid (Depakene, Depakote)	1, 2	Hepatic	80–95%	6–15	P: 30–80 mg/kg A: 1–3 g
Gabapentin (Neurontin)	6	Renal	None	6–8	P: 30–60 mg/kg A: 1800–3600 mg
Lamotrigine (Lamictal)	1, 3	Hepatic	55%	12–48‡	P: 5–15 mg/kg A: 200–700 mg
Felbamate (Felbatol)	1, 3	Hepatic	25%	20–23	P: 15–45 mg/kg A: 1800–4800 mg
Topiramate (Topamax)	1, 2, 3, 4	Renal	15%	12–23	P: 5–10 mg/kg A: 100–400 mg
Tiagabine (Gabitril)	2	Hepatic	96%	7–9	P: 0.5–0.8 mg A: 32–56 mg
Vigabatrin (Sabril)	2	Renal	None	7	P: 50–60 mg/kg A: 2–5 g
Ezogabine (Potiga)	7, 8	Hepatic	45–80%	6–10	P: not established A: 600–1200 mg
Zonisamide (Zonegran)	9, 5 (6?)	Hepatic	40%	63 (50–68)	P: 200–400 mg A: 200–400 mg
Lacosamide (Vimpat)	9.a, 18	Hepatic	<15%	13	P: 200–400 mg A: 200–400 mg
Levetiracetam (Keppra)	15 (6?)	Hepatic	<10%	7	P: 60 mg/kg or 3000 mg A: 1000–3000 mg
Rufinamide (Banzel)	1 (6?)	Hepatic	34%	6–10	P: 45 mg/kg or 3200 mg A: 1600–3200 mg
Ethotoin (Peganone)	1 (6?)	Hepatic		3–9	P: 500–1000 mg A: 2–3 g
Primidone (Mysoline)	1 (6?)	Hepatic	25%	10–12	P: 750 mg or 10–25 mg/kg A: 750 mg–2 g
Methsuximide (Celontin)	16, 17	Hepatic	not significant	3	P: 600 mg–1.2 g A: 600 mg–1.2 g

(*continued*)

Table 43.2 (CONTINUED)

DRUG	MECHANISM	METABOLISM	PROTEIN BINDING	HALF LIFE (HOURS)*	DOSE (P–PEDIATRIC; A–ADULT)
Oxcarbazepine (Trileptal, Novartis)	9.b, 1, 12	Hepatic	40%	2–9	P: 900–1800 mg A: 1200–2400 mg
Pregabalin (Lyrica)	6, 13	Negligible/minimal (<2%)	None	6.3	P: not established A: 300–600 mg
Clobazam (Frisium)	14 (6?)	Hepatic	80–90%	36–42	P: 20 mg A: 20–40 mg

*Half-lives in children are typically 50% of adult.

‡Dependent on co-therapy.

1. Stabilizes voltage-dependent sodium channel.

2. Enhances GABA-ergic inhibition.

3. Glutamate receptor antagonist.

4. Carbonic anhydrase inhibitor.

5. Inhibits T-calcium currents.

6. Unknown.

7. Augmentation of GABA-mediated currents.

8. Opens potassium-channels.

9. Inhibits sodium channels. (9.a. Inactivates sodium-channels).

10. Modulation of collapsing response mediator protein-2.

11. Prolongation of inactive state of sodium-channel.

12. Increased potassium conductance.

13. Binds to α2-delta site (voltage-gated calcium channels).

14. Opening of GABA channel.

15. Inhibits burst firing.

16. Suppresses paroxysmal three cycle/second spike and wave activity.

17. Depresses motor cortex evaluation of CNS threshold to convulsive stimuli.

18. Binding to collapsing response mediator protein-2 (CRMP-2).

Some General Principles in Addressing Psychiatric Aspects of Epilepsy

A recent consensus statement from representatives from the International League Against Epilepsy underscored the importance of the neuropsychiatric aspects of epilepsy and treatment approaches (Kerr et al., 2011). The evaluation of any type of psychopathology in PWE must be approached with the following questions in mind.

1. Is this psychiatric disturbance temporally related to the occurrence of seizures?

2. Is the onset of psychiatric symptoms associated with the remission of seizures?

   We consider the peri-ictal psychiatric symptoms (pre-ictal and post-ictal) as well as inter-ictal symptoms associated with the onset or remission of seizures as an expression of a para-ictal process.

3. Are the psychiatric symptoms the result of the introduction of an anti-epileptic drug (AED) with potential

Table 43.3 PREVALENCE OF PSYCHIATRIC DISORDERS IN EPILEPSY AND THE GENERAL POPULATION

PSYCHIATRIC DISORDER	PREVALENCE	
	Epilepsy	*General Population*
Depression	11–80%	3.3%: Dysthymia 4.9–17%: Major Depression
Psychosis	2–9.1%	1%: Schizophrenia 0.2%: Schizophreniform Disorder
Generalized Anxiety Disorders	15–25%	5.1–7.2%
Panic Disorder	4.9–21%	0.5–3%
ADHD	12–37%	4–12%
Psychogenic Non-Epileptic Seizures	10–20%	.03%

negative psychotropic properties, or did they appear after discontinuation of an AED with positive psychotropic properties (mood stabilizing, antidepressant, and anxiolytic properties)?

4. Do the symptoms meet diagnostic criteria of the DSM-IV or the *International Classification of Diseases* (ICD), or do these symptoms present as an atypical disorder?

5. What is the impact of the psychiatric disorder at hand on the quality of life of patients?

6. What is the treatment for the psychiatric disorder? If pharmacotherapy is required, how do psychotropic drugs interact with AEDs, and what is the impact of psychotropic drugs on the seizure threshold?

Tables 43.4–43.7 summarize side effects and interactions of AEDs and psychotropic medications.

Psychiatric comorbid diagnoses have had a noted association with focal epilepsy—in particular, temporal and frontal lobe epilepsies—while little attention has been paid to comorbid psychiatric conditions in idiopathic generalized epilepsy (IGE). In fact, some researchers have hypothesized that patients with temporal lobe epilepsy (TLE) with involvement of temporomesial limbic structures show more psychiatric symptoms compared with extra-TLE patients. While some researchers showed higher depression scores in localization related epilepsies (Quiske, Helmstaedter, Lux, & Elger, 2000), other researchers did not find symptomatic differences between patients with TLE and extra-TLE patients (Swinkels, van Emde Boas, Kuyk, van Dyck, & Spinhoven, 2006). Furthermore, an increasing literature has shown a relatively high prevalence of psychiatric comorbidities in pediatric and adult patients with IGE. For example, in a comparison

of 100 patients with juvenile myoclonic epilepsy (JME) with 100 healthy controls, psychiatric diagnoses were found in 49 patients with JME. Anxiety and mood disorders, present in 23 and 19 patients, respectively, were the most frequently observed, and 20 of the JME group had personality disorders (de Araujo Filho et al., 2007). Psychiatric comorbidity has been associated with the frontal lobe dysfunction found in JME and other types of IGE, such as childhood and juvenile absence epilepsy.

DEPRESSION IN EPILEPSY

Depression is the most frequent psychiatric disorder in PWE. In three community-based studies, prevalence rates of depression ranged between 21% and 33% among patients with persistent seizures and from 4–6% among seizure-free patients (Edeh & Toone, 1987; Jacoby et al., 1996; O'Donoghue et al., 1999). Similar results were found in a recent Canadian population-based study of psychiatric disorders in PWE (Tellez-Zenteno, Patten, Jette, Williams, & Wiebe, 2007). Ettinger et al. reported the results of a population-based survey that investigated a lifetime prevalence of depression, epilepsy, diabetes, and asthma in 185,000 households (Ettinger, Reed, & Cramer, 2004). Among the 2,900 PWE, 32% reported having experienced at least one episode of depression. This contrasted with 8.6% prevalence among healthy respondents, 13% among patients with diabetes, and 16% among people with asthma. Using the same population, these investigators found that 13% of patients with epilepsy had experienced symptoms of manic-depressive illness, compared to 2% of healthy controls (Ettinger, Reed, Goldberg, & Hirschfeld, 2005).

Depression is more common in patients with partial seizure disorders of temporal or frontal lobe origin and among patients with poorly controlled seizures (Edeh & Toone, 1987; Jacoby et al., 1996; Mendez et al., 1986; O'Donoghue et al., 1999). Yet depression is also a predictor of worse seizure control, both with pharmacotherapy with AEDs and epilepsy surgery. For example, in a study of 780 patients with new-onset epilepsy, individuals with a history of psychiatric disorders, and particularly depression, were half as likely to be seizure-free with AEDs after a median follow-up period of 79 months, compared to patients without a psychiatric history (Hitiris, Mohanraj, Norrie, Sills, & Brodie, 2007). Likewise, in a prospective study of 138 patients with new-onset epilepsy, those with symptoms of depression and anxiety at the time of diagnosis of epilepsy were significantly less likely to be seizure-free at the one-year follow-up evaluation (Petrovski et al., 2010).

Several studies have found a worse post-surgical seizure outcome in patients with a lifetime history of psychiatric disorders and, in particular, depression. For example, in a study of 100 consecutive patients with treatment-resistant TLE who had an antero-temporal lobectomy, those with a lifetime history of depression were significantly less likely to achieve complete freedom from auras and disabling seizures (Kanner, Byrne, Chicharro, Wuu, & Frey, 2009).

Table 43.4 MAJOR PRESCRIPTION MEDICATIONS THAT MAY CAUSE SEIZURES OR SYNCOPE

Seizures	*Syncope*
Antihistamines	Beta blockers
Penicillin	Calcium channel blockers
Beta blockers	Nitrates
Baclofen	Tricyclic antidepressants
Theophylline	Clonidine
Tricyclic antidepressants	Clozapine
Sympathomimetics	Trazodone
Isoniazid	Thioridazine
Chlorpromazine	Chlorpromazine
Amoxapine	
Loxapine	
Clozapine	
Maprotiline	
Meperidine	

Table 43.5 NEUROPSYCHIATRIC SIDE EFFECTS OF ANTIEPILEPTIC DRUGS (MOST DOSE-DEPENDENT)

Clonazepam	Lethargy, ataxia, irritability, depression, psychosis
Ethosuximide	Psychosis, Parkinsonian changes
Phenobarbital	Lethargy, depression, memory loss, irritability, paradoxic excitation/agitation
Phenytoin	Lethargy. When toxic—delirium, seizures, psychosis, choreoathetosis
Carbamazepine	Lethargy, depression, irritability, agitation, psychosis, delirium, seizures, aggression
Valproic acid/Valproate	Lethargy, depression, hallucinosis, delirium, pseudodementia, hearing loss
Felbamate	Insomnia, fatigue anxiety, depression, agitation
Gabapentin	Lethargy, fatigue, aggression
Lamotrigine	Dizziness, lethargy, insomnia, seizures, agitation
Topiramate	Lethargy, confusion, trouble concentrating, word-finding difficulties
Tiagabine	Dizziness, fatigue, lethargy, nervousness, irritability, difficulty with concentration, depression
Vigabatrin	Lethargy, psychosis, depression anxiety, irritability, confusion, hyperactivity (children)
Ezogabine	Dizziness, somnolence, fatigue, confusion, asthenia, psychotic symptoms, hallucinations
Zonisamide	Dizziness, ataxia, concentration/ memory difficulties, agitation/ irritability, insomnia, somnolence, fatigue, depression, anxiety, speech problems
Levetiracetam	Somnolence, asthenia, dizziness, nervousness, vertigo, ataxia, irritability, depression, fatigue, coordination difficulties and abnormalities
Rufinamide	Somnolence, fatigue, dizziness, tremor, ataxia, blurred vision, coordination abnormalities, gait disturbances
Ethotoin	Ataxia, dizziness, fatigue, insomnia
Lacosamide	Dizziness, fatigue, vertigo, somnolence, ataxia, tremor, balance disorder, blurred vision
Primidone	Ataxia, vertigo, irritability, drowsiness, dizziness
Methsuximide	Drowsiness, ataxia, dizziness, seizures
Oxcarbazepine	Dizziness, somnolence, fatigue, ataxia, tremor, abnormal vision, abnormal gait
Pregabalin	Somnolence, dizziness, ataxia, blurred vision, abnormal thinking, fatigue, euphoric mood
Clobazam	Dizziness, agitation, fatigue, slurred speech, somnolence, aggression, irritability, insomnia, ataxia

The Neurological Disorders Depression Inventory for Epilepsy (NDDI-E), a brief six-item self-report screening tool for depression in epilepsy, has been shown to identify depressive symptoms exclusive of the neurovegetative side effects of AEDs (Gilliam et al., 2006). Screening questions include: Everything is a struggle, Nothing I do is right, Feel guilty, Better off dead, Frustrated, and Difficulty finding pleasure.

SUICIDALITY IN PATIENTS WITH EPILEPSY

The suicide rate in depressed PWE is 9–25 times higher in patients with partial seizures of temporal lobe origin than expected in the overall population (Nilsson, Tomson, Farahmand, Diwan, & Persson, 1997; Rafnsson, Olafsson, Hauser, & Gudmundsson, 2001; Robertson, 1997). In a Danish population-based study, patients with epilepsy had twice the risk of committing suicide in the absence of any psychosocial obstacles. A comorbid mood disorder increased the risk by 32-fold, while an anxiety disorder increased the risk by 12-fold. The highest risk of suicide in PWE occurred within six months after a new diagnosis of epilepsy was made (Christensen, Vestergaard, Mortensen, Sidenius, & Agerbo, 2007). In a review of the literature, Gilliam and Kanner concluded that suicide has one of the highest standardized mortality rates (SMR) of all causes of death in PWE (Gilliam & Kanner, 2002). Robertson reviewed 17 studies pertaining to mortality in epilepsy and found that suicide was ten times more frequent than in the general population (Robertson, 1997). Rafnsson et al. reported the results of a population-based incidence cohort study in PWE from Iceland in which suicide had the highest SMR (5.8) of all causes of death (Rafnsson et al., 2001). A Swedish study of cause specific mortality among 9,000 previously hospitalized PWE found an SMR of 3.5 (Nilsson et al., 1997).

Table 43.6 ANTI-EPILEPTIC DRUG (AED) INTERACTIONS

AED	DECREASE	INCREASE
Phenobarbital (PB)	DPH[1], CBZ[1], VPA, ESX, CZP, TGB, OXC, RFM, ZNS	
Clonazepam (CZP)	No consistent changes. OXC ZNS	No consistent changes
Ethosuximide (ESX)		DPH
Phenytoin (DPH)	PB[1], CBZ[1], VPA[1], TPX, ESX, TGB, FBM, LTG, OXC, RFM, EZG, ZNS	PRM
Carbamazepine (CBZ)	PB[1], DPH[1], VPA, TPX, LTG, FBM, TGB, ESX RFM, EZG, OXC, ZNS[6]	PRM
Valproate (VPA)	DPH[1], TPX, RFM[5]	CBZ[2], PB, LTG, TGB[3], RFM
Felbamate (FBM)	CBZ, OXC	DPH, VPA, PB, CBZ[2]
Gabapentin (GBP)	PGB	None
Lamotrigine (LTG)	VPA, RFM, EZG	CBZ[2]
Topiramate (TPX)	VPA	DPH[4]
Tiagabine (TGB)	VPA	
Vigabatrin (VGB)	DPH	
Rufinamide (RFM)	LTG, CBZ, CYP3A4 substrates, CBZ	PB, DPH, VPA
Ezogabine (EZG)	LTG	DPH
Zonisamide (ZNS)	DPH, CBZ, VPA, PB, PRM	
Oxcarbazepine (OXC)	CBZ, LTG	PB, DPH
Methsuximide (MSM)		PB, DPH
Primidone (PRM)	ZNS, RFM	LTG[5], VPA[5], PB[5], DPH[5], CBZ[5], TPX[5], TGB[5]
Valproic Acid		OXC, PRM
Clobazam (CLB)	PRM	

[1] Variable effects reported.

[2] Increases epoxide metabolite.

[3] Increased free Tiagabine (TGB).

[4] No change or increase.

[5] Decreased clearance.

[6] Decreased clearance of effect.

Key: Phenobarbital (PB), Clonazepam (CZP), Ethosuximide (ESX), Phenytoin (DPH), Carbamazepine (CBZ), Valproate (VPA), Felbamate (FBM), Gabapentin (GBP), Lamotrigine (LTG), Topiramate (TPX), Tiagabine (TGB), Vigabatrin (VGB), Rufinamide (RFM), Ezogabine (EZG), Zonisamide (ZNS), Oxcarbazepine (OXC), Methsuximide (MSM), Primidone (PRM), Clobazam (CLB).

DEPRESSION AS A PARA-ICTAL PHENOMENON

Pre-ictal symptoms of depression and depressive episodes typically present as a dysphoric mood in which the prodromal symptoms may extend for hours or even one to three days prior to the onset of a seizure. In children, this dysphoric mood often takes the form of irritability, poor frustration tolerance, and aggressive behavior. Blanchet and Frommer (1986) assessed mood changes during 56 days in 27 PWE who rated their mood on a daily basis. Mood ratings pointed to a dysphoric state three days prior to a seizure in 22 (81%) patients. This change in mood was greatest during the 24 hours preceding the seizure. Patients or parents of children

Table 43.7 SOME REPORTED PHARMACOKINETIC INTERACTIONS BETWEEN PSYCHOTROPIC DRUGS AND AEDS

DRUG	EFFECT ON BLOOD LEVELS OF DRUG LISTED BELOW RESULTING FROM INTERACTION WITH DRUG LISTED ON THE LEFT	AFFECTED MEDICATION
Fluoxetine	↑	CBZ, DPH,
Fluvoxamine	↑	CBZ, DPH, PB, LCM, ZNS
Nefazodone	↑	DPH
Paroxetine	↑	CBZ, DPH
Sertraline	↑	CBZ, DPH
Trazadone	↑	CBZ
Viloxazine	↑	CBZ
Carbamazepine (CBZ)	↓	Haloperidol, tricyclic antidepressants (TCA)
Phenobarbital (PB)	↓	Mirtazapine, olanzapine, TCA
Phenytoin (DPH)	↓	Mirtazapine, olanzapine, TCA
Rufinamide	↓	Dihydroergotamine, ergotamine, sertindole, almotriptan, alprazolam, aripiprazole, buspirone, clozapine, diazepam, eletriptan, iloperidone, quetiapine, trazadone, triazolam
Primidone	↓	Protriptyline

Key: Phenobarbital (PB), Lacosamide (LCM), Phenytoin (DPH), Carbamazepine (CBZ), Zonisamide (ZNS), Tricyclic Antidepressants (TCA).

with epilepsy often report that dysphoric symptoms completely resolve the day after the ictus.

Post-ictal symptoms of depressive and depressive episodes have been recognized for decades but have been investigated in a systematic manner in only one study (Kanner, Soto, & Gross-Kanner, 2004). The presence of post-ictal symptoms of depression was identified in 43 of 100 consecutive patients with refractory partial seizure disorders. These symptoms occurred after more than 50% of seizures, and their duration ranged from 0.5–108 hours, with a median duration of 24 hours. Other studies have shown that symptoms of depression can outlast the ictus for up to two weeks, and, at times, have led patients to suicide (Anatassopoulos & Kokkini, 1969; Hancock & Bevilacqua, 1971). Likewise, inter-ictal symptoms can worsen in severity during the post-ictal period. For example, in the study by Kanner et al. (Kanner et al., 2004) post-ictal exacerbation in severity of inter-ictal symptoms was identified in up to 30% of patients. In fact, some patients whose inter-ictal mood disorder was in remission with antidepressant medication experienced breakthrough symptoms of depression in the post-ictal period.

Ictal symptoms of depression or a depressive episode are the clinical expression of a simple partial seizure in which the depressive symptoms are the sole (or predominant) semiology. Ictal symptoms of depression ranked second after symptoms of anxiety or fear as the most common type of ictal affect in one study (Williams, 1956). This presentation occurred in 21% of 100 PWE who reported auras consisting of psychiatric symptoms (Daly, 1958; Weil, 1955). Yet, the actual prevalence of ictal symptoms of depression is yet to be established in larger studies. The most frequent symptoms include feelings of anhedonia, guilt, and suicidal ideation. Such mood changes are typically brief, stereotypical, occur out of context, and are associated with other ictal phenomena. More typically, however, ictal symptoms of depression are followed by an alteration of consciousness as the ictus evolves from a simple to a complex partial seizure.

DEPRESSION AS COMORBID DISORDER: INTER-ICTAL DEPRESSIVE DISORDERS

Inter-ictal forms of depression in epilepsy can be identical to depressive disorders described in non-epileptic patients (i.e., major depression, bipolar disorder, cyclothymia, dysthymia, and minor depression). Nevertheless, a review of the literature has clearly shown an atypical clinical presentation of inter-ictal depressive episodes that fail to meet any of the DSM categories. Blumer coined the term "inter-ictal dysphoric disorder" to describe this atypical presentation, found in about one-third of patients with mood disorders in epilepsy (Blumer, Altshuler, 1998). It is characterized by a chronic "dysthymic-like" state, where symptoms tend to occur intermittently, intermixed with brief euphoric moods, explosive irritability, anxiety, paranoid feelings, and somatoform symptoms (anergia, atypical pain, and insomnia). This type of depression is often unrecognized.

A significant number of patients with epilepsy present with depressive episodes that fail to meet the DSM diagnostic criteria and often present as sub-syndromic episodes. Even though this may be a less severe form of depression than a major depressive episode, sub-syndromic depressive episodes have a very negative impact on the quality of life of people with epilepsy (Kanner, Barry, Gilliam, Hermann, & Meador, 2010).

Depressive disorders often occur along with anxiety disorders. For example, in a study of 188 consecutive patients with epilepsy, 31 patients met DSM-IV criteria of a current major depressive episode (MDE). Twenty-one of these patients had a mixed MDE and an anxiety disorder (Kanner et al., 2010). Recognition of such comorbidity is of the essence, as failure to target the anxiety disorder in the treatment of these patients can result in recurrence of the depressive disorder. In addition, comorbid depressive and anxiety disorders in patients with and without epilepsy are associated with a worse course of the depressive disorder.

DEPRESSION AS AN IATROGENIC PROCESS

AEDs can cause psychiatric symptoms (McConnell & Duncan, 1998). AEDs with GABA-ergic properties, primarily phenobarbital, primidone, the benzodiazepines, tiagabine, and vigabatrin are more likely to cause depression (Barabas & Matthews, 1988; Brent, Crumrine, Varma, Allan, & Allman, 1987; Ferrari, Barabas, & Matthews, 1983; Ring & Reynolds, 1990; Smith et al., 1987). Other AEDs that have been linked to depression include felbamate, topiramate, levetiracetam, and zonisamide (Kanner, Faught, French, et al., 2000; McConnell et al., 1996; Mula & Trimble, 2003). A careful review of the data suggests that the occurrence of psychiatric adverse events is more likely to be identified in patients susceptible to developing psychiatric disorders, such as patients with a past psychiatric history or with a family psychiatric history (Mula & Trimble, 2003).

The addition of AEDs with mood-stabilizing properties, such as carbamazepine, valproic acid, and lamotrigine, can occasionally cause depressive episodes, albeit with a significantly lower frequency than other AEDs. More often than not, these AEDs are associated with the occurrence of depression *upon their discontinuation* in patients with a prior history of depression or panic disorder, which had been kept in remission by these AEDs (Ketter et al., 1994).

The Food and Drug Administration (FDA) announced in 2008 that it would require manufacturers of AEDs to add a warning to their labeling indicating that use of the drugs increases risk for suicidal thoughts and behaviors (Barclay, 2008). The announcement was based on an FDA review of 199 clinical trials of 11 AEDs, which reported risk for suicidal behavior or thoughts was nearly doubled for patients receiving AEDs vs. placebo (0.43% vs. 0.24%). A critique of the FDA analysis included the fact that the methodological approach including lumping all AEDs, which have different mechanisms of action, into one class, and basing the recommendation on adverse-event data rather than on systematically acquired data (Hesdorffer & Kanner, 2009). The authors concluded that the risk of adverse effects from uncontrolled seizures almost certainly outweighs the small risk of suicidality, and they emphasized the need for practitioners to screen for mood and anxiety disorders in PWE. Furthermore, attempts to replicate the data from the FDA meta-analysis in five large studies yielded contradictory findings. Therefore, certain, but not all, AEDs can cause psychiatric adverse events that can lead to suicidal ideation and behavior, but this is likely to occur in patients with a predisposition for psychiatric illness. Thus, before starting an AED like topiramate, zonisamide, vigabatrin, barbiturate, or levetiracetam, it is essential to inquire about a prior personal or psychiatric history.

DEPRESSION FOLLOWING EPILEPSY SURGERY

There has been an increasing number of reports of depressive disorders following an antero-temporal lobectomy (Savard, Andermann, Reutens, & Andermann, 1998). It is not unusual to see "mood lability" within the initial six weeks to three months after surgery. Often these symptoms subside, but in up to 30% of patients, overt symptoms of depression become apparent within the first six months. Characteristically, symptoms of depression vary in severity from mild to very severe, including suicidal attempts. In most instances, these depressive disorders respond readily to pharmacological treatment with antidepressant drugs (see depression treatment section). Patients with a prior history of depression are at greater risk. A German study found that patients with personality disorders are at higher risk of suffering from postoperative psychiatric complications compared with patients with other preoperative psychiatric conditions (such as depression) or with patients with no preoperative psychiatric diagnosis whatsoever (Koch-Stoecker, 2002). While some studies have not found a relationship between depression with the post-surgical control of seizures, others have (Kanner & Balabanov, 2008; Pintor et al., 2007). All patients undergoing epilepsy surgery, therefore, should be advised of this potential complication, *prior to surgery*.

TREATMENT OF DEPRESSION IN EPILEPSY

There is a lack of controlled studies on the treatment of depression in epilepsy. In their absence, a consensus statement has been published, outlining pharmacological and psychotherapeutic approaches for PWE with affective disorders (Barry, Ettinger, et al., 2008). Before starting a patient on an antidepressant drug (AD), it is important to determine if the seizures may be related to starting or stopping an AED.

In all cases inquiry into suicidality is mandatory.

Do antidepressant drugs worsen seizures? A review of the literature has found an increased incidence of seizures with the use of four specific antidepressant drugs. These are: maprotiline, amoxepine, clomipramine, and bupropion (McConnell & Duncan, 1998; Swinkels, Jonghe, 1995). Increased seizures have been identified in patients without epilepsy taking tricyclic antidepressants (TCA), but these seizures have been associated with the following variables: (1) Overdoses and/or high plasma serum concentrations, (2) rapid dose increments, (3) the presence of other drugs with pro-convulsant properties, and (4) the presence of central nervous system (CNS) pathology, abnormal EEG, and personal and family history of epilepsy (Curran & de Pauw, 1998; Preskorn & Fast, 1992; Rosenstein, Nelson, & Jacobs, 1993; Swinkels, Jonghe, 1995). Based on the evidence suggesting a bidirectional relationship between depression and epilepsy, and a higher incidence of seizures in patients with depression, it is important to reconsider the question of whether antidepressants increase the risk of seizures, or whether we are identifying the seizure occurrence associated with such increased risk. A study appears to challenge the notion of proconvulsant effect of antidepressants. Alper et al. (Alper, Schwartz, Kolts, & Khan, 2007) compared the incidence of seizures between depressed patients in trials randomized to selective serotonin-reuptake inhibitors (SSRIs), serotonin-norepinephrine reuptake inhibitors (SNRIs), mirtazapine, or placebo in the course of multicenter placebo-controlled studies of these drugs submitted to the FDA for approval. Compared to the expected incidence of seizures of the general population, all depressed patients had a higher incidence of seizures. Nonetheless, patients randomized to placebo had a significantly higher incidence of seizures than those treated with the actual antidepressant drug.

In general, the SSRI class of drugs is safe in patients with epilepsy. In one study, sertraline was found to *definitely* worsen seizures in *only one* out of 100 patients with refractory epilepsy (Kanner, Kozak, & Frey, 2000). Blumer has also reported using TCAs alone and in combination with SSRIs in epileptic patients, without seizure exacerbation (Blumer, Zielinksi, 1988). Monoamine-oxidase inhibitors (MAO-I) are not known to cause seizures in patients without epilepsy. Patients treated with TCAs should be started at low doses with small increments until the desired clinical response is reached. This will minimize the risk of causing or exacerbating seizures. (See Table 43.4.)

PHARMACOKINETIC INTERACTIONS BETWEEN ANTIDEPRESSANT DRUGS AND AEDS

Most antidepressants are metabolized in the liver, and their metabolism is accelerated in the presence of AEDs with enzyme-inducing properties, which include phenytoin, carbamazepine, phenobarbital, primidone at regular doses, and oxcarbazepine and topiramate at doses above 900 mg/day and 300 mg/day, respectively. This pharmacokinetic effect is not observed with the new AEDs gabapentin, lamotrigine, tiagabine, levetiracetam, zonisamide, pregabalin, vigabatrin, and ezogabine. Conversely, some of the SSRIs are inhibitors of one or more isoenzymes of the cytochrome P450 (CYP 450) system. These include fluoxetine, paroxetine, fluvoxamine,

and, to a lesser degree, sertraline (Fritze, Unsorg, & Lanczik, 1991; Grimsley, Jann, Carter, D'Mello, & D'Souza, 1991; Pearson, 1990). Citalopram, on the other hand, does not have pharmacokinetic interactions with AEDs (McConnell & Duncan, 1998). Sertraline has been shown rarely to increase phenytoin levels, and this is thought to be associated with displacement by tight protein binding, or by inhibition of the CYP 450 system (Haselberger, Freedman, & Tolbert, 1997; Thomson, 2006).

CHOICE OF ANTIDEPRESSANT

The SSRI class of drugs should be considered the first-line treatment in depressed PWE. They are safe with respect to seizure propensity, are less likely to result in fatalities after an overdose, and generally have a favorable adverse-effects profile. Furthermore, their efficacy in dysthymic disorders and in symptoms of irritability and poor frustration tolerance makes this class of AEDs more attractive among PWE who have atypical forms of depression. SSRIs with no or minimal effects on CYP 450 isoenzymes, such as citalopram and sertraline, should be considered in patients taking hepatically metabolized AEDs to avoid pharmacokinetic interactions.

In open, uncontrolled trials, TCAs have also been reported to yield a good clinical response, but the cardiotoxic effects and severe complications seen in overdose make these drugs a second-line antidepressant choice. Blumer has anecdotal reports of the utility of low-dose TCAs in PWE and inter-ictal dysphoric disorder (Blumer, Zielinksi, 1988).

A cautionary note is in order. Before starting an antidepressant, clinicians must rule out a history of any manic or hypomanic episodes that may be suggestive of a bipolar disorder, as antidepressants can potentially trigger a manic or hypomanic episode in the short term, and they may worsen the course of the bipolar disorder in the long term, particularly in the case of rapidly cycling bipolar disease. In such cases, an AED with mood-stabilizing and antidepressant properties such as lamotrigine must be considered. Carbamazepine and valproate may be added in case of persistent symptoms. Lithium should be considered if these AEDs cannot yield a euthymic state. If an antidepressant is required, it should not be started in the absence of a mood-stabilizing drug.

OTHER TYPES OF PSYCHIATRIC TREATMENTS

Lithium was the first mood-stabilizing drug used for the treatment of patients with bipolar disorder. Its use in epileptic patients with affective disorders, however, has been fraught with several problems, including changes in EEG recordings and pro-convulsant effects at therapeutic serum concentrations in patients without epilepsy (Bell, Cole, Eccleston, & Ferrier, 1993). Lithium's neurotoxicity and related increase in seizure risk are exacerbated with the concurrent use of neuroleptic drugs, in the presence of EEG abnormalities, and with a history of a central nervous system disorder.

Electroconvulsive therapy (ECT) is *not* contraindicated in depressed PWE (Fink, Kellner, & Sackeim, 1999; Regenold, Weintraub, & Taller, 1998; Sackeim, Decina, Prohovnik,

Malitz, & Resor, 1983). It is a well-tolerated treatment and is worth considering in PWE with very severe depression that fails to respond to antidepressant drugs. Furthermore, there is no evidence that ECT increases the risk of epilepsy (Blackwood, Cull, Freeman, Evans, & Mawdsley, 1980).

Vagal nerve stimulation (VNS) is used as adjunctive treatment for epilepsy and has also shown longer-term mood effects (Marangell et al., 2002). The impact of other neurostimulation interventions, such as deep brain stimulation (DBS) or transcranial magnetic stimulation (TMS), on mood in patients with epilepsy has not been studied in controlled trials.

In addition to pharmacological intervention, the value of psychotherapy for the treatment of depression in PWE should not be overlooked. Surveys reveal that fear of the next seizure is rated as the greatest concern in PWE (Fisher et al., 2000). Counseling and psychotherapy can be useful in helping the patient deal with the stresses and limitations of living with epilepsy (Ramaratnam, Baker, & Goldstein, 2008).

ANXIETY DISORDERS IN EPILEPSY

Anxiety is the second most common psychiatric comorbid diagnosis in PWE, with an estimated prevalence between 15% and 25% (Edeh & Toone, 1987; Jacoby et al., 1996; Jones et al., 2003; O'Donoghue et al., 1999; Vazquez & Devinsky, 2003). In 174 consecutive patients with epilepsy from five epilepsy centers, a current DSM-IV diagnosis of anxiety disorder was found in 30% of patients (Jones et al., 2003).

The various forms of anxiety disorders (generalized anxiety disorder, panic disorder, phobias, obsessive-compulsive disorder, and post-traumatic stress disorder) can present *inter-ictally* with the same clinical manifestations as anxiety disorders in the general population. The peri-ictal presentations of anxiety symptoms often differ from their inter-ictal manifestations, however.

ANXIETY EPISODES AS PARA-ICTAL PROCESSES

Ictal fear or panic is the most frequent ictal psychiatric symptom. It is the sole or predominant clinical expression of a simple partial seizure (aura) or the initial symptom of a complex partial seizure, and it usually has a mesial temporal lobe origin. Seizures of mesial frontal origin involving the cyngulate gyrus can also be associated with an anxious feeling, but not a panic attack, as an expression of the aura. Relying on electrographic inter-ictal and ictal data to document a diagnosis often yields false negative results. Indeed, simple partial seizures originating from mesial frontal regions are often undetected in scalp EEG recordings, as the location of the epileptogenic zone (in cyngulate gyrus) relative to the angle subtended by scalp electrodes positioned at the midline and over suprasylvian regions may not permit the detection of the epileptiform discharges or ictal patterns. Likewise, scalp recordings are unlikely to detect any epileptiform activity from simple partial seizures of mesial temporal lobe origin, particularly those in which the epileptogenic area is in the amygdala, as this structure

generates epileptiform discharges with a very narrow electric field. By the same token, inter-ictal recordings may fail to recode any inter-ictal discharges, even with the use of basal and antero-temporal electrodes. In these instances, the use of sphenoidal electrodes placed under fluoroscopic guidance will be necessary. It should be emphasized that the placement of sphenoidal electrodes without fluoroscopic guidance does not yield any advantage over antero-temporal and basal temporal electrodes (Kanner & Jones, 1997).

A careful history can help distinguish inter-ictal from ictal panic. Ictal panic is typically less than 30 seconds in duration, is stereotypical, occurs out of the context of concurrent events, and is associated with other ictal phenomena such as periods of confusion of variable duration and subtle or overt automatisms. The intensity of the sensation of fear is mild to moderate and rarely reaches the intensity of a panic attack. On the other hand, inter-ictal panic attacks consist of episodes of 5–20 minutes' duration, which at times may persist for several hours. The feeling of fear or panic is very intense ("feeling of impending doom") and is associated with a variety of autonomic symptoms, including tachycardia, diffuse diaphoresis, and dyspnea. Patients may become so completely absorbed by the panic that they may not be able to report what is going on around them; however, there is no confusion or loss of consciousness, as seen in complex partial seizures. It is not infrequent for patients to develop agoraphobia due to the fear of experiencing a panic attack. As stated above, EEG recordings with sphenoidal electrodes placed under fluoroscopic guidance may be necessary to demonstrate the mesial temporal lobe epileptiform activity that generates ictal panic (Kanner & Jones, 1997; Kanner, Ramirez, & Jones, 1995).

Patients with ictal panic may also suffer from inter-ictal panic attacks, which have been identified in up to 25% of patients with epilepsy (Vazquez & Devinsky, 2003).

Post-ictal symptoms of anxiety can be relatively frequent among patients with refractory partial epilepsy. In a study of 100 consecutive patients with pharmaco-resistant partial epilepsy, we identified a mean of 2 ± 1 post-ictal symptoms of anxiety (range: 1–5; median = 2) in 45 patients (Kanner et al., 2004). These symptoms occurred after more than 50% of their seizures and had a median duration of 24 hours (range: 0.5–148.0 hours). Thirty-two patients reported symptoms of generalized anxiety and/or panic; an additional ten patients also reported symptoms of compulsions, and 29 patients experienced post-ictal symptoms of agoraphobia. In 44 of these 45 patients, post-ictal symptoms of depression were also reported, which included anhedonia, feelings of helplessness, crying bouts, suicidal ideation, and feelings of guilt.

TREATMENT OF ANXIETY DISORDERS IN EPILEPSY

Antidepressants belonging to the SSRI class can prevent the occurrence of inter-ictal panic attacks as well as treat generalized anxiety disorders. On the other hand, there is as of yet no evidence that these drugs have any impact on post-ictal psychiatric symptoms. Antidepressant drugs of the SNRI family have been also been used with success, but no controlled studies exist in patients with epilepsy. Benzodiazepines have been used for years in the management of anxiety disorders. We do not recommend their chronic use because of the development of tolerance and sedating adverse events. However, short trials with clonazepam can be quite effective.

PSYCHOSIS OF EPILEPSY

Psychotic disorders are more frequent in PWE than in the general population, with some studies suggesting prevalence rates of up to 10%. Psychotic disorders can present as a schizophreniform disorder, indistinguishable from those of patients without epilepsy. However, the term "psychosis of epilepsy" implies the presence of certain characteristics that distinguish these disorders from those of patients without epilepsy.

POST-ICTAL PSYCHOTIC SYMPTOMS AND PSYCHOTIC EPISODES

Post-ictal psychotic phenomena can present in the form of isolated symptoms or as psychotic episodes, defined as a cluster of symptoms of at least 24 hours' duration. The prevalence of post-ictal psychotic disorders in PWE is yet to be established, but has been estimated to range between 6% and 10% (Dongier, 1959; Kanner, Stagno, Kotagal, & Morris, 1996). Recurrent post-ictal psychotic symptoms have been found in 7% of 100 consecutive patients with refractory partial epilepsy (Kanner et al., 2004). Common findings include:

1. A delay between the onset of psychiatric symptoms and the time of the last seizure.

2. A relatively short duration (from hours up to a few weeks long).

3. An affect-laden symptomatology.

4. The clustering of symptoms into delusional and affective-like psychosis.

5. An increase in the frequency of secondarily generalized tonic-clonic seizures preceding the onset of post-ictal psychosis (PIP).

6. The onset of PIP after having seizures for a mean period of more than ten years.

7. A prompt response to low-dose neuroleptic medication or benzodiazepines (Devinsky et al., 1995; Kanner et al., 1996; Lancman, Craven, Asconape, & Penry, 1994; Logsdail & Toone, 1988; Umbricht et al., 1995).

In a study with eight years of follow-up on patients with PIP, 3 developed chronic psychosis and 4 of 14 patients died (Logsdail & Toone, 1988).

In most cases, insomnia is the initial presenting symptom. In patients with recurrent post-ictal psychotic episodes, families need to learn to recognize these symptoms so that a timely administration of 1–2 mgs of risperidone may avert the episode. It should be given for two to five days and then discontinued.

The occurrence of post-ictal psychotic episodes also has important localizing implications. PIP suggests the presence of bilateral independent ictal *foci* (Devinsky et al., 1995; Logsdail & Toone, 1988; Umbricht et al., 1995). A 2008 study (Kanner & Ostrovskaya, 2008a) demonstrated that the presence of post-ictal psychotic episodes (PIPE) suggests the presence of bilateral ictal foci in close to 90% of patients with refractory partial epilepsy. Accordingly, patients undergoing surgical evaluation may require longer video EEG (vEEG) monitoring studies and possibly the use of intracranial electrodes. If recordings with depth or subdural electrodes are used, prophylactic treatment with low-dose risperidone or haloperidol can avert the occurrence of such episodes during the invasive vEEG monitoring studies (Kanner et al., 1996).

PIP can also lead to the development of inter-ictal psychotic episodes (IPE). Various authors have reported on the development of IPE following PIPE (Adachi et al., 2003; Adachi et al., 2002; Tarulli, Devinsky, & Alper, 2001). For example, Tarulli et al. found that 6 of 43 patients with PIPE met all the criteria for both PIPE and IPE (Tarulli et al., 2001). Five of the six patients had multiple documented PIPEs before they became chronically psychotic. The range of length of time between PIPE and IPE was 7 to 96 months. Kanner and Ostrovskaya found that 7 of 18 patients with PIPE went on to develop IPE, compared to 1 of 18 controls (Kanner & Ostrovskaya, 2008b). Other investigators have reported PIPEs preceding and/or following the occurrence of IPE (Adachi et al., 2003; Adachi et al., 2002).

Ictal psychotic symptoms or episodes should always be considered in the differential diagnosis of PIP and psychosis of epilepsy, as a whole. It is typically due to non-convulsive status epilepticus. The presence of unresponsiveness and automatisms should increase the suspicion. Yet confirmation with EEG recordings is of the essence, as certain psychotic processes, such as catatonic states, can be associated with unresponsiveness and mannerisms that mimic automatisms.

ALTERNATIVE PSYCHOSIS OR "FORCED NORMALIZATION"

The concept of alternative psychosis, developed from observations by Landoldt in 1953, (Landoldt, 1953; Blanchet & Frommer, 1986) implies an inverse relationship between seizure control and psychotic symptom occurrence. He described a "normalization" of EEG recordings with the appearance of psychiatric symptoms and coined the term "forced normalization." Forced normalization has been reported in patients with TLE and generalized epilepsies. Dongier reported the disappearance of a focal discharge during a psychotic episode in 15% of 318 patients with peri-ictal psychoses (Dongier, 1959). Prevalence rates of alternative psychosis are reported to be 11–25% (Janz, 2002). As with other forms of psychosis of epilepsy, the psychotic manifestations were identified after a 15-year history of epilepsy in 23 patients reported by Wolf (Wolf & Trimble, 1985). The dopamine (DA) system has been implicated in forced normalization. DA antagonists provoke seizures, and DA agonists have anticonvulsant properties but may precipitate psychosis. Both Landoldt and Wolf reported a pleomorphic clinical presentation with a paranoid psychosis without clouding of consciousness as being the most frequent manifestation. A premonitory phase involving insomnia, anxiety, a feeling of oppression, and social withdrawal may occur in a prodromal phase. Forced normalization may then manifest as psychosis, conversion symptoms, hypochondriasis, depression, or mania.

Inter-ictal psychotic disorders can present with delusions, hallucinations, referential thinking, and thought disorders, as in patients without epilepsy. Slater coined the term "inter-ictal psychosis of epilepsy" (POE) to describe certain clinical characteristics, particularly psychotic episodes seen inter-ictally in patients with chronic epilepsy (Slater, Beard, & Glithero, 1963). The description of these cases is remarkable for *the absence* of negative symptoms, better premorbid history, and less common deterioration of the patients' personality. The psychosis is less severe and more responsive to therapy.

IATROGENIC PSYCHOTIC DISORDERS

AED-RELATED PSYCHOSIS

Psychotic disorder as an expression of a drug toxicity has been reported with several AEDs, most prominently ethosuximide, phenobarbital, and primidone, as well as the newer AEDs topiramate and levetiracetam (McConnell & Duncan, 1998). Psychotic disorders can occasionally follow the discontinuation of AEDs, particularly those with mood-stabilizing properties. Ketter et al. reported the development of some cases of psychosis among 32 inpatients who were withdrawn from carbamazepine, phenytoin, and valproic acid (Ketter et al., 1994). Acute withdrawal from benzodiazepines is well known to result sometimes in an acute psychotic episode (Sironi, Franzini, Ravagnati, & Marossero, 1979).

PSYCHOSIS FOLLOWING TEMPORAL LOBECTOMY

Temporal lobectomy has been associated with postoperative psychosis. In a series of 100 of Falconer's patients, Taylor reported seven with *de novo* postoperative psychosis (Taylor, 1972). Jensen and Vaernet reported *de novo* psychotic disorders in 9 of 74 patients (Jensen & Vaernet, 1977). Trimble calculated postoperative *de novo* psychoses to range between 3.8–35.7% (mean, 7.6%) of patients and suggested that, in at least some cases, a causal relationship by way of forced normalization was possible (Trimble, 1992).

Many epilepsy centers currently do not consider patients with a preoperative history of psychosis to be candidates for epilepsy surgery. Thus, more recent reports of postsurgical psychosis in patients are primarily *de novo* psychoses, which would be expected to be of lower incidence than postoperative exacerbations of preexisting psychosis. Yet a history of psychosis should not be considered an absolute contraindication to epilepsy surgery, provided that the patient can cooperate during the presurgical evaluation, has a clear understanding of the nature of the surgical procedure, and can provide a fully informed consent.

DRUG TREATMENT OF PSYCHOSIS IN EPILEPSY PATIENTS

Antipsychotic drugs (APD) are necessary in the management of psychotic disorders in epilepsy patients, despite their proconvulsant properties. While the risk of seizure occurrence must always be carefully considered when starting antipsychotic drugs in these patients, it should never be a reason not to treat a patient in need of antipsychotic medication. Antipsychotic drugs can be separated into two classes: the typical antipsychotic drugs, and the atypical. The former include 18 drugs developed between the 1950s and the 1970s. Their mechanism of action resides in their ability to block dopamine (DA-2) receptors, at the level of meso-cortical, nigrostriatal, and tubero-infundibular DA pathways (Stahl, 2000). Blockade of the DA receptors at the former pathways is responsible for their antipsychotic effect, but it results as well in emotional blunting and cognitive symptoms that often lead to confusion with the negative symptoms of schizophrenia. Blockade at the nigrostriatal pathways results in acute and chronic movement disorders, presenting as Parkinsonian symptoms, as well as dystonic and dyskinetic movements, while blockade at the tubero-infundibular pathways results in increased secretion of prolactin. In addition to their DA-blockade properties, most of the typical antipsychotics have muscarinic cholinergic, alpha-1, and histaminic blocking properties, responsible for anticholinergic adverse effects, weight gain, sedation, dizziness, and orthostatic hypotension.

Atypical antipsychotic drugs (AAPD) are dopamine-serotonin antagonists that target DA-2 and 5HT-2A receptors (Stahl, 2000). Their main difference with conventional antipsychotic drugs (CAPDs) is the absence or mild occurrence of extrapyramidal adverse events and of hyperprolactinemia. In addition, this class of drugs has a lesser blunting of affect, and several of these AAPDs have mood-stabilizing properties. Hence, AAPDs have in large part replaced CAPDs. Today, six AAPDs have been introduced in the United States: clozapine (Clozaril), risperidone (Risperidal), olanzapine (Zyprexa), ziprasidone (Geodon), quetiapine (Seroquel), and aripiprazole (Abilify).

The seizure rate associated with the use of antipsychotic drugs has ranged from 0.5% to 1.2% among non-epileptic patients (Whitworth & Fleischhacker, 1995). The risk is higher with certain drugs, and higher in the presence of the following factors: (1) a history of epilepsy; (2) abnormal EEG recordings; (3) history of central nervous system disorder;

(4) rapid titration of the APD dose; (5) high doses of antipsychotic drugs; and (6) the presence of other drugs that lower the seizure threshold (McConnell & Duncan, 1998). For example, when chlorpromazine is used at doses above 1000 mgs/day, the incidence of seizures was reported to increase to 9%, in contrast to a 0.5% incidence when lower doses are taken (Logothetis, 1967). Clozapine has been reported to cause seizures in 4.4% when used at doses above 600 mgs/day, while at a doses lower than 300 mgs, the incidence of seizures is less than 1% (Toth & Frankenburg, 1994). While these two drugs have been associated with the higher frequencies of seizures, most antipsychotic drugs have been associated with seizure occurrence in the presence of the risk factors cited above.

With the exception of clozapine, atypical antipsychotic drug–related seizure incidence has not been higher than expected in the general population (Toth & Frankenburg, 1994). This finding was confirmed by Alper et al. in a study comparing the incidence of seizures of psychotic patients without epilepsy randomized to either placebo or one of the atypical antipsychotic drugs (risperidone, olanzapine, quetiapine, and aripiprazole) in regulatory studies submitted to the FDA. Thus, during pre-marketing studies of non-epilepsy patients taking antipsychotic drugs, seizures were reported in 0.3% of patients given risperidone, 0.9% given olanzapine, 0.8% given quetiapine (vs. 0.5% on placebo), and 0.4% of patients treated with ziprasidone (data in PDR, 2002).

The risk of seizure occurrence or worsening of seizures with atypical antipsychotic drugs in PWE has not been well studied. Pacia and Devinsky reviewed the incidence of seizures among 5,629 patients treated with clozapine (Pacia & Devinsky, 1994). Sixteen of these patients had epilepsy before the start of this antipsychotic drug, and all patients experienced worsening of seizures while on the drug: eight patients at doses lower than 300 mgs/day, three patients at doses between 300 and 600 mgs/day, and five at doses higher than 600 mgs/day. Higher doses of clozapine were associated with greater risk of seizures than lower dose therapy (Pacia & Devinsky, 1994). It goes without saying that clozapine should be avoided, or used in exceptional circumstances with extreme caution, in patients with epilepsy.

Most antipsychotic drugs can cause EEG changes consisting of slowing of the background activity, particularly when used at high doses. In addition, some of these drugs, particularly clozapine, can cause paroxysmal electrographic changes in the form of inter-ictal sharp waves and spikes. This type of epileptiform activity, however, is not predictive of seizure occurrence. Data from studies by Tiihonen et al. suggest that a severe disorganization of the EEG recordings is a better predictor of seizure occurrence (Tiihonen et al., 1991).

Clozapine followed by chlorpromazine and loxapine are the three antipsychotic drugs with the highest risk of seizure occurrence. Those with a lower seizure risk include haloperidol, molindone, fluphenazine, perphenazine, trifluoperazine, and the atypical, risperidone. The PDR data available on the atypicals report seizures during clinical trials occurring with olanzapine (0.9%), quetiapine (0.8%), risperidone (0.3%), and ziprasidone (0.4%) (PDR, 2002). Whether the presence of AEDs at adequate levels protects patients with epilepsy from breakthrough seizures upon the introduction of antipsychotic drugs with proconvulsant properties is yet to be established. AEDs are sometimes started when clozapine is used at greater than 600 mg/d.

In addition to the proconvulsant properties of antipsychotic drugs, clinicians must also consider the pharmacokinetic and pharmacodynamic interactions between these and AEDs. Induction of hepatic enzymes upon the introduction of enzyme-inducing AEDs may result in an increase of the clearance of most antipsychotics. By the same token, discontinuation of an AED with enzyme-inducing properties may result in a decrease in the clearance of the antipsychotic drug, which in turn can lead to extrapyramidal side effects caused by an increase of their serum concentrations. Finally, certain antiepileptic drugs, like valproic acid, can inhibit the glucuronidation metabolism of APDs like clozapine.

ATTENTION-DEFICIT DISORDERS AND BEHAVIOR DISTURBANCES

While the adult epilepsy literature has characterized the full spectrum of DSM- and ICD-defined psychiatric disorders (Swinkels, Kuyk, van Dyck, & Spinhoven, 2005), similar efforts in the pediatric epilepsy literature have essentially just begun (Caplan et al., 2005; Jones, Watson, et al., 2007; McLellan et al., 2005; Ott et al., 2001), again with a focus on children with chronic epilepsy. Of the potential psychiatric comorbid diagnoses of childhood epilepsy, attention-deficit hyperactivity disorder (ADHD) has been of longstanding interest. Ounsted (1955) was among the first to call attention to the syndrome of hyperkinetic disorder and its complications in children with epilepsy. A growing literature has characterized disorders of attention in youth with epilepsy using diverse methods, including proxy (parent, teacher) rating scales, behavioral checklists, or formal cognitive tests (Dunn & Kronenberger, 2005). However, only three investigations determined the rate of ADHD and its subtypes in pediatric epilepsy using contemporary diagnostic criteria that now recognize specific subtypes of the disorder (DSM-IV) (Task Force on DSM-IV, 1994). One of these studies was population-based (Hesdorffer et al., 2004), while the others were derived from tertiary care clinical settings (Dunn, Austin, Harezlak, & Ambrosius, 2003; Sherman, Slick, Connolly, & Eyrl, 2007). All studies reported a significantly elevated rate of ADHD in childhood epilepsy with an over-representation of the inattentive subtype; a distribution that appears different from clinically derived samples of ADHD children seen in tertiary care centers where the combined subtype predominates (Barkley, 2006). None of the studies of ADHD in epilepsy examined the neurobehavioral or neuroradiological complications compared to children with epilepsy without ADHD or healthy controls.

In a population-based study carried out in the Isle of Wight in Great Britain, Rutter and collaborators found behavioral disorders in 28.6% of children with uncomplicated seizures, and 58.3% of children with both seizures and additional central nervous system pathology (Rutter, 1970). In a separate, population-based study of children with seizures, cardiac disorders, and controls, McDermott and collaborators found that children with epilepsy had more behavioral problems than either the children with cardiac disease or the controls. The children with epilepsy presented with higher rates of hyperactive behavior (28.1% vs. 12.6% in cardiac children and 4.9% in controls), headstrong or oppositional behavior (28.1% vs. 18.3% of cardiac children and 8.6% of controls), and antisocial behavior (18.2% vs. 11.6% of cardiac children and 8.8% of controls) (McDermott, 1995).

PRE-ICTAL SYMPTOMS AND EPISODES

Pre-ictal irritability, impulsive behavior, and poor frustration tolerance have been frequently reported by parents of children with epilepsy without ADHD. Their actual prevalence rates have yet to be established, however. Blanchet and Frommer identified pre-ictal irritability as a prominent symptom, associated with symptoms of depression (Blanchet & Frommer, 1986). These changes were more accentuated during the 24 hours preceding the seizure.

POST-ICTAL SYMPTOMS OF ADHD AND BEHAVIORAL DISTURBANCES

In the study on clinical characteristics and prevalence of post-ictal psychiatric symptoms cited above (Kanner et al., 2004), we found post-ictal irritability in 30 patients and poor frustration tolerance in 36, with a median duration of 24 hours for each symptom (range: 0.5–108 hours).

ADHD AND BEHAVIOR DISTURBANCES AS AN EXPRESSION OF PARA-ICTAL PROCESSES

Behavior disturbances and ADHD are frequent expressions of para-ictal processes, remitting or improving significantly upon reaching seizure control. Examples include "epileptic encephalopathies" such as the acquired epileptic aphasia of childhood (also known as Landau-Kleffner syndrome) (Morrell et al., 1995).

Aggressive behavior and ADHD can be seen in children with gelastic seizures associated with hypothalamic hamartomas. These psychiatric symptoms remit with cessation of epileptic seizures (Fohlen, Lellouch, & Delalande, 2003).

ADHD AND BEHAVIORAL DISTURBANCES AS AN INTER-ICTAL COMORBID DISORDER

The prevalence of ADHD in PWE is reported to range between 10 and 40% (McDermott, 1995; Rutter, 1970; Semrud-Clikeman & Wical, 1999). These data reflect statistics from pediatric populations with epilepsy. In fact, there are no data on the incidence or prevalence of ADHD in adults with epilepsy. Theoretically, if ADHD were to follow the same natural course in PWE than primary ADHD, 50% to 75% of children with epilepsy and ADHD would be expected to display symptoms of ADHD when entering adulthood. This question will need to be answered in future studies. Furthermore, the clinical manifestations of ADHD in adults with epilepsy are yet to be described in a systematic manner (see Chapter 50 on ADHD).

IATROGENIC ADHD

Many of the AEDs can cause symptoms of behavioral disturbances. The most frequent offenders include GABA-ergic drugs such as the barbiturates, benzodiazepines, and vigabatrin. Among the newer AEDs, topiramate and levetiracetam have been implicated. Valproic acid can cause behavioral disturbances at higher doses, and encephalopathy even with therapeutic doses.

TREATMENT OF ADHD IN PEOPLE WITH EPILEPSY

The pharmacological treatment of ADHD in PWE is the same as that of patients without seizures. In general, there is no pharmacokinetic interaction between CNS stimulants and AEDs, though there have been two reports that methylphenidate can increase blood levels of phenytoin and phenobarbital (McConnell & Duncan, 1998).

PSYCHOSOCIAL CONSEQUENCES FOR PEOPLE WITH EPILEPSY

IMPACT OF DEPRESSION ON QUALITY OF LIFE IN EPILEPSY PATIENTS

Psychiatric symptoms in general are found to have a greater impact on quality of life in patients with TLE than in healthy controls (Hermann et al., 2000). Depression, specifically, has a significantly negative impact on the quality of life of PWE. Lehrner et al. (Lehrner et al., 1999) found that depression was the single strongest predictor for each domain of health-related quality of life that persisted after controlling for seizure frequency, seizure severity, and other psychosocial variables. Perrine et al. (Perrine et al., 1995) found that mood had the highest correlations with scales of the Quality of Life in Epilepsy Inventory–89 (QOLIE-89) and was the strongest predictor of poor quality of life in regression analyses. In a study of patients with pharmaco-resistant TLE, Gilliam et al. found that high ratings of depression and neurotoxicity from AEDs were the only independent variables significantly associated with poor quality of life scores on the QOLIE-89 summary score. The authors *did not* find any correlation between the type and/or the frequency of seizures. Gilliam et al. also found that mood status was the strongest predictor of the patients' assessment of their own health status in a group of 125 patients more than one year after temporal lobe surgery (Gilliam, 2002; Gilliam et al., 1997). In a recent study, Kanner et al. (Kanner et al., 2010) found that sub-syndromic forms of depression had as negative an impact on quality of life as major depressive episodes and anxiety disorders. Furthermore, the comorbidity of a major depressive episode and more than one anxiety disorder was associated with a worse impact on quality of life.

STIGMA

The statement that "treating the seizure is not the sum of treating the patient with epilepsy" is most apparent in the psychosocial consequences and familial impact of epilepsy. While the practice of "sterilization of the epileptic" seems archaic, laws were in place in four American states in the early twentieth century that ratified this policy (Friedlander, 2001). Sadly, in the twenty-first century, research in developing countries reveals that the stigma of epilepsy still affects women. Santosh et al. point out that "The psychosocial consequences of the stigma potentials of epilepsy are nowhere more evident than in the case of women with epilepsy of the marriageable age in a developing country." They examined the prevalence of concealment or disclosure of the history of epilepsy and its consequences on the married life of women with epilepsy in southern India (Santosh, Kumar, Sarma, & Radhakrishnan, 2007). The authors found that 55% of 82 women with epilepsy concealed their history of epilepsy before marriage, and 38% of those who concealed it were separated or divorced. Concealment was described as a coping strategy for anticipated negative consequences of disclosure of the stigmatized disease. Unfortunately, this attitude is not solely a reflection of a developing country's practice. Researchers in Japan who studied marital statistics in a population of 278 patients with epilepsy found that in one-quarter of PWE who divorced, the reason for divorce was epilepsy (Wada et al., 2004). Kleinman et al. found that family, marriage, financial, and moral consequences of the social experience of epilepsy as a chronic disease demonstrated the importance of the social impact of epilepsy (Kleinman et al., 1995).

Along with the stigma of epilepsy itself, the comorbidities of epilepsy, including depression, anxiety, and non-epileptic seizures, impose a psychosocial burden themselves. Because of stigmatizing attitudes, patients may avoid or delay medical care and treatment for their mental health problems (Andrews, Henderson, & Hall, 2001). In a survey of 1,400 respondents with depression and anxiety, one-quarter of individuals did not present their symptoms to a physician, with reasons including fear of stigma (Meltzer et al., 2003). The importance of early detection of mental illness in patients with chronic somatic disorders is paramount in order to initiate psychiatric treatment to prevent chronification (Gatchel, Polatin, & Kinney, 1995). Freidl et al. investigated the impact of perceptions of stigma in patients with epilepsy, with non-epileptic seizures, and somatoform pain disorders in 101 inpatients and outpatients (Freidl et al., 2007). The authors found a high stigmatization concerning psychiatry, even in patients with epilepsy and somatoform/dissociative symptoms with psychiatric comorbidity, and concluded that perceived stigma is a barrier to recovery. In the next section, another significant comorbidity in epilepsy, non-epileptic seizures, is discussed.

NON-EPILEPTIC SEIZURES

Non-epileptic events are either physiological or psychological in origin (Schachter & LaFrance Jr., 2010). Psychogenic non-epileptic seizures (NES) resemble epileptic seizures presenting as a sudden, involuntary, time-limited alteration in behavior, motor activity, autonomic function, consciousness, or sensation. However, unlike epilepsy, NES do not result from epileptogenic pathology and are not accompanied by an epileptiform electrographic ictal pattern. Patients with NES are often disabled and difficult to treat.

EPIDEMIOLOGY AND COSTS

Of the 1% of the U.S. population diagnosed with epilepsy, 5–20% have NES (Gates, Luciano, & Devinsky, 1991). They are usually women (~80%) and most are between 15 and 35 years old (~80%) (Shen, Bowman, & Markand, 1990), though young children and the elderly can develop NES. The patients, their families, and society bear an enormous cost if psychiatric care is not provided or if inappropriate neurological therapy is instituted (LaFrance & Benbadis, 2006). Patients with NES take double the number of medications compared to patients with epilepsy (Hantke, Doherty, & Haltiner, 2007), and while NES are not responsive to AEDs, most patients with NES receive unnecessary AEDs (de Timary et al., 2002), having been presumed epileptic. Extensive observational data suggest that AEDs are ineffective or may even worsen NES (Krumholz, Niedermeyer, Alkaitis, & Morel, 1980). In some cases, potentially dangerous invasive diagnostic studies, toxic parenteral medications, or emergency intubation are administered. Diagnostic and therapeutic challenges are complicated by the 10–30% rate of comorbid NES and epileptic seizures (ES). Misdiagnosis and mistreatment of NES as ES costs an estimated $110–$920 million annually on diagnostic evaluations, inappropriate administration of AEDs, and emergency department utilization (Martin, Gilliam, Kilgore, Faught, & Kuzniecky, 1998).

PATHOLOGY OF NON-EPILEPTIC SEIZURES

While there is not a specific focal "lesion" that produces NES, we do have an understanding of the comorbid psychopathology in patients with NES. The phenomenology of NES, formerly referred to as "pseudoseizures," is well defined, with systematic assessments of diagnostic comorbidities and psychological testing (Gates & Rowan, 2000; Gram, Johannessen, Oterman, & Sillanpää, 1993). Studies have informed us of risk factors for NES (e.g., sexual or physical abuse, head injury) (Alper, Devinsky, Perrine, Vazquez, & Luciano, 1993; Westbrook, Devinsky, & Geocadin, 1998), and good prognostic features for NES resolution (e.g., female, independent lifestyle, short duration of NES) (Chabolla, Krahn, So, & Rummans, 1996; Bowman, 1999; Barry, 2001; Ettinger, Dhoon, Weisbrot, & Devinsky, 1999). Negative prognostic factors include longer duration of NES, comorbid neurological and/or psychiatric disease, and pending litigation, among others. Interestingly, CNS pathology and abnormal EEG did not predict outcome in two studies (Lelliott & Fenwick, 1991; Kanner et al., 1999).

There are two main "causes" of NES: post-traumatic and developmental (Kalogjera-Sackellares, 1996). Post-traumatic NES are thought to develop in response to acute or chronic exposure to traumatic experience(s), such as physical or psychological trauma, and sexual or physical abuse. "Developmental NES" refers to coping difficulties with tasks and milestones along the individual's continuum of psychosocial development. NES are clinically classified under different DSM-5 diagnoses, including *Conversion*, and *Dissociation disorders*. A much smaller percentage (<5%), present as *Factitious disorder and malingering*. A psychosocial stressor (e.g., sexual or physical abuse, loss of a relationship, work stress, parental divorce) (Wyllie, Glazer, Benbadis, Kotagal, & Wolgamuth, 1999) is often identified but may take time to uncover. Many patients with NES also suffer from mood (12–100%), anxiety (11–80%), personality (33–66%), non-seizure conversion/somatoform (20–100%), and non-seizure dissociative disorders (up to 90%) co-occurring with their primary NES diagnosis of conversion, somatoform, or dissociative disorder (Bowman, 1999).

DIAGNOSIS OF NON-EPILEPTIC SEIZURES

Obtaining an accurate diagnosis of NES is the essential first step for instituting proper therapy and avoiding unnecessary and potentially dangerous therapies. Clinical features of ES and NES overlap, however, and there is no one clinical feature that reliably distinguishes ES from NES. Subjective visceral, sensory, or psychic phenomena, alterations in responsiveness, and convulsive motor activity can be present in both disorders. Ictal presentations range from uncoordinated, disorganized motor activity to unresponsiveness without motor signs in NES. Clinical differentiation between NES and epilepsy has also been based on other identifiers such as the presence of pre-ictal pseudosleep (where the patient reports being asleep but EEG shows them to be awake), geotropic eye movements (forced downward deviation of the eyes toward the floor, with head turning), eye closure and post-ictal whispering with NES, and the presence of post-ictal headache and post-ictal nose rubbing with epilepsy. The use of suggestion to both provoke and stop NES is documented. With the issue of disclosure and informed consent, provocative procedures (e.g., saline injection) have drawn fire recently as a potentially unethical intervention (Smith et al., 1997). However, it is argued that when properly employed, seizure induction can act as a "stepping stone" to appropriate treatment if the patient develops insight into the events (i.e., that they are not epileptic) (Devinsky & Fisher, 1996). The distinction between physiological non-epileptic events and psychological NES is based on the combination of thorough history, physical exam in the peri-ictal period, and neurophysiological monitoring (Benbadis & LaFrance Jr., 2010). (See Table 43.8.)

Video-electroencephalographic monitoring (vEEG) led to an explosion of NES knowledge beginning in the 1980s (Boon & Williamson, 1993; Desai, Porter, & Penry, 1979; Jedrzejczak, Owczarek, & Majkowski, 1999; Penin, 1968).

An article reviewing the diagnostic tests, including EEG, neuroimaging, prolactin levels, and personality testing, provides the sensitivities and specificities for each of these tests (Cragar, Berry, Fakhoury, Cibula, & Schmitt, 2002). It was once thought that absence of physical injury sustained during a seizure was a diagnostic indicator differentiating NES from ES; however, more than half of all patients with NES actually do have physical injuries associated with their NES (Kanner, 2003). Other injuries occur as a result of iatrogenic issues, which are also prevalent in NES, and death has resulted from medically aggressive treatment of NES (Reuber, Baker, Gill, Smith, & Chadwick, 2004). Up to half of NES patients have had "non-epileptic psychogenic status" (Dworetzky, Bubrick, & Szaflarski, 2010), and 27.8% of patients with NES are admitted to intensive care units inappropriately for treatment (Reuber et al., 2003).

NES are not associated with epileptiform discharges on vEEG recordings, the gold standard for NES diagnosis (Ghougassian, d'Souza, Cook, & O'Brien, 2004). Studies of inter-rater reliability (IRR) in vEEG show moderate to excellent IRR for NES diagnosis (Benbadis et al., 2009; Syed et al., 2011). Humility in diagnosing NES without vEEG—and sometimes with vEEG—is critical. In one study, prediction of the nature of unusual seizures by the admitting neurologist was accurate in only 67% of cases. When observing these events without accompanying EEG, determination from observations of unit personnel and neurologists was correct in less than 80% of episodes (King et al., 1982). Lancman et al. strongly assert that "No matter how suggestive the clinical manifestation of a paroxysmal event may be of pseudoseizures, such diagnosis should never be made without electrographic confirmation" (Lancman, Lambrakis, & Steinhardt, 2001). The co-occurrence of ES and NES in a patient, present in 10% of patients with NES (Benbadis et al., 2001), further potentially complicates diagnosis and therapy. The diagnosis comes through careful history and thorough review of medical records that can identify different episode types and assess the supportive data.

EEG abnormalities in patients with NES do not necessarily confirm the diagnosis of ES. For example, EEGs showing "sharpish waves" or paroxysmal slowing provide little support of ES. Normal variants are also misinterpreted as inter-ictal epileptiform discharges in patients without epilepsy (Benbadis & Lin, 2008). A positive neurological history was present in a quarter of patients with NES, and a positive family history of epilepsy was present in 37.6% of NES patients (Lancman, Brotherton, Asconape, & Penry, 1993). While neurological signs, symptoms, and history are important to note in seizure patients, they are in no way pathognomonic in distinguishing NES from ES. A 2004 paper described three criteria in NES patients admitted for vEEG, yielding a positive predictive value of 85% (Davis, 2004). The criteria were (1) at least two NES per week, (2) refractory to at least two AEDs, and (3) at least two EEGs without epileptiform activity. Using "the rule of 2's" documenting seizure frequency, EEG abnormalities, and drug-treatment response prior to vEEG may help with definitive diagnosis of NES. An International League Against Epilepsy commissioned paper provided diagnostic

Table 43.8 BEHAVIORS TO HELP DISTINGUISH PSYCHOGENIC NON-EPILEPTIC AND EPILEPTIC SEIZURES

	PSYCHOGENIC NON-EPILEPTIC SEIZURES	EPILEPTIC SEIZURES
Observation		
Situational onset	Occasional	Rare
Gradual onset	Common	Rare
Precipitated by stimuli (noise, light)	Occasional	Rare
Purposeful movements	Occasional	Very rare
Opisthotonus "*arc de cercle*"	Occasional	Very rare
Tongue biting (tip)	Occasional	Rare
Tongue biting (side)	Rare	Common
Prolonged ictal atonia	Occasional	Very rare
Vocalization during "tonic-clonic" phase	Occasional	Very rare
Reactivity during "unconsciousness"	Occasional	Very rare
Rapid post-ictal reorientation	Common	Unusual
Undulating motor activity	Common	Very rare
Asynchronous limb movements	Common	Rare
Rhythmic pelvic movements	Occasional	Rare
Side-to-side head shaking	Common	Rare
Ictal crying	Occasional	Very rare
Ictal stuttering	Occasional	Rare
Post-ictal whispering	Occasional	Not present
Closed mouth in "tonic phase"	Occasional	Very rare
Closed eyelids during seizure onset	Very common	Rare
Convulsion >2 minutes	Common	Very rare
Resisted lid opening	Common	Very rare
Pupillary light reflex	Usually retained	Commonly absent
Lack of cyanosis	Common	Rare
Ictal grasping	Rare	Occurs in FLE and TLE
Post-ictal nose rubbing	Not present	Can occur in TLE
Stertorous breathing post-ictally	Not present	Common
Self-injury	May be present (especially excoriations)	May be present (especially lacerations)
Incontinence	May be present	May be present

Abbreviations: FLE, frontal lobe epilepsy; TLE, temporal lobe epilepsy.

Source: from Benbadis, S. R., & LaFrance Jr., W. C. (2010). Chapter 4. Clinical features and the role of video-EEG monitoring. In S. C. Schachter & W. C. LaFrance, Jr. (Eds.), *Gates and Rowan's Nonepileptic Seizures* (3rd ed., p. 41). Cambridge; New York: Cambridge University Press.

levels of certainty for NES based on history, event semiology and studies (with vEEG being the gold standard) (LaFrance et al., 2013).

TREATMENT LITERATURE

Along with diagnostic advances and a solid understanding of NES phenomenology, there is a growing evidence base for treatments for NES. Historically, the literature provided divergent views on natural history and outcome, as well as the value of psychotherapy, psychotropic medication, and other interventions for NES (Barry, 2001; Ramani, 2000; Aboukasm, Mahr, Gahry, Thomas, & Barkley, 1998; Walczak et al., 1995). More than a century after this disorder was clearly identified, there is now only one Class I, randomized, clinical trial (RCT) for treatment of NES (LaFrance et al., 2014) (discussed below). More controlled studies on treating this costly and disabling disorder are needed.

The NES treatment literature has been systematically reviewed (LaFrance & Devinsky, 2004; LaFrance & Barry, 2005; Baker, Brooks, Goodfellow, Bodde, & Aldenkamp, 2007; LaFrance, Reuber & Goldstein, 2013). There is a growing number of prospective series in the NES treatment literature published. Ataoglu et al. (Ataoglu, Ozcetin, Icmeli, & Ozbulut, 2003) randomized 30 patients with NES: half to paradoxical intention (PI) inpatient psychotherapy, and the other half to oral benzodiazepine therapy. PI consists of the therapist's suggesting that the patient engage in the undesired activity intentionally. The authors found greater improvements in anxiety scores and mildly better seizure control in the PI group than in the diazepam group. More recently, two prospective open trials of cognitive behavioral therapy (CBT) (Goldstein, Deale, Mitchell-O'Malley, Toone, & Mellers, 2004; LaFrance et al., 2009) and another two using group psychotherapy showed reduction in NES frequency and post-traumatic symptoms, respectively (Barry, Wittenberg, et al., 2008; Zaroff, Myers, Barr, Luciano, & Devinsky, 2004).

In a follow-up cohort study, 11 of 14 (79%) inpatients with NES experienced cessation or significant improvement after receiving a combination of hypnosis, group therapy, family therapy, and individual therapy (Kim, Barry, & Zeifert, 1998). A follow-up study at a comprehensive epilepsy center (CEP) (Aboukasm et al., 1998) suggested that CEP psychotherapists and CEP neurologists have similar favorable treatment outcomes, underscoring the beneficial impact of continuity of care and explanation of the nature of the seizures. The study also showed that the absence of communication with a NES patient about the diagnosis yields no improvement or worsening in their seizures. Rusch et al. (Rusch, Morris, Allen, & Lathrop, 2001) found that matching specific psychotherapies to the patient's comorbid diagnoses produced greater seizure-free rates, with 21 of 33 patients (63%) reaching event-free status at the end of treatment.

Moving beyond open-label data, more recently, two pilot RCTs were published comparing treatments to control groups. Goldstein et al. enrolled 66 patients with NES who were randomized to either CBT (plus standard medical care [SMC])

or SMC alone, scheduled to occur over four months. They found a reduction in the CBT-treated group, compared to the SMC group (Goldstein et al., 2010). LaFrance et al. enrolled 38 patients with NES in a double-blind pilot RCT who were randomized to either flexible-dose sertraline or placebo. They found a 45% reduction in NES in the SSRI-treated group and an 8% increase in the placebo group (LaFrance et al., 2010). As noted above, a multicenter pilot RCT enrolling 38 patients compared a CBT-informed psychotherapy (CBT-ip), CBT-ip and sertraline, sertraline alone and Treatment As Usual (TAU/SMC) and found the two psychotherapy arms showed a significant reduction in NES, comorbid symptoms (depression and anxiety) and improvement in functioning and quality of life. Ements in depression. Medication alone showed improvements in depression. The TAU/SMC arm showed no improvement in NES or secondary measures (LaFrance et al., 2014). Along with providing evidence for a manualized therapy for NES (Reiter et al., 2015), the study underscored that the current standard is not adequately treating patients with NES. More large-scale clinical trials are greatly needed to provide more Class I efficacy data for treatments for NES.

TREATMENT OF NON-EPILEPTIC SEIZURES

Prior to recent years, there was a lack of systematic intervention studies for NES. The void of generalizable, effective treatments for NES left only consensus recommendations (Ramani, 2000). Although psychotherapy is the mainstay of treatment recommendations, (Ramani, 2000; Aboukasm et al., 1998) its efficacy had been unproven with controlled data. Furthermore, no medications had proven effective in the treatment of NES. Clinicians do, however, use psychotropic medications to treat comorbid mood, anxiety, and elements of personality disorders, which often occur in patients with NES.

TREATMENT THEORIES

Etiological approaches for NES include *biomedical, psychodynamic, cognitive behavioral,* and *family theory* models (Ziegler & Imboden, 1962; Swingle, 1998; Krawetz et al., 2001). Precursors to psychogenic NES include childhood sexual abuse, physical abuse, comorbid psychiatric conditions, minor head trauma, disability claims, and reinforced behavioral patterns, among others. In identifying signs, symptoms, and situations that are associated with NES in a patient, we can formulate predisposing, precipitating and perpetuating factors that then inform interventions to promote the mental, physical, and social health of the patient (LaFrance & Devinsky, 2002).

Biomedical approaches highlight the absence of epileptiform activity during NES, demonstrating a functional-neuroanatomical dissociation model for NES (Brown & Trimble, 2000; Blumer, 2000). AEDs do not treat NES, and in some patients can worsen NES (Niedermeyer, Blumer, Holscher, & Walker, 1970). Conversely, withdrawal of AEDs has been shown to be safe in patients with lone NES (Oto, Espie, Pelosi, Selkirk, & Duncan, 2005). Anti-depressant, anti-anxiety, and antipsychotic therapies (e.g., medication, relaxation techniques) can treat symptomatic comorbid disorders and are currently being studied to evaluate whether medications may indirectly improve NES frequency or severity (LaFrance, Blum, Miller, Ryan, & Keitner, 2007).

NES are currently treated as a neuropsychiatric illness with psychological underpinnings. Both psychotherapeutic and psychopharmacological interventions are used to treat psychological conflicts and to treat the psychiatric comorbid diagnoses. These approaches fall under the headings of psychodynamic psychotherapy, cognitive behavioral therapies, family systems therapies, behavioral modification (mainly for mentally handicapped individuals), and biological psychiatric treatments.

CONCEPTUALIZATION FOR TREATMENT RECOMMENDATIONS

Bowman recommends the "4 E's" for interventions by neurologists: Explanation, Exploration, Exportation (for treatment), and do not Exile. The circumspect neurologist will exercise caution when deciding whether or not to "explore" a patient's trauma history. The "exile" issue is of greatest importance because it must be realized that once the vEEG diagnosis of NES is confirmed by the neurologist, the difficult work of collaboratively treating the patient with psychiatry has just begun.

Treatment and outcome vary considerably with the underlying psychopathology. Patients with NES generally have poor to fair treatment outcomes, but children and adolescents tend to do better than adults. In one study, outcome was significantly better for the younger patients at 1, 2, and 3 years after diagnosis (seizure-free percentages: children, 73%, 75%, 81%; and adults, 25%, 25%, 40%, respectively). The authors proposed that different psychological mechanisms at different ages of onset and greater effectiveness with earlier intervention may be factors leading to better outcome for children and adolescents (Wyllie et al., 1991).

The higher success rates are noted in the treatment articles and chapters describing longer inpatient admissions where patients were managed by a multidisciplinary team familiar with NES (Ramani & Gumnit, 1982). More recent reviews, however, reveal that roughly one-third of the patients have NES cessation, and another third have reduction in their NES (Reuber & Elger, 2003). In one NES outcome study, 71% of patients reported persistence of their seizures, in spite of 41% of the patients' having had inpatient psychiatric treatment (Reuber et al., 2003). Of the patients with lone NES, 40% continued to receive AEDs inappropriately, impacting their quality of life. Patients with NES rate their quality of life more poorly than those with epilepsy (Testa, Schefft, Szaflarski, Yeh, & Privitera, 2007). Quigg et al. found that quality of life measures improve, however, when patients reach NES freedom, and not when their NES are merely reduced (Quigg, Armstrong, Farace, & Fountain, 2002). Even with NES improvement, up to half of the patients remain on government or family support and are unemployed (Krawetz et al., 2001), and patients with NES generally do not expect

to return to work (Pestana, Foldvary-Shaefer, Marsillio, & Morris, 2003). One study found that patients with NES scored higher on hypochondriasis and somatic-complaint scales of the Minnesota Multiphasic Personality Inventory (MMPI) compared with patients with epilepsy, reflective of a focus on bodily function and neurological complaints (Owczarek, 2003). Poor quality of life in patients with NES may partly result from their somatic focus. A factor analysis of predictors of health-related quality of life revealed that patients with NES had more bodily concern than those with epilepsy (Testa, Szaflarski, Fargo, Dulay, & Schefft, 2003), and that somatic focus may influence health-related quality of life.

Noting the good prognosis if NES has a recent onset, Gates suggested that psychiatric treatment be based on NES chronicity: short-term psychotherapy for those with NES for less than six months, and more intensive inpatient therapy for those with longstanding NES (Gates, 1998). Although patients who receive feedback about their diagnosis and psychotherapy have better outcomes than those who do not (Aboukasm et al., 1998), the difference may reflect baseline characteristics of the groups, rather than the effects of intervention.

Based on the clinical and research reports to date, we suggest the following assessment and treatment approach by a multi-specialty neuropsychiatric team:

1. Proper diagnosis—vEEG for each patient with suspected NES, refractory, or pharmaco-resistant seizures.

2. Presentation—explain the NES diagnosis in a clear, positive, non-pejorative manner. The patient may make the diagnosis presentation to the family members if cognitively and emotionally capable. This process helps reveal the level of understanding and initial acceptance of the diagnosis by the patient. Clarifications can be made by the physician who is present. Communicate the diagnosis unambiguously to the referring physician and explain the need to eliminate unnecessary medications.

3. Psychiatric treatment—conduct a thorough psychiatric assessment to identify predisposing factors (including comorbid psychiatric disorders), seizure precipitants, and perpetuating factors. As diagnosis informs treatment, a dual-armed approach ensues with pharmacotherapy and/or psychotherapy, as indicated by the individual needs of the patient with NES.

Psychopharmacology begins with tapering and discontinuing ineffective AEDs for patients with lone NES, unless a specific AED has a documented beneficial psychopharmacological effect in the patient. In patients with mixed ES/NES, reduce high-dose or multiple AED therapy if possible. Use psychopharmacological agents to treat mood, anxiety, or psychotic disorders (LaFrance & Devinsky, 2002).

Psychogenic NES are likely to be the result of a complex interaction between psychiatric disorders, psychosocial stressors, dysfunctional coping styles, and CNS vulnerability (Mökleby et al., 2002). Identifying the underlying stressors and providing supportive psychotherapy can help some patients, but this is often insufficient or ineffective. Studies consistently identify three main comorbid diagnoses in patients with NES: *Major depressive disorder, Post-traumatic stress disorder*, and *Cluster B personality traits characterized by impulsivity/hostility* (Bowman & Markand, 1996), (Rechlin, Loew, & Joraschky, 1997). Three additional critical areas of dysfunction in the NES population are emotion regulation, family dynamics, and unemployment/disability (Walczak et al., 1995; Holmes et al., 2001; Griffith, Polles, & Griffith, 1998). Poorer outcomes of treatment may be associated with the high number of comorbid psychiatric disorders and psychosocial stressors (Carson, Ringbauer, MacKenzie, Warlow, & Sharpe, 2000). Therefore, therapy for patients with NES may require combined psychological education, psychotherapy, and pharmacotherapy, while simultaneously eliminating ineffective AEDs. A National Institute of Neurological Disorders and Stroke (NINDS)/National Institute of Mental Health (NIMH)/American Epilepsy Society (AES) workshop emphasized that there is a great need for these interventions to be studied in randomized, controlled trials (LaFrance et al., 2006).

Prior published treatment reports reveal that coordination between neurologists and psychiatrists/psychologists with accurate diagnosis and prompt initiation of psychotherapy and communication between care providers, patients and families yields higher treatment success.

SUMMARY

In conclusion, a significant number of PWE have psychiatric disorders that accompany their seizures, and/or integrated mood/anxiety/psychotic and personality integrated symptoms secondary to their epilepsy. Quality of life and stigma associated with epilepsy have a significant impact on the lives of PWE. Management of epilepsy is also complicated by the presence of NES. Further research in these areas is needed to inform diagnosis, pathophysiology, and treatment of these neuropsychiatric aspects of epilepsy.

CLINICAL PEARLS

- Among the physiological non-epileptic events that must be considered in the differential diagnosis of treatment-resistant epilepsy are several sleep disorders, syncope, migraines, or transient ischemic attacks.

- Comorbid psychiatric disorders commonly occur in patients with epilepsy.

- The evaluation of any type of psychopathology in patients with epilepsy must be approached with the following questions in mind:

  - Is this psychiatric disturbance temporally related to the occurrence of seizures? Is the onset of psychiatric symptoms associated with the remission of seizures? (We consider the peri-ictal psychiatric symptoms (pre-ictal and post-ictal) as well as inter-ictal symptoms

associated with the onset or remission of seizures an expression of a para-ictal process.)

- Are the psychiatric symptoms the result of the introduction of an antiepileptic drug (AED) with potentially negative psychotropic properties, or did they appear after discontinuation of an AED with positive psychotropic properties (mood stabilizing, antidepressant, and anxiolytic properties)?

- Do the symptoms meet diagnostic criteria of the DSM or the ICD, or do these symptoms present as an atypical disorder?

- What is the impact of the psychiatric disorder at hand on the quality of life of patients?

- What is the treatment for the psychiatric disorder?

- If pharmacotherapy is required, how do psychotropic drugs interact with AEDs, and what is the impact of psychotropic drugs on the seizure threshold?

- Depression is the most frequent psychiatric disorder in patients with epilepsy: more common in patients with partial seizure disorders of temporal or frontal lobe origin and among patients with poorly controlled seizures (Edeh & Toone, 1987; Jacoby et al., 1996; Mendez et al., 1986; O'Donoghue et al., 1999).

- The suicide rate in depressed PWE is 9–25 times higher in patients with partial seizures of temporal lobe origin than expected in the overall population (Nilsson, Tomson, Farahmand, Diwan, & Persson, 1997; Rafnsson, Olafsson, Hauser, & Gudmundsson, 2001; Robertson, 1997).

- Pre-ictal symptoms of depression and depressive episodes typically present as a dysphoric mood in which the prodromal symptoms may extend for hours or even one to three days prior to the onset of a seizure.

- Depressive disorders often occur with anxiety disorders. Recognition of such comorbidity is critical, as failure to target the anxiety disorder in the treatment of these patients can result in recurrence of the depressive disorder.

- The addition of AEDs with mood-stabilizing properties, such as carbamazepine, valproic acid, and lamotrigine, can occasionally cause depressive episodes, albeit with a significantly lower frequency than other AEDs. More often than not, these AEDs are associated with the occurrence of depression *upon their discontinuation* in patients with a prior history of depression or panic disorder, which had been kept in remission by these AEDs (Ketter et al., 1994).

- Depressive disorder may follow antero-temporal lobectomy (Savard, Andermann, Reutens, & Andermann, 1998); patients with a prior history of depression are at greater risk.

- SSRIs are safe in general in patients with epilepsy.

- Most antidepressants are metabolized in the liver, and their metabolism is accelerated in the presence of AEDs with enzyme-inducing properties, which include phenytoin, carbamazepine, phenobarbital, primidone at regular doses, and oxcarbazepine and topiramate at doses above 900 mg/day and 300 mg/day, respectively. This pharmacokinetic effect is not observed with the new AEDs gabapentin, lamotrigine, tiagabine, levetiracetam, zonisamide, pregabalin, vigabatrin, and ezogabine.

- Electroconvulsive therapy (ECT) is not contraindicated in depressed PWE (Fink, Kellner, & Sackeim, 1999; Regenold, Weintraub, & Taller, 1998; Sackeim, Decina, Prohovnik, Malitz, & Resor, 1983).

- Vagal nerve stimulation (VNS) is used as adjunctive treatment for epilepsy and has also shown longer-term mood effects (Marangell et al., 2002).

- Ictal fear or panic is the most frequent ictal psychiatric symptom. It is the sole or predominant clinical expression of a simple partial epileptic seizure (aura) or the initial symptom of a complex partial epileptic seizure, and it usually has a mesial temporal lobe origin.

- A careful history can help distinguish inter-ictal from ictal panic. Ictal panic is typically less than 30 seconds in duration, is stereotypical, occurs out of context with concurrent events, and is associated with other ictal phenomena, such as periods of confusion of variable duration and subtle or overt automatisms. The intensity of the sensation of fear is mild to moderate and rarely reaches the intensity of a panic attack.

- SSRIs can prevent the occurrence of inter-ictal panic attacks and generalized anxiety disorder, but there is as of yet no evidence that these drugs have any impact on post-ictal psychiatric symptoms.

- In most cases, insomnia is the initial presenting symptom. In patients with recurrent post-ictal psychotic episodes, families need to learn to recognize these symptoms so that a timely administration of 1–2 mgs of risperidone may avert the episode. It should be given for two to five days and then discontinued.

- *Ictal psychotic symptoms or episodes* should always be considered in the differential diagnosis of post-ictal psychosis and psychosis of epilepsy as a whole.

- Psychotic disorder as an expression of a drug toxicity has been reported with several AEDs, most prominently ethosuximide, phenobarbital, and primidone, as well as the newer AEDs topiramate and levetiracetam (McConnell & Duncan, 1998). Psychotic disorders can occasionally follow the discontinuation of AEDs, particularly those with mood-stabilizing properties.

- Antipsychotic drugs (APD) are necessary in the management of psychotic disorders in epilepsy patients despite their proconvulsant properties. While the risk of seizure occurrence must always be carefully considered when starting antipsychotic drugs in these patients, it should never be a reason not to treat a patient in need of antipsychotic medication.

- There is no pharmacokinetic interaction between CNS stimulants and most AEDs.

- Clinical differentiation between non-epileptic seizures and epilepsy has also been based on other identifiers such as the presence of pre-ictal pseudosleep (where the patient reports being asleep but EEG shows them to be awake), geotropic eye movements (forced downward deviation of the eyes toward the floor with head turning), eye closure, and post-ictal whispering with NES; and the presence of post-ictal headache and post-ictal nose-rubbing with epilepsy.

- Non-epileptic seizures are currently treated as a neuropsychiatric illness with psychological underpinnings. Psychotherapeutic interventions are used to address psychological conflicts, and psychopharmacological interventions are used to treat comorbid psychiatric diagnoses.

- Validated, manualized treatment for patients with NES has been shown to reduce NES frequency, improve comorbid symptoms, quality of life and functioning.

DISCLOSURE STATEMENTS

Dr. LaFrance has received research support from the National Institutes of Health (NINDS 5K23NS45902 [PI]), the American Epilepsy Society, the Epilepsy Foundation, Rhode Island Hospital, and the Siravo Foundation; has acted a legal expert; serves on the editorial board of *Epilepsy & Behavior*; is chair of the American Epilepsy Society (AES) and International League Against Epilepsy (ILAE) NES Task Forces; and receives royalties from the publication of *Gates and Rowan's Nonepileptic Seizures,* 3rd ed. (New York: Cambridge University Press, 2010). Dr. Kanner has received research funding from Pfizer Laboratories.

REFERENCES

Aboukasm, A., Mahr, G., Gahry, B. R., Thomas, A., & Barkley, G. L. (1998). Retrospective analysis of the effects of psychotherapeutic interventions on outcomes of psychogenic nonepileptic seizures. *Epilepsia, 39*(5), 470–473.

Adachi, N., Kato, M., Sekimoto, M., Ichikawa, I., Akanuma, N., Uesugi, H., et al. (2003). Recurrent postictal psychosis after remission of interictal psychosis: further evidence of bimodal psychosis. *Epilepsia, 44*(9), 1218–1222.

Adachi, N., Matsuura, M., Hara, T., Oana, Y., Okubo, Y., Kato, M., et al. (2002). Psychoses and epilepsy: Are interictal and postictal psychoses distinct clinical entities? *Epilepsia, 43*(12), 1574–1582.

Alper, K., Devinsky, O., Perrine, K., Vazquez, B., & Luciano, D. (1993). Nonepileptic seizures and childhood sexual and physical abuse. *Neurology, 43*(10), 1950–1953.

Alper, K., Schwartz, K. A., Kolts, R. L., & Khan, A. (2007). Seizure incidence in psychopharmacological clinical trials: An analysis of Food and Drug Administration (FDA) summary basis of approval reports. *Biological Psychiatry, 62*(4), 345–354.

Anatassopoulos, G., & Kokkini, D. (1969). Suicidal attempts in psychomotor epilepsy. *Behavioral Neuropsychiatry, 1*(9), 11–16.

Andrews, G., Henderson, S., & Hall, W. (2001). Prevalence, comorbidity, disability and service utilisation. Overview of the Australian National Mental Health Survey. *British Journal of Psychiatry, 178,* 145–153.

Ataoglu, A., Ozcetin, A., Icmeli, C., & Ozbulut, O. (2003). Paradoxical therapy in conversion reaction. *Journal of Korean Medical Science, 18*(4), 581–584.

Baker, G. A., Brooks, J. L., Goodfellow, L., Bodde, N., & Aldenkamp, A. (2007). Treatments for non-epileptic attack disorder. *Cochrane Database of Systematic Reviews,* (1), CD006370.

Barabas, G., & Matthews, W. S. (1988). Barbiturate anticonvulsants as a cause of severe depression. *Pediatrics, 82*(2), 284–285.

Barclay, L. (2008). FDA requires warnings about suicidality risk with antiepileptic drugs. *Medscape Medical News,* http://www.medscape.com/viewarticle/585541.

Barry, J. J. (2001). Nonepileptic seizures: An overview. *Central Nervous System Spectrums, 6*(12), 956–962.

Barry, J. J., Ettinger, A. B., Friel, P., Gilliam, F. G., Harden, C. L., Hermann, B., et al. (2008). Consensus statement: The evaluation and treatment of people with epilepsy and affective disorders. *Epilepsy & Behavior, 13*(Suppl 1), S1–S29.

Barry, J. J., Wittenberg, D., Bullock, K. D., Michaels, J. B., Classen, C. C., & Fisher, R. S. (2008). Group therapy for patients with psychogenic nonepileptic seizures: A pilot study. *Epilepsy & Behavior, 13*(4), 624–629.

Bell, A. J., Cole, A., Eccleston, D., & Ferrier, I. N. (1993). Lithium neurotoxicity at normal therapeutic levels. *British Journal of Psychiatry, 162,* 689–692.

Benbadis, S. R., Agrawal, V., & Tatum, W. O. IV (2001). How many patients with psychogenic nonepileptic seizures also have epilepsy? *Neurology, 57*(5), 915–917.

Benbadis, S. R., & Hauser, W. A. (2000). An estimate of the prevalence of psychogenic non-epileptic seizures. *Seizure, 9*(4), 280–281.

Benbadis, S. R., & LaFrance, W. C. Jr (2010). Chapter 4. Clinical features and the role of video-EEG monitoring. In S. C. Schachter & W. C. LaFrance, Jr. (Eds.), *Gates and Rowan's nonepileptic seizures* (3rd ed., pp. 38–50). Cambridge; New York: Cambridge University Press.

Benbadis, S. R., LaFrance, W. C., Jr., Papandonatos, G. D., Korabathina, K., Lin, K., & Kraemer, H. C. (2009). Interrater reliability of EEG-video monitoring. *Neurology, 73*(11), 843–846.

Benbadis, S. R., & Lin, K. (2008). Errors in EEG interpretation and misdiagnosis of epilepsy. Which EEG patterns are overread? *European Neurology, 59*(5), 267–271.

Blackwood, D. H., Cull, R. E., Freeman, C. P., Evans, J. I., & Mawdsley, C. (1980). A study of the incidence of epilepsy following ECT. *Journal of Neurology, Neurosurgery, & Psychiatry, 43*(12), 1098–1102.

Blanchet, P., & Frommer, G. P. (1986). Mood change preceding epileptic seizures. *Journal of Nervous and Mental Disease, 174*(8), 471–476.

Blumer, D. (2000). Chapter 24. On the psychobiology of non-epileptic seizures. In J. R. Gates & A. J. Rowan (Eds.), *Non-epileptic seizures* (2nd ed., pp. 305–310). Boston: Butterworth-Heinemann.

Blumer, D., & Altshuler, L. L. (1998). Affective disorders. In J. Engel & T. A. Pedley (Eds.), *Epilepsy: A comprehensive textbook* (2nd ed., pp. 2083–2099). Philadelphia: Lippincott-Raven.

Blumer, D., & Zielinksi, J. (1988). Pharmacologic treatment of psychiatric disorders associated with epilepsy. *Journal of Epilepsy, 1,* 135–150.

Boon, P. A., & Williamson, P. D. (1993). The diagnosis of pseudoseizures. *Clinical Neurology & Neurosurgery, 95*(1), 1–8.

Bowman, E. S. (1999). Nonepileptic seizures: Psychiatric framework, treatment, and outcome. *Neurology, 53*(5 Suppl 2), S84–88.

Bowman, E. S., & Markand, O. N. (1996). Psychodynamics and psychiatric diagnoses of pseudoseizure subjects. *American Journal of Psychiatry, 153*(1), 57–63.

Bredkjaer, S. R., Mortensen, P. B., & Parnas, J. (1998). Epilepsy and non-organic non-affective psychosis. National epidemiologic study. *British Journal of Psychiatry, 172,* 235–238.

Brent, D. A., Crumrine, P. K., Varma, R. R., Allan, M., & Allman, C. (1987). Phenobarbital treatment and major depressive disorder in children with epilepsy. *Pediatrics, 80*(6), 909–917.

Brown, R. J., & Trimble, M. R. (2000). Editorial: Dissociative psychopathology, non-epileptic seizures, and neurology. *Journal of Neurology, Neurosurgery, & Psychiatry, 69*(3), 285–288.

Brown, R. T., Freeman, W. S., Perrin, J. M., Stein, M. T., Amler, R. W., Feldman, H. M., et al. (2001). Prevalence and assessment of attention-deficit/hyperactivity disorder in primary care settings. *Pediatrics, 107*(3), E43.

Caplan, R., Siddarth, P., Gurbani, S., Hanson, R., Sankar, R., & Shields, W. D. (2005). Depression and anxiety disorders in pediatric epilepsy. *Epilepsia, 46*(5), 720–730.

Carson, A. J., Ringbauer, B., MacKenzie, L., Warlow, C., & Sharpe, M. (2000). Neurological disease, emotional disorder, and disability: They are related: A study of 300 consecutive new referrals to a neurology outpatient department. *Journal of Neurology, Neurosurgery, & Psychiatry, 68*(2), 202–206.

Chabolla, D. R., Krahn, L. E., So, E. L., & Rummans, T. A. (1996). Psychogenic nonepileptic seizures. *Mayo Clinic Proceedings, 71*(5), 493–500.

Christensen, J., Vestergaard, M., Mortensen, P. B., Sidenius, P., & Agerbo, E. (2007). Epilepsy and risk of suicide: A population-based case-control study. *Lancet Neurology, 6*(8), 693–698.

Cragar, D. E., Berry, D. T., Fakhoury, T. A., Cibula, J. E., & Schmitt, F. A. (2002). A review of diagnostic techniques in the differential diagnosis of epileptic and nonepileptic seizures. *Neuropsychology Review, 12*(1), 31–64.

Curran, S., & de Pauw, K. (1998). Selecting an antidepressant for use in a patient with epilepsy. Safety considerations. *Drug Safety, 18*(2), 125–133.

Currie, S., Heathfield, K. W., Henson, R. A., & Scott, D. F. (1971). Clinical course and prognosis of temporal lobe epilepsy. A survey of 666 patients. *Brain, 94*(1), 173–190.

Daly, D. (1958). Ictal affect. *American Journal of Psychiatry, 115*(2), 97–108.

Davis, B. J. (2004). Predicting nonepileptic seizures utilizing seizure frequency, EEG, and response to medication. *European Neurology, 51*(3), 153–156.

de Araujo Filho, G. M., Pascalicchio, T. F., Sousa Pda, S., Lin, K., Ferreira Guilhoto, L. M., & Yacubian, E. M. (2007). Psychiatric disorders in juvenile myoclonic epilepsy: A controlled study of 100 patients. *Epilepsy & Behavior, 10*(3), 437–441.

de Timary, P., Fouchet, P., Sylin, M., Indriets, J. P., De Barsy, T., Lefebvre, A., et al. (2002). Non-epileptic seizures: Delayed diagnosis in patients presenting with electroencephalographic (EEG) or clinical signs of epileptic seizures. *Seizure, 11,* 193–197.

Desai, B. T., Porter, R. J., & Penry, J. K. (1979). Abstract GS 43: The psychogenic seizure by videotape analysis: A study of 42 attacks in 6 patients. *Neurology (Minneapolis), 29,* 602.

Devinsky, O., Abramson, H., Alper, K., FitzGerald, L. S., Perrine, K., Calderon, J., et al. (1995). Postictal psychosis: A case control series of 20 patients and 150 controls. *Epilepsy Research, 20*(3), 247–253.

Devinsky, O., & Fisher, R. (1996). Ethical use of placebos and provocative testing in diagnosing nonepileptic seizures. *Neurology, 47*(4), 866–870.

Dongier, S. (1959). Statistical study of clinical and electroencephalographic manifestations of 536 psychotic episodes occurring in 516 epileptics between clinical seizures. *Epilepsia, 1,* 117–142.

Dunn, D. W., Austin, J. K., Harezlak, J., & Ambrosius, W. T. (2003). ADHD and epilepsy in childhood. *Developmental Medicine & Child Neurology, 45*(1), 50–54.

Dunn, D. W., & Kronenberger, W. G. (2005). Childhood epilepsy, attention problems, and ADHD: Review and practical considerations. *Seminars in Pediatric Neurology, 12*(4), 222–228.

Dworetzky, B. A., Bubrick, E. J., & Szaflarski, J. P. (2010). Nonepileptic psychogenic status: Markedly prolonged psychogenic nonepileptic seizures. *Epilepsy & Behavior, 19*(1), 65–68.

Edeh, J., & Toone, B. (1987). Relationship between interictal psychopathology and the type of epilepsy. Results of a survey in general practice. *British Journal of Psychiatry, 151,* 95–101.

Ettinger, A., Reed, M., & Cramer, J. (2004). Depression and comorbidity in community-based patients with epilepsy or asthma. *Neurology, 63*(6), 1008–1014.

Ettinger, A. B., Dhoon, A., Weisbrot, D. M., & Devinsky, O. (1999). Predictive factors for outcome of nonepileptic seizures after diagnosis. *Journal of Neuropsychiatry & Clinical Neurosciences, 11*(4), 458–463.

Ettinger, A. B., Reed, M. L., Goldberg, J. F., & Hirschfeld, R. M. (2005). Prevalence of bipolar symptoms in epilepsy vs other chronic health disorders. *Neurology, 65*(4), 535–540.

Ferrari, M., Barabas, G., & Matthews, W. S. (1983). Psychological and behavioral disturbance among epileptic children treated with barbiturate anticonvulsants. *American Journal of Psychiatry, 140*(1), 112–113.

Fink, M., Kellner, C. H., & Sackeim, H. A. (1999). Intractable seizures, status epilepticus, and ECT. *Journal of ECT, 15*(4), 282–284.

Fisher, R. S., Vickrey, B. G., Gibson, P., Hermann, B., Penovich, P., Scherer, A., et al. (2000). The impact of epilepsy from the patient's perspective, I. Descriptions and subjective perceptions. *Epilepsy Research, 41*(1), 39–51.

Fohlen, M., Lellouch, A., & Delalande, O. (2003). Hypothalamic hamartoma with refractory epilepsy: Surgical procedures and results in 18 patients. *Epileptic Disorders, 5*(4), 267–273.

Forsgren, L., & Nystrom, L. (1990). An incident case-referent study of epileptic seizures in adults. *Epilepsy Research, 6*(1), 66–81.

Fountain, N. B., Van Ness, P. C., Swain-Eng, R., Tonn, S., & Bever, C. T., Jr. (2010). Quality improvement in neurology: AAN Epilepsy Quality Measures: Report of the Quality Measurement and Reporting Subcommittee of the American Academy of Neurology. *Neurology, 76*(1), 94–99.

Freidl, M., Spitzl, S. P., Prause, W., Zimprich, F., Lehner-Baumgartner, E., Baumgartner, C., et al. (2007). The stigma of mental illness: Anticipation and attitudes among patients with epileptic, dissociative or somatoform pain disorder. *International Review of Psychiatry, 19*(2), 123–129.

Friedlander, W. J. (2001). Chapter 9. Societal aspects. *The history of modern epilepsy: The beginning, 1865–1914* (vol. 45, pp. 239–275). Westport, CT: Greenwood Press.

Fritze, J., Unsorg, B., & Lanczik, M. (1991). Interaction between carbamazepine and fluvoxamine. *Acta Psychiatrica Scandinavica, 84*(6), 583–584.

Gatchel, R. J., Polatin, P. B., & Kinney, R. K. (1995). Predicting outcome of chronic back pain using clinical predictors of psychopathology: A prospective analysis. *Health Psychology, 14*(5), 415–420.

Gates, J. R. (1998). Chapter 8. Diagnosis and treatment of nonepileptic seizures. In H. W. McConnell & P. J. Snyder (Eds.), *Psychiatric comorbidity in epilepsy. Basic mechanisms, diagnosis, and treatment* (1st ed., pp. 187–204). Washington, DC: American Psychiatric Press.

Gates, J. R., Luciano, D., & Devinsky, O. (1991). Chapter 18. The classification and treatment of nonepileptic events. In O. Devinsky & W. H. Theodore (Eds.), *Epilepsy and behavior* (vol. 12, pp. 251–263). New York: Wiley-Liss.

Gates, J. R., & Rowan, A. J. (Eds.). (2000). *Non-epileptic seizures* (2nd ed.). Boston, MA: Butterworth-Heinemann.

Ghougassian, D. F., d'Souza, W., Cook, M. J., & O'Brien, T. J. (2004). Evaluating the utility of inpatient video–EEG monitoring. *Epilepsia, 45*(8), 928–932.

Gilby, K. L., Sydserff, S., Patey, A. M., Thorne, V., St.-Onge, V., Jans, J., et al. C. (2009). Postnatal epigenetic influences on seizure susceptibility in seizure-prone versus seizure-resistant rat strains.. *Behavioral Neuroscience, 123*(2), 337–346. doi: 10.1037/a0014730

Gilliam, F. (2002). Optimizing health outcomes in active epilepsy. *Neurology, 58*(8 Suppl 5), S9–S20.

Gilliam, F., & Kanner, A. M. (2002). Treatment of depressive disorders in epilepsy patients. *Epilepsy & Behavior, 3*(5 Suppl 1), S2–S9.

Gilliam, F., Kuzniecky, R., Faught, E., Black, L., Carpenter, G., & Schrodt, R. (1997). Patient-validated content of epilepsy-specific quality-of-life measurement. *Epilepsia, 38*(2), 233–236.

Gilliam, F. G., Barry, J. J., Hermann, B. P., Meador, K. J., Vahle, V., & Kanner, A. M. (2006). Rapid detection of major depression in epilepsy: A multicentre study. *Lancet Neurology, 5*(5), 399–405.

Goldstein, L. H., Chalder, T., Chigwedere, C., Khondoker, M. R., Moriarty, J., Toone, B. K., et al. (2010). Cognitive-behavioral therapy for psychogenic nonepileptic seizures: A pilot RCT. *Neurology, 74*(24), 1986–1994.

Goldstein, L. H., Deale, A. C., Mitchell-O'Malley, S. J., Toone, B. K., & Mellers, J. D. C. (2004). An evaluation of cognitive behavioral therapy as a treatment for dissociative seizures: A pilot study. *Cognitive & Behavioral Neurology, 17*(1), 41–49.

Gram, L., Johannessen, S. I., Oterman, P. O., & Sillanpää, M. (Eds.) (1993). *Pseudo-epileptic seizures* (1st ed.). Petersfield, UK: Wrightson Biomedical Publishing, Ltd.

Griffith, J. L., Polles, A., & Griffith, M. E. (1998). Pseudoseizures, families, and unspeakable dilemmas. *Psychosomatics, 39*(2), 144–153.

Grimsley, S. R., Jann, M. W., Carter, J. G., D'Mello, A. P., & D'Souza, M. J. (1991). Increased carbamazepine plasma concentrations after fluoxetine coadministration. *Clinical Pharmacology & Therapeutics, 50*(1), 10–15.

Hancock, J. C., & Bevilacqua, A. R. (1971). Temporal lobe dysrhythmia and impulsive or suicidal behavior: Preliminary report. *Southern Medical Journal, 64*(10), 1189–1193.

Hantke, N. C., Doherty, M. J., & Haltiner, A. M. (2007). Medication use profiles in patients with psychogenic nonepileptic seizures. *Epilepsy & Behavior, 10*, 333–335.

Haselberger, M. B., Freedman, L. S., & Tolbert, S. (1997). Elevated serum phenytoin concentrations associated with coadministration of sertraline. *Journal of Clinical Psychopharmacology, 17*(2), 107–109.

Hermann, B. P., Seidenberg, M., Bell, B., Woodard, A., Rutecki, P., & Sheth, R. (2000). Comorbid psychiatric symptoms in temporal lobe epilepsy: Association with chronicity of epilepsy and impact on quality of life. *Epilepsy & Behavior, 1*(3), 184–190.

Hesdorffer, D. C., Hauser, W. A., Annegers, J. F., & Cascino, G. (2000). Major depression is a risk factor for seizures in older adults. *Annals of Neurology, 47*(2), 246–249.

Hesdorffer, D. C., Hauser, W. A., Olafsson, E., Ludvigsson, P., & Kjartansson, O. (2006). Depression and suicide attempt as risk factors for incident unprovoked seizures. *Annals of Neurology, 59*(1), 35–41.

Hesdorffer, D. C., & Kanner, A. M. (2009). The FDA alert on suicidality and antiepileptic drugs: Fire or false alarm? *Epilepsia, 50*(5), 978–986.

Hesdorffer, D. C., Ludvigsson, P., Olafsson, E., Gudmundsson, G., Kjartansson, O., & Hauser, W. A. (2004). ADHD as a risk factor for incident unprovoked seizures and epilepsy in children. *Archives of General Psychiatry, 61*(7), 731–736.

Hitiris, N., Mohanraj, R., Norrie, J., Sills, G. J., & Brodie, M. J. (2007). Predictors of pharmacoresistant epilepsy. *Epilepsy Research, 75*(2–3), 192–196.

Holmes, M. D., Dodrill, C. B., Bachtler, S., Wilensky, A. J., Ojemann, L. M., & Miller, J. W. (2001). Evidence that emotional maladjustment is worse in men than in women with psychogenic nonepileptic seizures. *Epilepsy & Behavior, 2*, 568–573.

Jacoby, A., Baker, G. A., Steen, N., Potts, P., & Chadwick, D. W. (1996). The clinical course of epilepsy and its psychosocial correlates: Findings from a U.K. Community study. *Epilepsia, 37*(2), 148–161.

Janz, D. (2002). Chapter 4. The psychiatry of idiopathic generalized epilepsy. In M. R. Trimble & B. Schmitz (Eds.), *The neuropsychiatry of epilepsy* (pp. 41–61). New York: Cambridge University Press.

Jedrzejczak, J., Owczarek, K., & Majkowski, J. (1999). Psychogenic pseudoepileptic seizures: Clinical and electroencephalogram (EEG) video-tape recordings. *European Journal of Neurology, 6*(4), 473–479.

Jensen, I., & Vaernet, K. (1977). Temporal lobe epilepsy. Follow-up investigation of 74 temporal lobe resected patients. *Acta Neurochirurgica (Vienna), 37*(3–4), 173–200.

Jobe, P. C. (2006). Affective disorder and epilepsy comorbidity in the genetically epilepsy prone-rat (GEPR). In F. G. Gilliam, A. M. Kanner, & Y. I. Sheline (Eds.), *Depression and brain dysfunction* (pp. 121–157). London: Taylor & Francis.

Jobe, P. C., Mishra, P. K., Browning, R. A., Wang, C., Adams-Curtis, L. E., Ko, K. H., et al. (1994). Noradrenergic abnormalities in the genetically epilepsy-prone rat. [Research Support, U.S. Gov't, P.H.S. Review]. *Brain Research Bulletin, 35*(5–6), 493–504.

Jones, J. E., Bell, B., Fine, J., Rutecki, P., Seidenberg, M., & Hermann, B. (2007). A controlled prospective investigation of psychiatric comorbidity in temporal lobe epilepsy. *Epilepsia, 48*(12), 2357–2360.

Jones, J. E., Hermann, B. P., Barry, J. J., Gilliam, F. G., Kanner, A. M., & Meador, K. J. (2003). Rates and risk factors for suicide, suicidal ideation, and suicide attempts in chronic epilepsy. *Epilepsy & Behavior, 4*(3), 31–38.

Jones, J. E., Watson, R., Sheth, R., Caplan, R., Koehn, M., Seidenberg, M., et al. (2007). Psychiatric comorbidity in children with new onset epilepsy. *Developmental Medicine & Child Neurology, 49*(7), 493–497.

Jones, N. C., Kumar, G., O'Brien, T. J., Morris, M. J., Rees, S. M., & Salzberg, M. R. (2009). Anxiolytic effects of rapid amygdala kindling, and the influence of early life experience in rats. *Behavioural Brain Research, 203*(1), 81–87. doi: 10.1016/j.bbr.2009.04.023

Jones, N. C., Salzberg, M. R., Kumar, G., Couper, A., Morris, M. J., & O'Brien, T. J. (2008). Elevated anxiety and depressive-like behavior in a rat model of genetic generalized epilepsy suggesting common causation.. *Experimental Neurology, 209*(1), 254–260.

Kalogjera-Sackellares, D. (1996). Chapter 10. Psychological disturbances in patients with pseudoseizures. In J. C. Sackellares & S. Berent (Eds.), *Psychological disturbances in epilepsy* (pp. 191–217). Oxford, England: Butterworth Heinemann.

Kanner, A. M. (2003). Psychogenic nonepileptic seizures are bad for your health. *Epilepsy Currents, 3*(5), 181–182.

Kanner, A. M., & Balabanov, A. J. (2008). Chapter 133a. Psychiatric outcome of epilepsy surgery. In H. O. Lüders, W. Bongaman, & I. M. Najim (Eds.), *Textbook of epilepsy surgery* (3rd ed., pp. 1254–1262). London: Informa Healthcare.

Kanner, A. M., Barry, J. J., Gilliam, F., Hermann, B., & Meador, K. J. (2010). Anxiety disorders, subsyndromic depressive episodes, and major depressive episodes: Do they differ on their impact on the quality of life of patients with epilepsy? *Epilepsia, 51*(7), 1152–1158.

Kanner, A. M., Byrne, R., Chicharro, A., Wuu, J., & Frey, M. (2009). A lifetime psychiatric history predicts a worse seizure outcome following temporal lobectomy. *Neurology, 72*(9), 793–799.

Kanner, A. M., Faught, E., French, J., et al. (2000). Psychiatric adverse events caused by topiramate and lamotrigine: A postmarketing prevalence and risk factor study. *Epilepsia, 41*(Suppl 7), 169.

Kanner, A. M., & Jones, J. C. (1997). When do sphenoidal electrodes yield additional data to that obtained with antero-temporal electrodes? *Electroencephalography & Clinical Neurophysiology, 102*(1), 12–19.

Kanner, A. M., Kozak, A. M., & Frey, M. (2000). The use of sertraline in patients with epilepsy: Is it safe? *Epilepsy & Behavior, 1*(2), 100–105.

Kanner, A. M., & Ostrovskaya, A. (2008a). Long-term significance of postictal psychotic episodes, I. Are they predictive of bilateral ictal foci? *Epilepsy & Behavior, 12*(1), 150–153.

Kanner, A. M., & Ostrovskaya, A. (2008b). Long-term significance of postictal psychotic episodes, II. Are they predictive of interictal psychotic episodes? *Epilepsy & Behavior, 12*(1), 154–156.

Kanner, A. M., Parra, J., Frey, M., Stebbins, G., Pierre-Louis, S., & Iriarte, J. (1999). Psychiatric and neurologic predictors of psychogenic pseudoseizure outcome. *Neurology, 53*(5), 933–938.

Kanner, A. M., Ramirez, L., & Jones, J. C. (1995). The utility of placing sphenoidal electrodes under the foramen ovale with fluoroscopic guidance. *Journal of Clinical Neurophysiology, 12*(1), 72–81.

Kanner, A. M., Soto, A., & Gross-Kanner, H. (2004). Prevalence and clinical characteristics of postictal psychiatric symptoms in partial epilepsy. *Neurology, 62*(5), 708–713.

Kanner, A. M., Stagno, S., Kotagal, P., & Morris, H. H. (1996). Postictal psychiatric events during prolonged video-electroencephalographic monitoring studies. *Archives of Neurology, 53*(3), 258–263.

Kaplan, P. W., & Fisher, R. S. (Eds.). (2005). *Imitators of epilepsy* (2nd ed.). New York: Demos.

Kerr, M. P., Mensah, S., Besag, F., de Toffol, B., Ettinger, A., Kanemoto, K., et al. (2011). International consensus clinical practice statements for the treatment of neuropsychiatric conditions associated with epilepsy. *Epilepsia, 52*(11), 2133–2138.

Kessler, R. C., McGonagle, K. A., Zhao, S., Nelson, C. B., Hughes, M., Eshleman, S., et al. (1994). Lifetime and 12-month prevalence of DSM-III-R psychiatric disorders in the United States. Results from the National Comorbidity Survey. *Archives of General Psychiatry, 51*(1), 8–19.

Ketter, T. A., Malow, B. A., Flamini, R., White, S. R., Post, R. M., & Theodore, W. H. (1994). Anticonvulsant withdrawal-emergent psychopathology. *Neurology, 44*(1), 55–61.

Kim, C. M., Barry, J. J., & Zeifert, P. A. (1998). Abstract 7.078. The use of inpatient medical psychiatric treatment for nonepileptic events. *Epilepsia, 39*(Suppl 6), 242–243.

King, D. W., Gallagher, B. B., Murvin, A. J., Smith, D. B., Marcus, D. J., Hartlage, L. C., et al. (1982). Pseudoseizures: Diagnostic evaluation. *Neurology, 32*(1), 18–23.

Kleinman, A., Wang, W. Z., Li, S. C., Cheng, X. M., Dai, X. Y., Li, K. T., et al. (1995). The social course of epilepsy: Chronic illness as social experience in interior China. *Social Science & Medicine, 40*(10), 1319–1330.

Koch-Stoecker, S. (2002). Personality disorders as predictors of severe postsurgical psychiatric complications in epilepsy patients undergoing temporal lobe resections. *Epilepsy & Behavior, 3*(6), 526–531.

Kogeorgos, J., Fonagy, P., & Scott, D. F. (1982). Psychiatric symptom patterns of chronic epileptics attending a neurological clinic: A controlled investigation. *British Journal of Psychiatry, 140*, 236–243.

Krawetz, P., Fleisher, W., Pillay, N., Staley, D., Arnett, J., & Maher, J. (2001). Family functioning in subjects with pseudoseizures and epilepsy. *Journal of Nervous and Mental Disease, 189*(1), 38–43.

Krumholz, A., Niedermeyer, E., Alkaitis, D., & Morel, R. (1980). Abstract: Psychogenic seizures: A 5-year follow-up study. *Neurology, 30*, 392.

LaFrance, W. C., Jr., Alper, K., Babcock, D., Barry, J. J., Benbadis, S., Caplan, R., et al. (2006). Nonepileptic seizures treatment workshop summary. *Epilepsy & Behavior, 8*(3), 451–461.

LaFrance, W. C., Jr., Baird, G. L., Barry, J. J., Blum, A. S., Frank Webb, A., Keitner, G. I., et al. (2014). Multicenter pilot treatment trial for psychogenic nonepileptic seizures: a randomized clinical trial. *JAMA Psychiatry, 71*(9), 997–1005.

LaFrance, W. C., Jr., Baker, G. A., Duncan, R., Goldstein, L. H., & Reuber, M. (2013). Minimum requirements for the diagnosis of psychogenic nonepileptic seizures: a staged approach: a report from the International League Against Epilepsy Nonepileptic Seizures Task Force. *Epilepsia, 54*(11), 2005–2018.

LaFrance, W. C., Jr., & Barry, J. J. (2005). Update on treatments of psychological nonepileptic seizures. *Epilepsy & Behavior, 7*(3), 364–374.

LaFrance, W. C., Jr., & Benbadis, S. R. (2006). Avoiding the costs of unrecognized psychological nonepileptic seizures. *Neurology, 66*(11), 1620–1621.

LaFrance, W. C., Jr., Blum, A. S., Miller, I. W., Ryan, C. E., & Keitner, G. I. (2007). Methodological issues in conducting treatment trials for psychological nonepileptic seizures. *Journal of Neuropsychiatry & Clinical Neurosciences, 19*(4), 391–398.

LaFrance, W. C., Jr., & Devinsky, O. (2002). Treatment of nonepileptic seizures. *Epilepsy & Behavior, 3*(5 Suppl 1), S19–S23.

LaFrance, W. C., Jr., & Devinsky, O. (2004). The treatment of nonepileptic seizures: Historical perspectives and future directions. *Epilepsia, 45*(Suppl 2), 15–21.

LaFrance, W. C., Jr., Keitner, G. I., Papandonatos, G. D., Blum, A. S., Machan, J. T., Ryan, C. E., et al. (2010). Pilot pharmacologic randomized controlled trial for psychogenic nonepileptic seizures. *Neurology, 75*(13), 1166–1173.

LaFrance, W. C., Jr., Miller, I. W., Ryan, C. E., Blum, A. S., Solomon, D. A., Kelley, J. E., et al. (2009). Cognitive behavioral therapy for psychogenic nonepileptic seizures. *Epilepsy & Behavior, 14*(4), 591–596.

LaFrance, W. C., Jr., Reuber, M., & Goldstein, L. H. (2013). Management of psychogenic nonepileptic seizures. *Epilepsia*, *54*(Suppl 1), 53–67.

Lancman, M. E., Brotherton, T. A., Asconape, J. J., & Penry, J. K. (1993). Psychogenic seizures in adults: A longitudinal analysis. *Seizure*, *2*(4), 281–286.

Lancman, M. E., Craven, W. J., Asconape, J. J., & Penry, J. K. (1994). Clinical management of recurrent postictal psychosis. *Journal of Epilepsy*, *7*, 47–51.

Lancman, M. E., Lambrakis, C. C., & Steinhardt, M. I. (2001). Chapter 24. Psychogenic pseudoseizures: A general overview. In A. B. Ettinger & A. M. Kanner (Eds.), *Psychiatry issues in epilepsy: A practical guide to diagnosis and treatment* (1st ed., pp. 341–354). Philadelphia, PA: Lippincott, Williams & Wilkins.

Landoldt, H. (1953). Some clinical electroencephalographical correlations in epileptic psychosis (twilight states). *Electroencephalography & Clinical Neurophysiology*, *5*, 121 (abstract).

Lehrner, J., Kalchmayr, R., Serles, W., Olbrich, A., Pataraia, E., Aull, S., et al. (1999). Health-related quality of life (HRQOL), activity of daily living (ADL) and depressive mood disorder in temporal lobe epilepsy patients. *Seizure*, *8*(2), 88–92.

Lelliott, P. T., & Fenwick, P. (1991). Cerebral pathology in pseudoseizures. *Acta Neurologica Scandinavica*, *83*(2), 129–132.

Logothetis, J. (1967). Spontaneous epileptic seizures and electroencephalographic changes in the course of phenothiazine therapy. *Neurology*, *17*(9), 869–877.

Logsdail, S. J., & Toone, B. K. (1988). Post-ictal psychoses. A clinical and phenomenological description. *British Journal of Psychiatry*, *152*, 246–252.

Marangell, L. B., Rush, A. J., George, M. S., Sackeim, H. A., Johnson, C. R., Husain, M. M., et al. (2002). Vagus nerve stimulation (VNS) for major depressive episodes: One year outcomes. *Biological Psychiatry*, *51*(4), 280–287.

Martin, R. C., Gilliam, F. G., Kilgore, M., Faught, E., & Kuzniecky, R. (1998). Improved health care resource utilization following video-EEG-confirmed diagnosis of nonepileptic psychogenic seizures. *Seizure*, *7*(5), 385–390.

Mazarati, A., Siddarth, P., Baldwin, R. A., Shin, D., Caplan, R., & Sankar, R. (2008). Depression after status epilepticus: Behavioural and biochemical deficits and effects of fluoxetine. *Brain*, *131*(Pt 8), 2071–2083. doi: 10.1093/brain/awn117

McAfee, A. T., Chilcott, K. E., Johannes, C. B., Hornbuckle, K., Hauser, W. A., & Walker, A. M. (2007). The incidence of first provoked and unprovoked seizure in pediatric patients with and without psychiatric diagnoses. *Epilepsia*, *48*(6), 1075–1082.

McConnell, H., & Duncan, D. (1998). Chapter 10. Treatment of psychiatric comorbidity in epilepsy. In H. McConnell & P. Snyder (Eds.), *Psychiatric comorbidity in epilepsy* (pp. 245–361). Washington, DC: American Psychiatric Press.

McConnell, H., Snyder, P. J., Duffy, J. D., Weilburg, J., Valeriano, J., Brillman, J., et al. (1996). Neuropsychiatric side effects to treatment with Felbamate. *Journal of Neuropsychiatry & Clinical Neurosciences*, *8*(3), 341–346.

McDermott, S., Mani, S., & Krishnaswami, S. (1995). A population-based analysis of specific behavior problems associated with childhood seizures. *Journal of Epilepsy*, *8*, 100–110.

McLellan, A., Davies, S., Heyman, I., Harding, B., Harkness, W., Taylor, D., et al. (2005). Psychopathology in children with epilepsy before and after temporal lobe resection. *Developmental Medicine & Child Neurology*, *47*(10), 666–672.

Meltzer, H., Bebbington, P., Brugha, T., Farrell, M., Jenkins, R., & Lewis, G. (2003). The reluctance to seek treatment for neurotic disorders. *International Review of Psychiatry*, *15*(1–2), 123–128.

Mendez, M. F., Cummings, J. L., & Benson, D. F. (1986). Depression in epilepsy. Significance and phenomenology. *Archives of Neurology*, *43*(8), 766–770.

Mökleby, K., Blomhoff, S., Malt, U. F., Dahlström, A., Tauböll, E., & Gjerstad, L. (2002). Psychiatric comorbidity and hostility in patients with psychogenic nonepileptic seizures compared with somatoform disorders and healthy controls. *Epilepsia*, *43*(2), 193–198.

Morrell, F., Whisler, W. W., Smith, M. C., Hoeppner, T. J., de Toledo-Morrell, L., Pierre-Louis, S. J., et al. (1995). Landau-Kleffner syndrome. Treatment with subpial intracortical transection. *Brain*, *118*(Pt 6), 1529–1546.

Mula, M., & Trimble, M. R. (2003). The importance of being seizure free: Topiramate and psychopathology in epilepsy. *Epilepsy & Behavior*, *4*(4), 430–434.

Niedermeyer, E., Blumer, D., Holscher, E., & Walker, B. A. (1970). Classical hysterical seizures facilitated by anticonvulsant toxicity. *Psychiatric Clinics (Basel)*, *3*(2), 71–84.

Nilsson, L., Tomson, T., Farahmand, B. Y., Diwan, V., & Persson, P. G. (1997). Cause-specific mortality in epilepsy: A cohort study of more than 9,000 patients once hospitalized for epilepsy. *Epilepsia*, *38*(10), 1062–1068.

O'Donoghue, M. F., Goodridge, D. M., Redhead, K., Sander, J. W., & Duncan, J. S. (1999). Assessing the psychosocial consequences of epilepsy: A community-based study. *British Journal of General Practice*, *49*(440), 211–214.

Onuma, T., Adachi, N., Ishida, S., Katou, M., & Uesugi, S. (1995). Prevalence and annual incidence of psychosis in patients with epilepsy. *Psychiatry & Clinical Neurosciences*, *49*(3), S267–S268.

Oto, M., Espie, C., Pelosi, A., Selkirk, M., & Duncan, R. (2005). The safety of antiepileptic drug withdrawal in patients with non-epileptic seizures. *Journal of Neurology, Neurosurgery, & Psychiatry*, *76*(12), 1682–1685.

Ott, D., Caplan, R., Guthrie, D., Siddarth, P., Komo, S., Shields, W. D., et al. (2001). Measures of psychopathology in children with complex partial seizures and primary generalized epilepsy with absence. *Journal of the American Academy of, Child & Adolescent Psychiatry*, *40*(8), 907–914.

Ounsted, C. (1955). The hyperkinetic syndrome in epileptic children. *Lancet*, *269*(6885), 303–311.

Owczarek, K. (2003). Somatisation indexes as differential factors in psychogenic pseudoepileptic and epileptic seizures. *Seizure*, *12*(3), 178–181.

Pacia, S. V., & Devinsky, O. (1994). Clozapine-related seizures: Experience with 5,629 patients. *Neurology*, *44*(12), 2247–2249.

Pariente, P. D., Lepine, J. P., & Lellouch, J. (1991). Lifetime history of panic attacks and epilepsy: An association from a general population survey. *Journal of Clinical Psychiatry*, *52*(2), 88–89.

PDR (2002). *Physicians' Desk Reference* (56th ed.). Montvale, NJ: Medical Economics Co.

Pearson, H. J. (1990). Interaction of fluoxetine with carbamazepine. *Journal of Clinical Psychiatry*, *51*(3), 126.

Penin, H. (1968). Elektonische Patientenuberwachung in der Nervenklinik Bonn [Electronic patient monitoring in the Neurological Hospital of Bonn]. *Umschau in Wissenschaft und Technik*, *7*, 211–212.

Perini, G. I., Tosin, C., Carraro, C., Bernasconi, G., Canevini, M. P., Canger, R., et al. (1996). Interictal mood and personality disorders in temporal lobe epilepsy and juvenile myoclonic epilepsy. *Journal of Neurology, Neurosurgery, & Psychiatry*, *61*(6), 601–605.

Perrine, K., Hermann, B. P., Meador, K. J., Vickrey, B. G., Cramer, J. A., Hays, R. D., et al. (1995). The relationship of neuropsychological functioning to quality of life in epilepsy. *Archives of Neurology*, *52*(10), 997–1003.

Pestana, E. M., Foldvary-Shaefer, N., Marsillio, D., & Morris, H. H., III. (2003). Abstract [P05.023]: Quality of life in patients with psychogenic seizures. *Neurology*, *60*(5 Suppl 1), A355.

Petrovski, S., Szoeke, C. E., Jones, N. C., Salzberg, M. R., Sheffield, L. J., Huggins, R. M., et al. (2010). Neuropsychiatric symptomatology predicts seizure recurrence in newly treated patients. *Neurology*, *75*(11), 1015–1021. doi: 10.1212/WNL.0b013e3181f25b16

Pintor, L., Bailles, E., Fernandez-Egea, E., Sanchez-Gistau, V., Torres, X., Carreno, M., et al. (2007). Psychiatric disorders in temporal lobe epilepsy patients over the first year after surgical treatment. *Seizure*, *16*(3), 218–225.

Preskorn, S. H., & Fast, G. A. (1992). Tricyclic antidepressant-induced seizures and plasma drug concentration. *Journal of Clinical Psychiatry*, *53*(5), 160–162.

Quigg, M., Armstrong, R. F., Farace, E., & Fountain, N. B. (2002). Quality of life outcome is associated with cessation rather than reduction of psychogenic nonepileptic seizures. *Epilepsy & Behavior*, 3(5), 455–459.

Quiske, A., Helmstaedter, C., Lux, S., & Elger, C. E. (2000). Depression in patients with temporal lobe epilepsy is related to mesial temporal sclerosis. *Epilepsy Research*, 39(2), 121–125.

Rafnsson, V., Olafsson, E., Hauser, W. A., & Gudmundsson, G. (2001). Cause-specific mortality in adults with unprovoked seizures. A population-based incidence cohort study. *Neuroepidemiology*, 20(4), 232–236.

Ramani, V. (2000). Chapter 25: Treatment of the adult patient with non-epileptic seizures. In J. R. Gates & A. J. Rowan (Eds.), *Non-epileptic seizures* (2nd ed., pp. 300–316). Boston, MA: Butterworth-Heinemann.

Ramani, V., & Gumnit, R. J. (1982). Management of hysterical seizures in epileptic patients. *Archives of Neurology*, 39(2), 78–81.

Ramaratnam, S., Baker, G. A., & Goldstein, L. H. (2008). Psychological treatments for epilepsy. *Cochrane Database of Systematic Reviews*, (3), CD002029.

Rechlin, T., Loew, T. H., & Joraschky, P. (1997). Pseudoseizure "status." *Journal of Psychosomatic Research*, 42(5), 495–498.

Regenold, W. T., Weintraub, D., & Taller, A. (1998). Electroconvulsive therapy for epilepsy and major depression. *American Journal of Geriatric Psychiatry*, 6(2), 180–183.

Regier, D. A., Farmer, M. E., Rae, D. S., Myers, J. K., Kramer, M., Robins, L. N., et al. (1993). One-month prevalence of mental disorders in the United States and sociodemographic characteristics: The Epidemiologic Catchment Area study. *Acta Psychiatrica Scandinavica*, 88(1), 35–47.

Reiter, J., Andrews, D., Reiter, C., LaFrance, W. C. Jr. (2015). *Taking control of your seizures: Workbook*. New York: Oxford University Press.

Reuber, M., Baker, G. A., Gill, R., Smith, D. F., & Chadwick, D. W. (2004). Failure to recognize psychogenic nonepileptic seizures may cause death. *Neurology*, 62(5), 834–835.

Reuber, M., & Elger, C. E. (2003). Psychogenic nonepileptic seizures: Review and update. *Epilepsy & Behavior*, 4(3), 205–216.

Reuber, M., Pukrop, R., Bauer, J., Helmstaedter, C., Tessendorf, N., & Elger, C. E. (2003). Outcome in psychogenic nonepileptic seizures: 1 to 10-year follow-up in 164 patients. *Annals of Neurology*, 53(3), 305–311.

Ring, H. A., & Reynolds, E. H. (1990). Vigabatrin and behaviour disturbance. *Lancet*, 335(8695), 970.

Robertson, M. M. (1997). Suicide, parasuicide, and epilepsy. In T. Pedley & J. Engel (Eds.), *Epilepsy: A comprehensive textbook*. Philadelphia: Lippincott-Raver. pp. 2141–2151.

Rosenstein, D. L., Nelson, J. C., & Jacobs, S. C. (1993). Seizures associated with antidepressants: A review. *Journal of Clinical Psychiatry*, 54(8), 289–299.

Roy-Byrne, P. P., Stein, M. B., Russo, J., Mercier, E., Thomas, R., McQuaid, J., et al. (1999). Panic disorder in the primary care setting: Comorbidity, disability, service utilization, and treatment. *Journal of Clinical Psychiatry*, 60(7), 492–499; quiz, 500.

Rusch, M. D., Morris, G. L., Allen, L., & Lathrop, L. (2001). Psychological treatment of nonepileptic events. *Epilepsy & Behavior*, 2, 277–283.

Rutter, M., Graham, P., & Yule, W. (1970). *A neuropsychiatric study in childhood*. Philadelphia: J. B. Lippincott.

Sackeim, H. A., Decina, P., Prohovnik, I., Malitz, S., & Resor, S. R. (1983). Anticonvulsant and antidepressant properties of electroconvulsive therapy: A proposed mechanism of action. *Biological Psychiatry*, 18(11), 1301–1310.

Salzberg, M., Kumar, G., Supit, L., Jones, N. C., Morris, M. J., Rees, S., et al. (2007). Early postnatal stress confers enduring vulnerability to limbic epileptogenesis. *Epilepsia*, 48(11), 2079–2085. doi: 10.1111/j.1528-1167.2007.01246.x

Santosh, D., Kumar, T. S., Sarma, P. S., & Radhakrishnan, K. (2007). Women with onset of epilepsy prior to marriage: Disclose or conceal? *Epilepsia*, 48(5), 1007–1010.

Savard, G., Andermann, L. F., Reutens, D., & Andermann, F. (1998). Epilepsy, surgical treatment and postoperative psychiatric complications: A re-evaluation of the evidence. In M. Trimble & B. Schmitz (Eds.), *Forced normalization and alternative psychosis of epilepsy* (pp. 179–192). Petersfield, UK: Writson Biomedical Publishing, Ltd.

Schachter, S. C., & LaFrance, W. C. Jr. (Eds.). (2010). *Gates and Rowan's nonepileptic seizures* (3rd ed.). New York: Cambridge University Press.

Schmitz, B., & Wolf, P. (1995). Psychosis in epilepsy: Frequency and risk factors. *Journal of Epilepsy*, 8, 295–305.

Semrud-Clikeman, M., & Wical, B. (1999). Components of attention in children with complex partial seizures with and without ADHD. *Epilepsia*, 40(2), 211–215.

Shen, W., Bowman, E. S., & Markand, O. N. (1990). Presenting the diagnosis of pseudoseizure. *Neurology*, 40(5), 756–759.

Sherman, E. M., Slick, D. J., Connolly, M. B., & Eyrl, K. L. (2007). ADHD, neurological correlates and health-related quality of life in severe pediatric epilepsy. *Epilepsia*, 48(6), 1083–1091.

Sillaber, I., Holsboer, F., & Wotjak, C. T. (2009). Chapter 27: Animal models of mood disorders. In D. S. Charney & E. J. Nestler (Eds.), *Neurobiology of mental illness* (3rd ed., pp. 378–391). New York: Oxford University Press.

Sironi, V. A., Franzini, A., Ravagnati, L., & Marossero, F. (1979). Interictal acute psychoses in temporal lobe epilepsy during withdrawal of anticonvulsant therapy. *Journal of Neurology, Neurosurgery, & Psychiatry*, 42(8), 724–730.

Slater, E., Beard, A. W., & Glithero, E. (1963). The schizophrenialike psychoses of epilepsy. *British Journal of Psychiatry*, 109, 95–150.

Smith, D. B., Mattson, R. H., Cramer, J. A., Collins, J. F., Novelly, R. A., & Craft, B. (1987). Results of a nationwide Veterans Administration Cooperative Study comparing the efficacy and toxicity of carbamazepine, phenobarbital, phenytoin, and primidone. *Epilepsia*, 28 (Suppl 3), S50–S58.

Smith, M. L., Stagno, S. J., Dolske, M., Kosalko, J., McConnell, C., Kaspar, L., et al. (1997). Induction procedures for psychogenic seizures: Ethical and clinical considerations. *Journal of Clinical Ethics*, 8(3), 217–229.

Stahl, S. M. (2000). *Essential psychopharmacology: Neuroscientific basis and practical applications* (2nd ed.). New York: Cambridge University Press.

Swingle, P. G. (1998). Neurofeedback treatment of pseudoseizure disorder. *Biological Psychiatry*, 44(11), 1196–1199.

Swinkels, J., Jonghe, F. (1995). Safety of antidepressants. *International Clinical Psychopharmacology*, 9(Suppl 4), 19–25.

Swinkels, W. A., Kuyk, J., van Dyck, R., & Spinhoven, P. (2005). Psychiatric comorbidity in epilepsy. *Epilepsy & Behavior*, 7(1), 37–50.

Swinkels, W. A., van Emde Boas, W., Kuyk, J., van Dyck, R., & Spinhoven, P. (2006). Interictal depression, anxiety, personality traits, and psychological dissociation in patients with temporal lobe epilepsy (TLE) and extra-TLE. *Epilepsia*, 47(12), 2092–2103.

Syed, T. U., LaFrance, W. C., Jr., Kahriman, E. S., Hasan, S. N., Rajasekaran, V., Gulati, D., et al. (2011). Can semiology predict psychogenic nonepileptic seizures? A prospective study. *Annals of Neurology*, 69(6), 997–1004.

Tarulli, A., Devinsky, O., & Alper, K. (2001). Progression of postictal to interictal psychosis. [Case Reports]. *Epilepsia*, 42(11), 1468–1471.

Task Force on DSM-IV. (1994). *Diagnostic and Statistical Manual of Mental Disorders: DSM-IV* (4th ed.). Washington, DC: American Psychiatric Association.

Taylor, D. C. (1972). Mental state and temporal lobe epilepsy. A correlative account of 100 patients treated surgically. *Epilepsia*, 13(6), 727–765.

Tellez-Zenteno, J. F., Patten, S. B., Jette, N., Williams, J., & Wiebe, S. (2007). Psychiatric comorbidity in epilepsy: A population-based analysis. *Epilepsia*, 48(12), 2336–2344.

Testa, S. M., Schefft, B. K., Szaflarski, J. P., Yeh, H. S., & Privitera, M. D. (2007). Mood, personality, and health-related quality of life in epileptic and psychogenic seizure disorders. *Epilepsia*, 48(5), 973–982.

Testa, S. M., Szaflarski, J. P., Fargo, J. D., Dulay, M. F., & Schefft, B. K. (2003). Abstract [P05.097] Psychological correlates of health-related quality of life (HRQOL) in epileptic and nonepileptic seizures. *Neurology, 60*(5 Suppl 1), A383.

Thomson, P. (2006). *Physicians' Desk Reference* (60th ed.). Montvale, NJ: Thomson PDR.

Tiihonen, J., Nousiainen, U., Hakola, P., Leinonen, E., Tuunainen, A., Mervaala, E., et al. (1991). EEG abnormalities associated with clozapine treatment. *American Journal of Psychiatry, 148*(10), 1406.

Toth, P., & Frankenburg, F. R. (1994). Clozapine and seizures: A review. *Canadian Journal of Psychiatry, 39*(4), 236–238.

Trimble, M. R. (1992). Behaviour changes following temporal lobectomy, with special reference to psychosis. *Journal of Neurology, Neurosurgery, & Psychiatry, 55*(2), 89–91.

Umbricht, D., Degreef, G., Barr, W. B., Lieberman, J. A., Pollack, S., & Schaul, N. (1995). Postictal and chronic psychoses in patients with temporal lobe epilepsy. *American Journal of Psychiatry, 152*(2), 224–231.

Vazquez, B., & Devinsky, O. (2003). Epilepsy and anxiety. *Epilepsy & Behavior, 4*(Suppl 4), S20–25.

Wada, K., Iwasa, H., Okada, M., Kawata, Y., Murakami, T., Kamata, A., et al. (2004). Marital status of patients with epilepsy with special reference to the influence of epileptic seizures on the patient's married life. *Epilepsia, 45* (Suppl 8), 33–36.

Walczak, T. S., Papacostas, S., Williams, D. T., Scheuer, M. L., Lebowitz, N., & Notarfrancesco, A. (1995). Outcome after diagnosis of psychogenic nonepileptic seizures. *Epilepsia, 36*(11), 1131–1137.

Walsh, J. C., Vignaendra, V., Burrows, S., Healy, L., McCue, M., & Patterson, J. (1986). The application of prolonged electroencephalographic monitoring and video recording to the diagnosis of epilepsy. *Medical Journal of Australia, 144*(8), 401–404.

Weil, A. A. (1955). Depressive reactions associated with temporal lobe-uncinate seizure. *Journal of Nervous and Mental Disease, 121*(6), 505–510.

Westbrook, L. E., Devinsky, O., & Geocadin, R. (1998). Nonepileptic seizures after head injury. *Epilepsia, 39*(9), 978–982.

Whitworth, A. B., & Fleischhacker, W. W. (1995). Adverse effects of antipsychotic drugs. *International Clinical Psychopharmacology, 9*(Suppl 5), 21–27.

Williams, D. (1956). The structure of emotions reflected in epileptic experiences. *Brain, 79*(1), 29–67.

Wolf, P., & Trimble, M. R. (1985). Biological antagonism and epileptic psychosis. *British Journal of Psychiatry, 146*, 272–276.

Wyllie, E., Friedman, D., Luders, H., Morris, H., Rothner, D., & Turnbull, J. (1991). Outcome of psychogenic seizures in children and adolescents compared with adults. *Neurology, 41*(5), 742–744.

Wyllie, E., Glazer, J. P., Benbadis, S., Kotagal, P., & Wolgamuth, B. (1999). Psychiatric features of children and adolescents with pseudoseizures. *Archives of Pediatric & Adolescent Medicine, 153*(3), 244–248.

Zaroff, C. M., Myers, L., B. Barr, W., Luciano, D., & Devinsky, O. (2004). Group psychoeducation as treatment for psychological nonepileptic seizures. *Epilepsy & Behavior, 5*(4), 587–592.

Ziegler, F. J., & Imboden, J. B. (1962). Contemporary conversion reactions. II. A conceptual model. *Archives of General Psychiatry, 6*, 279–287.

44.

DIAGNOSIS AND TREATMENT OF HEADACHE

Elizabeth W. Loder

INTRODUCTION

Mild, occasional headaches are among the common aches and pains of life. These ordinary headaches are infrequent, respond well to simple over-the-counter treatments and do not require medical attention. When headaches are severe, frequent, or disabling, however, sufferers often seek medical care. Headache is among the most common outpatient complaints and a common reason for emergency department visits. Physicians in nearly every specialty can expect to encounter patients with troublesome headaches. Because a number of chronic headache conditions are comorbid with certain psychiatric disorders, however, psychiatrists are especially likely to encounter patients with complaints of headache. This chapter focuses on the diagnosis and management of recurrent headache.

HEADACHE DIAGNOSIS

Headache diagnosis depends heavily upon the patient's description of typical headache features. *The International Classification of Headache Disorders* (ICHD) has many features in common with the diagnostic system used in psychiatry: diagnosis is clinical, and is based on inclusion and exclusion criteria (Headache Classification Subcommittee of the International Headache Society, 2013). The diagnostic criteria focus on headache location, intensity, duration, and the presence or absence of typical aggravating or associated features. In addition to inquiring about these characteristics of headache, a complete headache history should include information about prescription and non-prescription medicines used now and in the past to treat headaches, a family history of headaches, and other medical conditions and medications.

ICHD divides headaches into two major categories. *Primary* headaches are those for which no other disorder can be identified as responsible for the headache. The three major primary headache disorders are migraine, tension-type, and cluster headaches. Boxes 44.1–44.3 list diagnostic criteria for these disorders. A fourth group of "other" primary headaches includes less common syndromes such as hemicrania continua and new daily persistent headache. When patients meet criteria for a primary headache disorder and have a normal neurological examination, additional testing generally is not needed or recommended (Bartleson, 2006).

Secondary headaches, in contrast, are those in which the headache is due to an underlying problem such as head injury, tumor, or infection. When there is suspicion of a secondary headache disorder on the basis of the history or physical examination, additional investigation is needed (Detsky et al., 2006). Table 44.1 lists worrisome or "red flag" symptoms or signs that generally should prompt further testing, and the specific diagnoses of concern. The testing necessary depends upon the disorder that is suspected, and might include computed tomography (CT) or magnetic resonance imaging (MRI) of the head or cervical spine, blood tests, or a lumbar puncture to assess cerebrospinal fluid pressure and composition (Evans & Silberstein, 2002). With the exception of situations in which acute cerebral bleeding or other unusual problems are suspected, MRI is the preferred imaging test. MRI is more sensitive than CT for a variety of abnormalities, and provides a better look at posterior brain structures. An MR angiogram (MRA) or venogram (MRV) can be useful to detect arterial or venous abnormalities responsible for headache (Mehndiratta, Garg, & Gurnani, 2006).

HEADACHE MISDIAGNOSIS AND TREATMENT ERRORS

It can sometimes be difficult to distinguish between primary and secondary disorders, and the two may coexist. Because the primary headache disorder of migraine is so common in the population, for example, many people who experience head trauma have a prior history of migraine, which may worsen in relation to the head injury. It can be difficult to distinguish the relative contributions of the two problems in such cases. Primary headache disorders such as migraine are often incorrectly attributed to medical disorders such as sinus pathology. The misdiagnosis of migraine as "sinus" headache is a well-known phenomenon (Silberstein, 2004a). In clinical practice it is not uncommon to see patients who have had multiple unsuccessful sinus surgeries for recurrent or frequent headaches, and who respond well to triptans or other specific anti-migraine therapies when those are tried. The confusion between sinus headaches and migraine probably stems from the fact that migraine can be accompanied by nasal congestion or stuffiness and can also produce facial pain. Migraine attacks can last several days, and if the symptoms are incorrectly attributed to sinus pathology, a course of antibiotics may be started

Infrequent episodic tension-Type headache

A. At least ten episodes occurring on <1 day per month on average (<12 days per year) and fulfilling criteria B–D

B. Headache lasting from 30 minutes to 7 days

C. Headache has at least two of the following characteristics:

1. Bilateral location
2. Pressing/tightening (non-pulsating) quality
3. Mild or moderate intensity
4. Not aggravated by routine physical activity such as walking or climbing stairs

D. Both of the following:

1. No nausea or vomiting (anorexia may occur)
2. No more than one of photophobia or phonophobia
E. Not better accounted for by another ICHD-3 diagnosis

Frequent episodic tension-Type headache

Like *Infrequent episodic tension-type headache*, except for:

A. At least ten episodes occurring on ≥1 but <15 days per month for at least 3 months (≥12 and <180 days per year) and fulfilling criteria B–D

Chronic tension-Type headache

A. Headache occurring on ≥15 days per month on average for >3 months (≥180 days per year)[1] and fulfilling criteria B–D

B. Headache lasts hours to days or may be unremitting

C. Headache has at least two of the following characteristics:

1. Bilateral location
2. Pressing/tightening (non-pulsating) quality
3. Mild or moderate intensity
4. Not aggravated by routine physical activity such as walking or climbing stairs

D. Both of the following:

1. No more than one of photophobia, phonophobia or mild nausea
2. Neither moderate nor severe nausea, nor vomiting

E. Not attributed to another ICHD-3 diagnosis

Note: Code 2.3, *Chronic tension-type headache*, evolves over time from episodic tension-type headache; when these criteria A–E are fulfilled by headache that, unambiguously, is daily and unremitting within three days of its first onset, code as 4.8, *New daily-persistent headache*.

Migraine without aura

A. At least five attacks fulfilling criteria B–D

B. Headache lasting 4 to 72 hours (untreated or unsuccessfully treated)

C. Headache has at least two of the following characteristics:

1. Unilateral location
2. Pulsating quality
3. Moderate or severe pain intensity (inhibits or prohibits daily activities)
4. Aggravation by, or causing avoidance of, routine physical activity such as walking stairs or similar routine physical activity

D. During headache, at least one of the following occurs:

1. Nausea and/or vomiting
2. Photophobia and phonophobia

E. At least one of the following is present:

1. History and physical and neurological examinations do not suggest an organic disorder
2. History and/or physical and/or neurological examinations do suggest such disorder, but it is ruled out by appropriate investigations
3. Such disorder is present, but migraine attacks do not occur for the first time in close temporal relation to the disorder

Migraine with aura

A. At least two attacks fulfilling criteria B and C

B. One or more of the following fully reversible aura symptoms:

1. Visual
2. Sensory
3. Speech and/or language
4. Motor
5. Brainstem
6. Retinal

C. At least two of the following four characteristics are present:

1. At least one aura symptom *develops gradually* over more than 5 minutes, and/or two or more symptoms occur in succession
2. No single aura symptom *lasts less than 5 minutes or more than 60 minutes*
3. At least one aura symptom is unilateral

4. *Headache follows aura* with a free interval of less than 60 minutes (it also may begin before or simultaneously with the aura)

D. Not better accounted for by another ICHD-3 diagnosis, and history, physical examination, and, where appropriate, diagnostic tests exclude a secondary cause

Chronic migraine

DIAGNOSTIC CRITERIA

A. Headache fulfilling criteria B and C for 1.1, *Migraine without aura*, on ≥15 days/month for >3 months which has the features of migraine headache on ≥8 days/month

B. Not better accounted for by another ICHD-3 diagnosis

Note:

1. History and physical and neurological examinations do not suggest any of the disorders listed in groups 5–12, or history and/or physical and/or neurological examinations do suggest such disorder, but it is ruled out by appropriate investigations, or such disorder is present, but headache does not occur for the first time in close temporal relation to the disorder.

2. When medication overuse is present and fulfils criterion B for any of the subforms of 8.2 *Medication-overuse headache*, it is uncertain whether this criterion B is fulfilled until 2 months after medication has been withdrawn without improvement (see *Comments*).

Comments:

Most cases of chronic migraine start as 1.1 *Migraine without aura*. Therefore, chronicity may be regarded as a complication of episodic migraine. As chronicity develops, headache tends to lose its attack-wise (episodic) presentation, although it has not been clearly demonstrated that this is always so.

and appear to be effective when the headache naturally wanes. Additionally, vasoconstrictive decongestant medications and mild analgesics contained in over-the-counter sinus medications can also be effective for migraine, which then reinforces the idea that the problem was due to sinus pathology.

Migraine is also often misdiagnosed as tension-type headache. In patients who develop daily or near-daily headache, there may be an evolution in headache characteristics over time. Typically, accompanying symptoms such as nausea and vomiting become less prominent as patients get older and as headache frequency increases. The clinical picture can be mistaken for tension-type headache if a full history of early attack characteristics is not obtained. One study carried out in general practice showed that most physician diagnoses of tension-type headache turned out to be incorrect. When longitudinal diary information was obtained, most patients initially diagnosed with tension-type headache turned out to have migraine (Lipton, Cady, Stewart, Wilks, & Hall, 2002).

Diagnostic delay is common in cluster headache. In one study, the mean delay before correct diagnosis was 2.6 years, and patients consulted an average of three physicians before a correct diagnosis was identified (Bahra & Goadsby, 2004). The most common misdiagnosis of cluster headache is migraine; there is

Episodic Cluster Headache

A. At least five attacks fulfilling criteria B–D

B. Severe or very severe unilateral orbital, supraorbital, and/or temporal pain lasting 15–180 minutes if untreated

C. Either or both of the following:

1. At least one of the following symptoms or signs ipsilateral to the headache:

   a. Ipsilateral conjunctival injection and/or lacrimation

   b. Ipsilateral nasal congestion and/or rhinorrhea

   c. Ipsilateral eyelid edema

   d. Ipsilateral forehead and facial sweating

   e. Ipsilateral forehead and facial flushing

   f. Sensation of fullness in the ear

   g. Ipsilateral miosis and/or ptosis

2. A sense of restlessness or agitation

D. Attacks have a frequency from one every other day to eight per day

E. Not attributed to another disorder

Chronic Cluster Headache

A. Attacks fulfilling criteria A–E for 3.1 *Cluster headache*

B. Attacks recur over >1 year without remission periods or with remission periods lasting <1 month

Comments:

Chronic cluster headache may arise *de novo* (previously referred to as *Primary chronic cluster headache*) or evolve from the episodic subtype (previously referred to as *Secondary chronic cluster headache*). Some patients may switch from chronic to episodic cluster headache.

some overlap in treatments for the two conditions (sumatriptan is effective for acute treatment of both disorders, for example), but there are also many differences. Preventive treatments such as beta blockers that are helpful for migraine are not effective for cluster headache, so diagnostic delay exposes some patients to many years of ineffective treatments. Patients with cluster headaches are also often thought to have dental problems, and many undergo unnecessary tooth extractions.

Misdiagnosis of headaches can lead to inappropriate treatment or missed treatment opportunities. Other causes

Table 44.1 "RED FLAG" OR WORRISOME HEADACHE FEATURES AND SUGGESTED EVALUATION

WORRISOME FEATURE	DIFFERENTIAL DIAGNOSIS	POSSIBLE EVALUATION
Acute onset of extremely severe headache	Subarachnoid hemorrhage, cerebral venous thrombosis, reversible cerebral vasoconstrictive syndrome	Computed tomography (CT) scan followed by a lumbar puncture if negative; Magnetic resonance angiography (MRA), Magnetic resonance venography (MRV), or CT angiogram in selected patients
Aura symptoms lasting longer than an hour	Stroke	MRI or CT scan to assess for ischemic lesion
New headache in a patient over 50	Temporal arteritis, neoplasm, other secondary headaches	Detailed history, CT or MRI, as well as selected blood tests
Headache with Valsalva, cough, sneezing	Chiari malformation or other occipital lesion	MRI
Progressive headache with focal neurological findings	Intracranial neoplasm	Detailed examination and CT or MRI
Chronic headache with tinnitus and transient visual disturbances	Idiopathic intracranial hypertension	MRA, MRV, followed by lumbar puncture to assess cerebrospinal fluid (CSF) pressure

of treatment errors include drug interactions, serious side effects, and inappropriate medication use in pregnant women. Perhaps the most common treatment errors in headache stem from prolonged use of nonsteroidal anti-inflammatory medications, with resulting gastrointestinal toxicity and bleeding. Vasoactive medications such as triptans and ergot compounds can occasionally produce vasoconstrictive complications, including myocardial infarction. Drug dependence and addiction syndromes can develop in patients who are prescribed habit-forming medications such as barbiturate-containing combination medications or opioids for the treatment of headache. Barbiturate dependence and addiction is no longer as common a problem as it was prior to the advent of the triptan medications for migraine treatment; opioid dependence and addiction, however, has increased in frequency among headache patients over the last decade (Loder, 2006). This coincides with a movement to use these medications more liberally for the treatment of chronic, non-malignant pain syndromes.

HEADACHE EPIDEMIOLOGY AND GENETICS

Most forms of headache are more common in women than in men, and women far outnumber men among those who seek specialty care for headache. This is because the clinical expression of the most common form of benign recurrent headache—migraine—is strongly influenced by cycling ovarian steroid hormone levels. At all ages past puberty, for example, the prevalence of migraine is higher in females than in males, and women are more likely than men to experience longer, more intense headaches and to be more disabled by migraine. The prevalence of headache also varies with age. In both sexes, the prevalence of primary headache disorders such as migraine increases throughout early adulthood, plateaus in the middle years, and gradually declines thereafter. Secondary headaches become relatively more common as people age (Lipton & Bigal, 2005). It is unusual for primary headache disorders to begin after the age of 50, and new onset headaches in someone over this age require a thoughtful work-up to exclude dangerous underlying sources of pain.

Many of the primary headache disorders have a genetic basis. The familial form of a rare subtype of migraine with aura, known as familial hemiplegic migraine, is an autosomal dominant condition. Three mutations that can lead to this disorder have been identified. These appear to increase brain susceptibility to cortical spreading depression, a neurological event that is thought to underlie migraine aura (Russell & Ducros, 2011). Genome-wide association and other studies have identified other loci that may be involved in more common forms of migraine (Anttila et al., 2010; Ligthart et al., 2011). At present, these findings have few clinical implications, but they are exciting because they validate the biological underpinnings of some of the primary headache disorders. They also provide targets for the development of drugs to treat these disorders.

PSYCHIATRIC DISORDERS AND HEADACHE

Psychiatric disorders are common in patients who are referred to specialty headache care. This may reflect an increased occurrence of headache in patients with chronic headache disorders. It may also reflect the fact that psychiatric disorders may interfere with adherence to recommended headache treatments or the development of a good working relationship with physicians (Saper & Lake, 2002). The term "comorbidity" is commonly used to indicate a clinical situation in which two disorders coexist at a frequency greater than would be expected based on chance alone. Affective disorders such as anxiety disorders and depression are more common in patients who have migraine, and the reverse situation is also true. This bidirectional association of affective spectrum disorders and migraine strongly suggests an underlying shared predisposition to both disorders, perhaps based on serotonergic abnormalities in the central nervous system. A longitudinal cohort study suggested that these disorders, when they coexist, appear in a fixed order, with the onset of anxiety preceding that of migraine, which in turn precedes the onset of depression (Merikangas, Whitaker, Isler, & Angst, 1994).

Psychiatric comorbidity has been most extensively studied in patients with migraine. Studies suggest that the odds of having major depression are roughly in the range of 2–4 for those with migraine compared with non-migraineurs. The risk of other affective spectrum disorders such as generalized anxiety disorder, bipolar disorder, or panic attacks is also increased in those who have migraine compared with those who do not. Suicide also appears to be more common in migraineurs compared with non-migraineurs (Breslau, Merikangas, & Bowden, 1994; Breslau, Chilcoat, & Andreski, 1996; Breslau, 1998; Breslau, Schultz, Stewart, Lipton, & Welch, 2001). The risk of depression and anxiety may be elevated in those with high-frequency migraine (Zwart et al., 2003).

The presence of a psychiatric disorder in a patient with headache can complicate treatment. Certain antidepressants may trigger a manic or hypomanic episode. There is also concern about the possibility of "serotonin syndrome" with combined use of triptans and selective serotonin reuptake inhibitors (SSRI) or selective serotonin norepinephrine reuptake inhibitors (SNRI). Serotonin syndrome has also been reported with triptan monotherapy (Soldin, Tonning, & Obstetric-Fetal Pharmacology Research Unit Network, 2008). The risk appears low, and the number of case reports is low and of variable credibility (Evans, 2007, 2008). However, the Food and Drug Administration (FDA) has issued an advisory regarding the possibility of serotonin syndrome with combined triptan and SSRI or SNRI treatment. A position paper from the American Headache Society concludes that available evidence is not sufficient to warrant limiting the use of these drugs; however, they recommend that clinicians using the combination be "vigilant" for signs or symptoms of serotonin syndrome (Evans, Tepper, Shapiro, Sun-Edelstein, & Tietjen, 2010).

Case reports and adverse event information from clinical trials suggest that certain medications used for psychiatric conditions may occasionally produce headache as a side effect, or aggravate preexisting headache. Low-grade, featureless headache or worsening of migraine have been reported as side effects of SSRI or SNRI therapy, for example (Bickel, Kornhuber, Maihofner, & Ropohl, 2005). There are no evidence-based strategies or treatments for this complication, but clinical experience suggests that the headache may wane over time, even if the patient remains on the offending drug; alternatively, switching to another drug in the same class may relieve the headache. On the other hand, there is some evidence that certain antidepressants can be helpful as treatment for headache, though none is FDA-approved for that purpose (Tarlaci, 2009).

GENERAL PRINCIPLES OF HEADACHE MANAGEMENT

Most patients with headaches should be encouraged to keep a simple headache diary where they record the frequency and severity of the headaches and any medications used to treat them (Russell et al., 1992). In general a single daily composite rating of headache intensity is sufficient to guide treatment decisions. More complex diaries that require multiple daily entries have not been shown to be superior to simpler diaries, and may promote somatic preoccupation. The website of the American Headache Society provides several simple diaries that can be easily downloaded.

Patients prone to recurrent, troublesome headaches should be advised to get sufficient and regular amounts of sleep, eat regular meals, and get regular exercise. Sleep disruption, emotional upset, hormonal fluctuations, and alcohol may trigger migraine attacks. Alcohol and napping are triggers for cluster headache. There is good evidence that relaxation training, biofeedback, and stress-management techniques may be useful adjuncts to an overall management plan for migraine and tension-type headache, but they are less useful for cluster headache (Sandor & Afra, 2005).

Many patients with primary headache disorders can be treated successfully in general practice. Referral to a headache specialist should be considered when the patient has complex medical comorbidities, unusually frequent or debilitating headaches, or is poorly responsive to treatment attempts.

TENSION-TYPE HEADACHE

Tension-type headache (TTH) is a mild or moderate, nondescript headache that is usually bilateral, with pain that is "pressing" or "tightening." It is usually not associated with migrainous features such as nausea or vomiting, or photo- or phonophobia (Table 44.2). It is divided into episodic and chronic forms, depending on the frequency of headaches. The second edition of the ICHD provides criteria for: (1) infrequent episodic TTH (fewer than 12 headache days per year), (2) frequent episodic TTH (between 12 and 180 days per year) and (3) chronic TTH (at least 180 days per year). These can be further subdivided according to the presence or absence of muscle tenderness. Although the name implies that muscle or emotional tension might be the underlying

Table 44.2 ABORTIVE AND PREVENTIVE TREATMENT OPTIONS FOR TENSION-TYPE HEADACHE

ABORTIVE AGENTS
Over-the-counter drugs
Aspirin
Acetaminophen
Ketoprofen
Naproxen sodium
Aspirin-acetaminophen-caffeine
Prescription drugs
Tramodol
Aspirin (or acetaminophen)-butalbital-caffeine combinations
Preventive agents for tension-type headache
Agent: Typical dose
Amitriptyline: 25–100 mg/day
NSAIDs, e.g. naproxen sodium: 550 mg bid

cause of these headaches, evidence is lacking to support this view. For example, people with migraine have higher muscle tension on average than do those who meet criteria for tension-type headache. Because TTH can mimic secondary types of headache, it is a diagnosis that should be made only after consideration has been given to organic disorders. This requires a general and neurological examination and in some cases the examination of headache diaries. It is a clinical diagnosis; there are no laboratory or radiological studies that can rule in a diagnosis of TTH. Manual palpation of the pericranial muscles and their insertions can sometimes demonstrate muscle pathology that is contributing to the headaches (Couppe, Torelli, Fuglsang-Frederiksen, Andersen, & Jensen, 2007; Jensen, 1999; Bendtsen, 2000).

It can sometimes be difficult to distinguish tension-type headaches from migraine. Almost all patients with migraine also experience at least occasional TTH, and roughly half have frequent TTH (Lyngberg, Rasmussen, Jorgensen, & Jensen, 2005a). Migraine and tension-type headache share many common triggers, such as lack of sleep and emotional stress or tension (Rasmussen, 1993). In contrast to migraine, which is a severe headache (if untreated), tension-type headaches may interfere with function but are rarely incapacitating. Occasional tension-type headaches are generally self-managed; most tension-type headache sufferers who seek care do so because the headaches are very frequent. Also in contrast to migraine, tension-type headaches are not associated with prominent associated features such as nausea, vomiting, or photo- or phonophobia.

Tension-type headache is the most prevalent form of primary headache, with a lifetime prevalence above 90%. For the individual sufferer, it is less severe and disabling than migraine, but at the population level, it is responsible for a substantial amount of missed work and decreased work function simply because it is so common (Lyngberg, Rasmussen, Jorgensen, & Jensen, 2005b; Lyngberg, Rasmussen, Jorgensen, & Jensen, 2005c). A recent comprehensive review showed that disability attributable to TTH exceeds that due to migraine, and several studies show a higher number of missed workdays due to TTH compared with migraine (Schwartz, Stewart, & Lipton, 1997; Stovner & Hagen, 2006). Unsurprisingly, this burden is concentrated in the small proportion of patients who have TTH and comorbidities. Most sufferers do not seek medical attention unless headaches are chronic or associated with other disorders such as depression, which may render the additional burden of headache more difficult to tolerate (Holroyd et al., 2000).

TREATMENT OF TENSION-TYPE HEADACHE

Far less research attention has been devoted to the development of treatments for tension-type headache than to migraine. Table 44.3 lists commonly used abortive and preventive medications for tension-type headache. There is relatively old evidence suggesting that tricyclic antidepressants are probably effective, with amitriptyline being the best studied and therefore the most commonly used (Bendtsen & Jensen, 2000; Bryson & Wilde, 1996; Diamond & Baltes, 1971). The doses used are lower than those used for the treatment of

Table 44.3 ABORTIVE AND PREVENTIVE TREATMENT OPTIONS FOR MIGRAINE

ABORTIVE AGENTS

Over-the-counter drugs for mild–moderate attacks

Aspirin

Acetaminophen

Ketoprofen

Naproxen sodium

Aspirin-acetaminophen-caffeine

Prescription drugs for mild–moderate attacks

Tramadol

Aspirin (or acetaminophen)-butalbital-caffeine combinations

Prescription drugs for moderate–severe attacks

Sumatriptan

Rizatriptan

Zolmitriptan

Eletriptan

Almotriptan

Naratriptan

Frovatriptan

Ergotamine preparations

Opioids

Drugs to treat associated nausea/vomiting

Metoclopramide

Hydroxyzine

Prochlorperazine

Preventive agents for migraine

Agent	Typical dose
Low-dose tricyclic antidepressants, e.g. amitriptyline	25–100 mg/day
Beta blockers, e.g. propranolol*	80–160 mg/day
Divalproex sodium*	250 mg bid–500 mg bid
Topiramate*	15–25 mg po q hs to initiate; increase as tolerated to 50 mg po bid
Calcium blockers, e.g. verapamil	80–240 mg/day
Cyproheptadine	4–8 mg bid

(*continued*)

Table 44.3 (CONTINUED)

ABORTIVE AGENTS

NSAIDs, e.g. naproxen sodium	550 mg bid
Lisinopril/Candesartan	5–10 mg qd/20 mg qd
Onabotulinum toxin type A injections*	155 units IM in pericranial muscles

* Approved by the FDA for prevention of migraine

depression, and are typically in the range of 25 mg to 100 mg per day, generally given as a single dose in the evening.

Anticholinergic side effects such as dry mouth, sedation, and constipation may be treatment-limiting. Appetite increase and weight gain are particularly troublesome long-term side effects. Starting with a low dose of medication, such as 10 mg nightly, and working up slowly to a higher dose is helpful, since some patients develop tolerance to these effects. A "start low and go slow" approach also enables patients to identify the lowest dose that successfully treats their problem. Preventive medications for headache commonly take weeks to months to show their full benefits, however. As is true in other headache disorders, treatment benefits are best identified through the use of carefully kept headache diaries or calendars. Total eradication of headache is unlikely; instead, the goal of treatment is to reduce headaches to a manageable frequency. If amitriptyline is effective for headache but poorly tolerated, it may be worthwhile to systematically try other tricyclics, which may have fewer side effects. Although many of them have not been systematically studied for the treatment of headache, there is a strong clinical impression that they are effective.

In contrast to the tricyclic antidepressants, there is not strong evidence to support the use of SSRIs or SNRIs for the treatment of chronic tension-type headache, although fluvoxamine may be an exception (Langemark & Olesen, 1994; Manna, Bolino, & Di Cicco, 1994).

Non-pharmacological treatments such as physical therapy or other physical treatments are commonly used for tension-type headaches. These include the use of heat, cold, massage, and exercise-based physical treatments. In general, there is no strong evidence to support or refute the benefits of such treatments, but they do not appear to be harmful.

Relaxation therapies such as biofeedback training may be useful for tension-type headache. Biofeedback training provides the patient with feedback about muscle tension or finger temperature. Lower levels of muscle tension or higher finger temperatures are generally correlated with a more relaxed state; over time, with such feedback most patients are able to achieve a state of relaxation. Typically, they are then expected to practice biofeedback techniques daily (Nicholson, Buse, Andrasik, & Lipton, 2011).

MIGRAINE

Migraine is also a highly prevalent primary headache disorder, with a cumulative lifetime incidence of 43% in women and 28% in men. This high disease burden is explained by the fact that migraine is a chronic condition of long duration, with peak incidence in the late teens or early twenties (Stewart et al., 2008). Migraine is more prevalent than many other conditions commonly seen in neurology, yet it is often missed or incorrectly diagnosed as "sinus" or "tension" headache. In contrast to tension-type headaches, the pain of migraine is usually moderate or severe in intensity, and the headaches are usually associated with accompanying symptoms such as nausea, vomiting, photophobia, or phonophobia. Headaches can last up to 72 hours (and occasionally even longer, a situation known as *status migrainosus*). In a subset of patients with migraine, the disorder is progressive, and over time, intermittent attacks may become more frequent and develop into *chronic migraine,* a condition in which attacks occur 15 or more days per month (Lipton, 2009) (Table 44.4).

Migraine pain is often experienced on one side of the head, usually in the temporal area, and the affected side may vary from attack to attack. Most patients report that the pain is "throbbing" or "pulsating." Sensitivity to sound and light are common, and some patients report that strong sensory experiences (smells, sound, light) can trigger an attack. The pain is commonly aggravated by physical activity, and sufferers generally prefer to lie still, often in a dark, quiet room. Migraine attacks in children may be shorter than those in adults, and vomiting is often a more prominent symptom. Many children and some adults report that vomiting partially relieves the headache.

Migraine, especially migraine with aura, is increasingly recognized to have medical implications. It is associated with an increased prevalence of ischemic stroke, coronary heart disease, patent foramen ovale, and affective disorders such as depression and anxiety (Breslau et al., 1994; Diener, Kurth, & Dodick, 2007; Kurth, 2010; Kurth, Kase, Schurks, Tzourio, & Buring, 2010; Schurks et al., 2009). In women, it is associated with an increased risk of preeclampsia and peri-pregnancy stroke (Bushnell, Jamison, & James, 2009; Facchinetti et al., 2009; James, Bushnell, Jamison, & Myers, 2005). It is a relative contraindication to the use of exogenous estrogens after the age of 35, or at any age when aura is present (Loder, Buse, & Golub, 2005).

Many women with migraine report that headaches are more common, severe, and long-lasting around the time of menstruation. This menstrual susceptibility to headache is probably caused by declining estrogen levels. Headaches seem particularly likely to occur when these falling estrogen levels occur after a prolonged period of relatively high levels of estrogen. Some evidence suggests that efforts to minimize or eliminate this drop in estrogen levels (for example, continuous rather than interrupted oral contraceptive regimens) may reduce the frequency or intensity of menstrual migraines. At present, however, the harm-to-benefit balance of such treatment has not been carefully studied, and there are no hormonal treatment regimens that have an FDA indication for the treatment of migraine (Loder, 2004).

Emotional stress or tension is among the most commonly mentioned triggers of migraine attacks. A hallmark of migraine is that the headache often comes *after* rather than *during* a stressful event (Kelman, 2007) (AMPP) (Peatfield,

Table 44.4 NEWER PRESCRIPTION MEDICATIONS FOR TREATMENT OF MIGRAINE

DRUG	ADVANTAGES	SIDE EFFECTS	INTERACTIONS WITH PSYCHOPHARMACOLOGICAL MEDICATIONS	COMMENT
Candesartan	Can be useful in patients with concomitant hypertension	Hypotension, fatigue	Few that are clinically important, although many CNS drugs such as anxiolytics or sedatives can produce hypotensive or orthostatic side effects; additive effects may occur when they are used with blood pressure medications	Not FDA-approved for migraine prevention, but use is supported by randomized trials
Lisinopril	Can be useful in patients with concomitant hypertension	Pedal edema, chronic cough, angioedema (rare)	As above	Not FDA-approved for migraine prevention, but use is supported by randomized trials
Topiramate	Reduction of migraine frequency and severity in roughly half of trial subjects; not associated with weight gain	Memory and word-finding difficulties; paresthesias; kidney stones; acute glaucoma (rare); associated with cleft deformities when used in pregnancy	Caution recommended when used in conjunction with other CNS depressants; no specific reported interactions with antidepressants	FDA-approved for migraine prevention. Used off-label for mood stabilization. Psychiatric adverse effects have been reported, including acute mood changes and suicidal thoughts. The package insert states that "Antiepileptic drugs (AEDs), including Topiramate, increase the risk of suicidal thoughts or behavior in patients taking these drugs for any indication. Patients treated with any AED for any indication should be monitored for the emergence or worsening of depression, suicidal thoughts or behavior, and/or any unusual changes in mood or behavior."
Onabotulinum toxin type A	Administered as intramuscular injections to sites in the head and neck every three months; no need to take daily oral medications	Local irritation, injection reactions. Muscle weakness is expected and can occasionally produce unwanted ptosis or neck pain that improve as the medication wears off over 2–3 months. Rare cases reported of possible toxin spread with botulism-like symptoms—none in patients who have received treatment for headache	None	FDA-approved for treatment of chronic migraine (migraine 15 or more days per month). Not effective in episodic forms of the disorder

1995). Other commonly mentioned triggers of migraine include dietary substances such as alcohol, aged cheeses, chocolate, or food additives, especially monosodium glutamate. It is difficult to establish the relationship between dietary practices and headache. Patients with migraine vary in their susceptibility to dietary triggers. Strict elimination diets to treat headaches, although popular, lack strong scientific support for their specific benefits (Blau, 1992; Mitchell et al., 2011; Zencirci, 2010).

Caffeine is a special case, since it can be a treatment for headache, or, when it is withdrawn, a cause of headache. In small amounts, caffeine augments the effects of mild analgesics such as aspirin or acetaminophen, and it is a common ingredient in both over-the-counter and prescription combination headache medications. Taken too frequently, however, caffeine is suspected of aggravating migraine, and its abrupt withdrawal may produce a caffeine-withdrawal headache (Wolpow, 2010). It has even been suggested that caffeine is the "trigger" for ischemic stroke associated with migraine, and caffeine intake is associated with the development of chronic daily headache (Logroscino & Kurth, 2010; Scher, Stewart, & Lipton, 2004). For all of these reasons, it should be used judiciously in people with migraine, whether it is ingested as a drug or in drinks.

Physical activity or exertion, including sexual activity, can also aggravate or trigger headache in those with migraine. Exercise-induced migraine usually comes on after sustained exertion, rather than immediately upon onset of exercise, and can sometimes be modified or eliminated by a change in exercise routine or intensity. A variety of serious causes of exertional headaches must be ruled out by appropriate investigation (Mokri, 2002).

MIGRAINE AURA

Only about a third of migraineurs experience the focal neurological symptoms that constitute aura. Visual aura is by far the most common form of aura, followed by auras consisting of sensory or speech disturbances. In typical visual aura, the visual symptoms precede the headache, come on gradually, and fade away within an hour as the headache begins. They may consist of partial or complete homonymous loss of vision, or visual abnormalities such as flickering, glittery zig-zag lines, sometimes referred to as a "scintillating scotoma." These abnormalities usually begin near the center of the visual field, then expand and enlarge before fading away (Eriksen, Thomsen, & Olesen, 2005).

Sensory auras often consist of paresthesias, commonly beginning in one hand and traveling upwards to the arm and face on the same side. This stereotyped "march" of symptoms is sometimes referred to as the "cheiro-oral syndrome." In this case, too, symptoms usually develop and fade away gradually, to be followed by the headache. It can be difficult for patients to distinguish between numbness and weakness.

Aura can also take the form of muscle weakness, usually unilateral, and patients may experience a dense and sometimes prolonged hemiplegia. These syndromes, although rare, are of interest because they are frequently familial, with autosomal dominant inheritance. Three genes associated with these rare hemiplegic migraine syndromes have been identified, all of which appear to affect neuronal excitability (Russell & Ducros, 2011).

The underlying cause of migraine aura is thought to be a process called *cortical spreading depression*. This term refers to a wave of initial activation of neurons, followed by a prolonged depression of neuronal activity. This process spreads across the surface of the brain at a rate of approximately 3 mm per minute, a time course consistent with the progression of the neurological events of aura. A decrease in cerebral blood flow may occur, but it is thought to reflect these changes in neuronal activity rather than produce them. These decreases in blood flow rarely reach a level sufficient to cause ischemia of brain tissue (Sanchez-Del-Rio, Reuter, & Moskowitz, 2006).

There is, however, a small increased risk of ischemic stroke in people who have migraine with aura. Whether this is due to rare circumstances in which dehydration or platelet activation are sufficient to aggravate low blood-flow levels is not entirely clear. While the elevated risk of ischemic stroke in migraineurs with aura is high relative to that in people without migraine (or even those who have migraine without aura), the absolute risk of stroke is low, meaning that patients should not panic. Rather, it is reason to emphasize the importance of minimizing other risk factors for stroke such as smoking or hypertension. In women of childbearing age, the combined stroke risk from aura and the use of estrogen-containing contraceptives is generally felt to be unacceptable; official guidelines from a number of authoritative bodies recommend that women with aura should not use estrogen-containing contraceptives or other forms of exogenous estrogen (Loder, 2009).

TREATMENT TO ABORT A MIGRAINE ATTACK

Treatment for migraine can be aimed at terminating an individual attack (abortive treatment) or at preventing migraine attacks (preventive treatment). Many patients need both forms of treatment. Abortive treatment alone is appropriate for patients who have intermittent attacks of migraine, whereas those who have frequent attacks are candidates for preventive treatment in addition to abortive therapy. There are no hard and fast rules about when preventive treatment should be considered; in general, patients are candidates for preventive treatment if they have more than one attack of migraine a week, or do not respond to or cannot tolerate abortive therapy.

Abortive treatment of migraine is initiated at the onset of or during an attack. The primary goals of acute treatment are to resolve headache pain and associated symptoms as rapidly as possible and restore function with minimal side effects. Some older medications relieve pain but can worsen disability because they produce sedation or side effects such as nausea and vomiting. Secondary goals of acute treatment include minimization of the need for rescue medication (backup medications used at home by patients when the usual treatment fails to relieve pain) and trips to the doctor's office or emergency department.

Abortive treatment is most effective when used early in an attack while pain is still mild (Foley et al., 2005). This approach should be recommended in patients who have intermittent attacks of headache. An emphasis on early treatment can backfire, however, in patients who have frequent attacks of headache, since it may lead to medication overuse. Patients with frequent headaches need to limit use of abortive medications and may need to pick and choose which attacks are treated pharmacologically. Some patients, particularly those with anxiety disorders, may medicate in anticipation of headache, another situation that can easily lead to medication overuse. They may need instructions to postpone treatment until headache reaches a predetermined pain intensity.

Table 44.5 lists commonly used abortive treatments for migraine. Abortive treatments for migraine can be divided into nonspecific and specific medications. Nonspecific medications are those that are effective for many different kinds of pain, not just migraine. These include nonsteroidal anti-inflammatory agents (NSAIDs), acetaminophen, opioids, and various combination analgesics such as the barbiturate-containing medications (e.g., Fiorinal, Esgic, Phrenelin) (Cutrer, Mitsikostas, Ayata, & Sanchez-del-Rio, 1999; Mett & Tfelt-Hansen, 2008; Tfelt-Hansen, 2008).

Table 44.5 ACUTE AND PREVENTIVE TREATMENT OPTIONS FOR CLUSTER HEADACHE

ABORTIVE AGENTS FOR CLUSTER HEADACHE		
Parenteral sumatriptan*, nasal spray triptans, or dihydroergotamine		
100% oxygen at 10–12 liters via face mask		
Preventive Agents Commonly Used for Cluster Headache		
Agent	Typical dose	
Verapamil	240 mg SR daily or above	240 SR po qd-bid (check EKG)
Lithium	Lithium carbonate 300 mg po tid; dose adjusted to achieve response	

* FDA-approved for cluster headache treatment

These medications, particularly NSAIDs, can be effective for migraine, but the combination medications and opioids are associated with overuse, dependence, and addiction. The combination medications and opioids also may produce sedation that limits the ability of patients to carry out daily activities or remain at work (Martin & Goldstein, 2005; Silberstein & McCrory, 2001). Isometheptene-containing combination medications are an exception to this rule, as they usually do not produce substantial fatigue. Isometheptene is a vasoconstrictive agent that is usually combined with acetaminophen and the mildly sedative medication dichloralphenazone (Freitag et al., 2001). However, isometheptene combination products are now difficult to obtain from commercial sources. At the time of this writing, only one company is manufacturing the drug, although it can be compounded.

Nausea and vomiting are prominent symptoms of migraine and can be debilitating in their own right. They are thus sometimes targets of treatment. For many patients, triptans successfully treat the nausea associated with migraine. When that is not the case, nausea can be treated with the use of the prokinetic dopamine antagonist metoclopramide, or with ondansetron, which is a serotonin agonist. These two medications typically do not produce sedation, and they can be taken early in an attack to help prevent or minimize the development of nausea. There is some evidence that metoclopramide or other anti-dopaminergic anti-nausea medications are effective for migraine pain in addition to their effects on nausea (Allena, Magis, & Schoenen, 2005; Azzopardi & Brooks, 2008; Friedman et al., 2005).

Specific medications are those that are effective for migraine or related headache disorders but are generally ineffective for other types of pain. The two categories of specific migraine medications in use are the ergots and triptans. Ergotamine and its derivatives, such as dihydroergotamine, have a complex pharmacology. In many cases, side effects such as nausea and vasoconstrictive complications limit their usefulness (Tfelt-Hansen & Koehler, 2008). The triptans are selective serotonin 5-hydroxytryptamine (5HT) 1B/D agonists. The $5HT_{1B}$ receptors are located postsynaptically on the cerebral blood vessel's smooth muscle. Stimulation of these receptors by triptans produces cranial vasoconstriction. The $5HT_{1D}$ receptors are located presynaptically on the nerve fibers, and stimulation of these receptors inhibits the release of inflammatory neurotransmitters. Although the triptans are highly selective for the cerebral vasculature, a small degree of coronary arterial constriction can occur, possibly through their activity with $5HT_{2A}$ receptors. For this reason, they should generally not be used in patients who have underlying coronary artery disease or who are at high risk for occult coronary artery disease, on the basis of risk-factor stratification. In cases where there is doubt about the patient's coronary status, evaluation prior to triptan prescription may be prudent; however, there is no clear evidence to underpin the decision about what sort of evaluation is needed.

The triptans came into widespread use in the 1990s and are the abortive treatment of choice for patients without cardiovascular disease. Seven triptans are available in the United States (Table 44.5). All are available as oral tablets. Only one, sumatriptan, is available in a parenteral formulation, which is ideal for patients with rapid onset, severe headaches or those in whom nausea or vomiting preclude the use of oral medication. Two triptans are available as nasal sprays; two as orally dissolving tablets. Nasal spray administration of triptans has the advantage of convenience, but much of the dose is actually swallowed and absorbed orally, so the pharmacokinetic advantages of this route of administration are slight. Some of the medication drips down the back of the throat, and many patients complain of a bitter taste from the medication. Orally dissolving tablets are placed on the tongue and can be taken without water. Although patients perceive that these tablets work more quickly than those that are swallowed, objective measures of drug absorption do not clearly support the idea that this is so. The choice of formulation and dose depends upon patient preference and the circumstances of headaches. Most oral triptans can be repeated after two hours; the maximum daily dose varies, depending upon the drug (Loder, 2010).

Most patients who use triptans have a strong preference for oral treatment. A meta-analysis that compared the seven orally available triptans showed comparable efficacy for the marketed doses of most of them; the exceptions were naratriptan and frovatriptan. The marketed doses of those two drugs have lower rates of pain relief than do the others. They have the advantage of longer half-lives, however, so that duration of action may be prolonged, making them reasonable treatment choices for patients with long-duration moderate headaches (Mett & Tfelt-Hansen, 2008).

In general the triptans are well tolerated. Common nonserious side effects include occasional fatigue or nausea. So-called triptan sensations are more common with injectable sumatriptan, probably because of the rapid increase in plasma levels of the drug. This can include transient neck or chest tightness. If patients are unprepared for this side effect, they may worry that they are experiencing cardiac problems; however, studies of coronary perfusion do not support the idea that these side effects reflect decreased coronary perfusion.

Several drug–drug interactions are worth noting. Of most relevance to psychiatrists, the U.S. Food and Drug Administration issued an advisory regarding the concomitant use of triptans and other serotonergic drugs (e.g., lithium, SSRIs, or SNRIs). In clinical practice, however, this side effect appears to be extremely rare and should not inhibit use of these drugs; rather, vigilance for this complication should be maintained (Evans et al., 2010).

If oral treatment of a migraine attack is not successful, non-oral routes of administration should be considered. Injectable treatment with subcutaneous sumatriptan is one option; sumatriptan comes in an autoinjector that can be easily used by most patients, even those with no medical experience. Prefilled cartridges are inserted into the reusable autoinjector. When the medication first came onto the market, these cartridges contained 6 mg of sumatriptan; recently, cartridges containing 4 mg of the medication have become available (Wendt et al., 2006). The efficacy of the sumatriptan 6 mg injection is 77% when evaluated as the proportion of patients who have a decrease from moderate or severe headache to mild or no headache within 1 hour of treatment (Cady et al., 1991). The injection can be repeated, if necessary, after 1 hour. When administered during migraine aura, the sumatriptan injection does not prolong aura but may not be optimally effective for the subsequent headache (Aurora, Barrodale, McDonald, Jakubowski, & Burstein, 2009; Bates et al., 1994). Consequently, many physicians instruct patients with aura who use the sumatriptan injection to delay dosing until headache is present.

Ketorolac is also available in prefilled syringes (though not in an autoinjector). It must be given intramuscularly; consequently, its use is limited to patients who have some medical training or who are willing and able to learn intramuscular injection technique.

Rectal suppositories are another possible treatment approach. Indomethacin is available as a 50 mg rectal suppository and is a highly effective treatment for many patients (Sah & Saini, 2008). It is well to remember that administration of NSAIDs through non-oral routes does not reduce the risk of gastrointestinal complications or bleeding; those side effects are mediated systemically and not through direct mucosal irritation. Dihydroergotamine (DHE) is available as a nasal spray, but its administration is cumbersome, and as with the triptan nasal spray, many patients complain of a bad taste (Ziegler et al., 1994).

A pulmonary inhaler version of DHE may soon become commercially available, but at the time of this writing it has not yet been approved by the FDA. DHE has vasoconstrictive properties and, like the triptans and other ergot preparations, should not be used in patients with known coronary artery disease or those who are at high risk for cardiovascular disease (Aurora, Rozen, Kori, & Shrewsbury, 2009; Shrewsbury, Kori, Miller, Pedinoff, & Weinstein, 2008).

RESCUE TREATMENT FOR MIGRAINE

Headache attacks vary in intensity, and there are times when abortive medication is ineffective. If patients have backup rescue treatment they can self-administer, they may be able to avoid a trip to the physician's office or emergency department. Non-oral rescue therapies are typically used where possible, to reduce the risk that nausea or vomiting will interfere with use. Opioids have a place as rescue treatment for patients with contraindications to triptan use, but in general they should be used only occasionally. Options for rescue therapy include subcutaneous sumatriptan or dihydroergotamine-45, injectable ketorolac, butorphanol nasal spray, hydromorphone suppositories, acetaminophen in combination with opioids, and phenothiazine suppositories (Whyte, Tepper, & Evans, 2010).

PREVENTIVE MIGRAINE TREATMENT

Only a subset of patients with migraine will be candidates for preventive (prophylactic) treatments. These are medications that are administered on a daily basis with the intention of reducing the frequency, duration, or severity of migraine overall. In general, currently available medications rarely eliminate all migraine attacks; rather, a common standard applied to indicate success with preventive migraine therapy is a reduction in attack frequency of 50%. Preventive medications are used by only about 5% of migraineurs (Diamond et al., 2007).

Preventive treatment should usually be offered to patients who cannot use or who do not benefit from abortive therapy, as well as those who have frequent headaches. A commonly used cutoff point for headache frequency at which prevention should be considered is one headache per week. Other special circumstances, such as prolonged headaches, even if infrequent, may merit consideration of prophylactic therapy as well. In general, treatment choices are based on a consideration of side effect profiles and any other benefits that might be obtained from a particular medication. For example, in patients with hypertension, one of the antihypertensive medications with anti-migraine efficacy may be a good choice.

While no preventive medication is effective for every patient in whom it is tried, a common reason for failure is an inadequate trial of the drug. Preventive medications for migraine typically take effect over weeks or even months. Migraine is a condition that naturally waxes and wanes, so that it can be difficult to distinguish true drug effects from the natural history of the illness.

Five drugs are approved by the U.S. Food and Drug Administration for the prevention of migraine (Table 44.5). These are timolol, propranolol, methysergide, divalproex sodium, and topiramate (Bigal & Lipton, 2006). Methysergide is no longer commercially available, and timolol is rarely used. Fibrotic complications curbed enthusiasm for use of methysergide, which was otherwise a remarkably effective drug. The remaining medications seem to have roughly similar efficacy in clinical practice; that is, in about half of patients they reduce headache frequency by roughly 50%. Treatment is usually attempted with a single drug, but combinations of drugs can be tried in refractory cases. No clinical trials support this practice, however, and it is important to note that a recent trial of the combination of topiramate and propranolol failed to show any augmented benefit from the combination over topiramate alone.

Table 44.6 lists selected newer agents used for prevention of migraine, and provides additional details about drug-specific characteristics. Onabotulinum toxin type A is approved for the prevention of chronic migraine, which is migraine occurring 15 or more days per month. It does not appear to be effective for the prevention of episodic migraine, which suggests that mechanisms targeted by the drug become active only after the

transition to the chronic form of the disorder (Dodick et al., 2005; Gobel & Heinze, 2011). Other drugs are used off-label, with varying degrees of evidence of benefit. Commonly used off-label treatments include amitriptyline, verapamil, gabapentin, lisinopril, riboflavin (vitamin B2) and cyproheptadine. Preventive medication must be used sparingly and with great caution in women likely to become pregnant. Some, such as divalproex and topiramate, are teratogenic.

The mechanisms of action of preventive treatments for migraine are not firmly established. Many probably work to inhibit cortical spreading depression, but some may also block neurogenic inflammation or peripheral or central sensitization. Table 44.7 lists some commonly used preventive agents

Table 44.6 NEWER PRESCRIPTION MEDICATIONS FOR TREATMENT OF MIGRAINE

DRUG	ADVANTAGES	SIDE EFFECTS	INTERACTIONS WITH PSYCHOPHARMACOLOGIC MEDICATIONS	COMMENT
Candesartan	Can be useful in patients with concomitant hypertension	Hypotension, fatigue	Few that are clinically important, although many CNS drugs such as anxiolytics or sedatives can produce hypotensive or orthostatic side effects; additive effects may occur when they are used with blood pressure medications.	Not FDA approved for migraine prevention, but use is supported by randomized trials
Lisinopril	Can be useful in patients with concomitant hypertension	Pedal edema, chronic cough, angioedema (rare)	As above.	Not FDA approved for migraine prevention, but use is supported by randomized trials
Topiramate	Reduction of migraine frequency and severity in roughly half of trial subjects; not associated with weight gain	Memory and word-finding difficulties; paresthesias; kidney stones; acute glaucoma (rare); associated with cleft deformities when used in pregnancy	Caution recommended when used in conjunction with other CNS depressants; no specific reported interactions with antidepressants	FDA approved for migraine prevention. Used off-label for mood stabilization. Psychiatric adverse effects have been reported, including acute mood changes and suicidal thoughts. The package insert states that "Antiepileptic drugs (AEDs), including Topiramate, increase the risk of suicidal thoughts or behavior in patients taking these drugs for any indication. Patients treated with any AED for any indication should be monitored for the emergence or worsening of depression, suicidal thoughts or behavior, and/or any unusual changes in mood or behavior."
Onabotulinum toxin type A	Administered as intramuscular injections to sites in the head and neck every three months; no need to take daily oral medications.	Local irritation, injection reactions. Muscle weakness is expected and can occasionally produce unwanted ptosis or neck pain that improve as the medication wears off over 2-3 months. Rare cases reported of possible toxin spread with botulism-like symptoms – none in patients who have received treatment for headache	None	FDA approved for treatment of chronic migraine (migraine 15 or more days per month). Not effective in episodic forms of the disorder.

for migraine, while Table 44.8 provides more detail on newer preventive treatments that have come into use in the last decade.

Beta Blockers

Although propranolol and timolol are the beta blockers that are approved by the FDA for migraine prevention, some clinicians use atenolol, metoprolol, or nadolol. The typical dose range for propranolol is between 60 mg and 160 mg daily. Beta blockers with intrinsic sympathomimetic activity, such as pindolol, do not appear to be effective for migraine prevention. Beta blockers are a good choice in patients with concomitant hypertension, tremor disorders, mitral valve prolapse, or anxiety. They are typically avoided in patients who have asthma or Raynaud's syndrome.

Table 44.7 **DIAGNOSTIC CRITERIA FOR EPISODIC AND CHRONIC CLUSTER HEADACHE (ICHD-II) (HEADACHE CLASSIFICATION SUBCOMMITTEE OF THE INTERNATIONAL HEADACHE SOCIETY 2004). (HEADACHE CLASSIFICATION SUBCOMMITTEE OF THE INTERNATIONAL HEADACHE SOCIETY, 2004)**

Episodic cluster headache

A. At least 5 attacks fulfilling criteria B-D

B. Severe or very severe unilateral orbital, supraorbital and/or temporal pain lasting 15–180 minutes if untreated

C. Headache is accompanied by at least one of the following:

    1. ipsilateral conjunctival injection and/or lacrimation

    2. ipsilateral nasal congestion and/or rhinorrhoea

    3. ipsilateral eyelid edema

    4. ipsilateral forehead and facial sweating

    5. ipsilateral miosis and/or ptosis

    6. a sense of restlessness or agitation

D. Attacks have a frequency from one every other day to 8 per day

E. Not attributed to another disorder

Chronic Cluster Headache

A. Attacks fulfilling criteria A-E for 3.1 Cluster headache

B. Attacks recur over >1 year without remission periods or with remission periods lasting <1 month

Comments:

Chronic cluster headache may arise de novo (previously referred to as primary chronic cluster headache) or evolve from the episodic subtype (previously referred to as secondary chronic cluster headache). Some patients may switch from chronic to episodic cluster headache.

Table 44.8 **ACUTE AND PREVENTIVE TREATMENT OPTIONS FOR CLUSTER HEADACHE**

Abortive Agents for Cluster Headache

Parenteral sumatriptan*, nasal spray triptans or dihydroergotamine

100% oxygen at 10-12 liters via face mask

Preventive Agents Commonly Used for Cluster Headache

Agent	Typical dose
Verapamil	240 mg SR daily or above 240 SR po qd-bid (check EKG)
Lithium	Lithium carbonate 300 mg po tid; dose adjusted to achieve response

Antidepressants

Antidepressants are commonly used for migraine prevention despite the fact that none has an FDA indication for the disorder. The best evidence is for amitriptyline (Buchanan & Ramadan, 2006). Doses used to prevent migraine are typically in the range of 25–100 mg daily, much lower than those used to treat depression. The anti-migraine effect of amitriptyline is independent of its effects on depression. The medication is commonly given in a single daily dose at bedtime. Side effects are frequently treatment-limiting; they include sedation, weight gain, dry mouth, hypotension, and constipation.

SSRIs do not seem effective as migraine preventive agents. Fluoxetine appeared helpful in one small study, but a larger trial showed no benefit (Adly, Straumanis, & Chesson, 1992; Saper, Silberstein, Lake, & Winters, 1995). Some of the SNRIs may be effective. Trials suggesting this are small, however, and suffer from a number of methodological problems. An additional problem with using antidepressants to prevent migraine is the theoretical risk of serotonin syndrome when these drugs are used concomitantly with triptans.

Monoamine oxidase inhibitors have been used in the preventive treatment of migraine, but this is no longer common practice, probably owing to concern about side effects and the availability of newer preventive drugs such as topiramate (Silberstein, 2006). Lithium is another drug that has been used in the past but is no longer commonly employed for migraine, although it remains useful in cluster headache.

Anticonvulsants

Various anti-seizure medications are effective for migraine prevention. Divalproex sodium and topiramate are FDA-approved for this indication. The typical daily dose of divalproex for migraine ranges from 500 mg to 1500 mg per day, lower doses than are typically used for epilepsy. An extended-release version of the drug is available that allows once-daily dosing. Drug levels can be checked, but efficacy does not correlate with blood levels. Common side effects include weight gain, hair loss, and gastrointestinal problems such as nausea. Hepatotoxicity and pancreatitis are rare side effects. Divalproex is a known teratogen and thus a last resort in women of childbearing age, who should be strongly cautioned against becoming pregnant while on the drug (Modi & Lowder, 2006).

The target dose for topiramate is in most cases 100 mg per day, given as 50 mg twice daily. Most patients cannot tolerate this as a starting dose, however. A common practice is to begin with 25 mg at bedtime daily for a week, and then to increase the dose in 25 mg increments each week until the target level is achieved. Doses of 50 mg per day and up to 200 mg per day were evaluated in clinical trials and were more effective than placebo; in clinical practice, some patients do best at these extremes of the dosing range (Silberstein, 2004b).

Gabapentin does not have FDA approval for treatment of migraine, but is commonly used, perhaps because it is well tolerated and has few drug interactions. Side effects include fatigue. Typical doses range from 300 mg to 1200 mg, three times a day (Young, Siow, & Silberstein, 2004). Lamotrigine does not appear to be effective for prevention of migraine headaches, but it may have efficacy against aura; it is not FDA-approved for this indication, however, and the rare but serious side effect of Stevens-Johnson syndrome argues against its routine use for this purpose. Zonisamide is sometimes used off-label, as is levatiracetam (Young et al., 2004).

Calcium Channel Antagonists

No calcium channel antagonist is FDA-approved for migraine prevention. Verapamil, however, is frequently used and generally well tolerated. It is usually given in a dose of 120–240 mg per day in a sustained-release formulation. The most common side effect is constipation; peripheral edema can also occur (Black, 2006).

Several double-blind, placebo-controlled trials support the use of lisinopril for migraine prophylaxis. There is also some evidence for the angiotensin receptor blocker candesartan. These drugs are not, however, FDA-approved for migraine. They can cause fetal renal abnormalities when used during pregnancy, so must be used with caution in women of childbearing age (Gales, Bailey, Reed, & Gales, 2010).

Miscellaneous

Cyproheptadine is commonly used for pediatric migraine prevention, although evidence supporting this practice is sparse; the drug is, however, somewhat similar to methysergide in being a serotonin antagonist, and is well tolerated. It also has antihistaminic effects and is a modest calcium channel blocker (Rao, Das, Taraknath, & Sarma, 2000).

Vitamin B2 in doses of 400 mg once daily has demonstrated some migraine preventive effects in two double-blind, randomized trials. It turns the urine bright yellow but is well tolerated. There is likewise some modest evidence supporting the use of the herb butterbur for migraine prevention; a recent meta-analysis suggested that the herb feverfew, long popular as a migraine preventive treatment, is probably ineffective. Evidence for the benefits of oral magnesium is mixed, and diarrhea is a treatment-limiting side effect (Evans & Taylor, 2006).

CLUSTER HEADACHE

Cluster headache is a distinct type of headache that is more common in men than in women. It is a relatively rare headache disorder, with estimates of its prevalence given as roughly 70 per 100,000. In contrast to migraine, cluster headache is a short-lived headache, with duration not exceeding three hours. It is a strictly unilateral headache with severe, stabbing pain localized in and behind the eye. It can, however, switch sides from one attack to the next, and occasionally even within an attack. It is associated with autonomic features on the same side as the pain, which can include ptosis, meiosis, and nasal stuffiness or rhinorrhea (Table 44.7). Nausea, vomiting, photophobia and phonophobia, which are common accompaniments to headache in migraineurs, are not common in cluster headache. Aura has been reported in association with cluster headache but is not the rule (Kudrow, 1979).

Multiple attacks of cluster headache can occur per day. Cluster headache is so-called because attacks of headache cluster together for weeks to months in cluster "periods" or "episodes." Most sufferers have episodic cluster headache and will have daily or near-daily attacks for several months, interspersed with remission periods during which they are headache-free for intervals of months to years. About 15% of sufferers, however, have chronic cluster headache, in which there are no or very short remission periods (Kudrow, 1982).

During a cluster episode, patients are commonly susceptible to a number of environmental triggers that can cause individual attacks of headache to occur. For example, ingestion of alcohol is commonly reported to trigger cluster headaches during a cluster period, while during remission periods, patients can drink with impunity. Many patients also experience cluster attacks in conjunction with rapid-eye-movement (REM) sleep, so that cluster headache is sometimes considered a parasomnia. Patients with cluster headache are usually physically restless during an attack, in contrast to migraine patients, who prefer to lie quiet and avoid motion.

TREATMENT OF CLUSTER HEADACHE

Patients with cluster headache usually do not have to be told to avoid triggers such as alcohol and napping during a cluster episode. Again in contrast to migraine, trigger avoidance and lifestyle alterations are not notably effective treatments for cluster headache. Because the headache occur daily, sometimes multiple times per day, reliance on abortive therapy alone is typically not recommended; essentially, all patients with cluster headache should be offered concomitant preventive therapy in addition to abortive therapy of individual attacks. Table 44.8 lists commonly used treatments for cluster headache.

The sumatriptan injection is FDA-approved for the treatment of cluster headache. The 6 mg dose of sumatriptan aborts about three-quarters of cluster headaches within 15 minutes of treatment (Capobianco & Dodick, 2006). Side effects are those observed in the migraine trials and are mostly nonserious events such as flushing or nausea. As in migraine patients, triptans are contraindicated in uncontrolled hypertension and coronary artery disease. Although there is some evidence that nasal or oral administration of triptans is more effective than placebo for cluster headache, they are not preferred agents. Their onset of action is relatively slow, and the patient may suffer needlessly while waiting for them to take effect. Nonetheless, there may be some circumstances where these are appropriate therapies. Ergots, including DHE, can also be used, but there are few circumstances where they are preferred to the triptans.

Indomethacin suppositories can also be tried for patients with cluster headache, and they may be particularly helpful for patients who cannot take or do not benefit from sumatriptan injections. Oxygen inhalation has been shown to be effective for abortive treatment of cluster headache in two controlled trials; typically the oxygen should be administered through a non-rebreather mask at a rate of 8–10 liters per minute for 10–15 minutes at the onset of the attack. Roughly 80% of patients report benefit from oxygen treatment, and there are no major contraindications to its use aside from severe chronic obstructive pulmonary disease with carbon dioxide retention (Cohen, Burns, & Goadsby, 2009).

Preventive treatment of cluster headache is often remarkably effective. Unlike patients with migraine, those with cluster headache are commonly rendered headache-free by prophylaxis. There is good evidence of benefit for the preventive use of verapamil and lithium in the treatment of cluster headache, although neither is FDA-approved for treatment of cluster headache. Verapamil is effective for about three-quarters of patients with episodic cluster headache and slightly more than half with chronic cluster headache (Gabai & Spierings, 1989). The doses necessary to achieve benefit can be quite high, however—often in the range of 240 mg or above per day—and it is prudent to monitor the electrocardiogram to assess for conduction delay.

Lithium is effective in 87% of patients (Kudrow, 1977). It is typically given as lithium carbonate at a starting dose of 300 mg three times daily; most patients respond well to this dose and do not need upward titration. Monitoring of serum levels is not useful to guide therapy, which is based on clinical response, but can help avoid toxicity. Caution should be used if lithium is administered with diuretics or NSAIDs. Nausea and tremor are common side effects. Prolonged use can affect kidney and thyroid function. Fortunately, many patients need the medication for relatively short periods of time, thus minimizing the likelihood of toxicity with prolonged use.

Steroids such as prednisone are highly effective in the treatment of cluster headache, but serious side effects such as osteonecrosis limit the duration of their use. Therefore, they are most commonly employed as "bridging therapy" to cover the patient while he waits for preventive medication with lithium or verapamil to become effective. Suppression of headaches may be dose-dependent, so that when patients taper from a high to a low dose of prednisone, for example, headaches may resume with dose reduction (Gaul, Diener, & Muller, 2011). Potential side effects are stomach pain, fluid retention, and insomnia.

Two promising new therapies are under investigation for medically refractory cluster headache. Occipital nerve blocks can temporarily relieve cluster headache, so trials are underway to see if implantable occipital nerve stimulators might provide longer lasting relief; results so far are encouraging but not definitive. Lead migration is the most common problem with the procedure, and infection is also a concern (Dodick, 2011; Leroux et al., 2011; Strand, Trentman, Vargas, & Dodick, 2011). Deep brain stimulation of the hypothalamus with implantable electrodes also appears effective in several case series, but severe complications can occur with this surgery; it is unlikely that this will ever be anything other than a last resort for treatment (Leone, Franzini, Cecchini, Broggi, & Bussone, 2010).

PAROXYSMAL HEMICRANIA

A variety of other headache syndromes have similarities to cluster headache. One is paroxysmal hemicranias, a condition in which headaches are unilateral and associated with autonomic features but briefer (10–30 minutes) and more frequent (up to 15 times daily) than cluster headache (Matharu, Boes, & Goadsby, 2003). These headaches are important to diagnose because they are very sensitive to scheduled treatment with indomethacin. Indomethacin is usually given initially as 25 mg orally, three times daily; the dose is doubled every three days until relief occurs or a maximum of 75 mg three times daily is reached. Drug benefit occurs quickly in susceptible patients, so that an indomethacin treatment trial can be completed within nine days. If indomethacin is not effective or tolerated, other treatments effective in cluster headache can be tried but do not commonly meet with success.

IDIOPATHIC STABBING HEADACHE

Patients with idiopathic stabbing headache, sometimes referred to as "icepick headache" or "jabs and jolts," complain of short, sharp episodes of very intense pain, usually in the temples. Occasional jabs of pain are not uncommon in patients who have migraine, but these stabbing pains can also occur in isolation from other forms of headache. When they are only occasional, the only treatment needed is reassurance. Frequent volleys of pain, however, can be disabling. They usually respond well to treatment with indomethacin or sometimes other NSAIDs. Because they are so brief and can occur unpredictably throughout the day, this treatment must be administered on a continuous basis. A common practice is to give indomethacin 25 mg orally, three times daily, for several weeks. In many cases, when this treatment is withdrawn, the headaches will not recur (Mukharesh & Jan, 2011).

This condition should be distinguished from short, sharp jabs of pain in the face, a situation in which trigeminal neuralgia must be considered. Trigeminal neuralgia is most common in older patients. Often the pain can be triggered by chewing or exposure to wind or cold. This triggerability is not a feature of idiopathic stabbing headaches. Medical treatment of trigeminal neuralgia usually consists of carbamazepine or other anticonvulsant medications. Some cases of ectatic blood vessels' compressing the nerve have been reported, and surgical decompression for such patients can be effective (Feinmann & Peatfield, 1993).

NEW DAILY PERSISTENT HEADACHE

New daily persistent headache (NDPH) is a headache that is constant from onset or within three days of onset, and continues for at least three months. It is defined as a headache that has few if any associated features such as nausea, or photo- or phonophobia, although a migrainous form is increasingly recognized. It is bilateral, pressing or tightening in quality, and mild to moderate in intensity. Its cause is unknown, although in some patients it is preceded by infection. Although it is similar in many ways to chronic tension-type headache, it is distinguished from that disorder by its sudden onset. There are no established treatments for NDPH, so treatment is usually that used for other headache disorders such as migraine or tension-type headache. Unfortunately, treatment is often ineffective (Goadsby & Boes, 2002).

HYPNIC HEADACHE

Hypnic headache is a dull headache that wakens the patient, usually over the age of 50, from sleep. It occurs 15 or more days a month and lasts at least 15 minutes. It is not associated with autonomic signs or symptoms, and is not associated with prominent migrainous features such as nausea, or photo- or phonophobia. It can be distinguished from cluster headache by its moderate intensity and lack of autonomic features. It often responds to caffeine or lithium carbonate 300 mg administered at bedtime. Indomethacin and melatonin can also be tried (Evers & Goadsby, 2003).

HEMICRANIA CONTINUA

Hemicrania continua is, as its name implies, a unilateral headache that is daily and continuous without pain-free periods or side-shift for at least three months. It is typically moderate in intensity, but most patients experience periodic exacerbations. During these periods of worsening, autonomic signs occur on the side of the pain. These may include conjunctival injection, tearing, nasal congestion, or ptosis. This is a headache that typically responds to indomethacin; in fact, diagnostic criteria require indomethacin response in order to make a definite diagnosis (Silberstein & Peres, 2002).

MEDICATION OVERUSE HEADACHE AND DRUG-INDUCED HEADACHE

Daily or near-daily intake of symptomatic pain medications is common in people with frequent headaches. This is undesirable for a number of reasons. Many commonly used symptomatic headache medications contain barbiturates or opioids, which can be habit-forming and produce sedation or impaired judgement that interfere with daily activities. The adverse effects of daily use of even simple analgesics such as acetaminophen or NSAIDs can also be important, and include abnormalities of liver or kidney function as well as gastrointestinal bleeding.

Finally, considerable observational evidence suggests that frequent use of short-acting pain-relieving medications can produce or perpetuate headache disorders, a clinical situation known as "medication overuse headache" (Bigal et al., 2008). Those with preexisting headache disorders seem most susceptible. This observational evidence, however, is likely to be confounded by severity of illness.

From a scientific point of view, it remains uncertain whether medication use drives headache progression, or whether those with severe progressive headaches are simply using a great deal of medication in response to their pain. A combination of these things is also possible, and it may be the case that only some headache patients are vulnerable to the disease-aggravating effects of too-frequent use of pain relievers. It is also unclear whether all short-term symptomatic medications are implicated in headache progression, or just some of them. Some experts, for example, believe that plain NSAIDs are unlikely to produce medication overuse headache (as opposed to combination medications that may contain NSAIDs along with other ingredients such as caffeine). Analysis of data from one longitudinal study, for example, suggested that regular use of aspirin might actually protect against the progression from episodic to chronic forms of headache (Ashina, Zeeberg, Jensen, & Ashina, 2006).

It is also uncertain whether overuse of symptomatic medications interferes with or prevents benefit from longer-term preventive headache strategies. There has long been a strong clinical impression that this is the case, with some experts claiming preventive treatment can only be effective once patients are withdrawn from overused short-term medications. Recent analyses of data from trials of preventive treatment with topiramate and onabotulinum toxin type A, however, did not show reduced benefit of those prophylactic treatments in subjects who were overusing short-acting headache relief medications. This suggests that not all patients must be withdrawn from overused medications in order to benefit from preventive headache therapy. There are still many other reasons, however, to attempt medication reduction or withdrawal in patients who are using these treatments frequently (Katsarava et al., 2005).

ICHD criteria for the diagnosis of medication overuse headache have frequently been altered, and expert opinion remains divided on the amount and type of symptomatic headache medication that is needed to produce medication overuse headache. From a practical clinical point of view, a reasonable practice is to restrict the use of symptomatic medication to no more than three days of use per week (Silberstein et al., 2005).

It can be difficult to help patients with chronic headache disorders maintain reasonable limits on the use of symptomatic headache-relief medications. There is a tension between the desire for pain relief for individual headaches and the longer-term goal of prevention of headache worsening or the development of treatment-related morbidities. Disagreement between patients and their physicians about the type and amount of medication that should be used to treat individual headache episodes is a common cause of treatment difficulty. Treatment strategies that are appropriate for patients with occasional headaches—in particular, the emphasis on early, aggressive treatment of individual headache attacks—can be counterproductive for patients who have frequent headaches. Over time, some patients develop maladaptive beliefs and behaviors regarding medications; a common example is the belief that only a certain medication (such as meperidine) will help a bad headache (Kavuk et al., 2004; Usai et al., 2004).

Treatment agreements that limit the monthly amount of short-term pain medications that can be used by the patient are often the most successful approach to preventing medication overuse. Patients with chronic headache should be encouraged to use non-medication strategies to augment pharmacological treatment of headaches, and should understand that they may have to pick and choose which headaches to treat.

Treatment of patients whose medication overuse is an entrenched behavior can be difficult. It is not always easy to obtain an accurate history of medication intake. Patients may not disclose use of over-the-counter medications unless asked, for example. Thus it is essential that patients with frequent headaches, even those that are mild, be asked specifically about prescription and non-prescription medications, including details about the number of tablets taken and the number of times per day they are used. When medication reduction or withdrawal is necessary, the methods used depend upon the drug(s) being taken. If patients also are heavy consumers of caffeine in the form of caffeine-containing headache medications, cola drinks, energy drinks, or coffee, headache from caffeine withdrawal will make the treatment more difficult. In such cases, it may be worthwhile to taper and discontinue caffeine prior to beginning the rest of the medication taper.

From a behavioral point of view, non-barbiturate or non-opioid medications are best discontinued abruptly, in order to avoid perpetuating medication-taking behavior. Opioid or barbiturate withdrawal syndromes can be severe, and these medications must be withdrawn more slowly to avoid precipitating withdrawal seizures. Patients using these medications on an "as needed" basis should be converted to a regular schedule of use and the dose reduced gradually (Paemeleire, Crevits, Goadsby, & Kaube, 2006).

Severe withdrawal headache may occur when regular use of short-acting pain medications is discontinued. Typically, these withdrawal headaches will last two to three days. They may respond to the use of steroids such as decadron 4 mg three times daily for three days. Strong sedatives such as prochlorperazine can be used to help patients tolerate the withdrawal headache and any nausea; they are particularly effective when given as rectal suppositories.

Following medication withdrawal, patients typically need considerable emotional support to avoid returning to previous patterns of medication use. Preventive treatments, including non-pharmacological methods of headache management, must be emphasized. Patients who are unable to withdraw on an outpatient basis from overused medications may require hospitalization. The most successful approach involves hospitalization in a dedicated headache unit, where the underlying headache disorder can be managed in addition to accomplishing medication withdrawal. Unfortunately, there are only a few such dedicated hospital programs remaining in the United States. The majority of headache patients requiring hospitalization for medication withdrawal will thus need to be treated in a general medical or detoxification unit or on an outpatient basis.

TREATMENT OF MEDICALLY REFRACTORY HEADACHE DISORDERS

The long-term management of patients with refractory benign headache is challenging. Organic causes must be ruled out before chronic daily headache can be considered a primary headache problem. These recommendations do not apply to patients who have chronic headache on the basis of head trauma, surgery, or other medical conditions. The following management principles can be helpful in treating patients whose headaches respond poorly to aggressive treatment.

The first principle is to rethink the goals of treatment, which should shift from the idea that a cure is possible and towards a philosophy of symptom management and preservation of functioning and quality of life. Depression, somatic preoccupation, inactivity, and medication overuse are important treatment targets. Patients who can tolerate the medications should be on prophylaxis for their condition, even in the absence of a clear decrease in headache frequency or severity. This may prevent worsening of headache and disease progression. A simple headache calendar can help guide treatment.

Use of most abortive medications for headache should be limited to two or three days per week. Disease-specific medications such as the triptans and ergots are preferable; opioids and barbiturate-containing drugs should be used with caution. Medications such as hydroxyzine, promethazine, or 4% lidocaine drops, and non-pharmacological methods of management (ice, heat, massage) can be used more often.

The role of maintenance opioids in chronic, benign headache is controversial. The only two long-term studies show benefit (as measured by decreased pain levels, decreased use of emergency department [ED]) in only 25% of patients; no reductions in abortive medication use, returns to work, or improvements in mood were found (Rothrock, 1999; Saper et al., 2004; Saper et al., 2010). Scheduled use of long-acting opioids may be most helpful as a time-limited bridging or respite treatment for three to six months in carefully selected patients. Considerable clinical experience is needed to select patients with chronic headache who might benefit from opioid maintenance treatment (Saper et al., 2010).

CLINICAL PEARLS

- The misdiagnosis of migraine as "sinus" headache is a well-known phenomenon (Silberstein, 2004a).

- Preventive treatments, such as beta blockers, that are helpful for migraine are not effective for cluster headache, so diagnostic delay exposes some patients to many years of ineffective treatments.

- Perhaps the most common treatment errors in headache stem from prolonged use of nonsteroidal anti-inflammatory medications, with resulting gastrointestinal toxicity and bleeding.

- It is unusual for primary headache disorders to begin after the age of 50.

- Affective disorders such as anxiety disorders and depression are more common in patients who have migraine, and the reverse situation is also true.

- Studies suggest that the odds of having major depression are roughly in the range of 2–4 for those with migraine compared with non-migraineurs.

- Serotonin syndrome has also been reported with triptan monotherapy (Soldin, Tonning, & Obstetric-Fetal Pharmacology Research Unit Network, 2008). The risk appears low, and the number of case reports is low and of variable credibility (Evans, 2007, 2008). However, the FDA has issued an advisory regarding the possibility of serotonin syndrome with combined triptan and SSRI or SNRI treatment. A position paper from the American Headache Society concludes that available evidence is not sufficient to warrant limiting the use of these drugs; however, they recommend that clinicians using the combination be "vigilant" for signs or symptoms of the disorder (Evans, Tepper, Shapiro, Sun-Edelstein, & Tietjen, 2010).

- Low-grade, featureless headache or worsening of migraine have been reported as side effects of SSRI or SNRI therapy (Bickel, Kornhuber, Maihofner, & Ropohl, 2005). Clinical experience suggests that the headache may wane over time, even if the patient remains on the offending drug; alternatively, switching to another drug in the same class may relieve the headache.

- Unlike patients with migraine, those with cluster headache are commonly rendered headache-free by prophylaxis.

- Although the name implies that muscle or emotional tension might be the underlying cause of tension-type headaches, evidence is lacking to support this view.

- There is relatively old evidence suggesting that tricyclic antidepressants are probably effective for tension-type headaches, with amitriptyline being the best studied and

therefore the most commonly used (Bendtsen & Jensen, 2000; Bryson & Wilde, 1996; Diamond & Baltes, 1971).

- A hallmark of migraine is that the headache often comes after, rather than during, a stressful event.

- In women of childbearing age, the combined stroke risk from aura and the use of estrogen-containing contraceptives is generally felt to be unacceptable.

- So-called triptan sensations are more common with injectable sumatriptan, probably because of the rapid increase in plasma levels of the drug. This can include transient neck or chest tightness. If patients are unprepared for this side effect, they may worry that they are experiencing cardiac problems; however, studies of coronary perfusion do not support the idea that these side effects reflect decreased coronary perfusion.

- Opioid or barbiturate withdrawal syndromes can be severe, and these medications must be withdrawn more slowly to avoid precipitating withdrawal seizures. Patients using these medications on an "as needed" basis should be converted to a regular schedule of use and the dose reduced gradually (Paemeleire, Crevits, Goadsby, & Kaube, 2006).

DISCLOSURE STATEMENT

Dr. Loder is a research editor for the British Medical Journal. She has no financial connections with pharmaceutical or device companies.

REFERENCES

Adly, C., Straumanis, J., & Chesson, A. (1992). Fluoxetine prophylaxis of migraine. *Headache, 32*(2), 101–104.

Allena, M., Magis, D., & Schoenen, J. (2005). A trial of metoclopramide vs. sumatriptan for the emergency department treatment of migraines. *Neurology, 65*(8), 1339–1340; author reply, 1339–1340.

Anttila, V., Stefansson, H., Kallela, M., Todt, U., Terwindt, G. M., Calafato, M. S., et al. (2010). Genome-wide association study of migraine implicates a common susceptibility variant on 8q22.1. *Nature Genetics, 42*(10), 869–873.

Ashina, S., Zeeberg, P., Jensen, R. H., & Ashina, M. (2006). Medication overuse headache [Medicinoverforbrugshovedpine]. *Ugeskrift for Laeger, 168*(10), 1015–1019.

Aurora, S. K., Barrodale, P. M., McDonald, S. A., Jakubowski, M., & Burstein, R. (2009). Revisiting the efficacy of sumatriptan therapy during the aura phase of migraine. *Headache, 49*(7), 1001–1004.

Aurora, S. K., Rozen, T. D., Kori, S. H., & Shrewsbury, S. B. (2009). A randomized, double blind, placebo-controlled study of MAP0004 in adult patients with migraine. *Headache, 49*(6), 826–837.

Azzopardi, T. D., & Brooks, N. A. (2008). Oral metoclopramide as an adjunct to analgesics for the outpatient treatment of acute migraine. *The Annals of Pharmacotherapy, 42*(3), 397–402.

Bahra, A., & Goadsby, P. J. (2004). Diagnostic delays and mis-management in cluster headache. *Acta Neurologica Scandinavica, 109*(3), 175–179.

Bartleson, J. D. (2006). When and how to investigate the patient with headache. *Seminars in Neurology, 26*(2), 163–170.

Bates, D., Ashford, E., Dawson, R., Ensink, F. B., Gilhus, N. E., Olesen, J., et al. (1994). Subcutaneous sumatriptan during the migraine aura. Sumatriptan Aura Study Group. *Neurology, 44*(9), 1587–1592.

Bendtsen, L., & Jensen, R. (2000). Amitriptyline reduces myofascial tenderness in patients with chronic tension-type headache. *Cephalalgia: An International Journal of Headache, 20*(6), 603–610.

Bickel, A., Kornhuber, J., Maihofner, C., & Ropohl, A. (2005). Exacerbation of migraine attacks during treatment with the selective serotonin reuptake inhibitor sertraline. A case report. *Pharmacopsychiatry, 38*(6), 327–328.

Bigal, M. E., & Lipton, R. B. (2006). The preventive treatment of migraine. *Neurologist, 12*(4), 204–213.

Bigal, M. E., Serrano, D., Buse, D., Scher, A., Stewart, W. F., & Lipton, R. B. (2008). Acute migraine medications and evolution from episodic to chronic migraine: A longitudinal population-based study. *Headache, 48*(8), 1157–1168.

Black, D. F. (2006). Sporadic and familial hemiplegic migraine: Diagnosis and treatment. *Seminars in Neurology, 26*(2), 208–216.

Blau, J. N. (1992). Migraine triggers: Practice and theory. *Pathologie-Biologie, 40*(4), 367–372.

Breslau, N. (1998). Psychiatric comorbidity in migraine. *Cephalalgia: An International Journal of Headache, 18*(Suppl 22), 56–58; discussion, 58–61.

Breslau, N., Chilcoat, H. D., & Andreski, P. (1996). Further evidence on the link between migraine and neuroticism. *Neurology, 47*(3), 663–667.

Breslau, N., Merikangas, K., & Bowden, C. L. (1994). Comorbidity of migraine and major affective disorders. *Neurology, 44*(10 Suppl 7), S17–S22.

Breslau, N., Schultz, L. R., Stewart, W. F., Lipton, R., & Welch, K. M. (2001). Headache types and panic disorder: Directionality and specificity. *Neurology, 56*(3), 350–354.

Bryson, H. M., & Wilde, M. I. (1996). Amitriptyline. A review of its pharmacological properties and therapeutic use in chronic pain states. *Drugs & Aging, 8*(6), 459–476.

Buchanan, T. M., & Ramadan, N. M. (2006). Prophylactic pharmacotherapy for migraine headaches. *Seminars in Neurology, 26*(2), 188–198.

Bushnell, C. D., Jamison, M., & James, A. H. (2009). Migraines during pregnancy linked to stroke and vascular diseases: US population based case-control study. *British Medical Journal (Clinical Research Edition), 338*, b664.

Cady, R. K., Wendt, J. K., Kirchner, J. R., Sargent, J. D., Rothrock, J. F., & Skaggs, H., Jr. (1991). Treatment of acute migraine with subcutaneous sumatriptan. *JAMA: The Journal of the American Medical Association, 265*(21), 2831–2835.

Capobianco, D. J., & Dodick, D. W. (2006). Diagnosis and treatment of cluster headache. *Seminars in Neurology, 26*(2), 242–259.

Cohen, A. S., Burns, B., & Goadsby, P. J. (2009). High-flow oxygen for treatment of cluster headache: A randomized trial. *JAMA: The Journal of the American Medical Association, 302*(22), 2451–2457.

Couppe, C., Torelli, P., Fuglsang-Frederiksen, A., Andersen, K. V., & Jensen, R. (2007). Myofascial trigger points are very prevalent in patients with chronic tension-type headache: A double-blinded controlled study. *The Clinical Journal of Pain, 23*(1), 23–27.

Cutrer, F. M., Mitsikostas, D. D., Ayata, G., & Sanchez del Rio, M. (1999). Attenuation by butalbital of capsaicin-induced c-fos-like immunoreactivity in trigeminal nucleus caudalis. *Headache, 39*(10), 697–704.

Detsky, M. E., McDonald, D. R., Baerlocher, M. O., Tomlinson, G. A., McCrory, D. C., & Booth, C. M. (2006). Does this patient with headache have a migraine or need neuroimaging? *JAMA: The Journal of the American Medical Association, 296*(10), 1274–1283.

Diamond, S., & Baltes, B. J. (1971). Chronic tension headache—treated with amitriptyline—a double-blind study. *Headache, 11*(3), 110–116.

Diamond, S., Bigal, M. E., Silberstein, S., Loder, E., Reed, M., & Lipton, R. B. (2007). Patterns of diagnosis and acute and preventive treatment for migraine in the United States: Results from the American Migraine Prevalence and Prevention Study. *Headache, 47*(3), 355–363.

Diener, H. C., Kurth, T., & Dodick, D. (2007). Patent foramen ovale, stroke, and cardiovascular disease in migraine. *Current Opinion in Neurology, 20*(3), 310–319.

Dodick, D. W. (2011). Suboccipital steroid injections for cluster headache. *Lancet Neurology, 10*(10), 867–869.

Dodick, D. W., Mauskop, A., Elkind, A. H., DeGryse, R., Brin, M. F., Silberstein, S. D., et al. (2005). Botulinum toxin type A for the prophylaxis of chronic daily headache: Subgroup analysis of patients not receiving other prophylactic medications: A randomized double-blind, placebo-controlled study. *Headache, 45*(4), 315–324.

Eriksen, M. K., Thomsen, L. L., & Olesen, J. (2005). The Visual Aura Rating Scale (VARS) for migraine aura diagnosis. *Cephalalgia: An International Journal of Headache, 25*(10), 801–810.

Evans, R. W. (2007). The FDA alert on serotonin syndrome with combined use of SSRIs or SNRIs and triptans: An analysis of the 29 case reports. *MedGenMed: Medscape General Medicine, 9*(3), 48.

Evans, R. W. (2008). Concomitant triptan and SSRI or SNRI use: What is the risk for serotonin syndrome? *Headache, 48*(4), 639–640.

Evans, R. W., & Silberstein, S. D. (2002). Diagnostic testing for chronic daily headache. *Headache, 42*(6), 556–559.

Evans, R. W., & Taylor, F. R. (2006). "Natural" or alternative medications for migraine prevention. *Headache, 46*(6), 1012–1018.

Evans, R. W., Tepper, S. J., Shapiro, R. E., Sun-Edelstein, C., & Tietjen, G. E. (2010). The FDA alert on serotonin syndrome with use of triptans combined with selective serotonin reuptake inhibitors or selective serotonin-norepinephrine reuptake inhibitors: American Headache Society position paper. *Headache, 50*(6), 1089–1099.

Evers, S., & Goadsby, P. J. (2003). Hypnic headache: Clinical features, pathophysiology, and treatment. *Neurology, 60*(6), 905–909.

Facchinetti, F., Allais, G., Nappi, R. E., D'Amico, R., Marozio, L., Bertozzi, L., et al. (2009). Migraine is a risk factor for hypertensive disorders in pregnancy: A prospective cohort study. *Cephalalgia: An International Journal of Headache, 29*(3), 286–292.

Feinmann, C., & Peatfield, R. (1993). Orofacial neuralgia. Diagnosis and treatment guidelines. *Drugs, 46*(2), 263–268.

Foley, K. A., Cady, R., Martin, V., Adelman, J., Diamond, M., Bell, C. F., et al. (2005). Treating early versus treating mild: Timing of migraine prescription medications among patients with diagnosed migraine. *Headache, 45*(5), 538–545.

Freitag, F. G., Cady, R., DiSerio, F., Elkind, A., Gallagher, R. M., Goldstein, J., et al. (2001). Comparative study of a combination of isometheptene mucate, dichloralphenazone with acetaminophen and sumatriptan succinate in the treatment of migraine. *Headache, 41*(4), 391–398.

Friedman, B. W., Corbo, J., Lipton, R. B., Bijur, P. E., Esses, D., Solorzano, C., et al. (2005). A trial of metoclopramide vs. sumatriptan for the emergency department treatment of migraines. *Neurology, 64*(3), 463–468.

Gabai, I. J., & Spierings, E. L. (1989). Prophylactic treatment of cluster headache with verapamil. *Headache, 29*(3), 167–168.

Gales, B. J., Bailey, E. K., Reed, A. N., & Gales, M. A. (2010). Angiotensin-converting enzyme inhibitors and angiotensin receptor blockers for the prevention of migraines. *The Annals of Pharmacotherapy, 44*(2), 360–366.

Gaul, C., Diener, H. C., & Muller, O. M. (2011). Cluster headache: Clinical features and therapeutic options. *Deutsches Arzteblatt International, 108*(33), 543–549.

Goadsby, P. J., & Boes, C. (2002). New daily persistent headache. *Journal of Neurology, Neurosurgery, and Psychiatry, 72*(Suppl 2), ii6–ii9, p. ii7.

Gobel, H., & Heinze, A. (2011). Botulinum toxin type A in the prophylactic treatment of chronic migraine [Prophylaxe der chronischen Migrane mit Botulinumtoxin Typ A]. *Schmerz (Berlin, Germany), 25*(5), 563–570; quiz, 571.

Headache Classification Subcommittee of the International Headache Society. (2004). The International Classification of Headache Disorders: 2nd edition. *Cephalalgia 24*(Suppl 1), 9–160.

Headache Classification Subcommittee of the International Headache Society. (2013) The International Classification of Headache Disorders: 3rd edition (beta version). *Cephalalgia, 33*, 629–808.

Holroyd, K. A., Stensland, M., Lipchik, G. L., Hill, K. R., O'Donnell, F. S., & Cordingley, G. (2000). Psychosocial correlates and impact of chronic tension-type headaches. *Headache, 40*(1), 3–16.

James, A. H., Bushnell, C. D., Jamison, M. G., & Myers, E. R. (2005). Incidence and risk factors for stroke in pregnancy and the puerperium. *Obstetrics and Gynecology*, *106*(3), 509–516.

Katsarava, Z., Muessig, M., Dzagnidze, A., Fritsche, G., Diener, H. C., & Limmroth, V. (2005). Medication overuse headache: Rates and predictors for relapse in a 4-year prospective study. *Cephalalgia: An International Journal of Headache*, *25*(1), 12–15.

Kavuk, I., Katsarava, Z., Selekler, M., Sayar, K., Agelink, M. W., Limmroth, V., et al. (2004). Clinical features and therapy of medication overuse headache. *European Journal of Medical Research*, *9*(12), 565–569.

Kelman, L. (2007). The triggers or precipitants of the acute migraine attack. *Cephalalgia: An International Journal of Headache*, *27*(5), 394–402.

Kudrow, L. (1977). Lithium prophylaxis for chronic cluster headache. *Headache*, *17*(1), 15–18.

Kudrow, L. (1979). Cluster headache: Diagnosis and management. *Headache*, *19*(3), 142–150.

Kudrow, L. (1982). Cluster headache. Clinical, mechanistic, and treatment aspects. *Panminerva Medica*, *24*(1), 45–54.

Kurth, T. (2010). The association of migraine with ischemic stroke. *Current Neurology and Neuroscience Reports*, *10*(2), 133–139.

Kurth, T., Kase, C. S., Schurks, M., Tzourio, C., & Buring, J. E. (2010). Migraine and risk of haemorrhagic stroke in women: Prospective cohort study. *British Medical Journal (Clinical Research Edition)*, *341*, c3659.

Langemark, M., & Olesen, J. (1994). Sulpiride and paroxetine in the treatment of chronic tension-type headache. an explanatory double-blind trial. *Headache*, *34*(1), 20–24.

Leone, M., Franzini, A., Cecchini, A. P., Broggi, G., & Bussone, G. (2010). Hypothalamic deep brain stimulation in the treatment of chronic cluster headache. *Therapeutic Advances in Neurological Disorders*, *3*(3), 187–195.

Leroux, E., Valade, D., Taifas, I., Vicaut, E., Chagnon, M., Roos, C., et al. (2011). Suboccipital steroid injections for transitional treatment of patients with more than two cluster headache attacks per day: A randomised, double-blind, placebo-controlled trial. *Lancet Neurology*, *10*(10), 891–897.

Ligthart, L., de Vries, B., Smith, A. V., Ikram, M. A., Amin, N., Hottenga, J. J., et al. (2011). Meta-analysis of genome-wide association for migraine in six population-based European cohorts. *European Journal of Human Genetics: EJHG*, *19*(8), 901–907.

Lipton, R. B. (2009). Tracing transformation: Chronic migraine classification, progression, and epidemiology. *Neurology*, *72*(5 Suppl), S3–S7.

Lipton, R. B., & Bigal, M. E. (2005). The epidemiology of migraine. *The American Journal of Medicine*, *118*(Suppl 1), 3S–10S.

Lipton, R. B., Cady, R. K., Stewart, W. F., Wilks, K., & Hall, C. (2002). Diagnostic lessons from the spectrum study. *Neurology*, *58*(9 Suppl 6), S27–S31.

Loder, E. (2004). Menstrual migraine: Timing is everything. *Neurology*, *63*(2), 202–203.

Loder, E. (2006). Post-marketing experience with an opioid nasal spray for migraine: Lessons for the future. *Cephalalgia: An International Journal of Headache*, *26*(2), 89–97.

Loder, E. (2009). Migraine with aura and increased risk of ischaemic stroke. *British Medical Journal (Clinical Research Edition)*, *339*, b4380.

Loder, E. (2010). Triptan therapy in migraine. *The New England Journal of Medicine*, *363*(1), 63–70.

Loder, E. W., Buse, D. C., & Golub, J. R. (2005). Headache and combination estrogen-progestin oral contraceptives: Integrating evidence, guidelines, and clinical practice. *Headache*, *45*(3), 224–231.

Logroscino, G., & Kurth, T. (2010). Ischemic stroke: Coffee may pull the trigger. *Neurology*, *75*(18), 1576–1577.

Lyngberg, A. C., Rasmussen, B. K., Jorgensen, T., & Jensen, R. (2005a). Incidence of primary headache: A Danish epidemiologic follow-up study. *American Journal of Epidemiology*, *161*(11), 1066–1073.

Lyngberg, A. C., Rasmussen, B. K., Jorgensen, T., & Jensen, R. (2005b). Prognosis of migraine and tension-type headache: A population-based follow-up study. *Neurology*, *65*(4), 580–585.

Lyngberg, A. C., Rasmussen, B. K., Jorgensen, T., & Jensen, R. (2005c). Secular changes in health care utilization and work absence for migraine and tension-type headache: A population based study. *European Journal of Epidemiology*, *20*(12), 1007–1014.

Manna, V., Bolino, F., & Di Cicco, L. (1994). Chronic tension-type headache, mood depression and serotonin: Therapeutic effects of fluvoxamine and mianserine. *Headache*, *34*(1), 44–49.

Martin, V. T., & Goldstein, J. A. (2005). Evaluating the safety and tolerability profile of acute treatments for migraine. *The American Journal of Medicine*, *118*(Suppl 1), 36S–44S.

Matharu, M. S., Boes, C. J., & Goadsby, P. J. (2003). Management of trigeminal autonomic cephalalgias and hemicrania continua. *Drugs*, *63*(16), 1637–1677.

Mehndiratta, M. M., Garg, S., & Gurnani, M. (2006). Cerebral venous thrombosis—clinical presentations. *JPMA: The Journal of the Pakistan Medical Association*, *56*(11), 513–516.

Merikangas, K. R., Whitaker, A. E., Isler, H., & Angst, J. (1994). The Zurich Study: XXIII. Epidemiology of headache syndromes in the Zurich cohort study of young adults. *European Archives of Psychiatry and Clinical Neuroscience*, *244*(3), 145–152.

Mett, A., & Tfelt-Hansen, P. (2008). Acute migraine therapy: Recent evidence from randomized comparative trials. *Current Opinion in Neurology*, *21*(3), 331–337.

Mitchell, N., Hewitt, C. E., Jayakody, S., Islam, M., Adamson, J., Watt, I., et al. (2011). Randomised controlled trial of food elimination diet based on IgG antibodies for the prevention of migraine-like headaches. *Nutrition Journal*, *10*, 85.

Modi, S., & Lowder, D. M. (2006). Medications for migraine prophylaxis. *American Family Physician*, *73*(1), 72–78.

Mokri, B. (2002). Spontaneous CSF leaks mimicking benign exertional headaches. *Cephalalgia: An International Journal of Headache*, *22*(10), 780–783.

Mukharesh, L. O., & Jan, M. M. (2011). Primary stabbing "ice-pick" headache. *Pediatric Neurology*, *45*(4), 268–270.

Nicholson, R. A., Buse, D. C., Andrasik, F., & Lipton, R. B. (2011). Nonpharmacologic treatments for migraine and tension-type headache: How to choose and when to use. *Current Treatment Options in Neurology*, *13*(1), 28–40.

Paemeleire, K., Crevits, L., Goadsby, P. J., & Kaube, H. (2006). Practical management of medication-overuse headache. *Acta Neurologica Belgica*, *106*(2), 43–51.

Peatfield, R. C. (1995). Relationships between food, wine, and beer-precipitated migrainous headaches. *Headache*, *35*(6), 355–357.

Rao, B. S., Das, D. G., Taraknath, V. R., & Sarma, Y. (2000). A double blind controlled study of propranolol and cyproheptadine in migraine prophylaxis. *Neurology India*, *48*(3), 223–226.

Rasmussen, B. K. (1993). Migraine and tension-type headache in a general population: Precipitating factors, female hormones, sleep pattern and relation to lifestyle. *Pain*, *53*(1), 65–72.

Rothrock, J. F. (1999). Management of chronic daily headache utilizing a uniform treatment pathway. *Headache*, *39*(9), 650–653.

Russell, M. B., & Ducros, A. (2011). Sporadic and familial hemiplegic migraine: Pathophysiological mechanisms, clinical characteristics, diagnosis, and management. *Lancet Neurology*, *10*(5), 457–470.

Russell, M. B., Rasmussen, B. K., Brennum, J., Iversen, H. K., Jensen, R. A., & Olesen, J. (1992). Presentation of a new instrument: The diagnostic headache diary. *Cephalalgia: An International Journal of Headache*, *12*(6), 369–374.

Sah, M. L., & Saini, T. R. (2008). Formulation development and release studies of indomethacin suppositories. *Indian Journal of Pharmaceutical Sciences*, *70*(4), 498–501.

Sanchez-Del-Rio, M., Reuter, U., & Moskowitz, M. A. (2006). New insights into migraine pathophysiology. *Current Opinion in Neurology*, *19*(3), 294–298.

Sandor, P. S., & Afra, J. (2005). Nonpharmacologic treatment of migraine. *Current Pain and Headache Reports*, *9*(3), 202–205.

Saper, J. R., & Lake, A. E., 3rd. (2002). Borderline personality disorder and the chronic headache patient: Review and management recommendations. *Headache, 42*(7), 663–674.

Saper, J. R., Lake, A. E., 3rd, Bain, P. A., Stillman, M. J., Rothrock, J. F., Mathew, N. T., et al. (2010). A practice guide for continuous opioid therapy for refractory daily headache: Patient selection, physician requirements, and treatment monitoring. *Headache, 50*(7), 1175–1193.

Saper, J. R., Lake, A. E., 3rd, Hamel, R. L., Lutz, T. E., Branca, B., Sims, D. B., et al. (2004). Daily scheduled opioids for intractable head pain: Long-term observations of a treatment program. *Neurology, 62*(10), 1687–1694.

Saper, J. R., Silberstein, S. D., Lake, A. E., 3rd, & Winters, M. E. (1995). Fluoxetine and migraine: Comparison of double-blind trials. *Headache, 35*(4), 233.

Scher, A. I., Stewart, W. F., & Lipton, R. B. (2004). Caffeine as a risk factor for chronic daily headache: A population-based study. *Neurology, 63*(11), 2022–2027.

Schurks, M., Rist, P. M., Bigal, M. E., Buring, J. E., Lipton, R. B., & Kurth, T. (2009). Migraine and cardiovascular disease: Systematic review and meta-analysis. *British Medical Journal (Clinical Research Edition), 339*, b3914.

Schwartz, B. S., Stewart, W. F., & Lipton, R. B. (1997). Lost workdays and decreased work effectiveness associated with headache in the workplace. *Journal of Occupational and Environmental Medicine / American College of Occupational and Environmental Medicine, 39*(4), 320–327.

Shrewsbury, S. B., Kori, S. H., Miller, S. D., Pedinoff, A., & Weinstein, S. (2008). Randomized, double-blind, placebo-controlled study of the safety, tolerability and pharmacokinetics of MAP0004 (orally-inhaled DHE) in adult asthmatics. *Current Medical Research and Opinion, 24*(7), 1977–1985.

Silberstein, S. D. (2004a). Headaches due to nasal and paranasal sinus disease.

Silberstein, S. D. (2004b). Topiramate in migraine prevention: Evidence-based medicine from clinical trials. *Neurological Sciences: Official Journal of the Italian Neurological Society and of the Italian Society of Clinical Neurophysiology, 25*(Suppl 3), S244–S245.

Silberstein, S. D. (2006). Preventive treatment of migraine. *Trends in Pharmacological Sciences, 27*(8), 410–415.

Silberstein, S. D., & McCrory, D. C. (2001). Butalbital in the treatment of headache: History, pharmacology, and efficacy. *Headache, 41*(10), 953–967.

Silberstein, S. D., & Peres, M. F. (2002). Hemicrania continua. *Archives of Neurology, 59*(6), 1029–1030.

Silberstein, S. D., Olesen, J., Bousser, M. G., Diener, H. C., Dodick, D., First, M., et al. (2005). The International Classification of Headache Disorders, 2nd edition (ICHD-II)—revision of criteria for 8.2, medication-overuse headache. *Cephalalgia: An International Journal of Headache, 25*(6), 460–465.

Soldin, O. P., Tonning, J. M., & Obstetric-Fetal Pharmacology Research Unit Network. (2008). Serotonin syndrome associated with triptan monotherapy. *The New England Journal of Medicine, 358*(20), 2185–2186.

Stewart, W. F., Wood, C., Reed, M. L., Roy, J., Lipton, R. B., & the American Migraine Prevalence and Prevention (AMPP) Advisory Group. (2008). Cumulative lifetime migraine incidence in women and men. *Cephalalgia: An International Journal of Headache, 28*(11), 1170–1178.

Stovner, L. J., & Hagen, K. (2006). Prevalence, burden, and cost of headache disorders. *Current Opinion in Neurology, 19*(3), 281–285.

Strand, N. H., Trentman, T. L., Vargas, B. B., & Dodick, D. W. (2011). Occipital nerve stimulation with the Bion® microstimulator for the treatment of medically refractory chronic cluster headache. *Pain Physician, 14*(5), 435–440.

Tarlaci, S. (2009). Escitalopram and venlafaxine for the prophylaxis of migraine headache without mood disorders. *Clinical Neuropharmacology, 32*(5), 254–258.

Tfelt-Hansen, P. (2008). Triptans vs. other drugs for acute migraine: Are there differences in efficacy? A comment. *Headache, 48*(4), 601–605.

Tfelt-Hansen, P. C., & Koehler, P. J. (2008). History of the use of ergotamine and dihydroergotamine in migraine from 1906 and onward. *Cephalalgia: An International Journal of Headache, 28*(8), 877–886.

Usai, S., Grazzi, L., Andrasik, F., D'Amico, D., Rigamonti, A., & Bussone, G. (2004). Chronic migraine with medication overuse: Treatment outcome and disability at 3 years follow-up. *Neurological Sciences: Official Journal of the Italian Neurological Society and of the Italian Society of Clinical Neurophysiology, 25*(Suppl 3), S272–S273.

Wendt, J., Cady, R., Singer, R., Peters, K., Webster, C., Kori, S., et al. (2006). A randomized, double-blind, placebo-controlled trial of the efficacy and tolerability of a 4-mg dose of subcutaneous sumatriptan for the treatment of acute migraine attacks in adults. *Clinical Therapeutics, 28*(4), 517–526.

Whyte, C., Tepper, S. J., & Evans, R. W. (2010). Expert opinion: Rescue me: Rescue medication for migraine. *Headache, 50*(2), 307–313.

Wolpow, E. (2010). By the way, doctor: If coffee constricts blood vessels, why would it help migraine sufferers, since the constriction curtails blood flow, which would seem to cause more pain? *Harvard Health Letter / from Harvard Medical School, 35*(7), 4.

Young, W. B., Siow, H. C., & Silberstein, S. D. (2004). Anticonvulsants in migraine. *Current Pain and Headache Reports, 8*(3), 244–250.

Zencirci, B. (2010). Comparison of the effects of dietary factors in the management and prophylaxis of migraine. *Journal of Pain Research, 3*, 125–130.

Ziegler, D., Ford, R., Kriegler, J., Gallagher, R. M., Peroutka, S., Hammerstad, J., et al. (1994). Dihydroergotamine nasal spray for the acute treatment of migraine. *Neurology, 44*(3 Pt 1), 447–453.

Zwart, J. A., Dyb, G., Hagen, K., Odegard, K. J., Dahl, A. A., Bovim, G., et al. (2003). Depression and anxiety disorders associated with headache frequency. The Nord-Trondelag Health Study. *European Journal of Neurology: The Official Journal of the European Federation of Neurological Societies, 10*(2), 147–152.

45.

TRAUMATIC BRAIN INJURY

EVALUATION AND MANAGEMENT FOR THE PSYCHIATRIC PHYSICIAN

Gregory J. O'Shanick, George T. Moses, and Nils R. Varney

INTRODUCTION

All psychiatrists practicing in medical settings, and most psychiatrists in community practice, will encounter patients who have sustained traumatic brain injuries (TBI) in their clinical practices. While in some situations the TBI is the cause for the initial psychiatric evaluation, frequently the TBI is not the presenting concern, but is an aspect of the medical history that has been neglected, or is unrecognized by the patient, their family, or their healthcare team. The presence of a prior neurological injury is always relevant information to be ascertained by the consulting psychiatric physician, who frequently is the only person caring for a patient who will take a sufficiently detailed history and perform a sufficiently detailed neurocognitive examination to establish the presence and relevance of TBI to the patient's condition (Table 45.1). The examination required once TBI is under consideration includes the assessment of auditory, visual perceptive, vestibular, and language functions. Absent such a focused neurological examination, deficits in these areas may go undetected. Without an appreciation of the context of a prior TBI, the deficits that are found might be misattributed to a primary psychiatric disorder or malingering. This chapter will assist the reader in the recognition of those salient post-TBI neuropsychiatric and neurosensory manifestations often seen, but under-recognized in these patients, and will focus on the recognition and management of late effects of TBI as they are encountered in psychiatric practice.

TBI has a far more important role for clinical psychiatry than determination of disability, as it causes or alters the symptoms of mood disorders. Seventeen to 61% of all TBI patients develop depression within two years of injury (Rapoport, 2012) and seek psychiatric care without considering the relevance of TBI. TBI-related mood disorders offer different diagnostic challenges, respond differently to medications, and can have substantially different outcomes than do "conventional" mood disorders. In an ideal setting, the patient's reporting that they have memory trouble, episodes of confusion, or anger problems would be adequate history from which to proceed. However, TBI patients may be involved in litigation, so clinical caution is necessary. Unfortunately, the issues generated by caution may produce wrong answers of their own. For example, the same TBI patient who has suffered only a brief loss of consciousness (LOC) and has a normal magnetic resonance imaging (MRI) could be the same patient who experienced an intermittent post-traumatic amnesia (PTA) lasting three days and a quantitative PET scan showing right fronto-temporal hypometabolism (cf. Bigler, 2008). Thus, as diagnostic errors can cut either way, balanced caution is advisable.

CONTEXT OF TRAUMATIC BRAIN INJURY

TBI occurs in a variety of contexts (Faul, Xu, Wald, & Coronado, 2010). Falls remain the leading cause of TBI among civilians followed by motor vehicle accidents (MVA) and other blows to the head, including sports injuries and assaults. Assaults may be due to blunt objects such as body parts (fists, feet, elbows, knees, heads, etc.), edged weapons, or firearms. Penetrating TBI are associated with lower Glasgow Coma Scores (GCS) and higher acute mortality rates. The vast majority of TBI are closed, meaning no breach of the dura has occurred. TBI from MVA result from rapid acceleration/deceleration forces causing micro-shearing and diffuse axonal injury (DAI). DAI may appear on MRI as numerous, small, white matter lesions. Ischemic injury of brain tissue also can occur due to vasospasm, microvascular

Table 45.1 ESSENTIAL EQUIPMENT FOR TBI NEUROLOGICAL EXAMINATION

Penlight	Pupillary size, reactivity, tracking (monocular and binocular), eye teaming, palatal elevation, saccades
Peanut butter	Assess olfactory functioning for unilateral anosmia
Tuning fork	Assess CN VIII by Weber and Rinne; assess vibratory sensation for distal neuropathy and dorsal column/proprioception assessment
Blindfold	BESS and Fukuda Stepping Test for vestibular dysfunction
Reflex hammer	Deep tendon reflex assessment

occlusion, and/or the rupture of blood vessels. Intravascular coagulopathy, either immediate or delayed, is common in more severe cases of TBI, which adds an additional mechanism of injury (Stein, Chen, Sinson, & Smith, 2002; Harhangi, Kompanje, Leebeek, & Maas, 2008; Greuters, van den Berg, Franschman, Viersen, Beishuizen, Peerdeman, & Boer, 2011). With the exception of mine workers, injury from blast waves is uncommon among the civilian population. As a consequence of the high incidence of blast-induced neurotrauma among combat veterans, significant research efforts are now underway regarding this form of TBI (Cernak & Noble-Haeusslein, 2009; Lippa, Pastorek, Benge, & Thornton, 2010; Luethcke, Bryan, Morrow, & Isler, 2011).

TBI can also be subdivided into primary and secondary brain injuries. The primary injuries occur at the time of the trauma. The secondary brain injuries are the result of a cascade of molecular injury mechanisms that unfold over hours and sometimes days following the acute event. This separation is likely an oversimplification, since secondary injury likely begins at the time of the mechanical injury and primary injury is often modulated by the immediate treatments (Moppett, 2007). Secondary injuries can occur following even mild TBI, and variability in their scope and severity is an important reason for the wide variation in symptoms and impairments that follow mild TBI (cf. Bigler & Maxwell, 2012). Inflammatory responses and glutamate-related excitotoxicity (including oxidative stress and damage to cell membranes by free radicals) are well-established mechanisms of secondary injury. Neuronal death by apoptosis following TBI has been demonstrated in animal models; it may be relevant to secondary injury in humans, particularly following severe TBI. Electrolyte imbalances are often the cause of secondary injury in severe head traumas. This injurious cascade continues for hours and potentially days. Inflammatory responses as well as glutamate mediated excitotoxicity causing free radical damage to cell membranes become part of the secondary TBI. The mechanism of trauma-related neuronal apoptosis remains to be definitively elucidated in humans.

EPIDEMIOLOGY

TBI remains a leading cause of injury, death, and disability in the United States. Persons of all ages, races, and socioeconomic backgrounds are at risk for TBI. From 1997 through 2007, the average annual incidence in US civilians of TBI severe enough to warrant medical attention or to contribute to mortality was 1.7 million. According to the Centers for Disease Control and Prevention (Faul et al., 2010), TBI contributes to over 52,000 deaths annually—about one-third of all deaths related to trauma. Annual emergency department (ED) visits due to TBI number over 1.3 million, which result in approximately 275,000 hospitalizations. The age groups most affected are children under 4, adolescents in their late teens, and older adults (over 65).

The incidence of TBI among active duty U.S. military personnel is quadruple the civilian rate, approximately 23 TBIs per 1000 service members. The majority of these injuries are non-combat related, and over 80% are classified as mild. The incidence of TBI in the military has tripled since the beginning of this century with mild injuries accounting for almost all of the increase. The increasing incidence is due partly to increased ascertainment of TBI and improvements in body armor that now allow combatants to survive injuries that previously would have been lethal (Belmont, Schoenfeld, & Goodman, 2010; Capehart & Bass, 2011).

PROBABILITY ISSUES REGARDING TRAUMATIC BRAIN INJURY'S SIGNIFICANCE IN MENTAL HEALTH POPULATIONS

While it is commonly agreed that 2-million persons sustain mild TBIs annually, only 5% of these have significant residual mental status problems. However, it does not follow that only 5% of prospective psychiatric patients with mild TBI have "real" problems. These individuals are a self-selected subgroup because they are seeking and paying for psychiatric care rather than being selected at random from among the 2 million with mild TBI. In addition, this group would include the 100,000 persons who are expected to have neuropsychiatric symptoms each year, which is five percent of two million mild TBIs. From this perspective, the base rate of real patients with treatable symptoms is far higher than 5%.

DETERMINING SEVERITY

Three commonly used means for rating the severity of a TBI exist: The Glasgow Coma Scale (Teasdale & Jennett, 1974), the standards set by the American College of Rehabilitation Medicine (ACRM, 1993) and clinical, post-hoc observation. Each procedure employs highly selective rigorous inclusion criteria for moderate and severe TBI so that there can be no question about the reliability of each diagnosis. However, it does not follow that failure to meet these criteria demonstrates that a TBI is either mild or inconsequential.

GLASGOW COMA SCALE

This rating scale is based on best observed, verbal and motor responses recorded 30 minutes after a TBI occurs. However, as Teasdale, who co-authored the GCS, wrote, "the Glasgow Coma Scale was designed and should be used to assess the depth and duration coma (Teasdale et al., 1978). It is not, therefore, appropriate for determining the severity of TBIs in general. On the GCS, a TBI is rated as mild if the sum of points obtained regarding eye, motor, and speech responses is between 13 and 15. All such patients have their eyes open; the highest rated eye response. This would seem appropriate for the designation of mild for a coma, but does not indicate that the patient is capable of tracking a visual target or reading. In addition, patients with GCS scores of 13 could be insensible, disoriented and incoherent. A patient with a score of 14 would be much more responsive, but would remain confused.

A patient with an errorless score of 15 would be responsive and capable of comprehensible speech, but still might have conspicuous problems with thinking and memory, severe headache, or even such major symptoms as intermittent seizures or "organic" hallucinosis. Thus, while the GCS may have utility in an ED for triage and in an intensive care unit (ICU) for tracking a patient's progress, a normal GCS score denotes only the absence of a coma and does not exclude a wide variety of major neurocognitive, neurosensory and neuropsychiatric symptoms.

AMERICAN CONGRESS OF REHABILITATION MEDICINE CRITERIA

Most TBIs are classified as mild to severe by standards set by the ACRM in 1993. Indeed, these could be regarded as the "gold standard" of TBI classification. These diagnostic criteria are based on duration of LOC or of PTA. In our experience, the diagnostic criteria based on PTA are neglected by many clinicians, who classify a TBI as more than mild only if the LOC is greater than 30 minutes. However, the ACRM criteria mandate that a TBI be rated as moderately severe if a patient has a PTA or period of altered consciousness lasting 24 hours or more. As a result of this oversight, the erroneous diagnosis of mild TBI is commonly made in patients who in actuality have sustained a moderately severe TBI, where lasting post-concussive symptoms are probable rather than rare (Bigler, 1990; Lezak et al., 2004).

Determining the duration of PTA can also be done incorrectly if the duration of PTA is determined by the patient's first memory. It is not at all uncommon for patients to have shards of memory during the immediate post-impact stage of a PTA, or even over the next few days of recovery (especially memories of physical pain). Ritchie Russell (Russell & Smith, 1961), who defined PTA, said that PTA was over when continuous memory was restored; however, the presence of bits of recollection here and there are permitted and do not reflect resolution of PTA. Failure to consider PTA in rating a TBI can result in misclassification of moderate TBI as "mild." This is particularly important with regard to TBIs from the wars in Iraq and Afghanistan, which are primarily the result of blast. Blast inflicts brain injury by passing through the body and thus rarely results in prolonged LOC, despite frequently causing prolonged PTA. (MacDonald et al., 2011).

CLINICAL OBSERVATION OF OUTCOME

Following TBI, patients improve to varying degrees. However, improvement does not alter the classification of the original injury as mild, moderate, or severe. This apparently obvious point, like the importance of PTA to rating TBI severity, frequently appears to be neglected in practice. The severity in the initial injury remains the best predictor of long-term prognosis; while at a particular point in recovery a patient with a moderate TBI may resemble one with a mild TBI, the likelihood of residual symptoms or impairments will be much higher in the former.

Kinematics

The debate over PTA and LOC in the classification of TBI severity overlooks a critical point; namely, that each is an outcome variable that is dependent. The independent variable that actually reflects the severity of physical impact to the brain should be expressed with reference to *kinematics*, the branch of physics concerned with objects in motion. That is, accelerations and decelerations expressed as g-forces describe and quantify the forces that cause a brain injury (Varney & Varney, 1995). The basic formula for describing the forces of a TBI as it affects the brain, derived from Newtonian physics, is: $\mathbf{a = v^2/(2s)}$. This is a direct reflection of a law of physics (Newton's Third Law), not an engineering formula. This numerical result is expressed in g-forces. That is, the severity of a TBI is a result both of how fast you were going and of how quickly you stop (Varney & Roberts, 1999). The relationship between velocity, stopping distance, and acceleration is shown in Figure 45.1. In this figure, stopping distance reflects the vehicle's front-end collapse distance. Automakers such as Mercedes-Benz have developed break-away frame assemblies that cause the front end to collapse by up to four feet in a head-on impact. As shown in Figure 45.1, at 50 miles per hour, approximately 10 g's are generated when the front end collapses to absorb the kinetic force, and this represents a safe amount for the occupants to experience. The car, however, would be a total wreck. Conversely, a vehicle with only a 0.5-foot collapse zone, such as would be seen in an armored car, would generate 200 g's if it were to experience a front-end collision at 50 miles per hour. This is more than adequate for a serious brain damage to occur in the occupants of the vehicle. In this case, the vehicle would appear to be relatively undamaged. As the car absorbs more force, less force affects those inside. Until TBI classification reflects the forces that cause brain injury, and not outcome variables such as LOC and PTA, determination of the initial severity of TBI will remain inexact and imprecise.

IMAGING

Anatomic neuroimaging, computerized tomography (CT), and MRI of patients with acute TBI is the standard for the diagnosis of gross injuries and complications of neurosurgical

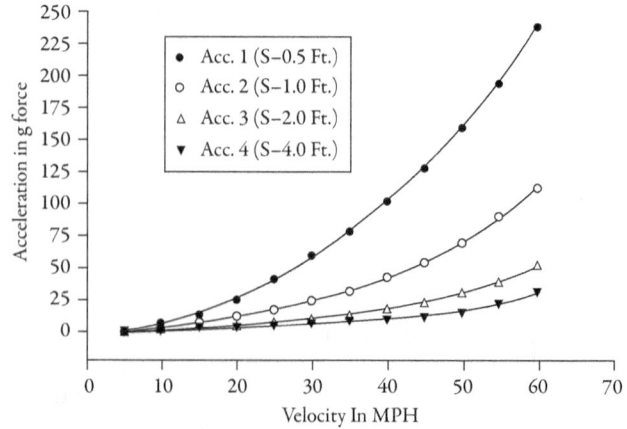

Figure 45.1 Acceleration as function of velocity.

magnitude such as subdural and epidural hematomas and life-threatening cerebral edema. However, their limited spatial resolution (CT, 2–3 mm; 1.5 Tesla MRI, 1 mm; 3 Tesla MRI–0.5 mm) makes them insensitive to two common consequences of closed TBI—cavitation and micro-shearing. These injuries have been observed in post-mortem studies of patients with TBI who have died from other causes (Bigler, 2004).

Anatomical neuroimaging offers no information about abnormal metabolic activity of injured neurons. Following brain contusions, the cortex shows diminished metabolic activity with associated cognitive impairments. Contusions may also produce irritable foci that result in intermittent sensory phenomena or memory disruption; metabolism in these areas may be increased either persistently or episodically. In the latter case, even functional imaging may miss a clinically significant lesion.

In the context of neuropsychiatric evaluation and treatment of patients with mild TBI, the limitations of neuroanatomical imaging frequently predominate, with "normal" structural studies as the usual finding in the face of unequivocally "organic" symptoms (cf. Shenton et al., 2012). Confident diagnoses can nonetheless be made without corroboration from neuroanatomical imaging, as indeed they were for most neurological disorders in the era that preceded the advent of CT scanning. The occurrence of typical constellations of symptoms, unfolding of the clinical course along typical lines, stereotypical symptoms (semiology), and valid and confirmatory neuropsychological test findings can add up to diagnostic confidence. Nonetheless, clinicians treating TBI patients frequently encounter the prejudice that neuroanatomical imaging is "objective" and all else is "subjective."

ORBITAL FRONTAL PATIENTS: THE OTHER MASK OF SANITY

The most common area of tissue damage in typical closed TBI is the orbital frontal cortex, usually via lacerations, abrasions, and contusions of the cortex caused by friction of the ventral surface of the frontal lobe against the sharp, irregular ridges of the cribriform plate. Clinical awareness of this site of injury often is absent early on, because the symptoms and signs of orbital frontal injury may not be manifest in a typical diagnostic evaluation by an emergency medicine physician or even a general neurologist or psychiatrist. Patients with orbital frontal injury may have no conspicuous abnormality on mental status examination, may appear euthymic, and may have few spontaneous complaints (see Chapter xx on frontal lobe disorders, and the discussion of frontotemporal degeneration in Chapter xx on dementia). The seeming invisibility of the orbital frontal syndrome is caused by alexithymia, a condition of pathologically limited insight and self-perception. Patients with alexithymia either do not realize that they have psychological symptoms, or they simply do not care. They can be quite illogical in doing so. For example, patients may report suicidal ideation when asked (never with a specific plan), but then deny dysphoria. Typically, they fail to report symptoms

other than those that are immediately present, such as localized pain, and overlook severe migraine headaches, for example, that are not occurring at the time of the interview. An easy screening procedure for suspected alexithymia is to ask for the chief complaints without any prior discussion (i.e., no hints). The list generated independently by the patient will be badly impoverished, particularly regarding already documented problems such as headache, insomnia, temper, impotence, unemployment, and the like.

Experiencing alexithymia creates an interesting scenario with regard to evidence of malingering. Malingering, after all, is something that requires intact executive functioning to plan and execute a plausible symptom complaint. Although the alexithymic patient is not aware of his problems, he is still potentially influenced by the temptation of unearned money (as in a personal injury, disability determination, or worker's compensation setting), but cannot generate an effective plan to fake symptoms. Thus, his alexithymia and executive dysfunction result in unnecessary and poorly executed transparent attempts at malingering (Ju & Varney, 2000).

The core disability of orbital frontal patients is that they think less (Varney & Menafee, 1993). Spontaneous decision-making becomes labored, less frequent, and less reliable, particularly with the multiple small decisions of ordinary life, such as deciding what to do next (Varney, 1999). Emotional responses are muted, and indifference is manifest. While this is virtually invisible to non-family members, these symptoms are wrenching to those who previously have enjoyed a close relationship with the patient. Severe anxiety and associated autonomic stress-related physical disorders are very common among family members (Chwalisz, 1999). Even among family members, long-delayed full recognition can take two or more years (Siders, 1999). Even the milder varieties of frontal symptoms may cause a disability based on problems with productivity and reliability of work product (Varney, 1988) without any loss of vocational knowledge.[1] Unfortunately, this is often viewed as the result of poor motivation; or, when legal or disability issues are involved, desire for "secondary gain" is suspected.

Patients with damage largely confined to the orbital frontal region and its connections typically do very well on conventional neuropsychological testing (Varney & Stewart, 2004), as many of the neuropsychological tests aimed at identifying frontal lobe disorders are more sensitive to dorsolateral frontal than to orbital frontal functioning. As stated by Heilman and Valenstein (2012), "unlike most artificial problems posed by neuropsychological tests, the relevant issues, rules of engagement and endpoints are not always clearly identified. Patients with frontal lobe damage who despite good IQ scores, cannot effectively deploy their intelligence in real world situations."

With no obvious symptoms and no expressed complaints, orbital frontal patients can prove difficult to assess without also interviewing a collateral source such as a spouse, domestic

---

1. Eighty percent productivity and 5% errors of omission add up to a disability in most jobs. For example, a hotel housekeeper with 20 rooms to clean and 20 things to do in each room would be unable to clean more than 16 rooms and would overlook at least one important duty in each room.

partner, parent, or sibling. Ideally, this will be done apart from the patient, but with the patient's consent. The spontaneous complaints offered by the collateral source typically describe the syndrome and its impact on the family. Families may offer accounts of extreme behavior that are striking in view of the bland presentation of the patient; for example, a patient may watch television all day, literally without doing anything else—not even changing channels or eating.

Orbital frontal symptoms relating to activities of daily living (e.g., indecisiveness, mental inertia) and psychosocial symptoms (poor empathy, indifference) can be reliably determined by structured interview of a collateral informant (Varney, 1991). In functional neuroimaging studies (Varney & Bushnell, 1998; Varney et al., 1995; Varney et al., 2001), the correlation coefficient of gamma rays per voxel from the orbital frontal region and the interview test score was −.61.[2] Interview results did not correlate significantly with any other region. No score from seven neuropsychological measures of executive function correlated with orbital frontal activity, but each correlated significantly with metabolic activity in other frontal areas. Thus, with regard to descriptive symptoms not appropriate for formal neuropsychological testing, the relationship with orbital frontal activity was significant and specific.

Executive disability in patients with orbital frontal injury involves problems not detected by conventional neuropsychological testing (Martzke et al., 1991) which isolates individual abilities for testing. These injuries create problems with independent living due to several factors, including:

1. inability to recognize the need to execute daily activities such as meal planning and preparation, money management, and safety awareness;

2. inability to generate an internal means of goal-directed activity, such that they are directionless, and living on their own becomes bewildering;

3. vulnerability to exploitation and victimization, as they require others (who are often unscrupulous and predatory due to impaired risk-assessment by the patient) to assist them in decision-making and providing external structure; and

4. impaired insight into their own limitations and adaptability.

Neuropsychological testing in the typical structured format of assessment fails to demonstrate such relevant "real world" disability. To further complicate matters, seemingly similar tests of dysexecutive disability are not closely related to real-world functional independence and success in some patients (Varney & Stewart, 2004).

Psychological tests to demonstrate executive disability in orbital frontal patients are a relatively new area of assessment in which there are no tests with high "hit rates" as validated against the patient's activities of daily living or a specific locus of lesion such as orbital frontal cortex. Lezak's Tinker Toy Test (Lezak et al., 2012) is an unconventional, but accurate, means of testing executive functioning. Superficially, this assessment appears so simple that most preschool age children could make a passing construction. The elements that render this test difficult for the patient with executive disability are (1) there are 100,000 potential "right answers" from which to select, and (2) the patient must independently choose one and persevere to its completion to "pass." By contrast, Block Design, no matter how difficult, has only one correct solution. With indecisiveness being the hallmark of impaired executive functioning, the Tinker Toy Test can be failed by individuals who otherwise appear to be quite intelligent. Because of the elementary nature of the task, failure is a quite conspicuous and remarkable symptom with well-established prognostic significance (Bayless et al., 1989).

NEUROPSYCHOLOGICAL ASSESSMENT IN TRAUMATIC BRAIN INJURY: A CONSUMER'S GUIDE

A fundamental problem with contemporary neuropsychological assessment arises when an abnormal test score is viewed as a primary symptom rather than an indication of a known symptom. Tests are psychometric inventions that can be failed for a variety of reasons. For example, it might be correct to describe Block Design as a measure of non-verbal problem-solving; however, a defective Block Design score could reflect a variety of problems with no relevance to intelligence, such as confusion, constructional apraxia, optic ataxia, bradyphrenia, unilateral visual neglect, absence spells, poor mental focus, or morphopsia. The great majority of neuropsychologists now performing TBI assessments use the Wechsler tests to measure IQ and memory; new versions of these tests are published every five years.

The Wechsler Adult Intelligence Scale, Version IV (WAIS-IV) consists of a wide variety of different subtests, each of which measures a different ability. The results of each test are then converted into a scaled score, a statistical representation of each test performance that permits direct comparison of individual test scores. Averaging these test scores determines overall IQ, with selected groups of subtests defining verbal and performance IQ, and subsidiary index scoring such areas as verbal comprehension, working memory, or perceptual reasoning.

WAIS-IV presents a number of problems, including the following:

1. IQ and other composite scores can be misleading, as they average multiple individual test scores. While this may be useful in the assessment of normal school children for class placement, it can be misleading with a TBI patient. Put simply, various specific mental abilities can be selectively impaired from focal brain lesions such that averaging scores can obscure the presence of a specific symptom.

---

2. This Iowa Collateral Head Injury Interview measure looks for mild symptoms described following transorbital frontal leucotomy. This particular measure is standardized and covers well-established orbital frontal symptoms as described, including those that are much milder in transorbital frontal lobotomy patients.

2. A test score can be interpreted as being "within normal limits" if it falls above the ninth percentile, the very low end of normal (i.e., just above the level for mild mental retardation). It would follow, therefore, that 91% of testing subjects should score above the ninth percentile, making such a very low score acceptable for all of them as individuals. Consequently, the designation of a score as being "within normal limits" provides no diagnostically relevant information for the top half of the distribution of an individual ability.

3. It should be noted that the Wechsler tests are commercial products, developed and published by a for-profit company. As such, they do not reflect unbiased consensus within the scientific community as would be achieved in a non-profit setting (e.g., just as procedures for assessing and interpreting thyroid function are established separately from machinery to perform these assessments). Nevertheless, neuropsychology's ethical guidelines state that it is "unethical" not to purchase the latest models from this line of products.

The Wechsler Memory Scale, Version IV (WMS-IV) is also made up of a number of specific subtests that measure immediate and delayed recall on a variety of verbal and non-verbal subtests. These test results can also be converted to scale scores and used in a manner similar to those described with regard to IQ. Most of the tasks that make up this battery involve memorization. This creates four problems:

1. They lack ecological validity because they are irrelevant to what a patient is expected to remember outside the clinic.

2. They are boring for patients to take, so there are no natural incentives to learn.

3. They offer no opportunity to assess the role of autonomic activation for memory retention and implicit memory.

4. They do not address issues that affect memory encoding, such as absentmindedness, distractibility, and fatigue.

Other controversies exist regarding evaluative methods commonly employed by neuropsychologists. The first involves effort or malingering testing. On the basis of one or more such tests, a patient may be labeled as deliberately producing poor scores or putting forth a suboptimal effort: such tests are purported to be essential in settings with the potential for personal injury litigation. A number of issues exist concerning the validity or fairness of these tests, resulting in their exclusion from assessments utilized for Social Security disability determination, where regulations specifically state, "Remove malingering and credibility tests from the list of test options (e.g., Test of Memory Malingering, Minnesota Multiphasic Personality Inventory [MMPI])" (Disability Determination Services Administrators' Guide (DDSA), 2012). A similar prohibition against their utilization has been instituted by the United States Army (Office of the Surgeon General/US Army Medical Command [OTSG/MEDCOM] Policy 11-076, 2011).

The use of the MMPI as a measure of "emotional functioning" is another area of controversy in assessment of those with TBI. The test purports to assess a variety of different dimensions of abnormal psychology (e.g., depression, hypochondriasis) to derive a profile that supports various psychological diagnoses. Many of these subsets generate inaccurate descriptions of the TBI patient's psychiatric state, prognosis, and *Diagnostic and Statistical Manual of Mental Disorders* (DSM-IV) diagnosis. The fundamental problem stems from the original intention of the MMPI, which was not for use with neuropsychiatric populations. Many items used to identify somatoform disorder, psychoses, and faking involve well-established neuropsychiatric symptoms such as absence spells or visual illusions associated with migraine headaches (Roberts et al., 1989). Thus, the misuse of the MMPI with TBI patients can result in highly pejorative psychiatric and psychological diagnoses for illness-appropriate symptoms.

SEIZURES

Although generalized tonic-clonic seizures are readily recognized, the existence of seizure events with absent or less overt motor manifestations may be overlooked in those with a history of TBI. Initial seizures following the acute TBI event occur in 10–15% of adults in the first week following severe TBI (Langendorf & Pedley, 1997). While less commonly than with severe TBI, both moderate and mild TBIs can precipitate acute seizure episodes. Similarly, the potential for late seizures is not limited to those with severe TBI. Longitudinal studies define increased lifetime seizure risk for those with mild, moderate, or severe TBI across the lifespan as ranging from a relative risk of 2.22 in those with mild closed TBI, to 7.4 in severe brain injury, to 2.17 in those with skull fracture (Christensen, Pedersen, Pedersen, Sidenius, Olsen, & Vestergaard, 2009). Evaluation of these events generally begins with either a routine or sleep-deprived electroencephalogram (EEG), the latter evaluation being more sensitive because of the effect of sleep deprivation on seizure threshold. While the specificity of EEG is high, the sensitivity is low, with studies indicating only a 30% likelihood of capturing an actual seizure discharge, even in those with diagnosed epilepsy. More extended EEG monitoring with either ambulatory recording or inpatient telemetry can be effective; however, in situations where the irritable focus is in either the frontal lobe or deep temporal regions, surface electrodes may still fail to detect abnormalities. The use of a structured diagnostic interview, such as the 40-item Iowa Inventory for Partial Seizure-like Symptoms (Roberts, 1999), will not only identify those whose events may be misdiagnosed, but, as it can be serially administered, it will also allow a method of tracking the therapeutic impact of anticonvulsant treatment over time. Table 45.2 outlines the historical elements that are of significance in assessing seizure presence.

NEUROPROTECTION

Using neuroprotective agents to mitigate the degree of residual damage after TBI has been the "Holy Grail" of neurotraumatologists since the 1980s saw the establishment of the

Table 45.2 "RED FLAG" SYMPTOM FREQUENCY RESPONSES FOR PARTIAL SEIZURES FROM IIPSS (ESTABLISHED WITH 5000 CONTROL SUBJECTS)

Essential symptoms	Episodic gaps in memory lasting over 5 minutes
	Absence spells (others noting transient "blank look" or reporting "spacing out" episodes watching TV)
Corroborative symptoms	Any symptom occurring more than once per week
	Sensory hallucinations (olfactory, gustatory, kinesthetic, tactile, visual, etc.) occurring more than once a week
	Unrecalled anger episodes occurring more than once a month

multi-center Traumatic Coma Data Bank. While the shearing effects of head impact or acceleration and deceleration forces created DAI in the acute phase (so-called cell murder), a delayed disconnection of axons from the cell body was recognized and termed "programmed cell death" or apoptosis (Povlishock & Katz, 2005). This secondary cause of DAI, termed "cell suicide" (Ucker, 1991), was recognized as a potential opportunity for secondary prevention of white matter damage and consequent disconnection of cortical regions. Unfortunately, large scale multi-centered international studies failed to define a universally effective pharmacological intervention that could be administered post-event. Lyeth and colleagues (1988) identified that the pre-injury use of an anticholinergic agent in a rat model of TBI would reduce injury severity, duration of coma, and favorably affect outcome. Unfortunately, this had little practical application in neurotrauma settings, as no benefit was obtained with post-injury administration. Only one study to date has shown efficacy of an agent when given to humans in clinical settings *following* TBI. The use of naturally derived progesterone was explored by Stein (2011) over a several-decade span in non-human settings and resulted in a large, multi-center study that defined significant benefit from post-injury–administered progesterone in severe TBI. In that study, progesterone's neuroprotective benefits were realized even when the drug was administered 8 hours post-injury. Current multi-center studies aim to better define the parameters and limitations of progesterone therapy.

POST-TRAUMATIC HEADACHES AND VERTIGO

Hines (1999), in his seminal treatise on post-traumatic headache (PTHA), identified six subtypes: (1) tension type, (2) local injury or scar-related pain, (3) migraine, (4) dysautonomic cephalgia, (5) cervicogenic, and (6) neuralgic. (Many patients have more than one mechanism for their headaches, and dissecting them may be difficult in patients who do not spontaneously provide an accurate and comprehensive account of their symptoms.) As with assessment of other neuropsychiatric symptoms following TBI, it is usually necessary

to interview collateral sources to fill in the history. In addition, a particularly careful physical and neurological examination of the head and neck may reveal findings not noted in a more cursory examination by a generalist physician. As atypical as this may seem for the psychiatrist, facility with evaluating temporomandibular joint functioning; assessing trigger points at the greater occipital notches, levator scapulae, and insertion of the splenius capitus; and evaluating deficits in oculomotor control, including teaming and saccades, will increase capture of subtle triggers of PTHA and permit more definitive intervention and symptom relief. Fatigue and poor sleep architecture further contribute to and complicate pain tolerance. Optimizing sleep efficiency to improve restorative sleep is essential to the comprehensive treatment of post-traumatic pain disorders, including headache.

NEUROSENSORY DEFICITS

Failure to appreciate neurosensory abnormalities following TBI can result in its misdiagnosis as a primary psychiatric syndrome and thus lead to ineffective and potentially damaging treatment. To identify these abnormalities, the psychiatric physician must be capable of performing a competent and accurate cranial nerve examination, including assessment of olfactory functioning. Visuo-perceptual dysfunctions and lateralized loss of visual awareness (due to non-dominant temporal-parietal damage) results in increased startle and reaction when the patient is approached from the dysfunctional side. Over time, this evolves into a subtle form of hypervigilance that may resemble paranoia. Coexistent orbital frontal damage results in faulty problem-solving/threat assessment, and potentially impulsive reactions may occur.

Damage to anterior or posterior tracts in the non-dominant hemisphere involved in prosodic aspects of language may be misattributed to either a severe depressive or even a schizophreniform loss of affective tone. Some patients with these deficits punctuate their communication with expletives, use physical gestures, or deliberately increase the volume of their speech in order to convey their intended affect. Damage to the dominant superior temporal gyrus creates an alteration in auditory processing that may resemble a primary attention-deficit disorder. Individuals with such asymmetrical functioning retain the capacity for focused attention in visual domains, but evidence problems with auditory figure–ground differentiation, sound localization, and sustained auditory attention. While such an auditory-processing dysfunction may be seen as a developmental issue in 10–20% of men (Cooper & Gates, 1991), its presence in women implies a high probability of some form of acquired central nervous system dysfunction. In addition, when auditory-processing disorders are misdiagnosed as a primary attention-deficit hyperactivity disorder (ADHD) and treated with stimulants, they may actually get worse.

Frequently seen with auditory-processing deficits, subtle balance disorders may result in the individual's limiting social activities, especially in settings of visual complexity and movement. Normal balance functioning requires the integration of vestibular, visual, and proprioceptive functions; at least two of the three must be functional for normal balance. Usually, vestibular functioning is the constant component and thus permits balance in settings of darkness (vestibular and proprioceptive) or shifting or soft surfaces (vestibular and visual). When vestibular asymmetry occurs following TBI, the individual is rendered reliant on vision and proprioceptive functions for all balance. Thus, one is unable to close one's eyes in the shower when shampooing, as the vestibular system is faulty. Such a "visually dependent" balance will result in patients' avoiding crowded settings such as grocery stores, where their point of visual fixation is intermittently blocked by passers-by. The internal signal of apprehension at loss of balance results in withdrawal from the setting, followed by relief from anxiety. This may be misinterpreted as agoraphobia, unless a thorough neurological examination is conducted, including the use of the Balance Error Scoring System (Riemann & Guskiewicz, 2000) or the Fukuda Stepping Test (Fukuda, 1959).

POST-TRAUMATIC HYDROCEPHALUS

Neurosurgeons and neurologists are the principal managers of post-traumatic hydrocephalus (PTH) developing in the acute phase following TBI. Psychiatric physicians more typically encounter PTH as a cause of progressive cognitive impairment in their differential diagnosis of any patient who presents with a dementing disorder who also has a history of intracranial hemorrhage of any type and severity. Chronic mismatch between normal rates of cerebrospinal fluid (CSF) production and reduced drainage (due to partial occlusion by residual blood products of arachnoid granulations, which are villous enlargements that protrude into dural sinuses or diploic veins and drain CSF) will not be evident immediately. Rather, much like the hair collected in the bottom of the shower drain, the longer the shower runs, the more the water backs up on the floor. The importance of this diagnosis is its usually gratifying response to lumbar drainage of CSF and definitive neurosurgical intervention, usually an extracranial shunt.

A diagnosis of PTH should be entertained whenever the patient presents with any evidence of the cardinal triad of urinary incontinence, cognitive decline, and balance disorder ("wet, weird, and wobbly"). Severity of urinary incontinence may range from slight leakage while sleeping or with coughing or sneezing, to more significant loss of control. This probably reflects subtle pressure effects in the mid-sagittal region of the frontal lobes. Balance disorder may appear initially to be suggestive of early Parkinsonian gaits, with reduced upper extremity–associated movements while walking, en bloc turning, petit march, and festination. Cog-wheeling elicited spontaneously or with recruitment may be an initial finding as well. Cognitive deficits may include impaired short-term memory, poor performance on multitasking, and apathy (see Chapter xx on apathy).

While fundoscopic examination may find papilledema or loss of previously present spontaneous venous pulsations, neuroimaging by CT scan is the initial diagnostic study of choice.

The presence of symmetrical ventriculomegaly, while consistent with PTH, is still not diagnostic, as following TBI the post-traumatic loss of cerebral tissue can result in *hydrocephalus ex vacuo*. CSF drainage in that setting would not help, and could even precipitate intracranial bleeding. Comparison with earlier CT scans is the best way to confirm progressive ventricular enlargement, making it worthwhile to track down scans that may have been done years ago, at other sites of care. Another option is the use of a computer-assisted volumetric measurement, NeuroQuant' (FDA 510(k)K061855, Cortech Labs, La Jolla, California), that uses a database of normal controls aged 50 to 100 to compare ventricular and regional volumes and express that as an age-based percentile. This software also permits intra-subject comparison of bilateral structures to assess for asymmetrical focal atrophy or ventriculomegaly. Generally, left and right volumetric measurements should vary no more than 30%, and findings in excess of this are reasonably viewed as evidence of asymmetry. In most hospital settings, serial lumbar drainage comparing baseline assessments of gait/balance and mental status for improvement is the next step in the evaluation and treatment of PTH. Videotaping gait pre- and post-drainage can detect subtle changes not appreciated in the immediate examination setting. The use of a structured mental status exam with alternate forms is necessary when mental status rather than gait or continence is the primary manifestation of the suspected hydrocephalus.

Select academic institutions with specialized hydrocephalus treatment programs will have available a more sophisticated computer-assisted analysis of CSF dynamic cerebral compliance through the use of a pressure volume infusion (PVI) study. This represents the ultimate "gold standard" for PTH diagnosis. In this procedure, CSF pressure is measured using an attached transducer at opening, after withdrawal of a quantity of CSF, and after the infusion of a small quantity of fluid isotonic with CSF. These three measurements then are used to calculate the "compliance," which is a reflection of the drainage capacities of the arachnoid granulations. PVI calculations then assist with determining the degree of shunt flow and which form of shunting is optimal for a given patient (cf. Czosnyka & Whitfield, 2006).

TAU NEURODEGENERATION

Dementia pugilistica, first described in 1928 by forensic pathologist Harrison Stanford Martland, remains the prototype for dementia seen following multiple concussive injuries. When compared to Alzheimer's-type dementia, the lack of beta-amyloid deposition on neuropathological study is the distinguishing difference in dementia known as chronic traumatic encephalopathy (CTE) (cf. Shively, Scher, Perl, & Diaz-Arrastia, 2012). While public attention regarding CTE has been drawn to tragic deaths seen in professional athletes, tau deposition has been seen at autopsy in youths in their teens with histories of far fewer concussive events. The lack of data regarding individual recovery variability and threshold for symptom development creates a conundrum for the psychiatrist confronted with the youth athlete who has sustained a series of sports-related concussions that result in a persistence of post-concussive deficits. Apprehensive parents often expect the clinician to be the referee in deciding whether or not to end participation in contact sports. Unfortunately, no good data exist regarding cumulative risk for a given individual, although some effort has been made to generate a "hit count" (much like a "pitch count" for pitchers whose upper extremity is not fully developed) to limit exposure (Cantu & Nowinski, 2012).

In settings where the clinical history and examination is suggestive for CTE, no definitive treatment is currently available. Attention to factors that exacerbate cognitive dysfunction may help, including sleep quantity and quality, depression, pain, nutritional status, and endocrine status. Functional neuroimaging with PET usually does not show the biparietal hypometabolism typical of Alzheimer's disease, but rather shows a multifocal, asymmetrical pattern of glucose hypometabolism consistent with multiple concussive events inflicted from multiple directions.

Pharmacological stabilization appears to be prudent in enhancing nutritional and vitamin stability, including the use of supplemental vitamin D, B$_{12}$, and tetrahydrofolate. Treatment of endocrine deficiencies such as thyroid, testosterone, insulin-like growth factor (IGF-1), and growth hormone may also be initiated, although no definitive data exist on their efficacy in delaying decline. Treatment with either N-Methyl-D-aspartate (NMDA) antagonists and/or cholinesterase inhibitors theoretically may slow the rate of decline, but no definitive studies have been done to date.

BRAIN INJURY AS A CHRONIC DISEASE

The majority of TBIs resolve without any noticeable residual symptoms. Despite this, even mild TBI results in temporary disruption in cognitive functioning and not infrequently produces some degree of permanent disability. After a mild TBI, some groups have reported that up to half are left with a moderate or severe disability (Thornhill et al., 2000; Moppett, 2007). This is primarily true for recurrent episodes of TBI, but it is much more common for moderate and severe TBI to result in significant, permanent disability. The disability resulting from TBI may be anything from a slight decrement in fine-motor coordination to quadriplegia with severe cognitive impairments. As the severity of the impairment increases, so do the comorbid medical and psychiatric problems. TBI patients frequently suffer with chronic pain, planning and motivation problems, depression, anxiety, or even psychosis. Patients with persistent symptoms of TBI may have a decreased ability and desire to engage in their usual socialization. As a result, many of these patients do not engage in regular exercise or consume a rational diet. Lacking the typical social support and feedback mechanisms to correct these deficiencies, they become long-term problems. The subsequent loss of muscle tone and weight gain predispose them to additional injuries, hypertension, diabetes, dyslipidemia, coronary artery disease, and gastrointestinal problems. TBI, along with the aforementioned problems, also predisposes these individuals to many

sleep-related problems. These factors combined result in a general decrease in the perceived quality of their lives, further exacerbating problems with motivation and resulting in a downward health spiral. In 2012, it was estimated that there were between 3 and 5 million persons in the United States living with significant long-term TBI-related disabilities. Conceptualizing TBI as a chronic disease that occurs in staggering numbers makes it easy to see how the economic cost of TBI in the United States reaches $60 billion annually (cf. Masel & DeWitt, 2010).

LABORATORY EVALUATION OF TRAUMATIC BRAIN INJURY

When a patient presents with TBI acquired under suspicious circumstances (e.g., a serious fall in a person without a sensory or coordination problem or trauma from a single-car motor vehicle accident [MVA]), the laboratory evaluation should include levels of substances that are commonly used in suicide attempts. Such substances include not only sedatives and drugs of abuse but also acetaminophen, salicylates, and tricyclic antidepressants (TCA). Urine qualitative tests of TCA compounds and their metabolites are readily available in most hospital laboratories. They are not as sensitive or specific as the serologic tests but serve adequately as initial screening tests. An example of a potential confounding factor from using the less specific screen is that cyclobenzaprine may cause a positive TCA result.

Acute laboratory evaluation of the severe TBI patient will not be addressed other than as noted above since that is likely to be handled by an intensivist in the ICU. Specific laboratory evaluation of a patient with TBI will depend on the setting and the chronicity of the TBI.

In the acute setting, gonadotropic hormone levels will not be followed since they frequently are low but most commonly return to premorbid levels within a few months while even more return to normal within a year. During the rehabilitation phase, and certainly in a debilitated patient with a remote history of TBI, persistent hormonal deficiencies become more of a concern. Posterior pituitary damage is most often obvious in the acute stage, though it can manifest days after the initial trauma. This occasionally happens in those deemed to have only a mild TBI and turns what was thought to be a routine concussion into a life-threatening emergency. A screening battery is outlined in Box 45.1 (Elovic et al., 2005). Current guidelines suggest serial neuroendocrine evaluations annually for five years following TBI (Ghigo et al., 2005).

Studies relating to the incidence of TBI-associated anterior pituitary and pituitary stalk damage vary widely. Near universal agreement exists that there is a possibility of some degree of hypopituitarism after any TBI. Due to the compromise of anterior pituitary vascular structures, specific deficiencies can occur without panhypopituitarism such as hypothyroidism, hypogonadism, growth hormone deficiency, and adrenal failure with elevated prolactin. Growth hormone hyposecretion results in age-related IGF-1 deficiencies and may be the first anterior pituitary hormone deficiency seen in

Box 45.1 PITUITARY ASSESSMENT PROTOCOL
(ALL DRAWN AT 0800)

Cortisol levels (<12 mcg/dl → follow-up)
TSH—thyroid-stimulating hormone
Free T4—free thyroxin
LH—luteinizing hormone
FSH—follicle stimulating hormone
Testosterone (free and weakly bound)—males only
Estradiol—females only
IGF-1—insulin-like growth factor (<165 nG/mL in
<40 yo → follow-up)

non-acute TBI. When sex hormones are low due to TBI, the gonadotropins will not be elevated, highlighting the importance of ordering follicle-stimulating hormone (FSH) and luteinizing hormone (LH) when evaluating low testosterone or estradiol. When checking sex hormones, it is important to include the sex hormone-binding globulin (SHBG) to indicate the relative quantity of usable testosterone and estradiol. Elevated SHBG is also an important measure of risk for osteoporosis in men. (Note: SHBG may not be elevated in certain conditions, such as type II diabetes.)

Ordering only basal hormone studies will miss many neuroendocrine dysfunctions, though it will result in a significant increase in the number of such deficiencies that are identified. Most often, provocative testing is left to the endocrinologist.

Studies have shown that neuroendocrine disorders are common after TBI of any severity, with the majority resolving after 12 months. Any history of severe TBI should prompt a neuroendocrine evaluation, especially in patients that experience increased intracranial pressure (Klose, Juul, Poulsgaard, Kosteljanetz, Brennum, & Feldt-Rasmussen, 2007). Additionally, any history of TBI with severe residual symptoms that could be attributable to the neuroendocrine axis also warrants further investigation. Some authors advocate that "pituitary function after TBI should be assessed in all patients, regardless of the severity of the trauma" (Schneider, 2006).

Elevations in either creatine kinase (CK) and/or prolactin may occur during seizure activity. Both of these tests will be elevated after tonic-clonic seizures, though the prolactin level begins to fall approximately 20 minutes into the postictal state. The CK will also be elevated in patients fighting against physical restraints and in those that have experienced a dystonic reaction. Any patient with significant physical trauma will have elevated CK. Serially following of CK levels will give an objective measure of the healing process. If levels remain high, then neuropsychiatric manifestations can be expected since this is a measure of the severity of trauma to the entire individual.

Low levels of magnesium are associated with seizure activity, alcoholism, delirium, and agitation. Lactate dehydrogenase (LDH) is elevated in cerebral damage, seizures, megaloblastic anemia, hepatic disease, and infarctions of the heart, lungs, and kidneys. Improper handling of the blood specimen may also elevate LDH. In many institutions, after the patient leaves the ICU arterial blood gasses are rarely performed. A normal pulse oximetry does not rule out cerebral hypercapnia, though this is more often a problem in early management of severe TBI. Sleep disorders of most types are increased in TBI, with hypercapnia occurring in many of these. Rarely is this sufficient to cause significant problems with mental status, but it is certainly worth considering when unexpected mental status changes occur.

Sleep disorders following any degree of TBI are the rule rather than the exception. Decreased CSF levels of hypocretin-1, a wakefulness-promoting neurotransmitter, have been observed in the acute TBI setting but tend to resolve within 6 months (Baumann, Werth, Stocker, Ludwig, Bassetti, 2007). Despite this, many patients suffer with hypersomnia, excessive daytime sleepiness, and fatigue after TBI. Overnight pulse oximetry is a convenient and inexpensive test that yields clinically useful information. If oxygen saturations fall below 88% throughout the night or if a significant drop in oxygen saturation occurs, intervention is needed. This can be in the form of continuous positive airway pressure (CPAP), supplemental oxygen, or an oral appliance that advances the mandible. Failure to correct aberrant cerebral oxygen and carbon dioxide levels may lead to useless and damaging treatments while the patient continues to fail.

Numerous biomarkers have been studied in TBI patients in attempts to predict morbidity, mortality, and effective rehabilitation strategies. Concentrations of neuron-specific enolase, S100B, myelin basic protein, cleaved tau, and brain natriuretic peptide as well as others have been followed serially in TBI patients. The usefulness of these biomarkers remains to be definitively elucidated (cf. Dash, Zhao, Hergenroeder,& Moore, 2010).

PSYCHOPHARMACOLOGY OF SUBACUTE AND CHRONIC TRAUMATIC BRAIN INJURY SEQUELAE

Currently, no FDA-approved pharmacological interventions exist for subacute and chronic TBI sequelae. Nonetheless, multiple treatment options exist that are "off-label." Considering the frequency of these conditions, as well as the numerous medical and psychiatric sequelae associated with them, it is logical to presume that many hospitalized individuals suffer from TBI sequelae. As has been stated, the reason for the consult will probably not state an association with TBI, but the astute psychiatric physician must illuminate the true source of the malady resulting in a psychiatric consult for the medical patient.

Basic principles of psychopharmacology need to be observed when prescribing medications for TBI. Most medications used by psychiatrists lower the seizure threshold, which can be problematic for this population. Such medications may still be beneficial, but dosages may need to be lower than usually prescribed. While in the hospital, access to the complete medication list is readily available, which is rarely the case after discharge. When seen as an out patient, even if you have been following the patient, another physician may have ordered or the patient may have started something new without informing you. When the full medication list is seen, it often contains potentially dangerous combinations.

BENZODIAZEPINES

Generally speaking, there is no role for the chronic use of benzodiazepines in patients with TBI-related sequelae, with the possible exception of clonazepam due primarily to its anti-epileptic properties and benefit for restless leg syndrome. One of the many problems with benzodiazepines is that once they are started the patients rarely want to stop them. If never started, no fight will occur with the patient about stopping a medication that is "working so well." Frequently, patients with histories of alcohol and sedative abuse will be the ones that find them most "effective" and there are many less problematic options. An even more common problem associated with this class of medication is the cognitive slowing and associated memory impairment. This is especially problematic in patients with TBI who may be less able to articulate the decline they experience as a result of benzodiazepines. Often the spouse or other collateral informant will be the one to point out the decline associated with these or any other changes. Even typically well-tolerated benzodiazepines may be overly sedating in this population or cause unacceptable cognitive impairment.

ANTIPSYCHOTICS

As with benzodiazepines, antipsychotics play only a minor role in the treatment of TBI. Although they are effective chemical restraints, dopamine antagonists decrease neuronal regeneration (Feeney, Gonzalez, & Law, 1982), which may cause problems even a year after the initial insult. Use of antipsychotics is generally not advocated except in life-threatening settings where an actively violent patient is trying to harm himself or others, as may occur in the immediate post-acute phase. In those cases, antipsychotics commonly used in similar situations are appropriate with the added caveat of "start low and go slow." Previously existing psychiatric conditions do not disappear once a person sustains a TBI and many predispose a person to incurring TBIs. Some believe that in the case of substance addiction, TBI should be assumed since rarely does such a person retain perfect memory of their traumatic experiences. If the patient had a condition that warranted antipsychotic use prior to TBI, it is certainly appropriate to continue such use. It should be noted that TBI often alters the way a person's brain responds to certain medications, so previously effective medications may become ineffective or even intolerable.

SOPORIFICS

Sedative-hypnotics should be used sparingly in persons after TBI and in anyone in general. Sleep hygiene is always the first step in addressing insomnia. When starting a soporific agent, the patient should always be informed that it is a short-term solution and that other agents or actions are more appropriate for chronic insomnia. While it has been shown in general populations that counseling is as effective as medication for sleep, similar studies in TBI populations are lacking. Anti-epileptic drugs or sedating antidepressants may be more beneficial in this population. Benzodiazepine derivatives often lose effectiveness quickly and should always be used with caution if an underlying sleep apnea is suspected as they will decrease muscle tone and worsen hypoxemia. Any soporific can be habit-forming, but zolpidem may be more problematic than other modern sleep aids in this respect. It may also cause more Zolpidem may be better at maintaining normal sleep architecture, but may cause amnesia and hallucinations than zaleplon or eszopiclone though may be better at maintaining normal sleep architecture. All of these can be effective in achieving sleep for brief, well-circumscribed periods. Although nightmares may occur with TBI, the patient with post-traumatic stress disorder (PTSD), which is not an uncommon comorbidity, is at greater risk. When this is the case, prazosin or clonidine may be useful for achieving sleep restoration and suppressing nightmares. If used during the day, they may also help curb the autonomic hyperreactivity often seen as a chronic symptom of TBI.

ANTIDEPRESSANTS

Older antidepressants, with the exception of trazodone, should generally be avoided in TBI patients. Low-dose tricyclics can be helpful in treating certain types of post-traumatic headaches and sleep, but the antidepressant doses are most often excessively anticholinergic, which limits their usefulness. Even the selective serotonin reuptake inhibitor (SSRI) and serotonin—norepinephrine reuptake inhibitor (SNRI) antidepressants are often not as beneficial as might be expected. Bupropion can be helpful for improving energy, concentration, mood, and motivation, but in doses above 300 mg it has more chance of lowering the seizure threshold than most other antidepressants. Patients being started on bupropion should be warned that the drug may cause them to be nervous, anxious, jittery, or "mean." Generally, people who start out "mean" do not get "meaner" and often become calmer. Anxiety symptoms should be addressed with the SSRI or SNRI medications as opposed to the benzodiazepines or bupropion due to the considerations noted above.

PSYCHOSTIMULANTS

Various psychostimulants have been utilized to address post-TBI hypersomnia, inattention, and apathy. These attempts occasionally result in full resolution of symptoms, but this is very rare. Frequently there is little or no benefit and some symptoms may be worsened. When the hypersomnia, inattention, or apathy are severe and not addressed adequately by sleep hygiene, soporifics, antidepressants, and other treatments, then a trial of a psychostimulant or amantadine (an antiviral drug with stimulant properties in some individuals) is reasonable. As always in this population, starting at a lower than usual dosage is advisable, and the titration schedule should also be conservative. It is common for a patient to report fabulous results initially only to report severe side effects at the next visit. Having an objective collateral source of information is invaluable in these situations. Any of the stimulants is a potential candidate for a trial with the patient exhibiting the above symptoms with the key to success often being the prescriber's comfort and confidence with a given stimulant. The wakefulness-promoting agents modafinil and armodafinil may offer a reasonable initial strategy for fatigue, though insurance considerations may prevent these as first-line agents as no supportive clinical research exists. Dextroamphetamine, mixed amphetamine salts, as well as the various methylphenidate compounds are all options.

COGNITIVE ENHANCERS

Acetylcholinesterase inhibitors—rivastigmine, donepezil, and galantamine—have demonstrated some degree of benefit in studies of TBI-related cognitive disorders. They may also improve apathy and fatigue associated with TBI. While the mechanisms for these benefits are unclear, some evidence indicates it is from an increase in IGF-1. Memantine, an NMDA-receptor antagonist with antagonistic effects at the 5-Hydroxytryptophan (5-HTP) receptor and nicotinic acetylcholine receptors, may also be tried. The proposed benefit in TBI is mainly from blocking the NMDA receptors from persistent activation by the excitatory amino acid glutamate, though the other mechanisms of action probably also play a role. Studies have shown that blocking glutamate activity early after TBI is counterproductive, but persistent activation of the NMDA receptors by glutamate is thought to play a role in secondary injury in TBI. Prescribing acetylcholinesterase inhibitors and memantine generally is not based on any empirical evidence, but more on logic and the symptom complex that is presented. If resources are no impediment, then serial neuropsychological testing can be utilized to determine the effectiveness of these strategies. If time and financial constraints are a problem, then patient reports, collateral interviews, and personal observations can suffice.

ANTI-EPILEPTIC DRUGS

Anti-epileptic drugs (AED) are often the best choice for TBI-related symptoms. Depending on the choice of AED, they may have efficacy for mood lability, migraine and other headache prophylaxis, sleep, restless leg/periodic limb movement syndromes, neuropathic pain, anxiety, etc. As with many psychotropic medications, they do not work immediately. The patients must be educated about this, since many will stop their medications after a few days since they are not seeing benefits or are having mild side effects without commensurate symptom relief. An undervalued AED is gabapentin, often a better choice for treating restless leg syndrome than clonazepam. While it may not be as rapidly effective as clonazepam, on occasion a first-night benefit is observed. Rarely, patients may find gabapentin stimulating and hence abusable, but the abuse risks are much less than

with the benzodiazepines. The same caution applies to pregabalin, with the added concern that it may cause teratogenesis via spermatic mechanisms. (Note: barrier protection is mandatory for sexually active males with fertile partners.) In many TBI patients, gabapentin can be especially helpful for concentration, although this is not often seen in the non-TBI population. Patients with other forms of cerebral insults, such as anoxia or febrile brain injury, may also find similar benefits. This is not a benefit that occurs reliably, but it is not unusual either. Gabapentin, pregabalin, and tiagabine may also help a patient achieve deeper stages of sleep. Considering the restorative benefits of sleep as well as the hormonal benefits of deep sleep in light of the chronic sleep disturbances in this population, these are certainly good choices for many. Frequently, AED combinations are required. Certain combinations seem more helpful than others. Gabapentin and tiagabine tend to have a synergistic effect, as does gabapentin and levetiracetam. Pregabalin and gabapentin also do well together, despite their similar-sounding names. Older AEDs are also very effective, but they have more side effects and more requirements for monitoring. Often these older medications are necessary since they are much more affordable than branded formulations. Encouraging patients without medication coverage to shop for the best price at local pharmacies, discount super stores, and member warehouse stores is also a beneficial intervention to suggest as frontal lobe problem-solving strategies may be impaired.

OVER THE COUNTER (OTC) PREPARATIONS

Melatonin is often a good choice when dealing with sleep-related issues shortly after TBI. Patients are usually comfortable with using an OTC preparation and often do not require more intervention than this. Dosages can range from 3–10 mg at bedtime and can be repeated if middle insomnia occurs. Rarely is residual daytime sedation observed, although it is not unheard of. It is not recommended in pregnancy, but few other restrictions apply. Melatonin may even be effective in chronic TBI for achieving sleep and for ameliorating middle insomnia, if taken when the awakening occurs. Valerian root does not have significant literature to substantiate its use in insomnia from any condition. Despite this, many tout its therapeutic properties in decreasing anxiety and insomnia. When used in recommended dosages and for short periods of time, some TBI patients may find it effective. Caution with the concomitant use of AEDs is advised. Typical OTC sleep aids contain diphenhydramine and are generally not recommended. As with prescription anticholinergic agents, diphenhydramine may worsen some cognitive symptoms associated with TBI. Despite this warning, some find it to be very helpful in the short term, and diphenhydramine is usually acceptable in pregnancy. In a patient unwilling to take prescription sleep aids, preferring OTC agents, or with positive expectations of success due to pre-TBI response, a trial may be appropriate with the patient being well aware of the risks and following a clear documentation of the discussion.

SPECIAL CONSIDERATIONS

The elderly always present special challenges, and TBI is no exception. While moderate and severe TBI are associated with a higher statistical likelihood of dementia, the precise mechanism is unknown. As discussed above, CTE, following multiple repetitive concussive injuries, is known to induce a tau-opathy.

TBI may also result in side effects to previously well-tolerated medications and alter alcohol tolerance. These issues are confusing to patients and often result in questions about losing their sanity. Sometimes these changes are temporary, but occasionally they become longstanding. Either way, reassurance will go far to comfort the elderly TBI patient. Depending on the acuity and severity of the TBI, the reassurance may need to be repeated often.

As previously noted, when a person with any psychiatric condition sustains a TBI, their psychiatric condition does not disappear. It is not unusual for the premorbid condition to be changed, but it will not disappear, unless the TBI is so severe as to render the person insensible. Frequently, the premorbid condition will be relegated to a less prominent position during the early stages of TBI, but it may later become more severe than it was premorbidly. Frequently, the person with a mild TBI who does not return to baseline will experience further psychiatric symptoms and possibly an entirely new condition. These nascent conditions must be dealt with in the appropriate clinical fashion, while keeping in mind the aforementioned precautions.

SUMMARY

Given the known epidemiology of TBI, it is certain that individuals with a history of TBI will be evaluated by the practicing psychiatrist. Such a past event may influence treatment response to conventional interventions, be misclassified as denial or treatment resistance, or be erroneously labeled as noncompliance or malingering. It is incumbent upon the psychiatric physicians to familiarize themselves with the evaluation and treatment of these organically based disorders to prevent needlessly increasing morbidity and mortality for the patients they serve.

CLINICAL PEARLS

- The examination required once TBI is under consideration includes assessment of auditory, visual perceptive, vestibular, and language function.

- Seventeen to 61% of all TBI patients develop depression within two years of injury (Rapoport, 2012) and seek psychiatric care without considering the relevance of TBI.

- Falls remain the leading cause of TBI among civilians, followed by motor vehicle accidents and other blows to the head, including sports injuries and assaults.

- TBI from motor vehicle accidents results from rapid acceleration and deceleration forces causing micro-shearing and DAI. DAI may appear on MRI as numerous small white matter lesions.

- Secondary brain injuries are the result of a cascade of molecular injury mechanisms that unfold over hours and sometimes days following the acute event.

- The Glasgow Coma Scale was designed and should be used to assess the depth and duration coma (Teasdale et al., 1978). It is not, therefore, appropriate for determining the severity of TBIs in general.

- ACRM criteria mandate that a TBI be rated as moderately severe if a patient has a PTA or a period of altered consciousness lasting 24 hours or more.

- The severity of the initial injury remains the best predictor of long-term prognosis.

- The basic formula for describing the forces of a TBI as it affects the brain is derived from Newtonian physics: $\mathbf{a = v^2/(2s)}$. This means that the severity of a TBI is a result both of how fast you were going and of how quickly you stop.

- Head CT and MRI are insensitive to two common consequences of closed TBI—cavitation and micro-shearing.

- Following brain contusions, the cortex shows diminished metabolic activity with associated cognitive impairments. Contusions may also produce irritable foci that result in intermittent sensory phenomena or memory disruption.

- The most common area of tissue damage in typical closed TBI is the orbital frontal cortex, usually via lacerations, abrasions, and contusions of the cortex caused by friction of the ventral surface of the frontal lobe against the sharp, irregular ridges of the cribriform plate.

- The core disability of orbital frontal patients is that they think less (Varney & Menafee, 1993). Spontaneous decision-making becomes labored, less frequent, and less reliable, particularly with the multiple small decisions of ordinary life, e.g., "what to do next" (Varney, 1999).

- Orbital frontal symptoms relating to activities of daily living (e.g., indecisiveness, mental inertia) and psychosocial symptoms (poor empathy, indifference) can be reliably determined by structured interview of a collateral informant (Varney, 1991).

- Executive disability in patients with orbital frontal injury involves problems not detected by conventional neuropsychological testing (Martzke et al., 1991), which isolates individual abilities for testing.

- Initial seizures following the acute TBI event occur in 10–15% of adults in the first week following severe TBI (Langendorf & Pedley, 1997).

- Longitudinal studies define increased lifetime seizure risk for those with mild, moderate, or severe TBI across the lifespan ranging from a relative risk of 2.22 in those with mild closed TBI, to 7.4 in severe brain injury, to 2.17 in those with skull fracture (Christensen et al., 2009).

- To identify neurosensory dysfunction, the psychiatric physician must be capable of performing a competent and accurate cranial nerve examination, including assessment of olfactory functioning.

- Visuo-perceptual dysfunctions and lateralized loss of visual awareness (due to non-dominant temporal-parietal damage) results in increased startle and reaction when the patient is approached from the dysfunctional side. Over time, this evolves into a subtle form of hypervigilance that may resemble paranoia.

- When auditory-processing disorders are misdiagnosed as a primary ADHD and treated with stimulants, they may actually get worse.

- When vestibular asymmetry follows TBI, the individual must rely on vision and proprioceptive functions for all balance. Such a visually dependent balance will result in patients' avoiding crowded settings such as grocery stores, where the point of visual fixation is intermittently blocked by passers-by.

- Current guidelines suggest serial neuroendocrine evaluations annually for five years following TBI (Ghigo et al., 2005).

- Sleep disorders following any degree of TBI are the rule rather than the exception.

- Generally speaking, there is no role for chronic use of benzodiazepines in patients with TBI-related sequelae.

- When hypersomnia, inattention, or apathy are severe and not addressed adequately by sleep hygiene, soporifics, antidepressants, and other treatments, then a trial of a psychostimulant or amantadine (an antiviral drug with stimulant properties in some individuals) is reasonable.

DISCLOSURE STATEMENTS

Dr. O'Shanick has served as a consultant and expert for Avanir, Cephalon, and Ceretec and has received payment for those services. He is also the sole owner of a private outpatient brain injury medicine program (Center for Neurorehabilitation Services, PC) in Richmond, Virginia.

Dr. Moses has received speaker bureau fees from Pamlabs, Inc, maker of Cerefolin NAC, Deplin & Metanx.

Dr. Varney has nothing to disclose.

REFERENCES

American Congress of Rehabilitation Medicine (1993). Definition of mild traumatic brain injury. *Journal of Head Trauma Rehabilitation*, *8*(3), 86–87.

Baumann, C. R., Werth, E., Stocker, R., Ludwig, S., & Bassetti, C. L. (2007). Sleep-wake disturbances 6 months after traumatic brain injury: a prospective study. *Brain*, *130*(7), 1873–1883.

Bayless, J. D., Roberts, R., & Varney, N. R. (1989). Tinker Toy™ performance of patients with closed head trauma. *Journal of Clinical and Experimental Neuropsychology*, *11*, 913–917.

Belmont, P. J., Schoenfeld, A. J., & Goodman, G. (2010). Epidemiology of combat wounds in Operation Iraqi Freedom and Operation Enduring Freedom: Orthopedic burden of disease. *Journal of Surgical Orthopaedic Advances*, *19*(1), 2–7.

Bigler, E. D. (1990) Neuropathology of traumatic brain injury. In E. D. Bigler (Ed.), *Traumatic brain injury*. Austin, TX: Pro-Ed.

Bigler, E. D. (2004). Neuropsychological results and neuropathological findings at autopsy in a case of mild traumatic brain injury. *Journal of the International Neuropsychological Society*, *10*(5), 794–806.

Bigler, E. D. (2008). Critical review: Neuropsychology and clinical neuroscience of persistent post-concussive syndrome. *Journal of the International Neuropsychological Society*, *14*, 1–22.

Bigler, E. D., & Maxwell, W. L. (2012). Neuropathology of mild traumatic brain injury: relationship to neuroimaging findings. *Brain Imaging and Behavior*, DOI 10.1007/s11682-011-9145-0, published online 21 March 2012.

Cantu, R., & Nowinski, C. (2012). *Hit count*. Boston: Sports Legacy Institute,.

Capehart, B., & Bass, D. (2011). The aftermath of war: traumatic brain injury among veterans returning from Afghanistan and Iraq. Strategies for diagnosis and treatment. *Psychiatric Times*, *28*(7), 1–6.

Cernak, I., & Noble-Haeusslein, L. J. (2009). Traumatic brain injury: an overview of pathobiology with emphasis on military populations. *Journal of Cerebral Blood Flow and Metabolism*, *30*, 255–266.

Christensen, J., Pedersen, M. G., Pedersen, C. B., Sidenius, P., Olsen, J., & Vestergaard, M. (2009). Long-term risk of epilepsy after traumatic brain injury in children and young adults: a population-based cohort study. *Lancet 373*(9669), 1105–1110.

Chwalisz, K. (1999). The problem of comorbidity in spouses. In N. R. Varney & T. J. Roberts, *Evaluation and treatment of mild traumatic brain injury*. Mahwah, NJ: Lawrence Erlbaum.

Cooper, J. C., & Gates, G. A. (1991). Hearing in the elderly—the Framingham cohort, 1983–1985: Part II. Prevalence of central auditory processing disorders. *Ear & Hearing*, *12*(5), 304–311.

Czosnyka, M., & Whitfield, P. (2006). Hydrocephalus. A practical guide to CSF dynamics and ventriculoperitoneal shunts. *Advances in Clinical Neuroscience and Rehabilitation*, *6*(3), 14–17.

Dash, P. K., Zhao, J., Hergenroeder, G., & Moore, A. N. (2010). Biomarkers in the diagnosis, prognosis, and evaluation of treatment efficacy for traumatic brain injury. *Neurotherapeutics*, *7*(1), 100–114.

Disability Determination Services Administrators' Letter No. 866 (Jan. 26, 2012).

Elovic E., Perrone K., Stalla G., Thompson C., & Urban, R. (2005). Consensus guidelines on screening for hypopituitarism following traumatic brain injury. On behalf of participants in the hypopituitarism following traumatic brain injury consensus workshop. *Brain Injury*, *19*, 711–724.

Faul, M., Xu, L., Wald, M. M., & Coronado, V. G. (2010). *Traumatic brain injury in the United States: emergency department visits, hospitalizations, and deaths*. Atlanta: Centers for Disease Control and Prevention, National Center for Injury Prevention and Control.

Feeney, D. M., Gonzalez, A., & Law, W. A. (1982). Amphetamine, haloperidol, and experience interact to affect rate of recovery after motor cortex injury. *Science*, *217*(4562), 855–857.

Fukuda, T. (1959). The stepping test: Two phases of the labyrinthine reflex. *Acta Oto-laryngologica*, *50*(1–2), 95–108.

Ghigo, E., Masel, B., Aimaretti, G., Léon-Carrión, J., Casanueva, F. F., Dominguez-Morales, M. R., Elovic, E., et al. (2005). Consensus guidelines on screening for hypopituitarism following traumatic brain injury. *Brain Injury, 19*(9), 711–724.

Greuters, S., van den Berg, A., Franschman, G., Viersen, V. A., Beishuizen, A., Peerdeman, S. M., et al. (2011). Acute and delayed mild coagulopathy are related to outcome in patients with isolated traumatic brain injury. *Critical Care, 15*(1), R2.

Harhangi, B. S., Kompanje, E. J., Leebeek, F. W., & Maas, A. I. (2008). Coagulation disorders after traumatic brain injury. Acta Neurochir (Wien), 150(2), 165.

Heilman, K. M., & Valenstein, E. (2012). *Clinical neuropsychology* (5th ed.). New York: Oxford University Press.

Hines, M. E. (1999). Posttraumatic headaches. In N. R. Varney & T. J. Roberts, *Evaluation and treatment of mild traumatic brain injury.* Mahwah, NJ: Lawrence Erlbaum.

Ju, D., & Varney, N. R. (2000). Can head injury patients simulate malingering? *Applied Neuropsychology: Adult, 7*(4), 201–207.

Klose, M., Juul, A., Poulsgaard, L., Kosteljanetz, M., Brennum, J., & Feldt-Rasmussen, U. (2007). Prevalence and predictive factors of post-traumatic hypopituitarism. *Clinical Endocrinology (Oxford), 67*(2), 193–201.

Langendorf, F., & Pedley, T. A. (1997). *Epilepsy: A comprehensive textbook.* Philadelphia: Lippincott-Raven.

Lezak, M. D., Howieson, D. B., Bigler, E. D., & Tranel, D. (eds.) (2012). *Neuropsychological assessment.* New York: Oxford University Press, for a complete discussion of the test's various uses.

Lezak, M. D., Howieson, D. B., Loring, D. W., Hannay, H. J., & Fischer, J. S. (2004). *Neuropsychological assessment* (4th ed.; pp. 160–161). New York: Oxford University Press.

Lippa, S. M., Pastorek, N. J., Benge, J. F., & Thornton, G. M. (2010). Postconcussive symptoms after blast and non-blast-related mild traumatic brain injuries in Afghanistan and Iraq war veterans. *Journal of the International Neuropsychological Society, 16,* 856–866.

Luethcke, C. A., Bryan, C. J., Morrow, C. E., & Isler, W. C. (2011). Comparison of concussive symptoms, cognitive performance, and psychological symptoms between acute blast versus non-blast-induced mild traumatic brain injury. *Journal of the International Neuropsychological Society, 17,* 36–45.

Lyeth, B. G., Dixon, C. E., Hamm, R. J., Jenkins, L. W., Young, H. F., Stonnington, H. H., et al. (1988). Effects of anticholinergic treatment on transient behavioral suppression and physiological responses following concussive brain injury to the rat. *Brain Research, 448*(1), 88–97.

MacDonald, C. L., Johnson, A. M., Cooper, D., Nelson, E. C., Werner, N. J., Shimony, J. S., et al. (2011). Detection of blast-related traumatic brain injury in US military personnel. *New England Journal of Medicine, 364,* 2091–100.

Martland, H. S. (1928). Punch drunk. *Journal of the American Medical Association,* 91 (15): 1103–1107.

Martzke, J., Swan, C., & Varney, N. R. (1991). Post-traumatic anosmia and orbital frontal damage neuropsychological and neuropsychiatric correlates. *Neuropsychology,* 1991, 5, 213–225.

Masel, B. E., & DeWitt, D. S. (2010). Traumatic brain injury: a disease process, not an event. *Journal of Neurotrauma, 27*(8), 1529–1540.

Moppett, I. K. (2007). Traumatic brain injury: assessment, resuscitation and early management. *British Journal of Anaesthesia, 99*(1),18–31.

Office of the Surgeon General/US Army Medical Command (OTSG/MEDCOM) (2011). Policy Memo 11-076, Sept. 11, 2011: subject: "Optimal Use of Psychological/Neuropsychological Assessment."

Povlishock, J. T., & Katz, D. I. (2005). Update of neuropathology and neurological recovery after traumatic brain injury. *Journal of Head Trauma Rehabilitation* 20(1), 76–94.

Rapoport, M. J. (2012). Depression following traumatic brain injury: Epidemiology, risk factors, and management. *CNS Drugs, 26*(2), 111–121.

Riemann, B. L., & Guskiewicz, K. M. (2000). Effects of mild head injury on postural stability as measured through clinical balance testing. *Journal of Athletic Training* 35(1), 19–25.

Roberts, R. J. (1999). Epilepsy spectrum disorder in the context of mild traumatic brain injury. In N. R. Varney & T. J. Roberts, *Evaluation and treatment of mild traumatic brain injury.* Mahwah, NJ: Lawrence Erlbaum.

Roberts, R. J., Paulsen, J. S., Marchman, J. N., & Varney, N. R. (1989). MMPI profiles of patients who endorse multiple partial seizure symptoms. *Neuropsychology,* 2, 183–198.

Russell, W. R., & Smith, A. (1961). Post-traumatic amnesia in closed head injury. *Archives of Neurology, 5*(1), 4–7.

Schneider, H. J. (2006). Prevalence of anterior pituitary insufficiency 3 and 12 months after traumatic brain injury. *European Journal of Endocrinology, 154*(2), 259–265.

Shenton, M. E., Hamoda, H. M., Schneiderman, J. S., Bouix, S., Pasternak, O., Rathi, Y., et al. (2012). A review of magnetic resonance imaging and diffusion tensor imaging findings in mild traumatic brain injury. *Brain Imaging and Behavior,* published online 22 March 2012.

Shively, S., Scher, A. I., Perl, D. P., & Diaz-Arrastia R (2012). Dementia resulting from traumatic brain injury: What is the pathology? *Archives of Neurology.* Published online July 9, 2012. doi:10.1001/archneurol.2011.3747

Siders, T. K. (1999). Therapy for spouses of head injured patients. In N. R. Varney & T. J. Roberts, *Evaluation and treatment of mild traumatic brain injury.* Mahwah, NJ: Lawrence Erlbaum.

Stein, D. G. (2011). Is progesterone a worthy candidate as a novel therapy for traumatic brain injury? *Dialogues in Clinical Neuroscience, 13*(3), 352–359.

Stein, S. C., Chen, X. H., Sinson, G. P., & Smith, D. H. (2002). Intravascular coagulation: a major secondary insult in nonfatal traumatic brain injury. *Journal of Neurosurgery, 97*(6),1373.

Teasdale, G., & Jennett, B. (1974). Assessment of coma and impaired consciousness. A practical scale. *Lancet, 2*(7872), 81–84.

Teasdale, G., Kril-Jones, R., & van der Sande, J. (1978). Observer variability in assessing impaired consciousness and coma. *Journal of Neurology, Neurosurgery & Psychiatry, 41,* 603–610.

Thornhill, S., Teasdale, G. M., Murray, G. D., McEwen, J., Roy, C. W., & Penny, K. I. (2000). Disability in young people and adults one year after head injury: prospective cohort study. *British Medical Journal, 320*(7250),1631–1635.

Ucker, D. S. (1991). Death by suicide: One way to go in mammalian development? *New Biologist, 3,* 103–109.

Varney, N. R. (1988). The prognostic significance of anosmia in patients with closed head trauma. *Journal of Clinical and Experimental Neuropsychology, 10,* 250–254.

Varney, N. R. (1991). Iowa Collateral Head Injury Interview. (1989). Reprinted in *Neuropsychology,* 1991, 5, 223–225.

Varney, N. R. (1999). Post traumatic anosmia and orbital fronal injury. In N. R. Varney & T. J. Roberts, *Evaluation and treatment of mild traumatic brain injury.* Mahwah, NJ: Lawrence Erlbaum.

Varney, N. R., & Bushnell, D. (1998). NeuroSPECT findings in patients with post-traumatic anosmia: a quantitative analysis. *Journal of Head Trauma Rehabilitation, 13,* 63–72.

Varney, N. R., & Menefee, L. (1993). Psychosocial and executive deficits following closed head injury: implications for orbital frontal cortex. *Journal of Head Trauma Rehabilitation, 8*(1), 32–44.

Varney, N. R., & Roberts, R. J. (1999). Forces and accelerations in car accidents and resultant head injuries. In N. R. Varney & T. J. Roberts, *Evaluation and treatment of mild traumatic brain injury.* Mahwah, NJ: Lawrence Erlbaum.

Varney, N. R., & Stewart, H. (2004). Is impaired executive function a single or multidimensional disability? A beginning. *Applied Neuropsychology, 18,* 229–235.

Varney, N. R., & Varney, R. N. (1995). Brain injury without head injury: Some physics of automobile collisions with particular reference to brain injuries occurring without physical head trauma. *Applied Neuropsychology, 2,* 47–62.

Varney, N. R., Bushnell, D., Nathan, M., Kahn, D., Roberts, R., & Rezai, K., et al. (1995). NeuroSPECT correlates of disabling "mild" head injury: Preliminary findings. *Journal of Head Trauma Rehabilitation, 10,* 18–28.

Varney, N. R., Pinkston, J., & Wu, J. (2001). Quantitative PET scan findings 14 patients with posttraumatic anosmia. *Journal of Head Trauma Rehabilitation, 16,* 253.

46.

FRONTAL SYSTEMS AND DYSFUNCTIONS

Kimiko Domoto-Reilly, Paul Malloy, Deborah A. Cahn-Weiner, and Thomas Markham Brown

INTRODUCTION

The frontal lobes comprise about one-third of the cerebrum and have extensive connections with other brain regions. Frontal systems, therefore, are susceptible to injury from a wide variety of diseases and insults; because the frontal lobes are responsible for orchestrating many higher cognitive abilities, impairment may result in devastating effects on socially adaptive behavior. This chapter reviews the functional neuroanatomy of the frontal lobes, the cognitive and behavioral features of frontal lobe syndromes, evaluation techniques, and treatment options. Social and legal implications are also briefly discussed.

CAUSES OF FRONTAL SYSTEM DYSFUNCTION

Degenerative disorders can have their earliest and most dramatic effects on the frontal lobes, including frontotemporal dementia and Alzheimer's disease. A number of the so-called subcortical dementias disturb both motor and executive/frontal systems (e.g., Parkinson's, Huntington's disease; Goldberg et al., 1990; Gotham, Brown, & Marsden, 1988). Some developmental conditions such as attention-deficit hyperactivity disorder (ADHD) and autism spectrum disorders feature prominent frontal system disruption. Many psychiatric illnesses are associated with frontal system dysfunction, including but not limited to: Tourette's syndrome, major depression, schizophrenia, and obsessive-compulsive disorder.

The frontal lobes are often involved in stroke. The middle cerebral artery serves the frontal convexity and is the most common territory for large vessel ischemic stroke. The anterior communicating artery is a common site for aneurysm, and hemorrhage can cause a severe frontal syndrome due to mesial and basal frontal damage. The watershed zone between the anterior and middle cerebral arteries is also at risk in settings of decreased intracranial blood flow, such as in cardiac arrest.

Other disorders may not affect frontal cortex directly but will disrupt frontal systems through destruction of white matter connections to posterior and subcortical structures (e.g., multiple sclerosis, small vessel cerebrovascular disease). These diffuse connections render the frontal systems particularly vulnerable to so-called toxic/metabolic dysfunction, which can have multiple etiologies, including sepsis, sleep deprivation, medications, seizures, and intoxication. Infections such as HIV and syphilis (tertiary) produce frontal system dysfunction. Mass lesions such as tumors can exert local and/or diffuse effects via focal expansion, axonal disruption, and hydrocephalus. Treatment with radiation and/or chemotherapy can result in delayed degenerative effects. The frontal lobes are also particularly prone to damage in head injury, due to the high incidence of direct contusion and of disruption of critical connections from other regions of the brain. Normal aging also contributes to frontal system dysfunction (D'Esposito & Gazzaley, 2011; Prakash et al., 2009).

FUNCTIONAL NEUROANATOMY OF THE FRONTAL LOBES

The functional subdivisions of the frontal lobes include the primary motor area, premotor area, frontal eye fields, dorsolateral area, orbital/basal area, and anterior cingulate gyrus/supplementary motor areas (SMA). The primary motor area subserves pyramidal motor functions; the premotor area is involved in sensorimotor integration and praxis; and the frontal eye fields control volitional eye movement and visual search. Damage to these zones generally results in relatively simple disorders of motor functioning (e.g., hemiparesis, volitional gaze disturbance). The dorsolateral, orbital, and mesial (cingulate/SMA) subdivisions are involved in higher cognitive functions. These *prefrontal* cortical regions have been of greatest interest to psychiatrists, behavioral neurologists, and neuropsychologists because of the striking personality and behavioral changes that can result from insults to these areas.

Each prefrontal zone has extensive connections with posterior cortical, thalamic, and basal ganglia structures that play an important role in their expression of complex behavioral patterns. The dorsolateral and orbital frontal areas, for example, receive input from distinct posterior association areas in each sensory modality. Parallel but separate subcortical connections exist as well (e.g., the dorsolateral area is connected to dorsolateral caudate nucleus, while the orbital area is connected to ventromedial caudate). The insular cortex, the ancient "hidden lobe of the brain" buried under the frontal and temporal opercula, has emerged as an area intimately connected with the frontal lobe, and contributing to interoception, emotional awareness, and cognitive abilities traditionally ascribed to the frontal lobe such as performance-monitoring and decision-making (Craig, 2009). Thus, frontal cortical areas act in concert with other cortical and subcortical structures to form distinct frontal systems (Cummings, 1993). Current models of cognition consider behavior in the setting of networks, reflecting the functional connectivity of specific, distributed brain regions implicated in task performance.

SPECIFIC FRONTAL LOBE SYNDROMES

For practical teaching purposes, this section will treat the syndromes of frontal lobe damage as though each were distinct. The reader must keep in mind, however, that patients may suffer damage to multiple frontal zones as well as damage to other cortical and subcortical areas, and hence may display deficits reflecting disruption of several behavioral subsystems. Furthermore, these subsystems act in concert (not isolation) in facilitating normal behavior.

EXECUTIVE FUNCTION

Dysexecutive syndrome refers to cognitive and organizational functions subserved primarily by dorsolateral frontal systems. Executive functions include the ability to integrate sensory information from multiple modalities, formulate goals with due regard for long-term consequences, generate multiple response alternatives, and choose appropriate goal-directed behavior. As a behavior sequence progresses, executive functions continue to play a role in self-monitoring of the adequacy and correctness of the behavior, and to modify behaviors when conditions change. Executive abilities allow us either to change a plan or to persist in the face of distractions and shifting circumstances.

Lesions of the dorsolateral prefrontal region can result in a stereotyped or limited response repertoire, easy loss of task set, perseverative or inflexible behavior, inability to integrate disparate sensory elements into a coherent whole, and lack of self-monitoring of errors. Problems with behavioral switching can cause a lack of response flexibility, such that the patient becomes rigidly "stuck in set" (i.e., stuck in a set of behaviors; Luria, 1980; Stuss, 1993). It is not difficult to see how such problems could interfere with one's ability to problem-solve when task demands are high.

Dysexecutive problems may affect performance in other cognitive domains. For example, poor organization may lead the patient with frontal lobe functional injury to fail clock-drawing tests, by drawing a series of numbers around the periphery without concern for spatial placement, or continuing beyond 12 due to poor self-monitoring. Patients with frontal dysfunction may also make concrete errors in setting the hands on the clock face (for example, when asked to set the hands to "ten after eleven," the patient may draw the hands to the "10" and the "11"). Perseverative tendencies may cause patients to reuse an earlier item or response during a later task. For example, when asked to name a book and then name a house, the patient may say "book." The examiner must be aware of the underlying frontal deficit so that these errors are not mistaken for primary difficulties in language functions. Hence, it is usually desirable to interrogate frontal functions early in the assessment.

Executive deficits may also affect memory performance. Frontal system damage can result in inefficient learning due to failure to make use of active learning strategies, reduced memory for temporal/situational context, and a tendency to make perseverative errors (Vilkki, 1989). These deficits have usually been characterized as a failure of working memory. *Working memory* is thought of as the ability to take information in for short-term storage, manipulate it over a brief period of time, and organize it for permanent memory encoding. Frontal system injury patients perform particularly poorly when the memory task includes test-controlled distractions or interference techniques (Parkin & Walter, 1992) because they are unable to simultaneously hold the items in temporary storage and ignore the distraction.

DISINHIBITION SYNDROME

Disinhibited behavior is commonly associated with damage to the orbital area, which is thought to result in disruption of frontolimbic connections. Disinhibited personality changes, amnesia with confabulation, and failure on neuropsychological tests of inhibition are signs of orbitofrontal damage (Malloy et al., 1993). Lesions of this subsystem result in disruption of inhibitory and emotional mechanisms, with consequent impulsive and socially inappropriate behavior. A patient may be aware that a particular behavior is inappropriate, but may still be unable to inhibit the behavior. Disorders of emotional reactivity can include emotional incontinence, mood lability, and irritability, culminating in situationally inappropriate reactions. Disinhibition can also result in "stimulus-bound behavior," in which the patient is unable to control the attentional "pull" to a stimulus. The patient may also exhibit increased distractibility by irrelevant stimuli, paralleled by diminished sustained attention.

Disinhibition is perhaps most disruptive and embarrassing to the patient's caregiver, particularly because the patient often lacks insight into the inappropriateness of the behavior. Some family members may be confused and disturbed by a patient's sudden irritability and insensitivity towards them, in contrast to their previous mild-mannered personality. Unfortunately, this behavior can sometimes be misinterpreted as intentionally provocative and malicious.

APATHETIC/AKINETIC SYNDROME

Akinetic syndromes most often result from damage to the mesial cingulate-supplementary motor system subserving drive and motivation. Lesions to the anterior cingulate gyrus can result in *akinetic mutism,* in which the patient fails to respond to environmental stimuli and remains inert. Bilateral lesions frequently result in persistent akinesia, whereas unilateral lesions produce typically transient akinetic symptoms. Lesions to the supplementary motor area and corpus callosum can result in "alien hand syndrome" in which the patient may seize objects, throw things, or otherwise explore the environment in a disinhibited fashion (typically with the non-dominant hand) (Goldberg & Bloom, 1990). The patient may report having no control over movements of the hand. Such behavior is likely attributable to initiation of action by the right hemisphere while disconnected from the verbal left hemisphere.

Diminished responsiveness can manifest itself in problems with initiating or persisting in behavior, without reaching the severity of akinetic mutism. Patients with frontal lobe damage may often begin a task correctly, but then stop prior to completion, requiring repeated prompts from the examiner to continue. *Impersistence* refers to the failure to maintain a particular response despite reinforcement, feedback, cues, or other signals indicating that additional responses are necessary. The patient may be described as not "following through" with chores or tasks at work.

Flat or diminished affect may be seen. Some patients become docile, apathetic, abulic, or even akinetic. Patients may have lowered responsiveness to environmental triggers, or may have a preserved motivation to act, but be unable to organize these impulses into directed drives, action plans, or response sequences. Such changes often lead to profound disruption of interpersonal relationships.

ADDITIONAL BEHAVIORAL FINDINGS

Anosognosia and neglect are other common behavioral features. *Anosognosia* refers to patients' lack of awareness, or disregard, of their deficits. Patients with frontal dysfunction vary in their degree of awareness of their deficit. Such deficits can profoundly affect treatment and responsiveness to rehabilitative efforts. *Neglect* is the inability to attend to a particular aspect of one's environment. Neglect can be specific to a body part or space, and has been reported in association with right dorsolateral prefrontal and anterior cingulate lesions in humans (Heilman & Valenstein, 1972).

Environmental dependency is a syndrome in which the patient responds in a habitual or perseverative way to stimuli in the surrounding area, without regard to the necessity or appropriateness of the response. *Utilization behavior* is a subtype of environmental dependency in which the patient uses encountered objects without a specific goal or need (e.g., donning a stethoscope left on the table in the examination room). Environmental dependency has been conceptualized as the release of parietal lobe exploratory behavior due to absence of frontal inhibition (Lhermitte, 1986). In a somewhat similar fashion, with *imitation behavior*, the patient may find it difficult to stop himself from mimicking the actions of the examiner, even when specifically instructed not to do so.

Various psychiatric symptoms can also emerge. Patients with frontal lobe damage are at greater risk to develop disturbances of mood and affective expression, ranging from intermittent mood lability to major depression or mania (Mayberg, 1994; Robinson et al., 1988). The challenge for the clinician is to differentiate these possible affective disturbances from the frontal lobe syndromes of apathy and disinhibition. Damage to structures functionally connected to the orbitofrontal cortex, mainly in the right hemisphere, seems to be associated with secondary mania in traumatic brain injury (Starkstein et al., 1988). New onset of anxiety disorders, personality disorders, sexual dysfunction, and obsessive-compulsive disorder have also been reported after closed head injury (Max et al., 1995; van Reekum et al., 1996; Bryant & Harvey, 1998).

DISEASE FOCUS: FRONTOTEMPORAL DEMENTIA

Frontotemporal dementia (FTD) is a neurodegenerative disease characterized by progressive atrophy of the frontal and anterior temporal lobes. FTD can present with several distinct clinical syndromes involving disturbances in personality, judgement and insight, and/or language function (Gorno-Tempini et al., 2011; Rascovsky et al., 2011). Roughly 15% of all patients with dementia carry a diagnosis of FTD; among patients under 65 years old, it has been estimated that FTD is as common as Alzheimer's disease (Rascovsky et al., 2005). Current classification comprises a behavioral variant (bvFTD), which accounts for roughly 50% of FTD cases, and two language subtypes. This disease has proven to be a heartbreaking demonstration of the profound disabilities rendered by progressive dissolution of frontal systems. Patients can present with insidious onset of abnormal social behaviors, including poor hygiene, inappropriate remarks, increased risk-taking (gambling, stealing, speeding), diminished social engagement, and ritualistic behaviors. Involvement of the insula is thought to account in part for dietary changes such as binge eating. Language disturbances related to frontal lobe atrophy include speech apraxia and agrammatism.

ASSESSMENT OF FRONTAL SYSTEMS

This section provides a brief overview of clinical assessment techniques for evaluating patients with frontal lobe syndromes. The interested reader is referred to more comprehensive articles on assessment such as those by Levin and Malloy (Levin & Kraus, 1994; Malloy & Richardson, 1994).

The clinical interview can provide a great deal of information about the integrity of frontal systems. A relatively unstructured initial interview may be very useful in eliciting abnormal behaviors such as reduced initiative and drive, poor insight into deficits, inappropriate social behavior, environmental dependency, poor self-monitoring of errors, and labile affect. A disinhibited personality may become apparent during the interview, with the patient interrupting with inappropriate questions or intrusive comments. The patient may be distracted by extraneous stimuli in the environment, or require repeated reminders to answer a specific question, because of either off-topic remarks or lack of response.

The examiner should pay particular attention to discrepancies between patients' and caregivers' reports of problems. An important caveat is that some patients respond well to the formal clinical setting, and may perform well in such a structured environment; the family's description of the patient's daily behavior in various daily social settings provides valuable insight. Obtaining a comprehensive history from a close informant is essential, as the patient may be unable to recount the complete history of events or to provide a valid report of behavioral changes. Asking specifically about risky and inappropriate behaviors such as gambling or sexual exploits is also important, as families are sometimes reluctant to volunteer such information, or do not realize that it is relevant.

Physical appearance may provide the clinician with some information about a patient's executive functioning and reflective insight. For example, patients may wear clothes that are mismatched or inappropriate for the season, neglect personal hygiene, or show no concern over incontinence. Some patients may develop perseverative or stereotyped behaviors, such as finger tapping, pacing, or phrase repetition. Altered food preferences and binge eating may lead to significant weight gain; some patients may attempt to consume non-food items.

Neurological assessment, including the elicitation of "frontal release signs" (e.g., grasp, snout, palmomental), can be useful for the assessment of frontal lobe dysfunction. The presence of these "primitive" reflexes may be an indication that motor/premotor portions of the frontal lobe have been damaged; however, these reflexes can often be seen in elderly individuals without neurological disease (Tweedy et al., 1982). Patients may have difficulty initiating or inhibiting eye movements towards a target, or sustaining fixation; frontal eye fields in particular are implicated in antisaccade abilities (Everling et al., 1998). Basic language assessment of patients with frontal lobe dysfunction can reveal dysarthria, grammatical errors in production and comprehension, and variable but effortful production of speech sounds and prosody (speech apraxia), especially with increasing articulatory complexity (Brazis et al., 2007).

Difficulties with motor programming can be observed with motor impersistence (e.g., unable to keep eyes closed or tongue protruded for 10 seconds), gait disturbance (e.g., initiation and continued ambulation, foot elevation and forward propulsion), despite the preservation of isolated components of the motor sequence. Patients may have difficulty coordinating bimanual movements, or inhibiting movements of the contralateral limb. Traditional motor assessment often includes Luria sequencing (three meaningless hand movements performed in sequence) and ramparts drawing (see Figure 46.1a), which are often useful means of assessing patients with diffuse brain damage, as the demand on language comprehension is minimal. Frontal system dysfunction errors on these tasks include perseveration and pull to stimulus (e.g., grasping at the examiner's hands, or copying directly over a figure; see Figure 46.1b).

Although a formal mental status examination may provide additional useful information, the bedside evaluation of frontal dysfunction should not be limited to such instruments. Measures such as the Mini-Mental State Examination (MMSE) have been shown to be inadequate and inexact for assessment of frontal/executive abilities (Malloy et al., 1998; Royall et al., 1992). It is also important to recognize that large frontal lesions may be relatively clinically silent, and only revealed with skilled evaluation, including a detailed history of social and interpersonal changes.

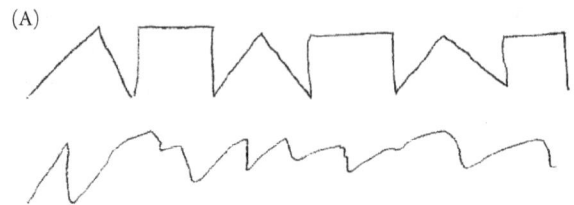

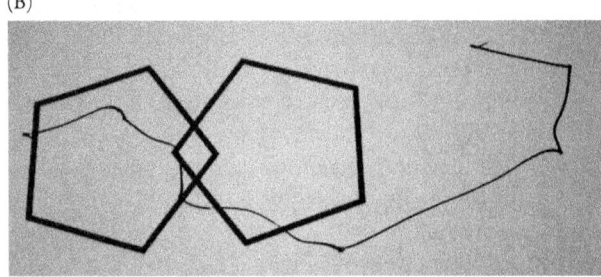

Figure 46.1 Examples of frontal-system errors on ramparts drawing (A), demonstrating set loss, and figure copying (B), demonstrating pull to stimulus.

Tests commonly used by neuropsychologists to evaluate the integrity of frontal systems include the Controlled Oral Word Association test (COWA) (Benton, 1968), which requires the patient to produce as many words as possible in one minute beginning with specified letters. This task requires multiple-response generation as well as maintenance of a complex task set, and permits the examiner to observe perseverative and intrusive response styles. The Stroop Test, requiring the patient to name the color of the ink in which color names are printed, measures selective attention and cognitive flexibility, and gives information about the patient's ability to inhibit a habitual response (Golden, 1976). These tests represent only a few of the numerous tests available to neuropsychologists in the assessment of frontal systems. More detailed description of the neuropsychological assessment can be found in Chapter <<??>>.

Neuroimaging can be extremely useful in determining the location and extent of frontal damage. A brief overview is offered here regarding imaging techniques that would be most commonly encountered in the clinical setting; technical capabilities, especially in structural and functional MRI, are rapidly expanding. Computed tomography (CT) scan may be the first structural imaging method employed, as it is typically easily tolerated and is usually adequate for the detection of large contusions, hemorrhage, hydrocephalus, and projectile wounds. Metal artifacts may obscure specific structures, however, and the resolution of routine clinical CT scans limits detection of small lesions and subtler atrophy patterns.

Diffuse axonal injuries, for example, are better seen on T2-weighted MRI scans as small areas of hyperintensity in the cerebral white matter. Diffusion tensor imaging is emerging as a specific MR sequence for assessment of white matter tract integrity. MRI is superior in detecting cerebral edema as well as earlier detection of ischemic injury and malignancies (the latter with contrast media). MRI is also superior in imaging lesions close to bone (e.g., orbitofrontal areas) due to beam-hardening artifact on CT scan.

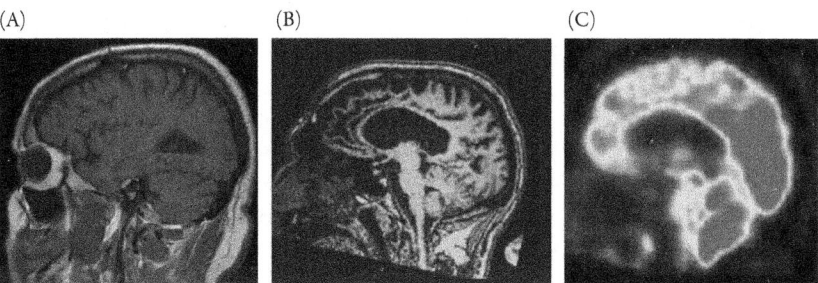

Figure 46.2 Structural (MR) and functional (PET) imaging findings in a patient with frontotemporal dementia, with sagittal views of focal frontal atrophy (B) and hypometabolism (C), respectively, in comparison to a healthy individual (A).

In addition to the structural findings on CT and MRI (compare the brain MRI of a healthy individual (Figure 46.2a) to the profound frontal lobe atrophy of an individual with FTD (Figure 46.2b)), functional imaging scans such as single-photon emission computed tomography (SPECT) and positron emission tomography (PET) can provide important diagnostic insights. Each of these technologies requires administration of a radioactively tagged nucleotide. Spatial resolution is superior with PET, but SPECT radiotracers typically have longer half-lives and thus may be more readily accessible in the clinical setting (Wahl et al., 2011). Relevant findings on these scans include increased tracer uptake in tumors, regional hypometabolism in neurodegenerative diseases (see Figure 46.2c for an illustration of frontal lobe hypometabolism in a patient with FTD), and peri-ictal hyperperfusion in focal epilepsy.

Additional clinical assessment may include laboratory testing for suspected toxic or disease exposure. Patients suspected of obstructive sleep apnea or other sleep disorders should undergo a polysomnogram. Electroencephalogram (EEG) is indispensable in the work-up of suspected seizures; frontal lobe seizures in particular have a heterogeneous semiology, including fencing posture, pelvic thrusting, motor automatisms, olfactory hallucinations, speech arrest, bipedal movements, and urinary incontinence (O'Muircheartaigh & Richardson, 2012).

TREATMENT STRATEGIES

Treatments have primarily been aimed at reducing undesirable or disruptive behaviors, based on hypotheses about underlying neurophysiological substrates.

PHARMACOLOGICAL TREATMENT

The treatment of behavioral, emotional, and cognitive disturbances in frontal systems dysfunction can be complicated by the abnormal condition of the tissues that are the targets of pharmacological interventions. Damaged brain tissue may disrupt circuits necessary not just for normal functioning, but also for normal responses to medication. Additionally, thorough and ongoing review of the patient's medications is necessary to ensure that substances that can contribute to cognitive dysfunction are eliminated. Targeted neurotransmitter enhancements include norepinephrine for arousal, dopamine

for motivation and working memory, and acetylcholine for attention (Daffner & Wolk, 2010). The clinician must be careful to distinguish between behavioral symptomatology and mood disorders in order to direct treatment appropriately.

AGGRESSION AND IMPULSIVITY

Inappropriate jocularity, disinhibition, and aggression may result from a decreased ability to recognize and respond appropriately to social cues. In addition, such behaviors may be the secondary products of depression, mania, anxiety, or psychosis. The clinician must determine the origin of the disturbed behavior and intervene accordingly. Beta blockers, usually in high dose ranges, have proven effective, although onset of action may be delayed. Valproic acid can also be helpful, and often is well tolerated; it has been shown to be effective in reducing destructive and aggressive behaviors in patients with brain injury and dementia, although results are mixed and side effects such as over-sedation and lightheadedness can occur (Dolder & McKinsey, 2010; Wroblewski et al., 1993). Selective serotonin-reuptake inhibitors (SSRIs) can be helpful in neurodegenerative conditions such as FTD (Vossel & Miller, 2008); conversely, cholinesterase inhibitors may exacerbate disinhibition, irritability, and impulsivity in FTD (Mendez et al., 2007).

DEPRESSION AND MANIA

The choice of agent is guided mainly by side effects and the particular neurological susceptibilities of the patient in question. Depression may respond to SSRIs, and mood lability may respond well to mood stabilizers such as lithium, carbamazepine, and sodium valproate (Sloan et al., 1992; Wroblewski et al., 1996). Mania in patients with traumatic brain injury (TBI) has been successfully treated with lithium carbonate, carbamazepine, valproic acid, clonidine, and electroconvulsive therapy (ECT). Lithium management requires careful oversight; the risks of confusion, nausea, tremor, ataxia, and lethargy in a patient with frontal system dysfunction are worth considering carefully (Brown & Stoudemire, 1998; Schiff et al., 1982). Lithium may also lower the seizure threshold (Massey & Folger, 1984). Under controlled circumstances in which the drug may be reliably administered and serum levels monitored closely, lithium can prove quite effective for behavioral problems, but benefits should be weighed against the risk of an exacerbation of cognitive dysfunction.

ATTENTION AND AROUSAL

Patients with frontal lobe syndrome can display severe decrements in arousal, energy, and motivation. Apathy may become pathological, and can interfere with attempts at rehabilitation. It has been hypothesized that such apathetic behaviors result from dysfunction of the mesolimbic/mesocortical dopamine projections to the frontal lobes. Hence, pharmacotherapy for patients with decreased energy and motivation has frequently involved the use of dopamine-system–enhancing agents such as bromocriptine and pramipexole. Amantadine, an N-methyl-D-aspartate (NMDA) receptor antagonist, may also enhance dopaminergic systems via indirect mechanisms; a recent study in patients with severe, non-penetrating TBI and prolonged disturbances in level of consciousness suggests that amantadine may increase the rate of behavioral recovery (Giacino et al., 2012). One potential consequence of using dopamine agonists in this patient population, however, is a risk of developing psychosis or other hypervigilant states (Gualtieri & Evans, 1988). Therefore, these medications should be administered with careful dose escalation and monitoring for emergent psychotic behavior.

Additional problems include disruptions of impulsivity, disinhibition, and planning, and it has been theorized that dopaminergic agents may be useful in minimizing these behavioral disturbances and in improving attention span and information processing speed. At least some studies have reported positive effects on cognitive functioning with dopaminergic agents (Kraus & Maki, 1997a, 1997b).

Some studies have found that stimulant medications, such as methylphenidate and dextroamphetamine, result in improved cognitive functioning (Gualtieri & Evans, 1988; Wroblewski, 1993), although findings have been mixed (Speech et al., 1993). Modafinil is a newer agent with a different (and incompletely understood) mechanism of action, and may be better tolerated.

Acetylcholine is known to play a role in attentional systems, although the precise mechanisms remain unclear (Furey et al., 2008; Taverni et al., 1998), and studies involving cholinesterase inhibitors such as donepezil or rivastigmine have produced mixed results. Patients with multiple sclerosis often complain of cognitive fatigue and have difficulties with tasks requiring sustained attention (Kujala et al., 1995), and a recent study investigating administration of rivastigmine showed improvement in processing speed (Huolman et al., 2011). Anticholinergic agents such as bladder antispasmodics may exacerbate cognitive impairments and should be carefully screened for in medication review.

BEHAVIORAL TREATMENT

Sohlberg and colleagues (Sohlberg et al., 1993) have presented a model for rehabilitation following TBI that provides a theoretical framework for understanding the patient's executive deficits. These authors also identify intervention options for managing executive dysfunction and provide decision rules for selecting the most appropriate interventions for these patients. Briefly, their treatment model includes environmental modification (e.g., labeling cupboard contents and organizing physical space), specific skill training (e.g., using a written or computerized organizational system), communication skills (e.g., turn taking), overtraining task-specific routines (e.g., grooming), external compensatory training (e.g., organizational or memory books), and training in metacognitive skills. Sohlberg's work represents a pioneering effort in devising a behavioral treatment program for patients with frontal lobe injuries secondary to TBI.

Socially inappropriate or disruptive behaviors may respond well to behavior modification techniques such as *response cost* and *differential reinforcement of other behaviors* (DRO). Response cost involves defining situations in which certain responses will cost the patient opportunities for other reinforcers. For example, "If you interrupt other group members during meeting, you will not be allowed to watch television in the afternoon." DRO involves positively reinforcing an alternative, appropriate behavior. Differential reinforcement can be geared towards any other behavior that takes up time (e.g., any interaction with a stranger that is not sexual), a specific alternative behavior (e.g., shaking hands with a stranger), or an incompatible behavior (e.g., not speaking with the stranger). It is generally most practical to first use behavioral modification for those with disinhibitory behavior, and apply specific cognitive rehabilitation techniques to those with obvious specific deficits after problem behaviors have decreased. There is some evidence that cognitive-behavioral interventions, at least in patients with mild TBI, can shorten the duration of symptoms following injury (Mittenberg et al., 1996).

Behavioral interventions include the development of compensatory strategies and the manipulation of the patient's environment in an attempt to reduce unwanted behaviors and shape more desirable ones. These techniques can be helpful not only in eliminating problem behaviors but also in reducing caregiver burden. Many patients find comfort in daily routines; indeed, disruption can lead to behavioral outbursts. If the cognitive impairment or behavioral issues necessitate institutionalization, the family may be pleasantly relieved to find that the patient is much more at ease in the standardized predictability.

ENVIRONMENTAL INTERVENTIONS

Clinicians have also devised interventions based on the knowledge that patients with frontal systems dysfunction tend to respond impulsively in many situations and fail on tasks when working memory is taxed. Clinicians can restructure the environment to provide salient operant cues and greater external executive control, and work with patients on overlearning adaptive responses so they have a high probability of occurring in problem situations. External or environmental interventions can be particularly effective with severely impaired patients who cannot benefit from cognitive retraining. An example of a simple environmental intervention would be setting a timer alarm on an electronic watch as a reminder to check an assignment book.

With recent advances in technology, there has been a proliferation of rehabilitative devices and technologies. Such developments include computer-assisted cognitive rehabilitation (Chen et al., 1997), electronic reminder devices for patients with planning and organizational disabilities secondary to frontal lobe damage (Wilson et al., 1997), and telephone intervention and follow-up (Dombovy & Olek, 1997). Microcomputer devices show great promise as executive prosthetic devices, which can provide the organization and self-monitoring skills that many frontal patients lack. Chute and colleagues have done extensive work on computerized speech devices and computer-controlled household devices (Chute, 2002). For example, a computer attached to a wheelchair can provide synthetic speech cues to guide patients through a task step-by-step, prompting them to check the correctness of each response against a model. Unfortunately, little research has been conducted in the area of executive prosthetics, and user-friendly interfaces are still lacking.

LEGAL IMPLICATIONS AND CAREGIVER BURDEN

As described above, patients with frontal lobe disorders are often unaware of their deficits. Additionally, even when help is offered, patients may either not understand why it is necessary, or may outright refuse intervention. Some patients only come to medical attention after breaking the law, such as with reckless driving or illicit drug use. Families may become bankrupt if the patient makes impulsive or irrational decisions with investments. Decision-making competence entails an ability to understand the situation at hand and the implications of the consequences, and to behave according to the expressed reasoning behind a decision. Impaired decision-making can lead to life-threatening situations, as illustrated by the following story: a patient with bvFTD was speaking with her husband on the phone, and he heard an alarm in the background. When he asked her what the sound was, she reported that the fire alarm was going off; he had to instruct her to leave the house (which unfortunately burned to the ground). The fire had been set by her cigarette, as she had been compulsively smoking. Standardized tests such as the MMSE often do not capture executive dysfunction, and thus the clinician must be attuned to the appropriate assessment of such impairments.

CLINICAL PEARLS

• Patients with frontal lobe damage may often begin a task correctly, but then stop prior to completion, requiring repeated prompts from the examiner to continue. *Impersistence* refers to the failure to maintain a particular response despite reinforcement.

• In frontotemporal dementia (FTD), patients can present with insidious onset of abnormal social behaviors, including poor hygiene, inappropriate remarks, increased risk-taking (gambling, stealing, speeding), diminished social engagement, and ritualistic behaviors.

• *Anosognosia* refers to patients' lack of awareness or disregard of their deficits. Patients with frontal dysfunction vary in their degree of awareness of their deficit. Such deficits can profoundly affect treatment and responsiveness to rehabilitative efforts.

• Clinicians can restructure the environment to provide salient operant cues and greater external executive control, and work with patients on overlearning adaptive responses so they have a high probability of occurring in problem situations.

DISCLOSURE STATEMENTS

This chapter is a modification of Chapter 41, "Frontal Lobe Syndromes and Traumatic Brain Injury," by Paul Malloy, Deborah Cahn-Weiner, and Thomas Markham Brown, from *Psychiatric Care of the Medical Patient*, Second Edition.

Dr. Domoto-Reilly has nothing to disclose.

Dr. Malloy

Dr. Cahn-Weiner

Dr. Brown

REFERENCES

Benton, A. (1968). Differential behavioral effects in frontal lobe disease. *Neuropsychologia, 6,* 53–60.

Brazis, P. W., Masdeau, J. C., & Biller, J. (2007). *Localization in Clinical Neurology* (5th ed.). Philadelphia, PA: Lippincott Williams & Wilkins.

Brown, T. M., & Stoudemire, A. (1998). *Psychiatric side effects of prescription and over-the-counter medications: Recognition and management* (1st ed.). Washington, DC: American Psychiatric Press.

Chen, S. H., Thomas, J. D., Glueckauf, R. L., & Bracy, O. L. (1997). The effectiveness of computer-assisted cognitive rehabilitation for persons with traumatic brain injury. *Brain Injury, 11*(3), 197–209.

Chute, D. L. (2002). Neuropsychological technologies in rehabilitation. *Journal of Head Trauma Rehabilitation, 17*(5), 369–377.

Craig, A. D. (2009). How do you feel—now? The anterior insula and human awareness. *Nature Reviews Neuroscience, 10*(1), 59–70.

Cummings, J. L. (1993). Frontal-subcortical circuits and human behavior. *Archives of Neurology, 50*(8), 873–880.

D'Esposito, M., & Gazzaley, A. (2011). Can age-associated memory decline be treated? *New England Journal of Medicine, 365,* 1346–1347.

Daffner, K. R., & Wolk, D. A. (2010). Behavioral neurology and dementia. In M. A. Samuels & A. H. Ropper (Eds.), *Samuels's manual of neurologic therapeutics* (3rd ed.; 418–457). Philadelphia, PA: Lippincott Williams & Wilkins.

Dolder, C., & McKinsey, J. (2010). Low-dose divalproex in agitated patients with Alzheimer's disease. *Journal of Psychiatric Practice, 16*(1), 63–67.

Dombovy, M. L., & Olek, A. C. (1997). Recovery and rehabilitation following traumatic brain injury. *Brain Injury, 11*(5), 305–318.

Everling, S., & Fischer, B. (1998). The antisaccade: A review of basic research and clinical studies. *Neuropsychologia, 36,* 885–899.

Furey, M. L., Pietrini, P., Haxby, J. V., & Drevets, W. C. (2008). Selective effects of cholinergic modulation on task performance during selective attention. *Neuropsychopharmacology, 33*(4), 913–923.

Giacino, J. T., Whyte, J., Bagiella, E., Kalmar, K., Childs, N., Khademi, A., et al. (2012). Placebo-controlled trial of amantadine for severe traumatic brain injury. *New England Journal of Medicine, 366*(9), 819–826.

Goldberg, G., & Bloom, K. K. (1990). The alien hand sign. Localization, lateralization and recovery. *American Journal of Physical Medicine & Rehabilitation, 69*(5), 228–238.

Goldberg, T. E., Berman, K. F., Mohr, E., & Weinberger, D. R. (1990). Regional cerebral blood flow and cognitive function in Huntington's disease and schizophrenia. A comparison of patients matched for performance on a prefrontal-type task. *Archives of Neurology, 47*(4), 418–422.

Golden, C. J. (1976). Identification of brain disorders by the Stroop Color and Word Test. *Journal of Clinical Psychology, 32*(3), 654–658.

Gorno-Tempini, M. L., Hillis, A. E., Weintraub, S., Kertesz, A., Mendez, M., Cappa, S. F., et al. (2011). Classification of primary progressive aphasia and its variants. *Neurology, 76*(11), 1006–1014.

Gotham, A. M., Brown, R. G., & Marsden, C. D. (1988). "Frontal" cognitive function in patients with Parkinson's disease "on" and "off" levodopa. *Brain, 111*(Pt 2), 299–321.

Gualtieri, C. T., & Evans, R. W. (1988). Stimulant treatment for the neurobehavioural sequelae of traumatic brain injury. *Brain Injury, 2*(4), 273–290.

Harvey, A. G., & Bryant, R. A. (1998). Acute stress disorder after mild traumatic brain injury. *Journal of Nervous & Mental Disease, 186*(6), 333–337.

Heilman, K. M., & Valenstein, E. (1972). Frontal lobe neglect in man. *Neurology, 22*(6), 660–664.

Huolman, S., Hämäläinen, P., Vorobyev, V., Ruutiainen, J., Parkkola, R., Laine, T., et al. (2011). The effects of rivastigmine on processing speed and brain activation in patients with multiple sclerosis and subjective cognitive fatigue. *Multiple Sclerosis*, Nov., *17*(11), 1351–1361.

Kraus, M. F., & Maki, P. M. (1997a). The combined use of amantadine and l-dopa/carbidopa in the treatment of chronic brain injury. *Brain Injury, 11*(6), 455–460.

Kraus, M. F., & Maki, P. M. (1997b). Effect of amantadine hydrochloride on symptoms of frontal lobe dysfunction in brain injury: case studies and review. *Journal of Psychiatry and Clinical Neuroscience, 9*(2), 222–230.

Kujala, P., Portin, R., Revonsuo, A., & Ruutiainen, J. (1995). Attention related performance in two cognitively different subgroups of patients with multiple sclerosis. *Journal of Neurology, Neurosurgery & Psychiatry, 59*(1), 77–82.

Levin, H., & Kraus, M. F. (1994). The frontal lobes and traumatic brain injury. *Journal of Psychiatry and Clinical Neuroscience, 6*(4), 443–454.

Lhermitte, F. (1986). Human autonomy and the frontal lobes. Part II: Patient behavior in complex and social situations: The "environmental dependency syndrome." *Annals of Neurology, 19*(4), 335–343.

Luria, A. R. (1980). *Higher cortical functions in man* (1st ed.). New York: Basic Books.

Malloy, P. F., & Aloia, M. (1998). Frontal lobe dysfunction in traumatic brain injury. *Seminars in Clinical Neuropsychiatry, 3*(3), 186–194.

Malloy, P. F., & Richardson, E. D. (1994). Assessment of frontal lobe functions. *Journal of Psychiatry and Clinical Neuroscience, 6*(4), 399–410.

Malloy, P., Bihrle, A., Duffy, J., & Cimino, C. (1993). The orbitomedial frontal syndrome. *Archives of Clinical Neuropsychology*, May, *8*(3), 185–201.

Massey, E. W., & Folger, W. N. (1984). Seizures activated by therapeutic levels of lithium carbonate. *Southern Medical Journal, 77*(9), 1173–1175.

Max, J. E., Smith, W. L. Jr., Lindgren, S. D., Robin, D. A., Mattheis, P., Stierwalt, J., et al. (1995). Case study: obsessive-compulsive disorder after severe traumatic brain injury in an adolescent. *Journal of the American Academy of Child & Adolescent Psychiatry, 34*(1), 45–49.

Mayberg, H. S. (1994). Frontal lobe dysfunction in secondary depression. *Journal of Psychiatry and Clinical Neuroscience, 6*(4), 428–442.

Mendez, M. F., Shapira, J. S., McMurtray, A., & Licht, E. (2007). Preliminary findings: behavioral worsening on donepezil in patients with frontotemporal dementia. *American Journal of Geriatric Psychiatry, 15*(1), 84–87.

Mittenberg, W., Tremont, G., Zielinski, R. E., Fichera, S., & Rayls, K. R. (1996). Cognitive-behavioral prevention of postconcussion syndrome. *Archives of Clinical Neuropsychology, 11*(2), 139–145.

O'Muircheartaigh, J., & Richardson, M. P. (2012). Epilepsy and the frontal lobes. *Cortex, 48*(2), 144–155.

Parkin, A. J., & Walter, B. M. (1992). Recollective experience, normal aging, and frontal dysfunction. *Psychology and Aging, 7*(2), 290–298.

Prakash, R. S., Erickson, K. I., Colcombe, S. J., Kim, J. S., Voss, M. W., & Kramer, A. F. (2009). Age-related differences in the involvement of the prefrontal cortex in attentional control. *Brain and Cognition, 71*(3), 328–335.

Rascovsky, K., Hodges, J. R., Knopman, D., Mendez, M. F., Kramer, J. H., Neuhaus, J., et al. (2011). Sensitivity of revised diagnostic criteria for the behavioural variant of frontotemporal dementia. *Brain, 134*(Pt 9), 2456–2477.

Rascovsky, K., Salmon, D. P., Lipton, A. M., Leverenz, J. B., DeCarli, C., Jagust, W. J., et al. (2005). Rate of progression differs in frontotemporal dementia and Alzheimer disease. *Neurology, 65*(3), 397–403.

Robinson, R. G., Boston, J. D., Starkstein, S. E., & Price, T. R. (1988). Comparison of mania and depression after brain injury: Causal factors. *American Journal of Psychiatry, 145*(2), 172–178.

Royall, D. R., Mahurin, R. K., & Gray, K. F. (1992). Bedside assessment of executive cognitive impairment: The executive interview. *Journal of the American Geriatric Society, 40*(12), 1221–1226.

Schiff, H. B., Sabin, T. D., Geller, A., Alexander, L., & Mark, V. (1982). Lithium in aggressive behavior. *American Journal of Psychiatry, 139*(10), 1346–1348.

Sloan, R. L., Brown, K. W., & Pentland, B. (1992). Fluoxetine as a treatment for emotional lability after brain injury. *Brain Injury, 6*(4), 315–319.

Sohlberg, M. M., Mateer, C. A., & Stuss, D. T. (1993). Contemporary approaches to the management of executive control dysfunction. *Journal of Head Trauma Rehabilitation, 8*, 45–58.

Speech, T. J., Rao, S. M., Osmon, D. C., & Sperry, L. T. (1993). A double-blind controlled study of methylphenidate treatment in closed head injury. *Brain Injury, 7*(4), 333–338.

Starkstein, S. E., Boston, J. D., & Robinson, R. G. (1988). Mechanisms of mania after brain injury. 12 case reports and review of the literature. *Journal of Nervous & Mental Disease, 176*(2), 87–100.

Stuss, D. T. (1993). Assessment of neuropsychological dysfunction in frontal lobe degeneration. *Dementia, 4*(3–4), 220–225.

Taverni, J. P., Seliger, G., & Lichtman, S. W. (1998). Donepezil medicated memory improvement in traumatic brain injury during post acute rehabilitation. *Brain Injury, 12*(1), 77–80.

Tweedy, J., Reding, M., Garcia, C., Schulman, P., Deutsch, G., & Antin, S. (1982). Significance of cortical disinhibition signs. *Neurology, 32*(2), 169–173.

van Reekum, R., Bolago, I., Finlayson, M. A., Garner, S., & Links, P. S. (1996). Psychiatric disorders after traumatic brain injury. *Brain Injury, 10*(5), 319–327.

Vilkki, J. (1989). Perseveration in memory for figures after frontal lobe lesion. *Neuropsychologia, 27*(8), 1101–1104.

Vossel, K. A., & Miller, B. L. (2008). New approaches to the treatment of frontotemporal lobar degeneration. *Current Opinion in Neurology, 21*(6), 708–716.

Wahl, R. L., Herman, J. M., & Ford, E. (2011). The promise and pitfalls of positron emission tomography and single-photon emission computed tomography molecular imaging-guided radiation therapy. *Seminars in Radiation Oncology, 21*(2), 88–100.

Wilson, B. A., Evans, J. J., Emslie, H., & Malinek, V. (1997). Evaluation of NeuroPage: A new memory aid. *Journal of Neurology, Neurosurgery, & Psychiatry, 63*(1), 113–115.

Wroblewski, B. (1993). Use of anticonvulsants in traumatic brain injury. *Archives of Physical Medicine & Rehabilitation, 74*(2), 224–225.

Wroblewski, B. A., Joseph, A. B., & Cornblatt, R. R. (1996). Antidepressant pharmacotherapy and the treatment of depression in patients with severe traumatic brain injury: A controlled, prospective study. *Journal of Clinical Psychiatry, 57*(12), 582–587.

47.

MOVEMENT DISORDERS

Shreya Raj and Jeremiah M. Scharf

INTRODUCTION

The basal ganglia are composed of deep subcortical nuclei (caudate, putamen, globus pallidus, subthalamic nucleus, substantia nigra, nucleus accumbens, and extended amygdala) that participate in action selection and reinforcement learning. Disorders of basal ganglia circuits are classically defined based on resulting motor output, where disruptions cause either too little movement (hypokinetic disorders, e.g., Parkinsonism) or too much movement (hyperkinetic disorders, e.g., chorea, dystonia, myoclonus, and tics) (Albin, Young, & Penney, 1989). For many years, movement disorders were thought to be entirely motor phenomena; however, it is now known that the basal ganglia also mediate selection and regulation of cognitive, behavioral, and affective processes via parallel loops of cortico-striato-thalamo-cortical (CSTC) circuits (Alexander, DeLong, & Strick, 1986). Subsequently, clinical researchers have demonstrated that disorders arising from basal ganglia dysfunction have cognitive, behavioral, and affective symptoms that parallel their motor abnormalities. Until recently, these symptoms have been overlooked, but they can often cause significant morbidity unless treated. In this chapter, we highlight psychiatric features of three paradigmatic basal ganglia disorders (Huntington disease, Parkinson disease, Tourette syndrome); however, any neurological or systemic conditions that affect basal ganglia function (e.g., focal stroke, trauma, infection, neoplasm, toxic/metabolic injury, endocrine disturbances) will also cause psychiatric disturbances that require evaluation and treatment.

HUNTINGTON DISEASE

Huntington disease (HD) is a progressive, inherited neuropsychiatric illness with characteristic motor, cognitive, and psychiatric dysfunction. It has a prevalence of 4 to 10 per 100,000 in populations of European ancestry, and equal rates among men and women (Ross & Tabrizi, 2011). The mean age of onset is approximately 40 years old, and death typically occurs 15 to 20 years after diagnosis. However, there is a juvenile form, the Westphal variant, which is associated with slowed movements, rigidity, dystonia, myoclonus, seizures, and a more rapidly progressive course.

ETIOLOGY

HD is an autosomal dominant genetic disorder caused by an expanded CAG trinucleotide repeat within the huntingtin (*HTT*) gene on chromosome 4. The *HTT* gene codes for the protein huntingtin, and CAG expansion results in long stretches of poly-glutamine repeats within this protein. The functions of both normal and mutant huntingtin are still unclear, though the CAG expansion appears to cause a gain-of-function toxicity to neurons that results in neurodegeneration. While unaffected individuals have up to 36 CAG repeats within the *HTT* gene, individuals with CAG repeat lengths above 36 are at risk for developing HD. People with repeat CAG lengths of 36 to 39 may or may not develop HD, whereas individuals with 40 or more will almost certainly develop the disease by age 65. In general, longer CAG repeat lengths are associated with earlier disease onset, and also associated to a lesser degree with motor and cognitive disease progression (Rosenblatt et al., 2012). However, neither the type nor the severity of associated behavioral or psychiatric syndromes is associated with repeat codon length (Weigell-Weber, Schmid, & Spiegel, 1996; Zappacosta et al., 1996). The number of CAG repeats can increase with successive generations, resulting in an earlier age of onset in children of affected parents, a process called "genetic anticipation."

CLINICAL FEATURES

HD is characterized by symptoms in the motor, cognitive, and psychiatric domains. Disease onset is declared when motor symptoms develop. However, many patients may go through a "prodromal period," experiencing substantial cognitive or behavioral disturbances years before motor signs become evident.

MOTOR SIGNS

Motor signs can be classified as (1) involuntary movements, specifically chorea, and (2) altered voluntary movements. Chorea is commonly treated with dopamine-blocking (antipsychotic) or dopamine-depleting (tetrabenazine) drugs. Tetrabenazine is the only U.S. Food and Drug Administration (FDA) approved drug for HD, with an indication for chorea (Frank & Jankovic, 2010). Its mechanism of action is dopamine depletion at the presynaptic vesicles.

Common adverse side effects include sedation, insomnia, weight gain, depressed mood, akathisia, and Parkinsonism. All patients on tetrabenazine should be monitored for signs of depression, which can occur in 15–20% of patients on the medication (Kenney, Hunter, Mejia, & Jankovic, 2006), as well as for suicidality. Although both typical and atypical neuroleptics are also used in clinical practice, there are few double-blind, placebo-controlled studies evaluating the efficacy and safety of neuroleptic medications in HD. These medications may also cause apathy and akathisia, both of which can be difficult to distinguish from the "organic" effects of HD. Atypical antipsychotics may be better tolerated than typical neuroleptics, and small studies have looked at olanzapine, quetiapine, clozapine, and aripiprazole. Clozapine usage was complicated by drowsiness, fatigue, anticholinergic side effects, and exacerbation of gait problems. Aripiprazole was found to help with chorea at a level comparable to tetrabenazine but has not been tested in larger, randomized trials. Other medications studied for management of chorea include amantadine and benzodiazapines. Amantadine, an N-methyl-D-aspartate (NMDA)-receptor antagonist, significantly reduced chorea in one of two studies, but has been associated with increased irritability, aggression, and hallucinations (Armstrong & Miyasaki, 2012). Benzodiazepines can be helpful with anxiety and chorea, but require higher doses that risk sedation.

COGNITIVE SYMPTOMS

Cognitive symptoms in HD patients often begin before motor findings are recognized, and include impairment in memory, concentration, judgement, insight, and learning (Jason et al., 1997; Salmon, Granholm, McCullough, Butters, & Grant, 1989). HD patients characteristically describe problems with attention and executive function early in the disease (e.g., multitasking, sustained attention). A 2010 study compared 575 pre-motor HD patients to 160 non-CAG expansion controls in various neuropsychological tests of executive functioning, memory, visuospatial perception, and processing speed (Duff et al., 2010). They found approximately 40% of pre-HD individuals met criteria for mild cognitive impairment (MCI), and individuals closer to HD diagnosis had higher rates of MCI. Within this group, non-amnestic MCI was more common than amnestic MCI, and single-domain MCI was more common than multiple-domain MCI. In the non-amnestic single-domain subtype, impairments in processing speed were most frequent.

PSYCHIATRIC

There is a wide range of psychiatric syndromes found in patients with HD, which can often precede diagnosis and be a major source of functional impairment throughout the disease. In general, there is a lack of controlled clinical trials for treatment of HD-related psychiatric symptoms; thus, most recommendations come from case reports and clinician experience.

DEPRESSION

Depression is the most common psychiatric disorder in HD. A 2005 study involving 2,835 patients with an established diagnosis of HD found over 40% of subjects endorsed significant depressive symptoms, and more than half had sought treatment for depression in the past (Paulsen et al., 2005). Many studies cite a lifetime prevalence of 30–40% (Rosenblatt, 2007). Diagnosis can be complicated by the overlap between symptoms of HD and depression—namely, fatigue, cognitive problems, weight loss, and apathy.

A critical feature of depression in HD is the increased suicide rate among individuals with HD, which has been estimated to be 4 to 6 times higher than found in the general population (Roos, 2010). Suicidal behavior is likely to be impulsive, and at times may even occur in the absence of active depression. Two particularly risky times for suicide attempts are around the gene test and when increased symptom severity leads to loss of independence.

Despite the high prevalence of depression in HD, there is a general lack of controlled clinical trials to guide its treatment, and the majority of treatment recommendations come from case studies. In general, management recommendations adhere to those in non-HD depression. Selective-serotonin reuptake inhibitors (SSRI) are commonly used as first-line treatment, given the relatively benign side-effect profile and safety in overdose. One caveat is that individuals with HD tend to be more sensitive to medication side effects, so therapies should be started at low doses and titrated slowly. In addition, mediations with anticholinergic properties may worsen motor function due to changes in the dopaminergic–cholinergic balance. If trials of SSRIs are ineffective, one could consider venlafaxine or mirtazapine. Electroconvulsive therapy (ECT) is also an accepted therapy for depression in HD.

APATHY

Apathy is highly associated with HD. Unlike depression and anxiety, its progression can be related to disease stage. Apathy is so characteristic of HD that the disease has been termed the "apathetic dementia" (Burns, Folstein, Brandt, & Folstein, 1990). Inertia, lack of interest, impersistence, and lack of initiative may precede other signs by years. Progression of apathy to a terminal state of global self-neglect, inertness, and mutism may leave the patient completely inaccessible. Apathy in HD is usually attributed to the impaired arousal, attention, and concentration that mark relative disconnection of the frontal lobes and the striatum (Caine & Shoulson, 1983).

There have been no gold-standard, or even particularly efficacious, treatments identified thus far for apathy (see Chapter 34). A literature review reveals anecdotal reports about use of amantadine, amphetamines, bromocriptine, buproprion, methylphenidate, and selegiline. One could also consider non-sedating SSRIs like fluoxetine, sertraline, or citalopram. Non-pharmacological interventions include avoiding open-ended questions, providing cues, maintaining a regular schedule, increasing environmental stimulation, and limiting expectations of the patient.

IMPULSE DYSCONTROL

Irritability and aggression are also often seen in HD patients. Again, there are no controlled clinical trials to guide treatment. However, physicians use a wide variety of medication classes, including neuroleptics, mood stabilizers, and SSRIs, to manage these symptoms. Beta blockers have been used to decrease autonomic arousal. Pindolol may be better tolerated than propranolol, as the latter can cause bradycardia and hypotension (Abrahamsen, Digranes, & Gisholt, 1990).

MANIA

The lifetime prevalence estimate of mania in HD is between 5% and 10% (Rosenblatt, 2007). Mainstays of treatment are anticonvulsants or neuroleptics. Interestingly, lithium does not seem to work in HD patients; there is a poor response, and HD patients are at greater risk for lithium toxicity. Better choices may be valproate, lamotrigine, or carbamazepine (Novak & Tabrizi, 2010).

PSYCHOSIS

Psychosis can manifest as delusions or hallucinations. The most common psychotic presentation in HD is of poorly organized paranoia, and it may be considered part of executive dysfunction seen in the disease. Any sort of psychotic symptoms are usually treated with neuroleptics, and atypicals are preferred due to the more tolerable side-effect profile.

OBSESSIVE-COMPULSIVE DISORDER

Obsessive-compulsive disorder (OCD) does not have a clearly defined prevalence in HD, but studies have shown 22–50% of patients endorsing some kind of obsession or compulsion. Pharmacological agents used include SSRIs and clomipramine, while non-pharmacological behavioral management techniques utilize distraction, setting a routine, and cognitive behavioral therapy (CBT; although CBT may become impossible as cognitive dysfunction worsens).

ALCOHOLISM

Increased rates of alcoholism have been associated with HD, but most reports are methodologically flawed (Mayeux, 1984). The best studies report figures that match rates found in contemporaneous control populations (King, 1985).

PARKINSON DISEASE

There are numerous psychiatric and cognitive disturbances seen in Parkinson disease (PD). Some of the more common include depression, anxiety, apathy, psychosis, and dementia/dysexecutive syndromes. Diagnosing mood disorders in PD can be complicated by the fact that many of the disorder's cardinal features often mimic the somatic symptoms of psychiatric disorders. These include apathy, fatigue, sleep disturbances, motor slowing/retardation, weight gain/loss, and changes in appetite. Mood symptoms can also be caused or exacerbated by the dopaminergic medications commonly used for PD treatment.

DEPRESSION

In a systematic review of 36 PD studies, the average prevalence of major depressive disorder (MDD) was 17%, minor depression was 22%, and 13% of patients had dysthymia. Clinically significant depressive symptoms (irrespective of a *Diagnostic and Statistical Manual of Mental Disorders* [DSM] diagnosis) were endorsed by 35% of PD patients (Reijnders, Ehrt, Weber, Aarsland, & Leentjens, 2008). The DSM IV maintains that any symptoms associated with a "general medical condition" must be excluded when assessing for depression. However, this requirement runs the risk of missing clinically significant mood disorders that often adversely affect the lives and functionality of PD patients. In 2006, a workgroup put together by the National Institute of Neurologic Diseases and Stroke (NINDS) and National Institute of Mental Health (NIMH) recommend eliminating this DSM IV exclusion criterion in the assessing for depression in PD (Blonder & Slevin, 2011).

Risk factors for depression in PD include female sex, a personal or family history of depression, early-onset PD, "atypical" Parkinsonism, and the presence of other psychiatric comorbidities. Compared to non-PD depression, affected Parkinson's patients may have higher rates of anxiety, pessimism, and suicidal ideation, but less guilt or self-reproach (Weintraub & Burn, 2011).

There are no clear guidelines as to which treatment is most efficacious in PD depression. A National Institutes of Health (NIH)–funded eight-week, randomized, and placebo-controlled pilot study by Menza and colleagues (Menza et al., 2009) involved 52 PD patients with major depression or dysthymia. They were given paroxetine controlled release (CR), nortriptyline, or placebo. Nortriptyline was effective at reducing depressive symptoms, while paroxetine CR was not different from placebo. A randomized, placebo-controlled pilot study by Devos and colleagues (Devos et al., 2008) of 48 PD patients with major depression compared the effects of citalopram, desipramine, and placebo. The results suggested that both citalopram and desipramine were more effective than placebo at the end of the 30-day trial. Although desipramine showed a greater reduction in depressive symptoms at the study midpoint (day 14) relative to citalopram, this difference did not persist at the end of the trial, and desipramine was not as well tolerated overall, primarily due to anticholinergic side effects such as dry mouth, constipation, and orthostatic hypotension. There is still a dearth of published serotonin-norepinephrine reuptake inhibitor (SNRI) studies, although a recent NINDS-funded study comparing paroxetine and extended-release venlafaxine (Richard et al., 2012) found evidence of efficacy for both medications.

Some treatment considerations for depression in PD include the side-effect profile of various antidepressant classes. PD patients are already at risk of dysautonomic symptoms, and the anticholinergic properties of tricyclic antidepressants may exacerbate these symptoms, in particular constipation and orthostatic hypotension. In addition, anticholinergic agents can worsen cognitive impairment and predispose PD patients to delirium. In general, most treaters start with an SSRI given the relatively benign side-effect profiles and track record with non-PD patients (Blonder & Slevin, 2011), though SSRIs can worsen bradykinesia or apathy in some cases (Gerber & Lynd, 1998). Although SSRIs given in conjunction with monoamine oxidase B (MAO-B) inhibitors (such as selegiline and rasagiline) theoretically increase the risk of serotonin syndrome, in practice this is rarely observed, as there is not significant MAO-A inhibition at therapeutic doses of selective MAO-B inhibitors (Gallagher & Schrag, 2012).

ANXIETY

Up to 40% of PD patients report anxiety symptoms. In fact, anxiety disorders may predate diagnosis of a movement disorder by up to 20 years, possibly due to reduction of dopaminergic neurons in the earliest stages of the disease (Gallagher & Schrag, 2012). Commonly seen diagnoses include panic disorder, social phobia, generalized anxiety disorder, and anxiety not otherwise specified (NOS). There are correlations to the on/off phenomenon observed with the motor fluctuations; anxiety is most often associated with "off" periods. The prevalence of anxiety in PD patients exceeds that seen in both the general population and in patients with other chronic medical conditions; as such, it cannot be explained away simply as a reactive phenomenon. In addition, rates of anxiety in relatives of PD are also greater than those observed in the general population (Arabia et al., 2007). There are no systematic assessments or large placebo-controlled trials for the management of anxiety in PD. Various drug classes have been used in everyday practice, including benzodiazepines, tricyclic antidepressants (TCAs), SSRIs, atypical cyclic antidepressants (such as trazodone), non-selective monoamine oxidase inhibitors (MAOIs), and buspirone. When choosing a pharmacological strategy, the major consideration is side effects of certain medications. For example, benzodiazepines are commonly used for anxiety in the general population; in PD patients, however, their sedative and autonomic effects can be troublesome. TCAs have anticholinergic side effects that can dull cognition or exacerbate PD-associated dysautonomia. SSRIs are well tolerated and have a relatively benign side-effect profile, but there are no studies clearly demonstrating their efficacy in PD anxiety.

APATHY

Parkinsonian apathy is recognized as a distinct clinical entity from depression. It is highly prevalent in its own right, affecting up to 60% of PD patients (Gallagher & Schrag, 2012). It is generally characterized by a diminishment in goal-directed behavior, speech, and emotional engagement. Comorbidities of Parkinsonian apathy include depression, cognitive impairment, and dysexecutive syndromes. Apathy may also be associated with a more rapid progression in motor and cognitive decline (Blonder & Slevin, 2011).

In treating apathy, one should first address any depressive symptoms beforehand, as the two are so closely related. Beyond that, treatment guidelines are based on a number of case reports and smaller studies. Pharmacological agents studied include cholinesterase inhibitors, stimulants, and testosterone replacement. McKeith and colleagues performed a double-blind, placebo-controlled study that demonstrated improvement in apathy and indifference in patients with dementia with Lewy bodies (DLB) using rivastigmine (McKeith et al., 2000). In 2004, Ready and colleagues (Ready, Friedman, Grace, & Fernandez, 2004) showed a significant inverse correlation between free testosterone levels and apathy in elderly male PD patients. This was independent of disease severity, suggesting a possible role for testosterone replacement. Unfortunately, this hypothesis was not confirmed in later studies. Chatterjee and Fahn successfully alleviated apathy with methylphenidate, but this was a single case study (Chatterjee & Fahn, 2002).

PSYCHOSIS

Psychotic symptoms such as hallucinations and delusions are common in PD patients, although they tend to arise late in the course of the disease (on average, after ten years) (Zahodne & Fernandez, 2008). The estimated prevalence of visual hallucinations is 22–38%. Other examples include minor psychotic symptoms (for example, illusions of presence and visual illusions) in 17–72% and delusions in 1–7% (Gallagher & Schrag, 2012). Risk factors include cognitive impairment, age greater than 65, advanced disease status, concurrent sleep disorders or depression, and use of dopamine agonists (Eng & Welty, 2010). The first step in addressing psychotic symptoms is the reduction of any nonessential PD medications. If the patient is on multiple agents, one could try reducing or removing PD medications in the following order (from first discontinuation to last): anticholinergics, selegiline, amantadine, dopamine agonists, catechol-O-methyltransferase (COMT) inhibitors, and lastly, levodopa (Zahodne & Fernandez, 2008). Antipsychotics can be used in refractory cases. Although both quetiapine and clozapine are commonly used in practice, only the latter is recommended by the American Academy of Neurology guidelines (Miyasaki et al., 2006). These guidelines recommend avoiding olanzapine, as it has failed to show benefit, and worsened PD symptoms in some studies. Of note, PD patients can experience therapeutic benefit at clozapine doses as low as 6.25 mg/day (Zahodne & Fernandez, 2008). At higher doses, patients may experience sedation, orthostatic hypotension, and sialorrhea due to the anticholinergic effects of clozapine.

DEMENTIA/DYSEXECUTIVE SYNDROMES

Cognitive dysfunction is a frequently seen outcome in PD. Up to 80% of PD patients may experience cognitive decline as the disease progresses, and up to 25% of non-demented PD patients can meet MCI criteria (Weintraub & Burn, 2011). There can be measurable cognitive deficits even prior to the diagnosis of PD, which often involve executive and visuospatial dysfunction. Despite the widespread prevalence of PD

MCI and dementia, there have been few trials demonstrating efficacious treatment with cognitive enhancers. Emre and associates showed statistically significant but clinically modest cognitive improvement in PD patients on rivastigmine (Emre et al., 2004). Trials of donepezil have not shown sufficient evidence for treatment of PD dementia based on primary endpoints (Alzheimer Disease Assessment Scale-Cognitive [ADAS-Cog]), but the American Academy of Neurology (AAN) Practice Parameter concluded that donepezil is "probably effective," based on secondary endpoint improvements in Mini-Mental Status Exam (MMSE) (Dubois et al., 2012; Miyasaki et al., 2006).

IMPULSE CONTROL DISORDERS

Impulse control disorders (ICD) in PD are common, with an incidence of 13.7%. Subtypes include problematic and pathological gambling, compulsive sexual behavior, compulsive buying, and binge-eating disorders. There is an association between ICDs and dopamine agonists, as patients on dopaminergic medications are up to 3.3 times more likely to have an ICD than those who are not taking them (Weintraub et al., 2010). Risk factors for the development of ICDs include early onset of disease, younger age, higher doses of dopaminergic drugs (especially dopamine agonists), history of psychiatric disorder, and recreational drug or alcohol abuse (Kummer & Teixeira, 2009). Careful evaluation and psychoeducation before starting dopaminergic medications may be helpful in staving off an ICD. Patients and caregivers should be advised of the warning signs at the start of treatment, and again at follow-up. This is especially important if the patient has a history of behavioral or substance addictions (Voon et al., 2011). If an ICD does develop, the first step should be to reduce dopaminergic medications where possible. Close monitoring is needed, as patients who have been exposed to high doses of dopamine agonists are at risk of a withdrawal syndrome, characterized by anxiety, dysphoria or depression, fatigue, autonomic symptoms, and drug cravings (Rabinak & Nirenberg, 2010).

PUNDING

Punding refers to a diverse set of non-goal-directed, stereotyped actions or behaviors. The type of behavior is often related to the individual's interests or former occupation: for example, an office worker repetitively shuffling papers, or a beautician brushing hair (Spencer, Rickards, Fasano, & Cavanna, 2011). Other common examples include sorting buttons and assembling or disassembling watches or other household items. Punding has been associated with dopaminergic therapy, although there is no clear pathophysiology established. Punding behaviors are most often described in the PD literature, but they have also been observed in other patient groups on dopaminergic drugs (e.g., patients treated for restless leg syndrome) (Spencer et al., 2011). While there are superficial similarities to the compulsions observed in OCD, punding behaviors lack a distressing ego-dystonic quality. Rather, PD patients appear to find them soothing.

Problems arise with the amount of time devoted to punding, which can lead to social withdrawal or ignoring of other important activities of daily living. Like ICDs, there are no clear treatment guidelines for punding other than decreasing dopaminergic medications.

DEMENTIA WITH LEWY BODIES

DLB and dementia associated with Parkinson disease (PDD) have traditionally been considered different disorders, but it is more likely that they represent two conditions along a disease continuum rather than distinct entities. The differentiation between DLB and PDD is made on the basis of the onset of cognitive dysfunction relative to onset of motor symptoms: DLB should be diagnosed when dementia occurs before or concurrently with the onset of Parkinsonism, while PDD requires that the dementia develop in the context of an established PD (classically, more than one year after onset of motor symptoms) (McKeith et al., 2005).

DLB is formally characterized by cognitive fluctuations, visual hallucinations, and Parkinsonism. Fluctuations take the form of changes in alertness or attention. These may be difficult to observe during a time-limited office visit, so collateral information from family members or a caregiver is crucial. The visual hallucinations are generally well formed and often non-frightening to the patient. Motor symptoms, similar to those found in PD, include bradykinesia, rigidity, postural instability, and masked facies. A tremor may also be present, although often not as pronounced as in PD. Motor symptoms may also be more symmetrical in DLB patients compared to those with PD, and responses to levodopa are often less robust (see also Chapter 42).

Another hallmark of DLB is exquisite sensitivity to neuroleptics. Reactions may include delirium, acute psychosis, and exacerbation of Parkinsonian motor symptoms. On the other hand, DLB patients typically have a very good response to cholinesterase inhibitors. These agents can dramatically improve cognition (to a degree beyond what is observed in Alzheimer's disease patients), and may alleviate visual hallucinations by improving attentional systems (McKeith, Wesnes, Perry, & Ferrara, 2004). Both the marked response to cholinesterase inhibitors and the sensitivity to anticholinergic drugs are thought to be related to a pathological deficit of cortical cholinergic function in DLB (Tiraboschi et al., 2000).

ATYPICAL PARKINSON SYNDROMES

Atypical Parkinsonian syndromes include DLB, progressive supranuclear palsy (PSP), corticobasal syndromes (CBS), and multiple system atrophy (MSA), the latter of which is divided into three subtypes based on whether the predominant symptom is Parkinsonism (MSA-P, previously called striatonigral degeneration), cerebellar (MSA-C, also known as olivopontocerebellar atrophy), or dysautonomic (MSA-A, also known as Shy-Drager syndrome). Clinical features that can help differentiate an atypical syndrome from primary

PD include symmetry of motor symptoms at onset, a more rapid course of progression, early dysautonomia and postural instability, as well as partial or non-responsiveness to dopaminergic medications. Careful consideration of these syndromes is important not only for precise diagnosis, but also to guide treatment choices. In particular, patients with atypical Parkinsonian syndromes often have significant sensitivity to the side effects of anticholinergic medications, including exacerbation of constipation, orthostatic hypotension, and postural instability leading to an increased rate of falls. Furthermore, urinary frequency or urgency is commonly observed in PD and atypical PD-related dysautonomia, but most of the anticholinergic medications that are typically used as anti-spasmodic agents can worsen cognitive dysfunction. Thus, treatment of PD-related bladder dysfunction should be limited to the agents with the least central nervous system penetration, such as darifenacin or trospium chloride.

TOURETTE SYNDROME

Tourette syndrome (TS) is a childhood-onset neurodevelopmental disorder characterized by the presence of waxing and waning motor and vocal tics. *Tics* are classically described as brief, rapid, non-rhythmic, involuntary movements or sounds. They may be simple (e.g., eye blinking, grimacing, coughing, sniffing, or grunting) or complex. Complex tics vary widely and include coordinated movements of multiple muscle groups, slower dystonic (posturing) movements; more purposeful-appearing movements with compulsive (touching/tapping) or aggressive/self-injurious (poking or punching) features; as well as syllables, words, phrases, and complex utterances such as repeating oneself (palilalia), repeating others (echolalia), and socially inappropriate utterances (coprolalia). Of note, coprolalia is only present in 10–20% of TS patients (McNaught & Mink, 2011). Tics are most commonly associated with an uncomfortable premonitory sensation/urge and are briefly suppressible, with subsequent buildup of the urge until the tic is released. Tics can worsen with a variety of external triggers, including stress, anxiety, excitement, or systemic infection.

Current DSM classification separates tic disorders based on length of symptoms, age of onset, and tic types (American Psychiatric Association [APA], 2000). Transient tic disorder (TTD) (now called *Provisional tic disorder* in DSM-5) requires that single or multiple tics be present for more than four weeks, but less than one year. Chronic motor or vocal tic disorder (CT) is defined by the presence of either multiple motor or vocal tics (but not both) that are present for more than one year, while TS (*Tourette disorder* in DSM-IV-TR and DSM-5) requires that both motor and vocal tics be present, though not necessarily concurrently. This distinction between CT and TS is somewhat arbitrary, since vocal tics are merely motor contractions of oropharyngeal, laryngeal, and diaphragmatic muscles resulting in sounds (Singer, 2010). Thus TS and CT may best be considered part of a continuous spectrum of developmental tic disorders. Lastly, TTD,

CT, and TS are required to have onset prior to age 18; otherwise they are classified as *Tic disorder, not otherwise specified* (TD-NOS).

TS prevalence estimates have ranged widely between 0.05–3% of the pediatric population, though more recent community-based studies using larger sample sizes and multistage assessment procedures have provided more consistent estimates of 0.3–0.7% in school-age children ("Prevalence of diagnosed Tourette syndrome in persons aged 6–17 years—United States, 2007," 2009). Higher rates are observed in special education populations. The average onset age of tics is 5–7 years old, with peak severity typically in early adolescence (mean age of 10, with significant variability between individual patients). The majority of TS patients experience reduction in symptoms in late adolescence or early adulthood (Leckman et al., 1998). Singer's "rule of thirds" estimates that, by early adulthood, a third of tic disorders have disappeared, a third have improved, and the final third continue or worsen (Singer, 2006). Approximately 15% have persistent, disabling tics as adults (Bloch, Peterson, et al., 2006).

The etiology of TS and other developmental tic disorders is still unclear, though imaging studies have implicated dysfunction in CSTC circuitry, in particular impaired frontal CSTC circuits mediating cognitive control as well as overactive motor CSTC circuits (Wang et al., 2011). Although the presence of high rates of TS, CMT, and OCD in first-degree relatives of TS patients indicates a significant genetic predisposition, researchers have thus far only identified a small number of strong candidate susceptibility genes (O'Rourke, Scharf, Yu, & Pauls, 2009). Many environmental risk factors have been proposed, but none have been consistently replicated across studies.

TREATMENT

The decision to treat tics is based on the extent to which tics cause impairment in physical, social, educational, or occupational functioning. Medication choice can be guided by the severity of tics and effectiveness in treating comorbid conditions (Singer, 2010). Treatment algorithms generally aim to use a step-wise approach, with the goal of using medications with the lowest side-effect risk first, as described in the tiers below.

Tier 1: Alpha-2 Agonists

Alpha-2 agonists, including clonidine or guanfacine, should be the first-line treatment, especially for tics of mild severity. Guanfacine is sometimes better tolerated due to less sedation and a longer half-life. However, clonidine may be more effective in some patients, based on anecdotal experience. Both agents can reduce hyperactivity and impulsivity and can improve attention to some degree, and therefore can be helpful in patients with TS and attention-deficit hyperactivity disorder (ADHD). Alpha-2 agonist side effects include sedation, dry mouth, stomachaches, headaches, hypotension/dizziness, and (rare) bradyarrhythmias.

Tier 2: Atypical Neuroleptics

Neuroleptics (dopamine D2 receptor antagonists) may be necessary for more severe or refractory tics. In general, higher D2-blockade correlates with increased efficacy in tic reduction. Common side effects of atypical neuroleptics include weight gain, hyperlipidemia, impaired glucose tolerance, and sedation. Less often, they can cause Parkinsonism, acute dystonic reactions, akathisia, and tardive dyskinesia. Patients on atypical neuroleptics should have fasting lipids and glucose levels checked prior to initiation, and every three to six months, depending on the clinical context.

Tier 3: Typical Neuroleptics

The only FDA-approved medications for tics are haloperidol and pimozide, which along with fluphenazine are the three typical neuroleptics with the highest D2-receptor potency. Typical neuroleptics can be highly effective in treating tics, but are often not tolerated due to their severe side-effect profiles, including weight gain, cognitive dulling, extrapyramidal symptoms, akathisia, and tardive dyskinesia. In general, typical neuroleptics should be reserved for refractory tics.

Other medications also used to treat tics include clonazepam, topiramate, baclofen, levetiracetam, dopamine agonists (ropinirole and pramipexole), and tetrabenazine. Clonazepam is sedating, which often limits its use and can be associated with physiological dependence. Topiramate may be considered as an alternate Tier 1 medication prior to a neuroleptic trial, though it can exacerbate executive dysfunction in patients with comorbid ADHD and can cause (reversible) word-finding difficulties. Tetrabenazine, an inhibitor of the vesicular monoamine transporter (VMAT) resulting in presynaptic dopamine depletion, can be very effective in treating tics, and has a lower risk of tardive dyskinesia than neuroleptics. However, it can also cause significant weight gain, sedation, and reversible Parkinsonism, as well as depression in up to 25% of patients. It is contraindicated in patients who are actively suicidal, have impaired hepatic function, or are taking MAOIs (Lyon, Shprecher, Coffey, & Kurlan, 2010). For the latter, there should be a minimum two- to three-week "washout" period between use of MAOIs and tetrabenazine to avoid hypertensive crises. Neurologists have also had success with use of botulinum toxin in treating eye blinking and neck tics as well as simple vocal tics, in collaboration with specialists in otorhinolaryngology.

Behavioral Therapy

Given that tics are preceded by a premonitory sensory urge that is temporarily relieved by tic completion, behavioral therapy—specifically habit-reversal training (HRT)—can be an effective, non-pharmacological treatment for tics. Based on the known role of the basal ganglia in both motor learning and reinforcement learning of "habits," HRT teaches patients to respond to a premonitory urge with a "competing response" (CR) that is physically incompatible with the tic (Azrin & Peterson, 1988). While urges temporarily increase with CR implementation, over time, premonitory urges habituate in a manner akin to reduction of obsessive-compulsive symptoms in exposure-ritual prevention therapy for OCD. HRT has been demonstrated to be effective in reducing tics in multiple randomized clinical trials, in both children and adults (Wilhelm et al., 2012; Piacentini et al., 2010) and currently is formulated in the context of a "comprehensive behavioral intervention for tics (CBIT)," which incorporates several modalities, including psychoeducation, relaxation training, functional analysis to identify and mitigate common tic triggers, and HRT (Piacentini et al., 2010).

NEUROPSYCHIATRIC COMORBIDITIES

TS rarely occurs as an isolated tic disorder. A large, clinic-based, multi-center registry study of 3,500 patients found only 12% of TS patients without any comorbidities (Freeman et al., 2000). The most common neuropsychiatric comorbidities in TS are ADHD and OCD. Other co-occurring conditions include ICD, anxiety and mood disorders, sleep disorders, and learning disabilities. For the sake of concision, we have limited the review below to the more frequently found conditions.

Attention-Deficit Hyperactivity Disorder

ADHD is characterized either by an impaired ability to sustain attention (inattentive subtype), by the presence of impulsivity and hyperactivity (hyperactive/impulsive subtype), or by both sets of symptoms (combined subtype) (APA, 2000). It is the most common comorbid disorder in TS, with a prevalence of up to 60–80% of clinically referred patients (Cavanna, Servo, Monaco, & Robertson, 2009). ADHD usually precedes onset of tics by two or three years. Comorbid TS and ADHD are associated with increased tic severity and impairment. In addition, patients with TS plus ADHD often have additional comorbid disorders, including oppositional defiant disorder, conduct disorder, and episodic explosive episodes ("rage" attacks). A 2006 study comparing behavioral symptoms in children with TS alone, TS plus ADHD, ADHD alone, and an unaffected population found that while children with TS alone did not differ from unaffected children with respect to aggression, delinquency, or conduct difficulties, children with TS plus ADHD had significantly higher scores on indices of disruptive behaviors and scored similarly to children with ADHD alone (Sukhodolsky et al., 2003). Diagnosing ADHD within the TS population requires a careful assessment of other potential causes of executive dysfunction that can mimic ADHD, such as constant inward focus on tic suppression, prominent obsessional or non-obsessional anxiety, and sedative side effects of many tic-suppressant medications.

Stimulants are the treatment of choice in ADHD, but many physicians remain leery of using them in patients with tics disorders for fear of worsening tics. However, controlled clinical trials have found that this concern is unwarranted for most TS patients. The 2002 Treatment of ADHD in Children with Tics (TACT) study randomized 136 children with comorbid chronic tic disorder and ADHD into four treatment groups: (1) clonidine, (2) methylphenidate, (3) methylphenidate and clonidine, and (4) placebo (Tourette Syndrome Study Group [TSSG], 2002). For ADHD symptoms, all three medication arms were significantly improved compared to placebo at the end of the 16-week trial, but the greatest improvement was observed in the combined methylphenidate and clonidine group. A secondary measure of tic severity also demonstrated decreased tic severity in all three treatment groups (including methylphenidate alone) compared to placebo. Lastly, tic-worsening occurred in the same number of children in each group (20% on methylphenidate, 26% on clonidine, and 22% on placebo).

These data suggest that stimulants are not contraindicated in patients with tic disorders, and, when started at low doses and titrated up slowly, can successfully treat ADHD without concomitant tic-worsening. Another randomized controlled trial has demonstrated success in treating ADHD symptoms with the non-stimulant medication atomoxetine without associated tic-worsening (Allen et al., 2005).

Obsessive-Compulsive Disorder

The lifetime prevalence of OCD in the general population is thought to be between 1.9% and 3.2%. However, OCD has been observed at much higher rates in TS patients, though prevalence estimates vary widely (20–89%) (Singer, 2010). There is a preponderance of evidence to suggest a shared genetic susceptibility between OCD and tic disorders (Pauls et al., 1986; Pauls, Raymond, Stevenson, & Leckman, 1991). OCD symptoms generally emerge several years after the onset of tics and are more likely to persist over time than tics (Bloch, Peterson, et al., 2006). OCD symptoms in TS usually include a need for order or routine, a requirement for things to be symmetrical or "just so," and "evening-up" rituals (Cavanna et al., 2009). Some compulsions overlap with complex tics, requiring a mindful evaluation and in many cases treatment targeting both OCD and tic suppression. Studies have also described phenomenological differences between OCD alone and OCD with comorbid TS. For example, individuals with OCD in the absence of tics tend to have cognitive obsessions preceding compulsions; while individuals with both TS and OCD more often have a sensorimotor phenomenon, such as focal or generalized body sensations (usually tactile, musculoskeletal/visceral, or both, often described as feelings of pressure, aching, itching, or tension) occurring either before or during the patient's performance of the repetitive behaviors (Ferrao et al., 2012; Leckman et al., 1993; Miguel et al., 2000). Mental sensations, defined as "general, uncomfortable feelings or perceptions" (Miguel et al., 2000) (including urge only, energy release, sense of incompleteness, and just-right perceptions) were also observed at higher rates in patients with TS and OCD than in those with OCD only. Another study noted that obsessions in OCD and TS tended to include sexual, religious, aggressive, and symmetrical themes, while individuals with OCD were more likely to report obsessions related to contamination, bad things happening, or becoming ill (Leckman et al., 1994).

The pharmacological first-line treatment for concurrent OCD and TS is SSRIs (Goodman, Storch, Geffken, & Murphy, 2006; Lombroso & Scahill, 2008). Patients with OCD will typically need higher doses than one would normally use for depression, and up to 25% of OCD patients show no meaningful improvement on SSRIs alone and may require augmentation. In such cases, neuroleptics are often the agent of choice. A 2006 systematic review and meta-analysis of antipsychotic augmentation studies in adults with refractory OCD demonstrated a significant benefit of neuroleptic augmentation, particularly in patients with comorbid tic disorders (Bloch, Landeros-Weisenberger, et al., 2006). Clomipramine continues to remain the most effective pharmacological treatment for OCD, though it is usually used as a second-line agent due to its side-effect profile (weight gain, anticholinergic side effects, electrocardiogram QT interval prolongation).

Psychotherapeutic interventions, specifically CBT involving exposure and ritual prevention (ERP), have been demonstrated in multi-center randomized controlled trials to be effective treatments for OCD both in children and adults. These studies suggest that the combination of CBT and medications (either SSRIs or clomipramine) may be more effective than either treatment alone. Current guidelines recommend initial non-pharmacological interventions for mild-to-moderate OCD, with the addition of medications in refractory or more severe cases ("Treatment of Obsessive-Compulsive Disorder," 1997).

Anxiety/Depression

Non-obsessional anxiety and depression frequently co-occur in patients with TS and chronic tic disorder, with estimates in the TS clinical population averaging roughly 20% for both anxiety and depression, but as high as 40% each in some clinical cohorts (Freeman et al., 2000). In general, anxiety and depression are treated with the same interventions in tic disorder patients as they are in the general population (i.e., CBT and pharmacotherapy). However, they are important to evaluate and monitor, since untreated depression and anxiety can increase tic severity; therefore, targeting these two common psychiatric disorders can sometimes reduce mild tics to such a degree that tic-specific treatments are not necessary. Given the high rates of comorbid OCD, SSRIs are often the pharmacological therapy of choice for TS-related anxiety and depression. Caution may also be needed when prescribing antidepressants with noradrenergic activity, such as SNRIs or buproprion, both of which can exacerbate tics. Lastly, physicians should be aware of the pharmacokinetic interactions between many SSRIs and the common dopamine antagonists used for tic suppression, such as fluoxetine, paroxetine, or buproprion with aripiprazole (via the CYP2D6 enzyme), fluoxetine with haloperidol (via CYP2D6), and fluoxetine, fluvoxamine, citalopram/escitalopram or (to a lesser degree) sertraline with pimozide (via CYP1A2 and/or CYP3A4).

Episodic Dyscontrol/Intermittent Explosive Disorder (IED)

Explosive outbursts are characterized by unpredictable and abrupt displays of aggression out of proportion to provoking stimuli (Budman, Bruun, Park, Lesser, & Olson, 2000).

There is often a preceding sense of tension or increased arousal, relieved by the outburst. They can be present in 15–30% of TS patients and can often be the most impairing symptom of the disorder. Explosive outbursts are associated with high family distress, problematic interpersonal relationships, impaired functioning, and increased rates of psychiatric hospitalization (Budman et al., 2008). A 2000 study by Budman and colleagues found the probability of explosive outburst in TS was greatly associated with comorbid disorders (including ADHD and OCD), and its likelihood rose with the number of comorbidities. Neither the presence of mood disorders nor tic severity was correlated with the number of explosive episodes in the population studied (Budman et al., 2000). While no randomized controlled trials have been conducted on treatment of IED in patients with tic disorders, experts currently recommend the following: (1) treatment of underlying triggers that may exacerbate outbursts (untreated/incompletely treated tics, OCD, ADHD, depression or non-obsessional anxiety); (2) behavioral therapy targeting anger; and (3) pharmacotherapy, including SSRIs and atypical neuroleptics.

In the same vein, TS patients have higher rates of self-injurious behaviors (SIB) than found in the general population. SIBs have been observed in up to 33% of TS patients (Robertson, Trimble, & Lees, 1989). Although the range of severity varies, some patients do have very serious manifestations that result in injury or even life-threatening consequences. A study of 332 TS patients seen at a single clinic during a three-year period found that 5.1% met criteria for "malignant TS," defined as two or more emergency-room visits or one or more inpatient admissions for TS-related issues (Cheung, Shahed, & Jankovic, 2007).

CLINICAL PEARLS

- Apathy is so characteristic of Huntington's disease that it has been termed the "apathetic dementia" (Folstein, 1989). Inertia, lack of interest, impersistence, and lack of initiative may precede other signs by years.

- A critical feature of depression in Huntington's disease is the increased suicide rate among individuals with HD, which has been estimated to be four to six times higher than found in the general population. Suicidal behavior is likely to be impulsive, and at times may even occur in the absence of active depression. Two particularly risky times for suicide attempts are around the gene test, and when increased symptom severity leads to loss of independence.

- OCD does not have a clearly defined prevalence in HD, but studies have shown 22% to 50% of patients endorsing some kind of obsession or compulsion.

- In general, most treaters of depression in Parkinson's disease start with an SSRI, though SSRIs can worsen bradykinesia or apathy in some cases. Although SSRIs given in conjunction with MAO-B inhibitors (such as selegiline and rasagiline) theoretically increase the risk of serotonin syndrome, in practice this is rarely observed, as there is not significant MAO-A inhibition at therapeutic doses of selective MAO-B inhibitors.

- Punding is a diverse set of non-goal-directed, stereotyped actions or behaviors associated with dopaminergic therapy, although there is no clear pathophysiology established. PD patients appear to find punding soothing. The type of behavior is often related to the individual's interests or former occupation: for example, an office worker repetitively shuffling papers or a beautician brushing hair. Like ICD, there are no clear treatment guidelines for punding other than decreasing dopaminergic medications.

- Up to 40% of PD patients report anxiety symptoms. In fact, anxiety disorders may predate diagnosis of a movement disorder by up to 20 years.

- Comorbidities of Parkinsonian apathy include depression, cognitive impairment, and dysexecutive syndromes. Apathy may also be associated with a more rapid progression in motor and cognitive decline.

- Although both quetiapine and clozapine are commonly used in practice for PD dementia, only the latter is recommended by the American Academy of Neurology guidelines (Miyasaki et al., 2006). These guidelines recommend avoiding olanzapine, as it has failed to show benefit and even worsened PD symptoms in some studies. Of note, PD patients can experience therapeutic benefit at clozapine doses as low as 6.25 mg/day.

- McKeith and colleagues performed a double-blind, placebo-controlled study that demonstrated improvement in apathy and indifference in patients with DLB using rivastigmine.

- DLB is formally characterized by cognitive fluctuations, visual hallucinations, and Parkinsonism. Fluctuations take the form of changes in alertness or attention. These may be difficult to observe during a time-limited office visit, so collateral information from family members or a caregiver is crucial. The visual hallucinations are generally well formed and often non-frightening to the patient.

- Another hallmark of DLB is exquisite sensitivity to neuroleptics. Reactions may include delirium, acute psychosis, and exacerbation of Parkinsonian motor symptoms. On the other hand, DLB patients typically have a very good response to cholinesterase inhibitors.

- Patients with atypical Parkinsonian syndromes often have significant sensitivity to the side effects of anticholinergic medications, including exacerbation of constipation, orthostatic hypotension, and postural instability leading to an increased rate of falls.

- Of note, coprolalia is only present in 10–20% of TS patients.

- Alpha-2 agonists, including clonidine or guanfacine, should be the first-line pharmacological treatment for TS, especially for tics of mild severity. While haloperidol and pimozide are the only two FDA-approved medications for tics, they are now considered third-line agents due to their side-effect profile.

- Cognitive Behavioral Intervention for Tics (CBIT), which includes Habit Reversal Training (HRT) has been demonstrated in multi-center randomized controlled trials to be effective for reducing tics both in children and adults and should also be considered first-line treatment when available.

- Pimozide (Orap) is not clearly more effective than haloperidol and fluphenazine, since all three have equally high D2-receptor potency; pimozide has many drug–drug interactions that affect the QT interval, which limits its utility in practice.

- The most common neuropsychiatric comorbidities in TS are ADHD and OCD, though anxiety, depression, and impulse dyscontrol/anger outbursts also frequently occur and often cause more impairment than the tics themselves.

- Diagnosing ADHD within the TS population requires a careful assessment of other potential causes of executive dysfunction that can mimic ADHD, such as constant inward focus on tic suppression, prominent obsessional or non-obsessional anxiety, and sedative side effects of many tic-suppressant medications.

- Stimulants are the treatment of choice in ADHD, but many physicians remain leery of using them in patients with tics disorders for fear of worsening tics. However, controlled clinical trials have found that this concern is unwarranted for most TS patients.

DISCLOSURE STATEMENTS

Dr. Raj has no potential conflicts to disclose.

Dr. Scharf has received grant support from the American Academy of Neurology Brain Foundation, the Tourette Syndrome Association, the Trichotillomania Learning Center, National Human Genome Research Institute (NHGRI), National Institute of Mental Health (NIMH) and NINDS. He has also received travel support from a joint education grant from the Tourette Syndrome Association and Centers for Disease Control and is a member of the Tourette Syndrome Association Scientific Advisory Board. He has no other potential conflicts to disclose.

REFERENCES

Abrahamsen, A. M., Digranes, O., & Gisholt, K. (1990). Comparison of the side-effects of pindolol and atenolol in the treatment of hypertension. *Journal of Internal Medicine, 228*(3), 219–222.

Albin, R. L., Young, A. B., & Penney, J. B. (1989). The functional anatomy of basal ganglia disorders. *Trends in Neuroscience, 12*(10), 366–375.

Alexander, G. E., DeLong, M. R., & Strick, P. L. (1986). Parallel organization of functionally segregated circuits linking basal ganglia and cortex. *Annual Review of Neuroscience, 9*, 357–381.

Allen, A. J., Kurlan, R. M., Gilbert, D. L., Coffey, B. J., Linder, S. L., Lewis, D. W., et al. (2005). Atomoxetine treatment in children and adolescents with ADHD and comorbid tic disorders. *Neurology, 65*(12), 1941–1949.

American Psychiatric Association (2000). *Diagnostic and Statistical Manual of Mental Disorders* (4th ed., text revision [DSM-IV-TR]). Washington, DC: American Psychiatric Association.

Arabia, G., Grossardt, B. R., Geda, Y. E., Carlin, J. M., Bower, J. H., Ahlskog, J. E., et al. (2007). Increased risk of depressive and anxiety disorders in relatives of patients with Parkinson disease. *Archives of General Psychiatry, 64*(12), 1385–1392.

Armstrong, M. J., & Miyasaki, J. M. (2012). Evidence-based guideline: Pharmacologic treatment of chorea in Huntington disease. Report of the Guideline Development Subcommittee of the American Academy of Neurology. *Neurology, 79*(6), 597–603.

Azrin, N. H., & Peterson, A. L. (1988). Habit reversal for the treatment of Tourette syndrome. *Behaviour Research and Therapy, 26*(4), 347–351.

Bloch, M. H., Landeros-Weisenberger, A., Kelmendi, B., Coric, V., Bracken, M. B., & Leckman, J. F. (2006). A systematic review: Antipsychotic augmentation with treatment refractory obsessive-compulsive disorder. *Molecular Psychiatry, 11*(7), 622–632.

Bloch, M. H., Peterson, B. S., Scahill, L., Otka, J., Katsovich, L., Zhang, H., et al. (2006). Adulthood outcome of tic and obsessive-compulsive symptom severity in children with Tourette syndrome. *Archives of Pediatrics & Adolescent Medicine, 160*(1), 65–69.

Blonder, L. X., & Slevin, J. T. (2011). Emotional dysfunction in Parkinson's disease. *Behavioural Neurology, 24*(3), 201–217.

Budman, C., Coffey, B. J., Shechter, R., Schrock, M., Wieland, N., Spirgel, A., et al. (2008). Aripiprazole in children and adolescents with Tourette disorder with and without explosive outbursts. *Journal of Child & Adolescent Psychopharmacology, 18*(5), 509–515.

Budman, C. L., Bruun, R. D., Park, K. S., Lesser, M., & Olson, M. (2000). Explosive outbursts in children with Tourette's disorder. *Journal of the American Academy of Child & Adolescent Psychiatry, 39*(10), 1270–1276.

Burns, A., Folstein, S., Brandt, J., & Folstein, M. (1990). Clinical assessment of irritability, aggression, and apathy in Huntington and Alzheimer disease. *Journal of Nervous & Mental Diseases, 178*(1), 20–26.

Caine, E. D., & Shoulson, I. (1983). Psychiatric syndromes in Huntington's disease. *American Journal of Psychiatry, 140*(6), 728–733.

Cavanna, A. E., Servo, S., Monaco, F., & Robertson, M. M. (2009). The behavioral spectrum of Gilles de la Tourette syndrome. *Journal of Neuropsychiatry and Clinical Neurosciences, 21*(1), 13–23.

Chatterjee, A., & Fahn, S. (2002). Methylphenidate treats apathy in Parkinson's disease. *Journal of Neuropsychiatry and Clinical Neurosciences, 14*(4), 461–462.

Cheung, M. Y., Shahed, J., & Jankovic, J. (2007). Malignant Tourette syndrome. *Movement Disorders, 22*(12), 1743–1750.

Devos, D., Dujardin, K., Poirot, I., Moreau, C., Cottencin, O., Thomas, P., et al. (2008). Comparison of desipramine and citalopram treatments for depression in Parkinson's disease: A double-blind, randomized, placebo-controlled study. *Movement Disorders, 23*(6), 850–857.

Dubois, B., Tolosa, E., Katzenschlager, R., Emre, M., Lees, A. J., Schumann, G., et al. (2012). Donepezil in Parkinson's disease dementia: A randomized, double-blind efficacy and safety study. *Movement Disorders, 27*(10), 1230–1238.

Duff, K., Paulsen, J., Mills, J., Beglinger, L. J., Moser, D. J., Smith, M. M., et al. (2010). Mild cognitive impairment in prediagnosed Huntington disease. *Neurology, 75*(6), 500–507.

Emre, M., Aarsland, D., Albanese, A., Byrne, E. J., Deuschl, G., De Deyn, P. P., et al. (2004). Rivastigmine for dementia associated with Parkinson's disease. *New England Journal of Medicine, 351*(24), 2509–2518.

Eng, M. L., & Welty, T. E. (2010). Management of hallucinations and psychosis in Parkinson's disease. *American Journal of Geriatric Pharmacotherapy, 8*(4), 316–330.

Ferrao, Y. A., Shavitt, R. G., Prado, H., Fontenelle, L. F., Malavazzi, D. M., de Mathis, M. A., et al. (2012). Sensory phenomena associated with repetitive behaviors in obsessive-compulsive disorder: An exploratory study of 1001 patients. *Psychiatry Research, 197*(3), 253–258.

Folstein, S. (1989). *Huntington's disease: A disorder of families*. Baltimore, MD: Johns Hopkins University Press.

Frank, S., & Jankovic, J. (2010). Advances in the pharmacological management of Huntington's disease. *Drugs, 70*(5), 561–571.

Freeman, R. D., Fast, D. K., Burd, L., Kerbeshian, J., Robertson, M. M., & Sandor, P. (2000). An international perspective on Tourette syndrome: Selected findings from 3,500 individuals in 22 countries. *Developmental Medicine & Child Neurology, 42*(7), 436–447.

Gallagher, D. A., & Schrag, A. (2012). Psychosis, apathy, depression and anxiety in Parkinson's disease. *Neurobiology of Disease, 46*(3), 581–589.

Gerber, P. E., & Lynd, L. D. (1998). Selective serotonin-reuptake inhibitor-induced movement disorders. *Annals of Pharmacotherapy, 32*(6), 692–698.

Goodman, W. K., Storch, E. A., Geffken, G. R., & Murphy, T. K. (2006). Obsessive-compulsive disorder in Tourette syndrome. *Journal of Child Neurology, 21*(8), 704–714.

Jason, G. W., Suchowersky, O., Pajurkova, E. M., Graham, L., Klimek, M. L., Garber, A. T., et al. (1997). Cognitive manifestations of Huntington disease in relation to genetic structure and clinical onset. *Archives of Neurology, 54*(9), 1081–1088.

Kenney, C., Hunter, C., Mejia, N., & Jankovic, J. (2006). Is history of depression a contraindication to treatment with tetrabenazine? *Clinical Neuropharmacology, 29*(5), 259–264.

King, M. (1985). Alcohol abuse in Huntington's disease. *Psychological Medicine, 15*(4), 815–819.

Kummer, A., & Teixeira, A. L. (2009). Neuropsychiatry of Parkinson's disease. *Arquivos de Neuro-Psiquiatria, 67*(3B), 930–939.

Leckman, James F., Walker, David E., Cohen, Donald J. (1993). Premonitory urges in Tourette's syndrome. *The American Journal of Psychiatry, 150*(1), 98–102.

Leckman, J. F., Grice, D. E., Barr, L. C., de Vries, A. L., Martin, C., Cohen, D. J., et al. (1994). Tic-related vs. non-tic-related obsessive compulsive disorder. *Anxiety, 1*(5), 208–215.

Leckman, J. F., Zhang, H., Vitale, A., Lahnin, F., Lynch, K., Bondi, C., et al. (1998). Course of tic severity in Tourette syndrome: The first two decades. *Pediatrics, 102*(1 Pt 1), 14–19.

Lombroso, P. J., & Scahill, L. (2008). Tourette syndrome and obsessive-compulsive disorder. *Brain Development, 30*(4), 231–237.

Lyon, G. J., Shprecher, D., Coffey, B., & Kurlan, R. (2010). Tourette's disorder. *Current Treatment Options in Neurology, 12*(4), 274–286.

Mayeux, R. (1984). Behavioral manifestations of movement disorders. Parkinson's and Huntington's disease. *Neurologic Clinics, 2*(3), 527–540.

McKeith, I., Del Ser, T., Spano, P., Emre, M., Wesnes, K., Anand, R., et al. (2000). Efficacy of rivastigmine in dementia with Lewy bodies: a randomised, double-blind, placebo-controlled international study. *Lancet, 356*(9247), 2031–2036.

McKeith, I. G., Dickson, D. W., Lowe, J., Emre, M., O'Brien, J. T., Feldman, H., et al. (2005). Diagnosis and management of dementia with Lewy bodies: Third report of the DLB Consortium. *Neurology, 65*(12), 1863–1872.

McKeith, I. G., Wesnes, K. A., Perry, E., & Ferrara, R. (2004). Hallucinations predict attentional improvements with rivastigmine in dementia with Lewy bodies. *Dementia & Geriatric Cognitive Disorders, 18*(1), 94–100.

McNaught, K. S., & Mink, J. W. (2011). Advances in understanding and treatment of Tourette syndrome. *Nature Reviews Neurology, 7*(12), 667–676.

Menza, M., Dobkin, R. D., Marin, H., Mark, M. H., Gara, M., Buyske, S., et al. (2009). A controlled trial of antidepressants in patients with Parkinson disease and depression. *Neurology, 72*(10), 886–892.

Miguel, E. C., do Rosario-Campos, M. C., Prado, H. S., do Valle, R., Rauch, S. L., Coffey, B. J., et al. (2000). Sensory phenomena in obsessive-compulsive disorder and Tourette's disorder. *Journal of Clinical Psychiatry, 61*(2), 150–156; quiz, 157.

Miyasaki, J. M., Shannon, K., Voon, V., Ravina, B., Kleiner-Fisman, G., Anderson, K., et al. (2006). Practice parameter: Evaluation and treatment of depression, psychosis, and dementia in Parkinson disease (an evidence-based review): Report of the Quality Standards Subcommittee of the American Academy of Neurology. *Neurology, 66*(7), 996–1002.

Novak, M. J., & Tabrizi, S. J. (2010). Huntington's disease. *British Medical Journal, 340*, c3109.

O'Rourke, J. A., Scharf, J. M., Yu, D., & Pauls, D. L. (2009). The genetics of Tourette syndrome: A review. *Journal of Psychosomatic Research, 67*(6), 533–545.

Pauls, D. L., Hurst, C. R., Kruger, S. D., Leckman, J. F., Kidd, K. K., & Cohen, D. J. (1986). Gilles de la Tourette's syndrome and attention deficit disorder with hyperactivity. Evidence against a genetic relationship. *Archives of General Psychiatry, 43*(12), 1177–1179.

Pauls, D. L., Raymond, C. L., Stevenson, J. M., & Leckman, J. F. (1991). A family study of Gilles de la Tourette syndrome. *American Journal of Human Genetics, 48*(1), 154–163.

Paulsen, J. S., Nehl, C., Hoth, K. F., Kanz, J. E., Benjamin, M., Conybeare, R., et al. (2005). Depression and stages of Huntington's disease. *Journal of Neuropsychiatry and Clinical Neurosciences, 17*(4), 496–502.

Piacentini, J., Woods, D. W., Scahill, L., Wilhelm, S., Peterson, A. L., Chang, S., et al. (2010). Behavior therapy for children with Tourette disorder: A randomized controlled trial. *Journal of the American Medical Association, 303*(19), 1929–1937.

Prevalence of diagnosed Tourette syndrome in persons aged 6–17 years—United States, 2007 (2009). *MMWR Morbidity & Mortality Weekly Report, 58*(21), 581–585.

Rabinak, C. A., & Nirenberg, M. J. (2010). Dopamine agonist withdrawal syndrome in Parkinson disease. *Archives of Neurology, 67*(1), 58–63.

Ready, R. E., Friedman, J., Grace, J., & Fernandez, H. (2004). Testosterone deficiency and apathy in Parkinson's disease: A pilot study. *Journal of Neurology, Neurosurgery, & Psychiatry, 75*(9), 1323–1326.

Reijnders, J. S., Ehrt, U., Weber, W. E., Aarsland, D., & Leentjens, A. F. (2008). A systematic review of prevalence studies of depression in Parkinson's disease. *Movement Disorders, 23*(2), 183–189; quiz 313.

Richard, I. H., McDermott, M. P., Kurlan, R., Lyness, J. M., Como, P. G., Pearson, N., et al. (2012). A randomized, double-blind, placebo-controlled trial of antidepressants in Parkinson disease. *Neurology, 78*(16), 1229–1236.

Robertson, M. M., Trimble, M. R., & Lees, A. J. (1989). Self-injurious behaviour and the Gilles de la Tourette syndrome: A clinical study and review of the literature. *Psychological Medicine, 19*(3), 611–625.

Roos, R. A. (2010). Huntington's disease: A clinical review. *Orphanet Journal of Rare Diseases, 5*(1), 40.

Rosenblatt, A. (2007). Neuropsychiatry of Huntington's disease. *Dialogues in Clinical Neuroscience, 9*(2), 191–197.

Rosenblatt, A., Kumar, B. V., Mo, A., Welsh, C. S., Margolis, R. L., & Ross, C. A. (2012). Age, CAG repeat length, and clinical progression in Huntington's disease. *Movement Disorders, 27*(2), 272–276.

Ross, C. A., & Tabrizi, S. J. (2011). Huntington's disease: From molecular pathogenesis to clinical treatment. *Lancet Neurology, 10*(1), 83–98.

Salmon, D. P., Granholm, E., McCullough, D., Butters, N., & Grant, I. (1989). Recognition memory span in mildly and moderately demented patients with Alzheimer's disease. *Journal of Clinical & Experimental Neuropsychology, 11*(4), 429–443.

Singer, H. S. (2006). Discussing outcome in Tourette syndrome. *Archives of Pediatrics & Adolescent Medicine, 160*(1), 103–105.

Singer, H. S. (2010). Treatment of tics and Tourette syndrome. *Current Treatment Options in Neurology, 12*(6), 539–561.

Spencer, A. H., Rickards, H., Fasano, A., & Cavanna, A. E. (2011). The prevalence and clinical characteristics of punding in Parkinson's disease. *Movement Disorders, 26*(4), 578–586.

Sukhodolsky, D. G., Scahill, L., Zhang, H., Peterson, B. S., King, R. A., Lombroso, P. J., et al. (2003). Disruptive behavior in children with Tourette's syndrome: Association with ADHD comorbidity, tic severity, and functional impairment. *Journal of the American Academy of Child & Adolescent Psychiatry, 42*(1), 98–105.

Tiraboschi, P., Hansen, L. A., Alford, M., Sabbagh, M. N., Schoos, B., Masliah, E., et al. (2000). Cholinergic dysfunction in diseases with Lewy bodies. *Neurology, 54*(2), 407–411.

Treatment of obsessive-compulsive disorder (1997). *The Expert Consensus Guideline Series,* from http://web.archive.org/web/20070219114941/http:/www.psychguides.com/ocgl.html.

Tourette Syndrome Study Group (TSSG) (2002). Treatment of ADHD in children with tics: A randomized controlled trial. *Neurology, 58*(4), 527–536.

Voon, V., Sohr, M., Lang, A. E., Potenza, M. N., Siderowf, A. D., Whetteckey, J., et al. (2011). Impulse control disorders in Parkinson disease: A multicenter case–control study. *Annals of Neurology, 69*(6), 986–996.

Wang, Z., Maia, T. V., Marsh, R., Colibazzi, T., Gerber, A., & Peterson, B. S. (2011). The neural circuits that generate tics in Tourette's syndrome. *American Journal of Psychiatry, 168*(12), 1326–1337.

Weigell-Weber, M., Schmid, W., & Spiegel, R. (1996). Psychiatric symptoms and CAG expansion in Huntington's disease. *American Journal of Medical Genetics, 67*(1), 53–57.

Weintraub, D., & Burn, D. J. (2011). Parkinson's disease: The quintessential neuropsychiatric disorder. *Movement Disorders, 26*(6), 1022–1031.

Weintraub, D., Koester, J., Potenza, M. N., Siderowf, A. D., Stacy, M., Voon, V., et al. (2010). Impulse control disorders in Parkinson disease: A cross-sectional study of 3090 patients. *Archives of Neurology, 67*(5), 589–595.

Wilhelm, S., Peterson, A. L., Piacentini, J., Woods, D. W., Deckersbach, T., Sukhodolsky, D. G., et al. (2012). Randomized trial of behavior therapy for adults with Tourette syndrome. *Archives of General Psychiatry, 69*(8), 795–803.

Zahodne, L. B., & Fernandez, H. H. (2008). Pathophysiology and treatment of psychosis in Parkinson's disease: A review. *Drugs & Aging, 25*(8), 665–682.

Zappacosta, B., Monza, D., Meoni, C., Austoni, L., Soliveri, P., Gellera, C., et al. (1996). Psychiatric symptoms do not correlate with cognitive decline, motor symptoms, or CAG repeat length in Huntington's disease. *Archives of Neurology, 53*(6), 493–497.

48.

NEUROPSYCHIATRIC ASPECTS OF FOCAL NEUROLOGICAL DISEASE

CEREBROVASCULAR DISEASE AND MULTIPLE SCLEROSIS

Ruchi Aggarwal and Mario F. Mendez

INTRODUCTION

For most of the last century, brain injury has been about location. The specific focal area of a brain injury primarily determines the manifestations of the neurological disease, regardless of the pathophysiological process. Basic brain–behavior principles include cerebral dominance and hemispheric specialization. Lesions in the left hemisphere result in aphasias, alexias, agraphias, ideomotor apraxia, and forms of acalculia. Some left-hemisphere lesions alter the ability to localize sensations on one's body or to recognize objects by looking at them. In contrast, lesions in the right hemisphere result in visuospatial difficulties, face-discrimination problems, environmental disorientation, and even amusias (the inability to recognize musical tones or to reproduce them). Disturbances in the frontal lobes can produce executive and personality changes; in the temporal lobes, memory and language changes; and in the parietal lobe, spatial and attentional changes. Although we now know that cognition is organized in more distributed and interactive networks throughout the brain, we still use these basic brain–behavior principles to localize and understand the consequences of focal neurological disease.

In contrast to cognitive deficits, clinicians and investigators are less aware of the focal psychiatric manifestations of brain lesions. As a general rule, any cognitive deficit can result from any focal neurological disease, depending on the focality and location. Psychiatric symptoms, however, may be more complicated. Yet psychiatric symptoms may be just as common as cognitive dysfunction. For example, common neurological causes of depression include left frontal strokes, multiple sclerosis, Parkinson's disease, Huntington's disease, Alzheimer's disease and other dementias, and epilepsy. Neurological causes of mania are right-hemisphere strokes, multiple sclerosis, Parkinson's disease after dopaminergic treatment, Huntington's disease, and trauma. Delusions and obsessive-compulsive symptoms may result from many of these disorders as well as from other neurological diseases.

This chapter focuses on the psychiatric manifestations of stroke and other cerebrovascular diseases and on multiple sclerosis, disorders that exemplify focal and multifocal diseases of the brain. While the effect on basic cognition is highly dependent on the location of the lesions, the psychiatric manifestations may result from other mechanisms as well. An understanding of these behaviors and their causes, and the need to evaluate neurological patients for psychiatric symptoms, can greatly facilitate the management of these patients.

CEREBROVASCULAR DISEASE

Cerebrovascular disease is associated with depression, mania, and a range of other psychiatric symptoms (see Table 48.1). In the United States, cerebrovascular disease is the third leading cause of mortality among those age 50 and older, preceded only by heart disease and cancer. Cerebrovascular disease encompasses a range of disorders, most prominently stroke, or a sudden loss of blood supply to the brain leading to permanent tissue damage. According to the American Stroke Association, approximately 795,000 Americans each year will suffer a new or recurrent stroke. Although other forms of cerebrovascular disease, including transient ischemic attack and chronic subcortical white matter change, may display neuropsychiatric symptoms, the systematic study and review of psychiatric disease in stroke has been the overwhelmingly predominant theme in the literature and will therefore be the focus of our review.

Strokes are often divided in terms of their pathophysiology, or, alternatively, by the site of damage. The pathophysiology of stroke can be ischemic (both thrombotic and embolic events) or hemorrhagic. Ischemic events constitute approximately 85% of cerebrovascular accidents, while hemorrhagic events are estimated to make up the rest. No matter what the cause of stroke, psychiatric manifestations are a well-recognized consequence.

DEPRESSION

PREVALENCE

Among all the possible psychiatric or behavioral manifestations post-stroke, depression is consistently the most prevalent. The prevalence of post-stroke depression (PSD) is approximately 33%, a rate much higher than that of depression in the

Table 48.1 NEUROPSYCHIATRIC SYMPTOMS ASSOCIATED WITH STROKE

SYNDROME	CLINICAL SYMPTOM	ASSOCIATED LESION LOCATION	COURSE AND PROGNOSIS	TREATMENT
Vascular Dementia	Cognitive decline demonstrated by loss of memory and at least one other deficit in domain of aphasia, apraxia, agnosia, or executive function	Multiple ischemic lesions	Current stroke with associated deterioration of cognitive function; influenced by: hypertension, hypotension, atherosclerotic heart disease, cigarette smoke, hyperlipidemia, diabetes	Anticoagulation effective to reduce risk of recurrence, antiplatelet aggregate drugs effective in secondary prevention of stroke, antihypertensives, lipid-lowering agents, smoking cessation, and prevention or management of diabetes mellitus; for pre-dementia (history of transient ischemic attacks, stroke, previous cognitive impairment), prevention may include carotid endarterectomy (when carotid stenosis is from 70–99%); patients in dementia stage (cognitive decline in several areas of intellectual functioning) treatment may include antidepressants, antihypertensive, cholinergic agonists, antiplatelet aggregation agents, statins, and neurotrophic factors
Major Depression	Depressed mood, diurnal mood variation, loss of energy, anxiety, restlessness, worry, weight loss, decreased appetite, early-morning awakening, delayed sleep onset, social withdrawal, and irritability	Left frontal lobe or left basal ganglia during first 2 mos. post-stroke	Mean duration of 40 weeks, minority develop long prolonged depression post-stroke, increased mortality	Nortriptyline showed significantly greater improvement in Hamilton Rating Scale for Depression (HAMD) vs. placebo but side effects were severe enough to require discontinuation; Citalopram (SSRI) showed a response rate of 59% to placebo 28% on HAMD: Recent study showed that patients treated with nortriptyline showed significantly greater decrease in HAMD score than either placebo or fluoxetine treated patients, no significant difference between fluoxetine and placebo
Minor Depression	See Major Depression; less severe; no suicidal ideation	Right basotemporal or right orbitofrontal lesions; right subcortical lesions; left posterior lesions	Mean duration of 12 weeks, increased mortality	See Major Depression
Mania	Elevated mood, increased energy, decreased sleep, feelings of well-being, pressured speech, flight of ideas, grandiose thoughts	Right basotemporal or right orbitofrontal lesions or right subcortical lesions	Not systematically studied	Effective treatments have not been established

Disorder	Symptoms	Lesion Location	Clinical Course	Treatment
Anxiety Disorder	Symptoms of major depression, intense worry, and anxious foreboding in addition to depression, associated light-headedness or palpitations and muscle tension or restlessness, and difficulty concentrating or falling asleep	Left cortical lesions, usually dorsal lateral frontal lobe; anxiety alone with right hemisphere lesions	Early onset (during acute in-hospital evaluation) but not late onset associated with psychiatric history including alcohol abuse, with mean duration of 15 months, delayed generalized onset mean duration of 3 months; Patients with GAD and depression had mean duration of depression significantly longer than duration of depression without GAD	SSRIs; benzodiazepines common for GAD, very conservative dosage and careful monitoring must be used; patients receiving nortriptyline treatment showed significantly greater improvement in HAMA and Hamilton Rating Scale for Anxiety (HAMA) scales than placebo group; furthermore, anxiety symptoms showed earlier improvement than depressive symptoms; buspirone may be useful in reducing anxiety without many of the adverse side effects, such as sedation, and without the risk of development of tolerance; however, this medication has not been empirically evaluated to treat post-stroke anxiety disorders
Psychotic Disorder	Hallucinations or delusions	Right temporal parietal occipital junction	Not systematically studied	No controlled treatment trials; anecdotal reports suggest two basic approaches, one using anticonvulsant therapy and the other neuroleptic therapy (use of anticonvulsants has its rationale in the frequent coexistence of seizures with psychotic disorders after stroke)
Apathy	Loss of drive, motivation, interest, low energy, unconcern	Posterior internal capsule or cingulate gyrus ventral striation and dorsomedial thalamus	Not systematically studied	No controlled trials for treatment; Patients have been treated with nortriptyline, apomorphine, and amphetamine with some success
Catastrophic Reaction	Anxiety, reaction, tears, aggressive behavior, swearing, refusal, renouncement, and compensatory boasting	Left anterior subcortical	Not systematically studied	Effective treatments have not been established
Pathological Laughing and Crying	Frequent, usually brief laughing or crying; crying not caused by sadness or out of proportion to it; and social withdrawal secondary to emotional outbursts	Frequently bilateral hemispheric lesions; lesions involving the frontopontine cerebellar pathways with almost any lesion location	Not systematically studied	Patients on nortriptyline showed significantly greater improvement in Pathological Laughter and Crying Scale (PLACS) compared to placebo group, significant improvements in depression scores were also observed; however, PLACS scores were significant for both depressed and non-depressed patients; All citalopram-treated patients reported greater than 50 percent reduction in the number of crying episodes; Hamilton scores dropped significantly during treatment as well

general population. Patients hospitalized at the time of a survey tended to have a higher frequency of PSD, at about 40%, as compared to community samples where the frequency was about 20% (Kaplan & Sadock, 1995). The prevalence of PSD among patients with left anterior strokes is as high as 70% (Robinson, 1986).

RISK FACTORS

Investigators have studied many risk factors for PSD. The significance of individual risk factors varies from study to study, probably reflecting the multifactorial nature of PSD. In addition, there is a bidirectional relationship or reciprocal correlation between stroke and depression. In other words, depression itself has also been found to be associated with an increased risk of stroke (Dong, Zhang, et al., 2011).

Among the identified risk factors, the presence of left anterior stroke lesions may be the most important. Clinicians have long observed a relationship between left-sided lesions and depression and between right-sided lesions and mania. The high prevalence of PSD allows for greater certainty of a relationship with left-sided lesions, but the relationship of mania to right-sided lesions is not as firm. Furthermore, the severity of depression in the acute post-stroke period is related to distance of the anterior border of the lesion from the left frontal pole (Robinson, Kubos, et al., 1984; Kaplan & Sadock, 1995; Narushima, Kosier, et al., 2003). Conversely, in the case of late-onset PSD, evidence for an association with lesion location has not held true in meta-analysis (Carson, MacHale, et al., 2000) (see Figure 48.1).

Other variables that may increase the risk for PSD include generalized cerebral atrophy, subcortical atrophy, dysphasia, living alone or with poor social support, pre-stroke psychopathology, and low level of functioning (Astrom, Adolfsson, et al., 1993). The relationship with impaired level of functioning is particularly evident among hospitalized patients. However, the relationship here is also bidirectional in that depression leads to poor performance in activities of daily living (ADLs) and decreased participation in rehabilitation (Parikh, Robinson, et al., 1990). A self-defeating cycle of depression, poor recovery, and worsening depression can be an unfortunate and dangerous consequence of untreated PSD. In contrast, severity of stroke has not been consistently correlated with the development of PSD.

DIAGNOSIS

The diagnosis of PSD can be challenging. This helps explain the varied rates of depression found across studies. PSD is can be very similar to primary depression, except that the patient exhibits less guilt and more somatic or vegetative symptoms (Lokk & Delbari, 2010). In some cases, however, it may be impossible to know if somatic symptoms such as low energy, insomnia, poor appetite, and cognitive dysfunction are related to depression or to other factors such as the physical sequelae of stroke itself, medications being used, or comorbid medical illnesses. In addition, deficits such as aphasia, dysarthria, neglect, and anosognosia (the lack of awareness of deficit) complicate the ability of stroke survivors to communicate their symptoms. Patients with depression specifically associated with cerebral microvascular disease or extensive deep white matter and periventricular hyperintensities on magnetic resonance imaging (MRI) have prominent psychomotor slowing, executive function deficits, and relatively poor long-term outcomes (Yamashita, Fujikawa, et al., 2010).

The *Diagnostic and Statistical Manual of Mental Disorders–IV* (DSM-IV) criteria for *Depression secondary to a general medical condition* provide some general guidance for the diagnosis of PSD. For a diagnosis of *Major depression*, patients must demonstrate a depressed mood and four

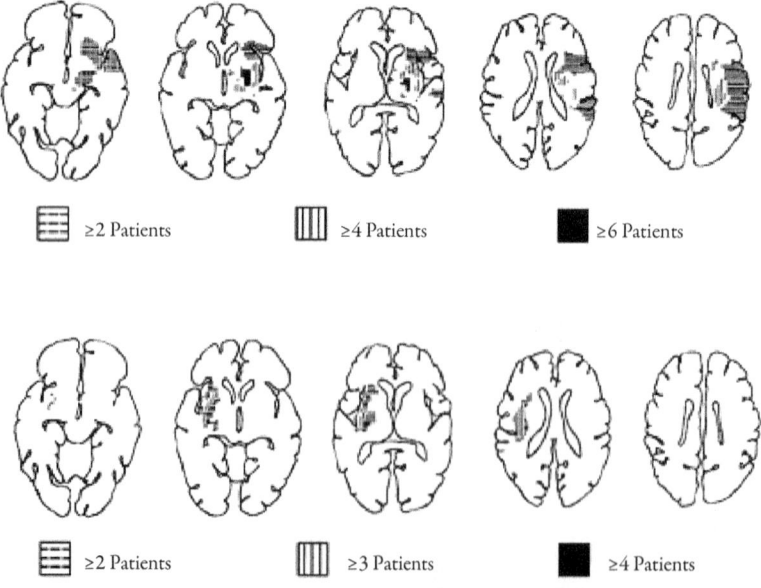

Figure 48.1 Schematic representation of superimposed lesions in patients with depressive disorders after stroke. *Top*, Nine patients with major depression and left hemisphere stroke. *Bottom*, Five patients with "minor depression" and right hemisphere stroke. Reproduced with permission (Herrmann, Bartels, et al., 1995).

additional symptoms from the following list: change in appetite, insomnia or hypersomnia, decreased interest or pleasure, psychomotor changes, decreased energy, feelings of guilt or worthlessness, poor concentration, and suicidal thoughts. *Minor depression* requires at least two but fewer than four of the above criteria, along with depressed mood or loss of interest. For *Dysthymia*, the DSM-IV criteria specify minor depression with a duration of at least two years (American Psychiatric Association Task Force on DSM-IV, 2000).

Several scales or screening instruments are available to measure and monitor depression severity. The Geriatric Depression Scale (Yesavage, Brink, et al., 1982) may be beneficial in the diagnosis of depression after a stroke as it focuses more on core symptoms of depression than on somatic symptoms alone. It is not designed for use in patients with cognitive impairment or aphasia. Other screening instruments include the Patient Health Questionnaire (PHQ-9), the Montgomery-Asberg Depression Rating Scale (MADRS), and the Hamilton Rating Scale for Depression (HRSD). Although all of these scales are acceptable screening instruments in PSD, their sensitivity and specificity are difficult to determine as there is no existing gold standard for the diagnosis of PSD beyond DSM-IV criteria. The Aphasic Depression Rating Scale (ADRS) is a useful tool and has been validated in patients both with and without aphasia (Benaim, Cailly, et al., 2004). It can be administered by the treating or rehabilitation team as it is based on observable behaviors, and therefore does not depend on the input of a family member or the patient. Finally, the Stroke Inpatient Depression Inventory (SIDI) is a scale specifically designed for PSD (Roger & Johnson-Greene, 2009). It is helpful even in the acute hospital setting, where questions regarding decreased interest in usual activities may be difficult to interpret, or even meaningless.

No matter what technique is used to evaluate PSD, the screening of all stroke patients for depression is better than the common practice of evaluating patients only if they display obvious symptomatology. In addition, evaluation of depression post-stroke should always include evaluation for suicidal ideation, plans, and intent. Suicidal thoughts are frequent after a stroke, as evidenced by an overall rate of suicidal ideation of 15% (Santos, Caeiro, et al., 2012).

CLINICAL COURSE

Acute-onset PSD occurring days to less than three months after a stroke may remit; however, late-onset PSD occurring after three months is likely to persist and display a more chronic course (Lokk & Delbari, 2010). The duration of post-stroke major versus minor depression is variable across studies. In general, whether acute-onset or late-onset, of minor or major intensity, PSD has the potential to become chronic, with symptoms lasting up to or more than three years. In one longitudinal study of post-stroke major depression, researchers found that, among patients with acute depression immediately following stroke, 60% had remission of symptoms by the one-year follow-up (Astrom, Adolfsson, et al., 1993). In this same study, if not remitted by one to two years, patients were unlikely to be remitted at the three-year follow-up.

Finally, PSD has an impact on ADLs and functional recovery, and PSD increases the risk of death (Morris, Robinson, et al., 1993).

ETIOLOGY

The different course, prognosis, and risk factors in acute-onset PSD versus late-onset PSD suggest a different underlying pathophysiology in these conditions. Acute-onset PSD may be more biologically mediated, while late-onset or chronic forms of PSD may be more psychologically mediated. Major and minor depressions have also been proposed to have different etiologies. A study conducted by Robinson and colleagues found that major depression was more likely to be found after left anterior lesions, whereas left posterior lesions were more likely to account for the emergence of minor depression after stroke (Robinson, Kubos, et al., 1984). While psychosocial factors certainly play a role in the etiology of PSD, biological factors are of key importance.

Disruption in corticolimbic circuits, especially with left anterior lesions, is a proposed mechanism for PSD. Numerous researchers have found a strong correlation between a left-sided frontal or left basal ganglia location of strokes and acute-onset PSD. Destruction of neurons and circuits in this area may lead to decreased ability to produce neurotransmitters, including serotonin (Narushima, Kosier, et al., 2003). Patients with PSD have reduced levels of 5-hydroxyindoleacetic acid (5-HIAA) in their cerebrospinal fluid (CSF) compared to matched controls (Spalletta, Bossu, et al., 2006).

An increase in the production and circulation of cytokines forms the basis of another major theory for PSD. As part of the inflammatory response, certain proinflammatory cytokines are increased after an acute stroke. Specifically, cytokine interleukin-1 (IL-1) plays an important role in the initiation and maintenance of inflammatory and immune responses following ischemic injury (Spalletta, Bossu et al., 2006). Additional cytokines involved in this acute response may include tumor necrosis factor alpha (TNF-alpha), IL-6, IL-8, and IL-18 and may be overproduced in patients with depression. Other cytokines, when administered to mice, can induce a syndrome similar to depression. The proposed mechanisms by which these cytokines lead to depressive symptoms include theories on alterations in the hypothalamic-pituitary-adrenal (HPA) axis with decreased production or change in neurotransmitters. Some of the cytokines, IL-1 included, are indeed potent stimulators of the HPA axis. Other cytokines may cause increased degradation or metabolism of tryptophan, resulting in a reduced ability to produce serotonin. Spalletta and colleagues have discussed a "cytokine–serotonin interaction" and the cycle that may lead to decreased overall production of serotonin, thus leading to depression (Spalletta, Bossu, et al., 2006).

The presence of genetic vulnerability is a further biological factor in PSD. Recent findings indicate that PSD is more common in those patients with certain serotonin transporter (*SERT*) gene polymorphisms (Kohen, Cain, et al., 2008). The *SERT* gene is located on chromosome 17q and encodes for the SERT protein. This SERT protein is located on presynaptic membranes of serotonergic neurons and controls serotonergic signaling by uptake of serotonin into the synapse. Therefore, variations in expression of this gene may lead to increased susceptibility of mental illnesses, including major depressive disorder (Kohen, Cain, et al., 2008).

TREATMENT

The literature on treatment of PSD includes several randomized control trials with selective serotonin-reuptake inhibitors (SSRIs) and with nortriptyline (Kaplan & Sadock, 1995). Both types of antidepressants have shown promising results in the treatment of PSD, with findings of improved level of functioning compared to untreated depressed patients. Additionally, research suggests the long-term benefit of treating depression immediately after stroke (Kaplan & Sadock, 1995) (see Figure 48.2).

Due to the high prevalence of PSD and the improvement in prognosis with antidepressants, some researchers have studied the prophylactic use of antidepressants in stroke. Their findings indicate a possible benefit of antidepressants, even in patients who were not found to have clinical depression (Chen, Patel, et al., 2007). However, not enough data are available to recommend the use of antidepressants as prophylactic agents in stroke patients.

Stimulant medications are also used in PSD, especially in patients with comorbid apathy and fatigue. For patients whose participation in rehabilitation is essential to good recovery and where quick onset is needed, stimulant medication may be the best option. The most studied stimulant is methylphenidate, with data supporting its use with a low incidence of side effects (Lokk & Delbari, 2010).

Nonpharmacological strategies include social support, cognitive-behavioral therapy, behavioral activation therapy, electroconvulsive therapy, and rehabilitation strategies. Given that poor social support or living alone are consistent risk factors for chronic depression in the literature, social support and the involvement of family or other support networks is vital. Psychological interventions such as behavioral activation therapy remain the treatment of choice for minor depression or for those who cannot tolerate antidepressants (Lokk & Delbari, 2010). Cognitive-behavioral therapy in the treatment of PSD has not shown a robust response, and it is of limited use in those whose cognitive impairment or aphasia is too severe for them to actively participate. Although electroconvulsive therapy is often effective in severe or treatment-resistant cases, adverse events and risks in the post-stroke period limit its use (Lokk & Delbari, 2010).

MANIA

Prevalence

As post-stroke mania is much less frequent than PSD, data on its prevalence rates, etiology, risk factors, and treatment are limited. Estimated prevalence rates are less than 1% (Santos, Caeiro, et al., 2011). Nevertheless, given a high prevalence of silent stroke and the possibility for mania to present late after a stroke, post-stroke mania should be in the differential diagnosis of late-onset bipolar disorders. In fact, among patients with new-onset mania after the age of 50, more than half have "asymptomatic" or "silent" cerebral infarctions on MRI of the brain (Fujikawa, Yamawaki, et al., 1995).

Risk Factors

Stroke location, but not family history, may predispose to post-stroke mania (Santos, Caeiro, et al., 2011). Despite debate, mania after stroke tends to be more frequent after right-sided lesions involving frontal lobe, temporal lobe, or caudate nucleus. These lesions may be evident on MRI but not on computerized tomography (Cummings & Mendez, 1984). As with many of the other psychiatric manifestations post-stroke, subcortical atrophy may pose an increased risk for development of mania (Robinson & Starkstein, 1989). As with PSD, mania after stroke is not clearly related to a family history of affective and bipolar disorder. Although several reports suggested an increased risk of post-stroke mania in those with a positive family history of bipolar disorder, a recent review of the literature by Santos and colleagues (2011) did not support such a relationship.

Diagnosis

Case reports have described the symptoms of post-stroke mania as indistinguishable from those seen in patients with primary mania. DSM-IV criteria for *Manic episode* provide a useful guideline. Criteria include elevated, expansive, or irritable mood lasting for at least one week, accompanied by at least three (four if the mood is only "irritable") of the following symptoms: inflated self-esteem or grandiosity, decreased need for sleep, more talkative or pressure to keep talking, flight of ideas or racing thoughts, distractibility, increase in goal-directed activity or psychomotor agitation, and excessive

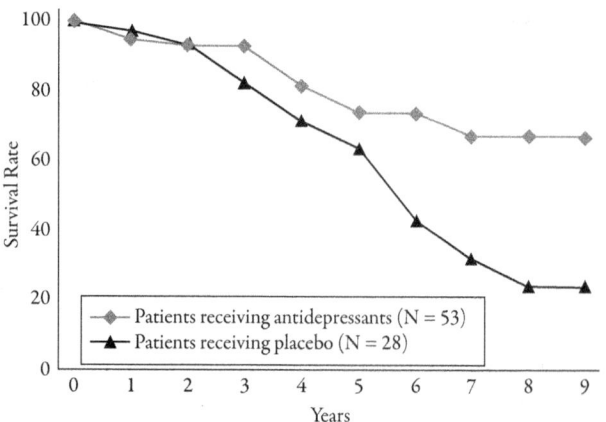

Figure 48.2 Survival rates over 9-year follow-up of acute stroke patients who received a 12-week post-stroke course of antidepressants or placebo. Reproduced with permission (Jorge, Robinson, et al., 2003).

involvement in pleasurable activities that have high potential for negative consequences (American Psychiatric Association Task Force on DSM-IV, 2000).

Another diagnostic tool is the criteria for secondary mania proposed by Krauthammer and Klerman (1978). The core criteria are similar to that of mania as diagnosed by DSM-IV, with the addition of the requirement that there be no prior history of mania or affective illness (Krauthammer & Klerman, 1978). As with DSM-IV criteria for *Mood disorder due to a general medical condition*, the symptoms cannot be present during the course of a delirium alone.

Clinical Course

The temporal relationship of mania or bipolar spectrum illness after stroke can vary from a very acute presentation to delayed mania for up to two years. The majority of cases do appear immediately after the stroke, with approximately 53% occurring in the first few days (Santos, Caeiro, et al., 2011). Another 23% of mania cases occur within the first month following the stroke (Santos, Caeiro, et al., 2011). Secondary mania associated with stroke or "vascular mania" is more difficult to treat than primary mania, as it may not respond to conventional mood stabilizers or antipsychotic medications. However, the mania often resolves without recurrence of further manic episodes (Cummings & Mendez, 1984). In the majority of cases reviewed in the literature, manic symptoms lasted from 1 to 12 weeks (Santos, Caeiro, et al., 2011).

Etiology

The increased risk with right-sided lesions is consistent with studies of primary mania showing decreased perfusion in the right hemisphere (Migliorelli, Starkstein, et al., 1993). Predominantly, right-sided lesions in the frontal lobe, especially in the orbitofrontal cortex, temporal lobe, caudate nucleus, and thalamus, are all implicated in the etiology for post-stroke mania. Consequently, a leading hypothesis for the origin of post-stroke mania is the interruption or dysfunction of frontolimbic circuits necessary for mood regulation (Santos, Caeiro, et al., 2011). Increase in serotonin receptor binding found after right-sided, but not left-sided, strokes has been one proposed mechanism for the development of mania in this population (Robinson & Starkstein, 1989).

Treatment

No randomized control studies are available for treatment of mania after stroke. Case reports do describe the resolution of symptoms with mood stabilizers, as used in primary mania (Cummings & Mendez, 1984). Mood stabilizers such as lithium or valproic acid and atypical antipsychotics for mania with psychotic features may be effective (Santos, Caeiro, et al., 2011). As the majority of the cases of post-stroke mania are thought to remit without recurrence, prolonged treatment is usually unnecessary.

ANXIETY

Prevalence

The rate of anxiety after stroke is about 25% across studies. The most likely anxiety diagnosis given is generalized anxiety disorder (GAD) or GAD due to stroke. As in primary anxiety, post-stroke anxiety is often comorbid with depression. Of those with post-stroke anxiety, approximately 75% are felt to have concomitant depression (Chemerinski & Levine, 2006). If anxiety and depression are comorbid, the severity and prognosis of depression is worse (Astrom, 1996). Studies on anxiety after stroke are few, with work focusing almost exclusively on GAD.

Risk Factors

Risk factors for anxiety after stroke, especially in chronic anxiety, include both predisposing factors and either cortical or subcortical atrophy (Astrom, Adolfsson, et al., 1993; Astrom, 1996). Patients with early-onset anxiety after stroke often have a previous psychiatric history or a history of alcohol abuse (Castillo, Starkstein, et al., 1993). Lesion location may also have an associated risk, with findings that right-hemisphere strokes are more likely to present with anxiety alone versus left-hemisphere strokes that present with both anxiety and depression (Castillo, Starkstein, et al., 1993).

Diagnosis and Clinical Course

DSM-IV criteria form the basis for diagnosis in GAD secondary to stroke. Excessive worrying for at least six months, with related symptoms including restlessness, decreased energy, concentration difficulties, irritability, muscle tension, and/or sleep disturbances, make up the diagnostic criteria (American Psychiatric Association Task Force on DSM-IV, 2000). Anxiety has approximately the same time course and presentation of symptoms after stroke as with depressive disorders.

Treatment

As with the other psychiatric manifestations related to stroke, treatment is currently guided and limited to what is known for primary psychiatric disorders. SSRIs are the primary treatment of choice, and buspirone may be helpful as well. Benzodiazepines, although effective in some cases, should be used with caution due to side effects, especially in an elderly population (Chemerinski & Levine, 2006).

APATHY

Prevalence

Although apathy, defined as lack of motivation or reduced goal-directed behaviors and cognition, can be associated with depression, it is often a separate condition. Apathy or abulia is frequently the first or most prominent sign of the development of vascular dementia. The frequency of apathy following stroke is 20–25% (Jorge, Starkstein, et al., 2010).

Risk Factors

There are several risk factors for post-stroke apathy. It is most frequent among patients with some degree of cognitive impairment, as demonstrated by lower scores on the Mini-Mental State Examination (Jorge, Starkstein, et al., 2010). However, there is not a direct correlation here, as even patients with severe dementia may not be apathetic. Other factors associated with apathy may include older age, impairment in ADLs, and frontal lobe and other lesion locations.

Diagnosis

Clinicians can document the signs of decreased spontaneous behavior and engagement with an apathy scale. The Apathy Evaluation Scale by Marin and colleagues is one such reliable measure for apathy (Marin, Biedrzycki, et al., 1991). It has three available versions, with one version a self-rated scale to be filled out by the patient, another a caregiver scale, and a third version a clinician-administered scale. There are 18 items designed to measure signs and symptoms associated with apathy, including reduced levels of goal-directed behavior; reduced goal-directed cognition, such as decreased interests, lack of plans and goals, and lack of concern about one's own health or functional status; and reduced emotional expressions as manifested by flat affect, indifference, and restricted responses to events. Alternative apathy measures include the Starkstein Structured Interview for Apathy (Jorge, Starkstein, et al., 2010).

Clinical Course and Etiology

Apathy occurs most often as a late presentation after stroke and seems to have a chronic course. The chronic nature of apathy is also associated with continued decline in level of functioning and poor recovery. Strokes involving the medial frontal region and anterior cingulate and the caudate nuclei can result in a frontal apathic-abulic state. After finding that lesions of the posterior limb of the internal capsule were also associated with apathy, Starkstein and colleagues concluded that damage to the frontal-subcortical networks plays a prominent role in the development of this condition (Jorge, Starkstein, et al., 2010).

Treatment

The literature on treatment of apathy is mostly limited to case reports. The mainstays of pharmacological treatment have been dopamine agonists or stimulant medications (Jorge, Starkstein, et al., 2010). Unfortunately, although apathy is often associated with depression, use of antidepressant medications such as SSRIs may worsen the symptoms of apathy.

Other Neuropsychiatric Manifestations

Other neuropsychiatric manifestations of cerebrovascular disease include catastrophic reaction, pathological laughter and crying, psychosis, anosognosia, irritability/agitation, disinhibition, and cognitive deficits, including vascular dementia (Kaplan & Sadock, 1995; Chemerinski & Levine, 2006) (see Table 48.2).

MULTIPLE SCLEROSIS

Multiple sclerosis (MS) is a chronic, often unpredictable, autoimmune, demyelinating neurological illness. After trauma, MS is the most common cause of neurological disability in young and middle-aged adults. The prevalence of MS is approximately 1 per 1,000 in the United States population, with about twice as many women affected as men (Vattakatuchery, Rickards, et al., 2011). Curiously, the prevalence of MS increases as the distance from the equator increases (Kaplan & Sadock, 1995). As any of the myelin sheaths in the central nervous system is susceptible to destruction by this disease, MS can have a variety of presentations and manifestations (see Table 48.2). The diagnosis requires at least two episodes of neurological disturbance with lesions separated in time and space (see Table 48.3).

The three main types of MS are divided by their clinical course into relapsing-remitting, secondary progressive, and primary progressive multiple sclerosis. Another category of multiple sclerosis, which is less studied, is "benign MS." Neuropsychiatric symptoms can occur any time in the course of the illness, with some case reports describing behavioral manifestations as the only presenting symptom. Comorbid psychiatric diagnoses are common and have long been recognized as part of the disease. In fact, as early as 1877, Jean-Martin Charcot first described a common presentation he observed in MS patients as "cheerful indifference."

DEPRESSION

Prevalence

Historically, early investigators and clinicians described MS as resulting in eutonia or euphoria with relative immunity from depression. This has subsequently proven to be incorrect. As in stroke, depression is one of the most common neuropsychiatric manifestations of MS, with an estimated 50% of MS patients suffering from depression across studies (Feinstein, 2004). The prevalence of depression is in fact more common in MS than in several other neurological diseases, even in diseases with comparable or similar amounts of loss in function, suggesting that a biological mechanism is involved. In addition, risk of suicide is unfortunately high compared with other neurological disorders (Goldman Consensus Group, 2005).

Risk Factors

Lesion load, location of lesion, and brain involvement may be risk factors for depression in MS. In this disorder, patients with brain involvement are more likely to be depressed than patients with spinal cord lesions alone (Schiffer, Caine, et al., 1983). Poor functional status and cognitive impairment are other risk factors for depression. In some samples, younger

Table 48.2 NEUROPSYCHIATRIC MANIFESTATIONS OF MULTIPLE SCLEROSIS

SYNDROME	LIFETIME PREVALENCE	CLINICAL SYMPTOMS	TREATMENT
Depression	50%	Depressed mood and other symptoms of primary depression, irritability, less guilt	SSRIs as first line; treatment guided by what is known for primary depression
Mania and Bipolar Disorders	2% (approximately twice that of general population)	Similar to primary mania: flight of ideas, expansive mood, reduced sleep, grandiosity, etc.	Mood stabilizers; antipsychotics; immunomodulatory/ disease-modifying therapies
Euphoria	15–25%; more common in patients with cognitive dysfunction and heavier lesion load, esp. in frontal lobes	State of mental and physical (eutonia, sclerotic) well-being or optimism despite significant disability; "cheerful indifference"	No recommended pharmacological treatment for euphoria alone
Anxiety	14–40%	Similar to primary anxiety disorders	SSRIs
Fatigue	75%–90%	Divided into: – motor fatigue: physical weakness following sustained activity –mental fatigue: feeling tired or exhausted out of proportion to level of activity	Dopamine agonists, amantadine, modafinil; exercise training programs Also, treat any underlying sleep disorders, pain, or comorbid depression
Psychosis	1–2% (controversial as to whether it is more prevalent than in the general population)	Hallucinations/delusions	Antipsychotics
Pathological Laughter and Crying (PLC)	10%	Spontaneous, uncontrollable outbursts of either crying or laughing, often inappropriate to situation or incongruent with actual mood	SSRIs; nortriptyline; dextromethorphan-quinidine
Cognitive Impairments	43–70%	Deficits in complex attention, information processing and speed, executive functioning, encoding, visual processing; can progress to subcortical dementia; language may be spared	Acetylcholinesterase inhibitors; disease-modifying therapies incl. INF-β Cognitive rehabilitation programs

age of onset and recent diagnosis (shorter disease duration) of MS are also associated with increased risk of depression (Paparrigopoulos, Ferentinos, et al., 2010).

Risk factors for suicide and suicidal ideation are similar to those seen in the general population and include male gender, social isolation, substance abuse, and younger age of onset of MS (Paparrigopoulos, Ferentinos, et al., 2010). The most important risk factor for completed suicide in MS is depression, underscoring the importance of detecting depression in this disorder (Goldman Consensus Group, 2005).

Diagnosis

As is the case for stroke and other neurological diseases, depression in MS can be a diagnostic challenge. Many of the symptoms that may be inherent with MS, including fatigue, appetite changes, insomnia, and problems with concentration or cognition, overlap with the symptoms of depression. This may account for the missed diagnosis of depression among known MS patients as "just a natural part of their illness" or, alternatively, the misdiagnosis of MS as depression.

Depression in MS often presents with less guilt than seen in primary depression. In addition, MS-related depression may present with more irritability, discouragement, and frustration (Feinstein, 2004).

Diagnosis is again guided by DSM-IV criteria for *Mood disorder secondary to a general medical condition*. Scales used in measuring primary depression are also used in the study of depression in MS. Examples of scales used include the Beck Depression Inventory and the Hamilton Depression Rating Scale. According to the Goldman Consensus Group, the best approach to screening depression in MS is by using the Beck Inventory, with a cutoff score of 13 indicating depression (Goldman Consensus Group, 2005). Concern about over-diagnosis of depression in MS has led to the development and administration of scales that can separate vegetative symptoms from other symptoms of depression. For example, the Chicago Multiscale Depression Inventory may be useful in patients with medical illnesses such as MS, as it has three separate sub-scales to evaluate depression, including vegetative, mood, and evaluative/ cognitive scales. It is self-administered by patients and asks them to score how closely a given statement or phrase describes them

Table 48.3 MULTIPLE SCLEROSIS

Multiple Sclerosis	Clinical Definition		Etiology
	The presence of two attacks, involving different parts of the CNS, separated by a period of at least 1 month, and lasting a minimum of 24 hours		T cells, and to a lesser extent, B lymphocytes invade the CNS, destroying axons; damage to myelin leads to an inflammatory reaction, and resolution of this to plaque formation
Symptoms	*Initial symptoms*	*Motor symptoms*	*Symptoms of cerebellar dysfunction*
	Heterogeneous; may include a broad range of somatosensory, ocular, and motor symptoms	Include transient hemiparesis and various forms of seizure, among others	May occur, including scanning speech, gait ataxia, and various tremors
Common Courses	*Relapsing-remitting form*	*Secondary progressive form*	*Primary progressive type*
	Most common; patient has relapses of illness that can present with a broad range of neurological symptoms leading to remission and almost complete recovery with each episode	May evolve from relapsing-remitting form, leading to incomplete recovery after acute exacerbation of illness	Quite uncommon, occurring in no more than 10% of cases; steady worsening of course from the outset of the disease; may be rapidly progressing and is rarely seen in patients younger than 40 years of age
Treatment	*Nonspecific symptomatic treatments*		*Interferon (immunosuppressive/immunomodulatory agents)*
	Neuropsychiatric symptom treatment as per Table 48.1; Glucocorticoids used to treat acute inflammatory responses associated with damage to the myelin sheath; although causing symptomatic relief, they do not impact the long-term course or outcome of the disorder		*Interferon- β-1b*: shown to reduce annual relapse rates, in addition to changing the course of the disorder, there are preliminary data that this compound may also ameliorate the cognitive symptoms associated with MS; *Interferon- β-1a*: shown to reduce disability and relapse in patients, and may also have beneficial effects on cognitive function; *Glatiramer acetate*: effects on reducing relapse and improving disability, and, like the others, also has stabilizing effects on MRI changes

(Arnett & Randolph, 2006). The limitation of using screening instruments to diagnose depression in any condition, including MS, emphasizes that depression is a clinical diagnosis, and good clinical judgement in conjunction with instruments is the ideal approach. Finally, failure to suppress in the dexamethasone suppression test in MS is similar to findings seen in primary major depressive disorder (Goldman Consensus Group, 2005).

Clinical Course

According to the Goldman Consensus Group statement on depression in MS, depression does contribute to functional impairment in this disorder (Goldman Consensus Group, 2005). Study findings vary on the amount of functional impairment caused. There are reported associations with depression and decreased compliance with medications, decreased cognitive function, increased time off from work and disability, and disruption in family support systems. It is still not clear if emotional stress or depression can actually lead to increased progression of MS as measured by new gadolinium-enhancing lesions on MRI (2005). Unlike after acute stroke, depression in MS seems to have a chronic and possibly even worsening progressive course (2005).

Etiology

Depression in MS may be multifactorial. There are studies of lesion-related anatomical, autoimmune, inflammatory, and psychological factors (Vattakatuchery, Rickards, et al., 2011). Given evidence for and against the many different proposed mechanisms, it is very likely that the etiology of depression differs from patient to patient and that multiple factors may be involved even in the same patient.

Study findings on the correlation of depression with lesion location are inconsistent. Some report a correlation of depression with left-sided lesions, others with right-sided lesions, and others find no correlation at all (Vattakatuchery, Rickards, et al., 2011). Improvement in imaging techniques for MS and future studies may help clarify the relationship between lesion location and depressive symptomatology. Among the studies that have found a correlation with lesion location, the left arcuate fasciculus, the right parietal lobe, periventricular and frontal areas, temporal lobes, right frontal lobe, left medial inferior frontal cortex, and right medial inferior frontal regions have been variably implicated (Vattakatuchery, Rickards, et al., 2011). Brain atrophy, especially in the frontal lobes, could also play a role in increased risk of depression (Vattakatuchery, Rickards, et al., 2011) (see Figure 48.3, left and right).

Inflammatory and immune mechanisms may be the common link between the pathogenesis of depression and MS, as was suggested in the case of stroke. Proinflammatory cytokines are increased in patients with MS as well as in patients with primary depression (Vattakatuchery, Rickards, et al., 2011). Although small sample sizes limit definitive

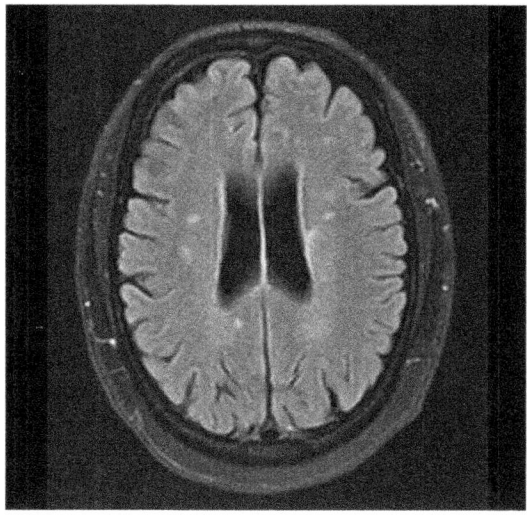
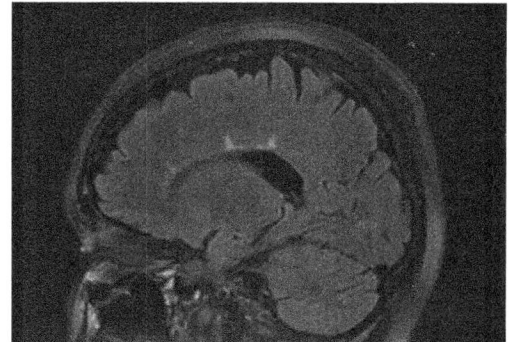

Figure 48.3 Patient with chronic dysthymia and multiple sclerosis. MRI on left shows axial flair image; MRI on right shows coronal T1 image.

conclusions, a few studies have found a correlation between the production of interferon gamma (INF-γ) and TNF-α in MS-related depression (Kahl, Kruse, et al., 2002). The mechanism by which cytokines cause depression may be related to cytokine modulation of serotonin. In animal and experimental models, cytokines such as TNF-α are found to upregulate the expression of the SERT protein, which in turn decreases availability of serotonin in the synapse (Vattakatuchery, Rickards, et al., 2011).

Complicating the relationship between depression and MS is the finding of worsening depression in patients treated with interferon. Immunomodulatory therapies remain a mainstay of treatment of MS, and one of these treatments, INF-β, had been associated with an increased risk of depression. While subsequent studies have not shown INF-beta to cause depression, INF-α used in treatment of diseases such as hepatitis C does result in depression in some patients (Myint, Schwarz, et al., 2009). These findings help support the idea that cytokines are involved in etiology of depression. In addition, the finding that this is specific to certain interferon treatments, but not to INF-β used in MS, helps differentiate MS-related depression from iatrogenic or treatment-induced depression (Vattakatuchery, Rickards, et al., 2011).

There are additional psychological factors in the etiology of MS-related depression. Although studies investigating a relationship between severity of illness and depression have found conflicting results, there is no doubt that MS leads to loss of functioning and that the unpredictable nature of the illness can leave patients feeling hopeless or out of control (Vattakatuchery, Rickards, et al., 2011). The types of coping strategies employed by patients can have a significant impact on the development of depression. Specifically, escape-avoidance strategies lead to higher incidence of depression, compared to cognitive reframing and active problem-solving strategies that lead to decreased depression (Mohr, Goodkin, et al., 1997). The finding that anxiety and depression are higher in patients during the first year after the diagnosis of MS supports the

"illness representation" model of dealing with disease. In other words, the patient's view of the illness and beliefs about their own personal identity can influence the likelihood of developing anxiety and depression (Vattakatuchery, Rickards, et al., 2011).

Treatment

The Goldman Consensus Group statement on depression in MS advocates a combined psychotherapeutic and pharmacological approach to this disease (Goldman Consensus Group, 2005). As with primary depression, cognitive-behavioral therapy can play an important therapeutic role (Larcombe & Wilson, 1984). In moderate to severe cases of major depressive disorder in MS, antidepressants are recommended and usually effective; however, the only two double-blind randomized placebo-controlled trials of antidepressants in MS-related depression, one with desipramine and one with paroxetine, showed only modest to questionable benefit (Koch, Glazenborg, et al., 2011). Tolerability may have been a limiting factor in these studies; tricyclic antidepressants (TCAs) such as desipramine and paroxetine are often associated with more side effects than non-paroxetine SSRIs. In general, tolerability of the anticholinergic properties of TCAs may be an issue in MS patients, many of whom already deal with bladder dysfunction. The sexual dysfunction related to SSRIs can also pose a problem in this sensitive patient population.

Electroconvulsive therapy (ECT) has alleviated depression in some patients with MS. Although the majority of case studies suggest that ECT is safe, effective, and well tolerated in this population (Rasmussen & Keegan, 2007; Pontikes & Dinwiddie, 2010), there is one report of a depressed patient with active MS lesions who had a worsened neurological outcome after ECT. Before the use of ECT for MS-related depression, patients should undergo a gadolinium-enhanced MRI scan to rule out active lesions (Mattingly, Baker, et al., 1992).

MANIA

Prevalence and Risk Factors

The rates of bipolar disorder and mania are estimated to be twice as common, at approximately 2% in MS versus 1% in the general population. Although other symptoms in MS, such as pathological laughter and crying, euphoria, and corticosteroid-induced mania, may be mistakenly diagnosed as bipolar disorder, studies that have taken this into account still find higher rates of bipolar illness among patients with MS (Iacovides & Andreoulakis, 2011). Unlike in the case of depression, bipolar disorder in MS does seem to be more prevalent in those with a family history of bipolar disease (Feinstein, 2004).

Diagnosis and Clinical Course

Mania in MS may be indistinguishable from mania in primary bipolar disorder. There are several case reports describing patients with the initial presentation of mania who were misdiagnosed with primary bipolar disorder. A key study by Lyoo and colleagues (1996) found that, of 2,783 patients admitted to a mental hospital over a six-year period, 23 (0.83%) had findings consistent with MS on MRI. Many of these patients had mania or bipolar symptoms. The authors also found that the patients with likely MS had a greater length of hospital stay on index admission compared to those without the MS lesion findings (Lyoo, Seol, et al., 1996). This result suggests that, in patients whose manic symptoms do not resolve within expected time frames, a search for secondary causes such as MS is indicated.

Several case reports indicate the resolution of manic episodes with traditional treatments for bipolar disorder, including mood stabilizers. Unlike in stroke patients, mania can be part of a bipolar course with multiple episodes of mania occurring throughout the lifetime. Manic and euphoric episodes in MS are also associated with increased cognitive decline (Feinstein, 2004).

Etiology

As is the case with all psychiatric disorders, including bipolar disorder, found in the setting of MS, the etiology is likely to be multifactorial. Genetic predisposition, lesion location, and cortical atrophy all play a role. Genetic factors include the presence of certain Human Leukocyte Antigen (HLA) antigens in families with both MS and bipolar illness (Schiffer, Weitkamp, et al., 1988; Bozikas, Anagnostouli, et al., 2003). While studies are inconclusive, psychotic mania appears to be associated with MS plaques in the bilateral temporal lobes, possibly due to limbic involvement (Paparrigopoulos, Ferentinos, et al., 2010). As with stroke, lesions of the right frontal lobe can result in manic symptoms. In addition, the demyelination of orbitofrontal circuits can lead to mania-like behavior from disinhibition, impulsivity, and socially inappropriate acts (Asghar-Ali, Taber, et al., 2004). There may be a further association between cortical atrophy and reduced overall gray matter volume and the development of euphoria in MS (Paparrigopoulos, Ferentinos, et al., 2010).

Treatment

Mood stabilizers and antipsychotics are the primarily interventions for MS-related mania. Lithium has been effective in managing mania in many patients with MS. In contrast, patients with mania due to MS may show delayed or limited response to conventional psychotropic medications (Asghar-Ali, Taber, et al., 2004). There may be an additional benefit of treating the underlying MS with high-dose corticosteroids or immunomodulatory therapies (Asghar-Ali, Taber, et al., 2004; Thone & Kessler, 2008). Euphoria by itself, without mania or pathological affect, a much more frequent presentation of MS, may not require or respond to psychopharmacological intervention (Feinstein, 2004).

FATIGUE

Prevalence and Diagnosis

Perhaps the most common symptom of MS is fatigue, occurring in at least 75% of patients at some point in the course of their illness (Braley & Chervin, 2010). Fatigue contributes to substantial disability and loss of work hours. No universal definition of fatigue exists, as it is more of a subjective experience. Some definitions found in the literature include a "subjective feeling of exhaustion, not improved by bed rest," "lack of energy," and "tiredness." Many authors divide fatigue into mental and physical varieties. Alternatively, fatigue can be divided into central and peripheral types, with MS fatigue representing a central fatigue because it results from central nervous system disease (Cantor, 2010). In contrast, peripheral nervous system fatigue, such as that found in myasthenia gravis, is more easily understood and quantified (Cantor, 2010).

In asking patients about fatigue, a positive answer should be followed by questions to look for depression or primary sleep disorders. Scales for fatigue can be helpful, such as the Krupp's Fatigue Severity Scale and the Modified Fatigue Impact Scale, both of whom have been validated in MS patients; the Epworth Sleepiness Scale; and the Chalder Fatigue Scale (Braley & Chervin, 2010). After other conditions are ruled out, one of these above scales may be useful to monitor the level of fatigue and the treatment response.

Etiology

Among patients with MS, some of the same mechanisms involved in the production of depression play a role in their fatigue. These include cytokine and endocrine changes. Among the cytokines, INF-γ and TNF-α are potential contributors to fatigue as they are increased in MS patients with fatigue compared to those without fatigue (Braley & Chervin, 2010). The HPA axis is also implicated, as low cortisol and Dehydroepiandosterone (DHEA) levels occur in chronic fatigue syndrome. Axonal loss with resulting decreased or altered cerebral metabolism can contribute to fatigue (Braley & Chervin, 2010). MRI studies suggest that frontal or parietal cortical atrophy plays a role in MS-related fatigue (Pellicano, Gallo, et al., 2010). Positron emission tomography (PET) imaging shows decreased glucose metabolism in frontal cortex and basal ganglia in MS patients with fatigue compared to those without fatigue (Roelcke, Kappos, et al., 1997).

Sleep disorders are another potential contributor to fatigue, with poor-quality sleep leading to daytime fatigue. The prevalence of restless leg syndrome in MS is greater than that of the general population, and this contributes to disrupted sleep. If an MS lesion is located in the medullary respiratory centers of the reticular formation, it can lead to central type sleep apnea (Braley & Chervin, 2010). Sleep disruption is also related to medications, pain, depression, anxiety, and spasticity (Braley & Chervin, 2010).

Treatment

There have been several studies investigating amantidine, modafinil, pemoline, and other medications for the treatment of fatigue in MS. Pemoline has not proven to be of any benefit in this condition, but studies with this drug are limited. Placebo-controlled trials for both amantadine and modafinil show some modest, but positive results (Braley & Chervin, 2010). There are no clear data on the use of methylphenidate or amphetamine in MS-related fatigue. The effectiveness of these medications can be enhanced in combination with non-pharmacological interventions, including exercise programs and cooling devices (Braley & Chervin, 2010).

OTHER NEUROPSYCHIATRIC MANIFESTATIONS

Other behavioral manifestations of MS are catatonia, pathological laughter and crying, euphoria, anxiety, psychosis, and personality changes beyond eutonia or euphoria (Feinstein, 2004). In addition, cognitive dysfunction is a key neuropsychiatric complication of MS (Kaplan & Sadock, 1995; Feinstein, 2004).

CLINICAL PEARLS

- Common neurological causes of depression include left frontal strokes, MS, Parkinson's disease, Huntington's disease, Alzheimer's disease and other dementias, and epilepsy.

- Neurological causes of mania are right hemisphere strokes, MS, Parkinson's disease after dopaminergic treatment, Huntington's disease, and trauma.

- Among all the possible psychiatric or behavioral manifestations, post-stroke, depression is consistently the most prevalent. The prevalence of PSD is approximately 33%, a rate much higher than in the general population.

- Depression itself has also been found to be associated with an increased risk of stroke (Dong, Zhang, et al., 2011).

- The severity of depression in the acute post-stroke period is related to distance of the anterior border of the lesion

from the left frontal pole (Robinson, Kubos, et al., 1984; Kaplan & Sadock, 1995; Narushima, Kosier, et al., 2003).

- Patients with depression specifically associated with cerebral microvascular disease or extensive deep white matter and periventricular hyperintensities on MRI have prominent psychomotor slowing, executive function deficits, and relatively poor long-term outcome (Yamashita, Fujikawa, et al., 2010).

- The SIDI is a scale specifically designed for PSD (Roger & Johnson-Greene, 2009).

- Acute-onset PSD occurring days to less than three months after a stroke may remit; however, late-onset PSD occurring after three months is likely to persist and display a more chronic course (Lokk & Delbari, 2010).

- Suicidal thoughts are frequent after a stroke, as evidenced by an overall rate of suicidal ideation of 15% (Santos, Caeiro et al., 2012).

- PSD is more common in those patients with certain *SERT* gene polymorphisms (Kohen, Cain, et al., 2008).

- Despite debate, mania after stroke tends to be more frequent after right-sided lesions involving frontal lobe, temporal lobe, or caudate nucleus.

- The majority of cases of mania appear immediately after the stroke, with approximately 53% occurring in the first few days. Another 23% of mania cases occur within the first month following the stroke (Santos, Caeiro, et al., 2011).

- Strokes involving the medial frontal region and anterior cingulate and the caudate nuclei can result in a frontal apathic-abulic state. After finding that lesions of the posterior limb of the internal capsule were also associated with apathy, Starkstein and associates concluded that damage to the frontal-subcortical networks plays a prominent role in the development of this condition (Jorge, Starkstein, et al., 2010).

- The prevalence of depression is more common in MS than in several other neurological diseases, even in diseases with a comparable amount of loss in function, suggesting that a biological mechanism is involved. In addition, risk of suicide is unfortunately high compared with other neurological disorders (Goldman Consensus Group, 2005).

- Although other symptoms in MS, such as pathological laughter and crying, euphoria, and corticosteroid-induced mania, may be mistakenly diagnosed as bipolar disorder, studies that have taken this into account still find higher rates of bipolar illness among patients with MS (Iacovides & Andreoulakis, 2011).

- Demyelination of orbitofrontal circuits can lead to mania-like behavior from disinhibition, impulsivity, and socially inappropriate acts (Asghar-Ali, Taber, et al., 2004).

- Prevalence of restless leg syndrome in MS is increased compared to that of the general population.

- In MS-related fatigue, placebo-controlled trials for both amantadine and modafinil show some modest, but positive results (Braley & Chervin, 2010). There are no clear data on the use of methylphenidate or amphetamine in MS-related fatigue.

DISCLOSURE STATEMENTS

Dr. Aggarwal has no conflicts of interest to disclose.

Dr. Mendez has no conflicts of interest to disclose.

REFERENCES

Goldman Consensus Group. (2005). The Goldman Consensus statement on depression in multiple sclerosis. *Multiple sclerosis, 11*(3), 328–337.

American Psychiatric Association Task Force on DSM-IV (2000). *Diagnostic and statistical manual of mental disorders: DSM-IV-TR.* Washington, DC: American Psychiatric Association.

Arnett, P. A., & Randolph, J. J. (2006). Longitudinal course of depression symptoms in multiple sclerosis. *Journal of neurology, neurosurgery, and psychiatry, 77*(5), 606–610.

Asghar-Ali, A. A., Taber, K. H., et al. (2004). Pure neuropsychiatric presentation of multiple sclerosis. *The American journal of psychiatry, 161*(2), 226–231.

Astrom, M. (1996). Generalized anxiety disorder in stroke patients. A 3-year longitudinal study. *Stroke; a journal of cerebral circulation, 27*(2), 270–275.

Astrom, M., Adolfsson, R., et al. (1993). Major depression in stroke patients. A 3-year longitudinal study. *Stroke; a journal of cerebral circulation, 24*(7), 976–982.

Benaim, C., Cailly, B., et al. (2004). Validation of the Aphasic Depression Rating Scale. *Stroke; a journal of cerebral circulation, 35*(7), 1692–1696.

Bozikas, V. P., Anagnostouli, M. C., et al. (2003). Familial bipolar disorder and multiple sclerosis: a three-generation HLA family study. *Progress in neuro-psychopharmacology & biological psychiatry, 27*(5), 835–839.

Braley, T. J., & Chervin, R. D. (2010). Fatigue in multiple sclerosis: mechanisms, evaluation, and treatment. *Sleep, 33*(8), 1061–1067.

Cantor, F. (2010). Central and peripheral fatigue: exemplified by multiple sclerosis and myasthenia gravis. *PM & R: the journal of injury, function, and rehabilitation, 2*(5), 399–405.

Carson, A. J., MacHale, S., et al. (2000). Depression after stroke and lesion location: a systematic review. *Lancet, 356*(9224), 122–126.

Castillo, C. S., Starkstein, S. E., et al. (1993). Generalized anxiety disorder after stroke. *The Journal of nervous and mental disease, 181*(2), 100–106.

Chemerinski, E., & Levine, S. R. (2006). Neuropsychiatric disorders following vascular brain injury. *The Mount Sinai journal of medicine, New York, 73*(7), 1006–1014.

Chen, Y., & Patel, N. C., et al. (2007). Antidepressant prophylaxis for poststroke depression: a meta-analysis. *International clinical psychopharmacology, 22*(3), 159–166.

Cummings, J. L., & Mendez, M. F. (1984). Secondary mania with focal cerebrovascular lesions. *The American journal of psychiatry, 141*(9), 1084–1087.

Dong, J. Y., Zhang, Y. H., et al. (2011). Depression and risk of stroke: A meta-analysis of prospective studies. *Stroke; a journal of cerebral circulation, 43*(1), 32–37.

Feinstein, A. (2004). The neuropsychiatry of multiple sclerosis. *Canadian journal of psychiatry. Revue canadienne de psychiatrie, 49*(3), 157–163.

Fujikawa, T., Yamawaki, S., et al. (1995). Silent cerebral infarctions in patients with late-onset mania. *Stroke; a journal of cerebral circulation, 26*(6), 946–949.

Herrmann, M., Bartels, C., et al. (1995). Poststroke depression. Is there a pathoanatomic correlate for depression in the postacute stage of stroke? *Stroke; a journal of cerebral circulation, 26*(5), 850–856.

Iacovides, A., & Andreoulakis, E. (2011). Bipolar disorder and resembling special psychopathological manifestations in multiple sclerosis: a review. *Current opinion in psychiatry, 24*(4), 336–340.

Jorge, R. E., Robinson, R. G., et al. (2003). Mortality and poststroke depression: a placebo-controlled trial of antidepressants. *The American journal of psychiatry, 160*(10), 1823–1829.

Jorge, R. E., Starkstein, S. E., et al. (2010). Apathy following stroke. *Canadian journal of psychiatry. Revue canadienne de psychiatrie, 55*(6), 350–354.

Kahl, K. G., Kruse, N., et al. (2002). Expression of tumor necrosis factor-alpha and interferon-gamma mRNA in blood cells correlates with depression scores during an acute attack in patients with multiple sclerosis. *Psychoneuroendocrinology, 27*(6), 671–681.

Kaplan, H. I., & Sadock, B. J. (1995). *Comprehensive textbook of psychiatry/VI.* Baltimore, MD: Williams & Wilkins.

Koch, M. W., Glazenborg, A., et al. (2011). Pharmacologic treatment of depression in multiple sclerosis. *Cochrane database of systematic reviews*(2), CD007295.

Kohen, R., Cain, K. C., et al. (2008). Association of serotonin transporter gene polymorphisms with poststroke depression. *Archives of general psychiatry, 65*(11), 1296–1302.

Krauthammer, C., & Klerman G. L. (1978). Secondary mania: manic syndromes associated with antecedent physical illness or drugs. *Archives of general psychiatry, 35*(11), 1333–1339.

Larcombe, N. A., & Wilson, P. H. (1984). An evaluation of cognitive-behaviour therapy for depression in patients with multiple sclerosis. *The British journal of psychiatry: the journal of mental science, 145,* 366–371.

Lokk, J., & Delbari, A. (2010). Management of depression in elderly stroke patients. *Neuropsychiatric disease and treatment, 6,* 539–549.

Lyoo, I. K., Seol, H. Y., et al. (1996). Unsuspected multiple sclerosis in patients with psychiatric disorders: a magnetic resonance imaging study. *The Journal of neuropsychiatry and clinical neurosciences, 8*(1), 54–59.

Marin, R. S., Biedrzycki, R. C., et al. (1991). Reliability and validity of the Apathy Evaluation Scale. *Psychiatry research, 38*(2), 143–162.

Mattingly, G., Baker, K., et al. (1992). Multiple sclerosis and ECT: possible value of gadolinium-enhanced magnetic resonance scans for identifying high-risk patients. *The Journal of neuropsychiatry and clinical neurosciences, 4*(2), 145–151.

Migliorelli, R., Starkstein, S. E., et al. (1993). SPECT findings in patients with primary mania. *The Journal of neuropsychiatry and clinical neurosciences, 5*(4), 379–383.

Mohr, D. C., Goodkin, D. E., et al. (1997). Depression, coping and level of neurological impairment in multiple sclerosis. *Multiple sclerosis, 3*(4), 254–258.

Morris, P. L., Robinson, R. G., et al. (1993). Association of depression with 10-year poststroke mortality. *The American journal of psychiatry, 150*(1), 124–129.

Myint, A. M., Schwarz, M. J., et al. (2009). Neuropsychiatric disorders related to interferon and interleukins treatment. *Metabolic brain disease, 24*(1), 55–68.

Narushima, K., Kosier, J. T., et al. (2003). A reappraisal of poststroke depression, intra- and inter-hemispheric lesion location using meta-analysis. *The Journal of neuropsychiatry and clinical neurosciences, 15*(4), 422–430.

Paparrigopoulos, T., Ferentinos, P., et al. (2010). The neuropsychiatry of multiple sclerosis: focus on disorders of mood, affect and behaviour. *International review of psychiatry, 22*(1), 14–21.

Parikh, R. M., Robinson, R. G., et al. (1990). The impact of poststroke depression on recovery in activities of daily living over a 2-year follow-up. *Archives of neurology, 47*(7), 785–789.

Pellicano, C., Gallo, A., et al. (2010). Relationship of cortical atrophy to fatigue in patients with multiple sclerosis. *Archives of neurology, 67*(4), 447–453.

Pontikes, T. K., & Dinwiddie, S. H. (2010). Electroconvulsive therapy in a patient with multiple sclerosis and recurrent catatonia. *The journal of ECT 26*(4), 270–271.

Rasmussen, K. G., & Keegan, B. M. (2007). Electroconvulsive therapy in patients with multiple sclerosis. *The journal of ECT 23*(3), 179–180.

Robinson, R. G. (1986). Post-stroke mood disorders. *Hospital practice, 21*(4), 83–89.

Robinson, R. G., & Starkstein, S. E. (1989). Mood disorders following stroke: new findings and future directions. *Journal of geriatric psychiatry, 22*(1), 1–15.

Robinson, R. G., Kubos, K. L., et al. (1984). Mood disorders in stroke patients. Importance of location of lesion. *Brain: a journal of neurology, 107*(Pt 1), 81–93.

Roelcke, U., Kappos, L., et al. (1997). Reduced glucose metabolism in the frontal cortex and basal ganglia of multiple sclerosis patients with fatigue: a 18F-fluorodeoxyglucose positron emission tomography study. *Neurology, 48*(6), 1566–1571.

Roger, P. R., & Johnson-Greene, D. (2009). Comparison of assessment measures for post-stroke depression. *The Clinical neuropsychologist, 23*(5), 780–793.

Santos, C. O., Caeiro, L., et al. (2011). Mania and stroke: a systematic review. *Cerebrovascular diseases, 32*(1), 11–21.

Santos, C. O., Caeiro, L., et al. (2012). A Study of suicidal thoughts in acute stroke patients. *Journal of stroke and cerebrovascular diseases: the official journal of National Stroke Association, 21*(8), 749–754.

Schiffer, R. B., Caine, E. D., et al. (1983). Depressive episodes in patients with multiple sclerosis. *The American journal of psychiatry, 140*(11), 1498–1500.

Schiffer, R. B., Weitkamp, L. R., et al. (1988). Multiple sclerosis and affective disorder. Family history, sex, and HLA-DR antigens. *Archives of neurology, 45*(12), 1345–1348.

Spalletta, G., Bossu, P., et al. (2006). The etiology of poststroke depression: a review of the literature and a new hypothesis involving inflammatory cytokines. *Molecular psychiatry, 11*(11), 984–991.

Thone, J., & Kessler, E. (2008). Improvement of neuropsychiatric symptoms in multiple sclerosis subsequent to high-dose corticosteroid treatment. *Primary care companion to the Journal of clinical psychiatry, 10*(2), 163–164.

Vattakatuchery, J. J., Rickards, H., et al. (2011). Pathogenic mechanisms of depression in multiple sclerosis. *The Journal of neuropsychiatry and clinical neurosciences, 23*(3), 261–276.

Yamashita, H., Fujikawa, T., et al. (2010). Long-term prognosis of patients with major depression and silent cerebral infarction. *Neuropsychobiology, 62*(3), 177–181.

Yesavage, J. A., Brink, T. L., et al. (1982). Development and validation of a geriatric depression screening scale: a preliminary report. *Journal of psychiatric research, 17*(1), 37–49.

49.

BRAIN TUMOR

Donna B. Greenberg

INTRODUCTION

Patients with brain tumors face the emotional challenge of cancer and mortality along with a threat to their neurological function and their very identity. The great variability in the likelihood of tumor progression and its pace brings anxiety and uncertainty. Some brain tumors have a relatively benign prognosis and cause problems disproportionately less than the fears they engender in patients and their families. The poor prognosis of others makes palliative care an early consideration. Finally, brain tumors can be histologically benign but cause major symptoms and functional impairments because of their location in the brain.

PRIMARY BRAIN TUMORS

Primary brain and other nervous system tumors are relatively rare (incidence of 8 per 100,000) compared to lung cancer, for instance (85 per 100,000). More than 213,500 primary brain and nervous system tumors were diagnosed between 2004 and 2007, and 36% were malignant. The incidence of neuroepithelial malignant brain and nervous system tumors has been essentially stable over the 20 years from 1987 to 2007. Risk is related to hereditary tumor syndromes like neurofibromatosis, increased familial risk, and ionizing radiation (Kohler et al., 2011). There is no evidence for short-term risk of cellular telephones producing brain cancer, and the long-term risk is yet to be fully studied (Corle et al., 2012). The known risk factors highlight the importance of family history and personal history of brain cancer as well as history of radiation exposure in judging who would be more likely to develop a brain tumor.

Primary neuroepithelial tumors include astrocytic, oligodendroglia, and oligoastrocytic tumors, and ependymal and choroid plexus tumors. There are also neuronal and mixed neuronal-glial tumors, pineal tumors, embryonal tumors like medulloblastoma, and primitive neuroectodermal tumors (PNET). In addition, lymphomas and germ-cell tumors can present in the central nervous system (CNS); and craniopharyngiomas develop in the region of the sella. Here we will focus on primary meningiomas and gliomas, then CNS lymphoma, and brain metastases.

MENINGIOMAS

Meningiomas are the most common primary brain tumor. They arise from the dura and most are intracranial. The majority are found in parasagittal regions, the sphenoid ridge, tubercule of the sella turcica, and in the convexity of the brain. The lateral ventricle, olfactory groove, falx, cerebellar tentorium, middle fossa, and orbits are less common sites (Fathi & Roelcke, 2013). The incidence rises with advancing age (Niiro et al., 2000; Go, Taylor, & Kimmel, 1998). Most are asymptomatic and remain the same size or grow very slowly. They are resected for symptoms. Meningiomas may recur once resected and may (rarely) be malignant. Half of patients with neurofibromatosis type 2 develop meningiomas. Those that grow large may have diffuse effects and behavioral symptoms, especially when affecting the frontal or temporal lobe. While patients are anxious before surgery, rates of depression after successful surgery are similar to population norms (Goebel & Mehdorn, 2013).

GLIOMAS

Gliomas are tumors of the neuroglia, the cells that surround and support the neurons of the brain. Gliomas are graded according to their histology and described by their location, size, and grade. Gliomas can begin as low-grade tumors that grow slowly over many years, then transform into (secondary) highly malignant, rapidly progressive tumors. Gliomas infiltrate the brain, so that resection of the visible tumor often is insufficient to completely remove the malignancy. These low-grade gliomas (World Health Organization [WHO] grades I and II)—diffuse astrocytomas, oligodendrogliomas, and mixed oligoastrocytomas—include about 15% of primary brain tumors. The 10-year cumulative survival of supratentorial low-grade gliomas is 43%, and 20-year survival is 26%, so for many they act as a chronic neurological disease (Claus & Black, 2006). The best prognosis occurs with complete resection and with frontal and parietal locations. Low-grade gliomas may be biopsied, resected (Batchelor, 2014), followed with imaging, and treated with chemotherapy intermittently when growth is noted. More rapid growth may occur as time goes on, and then chemotherapy treatments are intensified.

High-grade, rapidly progressive gliomas include anaplastic oligodendroglioma, mixed anaplastic oligoastrocytoma, anaplastic astrocytomas (WHO grade III), and glioblastoma (WHO grade IV). Pure oligodendroglioma has the best outcome and responsiveness to treatment (Stupp et al., 2014). Isocitrate dehydrogenase gene (IDH) mutations are associated with better prognosis. The standard of care for aggressive tumors like glioblastoma includes immediate upfront multi-modal treatment with surgery, radiation, and chemotherapy.

CNS LYMPHOMA

Primary CNS lymphoma represents 4% of newly diagnosed brain tumors. Because lymphoma occurs in the setting of immunodeficiency, the incidence rose when HIV/AIDS was more rampant and untreated, peaking in the mid-1990s. Psychiatric presentations occur in 43% as insidious personality changes, depression, apathy, psychosis, or confusion. Visual hallucinations may be related to infiltration of visual pathways, eye, or leptomeninges (Bataille et al., 2000; Hochberg et al., 2014). If primary CNS lymphoma is suspected, a brain biopsy should precede use of corticosteroids that might alter the biopsy, preventing specific diagnosis.

BRAIN METASTASES

More than half of all brain tumors are metastases from a primary tumor. Now that systemic treatment has improved, and patients live longer, there is more opportunity for brain metastases to develop. The majority occur in the cerebral hemispheres. Metastases occur preferentially at the junction of gray and white matter where the diameter of vessels decreases and traps clumps of tumor cells. They are more common in the watershed areas or border zones between areas of cerebral circulation (Gavrilovic & Posner, 2005).

The rate that brain metastases are diagnosed in life is 20% for lung cancer, 7% for melanoma and renal, 5% for breast, 1–2% in colorectal cancers (Barnholtz-Sloan et al., 2004). The metastatic brain tumors most likely to bleed and therefore to present with stroke are melanoma, choriocarcinoma, thyroid, and renal cancers (Lacy et al., 2012). Brain metastases occur rarely in ovarian cancer, prostate cancer, testicular cancer, esophageal cancer, soft tissue sarcoma, and thyroid cancer (Gavrilovic & Posner, 2005).

PRESENTING SYMPTOMS OF BRAIN TUMORS

Headache occurs in almost half of patients with primary brain tumor, most often tension-type headache, more rarely migrainous headache, typically bifrontal but worse on one side. Nausea and vomiting, a change in headache characteristics or temporal pattern from those the patient has had in the past, and positional worsening with bending forward are clues to a mass. Classic early morning headaches are uncommon as a presenting sign (Forsyth & Posner, 1993), but the headache may awaken the patient from sleep (Omuro & De Angelis, 2013). Change in personality or memory problems are presenting factors in 30–35% (Chang et al., 2005). Less often, stroke from hemorrhage is a presenting symptom in tumors with the tendency to bleed. Nausea, vomiting, papilledema, lethargy, confusion, and signs of increased intracranial pressure require imaging to rule out brain tumor regardless of age (Sivani et al., 2011).

TUMORS HIDDEN BEHIND PSYCHIATRIC ILLNESS

To the extent that patients with brain tumors can present with psychiatric syndromes and a relative absence of neurological findings, psychiatrists are concerned about missing the diagnosis. Chronic persistent headache, a change in headache, or cognitive impairment—slowed thinking, memory loss, and difficulty with multitasking—accompanying more common affective symptoms may be clues. Atypical presentations of typical psychiatric syndromes, treatment resistance, and a recent change in psychiatric presentation should add to suspicion (Madhusoodanan et al., 2007). The availability of imaging in the modern day may have eased worry about a missed diagnosis, but some patients are labeled as having non-organic psychiatric illness without brain imaging, and it is the psychiatrist who must make a decision to look at the patient with a full neurological examination, neuropsychiatric testing, neurological consultation, or to get a brain MRI with contrast. A recent large meta-analysis of published case studies (Subramoniam et al., 2010) did not find a link between specific psychiatric symptoms and location of the tumor in most cases, but found that early mental symptoms occurred in 18% of patients with supratentorial tumors and 5% of infratentorial tumors. Anorectic symptoms and consideration of anorexia nervosa were significantly associated with hypothalamic tumors (Goddard et al., 2013). The neurobehavioral findings of patients with frontal lobe tumors include abulia, personality change, and depression, in contrast to patients with temporolimbic tumors, who present with auditory and visual hallucinations, mania, panic attacks, or amnesia (Filley & Kleinschmidt-DeMasters, 1995).

TREATMENT

SURGERY

The neurosurgeon in planning treatment for a brain tumor considers the anatomy and the tumor's proximity to vital structures. The quality of a biopsy is key to treatment planning in the modern day—for both reliable tumor-grading and for full molecular characterization. In glioblastoma patients, resection is the first goal; the extent of resection is a predictor of survival (Huang et al., 2013). Surgical resection leads to the best outcome for low-grade glioma as well (Jakola et al., 2012). In patients with benign tumors, the decision for resection depends on whether symptoms can be alleviated and comorbid complications minimized.

Surgery is a consideration for an isolated brain metastasis in the setting of a younger patient with good function (Kalkanis et al., 2010). Furthermore, resection of multiple lesions or recurrent lesions is a consideration with or without whole-brain radiation treatment if the tumor is causing a mass effect, if it is accessible, and if it is larger than 30–40 mm. Surgery is coordinated with options for radiation treatment. It is also used when the diagnosis is uncertain and the pathology is known to be radiation-resistant (Owonikoko et al., 2014). Surgical resection may be the only approach to cerebellar lesions particularly if they are large and threaten to cause herniation.

Advances including the use of an operating microscope, real-time correlation of intra-operative findings with intra-operative MRI, and intra-operative dyes that highlight neoplastic tissue have refined the precision of biopsy and tumor removal. Language centers can be preserved if identified by cortical mapping and stimulation when the patient is awake and asleep. Subcortical mapping and diffusion tensor imaging-based tractography map motor pathways.

RADIATION TREATMENT

External beam radiation treatment (RT) requires positioning of the patient on a flat table and immobilization with a thermoplastic mask. The table can move such that more than one beam can aim at the targeted tumor, with the most intense radiation occurring at the intersection of the beams (Huang et al., 2013). Computerized tomography information describes the shape of the tumor and relative density of tissues, so that an RT-planning computer can devise the program. Three-dimensional conformal RT or intensity modulated radiation treatment (IMRT) modulates the intensity of each beam and delivers doses that match complex tumor shapes to reduce damage to healthy tissues near the tumor. Thin beams of radiation of different intensities are aimed at the tumor from many angles. Imaging techniques can be combined with planning to offer image-guided radiotherapy. This treatment is typically done five days per week for several weeks. Stereotactic radiosurgery (SRS) is a form of RT, delivering high doses with precision, using a rigid immobilization device, like a head frame or face mask. The goal is obliteration of a tumor less than 3 cm in a one- to five-day treatment. Sometimes automated robotic devices adjust the patient's position (Huang et al., 2013). SRS is used on focal metastatic lesions to limit or to delay toxicity from whole-brain radiation. It has shown benefit for patients with one to three lesions and is considered for patients with more than three (Owonikoko et al., 2014).

These treatments are difficult for patients who have claustrophobia or anxiety about being immobilized. Several technical modifications for claustrophobic patients have been evaluated (Kim et al., 2004). Relaxation training, urgent behavioral treatments, and/or premedication with benzodiazepines can help phobic patients tolerate the treatment. All these psychological modalities may be used in advance to reduce anticipatory anxiety and to facilitate treatment as it is planned.

CHEMOTHERAPY

Some chemotherapy drugs, like temozolomide, cross the blood–brain barrier, but others have been delivered by intrathecal or intraventricular methods or by chemotherapy-impregnated wafers.

Glioblastoma

In a practice-changing study in 2005, the addition of temozolomide to radiotherapy for newly diagnosed glioblastoma led to a clinically meaningful and statistically significant survival benefit with minimal toxicity (Stupp et al., 2005). That regimen of chemoradiation—post-operative radiation (60 gray [Gy] divided in 30 fractions) with temozolomide initially and then adjuvant six cycles of five days of temozolomide every four weeks—prolonged progression-free and overall survival and is currently the preferred treatment for all age groups (Stupp et al., 2005; Stupp et al., 2009; Hart et al., 2013). In the signal study, with radiation and chemotherapy, the two-year survival rate was 27%, versus 10% with only radiotherapy. The prognosis is still poor, however, with a five-year survival rate of 17% in patients younger than 50. Tumors with methylation of the promoter for methylguanine methyltransferase (MGMT) were more responsive to temozolomide. The outcome for glioblastoma with radiation and temozolomide for the MGMT-positive group was a 49% two-year survival (Stupp et al., 2009). A similar treatment is often recommended for anaplastic astrocytoma, but the contributions of chemotherapy and/or radiation treatment are not yet clear. The third category, anaplastic oligodendroglioma, has a somewhat better prognosis than anaplastic astrocytoma (Batchelor, 2014; Stupp et al., 2014). Salvage chemotherapy includes bevacizumab; temozolomide again; carmustine, lomustine, and carboplatin (Omuro & De Angelis, 2013). Other targeted drugs are under development.

Half of patients with glioblastoma are over age 65, and their prognosis is related to performance status and age. For the older patient with other medical comorbidities, treatment can include temozolomide alone, hypofractionated RT alone, best supportive care, or whole-brain RT for urgent relief of symptoms (Arvold & Reardon, 2014).

Primary CNS Lymphoma

Methotrexate, high-dose systemic treatment, is the backbone of induction treatment for CNS lymphoma. This may be combined with cytarabine, or a combination of rituximab and temozolomide (Hochberg & Batchelor, 2014). RT is deferred.

Brain Metastases

Systemic chemotherapy and targeted drugs that offer hope of treating brain metastases, often as part of the treatment for systemic disease, include gefitinib, erlotinib, and crizotinib in non–small cell lung cancer; and lapatinib and capecitabine for human epidermal growth factor receptor (HER)-2 positive breast cancer. Dabrafenib and vemurafenib,

(BRAF)-inhibitors used for BRAF-mutant melanoma and ipilimumab, have shown promise in treating CNS disease in melanoma (Owonikoko, 2014).

ISSUES IN CARE

PROGRESSION VS. PSEUDOPROGRESSION

One of the difficulties of care for patients with glioblastoma and their physicians is that the assessment of the response to treatment or the progression of tumors can be ambiguous. *Pseudoprogression* is transient radiographic worsening occurring up to four months after RT. This occurred in 21% of patients in the glioblastoma treatment study (Stupp et al., 2005) with RT and temozolomide compared to 90% with RT alone. More pseudoprogression is seen in MGMT-positive patients. Treatment is often continued if progression is not definitive (Batchelor & Loeffler, 2014). The patient has regularly repeated scans to assess the state of the tumor, and coping with ambiguity and uncertainty is a regular challenge for the patient and family.

THROMBOEMBOLIC DISEASE

Patients with brain tumor are at greater risk of veno-occlusive disease and pulmonary embolism. Therefore, clinicians should be alert to signs of clots. The risk of spontaneous bleeding in the tumor is low, except in patients with metastases of tumors prone to hemorrhage, including melanoma, choriocarcinoma, thyroid carcinoma, and renal carcinoma. Prophylactic anticoagulation is not recommended but the presence of a brain tumor does not contraindicate anticoagulant treatment for thrombosis that has been proven (Jenkins et al., 2010; Gerber et al., 2006; Stupp et al., 2014).

SEIZURES

Brain tumor patients present with a seizure 20–40% of the time, and another 20% have at least one or more during their course of treatment. Primary tumors are more apt to cause seizure than metastases (Wen, 2006; Lacy et al., 2012). The most benign neuroepithelial tumors have the highest risk of seizure. If the tumor is in the temporal and insular cortex, the rate of developing epilepsy is higher (Kerkhof & Vecht, 2013).

Low-grade gliomas have a 70–90% incidence of seizure, while glioblastoma rates of seizure range from 30% to 62% (Kerkhof & Vecht, 2013; Lote et al., 1998). Both simple and complex seizures with or without generalization are seen. An electroencephalogram has two roles: to see if unexplained symptoms may be caused by subclinical seizures and to determine if delirium is caused by status epilepticus (Omuro & De Angelis, 2013). Management of persistent seizures is key to quality of life in low-grade glioma patients who have a chronic course (Shields & Choucair, 2014).

Short-term prophylaxis with a newer anti-epileptic drug is appropriate for patients having brain surgery, to prevent early post-operative seizures (Rossetti & Stupp, 2010; Glantz et al., 2000). Levetiracetam is the most common drug currently used. How long the drug is continued is not well defined, (Chang et al., 2005), but generally anti-seizure drugs are tapered beginning one or two weeks after tumor resection and discontinued in those who do not have a seizure (Kuijlen et al., 1996; Chang et al., 2008; Fuller et al., 2013).

In patients with brain tumors who have not had a seizure, anti-epileptic drugs are not recommended, as there is no evidence of prophylactic benefit (Sirven et al., 2004; Mikkelsen et al., 2010; Tremont-Lukats et al., 2008; Stupp et al., 2014). Anti-epileptic drugs are not required for posterior fossa tumors (Wen et al., 2006). For those who have had a seizure, anticonvulsants are continued as long as the brain tumor is present, better at low doses in the setting of partial resection, with stable and controlled seizures (Rossetti & Stupp, 2010; Drappatz et al., 2014).

When anticonvulsants are required, levetiracetam, pregabalin, lamotrigine, lacosamide, and topiramate are preferred rather than older anticonvulsants like valproate that affect the cytochrome P450 system and have more drug interactions and toxicity (Lacy et al., 2012).

For the psychiatrist following a patient with a brain tumor who is on levetiracetam, the most common clinical question is whether irritability is due to this drug and whether an anticonvulsant switch is warranted. Irritability is reported in 6–12% of patients on levetiracetam. In a study comparing phenytoin and levetiracetam perioperatively, levetiracetam had only mild mood effects (Fuller et al., 2013). Helmstaedter and colleagues (2008) found a moderate increase in aggression, loss of self-control, restlessness, and sleep problems in 25 percent of 288 consecutive epilepsy patients taking levetiracetam and more severe symptoms in 12%. These symptoms were independent of dose, but associated with poorer seizure control, mental retardation, and a psychiatric disposition of impulsivity. When irritability and aggression are problematic symptoms in patients with brain tumors, it is worth considering a change of anticonvulsant; however, the ease of treatment with levetiracetam, and the lack of need for frequent blood levels, has made it the default choice. Lamotrigine is an alternative that has beneficial effects on mood. Reports related to anxiety for most anticonvulsants are mixed (Piedad et al., 2012).

CEREBRAL EDEMA

Cerebral edema comes with tumor presentation, tumor progression, RT, and steroid withdrawal. The vessels in the brain are more permeable when the blood–brain barrier is disrupted, so that plasma fluid and proteins move into the brain parenchyma and interstitial fluid. Headache, lethargy, and confusion are symptoms. The symptom of dizziness can increase with the Valsalva maneuver or upon standing, due to transient increases in pressure associated with near syncope. The risk is herniation of the cerebellar tonsils through the foramen magnum and death (Lacy et al., 2012). Disruption of the blood–brain barrier is noted when gadolinium seeps through breaks in blood–brain barrier into areas of parenchymal enhancement noted on post-contrast T1 sequences of the MRI. Edema is seen as hyperintensity on T2 images and fluid attenuated inversion recovery (FLAIR) sequences without contrast. To complicate matters, hyperintensity is also seen with infiltrative non-enhancing tumor or post-treatment gliosis (Lacy et al., 2012).

CORTICOSTEROIDS

Dexamethasone is the treatment of choice for cerebral edema. Dexamethasone 4 mg orally every 6 hours is usually given for moderate symptoms. If herniation is not a risk, 4 mg or 8 mg per day may work and can be used for mild symptoms (Vecht et al., 1994). The half-life of dexamethasone is actually longer than six hours. Improvement occurs within hours to several days. A taper should occur at 50% reduction of the previous dose, tapered to the dose that preserves neurological function.

Toxicity of steroids is related to dose and duration. After 7 or 28 days of the full dose of 16 mg per day, brain tumor patients suffer proximal weakness (38%), peripheral edema (26%), hypertension 26%, gastrointestinal (GI) side effects, and change in mental status 21% (Vecht et al., 1994). Hyperglycemia is common.

Gastrointestinal Side Effects

Proton pump inhibitors as prophylaxis against ulcer or gastritis are preferred for patients with a history of ulcer, in the perioperative period and in patients taking non-steroidal anti-inflammatory agents (Kostaras et al., 2014; Lacy et al., 2012).

Psychiatric Side Effects

The medical psychiatrist can be helpful in evaluation and treatment of psychiatric side effects of corticosteroids. With steroids alone, in the absence of the trauma and disability of a brain tumor, patients can develop insomnia, manic-like symptoms, psychosis, and depression. Mood stabilizers like atypical antipsychotics may be helpful for emotional lability. Antidepressants may be necessary for typical syndromes of major depressive disorder. Cessation of steroids does not cause immediate improvement of psychiatric side effects, so psychotropic drugs have a role in the interval.

Steroid Myopathy

Steroid myopathy correlates with Cushingoid appearance and tends to occur after two to twelve weeks of treatment. Weakness is seen in proximal muscles bilaterally, in the legs more than in the arms. Therefore, patients may need help getting up from a low seat and have trouble climbing stairs; they may have difficulty doing things with their arms above their heads. Although the role of exercise in repair of myopathy is limited, physical therapy may be an important factor in the maintenance of mobility and quality of life (Pereira & de Carvalho, 2010).

Pneumocystis Prophylaxis

Patients under treatment with chemotherapy and RT, often also on corticosteroids, are immunodeficient and prone to pneumocystis pneumonia. Prophylaxis against pneumocystis makes trimethoprim-sulfamethoxazole, atovaquone, dapsone, or pentamidine a recommended part of the treatment (Kelly & Cronin, 2014).

COMPLICATIONS OF SURGERY

Infection and hematoma are common complications of surgery; others (less common) are hydrocephalus, pseudomeningocele, and posterior fossa syndrome (mutism, emotional lability, difficulties initiating movement). Posterior fossa syndrome is seen mostly in children after posterior fossa surgery; for instance, for medulloblastoma. Children with midline tumors and brainstem invasion are more at risk. Language, thinking, and balance disturbances may persist beyond one year, with incomplete recovery (Korah et al., 2010). Risperidone has been used in these children for irritability and difficulty with speech; study of its benefit is in progress.

COMPLICATIONS OF RADIATION TREATMENT

Side effects of RT depend on treatment location, fraction size, total dose, target volume, and technique. The dose and type of radiation are defined to minimize injury to normal tissue. Radiation is avoided in children less than three years old. Partial brain radiotherapy with doses of 50 to 60 Gy is associated with a low incidence of late neurocognitive decline (Armstrong et al., 2002; Brown, 2003). SRS treatment without whole-brain radiation causes less neurocognitive decline in function than does whole-brain RT with SRS (Tsao et al., 2012). Studies of hippocampal-sparing techniques are now in progress to reduce the neurocognitive toxicity of whole-brain radiation (Gondi et al., 2010; 2012).

The acute side effects of brain radiation include cerebral edema, and then within a few weeks, early demyelination. Corticosteroids are the main treatment for the symptoms of headache, neurocognitive and focal neurological deficits, and seizures. Patients can develop a transient cognitive decline, fatigue during treatment, and somnolence, which can persist for several months. Pseudoprogression, as noted above, is a radiation effect that tends to occur in the first three months after treatment, sometimes with neurological findings. Because the symptoms are sleepiness and exacerbation of tumor-related symptoms, the syndrome is difficult to distinguish from tumor growth (Wen et al., 2010; Patel et al., 2011). Complications six months to three years after whole-brain RT include asymptomatic white matter lesions, and diffuse white matter injury.

Leukoencephalopathy after whole-brain RT has an incidence of 34% if the patient is followed for more than six months; older age is a risk factor (Ebi et al., 2013). The process is thought to be related to accelerated atherosclerosis and mineralizing microangiopathy from small-vessel disease.

Gradual pituitary-hypothalamus dysfunction, hypothyroidism, hypogonadism, and growth hormone deficiency are also seen as a consequence of radiation. An endocrinologist is often consulted for management of thyroid hormones, reproductive hormones, corticosteroids, and growth hormone replacement. Brain tumor survivors who suffered growth hormone deficiency after treatment have been shown to be similar to patients with growth hormone deficiency from other pituitary pathologies. Their quality of life improved when growth hormone was replaced (Mukherjee et al., 2005).

Radiation necrosis with mass effect and associated progressive neurological dysfunction (Fink et al., 2012) is related to microvascular degeneration and loss of capillary endothelial cells. On imaging, white matter change, ventricular dilatation, and cortical atrophy are noted. While the first treatment for radiation necrosis is typically corticosteroids or sometimes surgery for symptoms, bevacizumab at doses lower than the anti-tumor dose for four treatments has been used (Levin et al., 2011).

Vascular effects of radiation may present as stroke-like migraine attacks. These effects are due to radiation injury, endothelial injury, and their direct effect on oligodendritic progenitor cells (Lacy et al., 2012).

BEVACIZUMAB

Bevacizumab is an antiangiogenic medication often used in the setting of malignant glioma in the hope of blocking microvessel sprout growth and proliferation of endothelial cues in the tumor. In the treatment of recurrent glioblastoma, contrast enhancement can be reduced in hours or days after initiation of bevacizumab. It is unclear whether this is related to tumor response or to treatment-induced reduction of the blood–brain barrier, or both. Furthermore, it is unclear if this drug will alter the pattern of spread of the tumor (Armstrong et al., 2012).

Side effects of bevacizumab include hypertension and proteinuria. Hypertension is best treated with the same principles as general hypertension. The preferred antihypertensive drugs (due to a lack of drug interactions) are amlodipine and felodipine. Angiotensin-converting enzyme (ACE) inhibitors are used when hypertension requires rapid response, and this class of drugs is useful for proteinuria as well.

A complication of bevacizumab is posterior reversible encephalopathy syndrome (PRES). This syndrome is associated with VEGF-sequestering agents and with tyrosine kinase inhibitors targeting VEGF. It resolves with treatment of hypertension and removal of the causative agent. It presents with headache, seizure, confusion, and often cortical blindness. MRI shows T2/FLAIR hyperintensities, mostly in white matter. Lesions are more often seen in the posterior cerebral hemisphere or posterior fossa. The pathogenesis is presumed to be related to cerebral vasomotor autoregulation or preeclampsia-like endothelial damage.

The risk of hemorrhage is increased with bevacizumab. This ranges from epistaxis to more serious bleeding. The risk of intracerebral hemorrhage remains low in patients with brain metastasis, with the exception of tumors like melanoma that have higher rates of hemorrhage. Because of impaired wound healing, bevacizumab is stopped around surgery. Venous and arterial thromboembolism and bowel perforation are also considerations.

PSYCHIATRIC SIDE EFFECTS AND THEIR TREATMENTS

DEPRESSION AND ANXIETY

Depressive symptoms are common in patients with brain tumors, as many of the symptoms of the tumor or treatment include fatigue, poor concentration, and the challenge of coping with the predicament of diagnosis; as many at 44% are reported to be depressed (Ford et al., 2012). In one series of about 600 patients with high-grade gliomas, 93% reported depressive symptoms (Litofsky et al., 2004). About 15% reported explicitly that they were depressed, and their symptoms increased after surgery. Patients with high-grade gliomas worry about starting treatment and what will ensue; they are demoralized by hair loss, weight gain, fatigue, and lower function (Kilbride et al., 2007). Loss of autonomy is a major difficulty for many patients (Sterckx et al., 2013). In the first six months, radiation effect complicates the diagnosis of major depressive disorder.

Preoperative depression was independently associated with decreased survival in a retrospective review of more than 1,000 astrocytoma patients (Gathinji et al., 2009; and depressive symptoms have also been linked to shorter survival among patients with low-grade glioma (Mainio et al., 2005; Mainio et al., 2006). Patients with low-grade gliomas also have a high prevalence of generalized anxiety, phobia and obsessionality (Arnold et al., 2008; Mainio, 2011). The risk of hospitalization for depression in the first year after a cancer diagnosis was highest for men with brain cancer in a nationwide, population based study of cancer patients in Denmark (Dalton et al., 2009).

COGNITIVE IMPAIRMENT AND INATTENTION

Cognitive impairment may come with subclinical tumor progression and before radiological changes, interfering with patients' communication and ability to make decisions (Ford et al., 2012). The specific impairments vary according to location of the tumor and treatment. One study of patients with brain metastases documented deficits in 91% of patients at baseline, with some improvement in executive function and memory after treatment with fractionated whole-brain radiation. Cognitive function before treatment was inversely related to tumor volume and correlated with better survival (Meyers et al., 2004).

Patients with low-grade gliomas experience long-term cognitive deficits related to the tumor, but also to epilepsy, disease progression, surgery, and radiation therapy (Surma-aho et al., 2001; Taphoorn, 2003). In patients with CNS lymphoma, the cognitive deficits associated with methotrexate-induced leukoencephalopathy, especially when combined with radiation, have been followed with a standardized battery measuring attention, executive function, memory, and psychomotor speed (Correa et al., 2007).

Patients with tumors in the frontal and temporal lobes are often referred to psychiatry because of the behavioral symptoms and poor executive function that may be associated with their lesion. Disability often leads to loss of a job or profession. Neuropsychiatric testing can highlight particular deficits in memory or attention. The combined power of cognitive rehabilitation, vocational rehabilitation, and individualized psychopharmacological treatment of depression, anxiety, and irritability can be brought to bear by the medical psychiatrist. In children who had multi-modal treatment for brain tumors, cognitive rehabilitation (including attention process training, strategy acquisition, and cognitive behavioral therapy) has been shown to improve academic achievement (Lagenbahn et al., 2013). The data for adults are also suggestive (Butler & Copeland, 2002; Butler & Copeland, 2008; Gehring et al., 2009). Both cognitive deficits and behavioral challenges, including inertia, anger, and inappropriate behavior, have been tackled by teaching the patient self-management skills and compensatory strategies and educating the family and staff, the people around the patient, techniques of behavioral management (Whiting et al., 2012).

Modafinil (Kaleita et al., 2006) has been used for attention and energy (Gehring et al., 2012; Meyers et al., 1998; Weitzner et al., 1995). However, one recent multi-center randomized controlled trial with a crossover design evaluating modafinil up to 400 mg per day did not find that modafinil improvement exceeded that of placebo (Boele et al., 2013).

Methylphenidate has improved attention and energy in adult brain tumor survivors and has also been shown to have benefits of sustained attention over a year for childhood cancer survivors (Conklin et al., 2010). A randomized, double-blind, placebo-controlled crossover trial of methylphenidate in child cancer survivors identified as having attention deficits and learning problems showed a better response with moderate-dose methylphenidate (0.6 mg/kg) in the patients whom parents and teachers noted as having more problems.

Donepezil, an anticholinesterase (AChE) inhibitor, has been tested for treatment of cognitive impairment after radiation. Survivors who have had brain radiation complain of decreased attention and concentration, poor short-term memory, and difficulty with expressive language. A pilot study of patients, mostly with low-grade glioma, more than six months after treatment, given donepezil 5 mg per day for six weeks and then 10 mg per day for 18 weeks, found improved attention/concentration, verbal memory and figural memory, and a trend for verbal fluency (Shaw et al., 2006). Another small, open-trial pilot study of childhood brain tumor survivors more than one year from cancer treatment who had received cranial radiation found that donepezil led to executive function and memory improvements. Some had initial vomiting and diarrhea (Castellino et al., 2012).

Memantine acts as an N-methyl-D-aspartate (NMDA) receptor antagonist and is used for Alzheimer's disease. The Radiation Therapy Oncology Group (RTOG) compared whole-brain radiation treatment with memantine to whole-brain radiation treatment with placebo, and found less neurocognitive decline in the memantine group (Brown et al., 2013). The dose of memantine began with 5 mg the first week and was increased to 5 mg twice daily in week 2, 10 mg in the mornings and 5 mg in the evenings in week 3, until the 10 mg twice-a-day dose was reached at week 4. That full dose was continued for 24 weeks. Those taking memantine had delayed decline in cognition over time in memory, executive function, and processing speed.

CARE OF CAREGIVERS

The mental well-being of caregivers has a profound effect on the well-being of patients with brain tumors, so consideration of caregiver mental health is an important aspect of psychiatric care. More than 40% of caregivers have depression and anxiety, and patients' mood correlates with their caregivers' mood. Caregivers report challenges like the difficulty of telling others about the diagnosis, and worrying about their role change in a marriage. Relationships have to be renegotiated. Caregivers worry that their loved one might have recurrent seizures and therefore sometimes limit their activities with the patient for fear of seizures. They often find the patient's mood change, change of personality, and cognitive decline more difficult to bear than their physical disabilities. Cognitive impairment increases as the disease progresses, and the loss of the loved one's identity, memory, and awareness, the sense that the patient is "absent," is a major source of grief (Schmer et al., 2008; McConigley et al., 2010; Sterckx et al., 2013).

END OF LIFE

Drowsiness and loss of consciousness are the most common symptoms in the last weeks; in addition, poor communication, focal neurological deficits, seizures, dysphagia, and headaches are frequent (Walbert & Khan, 2014). Steroids are often used in the last weeks. Anticonvulsants may be compounded as a rectal suppository; intranasal or buccal midazolam has also been used to stop seizures (Nakken & Lossius, 2011). Decisions are required around tube feeding, hydration, steroid discontinuation, and palliative sedation (Pace et al., 2009). Dissolving wafers, sublingual and transdermal medications are important in the last days when dysphagia is prominent. Headaches are treated with non-steroidal medications and steroids. Most patients are not deemed competent for decisions in the last weeks. Dying with dignity depends on timely treatment of symptoms, good communication, defining preferences before the patient can no longer communicate, and fewer transitions in the last month of life (Sizoo et al., 2013).

CONCLUSION

In sum, the medical psychiatrist and psychologist have the role of helping the patient deal with existential anxiety in the setting of a malignant brain tumor diagnosis, whether preparing for a short or long course. They remain alert to pharmacological treatment of major depressive disorder as it occurs in this stressful setting. Distinct attention to the psychiatric side effects of corticosteroids and treatment with mood stabilizers may be critical at times. The organizing structure of physical therapy, particularly for steroid myopathy as the steroids are tapered, can make a difference in the patients' quality of life. Psychotherapeutic discussion includes grief, anger at the illness or between loved ones, adjustments in lifestyle, conservation of emotional and physical energy, and the need to "put things in order" in the context of the patient's values. The factors that sustain a patient's ability to drive a car or require adjustment to the loss of driving, even temporarily, are pertinent. Treatments of anxiety, behavioral and pharmacological, may be particularly important in patients with low-grade tumors who face a chronic course. Anxiety disorder may predate the brain tumor, and the added contribution to the patient's current anxiety may not be as evident to the medical team. For patients who have cognitive deficits after tumor resection or radiation, psychiatrists optimize treatment of depression, clarify cognitive deficits, and make referrals for cognitive rehabilitation. Methylphenidate and modafinil have a role, especially for attentional deficits in survivors. Pituitary dysfunction should not be missed; consideration of hypothyroidism, hypogonadism, adrenal dysfunction, or growth hormone deficiency is something to remember for survivors. The role of memantine and donepezil for preserving or improving memory after brain radiation is under further study.

CLINICAL PEARLS

- The incidence of meningioma rises with advancing age (Niiro et al., 2000; Go et al., 1998). Most are asymptomatic and remain the same size or grow very slowly.

- The rate of brain metastases diagnosed in life is 20% for lung, 7% for melanoma and renal, 5% for breast, 1–2% in colorectal cancers (Barnholtz-Sloan, 2004).

- The metastatic brain tumors most likely to bleed and therefore to present with stroke are melanoma, choriocarcinoma, and thyroid and renal tumors (Lacy et al., 2012).

- Headache, occurring in almost half of patients with primary brain tumor, is most often a tension-type headache, (more rarely) migrainous headache, typically bifrontal but worse on one side. Nausea and vomiting, a change in headache characteristics or temporal pattern from those the patient has had in the past, and positional worsening with bending forward are clues to a mass (Forsyth & Posner, 1993).

- Anti-seizure medication to prevent seizure in a patient with a brain tumor who never had a seizure is not necessary.

- Memantine may have a role in preventing cognitive decline from whole-brain radiation.

- Attentional deficits after treatment may be treated with cognitive rehabilitation and stimulants.

- Hormonal deficits like thyroid, growth hormone, corticosteroids, and reproductive hormones warrant monitoring and endocrine referral after treatment for brain tumor.

DISCLOSURE STATEMENT

Dr. Greenberg has no conflicts of interest to disclose.

REFERENCES

Arvold, N. D., & Reardon, D. A. (2014). Treatment options and outcomes for glioblastoma in the elderly patient. *Clinical Interventions in Aging, 9,* 357–367.

Armstrong, C. L., Hunter, J. V., Ledakis, G. E., et al. (2002). Late cognitive and radiographic changes related to radio therapy: initial prospective findings. *Neurology, 59,* 40–48.

Armstrong, T. S., Wen, P. Y., Gilbert, M. R., & Schiff, D. (2012). Management of treatment associated toxicity of anti-angiogenic therapy in patients with brain tumors. *Neuro-Oncology, 14*(10), 1203–1214.

Arnold, S. D., Forman, L. M., Brigidi, B. D., Carter, K. E., et al. (2008). Evaluation and characterization of generalized anxiety and depression in patients with primary brain tumors. *Neuro-Oncology, 10,* 171–181.

Bataille, B., Delwail, V., Menet, E., et al. (2000). Primary intracerebral malignant lymphoma: report of 248 cases. *Journal of Neurosurgery, 92,* 261.

Barnholtz-Sloan, J. S., Sloan, A. E., Davis, F. G., Vigneau, F. D., Lai, P., & Sawaya, R. E. (2004). Incidence proportions of brain metastases in patients diagnosed (1973 to 2001) in the Metropolitan Detroit Cancer Surveillance system. *Journal of Clinical Oncology, 22,* 2865–2872.

Batchelor, T. (2014). Adjuvant chemotherapy for glioblastoma and anaplastic astrocytoma malignant gliomas. *Up-To-Date.* Basow, DS (Ed), Waltham MA, UpToDate.

Boele, F. W., Douw, L., de Groot, M., et al. (2013). The effect of modafinil on fatigue, cognitive functioning, and mood in primary brain tumor patients: a multicenter randomized controlled trial. *Neuro-Oncology, 15,* 1420–1428.

Brown, P. D., Buckner, J. C., O'Fallon, J. R., et al. (2003). Effects of radiotherapy on cognitive function in patients with low-grade glioma measured by the Folstein Mini-Mental State Examination. *Journal of Clinical Oncology, 21,* 2519–2524.

Brown, P. D., Pugh S., Laack N. N., et al. (2013). memantine for the prevention of cognitive dysfunction in patients receiving whole-brain radiotherapy: a randomized, double blind, placebo controlled trial. *Neuro-Oncology, 15,* 1429–1437.

Butler, R. W., Copeland, D. R., Fairclough, D. L., et al. (2008). A multicenter, randomized clinical trial of a cognitive remediation program for childhood survivors of a pediatric malignancy. *Journal of Consulting Clinical Psychology, 76,* 367–378.

Butler, R. W., Copeland DR. (2002). Attentional processes and their remediation in children treated for cancer a literature review and the development of a therapeutic approach *Journal of the International Neuropsychology Society, 8,* 115–124.

Castellino, S. M., Tooze, J. A., Lowers, L., et al. (2012). Toxicity and efficacy of the acetylcholinesterase (AChE) inhibitor donepezil in childhood brain tumor survivors: a pilot study. *Pediatric Blood & Cancer, 59,* 540–547.

Chang, S., Parney, I. F., Huang, W., et al. (2005). Patterns of care for adults with newly diagnosed malignant glioma. *Journal of the American Medical Association, 293,* 557–564.

Chang, E. F., Potts, M. B., Keles, G. E., et al. (2008). Seizure characteristics and control following resection in 332 patients with low grade gliomas. *Journal of Neurosurgery, 108,* 227–235.

Claus, E. B., & Black, P. M. (2006). Survival rates and patterns of care for patients diagnosed with supratentorial low-grade gliomas: data from the SEER [Surveillance Epidemiology and End Results] program, 1973–2001. *Cancer, 106*, 1358–63.

Conklin, H. M., Reddick, W. E., Ashford, J., et al. (2010). Long-term efficacy of methylphenidate in enhancing attention regulation, social skills and academic abilities of childhood cancer survivors. *Journal of Clinical Oncology, 28*, 4465–4472.

Correa, D. D., Maron, L., Harder, H., et al. (2007). Cognitive functions in primary central nervous system lymphoma: literature review and assessment guidelines. *Annals of Oncology, 18*, 1145.

Corle, C., Makale, M., & Keari, S. (2012). Cell phones and glioma risk: a review of the evidence. *Journal of Neurooncology, 106*, 1–113.

Dalton, S. O., Laursen, T. M., Ross, L., et al. (2009). Risk for hospitalization with depression after a cancer diagnosis: a nationwide, population based study of cancer patients in Denmark from 1973–2003. *Journal of Clinical Oncology, 27*(9), 1440–1445.

Drappatz, J., Wen, P. Y., Avila, E. K., et al. (2014). Seizures in patients with primary and metastatic brain tumors. In: *UpToDate*, Baslow DS (Ed), Waltham MA, UpToDate, 2014.

Ebi, J., Sato, H., Nakajima, M., & Shishido, F. (2013). Incidence of leukoencephalopathy after whole-brain radiation therapy for brain metastases. *International Journal of Radiation Oncology Biology Physics, 85*, 1212–1217.

Fathi, A.-R., & Roelcke, U. (2013). Meningioma. *Current Neurology & Neuroscience Reports, 13*, 337–315.

Filley, C. M., & Kleinschmidt-DeMasters, B. K. (1995). Neurobehavioral presentations of brain neoplasms. *Western Journal of Medicine, 163*, 19–25.

Fink, J., Born, D., & Chamberlain, M. C. (2012). Radiation necrosis: relevance with respect to treatment of primary and secondary brain tumors. *Current Neurology & Neuroscience Reports, 12*, 276–285.

Ford, E., Catt, S., Chalmers, A., & Fallowfield, L. (2012). Systematic review of supportive care needs in patients with primary malignant brain tumors. *Neuro-Oncology, 14*(4), 392–404.

Forsyth, P. A., & Posner, J. B. (1993). Headaches in patients with brain tumors: a study of 111 patients. *Neurology, 43*, 1678–1683.

Fuller, K. L., Wang, Y. Y., Cook, M. J., et al. (2013). Tolerability, safety, and side effects of levetiracetam versus phenytoin in intravenous and total prophylactic regimen among craniotomy patients: a prospective randomized study. *Epilepsia, 54*, 45.

Gathinji, M., McGirt, M., Attenello, F., et al. (2009). Association of preoperative depression and survival after resection of malignant brain astrocytoma. *Surgical Neurology, 71*(3), 299–303.

Gavrilovic, I. T., & Posner, J. B. (2005). Brain metastases: epidemiology and pathophysiology. *Journal of Neuro-Oncology, 75*, 5–14.

Gehring, K., Patwardhan, S. Y., Collins, R., et al. (2012). A randomized trial on the efficacy of methyphenidate and modafinil for improving cognitive functioning and symptoms in patients with a primary brain tumor. *Journal of Neurooncology, 107*(1), 165–174.

Gehring, K., Sitskoorn, M. M., Gundy, C. M., et al. (2009). Cognitive rehabilitation in patients with gliomas: a randomized, controlled trial. *Journal of Clinical Oncology, 27*, 3712–3722.

Gerber, D. E., Grossman, S. A., & Streiff, M. D. (2006). Management of venous thromboembolism in patients with primary and metastatic brain tumors. *Journal of Clinical Oncology, 24*, 1310–1318.

Glantz, M. J., Cole, B. F., Forsyth, P. A., et al. (2000). Practice parameter: anticonvulsant prophylaxis in patients with newly diagnosed brain tumors. Report of the Quality Standards Subcommittee of the American Academy of Neurology. *Neurology, 54*, 1886–1893.

Go, R. S., Taylor, B. V., & Kimmel, D. W. (1998). The natural history of asymptomatic meningiomas in Olmsted County, Minnesota. *Neurology, 51*, 1718.

Goddard, E., Ashkan, K., Farrimond, S., Bunnage, M., & Treasure, J. (2013). Right frontal lobe glioma presenting as anorexia nervosa: further evidence implicating dorsal anterior cingulate as an area of dysfunction. *International Journal of Eating Disorders, 46*, 189–192.

Goebel, S., & Mehdorn, H. M. (2013). Development of anxiety and depression in patients with benign intracranial meningiomas: a prospective long-term study. *Supportive Care in Cancer, 21*, 1365–1372.

Gondi, V., Hermann, B. P., Mehta, M. P., & Tome, W. A. (2012). Hippocampal dosimetry predicts neurocognitive function impairment after fractionated stereotactic radiotherapy for benign or low-grade adult brain tumors. *International Journal of Radiation Oncology Biology Physics, 83*, e487–e493.

Gondi, V., Tolakanahalli, R., Mehta, M. P., et al. (2010). Hippocampalsparing whole-brain radiotherapy: a how-to technique using helical tomography and linear accelerator-based intensity modulated radiotherapy. *International Journal of Radiation Oncology Biology Physics, 78*, 1244–1252.

Hart, M. G., Garside, R., Rogers, G., et al. (2013). Temozolomide for high grade glioma. *Cochrane Database of Systematic Reviews, 4*, CD007415.

Helmstaedter, C., Fritz, N. E., Kockelmann, E., Kosanetzky, N., & Elger, C. E. (2008). Positive and negative psychotropic effects of levetiracetam. *Epilepsy and Behavior, 13*, 535–541.

Hochberg, F. H., Batchelor, T. (2014). Treatment and prognosis of primary central nervous system lymphoma. *UpToDate*, Basow, DS (Ed), Waltham, MA, UpToDate.

Hochberg, F. H., Batchelor, T., Loeffler, J. S. (2014). Clinical presentation, pathologic features, and diagnosis of primary central nervous system lymphoma. *UpToDate*. Basow, DS (Ed), Waltham, MA, UpToDate.

Huang, T., Mueller, S., Rutkowski, M. J., et al. (2013). Multidisciplinary care of patients with brain tumors. *Surgical Oncology Clinics of North America, 22*, 161–178.

Jakola, A. S., Myrmel, K. S., Kloster, R., et al. (2012). Comparison of a strategy favoring early surgical resection vs. a strategy favoring watchful waiting in low-grade gliomas. *Journal of the American Medical Association, 308*, 1881–1888.

Jenkins, E. O., Schiff, D., Mackman, N., et al. (2010). Venous thromboembolism in malignant gliomas. *Journal of Thrombosis & Haemostasis, 8*, 221–227.

Kaleita, T. A., Wellisch, D. K., Graham, C. A., et al. (2006). Pilot study of modafinil for treatment of neurobehavioral dysfunction and fatigue in adult patients with brain tumors. *Proceedings of the Annual Meeting of the American Society of Clinical Oncology, 24*(18S), A1503.

Kalkanis, S. N., et al. (2010). The role of surgical resection in the management of newly diagnosed brain metastases: a systematic review and evidence-based clinical practice guideline. *Journal of Neurooncology, 96*, 33–43.

Kelly, D. M., & Cronin S. (2014). PCP prophylaxis with use of corticosteroids by neurologists. *Practice Neurology 14*, 74–76.

Kerkhof, M., & Vecht, C. J. (2013). Seizure characteristics and prognostic factors of gliomas. *Epilepsia, 54*(Suppl), 12–17.

Kilbride, L., Smith, G., & Grant, R. (2007). The frequency and cause of anxiety and depression amongst patients with malignant brain tumours between surgery and radiotherapy. *Journal of Neurooncology, 84*, 297–304.

Kim, S., Akpati, H. C., Li, J. G., Liu, C. R., Amdur, R. J., & Palta, J. R. (2004). An immobilization system for claustrophobic patients in head-and-neck intensity-modulated radiation therapy. *International Journal of Radiation Oncology Biology Physics, 59*, 1531–1539.

Korah, M. P., Esiashvili, N., Mazewski, C. M., et al. (2010). Incidence, risks and sequelae of posterior fossa syndrome in pediatric medulloblastoma. *International Journal of Radiation Oncology Biology Physics, 77*, 106–112.

Kohler, B. A., Ward, E., McCarthy, B. J., et al. (2011). Annual report to the nation on the status of cancer, 1975–2007, featuring tumors of the brain and other nervous system. *Journal of the National Cancer Institute, 103*, 714–736.

Kostaras, X., Cusano F., Klin G. A., Roa W., and Easaw, J. Use of dexamethasone in patients with high-grade glioma: a clinical practice guideline. *Current Oncology, 21*, e493–e503.

Kuijlen, J. M., Teernstra, O. P., Kessels, A. G., et al. (1996). Effectiveness of antiepileptic prophylaxis used with supratentorial craniotomies: a meta-analysis. *Seizure, 5*, 291–298.

Lacy, J., Saadati, H., & Yu, J. B. (2012). Complications of brain tumors and their treatment. *Hematology/Oncology Clinics of North America*, *26*, 779–796.

Lagenbahn, D. M., Ashman, T., Cantor, J., & Trott, C. (2013). An evidence-based review of cognitive rehabilitation in medical conditions affecting cognitive function. *Archives of Physical Medicine and Rehabilitation*, *94*, 271–286.

Levin, V. A., Bidaut, L., Hou, P., et al. (2011). Randomized double-blind placebo-controlled trial of bevacizumab therapy for radiation necrosis of the central nervous system. *International Journal of Radiation Oncology Biology Physics*, *79*, 1487–1495.

Litofsky, N. S., Farace, E., Anderson, F. Jr., et al. (2004). Depression in patients with high-grade glioma: results of the Glioma Outcomes Project. *Neurosurgery*, *54*, 358–366.

Lote, K., Stenwig, A. E., Skullerud, K., et al. (1998). Prevalence and prognostic significance of epilepsy in patients with gliomas. *European Journal of Cancer*, *17*, 479–482.

Madhusoodanan, S., Danan, D., & Moise, D. (2007). Psychiatric manifestations of brain tumors: diagnostic implications. *Expert Review of Neurotherapeutics*, *4*, 343–349.

Mainio A, Hakko H, Niemala A et al. (2011) Depression in relation to anxiety, obsessionality and phobia among neurosurgical patients with brain tumors: a 1-year follow-up study. *Clincal Neurology Neurosurgery*, *113*, 649–653.

Mainio, A., Hakko, H., Niemela, A., et al. (2005). Depression in relation to survival among neurosurgical patients with a primary brain tumor: a 5-year follow-up study. *Neurosurgery*, *56*, 1234–1241.

Mainio, A., Tuunanen, S., Hakko, H., et al. (2006). Decreased quality of life and depression as predictors for shorter survival among patients with low-grade gliomas: a follow-up from 1990–2003. *European Archives of Psychiatry & Clinical Neurosciences*, *256*(8), 516–521.

McConigley, R., Halkett, G., Lobb, E., & Nowak, A. (2010). caring for someone with high-grade glioma: a time of rapid change for caregivers. *Palliative Medicine*, *24*, 473–479.

Meyers, C. A., & Hess, K. R. (2003). Multifaceted end points in brain tumor clinical trials: cognitive deterioration precedes MRI progression. *Neuro-Oncology*, *5*, 89–95.

Meyers, C. A., Hess, K. R., Yung, W. K., et al. (2000). Cognitive function as a predictor of survival in patients with recurrent malignant glioma. *Journal of Clinical Oncology*, *18*, 646–650.

Meyers, C. A., Smith, J. A., Bezjak, A., et al. (2004). Neurocognitive function and progression in patients with brain metastases treated with whole-brain radiation and motexafin gadolinium: Results of a randomized phase III trial. *Journal of Clinical Oncology*, *22*, 157–165.

Meyers, C. A., Weitzner, M. A., Valentine, A. D., et al. (1998). Methylphenidate therapy improves cognition, mood, and function of brain tumor patients. *Journal of Clinical Oncology*, *16*(7), 2522–2527.

Mikkelsen, T., Paleologos, N. A., Robinson, P. D., et al. (2010). The role of prophylactic anticonvulsants in the management of brain metastases: a systematic review and evidence-based clinical practice guideline. *Journal of Neurooncology*, *96*, 97–102.

Mukherjee, A., Tolhurst-Cleaver, S., Ryder, W. D., et al. (2005). the characteristics of quality of life impairment in adult growth hormone deficient survivors of cancer and their response to GH replacement therapy. *Journal of Clinical Endocrinology & Metabolism*, *90*, 1542–1529.

Nakken, K. O., & Lossius, M. I. (2011). Buccal midazolam or rectal diazepam for treatment of residential adult patients with serial seizures or status epilepticus. *Acta Neurologica Scandinavica*, *124*, 99–103.

Niiro, M., Yatsushiro, K., Nakamura, K., et al. (2000). Natural history of elderly patients with asymptomatic meningiomas. *Journal of Neurology, Neurosurgery & Psychiatry*, *68*, 25.

Omuro, A., & De Angelis, L. M. (2013). Glioblastoma and other malignant gliomas: a clinical review. *Journal of the American Medical Association*, *310*, 1842–1850.

Owonikoko, T. K., Arbiser, J., Zelnak, A., et al. (2014). Current approaches to the treatment of metastatic brain tumours. *Nature Reviews Clinical Oncology*, *11*, 203–222.

Pace, A., Di Lorenzo, C., Guariglia, L., Jandolo, B., Carapella, C. M., & Pompili, A. (2009). End of life issues in brain tumor patients. *Journal of Neurooncology*, *91*, 39–43.

Patel, T. R., McHugh, B. J., Bi, W. L., et al. (2011). a comprehensive review of MR imaging changes following radiosurgery to 500 brain metastases. *AJNR: American Journal of Neuroradiology*, *32*, 1885–1892.

Piedad, J., Rickards, H., Besag, F. M. C., & Cavanna, A. E. (2012). Beneficial and adverse psychotropic effects of antiepileptic drugs in patients with epilepsy. *CNS Drugs*, *26*, 319–335.

Pereira R. M. R., de Carvalho J. F. (2011). Glucocorticoid-inuced myopathy. *Joint Bone Spine*, *78*, 41–44.

Rossetti, A. O., & Stupp, R. (2010). Epilepsy in brain tumor patients. *Current Opinion in Neurology*, *23*, 603–609.

Ruden, E., Reardon, D. A., Coan, A. D., et al. (2011). Exercise behavior, functional capacity and survival in adults with malignant recurrent glioma. *Journal of Clinical Oncology*, *29*(21), 2918–2923.

Schmer, C., Ward-Smith, P., Latham, S., & Salacz, M. (2008). when a family member has a malignant brain tumor: the caregiver perspective. *Journal of Neuroscience Nursing*, *40*, 78–84.

Shaw, E. G., Rosdhal, R., D'Agostino, R. B. Jr., et al. (2006). Phase II study of donepezil in irradiated brain tumor patients: effect on cognitive function, mood and quality of life. *Journal of Clinical Oncology*, *24*(9), 1415–1420.

Shields, L. B. E., & Choucair, A. K. (2014). Management of low-grade gliomas—A review of patient perceived quality of life and neurocognitive outcome. *World Neurosurgery*. doi:10.1016/j.wneu.2014.02.033

Silvani, A., Gaviani, P., Lamperti, E., et al. (2011). Malignant gliomas: early diagnosis and clinical aspects. *Neurological Sciences*, *32*(Supp 2), S213–215.

Sirven, J. I., Wingerchuk, D. M., Drazkowski, J. F., et al. (2004). Seizure prophylaxis in patients with brain tumors: a meta-analysis. *Mayo Clinic Proceedings*, *79*, 1489–1494.

Sizoo, E. M., Taphoorn, M. J., Uitdehaag, B., Heimans, J. J., Deliens, L., Reijneveld, J. C., Pasman, H. R. (2013). The end-of-life phase of high-grade glioma patients: dying with dignity? *Oncologist*, *18*, 198–203.

Sterckx, W., Coolbrandt, A., de Casterle B. D., et al. (2013). The impact of a high-grade glioma on everyday life: A systematic review from the patient's and caregiver's perspective. *European Journal of Oncology Nursing*, *17*, 107–117.

Stupp, R., Hegi, M. E., Mason, W. P., et al. (2009). Effects of radiotherapy with concomitant and adjuvant temozolomide versus radiotherapy alone on survival in glioblastoma in a randomised phase III study: 5-year analysis of the EORTC-NCIC[European Oranization for Research and Treatment of Cancer-National Cancer Institute of Canada] trial. *Lancet Oncology*, *10*, 459.

Stupp, R., Mason, W. P., van den Bent, M. J., et al. (2005). Radiotherapy plus concomitant and adjuvant temozolomide for glioblastoma. *New England Journal of Medicine*, *352*, 987.

Stupp, R., Brada, M., van den Bent, M. J., et al. (2014). High-grade malignant glioma: ESMO [European Society for Medical Oncology] Clinical Practice guidelines for diagnosis, treatment and follow-up. *Annals of Oncology*, *00*, 1–9. doi:10,1093/annonc/mdu050

Surma-aho, O., Niemela, M., Vikki, J., et al. (2001). adverse long-term effects of brain radiotherapy in adult low-grade glioma patients. *Neurology*, *56*, 1285–1290.

Taphoorn, M. J. (2003). Neurocognitive sequelae in the treatment of low-grade gliomas. *Seminars in Oncology*, *30*, 45–48.

Tremont-Lukats, I. W., Ratilal, B. O., Armstrong, T., & Gilbert, M. R. (2008). Antiepileptic drugs for preventing seizures in people with brain tumors. *Cochrane Database of Systematic Reviews*, CD004424.

Tsao, M., Xu, W., & Sahgal, A. (2012). A meta-analysis evaluating stereotactic radiosurgery, whole-brain radiotherapy, or both for patients presenting with a limited number of brain metastases. *Cancer*, *118*, 2486–2493.

Vecht, C. J., Hovestadt, A., Verbiest, H. B., et al. (1994). Dose-effect relationship of dexamethasone on Karnofsky performance in metastatic brain tumors: a randomized study of doses of 4, 8, and 16 mg per day. *Neurology*, *44*, 675–680.

Walbert, T., & Khan, M. (2014). End of life symptoms and care in patients with primary malignant brain tumors: a systematic literature review. *Journal of Neurooncology, 117,* 217–214.

Weitzner, M. A., Meyers, C. A., & Valentine, A. D. (1995). Methylphenidate in the treatment of neurobehavioral slowing associated with cancer and cancer treatment. *Journal of Neuropsychiatry & Clinical Neurosciences, 7,* 347–350.

Wen, P. Y., MacDonald, D. R., Reardon, D. A., et al. (2010). Updated response assessment criteria for high-grade gliomas: response assessment in neurooncology working group. *Journal of Clinical Oncology, 28,* 1963.

Wen, P. Y., Schiff, D., Kesari, S., Drappatz, J., Gigas, D. C., & Doherty, L. (2006). Medical management of patients with brain tumors. *Journal of Neurooncology, 80,* 313–332.

Whiting, D. L., Simpson G. K., Koh E.-S., et al. (2012). A multi-tiered intervention to address behavioural and cognitive changes after diagnosis of primary brain tumour: a feasibility study. *Brain injury, 26,* 950–961.

50.

ATTENTION-DEFICIT HYPERACTIVITY DISORDER IN MEDICAL ILLNESS

Anna M. Georgiopoulos and Craig B. H. Surman

INTRODUCTION

Attention-deficit hyperactivity disorder (ADHD) is a syndrome involving broad impairment in self-regulation and impacting many dimensions of life pertinent to the comprehensive management of medical patients. ADHD is diagnosed by the presence of functionally impairing inattention, impulsivity, and/or hyperactivity, and its biological basis has been elucidated at a genetic, neurostructural, and neurofunctional level. ADHD occurs in up to 7–9% of children and adolescents (American Psychiatric Association [APA], 2000; Faraone, Sergeant, Gillberg, & Biederman, 2003) and 4–5% of adults (Kessler et al., 2006), but it may be more common in some medically ill populations. In addition to its impact on educational, occupational, and social functioning, ADHD can create barriers to adherence with medical treatment and difficulties in navigating medical systems of care. Psychopharmacological and non-psychopharmacological therapies can substantially reduce associated morbidity.

ADHD DIAGNOSIS ACROSS THE LIFESPAN

The diagnosis of ADHD using *Diagnostic and Statistical Manual of Mental Disorders–5* (DSM-5) criteria requires impairment in two or more life settings (such as school, work, home, or social environments) due to persistent symptoms of inattention, impulsivity, and/or hyperactivity. Symptoms must begin in childhood and not be caused by another medical or psychiatric condition. Diagnostic criteria for ADHD continue to evolve. The majority of intervention research has relied on the DSM-IV definition, which specifically required onset of symptoms by age seven, and at least six current inattentive or impulsive/hyperactive symptoms. Inattentive symptoms include having trouble keeping focused attention on tasks, distractibility, being prone to careless mistakes, appearing not to listen in conversation, lack of follow-through, trouble with organizing activities, avoidance of effortful activities such as homework, losing things, and forgetfulness. Hyperactive symptoms include fidgetiness, having trouble remaining seated, motor restlessness, trouble playing or relaxing quietly, feeling "on the go," and talkativeness. Impulsivity can manifest verbally or behaviorally, and includes interrupting, becoming highly impatient when needing to wait, and blurting things out (American Psychiatric Association, 2000).

Third-party reports are useful in understanding the impact of ADHD in both children and adults but are essential to its identification in children; young children, along with some adolescents and adults, may have limited insight into their ADHD symptoms. In addition, adults often cannot fully recall childhood symptoms. Difficulties beyond those described in the core symptoms commonly occur, including sleep dysregulation, emotional reactivity, and poor organizational behavior (Biederman, Petty et al., 2006; Murphy, Barkley, & Bush, 2001; Surman et al., 2009; Surman et al., 2011).

The chief complaints of individuals with ADHD are diverse due to the heterogeneity of the functional problems they face. Children with ADHD are often brought to clinical attention for disruptive behavior or academic difficulty at school, or for impulsive or seemingly oppositional behaviors at home. Symptoms of impulsivity and hyperactivity typically decrease across the lifespan. While physical restlessness, talkativeness, and impatience commonly occur in both children and adults with ADHD, adults tend to have more socially acceptable manifestations. For example, while a child with ADHD may be out of his seat frequently during class time, as an adult he may be able to stay seated through a meeting but report feeling bored, restless, and "tuned out," missing important material due to disengagement, or stepping out to answer non-urgent calls. Similarly, a teenager with ADHD may constantly interrupt family conversations and be disruptively loud in the library; as an adult, she may alienate coworkers by persisting with social conversation at unwelcome times or talking so much during work meetings that it is difficult for others to participate.

Compensatory capacities and effort may mask the burden of ADHD. While it is adaptive for individuals to learn ways to get tasks done despite their ADHD-related challenges, such compensatory efforts may require large investments of time and energy. An individual with ADHD may be able to accomplish tasks requiring attention and control of behavior only with great difficulty, often needing to work harder or differently than his peers in order to achieve the same goals. Patients may spend longer hours than peers at study or work due to wandering thoughts, frequent breaks, or time spent checking for mistakes. Disorganization and forgetfulness may require heavy reliance on organizational systems, such as extensive checklists to ensure completion of simple tasks such as small shopping trips, or frequent use of alarms as reminders of appointments or tasks. Reliance on others is another form of compensatory burden. A patient who accomplishes the seemingly routine task of arriving at a scheduled medical appointment on time, for example, may be straining his marital relationship because he is reliant on his wife to call the medical office to schedule the follow-up visit, enter the information into the family calendar, and remind him repeatedly on the day of the appointment. Medical patients with ADHD with poorer compensatory supports may not follow through with care and become lost to follow-up.

The burden of ADHD also includes tendency to defer or avoid activities that strain an individual's capacities. For example, an individual with impulsive/hyperactive traits may avoid jobs requiring prolonged sitting, or drive longer and more time-consuming routes to avoid waiting in traffic. The otherwise capable individual may also simply avoid pursuing a promotion, higher education, or relationship that would tax his or her capacities.

The manifestation of ADHD symptoms varies according to each individual's challenges, strengths, and evolving psychosocial context. For example, a student with ADHD who also struggles with learning disabilities or low cognitive abilities may disengage from class more frequently, particularly without sufficient educational accommodations. A relative strength in academic performance may mask the impact of ADHD until vulnerable capacities—such as relative weaknesses in executive functioning—are strained by new demands (Antshel et al., 2009; Antshel et al., 2010). In many cases of apparently late-onset ADHD, childhood symptoms, while present, had been well compensated for by caregiving adults in highly structured environments, minimizing apparent functional impairment. While it is common for ADHD to be diagnosed for the first time following the transition to middle school, high school, college, or a new job, transfer to an educational or occupational setting that better fits an individual's strengths can also result in fewer impairing symptoms. The need for support should be reevaluated over time and at new developmental stages.

Revisions to the DSM-IV diagnostic criteria for ADHD during the 2013 update to the psychiatric diagnostic manual, DSM-5, included:

1. Moving away from separate diagnostic categories for subtypes of ADHD in DSM-IV (inattentive, impulsive/hyperactive, combined), and instead conceptualizing these to all be different "presentations" of ADHD, by using specifiers to note these symptom patterns;

2. Adopting onset before age twelve as a more appropriate historical criterion than on set before age seven;

3. Allowing simultaneous diagnosis of ADHD and pervasive developmental disorders or autism;

4. Enhancing descriptions of ADHD symptoms (American Psychiatric Association, 2013);

5. Reduction of number of current symptoms of either the inattentive presentation or impulsive/hyperactive presentation required in individuals over age 17, from 6 to 5.

It is clinically relevant to consider the reason for reduction of current symptom threshold for adult diagnosis in DSM-5. When children with full ADHD grow to have fewer than six current symptoms within an ADHD subtype category as adults, functional impairment may nevertheless remain significant (Faraone, Biederman, & Mick, 2006). Patients with onset by adolescence and four or more current symptoms in the "inattentive" or "hyperactive" category also often have effectively the same life problems as those with full ADHD (Barkley, Murphy, & Fischer, 2008; Faraone, Biederman, Spencer, et al., 2006). ADHD presentations that are clearly impairing but sub-threshold for full diagnostic criteria because of fewer current symptoms or difficulty in documenting age of onset may often warrant intervention. Under the new DSM-5 classification system, these presentations can be categorized as *ADHD not elsewhere classified*. The utility and implications of the DSM-5 revisions to ADHD diagnostic criteria will emerge with further research.

ASSESSMENT OF ADHD

Table 50.1 summarizes several rating scales that may be used for assessing baseline symptoms and tracking treatment progress. In children, a variety of ADHD measures is available for clinical use, including the ADHD-Rating Scale (DuPaul, Power, Anastopoulos, & Reed, 1998; Faries, Yalcin, Harder, & Heiligenstein, 2001), the Vanderbilt ADHD Parent Rating Scale (Wolraich et al., 2003), and Conners' Parent Rating Scale—Revised (S) (Conners, 1997). Self-report scales that offer indication of likelihood of diagnosis of ADHD are also available for children and adults (Brown, 1995; Conners, Erhardt, & Sparrow, 1999). The websites Schoolpsychiatry.org and CAPPCNY.org contain information and links to ADHD scales. A useful screening tool for adults, the Adult ADHD Self Report Scale (ASRS–v1.1), has been adopted by the World Health Organization (WHO; Kessler, Adler, Ames, Demler et al., 2005) (Figure 50.1). Like all disease-specific rating scales, it could be more likely to produce false positives in populations with high rates of comorbidity. The ASRS screener is a 6-item subset of the ASRS 18-item self-report form, which has a question for each of the 18 symptoms of inattention or impulsivity/hyperactivity.

Screening tools and rating scales should be supplemented with interviews and the collection of related information to confirm that an individual meets full criteria for

Table 50.1 SELECTED ADHD RATING SCALES

RATING SCALE	AGE GROUPS	REFERENCES	AVAILABILITY	FORMAT	ADVANTAGES/ DISADVANTAGES
ADHD-Rating Scale–IV	Pediatric	DuPaul 1998, Faries 2001	Purchase online, includes permission to reproduce forms	Parent and teacher versions	Maps onto DSM-IV-TR criteria.
Vanderbilt	Pediatric	Wolraich 2004	Free online at www.cappcny.org or www.schoolpsychiatry.org	Parent and teacher versions	Some items track non-ADHD disruptive symptoms (oppositional-defiant/conduct), anxiety and mood.
Conners	Pediatric Adult	Conners 1997, Conners 1999	Purchase online	Parent, teacher, and self-report versions	Short and long versions. Clearly delineated subscales for non-ADHD disruptive symptoms (oppositional-defiant/conduct).
Brown	Preschool through Adult	Brown 1995	Purchase online	Parent, teacher, and self-report versions	Scoring correlates with clinical diagnosis. Items emphasize organizational difficulties.
Adult ADHD Self-Report Scale (ASRS-v1.1)	Adult	Kessler 2005	Free online at www.cappcny.org	Self-report	First six items can be used as a screener. Full 18-item version useful for review of DSM-IV-TR current symptoms.

Please answer the questions below, rating yourself on each of the criteria shown using the scale on the right side of the page. As you answer each question, place an X in the box that best describes how you have felt and conducted yourself over the past 6 months. Please give this completed checklist to your healthcare professional to discuss during today's appointment	Never	Rarely	Sometimes	Often	Very Often
1. How often do you have trouble wrapping up the final details of a project, once the challenging parts have been done?					
2. How often do you have difficulty getting things in order when you have to do a task that requires organization?					
3. How often do you have problems remembering appointments or obligations?					
4. When you have a task that requires a lot of thought, how often do you avoid or delay getting started?					
5. How often do you fidget or squirm with your hands or feet when you have to sit down for a long time?					
6. How often, do you feel overly active and compellled to do things, like you were driven by a motor?					

Figure 50.1 Adult ADHD Self-Report Scale (ASRS-v1.1) Symptom Checklist. If four or more marks appear in the darkly shaded boxes within Part A, then the patient has symptoms highly consistent with ADHD in adults and further investigation iswarranted (Kessler, Adler, Ames, Demler et al., 2005; World Health Organization, 2005).

ADHD. There is no "test" for ADHD. The clinical diagnosis of ADHD can be made by any clinician who is familiar with the syndrome and familiar with alternative explanations of mental and behavioral problems (Subcommittee on Attention-Deficit/Hyperactivity Disorder, 2011). In cases with complex psychiatric or psychosocial comorbidity, or when standard treatments have not been effective, psychiatric consultation may be helpful to confirm the diagnosis. While neuropsychological testing is highly useful for characterization of learning disabilities or cognitive impairments and may be required by schools or other institutions for disability documentation, it demonstrates significant deficits in only a subset of clinically confirmed cases of ADHD Seidman, 2006) and is not required to make the clinical diagnosis of ADHD.

NEUROBIOLOGY

Converging evidence demonstrates that ADHD has a heterogeneous etiology. Structural and functional differences from controls have been found using imaging techniques in children and adults with ADHD, including prefrontal, cingulate, basal ganglia, and cerebellar regions (Bush, 2011; Seidman, Valera, & Bush, 2004). The efficacy of catecholaminergic pharmacotherapies and imaging studies implicate deficits in dopamine and norepinephrine pathways and also a role of these pathways in the effects of pharmacotherapies. ADHD is a genetic condition, as demonstrated by high familiality: the heritability coefficient is 0.76 based on twin studies (Faraone et al., 2005). Individual genes appear to contribute low risk for ADHD, but multiple genes, including those expressing catecholaminergic pathway components, may contribute to ADHD. Environmental (Banerjee, Middleton, & Faraone, 2007) and familial factors may have an impact on the expression of ADHD (Faraone, 2004). ADHD probably has heterogeneous neurobiological trajectories, and initial research demonstrates that genetic variation between individuals contributes to these trajectories (Shaw et al., 2007).

FUNCTIONAL IMPAIRMENT

ADHD is associated with significant deficits in both children and adults, including educational and occupational underperformance (Loe & Feldman, 2007); low frustration tolerance and antisocial behavior; poor relationships with peers, family members, and authorities; and more frequent traffic violations, accidents, and injuries (Barkley, 1997, 2004; Barkley, Guvremont, Anastopoulos, DuPaul, & Shelton, 1993; Barkley, Murphy, & Kwasnik, 1996; Barkley & Cox, 2007; Barkley & Murphy, 2010; Barkley et al., 2008; Biederman & Faraone, 2006; Biederman et al., 2006; Brown, 2000; Weiss & Hechtman, 1993). Between absence and underperformance at work, ADHD is associated with workforce inefficiency that costs the United States $19.6 billion (Kessler, Adler, Ames, Barkley, et al., 2005) to $116 billion (Biederman & Faraone, 2005) per year. A case-control study of 173 adults with and 134 adults without ADHD demonstrated a large impact of ADHD on overall quality of life (Mick, Spencer, Faraone, Biederman, & Zhang, 2007). The National Comorbidity Survey Replication (Kessler et al., 2006) confirmed on an epidemiological level that ADHD confers significant disability in all dimensions of functioning considered: self-care, mobility, cognition, days out of role, productive role functioning, and social role functioning.

PSYCHIATRIC COMORBIDITY AND DIFFERENTIAL DIAGNOSIS

Psychiatric comorbidity is common in both children and adults with ADHD (Barkley, 1997; Biederman et al., 1999; Kessler et al., 2006). Oppositional defiant disorder, conduct disorder, and developmental disorders such as Tourette's syndrome, enuresis/encopresis, and learning disabilities are common in children with ADHD (Biederman et al., 2010; Germano, Gagliano, & Curatolo, 2010). Pediatric ADHD confers higher risk for the onset of antisocial, mood, anxiety, substance use, and eating disorders as children age into adolescence and adulthood (Biederman et al., 2010). Case-control studies also demonstrate higher rates of antisocial, mood, anxiety, and substance abuse disorders in adults with ADHD (Biederman et al., 2004; Biederman et al., 1994; McGough et al., 2005). ADHD may increase risk for bulimia nervosa (Surman, Randell, & Biederman, 2006). Sleep disorders are strongly associated with ADHD across the lifespan (Choi, Yoon, Kim, Chung, & Yoo, 2010; Cortese, Faraone, Konofal, & Lecendreux, 2009; Surman et al., 2009). Because of the high rates of comorbid mental health disorders in ADHD patients, and of ADHD in patients with other mental health disorders, ADHD patients should be screened for co-occurring mental health conditions, and ADHD should be considered in patients presenting with other psychiatric concerns. If potential concern for ADHD is raised by a review of a patient's social history (i.e., history of educational, occupational, or legal difficulties) or by such symptoms as poor concentration, distractibility, or impulsive behavior on psychiatric review of systems, more detailed evaluation for ADHD should be conducted.

When another condition that robustly impairs concentration and controlled behavior is present—such as major depression, acute agitation or panic, mania/hypomania, or substance intoxication—it is typically appropriate to defer confirmation of ADHD and address the priority condition first. The diagnosis of ADHD is facilitated by identifying that the criteria are fully met, and that the hallmarks of alternate conditions are absent. Examples of conditions that can present with symptoms similar to ADHD are presented in Table 50.2. ADHD may often be differentiated from other mental health conditions by the persistence of symptoms since childhood, continuation of ADHD symptoms during non-comorbid periods (i.e., when the patient is in full remission from depression), and the presence of non-overlapping symptoms. In the differential diagnosis of ADHD and bipolar disorder, for example, talkativeness, impulsivity, tangential speech, physical restlessness, and high energy occur in both conditions. However, impairing mood elevation or irritability, grandiosity, hypersexuality, and psychosis are hallmarks of bipolar disorder, not ADHD. When impulsivity, the amount or rapidity of speech, or other overlapping symptoms are not consistently present over time and seem largely driven by mood state, bipolar disorder should be considered. While sleep can be chronically dysregulated in ADHD patients, a change in sleep patterns may also signal a mood disorder. The sudden development of early morning insomnia is uncommon in ADHD, but it is a hallmark of major depression. Decreased need for sleep (total sleep time substantially decreased from a patient's own baseline without effort to stay awake, or daytime sleepiness) is uncommon in ADHD but can be indicative of mania.

Low mood or anxiety can create internal distraction, complicating the diagnosis of ADHD. For example, a patient who reports having trouble paying attention in conversations at work might further explain that he is thinking constantly about whether people respect or like him; prior to treating him for ADHD, it would be important to build evidence that ADHD symptoms were present in contexts less vulnerable to

Table 50.2 DIFFERENTIAL DIAGNOSIS: OTHER CONDITIONS PRESENTING WITH ADHD-LIKE TRAITS

CONDITION	DIFFERENTIATING DIAGNOSTIC TOOLS	DIFFERENTIATING FEATURES ON HISTORY, EXAMINATION
Autism spectrum disorder	Standardized diagnostic interview	Social reciprocity deficits
Dementia	Neuropsychological testing	Late onset; worsening course; memory impairment
Delirium	Diagnostic evaluation for occult medical conditions (e.g., chest X-ray, urinalysis)	Change in level of consciousness; waxing and waning symptoms; physical illness
Executive dysfunction without ADHD	Neuropsychological testing and behavioral interview	Absence of full ADHD criteria; prominent disorganization
Genetic, metabolic, or other acquired neurological syndromes (e.g., fetal alcohol syndrome)	Brain imaging, genetic testing, laboratory evaluation as suggested by symptoms	Temporal pattern; family history; developmental delay; mental status severity; neurological findings
Learning disability	Neuropsychological testing	Impairment in particular academic skills
Mental illness (e.g., mood, anxiety, psychotic disorders)	Psychiatric screening instruments	New onset; intermittent or worsening course; non-ADHD psychiatric symptoms, family history
Movement disorders (e.g., ataxias, chorea)	Electromyography, laboratory evaluations	Motor activity pattern; neurological findings
Poisoning (e.g., lead, pesticide)	Toxicology screen	Environmental exposure; new onset; associated symptoms
Seizure disorder (e.g., absence, partial seizure)	Sleep-deprived electroencephalography	New onset; intermittent symptoms; inability to respond during symptoms
Sensory impairment	Hearing, vision testing	Contextual symptoms (e.g., when seated in back of classroom only)
Sleep disorder (e.g., insomnia, restless leg syndrome, sleep apnea, narcolepsy)	Sleep study, sleep diary	Temporal pattern; associated symptoms (e.g., snoring, daytime somnolence)
Substance abuse	Toxicology screen	Worsening course; substance-centered behavior
Thyroid disorder	Laboratory testing	Cognitive decline; physical symptoms (e.g., weight change, heat/cold intolerance, poor growth)
Traumatic brain injury; post-concussive symptoms	Brain imaging	History of head trauma; acute onset

his self-critical and socially anxious mindset. Other neuropsychiatric challenges, such as learning disabilities, can also exacerbate or mimic ADHD traits. A student with dyslexia may find it harder to concentrate on reading, for example, regardless of the presence of ADHD.

Psychological distress not severe enough to merit diagnosis with another major psychiatric disorder is also common in ADHD patients. Circumscribed feelings of guilt, sadness, lack of hope, lack of interest, or anxiety may all be experienced relative to the domains of life that are a struggle for patients with ADHD. In some cases of highly impairing ADHD, successful treatment of comorbid psychiatric conditions can prove difficult until ADHD is appropriately addressed. When prioritizing the order of psychopharmacology interventions, typically depression or anxiety should be treated before comorbid ADHD. However, when impairment from ADHD is judged to be much more longstanding and severe, and when symptoms of anxiety or dysphoria seem related substantially to sequelae of ADHD, initiating ADHD treatment first can be an effective strategy that minimizes the need for additional medication to treat mood and anxiety. Very limited evidence supports the cautious introduction of ADHD pharmacotherapy in children or adults with bipolar illness and comorbid ADHD, but typically this should be attempted only once their mood has been well stabilized (Bond et al., 2012; Chang, Nayar, Howe, & Rana, 2009; Joshi & Georgiopoulos, 2012).

PHARMACOLOGICAL TREATMENT

All agents approved by the Food and Drug Administration (FDA) to treat ADHD (Table 50.3) have catecholaminergic properties and are thought to work by increasing available norepinephrine or dopamine, particularly in prefrontal regions. Patients should always be warned that distressing

Table 50.3 FDA-APPROVED MEDICATIONS FOR ADHD

MEDICATION	FDA STARTING DOSE	FDA MAXIMUM DAILY DOSE	AACAP OFF-LABEL MAXIMUM DAILY DOSE[a]	TYPICAL DURATION OF EFFECT[b]	REPRESENTATIVE BRAND NAMES/ COMMENTS
Stimulants: Amphetamines					
Dextroamphetamine (immediate release)	2.5 mg (age 3–5) 5 mg (age 6+)	40 mg	60 mg	5 h	Dexedrine Dextrostat Liquadd (liquid formulation)
Dextroamphetamine ER	5 mg qam	40 mg	60 mg	8 h	Dexedrine Spansules (capsule can be opened and sprinkled)
Mixed amphetamine salts (immediate release)	2.5 mg (age 3–5) 5 mg (age 6+)	40 mg	60 mg	5 h	Adderall
Mixed amphetamine salts extended release*	10 mg qam	30 mg	60 mg	12 h	Adderall XR (capsule can be opened and sprinkled) Consider 5 mg starting dose for smaller children
Lisdexamfetamine*	30 mg qam	70 mg	n/a	12 h	Vyvanse: Consider 20 mg starting dose for smaller children
Stimulants: Methylphenidates					
Methylphenidate (immediate release)	5 mg bid	60 mg in divided doses	100 mg	4 h	Ritalin Methylin (includes chewable and liquid formulations)
Dexmethylphenidate (immediate release)	2.5 mg bid	10 mg bid	50 mg	5 h	Focalin
Methylphenidate SR/ER	10–20 mg qam	60 mg	100 mg	8 h	Metadate CD (capsule can be opened and sprinkled) Metadate ER Methylin ER Ritalin SR Ritalin LA
OROS methylphenidate*	18 mg qam (pediatric) 18–36 mg qam (adult)	54 mg (age 6–12) 72 mg (age 13+)	108 mg	12 h	Concerta
Dexmethylphenidate extended release*	5 mg qam (age 6–17) 10 mg qam (adult)	30 mg (age 6–17) 40 mg (adult)	50 mg	12 h	Focalin XR
Methylphenidate patch	10 mg qam	30 mg	n/a	9–12 h	Daytrana (patch may be removed early to shorten duration)
Non-stimulants					
Atomoxetine*	Pediatric: 0.5 mg/kg/day Adult: 40 mg/day	Lesser of 1.4 mg/ kg or 100 mg	Lesser of 1.8 mg/kg or 100 mg	24 h	Strattera 25–50% dose-reduction in hepatic impairment
Clonidine extended-release	0.1 mg qhs	0.2 mg bid	n/a	24 h	Kapvay ER (immediate-release and patch formulations may be used off-label)
Guanfacine extended-release	1 mg	4 mg or 0.12 mg/ kg/ day	n/a	24 h	Intuniv (immediate-release formulation may be used off-label)

* Indicates FDA approval in adults as well as in children; other listed medications are FDA-approved in children only but are commonly used off-label in adults.

[a] Adapted from AACAP ADHD Practice Parameter for pediatric care (Pliszka, 2007). In clinical practice, doses of stimulants above FDA limits may be indicated where meaningful incremental benefit has occurred with dose increase. Experience suggests that doses of most racemic methylphenidates up to 2 mg/kg/day, and doses of amphetamines (and dexmethylphenidate) up to 1 mg/kg/day may be well tolerated.

[b] Based on average clinical duration; may vary in individuals.

thoughts and feelings (i.e., anxiety, irritability, agitation, or suicidal thoughts) as well as physical discomforts are possible side effects of medications that work on the brain. These agents also have peripheral nervous system side effects. Some medications commonly used for ADHD do not carry an FDA indication for use in adults, and others are commonly used off-label (i.e., without an FDA approval for use in ADHD), even in children and adolescents; the American Academy of Child and Adolescent Psychiatry ADHD Practice Parameter contains specific information about medications often used off-label for ADHD (Pliszka &AACAP, 2007). Before prescribing ADHD therapies, particularly non-stimulants, to patients taking other medications, it is advisable to check for specific drug–drug interactions (Table 50.4).

STIMULANT TREATMENT

In an ADHD patient with no contraindicating conditions, stimulants are typically the first choice over non-stimulant medications because of their more robust efficacy for ADHD management. A meta-analysis of adult trials showed greater effect size for stimulants (0.91 for immediate-release and 0.95 for long-acting) than for non-stimulant treatments (0.62) (Faraone, Biederman, Spencer, & Aleardi, 2006). Several methylphenidate and amphetamine drug products are available, with differing release patterns and duration of effect. For example, long-acting methylphenidate products typically acting for 12 hours include osmotic-release, layered bead, and patch formulations. Individuals may tolerate one formulation of a stimulant agent better than another.

Long-acting stimulants are preferable to immediate-release agents for many patients. Stimulants can be misused or abused. Among college-age individuals, studies suggest that

5–35% misuse non-prescribed stimulants, but long-acting agents are less likely to be abused (Wilens et al., 2008). An extended-release form of dextroamphetamine, lisdexamfetamine, is a pro-drug requiring enzymatic activation, which may further decrease its potential for abuse. Due to the convenience of once-daily dosing, long-acting formulations may also be preferable to promote treatment adherence. For young children or others unable to swallow pills, liquid formulations, extended-release formulations with capsules that may be opened and sprinkled on food, crushable short-acting agents, or the methylphenidate patch may be helpful.

While stimulants are typically well tolerated in use with other medications, some interactions are possible. Stimulants should be avoided for patients taking monoamine-oxidase (MAO)-inhibitor antidepressants. Methylphenidate may increase the effects of warfarin, phenobarbital, phenytoin, and primidone. The plasma level of amphetamine agents is lowered by acidifying agents, and treatments that lower acidity, such as proton pump inhibitors, can increase serum levels. This may vary by release mechanism, as a study demonstrated, for example, that levels of lisdexamfetamine were not changed in the presence of omeprazole, but that extended-release mixed amphetamine salts had a different time to maximum concentration in half of subjects studied (Haffey et al., 2009). Stimulants can also potentiate the effects of opiates, but they have not been proven to cause significant interaction when used with methadone or buprenorphine (McCance-Katz, 2009).

NON-STIMULANT TREATMENT

Because of their lower potential for abuse, non-stimulants are favorable for treatment of ADHD when the patient also has an active problem with substance abuse or dependence. Most also

Table 50.4 DRUG–DRUG INTERACTIONS IN ADHD AND MEDICAL ILLNESS

MEDICATION	ADHD PHARMACOTHERAPY	INTERACTION
MAO-inhibitor antidepressant	Stimulants, atomoxetine, bupropion	Contraindicated due to hypertensive reaction.
MAO-inhibitor antidepressant	Tricyclic antidepressants (desipramine, imipramine, nortriptyline)	Contraindicated due to hypertensive reaction, serotonin syndrome.
Linezolid (weak MAO-inhibitor)	Stimulants, atomoxetine, bupropion, tricyclic antidepressants (desipramine, imipramine, nortriptyline)	Risk of hypertensive reaction, serotonin syndrome. Use with caution and informed consent when clinically necessary.
Warfarin, phenobarbital, phenytoin, primidone	Methylphenidate	Stimulant increases effects of other medication; adjust doses as needed.
Proton pump inhibitors	Amphetamines	Increased serum levels of stimulant; adjust doses as needed.
Fluoxetine, paroxetine, quinidine, and other CYP2D6 inhibitors	Atomoxetine	Increased levels of atomoxetine; reduce atomoxetine dose as needed.
Fluoxetine, paroxetine, quinidine, other CYP2D6 inhibitors	Tricyclic antidepressants (desipramine, imipramine, nortriptyline)	Increased levels of tricyclic antidepressant, narrow therapeutic margin, fatal in overdose. Reduce tricyclic dose and monitor EKG and blood levels if concomitant use cannot be avoided.

have the advantage of 24-hour duration of effect. Atomoxetine is the only non-stimulant FDA-approved to treat ADHD in both children and adults. Slow titration and nighttime dosing can minimize the risk of sedation and gastrointestinal intolerance. Atomoxetine carries warnings about (very rare) liver failure, and the possibility of emerging suicidal ideation (Eli Lilly & Company, 2011). Atomoxetine is metabolized through the cytochrome P450 2D6 pathway, so other medicines using this pathway may affect atomoxetine levels; atomoxetine doses commonly need to be reduced by more than half when used concomitantly with fluoxetine, for example. Atomoxetine has anxiety-reducing properties for some patients, and one study demonstrated its efficacy for ADHD comorbid with social anxiety (Adler, Rubin, Qiao, Heinloth, & Durell, 2010).

While guanfacine and clonidine have been used off-label for ADHD in children for many years, newer extended-release formulations of both have received FDA approval. To date they have not been studied in adults. These agents are agonists at the alpha-2 adrenergic receptor, stimulation of which is thought to increase catecholaminergic activity in frontal regions. Side effects of short-acting alpha-2 agonists may include sedation, hypotension, and rebound hypertension, which can be minimized by gradual dose change for initiation or discontinuation. Short-acting preparations may be used for late-day ADHD symptoms interfering with bedtime routines. Extended-release formulations tend to be less sedating and provide 24-hour symptom coverage. They can be used as ADHD monotherapy, particularly in patients unable to tolerate stimulants due to exacerbation of comorbid anxiety, mania or tic disorders, low appetite, or insomnia.

The antidepressant bupropion (Wilens et al., 2005; Wilens et al., 2001) has demonstrated efficacy for ADHD in adults in double-blind clinical trials. Bupropion's efficacy for depression may make it an attractive option for patients presenting with both ADHD and impairing depressive symptoms. Bupropion should be avoided in patients at high risk for seizure, including binge drinkers and patients with bulimia nervosa.

There is also evidence to support the off-label use of tricyclic antidepressants for ADHD, including desipramine (Pataki, Carlson, Kelly, Rapport, & Biancaniello, 1993; Wilens et al., 1996), nortriptyline (Prince et al., 2000; Spencer, Biederman, Wilens, Steingard, & Geist, 1993; Wilens, Biederman, Geist, Steingard, & Spencer, 1993), or imipramine (Pliszka & AACAP, 2007). These medications can prolong the QT interval, be fatal in overdose, be subject to significant drug–drug interactions, and be associated with sedation and orthostatic hypotension (Riddle, Geller, & Ryan, 1993). As a result, tricyclics are most often considered in ADHD patients who cannot tolerate stimulants and FDA-approved non-stimulants, or in those with comorbid depression or anxiety. More commonly, however, a patient with comorbid depression and anxiety would be tried first with a combination of a selective serotonin reuptake inhibitor (SSRI) and a stimulant.

While modafinil has not been FDA-approved for ADHD, there is one published trial that demonstrates its efficacy in adults (Turner, Clark, Dowson, Robbins, & Sahakian, 2004). The side effects of this agent are similar to those of other sympathomimetics (Provigil, 1999), but it also carries warnings

of (rare) Stevens-Johnson syndrome, may not provide 24-hour symptom control, and can interfere with the effectiveness of oral contraceptives.

Like stimulants, atomoxetine, tricyclic antidepressants, and bupropion should be avoided in patients taking MAO-inhibitor antidepressants. While the antibiotic linezolid is a weak MAO-inhibitor with potential for interaction with psychotropic medications, a retrospective review revealed that only 1 out of 53 cases (1.8%) in which SSRIs were co-administered with linezolid experienced a serotonin syndrome (Lorenz, Vandenberg, & Canepa, 2008). In general, the combination is relatively well tolerated. Use of concomitant linezolid and ADHD medications may be considered with informed consent regarding the possibility of hypertensive reaction and/or serotonin syndrome, and if the risk–benefit ratio is favorable for a particular patient. If the use of linezolid will be time-limited and administered in a setting in which medical treatment adherence is unlikely to be affected by discontinuation of ADHD treatment (i.e., under parental supervision or in a hospital), the ADHD medication can readily be discontinued for the duration of linezolid therapy. However, when linezolid needs to be used over extended periods of time in patients with chronic infections or where underlying ADHD is so severe that discontinuation of ADHD pharmacotherapy is likely to result in non-adherence with life-saving medical treatment, a cautious trial of concomitant use of linezolid and ADHD medication may be necessary.

COMBINATION PHARMACOTHERAPY FOR ADHD

ADHD monotherapy may be ineffective in 30–40% of children (Wilens & Biederman, 1992). Combination therapies for ADHD (Hammerness, Georgiopoulos, et al., 2009; Pohl, Van Brunt, Ye, Stoops, & Johnston, 2009; Wilens et al., 2009) may be useful when monotherapies are only partially effective, when psychiatric comorbidities also require treatment, or to permit dose-reduction of one or both agents to minimize side effects. In addition to use as monotherapy, both extended-release guanfacine and clonidine have demonstrated effectiveness and recently received FDA approval as adjunctive agents in combination with stimulants (Palumbo et al., 2008; Spencer, Greenbaum, Ginsberg, & Murphy, 2009). In one study, significant improvement in ADHD with good tolerability was noted when osmotic controlled release oral delivery system (OROS) methylphenidate (OROS-MPH) was added in children who were partial responders to atomoxetine (Hammerness, Georgiopoulos et al., 2009; Wilens et al., 2009).

CARDIAC CONSIDERATIONS IN ADHD PHARMACOTHERAPY

The catecholaminergic effects of ADHD pharmacotherapies on heart rate, cardiac contractility, and blood pressure should be considered before administration. In most patients, increased blood pressure and heart rate are not clinically significant, but some patients can be particularly vulnerable to them and require dose-reduction or discontinuation (Hammerness, Wilens et al., 2009). With the exception of the tricyclic antidepressants, there is little evidence of QT-prolongation from these agents. Coexisting conditions that could be exacerbated by sympathomimetic activity should be identified (Table 50.5). Depending on the potential consequences of exacerbation, these may represent absolute or relative contraindications.

Sudden death has been reported in individuals receiving stimulants or atomoxetine, and FDA-approved package inserts for these agents note this. The rate of sudden death while taking stimulant medication may be higher in patients with preexisting structural heart defects (Vetter et al., 2008), but an increase in the rate of sudden death has not been documented in otherwise healthy patients. Large retrospective population-based studies of pediatric and adult patients receiving ADHD pharmacotherapy showed no association with serious cardiovascular events, including myocardial infarction, stroke, and death (Cooper et al., 2011; Habel et al., 2011). The advisability of routine screening electrocardiograms to identify cardiac risk factors in children and adolescents has been debated (American Academy of Pediatrics, 2000; Perrin, Friedman, & Knilans, 2008). Evaluation prior to initiating therapy for ADHD medication should include physical examination; personal history of cardiac symptoms such as chest pain, syncope or palpitations; and family history of pertinent cardiac risk factors, including hypertrophic cardiomyopathy, long QT syndrome, Wolff-Parkinson-White syndrome, or sudden death at an early age. Depending on these findings, electrocardiogram (EKG), echocardiography, or cardiology consultation may be indicated in some cases prior to initiating ADHD pharmacotherapy. The onset of symptoms suggestive of cardiac disorders during treatment for ADHD should lead to prompt evaluation (Hammerness, Perrin, Shelley-Abrahamson, & Wilens, 2011). Relatively few children (1–3%) will have persistent elevations of blood pressure or pulse while taking stimulants, but more research is required regarding the clinical significance over long-term use of stimulants in these outliers (Hammerness et al., 2011).

Sudden death, stroke, and myocardial infarction are more common in adults than in children, as are baseline cardiac risk factors. Particular caution is advised with ADHD pharmacotherapy in cases of poorly controlled hypertension, heart failure, recent myocardial infarction, or arrhythmia. One open-label study demonstrated that extended-release mixed amphetamine salts for ADHD were well tolerated by a small group of adults who were also taking anti-hypertensive treatment (Wilens et al., 2006). In adults, the most common condition that emerges during ADHD treatment and requires modification of therapeutic approach is the emergence of hypertension. When this occurs, there are several reasonable strategies, depending on the individual clinical scenario, including ADHD severity and other medical factors contributing to hypertension. These include dose-reduction of ADHD medication, use of the alpha-agonist ADHD treatments guanfacine or clonidine (indicated for hypertension but off-label in adults for ADHD, and requiring cautious monitoring for rebound hypertension in withdrawal), or treatment with other anti-hypertensive agents and continuation of stimulant medication.

Table 50.5 POTENTIAL CONTRAINDICATIONS TO ADHD PHARMACOTHERAPIES*

TYPE OF CONTRAINDICATION	RELEVANT AGENTS
Personal or family history of structural cardiac defect or arrhythmia	Tricyclic antidepressants may prolong QT interval; stimulants and atomoxetine may increase heart rate; alpha agonists may cause syncope, hypotension, bradycardia.
Agents with interaction/additive effects	MAOI antidepressants; sympathomimetics (e.g., caffeine, theophylline, pseudoephedrine).
Past or current psychosis (hallucinations, paranoia)	Stimulants and atomoxetine may exacerbate.
Past or current hypomania/mania	Stimulants, atomoxetine, and antidepressants may exacerbate.
Narrow angle glaucoma	Stimulants and atomoxetine may exacerbate.
Substance use or abuse	Stimulants may be abused.
Tic disorder	Stimulants (and rarely atomoxetine) may exacerbate; May improve with alpha-2 agonists.
Untreated hyperthyroidism	Stimulants and atomoxetine may exacerbate.
Untreated hypertension	Stimulants and atomoxetine may exacerbate.

*Incomplete list—stimulants may be contraindicated in any condition potentially exacerbated by sympathomimetic effects. Specialty consultation or management may allow safe treatment.

TREATMENT GOALS

It is useful to agree on treatment goals with a patient to focus treatment efforts. Asking a patient to identify the most important daily life tasks that would benefit from increased focus and reduced restlessness can generate treatment targets that can be tracked during intervention. Reasonable targets for ADHD pharmacotherapy include reduction of time spent looking for misplaced items; increased duration of concentration in reading, studying, or meetings; or reduction in missed content of conversations. Although pharmacotherapies for ADHD may robustly improve patients' capacities for attention and engagement, there are ADHD-related traits such as organizational abilities that may not benefit. An additional important goal is to learn to compensate for lack of these native skills. It may be useful to ask patients what they do to organize their lives, such as setting aside time for planning and using a reminder system, and to encourage them to practice these skills. For example, a college student might ask his roommate to send him a reminder text message 30 minutes before a scheduled midterm examination, because he is afraid he will forget when it is scheduled or get distracted and miss it. With help, he may develop a system of entering such reminders into his cellphone, decreasing his dependence on others and increasing his consistency in meeting his obligations. Formation of new habits may be optimized by utilizing what has motivated behavior change and held the patient accountable in the past.

INITIATING PHARMACOTHERAPY

Rapid adjustment of medication occurs best with frequent visits at the outset of treatment. Gradually increasing sympathomimetic agents allows accommodation to peripheral effects such as dry mouth or decreased appetite. Some infrequent side effects of stimulants, such as mood or personality changes or muscle tension, are often reported only after several days of exposure. A typical dosing schedule calls for incremental increases in dose every few days to weeks, giving a long enough time for the patient and caregivers to monitor benefits and side effects of each dose. The rating scales described above, including the Conners, Vanderbilt, or ADHD-RS for children, or the 18-item ASRS for adults, may be used to monitor treatment response over time.

While the effects of stimulants may be experienced the same day they are taken, for non-stimulant agents, time to effect can vary from days to weeks. A typical strategy for atomoxetine is to start below 0.5 mg/kg/day, and increase every three to seven days, up to a maximum of 1.4 mg/kg/day. Because bupropion is thought to increase risk for seizures, it may be advisable to evaluate response at lower doses for several weeks before increasing the dose to a maximum of the 400–450 mg/day doses that have been studied in adults in clinical trials, or 6 mg/kg or 300 mg (whichever is lowest) if used off-label in children; if short-acting or sustained-release (SR) bupropion is used, split dosing with no single dose above 200 mg (150 mg in children) may also reduce this risk (Pliszka & AACAP, 2007).

Adults may require doses above FDA-approved limits for effective control of ADHD (Spencer et al., 2005). Limited study suggests that children requiring high doses do not demonstrate excessive plasma levels (Stevens, George, Fusillo, Stern, & Wilens, 2010). While optimal dosing cannot be predicted based on patient weight, it is reasonable to use weight to guide estimation of *maximum* dosing for stimulant treatment. Based on clinical experience, doses of methylphenidate up to 2 mg/kg/day, of dexmethylphenidate up to 1 mg/kg/day, and of amphetamine formulations up to 1 mg/kg/day may be well tolerated. However, it is advisable to increase the dose slowly, allowing several days to evaluate patient response carefully, particularly below or at the level of one-half of these suggested safety maximums. Further increase may be most prudent where there is incremental benefit at lower strengths.

Blood levels of stimulants are not typically monitored in clinical settings and may not be easily obtained from clinical laboratories.

MAINTAINING PHARMACOTHERAPY

Once treatment is stable, follow-up should occur on a time frame dictated by the outcomes being tracked. Uncomplicated patients can be followed every few months, or as dictated by local regulations for the monitoring of the medication employed. It is advisable to reevaluate need for medication treatment periodically. If patients have a change in circumstance that minimizes ADHD-related challenges, such as increase in how engaging or structured their daily activities are, this should also prompt reevaluation of need for ongoing treatment.

Some patients experience a change in the level of benefit over time. New environmental demands that render compensatory habits insufficient may merit stronger medication support. Weight gain, sleep deprivation, or decreased frequency of exercise (e.g., at the end of a sports season) may prompt reports of a changing level of benefit from treatment. Physiological transitions also necessitate alertness to possible need for dose adjustments. Pubertal patients may require increased doses due to their rapid increase in body size and environmental demands, or decreased doses, possibly due to frontal lobe maturation or slower medication clearance. Menopausal patients may complain of poorer attention and memory at menopause. Individuals may develop increased sensitivity to side effects or a need for dose-reduction with aging. Occasionally, patients appear to have tachyphylaxis to the effects of stimulants. Before raising dose in an established treatment, it is reasonable to address apparent tolerance by having patients take brief medication holidays. Patients who experience initiation or discontinuation side effects may need to taper doses up or down when there are breaks in treatment. Other patients with tachyphylaxis will benefit from switching at least temporarily to a different stimulant or to a non-stimulant. It is also important to consider the possibility that emerging psychiatric comorbidities such as depression could be resulting in a pattern of apparent loss of efficacy.

MONITORING AND MANAGING SIDE EFFECTS

Physical effects such as dry mouth, decreased appetite, insomnia, gastrointestinal upset, or other perturbations of peripheral nervous system function often occur with ADHD pharmacotherapies, and sometimes improve or resolve over a several-day period at a steady dose. Minimizing caffeine and sympathomimetic agents sometimes eliminates or reduces side effects, particularly early in a medication trial. Growth monitoring may prompt treatment holidays or non-stimulant treatment in children, as some studies associate stimulant treatment with effects on weight and height (Pliszka & AACAP, 2007). Blood pressure and heart rate should be monitored during the course of ADHD pharmacotherapy. Patients should be prompted to report any detrimental changes in mood, thoughts, personality, mental function, or tics; these are expected to resolve with termination of treatment.

Some side effects may be managed by changing to an alternate form of the same active agent. For example, dry mouth may be less prominent on one form of long-acting methylphenidate than another for an individual patient, but switching between agents may also produce a new side effect. If a stimulant side effect occurs most at a particular time of day, changing to a different release pattern, or delaying the second daily dose by a small interval may eliminate the side effect. Tapering off stimulant doses by adding a smaller second dose later in the day to a long-acting agent given in the morning may limit wear-off effects such as fatigue or irritability. Changing the time of dose or dividing the dose can mitigate atomoxetine side effects, such as fatigue, sleep interruption, or gastrointestinal distress, in some cases.

NON-PSYCHOPHARMACOLOGICAL TREATMENT

While medications are often effective for reducing ADHD symptoms, non-medication interventions are important in order to minimize functional impairment and ADHD-related challenges such as executive function difficulties, distress over the consequences of ADHD, and comorbid mental health problems. Non-medication approaches to ADHD management include psychoeducation, cognitive-behavioral and parent training therapies, ADHD coaching, and disability accommodations. Effective pharmacotherapy may greatly facilitate adherence to non-medication interventions, and vice versa.

Patients benefit significantly from considering how ADHD impacts their lives via psychoeducation. Acknowledgement that ADHD is neurobiological condition that can be understood and compensated for can be very powerful for patients who have blamed themselves for a lifetime of underperformance relative to their potential. Helping loved ones understand how ADHD impacts their relationship, and how to best nurture the relationship given those challenges, can be very valuable. Community resources with helpful websites include organizations such as Children and Adults with ADHD (CHADD), and the Attention Deficit Disorder Association.

Structured cognitive-behavioral therapies (CBT) offer techniques to improve patients' compensatory strategies and change unhelpful beliefs (Safren et al., 2005; Safren et al., 2010; Solanto et al., 2010). A therapist's manual and client workbook are available (Safren, 2005a, 2005b). Training family members and teachers how to respond to behavior resulting from ADHD can be helpful. Parent training, for example, improved both child and parent functioning in some studies (Barkley, 2002; Pelham & Fabiano, 2008). Therapies and coaching for ADHD that foster new habits rely in part on establishing accountability. Groups can be another powerful context in which to teach new skills (Solanto et al., 2010).

Under the Americans with Disabilities Act, individuals with ADHD have a right to reasonable accommodations in work and school environments. Patients should be encouraged to explore what may be available for accommodation through the special education eligibility evaluation process in school districts, the college disability services office, or the human resources department at their job. Although neuropsychological testing is not necessary to confirm a DSM-IV diagnosis of ADHD, it can be a powerful tool for guiding patients toward interventions that will capitalize on their strengths and is often required to help secure educational or occupational accommodations.

MEDICAL SEQUELAE OF ADHD

Undiagnosed ADHD can significantly impact patients presenting for treatment of physical concerns. The impulsivity and lack of planning common in patients with ADHD may increase their risk for engaging in unhealthy behavior patterns. Impulsivity is linked to a shortened life expectancy (Friedman et al., 1995). ADHD is linked to higher rates of substance abuse, with lower quit rates, and thus to related medical sequelae (Biederman, Monuteaux, et al., 2006; Biederman et al., 1995; Pomerleau, Downey, Stelson, & Pomerleau, 1996; Wilens, 2006). ADHD may be associated with obesity in children (Kim, Mutyala, Agiovlasitis, & Fernhall, 2011) and adults (Cortese et al., 2008; Fleming, Levy, & Levitan, 2005).

Patients seen in urgent and emergency care settings for trauma secondary to poorly regulated behavior may be suffering from ADHD. Preschool children hospitalized for mild traumatic brain injury are at increased risk for ADHD persisting through adolescence (McKinlay, Grace, Horwood, Fergusson, & MacFarlane, 2009). Children with ADHD symptoms are more likely to experience physical injuries (Schwebel et al., 2011). Older adolescents and young adults with ADHD are more likely to get into motor vehicle accidents (Barkley & Cox, 2007; Barkley, Murphy, Dupaul, & Bush, 2002). The possibility of ADHD should be considered in patients with reckless behavior and poor judgement—for example, a child on a burn unit who has been injured playing with firecrackers—but also in patients accidentally injured during repetitive or routine tasks that require sustained attention, such as a construction worker who shoots himself in the hand with a nail gun.

PREVALENCE OF ADHD IN MEDICAL ILLNESS

Patients with chronic medical illness are at increased risk for psychiatric illness (Wells, Golding, & Burnam, 1988). One study of psychiatric disorders in chronically ill children between 4 and 16 years of age revealed the presence of ADHD in 9.2%, versus 4.3% in controls (Cadman, Boyle, Szatmari, & Offord, 1987). While ADHD is strongly familial (Faraone, 2004), early medical insults could increase the likelihood of phenotypical expression of ADHD in genetically predisposed patients. Plausible contributory factors include intrauterine growth retardation (Heinonen et al., 2010), perinatal hypoxia (Boksa & El-Khodor, 2003), malnutrition, and failure to thrive (Galler & Ramsey, 1989; Giglio, Candusso, D'Orazio, Mastella, & Faraguna, 1997), and tobacco, lead, or other environmental exposures (Froehlich et al., 2009). Psychosocial stressors resulting from chronic illness could also exacerbate functional impairment in patients with comorbid ADHD.

Differences in how cases have been ascertained in studies of ADHD across medical illness categories may be responsible for the high variability in ADHD prevalence rates found in pediatric cohorts (see Table 50.6). The high prevalence of ADHD in patients with some genetic syndromes (Lo-Castro, D'Agati, & Curatolo, 2010) raises the possibility of a common etiology. ADHD may be associated with particular alleles of the androgen receptor gene (Comings, Chen, Wu, & Muhleman, 1999). Specific patterns of increased ADHD symptoms may emerge in some medical illnesses. For example, inattentive symptoms may be more common in epileptic children (Bennett-Back, Keren, & Zelnik, 2011) and children with asthma (Yuksel, Sogut, & Yilmaz, 2008). On the other hand, pediatric migraine was found to be associated with hyperactive-impulsive, but not inattentive, ADHD symptoms(Bigal & Arruda, 2010).

ADHD-LIKE SYMPTOMS DUE TO MEDICAL ILLNESS OR TREATMENT

Neurocognitive effects of medical illness or its treatment, such as those experienced in HIV/AIDS, cancer, rheumatic conditions, endocrine disorders, and sleep disorders, may also result in impairment that should not be mistaken for ADHD. Hypertension may be associated with an increase in executive function and attentional difficulties in adult and pediatric patients (Adams, Szilagyi, Gebhardt, & Lande, 2010). Options to address these conditions include improving treatment of the underlying medical illness (e.g., using an HIV medication that better penetrates the blood–brain barrier), altering medical treatments causing cognitive side effects (e.g., reducing steroid dose in inflammatory bowel disease), or by symptomatic treatment with stimulant (Conklin et al., 2009) or non-stimulant ADHD medications when appropriate.

It may sometimes be challenging to distinguish among symptoms related to the underlying medical disorder, side effects of medications, or comorbid ADHD. In the case of epilepsy, for example, comorbid ADHD is common, but imperfectly controlled seizures or anticonvulsants such as topiramate can also impair cognition and mimic or exacerbate inattentive symptoms. Family history of ADHD and documentation of ADHD symptom-onset prior to medical illness, when available, can be helpful in establishing ADHD as a separate comorbidity, but these factors are not clear or applicable in every medically complex case. Prospective tracking of ADHD-like symptoms with ADHD rating scales during systematic and, when possible, sequential rather than simultaneous trials of changes in medical treatments (e.g., increase, decrease, or change in anticonvulsant) or psychotropic treatments (e.g., empirical trial of an ADHD medication) can help to disentangle these effects and guide treatment.

ADHD DIAGNOSIS IN THE CONTEXT OF MEDICAL ILLNESS

ADHD may be challenging to diagnose in patients with chronic medical illness. Caregivers may fail to consider ADHD in medically ill children and adults, even when they

Table 50.6 VARIABILITY OF ADHD PREVALENCE IN PEDIATRIC MEDICAL ILLNESS

PEDIATRIC MEDICAL ILLNESS	PREVALENCE OF ADHD	REFERENCES
Fetal alcohol syndrome	>50%	Peadon 2010
Congenital heart disease	40–50%	Vetter 2008
Familial male precocious puberty	44.4%	Mueller 2010
Chromosome 18 abnormalities	41.7%	Zavala 2010
Velocardiofacial syndrome (22q11.2 deletion)	38%	Jolin 2009
Migraine	23.7% (hyperactive type only)	Bigal 2010
Congenital adrenal hyperplasia (males)	18.2%	Mueller 2010
Alopecia areata	14.3%	Ghanizadeh 2008
Complicated epilepsy	12.0%	Davies 2003
Cystic fibrosis	21% (disruptive behavior disorder) 9.6%	White 2009, Georgiopoulos 2011
Diabetes	2.1% 4%	Davies 2003, Levitt-Katz 2005

are having significant difficulty. In complex patients with medical illness, ADHD-related functional impairment may be misunderstood as being solely due to missing school or work frequently when ill, or to medical symptoms or treatment side effects such as pain or fatigue. A systematic search for persistent ADHD symptoms in multiple contexts over time will help establish the diagnosis.

<hr/>

CASE VIGNETTE

A six-year-old girl with cystic fibrosis (CF) is at nutritional risk due to poor weight gain. Pulmonary function tests cannot be completed reliably due to hyperkinesis. When specifically asked about her behavior in other settings, her mother reports that she won't sit at the table long enough to eat full meals; her teacher is concerned about inattention, and redirects her frequently in the classroom. On further assessment, she is found to meet criteria for *ADHD, combined type.* Atomoxetine improves her engagement at school, at home, and in medical care.

<hr/>

Adolescents with chronic illness may report lower rates of risky behavior than do adolescents in the general population (Britto et al., 1998). When these behaviors emerge in the setting of chronic illness, the presence of ADHD, some other psychiatric illness, or psychosocial stressors should be considered. Early identification and management of ADHD may better prepare children with chronic illness to pass through the high-risk stage of adolescence. The ability to meet educational and occupational demands is of key importance in the medically ill. In adults with CF, for example, psychological health and educational attainment may be more salient than pulmonary function for quality of life and the ability to continue working as they age and become sicker (Burker, Sedway, & Carone, 2004; Riekert, Bartlett, Boyle, Krishnan, & Rand, 2007).

<hr/>

CASE VIGNETTE

A 16-year-old boy with Crohn's disease is brought to psychiatric attention for the first time and diagnosed with longstanding ADHD, oppositional defiant disorder, and possible learning disabilities. He refuses neuropsychological evaluation or ADHD treatment, stating that he is on too many medicines and sees too many doctors already. Within a year, he has dropped out of high school and is using marijuana daily and abusing alcohol in a binge pattern. He experiments with opiates, which he justifies as an attempt to manage his chronic diarrhea, coinciding with medical and functional decline with repeated inpatient medical hospitalization in young adulthood.

<hr/>

IMPACT OF ADHD ON MEDICAL TREATMENT ADHERENCE

In addition to school or work, home, and the social arena, patients with medical illness have an extra domain of functioning that may be pervasively affected by ADHD: medical self-care. Forgetfulness, avoidance, distractibility, and impulsive, restless behavior interfering with medical care

should prompt consideration of the presence of ADHD. Oppositional or defiant behavior, which often accompanies ADHD in childhood and may persist into adulthood (Harpold et al., 2007), can similarly confound consistent follow-through with medical recommendations.

Treatment adherence is often poor in chronic illness (Brown & Bussell, 2011; Modi et al., 2006; Zindani, Streetman, Streetman, & Nasr, 2006). There has been increasing recognition in the literature of psychological factors such as depression that may exacerbate non-adherence and affect medical outcomes (Cruz, Marciel, Quittner, & Schechter, 2009; Gonzalez et al., 2008; Kettler, Sawyer, Winefield, & Greville, 2002; Safren et al., 2009; Smith & Wood, 2007). Less studied are the effects of ADHD on adherence to medical care. Common barriers to adherence in chronic illness include oppositional behaviors, forgetting, and time-management difficulties, all of which are also prominent in ADHD (Dziuban, Saab-Abazeed, Chaudhry, Streetman, & Nasr, 2010; Modi & Quittner, 2006; Simons, McCormick, Devine, & Blount, 2010). The distractibility, avoidance of unpleasant tasks, and impairments in organization associated with ADHD may exacerbate the burden of medical self-care in chronic illness.

A trend between presence of externalizing disorders and non-adherence was noted in one study of children with CF (White, Miller, Smith, & McMahon, 2009). Georgiopoulos and Hua found that 61% of 18 pediatric CF patients with ADHD had non-adherence among the chief complaints at the time of initial evaluation; when effective ADHD treatment could be implemented, medical adherence often improved (Georgiopoulos & Hua, 2011). Examples of difficulties with medical adherence and navigating through systems of care that may be more common in patients with ADHD are found in Table 50.7.

ADHD TREATMENT IN THE MEDICALLY ILL PATIENT

The decision about whether and how to treat ADHD in medical illness requires careful consideration of each patient's psychiatric and medical status. There are limited data to suggest differential effectiveness of particular ADHD treatments in the context of medical illness. For example, there is preliminary evidence that stimulants, non-stimulants, and combination therapies are all useful treatment options in children with CF (Georgiopoulos & Hua, 2011).

Clinicians should consider that ADHD treatments could have unique adverse effects in patients with concurrent illness. In particular, some conditions could be exacerbated by their sympathomimetic activity. ADHD medication side effects should be considered if the intensity or character of symptoms differs from a patient's usual pattern or correlates with a new medication trial or dose adjustment. In cases of uncertain etiology of such symptoms, an on–off–on trial or dose-reduction of ADHD medication may be useful.

In medically ill patients, ADHD medication side effects may alter the usual risk–benefit ratios for these treatments on a case-by-case basis. For example, tricyclic antidepressants

Table 50.7 TYPICAL MANIFESTATIONS OF ADHD IN MEDICAL SETTINGS

ADHD SYMPTOM	SAMPLE MANIFESTATIONS IN MEDICAL SETTING
Forgetful	Forgets to do treatments.
	Forgets to refill medication or ask for refills at time of visit.
	Forgets to come to appointments.
	Vague historian.
	Forgets to pay bills or do insurance paperwork.
Loses things	Misplaces prescriptions, medications, or important medical equipment.
	Loses medical correspondence, lab results.
	Loses cell phone, wallet with insurance cards, appointment cards.
Leaves tasks unfinished	Intends to but doesn't make follow-up appointments.
	Doesn't follow through on referrals or medical tests.
	Agrees to treatment plan but can't seem to follow through.
Executive dysfunction (poor organization, time management, planning)	Last-minute refill requests (i.e., runs out while on vacation).
	Doesn't anticipate adjustments in insurance, treatment providers, or treatment plan needed for major changes (moving to a new city, birth of child).
	Financial difficulties, runs out of money to buy medicines or make copays.
	Can't prioritize well in making medical decisions, seems to have poor "common sense."
	Late for appointments.
	Comes at wrong day or time.
	Difficult to determine chief complaint or main priority for visit.
On the go, restless; inability to stay seated	Doesn't comply with activity restrictions.
	Can't sit still for treatments.
	Leaves without treatment when has to wait.
Poor listening and easily distracted	Leaves office without fully understanding care instructions.
	Needs to hear or read instruction multiple times to retain information.
	Asks care providers to repeat instructions.
Avoids difficult tasks	Puts off medical treatments or important paperwork.
	Complexity of treatment plan feels overwhelming to patient.
Talkativeness/interrupting	Hard to keep conversation on track during visit.
Trouble waiting their turn	Excessive impatience or irritability with long waits.
	Heightened sense of urgency, demanding immediate intervention for medical problem.
Careless mistakes	Takes medication at wrong doses.
	Takes previously discontinued medication from wrong bottles.
	Injured or ill because of careless/risky behavior.
	Misses key steps of treatment plan.

are often considered third-line ADHD agents, after stimulants and FDA-approved non-stimulants (Pliszka & AACAP, 2007), due to the potential for lethal overdose and cardiac side effects. The risk–benefit ratio for the use of tricyclics to treat ADHD would be even less favorable than usual in patients with unstable cardiac illness, but more favorable in the setting of medical illnesses like CF in which weight gain is welcome (Pedreira et al., 2005) and comorbid anxiety and depression are common.

Body mass index (BMI) percentile and gastrointestinal side effects should be carefully monitored in medically ill patients at high risk for weight loss and its consequences—as with some malignancies or gastrointestinal illnesses—who elect to try stimulants. Cyproheptadine (Daviss & Scott, 2004) or other agents can be added to increase appetite, and actively countering constipation, improving gastric motility, and/or better addressing malabsorption may be helpful. Nutritional consultation can be helpful in patients who need additional strategies to increase caloric intake—for example, by increasing caloric density, increasing frequency of food intake, or adding nutritional supplements. Alternatively, the combination of a non-stimulant and a stimulant may provide enough additional ADHD benefit to permit lowering the stimulant dose to stabilize weight.

Abdominal pain and nausea are common side effects of stimulants, atomoxetine, bupropion, and tricyclic antidepressants; in the presence of preexisting gastrointestinal disease, these side effects may be more bothersome and could contribute to unwanted appetite suppression. In addition, as noted above, there are reports of liver abnormalities with atomoxetine; it may be prudent to avoid introducing atomoxetine in patients with significant or unstable liver disease, and to consider active monitoring in patients who are also at risk of developing liver abnormalities due to their primary medical illness or the medications used to treat it. To prevent bowel obstruction, medications delivered with non-deformable capsules are not advised in the presence of preexisting severe gastrointestinal narrowing such as may occur, for example, in inflammatory bowel disease (McNeil Pediatrics, 2010).

Occasionally, normally minor side effects of ADHD medication can become significant due to medical comorbidity. Exacerbation of dry mouth by a stimulant or tricyclic antidepressant could be intolerable in a patient with Sjögren's syndrome. Muscle tension from a stimulant could exacerbate musculoskeletal pain. Urinary retention may be a positive side effect of atomoxetine for a child with nocturnal enuresis (Sumner, Schuh, Sutton, Lipetz, & Kelsey, 2006), but not for a middle-aged man with benign prostatic hypertrophy.

Patients with comorbid epilepsy and ADHD should be stabilized on anti-epileptic treatment to the extent possible prior to initiation of ADHD treatment. Such patients should be both cautioned about and monitored for any increase in seizure activity during therapy, as ADHD medications, like many drugs, may lower the seizure threshold. Similarly, patients with stable congenital cardiac malformations may tolerate ADHD treatment but should be closely monitored during treatment (Vetter et al., 2008).

ADHD TREATMENT IN PREGNANCY

Because there is potential risk to a developing fetus or infant with exposure to pharmacotherapies, pharmacotherapy should be used during pregnancy and lactation only in severe cases, where the mother's safety or well-being would be significantly compromised otherwise. When necessary, exposure should be minimized through as much of pregnancy as possible. Pregnancy may be an ideal time to explore and practice non-pharmacological strategies. Although stimulant abuse appears to correlate with adverse reproductive outcomes (Debooy, Seshia, Tenenbein, & Casiro, 1993; Golub et al., 2005; Plessinger & Woods, 1993), there are limited data to support the reproductive safety of use of amphetamines at doses prescribed for therapeutic use in humans (Golub et al.). While there are over 1,500 exposures to amphetamines during pregnancy reported in the literature, there is less evidence on the safety of methylphenidate, with reports of less than 70 cases in the literature (Humphreys, Garcia-Bournissen, Ito, & Koren, 2007). In one study of 237 pregnant women who took dextroamphetamine to control weight gain, birth weights were 4% lower than in non-users when the medication was used in the thirdtrimester, but there was no increase in perinatal mortality (Naeye, 1983). In one observational study, amphetamines prescribed in the first trimester may have increased the occurrence of oral clefts, but not of severe congenital anomalies (Milkovich & van der Berg, 1977).

However, given the paucity of evidence regarding the safety of ADHD medication in pregnancy, discontinuation of ADHD medication is prudent in most pregnant women. For those with severely impairing symptoms, a switch from a stimulant to a tricyclic antidepressant, clonidine, guanfacine, or bupropion, for which there is more experience with use during pregnancy, could be considered (Milanovic, 2010). If a stimulant were required during pregnancy, an amphetamine product may be preferred to methylphenidate. Given the very limited data available for atomoxetine, it may be best avoided in pregnancy. Ideally, a strategy to switch ADHD medication during pregnancy would be developed during pre-conception planning and tested prior to pregnancy to avoid fetal exposure to a medication that may ultimately be ineffective for a given woman.

ADAPTING MEDICAL CARE TO PATIENTS WITH ADHD

ADHD can affect how patients care for themselves and interact with medical systems of care. Therapeutic interventions should target self-care behaviors with sensitivity to the impact of ADHD in patients with chronic medical illness (Table 50.8). Strategies for maintaining healthy sleep patterns, eating, exercise, and treatment adherence will foster health and minimize the burden of chronic illness. In patients with ADHD, adopting new or consistent routines may be particularly challenging. Difficulty initiating tasks, following through, and organizing behavior will have an impact on the ability of these patients to establish healthy routines.

Table 50.8 ADAPTATIONS TO MEDICAL CARE FOR PATIENTS WITH ADHD

ADHD-RELATED IMPAIRMENT	SAMPLE STRATEGIES TO ADAPT CARE FOR ADHD PATIENT
Inattention	— Expect inattention to interfere with verbal communication in your office. Ask the patient to repeat the treatment plan back to you to assess completeness of understanding.
Poor memory	— Write down instructions. Ask what reminder systems patients already use or can create, and apply them to medical self-care. — Expect details to be missed or avoided. Coach the patient on procedures for insurance approvals or refills.
Poor attention to detail	— Understand that medical treatment adherence may be difficult. Anticipate missed or late doses. When possible, select medicines that are less dangerous or ineffective when doses are missed.
Poor executive function	— Expect organizational challenges. At each visit, foster engagement in the organizational systems and social supports the patient needs to stay adherent.
Task avoidance, poor follow-through	— Expect motivation or interest in new strategies to decrease over time. — Help patients self-monitor their compliance with your recommendations, and establish external accountability for goals: computer or phone-based reminders, more frequent check-ins with your office, and the support of significant others may facilitate adherence.

- Expect inattention to interfere with verbal communication in your office. Ask the patient to repeat the treatment plan back to you to assess completeness of understanding.

- Expect memory challenges. Write down instructions for patients. Ask what reminder systems patients already use or can create, and apply them to medical self-care.

- Expect details to be missed or avoided. Coach the patients on procedures for insurance approvals or refills.

- Expect organizational challenges. At each visit, foster engagement in the organizational systems and social supports the patient needs to stay adherent.

- Understand that medical treatment adherence may be difficult. Anticipate missed or late doses. When possible, prescribe medicines which are less dangerous or ineffective when doses are missed.

- Expect their interest in or motivation with new strategies to decrease over time. Help patients self-monitor their compliance with your recommendations, and establish external accountability for goals: computer or phone-based reminders, more frequent check-ins with your office, and the support of significant others may facilitate adherence.

SUMMARY

ADHD is a common and well-characterized syndrome of self-regulatory difficulties with a high degree of familiality and individual variation in presentation. A variety of screening and diagnosis instruments are available that are appropriate to help detect ADHD. The biological underpinnings of ADHD are becoming increasingly understood at the genetic, neurostructural, and neurofunctional levels. Pharmacological and psychosocial treatments can minimize the impact of the inattention, impulsivity, and hyperactivity associated with the syndrome. The functional impairments seen in medically ill patients with ADHD may include challenges in self-care that can adversely affect physical health. Adaptations in the delivery of medical care may help increase medical treatment adherence in patients with ADHD.

CLINICAL PEARLS

- Methylphenidate may increase the effects of warfarin, phenobarbital, phenytoin, and primidone.

- The plasma level of amphetamine agents may be lowered by acidifying agents, and treatments that lower acidity, such as proton pump inhibitors, can increase serum levels.

- While optimal dosing cannot not be predicted based on weight, it is reasonable to use weight to guide your estimation of *maximum* dosing for stimulant treatment. Based on clinical experience, doses of methylphenidate up to 2 mg/kg/day, of dexmethylphenidate up to 1 mg/kg/day, and of amphetamine formulations up to 1 mg/kg/day may be well tolerated. However, it is advisable to increase the dose slowly, allowing several days to evaluate patient response carefully, particularly below or at the level of one-half of these suggested safety maximums. Further increase may be most prudent where there is incremental benefit at lower strengths.

- Therapies and coaching for ADHD that foster new habits rely in part on establishing accountability.

- The possibility of ADHD should be considered in patients with reckless behavior and poor judgement—for example, a child on a burn unit who has been injured playing with firecrackers—but also in patients accidentally injured during repetitive or routine tasks that require sustained attention, such as a construction worker who shoots himself in the hand with a nail gun.

- Patients should be encouraged to explore what may be available for accommodation through the special education eligibility evaluation process in school districts, college disability services offices, or the human resources department at their job.

- Pediatric migraine was found to significantly increase the risk of hyperactive-impulsive, but not inattentive, ADHD symptoms.

- When risky behaviors emerge in the setting of chronic illness, the presence of ADHD, other psychiatric illness, or psychosocial stressors should be considered.

- Forgetfulness, avoidance, distractibility, and impulsive, restless behavior interfering with medical care should prompt consideration of the presence of ADHD.

- Ideally, a strategy to discontinue or switch ADHD medication during pregnancy would be developed during pre-conception planning and tested prior to pregnancy to avoid fetal exposure to a medication that may ultimately be ineffective for a given woman.

DISCLOSURE STATEMENT

Dr. Georgiopoulos has the following relationships to disclose during the period from July 2011–July 2014. Cystic Fibrosis Foundation: grant support, committee service, honoraria, travel reimbursement. European Cystic Fibrosis Society: committee service, travel reimbursement. U.S. Food and Drug Administration: employed for work unrelated to this chapter. Lippincott, Williams & Wilkins: royalties.

Craig Surman, MD discloses the following relationships through July 2014: Speaking or education supported by McNeil, Janssen, Janssen-Ortho, Novartis, Shire, and Reed/ MGH Academy (funded by multiple companies). Consulting to McNeil, Nutricia, Pfizer, Takeda, Shire, Somaxon. Research Support at the MGH Adult ADHD Program from Abbot, Cephalon, Hilda and Preston Davis Foundation, Eli Lilly, Magceutics, J & J / McNeil, Merck, Nordic Naturals, Nutricia, Pamlab, Pfizer, Organon, Shire, and Takeda. Royalties from Berkeley/Penguin for "FASTMINDS How to Thrive If You Have ADHD (or think you might)", and from Humana/Springer for "ADHD in Adults: A Practical Guide to Evaluation and Management".

REFERENCES

Adams, H. R., Szilagyi, P. G., Gebhardt, L., & Lande, M. B. (2010). Learning and attention problems among children with pediatric primary hypertension. *Pediatrics*, 126(6), e1425–e1429.

Adler, L. A., Rubin, R., Qiao, M., Heinloth, A. N., & Durell, T. M. (2010). Patient characteristics and treatment response to atomoxetine in adults with ADHD versus ADHD comorbid with social anxiety disorder. *Journal of ADHD and Related Disorders*, 1(3), 5–15.

American Academy of Pediatrics (2000). Diagnosis and evaluation of the child with attention-deficit/hyperactivity disorder. *Pediatrics*, 105(5), 1158–1170.

American Psychiatric Association (2000). *Diagnostic and statistical manual of mental disorders: DMS-IV-TR*. Washington, DC: American Psychiatric Press.

American Psychiatric Association (2013). *Diagnostic and statistical manual of mental disorders (5th ed.)*. Arlington, VA: American Psychiatric Publishing.

Antshel, K. M., Faraone, S. V., Maglione, K., Doyle, A., Fried, R., Seidman, L., et al. (2009). Is adult attention deficit hyperactivity disorder a valid diagnosis in the presence of high IQ? *Psychological Medicine*, 39(8), 1325–1335.

Antshel, K. M., Faraone, S. V., Maglione, K., Doyle, A. E., Fried, R., Seidman, L. J., et al. (2010). Executive functioning in high-IQ adults with ADHD. *Psychological Medicine*, 40(11), 1909–1918.

Banerjee, T. D., Middleton, F., & Faraone, S. V. (2007). Environmental risk factors for attention-deficit hyperactivity disorder. *Acta Paediatrica*, 96(9), 1269–1274.

Murphy, K., Barkley, R. (1997) Attention deficit hyperactivity disorder adults: Comorbidities and adaptive impairments.*Comprehensive Psychiatry*, 37(6), 3937(6).

Barkley, R. (2002). Psychosocial treatments for attention-deficit hyperactivity disorder in children. *Journal of Clinical Psychiatry*, 63(Suppl 12), 36–43.

Barkley, R. (2004). Driving impairments in teens and adults with attention-deficit/hyperactivity disorder. *Psychiatric Clinics of North America*, 27, 233–260.

Barkley, R., Guvremont, D., Anastopoulos, A., DuPaul, G., & Shelton, T. (1993). Driving-related risks and outcomes of attention deficit hyperactivity disorder in adolescents and young adults: A 3- to 5-year follow-up survey. *Pediatrics*, 92(2), 212–218.

Barkley, R., Murphy, K., & Kwasnik, D. (1996). Motor vehicle driving competencies and risks in teens and young adults with attention deficit hyperactivity disorder. *Pediatrics*, 98(6), 1089–1095.

Barkley, R. A., & Cox, D. (2007). A review of driving risks and impairments associated with attention-deficit/hyperactivity disorder and the effects of stimulant medication on driving performance. *Journal of Safety Research*, 38(1), 113–128.

Barkley, R. A., & Murphy, K. R. (2010). Impairment in occupational functioning and adult ADHD: The predictive utility of executive function (EF) ratings versus EF tests. *Archives of Clinical Neuropsychology*, 25(3), 157–173.

Barkley, R. A., Murphy, K. R., Dupaul, G. I., & Bush, T. (2002). Driving in young adults with attention deficit hyperactivity disorder: knowledge, performance, adverse outcomes, and the role of executive functioning. *Journal of the International Neuropsychology Society*, 8(5), 655–672.

Barkley, R. A., Murphy, K. R., & Fischer, M. (2008). *ADHD in adults: What the science says*. New York: Guilford Press.

Bennett-Back, O., Keren, A., & Zelnik, N. (2011). Attention-deficit hyperactivity disorder in children with benign epilepsy and their siblings. *Pediatric Neurology*, 44(3), 187–192.

Biederman, J., & Faraone, S. V. (2005). Economic impact of adult ADHD. Paper presented at the 158th Annual Meeting of the American Psychiatric Association,May 21–26, 2005. Atlanta, GA.

Biederman, J., & Faraone, S. V. (2006). The effects of attention-deficit hyperactivity disorder on employment and household income. *Medscape General Medicine*, 8(3), 12.

Biederman, J., Faraone, S. V., Mick, E., Williamson, S., Wilens, T. E., Spencer, T. J., et al. (1999). Clinical correlates of ADHD in females: findings from a large group of girls ascertained from pediatric and psychiatric referral sources. *Journal of the American Academy of Child & Adolescent Psychiatry*, 38(8), 966–975.

Biederman, J., Faraone, S. V., Monuteaux, M. C., Spencer, T., Wilens, T., Bober, M., et al. (2004). Gender effects of attention deficit hyperactivity disorder in adults, revisited. *Biological Psychiatry*, 55(7), 692–700.

Biederman, J., Faraone, S. V., Spencer, T., Wilens, T., Mick, E., & Lapey, K. A. (1994). Gender differences in a sample of adults with attention deficit hyperactivity disorder. *Psychiatry Research*, 53(1), 13–29.

Biederman, J., Monuteaux, M., Mick, E., Spencer, T., Wilens, T., Silva, J., et al. (2006). Young adult outcome of attention deficit hyperactivity disorder: A controlled 10-year prospective follow-up study. *Psychological Medicine*, 36(2), 167–179.

Biederman, J., Monuteaux, M., Mick, E., Wilens, T., Fontanella, J., Poetzl, K. M., et al. (2006). Is cigarette smoking a gateway drug to subsequent alcohol and illicit drug use disorders? A controlled study of youths with and without ADHD. *Biological Psychiatry, 59*(3), 258–264.

Biederman, J., Petty, C., Fried, R., Fontanella, J., Doyle, A. E., Seidman, L. J., et al. (2006). Impact of psychometrically defined deficits of executive functioning in adults with attention deficit hyperactivity disorder. *American Journal of Psychiatry, 163*(10), 1730–1738.

Biederman, J., Petty, C. R., Monuteaux, M. C., Fried, R., Byrne, D., Mirto, T., et al. (2010). Adult psychiatric outcomes of girls with attention deficit hyperactivity disorder: 11-year follow-up in a longitudinal case-control study. *American Journal of Psychiatry, 167*(4), 409–417.

Biederman, J., Wilens, T., Mick, E., Milberger, S., Spencer, T., & Faraone, S. (1995). Psychoactive substance use disorder in adults with attention deficit hyperactivity disorder: effects of ADHD and psychiatric comorbidity. *American Journal of Psychiatry, 152*(11), 1652–1658.

Bigal, M. E., & Arruda, M. A. (2010). Migraine in the pediatric population—evolving concepts. *Headache, 50*(7), 1130–1143.

Boksa, P., & El-Khodor, B. F. (2003). Birth insult interacts with stress at adulthood to alter dopaminergic function in animal models: possible implications for schizophrenia and other disorders. *Neuroscience & Biobehavioral Reviews, 27*(1–2), 91–101.

Bond, D. J., Hadjipavlou, G., Lam, R. W., McIntyre, R. S., Beaulieu, S., Schaffer, A., et al. (2012). The Canadian Network for Mood and Anxiety Treatments (CANMAT) Task Force recommendations for the management of patients with mood disorders and comorbid attention-deficit/hyperactivity disorder. *Annals of Clinical Psychiatry, 24*(1), 23–37.

Britto, M. T., Garrett, J. M., Dugliss, M. A., Daeschner, C. W., Jr., Johnson, C. A., Leigh, M. W., et al. (1998). Risky behavior in teens with cystic fibrosis or sickle cell disease: a multicenter study. *Pediatrics, 101*(2), 250–256.

Brown, M. T., & Bussell, J. K. (2011). Medication adherence: WHO cares? *Mayo Clinic Proceedings, 86*(4), 304–314.

Brown, T. (1995). *Brown Attention Deficit Disorder Scales*. San Antonio, TX: The Psychological Corporation.

Brown, T. E. (Ed.). (2000). *Attention-deficit disorders and comorbidities in children, adolescents, and adults*. Washington, DC: American Psychiatric Press.

Burker, E. J., Sedway, J., & Carone, S. (2004). Psychological and educational factors: better predictors of work status than FEV1 in adults with cystic fibrosis. *Pediatric Pulmonology, 38*(5), 413–418.

Bush, G. (2011). Cingulate, frontal, and parietal cortical dysfunction in attention-deficit/hyperactivity disorder. *Biological Psychiatry, 15;69*(12), 1160–1167.

Cadman, D., Boyle, M., Szatmari, P., & Offord, D. (1987). Chronic illness, disability, and mental and social well-being: Findings of the Ontario Child Health Study. *American Academy of Pediatrics, 79*, 805–813.

Chang, K., Nayar, D., Howe, M., & Rana, M. (2009). Atomoxetine as an adjunct therapy in the treatment of co-morbid attention-deficit/hyperactivity disorder in children and adolescents with bipolar I or II disorder. *Journal of Child & Adolescent Psychopharmacology, 19*(5), 547–551.

Choi, J., Yoon, I. Y., Kim, H. W., Chung, S., & Yoo, H. J. (2010). Differences between objective and subjective sleep measures in children with attention deficit hyperactivity disorder. *Journal of Clinical Sleep Medicine, 6*(6), 589–595.

Comings, D. E., Chen, C., Wu, S., & Muhleman, D. (1999). Association of the androgen receptor gene (AR) with ADHD and conduct disorder. *Neuroreport, 10*(7), 1589–1592.

Conklin, H. M., Lawford, J., Jasper, B. W., Morris, E. B., Howard, S. C., Ogg, S. W., et al. (2009). Side effects of methylphenidate in childhood cancer survivors: a randomized placebo-controlled trial. *Pediatrics, 124*(1), 226–233.

Conners, C.K. (1997). *Conners Rating Scales—Revised*. North Tonawanda, NY: Multi-Health Systems.

Conners, C.K., Erhardt, D., & Sparrow, E. (1999). *Conners' Adult ADHD Rating Scales (CAARS)*. North Tonawanda, NY: Multi-Health Systems.

Cooper, W. O., Habel, L. A., Sox, C. M., Chan, K. A., Arbogast, P. G., Cheetham, T. C., et al. (2011). ADHD drugs and serious cardiovascular events in children and young adults. *New England Journal of Medicine, 365*(20), 1896–1904.

Cortese, S., Angriman, M., Maffeis, C., Isnard, P., Konofal, E., Lecendreux, M., et al. (2008). Attention-deficit/hyperactivity disorder (ADHD) and obesity: a systematic review of the literature. *Critical Reviews in Food Science & Nutrition, 48*(6), 524–537.

Cortese, S., Faraone, S. V., Konofal, E., & Lecendreux, M. (2009). Sleep in children with attention-deficit/hyperactivity disorder: meta-analysis of subjective and objective studies. *Journal of the American Academy of Child & Adolescent Psychiatry, 48*(9), 894–908.

Cruz, I., Marciel, K. K., Quittner, A. L., & Schechter, M. S. (2009). Anxiety and depression in cystic fibrosis. *Seminars in Respiratory & Critical Care Medicine, 30*(5), 569–578.

Daviss, W. B., & Scott, J. (2004). A chart review of cyproheptadine for stimulant-induced weight loss. *Journal of Child & Adolescent Psychopharmacology, 14*(1), 65–73.

Debooy, V. D., Seshia, M. M., Tenenbein, M., & Casiro, O. G. (1993). Intravenous pentazocine and methylphenidate abuse during pregnancy. Maternal lifestyle and infant outcome. *American Journal of Diseases of Children, 147*(10), 1062–1065.

DuPaul, G. I., Power, T. J., Anastopoulos, A., & Reed, R. (1998). *The ADHD Rating Scale-IV Checklist, Norms and Clinical Interpretation*. New York: Guilford Press.

Dziuban, E. J., Saab-Abazeed, L., Chaudhry, S. R., Streetman, D. S., & Nasr, S. Z. (2010). Identifying barriers to treatment adherence and related attitudinal patterns in adolescents with cystic fibrosis. *Pediatric Pulmonology, 45*(5), 450–458.

Eli Lilly & Company. (2011). Atomoxetine package insert.

Faraone, S., Biederman, J., & Mick, E. (2006). The age-dependent decline of attention-deficit/hyperactivity disorder: A meta-analysis of follow-up studies. *Psychological Medicine, 36*(2), 159–165.

Faraone, S. V. (2004). Genetics of adult attention-deficit/hyperactivity disorder. *Psychiatric Clinics of North America, 27*(2), 303–321.

Faraone, S. V., Biederman, J., Spencer, T., Mick, E., Murray, K., Petty, C., et al. (2006). Diagnosing adult attention deficit hyperactivity disorder: Are late onset and subthreshold diagnoses valid? *American Journal of Psychiatry, 163*(10), 1720–1729; quiz, 1859.

Faraone, S. V., Biederman, J., Spencer, T. J., & Aleardi, M. (2006). Comparing the efficacy of medications for ADHD using meta-analysis. *MedGenMed: Medscape General Medicine, 8*(4), 4.

Faraone, S. V., Perlis, R. H., Doyle, A. E., Smoller, J. W., Goralnick, J. J., Holmgren, M. A., et al. (2005). Molecular genetics of attention-deficit/hyperactivity disorder. *Biological Psychiatry, 57*(11), 1313–1323.

Faraone, S. V., Sergeant, J., Gillberg, C., & Biederman, J. (2003). The worldwide prevalence of ADHD: Is it an American condition? *World Psychiatry, 2*(2), 104–113.

Faries, D., Yalcin, I., Harder, D., & Heiligenstein, J. (2001). Validation of the ADHD Rating Scale as a clinician administered and scored instrument. *Journal of Attention Disorders, 5*(2), 107–115.

Fleming, J. P., Levy, L. D., & Levitan, R. D. (2005). Symptoms of attention deficit hyperactivity disorder in severely obese women. *Eating & Weight Disorders, 10*(1), e10–e13.

Friedman, H. S., Tucker, J. S., Schwartz, J. E., Tomlinson-Keasey, C., Martin, L. R., Wingard, D. L., et al. (1995). Psychosocial and behavioral predictors of longevity. The aging and death of the "termites." *American Psychologist, 50*(2), 69–78.

Froehlich, T. E., Lanphear, B. P., Auinger, P., Hornung, R., Epstein, J. N., Braun, J., et al. (2009). Association of tobacco and lead exposures with attention-deficit/hyperactivity disorder. *Pediatrics, 124*(6), e1054–e1063.

Galler, J. R., & Ramsey, F. (1989). A follow-up study of the influence of early malnutrition on development: behavior at home and at school. *Journal of the American Academy of Child & Adolescent Psychiatry, 28*(2), 254–261.

Georgiopoulos, A. M., & Hua, L. L. (2011). The diagnosis and treatment of attention deficit-hyperactivity disorder in children and adolescents with cystic fibrosis: a retrospective study. *Psychosomatics, 52*(2), 160–166.

Germano, E., Gagliano, A., & Curatolo, P. (2010). Comorbidity of ADHD and dyslexia. *Developmental Neuropsychology, 35*(5), 475–493.

Giglio, L., Candusso, M., D'Orazio, C., Mastella, G., & Faraguna, D. (1997). Failure to thrive: the earliest feature of cystic fibrosis in infants diagnosed by neonatal screening. *Acta Paediatrica, 86*(11), 1162–1165.

Golub, M., Costa, L., Crofton, K., Frank, D., Fried, P., Gladen, B., et al. (2005). National Toxicology Program-Center for the Evaluation of Risks to Human Reproduction [NTP-CERHR] Expert Panel Report on the reproductive and developmental toxicity of amphetamine and methamphetamine. *Birth Defects Research. Part B, Developmental and Reproductive Toxicology, 74*(6), 471–584.

Gonzalez, J. S., Safren, S. A., Delahanty, L. M., Cagliero, E., Wexler, D. J., Meigs, J. B., et al. (2008). Symptoms of depression prospectively predict poorer self-care in patients with Type 2 diabetes. *Diabetic Medicine, 25*(9), 1102–1107.

Habel, L. A., Cooper, W. O., Sox, C. M., Chan, K. A., Fireman, B. H., Arbogast, P. G., et al. (2011). ADHD medications and risk of serious cardiovascular events in young and middle-aged adults. *Journal of the American Medical Association, 306*(24), 2673–2683.

Haffey, M. B., Buckwalter, M., Zhang, P., Homolka, R., Martin, P., Lasseter, K. C., et al. (2009). Effects of omeprazole on the pharmacokinetic profiles of lisdexamfetamine dimesylate and extended-release mixed amphetamine salts in adults. *Postgraduate Medicine, 121*(5), 11–19.

Hammerness, P., Georgiopoulos, A., Doyle, R. L., Utzinger, L., Schillinger, M., Martelon, M., et al. (2009). An open study of adjunct OROS-methylphenidate in children who are atomoxetine partial responders: II. Tolerability and pharmacokinetics. *Journal of Child & Adolescent Psychopharmacology, 19*(5), 493–499.

Hammerness, P., Wilens, T., Mick, E., Spencer, T., Doyle, R., McCreary, M., et al. (2009). Cardiovascular effects of longer-term, high-dose OROS methylphenidate in adolescents with attention deficit hyperactivity disorder. *Journal of Pediatrics, 155*(1), 84–89, 89 e81.

Hammerness, P. G., Perrin, J. M., Shelley-Abrahamson, R., & Wilens, T. E. (2011). Cardiovascular risk of stimulant treatment in pediatric attention-deficit/hyperactivity disorder: update and clinical recommendations. *Journal of the American Academy of Child & Adolescent Psychiatry, 50*(10), 978–990.

Harpold, T., Biederman, J., Gignac, M., Hammerness, P., Surman, C., Potter, A., et al. (2007). Is oppositional defiant disorder a meaningful diagnosis in adults? Results from a large sample of adults with ADHD. *Journal of Nervous & Mental Diseases, 195*(7), 601–605.

Heinonen, K., Raikkonen, K., Pesonen, A. K., Andersson, S., Kajantie, E., Eriksson, J. G., et al. (2010). Behavioural symptoms of attention deficit/hyperactivity disorder in preterm and term children born small and appropriate for gestational age: a longitudinal study. *Biomed Central Pediatrics, 10*, 91.

Humphreys, C., Garcia-Bournissen, F., Ito, S., & Koren, G. (2007). Exposure to attention deficit hyperactivity disorder medications during pregnancy. *Canadian Family Physician, 53*(7), 1153–1155.

Joshi, G., & Georgiopoulos, A. (2012). Combination pharmacotherapy for psychiatric disorders in children and adolescents. In D. Rosenberg & S. Gershon (Eds.), *Pharmacotherapy of child and adolescent psychiatric disorders* (3rd ed., pp. 421–438). Hoboken, NJ: John Wiley & Sons.

Kessler, R. C., Adler, L., Ames, M., Barkley, R. A., Birnbaum, H., Greenberg, P., et al. (2005). The prevalence and effects of adult attention deficit/hyperactivity disorder on work performance in a nationally representative sample of workers. *Journal of Occupational & Environmental Medicine, 47*(6), 565–572.

Kessler, R. C., Adler, L., Ames, M., Demler, O., Faraone, S., Hiripi, E., et al. (2005). The World Health Organization Adult ADHD Self-Report Scale (ASRS): a short screening scale for use in the general population. *Psychological Medicine, 35*(2), 245–256.

Kessler, R. C., Adler, L., Barkley, R., Biederman, J., Conners, C. K., Demler, O., et al. (2006). The prevalence and correlates of adult

ADHD in the United States: results from the National Comorbidity Survey Replication. *American Journal of Psychiatry, 163*(4), 716–723.

Kettler, L. J., Sawyer, S. M., Winefield, H. R., & Greville, H. W. (2002). Determinants of adherence in adults with cystic fibrosis. *Thorax, 57*(5), 459–464.

Kim, J., Mutyala, B., Agiovlasitis, S., & Fernhall, B. Health behaviors and obesity among US children with attention deficit hyperactivity disorder by gender and medication use. *Preventive Medicine, 52*(3–4), 218–222.

Lo-Castro, A., D'Agati, E., & Curatolo, P. (2010). ADHD and genetic syndromes. *Brain Dev.*

Loe, I. M., & Feldman, H. M. (2007). Academic and educational outcomes of children with ADHD. *Ambulatory Pediatrics, 7*(1 Suppl), 82–90.

Lorenz, R. A., Vandenberg, A. M., & Canepa, E. A. (2008). Serotonergic antidepressants and linezolid: a retrospective chart review and presentation of cases. *International Journal of Psychiatry Medicine, 38*(1), 81–90.

McCance-Katz, E. F. (2011). Drug interactions associated with methadone, buprenorphine, cocaine, and HIV medications: Implications for pregnant women. *Life Science, 88*(21–22), 953–958.

McGough, J. J., Smalley, S. L., McCracken, J. T., Yang, M., Del'Homme, M., Lynn, D. E., et al. (2005). Psychiatric comorbidity in adult attention deficit hyperactivity disorder: findings from multiplex families. *American Journal of Psychiatry, 162*(9), 1621–1627.

McKinlay, A., Grace, R., Horwood, J., Fergusson, D., & MacFarlane, M. (2009). Adolescent psychiatric symptoms following preschool childhood mild traumatic brain injury: evidence from a birth cohort. *Journal of Head Trauma Rehabilitation, 24*(3), 221–227.

McNeil Pediatrics. (2010). Concerta Medication Guide. Retrieved May 25, 2011, from http://www.concerta.net/assets/Prescribing_Info-short.pdf.

Mick, E., Spencer, T., Faraone, S. V., Biederman, J., & Zhang, H. F. (2008). Assessing the validity of the Quality of Life Enjoyment and Satisfaction Questionnaire Short Form in adults with ADHD. *Journal of Attention Disorders, 11*(4), 504–509.

Milanovic, S. (2010). Clinical update: Use of stimulant medications in pregnancy. Publication. Retrieved October 26, 2010, from http://www.womensmentalhealth.org/posts/clinical-update-use-of-stimulant-medications-in-pregnancy/.

Milkovich, L., & van der Berg, B. J. (1977). Effects of antenatal exposure to anorectic drugs. *American Journal of Obstetrics & Gynecology, 129*(6), 637–642.

Modi, A. C., Lim, C. S., Yu, N., Geller, D., Wagner, M. H., & Quittner, A. L. (2006). A multi-method assessment of treatment adherence for children with cystic fibrosis. *Journal of Cystic Fibrosis, 5*(3), 177–185.

Modi, A. C., & Quittner, A. L. (2006). Barriers to treatment adherence for children with cystic fibrosis and asthma: What gets in the way? *Journal of Pediatric Psychology, 31*(8), 846–858.

Murphy, K. R., Barkley, R. A., & Bush, T. (2001). Executive functioning and olfactory identification in young adults with attention deficit-hyperactivity disorder. *Neuropsychology, 15*(2), 211–220.

Naeye, R. L. (1983). Maternal use of dextroamphetamine and growth of the fetus. *Pharmacology, 26*(2), 117–120.

World Health Organization. (2005). Adult ADHD Self-Report Scale (ASRS). Retrieved September 4, 2012, from www.hcp.med.harvard.edu/ncs/asrs.php.

Palumbo, D. R., Sallee, F. R., Pelham, W. E., Jr., Bukstein, O. G., Daviss, W. B., & McDermott, M. P. (2008). Clonidine for attention-deficit/hyperactivity disorder: I. Efficacy and tolerability outcomes. *Journal of the American Academy of Child & Adolescent Psychiatry, 47*(2), 180–188.

Pataki, C., Carlson, G., Kelly, K., Rapport, M., & Biancaniello, T. (1993). Side effects of methylphenidate and desipramine alone and in combination in children. *American Journal of Psychiatry, 32*(5), 1065–1072.

Pedreira, C. C., Robert, R. G., Dalton, V., Oliver, M. R., Carlin, J. B., Robinson, P., et al. (2005). Association of body composition and lung function in children with cystic fibrosis. *Pediatric Pulmonology, 39*(3), 276–280.

Pelham, W. E., Jr., & Fabiano, G. A. (2008). Evidence-based psychosocial treatments for attention-deficit/hyperactivity disorder. *Journal of Clinical Child & Adolescent Psychology, 37*(1), 184–214.

Perrin, J. M., Friedman, R. A., & Knilans, T. K. (2008). Cardiovascular monitoring and stimulant drugs for attention-deficit/hyperactivity disorder. *Pediatrics, 122*(2), 451–453.

Plessinger, M. A., & Woods, J. R., Jr. (1993). Maternal, placental, and fetal pathophysiology of cocaine exposure during pregnancy. *Clinical Obstetrics & Gynecology, 36*(2), 267–278.

Pliszka, S., & AACAP Workgroup on Quality Issues (2007). Practice parameter for the assessment and treatment of children and adolescents with attention-deficit/hyperactivity disorder. *Journal of the American Academy of Child & Adolescent Psychiatry, 46*(7), 894–921.

Pohl, G. M., Van Brunt, D. L., Ye, W., Stoops, W. W., & Johnston, J. A. (2009). A retrospective claims analysis of combination therapy in the treatment of adult attention-deficit/hyperactivity disorder (ADHD). *BMC Health Services Research, 9*, 95.

Pomerleau, O., Downey, K., Stelson, F., & Pomerleau, C. (1996). Cigarette smoking in adult patients diagnosed with ADHD. *Journal of Substance Abuse, 7*, 373–378.

Prince, J. B., Wilens, T. E., Biederman, J., Spencer, T. J., Millstein, R., Polisner, D. A., et al. (2000). A controlled study of nortriptyline in children and adolescents with attention deficit hyperactivity disorder. *Journal of Child and Adolescent Psychopharmacology, 10*(3), 193–204.

Cephalon. (1999). Provigil package insert.

Riddle, M., Geller, B., & Ryan, N. (1993). Case study:Another sudden death in a child treated with desipramine. *Journal of the American Academy of Child and Adolescent Psychiatry, 32*(4), 792–797.

Riekert, K. A., Bartlett, S. J., Boyle, M. P., Krishnan, J. A., & Rand, C. S. (2007). The association between depression, lung function, and health-related quality of life among adults with cystic fibrosis. *Chest, 132*(1), 231–237.

Safren, S. A. (2005a). *Mastering your adult ADHD: a cognitive-behavioral treatment program: Client workbook.* New York: Oxford University Press.

Safren, S. A. (2005b). *Mastering your adult ADHD: A cognitive-behavioral treatment program: therapist guide.* New York: Oxford University Press.

Safren, S. A., O'Cleirigh, C., Tan, J. Y., Raminani, S. R., Reilly, L. C., Otto, M. W., et al. (2009). A randomized controlled trial of cognitive behavioral therapy for adherence and depression (CBT-AD) in HIV-infected individuals. *Health Psychology, 28*(1), 1–10.

Safren, S. A., Otto, M. W., Sprich, S., Winett, C. L., Wilens, T. E., & Biederman, J. (2005). Cognitive-behavioral therapy for ADHD in medication-treated adults with continued symptoms. *Behavior Research and Therapy, 43*(7), 831–842.

Safren, S. A., Sprich, S., Mimiaga, M. J., Surman, C., Knouse, L., Groves, M., et al. (2010). Cognitive behavioral therapy vs relaxation with educational support for medication-treated adults with ADHD and persistent symptoms: a randomized controlled trial. *Journal of the American Medical Association, 304*(8), 875–880.

Schwebel, D. C., Roth, D. L., Elliott, M. N., Visser, S. N., Toomey, S. L., Shipp, E. M., et al. (2011). Association of externalizing behavior disorder symptoms and injury among fifth graders. *Academic Pediatrics, 11*(5), 427–431.

Seidman, L. J. (2006). Neuropsychological functioning in people with ADHD across the lifespan. *Clinical Psychology Review, 26*(4), 466–485.

Seidman, L. J., Valera, E., & Bush, G. (2004). Brain function and structure in adults with attention-deficit/hyperactivity disorder. *Psychiatric Clinics of North America, 27*(2), 323–347.

Shaw, P., Gornick, M., Lerch, J., Addington, A., Seal, J., Greenstein, D., et al. (2007). Polymorphisms of the dopamine D4 receptor, clinical outcome, and cortical structure in attention-deficit/hyperactivity disorder. *Archives of General Psychiatry, 64*(8), 921–931.

Simons, L. E., McCormick, M. L., Devine, K., & Blount, R. L. (2010). Medication barriers predict adolescent transplant recipients' adherence and clinical outcomes at 18-month follow-up. *Journal of Pediatric Psychology, 35*(9), 1038–1048.

Smith, B. A., & Wood, B. L. (2007). Psychological factors affecting disease activity in children and adolescents with cystic fibrosis: medical adherence as a mediator. *Current Opinion in Pediatrics, 19*(5), 553–558.

Solanto, M. V., Marks, D. J., Wasserstein, J., Mitchell, K., Abikoff, H., Alvir, J. M., et al. (2010). Efficacy of meta-cognitive therapy for adult ADHD. *American Journal of Psychiatry, 167*(8), 958–968.

Spencer, T., Biederman, J., Wilens, T., Faraone, S. V., Doyle, R. D., Surman, C., et al. (2005). A large, double-blind, randomized clinical trial of methylphenidate in the treatment of adults with attention-deficit/hyperactivity disorder. *Biological Psychiatry, 57*(5), 456–463.

Spencer, T., Biederman, J., Wilens, T., Steingard, R., & Geist, D. (1993). Nortriptyline treatment of children with attention-deficit hyperactivity disorder and tic disorder or Tourette's syndrome. *Journal of the American Academy of Child & Adolescent Psychiatry, 32*(1), 205–210.

Spencer, T., Greenbaum, M., Ginsberg, L. D., & Murphy, W. R. (2009). Safety and effectiveness of coadministration of guanfacine extended release and psychostimulants in children and adolescents with attention-deficit/hyperactivity disorder. *Journal of Child & Adolescent Psychopharmacology, 19*(5), 501–510.

Stevens, J., George, R. A., Fusillo, S., Stern, T., & Wilens, T. E. (2010). Plasma methylphenidate concentrations in youths treated with high-dose osmotic release oral system formulation. *Journal of Child & Adolescent Psychopharmacology, 20*(1), 49–54.

Subcommittee on Attention-Deficit/Hyperactivity Disorder, Steering Committee on Quality Improvement and Management. Evaluation, and Treatment of Attention-Deficit/Hyperactivity Disorder in Children and Adolescents (2011). Clinical practice guideline for the diagnosis,evaluation, and treatment of attention-deficit/hyperactivity disorder in children and adolescents. *Pediatrics, 128*(5), 1007–1022.

Sumner, C. R., Schuh, K. J., Sutton, V. K., Lipetz, R., & Kelsey, D. K. (2006). Placebo-controlled study of the effects of atomoxetine on bladder control in children with nocturnal enuresis. *Journal of Child & Adolescent Psychopharmacology, 16*(6), 699–711.

Surman, C., Randell, E., & Biederman, J. (2006). Association between attention-deficit/hyperactivity disorder and bulimia nervosa: Analysis of 4 case-control studies. *Journal of Clinical Psychiatry, 67*(3), 351–354.

Surman, C., Adamson, J., Petty, C., Biederman, J., Kenealy, D. C., Levine, M., et al. (2009). Association between attention-deficit/hyperactivity disorder and sleep impairment in adulthood: evidence from a large controlled study. *Journal of Clinical Psychiatry, 70*(11), 1523–1529.

Surman, C., Biederman, J., Spencer, T., Yorks, D., Miller, C. A., Petty, C. R., et al. (2011). Deficient emotional self-regulation and adult attention deficit hyperactivity disorder: a family risk analysis. *American Journal of Psychiatry, 168*(6), 617–623.

Turner, D. C., Clark, L., Dowson, J., Robbins, T. W., & Sahakian, B. J. (2004). Modafinil improves cognition and response inhibition in adult attention-deficit/hyperactivity disorder. *Biological Psychiatry, 55*(10), 1031–1040.

Vetter, V. L., Elia, J., Erickson, C., Berger, S., Blum, N., Uzark, K., et al. (2008). Cardiovascular monitoring of children and adolescents with heart disease receiving medications for attention deficit/hyperactivity disorder [corrected]: a scientific statement from the American Heart Association Council on Cardiovascular Disease in the Young Congenital Cardiac Defects Committee and the Council on Cardiovascular Nursing. *Circulation, 117*(18), 2407–2423.

Weiss, G., & Hechtman, L. (1993). Hyperactive children grown up. *ADHD in children, adolescents, and adults* (2nd ed.). New York: Guilford Press.

Wells, K. B., Golding, J. M., & Burnam, M. A. (1988). Psychiatric disorder in a sample of the general population with and without chronic medical conditions. *American Journal of Psychiatry, 145*(8), 976–981.

White, T., Miller, J., Smith, G. L., & McMahon, W. M. (2009). Adherence and psychopathology in children and adolescents with cystic fibrosis. *European Child & Adolescent Psychiatry, 18*(2), 96–104.

Wilens, T., Adler, L. A., Adams, J., Sgambati, S., Rotrosen, J., Sawtelle, R., et al. (2008). Misuse and diversion of stimulants prescribed for

ADHD: A systematic review of the literature. *Journal of the American Academy of Child & Adolescent Psychiatry, 47*(1), 21–31.

Wilens, T., & Biederman, J. (1992). The stimulants. In D. Schaffer (Ed.), *Psychiatric Clinics of North America* (Vol. 15, pp. 191–222). Philadelphia, PA: W. B. Saunders.

Wilens, T., Haight, B. R., Horrigan, J. P., Hudziak, J., Rosenthal, N. E., Connor, D., et al. (2005). Bupropion XL in adults with ADHD: A randomized, placebo-controlled study. *Biological Psychiatry, 57*(7), 793–801.

Wilens, T., Zusman, R. M., Hammerness, P. G., Podolski, A., Whitley, J., Spencer, T., et al. (2006). An open-label study of the tolerability of mixed amphetamine salts in adults with ADHD and treated primary essential hypertension. *Journal of Clinical Psychiatry, 67*(5), 696–702.

Wilens, T. E. (2006). Attention deficit hyperactivity disorder and substance use disorders. *American Journal of Psychiatry, 163*(12), 2059–2063.

Wilens, T. E., Biederman, J., Geist, D. E., Steingard, R., & Spencer, T. (1993). Nortriptyline in the treatment of attention deficit hyperactivity disorder: A chart review of 58 cases. *Journal of the American Academy of Child and Adolescent Psychiatry, 32*(2), 343–349.

Wilens, T. E., Biederman, J., Prince, J., Spencer, T. J., Faraone, S. V., Warburton, R., et al. (1996). Six-week, double-blind, placebo-controlled study of desipramine for adult attention deficit hyperactivity disorder. *American Journal of Psychiatry, 153*(9), 1147–1153.

Wilens, T. E., Hammerness, P., Utzinger, L., Schillinger, M., Georgiopoulous, A., Doyle, R. L., et al. (2009). An open study of adjunct OROS-w. *Journal of Child & Adolescent Psychopharmacology, 19*(5), 485–492.

Wilens, T. E., Spencer, T. J., Biederman, J., Girard, K., Doyle, R., Prince, J., et al. (2001). A controlled clinical trial of bupropion for attention deficit hyperactivity disorder in adults. *American Journal of Psychiatry, 158*(2), 282–288.

Wolraich, M. L., Lambert, W., Doffing, M. A., Bickman, L., Simmons, T., & Worley, K. (2003). Psychometric properties of the Vanderbilt ADHD Diagnostic Parent Rating Scale in a referred population. *Journal of Pediatric Psychology, 28*(8), 559–567.

Yuksel, H., Sogut, A., & Yilmaz, O. (2008). Attention deficit and hyperactivity symptoms in children with asthma. *Journal of Asthma, 45*(7), 545–547.

Zindani, G. N., Streetman, D. D., Streetman, D. S., & Nasr, S. Z. (2006). Adherence to treatment in children and adolescent patients with cystic fibrosis. *Journal of Adolescent Health, 38*(1), 13–17.

51.

THE PSYCHIATRIC CARE OF MEDICAL PATIENTS WITH AUTISM

Robert L. Doyle

At present, an estimated 1% of the general population suffers with some form of pervasive developmental disorder (Pasco, 2010). The spectrum of autistic people ranges from severely impaired individuals who appear aloof and apart from the world around them to those who are considered high-functioning and able to compensate for their social impairments by their substantial strength in other areas of life. At one end of this spectrum, the diagnosis is difficult to miss; but the higher functioning individuals may not be as easy to recognize, and their peculiar and concrete ways of dealing with the world can complicate medical care.

The disorders of the autism spectrum include pervasive difficulties in the domains of social interaction and communication, and stereotyped or restrictive repetitive behaviors, interests, and activities. The spectrum also includes what had been called Asperger's syndrome (AS), a condition with normal communication development but difficulties of social interaction and repetitive behaviors. Pervasive disorder not otherwise specified (PDD NOS) refers to patients with impairments in the three domains, but not sufficient to called autism and not meeting criteria for an alternative psychiatric diagnosis. Also in the spectrum is an uncommon condition that had been called "child disintegrative disorder" (CDD), characterized by loss in two autistic domains after two years of normal development. These children also had significant deficits in motor skills, bowel or bladder control, adaptive skills, or play before the age of ten years old. The autistic spectrum is more common in males.

Those who do not have stereotyped behaviors but have deficits in social communication are now diagnosed separately with "social communication disorder."

Rett's disorder, which was also grouped with autistic disorders, is characterized by social deficits and expressive and receptive language impairments that occurred after five months of normal development. Physical exam findings then included deceleration of head growth up to the age of four years, loss of purposeful hand movements until two and a half years old, along with gait or trunk coordination problems. It is distinct because it occurs almost exclusively in females.

Some cases of Rett's syndrome have been attributed to a mutation in the *MeCP2* gene, so these cases may eventually be categorized as a genetic disorder with autistic features, as has been the case with fragile X syndrome (Amir et al.,

1999). Since Rett's and childhood disintegrative disorders are "rare" to "very rare," the treatment studies have been scant and probably cannot be generalized. Therefore, clinicians often extrapolate information from larger studies on autism, which sometimes include individuals with Rett's disorder or childhood integrative disorder, but such extrapolations pose obvious shortcomings (APA, 2000). Due to the dearth of well-designed treatment studies on the rare conditions of Rett's disorder and childhood disintegrative disorder, this chapter will focus on treatments of the more commonly encountered diagnoses on the autism spectrum.

Psychiatrists, neurologists, and developmental pediatricians who specialize in treating children and adolescents routinely probe for symptoms all along the spectrum of autism. General psychiatrists and other physicians who exclusively treat adult patients encounter more difficulty with the nuanced presentations of autism in the higher functioning range, such as the individuals with Asperger's disorder or PDD NOS. Sometimes these very individuals slip through their childhood and adolescence without being formally diagnosed as belonging somewhere along the autism spectrum. Although the study of autism remains in its infancy, new information about the underpinnings of autism exponentially expands our understanding of this condition in each passing year. Nonetheless, no medication yet exists that can treat the core symptoms of the disorder.

Despite a lack of any behavioral or pharmacological treatment that shows robust improvements in the core symptoms, peripheral problems associated with autism can be improved with some existing interventions. Peripheral problems include common, co-occurring symptoms, such as self-injurious behaviors, poor concentration, insomnia, sensory integration issues, and even comorbid psychiatric conditions. Psychiatric disorders may be more difficult to recognize, due to communication problems that impair accurate descriptions of internal states in persons with autism. In addition, these psychiatric conditions may not respond as well to accepted treatments in the context of autism spectrum disorders, yet the same holds true whenever comorbid psychiatric conditions exist in the same person. Treating comorbid psychiatric conditions can be challenging and the outcomes suboptimal, but some improvement in the psychiatric symptoms can result in significant improvement in functioning.

At the very least, awareness of these problems will help develop more holistic treatment plans that will support patient adherence to the clinician's recommendations for care. For example, sensory integration issues related to tastes or textures could pose major challenges for persons on the autistic spectrum who are prescribed oral medications. The astute clinician treating autistic patients will have a close relationship with a compounding pharmacist, who can convert certain medications from pill form to solutions or suppository. The author recently evaluated two adolescent sisters with autism who have never been able to take oral medication due to sensory issues. Injections are not an option with their extreme needle phobia, but their aggressive behaviors have been successfully managed using specially compounded suppositories of risperidone.

This chapter will offer some advice on caring for patients with autism in the medical setting, but it cannot cover all scenarios that a clinician will encounter. Therefore, the reader is encouraged to consider creative ways to deal with the unique difficulties of autism while remembering that a simple and commonsense approach often gives the best outcome.

A cure for autism remains on the distant horizon; however, a number of interventions exist today that address coexisting problems as well as possible comorbid psychiatric disorders. Although treating "around the edges" may not improve core symptoms of autism per se, this approach can certainly improve the quality of life for persons with autism and the families who care for them. This chapter aims to address several common problems associated with autism spectrum disorder (ASD) that impair the delivery of optimal care in the medical setting.

AGGRESSION AND SELF-MUTILATION

First, aggression and self-mutilation occur frequently in persons with autism, and the *Diagnostic and Statistical Manual of Mental Disorders IV* (DSM-IV-TR) (APA, 2000) conceptualized these behaviors as core stereotypical symptoms. Nonetheless, such behaviors often increase during periods of medical illness, thereby serving as a sentinel of an underlying disease process. An exacerbation in self-injurious or aggressive behaviors without any recent change in the environment should warrant a medical work-up. The aggression and self-mutilation may be driven by the patient's need for medical attention, since he or she may not be able to communicate pain or distress verbally. As with delirium, the definitive treatment lies in treating the underlying medical condition as soon as possible.

ASSESSMENT OF COMORBID PSYCHIATRIC CONDITIONS

Second, assessing and treating comorbid conditions will be discussed. Failure to treat comorbid psychiatric conditions often sabotages medical treatments because far too often they go undiagnosed. Part of the problem lies in the tendency to attribute many difficult behaviors or other psychiatric symptoms to the pervasive developmental disorder

(PDD). Perhaps the term *pervasive developmental disorder* tricks one into thinking that every symptom or problem must be attributed to the pervasive nature of autism. Of course, teasing out the symptoms of other comorbid psychiatric disorders from a morass of autistic symptoms is more tedious than diagnosing these conditions in normally developing individuals, but the approach pays off with a better quality of life once the psychiatric condition is in remission. Consider the burden of untreated depression in persons with diabetes. That burden of illness becomes magnified if the person has autism in addition to the depression and diabetes, because the depression often goes unrecognized.

INSOMNIA

Insomnia is a third area that can complicate medical treatment. Sleep problems can be part of a comorbid psychiatric disorder, but most of the time insomnia occurs in the absence of comorbid psychopathology. Poor sleep leads to low energy, poor concentration, and, sometimes, increased irritability, so correcting sleep problems can be crucial to providing optimal medical care.

SENSORY INTEGRATION ISSUES

Children with autism sometimes have symptoms that are thought to be related to disruptions in how the children process and integrate information from other senses. Sensory integration theory suggests that inappropriate or deficient sensory processing is a developmental disorder or part of a developmental disorder amenable to treatment, and often referred to occupational therapists. A standard profile reporting children's sensory experiences illustrate how these symptoms present in children. Both social and non-social dimensions are noted. On the hyposensory-social dimension, children do not respond to their name, ignore new persons, or seek rough-housing play. On the hyposensory-non-social dimension, children stare at lights or objects; flap their arms, do not pay attention to novel objects, mouth objects, ignore loud noises, smell objects, do not respond to pain, and crave movement. The hypersensory-social dimension is captured in children who dislike being held, are distressed during grooming, are averse to social touch, avoid eye contact, and dislike tickling. The hypersensory-non-social children are sensitive to loud noises, avoid textures, are sensitive to light, averse to water, and avoid food with a strong taste/texture (Baranek, 2006). In order to deliver medical care to patients with milder forms of sensory idiosyncrasies, these traits can be taken into consideration. Patients may have distinct responses to restraints, to touching, to specific types of foods. Understanding this aspect of their makeup can facilitate care.

Occupational therapists have developed treatments for these symptoms. They use brushes, swings, balls, and other equipment with the hope of organizing sensory inputs and clarifying their role in developmental disorder and adaptation. The American Academy of Pediatrics (AAP) has written a policy statement to clarify the role of these treatments (AAP, 2012).

Before beginning, the clinician must be aware that persons with autism frequently exhibit finicky eating patterns. Sometimes these relate to sensory integration issues, as in the case of the sisters already mentioned. At other times, restricted or repetitive behaviors at the core of autism could result in a peculiar dietary regimen. For instance, a person on the autism spectrum may be stuck on foods of a certain color and end up eating a "beige" diet. Such restricted diets can lead to nutritional deficiencies, which could cause medical problems or slow recovery from a medical condition.

DIFFICULTY EXPRESSING INNER STATES

Since autism runs the range from nonverbal to the precocious verbal skills that some persons with Asperger's disorder exhibit, a clinician may struggle to obtain information from most patients. Even those with impressive vocabularies might have great difficulty expressing their feelings or internal states. Any technique or technology that facilitates communication will make history-taking easier. This is not to be confused with "facilitated communication," a therapy that once seemed to be a breakthrough in autism. "Facilitated communication" trained therapists to help guide the patient's hand over a keyboard so that thoughts that could not be expressed verbally could be typed. The rationale was that the therapist could help the patients compensate for their fine motor deficits, but "facilitated communication" eventually fell from favor after scientific scrutiny showed significant flaws in its effectiveness. Nevertheless, numerous electronic devices have been invented to help nonverbal or nearly nonverbal persons with autism express themselves. As technology advances, these devices are becoming less expensive, more reliable, more compact, and easier to operate. At first, these devices were designed specifically for persons with communication problems and were limited to this application. Now, software programs can be downloaded into electronic pads and even pocket-sized smartphones with touchpad technologies. These can help in gathering more accurate histories and augment incomplete information provided by caregivers.

CONCRETE THINKING PATTERNS

Even persons on the autism spectrum without speech delays might still struggle with communication issues, given their concrete thinking patterns. Clinicians should remain aware that their patients with higher functioning autism are likely to interpret conversations in literal terms. The author recalls an interview in medical school in which the silver-haired and seasoned psychiatrist asked a patient if he heard voices. The patient responded, "Of course I do, how else could I be answering all your questions?" Although concrete and literal ways of thinking make for amusing moments, this sort of thinking may result in unintentional miscommunication of relevant clinical information. Therefore, carefully framing questions and accepting that responses may come from a person with a different frame of mind makes for more effective communication with the patient.

PROBLEMS IN THE LITERATURE

Even though research into ASDs has made many recent gains, most of the literature on treatment interventions suffers from a number of shortcomings. For instance, many studies include heterogeneous groups of patients on the autism spectrum, and the heterogeneity waters down results, thereby obscuring conclusive evidence that a homogeneous selection of patients would offer. Other studies are too poorly powered to make any clear assumptions about effectiveness, so the literature limps along, only hinting at the benefits of one treatment over another. Another common problem, which is magnified in poorly designed studies, is the high rate of placebo response in the autistic population. Several factors, such as reliance on caregiver's reports and using inadequate rating scales that cannot accurately capture changes in autism symptoms over the short course of a clinical trial contributes to the placebo response problem. Some studies attempt to assess the treatment outcomes of comorbid conditions, such as depression or anxiety, but the standard rating scales that work well for the general population with depression or anxiety have not been validated in the autistic population. Moreover, most of the research into autism focuses on younger populations. Many other deficiencies exist; however, a few studies have met the gold standard seen in other areas of psychiatric research. These studies have provided the first two FDA-approved treatments for people with autism, even though these treatments do not treat the core symptoms of autism.

MEDICATIONS

IRRITABILITY, AGGRESSION, SELF-INJURIOUS BEHAVIORS

Two atypical antipsychotic agents, risperidone and aripiprazole, are approved for the treatment of "irritability," defined as tantrums, aggressive behaviors, and self-mutilation in children with autism. These medications have improved the quality of life for these children and their families, but the core symptoms of autism, for the most part, remain unchanged. Although risperidone and aripiprazole do not improve the social and communication problems common to autism, one might argue that a reduction in certain forms of aggression or self-mutilation represents an improvement in stereotypical behaviors. Nevertheless, the medications target irritability, and some aspects of irritability are rhythmic and repetitive in the realm of stereotypies, or occur if such stereotypical behaviors are blocked (Aman et al., 2009; Marcus et al., 2009; Owen et al., 2009; Stigler et al., 2009). Take, for example, head banging, which fits criteria for stereotypy and improves with atypical neuroleptic treatment.

ATYPICAL NEUROLEPTICS
Risperidone

Risperidone was the first medication approved specifically for patients with autism. Information from several case series and double-blind, placebo-controlled studies indicated that risperidone was effective in reducing irritability in children and adolescents with autism and related disorders (Posey & McDougle, 2008). The Research Units of Pediatric Psychopharmacology (RUPP) Autism Network showed foresight in conducting the first double-blind, placebo-controlled trial of risperidone in children and adolescents with autism. The eight-week study followed 101 youths (mean age, 8.8 years) who were randomly assigned to either risperidone or placebo. Subjects had "significant irritability," defined by a score of 18 or greater on the Aberrant Behavior Checklist (ABC) Irritability subscale. A mean dosage of 1.8 mg per day provided a 57% reduction on the ABC Irritability subscale score, compared with a 14% in the placebo group (RUPP Autism Network, 2005a; Aman et al., 1985). With "response" defined as greater than 25% improvement on the ABC Irritability subscale score and a rating of "much improved" or "very much improved" on the Clinical Global Impressions–Improvement (CGI-I) scale, 69% on risperidone and 12% on the placebo were responders. An effect size of d = 1.2 in favor of risperidone on the main outcome measure was documented by the Research Units in Pediatric and Psychopharmacology (RUPP) Autism Network (Arnold et al., 2010). Even though improvements were seen on the Social Withdrawal and Inappropriate Speech subscales, these were not statistically significant. Risperidone was associated with a mean weight gain of 5.8 lbs., while the placebo group experienced a mean weight gain of 1.8 lbs. Drooling occurred more frequently with risperidone, yet extrapyramidal symptoms (EPS) and tardive dyskinesia (TD) showed no significant differences between the risperidone- and placebo-treated groups (RUPP Autism Network, 2005a).

An analysis of secondary outcome measures showed significant improvements in sensorimotor behaviors, affective reactions, and sensory responses on the modified Ritvo-Freeman Real Life Rating Scale (R-F RLRS), but no significant change appeared on the Social Relationship to People or Language subscales (McDougle et al., 2005; Freeman et al., 1986). The analysis of the Children's Yale-Brown Obsessive Compulsive Scale (CY-BOCS) found risperidone to be more efficacious than placebo for reducing interfering repetitive behaviors (Scahill et al., 1997).

After the acute eight-week phase of the study, 63 responders entered the extended 16-week, open-label phase of the study (RUPP Austism Network, 2005a). Over the course of 16 weeks, two subjects discontinued taking the drug due to loss of effectiveness, and one due to an adverse event. The remainder of the subjects showed no clinically significant worsening of target symptoms while the mean dosage remained stable. Weight gain averaged 11.2 lbs. during the six months of risperidone treatment. Following the 16-week open-label phase, the 32 subjects who continued to be responders were randomized to either continued risperidone treatment or gradually switch to placebo over the course of three weeks. Of the 16 subjects switched to placebo, 62.5% showed significant worsening of symptoms, while only 12.5% of those continuing on risperidone worsened. Therefore, these results, along with those of another placebo-controlled discontinuation study, suggest that risperidone treatment beyond six months is probably necessary to prevent relapse (RUPP Autism Network, 2005a).

Recently, intention-to-treat (ITT) analyses were performed with suspected moderators and mediators entered into the regression equations (Arnold et al., 2010). The benefit–risk ratio of risperidone appeared better with greater symptom severity prior to treatment. Weight gain was not required for risperidone response, and it might even detract from it. Also, socioeconomic advantage, low prolactin, and absence of comorbid problems non-specifically gave better outcome (Arnold et al., 2010).

In addition to the RUPP study, a second multicenter, placebo-controlled study of risperidone in children and adolescents with PDDs completed the database needed to demonstrate requisite efficacy and tolerability to secure FDA approval (Posey & McDougle, 2008; Shea et al., 2004). This second study included 79 youths (mean age, 7.5 years) randomly assigned to risperidone (mean dose, 1.2 mg/d) or placebo (Shea et al., 2004). All subjects met criteria for PDD and scored greater than 30 on the Childhood Autism Rating Scale (CARS) (Shea et al., 2004; Shopler et al., 1980). The mean baseline score on the ABC Irritability subscale was 20. Risperidone-treated subjects experienced a 64% reduction in the ABC Irritability subscale score, while scores for subjects on placebo only decreased by 31%. Moreover, 53% of subjects on risperidone versus 18% on placebo showed an adequate response to the assigned treatment. Subjects given risperidone gained more weight than those given placebo (5.9 lbs. versus 2.2 lbs.), but extrapyramidal symptoms did not differ between groups over the eight-week study period (Shea et al., 2004).

In smaller study of 30 youths (ages, 8–18 years) treated with risperidone (0.01 mg/kg/d) versus haloperidol (0.01 mg/kg/d) under double-blinded conditions, the risperidone group showed significantly greater reductions in the total ABC scores, along with greater improvements in general behavior compared to a haloperidol group (Posey & McDougle, 2008; Miral et al., 2008). Subjects on risperidone experienced significant increases in prolactin levels (Posey& McDougle, 2008; Miral et al., 2008).

Although controlled studies of risperidone in adults with ASDs are needed, a placebo-controlled study of risperidone did focus on children down to the very young age of two years old (Nagaraj, Singhi, & Malhi, 2006). Children aged two to nine years received risperidone (1 mg/day) or placebo. Scores on the CARS and Children's Global Assessment Scale showed risperidone to be highly efficacious (Posey & McDougle, 2008; Nagaraj, Singhi, & Malhi, 2006). On the other hand, a six-month, placebo-controlled study of 24 children with PDDs under six years old showed the risperidone dose range of 0.5–1.5 mg/day to be only minimally efficacious compared to placebo (Posey & McDougle, 2008; Luby et al., 2006). The low level of baseline irritability may have dampened the effect seen in other studies in which baseline irritability started substantially higher (Posey, 2008).

Emerging research involving 45 autistic patients treated for up to a year with risperidone monotherapy suggests that polymorphisms on certain candidate genes may help predict clinical improvement with risperidone (Corriea et al., 2010). Corriea and colleagues also found that polymorphisms on particular genes were associated with risperidone-induced increases in prolactin levels and body mass index (BMI) (Corriea et al., 2010). These associations will require replication, but this early work may eventually lead to routine clinical tests that identify the drug that will work best with the fewest risks of adverse events for a given individual with autism.

Aripiprazole

The second medication approved for aggression and irritability in children with PDDs was aripiprazole. To evaluate the short-term efficacy and safety of aripiprazole in the treatment of irritability associated with autism, 218 children and adolescents (aged 6–17 years) were randomized 1:1:1:1 to aripiprazole (5, 10, 15 mg/day) or placebo in a double-blind, randomized, placebo-controlled, parallel group, eight-week study (Marcus et al., 2009). The efficacy was assessed with the (ABC) Irritability subscale (primary efficacy measure) and the clinician-rated Clinical Global Impression–Improvement score. All aripiprazole doses showed significantly better ABC Irritability subscale scores (5 mg/day, –12.4; 10 mg/day, –13.2; 15 mg/day, –14.4; versus placebo, –8.4; all, p < 0.05). Additionally, all aripiprazole doses delivered significantly greater improvements in the mean Clinical Global Impression–Improvement scores than the placebo group at week 8. Sedation was the most common cause for discontinuation. Mean weight gain was approximately 1 kg greater in each aripiprazole group (5 mg/day, 1.3 kg; 10 mg/day, 1.3kg; 15 mg/day, 1.5 kg) compared to placebo (0.3 kg). Two serious adverse events—presyncope (5 mg/day) and aggression (10 mg/day)—occurred during the treatment phase. Overall, aripiprazole showed efficacy and was generally well tolerated (Marcus et al., 2009).

An eight-week double-blind, placebo-controlled trial of aripiprazole in 98 youths (aged 6–17 years) showed significantly greater improvement on the ABC Irritability subscale with aripiprazole treatment in a flexible dose range of either 5, 10, or 15 mg/day (Owen et al., 2009).

In a 14-week prospective open-label trial in patients with PDD NOS or Asperger's disorder, Stigler and colleagues noted significant improvement in 22 of 25 (88%) subjects with a dose range of 2.5 to 15 mg in 5–17-year-olds (Stigler et al., 2009). The ABC Irritability subscale dropped from a mean score of 29 at study start to 8.1 at study endpoint (Stigler et al., 2009). Weight gain was the most common adverse event (19/25 subjects, mean +2.3 lbs.) followed by tiredness (16/25 subjects, mild; 1/25 subjects, moderate) and extrapyramidal side effects (EPS) (9/25 subjects, mild) (Stigler et al., 2009).

The RUPP Autism Network implemented an elegantly designed multiple-site study with 124 children aged 4 to 13 who were diagnosed with PDDs accompanied by frequent tantrums, aggression, or self-injury (Aman et al., 2009). Subjects were randomly assigned to either risperidone monotherapy ranging from 0.5 to 3.5 mg/day (MED) or risperidone along with an average of 10.9 sessions of parent training (COMB). A positive clinical response was defined as a rating of "much or very much improved" on the Clinical Global Impression–Improvement subscale plus at least 25% reduction on the ABC Irritability subscale. If clinical response was not reached by week 8, the risperidone was phased out and replaced with aripiprazole. The study sample was composed of 105 (85%) boys and 19 (15%) girls, with groups similar in terms of household income, parental education, and educational placement; however, the MED group had lower functional skills and was more likely to be treated with anticonvulsants. The COMB group's Home Situations Questionnaire Severity score decreased 71% compared to the MED groups score, resulting in an effect size of 0.34 by week 24. The effect-size differences between the MED and COMB groups were small up to week 16, but by week 24, the effect-size differences were in the medium range and favored the COMB group for the ABC Irritability and Hyperactivity/Noncompliance subscales (Aman et al., 2009a).

Olanzapine

Evidence for olanzapine's effectiveness is limited to one small placebo-controlled study and three open-label trials (Posey, 2008). The small, eight-week, placebo-controlled study enrolled 11 subjects (aged 6–14) randomly assigned to olanzapine (mean dose, 10 mg/day) or placebo (Hollander et al., 2006). While three of six (50%) subjects on olanzapine responded, one of 5 (20%) on placebo met response criteria. The olanzapine group gained substantially more weight (mean weight gain, 7.5 lbs., versus 1.5 lbs. on placebo) (Hollander et al., 2006).

A 12-week open-label study of olanzapine (mean dose, 7.8 mg/day) in eight individuals (mean age, 20.9 years; age range, 5–42 years) reported significant improvement irritability in six of the seven (86%) subjects completing the study (Potenza et al., 1999). Weight gain was significant in six subjects (mean weight gain, 18.4 lbs.), while three subjects experienced sedation (Potenza et al., 1999). Another six-week open-label study used a parallel group design to compare olanzapine (mean dose, 7.9 mg/day) versus haloperidol (mean dose, 1.4 mg/day) in 12 children with autism (mean age, 7.8 years) (Malone et al., 2001). Five of six (83%) subjects on olanzapine responded to treatment, whereas three of six (50%) improved on haloperidol. The olanzapine-treated subjects gained more weight (mean, 9 lbs.; range 5.9 to 15.8 lbs.) compared to those on haloperidol (mean 3.2 lbs.; range, –5.5 to +8.8 lbs.) (Malone et al., 2001).

On the other hand, a three-month open-label study of olanzapine (mean dose, 10.7 mg/day) in 25 children (mean age, 11.2 years) with PDD found it to be effective in only three (12%) subjects. As was the case in preschool-aged children treated with risperidone, low baseline scores on the ABC Irritability subscale may have contributed to the limited improvement in this study (Posey, 2008).

Quetiapine

Only two prospective and two retrospective studies have examined the benefits of quetiapine in persons with PDD (Posey & McDougle, 2008). In a 16-week open-label study (mean dose, 225mg/day), two of six (33%) of the youths (ages, 6–15 years) responded to treatment (Martin et al., 1999).

Of the nine subjects originally enrolled, two discontinued due to sedation or lack of response, and one due to a possible seizure (Martin et al., 1999). Weight gain ranged from 2 to 18 lbs. The other prospective study enrolled nine adolescents (age range, 12–17 years) for a 12-week trial on quetiapine (mean dose, 292 mg/day). Again, only six of nine subjects completed the study, with a mere two (22%) subjects considered responders (Findling et al., 2004). One of the subjects discontinued due to agitation and aggression, and weight gain and sedation were the most common adverse events in other subjects (Findling et al., 2004).

In the first published retrospective study, 20 subjects (mean age, 12.1 years; range 5–28 years) received monotherapy with quetiapine (mean dose, 249 mg/day; range, 25–600 mg/day) for at least four weeks (mean duration, 59.8 weeks; range, 4–180 weeks) (Corson et al., 2004). Although eight (40%) subjects responded, 15% of the subjects discontinued, while 50% reported adverse events (Corson et al., 2004). The other retrospective review included ten subjects (ages, 5–19 years) who were diagnosed with PDD and mental retardation (MR) (Hardan, Jou, & Handen, 2005). The mean dose of quetiapine was 477 mg/day, and concomitant medications were allowed as long as the dosages did not change during the period of observation on quetiapine. A response rate of 60% resulted from the intervention, with mild sedation, excessive salivation, and weight gain reported as adverse events (Hardan, Jou, & Handen, 2005).

Ziprasidone

Evidence for ziprasidone in treating irritability associated with PDD is limited to three published papers (Posey & McDougle, 2008). One six-week, prospective, open-label study of ziprasidone enrolled 12 adolescents (mean age, 14.5 years; range 12–18 years) with autism who were treated with ziprasidone (mean dose, 98.3 mg/day; range 20–160 mg/day) (Malone et al., 2007). At the study endpoint, 9 of the 12 subjects responded to treatment with reduction in irritability, aggression, and hyperactivity. Acute dystonic reaction occurred in two subjects, but ziprasidone treatment appeared to be weight-neutral. Electrocardiography recorded a mean prolongation in QTc of 14.7 milliseconds which should be considered in the context of the FDA warning about using ziprasidone with other drugs that may prolong QTc in individuals with known cardiac arrhythmias or a long QT syndrome. Total cholesterol decreased without any change in prolactin levels (Posey & McDougle, 2008; Malone et al., 2007).

The first retrospective review reported on 12 subjects (mean age, 11.6 years; range 8–20 years) receiving open-label treatment with ziprasidone (mean dose, 59.2 mg; range, 20–120 mg/day) for at least six weeks (mean duration, 14.2; range, 6–30 weeks) (McDougle, Kem, & Posey, 2002). Aggression, agitation, and irritability improved in six (50%) of the 12 subjects. Transient sedation was the most common adverse event, and no untoward cardiac effects were reported or observed. Although a mean weight loss of 5.8 lbs. (range, –35 to +6 lbs.) was documented, this probably occurred as a result of subjects'

being switched from other medications known to cause significant weight gain (McDougle, Kem, & Posey, 2002). The second retrospective study involved ten adults with autism and mental retardation who switched from clozapine, risperidone, or quetiapine to ziprasidone (Cohen et al., 2004). Weight gain most often prompted the switch, and ziprasidone resulted in a significant mean weight loss of 9.5 lbs. after six months of treatment. Maladaptive behaviors improved in six subjects, while three subjects experienced worsening, and one remained unchanged with respect to the maladaptive behaviors (Cohen et al., 2004).

Paliperidone

Paliperidone, approved by the FDA for schizophrenia in adults, is the major active metabolite of risperidone and the only atypical antipsychotic agent to use the Osmotic [Controlled] Release Oral System (OROS™) technology (Stigler et al., 2010). Unlike risperidone, cytochrome P450 2D6 (CYP2D6) has a limited role in the elimination of paliperidone, and most of the drug is excreted mainly unchanged in the urine. Recently, case reports of a 16-year-old Caucasian female and a 20-year-old Caucasian male with DSM-IV-TR–defined autism suggested that paliperidone may be an effective and well-tolerated treatment for severe irritability in adolescent and adult patients with autism (Stigler et al., 2010).

Clozapine

At the end of the list of atypical antipsychotic agents is clozapine. It rounds off the list as one the last medications to try, due to factors that make it an end-of-the-line treatment for schizophrenia. The main reason it is reserved as a last-ditch treatment is the risk of agranulocytosis. Many patients with autistic spectrum disorder struggle with venipuncture in conjunction with their yearly physical, so biweekly blood work would be out of the question. Since the prevalence of seizures ranges between 20% and 35% in adults and 17% and 14% in children and adolescents with ASD (Minshew, Sweeney, & Bauman, 1997; Rapin, 1996), clozapine would not be a first-line choice given its propensity to lower the seizure threshold (Posey & McDougle, 2008). Moreover, the literature only documents three reports of the use of clozapine in individuals with ASD. Three children ages 8 to 12 received treatment with clozapine 200-450 mg/day after they failed haloperidol treatment for eight months. Zudda and colleagues reported that decrease in aggression, hyperactivity, and negativism was sustained in two of the children, while the third child relapsed after five months (Zudda et al., 1996). These three children experienced transient sedation and enuresis (Zudda et al., 1996). Chen and colleagues treated a 17-year-old male inpatient with clozapine 275 mg/day and showed significant reduction in "overt tension," hyperactivity, and stereotypies; however, the period of observation was only 15 days (Chen et al., 2001). A case report on a 32-year-old male patient with autism and profound mental retardation treated with clozapine 300 mg/day showed marked improvement in treatment-refractory aggression and social interactions over two months, with further improvements over five years of treatment (Gobbi & Pulvirenti, 2001). This individual did not develop extrapyramidal syndrome (EPS) or agranulocytosis over the five years of treatment, but literature on clozapine's use in autistic spectrum disorder is scant and the risk of agranulocytosis serious, albeit uncommon, so it should remain delegated to a last-resort treatment until more substantial data are available.

On the other hand, EPS is much more common with typical antipsychotic agents, but they have been a mainstay of managing certain psychiatric conditions in the medical setting. The typical antipsychotic agents have a track record for rapid and reliable treatment stretching back decades. The typical antipsychotic agents often served as first-line treatments for aggression and agitation associated with delirium, psychotic disorders, and mania in the medical setting, given that they were less expensive than their non-generic atypical counterparts. In recent years, generic versions of atypical neuroleptics narrowed the price gap between the typical and atypical antipsychotic agents, so hospital formularies usually offer easy access to first-generation atypical agents, from aripiprazole to ziprasidone. Nonetheless, the typical antipsychotic agents still maintain an edge in the medical setting, because they can be rapidly titrated, and, in certain situations, intramuscular formulations can be used to expedite an effective dosage and thereby reduce patients' length of stay.

TYPICAL NEUROLEPTICS

Haloperidol

In hindsight, many of the earliest studies using typical antipsychotic agents to treat self injurious behaviors (SIB) and aggression in individuals with autism contained flaws in methodology or diagnostic accuracy. The first well-designed research studies in this vein came from Campbell and colleagues, who systematically evaluated haloperidol in children with autism (Campbell et al., 1978). They first studied children with autism aged 2.6 to 7.2 years treated with haloperidol (mean dosage 1.7 mg/day) versus placebo in combination with one of two language-based training groups. Although sedation occurred in 12 and dystonia in 2 of the 20 subjects on haloperidol, significant improvement was noted in symptoms of withdrawal and stereotypy in the youths aged 4.5 years and older who were randomized to medication treatment (Campbell et al., 1978). Other studies showed that haloperidol targeted a range of maladaptive behaviors in youths, but acute dystonic reactions and dyskinesias consistently appeared in this treatment population (Posey & McDougle, 2008). Two larger studies focused on the association between haloperidol treatment and the frequency of dyskinesias. One study enrolled 60 children aged 2.3 to 7.9 years and randomly assigned them to either continuous or discontinuous (5 days on and 2 days off) treatment with haloperidol for six months, followed by one month on placebo. The other treated 118 children aged 2.3 to 8.2 years with haloperidol for six months, followed by one month on placebo. In both studies, withdrawal dyskinesias occurred more frequently and tended to be reversible; however, nine of ten subjects treated with the higher mean dosage of haloperidol 3.4 mg/

day developed dyskinesia in the latter study (Posey, 2008). In general, children and adolescents experience more movement disorders with the high-potency typical antipsychotic agents than do adult patients. Unfortunately, the high-potency typical neuroleptics such as haloperidol have not been studied systematically in adults with autism. Poor tolerability in terms of dyskinesias limits the use of high-potency and sedation the use of low-potency antipsychotic agents in children; however, the high-potency typical neuroleptics may have a role in the treatment of adults with autism, given that they have a long and successful history of treating agitation and aggression secondary to other conditions in adults.

ALPHA-2 ADRENERGIC AGONISTS

Guanfacine and Clonidine

Since irritability, agitation, and self-injurious behaviors cause such problems for persons with autism or those who care for them, a number of other medications have been studied. These medications may have offered a better side effect profile, but they proved to be less effective than the two FDA-approved atypical neuroleptics. Moreover, shortcomings in the design of these published reports limit one's ability to generalize the results. The largest of these studies retrospectively analyzed guanfacine (mean dosage 2.6 mg/day) treatment in 80 subjects aged 3 to 18 years (mean age 7.7 years) with PDD (Posey et al., 2004). Subjects diagnosed with Asperger's disorder or PDD NOS showed a greater response than those with autism; however, guanfacine was only effective in 10 of 69 (14%) subjects with significant aggression (Posey et al., 2004). In a six-week, double-blind, placebo-controlled crossover trial of clonidine (dosage range 0.04–0.10 mg/kg/day) in eight youths aged 5 to 13 (mean age, 8.1 years) with autism, significant improvements were noted on the Autism Behavior Checklist by teacher and parent ratings, but not by the clinician (Posey, 2008). A similarly designed four-week study with transdermal clonidine (dosage range 0.16 to 0.48 mg/day) in nine individuals aged 5 to 33 (mean age, 12.9 years) appeared beneficial for impulsivity, hyperarousal, and self-stimulation (Posey& McDougle, 2008). Sedation was the most common side effect in all the above studies with alpha-2 adrenergic agonists (Posey, 2008). Presently, long-acting formulations of guanfacine and clonidine have been approved for the treatment of attention-deficit hyperactivity disorder (ADHD) in children, and these may offer a better pharmacokinetic profile for individuals with autism. Nevertheless, these long-acting alpha-2 adrenergic agonists have not been systematically studied in the autistic population. Again, except for the few adult patients in the transdermal clonidine study above, the literature remains limited to the children and adolescents with autism.

ANTICONVULSANTS AND MOOD STABILIZERS

Divalproex

Given that mood stabilizers and certain anticonvulsants show efficacy in controlling agitation in manic states, these were a logical choice for possibly controlling agitated, aggressive states in persons with autism. The most well-designed study of this group was an eight-week double-blind, placebo-controlled study of divalproex sodium in 30 subjects aged 6 to 20 years with PDD and significant aggression. Despite a mean serum trough level of 77.8 ug/mL, no significant difference between treatment and placebo groups was noted on the ABC Irritability subscale (Hellings et al., 2005). A smaller, open-label study of divalproex sodium (mean dosage, 768 mg/day) resulted in CGI-I ratings of "much improved" or "very much improved" in 10 of 14 subjects. Improvement was noted in impulsivity, aggression, and affective instability (Posey, 2008).

Lamotrigine

Although 8 of 13 (62%) youths initially prescribed lamotrigine for intractable epilepsy experienced a reduction in interfering behavioral symptoms, a double-blind, placebo-controlled trial in 14 youths aged 3 to 11 with autism demonstrated no differences between lamotrigine (5 mg/kg/d) and placebo groups on the Autism Behavior Checklist over the four weeks of treatment (Posey, 2008). In a small, naturalistic study of five patients aged 9 to 13 treated from 10 to 33 weeks (mean duration, 22 weeks) two of five responded with CGI-I ratings of "much improved" or "very much improved" for irritability, anger, and hyperactivity. Of note, two study patients received add-on sertraline at six months for obsessive behaviors, while another one was on long-term treatment with risperidone (Mazzone et al., 2006).

Levetiracetam

Rugino and colleagues investigated levetiracetam for the treatment of aggression, hyperactivity, mood lability, and impulsivity in ten children aged 4 to 10 with autism (Rugino & Samsock, 2002). Over the course of four weeks of treatment, only the subjects who were not recently weaned from drugs targeting aggression showed significant improvement in aggression. Nevertheless, a ten-week, double-blind, placebo-controlled study of levetiracetam (mean dosage, 862.5 mg/day) in 20 youths (age range, 5–17 years) with autism found no significant difference in parent and teacher ratings on the Autism Behavior Checklist between the levetiracetam and placebo group (Wasserman et al., 2006).

With estimates of seizure disorders of up to 35% of adults and 14% of children with autism, the appropriate anticonvulsant can be life-saving and offer improvement in functioning, but as a treatment solely targeting aggression and self-injurious behaviors without a comorbid seizures, these medications have shown inconsistent results (Bauman, 2010). At any rate, new-onset disruptive behaviors should make one consider the possibility that a seizure disorder might be emerging, particularly if caregivers cannot identify any changes in the environment or clinicians do not observe any other common medical issues that might provoke the change in behavior. Sensory issues may pose challenges to obtaining electroencephalography (EEG) in some individuals with autism, but the results can be a useful guide to the type of medication that should be employed, if EEG abnormalities appear. Be aware that the partial complex seizures occur most frequently in individuals with ASD, and atypical behaviors and body movements associated with this type of seizure may be attributed to ASD. Temporal lobe seizures sometimes escape detection on regular EEG recordings, so clinical judgement should guide whether the patient could tolerate continuous monitoring with videography or the use of nasopharyngeal leads to confirm seizure activity.

Nonetheless, not all odd movements and mannerisms arise from abnormal EEG activity or stereotypical ASD symptoms. Other medical conditions, ranging from asthma to gastric reflux to acute sinusitis, could manifest in abnormal behaviors, particularly if the person with ASD struggles with expressing pain and distress (Buie, 2005).

Lithium

Lastly, one case report of lithium (900 mg/day) augmenting fluvoxamine therapy in an autistic patient without comorbid mania or bipolar disorder resulted in a marked decrease in aggression and impulsivity after two weeks of treatment (Epperson et al., 1994).

COMORBIDITY

Often, autistic symptoms predominate in the clinical picture, which causes clinicians and caregivers to overlook comorbid psychiatric and medical conditions and mistakenly attribute these to autism. A condition that could be addressed in conventional ways goes unrecognized and untreated. In the case of psychiatric disorders, a strong family history of mood, anxiety, or psychotic disorders should make clinicians vigilant to the emergence of such disorders in their patient with ASD.

For persons of normal intelligence with ASDs, estimates of coexisting psychiatric conditions vary considerably, from 9% to 89% (Hofvander et al., 2009). Hofvander and colleagues examined a sample of normal-intelligence individuals with ASD (n = 122) and noted that 80% of the of adult subjects met criteria for at least one other major Axis-I disorder, whereas all subjects in the Asperger's syndrome and PDD NOS subgroups carried at least one other comorbid Axis-I diagnosis (Hofvander et al., 2009). Several studies cite mood disorders along with anxiety disorders as common co-morbid psychiatric conditions (Hofvander et al., 2009). A lifetime incidence of mood disorder ranked highest of the comorbid psychiatric conditions (n = 65, 53%) with a third of the subjects (n = 42, 34%) having been prescribed antidepressant medications at least once in their lives, according to Hofvander's more recent work (Hofvander et al., 2009). Approximately 8% (n = 10) of the subjects with AS or PDD NOS in Hofvander's sample met criteria for bipolar disorder (Hofvander et al., 2009). The small sample size of subjects with ASD in this study prevented any accurate prediction of incidence rates in the larger population with ASD.

Anxiety disorders followed as the second most commonly encountered DSM-IV condition in individuals with normal intelligence and ASDs in Hofvander's study (Hofvander et al., 2009). The anxiety disorders in this sample included: generalized anxiety disorder (n = 18, 15%), social phobia (n = 16,

13%), panic disorder ($n = 13$, 11%), specific phobia ($n = 7$, 6%), post-traumatic stress disorder (PTSD) ($n = 2$, <2%), and anxiety disorder NOS ($n = 1$, <1%). Other studies note high rates of tic disorders, but tics are sometimes difficult to distinguish from stereotypical movements associated with ASDs (Posey, 2008). Substance use disorder (SUD) was more common in the PDD NOS group than the AD group, with alcohol listed as the most frequently abused substance (Hofvander et al., 2009). Fifteen percent ($n = 19$) of the subjects met criteria for SUD, while 12% ($n = 15$) reported alcohol as the substance of choice (Hofvander et al., 2009). Intermittent explosive disorder ranked at the top of the list for impulse control disorders, with an incidence rate of 6% ($n = 7$) (Hofvander et al., 2009). According to Hofvander and colleagues, about 12% ($n = 15$) of the adults in this sample met criteria for a psychotic disorder, and 15% ($n = 18$) had received neuroleptic medication at least once in their lives (Hofvander et al., 2009). In Hofvander and colleagues' sample, a substantial proportion ($n = 52$, 43%) met DSM-IV criteria for ADHD. The PDD NOS subgroup exhibited more symptoms of inattention and hyperactivity/impulsivity than their AS counterparts. About 14% ($n = 16$) had a reading disorder in combination with a disorder of written expression.

Larger prospective studies may provide more precise estimations of comorbid conditions in the future. At the present time, clinicians should be aware that comorbid conditions are a logical target for psychopharmacological interventions, even if this means extrapolating information from treatment studies performed on persons with various psychiatric disorders who were not diagnosed with an ASD.

Sometimes sorting out symptoms related to autism and those related to other comorbid conditions proves difficult. For instance, restrictive, repetitive behaviors and interests (RRBIs) resemble obsessions and compulsions typical of obsessive-compulsive disorder (OCD). The DSM-IV defines RRBIs as follows:

> A preoccupation with stereotyped and restricted patterns of interest;
> Inflexibility in adhering to routines and rituals;
> Stereotyped and repetitive motor mannerisms;
> Persistent preoccupations with parts of objects.
>
> *(Soorya, Kiarashi, & Hollander, 2008)*

Neuropsychological, behavioral, and biological theories have been proposed to explain repetitive and restrictive behaviors in ASD. This chapter focuses on the biological theories, since double-blind, placebo-controlled trials of medications have tried to target the proposed dysregulation of serotonin or sensitivity to dopamine or endogenous opioids.

As for the RRBIs seen in autism, McDougle and colleagues reported differences in the Yale-Brown Obsessive Compulsive Scale (YBOCS) in autistic adults compared to those with OCD (Soorya, Kiarashi, & Hollander, 2008). Those with autism exhibited more compulsive behaviors than obsessions, and their obsessions were less likely to involve sex, religion, symmetry, contamination, and aggression compared to adults with only OCD (Soorya, Kiarashi, & Hollander, 2008). With

the similarities between RRBIs and OCD symptoms, drugs used for OCD treatment were tried for RRBIs in autistic individuals. A study by Shain, Freedman, and colleagues as well as other subsequent studies indicate that approximately a third of individuals with autism express elevated platelet levels of serotonin (Soorya, Kiarashi, & Hollander, 2008; Cook & Leventhal, 1996). McDougle and colleagues demonstrated that tryptophan depletion in adults with autism led to their exhibiting more repetitive behaviors such as whirling, flapping, pacing, banging, rocking, and self-injury. In addition, they showed that the sensitivity of the 5-HT1d receptor positively correlated with the severity of repetitive behaviors (Soorya, Kiarashi, & Hollander, 2008). With this evidence, serotonin-reuptake inhibitors (SRIs) and selective serotonin-reuptake inhibitors (SSRIs) reuptake inhibitors received attention as possible interventions for the RRBIs associated with autism.

SEROTONIN-REUPTAKE INHIBITORS

Despite significant improvement in RRBIs in the double-blind, placebo-controlled trials of clomipramine, they lack approval for the treatment of the repetitive and restrictive aspects of autism due to the small size of the studies and tolerability issues. An early randomized, crossover study of children with autism started with a two-week single-blind placebo phase followed by a crossover to ten weeks in either the clomipramine/placebo ($n = 12$) or the clomipramine/desipramine arm ($n = 12$). Clomipramine performed better than desipramine and placebo, as measured by the Autism subscale of the Children's Psychiatric Rating Scale and several outcome measures of OCD (Gordon et al., 1993). Although adverse events paralleled those seen in the treatment of OCD, one subject was dropped due to a seizure (Gordon et al., 1993). Other open-label and placebo-controlled studies showed less favorable outcomes (Posey, 2008). For example, clomipramine failed to separate from placebo in terms of decreased stereotypy on the ABC in a double-blind, placebo-controlled crossover trial of clomipramine, haloperidol, and placebo (Remington et al., 2001). High dropout rates occurred, with 20 of 32 subjects prematurely terminating in the clomipramine arm, vs. 10 out of 32 of those receiving haloperidol (Remington et al., 2001). Those receiving clomipramine reported high rates of fatigue, tremors, tachycardia, diaphoresis, and behavior problems (Remington et al., 2001). The need to monitor serum levels and electrocardiograms during treatment especially complicates treatment with SRI agents.

SELECTIVE SEROTONIN-REUPTAKE INHIBITORS

Since SSRI medications offered a more favorable side effect profile, a number of open-label studies with sertraline, citalopram, escitalopram, fluvoxamine, and fluoxetine attempted to demonstrate improvement in RRBIs associated with autism (Posey & McDougle, 2008). These open-label studies incorporated various designs, sample sizes, and durations of treatment, but results tended to be positive in terms of decreasing RRBIs (Posey & McDougle, 2008). Of note, the literature lacks studies of citalopram and escitalopram in adults with ASDs.

At present, double-blind placebo-controlled trials of fluvoxamine ($n = 30$) and fluoxetine ($n = 6$) in adults and fluoxetine ($n = 45$) in children and adolescents reported significant improvement in repetitive behaviors on YBOCS or Children's YBOCS (C-YBOCS), depending on the age group (Posey & McDougle, 2008). However, a double-blind, placebo-controlled study of fluvoxamine in children and adolescents ($n = 18$, mean age 9.5 years) with ASDs showed a poor response, with 14 of the subjects reporting notable adverse events (Posey & McDougle, 2008).

Unfortunately, limited information is available about the effect size, response rates, and other clinically pertinent points related to SSRIs in the treatment of major depression and other anxiety disorders. The same holds true for other classes of medications for mood disorders, including norepinephrine-reuptake inhibitors, tricyclic antidepressants, and monoamine oxidase inhibitors. Although not specifically studied in individuals with autism, the sedating properties of some of these classes of medication may address insomnia. For example, fluvoxamine, mirtazapine, and other medications could improve insomnia; however, trazodone probably should be avoided in males who cannot communicate, given the risk that priapism could occur and go untreated.

BENZODIAZEPINES

Clonazepam can be effective for non–rapid-eye-movement (REM) arousal disorders. It may be particularly helpful for individuals who exhibit repetitive, stereotyped, and rhythmic motor behaviors that impair their transition to sleep. Even though clonazepam does not always improve non-REM sleep disorder behaviors, it often helps REM sleep behavior disorders. Nonetheless, the use of benzodiazepines has not been extensively studied in persons with autistic spectrum disorders. Therefore, one must infer the benefits of benzodiazepines from studies performed with persons without autism. On the other hand, the risks, such as dependence, cognitive slowing, and reduced respiratory drive, are assumed to be at least as prevalent in persons with autism as in those without PDD. Paradoxical reactions can occur with benzodiazepines, and this may happen somewhat more frequently in persons with autism in this author's experience. Therefore, start benzodiazepines at a low dosage, and watch for disinhibition as the medication is slowly titrated.

Of course, non-pharmacological approaches to insomnia, such as attention to sleep hygiene, should be tried before turning to medications. Should these fail, a number of other prescription medications are now FDA-approved for the treatment of insomnia in adults, but few if any of the subjects in the studies had an ASD. Although no medication has FDA approval for the treatment of insomnia in children, two open-label trials of melatonin, one with immediate release (3 mg, $n = 15$), another combining immediate and controlled release (3–6 mg, $n = 16$), and a retrospective trial of melatonin ($n = 100$) in

children with ASD suggest that this supplement could reduce time to sleep onset and increase total sleep time (Posey, 2008). Like other over-the-counter supplements and herbal remedies, the purity and bioavailability of melatonin products may vary widely, as these are not regulated by the FDA.

DIETARY SUPPLEMENTS

Thus far, the literature on dietary supplements appears weak, and the few positive studies usually suffer from methodological flaws or small sample sizes. One of the better studies was a double-blind, placebo-controlled trial of l-carnitine 800 mg/day in 31 children with autism. In this study, a substantial improvement on the Gilliam Autism Rating Scale was seen over the eight-week trial (Crill & Helms, 2007). Although tryptophan depletion in adults diagnosed with autism resulted in worsening of their symptoms, no convincing evidence exists to suggest that supplementing with tryptophan or other amino acids improves autism symptoms. A 30-week, double-blind, placebo-controlled trial of vitamin C in 18 children with ASD showed positive results. A double-blind, placebo-controlled trial ($n = 18$ children) of supplementation with vitamin C for 30 weeks resulted in a reduction in stereotyped behaviors (Dolske et al., 1993). Another randomized, double-blind, placebo-controlled trial ($n = 13$ children) of omega 3 fatty acids reduced severe behavioral difficulties (Amminger et al., 2007). Supplementation with vitamin B_6 plus magnesium showed improvement in IQ and social quotient in one small study ($n = 8$); no change was noted in a slightly larger randomized, double-blind, placebo-controlled study ($n = 12$). Even though an open-label study of 33 children also showed improvement, all three studies contained methodological shortcomings (Posey & McDougle, 2008). Moreover, studies with supplements primarily focused on children, so even less is known about the use of dietary supplements in adults with autism. On the other hand, the use of vitamins and other supplements whenever a specific deficiency is present makes good clinical sense.

PSYCHOSTIMULANTS

In general, psychostimulants lack the robust effectiveness in treating attention deficits and impulsive behaviors in persons with ASD compared to those with typical ADHD, and side effects tend to be more common in the ASD group. Nonetheless, psychostimulants could improve adherence to treatment and increase functioning in some individuals on the ASD spectrum. Given the problems with tolerability, trials with psychostimulants should be deferred until after episodes of acute medical illness resolve. Patients in pain or distress from acute illnesses typically exhibit a reduced capacity for concentration, and their hyperactivity might be an attempt to find a body position that minimizes their physical discomfort. As always, clinicians should use every means available to ascertain whether a patient with ASD is suffering, then make every effort to relieve the physical pain. Once the patient is fully recovered from an illness, a reexamination of his level of inattention, hyperactivity, and impulsivity can be considered.

The preponderance of studies on the benefits of stimulants in children with ASD was done with younger subjects, so scant information is available about the ways that adolescents or adults with ASD might respond to such treatments. The RUPP Autism Network conducted the best of these studies to date. The RUPP study sample included 72 youths between the ages of 5 and 14 years (RUPP Autism Network, 2005b). About 74% of the sample carried the diagnosis of autism, while another 26% had PDD NOS or Asperger's disorder as their diagnosis (RUPP Autism Network, 2005b). This double-blind, crossover, placebo-controlled study used one-week treatment phases with doses of methylphenidate (immediate release) approximating 0.125, 0.25, and 0.5 mg/kg (RUPP Autism Network, 2005b). The first two doses of the day were the same, while the last dose, given in the late afternoon, was smaller to improve tolerability (RUPP Autism Network, 2005b). The ABC as scored by parents served as the main outcome measure (RUPP Autism Network, 2005b). About half of the subjects (39/72) responded favorably to the methylphenidate, whereas 18% (13/72) dropped out of this study due to side effects (RUPP Autism Network, 2005b). Parent ratings showed significant improvement in their children on the Hyperactivity subscale, while their ratings on the Withdrawal subscale of the ABC was significantly worse on the higher dosage (RUPP Autism Network, 2005b). A subsequent analysis by Posey and his colleagues of those who completed the Swanson, Nolen, and Pelham (SNAP) rating scale reported that parents saw significant improvement at all three dosages, while teachers only appreciated significant improvement in the youths at the medium and high dosages on the Hyperactivity subscale (Posey, 2008). Irritability, emotional outbursts, and initial insomnia associated with methylphenidate caused the most problems for those who experienced side effects (Posey, 2008).

Beyond the RUPP study, the literature remains weak, with two small double-blind, placebo-controlled, crossover studies of methylphenidate ($n = 10$, mean age 8.5 years; $n = 13$, mean age 7.4 years), which suggested a trend toward improvement compared to placebo (Posey, 2008). In the smaller study of the two, a significant but modest improvement was noted on the Conners' Parent and Teacher Rating Scales and the clinician-completed ABC Hyperactivity subscale (Posey, 2008). The other study focused on results from the Conners' Abbreviated Symptom Questionnaire and the ABC Hyperactivity subscale completed by teachers (Posey, 2008). A few other small ($n = 9$ to 15), open-label studies with methylphenidate using Conners' Rating Scales or other instruments reported similar results compared to those above (Posey, 2008). Of note, two older studies in children ages 3 to 6 years using amphetamines (d-amphetamine, $n = 16$; and l-amphetamine, $n = 11$) were conducted with autistic children during inpatient hospitalizations (Posey, 2008). The d-amphetamine study employed an open-label design, while the l-amphetamine used a crossover design with levodopa; however, both studies showed worsening in the majority of the patients on the CGI scale (Posey & McDougle, 2008).

About half of the individuals with "ADHD but not PDD" continue to have symptoms as adults. With this in mind, one could expect that a number of adults with PDD and ADHD symptoms would follow a similar pattern and perhaps require treatment into adulthood. The bulk of research on stimulant use in persons with PDD focused on children and adolescents. If using stimulants in adults with PDD, be aware that this class of medication reliably increases blood pressure and pulse. This may cause problems in individuals with hypertension or borderline hypertension. The elevated heart rate could be construed as an anxiety symptom as well. Nevertheless, carefully monitoring adult patients who are prescribed stimulants provides the optimal level of care and predicts a better outcome.

Atomoxetine

The norepinephrine-reuptake inhibitor atomoxetine offers another approach to treating ADHD symptoms in the context of PDD. Arnold and colleagues used a randomized, double-blind, placebo-controlled, crossover design in their study with a one-week washout period (Posey & McDougle, 2008). Of the 16 children enrolled, one discontinued early due to adverse events, and two others due to lack of effect (Posey, 2008). Responder status (25% reduction on the ABC Hyperactivity subscale and a 1 or 2 on the CGI) was achieved by 56% ($n = 9$) of the children while 25% ($n = 4$) responded to placebo (Posey & McDougle, 2008). Although the response rate was lower than that found in larger studies of children with ADHD who did not have PDD, it produced a slightly better response rate than the RUPP study using methylphenidate cited above (Posey, 2008). Several small open-label studies using atomoxetine in children with ASD showed significant improvement on the Conners' Parent Rating Scale (Jou, Harden, & Handen, 2005), the parent-rated investigator-scored ADHD Rating Scale–IV (ADHD RS), and the ABC (Troost et al., 2006), and the CGI and SNAP (Posey, Wiegan, & Wilkerson, 2006). Although the literature is limited and mainly confined to studies of younger subjects, improving ADHD symptoms may be helpful in a number of ways.

SUMMARY

Given the paucity of effective treatments for persons with autism, clinicians face special challenges whenever they encounter persons on the autistic spectrum who present with medical problems. This chapter presents a few interventions that may lessen this challenge and provide better care for this population of patients. A major obstacle includes the difficulty of obtaining an accurate history. Verbal communication skills range from nonverbal on the severely autistic side of the spectrum, to those with precocious vocabularies at the Asperger's disorder end of the spectrum. Despite their impressive vocabularies, most of these patients still struggle with expressing internal states. This lack of a first-person description of internal states often obscures the clinical picture and can hinder accurate reporting of adverse events. Since many young people show difficulty expressing internal states, child and adolescent psychopharmacologists adhere to the adage "Start low and go slow." In treating persons of any age who carry a diagnosis of ASD, the prescribing clinician would be wise to start very low and go very slow, if possible.

Although studies can help guide treatment in youths with PDD and disruptive behaviors, the literature has neglected adults who continue to meet criteria for PDD and consistently or intermittently display aggressive, irritable, or disruptive behaviors. The clinician treating these issues in older persons on the PDD spectrum must rely on safety data from studies of these drugs in adults with other psychiatric disorders and presume that some measure of effectiveness of these drugs in dampening disruptive behaviors in children and adolescents will also apply to adults. Until well-controlled studies in the adults with PDD are done, extrapolating results from studies of youths with autism will be the best approach.

Lastly, less is known about the effective treatments for psychiatric disorders co-morbid with autism spectrum disorder. Study size, design flaws, and other limitations mean that clinicians will need to carefully extrapolate information from the scientific literature as they try to apply study results to the clinical setting. Of note, medications approved for certain psychiatric disorders show less robust response rates or appear less effective in studies that target mood, anxiety, or other psychiatric conditions in persons with autism. The population with PDD also experiences more adverse event in clinical trials compared to subjects in studies recruited from the general population. Despite these limitations, clinicians should take care to thoroughly asses their patients with autism to make sure that co-morbid psychiatric and medical conditions are appropriately diagnoses and adequately treated.

CLINICAL PEARLS

- Common symptoms occur with pervasive developmental disorder (PDD): self-injurious behaviors, poor concentration, insomnia, sensory integration issues, and other comorbid psychiatric conditions. These deserve separate consideration and attention.

- Sensory integration issues include:
  - Hyposensory-social: does not respond to own name, ignores new persons, seeks rough-housing play
  - Hyposensory-nonsocial: stares at lights/objects; flaps arms, does not give attention to novel objects, mouths objects, ignores loud noises, smells objects, does not respond to pain, craves movement
  - Hypersensory-social: dislikes being held, is distressed during grooming, is averse to social touch, avoids eye contact, dislikes tickling
  - Hypersensory-nonsocial: is sensitive to loud noises, avoids textures, is sensitive to lights, is averse to water, avoids food taste/texture (Baranek, 2006)

- Clinicians must be aware that people with autism frequently exhibit finicky eating patterns because of sensory integration issues or restrictive behavior. They are sensitive to tastes and textures of food.

- A person with autism may be "stuck" on eating foods of a certain color and stick to a "beige" diet. Such restricted diets can lead to dietary deficiencies.

- The astute clinician treating patients with autism should have a close relationship with a compounding pharmacist who can convert certain medications from pill form to solutions or suppositories.

- Even patients with autism who possess impressive vocabularies might display great difficulty in expressing their feelings or internal states.

- Clinicians should remain aware that their patients with higher functioning autism probably interpret conversations in literal terms with concrete thinking.

- Mood, anxiety, and other psychiatric disorders often go undiagnosed in the patient with autism.

- Alcohol is the most common substance abused among those with autism. ADHD is common.

- Repetitive behaviors include whirling, flapping, pacing, head banging, rocking, and self-injury.

- Insomnia is common and should be treated as a separate problem or as a component of a comorbid psychiatric disorder.

- Partial complex seizures and other seizures occur more frequently in individuals with autism spectrum disorder (ASD).

- Stimulants are not as effective in ASD as they are in attention-deficit disorder.

- Atypical antipsychotic agents can diminish disruptive behavior in patients with ASD.

- Restrictive repetitive behaviors and interests (RRBIs) resemble obsessions and compulsions typical of obsessive compulsive disorder (OCD). These include: a preoccupation with stereotyped and restricted patterns of interest; inflexibility in adhering to routines and rituals; stereotyped and repetitive motor mannerisms; and persistent preoccupations with parts of objects.

DISCLOSURE STATEMENT

Dr. Doyle has received honoraria for lectures presented at the Universite di Chieti in Italy and the Conferencia de Neurosciencias in Bogata, Colombia. He also is a paid presenter for the American Physician's Institute Beat the Boards CME courses. Dr. Doyle also receives royalties from his book, Almost Alcoholic.

REFERENCES

Aman, M. G., McDougle, C. J., Scahill, L., et al., & the RUPP Autism Network (2009). Medication and parent training in children with pervasive developmental disorders and serious behavior problems: Results from a randomized clinical trial. *Journal of the American Academy of Child & Adolescent Psychiatry, 48*, 1143–1154.

Aman, M. G., Singh, N. N., Stewart, A. W., & Field, C. J. (1985). The aberrant behavior checklist: a behavior rating scale for the assessment of treatment effects. *American Journal of Mental Deficiency, 5*, 485–491.

American Academy of Pediatrics (2012). Section on complementary and integrative medicine and council on children with disabilities. In M. Zimmer, L. Desch (Eds.), Sensory integration therapies for children with developmental and behavioral disorders. *Pediatrics, 129*, 1186–1189.

American Psychiatric Association (2000). *Diagnostic and Statistical Manual, 4th ed., Text Revision*. Washington, DC: American Psychiatric Association.

Amir, R., Van den Veyver, I. B., Wan, M., et al. (1999). Rett syndrome is caused by a mutation in X-linked *MeCP2*, encoding methyl CpG binding protein 2. *Nature Genetics, 23*, 185–188.

Amminger, G., Berger, G. E., Schafer, M. R., et al. (2007). Omega-3 supplementation in children with autism: a double-blind randomized, placebo-controlled pilot study. *Biological Psychiatry, 61*, 551–553.

Arnold, L. E., Farmer, C., Kraemer, H. C., et al. (2010). Moderators, mediators, and other predictors of risperidone response in children with autistic disorder and irritability. *Journal of the American Academy of Child & Adolescent Psychopharmacology, 20*(2), 83–93.

Baranek, G. T., Fabian, J. D., Poe, M. D. Stone, W. L., & Watson, L. R. (2006). Sensory experiences questionnaire: discriminating sensory features in young children with autism, developmental delays and typical development. *Journal of Child Psychology and Psychiatry, 47*, 591–601.

Bauman, M. (2010). Autism spectrum disorders: Clinical and medical perspectives. In G. Blatt (Ed.), *The neurochemical basis of autism* (pp. 4–8). New York: Springer Science + Business Media.

Buie, T. (2005). Gastrointestinal issues encountered in autism. In M. A. K. Bauman, T. L. Kemper (Eds.), *The neurobiology of autism* (pp. 103–120). Baltimore, MD: Johns Hopkins University Press.

Campbell, M., Anderson, L. T., Meier, M., et al. (1978). A comparison of haloperidol and behavioral therapy and their interaction in autistic children. *Journal of the American Academy of Child & Adolescent Psychiatry, 17*, 640–655.

Chen, N., Bedair, H. S., McKay, B., et al. (2001). Clozapine in the treatment of aggression in an adolescent with autistic disorder. *Journal of Clinical Psychiatry, 62*(6), 479–480.

Cohen, S. A., Fitzgerald, B. J., Khan, S. R., & Khan A. (2004). The effect of a switch to ziprasidone in an adult population with autistic disorder: chart review of naturalistic, open-label treatment. *Journal of Clinical Psychiatry, 65*, 110–113.

Cook, E., & Leventhal, B. L. (1996). The serotonin system in autism. *Current Opinion in Pediatrics, 9*(4), 384–354.

Corriea, C. T., Almeida, J. P., Santos, P. E., et al. (2010). Pharmacogenetics of risperidone therapy in autism: association analysis of eight candidate genes with drug efficacy and adverse drug reactions. *The Pharmacogenomics Journal, 10*, 418–430.

Corson, A. H., Barkenbus, J. E., Posey, D. J., Stigler, K. A., & McDougle, C. J. (2004). A retrospective analysis of quetiapine in the treatment of pervasive developmental disorders. *Journal of Clinical Psychiatry, 65*, 1631–1536.

Crill, C., & Helms, R. A. (2007). The use of carnitine in pediatric nutrition. *Nutrition in Clinical Practice, 22*, 204–213.

Dolske, M. C., Spollen, J., McKay, S., Lancashire, E., & Tolbert, L. (1993). A preliminary trial of ascorbic acid as supplemental therapy for autism. *Progress in Neuropsychopharmacology & Biological Psychiatry, 17*, 765–774.

Epperson, C., McDougle, C. J., Anand, A., et al. (1994). Lithium augmentation of fluvoxamine in autistic disorder: A case report. *Journal of Child & Adolescent Psychopharmacology, 4*, 201–207.

Findling, R. L., McNamara, N. K., Gracious, B. L., et al. (2004). Quetiapine in nine youths with autistic disorder. *Journal of the American Academy of Child & Adolescent Psychopharmacology, 14*, 287–294.

Freeman, B. J., Ritvo, E. R., Yakota, A., & Ritvo A. (1986). A scale for rating symptoms of patients with the syndrome of autism in real life settings. *Journal of the American Academy of Child & Adolescent Psychiatry, 25*, 130–136.

Gobbi, G., & Pulvirenti, L. (2001). Long-term treatment with clozapine in an adult with autistic disorder accompanied by aggressive behavior. *Journal of Psychiatry and Neuroscience, 26*, 340–341.

Gordon, C., State, R. C., Nelson, J. E., et al. (1993). A double-blind comparison of clomipramine, desipramine, and placebo in the treatment of autistic disorder. *Archives of General Psychiatry, 50*(6), 441–447.

Hardan, A. Y., JouR. J., & Handen, B. L. (2005). Retrospective study of quetiapine in children and adolescents with pervasive developmental disorder. *Journal of Autism & Developmental Disorders, 35*, 387–391.

Hellings, J., Weckbaugh, M., Nickel, E. J., et al. (2005). A double-blind, placebo-controlled study of valproate for aggression in youth with pervasive developmental disorder. *Journal of Child & Adolescent Psychopharmacology, 15*(4), 682–692.

Hofvander, B., Delorme, R., Chaste, P., et al. (2009). Psychiatric and psychosocial problems in adults with normal-intelligence autism spectrum disorders. *BMC Psychiatry, 9*(35), 1–11.

Hollander, E., Wasserman, S., Swanson, E. N., et al. (2006). A double-blind placebo-controlled pilot study of olanzapine in childhood/adolescent pervasive developmental disorder. *Psychopharmacology, 16*, 541–548.

Jou, R. J., Handen, B. L., & Hardan, A. Y. (2005). Retrospective assessment of atomoxetine in children and adolescents with pervasive developmental disorder. *Journal of Child & Adolescent Psychopharmacology, 15*, 225–230.

Luby, J., Mratkosky, C., Stalets, M. M., et al. (2006). Risperidone in preschool children with autistic spectrum disorders: an investigation of safety and efficacy. *Journal of Child & Adolescent Psychopharmacology, 16*, 575–587.

Malone, R. P., Cater, J., Sheikh, R. M., Choudhury, M. S., & Delaney, M. A. (2001). Olanzapine versus haloperidol in children with autistic spectrum disorder: an open pilot study. *Journal of the American Academy of Child & Adolescent Psychiatry, 40*, 887–894.

Malone, R. P., Delaney, M. A., Hyman, S. B., & Cater, J. (2007). Ziprasidone in adolescents with autism: and open-label pilot study. *Journal of the American Academy of Child & Adolescent Psychiatry, 17*(6), 779–790.

Marcus, R. N., Randall, O., Kamen, L., et al. (2009). A placebo-controlled, fixed-dose study of aripiprazole in children and adolescents with irritability associated with autistic disorder. *Journal of the American Academy of Child & Adolescent Psychiatry, 48*(11), 1110–1119.

Martin, A., Koenig, K., Scahill, L., & Bregman, J. (1999). Open-label quetiapine in the treatment of children and adolescents with autistic disorder. *Journal of the Canadian Academy of Child & Adolescent Psychopharmacology, 9*, 99–107.

Mazzone, L., & Ruta, L. (2006). Topirimate in children with autistic spectrum disorders. *Brain Development, 28*(10), 668.

McDougle, C. J., Kem, D. L., & Posey, D. J. (2002). Case series: use of ziprasidone for maladaptive symptoms in youths with autism. *Journal of the American Academy of Child & Adolescent Psychiatry, 41*, 921–927.

McDougle, C. J., Scahill, L., Aman, M. G., et al. (2005). Risperidone for the core symptom domains of autism: results from the study by the autism network of the Research Units on Pediatric Psychopharmacology. *American Journal of Psychiatry, 162*, 1142–1148.

Minshew, N., Sweeney, J. A., & Bauman, M. L. (1997). Neurologic aspects of autism. In D. J. Cohen, F. R. Volkmar (Eds.), *Handbook of autism and pervasive developmental disorders* (2nd ed., p. 344–369). New York: Wiley.

Miral, S., Genser O., Inal-Erimoglu, F. N., et al. (2008). Risperidone versus haloperidol in children and adolescents with AD: a randomized, controlled, double-blind trial. *European Child & Adolescent Psychiatry, 17,* 1–8.

Nagaraj, R., Singhi, P., & Malhi, P. (2006). Risperidone in children with autism: randomized, placebo-controlled, double-blind study. *Journal of Child Neurology, 21,* 450–455.

Owen, R., Sikich, L., Marcus, R. N., et al. (2009). Aripiprazole in the treatment of irritability in children and adolescents with autistic disorder. *Pediatrics, 124*(6), 1533–1540.

Pasco, G. (2010). Identification and diagnosis of autism spectrum disorders: An update. *Pediatric Health, 4*(1), 107–114.

Posey, D. J., & McDougle, C. J. (2008). Treating autism spectrum disorders. *Child and Adolescent Psychiatric Clinics of North America, 17*(4), 742.

Posey, D. J., Wiegand, R. E., & Wilkerson, J. (2006). Open-label atomoxetine for attention-deficit/hyperactivity disorder symptoms associated with high-functioning pervasive developmental disorders. *Journal of Child & Adolescent Psychopharmacology, 16,* 599–610.

Posey, D., Decker, J., Sasher, T. M., et al. (2004). Guanfacine treatment of hyperactivity and inattention in autism: a retrospective analysis of 80 cases. *Journal of Child & Adolescent Psychopharmacology, 14,* 233–241.

Potenza, M. N., Holmes, J. P., Kanes, S. J., et al. (1999). Olanzapine treatment of children, adolescents, and adults with pervasive developmental disorders: an open-label pilot study. *Journal of Clinical Psychopharmacology, 19,* 37–45.

Rapin, I. (1996). Neurological examination. In I. Rapin (Ed.), *Preschool children with inadequate communication* (pp. 98–122). London: MacKeith.

Remington, G., Sloman, L., Konstantareas, M., et al. (2001). Clomipramine versus haloperidol in the treatment of autistic disorder: A double-blind, placebo-controlled, crossover study. *Journal of Clinical Psychopharmacology, 21*(4), 440–444.

Research Units on Pediatric Psychopharmacology (RUPP) Autism Network (2002). Risperidone in children with autism and serious behavioral problems. *New England Journal of Medicine, 347,* 314–321.

Research Units on Pediatric Psychopharmacology (RUPP) Autism Network (2005a). Risperidone treatment of autistic disorder: longer-term benefits and blinded discontinuation after 6 months. *American Journal of Psychiatry, 162,* 1361–1369.

Research Units on Pediatric Psychoharmacology (RUPP) Autism Network (2005b). A randomized, double-blind, placebo-controlled, crossover trial of methylphenidate in children with hyperactivity associated with developmental disorders. *Archives of General Psychiatry, 62,* 1266–1274.

Rugino, T., & Samsock, T. C. (2002). Levetiracetam in autistic children: an open-label study. *Journal of Developmental & Behavioral Pediatrics, 23*(4), 225–230.

Scahill, L., Riddle, M. A., McSwiggin-Hardin, M., et al. (1997). Children's Yale-Brown Obsessive Compulsive Scale: reliability and validity. *Journal of the American Academy of Child & Adolescent Psychiatry, 36,* 844–852.

Schopler, E., Reichler, R. J., DeVellis, R. F., et al. (1980). Toward objective classification of childhood autism: childhood Autism Rating Scale (CARS). *Journal of Autism & Developmental Disorders, 10,* 91–103.

Shea, S., Turgay, A., Carrol, A., et al. (2004). Risperidone in the treatment of disruptive behavioral symptoms in children with autistic and other pervasive developmental disorders. *Pediatrics, 114,* e634–e641.

Soorya, L., Kiarashi, J., & Hollander, E. (2008). Psychopharmacologic interventions for repetitive behaviors in autism spectrum disorders. *Child & Adolescent Psychiatric Clinics of North America, 17,* 753–771.

Stigler, K. A., Diener, J. T., Kohn, A. E., Li, L., et al. (2009). Aripiprazole in pervasive developmental disorder not otherwise specified and Asperger's disorder: a 14-week, prospective, open-label study. *Journal of Child & Adolescent Psychopharmacology, 19,* 265–274.

Stigler, K. A., Erickson, C. A., Mullett, J. E., Posey, D. J., & McDougle, C. J. (2010). Paliperidone for irritability in autistic disorder. *Journal of the American Academy of Child & Adolescent Psychopharmacology, 20*(1), 75–78.

Troost, P., Steenhuis, M., Tuynman, H., et al. (2006). Atomoxetine for attention-deficit/hyperactivity disorder symptoms in children with pervasive developmental disorders: a pilot study. *Journal of Child & Adolescent Psychopharmacology, 16,* 611–619.

Wasserman, S., Iyengar, R., Chaplin, W. F., et al. (2006). Levetiracetam versus placebo in childhood and adolescent autism: a double-blind, placebo controlled study. *International Clinical Psychopharmacology, 21*(6), 363–367.

Zudda, A., Ledda, M. G., Fratta, A., et al. (1996). Clinical effects of clozapine on autistic disorder. *American Journal of Psychiatry, 153*(5), 738.

PART VI

MEDICAL SPECIALTIES

52.

PSYCHIATRIC CARE OF THE PATIENT WITH HEART DISEASE

W. Victor R. Vieweg and Mehrul Hasnain*

INTRODUCTION

Depression will soon join atherosclerotic coronary artery disease (CAD) to produce the two leading causes of disability in the developed world (Murray & Lopez, 1997). When CAD expresses itself as coronary heart disease (CHD) clinically in the forms of angina pectoris, acute coronary syndrome (ACS), myocardial infarction (MI), and heart failure (HF), it may lead to interventions such as coronary arteriography, angioplasty and stent placement, coronary artery bypass graft (CABG) surgery, and cardiac transplantation. Recognized risk factors for CAD have largely remained stable over the past several decades. Those risk factors that may be altered include: (1) elevated low-density lipoprotein (LDL) cholesterol and fasting triglycerides, (2) hypertension, (3) diabetes mellitus (DM) and prediabetes, (4) overweight and obesity, (5) smoking, (6) lack of physical activity (sedentary lifestyle), (7) unhealthful diet, and (8) stress (variously defined and understood). Risk factors that cannot be altered include (9) age, (10) sex, and (11) family history.

The psychiatrist is commonly asked to evaluate and treat the depressed patient with CHD. Thus, depression will be the prototypical psychiatric syndrome and CHD the prototypical heart disease reviewed in this chapter. The same general principles will apply for CHD patients with anxiety disorders. Because atypical antipsychotic drugs raise many concerns and questions exist about cardiometabolic problems, we will discuss their use in patients with heart disease, even though psychosis is much less common in the general population than are depression and anxiety. Discussion of cardiac toxicity associated with antidepressant and antipsychotic medications will follow, with a focus on arrhythmias associated with these medications.

Additional issues we cover concern psychiatric aspects of arrhythmias, cardiac pacemakers, cardioverter defibrillators, and sudden cardiac death (SCD); hypotension, presyncope (symptomatic lightheadedness), and syncope (fainting); valvular heart disease; congenital heart disease; and pregnancy and heart disease.

BRAIN-HEART CONNECTION

Awareness of a connection between the heart and the mind dates to antiquity. Over 150 years ago, Claude Bernard hypothesized that the connection between these two organs was mediated via the vagus nerve (Thayer & Lane, 2009). The basis of this connection are now better understood. Functional neuroimaging suggests that the central neural circuitry of the brain–heart axis is the dorsal and subgenual regions of the anterior cingulated cortex, the insular cortex, and, to a lesser extent, the amygdala and basal ganglia. Brainstem regions, including the periaqueductal gray and the parabrachial nucleus, integrate afferent baroreceptor and mechanoreceptor information to shape the descending autonomic drive to the heart (Taggart, Critchley, & Lambiase, 2011).

We know that stress hormones, the autonomic nervous system, and inflammation play important roles in the bidirectional heart–brain association. Precise neurohormonal mechanisms linking heart and mind are still unknown, but stress is probably the shared underlying mechanism. In reviewing the influence of stress on heart disease, we (Vieweg et al., 2011a) reviewed the stressor effects of earthquakes on patients with and without CAD. For instance, earthquake victims experiencing SCD invariably had advanced atherosclerotic CAD. In contrast, patients developing stress-induced Takotsubo cardiomyopathy, a generally reversible cardiomyopathy (also known as left ventricular apical ballooning syndrome or broken heart syndrome—often precipitated by learning of an unexpected death of a loved one), were free of any form of CAD and most often survived the stressful event. These patients presented with symptoms and signs of MI and left ventricular hypokinesis, but recovery from stress-induced cardiomyopathy mediated by catecholamines commonly occurred during the weeks following its development. We hypothesized that stress was largely similar in both conditions but that the pre-morbid condition of the coronary arteries was distinctly different; that is, the pre-stress medical state better predicted the clinical outcome than the nature or magnitude of the stress.

---

* W. Victor Vieweg, MD, an author on this book chapter, died on October 7, 2013, in Charlottesville, Virginia. Dr. Vieweg, who began his career as a cardiologist, later specialized in psychiatry. He was a prolific researcher, especially in the interface of psychiatry and medicine, and often ahead of the times in conceptualizing disease and treatment models. In his death, both psychiatry and medicine have lost a great scholar and teacher.

Mind–heart connection also occurs at the behavioral level. Patients with mental illness are more likely to smoke, eat poorly, and exercise less than healthy individuals. There may be a genetic link to glucose dysregulation among individuals with major mental illness. The potentially adverse cardiometabolic effects of psychotropic medications further contribute to the link between brain and heart and will be emphasized in this chapter.

PSYCHOSOCIAL STRESSORS AND THE HEART

In the late eighteenth century, Dr. John Hunter, suffering from angina pectoris and CAD, stated "My life is at the mercy of any rogue who chooses to provoke me" (Skandalakis & Skandalakis, et al., 1992). Since at least the eighteenth century, clinicians have been interested in the relationship between psychosocial stressors and heart disease. We know that many psychosocial states may cause or contribute to adverse cardiac events, including: anger (Denollet et al., 2010), anger and hostility (Chida & Steptoe, 2009), anhedonia (Davidson et al., 2010), anxiety (Shen et al., 2008; Roest et al., 2010), anxiety-prone disposition (Shen et al., 2008), bereavement (Buckley et al., 2009), cynical hostility (Tindle et al., 2009), depression (Wulsin & Singal, 2003; Barth, Schumacher, & Herrmann-Lingen, 2004), depression and pain (Morone et al., 2010), early-onset anxiety (Janszky et al., 2010), episodic physical and sexual activity (Dahabreh & Paulus, 2011), generalized anxiety disorder (Martens et al., 2010a), natural and unnatural stress (such as naturally induced earthquakes and blizzards and humanly induced holiday events such as Christmas and New Year; Kloner, 2006), overtime work (Virtanen et al., 2010), panic disorder (Soh & Lee, 2010), phobia (Kawachi et al., 1994), phobic anxiety (Albert et al., 2005), post-traumatic stress disorder (Ahmadi et al., 2011), somatic symptoms of anxiety (Nabi et al., 2010), suppressed anger (Denollet et al., 2010), the "distressed" (Type D) personality (tendency towards negative affectivity and social inhibition (Denollet et al., 2009; Denollet, Schiffer, & Spek, 2010; Martens et al., 2010b), stressful work environment (Allesøe et al., 2010), and mixtures of anxiety and depression (Frasure-Smith & Lespérance, 2008). Not only may stress syndromes cause or exacerbate adverse cardiac events, but a panic attack may also mimic ACS or severe cardiac arrhythmia so well that they are indistinguishable from an actual cardiac event (Soh & Lee, 2010). Although better understanding of the impact of psychosocial stressors on the heart is still needed (Figueredo, 2009), Frasure-Smith and Lespérance (Frasure-Smith & Lespérance, 2008) have argued that a more general distress disorder may be the best way to link mental disorders and CHD.

CORONARY HEART DISEASE AND DEPRESSION

Depression is the most common stressor linked to CHD. This topic has been studied and reviewed frequently and may be found in both the psychiatric and the medical literature. (Lespérance & Frasure-Smith, 2000; Frasure-Smith & Lespérance, 2006; de Jonge et al., 2006; Glassman, 2007; Marano et al., 2009; Pozuelo et al., 2009; Linke et al., 2009; Vieweg et al., 2010a; Vieweg et al., 2010b; Zuidersma, Thombs, & de Jonge, 2011). Several important points can be drawn from this literature.

1. Depression is about three times more common in patients after MI than the general population.

2. 15–20% of patient after MI meet *Diagnostic and Statistical Manual of Mental Disorders IV* (DSM-IV-TR) (American Psychiatric Association [APA], 2000) criteria for major depressive disorder and even a larger percentage will manifest depressive symptoms.

3. Women are at particularly high risk for depression following acute MI.

4. Major depressive disorder and elevated depressive symptoms link to a worse prognosis in patients with CHD in a dose-dependent manner.

5. Although it is suggested that ACS patients with first-time and new-onset depression are at particularly increased risk of worse prognosis, there is no consistent evidence to support such statements.

6. The nebulous boundaries of depression and the mismatch between the precision and reliability of instruments used to assess depression and those used to assess CHD are barriers to a better understanding of any link between depression and CHD.

7. Somatic symptoms of depression (in particular, sleep disturbances, fatigue, and appetite problems) have a stronger association with CHD prognosis than the cognitive symptoms.

8. Both biological and behavioral mechanisms have been offered to explain the link between depression and comorbid CHD.

9. Depressed patients with comorbid CHD have reduced medication compliance.

10. Screening for depression in CHD subjects is recommended (although we have argued for additional evidence before implementing such screening. (Hasnain et al., 2011).

11. The Patient Health Questionnaire (PHQ-2) (Wooley & Simon, 2000) provides two screening questions and may be followed by the PHQ-9 (Kroenke, Spitzer, & Williams, 2001) if either answer is positive.

12. If the PHQ-9 is consistent with a high probability of depression, the patient should be assessed further for depression.

13. Cardiologists should take depression into account when managing patients with CHD.

14. About one-half of cardiologists report that they treat depression in their patients.

15. There is no current evidence that screening for depression improves outcome in CHD patients.

16. Treatment options for major depression in patients with CHD include antidepressant drugs, cognitive behavioral therapy, and physical activity.

17. Interest is emerging in understanding the role of depressive symptoms in the pathogenesis of cardiovascular disease (CVD) among adolescents (Dietz & Matthews, 2011).

SCREENING FOR DEPRESSION AMONG PATIENTS WITH CHD

Depressed patients with CHD will reach the psychiatrist in a variety of ways. Probably, the most controversial pathway is screening CHD patients for depression. We discuss this topic because the psychiatrist may be asked by the cardiologist, internist, or primary care physician to assist in the screening process.

In 2008, the American Heart Association (AHA) Science Advisory published "Depression and Coronary Heart Disease: Recommendations for Screening, Referral, and Treatment" (Lichtman et al., 2008). This document arose from concerns that depression was highly prevalent in patients with CHD and was associated with suffering, poor CHD prognosis, and poor treatment compliance. It recommended initial screening using the PHQ-2 (Whooley & Simon, 2000; Kroenke, Spitzer, & Williams, 2003): [Over the past two weeks, how often have you been bothered by any of the following problems? (1) Little interest or pleasure in doing things. (2) Feeling down, depressed, or hopeless.] If the answer to either question is "yes," then refer the patient for a more complete evaluation by a mental healthcare profession or screening with the PHQ-9 (Kroenke, Spitzer, & Williams, 2001) that employs the nine major items used in the DSM-IV-R (American Psychiatric Association [APA], 2000) to diagnose major depressive disorder. The AHA advisory acknowledged the lack of data showing that screening led to improved outcome of patients with CHD. A meta-analysis underscored this point (Thombs et al., 2008). One difficulty is that 12% of patients report suicidal ideation on the PHQ-9, but only 0.45% will turn out to have suicidal intent (Shemesh et al., 2009). Having to immediately evaluate more than 10% of cardiology clinic patients for suicidal intent may place an enormous burden on cardiology clinic staff. As pointed out by Thombs et al. (Thombs et al., 2008) in their systematic review of screening for depression in cardiac patients, no studies have shown that screening for depression improves symptoms of depression or cardiac outcomes in patients with cardiac disease.

For readers having to grapple with this issue in more depth, see articles by Whooley, 2009; Ziegelstein et al., 2009; Larsen et al., 2010; Williams, 2010; Hasnain et al., 2011; Holmes, 2011; Ziegelstein & Thombs, 2011; Jelinek, 2011; and Huffman et al., 2011.

PSYCHOSOCIAL ADJUSTMENT AFTER ONSET OF ACS

Onset of ACS can be quite distressing and may generate grief-like symptoms. Higgins et al. (Higgins et al., 2007) conducted a semi-structured interview of 14 psychologists and social workers with extensive experience managing cardiac patients. The clinicians described the interactions among anxiety, depression, grief, loss, and denial; they also identified trauma, guilt, and anger as issues of concern in some patients. The perception of low support is associated with poor prognosis in patients with CHD, acts synergistically with depression, and may be more prominent in women (Lett et al., 2007; Leifheit-Limson et al., 2010; Chung et al., 2011). Psychoeducation and supportive counseling helps patients adjust after the onset of ACS. There is growing interest in home-based or telephone-delivered nursing psychosocial support interventions for patients post-ACS, but results have been mixed and inconclusive (Frasure-Smith et al., 1997; Cosette, Frasure-Smith, & Lespérance, 2001; Gallagher, McKinley, & Dracup, 2003; Bambauer et al., 2005). Face-to-face counseling offered in mental health or collaborative care settings is currently the best intervention for patients experiencing psychosocial adjustment difficulties after ACS (Huffman et al., 2011).

DEPRESSION AND HEART FAILURE

What used to be called congestive heart failure (CHF) is now called, for the most part, HF because "congestion" has been better managed (with diuretics and preload and afterload reduction) in HF (Braunwald & Bristow, 2000; Braunwald, 2008). Depression in HF patients with and without atrial fibrillation is associated with increased cardiac morbidity and mortality (Frasure-Smith et al., 2009; Sherwood et al., 2011). Persistent depression remains a major problem after implantable cardioverter defibrillator placement in HF patients (Pedersen et al., 2011). Shimizu et al. (Shimuzu et al., 2011) recommend targeted treatment of depression in chronic HF as a strategy to improve cardiac function. Depression, but not treatment with antidepressant drugs, may be associated with increased mortality in HF patients (O'Connor et al., 2008). Conversely, HF is a risk factor for depression among the elderly (Luijendijk et al., 2010).

Depression reduces the effectiveness of a disease-management program in HF patients (Jaarsma et al., 2010); managing depression in HF patients is a formidable challenge for psychiatrists, even when working with a cardiologist who is both knowledgeable about and interested in the brain–heart interface. Side effects from antidepressants and antipsychotics drugs include: (1) hypotension, (2) hypertensive crisis, (3) arrhythmias such as those derived from QTc interval prolongation and bradycardia/tachycardia syndromes, (4) increases and decreases in prothrombin time and other parameters of anticoagulation monitoring, and (5) increases and decreases in myocardial contractility (Dimos et al., 2009; Silver, 2010). In the Sertraline AntiDepressant Heart Attack Randomized Trial-Congestive Heart Failure

(SADHART-CHF) study, sertraline was found safe but ineffective among depressed cardiac patients with HF and did not improve cardiac outcome (O'Connor et al., 2010). Tousoulis et al. (Tonsoulis et al., 2010) speculated that selective serotonin reuptake inhibitors (SSRIs) may improve depression in HF patients.

DEPRESSION AFTER CORONARY ARTERY BYPASS SURGERY (CABG)

In a randomized controlled trial of nonpharmacological interventions in patients developing major or minor depression within a year of CABG, Freedland et al. (Freedland et al., 2009) found that both cognitive behavioral therapy (CBT) and supportive stress management, compared with usual care, improved depressive symptoms. CBT had greater and more durable effects on depression than did supportive stress management. The authors did not assess cardiac outcome.

Rollman et al. (Rollman et al., 2009), in a randomized, controlled trial, reported that telephone-delivered collaborative care to treat post-CABG depression, compared with usual care, improved depressive symptoms, mental health–related quality of life, and physical functioning at eighth-month follow-up. However, a substantial number of study patients did not benefit from this intervention. The authors argued for additional studies to better define favorable patient characteristics.

DEPRESSION AND CARDIAC REHABILITATION

The Ochsner Heart and Vascular Institute assessed the impact of cardiac rehabilitation on depression and CHD rehabilitation–associated mortality on consecutive CHD patients (Milani & Lavie, 2007). Cardiac rehabilitation reduced both depressive symptoms and excess CHD mortality (Milani & Lavie, 2007) in patients following major coronary events. In an earlier study (Lavie & Milani, 2006), the same group showed that young CHD patients with adverse psychological and coronary risk profiles benefited from a formal cardiac rehabilitation program. Specifically, metabolic syndrome parameters and psychological stress profiles among the study patients improved in response to a formal cardiac rehabilitation program. Participation in physical activity and improved physical fitness may explain the beneficial effects on both depression and CHD (Milani & Lavie, 2007).

In a prospective study of 195 patients entering outpatient cardiac rehabilitation, participants were screened by a trained researcher for depression with "The Structured Clinical Interview for DSM-IV Axis I Disorders, Nonpatient Edition" under the supervision of a psychiatrist to ascertain the diagnosis of major depression (Swardfager et al., 2011). Patients with Center for Epidemiological Studies of Depression (CES-D) scores ≥16, those voicing subjective mood complaints, or those showing objective signs of depression during cardiac rehabilitation visits were referred to a staff psychologist. Psychosocial interventions included stress management seminars, group therapy sessions, individual counseling, and/or psychiatric referral as appropriate. Comprehensive lifestyle management resources were offered to all participants. Major depression was diagnosed in 22.1% and was associated with high rates of non-completion (44.2% versus 28.9%) and non-adherence (53% versus 34.9%). Also, individuals with major depression achieved poorer cardiopulmonary fitness increases and poorer body fat outcomes than individuals without major depression. Authors highlighted that, despite depression screening and structured psychosocial support, major depression remained a significant barrier to effective cardiac rehabilitation.

HEART RATE VARIABILITY (HRV) IN DEPRESSED CHD PATIENTS

Glassman et al (Glassman et al., 2007) sought to assess the influence of sertraline and mood improvement on heart rate variability (HRV) in ACS patients with major depressive disorder. Study subjects in the Sertraline AntiDepressant Heart Attack Randomized Trial (SADHART) underwent 24-hour Holter monitor electrocardiographic (EKG) assessment at baseline and at 16-week following up after randomization to sertraline or placebo. The authors found that both treatment with sertraline and depressive symptom improvement were associated with increased (improved) HRV. However, the clinical utility of this observation remains to be determined.

DIABETES MELLITUS (DM) AND CAD EQUIVALENT

In an often-referenced study published in 1998, Haffner et al. (Haffner et al., 1998) reported that patients with DM free of previous MI have as great a risk of a new MI as patients free of DM but with a previous MI. From these data flows the argument that treating risk factors for CAD is as important in patients with DM free of CHD as in patients with established CAD. Scherrer et al. (Scherrer et al., 2011), in a very large Department of Veterans Affairs database, showed that patients with combined type 2 DM and depression were at 30% increased likelihood of developing new-onset MI, compared with patients who only had type 2 DM or patients who only had major depressive disorder. This finding was undercut by a more recent meta-analysis of 45,000 subjects followed for 5 to 25 years showing that patients with DM without prior MI had a 43% lower risk of developing CHD than patients with previous MI free of DM (Bulugahapitiya et al., 2009). For purposes of this chapter about psychiatric patients with heart disease, we will not separate our remarks based on whether they do or do not have comorbid DM.

Less controversial is the observation that patients with depression and DM have increased CHD and all-cause morbidity and mortality (Katon et al., 2008; Pan et al., 2011). Given the overlap of psychotropic drug-induced weight gain, obesity, DM, and metabolic syndrome, the psychiatrist faces the challenge of treating patients with psychiatric problems and various metabolic disturbances.

PSYCHOTHERAPY IN CHD PATIENTS WITH DEPRESSION

Enhancing Recovery in Coronary Heart Disease (ENRICHD) study tested the hypothesis that, in patients with acute MI and either low social support or depression, CBT would reduce the rates of subsequent deaths and recurrent MIs compared with patients receiving usual care (Writing Committee, 2003). The CBT intervention was delivered in individual or group treatment, or both. Most patients received between six and ten sessions of treatment. The treatment involved traditional elements of CBT, including cognitive restructuring, relaxation and skills training, and behavioral activation. With 2,481 patients, 334 of whom had a history of CHF, ENRICHD was, to date, the largest trial by far in psychosomatic cardiology. While the primary trial hypothesis was not supported—there was no difference in mortality or the composite event rate—there was a small benefit of the CBT intervention regarding depression symptoms. Intervention-treated patients experienced a decline of about 10.1 points on the Hamilton Rating Scale for Depression, compared to about 8.4 points for patients in the usual care arm.

Cardiac Randomized Evaluation of Antidepressant and Psychotherapy Efficacy (CREATE) trial included depressed patients with stable CAD and sought to compare both the effects of citalopram versus placebo and the effects of interpersonal psychotherapy (IPT) versus clinical management (Lespérance et al., 2007). In IPT, treatment focuses on an interpersonal problem area associated with depression. Typically, these problems fall within the domains of grief, role disputes, role transitions, or interpersonal deficits. One or more domains may be targeted for intervention in patients with CHD. In CREATE, citalopram was more effective than placebo in reducing depressive symptoms and in achieving response and remission. In contrast, the patients who had IPT did not separate from clinical management (Lespérance et al., 2007).

ELECTROCONVULSIVE THERAPY (ECT) IN CHD PATIENTS WITH DEPRESSION

Electroconvulsive therapy (ECT) may be indicated in CHD patients with depression who are not responding to pharmacotherapy, when depressive symptoms pose a significant barrier to care, or when a patient prefers ECT to pharmacotherapy. ECT is associated with a transient increase in heart rate and blood pressures and a decrease in HRV. Although rare, adverse cardiovascular events during ECT are important causes of morbidity and mortality. Zielinski et al. (Zielinski et al., 1993) compared the rate of ECT-related cardiac complications in 40 patients with major depression and left ventricular impairment, ventricular arrhythmias, and/or conduction delay with a matched comparison group of 40 depressed patients without cardiac disease. The rate of complications (ventricular or arterial arrhythmias, bradycardia and/or ischemic event) was significantly higher in patients with cardiac disease than controls, but most of the complications

were transitory and did not prevent the completion of ECT (38 of the 40 cardiac patients completed the course of ECT). Case reports and case series describe successful ECT in patients with recent MI (Magid et al., 2005), recent CABG (Riesenman & Scanlan, 1995), hypertrophic cardiomyopathy (Adabag, Kim, & Aloul, 2008), cardiac pacemakers and implantable cardioverter defibrillators (Dolenc et al., 2004), and CHF and valvular diseases (Rayburn, 1997). Overall, ECT can be performed safely in most patients with underlying cardiac conditions, as long as such patients are identified ahead of time and are closely monitored for potential complications.

OBESITY, SICK FAT, GLUCOSE AND LIPID DYSREGULATION, AND THE METABOLIC SYNDROME

The major portion of this chapter focuses on the adverse cardiometabolic effects of antidepressant and antipsychotic drugs, with emphasis on those adverse effects among psychiatric patients with heart disease. In the United States, morbidity and mortality from CAD is decreasing, while both the prevalence of and mortality from schizophrenia have remained stable over the past several decades (Tiihonen et al., 2009) with life-expectancy shortened by 25 years or more, with most of this reduction due to CHD (Newcomer & Hennekens, 2007). This differential mortality gap is widening (Saha, Chant, & McGrath, 2007). Risk factors for CHD morbidity and mortality are more common in subjects with schizophrenia compared with the general population and include smoking, DM, dyslipidemia, hypertension, and obesity. Many of these risk factors appear as part of the metabolic syndrome, with its increased prevalence in schizophrenia (Meyer & Stahl, 2009). Thus, psychiatrists face the daunting task of improving the mental health of the many subjects suffering from depression, schizophrenia, and other psychiatric illnesses while employing psychotropic agents with substantial adverse cardiometabolic effects.

OBESITY

The most common parameter defining obesity in the United States is body mass index (BMI). In the metric system, BMI is determined by dividing body weight by body height squared (kg/m^2). When weight is measured in pounds, and height in feet and inches, BMI in kg/m^2 is [weight (pounds)/height^2 (inches)] × 703.07. A BMI less than 18.5 kg/m^2 is considered "underweight." The "normal" range for BMI is 18.5 to 25 kg/m^2. A BMI greater than 25 kg/m^2 but less than 30 kg/m^2 is considered "overweight." BMI ≥30 kg/m^2 is considered "obese." Obesity may be graded [Grade 1, BMI <35 kg/m^2; Grade 2, BMI <40 kg/m^2; and Grade 3, BMI ≥40 kg/m^2 (morbid obesity)]. BMI in children and adolescents is measured as a percentile to adjust for the changes associated with growth. A variety of BMI calculators is available on the Internet, including BMI percentile charts for children and adolescents.

Because abdominal fat (apple shape) more than hip fat (pear shape) better links to cardiovascular morbidity and mortality, abdominal circumference may be a better index of sickness-related excess weight. Abdominal circumference is measured at the level of the umbilicus. For Caucasian adult men, at-risk abdominal circumference is 40 inches (102 cm). For Caucasian adult women, this value is 35 inches (88 cm). For Asian men and women, comparable values are 35 inches (88 cm) and 32 inches (80 cm), respectively.

SICK FAT

Adiposopathy ("sick fat"), as described in historical perspective by Bays (Bays, 2011), comprises pathogenic anatomical adipose tissue changes occurring with positive caloric balance (when caloric intake is greater than body requirements), resulting in pathophysiological endocrine and immune responses and subsequent metabolic disease. Visceral or abdominal fat arises within the abdominal cavity and embraces the stomach, liver, intestines, kidneys, etc. It differs from subcutaneous fat located under the skin and intramuscular fat located in skeletal muscles. Excess visceral fat explains central obesity and the protuberant abdomen. Central obesity is linked to CVD and type 2 DM, insulin resistance, inflammatory diseases, and other obesity-related conditions. Although pericardial fat is located in the thorax rather than the abdomen, it can be considered another form of visceral fat.

Among younger women, fat is commonly stored in the buttocks, thighs, and hips (pear shape) due to female sex hormones. When women reach menopause and estrogen production declines, fat migrates from their buttocks, hips, and thighs to the waist. Among men, fat is more commonly stored in the abdomen (apple shape) because of sex hormone differences. High-intensity exercise may reduce total abdominal (visceral) fat.

Operationally, obtaining patients' weight and height is the most common practice to determine obesity and BMI. Obtaining vital signs, fasting glucose, fasting lipids, and triglycerides should be routine practice. Measurement of abdominal circumference can also be added. These findings will help determine patient education, drug selection, and extent of monitoring for CVD risk factors.

All too commonly, psychiatrists and other clinicians describe DM and hypertension as adequately controlled if "the numbers look good," even among patients who are overweight or obese. The Food and Drug Administration (FDA) and pharmaceutical industry have selected "≥7% increase in body weight" to define excessive weight gain in phase 2 and phase 3 drug studies (Vieweg et al., 2011b). Thus, both individual clinicians and federal agencies may downplay the importance of reducing body fat, particularly visceral fat.

It is likely that personalized medicine will soon reach a level of sophistication and application warranting a detailed understanding of the role that obesity, visceral fat, and psychotropic drug-induced obesity play in psychiatric conditions with comorbid medical problems. Even at this point, casual acceptance of "modest" psychotropic drug-induced weight gain is no longer clinically appropriate in most cases.

GLUCOSE DYSREGULATION

The definition of DM is in transition (Table 52.1). Hemoglobin A1c (HbA1c) is gaining traction as another benchmark to diagnose DM (Malkani & Mordes, 2011). Table 52.2 depicts the correlation between HbA1c and mean serum glucose values over the preceding several weeks. HbA1c greater than or equal to 6.5% (≥48 mmol/mol in IFCC-standardized units) in Diabetes Control and Complications Trial (DCCT)-aligned units is a convenient benchmark to diagnose this condition. However, compared with fasting serum glucose or oral glucose-tolerance testing, it will miss some cases of DM. Thus, the presence of an elevated HbA1c is very useful to diagnosis DM, but the absence of an elevated value is not necessarily reassuring, and testing should move to fasting serum glucose measurements and glucose-tolerance testing.

METABOLIC SYNDROME

Reaven (Reaven, 1997; 2006) noted that several of the CVD risk factors (dyslipidemia, hypertension, hyperglycemia) commonly occur together and introduced the term *syndrome X* to describe this clustering. The syndrome, characterized by insulin resistance, is now called the *metabolic syndrome*. Its core features are obesity, atherogenic dyslipidemia (elevated triglycerides and low high-density lipoprotein [HDL] cholesterol), disturbed insulin and glucose metabolism, and

Table 52.1 SERUM GLUCOSE AND HBA1C VALUES FOR PREDIABETES AND DIABETES, AS DEFINED BY THE AMERICAN DIABETES ASSOCIATION (ADA, 2014)

CARBOHYDRATE LOADED STATE	SERUM GLUCOSE VALUES	DESCRIPTIVE STATE
Fasting glucose		
	100 mg/dl to 125 mg/dl	Prediabetes
	≥126 mg/dl	Diabetes
Random glucose		
	≥200 mg/dl	Diabetes
2-hour post Oral Glucose Tolerance Test (OGTT)		
	140 to 199 mg/dl	Prediabetes
	≥200 mg/dl	Diabetes
HbA1c		
	5.7 to 6.4%	Prediabetes
	≥ 6.5%	Diabetes

For clinicians using mmol/l (molarity) instead of mg/dl (weight dimension) to report serum glucose measurements, use the following principles of conversion:

Mg/dl × 0.0555 = mmol/l

Mmol/l × 18.0182 = mg/dl

Table 52.2 ESTIMATED MEAN SERUM GLUCOSE
MEASUREMENTS OVER PRECEDING SEVERAL
WEEKS BASED ON HBA1C DETERMINATIONS
(NATHAN ET AL., 2008)

HBA1C	ESTIMATED MEAN SERUM GLUCOSE (MG/DL)
5	97 (76–120)
6	126 (100–152)
7	154 (123–185)
8	183 (147–217)
9	212 (170–249)
10	240 (193–282)
11	269 (217–314)
12	298 (240–347)

hypertension (Grundy, 2007; 2008). Individuals with these characteristics commonly manifest prothrombotic and pro-inflammatory states. It is associated with increased risk of type 2 DM, CVD (to a lesser extent), and all-cause mortality. However, the metabolic syndrome does not necessarily predict these adverse health risks to a greater extent than do the additive effects of its individual components. This observation has generated debate about its clinical utility (Sattar et al., 2008; Simmons et al., 2010).

DRUG-INDUCED WEIGHT GAIN AND OTHER METABOLIC PROBLEMS ASSOCIATED WITH ANTIDEPRESSANT AND ANTIPSYCHOTIC DRUG ADMINISTRATION

In recent publications (Vieweg et al., 2011b; Vieweg et al., 2008), we developed drug-induced weight gain tables comparing various psychotropic drugs, with a focus on antidepressant and antipsychotic drugs and drawing on information from more than 50 publications. These tables have been further modified and appear in Table 52.3. There has been much more interest in antipsychotic drug-induced weight gain than in antidepressant drug-induced weight gain, but management principles are the same for both drug types. Readers looking for a more detailed review of weight gain and glucose dysregulation with antidepressant and antipsychotic drugs are invited to a recent review by our group (Hasnain, Vieweg, & Hollett, 2012).

In 2004, the American Diabetes Association, the American Psychiatric Association, the American Association of Clinical Endocrinologists, and the North American Association for the Study of Obesity published the Consensus Development Conference on Antipsychotic Drugs and Obesity and Diabetes (American Diabetes Association et al., 2004). This consensus statement was an outgrowth of a variety of factors. The arrival of the second-generation (atypical) antipsychotic drugs (clozapine

in 1989, risperidone 1993, olanzapine 1996, quetiapine 1997, ziprasidone 2001, aripiprazole 2002, paliperidone 2006, iloperidone 2009, asenapine 2009, and lurasidone 2010) was thought to bring a more favorable side-effect profile than commonly used first-generation (typical) antipsychotic drugs such as chlorpromazine, perphenazine, trifluoperazine, thiothixene, haloperidol, and fluphenazine. However, emerging evidence revealed that serious problems with second-generation antipsychotic drugs included drug-induced weight gain. Opinions differ about the forthrightness of the pharmaceutical companies advising treating physicians and patients of this problem, and litigation has ensued (Berenson, 2007).

Antipsychotic drugs differ in their metabolic liability. Table 52.4 provides approximate relative likelihood of second-generation antipsychotic drugs' causing specific metabolic disturbances (Hasnain, Vieweg, & Hollett, 2012; Hasnain et al., 2009). Despite these differences, the FDA requires that all the manufacturers of second-generation antipsychotic drugs warn prescribers and patients of the potential for their drugs to induce hyperglycemia and DM (usually accompanied by weight gain). Table 52.5 outlines screening and monitoring guidelines for patients taking second-generation antipsychotic drugs.

RISK FACTORS FOR WEIGHT GAIN

Young age, low BMI at baseline, diagnosis of non-affective psychosis, and limited or no previous exposure to antipsychotic medications are predictors of weight gain (Álvarez-Jiménez et al., 2008; Saddicha, Ameen, & Akhtar, 2008; Gebhardt et al., 2009). Early weight gain may predict long-term weight gain (Kinon et al., 2005). Vigilant monitoring of weight gain early during antipsychotic drug treatment and appropriate interventions as indicated can limit long-term obesity and obesity-related complications. Education and encouraging a healthy lifestyle should be offered to all patients receiving antipsychotic medications. The suggested pharmacological intervention for patients who gain weight or develop metabolic complications is to switch the antipsychotic medication to one with lower metabolic liability (American Diabetes Association et al., 2004). Numerous anti-obesity and insulin-sensitizing agents have been studied for antipsychotic-induced weight gain and glucose metabolism dysregulation, but data do not support their routine use (Faulkner & Cohn, 2006; Baptista et al., 2008). Several recent studies suggest metformin may be a suitable option in young, high-risk patients who show a pattern of rapid weight gain early during treatment. For specific discussion on this topic, readers are invited to consult two recent publications by our group (Hasnain, Vieweg, & Fredrickson, 2010; Hasnain, Fredrickson, & Vieweg, 2011).

DIABETIC KETOACIDOSIS

Life-threatening hyperglycemia, with or without complications (diabetic ketoacidosis [DKA]), may appear after antipsychotic drug administration. Patients with DKA may be younger, less overweight at baseline, and, more commonly, female (Scheen & De Hert, 2007). The associated ranking

Table 52.3 PSYCHOTROPIC DRUG-INDUCED WEIGHT CHANGES SHOWING EXPECTED RELATIVE (WEIGHT BURDEN SCALE) AND APPROXIMATE ABSOLUTE (WEIGHT CHANGE/YEAR) WEIGHT ALTERATIONS (AFTER VIEWEG ET AL., 2011B)

WEIGHT BURDEN SCALE	-0.5	0	+0.5	+1.0	+1.5	+2.0
Potential weight change in a year (lb.)	-5–0	0	1–5	6–10	11–15	>15
Antidepressant drugs						
SSRI	Fluoxetine	Citalopram Escitalopram Fluvoxamine Sertraline	Paroxetine			
TCA			Desipramine Nortriptyline Protriptyline	Amitriptyline Doxepin Imipramine		
MAOI		Selegiline		Phenelzine Tranylcypromine		
SNRI		Duloxetine Venlafaxine				
Other	Bupropion	Nefazodone Trazodone		Mirtazapine		
Antipsychotic drugs						
Typical	Molindone		Fluphenazine Haloperidol Perphenazine	Thioridazine		
Atypical		Aripiprazole Ziprasidone	Paliperidone	Quetiapine Risperidone		Clozapine Olanzapine
Mood-stabilizing drugs						
Antiseizure	Topiramate	Lamotrigine Oxcarbazepine	Carbamazepine	Gabapentin	Valproate	
Other		Modafinil			Lithium	
Stimulant drugs	Amphetamine Atomoxetine Methylphenidate Pemoline					
Sedative-hypnotic drugs		Benzodiazepines Buspirone Diphenhydramine				

Table 52.4 APPROXIMATE RELATIVE LIKELIHOOD OF ATYPICAL ANTIPSYCHOTIC MEDICATIONS TO CAUSE VARIOUS METABOLIC DISTURBANCES (HASNAIN, VIEWEG, & HOLLETT, 2012; HASNAIN ET AL., 2009)

MEDICATION	WEIGHT GAIN	GLUCOSE METABOLISM ABNORMALITIES	DYSLIPIDEMIA	METABOLIC SYNDROME
▼ Amisulpride	Low	Low	Low	———
Aripiprazole	Low	Low	Low	Low
Asenapine	Low	Low	———	———
Clozapine	High	High	High	High
Iloperidone	Medium	Low	———	———
Lurasidone	Low	Low	———	———
Olanzapine	High	High	High	High
Paliperidone	Medium	Low	———	———
Risperidone	Medium	Medium to low	Low	———
Quetiapine	Medium	Medium to low	High	———
▼ Sertindole	Low	———	———	———
Ziprasidone	Low	Low	Low	Low
▼ Zotepine	Medium	———	———	———

▼ Antipsychotic drugs that are investigational and/or not available in the United States

– indicates lack of data

Table 52.5 SCREENING AND MONITORING GUIDELINES DURING ANTIPSYCHOTIC TREATMENT

RISK FACTOR	CONSENSUS STATEMENT FROM UNITED STATES	CONSENSUS STATEMENT FROM AUSTRALIA
Background risk assessment	Personal and family history of obesity, diabetes, dyslipidemia, hypertension, or CVD.	Assess risk factors for DM: Older age, family history of DM, CVD, or other cardiovascular risk factors, personal history of gestational DM or polycystic ovary syndrome, ethnic predisposition (e.g., indigenous Australian, Pacific Islander, Asian, African-American), lack of exercise, poor diet, obesity
Obesity	Measure weight, BMI, and waist circumference at baseline. Monitor weight and BMI every 4 weeks for 12 weeks, then quarterly. Monitor waist circumference annually.	Measure BMI and waist–hip ratio every visit or every 3 months
Glucose dysregulation	Check fasting serum glucose at baseline. Monitor at 12 weeks and then annually.	Measure serum glucose level (random or fasting): • Immediately on starting or changing antipsychotic medication and then every 3–6 months (ideally every month for 6 months) • Then minimum of twice yearly • Reassess earlier or more frequently if rapid weight gain/loss, polydipsia, or polyuria occur • Perform oral glucose tolerance test (OGTT) if fasting serum glucose 99.1–126.1 mg/dl (5.5–7.0 mmol/l) or random serum glucose 99.1–198.2 mg/dl (5.5–11.0 mmol/l)
Dyslipidemia	Check lipid profile at baseline. Monitor after 12 weeks and then every 5 years.	Check lipid profile every 6 months
Blood pressure	Measure blood pressure at baseline. Monitor after 12 weeks and then annually.	Blood pressure measurement every 6 months

Both guidelines advise intense monitoring in high-risk patients (American Diabetes Association et al., 2004; Lambert & Chapman, 2004).

strength is strong for clozapine and olanzapine, medium for quetiapine and risperidone, and low for ziprasidone and aripiprazole (DuMouchel et al., 2008). Educate patients about, and look for, symptoms and signs of DM and DKA during the first several months, especially in patients taking clozapine, olanzapine, quetiapine, or risperidone. The risk of new-onset DM persists throughout the course of therapy and is not necessarily restricted to the first few months or years of treatment. While weight gain usually precedes the development of glucose dysregulation, DM and DKA may develop in the absence of weight gain. Emerging weight loss is not necessarily a sign of metabolic improvement, but may be the harbinger of worsening glucose dysregulation. Remind patients that new-onset polydipsia and polyuria may be an early sign of DM.

ADVERSE CARDIAC EFFECTS OF ANTIDEPRESSANT AND ANTIPSYCHOTIC DRUGS

CHEMICAL CARDIOMYOPATHIES

Factors that determine cardiac vulnerability to the cardio-toxic effects of various medications and non-prescribed drugs, include: (1) direct toxic effects on myocyte structure and function, (2) pathological increases in sympathetic activation, and (3) myocyte oxidative stress (Figueredo, 2011). Drugs such as methamphetamine, clozapine, and methylphenidate are implicated in cardiomyopathy (Figueredo, 2011). Other agents used by psychiatric patients implicated in chemical cardiomyopathies are anabolic/androgenic steroids, catechol-amines, cocaine, ethanol, and ma huang (ephedra). For a fuller list, see the table in the paper by Figueredo (Figueredo, 2011).

PROARRHYTHMIC EFFECTS OF ANTIDEPRESSANT AND ANTIPSYCHOTIC DRUGS

Box 52.3 provides detailed commentary on antidepressant and antipsychotic drug-induced EKG changes, including QTc interval prolongation, polymorphic ventricular tachy-cardia (PVT), and *torsade de pointes* (*TdP*). We encourage the reader to review this appendix at this time to better under-stand our comments below. Those interested in even more detail are referred to several of our recent papers on this topic (Vieweg et al., 2009; Vieweg et al., 2011c; Vieweg et al., 2012; Vieweg et al., 2013c; Hasnain et al., 2014).

General Comments

Case-control studies have produced conflicting evidence that tricyclic antidepressants (TCAs) and SSRIs lead to an increased risk of CVD (Meier, Schlienger, & Jick, 2001; Hippisley-Cox, et al., 2001; Sauer, Berlin, & Kimmel, 2003; Monster et al., 2004; Schlienger et al., 2004; Tata et al., 2005; Reid & Barbui, 2010). A paper by Hamer et al. (Hamer et al., 2011) described a prospective cohort study of 14,784 middle-aged adults free of CVD drawn from the Scottish Health Surveys. About 5% had used antidepressant drugs. Over an eight-year follow-up, TCAs were linked (hazard ratio [HR] 1.35, 95% confidence interval [CI], 1.03–1.77) to an increased risk of new-onset CVD. The link (HR 1.24, 95% CI, 0.87–1.75) between TCAs and CHD events did not reach statistical significance. SSRI use did not link to CVD. While recommending replication of this important prospective study showing a link between TCAs and CVD, the authors concluded that existing mental illness did not explain this link. Rather, TCA administration best explained the excess disease burden.

ANTIPSYCHOTIC DRUGS AND CARDIAC TOXICITY

Evidence linking antipsychotic drugs to SCD is compel-ling. In 2001, Ray et al. (Ray et al., 2001) studied 481,744 Tennessee Medicaid enrollees from January 1, 1988, through December 31, 1993 (before the introduction of risperidone and other newer [atypical] antipsychotic drugs) with 26,749 person-years for current moderate-dose antipsy-chotic drug use (>100 mg thioridazine equivalents), 31,864 person-years for current low-dose antipsychotic drug use (<100 mg thioridazine equivalents), 37,881 person-years for use in the past year only, and 1,186,501 person-years for no antipsychotic drug use. There were 1,487 confirmed SCDs in this cohort. Current moderate-dose use compared with nonuse yielded a risk ratio of 2.39 (95% CI, 1.77–3.22; p < 0.001). This risk ratio was greater than for current low-dose (1.30; 95% CI, 0.98–1.72; p = 0.003) and former use (1.20; 95% CI, 0.91–1.58; p < 0.001). However, among current moderate-dose users with severe CVD, the risk ratio was 3.53 (95% CI, 1.66–7.51), yielding an additional 367 SCDs per 10,000 person-years of follow-up. In an accompanying editorial, Zarate and Patel (Zarate & Patel, 2001) pointed out the following:

1. Newer antipsychotic drugs are no less cardiotoxic than older ones;

2. Antipsychotic drug cardiotoxicity may be missed in phase 2 and phase 3 clinical trials because of the small number of patients and short trial duration;

3. Psychotropic drugs, including TCAs and some antipsy-chotic drugs (particularly thioridazine), are known to prolong the EKG QTc interval (see Box 52.3) and may produce PVT and its subtype *TdP*;

4. QTc interval prolongation may be found in up to 8% of psychiatric patients with women and older patients at the greatest risk;

5. Antipsychotic drug-induced ventricular fibrillation is thought to be the main contributor to SCD among patients taking TCAs and antipsychotic drugs;

6. Additional risk factors including hypokalemia, hypo-magnesemia, hypocalcemia, bradycardia, preexisting

CVD, congenital QTc interval prolongation, female sex, advancing age, baseline QTc interval prolongation, and co-administration of non-psychotropic drugs were associated with QTc interval prolongation;

7. Chronically psychotic patients have reduced life-expectancy independent of any drug administration; and

8. Depression may accompany psychosis and not be recognized, or depression may itself be a cardiovascular risk factor independent of antipsychotic drug treatment and contribute importantly to cardiac toxicity.

Strikingly absent from this editorial (written in 2001) is weight gain commonly associated with antidepressant and antipsychotic drug administration. In our observation, malpractice litigation is more likely to arise from psychotropic drug-induced metabolic problems than from psychotropic drug-induced cardiac arrhythmias.

In a 2009 paper, Ray et al. (Ray et al., 2009) extended their earlier work to look at patients taking newer (second-generation, atypical) antipsychotic drugs. They conducted a primary analysis in a retrospective cohort study of Tennessee Medicaid enrollees that included 44,218 and 46,089 baseline users of single typical and atypical antipsychotic drugs, respectively, and 186,600 matched nonusers. The authors performed a secondary analysis of users of antipsychotic drugs free of a baseline diagnosis of schizophrenia or related psychoses, and with whom nonusers were matched according to propensity score, to assess residual confounding due to factors linked to antipsychotic drug use. Ray et al. (Ray et al., 2009) found that current typical and atypical antipsychotic drug users had higher rates of SCD than did nonusers (adjusted incidence-rate ratio of 1.99; 95% CI, 1.68–2.34 and 2.26; 95% CI, 1.88–2.72, respectively). Users of atypical compared with typical antipsychotic drug users showed an incidence-rate ratio of 1.14 (95% CI, 0.94–1.39). There was no significantly increased risk of SCD for former antipsychotic drug users 1.13 (95% CI, 0.98–1.30). For both typical and atypical current antipsychotic drug users, the risk of SCD increased significantly with increasing dose. The incidence-rate ratios increased (p < 0.001) from 1.31 (95% CI, 0.97–1.77) for those taking low doses, to 2.42 (95% CI, 1.91–3.06) for those taking high doses of typical antipsychotic drugs. The incidence-rate ratios increased (p = 0.01) from 1.59 (95% CI, 1.03–2.46) for those taking low doses, to 2.86 (95% CI, 2.25–3.65) for those taking high doses of atypical antipsychotic drugs. In the cohort matched for propensity score, findings were similar. The authors concluded that both typical and atypical antipsychotic drug users had similar, dose-related increased risk of SCD.

Thus, a series of studies argues that psychiatrists and their patients face formidable cardiac challenges when considering prescribing and receiving TCAs and antipsychotic drugs. We review management approaches to those cardiac challenges in the following sections.

BRUGADA SYNDROME, SUDDEN CARDIAC DEATH, AND ANTIDEPRESSANT AND ANTIPSYCHOTIC DRUGS

We will briefly review antidepressant and antipsychotic drug–induced SCD in the Brugada syndrome (Sicouri & Antzelevitch, 2008). Brugada syndrome was first described in 1992 as a distinct EKG and clinical syndrome characterized by right bundle branch block (RBBB) and persistent ST-segment elevation in the right precordial leads plus SCD (Brugada & Brugada, 1992). Drug-induced Brugada syndrome is of intense interest (Postema et al., 2009; Yap, Behr, & Camm, 2009), with the website Brugada Drugs (www.brugadadrugs. org) dedicated to the drug-induced aspects of this syndrome. Drugs to be avoided or preferably avoided by Brugada syndrome patients are listed in Box 52.1 (Postema et al., 2009).

EKG manifestations of this syndrome may be intermittent. Therefore, a normal EKG does not rule it out. Fever and low heart rates may allow this syndrome to become manifest, and provocative testing with infusions of sodium channel (fast-channel) blocking drugs (flecainide, ajmaline, procainamide) may uncover the diagnostic EKG pattern. Drugs (e.g., quinidine) that block the myocardial cell action potential transient outward potassium current (see Vieweg et al., 2009) appear to reduce arrhythmias.

To diagnose an individual with the Brugada syndrome, look for the EKG pattern described above, with at least one clinical feature, including syncope, prior cardiac arrest, PVT or ventricular fibrillation, and/or a family history of SCD in member[s] under 45 years of age (Yap, Behr, & Camm, 2009). This syndrome is familial (more common among men, contrasted with *TdP*, more common among women), displaying an autosomal dominant transmission mode, with incomplete penetrance and an incidence of 5–66/10,000.

The Brugada syndrome is one of the ion-channel disorders, the so-called channelopathies, usually found in structurally normal hearts. Early interest was in the congenital long QT syndrome (Vincent, 1999), with subsequent attention paid to the Brugada syndrome. Now there is a short QT syndrome (Patel & Pavri, 2008), but this syndrome has not been linked to psychotropic drug administration.

CARDIAC RISKS OF ANTIDEPRESSANT DRUGS

Several years ago, we reviewed the cardiovascular side effects of newer antidepressant drugs (primarily SSRIs) (Fernandez, 2007) and pointed their superior cardiovascular safety

---

Box 52.1 DRUGS TO AVOID IN PATIENTS WITH BRUGADA SYNDROME (POSTEMA ET AL., 2009)

AVOID: amitriptyline, clomipramine, desipramine, lithium, loxapine, nortriptyline, trifluoperazine

Preferably AVOID: carbamazepine, cyamemazine, doxepin, fluoxetine, imipramine, maprotiline, perphenazine, phenytoin, thioridazine, antianginal drugs, and others.

compared with older antidepressant drugs, particularly TCAs. In this review, we described complications of SSRI administration, including the serotonin syndrome, tachycardia, arrhythmias, and other cardiovascular findings.

We reviewed antidepressant drug–induced blood pressure changes and their management in 1996 (Vieweg & Nicholson, 1996; Vieweg, 1996). TCAs have the most significant cardiovascular side effects of any of the antidepressant drugs currently available in the United States. These side effects are most manifest in subjects with preexisting CVD. Hypotension, with or without orthostasis, is the most common cardiovascular adverse effect, and conduction disturbances and ventricular arrhythmias are the most life-threatening side effects. TCAs' quinidine-like action accounts for conduction and rhythm disturbances. Monoamine oxidase inhibitors (MAOIs) commonly induce hypotension, with or without orthostasis. Hypertensive crises and the serotonin syndrome are the most serious cardiac adverse effects associated with MAOI administration, and patients using these agents require dietary and concomitant drug restrictions to minimize adverse effects. Rarely, spontaneous severe hypertension may occur without dietary or drug–drug interaction. Bupropion may increase blood pressure, particularly in those with preexisting hypertension. Trazodone may be associated with ventricular arrhythmias. Nefazodone (no longer used much in the U.S. because of adverse liver effects) and SSRIs may contribute to adverse cardiac drug–drug interactions. Co-administration of SSRIs and MAOIs may produce the serotonin syndrome and vasomotor instability. Venlafaxine may increase supine diastolic blood pressure, and, according to the manufacturer, such subjects require blood pressure monitoring. Periodic blood pressure assessment should probably be a routine part of patient care among those taking antidepressant drugs—particularly elderly patients. Recently, Mark et al. (Mark et al., 2011) documented that about half of geriatric patients receiving antidepressant drugs face drug–drug interactions.

QT INTERVAL PROLONGATION AND TDP WITH NEWER ANTIPSYCHOTIC ANTIDEPRESSANT DRUGS

Well known to be associated with some of the older antipsychotic and antidepressant drugs such as haloperidol and amitriptyline, QTc interval prolongation and *TdP* are also associated with some of the newer drugs from these categories. In 2011, an FDA Safety Announcement advised health care professionals and patients that citalopram should no longer be used at doses above 40mg/day because in higher doses the drug can unfavorably alter the electrical activity of the heart, and higher doses provide no additional benefit in the treatment of depression. The same year, the FDA directed the manufacturer to add a warning to the quetiapine (Seroquel) labeling about quetiapine-induced QTc interval prolongation and the potential for drug-induced *TdP*. Ziprasidone was associated with a dose-dependent QTc interval prolongation in the Pfizer 054 study specifically designed for this purpose (Psychopharmacological Drugs Advisory Committee, 2000). In a recent study (Potkin et al., 2013), iloperidone was associated with a greater increase

in QTc interval than competitor drugs (quetiapine and ziprasidone), but the increase was not clinically significant. Readers interested in more information are invited to the review by Hasnain and Vieweg (Hasnain & Vieweg, 2014).

Both citalopram and escitalopram cause dose-dependent QTc interval prolongation, which is greater for citalopram than escitalopram. While the FDA issued warning only for citalopram, the Medicines and Healthcare Products Regulatory Agency (MHRA) of the United Kingdom issued the same safety warning for both citalopram and escitalopram (Medicines and Healthcare Products Regulatory Agency 2011). The threshold for clinical significance of the QTc interval is an absolute duration of more than 500 milliseconds, or a change from baseline of more than 60 milliseconds (FDA, 2005). The warnings did not specify whether any subjects exceeded these thresholds for either drug.

We reviewed the literature and found no cases of citalopram-induced SCD among patients taking up to 60 mg/day of citalopram and free of risk factors for QTc interval prolongation and *TdP* (Vieweg et al., 2012). About 500 escitalopram overdoses and nearly 600 citalopram overdoses have been described, without serious cardiac sequelae or deaths due to either drug (Howland, 2011a; Howland, 2011b). Less than one-third of citalopram overdoses presented with QTc interval prolongation. In one study, 14% of escitalopram overdoses presented with QTc interval prolongation. In another study, the proportion of prolonged QTc intervals associated with escitalopram overdoses (1.7%) was not significantly different from that associated with citalopram overdoses (3.7%).

In several reviews of psychotropic drug–associated QTc interval prolongation and *TdP*, we noted that, while a drug may be associated with QTc interval prolongation, *TdP* occurs mostly when other risk factors besides the drug are present (Vieweg et al., 2012; Vieweg et al., 2013c; Kogut et al., 2013; Vieweg et al., 2013b, Hasnain & Vieweg, 2014). Box 52.2 lists the important risk factors. We will review each below.

Age

Su et al. (Su et al., 2006) assessed QT interval aging trends in healthy elderly Taiwanese. They manually measured the QT

Box 52.2 **RISK FACTORS FOR QT INTERVAL PROLONGATION**

1. Age—elderly at greatest risk

2. Circadian variation—nighttime period of greatest risk

3. Sex—women more vulnerable than men

4. Cardiovascular disease—presence considerably increases risk

5. Electrolyte abnormalities—particularly hypokalemia and hypomagnesemia

6. Pharmacodynamic and pharmacokinetic factors—drug–drug interaction, concomitant use of QTc interval-prolonging drugs, hepatic impairment, and poor metabolizer status

interval from the beginning of the QRS complex to the end of the T-wave. Study subjects comprised 115 persons (90 men and 25 women). Serial QTc interval measurements at baseline, two years, and four years were 422 ± 20, 425 ± 21, and 429 ± 27 msec, respectively. The QTc interval increased significantly during the four year follow-up (p = 0.001). The authors concluded that the QTc interval increases progressively with age.

However, conclusions and regulatory guidelines about drug-induced QTc interval prolongation in studies and clinical practice comprise periods of weeks and months, not years. Even though the FDA wants drug-induced group mean QTc interval lengthening not to exceed five msec before approving a medication for marketing (Darpo, Nebout, & Sager, 2006), individual patient/drug changes of less than 20 msec may not be clinically significant, due, in part, to differences in individual measurements (Camm, Malik, & Yap, 2004). Thus, changes in the QTc interval over four years as documented by Su et al. (Su et al., 2006) may have limited clinical utility.

Circadian Variation

The QTc interval varies throughout the day and night, with nighttime values about 20 msec longer than daytime measurements, due to differences in sympathetic and parasympathetic tone (Browne et al., 1983; Morganroth et al., 1991). In 20 normal subjects, daily QTc interval variation was 76 ± 19 msec (range 35–108 msec). However, CVD may increase this range (Morganroth et al., 1991).

Sex

Before puberty, the QTc interval is the same for both sexes (Tutar et al., 1998). Compared with adolescent girls, the QTc interval in boys shortens by about 20 msec at puberty and this shortening appears to be androgen-driven. This sex difference remains until ages 50–55 years, when declining male testosterone values narrow these differences, but differences may continue even into old age. Based on the usual cardiovascular risk factors, we would expect about 45% of cases of *TdP* to occur in women; but, about 70% of cases of *TdP* occur in women, particularly older women (Vincent, 1999). In a recent review of subjects 60 years or older who developed QTc interval prolongation, PVT/*TdP*, and/or SCD while taking antidepressant or antipsychotic drugs or a combination of them, almost four-fifths of subjects were women (Vieweg et al., 2009).

Age and Cardiovascular Disease

Elderly men and women tend to have longer QTc intervals than their younger counterparts, even when both groups are free of CVD (Khan et al., 1998). Age-matched patients with CVD tend to have longer QTc intervals than those free of CVD (Khan et al., 1998).

Electrolytes

Electrolyte abnormalities, especially hypokalemia and hypomagnesemia, may cause or worsen QTc interval prolongation (Compton et al., 1996; Hatta et al., 1999; Hatta et al., 2000). Hypokalemia prolongs the cardiac action potential and may cause early afterdepolarizations (EADs) leading to *TdP* (see Box 52.3). Diuretics, especially the thiazides, are the most common cause of hypokalemia. Other causes include vomiting, diarrhea, postprandial states, exercise, and agitation.

Box 52.3 BASIC CARDIAC ELECTROPHYSIOLOGY FOR QTC INTERVAL PROLONGATION AND POLYMORPHIC VENTRICULAR TACHYCARDIA/*TORSADE DE POINTES*

Much of the material reported below is drawn from "Proarrhythmic Risk with Antipsychotic and Antidepressant Drugs: Implications in the Elderly" (Vieweg et al., 2009).

The Cardiac Conduction System and the Electrocardiogram

The heart has three important systems: (1) an energy system providing the force necessary to deliver cardiac contraction, (2) a conduction system consisting of special cardiac cells that electrically coordinate cardiac contraction to optimize cardiac output, and (3) the pump or (mechanical) pumping action itself. Antidepressant and antipsychotic drugs may have an impact on cardiac performance by altering any or all of these three systems. However, for purposes of this discussion, we will largely focus on the cardiac conduction system. This review is a condensation of several of our earlier publications on this topic (Vieweg et al., 2009; Vieweg et al., 2011c; Vieweg, 2002, Vieweg, 2003; Vieweg & McDaniel, 2003a; Vieweg & McDaniel, 2003b; Vieweg & McDaniel, 2003c; Vieweg & McDaniel, 2003d; Vieweg & Wood, 2004).

FIGURE 52.1

The standard EKG intervals (PR, QRS, and QT intervals) are usually best seen in limb lead II (voltage between the left leg electrode and the right arm electrode) and appear in Figure 52.1. The summed electrical charges generated within myocardial cells produce these EKG intervals. The QT interval and the effects that antidepressant and antipsychotic drugs have on it are of great interest to the psychiatrist.

(continued)

Box 52.1 (CONTINUED)

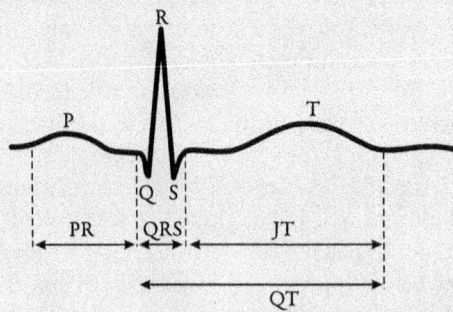

Figure 52.1 Representative lead II EKG showing standard intervals. The "P" wave is atrial electrical *depolarization* and just precedes mechanical right and left atrial contraction. The "QRS" interval is electrical ventricular *depolarization* and just precedes mechanical left and right ventricular contraction. The "ST" segment is the isoelectric portion of ventricular *repolarization,* and the "T" wave is the directional component of ventricular *repolarization.* The "QRS" interval, "ST" segment, and "T" wave on the surface EKG make up the "QT interval." This interval consists of the "QRS" interval and "JT interval" ("ST" segment and "T" wave). Most of the "QT interval" represents ventricular *repolarization.*

FIGURE 52.2

The tangent method is the most popular way to calculate or measure the QT interval (Figure 52.2) (Postema et al., 2008). Not defined in the caption are U waves that are associated with hypokalemia and may fuse with the T-wave in severe hypokalemia (El-Sherif & Turitto, 2011). We know empirically that the length of the QT interval varies inversely with heart rate: the slower the heart rate, the longer the QT interval. Several group-derived formulae are used to correct (normalize) the QT interval (QTc interval) for heart rate (Goldenberg, Moss, & Zareba, 2006). The Bazett formula (Bazett, 1920) (QTc interval = QT interval in seconds divided by the square root of the RR interval in seconds) is the most popular current method used to calculate the QTc interval. The recommended Bazett-corrected QTc interval measurements in adults appear in Table 52.6 (Goldenberg, Moss, & Zareba, 2006). While seemingly beyond the expertise of the psychiatrist, accurately measuring the QTc interval may even be challenging for the internist or cardiologist (Viskin et al., 2005). Therefore, it behooves the psychiatrist to be familiar with the issues and language surrounding QTc interval calculation so as to best engage the assistance of the interested cardiac electrophysiologist as necessary.

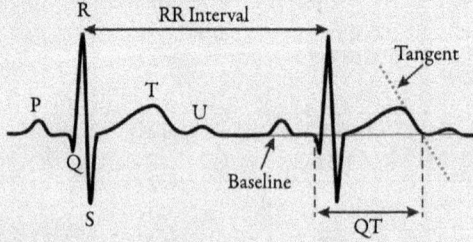

Figure 52.2 Shown is the tangent method of measuring the QT interval using EKG lead II. See Figure 52.1 for definitions appearing in Figure 52.2 except for the "U" wave (see text). Draw a tangent to the steepest slope of the last limb of the "T" wave. The intersection of the tangent with the baseline defines the end of the "QT" interval. (Figure after Postema et al., 2008.)

Table 52.6 RECOMMENDED BAZETT-CORRECTED QTC MEASUREMENTS TO DIAGNOSE QT INTERVAL PROLONGATION, ACCORDING TO GOLDENBERG AND COLLEAGUES (GOLDENBERG, MOSS, & ZAREBA, 2006)

RATING	ADULT MEN (MSEC)	ADULT WOMEN (MSEC)
Normal	<430	<450
Borderline	430–450	450–470
Prolonged	>450	>470

(continued)

Box 52.1 (CONTINUED)

FIGURE 52.3

The action potential of a single ventricular muscle appears in Figure 52.3. Sodium (Na⁺), calcium (Ca²⁺), and potassium (K⁺) ionic movements are very important in understanding the shape and direction of a cardiac cell action potential. These ions are unevenly distributed between the interstitium and interior of the cardiac myocyte due to its cell membrane that selectively limits ionic movement between the cell and interstitium (Fu, Clemo, & Ellenbogen, 1998). Ion channels are made of specialized proteins selective for certain ions. Ion channel activity is influenced by such factors as membrane potential, neurohormones, adenosine triphosphate supply, and certain drugs.

Cell *depolarization* (QRS interval or duration on the surface EKG; Figure 52.1) derives from a net inward flux of sodium and then calcium ions. Cell *repolarization* (JT interval on the surface EKG; Figure 52.1) derives from a net outward flux of potassium, mainly via the rapid delayed rectifier potassium channels (I_{Kr}). Reducing or slowing outward potassium currents by any agent, drug, condition, or process may prolong (lengthen or delay) *repolarization*, leaving the patient vulnerable to PVT or *TdP*.

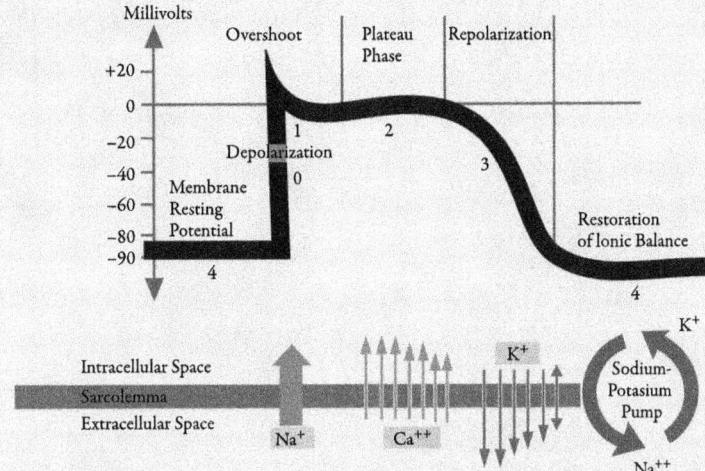

Figure 52.3 Myocardial action potential. Shown is the action potential of a ventricular muscle cell. The numbers 0, 1, 2, 3, and 4 represent the phases of the action potential. The membrane resting potential is largely determined by the ratio of extracellular to intracellular potassium (phase 4). This phase is associated with ventricular diastole. The sudden surge of sodium (sodium "fast" channel) into the ventricular muscle cell (phase 0) represents the onset of cellular *depolarization* and is the rapid *depolarization* phase. The slope of phase 0 represents the maximum rate of *depolarization* of the cell and is known as Vmax. Phase 0 is due to the opening of the fast sodium channels causing a rapid increase in the membrane conductance to sodium and the rapid influx of sodium ions into the cell, creating sodium current. The QRS interval (ventricular *depolarization*) on the surface EKG (see Figure 52.1) represents the initial electrical energy of the action potential of all the myocardial muscle cells.

Phase 1 of the action starts with the inactivation of the fast sodium channel. Following this phase, the "plateau" phase appears (phase 2) and is sustained by the inward movement of calcium (calcium "slow" channels) and outward movement of potassium through the slow, delayed rectifier potassium channels. During phase 3 (*repolarization*), the outward flow of potassium using the rapid delayed rectifier potassium channel (I_{Kr}) is the main ion channel causing the cell to repolarize and return to the membrane resting potential (phase 4).

FIGURE 52.4

Sequential changes on the surface EKG and cardiac cell action potential leading to PVT/*TdP* appear in Figure 52.4 (Viskin et al., 2003). Enhancing inward sodium or calcium currents or decreasing outward potassium currents may lead to QT interval prolongation (Tan et al., 1995). The most common mechanism of drug-induced PVT and *TdP* is potassium channel blockade.

The antipsychotic drug thioridazine of the phenothiazine family primarily blocks the rapid component (I_{Kr}) of outward potassium flow, causing inhomogeneous lengthening of the cardiac cell action potential, QT interval prolongation, early after depolarizations (EADs), and *TdP* (Yap & Camm, 2000). The quinidine-like (ion blocking) properties of TCAs primarily act on sodium influx during the early phase of the cardiac cell action potential (phase "0" or sodium "fast" channel) and may produce QRS widening as found in TCA overdose (Boehnert & Lovejoy, 1985). Secondarily, TCAs may block calcium influx (calcium "slow" channel) and potassium efflux during phase 3 (Figure 52.3) of the cardiac myocyte action potential, leading to JT interval (Figure 52.1) lengthening with subsequent prolongation of the QT interval. Therefore, QT interval prolongation may occur after TCA administration by at least two mechanisms: (1) widening of the

(*continued*)

Box 52.1 (CONTINUED)

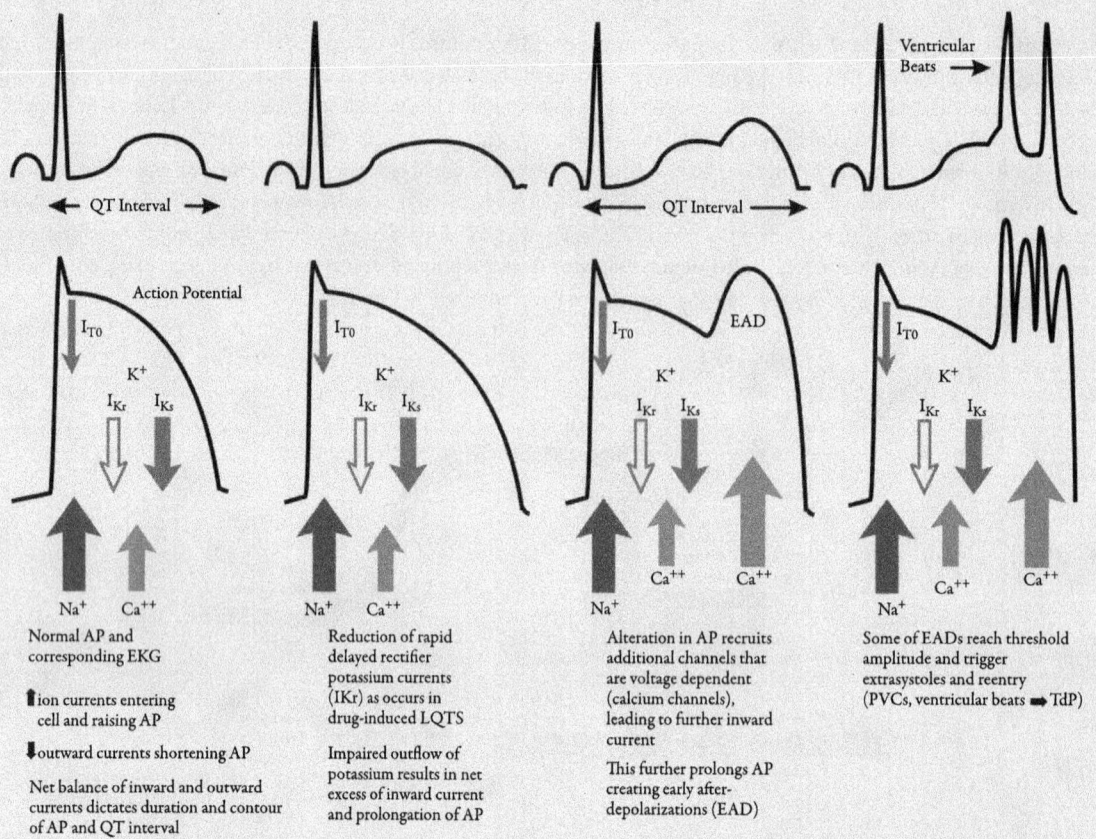

Figure 52.4 EKG, myocardial cell action potential, and *TdP* (data from Viskin et al., 2003). *Abbreviations*: EKG = electrocardiogram; AP = action potential; Na⁺ = sodium; K⁺ = potassium; Ca²⁺ = calcium; I_{To} = transient outward potassium current; I_{Kr} = rapid delayed rectifier potassium current; I_{Ks} = slow delayed rectifier potassium current; LQTS = long QT syndrome; EAD = early after depolarization of the AP; PVC = premature ventricular contraction

QRS interval during *depolarization*, and (2) lengthening of the JT interval during *repolarization*. It is lengthening of the JT interval rather than widening of the QRS complex that leaves the patient vulnerable to PVT and *TdP*. Summation of TCA secondary effects on the QT interval and thioridazine-like primary effects on the QT interval may act together to further lengthen the QT interval and lead to PVT and *TdP*.

FIGURE 52.5

The typical EKG features of PVT of the *TdP* type appear in Figure 52.5. The ventricular complexes appear wide and ventricular beats appearing close together. Cyclic alterations of the QRS electrical axis (due to migrating electrical foci) best explain the varying QRS morphology (twisting of the points—*torsade de pointes*) in *TdP*. Both the QT and QTc interval commonly exceed 500 ms in *TdP* (Bednar et al., 2001), and the most common QTc interval is 600–649 msec.

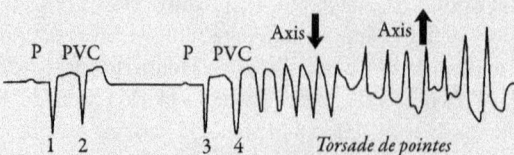

Figure 52.5 *Torsade de pointes.* Shown is the typical pattern found in *TdP* type of PVT. A sinus beat with a normal QRS interval (1) is followed by premature ventricular contraction (PVC) (2) with a short coupling interval. After a compensatory pause, another sinus beat (3) with a normal QRS interval is followed by another PVC (4) with a short coupling interval. The second PVC (4) is the first beat in a PVT of the *TdP* type. The sequence of beats 1–4 comprises the typical EKG features of short-long-short R-R intervals followed by *TdP*.

Pharmacodynamic and Pharmacokinetic Factors

Pharmacokinetic and pharmacodynamic factors that may potentiate (or inhibit) the effect of a drug are of utmost importance when prescribing drugs associated with QTc interval prolongation. Combining drugs with a potential to cause QTc interval prolongation would theoretically increase the risk of QTc prolongation and should be avoided. Metabolic inhibition of a drug would increase its blood level and thus increase the risk of toxicity (except in rare cases when a metabolite is associated with the risk). Drug–drug interactions are the most common reason for metabolic inhibition. Hepatic impairment is another reason for metabolic inhibition. Renal impairment would be pertinent to consider for drugs primarily excreted renally. Five to 10% of European Americans are "poor metabolizers" (pharmacokinetic factor) for certain drugs, with the CYP450 isoenzyme 2D6 most commonly explaining these differences in metabolism. This possibility should be entertained if a patient does not tolerate the usual doses of a drug well.

HOSPITAL SETTINGS

Recently, a scientific statement from the American Heart Association and the American College of Cardiology Foundation that focused on prevention of *TdP* in hospital settings was published jointly in *Circulation* (Drew et al., 2010a) and the *Journal of the American College of Cardiology* (Drew et al., 2010b). Box 52.4 provides their list of drugs having a risk of causing *TdP*. For readers interested in a more detailed list of medications associated with QTc interval prolongation and risk of *TdP*, visit the CredibleMeds website, www.qtdrugs.org, provided by the Arizona Center for Education and Research on Therapeutics (AZCERT) website.

Box 52.4 **DRUGS THAT HAVE A RISK OF CAUSING *TDP* (DREW ET AL., 2010A; DREW ET AL., 2010B)**

GENERIC NAME	BRAND NAME(S)	CLINICAL USE
Arsenic trioxide	Trisenox	Cancer/leukemia
Bepridil	Vascor	Antianginal
Chloroquine	Aralen	Antimalarial
Chlorpromazine	Thorazine	Antipsychotic, schizophrenia, antiemetic
Cisapride	Propulsid	Gastrointestinal stimulant
Clarithromycin	Biaxin	Antibiotic
Disopyramide	Norpace	Antiarrhythmic
Dofetilide	Tikosyn	Antiarrhythmic
Droperidol	Inapsine	Sedative, antiemetic
Erythromycin	E.E.S., Erythrocin	Antibiotic, increase gastrointestinal motility
Halofantrine	Halfan	Antimalarial
Haloperidol	Haldol	Antipsychotic, schizophrenia, agitation
Ibutilide	Covert	Antiarrhythmic
Levomethadyl	Orlaam	Opiate agonist, pain control, narcotic dependence
Mesoridazine	Serentil	Antipsychotic, schizophrenia
Methadone	Dolophine, Methadose	Opiate agonist, pain control, narcotic dependence
Pentamidine	NebuPent, Pentam	Antiinfective, pneumocystis pneumonia
Pimozide	Orap	Antipsychotic, Tourette tics
Procainamide	Pronestyl, Procan	Antiarrhythmic
Quinidine	Quinaglute, Cardioquin	Antiarrhythmic
Sotalol	Betapace	Antiarrhythmic
Sparfloxacin	Zagam	Antibiotic
Thioridazine	Mellaril	Antipsychotic, schizophrenia

HYPERTROPHIC CARDIOMYOPATHY

Although not traditionally considered a risk factor for QTc interval prolongation among subjects receiving antidepressant and antipsychotic drugs, cardiac hypertrophy and left ventricular outflow tract obstruction may delay ventricular depolarization and repolarization, thereby prolonging the QT and QTc intervals (Johnson et al., 2011). Johnson et al. (Johnson et al., 2011) found QTc interval prolongation (>480 msec) in one out of eight subjects with hypertrophic cardiomyopathy. Therefore, when considering administration of psychotropic drugs with the potential to prolong the QTc interval to subjects with hypertrophic cardiomyopathy, obtain a baseline EKG.

ILLNESS SEVERITY

Recently, our group has looked at macrolide antibiotics and their relationship with QTc interval prolongation and *TdP* in an effort to study a more uniform population (Vieweg et al., 2013a; Hancox et al., 2013a; Hancox et al., 2013b). These papers include more than 60 case reports. Elderly women with heart disease are particularly vulnerable to QTc interval prolongation and *TdP*. Also, we developed an illness severity scale, as follows: (1) 1+ managed as outpatient, (2) 2+ required hospitalization, (3) 3+ required admission to the ICU and/or careful cardiac monitoring, and (4) 4+ required some aspect of life support other than cardioversion. Illness severity is highly predictive of drug-related QTc interval prolongation and *TdP*, and more predictive than prevalence/incidence studies employing principles of parametric statistics. Of course, illness severity incorporates risk factors, but it seems to be a new way to think about drug-related QTc interval prolongation and *TdP*. Further studies are needed to help understand this possible association.

SPECIAL TOPICS IN PSYCHOSOMATIC MEDICINE AND THE HEART

SSRIs, PREGNANCY, AND CONGENITAL CARDIAC MALFORMATIONS

About 10–15% of women experience depression during pregnancy, and 3–6% of women use SSRIs during pregnancy (Wichman et al., 2009). Untreated depression during pregnancy may link to low birth weight, preterm delivery, and lower Apgar scores; poor prenatal care; not recognizing or reporting signs of labor; and increased risk of fetal abuse, neonaticide, and maternal suicide (Wichman et al., 2009). There has been a flurry of recent interest in the risk of cardiac malformations among women taking SSRIs during pregnancy.

Alwan & Friedman (Alwan & Friedman, 2009) comprehensively reviewed the literature on exposure to SSRIs during the first trimester of pregnancy and fetal malformations. They grouped the available literature into four categories: (1) exposure Cohort (teratogen information service) studies, (2) studies based on linked administrative records, (3) population-based prospective cohort studies, and (4) retrospective case-control

studies. They concluded that that first-trimester maternal paroxetine treatment may increase the risk for cardiac anomalies about 1.5-fold to about 1%, considering a general population incidence of approximately 0.7% for the occurrence of congenital heart defects. The authors noted that it was difficult to determine the magnitude of risk for major malformations more generally or the risks associated with use of other SSRIs, as available data were inconsistent. More recently, Gentile (Gentile, 2011) specifically looked at the methodological quality of the data on the potential teratogenic effects of SSRIs. He identified 16 peer-reviewed studies suggesting an SSRI-associated teratogenic risk. He noted several limitations in the available data and concluded that the hypothesized teratogenicity of SSRIs remains undemonstrated.

Paroxetine

Among the SSRIs, paroxetine has received particular attention. Wurst et al. (Wurst et al., 2009) undertook a meta-analysis with a focus on first-trimester use of paroxetine and the prevalence of congenital, specifically cardiac, defects. The authors found an increased prevalence of aggregated congenital defects (prevalence odds ratio [POR] 1.24; 95% CI, 1.08–1.43) with paroxetine use. However, the increased prevalence of combined cardiac defects (POR 1.46; 95% CI, 1.17–1.82) may best explain this association. The small proportion of studies reporting specific cardiac lesions precluded statistical analysis. However, Wurst et al. (Wurst et al., 2009) tabulated the POR of selected reported specific cardiac defects and first-trimester use of paroxetine. Specific cardiac defects included (1) septal defects (atrial septal defect and ventricular septal defect), (2) bulbus cordis anomalies and anomalies of cardiac septal closure, (3) ventricular septal defect, (4) right ventricular outflow tract obstruction defects, (5) conotruncal defects, and (6) left ventricular outflow obstruction defects.

In a population-based case-control study, Bakker et al. (Bakker et al., 2010) evaluated the association of first-trimester paroxetine use and congenital cardiac defects (678 cases of isolated cardiac defects [first-trimester paroxetine exposure 1.5%] and 615 controls [first-trimester paroxetine exposure 1.0%]). After excluding mothers who used paroxetine outside the first trimester, or were exposed to another SSRI, the authors found no significantly increased risk for cardiac defects overall but did find a significantly increased risk for atrial septal defects (3 exposed cases; adjusted odds ratio, 5.7; 95% CI, 1.4–23.7).

General Comment

Scialli (Scialli, 2010) noted that the U.S. Food and Drug Administration and the manufacturer of paroxetine (brand name Paxil) agreed to classifying this drug as Pregnancy Category D (positive evidence of human fetal risk based on adverse reaction data from investigational or marketing experience or studies in humans, but potential benefits may warrant use of the drug in pregnant women despite potential risks). The package insert stated that epidemiology studies had shown that infants born to women exposed to paroxetine during the first trimester had increased cardiovascular malformations, particularly atrial septal defects. Scialli (Scialli, 2010) pointed out that septal defects are prone to diagnostic bias. For example, ventricular septal defects may be found in up to 5% of newborns, with the vast majority of the defects representing small muscular defects that close spontaneously without intervention. Scialli (Scialli, 2010) then remarked, based on the evidence reviewed by Wurst et al. (Wurst et al., 2009) and others, that the scientific evidence does not support the conclusion that paroxetine causes cardiac defects.

HOW DO WE MOVE BEYOND QTC INTERVAL PROLONGATION AS THE BEST ESTIMATE OF THE RISK FOR PSYCHOTROPIC DRUG–INDUCED PVT/*TdP*?

By mid-2011, AstraZeneca, in concert with the FDA, altered the package insert for Seroquel (quetiapine) to reflect new concerns about the capacity of this drug to induce QTc interval prolongation. The package insert was changed after the FDA learned of reports of ventricular arrhythmias in 17 patients who took more than the recommended dose of quetiapine. Though QTc interval prolongation should not be problematic at recommended doses, quetiapine should be avoided in combination with at least 12 other medications linked to cardiac arrhythmias associated with SCD. Drugs not to be co-administered with quetiapine include: (a) the antiarrhythmic agents amiodarone, procainamide, quinidine, and sotalol; (b) antimicrobial medications gatifloxacin, moxifloxacin, and pentamidine; (c) synthetic opioids levomethadyl acetate and methadone; and (d) the antipsychotic drugs chlorpromazine, thioridazine, and ziprasidone. The package insert offers a note of caution in administering quetiapine to the elderly and patients with heart disease.

In our earlier section on QTc interval prolongation and PVT/*TdP*, we listed a series of risk factors for these EKG changes: hypokalemia or hypomagnesemia, female sex, old age, presence of congenital QTc interval prolongation, personal history of presyncope or syncope, family history of SCD, and bradycardia. We pointed out that even among drugs known to induce QTc interval prolongation and PVT/*TdP*, one or more of the above risk factors are almost always present when PVT/*TdP* is found. That is, the drug alone is highly unlikely to lead to serious cardiac arrhythmias or SCD when taken as prescribed in an otherwise healthy person.

Concerns about QTc interval prolongation embrace general principles of medicine. That is, the more immediately serious the illness, the more willing we are to try interventions with significant side effects; and the less immediately serious the illness, the less willing we are to use drugs with significant adverse effects. The incidence of drug-induced proarrhythmias with non-cardiovascular drugs is quite low (≤1 in 100,000) (Darpo, 2010). A drug at substantive risk to prolong the QTc interval may still be approved by regulatory agencies if the medical condition it treats has immediate life-threatening or life-shortening dimensions. This principle applies to some currently approved antiarrhythmic agents.

Although clinicians are generally most familiar with the Bazett formula (QTc = QT/RR$^{0.5}$, discussed earlier) in estimating the QTc interval, the Fridericia correction (QTc = QT/RR$^{0.33}$) is the method recommended by the FDA in clinical trials of non-antiarrhythmic drugs (FDA, 2005). Our understanding of the cardiac pathophysiology underlying QTc interval prolongation continues to advance. The congenital long QT syndromes represent rare genetic disorders deriving from gene mutations encoding cardiac ion channels and lead to ventricular action potential prolongation and repolarization delay, resulting in great risk for life-threatening PVT/*TdP* (Hedley et al., 2009). Mutations disrupting a variety of ion currents, including I_{Ks}, I_{Kr}, and I_{Na}, cause long congenital QT syndromes. Drug-induced QTc interval prolongation, in contrast, almost always involves I_{Kr} (rapid component of the delayed rectifier potassium current). Drugs with diverse structures block this KCNH2 channel. Those drug classes include antiarrhythmic drugs, antipsychotic medications, antibiotic and antimicrobial drugs, and antihistamines, and can exhibit a phenotype similar to that of carriers of KCNH2 (congenital long QT syndrome 2) (Mohammad et al., 1997; Kannankeril, Roden, & Darbar, 2010). The FDA has emphasized the need to find new methods of recognizing and measuring the QTc interval–prolonging effect of new drugs. Recently, more than 50 prescription drugs have been found to prolong the QTc interval, and more than 30 of them have been associated with PVT/*TdP* (Parvez & Darbar, 2011). Great attention has been given to the QTc interval because it is a surrogate marker of I_{Kr}. Blocking this ion channel may lead to QTc interval prolongation and possibly, progression to PVT/*TdP*. However, the QT interval is a marker for the total duration of ventricular repolarization and ignores abnormalities of the repolarization sequence. Also, the QTc interval requires normalization for heart rate because of the inherent confounding phenomena such as QT lag and hysteresis (Franz et al., 1988; Pueyo et al., 2003).

Digital EKGs have become available in recent years. Using this technology to assess T-wave morphology has become more important in predicting adverse cardiac events among patients with both the congenital and acquired (drug-induced) forms of the long QT syndrome (Couderc, 2009). Recently, Couderc et al. (Couderc et al., 2011) investigated repolarization morphology in both congenital and acquired forms of long QT syndrome and showed that phenotypical expression of KCNH2 mutations and the effect of I_{Kr}-inhibitory drugs are specific on the surface EKG (model for the LQT2 showed that left slope was associated with the presence of the KCNH2 mutation). This opens an exciting frontier for clinicians and investigators interested in psychotropic drug-induced or drug-associated PVT/*TdP* to better predict the drugs and circumstances placing psychiatric patients at increased risk for life-threatening cardiac arrhythmias.

DOES AGE ALONE EXPLAIN INCREASED RISK OF SERIOUS ADVERSE CARDIAC EVENTS IN ELDERLY RECEIVING ANTIPSYCHOTIC DRUGS?

In 2005, the FDA issued an advisory stating that atypical (second-generation) antipsychotic drugs, versus placebo, significantly increased the risk of death among the cognitively impaired elderly (FDA, 2005). Typical (first generation) antipsychotic drugs were subsequently included in this concern.

Wang et al. (Wang et al., 2007) studied a large population of elderly from the Pennsylvania Pharmaceutical Assistance Contract for the Elderly Program using these outcome variables: (1) acute MI, (2) ventricular arrhythmia, (3) cerebrovascular events, (4) CHF, (5) pneumonia, and (6) other serious bacterial infections. The authors sought to determine whether the elderly newly started on typical versus atypical antipsychotic drugs had greater risks of adverse cardiac, cerebrovascular, and infection outcomes. They found that typical antipsychotic drugs had a modestly increased risk of developing ventricular arrhythmias and cerebrovascular events compared with atypical antipsychotic drugs.

In 2008, Setoguchi et al. (Setoguchi et al., 2008) sought to determine potential causes of higher mortality among elderly patients taking typical and atypical antipsychotic drugs among all British Columbia residents aged 65 years and older who started any antipsychotic drug between 1996 and 2004. The authors found that the greater risk of cardiovascular death best explained about half of the excess mortality among those elderly taking typical antipsychotic drugs.

Mehta et al. (Mehta et al., 2011) compared the risk of serious adverse cardiac events in the elderly taking typical and atypical antipsychotic drugs. They found a moderate increased risk of serious adverse cardiac events among elderly adults taking typical antipsychotic drugs compared with those taking atypical agents. The authors emphasized the need for health care professionals to carefully evaluate the risk–benefit ratio of antipsychotic drugs before prescribing these drugs to a vulnerable population. Psychiatry Drug Alerts (Anonymous, 2011) hypothesized that this finding may be explained by the greater risk of QTc interval prolongation and subsequent ventricular arrhythmias of typical compared with atypical antipsychotic drugs.

When asked for inpatient consultation, the referring clinician invariably wants a quick fix and does not want a recommendation to put the patient under one-on-one nursing observation and withhold medications. Medications then narrow down to sedatives (usually benzodiazepines) and antipsychotic drugs (both typical and atypical agents). Surgeons are most familiar with the typical antipsychotic drug haloperidol and hope that will be your recommendation. If sedation is important, haloperidol would be a poor choice since it is one of the less sedating typical antipsychotic agents. This property likely accounts for haloperidol's increased risk, particularly when administered intravenously in high doses, of inducing QTc interval prolongation and PVT/*TdP* (Vieweg et al., 2009).

In the outpatient setting, behavioral problems in the nursing home are a common stimulus for psychiatric consultation. Behavioral psychologists are becoming more available for nursing home consultation, and a behavioral approach to agitation may be the best initial intervention if time permits (Snowden, Sato, & Roy-Byrne, 2003).

PANIC ATTACKS, THE CARDIOLOGIST, AND THE PSYCHIATRIST

An all-too-common problem is to receive a phone call from a patient with known heart disease and/or cardiac arrhythmias complaining of new-onset "panic attacks" with fear or a sense of impending doom, racing heart, and difficulty breathing. The patient may ask the psychiatrist or cardiologist to phone in an antianxiety agent.

Thavendiranathan et al. (Thavendiranathan et al., 2009) systematically reviewed the accuracy of historical features, physician examination, and cardiac testing to identify a cardiac arrhythmia in a patient complaining of palpations. The authors concluded that even with the presence of a regular rapid-pounding sensation in the neck or visible neck pulsations consistent with atrio-ventricular nodal reentry tachycardia, clinical examination is not sufficiently accurate to exclude clinically significant arrhythmias in most patients. Therefore, in the patient described above, the clinician must either send the patient to the emergency room or examine the patient electrocardiographically and with other tests as appropriate.

In about half of the cases, chest pain is of cardiac origin. Lenfant (Lenfant, 2010) reviewed chest pain of cardiac and non-cardiac origin—either ischemic or nonischemic. Among the non-cardiac causes, primary esophageal disorder rises to the top of the list. Psychological and psychiatric factors may play a significant role in the perception and severity of the chest pain regardless of its cause, with depression and panic attack or disorder commonly present. Careful evaluation is indicated whatever the cause[s] of a sense of impending doom, racing heart, and difficulty breathing.

MITRAL VALVE PROLAPSE (MVP) AND PANIC DISORDER

Perhaps the most representative prevalence study of MVP was conducted by Procacci et al. (Procacci et al., 1976). These investigators were on active duty in the U.S. Air Force during the Vietnam War and were stationed at Edwards Air Force Base in California. Dependent wives ($n = 1,169$) of Air Force personnel were urged to undergo a physical examination that included cardiac auscultation in the supine, left lateral decubitus, standing, and squatting positions as part of a "Women's Health Week." All women found to have non-ejection clicks or late systolic murmurs (or both) on cardiac auscultation underwent reexamination and M-mode echocardiography. Of the 1,169 study subjects, 74 (6.3%) were considered to have MVP. Thus, MVP is a very common condition.

There remains interest in how frequently cardiac arrhythmias are associated with MVP, and in the association of MVP, cardiac arrhythmias, and panic attacks. Kramer el al. (Kramer et al., 1984) compared ambulatory arrhythmias in 63 subjects with MP and 28 control subjects with matched symptoms. The authors found no statistically significant difference in atrial and ventricular arrhythmias between study subjects and controls. Alpert, in an accompanying editorial (Alpert, 1984), made the observation that it was premature to conclude that MVP was not, in and of itself, a cause of cardiac arrhythmias but asked the clinician to avoid raising the specter of SCD in this population. He carefully outlined his clinical approach to these patients.

Margraf et al. (Margraf, Ehlers, & Roth, 1988) undertook an extensive review of MVP and panic disorder, pointing out that the link between these two conditions remains uncertain and that cardiac complaints occur with some frequency among patients with panic disorder. Also, panic attacks are sometimes accompanied by palpitations and rapid heart rate. Panic disorder patients and those with MVP may complain of chest pain, dizziness, dyspnea, fatigue, and presyncope and syncope, raising the question of whether the cardiac condition may be a cause of this anxiety disorder. The authors quote a prevalence of MVP of 4–21% and the prevalence of MVP in patients with panic attacks ranging on the low side 0–8% and on the high side 24–35%, with these variations demonstrating a bimodal distribution. Margraf et al. (Margraf, Ehlers, & Roth, 1988) state that there is no increased prevalence of panic attacks in patients with MVP compared with controls with other cardiac complaints.

Margraf et al. (Margraf, Ehlers, & Roth, 1988) concluded that available information neither supports nor excludes a greater frequency of MVP in patients with panic disorder. If there is an association, it is quite small. Perhaps the best course of action is to borrow Dr. Alpert's recommendations (Alpert, 1984) for patients with MVP and cardiac arrhythmias:

1. Avoid creating an incapacitating anxiety disorder by placing emphasis on SCD among patients with MVP;

2. Carefully assess MVP patients at high risk for significant cardiac arrhythmias, using studies including ambulatory EKG monitoring, exercise stress testing, and invasive electrophysiological studies;

3. Treat high-risk MVP patients who have high-grade, potentially malignant cardiac arrhythmias;

4. After initiating therapy, monitor carefully and accomplish further arrhythmia testing as necessary; and

5. Pursue treatment until cardiac and panic complaints are adequately controlled.

ANXIETY SENSITIVITY, ATRIAL FIBRILLATION, AND HEART FAILURE

Anxiety sensitivity—the tendency to fear bodily sensations associated with anxiety: sweaty palms, shallow breathing, and rapid pulse—is a trait seen in patients with panic disorder. This sensitivity complicates quality of life in patients with atrial fibrillation who may be sensitive to their heartbeats and reactivity. In a large sample of patients with atrial fibrillation and HF, the patients with anxiety sensitivity who were treated with rhythm- rather than rate-control had a better long-term prognosis (Frasure-Smith et al., 2012).

IMPLANTABLE CARDIOVERTER DEFIBRILLATOR

Patients who have severe left ventricular dysfunction or who have survived life-threatening cardiac arrhythmias are currently treated with an implantable device that can deliver electric shock for life-threatening arrhythmias. Most patients adjust to the implantable cardioverter defibrillator (ICD), and the course of anxiety usually improves over the first year (Pedersen et al., 2010; Kapa et al., 2010). The experience of the shock has been compared to getting kicked in the chest by a horse. Sometimes the defibrillator fires inappropriately. At 18 months post-implantation in one Dutch study, 8% of nearly 400 patients qualified for a diagnosis of post-traumatic distress disorder (PTSD). These were patients more anxious at baseline and more apt to have Type D personality (traits of social inhibition and high negative affect). Shocks per se did not predict PTSD (Habibovic et al., 2012). Phantom shocks (the perceptions of a shock when the device has not fired) are most often seen in ICD patients who had prior exposure to traumatic device shocks and are more common in patients with a history of depression, anxiety, and cocaine use (Jacob et al., 2012). CBT has been shown to reduce PTSD symptoms in patients with acute cardiovascular events and high-baseline PTSD, though not specifically with ICDs (Shemesh et al., 2011).

SUMMARY

Antidepressant and antipsychotic drugs represent a remarkable advance in our treatment of various psychiatric conditions, especially depression and psychosis.

We have focused on two main areas of cardiotoxicity: (1) drug-induced weight gain and other metabolic problems, and (2) drug-induced EKG changes, especially life-threatening ventricular arrhythmias. In discussing weight gain and some of its complications, we have not discussed the capacity of several of the second-generation antipsychotic drugs to induce metabolic problems, including DM, without inducing weight gain. That is a topic for another paper and has been discussed by a number of investigators, including Newcomer (Newcomer et al., 2002).

Antidepressant and antipsychotic drug-induced life-threatening ventricular arrhythmias almost invariably occur among patients (especially women) with existing risk factors for QTc interval prolongation. We have not discussed congenital QT interval prolongation or the rare case of comorbid congenital and acquired (drug-induced) QTc interval prolongation. We did cite such an instance in one of our reviews (Vieweg et al., 2009).

As is the case in so many other aspects of medicine, we recognize what we know and tend to use pattern-recognition in both diagnosing and treating various psychiatric conditions. The tables and figures we offer are our attempt to provide a "picture" clinicians may use in their evaluation and treatment of psychiatric patients. Ready consultation with both the primary care physician and the cardiologist will enhance the cardiac care of patients receiving antidepressant and antipsychotic drugs. However, a burden does fall on the psychiatrist prescribing antidepressant and antipsychotic drugs to identify a cardiology colleague with sufficient expertise and interest in drug-induced QTc interval prolongation and the potential arrhythmias that may follow, given the observation by Viskin et al. (Viskin et al., 2005) that most physicians and many cardiologists fail to accurately calculate a QTc interval or correctly identify a prolonged QTc interval.

Clinicians may overly rely on computerized interpretations of the EKG (Hongo & Goldschlager, 2004), and cardiac electrophysiologists continue to debate whether QT interval prolongation is a reliable predictor of ventricular arrhythmias (Hondeghem, 2008; Roden, 2008). Malik (Malik et al., 2008) argues that the Bazett formula (QTc = QT/square root of the RR interval) is "clearly one of the worst options" to assess QTc interval prolongation. He used the Fridericia formula (QTc = QT/cube root of the RR interval) modified by individually optimized curvature correction as an accurate measurement of the QTc interval throughout the 24-hour cycle (Malik et al., 2008). This method is labor-intensive and unlikely to be adopted on a large scale any time soon. Franz (Franz, 2008), in an editorial comment, noted that in the best of circumstances QTc interval prolongation is a poor predictor of *TdP* unless it is very long.

A guideline useful to the psychiatrist, is that as long as the heart rate is 70 beats per minute or more, the QTc interval will be normal if the QT interval is less than one-half of the RR interval (Phoon, 1998). We should study carefully QT intervals that are one-half or more of the RR interval. We recommend that non-cardiologists prescribing antipsychotic and antidepressant drugs in the elderly that may prolong the QTc interval should obtain a baseline EKG for female patients with additional risk factors such as personal or family history of presyncope or syncope, electrolyte disturbance, and CVD. Elderly male patients with similar risk factors are also at increased risk for QTc interval prolongation and *TdP*. Inspect the EKG yourself using the Phoon shorthand rule (Phoon, 1998).

Familiarity of psychiatrists with cardiometabolic risk factors and close collaboration with other healthcare professionals will facilitate optimal psychiatric and cardiometabolic care of patients with major mental illness. A patient-centered approach that emphasizes coordination between health professionals will improve metabolic and cardiovascular care and outcome of patients suffering from depression or schizophrenia and needing treatment with antidepressant and antipsychotic drugs.

CLINICAL PEARLS

- Depression is about three times more common in patients after MI than the general population.

- Fifteen to 20% of patients after MI meet DSM-IV-TR (American Psychiatric Association, 2000) criteria for major depressive disorder, and an even larger percentage will manifest depressive symptoms.

- Women are at particularly high risk for depression following acute MI.

- Major depressive disorder and elevated depressive symptoms link to a worse prognosis in patients with CHD in a dose-dependent manner.

- Although it is suggested that ACS patients with first-time and new-onset depression are at particularly increased risk of worse prognosis, there is no consistent evidence to support such statements.

- Somatic symptoms of depression (in particular, sleep disturbances, fatigue, and appetite problems associated with anhedonia) have a stronger association with CHD prognosis than do the cognitive symptoms.

- Depressed patients with comorbid CHD have reduced medication compliance.

- Screening for depression in CHD subjects is recommended (although the authors have argued for additional evidence before implementing such screening [Hasnain et al., 2011]).

- The Patient Health Questionnaire (PHQ-2) (Wooley & Simon, 2000) provides two screening questions and may be followed by the PHQ-9 (Kroenke, Spitzer, & Williams, 2001) if either answer on the PHQ-2 is positive. If the PHQ-9 is consistent with a high probability of depression, the patient should be assessed further for depression.

- Shimizu et al. (Shimuzu et al., 2011) recommend targeted treatment of depression in chronic HF as a strategy to improve cardiac function.

- Depression, but not treatment with antidepressant drugs, may be associated with increased mortality in HF patients (O'Connor et al., 2008).

- Conversely, HF is a risk factor for depression among the elderly (Luijendijk et al., 2010).

- ENRICHD tested the hypothesis that, in patients with acute MI and either low social support or depression, CBT would reduce the rates of subsequent deaths and recurrent MIs, compared with patients receiving usual care. With 2,481 patients, including 334 patients with a history of CHF, ENRICHD was the largest trial to date by far in psychosomatic cardiology. While the primary trial hypothesis was not supported—there was no difference in mortality or the composite event rate—there was a small benefit of the CBT intervention regarding depression symptoms.

- In the CREATE trial, which included depressed patients with stable CAD, investigators sought to compare both the effects of citalopram versus placebo and the effects of IPT versus clinical management

(Lespérance et al., 2007). Citalopram was more effective than placebo in reducing depressive symptoms and in achieving response and remission. In contrast, IPT did not separate from clinical management.

- ECT can be safely done in patients with cardiac disease.

- Operationally, obtaining patients' weight and height is the most common practice to determine BMI. Obtaining vital signs, fasting glucose (or HbA1c), fasting lipids, and triglycerides should be routine practice. Measurement of abdominal circumference can also be added.

- Early weight gain may predict long-term weight gain (Kinon et al., 2005).

- Vigilant monitoring of weight gain early during antipsychotic drug treatment and appropriate interventions as indicated can limit long-term obesity and obesity-related complications.

- For patients who gain weight or develop metabolic complications, switch the antipsychotic medication to one with lower metabolic liability.

- Physicians should be aware, not just of the potential cardiac effects of a drug, but also of all non-drug risk factors that are associated with adverse cardiac events, and on-drug risk factors that prolong QTc interval marginally. Citalopram should not be used in patients with congenital long QT syndrome. Hypokalemia and hypomagnesemia should be corrected and periodically monitored. Electrocardiographic monitoring is recommended in patients with HF, bradyarrhythmias, or patients on other medications that prolong the QTc interval.

- In a large sample of patients with atrial fibrillation and HF, those patients with anxiety sensitivity who were treated with rhythm- rather than rate-control had a better long-term prognosis (Frasure-Smith, et al., 2012).

DISCLOSURES

Dr. Vieweg no conflict of interest to disclose.

Dr. Hasnain no conflict of interest to disclose.

REFERENCES

Adabag, A. S., Kim, H. G., & Al Aloul, B. (2008). Arrhythmias associated with electroconvulsive therapy in hypertrophic cardiomyopathy. *Pacing & Clinical Electrophysiology, 31*, 253–255.

Ahmadi, N., Hajsadeghi, F., Mirshkarlo, H. B., Budoff, M., Yehuda, R., & Ebrahimi R. (2011). Post-traumatic stress disorder, coronary atherosclerosis, and mortality. *American Journal of Cardiology, 108*, 29–33.

Albert, C. M., Chae, C. U., Rexrode, K. M., Manson, J. E., & Kawachi I. (2005). Phobic anxiety and risk of coronary heart disease and sudden cardiac death among women. *Circulation, 111*, 480–487.

Ali, S., Stone, M. A., Peters, J. L., Davies, M. J., & Khunti K. (2006). The prevalence of co-morbid depression in adults with Type 2 diabetes: a systematic review and meta-analysis. *Diabetic Medicine, 23*(11), 1165–1173.

Allesøe, K., Hundrup, Y. A., Thomsen, J. F., & Osler M. (2010). Psychosocial work environment and risk of ischaemic heart disease in women: the Danish Nurse Cohort Study. *Occupational & Environmental Medicine, 67*, 318–322.

Alpert, J. S. (1984). Association between arrhythmias and mitral valve prolapse. *Archives of Internal Medicine, 144*, 2333–2334.

Álvarez-Jiménez, M., González-Blanch, C., Crespo-Facorro, B., et al. (2008). Antipsychotic-induced weight gain in chronic and first-episode psychotic disorders: a systematic critical reappraisal. *CNS Drugs, 22*, 547–562.

Alwan, S., & Friedman, J. M. (2009). Safety of selective serotonin reuptake inhibitors in pregnancy. *CNS Drugs, 23*, 493–509.

American Diabetes Association (2009). Standards of medical care in diabetes—2014. *Diabetes Care,* Jan;37(Suppl 1), S14–S80.

American Diabetes Association, APA, American Association of Clinical Endocrinologists, North American Association for the Study of Obesity (2004). Consensus development conference on antipsychotic drugs and obesity and diabetes. *Diabetes Care, 27*, 596–601.

American Psychiatric Association (2000). *DSM-IV-TR Diagnostic and Statistical Manual of Mental Disorders* (4th ed., Text Revision). Washington, DC: American Psychiatric Association.

Anonymous (2011). Cardiac risks of antipsychotics in older adults. *Psychiatry Drug Alerts, 25*, 41–42.

Bakker, M. K., Kerstjens-Frederikse, W. S., Buys C. H. C. M., de Walle, H. E. K., & de Jong-van den Berg, L. T. W. (2010). First-trimester use of paroxetine and congenital heart defects: A population-based case-control study. *Birth Defects Research (Part A), 88*, 94–100.

Bambauer, K. Z., Aupont, O., Stone, P. H., et al. (2005). The effect of a telephone counseling intervention on self-rated health of cardiac patients. *Psychosomatic Medicine, 67*, 539–545.

Baptista, T., El Fakih, Y., Uzcategui, E., et al. (2008). Pharmacological management of atypical antipsychotic-induced weight gain. *CNS Drugs, 22*, 477–495.

Barth, J., Schumacher, M., & Herrmann-Lingen C. (2004). Depression as a risk factor for mortality in patients with coronary heart disease: a meta-analysis. *Psychosomatic Medicine, 66*, 802–813.

Bays, H. E. (2011). Adiposopathy: Is "sick fat" a cardiovascular disease? *Journal of the American College of Cardiology, 57*, 2461–2473.

Bazett, H. C. (1920). An analysis of the time-relations of electrocardiograms. *Heart, 7*, 353–370.

Bednar, M. M., Harrigan, E. P., Anziano, R. J., Camm, A. J., & Ruskin, J. N. (2001). The QT interval. *Progress in Cardiovascular Diseases, 43*(5 Suppl 1), 1–45.

Berenson, A. (2007). Lilly settles with 18,000 over Zyprexa. *New York Times,* January 5, 2007. http://query.nytimes.com/gst/fullpage.htm l?res=9F00E5DB1430F936A35752C0A9619C8B63

Boehnert, M. T., & Lovejoy, F. H., Jr. (1985). Value of the QRS duration versus the serum drug level in predicting seizures and ventricular arrhythmias after an acute overdose of tricyclic antidepressants. *New England of Medicine, 313*, 474–479.

Braunwald E. (2008). Biomarkers in heart failure. *New England Journal of Medicine, 358*, 2148–2159.

Braunwald, E., & Bristow, M. R. (2000). Congestive heart failure: Fifty years of progress. *Circulation, 102*(IV), 14–23.

Browne, K., Prystowsky, E., Heger, J. J., Chilson, D. A., & Zipes, D. P. (1983). Prolongation of the Q-T interval in man during sleep. *American Journal of Cardiology, 52*, 55–59.

Brugada, P., & Brugada, J. (1992). Right bundle branch block, persistent ST segment elevation and sudden cardiac death: a distinct clinical and electrocardiographic syndrome: a multicenter report. *Journal of the American College of Cardiology, 20*, 1391–1396.

Buckley, T., McKinley, S., Tofler, G., Bartrop R. (2009). Cardiovascular risk in early bereavement: a literature review and proposed mechanisms. *International Journal of Nursing Studies, 47*, 229–238.

Bulugahapitiya, U., Siyambalapitiya, S., Sithole, J., & Idris, I. (2009). Is diabetes a coronary risk equivalent? Systematic review and meta-analysis. *Diabetic Medicine*, 26, 142–148.

Camm, A. J., Malik, M., & Yap, Y. G. (2004). *Acquired long QT syndrome*. London: Blackwell Futura.

Chida, Y., & Steptoe A. (2009). The association of anger and hostility with future coronary heart disease: A meta-analytic review of prospective evidence. *Journal of the American College of Cardiology*, 53, 936–946.

Chung, M. L., Lennie, T. A., Dekker, R. L., Wu, J.-R., & Moser, D. K. (2011). Depressive symptoms and poor social support have a synergistic effect on event-free survival in patients with heart failure. *Heart & Lung: The Journal of Acute and Critical Care*, 40(6), 492–501.

Compton, S. J., Lux, R. L., Ramsey, M. R., et al. (1996). Genetically defined therapy of inherited long-QT syndrome. Correction of abnormal repolarization by potassium. *Circulation*, 94, 1018–1022.

Cossette, S., Frasure-Smith, N., & Lespérance, F. (2001). Clinical implications of a reduction in psychological distress on cardiac prognosis in patients participating in a psychosocial intervention program. *Psychosomatic Medicine*, 63, 257–266.

Couderc, J. P. (2009). Measurement and regulation of cardiac ventricular repolarization: from the QT interval to repolarization morphology. *Philosophical Transactions of the Royal Society, A: Mathematical, Physical, & Engineering Sciences*, 367, 1283–1299.

Couderc, J. P., Xia, X., Peterson, D. R., et al. (2011). T-wave morphology abnormalities in benign, potent, and arrhythmogenic Ikr inhibition. *Heart Rhythm*, 8, 1036–1043.

Dahabreh, I. J., & Paulus, J. K. (2011). Association of episodic physical and sexual activity with triggering of acute cardiac events. *Journal of the American Medical Association*, 305, 1225–1233.

Darpo, B. (2010). The thorough QT/QTc study 4 years after the implementation of the ICH E14 guidance. *British Journal of Pharmacology*, 159, 49–57.

Darpo, B., Nebout, T., & Sager, P. T. (2006). Clinical evaluation of QT/QTc prolongation and proarrhythmic potential for nonantiarrhythmic drugs: The International Conference on Harmonization of Technical Requirements for Registration of Pharmaceuticals for Human Use E14 Guideline. *Journal of Clinical Pharmacology*, 46, 498–507.

Davidson, K. W., Burg, M. M., Kronish, I. M., et al. (2010). Association of anhedonia with recurrent major adverse cardiac events and mortality 1 year after acute coronary syndrome. *Archives of General Psychiatry*, 67, 480–488.

de Jonge, P., Ormel, J., van den Brink, R. H. S., et al. (2006). Symptom dimensions of depression following myocardial infarction and their relationship with somatic health status and cardiovascular prognosis. *American Journal of Psychiatry*, 163, 138–144.

Denollet, J. P., Schiffer, A. A. P., & Spek, V. P. (2010). A general propensity to psychological distress affects cardiovascular outcomes: Evidence from research on the Type D (distressed) personality profile. [Review]. *Circulation: Cardiovascular Quality & Outcomes*, 3, 546–557.

Denollet, J., de Jonge, P., Kuyper, A., et al. (2009). Depression and Type D personality represent different forms of distress in the Myocardial INfarction and Depression–Intervention Trial (MIND-IT). *Psychological Medicine*, 39, 749–756.

Denollet, J., Gidron, Y., Vrints, C. J., & Conraads, V. M. (2010). Anger, supressed anger, and risk of adverse events in patients with coronary artery disease. *American Journal of Cardiology*, 105, 1555–1560.

Dietz, L. J., & Matthews, K. A. (2011). Depressive symptoms and subclinical markers of cardiovascular disease in adolescents. *The Journal of Adolescent Health*, 48, 579–584.

Dimos, A. K., Strougiannos, P. N., Kakkavas, A. T., & Trikas, A. G. (2009). Depression and heart failure. *Hellenic Journal of Cardiology*, 50, 410–417.

Dolenc, T. J., Barnes, R. D., Hayes, D. L., & Rasmussen, K. G. (2004). Electroconvulsive therapy in patients with cardiac pacemakers and implantable cardioverter defibrillators. *Pacing & Clinical Electrophysiology*, 27, 1257–1263.

Drew, B. J., Ackerman, M. J., Funk, M. R., et al. (2010a). Prevention of *torsade de pointes* in hospital settings: a scientific statement from the American Heart Association and the American College of Cardiology Foundation. *Circulation*, 121, 1–14.

Drew, B. J., Ackerman, M. J., Funk, M., et al. (2010b). Prevention of *torsade de pointes* in hospital settings: a scientific statement from the American Heart Association and the American College of Cardiology Foundation. *Journal of the American College of Cardiology*, 55, 934–947.

DuMouchel, W., Fram, D., Yang, X., et al. (2008). Antipsychotics, glycemic disorders, and life-threatening diabetic events: a Bayesian data-mining analysis of the FDA adverse event reporting system (1968–2004). *Annals of Clinical Psychiatry*, 20, 21–31.

El-Sherif, N., & Turitto, G. (2011). Electrolyte disorders and arrhythmogenesis. *Cardiology Journal*, 18, 233–245.

Faulkner, G., & Cohn, T. A. (2006). Pharmacologic and nonpharmacologic strategies for weight gain and metabolic disturbance in patients treated with antipsychotic medications. *Canadian Journal of Psychiatry*, 51, 502–511.

FDA (2005). Public Health Advisory: Deaths with antipsychotics in elderly patients with behavioral disturbances. Available at the FDA website, www.fda.gov/Drugs/DrugSafety/PostmarketDrugSafetyInformationforPatientsandProviders/DrugSafetyInformationforHeathcareProfessionals/PublicHealthAdvisories/ucm053171.htm. Accessed July 24, 2011.

Fernandez, A., Bang, S. E., Srivathsan, K., & Vieweg, W. V. R. (2007). Cardiovascular side effects of newer antidepressants. *Anadolu Kardiyoloji Dergisi*, 7, 305–309.

Figueredo, V. M. (2009). The time has come for physicians to take notice: the impact of psychosocial stressors on the heart. *American Journal of Medicine*, 122, 704–712.

Figueredo, V. M. (2011). Chemical cardiomyopathies: The negative effects of medications and nonprescribed drugs on the heart. *The American Journal of Medicine*, 124, 480–488.

Food and Drug Administration (2005). Guidance for industry. E14 Clinical evaluation of QT/QTc interval prolongation and proarrhythmic potential for non-antiarrhythmic drugs. Available at FDA website, http://www.fda.gov/RegulatoryInformation/Guidances/ucm129335.htm.

Franz, M. R. (2008). Bazett, Fridericia, or Malik? *Heart Rhythm*, 5, 1432–1433.

Franz, M. R., Swerdlow, C. D., Liem, L. B., & Schaefer, J. (1988). Cycle length dependence of human action potential duration in vivo. Effects of single extrastimuli, sudden sustained rate acceleration deceleration, and different steady state frequencies. *Journal of Clinical Investigation*, 82, 972–979.

Frasure-Smith, N., & Lespérance, F. (2006). Recent evidence linking coronary heart disease and depression. *Canadian Journal of Psychiatry*, 51, 730–737.

Frasure-Smith, N., & Lespérance, F. (2008). Depression and anxiety as predictors of 2-year cardiac events in patients with stable coronary artery disease. *Archives of General Psychiatry*, 65, 62–71.

Frasure-Smith, N., Lesperance, F., Prince, R. H., et al. (1997). Randomised trial of home-based psychosocial nursing intervention for patients recovering from myocardial infarction. *Lancet*, 350, 473–479.

Frasure-Smith, N., Lespérance, F., Talajic, M., et al. (2012). Anxiety sensitivity moderates prognostic importance of rhythm-control versus rate-control strategies in patients with atrial fibrillation and congestive heart failure: insights from the Atrial Fibrillation and Congestive Heart Failure Trial. *Circulation, Heart Failure*, 5, 322–330.

Frasure-Smith, N., Lespérance, J., Habra, M., et al. (2009). Elevated depression symptoms predict long-term cardiovascular mortality in patients with atrial fibrillation and heart failure. *Circulation*, 120, 134–140.

Freedland, K. E., Skala, J. A., Carney, R. M., et al. (2009). Treatment of depression after coronary artery bypass surgery. A randomized controlled trial. *Archives of General Psychiatry*, 66, 387–396.

Fu, E. Y., Clemo, H. F., & Ellenbogen, K. A. (1998). Acquired QT prolongation. Mechanisms and implications. *Cardiology Review, 6*, 319–324.

Gallagher, R., McKinley, S., & Dracup K. (2003). Effects of a telephone counseling intervention on psychosocial adjustment in women following a cardiac event. *Heart & Lung: The Journal of Acute and Critical Care, 32*, 79–87.

Gebhardt, S., Haberhausen, M., Heinzel-Gutenbrunner, M., et al. (2009). Antipsychotic-induced body weight gain: predictors and a systematic categorization of the long-term weight course. *Journal of Psychiatric Research, 43*, 620–626.

Gentile, S. (2011). Selective serotonin reuptake inhibitor exposure during early pregnancy and the risk of birth defects. *Acta Psychiatrica Scandinavica, 123*, 266–275.

Glassman, A. H. (2007). Depression and cardiovascular comorbidity. *Dialogues in Clinical Neuroscience, 9*, 9–17.

Glassman, A. H., Bigger, J. T., Gaffney, M., & Van Zyl, L. T. (2007). Heart rate variability in acute coronary syndrome patients with major depression: Influence of sertraline and mood improvement. *Archives of General Psychiatry, 64*, 1025–1031.

Goldenberg, I., Moss, A. J., & Zareba, W. (2006). QT interval: how to measure it and what is "normal." *Journal of Cardiovascular Electrophysiology, 17*, 333–336.

Grundy, S. M. (2007). Cardiovascular and metabolic risk factors: How can we improve outcomes in the high-risk patient? *The American Journal of Medicine, 120*(9 Suppl 1), S3–S8.

Grundy, S. M. (2008). Metabolic syndrome pandemic. *Arteriosclerosis, Thrombosis, & Vascular Biology, 28*, 629–636.

Habibovic, M., van den Broek, K. C., Alings, M., Van der Voort, P. H., & Denollet, J. (2012). Posttraumatic stress 18 months following cardioverter defibrillator implantation: shocks, anxiety, and personality. *Health Psychology, 31*, 186–193.

Haffner, S. M., Lehto, S., Rönnemaa, T., Pyörälä, K., & Laakso, M. (1998). Mortality from coronary heart disease in subjects with type 2 diabetes and in nondiabetic subjects with and without prior myocardial infarction. *New England Journal of Medicine, 339*, 229–234.

Hamer, M., David Batty, G., Seldenrijk, A., Kivimaki M. (2011). Antidepressant medication use and future risk of cardiovascular disease: the Scottish Health Survey. *European Heart Journal, 32*, 437–442.

Hancox, J. C., Hasnain, M., Vieweg, W. V. R., Crouse, E. B., & Baranchuk, A. (2013). Azithromycin, cardiovascular risks, QTc interval prolongation, *torsade de pointes*, and regulatory issues. A narrative review based on the study of case reports. *Therapeutic Advances in Infectious Disease, 1*(5), 155–165.

Hancox, J. C., Hasnain, M., Vieweg, W. V. R., Gysel, M., Methot, M., & Baranchuk, A. (2014). Erythromycin, QTc interval prolongation, and *torsade de pointes*: Case reports, major risk factors and illness severity. *Therapeutic Advances in Infectious Disease, 2*(2), 47–59.

Hasnain, M., Fredrickson, S. K., & Vieweg, W. V. R. (2011). Metformin for obesity and glucose dysregulation in patients with schizophrenia receiving antipsychotic drugs. *Journal of Psychopharmacology, 25*, 715–721.

Hasnain, M., Vieweg, W. V. (2014). QTc interval prolongation and torsade de pointes associated with second-generation antipsychotics and antidepressants: a comprehensive review. *CNS Drugs, Oct;28*(10), 887–920.

Hasnain, M., Vieweg, W. V. R., Fredrickson, S. K., Beatty-Brooks, M., Fernandez, A., & Pandurangi, A. K. (2009). Clinical monitoring and management of the metabolic syndrome in patients receiving atypical antipsychotic medications. *Primary Care Diabetes, 3*, 5–15.

Hasnain, M., Vieweg, W. V. R., Howland, R., et al. (2014). Quetiapine and the need for a thorough QT/QTc study. *Journal of Clinical Psychopharmacology, 34*(1), 3–6.

Hasnain, M., Vieweg, W. V. R., Lesnefsky, E. J., & Pandurangi, A. K. (2011). Depression screening in patients with coronary heart disease: a critical evaluation of the AHA guidelines. *Journal of Psychosomatic Research, 71*, 6–12.

Hasnain, M., Vieweg, W. V., & Fredrickson, S. K. (2010). Metformin for atypical antipsychotic-induced weight gain and glucose metabolism dysregulation: review of the literature and clinical suggestions. *CNS Drugs, 24*, 193–206.

Hasnain, M., Vieweg, W. V., & Hollett, B. (2012). Weight gain and glucose dysregulation with second-generation antipsychotics and antidepressants: a review for primary care physicians. *Postgraduate Medicine, 124*, 154–167.

Hatta, K., Takahashi, T., Nakamura, H., Yamashiro, H., Asukai, N., & Yonezawa, Y. (1999). Hypokalemia and agitation in acute psychotic patients. *Psychiatry Research, 86*, 85–88.

Hatta, K., Takahashi, T., Nakamura, H., Yamashiro, H., & Yonezawa, Y. (2000). Prolonged QT interval in acute psychotic patients. *Psychiatry Research, 94*, 279–285.

Hedley, P. L., Jørgensen, P., Schlamowitz, S., et al. (2009). The genetic basis of long QT and short QT syndromes: A mutation update. *Human Mutation, 30*, 1486–1511.

Higgins R. O., Murphy, B. M., Nicholas, A., Worcester, M. U., & Lindner, H. (2007). Emotional and adjustment issues faced by cardiac patients seen in clinical practice: a qualitative survey of experienced clinicans. *Journal of Cardiopulmonary Rehabilitation & Prevention, 27*, 291–297.

Hippisley-Cox, J., Pringle, M., Hammersley, V., et al. (2001). Antidepressants as risk factor for ischaemic heart disease: case-control study in primary care. *British Medical Journal, 323*, 666–669.

Holmes, S. D. (2011). American Heart Association guidelines for depression screening in heart disease: Call to action for the research community? *Journal of Psychosomatic Research, 71*, 1–2.

Hondeghem, L. M. (2008). QT prolongation is an unreliable predictor of ventricular arrhythmia. *Heart Rhythm, 5*, 1210–1212.

Hongo, R. H., & Goldschlager, N. (2004). Overreliance on computerized algorithims to interpret electrocardiograms. *American Journal of Medicine, 117*, 706–708.

Howland, R. H. (2011a). A critical evaluation of the cardiac toxicity of citalopram. Part 2. *Journal of Psychosocial Nursing & Mental Health Services, 49*, 13–16.

Howland, R. H. (2011b). A critical evaluation of the cardiac toxicity of citalopram. Part 1. *Journal of Psychosocial Nursing & Mental Health Services, 49*, 13–16.

Huffman, J. C., Mastromauro, C. A., Sowden, G. L., Wittmann, C., Rodman, R., & Januzzi, J. L. (2011). A collaborative care depression management program for cardiac inpatients: depression characteristics and in-hospital outcomes. *Psychosomatics, 52*, 26–33.

Jaarsma, T., Lesman-Leegte, I., Hillege, H. L., Veeger, N. J., Sanderman, R., & van Veldhuisen, D. J. (2010). Depression and the usefulness of a disease management program in heart failure: Insights from the COACH (Coordinating study evaluating Outcomes of Advising and Counseling in Heart failure) Study. *Journal of the American College of Cardiology, 55*, 1837–1843.

Jacob, S., Panaich, S. S., Zalawadiya, S. K., et al. (2012). Phantom shocks unmasked: clinical data and proposed mechanism of memory reactivation of past traumatic shocks in patients with implantable cardioverter defibrillators. *Journal of Interventional Cardiac Electrophysiology, 34*, 205–213.

Janszky, I., Ahnve, S., Lundberg, I., & Hemmingsson T. (2010). Early-onset depression, anxiety and risk of subsequent coronary heart disease. *Journal of the American College of Cardiology, 56*, 31–37.

Jelinek, K. (2011). Screening for depression in coronary heart disease: the perfect Hegelian dialectic? A short commentary on "Beyond the blues: the need for integrated care pathways." *European Journal of Cardiovascular Prevention & Rehabilitation, 18*, 222–223.

Johnson, J. N., Grifoni, C., Bos, J. M., et al. (2011). Prevalence and clinical correlates of QT prolongation in patients with hypertrophic cardiomyopathy. *European Heart Journal, 32*(9), 1114–1120.

Kannankeril, P., Roden, D. M., & Darbar, D. (2010). Drug-induced long QT syndrome. *Pharmacology Review, 62*, 760–781.

Kapa, S., Rotondi-Trevisan, D., Mariano, Z., et al. (2010). Psychopathology in patients with ICDs over time: results of a prospective study. *Pacing & Clinical Electrophysiology, 33*, 198–208.

Katon, W., Fan M-Y, Unützer, J., Taylor, J., Pincus, H., & Schoenbaum, M. (2008). Depression and diabetes: A potentially lethal combination. *Journal of General Internal Medicine, 23*, 1571–1575.

Kawachi, I., Colditz, G. A., Ascherio, A., et al. (1994). Prospective study of phobic anxiety and risk of coronary heart disease in men. *Circulation, 89*, 1992–1997.

Khan, S. P., Dahlvani, S., Vieweg, W. V. R., Bernardo, N. L., & Lewis, R. E. (1998). Electrocardiographic QT interval in a geropsychiatric inpatient population: a preliminary study. *Medicine + Psychiatry, 1*, 71–74.

Kinon, B. J., Kaiser, C. J., Ahmed, S., Rotelli, M. D., & Kollack-Walker, S. (2005). Association between early and rapid weight gain and change in weight over one year of olanzapine therapy in patients with schizophrenia and related disorders. *Journal of Clinical Psychopharmacology, 25*, 255–258.

Kloner, R. A. (2006). Natural and unnatural triggers of myocardial infarction. *Progress in Cardiovascular Diseases, 48*, 285–300.

Kogut, C., Crouse, E. B., Vieweg, W. V. R., et al. (2013). Selective serotonin reuptake inhibitors and *torsade de pointes*: new concepts and new directions derived from a systematic review of case reports. *Therapeutic Advances in Drug Safety, 4*(5), 189–198.

Kramer, H. M., Kligfield, P., Devereux, R. B., Savage, D. D., & Kramer-Fox, R. (1984). Arrhythmias in mitral valve prolapse: effect of selection bias. *Archives of Internal Medicine, 144*, 2360–2364.

Kroenke, K., Spitzer, R. L., & Williams, J. B. (2003). The Patient Health Questionnaire–2: validity of a two-item depression screener. *Medical Care, 41*, 1284–1292.

Kroenke, K., Spitzer, R., Williams J. (2001). The PHQ-9. *Journal of General Internal Medicine, 16*, 606–613.

Lambert, T. J., & Chapman, L. H. (2004). Diabetes, psychotic disorders and antipsychotic therapy: a consensus statement. *Medical Journal of Australia, 181*, 544–548.

Larsen, K. K., Agerbo, E., Christensen, B., Sondergaard, J., & Vestergaard, M. (2010). Myocardial infarction and risk of suicide: a population-based case-control study. *Circulation, 122*(23), 2388–2393.

Lavie, C. J., & Milani, R. V. (2006). Adverse psychological and coronary risk profiles in young patients with coronary artery disease and benefits of formal cardiac rehabilitation. *Archives of Internal Medicine, 166*, 1878–1883.

Leifheit-Limson, E. C., Reid, K. J., Kasl, S. V., et al. (2010). The role of social support in health status and depressive symptoms after acute myocardial infarction: evidence for a stronger relationship among women. *Circulation: Cardiovascular Quality & Outcomes, 3*, 143–150.

Lenfant, C. (2010). Chest pain of cardiac and noncardiac origin. *Metabolism, 59*(Suppl 1), S41–S46.

Lespérance, F., & Frasure-Smith N. (2000). Depression in patients with cardiac disease: a practical review. *Journal of Psychosomatic Research, 48*, 379–391.

Lespérance, F., Frasure-Smith, N., Koszycki, D., et al. (2007). Effects of citalopram and interpersonal psychotherapy on depression in patients with coronary artery disease. The Canadian Cardiac Randomized Evaluation of Antidepressant and Psychotherapy Efficacy (CREATE) trial. *Journal of the American Medical Association, 297*, 367–379.

Lett, H. S., Blumenthal, J. A., Babyak, M. A., et al. (2007). Social support and prognosis in patients at increased psychosocial risk recovering from myocardial infarction. *Health Psychology, 26*, 418–427.

Lichtman, J. H., Bigger, J. T., Blumenthal, J. A., et al. (2008). Depression and coronary heart disease. Recommendations for screening, referral, and treatment. A Science Advisory from the American Heart Association Prevention Committee of the Council on Cardiovascular Nursing, Council on Clinical Cardiology, Council on Epidemiology and Prevention, and Interdisciplinary Council on Quality of Care and Outcomes Research. Endorsed by the American Psychiatric Association. *Circulation, 118*, 1768–1775.

Linke, S. E., Rutledge, T., Johnson, B. D., et al. (2009). Depressive symptom dimensions and cardiovascular prognosis among women with suspected myocardial ischemia. A report from the National Heart, Lung, and Blood Institute–sponsored Women's Ischemia Syndrome Evaluation. *Archives of General Psychiatry, 66*, 499–507.

Luijendijk, H. J., Tiemeier, H., van den Berg, J. F., Bleumink, G. S., Hofman, A., & Stricker, B. H. C. (2010). Heart failure and incident late-life depression. *Journal of the American Geriatric Society, 58*, 1441–1448.

Magid, M., Lapid, M. I., Sampson, S. M., & Mueller, P. S. (2005). Use of electroconvulsive therapy in a patient 10 days after myocardial infarction. *Journal of ECT*, Sept. 21, 182–185.

Malik, M., Hnatkova, K., Schmidt, A., & Smetana, P. (2008). Accurately measured and properly heart-rate corrected QTc intervals show little daytime variability. *Heart Rhythm, 5*, 1424–1431.

Malkani, S., & Mordes, J. P. (2011). Implications of using hemoglobin A1C for diagnosing diabetes mellitus. *The American Journal of Medicine, 124*, 395–401.

Marano, G., Harnic, D., Lotrionte, M., et al. (2009). Depression and the cardiovascular system: increasing evidence of a link and therapeutic implications. *Expert Review of Cardiovascular Therapy, 7*, 1123–1147.

Margraf, J., Ehlers, A., & Roth, W. T. (1988). Mitral valve prolapse and panic disorder: a review of their relationship. *Psychosomatic Medicine, 50*, 93–113.

Mark, T. L., Joish, V. N., Hay, J. W., Sheehan, D. V., Johnston, S. S., & Cao, Z. (2011). Antidepressant use in geriatric populations: The burden of side effects and interactions and their impact on adherence and costs. *American Journal of Geriatric Psychiatry, 19*, 211–221.

Martens, E. J., de Jonge, P., Na, B., Cohen, B. E., Lett, H., & Whooley, M. A. (2010a). Scared to death? Generalized anxiety disorder and cardiovascular events in patients with stable coronary heart disease. *Archives of General Psychiatry, 67*, 750–758.

Martens, E. J., Mols, F., Burg, M. M., & Denollet J. (2010b). Type D personality predicts clinical events after myocardial infarction, above and beyond disease severity and depression. *Journal of Clinical Psychiatry, 71*, 778–783.

Medicines and Healthcare Products Regulatory Agency (MHRA) (2011). Citalopram and escitalopram: QT interval prolongation—new maximum daily dose restrictions (including in elderly patients), contraindications, and warnings. Available at Medicines and Healthcare Products Regulatory Agency UK website, http://www.mhra.gov.uk/Safetyinformation/DrugSafetyUpdate/CON137769.

Mehta, S., Chen, H., Johnson, M., & Aparasu, R. R. (2011). Risk of serious cardiac events in older adults using antipsychotic agents. *American Journal of Geriatric Pharmacotherapy, 9*, 120–132.

Meier, C. R., Schlienger, R. G., & Jick, H. (2001). Use of selective serotonin reuptake inhibitors and risk of developing first-time acute myocardial infarction. *British Journal of Clinical Pharmacology, 52*, 179–184.

Meyer, J. M., & Stahl, S. M. (2009). The metabolic syndrome and schizophrenia. *Acta Psychiatrica Scandinavica, 119*, 4–14.

Milani, R. V., & Lavie, C. J. (2007). Impact of cardiac rehabilitation on depression and its associated mortality. *American Journal of Medicine, 120*, 799–806.

Mohammad, S., Zhou, Z., Gong, Q., & January, C. T. (1997). Blockage of the HERG human cardiac K+ channel by the gastrointestinal prokinetic agent cisapride. *American Journal of Physiology—Heart and Circulatory Physiology, 273*, H2534–H2538.

Monster, T. B. M., Johnsen, S. P., Olsen, M. L., McLaughlin, J. K., & Sørensen, H. T. (2004). Antidepressants and risk of first-time hospitalization for myocardial infarction: A population-based case-control study. *American Journal of Medicine, 117*, 732–737.

Morganroth, J., Brozovich, F. V., McDonald, J. T., & Jacobs, R. A. (1991). Variability of the QT measurement in healthy men, with implications for selection of an abnormal QT value to predict drug toxicity and proarrhythmia. *American Journal of Cardiology, 67*, 774–776.

Morone, N. E., Weiner, D. K., Herbeck Belnap, B. H., et al. (2010). The impact of pain and depression on recovery after coronary artery bypass grafting. *Psychosomatic Medicine, 72*, 620–625.

Murray, C. J. L., & Lopez, A. D. (1997). Alternative projections of mortality and disability by cause 1990–2020: Global Burden of Disease Study. *Lancet, 349*(9064), 1498–1504.

Nabi, H., Hall, M., Koskenvuo, M., et al. (2010). Psychological and somatic symptoms of anxiety and risk of coronary heart disease: the Health and Social Support Prospective Cohort Study. *Biological Psychiatry, 67,* 378–385.

Nathan, D. M., Kuenen, J., Borg, R., Zheng, H., Schoenfeld, D., & Heine, R. J. (2008). Translating the A1C assay Into estimated average glucose values. *Diabetes Care, 31,* 1473–1478.

Newcomer, J. W., & Hennekens, C. H. (2007). Severe mental illness and risk of cardiovascular disease. *Journal of the American Medical Association, 298,* 1794–1796.

Newcomer, J. W., Haupt, D. W., Fucetola, R., et al. (2002). Abnormalities in glucose regulation during antipsychotic treatment of schizophrenia. *Archives of General Psychiatry, 59,* 337–345.

O'Connor, C. M., Jiang, W., Kuchibhatla, M., et al. (2008). Antidepressant use, depression, and survival in patients with heart failure. *Archives of Internal Medicine, 168,* 2232–2237.

O'Connor, C. M., Jiang, W., Kuchibhatla, M., et al. (2010). Safety and efficacy of sertraline for depression in patients with heart failure: Results of the SADHART-CHF (Sertraline Against Depression and Heart Disease in Chronic Heart Failure) trial. *Journal of the American College of Cardiology, 56,* 692–699.

Pan, A., Lucas, M., Sun, Q., et al. (2011). Increased mortality risk in women with depression and diabetes mellitus. *Archives of General Psychiatry, 68,* 42–50.

Parvez, B., & Darbar, D. (2011). Novel ECG markers for ventricular repolarization: Is the QT interval obsolete? *Heart Rhythm, 8,* 1044–1045.

Patel, U., & Pavri, B. B. (2008). Short QT syndrome. *Cardiology in Review, 17,* 300–3003.

Pedersen, S. S., Hoogwegt, M. T., Jordaens, L., & Theuns, D. A. (2011). Relation of symptomatic heart failure and psychological status to persistent depression in patients with implantable cardioverter-defibrillator. *The American Journal of Cardiology, 108,* 69–74.

Pedersen, S. S., Theuns, D. A., Jordaens, L., & Kupper, N. (2010). Course of anxiety and device-related concerns in implantable cardioverter defibrillator patients the first year post implantation. *Europace: European pacing, arrhythmias, and cardiac electrophysiology: journal of the working groups on cardiac pacing, arrhythmias, and cardiac cellular electrophysiology of the European Society of Cardiology, 12,* 1119–1126.

Phoon, C. K. L. (1998). Mathematical validation of a shorthand rule for calculating QTc. *American Journal of Cardiology, 82,* 400–402.

Postema, P. G., De Jong J. S., Van der Bilt, I. A. C., & Wilde, A. A. M. (2008). Accurate electrocardiographic assessment of the QT interval: teach the tangent. *Heart Rhythm, 5,* 1015–1018.

Postema, P. G., Wolpert, C., Amin, A. S., et al. (2009). Drugs and Brugada syndrome patients: Review of the literature, recommendations, and an up-to-date website (www.brugadadrugs.org). *Heart Rhythm, 6,* 1335–1341.

Potkin, S. G., Preskorn, S., Hochfeld, M., & Meng, X. (2013). A thorough QTc study of 3 doses of iloperidone including metabolic inhibition via CYP2D6 and/or CYP3A4 and a comparison to quetiapine and ziprasidone. *Journal of Clinical Psychopharmacology, 33,* 3–10.

Pozuelo, L., Zhang, J., Franco, K., Tesar, G., Penn, M., & Jiang, W. (2009). Depression and heart disease: what do we know, and where are we headed? *Cleveland Clinic Journal of Medicine, 76,* 59–70.

Procacci, P. M., Savran, S. V., Schreiter, S. L., & Bryson, A. L. (1976). Prevalence of clinical mitral-valve prolapse in 1169 young women. *New England Journal of Medicine, 294,* 1086–1088.

Psychopharmacological Drugs Advisory Committee (PDAC) (2000). July 19 Briefing Document for ZELDOX® CAPSULES (Ziprasidone HCl), Pfizer: www.fda.gov/ohrms/dockets/ac/00/backgrd/3619b1a.pdf (accessed January 7, 2012), 1–173.

Pueyo, E., Smetana, P., Laguna, P., & Malik, M. (2003). Estimation of the QT/RR hysteresis lag. *Journal of Electrocardiology, 36*(Suppl), 187–190.

Ray, W. A., Chung, C. P., Murray, K. T., Hall, K., & Stein, C. M. (2009). Atypical antipsychotic drugs and the risk of sudden cardiac death. *New England Journal of Medicine, 360,* 225–235.

Ray, W. A., Meredith, S., Thapa, P. B., Meador, K. G., Hall, K., & Murray, K. T. (2001). Antipsychotics and the risk of sudden cardiac death. *Archives of General Psychiatry, 58,* 1161–1167.

Rayburn, B. K. (1997). Electroconvulsive therapy in patients with heart failure or valvular heart disease. *Convulsive Therapy, 13,* 145–156.

Reaven, G. M. (1997). Banting Lecture, 1988. Role of insulin resistance in human disease. *Nutrition, 13,* 64–66.

Reaven, G. M. (2006). The metabolic syndrome: is this diagnosis necessary? *American Journal of Clinical Nutrition, 83,* 1237–1247.

Reid, S., & Barbui, C. (2010). Long term treatment of depression with selective serotonin reuptake inhibitors and newer antidepressants. *British Medical Journal, 340,* 752–756.

Riesenman, J. P., & Scanlan, M. R. (1995). ECT 2 weeks post coronary artery bypass graft surgery. *Convulsive Therapy, 11,* 262–265.

Roden, D. M. (2008). Keep the QT interval: it is a reliable predictor of ventricular arrhythmias. *Heart Rhythm, 5,* 1213–1215.

Roest, A. M., Martens, E. J., de Jonge, P., & Denollet, J. (2010). Anxiety and risk of incident coronary heart disease. *Journal of the American College of Cardiology, 56,* 38–46.

Rollman, B. L., Belnap, B. H., LeMenager, M. S., et al. (2009). Telephone-delivered collaborative care for treating post-CABG depression. *Journal of the American Medical Association, 302,* 2095–2103.

Saddichha, S., Ameen, S., & Akhtar, S. (2008). Predictors of antipsychotic-induced weight gain in first-episode psychosis: conclusions from a randomized, double-blind, controlled prospective study of olanzapine, risperidone, and haloperidol. *Journal of Clinical Psychopharmacology, 28,* 27–31.

Saha, S., Chant, D., & McGrath, J. (2007). A systematic review of mortality in schizophrenia: Is the differential mortality gap worsening over time? *Archives of General Psychiatry,* October 1, *64*(10), 1123–1131.

Sattar, N., McConnachie, A., Shaper, A. G., et al. (2008). Can metabolic syndrome usefully predict cardiovascular disease and diabetes? Outcome data from two prospective studies. *Lancet, 371,* 1927–1935.

Sauer, W. H., Berlin, J. A., & Kimmel, S. E. (2003). Effect of antidepressants and their relative affinity for the serotonin transporter on the risk of myocardial infarction. *Circulation, 108,* 32–36.

Scheen, A. J., & De Hert, M. A. (2007). Abnormal glucose metabolism in patients treated with antipsychotics. *Diabetes & Metabolism, 33,* 169–175.

Scherrer, J. F., Garfield, L. D., Chrusciel, T., et al. (2011). Increased risk of myocardial infarction in depressed patients with type 2 diabetes. *Diabetes Care, 34*(8), 1729–1734.

Schlienger, R. G., Fischer, L. M., Jick, H., & Meier, C. R. (2004). Current use of selective serotonin reuptake inhibitors and risk of acute myocardial infarction. *Drug Safety, 27,* 1157–1165.

Scialli, A. R. (2010). Paroxetine exposure during pregnancy and cardiac malformations. *Birth Defects Research, Part A, Clinical and Molecular Teratolology, 88,* 175–177.

Setoguchi, S., Wang, P. S., Alan Brookhart, M., Canning, C. F., Kaci, L., & Schneeweiss, S. (2008). Potential causes of higher mortality in elderly users of conventional and atypical antipsychotic medications. *Journal of the American Geriatric Society, 56,* 1644–1650.

Shemesh, E., Annunziato, R. A., Rubinstein, D., et al. (2009). Screening for depression and suicidality in patients with cardiovascular illnesses. *American Journal of Cardiology, 104,* 1194–1197.

Shemesh, E., Annunziato, R. A., Weatherley, B. D., et al. (2011). A randomized controlled trial of the safety and promise of cognitive-behavioral therapy using imaginal exposure in patients with posttraumatic stress disorder resulting from cardiovascular illness. *Journal of Clinical Psychiatry, 72,* 168–174.

Shen, B., Avivi, Y. E., Todaro, J. F., et al. (2008). Anxiety characteristics independently and prospectively predict myocardial infarction in men. The unique contribution of anxiety among psychological factors. *Journal of the American College of Cardiology, 51,* 113–119.

Sherwood, A., Blumenthal, J. A., Hinderliter, A. L., et al. (2011). Worsening depressive symptoms are associated with adverse clinical outcomes in patients with heart failure. *Journal of the American College of Cardiology, 57,* 418–423.

Shimizu, Y., Yamada, S., Miyake, F., & Izumi T. (2011). The effects of depression on the course of functional limitations in patients with chronic heart failure. *Journal of Cardiac Failure, 17*, 503–510.

Sicouri, S., & Antzelevitch, C. (2008). Sudden cardiac death secondary to antidepressant and antipsychotic drugs. *Expert Opinion on Drug Safety, 7*, 181–194.

Silver, M. A. (2010). Depression and heart failure: An overview of what we know and don't know. *Cleveland Clinic Journal of Medicine, 77*(Suppl 3), S7–S11.

Simmons, R. K., Alberti, K. G., Gale, E. A., et al. (2010). The metabolic syndrome: useful concept or clinical tool? Report of a WHO Expert Consultation. *Diabetologia, 53*, 600–605.

Skandalakis, M. C., & Skandalakis, J. E. (1992). John Hunter (1728–1793). *Clinical Cardiology, 15*, 134–135.

Snowden, M., Sato, K., & Roy-Byrne, P. (2003). Assessment and treatment of nursing home residents with depression or behavioral symptoms associated with dementia: a review of the literature. *Journal of the American Geriatric Society, 51*, 1305–1317.

Soh, K. C., & Lee C. (2010). Panic attack and its correlation with acute coronary syndrome—more than just a diagnosis of exclusion. *Annals of the Academy of Medicine, Singapore, 39*, 197–202.

Su, H. M., Chiu, H. C., Lin, T. H., Voon, W. C., Liu, H. W., & Lai, W. T. (2006). Longitudinal study of the ageing trends in QT interval and dispersion in healthy elderly subjects. *Age & Ageing, 35*, 636–638.

Swardfager, W., Herrmann, N., Marzolini, S., et al. (2011). Major depressive disorder predicts completion, adherence, and outcomes in cardiac rehabilitation: a prospective cohort study of 195 patients with coronary artery disease. *Journal of Clinical Psychiatry, 72*(9), 1181–1188.

Taggart, P., Critchley, H., & Lambiase, P. D. (2011). Heart-brain interactions in cardiac arrhythmia. *Heart, 97*, 698–708.

Tan, H. L., Hou, C. J. Y., Lauer, M. R., & Sung, R. J. (1995). Electrophysiologic mechanisms of the long QT interval syndromes and *torsade de pointes. Annals of Internal Medicine, 122*, 701–714.

Tata, L. J., West, J., Smith, C., et al. (2005). General population based study of the impact of tricyclic and selective serotonin reuptake inhibitor antidepressants on the risk of acute myocardial infarction. *Heart, 91*, 465–471.

Thavendiranathan, P., Bagai, A., Khoo, C., Dorian, P., & Choudhry, N. K. (2009). Does this patient with palpitations have a cardiac arrhythmia? *Journal of the American Medical Association, 302*, 2135–2143.

Thayer, J. F., & Lane, R. D. (2009). Claude Bernard and the heart-brain connection: further elaboration of a model of neurovisceral integration. *Neuroscience & Biobehavioral Reviews, 33*, 81–88.

Thombs, B. D., de Jonge, P., Coyne, J. C., et al. (2008). Depression screening and patient outcome in cardiovascular care. A systematic review. *Journal of the American Medical Association, 300*, 2161–2171.

Tiihonen, J., Lönnqvist, J., Wahlbeck, K., et al. (2009). Eleven-year follow-up of mortality in patients with schizophrenia: a population-based cohort study (FIN11 study). *Lancet, 374*(9690), 620–627.

Tindle, H. A., Chang, Y-FP, Kuller, LHMDD, et al. (2009). Optimism, cynical hostility, and incident coronary heart disease and mortality in the Women's Health Initiative. *Circulation, 120*, 656–662.

Tousoulis, D., Antonopoulos, A. S., Antoniades, C., et al. (2010). Role of depression in heart failure—Choosing the right antidepressive treatment. *International Journal of Cardiology, 140*, 12–18.

Tutar, H. E., Öcal, B., Imamoglu, A., & Atalay, S. (1998). Dispersion of QT and QTc interval in healthy children, and effects of sinus arrhythmia on QT dispersion. *Heart, 80*, 77–79.

Vieweg, W. V. R. (1996). Antidepressant drug-induced blood pressure changes and their management. *Medical Update for Psychiatrists, 1*(5), 161–164.

Vieweg, W. V. R. (2002). Mechanisms and risks of electrocardiographic QT interval prolongation when using antipsychotic drugs. *Journal of Clinical Psychiatry, 63*(suppl 9), 18–24.

Vieweg, W. V. R. (2003). New generation antipsychotic drugs and QTc interval prolongation. *Primary Care Companion to the Journal of Clinical Psychiatry, 5*, 205–215.

Vieweg, W. V. R., & McDaniel, N. L. (2003a). Drug-induced QT interval prolongation and *torsade de pointes* in children and adolescents. Part I of a four-part series. *Child and Adolescent Psychopharmacology News, 8*(1), 1–7.

Vieweg, W. V. R., & McDaniel, N. L. (2003b). Drug-induced QT interval prolongation and *torsade de pointes* in children and adolescents. Part II of a four-part series. *Child and Adolescent Psychopharmacology News, 8*(2), 1–5.

Vieweg, W. V. R., & McDaniel, N. L. (2003c). Drug-induced QT interval prolongation and torsade de pointes in children and adolescents. Part III of a four-part series. *Child and Adolescent Psychopharmacology News, 8*(3), 1–4.

Vieweg, W. V. R., & McDaniel, N. L. (2003d). Drug-induced QT interval prolongation and *torsade de pointes* in children and adolescents. Part IV of a four-part series. *Child and Adolescent Psychopharmacology News, 8*(4), 1–4.

Vieweg, W. V. R., & Nicholson, C. S. (1996). Antidepressant drugs and the cardiovascular system. *Medical Update for Psychiatrists, 1*, 154–160.

Vieweg, W. V. R., & Wood, M. A. (2004). Tricyclic antidepressants, QT interval prolongation, and *torsade de pointes. Psychosomatics, 45*, 371–377.

Vieweg, W. V. R., Levy, J. R., Fredrickson, S. K., et al. (2008). Psychotropic drug considerations in depressed patients with metabolic disturbances. *American Journal of Medicine, 121*, 647–655.

Vieweg, W. V. R., Wood, M. A., Fernandez, A., Beatty-Brooks, M., Hasnain, M., & Pandurangi, A. K. (2009). Proarrhythmic risk with antipsychotic and antidepressant drugs: implications in the elderly. *Drugs & Aging, 26*, 997–1012.

Vieweg, W. V. R., Hasnain, M., Pandurangi, A. K., & Lesnefsky, E. J. (2010a). Major depression and coronary artery disease. *Archives of General Psychiatry, 67*, 653.

Vieweg, W. V. R., Hasnain, M., Lesnefsky, E. J., Turf, E. F., & Pandurangi, A. K. (2010b). Assessing the presence and severity of depression in subjects with comorbid coronary heart disease. *American Journal of Medicine, 123*, 683–690.

Vieweg, W. V. R., Hasnain, M., Mezuk, B., Levy, J., Lesnefsky, E. J., Pandurangi, A. K. (2011a). Depression, stress, and heart disease in earthquakes and Takotsubo cardiomyopathy. *American Journal of Medicine, 124*, 900–907.

Vieweg, W. V. R., Hasnain, M., Wood, M. A., Fernandez, A., Lesnefsky, E. J., & Pandurangi, A. K. (2011b). Cardiometabolic risks of antidepressant and antipsychotic drugs, Part 2. Metabolic risks of antidepressant and antipsychotic drugs. *Psychiatric Times, 28*(May), 68–71.

Vieweg, W. V. R., Hasnain, M., Wood, M. A., Fernandez, A., Lesnefsky, E. J., & Pandurangi, A. K. (2011c). Cardiometabolic risks of antidepressant and antipsychotic drugs, Part 1. Proarrhythmic risks of antidepressant and antipsychotic drugs. *Psychiatric Times, 28*(April), 50–55.

Vieweg, W. V., Hasnain, M., Howland, R. H., et al. (2012). Citalopram, QTc interval prolongation, and *torsade de pointes*. How should we apply the recent FDA ruling? *American Journal of Medicine, 125*, 859–868.

Vieweg, W. V., Hasnain, M., Hancox, J. C., et al. (2013). Risperidone, QTc interval prolongation, and torsade de pointes: a systematic review of case reports. *Psychopharmacology (Berl), 228*(4), 515–524.

Vieweg, W. V. R., Hancox, J. C., Hasnain, M., Koneru, J. N., Gysel, M., & Baranchuk, A. (2013a). Clarithromycin, QTc interval prolongation, and *torsades de pointes*: the need to study case reports. *Therapeutic Advances in Infectious Disease, 1*, 121–138.

Vieweg, W. V. R., Hasnain, M., Howland, R. H., et al. (2013b). Methadone, QTc interval prolongation and torsade de pointes: Case reports offer the best understanding of this problem. *Ther Adv Psychopharmacol, 3*(4), 219–232.

Vieweg, W. V., Hasnain, M., Hancox, J. C., et al. (2013c). Risperidone, QTc interval prolongation, and *torsade de pointes*: a systematic review of case reports. *Psychopharmacology (Berlin)*, June 30. [Epub ahead of print].

Vincent, G. M. (1999). Long QT syndrome. *Cardiology Clinics,18*, 309–325.

Virtanen, M., Ferrie, J. E., Singh-Manoux, A., et al. (2010). Overtime work and incident coronary heart disease: the Whitehall II prospective cohort study. *European Heart Journal, 31*, 1737–1744.

Viskin, S., Justo, D., Halkin, A., & Zeltser, D. (2003). Long QT syndrome caused by non-cardiac drugs. *Progress in Cardiovascular Diseases, 45*, 415–427.

Viskin, S., Rosovski, U., Sands, A. J., et al. (2005). Inaccurate electrocardiographic interpretation of long QT: the majority of physicians cannot recognize a long QT when they see one. *Heart Rhythm, 2*, 569–574.

Wang P. S., Schneeweiss S., Setoguchi S., et al. (2007). Ventricular arrhythmias and cerebrovascular events in the elderly using conventional and atypical antipsychotic medications. *Journal of Clinical Psychopharmacology, 27*, 707–710.

Whooley, M. A. (2009). To screen or not to screen? Depression in patients with cardiovascular disease. *Journal of the American College of Cardiology, 54*, 891–893.

Whooley, M. A., & Simon, G. E. (2000). Managing depression in medical outpatients. *New England Journal of Medicine, 343*, 1942–1950.

Wichman, C. L., Moore, K. M., Lang, T. R., St. Sauver, J. L., Heise, R. H., & Watson, W. J. (2009). Congenital heart disease associated with selective serotonin reuptake inhibitor use during pregnancy. *Mayo Clinic Proceedings, 84*, 23–27.

Williams, R. B. (2010). Myocardial infarction and risk of suicide: another reason to develop and test ways to reduce distress in postmyocardial-infarction patients? *Circulation, 122*(23), 2356–2358.

Wooley, M. A., & Simon, G. E. (2000). Managing depression in medical outpatients. *New England Journal of Medicine, 343*, 1942–1950.

Writing Committee for the ENRICHD Investigators (2003). Effects of treating depression and low perceived social support on clinical events after myocardial infarction. The Enhancing Recovery in Coronary Heart Disease Patients (ENRICHD) randomized trial. *Journal of the American Medical Association, 289*, 3106–3116.

Wulsin, L. R., & Singal, B. M. (2003). Do depressive symptoms increase the risk for the onset of coronary disease? A systematic quantitative review. *Psychosomatic Medicine, 65*, 201–210.

Wurst, K. E., Poole, C., Ephross, S. A., & Olshan, A. F. (2009). First trimester paroxetine use and the prevalence of congenital, specifically cardiac, defects: a meta-analysis of epidemiological studies. *Birth Defects Research, Part A, Clinical and Molecular Teratolology, 88*, 159–170.

Yap, Y. G., & Camm, J. (2000). Risk of *torsade de pointes* with non-cardiac drugs. *British Medical Journal, 320*, 1158–1159.

Yap, Y. G., Behr, E. R., & Camm, A. J. (2009). Drug-induced Brugada syndrome. *Europace: European pacing, arrhythmias, and cardiac electrophysiology: journal of the working groups on cardiac pacing, arrhythmias, and cardiac cellular electrophysiology of the European Society of Cardiology, 11*, 989–994.

Zarate, C. A., & Patel, J. (2001). Sudden cardiac death and antipsychotic drugs: do we know enough? *Archives of General Psychiatry, 58*, 1168–1171.

Ziegelstein, R. C., & Thombs, B. D. (2011). Is routine screening a parachute for heart disease patients with depression? *Journal of Psychosomatic Research, 71*, 3–5.

Ziegelstein, R. C., Thombs, B. D., Coyne, J. C., & de Jonge, P. (2009). Routine screening for depression in patients with coronary heart disease: Never mind. *Journal of the American College of Cardiology, 54*, 886–890.

Zielinski, R. J., Roose, S. P., Devanand, D. P., Woodring, S., & Sackeim, H. A. (1993). Cardiovascular complications of ECT in depressed patients with cardiac disease. *American Journal of Psychiatry, 150*, 904–909.

Zuidersma, M., Thombs, B. D., & de Jonge P. (2011). Onset and recurrence of depression as predictors of cardiovascular prognosis in depressed acute coronary syndrome patients: A systematic review. *Psychotherapy & Psychosomatics, 80*, 227–237.

53.

MULTIDIMENSIONAL BEHAVIORAL MEDICINE STRATEGIES

MANAGEMENT OF TOBACCO USE AND OBESITY

Michael G. Goldstein and Margaret Dundon

INTRODUCTION

Behavioral medicine is the interdisciplinary field concerned with the development and integration of behavioral, psychosocial, and biomedical science knowledge and techniques relevant to the understanding of health and illness, and the application of this knowledge and these techniques to prevention, diagnosis, treatment and rehabilitation (Society of Behavioral Medicine, 2012). Behavioral Medicine interventions may be applied at the clinical, population or community level. In this chapter, we will focus on the application of Behavioral Medicine interventions within clinical settings and will emphasize the integration of these interventions within a Patient-Centered Medical Home model. The Patient-Centered Medical Home (PCMH) is an approach to organizing primary care that has been advocated by the Institute of Medicine, the United States Agency for Healthcare Research and Quality (AHRQ), the National Committee on Quality Assurance and a wide range of primary care medical societies and organizations (Carrier, Gourevitch, & Shah, 2009; Rosenthal, 2008). To meet the AHRQ definition of a PCMH, a health care system must: deliver patient-centered, comprehensive and coordinated care; provide superb access; and employ a system-based approach to quality and safety (Agency for Healthcare Research and Quality, 2012).

Delivering evidence-based preventive care is a critical element of a comprehensive PCMH and promoting positive health behaviors is critical to preventing illness and optimizing patient health and wellbeing. Health behaviors accounted for almost 50% of mortality in the United States in 2000 (Mokdad, Marks, Stroup, & Gerberding, 2004). Among all causes of death, the leading causes were tobacco (435,000 deaths; 18.1% of total US deaths) and poor diet and physical inactivity (365,000 deaths; 15.2%) (Mokdad et al., 2004). This chapter focuses on tobacco use and obesity, two conditions that have strong behavioral and psychosocial determinants. In the sections that follow, we will describe how to apply a multi-dimensional behavioral medicine approach to the management of these conditions and will illustrate how to integrate assessment and treatment of tobacco use and obesity within the emerging Patient-Centered Medical Home model. We will focus our attention on the assessment and treatment of tobacco use and obesity in adults.

TOBACCO USE AND DEPENDENCE

Cigarette smoking remains the single greatest preventable cause of premature death, disability, and unnecessary expense in the United States (U.S. Department of Health and Human Services, 2010). Currently, about 44 million adults, or about 19% of the U.S. adult population, smoke cigarettes (B. A. King, Dube, & Tynan, 2012) and 70% of smokers report wanting to quit (M. Fiore et al., 2008). Cigarette use, along with other forms of tobacco use such as smokeless tobacco and cigars, is responsible for nearly one in five deaths (443,000) annually in the US, and for $100 billion annually of direct medical costs and $97 billion in lost productivity (M. C. Fiore & Baker, 2011). Though most smokers want to quit, quitting smoking can be very difficult, especially for the heavily dependent smoker. Data from the 2010 National Health Interview Survey revealed that 52% of adult smokers had made a quit attempt in the past year, but only 6% were able to successfully quit (CDC, 2011). Biological, psychological, behavioral, and socioenvironmental factors all play a role in the development and maintenance of dependence on tobacco products (D. B. Abrams et al., 2003; Benowitz, 2010; U.S. Department of Health and Human Services, 2010). Smoking prevalence is particularly high among several subgroups including those with low educational attainment, low socioeconomic status, and individuals with psychiatric disorders, including substance use disorders (B. A. King et al., 2012; McClave, McKnight-Eily, Davis, & Dube, 2010; Ziedonis et al., 2008).

The 2008 US Public Health Service (PHS) Clinical Practice Guideline for Treating Tobacco Use and Dependence (CPG) (M. Fiore et al., 2008) (available at http://www.ahrq.gov/professionals/clinicians-providers/guidelines-recommendations/tobacco/clinicians/update/treating_tobacco_use08.pdf) identifies multiple effective smoking cessation

To successfully quit tobacco use, consider all of the factors that contribute to your use of tobacco. It can be helpful to group these factors into three main categories: physical factors, habits, and psychological factors (i.e., your thoughts and emotions).

Physically, nicotine is the most addictive substance on the planet. Your medical provider will tell you whether it is appropriate for you to use a nicotine replacement product, such as the patch or gum. Some medications, like Zyban, are very helpful to some people but don't seem to help other people with their nicotine cravings. Sometimes, using two products together can help relieve cravings and withdrawal symptoms better. It is best to work closely with your medical provider to choose the best medication or combination of medications which may be right for you. These products have been proven to help people quit and are often key to success. People who use medication have much higher rates of success in quitting.

Behaviorally, you will need to change your habits and the situations that you typically associate with tobacco. Undoubtedly, you will experience situations that cause you to crave tobacco, but you can learn skills that will help you choose alternatives other than using tobacco. Practical counseling and support are available to help you through this process and can help you recognize situations that tempt you to use tobacco, problem-solve and develop skills to cope with these situations. Even brief counseling greatly increases the success of a quit attempt. Also, if you would find telephone counseling supportive, you can call 1-800-Quit-Now to get connected to your state telephone quit line.

Thoughts and emotions are some of the hardest aspects of tobacco use to change. Changing thoughts to cope with stress and negative emotions is an essential aspect of successful tobacco cessation. One helpful strategy is to list your top 3 reasons for quitting, and remind yourself of them as a way to stay strong if you need a boost along the way. Take a moment to list *your* main reasons for quitting:

1. _____

2. _____

3. _____

Preparing to Quit

Your Quit Date

When is the last day and time that you are going to use tobacco?
Month_____ Day_____ Year_____ Time_____

Preparing Your Surroundings

What are the things that remind you to use tobacco? It is important to change your surroundings so that you won't be reminded about tobacco use as frequently. Before your quit date consider the following:

- Don't buy tobacco in bulk (e.g., don't buy cartons).

- Find all of your hidden stashes of tobacco or supplies (ashtrays etc.) and dispose of them.

- Prepare family and friends. Let them know that you are planning to quit and ask for their help. If you have friends and family who do use tobacco, ask if they would avoid using tobacco around you.

- Prepare and develop a plan for coping with cravings and withdrawal symptoms. Use the combination of strategies that works for you.

- Choose a method to quit. There are several ways to consider quitting, but one of the most important is to use medications and prepare for coping with urges as well as stress.

Quitting is difficult and many people find it to be challenging. Preparing can help you succeed. What do you expect to be the most difficult challenge for you as you quit? Will it be going without a cigarette with your morning coffee? Will it be not smoking when your spouse or friends light up? Anticipating and having a plan for how to handle these challenges will increase your success.

As you prepare to quit there are other things in your life that you can do a little bit differently that will help you to be successful. There may be places you should avoid or things you should do differently.

Using the Four A's to Outsmart Tobacco Urges

Avoid. What are the situations or places that you need to avoid over the next month?

1. _____

2. _____

Figure 53.1 Tobacco Cessation: How to Change?

Alter. What situations will you need to change to help you be more successful?

1. _____

2. _____

Alternatives. What can you put in your mouth or hands instead of using tobacco?

1. _____

2. _____

Action. When you get an urge to use tobacco, what can you do to be active or busy?

1. _____

2. _____

Follow-Up Plan:

_____

_____

_____

Adapted from: Hunter, C. L., Goodie, J. L., Oordt, M. S., & Dobmeyer, A. C. (2009). Integrated *Behavioral Health in Primary Care: Step-by-step Guidance for Assessment and Intervention.* Washington, DC: American Psychological Association.

Figure 53.1 Continued

treatments, including both behavioral and pharmacologic interventions. As we will stress in the discussion below, treatment that combines behavioral and pharmacologic intervention elements is more effective than either behavioral or pharmacologic treatment alone (M. Fiore et al., 2008; M. C. Fiore & Baker, 2011). However, less than a third of smokers will utilize either medication or counseling in their efforts to stop smoking (CDC, 2011). Even a small increase in the percentage of people who use effective treatments during efforts to quit can have a significant impact on smoking cessation rates. Because more than 70% of smokers see a physician or other health care clinician each year, clinicians have multiple opportunities to offer tobacco cessation interventions and encourage patients who want to quit to employ effective treatments (M. Fiore et al., 2008; M. C. Fiore & Baker, 2011; Jamal, Dube, Malarcher, Shaw, & Engstrom, 2012; Rigotti, 2012). The CPG also frames tobacco dependence as a chronic condition, with most smokers experiencing periods of remission and relapse and requiring multiple quit attempts before achieving stable maintenance of abstinence. As with other chronic conditions, such as diabetes and hypertension, clinicians should consider taking a long term view marked by repeated efforts to offer patient education, counseling and intervention.

In the sections that follow, we will first summarize evidence regarding the factors that contribute to tobacco use and dependence that impact treatment decisions. Then, we will outline evidence-based interventions for tobacco use and dependence, emphasizing the recommendations of the US PHS Clinical Practice Guideline (M. Fiore et al., 2008). We will also offer guidance for implementing a patient-centered approach to tobacco use treatment in health care settings, particularly within the context of a PCMH.

GENERAL CONSIDERATIONS FOR TREATMENT

NICOTINE DEPENDENCE AND NICOTINE'S EFFECTS

Nicotine dependence, like other forms of substance use dependence, results from a complex interplay of pharmacology, learned or conditioned factors, genetics, and social and environmental factors (Benowitz, 2010). Nicotine is a powerful pharmacologic agent with a wide variety of stimulant and depressant effects involving the central and peripheral nervous, cardiovascular, endocrine, and other systems (Benowitz, 2010; U.S. Department of Health and Human Services, 1988, 2010). Release of brain dopamine, glutamate, and GABA is particularly important in the development of nicotine dependence (Benowitz, 2010). Reinforcement of nicotine use results from nicotine's "positive" effects, including arousal, increased concentration and enhancement of mood, while negative reinforcement occurs when nicotine use leads to avoidance of withdrawal symptoms after periods of abstinence (Benowitz, 2010). The very rapid speed of nicotine delivery to the lung alveoli and to the brain (7 to 10 seconds post inhalation) contributes to nicotine's reinforcing effects, as well as to behavioral conditioning resulting from the strong association between cues associated with smoking (i.e., situations, taste, smell, handling) and reinforcement (Benowitz, 2010).

Significant nicotine withdrawal symptoms occur among at least 50% of smokers who try to quit (J. R. Hughes, 2007). The signs and symptoms of nicotine withdrawal can appear within 2 to 6 hours after the last use of tobacco, usually peak between 24 and 48 hours after cessation, and last from a few days to a few weeks (Benowitz, 2010; J. Hughes & Hatsukami, 1992). Withdrawal symptoms include craving or urges to use nicotine, dysphoric or depressed mood, irritability, frustration, anger, anxiety, difficulty concentrating, restlessness, decreased heart rate and increased appetite or weight gain (J. Hughes & Hatsukami, 1992). Some smokers experience episodic response to tobacco cues, and urges to smoke, years after quitting (Ferguson & Shiffman, 2009; R. S. Niaura et al., 1988). There is a continuum of nicotine dependence, from mild to severe, among the population of smokers (R. Niaura & Shadel, 2003). Genetic studies indicate that nicotinic receptor subtypes and the genes involved in neuroplasticity play a role in the development of dependence, while other studies suggest that people with psychiatric or substance-abuse disorders have an increased susceptibility to tobacco dependence (Benowitz, 2010). The experience of serious withdrawal symptoms after quitting, smoking more than 25 cigarettes per day or smoking a cigarette within 15 to 30 minutes after awakening suggest higher levels of nicotine dependence, and more difficulty with unaided quitting (Benowitz, 2010; Rigotti, 2012).

PSYCHIATRIC COMORBIDITY

Individuals with comorbid psychiatric disorders, especially anxiety, mood disorders, other substance abuse disorders, and schizophrenia, are associated with increased prevalence of smoking, higher levels of nicotine dependence and more difficulty achieving abstinence from tobacco use (Hitsman, Moss, Montoya, & George, 2009; Kalman, Morissette, & George, 2005; Ziedonis et al., 2008). Nicotine use in these individuals is impacted by a complex interplay of factors, including increased vulnerability to nicotine's effects, nicotine's effects on psychiatric symptoms, challenges managing craving and nicotine withdrawal symptoms, and interactions between nicotine, psychiatric medications and other psychoactive substances (Hitsman et al., 2009; Kalman et al., 2005; Ziedonis et al., 2008). Therefore, more intensive and tailored interventions are needed for individuals with these comorbid conditions (Kalman et al., 2005; Ziedonis et al., 2008). For example, it may be critical to understand an individual's reasons and triggers for smoking in order to better prepare them for quitting. It may also be important to address underlying issues such as depression or anxiety or alcohol abuse, before, or at least concurrently with tobacco cessation in order to enhance the effectiveness of treatment interventions for these patients (Hitsman et al., 2009; McFall et al., 2007; McFall et al., 2005; Ziedonis et al., 2008).

MEDICAL COMORBIDITY AND NICOTINE DEPENDENCE

There is no safe level of smoking and no safe tobacco product. The scientific evidence of bodily damage from smoking has grown steadily for more than 50 years and is documented in 30 Surgeon General Reports. The 2010 report lists 13 cancers causally linked to smoking and over 12 additional chronic diseases (U.S. Department of Health and Human Services, 2010).

Tobacco inhalation includes over 7,000 chemicals, 69 of which are known carcinogens. The cellular changes related to absorption of these toxic chemicals lead to disease, particularly cancer, cardiovascular and pulmonary diseases. Disease mechanisms include DNA damage, inflammation, and oxidative stress (U.S. Department of Health and Human Services, 2010).

REPRODUCTIVE AND POST-PARTUM EFFECTS

Tobacco smoke exposure has been linked to multiple adverse reproductive outcomes (U.S. Department of Health and Human Services, 2010). They include low birth weight, possible cognitive and neurobehavioral deficits, cleft lip with or without cleft palate, histopathologic changes in the lung and brain of the fetus from maternal smoking, reduced gestation and possible miscarriage (U.S. Department of Health and Human Services, 2010). Maternal smoking is clearly linked to transient increases in heart rate and blood pressure, placental problems, immunosuppressive effects that may lead to miscarriage and preterm delivery, and diminished oviductal functioning which could impair fertilization (U.S. Department of Health and Human Services, 2010). In addition, paternal smoking is linked to DNA damage in sperm and reduced fertility, pregnancy viability issues and anomalies in offspring (U.S. Department of Health and Human Services, 2010).

Utilizing intensive behavioral counseling interventions with pregnant smokers is extremely important and should continue throughout pregnancy and postpartum (M. Fiore et al., 2008) as smoking in households with young children results in significant increases in the prevalence of asthma, upper respiratory and ear infections, and doubles the risk of sudden infant death syndrome (SIDS) (U.S. Department of Health and Human Services, 2010). The safety and effectiveness of nicotine replacement medication and other cessation medications in pregnancy is unclear (M. Fiore et al., 2008). Because of some evidence that nicotine replacement use during pregnancy may be associated with small risks to the fetus, and because trials assessing the effectiveness of NRT among pregnant women are inconclusive, NRT during pregnancy was not recommended by the CPG (M. Fiore et al., 2008). Encouraging pregnant smokers who are reluctant to quit to, at a minimum, reduce their smoking rate, is likely to have beneficial effects, as a dose-response relationship between smoking rate and birth weight has been observed (M. Fiore et al., 2008).

FEAR OF POST-CESSATION WEIGHT GAIN

There is substantial evidence that cigarette smoking is associated with lower body weight on average, and that smoking cessation is associated with weight gain, generally under 10 pounds (M. Fiore et al., 2008). However, as many as 10% of quitters gain as much as 30 pounds and some smokers, especially women, smoke to prevent weight gain despite the risks (Kleges & Kleges, 1988). In addition, some data suggest that fear of post-cessation weight gain may decrease rates of smoking cessation (Pomerleau & Saules, 2007). Smoking cessation programs that have added a weight control component have not been successful at decreasing post-cessation weight gain or enhancing achievement of smoking cessation, though they also do not appear to reduce cessation success (M. Fiore et al., 2008; Spring et al., 2009). Use of 4 mg nicotine gum and lozenge, and Bupropion SR delay but do not prevent post-cessation weight gain (M. Fiore et al., 2008). One promising approach to minimizing the weight gain associated with smoking cessation is to increase physical activity (Marcus et al., 2005). Others have suggested that rather than try to combat post-cessation weight gain, it might be more effective to help ex-smokers accept the weight gain (M. Fiore et al., 2008). A table outlining suggested clinician statements to help a patient prepare for post-cessation weight gain is available in the PHS CPG—(Table 7.9) (M. Fiore et al., 2008).

MOTIVATION

Though 70% of smokers express an interest in quitting smoking, only about 20% of smokers are ready to attempt to quit at any given time (M. C. Fiore & Baker, 2011). Thus, exploration of motivation is a key element of tobacco use cessation efforts (M. Fiore et al., 2008). A variety of factors may contribute to smokers' low motivation or ambivalence regarding quitting, including limited understanding about the risks of smoking or the benefits of quitting, concerns about the effects of quitting (e.g., withdrawal symptoms, dysphoria, and weight gain) and lack of confidence in their ability to quit. Providing advice or admonitions to quit to patients who are not ready is usually not effective and may harden ambivalence or produce discord. In contrast, Motivational Interviewing (MI), a collaborative patient-centered approach that seeks to explore ambivalence and elicit and strengthen the individual's intrinsic motivation, is associated with an increase in both quit attempts and a modest but significant increase in abstinence from smoking (Lai, Cahill, Qin, & Tang, 2010). Several of the strategies described in the MI chapter in this textbook can be used to enhance motivation among ambivalent smokers.

RECOMMENDATIONS FOR INTERVENTIONS IN HEALTH CARE SETTINGS

Based on an extensive review of the research literature, the 2008 update of the US Public Health Service Treating Tobacco Use and Dependence Clinical Practice Guideline (M. Fiore et al., 2008) made the following 10 key findings and recommendations:

1. Tobacco dependence is a chronic disease that often requires repeated intervention and multiple attempts to quit. Effective treatments exist, however, that can significantly increase rates of long-term abstinence.

2. It is essential that clinicians and health care delivery systems consistently identify and document tobacco use status and treat every tobacco user seen in a health care setting.

3. Tobacco dependence treatments are effective across a broad range of populations. Clinicians should encourage every patient willing to make a quit attempt to use the counseling treatments and medications recommended in this Guideline.

4. Brief tobacco dependence treatment is effective. Clinicians should offer every patient who uses tobacco at least the brief treatments shown to be effective in this Guideline (see recommendation #4 as well as the discussion below).

5. Individual, group, and telephone counseling are effective, and their effectiveness increases with treatment intensity. Two components of counseling are especially effective, and clinicians should use these when counseling patients making a quit attempt: (a) practical counseling (problem solving/skills training), and (b) social support delivered as part of treatment.

6. Numerous effective medications are available for tobacco dependence, and clinicians should encourage their use by all patients attempting to quit smoking—except when medically contraindicated or with specific populations for which there is insufficient evidence of effectiveness (i.e., pregnant women, smokeless tobacco users, light smokers, and adolescents). Seven first-line medications (5 nicotine and 2 non-nicotine) reliably increase long-term smoking abstinence rates:

   - Bupropion SR
   - Nicotine gum
   - Nicotine inhaler
   - Nicotine lozenge
   - Nicotine nasal spray
   - Nicotine patch
   - Varenicline

   Clinicians also should consider the use of certain combinations of medications identified as effective in this Guideline (see discussion below).

7. Counseling and medication are effective when used by themselves for treating tobacco dependence. The combination of counseling and medication, however, is more effective than either alone. Thus, clinicians should encourage all individuals making a quit attempt to use both counseling and medication.

8. Telephone quitline counseling is effective with diverse populations and has broad reach. Therefore, both clinicians and health care delivery systems should ensure patient access to quitlines and promote quitline use.

9. If a tobacco user currently is unwilling to make a quit attempt, clinicians should use the motivational methods shown in this Guideline to be effective in increasing

future quit attempts (see section on Motivation in this chapter and discussion below).

10. Tobacco dependence treatments are both clinically effective and highly cost-effective relative to interventions for other clinical disorders. Providing coverage for these treatments increases quit rates. Insurers and purchasers should ensure that all insurance plans include the counseling and medication identified as effective in this Guideline as covered benefits.

As noted in the CPG, evidence is clear and compelling that health care providers should routinely ask patients about their tobacco use status and document it in the medical record (M. Fiore et al., 2008; M. C. Fiore & Baker, 2011). Clinic-based reminders that prompt clinic staff to ask about smoking status increase rates of screening and intervention and should be implemented in all health care settings (M. Fiore et al., 2008; M. C. Fiore & Baker, 2011). Further, brief clinician intervention increases abstinence rates, even if delivered during an interaction lasting 3 minutes or less (M. Fiore et al., 2008; M. C. Fiore & Baker, 2011). However, because there is a dose-response relationship between intensity of intervention and abstinence rates, more intensive interventions (i.e., at least 4 sessions for a total of at least 20 minutes) should be made available to smokers who want assistance in quitting (M. Fiore et al., 2008; M. C. Fiore & Baker, 2011).

The following section of this chapter outlines core elements for a stepped care, comprehensive, patient-centered approach for tobacco cessation programming that is consistent with the CPG and current evidence. It is designed to take advantage of multiple members of a health care team so no one member is saddled with all the responsibility for assessment and intervention. Readily accessible treatment, at the intensity desired by the patient, promotes patient engagement and is an essential feature of this approach (M. C. Fiore & Baker, 2011).

Despite convincing evidence for the effectiveness of tobacco cessation intervention in health care settings, recent evidence indicates that, although tobacco use screening occurred during the majority of adult visits to outpatient physician offices during 2005–2008 (62.7%), among patients who were identified as current tobacco users, only 20.9% received tobacco cessation counseling (Jamal et al., 2012). The approach outlined in this chapter may help clinicians to overcome barriers to implementation so they might intervene more consistently and effectively.

FIVE STRATEGIES (THE 5 A'S) AND THREE LEVELS OF CARE

The intervention approach described below is based on the "5A's" approach to addressing tobacco use that is described in detail in the PHS CPG (M. Fiore et al., 2008) and outlined below (Table 53.1). This CPG version of the 5 A's differs slightly from the subsequent version that was recommended by the Counseling and Behavioral Interventions Work Group of the U.S. Preventive Services Task Force (USPSTF) in 2002 (E. P. Whitlock, Orleans,

Table 53.1 THE 5 A'S MODEL FOR TREATING TOBACCO USE AND DEPENDENCE

Ask about tobacco use	Identify and document tobacco use status for every patient at every visit. (Strategy A1)
Advise to quit	In a clear, strong, and personalized manner, urge every tobacco user to quit (Strategy A2)
Assess willingness to make a quit attempt	Is the tobacco user willing to make a quit attempt at this time? (Strategy A3)
Assist in quit attempt	For the patient willing to make a quit attempt, offer medication and provide or refer for counseling or additional treatment to help the patient quit. (Strategy A4)
	For patients unwilling to quit at the time, provide interventions designed to increase future quit attempts. (Strategies B1 and B2)
Arrange followup	For the patient willing to make a quit attempt, arrange for followup contacts, beginning within the first week after the quit date. (Strategy A5)
	For patients unwilling to make a quit attempt at the time, address tobacco dependence and willingness to quit at next clinic visit.

From PHS Treating Tobacco Use and Dependence" is an acknowledgment that table 53.1 was reproduced from the PHS CPG (M. Fiore et al., 2008 (May)

Pender, & Allan, 2002). The USPSTF recommended adoption of the "5 A's" construct as a unifying conceptual framework for evaluating and describing health behavior counseling interventions in clinical settings (E. P. Whitlock et al., 2002). When we address the 4th A, Assist, we will describe 3 "levels" of intervention (i.e., brief, moderate, intensive) which may applied in a "stepped-care" manner. In the obesity section of this chapter we will specify the minor differences between the USPSTF version of the 5A's and the version used in the CPG.

A1. Ask about tobacco- Identify and document tobacco use status for every patient at every visit. Structuring a clinic system to systematically identify all tobacco users at every visit is associated with increased tobacco use counseling (M. Fiore et al., 2008). This may be accomplished through electronic clinical reminders or with expanded vital signs documentation to include tobacco use. The responsibility for documenting tobacco status can be shared across the clinic team but should be explicitly determined.

A2. Advise to quit- Offer clear and unambiguous advice to quit, preferably tied to the individual patient's health concerns. For example, "As your clinician, I must tell you that quitting smoking is one of the most important things you can do to protect your health, now and in the future. Continuing to smoke makes your asthma worse, and quitting will dramatically improve your health". Before providing advice, it is helpful to ask the patient about their understanding of the impact of smoking on their health. Clinician use of this patient-centered strategy promotes patient engagement, limits unnecessary information sharing and provides an opportunity for the clinician to reinforce the patient's understanding. When providing information and advice, it is also useful to ask permission first, (e.g., "Would it be ok if I shared some information about the benefits of quitting smoking?"). Asking permission before providing advice is not only respectful, it supports patient autonomy, which is especially important when patients are not ready for taking action (Miller & Rollnick, 2013; S. Rollnick, Mason, & Butler, 1999; G. C. Williams et al., 2006). See below, under A4, for a more extensive discussion of motivational strategies.

A3. Assess willingness to quit—Assessment of the patient's interest in and motivation for quitting is a key step. Simply asking, "What are your thoughts about quitting?" may start a productive conversation that allows the clinician to tailor intervention based on the patient's motivation.

A4. Assist the patient. Assistance is tailored to the patient based on their willingness to quit.

A4.1. For those patients clearly unwilling to pursue quitting at that time, future treatment engagement will be more likely if the clinician offers a non-judgmental, supportive response such as, "It doesn't sound like you are interested in quitting right now. If you decide you want to consider quitting in the future, I will be happy to help you." For those patients who are ambivalent about quitting, use of motivational strategies can be productive and can increase the likelihood of making a quit attempt in the future (M. Fiore et al., 2008). The use of Motivational Interviewing (MI), a specific person-centered clinical method for enhancing motivation by addressing ambivalence about change (Miller & Rollnick, 2013; S. Rollnick et al., 1999), increases tobacco cessation rates more than advice alone (M. C. Fiore & Baker, 2011; Lai et al., 2010). Training is needed for clinicians to develop and effectively apply MI skills (Miller & Rollnick, 2013). However, even without specific training in MI, use of a patient-centered approach that supports patient autonomy, builds trust, affirms existing kernels of motivation and avoids shaming, directing and judging is much more effective at building motivation than more directive or confrontational approaches (Miller & Rollnick, 2013; S. Rollnick et al., 1999; G. C. Williams et al., 2006).

The 5 R's approach described in the PHS CPG is useful for framing brief motivational elements. The 5 R's are: identify personally *R*elevant reasons to quit, review perceived *R*isks of smoking; identify *R*ewards for quitting, explore potential *R*oadblocks to success; and address motivation through *R*epetition at subsequent visits (See also the chapter in this text on Motivational Interviewing) see Table 53.2.

A4.2. For those patients who are willing to make a quit attempt, the clinician should offer a menu of treatment options that include medication, brief behavioral counseling, or an intensive group program (See below for a discussion about varying the intensity of intervention to accommodate both patient preferences and typical clinic constraints.). For those patients who are willing to consider a quit attempt, asking permission to share treatment options may set a productive and collaborative tone. "Would you be interested in talking about treatment options?" is one such example. The discussion of treatment options should include a range of choices to accommodate patient preferences as well as maximize success.

A4.3. For patients willing to make a quit attempt, we describe three levels of intensity of tobacco cessation treatment (in terms of duration of treatment and number of contacts): brief, intermediate and intensive. The choice among levels of treatment intensity is largely determined by patient preference, though clinical constraints due to limited staffing and lack of resources may also influence the choice of treatment intensity. As emphasized in the PHS CPG, the combination of pharmacological and behavioral interventions produces higher quit rates than either element alone (M. Fiore et al., 2008 (May); M. C. Fiore & Baker, 2011; Rigotti, 2012). Thus, even brief interventions should offer 3 elements: medication, a behavioral component that addresses triggers for smoking and barriers to quitting; and educational resources. According to a meta-analysis of 35 randomized trials, there is a dose-response relationship between the minutes of total counseling contact and 6-month abstinence rates: about 14% for 1 to 3 minutes of counseling, 19% for 4 to 30 minutes of counseling, and 27% for 31 to 90 minutes of counseling, versus 11% for no counseling (M. Fiore et al., 2008 (May)). (Some studies included pharmacotherapy across all counseling conditions, so medication contributed to these success rates.). A 2012 Cochrane review of the benefits of combining behavioral counseling and medication found a 70 to 100% increase in quit rates when pharmacotherapy was combined with intensive behavioral compared to usual care, brief intervention or minimal behavioral counseling (Stead & Lancaster, 2012). Because intensive interventions that offer multiple contacts and more minutes of behavioral counseling produce the best outcomes, all patients who are interested in intensive treatment should have access to this level of treatment (M. Fiore et al., 2008 (May)). Patients with higher degrees of nicotine dependence, those with co-morbid mental health conditions and substance abuse, and those who have struggled to quit using less intensive interventions are likely to derive the greatest benefit from more intensive interventions, though all populations of smokers fare better when receiving intensive vs. briefer treatments (M. Fiore et al., 2008 (May)). However, many patients are not able to commit to intensive intervention or prefer less intensive interventions. As noted in the PHS CPG, even very brief interventions enhance quit rates when compared to no intervention.

Table 53.2 ENHANCING MOTIVATION TO QUIT TOBACCO—THE 5 R'S

Relevance	Encourage the patient to indicate why quitting is personally relevant, being as specific as possible. Motivational information has the greatest impact if it is relevant to a patient's disease status or risk, family or social situation (e.g., having children in the home), health concerns, age, gender, and other important patient characteristics (e.g., prior quitting experience, personal barriers to cessation).
Risks	The clinician should ask the patient to identify potential negative con-sequences of tobacco use. The clinician may suggest and highlight those that seem most relevant to the patient. The clinician should emphasize that smoking low-tar/low-nicotine cigarettes or use of other forms of tobacco (e.g., smokeless to bacco, cigars, and pipes) will not eliminate these risks. Examples of risks are: • *Acute risks*: Shortness of breath, exacerbation of asthma, increased risk of respiratory infections, harm to pregnancy, impotence, infertility. • *Long-term risks:* Heart attacks and strokes, lung and other cancers (e.g., larynx, oral cavity, pharynx, esophagus, pancreas, stomach, kidney, bladder, cervix, and acute myelocytic leukemia), chronic obstructive pulmonary diseases (chronic bronchitis and emphysema), osteoporosis, long-term disability, and need for extended care. • *Environmental risk:* Increased risk of lung cancer and heart disease in spouses; Increased risk for low birth-weight, sudden infant death syndrome (SIDS), asthma, middle ear disease, and respiratory infec-tions in children of smokers.
Rewards	The clinician should ask the patient to identify potential benefits of stopping tobacco use. The clinician may suggest and highlight those that seem most relevant to the patient. Examples of rewards follow: • Improved health • Food will taste better • Improved sense of smell • Saving money • Feeling better about oneself • Home, car, clothing, breath will smell better • Setting a good example for children and decreasing the likelihood that they will smoke • Having healthier babies and children • Feeling better physically • Performing better in physical activities • Improved appearance, including reduced wrinkling/aging of skin and whiter teeth
Roadblocks	The clinician should ask the patient to identify barriers or impediments to quitting and provide treatment (problem solving counseling, medication) that could address barriers. Typical barriers might include: • Withdrawal symptoms • Fear of failure • Weight gain • Lack of support • Depression • Enjoyment of tobacco • Being around other tobacco users • Limited knowledge of effective treatment options
Repetition	The motivational intervention should be repeated every time an unmotivated patient visits the clinic setting. Tobacco users who have failed in previous quit attempts should be told that most people make repeated quit attempts before they are successful.

From the PHS CPG (M. Fiore et al., 2008 (May)).

A4.3. Level One: Brief Intervention Brief intervention may be delivered in a single session. As noted previously, all interventions should offer effective tobacco cessation medications plus behavioral strategies as offering both elements together significantly enhances success (M. Fiore et al., 2008 (May); M. C. Fiore & Baker, 2011). Thus, at a minimum, a brief intervention should include identifying a quit date, removing tobacco use cues, choosing a medication (unless the patient does not want medication) and making a referral to other cessation resources that offer behavioral counseling. This very brief approach, which may be delivered with minimum staffing and resources, has been called AAR (Ask, Advise, Refer) (Rigotti, 2012; Schroeder, 2012). The additional resources might include written guides, online resources or telephone or online counseling (see also Level Two section below). The referral process can be simplified further by using templated fax forms or referral cards. Key behavioral strategies include: selecting a quit date, encouraging patients to share quit plans with others to solicit support for quitting; and helping the patient to employ specific strategies to anticipate and prepare for barriers and challenges to quitting. Exploring previous experience with quitting helps patients to identify triggers for smoking and potential relapse situations while also identifying strategies that helped them to successfully cope with urges, triggers and challenges. Brief advice for managing triggers includes 3 simple and practical behavioral strategies:1)advising *removal* of all nicotine use-related items (cigarettes, lighters etc.) prior to quitting; 2) *avoiding* or *altering* situations associated with urges or previous lapses; and3) *problem-solving* to identify possible substitutes for situations or emotions associated with urges or previous lapses. A sample planning sheet is provided in table *53.3*. In addition, there is an online guide to quitting available free of charge at www.smokefree.gov.

A4.3 Level Two: Moderate Intervention. This mid-level intervention offers more than brief intervention, and may include up to 3 individual contacts. The contacts may be delivered in a variety of modalities including face-to-face appointments with a trained member of the clinic team, such as a nurse, a behaviorist (most often psychologist or social worker), or a pharmacist. Alternatively, effective counseling may be delivered via telephone (M. Fiore et al., 2008 (May); M. C. Fiore & Baker, 2011) and can be accessed via state quitlines (1-800 QUIT NOW) or through the Tobacco Control Research Branch of the National Cancer Institute (NCI) (1-877-44U-QUIT). The expansion of interactive computer and smart phone technology has great potential to support cessation efforts and reach the 75% of US adults who are on-line (Whittaker et al., 2012) though the evidence for the effectiveness of this modality of intervention is not as strong as for face-to-face

and telephone-based live counseling (M. C. Fiore & Baker, 2011). NCI is currently testing the effectiveness of LiveHelp, an online health program that uses social media and text messaging. Emerging technologies such as smart phone "apps" are also showing promise in supporting cessation success. Currently, there are at least a dozen versions of mobile apps available to support quitting. Many of these electronic approaches are expected to be particularly appealing to young smokers, though their effectiveness still needs to be studied.

A4.3. Level Three—Intensive Intervention: The most intensive level of treatment is face-face individual or group treatment with at least 4 sessions. Group intervention is widely available in a variety of standardized formats through agencies such The American Lung Association (ALA), the American Cancer Society (ACS) and the proprietary sector. These programs can be offered within the clinic or, patients may be referred to community offerings. As noted previously, key elements of intensive intervention include pharmacotherapy, practical problem-solving behavioral counseling and educational tools and resources. Offering multiple sessions provides an opportunity to deliver tailored treatment across the three phases of treatment: preparation, quitting and maintenance/preventing relapse (Brown, 2003). The behavioral treatment elements included in intensive treatment are discussed in more detail below in section on specific smoking cessation counseling strategies.

A5. Arrange for follow-up contacts, either in person on the phone, or through one of the new technological options such as a smartphone application. While follow-up is a core element of any moderate or intensive program, follow-up contact is also recommended for brief intervention and even after a motivational intervention for patients not ready to quit (M. Fiore et al., 2008 (May); M. C. Fiore & Baker, 2011). If a quit attempt is planned, initial follow-up should occur shortly after quitting tobacco, preferably within 3–7 days. A system for follow-up could include secure e-mail, telephone follow-up with administrative support staff, or, if time permits, a phone call from a clinical team member to inquire about the patient's experience. Implementing a health system approach that triggers assessment of smoking status at every visit provides opportunities to provide follow-up even when specific encounters for tobacco cessation are not planned. This systems-based approach, together with the chronic, relapsing nature of tobacco dependence, provides multiple opportunities to support abstinence, encourage additional quit attempts or make adjustments to current strategies as needed. For example, if patients who have quit are still struggling with strong urges, or using nicotine replacement months after quitting, the clinician may add additional pharmacological or behavioral interventions to help the patient maintain abstinence.

PHARMACOTHERAPY

Medications for tobacco use cessation reduce withdrawal symptoms and increase achievement of successful abstinence, even when used with minimal counseling (M. Fiore et al., 2008; M. C. Fiore & Baker, 2011; Rigotti, 2012). Medications for smoking cessation have been shown to be effective when used in a variety of health care settings and with smokers with coexisting conditions (e.g., substance abuse and depression) (M. Fiore et al., 2008; M. C. Fiore & Baker, 2011; Rigotti, 2012). Therefore, the PHS CPG recommends medication for all smokers who are willing to commit to quitting, with only some minor exceptions (M. Fiore et al., 2008; M. C. Fiore & Baker, 2011; Rigotti, 2012). See Table 53.3—VHA Tobacco Use Cessation Treatment Guidance—*Part 3: Medications for Tobacco Use Cessation* for an overview of the most commonly used effective medications. Selection of medication should be done collaboratively with the patient, considering past successes, current preferences, and the pros and cons of available options. Because is not uncommon for patients to misperceive medication use as a sign of weakness, discussion of this concern can be helpful, along with a discussion of the benefits of medication use and a reiteration of the very large health benefits of quitting.

Seven medications have been approved by the FDA including five forms of nicotine replacement, bupropion and varenicline. The evidence reviewed for the PHS CPG strongly shows that abstinence rates are higher among patients using medications than among those who do not (M. Fiore et al., 2008; M. C. Fiore & Baker, 2011; Rigotti, 2012). A meta-analytic study of 83 RCTs studying the effects of various medications on 6 month abstinence rates found that most of them doubled the odds of achieving abstinence compared to placebo and minimal counseling (M. Fiore et al., 2008; M. C. Fiore & Baker, 2011; Rigotti, 2012). Combination therapies (i.e., combining nicotine patch with either lozenge or gum; combining bupropion and nicotine patch) are effective alternatives to monotherapies, though only the combination of nicotine patch plus bupropion is currently approved by the Food and Drug Administration (M. Fiore et al., 2008; M. C. Fiore & Baker, 2011; Rigotti, 2012). Each of the medications has contraindications and potential side effects, which are outlined in Table 53.3–VHA Tobacco Use Cessation Treatment Guidance—*Part 3: Medications for Tobacco Use Cessation*. Additionally, individual factors such as the presence of conditions which may increase the likelihood of adverse effects (e.g., dental conditions, dentures or jaw pain when considering gum; dermatitis when considering the patch; hypertension when considering bupriopion; mental health conditions when considering varenicline) should be considered when choosing a specific pharmacologic agent. It is helpful to explore past successes, and identify what, if any, medication was helpful to a patient in the past and what medication they feel most confident about using. Importantly, clear, reading level appropriate patient education materials with instructions for use should be made available to all patients.

Nicotine replacement. The principle of nicotine replacement therapy (NRT) is to provide the patient with a more manageable and safer form of nicotine to ameliorate withdrawal symptoms and allow the patient to gradually reduce and then discontinue use of the drug (Benowitz, 2010; M. Fiore et al., 2008). Replacement therapy also provides an opportunity for the patient to develop and practice strategies to deal with behavioral or learned components of the drug dependence while controlling the physiologic "need" for the drug. Nicotine replacement therapy has been shown to be an effective aid to smoking cessation approximately doubling the quit rate compared with placebo (M. Fiore et al., 2008; M. C. Fiore & Baker, 2011; Rigotti, 2012). The combination of nicotine patches with other forms of NRT, such as gum or lozenge, added on as needed basis for breakthrough urges, further increases effectiveness (M. Fiore et al., 2008; M. C. Fiore & Baker, 2011; Rigotti, 2012). Since publication of the PHS CPG in 2008, evidence is accumulating that novel ways of administering NRT can improve quit rates, including prolonging treatment beyond the standard 12 weeks of treatment, continuing rather than discontinuing NRT use after a lapse and starting NRT 2 weeks before the quit day rather than on the quit day (M. C. Fiore & Baker, 2011; Rigotti, 2012). Preliminary evidence also suggests that offering NRT to smokers who want to cut down but not to quit might increase quitting rates (M. C. Fiore & Baker, 2011; Rigotti, 2012). However, the FDA label for NRT warns smokers against combining products, starting NRT before the quit date, and smoking while using NRT. These restrictions reflect some concerns about causing nicotine overdose or sustaining dependence that appear to be unfounded (Rigotti, 2012). In the United Kingdom, NRT is licensed for combination use and for reducing smoking prior to cessation.

When considering NRT for patients with cardiovascular disease, it is important to be aware of the relative risks of NRT use versus continued smoking in these patients. The PHS CPG notes that systematic study of the use of NRT in patients with cardiovascular disease has not found an association between nicotine patch use and cardiovascular events, even in patients who continue to smoke while using the patch (M. Fiore et al., 2008; Rigotti, 2012). Nicotine replacement is likely to be less dangerous to a patient with cardiovascular disease than smoking because NRT does not produce the peak nicotine levels associated with smoking and does not decrease oxygen-carrying capacity. However, as noted in the CPG, "NRT should be used with caution among particular cardiovascular patient groups: those in the immediate (within 2 weeks) post-myocardial infarction period, those with serious arrhythmias, and those with unstable angina pectoris." (M. Fiore et al., 2008)

Nicotine patches. The nicotine patch delivers nicotine through the skin in 21, 14 and 7 mg doses. Patch use is recommended for an initial 8–12 weeks after quitting. The highest dose is recommended if the patient smokes 10 or more cigarettes a day. Nicotine patches reduce some but not all nicotine withdrawal symptoms. They are easy to use, are available over-the-counter and are generally well-tolerated. Mild skin rashes and irritation occur in up to 50% of patients.

Table 53.3 VHA TOBACCO USE CESSATION TREATMENT GUIDANCE—*PART 3: MEDICATIONS FOR TOBACCO USE CESSATION*

DESCRIPTION & EXAMPLES	PROS & CONS	COMMENTS / LIMITATIONS	DOSING RECOMMENDATIONS
Nicotine Patch **24-hour delivery systems** *21, 14, 7 mg/24 hr* **16-hour delivery systems** *15 mg/16 hr* *(Generic available, over-the-counter (OTC))* *Delivers nicotine directly through the skin.*	**PROS** • Achieve constant levels of replacement • Easy to use • Only needs to be applied once a day • Few side effects **CONS** • Less-flexible dosing—cannot titrate dose to acutely manage withdrawal symptoms • Slow onset of delivery • Mild skin rashes and irritation	• Patches vary in strengths and the length of time over which nicotine is delivered. • Patches may be placed anywhere on the upper body including arms and back. Avoid hairy areas. • Rotate the patch site each time a new patch is applied.	• ≥10 cigs/day = 21 mg/day × 4–6 wks, then 14mg/day × 2–3 wks, then 7mg/day × 2–3 wks. • <io cigs/day = 14 mg/day × 6wks, then 7mg/day × 2 wks. • Adjust based on withdrawal symptoms, urges, and comfort. After 4–6 weeks of abstinence, taper every 2–4 weeks in 7–14 mg steps as tolerated. **DURATION** • 8–12 weeks
Nicotine Lozenge *2 mg, 4 mg* *(OTC)* *Delivers nicotine through the lining of the mouth while the lozenge dissolves.*	**PROS** • Easy to use • Can titrate to manage withdrawal symptoms • May satisfy oral cravings • Delivers doses of nicotine approximately 25% higher than nicotine gum **CONS** • Should not eat or drink 15 minutes before or during use; avoid acidic beverages • Should not be chewed or swallowed • Need for frequent dosing can compromise compliance • Nausea frequent (12–15%)	• Use at least 8–9 lozenges/day initially. • Instruct patients to allow lozenge to dissolve slowly over 20–30 minutes. • Rotate to different sites of the mouth. • Nicotine release may cause a warm, tingling sensation. • Maximum 20 lozenges/day • Efficacy and frequency of side-effects related to amount used. • Review package directions carefully to maximize benefit of product.	• Based on time to first cigarette of the day: <30 minutes = 4 mg >30 minutes = 2 mg • Based on cigarettes/day: >20 cigs/day = 4 mg <20 cigs/day = 2 mg • Initial dosing = 1–2 lozenges every 1–2 hours (minimum 9/day) × 6wks, then 1 q2–4hrs × 3wks, then 1 q4–8hrs x 3wks. • Taper as tolerated. **DURATION** • 12 weeks
Nicotine Gum *2mg, 4mg* *(Generic available, OTC)* *Delivers nicotine through the lining of the mouth while gum is parked between cheek and gum.*	**PROS** • Convenient/flexible dosing that allows for titration to manage withdrawal symptoms • Faster delivery of nicotine than the patches • Might satisfy oral cravings **CONS** • May be inappropriate for people with dental problems and those with temporomandibular joint (TMJ) syndrome • Should not eat or drink 15 minutes before or during use; avoid acidic beverages • Frequent use during the day required to obtain adequate nicotine levels—may compromise compliance • Requires proper chewing technique for maximum benefit and to minimize adverse effects	• The term "gum" is misleading; it is not chewed like regular gum. • Many people use this medication incorrectly. • Advise patients to chew each piece slowly. • Chew for 15–30 chews and park between cheek and gum when peppery or tingling sensation appears. • Rotate to different sites of the mouth. • Resume chewing when taste or tingle fades. • Repeat chew/park steps until taste or tingle does not return (about 30 minutes). • Review package directions carefully to maximize benefit of product.	• Based on cigarettes/day: >20 cigs/day = 4 mg gum <20 cigs/day = 2 mg gum • Based on time to first cigarette of the day: <30 minutes = 4 mg >30 minutes = 2 mg • Initial dosing = 1–2 pieces every 1–2 hrs (10–12 pieces/day) × 6 wks, then 1 piece every 2–4 hours × 3 wks, then 1 piece every 4–8 hours x 3 wks. • Taper as tolerated. **DURATION** • Standard duration is up to 12 weeks. Longer durations have been studied and associated with better abstinence rates.

Combination Nicotine Replacement Therapy (NRT)
Nicotine patch + Nicotine gum PRN
Nicotine patch + Nicotine lozenge PRN

- Providing two types of delivery system, one passive and one active, appears to be more efficacious.
- Should be considered for those who have failed single therapy in the past or those considered highly tobacco dependent.
- Considered a first-line treatment in the 2008 Update USPHS Clinical Practice Guidelines.
- Not a FDA-approved strategy.

- Dose patch as described above.
- Prescribe 2 mg or 4 mg gum or lozenge (according to dose-dependence level described above) on an as-needed basis when acute withdrawal symptoms and urges to use tobacco occur. (Initially most patients require about 6–8 pieces of gum or lozenges/day)
- Nicotine patch dose may be increased if patient is requiring more frequent use of PRN gum or lozenge after patch taper.

DURATION
- Patch: 8–10 weeks (with lozenge) or 8–24 weeks (with gum)
- Gum: 26–52 weeks
- Lozenge: 12 weeks

PROS
- Permits sustained levels of nicotine (patch) with rapid adjustment for acute cravings and urges (PRN gum or lozenge)
- More efficacious than monotherapy

CONS
- May increase risk of nicotine toxicity
- Added cost of two NRT products versus one

NON-NICOTINE MEDICATION
Bupropion SR
(Generic available)

- Treatment should be initiated 1 week prior to quit date and titrated.
- Avoid bedtime dosing to minimize insomnia, but allow 8 hours between doses.
- Use with caution in patients with liver disease (dose adjustment necessary).
- A slight risk of seizure (1:1000) is associated with use of this medication.
  - Assess seizure risk and avoid if:
  - Personal history of seizures
  - Significant head trauma/brain injury
  - Anorexia nervosa or bulimia
  - Abrupt discontinuation of alcohol or sedatives
  - Concurrent use of medications that lower the seizure threshold

- Start medication 1 week prior to the quit date:
- 150 mg QD × 3 days, then
- 150 mg BID × 4 days, then
- On quit date STOP SMOKING
- Continue at 150 mg BID × 8–12 weeks.
- If patient has been successful at quitting, an additional 12 weeks may be considered.
- May stop abruptly.
- No need to taper.

PROS
- Easy to use
- Pill form—may be associated with better compliance
- Few side effects
- May be beneficial in patients with depression
- May be used in combination with NRT

CONS
- Contraindicated with certain medical conditions and medications
- Increased seizure risk

COMBINATION MEDICATION
Bupropion SR + Nicotine Patch

- Should be considered for those who have failed single therapy in the past or those considered highly tobacco dependent.
- Considered a first-line treatment in the 2008 Update USPHS Clinical Practice Guidelines.

- Use standard doses and duration.
- Bupropion: See bupropion dosing above; continue for 8–12 weeks.
- If patient has been successful at quitting, an additional 12 weeks may be considered.
- Nicotine patch: Dose patch as described above for total duration of 8–12 weeks.

PROS
- Easy-to-use combination (FDA approved)
- Uses agents with two different mechanisms of action

CONS
- Does not allow for adjustment of acute cravings or urges
- Added cost of two NRT products versus one
- May be associated with more side effects than monotherapy

(continued)

Table 53.3 (CONTINUED)

DESCRIPTION & EXAMPLES	PROS & CONS	COMMENTS / LIMITATIONS	DOSING RECOMMENDATIONS
COMBINATION MEDICATION Bupropion SR + Nicotine Lozenge or Gum	**PROS** • Uses agents with two different mechanisms of action • Allows for rapid adjustment for acute cravings and urges (PRN gum or lozenge) • More efficacious than monotherapy **CONS** • Added cost of two NRT products versus one • May be associated with more side effects than monotherapy	• Providing two types of mechanisms of action, including an active delivery system, appears to be more efficacious. • Should be considered for those who have failed single therapy in the past or those considered highly tobacco dependent. • Though not included in the 2008 Update USPHS Clinical Practice Guidelines, data published after the Update supports this combination. • Not a FDA-approved strategy.	• Use standard doses and duration. • **Bupropion:** See bupropion dosing above; continue for 8–12 weeks. • If patient has been successful at quitting, an additional 12 weeks may be considered. • Prescribe 2 mg or 4 mg gum or lozenge (according to dose-dependence level described above) on an as-needed basis when acute withdrawal symptoms and urges to use tobacco occur. (Initially, most patients require about 6–8 pieces of gum or lozenges/day)
NON-NICOTINE MEDICATION Varenicline	**PROS** • Easy to use • Pill form—may be associated with better compliance • No known drug interactions • Unique mechanism of action **CONS** • Nausea common in up to 1/3rd of patients • Severe neuropsychiatric symptoms may occur • Safety and efficacy have not been established in patients with serious psychiatric illness	• Treatment should be initiated 1 week prior to quit date and titrated. • Taking the medication with food and titrating the dose as directed may help with nausea. • Take with a full glass of water. • Varenicline should not be used in combination with NRT. • Dose must be adjusted if kidney function is impaired. • VHA-specific varenicline prescribing guidelines at: *www.pbm.va.gov/Clinical Guidance/Criteria For Use/Varenicline Criteria for Prescribing.doc*	• TAKE WITH FOOD and full glass of water • Start medication one week prior to the quit date: • 0.5 mg QD × 3 days, then • 0.5 mg BID × 4 days, then • On quit date STOP SMOKING and • Take 1.0 mg BID × 11 weeks • If not smoking at the end of twelve weeks, may continue for an additional 12 weeks. • May stop abruptly. • No need to taper.

Reproduced from: "The US Department of Veteran Affairs Office of Public Health and Environmental Hazards (138), Public Health Strategic Health Care Group, July, 2010.

These tend to self-limiting but sometimes worsen and may be treated with hydrocortisone cream (1%) or triamcinolone cream (0.5%) as well as rotating the patch site to minimize irritation. Insomnia and/or vivid dreams also may also occur. Dosing guidelines are available in Table 53.3—VHA Tobacco Use Cessation Treatment Guidance—*Part 3: Medications for Tobacco Use Cessation* and most follow a recommended dosage step-down process. Some preparations of patches are effective when used in a single dose.

Nicotine gum. Nicotine gum, which is available in 2 and 4 mg doses, delivers nicotine through the lining of the mouth while the gum is parked between gums and cheek. The 4 mg gum is recommended for more highly dependent smokers (e.g., smoking 25 or more cigarettes per day) (M. Fiore et al., 2008; M. C. Fiore & Baker, 2011; Rigotti, 2012). Gum can be used as a stand-along medication or as an adjunct to patches. It allows for rapid titration of nicotine withdrawal and can be used flexibly by patients to self-manage control of withdrawal symptoms. Patients must learn a specific technique (chew slowly, park and chew) to achieve successful nicotine replacement and limit side effects. Use of nicotine gum may not be appropriate for denture wearers. Common side effects include mouth soreness, hiccups, dyspepsia, and jaw ache. These tend to be mild and manageable, often improving with guidance about chewing technique. Acidic beverages can interfere with absorption of the nicotine and should be avoided 15 minutes prior to or during chewing. It is common for patients to use insufficient gum to achieve optimal benefit. The CPG recommends a fixed schedule of at least one piece of gum every 1–2 hours for the first 1–3 months after quitting smoking. See Table 53.3—VHA Tobacco Use Cessation Treatment Guidance—*Part 3: Medications for Tobacco Use Cessation* for more detailed guidance.

Nicotine lozenge. Similar to the gum, the nicotine lozenge is available in 4 mg and 2 mg doses, and the higher dose is recommended for more heavily dependent smokers who smoke within 30 minutes after awakening (M. Fiore et al., 2008; M. C. Fiore & Baker, 2011; Rigotti, 2012). Like the gum, the lozenge allows for rapid self-titration. It can be used as a stand-along medication or in combination with patches. The lozenge should be allowed to dissolve in the mouth rather than be chewed or swallowed. Patients are advised to use at least 9 lozenges per day for the first 6 weeks but no more than 20 per day. Like the gum, under-dosing is common. Common side effects are nausea, hiccups and heartburn as well as headache and coughing. Acidic beverages can interfere and should be avoided 15 minutes prior to and during use. Pattern of use and possible underuse should be explored if patients are struggling to stay quit or have relapsed. See table See Table 53.3—VHA Tobacco Use Cessation Treatment Guidance—*Part 3: Medications for Tobacco Use Cessation* for more detailed guidance.

Nicotine spray. The nicotine spray is available as an additional NRT option with one 0.5 mg squirt per nostril equaling one dose. The recommendation for use is 1–2 doses per hour with a maximum of 40 doses per day (M. Fiore et al., 2008; M. C. Fiore & Baker, 2011; Rigotti, 2012). Nasal irritation is a very common side effect, with 94% of users reporting moderate-severe nasal irritation in the first 2 days of use. The frequency of irritation goes down to 81% after 3 weeks and typically becomes mild to moderate over time. Additional concerns include nasal congestion and transient changes in smell or taste. Spray is not recommended for patients with severe reactive airway disease. Dependency is more common with the nasal spray, as it produces higher peak nicotine levels than other forms of NRT. The CPG reports 15–20% of patients use the active spray for longer than 6–12 months and 5% use higher than recommended doses. See table See Table 53.3—VHA Tobacco Use Cessation Treatment Guidance—*Part 3: Medications for Tobacco Use Cessation* for more details.

Nicotine inhaler. The nicotine inhaler is a cartridge delivery system with each puff or inhalation constituting a dose from the 4 mg device. Each inhaler delivers 80 inhalations and recommended dosing is 6–16 cartridges daily (M. Fiore et al., 2008; M. C. Fiore & Baker, 2011; Rigotti, 2012). Local irritation of the mouth and throat is reported by 40% of patients, followed by coughing (32%) and rhinitis (23%). All generally mild and all remit with continued use. Ambient temperature impacts delivery which declines below 40 degrees. Acidic beverages interfere much like they do with gum or lozenge, and should be avoided 15 minutes prior to or during use. As with gum and lozenges, patients frequently under-utilize the inhaler and do not use enough as needed NRT for optimal effect. At least 6 cartridges daily are recommended. See Table 53.3—VHA Tobacco Use Cessation Treatment Guidance—*Part 3: Medications for Tobacco* for details.

Bupropion Sustained Release (brand name, Zyban) is one of the 2 FDA approved pharmacological alternatives to NRT (M. Fiore et al., 2008; M. C. Fiore & Baker, 2011; Rigotti, 2012). Bupropion is an antidepressant medication that is generally well-tolerated with occasional reports of hypertension. Most common side effects are insomnia (35–40%) and dry mouth (10%). Insomnia may improve by shifting the second daily dose to an earlier time, but still 8 hours after the first dose. Use is contraindicated in patients with a history of seizures or eating disorders. In 2009, the FDA issued a boxed warning in bupropion's packaging insert as a result of many reports of changes in behavior, including hostility, agitation, depressed mood and suicidal ideation (M. C. Fiore & Baker, 2011; Rigotti, 2012). Therefore, caution and careful monitoring is recommended for patients with psychiatric conditions. Patients are instructed to begin use 1–2 weeks prior to quitting. Dosing involves 150 mg each morning for 3 days, then increase to twice daily for a total maximum of 300 mg per day for 7–12 weeks. At times, patients stop or reduce smoking spontaneously, reporting lost desire and pleasure in tobacco. Alcohol should only be used in moderation. Bupropion blunts the weight gain usually seen post smoking cessation attempts, though the difference in weight gain disappears after bupropion is discontinued (Rigotti, 2012). If there are no contraindications or cautions, bupropion can be considered a first-line agent if a patient has a preference for a medication other than nicotine replacement therapy. It may also be considered when (1) patients have concerns about weight gain post quitting;

(2) patients have a history of mild or moderate depression or previous smoking cessation attempts were associated with prominent depressive symptoms; or (3) previous attempts at cessation using behavioral interventions and nicotine replacement agents have failed. However, as noted previously, if used in a patient with a previous psychiatric disorder, close monitoring is required. See Table 53.3—VHA Tobacco Use Cessation Treatment Guidance—*Part 3: Medications for Tobacco* for guidelines for prescribing bupropion.

Varenicline (brand name, Chantix), a partial nicotine receptor agonist, is also FDA approved for treatment of tobacco dependence and is also recommended as a possible first line agent by the CPG (M. Fiore et al., 2008; M. C. Fiore & Baker, 2011; Rigotti, 2012). Varenicline efficacy is the highest of any of the medications when used alone, with 33% of smokers achieving abstinence 6 months post quit attempt (M. Fiore et al., 2008; M. C. Fiore & Baker, 2011; Rigotti, 2012). However, varenicline carries the strongest warnings of any of the medication options, including caution for those with significant kidney disease or who are on dialysis. As with bupropion, reports of depressed mood, agitation, behavior changes, suicidal ideation and suicide behavior have prompted an FDA warning for use since 2009 (M. C. Fiore & Baker, 2011; Rigotti, 2012). Side effects include nausea, sleep difficulty, and abnormal/vivid dreams. Dosing starts 1 week prior to quit date at 0.5 mg in the morning for 3 days followed by 0.5 mg twice daily on days 4–7, and finally 1 mg twice daily from days 8 to end of treatment, which is in 3–6 months. Because of reports of neuropsychiatric adverse effects, a careful psychiatric history should be gathered, and ongoing monitoring for changes in mood or behavior is recommended during and immediately after a course of treatment. One recent RCT evaluating safety and efficacy of varenicline in patients with cardiovascular disease suggested it may be associated with a small increased risk of events including heart attack (M. C. Fiore & Baker, 2011). Providers are encouraged to weigh the costs and potential benefits of varenicline for each individual patient. As noted below, the combination of nicotine patches and supplemental nicotine gum or lozenge achieves a rate of abstinence that compares favorably with varenicline as a monotherapy. See Table 53.3—VHA Tobacco Use Cessation Treatment Guidance—*Part 3: Medications for Tobacco* for further guidance.

Combination Medication Treatment: Improvements in smoking cessation outcomes in recent years have often been due to combined medication approaches. While most all individual medications double the odds of abstinence, compared to placebo, to reach 19–26% abstinence at 6 months post quit date, the combination of nicotine patches and supplemental nicotine gum or lozenge achieve abstinence rates as high as 37% at 6 months (M. Fiore et al., 2008; M. C. Fiore & Baker, 2011; Rigotti, 2012). The patch provides a steady dose of nicotine, limiting withdrawal symptoms, while the as-needed use of gum or lozenge allows the patient to obtain an added bolus of nicotine when needed to address breakthrough withdrawal or craving in response to a trigger. See Table 53.3—VHA Tobacco Use Cessation Treatment Guidance—*Part 3: Medications for Tobacco* for additional guidance on approved combination therapies.

OTHER MEDICATIONS

The PHS CPG identified 2 additional medications as "second-line" pharmacologic agents for smoking cessation, clonidine and nortriptyline (M. Fiore et al., 2008). Though these medications produce enhanced abstinence rates in controlled trials, they are not approved by FDA for a tobacco cessation indication and have relatively high rates of adverse effects (Rigotti, 2012). Therefore, we do not recommend their routine use for treatment of tobacco dependence. A nicotinic receptor partial agonist, cytosine, has shown promise, (West et al., 2011) though more research is needed to determine its place among pharmacologic agents for treating nicotine use and dependence.

COUNSELING ELEMENTS AND STRATEGIES

Behavioral treatment strategies are essential components of tobacco use and dependence treatment (D. B. Abrams et al., 2003; Brown, 2003; M. Fiore et al., 2008). The expert panel that reviewed and synthesized scores of controlled trials of psychosocial and behavioral treatments for tobacco use cessation identified two key components of effective tobacco use counseling programs: a "practical" problem-solving/skills training counseling approach and social support as part of treatment (M. Fiore et al., 2008).

Practical problem-solving/skills training is an integral element of several health behavior change theoretical models, including Social Cognitive Theory, which suggests that behavior change and maintenance are a function of an individual's learning history, shaped by classical and operant conditioning, as well as the individuals outcome expectations (i.e., beliefs about outcomes that result from engaging in a behavior) and self-efficacy (i.e., beliefs and confidence in one's capacity to carry out specific behaviors in specific situations) (Bandura, 2004; Brown, 2003). Behavioral counseling provides smokers with opportunities to learn and practice skills to break the learned/automatic chain of events associated with smoking (Antecedent → Behavior → Consequences) and replacing smoking with more adaptive behaviors and coping strategies. Learning and practicing self-control strategies (e.g., goal setting, self-monitoring, self-evaluation and self-correction) and problem-solving and coping strategies (e.g., using a relaxation exercise to manage anxiety as an alternative to smoking) builds small successes which, in turn, builds self-efficacy and positive outcome expectations (Brown, 2003). Removing cues to smoking and avoiding or altering situations that are associated with smoking (e.g., taking a walk instead of a smoking break; having morning coffee in the bedroom rather than the kitchen) break learned links and establishes new routines that are not linked to smoking (Brown, 2003). The environment also exerts an effect on behavior through modeling (Brown, 2003). Thus, repeated exposure to positive role models, such as clinicians who engage in healthy behaviors or peers with effective coping repertoires, may promote adoption and maintenance of healthy behaviors.

The CPG specifies the key problem-solving/skills training elements that should be included in the behavioral counseling components of smoking cessation interventions. These are: 1) recognize danger situations—identify events, internal states or activities that increase the risk of smoking or relapse: 2) develop and practice coping and problem-solving skills to cope with danger situations; 3) provide basic information about the process and course of quitting, including and the risks of having even a single puff, as well as the benefits of reframing slips as a learning experience, rather than a failure (M. Fiore et al., 2008). It is helpful to consider treatment of tobacco dependence as akin to management of a chronic disease, with a need for repeated quit attempts and understandable lapses and relapses before long-term abstinence is achieved. Lapses can actually help to inform treatment needs and can be reframed as learning opportunities that can guide choice of behavioral strategies during subsequent efforts to quit and maintain abstinence.

SPECIFIC ELEMENTS OF PRACTICAL PROBLEM-SOLVING/SKILLS TRAINING (SEE TABLE 53.4—ELEMENTS OF PRACTICAL PROBLEM SOLVING/SKILLS TRAINING)

As noted previously in the discussion of the 5A's approach to intervention, it is useful for patients to establish a *target quit date* that is soon enough to build on motivation to quit while also providing an opportunity for the patient to prepare for quitting. Patients may use the time before the quit date to obtain medication, arrange sources of social support, and learn and practice problem-solving and coping skills to address anticipated barriers and challenges. If an intermediate or intensive form of treatment is chosen, the planning phase may include a period of self-monitoring to identify key smoking triggers and situations that may prompt relapse. The time prior to the target quit date may also be used to reduce nicotine consumption by changing brands or by reducing the number of cigarettes smoked per day.

Behavioral counseling includes developing a *specific plan* to address barriers to quitting and to cope with urges to smoke. As noted previously, the plan should include: removing all nicotine use-related items (cigarettes, lighters etc.) prior to quitting; avoiding or altering situations associated with urges or previous lapses; and 3) specifying possible substitutes or alternative behaviors or coping strategies for situations or emotions associated with urges or previous lapses. General stress management strategies (e.g., relaxation exercises, cognitive reframing, use of a stress ball) may help the patient to cope with common emotional and cognitive triggers. The plan should also include strategies for identifying and managing nicotine withdrawal symptoms and cravings to smoke, which might include use of as needed doses of nicotine gum, lozenge or inhaler.

Management of lapses (relapse prevention) is another key element of behavioral counseling. Because most treated smokers resume smoking within hours or days to several months after quitting, relapse prevention or management is a critical issue in smoking cessation. When lapses occur, patients

Table 53.4 ELEMENTS OF PRACTICAL PROBLEM SOLVING/SKILLS TRAINING

STRATEGY	EXAMPLES
Identify a Specific Quit Day	• Soon enough to build upon motivation • Provide opportunity to prepare and practice skills • Consider self-monitoring as a strategy for identifying triggers and barriers
Identify strategies for managing triggers to smoke and relapse situations	• Explore past experience to identify strategies that were successful • Remove smoking-related items • Develop plan for avoiding or altering trigger/relapse situations • Identify substitute behaviors to use in place of smoking for triggers and relapse situations • Teach/practice stress management skills
Managing lapses	• Reframe lapses as an opportunity for learning and problem-solving • Challenge self-blame, guilt, other negative emotions and cognitive distortions associated with lapses • After lapses occur, develop a revised plan to address lapse/relapse situations • Consider specific therapeutic interventions and coping strategies to address emergent challenges (e.g., anxiety or depressive symptoms, weight gain)

and clinicians need to guard against what has been called the "abstinence violation effect" (e.g., excess guilt, shame, pessimism and reduced confidence for change) (Baer & Marlatt, 1991; Ockene et al., 2000). As noted repeatedly, most successful quitters have made repeated attempts to quit. Health care providers can support a more positive approach by framing lapses and relapses as a normal, expected part of the process of learning to become a nonsmoker. Moreover, treating tobacco dependence is often a complex process that may require sustained and coordinated care, especially if the patient has coexisting medical and psychiatric comorbidity. Slips or full relapses should be met with non-judgmental, supportive problem-solving and an assessment of factors which may be contributing to difficulty quitting, including coexisting depressive or anxiety symptoms, the use or abuse of other psychoactive substances, or concerns about weight gain (Rigotti, 2012).

Supportive elements. The critical value of supportive elements in smoking cessation treatment is consistent with psychotherapy research that has identified "common factors" associated with positive outcomes of a wide variety of psychotherapeutic interventions across a range of conditions (Brown, 2003; M. Fiore et al., 2008; Miller, 2000; Orlinsky, Grawe, & Parks, 1994; Squier, 1990). These factors include a caring, empathic, collaborative, nonjudgmental, patient-centered approach that fosters patient engagement, activation and empowerment and supports patient autonomy (Goldstein, DePue, & Kazura, 2008; Miller, 2000; Miller & Rollnick, 2013; Orlinsky et al., 1994; Squier, 1990; Williams et al., 2002). Operationally, social support in treatment means: eliciting patient concerns and worries as well as reasons for quitting and successes; communicating caring and concern; offering treatment choices and options; engaging in shared decision-making; and encouraging the patient in their efforts to quit (M. Fiore et al., 2008; Goldstein et al., 2008).

As noted previously, there is a dose-response relationship between the intensity of tobacco cessation treatment and treatment outcome (M. Fiore et al., 2008). Evidence from meta-analyses conducted by the PHS CPG indicate that intensive treatment should include the following counseling elements: at least 4 sessions, each at least 10 minutes in duration; individualized assessments of motivation, beliefs, past experience, nicotine dependence, triggers and relapse situations; inclusion of practical problem-solving/skills training and in-treatment support; integration with pharmacotherapy; and ideally, involvement of multiple clinicians and intervention team members from a variety of disciplines (M. Fiore et al., 2008).

OTHER NON-PHARMACOLOGIC TREATMENT APPROACHES

The PHS CPG reviewed a number of additional non-pharmacologic treatment approaches, including acupuncture, hypnosis, exercise, aversive treatments and strategies to prevent weight gain after quitting smoking found there was either no evidence or insufficient evidence to support the use of these interventions (M. Fiore et al., 2008). Subsequent reviews have not revealed sufficient evidence to recommend these treatment modalities (Spring et al., 2009; Ussher, Taylor, & Faulkner, 2012; Barnes et al., 2010; White, Rampes, & Ernst, 2002).

OBESITY

As noted in the introductory section of this chapter, after tobacco, poor diet and decreased activity is the second highest cause of deaths in the United States each year (365 000 deaths) (Mokdad et al., 2004). The development of obesity is closely linked to these 2 behaviors, though obesity, like tobacco use is a biopsychosocial condition that has multiple contributing factors.

Obesity is identified based on measurement of Body Mass Index (BMI), defined as an individual's weight in kilograms divided by the square of their height in meters (kg/m^2). The United States Preventive Services Task Force (USPSTF) and US government health care agencies uses the following terms to define categories of increased BMI: overweight is defined as a BMI of 25 to 29.9 kg/m^2, and obesity is defined as a BMI of 30 kg/m^2 or higher (Moyer, 2012).

Epidemiological studies have demonstrated links between obesity and increased risk of death, particularly in adults younger than age 65 years. The impact of obesity on mortality is large; obesity reduces life expectancy by 6 to 20 years depending on age and race (Fontaine, Redden,

Wang, Westfall, & Allison, 2003; E. LeBlanc, E. O'Connor, E. P. Whitlock, C. Patnode, & T. Kapka, 2011). The leading causes of death in persons who are obese are ischemic heart disease, diabetes, cancer (especially liver, kidney, breast, endometrial, prostate, and colon), and respiratory diseases (G. Whitlock et al., 2009). It is less clear whether being overweight is associated with an increased mortality risk (E. LeBlanc et al., 2011).

Data from the 2009–2010 National Health and Nutrition Exam Survey indicated that the prevalence of obesity in the United States now exceeds 33% in most age- and sex-specific groups (Flegal, Carroll, Kit, & Ogden, 2012). Thirty-five and one half percent of U.S. adult men and 35.8% of U.S. women were obese and an additional 38% of men and 28% of women were overweight (Flegal et al., 2012). Moreover, about 1 in 20 Americans has a Body Mass Index (BMI) of >40 kg/m^2, which is class III obesity (Flegal et al., 2012). Alarmingly, the prevalence of obesity and overweight has increased by 134 % and 48%, respectively, since 1976 (Stein & Colditz, 2004). If current trends continue, researchers have estimated that, by 2030, 86.3% adults will be overweight or obese; and 51.1%, obese (Wang, Beydoun, Liang, Caballero, & Kumanyika, 2008).

Obesity increases the risk of coronary heart disease by almost 50% even after adjustment for other established risk factors (E. LeBlanc et al., 2011), while obese men and obese women have a 6.7-fold and 12.4-fold greater risk, respectively, of developing type 2 diabetes compared with normal weight men and women (Guh et al., 2009). Other diseases that have been associated with obesity include ischemic stroke, heart failure, dementia, venous thrombosis, gallstones, gastroesophageal reflux disease, renal disease, sleep apnea, osteoarthritis, and adverse pregnancy outcomes (E. LeBlanc et al., 2011).

Though obesity poses great health risks to obese individuals, the good news is that loss of as little as 5–10% of body weight, achievable with multi-component behavioral intervention programs, is associated with numerous health benefits, including reduction in the risk of heart disease and diabetes and better control of chronic conditions (E. LeBlanc et al., 2011; E. S. Leblanc, E. O'Connor, E. P. Whitlock, C. D. Patnode, & T. Kapka, 2011; Wing, 2010; Wing & Gorin, 2003).

FACTORS CONTRIBUTING TO OBESITY

Energy balance. Weight status is largely a function of the amount of calories consumed (intake) and the amount of calories burned (output). Positive energy balance exists when more calories are consumed than are burned, and this imbalance will result in obesity if even a small positive energy balance is maintained over time. As a general rule, an individual will gain one pound whenever they consume 3500 calories more than they burn (D. Abrams et al., 2000; Katz, 2001). Thus, consuming 100 additional calories daily will produce a 1 pound weight gain after 5 weeks, about a 10 pound weight gain after a year, and a 100 pound weight

Background. The Five As were developed by the National Cancer Institute and later adopted by the Canadian Task Force on Preventive Healthcare, as a way to organize a general approach to counseling patients to address health behavior change. The 5As construct has been used in clinical trials for smoking cessation and other primary care-based interventions for a variety of behaviors.

Application: The content of each step in the Five As varies from behavior to behavior, though clinical intervention targeting change in any behavior can be described using these five intervention components.

The Five As

Assess	Ask about—and assess behavioral health risks and factors that affect choice of behavior change goals and methods. • Assessing behavioral risk factors identifies patients in need of intervention. • Assess beliefs, behaviors, knowledge, motivation and past experience.
Advise	Give clear, specific, well-timed and behavior change advice, including personalized information about health harms and benefits. • Clinician advice establishes behavioral issues as an important part of health care. • Advise in a non-coercive, non-judgmental manner that respects readiness for change and patient autonomy. • Advice is most powerful when linked to the patient's own health concerns, past experiences, family / social situations, and level of health literacy.
Agree	Collaboratively select appropriate goals and methods based on the patient's interest in and willingness to change the behavior. • Collaborate to find common ground and to specify behavior change goals and methods. • Shared decision-making is especially recommended for interventions that involve significant risk-benefit tradeoffs. • Shared decision-making about behavior change results in a greater patient autonomy choices based on patient values, improved patient follow through and time saved in the exam room.
Assist	Using self-help resources and/or counseling, help the patient to achieve goals by enhancing skills, confidence, and social and environmental supports for behavior change. • Health care staff provide motivational interventions, address barriers to change, and/or secure support needed for successful change. • Effective interventions support self-management and enhance problem-solving or coping skills that enable patients to take the next immediate steps toward targeted behavior change. • An action plan is developed that lists goals, barriers and strategies, and specifies follow-up.
Arrange	Schedule follow-up (in person or by phone or secure messaging) to provide ongoing assistance and support and to adjust the plan as needed, including referral to more specialized or intensive intervention. • **Consider behavioral risk factors as chronic conditions that ebb and flow over time.** • Routine follow-up assessment and support is usually necessary to promote and maintain behavior change.

Adapted from Whitlock, P, Orleans, C.T., Pender, N., and Allan, J (2002). *EvaluatingPrimary Care Behavioral Counseling Interventions: An Evidence-based Approach*, American Journal of Preventive Medicine and reproduced from Goldstein et al., AJPM, 2004.

gain over a decade. To underscore how easily this can happen, consider that 2 cookies, 1 banana, or 6 oz. of juice are examples of foods that contain about 100 calories. Overall caloric intake intake appears to be a more important factor than macronutrient composition in the development or maintenance of obesity (Wadden et al., 2012). However, it is harder to achieve energy balance on diets that are high in energy-dense foods, such as fats. Low-fat diets that also feature increased plant-based foods (e.g., grains, fruits and vegetables) yield a low-energy-density diet that may improve satiety because of the larger volume of food that may be consumed while still maintaining energy balance (Wadden et al., 2012).

Energy expenditure. Epidemiologic studies have consistently shown that the level of physical activity is inversely related to weight (D. Abrams et al., 2000; Katz, 2001).

However, decreased physical activity may be both a cause and a consequence of obesity. Moreover, the associations between physical activity and weight are confounded by associations between sedentary behavior and increased caloric and fat intake (Katz, 2001). However, physical activity increases energy expenditure both directly (15 minutes of brisk walking burns approximately 100 calories) and indirectly, through physical activity's effect on lean body mass, which increases basal metabolic rate, the largest contributor to daily energy expenditure (Katz, 2001). Increased physical activity is an essential element of successful weight loss and weight maintenance programs, to be discussed below (Thompson, Cook, Clark, Bardia, & Levine, 2007; Wing & Gorin, 2003).

Psychological factors. Depressive symptoms and obesity frequently coexist and there is an increased prevalence of depressive and anxiety disorders in patients with obesity (Simon et al., 2006). The relationship between depression and obesity appears to be bidirectional (Ball, Burton, & Brown, 2009; Konttinen, Silventoinen, Sarlio-Lahteenkorva, Mannisto, & Haukkala, 2010; Thompson et al., 2007; Zhao et al., 2011). For example, individuals with depressive symptoms are more likely to report emotional eating or binge eating and also are less likely to engage in physical activity, putting them at increased risk of developing obesity (Konttinen et al., 2010). The rates of binge eating in an obese population seeking treatment for weight control is as high as 20% to 50% (Thompson et al., 2007). In cross-sectional studies of overweight and obese adults, waist circumference or abdominal obesity was significantly associated with increased likelihood of having major depressive symptoms or moderate-to-severe depressive symptoms (Zhao et al., 2011). Prospective studies have shown an increased risk of developing depressive symptoms among individuals who are overweight (Ball et al., 2009; Needham, Epel, Adler, & Kiefe, 2010).

Genetic factors. Though heritability of obesity has been estimated to range from 40–70%, (Herrera, Keildson, & Lindgren, 2011) the search for genetic variants contributing to susceptibility has been challenging task. For example, the candidate gene Ob and its product leptin received significant attention when obese Ob/Ob mice were found to be deficient in leptin (Mutch & Clement, 2006). However, leptin and melanocortin, previously assumed to be controlled by a single gene appear to be regulated by multiple interacting genetic and environmental elements (Mutch & Clement, 2006). More recently, genome wide association (GWA) studies have identified more than 40 genetic variants that have been associated with obesity and fat distribution, (Herrera et al., 2011) though the effect sizes of the established loci are small, and combined they explain only a fraction of the inter-individual variation in BMI (Day & Loos, 2011). Though their value in guiding clinical interventions will be limited in the short term, genetic variants are likely to provide new insights into body weight regulation (Day & Loos, 2011). Experts, after reviewing the genetic and environmental influences on obesity, have concluded that genetics most likely contribute to the propensity for obesity, while environmental, behavioral, social and psychological factors determine the severity of obesity (D. Abrams et al., 2000).

MANAGEMENT/TREATMENT OF OBESITY

GENERAL CONSIDERATIONS

Like tobacco use, obesity is best viewed as a chronic, relapsing condition. The vast majority of obese individuals have engaged in serious weight loss efforts. Fifty-eight percent of obese adult women and 50% of adult obese men participating in the 1998 National Health Interview Study reported attempts to lose weight within the past year (Kruger, Galuska,

Serdula, & Jones, 2004). Using data from the Behavioral Risk Factor Surveillance System, investigators noted that adults who had a routine physician checkup in the previous year and reported receiving advice to lose weight had a higher prevalence of trying to lose weight (81% of women and 77% of men) when compared with adults who had a health care visit and reported no advice (41% of women and 28% of men, respectively).

Though many are successful at losing weight, recidivism following successful weight loss is extremely high (DePue, Clark, Ruggiero, Medeiros, & Pera, 1995). To learn about factors associated with enhanced maintenance of weight loss, researchers created a National Weight Control Registry (NWCR) of women and 155 men who lost an average of 30 kg and had maintained a weight loss of at least 13.6 kg for at least 5 years (Klem, Wing, McGuire, Seagle, & Hill, 1997). Researchers were interested in identifying the strategies used by successful maintainers. Initial studies indicated that maintainers modified both their dietary intake and physical activity level to lose weight. The three most commonly used strategies to change diet were limiting the intake of certain foods, limiting the quantities of food, and counting calories (Klem et al., 1997).

A prospective study examined behavioral and psychological predictors of weight regain in 261 successful weight losers who completed an 18-month trial of weight regain prevention (Wing et al., 2008). Decreases in physical activity were related to weight regain while increased frequency of self-weighing was protective in the 2 intervention groups, but not in the control group (Wing et al., 2008). This finding is consistent with a prospective study of participants in the NWCR who had lost > 30 pounds and kept it off for at least 1 year (Butryn, Phelan, Hill, & Wing, 2007). Consistent self-weighing in this cohort was associated was associated with decreased weight gain over the subsequent year (Butryn et al., 2007). Investigators hypothesized that self-weighing may help individuals maintain their successful weight loss by allowing them to catch weight gains before they escalate and by making behavior changes to prevent additional weight gain (Butryn et al., 2007). Of note, in another study, increases in self-weighing was associated with increases in dietary restraint, decreases in disinhibition and decreases in depressive symptoms (Wing et al., 2007).

An American College of Sports Medicine (ACSM) Position Statement, published in 2009, reviewed the evidence regarding the role of physical activity as a weight maintenance strategy after weight loss (Donnelly et al., 2009). Both cross-sectional and prospective studies suggest that after weight loss, weight maintenance is improved with more than 250 minutes of physical activity per week, (Donnelly et al., 2009) considerably more than the 150 minutes of moderate physical activity per week recommended by ACMS and other bodies to get health benefits from physical activity (Haskell et al., 2007). However, there is insufficient evidence from well-designed randomized controlled trials to judge the effectiveness of physical activity for prevention of weight regain after weight loss.

Providing some form of long term follow-up contact may also enhance maintenance after a successful weight loss intervention. In a controlled trial of 2 forms of a maintenance intervention after a 6 month weight loss intervention, providing access to monthly personal contact was effective in helping to sustain weight loss, while an interactive technology-based intervention provided only transient benefit (Svetkey et al., 2008).

Obesity researchers and practitioners have also found value in focusing on challenging patients' unrealistic outcome expectations. If individuals are disappointed in their ability to reach their goal weight or discouraged with their new weight, these negative emotions may reduce motivation and trigger overeating episodes that lead to a full relapse (Thompson et al., 2007).

Though long-term maintenance of weight loss is challenging, as noted previously, the good news is that loss of as little as 5–10% of body weight, achievable with multi-component behavioral intervention programs, is associated with numerous health benefits (E. LeBlanc et al., 2011; Wing & Gorin, 2003).

PRIMARY CARE-BASED INTERVENTIONS

As with tobacco use, there is great opportunity to address obesity within health care settings, and in particular within primary care settings that have adopted the Patient-Centered Medical Home (PCMH). However, in most health care organizations, assessment and intervention for obesity is very limited. Despite the ease of determining BMI, surveys of patients have indicated that only 38 to 66% of overweight or obese patients report that they have received diagnoses of overweight or obesity, and less than half of obese patients report that their physicians have advised them to lose weight or provided specific information about how to lose weight (E. LeBlanc et al., 2011). Even among those who suffer from obesity-related comorbidities, only 52% were screened for obesity, 34% were diagnosed with obesity, and 46% were counseled about their obesity (E. LeBlanc et al., 2011). Moreover, only 24% of obese Americans were referred by their physician to a dietician or nutritionist and only 11% received a recommendation to attend a formal weight management program (Ma, Xiao, & Stafford, 2009). Surveys of obese patients indicate that 4–10% of obese adults received a prescription for weight loss medication, though less than half of the patients who were prescribed weight loss medication reported that they received the behavioral counseling and support that should accompany medication management (Shiffman et al., 2009).

The low rates of assessment and intervention for obesity within primary care settings suggests the need for systematic approaches to support clinician use of educational and counseling interventions that enhance patient engagement in weight management and participation in effective obesity treatment programs. The adoption of systematic approaches for addressing tobacco use interventions in health care settings (discussed in the section of this chapter on tobacco use treatments) may serve as a model for interventions to address obesity. For example, the 5 As behavioral counseling approach that was developed for smoking cessation interventions in health care settings, may be adapted to address obesity,

healthy eating, physical activity and other health risk behaviors (Glassgow & Goldstein, 2008; Goldstein, Whitlock, & DePue, 2004; E. P. Whitlock et al., 2002). See Box 53.1 for an adapted version of the 5 As that may be used for this purpose. Note that version of the 5 As (Assess, Advise, Agree, Assist, Arrange) omits the Ask step (actually combined with Assess) and adds the Agree step to emphasize the importance of addressing patient motivation and readiness for making a health behavior change. The collaborative Agree step supports patient autonomy and may contribute to building patient motivation and commitment to taking action, (S Rollnick, Miller, & Butler, 2008; Williams et al., 2002) as specified in the Assist step.

Obesity interventions in primary care settings may be spurred by a change in the United States Preventive Services Task Force's recommendations for management of obesity in health care settings. In 2012, after an extensive review of the impact of screening and weight loss interventions, the USPSTF recommended BMI screening of adult patients and offering or referring patients with a body mass index (BMI) of 30 kg/m^2 or higher to intensive, multicomponent behavioral interventions (E. S. Leblanc et al., 2011; Moyer, 2012). The USPSTF concluded that "adequate evidence indicates that intensive, multicomponent behavioral interventions for obese adults can lead to weight loss, as well as improved glucose tolerance and other physiologic risk factors for cardiovascular disease." (Moyer, 2012). The USPSTF also concluded that the possible harms of screening and behavioral weight-loss interventions (i.e., decreased bone mineral density and increased fracture risk, injuries from increased physical activity, increased risk of eating disorders) were small (Moyer, 2012). USPSTF rated the strength of evidence supporting this recommendation as "B," indicating "high certainty that the net benefit is moderate or there is moderate certainty that the net benefit is moderate to substantial." (Moyer, 2012). The B rating was provided even though the USPSTF noted that there was inadequate evidence about the effectiveness of behavioral weight loss interventions on long-term health outcomes, including mortality, cardiovascular disease, and hospitalizations (E. S. Leblanc et al., 2011; Moyer, 2012).

The evidence review utilized by the AHRQ for the USPSTF included a total of 58 weight-loss intervention trials with a total of more than 27,000 participants (E. S. Leblanc et al., 2011; Moyer, 2012). All of the trials included a strong behavioral component, while 21 also included a medication for weight management (either orlistat or metformin) (E. S. Leblanc et al., 2011; Moyer, 2012). Behavioral intervention participants lost an average of 6% of their baseline weight (4 to 7 kg), compared with little or no weight loss in control group participants (E. S. Leblanc et al., 2011; Moyer, 2012). A 5% weight loss is considered clinically important by the U.S. Food and Drug Administration (FDA). The Task Force's evidence review also concluded that weight loss outcomes were greatest when interventions involved more sessions (12 to 26 sessions) (E. S. Leblanc et al., 2011; Moyer, 2012).

The Diabetes Prevention Program (DPP) is a particularly strong example of the effectiveness of a multicomponent behavioral intervention program (Diabetes Prevention Program

Research Group, 2002). The DPP was a multi-centered randomized controlled trial that was designed to test whether a behavioral intervention or metformin, a antihyperglycemic agent, could prevent or delay the onset of diabetes among adults at risk for the development of type 2 diabetes (Diabetes Prevention Program Research Group, 2002). The behavioral "lifestyle" intervention consisted of an individualized 16-lesson curriculum addressing diet, weight loss and physical activity, delivered by case managers (Diabetes Prevention Program Research Group, 2002). Over 3,200 individuals were randomized to one of three conditions: lifestyle recommendations plus metformin; lifestyle recommendations plus placebo; or the intensive lifestyle intervention. After an average follow-up of 2.8 years, the lifestyle intervention reduced the incidence of diabetes by 58% compared with placebo, while metformin reduced the incidence of diabetes by 31% (Diabetes Prevention Program Research Group, 2002). Both the intensive behavioral intervention condition and metformin intervention outperformed the placebo control group, and the behavioral intervention was significantly more effective than metformin in preventing diabetes (Diabetes Prevention Program Research Group, 2002). The behavioral intervention also produced significantly greater weight loss and greater increases in physical activity than metformin or placebo (Diabetes Prevention Program Research Group, 2002).

Although the 21 trials in the USPSTF evidence review that combined pharmacologic agents (orlistat or metformin) with behavioral interventions resulted in significant weight loss and improvement in physiologic outcomes, the USPSTF elected to withhold a recommendation for use of medication to treat obesity because of concerns about the safety of orlistat and insufficient data on maintenance of weight loss after discontinuation of medications (E. S. Leblanc et al., 2011; Moyer, 2012). See the section on pharmacotherapy below for more on use of medications to treat obesity.

COMPONENTS OF INTENSIVE MULTICOMPONENT TREATMENT PROGRAMS TO MANAGE OBESITY

Based on their review of the research literature, the USPSTF specified that intensive, multicomponent behavioral interventions for obesity should include the following components:

- Behavioral management activities, such as setting weight-loss goals;
- Improving diet or nutrition and increasing physical activity;
- Addressing barriers to change;
- Self-monitoring; and
- Strategizing how to maintain lifestyle changes (Leblanc et al., 2011; Moyer, 2012).

The basic premise of the behavioral components included in multicomponent programs is that, in order to lose weight and keep it off, individuals must gradually replace current maladaptive eating behaviors and sedentary behavior with healthy eating behaviors and physical activity habits that can be incorporated into their lifestyles and maintained indefinitely (D. Abrams et al., 2000; Thompson et al., 2007).

Behavioral program elements for weight management include self-monitoring (keeping a daily record of food or calorie intake or both), stimulus control procedures (i.e., rearranging the environment in order to eliminate unhealthy food cues), goal setting, self-reinforcement to help shape new behaviors (e.g., slower eating), cognitive restructuring (e.g., changing maladaptive thinking regarding eating and dieting), an emphasis on a gradual increase and then maintenance of physical activity, assertiveness training focused on weight loss issues (e.g., food refusal), facilitation of social support for weight loss efforts, and relapse prevention training (D. Abrams et al., 2000; Thompson et al., 2007).

ASSESSMENT

When deciding when and how to intervene to treat obesity, several dimensions of patient characteristics may be evaluated: (1) psychological and medical findings; (2) cognitive-behavioral and social factors; and (3) patient motivation and preferences (D. Abrams et al., 2000; Thompson et al., 2007).

Psychological evaluation. Some obese patients have psychiatric comorbidity or psychosocial factors that warrant individualized treatment. Therefore, obese patients should ideally be screened for the presence of a co-morbid psychiatric disorder. Special attention should be placed on assessing the presence of an eating disorder, substance abuse or dependence, body image disturbance, depression, anxiety, binge eating disorder, history of sexual abuse, or a personality disorder (D. Abrams et al., 2000; Thompson et al., 2007).

Patients with an active substance abuse problem or eating disorder are best managed by being offered specific services for these problems. Patients with other co-morbid psychiatric disorders may be appropriate for participation in a weight management program if they are in simultaneous treatment for their comorbid psychiatric disorder, and if their current level of functioning would not prohibit their ability to adhere to weight management interventions (D. Abrams et al., 2000; Thompson et al., 2007).

In addition, we recommend that clinicians inquire about cognitive-behavioral factors specific to treatment planning, such as previous weight loss attempts, current eating habits, motivation for weight loss, body image, positive aspects of their obesity (secondary gain), binge eating, weight goal, expectations, high risk for relapse situations, and willingness to make long-term lifestyle changes (D. Abrams et al., 2000; Thompson et al., 2007). To assess binge eating, patients should be asked about the occurrence of binge episodes (rapid consumption of a large amount of food accompanied by a loss of control), frequency of binge episodes, history of binge eating, cognition during a binge (perceived loss of control of their eating), physical distress following a binge, negative affect or cognition following a binge episode (D. Abrams et al., 2000; Thompson et al., 2007). (See Chapter on Eating Disorders in this text.)

If a patient has a history of having been sexually abused, the trauma may or may not be related to the patient's current weight status (D. Abrams et al., 2000; Thompson et al., 2007). However, women in a weight management program who reported a history of being the victim of sexual abuse lost less weight and reported more nonadherence compared to women matched on BMI and age who denied a history of abuse (Clark et al., 2007; T. K. King, Clark, & Pera, 1996). For such patients, clinicians should additionally attempt to assess how likely it is that weight loss will: (1) trigger memories of sexual abuse (based on a return to a lower weight, which may coincide with the weight at which the patient was abused); (2) cause problematic disruptions in their relationships secondary to potential increased sexual attention or demands from others; or (3) lead to feelings of vulnerability (D. Abrams et al., 2000; Thompson et al., 2007). These areas are difficult to assess but may affect treatment; therefore, we recommend that clinicians are trained in this area or maintain a close referral relationship with a program and clinicians who specialize in sexual abuse issues (D. Abrams et al., 2000; Thompson et al., 2007).

Increasing physical activity. Engagement in regular physical activity is a key component of successful weight loss interventions (Jakicic & Davis, 2011; Leblanc et al., 2011; Wing & Gorin, 2003). Physical activity includes both structured exercise as well as lifestyle activity. Regular physical activity is useful in a variety ways: it increases energy expenditure, raises basal metabolic rate, suppresses appetite, counteracts some of the deleterious effects of obesity and sedentary behavior (e.g., improves cardiac efficiency), and minimizes the loss of lean tissue during weight loss (Jakicic & Davis, 2011; Thompson et al., 2007). Researchers have found that both aerobic exercise and strength training are beneficial and that home-based exercise improves long-term adherence compared to on-site exercise programs (Ashworth, Chad, Harrison, Reeder, & Marshall, 2005; Perri, Martin, Leermakers, Sears, & Notelovitz, 1997). The adherence advantages of home based activity may allow unstructured moderate exercise to be used as a viable alternative to structured program. Thus, obese individuals should be encouraged not only to increase their energy expenditure through regular structured exercise (e.g., walking, swimming, aerobics), but also to increase their level of lifestyle activity (e.g., using stairs rather than elevators, walking to the corner store instead of driving). Furthermore, there is evidence that increase in fitness associated with regular physical activity enhances outcomes even when patients remain obese (McAuley & Blair, 2011).

Nutritional education and use of a balanced-deficit diet. It is important to include a nutritional education component in all obesity treatment programs. Though many different diets have been advocated for weight loss, there is little scientific evidence to recommend one diet over another (Katz, 2001; Thompson et al., 2007). A trial that compared 4 approaches,

the Atkins (low carbohydrate), Zone (high protein, low carbohydrate), Ornish (very low fat), and Weight Watchers diets, found no significant difference in weight loss at 1 year (Dansinger, Gleason, Griffith, Selker, & Schaefer, 2005). An ideal nutritionally balanced diet consists of approximately 50% to 60% of calories from carbohydrates, no more than 30% from fat, and 15% to 20% from protein (D. Abrams et al., 2000; Katz, 2001; Thompson et al., 2007).

Long-term weight loss and weight maintenance usually requires both a reduction in energy intake as well as an increase in energy expenditure. A balanced-deficit diet provides nutritionally balanced daily meals with a caloric intake level below the individual's caloric expenditure level. Decreasing daily caloric intake by 500 kcal below that necessary for weight maintenance generally yields a 1 lb weight loss per week. Generally these diets are 1200 kcal per day for women and 1500 kcal per day for men. It is generally recommended that mildly obese individuals lose 1.0 to 1.5 lb per week (Thompson et al., 2007). A useful and practical approach to reducing caloric intake includes a combination of reducing total fat intake, reducing portion size, reducing energy density, and increasing fruit and vegetable intake (Katz, 2001; Thompson et al., 2007).

Low-calorie and very-low-calorie diets. Two more intense levels of caloric restriction are used in some settings to produce more rapid weight loss: the low-calorie diet (LCD) of about 1000 calories per day and the very-low-calorie diet (VLCD) of 800 or fewer calories per day. Both diets may produce adverse side effects, including excessive loss of lean body mass; therefore, prior to participating in one of these diets, patients must undergo a thorough medical evaluation by a trained physician (D. Abrams et al., 2000; Thompson et al., 2007). A review of VLCDs concluded that they did not produce greater long-term weight losses than LCDs (Tsai & Wadden, 2006). The use of liquid meal replacements as part of a 1000 to 1500 kcal/d diet may provide an effective, safer and less expensive alternative to VLCDs (Tsai & Wadden, 2006).

Interactive computer-based programs. A Cochrane review of 14 interactive computer-based interventions to manage obesity found that, when compared to no intervention or minimal interventions (pamphlets, usual care), these interventions are effective for weight loss and weight maintenance. Compared to infrequent in-person interventions, interactive computer-based interventions result in smaller weight losses and lower levels of weight maintenance, though the greater accessibility and convenience of the computer-based interventions make them an attractive alternative, especially for patients unwilling to commit to in-person care (Wieland et al., 2012).

Pharmacotherapy. The role of medications to treat obesity is an area of considerable interest and research (Colman et al., 2012). However, it should be noted that virtually all medications that have been approved by the FDA for the management of obesity must be paired with behavioral and nutritional intervention elements, as medications alone have not been shown to produce long-term weight loss. Moreover, studies have clearly demonstrated that weight is usually regained when pharmacologic agents are discontinued (Katz, 2001).

Unfortunately, several effective pharmacologic aids to treatment obesity drugs have been abandoned or withdrawn from the market because of serious toxicity: fenfluramine and dexfenfluramine (due to valvulopathy); sibutramine (myocardial infarction and stroke); phenylpropanolamine (stroke); aminorex (pulmonary hypertension; and rimonabant (suicidal ideation and behavior) (Colman et al., 2012). By mid-2012, orlistat was the only prescription drug approved for the long-term treatment of obesity.

Orlistat prevents absorption of fats in the gastrointestinal tract by inhibiting lipases. Multiple placebo-controlled trials have demonstrated orlistat's efficacy when combined with nutritional and behavioral counseling and it has been approved by the FDA for treatment of obesity for up to 2 years (Colman et al., 2012). All trials included elements of nutritional or behavioral counseling. Meta-analyses suggest that the mean weight loss with orlistat is 2.89 kg (Li et al., 2005). Patients switched to a weight maintenance diet after weight loss regain less weight if they continue on orlistat compared to placebo (Davidson et al., 1999). Orlistat needs to be taken in advance of meals containing fats and its use is limited by common gastrointestinal side effects (cramping, diarrhea, oily stool) secondary to fat malabsorption. Vitamin supplementation with lipid soluble vitamins is required. As a result, orlistat is most likely to be useful for patients who can follow a low-fat diet and who are willing to tolerate the side effects (D. Abrams et al., 2000).

In late 2012, the FDA approved two new medications for treating obesity: lorcaserin, and phentermine/topiramate combination (Colman et al., 2012). Both are approved as adjuncts to a reduced-calorie diet and increased physical activity for chronic weight management in adults who are either obese (BMI ≥30), or overweight (BMI ≥27) with at least one weight-related condition (Colman et al., 2012). Both new medications were assessed in placebo-controlled clinical trials in which all participants also received behavioral counseling. It should be noted that both of these new medications were approved despite safety concerns that are noted in the discussion below.

The efficacy of locaserin and phentermine/topiramate were demonstrated in placebo-controlled trials. At the end of 1 year, participants in trials of lorcaserin and phentermine/topiramate who were assigned to the active drug conditions were significantly more likely to achieve at least a 5% weight loss than those on placebos (For lorcaserin, the difference in was 38–47% vs. 16–23%; for phentermine/topiramate, 62–70% vs. 16–21%) (Colman et al., 2012).

Lorcaserin is a selective agonist of the serotonin 2C receptor. Serotonin is a neurotransmitter that affects mood and also a number of physiologic drives including food intake and satiety. Because lorcaserin shares a serotinergic mechanism with the withdrawn agents fenfluramine and dexfenfluramine, questions were raised about lorcaserin's effects on heart valves. However, locaserin has low affinity for the 2B serotonergic receptor (Colman et al., 2012). Fenfluramine's and dexfenfluamine's affinity for the 2B receptor is believed to be responsible for the toxic heart valve effects that led to the withdrawal of those agents (Colman et al., 2012). Before FDA approval, lorcaserin's manufacturer completed an echocardiographic safety study that found no significant increase in valvulopathy in patients on lorcaserin (Colman et al., 2012). Though concerns about lorcaserin's propensity to increase tumor types in rats were also identified, these fears were allayed by subsequent studies (Colman et al., 2012). In addition, lorcaserin may increase the risk of psychiatric, cognitive, and serotonergic adverse effects (Colman et al., 2012).

Phentermine, a sympathomimetic, and extended-release topiramate, an anticonvulsant with anorectic properties, are combined in a fixed-dose preparation. Because of the potential for cardiovascular toxicity, the effects of this combination on cardiac function were scrutinized by the FDA (Colman et al., 2012). At doses of 7.5 mg/46 mg and 15 mg/92 mg, phentermine/topiramate was associated with mean increases in heart rate of 0.6 bpm and 1.6 bpm, respectively, as compared with placebo (Colman et al., 2012). However, this effect on heart rate was offset by greater mean reductions in blood pressure on active drug than on placebo (Colman et al., 2012). Taking into account the magnitude of weight loss and the favorable changes in blood pressure, the FDA concluded that the benefit–risk balance was positive and supported the approval (Colman et al., 2012). Because topiramate use during pregnancy is associated with an increased incidence of oral-facial clefts in pregnancy, FDA approval of phentermine/topiramate required a risk evaluation and mitigation strategy (REMS) that includes a training program for prescribers, a medication guide and a patient brochure that stresses the need for women of reproductive potential to use effective forms of contraception (Colman et al., 2012). Phentermine/topiramate may also increase the risk of metabolic acidosis, glaucoma, and psychiatric and cognitive adverse effects (Colman et al., 2012). The REMS also specifies that only specially certified pharmacies will be able to dispense phentermine/topiramate (Colman et al., 2012).

Because these new medications are associated with potentially serious risks and the FDA has stressed that it is important that their use be limited to patients who are obese, or overweight (BMI ≥27) with at least one weight-related condition (Colman et al., 2012). Prescribers should also adhere to the recommendations in the labels regarding patients' initial weight loss response to treatment (Colman et al., 2012). If, after 12 weeks of treatment with lorcaserin, a patient has not lost at least 5% of the baseline body weight, use of the drug should be discontinued, since results from the initial trials suggest that it is unlikely that the patient will achieve meaningful weight loss with continued treatment (Colman et al., 2012). Similarly, if after 12 weeks of treatment with phentermine–topiramate at the 7.5 mg/46 mg dose, a patient has not lost at least 3% of the baseline weight, either the drug should be discontinued or the dose increased (Colman et al., 2012). If the latter option is chosen and the patient does not lose at least 5% of the baseline weight during an additional 12 weeks of treatment, the drug should be discontinued, because the patient is unlikely to achieve meaningful weight loss with continued treatment (Colman et al., 2012). Finally, the FDA is also requiring that the manufacturers of both lor-caserin and phentermine/topiramate conduct a number of postapproval clinical trials, including a "rigorous assessment of long-term cardiovascular safety in overweight and obese patients" (Colman et al., 2012).

In summary, medications have a place in the management of obesity. Three medications, orlistat, lorcaserin and phenter-mine/topiramate, are efficacious when combined with behav-ioral and nutritional intervention elements. However, there are questions regarding their long term safety and efficacy. Longer-term studies with large numbers of subjects may be necessary to further define exactly what role medications will play in the treatment of obesity in the future.

SURGERY

Surgery for obesity, also known as bariatric surgery, has been reported to result in substantial 10-year weight loss (Maggard et al., 2005). Currently accepted criteria for consideration of bariatric surgery include a body mass index (calculated as weight in kilograms divided by the square of height in meters) of 40 kg/m² or greater (or >35 kg/m² with obesity-related comorbidities), patient readiness to participate in dietary, physical activity and self-care activities, and acceptable medi-cal and surgical risk (Collazo-Clavell, Clark, McAlpine, & Jensen, 2006). In a 2004 review and meta-analysis of the health benefits of bariatric surgery, investigators reported that diabetes, hyperlipidemia, hypertension, and obstructive sleep apnea resolved or improved in more than half of the patients who had these conditions preoperatively (Buchwald, et al., 2004). A subsequent meta-analysis of bariatric surgery involv-ing over 7,000 patients with diabetes found 78.1% of diabetic patients had complete resolution, and diabetes was improved or resolved in 86.6% of patients (Buchwald et al., 2009). Weight loss and diabetes resolution were greatest for patients undergoing biliopancreatic diversion/duodenal switch, fol-lowed by gastric bypass, and least for banding procedures (Buchwald et al., 2009).

A 2005 meta-analysis and review found that common bariatric procedures (gastric bypass, laparoscopic adjustable gastric band, vertical banded gastroplasty, and biliopancreatic diversion and switch) have been performed with an overall mortality rate of less than 1%, and with adverse events occur-ring in about 20% of cases (Maggard et al., 2005). Though gas-tric bypass (GBP) procedures result in more weight loss than gastroplasty, laparoscopic approaches result in fewer wound complications than an open approach (Maggard et al., 2005). A systematic review indicated that laparoscopic isolated sleeve gastrectomy (LISG) was more effective than adjustable gastric banding (AGB). GBP and banded GBP led to similar weight loss and results for GBP versus LISG and VBG versus AGB were equivocal (Picot et al., 2009).

An interdisciplinary team approach, including surgeons, primary care clinicians, psychologists and nutritionists, is essential for achieving both good and safe long-term outcomes of bariatric surgery (McMahon et al., 2006). Careful screening of suitable candidates is useful, including a psychological and

Box 53.2 CRITERIA FOR BARIATRIC SURGERY

- Body mass index of 40 kg/m² or more (approximately 45 kg overweight for men and 36 kg for women) *or*
- Body mass index between 35 and 39.9 kg/m² and a serious obesity-related health problem such as type 2 diabetes, heart disease, or severe sleep apnea
- The patient should understand the operation and the lifestyle changes that will be needed
- Be unlikely to lose weight or maintain weight loss long term with nonsurgical measures
- Be well informed about the surgical procedure and the effects of treatment
- Be motivated to lose weight and improve health
- Be aware of how life may change after the operation (e.g., the need to chew food well and the inability to eat large meals)
- Have no psychological contraindications to obesity surgery such as untreated depression or personality disorders
- Be aware of the potential for serious complications, dietary restrictions, and occasional failures
- Be committed to lifelong medical follow-up and vitamin/ mineral supplementation
- Realize that no method, including surgery, is guaranteed to produce and maintain weight loss and that success is possible only with long-term commitment to behavioral change and medical follow-up

Adapted from the National Institute of Diabetes and Digestive and Kidney Diseases, National Institutes of Health. *Gastrointestinal Surgery for Severe Obesity*. Bethesda, Md: National Institutes of Health; December 2004. NM Publication No. 04-4006.

behavioral assessment of the patient's capacity to manage self-care, behavioral change and nutritional needs before and after surgery (See Box 53.2). Understanding of potential vitamin and mineral deficiencies, effects of weight loss on medical co-morbid conditions, and common postoperative surgical issues are quite important (McMahon et al., 2006). Educational and behavioral interventions are also essential, as the long-term success of bariatric surgery relies on patients' ability to make sustained lifestyle changes in nutrition and physical activity (McMahon et al., 2006). Moreover, collaborative longitudi-nal care allows prompt and frequent adjustment as weight loss occurs and nutritional and behavioral elements are adapted to current needs (McMahon et al., 2006).

SUMMARY—OBESITY ASSESSMENT AND MANAGEMENT

The prevalence of obesity, a major contributor to morbidity and mortality, is increasing at an alarming rate. Obesity is a complex biopsychosocial condition that, like tobacco use, is best considered as a chronic relapsing condition that usually requires multiple treatment courses. Because of the complex interactions of factors that underlie and contribute to obesity, and the recidivism that commonly occurs after treatment, the management of obesity requires close attention to not only weight loss, but life-long maintenance of weight. Obesity management should include multiple intervention components including caloric restriction and nutritional education, cognitive-behavioral strategies, a physical activity element, and support of maintenance strategies. Pharmacotherapy and surgical interventions are effective, though they must be closely integrated with behavioral, physical activity and nutritional elements to achieve successful long-term outcomes.

SUMMARY

In this chapter, we have described and illustrated behavioral medicine treatment approaches for two critical conditions: tobacco use and obesity. We applied a multidimensional biopsychosocial approach to the assessment and treatment of tobacco use and obesity and illustrated strategies for integrating this approach within the emerging Patient-Centered Medical Home model. We reviewed the evidence-based recommendations of the PHS Clinical Practice Guideline for Treating Tobacco Use and Dependence and recommendations of the US Preventive Services Task Force regarding Screening for and Managing Obesity. These guidelines both emphasize the importance of a multidimensional approach that integrates motivational strategies, cognitive-behavioral interventions, education elements, medication management and, in the case of obesity, surgical approaches. Though intensive multicomponent multisession interventions produce the best outcomes for both tobacco use and obesity, we have also shared strategies for delivering brief and less intensive interventions (e.g., 5As counseling) that are widely applicable in primary care and other medical settings. Since up to 75% of Americans visit a health care provider each year, clinicians in these setting have the potential to play a central role in addressing health behaviors that are critical to preventing illness and promoting health, functioning and wellbeing.

CLINICAL PEARLS

- Less than a third of smokers will utilize either medication or counseling in their efforts to stop smoking (CDC, 2011).

- In tobacco addiction, as with other chronic conditions such as diabetes and hypertension, clinicians should consider taking a long term view marked by repeated efforts to offer patient education, counseling and intervention.

- The signs and symptoms of nicotine withdrawal can appear within 2 to 6 hours after the last use of tobacco, usually peak between 24 and 48 hours later, and last from a few days to a few days to a few weeks (Benowitz, 2010; Hughes & Hatsukami, 1992). Withdrawal symptoms include psychological symptoms of craving or urges to use nicotine, dysphoric or depressed mood, irritability, frustration, anger, anxiety, difficulty concentrating,

restlessness, decreased heart rate and increased appetite or weight gain (Hughes & Hatsukami, 1992).

- Encouraging pregnant smokers who are reluctant to quit to, at minimum, reduce their smoking rate is likely to have beneficial effects, as a dose-response relationship between smoking rate and birth weight has been observed (M. Fiore et al., 2008).

- Smoking cessation is generally associated with under 10 pounds of weight gain (Fiore et al., 2008); however, as many as 10% of quitters gain as much as 30 pounds.

- Brief tobacco dependence treatment is effective. Two components of counseling are especially effective and should be used when counseling patients making a quit attempt: practical counseling (problem solving/skills training) and social support delivered as part of treatment.

- Drugs that support nicotine cessation include bupropion SR, nicotine gum, nicotine inhaler, nicotine lozenge, nicotine nasal spray, nicotine patch, and varenicline.

- Nicotine replacement therapy provides an opportunity for the patient to practice strategies to deal with behavioral or learned components of drug dependence while controlling the physiologic "need" for the drug.

- Novel ways of administering nicotine replacement treatment (NRT) that can improve quit rates, include prolonging treatment beyond the standard 12 weeks of treatment; continuing rather than discontinuing NRT use after a lapse; and starting NRT 2 weeks before the quit day rather than on the quit day (Fiore & Baker, 2011; Rigotti, 2012).

- It is common for patients to use insufficient gum to achieve optimal benefit. The CPG recommends a fixed schedule of at least one piece of gum every 1–2 hours for the first 1–3 months after quitting smoking.

- Insomnia with bupropion SR may improve by shifting the second daily dose to an earlier time, but still 8 hours after the first dose.

- Recognize danger situations—identify events, internal states or activities that increase the risk of smoking or relapse.

- When lapses occur, patients and clinicians need to guard against what has been called the "abstinence violation effect" (e.g., excess guilt, shame, pessimism and reduced confidence for change) (Baer & Marlatt, 1991; Ockene et al., 2000).

- Loss of as little as 5–10% of body weight, achievable with multicomponent behavioral intervention programs, is associated with numerous health benefits.

- Ask about previous (a) weight loss attempts, (b) current eating habits, (c) motivation for weight loss, (d) body image, (e) positive aspects of their obesity (secondary gain), (f) binge eating, (g) weight goal, (h) expectations,

(i) high risk for relapse situations, and (j) willingness to make long-term lifestyle changes.

DISCLOSURE STATEMENTS

Dr. Goldstein has no conflicts to disclose. He is an employee of the US Veterans Health Administration. His contributions to this publication are his own and do not represent the views, positions or policies of the Veterans Health Administration.

Dr. Dundon has no conflicts to disclose. She is an employee of the US Veterans Health Administration. Her contributions to this publication are her own and do not represent the views, positions or policies of the Veterans Health Administration.

REFERENCES

Abrams, D., King, T., Clark, M., Forsyth, L., Pera Jr., V., & Goldstein, M. (2000). Behavioral medicine strategies: management of nicotine dependence, obesity, and cardiopulmonary rehabilitation exercise. In A. Stoudemire, B. Fogel & D. Greenberg (Eds.), *Psychiatric Care of the Medical Patient* (Second ed., pp. 519–544). New York: Oxford University Press.

Abrams, D. B., Niaura, R., Brown, R. A., Emmons, K. M., Goldstein, M. G., & Monti, P. M. (Eds.). (2003). *The Tobacco Dependence Treatment Handbook: A Guide to Best Practices.* New York: Guilford.

Agency for Healthcare Research and Quality, P. H. S., USDHHS (2012). Patient-Centered Medical Home Resource Center.

Ashworth, N. L., Chad, K. E., Harrison, E. L., Reeder, B. A., & Marshall, S. C. (2005). Home versus center based physical activity programs in older adults. *Cochrane Database SystRev* (1), CD004017.

Baer, J. S., & Marlatt, G. A. (1991). Maintenance of smoking cessation. *Clin Chest Med, 12*(4), 793–800.

Ball, K., Burton, N. W., & Brown, W. J. (2009). A prospective study of overweight, physical activity, and depressive symptoms in young women. *Obesity (Silver Spring), 17*(1), 66–71.

Bandura, A. (2004). Health promotion by social cognitive means. *Health EducBehav, 31*(2), 143–164.

Barnes, J., Dong, C. Y., McRobbie, H., Walker, N., Mehta, M., & Stead, L. F. (2010). Hypnotherapy for smoking cessation. *Cochrane Database of Systematic Reviews*, Issue 10. Art. No.: CD001008. doi: 10.1002/14651858.CD001008.pub2

Benowitz, N. L. (2010). Nicotine addiction. *N Engl J Med, 362*(24), 2295–2303.

Brown, R. (2003). Intensive Behavioral Treatment. In D. B. Abrams, R. Niaura, R. A. Brown, K. M. Emmons, M. G. Goldstein & P. M. Monti (Eds.), *The Tobacco Dependence Treatment Handbook: A Guide to Best Practices.* New York: Guilford.

Buchwald, H., Avidor, Y., Braunwald, E., Jensen, M. D., Pories, W., Fahrbach, K., et al. (2004). Bariatric surgery: a systematic review and meta-analysis. *Jama, 292*(14), 1724–1737.

Buchwald, H., Estok, R., Fahrbach, K., Banel, D., Jensen, M. D., Pories, W. J., et al. (2009). Weight and type 2 diabetes after bariatric surgery: systematic review and meta-analysis. *Am J Med, 122*(3), 248–256 e245.

Butryn, M. L., Phelan, S., Hill, J. O., & Wing, R. R. (2007). Consistent self-monitoring of weight: a key component of successful weight loss maintenance. *Obesity (Silver Spring), 15*(12), 3091–3096.

Carrier, E., Gourevitch, M. N., & Shah, N. R. (2009). Medical homes: challenges in translating theory into practice. *Med Care, 47*(7), 714–722.

CDC (2011). Quitting smoking among adults—United States, 2001–2010. *MMWR Morb Mortal Wkly Rep, 60*(44), 1513–1519.

Clark, M. M., Hanna, B. K., Mai, J. L., Graszer, K. M., Krochta, J. G., McAlpine, D. E., et al. (2007). Sexual abuse survivors and psychiatric hospitalization after bariatric surgery. *Obes Surg, 17*(4), 465–469.

Collazo-Clavell, M. L., Clark, M. M., McAlpine, D. E., & Jensen, M. D. (2006). Assessment and preparation of patients for bariatric surgery. *Mayo Clin Proc, 81*(10 Suppl), S11–S17.

Colman, E., Golden, J., Roberts, M., Egan, A., Weaver, J., & Rosebraugh, C. (2012). The FDA's assessment of two drugs for chronic weight management. *N Engl J Med, 367*(17), 1577–1579.

Dansinger, M. L., Gleason, J. A., Griffith, J. L., Selker, H. P., & Schaefer, E. J. (2005). Comparison of the Atkins, Ornish, Weight Watchers, and Zone diets for weight loss and heart disease risk reduction: a randomized trial. *Jama, 293*(1), 43–53.

Davidson, M. H., Hauptman, J., DiGirolamo, M., Foreyt, J. P., Halsted, C. H., Heber, D., et al. (1999). Weight control and risk factor reduction in obese subjects treated for 2 years with orlistat: a randomized controlled trial. *Jama, 281*(3), 235–242.

Day, F. R., & Loos, R. J. (2011). Developments in obesity genetics in the era of genome-wide association studies. *J Nutrigenet Nutrigenomics, 4*(4), 222–238.

DePue, J. D., Clark, M. M., Ruggiero, L., Medeiros, M. L., & Pera, V., Jr. (1995). Maintenance of weight loss: a needs assessment. *Obes Res, 3*(3), 241–248.

Diabetes Prevention Program Research Group (2002). Reduction in the Incidence of Type 2 Diabetes with Lifestyle Intervention or Metformin. *N Engl J Med, 346*(6), 393–403.

Donnelly, J. E., Blair, S. N., Jakicic, J. M., Manore, M. M., Rankin, J. W., & Smith, B. K. (2009). American College of Sports Medicine Position Stand. Appropriate physical activity intervention strategies for weight loss and prevention of weight regain for adults. *Med Sci Sports Exerc, 41*(2), 459–471.

Ferguson, S. G., & Shiffman, S. (2009). The relevance and treatment of cue-induced cravings in tobacco dependence. *J Subst Abuse Treat, 36*(3), 235–243.

Fiore, M., Jaén, C., Baker, T., Bailey, W., Benowitz, N., Curry, S., et al. (2008). *Treating Tobacco Use and Dependence: 2008 Update. Clinical Practice Guideline.* Rockville, MD: Public Health Service.

Fiore, M. C., & Baker, T. B. (2011). Clinical practice. Treating smokers in the health care setting. *N Engl J Med, 365*(13), 1222–1231.

Flegal, K. M., Carroll, M. D., Kit, B. K., & Ogden, C. L. (2012). Prevalence of obesity and trends in the distribution of body mass index among US adults, 1999–2010. *Jama, 307*(5), 491–497.

Fontaine, K. R., Redden, D. T., Wang, C., Westfall, A. O., & Allison, D. B. (2003). Years of life lost due to obesity. *Jama, 289*(2), 187–193.

Glassgow, R. E., & Goldstein, M. G. (2008). Introduction to the Principles of Health Behavior Change. In S. H. Woolf, S. Jonas & E. Kaplan-Liss (Eds.), *Health Promotion and Disease Prevention in Clinical Practice* (Second ed., pp. 129–147). Philadelphia: Lippincott Williams & Wilkins

Goldstein, M. G., DePue, J., & Kazura, A. (2008). Models of Provider-Patient Interaction and Shared Decision Making. In S. A. Shumaker, J. K. Ockene & K. A. Riekert (Eds.), *Handbook of Health Behavior Change* (Third ed., pp. 107–126). New York: Springer Publishing Company.

Goldstein, M. G., Whitlock, E. P., & DePue, J. (2004). Multiple behavioral risk factor interventions in primary care; Summary of research evidence. *Am J Prev Med, 27*(2 Suppl), 61–79.

Guh, D. P., Zhang, W., Bansback, N., Amarsi, Z., Birmingham, C. L., & Anis, A. H. (2009). The incidence of co-morbidities related to obesity and overweight: a systematic review and meta-analysis. *BMC Public Health, 9*, 88.

Haskell, W. L., Lee, I. M., Pate, R. R., Powell, K. E., Blair, S. N., Franklin, B. A., et al. (2007). Physical activity and public health: updated recommendation for adults from the American College of Sports Medicine and the American Heart Association. *Circulation, 116*(9), 1081–1093.

Herrera, B. M., Keildson, S., & Lindgren, C. M. (2011). Genetics and epigenetics of obesity. *Maturitas, 69*(1), 41–49.

Hitsman, B., Moss, T. G., Montoya, I. D., & George, T. P. (2009). Treatment of tobacco dependence in mental health and addictive disorders. *Can J Psychiatry, 54*(6), 368–378.

Hughes, J., & Hatsukami, D. (1992). The nicotine withdrawal syndrome: a brief review and update. *International Journal of Smoking Cessation, 1*, 21–26.

Hughes, J. R. (2007). Effects of abstinence from tobacco: etiology, animal models, epidemiology, and significance: a subjective review. *Nicotine Tob Res, 9*(3), 329–339.

Jakicic, J. M., & Davis, K. K. (2011). Obesity and physical activity. *Psychiatr Clin North Am, 34*(4), 829–840.

Jamal, A., Dube, S. R., Malarcher, A. M., Shaw, L., & Engstrom, M. C. (2012). Tobacco use screening and counseling during physician office visits among adults—National Ambulatory Medical Care Survey and National Health Interview Survey, United States, 2005–2009. *MMWR Morb Mortal Wkly Rep, 61 Suppl*, 38–45.

Kalman, D., Morissette, S. B., & George, T. P. (2005). Co-morbidity of smoking in patients with psychiatric and substance use disorders. *Am J Addict, 14*(2), 106–123.

Katz, D. L. (2001). Diet, Obesity, and Weight Regulation. In D. L. Katz (Ed.), *Nutrition in Clinical Practice: A Comprehensive, Evidence-Based Manual for the Practitioner* (pp. 37–62). Philadelphia: Lippincott Williams & Wilkins.

King, B. A., Dube, S. R., & Tynan, M. A. (2012). Current tobacco use among adults in the United States: findings from the national adult tobacco survey. *Am J Public Health, 102*(11), e93–e100.

King, T. K., Clark, M. M., & Pera, V. (1996). History of sexual abuse and obesity treatment outcome. *Addict Behav, 21*(3), 283–290.

Kleges, R., & Kleges, L. (1988). Cigarette smoking as a dieting strategy in a university population. *International Journal of Eating Disorders, 7*, 413–419.

Klem, M. L., Wing, R. R., McGuire, M. T., Seagle, H. M., & Hill, J. O. (1997). A descriptive study of individuals successful at long-term maintenance of substantial weight loss. *Am J ClinNutr, 66*(2), 239–246.

Konttinen, H., Silventoinen, K., Sarlio-Lahteenkorva, S., Mannisto, S., & Haukkala, A. (2010). Emotional eating and physical activity self-efficacy as pathways in the association between depressive symptoms and adiposity indicators. *Am J Clin Nutr, 92*(5), 1031–1039.

Kruger, J., Galuska, D. A., Serdula, M. K., & Jones, D. A. (2004). Attempting to lose weight: specific practices among U.S. adults. *Am J Prev Med, 26*(5), 402–406.

Lai, D. T., Cahill, K., Qin, Y., & Tang, J. L. (2010). Motivational interviewing for smoking cessation. *Cochrane Database SystRev*(1), CD006936.

LeBlanc, E., O'Connor, E., Whitlock, E. P., Patnode, C., & Kapka, T. (2011). Screening for and Management of Obesity and Overweight in Adults. *Evidence Report No. 89*. AHRQ Publication No. 11-05159-EF-1. Rockville, MD: Agency for Healthcare Research and Quality; 2011.

Leblanc, E. S., O'Connor, E., Whitlock, E. P., Patnode, C. D., & Kapka, T. (2011). Effectiveness of primary care-relevant treatments for obesity in adults: a systematic evidence review for the U.S. Preventive Services Task Force. *Ann Intern Med, 155*(7), 434–447.

Li, Z., Maglione, M., Tu, W., Mojica, W., Arterburn, D., Shugarman, L. R., et al. (2005). Meta-analysis: pharmacologic treatment of obesity. *Ann Intern Med, 142*(7), 532–546.

Ma, J., Xiao, L., & Stafford, R. S. (2009). Adult obesity and office-based quality of care in the United States. *Obesity (Silver Spring), 17*(5), 1077–1085.

Maggard, M. A., Shugarman, L. R., Suttorp, M., Maglione, M., Sugerman, H. J., Livingston, E. H., et al. (2005). Meta-analysis: surgical treatment of obesity. *Ann Intern Med, 142*(7), 547–559.

Marcus, B. H., Lewis, B. A., Hogan, J., King, T. K., Albrecht, A. E., Bock, B., et al. (2005). The efficacy of moderate-intensity exercise as an aid for smoking cessation in women: a randomized controlled trial. *Nicotine Tob Res, 7*(6), 871–880.

McAuley, P. A., & Blair, S. N. (2011). Obesity paradoxes. *J Sports Sci, 29*(8), 773–782.

McClave, A. K., McKnight-Eily, L. R., Davis, S. P., & Dube, S. R. (2010). Smoking characteristics of adults with selected lifetime mental illnesses: results from the 2007 National Health Interview Survey. *Am J Public Health, 100*(12), 2464–2472.

McFall, M., Saxon, A. J., Thaneemit-Chen, S., Smith, M. W., Joseph, A. M., Carmody, T. P., et al. (2007). Integrating smoking cessation into mental health care for post-traumatic stress disorder. *Clin Trials, 4*(2), 178–189.

McFall, M., Saxon, A. J., Thompson, C. E., Yoshimoto, D., Malte, C., Straits-Troster, K., et al. (2005). Improving the rates of quitting smoking for veterans with posttraumatic stress disorder. *Am J Psychiatry, 162*(7), 1311–1319.

McMahon, M. M., Sarr, M. G., Clark, M. M., Gall, M. M., Knoetgen, J., 3rd, Service, F. J., et al. (2006). Clinical management after bariatric surgery: value of a multidisciplinary approach. *Mayo ClinProc, 81*(10 Suppl), S34–45.

Miller, W. R. (2000). Rediscovering fire: small interventions, large effects. *Psychol Addict Behav, 14*(1), 6–18.

Miller, W. R., & Rollnick, S. (2013). *Motivational Interviewing: Helping People Change* (Third ed.). New York: The Guilford Press.

Mokdad, A. H., Marks, J. S., Stroup, D. F., & Gerberding, J. L. (2004). Actual causes of death in the United States, 2000. *Jama, 291*, 1238–1245.

Moyer, V. A. (2012). Screening for and management of obesity in adults: U.S. Preventive Services Task Force recommendation statement. *Ann Intern Med, 157*(5), 373–378.

Mutch, D. M., & Clement, K. (2006). Genetics of human obesity. *Best Pract Res Clin Endocrinol Metab, 20*(4), 647–664.

Needham, B. L., Epel, E. S., Adler, N. E., & Kiefe, C. (2010). Trajectories of change in obesity and symptoms of depression: the CARDIA study. *Am J Public Health, 100*(6), 1040–1046.

Niaura, R., & Shadel, W. G. (2003). Assessment to Inform Smoking Cessation Treatment. In D. B. Abrams, R. Niaura, R. A. Brown, K. M. Emmons, M. G. Goldstein & P. M. Monti (Eds.), *The Tobacco Dependence Treatment Handbook: A Guide to Best Practices* (pp. 27–72). New York: The Guilford Press.

Niaura, R. S., Rohsenow, D. J., Binkoff, J. A., Monti, P. M., Pedraza, M., & Abrams, D. B. (1988). Relevance of cue reactivity to understanding alcohol and smoking relapse. *J Abnorm Psychol, 97*(2), 133–152.

Ockene, J. K., Emmons, K. M., Mermelstein, R. J., Perkins, K. A., Bonollo, D. S., Voorhees, C. C., et al. (2000). Relapse and maintenance issues for smoking cessation. *Health Psychol, 19*(1 Suppl), 17–31.

Orlinsky, D., Grawe, K., & Parks, B. (1994). Process and outcome in psychotherapy—nocheinmal. In A. Bergin & S. Garfield (Eds.), *Handbook of Psychotherapy and Behavior Change* (4th ed., pp. 270–378). New York: Wiley.

Perri, M. G., Martin, A. D., Leermakers, E. A., Sears, S. F., & Notelovitz, M. (1997). Effects of group- versus home-based exercise in the treatment of obesity. *J Consult Clin Psychol, 65*(2), 278–285.

Picot, J., Jones, J., Colquitt, J. L., Gospodarevskaya, E., Loveman, E., Baxter, L., et al. (2009). The clinical effectiveness and cost-effectiveness of bariatric (weight loss) surgery for obesity: a systematic review and economic evaluation. *Health Technol Assess, 13*(41), 1–190, 215–357, iii-iv.

Pomerleau, C. S., & Saules, K. (2007). Body image, body satisfaction, and eating patterns in normal-weight and overweight/obese women current smokers and never-smokers. *Addict Behav, 32*(10), 2329–2334.

Rigotti, N. A. (2012). Strategies to help a smoker who is struggling to quit. *JAMA, 308*(15), 1573–1580.

Rollnick, S., Mason, P., & Butler, C. (1999). *Health Behavior Change: A Guide for Practitioners*. Edinburgh: Churchill Livingstone.

Rollnick, S., Miller, W. R., & Butler, C. C. (2008). *Motivational Interviewing in Health Care: Helping Patients Change Behavior*. New York: The Guilford Press.

Rosenthal, T. C. (2008). The medical home: growing evidence to support a new approach to primary care. *J Am Board Fam Med, 21*(5), 427–440.

Schroeder, S. A. (2012). How clinicians can help smokers to quit. *Jama, 308*(15), 1586–1587.

Shiffman, S., Sweeney, C. T., Pillitteri, J. L., Sembower, M. A., Harkins, A. M., & Wadden, T. A. (2009). Weight management advice: what do doctors recommend to their patients? *Prev Med, 49*(6), 482–486.

Simon, G. E., Von Korff, M., Saunders, K., Miglioretti, D. L., Crane, P. K., van Belle, G., et al. (2006). Association between obesity and psychiatric disorders in the US adult population. *Arch Gen Psychiatry, 63*(7), 824–830.

Society of Behavioral Medicine (2012). Definition of Behavioral Medicine Retrieved November 16, 2012, from http://www.sbm.org/about

Spring, B., Howe, D., Berendsen, M., McFadden, H. G., Hitchcock, K., Rademaker, A. W., et al. (2009). Behavioral intervention to promote smoking cessation and prevent weight gain: a systematic review and meta-analysis. *Addiction, 104*(9), 1472–1486.

Squier, R. W. (1990). A model of empathic understanding and adherence to treatment regimens in practitioner-patient relationships. *Soc Sci Med, 30*(3), 325–339.

Stead, L. F., & Lancaster, T. (2012). Combined pharmacotherapy and behavioural interventions for smoking cessation. *Cochrane Database Syst Rev, 10*, CD008286.

Stein, C. J., & Colditz, G. A. (2004). The epidemic of obesity. *J Clin Endocrinol Metab, 89*(6), 2522–2525.

Svetkey, L. P., Stevens, V. J., Brantley, P. J., Appel, L. J., Hollis, J. F., Loria, C. M., et al. (2008). Comparison of strategies for sustaining weight loss: the weight loss maintenance randomized controlled trial. *Jama, 299*(10), 1139–1148.

Thompson, W. G., Cook, D. A., Clark, M. M., Bardia, A., & Levine, J. A. (2007). Treatment of obesity. *Mayo ClinProc, 82*(1), 93–101; quiz 101–102.

Tsai, A. G., & Wadden, T. A. (2006). The evolution of very-low-calorie diets: an update and meta-analysis. *Obesity (Silver Spring), 14*(8), 1283–1293.

U.S. Department of Health and Human Services (1988). The Health Consequences of Smoking: Nicotine Addiction. A Report of the Surgeon General. Rockville: U.S. Department of Health and Human Services, Public Health Service, Centers for Disease Control. DHHS Publication no (CDC) 88-8406.

U.S. Department of Health and Human Services (2010). *How Tobacco Smoke Causes Disease: The Biology and Behavioral Basis for Smoking-Attributable Disease: A Report of the Surgeon General.* Atlanta, GA: Centers for Disease Control and Prevention, National Center for Chronic Disease Prevention and Health Promotion, Office on Smoking and Health.

Ussher, M. H., Taylor, A., & Faulkner, G. (2012). Exercise interventions for smoking cessation. *Cochrane Database Syst Rev, 1*, CD002295.

Wadden, T. A., Webb, V. L., Moran, C. H., Bailer, B. A. (2012). Lifestyle modification for obesity: New developments in diet, physical activity, and behavior therapy. Circulation, 125, 1157–1170.

Wang, Y., Beydoun, M. A., Liang, L., Caballero, B., & Kumanyika, S. K. (2008). Will all Americans become overweight or obese? estimating the progression and cost of the US obesity epidemic. *Obesity (Silver Spring), 16*(10), 2323–2330.

West, R., Zatonski, W., Cedzynska, M., Lewandowska, D., Pazik, J., Aveyard, P., et al. (2011). Placebo-controlled trial of cytisine for smoking cessation. *N Engl J Med, 365*(13), 1193–1200.

White, A. R., Rampes, H., & Ernst, E. (2002). Acupuncture for smoking cessation. *Cochrane Database SystRev*(2), CD000009.

Whitlock, E. P., Orleans, C. T., Pender, N., & Allan, J. (2002). Evaluating primary care behavioral counseling interventions: an evidence-based approach. *Am J Prev Med, 22*(4), 267–284.

Whitlock, G., Lewington, S., Sherliker, P., Clarke, R., Emberson, J., Halsey, J., et al. (2009). Body-mass index and cause-specific mortality in 900 000 adults: collaborative analyses of 57 prospective studies. *Lancet, 373*(9669), 1083–1096.

Whittaker, R., McRobbie, H., Bullen, C., Borland, R., Rodgers, A., & Gu, Y. (2012). Mobile phone-based interventions for smoking cessation. *Cochrane Database of Systematic Reviews*, (11). Retrieved from http://onlinelibrary.wiley.com/doi/10.1002/14651858.CD006611.pub3/abstract. doi:10.1002/14651858.CD006611.pub3

Wieland, L. S., Falzon, L., Sciamanna, C. N., Trudeau, K. J., Brodney, S., Schwartz, J. E., et al. (2012). Interactive computer-based interventions for weight loss or weight maintenance in overweight or obese people. *Cochrane Database Syst Rev, 8*, CD007675.

Williams, G. C., McGregor, H. A., Sharp, D., Levesque, C., Kouides, R. W., Ryan, R. M., et al. (2006). Testing a self-determination theory intervention for motivating tobacco cessation: supporting autonomy and competence in a clinical trial. *Health Psychol, 25*(1), 91–101.

Williams, G. C., Minicucci, D. S., Kouides, R. W., Levesque, C. S., Chirkov, V. I., Ryan, R. M., et al. (2002). Self-determination, smoking, diet and health. *Health Educ. Res., 17*(5), 512–521.

Wing, R. R. (2010). Long-term effects of a lifestyle intervention on weight and cardiovascular risk factors in individuals with type 2 diabetes mellitus: four-year results of the Look AHEAD trial. *Arch Intern Med, 170*(17), 1566–1575.

Wing, R. R., & Gorin, A. A. (2003). Behavioral techniques for treating the obese patient. *Prim Care, 30*(2), 375–391.

Wing, R. R., Papandonatos, G., Fava, J. L., Gorin, A. A., Phelan, S., McCaffery, J., et al. (2008). Maintaining large weight losses: the role of behavioral and psychological factors. *J Consult Clin Psychol, 76*(6), 1015–1021.

Wing, R. R., Tate, D. F., Gorin, A. A., Raynor, H. A., Fava, J. L., & Machan, J. (2007). STOP regain: are there negative effects of daily weighing? *J Consult ClinPsychol, 75*(4), 652–656.

Zhao, G., Ford, E. S., Li, C., Tsai, J., Dhingra, S., & Balluz, L. S. (2011). Waist circumference, abdominal obesity, and depression among overweight and obese U.S. adults: National Health and Nutrition Examination Survey 2005–2006. *BMC Psychiatry, 11*, 130.

Ziedonis, D., Hitsman, B., Beckham, J. C., Zvolensky, M., Adler, L. E., Audrain-McGovern, J., et al. (2008). Tobacco use and cessation in psychiatric disorders: National Institute of Mental Health report. *Nicotine Tob Res, 10*(12), 1691–1715.

54.

PSYCHIATRIC ASPECTS OF PULMONARY DISEASE

Richard Kradin

INTRODUCTION

Like facial expressions, ventilation can serve as a window into the domain of psychological affects. The physiology of respiration is closely integrated with psychoneurobiological activities (Caruana-Montaldo, Gleeson, & Zwillich, 2000), yielding bidirectional changes. Both conscious and unconscious motivation systems can affect the ventilatory centers of the central nervous system (CNS); in turn, biochemical imbalances that result from abnormal respiration may alter cognitions, mood, and behaviors (Heaton, Grant, McSweeney, & al, 1983; Prigatano, Parson, Wright, & Hawrylak, 1983).

For this reason, conscious attention to the breath has served as a fundamental technique in the meditation practices of many ancient religious traditions (Mijares, 2009). In attending effortlessly to the breath, it is possible to reach profound levels of relaxation and a sense of well-being. Modern secular practices of relaxation, respiratory physical therapy, and behavioral treatments of anxiety, all continue to adopt awareness of breathing as a means of reducing physiological arousal.

PULMONARY PHYSIOLOGY

In order to better appreciate the links between pulmonary and neurophysiology, it is helpful to review some of the basic features of breathing. The respiratory system has evolved primarily in the service of the exchange of the gases that are critical for vital metabolism. Ventilation—the bellows function of the lungs that results in inspiration and expiration—is homeostatically tightly controlled to meet the oxygen requirements required for both basal metabolism and strenuous exercise. The normal resting breath or tidal volume (Vt) is approximately 500 ml of air with a resting respiratory rate (RR) of 12–15/min. This yields minute ventilation (VE) between 6–7.5 L/min.

1) $$(VE = RR \times Vt)$$

The primary controllers of ventilation include arterial pCO_2 and arterial pH, but an arterial pO_2 of less than 65 mm/Hg can also drive ventilation. Ventilatory failure is defined as a pCO_2 greater than 45mm/Hg. Elevation of the alveolar pCO_2, or alveolar hypoventilation, leads to respiratory acidosis, which, when inadequately compensated by the renal absorption of bicarbonate, can rapidly result in life-threatening peripheral blood acidemia.

2) $$[H^+] = 24 \times pCO2/[HCO3^-]$$

Breathing elevated concentrations of pCO_2 normally yields a rapid rise in minute ventilation. However, patients with central nervous system (CNS) abnormalities, hypothyroidism, severe hepatic failure, who are receiving respiratory depressants following carotid endarterectomy, and those who suffer from major vegetative depression, can all show blunted ventilatory responses to breathing elevated concentrations of carbon dioxide (CO_2) (Bone, 1993). On the other hand, patients with panic anxiety frequently exhibit attacks triggered by breathing elevated concentrations of pCO_2, a finding that prompted Donald Klein and co-workers to postulate that panic anxiety may result from an overly sensitive CNS "suffocation alarm" (Klein, 1999).

Sensors for the control of ventilation are located in the arterial chemoreceptors of the carotid body and in the pontomedullary areas of the brainstem (Caruana-Montaldo et al., 2000). The central respiratory controllers include pneumotaxic, apneustic, and medullary centers, whose roles are to initiate inspiration and to signal the beginning of exhalation. The pneumotaxic center is located both in the *nucleus parabrachialis* and in the *Kolliker-Fuse* nucleus of the pons, whereas the apneustic center is found in the lower pons. The medullary center includes the inspiratory dorsal respiratory group (DRG) of *nucleus tractate salivarius* and the expiratory ventral respiratory group (VRG). These groups project axons into the ventrolateral columns of the spinal cord, the phrenic nerves that innervate the diaphragm, and intercostal nerves that supply the muscles of the chest wall.

Changes in pCO_2 and the acid–base balance have marked effects on both cerebral blood flow and neuronal function. An acute elevation in pCO_2 due to ventilatory failure results in cerebral vasodilatation and brain edema, which can compromise levels of consciousness and mental acuity. Acute ventilatory failure always implies the inability of the ventilatory system to meet the demands of elevated levels of CO_2. This may be due to a cerebrovascular accident, the obesity-hypoventilation (Pickwickian) syndrome, or the absence of primary inspiratory drive (Ondine's curse). More commonly, acute respiratory failure reflects an increase in the work of breathing due to increased airways resistance, as in chronic obstructive pulmonary disease (COPD) or asthma, unmatched ventilatory energy requirements secondary to pulmonary interstitial and vascular disease, or a failure of the mechanical bellows function due to muscle weakness caused by diffuse myopathies, motor neuron disease, peripheral neuropathy, the Guillain-Barré syndrome, or myasthenia gravis.

Chronic respiratory failure is normally compensated for by a metabolic alkalosis, so that in the absence of blood-volume contraction, elevated serum HCO^{3-} concentrations are a reliable clue to the presence of underlying ventilatory failure. But despite maintenance of near-normal arterial blood pH, persistent chronic elevations of pCO_2 can produce cerebral vasodilatation and edema with headache and stuporous mental states (Burns & Howell, 1969).

Hypocapnea reflects increased ventilatory rates. It may be due to primary neuropsychiatric disorders or compensatory for a metabolic acidosis, as can be seen in an anion gap acidosis. In addition to lowering the threshold for musculoskeletal tetany, respiratory alkalosis also diminishes cognitive and memoric processes (Posner, 1972).

Hypoxemia is due to decreased levels of arterial pO_2 attributable to one or more of the following four basic mechanisms: (1) hypoventilation; (2) a mismatch of pulmonary ventilation and perfusion (V/Q abnormality); (3) intrapulmonary shunting, in which alveolar blood flow persists despite the absence of oxygenation (V/Q = 0), or when there is shunting of deoxygenated venous blood to the left side of the heart; or (4) alveolar-capillary block due to scarring or infiltration of the alveolar gas-exchange surface, which limits the diffusion of oxygen and carbon monoxide (DLCO) across the air–blood barrier, especially with decreased capillary transit times that are seen with exercise.

DYSPNEA

A cardinal symptom of respiratory disease is dyspnea, which can be defined as the *subjective* apperception of air hunger. For this reason, it is often not possible to accurately assess the appropriateness of an individual's shortness of breath in the absence of detailed physiological testing. Dyspnea occurs when the mechanical work of breathing increases beyond the limits of ventilation, and may be expected when the forced expiratory volume in the first second of exhalation (FEV_1) is reduced to less than 1 liter (Rock & Schwartzstein, 2007). The afferent sensory information that is interpreted centrally

as dyspnea appears to be mediated primarily by neural receptors in the lung and chest wall (Killian & Campbell, 1983).

The normal work of breathing accounts for about 5% of total O_2 consumption, but this can increase dramatically during exercise or in the presence of underlying cardiopulmonary disease. A measure of the work of breathing is the maximum voluntary ventilation (MVV); that is, the maximum amount of air that can be moved in and out of the lungs during a defined interval. This can be empirically approximated from the FEV_1 (Caruana-Montaldo et al., 2000).

$$3) \qquad MVV = FEV_1 \times 40$$

Ventilation is normally an energy-dependent process only during inspiration, which relies on the pressure-volume work done by the diaphragm and the inspiratory muscles of the chest wall. On the other hand, exhalation results from the passive elastic recoil of the lung. But when airway resistance is increased, as it is in asthma and COPD either due to the accumulation of viscid lumenal secretions, or by loss of the tethering function of the airways by pulmonary elastic tissue, then the work of breathing may extend to include the expiratory phase. This increased energy demand is sensed as dyspnea, especially during exercise. It is important to recognize that severe dyspnea can be reported in patients with normal arterial pO_2 levels due to an increase in the work of breathing or may be disproportionate to physiological abnormalities, as is often the case when there is a comorbid contribution by psychogenic dyspnea. In addition to increased work of breathing, marked hypoxemia, abnormal afferent stimulation from an inflamed esophagus due to reflux, mechanical compression of the lungs by increased abdominal pressure due to intra-abdominal tumor or fluid, gastric distention (*magenblase*) due aerophagia in anxious patients, and intense fear can also produce dyspnea. Although efforts have been made to correlate the language used by patients to describe dyspnea with known causes, in practice there is considerable overlap in how dyspnea is communicated (Mahler, Harver, Lentine, Scott, Beck, & Schwartzstein, 1996).

PHYSIOLOGICAL CATEGORIES OF RESPIRATORY DISEASE

Abnormalities in the compartmental anatomy of the lung determine the physiological changes seen in disease and also play a role in the types of psychological changes that accompany them. Diseases of the pulmonary airways result in diminished airflow due to increased resistance and are physiologically referred to as *obstructive lung disease*. These include asthma, defined as reversible airways narrowing; chronic bronchitis, defined by a clinical increase in airway secretions; and emphysema, which is defined as loss of the alveolar elastic tissue that normally tethers small conducting airways, leading to their narrowing; and bronchiectasis, which may reflect a variety of pathologies of the airways that lead to a loss of the normal cartilaginous support and to airway collapse during expiration. With the exception of asthma, all of the above disorders are often grouped generically as COPD.

Patients with COPD often exhibit one of two distinct phenotypes. Patients with Type A COPD have primarily emphysematous changes and are most often asthenic and exhibit purse-lipped breathing; consequently, they are referred to as "pink-puffers." Type B COPD patients often show truncal obesity, hypoventilation, and are both cyanotic and edematous due to right heart failure or *cor pulmonale*; and they are referred to as "blue bloaters."

Interstitial disease is due to a variety of conditions that primarily affect the alveolar wall. It produces diminished compliance of the lung with matched reductions in FEV_1 and the forced vital capacity (FVC), so that the ratio of FEV_1/FVC is maintained as near-normal. The chronic interstitial pneumonias produce alveolar scarring and lead to a loss of gas-exchange surface, as evidenced by reduced diffusion capacity (DLCO), although a decreased DLCO is also a hallmark of both emphysema and primary pulmonary vascular disease. Patients with these abnormalities tend to complain of dyspnea on exertion early in the course of their disease that is accompanied by rapid O_2 desaturation of the arterial blood with exercise. Physiologically, patients with chronic interstitial disease also have pulmonary restriction due to a decrease in their total lung capacity (TLC). However, restriction can also result from abnormalities of the pleura, chest wall, and thoracic musculature, although in these cases the DLCO when corrected for alveolar volume DLCO/VA is near normal.

THE NEUROBIOLOGY OF VENTILATION AND AFFECT

Neuronal networks that control the rate and depth of ventilation are integrated with the pontine reticular activating formation, so that CNS arousal increases ventilation. Ventilation varies within the normal sleep cycle, and decreased ventilation during sleep, either related to a central CNS deficit or obstruction of the upper airways, is the *sine qua non* of the sleep apnea syndromes.

The lung is richly innervated by cholinergic fibers from cranial nerve X (vagus), but sympathetic adrenergic nerves, although less plentiful, can also be identified in the pulmonary bronchovascular septa. A variety of neurotransmitters modulates the activity of the CNS respiratory control centers. Cholinergic neurons are the primary excitatory neurons for the effector motor pacemakers of breathing (Burton, Johnson, & Kazemi, 1989). Gamma-aminobutyric acid (GABA)-ergic neurons inhibit firing of the pacemaker center (Hedner, Hedner, Wessberg, & Jonason, 1984), and adrenergic neurotransmitters augment the output of cholinergic neurons. Finally, noradrenergic noncholinergic (NANC) neuropeptides, including the tachykinins, can modulate the activation of ventilatory neurons (Lindefors, Yamamoto, Pantaleo, Lagercrantz, Brodin, & Ungerstedt, 1986). In addition, endocrine hormones, including thyroxine and progesterone (Fadel, Northrop, Misenhimer, & Harp, 1979) can directly increase the firing of respiratory center neurons, and the latter contribute to the hyperventilation that is observed during pregnancy.

PSYCHIATRIC CONTRIBUTIONS TO DYSPNEA

The subjective assessment of the severity of dyspnea affects quality of life and functional status. The apperception of severity correlates with mood, catastrophic cognitions, phobic concerns with respect to dyspnea, and its intrapsychic meaning (Carr, Lehrer, Rausch, & Hochron, 1994; Preter & Klein, 2008). Emotions affect breathing; breathing affects emotion; as such, they are inextricably linked.

EXERCISE TESTING

Many hospital centers provide sophisticated methods of assessing pulmonary and cardiac physiology, both at rest and with exercise (Wassermann, Hansen, Sue, Casaburi, & Whipp, 1999). These can be measured concomitantly with real-time measurements of arterial blood gases, ventilation, and serum lactate during exercise. Pulmonary exercise testing offers an accurate assessment of the functional limitation during exercise and insight into its cause. Normally, with exercise an anaerobic threshold (AT) is achieved based on the cardiopulmonary limit of O_2 delivery to the tissues, which can be correlated with the minute ventilation and heart rate. As a consequence, one can usually determine whether there is a primary pulmonary or cardiac limit to exercise, based on the patient's simultaneous reporting of dyspnea and fatigue. Exercise testing is an invaluable tool for parsing the contributions by heart and lung to dyspnea, and yields insight into the presence of physical deconditioning and underlying psychiatric disorders, in which dyspnea is reported without achieving either an anaerobic threshold or maximum ventilatory effort. These tests vary in their level of invasiveness (Table 54.1); however, a basic non-invasive study, in the appropriate setting, will often suffice in excluding serious underlying pathology.

ASTHMA

Asthma is a syndrome characterized by reversible bronchoconstriction. It is the most common chronic respiratory disease, affecting about 6% of the U.S. population (American Lung Association [ALA], 2012). Asthma generally begins in childhood, with a second peak of incidence later in life. Most cases of asthma are attributable to atopic disease, and related to abnormalities of the T-helper (Th-2) immune system in response to common environmental allergens. However, some cases of asthma, so called "intrinsic" asthma, are unrelated to atopy. In addition, asthma attacks may be triggered by drugs, including aspirin; or by exercise, exposure to cold, isothiocyanates, or strong emotions.

PSYCHOLOGICAL FACTORS IN ASTHMA

French and Alexander considered asthma to be a psychosomatic disorder. They postulated a psychodynamic cause reflecting unconscious dependency on the mother and triggered by separation anxiety (French & Alexander, 1939–1941). It was suggested metaphorically that asthma was also the patient's unconscious wish to "have the last word" in the

Table 54.1 ROLE OF CARDIOPULMONARY EXERCISE TESTING (CPET) IN EVALUATION OF DYSPNEA

CARDIOPULMONARY EXERCISE TESTING (CPET)	
Level 1	Non-invasive basic cardiopulmonary screening test. Consider for dyspnea, fatigue of unknown origin, heart versus lung as cause of symptoms
Level 2	Level 1 with radial arterial line. Consider to confirm non-invasive arterial desaturation, suspected pulmonary vascular disease, hyperventilation syndromes
Level 3	Level 2 plus pulmonary arterial catherization. Consider to confirm pulmonary arterial hypertension, dynamic congestive heart failure including left ventricular diastolic dysfunction, valvular heart disease, and oxidative myopathies with abnormal systemic oxygen extraction.

First-pass nuclear ventriculography should be part of most CPET studies as it allows differentiation between cardiac dysfunction and detraining.

CPET studies may vary in their sophistication, depending on the center. The designations above reflect the practice at the Massachusetts General Hospital but are available at most academic medical centers.

struggle for autonomy. While current concepts in both psychiatry and pulmonary medicine do not include a primary psychogenic causative role for most cases of asthma, it is evident that stress and strong affect can trigger or exacerbate episodes of asthma disease. Emotional arousal, anxiety, fear, and anger can yield an increase in bronchomotor tone. Stress can also promote the Th2 immune system response (Cormier, Yuan, Crosby, Protheroe, Dimina, Hines, et al., 2002; Shen, Ochkur, McGarry, Crosby, Hines, Borchers, et al., 2003). Airway reactivity to emotion may be mediated by the vagus nerve (Isenberg, Lehrer, & Hochron, 1992), and there is evidence that emotion may preferentially affect large-caliber airways (Lehrer, Hochron, McCann, Swartzman, & Reba, 1986) innervated by cholinergic neurons.

Both acute and chronic stress have been demonstrated to affect the pathways that mediate asthma (Greenberg & Kradin, 1996). Stress has been correlated with increased levels of atopic cytokines and decreased expression of adrenergic and corticosteroid receptors (Hoshino, Suzuki, Yamauchi, & Inoue, 2008; Wolf, Nicholls, & Chen, 2008). Although emotions are currently not thought to be causative, comorbidity with both anxiety and depressive disorders is high. In one major study at tertiary care centers, comorbid depression was present in almost half of asthma patients (Van Lieshout, Bienenstock, & MacQueen, 2009). There is also an increased prevalence of general anxiety disorder, panic disorder, and phobic disorders in asthmatics (Rosenkranz & Davidson, 2009). Underlying psychopathology may have deleterious consequences on the prognosis in asthma, as it can limit patient compliance with medications, lead to smoking and other risk-taking behaviors, and result in increased utilization of emergency room visits and hospitalizations (Richardson, Russo, Lozano, McCauley, & Katon, 2008; Strine, Mokdad, Balluz, Berry, & Gonzalez, 2008).

The role of anxiety in asthma is both multifactorial and complex (ten Thoren & Petermann, 2000). Anxiety can trigger an acute attack of asthma or exacerbate an established one. In addition, increased anxiety can be fostered by sensations of decreased airflow, and phobic anxieties conditioned by repeated attacks of breathlessness (Goodwin, Jacobi, & Thefeld, 2003). Some patients with panic attacks are erroneously diagnosed with asthma when dyspnea is a prominent symptom of the attack. Unlike asthma, panic attacks will generally resolve within 30 minutes, and wheezing is generally not present. If doubt persists, once the acute symptoms have resolved, methacholine-challenge testing, which is based on the ability of a cholinergic stimulus to hyperconstrict irritable airways, should be performed (Schmaling, 1999).

Anxiety, depression, and psychosocial factors all contribute to the severity of asthma. Adverse circumstances in childhood appear to be an excellent predictor of the risk of developing adult asthma (Scott, Von Korff, Alonso, Angermeyer, Benjet, Bruffaerts, et al., 2008; Turyk, Hernandez, Wright, Freels, Slezak, Contraras, et al., 2008). Anxiety and depression both increase the severity of attacks, their frequency, and time spent in hospital, and diminish the quality of life (Marsac, Funk, & Nelson, 2007).

Acute traumatic events can exacerbate asthma. In a study of respiratory complaints following the September 11, 2001, terror attacks in New York City, there was a 27% increase in asthmatic symptoms in the ensuing two months (Fagan, Galea, Ahern, Bonner, & Vlahov, 2003). Physical and sexual abuse also were shown to increase the risk of developing asthma in a study of Puerto Rican children (Cohen, Canino, Bird, & Celedon, 2008). Negative and catastrophic cognitions can exacerbate asthma by leading to irritability, panic, and hyperventilation.

TREATMENT OF ASTHMA

The current pharmacological management of asthma is based on the administration of adrenergic and anticholinergic bronchodilators, drugs like salmeterol that tend to stabilize the airways, and inhaled corticosteroids. Most patients can be treated effectively with hand-held nebulizers. Patients with more severe disease may benefit from leukotriene inhibitors. Aminophylline, once a mainstay in the management of asthma, has largely fallen out of favor due to its toxicities and the need to monitor blood levels.

The vast majority of asthmatics can be managed without hospitalization; however, others will require frequent visits to the emergency room and in-hospital stays. In patients with severe atopic asthma, efforts should be made to identify an offending environmental antigen and to exclude allergic bronchopulmonary aspergillosis due to aspergillus mold colonizing the proximal airways. These patients may benefit from additional antifungal treatment.

The mainstay in the treatment of severe asthma is the judicious use of oral or intravenous corticosteroids. However, corticosteroids have panoply of metabolic side effects and can aggravate underlying mood disorders. The common side effects of anti-asthmatic drugs include jitteriness, palpitations, and insomnia, but more serious side effects can at times be observed (Greenberg & Kradin, 1996). Table 54.2 summarizes the adverse effects of pulmonary medications in patients with psychiatric disorders.

Psychoeducation, relaxation, biofeedback, perception, cognitive-behavioral therapy (CBT), yoga, and family therapy may have a role in the care of asthma patients (Lehrer, Sargunaraj, & Hochron, 1992). Weiss (Weiss, 1994) described a detailed behavioral management program for asthma that included a checklist to assess asthma medications, early signs of wheezing, triggers of an attack, individual behavior and behavior of other people during an attack, and the effects of asthma on social development, school, and the family. Asking patients to maintain a daily diary of their symptoms may provide an additional resource for diagnosis and management.

Identifying core psychological issues that might prevent the patient from attending to early warning signals or from taking medication appropriately is an important strategy. These include fear of inadequacy, fear of social rejection, or a drive to excel athletically, all of which can be motives for hiding vulnerability with respect to the severity of asthma, especially in teenagers. Weiss's treatment approach included knowing the facts and fallacies about asthma, identifying emotional and physical factors that precipitate or aggravate attacks, recognizing the early warning signs of an attack and knowing what to do about them, and learning to relax via focusing on abdominal breathing.

Asthma exhibits a spectrum of severity. Whereas most patients can be well controlled with inhaled corticosteroids and the periodic use β-adrenergic inhalers, others suffer from repeated episodes that are difficult to control. Attack severity has been linked to major depression, panic attacks, number of emergency room visits, and self-assessment of risk of death. Boner and colleagues (Boner, Vallone, Chiesa, Spezia, Fambri, & Sette, 1992) found that patients make judgements about their condition, assessments that correlate with objective markers of increased mortality risk and increased severity. Those who become phobic with respect to the dysphoria of dyspnea may overuse bronchodilator inhalers. Alexithymia, the inability to "read interoceptive cues," may be a prominent cause of excessive inhaled adrenergic use, as in the at-times-fatal error of underrating the severity of status asthmaticus. A role for antidepressants, including selective serotonin-reuptake inhibitors (SSRIs) and buproprion in the absence of underlying comorbid depression or panic disorder has not been demonstrated (Melien, 2005; Brown, Vornik, Khan, & Rush, 2007).

FACTITIOUS ASTHMA

Occasionally, asthma may be a factitious illness. The distinguishing clinical and physiological features were documented in three cases reported by Downing et al. (Downing, Braman, Fox, & Corrao, 1982). These patients, all of whom had a history of underlying psychiatric illness, exhibited frequent emergency room visits for asthma, no clinical response to bronchodilators, no evidence of hypoxemia or hyperinflation on chest radiographs, and no airway dysfunction on pulmonary function testing shortly after the attack. Methacholine-challenge testing, a sensitive method for excluding asthma, should be utilized when the diagnosis is in doubt (Schmaling, 1999).

Self-induced wheezing in factitious cases is loudest over the neck, with transmission to the chest wall on auscultation. Bronchial wheezes can be mimicked by maneuvers that include holding the vocal cords in apposition. However, one must first exclude vocal cord dysfunction and other causes of intrathoracic and extrathoracic upper airway obstruction (Bahrainwala & Simon, 2001). Intentional malingering is rare. However, "asthma" as a feature of panic disorder is well recognized and should be excluded by careful history-taking and auscultation of the chest.

CHRONIC OBSTRUCTIVE PULMONARY DISEASE (COPD)

COPD is the fourth major cause of death in the United States and affects 16 million people, the vast majority having clinical evidence of chronic bronchitis (Lindberg, Jonsson, Ronmark, Lundgren, Larsson, & Lundback, 2005). The definitions of these disorders are based on clinical, anatomical, and physiological criteria. Chronic bronchitis is diagnosed clinically as the presence of increased sputum production for at least three

Table 54.2 NEUROPSYCHIATRIC SIDE EFFECTS OF DRUGS USED IN THE TREATMENT OF PULMONARY DISORDERS

Anticholinergics	Delirium, amnesia, paranoia, hallucinations
Leukotriene antagonists	Anxiety, vasculitis
Beta-agonists	Anxiety, tremulousness
Corticosteroid inhalers	None
Oral corticosteroids	Irritability, depression, mania, paranoia
Theophylline	Anxiety, tremor, irritability, delirium, insomnia

months of at least two consecutive years, whereas emphysema is diagnosed by evidence of alveolar loss, as reflected by radiographic imaging and decreased DLCO. These diseases develop in a dose-dependent manner with cigarette consumption, and more than 80% of cases of COPD are attributable to cigarette smoking (Tashkin, Kanner, Bailey, Buist, Anderson, Nides, et al., 2001). A subset of patients with emphysema may have an associated deficiency in α-1 antiprotease, which can yield severe panacinar emphysema even with light cigarette consumption.

The disease develops progressively, beginning with inflammation in the small airways less than 2 mm in diameter. In patients with COPD, even mild chronic hypoxia can compromise cognitive capacities, lead to mood lability, and lead to restrictions in daily activities (Lishman, 1987). Patients with COPD have impaired abstracting ability and complex perceptual motor integration. These are impaired more than motor speed, strength, or gross coordination. COPD is associated with a significant decline in cognitive function over time, and cerebral hypoperfusion has been documented in patients with COPD who are also hypoxemic. Morbidity in COPD is complex; and contrary to expectations, patients with mild reductions of FEV1 may show levels of diminished health-related quality of life that are comparable to those in patients with severe deficits.

DEPRESSION IN COPD

Major depression is common in heavy smokers. In one study, almost 50% of smokers met criteria for depression, whereas only 20% were being treated with antidepressants, and a national multidisciplinary workshop concluded that depression remains underdiagnosed and undertreated, particularly in men with COPD. Borson and McDonald (Borson, Claypoole, & McDonald, 1998) suggested that clues to the diagnosis of major depressive disorder in patients with COPD include the perception of activity as effortful, pervasive pessimism, diurnal mood variation with morning worsening, and early-morning awakening. In an autopsy-documented community study of suicide in men older than 65, Horton-Deutsch and colleagues found that 14 of 73 patients had a chief complaint of dyspnea and undiagnosed major depressive disorder (Horton-Deutsch, Clark, & Farran, 1992).

ANXIETY IN COPD

Anxiety is likewise common in COPD. It has been suggested that as many as 44% of patients with severe COPD have comorbid panic disorder, and panic symptoms may be linked to depression (Light, Merrill, Despars, Gordon, & Mutalipassi, 1985). Although the presence of underlying lung disease tends to disqualify this group from a diagnosis of primary panic disorder, it is likely that the experience of panic is similar, particularly with respect to the catastrophic interpretation of interoceptive cues. Whereas both anxiety and depression can produce reports of dyspnea, only depression has been linked to reduced exercise tolerance (Funk, Kirchheiner, Burghuber, & Hartl, 2009).

TREATMENT OF COPD

The treatment of COPD relies primarily on smoking cessation and on the treatment of exacerbations with steroids and antibiotics. Psychoeducation, psychotherapy, physical therapy, and nutritional therapy can be useful in the setting of COPD and may best be delivered in the setting of an established pulmonary rehabilitation program (Coventry & Hind, 2007; Lacasse, Brosseau, Milne, Martin, Wong, Guyatt, et al., 2002). When present, the treatment of concomitant anxiety and mood disorders is indicated.

Supplemental O_2 is required when O_2 saturations fall to less than 88% either at rest or with ambulation. Continuous O_2 supplementation should be prescribed during sleep as O_2 saturations normally decrease during sleep, which can aggravate pulmonary vasoconstriction, cerebral blood flow, and cardiac output. Continuous oxygen treatment improves quality of life, neuropsychiatric function, and longevity better than nocturnal-only treatment (Group, 1980; Prigatano et al., 1983; Group, 1980). Neuropsychiatric changes were documented in a six-center trial of more than 200 patients, in which continuous versus nocturnal supplemental oxygen administration was compared in subjects with a pO_2 of less than 55 mmHg or incipient right heart failure, although no change in mood was documented (Grant, Chittleborough, Taylor, Dal Grande, Wilson, Phillips, et al., 2006).

However, the benefits of supplemental oxygen come with a psychological cost. The use of supplemental oxygen use may be experienced as social embarrassment. Some patients feel that the need for home oxygen marks the beginning of terminal illness, and become depressed and socially withdrawn. Others may become psychologically dependent on the oxygen supply even when it is not physiologically required. Some patients may phobically limit emotional expression in order not to tax their breathing. Sexual dysfunction, inhibited sexual excitement, premature ejaculation, and avoidance of intimacy, have all been noted in patients with chronic lung disease (Thompson, 1982). The consequent deconditioning, and associated anxiety and depression, only serve to compound the already severe shortness of breath reported by patients with COPD. The introduction of portable lightweight O_2 delivery systems that are less conspicuous and may lead to less social anxiety and stigma than in the past has been a great boon for patients who require supplemental oxygen (Stoller, Panos, Krachman, Doherty, & Make, 2010).

The treatment of anxiety and mood disorders in patients with COPD has certain challenges. Benzodiazepines can suppress the respiratory pacemaker, but they can be used effectively in COPD when pCO_2 retention is either absent or mild, and when they are prescribed judiciously. As a rule, they should be avoided during acute exacerbations. Compared to the benzodiazepines, buspirone is a relatively weak anxiolytic. Its use should be limited to cases where benzodiazepines are contraindicated.

SSRIs are useful in the management of both depression and panic disorder. In a pilot study, seven patients with mild to severe COPD that was largely intractable to standard medical therapies reported substantially diminished dyspnea after receiving sertraline (25–100 mg/day), with no apparent change in pulmonary function (Smoller, Pollack, Otto, Rosenbaum, & Kradin, 1996; Smoller, Pollack, Systrom, & Kradin, 1998). To diminish fear and agitation without risking respiratory suppression, neuroleptic medications can also be beneficial, in low doses.

Protriptyline, a stimulating tricyclic antidepressant, improves diurnal and nocturnal hypoxemia at a dose of 20 mg in a small percentage of patients with COPD. This effect appears to be unrelated to pulmonary mechanics but may correlate with decreased rapid eye movement (REM) sleep (Series, Cormier, & La Forge, 1990). Protriptyline has also been shown to be beneficial in treating patients with sleep apnea; however, its effect on mood has not been clarified. Borson and McDonald (Borson et al., 1998) reported preliminary data from a trial of nortriptyline in patients with COPD and major depressive disorder. There was a notable risk of hypotension, especially when other antihypertensive medications were used concomitantly.

Some patients with COPD benefit clinically from corticosteroids, and the acute treatment of COPD exacerbations includes high-dose steroids together with antibiotics. However, corticosteroids can exacerbate depression, emotional lability, and irritability, especially in patients with a bipolar diathesis. The psychiatric side effects of steroids are dose-related, and agitation and mania can be misattributed to the effects of hypoxemia unrecognized in this acute setting. Steroid side effects may respond acutely to low-dose neuroleptics.

SMOKING AND SMOKING CESSATION

For historical and practical reasons, cigarette smoking was largely unaddressed by members of the psychiatric community, despite considerable evidence that nicotine was addictive. It has been argued that Freud's compulsive cigar-smoking disposed psychotherapists to excuse the smoking habit in their patients. In addition, the extraordinarily high prevalence of cigarette smoking in hospitalized patients with chronic psychosis and substance-related disorders has been tacitly accepted (Goff, Henderson, & Amico, 1992). Although cigarette smoke contains hundreds of bioactive substances, nicotine appears to be the major component that has both central and peripheral neuroactivities. Nicotine, which increases heart rate and blood pressure, acts as an acute stimulus for breathing. Nicotine also increases dopamine release in the prefrontal cortex and nucleus accumbens (Mifsud, Hernandez, & Hoebel, 1989). Other addictive agents such as opiates, amphetamines, and cocaine also release dopamine (Kradin, 2008).

Several large studies (Anda, Williamson, Escobedo, Mast, Giovino, & Remington, 1990; Glassman, Helzer, Covey, Cottler, Stetner, Tipp, et al., 1990) have found that cigarette smoking is associated with a history of major depression and with other negative states. In a review of this subject, Glassman (Glassman, 1993) made a convincing argument that depressive illness is highly correlated with having ever smoked, with addictive smoking, and with substantial difficulty with smoking cessation. Based on these highly significant correlations, it has been suggested that smokers may share a genetic vulnerability toward both behaviors, because little evidence suggests that smoking alone can predispose to depression. Alcoholism (Covey, Glassman, Stetner, & Becker, 1993), generalized anxiety disorder, and panic disorder all show an increased association with cigarette smoking (Glassman, 1993). Most anxious smokers report that cigarette smoking allays anxiety, despite experimental models that do not support this observation (Frederick, Frerichs, & Clark, 1988).

The association between smoking and depression remains even when the variables of anxiety and alcoholism are controlled. Glassman (Glassman, 1993) pointed out that 75% of heavy cigarette smokers who attempt to quit will experience depressive symptoms. In some patients with severe psychiatric disease in remission, attempts at smoking cessation have led to severe exacerbations of symptoms that remitted with a return to smoking. Nevertheless, reasonable efforts should be made towards smoking abstinence whenever possible, due to the malignant complications of chronic tobacco use.

The effects of nicotine on dopaminergic pathways modulate dysphoric symptoms. Nicotine-induced firing of dopaminergic neurons that project to prefrontal areas may also antagonize the negative symptoms in patients with schizophrenia and could help explain the inordinately high prevalence of cigarette smoking in this population (Goff et al., 1992).

Fiore et al. found that 95% of former smokers who had been abstinent for 1–10 years had made an unassisted last quit attempt (Fiore & Baker, 2011). The most frequent unassisted methods were "going cold turkey" and smoking a "gradually decreased number" of cigarettes. However, only about 4% to 7% of people are able to quit smoking on any given attempt without medicines or other help.

A 2008 meta-analysis estimated that physician advice to quit smoking led to a quit rate of 10.2%, as opposed to a quit rate of 7.9% among patients who did not receive physician advice to quit smoking (Polito, 2008). But one study from Ireland involving vignettes found that physicians' probability of giving smoking cessation advice declines with the patient's age (Cahill & Perera, 2008), and another, from the United States, found that only 81% of smokers over age 50 had received advice on quitting from their physician in the preceding year (Ossip-Klein, McIntosh, Utman, Burton, Spada, & Guido, 2000).

The American Cancer Society estimates that "between about 25% and 33% of smokers who use medicines can stay smoke-free for over six months. Single medications include nicotine replacement therapy (NRT), as transdermal nicotine patches, sprays, and inhalers, but studies suggest that the vast majority of over-the-counter NRT users relapse within six months" (Ossip-Klein & McIntosh, 2003).

Bupropion is FDA-approved and marketed under the brand name Zyban. Bupropion is contraindicated in epilepsy, seizure disorder, anorexia/bulimia, recent monoamine oxidase (MAO) inhibitor use, and in patients undergoing abrupt discontinuation of ethanol or sedatives.

Varenicline tartrate (Chantix) decreases the urge to smoke and reduces withdrawal symptoms (Crain & Bhat, 2010). Varenicline appears to be more effective than either NRT or bupropion (Fiore & Baker, 2011). A 2 mg/day regimen of varenicline leads to the highest abstinence rate (33%) of any single therapy, while a 1 mg/day dosage yielded abstinence in 25%. However, a 2011 review suggests that varenicline also produces adverse cardiac and neuropsychiatric effects, including arrhythmias, suicidal ideation, and suicidal behavior.

VENTILATION IN CLINICAL DEPRESSION

Severe vegetative depression may contribute to respiratory acidosis and cor pulmonale, due to diminished ventilatory drive in response to the inhalation of pCO_2. Depressed and grieving patients manifest lower respiratory rates, lower resting-end tidal volumes, and elevated levels of pCO_2 (Damas-Mora, Souster, & Jenner, 1982). Patients who experience depression or grief do not increase their minute ventilation appropriately when they breathe a mixture of gas with either high pCO_2 or low O_2, indicating primary depression of the ventilatory neuronal centers (Jellinek, Goldenheim, & Jenike, 1985). Patients with depression who experience sleep disturbance are more vulnerable to CO_2 retention, so patients who have both depression and lung disease are at increased risk for complications of respiratory depression.

VENTILATION IN CLINICAL ANXIETY

Ventilatory patterns in anxiety disorders are characterized by dystaxic breathing. This may include a decreased Vt with rapid rates. Irregular breathing is common, including breath-holding, frequent sighs, and a tendency to breathe at higher lung capacities due to the inability to relax to the normal functional residual capacity (FRC) at end tidal volume. One can get an immediate sense of the psychological effects of dystaxic breathing on affect by grasping their chest and modeling one's own breath on the patients.

Hyperventilation is common in anxiety disorders, affecting as many as 15% in the general population, and it may be part of generalized anxiety or panic disorder (Lachman, Gielis, Thys, Lorimier, & Sergysels, 1992). Rapid respiratory rates can lead to a syndrome of hyperventilation characterized by respiratory alkalosis, dizziness, and syncope. Carpopedal spasms may result from abnormalities of calcium mobilization at high intramuscular pH.

The appearance of anxiety, and in particular panic attacks, can mimic major medical illnesses, such as pulmonary thromboembolic disease, myocardial infarction, diabetic ketoacidosis, carbon monoxide poisoning, vasovagal syncope, and drug overdose.

Hyperventilation can be seen as a secondary phenomenon in all of the above, as well as in CNS injury. A panic attack in the postoperative setting, or in a patient with phlebitis, should lead reflexively to a computerized tomography (CT)-angiogram, in order to exclude thromboembolic disease.

CYSTIC FIBROSIS

Once exclusively a disease of childhood, cystic fibrosis (CF) now includes a sizable number of survivors into adulthood, thanks to improved management of its metabolic and infectious complications. Most cases are due to a mutation of the *CFTR* gene ($\Delta 405$) that regulates chloride channels, but a variety of genetic variants have been reported. CF affects almost 20,000 children in the United States, with a frequency of 1 in 2,500 births. It is the most common autosomal recessive gene amongst Caucasians.

The disease is caused by the production of viscid mucous (mucoviscidosis) that leads to sinus obstruction, chronic cystic bronchiectasis, chronic pancreatitis with endocrine abnormalities, especially insulin-dependent diabetes, and infertility.

Treatment is complicated medically, and its difficulty is compounded by the young age of its victims. Prominent psychiatric issues may emerge related to anxiety, depression, borderline-spectrum behaviors, dependency, and drug addiction (Anderson, Flume, & Hardy, 2001). The incidence of drug addiction in this population has not been adequately addressed and requires more intensive study by addiction specialists.

One study showed that the levels of anxiety and depression did not parallel disease severity as evidenced by pulmonary function, but were more influenced by patient expectation and their perceived level of support (Wargnies, Houze, Vanneste, Perez, & Wallaert, 2002). Adult survivors tend to show less anxiety and depression and are more resilient. It is unclear whether this is due to selection bias or to the psychological effects of the disorder.

Relaxation techniques, biofeedback, and psychoeducation aimed at independent living can be helpful, and it is generally wise to have stable psychiatric input with these patients, especially during their teenage years. Unfortunately, despite improvements in care and the use of lung transplantation as definitive therapy, many patients with the disorder will die at a young age. Dealing with end-of-life issues is an important part of the care of this patient group and should take into account the patient's own wishes with respect to outcome, when it is judged that they are indeed mature enough to make such informed decisions (Chapman, Landy, Lyon, Haworth, & Bilton, 2005).

IDIOPATHIC PULMONARY FIBROSIS

A large number of disorders can produce interstitial disease with restrictive physiology and decreased alveolar gas exchange. Idiopathic pulmonary fibrosis (IPF) is the clinical moniker for a pathological syndrome termed *usual interstitial pneumonitis* (UIP), in which end-stage lung with progressive hypoxemia ensues with high five-year mortality. The incidence is approximated at 3–5 per hundred thousand; however, diagnostic mimics can confound its true prevalence. Unlike the obstructive lung disorders, relatively little emphasis has been directed at the psychiatric comorbidity in IPF (Martinez, Pereira, dos Santos, Ciconelli, Guimaraes, & Martinez, 2000).

Dyspnea is the dominant finding, but anxiety and depression may contribute to a diminished quality of life. Other biosocial factors, including diminished sleep, the inability to work, and diminished sexual activity, all contribute to the impaired quality of life in this disease (Mermigkis, Stagaki, Amfilochiou, Polychronopoulos, Korkonikitas, Mermigkis, et al., 2009).

There is no effective treatment for IPF, although a small percentage of patients do respond favorably to corticosteroids and other immunosuppressant agents. There is an increasing suspicion by pulmonologists that acid aspiration may contribute to the exacerbations of this disorder, at least in some patients. Lung orthotopic transplantation is the known effective treatment, but this intervention is generally not available to the older population in which the disease predominates.

SLEEP APNEA

Sleep apnea has become an increasingly recognized disorder that affects both adults and children. It manifests clinically as loud snoring, weight gain or loss, excessive daytime sleepiness, hypertension, altered cognitions, and difficulties in concentrating. Depression is common in sleep apnea. Ohayon and colleagues, in a study of more than 18,000 European subjects, showed that subjects with depression were five times more likely to have a breathing-related sleep disorder than non-depressed ones, a five-fold increase (Ohayon, 2003).

Sleep apnea may be divided into obstructive, central, and mixed types. During normal sleep, oxygenation falls and pCO_2 rises. In stage 4 sleep, breathing is regular (Cherniack, Mitra, Prabhakar, & Adams, 1988). During REM and stages 1 and 2 non-REM sleep, irregular breathing and apnea, either obstructive, central, or both, may occur.

The diagnosis of obstructive sleep apnea (OSA) is based on clinical symptoms and the results of a formal sleep study or polysomnogram. Testing identifies apnea events per hour of sleep (Apnea Hypopnea Index [AHI]), and events that exceed a formal threshold identify the patient as suffering from sleep apnea. Oximetry, which may be performed overnight in a patient's home, is an alternative to a formal sleep study.

Treatment often is initiated as behavioral therapy. For mild cases, it may include weight loss when obesity is judged to be a factor; or sleeping on one's side, which prevents the tongue and palate from falling backwards and blocking the airway. Patients should be counseled to avoid alcohol and sleeping pills, both of which relax the throat muscles, contributing to the collapse of the upper airway while sleeping.

Continuous positive airway pressure (CPAP) or automatic positive airway pressure (APAP) devices are the standard treatment modality, as they pressurize the patient's airway open during sleep (Kohler, Stoewhas, Ayers, Senn, Bloch, Russi, et al., 2011). CPAP is generally administered via a plastic facial mask, connected by a flexible tube to a small bedside CPAP machine. Advanced models warm and humidify the air to prevent excessive drying of mucosal membranes. Although CPAP therapy is extremely effective in reducing apneas and less expensive than other treatments, many patients find it extremely uncomfortable and either refuse the treatment

or fail to use their CPAP machines on a nightly basis. In a recent study, 57% of patients with OSA met concomitant criteria for major depression that was alleviated with CPAP. The authors concluded that CPAP should be considered as the first modality of treatment for depression in patients with OSA (El-Sherbini, Bediwy, & Et-Mitalli, 2011).

Oral appliance therapy (OAT) includes a custom-made mouthpiece that shifts the lower jaw forward, opening up the airway. It is usually successful in patients with mild to moderate obstructive sleep apnea. OAT is a relatively new treatment option for sleep apnea in the United States, but it is commonly used in Canada and Europe (Lettieri, Paolino, Eliasson, Shah, & Holley, 2011).

The Pillar procedure is a minimally invasive treatment for snoring and obstructive sleep apnea (Randerath, Verbraecken, Andreas, Bettega, Boudewyns, Hamans, et al., 2011). Dacron strips are inserted into the soft palate with a modified syringe and local anesthetic. After this brief outpatient procedure, the soft palate is rendered more rigid, and snoring and sleep apnea are reduced. Other, more-invasive procedures such as uvuloplasty have been administered with mixed success.

ACUTE LUNG INJURY

Acute lung injury (ALI) or the acute respiratory distress syndrome is a devastating disorder that leads to respiratory failure and the need for prolonged mechanical ventilation. Mortality has been markedly reduced due to mechanical ventilation and optimization of ventilator settings. However, with increased survival it has become apparent that there are neuropsychiatric complications attributable to the disease and the treatment setting. Cognitive disturbances are common and in one study led to occupational disability in 41% of affected survivors (Rothenhausler, Ehrentraut, Stoll, Schelling, & Kapfhammer, 2001). Clinical post-traumatic stress disorder (PTSD) occurs in 44% of survivors at the time of hospital discharge and persists in nearly one-quarter at 5–8 years (Davydow, Desai, Needham, & Bienvenu, 2008).

LUNG TRANSPLANTATION

Lung transplantation has become a widely available procedure, limited primarily by acceptable donor graft availability. The most common indication is severe COPD, but orthotopic lung transplantation has been performed in patients with cystic fibrosis, pulmonary hypertension, IPF, and other less common pulmonary disorders. The current one- and five-year survival rates following orthotopic lung transplantation are ~84% and 52%, respectively.

The pre-transplantation testing and post-transplant monitoring and immunosuppression regimens are rigorous and include the exclusion of patients who are judged to be less than optimal candidates for success. This may include patients with serious psychiatric disorders, those who are addicted to smoking or ethanol, non-compliance with treatment regimens, and poor psychosocial support systems.

During the candidate-screening process, mild to moderate depression was identified in over 50% of patients in one study

(Najafizadeh, Ghorbani, Rostami, Fard-Mausavi, Lorgard-Dezfuli-Nejad, Marashian, et al., 2009). Prolonged waiting times for an allograft are associated with increased stress, anxiety, and depression (Vermeulen, Bosma, Bij, Koeter, & Tenvergert, 2005). Complications from chronic hypoxemia are common, including diminished cognitive function and memory loss.

Despite the need for rigorous monitoring, following transplantation most patients report an improved quality of life, associated with diminished anxiety and depression; however, this tends to diminish with the development of chronic rejection after several years (Vermeulen, Ouwens, van der Bij, de Boer, Koeter, & TenVergert, 2003). The incidence of PTSD is also increased post-transplantation (Kollner, Einsle, Schade, Maulhardt, Gulielmos, & Joraschky, 2003). Candidates with psychosocial risks may benefit from cognitive behavioral interactions, and increased patient contact with members of the transplant staff (Blumenthal, Babyak, Keefe, Davis, Lacaille, Carney, et al., 2006). One study showed that having a pet increased the quality of life for patients post-transplantation (Irani, Mahler, Goetzmann, Russi, & Boehler, 2006).

SOMATIZATION AND LUNG DISEASE

An undetermined percentage of patients present to outpatient pulmonary clinics with pulmonary symptoms that have no demonstrable etiology. These most commonly include dyspnea, chronic cough, and chest pain. In a preliminary study at Massachusetts General Hospital (MGH), 100 patients who presented with pulmonary-related symptoms were assessed for depression, anxiety, and stress with a validated subjective scale, the Depression Anxiety Stress Scale (DASS) (Lovibond & Lovibond, 1995). The results of subjective reports were correlated with the impression of a psychiatrically trained pulmonary practitioner. Preliminary findings suggest that a substantial number of patients with objective evidence of pulmonary disease are either syndromally or subsyndromally anxious, depressed, or have been subject to nontrivial stressors. However, there is poor correlation with the subjective and objective assessments in more than half of cases. The following case reports illustrate the point.

CASE REPORT 1

A 55-year-old woman presented to the MGH Pulmonary Clinic with persistent shortness of breath and a diagnosis of asthma. She had previously been seen in various area emergency departments, and treated for asthma, but without sustained relief.

History revealed evidence of major developmental trauma and familial alcoholism. The patient was tense, guarded, and reticent about answering questions concerning possible ongoing stressors. She reported the sensation of a "lump in my throat," gastroesophageal reflux (GERD), irritable bowel syndrome, and fibromyalgia. Her physical examination was normal except for a resting tachycardia, and her resting pulmonary function tests showed no evidence of airway obstruction. However, she did have a positive methacholine-challenge test, implying an element of irritation in the airways. (The methacholine-challenge test assesses airway responsiveness. The patient has pulmonary function tests evaluated before and after inhaling an aerosol of different concentrations of methacholine in order to diagnose asthma or evaluate its severity.)

A cardiopulmonary exercise tolerance test (CPET) demonstrated no pulmonary limit to exercise, despite her report of being unable to walk more than several steps without becoming dyspneic. She scored low across all subscales of the DASS. When I suggested that emotional factors might be playing a role in her asthma, she became angered and chose to pursue her care at another hospital center, where she has been treated with combination immunosuppressive therapies, from which she suffered a serious opportunistic infection. There has been essentially no improvement in her pulmonary symptoms.

CASE REPORT 2

A 27-year-old woman presented with a recent exacerbation of her asthma. She had been treated as an outpatient for asthma, although no one had documented wheezing on physical examination. She reported low distress across the DASS subscales, although she appeared both depressed and anxious on interview and reported having difficulty finding employment post-graduation. Her physical examination and detailed pulmonary function tests were normal. She was referred for both a methacholine-challenge test and pulmonary exercise testing. The methacholine challenge test was positive, indicating an element of irritable airways; however, her CPET showed no pulmonary mechanical limit to exercise, but it did demonstrate abnormal hyperventilation. She presented to her follow-up visit with her mother. When I informed her of her results and again wondered whether anxiety and stress might be contributing to her symptoms, she began to cry and admitted that she had been suffering from numerous panic attacks and was very stressed about leaving home. She was treated with a bronchodilator as well as an SSRI and anxiolytic, with excellent response.

The above cases suggest that reliance on self-reporting can fail to identify patients whose symptoms are exacerbated by psychiatric factors. This may be due to alexithymia or reticence to admit psychological symptoms in a medical setting. Unfortunately, failure to address these symptoms may lead to iatrogenic complications when treatment is directed at organic factors exclusively.

The key to the proper identification of this population is better recognition by medical internists and pulmonologists of the role that psychological factors may play in the exacerbation of pulmonary disease, as well as education in how to identify these patients. In many cases, symptoms may have persisted for weeks to years without evidence of deleterious progression, which may be a clue to the psychological basis of symptoms. Poly-symptomatology is the rule in somatization, and a detailed review of systems will generally reveal other functional symptoms. In all cases, a brief developmental history should be elicited and efforts made to assess the patient's current and developmental level of stress. Physical exam often reveals depressed or flat affect, anxious responses, resting tachycardia, altered pupillary tone, dystaxic breathing, frequent sighing, tense musculature, and evidence of bruxism, all of which may point towards a diagnosis of somatization.

Subsequent diagnostic testing must be tailored to the patient's symptoms. For patients with complaints of dyspnea, an aerobic exercise history can help in ascertaining their level of fitness, and observations with respect to weight and body habitus are helpful. As noted, dynamic cardiopulmonary exercise testing (CPET) can determine the limits of exercise and correlated in real-time with symptoms of dyspnea or chest pain. For patients who show no apparent abnormality in pulmonary-function testing, a simple noninvasive exercise study may point to a cardiac or respiratory limit to exercise versus fatigue. Hyperventilation syndromes can be detected with the presence of an arterial line with frequent samplings of pCO_2 during the exam. More complex issues, including diastolic cardiac dysfunction, abnormal blood-shunting myopathy, and mitochondrial disorders, require sampling of central venous as well as arterial blood.

Cough is a complex problem with both anatomical and functional etiologies. Many cases are attributable to chronic post-nasal drip and allergies, but detailed imaging of the sinuses and upper airways should be performed in all cases, together with an otolaryngological examination. CT scans of the neck and chest may occasionally reveal a benign or low-grade neoplasm such as carcinoid as the cause of chronic cough. Asthma and gastroesophageal reflux (GERD) are common causes and should be excluded. Bronchoscopic examination is rarely indicated in the absence of other troublesome or constitutional symptoms. A recent study has demonstrated some efficacy for gabapentin in the treatment of chronic cough. When all reasonable diagnostic options have been excluded, a diagnosis of psychogenic cough can comfortably be established. Treatment is rarely effective.

Treatment of the somatization syndromes has recently been reviewed elsewhere, and there is limited evidence that drugs and targeted psychotherapies may be helpful (Kradin, 2012). But ultimately, treatment must depend on patient preference and their willingness to actively participate in their therapy. Whereas some patients clearly benefit from antidepressant and/or anxiolytic medications, most refuse both psychopharmacological interventions and psychotherapies. However, they may be willing to participate in behavioral modifications such as meditation, yoga, tai chi, and Pilates. Eliciting the patient's cooperation is most critical, but this is directly proportional to their level of insight.

DOCTOR AS PLACEBO

I have elsewhere discussed the substantial overlap between the placebo response and the therapeutic action of psychotherapy (Kradin, 2008). It is evidence that the factors that promote well-being via placebo mechanisms parallel those adopted in optimal interpersonal communications in the therapeutic setting. Active listening, empathy, mirroring attention, and time spent attending to the patient, all foster therapeutic alliances in both somatic and psychological therapies. At the same time, it is important to recognize that nocebo effects and help-rejecting behaviors are commonly seen in patients with somatization, complicating the therapeutic stance.

Somatizing patients represent a substantial challenge to the self-esteem of the medical practitioners, who often find themselves at a loss both with respect to diagnose symptoms or how to effectively alleviate them. Nevertheless, it is critically important to maintain a patient and empathic stance with these patients, who often view the medical practitioner as their only resource and may adamantly refuse any form of psychological counseling.

DRUG INTERACTIONS BETWEEN PSYCHOACTIVE AND PULMONARY DRUGS

Many of the commonly prescribed pulmonary drugs interact adversely with psychiatric medications, and these are listed in Table 54.3. As previously noted, corticosteroids may exacerbate both depression and mania. Psychotic effects of corticosteroids are dose-related, and they are rarely seen in patients receiving less than 40 mg a day of prednisone. However, physicians and family members must carefully monitor untoward psychiatric side effects, as corticosteroid therapy at times may be completely contraindicated in some patients. When immunosuppressant therapy is necessary, other medications, such as methotrexate, cyclophosphamide, or cyclosporine, may be alternative options.

Neuroleptic medications, when prescribed at high dosages, can produce laryngospasm, paradoxical movement of the chest wall musculature, and diaphragmatic tardive dyskinesia.

Table 54.3 POTENTIAL DRUG INTERACTIONS BETWEEN PULMONARY AND PSYCHIATRIC MEDICATIONS

BETA-AGONISTS	TRICYCLICS, MAO INHIBITORS	HYPERTENSIVE CRISIS
Sildenafil	Fluvoxamine	Increased vasodilatation
Theophylline	Alprazolam	Diminished benzodiazepine effect
Theophylline	Clozapine	Increased theophylline level
Theophylline	Fluvoxamine	Increased theophylline level
Theophylline	Lithium	Decreased lithium level
Theophylline	Carbamazepine	Decreased carbamazepine effect

Drugs with diminished incidence of extrapyramidal effects are preferred in chronic respiratory failure.

The β-adrenergic medications can induce anxiety and tremulousness. β2 selective agents should be routinely prescribed, as they reduce cardiac effects and the incidence of psychosis. Anticholinergics can lead to delirium, hallucinations, amnesia, paranoia, and depersonalization. Anxiety has been reported with leukotriene inhibitors. Theophylline, once a commonly prescribed medication for asthma and COPD, has fallen out of favor, in part due to its side effect profile and because of the need to monitor the patient's blood levels. However, it may still be used in resistant cases of asthma and in COPD at times to improve diaphragmatic function. It can cause anxiety, delirium, and tremors, especially when serum levels are in a toxic range.

Among the SSRIs, short-acting medications and those with a low incidence of interaction with pulmonary medications should be chosen. These include sertraline, citalopram, and escitalopram. The SSRIs have been shown to reduce dyspnea in patients with subsyndromal panic disorder. Tricyclic antidepressants (TCA) are as effective as the SSRIs in the treatment of depression but have a wider side-effect profile, including dry mouth, constipation, and cardiotoxic effects. QT-intervals should be checked by electrocardiogram prior to prescribing a TCA.

Short-acting benzodiazepines are preferred in patients with COPD and the elderly. Buspirone is a weak anxiolytic but can be used safely in patients with COPD and may improve exercise tolerance and dyspnea. β-blockers are relatively contraindicated in patients with asthma and COPD, due to their bronchoconstrictor properties.

Fluvoxamine can unpredictably promote the pulmonary vasodilatory effects of sildenafil and sodium nitroprusside by increasing half-life and venous dilatation.

SUMMARY

Mind and body may be nowhere more inextricably linked than in the physiological interactions between the nervous and respiratory systems. Severe chronic respiratory ailments invariably show neuropsychiatric effects, or may exhibit preexisting psychiatric disorders that require treatment. Conversely, primary psychiatric disorders are frequently complicated by addictions, such as smoking, which is the primary cause of COPD and the fourth most common cause of death in the United States, or they may exacerbate and confound the diagnosis and treatment of pulmonary disorders. There is a need for increased recognition of the complex interactions between mind and lung, as well as a team approach that includes pulmonologists, thoracic surgeons, and psychiatrists, in the optimal care of complex medical problems such as cystic fibrosis and lung transplantation. Drugs prescribed by psychiatrists and their medical counterparts can have complex and adverse interactions, so it is important to be aware of how to administer them in the least potentially toxic combinations. Finally, increased sensitivity to psychiatric issues in pulmonary disease has been convincingly demonstrated to improve the quality of care of individual patients and to reduce the overall costs of health care.

CLINICAL PEARLS

- Arterial pCO_2 and arterial pH are the primary controllers of ventilation, but an arterial pO_2 of less than 65 mm/Hg can also drive ventilation.

- Blunted ventilatory responses to breathing elevated concentrations of CO_2 are seen in patients who have clinical depression, CNS abnormalities, hypothyroidism, or severe hepatic failure. They also occur after carotid endarterectomy and in patients on respiratory depressants (Bone, 1993).

- In the absence of blood volume contraction, elevated serum HCO^{3-} concentrations are a reliable clue to the presence of underlying ventilatory failure.

- In addition to lowering the threshold for musculoskeletal tetany, respiratory alkalosis also diminishes cognitive and memoric processes (Posner, 1972).

- Dyspnea occurs when the mechanical work of breathing increases beyond the limits of ventilation and may be expected when the forced expiratory volume in the first second of exhalation (FEV_1) is reduced to less than 1 liter (Rock & Schwartzstein, 2007).

- A measure of the work of breathing is the maximum voluntary ventilation (MVV); that is, the maximum amount of air that can be moved in and out of the lungs during a defined interval. This can be empirically approximated from the FEV_1 (Caruana-Montaldo et al., 2000).

- The chronic interstitial pneumonias produce alveolar scarring and lead to a loss of gas-exchange surface, as evidenced by reduced diffusion capacity (DLCO), although a decreased DLCO is also a hallmark of both emphysema and primary pulmonary vascular disease. Patients with these abnormalities tend to complain of dyspnea on exertion early in the course of their disease that is accompanied by rapid O_2 desaturation of the arterial blood with exercise.

- Normally, with exercise, an anaerobic threshold (AT) is achieved based on the cardiopulmonary limit of O_2 delivery to the tissues, which can be correlated with the minute ventilation and heart rate. Physical deconditioning and psychiatric disorders might cause dyspnea in patients who do not show maximal effort on testing.

- Asthmatics have an increased prevalence of general anxiety disorder, panic disorder, and phobic disorders (Rosenkranz & Davidson, 2009).

- Adverse circumstances in childhood can predict adult asthma, and acute traumatic events can exacerbate asthma.

- Weiss (Weiss, 1994) described a detailed behavioral management program for asthma that included a checklist to assess asthma medications, early signs of wheezing, triggers of an attack, individual behavior and behavior of other people during an attack, and the effects of asthma on social development, school, and the family. Asking patients to maintain a daily diary with respect to symptoms may provide an additional resource for diagnosis and management (p. 13).

- Self-induced wheezing in factitious cases is loudest over the neck, with transmission to the chest wall on auscultation. Bronchial wheezes can be mimicked by maneuvers that include holding the vocal cords in apposition. However, one must first exclude vocal cord dysfunction and other causes of intrathoracic and extrathoracic upper airway obstruction (Bahrainwala & Simon, 2001).

- A panic attack in the postoperative setting, or in a patient with phlebitis, should lead reflexively to a CT-angiogram, in order to exclude thromboembolic disease.

- Symptoms that have persisted for weeks to years without evidence of deleterious progression may be a clue to the psychological basis of symptoms.

DISCLOSURE STATEMENT

Dr. Kradin has no conflicts to disclose.

ACKNOWLEDGMENTS

The author wishes to acknowledge Dr. Donna Greenberg for her assistance. I also thank Linda Arini for her help in compiling this manuscript.

REFERENCES

American Lung Association (ALA) (2012). Trends in Asthma Morbidity and Mortality. American Lung Association.

American Psychiatric Association (1994). *Diagnostic and statistical manual of mental disorders: DSM-IV* (4th ed.). Washington, DC: American Psychiatric Association.

Anda, R. F., Williamson, D. F., Escobedo, L. G., Mast, E. E., Giovino, G. A., & Remington, P. L. (1990). Depression and the dynamics of smoking. A national perspective. *Journal of the American Medical Association, 264*(12), 1541–1545.

Anderson, D. L., Flume, P. A., & Hardy, K. K. (2001). Psychological functioning of adults with cystic fibrosis. *Chest, 119*(4), 1079–1084.

Bahrainwala, A. H., & Simon, M. R. (2001). Wheezing and vocal cord dysfunction mimicking asthma. *Current Opinion in Pulmonary Medicine, 7*(1), 8–13.

Blumenthal, J. A., Babyak, M. A., Keefe, F. J., Davis, R. D., Lacaille, R. A., Carney, R. M., et al. (2006). Telephone-based coping skills training for patients awaiting lung transplantation. *Journal of Consulting Clinical Psychology, 74*(3), 535–544.

Bone, R. (Ed.). (1993). *Pulmonary and critical care medicine* (Vol. 1). St. Louis, MO: Mosby.

Boner, A. L., Vallone, G., Chiesa, M., Spezia, E., Fambri, L., & Sette, L. (1992). Reproducibility of late phase pulmonary response to exercise and its relationship to bronchial hyperreactivity in children with chronic asthma. *Pediatric Pulmonology, 14*(3), 156–159.

Borson, S., Claypoole, K., & McDonald, G. J. (1998). Depression and chronic obstructive pulmonary disease: Treatment trials. *Seminars in Clinical Neuropsychiatry, 3*(2), 115–130.

Brown, E. S., Vornik, L. A., Khan, D. A., & Rush, A. J. (2007). Bupropion in the treatment of outpatients with asthma and major depressive disorder. *International Journal of Psychiatry in Medicine, 37*(1), 23–28.

Burns, B. H., & Howell, J. B. (1969). Disproportionately severe breathlessness in chronic bronchitis. *Quarterly Journal of Medicine, 38*(151), 277–294.

Burton, M. D., Johnson, D. C., & Kazemi, H. (1989). CSF acidosis augments ventilation through cholinergic mechanisms. *Journal of Applied Physiology, 66*(6), 2565–2572.

Cahill, K., & Perera, R. (2008). Competitions and incentives for smoking cessation. *Cochrane Database of Systematic Reviews,* (3), CD004307.

Carr, R. E., Lehrer, P. M., Rausch, L. L., & Hochron, S. M. (1994). Anxiety sensitivity and panic attacks in an asthmatic population. *Behavior Research & Therapy, 32*(4), 411–418.

Caruana-Montaldo, B., Gleeson, K., & Zwillich, C. (2000). The control of breathing in clinical practice. *Chest, 117,* 205–225.

Chapman, E., Landy, A., Lyon, A., Haworth, C., & Bilton, D. (2005). End of life care for adult cystic fibrosis patients: Facilitating a good enough death. *Journal of Cystic Fibrosis, 4*(4), 249–257.

Cherniack, N. S., Mitra, J., Prabhakar, N. R., & Adams, E. M. (1988). Respiratory and vasomotor influences of the ventrolateral medulla. *Clinical & Experimental Hypertension A, 10*(Suppl 1), 1–9.

Cohen, R. T., Canino, G. J., Bird, H. R., & Celedon, J. C. (2008). Violence, abuse, and asthma in Puerto Rican children. *American Journal of Respiration & Critical Care Medicine, 178*(5), 453–459.

Cormier, S. A., Yuan, S., Crosby, J. R., Protheroe, C. A., Dimina, D. M., Hines, E. M., et al. (2002). T(H)2-mediated pulmonary inflammation leads to the differential expression of ribonuclease genes by alveolar macrophages. *American Journal of Respiratory Cell & Molecular Biology, 27*(6), 678–687.

Coventry, P. A., & Hind, D. (2007). Comprehensive pulmonary rehabilitation for anxiety and depression in adults with chronic obstructive pulmonary disease: Systematic review and meta-analysis. *Journal of Psychosomatic Research, 63*(5), 551–565.

Covey, L. S., Glassman, A. H., Stetner, F., & Becker, J. (1993). Effect of history of alcoholism or major depression on smoking cessation. *American Journal of Psychiatry, 150*(10), 1546–1547.

Crain, D., & Bhat, A. (2010). Current treatment options in smoking cessation. *Hospital Practice (Minneapolis), 38*(1), 53–61.

Damas-Mora, J., Souster, L., & Jenner, F. A. (1982). Diminished hypercapnic drive in endogenous or severe depression. *Journal of Psychosomatic Research, 26*(2), 237–245.

Davydow, D. S., Desai, S. V., Needham, D. M., & Bienvenu, O. J. (2008). Psychiatric morbidity in survivors of the acute respiratory distress syndrome: A systematic review. *Psychosomatic Medicine, 70*(4), 512–519.

Downing, E. T., Braman, S. S., Fox, M. J., & Corrao, W. M. (1982). Factitious asthma. Physiological approach to diagnosis. *Journal of the American Medical Association, 248*(21), 2878–2881.

El-Sherbini, A., Bediwy, A., & Et-Mitalli, A. (2011). Association between obstructive sleep apnea and depression and the effect of continuous positive airway pressure (CPAP) treatment. *Neuropsychiatric Disease and Treatment, 7,* 715–721.

Fadel, H. E., Northrop, G., Misenhimer, H. R., & Harp, R. J. (1979). Normal pregnancy: A model of sustained respiratory alkalosis. *Journal of Perinatal Medicine, 7*(4), 195–201.

Fagan, J., Galea, S., Ahern, J., Bonner, S., & Vlahov, D. (2003). Relationship of self-reported asthma severity and urgent health care utilization to psychological sequelae of the September 11, 2001, terrorist attacks on the World Trade Center among New York City area residents. *Psychosomatic Medicine, 65*(6), 993–996.

Fiore, M. C., & Baker, T. B. (2011). Clinical practice. Treating smokers in the health care setting. *New England Journal of Medicine, 365*(13), 1222–1231.

Frederick, T., Frerichs, R. R., & Clark, V. A. (1988). Personal health habits and symptoms of depression at the community level. *Preventive Medicine, 17*(2), 173–182.

French, T., & Alexander, F. (1939–41). Psychogenic Factors in bronchial asthma. *Psychosomatic Medicine, 4*, 1–96.

Funk, G. C., Kirchheiner, K., Burghuber, O. C., & Hartl, S. (2009). BODE index versus GOLD classification for explaining anxious and depressive symptoms in patients with COPD—a cross-sectional study. *Respiratory Research, 10*, 1.

Glassman, A. H. (1993). Cigarette smoking: Implications for psychiatric illness. *American Journal of Psychiatry, 150*(4), 546–553.

Glassman, A. H., Helzer, J. E., Covey, L. S., Cottler, L. B., Stetner, F., Tipp, J. E., et al. (1990). Smoking, smoking cessation, and major depression. *Journal of the American Medical Association, 264*(12), 1546–1549.

Goff, D. C., Henderson, D. C., & Amico, E. (1992). Cigarette smoking in schizophrenia: Relationship to psychopathology and medication side effects. *American Journal of Psychiatry, 149*(9), 1189–1194.

Goodwin, R. D., Jacobi, F., & Thefeld, W. (2003). Mental disorders and asthma in the community. *Archives of General Psychiatry, 60*(11), 1125–1130.

Grant, J. F., Chittleborough, C. R., Taylor, A. W., Dal Grande, E., Wilson, D. H., Phillips, P. J., et al. (2006). The North West Adelaide Health Study: Detailed methods and baseline segmentation of a cohort for selected chronic diseases. *Epidemiologic Perspectives & Innovations, 3*, 4.

Greenberg, D. B., & Kradin, R. L. (1996). Lung disorders. In *The American Psychiatric Press textbook of consultation–liaison psychiatry* (pp. 565–566). Washington, DC: American Psychiatric Press.

Group, N. O. T. (1980). Continuous or nocturnal oxygen therapy in hypoxemic COPD: A clinical trial. *Annals of Internal Medicine, 93*, 391–398.

Heaton, R., Grant, I., McSweeney, A., Adams, K., & Petty, T. L. (1983). Psychological effects of continuous and nocturnal oxygen therapy in hypoxemic chronic obstructive lung disease. *Archives of Medicine, 143*, 1941–1947.

Hedner, J., Hedner, T., Wessberg, P., & Jonason, J. (1984). An analysis of the mechanism by which gamma-aminobutyric acid depresses ventilation in the rat. *Journal of Applied Physiology, 56*(4), 849–856.

Horton-Deutsch, S. L., Clark, D. C., & Farran, C. J. (1992). Chronic dyspnea and suicide in elderly men. *Hospital & Community Psychiatry, 43*(12), 1198–1203.

Hoshino, K., Suzuki, J., Yamauchi, K., & Inoue, H. (2008). Psychological stress evaluation of patients with bronchial asthma based on the chromogranin a level in saliva. *Journal of Asthma, 45*(7), 596–599.

Irani, S., Mahler, C., Goetzmann, L., Russi, E. W., & Boehler, A. (2006). Lung transplant recipients holding companion animals: Impact on physical health and quality of life. *American Journal of Transplantation, 6*(2), 404–411.

Isenberg, S. A., Lehrer, P. M., & Hochron, S. (1992). The effects of suggestion and emotional arousal on pulmonary function in asthma: A review and a hypothesis regarding vagal mediation. *Psychosomatic Medicine, 54*(2), 192–216.

Jellinek, M. S., Goldenheim, P. D., & Jenike, M. A. (1985). The impact of grief on ventilatory control. *American Journal of Psychiatry, 142*(1), 121–123.

Killian, K. J., & Campbell, E. J. (1983). Dyspnea and exercise. *Annual Review of Physiology, 45*, 465–479.

Klein, D. F. (1999). Panic disorder. *Lancet, 353*(9149), 326–327.

Kohler, M., Stoewhas, A. C., Ayers, L., Senn, O., Bloch, K. E., Russi, E. W., et al. (2011). The effects of CPAP therapy withdrawal in patients with obstructive sleep apnea: A randomised controlled trial. *American Journal of Respiration & Critical Care Medicine, 33*, 2206–2212.

Kollner, V., Einsle, F., Schade, I., Maulhardt, T., Gulielmos, V., & Joraschky, P. (2003). [The influence of anxiety, depression and post-traumatic stress disorder on quality of life after thoracic organ transplantation]. *Zeitschrift fur Psychosomatische Medizin und Psychotherapie, 49*(3), 262–274.

Kradin, R. (2008). *The placebo response: Power of unconscious healing.* London: Routledge.

Kradin, R. (2012). *Pathologies of the mind–body interface: The curious domain of the psychosomatic symptom.* London: Routledge.

Lacasse, Y., Brosseau, L., Milne, S., Martin, S., Wong, E., Guyatt, G. H., et al. (2002). Pulmonary rehabilitation for chronic obstructive pulmonary disease. *Cochrane Database of Systematic Reviews* (3), CD003793.

Lachman, A., Gielis, O., Thys, P., Lorimier, P., & Sergysels, R. (1992). [Hyperventilation syndrome: Current advances]. *La Revue des Maladies Respiratoires, 9*(3), 277–285.

Lehrer, P. M., Hochron, S. M., McCann, B., Swartzman, L., & Reba, P. (1986). Relaxation decreases large-airway but not small-airway asthma. *Journal of Psychosomatic Research, 30*(1), 13–25.

Lehrer, P. M., Sargunaraj, D., & Hochron, S. (1992). Psychological approaches to the treatment of asthma. *Journal of Consulting Clinical Psychology, 60*(4), 639–643.

Lettieri, C. J., Paolino, N., Eliasson, A. H., Shah, A. A., & Holley, A. B. (2011). Comparison of adjustable and fixed oral appliances for the treatment of obstructive sleep apnea. *Journal of Clinical Sleep Medicine, 7*(5), 439–445.

Light, R. W., Merrill, E. J., Despars, J. A., Gordon, G. H., & Mutalipassi, L. R. (1985). Prevalence of depression and anxiety in patients with COPD. Relationship to functional capacity. *Chest, 87*(1), 35–38.

Lindberg, A., Jonsson, A. C., Ronmark, E., Lundgren, R., Larsson, L. G., & Lundback, B. (2005). Ten-year cumulative incidence of COPD and risk factors for incident disease in a symptomatic cohort. *Chest, 127*(5), 1544–1552.

Lindefors, N., Yamamoto, Y., Pantaleo, T., Lagercrantz, H., Brodin, E., & Ungerstedt, U. (1986). In vivo release of substance P in the nucleus tractus solitarii increases during hypoxia. *Neuroscience Letters, 69*(1), 94–97.

Lishman, W. A. (1987). *Organic psychiatry.* London, England: Blackwell.

Lovibond, P. F., & Lovibond, S. H. (1995). The structure of negative emotional states: Comparison of the Depression Anxiety Stress Scales (DASS) with the Beck Depression and Anxiety Inventories. *Behaviour Research and Therapy, 33*, 335–343.

Mahler, D. A., Harver, A., Lentine, T., Scott, J. A., Beck, K., & Schwartzstein, R. M. (1996). Descriptors of breathlessness in cardiorespiratory diseases. *American Journal of Respiration & Critical Care Medicine, 154*(5), 1357–1363.

Marsac, M. L., Funk, J. B., & Nelson, L. (2007). Coping styles, psychological functioning and quality of life in children with asthma. *Child: Care, Health & Development, 33*(4), 360–367.

Martinez, T. Y., Pereira, C. A., dos Santos, M. L., Ciconelli, R. M., Guimaraes, S. M., & Martinez, J. A. (2000). Evaluation of the short-form 36-item questionnaire to measure health-related quality of life in patients with idiopathic pulmonary fibrosis. *Chest, 117*(6), 1627–1632.

Mermigkis, C., Stagaki, E., Amfilochiou, A., Polychronopoulos, V., Korkonikitas, P., Mermigkis, D., et al. (2009). Sleep quality and associated daytime consequences in patients with idiopathic pulmonary fibrosis. *Medical Principles & Practice, 18*(1), 10–15.

Mifsud, J. C., Hernandez, L., & Hoebel, B. G. (1989). Nicotine infused into the nucleus accumbens increases synaptic dopamine as measured by in vivo microdialysis. *Brain Research, 478*(2), 365–367.

Mijares, S. (2009). S. Mijare (Ed.), *Revelation of the breath.* Albany, State University of New York Press Book.

Najafizadeh, K., Ghorbani, F., Rostami, A., Fard-Mausavi, A., Lorgard-Dezfuli-Nejad, M., Marashian, S. M., et al. (2009). Depression while on the lung transplantation waiting list. *Annals of Transplantation, 14*(2), 34–37.

Ohayon, M. M. (2003). The effects of breathing-related sleep disorders on mood disturbances in the general population. *Journal of Clinical Psychiatry, 64*(10), 1195–1200; quiz, 1274–1196.

Ossip-Klein, D. J., & McIntosh, S. (2003). Quitlines in North America: evidence base and applications. *American Journal of Medical Science, 326*(4), 201–205.

Ossip-Klein, D. J., McIntosh, S., Utman, C., Burton, K., Spada, J., & Guido, J. (2000). Smokers ages 50+: who gets physician advice to quit? *Preventive Medicine, 31*(4), 364–369.

Polito, J. R. (2008). Smoking cessation trials. *Canadian Medical Association Journal, 179*(10), 1037–1038; author reply, 1138.

Posner, J. B. (1972). Newer techniques of cerebral blood flow measurement. *Stroke, 3*(3), 227–237.

Preter, M., & Klein, D. F. (2008). Panic, suffocation false alarms, separation anxiety and endogenous opioids. *Progress in Neuro-Psychopharmacology & Biological Psychiatry, 32*(3), 603–612.

Prigatano, G., Parson, O., Wright, E., Hawrylak, G. (1983). Neuropsychological test performance in mildly hypoxemic patients with chronic obstructive pulmonary disease. *Journal of Consulting Clinical Psychology, 51*, 108–116.

Randerath, W. J., Verbraecken, J., Andreas, S., Bettega, G., Boudewyns, A., Hamans, E., et al. (2011). Non-CPAP therapies in obstructive sleep apnoea. *European Respiratory Journal, 37*(5), 1000–1028.

Richardson, L. P., Russo, J. E., Lozano, P., McCauley, E., & Katon, W. (2008). The effect of comorbid anxiety and depressive disorders on health care utilization and costs among adolescents with asthma. *General Hospital Psychiatry, 30*(5), 398–406.

Rock, L. K., & Schwartzstein, R. M. (2007). Mechanisms of dyspnea in chronic lung disease. *Current Opinion in Supportive & Palliative Care, 1*(2), 102–108.

Rosenkranz, M. A., & Davidson, R. J. (2009). Affective neural circuitry and mind-body influences in asthma. *NeuroImage, 47*(3), 972–980.

Rothenhausler, H. B., Ehrentraut, S., Stoll, C., Schelling, G., & Kapfhammer, H. P. (2001). The relationship between cognitive performance and employment and health status in long-term survivors of the acute respiratory distress syndrome: Results of an exploratory study. *General Hospital Psychiatry, 23*(2), 90–96.

Schmaling, K. B. (1999). Medical and psychiatric predictors of airway reactivity. *Respiratory Care, 44*, 1452–1457.

Scott, K. M., Von Korff, M., Alonso, J., Angermeyer, M. C., Benjet, C., Bruffaerts, R., et al. (2008). Childhood adversity, early-onset depressive/anxiety disorders, and adult-onset asthma. *Psychosomatic Medicine, 70*(9), 1035–1043.

Series, F., Cormier, Y., & La Forge, J. (1990). Influence of apnea type and sleep stage on nocturnal postapneic desaturation. *American Review of Respiratory Disease, 141*(6), 1522–1526.

Shen, H. H., Ochkur, S. I., McGarry, M. P., Crosby, J. R., Hines, E. M., Borchers, M. T., et al. (2003). A causative relationship exists between eosinophils and the development of allergic pulmonary pathologies in the mouse. *Journal of Immunology, 170*(6), 3296–3305.

Smoller, J. W., Pollack, M. H., Otto, M. W., Rosenbaum, J. F., & Kradin, R. L. (1996). Panic anxiety, dyspnea, and respiratory disease. Theoretical and clinical considerations. *American Journal of Respiration & Critical Care Medicine, 154*(1), 6–17.

Smoller, J. W., Pollack, M. H., Systrom, D., & Kradin, R. L. (1998). Sertraline effects on dyspnea in patients with obstructive airways disease. *Psychosomatics, 39*(1), 24–29.

Stoller, J. K., Panos, R. J., Krachman, S., Doherty, D. E., & Make, B. (2010). Oxygen therapy for patients with COPD: Current evidence and the long-term oxygen treatment trial. *Chest, 138*(1), 179–187.

Strine, T. W., Mokdad, A. H., Balluz, L. S., Berry, J. T., & Gonzalez, O. (2008). Impact of depression and anxiety on quality of life, health behaviors, and asthma control among adults in the United States with asthma, 2006. *Journal of Asthma, 45*(2), 123–133.

Tashkin, D., Kanner, R., Bailey, W., Buist, S., Anderson, P., Nides, M., et al. (2001). Smoking cessation in patients with chronic obstructive pulmonary disease: A double-blind, placebo-controlled, randomised trial. *Lancet, 357*(9268), 1571–1575.

ten Thoren, C., & Petermann, F. (2000). Reviewing asthma and anxiety. *Respiratory Medicine, 94*(5), 409–415.

Thompson, P. D. (1982). Cardiovascular hazards of physical activity. *Exercise & Sports Sciences Reviews, 10*, 208–235.

Turyk, M. E., Hernandez, E., Wright, R. J., Freels, S., Slezak, J., Contraras, A., et al. (2008). Stressful life events and asthma in adolescents. *Pediatric Allergy & Immunology, 19*(3), 255–263.

Van Lieshout, R. J., Bienenstock, J., & MacQueen, G. M. (2009). A review of candidate pathways underlying the association between asthma and major depressive disorder. *Psychosomatic Medicine, 71*(2), 187–195.

Vermeulen, K. M., Bosma, O. H., Bij, W., Koeter, G. H., & Tenvergert, E. M. (2005). Stress, psychological distress, and coping in patients on the waiting list for lung transplantation: An exploratory study. *Transplant International, 18*(8), 954–959.

Vermeulen, K. M., Ouwens, J. P., van der Bij, W., de Boer, W. J., Koeter, G. H., & TenVergert, E. M. (2003). Long-term quality of life in patients surviving at least 55 months after lung transplantation. *General Hospital Psychiatry, 25*(2), 95–102.

Wargnies, E., Houze, L., Vanneste, J., Perez, T., & Wallaert, B. (2002). [Depression, anxiety and coping strategies in adult patients with cystic fibrosis]. *La Revue des Maladies Respiratoires, 19*(1), 39–43.

Wassermann, K., Hansen, J., Sue, D., Casburi, R., & Whipp, B. (1994). *Principles of exercise testing and interpretation.* Philadelphia: Lea and Febiger.

Weiss, J. (1994). Behavioral management of asthma. In *Behavioral approaches to breathing disorders* (pp. 205–219). New York: Plenum.

Wolf, J. M., Nicholls, E., & Chen, E. (2008). Chronic stress, salivary cortisol, and alpha-amylase in children with asthma and healthy children. *Biological Psychology, 78*(1), 20–28.

55.

NEUROPSYCHIATRIC MANIFESTATIONS OF ENDOCRINE DISORDERS

Erin Sterenson, Christopher L. Sola, and Shirlene Sampson

INTRODUCTION

It has long been known that endocrine disorders are associated with neuropsychiatric symptoms. In 1786, Parry described psychotic symptoms associated with hyperthyroidism, and Graves first lectured on the psychiatric complications of hyperthyroidism in 1834. Other remote observations of psychiatric symptoms associated with endocrine disorders include reports by Addison in 1868, Cushing in 1932, and Sheehan in 1939 (Addison, 1868; Cushing, 1932; Sheehan, 1939).

Psychiatric symptoms can precede or present concurrently with the more typical physical symptoms of endocrine disease. These secondary disorders can be impossible to distinguish from primary psychiatric disorders, such as depression, mania, psychosis, anxiety, delirium, or dementia. Thus, testing for endocrine diseases should be routinely performed as part of the medical work up for these neuropsychiatric disorders.

In this chapter, we will review psychiatric syndromes associated with disorders of the thyroid, adrenal, pituitary, and parathyroid glands, as well as those associated with diabetes mellitus, hypoglycemia, and disturbances of gonadal hormones. For information related to the physical clinical presentations, medical evaluation, and management of endocrine disorders, we refer you to Chapter 6. When psychiatric symptoms are thought to be secondary to endocrine disease, the primary treatment focus remains correcting the endocrine disorder. That being said, there are times when the psychiatric symptoms are severe enough to warrant immediate intervention. This is clearly the case for mania, psychosis, and severe depression that could be life-threatening. The treatment intervention of choice for acute mania and psychosis remains the atypical antipsychotics, and antidepressant medications and interventions remain the treatment of choice for depression. When significant anxiety is present, benzodiazepines can be used to get symptoms under control in the short term, followed by serotonergic antidepressants if longer term drug treatment is needed.

THYROID DISORDERS

HYPERTHYROIDISM (THYROTOXICOSIS)

Numerous neuropsychiatric symptoms have been noted in patients with hyperthyroidism and include psychosis, depression, mania, anxiety, and cognitive dysfunction (Feldman et al., 2013). Neuropsychiatric symptoms can occur with primary hyperthyroidism (Graves disease), as well as with toxic nodular goiter and excessive consumption of exogenous thyroid hormone (Feldman et al., 2013; Brownlie et al., 2000). Brownlie and colleagues (2000) reported a series of 18 patients: seven presented with mania, seven with depression, three with psychosis, and one with delirium. Thus the range of neuropsychiatric symptoms seen with hyperthyroidism is quite broad. Of note, a case of subacute thyroiditis presenting with neuropsychiatric symptoms (acute psychosis) has also been reported (Lee et al., 2013).

The presenting neuropsychiatric symptoms of hyperthyroidism include emotional lability, poor impulse control, crying spells, euphoria, irritability, distractibility, reduced attention, impaired recall, and psychosis (delusions and hallucinations) (Esposito et al., 1997; Brownlie et al., 2000). A minority of patients can present with symptoms of depression, apathy, or lethargy. Treatment includes targeting the cause of hyperthyroidism and addressing the presenting neuropsychiatric symptoms as clinically indicated.

HYPOTHYROIDISM (MYXEDEMA)

Neuropsychiatric symptoms associated with hypothyroidism include cognitive dysfunction, affective disorders, and psychosis (Heinrich & Grahm, 2003). Early descriptions of psychiatric symptoms in hypothyroidism include reports by Gull in 1874 and Ord in 1887. The psychiatric presentation may be indistinguishable from a primary psychiatric disorder, thus reinforcing the importance of ruling out medical causes of psychiatric disorders. The onset of symptoms of hypothyroidism is often gradual, and slow progression is common, especially in the elderly, mimicking the development of a degenerative dementia. Common symptoms include slowed comprehension and impairment in attention, recent memory, and abstract thinking. In contrast to cortical dementias such as Alzheimer's disease and frontotemporal degeneration, the cognitive disorder of myxedema does not present with discrete cortical syndromes like aphasia, anomia, apraxia, and frontal disinhibition.

The most common affective disorder seen with hypothyroidism is depression, manifested most often as reduced mood, psychomotor retardation, sleep and appetite disturbances, anhedonia, reduced libido, and emotional lability. Suicidal thinking, delusions, and hallucinations can be present in more advanced illness. Thomsen et al. (2005) have reported that patients hospitalized for hypothyroidism had a greater risk of being admitted for the treatment of depression or bipolar disorder, and that this risk was greatest in the first year after index hospitalization.

A meta-analysis of individuals with treatment resistant depression demonstrated that approximately 50% had subclinical hypothyroidism, and the response to antidepressant therapy is known to be reduced if the thyroid disease is not treated (Howland, 1993; Pae et al., 2009). Demartini et al. (2010) found a prevalence of depressive symptoms in 63.5% of their subjects with subclinical hypothyroidism. In contrast, others have found no increase in neuropsychiatric symptoms in patients with subclinical hypothyroidism (Park et al., 2010). Although it is generally believed that treatment of the underlying hypothyroidism will treat the neuropsychiatric symptoms, Demartini et al. (2010) found that thyroid replacement alone was not effective in producing remission of the depressive symptoms. Evidence for benefit from thyroid replacement in depressed patients with subclinical hypothyroidism remains variable; therefore, the use of thyroid replacement in this patient population remains controversial (Feldman et al., 2013).

Compared to depression, mania is a much less common manifestation of hypothyroidism; however, there are a number of reported cases of hypothyroidism presenting with symptoms of mania (Stowell & Barnhill, 2005; Khaldi et al., 2006; Tor, 2007; Sathya et al., 2009). Patients can present with elevated mood and energy, irritability, psychomotor agitation, decreased need for sleep, increased goal-directed behavior, pressured speech, flight of ideas, grandiosity, hallucinations, and delusions.

Hypothyroidism has been associated with psychosis (myxedema madness), and there is no typical presentation of psychotic symptoms (Davis, 1989; Heinrich & Grahm, 2003), which can include delusions (paranoia), auditory and visual hallucinations, perseveration, and thought disorganization. Psychosis has been noted in 5–15% of patients with hypothyroidism (Hall, 1983).

ADRENAL DISORDERS

HYPERCORTISOLEMIA (CUSHING'S SYNDROME)

Psychiatric disturbances are common with Cushing's syndrome. Sonino and Fava (2001) reviewed the prevalence of psychiatric disorders in Cushing's syndrome and reported the presence of major depression was on average 57%, with a range of 50–80% across studies. Depression was significantly associated with older age, female gender, higher pretreatment urinary cortisol levels, a relatively more severe clinical condition, and the absence of pituitary adenoma. Patients with depression appeared to have a more severe clinical presentation and

have higher cortisol levels than patients with increased cortisol without depression.

Mania in Cushing's syndrome presents less commonly than depression, though approximately 30% of patients present with hypomanic or manic symptoms. Sustained elation is rare, with subclinical mood fluctuations being more common. Hypomania or mania may be some of the earliest signs of illness onset.

Anxiety can be commonly associated with Cushing's syndrome. The rate of generalized anxiety disorder has been noted to be as high as 79%, and panic disorder as high as 53%. The association between anxiety and Cushing's syndrome is complex, given that depression is common with Cushing's syndrome (50–80%), and anxiety is a common symptom of depression, even in patients with depression that is not caused by an endocrine disorder.

Cognitive dysfunction has been noted in approximately two-thirds of patients with Cushing's syndrome. Impairments can be seen in nonverbal, visual-ideational, visual-memory, and spatial-constructional abilities, as well as concentration, memory, reasoning ability, comprehension, and processing new information. Neuroimaging studies may reveal cerebral atrophy.

Although the successful control of hypercortisolism can result in a progressive improvement of psychiatric symptoms and cognitive function, this is not always the case. Pereira et al. (2010) describe a Cushing's syndrome cohort comprising 33 patients, with 67% having significant psychopathology (primarily depression). After cure of Cushing's syndrome, the prevalence of diagnosed psychopathology was 54% at three months, 36% at six months, and 24% at one year. They also report a 74-patient cohort that continued to experience impairments in memory and executive function despite long-term cure of the Cushing's disease.

ADRENAL INSUFFICIENCY (ADDISON'S DISEASE)

Compared to the neuropsychiatric effects of Cushing's syndrome, much less is known about the neuropsychiatric effects of Addison's disease, which results in deficiencies in glucocorticoids and mineralocorticoids. Anglin et al. (2006) reviewed the literature on neuropsychiatric symptoms associated with Addison's disease and reported a prevalence of neuropsychiatric symptoms of 64–84% in the four case series examined. Mild disturbances in mood, motivation, and behavior were described as core clinical symptoms. Psychosis and extensive cognitive changes, including delirium, were less common and associated with more severe disease. Catatonia and self-mutilation were still more rarely seen. Neuropsychiatric symptoms were noted before the diagnosis was made. Specific drug treatment of the neuropsychiatric symptoms was started in 80% of the cases.

The diagnosis of Addison's disease is commonly delayed. Bleicken et al. (2010) report a cohort of 216 patients with adrenal insufficiency in which 41% received a false diagnosis of a psychiatric illness. Thus it is important to have a low threshold for screening for Addison's disease, particularly with atypical presentations and treatment-resistant symptoms.

Adrenal insufficiency is generally treated by replacing hydrocortisone. Thomsen et al. (2006) note that patients with adrenal insufficiency may be at risk for developing severe affective disorders, and in particular may be at risk for developing elevated mood symptoms in the context of receiving hormone replacement.

DISORDERS OF THE PARATHYROID GLANDS

HYPERPARATHYROIDISM

Reports of the occurrence of psychiatric symptoms in patients with hyperparathyroidism vary widely and have been reported for decades, including in the medical school mnemonic "stones, bones, groans, and psychiatric overtones," referring to the renal or biliary stones, bone pain, abdominal discomfort (eliciting groans), and psychiatric sequelae (overtones) of hypercalcemia. Though it has been commonly held that neuropsychiatric symptoms tend to positively correlate with the degree of elevation of serum calcium (Brown, Fischman, & Showalter, 1987; Haden, Stoll, McCormick, Scott, & Fuleihan, 1997), many patients may tolerate significant elevations in serum calcium without any symptoms, and patients with relatively mild elevation of serum calcium may have significant psychiatric sequelae (McAllion & Paterson, 1989).

Historically, it has been suggested that in mild hypercalcemia, personality changes, irritability, decreased spontaneity, and lack of initiative are more commonly noted. Moderate hypercalcemia (12–16 mg/dl), is more likely to result in more frequent depressive symptoms, including dysphoria, anhedonia, apathy, anxiety, increased irritability, impaired concentration and recent memory, and sometimes suicidal ideation. In severe hypercalcemia (16–19 mg/dl)—or following a precipitous rise in serum calcium—psychosis and cognitive symptoms predominate, including auditory and visual hallucinations, delusions, confusion, disorientation, catatonia or agitation, and paranoid ideation. At levels above 19 mg/dl, stupor and coma are common.

However, this may not be the case. Some studies (McAllion, 1989; Hecht, Gershberg, & St. Paul, 1975) demonstrate "no relationship between the overall psychiatric score and serum levels of calcium." Increasingly, the literature has recognized that many patients may have atypical features, such as fatigue, generalized weakness, sleep disorders, and cognitive deficits leading to decreased ability to complete common tasks (Coker et al., 2005; Walker, Rubin, & Silverberg, 2013). Indeed, "nearly 80% of biochemically identified cases of primary hyperparathyroidism are 'asymptomatic' in terms of the classical symptoms" (Benge et al., 2009).

In view of the insidious onset and frequent lack of specific symptomatology, the diagnosis of hyperparathyroidism is often overlooked (Gatewood, Organ, & Mead, 1975; McAllion, 1989; Coker et al., 2005; Benge et al., 2009; Walker et al., 2013). For this reason, and because of its relatively low cost, a screening ionized calcium determination should be obtained for most psychiatric patients during their initial evaluation.

Common misdiagnoses include anxiety disorders, hypochondriasis, mood disorders, schizophrenia, and cognitive impairment disorders of other etiology. Correction of hypercalcemia generally results in rapid reversal of many of the psychiatric manifestations (Borer & Bhanot, 1985). Evidence regarding the reversibility of psychiatric symptoms following parathyroidectomy is conflicting (Heath, 1989; Walker et al., 2013), though there is some support in the literature for surgical intervention. Due to the high proportion of "asymptomatic" patients who are nonetheless suffering, which may be as much as 80% of patients with hyperparathyroidism, surgery can often, though not always, result in a demonstrable decrease in neuropsychiatric (emotional or cognitive) symptom burden (Heath et al., 1980; Joborn et al., 1988; Benge et al., 2009; Coker et al., 2005; Goyal et al., 2001; Solomon, Schaaf, & Smallridge, 1994; Roman et al., 2011; Walker et al., 2013); however, which symptom improves—and how much—is not predictable (Silverberg, 2013; Walker et al., 2013). Younger patients are thought to benefit more than older patients, and tend to tolerate the procedure better (Benge et al., 2009).

LITHIUM AND HYPERPARATHYROIDISM

Patients on chronic lithium therapy, though more likely to present with renal or thyroid dysfunction, may, more rarely, present a clinical picture indistinguishable from that of primary hyperparathyroidism (Mallette & Eichorn, 1986; Rifai, Moles, & Harrington, 2001). Discontinuation of lithium in these patients most often results in return of serum calcium levels to the normal range, though this is not always immediate (Rifai et al., 2001), and simple lithium cessation may not be sufficient in every case. If stopping the medication does not reverse the hypercalcemia, parathyroidectomy may be indicated (Duggal & Singh, 2007). One review highlighted the possibility that lithium "unmasks" native hyperparathyroidism, causes multiglandular parathyroid hyperplasia, or promotes the growth of existing parathyroid adenomas, and noted that women are four times more likely to present with this issue (Szalat, Mazeh, & Freund, 2009). It is vital that serum calcium be checked in delirious patients who are taking lithium, as hypercalcemia would suggest the need to immediately discontinue lithium (Rifai et al., 2001; Duggal & Singh, 2007). The pathophysiological mechanism of lithium-induced hyperparathyroidism is poorly understood. It has been postulated that lithium might directly stimulate parathyroid (PTH) production, that lithium-induced hypercalcemia could be related to hypocalciuria resulting from impaired renal function, or that lithium may interfere with calcium-mediated, transmembrane signal transduction by the calcium-sensing receptor, inducing a reduction in the set-point for PTH secretion. Lithium may magnify the set-point error in patients with primary hyperparathyroidism, may unmask preexisting changes in the parathyroid glands, or may cause mild, clinically insignificant hypercalcemia and hyperparathyroidism. Lithium-associated hypercalcemia can present a clinical dilemma in patients with bipolar disorder because of limitations in treatment options and the potential of hypercalcemia to exacerbate psychopathological symptoms

(McHenry & Lee, 1996). Because it may be difficult to simply discontinue the lithium, and surgical resection of the parathyroid gland is not indicated (Gregoor, 2007), some authors have explored the potential benefits of cinacalcet hydrochloride, an allosteric activator of the calcium-sensing receptor that decreases serum calcium (Sloand & Shelly, 2006; Gregoor, 2007).

HYPOPARATHYROIDISM

Psychiatric findings occur in 30–50% of hypoparathyroid patients (Popkin & Mackenzie, 1980; Wee-Kiat Ang et al., 1995). The rapidity of change in serum calcium and other electrolytes, especially magnesium, as well as vitamin D, seems to be the most important factor in determining the severity of complaints. As with hyperparathyroidism, symptoms may include anxiety, depression, irritability, emotional lability, social withdrawal, phobias, and obsessions; and, in severe cases, delirium with confusion, disorientation, agitation, and paranoia. Auditory and visual hallucinations may be present, especially in the context of delirium. Intellectual deterioration is found in one-third of patients with primary hypoparathyroidism, the result of a long duration of illness prior to diagnosis and treatment. "Up to 80% of cases studied by Denko and Kaelbling had intellectual impairment (IQ 40 to 90) as the sole or major psychiatric finding" (Hossain, 1970). With surgically induced hypoparathyroidism, cognitive changes are rare, as the condition is usually treated promptly and calcium levels are monitored more closely. Symptoms of hypoparathyroidism may be mistaken for anxiety disorders such as generalized anxiety disorder, hypochondriasis, conversion disorders, depression, schizophrenia, dementia, and cognitive impairment disorders. Normalization of serum calcium levels may result in resolution of symptoms, though this is often insufficient until any existing hypomagnesemia is corrected (Wee-Kiat Ang et al., 1995). When intellectual impairment is present, residual cognitive deficits often persist despite calcium and magnesium correction. In severe cases requiring antipsychotics, it is prudent to consider supplementing with both calcium and magnesium to mitigate the risk of extrapyramidal symptoms, a risk increased by hypomagnesemia and hypocalcemia.

DISORDERS OF PITUITARY FUNCTION

There is a significant literature on the influence of the hypothalamic-pituitary-thyroid and hypothalamic-pituitary-adrenal axes on emotional well-being. Discussion of each can be found in the end-organ (i.e., thyroid and adrenal) sections of this chapter, with specific attention here directed toward the effects of altered pituitary function not contained in those reviews.

HYPERPITUITARISM

The most common type of pituitary tumor is a prolactin-secreting adenoma (prolactinoma). Microadenomas (<1 cm in diameter) are more common in females, and macroadenomas (>1 cm, and more likely to invade or compress surrounding structures) have an equal gender distribution (Ali, Miller, & Freudenreich, 2010). Hyperprolactinemia can result in a wide variety of symptoms, including galactorrhea, gynecomastia, amenorrhea, decreased libido, and sexual dysfunction (Ali et al., 2010). Psychological disturbances including hostility, depression, and anxiety, as well as apathy, are seen often without dysphoric mood irritability and impulsivity (Fava et al., 1981; Cohen et al., 1984; Ali et al., 2010).

Categories of drugs associated with inducing hyperprolactinemia include antipsychotics (phenothiazines, butyrophenones, and risperidone), antidepressants (amitriptyline, imipramine, amoxapine), and dopamine-receptor antagonists (metoclopramide, domperidone, sulpiride). Of the atypical neuroleptics, risperidone has the greatest capacity for stimulating prolactin secretion (Ali et al., 2010). As a class, however, the atypical neuroleptics have less tendency to be associated with prolactin increases in the serum than the typical agents.

A common clinical dilemma is the psychotic patient on a neuroleptic drug who develops menstrual dysfunction, galactorrhea, or (in males) gynecomastia associated with an elevated serum prolactin concentration. Treatment requires a careful balancing act between the decreasing prolactin and maintenance of adequate control of the psychotic disorder. In such cases, it is reasonable to consider a switch to an alternative antipsychotic, such as quetiapine or olanzapine (Kane et al., 1997), which is less likely to exacerbate hyperprolactinemia. Consideration could also be given to the use of aripiprazole, which might actually decrease prolactin due to its mixed dopaminergic antagonism and agonism. However, metabolic syndrome or diabetes each confer a higher long-term risk than hyperprolactinemia, so it may be wise to introduce aripiprazole as an adjunct, and slowly cross-titrate the offending agent—most often risperidone or haloperidol—to optimize control of psychosis and minimize the effects of increased prolactin (Ali et al., 2010). If the serum prolactin level returns to normal when the offending agent is stopped, the possibility of a pituitary tumor is virtually excluded. If there is an adenoma, though, consideration must be given to surgical intervention, though surgery may not be persistently curative (Cohn et al., 1985; Perovich et al., 1989; Ali et al., 2010). The use of a dopamine agonist such as bromocriptine or cabergoline is potentially risky, as these may theoretically—though rarely—lead to worsened psychotic symptoms despite the patient's remaining on an antipsychotic (Rao, Hiemke, Grasmader, & Baumann, 2001; Konopelska, Quinkler, Strasburber, Ventz, 2008; Ali et al., 2010). In these cases it is useful to systematically track the psychiatric and endocrine symptoms, perhaps with rating scales as well as blood tests, to find the optimal balance of psychiatric and endocrine symptom control. In order for the psychiatrist and endocrinologist to work effectively together, it is helpful to have a common "dashboard" to which both can refer.

Acromegaly is the clinical syndrome that results from sustained hypersecretion of growth hormone, most often the result of a pituitary adenoma (Ezzat, 1997; Furman &

Ezzat, 1998). Personality changes, including apathy, lack of initiative and spontaneity, and mood lability (Bleuler, 1951), often in relationship to patients' altered physical appearance in active disease, have been reported for decades, albeit with little formal investigation. More recently, increased use of structured diagnostic interviews and validated surveys has generated more detailed descriptions of psychiatric disturbances associated with acromegaly, including depression, pathological gambling, psychosis, amotivational syndrome (De Sousa, 2009), harm avoidance, neurosis, anticipatory worry, pessimism, and reduced impulsivity and less novelty-seeking behaviors (Sievers et al., 2009). A relatively recent examination of 81 acromegalic patients revealed "increased lifetime rates of affective disorders," especially major depression and dysthymia, but not anxiety disorders, which persisted even after curative surgery. The same review revealed that radiotherapy, but not biochemical interventions, "was a predictor for an increased risk for DSM-IV mental disorders" (Sievers et al., 2009), supporting earlier work that demonstrated pituitary irradiation sometimes resulting in delayed cerebral radiation necrosis (DCRN), leading to "progressive dementia, blindness, status epilepticus, and stroke-like episodes" (Furman & Ezzat, 1998). Of note, most of the above-described traits have also been found in patients with nonfunctioning pituitary macroadenomas, though to a lesser degree (Sievers et al., 2009). Finally, 68 acromegalic patients "scored significantly worse on virtually all psychopathology questionnaires," including depression and anxiety scales, but did not score worse on cognitive tests when compared to healthy matched controls and patients treated for nonfunctioning pituitary macroadenomas (Tiemensma et al., 2010).

One pharmacological intervention, octreotide, has very few psychiatric side effects, although according to the package insert it may cause depressive symptoms in 1–4% of patients and, in fewer than 1% of patients, may cause anxiety, libido decrease, paranoia, or amnesia (Sandostatin package insert [Novartis—US], Rev., 01/97, Rec 02/23/99).

HYPOPITUITARISM

The infundibular-hypothalamic anatomy is relatively fragile, such that brain pathology, especially traumatic brain injury (TBI), subarachnoid hemorrhage, or brain tumors increase the risk of patients' developing hypopituitarism, including the first and most common sign of pituitary impairment, growth hormone deficiency (Aimaretti, et al., 2005). Regardless of etiology, the primary issue is the decreased hormonal output, and use of psychotropic agents directed at the nature of the presenting symptom (e.g., antidepressants for depression, anxiolytics for anxiety, or antipsychotics for psychosis) is suggested only after correction of the endocrine abnormality. Despite this final common pathway, much of the literature on the psychiatric sequelae of hypopituitarism is focused on the result of TBI, with estimates of post-TBI hypopituitarism as high as 25–50% (Urban, Harris, & Masel, 2005; Lane, 2010). Most references describe increased rates of depression (Rao et al., 2001; Popovic et al., 2004; Popovic,

Aimaretti, Casaneuva, & Ghigo, 2005; Bavisetty et al., 2008; Lane, 2010), and at least one suggesting an attempted suicide rate as high as 18% (Simpson et al., 2002) in untreated cases. Others describe amotivation, dysphoria, disturbed sleep pattern, personality change, affective blunting, and auditory and visual hallucinations (Chang, Tsai, & Tseng, 2006), and cognitive impairment, including visual and verbal memory impairment (Rao et al., 2001; Popovic et al., 2004) and decreased quality of life (Battisetty, 2008). In one study, nearly half of patients with post-traumatic hypopituitarism (as measured by hormone-level output) expressed symptoms of mild to moderate depression, and scales reflecting somatization and paranoid ideation were inversely correlated with pituitary hormone levels. Many neuropsychiatric symptoms significantly improved with hormone replacement (Popovic et al., 2004).

DISORDERS OF GLUCOSE METABOLISM

DIABETES MELLITUS

The interface of diabetes mellitus and psychiatric illness is of growing interest to psychiatrists, endocrinologists, and primary care providers alike. The comorbidity, however, is not new, and, in the seventeenth century, it was speculated that diabetes was caused by "long sorrow and other depressions." Likewise, in 1879, Sir Henry Maudsley asserted that "diabetes is a disease which often shows itself in families in which insanity prevails." As the comorbidity is examined in greater detail, it has become apparent that the relationship is bidirectional; both disorders and their treatment influence one another. Balhara suggests the association between the two illnesses is far more complex than previously thought (Balhara, 2011).

In this chapter, we will discuss type I and type II diabetes mellitus together. Only where the relationship to psychopathology is different will we specify the type of diabetes.

It is generally acknowledged that the presence of psychiatric illness in the context of diabetes mellitus can affect patient motivation and compliance with treatment recommendations. As such, psychiatric comorbidity is associated with decreased quality of life, increased cost of care, elevated glycosylated hemoglobin (HbA1c), and greater end organ damage, as well as increased healthcare service utilization, especially of emergency and hospital services. Given the frequency and consequences of the co-occurrence of diabetes and mental illness, many advocate for regular mental health screening measures in the diabetic population (Collins et al., 2009; Campayo et al., 2011; Balhara, 2011).

Diabetes Mellitus and Depression

Depression is nearly twice as common in individuals with diabetes as in those without (Sridhar, 2007; Campayo et al., 2011; Balhara, 2011). This relationship is felt to be bidirectional; having diabetes may increase one's risk of developing depression, and having depression may increase the likelihood of developing diabetes, especially type II diabetes (Sridhar, 2007; Campayo et al., 2011; Balhara, 2011).

The risk of developing diabetes appears to be greatest when the preexisting depression is non-severe, persistent, and untreated (Campayo et al., 2011; Balhara, 2011). The association involves both health-related behavior and physiological abnormalities in the hypothalamic-pituitary-adrenal and sympathoadrenal systems that increase insulin resistance (Campayo et al., 2011).

Given the consequences of these coexisting illnesses (i.e. increased morbidity, mortality, healthcare costs, and decreased quality of life), screening and treatment are vital (Campayo et al., 2011; Balhara, 2011). Successful detection and treatment of depression may prevent the development of type II diabetes in patients at risk. Patients were considered at risk if they had persistent, non-severe depression (Campayo et al., 2011). A study comparing the Patient Health Questionnaire (PHQ-9) and the Hospital Anxiety and Depression Scale (HADS-D), two common self-administered tests used to assess depression, suggested that both are reliable tools. The latter (HADS-D), however, appears to provide results less influenced by somatic symptoms often seen in patients with diabetes in the absence of depression, specifically fatigue, sleep disturbances, and changes in appetite (Reddy et al., 2010). Diagnosing depression without considering somatic symptoms is, however, controversial.

Treatment of depression in diabetics is much the same as in non-diabetics, though one must be aware that antidepressants may affect appetite and blood glucose. Likewise, once depressive symptoms are treated, the patient may reengage in physical activity, which may further influence glycemic control.

The selective serotonin-reuptake inhibitors (SSRIs) are the preferred treatment for depression in diabetics due to their lack of effect on glucose metabolism, lower incidence of weight gain and carbohydrate craving, as well as the lower, but not absent, risk of anticholinergic and cardiac side effects (Goodnick, 1997). However, SSRIs can suppress appetite, enhance insulin sensitivity, and lead to hypoglycemia if diet and medication (oral hypoglycemics, insulin) are not adjusted accordingly (Sridhar, 2007). Tricyclic antidepressants should be avoided in the treatment of depression in patients with diabetes, as studies show a correlation with impaired fasting glucose as well as increased appetite and carbohydrate craving (Goodnick, 1997; Sridhar, 2007).

Treatment for diabetes in light of mental illness should be considered carefully, recognizing that cognitive disorders and symptoms of depression, including low motivation and suicidal ideation, may affect a patient's ability and willingness to comply with recommendations. Likewise, patients with diabetes are at greater risk for suicide than the general population, raising the question about the safety of insulin or oral hypoglycemics for disease management. The frequency of suicide attempts via insulin overdose is unclear, and consequences range from mild to severe, including encephalopathy and death. Among antidiabetic agents used with lethal intent, sulfonylureas were responsible for the greatest number of deaths, though this may be related to the larger type II population, rather than to greater lethality. Medications should be monitored carefully in depressed diabetics, and some studies suggest discontinuation of insulin pumps during acute episodes of depression with suicidal ideation (Russell, Stevens, & Stern, 2009).

Diabetes Mellitus and Anxiety

The prevalence of anxiety disorders, specifically generalized anxiety disorder (GAD), in diabetics is two to three times that in non-diabetics (Collins et al., 2009; Balhara, 2011). As with depression, the presence of comorbid anxiety and diabetes mellitus is associated with elevated HbA1c levels (Balhara, 2011). Treatment of anxiety has been found, in some studies, to improve glycemic control (Grigsby, Anderson, Freedland, Clouse, & Lustman, 2002). It is important to note that the symptoms of anxiety disorders and depressive disorders often overlap, making a very distinct differentiation quite difficult. In most cases, though, treatment is very similar.

The relationship between anxiety and diabetes appears to be bidirectional in type II, but not type I diabetes; the risk of developing incident diabetes following a diagnosis of anxiety is far greater in type II diabetes. It is unclear if diagnosis of anxiety or presence of symptoms predicts onset of diabetes independently or through associated risk factors (later onset of illness, high-fat diet, smoking, etc.) (Engum, 2007).

Studies have shown the presence of incident anxiety in diabetic patients is independent of diabetes subtype. Risk factors associated with more severe anxiety in diabetics include: female gender, presence of diabetes complications, insulin use, unemployment, smoking, and past/present misuse of alcohol. Protective factors associated with a lower risk of developing comorbid anxiety include: older age, structured medical care, private medical insurance, and patient perception of adequate glycemic control (Collins et al., 2009).

In general, anxiety is treated much the same in diabetics as it is in non-diabetics, both pharmacologically and with cognitive behavioral therapy. Caution, however, should be used with pharmacotherapy, such as benzodiazepines and beta blockers, as they may mask the physiological symptoms of hypoglycemia, including tachycardia (Balhara, 2011). Studies suggest selective serotonin reuptake inhibitors are used with greatest frequency, owing to their potential synergistic effects; they have been found to provide adequate control of mood and anxiety symptoms while also improving diabetes self-care (Markowitz et al., 2011).

Diabetes, Eating Disorders, and Eating Disordered Behavior

Despite years of research, it remains controversial as to whether eating disorders, as classified by the DSM-III and DSM-IV TR, are more prevalent in diabetics than in non-diabetics (Herpertz et al., 2001). Some studies have found a high prevalence of eating disorders and subclinical eating disorders in young female diabetic patients (Lloyd et al., 1987; Rosmark et al., 1986; Goodwin, Hoven, & Spitzer, 2003; Larranaga, Docet, & Garcia-Mayor, 2011). A small study focusing on eating disorders and disordered eating habits in young women with type I diabetes showed an incidence of 25% (Pelever et al., 2005). Most studies on the topic focus on young women and adolescents with insulin-dependent diabetes, but more recent work has suggested eating disorders are equally likely in non-insulin-dependent diabetes, though the features of the illness may differ (Herpertz et al., 1998).

In addition to eating disordered behaviors employed by non-diabetics, those with insulin-dependent diabetes frequently turn to insulin omission or underuse as a means to prevent weight gain and/or to promote weight loss. This appears to be the most common disordered eating habit in diabetics, particularly young women with insulin-dependent diabetes (Rodin & Daneman, 1992; Crow et al., 1998; Herpertz et al., 1998, 2001; Peveler et al., 2005). Weight control via this method has been termed *diabulimia* in the literature, though it is not specifically named in the current diagnostic manuals. Some report that this behavior is present in 30% of females with type I diabetes and suggest the initial effect of this behavior is rapid weight loss via glycosuria (Peveler et al., 2005).

Many studies have shown that diabetics engaging in eating disordered behaviors, particularly insulin omission or underuse, are at particularly elevated risk of experiencing physical complications of diabetes. Glycemic control in this population, as measured by HbA1c, is generally poorer than in those without eating disorders or disturbed eating behaviors. Both short-term complications (severe hypoglycemia, diabetic ketoacidosis [DKA]) and long-term complications (growth retardation, neuropathy, nephropathy, cardiovascular disease) are found with higher prevalence in diabetics engaging in eating-disordered behaviors (Rodin & Daneman, 1992; Peveler et al., 2005).

Providers should be suspicious regarding the presence of an eating disorder or disturbance in patients with persistently poor glycemic control, repeated episodes of DKA, and elevated concerns of weight (Larranaga et al., 2011). Screening for eating disorders is difficult in diabetics, as current rating scales generally incorporate items measuring dietary concern that are often prescribed as part of diabetes self-management. Even in the absence of a diagnosed eating disorder or subclinical eating disorder, one would expect these markers to be elevated in diabetics (Crow et al., 1998). There is suspicion that diabetics are at greater risk than non-diabetics of developing eating disorder syndromes secondary to the perceived and actual dietary restraint necessitated by management of their illness. This is particularly true in patients who eat according to a predetermined meal plan rather than in response to hunger and satiety cues. At present, there are no validated screening measures to accurately detect eating disorders in diabetics, though many experts use tools designed for the general population (Larranaga et al., 2011).

There is little in the current literature about prevention of eating disorders in the diabetic population. For those with type I diabetes, particularly young females, some suggest that less restrictive and intensive dietary regimens may decrease their likelihood of developing disordered eating behaviors or diagnosable eating disorders. Others favor interventions aimed at increasing self-esteem and body acceptance, which are often compromised in those with chronic medical conditions (Larranaga et al., 2011). Treatment of eating disorders in those with diabetics is often complicated and is best delivered using a team approach, including physicians, diabetes educators, nutritionists, and therapists (Crow et al., 1998; Larranaga et al., 2011).

At present, there is no consensus about which—insulin pump therapy or multiple daily injections (MDI)—is more appropriate for those with comorbid diabetes mellitus and eating disorders. Recent studies, however, have shown that insulin pump therapy may decrease eating disordered behaviors and HbA1c, in comparison to MDI (Pinhas-Hamiel et al., 2010; Markowitz et al., 2013).

Diabetes Mellitus and Cognitive Changes

Many studies have shown an association between diabetes, both type I and type II, and the presence of cognitive decline (Christman et al., 2011). Cognitive status, as measured by the Mini Mental Status Examination (MMSE), appears to decline faster and further in diabetics in comparison to their non-diabetic cohorts. The most significant deficits were seen in tests of executive functioning and processing speeds (Ravona-Springer et al., 2010).

The exact cause of these cognitive changes remains unclear, and some studies have failed to reveal an association with HbA1c, the blood test reflective of long-term glucose control. Other studies, however, have found a correlation, but suggest that HbA1c is not the most significant predictor of cognitive decline in diabetic patients (Ravona-Springer et al., 2010). Current studies indicate that any of a number of mechanisms may lead to increased rate of cognitive decline, including rapid accumulation of advanced glycosylated end products (AGEs), which lead to tissue damage and inflammation, often in cerebral vasculature. In addition, it is thought that a state of hyperinsulinemia, seen in type II diabetics, may contribute to microvascular damage and may interfere with amyloid precursor protein metabolism, leading to cerebral beta amyloid deposits.

HYPOGLYCEMIA

Symptoms of hypoglycemia may be broken down into two distinct constellations: autonomic and neuroglycopenic effects. The autonomic effects are typically defined as adrenergic or catecholamine-mediated symptoms, including tachycardia, diaphoresis, tremor, weakness, hunger, irritability, and palpitations (McCrimmon, Frier & Deary, 1999; Frier, 2001; Graveling & Frier, 2009; Barendse, Singh, Frier, & Speight, 2012), and these hyperadrenergic symptoms can mimic a panic attack. An inadequate supply of glucose to the central nervous system (CNS), or neuroglycopenia, may result in faintness, headache, blurred vision, lethargy, confusion, dizziness, weakness, incoordination, bizarre behavior, reversible focal neurological findings, seizures, and coma, which typically abates with normalization of glucose levels (McCrimmon et al., 1999; Strachan, 2000; Frier, 2001; Barendse et al., 2012). On formal cognitive testing, "accuracy is often preserved at the expense of speed" (Frier, 2001; Graveling & Frier, 2009).

The brains of the young or the elderly are more vulnerable to longer-lasting effects, and the number of hypoglycemic episodes is predictive of more persistent cognitive deficits (Frier, 2008; Bauduceau, 2010). Additionally, chronic hypoglycemia can lead to considerable personal and familial stress, chronic anxiety, sadness, "tense-tiredness," overt pessimism, irritability, and anger (Frier, 2008). It is now commonly accepted that hypoglycemia is associated with negative mood states, and understood that negative mood states—including anxiety (such as fear of hypoglycemia) or depression—can worsen adherence to a diabetic regimen (Pirraglia & Gupta, 2007; Papelbaum et al., 2011; Rustad, Musselman, & Nemeroff, 2011).

The differential diagnosis of fasting hypoglycemia must include surreptitious administration of either insulin or an oral hypoglycemic agent. Factitious hypoglycemia secondary to one of these agents must be considered prior to pancreatic exploration for an islet cell tumor in any patient with hyperinsulinism. Up to 7% of patients on a sulfonylurea with adequate glycemic control and 25% of patients with type II diabetes on insulin experience one or more episodes of severe hypoglycemia per year (Barendse et al., 2012). The presence of anti-insulin antibodies or low C-peptide levels at the time of hypoglycemia strongly suggests a factitious etiology (Horwitz, 1989). Screening of urine or blood for sulfonylureas is available for patients suspected of surreptitious oral hypoglycemic-agent ingestion.

Historically, there was significant concern regarding the overdiagnosis of hypoglycemia (Cahill & Soeldner, 1974; Gastineau, 1983; Nelson, 1985), as "reactive hypoglycemia" was once a fashionable diagnosis to account for a variety of poorly defined physical and psychological ills (Yager & Young, 1974). The Minnesota Multiphasic Personality Inventory (MMPI) profiles of patients being evaluated for reactive hypoglycemia differed significantly from those of general medical patients, demonstrating the classic "conversion-V" triad (elevated scales Hs and Hy, and relatively lower scale D) suggestive of underlying emotional disturbance as the basis for their somatic complaints (Johnson et al., 1980). In recent years, however, it has become increasingly clear that the major clinical issue with hypoglycemia is the apparently cumulative effect of repeated hypoglycemic episodes, and that "the profound and negative effects of hypoglycemia on mood and emotion are often unrecognized" (Graveling & Frier, 2009). In a recent thorough review of the impact of hypoglycemia on quality of life, it was noted that "the detrimental impact of hypoglycemia extends beyond immediate physical consequences, and may include pervasive cognitive, behavioral, and emotional effects" (Barendse et al., 2012). This same review notes that "chronic mood changes, depression, and even phobia (of hypoglycemia) may be more common in those who have a history of recurrent severe hypoglycemia." This detrimental

impact on mood and quality of life has been noted repeatedly (Gold, MacLeod, Deary, & Frier, 1995; Merbis, Snoek, Kanc, & Heine, 1996; Gold, Frier, MacLeod, & Deary, 1997; Williams, 2010; Fidler, Elmelund Christensen, & Gillard, 2011; Korczak, Pereira, Koulajian, Matejcek, & Giacca, 2011).

An important issue in the psychopharmacological management of patients with hypoglycemia is the risk of beta-blocker therapy. Early misdiagnosis of hypoglycemia as an anxiety disorder and treatment with agents whose action blocks the normal response to hypoglycemia may prevent the subjective experience of potentially lethal hypoglycemia. This mimics, and can potentially accelerate, the impaired awareness of hypoglycemia that can develop and is more common in elderly patients who have a long history of diabetes. Additionally, there is some suggestion that the use of antidepressants can impair glycemic control (Dijkgraaf, 2008), leading to hyperglycemia or hypoglycemia (Khoza, 2011), so serum glucose levels should be monitored more closely if any medication is added.

DEVIATIONS IN GONADAL HORMONES

MALE HYPOGONADISM

Male hypogonadism of any etiology may cause significant psychological distress and impaired social adjustment. Low self-esteem and self-confidence and feelings of inadequacy, isolation, and alienation are common.

KLINEFELTER'S SYNDROME AND XXY KARYOTYPES

The XXY karyotypes, the most common human chromosomal abnormality, occur in 1 of 500 live male births (DeLisi et al., 2005). Individuals with XXY chromosomes are generally characterized by tall stature, abnormal spermatogenesis, small testes, and breast tissue development (DeLisi et al., 2005; Slim et al., 2009). Klinefelter's syndrome, and other XXY karyotypes, has been reported in association with a wide variety of psychiatric disorders, including mental retardation, personality disorders, depression, bipolar disorder, sexual deviance, neuroses, alcoholism, paranoid states, and schizophrenia (Caroff, 1978; Swanson & Stipes, 1969; DeLisi et al., 2005).

Studies have shown a four- to five-fold increase in the presence of schizophrenia in men with XXY karyotype in comparison to their XY cohorts. Interestingly, it is thought that auditory hallucinations, more than other psychotic symptoms, have been associated with the presence of a second X chromosome in men (DeLisi et al., 2005). The incidence of Klinefelter's syndrome is five times higher in males who are in the mental health and penal systems than in males in the general population (Smyth and Bremner, 1998).

The most consistent association is a form of personality disorder characterized by passivity, dependency, and low social drive; it is thought that such traits may be related to androgen deficiency, although the exact mechanism remains unclear (Swanson & Stipes, 1969). While major depressive disorder is seen in the XXY population, it is often difficult to separate this from personality traits characteristic of these people; namely, social isolation, passivity, and disinterest (Slim et al., 2009). In addition to standard treatment for depression in men with XXY genotypes, including psychotherapy and antidepressant medications, some studies have proven testosterone replacement therapy is effective in not only promoting development of secondary sexual characteristics, but also improving self-esteem, and, as a result, mood and anxiety (Smyth & Bremner, 1998). This remains controversial.

Cognitive and learning difficulties are common in patients with Klinefelter's. The deficits are seen most often in verbal IQ scores, speech and language acquisition and recognition, as well as in memory (DeLisi et al., 2005; Smyth & Bremner, 1998). Some studies have also shown a higher incidence of attention-deficit hyperactivity disorder (ADHD) and dyslexia in these males. The incidence of mental retardation increases with the number of supernumerary X chromosomes (Smyth & Bremner, 1998).

LOW TESTOSTERONE SYNDROME

Depression is often under-recognized and under-treated in the aging male population. It remains a serious problem, though, as evidenced by the increasing rates of suicide among this cohort. In the United States, suicide rates are highest in men over 65 years of age. This phenomenon is not unique to the United States. According to the World Health Organization (WHO), men over the age of 75 years had the highest rate of suicide in all but one country reporting. Experts remain unsure as to what predisposes this population to depression and suicide (Carnahan & Perry, 2004).

It remains controversial whether men, like women, experience "menopause." Literature within the fields of endocrinology, urology, and gerontology suggest that a male equivalent exists and have named it "the male climacteric," "andropause," and "low testosterone syndrome (LTS)" (Sternbach, 1998). For the purposes of this section, we will refer to it as LTS.

In healthy males, testosterone secretion peaks approximately at age 20 and steadily declines thereafter. Levels decrease more significantly after age 50 (Seidman & Walsh, 1999). The serum testosterone level at which one is diagnosed with LTS remains non-standardized, as the decline in hormone levels occurs gradually throughout life (Carnahan & Perry, 2004). Studies have shown up to 20% of males 60 years and older may have testosterone levels considered to be lower than normal (Seidman & Walsh, 1999).

The effect of declining testosterone levels on mood and anxiety continues to be unclear and inconsistent. Some have described a syndrome of depressed mood, increased anxiety, insomnia, irritability, and poor memory (Sternbach, 1998). Because of confounding factors, namely comorbid medical conditions, weight, alcohol, and tobacco use, and external stressors, it remains unclear if hypogonadism or LTS can cause depressed mood, increase stress-related vulnerability, or lead to resistance to standard antidepressant treatments (Carnahan & Perry, 2004).

Anecdotal reports suggest that testosterone replacement, orally, parenterally, or transdermally, can improve mood, energy, libido, sense of well-being, sleep, and appetite, in addition to other physical changes (Seidman & Walsh, 1999; Carnahan & Perry, 2004). There are, however, few long-term, placebo-controlled studies of testosterone replacement in elderly men, and it is important to note the treatment is not without potentially serious side-effects.

Given the overlap of symptoms in depressive syndromes and LTS, there is little evidence to support obtaining serum testosterone levels in all elderly men who present with depressed mood, low libido, and decreased energy (Sternbach, 1998). Testosterone testing and replacement may be reserved for men with treatment-refractory depression and/or dysthymia (Carnahan & Perry, 2004).

POLYCYSTIC OVARIAN SYNDROME

Polycystic ovarian syndrome (PCOS) is the most common reproductive endocrine condition in women and is characterized by chronic anovulation, obesity, insulin resistance, clinical hyperandrogenism, infertility, male-pattern baldness, and hirsutism (Rassi et al., 2010; Cipkala-Gaffin, Talbott, Song, Bromberger, & Wilson, 2012). It can affect 5–10% of women of reproductive age (Kerchner et al., 2009; Rassi et al., 2010; Cipkala-Gaffin et al., 2012).

Psychiatric illness, specifically major depression and bipolar disorder, are seen with high frequency in this population. Studies have shown the prevalence of depression can reach 50% in women with PCOS (Rassi et al., 2010). Additionally, higher rates of anxiety and body dissatisfaction with resultant eating disorders have been demonstrated (Himelein & Thatcher, 2006). Studies suggest that most of the physical manifestations of PCOS lead to anxiety and decreased health-related quality of life but do not, alone, account for the increased incidence of mood disorders in this population (Kerchner et al., 2009). Specifically, hirsutism and infertility were not correlated with increased levels of depression (Himelein & Thatcher, 2006). Increased weight and body mass index associated with PCOS, however, appear to increase a woman's risk of depression (Kerchner et al., 2009; Cipkala-Gaffin et al., 2012).

The comorbidity of bipolar disorder, types I and II, and PCOS is of high interest and may be bidirectional. Medications used to treat bipolar disorder, specifically valproate, may promote polycystic ovaries or lead to other menstrual irregularities (Himelein & Thatcher, 2006; Rassi et al., 2010). Rasgon and his colleagues completed a small outpatient study that suggested the menstrual irregularities and PCO symptoms seen in women with bipolar disorder are a result of hormonal abnormalities intrinsic to the mental illness, rather than of the treatment itself (Rasgon et al., 2000). Most studies to date have been small and inconclusive, and more research is warranted to better understand the complex relationship between bipolar disorder and polycystic ovarian syndrome (Himelein & Thatcher, 2006).

PCOS has also been associated with a higher prevalence of eating disorders, specifically bulimia nervosa and binge-eating disorder, in comparison to non-PCOS populations (Himelein & Thatcher, 2006; Kerchner et al., 2009). It is believed this is related to higher rates of body dissatisfaction (Himelein & Thatcher, 2006). Given the high rate of mental illness in women with PCOS, it is important to regularly screen for and aggressively treat these diseases in the PCOS population (Kerchner et al., 2009).

PRE-MENSTRUAL DYSPHORIC DISORDER

Pre-menstrual dysphoric disorder (PMDD) was classified as an official mood disorder and added to the appendix of the *Diagnostic and Statistical Manual of Mental Disorders IV* (DSM-IV) in 1994. It is classified as a *Depressive disorder not otherwise specified*, and the diagnosis remains controversial (Di Giulio & Reissing, 2006; Pearlstein & Steiner, 2008; Zukov et al., 2010). PMDD affects less than 10% of women (Zukov et al., 2010).

Diagnosis of PMDD requires five or more of 11 possible symptoms present during the late luteal phase, approximately days 21–28 of the menstrual cycle. At least one of the five symptoms must be depressed mood, anxiety, affective lability, or irritability. Other symptoms include anhedonia, poor concentration, decreased energy, a sense of being overwhelmed, changes in appetite with particular cravings, changes in sleep, headaches, joint/muscle pain, and abdominal bloating. For diagnosis, these symptoms must be of sufficient severity to cause functional impairment (Di Giulio & Reissing, 2006; Pearlstein & Steiner, 2008). In actively menstruating females, symptoms typically remit within one week of menses (Di Giulio & Reissing, 2006; Ptacek et al., 2010). PMDD is absent after menopause, during pregnancy, and in other situations that may interrupt the cycle of ovulation (Di Giulio & Reissing, 2006). The diagnosis and treatment of this disorder are discussed in detail in Chapter 67.

The cause of PMDD is as yet unknown, but research has focused on serotonin, gonadal and other hormones, as well as genetics and environmental stresses (Di Giulio & Reissing, 2006; Pearlstein & Steiner, 2008). Women with PMDD are more likely to have a history of depression and are more likely to develop subsequent depression following a diagnosis of PMDD (Di Giulio & Reissing, 2006).

Thus far, derangements and dysregulation of the serotonergic system are the most probable causes of PMDD. This is not surprising, giving the significant overlap in symptomatology in PMDD and other depressive illnesses. In addition to depressed mood, decreased serotonin levels have been found to be associated with symptoms more specific for PMDD, including mood swings, self-deprecation, poor impulse control, and decreased pain threshold (Di Giulio & Reissing, 2006).

Treatment studies also support the serotonin hypothesis of PMDD causality, as SSRIs have proven efficacious in decreasing symptoms. A systematic review demonstrated a response rate seven times greater in PMDD patients treated with an SSRI in comparison to those treated with placebo. Improvement of PMDD symptoms with SSRI treatment is far more rapid in comparison to major depressive disorder; women can experience improvements in symptoms within a few days of treatment initiation. As such, some experts opt to use SSRI medications three to seven days before the onset of menses and discontinue use at the onset of menstruation or shortly thereafter. Dosage requirements for women with PMDD are often lower than for those with depression. Studies comparing the efficacy of intermittent versus continuous use of SSRIs in the treatment of PMDD have, thus far, been inconclusive (Di Giulio & Reissing, 2006; Pearlstein & Steiner, 2008; Ptacek et al., 2010).

CONSULTATION BETWEEN ENDOCRINOLOGY AND PSYCHIATRY

Evaluation of endocrine disorders has traditionally occurred only after the demonstration of systemic signs and symptoms, including dermatological changes, electrolyte and metabolic disturbances, and other evidence of hormonal abnormalities, trigger the diagnostic workup. Expanding awareness of cognitive, affective, and behavioral changes associated with endocrinopathies should facilitate earlier recognition of these treatable disorders.

The personal experience of the psychiatrist determines his or her level of comfort and confidence when administering and interpreting endocrine tests. If a psychiatrist chooses not to pursue an endocrine evaluation when clinically indicated, the primary care physician should purse the endocrine consultation and serve as intermediary between the specialties if necessary. With collaboration, both the psychiatrist and the endocrinologist can define their limits of confidence with the evaluation and treatment of secondary mental disorders due to endocrine dysfunction. Certainly, having a specialist in each facet of the issue involved and communicating with each other would be expected to result in a better, more precise balance being achieved.

SUMMARY

Endocrine disturbances frequently mimic or exacerbate psychiatric disturbances, and psychiatric illness can clearly exacerbate endocrinological disease; if not directly, then as a result of decreased compliance with treatment. "High-risk" groups, which require careful endocrine and psychiatric evaluation, include the following:

- Patients with mood and other unusual behavioral symptoms and coexistent cognitive dysfunction, especially geriatric patients

- Patients with inconsistent or atypical presentations of psychiatric disorders

- Patients with mental symptoms that are refractory to standard psychiatric treatments

- Patients with symptoms of dementia or other cognitive dysfunction syndromes

- Patients with known preexisting endocrine abnormalities

- Patients with affective symptoms after closed-head injury

- Patients with a family history of either psychiatric or endocrine disorders

- Patients on medications known to affect endocrine functioning (amiodarone, lithium, antipsychotics)

- Patients with a history of brain tumor

CLINICAL PEARLS

- The onset of symptoms of hypothyroidism is often gradual and, especially in the elderly, mimics the development of a degenerative dementia.

- In contrast to cortical dementias such as Alzheimer's disease and frontotemporal degeneration, the cognitive disorder of myxedema does not present with discrete cortical syndromes like aphasia, anomia, apraxia, and frontal disinhibition.

- In Cushing's syndrome, depression is extremely common, and persistent elation rare.

- The majority of cases of primary hyperparathyroidism are asymptomatic (Benge et al., 2009).

- The diagnosis of Addison's disease commonly is delayed. In one cohort of 216 patients with adrenal insufficiency, 41% received a false diagnosis of a psychiatric illness (Bleiken et al., 2010).

- Risperidone is the atypical antipsychotic most likely to cause hyperprolactinemia.

- Acromegaly is associated with depression, psychosis, and amotivational syndrome (De Sousa, 2009).

- Those with insulin-dependent diabetes and eating disorders frequently turn to insulin omission or underuse as a means to prevent weight gain and to promote weight loss.

- The presence of anti-insulin antibodies or low C-peptide levels at the time of hypoglycemia strongly suggests a factitious etiology (Horwitz, 1989).

- Beta-blocker therapy may prevent the normal sympathetic response to potentially lethal hypoglycemia in insulin-dependent diabetics.

- In Klinefelter's syndrome, XXY, boys with hypogonadism, cognitive and learning difficulties are seen most often in verbal IQ scores, speech and language acquisition and recognition, as well as in memory (DeLisi et al., 2005; Smyth & Bremner, 1998).

DISCLOSURE STATEMENTS

Dr. Sterenson, Dr. Sola, and Dr. Sampson have no conflicts of interest. Dr. Sampson has research funded by the National Institute of Mental Health (NIMH) and has been involved in research with equipment support from Neuronetics, Inc.

REFERENCES

Addison, T. (1868). On the constitutional and local effects of disease of the suprarenal capsules. In S. Wilkes & E. Daldey (Eds.), *A collection of the unpublished writings of Thomas Addison* (Vol. 36). London: New Sydenham Society.

Aimaretti, G., Ambrosio, M.R., diSomma, C., Gasperi, M., Cannavo, S., et al. (2005). Residual pituitary function after brain injury-induced hypopituitarism: a prospective 12-month study. *Journal Clinical Endocrionology & Metabolism, 90,* 6085–6092.

Anglin, R. F., Rosebush, P. I., & Mazurek, M. F. (2006). The neuropsychiatric profile of Addison's disease: Revisiting a forgotten phenomenon. *Journal of Neuropsychiatry and Clinical Neurosciences, 18,* 450–459.

Balhara, Y. P. (2011). Diabetes and psychiatric disorders. *Indian Journal of Endocrinology & Metabolism, 15,* 274–283.

Barendse, S., Singh, H., Frier, B. M., & Speight, J. (2012). The impact of hypoglycaemia on quality of life and related patient-reported outcomes in Type 2 diabetes: a narrative review. *Diabetes Medicine, 29,* 293–302.

Bavisetty, S., Bavisetty, S., McArthur, D. L., Dusick, J. R., Wang, C., et al. (2008) Chronic hypopituitarism after traumatic brain injury: Risk assessment and relationship to outcome. *Neurosurgery, 62,* 1080–1093.

Benge, J. F., Perrier, N. D., Massman, P. J., Meyers, C. A., Kayl, A. E., & Wefel, J. S. (2009). Cognitivie and affective sequelae of primary hypeaparathyroidism and early response to parathyroidectomy. *Journal of International Neuropsychology Society, 15,* 1002–1011.

Bleicken, B., Hahner, S., Ventz, M. and Quinkler, M. (2010). Delayed diagnosis of adrenal insufficiency is common: A cross sectional study in 216 patients. *American Journal of the Medical Sciences, 339*(6), 525–531.

Bleuler, M. (1951). The psychopathology of acromegaly. *Journal of Nervous & Mental Disease, 113,* 497–511.

Borer, M. S., & Bhanot, V. K. (1985). Hyperparathyroidism: neuropsychiatric manifestations. *Psychosomatics, 26,* 597–601.

Brown, R. S., Fischman, A., & Showalter, C. R. (1987). Primary hyperparathyroidism, hypercalcemia, paranoid delusions, homicide, and attempted murder. *Journal of Forensic Science, 32,* 1460–1463.

Brownlie, B. E. W., Rae, A. M., Walshe, J. W. B., & Wells, J. E. (2000). Psychosis associated with thyrotoxicosis—"thyrotoxic psychosis." A report of 18 cases, with statistical analysis of incidence. *European Journal of Endocrinology, 142,* 438–444.

Cahill, G. F., Jr., & Soeldner, J. S. (1974). "A non-editorial on non-hypoglycemia." *New England Journal of Medicine, 291,* 905–906.

Campayo, A., Gomez-Biel, C. H., & Lobo, A. (2011). Diabetes and depression. *Current Psychiatry Reports, 13,* 26–30.

Carnahan, R. M., & Perry, P. J. (2004). Depression in aging men: The role of testosterone. *Drugs & Aging, 21,* 361–376.

Caroff, S. N. (1978). Klinefelter's syndrome and bipolar affective illness: A case report. *American Journal of Psychiatry, 135,* 748–749.

Chang, Y. C., Tsai, J. C., & Tseng, F. Y. (2006). Neuropsychiatric disturbances and hypopituitarism after traumatic brain injury in an elderly man. *Journal of Formosan Medical Association, 105,* 172–176.

Christman, A. L., Matsushita, K., Gottesman, R. F., Mosley, T., Alonso, A., Coresh, J., et al. (2011). Glycatedhaemoglobin and cognitive decline: The Atherosclerosis Risk in Communities (ARIC) study. *Diabetologia, 54,* 1645–1652.

Cipkala-Gaffin, J., Talbott, E. O., Song, M. K., Bromberger, J., & Wilson, J. (2012). Associations between psychological symptoms and life satisfaction in women with polycystic ovary syndrome. *Journal of Women's Health (Larchmont), 21,* 179–187.

Cohen, L. M., Greenberg, D. B., & Murray, G. B. (1984). Neuropsychiatric presentation of men with pituitary tumors (the 'Four A's'). *Psychosomatics, 25,* 925–928.

Cohn, J. B., Brust, J., DiSerio, F., & Singer, J. (1985). Effect of bromocriptine mesylate on induced hyperprolactinemia in stabilized psychiatric outpatients undergoing neuroleptic treatment. *Neuropsychobiology, 13,* 173–179.

Coker, L. H., Rorie, K., Cantley, L., Kirkland, K., Stump, D., Burbank, N., et al. (2005). Primary hyperparathyroidism, cognition, and health-related quality of life. *Annals Surgery, 242,* 642–650.

Collins, M. M., Corcoran, P., & Perry, I. J. (2009). Anxiety and depression symptoms in patients with diabetes. *Diabetes Medicine, 26,* 153–161.

Crow, S. J., Keel, P. K., & Kendall, D. (1998). Eating disorders and insulin-dependent diabetes mellitus. *Psychosomatics* , r39:233–243.

Cushing, H. (1932). The basophil adenomas of the pituitary body and their clinical manifestations. *Johns Hopkins Medical Journal, 50,* 137–195.

Davis, A. T. (1989). Psychotic states associated with disorders of thyroid function. *International Journal of Psychiatry & Medicine, 19,* 47–56.

DeLisi, L. E., Maurizio, A. M., Svetina, C., Ardekani, B., Szulc, K., Nierenberg, J., et al. (2005). Klinefelter's syndrome (XXY) as a genetic model for psychotic disorders. *American Journal of Medical Genetics Part B: Neuropsychiatric Genetics, 135B,* 15–23.

Demartini, B., Scarone, S., Pontiroli, A. E., & Gambini, O. (2010). Prevalence of depression in patients affected by subclinical hypothyroidism. *Panminerva Medica, 52,* 277–282.

De Sousa, A. (2009). Depression in acromegaly treated with escitalopram and cognitive therapy. *Indian Journal Psychological Medicine, 31,* 50–51.

Di Giulio, G., & Reissing, E. D. (2006). Premenstrual dysphoric disorder: Prevalence, diagnostic considerations, and controversies. *Journal of Psychosomatic Obstetrics & Gynaecology, 27,* 201–210.

Duggal, H. S., & Singh, I. (2007). Lithium-induced hypercalcemia and hyperparathyroidism presenting with delirium. *Progress in Neuropsychopharmacology Biological Psychiatry, 32,* 903–904.

Engum, A. (2007). The role of depression and anxiety in onset of diabetes in a large population-based study. *Journal of Psychosomatic Research, 62,* 31–38.

Esposito, S., Prange, A. J., & Golden, R. N. (1997). The thyroid axis and mood disorders: Overview and future prospects. *Psychopharmacology Bulletin, 33*(2), 205–217.

Ezzat, S. (1997). Acromegaly. *Endocrinology Metabolism Clinics of North America, 26,* 703–723.

Fava, G. A., Fava, M., Kellner, R., Serafini, E., & Mastrogiacomo, I. (1981). Depression, hostility and anxiety in hyperprolactinemic amenorrhea. *Psychotherapy & Psychosomatics, 36,* 122–128.

Feldman, A. Z., Shrestha, R. T., & Hennessey, J. V. (2013). Neuropsychiatric manifestations of thyroid disease. *Metabolism Clinics of North America, 42,* 453–476.

Fidler, C., Elmelund Christensen, T., & Gillard, S. (2011). Hypoglycemia: an overview of fear of hypoglycemia, quality-of-life, and impact on costs. *Journal of Medical Economics, 14,* 646–655.

Frier, B. M., (2001). Hypoglycaemia and cognitive function in diabetes. *International Journal of Clinical Practice Supplement, 123,* 30–37.

Furman, K., & Ezzat, S. (1998). Psychological features of acromegaly. *Psychotherapy & Psychosomatics, 67,* 147–153.

Gastineau, C. F. (1983). Is reactive hypoglycemia a clinical entity? *Mayo Clinic Proceedings, 58,* 545–549.

Gatewood, J. W., Organ, C. H., Jr., & Mead, B. T. (1975). Mental changes associated with hyperparathyroidism. *American Journal of Psychiatry, 132,* 129–132.

Gold, A. E., Frier, B. M., MacLeod, K. M., & Deary, I. J. (1997). A structural equation model for predictors of severe hypoglycaemia in patients with insulin-dependent diabetes mellitus. *Diabetes Medicine, 14,* 309–315.

Gold, A. E., MacLeod, K. M., Deary, I. J., & Frier, B. M. (1995). Hypoglycemia-induced cognitive dysfunction in diabetes mellitus: effect of hypoglycemia unawareness. *Physiological Behavior, 58,* 501–511.

Goodnick, P. J. (1997). Diabetes mellitus and depression: Issues in theory and treatment. *Psychiatric Annals, 27,* 353–359.

Goodwin, R. D., Hoven, C. W., & Spitzer, R. L. (2003). Diabetes and eating disorders in primary care. *International Journal of Eating Disorders, 33,* 85–91.

Goyal, A., Chumber, S., Tandon, N., Lal, R., Srivastava, A., & Gupta, S. (2001). Neuropsychiatric manifestations in patients of primary hyperparathyroidism and outcome following surgery. *Indian Journal of Medical Sciences, 55,* 677–686.

Graveling, A. J., & Frier, B. M. (2009). Dementia and hypoglycemic episodes in patients with type 2 diabetes mellitus. *Journal of the American Medical Association, 302,* 843.

Gregoor, P. S., & de Jong, G. M. (2007). Lithium hypercalcemia, hyperparathyroidism, and cinacalcet. *Kidney International, 71,* 470.

Grigsby, A. B., Anderson, R. J., Freedland, K. E., Clouse, R. E., & Lustman, P. J. (2002). Prevalence of anxiety in adults with diabetes: A systematic review. *Journal of Psychosomatic Research, 53,* 1053–1060.

Haden, S. T., Stoll, A. L., McCormick, S., Scott, J., & Fuleihan, G. el-H. (1997). Alterations in parathyroid dynamics in lithium-treated subjects. *Journal of Clinical endocrinology and Metabolism, 82,* 2844–2888.

Hall, R. C. (1983). Psychiatric effects of thyroid hormone disturbance. *Psychosomatics, 24,* 7–11, 15–18.

Heath, D. A. (1989). Primary hyperparathyroidism. Clinical presentation and factors influencing clinical management. *Endocrinology Metabolism Clinics of North America, 18,* 631–646.

Heath, D. A., Wright, A. D., Barnes, A. D., Oates, G. D., & Dorricott, N. J. (1980). Surgical treatment of primary hyperparathyroidism in the elderly. *British Medical Journal, 280,* 1406–1408.

Heath, H., 3rd, Hodgson, S. F., & Kennedy, M. A. (1980). Primary hyperparathyroidism. Incidence, morbidity, and potential economic impact in a community. *New England Journal of Medicine, 302,* 189–193.

Hecht, A., Gershberg, H., & St. Paul, H. (1975). Primary hyperparathyroidism. Laboratory and clinical data in 73 cases. *Journal of the American Medical Association, 233,* 519–526.

Heinrich, T. W., & Grahm, G. (2003). Hypothyroidism presenting as psychosis: Myxedema madness revisited. *Primary Care Companion Journal of Clinical Psychiatry, 5*(6), 260–266.

Herpertz, S., Albus, C., Kielmann, R., Hagemann-Patt, H., Lichtblau, K., Kohle, K., et al. (2001). Comorbidity of diabetes mellitus and eating disorders: A follow-up study. *Journal of Psychosomatic Research, 51,* 673–678.

Herpertz, S., Wagener, R., Albus, C., Kocnar, M., Wagner, R., Best, F., et al. (1998). Diabetes mellitus and eating disorders: A multicenter study on the comorbidity of the two diseases. *Journal of Psychosomatic Research, 44,* 503–515.

Himelein, M. J., & Thatcher, S. S. (2006). Polycystic ovary syndrome and mental health: A review. *Obstetric & Gynecological Survey, 61,* 723–732.

Howland, R. H. (1993). Thyroid dysfuncton in refractory dep0ression: implications for pathophysiology and treatment. *Journal of Clinical Psychiatry, 54*(2). 47–54.

Horwitz, D. L. (1989). Factitious and artifactual hypoglycemia. *Endocrinology Metabolism Clinics of North America, 18,* 203–210.

Joborn, C., Hetta, J., Johansson, H., Rastad, J., Agren, H., Akerstrom, G., et al. (1988). Psychiatric morbidity in primary hyperparathyroidism. *World Journal of Surgery, 12,* 476–481.

Johnson, D. D., Dorr, K. E., Swenson, W. M., & Service, F. J. (1980). Reactive hypoglycemia. *Journal of the American Medical Association, 243,* 1151–1155.

Kerchner, A., Lester, W., Stuart, S. P., & Dokras, A. (2009). Risk of depression and other mental health disorders in women with polycystic ovary syndrome: A longitudinal study. *Fertility & Sterility, 91,* 207–212.

Khaldi, S., Dan, B., Basiaux, P., De Nutte, N., Kornreich, C., & Gorman, J. M. (2006). Manic episode precipitated by withdrawal of hormone replacement therapy in severe hypothyroidism. *Journal of Psychiatric Practice, 12*(6), 409–410.

Konopelska, S., Quinkler, M., Strasburber, C. J., & Ventz, M. (2008). Difficulties in the medical treatment of prolactinoma in a patient with schizophrenia—a case report with a review of the literature. *Journal of Clinical Psychopharmacology, 28,* 120–122.

Korczak, D. J., Pereira, S., Koulajian, K., Matejcek, A., & Giacca, A. (2011). Type 1 diabetes mellitus and major depressive disorder: evidence for a biological link. *Diabetologia, 54,* 2483–2493.

Lane, J. (2010). Hypopituitarism after brain injury. *British Journal of Neurosurgery, 24,* 8.

Larranaga, A., Docet, M. F., & Garcia-Mayor, R. V. (2011). Disordered eating behaviors in type 1 diabetic patients. *World Journal of Diabetes, 2,* 189–195.

Lee, K. A., Park, K. T., Yu, H. M., Jin, H. Y., Baek, H. S., & Park, T. S. (2013). Subacute thyroiditis presenting as acute psychosis: A case report and literature review. *Korean Journal of Internal Medicine, 28*(2), 242–246.

Lloyd, G. G., Steel, J. M., & Young, R. J. (1987). Eating disorders and psychiatric morbidity in patients with diabetes mellitus. *Psychotherapy & Psychosomatics, 48,* 189–195.

Mallette, L. E. & Eichorn, E. (1986) Effects of lithium carbonae o human Calcium metabolism. *Archives of Internal Medicine, 146,* 770–776.

Markowitz, J. T., Alleyn, C. A., Phillips, R., Muir, A., Young-Hyman, D., & Laffel, L. M. (2013). Disordered eating behaviors in youth with type 1 diabetes: Prospective pilot assessment following initiation of insulin pump therapy. *Diabetes Technology & Therapeutics, 15,* 428–433.

Markowitz, S. M., Gonzalez, J. S., Wilkinson, J. L., & Safren, S. A. (2011). A review of treating depression in diabetes: Emerging findings. *Psychosomatics, 52,* 1–18.

McAllion, S. J., & Paterson, C. R. (1989). Psychiatric morbidity in primary hyperparathyroidism. *Postgraduate Medical Journal, 65,* 628–631.

Mc Crimmon, R. J., Frier, B. M., & Deary, I. J. (1999). Appraisal of mood and personality during hypogylaemia in human subjects. *Physiology & Behavior, 1,* 27–33.

McHenry, C. R., & Lee, K. (1996). Lithium therapy and disorders of the parathyroid glands. *Endocrine Practice, 2,* 103–109.

Merbis, M. A., Snoek, F. J., Kanc, K., & Heine, R. J. (1996). Hypoglycaemia induces emotional disruption. *Patient Education Counseling, 29,* 117–122.

Nelson, R. L. (1985). Hypoglycemia: Fact or fiction? *Mayo Clinic Proceedings, 60,* 844–850.

Pae, C., Mandelli, L., Han, C., Ham, B., Masand, P. S., Patkar, A. A., et al. (2009). Thyroid hormones affect recovery from depression during antidepressant treatment. *Psychiatry and Clinical Neurosciences, 63,* 305–313.

Papelbaum, M., Moreira, R. O., Coutinho, W., Kupfer, R., Zagury, L., et al. (2011). Depression, glycemic control and type 2 diabetes. *Diabetology & Metabolic Syndrome, 3,* 26.

Park, Y. J., Lee, E. J., Lee, Y. J., Choi, S. H., Park, J. H., Lee, S. B., et al. (2010). Subclinical hypothyroidism (SCH) is not associated with metabolic derangement, cognitive impairment, depression or poor quality of life (QoL) in elderly subjects. *Archives of Gerontology and Geriatrics, 50,* e68–e73.

Pearlstein, T., & Steiner, M. (2008). Premenstrual dysphoric disorder: Burden of illness and treatment update. *Journal of Psychiatry & Neuroscience, 33,* 291–301.

Pereira, A. M., Tiemensma, J., & Romijn, J. A. (2010). Neuropsychiatric disorders in Cushing's syndrome. *Neuroendocrinology, 92*(1), 65–70.

Perovich, R. M., Lieberman, J. A., Fleischhacker, W. W., & Alvir, J. (1989). The behavioral toxicity of bromocriptine in patients with psychiatric illness. *Journal of Clinical Psychopharmacology, 9,* 417–422.

Peveler, R. C., Bryden, K. S., Neil, H. A., Fairburn, C. G., Mayou, R. A., et al. (2005). The relationship of disordered eating habits and attitudes to clinical outcomes in young adult females with type 1 diabetes. *Diabetes Care, 28,* 84–88.

Pinhas-Hamiel, O., Graph-Barel, C., Boyko, V., Tzadok, M., Lerner-Geva, L., & Reichman, B. (2010). Long-term insulin pump treatment in girls with type 1 diabetes and eating disorder—is it feasible? *Diabetes Technology & Therapeutics, 12,* 873–878.

Pirraglia, P. A., & Gupta, S. (2007). The interaction of depression and diabetes: A review. *Current Diabetes Review, 3,* 249–251.

Popkin, M. K., & Mackenzie, T. B. (1980). Psychiatric presentations of endocrine dysfunction. In R. C. W. Hall (Ed.), *Psychiatric presentations of medical illness* (pp. 139–156). New York: Spectrum Publications.

Rasgon, N. L., Altshuler, L. L., Gudeman, D., Burt, V. K., Tanavoli, S., Hendrick, V., et al. (2000). Medication status and polycystic ovary syndrome in women with bipolar disorder: A preliminary report. *Journal of Clinical Psychiatry, 61,* 173–178.

Rassi, A., Veras, A. B., dos Reis, M., Pastore, D. L., Bruno, L. M., Bruno, R. V., et al. (2010). Prevalence of psychiatric disorders in patients with polycystic ovary syndrome. *Comprehensive Psychiatry, 51,* 599–602.

Rao, M. L., Hiemke, C., Grasmader, K., & Baumann, P. (2001). Olanzapine: pharmacology, pharmacokinetics and therapeutic drug monitoring. *Fortschritte der Neurologie Psychiatrie, 69,* 510–517.

Ravona-Springer, R., Luo, X., Schmeidler, J., Wysocki, M., Lesser, G., Rapp, M., et al. (2010). Diabetes is associated with increased rate of cognitive decline in questionably demented elderly. *Dementia & Geriatric Cognitive Disorders, 29,* 68–74.

Reddy, P., Philpot, B., Ford, D., & Dunbar, J. A. (2010). Identification of depression in diabetes: The efficacy of PHQ-9 and HADS-D. *British Journal of General Practice, 60,* e239–e245.

Rifai, M. A., Moles, J. K., & Harrington, D. P. (2001). Lithium-induced hypercalcemia and parathyroid dysfunction. *Psychosomatics, 43,* 359–361.

Rodin, G. M., & Daneman, D. (1992). Eating disorders and IDDM. A problematic association. *Diabetes Care, 15,* 1402–1412.

Roman, S. A., Sosa, J. A., Pietrzak, R. H., Snyder, P. J., Thomas, D. C., et al. (2011). The effects of serum calcium and parathyroid hormone changes on psychological and cognitive function in patients undergoing parathyroidectomy for primary hyperparathyroidism. *Annals Surgery, 253,* 131–137.

Rosmark, B., Berne, C., Holmgren, S., Lago, C., Renholm, G., & Sohlberg, S. (1986). Eating disorders in patients with insulin-dependent diabetes mellitus. *Journal of Clinical Psychiatry, 47,* 547–550.

Russell, K. S., Stevens, J. R., & Stern, T. A. (2009). Insulin overdose among patients with diabetes: A readily available means of suicide. *Primary Care Companion Journal of Clinical Psychiatry, 11,* 258–262.

Rustad, J. K., Musselman, D. L., & Nemeroff, C. B. (2011). The relationship of depression and diabetes: pathophysiological and treatment implications. *Psychoneuroendocrinology, 36,* 1276–1286.

Sathya, A., Radhika, R., Mahadevan, S., & Sriram, U. (2009). Mania as a presentation of primary hypothyroidism. *Singapore Medical Journal, 50*(2), e65–e67.

Seidman, S. N., & Walsh, B. T. (1999). Testosterone and depression in aging men. *American Journal of Geriatric Psychiatry, 7,* 18–33.

Service, F. J. (1997). Hypoglycemia. *Endocrinology Metabolism Clinics of North America, 26,* 937–955.

Sheehan, H. L. (1939). Simmonds disease due to post-partum necrosis of the anterior pituitary. *Quarterly Journal of Medicine, 8,* 277–307.

Sievers, C., Ising, M., Pfister, H., Dimopoulou, C., Schneider, H. J., et al. (2009). Personality in patients with pituitary adenomas is characterized by increased anxiety-related traits: comparison of 70 acromegalic patients with patients with non-functioning pituitary adenomas and age- and gender-matched controls. *European Journal of Endocrinology, 160,* 367–373.

Silverberg, S. J., Fitzpatrick, L. A., & Bilezikian, J. P. (1995). Primary hyperparathryoidism. In K. L. Becker (Ed.), *Principles and practice of endocrinology and metabolism* (pp. 512–520). Philadelphia, PA: Lippincott.

Silverberg, S. J., Walker, M. D., & Bilezikian, J. P. (2013). Asymptomatic primary hyperparathyroidism. *Journal of Clinical Densitometry, 16*, 14–21.

Popovic, V., Aimaretti, G., Casaneuva, F. F., & Ghigo, E. (2005). Hypopituitarism following traumatic brain injury. *Frontiers of Hormone Research, 33*, 33–44.

Popovic, V., Pekic, S., Pavlovic, D., Maric, N., Jasovic-Gasic, M., et al. (2004). Hypopituitarism as a consequence of traumatic brain injury (TBI) and its possible relation with cognitive disabilities and mental distress. *Journal Endocrinological Investigation, 27*, 1048–1054.

Simpson, H., Savine, R., Sonksen, P., Bengtsson, B. A., Carlsson, L., et al. (2002). Growth hormone replacement therapy for adults: ito the new millenium. *Growth Hormone and IGF Research 12*, 1–33.

Slim, I., Kissi, Y. E., Ayachi, M., Maaroufi-Beizig, A., Mlika, S., Ach, K., et al. (2009). Diagnosis and treatment difficulties of psychiatric symptoms in Klinefelter syndrome: A case report. *British Medical Journal Case Reports*, pii: bcr08.2008.0741. doi: 10.1136/bcr.08.2008.0741.

Sloand, J. A., & Shelly, M. A. (2006). Normalization of lithium-induced hypercalcemia and hyperparathyroidism with cinacalcet hydrochloride. *American Journal of Kidney Diseases, 48*, 832–837.

Smyth, C. M., & Bremner, W. J. (1998). Klinefelter syndrome. *Archives of Internal Medicine, 158*, 1309–1314.

Solomon, B. L., Schaaf, M., & Smallridge, R. C. (1994). Psychologic symptoms before and after parathyroid surgery. *American Journal of Medicine, 96*, 101–106.

Sonino, N., & Fava, G. A. (2001). Psychiatric disorders associated with Cushing's syndrome: Epidemiology, pathophysiology and treatment. *CNS Drugs, 15*(5), 361–373.

Sridhar, G. R. (2007). Psychiatric co-morbidity & diabetes. *Indian Journal of Medical Research, 125*, 311–320.

Sternbach, H. (1998). Age-associated testosterone decline in men: Clinical issues for psychiatry. *American Journal of Psychiatry, 155*, 1310–1318.

Stowell, C. P., & Barnhill, J. W. (2005). Acute mania in the setting of severe hypothyroidism. *Psychosomatics, 46*(3), 259–261.

Swanson, D. W., & Stipes, A. H. (1969). Psychiatric aspects of Klinefelter's syndrome. *American Journal of Psychiatry, 126*, 814–822.

Szalat, A., Mazeh, H., & Freund, H. R. (2009). Lithium-associated hyperparathyroidism: report of four cases and review of the literature. *European Journal Endocrinology, 160*, 317–323.

Thomsen, A. F., Kvist, T. K., Andersen, P. K., & Kessing, L. V. (2005). Increased risk of developing affective disorder in patients with hypothyroidism: A register-based study. *Thyroid, 15*(7), 700–707.

Tiemensma, J., Biermasz, N. R., van der Mast, R. C., Wassenaar, M. J., Middelkoop, H. A., et al. (2010). Increased psychopathology and maladaptive personality traits, but normal cognitive functioning, in patients after long-term cure of acromegaly. *Journal Clinical Endocrinology & Metabolism, 95*, E392–402.

Tor, P. C., Lee, H. Y., & Fones, C. S. L. (2007). Late-onset mania with psychosis associated with hypothyroidism in an elderly Chinese lady. *Singapore Medical Journal, 48*(4), 354–357.

Urban, R. J., Harris, P., & Masel, B. (2005). Anterior hypopituitarism following traumatic brain injury. *Brain Injury, 19*, 349–358.

Walker, M. D., Rubin, M., & Silverberg, S. J. (2013). Nontraditional manifestations of primary hyperparathyroidism. *Journal of Clinical Densitometry, 16*, 40–47.

Webb, E. A., O'Reilly, M. A., Clayden, J. D., Seunarine, K. K., Chong, W. K., Dale, N., et al. (2012). Effect of growth hormone deficiency on brain structure, motor function and cognition. *Brain, 135*, 216–227.

Yager, J., & Young, R. T. (1974). Non-hypoglycemia is an epidemic condition. *New England Journal of Medicine, 291*, 907–908.

Zukov, I., Ptacek, R., Raboch, J., Domluvilova, D., Kuzelova, H., Fischer, S., et al. (2010). Premenstrual dysphoric disorder—review of actual findings about mental disorders related to menstrual cycle and possibilities of their therapy. *Prague Medical Report, 111*, 12–24.

56.

GASTROENTEROLOGY

Donna B. Greenberg

THE BRAIN–GUT AXIS

For Franz Alexander, ulcerative colitis was one of the psychosomatic illnesses with chronic parasympathetic stimulation like asthma, as distinct from the chronic sympathetic stimulation of hypertension, diabetes, rheumatoid arthritis, and thyrotoxicosis. He thought that a specific conflict that could be expressed in overdrive of the parasympathetic or sympathetic nervous system could lead to specific diseases. "First, the functional disturbance of a vegetative organ is caused by chronic emotional disturbance; and second, the chronic functional disturbance gradually leads to tissue changes, and to irreversible organic disease" (Alexander, 1950). Engel pointed to a transient state of helplessness and hopelessness in patients with ulcerative colitis that could be alleviated but not cured with psychotherapy (Engel, 1958, 1961).

Gut feelings of anxiety, anguish, revulsion, or a need to flee—stomach butterflies, the lump in the throat, loss of appetite, nausea, or hyperactive bowels—are part of the human experience. The mind is connected to the gut. Nervous diarrhea was mentioned in nineteenth-century medical texts and reviewed in a 1936 *New England Journal of Medicine* paper (Aronowitz & Spiro, 1988; Sullivan, 1936). Selye (1956) linked stress and ulcers, but the role of *Helicobacter pylori* and the effectiveness of proton pump inhibitors pushed psychic causes of ulcer into the background. Nonetheless, peptic ulcer still has a psychosomatic component: patients with existing ulcers can become more symptomatic when they are under stress (Choung & Talley, 2008), and the questions remain as to why many more patients are infected with *H. pylori* than have ulcers, and how *H. pylori* and emotional factors interact in the production of non-ulcer dyspepsia. Emotion can increase gastric acid production (Wolff & Wolff, 1943; Brady et al., 1958), and animal studies have shown that an unpredictable, uncontrolled environment facilitates the development of ulcers. The availability of behavioral coping strategies can reduce vulnerability (Overmier & Murison, 2013). An epidemiological literature supports the relationship between life stress and peptic ulcer, its severity and tendency to recur. (Levenstein, 2002).

Since the time of Alexander, the neuroanatomy of the interactions between the brain and the enteric nervous system has been more clearly delineated (Mayer et al., 2006; Bonaz & Bernstein, 2013; Mayer et al., 2011). The *brain–gut axis,* better understood through functional neuroimaging studies, refers to the connection between the autonomous nervous system and circumventricular organs. The sensory circumventricular organs—the area postrema, the subfornical organ, and the organum vasculosum of the lamina terminalis—sense molecules in plasma and pass information to the rest of the brain and autonomic nervous system. The activity of the secretory component of the circumventricular organs (the subcommissural organ, the posterior pituitary, the pineal gland, median eminence and intermediate lobe of the pituitary) is based on feedback from the brain and external stimuli.

The central autonomic system integrates visceral information from the enteric nervous system embedded in the lining of the GI tract with sensory information from other peripheral sites and affective and sensory information from the limbic system. Homeostatic emotions—the motivations and feelings that come with changes in the body's condition—are associated with autonomic responses and behavior that corrects an imbalance: for instance, low glucose leads to hunger and eating behavior (Mayer et al., 2006). Other typical visceral sensations are thirst, vasomotor flush, satiation, fullness, and urgency. The proposed framework for this process is that homeostatic emotions have a sensory dimension processed in the anterior insula and an affective/motivational dimension processed in the dorsal anterior cingulate cortex. The right anterior insula seems to hold the subjective awareness of homeostatic emotions as well as emotions of anger, fear, disgust, happiness, trust, love, empathy, and social exclusion (Mayer et al., 2008). The sensory signals of hunger or pain usually remain in the background to modulate homeostasis and color the memories of experience. This system provides a context for visceral memories.

The parasympathetic nervous system includes the vagus nerves that innervate the foregut and the sacral nerves that innervate the hindgut. Sacral parasympathetic pelvic nerves and mixed splanchnic nerves with both afferent and efferent fibers communicate between the gut and the thoracolumbar and sacral spinal cord. The vagus nerves are 90% afferent, and vagal afferent neurons respond to both mechanical and chemical signals; for example, distention of the stomach or intestines and differences in the composition of food in the stomach. Vagal cholinergic efferents have anti-inflammatory actions as well as effects on gastrointestinal (GI) motility. The sympathetic nerves are half afferent and half efferent and transmit signals of visceral pain to the central nervous system. The sympathetic nervous system is typically pro-inflammatory.

Autonomic afferent axons, whether traveling through parasympathetic or sympathetic nerves, terminate in the nucleus tractus solitaries in the medulla.

Because the circumventricular organs are outside the blood–brain barrier, they are also sensitive to circulation of emetic stimuli and to the inflammatory cytokines that modulate the hypothalamic-pituitary-adrenal (HPA) axis and the production of glucocorticoids. The prefrontal-amygdaloid complex integrates the balance of sympathetic and parasympathetic activity and the HPA axis. The prefrontal cortex modulates the outflow of vagus nerve efferents. The hypothalamic corticoid releasing factor system adapts to chronic stress. This affects the intestinal response, including the intestinal barrier, luminal microbiota, and the intestinal immune response.

Mayer posits that interoceptive memories of complex homeostatic states with both affective and motivational dimensions like pain, nausea, hunger, and satiation may be encoded during development from infancy so that a child has a value-based map of the world analogous to Damasio's concept of "somatic markers." The somatic markers may be memories of body states encoded as meta-representations in the orbitofrontal cortex (Mayer, 2011). In this way, unconscious visceral memories may color current experience and decision making. These distresses may come to the foreground for functional GI patients who are more attentive, perhaps more able to perceive these signals, and more distressed by them.

FUNCTIONAL GASTROINTESTINAL DISORDERS

The functional gastrointestinal disorders identified by symptoms in the absence of known anatomical and biochemical abnormalities have been defined by consensus of a group of international clinical investigators and the third iteration, the Rome III criteria, were further developed with the hope that the definitions will lead to more clarity in the pathophysiology (Drossman, 2006). Rome III categories for functional gastrointestinal disorders (Tack et al., 2006) include:

1. *Functional esophageal disorders*: functional heartburn, chest pain of presumed esophageal origin, functional dysphagia and globus;

2. *Gastroduodenal disorders*: functional dyspepsia (postprandial distress and epigastric pain); belching disorders: aerophagia, excessive belching, and belching; nausea and vomiting disorders: chronic idiopathic nausea, functional vomiting, and cyclic vomiting syndrome;

3. *Functional bowel disorders*: irritable bowel syndrome, functional bloating, diarrhea, and constipation;

4. *Functional abdominal pain syndrome*;

5. *Functional gallbladder and sphincter of Oddi disorders*: gallbladder dysfunction, biliary sphincter of Oddi disorder, pancreatic sphincter of Oddi disorder; and

6. *Functional anorectal disorders*; fecal incontinence; anorectal pain (chronic proctalgia, levator ani syndrome, unspecified anorectal pain); functional defecation disorder (dyssynergic defecation and inadequate defecatory propulsion).

Historically, there has been an overlap between functional GI disorders and gastrointestinal motility disorders (Drossman et al., 2006; Ouyang & Locke, 2007). The functional disorders are contrasted to conditions with clear evidence for GI dysmotility like pelvic floor dyssynergia, Hirschsprung's disease, scleroderma, colonic inertia, and gastroparesis (Ouyang and Locke, 2007). The syndromes of pain in different functional disorders may not be distinct, as a patient may transition from one to another. The pattern of pain is similar to that in diabetic gastroparesis, celiac disease, and inflammatory bowel disease. These chronic GI disorders overlap with anxiety, depression, and somatization, and with other persistent pain disorders like painful bladder syndrome/interstitial cystitis, temporomandibular joint (TMJ) disorder, and fibromyalgia (Mayer & Tillisch, 2011).

The Rome group and others emphasized that effective treatment of patients with functional GI disorders requires an understanding of the psychosocial background against which symptoms occur (Jones et al., 2007). Patients do better who are not suffering from depression, panic, neurasthenia, a history of abuse, and illness worry. Histories of physical or sexual abuse are high (30–56%) in referral populations. A review of the psychosocial aspects of functional gastrointestinal disorders (Levy et al., 2006) highlighted the importance of the physician–patient relationship and a stepped-care approach, educating the patient about the condition, offering symptomatic treatment and simple behavioral or life style changes, and then the opportunity for a psychological assessment and assessment of psychiatric diagnoses. After medical therapies such as lifestyle changes, dietary manipulation, prokinetics, proton pump inhibitors, laxatives, bulking agents, antidiarrheals, and antispasmodics, relaxation therapies can be combined with an antidepressant medication (Jackson et al., 2000) and then more formal psychotherapies. Those with most evidence of depression, panic, history of abuse, and illness worry would benefit from the addition of thoughtful psychological care.

GLOBUS

Globus, the sensation of a lump in the throat, something stuck, or tightness in the throat, has been attributed to esophageal dysfunction. In some patients it may evolve into a fear of swallowing. The symptom is extremely common, mostly in women, and is often seen by otolaryngologists. Direct laryngoscopy and barium studies of swallowing are a critical part of the evaluation to rule out abnormalities, including cancer or other anatomical causes of the lump in the throat. Patients may try to dislodge the "lump" by swallowing repeatedly. Gastroesophageal reflux was noted in about 25% of patients with globus (Clouse et al., 1999), and patients are commonly treated with proton pump inhibitors. The term *globus hystericus* has evolved to *globus pharyngeus* (Lee & Kim, 2012). Historically, globus has been associated with anxiety, phobia, and grief. It has been the fourth most common symptom in somatization disorder. Antidepressants can be useful if there are other signs of panic disorder or depression (Clouse et al., 1999).

FUNCTIONAL DYSPEPSIA

Proton pump inhibitors and prokinetic drugs are often used for functional dyspepsia with consideration of gastroesophageal reflux disease and the possibility of delayed gastric emptying. Buspirone, the 5HT 1A-receptor agonist, has been shown to relax the proximal stomach in healthy subjects and to improve functional dyspepsia better than placebo (Tack et al., 2012). Venlafaxine also enhances gastric accommodation and reduces sensations of distension, but a randomized controlled study of venlafaxine did not find benefit for functional dyspepsia (van Kerkhoven et al., 2008). Particularly in women, tricyclic antidepressants reduce sensations in response to food, including nausea and delayed gastric emptying (Grover et al., 2013).

CYCLIC VOMITING SYNDROME

Cyclic vomiting syndrome (CVS) is a syndrome of three or more recurrent discrete episodes of vomiting, variable intervals of completely normal health between episodes, and stereotyped episodes repetitive in symptom onset and duration, with no laboratory or imaging findings suggesting another diagnosis. By contrast, functional vomiting occurs once or more per week without evidence of an eating disorder, rumination (a gastrointestinal disorder of effortless regurgitation), or another psychiatric diagnosis (Olden & Chepyala, 2008). CVS is mostly seen in children with a history or family history of migraine headaches. In adults, CVS like functional vomiting is rare. Both are associated with migraines. The prevalence of anxiety and depression is not elevated in CVS, but sometimes there is a distinct aura that precedes emesis like an aura often precedes a migraine. Triggers for this syndrome are like the triggers for migraine: menses, infection, motion sickness, sleep deprivation, infection, stress, and foods with high tyramine content such as cured meats, aged cheeses, and pickled meat or fish. Anti-migraine medications like low-dose propranolol, sumatriptan, cyproheptadine, valproic acid, carbamazepine, and phenobarbital have been used, as well as erythromycin as a prokinetic agent. There are no randomized studies of treatment, but low-dose tricyclic antidepressants have led to improvement in small studies. Zonisamide 400 mg/day or levetiracetam have been effective in some cases (Choung et al., 2008; Choung et al., 2013).

In the differential diagnosis of CVS is *cannabis hyperemesis syndrome*. In fact, CVS more than functional vomiting is associated epidemiologically with young men who use cannabis (Choung et al., 2008, Choung et al., 2013). Cannabis hyperemesis syndrome—recurrent episodes of severe nausea and intractable vomiting with colicky or epigastric pain—is associated with daily heavy cannabis use for years. Patients learn that relief comes with hot baths or showers and may compulsively bathe (Chepyala & Olden, 2008). Episodes last one to several days and may repeat over months. Relief comes with cessation of cannabis use. Patients are often constantly sipping water (Sullivan et al., 2010). The mechanism is unknown (Sontineni et al., 2009).

IRRITABLE BOWEL SYNDROME

Irritable bowel syndrome (IBS) is a condition of chronic abdominal pain and altered bowel habits categorized by the predominant pattern: diarrhea, constipation, or both. The definition suggests that symptoms occur at least three days per month and are associated with change in stool frequency or form and relief with defecation. IBS occurs in 10–15% of the population, 1.5 times as often in women; and only a small proportion of these (15%) seek care. Diarrhea is associated with cramps, urgency, frequent stools while awake, and mucus in the stool (American College of Gastroenterology [ACG] IBS Task Force, 2009).

Mechanisms

IBS is attributed to an interaction between intestinal microbiota, the mucosal barrier, and immune activation, nerve plasticity, visceral hypersensitivity, enteroendocrine factors, and the amplification of these contributors by anxiety and depression. Visceral hypersensitivity is thought to contribute to abdominal pain and reflect altered neurotransmission. Low thresholds to sensory perception have been found in esophagus, stomach, small bowel, and colon; however, only a portion of patients with IBS have such hypersensitivity. Gut enterochromaffin cells contain 90% of human serotonin (Barbara et al., 2011).

Visceral sensation is modulated by the 5-HT3 receptor and non 5-HT3 receptor–dependent mechanisms on vagal or spinal sympathetic afferent nerves; and mucosal 5HT may have a role in IBS. Some patients with IBS have an infectious trigger, with IBS following acute infectious enteritis. Abnormal microbiota may activate mucosal innate immune responses that increase epithelial permeability, activate nociceptive sensory pathways, and dysregulate the enteric nervous system (Simren et al., 2013). Some interventions to alter the intestinal microbiome—diet, probiotics, fiber, and non-absorbable antibiotics—have been used clinically; however, the significance of the flora for a particular patient cannot be defined clinically beforehand.

The role of altered motor function in the colon and the pelvic floor has gained importance. The disturbances of colonic motility can be documented by the radiopaque-marker transit time, scintigraphy, or wireless motility capsule (Rao et al., 2011). Pelvic-floor retraining for evacuation disorders can have a role for anismus (the failure of the pelvic floor muscles to relax with defecation), pelvic floor dyssynergia or puborectalis spasm, and descending perineum syndrome, all syndromes that meet criteria for IBS in adults. These may also cause bloating that worsens throughout the day (Camilleri & DiLorenzo, 2012).

Factors that should set off alarms about the diagnosis of IBS and warrant further workup are older age and male gender, weight loss, nocturnal symptoms, family history of colon cancer, anemia, rectal bleeding, and recent antibiotic use. (Spiller et al., 2007).

Interventions

A sequence of dietary changes is often one aspect of treatment. Food sensitivity—both immune-mediated and pseudo-allergic—can be considered (Bischoff & Crowe, 2005). Food elimination may begin with exclusion of gas-producing foods like onions. The role of dietary fermentable oligosaccharides, disaccharides, monosaccharides, and polyols (FODMAPs) in causing symptoms has led to exclusion of apples, cherries, peaches, nectarines, artificial sweeteners, most lactose-containing foods, legumes, broccoli, Brussels sprouts, cabbage, and peas (Halmos et al., 2013). A trial exclusion of gluten is also a consideration (Boettcher & Crowe, 2013).

The ACG review of the evidence on medications and strategies for treatment of IBS (ACG, 2009) supported short-term benefit of antispasmodics like hyoscine, cimetropium, pinaverium, and peppermint oil. Loperimide is effective for diarrhea. The benefit of fiber was not clear. Bifidobacteria and some combinations of probiotics have offered benefit, but lactobacilli has not.

Both 5HT3 antagonists and 5HT4 agonists have been used for IBS symptoms (Barbara et al., 2011). Of the drugs developed for IBS, alosetron, the 5-HT3 receptor antagonist, is only used in women with severe IBS and diarrhea who have not responded to other therapies. Lubiprostone, a selective C-2 chloride channel activator, has been useful at 8 mg bid in women with constipation. The 5-HT4 receptor agonist tegaserod helpful for female patients with constipation was taken off the market due to side effects.

THE PSYCHOLOGICAL DIMENSION

IBS is more common in families, presumably from both genetic and environmental factors. Parents can be role models for sickness behavior; also, parents' responses to a child's illness behavior can reinforce it. Diminishing this reinforcement can reduce recurrent abdominal pain in children (Levy et al., 2006). A history of sexual, physical, and/or emotional abuse is common in patients with functional gastrointestinal disorders as it is in other conditions of chronic pain. A history of trauma and current post-traumatic stress disorder is often found (Irwin et al., 1996). The connection between previous trauma and IBS has been attributed to concurrent psychiatric disorder, psychological distress, the tendency to report many somatic symptoms, increased hypervigilance about symptoms, maladaptive coping styles like catastrophic thinking, lack of social support, amplified sensory signals, and increased sympathetic function with hyperarousal (Levy et al., 2006; Halpert & Drossman, 2005). Many patients are depressed or anxious. IBS may overlap and co-occur with fibromyalgia or chronic fatigue syndrome and has been seen as one of the functional somatic syndromes with higher than expected psychiatric comorbidity (Barsky & Borus, 1999; Nater et al., 2013).

Gastroenterologists caring for IBS patients are encouraged to interview their patients in a comprehensive way, more typical of a psychiatric evaluation than a typical medical examination (Levy et al., 2006). This acknowledges that those who come for treatment are more chronically distressed, in more chronic pain, and that their nervous system and psychological context affect treatment outcome. Understanding patient's concerns, like fear of cancer, the impact of the disorder on their life, and the psychological context at times of exacerbations makes a difference. Treatment of anxiety and depression improves bowel and other symptoms. (Spiller et al., 2007).

Two recent meta-analyses have concluded that antidepressants are helpful for IBS (Ford et al., 2012; Ruepert et al., 2011). Both tricyclic antidepressants and selective serotonin-reuptake inhibitors (SSRIs) have shown benefit. Tricyclic antidepressants have a better record of treatment for visceral pain, and the analgesic effect occurs at doses below the usual antidepressant range. Most studies with SSRIs have used paroxetine or fluoxetine (Grover & Camilleri, 2013). Since the analgesic benefit of antidepressants comes with lower doses, an effect that may be separate from their effect on mood, clinicians can describe these drugs as central analgesics (Grover & Drossman, 2008).

Some psychotropic medications have been studied for specific effects on the gut. In regard to colonic motility, compliance, and sensation, buspirone had no effect. Venlafaxine increases colonic compliance, relaxes tone, reduces postprandial colonic contraction, and tends to increase thresholds for sensation and gas. It reduces pain-sensation ratings as provoked by graded distension. Venlafaxine does not alter colonic transit time nor does paroxetine or buspirone (Chial et al., 2003). Citalopram has been shown to reduce pain, bloating, and overall symptoms independent of anxiety, depression, and colonic sensorimotor function (Grover, 2013).

For the psychiatrist familiar with the profile of antidepressants, a reasonable strategy would be to use tricyclic antidepressants for their analgesic effects and constipating side effects as well as antidepressant effects in patients with IBS with prominent diarrhea. SSRIs may be neutral in the patients with more prominent constipation (Grover & Drossman, 2008). It is worth noting that a specific SSRI can occasionally make diarrhea worse; sertraline in depression studies caused diarrhea in 18% of subjects, compared to 9% in placebo (Micromedex, 2009). Both venlafaxine and duloxetine have about a 10% rate of constipation as an adverse effect, and paroxetine, although anticholinergic in part, has a similar rate of both constipation and diarrhea. Olanzapine has some benefit for nausea, and quetiapine 25–100 mg has had benefit for augmenting treatment in patients with severely refractory symptoms (Grover & Drossman, 2008).

Focused attention on antidepressant medication adherence, as practiced in collaborative care studies for depression and titration of medication in the context of the physician–patient relationship, would improve the outcome of IBS patients (Sayuk et al., 2007). One-quarter of outpatients seen by gastroenterologists do not adhere to the antidepressant regimens offered by the gastroenterologist for their IBS.

Interpersonal psychodynamic therapy has been shown to be beneficial in patients with severe IBS, reducing healthcare costs over the following year (Creed et al., 2003). Patients with social inhibition and dependency had a longer disease duration, and improvements in interpersonal difficulties independently predicted better health status (Hyphantis et al., 2009).

Behavioral therapy has also proven more effective than placebo at relieving individual IBS symptoms (Drossman et al., 2003; Spiller et al., 2007). Strategies of cognitive behavioral treatment include reframing maladaptive beliefs, reducing over-responsiveness to stress, changing catastrophizing, reducing anxiety about symptoms, reducing shame or guilt, and changing maladaptive behavior (Grover & Drossman, 2008). Benefits are reported with relaxation therapy, biofeedback, and hypnotherapy, which has shown benefit in otherwise refractory patients (Spiller et al., 2007).

While antidepressants are known to benefit these patients, ameliorating chronic pain and affective syndromes, the way these medications should interplay with other gastrointestinal medications and treatments is not clear (Wald, 2014). The medical psychiatrist and psychologist, watching more closely how the patients care for themselves and how their symptoms interact with the patients' roles and life stresses, have an opportunity to make psychotherapeutic interventions, especially in the most distressed patients.

FECAL INCONTINENCE

Fecal incontinence, the involuntary passage of stool or the inability to prevent expulsion of stool, is a serious cause of embarrassment, social isolation, and narrowing of the patient's world. In the elderly, it is sometimes a reason for nursing home placement. The incontinence may come as *urge incontinence* when the patient actively tries to prevent the stool from being released before reaching the bathroom; or passively as a consequence of involuntary loss without awareness. Sometimes patients' clothes are soiled by fecal seepage after normal evacuation (Shah et al., 2012). Patients may not mention incontinence to their physicians or may talk about it as fecal urgency or incomplete evacuation. Risk factors are history of pelvic radiation, obstetrical trauma, depression, chronic diarrhea, and urinary incontinence. In older patients, anatomical changes in the anorectal unit leading to decreased squeeze pressures come with age, stroke, dementia, and diabetes. Fecal incontinence due to seepage sometimes occurs from fecal impaction due to constipation.

Lactose, fructose, or sorbitol malabsorption can contribute to urgency. Sorbitol is an osmotic laxative found in dietetic foods that diabetics may seek out. Other contributors to incontinence are mental status changes that impair awareness or planning for getting to the bathroom in time. Conditions that impair peripheral nerve pathways like diabetes, polyneuropathies, cauda equina syndrome (compressing the sacral nerves), toxic neuropathy, and multiple sclerosis explain some of the loss of effective external and sphincter pressure. From the history, the clinician can gather information on stool consistency, urgency, lack of sensation of stool passage, and urinary incontinence. From the rectal examination, resting and squeezing anal sphincter tone, masses, hemorrhoids, prolapse, and intact sensation can be defined. Anorectal manometry and ultrasound are the most common tests if surgery is considered for sphincter injury (Lazarescu et al., 2009).

INFLAMMATORY BOWEL DISEASE

In the modern age, depression or anxiety are not seen simply to be risk factors for the development of ulcerative colitis or Crohn's disease. Perceived psychological stress and depression at the onset of illness, however, are risk factors for relapse of the disease. Patients with higher depressive scores at the time of a flare-up of inflammatory bowel disease were more apt to relapse sooner (Mittermaier et al., 2004). However, at least one study did not find that the diagnosis of major depressive disorder predicted relapse (Vidal et al., 2006).

Careful evaluation of depression and consideration of antidepressants has a key role in the care of patients with inflammatory bowel disease (Tache & Bernstein, 2009). Depressive disorder or generalized anxiety has been noted in 20% of patients with Crohn's disease or ulcerative colitis (van Assche et al., 2013), and depressive symptoms are associated with active disease (Hauser et al., 2011). Lifetime diagnosis of major depressive disorder is higher in IBD patients, and panic disorder is even more common. In one study, those with depression had developed the disease younger and been diagnosed younger. Depression often antedated the inflammatory disease by more than two years (Walker et al., 2008). Furthermore, in Crohn's disease, patients were more apt to achieve remission with infliximab if they did not have major depression (Persoons et al., 2005). While psychosocial treatment thus far has not prevented relapses, one study of psychodynamic psychotherapy and relaxation treatment in patients with Crohn's disease did show a reduction in healthcare utilization after psychological treatment (Deter et al., 2007).

About one-third of patients at a center for IBD feel the need of psychological treatment, especially if they are younger with limited social support. They benefit from relaxation exercises, adjunctive psychotherapy, and antidepressants. A retrospective case-control study suggests that cognitive behavioral therapy and antidepressants may improve the course of IBD, reducing relapse rates, the use of corticosteroids, and endoscopies (Goodhand et al., 2012). However, there has not been a definitive prospective study to show this. Corticosteroids are still used in flares of the disease and may contribute an element of affective instability.

IBS symptoms may also occur in the setting of healed anti-inflammatory disease (Mikocka-Walus et al., 2007), and gastroenterologists commonly use antidepressants to alleviate these symptoms in patients with IBD. The prevalence of depression in patients with IBD, and the suggestion that depression may interfere with remission or hasten relapse, argues for screening and treatment of depression in those with moderately severe IBD. The medical psychiatrist can contribute by championing multimodal treatment for depression and anxiety, paying attention to sleep and function, and using psychotherapies that facilitate coping.

CELIAC DISEASE AND NON-CELIAC GLUTEN SENSITIVITY

CELIAC DISEASE

In celiac disease, predisposed individuals cannot tolerate gluten, and gluten causes intestinal malabsorption, intestinal villi atrophy, and chronic inflammation of the jejunal mucosa. This is a genetically determined immune-mediated syndrome based on inappropriate response of T-lymphocytes to the gluten antigen. It affects multiple organs, including the skin, thyroid, heart, pancreas, spleen, liver, and nervous system. Patients with malabsorption, weight loss, steatorrhea, postprandial abdominal pain, and bloating should be tested for celiac disease.

Confirmation of a diagnosis of celiac disease should be based on a combination of findings from the medical history, physical examination, serology, and upper endoscopy with histological analysis of multiple biopsies of the duodenum. Both serology and biopsy should be performed while the patient is on a gluten-containing diet. Immunoglobulin-A (IgA) anti–tissue transglutaminase antibody (TTG) is the preferred single test for detection of celiac disease. A total IgA level is often obtained to eliminate the possibility that IgA itself is low. If IgA is low and the TTG is negative, then IgG TTG and deamidated gliadin peptide can be obtained. The test for antibodies against native gliadin is not recommended to detect the diagnosis, as it is less sensitive and is associated with too many false positives.

Patients with a first-degree family member who has a confirmed diagnosis of celiac disease should be tested if they show possible signs or laboratory evidence of celiac disease. Patients with type 1 diabetes who have some digestive symptoms should be tested for celiac disease. *HLA-DQ12/DQ8* genotyping should not be used routinely in the initial diagnosis of celiac disease but can be used to rule out the disease in patients with certain conditions like Down's syndrome. If the genotype is not *HLA-DQ12/DQ8*, then celiac disease in Down's syndrome patients is unlikely. This *HLA-DQ* typing test might also be used to try to exclude celiac disease prior to embarking on a formal gluten challenge (Rubio-Tapia et al., 2013).

Psychiatric symptoms in celiac disease include depression, anxiety, irritability, and apathy. Treatment with a gluten-free diet leads to recovery of the jejunum but may take years. In a cross-sectional survey of 2,265 adult patients with celiac disease in the Netherlands, the lifetime prevalence of self-reported depressive symptoms was 39%. Keeping a gluten-free diet for longer than five years was associated with a lower risk of current depressive symptoms, compared to the diet for less than two years (van Hees, 2013). Nutritional deficiencies—for instance, iron, folate, and vitamin D deficiency—should be considered as contributors to affective presentations in patients with this cause of malabsorption.

NON-CELIAC GLUTEN SENSITIVITY

A syndrome of gluten sensitivity in patients with IBS who do not have celiac disease has been suggested to cause GI symptoms, including bloating, abdominal pain, and persistent fatigue (Biesiekierski et al., 2011). Gluten sensitivity does not seem to have a familial risk or be associated with autoimmune disorders or intestinal malignancy (Biesiekierski, 2011; Lundin, 2012).

A diagnosis of non-celiac gluten sensitivity should be considered only after celiac disease has been excluded with appropriate testing (Rubio-Tapia, 2013). Non-celiac gluten sensitivity cannot be reliably differentiated from celiac disease, because the two syndromes overlap. Celiac serology (TTG) and small-intestinal histology, both obtained when the patient is consuming a gluten-rich diet, and *HLA-DQ* typing to rule out celiac disease if negative, are needed to differentiate between the two disorders.

The possibility of gluten sensitivity has led to the popularity of gluten-free diet trials; a growing number of people come to gastroenterologists with complaints of gluten intolerance. The cause of the sensitivity is not well understood (Mooney et al., 2013). Fermentable fructans present in wheat rather than gluten itself may provoke symptoms. Some patients who report gluten sensitivity respond to reduction of fermentable, poorly absorbed, short-chain carbohydrates (FODMAPs), or foods that cause gas (Biesiekierski et al., 2013b), rather than specifically to gluten-sparing diets.

The symptoms of non-celiac gluten sensitivity include abdominal discomfort, bloating, pain or diarrhea, and fatigue, and may extend to headaches, foggy mind, depression, musculoskeletal pains, and skin rash (Volta & De Giorgio, 2012; Sapone et al., 2012). As clinicians have been skeptical about the entity, some patients have been referred for psychiatric assessment (Mooney et al., 2013). In one study, somatization or abnormal personality traits were not found to explain symptoms (Brottveit et al., 2012). A gluten-free diet has also been suggested for autism and autism spectrum disorders, but a recent review documented that there is insufficient evidence to support this treatment (Buie, 2013).

One retrospective study found that patients with non-celiac gluten sensitivity were composed of two distinct groups: one with wheat sensitivity alone, and one associated with multiple-food hypersensitivity. The first seemed similar to celiac disease, and the second similar to patients with food allergy. Compared to controls with IBS, the whole group had a higher frequency of anemia, weight loss, self-reported wheat intolerance, and (in infancy) coexistent atopy and food allergy. The main histological feature is eosinophil infiltration of the duodenal and colon mucosa (Carroccio et al., 2012; Sanders & Aziz, 2012). Patients with non-celiac wheat sensitivity were those with IBS-like symptoms, negative TTG and anti-endomysium IgA antibodies, no villous atrophy on duo-denal histology, negative IgE-mediated immuno-allergy tests to wheat, and resolution of symptoms on a gluten-free diet and their reappearance on double-blind placebo-controlled wheat challenge. (This time-consuming double-blind placebo-controlled challenge has been used primarily as a research tool.)

The boundaries of the entity of gluten sensitivity have not been fully clarified. A response to a gluten-free diet or exacerbation of symptoms due to a gluten-containing diet is not sufficient to prove that these symptoms are due to specific effects of gluten (Biesiekierski et al., 2013a). Clarification of the disorder depends on further validation with diagnostic criteria and a better understanding of mechanisms of action.

HEPATIC ENCEPHALOPATHY

For the medical psychiatrist, hepatic encephalopathy (HE) is a diagnosis to consider in the confused patient, especially when asterixis is present and the patient has liver disease. In fact, when the syndrome is overt, there is marked confusion, incoherent speech, and altered consciousness, ranging from lethargy to coma. The mechanism of HE is not fully understood. However, the main explanation is that ammonia produced in the colon by intestinal bacteria gets into the systemic circulation when the liver is impaired and when portal-systemic shunts occur. Ammonia adversely affects neurotransmission, consciousness, and behavior. (Mas et al., 2006).

In the normal condition, ammonia is metabolized to urea by the liver; when the liver is injured, ammonia levels rise. Astrocyte swelling causes low-grade cerebral edema and a neuroinhibitory state related to elevated glutamine. The level of ammonia does not always correlate with the severity of encephalopathy. Elevated ammonia is only one component of the disorder; chronic inflammation and hyponatremia may also play a role.

Precipitants of overt encephalopathy are infection, GI bleeding, dehydration, hyponatremia, hypokalemia, metabolic alkalosis, renal failure, and constipation; benzodiazepines, narcotics, or alcohol; increase of protein intake; portal vein or hepatic vein thrombosis and portal-systemic shunts, the latter either spontaneous or iatrogenic. Treatment of acute HE requires general supportive care and a search for precipitants. Nutritional and metabolic precipitants should be corrected when feasible. Although proteins may be restricted initially, guidelines suggest that this restriction need not be prolonged (Blei et al., 2001).

Lactulose is a first-line treatment, facilitating the passage of ammonia into the colonic lumen. This drug can cause gas, abdominal cramping, and a sweet taste, as well as diarrhea. The dose is first hourly until the first evaluation, and then adjusted to achieve two to three soft bowel movements per day (Blei et al., 2001). Neomycin, a non-absorbable antibiotic, is also FDA-approved for the acute syndrome. Rifaximin has also been used in addition to lactulose for the overt syndrome but is primarily approved for secondary prevention. Percutaneous embolization of large portosystemic shunts has

been finding a place in treatment; and a molecular adsorbent recirculating system (MARS), designed to remove protein and albumin-bound toxins like bilirubin, bile acids, nitrous oxide, and endogenous benzodiazepines, but also removes non-protein-bound ammonia, has also been FDA-approved for overt HE. Probiotics have also been advantageous (McGee et al., 2011; Leise et al., 2014).

To prevent further episodes of HE, lactulose and rifaximin are recommended. How effective the treatment will be at preventing the next episode of encephalopathy is related to the patient's compliance and how well the patient is advised about lactulose and rifaximin. Furthermore, patients at risk for HE should be advised about driving, as some patients have impaired driving skills, and car accidents are common (Leise et al., 2014).

Agitation should not be treated with benzodiazepines, and sedatives are generally avoided. In patients awaiting liver transplantation, those taking SSRIs had better cognitive function and longer latency to encephalopathy (Bajaj et al., 2012). Limited data suggest that antipsychotics slow psychomotor speed but do not hasten encephalopathy (Bajaj et al., 2012).

Flumazenil, which blocks gamma aminobutyric acid (GABA), can bring temporary improvement in a few patients, but its value is to rule out possible previous administration of benzodiazepines. Bromocriptine or l-dopa are restricted to cases of extrapyramidal signs with chronic HE (Mas, 2006). A meta-analysis did not lend much support for the benefit of dopaminergic agents (Als-Nielsen et al., 2003).

COVERT HEPATIC ENCEPHALOPATHY

For the psychiatrist seeing a patient with liver disease in the office who is less ill, it may be more important to consider covert HE (Kappus & Bajaj, 2012). Covert HE combines patients who meet criteria for *minimal hepatic encephalopathy* (MHE) with those that have *Grade 1 hepatic encephalopathy* by West Haven criteria. Clinical recognition of the covert syndrome in patients with mild liver disease can have a significant impact. These patients are those with liver cirrhosis who have mild cognitive and attention deficits, compounded by response disinhibition, impaired working memory, and impaired coordination. The diagnosis requires neuropsychological and neurophysiological testing over and above a routine clinical assessment. These patients have difficulty sleeping, have poor executive function, suffer more falls, have difficulty driving, a poorer quality of life, and are destined to develop overt HE if they are not diagnosed and treated. Fifty-six percent of patients with MHE develop the overt syndrome in three years (Hartmann et al., 2000). Both lactulose and rifaximin have been shown to improve cognitive function in patients with MHE.

A psychometric hepatic encephalopathy score (PHES) has been recommended as a standard for following patients. Deficits in attention and processing speed are central to the diagnosis, with impairment of visuospatial function, attention, response time, and inhibition. The PHES includes the number connection test–A (NCT-A) and the number connection test–B (NCT-B) (These have also been called Trail Making Tests A and B (Weissenborn et al., 1998)); the digit symbol test (DST), the line-tracing test, and the serial dotting test. When a shorter test is required, the Working Group recommends two of the tests: NCT-A, NCT-B, the DST, and the block design test. The diagnosis is made by evidence of impairment on two of these tests, such that the patient scores two standard deviations below age-matched controls at the same education level (Kappus & Bajaj, 2012). The NCT-A tests psychomotor speed, and the NCT-B tests speed, set shifting, and divided attention. The DST tends to be sensitive and an early indicator of impairment. While these tests take a few minutes, the block design test is for visuospatial reasoning, praxis, and psychomotor speed, and takes 10–20 minutes (Kappus & Bajaj, 2012).

HEPATITIS C

Hepatitis C (HCV) infection is primarily the consequence of injection drug use, especially for the cohort born between 1945 and 1964. HCV is much less likely to be transmitted by sexual activity or transfusion than by drug injection. The prevalence of new infections dropped in the 1990s as drug users modified their behavior to prevent exposure to human immunodeficiency virus (HIV). Of the 1.6% of the U.S. population who had been infected with HCV (anti-HCV-positive), 1.3% were still positive for HCV riboneucleic acid (RNA) between 1999 and 2002. Those who still have active virus are prone to chronic liver disease, cirrhosis, and hepatocellular carcinoma (Armstrong et al., 2000). Chronic HCV is the most common reason for liver transplantation (Dienstag, 2006). In light of this and the evolution of new treatments for hepatitis C, screening is recommended for all patients born between 1945 and 1964.

HCV causes a flu-like syndrome acutely that may last 10–12 weeks. Only 20% of patients clear the infection the vast majority within 8–16 weeks of infection; the other 80% go on to develop chronic HCV lasting more than six months. The chronic phase is generally asymptomatic. Heavy alcohol use accelerates vulnerability to chronic liver disease. Chronic HCV itself has been associated with recurrent brief depression independent of treatment (Carta et al., 2012; Lim et al., 2010). Depression is more common in HCV- than in HBV-infected patients. Fatigue, the most common symptom, remits with antiviral treatment (Schaefer et al., 2012). Cognitive impairment also has a high prevalence in chronic HCV patients and raises the question of whether the virus can infect the central nervous system. Virus in human brain endothelial cells, a major component of the blood–brain barrier, may be a mechanism for entrance into the brain (Fletcher & McKeating, 2012).

The standard regimen for chronic HCV has included pegylated interferon and ribavirin. New protease inhibitors, including sofosbuvir and simeprevir, with ribavirin and with or without pegylated interferon have the potential to shorten treatment from 24 to 12 weeks. Ledipasvir and sofosbuvir have been given as one tablet with or without ribavirin in regimens as short as 8 weeks, and other direct-acting antiviral agents are on the way. The new agents may elevate the chance of successful treatment from 50% to more than 90%; however, the new drugs are very expensive, and the economic barriers may be the biggest challenge (Hoofnagle & Sherker, 2014). Actually, most patients with HCV have not received treatment (North et al., 2012; Volk, 2010; North et al., 2013), and psychiatric and medical syndromes have often made patients ineligible for treatment. One requirement has been to be sober from substance abuse for six months before starting treatment. In the real world, only 20% started treatment, and many did not finish. Patients with active injection drug use should not be systematically excluded (National Institutes of Health [NIH], 2002). It is worth noting that treatment of HCV, even in active drug users, can be as effective as it is in those in remission from drug use, particularly if there is specific support for psychiatric disorders and substance abuse (Zanini et al., 2010). Extra attention to treatment adherence, psychoeducation, and social support are critical (Grebely et al., 2010).

Patients with serious mental illness have a higher prevalence of HCV; for instance, among veterans the prevalence is 8% in bipolar patients and 7% in patients with schizophrenia (Himelhoch et al., 2009). In stable patients with bipolar disorder, interferon-related depressive disorder can be managed (Kelly et al., 2012).

The standard regimen for hepatitis C has included ribavirin and pegylated interferon alpha over 48 weeks. Interferon can cause malaise, major depressive disorder, anxiety, suicidal ideation, insomnia, anger, and irritability. The first 12 weeks of interferon treatment are the highest risk period for the emergence of suicidal ideation (Sockalingam et al., 2011; Lotrich, 2013). Depression is a cause of interferon dose reduction, and depression wanes after a few weeks off interferon. However, most patients who are depressed respond to SSRIs even as interferon is continued. Guideline suggestions include citalopram (Morasco et al., 2010), escitalopram, paroxetine, mirtazapine, sertraline, and others (Schaefer et al., 2012). Antidepressants given before interferon is started may reduce the psychiatric side effects of interferon given with ribavirin for hepatitis C treatment (Hou et al., 2013); however, the key point is that patients should be educated to report troubling dysphoric symptoms so that antidepressants can be initiated (Wise, 2011). Pre-treatment is recommended for those with chronic HCV infection who are depressed even before treatment begins (Raison et al., 2007) as well as for those with previous interferon- induced depression. Insomnia should be treated early and can be treated with mirtazapine, trazodone, antihistamines, or benzodiazepines. Guidelines suggest continuing antidepressants for 12 weeks after interferon is stopped. Psychosis and mania are rare. Cognitive function, particularly processing and reaction times, may be slowed, particularly with higher doses of interferon.

Thyroid function tests should be followed during interferon treatment. Interferon is associated with autoimmune thyroiditis, so hypothyroidism or hyperthyroidism and their psychiatric symptoms can complicate the psychiatric picture. Furthermore, hypothyroidism and interferon's inhibition of the P450 system can raise levels of antidepressants and thereby raise the risk of antidepressant drug–induced mania.

The website HCVguidelines.org has up-to-date recommendations for management, treatment, and screening. Resources are found at www.hepc123.org, the American Liver Foundation's dedicated online information center.

WILSON'S DISEASE

Wilson's disease is an autosomal recessive disorder of copper metabolism that presents with neuropsychiatric and/or hepatic symptoms. Three hundred discrete genetic mutations of the gene responsible for synthesis of the protein ATP7B for the transport of copper (Ala et al., 2007) have been found in patients with this disease (Ferenci, 2004).

Psychiatrists take note of the diagnosis in the differential of a new psychosis, especially when the psychosis is accompanied by a movement disorder. This is a critical diagnosis not to miss since the brain injury can improve with treatment, and the identification of vulnerable family members can prevent the disease. The full neurological syndrome of Wilson's disease is characterized by tremor, rigidity, dysarthria, dysphagia, and apraxia; the associated neuropathology includes signs of copper deposition in the basal ganglia, thalamus, and cerebellum. The dysarthria, one of the most common symptoms, can have dystonic (harsh, strained qualities) and ataxic irregularity of word spacing and volume. The tremor can take many forms, looking like essential, postural, or intentional tremor (Lorincz, 2010). Approximately one-third of cases of Wilson's disease present with neuropsychiatric rather than hepatic symptoms; the psychiatric symptoms include depression, labile mood, and functional consequences of impaired executive function (Frota et al., 2013). Cognitive symptoms may be mild, but both frontal syndromes and subcortical dementia can be seen. The onset is most often in patients under 35 years old (Lorincz, 2010).

The presence of liver disease may be the clue to the diagnosis. Of those with a neuropsychiatric presentation, 39% already have hepatic cirrhosis. In addition to cirrhosis, patients can present with fulminant liver failure or chronic hepatitis. One-third of the patients who present with hepatitis or liver failure will also have neuropsychiatric findings at the time of presentation. Sometimes these are misdiagnosed as having hepatic encephalopathy. Liver injury becomes evident in patients between 8 and 18 years old.

Kayser-Fleischer gray-green corneal rings are seen at the time of presentation in 95% of patients with nervous system disease, but only in half of those who present with liver abnormalities. This finding should be sought visually by ophthalmoscope and, if necessary, the patient should be referred to an ophthalmologist for a slit lamp exam. Neuropsychiatric assessment can document impairment, particularly in executive functions that correlate with MRI findings. The most common brain MRI findings are atrophy of the caudate, brainstem, and cerebral and cerebellar hemispheres, and both gray and white signal abnormalities (Frota et al., 2013).

Corneal rings and a low ceruloplasmin can make the diagnosis; however, a low ceruloplasmin level without Kayser-Fleischer rings is not sufficient. Ceruloplasmin may also be low in malnourished states and in autoimmune hepatitis. Some patients with Wilson's disease in the liver will have normal ceruloplasmin as it is an acute phase reactant that increases due to hepatic inflammation. Thus, a normal ceruloplasmin does not rule out the diagnosis.

A 24-hour urine copper test is the most useful screening procedure, and the gold standard for diagnosis is a quantitative measure of copper in a percutaneous liver biopsy.

The chelating agents penicillamine or trientine (the latter if the patient is intolerant to penicillamine) are the first treatment. Zinc is a useful alternative, as it disrupts intestinal absorption of copper and has been used for maintenance treatment and preventive treatment in presymptomatic patients (Lorincz, 2010). Liver transplantation is the treatment for liver failure; in some patients the neurological findings have improved post-transplant. Psychiatric syndromes may improve over the first two years of treatment (Akil & Brewer, 1995).

WHIPPLE'S DISEASE

Whipple's disease is a rare gastrointestinal syndrome of diarrhea, weight loss, and malabsorption, associated with psychiatric symptoms and cognitive impairment in 20%– of patients (Afshar et al., 2010; Fenollar et al., 2007). *Tropheryma whipplei*, a common gram positive bacterium, causes the disease, presumably in patients with special susceptibility. The presentation is associated with a prodrome of polyarticular arthritis after six to seven years of chronic diarrhea. The disease may be identified in the setting of rheumatological treatment with immunosuppressive therapy. (Fenollar et al., 2014). About one quarter of patients present with neurologic involvement, and depression and personality changes are seen in half of these (Lagier et al., 2010; Louis et al., 1996). Patients also can present with dementia, hemiparesis, ophthalmoplegia, Wernicke's encephalopathy, cranial nerve abnormalities, sensorimotor impairment, and cerebellar ataxia. A higher frequency of HLA DRB*13 and DQB *06 has been noted. Diagnosis depends usually on multiple intestinal biopsies and periodic acid-Schiff (PAS) stains with a polymerase chain reaction (PCR) analysis. Even if there are no central nervous system (CNS) findings, the cerebrospinal fluid (CSF) should be evaluated with PCR. Repeat study of CSF should be done after antibiotics. Relapses are common. Based on antibiotic susceptibilities, doxycycline and hydroxy-chloroquine are given for 12 months. Doxycycline may be continued life-long (Fenollar et al., 2014).

CLINICAL PEARLS

- Irritable bowel syndrome is attributed to an interaction between intestinal microbiota, the mucosal barrier, and immune activation, nerve plasticity, visceral hypersensitivity, enteroendocrine factors, and the amplification of these contributors by anxiety and depression.

- Buspirone 5HT-1A receptor agonist has been shown to relax the proximal stomach in healthy subjects and to improve functional dyspepsia better than placebo.

- In the differential diagnosis of cyclic vomiting is a syndrome associated with heavy and longtime cannabis use. Cessation of cannabis is the treatment.

- Lactose, fructose, or sorbitol malabsorption from dietetic foods may contribute to fecal urgency and incontinence.

- Two recent meta-analyses have concluded that antidepressants are helpful for IBS (Ford et al., 2012; Ruepert, 2011) but how these drugs related to other treatments and how they may be used for maximal benefit have not been fully defined.

- Patients with higher depressive scores at the time of a flare-up of inflammatory bowel disease were more apt to relapse sooner (Mittermaier, 2004).

- Recognizing that a patient with liver disease has covert hepatic encephalopathy can bring them to attention and treatment before they suffer the overt syndrome. They have deficits in attention and processing speed, with impairment of visuospatial function, attention, and response time, and are more prone to motor vehicle accidents.

- Immunoglobulin-A anti-tissue transglutaminase (TTG) antibody is the preferred single test for the detection of celiac disease.

- Antidepressants can prevent depression in the setting of interferon treatment for hepatitis C, and they may be continued for 12 weeks longer than the interferon.

- A diagnosis of non-celiac gluten sensitivity should be considered only after celiac disease has been excluded with appropriate testing (Rubio-Tapia, 2013).

- Wilson's disease is not the only thing that can cause a low ceruloplasm. It is also low in autoimmune hepatitis and malnourished states.

DISCLOSURE STATEMENT

Dr. Greenberg has no conflicts of interest to disclose.

REFERENCES

Afshar, P., Redfield, D. C., & Higginbottom, P. A. (2010). Whipple's disease: A rare disease revisited. *Current Gastroenterology Reports, 12*, 263–269.

Akil, M., & Brewer, G. J. (1995). Psychiatric and behavioral abnormalities in Wilson's disease. *Advances in Neurology, 65*, 171–178.

Ala, A., Walker, A. P., Ashkan, K., Dooley, J. S., & Schilsky, M. L. (2007). Wilson's disease. *Lancet, 369*, 397–408.

Alexander, F. (1950). *Psychosomatic medicine*. New York: Norton.

Als-Nielsen, B., Gluud, L., Gluud, C. (2004). Dopaminergic agonists for hepatic encephalopathy. *Cochrane Database of Systematic Reviews*, CD003047.

American College of Gastroenterology Task Force on Irritable Bowel Syndrome, Brandt, L. J., Chey, W. B., et al. (2009). An evidence-based position statement on the management of irritable bowel syndrome. *American Journal of Gastroenterology, 104*(Suppl 1), S1–S35.

Armstrong, G. L., Alter, M. J., McQuillan, G. M., Margolis, H. S. (2000). The past incidence of hepatitis C virus infection: Implications for the future burden of chronic liver disease in the United States. *Hepatology, 31*, 777–782.

Aronowitz, R., & Spiro, H. M. (1988). The rise and fall of the psychosomatic hypothesis in ulcerative colitis. *Journal of Clinical Gastroenterology, 10*, 298–305.

Bajaj, J. S., Thacker, L. R., Heumann, D. M., & Sterling, R. K. (2012). Cognitive performance as a predictor of hepatic encephalopathy in pretransplant patients with cirrhosis receiving psychoactive medications: A prospective study. *Liver Transplantation, 18*, 1179–1187.

Barbara, G., Cremon, C., DeGiorgio, R., et al. (2011). Mechanisms underlying visceral hypersensitivity in irritable bowel syndrome. *Current Gastroenterology Reports, 13*, 308–315.

Barsky, A. J., & Borus, J. F. (1999). Functional somatic syndromes. *Annals of Internal Medicine, 130*, 910–921.

Biesiekierski, J. R., Muir, J. G., & Gibson, P. R. (2013a). Is gluten a cause of gastrointestinal symptoms in people without celiac disease? *Current Allergy & Asthma Reports, 13*, 631–638.

Biesiekierski, J. R., Newnham, E. D., Irving, P. M., et al. (2011). Gluten causes gastrointestinal symptoms in subjects without celiac disease: A double blind randomized placebo-controlled trial. *American Journal of Gastroenterology, 106*, 508–514.

Biesiekierski, J. R., Peters, S. L., Newnham, E. D., et al. (2013b). No effects of gluten in patients with self-reported non-celiac gluten sensitivity after dietary reduction of fermentable, poorly absorbed, short-chain carbohydrates. *Gastroenterology, 145*, 320–328.

Bischoff, S., & Crowe, S. E. (2005). Gastrointestinal food allergy: New insights into pathophysiology and clinical perspectives. *Gastroenterology, 128*, 1089–1113.

Blei, A. T., & Cordoma, J., & The Practice Parameters Committee of the American College of Gastroenterology (2001). *American Journal of Gastroenterology, 96*, 1968–1976.

Boettcher, E., & Crowe, S. E. (2013). Dietary proteins and functional gastrointestinal disorders. *American Journal of Gastroenterology, 108*, 728–736.

Boettcher, E., & Crowe, S. E. (2013). Dietary proteins and functional gastrointestinal disorders. *American Journal of Gastroenterology, 108*, 728–736.

Bonaz, B. L., & Bernstein, C. N. (2013). Brain–gut interactions in inflammatory bowel disease. *Gastroenterology, 144*, 36–49.

Brady, J. V., Porter, R. W., Conrad, D. G., & Mason, J. W. (1958). Avoidance behavior and the development of gastroduodenal ulcers. *Journal of Experimental Analysis of Behavior*. doi:10.1901/jeab.19581, 69–72; doi:10.1901/jeab.19581515, 1–69.

Brottveit, M., Vandvik, P. O., Wojniusz, S., Lovik, A., Lundin, K. E., & Boye, B. (2012). Absence of somatization in non-coeliac gluten sensitivity. *Scandinavian Journal of Gastroenterology, 47*, 770–777.

Buie, T. (2013). The relationship of autism and gluten. *Clinical Therapeutics, 35*, 578–583.

Camilleri, M., & Di Lorenzo, C. (2012). Brain–gut axis: From basic understanding to treatment of IBS and related disorders. *Journal of Pediatric Gastroenterology & Nutrition, 54*, 446–453.

Carroccio, A., Mansuteo, P., Iacono, G., Soresi, M., D'Alcamo, A., et al. (2012). Non-celiac wheat sensitivity diagnosed by double-blind placebo-controlled challenge: Exploring a new clinical entity. *American Journal of Gastroenterology, 107*, 1898–1906.

Carta, M. G., Angst, J., Moro, M. F., Mura, G., Hardoy, M. C., et al. (2012). Association of chronic hepatitis C with recurrent brief depression. *Journal of Affective Disorders 141*, 361–366.

Chepyala, P., & Olden, K. W. (2008). Cyclic vomiting and compulsive bathing with chronic cannabis abuse. *Clinical Gastroenterology and Hepatology, 6*, 710–712.

Chial, H. J., Camilleri, M., Burton, D., Thomforde, G., Olden, K. W., & Stephens, D. (2003). Selective effects of serotonergic psychoactive agents on gastrointestinal functions in health. *American Journal of Physiology, 284*, G130–G137.

Choung, R. S., & Talley, N. J. (2008). Epidemiology and clinical presentation of stress-related peptic damage and chronic peptic ulcer. *Current Molecular Medicine, 9*, 253–257.

Choung, R. S., Locke, G. R. III, & Lee, R. M. (2012). Cyclic vomiting syndrome and functional vomiting in adults. Association with cannabis use in males. *Neurogastroenterology and Motility, 24*, 1 20–26 e1.

Clouse, R. E., Richter, J. E., Heading, R. C., Janassen, J., & Wilson, J. A. (1999). Functional esophageal disorder. *Gut, 45*(Suppl II), II131–II136.

Creed, F., Fernandes, L., Guthrie, E., et al. (2003). The cost effectiveness of psychotherapy and paroxetine for severe irritable bowel syndrome. *Gastroenterology, 124*, 303–317.

Creed, F., Ratcliffe, J., Ferndes, L., et al. (2005). Outcome in severe irritable bowel syndrome with and without accompanying depressive, panic and neurasthenic disorders. *British Journal of Psychiatry, 186*, 507–515.

Deter, H.-C., Keller, W., von Wietersheim, J., et al. (2007). Psychological treatment may reduce the need for healthcare in patients with Crohn's disease. *Inflammatory Bowel Diseases, 13*, 745–752.

Dienstag, J. L. (2006). Hepatitis C: A bitter harvest. *Annals of Internal Medicine, 144*, 770–771.

Dienstag, J. L., & McHutchison, J. G. (2006). American Gastroenterological Association technical review on the management of hepatitis C. *Gastroenterology, 130*, 231–264.

Drossman, D. A. (2006). The functional gastrointestinal disorders and the Rome III process. *Gastroenterology, 130*, 1377–1390.

Drossman, D. A., Toner, B. B., Whitehead, W. E., et al. (2003). Cognitive behavioral therapy versus education and desipramine versus placebo for moderate to severe functional bowel disorders. *Gastroenterology, 125*, 19–31.

Engel, G. (1958). Studies of ulcerative colitis, V. Psychological aspects and their implications for treatment. *American Journal of Digestive Diseases, 3*, 315–337.

Engel, G. (1961). Biologic and psychologic features of the ulcerative colitis patient. *Gastroenterology, 40*, 313.

Fenollar, F., Lagier, J-C, & Raoult, D, (2014). Tropheryma whjipplei and Whipple's disease. *Journal Infection, 69*, 103–112.

Fenollar, F., Puechal, X, & Raoult, D. (2007). whipple's disease. *New England Journal of Medicine, 356*, 55–66.

Ferenci, P. (2004). Review article: Diagnosis and current therapy of Wilson's disease. *Alimentary Pharmacology & Therapeutics, 19*, 157–165.

Fletcher, N. F., & McKeating, J. A. (2012). Hepatitis C virus and the brain. *Journal Viral Hepatitis, 19*, 301–306.

Ford, A. C., & Talley, N. J. (2012). Irritable bowel syndrome. *British Medical Journal, 345*, e5836.

Ford, A. C., Talley, N. J., Schoenfeld, P. S., et al. (2009). Efficacy of antidepressants and psychological therapies in irritable bowel syndrome: Systematic review and meta-analysis. *Gut, 58*, 367.

Frota, N. A., Barbosa, E. R., Porto, C. S., et al. (2013). Cognitive impairment and magnetic resonance imaging correlations in Wilson's disease. *Acta Scandivanica Neurolologica, 127*, 391–398.

Goodhand, J. R., Greig, F. I. S., Koodun, Y., et al. (2012). Do antidepressants influence the disease course in inflammatory bowel disease? A retrospective case-matched observational study. *Inflammatory Bowel Disease, 18*, 1232–1239.

Grebely, J., Knight, E., Genoway, K. A., et al. (2010). Optimizing assessment and treatment for hepatitis C virus infection in illicit drug users: A novel model incorporating multidisciplinary care and peer support. *European Journal Gastroenterology Hepatology, 22*, 270–277.

Grover, M., & Camilleri, M. (2013). Effects on gastrointestinal functions and symptoms of serotonergic psychoactive agents used in functional gastrointestinal disease. *Journal of Gastroenterology, 48*, 177–181.

Grover, M., & Drossman, D. A. (2008). Psychotropic agents in functional gastrointestinal disorder. *Current Opinion in Pharmacology, 8*, 715–723.

Halmos, E. P., Power, V. A., Shepherd, S. J., Gibson, P. R., & Muir, J. G. (2014). A diet low in FODMAPs reduces symptoms of irritable bowel syndrome. *Gastroenterology, 146*, 67–75e5.

Halpert, A., & Drossman, D. (2005). Biopsychosocial issues in irritable bowel syndrome. *Journal of Clinical Gastroenterology, 39*, 665–669.

Hartmann, I. J., Groeneweg, M., Quero, J. C., et al. (2000). The prognostic significance of subclinical hepatic encephalopathy. *American Journal of Gastroenterology, 95*, 2029–2034.

Hauser, W., Janke, K.-H., Klump, B., & Hinz, A. (2011). Anxiety and depression in patients with inflammatory bowel disease: Comparisons with chronic liver disease patients and the general population. *Inflammatory Bowel Diseases, 17*, 621–632.

Himelhoch, S., McCarthy, J. F., Ganoczy, D., Medoff, D., Kilbourne, A., Goldberg, R., et al. (2009). Understanding associations between serious mental illness and hepatitis C virus among veterans: A national multivariate analysis. *Psychosomatics, 50*, 30–37.

Hoofnagle, J. H., & Sherker, A. H. (2014). Therapy for hepatitis C—the costs of success. *New England Journal of Medicine, 370*, 1552–1553.

Hou, X. J., Xu, J. H., Wang, J., & Yu, Y. Y. (2013). Can antidepressants prevent pegylated interferon-alpha/ribavirin-associated depression in patients with chronic hepatitis C: Meta-analysis of randomized, double-blind, placebo-controlled trials? *PLoS One, 8*, e76799.

Hyphantis, T., Guthrie, E., Tomenson, B., & Creed, F. (2009). Psychodynamic interpersonal therapy and improvement in interpersonal difficulties in people with severe irritable bowel syndrome. *Pain, 145*, 196–2003.

Irwin, C., Flasetti, S. A., Lydiard, R. B., et al. (1996). Comorbidity of posttraumatic stress disorder and irritable bowel syndrome. *Journal of Clinical Psychiatry, 57*, 576–578.

Jackson, J. L., O'Malley, P. G., Tomkins, G., et al. (2000). Treatment of functional gastrointestinal disorders with antidepressant medications a meta-analysis. *American Journal of Medicine, 108*, 65–72.

Jones, M. P., Crowell, M. D., Olden, K. W., & Creed, F. (2007). Functional gastrointestinal disorders: An update for the psychiatrist. *Psychosomatics, 48*, 93–102.

Kappus, M. R., & Bajaj, J. S. (2012). Covert hepatic encephalopathy: Not as minimal as you might think. *Clinical Gastroenterology and Hepatology, 10*, 1208–1219.

Kelly, E. M., Corace, K., Emery, J., & Cooper, C. L. (2012). Bipolar patients can safely and successfully receive interferon-based hepatitis C antiviral treatment. *European Journal of Gastroenterology and Hepatology, 24*, 811–816.

Lagier, J. C., Lepidi, H., Raoult, D., & Fenollar, F. (2010). Systemic *Tropheryma whipplei*: Clinical presentation of 142 patients with infectins diagnosed or confirmed in a reference center. *Medicine (Baltimore), 89*, 337–345.

Lazarescu, A., Turnbull, G. K., & Vanner, S. (2009). Investigating and treating fecal incontinence: When and how. *Canadian Journal of Gastroenterology, 23*, 301–308.

Lee, B. E., & Kim, G. H. (2012). Globus pharyngeus: A review of its etiology, diagnosis and treatment. *World Journal of Gastroenterology, 18*, 2462–2471.

Leise, M. D., Poterucha, J. J., Kamath, P. S., & Kim, W. R. (2014). Management of hepatic encephalopathy in the hospital. *Mayo Clinic Proceedings, 89*, 241–253.

Levenstein, S. (2002). Psychosocial factors in peptic ulcer and inflammatory bowel disease. *Journal of Consulting and Clinical Psychology, 70*, 739–750.

Levy, R. L., Olden, K. W., Naliboff, B. D., Bradley, L. A., Francisconi, C., Drossman, D. A., et al. (2006). Psychosocial aspects of the functional gastrointestinal disorders. *Gastroenterology, 130*, 1447–1458.

Lim, C., Olson, J., Zaman, A., Phelps, J., & Ingram, K. D. (2010). Prevalence and impact of manic traits in depressed patients initiating interferon therapy for chronic hepatitis C infection. *Journal of Clinical Gastroenterology 44*, e141–e146.

Lorincz, M. T. (2010). Neurologic Wilson's disease. *Annals of the New York Academy of Sciences, 1184*, 173–187.

Lotrich, F. E. (2013). Psychiatric clearance for patients started on interferon-alpha-based therapies. *American Journal of Psychiatry, 170*, 592–595.

Louis, E. D., Lynch, T., Kauffmann, P., et al. (1996). Diagnostic guidelines in central nervous system Whipple's disease. *Annals of Neurology, 40*, 561–568.

Lundin, K. E., Alaedini, A. (2012). Non-celiac gluten sensitivity. *Gastrointestinal Endoscopy Clinics of North America, 22*, 723–734.

Mas, A. (2006). Hepatic encephalopathy: From pathophysiology to treatment. *Digestion, 73*(Suppl 1), 86–93.

Mayer, E. A. (2011). Gut feelings: The emerging biology of gut–brain communication. *Nature Reviews Neuroscience, 12*, 453–456.

Mayer, E. A., & Tillisch, K. (2011). The brain–gut axis in abdominal pain syndromes. *Annual Review of Medicine, 62*, 381–396.

Mayer, E. A., Nalibof, B., & Craig, D. B. (2006). Neuroimaging of the brain–gut axis: From basic understanding to treatment of functional GI disorders. Neuroimaging of the brain–gut axis: From basic understanding to treatment of functional GI disorders. *Gastroenterology, 131*, 1925–1942.

McGee, R. G., Bakens, A., Wiley, K., et al. (2011). Probiotics for patients with hepatic encephalopathy. *Cochrane Database of Systematic Reviews, 11*, CD008716.

Micromedex (2009). Zoloft, sertraline hydrochloride product information. New York: Pfizer, Inc.

Mikocka-Walus, A., Turnbull, D. A., Moulding, N. T., Wilson, I. G., Andrews, J. M., & Holtmann, G. J. (2007). It doesn't do any harm, but patients feel better: A qualitative exploratory study on gastroenterologists' perspectives on the role of antidepressants in inflammatory bowel disease. *BioMedCentral Gastroenterology, 7*, 38.

Mittermaier, C., Dejaco, C., Waldhoer, T., et al. (2004). Impact of depressive mood on relapse in patients with inflammatory bowel disease: A prospective 18 month follow-up study. *Psychosomatic Medicine, 66*, 79–84.

Mooney, P. D., Azziz, I., & Sanders, D. S. (2013). Non-celiac gluten sensitivity: Clinical relevance and recommendations for future research. *Neurogastroenterology & Motility, 25*, 864–871.

Morasco, B. J., Loftis, J. M., et al. (2010). Prophylactic antidepressant treatment in patients with hepatitis C on antiviral therapy: A double-blind, placebo-controlled trial. *Psychosomatics, 51*, 401–408.

Nater, U. M. (2013). Guest editorial: Functional somatic syndromes. *International Journal of Behavioral Medicine, 20*, 159–160.

North, C. S., Hong, B. A., & Kerr, T. (2012). Hepatitis C and substance use: New treatments and novel approaches. *Current Opinion in Psychiatry, 25*, 206–212.

North, S., Hong, B. A., Aewuyi, S. A., et al. (2013). Hepatitis C treatment and SVR: The gap between clinical trials and real-world treatment aspirations. *General Hospital Psychiatry, 35*, 122–128.

Olden, K. W., & Chepyala, P. (2008). Functional nausea and vomiting. *Nature, 5*, 202–206.

Ouyang, A., & Locke, R. (2007). Overview of neuro-gastroenterology-gastrointestinal motility and functional GI disorders: Classification, prevalence and epidemiology. *Gastroenterology Clinics of North America, 36*, 485–498.

Overmier, J. B., & Murison, R. (2013). Restoring psychology's role in peptic ulcer. *Applied Psychology, Health and Well-Being, 5*, 5–27.

Persoons, P., Vermeire, S., Bemyttenaere, K., et al. (2005). The impact of major depressive disorder on the short- and long-term outcome of Crohn's disease treatment with infliximab. *Alimentary Pharmacology & Therapeutics, 22*, 101–110.

Raison, C. L., Woolwine, B. J., Demetrashivli, M. F., Borisov, A. S., Weinreib, R., et al. (2007). Paroxetine for prevention of depressive symptoms induced by interferon-alpha and ribavirin for hepatitis c. aliment. *Pharmacology & Therapeutics, 25*, 1163–1174.

Rao, S. S., Camilleri, M., Hasler, W. L., Maurer, A. H., Parkman, H. P., Saad, R., et al. (2011). Evaluation of gastrointestinal transit in clinical practice: Position paper of the American and European Neurogastroenterology and Motility societies. *Neurogastroenterology & Motility, 23*, 8–23.

Rubio-Tapia, A., Hill, I. D., Kelly, C. P., Calderwood, A. H., & Murray, J. A. (2013). ACG Clinical Guidelines: Diagnosis and management of celiac disease. *American Journal of Gastroenterology, 108*, 656–676.

Ruepert, L., Quartero, A. O., deWit, N. J., et al. (2011). Bulking agents, antispasmodics and antidepressants for the treatment of irritable bowel syndrome *Cochrane Database of Systematic Reviews, 10*, CD003460.

Sanders, D. S., & Aziz, I. (2012). Non-celiac wheat sensitivity: Separating the wheat from the Chat. *American Journal of Gastroenterology, 107*, 1908–1912.

Sapone, A., Bai, J. C., Ciacci, C., et al. (2012). Spectrum of gluten-related disorders: Consensus on new nomenclature and classification. *BMC Medicine, 10*, 13.

Sayuk, G. S., Elwing, J. E., Lustman, P. J., & Clouse, R. E. (2007). Predictors of premature antidepressant discontinuation in functional gastrointestinal disorders. *Psychosomatic Medicine, 69*, 173–181.

Schaefer, M., Capuron, L., Friebe, A., Diez Quevedo, C., et al. (2012). Hepatitis C infection, antiviral treatment and mental health: A European expert consensus statement. *Journal of Hepatology, 57*, 1379–1390.

Selye, H. (1956). *The stress of life.* New York: McGraw-Hill.

Shah, B. J., Chokhavatia, S., & Rose, S. (2012). Fecal incontinence in the elderly: FAQ. *American Journal of Gastroenterology, 107*, 1635–1646.

Simren, M., Barbara, G., Flint, H. J., Spiegel, B. M. R., et al. (2012). Intestinal microbiota in functional bowel disorders: A Rome Foundation report. *Gut, 62*, 159–176.

Sockalingam, S., Links, P. S., & Abbey, S. E. (2011). Suicide risk in hepatitis C and during interferon-alpha therapy: A review and clinical update. *Journal of Viral Hepatitis, 18*, 153–60.

Sontineni, S. P., Chaudhary, S., Sontineni, V., & Lanspa, S. J. (2009). Cannabis hyperemesis syndrome: Clinical diagnosis of an under-recognized manifestation of chronic cannabis use. *World Gastroenterology, 15*, 1264–1266.

Spiller, R., Aziz, Q., Creed, F., Emmanuel, A., et al. (2007). Guidelines on the irritable bowel syndrome: Mechanisms and practical management. *Gut, 56*, 1770–1798.

Sullivan, A. J. (1936). Emotion and diarrhea. *New England Journal of Medicine, 214*, 299–305.

Sullivan, S. (2010). Cannabinoid hyperemesis. *Canadian Journal of Gastroenterology, 24*, 284–285.

Tache, Y., & Bernstein, C. N. (2009). Evidence for the role of the brain–gut axis in inflammatory bowel disease: Depression as cause and effect? *Gastroenterology, 136*, 2058–2060.

Tack, J., Janssen, P., Masaoka, T., Farre, R., & van Oudenhove, L. (2012). Efficacy of buspirone, a fundus-relaxing drug in patients with functional dyspepsia. *Clinical Gastroenterology and Hepatology, 10*, 1239–1245.

Tack, J., Talley, N. J., Camilleri, M., et al. (2006). Functional gastroduodenal disorders *Gastroenterology, 130*, 1466–1479 (the Rome III criteria).

Van Assche, G., Dignass, A., Bokemeyer, B., et al. (2013). Second European evidence-based consensus on the diagnosis and management of ulcerative colitis. Part 3: Special situations. *Journal of Crohn's and Colitis, 7*, 1–33.

Van Hees, N. J. M., van der Does, W., & Giltay, E. J. (2013). Coeliac disease, diet adherence and depressive symptoms. *Journal of Psychosomatic Research, 74*, 155–160.

Van Kerkhoven, L. A., Laheij, R. J., Aparicio, N., De Bower, W. A., van Den, H. S., Tan, A. C., et al. (2008). Effect of the antidepressant venlafaxine in functional dyspepsia: A randomized double-blind placebo-controlled trial. *Clinical Gastroenterology & Hepatology, 6*, 746–752.

Vidal, A., Gomez-Gil, E., Sans, M., Portella, M. J., Salamero, M., Pique, J. M., et al. (2006). Life events and inflammatory bowel disease relapse: A prospective study of patients enrolled in remission. *American Journal of Gastroenterology, 101*, 775–781.

Volk, M. L. (2010). Antiviral therapy for hepatitis C: Why are so few patients being treated? *Journal Antimicrobial Chemotherapy, 65*, 1327–1329.

Volta, U., & De Giorgio, R. (2012). New understanding of gluten sensitivity. *Nature Reviews Gastroenterology & Hepatology, 9*, 295–9.

Wald, A. (2014). Treatment of irritable bowel syndrome in adults. *UpToDate.*, Basow, D. S. (Ed.), Waltham MA: UpToDate.

Walker Jr, Ediger, J. P., Graff, L. A., et al. (2008). The Manitoba IBD Cohort study: A population-based study of the prevalence of lifetime and 12-month anxiety and mood disorders. *American Journal of Gastroenterology, 103*, 1989–1997.

Weissenborn, K., Ruckert, N., Hecker, H., & Manns, M. P. (1998). The number connection tests A and B: Interindividual variability and use for the assessment of early hepatic encephalopathy. *Journal of Hepatology, 28*, 646–653.

Wise, T. N. (2011). Prophylactic citalopram treatment in hepatitis patients on antiviral therapy: Will it limit drug-induced depression and enhance adherence? *Current Psychiatry Reports, 13*, 1–2.

Wolff, H. G., & Wolf, S. W. (1943). *Human gastric function: An experimental study of a man and his stomach.* New York: Oxford University Press.

Zanini, B., Covolo, L., Donato, F., & Lanzini, A. (2010). Effectiveness and tolerability of combination treatment of chronic hepatitis C in illicit drug users: meta-analysis of prospective studies. *Clinical Therapeutics, 32*, 2139–2159.

57.

PSYCHIATRIC CARE OF THE ONCOLOGY PATIENT

Donna B. Greenberg

The cancer patient is drafted into a complex series of diagnostic efforts to clarify his prognosis and medical plan, then a systematic series of upfront treatments, including surgery, radiation, and chemotherapy that may offer the best outcome. As patients comprehend the nature of their illness and adapt psychologically over time, they are moving through a sequence of assignments that also affect their symptoms and psyche. Because of the challenge of the illness and its dark history, individual and group psychosocial interventions have been developed to reduce the suffering of patients and to sustain their morale.

The medical psychiatrist meets the cancer patient where she is, grapples with the patient's requests as he discovers the patient's medical and personal saga. The clinician has a mission to hear the patient out and to support her, to clarify the medical predicament, and to help the patient break down the problem into smaller bits with appropriate priority. The specific course and implications of the cancer diagnosis and treatment interact with the individual psychological course. In consultation, the clinician may stabilize mood, anxiety, and clarity of thought, at the same time as he clarifies which symptoms have medical or psychiatric contributions.

The interview is the psychiatrist's trained method for assessing what is important to the patient, how he tolerates the threat of death, how the patient has begun to cope with the challenges of diagnosis and treatment, what bothers him the most, and what he fears. The medical facts as the clinician understands them are put in the context of the patient's experience of illness. In addition to the personal history, history of psychiatric syndromes, and developmental predicament, the patient may allow assessment of who is close to him, who can be relied upon for support, and who knows what is going on medically with the patient.

COPING WITH CANCER

Weisman (Weisman, 1974) outlined objectives that guided an approach to the patient coping with cancer. These were the objectives that came with the hope of an appropriate death—the death that we would choose if we had a choice. He defined as feasible:

1. Adequate medical care, alleviation of pain and suffering, full use of technical resources, prolongation of life but not prolongation of dying when recovery is wholly out of the question;

2. Informed collaboration between doctor and patient;

3. Encouragement of conscious, competent control; helping the patient use available, practical, and appropriate coping strategies;

4. Maintenance of behavior on as high a level as seems consistent with physical and psychological limitations;

5. Preservation and, if necessary, enhancement of self-esteem, an essential ingredient of a dignified death [and life];

6. Support of the significant key others, a gesture that helps them help the patient with gradual relinquishment of control to those who have shown themselves to be trustworthy;

7. Safe conduct in sustaining life until it ceases; and

8. Honest communication, designed to support acceptance, reduce bitterness, and replace denial with courage to confront what cannot be changed (pp. 188–189).

These principles can serve as a guide for good care.

In modern cancer treatment, the patient detours fairly abruptly from the preoccupation with her usual concerns to the challenge of diagnosis and biopsy and defining a complex medical plan. In many cases, the patient's ability to follow through with treatment over a long course will affect the outcome. The patient's family and extended supporters facilitate the urgent needs; and often in the emergency, subtler emotional concerns are left until later. The ability of the patient to cope over time and to use her support system strategically becomes critical.

As with any life-threatening illness, the patient faces an existential crisis, recognizing losses and mortality. The psychiatrist encounters the patient at a very vulnerable time, a moment when her relationships to the world are in critical transition. The psychiatrist, with patients and physicians, formulates the salient problems as succinctly as possible during continued patient care. The goal is to help the patient find the most efficient method of coping, with the best use of psychiatric knowledge for optimal oncological care.

It takes time for patients to metabolize the significance of the cancer. The course of acute distress has been described as taking 100 days (Weisman, Worden, 1976–1977); this three-month time frame can serve as a guide to the time course of acute adjustment.

Weisman highlighted the primary paradox that, in confronting a life-threatening illness, a dying man believes in the fact of his own death but hopes that he is an exception (Weisman, 1972, p. 13). In the setting of incurable cancer, clinicians set out a medical plan, standing by the patient as the patient fluctuates between acknowledgement and denial of his predicament. Denial has a social dimension. Patients tend to deny their knowledge of fatal illness to different people at different times; sometimes in order to preserve important relationships (Weisman, 1984, p. 83). The clinician can foster tactful discussion of mortality between a patient and his caretakers so that they may be responsive to each other as long as possible (Weisman, 1972, p. 18). Weisman described *middle knowledge* as the uncertain certainty that is "somewhere between open acknowledgement of death and its utter repudiation; middle knowledge is most evident particularly at serious transition points" (Weisman, 1972, p. 65). This concept of middle knowledge describes how patients often seemed to know and want to know about the gravity of their illness, yet often talked as if they did not know and did not want to be reminded (Weisman, 1972, p. 66). "Patients may deny facts, inferences, or extinction" (Weisman, 1972, p. 66). However, "denial is almost impossible to maintain; and inner perceptions force themselves on the most reluctant patient" (Weisman, 1972, p. 133). The balance between denial and acceptance evolves (Weisman, 1972, p. 112).

HOPE

The will to live is a combination of hope and the ability to put in effort (Weisman, 1972; Khan et al., 2010). Hope is related to a desirable self-image and a belief in one's personal ability to exert a degree of influence on the world (Weisman, 1972, p. 20), the conviction that a person may do something worth doing (Weisman, 1972, p. 21). That sense of purpose adds value to one's life regardless of the time frame. The clinician's respect for the patient sustains authentic hope.

The purpose of the treatment plan in the cancer setting is to facilitate coping. Faced with the conflict between sickness and responsibility, cancer patients by trial and error seek a way forward. Coping is a complicated mixture of cognitive appraisal and reappraisal, "first responses and corrected responses over a long time continuum" (Weisman, 1978, pp. 264–267). Simultaneously, the clinician assesses the contributions of demoralization, malaise, and major depressive disorder to the patient's presentation and judges how best to use the therapeutic armamentarium.

DEMORALIZATION

At times when the burden of illness is overwhelming and coping is difficult, patients can face existential despair, hopelessness, helplessness, and loss of meaning and purpose in life. This syndrome of demoralization has been seen as a normal response to the adversity of serious medical illness (Clark & Kissane, 2002) analogous to grief, echoing Frank's description of demoralization in combat soldiers and Schmale and Engel's "giving up–given up complex" (Frank, 1993; Schmale, 1972). The demoralized patients feel inhibited to act because they do not know what to do. They feel helpless and incompetent in the face of uncertainty. The focus is subjective incompetence rather than loss of pleasure. A scale of demoralization has distinct dimensions of loss of meaning, dysphoria, disheartenment, helplessness, and a sense of failure (Kissane et al., 2004). Helplessness, despair, or meaninglessness may combine to contribute to the sense of subjective incompetence, positioning a patient to retreat from the existential challenges of illness (Griffith & Gaby, 2005). Demoralization may be difficult to distinguish from clinical depression, as many feel more incompetent when their mood is persistently low. The clinician who recognizes demoralization must work with patients to promote a sense of mastery and return of hope regardless of what decision is made about medication treatments for depressive disorder (Shader, 2005).

In order to treat demoralization, Griffith and Gaby focus questions at the bedside to find the dominant existential theme in the patient's experience of illness; they then suggest nudging the patient forward with a series of questions oriented to attributes of resilience: coherence, communion, hope, agency, purpose, courage, and gratitude rather than their opposites: confusion, isolation, despair, helplessness, meaninglessness, cowardice, and resentment. They prod patients in interviews, as follows.

Coherence vs. Confusion

How do you make sense of what you are going through?
When you are uncertain how to make sense of it, how do you deal with feeling confused?
Whom do you turn to for help when you feel confused?
[For a religious patient] Do you have a sense that God has a way of making sense of it? Do you sense that God sees meaning in your suffering?

Communion vs. Isolation

Who really understands your situation?
When you have difficult days, whom do you talk with?
In whose presence do you feel a bodily sense of peace?
[For religious patients] Do you feel the presence of God? How? What does God know about your experience that other people may not understand?

Hope vs. Despair

From what sources do you draw hope?
On difficult days, what keeps you from giving up?
Who have you known in your life who would not be surprised to see you stay hopeful amid adversity? What did this person know about you that other people may not have known?

Purpose vs. Meaninglessness

What keeps you going on difficult days?

For whom, or for what, does it matter that you continue to live?

[For terminally ill patients] What do you hope to contribute in the time you have remaining?

[For religious patients] What does God hope you will do with your life in days to come?

Agency vs. Helplessness

What is your prioritized list of concerns/What concerns you the most? What the next most?

What most helps you stand strong against the challenges of this illness?

What should I know about you as a person that lies beyond your illness?

How have you kept this illness from taking charge of your entire life?

Courage vs. Cowardice

Have there been moments when you felt tempted to give up but didn't?

How did you make a decision to persevere?

If you were to see someone else taking such a step even though feeling afraid, would you consider that an act of courage?

If so, can you imagine viewing yourself as a courageous person? Is that a description of yourself that you would desire?

Can you imagine that others who witness how you cope with this illness might describe you as a courageous person?

Gratitude vs. Resentment

For what are you most deeply grateful?

Are there moments when you can still feel joy despite the sorrow you have been through?

If you could look back on this illness from some future time, what would you say that you took from the experience that added to your life?

Hopelessness and humiliation may be eased by psychotherapeutic interventions that sustain dignity and meaning (Chochinov et al., 2011; McClain et al., 2003). Group therapy for patients with metastatic cancer, a supportive-expressive approach, has reduced distress and facilitated the patients' confrontation with what had to be confronted (Spiegel et al., 2007; Spiegel et al., 2000). When the care of patients depends on spouse or family, the clinician can amplify the caregivers' understanding of the illness and support communication within a couple or family (Zaider & Kissane, 2010). Cognitive behavioral interventions, supportive psychotherapy, relaxation techniques, and mind–body medicine have all been found to reduce distress among cancer patients.

SYNDROMES OF ANXIETY

In the course of cancer treatment, anxiety is common. The medical team makes a plan for patients, informs them at each step what will happen, and pays attention to their comfort and the things that make them anxious.

CONDITIONED ANXIETY

Cancer treatment itself makes certain anxiety syndromes likely. The anticipatory anxiety associated with repeated painful procedures, anxiety about routine visits to oncologists, waits for results of studies redefining the stage of the cancer, and the worry about recurrence are typical elements of the oncology experience. A patient who has been at equilibrium may find that the experience of the first recurrent lesion, the medical event that changes the condition from curable to palliative is an alarm signal that is difficult to quiet. The patient may remain in a state of alarm for an extended period waiting for the next lesion; the patient's medical understanding of his continued vulnerability can perpetuate a chronic level of anxiety and contribute to "battle fatigue."

Historically, cancer chemotherapy has been associated with nausea and vomiting. Because of the power of vomiting as a visceral stimulus, emetic chemotherapy has provided a model for iatrogenic induction of conditioned anxiety. With repeated treatments associated with nausea and vomiting, patients can become conditioned to anticipate and to avoid the next chemotherapy or the sights, smells, and people that come with treatment. With highly emetic treatments, patients may vomit before they receive the treatment. With improvements in effective anti-emetic regimens and lorazepam infusions added to the chemotherapy protocol, conditioning has been reduced, but subclinical nausea may be a marker for this syndrome. With repetition of nauseating treatments, patients begin to have anxiety the day before or several days before treatment. Benzodiazepines used prophylactically as this syndrome evolves may reduce nausea and avoidance (Greenberg et al., 1987).

Keeping down the anxiety as patients go through treatment has a premium value as the best anti-emetic regimen and lessened anxiety help prevent visceral Pavlovian conditioning and subsequent anticipatory vomiting. Those with conditioned anxiety to the treatment are more apt to be reminded later by memories of the treatment, and respond with anticipatory anxiety to triggers of smells or residual symptoms like paresthesias of peripheral neuropathy (Greenberg et al., 1997; Kornblith, 2003). Persistent symptoms among survivors of Hodgkin's disease fitted with an explanatory model based on classical conditioning. Treatment-induced symptoms are less likely to persist if conditioning did not occur initially (Cameron et al., 2001). Younger patients, those with a history of motion sickness, and those with more emetic treatments are more at risk for conditioning (Andrykowski, 1990).

Claustrophobia can interfere with magnetic resonance imaging (MRI) scans and the preparation for radiation treatment. Benzodiazepines and behavioral treatments can be targeted for these procedures. The role of phobia and anxiety disorder in treatment is not always obvious, as embarrassed patients may disguise the degree of their disability. Anxiety about side effects often interferes with adherence to effective treatments. Patients with anxiety disorders are more likely to believe that oncologists would offer futile therapies and not adequately control their symptoms, and may have delayed diagnosis (Spencer et al., 2010). Among advanced cancer patients, those with panic disorder and post-traumatic stress disorder (PTSD) were more likely to report suicidal thoughts (Spencer et al., 2012). This fits with the recognition that patients with anxiety disorders in general have a greater independent risk of suicide (Sareen et al., 2005).

POST-TRAUMATIC STRESS DISORDER

Although the diagnosis of cancer can be traumatic, most cancer patients do not come to psychiatrists with the primary symptoms of flashbacks. They do experience intrusive thoughts and symptoms of acute stress as they go through complex cancer treatment, all the more if they have anxiety and depressive syndromes (Palgi et al., 2011). These symptoms most often ease with time, except in a small subset of patients. In breast cancer patients, post-traumatic stress symptomatology was noted at 18 months in 16% of patients, and those who met criteria for the disorder were more likely to have a history of violent trauma and anxiety disorder (Elklit et al., 2011; Shelby et al., 2009). In lung and head and neck patients, current cancer-related PTSD was noted in 22% six months after diagnosis and in 14% at 12 months (Kangas et al., 2005). Among more than 500 adult survivors of non-Hodgkin's lymphoma at least seven years from diagnosis, half reported no post-trauma symptoms, and 12% reported resolution of post-traumatic symptoms. (Smith et al., 2011).

Among more than 6,500 survivors of childhood cancer compared to sibling controls, Stuber et al. (2010) found only a minority (9%) who reported functional impairment and/or clinical distress and symptoms consistent with a full diagnosis of PTSD. Those most likely to have the full syndrome were more apt to have had more intensive treatment, to be less educated, and to be unemployed.

The concept of PTSD includes the avoidance of reminders of distress. Avoidance is often not immediately visible to the clinician, as patients avoid describing how they have narrowed their life. Psychosocial interventions have a role in enlarging a life constrained by cancer-related anxiety. Interventions like supportive-expressive group therapy (Spiegel et al., 2007) have strengthened patients' ability to confront, and cognitive behavioral therapy interventions activate patients and reduce avoidance.

Some medical problems masquerade as anxiety in cancer patients. Akathisia or restless leg syndrome is seen as an adverse reaction to anti-emetics, prochlorperazine, or perphenazine. Because patients use anti-emetics so commonly, they may even forget to mention the use of this medication. In the setting of chemotherapy, patients often have as-needed prescriptions of lorazepam 1 mg. If benzodiazepines have been used for a long period, patients may experience inter-dose jitteriness without recognizing any physiological dependence. Because pulmonary embolism is more common in cancer patients and may be heralded by obscure symptoms and anxiety, pulmonary embolism should be on the differential with pulmonary edema as a cause of anxiety and dyspnea.

SYNDROMES OF DEPRESSIVE SYMPTOMS

MALAISE

The flu-like syndrome of malaise, most associated with fever and acute illness—listlessness, poor concentration, hypersomnia, social withdrawal, anorexia, loss of interest, and poor grooming—has been described in animal models as "sickness behavior." This syndrome of fatigue associated with injury and inflammation triggers cytokines and mimics the vegetative somatic symptoms of major depressive disorder (Dantzer et al., 2008). A somatic fatigue syndrome predictably follows procedures like surgery, radiation treatment, and cumulative cycles of chemotherapy. After one year of complex, upfront, multimodal treatment for breast cancer, depressive symptoms were noted in 25% of patients and fatigue in 60%. Fatigue was associated with elevated levels of inflammatory-marker soluble tumor necrosis factor receptor II and with recent chemotherapy treatment. Depressive symptoms were associated with fatigue but not with inflammatory markers. These data support the idea that systemic adjuvant chemotherapy is followed over a year by a somatic fatigue syndrome related to inflammation and distinct from the fatigue of major depressive disorder (Bower et al., 2011). The fatigue of depression is associated with sleep disturbance, a sense of effort, and a dread of the day, rather than the lack of stamina that comes with the fatigue of sickness behavior. However, as the patient takes on pretreatment responsibilities, limited stamina can become a factor that undermines his self-esteem and adds to negative emotions and cognitions.

Clarifying the diagnosis of depression in cancer patients becomes more difficult when the burden of illness is greater and patients come closer to death. To put this in perspective, Lo et al. (2010) followed prospectively 365 patients with advanced gastrointestinal and lung cancer; depressive symptoms were assessed longitudinally every two months. At first, mild depressive symptoms were seen in 35% of patients; 16% had moderate to severe symptoms; and about 5% had persistent moderate to severe depressive symptoms. Compared to patients more than one year before death, the prevalence of moderate to severe symptoms tripled in the final three months of life. Those who were more apt to have depressive symptoms were younger, had a greater physical burden of disease, and had a closer proximity to death. They were the patients more apt to have been treated with antidepressants before the study and who had lower self-esteem, less sense of spiritual well-being, greater anguish about rejection and abandonment, and greater hopelessness.

The convergence of physical and mental symptoms was ultimately associated with the highest risk of depression (Lo et al., 2010), suggesting that the growing physical symptom burden over time is synergistic and demoralizing. Here depressive symptoms are seen as a final common pathway of distress, particularly in those who have psychosocial vulnerability and worse physical symptoms before death.

Depressive symptoms may reflect tumor-related systemic malaise and overlap clinically with the symptoms of major depressive disorder. The course of major depressive disorder in the normal population threads through symptomatic cancer patients as they are treated. For instance, men treated with androgen blockade were more likely to get depression if they had a history of depressive disorder (Pirl et al., 2008), and the rate of depression in cancer survivors seems to be the same as in the normal population (Pirl et al., 2009).

THE MOST VULNERABLE

The elements of psychosocial vulnerability identified in cancer patients in the 1970s—the characteristics that made some more apt to be distressed and more likely to benefit from psychosocial intervention with cancer treatment—showed a similar pattern to that of those most distressed in Lo's study (Weisman et al., 1980; Lo et al., 2010). Those at risk for more distress were more likely to have history of anxiety or depressive disorder; to have a greater burden of physical disease; to have the least social support; to be hopeless, despondent, helpless, anxious, exhausted; feeling worthless, with low self-esteem and a perspective that their time is short. They had more history of maladaptive coping, of being truculent and resentful, repudiating significant key others, and having lower ego strength (Weisman, 1984). The goal of treatment is to reduce tumor burden and medical symptoms, to treat psychiatric diagnoses, to minimize the behavior patterns that make coping inefficient, and to increase social support.

SUICIDAL THOUGHTS

The desire for hastened death, death sooner than natural disease progression, or passive or active suicidal wishes in the setting of advanced disease, comes with depressive disorder and hopelessness. Chochinov found 8.5% of those admitted to the hospital for terminal illness wished to die sooner, and most of these patients were clinically depressed (1998). Among 3,000 ambulatory cancer patients in Scotland, 8% reported that they had had thoughts in the previous two weeks that they would be better off dead, or had thoughts of hurting themselves (Walker et al., 2008). Those with suicidal thoughts were more apt to have clinically significant emotional distress,

substantial pain, and to a lesser extent, older age. A similar proportion, 8.9% of 700 advanced cancer patients, acknowledged the thought of suicide. By structured clinical interview, these patients were more apt to have current panic disorder and PTSD and more likely to be sad and to lack a sense of self-efficacy, spirituality, and a sense of being supported (Spencer et al., 2012).

In the setting of a cancer diagnosis, the likelihood of suicide is greatest when the diagnosis is new and when it seems to the patient more likely to be advanced and progressive: and therefore, more overwhelming. The cancers associated with the highest rates of suicide as determined by death certificate are lung, stomach, oral cavity and pharynx, larynx, and pancreatic cancer (Misono et al., 2008). Even with pancreatic cancer, however, suicide is extremely rare (Turaga et al., 2011). The presence of suicidal thoughts should lead directly to further assessment of the diagnosis of depressive disorder, to clarification of the medical predicament, and to attention for pain and other physically distressing symptoms.

HORMONAL CAUSES OF DEPRESSIVE SYMPTOMS

The diagnosis of depressive disorder is complicated by simultaneous hormonal changes.

Induction of Chemical Menopause

Many women in their forties or fifties or younger in the midst of cancer treatment develop temporary or permanent menopause as a side effect of treatment (Walsh et al., 2006). The symptoms of menopause—hot flashes, insomnia, dysphoria, and irritability—add to the psychic stress of coping with cancer and overlap with other depressive symptoms. The psychological adjustment is more difficult if women are younger and if they have rapid estrogen withdrawal. Reasons for estrogen withdrawal during cancer treatment are listed in Box 57.1.

Box 57.1 **CAUSES OF ESTROGEN WITHDRAWAL FROM CANCER TREATMENT**

1. Surgical oophorectomy.

2. Chemotherapy, particularly alkylating agents, can cause ovarian injury; so that women stop menses temporarily during treatment or come to menopause earlier than they would have otherwise. Permanent menopause is likelier if the woman is older or if the dose of the agent is higher.

3. Radiation treatment in the vicinity of ovaries can also lead to ovarian failure and hasten menopause.

4. Stopping estrogen replacement abruptly, particularly in women with newly diagnosed estrogen-positive breast cancer.

5. For women with estrogen receptor–positive tumors, the treatments with tamoxifen or aromatase inhibitors amplify menopausal symptoms.

Most women without cancer do not get depressed as they go through natural estrogen withdrawal, but some do. Clarification of menopausal symptoms like insomnia and hot flashes in the backdrop of cancer treatment may help women understand what they have been feeling. Risk of major depressive disorder is greater in perimenopause or the late menopausal transition (Schmidt et al., 2009). Estrogen withdrawal is more apt to induce depressive symptoms in women with a past history of perimenopausal depression than in those without such a history. Both tamoxifen and aromatase inhibitors, which suppress estradiol, have a risk of anxiety or depressive symptoms in a minority of women. In a large study comparing tamoxifen and anastrazole, an aromatase inhibitor, for instance, this rate of mood swings and irritability was about 10%, similar in both groups (Howell et al., 2005; Fallow field et al., 2004). Tamoxifen was associated with more disruptions in sleep and with hot flashes in 40–85% of women. Other menopausal symptoms, like vaginal dryness, low libido, dyspareunia, diarrhea, dizziness, and vaginal discharge, were worse over the first three months; thereafter, menopausal symptoms remained the same or improved.

One clinical strategy is to pay attention to the patient's quality of sleep. The risk of depression may be reduced by preserving the quality of sleep disrupted by estrogen deficiency (Joffe, 2006, 2010, 2011). Many psychotropic medications reduce the vasomotor symptoms of estrogen deficiency that disrupt sleep and may simultaneously treat anxiety or depression. These are gabapentin, venlafaxine, and serotonin reuptake inhibitors, especially citalopram, escitalopram, paroxetine. These have been more effective than sertraline or fluoxetine (Loprinzi, 2009). Escitalopram has also been shown to improve the quality of sleep in healthy menopausal women (Ensrud et al., 2012).

Postmenopausal women with hormone-sensitive breast cancer may have a choice of taking an aromatase inhibitor or tamoxifen; premenopausal women with estrogen-receptor-positive tumors may require tamoxifen as a component of anti-cancer treatment to lower the risk of relapse. Some have thought that the effectiveness of tamoxifen in preventing relapse of breast cancer hinges on the metabolism of tamoxifen to endoxifen by CYP 2D6 enzyme metabolism. Use of drugs that inhibit 2D6 has been discouraged, such as fluoxetine or paroxetine. Bupropion similarly inhibits 2D6 in some patients. Thus far, it has not been clear that the effectiveness of the CYP 2D6 enzyme actually affects the risk of relapse. In fact, there was no difference between rate of relapse compared by genetic CYP 2D profile in two large studies (Regan et al., 2012; Rae, 2010, 2012; Morrow et al., 2012; Lash et al., 2010, 2011). It may be that the other metabolites of tamoxifen are sufficiently anti-estrogen and variable in metabolism regardless of the 2D6 profile. It is cautious to use citalopram, escitalopram, or venlafaxine with tamoxifen to minimize the interaction. When bupropion is the drug of choice, the value of the dose and duration of treatment can be evaluated against the unproven relationship to 2D6 inhibition for tamoxifen.

The leutinizing hormone-releasing hormone (LHRH) agonist leuprolide that causes reversible inhibition of gonadotropin secretion and suppression of testosterone and ovarian function is used in breast cancer patients and prostate cancer patients. In breast cancer patients, it sustains a temporary menopause. Like other drugs that precipitate menopause, this drug can cause hot flashes, disturbed sleep, diminished libido, and poorer quality of orgasms in women, but significant depressive symptoms are less common (Schmidt, 2009; Ben Dor et al., 2013). In prostate cancer patients, this drug aids in androgen blockade. The risk of major depressive disorder in the setting of androgen blockade is related to a history of past depression (Pirl, 2008; Pirl et al., 2002; Roth et al., 1998).

Corticosteroids

Corticosteroids are mood destabilizers and the most common cause of mood lability in the course of cancer treatment. Psychiatric side effects are typically associated with the equivalent of prednisone 60 mg each day, and dexamethasone 9 mg is equivalent to 60 mg prednisone. To prevent vomiting with highly emetic chemotherapy drugs, dexamethasone 12 mg is often added on the day of treatment and in advance. Dexamethasone 8 mg twice daily has had a role in preventing delayed nausea, which occurs with doxorubicin, cisplatin, carboplatin, or oxaliplatin (Roscoe, 2012). Steroids prevent hypersensitivity from taxanes. Prednisone 100 mg per day for five days is a standard regimen in anti-lymphoma treatment, and dexamethasone is a treatment for myeloma. Steroids also prevent vomiting from visceral radiation treatment and reduce edema in the central nervous system.

Psychiatric side effects range from insomnia, jitteriness, and hyperactivity to depressed mood, emotional lability with tearfulness, and irritability, to psychotic and manic-like syndromes. The psychiatric side effects are not predictable from one time to another, but the risk is dose-related. Stopping the steroid may not relieve the psychiatric syndrome immediately, unless the syndrome is treated with psychotropic medication. Mood stabilizers can be used to advantage to minimize insomnia and mood lability, for instance brief use of atypical antipsychotics. Sometimes, a depressive syndrome comes with the cessation of steroids. In the setting of primary care, a history of using glucocorticoids increases the risk of suicidal behavior and neuropsychiatric disorders (Fardet et al., 2012).

Cushing's disease from a pituitary adenoma or adrenal malignancy is more likely to present with a depressive syndrome than hypomania. Ectopic adrenocorticotrophic hormone (ACTH) is a paraneoplastic non-pituitary cause of corticosteroid-induced psychiatric side effects. This condition accounts for about 10% of patients with Cushing's syndrome. About half present with psychiatric disorders. Ectopic ACTH is associated with carcinoid tumors, neuroendocrine tumors, small-cell lung cancer, pheochromocytoma, and medullary thyroid cancer (Ilias et al., 2005).

Hypothyroidism and Hyperthyroidism

Symptoms of hypothyroidism, such as fatigue, weakness, depression, memory loss, cold intolerance, and cardiovascular effects, can appear insidiously in patients with cancer. When hypothyroidism is not recognized, sedating medications can raise the risk of delirium, aspiration, and hypotension. An elevated thyroid stimulating hormone (TSH) will identify a patient with hypothyroidism from thyroidectomy, radiation to the thyroid, or radiation to the neck for lymphoma. However, TSH will be low or normal in patients who had pituitary radiation, and measures of free thyroxine will be required to document secondary hypothyroidism in a patient who has had radiation to the pituitary or brain. Iodinated contrast (from scans of organs for staging) can have acute effects on thyroid, in presence of autonomous nodules or mild Graves' disease, including transient hypothyroidism in patients with Hashimoto's thyroiditis. Hypothyroidism can also develop in patients on newer anti-cancer agents, immune modulators, tyrosine kinase inhibitors (Lodish et al., 2010), and lenalidomide. Thyroid function should be screened periodically in these patients and is an important differential diagnosis for major depressive disorder (Hamnvik et al., 2011).

Adrenal Insufficiency

Adrenal insufficiency may be another mimic of depression in patients with immune-mediated hypophysitis from anti-CTLA4 treatments, like iplimumab (Dillard et al., 2010; Weber et al., 2007).

Chemotherapy agents implicated in depressive syndromes are listed in Box 57.2.

TREATMENT

The medical psychiatrist's art is to tailor the type and timing of psychosocial interventions based on the diagnosis, the patient's willingness, and the data for the greatest clinical benefit to his psychological predicament and natural course of cancer illness. Since there is no laboratory test for the severity of major depressive disorder, an oncologist may not be evaluating the degree to which the patient's psychological suffering may be untreated, or related, for example, to a previous history of major depressive disorder and distinct from the course of cancer. In addition, patients with depression who also have anxiety syndromes are more difficult to treat, even when cancer is not an issue. It is helpful to use measures like the Patient Health Questionnaire 9 (PHQ9; Fann et al., 2009) as a screen and then to monitor outcome.

Pirl et al. (2012) found that lung cancer patients who met criteria for clinical depression in the two months following diagnosis had a worse prognosis. Patients often responded to clinical treatment for depression, but the data were not sufficient to show if successful antidepressant and psychosocial treatment improved their overall cancer prognosis. It is likely that both major depressive disorder and depressive- or malaise-like symptoms associated with the tumor contribute

---

Box 57.2 CHEMOTHERAPY AGENTS IMPLICATED IN DEPRESSIVE SYMPTOMS

Alkylating agents, sparse data for depressogenic effects (Celano et al., 2011)

Procarbazine (Deconti, 1971)
  Reported side effect of depression or lassitude
  Weak monoamine oxidase (MAO) inhibitor, inhibition of P450 enzymes
  Disulfiram reaction if patient drinks alcohol
  Rare cases of serotonin syndrome, mania

Vincristine and vinblastine—depressive reactions reported

Pemetrexed
  Depression reported (Cohen et al., 2005), an antifolate antimetabolite
  The drug is given with folate and vitamin B12 supplementation

L-asparaginase
  Irritability, depression, hallucination (Haskell et al., 1969; Oettgen et al., 1970)

Paclitaxel fatigue, given with steroids to prevent hypersensitivity

Docetaxel prominent fatigue, given with corticosteroids to prevent hypersensitivity (Thornton et al., 2008)

Imantinib, cetuximab, dasatinib, sorafenib, sunitinib (O'Brien, 2003; Quek, 2009; Pirl, 2009)
  Depression uncommon
  Consider hypothyroidism

Interleukin-2
  Dose-related depression scores (Walker et al., 1997)
  Correlated with increased cytokine levels (Capuron et al., 2001)

Interferon (Musselman, 2001; Kirkwood et al., 2002; Hauschild et al., 2008; Greenberg et al., 2000; Islam et al., 2002)
  Malaise and major depressive disorder common
  Inhibition of P450 enzymes
  Autoimmune changes in thyroid function
  Manic state has been observed, usually during interferon dose reductions, or pauses in therapy, or as interferon-induced depression is treated with antidepressants
  Nearly all patients develop adverse effects on memory after six doses of therapy in the dose used for advanced melanoma
  Generally mild to moderate neurospsychiatric symptoms that resolve in 2–3 weeks after interferon discontinuation

Tamoxifen, aromatase inhibitors, LHRH agonists, testosterone, anti-androgens
  Clinical depression related to hormonal change, history of depressive episodes, or history of mood vulnerability to hormonal change

Corticosteroids
  Affective change is dose related, most likely in equivalent of prednisone 60 mg or higher.
  Mood lability varying from anxiety, jitteriness, insomnia to hypomania and depression. Psychosis can occur. Mood stabilizers like atypical anti-psychotics are effective for lability as well as psychosis.
  Depression may occur after cessation of these drugs.

to the prognosis (Pirl et al., 2011). In these studies of advanced lung cancer patients, care was a collaboration between an oncology team and palliative care team who kept their eyes on depressive symptoms, provided antidepressants, and focused on other psychosocial issues (Yoong et al., 2013).

Collaborative care programs for psychosocial aspects of cancer treatment have been shown to be effective for treatment of depression in four other randomized controlled trials (Ell et al., 2008; Fann et al., 2012; Sharpe et al., 2004; Kroenke et al., 2010; Fann et al., 2009) in settings as diverse as the California public health sector, a cancer center in Scotland, primary care settings, and at home. These programs are structured with psychiatrists supervising care managers who hold a caseload of patients. The psychiatrists also consult to primary medical providers on the more challenging patients for additional specialty services, and see patients themselves when required. Care managers provide brief evidence-based psychosocial treatment. The emphasis is on a population-based approach to identifying needs, measuring outcomes, sustained follow-up, vigorous outreach, and treatment to remission. Measurement-based care and clinical rating scales identify patients who require treatment or are at risk.

Severity of depression is measured repeatedly, and the treatment is intensified to ensure targeted improvement. Of note, Ell found in a female, predominantly Hispanic population of cancer patients, including 114 with major depression, treated with antidepressant medication and/or problem-solving therapy, a response rate of 70% at six months. At 12 months, 14% relapsed, another 17% had responded, and 13% had not responded (Ell, 2008). Continuing attention to the instrument score measuring depressive symptoms is warranted.

When the rate of depressive disorder is high for specific anti-cancer treatments, antidepressants have prevented depression. Paroxetine given before a protocol of high-dose alpha interferon for melanoma reduced the rate of depression compared to placebo (Musselman et al., 2001). In head and neck cancer patients, escitalopram 10–20 mg compared to placebo given at the outset of multimodality treatment and continued for 16–17 weeks led to a reduction in the risk of depression by more than 50%. Better quality of life was reported for three months after cessation of the antidepressant in the treated group (Lydiatt et al., 2013).

The best treatments would combine protocols for affective psychiatric diagnoses with those that help patients tolerate cancer treatment. One recent trial combined a biobehavioral intervention for stress in cancer patients with cognitive behavioral treatment tailored specifically for depression, in order to treat cancer patients with depressive disorder who were already on antidepressant medication. Concurrent anxiety disorders and high levels of cancer stress were each associated with beginning and ending treatment with more depressive symptoms. The program included progressive muscle-relaxation training, emphasis on coping with the cancer crisis, behavioral activation, communication with healthcare providers, social support, cognitive reappraisal, communicating needs, problem solving, core beliefs, rhythmic walking, review of therapy components, and strategies

for successful maintenance (Brothers et al., 2011). The strategies of mind–body medicine used to foster healing in cancer patients were combined with evidence-based strategies for those with depression (see chapter 17).

Standard protocols for cognitive behavioral therapy for anxiety disorder or depression must be adapted to the realistic worries of the cancer patient who may face real progression toward feared events. Greer and colleagues (2012) have adapted a decisional model to help patients evaluate how much negative thoughts may contain both biased and realistic elements. Adaptive thinking skills may be supplemented with acceptance-oriented coping, like mindfulness for what seems realistic or getting more information when data is missing.

PSYCHOPHARMACOLOGY

Strategic use of pharmacology in cancer patients can make important contributions to their quality of life.

1. If patients have depressive disorder—particularly if they have a history of depressive disorder—the treatment of depression in the setting of cancer should be careful and persistent, with adequate and sequential trials of antidepressants and proactive monitoring for relapse.

2. Some patients undergoing recurrent cancer treatment will develop conditioned anxiety to procedures or traumas associated with treatment. When anxiety becomes chronic, antidepressants also have a role.

3. Anxious patients with depression do not respond as well to pharmacological treatment; multiple modalities of treatment and attention to specific anxiety, avoidance, and adherence may be particularly important.

4. Medications used for nausea with chemotherapy like olanzapine (Navari et al., 2013) or lorazepam may be used to advantage for anxiety or mood stabilization.

5. In the setting of estrogen withdrawal, serotonin reuptake inhibitors can suppress hot flashes as well as treat depression.

6. Gabapentin has benefit for neuropathic pain as well as hot flash suppression and the improvement of sleep or some types of anxiety (Pachman et al., 2012; Loprinzi et al., 2009). Duloxitene is useful both as an antidepressant and analgesic for chemotherapy-induced neuropathic pain (Lavoie-Smith et al., 2013).

7. Akathisia should not be missed when due to prochlorperazine.

8. Serotonin reuptake inhibitors can cause initial nausea and appetite suppression. This can be difficult in the anorectic patient, but ondansetron or another drug that offers 5HT3 blockade can be used as an antidote for the nausea until initial nausea dissipates and an anti-depressant response occurs.

9. Mirtazapine has an advantage in patients who wish for better sleep and appetite (Riechelmann et al., 2010).

10. Psychostimulants methylphenidate and dextroamphetamine have been used in the medically ill to improve concentration and attention, mood, and energy. They have the advantage of a quick effect. Recent meta-analyses have shown marginal improvement for depression or cancer-related fatigue, with more benefit in those more fatigued (Minton et al., 2011). Modafinil has also been useful to alert patients.

CANCER TREATMENT–ASSOCIATED COGNITIVE DECLINE

Since patients often have difficulty concentrating and thinking during chemotherapy treatment, they worry about permanent effects on the brain. The term "chemo-brain" suggests that chemotherapy puts cognitive functions at risk. Only a subset of patients has distress from clinically significant, persistent cognitive consequences.

Patients do not think as well as they face a series of infusions, recurrent inflammation, fatigue, and anemia. Anticholinergic medications, sedatives, corticosteroids, and narcotics that contribute to cognitive impairment are often added to the mix. Systemic illness with associated cytokines brings on a variety of cognitive complaints, fatigue, and low mood. Just as it takes time to recover from the fatigue associated with chemotherapy, it takes time to recover from the marathon of treatment. Breast cancer survivors, particularly those who had adjuvant chemotherapy, show improvement after a year; but markers for chronic inflammation and subjective cognitive complaints can persist (Bower, 2011).

Younger premenopausal women with breast cancer, three to four months after treatment with chemotherapy, had more difficulty with concentration, memory, processing speed, and more self-reported cognitive complaints of distraction, poor memory of names, and searching for words. Common complaints are being easily distracted, having difficulty concentrating and staying on task, and having difficulty recalling recent events or what was just said to them. The late transition to menopause even without cancer treatment is associated with temporary cognitive decrements in verbal memory, processing speed, and working memory (Greendale et al., 2009), and cognitive difficulties may be greater with the use of tamoxifen and chemotherapy compared to chemotherapy alone (Castellon et al., 2004) or tamoxifen compared to exemestane (Schilder et al., 2010; Janelsins et al., 2011). These hormonal effects may be more problematic in young patients.

The patients at risk for cognitive impairment from nonhormonal treatments may be older, may already have cognitive decline at cancer diagnosis, or may have genetic risk factors for cognitive impairment in cancer survivors like apolipoprotein E and catechol-0-methyltransferase (COMT) Val-allele genotypes. The more vulnerable patients may have less cognitive reserve, in terms of education, occupational attainment, and lifestyle.

Clinical depression, by itself associated with poor concentration, poor sleep, fatigue, and negative self-image, amplifies cognitive complaints. Neuropsychiatric testing does not typically document findings that parallel these complaints.

Patients who undergo hematopoietic stem cell transplantation (HCT) often develop delirium or seizures with significant cognitive impairment, gradually recovering after the procedure. About half have mild long-term deficits, and 20–28% have moderate long-term deficits, more than two standard deviations below population norms. The likelihood of persistent cognitive impairment is related to cumulative risk factors over time (Jim et al., 2012). These factors include history of cranial irradiation, intrathecal chemotherapy, total-body irradiation, multiple courses of standard-dose chemotherapy, baseline impairment, allogeneic rather than autologous transplantation, unrelated donor, and length of hospital stay. Hospital-stay duration is a proxy for complications of treatment like graft vs. host disease, or the use of steroids and narcotics. The domains most often impaired are memory and executive functioning, the ability to store and retrieve verbal and visual information, and the ability to plan higher order tasks. Cancer patients who receive standard-dose chemotherapy may have structural changes: for instance, reductions in gray matter, primarily in frontal structures and hippocampus, and white matter integrity (Ahles et al., 2012; Deprez et al., 2012).

The best clinical strategy for cognitive complaints is to simplify medication regimens, improve quality of sleep, and give the best treatment for depressive disorder. More thorough neuropsychological testing can offer objective data, clarifying particular deficits. Practice of compensatory strategies can lead to improvements in the range of 0.5 to 1.0 standard deviation on objective neuropsychological function and subjective description of function (Ferguson, 2007; or Ferguson et al., 2012). Cognitive rehabilitation, particularly in patients with brain tumors, has shown benefit (Langenbahn et al., 2013). Modafinil can make a positive contribution (Kohli, 2009; Lundorff et al., 2009).

Tests for cognitive impairment related to cancer should focus on the frontal subcortical profile, particularly the domains of learning, memory, processing speed, and executive function (more complex attention). A task force has suggested using standard tests: Hopkins Verbal Learning Test–Revised HVLT-R, Trail-Making Test (TMT), and the Controlled Oral Word Association (COWA) of the Multilingual Aphasia Examination. Tests for working memory like the auditory Consonant Trigrams, or Paced Auditory Serial Addition Test, Brief Test of Attention, and WAIS-III Letter-Number Sequencing may be added (Wefel, 2011).

PSYCHOSIS

It is uncommon for a patient to have a psychotic episode with hallucinations, delusions, and thought disorder from cancer alone. Delirium is the most common reason for delusion or hallucination. Corticosteroids given exogenously for treatment would be the most likely reason to see psychosis in cancer patients.

Tumors that produce corticosteroids also can lead to psychosis of Cushing's syndrome, including adrenocortical carcinoma, ACTH-producing tumor of the pituitary, and ectopic ACTH (Ilias, 2005). Antipsychotic medications may have some benefit as the tumor producing high levels of endogenous corticosteroid is treated. If the tumor continues to progress and psychotic symptoms persist, mifepristone can reduce psychiatric symptoms (Johanssen & Allolio, 2007).

There are case reports of psychosis occurring with carcinoid and thymoma. Chemotherapy has rarely led to psychosis; recent literature includes two cases associated with sunitinib, one with ifosfamide neurotoxicity (responsive to methylene blue), and one with 5-fluorouracil (5-FU) neurotoxicity. Neurotoxicity from 5-FU is worse in the setting of a vulnerable blood–brain barrier or dehydropyrimidine dehydrogenase (D6PD) deficiency. Sunitinib can cause cobalamin deficiency and hypothyroidism. An ifosfamide metabolite is thought to be the culprit in ifosfamide-induced encephalopathy.

Psychosis can be a late sequela of brain tumor treated in childhood or adolescence. Late-onset persistent psychosis may occur in survivors of childhood brain tumors at a rate of 2–3%. Many cases are associated with cognitive impairment and imaging showing diffuse, irregular, asymmetrical focal calcifications, glial scars, and multiple small areas of necrosis and infarction (Turkel, 2007). Survivors of cancer in childhood or adolescence ($n = 3700$) in a Danish population-based, retrospective cohort study, had no greater risk for psychiatric hospitalization for any psychiatric disorder; the rate of psychiatric hospitalization was only increased in survivors of brain tumors.

Patients with serious mental illness are more likely to present for care when they already have metastases, and to die of the cancer (Kisely et al., 2013). They do not have a greater incidence of cancer than the general population, and patients with schizophrenia may even have a *lower* risk for cancer (Bushe & Hodgson, 2010). However, once they have cancer they may not be offered treatments that require active compliance, and some refuse care (Hwang et al., 2012).

The key to management of cancer treatment in a patient with schizophrenia is coordinated care between psychiatric and oncology team. Psychotic symptoms should be stabilized before cancer treatment starts. The factors that make it more likely the patient will take psychotropic medications should be maximized. Complicating factors like depression and substance abuse should be considered and treated if possible. Because the patient with psychotic disorder may have cognitive deficits like concrete thinking, clinicians should avoid theoretical and statistical examples in talking to the patient about cancer and stick to basic facts about the specific patient. Attention should be paid to the possibility of delirium rather than psychosis complicating care during the course of the illness. Familiar staff and familiarizing the patient with the settings of radiation or chemotherapy can be helpful. When patients are assumed to have capacity to make decisions about their own care, they may still need extra help to follow up consistently with multiple medical appointments and to call with specific symptoms (Irwin et al., 2014).

USE OF CLOZAPINE

The neutropenia that results from chemotherapy for cancer has a different mechanism than neutropenia caused by clozapine. Clozapine is associated with a rare risk of idiosyncratic agranulocytosis. If a schizophrenic patient has been doing well on clozapine and now faces cancer chemotherapy, there is value in maintaining her clarity of thought and the remission of delusion and hallucination. Clozapine has been used even through the ablation chemotherapy and stem cell transplant for Hodgkin's lymphoma. The risks and benefits can be evaluated in each case (Rosenberg et al., 2007; Rosenstock, 2004; McKnight et al., 2011; Manu, 2012; Andres et al., 2008; Liu et al., 2010).

In practical terms, once started on chemotherapy, the patient will need to have white cell count, hematocrit, and platelets monitored just as with any chemotherapy. If the white count drops below 2000, or the absolute neutrophil count drops below 1000, any physician (oncology or psychiatry or primary care) can contact the clozapine registry and ask for a waiver (to be granted permission to continue clozapine treatment despite the expected granulocytopenia related to chemotherapy). The waiver is normally issued if the following elements are carefully documented:

1. The low absolute neutrophil count is not related to clozapine.

2. Clozapine treatment plus chemotherapy is needed to continue to treat the tumor.

3. There is a plan for the weekly monitoring of white count and absolute neutrophil count.

4. The method of support for the bone marrow has been defined should agranulocytosis develop.

The waiver cannot be issued in advance.

NEUROPSYCHIATRIC SYNDROMES AND SUBACUTE EMERGENCIES

Some emergencies in oncological care present with psychiatric symptoms, and it is useful for psychiatrists to keep in mind the subacute emergencies of the cancer patient.

METABOLIC ABNORMALITIES

Hypercalcemia presents with fatigue, constipation, thirst, cognitive impairment, and delirium. *Hyponatremia* due to the syndrome of inappropriate diuretic hormone (Smith et al., 2000) is a cause of confusion and seizure.

SPINAL CORD COMPRESSION

Spinal cord compression can present with symptoms that are gradual and not readily recognized: weakness in legs, falling, and incontinence associated with back pain. While not strictly psychiatric, the psychiatrist may hear about these embarrassing symptoms first.

BRAIN METASTASES

When a patient has a known cancer diagnosis, changes in mental status may signal brain metastases. The likelihood increases with the stage of cancer at first presentation and more common in some tumors than others. The total incidence proportion percentage of brain metastases was 10% for patients with primary lung, melanoma, breast, renal, or colorectal cancer. The rate was highest for lung (20%), then melanoma (7%), renal 7%, breast 5%, and colorectal cancers (2%) (Barnholtz-Sloan et al., 2004).

LEPTOMENINGEAL METASTASES

Leptomeningeal metastases may present with mental status changes and minimal brain MRI findings. Cancer spreads to the arachnoid and pia mater, the leptomeninges, surrounding the cerebrospinal fluid (CSF) in 5–8% of all patients with cancer. As treatments extend survival, the problem may become more common. Leptomeningeal metastases occur more often in breast cancer, particularly lobular, lung; melanoma, acute lymphoblastic leukemia, non-Hodgkin's lymphoma, and GI malignancies, but any cancer can spread to the leptomeninges (Groves, 2011). Patients usually present with cranial nerve and spinal nerve root dysfunction, but also mental status abnormalities, headache, syncope, seizures, balance problems, and nausea and vomiting. Diplopia, hearing changes and facial weakness may be signs of cranial nerve deficits. Diagnosis requires brain MRI with gadolinium and CSF evaluation for tumor cells. The entire neuraxis needs to be evaluated. Typically, the MRI shows contrast enhancement of the leptomeninges, subependyma, cranial and spinal nerves. It is not uncommon, however, for an MRI to be positive and the CSF negative or for the MRI to be normal in hematological cancers with leptomeningeal disease. Bevicizumab makes it harder to see the typical findings of leptomeningeal enhancement (Keinschimidet-DeMasters & Damek, 2010). If the patient presents with mental status changes deemed psychiatric and more subtle clinical findings, the psychiatrist's role may be to remain suspicious about cancer-related causes of deterioration.

PARANEOPLASTIC LIMBIC ENCEPHALITIS AND ENCEPHALOMYELITIS

A paraneoplastic autoimmune encephalitis in adults and children due to antibodies against neuronal cell surface antigens or immune reactions to intracellular antigens can present with psychiatric symptoms. Disseminated neuronal loss and inflammatory lesions in different parts of the nervous system, especially the hippocampus, the lower brainstem, spinal cord or doral root ganglia, characterize this syndrome. About half the patients with the syndrome associated with the onconeuronal antigen Hu-abs have a subacute sensory neuropathy, and some have cerebellar signs and limbic encephalitis. Most of these patients have small cell lung cancer (SCLC), and the course of the syndrome can improve with tumor treatment and relapse with tumor recurrence. Collapsin response mediator protein type 5 (CV2/CRMP5)-Abs and amphiphysin-abs are also implicated. Limbic encephalitis is now seen as part of a more disseminated encephalitis as more than the limbic system may be affected (Didelot & Honnorat, 2014).

Limbic encephalitis is characterized by short-term memory loss (an anterograde amnesia), behavioral disturbance, confusion, and seizures (Kayser et al., 2010). Irritability, depression, hallucinations, sleep disturbance, personality disturbances, and short-term memory loss progressing to dementia may be noted. In addition to a mild lymphocytic pleocytosis in the CSF, imaging may show medial temporal lobe hyperintensities on fluid-attenuated inversion recovery (FLAIR) and T2-weighted images with progressive hippocampal gyrus volume loss. The descriptions have ranged from psychosis to obsessive compulsive disorder. Abnormalities are noted in the limbic system and medial temporal lobe on MRI or positron emission tomography (PET). The presence of antibodies does not necessarily indicate that there is an underlying tumor. However, almost all patients with Hu-Abs have cancer after 5 years of follow-up. Ma2-Abs is associated with cancer in the majority of cases, mostly SCLC, but also testicular cancer. Antibodies to gamma aminobutyric acid-b receptor (GABAbR-ab) lead to limbic encephalitis in Hu-negative SCLC patients presenting with seizures (Boronat et al., 2011). Voltage gated potassium channel/ leucine rich glioma-inactivated 1 protein(VGKC/ LGI1) antibody-positive limbic encephalitis is associated with tumor in 12% of cases. The presentation includes hyponatremia, autonomic symptoms, and seizures, in addition to amnesia. Malignant thymoma as well as SCLC have been reported. Rarely limbic encephalitis associated with other antibodies have been linked to thymoma, breast cancer, lung cancer, or prostate cancer (Didelot & Honnorat, 2014).

Immunotherapy (intravenous immunoglobulin G (IgG) and/or plasma exchange at presentation for rapid antibody clearance, followed by six months of high-dose corticosteroids) may be helpful. Tumor resection, chemotherapy, or radiotherapy by reducing or removing the tumor can have benefit. Cortical atrophy is associated with persistent cognitive deficits, especially in verbal and visual memory.

Limbic encephalitis from antibodies to N-methyl-D-aspartate receptor (NMDAr-Abs) is a syndrome that psychiatrists should not miss. The antibody targets the N-terminal extracellular domain of the NR1 subunit of the glutamate receptor NMDA interfering with the glutamatergic pathway. It presents in the psychiatric setting as subacute atypical psychosis, irritability, catatonia, dyskinesia, autonomic instability, and central hypoventilation (Irani, 2011). This syndrome occurring predominantly in women, begins with psychiatric symptoms and seizures and progresses to movement disorders, loss of consciousness, and dysautonomia in one-third. In the first stage CSF lymphocytosis is noted; in the second oligoclonal bands are found in the CSF (Dalmau et al., 2014). It is associated with ovarian teratoma, and removal of the teratoma may be curative. The pertinent examination when this syndrome is suspected is transvaginal ultrasound and/ or pelvic MRI. This syndrome has been reported in children in association with teratoma and neuroblastoma (Didelot & Honnorat, 2011).

POSTERIOR REVERSIBLE ENCEPHALOPATHY SYNDROME (PRES)

Posterior reversible encephalopathy syndrome (PRES) is a syndrome of hypertension, headache, speech difficulty, altered consciousness, visual hallucinations, change in mental status, seizures, hallucinations, acute visual changes, and findings of symmetrical white matter lesions in parietal and occipital lobes (Hinchey, 1996).

The angiogenesis inhibitors put patients at risk for hypertension, alteration in the blood–brain barrier, capillary leakage, and vasogenic edema. The effects are more prominent posteriorly because of sparse sympathetic innervations of the vertebrobasilar system. Hypomagnesemia facilitates cortical spreading depression. Non-enhancing, confluent, periventricular white matter lesions, necrosis, ventriculomegaly, and cortical atrophy are seen with delayed onset of several months. An MRI with FLAIR images and diffusion-weighted sequences should be done. Treatment is control of blood pressure and management of seizures with anticonvulsants for three to six months. A specific offending agent should be discontinued. PRES is also one of the immune-related adverse events associated with some tyrosine kinase inhibitors.

CHEMOTHERAPY-INDUCED LEUKOENCEPHALOPATHY

Methotrexate leukoencephalopathy is precipitated in the setting of high-dose or intrathecal treatment, but it occurs later than PRES, resolves more slowly, and is associated with hemiparesis, paraparesis, and choreoathetoid movements. Visual disturbance and change in mental status are less prominent (Filley, 2005). Other chemotherapy agents known to cause leukoencephalopathy are cisplatin, ifosfamide, 5-fluoruracil, cytarabine, and carmustine. Delayed leukoencephalopathy syndrome mimicking stroke is seen mainly with methotrexate, 5-FU, and capecitabine.

Leukoencephalopathy Due to Radiation Treatment with or Without Chemotherapy

The combination of radiation treatment and intrathecal methotrexate increases the risk of cognitive impairment (Duffner, 2004; Crossen et al., 1994). Children treated for acute lymphocytic leukemia or a brain tumor with cranial irradiation are at risk for cognitive decline. Cognitive decline is progressive over at least ten years. A radiation-induced progressive microvasculopathy may account for this progression. Babies are particularly prone to radiotoxicity in the first two years of life because of the rapid growth of the brain and white matter development in those years. Cognitive defects have been seen in verbal comprehension, perceptual organization, distractibility, and memory in survivors of acute lymphocytic leukemia. Visuomotor integration, sequential memory, fine motor coordination, processing speed, and math abilities may also be affected. Risk factors include young age, female gender, and time since radiation. The volume and dose of radiation are also thought to be factors. Even with a relatively low dose of cranial radiation, deficits can persist, particularly in tasks involving rapid processing of information (Edelstein et al., 2011). Children exposed to cranial irradiation may also suffer hypothyroidism and growth hormone deficiency. Children who have been treated for leukemia or brain tumors should be monitored for cognitive and endocrine dysfunction.

CLINICAL PEARLS

- In confronting a life-threatening illness, the primary paradox is that a dying man believes in the fact of his own death but hopes that he is an exception (Weisman, 1972, p. 13).

- Hope is related to a desirable self-image and a belief in the personal ability to exert a degree of influence on the world (Weisman, 1972, p. 20); the conviction that a person may do something worth doing (p. 21).

- In order to treat demoralization, Griffith and Gaby focus questions at the bedside to find the dominant existential theme in the patient's experience of illness and then suggest nudging the patient forward with a series of questions oriented to attributes of resilience.

- Treatment-induced symptoms are less likely to persist if conditioning did not occur initially (Cameron, 2001). Younger patients, those with a history of motion sickness, and those with more emetic treatments are more at risk for conditioning (Andrykowski, 1990).

- Among more than 6,500 survivors of childhood cancer compared to sibling controls, Stuber et al. (2010) found only a minority (9%) who reported functional impairment and/or clinical distress and symptoms consistent with a full diagnosis of PTSD.

- The cancers most associated with the highest rates of suicide are lung, stomach, oral cavity and pharynx, larynx, and pancreatic cancer (Misono et al., 2008).

- Hypothyroidism can also develop in patients on newer anti-cancer agents, immune modulators, tyrosine kinase inhibitors (Lodish et al., 2010), and lenalidomide.

- Clozapine has been used even through the ablation chemotherapy and stem cell transplant for Hodgkin's lymphoma. The mechanism of agranulocytosis from clozapine is idiosyncratic and distinct from the mechanism of chemotherapy-induced leucopenia.

- Patients with serious mental illness are more likely to present for care when they already have metastases, and to die of the cancer (Kisely, 2013). They do not have a greater incidence of cancer than the general population, and patients with schizophrenia may even have a lower risk for cancer (Bushe et al., 2010); however, they present with more advanced disease.

- Collaborative care programs for psychosocial aspects of cancer treatment have been shown effective for treatment of depression in five randomized controlled trials (Ell, 2008; Fann, 2012; Sharpe, 2004; Kroenke, 2010; Fann, 2009).

- Antibodies against NMDA receptors (NMDAr-Abs) are associated with widespread encephalitis and paraneoplastic limbic encephalitis seen as subacute atypical psychosis, catatonia, dyskinesia, autonomic instability, and central hypoventilation. This syndrome is associated with ovarian teratoma, and removal of the teratoma may be curative.

DISCLOSURE STATEMENT

Dr. Greenberg has no conflicts of interest to disclose.

REFERENCES

Ahles, T. A., Root, J. C., & Ryan, E. L. (2012). Cancer- and center treatment–associated cognitive change: an update on the state of the science. *Journal of Clinical Oncology*, 30, 3675–3686.

Andres, E., & Maloisel, F. (2008). Idiosyncratic drug induced agranulocytosis or acute neutropenia review. *Current Opinion in Hematology*, 15, 15–21.

Andrykowski, M. A. (1990). The role of anxiety in the development of anticipatory nausea in cancer chemotherapy: A review and synthesis. *Psychosomatic Medicine*, 54, 458–475.

Barnholtz-Sloan, J. S., Sloan, A. E., Davis, F. G., Vigneau, F. D., Lai, P., & Sawaya, R. E. (2004). Incidence proportions of brain metastases in patients diagnosed (1973 to 2001) in the Metropolitan Detroit Cancer Surveillance system. *Journal of Clinical Oncology*, 22, 2865–2872.

Ben Dor, R., Harsh, V. L., Fortinsky, P., Koziol, D. E., Rubinow, D. R., & Schmidt, P. J. (2013). Effects of pharmacologically induced hypogonadism on mood and behavior in health young women. *American Journal of Psychiatry*, 170, 426–433.

Boronat, A., Sabater, L., Saiz, A., Dalmau, J., & Graus, F. (2011). GABAb receptor antibodies in limbic encephalitis and anti-GAD-associated neurologic disorder. *Neurology*, 76, 795–800.

Bower, J. E., Ganz, P. A., Irwin, M. R., et al. (2011). Inflammation and behavioral symptoms after breast cancer treatment: Do fatigue, depression, and sleep disturbance share a common underlying mechanism? *Journal of Clinical Oncology*, 29, 3517–3522.

Brothers, B. M., Yang, H. C., Strunk, D. R., & Andersen, B. L. (2011). Cancer patients with major depressive disorder: Testing a biobehavioral/cognitive behavior intervention. *Journal of Consulting Clinical Psychology*, 79, 253–260.

Bushe, C. J., & Hadgson, R. (2010). Schizophrenia and cancer: In 2010 do we understand the connection? *Canadian Journal of Psychiatry*, 55(12), 761–767.

Cameron, C. L., Cella, D., Herndon, J. E. 2nd, et al. (2001). Persistent symptoms among survivors of Hodgkin's disease: An explanatory model based on classical conditioning. *Health Psychology*, 20, 71–75.

Capuron, L., Ravaud, A., Gualde, N., et al. (2001). Association between immune activation and early depressive symptoms in cancer patients treated with interleukin-2-based therapy. *Psychoneuroendocrinology*, 26, 797–808.

Castellon, S. A., Ganz, P. A., Bower, J. E., et al. (2004). Neurocognitive performance in breast cancer survivors exposed to adjuvant chemotherapy and tamoxifen. *Journal of Clinical Experimental Neuropsychology*, 26, 955–969.

Celano, C. M., Freudenreich, O., Fernandez-Robles, C., et al. (2011). Depressogenic effects of medications: A review. *Dialogues in Clinical Neuroscience*, 13, 109–125.

Chochinov, H. M., Kristjanson, L. J., Breitbart, W., et al. (2011). Effect of dignity therapy on distress and end-of-life experience in terminally ill patients: A randomized controlled trial. *Lancet Oncology*, 12, 753–762.

Chochinov, H. M., Wilson, K. G., Enns, M., & Lander, S. (1998). Depression, hopelessness, and suicidal ideation in the terminally ill. *Psychosomatics*, 39, 366–370.

Clarke, D. M., & Kissane, D. W. (2002). Demoralization: Its phenomenology and importance. *Australia and New Zealand Journal of Psychiatry*, 36, 733–742.

Cohen, M. H., Johnson, J. R., Wang, Y. C., Sridhara, R., & Pazdur, R. (2005). FDA drug approval summary: Pemetrexed for injection (Alimta) for the treatment of non–small cell lung cancer. *Oncologist*, 10, 363–368.

Crossen, J. R., Garwood, D., Glatstein, E., & Neuwelt, E. A. (1994). Neurobehavioral sequelae of cranial irradiation in adults: A review of radiation-induced encephalopathy. *Journal of Clinical Oncology* 6, 1215–1228.

Dalmau, J., Lancaster, E., Martinez-Hernandez, E., et al. (2011). Clinical experience and laboratory investigations in patients with anti-NMDAr encephalitis. *Lancet Neurology*, 10, 63–74.

Dantzer, R., O'Connor, J. C., Freund, G. G., Johnson, R. W., & Kelley, K. W. (2008). From inflammation to sickness and depression: When the immune system subjugates the brain. *Nature Reviews Neuroscience*, 9, 46–57.

DeConti, R. C. (1971). Procarbazine in the management of late Hodgkin's disease. *Journal of the American Medical Association*, 215, 927–930.

Demopoulos, A. (2014). Pathophysiology, clinical features, and diagnosis of leptomeningeal metastases from solid tumors. In *UpToDate*, D. S. Basow (Ed.), Waltham MA, UpToDate.

Deprez, S., Amant, F., Smeets, A., et al. (2011). Longitudinal assessment of chemotherapy-induced structural changes in cerebral white matter and its correlation with impaired cognitive function. *Journal of Clinical Oncology*, 20, 274–281.

Didelot, A., & Honnorat, J. (2014). Paraneoplastic disorders of the central and peripheral nervous systems. In J. Biller & J. M. Ferro (Eds.), *Handbook of Clinical Neurology: Neurologic aspects of systemic disease Part III*. 121, 1159–1179.

Dillard, T. Yedinak, C. G., Alumkal, J., & Fleseriu, M. (2010). Anti-CTLA 4 antibody therapy associated autoimmune hypophysitis: Serious immune related adverse events across a spectrum of cancer subtypes. *Pituitary*, 12, 29–38.

Duffner, P. K. (2004). Long-term effects of radiation therapy on cognitive and endocrine function in children with leukemia and brain tumors. *The Neurologist*, 6, 293–310.

Edelstein, K., D'agostino, N., Bernstein, L. J., et al. (2011). Long-term neurocognitive outcomes in young adult survivors of childhood acute lymphoblastic leukemia. *Journal of Pediatric Hematology & Oncology*, 33, 450–458.

Elklit, A., & Blum, A. (2011). Psychological adjustment one year after the diagnosis of breast cancer: A prototype study of delayed post-traumatic stress disorder. *British Journal of Clinical Psychology*, 50, 350–363.

Ell, K., Xie, B., Quon, B., Quinn, D. J., Dwight-Johnson, M., & PeyJiuan, L. (2008). Randomized controlled trial of collaborative care management of depression among low-income patients with cancer. *Journal of Clinical Oncology*, 26, 4488–4496.

Ensrud, K. E., Joffe, H., Guthrie, K. A., et al. (2012). Effect of escitalopram on insomnia symptoms and subjective sleep quality in healthy perimenopausal and post-menopausal women with hot flashes: A randomized controlled trial. *Menopause*, 19, 848–855.

Fallowfield, L., Cella, D., Cuzick, J., et al. (2004). Quality of life of postmenopausal women in the Arimidex, Tamoxifen, Alone or in Combination (ATAC) adjuvant breast cancer trial. *Journal of Clinical Oncology*, 22, 4361–4271.

Fann, J. R., Berry, D. L., Wolpin, S., et al. (2009). Depression screening using the Patient Health Questionnaire–9 administered on a touch screen computer. *Psycho-Oncology*, 18, 14–22.

Fann, J. R., Ell, K., & Sharpe, M. (2012). Integrating psychosocial care into cancer services. *Journal of Clinical Oncology*, 30, 1178–1186.

Fann, J. R., Fan, M. Y., & Unutzer, J. (2009). Improving primary care for older adults with cancer and depression. *Journal of General Internal Medicine*, 24(Suppl 2), S417–S424.

Fardet, L., Petersen, I., & Nazareth, I. (2012). Suicidal behavior and severe neuropsychiatric disorders following glucocorticoid therapy in primary care. *American Journal of Psychiatry*, 169, 491–497.

Ferguson, R. J., McDonald, B. C., Rocque, M. A., et al. (2012). Development of CBT for chemotherapy-related cognitive change: Results of a waitlist control trial. *Psycho-Oncology*, 21, 176–186.

Filley, C. M. (2005). Neurobehavioral aspects of cerebral white matter disorders. *Psychiatric Clinics of North America*, 28, 685–700.

Frank, J. D. (1993). *Persuasion and healing* (2nd ed.). Baltimore, MD: The Johns Hopkins University Press.

Greendale, G. A., Huang, M. H., Wight, R. G., et al. (2009). Effects of the menopause transition and hormone use on cognitive performance in midlife women. *Neurology*, 72, 1850–1857.

Greenberg, D. B., Jonasch, E., Gadd, M. A., et al. (2000). Adjuvant therapy of melanoma with interferon alpha 2b associated with mania and bipolar syndromes, *Cancer*, 89, 356–362.

Greenberg, D. B., Kornblith, A. B., Herndon, J. E., et al. (1997). Quality of life for adult leukemia survivors treated on clinical trials of Cancer and Leukemia Group B during the period 1971–1988, predictors for later psychological distress. *Cancer*, 80, 1936–1944.

Greenberg, D. B., Surman, O. S., Clarke, J., et al. (1987). Alprazolam for phobic nausea and vomiting related to cancer chemotherapy. *Cancer Treatment Report*, 71, 549–550.

Greer, J. A., Traeger, L., Bemis, H., et al. (2012). A pilot randomized controlled trial of brief cognitive-behavioral therapy for anxiety in patients with terminal cancer. *Oncologist*, 17, 1337–1345.

Griffith, J. L., & Gaby, L. (2005). Brief psychotherapy at the bedside: Countering demoralization from medical illness. *Psychosomatics*, 46, 109–116.

Groves, M. D. (2011). Leptomeningeal disease. *Neurosurgical Clinics North America*, 22, 67–78.

Hamnvik, O. P., Larsen, P. R., & Marquesee, E. (2011). Thyroid dysfunction from antineoplastic agents (review). *Journal of the National Cancer Institute*, 103, 1572–1587.

Haskell, C. M., Canellos, G. P., Leventhal, B. G., et al. (1969). L-asparaginase: Therapeutic and toxic effects in patients with neoplastic disease. *New England Journal of Medicine*, 281, 1028–1034.

Hauschild, A., Goagas, H., et al. (2008). Practical guidelines for the management of interferon alpha 2 b side effects in patients receiving adjuvant treatment for melanoma. *Cancer*, 112, 982–984.

Hinchey, J., Chaves, C., Appignani, B., et al. (1996). A reversible posterior leukoencephalopathy syndrome. *New England Journal of Medicine*, 334, 494–500.

Howell, A., Cuzick, J., Baum, M., et al. (2005). Results of the ATAC (Arimidex, Tamoxifen, Alone or in Combination) trial after completion of 5 years' adjuvant treatment for breast cancer. *Lancet*, 365, 60–62.

Hwang, M., Farasatpour, M., Williams, C. D., et al. (2012). Adjuvant chemotherapy for breast cancer in patients with schizophrenia. *Oncology Letter*, 3, 845–850.

Ilias, I., Torpy, D. J., Pacak, K., et al. (2005). Cushing's syndrome due to ectopic corticotrophin secretion: Twenty years' experience at the National Institutes of Health. *Journal of Clinical Endocrinology & Metabolism*, 90, 4955–4962.

Irani, S. R., & Vincent, A. (2011). NMDA receptor antibody encephalitis. *Current Neurology and Neuroscience Reports*, 11, 298–304.

Irwin, K. E., Henderson, D. C., Knight, H. P., & Pirl, W. F. (2014). Cancer care for individuals with schizophrenia. *Cancer*, 120, 323–334.

Islam, M., Frye, R. F., Richards, T. J., et al. (2002). Differential effect of IFNalpha 2b on the cytochrome P450 enzyme system: A potential basis of IFN toxicity and its modulation by other drugs. *Clinical Cancer Research*, 8, 2480–2487.

Janelsins, M. C., Kohli, S., Mohile, S. G., Usuki, K., Ahles, T. A., & Morrow, G. R. (2011). An update on cancer- and chemotherapy-related cognitive dysfunction: Current status. *Seminars in Oncology*, 38, 431–438.

Janelsins, M. C., Kohli, S., Mohile, S. G., Usuki, K., Ahles, T. A., & Morrow, G. R. (2011). An update on cancer- and chemotherapy-related cognitive dysfunction: Current status. *Seminars in Oncology*, 38, 431–438.

Jim, H. S. L., Small, B., Hartman, S., et al. (2012). Clinical predictors of cognitive function in adults treated with hematopoietic cell transplantation. *Cancer*, 118, 3407–3416.

Joffe, H., Partridge, A., Giobbie-Hurder, A., et al. (2010). Augmentation of venlafaxine and selective serotonin reuptake inhibitors with zolpidem improves sleep and quality of life in breast cancer patients with hot flashes: A randomized, double-blind, placebo-controlled trial. *Menopause*, 17, 908–916.

Joffe, H., Petrillo, L. F., Koukopoulos, A., et al. (2011). Increased estradiol and improved sleep, but not hot flashes, predict enhanced mood during the menopausal transition. *Journal of Clinical Endocrinology & Metabolism*, 96, E1044–E1054.

Joffe, H., Hall, J. E., Gruber, S., et al. (2006). Estrogen therapy selectively enhances prefrontal cognitive processes: A randomized, double-blind, placebo-controlled study with functional magnetic resonance imaging in perimenopausal and recently postmenopausal women. *Menopause*, 12, 411–422.

Johanssen, S., & Allolio, B. (2007). Mifepristone (RU 486) in Cushing's syndrome. *European Journal of Endocrinology*. 157, 561–569.

Kangas, M., Henry, J. L., & Bryant, R. A. (2005). The relationship between acute stress disorder and posttraumatic stress disorder following cancer. *Journal of Consulting Clinical Psychology*, 73, 360–364.

Kayser, M. S. S., Kohler, C. G., & Dalmau, J. (2010). Psychiatric manifestations of paraneoplastic disorders. *American Journal of Psychiatry*, 167, 1039–1050.

Khan, L., Wong, R., Li, M., et al. (2010). Maintaining the will to live of patients with advanced cancer. *Cancer Journal*, 16, 524–531.

Kirkwood, J. M., Bender, C., Agarwala, S., et al. (2002). Mechanisms and management of toxicities associated with high-dose interferon alfa-2b therapy. *Journal of Clinical Oncology*, 20, 3703–3718.

Kisely, S., Crowe, E., & Lawrence, D. (2013). Cancer-related mortality in people with mental illness. *JAMA Psychiatry*, 70, 209–217.

Kissane, D. W., Wein, S., Love, A. L., et al. (2004). The Demoralization Scale: A report of its development and preliminary validation. *Journal of Palliative Care*, 20, 269–276.

Kleinschimidet-DeMasters, B. K., & Damek, D. M. (2010). The imaging and neuropathological effects of bevacizumab (Avastin) in patients with leptomeningeal carcinomatosis. *Journal of Neuro-oncology*, 96, 375.

Kohli, S. S., Fisher, S. G., Tra, Y., et al. (2009). The effect of modafinil on cognitive function in breast cancer survivors. *Cancer*, 115, 2605–2616.

Kornblith, A. B., Herndon, E. J. II, Weiss, R. B., et al., for the Cancer and Leukemia Group B [CALGB], Chicago, Ill. (2003). Long-term adjustment of survivors of early stage breast cancer 20 years after adjuvant chemotherapy. *Cancer*, 98, 679–689.

Kroenke, K., Theobald, D., Wu, J., et al. (2010). Effect of telecare management of pain and depression in patients with cancer: A randomized trial. *Journal of the American Medical Association*, 304, 163–171.

Lagenbahn, D. M., Ashman, T., Cantor, J., & Trott, C. (2013). An evidence-based review of cognitive rehabilitation in medical conditions affecting cognitive function. *Archives of Physical Medicine and Rehabilitation*, 94, 271–286.

Lash, T. L., & Rosenberg, C. L. (2010). Evidence and practice regarding the role for CYP2D6 inhibition in decisions about tamoxifen therapy. *Journal of Clinical Oncology*, 28, 1273–1275.

Lash, T. L., Cronin-Fenton, D., Ahern, T. P., et al. (2011). CYP2D6 inhibition and breast cancer recurrence in a population-based study in Denmark. *Journal of the National Cancer Institute*, 103, 489–500.

Lavoie Smith, E. M., Pang, H., Cirrincione, C., et al. (2013). Effect of duloxetine on pain, function, and quality of life among patients with chemotherapy-induced painful peripheral neuropathy. A randomized clinical trial. *Journal of the American Medical Association*, 309, 1359–1367.

Liu, F., Mahgoub, N. A., & Kotbi, N. (2010). Continue or stop clozapine when patient needs chemotherapy? *Journal of Neuropsychiatry & Clinical Neuroscience*, 22, e4–e5.

Lo, C., Zimmermann, C., Rydall, A., et al. (2010). Longitudinal study of depressive symptoms in patients with metastatic gastrointestinal and lung cancer. *Journal of Clinical Oncology*, 28, 3084–3089.

Lodish, M. B., & Stratakis, C. A. (2010). Endocrine side effects of broad-acting kinase inhibitors. *Endocrine Related Cancer*, 17(3), R233–R244.

Loprinzi, C. L., Sloan, J., Stearns, V., et al. (2009). Newer antidepressants and gabapentin for hot flashes: An individual patient pooled analysis. *Journal of Clinical Oncology*, 27, 2831–2837.

Lundorff, L. E., Jonsson, B. H., & Sjogren, P. (2009). Modafinil for attentional and psychomotor dysfunction in advanced cancer: A double-blind, randomized, cross-over trial. *Palliative Medicine*, 731–738.

Lydiatt, W. M., Bessette, D., Schmid, K. K., Sayles, H., & Burke, W. J. (2013). Prevention of depression with escitalopram in patients undergoing treatment for head and neck cancer. Randomized, double-blind, placebo-controlled clinical trial. *Journal of the American Medical Association: Otolaryngology—Head & Neck Surgery*, Jun 20, 1–9. doi: 10.1001/jamaoto.2013.3371. [Epub ahead of print].

Manu, P., Sarpal, D., Muir, O., et al. (2012). When can patients with potentially life-threatening adverse effects be rechallenged with clozapine? A systematic review of the published literature. *Schizophrenia Research*, 134, 180–186.

McClain, C. S., Rosenfeld, B., & Breitbart, W. (2003). Effect of spiritual well-being on end-of-life despair in terminally ill cancer patients, *Lancet*, 361, 1603–1607.

McKnight, C., Guirgis, H., & Votolato, N. (2011). Clozapine rechallenge after excluding the high-risk clozapine-induced agranulocytosis genotype of HLA=DQB1 6672G>C. *American Journal of Psychiatry*, 168, 1120.

Minton, O., Richardson, A., Sharpe, M., Hotopf, M., & Stone, P. C. (2011). Psychostimulants for the management of cancer-related fatigue: A systematic review and meta-analysis. *Journal of Pain & Symptom Management*, 41, 761–767.

Misono, S., Weiss, N. S., Fann, J. R., Redman, M., & Yueh, B. (2008). Incidence of suicide in persons with cancer. *Journal of Clinical Oncology*, 26, 4741–4738.

Morrow, P. K., Serna, R., Broglio, K., et al. (2012). Effect of CYP2D6 polymorphisms on breast cancer recurrence. *Cancer*, 118, 1221–1227.

Musselman, D. L., Lawson, D. H., Gumnick, J. F., et al. (2001). Paroxetine for the prevention of depression induced by high-dose interferon alfa. *New England Journal of Medicine*, 344, 961–966.

Navari, R. M., Nagy, C. K., & Gray, S. E. (2013). The use of olanzapine versus metoclopramide for the treatment of breakthrough chemotherapy-induced nausea and vomiting in patients receiving highly emetogenic chemotherapy. *Supportive Care in Cancer*, 21, 1655–1663.

O'Brien, S. G., Guilhot, F., Larson, R. A., et al. (2003). Imatinib compared with interferon and low-dose cytarabine for newly diagnosed chronic-phase chronic myeloid leukemia. *New England Journal of Medicine*, 348, 994–1004.

Oettgen, H. F., Stephenson, P. A., Schwartz, M. K., et al. (1970). Toxicity of E. coli L-asparaginase in man. *Cancer*, 25, 253–278.

Pachman, D. R., Barton, D. L., Swetz, K. M., & Loprinzi, C. L. (2012). Troublesome symptoms in cancer survivors: Fatigue, insomnia, neuropathy, and pain. *Journal of Clinical Oncology*, 30, 3687–3696.

Palgi, Y., Shrira, A., Haber, Y., et al. (2011). Comorbidity of posttraumatic stress symptoms and depressive symptoms among gastric cancer patients. *European Journal of Oncology Nursing*, 15, 454–458.

Pirl, W. F., Greer, J. A., Goode, M., & Smith, M. R. (2008). Prospective study of depression and fatigue in men with advanced prostate cancer receiving hormone therapy. *Psycho-Oncology*, 17, 148–153.

Pirl, W. F., Greer, J. A., Traeger, L., et al. (2012). Depression and survival in metastatic non-small-cell lung cancer: Effects of early palliative care. *Journal of Clinical Oncology*, 30, 1310–1315.

Pirl, W. F., Greer, J., Temel, J. S., Yeap, B. Y., & Gilman, S. E. (2009). Major depressive disorder in long-term cancer survivors: Analysis of the national co-morbidity survey replication. *Journal of Clinical Oncology*, 27, 4130–4134.

Pirl, W. F., Siegel, G. I., Goode, M. J., et al. (2002). Depression in men receiving androgen deprivation therapy for prostate cancer: A pilot study. *Psycho-oncology*, 11, 518–523.

Pirl, W. F., Solis, J., Greer, J., Sequist, L., Temel, J. S., & Lynch, T. J. (2009). Epidermal growth factor receptor tyrosine kinase inhibitors and depression. *Journal of Clinical Oncology*, 27, e49–e50; author reply, e1.

Pirl, W. F., Traeger, L., Greer, J. A., et al. (2011). Tumor epidermal growth factor receptor genotype and depression in stage IV non-small cell lung cancer. *Oncologist*, 16, 1299–1306.

Quek, R., Morgan, J. A., George, S., et al. (2009). Small molecule tyrosine kinase inhibitor and depression. *Journal of Clinical Oncology*, 27, 312–313.

Rae, J. M., Drury, S., Hayes, D. F., et al. (2012). ATAC trialists/ CYP2D6 and UGT287 genotype and risk of recurrence in tamoxifen-treated breast cancer patients. *Journal of the National Cancer Institute*, 104, 452–460.

Regan, M. M., Leyland-Jones, B., Bouzyk, M., et al. (2012). Breast International Group (BIG) 1-98 Collaborative Group. CYP2D6 genotype and tamoxifen response in postmenopausal women with endocrine-responsive breast cancer: The Breast International Group 1-98 trial. *Journal of the National Cancer Institute*, 104, 441–451.

Riechelmann, R. P., Burman, D., Tannock, I. F., Rodin, G., & Zimmermann, C. (2010). Phase II trial of mirtazapine for cancer-related cachexia and anorexia. *American Journal of Hospice & Palliative Medicine*, 27, 106–110.

Roscoe, J. A., Heckler, C. E., Morrow, G. R., et al. (2013). Prevention of delayed nausea: A University of Rochester Cancer Center Community Clinical Oncology Program study of patients receiving chemotherapy. *Journal of Clinical Oncology*, 31, 1378–1379.

Rosenberg, I., Mekinulov, B., Cohen, L. J., & Galynker, I. (2007). Restarting clozapine treatment during ablation chemotherapy and stem cell transplant for Hodgkin's lymphoma. *American Journal of Psychiatry*, 164, 1438–1439.

Rosenstock, J. (2004). Clozapine therapy during cancer treatment. *American Journal of Psychiatry*, 161, 175.

Roth, A. J., & Scher, H. I. (1998). Sertraline relieves hot flashes secondary to medical castration a treatment of advanced prostate cancer. *Psycho-oncology*, 2, 129–132.

Sareen, J., Cox, B. J., Afifi, T. O., et al. (2005). Anxiety disorders and risk for suicidal ideation and suicide attempts: A population-based longitudinal study of adults. *Archives of General Psychiatry*, 62(11), 1249–1257.

Schmale, A. H. (1972). Giving up as a final common pathway to changes in health. *Advances in Psychosomatic Medicine*, 8, 20–40.

Schmidt, P. J., & Rubinow, D. R. (2009). Sex hormones and mood in the perimenopause. *Annals of the New York Academy of Science*, 1179, 70–85.

Shader, R. I. (2005). Demoralization revisited. *Journal of Clinical Psychopharmacology*, 25, 291–292.

Sharpe, M., Strong, V., Allen, K., et al. (2004). Management of major depression in outpatients attending a cancer centre: A preliminary evaluation of a multi-component cancer nurse delivered intervention. *British Journal of Cancer*, 90, 310–313.

Shelby, R. A., Golden-Kreutz, D. M., & Andersen, B. L. (2009). PTSD diagnoses, subsyndromal symptoms, and comorbidities contribute to impairments for breast cancer survivors. *Journal of Traumatic Stress*, 21, 165–172.

Schilder, C. M., Seynaeve, C., Beex, L. V., et al. (2010). Effects of tamoxifen and exemestane on cognitive functioning of postmoenopausal patients with breast cancer: results from the neuropsychological side study of the tamoxifen and exemestane adjuvant multinational trial. *Journal Clinical Oncology*, 38, 1294–1300.

Smith, D. M., McKenna, K., & Thompson, C. J. (2000). Hyponatraemia. *Clinical Endocrinology*, 52, 667–678.

Smith, S. K., Zimmerman, S., Williams, C. S., et al. (2011). Posttraumatic stress symptoms in long-term non-Hodgkin's lymphoma survivors: Does time heal? *Journal of Clinical Oncology*, 29, 4526–4533.

Spencer, R. J., Nilsson, M., Wright, A., Pirl, W., & Prigerson, H. (2010). Anxiety disorders in advanced cancer patients: Correlates and predictors of end-of-life outcomes. *Cancer*, 116, 1810–1819.

Spencer, R. J., Ray, A., Pirl, W. F., & Prigerson, H. G. (2012). Clinical correlates of suicidal thoughts in patients with advanced cancer. *American Journal of Geriatric Psychiatry*, 20, 327–336.

Spiegel, D., & Classen, C. (2000). Group therapy for cancer patients: A research-based handbook of psychosocial care. New York: Basic Books.

Spiegel, D., Butler, L. D., Giese-Davis, J., et al. (2007). Effects of supportive expressive group therapy on survival of patients with metastatic breast cancer. A randomized prospective trial. *Cancer*, 110, 1130–1137.

Stuber, M. L., Meeske, K. A., Krull, K. R., et al. (2010). Prevalence and predictors of posttraumatic stress disorder in adult survivors of childhood cancer. *Pediatrics*, 125, e1124–e1134.

Thornton, L. M., Carson, W. E. 3rd, Shapiro, C. L., Farrar, W. B., Andersen, B. L. (2008). Delayed emotional recovery after taxane-based chemotherapy. *Cancer*, 113, 638–647.

Turaga, K. K., Malafa, M. P., Jacobsen, P. B., Schell, M. J., & Sarr, M. G. (2011). Suicide in patients with pancreatic cancer. *Cancer*, 117, 642–647.

Turkel, S. B., Tishler, D., & Tavare, C. J. (2007). Late onset psychosis in survivors of pediatric central nervous system malignancies. *Journal of Neuropsychiatry & Clinical Neuroscience*, 19, 293–297.

Walker, J., Waters, R. A., Murray, G., et al. (2008). Better off dead: Suicidal thoughts in cancer patients. *Journal of Clinical Oncology*, 26, 4725–4730.

Walker, L. G., Walker, M. B., Heys, S. D., Lolley, J., Wesnes, K., & Eremin, O. (1997). The psychological and psychiatric effects of rIL-2 therapy: A controlled clinical trial. *Psycho-oncology*, 6, 290–301.

Walker, L. G., Walker, M. B., Heys, S. D., Lolley, J., Wesnes, K., & Eremin, O. (1997). The psychological and psychiatric effects of rIL-2 therapy: A controlled clinical trial. *Psycho-Oncology*, 6, 290–301.

Walsh, J. M., Denduluri, N., & Swain, S. M. (2006). Amenorrhea in premenopausal women after adjuvant chemotherapy for breast cancer. *Journal of Clinical Oncology*, 24, 5769–5779.

Weber, J. (2007). Review: Anti-CTLA-4 antibody ipilimumab: Case studies of clinical response and immune-related adverse events. *The Oncologist*, 12, 864–872.

Wefel, J. S., Vardy, J., Ahles, T., & Schagen, S. B. (2011). International cognition and cancer task force recommendations to harmonize studies of cognitive function in patients with cancer. *Lancet*, 12, 703–708.

Weisman, A. D. (1972): *On denying and dying*. New York: Behavioral Publications, Inc.

Weisman, A. D. (1974). *The realization of death. A guide for the psychological autopsy*. New York: Jason Aronson, Inc.

Weisman, A. D. (1978). Coping with illness. In T. Hackett & N. H. Cassem (Eds.), *Massachusetts General Hospital Handbook of General Hospital Psychiatry* (pp. 264–275). St. Louis, MO: CV Mosby.

Weisman, A. D. (1984). *The coping capacity: On the nature of being mortal*. New York: Human Sciences Press.

Weisman, A. D., & Worden, J. W. (1976–1977). The existential plight in cancer: Significance of the first 100 days. *International Journal of Psychiatry in Medicine*, 7, 1–15.

Weisman, A. D., Worden, J. W., & Sobel, H. J. (1980). Psychosocial screening and intervention with cancer patients. Project Omega. NCI grant 19797 (1977–1980).

Yoong, J., Park, E. R., Greer, J. A., et al. (2013). Early palliative care in advanced lung cancer. *Journal of the American Medical Association: Internal Medicine*, 173, 283–290.

Zaider, T. I., & Kissane, D. W. (2010). Psychosocial interventions for couples and families coping with cancer. In J. C. Holland, W. S. Breitbart, P. B. Jacobsen, M. S. Lederberg, M. J. Loscalzo, & R. McCorkle (Eds.), *Psycho-oncology* (2nd ed.; pp. 483–487). New York: Oxford University Press.

58.

HEMATOLOGIC DISORDERS[*]

*Madeleine Becker, David J. Axelrod, Keira Chism, Tal E. Weinberger,
Dimitri Markov, Lex Denysenko, Christine Marchionni, Olu Oyesanmi,
Howard Field, and Elisabeth J. Shakin Kunkel*

INTRODUCTION

The psychiatric care of the patient with hematological illnesses is the focus of this chapter. This includes patients with anemia; and B12 and folate deficiency, patients with sickle cell disease, thalassemia; patients with clotting disorders and those who feign clotting disorders; and patients whose religion restricts the use of transfusions.

The making of hemoglobin requires iron, folate, and vitamin B12; the deficiency of these nutrients affects not only the blood but mood, cognition, and the development of the nervous system. Genetic disorders of hemoglobin and clotting factors lead to sickle cell anemia's vaso-occlusive crises, thalassemia's organ injury, hemophilia's risk of bleeding, and the psychological challenges for those who suffer with these disorders. The familial enzyme deficiencies of porphyrias that can lead to confusion and abdominal pain evolve from the neurotoxic effects of hepatic overproduction of metabolites in the heme biosynthetic pathway. Thrombocytopenic thrombotic purpura (TTP) and hyperviscosity syndrome are distinct hematological syndromes that can both present with signs of microangiopathic injury in the brain.

We also discuss agranulocytosis associated with clozapine, as well as bleeding risks with selective serotonin reuptake inhibitors (SSRIs). We review how to recognize patients with factitious disorder using anticoagulation as a means to become a patient. Patients who are Jehovah's Witnesses (who restrict the use of blood transfusions) face complex decisions in the setting of medical illness; and medical psychiatrists may be consulted.

IRON DEFICIENCY ANEMIA

David Axelrod

Iron deficiency, the world's most common nutritional deficiency, has a variety of psychiatric implications.

Besides anemia, iron deficiency is associated with pica and restless legs syndrome. Adequate iron, is critical for healthy brain development during gestation and the first months of life.

Iron, a component of hemoglobin, is essential to red blood cell production. Iron deficiency anemia, a hypochromic microcytic anemia, is an advanced state of iron deficiency, characterized by low or absent iron stores in the bone marrow. Laboratory measures show low serum iron concentration, low transferrin saturation, low serum ferritin, low hemoglobin concentration, and an associated elevation of free erythrocyte porphyrin and transferrin (Dorland, 2003).

Impaired iron intake, iron loss, or increased metabolic demand for iron can all lead to deficiency. The most common etiologies of iron deficiency anemia are chronic blood loss and, more rarely, decreased iron absorption. In men and in post-menopausal women, the first suspect is chronic bleeding from the gastrointestinal tract; in adults, the most common causes of gastrointestinal bleeding are peptic ulcer, reflux esophagitis, gastritis, hemorrhoids, vascular anomalies, diverticulitis, and neoplasms (Coban, 2003). In pre-menopausal women, heavy menstrual flow is a common cause of iron loss (Hallberg et al., 1995). The medical etiology for blood loss is always considered before blind iron replacement is prescribed.

In infants, iron deficiency anemia most often results from diets of milk that are not supplemented with adequate iron, or milk from lactating mothers already iron deficient. Most brands of infant formula are supplemented with iron. Premature infants are at even greater risk. For older children and young adults, an iron-poor diet may contribute to deficiency. Good sources of iron include animal-based foods such as beef, pork, poultry, fish, clams, and oysters. Plant sources of iron include leafy green vegetables, legumes, dried fruits, and molasses. Iron-enriched cereals, bread, and rice are other high iron sources. Coffee, tea, and cola may all interfere with iron absorption.

Due to poor nutrition, chronically mentally ill, homeless, and poverty-stricken patients all are at higher risk; as are young men, particularly during growth spurts; and pre-menopausal women with heavy menstrual flow (Hallberg,

---

[*] The following sections were reprinted and adapted with permission from the American Psychiatric Publishing's *Textbook of Psychosomatic Medicine: Psychiatric Care of the Medically Ill* (copyright, 2011).

1995). In pregnant women, iron-deficiency anemia has a high prevalence due to diversion of iron to the fetus and blood loss during delivery.

Daily iron demand dramatically increases during pregnancy and continues through to term. Breastfeeding leads to additional iron diversion to the baby, making iron deficiency common in the postpartum period (Milman, 2006).

Malabsorption of iron is uncommon, except after certain types of gastrointestinal surgery, especially gastrectomy or gastric bypass surgery, as the primary locus of absorption is the duodenum. In malabsorption syndromes, iron deficiency may take years to develop, due to the indolent nature of iron loss. Atrophic gastritis, *H. pylori* gastritis, and celiac disease are associated with iron malabsorption (Annibale et al., 2003; Dickey et al., 1999).

CLINICAL MANIFESTATIONS

Severe iron-deficiency anemia is associated with all of the various symptoms and signs of anemia, resulting from the body's response to hypoxia, including tachycardia with palpitations, pounding in the ears, headache, lightheadedness, and angina pectoris. Clinical symptoms of anemia include fatigue, tiredness, weakness, headache, irritability, and exercise intolerance. Glossal pain, reduced salivary flow with dry mouth and atrophy of tongue papillae, and alopecia may be more specific to iron deficiency (Osaki et al., 1999; Trost et al., 2006). Physical signs also include pallor, glossitis (smooth, red tongue), stomatitis, and angular cheilitis. Retinal hemorrhages and exudates may be seen in severely anemic patients. Koilonychia (dystrophy of the fingernails), a well-known finding in iron deficiency anemia, is uncommon (see Table 58.1).

NEUROPSYCHIATRIC MANIFESTATIONS

A hemoglobin level of less than 10 g/dL puts patients at risk of developing neuropsychiatric symptoms. Neuropsychiatric manifestations include depression, developmental delay, cognitive impairment, restless leg syndrome, and fatigue. Iron

Table 58.1 MANIFESTATIONS OF IRON DEFICIENCY ANEMIA

NEUROPSYCHIATRIC	NON-NEUROPSYCHIATRIC
Cognitive impairment	Alopecia
Depression	Angina
Developmental delay	Angular cheilitis
Fatigue	Exercise intolerance
Headache	Glossitis
Impaired auditory function	Koilonychia
Impaired vision	Pallor
Irritability	Stomatitis
Restless legs syndrome	Weakness

deficiency anemia may impair vision by causing occlusion of the central retinal artery, and can impair auditory function by an unknown mechanism. It has also been demonstrated to lead to decreased work and exercise performance, and to immune system abnormalities (Cook et al., 1989).

Iron is thought to play a crucial role in neurological development. Iron deficiency anemia is associated with both mental and motor developmental delays in infants and young children (Booth & Aukett, 1997). Many studies from all over the world have found that infants with iron deficiency anemia at 6–24 months old had poorer cognitive, motor, and social/emotional functioning. Although a few studies showed dramatic improvement after iron treatment, most have reported persistent deficit seven after three months of treatment (Lozoff, 2006). Children and adolescents with iron deficiency have been shown to have lower standardized math scores compared to children with normal iron status (Halterman et al., 2001). Long-lasting effects noted in the auditory and visual system function as well as memory and behavior have been attributed to iron's role in myelination and neurotransmitter synthesis (Algarin et al., 2003; Congdon et al., 2012). Less well established is the relationship of iron deficiency anemia to developmental deficits in adolescents and young adults.

In adults, iron deficiency anemia may impair cognitive function. In the postpartum period, when there is a high prevalence of iron deficiency, there is a strong association of low iron status with depression, stress, and impaired cognitive functioning in the mother (Beard et al., 2005). Women who have iron deficiency anemia are also more likely to have postpartum fatigue (Lee & Zaffke, 1999). In the elderly, anemic patients demonstrate significantly worse results on almost all measures of cognitive and functional assessments, mood, and quality of life (Lucca et al., 2008).

Patients with iron deficiency anemia may crave both food items and non-food substances. Pica, particularly the compulsive eating of clay, and pagophagia (ingesting extraordinary amounts of ice) are specific symptoms prevalent in patients with iron deficiency anemia (Rector, 1989; Reynolds et al., 1968; Kettaneh et al., 2005). Pica is more common in pregnant women and children. Why iron deficient patients eat ice or clay is not known, but treatment of the anemia seems to reduce the behavior (Coltman, 1969; Woods, 1970; Young, 2010).

Brain iron deficiency is suspected to play a role in restless leg syndrome (Krieger & Schroeder, 2001) by causing dopaminergic dysfunction (Connor et al., 2009). The severity of the syndrome has been demonstrated to correlate with serum ferritin levels (Sun et al., 1998). Some studies find that treatment with iron improves symptoms of restless legs syndrome (Krieger, 2001; O'Keeffe et al., 1994); however, a *Cochrane Review* of six studies found insufficient evidence to support this (Trotti et al., 2012).

DIAGNOSIS AND TREATMENT

Iron deficiency anemia often is discovered incidentally through screening laboratory tests. Plasma iron concentration and serum ferritin concentration are usually both low, and iron-binding capacity is increased. In inflammatory states, ferritin may be elevated.

All patients should be educated to maintain a diversified diet with adequate iron. Supplemental iron is almost always necessary for recovery. Iron supplementation can be replaced orally, parentally, or as a blood transfusion. The dosage in adults should be enough to provide between 150 mg and 200 mg of iron daily that may be taken in 3–4 doses one hour before meals. The effectiveness of oral iron is compromised by poor absorption, poor compliance, and side effects (e.g., constipation). Side effects, which limit compliance, are dose-dependent and may be ameliorated by choice of preparation. In one study, ferric disglycinate caused the lowest rate of side effects compared to other formulations (Melamed et al., 2007). The elderly are particular sensitive to side effects. Severe iron deficiency anemia can be treated with combined therapy of erythropoietin and intravenous iron (Breymann et al., 2001).

Symptom improvement is generally rapid after iron repletion. Headaches, fatigue, paresthesias, and pica rapidly resolve (Rector, 1989). There are conflicting data as to whether oral iron improves mental development in infants (Lozoff & Georgieff, 1982, 2006).

B_{12} AND FOLATE DEFICIENCY

Madeleine Becker

Many of the patients who are seen in the medical or psychiatric setting; older, malnourished, those with psychiatric disorders; strict vegans; and those who had gastric surgery are at high risk for both B_{12} and folic acid deficiency. Both folate and B_{12} deficiency are a consideration in patients with cognitive impairment, depression, and ataxia.

B_{12} and folate deficiency lead to megaloblastic anemia. Both B_{12} and folate are cofactors for the conversion of homocysteine to methionine, and are necessary for DNA synthesis (Andres et al., 2004). Deficiency of either B_{12} or folate correlates with high homocysteine levels, which is a risk factor for cardiovascular disease, stroke, dementia, and Alzheimer's disease (Carmel et al., 2003; Ravaglia et al., 2005; Reynolds et al., 2006; Seshadri et al., 2002). Elevated homocysteine level and high methylmalonic acid level indicate impairment in the cobalamin metabolic pathway. Both high homocysteine levels and deficiencies of B_{12} and folate have been associated with depression (Bottiglieri et al., 2000; Kim, 2008a). Multiple studies have shown a significant correlation between low levels of B_{12} and cognitive impairment and dementia (Vogel, 2009).

VITAMIN B_{12}

B_{12} is found in meat and dairy products, and in a variety of foods that are fortified with B_{12}, including fortified cereals and fortified nutritional yeast. The most common cause of B_{12} deficiency is pernicious anemia, an autoimmune disorder that causes loss of gastric parietal cells and an absence of intrinsic factor. Intrinsic factor is necessary for B_{12} absorption.

Pernicious anemia is often associated with other autoimmune disorders, including Hashimoto's thyroiditis, type 1 diabetes mellitus, Addison's disease, Graves' disease, vitiligo, myasthenia gravis, primary ovarian failure, and hypoparathyroidism (Carmel, 2003; Toh et al., 1997).

The prevalence of B_{12} deficiency in the elderly is common, about 20% (Andres, 2004; Vogel, 2009); and is often unrecognized because the clinical manifestations can be subtle. In the elderly, B_{12} deficiency is usually associated with pernicious anemia (20–30%), or food-cobalamin malabsorption (50–70%), mostly due to gastric atrophy (Andres et al., 2009). B_{12} malabsorption or gastric atrophy may be caused by *H. pylori* infection or intestinal overgrowth due to antibiotics.

Medications, including the chronic use of metformin (Bauman et al., 2000, Liu et al., 2006), antacids, H-2 receptor antagonists, and proton pump inhibitors also can cause B12 deficiency (Valuck et al., 2004). B_{12} malabsorption also can be caused by alcoholism, pancreatic failure, and Sjogren's syndrome. Vitamin B_{12} malabsorption also may result from gastrectomy, gastric bypass surgery (Malinowski, 2006), ileal diseases or resection, Crohn's disease, autoimmune deficiency syndrome (AIDS), or parasitic infestation with *Diphyllobothrium latum* (fish tapeworm) (Andres, 2004).

Dietary B_{12} deficiency is rare, but may occur in strict vegans. B_{12} deficiency also can occur in children who are exclusively breastfed and whose mothers are vegans (Chalouhi et al., 2008).

Abuse of nitrous oxide—"whippit" abuse—can cause neuropsychiatric signs of vitamin B_{12} deficiency when used chronically in patients with marginal levels of B_{12} (Sethi et al., 2006). The anesthetic inactivates cobalamin.

Neuropsychiatric Manifestations

Neurological and psychiatric symptoms are common in B_{12} deficiency, and may manifest before or without obvious hematological signs (Lindenbaum et al., 1988; Carmel, 2008). Peripheral neuropathy may present with paresthesias and numbness. A less common, but classic neurological manifestation is subacute combined degeneration of the spinal cord (Reynolds, 2006). This results in loss of vibration and position sense and ataxia (caused by posterior column disruption) and weakness, spasticity, and extensor plantar responses (caused by lateral column disruption) (Toh, 1997). Other, less common, manifestations of B_{12} deficiency include optic neuritis, optic atrophy, and incontinence.

In addition to neurological symptoms of ataxia and paresthesias, psychiatric symptoms may include mood changes, acute psychotic depression (Bar-Shai et al., 2012), psychosis (Rajkumar, 2008; Tufan et al., 2012; Hutto, 1997; Dogan et al., 2012), catatonia (Lewis et al., 2009), and obsessive-compulsive disorder (Sharma et al., 2012). No one symptom of psychosis is more commonly observed (Hutto, 1997).

B_{12} deficiency and high homocysteine have been associated with cognitive impairments (Selhub et al., 2000) and reversible dementia. B_{12} deficiency has also been associated with an increased rate of brain atrophy and damage to white matter (Smith et al., 2009). Multiple studies have shown an association with both B_{12} deficiency and high plasma homocysteine levels in patients with dementia; however, the relationship between vitamin B_{12} and dementia remains unclear (Andres, 2004; Reynolds, 2006; Vogel, 2009). In children, B_{12} deficiency may cause irritability, failure to thrive, apathy, anorexia, abnormal movements, and developmental regression, which are generally responsive to supplementation (Chalouhi, 2008).

Diagnosis and Treatment

A low-normal serum vitamin B_{12} level in the presence of megaloblastic cells and hypersegmented neutrophils, with or without anemia and/or the typical neuropsychiatric findings, should lead to further investigation for B_{12} deficiency. There is no "gold standard," and there are different normal values for cobalamin levels; however, a deficiency is usually defined as a B_{12} level less than 200 pg/ml (Schreir 2014). Elevated serum methylmalonic acid and elevated serum total homocysteine also can help establish if deficiency exists, as they are markers for functional B_{12} status (Smith, 2009). These tests should be done when the B_{12} level is found to be low or borderline. Tests for intrinsic factor antibody, serum gastrin, and a Schilling test may be used for diagnosing pernicious anemia. Identifying the cause of the B_{12} deficiency, however, yields important clinical information and can guide diagnosis and treatment (Carmel, 2003) .

Daily injections of 1000 mcg of cyanocobalamin are recommended for one week, then 1000 mcg every week for four weeks, then maintenance doses every 1–3 months, depending on the severity of the deficiency. Clinical evidence suggests that oral B_{12} replacement (1000 mcg) also is effective as a second-line therapy (Andres, 2009). Significant improvement of neuropsychiatric function has been shown after B12 administration (Andres 2009); the degree of recovery is correlated with symptom severity before treatment (Reynolds 2006). Neurological recovery is more variable than hematological improvement (Carmel, 2008). Continued maintenance therapy is recommended to fully replenish body stores. Administration of folate, without B_{12}, will reverse the hematological abnormalities, but if there is also an unrecognized B_{12} deficiency, neurological impairment may progress further, sometimes leading to irreversible deficits (e.g., subacute degeneration of the spinal cord) (Reynolds, 2006).

FOLIC ACID

Folic acid is found in both animal products and leafy green vegetables. Folate is important in mood, cognition, brain growth, and DNA synthesis and repair. These mechanisms are mediated through nucleotide synthesis and DNA transcription and integrity (Carmel, 2003; Duthie, 2011). Adequate folate levels may protect against certain cancers, neural tube defects (Lucock, 2004), and dementia (Ravaglia, 2005; Lushsinger, 2007), presumably by lowering homocysteine.

Inadequate diet, alcoholism, chronic illness, drugs that interfere with folate metabolism (phenytoin, valproic acid, lamotrigine, barbiturates, trimethoprim/sulfamethoxazole, oral contraceptives, and methotrexate), or malabsorption can cause folate deficiency (Reynolds et al., 2002). Folate deficiency is common in the elderly (Reynolds, 2006). Deficiency has been found to be relatively common in psychiatric patients, especially those with depression (Bottiglieri, 2000). This association is not entirely clear; it may in part be attributed to the use of psychotropic medications, especially anti-epileptic drugs and mood stabilizers, which are known to decrease folate levels, or to poor nutrition (Lerner et al., 2006).

Folate, by promoting conversion of homocysteine to methionine, catalyzes the production of s-adenosylmethionine (SAMe), which independently influences the rate of synthesis of serotonin and perhaps other transmitters like norepinephrine and dopamine. Recent research has exploited this benefit, and doctors have given folate in the form of 5-methyltetrahydrofolate (MTHF) and SAMe as supplements for treatment-resistant depression (Papakostas et al., 2012).

Clinical Manifestations

Symptoms of folate deficiency are similar to those of B_{12} deficiency; however, subacute combined degeneration of the spinal cord is specific to B_{12} deficiency. Depression has been associated with low baseline levels of both folate and B_{12} (Kim, 2008B), but the association is much more commonly seen with folate deficiency (Reynolds, 2006). The megaloblastic anemia is identical to that seen in B_{12} deficiency. Folate deficiency invariably is accompanied by an elevated plasma homocysteine level (Bottiglieri, 2000), which is associated with an increased risk of cardiovascular disease, dementia (Kim et al., 2008; Ravaglia, 2005), and depression (Bottiglieri, 2000; Kim, 2008b).

Insufficient folate during conception and early pregnancy results in neural tube defects. Since 1998, the U.S. Food and Drug Administration (FDA) mandated fortification of grains with folate in order to lower the risk of neural tube defects in women of childbearing age. This action led to a reduction in such defects and an improvement of blood folate status and homocysteine levels in adults in the United States (Jacques et al., 1999).

Diagnosis and Treatment

Low red blood cell folate combined with high plasma homocysteine is a good standard marker for the diagnosis of folate deficiency and is more accurate than measuring serum folate alone. Serum folate is quickly responsive to folate intake, but red blood cell folate offers a measure of folate presence over a longer time-average (Galloway, 2003).

If screening test for folate level is low or borderline, a homocysteine level should be checked. As mentioned before, B_{12} levels should also be checked when screening for folate deficiency so that cobalamin deficiency is not missed.

Full treatment response to folate supplementation takes many months. Although there are no clear guidelines for the dose or duration of folate therapy, treatment is recommended for at least six months (Reynolds, 2006). To treat folate deficiency, prescribing 1 mg daily for one to four months, or until hematological recovery is generally recommended (Schrier, 2014). For women of childbearing age, recommendations are 0.4 mg–0.8 mg daily (US Preventative Services Task Force, 2009). Higher doses are recommended for women at risk for folate deficiency or who already have had a child with a neural tube defect. Collaboration with an obstetrician is necessary. To lower homocysteine levels, 0.8 mg daily is typically required (Homocysteine Lowering Trialists' Collaboration, 2005). There has been some evidence that higher doses of folate may impair natural killer cell cytotoxicity, and possibly increase cardiac events (Smith, 2008).

B_{12} AND FOLATE AND LINKS TO DEMENTIA

The relationship between dementia and vitamin deficiency is complex and probably bidirectional. As low B_{12} levels and elevated homocysteine levels have been linked to cognitive impairment and dementia (Clark et al., 2007), there is controversy on whether supplementation of either folate or B_{12} (which lower homocysteine levels) has any effect on cognition or the development of dementia. A large, randomized double-blind placebo-controlled study found that memory, information-processing speed, and sensorimotor speed were improved in elderly people getting folic acid supplements (Durga et al., 2007). There is also evidence that B_{12} and folic acid supplementation can slow brain atrophy in elderly people with mild cognitive decline (Smith et al., 2010). However, findings to date have been inconsistent, and the association remains unclear. Although elevated plasma homocysteine levels are associated with dementia, there is no clear evidence that low B_{12} or folate vitamin levels are *independently* related to the risk of dementia (Seshardri, 2002). To date, Cochrane Reviews show that supplementation with folic acid, with or without B_{12}, provides no *consistent* evidence of a beneficial effect on cognition or the development of dementia in individuals with either normal or impaired cognitive functioning at baseline (Balk et al., 2007; Malouf et al., 2008; Vogel et al., 2009).

HEMOPHILIA

Dimitri Markov
Hemophilia is a bleeding disorder caused by a deficiency of one of the coagulation factors essential for blood clotting. Hemophilia A (factor VIII deficiency) and hemophilia B (factor IX deficiency) are the most common inherited bleeding disorders. Hemophilia A and B are clinically indistinguishable from each other.

Disease severity is related to the plasma concentrations of the clotting factors. Classification into *mild, moderate*, and *severe* hemophilia is useful for predicting prognosis and bleeding propensity (Bolton-Maggs et al., 2003; Casey et al., 2003; Manco-Johnson, 2005). Patients with severe hemophilia (clotting factor concentration less than 1% of normal) may bleed spontaneously into muscles, joints, and body cavities. Patients with moderate hemophilia (concentration of clotting factor 1–5% of normal) are typically diagnosed by the age of

five years and tend to bleed less frequently. Mild hemophilia (>5% of normal concentration) usually is diagnosed following trauma, surgery, or tooth extraction later in life. Patients with mild hemophilia rarely have spontaneous bleeding (Bolton-Maggs, 2003; Manco-Johnson, 2005). Most children with hemophilia are asymptomatic until they start to crawl or walk. These children may bruise easily and bleed after minor injuries. By the age of four years, many children with hemophilia have experienced a bleed into a joint. Families of these children may be inappropriately suspected of child abuse.

Purified factor VIII became commercially available in the 1960s. The use of purified factor VIII allowed for home-based infusions, improved the quality of life, and increased the life expectancy of patients with severe hemophilia. The use of purified factor VIII has reduced the frequency of bleeds into large joints and muscles, resulting in less joint injury and fewer patients with chronic pain. As a result of this advance, patients with severe hemophilia are much less likely to experience bleeding and its complications (Bolton-Maggs, 2003; Manco-Johnson, 2005). In the early 1980s, more than 80% of patients with severe hemophilia who were older than ten years of age were infected with viral illnesses, including hepatitis B, hepatitis C, and human immunodeficiency virus (HIV) from contaminated blood products. Beginning in the 1990s, the use of recombinant clotting factors almost eliminated the risk of acquiring viral infections.

The prevalence of psychiatric disorders in patients with hemophilia is not known. Children and adolescents with hemophilia have been reported to suffer higher rates of anxiety disorders than those with asthma (Bussing & Burket, 1993). Disease-related stressors pose challenges to children with hemophilia as they proceed toward developmental milestones. While facing chronic pain, disability, social ostracism, and job and insurance discrimination, adults living with hemophilia strive for a healthy identity, autonomy, and a good quality of life (Spilsbury, 2004).

Despite the severe pain associated with joint bleeds, some physicians are reluctant to prescribe opiate analgesics due to concerns about inducing opiate dependence; furthermore, some adult patients without opiate dependence report concerns about narcotic addiction (Elander & Barry, 2003). It is important to provide adequate analgesia to patients with hemophilia, and opiate analgesics may be prescribed safely. Healthcare providers should adequately address patient concerns about becoming opiate dependent.

Individual, family, and group psychotherapy are useful psychotherapeutic modalities for helping manage the stressors associated with hemophilia (Casey, 2003; Gerstner et al., 2006).

SICKLE CELL DISEASE

David Axelrod
Sickle cell disease is the most common hemoglobinopathy, presently affecting approximately 100,000 Americans (Hassell, 2010). The disease occurs primarily in those of African descent, but also afflicts people of Mediterranean,

Asian, and Middle Eastern origin. Eight percent of African-Americans in the United States carry the sickle cell trait, and approximately one out of three hundred have the disease. The disease is a classic example of a balanced polymorphism; the asymptomatic sickle cell trait provides a selective advantage against malaria, while the homozygous disease has devastating consequences. Medical advances have transformed the disease from what was once primarily a pediatric illness into a chronic disease of adults. Life expectancy has increased from a mean of 14 years in the 1970s to close to 50 years today (Platt et al., 1994).

The vaso-occlusive crisis is the hallmark event in sickle cell disease (SCD). These recurrent "crises," or "severe pain episodes," are the cause of acute episodes of intense pain and represent the most common reason patients seek medical care. Occlusion of macrovasculature and microvasculature produces pain and end-organ damage. All organ systems are potentially affected, but vascular occlusion particularly causes damage to bones, kidneys, lungs, eyes, and the central nervous system. Chronic pain becomes a problem for many patients. Neuropsychiatric manifestations of SCD can be grouped into three main categories:

1. Depression and anxiety resulting from living with a chronic, stigmatizing disease associated with unpredictable painful episodes, chronic pain, and high morbidity and mortality;

2. Problems from living with chronic and acute pain that is often undertreated and when treated with opioids can produce opioid tolerance, including pseudo-addiction and true opioid dependence;

3. Central nervous system damage resulting from cerebrovascular accidents, primarily during childhood.

Psychological and psychiatric complications in patients are common and contribute to impairment in functioning and quality of life. Psychological and psychiatric treatment is believed to improve outcomes, and many comprehensive SCD centers provide psychological and psychiatric care as a component of their treatment. A significant barrier to obtaining proper psychiatric treatment for patients with SCD is that African-Americans are often reluctant to see mental health specialists, attempting to overcome their mental health problems through self-reliance and determination (Snowden, 2001). In addition, lack of psychosocial resources and lower socioeconomic status may make it more difficult to access psychiatric care (Burlew et al., 2000).

Depression and anxiety are common in SCD and correlate with more daily pain and poorer physical and social quality of life (Levenson et al., 2008). The prevalence of any depressive syndrome in SCD approaches 30% (Burlew, 2000; Jenerette et al., 2005; Levenson et al., 2008). Potentially depression-inducing stressors in SCD include living with a chronic illness, chronic pain, developmental problems, and knowledge of a decreased life expectancy. The specific diagnoses of anemia, renal failure, and stroke all are independently associated with depression (Molock et al., 1994).

Children with SCD have a higher prevalence of excessive fatigue, physical complaints, impaired self-esteem, morbid ideation, and feelings of hopelessness (Anie, 2005; Yang, 1994). Adolescents with SCD have high rates of mental disorders; one study found a prevalence of 50% (Benton et al., 2011). The most common diagnoses in Benton's study were attention deficit disorder (40%), oppositional defiant disorder (22.5%), conduct disorder (17.5%), and major depressive disorder (12.5%). Adolescents with SCD frequently suffer from low self-esteem, heightened self-consciousness, dissatisfaction with body image, and social isolation (Morgan & Jackson, 1986).

CHRONIC AND ACUTE PAIN AND OPIOID USE

The most common reason that patients with SCD seek medical treatment is for management of pain. They have a tremendous pain burden; suffering from both episodes of acute, unpredictable, severe vaso-occlusive pain episodes, and also chronic daily pain. A recent prospective cohort study found that for these patients, pain is the rule rather than the exception. This study found that patients with SCD reported experiencing pain on more than half of the days in a year, and 29% had pain on more than 95% of the days (Smith et al., 2008).

For most cases of severe pain, nonsteroidal pain medications are inadequate. Treatment of sickle cell pain with opioids has now gained mainstream acceptance. Opioids help control pain, improve functional capacity, and decrease hospitalizations (Brookoff & Polomano, 1992; Smith et al., 2008). Chronic opioid use induces pharmacological tolerance and physiological dependence, and may lead to dysfunctional drug dependence and abuse. There is also evidence that chronic opioid use can produce cognitive deficits (Chapman et al., 2002). The few studies that address addiction in SCD report a low prevalence of addiction. Cocaine abuse may occur in up to 10% of patients with SCD who are treated with chronic opioids (Axelrod, 2011). Like patients with other chronically painful conditions, many with SCD use marijuana. In a questionnaire study from Great Britain, 36% of patients with SCD used cannabis in the previous 12 months to relieve symptoms of SCD. The main reasons for cannabis use were to reduce pain, to induce relaxation, or to relieve anxiety and depression (Howard et al., 2005).

Due to skepticism and fear of introducing iatrogenic addiction, many medical practitioners may under-treat pain in these patients (Labbe et al., 2005). Additionally, the medical literature supports the contention that African-Americans suffer from disparities of care in regards to pain management (Shavers et al., 2010). In cases of under-treatment of pain, patients may develop pseudo-addiction, where addiction-like behaviors occur in an attempt to obtain better pain control (Weissman & Haddox, 1989). Some patients seek out illegal narcotics in an attempt to better manage uncontrolled pain, and some patients use opioids to help non-pain symptoms such as depression, insomnia, and anxiety. These behaviors may lead to long-term problems with true addiction and illicit substance abuse (Alao et al., 2003). Careful monitoring with pain agreements, psychiatric evaluation, and urine drug testing mitigate the risks of opioid treatment.

CENTRAL NERVOUS SYSTEM DAMAGE

Central nervous system (CNS) complications of SCD frequently begin in childhood and often cause cognitive deficits. An estimated 25–33% of these children have CNS effects from the disease (Schatz & McClellan, 2006). Seizures occur in 12–14% of pediatric patients with SCD (Adams, 1994; Liu, 1994). Children suffering from strokes demonstrate intellectual deficits ranging from borderline to moderate mental retardation, reduced language function, and problems with adjustment (Hariman et al., 1991). Cognitive deficits in children with SCD may lead to learning problems, intellectual impairment, verbal problems, attention and concentration deficits, and dementia later in life (Anie, 2005). As early as kindergarten, patients with SCD had lower scores in language skills and auditory discrimination, compared to their peers, scores that could not be attributed to absence from school (Steen et al., 2002). Factors contributing to poorer cognitive function include degree of anemia and older age (Vichinsky et al., 2010).

THALASSEMIA

Keira Chism

Thalassemia is an inherited autosomal recessive disorder that causes changes to the globin chains of hemoglobin. Like sickle cell disease, thalassemia is believed to persist because the heterozygote state confers a selective advantage for survival in malarial areas. Adult hemoglobin consists of a tetramer, with two alpha and two beta chains. In patients with thalassemia, the decreased or absent production of alpha or beta globin chains results in the overproduction of the other chain, and to anemia, which in turn affects patients' development (Messina et al., 2008).

There are various forms of thalassemia, with various clinical consequences, The severest form, beta-thalassemia major, causes the greatest disability. Patients with beta-thalassemia major suffer from the effects of severe and chronic anemia, stigmata of chronic hemolysis, organ damage from transfusional iron overload, and local and systemic effects of rapidly expanding erythroid bone marrow progenitors. Damaged blood cells aggregate in the spleen, leading to splenomegaly, which causes increased red blood cell trapping and worsening anemia. An increase in erythropoiesis, albeit ineffective, leads to bony deformities, with severely disfigured pelvis, spine, and skull; facial deformities; and shortening of the limbs (Cunningham, 2008).

Individuals with severe forms of thalassemia (major and intermedia) require red blood cell transfusions to prevent growth retardation, severe bony defects, congestive heart failure, and endocrinopathies. High-risk periods such as pregnancy, growth spurts, and infection-associated aplastic crises demand more frequent transfusions. Regular blood transfusions lead to iron overload. Iron deposition causes cirrhosis,

diabetes, hypogonadism, secondary amenorrhea, short stature, congestive heart failure, and arrhythmias. To prevent these effects, patients with thalassemias undergo iron chelation therapy, in the form of defetoxamine infusion or oral deferasirox. Infusion is a rather onerous form of treatment, lasting throughout the night (Musallam, 2008). Side effects include neutropenia, shortness of breath, headaches, and dizziness (Abetz et al., 2006). Blood transfusions and chelation therapy have changed thalassemia from a fatal childhood illness to a chronic adult disease. Access to, and compliance with, hematological treatment allows 90% of children born with thalassemia major to survive past 40 years of age (Clarke et al., 2009).

PSYCHOLOGICAL ISSUES

The psychiatric sequelae of thalassemia arise from the chronic nature of the disease, from its association with developmental issues, and from the burden of treatment. Patients struggle with denial, acting out, concerns about body image, and low self-esteem (Messina, 2008). Patients may suffer from bony deformities, delayed or absent sexual development, and/or growth retardation, all of which can affect self-esteem. Children with thalassemia require frequent hospitalizations, transfusions, iron chelator therapy, and sometimes surgery. Given the intensive care needed to manage their disease, these children may suffer from the common psychological disturbances of any pediatric chronic disease: isolation, loss of autonomy, and overdeveloped identification with the sick role as well as with health professionals.

Both psychological problems and psychiatric illnesses are observed to be more common in patients with thalassemia than in the general population. Several studies show a higher incidence of anxiety and depressive disorders in these patients than in age-matched controls (Cakaloz et al., 2009).

Children with thalassemia may demonstrate cognitive dysfunction, including impaired abstract reasoning and deficits in attention and memory. They suffer from problems with visuospatial skills and executive functioning. Adults with thalassemia demonstrate similar deficits, as well as slower attention and processing speed, language skills, memory, and visual-constructional skills (Armstrong, 2008). Intellectual deficits, which include cognitive impairment and lack of access to education, are likely to accrue from a variety of etiologies: chronic anemia; missed schooling from illness and treatment; and complications from treatment itself. Iron deposits in the brain, resulting from transfusions, cause cognitive issues. Patients with thalassemia have a higher risk of transient ischemic attacks and microvascular ischemic disease, which contribute to cognitive deficits (Armstrong, 2008).

The complexity of psychosocial adjustment to the chronic disease, and its impact on individuals and their families throughout the lifespan, demand a multidimensional, multidisciplinary treatment strategy. Family counseling, clear communication between heathcare providers and patients, education, and frequent psychological assessments are crucial to good psychiatric, and therefore, hematological, outcomes in these individuals. In general, patients with psychiatric disorders have more difficulty adhering to chelation therapy. Finally, transitioning from pediatric to adult medicine also requires careful, multidisciplinary attention to foster ongoing compliance (Musallam, 2008).

PORPHYRIA

Tal Weinberger

The porphyrias are a group of eight rare metabolic disorders characterized by enzyme deficiencies in the heme biosynthesis pathway. Each porphyria is caused by deficiency of a different enzyme in the pathway, resulting in accumulation of specific toxic heme precursors. Heme is synthesized primarily in the erythropoetic cells for the production of hemoglobin, and in hepatic cells for synthesis of cytochromes and other proteins. The neuropsychiatric features of porphyria are thought to be due to neurotoxicity from hepatic overproduction of 5-aminolevulinic acid and other metabolites in this pathway (Puy et al., 2010).

Porphyrias are further categorized into "acute" (neuropsychiatric), cutaneous, and mixed forms. The four acute porphyrias are acute intermittent porphyria (AIP), variegate porphyria (VP), hereditary coproporphyria (HP), and aminolevulinic acid dehydratase deficiency porphyria (ADP). VP and hereditary coproporphyria are "mixed" porphyrias and can thus present with either neuropsychiatric or dermatological symptoms (which are characterized by a bullous or erythematous rash) (Crimlisk, 1997).

Patients with acute porphyria present with sudden, generally infrequent, crises. Clinical characteristics of these acute episodes are highly variable and can include mental status changes such as anxiety, depression, disorientation, hallucinations, and/or paranoia in 20–30% of patients. About 1% of acute attacks are fatal (Thadani et al., 2000). Most acute attacks present with severe abdominal pain (Puy et al., 2010). Muscular weakness is common, generally starting in the proximal muscles (Puy et al., 2010). In some cases, weakness can progress to quadriparesis and respiratory paralysis, resembling Guillain-Barré syndrome. Mild sensory symptoms can co-occur with a predominantly motor neuropathy (Thadani et al., 2000); motor neuropathies are unusual and thus, are a distinguishing feature of this illness. Other common symptoms include nausea, vomiting, constipation, tachycardia, and hypertension. Hyponatremia due to inappropriate antidiuretic hormone secretion occurs in 40% of cases. Seizures may occur secondary to electrolyte imbalances or as a direct manifestation of porphyria (Puy et al., 2010). The combination of acute mental status changes with acute weakness in a proximal greater than distal, neuropathic pattern is strongly suggestive of the diagnosis. AIP is the most common acute porphyria; it is caused by deficiency of porphobilinogen deaminase. It affects approximately 0.01% of the general population (Regan et al., 1999). The classic triad of symptoms in AIP consists of abdominal pain, mental status changes, and peripheral neuropathy; neuropsychiatric symptoms occur in 19–58% of patients during an acute episode (Regan et al., 1999). In addition to more obvious psychiatric symptoms such as psychosis

and agitation, AIP has also been associated with more subtle neuropsychiatric symptoms. Cases of panic attacks (Vgontzas et al., 1991) and obsessive-compulsive symptoms (Hamner, 1992) have been reported in patients with AIP. Increased incidence of generalized anxiety disorder was found in patients with both manifest and latent AIP, and the severity of anxiety symptoms was found to directly correlate with levels of porphyrin metabolites (Patience et al., 1994).

AIP, VP, and hereditary coproporphyria all have an autosomal dominant inheritance pattern with low penetrance. Only 10–15% of gene carriers ever become symptomatic (Thadani et al., 2000). Most symptomatic patients experience a few isolated attacks and then remain asymptomatic for the rest of their lives (Puy et al., 2010). As the disease remains latent in a large percentage of people carrying the gene, a third of patients have no family history. The clinical manifestations of porphyria vary dramatically. Some patients never develop symptoms, even when exposed to precipitating factors, while others have severe, life-threatening attacks without apparent triggers (Thadani et al., 2000). Acute episodes are rare before puberty and after menopause, most commonly occurring in the third decade (Puy et al., 2010). Women are four to five times more likely than men to develop the clinical syndrome (Thadani et al., 2000).

Acute episodes are precipitated by triggers that induce ALA synthase-1, the first enzyme in the heme biosynthesis pathway. As heme is necessary for the production of cytochrome P450 enzymes, the induction of these enzymes increases hepatic heme production. Most drugs that trigger acute attacks do so by inducing cytochrome P450 enzymes; since these enzymes are synthesized from heme, inducing them necessarily triggers heme synthesis. Many lists of medications considered unsafe in acute porphyria are available, but none is universally accepted. Some specific medications are widely regarded as safe, and some are generally accepted to be unsafe; however, for large number of drugs, safety data are unclear (Thadani et al., 2000). Drugs of abuse such as marijuana, Ecstasy (XTC), amphetamines, cocaine, smoking, and alcohol are also common triggers (Thadani et al., 2000). Fasting may induce hepatic amino levulinic acid (ALA) synthase, precipitating an acute attack (Crimlisk, 1997). Infectious and inflammatory processes can aggravate porphyria by inducing production of heme oxygenase 1, which catabolizes heme, thus indirectly stimulating increased heme production (Puy et al., 2010). Estrogen and progesterone can trigger acute attacks; hormone-related attacks most commonly occur during the luteal phase and during pregnancy (Crimlisk, 1997; Thadani et al., 2000). Emotional and physical stress can also induce an acute episode (Thadani et al., 2000), by unknown mechanism.

First-line diagnostic testing for porphyria includes urinalysis looking for increased porphobilinogen (PBG). Urinary 5-aminolevulinic acid (ALA) is also elevated in all three acute porphyrias (AIP, HP, and VP) during acute episodes (Puy et al., 2010). Urine can be dark due to the presence of porphyrins and other pigments. Between attacks, however, urinary concentration of PBG and ALA are often normal (Thadani et al., 2000). Measurement of urinary porphyrins can be misleading, as they are also elevated in other disorders; thus, this is not recommended as a first-line screening test (Puy et al., 2010). DNA analysis is useful only when the disease-specific mutation in an affected family member is known, as large numbers of mutations have been identified.

The diagnosis of porphyria may be missed for many reasons. As porphyria presents with symptoms that mimic other disorders, it may not even be considered in the differential diagnosis. Additionally, evaluation of the results of screening tests is complicated, and results may be misinterpreted (Crimlisk, 1997). On rare occasions, AIP can present exclusively with psychiatric symptoms. The literature describing this phenomenon consists primarily of case reports and small case series, with a wide variety of psychiatric symptoms (Ellencweig et al., 2006). Abrupt onset and resolution of symptoms, in the context of a known porphyrinogenic trigger, should prompt suspicion of and workup for this diagnosis in the psychiatric patient.

Intravenous hemin administration is the mainstay of treatment for an acute attack, as it inhibits the formation of ALA synthase, the rate-limiting enzyme in the synthesis of heme and the buildup of porphyrins toxic to the tissue. Intravenous glucose or food also reduces synthesis of aminolevulinic acid by shunting metabolism to the carbohydrate pathway, and can improve clinical symptoms; however, experts currently recommend initiating hemin treatment immediately, as it has been found to be more effective in reducing levels of heme precursors during an acute episode. If an attack of any acute porphyria is a consideration, urine urobilinogen can be sent, and distinctions among porphyrias can come later. Urgent use of hemin intravenously and dextrose 10% or food will limit the attack. Fasting state and delay of treatment put the patient at risk for the life-threatening consequences of an acute attack like progressive motor weakness, respiratory failure, and arrhythmias (www.porphyriafoundation.com).

THROMBOTIC THROMBOCYTOPENIC PURPURA (TTP)

Keira Chism

The fluctuating changes in mental status, confusion, or headache associated with microangiopathic injury can be a presenting feature of thrombotic thrombocytopenic purpura. Although the diagnosis of thrombotic thrombocytopenic purpura (TTP) and hemolytic uremic syndrome (TTP-HUS) no longer requires the classic pentad of microangiopathic hemolytic anemia, thrombocytopenia (low platelets with or without purpura), renal insufficiency (elevated creatinine), neurological abnormalities, and fever, some combination of microangiopathic hemolytic anemia and thrombocytopenia along with the other symptoms occurs in all patients. Together, hemolytic anemia and thrombocytopenia lead to a devastating and rapid multisystem coagulopathy, with deposition of platelet thrombi in arterioles and capillaries. These deposits lead to tissue ischemia and infarction. Renal insufficiency and CNS involvement are common; cardiac involvement also occurs (George, 2010).

TTP may be associated with infection, particularly enterohemorrhagic *E. coli*; malignancy; autoimmune diseases,

especially systemic lupus erythematosis; and a history of organ or stem cell transplantation. Exposure to some medications may lead to the development of TTP: chemotherapy; nonsteroidal immunosuppressants; quinine products; and some anti-platelet agents (George, 2010). Some case reports also link quetiapine with the development of TTP (Huynh et al., 2005). Up to one quarter of cases of TTP occur during pregnancy or the peripartum. Most cases of TTP are idiopathic. In these cases with no identifiable cause, molecular genetics reveals that the primary pathophysiology is deficiency or inactivity of ADAMTS13, an enzyme involved in the coagulation cascade (Meloni et al., 2001).

Psychiatric symptoms may herald the presentation of TTP. Sixty percent of patients have significant neurological changes at presentation, and up to 90% of patients develop such symptoms over the course of their illness (Meloni, 2001). Psychiatrists should consider workup for TTP in the context of unexplained change in mental status in context of low platelets and anemia. Prior to the use of plasmapheresis, TTP was associated with 95% mortality. Today, the treatment response rate, with attendant survival, reaches 80% (Meloni, 2001).

NEUROPSYCHIATRIC SYMPTOMS

TTP leads to a variety of neuropsychiatric symptoms, which can fluctuate throughout the course of the illness. Mild symptoms include headache and numbness. More serious symptoms include confusion, disorientation, paresis, aphasia, personality changes, mood changes, seizures, and coma. TTP can cause delirium, probably mediated by microvascular dysfunction and by the metabolic derangements associated with organ ischemia and failure (Meloni, 2001). One complication is nonconvulsive status epilepticus, which can occur with subtle or no motor manifestations. An electroencephalogram can be useful to make this diagnosis (Meloni, 2001). Neuroimaging rarely reveals infarct or hemorrhage, but MRI often shows findings consistent with reversible posterior leukoencephalopathy syndrome (PRES) (Burrus et al., 2009). Patients who have recovered from TTP may have subtle persistent cognitive abnormalities. Complaints of memory, concentration, and endurance difficulties may be related to measurable deficits in neuropsychological testing and may reflect the remnant of diffuse subcortical microvascular disease (Kennedy et al., 2009).

TREATMENT

Plasmapheresis is the mainstay of treatment in cases of idiopathic TTP. Cases associated with autoimmune conditions also benefit from brief pulses of high-dose corticosteroids. Testing for ADAMTS13 activity takes time. It is recommended not to wait for test results before making the diagnosis or starting treatment. With treatment, even severe neurological symptoms such as coma do resolve, with concomitant resolution of PRES findings on MRI. Patients with ADAMTS13 deficiency have higher rates of recurrence of TTP, especially during times of physiological stress such as illness or pregnancy.

HYPERVISCOSITY SYNDROME

Howard Field

Excessive blood viscosity is associated with a constellation of findings, together known as *hyperviscosity syndrome* (Sigle & Buser, 2011). These include bleeding diathesis, retinopathy with visual disturbances (Omoti et al., 2007), renal failure, cardiac decompensation (Corrigan, et al., 2010), and neurological symptoms, such as seizures, alteration of consciousness, and coma (*coma paraproteinaemicum*) (Kipps, 2001). Other symptoms, including fatigue, headache, vertigo, and cognitive impairment, are prominent (Stern et al., 1985; Gómez et al., 1999, 2000). Hyperviscosity is found in conditions that greatly increase either serum protein concentration or cell counts, including multiple myeloma (Barlogie et al., 2001), Waldenstrom's macroglobinemia (Kipps, 2001), leukemia (Pimental, 1993), polycythemia vera, sickle cell disease, AIDS (Gadaret et al., 2004), rheumatoid conditions, diabetes, and other illnesses (Rampling, 2003). The normal blood viscosity as measured by viscometer is 1.5 to 1.8 cP (centiPoises). A measurement of 4 cP or greater is an indication for further investigation. The neuropsychiatric symptoms like delirium are based on microangiopathic dysfunction. The finding of "sausaging" and retinal venous engorgement on ophthalmic exam can contribute to the diagnosis. Reducing the blood viscosity may be life-saving. Phlebotomy is used in polycythemia. Plasmapharesis (plasma exchange) is recommended for multiple myeloma (Teruya, 2002) and Waldentrom's macroglobulinemia (Drew, 2002). Where hyperviscosity is responsible, reduction in blood viscosity produces a prompt improvement in neuropsychiatric symptoms. Ultimately, treatment of the hyperviscosity syndrome is directed at the underlying condition.

HEMATOLOGICAL SIDE EFFECTS OF PSYCHOTROPIC MEDICATIONS

Olu Oyesanmi

AGRANULOCYTOSIS

Agranulocytosis, a life-threatening condition, occurs when the bone marrow stops production of granulocytes, leaving the body vulnerable to bacterial infection. Drug-induced agranulocytosis occurs as a rare idiosyncratic reaction related to the genetic vulnerability of the patient, traditionally thought to be a toxic or immune-mediated suppression of the bone marrow, although the mechanism is hard to pinpoint (Opgen-Rhein & Dettling, 2008; Tesfa et al., 2009; Chowdhury et al., 2011). This reaction is distinct from the low white count seen with direct cytotoxic effects of cancer chemotherapy agents.

Among the psychotropics, clozapine is the drug most often associated with this condition (Becker, 2007). In patients with agranulocytosis, absolute white blood cell (WBC) count is low (WBC < 500/mm³), and almost entirely composed of lymphocytes and monocytes. The hematocrit and platelet counts are normal. Patients with agranulocytosis frequently present with fever, headache, dry cough, sore throat, oral mucosa infection, bleeding gums, or sepsis.

Clozapine-induced agranulocytosis occurs in 1–2% of patients who are receiving clozapine. Total and differential WBC counts must be performed prior to the initiation of clozapine (package insert: see below, Chandrasekaran, 2008). Once clozapine is started, WBC counts must be monitored at least every week for the first 18 weeks, because the risk of agranulocytosis is greatest during this period. Subsequently, WBC counts must be performed at least every month during the entire duration of treatment and continued for one month after stopping treatment. Biweekly counts, however, may be done at total WBC < 3500/mm³ and/or absolute neutrophil count (ANC) < 1500/mm³, or in patients who develop infection. Following stoppage of clozapine, patients may resume treatment, provided that the total WBC > 3000/mm³ and ANC > 1500/mm³. Immediate withdrawal of clozapine is mandatory at total WBC < 3000/mm³ and/or ANC < 1500/mm³. Hematology consultation is advisable if, after stopping treatment, the total WBC count drops below 2000/mm³ and/or the ANC drops below 1000/mm³ (Teva Clozapine Monitoring Guidelines, 2008; Chandrasekaran, 2008). Support with hematopoietic growth factors like granulocyte-colony stimulating factor (G-CSF) and antibiotics would be considered.

In patients with clozapine-induced agranulocytosis, discontinuation of clozapine and a hematology consultation are recommended. Patients should be monitored until blood counts return to normal and for at least four weeks from the day the drug is stopped. Recommendations are daily monitoring until WBC > 3000/mm³ and ANC > 1500/mm³; then twice weekly until WBC > 3500/mm³ and ANC > 2000/mm³; then weekly after WBC > 3500/mm³ (Teva Clozapine Monitoring Guidelines, 2008; Chandrasekaran, 2008). Prior to discontinuing the blood monitoring, patients are educated on the symptoms of agranulocytosis and are advised to notify their medical provider should they experience any of these symptoms (Chandrasekaran, 2008).

Clozapine-induced agranulocytosis is an indication for hospitalization. During hospitalization, reverse isolation and a full septic workup should proceed. The associated risk of mortality is increased in patients who the develop infection prior to the discontinuation of clozapine. Treatment of agranulocytosis may include both the use of intravenous antibiotics and transfusion of granulocyte-stimulating factor. Following the exclusion of high-risk, clozapine-induced agranulocytosis patients with genotype HLA-DQB1 6672G>C, physicians may also reconsider clozapine rechallenge in refractory patients who responded to clozapine in the past (Manu et al., 2011; McKnight et al., 2011).

SELECTIVE SEROTONIN REUPTAKE INHIBITORS AND BLEEDING RISK

The SSRIs and serotonin norepinephrine reuptake inhibitors (SNRIs) are associated with increased upper gastrointestinal (GI) bleeding risk in relation to their serotonergic mechanisms (Meijer, 2004). The overall increased risk of upper GI bleeding, however, is low (Carvajal et al., 2011); for instance, compared to those not taking an SSRI, the risk was 3.1 per 1,000 treatment years in a Danish population study (Dalton et al., 2003). The risk of GI bleeding is greater in older patients taking nonsteroidal anti-inflammatory drugs (NSAIDs), low-dose aspirin, or anti-platelet drugs with SSRIs. Andrade et al. (2010) have suggested that the increase may be related to serotonergic increase in gastric acid production rather than platelet dysfunction. Proton pump inhibitors (PPI) are effective for reducing the risk of GI bleeding in those taking SSRIs. Most patients are restarted on the same antidepressant with a PPI (Dall et al., 2012).

Tendency to bleed had been presumed to be related to the effect on platelet function (Andrade et al., 2010; Wessinger et al., 2006). Patients chronically medicated with SSRIs exhibit lower platelet 5-HT content and reduced serotonergic platelet aggregation by ADP, collagen, and epinephrine (Bismuth-Evenzal et al., 2012). However, clotting parameters for patients on paroxetine, for instance, are not prolonged and do not vary by serotonin transporter polymorphism (Hougardy et al., 2008).

Patients taking warfarin with concomitant SSRIs also have an increased risk of clinically relevant bleeding (Wallerstedt et al., 2009; Cochran et al., 2011). Although not dose-related, an increased risk of bleeding in patients on any type of SSRIs/SNRIs and anticoagulants may be related to the inhibition of cytochrome $P_{450}2C9$ isoenzyme, as warfarin metabolism is principally mediated by this isoenzyme (de Abajo et al., 2006; Mansour et al., 2006). Bleeding may range from ecchymoses and bruising to gastrointestinal bleeding. In patients with a history of bleeding, SSRIs increased the risk of GI bleeding when used concurrently with nonsteroidal anti-infalmmatory drugs (Andrade, 2010).SSRIs do not seem to increase the risk of bleeding during procedures (Douglas et al., 2011; de Abajo et al., 2000, Andrade, 2010). In regard to brain hemorrhage, a recent meta-analysis found the absolute risk in those taking SSRIs was very low, although relative risk was slightly increased (Hackam & Mrkobrada, 2012).

SSRIs and SNRIs, then, should be administered with caution in patients receiving NSAIDs, aspirin, clopidogrel, warfarin, and enoxaparin (Kutscher et al., 2010; Hauta-Aho et al., 2009; Monastero et al., 2007; Wessinger, 2006; FDA.gov, 2011). Patients receiving anticoagulant therapy should receive careful coagulation-monitoring when SSRIs are initiated (Hauta-Aho, 2009; Holbrook et al., 2005). Andrade suggests that patients with a history of peptic ulcer disease or liver disease and those with a history of hemorrhages or GI bleeding might be at a higher risk of bleeding and should be monitored during treatment with fecal occult blood testing. Risk of bleeding usually returns to normal when the SSRI/SNRI is eliminated from the body following discontinuation (Andrade, 2010).

ANTICOAGULANTS AND MALINGERING

Howard Field

Confronted with hemorrhage that cannot be explained by medical conditions, clinicians may consider the possibility of self-induced bleeding. In malingering, the motivation is external (secondary gain); in factitious disorder, patients are motivated to assume the sick role (primary gain). Progress in pharmacology has provided many powerful drugs that can be used to feign a bleeding disorder (Misra et al., 2010; Weitzel et al., 1990). Warfarin and other, more powerful and long-acting warfarin-like anticoagulant agents (the "superwarfarins" brodifacoum or difenacoum) are easily obtained in hardware stores for the purpose of rodent control and at pharmacies by prescription. Elevated prothrombin times will point the clinician in the right direction. A normal factor V points to normal synthetic liver function and vitamin K deficiency. A plasma level for warfarin confirms the diagnosis. Active bleeding requires immediate treatment with vitamin K. In the case of superwarfarins, which also may be used to lace marijuana or crack cocaine, the warfarin level will be negative, and the serum level of the superwarfarin must be sought. Anticoagulation will last much longer and may be associated with thrombotic events as well.

In suspected malingering, a search for external gain factors can provide the clinician with an understanding of the diagnosis. Patients with factitious disorders often have masochistic and histrionic personality traits. Some fantasize about causing bleeding in others. Further exploration may reveal violent accounts of past bleeding episodes in family members or themselves (Feinsilver et al., 1983).

Once bleeding is corrected, the physician should gently discuss the situation with the patient. Initially, one can anticipate denial, rage, or other relatively primitive psychological defenses. It should be remembered that these patients have "selected" a maladaptive and dangerous means for coping with stress and for seeking attention, so a logical, rational response should not be expected. The patient should be encouraged to see a psychiatrist (with the primary physician present, if desired), who can do a comprehensive evaluation, including assessing whether the patient poses a danger to himself/herself or others, and whether psychotropic medication or hospitalization is warranted. Although integrated medical and psychiatric management is not always successful owing to the complexity of these patients, it continues to be the best available course. Factitious disorders by proxy (e.g., Munchausen's) involving children or frail elders must be reported to legal authorities and will entail the intervention of social service agencies (Meadow, 1977).

APPROACH TO THE JEHOVAH'S WITNESS PATIENT

Lex Denysenko and Chris Marchionni

According to their internal statistics, the Church of Jehovah's Witnesses has a global following of over 7.2 million people (Worldwide Report, 2010). Patients who are Jehovah's Witnesses believe eternal salvation comes through a literal interpretation of the Bible. The church's specific prohibition against blood transfusion is derived from an interpretation of various passages in the Bible prohibiting the "eating of blood," including Genesis 9:4, Leviticus 17:14, and Acts 15:29 (Hughes et al., 2008). Patients refuse treatment with blood products based on their religious beliefs, posing a challenge to physicians faced with diseases ordinarily requiring treatment with blood products. For decades, the church had a policy of excommunication, known as "disfellowing," of any member who accepted prohibited blood products. In 2000, the Watchtower Society, which is the corporation in charge of the church's legal, publishing, and administrative needs, published the following media statement:

> If a baptized member of the faith willfully and without regret accepts blood transfusions, he indicates by his own actions that he no longer wishes to be one of Jehovah's Witnesses. The individual revokes his own membership by his own actions, rather than the congregation initiating this step. . . . However, if such an individual later changes his mind, he may be accepted back as one of Jehovah's Witnesses. (Watchtower, Statement to the Media, 2000)

Although the church no longer initiates the judicial proceedings of disfellowing a member who accepts blood products, the current policy ensures that the member who is discovered to have accepted blood products, and who bears no remorse for his actions, will be immediately ostracized by his religious community (Muramoto, 2001).

An article in *The Watchtower*, the official magazine of the Watchtower Society, further explained that it is up to the individual to decide whether to accept or decline blood product fractions (e.g., hemoglobin or albumin, as well as erythropoietin and hemoglobin-based oxygen carriers; see Table 58.1) (Watchtower, Questions from Readers, 2000). In contrast, medical procedures that allow the blood to remain in circulation and do not separate the blood from the body are permitted, including hemodilution, intraoperative blood salvage, use of a heart-lung machine, hemodialysis, and plasmapheresis (Watchtower, October 2000).

A medical psychiatrist may be asked to evaluate a patient who is a Jehovah's Witness when their medical decision-making capacity is questioned, or if the wishes of the patient are discordant with those of family or hospital staff. The decision by a Jehovah's Witness to refuse a medical procedure normally meets criteria for rational decision-making if the decision is congruent with the patient's religious doctrine, and all other criteria are met for demonstrating capacity.

It may be difficult in some cases, however, to determine if the patient is refusing blood products on purely religious grounds, or whether the patient's decision to refuse life-saving treatment is under duress, fear of ostracism, and/or a desire to remain part of the religious community. Thus, involvement of hospital legal counsel and the hospital ethics committee may be needed in more complicated cases. For example, legal or ethical consultation may be warranted if the patient is believed to be lacking capacity; the patient is a minor; or the patient's wishes are inconsistent with the known method by which they practice their faith.

In 1964, the Washington, D.C., Appeals Court upheld Georgetown University Hospital's decision to transfuse blood against the known wishes of a critically ill patient (App. of Pres and Dir of Georgetown, 1964). The judge determined that the patient's wishes to not accept a transfusion were overshadowed by her decision to go to the hospital for medical care, an action that expressed a wish not to die, thereby overriding her religious beliefs. Furthermore, as the patient was "little able to competently decide for herself," the court determined that the hospital had the duty and responsibility to treat.

In an attempt to improve access to medical care for its congregation, the church established hospital liaison committees to assist communication between patients who are Jehovah's Witnesses and physicians who are willing to perform procedures without the use of blood transfusions. Advances in "bloodless medicine" have provided alternative management options for patients in some cases. The church has also instituted a "durable power of attorney wallet card" that followers can carry with them, listing their specific wishes about transfusion (Remmers et al., 2006).

The governing body of Jehovah's Witnesses continues to garner criticism from a vocal minority within its community who view themselves as "Reformed" Jehovah's Witnesses. One organization, the Associated Jehovah's Witnesses for Reform on Blood, seeks to reform the church's policy, and also to educate Jehovah's Witnesses about blood transfusions.

Finally, one should not assume that the personal beliefs of the Jehovah's Witness patient are the same as official church doctrine. As with all patients, the medical care of a Jehovah's Witness should be managed on a case-by-case basis, utilizing a multidisciplinary treatment approach, including engaging with the local Jehovah's Witness hospital liaison committee. Maintaining patient confidentiality is of paramount importance, because the patient may not wish to share their treatment decision with their family or their religious community.

CLINICAL PEARLS

- Iron deficiency is associated with pica and restless legs syndrome.

- Iron is critical for healthy brain development in gestation and the first months of life and prevents persistent emotional and cognitive neurodevelopmental deficits in children.

- In iron-deficiency anemia, plasma iron concentration and serum ferritin concentration are usually both low, and iron-binding capacity is increased. Ferritin is elevated in iron deficiency but also in inflammatory states.

- If the B12 level is found to be low or borderline, elevated serum methylmalonic acid and elevated serum total homocysteine also can help establish if a deficiency exists, as they are markers for functional B_{12} status (Smith, 2009).

- Administration of folate without B_{12} will reverse the hematological abnormalities, but if there is an unrecognized B$_{12}$ deficiency, neurological impairment may progress further, sometimes leading to irreversible deficits.

- Psychiatric aspects of sickle cell disease can be grouped into: (a) depression and anxiety from living with a chronic, stigmatizing disease associated with unpredictable pain, chronic pain, and high morbidity and mortality; (b) problems from living with chronic and acute pain that is often undertreated and when treated with opioids can produce opioid tolerance, including pseudo-addiction and true opioid dependence; and (c) central nervous system damage resulting from cerebrovascular accidents, primarily during childhood.

- People with thalassemia may demonstrate cognitive dysfunction, including impaired abstract reasoning and deficits in attention and memory. They suffer from problems with visuospatial skills and executive functioning.

- The classic triad of symptoms in acute intermittent porphyria consists of neuropathic severe abdominal pain, mental status changes, and peripheral neuropathy; neuropsychiatric symptoms occurs in 19-58% of patients in an acute episode (Regan et al., 1999).

- If an attack of any acute porphyria is a consideration, urine urobilinogen should be sent, and distinctions among porphyrias can come later. Urgent administration of hemin and dextrose 10%, or food will limit the attack. A fasting state and delay of treatment put the patient at risk for progressive motor weakness and respiratory failure.

- Thrombotic thrombocytopenic purpura (TTP) leads to a variety of neuropsychiatric symptoms that can fluctuate throughout the course of the illness. Mild symptoms include headache and numbness. Severe symptoms include delirium, paresis, aphasia, personality changes, mood changes, seizures, and coma. Treatment for idiopathic TTP is plasmapharesis.

- Hyperviscosity syndrome presents as bleeding diathesis, retinopathy with visual disturbances (Omoti, 2007), renal failure, cardiac decompensation (Corrigan, et al., 2010), and neurological symptoms, such as seizures, alteration of consciousness, and coma.

- Drug-induced agranulocytosis is a rare idiosyncratic reaction related to the genetic vulnerability of the patient, traditionally thought to be a toxic or immune-mediated suppression of the bone marrow (Opgen-Rhein, 2008; Tesfa, 2009; Chowdhury, 2011). This reaction is distinct from the low white count seen with the direct cytotoxic effects of cancer chemotherapy agents.

- Among Jehovah's Witnesses, it is up to the individual to decide whether to accept or decline blood product fractions (e.g., hemoglobin or albumin, as well as erythropoietin and hemoglobin-based oxygen carriers; see Table 58.1) (Watchtower, 2000b). Medical procedures like hemodilution, intraoperative blood salvage, use of a heart-lung machine, hemodialysis, and plasmapheresis that allow the blood to remain in circulation and do not separate the blood from the body are permitted (Watchtower, 2000c).

DISCLOSURE STATEMENTS

Dr. Becker has no conflicts to disclose.

Dr. Axelrod has no conflicts to disclose.

Dr. Chism has no conflicts to disclose.

Dr. Weinberger has no conflicts to disclose.

Dr. Markov has no conflicts to disclose.

Dr. Denysenko has no conflicts to disclose.

Dr. Marchionni has no conflicts to disclose.

Dr. Oyesanmi has no conflicts to disclose.

Dr. Field has no conflicts to disclose.

Dr. Kunkel has no conflicts to disclose.

REFERENCES

Iron Deficiency Anemia

Algarin, C., Peirano, P., Garrido, M., Pizarro, F., & Lozoff, B. (2003). Iron deficiency anemia in infancy: long-lasting effects on auditory and visual system functioning. *Pediatric Research, 53*, 217–223.

Annibale, B., Capurso, G., & Delle Fave, G. (2003). The stomach and iron deficiency anaemia: A forgotten link. *Digestive and Liver Disease: Official Journal of the Italian Society of Gastroenterology and the Italian Association for the Study of the Liver, 35*(4), 288–295.

Beard, J. L., Hendricks, M. K., Perez, E. M., et al. (2005). Maternal iron deficiency anemia affects postpartum emotions and cognition. *The Journal of Nutrition, 135*(2), 267–272.

Booth, I. W., & Aukett, M. A. (1997). Iron deficiency anaemia in infancy and early childhood. *Archives of Disease in Childhood, 76*(6), 549–553; discussion, 553–554.

Breymann, C., Visca, E., Huch, R., & Huch, A. (2001). Efficacy and safety of intravenously administered iron sucrose with and without adjuvant recombinant human erythropoietin for the treatment of resistant iron-deficiency anemia during pregnancy. *American Journal of Obstetrics and Gynecology, 184*(4), 662–667. doi: 10.1067/mob.2001.111717.

Coban, E., Timuragaoglu, A., & Meriç, M. (2003). Iron deficiency anemia in the elderly: prevalence and endoscopic evaluation of the gastrointestinal tract in outpatients. *Acta Haematologica, 110*(1), 25–28.

Coltman, C. A. (1969). Pagophagia and iron lack. *Journal of the American Medical Association, 207*, 513–516.

Congdon, E. L., Westerlund, A., Algarin, C. R., et al. (2012). Iron deficiency in infancy is associated with altered neural correlates of recognition memory at 10 years. *Journal of Pediatrics, 160,* (PII S0022-3476 (11)01261-3.

Connor, J. R., Wang, X.-S., Allen, R. P., et al. (2009). Altered dopaminergic profile in the putamen and substantia nigra in restless legs syndrome. *Brain, 132,* 2403–2412.

Cook, J. D., & Skikne, B. S. (1989). Iron deficiency: Definition and diagnosis. *Journal of Internal Medicine, 226*(5), 349–355.

Dickey, W., & McConnell, B. (1999). Celiac disease presenting as the Paterson-Brown Kelly (Plummer-Vinson) syndrome. *The American Journal of Gastroenterology, 94*(2), 527–529. doi: 10.1111/j.1572-02 41.1999.889_r.x.

Dorland, W. A. N. (2003). *Dorland's illustrated medical dictionary* (30th ed.). Philadelphia, PA: Saunders.

Hallberg, L., Hulthen, L., Bengtsson, C., Lapidus, L., & Lindstedt, G. (1995). Iron balance in menstruating women. *European Journal of Clinical Nutrition, 49*(3), 200–207.

Halterman, J. S., Kaczorowski, J. M., Aligne, C. A., Auinger, P., & Szilagyi, P. G. (2001). Iron deficiency and cognitive achievement among school-aged children and adolescents in the United States. *Pediatrics, 107*(6), 1381–1386.

Kettaneh, A., Eclache, V., Fain, O., et al. (2005). Pica and food craving in patients with iron-deficiency anemia: a case-control study in France. *American Journal of Medicine, 118,* 185–188.

Krieger, J., & Schroeder, C. (2001). Iron, brain and restless legs syndrome. *Sleep Medicine Reviews, 5*(4), 277–286. doi: 10.1053/ smrv.2001.0156.

Lee, K. A., & Zaffke, M. E. (1999). Longitudinal changes in fatigue and energy during pregnancy and the postpartum period. *Journal of Obstetric, Gynecologic, and Neonatal Nursing: JOGNN / NAACOG, 28*(2), 183–191.

Lozoff, B., Brittenham, G. M., Viteri, F. E., Wolf, A. W., & Urrutia, J. J. (1982). The effects of short-term oral iron therapy on developmental deficits in iron-deficient anemic infants. *The Journal of Pediatrics, 100*(3), 351–357.

Lozoff, B., & Georgieff, M. K. (2006). Iron deficiency and brain development. *Seminars in Pediatric Neurology, 13,* 158–165.

Lucca, U., Tettamanti, M., Mosconi, P., et al. (2008). Association of mild anemia with cognitive, functional, mood and quality of life outcomes in the elderly: The "health and anemia" study. *PLoS ONE, 3*(4), e1920. doi: 10.1371/journal.pone.0001920.

Melamed, N., Ben-Haroush, A., Kaplan, B., Yogev, Y. (2007). Iron supplementation in pregnancy—does the preparation matter? *Archives of Gynecology and Obstetrics, 276*(6), 601–604.

Milman, N. (2006). Iron and pregnancy—a delicate balance. *Annals of Hematology, 85*(9), 559–565. doi: 10.1007/s00277-006-0108-2.

O'Keeffe, S. T., Gavin, K., & Lavan, J. N. (1994). Iron status and restless legs syndrome in the elderly. *Age and Ageing, 23*(3), 200–203.

Osaki, T., Ueta, E., Arisawa, K., Kitamura, Y., & Matsugi, N. (1999). The pathophysiology of glossal pain in patients with iron deficiency and anemia. *The American Journal of the Medical Sciences, 318*(5), 324–329.

Rector, W. G. Jr. (1989). Pica: Its frequency and significance in patients with iron-deficiency anemia due to chronic gastrointestinal blood loss. *Journal of General Internal Medicine, 4*(6), 512–513.

Reynolds, R. D., Binder, H. J., Miller, M. B., Chang, W. W., & Horan, S. (1968). Pagophagia and iron deficiency anemia. *Annals of Internal Medicine, 69*(3), 435–440.

Sun, E. R., Chen, C. A., Ho, G., Earley, C. J., & Allen, R. P. (1998). Iron and the restless legs syndrome. *Sleep, 21*(4), 371–377.

Trost, L. B., Bergfeld, W. F., & Calogeras, E. (2006). The diagnosis and treatment of iron deficiency and its potential relationship to hair loss. *Journal of the American Academy of Dermatology, 54*(5), 824–844. doi: 10.1016/j.jaad.2005.11.1104.

Trotti, L. M., Bhaadriraju, S., & Becker, L. A. (2012). Iron for restless legs syndrome. *Cochrane Database of Systematic Reviews, 16*(5), CD007834.

Woods, S. C., & Weisinger, R. S. (1970). Pagophagia in the albino rat. *Science, 169,* 1334–1336.

Young, S. L. (2010). Pica in pregnancy: new ideas about an old condition. *Annual Review Nutrition, 30,* 403–422.

Andres, E., Dli-Youcef, N., Vogel, T., Serraj, K., & Zimmer, J. (2009). Oral cobalamin (vitamin B12) treatment. An update. *International Journal of Laboratory Hematology,* Feb; *31*(1), 1–8.

Andres, E., Loukili, N. H., Noel, E., et al. (2004). Vitamin B12 (cobalamin) deficiency in elderly patients. *Canadian Medical Association Journal, 171,* 251–259.

Balk, E. M., Raman, G., Tatsioni, A., Chung, M., Lau, J., & Rosenberg, I. H. (2007). Vitamin B6, B12, and folic acid supplementation and cognitive function: A systematic review of randomized trials. *Archives of Internal Medicine, 167,* 21–30.

Bar-Shai, M., Gott, D., & Marmor, S. (2011). Acute psychotic depression as a sole manifestation of vitamin B12 deficiency. *Psychosomatics, 52*(4), 384–386.

Bauman, W. A., Shaw, S., Jayatilleke, E., Spungen, A. M., & Herbert, V. (2000). Increased intake of calcium reverses vitamin B12 malabsorption induced by metformin. *Diabetes Care, 23,* 1227–1231.

Bottiglieri, T., Laundy, M., Crellin, R., Toone, B. K., Carney, M. W., & Reynolds, E. H. (2000). Homocysteine, folate, methylation, and monoamine metabolism in depression. *Journal of Neurology, Neurosurgery, & Psychiatry, 69,* 228–232.

Carmel, R. (2008). How I treat cobalamin (vitamin B12) deficiency. *Blood, 112*(6), 2214–2221.

Carmel, R., Green, R., Rosenblatt, D. S., & Watkins, D. (2003). Update on cobalamin, folate, and homocysteine. *Hematology: American Society of Hematology Education Program,* 62–81.

Chalouhi, C., Faesch, S., Anthoine-Milhomme, M. C., Fulla, Y., Dulac, O., & Cheron, G. (2008). Neurologic consequences of vitamin B12 deficiency and its treatment. *Pediatric Emergency Care,* Aug; *24*(8), 538–541.

Clark, R., Birks, J., Nexo, E., et al. (2007). Low vitamin B12 status and risk of cognitive decline in older adults. *American Journal of Clinical Nutrition,* Nov; *86*(5), 1384–1391.

Dogan, M., Ariyuca, S., Peker, E., et al. (2012). Psychotic disorder, hypertension and seizures associated with vitamin B12 deficiency: a case report. *Human & Experimental Toxicology, 31*(4), 410–413.

Durga, J., van Boxtel, M. P., Schouten, E. G., et al. (2007). Effect of 3 year folic acid supplementation on cognitive function in older adults in the FACIT trial: a randomised, double blind, controlled trial. *Lancet, 20,* 208–216.

Duthie, S. J. (2011). Folate and cancer: How DNA damage, repair and methylation impact on colon carcinogenesis. *Journal of Inherited Metabolic Disease,* Feb; *34*(1), 101–109.

Galloway, M., & Rushworth, L. (2003). Red cell or serum folate? Results from the National Pathology Alliance benchmarking review. *Journal of Clinical Pathology, 56,* 924.

Homocysteine Lowering Trialists' Collaboration (2005). Dose-dependent effects of folic acid on blood concentrations of homocysteine: A meta-analysis of the randomized trials. *American Journal of Clinical Nutrition, 82,* 806–812.

Hutto, B. R. (1997). Folate and cobalamin in psychiatric illness. *Comprehensive Psychiatry, 38,* 305–314.

Jacques, P., Selhub, J., et al. (1999). The effect of folic acid fortification on plasma folate and total homocysteine concentrations. *New England Journal of Medicine,* May 13; *340*(19), 1449–1454.

Kim, J. M., Stewart, R., Kim, S. W., Yang, S. J., Shin, I. S., & Yoon, J. S. (2008a). Predictive value of folate, vitamin B12 and homocysteine levels in late-life depression. *British Journal of Psychiatry,* Oct; *193*(4), 268–274.

Kim, J. M., Stewart, R., Kim, S. W., Shin, I. S., Yan, S. J., Shin, H. Y., & Yoon, J. S. (2008b). Changes in folate, vitamin B12 and homocysteine associated with incident dementia. *Journal of Neurosurgery & Psychiatry,* Aug; *79*(8), 864–868.

Lerner, V., Kanevsky, M., Dwolatzky, T., Rouach, T., Kamin, R., & Miodownik, C. (2006). Vitamin B12 and folate serum levels in newly admitted psychiatric patients. *Clinical Nutrition, 25,* 60–67.

Lewis, A. L., Pelic, C., & Kahn, D. A. (2009). Malignant catatonia in a patient with bipolar disorder, B12 deficiency and neuroleptic malignant syndrome: One cause or three? *Journal of Psychiatric Practice, 15*(5), 415–422.

Lindenbaum, J., Healton, E. B., Savage, D. G., et al. (1988). Neuropsychiatric disorders caused by cobalamin deficiency in the absence of anemia or macrocytosis. *New England Journal of Medicine, 318*, 1720–1728.

Liu, K. W., Dai, L. K., & Jean, W. (2006). Metformin-related vitamin B12 deficiency. *Age & Ageing, 35*, 200–201.

Luchsinger, J. A., Tang, M. X., Miller, J., Green, R., & Mayeux, R. (2007). Relation of higher folate intake to lower risk of Alzheimer disease in the elderly. *Archives of Neurology, 64*, 86–92.

Lucock, M. (2004). Is folic acid the ultimate functional food component for disease prevention? *British Medical Journal, 328*, 211–214.

Lushinger, J. A., Ming-Xin, T., Miller, J., Green, R., & Mayeux, R. (2007). Relation of higher folate intake to the lower risk of Alzheimer disease in the elderly. *Archives of Neurology, 64*(1), 86–92.

Malinowski, S. S. (2006). Nutritional and metabolic complications of bariatric surgery. *American Journal of the Medical Sciences*, Apr; *331*(4), 219–225.

Malouf, R., & Grimley, E. J. (2008). Folic acid with or without vitamin B12 for the prevention and treatment of healthy elderly and demented people. *Cochrane Database of Systematic Reviews*, Oct 8; (4), CD004514.

Nelson, J. C. (2012). The evolving story of folate in depression and the therapeutic potential of l-methylfolate. *American Journal of Psychiatry, 169*, 1223–1224.

Papakostas, G. I., Cassiello, C. F., & Iovieno, N. (2012). Folates and s-adenosylmethionine for major depressive disorder. *Canadian Journal of Psychiatry, 57*, 406–413.

Papakostas, G. I., Shelton, R. C., Zajcka, J. M., Etemad, B., Rickels, K., Clain, A., et al. (2012). L-methylfolate as adjunctive therapy for SSRI-resistant major depression: results of two randomized, double-blind, parallel-sequential trials. *American Journal of Psychiatry, 169*, 1267–1274.

Rajkumar, A. P., & Jebaraj, P. (2008). Chronic psychosis associated with vitamin B12 deficiency. *Journal of the Association of Physicians of India, 56*, 115–116.

Ravaglia, G., Forti, P., Maioli, F., et al. (2005). Homocysteine and folate as risk factors for dementia and Alzheimer's disease. *American Journal of Clinical Nutrition, 82*, 636–643.

Reynolds, E. H. (2002). Folic acid, ageing, depression, and dementia. *British Medical Journal, 324*, 1512–1515.

Reynolds, E. (2006). Vitamin B12, folic acid, and the nervous system. *Lancet Neurology, 5*, 949–960.

Roffman, J. L., Brohawn, D. G., Nitenson, A. Z., Macklin, E. A., Smoller, J. W., & Goff, D. C. (2013). Genetic variation throughout the folate metabolic pathway influences negative symptom severity in schizophrenia. *Schizophrenia Bulletin, 39*, 330–338.

Schrier, S. L. (2014). Diagnosis and treatment of vitamin B12 and folate deficiency June 2014.

Selhub, J., Bagley, L. C., Miller, J., & Rosenberg, I. H. (2000). B vitamins, homocysteine, and neurocognitive function in the elderly. *American Journal of Clinical Nutrition, 71*, 614S–620S.

Seshadri, S., Beiser, A., Selhub, J., Jacques, P. F., Rosenberg, I. H., D'Agostino, R. B., Wilson, P. W., & Wolf, P. A. (2002). Plasma homocysteine as a risk factor for dementia and Alzheimer's disease. *New England Journal of Medicine, 346*, 476–483.

Sethi, N. K., Mullin, P., Torgovnick, J., & Capasso, G. (2006). Nitrous oxide "whippit" abuse presenting with cobalamin responsive psychosis. *Journal of Medical Toxicology, 2*, 71–74.

Sharma, V., & Biswas, D. (2012). Cobalamin deficiency presenting as obsessive compulsive disorder: case report. *General Hospital Psychiatry, 34*(5), 578.e7–8.

Smith, A. D., Kim, Y. I., & Refsum, H. (2008). Is folic acid good for everyone? *American Journal of Clinical Nutrition*, Mar; *87*(3), 517–533.

Smith, A. D., & Refsum, H. (2009). Vitamin B12 and cognition in the elderly. *American Journal of Clinical Nutrition, 89*(Suppl), 707S–711S.

Smith, A. D., Smith, S. M., de Jager, C. A., et al. (2010). Homocysteine-lowering by B vitamins slows the rate of accelerated brain atrophy in in mild cognitive impairment: a randomized trial. *PLoS One*, Sep 8; *5*(9), e12244.

Stahl, S. M. (2008). Stahl's *Essential psychopharmacology* (3rd ed.; p. 628). New York: Cambridge University Press.

Toh, B. H., van Driel, I. R., & Gleeson, P. A. (1997). Pernicious anemia. *New England Journal of Medicine, 337*, 1441–1448.

Tufan, A. E., Bilici, R., & Usata, G. (2012). Mood disorder with mixed, psychotic features due to vitamin b12 deficiency in an adolescent: case report. *Child & Adolescent Psychiatry & Mental Health, 6*, 25.

US Preventative Services Task Force (2009). Folic acid for the prevention of neural tube defects: U.S. Preventative Services Task Force recommendation statement. *Annals of Internal Medicine, 150*(9), 626.

Valuck, R. J., & Ruscin, J. M. (2004). A case-control study on adverse effects: H2 blocker or proton pump inhibitor use and risk of vitamin B12 deficiency in older adults. *Journal of Clinical Epidemiology, 57*, 422–428.

Vogel, T., Dali-Youcef, N., Kaltenback, G., & Andres, E. (2009). Homocysteine, vitamin B12, folate and cognitive functions: a systematic and critical review of the literature. *International Journal of Clinical Practice*, Jul; *63*(7), 1061–1067.

Hemophilia

Bolton-Maggs, P. H., & Pasi, K. J. (2003). Haemophilias A and B. *Lancet, 361*, 1801–1809.

Bussing, R., & Burket, R. C. (1993). Anxiety and intrafamilial stress in children with hemophilia after the HIV crisis. *Journal of the America Academy of Child & Adolescent Psychiatry, 32*, 562–567.

Casey, R. L., & Brown, R. T. (2003). Psychological aspects of hematologic diseases. *Child & Adolescent Psychiatric Clinics of North America, 12*, 567–584.

Elander, J., & Barry, T. (2003). Analgesic use and pain coping among patients with haemophilia. *Haemophilia, 9*, 202–213.

Gerstner, T., Teich, M., Bell, N., et al. (2006). Valproate-associated coagulopathies are frequent and variable in children. *Epilepsia 47*, 1136–1143.

Manco-Johnson, M. (2005). Hemophilia management: optimizing treatment based on patient needs. *Current Opinion in Pediatrics, 17*, 3–6.

Spilsbury, M. (2004). Models for psychosocial services in the developed and developing world. *Haemophilia, 10*(Suppl 4), 25–29.

Sickle Cell Disease

Adams, R. J. (1994). Neurological complications. In N. Mohandas & M. H. Steinberg (Eds.), *Sickle cell disease: Basic principles and clinical practice* (pp. 599, 560–621). New York: Raven Press.

Alao, A. O., Westmoreland, N., & Jindal, S. (2003). Drug addiction in sickle cell disease: Case report. *International Journal of Psychiatry in Medicine, 33*(1), 97–101.

Anie, K. A. (2005). Psychological complications in sickle cell disease. *British Journal of Haematology*, June:*129*(6), 723–729.

Axelrod, D. J., & Wintersteen, M. (2011). Cocaine use in patients with sickle cell disease and chronic opioid treatment. Fifth Annual National Sickle Cell Disease Research and Educational Symposium and Annual Scientific Meeting, Hollywood, FL, April 11, 2011.

Benton, T. D., Boyd, R., Ifeagwu, J., Feldtmose, E., & Smith-Whitley, K. (2011). Psychiatric diagnosis in adolescents with sickle cell disease: A preliminary report. *Current Psychiatry Reports, 13*(2), 111–115. doi: 10.1007/s11920-011-0177-3

Brookoff, D., & Polomano, R. (1992). Treating sickle cell pain like cancer pain. *Annals of Internal Medicine, 116*(5), 364–368.

Burlew, K., Telfair, J., Colangelo, L., & Wright, E. C. (2000). Factors that influence adolescent adaptation to sickle cell disease. *Journal of Pediatric Psychology, 25*(5), 287–299.

Chapman, S. L., Byas-Smith, M. G., & Reed, B. A. (2002). Effects of intermediate- and long-term use of opioids on cognition in patients with chronic pain. *The Clinical Journal of Pain, 18*(4 Suppl), S83–S90.

Hariman, L. M., Griffith, E. R., Hurtig, A. L., & Keehn, M. T. (1991). Functional outcomes of children with sickle-cell disease affected by stroke. *Archives of Physical Medicine and Rehabilitation, 72*(7), 498–502. doi: 0003-9993(91)90195-O [pii].

Hassell, K. L. (2010). Population estimates of sickle cell disease in the U.S. *American Journal of Preventive Medicine, 38*(4 Suppl), S512–S521. doi: 10.1016/j.amepre.2009.12.022.

Howard, J., Anie, K. A., Holdcroft, A., Korn, S., & Davies, S. C. (2005). Cannabis use in sickle cell disease: A questionnaire study. *British Journal of Haematology, 31*(1), 123–128.

Jenerette, C., Funk, M., & Murdaugh, C. (2005). Sickle cell disease: A stigmatizing condition that may lead to depression. *Issues in Mental Health Nursing,* Dec 26(10), 1081–1101.

Labbe, E., Herbert, D., & Haynes, J. (2005). Physicians' attitude and practices in sickle cell disease pain management. *Journal of Palliative Care, 21*(4), 246–251.

Levenson, J. L., McClish, D. K., Dahman, B. A., et al. (2008). Depression and anxiety in adults with sickle cell disease: The PiSCES project. *Psychosomatic Medicine, 70*(2), 192–196. doi: 10.1097/PSY. 0b013e31815ff5c5.

Liu, J. E., Gzesh, D. J., & Ballas, S. K. (1994). The spectrum of epilepsy in sickle cell anemia. *Journal of the Neurological Sciences, 123*(1–2), 6–10.

Molock, S. D., & Belgrave, F. Z. (1994). Depression and anxiety in patients with sickle cell disease: Conceptual and methodological considerations. *Journal of Health & Social Policy, 5*(3–4), 39–53.

Morgan, S. A., & Jackson, J. (1986). Psychological and social concomitants of sickle cell anemia in adolescents. *Journal of Pediatric Psychology, 11*(3), 429–440.

Platt, O. S., Brambilla, D. J., Rosse, W. F., et al. (1994). Mortality in sickle cell disease: Life expectancy and risk factors for early death. *The New England Journal of Medicine, 330*(23), 1639–1644.

Schatz, J., & McClellan, C. B. (2006). Sickle cell disease as a neurodevelopmental disorder. *Mental Retardation and Developmental Disabilities Research Reviews, 12*(3), 200–207. doi: 10.1002/mrdd.20115 [doi].

Shavers, V. L., Bakos, A., & Sheppard, V. B. (2010). Race, ethnicity, and pain among the U.S. adult population. *Journal of Health Care for the Poor & Underserved, 21*(1), 177–210.

Smith, W. R., Penberthy, L. T., Bovbjerg, V. E., et al. (2008). Daily assessment of pain in adults with sickle cell disease. *Annals of Internal Medicine, 148*(2), 94–101.

Snowden, L. R. (2001). Barriers to effective mental health services for African Americans. *Mental Health Services Research, 3*(4), 181–187.

Steen, R. G., Hu, X. J., Elliott, V. E., Miles, M. A., Jones, S., & Wang, W. C. (2002). Kindergarten readiness skills in children with sickle cell disease: Evidence of early neurocognitive damage? *Journal of Child Neurology, 17*(2), 111–116.

Vichinsky, E. P., Neumayr, L. D., Gold, J. I., et al. (2010). Neuropsychological dysfunction and neuroimaging abnormalities in neurologically intact adults with sickle cell anemia. *Journal of the American Medical Association, 303*(18), 1823–1831. doi: 10.1001/jama.2010.562.

Weissman, D. E., & Haddox, J. D. (1989). Opioid pseudoaddiction—an iatrogenic syndrome. *Pain, 36*(3), 363–366.

Yang, Y. M., Cepeda, M., Price, C., Shah, A., & Mankad, V. (1994). Depression in children and adolescents with sickle-cell disease. *Archives of Pediatrics & Adolescent Medicine, 148*(5), 457–460.

Thalassemia

Abetz, L., Baladi, J., Jones, P., & Rofail, D. (2006). The impact of iron overload on quality of life: results from a literature review. *Health and Quality of Life Outcomes, 4,* 73.

Armstrong, F. D. (2008). Thalassemia and learning: neurocognitive functioning in children. *Annals of the New York Academy of Science, 1054,* 283–289.

Cakaloz, B., Cakaloz, I., Polat, A., et al. (2009). Psychopathology in thalassemia major. *Pediatrics International 51,* 825–828.

Clarke, S. A., Skinner, R., Guest, J., et al. (2009). Health-related quality of life and financial impact of caring for a child with thalassemia major in the UK. *Child: care, Health and Development, 36,* 118–122.

Cunningham, M. J. (2008). Update on thalassemia: clinical care and complications. *Pediatric Clinics of North America, 55,* 447–460; ix.

Messina, G., Colombo, E., Cassinerio, E., et al. (2008). Psychosocial aspects and psychiatric disorders in young adults with thalassemia major. *Internal & Emergency Medicine, 3,* 339–343.

Mussalam, K., Cappellini, M., & Taher, A. (2008). Challenges associated with prolonged survival of patients with thalassemia: transitioning from childhood to adulthood. *Pediatrics, 121,* E1426.

Porphyria

Anderson, K. E., Bloomer, J. R., Bonkovsky, H. L., et al. (2005). Recommendations for the diagnosis and treatment of the acute porphyrias. *Annals of Internal Medicine, 142,* 439–450.

Crimlisk, H. L. (1997). The little imitator—porphyria: a neuropsychiatric disorder. *Journal of Neurology, Neurosurgery, and Psychiatry, 62,* 319–328.

Ellencweig, N., Schoenfeld, N., & Zemishlany, Z. (2006). Acute intermittent porphyria: Psychosis as the only clinical manifestation. *Israel Journal of Psychiatry & Related Sciences, 43*(1), 52–56.

Hamner, M. B. (1992). Obsessive-compulsive symptoms associated with acute intermittent porphyria. *Psychosomatics, 33*(3), 329–331.

Patience, D. A., Blackwood, D. H. R., McColl, K. E. L., & Moore, M. R. (1994). Acute intermittent porphyria and mental illness—a family study. *Acta Psychiatrica Scandinavica, 89,* 262–267.

Puy, H., Gouya, L., & Deybach, J. C. (2010). Porphyrias. *Lancet, 375,* 924–937.

Regan, L., Gonsalves, L., & Tesar, G. (1999). Acute intermittent porphyria. *Psychosomatics, 40*(6), 521–523.

Thadani, H., Deacon, A., & Peters, T. (2000). Diagnosis and management of porphyria. *British Medical Journal, 320,* 1647–1651.

Vgontzas, A. N., Kales, J. D., et al. (1993). Porphyria and panic disorder with agoraphobia. *Psychosomatics, 34*(5), 440–443.

www.porphyriafoundation.com.

Thrombotic Thrombocytopenic Purpura (TTP)

Burrus, T., et al. (2009). Brain lesions are most often reversible in acute thrombotic thrombocytopenic purpura. *Neurology, 73,* 66–70.

George, J. N. (2010). How I treat patients with thrombotic thrombocytopenic purpura. *Blood, 116*(20), 4060.

Huynh, M., Chee, K., & Lau, D. H. (2005). Case report: TTP caused by quetiapine. *Annals of Pharmacotherapy,* Jul–Aug; 39(7–8), 1346–1348.

Kennedy, A. S., Lewis, Q. F., & Scott, J. G. (2009). Cognitive deficits after recovery from thrombotic thrombocytopenic purpura. *Transfusion, 49,* 1092–1101.

Meloni, G., Proia, A., et al. (2001). Thrombotic thrombocytopenic purpura: prospective neurologic, neuroimaging, and neurophysiologic evaluation. *Haematologica, 86,* 1194–1199.

Hyperviscosity Syndrome

Barlogie, B., Shaughnessy, J., Munshi, N., & Epstein, J. (2001). Plasma cell myeloma. In E. Beutler, B. S. Collier, M. A. Lichtman,

T. J. Kipps, & V. Seligsohn (Eds.), *Hematology* (6th ed.; Chap. 106). New York: McGraw-Hill.

Corrigan, F. E. 3rd, Leventhal, A. R., Khan, S., Rao, S., Christopher-Stine, L., & Schulman, S. P. (2010). A rare case of cardiac ischemia: systemic lupus erythematosus presenting as the hyperviscosity syndrome. *Annals of Internal Medicine,* Sep 21; *153*(6), 422–424.

Drew, M. J. (2002). Plasmapheresis in the dysproteinemias. *Therapeutic Apheresis & Dialysis,* Feb; *6*(1), 45–52.

Garderet, L., Fabiani, B., Lacombe, K., Girard, P. M., Fléjou, J. F., & Gorin, N. C. (2004). Hyperviscosity syndrome in an HIV-1–positive patient. *American Journal of Medicine,* Dec 1; *117*(11), 891–893.

Gómez, E., Roncero, C., de Pablo, J., & Bladé, J. (1999). [Acute confusion syndrome secondary to hyperviscosity in multiple myeloma]. *Medicina Clinica (Barcelona),* Nov 13; *113*(16), 635.

Gómez, E., Roncero, C., De Pablo, J., et al. (2000). Hyperviscosity syndrome and mental disorders. *Actas Espanolas de Psiquiatria,* Jul–Aug; *28*(4), 263–266.

Kipps, T. J. (2001). Waldstrom's macroglobulinemia. In E. Beutler, B. S. Collier, M. A. Lichtman, T. J. Kipps, & V. Seligsohn (Eds.), *Hematology* (6th ed.; Chap. 108, p. 1319). New York: McGraw-Hill.

Omoti, A. E., & Omoti, C. E. (2007). Ophthalmic manifestations of multiple myeloma. *West African Journal of Medicine,* Oct–Dec; *26*(4), 265–268.

Pimental, L. (1993). Medical complications of oncologic disease. *Emergency Medical Clinics of North America, 11*(2), 407–419.

Rampling, M. W. (2003). Hyperviscosity as a complication in a variety of disorders. *Seminars in Thrombosis & Hemostasis,* Oct; *29*(5), 459–465.

Sigle, J. P., & Buser, A. (2011). Hyperviscosity syndrome. *Blood,* Feb 3; *117*(5), 1446.

Stern, T. A., Purcell, J. J., & Murray, G. B. (1985). Complex partial seizures associated with Waldstrom's macroglobulinemia. *Psychosomatics, 26,* 890–892.

Stone, M. J., & Bogen, S. A. (2012). Evidence-based focused review of management of hyperviscosity syndrome. *Blood, 119,* 2205–2208.

Teruya J. (2002). Practical issues in therapeutic apheresis. *Therapeutic Apheresis & Dialysis,* Aug; *6*(4), 288–289.

Hematologic Side Effects

Andrade, C., Sandarsh, S., Chethan, K. B., & Nagesh, K. S. (2010). Serotonin reuptake inhibitor antidepressants and abnormal bleeding: a review for clinicians and a reconsideration of mechanisms. *Journal of Clinical Psychiatry, 71*(12), 1565–1575.

Becker, M., Axelrod, D. J., Oyesanmi, O., Markov, D. D., & Kunkel, E. J. (2007). Hematologic problems in psychosomatic medicine. *Psychiatric Clinics of North America, 30*(4), 739–759.

Bismuth-Evenzal, Y., Gonopolsky, Y., Gurwitz, D., et al. (2012). Decreased serotonin content and reduced agonist-induced aggregation in platelets of patients chronically medicated with SSRI drugs. *Journal of Affective Disorders, 136,* 99–103.

Bleeding; New molecular entities (NME) Review follow-up by the Department of Health and Human Services/Public Health Service/Food and Drug Administration/Center for Drug Evaluation and Research/Office of Surveillance and Epidemiology. Retrieved from http://www.fda.gov/downloads/Drugs/DrugSafety/PostmarketDrugSafetyInformationforPatientsandProviders/ucm103480.pd; accessed March 9, 2011.

Carvajal, A., Ortega, S., Del Olmo, L., et al. (2011). *PLoS One, 6,* 319819.

Chandrasekaran, P. K. (2008). Agranulocytosis monitoring with clozapine: To follow guidelines or to attempt therapeutic controversies? *Singapore Medical Journal, 49*(2), 96–99.

Chowdhury, N. I., Remington, G., & Kennedy, J. L. (2011). Genetics of antipsychotic-induced side effects and agranulocytosis. *Current Psychiatry Report, 13*(2), 156–165.

Cochran, K. A., Cavallari, L. H., et al. (2011). Bleeding incidence with concomitant use of antidepressants and warfarin. *Therapeutic Drug Monitoring, 33,* 433–438.

Dall, M., Schaffalitzky, de Mukadill, O. B., & Moller, H. J. (2011). *Heliobacter pylori* risk of gastrointestinal bleeding in users of serotonin reuptake inhibitors. *Scandinavian Journal of Gastroenterology, 46,* 1039–1044.

Dalton, S. O., Johansen, C., Mellemkjoer, et al. (2003). Use of selective serotonin reuptake inhibitors and risk of upper gastrointestinal tract bleeding. *Archives of Internal Medicine, 163,* 59–64.

De Abajo, F. J., Jick, H., Derby L et al. (2000). Intracranial haemorrhage and use of selective serotonin reuptake inhibitors. *British Journal of Clinical Pharmacology, 50,* 43–47.

de Abajo, F. J., Montero, D., Rodriguez, L., A., & Maddurga, M. (2006). Antidepressants and risk of upper gastrointestinal bleeding. *Basic & Clinical Pharmacology & Toxicology, 98*(3), 304–310.

Douglas, I., Smeeth, L., & Irvine, D. (2011). The use of antidepressants and the risk of haemorrhagic stroke: a nested case control study. *British Journal of Clinical Pharmacology, 71,* 116–120.

Hackam, D. G., & Mrkobrada, M. (2012). Selective serotonin reuptake inhibitors and brain hemorrhage: a meta-analysis. *Neurology,* Oct 30, *79*(18), 1862–1865. doi: 10.112/wnl.Ob013e318271f848. epub 2012; Oct 17.

Hauta-Aho, M., & Tirkkonen, T., & Vahlberg, T., & Laine, K. (2009). The effect of drug interactions on bleeding risk associated with warfarin therapy in hospitalized patients. *Annals of Medicine, 41*(8), 619–628.

Holbrook, A. M., Pereira, J. A., Labiris, R., et al. (2005). Systematic overview of warfarin and its drug and food interactions. *Archives of Internal Medicine, 165*(10), 1095–1106.

Hougardy, D. M. C., Egberts, T. C. G., van der Graaf, F., et al. (2008). Serotonin transporter polymorphism and bleeding time during SSRI therapy. *British Journal of Clinical Pharmacology, 65,* 761–766.

Kutscher, E. C., Leloux, M., & Lemon, M. (2010). Antidepressants in geriatric patients: reduce the risk of bleeding. *Current Psychiatry, 9*(11), 84–86.

Mansour, A., Pearce, M., Johnson, B., et al. (2006). Which patients taking SSRIs are at greatest risk of bleeding? [This is a short review.] *Journal of Family Practice, 55*(3), 206–208.

Manu, P., Sarpal, D., Muir, O., Kane, J. M., & Correll, C. U. (2011). When can patients with potentially life-threatening adverse effects be rechallenged with clozapine? A systematic review of the published literature. *Schizophrenia Research,* Feb; *134*(2-3), 180–186.

McKnight, C., Guirgis, H., & Votolato, N. (2011). Clozapine rechallenge after excluding the high-risk clozapine-induced agranulocytosis genotype of HLA-DQB1 6672G>C. *American Journal of Psychiatry, 168*(10), 1120.

Meijer, W. E., Heerdink, E. R., Nolen, W. A., et al. (2004). Association of risk of abnormal bleeding with degree of serotonin reuptake inhibition by antidepressants. *Archives of Internal Medicine, 164,* 2367–2370.

Micromedex Drug Information; Micromedex Healthcare Series (Version 2.0). Greenwood Village, CO: Thomson Healthcare.

Monastero, R., Camarda, R., & Camarda C. (2007). Potential drug–drug interaction between duloxetine and acenocoumarol in a patient with Alzheimer's disease. *Clinical Therapeutics, 29*(12), 2706–2709. http://www.fda.gov/downloads/Drugs/DrugSafety/PostmarketDrugSafetyInformationforPatientsandProviders/ucm103480.pd; accessed on March 9, 2011.

Opgen-Rhein, C., & Dettling, M. (2008). Clozapine-induced agranulocytosis and its genetic determinants. *Summary Pharmacogenetics, 9*(8), 1101–1111.

Tesfa, D., Keisu, M., & Palmbald, J. (2009). Idiosyncratic drug-induced agranulocytosis: possible mechanisms and management. *American Journal of Hematology, 84*(7), 428–434.

Teva Clozapine Monitoring Guidelines, retrieved on April 5, 2011, from https://www.clozapineregistry.com/Resuming_treatment_after_interruption.pdf.

Wallerstedt, S. M., Gleerup, H., Sundstrom, A., Stigendal, L., & Ny, L. (2009). Risk of clinically relevant bleeding in warfarin-treated patients—influence of SSRI treatment. *Pharmacoepidemiology & Drug Safety, 18*(5), 412–416.

Wessinger, S., Kaplan, M., Choi, L., et al. (2006). Increased use of selective serotonin reuptake inhibitors in patients admitted with gastrointestinal hemorrhage: a multicenter retrospective analysis. *Alimentary Pharmacology & Therapeutics, 23*(7), 937–944.

Malingering

Feinsilver, S. J., Raffin, T. A., Kornei, M. C., Sullivan, S. J., & Smith, M. A. (1983). Factitious hemoptysis: The case of the red towel. *Archives of Internal Medicine, 143*(3), 567–568.

Meadow, R. (1977). Munchausen syndrome by proxy: the hinterland of child abuse. *Lancet, 2*(8033), 343–345.

Misra, D., Bednar, M., Cromwell, C., Marcus, S., & Aledort, L. (2010). Manifestations of superwarfarin ingestion: a plea to increase awareness. *American Journal of Hematology, 85*(5), 391–393.

Weitzel, S. J., Sadowski, J. A., Furie, B. C., et al. (1990). Surreptitious ingestion of a long-acting vitamin K antagonist/rodenticide, brodifacoum: clinical and metabolic studies of three cases. *Blood, 76*(12), 2555–2559.

Jehovah's Witnesses

Application of the President and Directors of Georgetown College, United States Court of Appeals, District of Columbia Circuit. 118 U.S. App. D.C. 80; 331 F.2d 1000; (1964) U.S. App.

Hughes, D. S., Ullery, B. W., & Barrie, P. S. (2008). The contemporary approach to the care of Jehovah's Witnesses. *Journal of Trauma, 65*, 237–247.

Muramoto, O. (2001). Bioethical aspects of the recent changes in the policy of refusal of blood by Jehovah's Witnesses. *British Medical Journal, 322*, 37–39.

Remmers, P. A., & Speer, A. J. (2006). Clinical strategies in the medical care of Jehovah's Witnesses. *American Journal of Medicine, 119*, 1013–1018.

Watch Tower Bible and Tract Society (2000). Statement to the media. June 14. Retrieved from www.ajwrb.org/basics/jwpressrelease6-14-00.jpg (accessed May 18, 2011).

Watch Tower Bible and Tract Society of Pennsylvania (2011). *2010 Worldwide Report.* Retrieved from http://www.watchtower.org (accessed April 5, 2011).

Watch Tower Bible and Tract Society (2000). Questions from readers. *The Watchtower*, June 15, 29–31.

Watch Tower Bible and Tract Society (2000). *The Watchtower 2000*, Oct. 15, 30–31.

59.

END-STAGE RENAL DISEASE AND ITS TREATMENT

DIALYSIS AND TRANSPLANTATION

Gregory M. Gressel, Norman B. Levy, Michael J. Germain, and Lewis M. Cohen

INTRODUCTION

The term *psychonephrology* was coined by Levy to refer to the many complex psychiatric and psychological conditions associated with renal disease (Levy, 1978). Over the last three decades, the interaction between kidney failure, psychiatry, bioethics, geriatrics, social work, nursing, and other specialties has continued to challenge clinicians, patients, and families (Levy & Cohen, 2000).

Each year about 111,000 Americans develop end-stage renal disease (ESRD), and by the end of 2008, there were 548,000 people receiving dialysis, for a total national expenditure of $39.5 billion (Rettig, 2011; United States Renal Data System [USRDS], 2010). The number of patients receiving therapy for ESRD continues to increase at a rate of 5–7% per year (USRDS, 2009). Under a 1972 congressional amendment, Medicare covers the cost of ESRD care for most citizens, and this ranges from $26,668 per year for transplant recipients to $77,506 per year for patients receiving dialysis (Iglehart, 2011). The causes of renal failure include systemic illnesses such as diabetes, hypertension, generalized arteriosclerosis, AIDS, and lupus. Primary renal diseases include chronic glomerulonephritis, chronic interstitial nephritis, polycystic kidney disease, and other hereditary and congenital disorders. The national epidemic of obesity and type 2 diabetes has affected renal care and is responsible for the rapidly increasing numbers of patients with ESRD. The elderly (over 75 years of age) now constitute the fastest growing sector of the population (USRDS, 2009). Currently available treatments are kidney transplantation, dialysis, and conservative management (supportive care with no renal replacement therapies) (Murtagh et al., 2007).

DIALYSIS

Dialysis prevents derangements in extracellular volume and the accumulation of organic waste products that would normally be cleared by the kidneys in healthy people. Without dialysis, a patient with ESRD would become uremic and eventually expire.

Dialysis is usually initiated when the prominent symptoms of uremia, most notably lethargy and anorexia, progress to the point that they impair a patient's daily function. This is usually when the glomerular filtration rate approaches 7% of its normal value (Meyer & Hostetter, 2007). The evolution of uremic symptoms, including cognitive impairment, can be quite subtle and easily misdiagnosed as clinical depression.

The two most commonly employed methods of dialysis are peritoneal dialysis and hemodialysis. In peritoneal dialysis, dialysate fluid is introduced and removed from the peritoneal space via an indwelling catheter. The peritoneum serves as a semipermeable membrane through which fluid and wastes pass; they are removed together with dialysate. Peritoneal dialysis may be performed by a machine at home (continuous cycling peritoneal dialysis [CCPD]), or manually at home four to six times a day (continuous ambulatory peritoneal dialysis [CAPD]). Peritoneal dialysis now accounts for only 5–6% of all dialysis; this is a decrease from 13% in the early 1990s, which has taken place despite the fact that peritoneal dialysis is easier to perform at home and less costly than hemodialysis (USRDS, 2009). It is unclear why peritoneal dialysis is done less often than in the past, but it is probably a combination of economic variables and availability.

Hemodialysis may be performed at home or at dialysis units in which there are varying degrees of self-care. In hemodialysis, a fistula is produced by joining an artery and vein together in the arm or forearm. The vein is arterialized and thereby permits multiple venipunctures. Early placement of an arterio-venous (A-V) fistula allows the patient to prepare psychologically for the eventual initiation of dialysis.

If a fistula is not possible, an artificial graft or an indwelling venous catheter is used. This connects the patient's blood supply to a dialysis machine, and blood flows between the person and the mechanical device. Home dialysis can be done daily, three times a week, or during sleep (nocturnal dialysis). The patient can do his or her own treatments, but it is felt to be important that another person is present, for safety reasons.

Peritoneal dialysis can be performed by the patient even when living alone. This can be done nocturnally with an automated cycler or manual exchanges three to four times a day. Patients and their families frequently prefer peritoneal dialysis, as it affords them greater independence and freedom from hospitalization as well as a more liberal diet and latitude for fluid intake (Fan et al., 2008). Lately, there have been efforts aimed at encouraging nocturnal hemodialysis three to five times per week, either at home or in a dialysis center. Studies have reported improved quality of life ratings as well as better control of patient blood pressure, nutrition, and anemia (Rayment & Bonner, 2008; Pierratos, 2004). These advantages need to be balanced against the greater effort, time, and expense of this treatment approach.

Over the past few years, innovations have improved quality and safety of treatment. Hemodialysis membranes, dialysate buffers, electrolyte concentrations and temperature, prescription monitoring, volume ultrafiltration control, and arteriovenous-access monitoring have all been enhanced. Promising technologies include a wearable bioartificial kidney based on continuous hemofiltration and bioartificial tubules. Hopefully, with these advances, we may see a decrease in the morbidity and mortality associated with ESRD.

STRESS OF DIALYSIS

Chronic intermittent hemodialysis is associated with a low quality of life and high rates of morbidity and mortality. In-center hemodialysis forces patients to be unusually dependent on the technology and on the staff who are responsible for providing the procedure (Reichsmann & Levy, 1972). Treatment changes, such as switching from a dialysis center to home dialysis, or from peritoneal dialysis to hemodialysis (and vice versa), or from dialysis to a renal transplant, can be stressful for patients and their families. Patients who undergo hemodialysis may experience many tangible and symbolic losses secondary to their disease and treatment, including physical strength, employment, and social function. The cognitive and affective grief responses to loss have been collectively termed *kidney-disease-related losses* and have been extensively described (Chan et al., 2009). Applying a psychodynamic model to the somatic and psychological loss experienced by dialysis patients can help one understand the spectrum of reactions, from daily stress to clinical depression.

For example, emotional difficulties can ensue when highly independent patients receive treatment that requires them to be relatively passive (DeNour et al., 1968; Levy, 1976). Difficulties arise as a result of the conflict between the strong characterological need for independence in these people and the treatment modality, which places them in a situation of total dependence on a machine, a procedure, and medical personnel. Since traits such as hyperindependence are often refractory to psychological therapy, especially under the stress of medical illness, the more practical solution is to give such individuals a treatment modality (peritoneal, home hemodialysis, self-care center dialysis, or transplantation) that provides a greater amount of personal control. Conversely, dependent patients can have emotional problems if they are pushed into self-care, and such individuals often cope best when they are provided with ordinary in-center hemodialysis. Although transplantation affords an opportunity for a more independent lifestyle, it has its own set of challenges and responsibilities. Patients with renal disease should be provided with information about each treatment option by the renal team, and ideally, they should be permitted to choose a treatment modality that is best suited to their medical situation, social circumstances, personal preferences, and personality traits.

Another loss related to kidney disease that causes patients considerable distress is the unrelenting lack of respite from treatment and illness (Levy, 1976). Most other chronic illnesses afford their victims some break from continual awareness of the disease. For example, patients with cardiac conditions often have long periods of being asymptomatic, while patients with metastatic cancer may have substantial periods of remission or breaks in their therapy regimen during which time they do not have pain or require chemotherapy. However, patients with ESRD are constantly reminded of their illness by the need to take multiple medications throughout the day, adhere to a restrictive diet, and attend repetitive dialysis sessions. Furthermore, patients maintained on hemodialysis have to endure frequent hospitalizations and surgery for vascular access complications, while peritoneal dialysis patients often experience recurrent peritonitis.

Dialysis patients are often quite frail (Schell et al., 2010). The etiology of this is multifactorial, including the dialysis procedure itself, the chronic uremia, advanced age, and comorbidities. Although dialysis provides better filtration than the ESRD patient's failing kidneys, the filtration is incomplete, and the patient experiences partial and intermittently (between dialysis runs) treated uremia (Depner, 2001). The constant flux of extracellular fluid volume and exposure to bioincompatible compounds, in addition to the patient's ongoing acidemia and hyperphosphatemia, contribute to malnutrition, immunosuppression, low-grade serositis, impaired vascular function, and general malaise (Meyer & Hostetter, 2007). This overall feeling of low-grade illness may be particularly devastating to previously active individuals. Sleeplessness, fatigue, pain, and pruritis are very common among dialysis patients, and the overall symptom burden is comparable to that of oncological disease.

Patients on dialysis also experience a loss of freedom in what they can and cannot eat and drink, as they are placed on low-sodium, low-potassium, low-phosphate, high protein, and low fluid diets. Patients on peritoneal dialysis usually receive a more lenient diet since this treatment can remove more fluid and phosphate than hemodialysis. Many patients are non-adherent to the dietary regimen, in particular to low fluid intake. This is readily evident to dialysis staff, who can easily monitor and measure serum potassium levels and weight changes between dialysis treatments.

ESRD patients often experience marital tension as a result of their illness. It has been shown that spousal depressive affect correlates strongly with patient Beck Depression Inventory (BDI) scores (Daneker et al., 2001). Marriage can serve as a source of solace and comfort, or it can serve as a source of conflict and emotional stress. Well-adjusted couples negotiate various coping strategies to compensate for the time devoted to treatment and changes in family dynamics, employment, and sexual function. Emotional support has been correlated with decreased mortality secondary to ESRD (Gee et al., 2008). No major study has looked at divorce rates in the ESRD population compared to the general public. Compounding marital tension, patients on hemodialysis often experience a diminution in their ability to have, or interest in, sex (discussed later) (Finkelstein et al., 2007). When the patient's partner performs the dialysis treatment at home, this can lead to tension related to control issues and anger over complications of the treatment, placement of the needles in the fistula, and other issues.

The psychosocial disturbance experienced by patients extends into the realm of employment (Gutman et al., 1981). Prior to the initiation of dialysis, approximately 42% of patients are employed full- or part-time. This number decreases to 21% at dialysis initiation and to 6.6% at one year after initiation (Tappe et al., 2001). The resulting change in income, the loss of employment benefits, and additional expenses for medications, transportation, and special diets and equipment may have devastating economic effects on the family. For most people, work is not merely a source of income; self-esteem and identity are closely linked to work productivity in Western society (Bruce et al., 2009). Patients who are able to obtain late dialysis appointments, and who are on peritoneal dialysis or home hemodialysis are more likely to remain employed (Kutner et al., 2008). Although many dialysis facilities are attempting vocational rehabilitation, unemployment and its associated depressive symptoms remain an ongoing struggle (Kutner et al., 2010).

Despite the fact that peritoneal dialysis affords patients improved quality of life when compared with hemodialysis, it has special stresses of its own. Treatment distorts the patient's body by distending the abdomen. Patients also face the pain and discomfort of recurrent peritonitis with the ensuing need for hospitalizations. Hemodialysis patients may be similarly embarrassed at the appearance of their vascular access sites and the skin discoloration that is common with chronic treatment.

PSYCHOLOGICAL COMPLICATIONS OF DIALYSIS

Anxiety and depression are the most common psychological symptoms. Anxiety may be present during treatments, particularly in hemodialysis (Cukor et al., 2008). The fear of a medical emergency, such as significant blood loss or a cardiac event, may cause anxiety. Rapid removal of fluid and electrolytes may also produce anxiety, hypotension, nausea, vomiting, and muscular cramps. Anxiety is evident in the uncertainty many patients have about the future, fear about their sexual performance, and apprehension over their ability to cope with the ongoing demands of dialysis and the expectations of staff and family (Levy, 1983).

Evaluation of depression represents a diagnostic challenge, as the symptoms of ESRD along with its treatment may each produce the same somatic signs and symptoms that constitute the criteria of depression. *The Diagnostic and Statistical Manual of Mental Disorders* (DSM-IV) defines *Major depressive disorder* as a clinical syndrome wherein a patient experiences anhedonia and depression in conjunction with five of nine symptoms, including loss of interest or pleasure, depressed mood, appetite disturbance, sleep disturbance, psychomotor agitation or retardation, fatigue and tiredness, feelings of worthlessness, difficulty with concentration, or recurrent thoughts of death or suicide. These symptoms are not supposed to be attributable to a general medical condition, which complicates the diagnosis in ESRD. The symptoms of uremia, including fatigue, sleep disturbance, and anorexia, are common. "Criterion contamination" (Chilcot et al., 2008) refers to difficulty in assessing whether symptoms are the result of depression, somatic illness, or a combination of both.

Prevalence of major depression in the ESRD population is about 20–30%. The exact prevalence remains an issue of debate, as the literature has reported rates anywhere from 0–100%. This may be due, in part, to the numerous screening methods and diagnostic tools used in researching depression in this population. Self-administered questionnaires are commonly employed as a screening tool for the identification of depressive symptoms in the dialysis population. These tools include the Beck Depression Inventory (BDI), the Patient Health Questionnaire (PHQ), and the Center for Epidemiological Studies Depression Scale (CES-D). Self-screening tools tend to report large numbers of depressive symptoms in ESRD patients (Hedayati et al., 2009a). Structured screening by a physician remains the gold standard, but few studies have assessed the prevalence of clinical major depression using the DSM-IV for establishing the diagnosis.

Cohen's approach (1998) to diagnosing depression in these patients entails describing the criteria for major depression, eliciting patient opinion as to whether they believe they are depressed, and then documenting the existence of associated factors, such as depressive episodes prior to the onset of renal failure, a family history of depression, and past suicide attempts.

DEPRESSION, MORBIDITY, AND MORTALITY

Depressive symptoms as assessed by self-report questionnaires and retrospective analyses of maintenance dialysis patients are associated with increased hazard of death and risk of hospitalization. The formal diagnosis of depression by a DSM-IV-based, structured physician interview is also associated with poor outcomes (Hedayati et al., 2008). Patients on long-term hemodialysis with a clinical diagnosis of depression are twice as likely to die or require hospitalization within a year as those without depression. A depression diagnosis is independently associated with a 30% increase in both cumulative hospital days and the number of hospitalizations (Hedayati et al., 2009b).

Many theories exist as to why depressive symptoms are linked to poor patient outcomes, including decreased adherence to therapy, and metabolic changes in endocrine, neurological, hemodynamic, and immune functioning, which place a patient at increased risk for comorbidities (Watnick, 2009). Findings in cardiology disorders complement these conclusions (Boulware et al., 2006). It remains to be seen if successful treatment of depression in patients with ESRD will effectively reduce morbidity and mortality.

SUICIDE

When dialysis first became available in the 1960s, suicide mortality rates were calculated by combining data on deaths following dialysis discontinuation, treatment noncompliance, and clinical suicides. The result was an exaggerated conclusion that the risk of suicide was 400 times that of the general population (Cohen & Germain, 2005). The early estimates of suicide risk are no longer applicable, as dialysis withdrawal and treatment noncompliance are now widely believed to be distinctly different phenomena from clinical suicide.

Data from the USRDS indicates that suicide in ESRD occurs at a rate of two deaths per 10,000 patient-years—only a small increase compared with that of the general population. However, a study analyzed a national cohort of patients from 1995 to 2001 and determined the crude suicide rate to be 24.2 suicides per 100,000 patient-years, with a standardized incidence ratio of 1.84 (Kurella et al., 2005). Several independent predictors of suicide were identified, including older age, male gender, white race, substance abuse, and geographic region. Probability of suicidal behavior significantly increases among dialysis recipients who are single or divorced, who have low quality of life indices, and who perceive themselves as lacking friendship and familial support (Soykan et al., 2003). In contrast to patients who withdrew from dialysis, clinically suicidal patients were less malnourished and debilitated. Interestingly, in Western Europe, the dialysis discontinuation rate is a third of that in the United States, but the ESRD suicide rate is twice as high (Eiser, 1996). Lastly, it remains to be seen if the rates of suicide in the population can be decreased by systematic implementation of depression screening at dialysis facilities.

DIALYSIS CESSATION

Over the past twenty years, there has been growing societal awareness of end-of-life issues. Many religions, American jurisprudence, and mainstream medicine are more accepting of clinical practices that hasten death among the terminally ill, including withholding and withdrawal of life-prolonging treatments (Cohen, 2010). Despite improvements in the management of ESRD patients, the annual mortality rate remains high, and dialysis discontinuation is increasingly considered an option for patients by nephrologists (DeFrancisco & Pinera, 2006). Each year, older and sicker patients undergo dialysis; new advances in technology provide patients with extended life but do not necessarily ensure an acceptable quality of life. Accordingly, treatment decisions are increasingly complicated for practitioners and patients (Lowance,

1993). Paternalism is no longer an acceptable way to practice medicine. Physicians are increasingly involving their patients in treatment plans and encouraging them to make their own decisions about living and dying (Cohen et al., 2003).

Currently, the national withdrawal from dialysis accounts for 26% of ESRD deaths, 10% of deaths in patients age 20–26, and 46% of patients over age 85 (USRDS 2009). These patients are generally elderly, white, diabetic, and severely ill with multiple comorbidities (Bostwick & Cohen, 2009).

The decision to withdraw from dialysis is complicated and involves the patient, physicians, family members, and interdisciplinary teams. In a substantial number of these cases, nephrologists welcome psychiatric consultations. Most psychiatrists are unaccustomed to participating in these complex decisions, and the specialty of psychiatry as well as the rest of medicine and society has not yet sorted out the conflict over issues of physician-assisted dying and euthanasia (Cohen, 2010).

Withdrawal from dialysis allows patients who are terminally ill to shorten the time of suffering. Once dialysis is withdrawn, the mean time to death is 8.2 days (median, 6 days) (Cohen, Germain, et al., 2000). Dialysis withdrawal does not usually result in any pain or discomfort. Potentially, fluid gains could result in pulmonary edema and respiratory distress, but this occurs infrequently, and isolated ultrafiltration (fluid removal without toxin clearance) can be performed to treat these symptoms without prolonging the patient's suffering. Narcotics and sedatives can also be administered if the patient experiences respiratory distress.

The seminal study on dialysis withdrawal by Neu et al. (1986) reported withdrawal in 9% of 1,766 patients in a large regional program between 1966 and 1983; this accounted for 22% of all deaths. Although many were surprised at the high incidence of withdrawal reported by this study, these statistics are now validated and have since been exceeded by other reports and national data (USRDS, 2009). In New England over the past several years, over 40% of ESRD deaths are preceded by decisions to terminate dialysis.

An often-overlooked intervention is not starting dialysis in the chronically ill patient whose quality of life would not benefit from treatment (Murtagh et al., 2007). The incidence of "conservative management" is not known, but it is increasingly being employed in the United Kingdom and Europe. In the United States, there is a countervailing trend to give patients a trial of dialysis if there is a question as to whether they will benefit (Moss, 2001; Moss, 2011). This is carried out with the understanding that, if no benefits are apparent after the trial period, dialysis will then be withdrawn.

Dialysis patients and their families often have difficulty with end-of-life-issues, such as whether to perform cardiopulmonary resuscitation (CPR), or withdraw from dialysis, and decisions about ventilator and nutritional support. A survey of 121 dialysis patients demonstrated only 6% had advance (End of Life) directives. Seventy-four percent had never thought about the issue of dialysis withdrawal, and 84% had never discussed it with their nephrologist (Cohen et al., 1997). Dialysis patients have considerable denial surrounding these issues, and a minority prefer not to discuss

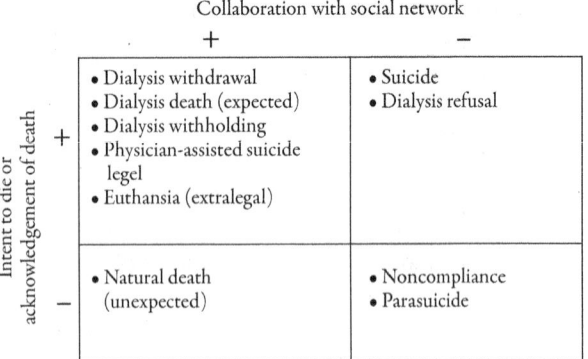

Collaboration with social network

	+	−
+	• Dialysis withdrawal • Dialysis death (expected) • Dialysis withholding • Physician-assisted suicide legel • Euthansia (extralegal)	• Suicide • Dialysis refusal
−	• Natural death (unexpected)	• Noncompliance • Parasuicide

Intent to die or acknowledgement of death

Figure 59.1 ESRD deaths can be categorized based on the patient's intent to die, their acknowledgement of death, and collaboration with the social network (Bostwick and Cohen, 2009).

it (Cohen et al., 1996)—although as many as 97% of some patient samples endorse that they want staff to communicate available prognostic information (Davison, 2010). One factor contributing to the hesitation to have dialysis discontinuation discussions is confusion over whether or not these practices constitute suicide. The renal community now largely sees cessation of dialysis, non-adherence to treatment, and clinical suicide as separate entities. To help physicians and their patients with these distinctions, Bostwick and Cohen (2009) have proposed an algorithm categorizing ESRD deaths based on the patient's intent to die, their acknowledgement of death, and collaboration with the social network (loved ones and staff) in making the decisions (See Figure 59.1).

The Baystate Dialysis Discontinuation Study has been the only prospective investigation analyzing the physical and psychosocial aspects of the dying process in patients who withdraw from dialysis. In the 79 patients from eight sites in the United States and Canada, 38% had "very good," 47% "good," and 15% "bad" deaths, as determined by a "quality of dying" score (Cohen et al., 1995). These findings stand in stark contrast to descriptions of families after a true suicide in which the death is overwhelmingly traumatic for everyone involved. In the ESRD discontinuation research, 57% of patients died within one week, and 75% within two weeks after dialysis withdrawal (Cohen & Germain, 2004).

The line between the presence of psychiatric disorders, such as depression, and patient capacity to refuse lifesaving therapies is sometimes blurred. Cohen has found that irrational thought processes rarely prompt requests for cessation of dialysis. In a few cases, psychopathology was obvious, and patients were strongly encouraged to continue dialysis while undergoing psychiatric treatment, including commitment to a hospital unit (Cohen, 1998). On the other hand, three studies have found an association between depression and patients' decisions to refuse or to terminate life-sustaining treatments (Brown et al., 1986; Ganzini et al., 1994; Sullivan & Younger, 1994). If there is concern that clinical depression may be influencing a patient's request to withdraw dialysis, this can usually be ascertained by seeking input from the family and treatment team.

In 2000, the Renal Physicians Association with the American Society of Nephrology published evidence-based guidelines entitled "Shared Decision-Making in the Appropriate Initiation of and Withdrawal from Dialysis" to aid practitioners and patients in their decisions (Moss, 2001). The guidelines were updated in 2010 (Moss, 2011), and they are the standard within the field.

The Renal Palliative Care Initiative (RPCI), a project funded by the Robert Wood Johnson foundation, was established to train a core group of physicians, nurses, and social workers in palliative medicine, and it charged them with the goals of developing and implementing innovative interventions. The RPCI's programs include: symptom-management protocols, advance care planning, and bereavement services for families and staff. The Initiative findings have been summarized by Poppel and associates (2003).

The Robert Wood Johnson ESRD End-Of-Life workgroup website offers information about additional programs, and the Kidney End-Of-Life coalition maintains an active website with useful resources for members of the health care team and patients (www.kidneyeol.org). A nephrology textbook on end-of-life care has now been published to assist clinicians in these efforts (Chambers et al., 2010). It is time for consultation psychiatrists to become further acquainted with the complexities of modern bioethics and master the techniques of compassionate palliative care (Cohen et al., 1995, Cohen et al., 2003).

SYMPTOM MANAGEMENT DURING DIALYSIS WITHDRAWAL

Historically, nephrology has focused on management of laboratory parameters and dialysis adequacy rather than on symptom assessment and quality of life. As the medical community comes to acknowledge the benefits of hospice and palliative medicine, more physicians are addressing the symptom burden in ESRD patients. Studies by Weisbord et al. (2005) and Davison (2003) have demonstrated that the symptoms experienced by dialysis patients are similar to those of other chronic disease states such as cancer. Pain, in particular, has been singled out as common, and recent studies demonstrate approximately 55% of patients experience an unacceptable degree of suffering in the last days of life. The World Health Organization has developed a three-step analgesic ladder that has been shown to adequately control pain symptoms in 96% of patients with ESRD (Barakzoy & Moss, 2006). The algorithm begins with acetaminophen for patients with mild pain and progresses to hydromorphone, methadone, fentanyl, and oxycodone for patients with severe pain. Narcotics are the mainstay of treatment for patients with extreme pain, and most patients on dialysis withdrawal are placed on a continuous drip, which is titrated as necessary. Respiratory failure is rare in most terminally ill patients receiving chronic opioids. Some authors have cautioned against the use of morphine in patients with CKD because of the side-effect profile (Angst et al., 2000; Dean, 2004; Davison, 2003). Dosing can be complicated by the multiple available preparations, and caution must be used when changing formulations and/or doses. With palliative care intervention, pain prevalence may decrease to 22% in the last 24 hours of life (Germain et al., 2007).

Other side-effects of dialysis-cessation and chronic kidney disease that cause patients discomfort must be anticipated by the physician and treated. As the patient becomes weaker, he or she may retain secretions and develop shortness of breath, which can be alleviated by anticholinergics such as transdermal scopolamine, and also proper positioning. Agitation and involuntary twitching from the buildup of toxins can be addressed with benzodiazepines, haloperidol, and atypical antipsychotics. Nausea, vomiting, and hiccoughs may be treated with traditional antiemetics such as metaclopramide, prochlorproperazine and ondansetron. Pruritis from accumulation of bile salts secondary to hepatorenal syndrome responds well to H1 antagonists and ondansetron. Thirst may be palliated with ice chips and mouth swabs. Palliative care principles applied throughout the patient's disease will help patients not only to live well, but also to die well.

SEXUAL DYSFUNCTION

Sexual dysfunction is prevalent in the ESRD population, with 40% of male patients and 55% of female patients reporting difficulty in achieving orgasm (Finkelstein et al., 2007). Men often complain of erectile dysfunction, premature or delayed ejaculation; women frequently report vaginal dryness or dyspareunia (Seethala, et al., 2010). Patients of both sexes have reduced libido, difficulty with sexual arousal, or inability to achieve orgasm. Younger men (under 50 years of age) are less likely to experience sexual dysfunction after the initiation of dialysis than older men (Stewart, 2006). A nationwide questionnaire study of dialysis patients was performed (Levy, 1973) comparing pre-uremic sexual functions of women with that which they experienced after being on dialysis or receiving a kidney transplant. It was found that women receiving dialysis have decreased libido and greater difficulty having orgasms during intercourse. Transplantation improved all of these sexual functions, but it did not bring them back to the level prior to the onset of renal failure.

The etiology of sexual dysfunction in patients with chronic kidney disease is multifactorial. As diabetes is the leading cause of kidney failure in the United States, it is understandable that the sexual dysfunction in these patients may be linked to vascular problems and neuropathy. One study examined ESRD patients using pharmacocavernostometry and pharmacocavernosography, and it found a 78% prevalence of cavernosal arterial occlusive disease (Kaufman et al., 1994). Autonomic neuropathy of pelvic organs also contributes to sexual dysfunction (Campese, 1990).

Uremic patients experience endocrinological derangements in the hypothalamic-pituitary axis (HPA). Male patients have decreased levels of testosterone and elevations in luteinizing hormone, follicular-stimulating hormone, and prolactin; these are accompanied by reductions in testicular size, impaired spermatogenesis, and weight gain. Women have similar hormone derangements, resulting in decreased libido, vaginal dryness, and inability to achieve orgasm (Finkelstein et al., 2007). Endocrinological changes rarely deviate sufficiently from the normal range to explain reduced sexual function on this basis alone.

Patients with ESRD are frequently placed on drug cocktails that interfere with sexual function. Diuretics, antihypertensives (Bailie et al., 2007), antidepressants, and histamine-receptor blockers may contribute to erectile dysfunction. Other drugs, such as spironolactone, ketoconazole, steroids, and cimetidine, interfere directly with the synthesis of sex hormones (Finkelstein et al., 2007).

Depression contributes to sexual dysfunction; it erodes self-esteem and causes marital difficulties. Patients with higher self-reported depressive symptoms appear to have higher degrees of sexual dysfunction (Peng et al., 2007). The three major physical functions of pre-menopausal women that distinguish them from men are menstruation, gestation, and lactation, and all are impaired in renal failure. Appearance remains an important aspect of femininity and is often compromised by renal failure and dialysis. In men, the actual or nearly total cessation of urination may compromise their sexual identity (Levy et al., 2006). Patients demonstrating pessimistic, anhedonic, or sad affects should be screened for the presence of sexual dysfunction.

There are now numerous treatments for impotence. A device consisting of a cylindrical pump placed over the penis can create a vacuum, which enables the penis to be engorged with blood and thereby become erect, and a rubber band-like instrument placed at the base of the penis prevents the egress of blood during sexual events. Prostaglandin may be inserted into the urethra or directly injected into the corpus cavernosa of the penis to create a temporary erection. Consideration should also be given to surgical approaches to intractable impotence through means of a penile prosthesis. Two systems involve either a silastic rod inserted in the body of the penis, or a hydraulic pump that the patient squeezes. Since these techniques involve destruction of erectile tissue, it is necessary to establish an organic cause prior to surgery by demonstrating the absence of nocturnal penile tumescence.

Less-invasive sexual therapies have demonstrated effectiveness, including in kidney transplantation (Espinoza et al., 2006; Muehrer, 2009; Ozdemir, 2007) where improvement rates are between 20–75% (Shamsa et al., 2005), and the use of medications. The last is the most commonly employed treatment approach, and pharmacotherapy research has largely focused on sildenafil (Viagra). Reported success rates in patients are between 60–80% (Turk et al., 2001; Chen et al., 2001). Studies of sildenafil in renal transplant recipients showed a satisfactory response in 60–81% of transplant patients with erectile dysfunction (Sharma et al., 2006). However, sildenafil is contraindicated in patients receiving medication for angina, and coronary artery disease is common among dialysis patients. Sildenafil and related medications are not covered by Medicare Part D, and the approximate retail cost of a single 100 mg tablet of Viagra is $18.

Currently, only 33% of dialysis centers have even limited educational programs that address sexual dysfunction

(Stewart, 2006). A more thorough initial evaluation is advisable as a screening tool to address all psychosocial and physiological concerns related to sexuality.

COGNITIVE IMPAIRMENT DISORDERS

The presence of cognitive impairment and its negative outcomes in ESRD have been largely neglected by clinicians and the academic community (Murray & Knopman, 2010). However, several studies now report a high frequency of moderate to severe cognitive impairment in these patients and an association with increased mortality. Even mild to moderate cognitive impairment of younger patients appears to increase the mortality rate (Griva et al., 2010). Dementia in dialysis patients increases the risk of hospitalization almost twofold, and a recent prognostic tool with very good validity to predict the likelihood of six-month mortality found dementia to be one of its five variables (Cohen et al., 2010). Cognitive impairment may lead to decreased medication and dietary adherence, and to increased risk of iatrogenic hospitalizations and death. Screening patients and identifying cognitive impairment may help clinicians and families design treatment plans to supervise medication administration, diet, and care plans, and to hold appropriate discussions regarding initiating and withdrawing from dialysis.

Just as ESRD patients have kidney damage from diabetes, cardiovascular disease, and hypertension, so, too, are their brains affected by microvascular pathological processes. If the brain and kidneys are equally thought of as target–end organs damaged by vascular disease, accelerated vascular cognitive impairment can be analogized to decreased glomerular filtration rate (GFR). It has been shown that as GFR decreases in CKD patients, the rate of global cognitive decline increases, as assessed by mental status examination (Murray, 2009). Patients with low levels of kidney function are more likely to have cognitive dysfunction compared with the general population, independent of prevalent cardiovascular disease and risk factors (Tamura et al., 2008). Furthermore, the incidence of clinically evident stroke is more common as CKD worsens in aging patients (15% per year, vs. 2.5% in the general Medicare population) (USRDS 2009).

Because of the higher incidence of organic brain syndromes and dementia, psychiatric hospitalization is 1.5 to 3 times higher in ESRD than in other chronic illnesses (Kimmel et al., 1998). Patients employed in intellectual occupations will tend to note progressive impairment as their day for dialysis approaches. Immediately after dialysis, they may experience a short period of delirium, termed "disequilibrium syndrome," caused by the rapid change of fluid and electrolytes that has taken place during the session. This syndrome may last from minutes to hours. Daily nocturnal hemodialysis may help prevent this syndrome (Pierratos, 2004). An electroencephalogram (EEG) can confirm the presence of a transient metabolic encephalopathy, especially if a baseline EEG is available for comparison; the typical finding is diffuse slowing. Computed tomography and magnetic resonance imaging do not help confirm a dialysis-related delirium but may be helpful in screening for opportunistic central nervous system infections of cerebrovascular events in patients with persistent changes in neurological function.

These acute changes are usually not seen in chronic ambulatory peritoneal dialysis, because this procedure is slow, continuous, and not accompanied by sudden fluxes of fluid and electrolytes. Single-photon emission tomography has been used to compare hemodialysis patients with matched controls, and dialysis patients appear to have reduced cerebral blood flow in the frontal cortex and thalamus (Fazekas et al., 1996).

Among the most serious cognitive disorders is "dialysis encephalopathy." This often-fatal neurological syndrome may occur in patients who have been on hemodialysis for at least two years. The early signs are dysarthria, stuttering speech, memory impairment, depression, and psychosis. Patients often develop choreoathetotic limb movements, asterixis, and generalized tremulousness. If not successfully treated, the disease is progressive and leads to neurological death. Its cause is not fully understood. Aluminum was at one time believed to be the etiological agent, and it was found in trace amounts in dialysate water and phosphate binding gels (Alfrey, 1986). Aluminum has since been removed from dialysate fluids; the incidence of "dialysis encephalopathy" has dropped significantly and is almost never seen clinically. Uremic encephalopathy is still found in patients with advanced uremia who have not been receiving dialysis. It progresses from subtle cognitive impairment, to seizures, coma, and then death.

TREATMENT OF DIALYSIS-INDUCED ANEMIA

Dialysis patients almost always experience severe anemia as a result of decreased endogenous erythropoietin production, decreased red blood cell survival, resistance to erythropoietin action, and impaired iron utilization. Erythropoietin is a glycoprotein hormone produced in the kidney and the liver that acts by stimulating red blood cell production in the bone marrow. ESRD patients experience profound anemia, which is cited as being an independent risk factor for increased weakness, fatigue, difficulty in concentrating, exercise intolerance, life dissatisfaction, and sexual dysfunction (Shah et al., 2009; Weisbord & Kimmel, 2008).

Recombinant human erythropoietin (rHuEpo) was introduced in 1988 for commercial use, and is now widely prescribed to ameliorate anemia. ESRD patients on rHuEpo have seen a drop in transfusion requirements from 16% to 3% per quarter, with less associated transfusion-related infections (Beusterien et al., 1996). Current guidelines advocate maintaining hematocrit levels between 11 and 12 g/dl (Spiegel, 2006). With relief of anemia, patients experience improvement in a wide variety of life functions and quality of life. The National Cooperative Recombinant Human Erythropoietin study demonstrated increased exercise capacity, decreased fatigue, as well as improvement on visual, conceptual, and auditory-verbal learning in patients on rHuEpo (Beusterien et al., 1996). RHuEpo has also been shown to improve erectile dysfunction in some male patients (Lawrence et al., 1997). Treatment with erythropoietin is widely prescribed except dialysis patients with polycythemia and some cases of uncontrolled hypertension.

TREATMENT OF HYPERPARATHYROIDISM

Virtually all patients with ESRD develop secondary and tertiary hyperparathyroidism that worsens as their renal function deteriorates. Hyperparathyroidism results from abnormalities in calcium, phosphorus, and vitamin D metabolism; increased parathyroid function prevents serum hypocalcemia. The end result is renal osteodystrophy secondary to bone resorption. Few studies have assessed the relationship between hyperparathyroidism and depression in ESRD; however, it has been shown that patients with cognitive disorders have higher levels of parathyroid hormone than do non-depressive patients (Driessen et al., 1995). Treatment of hyperparathyroidism involves the use of vitamin D and phosphate-binding agents, and the calcimimetic drug cincalcet (Goodman, 2003). Patients receiving these agents sometimes develop hypo- or hypercalcemia; this can lead to other neuropsychiatric conditions, such as delirium (Tanaka et al., 2007). The relationship between parathyroid hormone, calcium levels, and cognitive dysfunction in dialysis requires further analysis.

RENAL TRANSPLANTATION

In 2007, 17,500 patients with ESRD received kidney transplants, with 72,000 remaining on the waiting list (USRDS, 2009). Renal transplantation is the treatment of choice for many patients. Transplanted patients have improved health-related quality of life and fewer depressive symptoms compared to that of a well-matched sample of wait-listed hemodialysis patients (Kovacs et al., 2010; Szeifert et al., 2010). Kidneys may come from a living donor or be obtained by organ donation following death. Long-term kidney survival is greater with living donors. Most cadaveric kidneys are procured from brain-dead individuals following acute trauma, intracerebral bleeds, and cerebral vascular accidents.

There has been some debate in the transplant community concerning the use of living unrelated donors. Commercially available organs from individuals who were willing to sell their kidneys prompted an outcry, and these sales have been banned by federal statute in the United States and in many other countries. In India, living unrelated donors are not allowed due to past abuses. However, a long-standing critical shortage of cadaveric organs has led most transplant programs to liberalize requirements, and use of kidneys from living unrelated donors, such as a spouse, other relatives, and friends, have become increasingly common. Altruistic donation to an anonymous recipient also occurs, although this practice is controversial and sometimes clearly problematic. Psychiatric consultation is necessary in these latter cases, and psychiatrist and psychologists participate in many transplant programs.

Immunosuppressants are used postoperatively to inhibit rejection of the organ, and patients must remain on immunosuppressive therapy for the rest of their lives. The principal medications are cyclosporine, tacrolimus, sirolimus, mycophenolate mofetil, and steroids (prednisone). If Medicare is the primary insurance, it covers 80% of immunosuppressant medication costs in the initial 36 months, but this still leaves a substantial economic burden on patients and families.

Renal transplantation relieves many patients from the burdens and stresses that accompany dialysis. Diabetics may fare better with transplantation than dialysis, and one group of researchers has claimed that cognitive brain dysfunction associated with dialysis may be fully reversed by transplantation (Kramer et al., 1996). Children are fewer than 1% of the total number of people with renal failure, and have improved growth, development, independence, and quality of life following transplantation (Karrfelt & Berg, 2008).

Transplantation is certainly not a panacea (Cohen, 1996). In contrast with the prevailing belief, an elegant comparison study of men following transplantation matched with those continuing dialysis could not identify either improved psychological adjustment or vocational rehabilitation (Sayag et al., 1990). Transplant recipients face the same uncertainties about their health and future finances, in addition to medication side effects (Szeifert et al., 2010). Drawbacks of transplantation include the constant risk of rejection, the need to adhere to a complex regimen of medications that are capable of producing pronounced side effects, and the necessity for ongoing medical supervision (Fallon et al., 1997; Jindal et al., 2009; Pinsky et al., 2009). A recent prospective study of 840 renal transplant patients showed that depressive symptoms are an independent predictor of mortality in these people (Novak et al., 2010). Psychiatrists need to be alert to steroid-related changes in mood, as well as post-rejection depressions. Psychiatric screening of potential recipients is of value to avoid problems with post-transplant psychiatric complications and or lack of adherence to the post-transplant regime. A functional and histocompatible kidney for transplantation may become possible someday, given advances in organogenesis and therapeutic cloning (De Francisco & Pinera, 2006).

THE DONOR

Living donor-kidney transplants may come from related donors, or from unrelated living donors paired through a donor registry. The number of related donors has declined 18% from a high in 2001, while the number of unrelated living donors increased 125% between 2006 and 2007 (USRDS, 2009). Overall, living donor-kidney transplantations are increasingly performed and have excellent graft-survival outcomes. From a recipient perspective, it is preferable to receive a living donor-kidney transplant rather than waiting for a cadaveric transplant to materialize. In addition, a living donor allows for a pre-emptive transplant and avoids the need for dialysis with its complications. Wait-times on the transplant list continue to increase, with a median lag from registration to transplant of 2.8 years (USRDS, 2009). Studies are now focusing on the donor's well-being and quality of life after transplantation.

The selection of the donor can become a very complex matter, involving familial tension, personal anxiety, and emotional dilemmas. The patient expects that people will come forward voluntarily and without coaxing. It is uncommon for patients with renal failure to confront relatives with their need for a kidney. An intermediary, such as a family member, nurse, or physician, usually makes such requests. Parents, particularly mothers, often want to donate a kidney to their children. Children frequently wish to donate to their parents or siblings, but parents are often unwilling to accept the gift of a kidney.

Early analyses of psychosocial factors in organ donors claimed that they suffer long-term renal dysfunction, depression, and anger at being coerced to make the decision to donate (Saljiad et al., 2007). These data cause ambivalence among some physicians towards live organ donation. Newer studies refute these claims and demonstrate that donors are generally voluntarily forthcoming with their kidney, and after donation they experience good quality of life (Reimer et al., 2006).

In a study in Spain, 86% of donors voluntarily informed the recipient of their wish to donate a kidney; the other 14% were asked by a family member. Although 25% of patients claimed they suffered financially from the operation and were out of work for a mean of 58 days, 100% of the donors said they would favor donation a second time (Cabrer et al., 2003). A German study determined that most donors have an equal or better quality of life than that of the healthy population (Giessing et al., 2004).

Living related donor-kidney transplantation may also strengthen bonds between family members. Goetzmann et al. determined that 72% of patients feel a sense of responsibility toward the donor and the received organ; only 2.7% reported guilt for receiving the transplant (Goetzmann et al., 2008). Donors often feel a justifiable sense of pride, and families are relieved that their loved one has been spared a lifetime of dialysis. On the other hand, families may have unrealistic expectations of the positive ways donation will influence their relationship with the patient or be disappointed with the care provided to "their" kidney by the recipient.

Post-transplant psychosocial assessment of living kidney transplant donors is not yet the standard of care. Although most donors do not experience post-donation mental distress, many feel that psychiatric follow-up after their donation is inadequate (Giessing et al., 2004). Experts now advocate that transplant centers should monitor donors and perform routine psychosocial follow-ups of both recipients and donors of living kidney transplants while providing counseling to those in need (Saljiad et al., 2007).

PSYCHIATRIC SCREENING FOR ORGAN DONATION

Psychiatrists and social workers are members of many transplant teams, and may play an active role in screening donors and recipients. Although the presence of Axis I disorders (including psychotic disorders and substance abuse) do not represent contraindications to this procedure, they need to be considered in evaluating people considered for donation. Psychiatric disorders should be identified and managed prior to transplantation. It is our impression that screening by behaviorally trained professionals is a cost-effective method of reducing post-transplant complications. Surgery may need to be postponed until a sufficient period of time for sobriety or symptom control is achieved. Personality disorders pose a greater challenge, and they often require the involvement of the extended family. Transplantation is deferred when patients cannot emotionally or intellectually grasp the risks and responsibilities of surgery (Cohen, 1996). Since transplant organs are a precious resource, it is important that the patient will be adherent to the regimen and has no active psychiatric or abuse issues that could affect adherence.

Acute kidney rejection has fallen sharply, and now occurs in only 10% of patients (USRDS, 2009). Most recipients and donors have uncomplicated hospitalizations. However, renal transplant recipients have the lowest rates of adherence to postoperative immunosuppressive therapy among solid organ transplant recipients, and this has been correlated with graft loss (O'Grady et al., 2010). Like liver transplantation of people with alcoholic cirrhosis, people with kidney failure represent a skewed sample of the total population. They are overrepresented by people who are non-adherent to their diabetic and hypertensive medical regimens, as well as drug addicts with HIV. At least some degree of non-adherence in adult renal transplant recipients is estimated at about 22%, with graft failure increasing sevenfold among non-adherent versus adherent patients (Butler et al., 2004). Psychiatric screening needs to emphasize this risk factor. Surgery must be deferred until compliance is satisfactory, and these patients may require more intensive post-transplant psychiatric and psychotherapeutic treatment management.

In the past, people with a history of psychosis, sociopathy, and substance abuse were excluded from being kidney donors or recipients of renal transplants. Neuropsychiatric disorders are not currently considered contraindications to surgery, as graft survival is similar regardless of cognitive dysfunction. Many patients with major psychoses, depression, or bipolar disorder have undergone successful transplantation (Carrasco et al., 2009).

Psychiatric screening for organ transplantation should ensure that patients are able to give informed consent in order to understand the risks and benefits of the operation. Patient and professional education, reduction of polypharmacy and pill burden, and creating individualized patient adherence plans based on regular interviews starting before transplantation are of value towards optimizing adherence and reducing graft rejection (O'Grady et al., 2010).

POSTOPERATIVE PSYCHOLOGICAL PROBLEMS

Kidney transplant recipients often experience postoperative anxiety about losing their newfound freedom. As time goes on and rejection is not experienced, the recipient feels relatively relieved. The recipient is never, however, completely safe from the possibility of rejection, and diseases that caused the patient's initial renal failure can recur or affect the transplanted kidney.

Immunosuppressant medications may create difficulties. All transplant recipients must be placed on immunosuppressive therapy in order to reduce the risk of graft rejection. These drugs generally have narrow therapeutic windows, interact with other drugs, and have potentially deleterious physical, neuropsychological, and biochemical effects. The numerous psychiatric complications of steroids are well known. Corticosteroid-free regimens have been used successfully and are becoming increasingly common. Cyclosporine and tacrolimus have been associated with delirium, seizures, and tremors. They may interact with antidepressant medications in transplant recipients (Fireman et al., 2004). Little is known about the psychiatric manifestations of other immunosuppressants such as sirolimus, azathioprine, and mycophenalate, but it is clear that they also interact with other medications and may contribute to cognitive impairment.

New cognitive deficits in transplant recipients indicate the need for a careful workup, especially for infectious diseases. The psychiatrist can play a critical role in initiating the delirium evaluation by identifying the patient's mental symptoms as being of probable organic origin. Patients on prednisone and other immunosuppressants after transplantation are vulnerable to opportunistic pathogens and may have bacterial, fungal, and viral infections with fewer systemic signs than usual. In addition, neoplastic illnesses are slightly more common in these people than in the general population.

PSYCHOTROPIC MEDICATIONS IN RENAL FAILURE

Pharmacokinetics refers to the absorption, distribution, degradation, and excretion of drugs and their metabolites (McIntyre et al., 2008). Several of the factors constituting the pharmacokinetics of psychotropic medications can be altered in renal failure. However, few psychotropics are exclusively excreted by the kidneys; most are metabolized primarily by the liver, eliminated in the bile, and excreted by the gastrointestinal tract (Cohen, Ruthazer, et al., 2010). It is commonly recommended that psychotropic dosing be reduced because of renal failure. This recommendation is based on the fact that protein binding is an important part of the pharmacokinetics of psychotropic medications used in renal failure. People with this disorder have a marked decrease in the ability of their blood to bind protein, which is most likely due to decreased albumin, thereby making available more free medication in their blood for a given dose than in people with normal kidney functioning. Most studies on pharmacokinetics of psychotropics in the ESRD population have been inadequately powered and poorly controlled, and few *in vivo* studies have been performed (Cohen et al., 2004). Levy et al. (1996) performed a small double-blind, crossover study of fluoxetine (Prozac). Clinical evidence suggests that psychotropics are effective and may be safely used. Dosing requires trial and error, but most patients tolerate and require ordinary doses of psychotropic medications.

The bioavailability (drug absorption) of many psychotropics is decreased in patients with renal disease. Although not all psychotropics have been adequately evaluated in patients, it is known that many medications have diminished absorption from the small bowel because uremia results in excess gastric alkalinization and decreased gastrin levels (Mirot et al., 2008). Furthermore, dialysis patients frequently experience nausea and vomiting, and diabetic patients often have gastroparesis, all of which alters drug absorption and pharmacokinetics.

The distribution of psychiatric medications is altered in ESRD patients, as they are often malnourished and have less fluid and body mass in which a drug can diffuse. This theoretically decreases the volume of distribution and increases the potency of a single dose compared to that in a healthy person. The primary alteration in drug distribution is related to decreased serum protein binding of psychotropic drugs. Urea competes for plasma protein binding, decreasing binding of the drug, and resulting in elevated serum levels. Patients also usually have proteinuria that results in diminished protein binding and increased free drugs in the plasma. This is particularly important for drugs such as phenytoin and valproic acid, which normally have high levels of plasma protein binding (Cohen et al., 2004).

Patients also experience decreased degradation (breakdown) and clearance (excretion) of drugs from the body. As the GFR decreases, it is assumed that the rate of drug metabolism by the renal brush border will also decrease, leading to elevated levels in the plasma. It has been shown that ESRD patients have decreased levels of chemical reduction by hydrolysis but normal rates of glucoronidation, microsomal oxidation, and sulfate conjugation (Cohen et al., 2004). Finally, excretion is impaired in ESRD, because patients are unable to filter drugs or secrete their inactive metabolites into the renal tubules, thereby eliminating them from the body. Therefore, there are certain drugs that require altered dosing or should be avoided entirely.

ANTIDEPRESSANTS

Virtually all the antidepressants may be tried in renal failure, but some caution is required. Both SSRIs and tricyclic antidepressants (TCAs) have been demonstrated to be beneficial. Fluoxetine is the best studied of the SSRIs and appears to be well tolerated by patients with renal impairment (Levy et al., 1996). It has a very high therapeutic index, and the kinetic profile of single doses of fluoxetine is not changed in anephric patients, attesting to its safety for use in this population (McIntyre et al., 2008). Sertraline and citalopram are metabolized in the liver and are also widely prescribed without dose adjustment. Patients tend to have increased plasma levels of paroxetine, and the recommended initial dose is halved (10 mg) in the context of severe renal dysfunction (Cohen et al., 2004). TCAs should be reserved for treatment-resistant depression, although amitriptyline and imipramine are occasionally used for treatment of neuropathic pain, and trazodone is commonly tried for insomnia. Venlafaxine levels are markedly increased in patients with renal failure and should be dose-adjusted for ESRD patients. Buproprion may build up and predispose dialysis patients to seizures (Turpeinen et al., 2007), and this medication should be used cautiously. Little is known about nefazodone, and it should also be avoided as a first-line therapy since it may lead to hepatotoxicity (McIntyre et al., 2008).

MOOD STABILIZERS

Lithium has been used for years as the primary mood stabilizer for bipolar affective disorder. It is the only psychotropic medication associated with severe nephrotoxicity. Although there is a current trend to substitute less toxic anticonvulsants such as divalproex and carbamazepine, these drugs may not work as well in some patients as mood stabilizers. Lithium is completely dialyzable, and since it is entirely excreted by the kidneys, a single dose of 600 mg of lithium may be given after each dialysis run in patients with comorbid bipolar disorder and ESRD. After the dialysis session, the lithium level will remain unaltered because of the absence of any renal elimination. Smaller doses of lithium may be employed to augment antidepressant regimens (Mirot et al., 2008).

NEUROLEPTICS

Delirium and agitation are common comorbidities in ESRD patients, and clinicians regularly rely on typical neuroleptics, such as haloperidol (Cohen et al., 2004). The use of atypical neuroleptics is more complicated. Olanzapine is metabolized by the liver but excreted in urine. Studies suggest that special dosing is not required, but olanzapine may aggravate diabetes, a common comorbid disease in ESRD patients. Ziprasidone should probably be avoided because the frequent electrolyte shifts from dialysis may contribute to life-threatening arrhythmias related to QT prolongation. Risperidone clearance is decreased by 60% in patients with renal disease. Thioridazine and mesoridazine are more likely to cause life-threatening arrhythmias and should be avoided.

ANXIOLYTICS AND SEDATIVES

As has already been discussed, anxiety is common in ESRD patients, and pharmacological management is directed either at acute episodes of panic and anxiety or at more generalized nervousness. Benzodiazepines are hepatically metabolized, and dose-reduction is not necessary in ESRD—with the exception of midazolam and chlordiazepoxide, which have high plasma protein binding levels. Lorazepam, diazepam, alprazolam, and clonazepam can be administered in ordinary doses, and are often given at dialysis clinics immediately prior to sessions. The half-life of buspirone is prolonged in patients with renal dysfunction and can worsen dizziness and postural hypotension; the dose should be carefully titrated. Hypnotics such as temazepam or zolpidem may be used in normal doses in conjunction with behavioral management and sleep hygiene education to further prevent sleep disturbances (Cohen et al., 2004).

MEDICATION-RELATED PROBLEMS

ESRD patients have to take many medications several times a day, and they often face difficulties complying with the regimens. Most are elderly and have multiple comorbid conditions, such as diabetes, hypertension, and vascular disease, and this further compounds the medication problems encountered. The average hemodialysis patient is prescribed an average of 12 medications to treat a mean of six comorbid conditions (Manley et al., 2005). A recent retrospective study of 133 patients showed that 98% of patients had problems with medications, and that the number of medication-related problems in an individual patient increased directly with the number of comorbid conditions (Manley et al., 2003). The most frequent medication-related problems encountered are inappropriate laboratory monitoring, patients' not receiving medication for an indicated illness, and dosing errors (Manley et al., 2005). Responsibility to ameliorate these problems falls on physicians and pharmacists, who need to make sure patients are receiving the smallest effective doses, try to avoid polypharmacy, and ensure that medication instructions are clearly communicated.

PROFESSIONALS

Medicare has required all dialysis programs to include psychiatric social workers on their interdisciplinary teams, but only a small number of facilities have formed close working relationships with psychiatric consultants. Behaviorally trained professionals should ideally be involved in evaluating prospective patients for dialysis and transplantation. The data they gather may be useful in determining the modality of treatment that is most feasible each patient. They may give the nephrologist and transplant surgeon valuable information about what might be expected concerning compliance (based on character structure and past adherence), and identify individuals who require closer psychological attention. Professionals are occasionally valuable in managing patient or family requests for dialysis discontinuation. They certainly aid in the early diagnosis and treatment of psychiatric disorders, prevent major disruptions in therapy, and at times forestall hospitalizations. Although its cost-effectiveness has never been systematically studied, it is our impression that greater involvement of psychologically sophisticated clinicians should reduce the cost of caring for this population. Lastly, despite numerous technological advances in renal replacement therapies, treatments have not lived up to expectations that they will allow the majority of patients to return to work or to have satisfactory quality of life (Rettig, 2011). We believe it will require the addition of more behaviorally trained staff and a greater effort to establish more effective collaboration with psychiatric consultants before these important goals can be achieved.

CLINICAL PEARLS

- Dialysis is usually initiated when the prominent symptoms of uremia, most notably lethargy and anorexia, progress to the point that they impair a patient's daily function. This is usually when the glomerular filtration rate approaches 7% of its normal value (Meyer & Hostetter, 2007).

- The evolution of uremic symptoms, including cognitive impairment, can be quite subtle and easily misdiagnosed as clinical depression.

- Since traits such as hyperindependence are often refractory to psychological therapy, especially under the stress of medical illness, the more practical solution is to give such individuals a treatment modality (peritoneal, home hemodialysis; self-care center dialysis; or transplantation) that provides a greater amount of personal control.

- Conversely, dependent patients averse to being pushed into self-care often cope best when they are provided with ordinary in-center hemodialysis.

- The unrelenting lack of respite from treatment and illness in patients with end-stage kidney disease is a stress (Levy, 1976).

- An overall feeling of low-grade illness with sleeplessness, fatigue, pain, and pruritis is very common among dialysis patients.

- Cohen's approach (1998) to diagnosing depression in these patients entails describing the criteria for major depression, eliciting patients' opinion as to whether they believe they are depressed, and then documenting the existence of associated factors, such as depressive episodes prior to the onset of renal failure, a family history of depression, and past suicide attempts.

- Currently, the national withdrawal from dialysis accounts for 26% of ESRD deaths, 10% of deaths in patients age 20–26, and 46% of patients over age 85 (USRDS 2009). These patients are generally elderly, white, diabetic, and severely ill with multiple comorbidities (Bostwick & Cohen, 2009).

- Once dialysis is withdrawn, the mean time to death is 8.2 days (median, 6 days) (Cohen, Germain, et al., 2000).

- Pruritis from accumulation of bile salts secondary to hepatorenal syndrome responds well to H1 antagonists and ondansetron.

- As GFR decreases in CKD patients, the rate of global cognitive decline increases as assessed by mental status examination (Murray, 2009).

- Patients employed in intellectual occupations will tend to note progressive impairment as their day for dialysis approaches. Immediately after dialysis, they may experience a short period of delirium termed "disequilibrium syndrome," caused by the rapid change of fluid and electrolytes that has taken place during the session.

- Depressive symptoms are an independent predictor of mortality in renal transplant patients (Novak et al., 2010).

- Many patients with major psychoses, depression, or bipolar disorder have undergone successful transplantation (Carrasco et al., 2009).

DISCLOSURE STATEMENTS

Dr. Levy has no conflicts to disclose.

Dr. Gressel has no conflicts to disclose.

Dr. Germain has no conflicts to disclose.

Dr. Cohen has no conflicts to disclose.

REFERENCES

Alfrey, A. (1986). Dialysis encephalopathy. *Kidney International, 29*(Suppl), S53–S57.

American Psychiatric Association (1994). *Diagnostic and Statistical Manual of Mental Disorders* (4th ed.). Washington, DC: American Psychiatric Association.

Angst, M. S., Buhrer, M., & Lotsch, J. (2000). Insidious intoxication after morphine treatment in renal failure: Delayed onset of morphine-6-glucuronide action. *Anesthesiology, 92*, 1473–1476.

Bailie, G. R., Elder, S. J., Mason, N. A., et al. (2007). Sexual dysfunction in dialysis patients treated with antihypertensives or antidepressive medications: Results from the DOPPS. *Nephrology, Dialysis, Transplantation, 22*, 1163–1170.

Barakzoy, A. S., & Moss, A. H. (2006). Efficacy of the World Health Organization analgesic ladder to treat pain in end-stage renal disease. *Journal of the American Society of Nephrology, 17*, 3198–3203.

Beusterien, K. M., Nissenson, A. R., Port, F. K., et al. (1996). The effects of recombinant human erythropoietin on functional health and well-being in chronic dialysis patients. *Journal of the American Society of Nephrology, 7*, 763–773.

Bostwick, J. M., & Cohen, L. M. (2009). Differentiating suicide from life-ending acts and end-of-life decisions: a model based on chronic kidney disease and dialysis. *Psychosomatics, 50*, 1–7.

Boulware, L. E., Liu, Y., Fink, N. E., et al. (2006). Temporal relation among depression symptoms, cardiovascular disease events, and mortality in end-stage renal disease: Contribution of reverse causality. *Clinical Journal of the American Society of Nephrology, 1*, 496–504.

Brown, J. H., Henteleff, P., Barakat, S., & Rowe, C. J. (1986): Is it normal for terminally ill patients to desire death? *American Journal of Psychiatry, 143*, 208–211.

Bruce, M. A., Beech, B. M., Sims, M., et al. (2009). Social environmental stressors, psychological factors, and kidney disease. *Journal of Investigative Medicine, 57*(4), 583–589.

Butler, J. A., Roderick, P., Mullee, M., et al. (2004). Frequency and impact of nonadherence to immunosuppressants after renal transplantation: a systematic review. *Transplantation, 77*, 769.

Cabrer, C., Oppenheimer, F., Manyalich, M., et al. (2003). The living kidney donation process: the donor perspective. *Transplantation Proceedings, 35*, 1631–1632.

Campese, V. M. (1990). Autonomic nervous system dysfunction in uraemia. *Nephrology, Dialysis, Transplantation, 5*(Suppl 1), S98–S101.

Carrasco, F. R., Moreno, A., Ridao, N., et al. (2009). Kidney transplantation complications related to psychiatric or neurological disorders. *Transplantation Proceedings, 41*, 2430–2432.

Chambers, E. J., Germain, M., & Brown, E. (2010). *Supportive and palliative care for renal patients* (2nd ed.). Oxford, UK: Oxford University Press.

Chan, R., Brooks, R., Erlich, J., et al. (2009). The effects of kidney-disease-related loss on long-term dialysis patient's depression and quality of life: positive affect as a mediator. *Clinical Journal of the American Society of Nephrology, 4*, 160–167.

Chen, J., Mabjeesh, N. J., Greenstein, A., et al. (2001). Clinical efficacy of sildenafil in patients on chronic dialysis. *Journal of Urology, 165,* 819–821.

Chilcot, J., Wellsted, D., Da Silva-Gane, M., & Farrington, K. (2008). Depression on dialysis. *Nephron. Clinical Practice, 108,* 256–264.

Cohen, L. M. (1996). Renal disease. In J. R. Rundell & M. Wise (Eds.), *American Psychiatric Press textbook of consultation liaison psychiatry* (pp. 573–578). Washington, DC: American Psychiatric Press.

Cohen, L. M. (1998). Suicide, hastening death, and psychiatry. *Archives of Internal Medicine, 158,* 1973–1976.

Cohen, L. M. (2010). *No good deed: a story of medicine, murder accusations, and the debate over how we die.* New York: HarperCollins.

Cohen, L. M., & Germain, M. (2004). Measuring quality of dying in end-stage renal disease. *Seminars in Dialysis, 17,* 376–379.

Cohen, L. M., & Germain, M. J. (2005). The psychiatric landscape of withdrawal. *Seminars in Dialysis, 18*(2), 147–153.

Cohen, L. M., & Germain, M. J. (2006). Renal supportive care: view from across the pond: the United States perspective. *Journal of Palliative Medicine, 10*(6), 1241–1244.

Cohen, L. M., Fischel, S., Germain, M., et al. (1996). Ambivalence and dialysis discontinuation. *General Hospital Psychiatry, 18,* 431–445.

Cohen, L. M., Germain, M. J., & Poppel, D. M. (2003). Practical considerations in dialysis withdrawal: "To have that option is a blessing." *Journal of the American Medical Association, 289*(16), 2113–2119.

Cohen, L. M., Germain, M., Poppel, D. M., Woods, A., & Kjellstrand, C. M. (2000). Dialysis discontinuation and palliative care. *American Journal of Kidney Diseases, 36*(1), 140–144.

Cohen, L. M., McCue, J. D., Germain, M. J., et al. (1997). Denying the dying. *Psychosomatics, 38,* 27–34.

Cohen, L. M., McCue, J. D., Germain, M., et al. (1995). Dialysis discontinuation: A "good" death? *Archives of Internal Medicine, 155,* 42–47.

Cohen, L. M., Ruthazer, R., Moss, A. H., & Germain, M. J. (2010). Predicting six-month mortality for patients who are on maintenance hemodialysis. *Clinical Journal of the American Society of Nephrology, 5*(1), 72–79.

Cohen, L. M., Tessier, E. G., Germain, M. J., et al. (2004). Update on psychotropic medication use in renal disease. *Psychosomatics, 45,* 34–48.

Cukor, D., Coplan, J., Brown, C., et al. (2008). Course of depression and anxiety diagnosis in patients treated with hemodialysis: a 16-month follow-up. *Clinical Journal of the American Society of Nephrology, 3,* 1752–1758.

Daneker, B., Kimmel, P. L., Ranich, T., et al. (2001). Depression and marital dissatisfaction in patients with end-stage renal disease and in their spouses. *American Journal of Kidney Diseases, 38*(4), 839–846.

Davison, S. N. (2003). Pain in hemodialysis patients: prevalence, cause, severity and management. *American Journal of Kidney Diseases, 42,* 1239–1247.

Davison, S. N. (2010). End-of-life care preferences and needs: Perceptions of patients with chronic kidney disease. *Clinical Journal of the American Society of Nephrology,* ePress. Published on January 14, 2010, as doi: 10.2215/CJN.05960809

De Francisco, A. L. M., & Pinera, C. (2006). Challenges and future of renal replacement therapy. *Hemodialysis International, 10,* S19–S23.

Dean, M. (2004). Opioids in renal failure and dialysis patients. *Journal of Pain Symptom Management, 28,* 497–504.

DeNour, A. K., Shaltiel, J., & Czaczkeks, J. W. (1968). Emotional reactions of patients on chronic hemodialysis. *Psychosomatic Medicine, 30,* 521–533.

Depner, T. A. (2001). Uremic toxicity: urea and beyond. *Seminars in Dialysis, 14,* 246–251.

Driessen, M., Wetterling, T., Wedel, T., et al. (1995). Secondary hyperparathyroidism and depression in chronic renal failure. *Nephron, 70*(3), 334–339.

Eiser, A. R. (1996). Withdrawal from dialysis: the role of autonomy and community-based values. *American Journal of Kidney Diseases, 27*(3), 451–457.

Espinoza, R., Gracida, C., Cancio, J., et al. (2006). Prevalence of erectile dysfunction in kidney transplant recipients. *Transplantation Proceedings, 38,* 916–917.

Fallon, M., Gould, D., & Wainwright, S. P. (1997). Stress and quality of life in the renal transplant patient: a preliminary investigation. *Journal of Advances in Nursing, 25*(3), 562–570.

Fan, S. L., Sathick, I., McKitty, K., & Punzalan, S. (2008). Quality of life of caregivers and patients on peritoneal dialysis. *Nephrology, Dialysis, Transplantation, 23*(5), 1713–1719.

Fazekas, G., Fazekas, F., Schmidt, R., et al. (1996). Pattern of cerebral blood flow and cognition in patients undergoing chronic haemodialysis treatment. *Nuclear Medicine Communications, 17*(7), 603–608.

Finkelstein, F. O., Shirani, S., Wuerth, D., et al. (2007). Therapy insight: sexual dysfunction in patients with chronic kidney disease. *Nature Clinical Practice.* Nephrology, *3*(4), 200–207.

Fireman, M., DiMartini, A. F., Armstrong, S. C., et al. (2004). Immunosuppressants. *Psychosomatics, 45*(4), 354–360.

Francisco, A. L. M., & Pinera, C. (2006). Challenges and future of renal replacement therapy. *Hemodialysis International, 10,* S19–S23.

Ganzini, L., Lee, M. A., Heintz, R. T., Bloom, J. D., & Fenn, D. S. (1994). The effect of depression treatment on elderly patients' preferences for life sustaining medical therapy. *American Journal of Psychiatry, 151,* 1631–1636.

Gee, C. B., Howe, G. W., & Kimmel, P. L. (2008). Couples coping in response to kidney disease, a developmental perspective. *Seminars in Dialysis, 18*(2), 103–108.

Germain, M. J., Cohen, L. M., & Davison, S. N. (2007). Withholding and withdrawal from dialysis: what we know about how our patients die. *Seminars in Dialysis, 20*(3), 195–199.

Giessing, M., Reuter, S., Schonberger, B., et al. (2004). Quality of life of living kidney donors in Germany: a survey with the validated short form–36 and Giessen subjective complaints list–24 questionnaires. *Transplantation, 78*(6), 864–872.

Goetzmann, L., Sarac, N., Ambuhl, P., et al. (2008). Psychological response and quality of life after transplantation: a comparison between heart, lung, liver and kidney recipients. *Swiss Medical Weekly, 138*(33–44), 477–483.

Goodman, W. G. (2003). Medical management of secondary hyperparathyroidism in chronic renal failure. *Nephrology, Dialysis, Transplantation, 18*(Suppl 3), iii2–8.

Griva, K., Stygall, J., Hankins, M., Davenport, A., Harrison, M., & Newman, S. P. (2010). Cognitive impairment and 7-year mortality in dialysis patients. *American Journal of Kidney Diseases, 56*(4), 693–703.

Gutman, R. A., Stead, W., & Robinson, R. R. (1981). Physical activity and employment status of patients on maintenance dialysis. *New England Journal of Medicine, 304,* 309–313.

Hedayati, S. S., & Finkelstein, F. O. (2009). Epidemiology, diagnosis, and management of depression in patients with CKD. *American Journal of Kidney Diseases, 54*(4), 741–752.

Hedayati, S. S., Bosworth, H. B., Briley, L. P., et al. (2008). Death or hospitalization of patients on chronic hemodialysis is associated with a physician-based diagnosis of depression. *Kidney International, 74,* 930–936.

Hedayati, S. S., Minhajuddin, A. T., Toto, R. D., Morris D. W., & Rush, A. J. (2009a). Validation of depression screening scales in patients with CKD. *American Journal of Kidney Diseases, 54*(3), 433–439.

Hedayati, S. S., Minhajuddin, A. T., Toto, R. D., Morris, D. W., & Rush, A. J. (2009b). Prevalence of major depressive episode in CKD. *American Journal of Kidney Diseases, 54,* 424–432.

Iglehart, J. K. (2011). Bundled payment for ERSD: Including ESAs in Medicare's dialysis package. *New England Journal of Medicine, 364*(7), 593–595.

Jindal, R. M., Neff, R. T., Abbott, K. C., et al. (2009). Association between depression and nonadherence in recipients of kidney transplants: analysis of the United States Renal Data System. *Transplantation Proceedings, 41,* 3662–3666.

Karrfelt, H. M. E., & Berg, U. B. (2008). Long-term psychosocial outcome after renal transplantation during childhood. *Pediatric Transplantation, 12,* 557–562.

Kaufman, J. M., et al. (1994). Impotence and chronic renal failure: a study of the hemodynamic pathophysiology. *Journal of Urology, 151,* 612–618.

Kimmel, P. L., Thamer, M., Richard, C. M., et al. (1998). Psychiatric illness in patients with end-stage renal disease. *American Journal of Medicine, 105,* 214–221.

Kovacs, A. Z., Molnar, M. Z., Szeifer, L., et al. (2011). Sleep disorders, depressive symptoms and health-related quality of life—a cross-sectional comparison between kidney transplant recipients and waitlisted patients on maintenance dialysis. *Nephrology, Dialysis, Transplantation, 26,* 1058–1065.

Kramer, L., Madl, C., Stockenhuber, F., et al. (1996). Beneficial effect of renal transplantation on cognitive brain function. *Kidney International, 49*(3), 833–838.

Kurella, M., Kimmel, P. L., Young, B. S., et al. (2005). Suicide in the United States End-Stage Renal Disease Program. *Journal of the American Society of Nephrology, 16,* 774–781.

Kutner, N. G., Bowles, T., Zhang, R., et al. (2008). Dialysis facility characteristics and variation in employment rates: a national study. *Clinical Journal of the American Society of Nephrology, 3,* 111–116.

Kutner, N. G., Zhang, R., Huang, Y., & Johansen, K. L. (2010). Depressed mood, usual activity level, and continued employment after starting dialysis. *Clinical Journal of the American Society of Nephrology, 5,* 2040–2045.

Lawrence, I. G., Price, D. E., Howlett, T. A., et al. (1997). Erythropoietin and sexual dysfunction. *Nephrology, Dialysis, Transplantation, 12*(4), 741–747.

Levy, N. B. (1973). Sexual adjustment to maintenance hemodialysis and renal transplantation: national survey by questionnaire: preliminary report. *Transactions of the American Society of Artificial Internal Organs 19,* 138–142.

Levy, N. B. (1976). Coping with maintenance hemodialysis—psychological considerations in the care of patients. In S. G. Massry & A. L. Sellers (Eds.), *Clinical aspects of uremia and dialysis* (Chap. 3, pp. 53–68). Springfield, IL: Charles C. Thomas.

Levy, N. B. (1978). End-Stage Renal Disease and Its Treatment: Dialysis and Transplantation. First International Conference on Hemodialysis and Transplantation, Downstate Medical Center, Brooklyn, NY.

Levy, N. B. (1983). Sexual dysfunctions of hemodialysis. *Clinical & Experimental Dialysis & Apheresis, 7,* 275–288.

Levy, N. B., & Cohen, L. M. (2000). End-stage renal disease and its treatment: Dialysis and transplantation. In A. Stoudemire, B. S. Fogel, & D. Greenberg (Eds.), *Psychiatric care of the medical patient* (2nd ed.; pp. 791–800). London: Oxford University Press.

Levy, N. B., Blumenfield, M., Beasley, C. M., et al. (1996). Fluoxetine in depressed subjects with normal kidney function. *General Hospital Psychiatry, 18,* 8–193.

Levy, N. B., Cohen, L. M., & Tessier, E. G. (2006). Renal disease. In M. Blumenfield & J. Strain (Eds.), *Psychosomatic medicine* (pp. 157–175). Philadelphia, PA: Lippencott, Williams & Wilkins.

Lowance, D. L. (1993). The factors and guidelines to be considered in offering treatment to patients with end-stage renal disease: a personal opinion. *American Journal of Kidney Diseases, 21*(6), 679–683.

Manley, H. J., Cannella, C. A., Bailie, G. R., et al. (2005). Medication-related problems in ambulatory hemodialysis patients: a pooled analysis. *American Journal of Kidney Diseases, 46,* 669–680.

Manley, H. J., McClaran, M. L., Overbay, D. K., et al. (2003). Factors associated with medication-related problems in ambulatory hemodialysis patients. *Journal of Kidney Diseases, 41,* 386–393.

McIntyre, R. S., Baghdady, N. T., Banik, S., et al. (2008). The use of psychotropic drugs in patients with impaired renal function. *Primary Psychiatry, 15*(1), 73–88.

Meyer, T. W., & Hostetter, T. H. (2007). Uremia. *New England Journal of Medicine, 357,* 1316–1325.

Mirot, A. M., Tessier, E. G., Germain, M. G., & Cohen, L. M. (2008). Neuropsychiatric complications and psychopharmacology of end stage renal disease. In T. Berl, J. Himmelfarb, W. Mitch, et al. (Eds.), *Therapy in nephrology and hypertension: A companion to Brenner & Rector's The Kidney, 3rd Edition* (pp. 795–817). Philadelphia, PA: Saunders/Elsevier.

Moss, A. H. (2001). Shared decision-making in dialysis: the new RPA/ASN guidelines on appropriate initiation and withdrawal of treatment. *American Journal of Kidney Diseases, 37*(5), 1081–91.

Moss, A. H. (2011). Revised Dialysis Clinical Practice Guideline promotes more informed decision-making. *Clinical Journal of the American Society of Nephrology, 5:* 2380–2383.

Muehrer, R. J. (2009). Sexuality, an important component of the quality of life of the kidney transplant recipient. *Transplantation Reviews 23,* 214–223.

Murray, A. M. (2009). The brain and the kidney connection: a model of accelerated vascular impairment. *Neurology 73,* 916–917.

Murray, A. M., & Knopman, D. S. (2010). Cognitive impairment in CKD: No longer an occult burden. *American Journal of Kidney Diseases, 56*(4), 615–618.

Murtagh, F. E., Addington-Hall, J., & Higginson, I. J. (2007). The prevalence of symptoms in end-stage renal disease: a systematic review. *Advances in Chronic Kidney Disease, 14*(1), 82–99.

Novak, M., Molnar, M. Z., Szeifert, L., et al. (2010). Depressive symptoms and mortality in patients after kidney transplantation: a prospective prevalent cohort study. *Psychosomatic Medicine, 72,* 527–536.

O'Grady, J. G. M., Aserdakis, A., Bradley, R., et al. (2010). Multidisciplinary insights into optimizing adherence after solid organ transplantation. *Transplantation, 89,* 627–632.

Özdemir, C., Eryilmaz, M., Yurtman, F., et al. (2007). Sexual functioning after renal transplantation. *Transplantation Proceedings, 39,* 1451–1454.

Peng, Y., Chiang, C., Hung, K., et al. (2007). The association of higher depressive symptoms and sexual dysfunction in male haemodialysis patients. *Nephrology, Dialysis, Transplantation, 22,* 857–861.

Peng, Y., Chiang, C., Kao, T., et al. (2005). Sexual dysfunction in female hemodialysis patients: a multicenter study. *Kidney International, 68,* 760–765.

Pierratos, A. (2004). Daily nocturnal home hemodialysis. *Kidney International, 65,* 1975–1986.

Pinsky, B. W., Takemoto, S. K., Lentine, K. L., et al. (2009). Transplant outcomes and economic costs associated with patient noncompliance to immunosuppression. *American Journal of Transplantation, 9,* 2597–2606.

Poppel, D. M., Cohen, L. M., & Germain, M. J. (2003). The Renal Palliative Care Initiative. *Journal of Palliative Medicine, 6*(2), 321–326.

Rayment, G. A., & Bonner, A. (2008). Daily dialysis: Exploring the impact for patients and nurses. *International Journal of Nursing Practice 14*(3), 221–227.

Reichsmann, F., & Levy, N. B. (1972). Problems in adaptation to maintenance hemodialysis: a four-year study of 25 patients. *Archives of Internal Medicine, 130,* 850–865.

Reimer, J., Rensing, A., Haasen, C., et al. (2006). The impact of living-related kidney transplantation on the donor's life. *Transplantation, 81,* 1268–1273.

Rettig, R. A. (2011). Special treatment: The story of Medicare's ESRD entitlement. *New England Journal of Medicine, 364*(7), 596–598.

Saljiad, I., Baines, L. S., Salifu, M., et al. (2007). The dynamics of recipient–donor relationships in living kidney transplantation. *American Journal of Kidney Diseases, 50*(5), 834–854.

Sayag, R., Kaplan De-Nour, A., Shapira, Z., et al. (1990). Comparison of psychosocial adjustment of male nondiabetic kidney transplant and hospital hemodialysis patients. *Nephron, 54,* 214–218.

Schell, J., Finkelstein, F., Germain, M. J., & Cohen, L. M. (2010). An integrative approach to the elderly with advanced kidney disease. *Advances in Chronic Kidney Disease, 17*(4), 368–377.

Seethala, S., Hess, R., Bossola, M., et al. (2010). Sexual function in women receiving maintenance dialysis. *Hemodialysis International, 14,* 55–60.

Shah, R. C., Wilson, R. S., Tang, Y., et al. (2009). Relation of hemoglobin to level of cognitive function in older persons. *Neuroepidemiology, 32,* 40–46.

Shamsa, A., Motavalli, S. M., & Aghdam, B. (2005). Erectile function in end-stage renal disease before and after renal transplantation. *Transplantation Proceedings, 37,* 3087–3089.

Sharma, R. K., Prasad, N., Gupta, A., et al. (2006). Treatment of erectile dysfunction with sildenafil citrate in renal allograft recipients: a randomized, double-blind, placebo-controlled, crossover trial. *American Journal of Kidney Diseases, 48*(1), 128–133.

Soykan, A., Arapasian, B., & Kumbasar, H. (2003). Suicidal behavior, satisfaction with life, and perceived social support in end-stage renal disease. *Transplantation Proceedings, 35,* 1290–1291.

Spiegel, D. M. (2006). Anemia management in chronic kidney disease: what have we learned after 17 years? *Seminars in Dialysis, 19*(4), 269–272.

Stewart, M. (2006). Narrative literature review: sexual dysfunction in the patient on hemodialysis. *Nephrology Nursing, 33,* 631–641.

Sullivan, M. D., & Younger, S. D. (1994), Depression, competence, and the right to refuse lifesaving medical treatment. *American Journal of Psychiatry, 151,* 971–978.

Szeifert, L., Molnar, M. Z., Ambrus, C., et al. (2010). Symptoms of depression in kidney transplant recipients: a cross-sectional study. *American Journal of Kidney Diseases, 55*(1), 132–140.

Tamura, M. K., Wadley, V., Yaffe, K., et al. (2008). Kidney function and cognitive impairment in US adults: the Reasons for Geographic and Racial Differences in Stroke (REGARDS) Study. *American Journal of Kidney Diseases 52*(2), 227–234.

Tanaka, M., Yamazaki, S., Hayashino, Y., et al. (2007). Hypercalcaemia is associated with poor mental health in haemodialysis patients: results from Japan DOPPS. *Nephrology, Dialysis, Transplantation, 22*(6), 1658–1664.

Tappe, K., Turkelson, C., Doggett, D., et al., (2001). Disability under Social Security for patients with ESRD: an evidence-based review. *Disability & Rehabilitation, 23*(5), 177–185.

Turk, S., Karalezil, G., Tonbul, H. Z., et al. (2001). Erectile dysfunction and the effects of sildenafil treatment in patients on haemodialysis and continuous ambulatory peritoneal dialysis. *Nephrology, Dialysis, Transplantation, 16,* 1818–1822.

Turpeinen, M., Koivuviita, N., Tolonen, A., et al. (2007). Effect of renal impairment on the pharmacokinetics of buproprion and its metabolites. *British Journal of Clinical Pharmacology, 64*(2), 165–173.

United States Renal Data System: *USRDS 2009 Annual Data Report: Atlas of End-Stage Renal Disease in the United States.* Bethesda, MD: National Institutes of Health, National Institute of Diabetes and Digestive and Kidney Diseases, 2009.

United States Renal Data System: *USRDS 2010 Annual Data Report: vol. 2. Atlas of end-stage renal disease in the United States.* Bethesda, MD: National Institutes of Health, National Institute of Arthritis and Kidney Diseases, 2010.

Watnick, S. (2009). Quality of life and depression in CKD: improving hope and health. *American Journal of Kidney Diseases, 54,* 399–402.

Weisbord, S. D., & Kimmel, P. L. (2008). Health-related quality of life in the era of erythropoietin. *Hemodialysis International, 12,* 6–15.

Weisbord, S. D., Fried, L. F., Arnold, R. M., et al. (2005). Prevalence, severity, and importance of physical and emotional symptoms in chronic hemodialysis patients. *Journal of the American Society of Nephrology, 16,* 2487–2494.

60.

INFECTIOUS DISEASES

Scott R. Beach

INTRODUCTION

Infectious processes should be considered in the differential diagnosis of any patient presenting with neuropsychiatric symptoms. While many patients with infections will demonstrate additional signs or symptoms (fever, elevated white blood cell [WBC] count, rash, etc.), psychiatric symptoms may be the earliest or most prominent manifestation. As is the case for all psychiatric presentations, workup begins with a good history and physical. Risk factors leading to a potentially impaired immune response (e.g., human immunodeficiency virus [HIV] infection, immunosuppressant medications, substance abuse, extremes of age) should raise suspicion for infection. Behaviors, including hobbies, occupation, and sexual practices, may also influence risk. Geographic factors are of paramount importance, and birthplace, residence, and travel may represent the most essential components of the history in terms of evaluating an individual patient's risk for a particular infectious illness.

The history and physical should guide subsequent testing. Laboratory testing, including blood and urine cultures as well as serological tests for specific entities, may be indicated. Patients with new-onset psychiatric symptoms in the setting of other objective evidence of infection may require a lumbar puncture (LP) in order to analyze cerebrospinal fluid (CSF). Electroencephalogram (EEG) sometimes aids in localizing disease, while imaging of the brain and/or spinal cord may provide additional useful information. In rare cases, a brain biopsy may be indicated, though with advancing diagnostic techniques over the past decade, this is becoming a rarer necessity.

Many infectious processes have the potential to cause neuropsychiatric symptoms by leading to the development of delirium. Among these entities are typhoid fever, bacterial endocarditis, toxic shock syndrome (TSS), bacteremia, and occult infections (urinary tract infections, sinus infections, etc.). Encephalopathy may result from a variety of pathways, including direct invasion of the central nervous system (CNS) by the infectious organism, release of inflammatory cytokines, hypoxia, or edema. Presentations may include changes in mood, cognition, personality, or behavior, as well as psychosis. Like the canary in the mineshaft, the symptoms of delirium may be the first indication that something is amiss.

Other infectious agents may induce specific neuropsychiatric symptoms via direct invasion of the CNS, leading to meningitis, encephalitis, encephalomyelitis, or abscesses, as in Boxes 60.1 and 60.2. Still others, such as pediatric

autoimmune neuropsychiatric disorders associated with streptococcal infections (PANDAS) are thought to lead to CNS dysfunction by precipitating an immune reaction to natural brain proteins. Some entities, such as those in Box 60.3, may exist in a chronic form, sometimes controversial in nature, which may induce neuropsychiatric symptoms. Others, such as those in Box 60.4, are likely to be missed because they are more common in developing countries and more rarely seen by American physicians.

This chapter is organized by organism type, divided into sections on *bacteria, viruses, parasites*, and *fungi*. Entities lacking a well-defined subgroup—*prions* and *algae*—are presented towards the end. The chapter concludes with a discussion of some psychiatric concerns relating to the use of antimicrobial medications.

BACTERIAL INFECTIONS

SYPHILIS

Syphilis is a chronic systemic disease caused by the spirochetal bacterium *Treponema pallidum* and spread through contact with infectious lesions or body fluid, usually through

---

Box 60.1 INFECTIOUS DISEASES ASSOCIATED WITH ENCEPHALITIS

Bacteria:
  Lyme Disease
  Rocky Mountain Spotted Fever
  Typhus Fever
  Tuberculosis
Viral:
  Herpes Simplex Virus
  Arboviruses (West Nile, Eastern Equine, Western Equine, etc.)
  Cytomegalovirus
  Epstein-Barr Virus
  Varicella Zoster Virus
Parasites:
  Chagas' Disease
  Amoebiasis
Fungal:
  Histoplasmosis

---

sexual contact. Transmissibility is highest in the early stages of disease (Hook et al., 1992). As late as a hundred years ago, syphilis was the leading diagnosis in psychiatric inpatients; the incidence began to decline with the advent of penicillin and continued to decline with the institution of public health-control measures, reaching a nadir in 2000. In the past ten years, however, rates have begun to climb again, owing to a variety of factors such as increasingly unsafe sex practices, particularly among men who have sex with men (MSM), in the wake of available antiretroviral therapy for HIV. Furthermore, HIV-positive patients infected with syphilis are more likely to develop neurosyphilis (Chahine et al., 2011). With current trends, psychiatrists are obliged to relearn this disease.

Primary syphilis develops first as a small papule at the site of inoculation, which progresses to an ulcer or chancre. Secondary syphilis occurs four to ten weeks after the appearance of the chancre and can involve multiple organ systems. Onset of secondary syphilis is heralded by a macular rash in 70% of cases. Other symptoms are constitutional and include malaise, fatigue, anorexia, and weight loss. Secondary syphilis resolves without treatment but may recur in the next few years. If untreated, one-third of individuals develop later sequelae. Tertiary syphilis occurs years to decades after primary infection and can assume a benign (gummatous) form or affect the heart or CNS.

T. pallidum invades the CNS early in the disease course, and neurosyphilis can be seen at any of the three stages of illness. Early neurosyphilis, coexisting with primary or secondary syphilis, generally presents as meningitis or, less commonly, as meningovascular disease or stroke (Golden et al., 2003). Overall, rates of early neurosyphilis have increased in the HIV era. Late neurosyphilis, the most common form of tertiary syphilis, is rare but can affect the meninges, spinal cord, or brain parenchyma. The form best known to psychiatrists is general paresis, a rapidly progressing dementia, which may present with a host of psychiatric symptoms, including irritability, personality change, emotional lability, delirium, mania, or psychosis. A recent retrospective review suggests that a positive sucking reflex, Argyll-Robertson pupils that accommodate but do not react to light, and hyperreflexia are the most common signs (Zheng et al., 2011). Imaging commonly shows atrophy of the frontal and temporal lobes. Tabes dorsalis, marked by Argyll-Robertson pupils, sensory ataxia, and bowel and bladder dysfunction resulting from demyelination of the posterior columns and dorsal roots is the second potential form of late neurosyphilis.

Because *T. pallidum* cannot be cultured, diagnosis relies on serological testing. Workup for primary or secondary syphilis without presumed CNS involvement traditionally begins with a non-treponemal test, such as rapid plasma regain (RPR) or venereal disease research laboratory (VDRL), with positive results or high clinical suspicion leading to a treponemal test, such as *T. pallidum* particle agglutination (TPPA) or fluorescent treponemal antibodies (FTA-abs). Non-treponemal serological tests have a sensitivity of about 80% in primary syphilis, 100% in secondary syphilis, and 95% in latent syphilis. Acute false positives occur with non-treponemal tests after some immunizations, during acute infections, and in pregnancy.

Chronic false positives occur in autoimmune diseases (e.g., systemic lupus erythematosus [SLE]), in patients with leprosy, and in the elderly (Relman & Swartz, 1998). A prozone effect can also be seen, in which RPR is falsely negative because very high levels of antibodies interfere with the antigen–antibody interaction needed to visualize a positive reaction, and more commonly occurs in HIV-positive patients. Infection with HIV can cause false-positive or -negative results in non-treponemal tests. Although non-treponemal tests generally become negative after treatment and treponemal tests generally stay positive for life, this is not always the case. For further comparison of treponemal and non-treponemal tests, see Table 60.1.

As a result of these concerns, some have suggested a shift towards the use of treponemal-specific enzyme immunoassays (EIA) and chemiluminescence immunoassays (CIA) for initial screening, followed by a non-treponemal test in the setting of positive results.

The Centers for Disease Control and Prevention (CDC) has offered the following indications for LP in patients with syphilis: neurological or ocular symptoms, late latent syphilis or syphilis of unknown duration in patients with HIV, active tertiary syphilis (e.g., gumma, aortitis, iritis), or treatment failure for non-neurological syphilis. A positive CSF-VDRL establishes the diagnosis of neurosyphilis but has a sensitivity of 30–70% (Larsen et al., 1990). Conversely, a negative CSF-FTA-abs essentially excludes the diagnosis, but a positive result has low specificity.

Diagnosis of neurosyphilis can be difficult, particularly in its late stages. Current recommendations for the workup of neurosyphilis are summarized in Box 60.5 and begin with a serum treponemal test. Treponemal-specific tests should be positive in all patients with neurosyphilis. If positive, CSF-VDRL should be performed. If the CSF-VDRL is positive, diagnosis is established. If the result is negative, but the patient has a mild mononuclear pleocytosis, HIV-negative patients should be presumed to have neurosyphilis. Because HIV can cause a mild mononuclear pleocytosis as well, diagnosis in this population in the setting of a negative CSF-VDRL is further clarified via a CSF-FTA-abs. Some authors have recommended that asymptomatic patients without HIV be treated for neurosyphilis if they have a positive CSF-FTA-abs and either CSF pleocytosis or elevated CSF protein, while asymptomatic patients with HIV are treated on the basis of a positive CSF-FTA-abs and CSF pleocytosis.

Guidelines for treatment recommend a single dose of penicillin G for primary, secondary, or early latent syphilis. Late latent syphilis should be treated with a three-week course of penicillin G. Treatment for neurosyphilis involves a 10- to 14-day course of intravenous aqueous penicillin G. Within the first 24 hours of any treatment, an acute febrile illness associated with headache and myalgias, the Jarisch-Herxheimer reaction, may occur. All treated patients should have clinical and serological follow-up at 6 and 12 months, and HIV-positive patients should be followed for two years after treatment. All patients with neurosyphilis should have a repeat LP at three to six months, and then again every six months until the result is normal (Golden, 2003).

In late neurosyphilis, psychiatric symptoms frequently do not remit with antibiotic treatment. There have been case reports suggesting efficacy for most atypical antipsychotics in treating particular manifestations of neurosyphilis, especially in general paresis, though no controlled studies exist. Valproate has also been suggested to have some utility in terms of mood stabilization and controlling agitation in this population.

LYME DISEASE

Lyme disease (LD), caused by the spirochete *Borrellia burgdorferi* and transmitted by deer ticks, is a multisystem illness that can cause a variety of neuropsychiatric symptoms. LD is the most common tick-borne infection in the United States and is increasing in incidence and geographical spread, though risk remains highest in the Northeast. Erythema migrans, a large rash with central clearing, heralds the onset of the disease in over 90% of patients, though the rash may have an atypical appearance in more than half of those cases and may go unnoticed by the patient at the time (Schneider, Robinson & Levenson, 2002). Up to one-fifth of infected individuals have no further symptoms beyond the rash.

Three separate phases of disease progression have been described (acute, subacute, and chronic), and CNS involvement (Lyme neuroborreliosis) can occur in all of them. *B. burgdorferi* is rapidly disseminated in the body over the first month of illness and is known to invade the CNS

Table 60.1 TESTS FOR SYPHILIS

TYPE OF TEST	EXAMPLES	STATES CAUSING FALSE POSITIVE	STATES CAUSING FALSE NEGATIVE	EVOLUTION OF TEST RESULTS
Non-treponemal	RPR, VDRL	*Acute*: Immunizations, acute infections, pregnancy, HIV	Prozone effect (more common in patients with HIV)	Generally become negative after treatment
		Chronic: Autoimmune diseases, leprosy, elderly patients		
Treponemal	TPPA, FTA-abs	Autoimmune diseases	Unknown	Tend to stay positive for life

within the first few weeks after initial infection (Fallon et al., 2010). Common symptoms in the acute phase include fatigue, myalgias or arthralgias, headache, fever, and neck stiffness. Untreated LD may progress to subacute disease and affect other organ systems. Neurological symptoms during the subacute phase include Bell's palsy, radiculopathy, and meningitis. This is also the phase during which patients experience arthritis in a limited number of joints, usually including the knee. If patients remain untreated, chronic LD may develop, with further neuropsychiatric symptoms (chronic neuroborreliosis) that include cognitive dysfunction, fatigue, irritability, and depression. Lyme encephalopathy may include impairments in short-term memory, word-finding

difficulties, decreased processing speed, fatigue, and depressed mood. Lyme encephalomyelitis and cerebellitis have also been described. Stroke and hemorrhages are rare complications. Although the neuropsychiatric symptoms of chronic LD are relatively nonspecific, they are almost always preceded by classic early symptoms.

A variety of psychiatric symptoms, including mania, psychosis, catatonia, panic attacks, and personality change, have been described in the setting of LD, though causality has not been established. At least one study suggested no difference in neuropsychological testing between patients with LD at 10- to 20-year follow-up and normal controls, though it was noted that patients who had demonstrated Bell's palsy early in the course and had not received antibiotics were more likely to report sleep disturbances (Kalish et al., 2001). Nonetheless, neuropsychological testing is recommended for patients with chronic neuroborreliosis as a means of evaluating the presence and extent of cognitive dysfunction.

Diagnosis of LD should be made largely on clinical evaluation. If a patient has known exposure to an endemic area, history of a tick bite, history of rash, or symptoms in another involved system, in addition to new-onset or exacerbation of psychiatric symptoms, serological testing should be considered (Tugwell et al., 1997). Serological testing remains unreliable in many cases, with false positives occurring in the setting of other infections and true-positive tests only indicating a history of LD at some time in the past. If pursued, serological testing should involve an initial enzyme-linked immunoassay (ELISA) test, with positive results confirmed by a Western blot. Caveats include the fact that both tests may be negative within the first two to three weeks of infection, and early antibiotic treatment may lead to persistent false negatives (Bunikis & Barbour, 2002). Magnetic resonance imaging (MRI) may demonstrate white matter lesions in up to 25% of patients with chronic neuroborreliosis and may resemble a demyelinating process.

Treatment of LD is accomplished via a two- to four-week course of doxycycline or amoxicillin. Patients' symptoms sometimes worsen during the first few weeks in a phenomenon similar to the Jarisch-Herxheimer reaction seen in syphilis (Fallon et al., 1992). A two- to four-week course of intravenous (IV) ceftriaxone is recommended for neuroborreliosis. Antibiotic prophylaxis is not recommended after a tick bite because of the low risk of contracting LD. A vaccine for LD has been developed and has shown up to 90% protection after the first year (Sigal et al., 1998).

Recent years have seen a drastic increase in cases of post-treatment LD syndrome (PTLDS), colloquially labeled with the misnomer "chronic LD," with patients attributing a myriad of symptoms to LD and some physicians recommending indefinite courses of antibiotics for supposedly ongoing infection. Symptoms such as fatigue, sadness, and chronic nonspecific pain are common in such patients, and the spectrum of complaints overlaps significantly with those seen in chronic fatigue syndrome (CFS) and fibromyalgia. Clinical depression and somatization behavior are also common in this population. Most concerning is that some physicians, often labeling themselves as "Lyme experts," diagnose "chronic LD" without any objective evidence or through unvalidated tests such as Lyme urine antigen, and recommend unnecessary courses of antibiotics, which in some cases lead to "Lyme colitis."

Despite the controversy, the CDC has recognized PTLDS as an entity, though no treatment is recommended. A proposed definition includes established LD diagnosis, conclusion of an appropriate course of antibiotics with resolution or stabilization of objective manifestations of LD, and the presence of symptoms (fatigue, widespread pain, cognitive problems) more than six months after LD diagnosis. Exclusionary criteria include documented co-infection (*Babesia, Ehrlichia*), objective evidence of active LD, and preexisting conditions including CFS and fibromyalgia, thyroid disease, and psychiatric conditions (Wormser et al., 2006). It is estimated that up to 10% of patients with erythema migrans will have persistent or intermittent subjective symptoms 12 months after completion of appropriate therapy (Marques, 2008). Some have suggested that ongoing cytokine activation, including elevated interleukin-6 (IL-6), may contribute to persistent symptoms of pain, fatigue, and cognitive dysfunction in patients with prior LD (Fallon, 2010). It is further noted that patients with previously treated well-documented LD have a four-fold greater rate of concurrent depression than patients with medically unexplained symptoms who do not have a clear history for LD (Hassett et al., 2008).

The vast majority of patients who present with a diagnosis of "chronic LD" will have either symptoms of an unknown cause with no evidence of *Borrelia* infection or with a well-defined illness unrelated to *Borrelia* infection. In one study of patients presenting to a tertiary care center with a chief complaint of LD, 57% were found to not have LD and to have symptoms better explained by fibromyalgia and CFS. An additional 20% had evidence of prior LD without the need for further antibiotics (Steere et al., 1993). For psychiatrists who find themselves working with patients claiming to suffer from "chronic LD," evaluation for other underlying psychiatric and medical conditions is of paramount importance. It is also vital to educate patients that, although some physicians advocate long-term antibiotic treatment, all four randomized controlled trials of prolonged antimicrobial treatment have failed to demonstrate any lasting improvement, and many other open-label trials have failed to separate cases of well-documented LD from those without objective evidence (Halperin, 2008). Furthermore, such treatment carries significant risk in the form of complications related to catheters, biliary disease, *Clostridium difficile* infection, and promotion of antibiotic resistance. In the case of treatment with ceftriaxone, it is hypothesized that transient cognitive improvement seen in some subjects may be the result not of antimicrobial action but of neuroprotective effects involving the reduction of extracellular glutamate (Fallon et al., 2008). Patients may be encouraged by the fact that one-third of patients suffering from symptoms consistent with PTLDS improve regardless of treatment (Auwaerter, 2007).

ROCKY MOUNTAIN SPOTTED FEVER (RMSF)

Rocky Mountain spotted fever (RMSF), caused by *Rickettsia rickettsii*, is a tick-borne disease with a seasonal distribution paralleling human contact with ticks, peaking from May through September. Despite its name, RMSF is seen throughout the United States, with South Atlantic and Central states reporting the highest incidence between 2000 and 2007 (Openshaw et al., 2010). *R. rickettsii* enters the vascular endothelial cells, proliferates and disseminates, causing a diffuse vasculitis in many organ systems, including the CNS, skin, heart, and liver. Incubation period is typically seven days. As the name suggests, RMSF generally presents with fever and a rash characterized by erythematous macules that later progress to maculopapular lesions with central petechiae. The rash is notable in being one of the few diffuse rashes to involve the palms and soles (another being the rash of secondary syphilis). CNS involvement in the form of encephalitis occurs in 25% of all cases, and presents with lethargy, confusion, and occasionally seizures. Subtle changes such as irritability, personality changes, or apathy may occur before the rash, particularly in children.

While *R. rickettsii* may be demonstrated by direct immunofluorescence of skin biopsies, serology is the usual diagnostic method, though confirmation requires convalescent titers. The traditional Weil-Felix agglutination test lacks specificity and sensitivity, and indirect immunofluorescence (IFA), ELISA, or polymerase chain reaction (PCR) are preferred (Gunther & Haglund, 2005). Since mortality is high in untreated patients, a provisional clinical diagnosis (e.g., fever, rash, appropriate season and geographic setting) is sufficient to initiate definitive antimicrobial therapy. Only half of patients remember exposure to ticks. Doxycycline or chloramphenicol are the drugs of choice and are typically administered for two weeks.

OTHER TICK-BORNE ILLNESSES

Other tick-borne illnesses that may mimic LD in early stages include babesiosis and human granulocytic anaplasmosis (HGA), formerly known as *erlichiosis*. Both are transmitted by the same deer tick that transmits LD, and co-infection is possible. The number of reported cases of these illnesses is less than that of LD, though the geographic distribution is similar, with New England being the highest-incident area. Early symptoms of both illnesses may mimic those of LD, though neuropsychiatric symptoms are less common. Chronic babesiosis is not well described, and chronic HGA infection is said to not exist (Wormser, 2006). Diagnosis of babesiosis is based on epidemiological, clinical, and laboratory findings, the latter of which includes microscopic identification of organisms on Giemsa stains of thin blood smears or PCR detection. Diagnosis of HGA is made via identification of characteristic intragranulocytic inclusions on blood smear or by detection of antibodies to the infectious agent. A ten-day course of doxycycline is the recommended treatment for HGA and should treat coexistent LD as well. Treatment for babesiosis, on the other hand, most commonly involves a combination of atovaquone and azithromycin. Co-infection with LD should be considered in cases of treatment-resistant babesiosis.

PEDIATRIC AUTOIMMUNE NEUROPSYCHIATRIC DISORDERS ASSOCIATED WITH STREPTOCOCCAL INFECTIONS

PANDAS affect a subgroup of patients with obsessive-compulsive disorder (OCD) and tic disorders, including Tourette's disorder. The syndrome is defined by the presence of OCD and/or tic disorder according to DSM-IV (*Diagnostic & Statistical Manual of Mental Disorders–IV*) criteria; onset of symptoms between three years and onset of puberty; an episodic course characterized by abrupt onset of symptoms or by dramatic exacerbations; association with neurological abnormalities (especially tics); and temporal association with group A *b*-hemolytic streptococcal (GABHS) infections (most commonly pharyngitis), with at least two exacerbations occurring shortly after infection (Swedo et al., 1997). Classified in 1998, invocation of the diagnosis has risen dramatically in the past ten years, leading many to conclude that the phenomenon is over-diagnosed, while others question its existence altogether. It is suggested that the syndrome is often misdiagnosed in the community, and unrelated symptoms are inappropriately treated with antibiotics. Psychiatrists should be aware of the controversy and utilize a strict interpretation of criteria for diagnosis.

The age of onset for PANDAS is said to be younger by about three years than that for typical childhood-onset OCD and tic disorders. Including all children, boys outnumber girls by a ratio of 2.6:1; below the age of eight years, the ratio is 4.7:1. Preexisting psychiatric comorbidity is reportedly common (32–42%). Symptom exacerbations are thought to be sudden and dramatic, as distinct from the more gradual waxing and waning pattern of childhood-onset OCD. In addition to OCD symptoms and tics, other described symptoms include separation anxiety, personality changes, rage episodes, oppositional behaviors, cognitive dysfunction, and anorexia. Recently, particular attention has been paid to the presence of motoric hyperactivity, and some have argued that ADHD-like symptoms may be a very common manifestation of the disorder. Typical episodes are generally associated with an increase in anti-streptococcal antibody titers (Swedo et al., 1998). It has become clear recently that not all exacerbations are necessarily associated with GABHS infection, however, and other infectious agents are now being invoked as potential triggers. In cases that do demonstrate elevated titers, diagnosis is further supported by evidence of a decrease in titers with symptom remission.

Studies have suggested enlarged basal ganglia in patients with PANDAS, though neuroimaging is not currently part of the standard diagnostic workup. Pathogenesis has been thought to involve both genetic and environmental factors, with a possible aberrant immune response leading to antibodies against GABHS cross-reacting with basal ganglia neurons. This hypothesis has been challenged recently, however, by studies that have failed to demonstrate any correlation between clinical exacerbations and autoimmune markers (Singer et al., 2008). Treatment recommendations are not currently specific for this syndrome. Trials involving antibiotics as well as immunomodulatory treatments such as plasmapheresis and intravenous immunoglobulin (IVIG) are continuing, though with inconclusive results at this time. There is very little evidence from controlled trials to support the efficacy of standard psychopharmacological treatment for OCD or tic disorders (e.g., selective serotonin reuptake inhibitors [SSRIs], alpha-2 agonists) in PANDAS, but they are widely used, generally well tolerated, and most experts think they work (Martino et al., 2009).

TUBERCULOSIS

Tuberculosis (TB) remains a major world health problem and is endemic in many developing countries. Groups at high risk for TB include immunosuppressed patients, prisoners, institutionalized patients, immigrants, and the homeless. TB now represents the most common serious HIV-related complication worldwide. CNS TB accounts for 1% of all TB cases and disproportionately affects children and HIV-positive individuals, though alcoholism and immunocompromised states are also risk factors. In some cases, neuropsychiatric manifestations of TB may precede peripheral signs or symptoms. Tuberculous meningitis (TBM) is the most common form of CNS TB. The clinical presentation begins with low-grade fever, generalized malaise, and mild headache. Over the course of a week, symptoms progress to high-grade fever and severe nuchal rigidity. Fatigue, personality changes, and delirium are the most common early psychiatric symptoms. Later findings include vasculitis and cranial nerve involvement. A history of TB is elicited in only 10% of patients with TBM at the time of presentation, and tuberculin skin test may be positive in fewer than 50% of patients (Rock, 2008). CSF classically demonstrates low glucose and markedly elevated protein, with a moderate lymphocytic pleocytosis. Identification of acid-fast bacillus (AFB) in the CSF remains the most important diagnostic test. The presence of active pulmonary tuberculosis in patients with tuberculous meningitis ranges from 30–50%. Diffuse meningeal involvement by TB may be demonstrated on MRI (Gray, 1997). Other forms of CNS TB include tubercular encephalitis, intracranial tuberculoma, and tuberculous brain abscess.

Early treatment of CNS TB is essential, because delayed treatment is associated with higher morbidity and death. Current recommendations involve a two-month induction with isoniazid, rifampin, pyrazinamide, and ethambutol, followed by seven to ten additional months of isoniazid and rifampin (Rock et al., 2008). In many parts of the world, multi-resistant TB is rapidly emerging, requiring development and testing of novel drug combinations.

BACTERIAL CEREBRAL ABSCESS

Although rare in the United States, cerebral abscesses are serious and potentially life-threatening infections. Immunocompromised patients and those with uncontrolled diabetes are at highest risk for death or permanent neurological deficits, while delay in hospitalization and focal deficits on admission are also indicators of a poor prognosis. The pathogenesis of infection for brain abscesses includes hematogenous spread from a remote source, trauma (including neurosurgery), and most commonly, direct extension from another infected site. Non-pneumococcal streptococci account for the majority of cases, while *S. aureus* and anaerobes comprise most of the remaining cases. Other opportunistic pathogens, including *Nocardia*, TB (discussed above), and *Listeria* may affect immunocompromised patients.

The classic triad of headache, fever, and focal neurological deficits occurs in less than half of patients with this condition. Psychiatric symptoms, including personality change and encephalopathy, may be part of the initial presentation, and seizures are also common. Brain abscesses frequently mimic CNS tumors and other space-occupying lesions. Computed tomography scan (CT scan) with contrast is likely to reveal ring-enhancing lesions, though MRI remains the preferred imaging test. Prompt treatment includes empiric antibiotics, though attempts should be made to identify a pathogen prior to initiation (Honda & Warren, 2009). As abscesses are frequently polymicrobial, therapy should cover a range of organisms and is typically continued for six to eight weeks, though with individual variations. Most experts feel that abscesses greater than 2.5 cm in diameter should be surgically treated. Steroids and anticonvulsants are often used as adjuvant treatments.

Following successful treatment, a broad spectrum of psychiatric symptoms may persist, depending on the size and location of the abscess. Affective illness, cognitive dysfunction, psychosis, and aggression are the most common psychiatric complications.

BACTERIAL MENINGITIS

Bacterial meningitis is an acute, serious illness associated with significant morbidity and mortality. Annual incidence in the United States has not changed over the past decade, and *S. pneumoniae, N. meningitides,* and *L. monocytogenes* remain the most common pathogens. The *Haemophilus influenzae* type B vaccine has greatly reduced cases of meningitis caused by this agent (Schuchat et al., 1997). Nuchal rigidity, headache, nausea, vomiting, confusion, lethargy, and apathy may occur. Delirium is the most common psychiatric symptom. Symptom severity generally correlates with the magnitude of the host's immune response, and in elderly or immunocompromised patients the only clinical signs may be irritability or minor changes in mentation or personality (Weinstein, 1985; Segreti & Harris, 1996).

Once clinically suspected, the diagnosis is usually confirmed by examination of the CSF, typically revealing pleocytosis, low glucose, high protein, and evidence of the offending organism on appropriate staining. Neuroimaging rarely makes the diagnosis of bacterial meningitis. The morbidity and mortality of bacterial meningitis are associated with the time to treatment (Gray, 1997). Initially, antibiotics are chosen to cover a broad range of organisms common to the population in which the patient falls (e.g., age and immune status). Once a pathogen is identified, therapy can be modified. Physicians should be aware of the increasing resistance of *S. pneumoniae* to penicillins and cephalosporins.

VIRAL INFECTIONS

HERPES SIMPLEX VIRUS

Herpes encephalitis is caused by herpes simplex type 1 virus in 90% of cases. A bimodal distribution is seen with one-third of cases between ages 6 months to 20 years, and one-half of cases occurring in patients over 50 years old (Whitley, 2006). Herpes simplex virus (HSV) encephalitis differs from other types of viral meningoencephalitis in its greater likelihood to cause unilateral and focal findings and its predilection for temporoparietal involvement. Fever, headache, confusion, and seizures typically develop rapidly, over a matter of hours to days. Occasionally, onset may be heralded by the presence of olfactory or gustatory hallucinations. Other symptoms may include personality change, dysphasia, autonomic dysfunction, ataxia, and psychosis. Progressive obtundation and focal disturbances develop subsequently, and mortality approaches 70% if untreated. Lower initial level of consciousness and age over 30 are indicators of a poor prognosis. An additional possible, though rare, sequela of HSV encephalitis is Klüver-Bucy syndrome, which includes oral touching compulsions, hypersexuality, amnesia, placidity, agnosia, and bulimia (Thirunavukarasu, 2011).

MRI scans show abnormal signal in the medial temporal lobes and insula earliest on fluid-attenuated inversion recovery (FLAIR) sequences, diffusion-weighted imaging (DWI), and contrast-enhanced imaging, though most MRI scans are abnormal even without contrast or special sequencing once symptoms are apparent (Baringer, 2008). Early HSV encephalitis can be missed on CT scans. CSF typically shows pleocytosis, elevated protein, and normal glucose. PCR detection of HSV deoxyribonucleic acid (DNA) in the CSF has become the diagnostic method of choice, though it may be negative rarely in very early cases. It is widely available, and the time from LP to results is generally 24–72 hours. EEG may demonstrate slowing in frontal and temporal regions, but lacks the specificity of other tests. Brain biopsy is reserved for cases in which diagnostic confusion remains after other workup has been exhausted. Therapeutic decisions must be made within a matter of hours, because only early treatment improves outcome. The current recommendation is to initiate treatment with acyclovir while awaiting laboratory results, given the relatively low risk of the medication. If the PCR result returns negative, a decision regarding discontinuing therapy should be based on the clinical presentation and other diagnostic tests, with consideration given to repeating the CSF PCR study.

Following recovery from herpes encephalitis, psychiatric sequelae (especially mood disorders) are common and constitute a major cause of disability. Depression, hypomania, irritability, and psychosis have been noted months after recovery (Caparros-Lefebre et al., 1996). Neuropsychological testing is helpful in fully delineating the extent of cognitive damage. Depressive symptoms often respond to treatment with antidepressants or stimulants, but there are no controlled studies of their efficacy. Hypomania, irritability, and disinhibition have responded to mood stabilizers, and behavior modification may be helpful for aggressive and sexual behaviors (Vallini & Burns, 1987; Boulais et al., 1976).

VIRAL ENCEPHALITIS

Arboviruses are the most common cause of viral encephalitis worldwide, with Japanese encephalitis accounting for the most cases. In the United States, there are five common types: West Nile virus (WNV), St. Louis encephalitis, Eastern equine encephalitis (EEE), Western equine encephalitis, and California encephalitis. All are mosquito-borne, causing illness typically in the summer or fall. Of these, EEE causes the severest illness and has the highest fatality rate (Romero & Newland, 2003). Many survivors of neuroinvasive arboviruses have permanent sequelae.

WNV has been the most common cause of viral encephalitis in the United States over the past decade. Although identified in Uganda in 1937, WNV did not reach the United States until 1999, and between 2002 and 2003, 3,000 confirmed cases of neuroinvasive disease occurred. Despite this figure, neuroinvasive disease is thought to occur in only 1 in 150 individuals, and most cases of WNV are asymptomatic. Patients developing encephalitis are usually older and are often immunosuppressed or suffering from other medical illnesses such as diabetes. One study found a history of hypertension or cardiovascular disease to be associated with development of encephalitis, and the authors speculated that this might be due to increased penetrability of the blood–brain barrier in such states (Murray et al., 2006). The clinical presentation of WNV, like other arboviruses, involves an abrupt onset of fever, headache, nausea, photophobia, and vomiting. Psychiatric symptoms include confusion, cognitive changes, and psychosis. MRI will demonstrate areas of increased signal in the thalamus, basal ganglia, and upper brainstem in up to 75% of patients (Tyler, 2009). Diagnosis is typically based on serology with detection of WNV IgM antibodies in the CSF being diagnostic. Although there is no specific treatment available for viral encephalitis caused by arboviruses, rapid diagnosis is important for the institution of public health measures.

ACUTE DISSEMINATED ENCEPHALOMYELITIS

Acute disseminated encephalomyelitis (ADEM) has been described as occurring in the wake of a number of viral infections, including measles, mumps, rubella, varicella zoster (VZV),

Epstein-Barr virus (EBV), CMV, HSV, hepatitis A or B, Coxsackie virus, and influenza A or B (Huynh et al., 2008). Bacterial agents such as *Mycoplasma pneumoniae* and *Borrelia* have also been implicated. ADEM has additionally been described in the setting of immunization. The presumed mechanism is cell-mediated immunity to myelin basic protein, and clinical symptoms commonly include encephalopathy, fever, seizures, and meningismus. Changes in mood, as well as psychotic symptoms such as delusions and hallucinations, have also been reported in the absence of obviously altered sensorium (Krishnakumar, 2008). MRI is useful in diagnosis, revealing multifocal white matter and deep gray matter lesions, with lesion load typically greater than 50% of the total white matter volume (Menge et al., 2007). Options for treatment include corticosteroids, plasma exchange, and intravenous immunoglobulin.

HEPATITIS

Viruses including hepatitis A, B, C, D, or E; EBV; and CMV all cause hepatitis, an inflammation of the liver (see Chapter X). Hepatitis commonly presents with fatigue, malaise, and anorexia. Chronic forms of hepatitis-B and -C can lead to a secondary depression (Levenson & Fallon, 1993; Sharara, Hunt, & Hamilton, 1996). Treatment of viral hepatitis with interferon may cause a syndrome involving fatigue, apathy, and depressed mood, as well (see GI Chapter). Depression associated with interferon treatment is sometimes responsive to antidepressant therapy, though prophylaxis with antidepressants is not currently recommended.

EPSTEIN-BARR VIRUS

EBV, one of the herpes viruses, causes an acute lymphoproliferative disease called *infectious mononucleosis*, common in adolescents and young adults. The prodromal stage of infectious mononucleosis is characterized by headache, fatigue, and malaise, with progression to fever, sore throat, and lymphadenopathy. Diagnosis may be established on the basis of clinical presentation, the presence of atypical lymphocytes on peripheral blood smear, and a positive heterophile antibody (IgM) test, though the latter remains negative in 25% of patients during the first week of infection and in 5–10% during or after the second week (Luzuriaga & Sullivan, 2010). Definitive diagnosis requires testing for immunoglobulin-M (IgM) and IgG antibodies to viral capsid antigens, early antigens, and EBV nuclear antigen proteins. IgG antibodies to viral capsid antigens persist for life, while IgM antibodies typically disappear or decline significantly within four to eight weeks and are therefore diagnostic of primary EBV infection. Treatment is largely supportive.

Most cases of EBV completely resolve within one month, though the infection can recur in immunocompromised hosts. An entity known as *chronic active EBV* (CAEBV), involving recurrent symptoms of fever, hepatosplenomegaly, and lymphadenopathy, has also been defined in patients without apparent immunodeficiency and is diagnosed on the basis of extremely high titers of IgG antibody to viral capsid antigen and early antigen. Many patients who do not meet criteria for CAEBV, but who have experienced acute EBV infection, report ongoing symptoms of malaise and fatigue. A prospective study suggested that 9% of patients develop a syndrome of chronic fatigue up to six months after illness onset (White, 1998). A cohort study, however, concluded that, although many patients reported transient distress during acute infection, few subjects met criteria for a psychiatric disorder, and the vast majority demonstrated decreased impairment and distress at two- and six-month follow-ups (Katon et al., 1999).

The role of the psychiatrist in treating patients reporting chronic EBV symptoms is to aid in identifying those with an underlying psychiatric diagnosis, including a mood, anxiety, or somatoform disorder. The absence of any objective physical findings (e.g., significant lymphadenopathy, atypical lymphocytes, lymphocytosis, elevated erythrocyte sedimentation rate [ESR], fever, hepatosplenomegaly) raises suspicion for a primary psychiatric diagnosis but does not exclude the possibility of symptoms' being caused by EBV. Workup for CAEBV is appropriate, with patients failing to meet criteria considered to have CFS, an entity now thought to be unrelated to EBV.

EBV has been rarely associated with encephalitis and meningitis, with the findings indistinguishable from other viral causes. Laboratory diagnosis is enhanced by concomitant use of EBV-specific serology and PCR (Doja et al., 2012), though the pathogenesis may be either immune or viral; antiviral therapy has not shown clinical efficacy; and appropriate preferred diagnostic techniques are unclear, as EBV DNA is often detected in patients without neurological symptoms (Volpi, 2004).

CYTOMEGALOVIRUS

Like EBV, cytomegalovirus (CMV) is a common herpes virus, with infection rates ranging from 40–100% of the population, depending on geographic location. CMV infection occurs in a broad demographic age group. In addition to producing a syndrome similar to EBV mononucleosis, CMV may also cause hepatitis, retinitis, colitis, and pneumonitis. CNS involvement occurs most commonly in the immunocompromised host, particularly in HIV patients and solid-organ transplant recipients. Late-onset disease has also been described following allogenic stem-cell transplant (Reddy et al., 2010). CMV can cause encephalitis and has been implicated as a cause of depression and dementia in these populations. Diagnosis is most accurately made by PCR testing for viral DNA in the CSF. Treatment with ganciclovir or valganciclovir is preferred, with foscarnet reserved for resistant cases due to its toxicity (Griffiths, 2004). Antidepressant therapy may be needed if the patient develops a post-viral mood disorder.

VARICELLA ZOSTER VIRUS

Varicella zoster virus is the infectious agent that causes chickenpox (primary infection) and herpes zoster (HZ; reactivated virus). Prior to vaccine introduction in 1995, VZV was the most common etiological agent associated with meningitis, encephalitis, and myelitis. VZV continues to be associated with CNS disease despite an overall decrease in incidence. Manifestations in the post-vaccination era include encephalitis, meningitis, and ADEM. Meningitis is now the most common presentation in younger immunocompetent patients, in contrast to pre-vaccination observations that encephalitis was the typical manifestation in children. Encephalitis is now most common in immunocompromised patients or those over age 60, but it can also occur in younger immunocompetent patients (Pahud et al., 2011). Psychiatric symptoms may include depression, anxiety, or personality changes. CSF most commonly shows a lymphocytic predominance. Imaging is normal in 80% of patients, though some demonstrate diffuse meningeal enhancement. Occasionally, VZV may mimic HSV on imaging, showing abnormal enhancement in the temporal lobes. Classic HZ rash appears to be less commonly seen in recent cases. Six cases of vaccine-associated VZV CNS disease have also been reported in the literature.

Post-herpetic neuralgia, a chronic neuropathic pain that can develop following HZ, can substantially impact sleep and mood. First-line treatments include antidepressant medications such as selective norepinephrine reuptake inhibitors (SNRIs) or tricyclic antidepressants (TCAs), calcium channel α2-δ ligands like pregabalin or gabapentin, and topical lidocaine (Dworkin et al., 2012).

PROGRESSIVE MULTIFOCAL LEUKOENCEPHALOPATHY

Progressive multifocal leukoencephalopathy (PML) is an often-fatal demyelinating disease of the CNS usually affecting immunosuppressed patients and caused by the John Cunningham (JC) polyomavirus. It is seen in patients with HIV infection or lymphoid malignancies, transplant recipients, and in the context of treatment with monoclonal antibodies. Occasional cases have been reported in patients without overt immunosuppressive risk factors. Classically, clinical presentation varies with disease location and may include muscle weakness, sensory deficit, cognitive dysfunction, aphasia, and occasionally seizures. Multiple lesions are typically detected in the subcortical white matter or cerebral peduncles on CT scan or MRI, and are usually without evidence of edema or mass effect. Lesions may also be seen in the basal ganglia or thalami. Diagnosis is established by detection of JC virus DNA in CSF via PCR or detection of viral DNA or proteins on brain biopsy sample via *in situ* hybridization or immunohistochemistry. There is currently no specific antiviral medication for PML, and treatment is typically aimed at restoration of host immune defense. Interestingly, mirtazepine is being studied as a possible treatment because the JC virus has been found to enter cultured cells via the 5HT-2a receptor (Tan & Koralnik, 2010). Though still considered a life-threatening disease, positive prognostic factors in PML include a higher CD4+ T-cell count, and contrast enhancement on imaging have been associated with longer-term survival.

PML has also been described in the setting of immune reconstitution inflammatory syndrome (IRIS) following the initiation of therapy for HIV, and this may account for up to one-fourth of PML cases in HIV patients. In addition to PML, JC virus may also cause meningitis or encephalopathy.

RABIES

Rabies is a viral infection of mammals (rarely) transmitted to humans by bite. Bat-variant rabies strains have replaced carnivore-associated strains as the predominant cause of human rabies in the United States (Romero & Newland, 2003). Initial symptoms are nonspecific and include generalized anxiety, fever, melancholia, hyperesthesia, and abnormal sensations at the site of inoculation (e.g., pain, burning, cold, and pruritis). The neurological phase may present as an episodic encephalopathic form (furious rabies), involving agitation, hallucinations, and hydrophobia (an aversion to swallowing liquids secondary to the spasmodic contractions of the muscles of swallowing and respiration, resulting in pain and aspiration). Alternatively, patients may experience a paralytic (dumb rabies) phase, marked by ascending paralysis. The final phase in either case involves coma, usually two weeks after the onset of neurological symptoms, progressing to cardiorespiratory failure and death. Diagnosis is most reliable via either PCR detection from saliva or brain biopsy. However, if a potentially infected animal bites a person, the rabies vaccine should be given as soon as possible, as outcome is correlated with length of time to inoculation (Centers for Disease Control and Prevention, 1998). To date, there have been three reported cases of individuals' surviving symptomatic rabies without receiving the vaccine, though all suffered severe neurological injury. All survivors were treated with the Milwaukee Protocol, which involves placing patients in a medically induced coma and treating with ribavirin and amantadine (Hunter et al., 2010).

VIRAL MENINGITIS

Enteroviruses, mumps, and lymphocytic choriomeningitis primarily affect the meninges. Eighty percent of identifiable viral meningitis is caused by the enteroviruses. The clinical syndrome of viral, or aseptic meningitis includes headache, fever, nuchal rigidity, malaise, drowsiness, nausea, and photophobia. Typically, the CSF shows pleocytosis, elevated protein, and no evidence of an organism. PCR has become the gold standard for diagnosing viral meningitis. Treatment is generally supportive, though antiviral agents are paramount in the treatment of herpes meningitis. Correct early diagnosis is critical to a successful outcome (Deresiewicz et al., 1997).

PARASITIC INFECTIONS

NEUROCYSTICERCOSIS

The larvae (cysticerci) of the tapeworm *Taenia solium* cause an infection known as *cysticercosis*, which may progress to *neurocysticercosis* (NCC). NCC is the most frequent and widely disseminated human neuroparasitosis. It is particularly common in Latin America, Africa, and Asia, but endemic areas exist throughout the world. In the United States, NCC is reported in immigrants from and travelers to endemic areas. The American Southwest has seen a dramatic increase in reported cases since the mid-1970s. Humans acquire intestinal taeniasis (the tapeworm) by eating uncooked or undercooked pork infected with cysticerci, but only acquire cysticercosis by ingesting the eggs of *T. solium*. Contamination of food with the eggs of *T. solium* may occur indirectly via handling of the food by an infected person (Schneider et al., 2002). Hatched embryos penetrate the intestinal mucosa and enter the circulatory system where they are distributed to extra-enteric sites as cysticerci. In humans, the cysticerci locate primarily in skeletal muscles, but the recognition of disease usually occurs after CNS involvement.

The variable, nonspecific clinical spectrum is determined in part by the number of cysticerci, the location in the CNS (parenchymal, ventricular, subarachnoid, spinal), and the intensity of the host inflammatory response. The initial immune response to the cysticerci is minimal, which explains the potentially long asymptomatic latency period after infection. The inflammatory response is intensified when the cysticercus dies and releases a large number of antigens. The most frequent manifestation of NCC is seizures, commonly of the partial-complex variety, reported as the initial symptom in 66% of patients. Encephalitis, meningitis, and altered mental status are also commonly seen at presentation (Wallin et al., 2004). Dementia, other cognitive dysfunction, and a broad spectrum of other psychiatric manifestations, including depression and psychosis, have also been reported, but the literature consists of largely retrospective reports by non-psychiatric physicians. One study suggested that patients admitted to a chronic inpatient psychiatry unit in Venezuela, particularly those with mental retardation, were more likely to have a positive serology for *T. solium* than were healthy controls in the community (Meza et al., 2005).

Diagnosis is difficult because of the varied and nonspecific clinical presentation, and the only definitive method is biopsy. The diagnosis is often only considered after failed treatment. Diagnosis hinges on a high index of suspicion in a patient with new psychopathology and a history of exposure from an endemic area. MRI is superior to CT in demonstrating some cysticerci, small calcifications, and the inflammatory response. The cysticerci have a characteristic appearance of multiple cystic lesions with a denser central spot containing the scolex, though involvement of the subarachnoid or ventricular spaces may reveal only inflammation or calcification. The preferred test to detect antibodies is the enzyme-linked immunoelectrotransfer blot (EITB), which is more sensitive and specific than ELISA.

Treatment depends on symptoms, location of the cysticerci, stage of development, involution of the cysticerci, and inflammatory response. Surgery, antiepileptic drugs, glucocorticosteroids, and antihelmintic therapy are used with varying degrees of overlap. Although antihelmintics were once considered a key component of treatment, some have questioned their efficacy and potential propensity for side effects like edema and intracranial hypertension. Nonetheless, many experts continue to recommend their use in specific situations (Abba et al., 2010).

MALARIA

Malaria is the leading cause of morbidity in young children and pregnant women worldwide, and the incidence is increasing due to social and environmental changes as well as drug resistance. Co-infection with HIV is a risk factor for developing severe or complicated malaria. In the United States, cases occur in immigrants from and travelers to malarious areas. *Plasmodium* species are transmitted to humans by the bites of female mosquitoes. Erythrocytes infected with late maturing *Plasmodium* disappear from the peripheral blood and localize in the deep vascular beds of vital organs, in a process known as *sequestration*. In the life cycle, merozoites are released from erythrocytes, causing the paroxysms of chills and fever (in excess of 41°C [105°F]) typical of malaria. During the febrile stage, the patient may become encephalopathic. A relapsing pattern of high fever and chills with confusion points towards a diagnosis of malaria.

P. falciparum malaria may lead to a catastrophic complication known as *cerebral malaria*, thought to result from obstruction of the brain microvasculature due to sequestration of parasitized red blood cells. Cerebral malaria may present with disorientation, mild stupor, or even psychosis, within 24 hours of the first symptoms. It rapidly progresses to seizures and coma, sometimes with cranial nerve dysfunction and decerebrate posturing. The severity of the symptoms is correlated with the amount of sequestered parasitized red blood cells in the CNS (Turner, 1997). Definitive diagnosis of cerebral malaria is made by the identification of *Plasmodium* on the blood smear. In the setting of unarousable consciousness, neuroimaging may suggest cerebral edema.

Plasmodium is particularly adept at developing resistance to chemotherapy. Even treated individuals or those on prophylaxis may have active malaria. Antimalarial drugs, particularly mefloquine, also commonly cause psychiatric side effects, as outlined later in this chapter. Following treatment for cerebral malaria, neurological symptoms may resolve slowly, quickly, or not at all, and residual symptoms are described in up to 10% of immunocompetent patients. An entity known as *post-malaria neurological syndrome* has also been described in *P. falciparum* malaria, following or in the absence of cerebral malaria, occurring weeks to months after resolution of acute infection and involving seizures, cognitive dysfunction, and psychiatric manifestations (Walker et al., 2006). Proposed mechanisms for the syndrome include a delayed phenomenon similar to that occurring in cerebral malaria with sequestration of parasitized red blood cells, an immunological response, or perhaps a reaction to mefloquine that has been used earlier in the course for treatment in the majority of cases. Most patients recover from post-malaria neurological syndrome within ten days without specific treatment (Nguyen et al., 1996).

TOXOPLASMOSIS

Toxoplasmosis is caused by *Toxoplasma gondii*, a parasite affecting many mammals (especially cats) and some birds (Yermakov et al., 1982). Many healthy adults carry this protozoan asymptomatically, but immunocompromised individuals can develop serious disease. CNS toxoplasmosis is especially common in patients with AIDS, and may cause diffuse encephalitis or multiple brain abscesses. Toxoplasmosis is in fact the most frequent cause of CNS mass lesions in AIDS. Symptoms are nonspecific and reflect the location and extent of CNS involvement. Cognitive dysfunction, lethargy, confusion, and visual hallucinations are all common. Anxiety and paranoia may progress to delirium and obtundation. MRI is particularly valuable in the diagnosis of CNS toxoplasmosis, with ring-enhancing lesions in the basal ganglia or cerebrum very suggestive of the disease, though transplant recipients may show a variable enhancement pattern as compared to AIDS patients. While brain biopsy provides definitive diagnosis, most clinicians will initiate treatment in patients with suggestive neuroradiological findings and positive serology, reserving biopsy for those who fail to improve with treatment (Iacoangeli et al., 1994). Treatment of active CNS toxoplasmosis involves pyrimethamine, sulfadiazine, and folinic acid, followed by chronic maintenance treatment with any of several medical regimens (Walker & Zunt, 2005).

TRYPANOSOMIASIS

The family of protozoa Trypanosomatidae causes two clinically different syndromes: African trypanosomiasis (sleeping sickness) and American trypanosomiasis (Chagas' disease). African trypanosomiasis occurs in a number of sub-Saharan African countries. Few cases have been reported outside of tropical Africa, though numbers appear to be increasing in the Western hemisphere as a result of travel and migration. The disease is caused by a subspecies of *Trypanosoma brucei* and is transmitted to humans and animals by the bite of the blood-sucking tsetse fly. Early stages of the disease include headache, fever, malaise, weight loss, arthralgias, and myalgias, sometimes accompanied by a chancre at the site of inoculation. CNS symptoms begin in the second stage and may include excessive sleeping or sleep-phase reversal, abnormal gait or speech, and alterations in mood, including depression and mania. Later stages may include seizures or coma. Diagnosis relies on identification of the protozoa. CT is usually normal, but MRI may show hypointensity in the basal ganglia. Traditionally, melarsopol, which itself is fatal in some cases, was the only treatment available for CNS involvement, though newer evidence suggests that eflornithine and nifurtimox combined with eflornithine may be safer and effective (Lutje et al., 2010).

American trypanosomiasis, or Chagas' disease, is caused by *Trypanosoma cruzi*. *T. cruzi* is carried by Triatomine bugs, commonly called "kissing bugs" or "assassin bugs," which live in rural areas of Central and South America. Years of exposure are required to acquire the infection. CNS involvement is rare in the acute phase (seen mostly in children under two) and somewhat controversial in the chronic phase, though chronic Chagas' disease is thought to be an independent risk factor for vascular ischemic events (Carod-Artal, 2007). CNS involvement is most commonly seen during reactivation of disease in immunocompromised hosts, where it can involve meningoencephalitis and seizures. On CT scan of the brain, the lesions are indistinguishable from toxoplasmosis, and the organism is not seen on blood smear in chronic Chagas' disease, making diagnosis difficult. Two diagnostic tests based on different antigens or techniques are frequently used in combination (Bern, 2011). Treatment is recommended for chronic disease in patients under 50, but is frequently ineffective and carries significant risk of side effects.

SCHISTOSOMIASIS

Schistosomiasis is an infection caused by blood flukes (trematodes) of the genus *Schistosoma* and affecting 200 million people in 74 countries. Humans can be infected when skin comes in contact with the infective larval stage, usually while swimming in contaminated waters. Adult worms copulate and migrate to the intestines (*S. japonicum*, *S. mansoni*) or bladder (*S. haematobium*). Most infections are asymptomatic. CNS involvement is rare, though it may be more common than previously realized, affecting up to 4% of patients.

Psychiatric symptoms may occur at two distinct phases of infection. Acute toxemic schistosomiasis, seen in previously unexposed people such as travelers, produces symptoms of headache, malaise, and muscle aches several weeks after exposure and can progress to toxemia and associated encephalopathy. In chronically infected individuals, eggs deposited in ectopic locations, such as the CNS, induce a granulomatous reaction. The smaller eggs of *S. japonicum* may travel all the way to the brain, stimulating granuloma formation and leading to symptoms of increased intracranial pressure (e.g., headache, visual changes, nausea, and papilledema), seizures, and cranial nerve abnormalities. Conversely, the larger eggs of *S. mansoni* and *S. haematobium* are retained in the lower spinal cord, causing myelopathy (Ross et al., 2011). Diagnosis is typically based on clinical symptoms and exposure history, coupled with neuroimaging and the detection of schistosomal eggs in the urine or feces. Biopsy or necropsy demonstrating eggs and granulomas are the only definitive diagnostic methods. Drug treatment involving praziquantel and corticosteroids is effective except for rare cases requiring surgery.

TRICHINOSIS

Trichinosis is a worldwide disease caused by the ingestion of larvae encysted in the muscles of infected animals. In the United States and Europe, these parasites are most commonly found in pork, but 150 species of mammals from all latitudes may acquire the infection. Outbreaks of trichinosis are associated with ethnic groups that prefer raw or undercooked pork or horsemeat, or wild animals such as polar bear or walrus. Typical symptoms of infection include a febrile illness with myalgias and diarrhea. Ten to 24% of symptomatic cases have CNS involvement, usually developing three to four weeks after infection, and including headache,

delirium, insomnia, meningeal signs, and seizures (Taratuto & Venturiello, 1997). Some have suggested that there is a chronic form of trichinosis infection, involving persistent formication, numbness, and diaphoresis, but prospective studies have been unsupportive.

In patients with CNS involvement, CT scan shows multiple small, hypodense lesions with ring-like enhancement with contrast (Ellrodt et al., 1987). Diagnosis in humans is frequently based on clinical symptoms, known exposure, and eosinophilia, though ELISA is the most commonly used serodiagnostic method (Gottstein et al., 2009). A muscle biopsy, generally of the deltoid, demonstrating larvae is more definitive though invasive, and sensitivity is dependent on the size of the biopsy sampled. In the early stage of muscle invasion, it can be difficult to differentiate larvae from muscle fibers, though basophilic transformation of muscle cells may be apparent. Treatment in severe cases involves glucocorticosteroids for the inflammation and albendazole or mebendazole to kill the *Trichinella*. A pilot program for trichinella-free pig production has been developed in the United States, resulting in declining rates and changes in recommendations for cooking pork.

AMOEBIASIS

Several amoebas cause human disease, and all are ubiquitous in the environment worldwide. While CNS infection with amoebas remains uncommon in America, it is increasing, due largely to travel and immigration, though cases have also originated from bodies of water in the United States. Primary amoebic meningoencephalitis is produced by *Naegleria fowleri* in healthy, young individuals engaged in freshwater aquatic activities, particularly those in which water may forcibly enter the nasal passages, during the summer months. Its course is acute and fulminant, with headache, nausea, confusion, and a stiff neck, followed by coma and death in days. Treatment involves aggressive amphotericin therapy using intravenous and intrathecal routes, and swift diagnosis via visualization of the amoeba in the CSF is crucial, given that only ten survivors have been reported in the literature (Tuppeny, 2011). Clinical suspicion should be high in those presenting with fulminant meningitis and recent exposure to warm, inland waters.

Granulomatous amoebic encephalitis, caused by *Balamuthia mandrillaris* and some species of *Acanthamoeba*, usually occurs in debilitated, immunosuppressed (especially in AIDS), or malnourished individuals. The course is more chronic, with personality changes, confusion, and irritability, eventually progressing to seizures and death (Martinez & Visvesvara, 1997). Recent development of a multiplex real-time PCR test allows for the rapid detection of all free-living amoebae in a sample, thus potentially enhancing speed of diagnosis. Treatment remains empirical with poor penetration of the blood–brain barrier, though successful treatment following early diagnosis has been reported using fluconazole and sulfadiazine as well as a combination of trimethoprim-sulfamethoxazole, rifampin, and ketoconazole (Visvesvara, 2010).

FUNGAL INFECTIONS

CRYPTOCOCCOSIS

Cryptococcosis is an infection caused by *Cryptococcus* species, a pathogen distributed worldwide and found mainly in bird excreta and soil. *Cryptococcus* may act as a solo pathogen, but in up to 85% of cases, it is associated with another illness, and largely affects immunocompromised patients. In America, rates in AIDS patients have declined with the advent of highly active anti-retroviral therapy (HAART), though IRIS continues to account for many cases. The disease also affects up to 5% of solid-organ transplant recipients, and rates in developing countries remain high, with mortality in 50% of patients within three months (Cannon et al., 2009). The portal of entry is usually the respiratory tract, from which hematogenous spread occurs, though at the time of presentation pulmonary infection may not be evident. This pathogen has a predilection for the subarachnoid space, and *Cryptococcus* is the most common form of fungal meningitis (Sabetta & Andriole, 1985). Illness is typically insidious in onset and slowly progressive. Headache is present in up to 75% of the cases, and other findings include cerebellar signs, cranial nerve deficits, and motor deficits. Besides meningitis, chronic granulomas or cryptococcomas may occur in the parenchyma, and deep cerebral infarcts of the basal ganglia and thalamus may result from small-vessel arteritis.

Psychiatric presentations are broad in scope, ranging from irritability to mania to psychosis, all of which may be present prior to meningeal signs. Periods of remission and relapse are common in undiagnosed and untreated patients. The mean time from symptoms to diagnosis is six weeks. Imaging may be useful if it reveals clusters of pseudocysts in the basal ganglia and thalami, a fairly specific finding. Serological testing of patients with cryptococcal meningoencephalitis reveals cryptococcal antigen in serum, CSF, or both, 90% of the time, though serum testing is less specific in non-AIDS patients. Isolation of the fungi provides definitive diagnosis, and India ink staining is useful in highlighting the organism. Treatment is typically a prolonged course of an antifungal agent, and relapses are frequent. Permanent sequelae include dementia and personality changes (Mitchell et al., 1995). In HIV-negative patients, changes in diffusion tensor imaging in vulnerable brain regions have been shown to correspond to worse cognitive performance (Lu et al., 2011).

CANDIDIASIS

Candida causes limited local infections (cutaneous, vaginal, oral) in immunocompetent hosts, especially after broad-spectrum antibiotics. Disseminated candidiasis occurs only in the immunocompromised host. Psychiatric symptoms occur from the toxic effects of fungemia or from direct invasion of the CNS. Meningitis represents the most common form of CNS involvement, though microabscesses, macroabscesses, and vasculitis are also possible. Meningitis typically develops over several days to weeks, though an acute form resembling bacterial meningitis has been described, and *C. glabrata* may

cause a more insidious form evolving over weeks to months (Rauchway et al., 2010). Symptoms are nonspecific and include confusion, drowsiness, lethargy, and headache. Most diagnoses of CNS candidiasis are made at autopsy. However, CNS symptoms, radiographic changes (hydrocephalus, microabscesses) and isolation of *Candida* from a non-CNS site in an immunocompromised patient should lead to a presumptive diagnosis and prompt treatment with appropriate antifungal agents.

Candida infection has been alleged to be the cause of a wide array of somatic and psychological symptoms, comprising an entity known as *candidiasis hypersensitivity syndrome*. There is no scientific support for this theory or its associated treatments.

OTHER FUNGAL INFECTIONS

The frequency of fungal infection has steadily increased over the last three decades, primarily because of the HIV/AIDS epidemic, the availability of immunosuppressant drugs, and the increasing number of solid-organ transplantations. An aging population, increasing cancer rates, intravenous catheters, use of implantable medical devices, hyperalimentation, illicit drug use, the development of burn units, and the emergence of antifungal-resistant species have all also contributed to the increased frequency of fungal infection (Raman Sharma, 2010). For further details about other fungal infections, please see Table 60.2.

PRION DISEASES

Prion diseases are neurodegenerative diseases that have a broad spectrum of neuropsychiatric clinical manifestations. Human prion diseases include Creutzfeldt-Jakob disease (CJD, or "mad cow disease"), variant Creutzfeldt-Jakob disease (vCJD, also known as "new variant CJD"), Gerstmann-Sträussler-Scheinker syndrome (GSS), kuru, and fatal familial insomnia (FFI). Of these, CJD is the most common. All of the prion diseases are characteristically progressive and uniformly fatal. The incubation period can be months to years. The transmissible pathogen is a proteinaceous infectious particle (PrP) that does not have the structure of a virus, fails to produce an immune response, and is devoid of nucleic acid, and so is resistant to ribonucleic acid (RNA) and DNA destroying enzymes.

CJD can occur sporadically but may also be inherited or transmitted by intracerebral electrodes, dural grafts, corneal transplants, and human-derived growth hormone. It classically presents with confusion and memory loss progressing to a severe cortical dementia, usually accompanied by ataxia and myoclonus. Other symptoms, including rigidity, tremor, alien hand syndrome, and sensory disturbances have also been reported. The EEG pattern is distinctive, showing bilateral periodic discharges of triphasic or sharp wave bursts at 0.5–2Hz. Similar EEG changes can be seen in patients taking lithium, but will remit after discontinuation of the offending agent (Finelli, 1992). Routine CSF

Table 60.2 FUNGAL CENTRAL NERVOUS SYSTEM INFECTIONS

FUNGUS	WHERE IT LIVES	ROUTE OF TRANSMISSION	WHO IS AFFECTED?	CLINICAL FORMS	CNS SYMPTOMS	DIAGNOSIS	IMAGING	TREATMENT
Coccidiodomycosis	Soil	Inhalation; CNS involvement 1–3 months after initial infection, with insidious and chronic course[1]	Diabetics, Pregnant women, Immunocompromised patients	Meningitis, hydrocephalus, cerebral granulomas, abscesses	Confusion, restlessness, hallucinations, lethargy, and transient neurological signs[2]	Neuro-imaging and serological testing; culturing of the CSF; biopsy of infected tissue (usually skin nodules) is definitive	Meningeal enhancement, hydrocephalus	Oral fluconazole or itraconazole; amphotericin B for severe cases[3]
Aspergillosis	Soil, decaying vegetation	Infection of lung or GI tract; Extension to CNS via direct invasion from sinuses, hematogenous spread, or embolization	Immunocompromised patients	Meningitis, mycotic aneurysms, cerebritis, abscesses or infarcts	Confusion, headache, lethargy, focal neurological signs, seizures	Brain biopsy[4]; rarely isolated on CSF cultures	Localized edema; hemorrhagic lesions; Aspergillomas as low-density lesions in the cerebral hemisphere, basal ganglia, or thalami with little to no mass effect and no contrast enhancement on CT, often more numerous on MRI[5]	Voriconazole (response rates 35%); Amphotericin B
Histoplasmosis	Soil contaminated with bird or bat excreta	Inhalation	Immunocompromised; two peaks of distribution—infancy and 5th and 6th decades	Chronic meningitis; parenchymal brain lesions; stroke due to emboli; hydrocephalus; and diffuse encephalitis[3]	Extreme nervousness, irritability; lethargy; coma[6]	CSF can show pleocytosis with an elevated protein; most cultures are negative, though *Histoplasma* antigen may be detected in the serum, CSF, or urine; Brain biopsy in some cases	Usually normal	LF Amphotericin B for 4–6 weeks +Itraconazole for 1 year
Blastomycosis	Soil	Inhalation	Immuno-compromised or –competent	Meningitis, abscesses	Headache, focal neurological deficit, confusion, seizures	Detection of antigen in CSF; Brain biopsy	Dural-based granulomatous lesions; diffuse meningeal enhancement	LF Amphotericin B for 4–6 weeks +Itraconazole for 1 year
Mucormycosis	Common bread and fruit molds	Inhalation; rapid dissemination by attacking contiguous structures; Isolated CNS involvement can occur rarely[7]	Diabetic ketoacidosis, neutropenia, transplant patients, IV drug use[8]	Subdural abscesses; cavernous and occasionally sagittal sinus thrombosis; rarely meningitis[9]	Encephalopathy, facial pain, headache, ophthalmoplegia,	Biopsy, demonstration of mold in tissue	Various patterns; most commonly affects central gray matter	Aggressive debridement; LF Amphotericin B

1. Castleman, B., & McNeely, B. (Eds.) (1996). Case records of the Massachusetts General Hospital. Case 36-1971. *New England Journal of Medicine*, 285, 621–630.

2. Bañuelos, A. F., Williams, P. L., Johnson, R. H., et al. (1996). Central nervous system abscesses due to coccidioides species. *Clinical Infectious Diseases*, 22(2), 240–250.

3. Rauchway, A. C., Husain, S., & Selhorst, J. B. (2010). Neurologic presentations of fungal infections. *Neurologic Clinics*, 28(1), 293–309.

4. Hawkins, C., & Armstrong, D. (1984). Fungal infections in the immunocompromised host. *Clinical Haematology*, 13, 599–630.

5. Ruhnke, M., Kofla, G., Otto, K., et al. (2007). CNS aspergillosis: recognition, diagnosis and management. *Central Nervous System Drugs*, 21(8), 659–676.

6. Tan, V., Wilkins, P., Badve, S., et al. (1992). Histoplasmosis of the central nervous system. *Journal of Neurology, Neurosurgery, & Psychiatry*, 55(7), 619–622.

7. Siddiqi, I. U., & Freedman, J. D. (1994). Isolated central nervous system mucormycosis. *Southern Medical Journal*, 87(10), 997–1000.

8. Hopkins, R. J., Rothman, M., Fiore, A., et al. (1994). Cerebral mucormycosis associated with intravenous drug use: three case reports and review. *Clinical Infectious Diseases*, 19(6), 1133–1137.

9. Sun, H., & Singh, N. (2011). Mucormycosis: its contemporary face and management strategies. *Lancet Infectious Diseases*, 11(4), 301–311.

and other laboratory tests are almost always normal in CJD, but immunoassay detection of fragments 14-3-3, a normal brain protein, or elevated neuron-specific enolase is particularly useful in making the diagnosis. MRI classically shows hyperintensity in the basal ganglia or the so-called cortical ribbon. Cortical gray matter classically displays "spongiform degeneration" or vacuolation, though biopsy is not commonly performed, and most pathological diagnoses are made at autopsy (Brown & Mastrianni, 2010).

Compared to CJD, vCJD more commonly presents with psychiatric symptoms, particularly apathy and depression. Additionally, confusion, agitation, delusions, and hallucinations may be present. As a group, vCJD patients are younger (average age of 27 vs. 60), lack typical EEG findings, and experience a longer average time to death (14 months vs. 4 months) (Haywood, 1997). Variant CJD has been linked to the consumption of beef contaminated with bovine spongiform encephalopathy (BSE).

Kuru is the rarest of the prion diseases, with no new cases described in the past several decades. Kuru occurs only in Papua, New Guinea, and is spread by cannibalistic consumption of dead relatives during mourning rituals. GSS, a familial disease, commonly involves progressive cerebellar ataxia, corticospinal tract signs, dysarthria, nystagmus, and mild dementia. EEG shows diffuse slowing, and the duration of disease is typically much longer than with CJD. Finally, FFI is a genetically determined prion disease with a mutation in codon 178 of the PrP gene in which patients develop progressive insomnia with loss of the normal circadian sleep-activity pattern, which may manifest as a dreamlike confusional state during waking hours. Mental status and behavioral changes include inattention, hallucinations, confusion, and impaired concentration and memory, but overt dementia is rare. EEG shows diffuse slowing, but MRI is usually normal.

HARMFUL ALGAL BLOOM TOXINS

Many harmful algal bloom (HAB) toxins, produced by microalgae, are highly potent neurotoxins. These toxins can lead to massive fish kills, deaths of marine birds and other wildlife, and seafood contamination. Amnesic shellfish poisoning (ASP) involves the release of the toxin domoic acid during red tides, and human ingestion of contaminated shellfish can lead to headaches, memory loss, hemiparesis, seizures, and death (Friedman & Levin, 2005). The hallmark of the illness is a sustained anterograde memory deficit, possibly due to damage to the amygdala and hippocampus by the toxin.

Ciguatera fish poisoning, caused by the consumption of coral reef fish contaminated with ciguatoxin, is the most frequently reported food-poisoning illness caused by a marine toxin. Acute gastrointestinal symptoms are followed by fatigue, muscle weakness, hot–cold temperature reversal, and sustained memory and mood disturbances. Hallucinations are also frequently reported.

Pfiesteria piscicida, a dinoflagellate, can release a toxin capable of killing large numbers of fish. It occurs along the eastern coast of the United States from the Gulf of Mexico to Delaware Bay. An entity known as *possible estuary associated syndrome* (PEAS) is associated with exposure to *Pfiesteria*, though the specific toxin has not been identified, nor has it been confirmed that exposure leads to human illness. There have been reports of toxic effects in humans in Maryland and North Carolina, primarily in watermen exposed to large-scale fish kills and in researchers who cultured *Pfiesteria*. Prominent symptoms have included headache, skin lesions, burning sensation on contact with water, as well as reversible memory impairment improving months after cessation of exposure (Grattan et al., 1998).

ANTIMICROBIALS

Antimicrobial medications may cause psychiatric symptoms through a variety of mechanisms. The fluoroquinolones, particularly ciprofloxacin, have been commonly implicated as a cause of delirium. Despite some suggestion that this association has been exaggerated, this class of medications is noted to have a particular affinity for gamma-aminobutyric acid (GABA) and N-methyl D-aspartate (NMDA) receptors. It has been suggested that the mechanism for quinolone-associated delirium may be non-convulsive status epilepticus (NCSE) because of the known ability to lower seizure threshold and reports of abnormal EEGs in patients receiving the medications (Kiangkitiwan et al., 2008). Risk factors for development of neuropsychiatric side effects with quinolones appear to include impaired renal clearance, underlying CNS disease, and increased CNS penetrance due to inflammatory states. Physicians should also be aware of the potential for decreased metabolism of quinolones with certain cytochrome p450 alleles or due to p450-related interactions.

Delirium has also been associated with procaine penicillin, antimalarial drugs, and the antituberculous drug cycloserine. In evaluating the association between delirium and recent initiation of antimicrobial medication, psychiatrists should recall that the Latin dictum *Post hoc ergo propter hoc* ("after this, therefore because of this") does not always apply. Delirium may be driven instead by the underlying infection, with the temporal association of antibiotic therapy serving as a red herring.

Reports of secondary mania caused by antimicrobial drugs have increased significantly in the past fifteen years, presumably due to the increase in antibiotic prescriptions around the world, as well as the introduction of new classes of antibiotics. Clarithromycin and ciprofloxacin are the medications most commonly implicated (Abouesh et al., 2002). As with all cases of secondary mania, long-term prophylactic treatment may not be required, and overlap with delirium is unclear.

The antimalarial medication mefloquine (structurally related to fluoroquinolones) has been implicated in causing a variety of neuropsychiatric symptoms, including sleep disturbances, anxiety, depression, and frank psychosis. There is some suggestion that females and patients with low body mass index (BMI) are at the highest risk for experiencing adverse effects. Mechanisms may include interference with calcium homeostasis, acetylcholinesterase inhibition, and enhancement of striatal GABA (Toovey, 2009).

Many medications used to treat infections can prolong the QTc interval and therefore increase the risk of *torsades de pointes*, particularly if used in combination with psychiatric medications that also prolong the QTc interval (antipsychotics, TCAs, some SSRIs). These medications include chloroquine, macrolides (e.g., clarithromycin, erythromycin), pentamidine, and quinolones (Abramson et al., 2008). Macrolides, antifungal agents, chloramphenicol, and norfloxacin may additionally lead to QTc prolongation and predispose to ventricular arrhythmias by inhibiting the metabolism of other QTc-prolonging agents via their action on CYP3A4.

Linezolid, an oxazolidinone antibiotic widely used in hospitals for treatment of methicillin-resistant *Staphylococcus aureus* (MRSA) and vancomycin-resistant *Enterococcus* (VRE), is a mild, reversible, non-selective monoamine oxidase inhibitor (MAOI). If used in combination with serotonergic agents such as SSRIs, there is a small risk of precipitating serotonin syndrome. The standard recommendation is for a two-week washout period for patients taking serotonin agonists prior to initiating treatment with linezolid, but this may not always be prudent, given the potential seriousness of infections requiring linezolid. Most cases of toxicity occur within the first three weeks of treatment. Physicians should conduct a careful risk analysis to determine the relative danger of stopping as opposed to continuing serotonergic agents during linezolid therapy, particularly in patients with tenuous or potentially lethal mental illness (Quinn & Stern, 2009).

Amphotericin B, an antifungal agent, is at times associated with delirium and leukoencephalopathy. Voriconazole, an antifungal agent used for aspergillosis, can commonly (2–16%) cause hallucinations, especially when given intravenously. These are mostly visual and sometimes auditory. Visual hallucinations worsened when the patients' eyes closed to try to sleep, but the patient remained oriented and able to recognize the sensation as unreal (Zonios et al., 2008).

CLINICAL PEARLS

- In the past ten years, rates of syphilis have begun to climb again, owing to a variety of factors such as increasingly unsafe sex practices, particularly among men who have sex with men (MSM), in the wake of available antiretroviral therapy for HIV. HIV-positive patients infected with syphilis are more likely to develop neurosyphilis (Chahine, 2011).

- Secondary syphilis resolves without treatment but may recur in the next few years. If untreated, one-third of individuals develop later sequelae.

- A recent retrospective review of neurosyphilis in the modern age suggests that a positive sucking reflex, Argyll-Robertson pupils that accommodate but do not react to light, and hyperreflexia are the most common signs (Zheng et al., 2011).

- In late neurosyphilis, psychiatric symptoms frequently do not remit with antibiotic treatment.

- The rash of Rocky Mountain spotted fever is notable in being one of the few diffuse rashes to involve the palms and soles (another being the rash of secondary syphilis).

- Serological testing in Lyme disease remains unreliable in many cases, with false positives occurring in the setting of other infections and true-positive tests only indicating a history of LD at some time in the past.

- It is vital to educate patients that, although some physicians advocate long-term antibiotic treatment for post-treatment LD, all four randomized controlled trials of prolonged antimicrobial treatment have failed to demonstrate any lasting improvement, and many other open-label trials have failed to separate cases of well-documented LD from those without objective evidence (Halperin, 2008). Furthermore, such treatment carries significant risk in the form of complications.

- Symptom exacerbations of PANDAS are thought to be sudden and dramatic as opposed to the more gradual waxing and waning pattern of childhood-onset OCD.

- A history of TB is elicited in only 10% of patients with tubercular meningitis at the time of presentation, and the tuberculin skin test may be positive in fewer than 50% of patients (Rock, 2008).

- Herpes simplex virus (HSV) encephalitis differs from other viral meningoencephalities in its greater likelihood to cause unilateral and focal findings and its predilection for temporoparietal involvement.

- PCR detection of herpes simplex virus DNA in the CSF has become the diagnostic method of choice, though it may be negative rarely in very early cases. It is widely available, and the time from LP to results is generally 24–72 hours.

- The clinical symptoms of acute disseminated encephalomyelitis (ADEM), a cell-mediated immune reaction to myelin basic protein occurring in the wake of many viruses, commonly include encephalopathy, fever, seizures, and meningismus. Changes in mood, as well as psychotic symptoms such as delusions and hallucinations, have also been reported in the absence of obviously altered sensorium (Krishnakumar, 2008).

- The most frequent manifestation of neurocystocercosis is seizures, commonly of the partial-complex variety, reported as the initial symptom in 66% of patients. Encephalitis, meningitis, and altered mental status are also commonly seen at presentation (Wallin, 2004).

- *Plasmodium falciparum* malaria may lead to a catastrophic complication known as *cerebral malaria*, thought to result from obstruction of the brain microvasculature due to sequestration of parasitized red blood cells.

- *Cryptococcus* is the most common form of fungal meningitis and has a predilection for the subarachnoid space (Sabetta & Andriole, 1985). Psychiatric presentations are broad in scope, ranging from irritability to mania to psychosis, all of which may be present prior to meningeal signs.

- Voriconazole, an antifungal agent used for aspergillosis, can commonly (2–16%) cause hallucinations.

DISCLOSURE STATEMENT

Dr. Beach has no conflicts to disclose.

REFERENCES

Abba, K., Ramaratnam, S., & Ranganathan, L. N. (2010). Anthelmentics for people with neurocysticercosis. *Cochrane Database of Systematic Reviews*, (3), CD000215.

Abouesh, A., Stone, C., & Hobbs, W. R. (2002). Antimicrobial-induced mania (antibiomania): A review of spontaneous reports. *Journal of Clinical Psychopharmacology, 22*(1), 71–81.

Abramson, D. W., Quinn, D. K., & Stern, T. A. (2008). Methadone-associated QTc prolongation: A case report and review of the literature. *Primary Care Companion Journal of Clinical Psychiatry, 10*(6), 470–476.

Auwaerter, P. G. (2007). Point: Antibiotics therapy is not the answer for patients with persisting symptoms attributable to Lyme disease. *Clinical Infectious Diseases, 45*(2), 143–148.

Bañuelos, A. F., Williams, P. L., Johnson, R. H., et al. (1996). Central nervous system abscesses due to coccidioides species. *Clinical Infectious Diseases, 22*(2), 240–250.

Baringer, J. R. (2008). Herpes simplex infections of the nervous system. *Neurologic Clinics, 26*(3), 657–674.

Bern, C. (2011). Antitrypanosomal therapy for chronic Chagas' disease. *New England Journal of Medicine, 364*(26), 2527–2534.

Boulais, P., Delcros, J., Signoret, J. L., et al. (1976). Subacute excitation caused by probable herpetic encephalitis. Favorable effects of lithium. *Annales de Médicine Interne, 127*(5), 345–352.

Brown, K., & Mastrianni, J. A. (2010). The prion diseases. *Journal of Geriatric Psychiatry & Neurology, 23*(4), 277–298.

Bunikis, J., & Barbour, A. G. (2002). Laboratory testing for suspected Lyme disease. *Medical Clinics of North America, 86*(2), 311–340.

Cannon, R. D., Lamping, E., Holmes, A. R., et al. (2009). Efflux-mediated antifungal drug resistance. *Clinical Microbiology Reviews, 22*(2), 291–321.

Caparros-Lefebre, D., Girard-Buttaz, I., Reboul, S., et al. (1996). Cognitive and psychiatric impairment in herpes simplex virus encephalitis suggest involvement of the amygdalo-frontal pathways. *Journal of Neurology, 243*(3), 248–256.

Carod-Artal, F. J. (2007). Stroke: A neglected complication of American trypanosomiasis (Chagas' disease). *Transactions of the Royal Society of Tropical Medicine & Hygiene, 101*(11), 1075–1080.

Castleman, B., & McNeely, B. (Eds.) (1996). Case records of the Massachusetts General Hospital. Case 36–1971. *New England Journal of Medicine, 285*, 621–630.

Centers for Disease Control and Prevention (CDC) (1998). Human rabies—Texas and New Jersey, 1997. *Journal of the American Medical Association, 279*(6), 421–422.

Chahine, L. M., Khoriaty, R. N., Tomford, W. J., et al. (2011). The changing face of neurosyphilis. *International Journal of Stroke, 6*(2), 136–143.

Deresiewicz, R. L., Thaler, S. J., Hsu, L., et al. (1997). Clinical and neuroradiographic manifestations of Eastern equine encephalitis. *New England Journal of Medicine, 336*(26), 1867–1874.

Doja, A., Bitnun, A., Ford Jones, E. L., et al. (2006). Pediatric Epstein-Barr virus-associated encephalitis: 10 year review. *Journal of Child Neurology, 21*, 384–391.

Dworkin, R. H., Panarites, C. J., Armstrong, E. P., et al. (2012). Is treatment of postherpetic neuralgia in the community consistent with evidence-based recommendations? *Pain.* doi:10.1016/j.pain.2012.01.015

Ellrodt, A., Halfon, P., LeBras, P., et al. (1987). Multifocal central nervous system lesions in three patients with trichinosis. *Archives of Neurology, 44*(4), 432–434.

Fallon, B. A., Keilp, J. G., Corbera, K. M., et al. (2008). A randomized, placebo-controlled trial of repeated IV antibiotic therapy for Lyme encephalopathy. *Neurology, 70*(13), 992–1003.

Fallon, B. A., Levin, E. S., Schweitzer, P. J., et al. (2010). Inflammation and central nervous system Lyme disease. *Neurobiology of Disease, 37*(3), 534–541.

Fallon, B. A., Nields, J. A., Burrascano, J. J., et al. (1992). The neuropsychiatric manifestations of Lyme borreliosis. *Psychiatric Quarterly, 63*(1), 95–117.

Finelli, P. E. (1992). Drug-induced Creutzfeldt-Jakob-like syndrome. *Journal of Psychiatry & Neuroscience, 17*(3), 103–105.

Friedman, M. A., & Levin, B. E. (2005). Neurobehavioral effects of harmful algal bloom (HAB) toxins: a critical review. *Journal of the International Neuropsychological Society, 11*(3), 331–338.

Golden, M. R., Marra, C. M., & Holmes, K. K. (2003). Update on syphilis: Resurgence of an old problem. *Journal of the American Medical Association, 290*(11), 1510–1514.

Gottstein, B., Pozio, E., & Nockler, K. (2009). Epidemiology, diagnosis, treatment and control of trichinellosis. *Clinical Microbiology Reviews, 22*(1), 127–145.

Grattan, L. M., Oldachm D., Perl, T. M., et al. (1998). Learning and memory difficulties after environmental exposure to waterways containing toxin-producing Pfiesteria or Pfiesteria-like dinoflagellates. *Lancet 352*(9127), 532–539.

Gray, F. (1997). Bacterial infections. *Brain Pathology, 7*(1), 629–647.

Griffiths, P. (2004). Cytomegalovirus infection of the central nervous system. *Herpes, 11*(Suppl 2), 95A–104A.

Gunther, G., & Haglund, M. (2005). Tick-borne encephalopathies: Epidemiology, diagnosis, treatment and prevention. *Central Nervous System Drugs, 19*(12), 1009–1032.

Halperin, J. J. (2008). Prolonged Lyme disease treatment: Enough is enough. *Neurology, 70*(13), 986–987.

Hassett, A. L., Radvanski, D. C., Buyske, S., et al. (2008). Role of psychiatric comorbidity in chronic Lyme disease. *Arthritis & Rheumatology, 59*(12), 1742–1749.

Haywood, A. M. (1997). Transmissible spongiform encephalopathies. *New England Journal of Medicine, 337*(25), 1821–1828.

Honda, H., & Warren, D. K. (2009). Central nervous system infections: Meningitis and brain abscess. *Infectious Disease Clinics of North America, 23*(3), 609–623.

Hook, E. W. III, & Marra, C. M. (1992). Acquired syphilis in adults. *New England Journal of Medicine, 326*(16), 1060–1069.

Hopkins, R. J., Rothman, M., Fiore, A., et al. (1994). Cerebral mucormycosis associated with intravenous drug use: Three case reports and review. *Clinical Infectious Diseases, 19*(6), 1133–1137.

Hunter, M., Johnson, N., Hetterwick, S., et al. (2010). Immunovirological correlates in human rabies treated with therapeutic coma. *Journal of Medical Virology, 82*(7), 1255–1265.

Huynh, W., Cordato, D. J., Kehdi, E., et al. (2008). Post-vaccination encephalomyelitis: Literature review and illustrative case. *Journal of Clinical Neuroscience, 15*(12), 1315–1322.

Iacoangeli, M., Roselli, R., Antinori, A., et al. (1994). Experience with brain biopsy in acquired immune deficiency syndrome-related focal lesions of the central nervous system. *Journal of Brain Surgery, 81*(10), 1508–1511.

Kalish, R. A., Kaplan, R. F., Tayor, E., et al. (2001). Evaluation of study patients with Lyme disease, 10–20-year follow-up. *Journal of Infectious Diseases, 183*(3), 453–460.

Katon, W., Russo, J., Ashley, R. L., et al. (1999). Infectious mononucleosis: Psychological symptoms during acute and subacute phases of illness. *General Hospital Psychiatry, 21*(1), 21–29.

Kiangkitiwan, B., Doppalapudi, A., Fonder, M., et al. (2008). Levofloxacin-induced delirium with psychotic features. *General Hospital Psychiatry, 30*(4), 381–383.

Krishnakumar, P., Jayakrishnan, M. P., Beegum, M. N., et al. (2008). Acute disseminated encephalomyelitis presenting as acute psychotic disorder. *Indian Pediatrics, 45*(12), 999–1001.

Larsen, S. A., Kraus, S., & Whittington, W. (1990). Diagnostic tests. In S. A. Larsen, E. Hunter, & S. Kraus (Eds.), *A manual of tests for syphilis* (pp. 2–26). Washington, DC: American Public Health Association.

Levenson, J. L., & Fallon, H. J. (1993). Fluoxetine treatment of depression caused by interferon-alpha. *American Journal of Gastroenterology, 88*(5), 760–761.

Lu, C. H., Chen, H. L., Chang, W. N., et al. (2011). Assessing the chronic neuropsychologic sequelae of human immunodeficiency virus-negative cryptococcal meningitis by using diffusion tensor imaging. *AJNR: American Journal of Neuroradiology, 32*(7), 1333–1339.

Lutje, V., Seixas, J., Kennedy, A. (2010). Chemotherapy for second-stage human African trypanosomiasis. *Cochrane Database of Systematic Reviews,* (8), CD006201.

Luzuriaga, K., & Sullivan J. L. (2010). Infectious mononucleosis. *New England Journal of Medicine, 362*(21), 1993–2000.

Marques, A. (2008). Chronic Lyme disease: A review. *Infectious Disease Clinics of North America, 22*(2), 341–360.

Martinez, A. J., & Visvesvara, G. (1997). Free-living, amphizoic and opportunistic amebas. *Brain Pathology, 7*(1), 583–598.

Martino, D., Defazio, G., & Giovannoni, G. (2009). The PANDAS subgroup of tic disorders and childhood-onset obsessive-compulsive disorder. *Journal of Psychosomatic Research, 67*(6), 547–557.

Menge, T., Kiesseier, B. C., Nessler, S., et al. (2007). Acute disseminated encephalomyelitis: An acute hit against the brain. *Current Opinion in Neurology, 20*(3), 247–254.

Meza, N. W., Rossi, N. E., Galeazzi, et al. (2005). Cysticercosis in chronic psychiatric inpatients from a Venezuelan community. *American Journal of Tropical Medicine, 73*(3), 504–509.

Mitchell, D. H., Sorrell, T. C., Allworth, A. M., et al. (1995). Cryptococcal disease of the CNS in immunocompetent hosts: Influence of cryptococcal variety on clinical manifestations and outcome. *Clinical Infectious Diseases, 20*(3), 611–616.

Murray, K., Baraniuk, S., Resnick, M., et al. (2006). Risk factors for encephalitis and death from West Nile virus infection. *Epidemiology & Infection, 134*(6), 1325–1332.

Nguyen, T. H., Day, N. P., Ly, V. C., et al. (1996). Post-malaria neurologic syndrome. *Lancet, 348*(9032), 917–921.

Openshaw, J. J., Swerdlow, D. L., Krebs, J. W., et al. (2010). Rocky Mountain spotted fever in the United States, 2000–2007: Interpreting contemporary increases in evidence. *American Journal of Tropical Medicine and Hygiene, 83*(1), 174–182.

Pahud, B. A., Glaser, C. A., Dekker, C. L., et al. (2011). Varicella zoster disease of the central nervous system: Epidemiological, clinical, and laboratory features 10 years after the introduction of the Varicella vaccine. *Journal of Infectious Diseases, 203*(3), 316–323.

Quinn, D. K., & Stern, T. A. (2009). Linezolid and serotonin syndrome. *Primary Care Companion Journal of Clinical Psychiatry, 11*(6), 353–356.

Raman Sharma, R. (2010). Fungal infections of the nervous system: Current prospective and controversies in management. *International Journal of Surgery, 8*(8), 591–601.

Rauchway, A. C., Husain, S., & Selhorst, J. B. (2010). Neurologic presentations of fungal infections. *Neurologic Clinics, 28*(1), 293–309.

Reddy, S. M., Winston, D. J., Territo, M. C., et al. (2010). CMV central nervous system disease in stem-cell transplant recipients: An increasing complication of drug-resistant CMV infection and protracted immunodeficiency. *Bone Marrow Transplant 45*(6), 979–984.

Relman, D. A., & Swartz, M. N. (1988). Chapter IV. Syphilis and nonvenereal treponematoses. SAM-CD Annual.

Rock, R. B., Olin, M., Baker, C. A., et al. (2008). Central nervous system tuberculosis: Pathogenesis and clinical aspects. *Clinical Microbiology Reviews, 21*(2), 243–261.

Romero, J. R., & Newland, J. G. (2003). Viral meningitis and encephalitis: Traditional and emerging viral agents. *Seminars in Pediatric Infectious Diseases, 14*(2), 72–82.

Ross, A. G., McManus, D. P., Ferrar, J., et al. (2012). Neuroschistosomiasis. *Journal of Neurology, 259*(1), 22–32.

Ruhnke, M., Kofla, G., Otto, K., et al. (2007). CNS aspergillosis: Recognition, diagnosis and management. *Central Nervous System Drugs, 21*(8), 659–676.

Sabetta, J. R., & Andriole, V. T. (1985). Cryptococcal infection of the central nervous system. *Medical Clinics of North America, 69*(2), 333–344.

Schneider, R. K., Robinson, M. J., & Levenson, J. L. (2002) Psychiatric presentations of non-HIV infectious diseases: Neurocysticercosis, Lyme disease, and pediatric autoimmune neuropsychiatric disorder associated with streptococcal infection. *Psychiatric Clinics of North America, 25*(1), 1–16.

Schuchat, A., Robinson, K., Wenger, J. D., et al. (1997). Bacterial meningitis in the United States in 1995. *New England Journal of Medicine, 337*(14), 970–976.

Segreti, J., & Harris, A. A. (1996). Acute bacterial meningitis. *Infectious Disease Clinics of North America, 10*(4), 797–809.

Sharara, A. I., Hunt, C. M., & Hamilton, J. D. (1996). Hepatitis C. *Annals of Internal Medicine, 125*(8), 658–668.

Siddiqi, I. U., & Freedman, J. D. (1994). Isolated central nervous system mucormycosis. *Southern Medical Journal, 87*(10), 997–1000.

Sigal, L. H., Zahradnik, J. M., Lavin, P., et al. (1998). A vaccine consisting of recombinant *Borrelia burgdorferi* outer-surface protein A to prevent Lyme disease. *New England Journal of Medicine, 339*(4), 216–222.

Singer, H. S., Gause, C., Morris, C., et al. (2008). Serial immune markers do not correlate with clinical exacerbations in pediatric autoimmune neuropsychiatric disorders associated with streptococcal infection. *Pediatrics, 121*(6), 1198–1205.

Steere, A. C., Taylor, E., McHugh, G. L., et al. (1993). The overdiagnosis of Lyme disease. *Journal of the American Medical Association, 269*(14), 1812–1816.

Sun, H., & Singh, N. (2011). Mucormycosis: Its contemporary face and management strategies. *Lancet Infectious Diseases, 11*(4), 301–311.

Swedo SE, Leonard H. L., Garvey, M., et al. (1998). Pediatric autoimmune neuropsychiatric disorders associated with streptococcal infections: Clinical description of the first 50 cases. *American Journal of Psychiatry, 155*(2), 264–271.

Swedo, S. E., Leonard, H. L., Mittleman, B. B., et al. (1997). Identification of children with pediatric autoimmune neuropsychiatric disorders associated with streptococcal infections by a marker associated with rheumatic fever. *American Journal of Psychiatry, 154*(1), 110–112.

Tan, C. S., & Koralnik, I. J. (2010). Progressive multifocal leukoencephalopathy and other disorders caused by JC virus: Clinical features and pathogenesis. *Lancet Neurology, 9*(4), 425–437.

Tan, V., Wilkins, P., Badve, S., et al. (1992). Histoplasmosis of the central nervous system. *Journal of Neurology, Neurosurgery, & Psychiatry, 55*(7), 619–622.

Taratuto, A. L., & Venturiello, S. M. (1997). Trichinosis. *Brain Pathology, 7*(1), 663–672.

Thirunavukarasu, S. (2011). Temporal and pontine involvement in a case of herpes simplex encephalitis, presenting as Kluver Bucy syndrome—a case report. *Journal of Clinical Imaging Science, 1*(43), doi:10.4103/2156-7514.84318.

Toovey, S. (2009). Mefloquine neurotoxicity: A literature review. *Travel Medicine & Infectious Diseases, 7*(1), 2–6.

Tugwell, P., Dennis, D. T., Weinstein, A., et al. (1997). Laboratory evaluation in the diagnosis of Lyme disease. *Annals of Internal Medicine, 127*(12), 1109–1123.

Tuppeny M. (2011). Primary amoebic meningoencephalitis with subsequent organ procurement: A case study. *Journal of Neuroscience Nursing, 43*(5), 274–279.

Turner, G. (1997). Cerebral malaria. *Brain Pathology, 7*(1), 569–582.

Tyler, K. L. (2009). Emerging viral infections of the central nervous system, Part 1. *Archives of Neurology, 66*(8), 939–948.

Vallini, A. D., & Burns, R. L. (1987). Carbamazepine as therapy for psychiatric sequelae of herpes simplex encephalitis. *Southern Medical Journal, 80*(12), 1590–1592.

Visvesvara, G. S. (2010). Amebic meningoencephalitides and keratitis: Challenges in diagnosis and treatment. *Current Opinion in Infectious Diseases, 23*(6), 590–594.

Volpi, A. (2004). Epstein-Barr virus and human herpes virus type 8 infections of the central nervous system. *Herpes* 11(Suppl 2), 120A–127A.

Walker, M., & Zunt, J. R. (2005). Parasitic central nervous system infections in immunocompromised hosts. *Clinical Infectious Diseases, 40*(7), 1005–1015.

Walker, M., Kublin, J. G., & Zunt, J. R. (2006). Parasitic central nervous system infections in immunocompromised hosts: Malaria, microsporidiosis, leishmaniasis, and African trypanosomiasis. *Clinical Infectious Diseases, 42*(1), 115–125.

Wallin, M. T., & Kurtzke, J. F. (2004). Neurocysticercosis in the United States: Review of an important emerging infection. *Neurology, 63*(9), 1559–1564.

Weinstein, L. (1985). Bacterial meningitis. Specific etiologic diagnosis on the basis of distinctive epidemiologic, pathogenetic and clinical features. *Medical Clinics of North America, 69*(2), 219–229.

White, P. D., Thomas, J. M., Amess, D. H., et al. (1998). Incidence, risk and prognosis of acute and chronic fatigue syndromes and psychiatric disorders after glandular fever. *British Journal of Psychiatry, 173,* 475–481.

Whitley, R. J. (2006). Herpes simplex encephalitis: Adolescents and adults. *Antiviral Research, 71*(2–3), 141–148.

Wormser, G. P., Dattwyler, R. J., Shapiro, E. D., et al. (2006). The clinical assessment, treatment and prevention of Lyme disease, human granulocytic anaplasmosis, and babesiosis: Clinical practice guidelines by the Infectious Diseases Society of America. *Clinical Infectious Diseases, 43*(9), 1089–1134.

Yermakov, V., Rashid, R. K., Vuletin, J. C., et al. (1982). Disseminated toxoplasmosis. *Archives of Pathology & Laboratory Medicine, 106*(10), 524–528.

Zheng, D., Zhou, D., Zhao, Z., et al. (2011). The clinical presentation and imaging manifestation of psychosis and dementia in general paresis: A retrospective study of 116 cases. *Journal of Neuropsychiatry & Clinical Neurosciences, 23*(3), 300–307.

Zonios, D. I., Gea-Banacloche, J., Childs, R., & Bennett, J. E. (2008). Hallucinations during voriconazole therapy. *Clinical Infectious Diseases,* Jul 1; *47*(1), e7–e10.

61.

RHEUMATIC DISEASE, AUTOIMMUNE DISORDERS, AND ALLERGY

Sherese Ali

INTRODUCTION

Rheumatological disorders are grouped together, as they share an autoimmune basis and typically affect the skin, musculoskeletal system, and connective tissues. Although rheumatological disorders have specific antigens towards the musculoskeletal system, many of them feature multisystem effects, including effects on the central nervous system (CNS). When the CNS becomes affected, the brain effects may manifest as psychiatric symptoms. Secondly, as rheumatological disorders are chronic medical illnesses, these disorders also have a psychological impact on the patient. Thirdly, many of the medications used to treat rheumatological disorders are associated with side effects and adverse reactions that feature psychiatric symptoms. Thus, the psychiatrist managing a patient with rheumatological disorders may consider the etiology of psychiatric symptoms as (1) a direct biological effect of the underlying illness, (2) an indirect effect in terms of the mental health impact of the chronic illness, or (3) a medication effect. Finally, one may consider an independent psychiatric disorder that happens to be comorbid with a rheumatological disorder.

This chapter will focus on the psychiatric effects associated with the more common rheumatological disorders—systemic lupus erythematosus, rheumatoid arthritis, Sjögren's syndrome, and fibromyalgia—in terms of the first three etiologies of psychiatric symptoms in this patient population. (Autoimmune disorders that primarily affect the neurological system are classified as neurological disorders and are not discussed in this chapter.)

SYSTEMIC LUPUS ERYTHEMATOSUS

Systemic lupus erythematosus (SLE) is an inflammatory disorder that affects multiple systems. Its etiology is unknown, but aberrations in immunological function result in the production of certain antibodies that can result in cell damage, immune complex formation, or an inflammatory response. SLE affects women about nine times more frequently than men. It has been found to be three times more prevalent among blacks than among whites. The diagnosis of SLE is made by a set of criteria, outlined in Table 61.1, according to the American College of Rheumatology (ACR) in 1982 (Tan, 1982) and revised in 1997 (Hochbeg, 1997).

There are situations where the importance of knowing these diagnostic criteria is impressed upon the treating psychiatrist. In the author's experience, it is not uncommon to receive consultation requests on patients who have some symptoms not meeting full criteria for the diagnosis of SLE who are then referred for somatoform disorders or otherwise unexplained medical symptoms. Such patients may have subjective complaints without strong support for a diagnosis of SLE from objective tests. For example, a patient may be complaining of diffuse pain, fatigue, general malaise, and low-grade fever over the course of a few months, with a mild anemia, but otherwise normal investigations, including anti-nuclear antibody (ANA) profile and antibody screen. Such a patient would not have been diagnosed with lupus. When one closely examines the criteria, it is important to note that not all symptoms have to be present at the same time, and there is no one criterion that is absolutely essential for diagnosis (like anhedonia or depressed mood in major depression). There is therefore a risk of missing the diagnosis, particularly when objective tests are normal. In this diagnostic schema, a patient can have psychosis as the first presenting sign of lupus, but until other symptoms present over time, the diagnosis does not declare itself (Munoz-Malaga, 1999; Jghaimi, 2009; Simonin, 2004). Indeed, there is known to be a lag time of some years between the onset of the first symptom and the eventual diagnosis of lupus. Often, the significance of previous non-specific symptoms becomes recognized only in retrospect. In such patients, it may be left to the psychiatrist and/or primary care physician to monitor for new symptoms that might reach the threshold for a diagnosis of SLE. In this scenario, the psychiatrist can screen by periodically applying these diagnostic criteria, applying the SLE Disease Activity Index (Bombardier, 1992), and performing investigations including complete blood count (CBC), antibody screen, ANA profile, and urinalysis: every three to six months, at the onset of a worsening or new symptom, or if the psychiatric symptoms are atypical.

Table 61.1 PERCENT PREVALENCE OF NPSLE

	AINIALA ET AL. 2001 ($N = 46$)	BREY ET AL. 2002 ($N = 128$)	SANNA ET AL. 2003 ($N = 323$)	HANLY ET AL. 2004 ($N = 111$)	SIBBIT JR. 2002 ($N = 75$)
Cognitive disorder	80	79	11	3	55
Headache	54	57	24	25	72
Mood disorder	43	51	17	14	57
Cerebrovascular disease	15	2	15	5	12
Seizures	9	16	9	2	51
Polyneuropathy	28	22	3	2	15
Anxiety	13	24	4	1	21
Psychosis	0	5	8	3	12

NEUROPSYCHIATRIC SLE

DEFINITION

At first, only seizures or psychosis were listed as neuropsychiatric syndromes associated with lupus (criterion 8) in Box 61.1. These criteria were revised by the ACR in 1999 (ACR Ad Hoc Committee, 1999), and the neurological disorders were expanded from two syndromes (seizures and psychosis) to 19 syndromes that define neuropsychiatric SLE (NPSLE), as shown in Box 61.2.

EPIDEMIOLOGY OF NPSLE

Table 61.1 shows available data on the prevalence of some of the neuropsychiatric syndromes. The exact prevalence of psychiatric symptoms in SLE is not known. Prior to the 1999 revised ACR criteria, there was a broad range of prevalence of 14–75%. After the ACR 1999 revised criteria, five large studies (Ainali, 2001; Sibbit Jr., 2002; Brey, 2002; Sanna, 2003; Hanly, 2004) examined the prevalence of NPSLE among patients with SLE and produced an equally broad range of 37–95%. Among the 19 neuropsychiatric syndromes, cognitive impairment, headache, mood disorder, and cerebrovascular disease were the four most common, in descending order of prevalence. Among the psychiatric syndromes, cognitive disorder, mood disorder, anxiety disorder, and psychosis are thought to be the most common, in descending order of prevalence. Other studies were not uniform in their method of attribution of psychiatric symptoms to the direct biological effect of SLE versus an indirect psychological impact of the illness. It remains a clinical challenge to differentiate primary psychiatric from direct lupus-related etiologies of psychiatric syndromes in NPSLE. Of the four psychiatric syndromes, most studies have focused on lupus psychosis. From these epidemiological studies, lupus psychosis has a prevalence estimate of 8% of SLE patients. Prevalence rates for the remaining syndromes are estimated at less than 1%.

Box 61.1 ACR CRITERIA FOR THE DIAGNOSIS OF SLE

1. Malar rash: Fixed erythema, flat or raised, over the malar eminences

2. Discoid rash: Erythematous circular raised patches with adherent keratotic scaling and follicular plugging; atrophic scarring may occur

3. Photosensitivity: Exposure to ultraviolet light causes rash

4. Oral ulcers: Includes oral and nasopharyngeal ulcers, observed by physician

5. Arthritis: Non-erosive arthritis of two or more peripheral joints, with tenderness, swelling, or effusion

6. Serositis: Pleuritis or pericarditis documented by electrocardiogram or rub or evidence of effusion

7. Renal disorder: Proteinuria >0.5 g/d or 3+, or cellular casts

8. Neurological disorder: Seizures or psychosis without other causes

9. Hematological disorder: Hemolytic anemia or leukopenia (<4000/L), or lymphopenia (<1500/L), or thrombocytopenia (<100,000/L) in the absence of offending drugs

10. Immunological disorder: Anti-double stranded DNA antibody (Anti-dsDNA), anti-Smith antigen antibody (anti-Sm)), and/or anti-phospholipid antibody

11. Antinuclear antibodies: An abnormal titer of ANA by immunofluorescence or an equivalent assay at any point in time in the absence of drugs known to induce ANAs

Any combination of 4 or more of 11 criteria, well documented at any time during a patient's history, makes it likely that the patient has SLE (specificity and sensitivity are 95% and 75%, respectively).

ETIOLOGY AND PATHOGENESIS OF NPSLE

Three basic pathophysiological mechanisms for neuropsychiatric lupus have been purported: (1) autoantibodies, (2) vasculopathy, and (3) inflammation.

Over 150 articles have reported the involvement of several antibodies in the pathogenesis of NPSLE (Colasanti, 2009; Zandman-Goddard, 2006; Valesini, 2006). Some antibodies are CNS-specific, and others are systemic. CNS-specific antibodies are listed in Table 61.2.

Systemic antibodies implicated in NSPLE include anti-phospholipid antibody (anti-cardiolipin antibody and lupus anticoagulant), anti-β2 microglobulin antibody, anti-ribosomal P antibody, anti-Ro antibody, anti-Smith antibody, anti-endothelial cell antibody, and anti-Nedd 5′ antibody, to name a few.

In most cases, small numbers of studies involving small numbers of patients, with varying definitions of NPSLE and varying assays for detecting antibodies, have been carried out. Thus no single consistent biological marker for NPSLE has yet been found. In the case of NSPLE syndromes of stroke, transient ischemic attacks, seizure, and migraine, anti-phospholipid antibodies (anti-cardiolipin antibody and lupus anticoagulant) are by far the most widely investigated and are most consistently associated with these syndromes via their pro-thrombotic characteristics. There is also a lot of research implicating them in cognitive dysfunction, suggesting a pattern that is probably similar to that of vascular dementia.

Perhaps the most focus has been on anti-ribosomal P and anti-NMDA receptor antibodies for their role in lupus psychosis because of their apoptotic, rather than thrombotic or vasculitic, mechanism of cell death. Apoptosis and subsequent tissue necrosis have been the most common histopathological findings on biopsy (Johnson, 1968). Anti-ribosomal P antibody is the most studied antibody for lupus psychosis, but a meta-analysis (Reichlin, 2006) demonstrated that serum or CNS anti-ribosomal P antibody levels did not differentiate between different NPSLE syndromes or between organic versus primary psychiatric disease. The NMDA receptor antibody is the one most consistently associated with NPSLE (Fragoso-Loyo, 2008; Lauvsnes, 2011). In one study examining serum and CSF levels of five autoantibodies amongst patients with SLE, central NPLSE, peripheral NPSLE, and septic meningitis, only the anti-NMDA receptor antibody showed a distinctive distribution in central NPSLE, although it (and all other antibodies) was also elevated in patients with septic meningitis. The NMDA receptor binds glutamate and plays an important role in learning and memory. The anti-NMDA receptor antibody preferentially binds to the NMDA receptors in the hippocampus, resulting in the loss of hippocampal neurons via apoptosis, and therefore in memory impairment (Kowal, 2004; Kowal, 2006). Consequently, this raises the possibility of using NMDA receptor antagonists such as memantine as therapeutic intervention (Omdal, 2005; Colasanti, 2009), but efficacy studies are lacking.

Vasculopathy has been reported, a non-inflammatory vasculopathy involving the small vessels with vascular hyalinization, perivascular lymphocytosis, obliterative intimal fibrosis thrombosis, and leukagglutination (West, 1996; Pullman, 2004). The most predominant histopathological findings are reported to be multifocal, cerebral cortical micro-infarcts associated with microvascular injury. This vasculopathy causes decreased cerebral blood flow in several areas of the brain, including in the posterior cingulate and thalamus, as seen in psychotic disorders like schizophrenia. It is worth noting that an inflammatory process involving cerebral vessels, or vasculitis, is reported to be an extremely rare finding; therefore, the term "lupus cerebritis" is discouraged.

Some authors have reported increased cerebrospinal fluid (CSF) levels of inflammatory cytokines (Okamato, 2010); interleukins (IL) 1, 4, 6, 8, and 10; interferon α and γ; and tumor necrosis factor (TNF)-α; and chemokines: monocyte chemotactic protein-1 (MCP-1/CCL-2); interferon gamma inducible protein 10 (IP-10/CXCL-10); and Fractalkine (CX3CL1). It is thought that immune complex formation

Table 61.2 CNS-SPECIFIC AUTOANTIBODIES ASSOCIATED WITH NPSLE

CNS-SPECIFIC	NO. OF STUDIES SHOWING POSITIVE ASSOCIATION	CLINICAL SYMPTOMS ASSOCIATED WITH ANTIBODY
Antineuronal antibody	9	Cognitive impairment, non-focal NPSLE, psychosis (1 study, $N = 8$)
Anti-NMDA receptor antibody	4	Mood, cognition (by binding to NMDA receptor targets in hippocampus and causing cell death via apoptosis)
Anti-MAP-2 antibody	1	
Anti-neurofilament antibody	1	
Anti-ganglioside antibody	6 out of 8	Migraine, neuropathy, cognition, depression (1 study, $N = 448$)
Anti-CNS tissue antibody	2	
Anti-GFAP antibody	1	Non-specific NPSLE

NMDA–N-methyl D-aspartate; MAP-2–Microtubule Associated Protein-2; GFAP–Glial Fibrillary Acidic Protein

in the CNS stimulates a cascade of cytokine and chemokine activation, which in turn acts on monocytes, lymphocytes, and neutrophils and specific T cells to bring about CNS pathology resulting in NPSLE. Of the above cytokines implicated in the pathogenesis of NPSLE, IL-6 has the strongest positive correlation with lupus psychosis, in the context of preserved integrity of the blood–brain barrier. The significance of this is that the inflammatory response can occur in the CNS independent of systemic disease activity. Clinically, it aligns with the observation of CNS complaints in patients with otherwise "stable" disease. Such patients are typically referred to the psychiatrist, with a determination that their disease is stable, as serum investigations may also show that the systemic disease is quiescent. Their neuropsychiatric complaints may often get attributed to primary psychiatric illness or illness behavior. Increased levels of IL-6 mRNA have been found in hippocampus and cerebral cortex (Hirohata, 1999). However, not all studies have produced these results.

There is therefore insufficient evidence to support the routine use of lumbar puncture for CSF levels of these cytokines or autoantibodies in clinical practice as diagnostic tools in NPSLE, or of anti-ribosomal P or anti-NMDA receptor antibodies as a diagnostic tool for lupus psychosis.

CLINICAL FEATURES OF NPSLE

There is a significant paucity of studies looking at the phenomenology of psychiatric symptoms in NPSLE as a way of clinically differentiating between organic and non-organic disease in patients with SLE. Some anecdotes indicate that the hallucinations in NPLSE are more commonly visual, although they can certainly be auditory as well. Visual hallucinations have been described by several patients as typically involving faces distorting, animation of faces on wall pictures, or seeing a face or a person at the edge of the bed (observation from clinic population). Patients with stable, inactive SLE in the absence of other signs of NPSLE commonly report seeing nondescript black shadows transiently appearing in their peripheral field that disappear when they turn towards the perception.

There is no one pattern of cognitive impairment that defines SLE. Impairment can occur in one or more cognitive domains, and can be therefore termed *focal* or *multifocal* cognitive impairment. The specific cognitive domains include simple attention, complex attention, memory and learning, visuospatial function, reasoning and problem-solving, psychomotor speed, language (such as verbal fluency), and executive functioning (planning, sequencing, synthesis, drive). Cognitive impairment is defined as two or more standard deviations (SD) below the mean on neuropsychological testing, whereas a deficit of 1.5–1.9 SD below the mean is referred to as *cognitive decline* (Mikdashi, 2007). Cognitive impairment may follow a stepwise decline, with sharp decreases in function associated with acute flares, and an incomplete return to baseline upon flare remission. Thus the impairment becomes chronic, but static in between flares. Several patients describe this chronic, low-grade cognitive impairment as a "brain fog" and find it disabling. Although brain fog can occur in SLE patients with and without NPLSE, those with prior NPSLE are found to have more severe cognitive impairment (Hanly, 1997).

Symptoms of and criteria for depression in NPSLE are the same as those for a major depressive disorder. Symptom attribution becomes the key in differentiating the two, but this is a process riddled with subjectivity, particularly in the absence of a sensitive and specific biological marker for NPLSE. Features such as the presence of a contributory psychosocial history or the presence of a family history of psychiatric illness have not been shown to reliably help to differentiate organic from non-organic disease. In fact, many lupus flares are triggered by psychosocial stressors. There is an entire body of literature on the impact of psychological stress on cytokine activation, oxidative stress, and an inflammatory response. Thus the complex interplay of psychological factors with biological factors in depression in NPSLE makes it difficult to differentiate primary depression from mood disturbance due to a direct biological effect of lupus. An SLE Disease Activity Index (SLEDAI) (Gladman, 2002) can be applied in this circumstance. When there is no other systemic or serological sign of disease activity, it is thought that the symptoms are more likely to be attributable to a primary mental health problem rather than NPSLE. Thus the symptoms of depression and anxiety in NPSLE are phenomenologically similar to those in primary affective disorders in patients without SLE, and a history elucidating the temporal relationship of mood and anxiety symptoms with clinical and serological SLE disease activity may provide the only clue towards suspicion of NPSLE.

The occurrence of a single generalized seizure in patients with SLE does not necessitate anti-epileptic drug (AED) treatment, and does not necessarily mean that the patient will go on to have a recurrent seizure disorder. If the seizure is generalized and occurs in the context of a lupus flare without neurological localizing signs or focal damage on magnetic resonance imaging (MRI), treatment of the underlying lupus with prednisone and/or immunosuppressants such as intravenous methylprednisolone or intravenous cyclophosphamide is recommended (Barile-Fabris, 2005; Bertsias, 2010). If seizures are recurrent despite recovery from a lupus flare, or if seizures were partial with neurological localizing signs or focal lesions on MRI that raise suspicion of epileptic foci, then AEDs may be indicated.

Movement disorders occur more frequently, but not exclusively, in the subset of SLE patients who test positive for anti-phospholipid antibodies (Orzechowski, 2008) and have thrombotic events. The most commonly reported movement disorder in NPSLE is chorea (Cervera, 1997). It usually occurs as a single episode and subsides within weeks to months. MRI may still appear normal, as in most cases of NPSLE, and other imaging modalities that can detect altered function, such as positron emission tomography (PET) or single-photon emitted computed tomography (SPECT), are more likely to demonstrate changes in the basal ganglia. If generalized SLE activity is present, treatment with prednisone and immunosuppressants is recommended, with the addition of anticoagulation therapy if the patient is anti-phospholipid–antibody positive and other thrombotic manifestations are present (Bertsias, 2010).

IMAGING IN NPSLE

Computed tomography (CT) is of limited value in diagnosing NPSLE, unless an acute cerebral hemorrhage needs to be excluded. MRI is the current gold standard (Peterson, 2005; Stimmler, Coletti, & Quismorio [1993]) and should be done as part of the assessment of NPSLE. The MRI is, however, usually normal in NPSLE, and caution should be taken not to erroneously dismiss a possible diagnosis of NPSLE in the face of a normal MRI. Positive findings include transient, high-intensity, diffuse white matter lesions, more predominant in the frontoparietal area (Ishikawa, 1994; Jacobs, 1988; Chinn, 1997). Periventricular white matter lesions are thought to be associated more with anti-phospholipid–antibody syndrome. None of these findings, however, is specific for NPSLE, and similar findings are seen in other CNS disorders such as multiple sclerosis. They tend to occur early in the course of NPSLE and may resolve within the first 24 hours (Sibbit, 1999), and also resolve rapidly with corticosteroid

therapy (McCune, 1988; Sibbitt, 1989). MRI should therefore be done early in the course of illness, when NPSLE is suspected. The lesions are thought to represent edema and are therefore best visualized on T2-weighted images or fluid attenuated inversion recovery (FLAIR). FLAIR is more sensitive than T2-weighted MRI in NPSLE and is advantageous for use in clinical care (Sibbit, 2003). T1-weighted images will usually appear normal. Chronic lesions such as diffuse white matter disease, periventricular white matter hyperintensities, and focal subcortical lesions occur in about 25–50% of SLE patients without active NPSLE, and are more likely to be seen in patients with a history of more severe disease, in advanced age, and with a history of NPSLE (Jarek, 1994; Brooks, 1997; Rozell, 1998; Friedman, 1998; Hachulla, 1998). Lesion enhancement following gadolinium will help differentiate chronic from acute lesions (Miller, 1992), and radiologists also use certain morphological and intensity criteria of the lesions to help differentiate active NPLSE from non-specific white matter hyperintensities, from chronic SLE without CNS involvement, or from other causes such as hypertension.

Diffusion weighted imaging (DWI) and calculated the apparent diffusion coefficients (ADCs) show significant promise in NPSLE (Moritani, 2004; Welsh, 2007; Zhang, 2007) but are restricted to use in research as the data are limited. There are no studies comparing the sensitivity of FLAIR versus DWI. The same applies for diffusion tensor imaging (DTI), in which there are even fewer studies, but there is hope that it may help in diagnosis of NPSLE and even shed light on its pathogenesis in the future (Hughes, 2007).

Although functional MRI may detect the effects of SLE on cognition and brain function, it does not distinguish between chronic and acute effects, and there is no pattern of cognitive impairment that is specific for or suggestive of acute NPSLE. Serial testing to measure change might be more useful, but the degree of deterioration needed to be considered significant and the acuteness of the decline are not known factors and therefore make any such findings difficult to interpret. Such testing is not used in routine clinical practice and is still restricted to research or used for brain mapping, as in planning for neurosurgery and brain radiotherapy, or for documenting brain and cognitive deficits after traumatic or acquired brain injuries.

Therefore in the clinical setting, T2-weighted MRI is considered the gold standard, with FLAIR enhancing sensitivity and gadolinium enhancement helping to differentiate between acute and chronic lesions. Studies using DWI and DTI are promising but are in infancy stages and not used in routine clinical practice; there are no studies recommending these if MRI with T2, FLAIR, and gadolinium are negative. Functional MRI (fMRI) does not add any further value in the diagnosis of acute NPSLE.

Magnetic resonance spectroscopy (MRS) remains a research tool in NPSLE. It measures the levels of brain metabolites such as N-acetyl aspartate (NAA), total choline, and creatinine, to name a few. Brain NAA levels have been found to be reduced in NPLSE (Peterson, 2005), but again, this finding is not specific and can be seen in other disorders such as dementia of the Alzheimer's type, multiple sclerosis, and even obstructive sleep apnea (Fuller, 2004). It is also a transient finding, and its reversibility with treatment in cases such as epilepsy suggests reversible neuronal injury (Vermathen, 2002). There are no studies looking at whether NAA levels increase with treatment of NPSLE, and whether, therefore, MRS measuring NAA levels might be potentially useful for early diagnosis and monitoring response to treatment with the aim of preventing and/or predicting chronic CNS effects of NPSLE.

SPECT measures cerebral perfusion by detection of a radio-labelled tracer that is given intravenously prior to the procedure. There are several limitations with the use of SPECT. First of all, the studies are limited, and again, they mostly lack control or comparison groups. Secondly, the findings are variable. Altogether, the studies thus far suggest that SPECT is not very sensitive in detecting minor disease, but it has similar sensitivity to PET in detecting major CNS disease in NPSLE (Kao, 1999). A significant drawback is its high incidence of false positives (Borrelli, 2003). The most common finding is diffuse areas of hypoperfusion (Peterson, 2005). SPECT is, however, easier to administer and is appreciably cheaper than PET. It is often therefore the second modality used in clinical practice after, or in conjunction with, MRI.

PET measures metabolic activity in the brain by measuring glucose uptake and oxygen utilization. The most common observations on resting PET reported in patients with SLE are a higher frequency of gray matter than of white matter lesions, and hypometabolism in any part of the brain, but most frequently in the parieto-occipital and parietal areas (Otte, 1997; Weiner, 2000). Once again, these findings are not specific to NPSLE. PET has been demonstrated to have significantly higher sensitivity than MRI in detecting NPSLE, with several studies documenting normal MRIs where resting PET scans show hypometabolism, when both were done on the same patients at illness onset (Weiner, 2000; Otte, 1997; Kao, 1999), supporting the clinical observation of functional deficits in patients with subjective complaints of cognitive and/or psychiatric symptoms in the absence of structural deficits. Despite its greater sensitivity over MRI and consistent findings of parieto-occipital hypometabolism, there are not enough large studies to provide quantitative estimates of sensitivity and specificity. There are three studies in which resting PET abnormalities resolved with treatment and with clinical improvement of the NPSLE (Carbotte, 1992; Weiner, 2000; Otte, 1998), and a fourth study demonstrated correlation of PET findings with clinical course of the disease on longitudinal resting PET follow-up of 28 patients over a mean of 15 months (Weiner, 2000). Several other studies report resolution of PET findings with corticosteroid therapy or paralleling clinical improvement (Hiraiwa, 1983; Guttman, 1987; Otte, 1998; Meyer, 1989; Stoppe, 1990; Carbotte, 1992).

Although more sensitive than MRI in detecting NPSLE, resting PET has similar utility in helping to differentiate lupus-related from non-organic neuropsychiatric symptoms in patients with SLE (Weiner, 2000; Kao, 1999). Because of cost, invasiveness, and study limitations (such as lack of control groups in most studies), PET is not usually a first choice of imaging in routine clinical practice for evaluating NPSLE.

Its use is reserved for more complicated clinical pictures and clinical dilemmas, where MRI may have been normal or inconclusive and where PET results are likely to have practical implications for important treatment decisions.

In all imaging modalities, the findings of white or gray matter lesions are reported to be transient, and radiological findings on diffusion imaging modalities suggest that they most likely represent edema. Histopathological studies have consistently demonstrated a perivascular lymphocytic infiltration with increased capillary permeability and surrounding microedema, without antibody-complex formation or inflammatory changes. A true vasculitic picture is rarely found. For these reasons, the term "lupus cerebritis" is considered a misnomer, and "NPSLE" is the accepted term as it does not imply an etiopathogenesis, which is still unclear. Apart from the correlation of PET findings with clinical improvement and treatment response, the methodologies among the imaging studies are inconsistent in their reports of association with serology or symptoms, making it difficult to conclude whether the imaging findings correlate with serological activity, antibody type, symptom profile, or treatment response.

Thus MRI is the current gold standard imaging modality in the evaluation for NPSLE, and it should be done early, within 24 hours of suspicion of NPSLE. SPECT or PET may be done afterwards or in conjunction with MRI to further aid with diagnosis, depending on cost and availability.

TREATMENT OF NPSLE

Most psychotropic medications are safe in patients with lupus and the choice of medication should be individually tailored based on side effect profile, medical symptom complex, medication interactions, and phenotype of the psychiatric syndrome. For example, in depression, selective serotonin reuptake inhibitors (SSRIs) and serotonin and norepinephrine reuptake inhibitors (SNRIs) are safe to use, duloxetine may be particularly useful if chronic pain is comorbid, and bupropion may be chosen if fatigue is a prominent, but it may not be the first choice if the patient has symptoms of anxiety or NPSLE with seizures. If bupropion is being considered in a patient with a history of NPSLE, and there has never been a history of seizures, it is safe to use without need for a pre-treatment electroencephalogram (EEG). If there is a history of isolated seizure without focal brain damage, it is helpful to do an EEG prior to starting bupropion. If permanent focal brain damage accounts for the seizures, and if seizures are recurrent, bupropion is better avoided. The same is recommended if tricyclic antidepressants that lower the seizure threshold, such as clomipramine, imipramine, and amitriptyline, are being considered.

Psychosis, if determined to be due to NPSLE, will usually resolve with treatment of the lupus itself, but often adjunctive psychotropic medication is needed to expedite symptom control. The treatment of acute NPSLE with psychosis would assume the same hierarchy as treatment of an acute lupus flare, with preference for certain immunomodulators that have demonstrated specific efficacy for treatment of the psychosis. The hierarchy of treatment is as follows: oral high-dose prednisone, intravenous methylprednisolone, pulse cyclophosphamide, and rituximab (Trevisani, 2006; Tokunaga, 2007).

When patients are placed on high-dose steroids, a steroid psychosis may develop, which then complicates the clinical picture. A careful history must be taken to determine if the psychosis predated the initiation of steroid treatment, and to determine the temporal relationship between the development of psychotic symptoms and the initiation of steroid treatment. It is worth noting that the incidence of lupus psychosis in the pre-steroid era is not dissimilar to its incidence in the post-steroid era, after 1960 (Stern, 1960). Doses of oral prednisone of less than 40 mg are considered very unlikely to induce psychosis, while oral doses over 80 mg are considered more likely to induce psychosis. The phenomenology of steroid-induced psychosis is most similar to that of an affective psychosis seen in manic episodes. It is usually heralded by a brief period (24–48 hours) of insomnia and marked irritability. Despite these clinical clues, it is often difficult to make the differentiation between NPSLE psychosis and steroid-induced psychosis in the clinical setting, and often the addition of a psychotropic medication is necessary in either circumstance, as the underlying active lupus must be treated.

All neuroleptics are safe in NPSLE; again, paying attention to the individual patient in terms of medical comorbidity when choosing a specific medication. For example, in patients with pericarditis, care must be taken not to complicate the medical illness with psychotropics that have a high tendency to prolong the QTc interval. Risperidone, olanzapine, loxapine, and haloperidol are good first choices due to their higher affinity for the D2 receptor at fairly low doses, and to their tolerability, with predictable and easily manageable side effects. If agitation is an additional issue, a benzodiazepine can be added to the neuroleptic, which also facilitates response to lower doses of neuroleptics and helps reduce the incidence of extrapyramidal side effects. Quetiapine must be used in higher doses, which increases the risks of side effects of over-sedation and orthostatic changes in the blood pressure and heart rate. If insomnia is a prominent feature, however, the sedating side effects of quetiapine can be capitalized upon. Ziprasidone may exacerbate aggression and probably should not be first choice in patients with steroid-induced psychosis. Ziprasidone should be avoided in patients with pericarditis or pleuritis, as it raises the incidence of cardiac arrhythmias. The QTc interval should be monitored in the patient taking a neuroleptic, and patients should be examined for the emergence of extrapyramidal side effects. Dosing of neuroleptics is usually at a lower starting dose than usual, given the multisystem effects of the illness, with slow titration to clinical response tailored to the individual patient. Treatment should not be changed or altered prematurely, and medications should be given adequate time to have an effect while the lupus is also being treated. It usually takes several days to weeks for symptom control, and often the psychiatric symptoms lag behind the medical symptoms.

NPSLE syndromes, such as lupus psychosis, are not considered to be necessarily recurrent (Bertsias, 2010). Thus a patient with lupus psychosis does not require long-term antipsychotic treatment, which should be discontinued after the patient recovers and a period of stability has been achieved. Similar to seizures in NPSLE, lupus psychosis is not considered to be a chronic disorder, and patients and their families should be informed that full recovery from psychosis is expected (Pego-Reigosa, 2008). This is true for other affected organs as well, so that one episode of pericarditis does not necessarily mean permanent or recurrent cardiac pathology. There are only a few studies on long-term outcome of NPSLE. The available literature suggests that the natural course of SLE in patients with a history of NPSLE is not considered to be any different from the natural course of SLE in patients without such a history, as long as there was good immunosuppressive treatment of the NPSLE (Wang, 2012; Pego-Reigosa, 2008). The presence of NPSLE at presentation or during a lupus flare does not necessarily predict further NPSLE syndromes in subsequent flares. Few predictors of recurrent NPSLE have been found, and so far they are limited to the presence of anti-phospholipid antibodies, baseline severity of the disease, and the presence of permanent brain damage such as infarcts on MRI (Mikdashi, 2004).

OTHER PSYCHIATRIC DISTURBANCES IN SLE

ILLNESS BEHAVIOR AND SOMATIZATION IN SLE

Reaction to chronic illness and illness behavior in SLE reveals a fairly high incidence of somatization tendencies (Goodman, 2005). Most of these studies were in populations of young age, and early age of onset of illness. SLE, being a systemic disease, can affect any body system, any organ; and several symptoms are subjective. Even amongst the 19 NPSLE syndromes, symptoms can be vague and non-specific. The author has observed significant somatization tendencies; overreaction to vague, diffuse non-specific, non–life-threatening symptoms; and an apparently heightened perception of vague physical complaints in this population. A high level of alexithymia, which is commonly seen in patients with somatoform disorders, has been reported in this population (Barbosa, 2010).

Basic psychoeducation may be beneficial in some of these patients (Karlson, 2004). Stress-reduction strategies to target worry, fear, and illness anxiety may help. These include mindfulness-based stress reduction, breathing exercises, and progressive muscle relaxation. Basic support and education about coping with a chronic medical illness may also be helpful. As a general rule, patients with somatization tendencies or somatoform disorders take longer to respond to these treatment modalities, and improvement is even more difficult in a population with a known chronic medical illness. To avoid iatrogenic effects by secondary reinforcement of illness behavior and somatization, limited, regular, but not too frequent visits are suggested, such as once every one or two months, with focus on the above psychotherapeutic interventions and avoidance of over-investigation of multiple diffuse, vague, non-specific complaints. This is best done in a collaborative-care setting with close liaison between psychiatric and rheumatological services.

PSYCHOSOCIAL FACTORS IN SLE

The psychological impact of the illness includes high incidence of incomplete or interrupted education, threat to employability, difficulty securing relationships, difficulty bearing children, changes in physical appearance (moon-like facies, buffalo hump, and abdominal obesity associated with steroids; malar or "butterfly" rash; diffuse body rash with defacement and scarring), chronic fatigue, inability to fulfill life roles, social isolation, and impaired quality of life. These can all contribute to low self-esteem, self-rejection, and nihilism with increased risk of a clinical depression. The need for psychological support for coping with the impact of SLE should therefore always be assessed for these patients.

CHRONIC PAIN

Chronic pain can develop as a long-term sequela of SLE in the absence of active disease. In an acute flare, arthritis in SLE can affect any joint, most often the hands. Joints typically appear hot, red, and swollen. Treatment of the acute flare is often sufficient to treat the arthritis and associated pain. Avascular necrosis should be considered as a cause of acute pain in patients who are on long-term steroid treatment. Patients with SLE who have chronic pain often complain of diffuse muscle as well as joint pain. Some also complain of neuropathic pain. Often psychological factors are judged to be associated, and the presence of depression or maladaptive coping may heighten pain perception or increase the subjective burden and incurred disability of the chronic pain. Many of these patients may be diagnosed with fibromyalgia (discussed later in this chapter).

Chronic pain may be treated with basic analgesics such as acetaminophen or ibuprofen, on an as-needed or regular basis. Duloxetine and gabapentin, which have an effect on neuropathic pain, have also been successfully used. Referral to a pain specialist is frequently required, and many of these patients are often prescribed fentanyl patches, long-acting opioid preparations, and cannabinoids. This then complicates care due to controversies about drug-seeking behavior, dependence, and abuse versus bona fide need and therapeutic benefit. Sorting out the extent to which psychological and physical factors are contributing to the pain can be challenging, regardless of the underlying medical illness. Many patients request "medical marijuana," raising a lot of questions about the motives underlying these requests. Apart from clinical considerations, some physicians may struggle with moral or ethical issues surrounding this. Hesitation to prescribe can affect the therapeutic relationship and complicate the clinical encounter for both patient and physician. A systematic review of 18 trials of the efficacy of cannabinoids, including smoked cannabis and cannabis-based oral medicine, nabilone, and dronabinol, in patients with neuropathic pain, fibromyalgia (1 trial), rheumatoid arthritis (1 trial), and mixed chronic pain concluded that there is preliminary evidence of modest efficacy in fibromyalgia and rheumatoid arthritis (Lynch, 2011). The study's limitations were cited as short trial duration, small sample sizes, modest effect sizes, lack of examination of the potential for abuse, and patient attitudes about whether the modest reduction in pain intensity was clinically meaningful. Another review on the role of cannabinoids on chronic pain suggests that their efficacy and tolerability are still questionable, that they should not be considered first-line therapies where more supported and better-tolerated agents are available, and that they may be considered as adjunctive agents when other available treatments have failed (Turcotte, 2010). The latter is probably best done within a collaborative model with rheumatology and a comprehensive pain program, with one physician as designated prescriber to help monitor for misuse and avoid prescriptions from multiple sources. Mobility should be encouraged, and superimposed psychological factors—for example, coping mechanisms, acceptance of chronic illness, need for cognitive reframing, reactions to socio-occupational losses from the illness, and family support—should be addressed.

CHRONIC FATIGUE

Fatigue is a common complaint in patients with SLE. It can be acute and profound during a lupus flare, often being one of the presenting symptoms of a flare. Although withdrawal of steroid treatment after stabilization of a flare is very gradual, tapering over several months, secondary adrenal suppression during the steroid taper is a second possible cause of significant fatigue. Neither the dosage nor the duration of therapy is a reliable indicator of subsequent adrenal insufficiency, and it has been reported in courses of treatment as short as 14 days (Schlaghecke, 1992; Grinspoon, 1994; Oelkers, 1996; Henzen, 2000). Studies suggest it may take up to six months after steroid taper for the adrenal glands to recover full function (Morkane, 2011) and therefore for fatigue to improve. Also, fatigue can be chronic in patients with inactive disease who are otherwise stable. Individual- or group-graded exercise therapy can be recommended for chronic fatigue (White, 2011). If done in a group setting, the exercise prescription should be individually determined, based on the patient's exercise tolerance. It should be done by a qualified exercise therapist and planned jointly with the patient, increasing in duration and intensity every one to two weeks. The evidence is best for individual rather than group treatment.

Although stimulants such as modafinil and methylphenidate are not considered first-line treatments for fatigue, they have been safely used in this population. The doses are similar to those used in the psychiatric population, starting low and titrating slowly to clinical response. The author has used both medications in 15 patients, with about 50% of patients responding, as measured by subjective reports of some improvement in motivation and fatigue, coupled directly with improvement in occupational and daily function, as measured by task completion on a patient-generated task inventory (unpublished data). If there is no associated improvement in daily function, the medication is discontinued. Either medication can be chosen first, based on side effect profile and patient symptom complex. For example, if anxiety is comorbid, modafinil might be chosen over methylphenidate, due to the latter's risk of exacerbating anxiety.

Patients are informed that methylphenidate may suppress appetite, and this may be either an unwanted or a desirable side effect, depending on the individual patient. Modafinil is an inducer of cytochrome p450 3A4, and data on methylphenidate's effect on p450 enzymes are sparse and inconclusive, although it has been cited as an inhibitor of cytochrome p450 2D6 (Cozza, 2001). No drug interactions between either of these drugs with immunosuppressive SLE medications such as mycophenolate mofetil or hydroxychloroquine have been reported, but as in all patients taking multiple medications, caution must be exercised when prescribing, to be alert for potential drug interactions.

RHEUMATOID ARTHRITIS

Rheumatoid arthritis (RA) is a sporadically occurring disease of unknown cause. The strongest factors influencing disease expression are genetic and immunological. It affects women about twice as frequently as men. Although it can occur at any age, it has a peak age of onset in the fourth decade, with a sharp rise in incidence thereafter. It typically has a gradual onset, although both the course and clinical picture can be variable. This means that, despite the availability of diagnostic criteria, time for the evolution of symptoms is required before the diagnosis may actually be captured.

RA is a chronic inflammatory disorder affecting the joints. The process begins with inflammation of the synovium, which proliferates with each recurrence and eventually leads to bone erosion, destruction of joint cartilage, and loss of strength and elasticity of tendons and ligaments. One of the most common clinical features is diffuse, symmetrical joint pain and swelling affecting the small peripheral joints, such as the hands. Other affected joints include ankles, knees, wrists, and elbows. Joints may develop characteristic patterns of deformity (ulnar deviation of the fingers, swan-neck deformity, and boutonnière deformity), with or without subcutaneous nodules, often over the olecranon process and the ulna. This chronic inflammatory process can lead to mild illness with infrequent exacerbations and remissions, or it can follow a rapidly deteriorating course and lead to severe, disabling joint deformity and loss of physical function.

RA features extra-articular manifestations as well, such as fatigue, weight loss, fever, anorexia, and diffuse non-specific aching, and this may precede more characteristic joint symptoms. Some of these patients may be misdiagnosed with depression before the defining features of the illness reveal themselves. The effects of the disease are quite far-reaching, ranging from direct physical effects (from acute pain to chronic disability), to indirect physical and psychosocial effects (such as disturbances of sleep, fatigue, varying degrees of social and occupational impairment, and functional impairment in the instrumental and basic activities of daily living).

RA is a systemic illness, and cardiovascular disease is the leading cause of premature mortality. Cardiac complications include inflammation causing myocarditis and pericarditis, which lead to congestive heart failure, valvular insufficiency, and acceleration of atherosclerotic disease (Moreland, 2009).

Rheumatoid nodules may appear in lung parenchyma and in the airways, resulting in bronchial obstruction. Inflammation of the pleura can lead to pleurisy, and inflammation of lung parenchyma can lead to interstitial disease and progressive fibrosis (Amital, 2011). Gastroenterological manifestations occur usually as a complication of rheumatoid vasculitis, which develops in about 5% of RA patients. When vasculitis affects the intestinal tract, bowel ischemia and infarction may occur. Reduced esophageal motility can lead to dyspepsia and dysphagia. Mild pathological changes in the liver are seen in up to 92% of RA patients at autopsy (Ebert, 2011). Cases of autoimmune pancreatitis have been reported (Mustak, 2011). The eye may also be affected with scleritis and iridocyclitis. The nervous system is less commonly affected. Compression neuropathies can occur following joint deformities in the locale of major nerves, such as the peroneal, ulnar, and median nerves. CNS involvement is considered very rare. There has been one case of rheumatoid meningitis in a 66-year-old patient without a history of RA, but with high titers of rheumatoid factor and anti-cyclic citrullinated peptide antibody (Kim, 2011).

PSYCHIATRIC DISORDERS IN RA

Although RA is a systemic disease, direct neuropsychiatric complications are very rare (Moreland, 2009). More commonly, psychiatric disturbances occur as a consequence of coping with a chronic, disabling, and visibly deforming medical illness.

The prevalence of depression and anxiety in RA has been reported to be similar to that in other chronic medical illness, and is estimated at 21–34% (Creed, 1990; Pincus, 1996). The studies on which this figure is based took into account the somatic symptoms of depression that overlap with symptoms of RA, using an etiological approach, thus providing what is considered a more reliable and accurate estimate. Previous studies, which used an inclusive approach to diagnosing depression based on fulfilling a threshold number of depressive symptoms without consideration of symptom attribution, produced a much wider, and less accurate, range of 22–80% (Pincus, 1996). Psychosis as a consequence of RA is rare.

Most patients with RA will complain of symptoms of depression such as disturbed sleep, appetite, energy, and concentration, and reduced social activity. Sleep disturbance may be due to pain, while fatigue and anorexia may be systemic effects of the illness, and reduced social activity and engagement may be due to limitations imposed by physical disability rather than a low mood. When assessing for depression in patients with RA, therefore, it is helpful to consider the possibility of symptom contamination when applying diagnostic criteria for depression and anxiety. The Hospital Anxiety and Depression Scale (HADS) has attempted to capture depression and anxiety in medical patients while avoiding such symptom contamination, but there is still some debate about its psychometric properties and the advantages of other commonly used questionnaires (Bjelland, 2002). In routine clinical practice, however, symptom attribution, as in the etiological approach to using depression criteria in patients with medical illness (Koenig, 1997), might be adequate for diagnosis. This approach may be criticized for its subjectivity, but the role of sound clinical judgement and detailed clinical exploration of each depressive symptom in order to determine symptom attribution must not be overlooked. Furthermore, depression in RA may not present in its traditional manner. Patients with RA who are depressed often present to their rheumatologist with excessive complaints of pain and fatigue, anxiety about the disease, hypersensitivity to vague physical symptoms, frequent clinic visits, and increased complaints of disability (Hawley, 1988).

ETIOLOGY AND PATHOGENESIS OF PSYCHIATRIC DISTURBANCES IN RA

The similarity in the incidence of depression and anxiety between RA and other chronic medical illnesses suggests that the etiology of psychiatric symptoms in RA does not directly involve disease-specific factors. Several studies have examined the relationship between depression, anxiety, and various measures of disease activity and severity. In a review of studies examining the relationship of depression with disease severity and duration, there is a consistent finding of lack of direct correlation between measures of disease severity and activity (grip strength, erythrocyte sedimentation rate, total joint score, and duration of morning stiffness) or disease duration, and the presence or severity of depression and anxiety (Creed, 1990). Indeed, the determinants of depression in RA have been found to be the patients' attitude to illness, personality, and socioeconomic factors such as age, education level, marital status, and family income, rather than the disease's activity, duration, or its disabling effects (McFarlane, 1988; Hawley, 1988). These are similar to the determinants of anxiety and depression in patients without RA or a medical illness. Studies have documented that the presence of depression and anxiety in RA is significantly more reflective of lack of social support and experience of social stress, rather than the disabling effects of RA (Murphy, 1988; Creed, 1990). In addition, employment status correlates more with depression than with disease severity or activity. A past history of depression predicts greater complaints of pain in patients with RA. Such patients may receive a secondary diagnosis of fibromyalgia.

Depending on various parameters of personality, such as general response to stress, attitudes towards illness, and coping mechanisms, the patient may or may not react poorly to increasing physical disability. Therefore, these personality factors may shape the disease expression, rather than the disease's having a direct effect on personality, such as in some cases of temporal lobe epilepsy. Therefore, early views of the "rheumatoid personality" are no longer substantiated.

Lipowski wrote on coping mechanisms with regards to medical illness and classified them into "adaptive" and "maladaptive," based on their likelihood to result in psychopathology (Lipowski, 1970). This is shown in Box 61.3.

"Positively reappraising a situation" means to attempt to deliberately perceive it in a way that leads to more positive

action. Lipowski wrote about coping with medical illness by identifying perceptions of illness. If we perceive illness (for example) as a punishment, this is likely to lead to feelings of despair, low self-worth, hopelessness, and nihilism. If, on the other hand, we perceive illness as a challenge, it leads to feelings of wanting to rise above it, to take control and do whatever is necessary to manage it so we can move on with our regular activities as much as possible. Box 61.4 shows some examples of healthy versus unhealthy responses to illness, according to Lipowski.

Personality factors such as temperament, tendency towards dependency, and external locus of control may determine whether maladaptive coping mechanisms are utilized and whether unhealthy responses to illness are adopted. These are the factors that correlate with mood disturbance in patients with RA, rather than the disease severity, activity, or disabling consequences.

As in all cases of depression, socioeconomic factors may play a contributing or protective role. Lack of social support, lack of family support, and marginalization from society are important predisposing and perpetuating factors in depression in RA patients. Studies have shown that perceived spousal support plays a big role in depression and length of hospitalization after acute illness in RA (Creed, 1990). Loss of social function and reduced employability can lead to eroding self-esteem. Coping with fatigue can be emotionally taxing and can limit social engagement. Self-consciousness and negative self-perception from physical changes in joints and from steroid treatment contribute to social withdrawal and depression.

Perhaps because CNS abnormalities are so rare, there are few studies examining brain imagining and function in patients with RA. In a 2012 study (Hamed, 2012), the authors performed a battery of psychological tests, measured P300 amplitude in event-related potentials, and measured serum levels of neuronal cell markers. P300 latency and increased levels of neuronal cell markers correlated with poorer cognitive function, which was reported in 71% of their sample of 55 women. Only seven patients with cognitive dysfunction had MRIs showing white matter hyperintensities. The authors concluded that this was evidence that demyelination or vasculitis—the disease process—was directly affecting cognitive function in patients with RA. However, none of their outcome measures (P300 latency, serum levels of neuronal cell markers) are specific to RA, and cognitive dysfunction did not correlate with disease severity. Several confounding factors could have explained the fairly common finding of mild cognitive impairment and the observed MRI changes in middle age.

As of this writing, there are no reliable studies suggesting direct CNS involvement in patients with RA or outlining consistent CNS neuropathology, and it is still considered a rare entity. No specific pattern of cognitive deficit has been identified. Thus psychiatric CNS symptoms such as depression, anxiety, and cognitive complaints in RA have not been shown to correlate with disease activity or severity and can be thought of as resulting from a complex interplay of indirect consequences of RA, personality factors, psychosocial factors, and, to some extent, medication side effects.

TREATMENT

The treatment of depression and anxiety in patients with RA is similar to that in patients without RA, with a few additional considerations. Although SSRIs are generally safe, most patients with RA are on non-steroidal anti-inflammatory drug (NSAID) therapy for pain, and care must be taken to monitor for gastrointestinal (GI) bleeding. SSRIs induce increases in gastric acid secretion, causing one of their more common side effects, dyspepsia. It is thought that this, coupled with SSRIs' effects on platelet binding, increases the risk of GI bleeding. Although the absolute risk of GI bleeds with SSRIs is low, this risk increases twofold when SSRIs are combined with NSAIDs, anticoagulants, and antiplatelet agents, and is decreased by concurrent use of proton pump inhibitors (Andrade, 2010).

Drug–drug interactions must be taken into account when prescribing. There are no anti-rheumatic drugs that will be affected by prescription of psychotropics. Some potential interactions might include reduced efficacy of mycophenolate mofetil by CYP 3A4 induction by modafinil; or reduced efficacy of tricyclic antidepressants (TCAs), citalopram, or escitalopram via CYP 2C19 induction by prednisone. The clinical significance of these interactions is not known. One important clinically significant interaction is reduced efficacy of opioid analgesics when co-administered with potent CYP 2D6 inhibitors such as fluoxetine or paroxetine. These analgesics require metabolism by CYP 2D6 for conversion to active metabolites. SSRI-induced sexual dysfunction may add to problems that patients with RA already face in terms of limited sexual activity due to physical consequences of the illness. On the other hand, to the extent that decreased libido exists as a symptom of depression and anxiety, SSRIs may be helpful. Apart from these concerns, SSRIs are generally safe for use in patients with RA. Because patients with depression and anxiety have heightened pain perception, SSRIs may also be helpful in reducing complaints of pain. SSRIs also have a theoretical biological effect on pain as one of the two powerful descending pain-dampening or pain-modulating tracts that affect the ascending lateral spinothalamic tract as they carry pain sensations to the thalamus, is a serotonergic tract. Special consideration can be given to the use of the SNRI duloxetine for treatment of depression and anxiety in RA because of its demonstrated beneficial effects on pain in the clinical setting.

Bupropion may be chosen if fatigue, weight gain, apathy, or sexual dysfunction are prominent features of the depression. Mirtazapine is useful for anxiety and for depression with marked anorexia and insomnia, but weight should be monitored, as weight gain will exacerbate joint pain and instability, and some patients may be on concomitant steroids, already contributing to weight gain.

Patients should be screened for drug dependence before considering use of benzodiazepines, since patients can often be on several controlled narcotic analgesics for refractory pain. As is the case with most patients, benzodiazepines are better used in the short term rather than long-term, because of the risk of physical and psychological tolerance and dependence and risk of abuse.

Psychological therapies for RA include psychoeducation about the illness and its effects. Patients should have a clear understanding of the illness course and expectations of outcome. It is useful for the psychiatrist to be aware of such prognostic information, which is provided to the patient by the rheumatologist, as it would help guide therapy, for example, in terms of how much emphasis can be placed on acceptance of chronicity of a specific symptom, should that be the illness course in that particular patient. This is probably best facilitated via an educational support group run collaboratively between the rheumatology and psychiatry services. This also helps ensure that the patient is receiving consistent information from all care providers. This would help with their participation in the treatment, so as to avoid a complete external locus of control. In the latter case, such patients frequently complain about symptoms and project helplessness, which contributes significantly to poor social outcome and increased disability regardless of disease severity. Increased participation in their care and "self-regulation" (goal setting, planning, self-monitoring, feedback, and relapse prevention) has been found to be beneficial to many patients with RA and to play a role in reducing symptoms of anxiety and depression (Mulligan, 2003; Knittle, 2010).

Cognitive behavior therapy is useful for depression and anxiety if the patient is able to engage. Psychotherapies for anxiety such as mindfulness-based stress reduction, breathing exercises, and progressive muscle relaxation should be considered and can help with coping with pain as well. Alternative interventions like meditation and tai chi have been found to be helpful in the RA population, as they enhance cardiovascular fitness, muscle strength, balance, and physical function and are associated with reduction in stress, anxiety, and depression, and improved quality of life (Hewlett, 2011; Wang, 2011).

Patients with RA suffer varying degrees of social disadvantage, and RA has been associated with reduced employability. Embarrassment about physical changes in the body can lead to restriction of social activity. These factors can contribute to social isolation. Social support is an important determinant of psychiatric symptomatology and quality of life. While psychotherapy can help with coping, patients should be encouraged to mobilize social and family supports and remain engaged in their family and community. Social support can also occur via support groups or encouraging active participation in community activities. Volunteering has been shown to be very helpful for depression in patients with chronic medical illness (Thoits, 2001). Optimization of function is key. Physical therapy and rehabilitation may be helpful for joint and muscle function and for avoiding accelerated muscle atrophy. Physical exercise can be helpful for the physical effects of the illness (Knittle, 2010) as well as for depression, anxiety, stress, and cognitive function. It should be encouraged in all patients if possible. There are guidelines for prescribing physical exercise in patients with RA, and referral to a multidisciplinary clinic for rheumatological disorders should be considered where available.

SJÖGREN'S SYNDROME

Sjögren's syndrome (SJS) is an autoimmune illness in which antibodies are produced that target the exocrine glands, most commonly the lacrimal and salivary glands. The most common symptoms are therefore dry eyes and dry mouth. Specific antibodies, anti-Ro and anti-La, are associated with SJS.

Several other systemic manifestations can be present, including dyspepsia, myalgia, arthralgia, Raynaud's syndrome, dry skin with pruritus and photosensitivity, alopecia, vaginal dryness, and dyspareunia. Associated systemic diseases include pancreatic insufficiency, primary biliary cirrhosis, hypothyroidism, and scleroderma. CNS effects are controversial and are considered uncommon (Brito, Araujo, & Papi, 2002). However, several small studies demonstrate the mental impact of SJS (Gilberto, 2002; Mauch, 1994; Malinow, 1985; Andonopoulos, 1990). The spectrum of its mental impact can vary from strain from coping with a chronic medical illness, to clinical depression, anxiety, or cognitive effects.

PSYCHIATRIC DISORDERS IN SJÖGREN'S SYNDROME

The most common psychiatric complications of SJS have been identified as depression, anxiety, cognitive complaints, sleep disturbance, irritability, and headaches (Malinow, 1985; Gudbjörnsson, 1993; Valtýsdóttir, 2000). With respect to depression, low mood is the most common disturbance and has been found to correlate with fatigue (Rostron, 2002). Fatigue is a very serious problem in primary SJS and may be composed of different elements, including general fatigue, mental fatigue, physical fatigue, reduced activity, and reduced motivation. It may also be related to hypotension, which can develop from autonomic nervous system dysfunction from CNS SJS (Barendregt, 1998). Common symptoms of anxiety reported by patients with SJS include feeling more restless, feeling tense, having more difficulty relaxing, and having feelings of panic (Valtýsdóttir, 2000).

Patients with SJS tend to complain of "brain fog." The exact frequency of cognitive impairment in SJS is unknown, as the few available studies are limited by sample size and lack of standardized cognitive assessment. From some of the available data (Malinow, 1985; Spezialetti, 1993; Mauch, 1994; Lafitte, 2001; Segal, et al., 2012), the prevalence of cognitive impairment ranges from 20–70% (sample size range of 16–39) of patients with primary SJS without other CNS involvement, and from 27–35% (sample size range of 11–77) of patients with CNS SJS (Lafitte, 2001; Spezialetti, 1993). "Brain fog" in SJS is defined as a mild dysfunction of concentration, short-term memory, and cognitive-processing speed, which is disruptive to the patient's lifestyle. Patients often complain of having trouble concentrating, being forgetful, or finding that their memory is just not what it used to be, having difficulty finding words during conversation, having difficulty understanding information, feeling that they are just not a sharp as before, needing more time to process information, getting lost more frequently, and feeling the need to repeat things several times before understanding fully. Neuropsychological testing has documented impairment in attention and concentration, impaired associate learning, mild short-term-memory impairment, decreased perceptual speed, and difficulty with names, in the context of preserved generalized intelligence quotient (IQ) without any intellectual decline, except in one study showing mild intellectual decline compared to premorbid intellectual function in four out of 16 patients with primary SJS (Mauch, 1994).

Cognitive impairment can occur at any time during SJS. It has a very insidious onset, and may be chronic, recurrent, and in some cases may spontaneously remit. It is considered very rare that it would deteriorate into progressive memory impairment or dementia. In such progressive cases, it tends to be associated with active symptoms of SJS, and in those cases, treatment of the underlying disorder with prednisone or methylprednisolone usually also treats the cognitive impairment (Caselli, 1991; Alexander, 1992; Kawashima, 1993; Moll, 1993; Cox, 1999; Michel, 2011).

ETIOLOGY AND PATHOGENESIS OF PSYCHIATRIC DISTURBANCES IN SJÖGREN'S SYNDROME

In most cases, the psychosocial impact of the illness is the largest determinant of depression and anxiety. SJS can affect several aspects of life, including physical function, role function, social function, mental health, health perception, pain, and fatigue. These are all determinants of health-related quality of life, and therefore contribute to the overall mental impact of the disease.

Patients with SJS experience an inability to fulfill various role functions: work, family, social, and personal. Social interaction is at risk of being diminished because of issues around eating, swallowing, chewing food, and sustaining prolonged conversation. Fatigue, genitourinary sicca symptoms, and dyspareunia contribute to sexual dysfunction and affect intimate relationships. Lack of support or unsupportive environments can perpetuate low mood and anxiety.

Investigations into the role of biological factors have found inflammatory processes involving cytokines such as IL-6 and interferon-α to be associated with depression (Alexander, 1992). Although their involvement in depression in SJS has been postulated, it has not been empirically proven. One of the most common hypotheses is that neurological involvement in the form of autonomic neuropathy in SJS (Andonopoulos, 1995) leads to decreased levels of plasma norepinephrine. Correlation between decreased plasma norepinephrine levels and general fatigue, physical fatigue, and reduced activity has been reported. (Barendregt, 1998). In this study, there was no correlation between plasma norepinephrine levels and depression, but the patients with depression had added features of mental fatigue and reduced motivation. Based on this study, noradrenergic antidepressants might be chosen first, if medications are being considered.

Although a few antibodies have been reported to be involved, no one antibody has yet been isolated that is consistently associated with, or specific for, CNS symptoms in SJS such as depression, anxiety, or cognitive deficits.

No association has been found between cognitive deficits and anti-Ro or anti-La antibodies (Belin, 1999; Alexander, 1993). One of the more common findings in patients with cognitive deficits is a perivascular mononuclear inflammatory ischemic/hemorrhagic cerebral vasculopathy, causing ischemic damage (Alexander, 1993; Cox, 1999; Belin, 1999). This may be seen on an MRI as transient findings of multiple small areas of hyperintensity. SPECT studies have documented impairment of flow to certain parts of the brain, consistent with this hypothesis (Belin, 1999). However, such impairment of blood flow has been found to be quite mild.

TREATMENT

Depression, low mood, and anxiety negatively affect disease outcome by affecting compliance with treatment; decreasing physical, social, and mental activity; decreasing motivation; and compounding fatigue. Patients with depression are more likely to report decreased health-related quality of life, increased pain perception, and perception of illness burden. Depression slows recovery from physical illness because of its additive physical effects.

The treatment for depression in SJS is not different from that of depression in patients without medical illness. With respect to the pharmacotherapies, one consideration might be to avoid xerogenic antidepressants. Although most antidepressants have some xerogenic effects, TCAs, paroxetine, and high-dose venlafaxine carry the highest incidence, followed by bupropion and duloxetine. The last two antidepressants might be good choices due to their noradrenergic effects, and a risk–benefit ratio needs to be considered, based on the individual patient's symptoms and their tolerability. Serotonergic antidepressants with superior tolerability such as escitalopram or sertraline might be good first choices.

In cases where cognitive decline has been acute or subacute, progressive, and associated with other physical or neurological symptoms, case reports have reported improvement with corticotherapy, as mentioned above. One study examined the inhibiting effect of hydroxychloroquine on salivary gland cholinesterase and correlated an increase in salivary gland acetylcholine with clinical symptom improvement (Dawson, 2005). Surprisingly, however, there have been no studies examining the effect of cholinesterase inhibitors and other nootropic agents in treating the more common subtle cognitive decline of insidious onset in the absence of other symptoms of active SJS, referred to previously as "brain fog." Intuitively, these agents would seem useful because of their favorable effects on xerostomia and xeroopthalmia, two core symptoms of SJS.

Non-pharmacological intervention may include neuropsychological testing when indicated to document the deficits and explore the potential for cognitive rehabilitation, where strategies for optimizing current brain function can be taught. Physical activity has been associated with increased cerebral blood flow to the brain, including the parts that subserve memory, and it has been shown to be associated with documented improvement in cognitive function (Ratey, 2011). Social activity allows the practice of various cognitive domains such as thoughtful conversation, verbal fluency, comprehension, and cognitive processing. Physical activity and social engagement are also helpful for coexisting anxiety and depression, both of which can affect memory. Exercises such as creative writing, reading, and problem-solving serve to at least maintain brain function. Therefore, patients should be encouraged to keep socially, mentally, and physically active for positive effects on mood, anxiety, and cognitive function.

FIBROMYALGIA

DEFINITION

Fibromyalgia is a syndrome of widespread, diffuse, chronic pain associated with other features such as psychological factors, insomnia, and fatigue, and in which no organic cause for the symptoms can be identified. It affects about 2% of the population, with a female preponderance, and onsets between 30–50 years. The diagnosis has historically been controversial, and although it is gaining more acceptance by the medical community, patients with fibromyalgia still frequently report feeling stigmatized by physicians.

PATHOPHYSIOLOGY

Several factors have been implicated in the pathophysiology of the fibromyalgia syndrome, including (1) genetic factors; (2) altered pain processing at the level of the CNS; (3) altered pain perception at the level of the CNS (the latter two composing the central sensitization hypothesis); (4) viral causes; and (5) psychosocial factors.

Genetic factors are thought to play a role due to observation of familial clustering. First-degree relatives of affected patients are reported to have an eight-fold increase in the risk of expression of the syndrome (Arnold, 2004). Other studies have suggested a link with certain human lymphocyte antigen (HLA) types, (Yunnus, 1999), and others have found variations in genotype of different genes such as the promoter region of the serotonin transporter gene, polymorphisms in the $5HT_{2A}$ receptor gene, and in the dopamine D_4 gene (Ablin, 2009).

Pain processing has been frequently studied in fibromyalgia. Altered pain processing has been fairly consistently reported. Normally, peripheral nociceptors carrying pain stimuli arrive at the dorsal horn of the spinal cord via two afferent fibers: the small, thinly myelinated Aδ fibers and the small, unmyelinated C fibers. Using substance P, they synapse with interneurons that cross to the contralateral side and ascend via the lateral spinothalamic tract. The excitatory neurotransmitter glutamate is also released presynaptically and involved in central pain processing. Descending inhibitory fibers release serotonin at the same synapse before the interneurons cross over and ascend to carry pain signals to the brain. These descending pathways serve to modulate and dampen pain perception before the signal reaches the brain. In patients with chronic pain, both afferent input to the dorsal horn and levels of presynaptic substance P are increased (Bradley, 2009). What is not known is whether this represents cause or effect.

The response to pain in patients with fibromyalgia has been examined using functional MRI. Two major findings have been reported (Gracely, 2002). Firstly, increased signals in pain-responsive cerebral areas with lower pain stimuli were detected compared to controls, suggesting that patients with fibromyalgia have a lower threshold for perceiving pain and greater response to pain. Secondly, in the control groups, some areas of the brain showing increased signals were not active in patients with fibromyalgia. This led to the hypothesis that these areas may represent reduced activity in the descending inhibitory serotonergic pathways; however, the latter has not been demonstrated. Once again, whether these findings represent the cause of the altered response to pain or the effect of the classic response to pain in fibromyalgia, remains to be determined.

Taken together, the findings of increased central pain processing and increased pain signaling with lower pain stimuli is referred to as "central sensitization." It is currently the accepted theory accounting for chronic widespread pain in patients with fibromyalgia.

To date, no study has been able to make a direct causal link between viral infection and fibromyalgia. In several cases, patients report a preceding viral infection, but it is thought that this may represent a triggering factor for the expression of symptoms in the context of many other, usually psychosocial, factors, rather than a unifactorial direct cause of the illness. Limited data suggest increased prevalence of fibromyalgia in patients with HIV, HTLV-1, hepatitis B, and hepatitis C infections (Dinerman, 1992; Marquez, 2004; Cruz, 2006; Adak, 2005; Rivera 1007; Buskila, 1997). Even in these cases, associated psychosocial factors are significant and are thought to play an important role in symptom expression.

Psychosocial factors are usually quite prevalent in patients with fibromyalgia, although this history may be not elicited in early assessments. Patients may not be forthcoming about psychosocial factors, as many are aware of stigmatization and already feel rejected by the medical society. By the time they arrive at the liaison psychiatrist's office, they may have undergone various investigations and had some feedback about the diagnosis. Often the diagnosis is not well accepted, and some patients may insist on searching for a single cause. Studies have, however, recorded strong associations between fibromyalgia and a history of abuse, neglect, or a difficult childhood (Walker, 1997a). Fibromyalgia should also raise concern for physical abuse in adulthood, as an association has been demonstrated in one study (Walker, 1997b). Other frequently found external factors include preceding work-related injuries and poor job satisfaction, and a history of preceding motor vehicle accident and/or whiplash injury, although studies have produced mixed results of the prevalence of fibromyalgia in the latter population (Buskila, 1997; Harkness, 2004). Often there is a high incidence of underlying comorbid post-traumatic stress disorder and anxiety in patients with fibromyalgia (Jason, 2002).

Several other factors have been studied, but with limited results, thus their role in fibromyalgia remains unknown. These include levels of ferritin, magnesium, and zinc. The role of oxidative stress might be gaining more popularity.

CLINICAL FEATURES

The 1990 diagnostic criteria from the American College of Rheumatology (Wolfe, 1990) are shown in Box 61.5.

These diagnostic criteria highlight widespread musculoskeletal pain and tenderness, affecting both sides of the body, both below and above the hips, and including the axial skeleton as the classic features of fibromyalgia. A recent publication by the ACR (Wolfe, 2010) suggests that the tender-point exam may not be necessary for diagnosis, and provides revised preliminary diagnostic criteria for fibromyalgia that include not just chronic widespread pain as in the 1990 criteria, but also associated features that are commonly reported by patients with fibromyalgia, and a severity scale for those symptoms. These symptoms were so consistently prominent that they have come to be appreciated as key features of fibromyalgia. They include sleep disturbance, low energy, and complaints of memory impairment. The symptom severity scale attempts to address complaints of significant functional impairment and reduced quality of life as a result of these symptoms. Numerous general somatic symptoms with a severity scale are also included in the revised preliminary diagnostic criteria of 2010 (Box 61.6).

There are several studies examining the nature of sleep disturbance in fibromyalgia, and the full range has been reported: from difficulty initiating sleep, difficulty maintaining sleep, and early-morning awakening, to unrefreshing sleep. The most prominent type of sleep disturbance in fibromyalgia is non-restorative sleep. Although the DSM-IV defines this as "self-reported restless, light or poor quality sleep," the definition used in fibromyalgia studies is sleep that is subjectively unrefreshing regardless of sleep latency, duration, or continuity. Therefore, the 2010 preliminary diagnostic criteria list this symptom as "waking unrefreshed." Due to lack of consensus on the definition of non-restorative sleep in fibromyalgia studies, there are no reliable estimates of its prevalence. Non-restorative sleep is prevalent in mood and anxiety disorders—34.2% in one study (Taylor, 2005)—which are common comorbidities in fibromyalgia, and is also common in the general population after a stressful event in the absence of a diagnosable psychiatric disorder (Ohayon, 2005).

Many researchers have looked into the relationship between chronic widespread pain and quality of sleep in fibromyalgia. From the available studies, it is generally agreed that poor sleep predicts greater pain the following day, which negatively affects physical functioning and contributes to depression and worsening fatigue. The bidirectionality of the relationship between sleep quality and pain intensity, however, has not been demonstrated in all studies, so changes in pain intensity did not always correlate with changes in sleep quality in the same patient (Affleck, 1996).

A review of polysomnographic studies in patients with fibromyalgia (Spaeth, 2011) indicated that most studies have captured interruptions of slow wave sleep (SWS) by alpha EEG activity, called "alpha intrusions" or "EEG alpha sleep disorder" (16 studies). None of the polysomnographic findings is specific to or pathognomic for fibromyalgia, but the findings are as follows:

1. Alpha intrusions—pronounced EEG alpha activity during SWS (stages III and IV of non-rapid eye movement [REM] sleep)—corresponding to an increased number of arousals from SWS, characteristic of patients with fibromyalgia (16 studies)

2. Delayed sleep onset on EEG (1 study)

3. Reduced SWS and REM sleep (3 studies)

4. Poorer sleep efficiency (1 study)

Studies have documented certain pathophysiological effects of sleep on pain thresholds:

1. Restorative sleep is attributed to SWS. On a review of sleep in fibromyalgia (Spaeth, 2011), several studies have documented reduced pain threshold and induction of widespread musculoskeletal pain and fatigue upon total sleep-deprivation or experimental disruption of SWS, and one study documented reversal of pain with sleep restoration (Onen, 2001).

2. In line with the CNS sensitization hypothesis underlying pain in fibromyalgia, CNS hypersensitivity, as reflected in fibromyalgia patients by multiple somatic complaints and multiple sensitivities such as to sound or light, can be caused by fragmentation of SWS (Yunnus, 2007).

Criteria

All of the following three are met:

1. Widespread pain index (WPI) ≥7 and symptom severity (SS) scale score ≥5 or WPI 3–6 and SS scale score ≥9

2. Symptoms have been present at a similar level for at least three months

3. Absence of another disorder that would otherwise explain the pain

Ascertainment

1. WPI: Record the number of areas from 0–19 in which the patient has had pain over the past week.
   Left and right (2 points maximum for each):
      Shoulder girdle, Chest
      Upper arm, Abdomen
      Lower arm, Upper back
      Hip (buttock, trochanter), Lower back
      Upper leg, Neck
      Lower leg, Jaw

2. SS scale score = severity score for the three key associated symptoms + the extent of somatic symptoms; score range = 0–12
   3 key associated symptoms:
      Fatigue
      Waking unrefreshed
      Cognitive symptoms
   For each of the three symptoms above, indicate the level of severity over the past week using the scale below:
      0 = no problem
      1 = slight or mild problems, generally mild or intermittent
      2 = moderate, considerable problems, often present and/or at a moderate level
      3 = severe: pervasive, continuous, life-disturbing problems

Somatic symptoms:

Muscle pain, irritable bowel syndrome, fatigue/tiredness, thinking or remembering problem, muscle weakness, abdominal pain/cramps, numbness/tingling, dizziness, insomnia, depression, constipation, pain in upper abdomen, nausea, nervousness, chest pain, blurred vision, fever, diarrhea, dry mouth, itching wheezing, Raynaud's phenomenon, hives/welts, ringing in ears, vomiting, heartburn, oral ulcer, loss of/change in taste, seizures, dry eyes, shortness of breath, loss of appetite, rash, photosensitivity, hearing difficulties, easy bruising, hair loss, frequent urination, painful urination, and bladder spasms.

*For the somatic symptoms above, indicate whether the patient has:

0 = No symptoms

1 = Few symptoms

2 = A moderate number of symptoms

3 = A great deal of symptoms

*No numerical cut-off for the somatic symptom scale was indicated for determining "few" versus "moderate number" versus "great deal" of symptoms.

---

3. More than half of the total daily production of growth hormone (GH) occurs at the onset of SWS. Disruption of SWS is associated with decreased production of GH and insulin-like growth factor-1 (IGF-1).

Several studies have documented decreased GH and IGF-1 levels in patients with fibromyalgia (Bennett, 1997; Leal-Cerro, 1999; Yuen, 2007; Cuatrecasas, 2009; Cuatrecasas, 2010). GH and IGF-1 have an important role in the repair of microtrauma to muscle tissue, which occurs with the normal physical strain on muscle with daily activity. Thus SWS fragmentation has been found to be associated with chronic widespread pain via reduced muscle repair due to low GH and IGF-1 levels in patients with fibromyalgia, coupled with heightened pain sensitivity. Indeed, some studies have demonstrated improvement in pain with GH-replacement therapy (Bennett, 1998; Cuatrecasas, 2007).

The mechanism for alpha intrusions during SWS in patients with fibromyalgia has not been elucidated, but the roles of some of the same neurotransmitters involved in chronic widespread pain in fibromyalgia, particularly substance P and serotonin, have been studied. Studies in mice have shown increased sleep latency and an increased number of arousals after ventricular administration of substance P (Andersen, 2006). Animal and human studies have shown that decreased serotonin can induce insomnia (Moldofsky, 2009).

It is therefore recommended that assessment of the patient with fibromyalgia should include a detailed sleep history. The ACR, based on the 2010 revised preliminary diagnostic criteria, developed a visual analog scale as a patient-report measure of sleep disturbance, which may also be helpful in assessment. It is important to assess for other disorders associated with sleep disturbance such as mood disorders, periodic limb movement of sleep, sleep apnea, diabetes, and thyroid disorders, to name a few. Currently, there are insufficient data to suggest routine use of a polysomnogram in clinical practice, but it is recommended if a primary sleep abnormality is suspected. Sleep hygiene education, encouragement of physical activity, dietary contributions to sleep disturbance (caffeine, chocolate, cigarettes, alcohol), medication review, and treatment of comorbid disorders (e.g., depression, thyroid disorders) all are essential elements of assessment and management.

A significant proportion of patients with SLE and RA can meet criteria for fibromyalgia even before those diagnoses are made. Several patients will have symptoms of depression, anxiety (especially generalized anxiety disorder and post-traumatic stress disorder [PTSD]), and somatoform disorders (especially somatization disorder or undifferentiated somatoform disorder). Depending on how the diagnosis is presented, patients can be amenable to treatment by a psychiatrist for the underlying comorbid psychiatric disorders and associated psychosocial factors, and they may be receptive to taking antidepressants for helping with complaints of pain, sleep, and fatigue as well. Patients may be guarded about sharing their psychosocial history for fear of stigmatization. When job-related or legal factors are foremost, it can complicate case management, and features of malingering should be ruled out.

TREATMENT

Several systematic reviews have recently been undertaken, and some consensus has been reached on treatment recommendations for fibromyalgia (Garcia Campayo et al., 2010). Table 61.3 summarizes its pharmacological treatment, and Table 61.4 summarizes its non-pharmacological treatment.

Based on the proposed pathophysiological theories and the availability of evidence to support or refute them, antivirals, immunosuppressants, and steroid therapy have no role in the treatment of fibromyalgia to date. The aim of pharmacotherapy is control of the core and associated major symptoms, with a goal of improvement in quality of life and restoration of optimal function. The core symptoms that are the targets of pharmacotherapy are pain, sleep disturbance, fatigue, and depression. There is no specific treatment that is approved by the United States Food and Drug Administration (FDA) or the European Medicines Agency for the associated sleep disturbance, but several agents, including amitriptyline, gabapentin, and cyclobenzaprine, have been used off-label with reported benefit in sleep and pain, and trazodone has been used with reported benefit in sleep (Spaeth, 2011). Benzodiazepines carry a risk of tolerance with long-term use and are not associated

Table 61.3 PHARMACOLOGICAL TREATMENT OF FIBROMYALGIA

DRUG	AVAILABLE INFORMATION	RECOMMENDATION
Pregabalin	First medication FDA-approved for fibromyalgia; acts on VGCC in CNS; multiple robust studies (Mease, 2008) show reduction in pain, fatigue, sleep, and QOL; long-term studies (6 months) show efficacy; side effects include dizziness, somnolence, weight gain, and edema. Systematic review (Choy, 2011) confirms its therapeutic efficacy	Pregabalin is efficacious in the treatment of fibromyalgia and has shown improvement in pain, sleep, fatigue, and QOL; also indicated for hyperalgesia
Duloxetine	SNRI; systematic reviews (Choy, 2011) reveal several robust studies and confirm its therapeutic efficacy by measuring pain reduction and reduction in FIQ scores	Duloxetine 60–120 mg/day is the antidepressant of choice in the treatment of fibromyalgia for pain and depression
Milnacipran	SNRI (Europe and USA); studies show improvement in pain, fatigue, cognition, and FIQ scores both in short- and long-term (12 months) studies; well tolerated; headache and nausea are most common side effects (Mease, 2009; Branco, 2010); systematic review (Choy, 2011) confirms its therapeutic efficacy	Milnacipran is efficacious for the treatment of fibromyalgia without depression; it is not approved for the treatment of depression in the USA
SSRIs	increase serotonin at synapse) found helpful for pain regardless of depression (Goldenberg, 1996; Arnold, 2002); efficacy of fluoxetine + amitriptyline > amitriptyline = fluoxetine (Goldenberg, 1996); recent meta-analysis showed 2 out of 2 RCS with citalopram with negative results (Campayo, 2010)	Should be used for depression +/− pain after trying an SNRI; may be combined with a low-dose TCA; avoid citalopram

(continued)

Table 61.3 (CONTINUED)

DRUG	AVAILABLE INFORMATION	RECOMMENDATION
TCAs	Initial drug studied for fibromyalgia; increases levels of serotonin and norepinephrine; limited robust clinical data show short-term improvement in sleep, but long-term studies demonstrate limited efficacy; nortriptyline has the best side effect profile	Low-dose amitriptyline (25 mg – 50 mg) or nortriptyline may improve sleep, pain, fatigue, and QOL; high antidepressant dose limited by tolerability
Cyclobenzaprine	Skeletal muscle relaxant; similar pharmacological properties to TCAs; short-term studies show improvement in pain and fatigue; long-term studies showed no difference from placebo (Carette, 1994)	May be considered as a treatment option for pain in the short term
Gabapentin	Affects VGCC like pregabalin; studies show improvement in pain, sleep, and FIQ score; side effects include dizziness, lightheadedness, and sedation (Saxena & Solitar, 2010)	May be considered as a treatment option for pain in fibromyalgia; indicated in hyperalgesia
Sodium Oxybate	One open-label trial for narcolepsy suggested it was helpful; Three 8-week RCS showed improvement in FIQ score, pain and sleep (Russel, 2009; Saxena, 2010; Moldofsky, 2010)	May be considered as a treatment option for pain and sleep in fibromyalgia
Opiates	There is no evidence to inform the use of short- or long-term use but they are frequently prescribed. Some studies with limitations support use of the dual-action opiate, tramadol, a mu opioid agonist and SNRI (Saxena & Solitar, 2010)	No evidence to inform short- or long-term use. Dual-action tramadol may be considered for pain
NSAIDs and acetaminophen	Commonly prescribed; limited evidence for its use	Should not be prescribed unless other associated diseases justify their use
Oral steroids	One double-blind crossover trial of prednisone versus placebo showed no efficacy (Clark, 1985)	Not recommended
Nabilone	One RCS showed no change in tender points, but improvement in FIQ score, pain, and anxiety was reported (Skrabek, 2008)	Experimental; expert opinion and consensus reports recommend against experimental therapies
Naltrexone	One pilot study of 10 patients reported it was helpful (Younger, 2009)	Experimental; expert opinion and consensus reports recommend against experimental therapies

FDA: Food and Drug Administration; VGCC: voltage-gated calcium channels; QOL: quality of life; FIQ: fibromyalgia impact questionnaire; RCS: randomized controlled study; CNS: central nervous system

with specific benefit on sleep or pain. Zolpidem and zopiclone may lead to subjective reports of improvement in sleep and daytime fatigue but have no effect on pain and no demonstrated impact on the sleep architecture. Currently, pharmacotherapy in fibromyalgia is targeted at pain control via counteraction of central pain processing. The putative mechanism of pharmacotherapy in fibromyalgia, therefore, is by altering the levels of the implicated neurotransmitters; for example, pregabalin inhibiting presynaptic release of substance P and glutamate, and duloxetine and milnacipram, which are SNRIs (Rao, 2009; Hauser, et al., 2008). Duloxetine, milnacipram, and pregabalin, which are all FDA-approved for fibromyalgia, also have beneficial effects on fatigue and quality of sleep as well, but with inconsistent reports on associated changes in sleep architecture (Chalon, 2005; Kluge, 2007; Lemoine, 2004; Hindmarch, 2005).

Complementary and Alternative Medicine Treatments

The use of complementary and alternative medicine (CAM) is very common in fibromyalgia, with one study reporting up to 50% of fibromyalgia patients using some form of CAM therapy (Wahner-Roedler, 2005). Several studies have reported on various CAM modalities. These studies include clinical trials, reviews, and systematic reviews. Many of the studies on CAM therapy focus on just one or a few modalities, have variable response indicators, use different scales for the same outcome measures, use different criteria for diagnosis of fibromyalgia, and include mixed chronic pain populations, with several diagnoses other than fibromyalgia. The most recent systematic review on CAM in fibromyalgia (Terhorst et al., 2011) included only randomized control trials (RCTs) comparing CAM therapy to a control group, in patients with fibromyalgia only (as diagnosed by ACR 1990,

Table 61.4 NON-PHARMACOLOGICAL TREATMENT OF FIBROMYALGIA

INTERVENTION	AVAILABLE INFORMATION	RECOMMENDATION
Education	Meta-analysis and systematic reviews demonstrate increase in self-efficacy, reduced catastrophization, enhancement of QOL (Hauser, 2008)	Provide education about the diagnosis, course, and treatment; encourage patients to actively participate in their treatment
Cognitive Behavioral Therapy	Systematic review and meta-analysis of RCSs shows improvement in coping with pain, reduction of depression, reduction of healthcare-seeking behavior (Bernardy, 2010); Reduces catastrophization, which helps prognosis (Campayo, 2010)	CBT should be used in depressed patients with high levels of catastrophization
Exercise	Well-conducted meta-analysis and several systematic reviews show improvement in sense of well-being, physical performance, and pain (Busch, 2007) 1. Aerobic exercise (weight-bearing such as walking or dancing, and non-weight-bearing such as swimming or biking) 2. Muscle-strengthening exercises (weights or resistance training) 3. Stretching and flexibility exercises have been studied; the best evidence exists for aerobic exercise (Campayo, 2010)	Physical exercise should be one of the most basic treatments; prescribe or refer to supervised exercise program involving weight-bearing (walking) or non-weight-bearing (biking) aerobic activity

QOL: Quality of life; CBT—Cognitive Behavioral Therapy

Yunus, or Smythe criteria), with the specific outcome being the effect on pain, as measured by the Visual Analog Scale, the Fibromyalgia Impact Questionnaire (FIQ), and the McGill Pain Questionnaire. This systematic review also included every type of CAM modality published that met the inclusion criteria. The rating of the RCTs in this systematic review was as follows:

Good: 4–5 points

Moderate: 3 points

Low: 2 points

Very Low: 0–1 point

Points were awarded as follows:

One point each was received for (1) specific mention of randomization, (2) single-blinding, (3) intent-to-treat analysis for missing data/attrition, (4) appropriate data analysis for outcome measures, and (5) "other," i.e., no other methodological concerns.

No point was allotted if (1) randomization was mentioned but without specific details, (2) blinding was not mentioned at all, (3) there was minimal attrition and brief mention only about missing data, (4) there was a minor flaw in methodology.

One point each was subtracted for (1) randomization in the title, but not addressed at all in the manuscript, (2) large attrition rates without accounting for missing data, (3) concerns with thoroughness or adequacy of the results, (4) a

major flaw in methodology (e.g., use of prescription pain medication in conjunction with CAM therapy).

A summary of the data from this systematic review is shown in Table 61.5. It yielded findings compatible with previous systematic reviews (Baranowsky, 2009; Schneider, 2009), although not all forms of CAM modalities were reviewed in the latter studies.

The various forms of CAM therapies are as follows:

1. Hydrotherapy
   a. Balneotherapy—also known as spa therapy, medical hydrology, or thermal therapy—this refers to any type of bath including mineral baths and mud baths.
   b. Thalassotherapy—refers specifically to salt water baths versus pool water; a recent RCT on thalassotherapy examined the effect of underwater exercise in salt water versus pool water, but no significant difference in pain was found between groups (de Andrade, 2008), using the FIQ and number of tender points as outcome measures.

2. Massage Therapy
   a. Manipulative—includes osteopathic and chiropractic.

3. Vibration Therapy—this method involves use of a motor, such as in a vibration table, to apply a high-frequency vibration to the whole body or parts of the body.

4. Magnetic Therapy—this involves creation of an electromagnetic field around the person, such as via use of a magnetic pad.

5. Homeopathic/Nutritional Supplements—Homeopathic remedies include the use of highly diluted derivatives of animal, plant, mineral, or synthetic sources. Popular examples of such remedies used in fibromyalgia include *Rhus toxicodendron* (derived from poison ivy), *Lachesis muta* (derived from snake venom), opium, *Arnica montana* (a yellow flowering plant) and *Byronia alba* (a vine from the cucumber family). Nutritional supplements involve the use of several oral or topical compounds. Some of the more commonly utilized ones in fibromyalgia, and those that have been studied, include *Chlorella pyrenoidosa*, S-adenosyl methionine, Myer's cocktail, soy, anthocyanidins, and capsaicin.

6. Mind/Body Therapy—this includes techniques such as meditation, guided imagery, hypnosis, affective self-awareness, and biofeedback.

RHEUMATOLOGICAL MEDICATIONS AND THEIR NEUROPSYCHIATRIC EFFECTS

Medications used to treat the rheumatic diseases can be categorized as follows:

1. NSAIDs—indomethacin, ibuprofen, celecoxib, diclofenac

2. Acetaminophen

3. Opioid analgesics

4. Corticosteroids—prednisone, methylprednisolone

5. Sulfasalazine (5-aminosalicylic acid)

Table 61.5 COMPLEMENTARY AND ALTERNATIVE MEDICINE IN THE TREATMENT OF PAIN IN FIBROMYALGIA

CAM MODALITY	AVAILABLE DATA	CONCLUSION FROM AVAILABLE DATA
HYDROTHERAPIES:		
Balneotherapy	11 RCTS, only 8 with sufficient data to calculate effect size. 8/8 studies with mean effect size favoring tre atment group, but only 3/8 statistically significant. Of those 3 studies, 2 were Good quality (*N* = 69 and 16), although one combined balneotherapy with massage, and one Moderate quality (*N* = 40).	Positive effect based on available data, but paucity of good-quality data; underpowered studies. More studies needed to make a recommendation
Thalassotherapy	One RCT of moderate quality evaluating a combination of thalassotherapy, patient education and exercise on pain and FIQ score. It was included as one of the 8 balneotherapy studies above. Study showed no significant difference between treatment (n = 58) and control (n = 76) groups.	Insufficient evidence to make any recommendations
MASSAGE:	6 RCTs, 5 with sufficient data to calculate effect size, 3/5 with mean effect size favoring treatment group, only 1/3 statistically significant; Low quality, *N* = 23.	Current limited data show that massage therapy was not effective in reducing pain
Manipulative		
Chiropractic	2 RCTs, 2/2 with effect size favoring treatment group, but none statistically significant. Studies were Moderate and Low quality, *N* = 10 and 11	The limited evidence does not support its usefulness for pain
Osteopathic	1 RCT, insufficient data to calculate effect size; Low quality, *N* = 6	
Vibration	2RCTs, 1 with effect size favoring treatment group, but only when vibration was done in conjunction with exercise, and effects was not statistically significant; Good quality, *N* = 11; second study with effect size strongly favoring control group, effect statistically significant, Moderate quality, *N* = 13	The limited evidence does not support its usefulness for pain
MAGNETIC THERAPIES:	3RCTs, 1/3 with statistically significant effect size favoring treatment group (Good quality, *N* = 25). It was the only study using pulsed magnetic field rather than magnetic sleep pads	Insufficient evidence to support its usefulness for pain

(continued)

Table 61.5 (CONTINUED)

CAM MODALITY	AVAILABLE DATA	CONCLUSION FROM AVAILABLE DATA
HOMEOPATHIC AND NUTRITIONAL SUPPLEMENTS:	9 RCTs, 3 in homeopathy group (2 Good quality $N = 26, 20$; 1 Low quality, $N = 15$), 6 in nutritional supplements group (3 Good quality, $N = 15, 29, 12$; 2 Moderate quality, $N = 22, 37$; 1 Low quality, $N = 17$). 2/3 homeopathy studies had data to calculate effect size that showed no difference from control group. 5/6 nutritional supplement studies (including S-adenyl methionine, soy, chlorella, Myer's cocktail) with sufficient data to calculate effect size, none separated from placebo	Current data do not support the usefulness of homeopathic treatment and nutritional supplements for pain in fibromyalgia
MIND/BODY:	11 RCTs:	Positive effect based on available data, but paucity of good quality data; underpowered studies. More studies needed to make a recommendation
Biofeedback (EEG, heart-rate variability)	4 RCTs, 3 with effect size favoring treatment group (2 Moderate quality, 1 Low quality, $N = 15, 27, 38$), only 1 statistically significant (Very Low quality, $N = 6$)	
Hypnosis	2 RCTs (Moderate quality and Very Low quality, $N = 15, 20$), 1 with effect size favoring treatment group, but not statistically significant	
Meditation	2 RCTs, only 1 with sufficient data to calculate effect size (Moderate quality, $N = 51$), effect size favored treatment, but not statistically significant	
Guided Imagery	2 RCTs, both Moderate quality, $N = 17, 24$, both with statistically significant effect sizes favoring treatment group	
Affective Self-Awareness	1 RCT, Good quality, $N = 24$, effect size favors treatment, but not statistically significant	
MOVEMENT THERAPIES:	4 RCTs:	Positive effect based on limited data, but paucity of good quality data; underpowered studies. More studies needed to make a recommendation
Qigong	2 RCTs, 1 with effect size favoring treatment group, Low quality study, $N = 29$	
Tai Chi	2 RCTs, 1 with effect size favoring treatment group, Good quality study, $N = 30$	
ENERGY MEDICINE:	2 RCTs:	Limited evidence does not support the usefulness of energy medicine for pain in fibromyalgia
Reiki	1 RCT, Moderate quality, $N = 23$, no difference from sham Reiki	
Therapeutic Touch	1 RCT, Moderate quality, $N = 21$, no difference from placebo	
ACUPUNCTURE:	7 RCTs, 6 with sufficient data to calculate effect size. 4/6 with effect size favoring treatment, 3/4 statistically significant	Limited data show modest effect on pain; insufficient data to make recommendation. More studies needed
MISCELLANEOUS:		Inconclusive due to low-quality studies with insufficient data
Essential Oils	1 RCT, Low quality, $N = 65$, insufficient data to make calculations on effect size	
Wool Clothing	1 RCT, Low quality, $N = 25$, insufficient data to make calculations on effect size	

6. Disease-modifying anti-rheumatic drugs (DMARDs)
   a. Antimalarials—hydroxychloroquine
   b. Cytotoxics—mycophenolatemofetil, azathioprine, cyclophosphamide, methotrexate, leflunamide, cyclosporine A
   c. Biological response modifiers

   i. TNF-alpha blockers—etanercept, adalimumab, infliximab
   ii. IL-1 blockers—anakinra
   iii. T cell modifiers—abatacept
   iv. CD20+ B cell modifier—rituximab

Side effects of anti-rheumatic drugs are outlined in Table 61.6. Any of these drugs can cause delirium, but this is considered very rare and would be more common in toxicity. Delirium has never been reported with mycophenolatemofetil, or with leflunamide or any of the biological response modifiers, which are novel treatments and have not been in use for very long. There are rare reports (Van Royen, 2005; Pacchioarotti, 2007) of behavioral abnormalities, psychosis, vague mood alterations, and confusion associated with use of some of the cytotoxic drugs, but reports are extremely rare, and causal relationships were not confirmed. They are generally considered to be safe in terms of neuropsychiatric side effects. Cyclosporine A and corticosteroids are the drugs most commonly associated with neuropsychiatric side effects. Gold and penicillamine have never been associated with any neuropsychiatric side effects, but are essentially obsolete.

Corticosteroids more commonly cause mild symptoms of hypomania, usually insomnia, nervous tension, and irritability. Less commonly, but not too infrequently, this can take on a more severe form, and the patient may present with a maniform psychosis. The incidence of steroid psychosis is similar in the pre- and post-steroid era, at least in the SLE

Table 61.6 NEUROPSYCHIATRIC SIDE EFFECTS OF ANTI-RHEUMATIC DRUGS

ANTI-RHEUMATIC DRUG	NEUROPSYCHIATRIC SIDE EFFECTS
NSAIDs:	Reports of depression, anxiety, psychosis, hostility, delirium, confusion, and poor concentration at high doses
Acetaminophen	None reported
Opioid analgesics	Dependence, abuse, somnolence, apathy, euphoria
[†]Corticosteroids	Depression, mania with psychosis, hypomania, irritability, insomnia, fatigue, cognitive impairment
Sulfasalazine	Uncommon: mild headache and mood alterations (Amos, 1986)
Antimalarials: Hydroxychloroquine	Lower incidence of hallucinations, confusion, anxiety, nightmares compared to its non-hydroxylated form (http://www.ncbi.nlm.nih.gov/pubmed/15235536; Ferraro, 2004)
Cytotoxics:	Rare
Mycophenolatemofetil	None reported
Azathioprine	None reported
Cyclophosphamide	None reported
Methotrexate	
Immunosuppressants:	Anxiety
Leflunamide	Neurotoxicity at therapeutic levels (Telarovic, et al 2007; Gijtenbeek et al. (1999)
[‡]Cyclosporine A	
Biological Response Modifiers:	None reported

[†]Corticosteroids more commonly cause mild symptoms of hypomania, usually insomnia, nervous tension and irritability. Less commonly, but not too infrequently, this can take on a more severe form and the patient may present with a maniform psychosis. The incidence of steroid psychosis is similar in the pre- and post-steroid era at least in the SLE population. Steroid psychosis is usually associated with high doses of corticosteroids, such as oral prednisone > 60-80 mg /day. Depression is a more common side effect of corticosteroids and studies have found that the course of the depression in long-term corticosteroid treatment is variable, being influenced by many other psychosocial factors (Brown, 2007). Fatigue may occur from secondary adrenal suppression upon corticosteroid taper. Short-term use of corticosteroids cause cognitive dysfunction, usually noticeable and measurable decline in declarative memory without detectable changes in hippocampal volume (Hajek, 2006). Long-term corticosteroid treatment has been found to be associated with non-progressive declarative memory impairment with smaller amygdala volumes (Brown, 2008) andsmaller hippocampal volumes. There is little evidence about the reversibility of these neuroanatomical changes upon steroid withdrawal. However, the memory impairment is thought to be non-progressive without risk of dementia (Brown, 2007).

Indirect effect of steroids on mood involve feelings of low self-esteem, hopelessness and social withdrawal due to physical changes such as the classic buffalo hump, abdominal obesity, moon-like facies, alopecia and complications such as a vascular necrosis leading to physical disability and restricted mobility and independence.

Treatment of steroid-induced mood and memory impairment has been studied with acetaminophen (Brown, 2010), lamotrigine and leviteracetam (Brown, 2007), but none showed benefit. In one small placebo-controlled study of 39 patients phenytoin 300 mg /day was found to be helpful in preventing the hypomanic effects of corticosteroids but had no effect on memory (Brown, 2005).

[‡]There have been some reports of neurotoxicity with cyclosporine A. In one report (Palmer, 1991), 3 cases of cyclosporine A neurotoxicity in otherwise non-immuno compromised renal patients were described. One developed dementia, the second, a Guillain-Barré like syndrome with ascending motor neuropathy and the third, a flaccid hemiparesis. In all cases, levels of cyclosporine A were therapeutic.

One study (Meyer, 2002) used PET to determine the mechanism of cyclosporine A neurotoxicity in a 37-year-old patient with intention tremor and progressive psychiatric change (social withdrawal and flat affect) and found elevated blood glucose metabolism in the basal ganglia. The authors suggested that cyclosporine A neurotoxicity was mediated by metabolic abnormalities in the basal ganglia.

Side effects of cyclosporine A, though not rare, are usually mild, such as fine tremor, anxiety and hallucinations. There have been reports of exacerbation of paranoid schizophrenia, Di Nuzzo (2007) and depressive psychosis (Telarovic, 2007). Complex neurological side effects such as motor spinal cord and cerebellar syndromes are rare and more likely to be observed in the immuno compromised patient.

population. Steroid psychosis is usually associated with high doses of corticosteroids, such as oral prednisone >60–80 mg/day. Depression is a more common side effect of corticosteroids, and studies have found that the course of the depression in long-term corticosteroid treatment is variable, being influenced by many other psychosocial factors (Brown, 2007). Fatigue may occur from secondary adrenal suppression upon corticosteroid taper. Short-term use of corticosteroids causes cognitive dysfunction, usually noticeable and measurable decline in declarative memory, without detectable changes in hippocampal volume (Hajek, 2006). Long-term corticosteroid treatment has been found to be associated with non-progressive declarative memory impairment with smaller amygdala volumes (Brown, 2008) and smaller hippocampal volumes. There is little evidence about the reversibility of these neuroanatomical changes upon steroid withdrawal. However, the memory impairment is thought to be non-progressive and without risk of dementia (Brown, 2007).

Indirect effects of steroids on mood involve feelings of low self-esteem, hopelessness, and social withdrawal due to physical changes such as the classic buffalo hump, abdominal obesity, moon-like facies, alopecia, and complications such as avascular necrosis leading to physical disability and restricted mobility and independence.

Treatment of steroid-induced mood and memory impairment has been studied with acetaminophen (Brown, 2010), lamotrigine, and levetiracetam (Brown, 2007), but none showed benefit. In one small placebo-controlled study of 39 patients, phenytoin 300 mg/day was found to be helpful in preventing the hypomanic effects of corticosteroids, but it had no effect on memory (Brown, 2005).

There have been some reports of neurotoxicity with cyclosporine A. In one report (Palmer, 1991), three cases of cyclosporine A neurotoxicity in otherwise non-immunocompromised renal patients were described. One developed dementia; the second, a Guillain-Barré–like syndrome with ascending motor neuropathy; and the third, a flaccid hemiparesis. In all cases, levels of cyclosporine A were therapeutic.

One study (Meyer, 2002) used PET to determine the mechanism of cyclosporin A neurotoxicity in a 37-year-old patient with intention tremor and progressive psychiatric change (social withdrawal and flat affect) and found elevated blood-glucose metabolism in the basal ganglia. The authors suggested that cyclosporine A neurotoxicity was mediated by metabolic abnormalities in the basal ganglia.

Side effects of cyclosporin A, though not rare, are usually mild, such as fine tremor, anxiety, and hallucinations. There have been reports of exacerbation of paranoid schizophrenia (Di Nuzzo, 2007) and depressive psychosis (Telarovic, 2007). Complex neurological side effects such as motor spinal cord and cerebellar syndromes are rare and more likely to be observed in the immunocompromised patient.

CLINICAL PEARLS

- There is known to be a lag time of some years between onset of the first symptom and the eventual diagnosis of lupus. Often, the significance of previous non-specific symptoms becomes recognized only in retrospect.

- The psychiatrist can screen for SLE by periodically applying diagnostic criteria, applying the SLEDAI (Gladman, 2002; Bombardier, 1992), and by performing investigations including CBC, antibody screen, ANA profile, and urinalysis every three to six months or at the onset of a worsening or new symptom, or if the psychiatric symptoms are atypical.

- Lupus psychosis has a prevalence estimate of 8% of SLE patients. Prevalence rates for the remaining neuropsychiatric syndromes are estimated at less than 1%.

- No single consistent biological marker for NPSLE has yet been found.

- There is insufficient evidence to support the routine use of lumbar puncture for CSF levels of cytokines or autoantibodies as diagnostic tools for NPSLE, or of anti-ribosomal P or anti-NMDA receptor antibodies as a diagnostic tool for lupus psychosis.

- The occurrence of a single generalized seizure in patients with SLE does not necessitate AED treatment and does not necessarily mean that the patient will go on to have a recurrent seizure disorder.

- When NPSLE is suspected, a brain MRI should be done early in the course of illness.

- In the clinical setting, T2-weighted MRI remains the gold standard for assessing NPSLE, with FLAIR enhancing sensitivity and gadolinium enhancement helping to differentiate between acute and chronic lesions.

- SPECT or PET may be done following or in conjunction with MRI to further aid with diagnosis, depending on cost and availability.

- Psychosis, if determined to be due to NPSLE, will usually resolve with treatment of the lupus itself, but often adjunctive psychotropic medication is needed to expedite symptom control.

- The hierarchy of treatment is as follows: oral high-dose prednisone, intravenous methylprednisolone, pulse cyclophosphamide, and rituximab (Trevisani, 2006; Tokunaga, 2007).

- NPSLE syndromes, such as lupus psychosis, are not considered to be necessarily recurrent (Bertsias, 2010). Thus a patient with lupus psychosis does not require long-term antipsychotic treatment.

- Patients with lupus psychosis and their families should be informed that full recovery from psychosis is expected (Pego-Reigosa, 2008).

- Despite the availability of diagnostic criteria for RA, time for evolution of symptoms is required before the diagnosis may actually be captured.

- Since constitutional symptoms may predate joint symptoms and signs, some patients with RA may be misdiagnosed with depression before the defining features of the illness reveal themselves.

- The nervous system is less commonly affected in RA. Psychosis as a consequence of RA is rare.

- CNS effects are controversial and are considered uncommon in Sjögren's syndrome.

- Cognitive impairment can occur at any time during SJS. It has a very insidious onset; it may be chronic, recurrent, and in some cases may spontaneously remit. It is considered very rare that it would deteriorate into progressive memory impairment or dementia.

- The pain of fibromyalgia has been attributed to central sensitization.

- Based on the proposed pathophysiological theories and the availability of evidence to support or refute them, antivirals, immunosuppressants, and steroid therapy have no role in the treatment of fibromyalgia to date.

- The aim of pharmacotherapy in fibromyalgia is control of the core and associated major symptoms with a goal of improvement in quality of life and restoration of optimal function. Those core symptoms are pain, sleep disturbance, fatigue, and depression.

ADDENDUM

Arbuckle, M. R., McClain, M. T., Rubertone, M. V., Scofield, R. H., et al. (2003). Development of autoantibodies before the clinical onset of systemic lupus erythematosus. *New England Journal of Medicine, 349,* 1526–33.

In 115 of 130 patients with SLE (88%), at least one SLE autoantibody tested was present before the diagnosis (up to 9.4 years earlier; mean 3.3 years). Antinuclear antibodies were present in 78% at dilutions of 1:120 or more, anti-double stranded DNA antibodies in 55%, anti-Ro antibodies in 47%, anti-La antibodies in 34%, anti-Sm antibodies in 32%, antinuclear ribonucleoprotein antibodies in 26%, and anti-phospholipid antibodies in 18%. Antinuclear, anti-phospholipid antibodies, anti-Ro, and anti-La antibodies were present earlier than anti-Sm and antinuclear ribonucleoprotein antibodies (a mean of 3.4 years before the diagnosis vs 1.2 before the diagnosis). Anti-double-stranded DNA antibodies, with a mean onset 2.2 years before the diagnosis, were found later than ANA and earlier than ANRNP ab.

Autoantibodies are typically present many years before the diagnosis of SLE. Furthermore, the appearance of autoantibodies in patients with SLE tends to follow a predictable course, with a progressive accumulation of specific autoantibodies before the onset of SLE, while patients are still asymptomatic.

1. Some autoantibodies (antinuclear, anti-Ro, anti-La, and anti-phospholipid ab) usually precede the onset of SLE by many years.

2. Others (anti-Sm and antinuclear rnp ab) typically appear only months before the diagnosis, in the time of typical clinical manifestations.

3. Anti-Sm and anti-double-stranded DNA antibodies do not present before the clinical diagnosis.

4. Anti-Ro, anti-La, anti-phospholipid, and antinuclear antibodies are in fact relatively common in normal persons who never have clinical symptoms of rheumatic disease.

5. Anti-double-stranded DNA, anti-SM, and antinuclear ribonucleoprotein A/B are very rare in normal persons.

6. The presence of antinuclear antibodies at ratios of 1:120 or more, or anti-ro, anti-La, or anti-phospholipid ab appears to increase the risk by a factor of at least 40; however, their presence does not suggest that the onset of clinical illness is imminent.

Crescendo autoimmunity culminating in clinical illness however their presence alone does not suggest that the onset of clinical illness is imminent. Rather, there is crescendo immunity culminating in clinical illness.

DISCLOSURE STATEMENT

Dr. Ali, has no conflicts of interests and nothing to disclose.

REFERENCES

Ablin, J., Buskila, D., & Clauw, D. J. (2009). Biomarkers in fibromyalgia. *Current Pain & Headache Reports, 13,* 343–349.

ACR Ad Hoc Committee on Neuropsychiatric Lupus Nomenclature (1999). The American College of Rheumatology nomenclature and case definitions for neuropsychiatric lupus syndromes. *Arthritis and Rheumatism, 42*(4), 599–608.

Adak, B., Tekeoğlu, I., Ediz, L., Budancamanak, M., Yazgan, T., Karahocagil, K., et al. (2005). Fibromyalgia frequency in hepatitis B carriers. *Journal of Clinical Rheumatology, 11,* 157–159.

Affleck, G., Urrows, S., Tennen, H., Higgins, P., & Abeles, M. (1996). Sequential daily relations of sleep, pain intensity, and attention to pain among women with fibromyalgia. *Pain, 68*(2–3), 363–368.

Ainiala, H., Loukkola, J., Peltola, J., Korpela, M., & Hietaharju, A. (2001). The prevalence of neuropsychiatric syndromes in systemic lupus erythematosus. *Neurology, 57*(3), 496–500.

Alexander, E. L. (1992). Central nervous system disease in Sjögren's syndrome. New insights into immunopathogenesis. *Rheumatic Disease Clinics of North America, 18*(30), 637–672.

Alexander, E. L. (1993). Neurologic disease in Sjögren's syndrome: Mononuclear inflammatory vasculopathy affecting central/peripheral nervous system and muscle. A clinical review and update of immunopathogenesis. *Rheumatic Disease Clinics of North America, 19*(4), 869–908.

Amital, A., Shitrit, D., & Adir, Y. (2011). The lung in rheumatoid arthritis. *Petach Tikva, 40*(1 Pt 2), 31–48.

Amos, R. S., Pullar, T., Bax, D. E., Situnavake, D., Capell, H. A., & McConkey, B. (1986). Sulphasalazine for rheumatoid arthritis: Toxicity in 774 patients monitored for 1–11 years. *British Medical Journal, 293*, 420–423.

Andersen, M. L., Nascimento, D. C., Machado, R. B., Roizenblatt, S., Moldofsky, H., & Tufik, S. (2006). Sleep disturbance induced by substance P in mice. *Behavioural Brain Research, 167*(2), 212–218.

Andonopoulos, A. P., & Ballas, C. (1995). Autonomic cardiovascular neuropathy in primary Sjogren's syndrome. *Rheumatology International, 15*, 127–129.

Andonopoulos, A. P., Lagos, G., Drosos, A. A., & Moutsopoulos, H. M. (1990). The spectrum of neurological involvement in Sjögren's syndrome. *British Journal of Rheumatology, 29*, 21–23.

Andrade, C., Sandarsh, S., Chethan, K. B., & Nagesh, K. S. (2010). Serotonin reuptake inhibitor antidepressants and abnormal bleeding: A review for clinicians and a reconsideration of mechanisms. *Journal of Clinical Psychiatry, 71*(12), 1565–1575.

Arnold, L. M., Hess, E. V., Hudson, J. I., et al. (2002). A randomized, placebo controlled, double-blind, flexible-dose study of fluoxetine in the treatment of women with fibromyalgia. *American Journal of Medicine, 112*, 191–197.

Arnold, L. M., Hudson, J. I., Hess, E. V., Ware, A. E., Fritz, D. A., Auchenbach, M. B., et al. (2004). Family study of fibromyalgia. *Arthritis & Rheumatology, 50*, 944–952.

Baranowsky, J., Klose, P., Musial, F., Haeuser, W., Dobos, G., & Langhorst, J. (2009). Qualitative systemic review of randomized controlled trials on complementary and alternative medicine treatments in fibromyalgia. *Rheumatology International, 30*, 1–21.

Barbosa, F., Mota, C., Patrício, P., Alcântara, C., Ferreira, C., & Barbosa, A. (2011). The relationship between alexithymia and psychological factors in systemic lupus erythematosus. *Comprehensive Psychiatry, 80*, 123–124.

Barendregt, P. J., Visserm, M. R. M., Smetsm, E. M. A., Tulenm, J. H. M., van den Meirackerm, A. H., Boomsma, F., et al. (1998). Fatigue in primary Sjögren's syndrome. *Annals of the Rheumatic Diseases, 57*, 291–295.

Barile-Fabris, L., Ariza-Andraca, R., Olguín-Ortega, L., Jara, L. J., Fraga-Mouret, A., Miranda-Limón, J. M., et al. (2005). Controlled clinical trial of IV cyclophosphamide versus IV methylprednisolone in severe neurological manifestations in systemic lupus erythematosus. *Annals of the Rheumatic Diseases, 64*, 620–625.

Belin, C., Moroni, C., Caillat-Vigneron, N., Debray, M., Baudin, M., Dumas, J., et al. (1999). Central nervous system involvement in Sjögren's syndrome: Evidence from neuropsychological testing and HMPAO-SPECT. *Annales de Médecine Interne, 150*(8), 598–604.

Bennett, R. M., Clark, S. C., & Walczyk, J. (1998). A randomized, double-blind, placebo controlled study of growth hormone in the treatment of fibromyalgia. *American Journal of Medicine, 104*, 227–231.

Bennett, R. M., Cook, D. M., Clark, S. R., Burckhardt, C. S., & Campbell, S. M. (1997). Hypothalamic-pituitary-insulin-like growth factor 1–axis dysfunction in patients with fibromyalgia. *Journal of Rheumatology, 24*, 1384–1389.

Bernardy, K., Füber, N., Köllner, V., & Häuser, W. (2010). Efficacy of cognitive-behavioral therapies in fibromyalgia syndrome—a systematic review and metaanalysis of randomized controlled trials. *Journal of Rheumatology, 37*(10), 1991–2005.

Bertsias, G. K., Ioannidis, J. P.A., Aringer, M., Bollen, E., Bombardieri, S., Bruce, I. N., et al. (2010). EULAR recommendations for the management of systemic lupus erythematosus with neuropsychiatric manifestations: Report of a task force of the EULAR standing committee for clinical affairs. *Annals of the Rheumatic Diseases, 69*, 2074–2082.

Bjelland, I., Dahl, A. A., Haug, T. T., & Neckelmann, D. (2002). The validity of the Hospital Anxiety and Depression Scale: An updated literature review. *Journal of Psychosomatic Research, 52*, 69–77.

Bombardier, C., Gladman, D. D., Urowitz, M. B., Caron, D., & Chang, C. H. (1992). Derivation of the SLEDAI. A disease activity index for lupus patients. The Committee on Prognosis Studies in SLE. *Arthritis & Rheumatology, 35*(6), 630–640.

Borrelli, M., Tamarozzi, R., Colamussi, P., Govoni, M., Trotta F., & Lappi, S. (2003). Evaluation with MR, perfusion MR and cerebral flow SPECT in NPSLE patients. *Radiologica Medica, 105*(5–6), 482–489.

Bradley, L. A. (2009). Pathophysiology of fibromyalgia. *American Journal of Medicine, 122*(12 Suppl), S22–S30.

Branco, J. C., Zachrisson, O., Perrot, S., & Mainguy, Y. (2010). A European multicenter randomized double-blind placebo-controlled monotherapy clinical trial of milnacipran in the treatment of fibromyalgia. *Journal of Rheumatology, 37*, 851–859.

Brey, R. L., Holliday, S. L., Saklad, A. R., Navarrete, M. G., Hermosillo-Romo, D., Stallworth, C. L., et al. (2002). Neuropsychiatric syndromes in lupus: Prevalence using standardized definitions. *Neurology, 58*(8), 1214–1220.

Brito, G. H. O., Araujo, G. R. B., & Papi, A. (2002). Neuropsychological, neuroimage and psychiatric side aspects of primary Sjögren's syndrome. *Arquivos de Neuro-Psiquiatria, 60*(1), 28–31.

Brooks, W. M., Sabet, A., Sibbitt, W. L. Jr., Barker, P. B., van Zijl, P. C., Duyn, J. H., et al. (1997). Neurochemistry of brain lesions determined by spectroscopic imaging in systemic lupus erythematosus. *Journal of Rheumatology, 24*(12), 2323–2329.

Brown, E. S. (2009). Effects of glucocorticoids on mood, memory, and the hippocampus: Treatment and preventive therapy. *Annals of the New York Academy of Sciences, 1179*, 41–55.

Brown, E. S., Stuard, G., Liggin, J. D., Hukovic, N., Frol, A., Dhanani, N., et al. (2005). Effect of phenytoin on mood and declarative memory during prescription corticosteroid therapy. *Biological Psychiatry, 57*(5), 543–548.

Brown, E. S., Vera, E., Frol, A. B., Woolston, D. J., & Johnson, B. (2007). Effects of chronic prednisone therapy on mood and memory. *Journal of Affective Disorders, 99*(1), 279–283.

Brown, E. S., Woolston, D. J., & Frol, A. B. (2008). Amygdala volume in patients receiving chronic corticosteroid therapy. *Biological Psychiatry, 63*(7), 705–709.

Brown, E. S., Zaidel, L., Allen, G., McColl, R., Vazquez, M., & Ringe W. K. (2010). Effects of lamotrigine on hippocampal activation in corticosteroid-treated patients. *Journal of Affective Disorders, 126*(3), 415–419.

Busch, A. J., Barber, K. A., Overend, T. J., Peloso, P. M., & Schachter, C. L. (2007). Exercise for treating fibromyalgia syndrome. *Cochrane Database of Systematic Reviews, 17*(4), CD003786.

Buskila, D., Neumann, L., Vaisberg, G., Alkalay, D., & Wolfe, F. (1997). Increased rates of fibromyalgia following cervical spine injury. A controlled study of 161 cases of traumatic injury. *Arthritis & Rheumatology, 40*, 446–452.

Buskila, D., Shnaider, A., Neumann, L., (1997). Fibromyalgia in hepatitis C virus infection. Another infectious disease relationship. *Archives of Internal Medicine, 157*, 2497–2500.

Carbotte, R. M., Denburg, S. D., Denburg, J. A. (1992). Fluctuating cognitive abnormalities and cerebral glucose metabolism in neuropsychiatric systemic lupus erythematosus. *Journal of Neurology, Neurosurgery, & Psychiatry, 55*, 1054–1059.

Carette, S., Bell, M. J., Reynolds, W. J., Haraoui, B, McCain, G. A., Bykerk, V. P., et al. (1994). Comparison of amitriptyline, cyclobenzaprine, and placebo in the treatment of fibromyalgia. A randomized, double-blind clinical trial. *Arthritis & Rheumatology, 37*, 32–40.

Caselli, R. J., Scheithauer, B. W., Bowles, C. A., Trenerry, M. R., Meyer, F. B., Smigielski, J. S., et al. (1991). The treatable dementia of Sjögren's syndrome. *Annals of Neurology, 30*(1), 98–101.

Cervera, R., Asherson, R. A., Font, J., Tikly, M., Pallarés, L., Chamorro, A., et al. (1997). Chorea in the antiphospholipid syndrome. Clinical, radiologic, and immunologic characteristics of 50 patients from our clinics and the recent literature. *Medicine (Baltimore), 76*, 203–212.

Chalon, S., Pereira, A., Lainey, E., Vandenhende, F., Watkin, J. G., Staner, L., et al. (2005). Comparative effects of duloxetine and desipramine on sleep EEG in healthy subjects. *Psychopharmacology, 177*(4), 357–365.

Chinn, R. J. S., Wilkinson, I. D., Hall-Craggs, M. A., Paley, M. N. J., Shortall, E., Carter, S. J., et al. (1997). Magnetic resonance imaging of the brain and cerebral proton spectroscopy in patients with systemic lupus erythematosus. *Arthritis & Rheumatology, 40*, 36–46.

Clark, S., Tindall, E., & Bennett, R. M. (1985). A double blind cross-over trial of prednisone versus placebo in the treatment of fibrositis. *Journal of Rheumatology, 12*, 980–983.

Colasanti, T., Delumardo, F., Margutti, P., Vacirca, D., & Piro, E. (2009). Autoantibodies involved in neuropsychiatric manifestations associated with systemic lupus erythematosus. *Journal of Neuroimmunology, 212*, 3–9.

Cox, P. D., & Hales, R. E. (1999). CNS Sjögren's syndrome: An under-recognized and underappreciated neuropsychiatric disorder. *Journal of Neuropsychiatry & Clinical Neurosciences, 11*(2), 241–247.

Cozza, K. L., & Armstrong, S. C. (2001). *The cytochrome p450 system: Drug interaction principles for medical practice*. Washington, DC: American Psychiatric Publishing.

Creed, F. (1990). Psychological disorders in rheumatoid arthritis: A growing consensus? *Annals of the Rheumatic Diseases, 49*, 808–812.

Creed, F., Murphy, S., & Jayson, M. V. (1990). Measurement of psychiatric disorder in rheumatoid arthritis. *Journal of Psychosomatic Research, 34*(1), 79–87.

Cruz, B. A., Catalan-Soares, B., & Prioietti, F. (2006). Higher prevalence of fibromyalgia in patients infected with human T cell lymphotropic virus type I. *Journal of Rheumatology, 33*, 2300–2303.

Cuatrecasas, G. (2009). Fibromyalgic syndromes: Could growth hormone therapy be beneficial? *Pediatric Endocrinology Reviews, 6*(Suppl 4), 529–533.

Cuatrecasas, G., Gonzalez, M. J., Alegre, C., Sesmilo, G., Fernandez-Solá, J., Casanueva, F. F., et al. (2010). High prevalence of growth hormone deficiency in severe fibromyalgia syndromes. *Journal of Clinical Endocrinology & Metabolism, 95*(9), 4331–4337.

Cuatrecasas, G., Riudavets, C., Güell, M. A., & Nadal, A. (2007). Growth hormone as concomitant treatment in severe fibromyalgia associated with low IGF-1 serum levels. A pilot study. *BioMedCentral Musculoskeletal Disorders, 8*, 119.

Dawson, L. J., Caulfield, V. L., Stanbury, J. B., Field, A. E., Christmas, S. E., & Smith, P. M. (2005). Hydroxychloroquine therapy in patients with primary Sjögren's syndrome may improve salivary gland hypofunction by inhibition of glandular cholinesterase. *Rheumatology, 44*, 449–455.

de Andrade, S. C., de Carvalho, R. F. P. P., Soares, A. S., de Abreu Freitas, R. P., de Medeiros Guerra, L. M., & Vilar, M. J. (2008). Thalassotherapy for fibromyalgia: A randomized controlled trial comparing aquatic exercises in sea water and water pool. *Rheumatology International, 29*, 147–152.

Di Nuzzo, S., Zanni, M., & De Panfilis, G. (2007). Exacerbation of schizophrenia in a psoriatic patient after treatment with cyclosporine A, but not with etanercept. *Journal of Drugs in Dermatology, 6*(10), 1046–1047.

Dinerman, H., & Steere, A. C. (1992). Lyme disease associated with fibromyalgia. *Annals of Internal Medicine, 117*, 281–285.

Ebert, E. C., & Hagspiel, K. D. (2011). Gastrointestinal and hepatic manifestations of rheumatoid arthritis. *Digestive Diseases & Sciences, 56*(2), 295–302.

Ferraro, V., Mantoux, F., Denis, K., Lay-Macagno, M. A., Ortonne, J. P., & Lacour, J. P. (2004). Hallucinations during treatment with hydrochloroquine. *Annales de Dermatologie et de Vénéréologie, 131*(5), 471–473.

Fragoso-Loyo, H., Cabiedas, J., Orozco-Narváez, A., Dávila-Maldonado, L., Atisha-Fregoso, Y., Diamond, B., et al. (2008). Serum and cerebrospinal fluid autoantibodies in patients with neuropsychiatric lupus erythematosus. Implications for diagnosis and pathogenesis. *PLoS One, 3*(10), e3347.

Friedman, S. D., Stidley, C. A., Brooks, W. M., Hart, B. L., & Sibbitt, W. L. Jr. (1998). Brain injury and neurometabolic abnormalities in systemic lupus erythematosus. *Radiology, 209*, 79–84.

Fuller, R. A., Westmoreland, S. V., Ratai, E., Greco, J. B., Kim, J. P., Lentz, M. R., et al. (2004). A prospective longitudinal in vivo ^{1}H MR spectroscopy study of the SIV/macaque model of neuroAIDS. *BioMedCentral Neuroscience, 5*(1), 10.

García Campayo, J., Alegre de Miguel, C., Tomás Flórez, M., Gómez Arguelles, J. M., Blanco Tarrio, E., Gobbo Montoya, M., et al. (2010). Interdisciplinary consensus document for the treatment of fibromyalgia. *Actas Espanolas de Psiquiatria, 38*(2), 108–120.

Gijtenbeek, J. M. M., van den Bent, M. J., & Vecht, C. J. (1999). Cyclosporine neurotoxicity: a review. *Journal of Neurology, 246*, 339–346.

Gladman, D. D., Ibanez, D., & Urowitz, M. B. (2002). Systemic Lupus Erythematosus Disease Activity Index 2000. *Journal of Rheumatology, 29*(2), 288–291.

Goldenberg, D., Mayskiy, M., Mossey, C., Ruthazer, R., & Scmid, C. (1996). A randomized, double-blind crossover trial of fluoxetine and amitriptyline in the treatment of fibromyalgia. *Arthritis & Rheumatology, 39*, 1852–1859.

Goodman, D., Morrissey, S., Graham, D., & Bossingham, D. (2005). Illness representations of systemic lupus erythematosus. *Qualitative Health Research, 15*(5), 606–619.

Gracely, R. H., Petzke, F., Wolf, J. M., & Clauw, D. J. (2002). Functional magnetic resonance imaging evidence of augmented pain processing in fibromyalgia. *Arthritis & Rheumatology, 46*, 1333–1343.

Grinspoon, S. K., & Biller, B. M. (1994). Clinical Review 62: laboratory assessment of adrenal insufficiency. *Journal of Clinical Endocrinology and Metabolism, 79*, 923–931.

Gudbjörnsson, B., Broman, J. E., Hetta, J., & Hällgren, R. (1993). Sleep disturbance in patients with primary Sjögren's syndrome. *British Journal of Rheumatology, 32*, 1072–1076.

Guttman, M., Lang, A. E., Garnett, E. S., Nahmias, C., Firnau, G., Tyndel, F. J., et al. (1987). Regional cerebral glucose metabolism in SLE chorea: further evidence that striatal hypometabolism is not a correlate of chorea. *Movement Disorders, 2*, 201–210.

Hachulla, E., Michon-Pasturel, U., Leys, D., Pruvo, J. P., Queyrel, V., Masy, E., et al. (1998). Cerebral magnetic resonance imaging in patients with or without antiphospholipid antibodies. *Lupus, 7*, 124–131.

Hajek, T., Kopecek, M., Preiss, M., Alda, M., & Hoschl, C. (2006). Prospective study of hippocampal volume and function in human subjects treated with corticosteroids. *European Psychiatry, 21*, 123–128.

Hamed, S. A., Selim, Z. I., Elattar, A. M., Elserogy, Y. M., Ahmed, E. A., & Mohamed, H. O. (2012). Assessment of biocorrelates for brain involvement in female patients with rheumatoid arthritis. *Clinical Rheumatology 31*, 123–132.

Hanly, J. G., Cassell, K., & Fisk, J. D. (1997). Cognitive function in systemic lupus erythematosus: results of a 5-year prospective study. *Arthritis & Rheumatology, 40*(8), 1542–1543.

Hanly, J. G., McCurdy, G., Fougere, L., Douglas, J. A., & Thompson, K. (2004). Neuropsychiatric disease in systemic lupus erythematosus (SLE): attribution and clinical significance. *Journal of Rheumatology, 31*, 2156–2162.

Harkness, E. F., Macfarlane, G. J., Nahit, E., Silman, A. J., & Macbeth, J. (2004). Mechanical injury and psychosocial factors in the work place predict the onset of widespread body pain: a two-year prospective study among cohorts of newly employed workers. *Arthritis & Rheumatology, 50*:1357–1359.

Hauser, W., Arnold, B., Eich, W., Felde, E., Flügge, C., Henningsen, P., et al. (2008). Management of fibromyalgia syndrome—an interdisciplinary evidence-based guideline. *German Medical Science, 6*, Doc 14, 1612–3174.

Hawley, D. J., & Wolfe, F. (1988). Anxiety and depression in patients with rheumatoid arthritis: a prospective study of 400 patients. *Journal of Rheumatology, 15*, 932–941.

Henzen, C., Suter, A., Lerch, E., Urbinelli, R., Schorno, X. H., & Briner, V. A. (2000). Suppression and recovery of adrenal response after short-term, high-dose glucocorticoid treatment. *Lancet, 355*, 542–545.

Hewlett, S., Ambler, N., Almeida, C., Cliss, A., Hammond, A., Kitchen, K., et al. (2011). Self-management of fatigue in rheumatoid arthritis: a randomised control trial of group cognitive behaviour therapy. *Annals of the Rheumatic Diseases, 70*, 1060–1067.

Hindmarch, I., Dawson, J., & Stanley, N. (2005). A double-blind study in healthy volunteers to assess the effects on sleep of pregabalin compared with alprazolam and placebo. *Sleep, 28*(2), 187–93.

Hiraiwa, M., Nonaka, C., Abe, T., & Iio, M. (1983). Positron emission tomography in systemic lupus erythematosus: relation of cerebral vasculitis to PET findings. *American Journal of Radiology, 4,* 541–543.

Hirohata, S., & Hayakawa, K. (1999). Enhanced interleukin-6 messenger RNA expression by neuronal cells in a patient with neuropsychiatric systemic lupus erythematosus. *Arthritis and Rheumatism, 42*(12), 2729–2730.

Hochberg, M. C. (1997). Updating the American College of Rheumatology revised criteria for the classification of systemic lupus erythematosus. *Arthritis and Rheumatism, 40*(9), 1725.

Hoque, R., & Chesson, A. L. Jr. (2009). Zolpidem-induced sleepwalking, sleep-related eating disorder, and sleep-driving: Fluorine-1 8-flourodeoxyglucose positron emission tomography analysis, and a literature review of other unexpected clinical effects of zolpidem. *Journal of Clinical Sleep Medicine, 5*(5), 471–476.

Hughes, M., Sundgren, P. C., Fan, X., Foerster, B., Nan, B., Welsh, R. C., et al. (2007). Diffusion tensor imaging in patients with acute onset of neuropsychiatric systemic lupus erythematosus: a prospective study of apparent diffusion coefficient, fractional anisotropy values, and eigenvalues in different regions of the brain. *Acta Radiologica, 48*(2), 213–222.

Ishikawa, O., Ohnishi, K., Miyachi, Y., & Ishizaka, H. (1994). Cerebral lesions in systemic lupus erythematosus detected by magnetic resonance imaging: relationship to anticardiolipin antibody. *Journal of Rheumatology, 21,* 87–90.

Jacobs, L., Kinkel, P. R., Costello, P. B., Alukal, M. K., Kinkel, W. R., & Green, F. A. (1988). Central nervous system lupus erythematosus: the value of magnetic resonance imaging. *Journal of Rheumatology, 15,* 601–606.

Jarek, M. J., West, S. G., Baker, M. R., & Rak, K. M. (1994). Magnetic resonance imaging in systemic lupus erythematosus patients without a history of neuropsychiatric lupus erythematosus. *Arthritis & Rheumatology, 37,* 1609–1613.

Jason, L. A., Richman, J. A., Rademaker, A. W., Jordan, K. M., Plioplys, A. V., Taylor, R. R., et al. (1999). A community-based study of chronic fatigue syndrome. *Archives of Internal Medicine, 159*(18), 2129–2137.

Jghaimi, F., Kabbaj, A., & Essaadouni, L. (2009). Systemic lupus erythematous revealed by an acute psychotic episode. *Revue Neurologique (Paris), 165*(12), 1107–1110.

Johnson, R. T., & Richardson, E. P. (1968). The neurological manifestations of systemic lupus erythematosus: A clinical-pathological study of 24 cases and review of the literature. *Medicine (Baltimore), 47,* 337–369.

Kao, C. H., Ho, Y. J., Lan, J. L., Changlai, S. P., Liao, K. K., & Chieng, P. U. (1999). Discrepancy between regional cerebral blood flow and glucose metabolism of the brain in systemic lupus erythematosus patients with normal brain magnetic resonance imaging findings. *Arthritis & Rheumatology, 42,* 61–68.

Kao, C. H., Lan J. L., Chang Lai, S. P., Liao, K. K., Yen, R. F., & Chieng, P. U. (1999). The role of FDG-PET, HMPAO-SPECT and MRI in the detection of brain involvement in patients with systemic lupus erythematosus. *European Journal of Nuclear Medicine, 26*(2), 129–134.

Karlson, E. W., Liang, M. H., Eaton, H., Huang, J., Fitzgerald, L., Rogers, M. P., et al. (2004). A randomized clinical trial of a psycho-educational intervention to improve outcomes in systemic lupus erythematosus. *Arthritis & Rheumatology, 50*(6), 1832–1841.

Kawashima, N., Shindo, R., & Kohno, M. (1993). Primary Sjögren's syndrome with subcortical dementia. *Internal Medicine, 32*(7), 561–564.

Kim, H. Y., Park, J. H., Oh, H. E., Han, H. J., Shin, D. I., & Kim, M. H. (2011). A case of rheumatoid meningitis: Pathologic and magnetic resonance imaging findings. *Neurological Sciences, 32,* 1191–1194.

Kluge, M., Schussler, P., & Steiger, A. (2007). Duloxetine increases stage 3 sleep and suppresses rapid eye movement (REM) sleep in patients with major depression. *European Neuropsychopharmacology, 17*(8), 527–531.

Knittle, K., Maes, S., & de Gucht, V. (2010). Psychological interventions for rheumatoid arthritis: Examining the role of self-regulation with a systematic review and meta-analysis of randomized controlled trials. *Arthritis Care & Research, 62*(10), 1460–1472.

Koenig, H. G., George, L. K., Peterson, B. L., & Pieper, C. F. (1997). Depression in medically ill hospitalized older adults: Prevalence, characteristics, and course of symptoms according to six diagnostic schemes. *American Journal of Psychiatry, 154*(10), 1376–1383.

Kowal, C., DeGiorgio, L. A., Lee, J. Y., Edgar, M. A., Huerta, P. T., Volpe, B. T., et al. (2006). Human lupus autoantibodies against NMDA receptors mediate cognitive impairment. *Proceedings of the National Academy of Sciences, 103,* 19854–19859.

Kowal, C., DeGiorgio, L. A., Nakaoka, T., Hetherington, H., Huerta, P. T., Diamond, B., et al. (2004). Cognition and immunity; antibody impairs memory. *Immunity, 21,* 179–188.

Lafitte, C., Amoura, Z., Cacoub, P., Pradat-Diehl, P., Picq, C., Salachas, F., et al. (2001). Neurological complications of primary Sjögren's syndrome. *Journal of Neurology, 248*(7), 577–584.

Lauvsnes, M. B., & Omdal, R. (2011). Systemic lupus erythematosus, the brain, and anti-NR2 antibodies. *Journal of Neurology, 259,* 622–629.

Leal-Cerro, A., Povedano, J., Astorga, R. Gonzalez, M., Silva, H., Garcia-Pesquera, F., et al. (1999). The growth hormone (GH)-releasing hormone-GH-insulin-like growth factor-1 axis in patients with fibromyalgia syndrome. *Journal of Clinical Endocrinology & Metabolism, 84,* 3378–3381.

Lemoine, P., & Faivre, T. (2004). Subjective and polysomnographic effects of milnacipran on sleep in depressed patients. *Human Psychopharmacology, 19*(5), 299–303.

Lipowski, Z. J. (1970). Physical illness, the individual and the coping process. *Psychiatry in Medicine, 1,* 91–102.

Lynch, M. E., & Campbell, F. (2011). Cannabinoids for treatment of chronic non-cancer pain: A systematic review of randomized trials. *British Journal of Clinical Pharmacology, 72*(5), 735–744.

Malinow, K. L., Molina, R., Gordon, B., Selnes, O. A., Provost, T. T., & Alexander, E. L. (1985). Neuropsychiatric dysfunction in primary Sjögren's syndrome. *Annals of Internal Medicine, 103,* 344–349.

Marquez, J., Restrepo, C. S., Candia, L., Berman, A., & Espinoza, L. R. (2004). Human immunodeficiency virus–associated rheumatic disorders in the HAART era. *Journal of Rheumatology, 31,* 741–746.

Mauch, E., Völk, C., Kratzsch, G., Krapf, H., Kornhuber, H. H., Laufen, H., et al. (1994). Neurological and neuropsychiatric dysfunction in primary Sjögren's syndrome. *Acta Neurologica Scandinavica, 89,* 31–35.

McCune, W. J., MacGuire, A., Aisen, A., & Gebarski, S. (1988). Identification of brain lesions in neuropsychiatric systemic lupus erythematosus by magnetic resonance scanning. *Arthritis & Rheumatology, 31,* 159–166.

McFarlane, A. C., & Brooks, P. M. (1988). An analysis of the relationship between psychological morbidity and disease activity in rheumatoid arthritis. *Journal of Rheumatology, 15*(6), 926–931.

Mease, P. J., Clauw, D. J., Gendreau, R. M., Rao, S. G., Kranzler, J., Chen, W., et al. (2009). The efficacy and safety of milnacipran for treatment of fibromyalgia. A randomized, double-blind, placebo-controlled trial. *Journal of Rheumatology, 36,* 398–409.

Mease, P. J., Russel, I. J., Arnold, L. M., Florian, H., Young, J. P. Jr., Martin, S. A., et al. (2008). A randomized, doubleblind, placebo-controlled, phase III trial of pregabalin in the treatment of patients with fibromyalgia. *Nature Clinical Practice Rheumatology, 4,* 514–515.

Meyer, G. J., Schober, O., Stoppe, G., Wildhagen, K., Seidel, J. W., & Hundeshagen, H. (1989). Cerebral involvement in systemic lupus erythematosus (SLE): Comparison of positron emission tomography (PET) with other imaging methods. *Psychiatry Research, 29,* 367–368.

Meyer, M. A. (2002). Elevated basal ganglia glucose uptake metabolism in cyclosporine neurotoxicity: A positron emission tomography imaging study. *Journal of Neuroimaging, 12*(1), 92–93.

Michel L., Toulgoat, F., Desal, H., Laplaud, D. A., Magot, A., Hamidou, M., et al. (2001). Atypical neurologic complications in patients with primary Sjögren's syndrome: Report of 4 cases. *Seminars in Arthritis & Rheumatology, 40*(4), 338–342.

Mikdashi, J., & Handwerger, B. (2004). Predictors of neuropsychiatric damage in systemic lupus erythematosus: Data from the Maryland lupus cohort. *Rheumatology, 43*(12), 1555–1560.

Mikdashi, J., Esdaile, J. M., Alarcón, G. S., Crofford, L., Fessler, B. J., Shanberg, L., et al. (2007). Proposed response criteria for neurocognitive impairment in systemic lupus erythematosus clinical trials. *Lupus, 16*, 418–425.

Miller, D. H., Buchanan, N., Barker, G., Morrissey, S. P., Kendall, B. E., Rudge, P., et al. (1992). Gadolinium-enhanced magnetic resonance imaging of the central nervous system in systemic lupus erythematosus. *Journal of Neurology, 239*, 460–464.

Moldofsky, H. (2009). The significance of dysfunctions of the sleeping/waking brain to the pathogenesis and treatment of fibromyalgia syndrome. *Rheumatic Disease Clinics of North America, 35*(2), 275–283.

Moll, J. W. B., Markussse, H. M., & Pijnenburg, J. J. M. (1993). Antineuronal antibodies in patients with neurologic complications of primary Sjögren's syndrome. *Neurology, 43*, 2574–2581.

Moreland, L. W., & Curtis, J. R. (2009). Systemic nonarticular manifestations of rheumatoid arthritis: Focus on inflammatory mechanisms. *Seminars in Arthritis & Rheumatology, 39*(2), 132–143.

Moritani, T., Hiwatashi, A., Shrier, D. A., Wang, H. Z., Numaguchi, Y., & Westesson, P. L. (2004). CNS vasculitis and vasculopathy: Efficacy and usefulness of diffusion-weighted echoplanar MR imaging. *Clinical Imaging, 28*(4), 261–270.

Morkane, C., Gregory, J. W., Watts, P., & Warner, J. T. (2011). Adrenal suppression following intralesional corticosteroids for periocular hemangiomas. *Archives of Disease in Childhood, 96*(6), 587–589.

Mulligan, K., & Newman, S. (2003). Psychological interventions in rheumatic diseases: A review of papers published from September 2001 to August 2002. *Current Opinion in Rheumatology, 15*, 156–159.

Muñoz-Málaga, A., Anglada, J. C., Páez, M., Girón, J. M., & Barrera, A. (1999). Psychosis as the initial manifestation of systemic lupus erythematosus: The role of lupus band test and anti-ribosomal antibodies. *Revue Neurologique (Paris), 28*(8), 779–781.

Murphy, S., Creed, F., & Jayson M. I. V. (1988). Psychiatric disorder and illness behaviour in rheumatoid arthritis. *British Journal of Rheumatology, 27*, 357–363.

Mustak, M., Boltuch-Sherif, J., Horvath-Mechtler, B., Kowalski-Bodzenta, J., & Erlacher, L. (2011). Autoimmune pancreatitis associated with rheumatoid arthritis. *Deutsche Medizinische Wochenschrift, 136*(37), 1842–1844.

Oelkers, W. (1996). Adrenal insufficiency. *New England Journal of Medicine, 335*, 1206–1212.

Ohayon, M. M. (2005). Prevalence and correlates of nonrestorative sleep complaints. *Archives of Internal Medicine, 165*(1), 35–41.

Okamoto, H., Kobayashi, A., & Yamanaka, H. (2010). Cytokines and chemokines in neuropsychiatric syndromes of systemic lupus erythematosus. *Clinical Rheumatology, 23*(2), 97–101.

Omdal, R., Brokstad, K., Waterloo, K., Koldingsnes, W., Jonsson, R., & Mellgren, S. I. (2005). Neuropsychiatric disturbances in SLE are associated with Abs against NMDA receptors. *European Journal of Neurology, 12*, 392–398.

Onen, S. H., Alloui, A., Gross, A., Eschallier, A., & Dubray, C. (2001). The effects of total sleep deprivation, selective sleep interruption and sleep recovery on pain tolerance thresholds in healthy subjects. *Journal of Sleep Research, 10*(1), 35.

Orzechowski, N. M., Wolanskyj, A. P., Ahlskog, J. E., Kumar, N., & Moder, K. G. (2008). Antiphospholipid antibody associated chorea. *Journal of Rheumatology, 35*, 2165–2170.

Otte, A., Weiner, S. M., Hoegerie, S., Wolf, R., Juengling, F. D., Peter, H. H., et al. (1998). Neuropsychiatric systemic lupus erythematosus before and after immunosuppressive treatment: a FDG PET study. *Lupus, 7*(1), 57–59.

Otte, A., Weiner, S. M., Peter, H. H., Mueller-Brand, J., Goetze, M., Moser, E., et al. (1997). Brain glucose utilization in systemic lupus erythematosus with neuropsychiatric symptoms: A controlled positron emission tomography study. *European Journal of Nuclear Medicine, 24*, 787–791.

Palmer, B. F., & Toto R. D. (1991). Severe neurologic toxicity induced by cyclosporine A in three renal transplant patients. *American Journal of Kidney Diseases, 18*(1), 116–121.

Pego-Reigosa, J. M., & Isenberg, D. A. (2008). Psychosis due to systemic lupus erythematosus: Characteristics and long-term outcome of this rare manifestation of the disease. *Rheumatology, 47*(10), 1498–1502.

Pincus, T., Griffith, J., Pearce, S., & Isenberg, David. (1996). Prevalence of self-reported depression in patients with rheumatoid arthritis. *British Journal of Rheumatology, 35*, 879–883.

Rao, S. G. (2009). Current progress in the pharmacological therapy of fibromyalgia. *Expert Opinion on Investigational Drugs, 18*(10), 1479–1493.

Ratey, J. J., & Loehr, J. E. (2011). The positive impact of physical activity on cognition during adulthood: A review of underlying mechanisms, evidence and recommendations. *Reviews in the Neurosciences, 22*(2), 171–185.

Reichlin, M. (2006). Autoantibodies to the ribosomal P proteins in systemic lupus erythematosus. *Clinical & Experimental Medicine, 6*(2), 49–52.

Rivera, J., de Diego, A., Trinchet, M., & García Monforte, A. (1997). Fibromyalgia-associated hepatitis C virus infection. *British Journal of Rheumatology, 36*, 981–985.

Rood, M. J., Verschuuren, J. J. G. M., & van Duinen, S. G. (2000). CNS involvement in primary Sjögren's syndrome: a case with a clue for the pathogenesis. *Journal of Neurology, 247*, 63–64.

Rostron, J., Rogers, S., Longman, L., Kancy, S., & Field, E. A. (2002). Health-related quality of life in patients with primary Sjögren's syndrome and xerostomia: a comparative study. *Gerondontology, 19*(1), 54–59.

Rozell, C. L., Sibbitt, W. L. Jr., & Brooks, W. M. (1998). Structural and neurochemical markers of brain injury in the migraine diathesis of systemic lupus erythematosus. *Cephalalgia, 18*, 209–215.

Sanna, G., Bertolaccini, M. L., Cuadrado, M. J., Laing, H., Khamashta, M. A., Mathieu, A., et al. (2003). Neuropsychiatric manifestations in systemic lupus erythematosus: prevalence and association with antiphospholipid antibodies. *Journal of Rheumatology, 30*(5), 985–992.

Saxena, A., & Solitar, B. M. (2010). Fibromyalgia. Knowns, unknowns and current treatment. *Bulletin of the NYU Hospital for Joint Diseases, 68*(3), 157–161.

Schlaghecke, R., Kornely, E., Santen, R. T., & Ridderskamp, P. (1992). The effect of long-term glucocorticoid therapy on pituitary–adrenal responses to exogenous corticotrophin-releasing hormone. *New England Journal of Medicine, 326*, 226–230.

Schneider, M., Vernon, H., Ko, G., Lawson, G., & Perera, J. (2009). Chiropractic management of fibromyalgia syndrome: A systematic review of the literature. *Journal of Manipulative and Physiological Therapeutics, 32*(1), 25–40.

Segal, B. M., Pogatchnik, B., Holker, E., Liu, H., Sloan, J., Rhodus, N., et al. (2012). Primary Sjogren's syndrome: Cognitive symptoms, mood, and cognitive performance. *Acta Neurologica Scandinavica 125*, 272–278. doi:10.1111/j.1600-0404.2011.01530.x.].

Sibbit, W. L., Sibbit, R. R., & Brooks, W. M. (1999). Neuroimaging in neuropsychiatric systemic lupus erythematosus. *Arthritis & Rheumatism, 42*, 2026–2038.

Sibbitt, W. L. Jr, Sibbitt, R. R., Griffey, R. H., Eckel, C., & Bankhurst, A. D. (1989). Magnetic resonance and computed tomographic imaging in the evaluation of acute neuropsychiatric disease in systemic lupus erythematosus. *Annals of the Rheumatic Diseases, 48*, 1014–1022.

Sibbitt, W. L. Jr., Brandt, J. R., Johnson, C. R., Maldonado, M. E., Patel, S. R., Ford, C. C., et al. (2002). The incidence and prevalence of neuropsychiatric syndromes in pediatric onset systemic lupus erythematosus. *Journal of Rheumatology, 29*(7), 1536–1542.

Sibbitt, W. L. Jr., Schmidt, P. J., Hart, B. L., & Brooks, W. M. (2003). Fluid attenuated inversion recovery (FLAIR) imaging in neuropsychiatric systemic lupus erythematosus. *Journal of Rheumatology, 30*(9), 1983–1989.

Simonin, C., Devos, D., de Seze, J., Charpentier, P., Vaiva, G., Goudemand, M., et al. (2004). Systemic lupus erythematosus presenting with recurrent psychiatric disturbances. *Revue Neurologique (Paris), 160*(8–9), 811–816.

Skrabek, R. Q., Galimova, L., Ethans, K., & Perry, D. (2008). Nabilone for the treatment of pain in fibromyalgia. *Journal of Pain, 9,* 164–173.

Spaeth, M., Rizzi, M., & Sarzi-Puttini, P. (2011). Fibromyalgia and sleep. *Best Practice & Research Clinical Rheumatology, 25*(2), 227–239.

Spezialetti, R., Bluestein, H. G., Peter, J. B., & Alexander, E. L. (1993). Neuropsychiatric disease in Sjögren's syndrome: Anti-ribosomal P and anti-neuronal antibodies. *American Journal of Medicine, 95*(2), 153–160.

Stern, M., & Robbins, E. S. (1960). Psychoses in systemic lupus erythematosus. *Archives of General Psychiatry, 3,* 205–212.

Stimmler, M. M., Coletti, P. M., & Quismorio, F. P. Jr. (1993). Magnetic resonance imaging of the brain in neuropsychiatric systemic lupus erythematosus. *Seminars in Arthritis & Rheumatology, 22,* 335–349.

Stoppe, G., Wildhagen, K., Seidel, J. W., Meyer, G. J., Schober, O., Heintz, P., et al. (1990). Positron emission tomography in neuropsychiatric lupus erythematosus. *Neurology, 40,* 304–308.

Tan, E. M., Cohen, A. F., Fries, J. F., Masi, A. T., McShane, D. J., Rothfield, N. F., et al. (1982). The 1982 revised criteria for the classification of systemic lupus erythematosus. *Arthritis and Rheumatism, 25*(11), 1271–1277.

Taylor, D. J., Lichstein, K. L., Durrence, H. H., Reidel, B. W., & Bush, A. J. (2005). Epidemiology of insomnia, depression, and anxiety. *Sleep, 28*(11), 1457–1464.

Telarović, S., Telarović, S., & Mihanović, M. (2007). Cyclosporine-induced depressive psychosis in a liver transplant patient: A case report. *Lijec Vjesn, 129*(3–4), 74–76.

Terhorst, L., Schneider, M. J., Kim, K. H., Goozdich, L. M., & Stilley, C. S. (2011). Complementary and alternative medicine in the treatment of pain in fibromyalgia: A systematic review of randomized controlled trials. *Journal of Manipulative and Physiological Therapeutics, 34*(7), 483–496.

Thoits, P. A., & Hewitt, L. N. (2001). Volunteer work and well-being. *Journal of Health & Social Behavior, 42*(2), 115–131.

Tokunaga, M., Saito, K., Kawabata, D., Imura, Y., Fujii, T., Nakayamada, S., et al. (2007). Efficacy of rituximab (anti-CD20) for refractory systemic lupus erythematosus involving the central nervous system. *Annals of the Rheumatic Diseases, 66,* 470–475.

Trevisani, V. F. M., Castro, A. A., Neves Neto, J. F., & Atallah, A. N. (2006). Cyclophosphamide versus methylprednisolone for treating neuropsychiatric involvement in systemic lupus erythematosus. *Cochrane Database of Systematic Reviews, 19*(2), CD002265.

Turcotte, D., Le Dorze, J. A., Esfahani, F., Frost, E., Gomori, A., & Namaka, M. (2010). Examining the roles of cannabinoids in pain and other therapeutic indications: a review. *Expert Opinion on Pharmacotherapy, 11*(1), 17–31.

Valesini, G., Alessandri, C., Celestino, D., & Conti, F. (2006). Anti-endothelial antibodies and neuropsychiatric systemic lupus erythematosus. *Annals of the New York Academy of Sciences, 1069,* 118–128.

Valtýsdóttir, S. T., Gudbjörnsson, B., Lindqvist, U., Hällgren, R., & Hetta, J. (2000). Anxiety and depression in patients with primary Sjögren's syndrome. *Journal of Rheumatology, 27*(1), 165–169.

Van Royen, A. (2005). Probable psychiatric side effects of azathioprine. *Psychosomatic Medicine, 67,* 508.

Vermathen, P., Ende, G., Laxer, K. D., Walker J. A., Knowlton, R. C., Barbaro, N. M., et al. (2002). Temporal lobectomy for epilepsy: recovery of the contralateral hippocampus measured by ¹H MRS. *Neurology, 59*(4), 633–636.

Wahner-Roedler, D. L., Elkin, P. L., Vincent, A., Thompson, J. M., Oh, T. H., Loehrer, L. L., et al. (2005). Use of complementary and alternative medical therapies by patients referred to a fibromyalgia treatment program at a tertiary care center. *Mayo Clinic Proceedings, 80,* 55–60.

Walker, E. A., Keegan, D., Gardner, G., Sullivan, M., Bernstein, D., & Katon, W. J. (1997a). Psychosocial factors in fibromyalgia compared with rheumatoid arthritis, I: Sexual, physical, and emotional abuse and neglect. *Psychosomatic Medicine, 59*(6), 572–577.

Walker, E. A., Keegan, D., Gardner, G., Sullivan, M., Bernstein, D., & Katon, W. J. (1997b). Psychosocial factors in fibromyalgia compared with rheumatoid arthritis. II: Sexual, physical, and emotional abuse and neglect, *59,* 572–577.

Wang, C. (2011). Tai chi and rheumatic diseases. *Rheumatic Disease Clinics of North America, 37*(1), 19–32.

Wang, M., Gladman, D. D., Ibañez, D., & Urowitz, M. B. (2012). Long-term outcome of early neuropsychiatric events due to active disease in systemic lupus erythematosus. *Arthritis Care & Research.* doi:10.1002/acr.21624.

Weiner, S. M., Otte, A., Schumacher, M., Brink, I., Juengling, F. D., Sobanksi, T., et al. (2000). Alterations of cerebral glucose metabolism indicate progress to severe morphological brain lesions in neuropsychiatric systemic lupus erythematosus. *Lupus, 9*(5), 386–389.

Weiner, S. M., Otte, A., Scumacher, M., Klien, R., Gutfleisch, J., Brink, I., et al. (2000). Diagnosis and monitoring of central nervous system involvement in systemic lupus erythematosus: Value of F-18 fluorodeoxyglucose PET. *Annals of the Rheumatic Diseases, 59*(5), 377–386.

Welsh, R. C., Rahbar, H., Foerster, B., Thurnher, M., & Sundgren, P. C. (2007). Brain diffusivity in patients with neuropsychiatric systemic lupus erythematosus with new acute neurological symptoms. *Journal of Magnetic Resonance Imaging, 26*(3), 541–551.

West, S. G. (1996). Lupus and the central nervous system. *Current Opinion in Rheumatology, 8,* 408–414.

White, P. D., Goldsmith, K. A., Johnson, A. L., Potts, L., Walwyn, R., DeCesare, J. C., et al., & PACE Trial Management Group. (2011). Comparison of adaptive pacing therapy, cognitive behaviour therapy, graded exercise therapy, and specialist medical care for chronic fatigue syndrome (PACE): A randomised trial. *Lancet, 377*(9768), 823–836.

Wolfe, F., Clauw, D. J., Fitzcharles, M. A., Goldenberg, D. L., Katz, R. S., Mease, P., et al. (2010). The American College of Rheumatology preliminary diagnostic criteria for fibromyalgia and measurement of symptom severity. *Arthritis Care & Research, (Hoboken), 62*(5), 600–610.

Wolfe, F., Smythe, H. A., Yunus, M. B., Bennett, R. M., Bombardier, C., Goldenberg, D. L., et al. (1990). The American College of Rheumatology 1990 criteria for the classification of fibromyalgia. Report of the Multicenter Criteria Committee. *Arthritis & Rheumatology, 33*(2), 160–172.

Younger, J., & Mackey, S. (2009). Fibromyalgia symptoms are reduced by low-dose naltrexone: a pilot study. *Pain Medicine, 10,* 663–672.

Yuen, K. C., Bennett, R. M., Hryciw, C. A., Cook, M. B., Rhoads, S. A., & Cook, D. M. (2007). Is further evaluation for growth hormone (GH) deficiency necessary in fibromyalgia patients with low serum insulin-like growth factor (IGF-1) levels? *Growth Hormone & IGF Research, 17,* 82–88.

Yunnus, M. B., Khan, M. A., Rawlings, K. K., Green, J. R., Olson, J. M., & Shah, S. (1999). Genetic linkage analysis of multicase families with fibromyalgia syndrome. *Journal of Rheumatology, 26*(2), 408–412.

Yunus, M. B. (2007). Fibromyalgia and overlapping disorders: the unifying concept of central sensitivity syndromes. *Seminars in Arthritis & Rheumatism, 36*(6), 339–356.

Zammit, G. (2009). Comparative tolerability of newer agents for insomnia. *Drug Safety, 32*(9), 735–748.

Zandman-Goddard, G., Chapman, J., & Shoenfeld, Y. (2006). Autoantibodies involved in neuropsychiatric SLE and antiphospholipid syndrome. *Seminars in Arthritis & Rheumatology, 36,* 297–315.

Zhang, L., Harrison, M., Heier, L. A., Zimmerman, R. D., Ravdin, L., Lockshin, M., et al. (2007). Diffusion changes in patients with systemic lupus erythematosus. *Magnetic Resonance Imaging, 25*(3), 399–405.

62.

DERMATOLOGY

Joseph A. Locala

Who has the disease is as important as the disease they have.
—Hippocrates

INTRODUCTION

Erasmus Wilson published the initial writings in psycho-dermatology in 1867; he discussed nervous influences on skin function for multiple dermatological diseases. Almost a century elapsed before additional articles were published in the field, highlighted by a pivotal monograph on "psycho-physiological aspects of skin diseases" by Whitlock in 1976 (Medansky, 1981). Despite a relative upsurge in research and academic literature over the past 25 years, psychodermatology remains a narrow, subspecialty field with a limited group of clinicians dedicated to its practice worldwide.

With many psychiatric disorders, patients suffer internally, but their affliction is outwardly unrecognized. Patients with psychodermatological disorders face amplified stigma when they suffer both mental concerns and skin disease visible to others. They cannot keep their condition private, and others may remain distant due to fear of infection or just an uncertainty about how to react to their appearance. Indeed, some have theorized that the tendency for people without skin disease to avoid contact with the afflicted person results from transient identification and discomfort with this reminder of their own flaws and vulnerability (Walker, 2005; Updike, 1990). Studies have demonstrated increased prevalence of psychiatric morbidity in patients with lesions on exposed areas of the body. In an assessment of dermatology outpatients in Italy, women with skin lesions on their faces and hands had a greater prevalence of psychiatric disorders than patients with lesions elsewhere (Picardi, 2001). Persons with skin disorders may also develop their own avoidance behaviors, along with a diminished body image and lower self-esteem. Elpern (2010) has quite accurately described psychocutaneous disease as "darkness visible."

It should be no surprise that the mind affects the body in skin disorders and that the skin alters brain function through feedback loops. The skin is a primary organ for communication with the outside world. It serves as a vital barrier of defense for the organism and a crucial feedback mechanism to protect the body against trauma or external insults. As such, the skin is filled with dense afferent and efferent nervous system connections and is a target for stress hormones and immune modulators; its own feedback modifies the release of these chemicals. Disturbances in this delicately balanced system may morph into a myriad of disease states.

Dermatology is a discipline in which psychosomatic issues play a key role in the understanding of the etiology and progression of skin diseases as well as the determination of appropriate treatments. Psychodermatological disorders may be classified into several categories: primary psychiatric disorders associated with cutaneous symptoms; psychosocial factors affecting dermatological diseases, comorbid psychiatric and skin illnesses, and disorders related to medication use. Box 62.1 provides a list of diagnoses in each group.

This chapter will include discussion of selected psychodermatological disorders, review of psychiatric comorbidities, treatment approaches, medication issues, special areas of clinical concern, and, finally, a model for the establishment of a multidisciplinary care team.

PRIMARY PSYCHIATRIC DISORDERS MANIFESTED BY CUTANEOUS SYMPTOMS

Patients consult dermatologists with symptoms related to the hair or skin, but systemic disease or emotional illness actually causes or exacerbates many of these symptoms. This section will discuss a collection of skin disorders caused by a primary psychiatric illness; these run the gamut from frank psychosis, to self-inflicted lesions, to addiction and lifestyle choices.

DELUSIONAL PARASITOSIS

Patients with delusional parasitosis (DP), classified in the *Diagnostic & Statistical Manual of Mental Disorders* (DSM-IV) as a form of delusional disorder, somatic type, commonly presenting to dermatologists first because their skin complaints are the only manifestation of their illness. DP has been known by many names; these include: Ekbom's syndrome, parasitophobia, and Morgellons. As highlighted in a recent editorial in the *British Journal of Dermatology*, Freudenmann and Lepping's use of the name "delusional infestation" is more accurate, because patients believe worms, bacteria, parasites, insects, viruses, particles, fibers, and other agents may be responsible for their symptoms (Bewley, 2010).

This disorder is rare, with a prevalence of 80 cases per million people, and a bimodal age distribution with peaks from age 20–30 and over 50. In younger patients, there is an equal sex distribution, but in those over 50, it is three times more prevalent in women (Lyell, 1983). Five to 15% of persons close to patients with DP develop *folie à deux* (shared psychotic disorder) (Trabert, 1999; Wykoff, 1987). A recent study of 54 patients seen at the Mayo Clinic reported a 28% prevalence of shared psychotic disorder; in this group identified over a seven-year period, another striking finding was that 74% had a comorbid psychiatric disorder (depression, 45%; anxiety, 19%; drug dependence and abuse, 19%). Personality disorders were found to be uncommon (Hylwa, 2012). DP may be a primary delusional disorder or a disorder secondary to dementia, medication side effects (such as amantadine in Parkinson's), or drug intoxication or withdrawal (e.g., methamphetamine, cocaine, alcohol, marijuana) (Bewley, 2010).

Patients with DP have a specific fixed, false belief that they are infested with living organisms, and will offer samples of material as evidence of their disease. They commonly present to their physician collections of lint, skin crusts, and other debris, and the "matchbox sign" refers to the frequent use of small containers to carry this material. With the advent of smoking cessation and the disappearance of matchboxes, this author more commonly has seen patients arrive with plastic bags, bottles, and "specimens" taped to pieces of paper.

Symptoms of Morgellons disease closely match those of DP, with a greater emphasis on the extrusion of fibrous materials from the skin, rather than infestation with frank organisms. Morgellons disease was first described by physician Sir Thomas Browne, in a work posthumously published in 1690. It has been known by many names, and its existence as a genuine medical malady has been controversial. The dermatological community has long argued that Morgellons and delusions of parasitosis are one and the same disorder. The Centers for Disease Control (CDC) embarked on an epidemiological investigation in conjunction with Kaiser Permanente Northern California in 2008. After careful evaluation of 113 case subjects with Morgellons, "no single underlying medical condition or infectious source was identified." Most of the skin lesions were either arthropod bites or chronic excoriations, and fibers from patients' skin were identified as cellulose from clothing. No evidence was found for mycobacterial or parasitic infection. Furthermore, this population had significant rates of substance use, cognitive disorders, high somatic complaint scores, and greater functional disability, in line with those with major medical problems or significant psychiatric disorders (Pearson, 2012).

Often patients are very resistant to the notion that this problem is psychiatric in origin and will strongly defend their belief in an infectious etiology. Many refuse psychiatric evaluation, or if they attend one appointment, are often non-adherent with medication and follow-up. A useful approach is to target improvement of symptoms and quality of life as the goal of an initial treatment, without attempting to confront the question of the "infestation" directly. (Murase, Wu, & Koo, 2006).

Pimozide, a first-generation neuroleptic, has been a drug of choice for treating DP, potentially because of anti-pruritic action due to its effect on opioid pathways. However, pimozide has a risk for significant side effects, including QTc prolongation and cardiac arrhythmias. Risperidone, olanzapine, aripiprazole, and quetiapine have all shown efficacy in small studies or case reports in treatment of DP (Sandoz, 2008). Freudenmann (2008) reviewed case reports and identified full remission rates of 37% with atypical antipsychotics versus 51% with older antipsychotics (pimozide); the older antipsychotics were clearly associated with greater side effects. When adding both partial and full remission rates, atypical antipsychotics had better results against older agents (75% vs. 65%). Treatment with an atypical antipsychotic from the list above is a reasonable first-line therapy for DP. Some clinicians opt to initiate treatment without clear patient education about antipsychotics, with the hope that they will more readily accept medication. This approach is not advisable; when patients discover this deception, it will greatly erode the physician–patient alliance. A better approach is to inform patients of documented efficacy for this class of medication and instruct them that these medications will help allay the fears, stress, and anxiety associated with their illness.

TRICHOTILLOMANIA

Trichotillomania (TTM) is a disorder characterized by hair-pulling from regions such as the scalp, eyebrows, eyelashes, face, or pubic regions. Often hair is then chewed and/or ingested. Two specific subtypes of TTM have been identified: "Focused" hair pulling, which is very conscious and similar to compulsive behaviors, and "automatic," in which patients pull their hair with a decreased attention to their activity. DSM-IV-TR criteria for TTM include: "Recurrent pulling of one's hair resulting in noticeable hair loss and an increased sense of tension immediately before pulling…pleasure, gratification, or relief when pulling out the hair" (American Psychiatric Association, 2000). TTM tends to emerge in early childhood or adolescence, with average age of onset at 13 years. Later onset has been associated with greater symptom severity and treatment resistance. The bimodal onset and different characteristics lead some to believe there are "phenomenological differences between early and late onset" TTM (Mansueto, 2012). Prevalence rates vary by the criteria used for assessment. Two studies of different populations (student vs. general adult) both found prevalence rates of 0.6% using full DSM-IV-TR criteria. With expansion of those diagnostic criteria to include "clinically significant" hair-pulling and hair-pulling with noticeable hair loss, those rates increase to 1.2–2.5% (Christenson, 1999; Duke, 2009). As many as 57% of adults with TTM have a comorbid psychiatric disorder; most commonly major depressive disorder, other mood disorders, obsessive-compulsive disorder (OCD), or other mood or anxiety disorders (Flessner, 2012; Vythilingum & Stein, 2005).

The diagnostic criteria for TTM, and even use of the term "trichotillomania," have been recently debated. DSM-V includes a name change to "hair pulling disorder" and modified criteria to read: "Recurrent pulling out of one's hair resulting in hair loss; the hair-pulling causes clinically significant distress or impairment in social, occupational or other important areas of functioning." In DSM-IV-TR, it was classified as an impulse-control disorder. It has been argued that TTM could fit into one of three categories: obsessive-compulsive spectrum disorders, impulse-control disorders, or body-focused repetitive behavior disorders (Stein, 2010). As many as 57% of adults with TTM have a comorbid psychiatric disorder, the most common of which are major depression, other mood disorders, OCD, and other anxiety disorders. (Flessner, 2012) This pattern of comorbidity resembles that of patients with other body-focused repetitive behaviors.

A major hurdle in effective treatment is getting the patient's acknowledgement of a problem and a request for care; many persons in the population with TTM probably never seek clinical assistance. Psychotherapeutic approaches have been demonstrated to be valuable in TTM. Habit-reversal training (HRT) is a cognitive behavioral therapy (CBT) modality that has three stages: (1) Increase the awareness of pulling behaviors, (2) Engage in competing behavior that prevents pulling, and (3) Recruit a social support person to remind patients of their behavior. Stimulus control is a method by which patients identify situations that trigger hair-pulling and work with the therapist to find interventions that modify the setting or actions for pulling behavior. HRT has been combined with dialectical behavioral therapy, stimulus control therapy, acceptance and commitment therapy; all had favorable response rates (Woods, 2012).

Pharmacologically, there is limited positive evidence to support use of naltrexone, N-acetylcysteine, and olanzapine. Case reports and open-label studies suggest that other serotonin reuptake inhibitors (SSRIs), lithium, bupropion, topiramate, and other antipsychotics (haloperidol, pimozide, risperidone, quetiapine, and aripiprazole) may also be efficacious (Chamberlain, 2012; White, 2011).

EXCORIATION (SKIN-PICKING) DISORDER

Excoriation (skin-picking) disorder in DSM-V, also known as *neurotic excoriation* or *psychogenic excoriation*, or *pathological skin picking* (PSP), is a repetitive, compulsive picking of skin that causes actual damage. With pathological skin-picking (PSP), the patient is conscious of his/her behavior and will readily admit it. Often patients begin to pick or scratch an area due to initial itch or a perceived lesion or skin defect. Repetitive scratching initiates an itch-scratch cycle and perpetuates the behavior. A special form of skin-picking is acne excoriée, in which minimal acne lesions, typically on the face, are manipulated with fingers or sharp instruments to the point of ulcerations or erosions capable of scarring. PSP has similarities to trichotillomania and onchyphagia (nail-biting) and onchotillomania (peeling of the nail and cuticle); some authors consider these to be a group of pathological grooming behaviors. Another view is that PSP has a common etiology with obsessive-compulsive disorder because of similar clinical characteristics and the high comorbidity of OCD, as well as incidence of OCD in first-order relatives (Grant, 2010).

PSP has quite an extensive degree of psychiatric comorbidity, with lifetime rates of DSM-IV axis I diagnoses occurring with a range from 55% to 100%! The most common disorders identified have been major depressive disorder, bipolar disorder, anxiety disorders, OCD, eating disorders, alcohol abuse, and attention-deficit disorder (Odlaug et al., 2012). PSP occurs with TTM with lifetime prevalence of 38.3%, and with compulsive nail-biting, 31.7%. Patients with body dysmorphic disorder have lifetime rates of 44.9% with point prevalence of 36.9% (Odlaug et al., 2012). The significant overlap of disorders and symptoms paints a confusing clinical picture. Probably multiple different etiologies are involved, and with them, different required treatment modalities.

Small trials and case reports have suggested the efficacy of SSRIs, doxepin, aripiprazole, and olanzapine for PSP (Gupta, 2011). In a careful review of available double-blind, open-label studies and case reports, Chamberlain (2012) has identified fluoxetine as likely to be efficacious for PSP, whereas citalopram, escitalopram, fluvoxamine, and lamotrigene (Grant, 2010) had mixed results. With regard to psychotherapy, HRT alone or in conjunction with CBT, ACT alone or with HRT, may benefit persons with chronic skin-picking (Woods, 2012).

DERMATITIS ARTEFACTA

Dermatitis artefacta is a condition in which patients cause self-inflicted skin lesions, often without conscious awareness. Patients often deny recall of the event that caused lesions and may have dissociative episodes surrounding them. On interview, patients often are vague about symptoms, omit details, and appear emotionally disconnected as they discuss their illness. Dermatitis artefacta would typically be classified as a factitious disorder unless a clear secondary gain can be identified, in which case it would be malingering. Self-inflicted skin lesions may also occur as a symptom of several psychiatric disorders, such as severe personality disorders, dissociative disorders, and post-traumatic stress disorder (PTSD). Lesions are usually located in areas easily within reach and can imitate most forms of actual dermatological diseases. In order to create lesions, persons will bite, stab, apply pressure, create burns (thermal and chemical), introduce infectious material, and also inject covert medications such as heparin and insulin (Harth, 2009). Nielsen (2005) reported a retrospective analysis of 57 dermatitis artefacta patients seen over the course of 20 years in a dermatology department. Female to male ratio was 2.8:1, and median age was 39, with a range from 18 to 60 years. Two-thirds of patients initially denied self-infliction, and only one patient agreed to psychiatric consultation. Eighteen percent were diagnosed with psychiatric disorders. Multiple lesions were present in 88% of patients; the most common lesions were skin ulcers (72%), excoriations (46%), and erythema (30%).

Initial treatment of dermatitis artefacta consists of management of underlying psychiatric disorders with antidepressants or anxiolytics when appropriate. In a similar fashion to management of Munchausen's or factitious disorder, early intervention is crucial to avoid excessive utilization of medical resources and unnecessary or harmful treatments for the patient. Supportive psychotherapy has value, followed by a shift to behavioral, relaxation, and/or psychodynamic therapy when patients are ready to accept mental health intervention.

BODY DYSMORPHIC DISORDER

Body dysmorphic disorder (BDD) is a preoccupation with an imagined defect in appearance, or when an actual abnormality is present, the person's level of concern is excessive. Although classified as a somatoform disorder, BDD most certainly has characteristics of an obsessive-compulsive spectrum disorder as well. BDD affects approximately 1–2% of the American population. In dermatology clinics, incidence ranges from 12–16%, and in cosmetic dermatology offices, 15–46% (Malick, Howard, & Koo, 2008). Patients with BDD may focus on whole-body concerns such as aging, excessive hair, excessive sweating, or muscle mass; or regional concerns like the shape of specific body parts, scars, genitalia, hair-growth patterns, and so on. Approximately one-third of patients pick their skin to "improve" their physical appearance, sometimes using dangerous implements (Thomas, 2005). This author has cared for a patient who developed and sharpened homemade surgical instruments and spent significant periods of time doing intricate dissection of his face in order to remove perceived "small growths." He described in vivid detail the removal of pieces that sounded like lymphatic

system, subcutaneous fat, and blood vessels. Resultant poor wound healing led to infections, prolonged inpatient hospital stays, and repeated plastic surgery.

Malick and colleagues (2008) have written an excellent summary that outlines the process of screening for psychiatric issues in cosmetic surgery patients. They advocate screening for BDD, narcissistic personality disorder, and histrionic personality disorder, all of which are seen more commonly in cosmetic surgery populations; they also offer sets of diagnostic screening questions for clinical use. Interestingly, cosmetic dermatology patients have not been shown to have higher prevalence of psychotropic drug use compared to medical dermatology patients (18% vs. 17%), although both groups have much higher rates than the general population and a matched non–cosmetic surgery group (Orringer, 2006).

Treatment for BDD consists of psychotherapeutic and pharmacological interventions. SSRIs are effective, with case reports and open-label studies supporting use of fluvoxamine; a placebo-controlled study with fluoxetine (doses 20–80 mg daily) showed 53% response rate (Mackley, 2005). CBT has been proved efficacious; through a 12-week randomized, controlled study, Veale et al. (1996) demonstrated a 50% reduction in symptoms of BDD. Proper management of this disorder needs to address protection of the patient from unnecessary surgery or treatments for minimal or imagined deficits. It is also critical to screen for suicidal ideation or thoughts of self-harm, as patients with BDD are a high-risk group in dermatology.

TANNING ADDICTION

Despite society's increased awareness of the risks of ultraviolet (UV) exposure, such as premature aging and skin cancer, dermatologists continue to struggle with patients who engage in excessive tanning. Indoor tanning among young adults has increased from 1% to 27% between 1988 and 2007 (Robinson, 2008). Along with increased tanning, rates of skin cancer have increased in parallel. One study has shown an eightfold increase in melanoma rates in women under 40 between the years 1970 and 2009, and a fourfold increase for men under 40 (Reed, 2012). Ferrucci et al. (2011) recently reported a 69% increase in risk of early-onset basal cell carcinoma (under age 40) associated in a dose-dependent fashion with years of use of indoor tanning beds. One might hope that a history of skin cancer in the immediate family would dissuade younger persons from tanning; however, 35% of young adults from families at risk for melanoma use tanning beds. Indoor tanning prevalence is highest in young, white females, particularly those aged 18 to 29 (Heckman, 2008). This age group is at significantly higher risk for skin cancer; ten annual tanning visits per year doubles the risk for melanoma in those over 30, but the risk increases eightfold for those under age 30.

Frequent tanners have demonstrated the ability to discriminate between ultraviolet light (UV) versus non-ultraviolet light in a double-blind study, and chose to receive additional UV light 95% of the time. It is speculated that UV light stimulates production of beta-endorphin and acts as reinforcing stimulus for repeated tanning (Feldman, 2004). Naltrexone, an opioid antagonist, blocks the effect of UV light in frequent tanners and has caused withdrawal symptoms (nausea) (Kaur et al., 2006). Single photon-emission computed tomography (SPECT) identified regional cortical blood flow increases in the dorsal striatum, anterior insula, and medial orbitofrontal cortex, areas believed to be part of the reward circuits, when subjects were exposed to UV light vs. sham light (Harrington, 2012).

The concept that tanning may be a substance-related disorder is supported by the fact that frequent tanners have difficulty controlling their use, persist despite negative consequences, experience tolerance, and withdrawal, and have psychological dependence (Nolan, 2009). Mosher (2010) evaluated university students in the northeastern United States for prevalence of indoor tanning addiction and comorbidity with psychiatric disorders and substance use. Of these, 39.3% met DSM IV-TR criteria, and 36.6% met CAGE substance abuse screening tool criteria for addiction to indoor tanning, and within that group, scores were higher for drug and alcohol use and anxiety (but not depression). Perception of habitual tanning as an addiction may assist dermatologists in the goal of weaning patients. Mosher's data lend credence to the concept that tanning may be an addictive disorder, but also suggest that successful treatment needs to address substance use and anxiety disorders in this population. The obstacle to care is that most patients fail to understand the hazards of tanning or simply ignore them. Greater public education is necessary, and skin cancer prevention efforts that target school-age children would probably be beneficial. A number of localities worldwide and in the United States have set limits on minimum age for indoor tanning or have made it illegal.

PSYCHOSOCIAL FACTORS AFFECTING DERMATOLOGICAL DISORDERS

Emotional factors appear to significantly influence most skin diseases, and the correlation between stressful life events and disease flares is well recognized in dermatology. The skin is a target for stress hormones and immune modulators and also influences release of these mediators. The neuro-immuno-cutaneous-endocrine (NICE) model (O'Sullivan, 1998) explains the interplay between organ systems, neurotransmitters, hormones, and cytokines and the various feedback loops. Tausk (2008) has elegantly outlined the effects of chronic stress on the immune system, particularly with regard to skin diseases. The nervous system maintains a delicate balance between cell-mediated (Th1) and humoral (Th2) immune responses. When subject to acute stress, the hypothalamus is responsible for the release of corticotrophin-releasing hormone (CRH), adrenocorticotropic hormone (ACTH), noradrenaline (NE), and eventually cortisol, which result in an increase in immunity. Chronic stress may result in a decrease in overall immunity. The skin appears to have its own version of the hypothalamic-pituitary-axis (HPA), which Slominski (2000) called the "skin stress response system" (SSRS). The skin produces CRH, propiomelanocortin (POMC)-derived neuropeptides,

alpha-melanocyte stimulating hormone, ACTH, and beta-endorphin, and contains active receptors for CRH and POMC-peptides. The SSRS is believed to perform a "stress neutralizing activity" and limits disruptions of internal homeostasis. A similar localized system appears to be active in the hair follicles as well.

Specific sets of cytokines promote cell-mediated immunity, and other cytokines enhance humoral immunity. Cytokines are frequently regulated in cascades, where earlier cytokines serve to increase the production of later cytokines. Proinflammatory cytokines, such as interleukin-1 (IL-1), interleukin-6 (IL-6), and tumor necrosis factor (TNF) augment the immune response to speed elimination of pathogens and resolve inflammatory challenge, whereas anti-inflammatory cytokines, such as IL-4, IL-10, and IL-13, serve to dampen the immune response (Kronfol, 2000). Stress affects regulation of cytokines and may result in overexpression, a condition believed to be linked to a number of dermatological diseases.

Some studies have linked hyperactivity of the HPA and parallel increases in proinflammatory cytokines to the presence of major depression (Maes, 1995). Sickness behaviors (often associated with infection) include increased sleep, decreased appetite, and decreased sex drive; these may also be attributed to effects of the cytokines (Kronfol, 2000). Maes (2012) has recently reinforced the premise that depression and sickness behavior are "Janus-faced responses to shared inflammatory pathways." And yet, antidepressant therapy, despite effective treatment of depression, has failed to demonstrate decreases in proinflammatory cytokines as a class (although SSRIs as a subclass reduced TNF-alpha and IL-6) (Hannestad, 2011).

PSORIASIS

Psoriasis is a chronic, relapsing disease of the skin that affects approximately 2% of the United States population and 1–4% of people worldwide. It is considered to be an immune-mediated disorder with evidence for genetic risk. The clinical picture consists of papulosquamous plaques that are well delineated from surrounding normal skin. Plaques are red or salmon pink in color and are covered by white scales, with common areas of distribution on extensor aspects of elbows and knees, scalp, lumbosacral region, and umbilicus. Psoriasis has a several medical comorbidities, among them psoriatic arthritis (25%) and cardiovascular disease. Triggers for psoriasis flares include physical trauma or pressure (Koebner phenomenon), bacterial or viral infections, steroid withdrawal, and medications (for example, beta-blockers and lithium).

A well-established relationship exists between stress and exacerbations of psoriasis, and the degree of stress due to anticipation of others' perception of the psoriatic lesions is actually the greatest predictor of disability in these patients. Stress has been linked to onset of the initial episode of psoriasis in 44% of patients, and recurrent flares are attributed to stress in up to 80% of patients; patients who self-report high levels of stress are likely to have more severe skin and joint symptoms (Jafferany, 2007). A study of 1,580 psoriasis patients in 39 Italian dermatology centers revealed minor psychological distress in 46% of patients, and major distress, to the degree of psychopathology, in 11% (Finzi et al., 2007). Both types of distress were more frequent in women, and there was no correlation between degree of psoriasis severity and distress.

Pietrzak (2008) provides an excellent review of the role for overexpression of proinflammatory cytokines, particularly TNF, interleukins, and interferon gamma, in patients with psoriasis, as well as the utility of cytokines/anticytokines for treatment. TNF antagonists are cited as the most commonly used agents. Research has indicated that patients with psoriasis, particularly those whose disease appears stress-responsive, exhibit an altered HPA response to acute social stress, reflected by a diminished cortisol response. One group hypothesizes that the similarities are so "considerable" between depression and psoriasis—namely, elevated proinflammatory cytokines and acute-phase proteins—that both disorders can be considered immunologically mediated, inflammatory states (Filakovic, 2008). The most recent study to address HPA axis function in psoriasis found no significant correlation with neuroendocrine, psychiatric, and immune parameters in a sophisticated design with tracking of a number of hormonal and immune markers (Karanikas, 2009). Further investigation of the psychoneuroimmunology of psoriasis will be an important area for future research.

ATOPIC DERMATITIS

Atopic dermatitis (AD) is a form of eczema that affects between 5% and 30% of children and 2–3% of the adult population, and causes intense pruritus and inflammation, often complicated by excessive scratching. Most cases arise in childhood prior to age five, and AD may develop into a chronic, relapsing disorder. The itch-scratch cycle often results in excoriations, crusting, and areas of thickened skin (lichenification). Approximately half of all patients with AD will develop allergic asthma and/or allergic rhinitis. The severe itching often leads to sleep disturbance for patients, and in the case of children, for caretakers or family members. Thirty percent of patients notice exacerbations of AD with stress. Life-altering events may elicit itching or reduce the itching threshold. No specific personality type has been identified with AD.

Controlled studies have demonstrated that patients with AD are more anxious and depressed (Hashiro, 1997). Depression may worsen the perception of discomfort experienced with itching and also may be a contributor to the poor adherence to therapy often seen in patients with AD. Schmitt and colleagues (2009) utilized a multidisciplinary outpatient database in Germany to investigate the relationship between AD and multiple psychiatric disorders. AD was independently associated with affective disorders, schizophrenia, "neurotic" and stress-related disorders, somatoform disorders, and personality and "behavior disorders." Patients with stress- exacerbated AD have affected areas of the skin that contain fewer nerve fibers in the epidermis and an increase

in the epidermal fraction of 5-HT1A receptor and serotonin transporter (SERT) immunoreactivity in the involved skin (Lonne-Rahm, 2008). This research led to the hypothesis that changed innervation and modulation of the serotonergic system are implicated in AD and chronic stress, and future therapies targeting serotonin receptors and SERT may be efficacious.

Alternative therapies such as relaxation techniques and CBT, combined with antipruritics, antihistamines, and antidepressants/anxiolytics (when indicated) have the most value in treating this disorder.

ACNE

Acne is a papulopustular disease of the sebaceous glands with formation of comedones and secondary inflammation. Acne affects 90% of adolescents in puberty, but persistent acne (acne tarda) may continue into the fourth decade of life; 12% of adult women and 3% of adult men are affected. A genetic heritability is present, with an influence by androgen activity. The psychological impact of acne is significant, and emergence occurs at a period in life (adolescence and young adulthood) in which self-esteem, body image, and social functions are in stages of critical development. Significant comorbid depression, high stress levels, anxiety, social impairment, suicidality, and diminished quality of life are associated with acne. These factors may partly explain why acne patients are often poorly compliant with treatment regimens.

Gupta and Gupta (1998) cite a 5.6% prevalence of suicidal ideation, approximately double that of the general population. Compared to other skin disorders, the rates of suicidal ideation and depression were only greater in those with severe psoriasis. The highest rates of suicide in dermatology are in adolescent males with a severe form, acne conglomata. Acne is also associated with BDDs and eating disorders.

A topic for debate is the contribution of the acne treatment, isotretinoin, to the development of depression and suicidal thoughts. Hull et al. (2005) reviewed a number of studies, and concluded that both depression and anxiety occur at higher rates in acne patients without drug therapy. This article scrutinized existing treatment-cohort studies and large-scale population studies and concluded that the low number of cases of depression did not suggest a direct drug effect of isotretinoin. Magin et al. drew similar conclusions in a 2005 review of published database articles. Strahan (2006) published a rigorous review of available case reports, adverse drug event reports, prospective studies, and retrospective studies relating to psychiatric adverse events with isotretinoin. The analysis determined that a lack of solid scientific data "limits any conclusion that can be drawn about causal relationship between isotretinoin and psychiatric adverse events." Retinoids can influence central nervous system (CNS) functioning through effects on neuronal development and influence on transmitter receptors. Retinoids also cause hippocampal suppression, which is a known risk factor for depression (Strahan, 2006). The current consensus would appear to be that no definite conclusions can be made regarding risks of isotretinoin with regard to psychiatric side effects or suicidality. Patients should be made aware of potential risks and screened for history of mood or psychotic disorders, suicidal ideation, family psychiatric history, and current psychiatric symptoms prior to initiation of therapy and at each visit. The great value of isotretinoin for many patients with severe acne needs to be weighed against risk of a rare, and perhaps preventable, adverse event.

CHRONIC URTICARIA AND IDIOPATHIC PRURITUS

Idiopathic chronic urticaria (ICU) is defined by recurrent short-lived, itchy wheals and swelling of at least six weeks' duration for which no clear physical factor or cause can be identified. ICU is associated with high levels of anxiety and depression and diminished quality of life. Quality of life (QOL) has been correlated with mood symptoms more than with the extent of skin disease (Engin, 2007). Furthermore, patients with ICU and no comorbid axis I or axis II psychiatric disorder had a QOL similar to that of healthy controls (Uguz, 2008).

Idiopathic pruritus is defined as an itch that cannot be explained by an identified medical disorder and without a primary skin eruption. The presence of itching has been associated with psychosocial stressors, a variety of psychiatric conditions, and psychological features such as lack of emotional maturity, anxiety, and high subjective reaction to stress (Kretzmer et al., 2008). A study in hospitalized psychiatric inpatients revealed high incidence of idiopathic pruritus in 100 subjects (42% overall, 34% of men, 58% of women) and demonstrated higher levels in those without adequate social support and among those without regular employment (Karanikas, 2009). A total of 76% of regular opioid users experienced pruritus. Those treated with tricyclic antidepressants had much lower rates (14%) as opposed to those treated with other antidepressants (48%).

ALOPECIA AREATA

Alopecia areata is an abrupt loss of hair from round or oval patches, typically involving the scalp. Hair loss may occur in other regions, and a patient may present with loss of all scalp hair or all body hair.

Alopecia areata (AA) is presumed to be an autoimmune disease in which T-lymphocytes excrete cytokines that inhibit hair growth at the follicle (Willemsen, 2008). AA occurs in approximately 0.1–0.2% of the population. Up to 10% of patients will experience progression of hair loss, but for the majority, hair grows back after several months. AA has been linked to stressful life events (in the preceding 6 months to a year), higher anxiety and stress levels, alexithymia, avoidance of intimate or attached relationships, and poor social support (Willemsen, 2008). Significant percentages of patients with AA have psychiatric comorbidity. Koo et al. (1994) found rates of major depression, generalized anxiety disorder, social phobia, and paranoid disorders to be higher with AA patients than in the general population. A more recent study found a 66% rate of psychiatric comorbidity in persons with AA;

diagnoses were primarily adjustment disorder, depression, and anxiety (Ruiz Doblado, 2003).

COMORBID PSYCHIATRIC DISORDERS IN PATIENTS WITH SKIN DISEASE

Dermatology patients present with an overall estimated 30% prevalence of comorbid psychiatric and psychological disorders (Gupta, 2003). In outpatients in a dermatology clinic, Picardi et al. (2000) identified psychiatric disease in 25% of patients with vitiligo, 26% with psoriasis, 32% with acne, 34% with urticarial, and 35% with alopecia. Psychiatric comorbidities commonly observed in a dermatology practice include: depressive disorders, anxiety spectrum disorders, post-traumatic stress, BDD, and social anxiety. In a consecutively screened sample of 166 patients who presented to dermatology clinics, 24.7% met DSM-IV criteria for OCD. Only 14.6% of these patients had previously been diagnosed with OCD (Demet, 2005). PTSD, as a form of severe stressor, may be associated with exacerbation of psoriasis, AD, AA, and urticaria (Gupta, 2005). Social anxiety may be diagnosed in patients with disfiguring skin diseases, such as psoriasis or acne, particularly when they have received negative attention or ridicule earlier in life (Gupta, 2005). Patients with social anxiety or severe OCD may not be diagnosed due to their reluctance to leave home to attend doctor's appointments.

General adult dermatology patients were screened using the Patient Health Questionnaire in the clinic and found to have prevalence rates of 14% for anxiety and depressive disorders, and in the hospital setting had prevalence of 20% diagnosed anxiety and depressive disorders by Structural Clinical Interview for DSM disorders (SCID) (Picardi, 2004). This suggests that a higher acuity of skin disease is associated with more significant rates of psychiatric disorders.

Alexithymia is a personality trait that predisposes a person to have problems differentiating and describing feelings. A recent review of publications on alexithymia and dermatology concluded that alexithymia appears to be associated with AA, AD, psoriasis, vitiligo, and chronic urticaria (Willemsen, 2008). Alexithymia has been linked to changes in sympathetic activity, immunity, and brain activity. Alexithymia rates of 33% were found in a study of psoriasis patients using the Toronto Alexithymia Scale–20, equivalent to prevalence found in other severe chronic medical disease states; the researchers believe that alexithymia is not an acute coping strategy but rather a stable character trait (Richards, 2005). Seventy-five patients with chronic skin disorders, the majority hospitalized on a university dermatology inpatient service, were evaluated for depression, alexithymia, and degree of skin lesions. Significant correlations were found between score on the Toronto Alexithymia Scale, Hamilton Depression Scale, and the extent of skin lesions (Asri, 2008). For individual patients, the presence of alexithymia may give psychotherapists a target for treatment.

By and large, comorbid psychiatric disorders in the dermatology patient are treated with a similar array of antidepressants, anxiolytics, and antipsychotics as solo psychiatric disorders. Medications specifically identified as advantageous in skin disease are discussed later in this chapter. Use caution to avoid drug–drug interactions with dermatology medications, and observe the potential for exacerbation of underlying dermatological disorders by the psychiatric medications (consult Box 62.2). CBT or biofeedback are frequently recommended for patients with anxiety or depression issues. The majority of patients with stress-induced skin disorders would benefit from relaxation training and exercises. Breathing techniques, yoga, tai chi, relaxation tapes, physical exercise, proper nutrition, and so forth may all help to reduce stress levels. Hypnosis has been found to be of value for a number of disorders. Shenefelt (2000) performed a MEDLINE search and identified that hypnosis or alternative

---

Box 62.2   MEDICATION-RELATED ISSUES IN PSYCHODERMATOLOGY

Skin diseases caused or exacerbated by psychotropic medication:

Anticonvulsants—maculopapular eruptions, alopecia, pruritus, pigmentation, erythema multiforme, Stevens-Johnson syndrome, toxic epidermal necrolysis, exfoliative dermatitis, hyperhidrosis, psoriasis, acne eruptions, seborrheic dermatitis, photosensitivity, drug hypersensitivity syndrome (DRESS), alopecia (valproate)

Lithium—psoriasis, acne, alopecia, folliculitis, urticaria, maculopapular eruptions, drug hypersensitivity vasculitis, seborrheic dermatitis, exfoliative dermatitis

Antipsychotics—photosensitivity (particularly phenothiazines) and changes in pigmentation (particularly thioridazine and chlorpromazine), injection-site reactions with depot meds, acne, exfoliative dermatitis, seborrheic dermatitis (phenothiazines), hyperhidrosis, drug hypersensitivity vasculitis (clozapine), alopecia

Antidepressants—hyperhidrosis, bleeding, photosensitivity/hyperpigmentation with exposure (tricyclic antidepressants), acne, exfoliative dermatitis (TCAs), alopecia

Barbiturates and benzodiazepines—drug hypersensitivity vasculitis, porphyria photosensitivity

Any psychotropic medication—risk for allergic reaction and fixed drug eruption

Psychiatric adverse effects of dermatological medications:

Isotretinoin—depression

Interferon-alpha—depression, suicidal ideation, psychosis, cognitive disorders

UV light therapy—mood changes, hypomania

Methotrexate—mood disorders

Dapsone—psychosis

Immunosuppressants (cyclosporine, etc.)—psychosis, delirium

Antihistamines—delirium, CNS depression

Steroids—mood disorders or psychosis

Adapted from Locala, J. A. (2009). Current concepts in psychodermatology. *Current Psychiatry Reports, 11,* 211–218.

---

and complementary treatments were beneficial for patients with AD, psoriasis, AA, rosacea, vitiligo, and hyperhidrosis.

MEDICATION-RELATED ISSUES

SKIN DISEASES CAUSED OR EXACERBATED BY PSYCHOTROPIC MEDICATION

Any psychotropic medication may cause an allergic reaction or drug eruption. A myriad of other skin conditions are caused or exacerbated by psychotropics, as outlined in Box 62.2.

Mood stabilizers, including lithium and anticonvulsants, are the most common causes of dermatological conditions in the realm of psychotropics. Lamotrigine, with dosing precautions necessary to prevent rash and concern about potentially life-threatening Stevens-Johnson syndrome, has received the most attention; however, note that severe skin reactions may occur with *any* of the anticonvulsants. Mood stabilizers have the highest incidence of severe dermatological problems out of all of the psychiatric medications (Warnock, 2003). Lithium causes a variety of skin problems, including exacerbation of psoriasis. Lithium-induced psoriasis typically occurs in the first few years of treatment, resists traditional psoriasis regimens, and resolves after discontinuation of lithium (Krahn, 1994). For patients on an established regimen of lithium with good control of mood symptoms, change of psychotropic medications is not always an option. Wachter (2007) reported successful treatment of a patient with recalcitrant psoriasis and the need to continue lithium for control of his suicidality. He was treated with etanercept 50 mg subcutaneously twice weekly and sustained almost complete remission of psoriatic lesions after 12 weeks (Wachter, 2007).

PSYCHIATRIC DISORDERS SECONDARY TO DERMATOLOGICAL MEDICATIONS

Medications used for dermatological disorders may precipitate mania, depression, psychosis, or acute confusional states (delirium). Steroids, particularly when given above the equivalent of 40 mg oral prednisone daily, may cause anxiety, mania, psychosis, delirium, and depression. The link between interferon-alpha and severe depression has been well documented in the literature, and case reports of mania have been presented from interferon as well. Higher doses used for melanoma patients seem especially prone to causing psychiatric side effects. Rapid identification of these side effects is critical for management, and education of patients in advance of potential psychiatric adverse events will prepare them to report promptly. Selected specific medications and side effects are listed in Box 62.2.

PSYCHOTROPIC MEDICATIONS USED AS A PRIMARY TREATMENT FOR DERMATOLOGICAL CONDITIONS

Antidepressants are often used for treatment of skin disorders in the absence of psychiatric symptomatology. Doxepin actually has higher affinity for histamine receptors than classic antihistamines. It is commonly used to treat acute pruritus or chronic urticaria when other antihistamines have proven ineffective. The long half-life of doxepin allows it to offer relief for a more prolonged period than medications like diphenhydramine or hydroxyzine (Lee et al., 2008). Dose range for therapeutic effect is highly variable and should be adjusted on an individual basis. Often lower doses are effective for pruritus. Tricyclic antidepressants (TCAs) may be employed in skin conditions associated with acute or chronic pain.

Postherpetic neuralgia is a chronic, painful condition that becomes more common with increasing age and produces a burning, lancinating, or stabbing pain. TCAs have been a primary treatment for postherpetic neuralgia, with amitriptyline as a well-documented agent, in average dosage ranges from 25–75 mg daily (Koo, 2002). For patients who cannot tolerate the side effects of tricyclic antidepressants, serotonin-noradrenaline receptor inhibitors (SNRIs) such as venlafaxine or duloxetine may be considered. Gabapentin, an anticonvulsant, is also useful in treatment of postherpetic pain.

TCAs are effective in any dermatological conditions associated with stinging, chafing, or burning sensations (Szepietowski, 2007). One study evaluated efficacy of bupropion slow release (SR) in ten non-depressed patients with AD and ten with psoriasis. Of these, 60% of subjects with AD and 80% of those with psoriasis showed demonstrable improvement in affected body surface area after six weeks of therapy (3 weeks at 150 mg daily and 3 weeks at 300 mg daily). The average reduction in affected surface area was 50%, and patients returned to pre-study baseline after discontinuation of bupropion (Modell et al., 2002). It has been proposed that bupropion may have anti-TNF properties; additional investigation is required (Kast, 2005).

MEDICATIONS USED IN DERMATOLOGY AS POTENTIAL TREATMENTS FOR PSYCHIATRIC DISORDERS

Psoriasis, fatigue, and depression have been linked to proinflammatory cytokines (such as TNF). Etanercept binds and inhibits TNF and is used for plaque psoriasis and psoriatic and rheumatoid arthritis. Krishnan (2007) demonstrated improvement of depression (measured by the Beck Depression Inventory and Hamilton Depression Inventory) as well as fatigue during an initial 12-week therapy with etanercept vs. placebo; additional improvement was seen in both of these symptoms during a 96-week follow-up, and this improvement was also demonstrated in the arm of the study that crossed over from placebo to active drug. It is unclear whether the antagonism of TNF caused improvement in mood and fatigue directly, or whether this occurred via another mechanism of action.

SPECIAL CLINICAL CONSIDERATIONS IN DERMATOLOGICAL DISEASES

SUICIDALITY

The presence of combined psychiatric and dermatological disorders appears to be associated with higher rates of suicidality, and every encounter in dermatology warrants careful screening for suicidal thoughts, particularly during periods of acute exacerbation of illness. A study of 217 psoriasis patients with depression revealed 9.7% with a passive death wish and 5.5% with active suicidal ideation (Gupta, 1993). Cotterill and Cunliffe (1997) performed a retrospective review of 16 completed suicides over a 20-year period. The overall age range was 16 to 73 years, but in the seven suicides of acne patients, the mean age was 20.4 (range 16–24 years).

Groups at highest risk were patients with BDD, acne, long-standing and debilitating dermatological disease, and a history of severe comorbid psychiatric illness. Case reports have identified persons with certain dermatological disorders to be at higher risk; namely, those with acne, metastatic tumors (particularly melanoma), progressive scleroderma, and BDD (Harth, 2008). The majority of dermatology patients are not under the care of a psychiatrist. Patients seen in a dermatology office may not feel comfortable broaching the topic of self-harm; they need to be asked routinely about suicidal ideation and referred for additional mental health care as indicated (See Box 62.3).

SUBSTANCE USE DISORDERS

Alcohol, drug, and nicotine screening and abstinence education must be standard components of evaluation of patients with skin disease. Substance use accompanies skin disease to a significant degree and may precipitate the onset or worsen the progression of skin pathology.

Alcohol consumption is a risk factor for development of psoriasis, and patients with excessive alcohol intake have more severe psoriasis and a more distinct distribution of plaques on acral surfaces; they are also more likely to be treatment-resistant. Psoriasis patients who consume alcohol have greater levels of anxiety, depression, and psoriasis-associated disability (Kirby, 2007). Individuals who chronically abuse alcohol also have twice the risk for seborrheic dermatitis and increased risk for nummular eczema, tinea versicolor, hyperpigmentation, skin cancer, oral cancer, glossitis, pruritus, spider telangiectasia, and palmar erythema (Smith, 2000; Rao, 2004). Alcohol also causes flushing and may exacerbate rosacea due to vasodilatation.

Box 62.3 **GROUPS AT HIGHEST RISK FOR SUICIDE IN DERMATOLOGY**

Severe acne (particularly males)
    Metastatic melanoma
    Progressive scleroderma
    Body dysmorphic disorder
    Psoriasis

Harth, W. (2008). Psychosomatic dermatology (psychodermatology). *Journal der Deutschen Dermatolischen Gesellschaft 1*, 67–76.

Cotterill, J., & Cunliffe, W. (1997). Suicide in dermatological patients. *British Journal of Dermatology, 17*, 246–250.

Smoking in general is hazardous to the skin, causing premature aging and acceleration of skin damage from other causes. Alcohol-controlled studies suggest that women who smoke have a 3.3-fold increased risk of developing plaque-type psoriasis. Men do not show the same risk for onset; however, men who smoke more than ten cigarettes per day may have more severe psoriasis expression in the extremities (Behnam, 2005).

Cocaine use is associated with numerous cutaneous manifestations, including multiple vasculitides, palpable purpura, Stevens-Johnson syndrome, infections, and nondescript skin eruptions. Cocaine may also cause formication and psychosis; cases of DP have been attributed to cocaine use (Brewer, 2008). Methamphetamine users also experience formication—"crank bugs" or "meth mites"—and may open skin in an endeavor to remove, see, or feel the nonexistent bugs. Intravenous drug users will develop linear scars along their veins ("track marks") or deep round scars due to "skin popping." Skin infections such as cellulitis, impetigo, abscesses, and necrotizing fasciitis develop with high prevalence secondary to drug injection. Pruritus may occur with cocaine, methamphetamine, and opioid use (Liu, 2010). Screening for drug use should be part of the evaluation of any patient with significant dermatological disease; referrals for smoking cessation and substance abuse treatment are an important component for comprehensive care. Skin manifestations of drugs, alcohol, and tobacco may be considered an early warning sign and an opportunity for intervention.

SEXUAL DYSFUNCTION

Issues with sexual dysfunction are a common problem in dermatology patients, but often are not explored on interview or recognized clinically. Sexual dysfunction in both men and women has been described in patients with psoriasis, AD, neurodermatitis, and vitiligo (Ermertcan, 2006; Mercan, 2008; Sukan, 2007). Many factors may play a role in sexual issues: body image, confidence, mood, or anxiety disorders and relationship strain due to chronic illness. Diseases with disfigurement may have a greater effect on patients' social, relational, and sexual lives. Much of the research thus far into sexual function has been in psoriasis. Physical discomfort such as itching, burning, and bleeding may disrupt intimacy; lesions in genital areas have been identified as particularly linked to high sexual distress and worsened quality of life (Meeuwis, 2011). Some authors have speculated that depression may be the primary cause for sexual dysfunction in psoriasis (Mercan, 2008). Other studies have demonstrated no effect of depression on sexual dysfunction in psoriasis patients (Ermertcan, 2006). Sampogna et al. (2007) identified the combination of psoriasis severity and psychological factors as contributory to sexual impairment.

Ruiz-Villaverde (2011), in a pilot study, determined that treatment of psoriasis for a period of six months with biological agents (etanercept and adalimumab) significantly improved sexual function for both men and women as measured by the International Index of Erectile Function and Female Sexual Function Index, respectively. Patients with depression and alcohol abuse were excluded from the study. If these data extrapolate to a larger population, it would imply that the sexual dysfunction is significantly related to the physical issues in psoriasis patients.

Sexual dysfunction is most likely to be identified by a specific, structured survey. Quality of life surveys and general health surveys may ask basic questions about sexuality, but gender-specific, sexual function questionnaires are necessary. Ermertcan (2009) has proposed that the Female Sexual Function Index (FSFI) be used to screen for sexual dysfunction in females and the International Index of Erectile Function (IIEF) be used for males. Clinicians are not always diligent in asking patients about their sex life, and patients are not apt to spontaneously offer that history. It is critical for caregivers to discuss the impact of dermatological disease on sexual function with their patients.

ITCHING

Regardless of etiology for a specific skin disorder, the battle to combat itching is omnipresent. Itching, or pruritus, is an unpleasant sensation that leads a person to want to scratch, and this is commonly cited as a factor in reduced quality of life, disturbed sleep, inattention, diminished sexual function, and incidence of psychiatric comorbidity in chronic skin disorders. Itching can be a particularly challenging problem to treat and may require multiple trials of medications due to high rates of therapeutic failure. It has been demonstrated that depression appears to worsen pruritus perception, with resultant increased pruritus score in patients with AD, psoriasis, and chronic idiopathic urticaria (Gupta, 1994). This may explain the efficacy seen in treatment of pruritus with antidepressants, even those with less antihistaminic effect. Topical therapies are employed for localized, mild areas of pruritus. For moderate or severe itching and that which covers larger areas of the body, systemic therapy is the choice. Patel (2010) has written a nice review of the management of pruritus that is summarized in Box 62.4.

Use of systemic antihistamines can be approached in a stepwise fashion. First, attempt to obtain relief from non-sedating antihistamines, such as cetirizine, loratidine, and fexofenadine; progress as needed to sedating antihistamines, such as hydroxyzine, diphenhydramine, and clemastine. Finally, advance to psychotropics such as promethazine or doxepin. Phototherapy may also assist in management of severe pruritus (Harth, 2009).

CLINIC MODELS FOR TREATMENT OF THE PATIENT WITH PSYCHIATRIC AND DERMATOLOGICAL ISSUES

Optimal care of the dermatology patient should include careful screening for psychiatric issues and the mechanism for referral either to external mental health providers or to an on-site psychiatric liaison. The best model for care delivery consists of an interdisciplinary clinic in which

Topical preparations:
  Barrier cream and moisturizers
  Topical calcineurin inhibitors
  Doxepin cream
  Menthol cream or lotion
  Capsaicin cream
  Salicylic acid
  Local anesthetics
Systemic therapies:
  Antihistamines
  Antidepressants (SNRIs or SSRIs)
  Mu-opioid receptor agonists
  Gabapentin
  Immunosuppressants (cyclosporine or azathioprine)

Adapted from Patel, T., & Yosipovitch, G. (2010). Therapy of pruritus. *Expert Opinion on Pharmacotherapy, 11*, 1673–1682.

patients meet providers from multiple specialties as part of a treatment team, thus reducing the stigma associated with emotional issues. At University Hospitals Case Medical Center, we launched the first interdisciplinary psoriasis clinic in the country, the Murdough Family Center for Psoriasis (Locala, 2009). This clinic provides comprehensive, disease-specific care with a team of dermatologists, psychiatrists, rheumatologist, nutritionists, and nurses. Patients who were previously reluctant to accept psychiatric referral much more readily agreed when the psychiatrist accompanied the dermatologist into the exam room. Patients complete a comprehensive questionnaire prior to their appointment, which includes basic questions regarding emotional coping, psychiatric symptoms, and mental health history. Taken in the context of a request for information about general medical history, the psychiatric review of systems is elicited in a non-threatening fashion. A targeted or comprehensive psychiatric assessment is

Table 62.1 TOP REASONS FOR REFERRAL

PSYCHIATRY TO DERMATOLOGY	DERMATOLOGY TO PSYCHIATRY
Drug-related rash	Delusion of parasitosis
Acne	Neurotic excoriation
Psoriasis	Trichotillomania
Atopic dermatitis	Depression associated with skin disease
Alopecia areata	
	Skin-related obsessive-compulsive behaviors

Jafferany, M., Stoep, A., Dumitrescu, et al. (2010). The knowledge, awareness, and practice patterns of dermatologists toward psychocutaneous disorders: Results of a survey study. *International Journal of Dermatology, 49,* 784–789.

Jafferany, M., Stoep, A., Dumitrescu, et al. (2010). Psychocutaneous disorders: A survey study of psychiatrists' awareness and treatment patterns. *Southern Medical Journal, 103,* 1199–1203.

performed in the exam room, and treatment initiated as part of the treatment team plan. We recently established a "virtual" psychodermatology clinic for referrals of patients with other skin disorders. Appointments in the psychiatry clinic (in a different building) are reserved for last-minute dermatology referrals, and dermatologists can readily access psychiatry during the workday for curbside consultation and recommendations. This approach has been an effective means of collaborative care at times when a multidisciplinary clinic model is not practical (see Table 62.1).

CONCLUSION

It is critical to identify psychiatric comorbidity and psychosocial factors in patients with dermatological disease. In 2010, Jafferany set out to evaluate the level of awareness of psychocutaneous disorders among practicing psychiatrists and dermatologists via mail-in survey. Both groups concluded that knowledge about diagnosis, treatment, and/or appropriate referrals was lacking. A distinct lack of awareness about resources for patients and families with skin disease was also identified.

Additional education in psychodermatology would be beneficial for both specialties and should ideally be initiated in residency training. Early exposure to the interplay between psychiatric and dermatological diseases would hopefully foster collaborative clinical care and expand interdisciplinary research.

CLINICAL PEARLS

- Risperidone, olanzapine, aripiprazole, and quetiapine have all shown efficacy in small studies or case reports in treatment of delusional parasitosis (Sandoz, 2008). Compared to pimozide, they seem to have fewer side effects.

- The dermatological community has long argued that Morgellons and delusional parasitosis are one and the same disorder.

- Depression, anxiety, and drug dependence and abuse are common comorbid disorders with delusional parasitosis.

- Trichotillomania tends to emerge in early childhood or adolescence, with average age of onset at 13 years; later onset has been associated with greater symptom severity and treatment resistance.

- As many as 57% of adults with trichotillomania have a comorbid psychiatric disorder; the most common are major depression, other mood disorders, OCD, and other anxiety disorders (Flessner, 2012). This pattern of comorbidity resembles that of patients with other body-focused repetitive behaviors.

- Habit-reversal training is a cognitive behavioral therapy modality used for trichotillomania that has three stages: (1) Increase the awareness of pulling behaviors; (2) Engage in competing behavior that prevents pulling;

and (3) Recruit a social support person to remind patients of their behavior.

- Excoriation (skin-picking) disorder has similarities to trichotillomania and onchyphagia (nail-biting) and onchotillomania (peeling of nail and cuticle); some authors consider these to be a group of pathological grooming behaviors.

- In a careful review of available double-blind, open-label studies and case reports on pathological skin-picking, Chamberlain (2012) has identified fluoxetine as likely to be efficacious, whereas citalopram, escitalopram, fluvoxamine, and lamotrigene (Grant, 2010) had mixed results.

- The prevalence of indoor tanning is highest in young, white females, particularly those aged 18 to 29 (Heckman, 2008). This age group is at significantly higher risk for skin cancer; ten annual tanning visits per year double the risk for melanoma in those over 30, but the risk increases eightfold for those under age 30.

- Supporting the concept of tanning addiction, it is speculated that UV light stimulates production of beta-endorphin and acts as reinforcing stimulus for repeated tanning (Feldman, 2004).

- The skin appears to have its own version of the hypothalamic-pituitary-axis, which Slominski (2000) calls the "skin stress response system" (SSRS). The skin produces corticotrophin-releasing hormone (CRH), propiomelanocortin (POMC)-derived neuropeptides, alpha-melanocyte stimulating hormone, ACTH, and beta-endorphin, and contains active receptors for CRH and POMC-peptides.

- Triggers for psoriasis flares include physical trauma or pressure (Koebner phenomenon), bacterial or viral infections, steroid withdrawal, and medications (for example, beta-blockers and lithium).

- Approximately half of all patients with atopic dermatitis will develop allergic asthma and/or allergic rhinitis.

- The highest rates of suicide in dermatology are in adolescent males with a severe form, acne conglomata.

- For the majority with alopecia areata, hair grows back after several months.

- Comorbid psychiatric disorders in the dermatology patient are treated with a similar array of antidepressants, anxiolytics, and antipsychotics as solo psychiatric disorders.

- Lithium-induced psoriasis typically occurs in the first few years of treatment, resists traditional psoriasis regimens, and resolves after discontinuation of lithium (Krahn, 1994).

- Cocaine use is associated with numerous cutaneous manifestations including multiple vasculitides, palpable purpura, Stevens-Johnson syndrome, infections, and nondescript skin eruptions and formication.

DISCLOSURE STATEMENT

Dr. Joseph Locala has no conflicts to disclose. He receives no outside funding, and his salary is entirely from University Hospitals Case Medical Center.

REFERENCES

American Psychiatric Association (2000). *Diagnostic and Statistical Manual of Mental Disorders, 4th edition, Text Revision*. Washington, DC: American Psychiatric Publishing.

Asri, F., Akhdari, R., Chagh, R., et al. (2008). Alexithymy and depression in chronic dermatosis. *European Psychiatry, 23*, S242.

Behnam, S., Behanam, S. E., & Koo, J. (2005). Smoking and psoriasis. *SKINmed Journal, 4*, 174–176.

Bewley, A., Lepping, P., Freundenmann, R., et al. (2010). Delusional parasitosis: Time to call it delusional infestation. *British Journal of Dermatology, 163*, 1–2.

Brewer, J., Meves, A., Bostwick, M., et al. (2008). Cocaine abuse: dermatologic manifestations and therapeutic approaches. *Journal of the American Academy of Dermatology, 59*, 483–487.

Chamberlain, S., Fineberg, N., & Odlaug, B. (2012). In J. Grant (Ed.), *Trichotillomania, skin picking and other body-focused repetitive behaviors* (pp. 175–192). Arlington, VA: American Psychiatric Publishing.

Christenson, G., Mackenzie, T., Mitchell, J., et al. (1999). Characteristics of 60 adult chronic hair pullers. *American Journal of Psychiatry, 148*, 365–370.

Cotterill, J., & Cunliffe, W. (1997). Suicide in dermatological patients. *British Journal of Dermatology, 17*, 246–250.

Demet, M. M., Devecci, A., Taskin, O., et al. (2005). Obsessive compulsive disorder in a dermatology outpatient clinic. *General Hospital Psychiatry, 27*, 426–430.

Duke, D., Bodzin, D., Tavares, P., et al. (2009). The phenomenology of hair pulling in a community sample. *Journal of Anxiety Disorders, 23*, 1118–1125.

Elpern, D. (2010). Darkness visible: Psychocutaneous disease. *Southern Medical Journal, 103*, 1196.

Engin, B., Uguz, F., Yilmaz, E., et al. (2007). The levels of depression, anxiety and quality of life in patients with chronic idiopathic urticaria. *Journal of the European Academy of Dermatology and Venereology, 22*, 36–40.

Ermertcan, A. T. (2009). Sexual dysfunction in dermatological diseases. *Journal of the European Academy of Dermatology and Venereology, 23*, 999–1007.

Ermertcan, A., Temeltas, G., Deveci, A., et al. (2006). Sexual dysfunction in patients with psoriasis. *Journal of Dermatology, 33*, 772–778.

Feldman, S. R., Liguori, A., Kucenic, M., et al. (2004). Ultraviolet exposure is a reinforcing stimulus in frequent indoor tanners. *Journal of the American Academy of Dermatology, 51*, 45–51.

Ferrucci, L., Cartmel, B., Molinaro, A., et al. (2011). Indoor tanning and risk of early-onset basal cell carcinoma. *Journal of the American Academy of Dermatology, 67*, 552–562.

Filakovic, P., Biljan, D., & Petek, A. (2008). Depression in dermatology: An integrative perspective. *Psychiatrica Danubina, 20*, 419–425.

Finzi, A., Colombo, D., Andeassi, L., et al. (2007). Psychological distress and coping strategies in patients with psoriasis: The PSYCHAE study. *Journal of the European Academy of Dermatology and Venereology, 21*, 1161–1169.

Flessner, C. (2012). Diagnosis and comorbidity. In J. Grant (Ed.), *Trichotillomania, skin picking and other body-focused repetitive behaviors* (pp. 175–192). Arlington, VA: American Psychiatric Publishing.

Grant, J., Odlaug, B., Chamberlain, S., Kim, S. (2010). A double-blind, placebo-controlled trial of lamotrigene for pathological skin picking. *Journal of Clinical Psychopharmacology, 30*, 396–403.

Gupta, M. A., &, Gupta, A. K. (2003). Psychiatric and psychological co-morbidity in patients with dermatologic disorders. *American Journal of Clinical Dermatology, 4*, 833–842.

Gupta, M. A., Gupta, A. K., Ellis, C. N., et al. (2005). Psychiatric evaluation of the dermatology patient. *Dermatologic Clinics, 23,* 591–599.

Gupta, M. A., Lanius, R. A., & Van der Kol, B. A. (2005). Psychological trauma, posttraumatic stress disorder and dermatology. *Dermatologic Clinics, 23,* 649–656.

Gupta, M., & Gupta, A. (1994). Depression modulates pruritus perception: A study in psoriasis, atopic dermatitis and chronic idiopathic urticaria. *Psychosomatic Medicine, 56,* 36–40.

Gupta, M., & Levenson, J. (2011): Dermatology. In J. Levenson (Ed.), *Textbook of psychosomatic medicine* (p. 672). Arlington, VA: American Psychiatric Publishing.

Gupta, M., Schork, N., & Gupta, A. (1993). Suicidal ideation in psoriasis. *International Journal of Dermatology, 32,* 188–190.

Hannestad, J., DellaGiola, N., & Bloch, M. (2011). The effect of antidepressant medication treatment on serum levels of inflammatory cytokines: A meta-analysis. *Neuropsychopharmacology, 36,* 2452–2459.

Harrington, C. R., Beswick, T. C., Graves, M., et al. (2012). Activation of the mesostriatal reward pathway with exposure to ultraviolet radiation (UVR) vs. sham UVR in frequent tanners: A pilot study. *Addiction Biology, 17,* 680–686.

Harth, W. (2008). Psychosomatic dermatology (psychodermatology). *JDDG, 1,* 67–76.

Harth, W., Gieler, U., Kusnir, D., & Tausk, F. A. (2009). Self-inflicted dermatitis: Factitious disorders. In W. Harth (Ed.), *Clinical management in psychodermatology* (pp. 12–13). Berlin: Springer Verlag.

Hashiro, M., & Okumura, M. (1997). Anxiety, depression and psychosomatic symptoms in patients with atopic dermatitis: Comparison with normal controls and among groups of different degrees of severity. *Journal of Dermatological Science, 14,* 63–67.

Heckman, C. J., Coups, E. J., & Manne, S. L. (2008). Prevalence and correlates of indoor tanning among US adults. *Journal of the American Academy of Dermatology, 58,* 769–780.

Hull, P. R., & D'Arcy, C. D. (2005). Acne, depression and suicide. *Dermatologic Clinics, 23,* 665–674.

Hylwa, S., Foster, A., Bury, J., et al. (2012). Delusional infestation is typically comorbid with other psychiatric diagnoses: Review of 54 patients receiving psychiatric evaluation at Mayo Clinic. *Psychosomatics 53,* 258–265.

Jafferany, M. (2007). Psychodermatology: A guide to understanding common psychocutaneous disorders. *Primary Care Companion Journal of Clinical Psychiatry, 9,* 203–213.

Jafferany, M., Stoep, A., Dumitrescu, A., et al. (2010). Psychocutaneous disorders: A survey study of psychiatrists' awareness and treatment patterns. *Southern Medical Journal, 103,* 1199–1203.

Jafferany, M., Stoep, A., Dumitrescu, A., et al. (2010). The knowledge, awareness, and practice patterns of dermatologists toward psychocutaneous disorders: Results of a survey study. *International Journal of Dermatology, 49,* 784–789.

Karanikas, E., Harsoulis, F., Giouzepas, I., et al.(2009). Neuroendocrine stimulatory tests of hypothalamus-pituitary-adrenal axis in psoriasis and correlative implications with psychopathological and immune parameters. *Journal of Dermatology, 36,* 35–44.

Kast, R., & Altshuler, E. (2005). Anti-apoptosis function of TNF-alpha in chronic lymphocytic leukemia: Lessons from Crohn's disease and the therapeutic potential of bupropion to lower TNF-alpha. *Archivum Immunologiae et Therapiae Experimentalis, 53,* 143–147.

Kaur, M., Liguori, A., Fleischer, A., et al. (2005). Side effects of naltrexone observed in frequent tanners: Could frequent tanners have ultraviolet-induced high opioid levels? *Journal of the American Academy of Dermatology, 52,* 916.

Kaur, M., Liguori, A., Lang, W., et al. (2006). Induction of withdrawal-like symptoms in a small randomized, controlled trial of opioid blockade in frequent tanners. *Journal of the American Academy of Dermatology, 54,* 709–711.

Kirby, B., Richards, H., Mason, D., et al. (2007). Alcohol consumption and psychological distress in patients with psoriasis. *British Journal of Dermatology, 158,* 138–140.

Koo, J. Y., & Ng, T. C. (2002). Psychotropic and neurotropic agents in dermatology: Unapproved uses, dosages or indications. *Clinica in Dermatology, 20,* 582–594.

Koo, J. Y., Shellow, W. V., Hallman, C. P., et al. (1994). Alopecia areata and increased prevalence of psychiatric disorders. *International Journal of Dermatology, 33,* 849–50.

Krahn, L. E., & Goldberg, R. L. (1994). Psychotropic medications and the skin. In P. A. Silver (Ed.), *Psychotropic drug use in the medically ill* (pp. 90–106). Basel, Switzerland: S. Karger, A. G.

Kretzmer, G. E., Gelkopf, M., Kretzmer, G., et al. (2008). Idiopathic pruritus in psychiatric inpatients: An explorative study. *General Hospital Psychiatry, 30,* 344–348.

Kronfol, Z., & Remick, D. (2000). Cytokines and the brain: Implications for clinical psychiatry. *American Journal of Psychiatry, 158,* 683–694.

Lee, C. S., Accordino, R., Howard, J., et al. (2008). Psychopharmacology in dermatology. *Dermatologic Therapy, 21,* 69–82.

Liu, S., & Lien Mand Fenske, N. (2010). The effects of alcohol and drug abuse on skin. *Clinics in Dermatology, 28,* 391–399.

Locala, J. A. (2009). Current concepts in psychodermatology. *Current Psychiatry Reports, 11,* 211–218.

Lonne-Rahm, S. B., Rickberg, H., El Nour, H., et al. (2008). Neuroimmune mechanism in patients with atopic dermatitis during chronic stress. *Journal of the European Academy of Dermatology and Venereology, 22,* 11–18.

Lyell, A. (1983). Delusions of parasitosis. *Journal of American Academy of Dermatology, 8,* 895–897.

Mackley, C. (2005). Body dysmorphic disorder. *Dermatologic Surgery, 31,* 553–558.

Maes, M., Berk, M., Goehler, L., et al. (2012). Depression and sickness behavior are Janus-faced responses to shared inflammatory pathways. *BioMed Central Medicine, 10,* 66.

Maes, M., Meltzer, H., Bosmans, E., et al. (1995). Increased plasma concentrations of interleukin-6, soluble interleukin-6 receptor, soluble interleukin-2 receptor and transferrin receptor in major depression. *Journal of Affective Disorders, 34,* 301–309.

Magin, P., Pond, D., & Smith, W. (2005). Isotretinoin, depression and suicide: A review of the evidence. *British Journal of General Practice, 55,* 134–138.

Malick, F., Howard, J., & Koo, J. (2008). Understanding the psychology of the cosmetic patients. *Dermatologic Therapy, 21,* 47–53.

Mansueto, C., & Rogers, K. (2012). Trichotillomania. In J. Grant (Ed.), *Trichotillomania, skin picking and other body-focused repetitive behaviors* (pp. 175–192). Arlington, VA: American Psychiatric Publishing.

Medansky, R. S., & Handler, R. M. (1981). Dermatopsychosomatics: Classification, physiology and therapeutic approaches. *Journal of the American Academy of Dermatology, 5,* 125–136.

Meeuwis, K. A., deHullu, J. A., van de Nieuwenhof, H. P., et al. (2011). Quality of life and sexual health in patients with genital psoriasis. *British Journal of Dermatology, 164,* 1247–1255.

Mercan, S., Altunay, I. K., Demir, B., et al. (2008). Sexual dysfunctions in patients with neurodermatitis and psoriasis. *Journal of Sex and Marital Therapy, 34,* 160–168.

Modell, J.G., Boyce S., Taylor E., Katholi, C. (2002). Treatment of atopic dermatitis and psoriasis vulgaris with bupropion-SR: a pilot study. *Psychosomatic Medicine, 64,* 835–840.

Murase, J. E., Wu, J. J., & Koo, J. (2006). Morgellons disease: A rapport-enhancing term for delusions of parasitosis. *Journal of the American Academy of Dermatology, 55,* 913–914.

Nielsen, K., Jeppesen, M., Simmelsgaard, L., Rasmussen, M., & Thestrup-Pedersen, K. (2005). Self-inflicted skin diseases. A retrospective analysis of 57 patients with dermatitis artefacta seen in a dermatology department. *Acta Dermato-Venereologica, 85,* 512–515.

Nolan, B. V., & Feldman, S. R. (2009). Ultraviolet tanning addiction. *Dermatologic Clinics, 27,* 109–112.

Odlaug, B. L., Chamberlain, S. R., Harvanko, A. M., & Grant, J. E. (2012). Age at onset in trichotillomania: clinical variables and neurocognitive performance. *Primary Care Companion for CNS Disorders, 14,* PMC 3505138.

O'Sullivan, R. L., Lipper, G., & Lerner, E. A. (1998). The neuro-immuno-cutaneous-endocrine network: Relationship of mind and skin. *Archives of Dermatology, 134,* 1431–1435.

Orringer, J. S., Helfrich, Y. R., Hamilton, T., et al. (2006). Prevalence of psychotropic medication use among cosmetic and medical dermatology patients: A comparative study. *Journal of the American Academy of Dermatology, 54*, 416–419.

Patel, T., & Yosipovitch, G. (2010). Therapy of pruritus. *Expert Opinion on Pharmacotherapy, 11*, 1673–1682.

Pearson, M. L., Selby, J. V., Katz, K. A., et al. (2012). Clinical, epidemiologic, histopathologic and molecular features of an unexplained dermopathy. *PLoS One, 7*(1), e29908. doi:10.1371/journal.pone.0029908.

Picardi, A., Abeni, D., Melchi, C. F., et al. (2000). Psychiatric morbidity in dermatological outpatients: An issue to be recognized. *British Journal of Dermatology, 143*, 983–991.

Picardi, A., Amerio, P., Baliva, G., et al. (2004). Recognition of depressive and anxiety disorders in dermatological outpatients. *Acta Dermato-Venereologica, 84*, 213–217.

Pietrzak, A. T., Zalewska, A., Chodrowska, G., et al. (2008): Cytokines and anticytokines in psoriasis. *Clinica Chimica Acta, 394*, 7–21.

Rao, G. (2004). Cutaneous changes in chronic alcoholics. *Indian Journal of Dermatology, Venereology & Leprology, 70*, 79–81.

Reed, K., Brewer, J., Lohse, C., et al. (2012). Increasing incidence of melanoma among young adults: an epidemiological study in Olmsted County, Minnesota. *Mayo Clinic Proceedings, 87*, 328–334.

Richards, H. L., Fortune, D. G., Griffiths, C. E., et al. (2005). Alexithymia in patients with psoriasis. Clinical correlates and psychometric properties of the Toronto Alexithymia Scale 20. *Journal of Psychosomatic Research, 58*, 89–96.

Robinson, J. K., Kim, J., Rosenbaum, S., et al. (2008). Indoor tanning knowledge, attitudes and behavior among young adults from 1988 to 2007. *Archives of Dermatology, 144*, 484–488.

Ruiz-Doblado, S., Carrizosa, A., & García-Hernández, M. J. (2003). Alopecia areata: Psychiatric comorbidity and adjustment to illness. *International Journal of Dermatology, 42*, 434–437.

Ruiz-Villaverde, R., Sanchez-Cano, D., Ramirez Rodrigo, J., et al. (2011). Pilot study of sexual dysfunction in patients with psoriasis: Influence of biological therapy. *Indian Journal of Dermatology, 56*, 694–699.

Sampogna, F., Gisondi, P., Tabolli, S., et al. (2007). Impairment of sexual life in patients with psoriasis. *Dermatology, 214*, 144–150.

Sandoz, A., LoPiccolo, M., Kusnir, D., et al. (2008). A clinical paradigm of delusions of parasitosis. *Journal of the American Academy of Dermatology, 59*, 698–764.

Shenefelt, P. (2000). Hypnosis in dermatology. *Archives of Dermatology, 136*, 393–399.

Stein, D., Grant, J., Franklin, M., et al. (2010). Trichotillomania (hair pulling disorder), skin picking disorder, and stereotypic movement disorder: Toward DSM-V. *Depression and Anxiety, 27*, 611–626.

Strahan, J. E., & Raimer, S. (2006). Isotretinoin and the controversy of psychiatric adverse effects. *International Journal of Dermatology, 45*, 789–799.

Sukan, M., & Maner, F. (2007). The problems in sexual functions of vitiligo and chronic urticaria patients. *Journal of Sex and Marital Therapy, 33*, 55–64.

Szepietowski, J. C., Salomon, J., Pacan, P., et al. (2007). Body dysmorphic disorder and dermatologists. *Journal of the European Academy of Dermatology and Venereology, 22*, 795–799.

Tausk, F., Elenkov, I., & Moynihan, J. (2008). Psychoneuroimmunology. *Dermatologic Therapy, 21*, 22–31.

Thomas, I., Patterson, W. M., Szepietowski, J. C., et al. (2005). Body dysmorphic disorder: More than meets the eye. *Acta Dermatovenerologica Croatica, 13*, 50–53.

Trabert, W. (1999). Shared psychotic disorder in delusinal parasitosis. *Psychopathology, 32*, 30–34.

Uguz, F., Engin, B., & Yilmaz, E. (2008). Quality of life in patients with chronic idiopathic urticaria: The impact if axis I and axis II psychiatric disorders. *General Hospital Psychiatry, 30*, 453–457.

Updike, J. (1990). *Self-consciousness: Memoirs*. London: Penguin Books.

Veale, D., Gournay, K., Dryden, W., et al. (1997). Body dysmorphic disorder: A cognitive behavioral model and pilot randomized controlled trial. *Behaviour Research & Therapy, 34*, 717–729.

Vythilingum, B., & Stein, D. (2005). Obsessive-compulsive disorders and dermatologic disease. *Dermatologic Clinics, 23*, 675–680.

Wachter, T., Murach, W. M., Brocker, E. B., et al. (2007). Recalcitrant lithium-induced psoriasis in a suicidal patient alleviated by tumour necrosis factor-alpha inhibition. *British Journal of Dermatology, 157*, 627–629.

Walker, C. (2005). Psychodermatology in context. In C. Walker & L. Papadopoulos (Eds.), *Psychodermatology* (pp. 44–66). Cambridge, UK: Cambridge University Press.

Warnock, J. K., & Morris, D. (2003). Adverse cutaneous reactions to mood stabilizers. *American Journal of Clinical Dermatology, 4*, 21–30.

White, M., & Koran, L. (2011). Open label trial of aripiprazole in the treatment of trichotillomania. *Journal of Clinical Psychopharmacology, 31*, 503–506.

Whitlock, F. A. (1976). *Psychophysiological aspects of skin disease*. Saunders, Philadelphia.

Willemsen, R., & Vanderlinden, J. (2008). Hypnotic approaches for alopecia areata. *International Journal of Clinical and Experimental Hypnosis, 56*, 318–333.

Willemsen, R., Roseeuw, D., & Vanderkinden, J. (2008). Alexithymia and dermatology: The state of the art. *International Journal of Dermatology, 47*, 903–910.

Wilson, E. (1867). *Diseases of the skin*. London: J. and A. Churchill, Ltd.

Woods, D., Snorrason, I., & Espil, F. (2012). Cognitive-behavioral therapy in adults. In J. Grant (Ed.), *Trichotillomania, skin picking and other body focused repetitive behaviors* (pp. 175–192). Arlington, VA: American Psychiatric Publishing.

Wykoff, R. E. (1987). Delusions of parasitosis: A review. *Reviews of Infectious Diseases, 9*, 433–437.

63.

HIV AND AIDS

Philip A. Bialer and Joseph Z. Lux

INTRODUCTION

Thirty years and more have now passed since the first case reports of the human immunodeficiency virus (HIV) epidemic. In 1981, the *Morbidity and Mortality Weekly Report* (MMWR) reported the cases of five previously healthy homosexual men in Los Angeles who had developed *Pneumocystis carinii* (now *P. jiroveci*) pneumonia (PCP), a rare pneumonia seen in patients with profound immunodeficiency (Centers for Disease Control [CDC], 1981b). This initial report was soon followed by other published cases of both PCP and the cancer known as Kaposi's sarcoma (KS), an illness not previously seen in healthy men in the United States (CDC, 1981a; Gottlieb et al., 1981; Masur et al., 1981). Soon there were reports of individuals in other groups developing PCP and KS, including people receiving blood transfusions, Haitians, injection drug users, infants of infected mothers, and, eventually, heterosexual partners of infected individuals. Given the nature of the infections and cancer, it was quickly recognized that an epidemic related to some type of immunodeficiency, but with an unknown etiology, was occurring.

Various hypotheses for this immunodeficiency were raised, including environmental exposure, infection, and cancer. Over the next few years, a causative virus was identified, isolated by several groups of scientists and given the name *human immunodeficiency virus* (HIV) (Gallo et al., 1984; Gallo et al., 1983). Patients continued to die, and communities began to be ravaged. Given the uncertainty of transmission and the already existing stigma surrounding some of the groups acquiring the infection, panicked and unsympathetic reactions were not uncommon. People feared that they could acquire the infection from casual contact with HIV-infected persons, and some physicians completely refused to treat patients with the infection. The identification of the virus enabled its further study. Research efforts defined the steps in the life cycle of the virus: attachment, fusion, reverse transcription, integration, and proteolytic cleavage. With increased understanding of the HIV virus, there was hope that a vaccine could be synthesized to prevent new infections.

The first HIV vaccine trials took place in the 1980s, but they were unsuccessful. In 1987, the first antiretroviral medication, azidothymidine (AZT), was shown to be effective against HIV, finally giving cause for optimism. As AZT began to be used, however, patients receiving treatment had an early increase in their CD4 lymphocyte (CD4) count, followed by what appeared to be drug resistance and drug failure. Several other antiretroviral medications were soon developed, but these showed the same pattern of initial clinical and immunological improvement—then failure. It is now understood that combination antiretroviral treatment with three effective agents is optimal, and the use of one antiretroviral agent or the addition of a single new drug to a previously failing regimen leads to increased HIV drug resistance.

Another clinical milestone was the realization that the incidence of the opportunistic infections associated with HIV such as PCP and *Mycobacterium avium-intracellulare* (MAI) could be reduced with prophylactic antibiotics (CDC, 1989; Nightingale et al., 1993). Since the introduction of AZT, antiretroviral drug development has progressed, and nearly 30 medications (including combination pills) in six classes now exist as therapeutic options for HIV-infected persons. The treatment of HIV has now become largely that of a chronic illness.

EPIDEMIOLOGY

From the onset of the HIV epidemic through 2008, an estimated 617,000 people in the United States have died from AIDS. The CDC estimates that more than one million people in the United States are living with HIV infection, and approximately one-fifth of these are unaware of their HIV-positive status. Despite public health efforts to limit new HIV infections, an estimated 56,300 persons in the United States continue to be newly infected each year. Men who have sex with men (MSM) account for almost half of all people living with HIV, and more than half (53%) of all new infections in the U.S. each year. Individuals infected through heterosexual sex are 28% of the people living with HIV and 31% of those with new infections. Women account for 25% of people living with HIV and 27% of new infections. Injection drug users are 19% of those living with HIV infection and 12% of new HIV infections. African Americans are the most disproportionally affected and account for nearly half of new infections (45%) and nearly half of those living with HIV in the United States. Hispanics/Latinos are also infected at an elevated rate; the infection rate for Hispanic men is more than twice that of white men and Hispanic women acquire infection almost four times more than white women (CDC, 2011).

GLOBAL ISSUES

The HIV epidemic has affected all parts of the world, but particularly sub-Saharan Africa. After the onset of the epidemic in the 1980s, the rate of HIV infection in this region skyrocketed, spread primarily through heterosexual sex and mother-to-child transmission. Average life expectancies in some countries diminished to the mid-40s. For economic reasons, antiretroviral medications were largely unavailable in countries with the highest prevalence of the infection. Further complicating HIV prevention and antiretroviral treatment in Africa were ongoing controversies about the origins of HIV and arguments that HIV infection was not itself the cause of AIDS. Issues related to the rights of women and the women's inability within local cultures to negotiate condom use and safer sex also hampered HIV prevention efforts.

In the 1990s and 2000s, a growing recognition of the devastation that was occurring in other parts of the world led to increased international efforts. Organizations such as the Global Fund and the U.S. President's Emergency Plan for AIDS Relief (PEPFAR) made the global delivery of HIV medications an increasing reality. While these efforts and accomplishments have been significant—some 5 million people internationally are now on antiretroviral drugs (ARVs)—the percentage of people with CD4 counts below 200 who receive ARVs remains limited, and the percentage of those with CD4 counts below 500 receiving ARVs is even smaller (Joint United Nations Programme on HIV/AIDS[UNAIDS], 2010).

The global HIV AIDS epidemic now appears to have stabilized, though much remains to be done. Compared to the peak of the epidemic in the late 1990s, there are fewer new infections and AIDS-related deaths. In 2009, there were an estimated 2.6 million people newly infected with HIV, approximately 20% fewer than at the time of peak incidence of new HIV infection in 1997. In sub-Saharan Africa, an estimated 1.8 million people were newly infected in 2009. In 2008, an estimated 32.8 million people were living with HIV infection worldwide; 52% of them women. An estimated 2.5 million children in 2009 were estimated to be living with HIV infection. (UNAIDS, 2010).

HUMAN IMMUNODEFICIENCY VIRUSES

HIV is now understood to have two variants: HIV-1 and HIV-2. Both variants appear to have originated in West Africa and jumped species from non-human primates: HIV-1 from the chimpanzee and HIV-2 from the sooty mangabey, a monkey found in West Africa (Hahn, Shaw, De Cock, & Sharp, 2000; Keele et al., 2006). The first confirmed cases appear to have occurred in the 1950s, and increased urbanization caused the epidemic to accelerate. HIV-2 is mainly seen in parts of West Africa; it follows a more indolent course than HIV-1 even without ARVs. There are four subtypes of the HIV-1 virus: More than 90% of cases worldwide are from Subtype Group M and other than a handful of cases in Groups N and P, the remainder from Group O, which is mainly limited to west-central Africa.

HIV TESTING AND COUNSELING

HIV antibody testing utilizing an enzyme immunoassay (EIA) method was first licensed in the United States in 1985. Successive generations of tests were developed to reduce the time interval between HIV exposure and when HIV testing could detect infection (Perry, Ramskill, Eglin, Barbara, & Parry, 2008). First-generation testing used viral lysate to detect HIV antibodies in a sample of the patient's blood; it had a high false-positive rate so was mainly useful in populations with a high base rate of the disease. Western blot testing was used as a confirmatory tool. Second-generation testing using recombinant HIV antigens was developed, which permitted earlier detection of HIV infection with fewer false positives Third-generation testing used a "sandwich" technique to detect both Immunoglobulin G (IgG) and Immunoglobulin M (IgM) antibodies, allowing for even earlier detection of HIV infection. In 2010, the FDA approved the first fourth-generation HIV assay which detects IgG and IgM antibodies and as well as p24 viral antigen, reducing the window period sufficiently to pick up to 80% of acute HIV infections that were previously only detectable via HIV RNA assays (Pandori & Branson, 2010). Speeding up the testing process has important implications, as patients may not return for their HIV test results. Current rapid HIV tests can produce preliminary results in as little as one minute, increasing the likelihood that patients will know their HIV status and, if it is positive, receive care. Clinicians should be aware that individuals with acute HIV illness may present with a variety of symptoms, which include a flu-like syndrome, aseptic meningitis, lymphadenopathy, and rash. If there is a high suspicion of acute HIV illness, HIV RNA testing remains indicated.

Current CDC guidelines recommend routine testing of patients in all health care settings for patients age 13–64 years old, and that patients be informed verbally or in writing that they will be tested for HIV unless they decline or "opt out" (Branson et al., 2006). Separate written consent is not recommended by the CDC. The objective is to enhance earlier diagnosis of HIV infection and link patients to care. Patients with acute HIV infection often have extremely high viral loads with increased risk of transmission. Research has shown that most HIV transmission occurs with people who are unaware that they are HIV-positive.

CD4 COUNT

HIV targets CD4 cells resulting in progressive immune dysfunction. Earlier treatment with antiretrovirals may help maintain immune function and prevent the decline of the CD4 count and the emergence of HIV-associated infections and cancers. However, there are reasons to delay treatment with antiretrovirals for a HIV-infected individual, including potential toxicity, issues of drug resistance, uncomfortable side effects from medications, as well as lifestyle adjustments related to the challenges of taking a large numbers of pills. At different times in the epidemic, the recommended CD4 threshold for commencement of antiretroviral therapy for asymptomatic patients has been raised and lowered, based on the available evidence and treatment options. Current U.S. guidelines suggest treatment of all symptomatic patients and asymptomatic patients with CD4 counts less than 500, and consideration of antiretroviral treatment for asymptomatic patients with CD4 counts greater than 500 and treatment of asymptomatic patients at a CD4 count less than or equal to 500 (Department of Health and Human Services [DHHS], 2011a; Thompson et al., 2010). The guidelines further advise that HIV-infected individuals with significant medical conditions, including cardiovascular, hepatic, or renal diseases, and pregnant women, be treated with antiretrovirals at any CD4 count.

VIRAL LOAD

Measurement of the HIV RNA level (viral load) is used as a baseline value for the diagnosis of acute HIV illness, before a patient is treated with ARVs, and it is used to assess the success of ARV therapy. The viral load varies, depending on the point in infection. The viral load of patients with acute HIV infection is often extremely high before settling down to a lower viral set point and generally staying at that level until antiretroviral treatment is begun. The magnitude of this set point is influenced by a number of host and virus factors, and remains a focus of research.

With successful antiretroviral treatment, the CD4 count rises, and the plasma viral load becomes undetectable. Achievement of an undetectable HIV viral load has important implications for health and transmission risk. The sensitivity of assays has increased over time, and the newest assays often measure down to 50 or 20 copies per milliliter (mL) of blood, with some assays even measuring as little as one copy per mL. Despite the ability of successful antiretroviral treatment to lower HIV viral load below 50 copies, continued HIV viremia in the range of 1–50 copies is found in a majority of patients on highly active anti-retroviral therapy (HAART) (Chun et al., 2011). This very low level of HIV plasma viral load generally does not appear to cause viral load rebound and drug failure. However, even low-level viral loads in the range of 1–50 copies may be associated with a chronic inflammatory process that is linked to cardiovascular disease and other signs of accelerated aging (Kuller et al., 2008; Triant, Meigs, & Grinspoon, 2009). Additionally, antiretroviral therapy penetrates poorly into the central nervous system (CNS), and ongoing CNS HIV replication and neurocognitive effects may persist despite viral load suppression in other parts of the body.

Transmission risk is reduced as plasma viral load decreases. Studies have shown that serodiscordant couples with a HIV-positive partner and a high viral load transmit HIV to their HIV-negative partners at a much greater rate as compared to those in which the HIV-positive partner has a low viral load. Although more controversial, some studies looking at the average viral load of a community have found that new HIV infections decrease as the community viral load is reduced. Mathematical models also support the use of aggressive testing and treatment of HIV-infected persons as HIV prevention (Granich, Gilks, Dye, De Cock, & Williams, 2009). Based on this evidence, a potential prevention strategy is to implement an aggressive "test and treat strategy" in which all adults are offered testing, linked to care, and immediately offered ARV treatment as a means of reducing community viral load and curtailing the HIV epidemic.

HIV AND INFLAMMATION

Contributing to the current emphasis on earlier antiretroviral treatment is a growing recognition that untreated HIV-infected patients, even those with a high CD4 count, suffer ill effects of HIV replication, including immune dysregulation and associated inflammation. The presence of elevated levels of immune markers such as interleukin-6 (IL-6) and C-reactive protein (CRP) (Kuller, et al., 2008) support that patients with ongoing HIV viral replication have an ongoing inflammatory process associated with endothelial inflammation and increased end-organ damage. For instance, comorbid infections such as hepatitis B and hepatic C appear to progress more quickly with accelerated development of cirrhosis and hepatocellular cancer when patients with HIV are not treated with antiretroviral medications (Sulkowski, 2008; Thein, Yi, Dore, & Krahn, 2008; Thio et al., 2002).

HIV LATENCY AND CURE

Studies have shown that, despite suppression of HIV by successful ARV treatment, a small proportion of CD4 cells remain latently infected with the HIV virus, leading to viral load rebound and progression of HIV-associated illness in patients who stop their antiretrovirals (Chun, et al., 2011; Finzi et al., 1999). This HIV reservoir decays very slowly, even for patients treated with combination antiretrovirals for long periods of time, and effectively is never eradicated. A current research focus is on how to safely activate these resting cells so that antiretroviral treatment can eradicate these infected cells without causing excessive systemic immune activation. HIV vaccine efforts have generally been disappointing, with the exception of one modest positive result (Rerks-Ngarm et al., 2009). A case study in Germany, with still unclear implications, has rekindled excitement about a future cure (Allers et al., 2011). In this case, a patient who was HIV-positive for more than ten years developed acute myeloid leukemia and required a bone marrow transplant after relapse following chemotherapy. The patient was transplanted with stems cells from a donor screened for homozygosity for the *CCR5* homozygous deletion (HIV predominantly uses CCR5 as a co-receptor for entry into CD4 cells). In four years since the transplant occurred, the patient has remained off antiretrovirals, and no sign of active replicating HIV virus has yet been detected.

ANTIRETROVIRALS

There are almost 30 approved antiretroviral medications (including combination pills) in six drug classes: nucleoside/nucleotide reverse transcriptase inhibitors (NRTI), non-nucleoside reverse transcriptase inhibitors (NNRTI), protease inhibitors (PI), CCR5-receptor antagonists, integrase inhibitors, and fusion inhibitors. During the 1990s, a number of large randomized, controlled trials showed that patients on combination antiretroviral therapy did better, with more durable clinical improvement (Hammer et al., 1996; Hammer et al., 1997). The current strategy is to choose a regimen with at least two, and preferably three, potent antiretroviral medications.

The use of these medications is complicated and may have serious adverse effects, and it is recommended that they be used and monitored by experienced HIV clinicians. Side effects of the NRTIs can range from lactic acidosis and lipodystrophy to bone loss, renal failure, and a potentially lethal hypersensitivity reaction. The class of NNRTIs includes delavirdine, nevirapine, efavirenz, etravirine, and rilpivirine. Efavirenz is associated with neuropsychiatric side effects, which generally occur early in treatment and are time-limited. Common side effects of efavirenz may include dizziness, bad dreams, and anxiety, and there have been case reports of severe depression, mania, and psychosis (Arendt, de Nocker, von Giesen, & Nolting, 2007; Tozzi et al., 2007). The protease inhibitors are often co-administered with low doses of the PI ritonavir. Ritonavir, one of the early protease inhibitors, is now rarely used for its antiviral effect, but is used for its drug-boosting effect. It is a potent P450 inhibitor, particularly of 3A4, and many of the protease inhibitors use this isoenzyme pathway. The co-formulation increases the drug levels of the PIs, decreasing the likelihood that resistance will develop and allowing dosing schedules that are less frequent and onerous. The PIs are associated with hyperlipidemia (though less so with atazanavir), and some studies have shown an association with protease inhibitor use and increased cardiovascular events. The CCR5 antagonist maraviroc is the only antiretroviral medication that targets, not the HIV virus, but a human cell receptor. HIV uses either the coreceptor CCR5 or CXCR4 to gain entry into target cells, and maraviroc is a CCR5 antagonist. Most patients with early HIV infection have a virus that preferentially uses a CCR5 co-receptor rather than CXCR4. As HIV infection progresses and CD4 count declines, the HIV virus may mutate to a virus that uses the CXC4 receptor, and maraviroc is therefore ineffective. A commercially available assay can determine the type of co-receptor used by an individual patient's virus. The integrase inhibitor raltegravir is generally well tolerated, and minimal long-term problems have been identified to date. The fusion inhibitor enfuvirtide, the only injectable antiretroviral, is a twice-daily medication that causes local skin reactions at the injection and is poorly tolerated. It is often used only as an antiretroviral medication of last resort for patients with broad class resistance. For a comprehensive table of currently available antiretrovirals with dosing recommendations, common side effects, and potential drug interactions, the reader is referred to the AIDS Meds website, http://www.aidsmeds.com/articles/DrugChart_10632.shtml.

It is important to realize that, even in the current antiretroviral era, not every HIV-infected patient receives care or adheres to antiretroviral therapy. Patients may poorly tolerate or decline treatment with ARVs; have active mental illness, cognitive deficits, or substance use complicating adherence; or continue to have limited access to HIV care if living in resource-limited settings.

GENOTYPE AND PHENOTYPE TESTING

Genotype testing is a technique that screens for HIV virus polymorphisms associated with antiretroviral drug resistance. Genotype testing is generally performed before a patient starts on antiretroviral therapy and when a patient on treatment has viral load rebound. Genotype testing usually requires a viral load of about 500–1000 copies/mL for the test to be accurate. Antiretrovirals have different resistance patterns. In some instances, a single mutation, such as the *M184V* mutation with the NRTIs lamivudine and emtricitabine, and the *K103N* mutation with the NNRTIs nevirapine and efavirenz, can render a single medication or multiple medications within a drug class ineffective. By contrast, the newer protease inhibitor medications have a higher resistance barrier and may remain active even with a number of mutations in the protease enzymes. Deciphering a genotype can be complicated, and to aid interpretation, a virtual phenotype, which predicts drug susceptibility based on a resistance pattern databank, can assist clinicians and guide clinical decision making.

A phenotype test may also be ordered for patients with significant treatment experience and complicated genotypes. This entails, not HIV genetic testing, but a more traditional approach of culturing the virus with various antiretrovirals and determining the concentration of drug needed to inhibit HIV virus growth. Whatever test is used, one important consideration is that different HIV subpopulations may coexist in a certain individual—both "wild type" virus and subpopulations of HIV with drug resistance. A genotype or phenotype may not detect a resistant HIV virus subpopulation that is not currently under drug pressure, but will emerge in the presence of antiretroviral therapy.

PRE- AND POST-EXPOSURE PROPHYLAXIS

A major success in combating the HIV epidemic has been the reduction of perinatal HIV transmission. In 1994, the Pediatric Aids Clinical Trial Group (PACTG 076) trial showed a two-thirds reduction in mother-to-infant transmission, from 25.5% in the placebo-treated group to 8.3% in the AZT-treated group (Connor et al., 1994). The use of HIV screening for pregnant women, antiretroviral therapy, elective

Caesarian delivery for women with suboptimal HIV viral suppression, and exclusive bottle-feeding has reduced the rates of vertical transmission to less than 2% in the United States and Europe (DHHS, 2011b).

Sexually transmitted infections (STIs) such as herpes simplex appear to increase HIV transmission. To date, randomized clinical trials using STI treatment as a means of HIV prevention have not generally demonstrated significant results, but further research is ongoing (Padian, McCoy, Balkus, & Wasserheit, 2010). Conversely, clinical trials have shown that circumcision can reduce the HIV acquisition rates of heterosexual men by up to 60% (Auvert et al., 2005; Bailey et al., 2007; Gray et al., 2007). Despite the dramatic reduction of HIV rates in heterosexual men who are circumcised, increasing circumcision rates as a means of reducing HIV risk in endemic regions has been a challenge.

Women may have difficulty negotiating condom use. As a means of addressing this obstacle, numerous trials have looked at the use of non-specific vaginal microbicides, including chemical surfactants, as a means of preventing the acquisition of HIV. The trials have generally been disappointing, but a recent placebo-controlled trial in a high-HIV prevalence area of South Africa was encouraging, and showed that the use of tenofovir intravaginal gel inserted within 12 hours before or after sex reduced HIV acquisition by 54% in "high adherers" and 39% reduction in the overall group (Abdool Karim et al., 2010).

The use of antiretrovirals for occupational post-exposure HIV prophylaxis has reduced HIV transmission rates in the workplace. In the absence of post-exposure antiretroviral prophylaxis, the estimated HIV transmission risk for percutaneous exposure is 0.3%, and after a mucous membrane exposure, 0.09%. Only a handful of cases due to occupational exposure have been reported since the introduction of the first occupational exposure guidelines (Panlilio, Cardo, Grohskopf, Heneine, & Ross, 2005). Antiretroviral post-exposure prophylaxis may also be used for high-risk sexual and injection drug-use exposures with a 28-day course of HAART administered within 72 hours of exposure (Smith et al., 2005).

As antiretrovirals have become more tolerable and less toxic, there has been increasing interest in using ARVs for sexual pre-exposure prophylaxis in high-risk groups. A recent placebo-controlled, double-blind randomized trial involving men who have sex with men (MSM) and transgender women (genetic male) engaging in high-risk behaviors suggested that once-daily prophylactic use of tenofovir and emtricitabine (Truvada) can reduce the likelihood of HIV acquisition (Grant et al., 2010). Enrollment in the treatment arm of the trial provided a 44% reduction in the incidence of HIV acquisition. Based on this single study, the CDC issued interim guidelines on the use of pre-exposure prophylaxis with antiretrovirals (CDC, 2011). The CDC interim guideline suggests that providers might consider use of tenofovir-emtricitabine for high-risk MSM and transgender women in combination with other prevention strategies. It is important to recognize that this use of antiretrovirals for pre-exposure HIV prophylaxis remains off-label, and the emergence of drug resistance and long-term toxicity remains a real concern. There is emerging, but not unanimous, new evidence that pre-exposure prophylaxis may be also be helpful in reducing HIV infection among high-risk heterosexual men and women, but expert guidelines have not yet been established to guide this antiretroviral indication.

ANTIRETROVIRAL DRUG INTERACTIONS WITH PSYCHOTROPIC MEDICATIONS

The protease inhibitor ritonavir has significant CYP P450 interactions, and is an extremely potent cytochrome 3A4 inhibitor, but it also inhibits the cytochrome isoenzyme 2D6 and induces 2B6, 1A2, and glucuronyl transferase. Benzodiazepines that undergo metabolism through the 3A4 enzyme pathway, notably alprazolam, midazolam, and triazolam (the latter two have absolute contraindications), can have markedly elevated plasma levels with ritonavir use. Many selective serotonin-reuptake inhibitors (SSRIs) and tricyclic antidepressants undergo metabolism through the 2D6 pathway and may require a dose decrease when used with ritonavir. There have been case reports of serotonin syndrome with fluoxetine- and ritonavir-containing regimens due to P450 inhibition with ritonavir (DeSilva et al., 2001). Trazodone plasma levels may be markedly increased through 3A4 inhibition on ritonavir-containing regimens. Drug levels of bupropion may initially be increased when used with ritonavir and also with efavirenz because of an initial 2B6 inhibition that precedes 2B6 induction; in the longer term, bupropion levels may decrease (Park Wyllie & Antoniou, 2003). Most antipsychotics are CYP 2D6 and/or 3A4 substrates and may require a lower dose of, for example, risperidone, perphenazine, and thioridazine, if used with ritonavir-containing regimens; olanzapine is one exception, as its plasma levels are decreased through induction of 1A2. Ritonavir may lower plasma drug levels of the anticonvulsant/mood stabilizers valproic acid and lamotrigine.

Pharmacotherapy for opioid dependence may be affected by the use of antiretroviral therapy. Methadone serum levels may be decreased by the antiretrovirals ritonavir, efavirenz, and nevirapine. Treatment with buprenorphine and atazanavir or atazanavir/ritonavir may increase buprenorphine drug levels and cause sedation, possibly through 3A4 inhibition and phase II metabolism of buprenorphine by atazanavir, requiring a reduction in buprenorphine dose; but a 2007 observational trial suggested the combination can be safely used (Bruce & Altice, 2006; McCance-Katz et al., 2007) (see Table 63.1). Due to the large number of drugs prescribed to patients with HIV/AIDS, we recommend consulting with comprehensive websites such as the University of Liverpool's http://www.hiv-druginteractions.org/ to check for potential drug interactions when recommending the addition of a psychotropic to the medication regimen.

Table 63.1 PHARMACOKINETIC EFFECTS OF SOME HIV AND PSYCHOTROPIC MEDICATIONS THAT CAN POTENTIALLY LEAD TO DRUG–DRUG INTERACTIONS

PROTEASE INHIBITORS	CYP 3A4[a]	CYP 2D6[b]	COMMENTS
Ritonavir	Potent Inhibition Induction	Potent Inhibition	Midazolam, triazolam contraindicated Alprazolam—use with extreme caution Tricyclic antidepressants—blood levels may increase due to inhibition; monitor carefully Clozapine—use with extreme caution Pimozide—contraindicated Methadone—serum levels may decrease Thioridazine—avoid use SSRIs—monitor for increased side effects Trazodone—plasma levels may increase Olanzapine—blood levels may decrease secondary to 1A2 induction Antipsychotics (non-olanzapine)—monitor for increased side effects Valproic acid—plasma levels may decrease; monitor serum levels Lamotrigine—plasma levels may decrease
Amprenavir	Moderate Inhibition		Midazolam, triazolam, alprazolam—use with caution
Indinavir	Moderate Inhibition	Mild Inhibition	Midazolam, triazolam, alprazolam—use with caution
Nelfinavir	Moderate Inhibition	Mild Inhibition	Midazolam, triazolam, alprazolam—use with caution
Atazanavir	Moderate Inhibition		
NNRTIs			
Nevirapine	Induction		Methadone—serum levels may decrease
Efavirenz	Moderate Inhibition Induction		Methadone—serum levels may decrease
Etravirine	Induction		
PSYCHOTROPICS			
Nefazodone	Moderate Inhibition		May cause protease inhibitor levels to increase
Phenytoin Carbamazepine Phenobarbital	Induction		May *decrease* serum levels of protease inhibitors and lead to viral resistance
St. John's Wort	Induction		May *decrease* serum levels of protease inhibitors and lead to viral resistance
Modafinil	Induction (High Doses)		May *decrease* serum levels of protease inhibitors and lead to viral resistance

a Cytochrome P450 34A metabolic enzyme
b Cytochrome P450 2D6 metabolic enzyme

MANAGEMENT OF HIV AND PRIMARY CARE

As options for the treatment of HIV and the prophylaxis of opportunistic infections have improved, HIV-infected individuals are dying less frequently from AIDS, and also living longer (Hogg et al., 2008). Most HIV-infected patients on combination antiretroviral therapy can now achieve an undetectable viral load (Moore, Keruly, Gebo, & Lucas, 2005) and increased CD4 count, lowering the risk of acquiring AIDS-related opportunistic infections, such as PCP, MAI, toxoplasmosis, and cytomegalovirus, and cancers, such as invasive cervical cancer, KS, and non-Hodgkin's lymphoma (El-Sadr et al., 2006). As the clinical management of HIV has changed into that of a chronic illness, the HIV population is aging. HIV-infected patients may develop diabetes mellitus (Palacios, Santos, Ruiz, Gonzalez, & Marquez, 2003), hypertension, and age-related cancers, and there is increasing evidence that patients with HIV may have an increased risk of bone loss (Brown & Qaqish, 2006), cardiovascular disease (El-Sadr, et al., 2006), renal disease (Gupta et al., 2004), cognitive changes and dementia, liver disease (Sulkowski, 2008; Thein, et al., 2008; Thio, et al., 2002), and a frailty phenotype (Desquilbet et al., 2007). As a result of these changes, the management of HIV patients requires expertise in general medicine beyond just antiretroviral management.

NEUROPSYCHIATRY OF HIV INFECTION

HIV-ASSOCIATED NEUROCOGNITIVE DISORDERS

Neurocognitive disorders and subtle cognitive impairment are seen throughout the spectrum of HIV infection. Formal neuropsychological testing combined with clinical examination, lumbar puncture, and radiographic imaging provides the most useful means for evaluating cognitive decline (Box 63.1). Some of the earliest reports about HIV/AIDS indicated that the virus entered the central nervous system during initial infection and that this was a neurocognitive disease as much as it was an immunological disease. In 1991, the American Academy of Neurology published criteria to be used in the diagnosis of HIV-associated dementia (HAD) and the minor cognitive motor disorder (MCMD). These criteria indicated that HAD was an acquired abnormality in at least two cognitive areas, causing impairment in work or acitivites of daily living (ADLs), and that there was abnormality in motor function or abnormality in neuropsychiatric or psychosocial functioning leading to behavioral change. These criteria have been updated to cover a slightly broader range of HIV-associated neurocognitive disorders (HAND), which places a greater emphasis on cognitive impairment and behavioral abnormalities without any requirement of motor impairment. Suggestions are given for age- and education-appropriate normed neuropsychological testing of eight cognitive domains as well as psychosocial evaluation that must be performed in order to make a HAND diagnosis.

Box 63.1 EVALUATION OF ALTERED MENTAL STATUS IN PATIENTS WITH HIV/AIDS

Physical Neurological Exam

- Focal deficits may indicate space-occupying lesion; e.g., CNS lymphoma, toxoplasmosis, PML*
- Ataxia or changes in gait may indicate myelopathy associated with HAD
- Sensory changes indicative of peripheral neuropathy

Labs

- Complete blood count with differential
- Serum chemistries
- Arterial blood gas in patients with pneumonia
- Venereal Disease Research Laboratory (VDRL), Flourescent Treponemal Antibody (FTA)
- B_{12}, folate

Neuroradiology

- MRI to rule out space-occupying lesion, Progressive Multifocal Leukoencephalopathy PML

Lumbar Puncture

- To rule out acute infection; e.g., herpes, cryptococcal meningitis, syphilis, toxoplasmosis

Review of Medications

- Neuropsychiatric side effects of AIDS meds; drug interactions, especially with protease inhibitors

Neuropsychological Testing

- AIDS Dementia Rating Scale**
- Finger Tapping Test
- Trail Making Test

EEG

*PML—progressive multifocal leukoencephalopathy

**See Power et al. (1995) to obtain the AIDS Dementia Rating Scale

---

Three categories of HAND are defined:

1. Asymptomatic neurocognitive impairment (ANI), in which the patient scores one standard deviation below the mean in two cognitive areas, with no subjective or objective signs of impairment in functioning;

2. Mild neurocognitive disorder (MND), again scoring one standard deviation below the mean in two or more areas, but with some mild impairment; and

3. HIV-associated dementia (HAD), in which the patient scores two standard deviations below the mean on

normative neuropsychiatric tests and has moderate to severe impairment in functioning (Antinori et al., 2007).

HAD is most commonly seen in more advanced stages of HIV disease. In the pre-HAART era, some degree of cognitive impairment was reported to be found in up to 60–90% of individuals with advanced-stage disease, and HAD was diagnosed in 15–20% patients. The annual incidence of HAD was reported to be 7% (McArthur et al., 1993). Since the introduction of HAART, several studies have shown the yearly incidence of HAD to have dropped to approximately 1% (d'Arminio Monforte et al., 2004; McArthur & Brew, 2010; Sacktor et al., 2001). However, as patients live longer with HIV, and with the inclusion of asymptomatic states, the overall prevalence of HAND has increased. For patients stabilized on a HAART regimen with no detectable viral load, the current prevalence estimates of ANI ranges from 32–50%; for MND, 12–17%; and for HAD, approximately 2–3% (Heaton et al., 2010; Simioni et al., 2010). The prevalence rates of HAND rise in patients with poor immunological control, as seen particularly in resource-poor countries (Robertson et al., 2007).

The precise pathophysiology of HAND remains unclear, but it appears to be related to neurotoxins secreted by mononuclear phagocytes. Some of the cytokines implicated include tumor necrosis factor (TNF), interleukin 1 (IL-1) and the N-methyl-D-aspartate (NMDA) agonists quinolinic acid and arachidonic acid. The immune cascade hypothesis supposes that inflammation at the blood–brain barrier (BBB) allows more HIV to enter the CNS, which provokes primed and immune activate macrophages to secrete neurotoxins that affect neuronal functioning and cause CNS inflammation, leading to further breakdown of the BBB and perpetuation of the inflammatory cascade. This hypothesis also emphasizes the importance of maintaining good immunological control peripherally to minimize CNS malfunction.

The early symptoms of HAD are subtle, typically with subcortical brain dysfunction and overlapping with the cognitive impairment associated with depression. Common early features include apathy, memory loss, cognitive slowing, impaired concentration, psychomotor slowing and slowed information processing, social withdrawal, and dyscoordination (Ferrando & Lyketsos, 2008). Later features include psychosis, severe memory loss with attention-deficit disorder, gross ataxia, seizures, and mutism (Price & Spudich, 2008).

The diagnosis of HAD is basically one of exclusion, and the evaluation will involve ruling out other primary causes of cognitive dysfunction, such as opportunistic CNS infections or neoplasms. Since the introduction of HAART, confounding factors such as increased age, co-infection with hepatitis C, substance use disorders, endocrinological disorders, and mental illness play a greater role in causing cognitive impairment in long-term survivors of HIV/AIDS. Computed tomography (CT) and magnetic resonance imaging (MRI), although not diagnostic, usually show some degree of cortical atrophy, and subcortical or periventricular white matter changes. Lumbar puncture often reveals a mild increase in protein and mononuclear pleocytosis, and while not diagnostic of HAD, examination of the cerebrospinal fluid (CSF) is helpful in excluding opportunistic CNS infections such as cryptococcal meningitis and toxoplasmosis.

The HIV Dementia Rating Scale assesses psychomotor processing speed, verbal memory, constructional ability, and executive function, and is a useful instrument for screening cognitive impairment in HIV-positive patients. It is more sensitive than the Mini-Mental Status Exam (MMSE; Power, Selnes, Grim, & McArthur, 1995). A recent study indicates that a cutoff score of less than 14 is a good predictor that HAND will be diagnosed on full clinical assessment (Simioni, et al., 2010). Formal neuropsychological testing can provide detailed information on deficits in specific domains and can be very helpful in differentiating self-reports of cognitive impairment seen in depressed patients. Corroborative history from family and friends is extremely important in accurately characterizing functional impairment. Risk factors for HAD have been reported to include: increased viral load, decreased CD4, anemia, older age, decreased body mass, a history of persistent physical symptoms, anemia, female sex, and injection drug use (McArthur & Brew, 2010).

The primary choice of treatment for HAD, and possibly all HAND, is a regimen of HAART. One the earliest clinical trials looking at the treatment of HIV/AIDS found that high-dose AZT led to significant neuropsychological improvement (Schmitt et al., 1988). However, because these patients were receiving monotherapy, the physical and neurocognitive improvements were short-lived. Since these early studies, HAART regimens have been shown to lead to neuropsychiatric improvement, radiological improvement, and decreased CSF viral load, despite concerns about variable BBB penetrance of the antiretrovirals (Ferrando, Rabkin, van Gorp, Lin, & McElhiney, 2003; Filippi, Sze, Farber, Shahmanesh, & Selwyn, 1998; Price & Spudich, 2008). Some authors recommend using a regimen of four agents, with at least two that have relatively high BBB penetrance, such as zidovudine, nevirapine, atazanavir, inidinavir, and lopinavir, in order to maximize treatment of CNS infection; while others emphasize the importance of systemic immunological control to minimize the neurotoxic immune cascade.

Psychostimulant medications such as methylphenidate have been studied extensively in HIV-positive patients and have been found to be well tolerated and to lead to a decrease in cognitive dysfunction and depressive symptoms associated with dementia (Fernandez, Levy, & Ruiz, 1994). More recently, modafinil was shown to increase cognitive performance in HIV patients with complaints of fatigue (Rabkin, McElhiney, Rabkin, & McGrath, 2010). Other agents, such as memantine, selegiline, nimodipine, and peptide T, thought to have neuroprotective effects, have been studied but none have been found to significantly ameliorate HAND (Turchan, Sacktor, Wojna, Conant, & Nath, 2003).

With current treatment regimens, the course of HAND has become more variable over time, with fluctuations and at times nearly complete remission of symptoms.

DELIRIUM

Delirium occurs frequently among hospitalized HIV-infected patients, with reported prevalence rates ranging from 29% to 57% (Bialer, Wallack, Prenzlauer, Bogdonoff, & Wilets, 1996; Fernandez, Levy, & Mansell, 1989). AIDS patients may be especially susceptible to the development of delirium in the context of underlying HIV brain infection, the common use of multiple drugs, and the frequency of multiple medical complications. The etiology of delirium in this population is usually multifactorial, and while the causes of delirium are similar to those of any medically ill patient, some are more specific to the patient with AIDS (Box 63.2).

Evaluation and correction of the underlying medical cause of delirium is of primary importance, since there may be significant morbidity and mortality associated with this diagnosis (Uldall, Harris, & Lalonde, 2000; Uldall, Ryan, Berghuis, & Harris, 2000). Repeated mental status exams, a careful review of medications, thorough physical and neurological exams, a search for infections or metabolic abnormalities, neuroradiological exams, lumbar puncture, and electroencephalograms

---

Box 63.2 ETIOLOGIES OF DELIRIUM IN HIV/AIDS PATIENTS

Intracranial

Seizures and postictal states
  Infections
  Cryptococcal meningitis
  Encephalitis due to HIV, herpes, Cytomegalovirus (CMV)
  Progressive multifocal leukoencephalopathy (PML)
  Mass lesions
  Lymphoma
  Toxoplasmosis

Extracranial

Medications and drugs (not exhaustive):
  Amphotericin B: Sedative/hypnotics
  Acyclovir: Cycloserine
  Ganciclovir: Opiate analgesics
  Ethambutol: Isoniazid
  Trimethoprim/sulfamethoxazole: Rifampin
  Pentamidine: Zidovudine, Didanosine
  Foscarnet: Vincristine
  Ketoconazole: Dapsone
  Drug or alcohol withdrawal
  Infections/sepsis
  Endocrine dysfunction/metabolic abnormality
  Hypoglycemia due to pentamidine, protease inhibitors
  Liver failure due to comorbid hepatitis, medication toxicities
  Nutritional deficiencies
  Wasting syndrome
  Failure to replace trace elements or vitamins in total parenteral nutrition

---

(EEG) are all essential in the evaluation of the delirious AIDS patient (Table 63.1).

Prompt management of agitation due to delirium is extremely important because of the distress caused to the patient and families, the potential for self-harm, as well the potential for exposure of HIV to others. Neuroleptics are the mainstay of treatment of the agitated delirious patient, and low-dose haloperidol is often effective in the AIDS population. Intravenous haloperidol may be necessary in very agitated patients where the risk of needle-stick injury is high. However, patients with HIV/AIDS may be more susceptible to severe, extrapyramidal and sedative side effects, and extreme caution must be exercised (Breitbart, Marotta, & Call, 1988; Fernandez et al., 1989). Cardiac arrhythmias and lengthening of the Q-T interval on electrocardiogram (EKG) have also been reported with the use of high-dose intravenous haloperidol (Metzger & Friedman, 1993). Medically ill patients receiving intravenous haloperidol at any dose should be monitored with frequent EKGs.

In a double-blind study, Breitbart (Breitbart, Marotta, et al., 1996) demonstrated the usefulness of low-dose oral haloperidol or chlorpromazine in the treatment of delirious AIDS patients. Although chlorpromazine is generally not recommended for the management of agitated, delirious patients, low doses that should have relatively mild anticholinergic effects may be useful for HIV patients who are very sensitive to the extra-pyramidal symptoms EPS caused by high-potency neuroleptics. The use of lorazepam in this study appeared to make many patients worse and had to be discontinued.

Atypical neuroleptics such as aripiprazole, quetiapine, risperidone, and olanzapine have been shown to be useful in the management of delirium (Breitbart, Tremblay, & Gibson, 2002; Schwartz & Masand, 2002; Straker, Shapiro, & Muskin, 2006) and may also be helpful in managing AIDS patients who are not highly agitated. Clinical experience indicates that patients with HIV/AIDS may tolerate these medications with fewer side effects and less EPS than they have with high-potency neuroleptics.

MOOD DISORDERS

DEPRESSION

Depressive disorders are the most frequently diagnosed mental disorder among patients with HIV/AIDS, with prevalence rates ranging from 35–85% depending upon sampling criteria such as hospitalization status, HIV disease stage, and comorbid risk behaviors (Bing et al., 2001; Ickovics et al., 2001; Morrison et al., 2002; Rabkin, 2008). One of the largest surveys of mental disorders among HIV patients found a rate of 36% for major depressive disorder and 26.5% for dysthymia (Bing et al., 2001) and a meta-analysis of published studies about depressive disorders among HIV patients demonstrated that seropositive compared to seronegative subjects were twice as likely to be diagnosed with major depression (Ciesla & Roberts, 2001). Although depression has been described as a component of HAD, individuals are more likely to present with apathy as a component of cognitive decline, which may be typical of frontal lobe and subcortical dementias, misdiagnosed as major depression (Price & Spudich, 2008).

As HIV disease progresses, depressive symptoms are more likely to arise (Lyketsos et al., 1996). Many investigators have found an association between the severity of HIV-related physical symptoms and the severity of depressive symptoms (Belkin, Fleishman, Stein, Piette, & Mor, 1992; Burack et al., 1993); however, other studies have reported no such association (Ciesla & Roberts, 2001; Lyketsos et al., 1993). In another investigation, Mayne et al. (Mayne, Vittinghoff, Chesney, Barrett, & Coates, 1996) found that while depression was independent of physical symptoms, depressed mood was associated with higher mortality risk. Mayne and colleagues hypothesized that behaviors associated with depression (treatment nonadherence, substance abuse) may speed the progression of HIV disease. A more recent study indicated that women diagnosed with dysthymia were less likely to receive HAART (Turner & Fleishman, 2006). These findings underscore the critical importance of diagnosis and treatment of depression in this population.

A thorough evaluation for suicide risk should be part of the assessment of all depressed individuals with HIV infection. Although occasional, transient thoughts of suicide are not uncommon among individuals with HIV disease—pervasive suicidal ideation often accompanies HIV-related depressive syndromes and may be particularly prevalent among individuals who have recently tested positive for HIV (Perry, Jacobsberg, & Fishman, 1990).

Although HIV/AIDS may be more commonly viewed as a treatable disease in the age of HAART, some studies have shown suicidal ideation to still be highly prevalent, in the range of 17–38% (Goggin et al., 2000; Heckman et al., 2002; Kalichman, Heckman, Kochman, Sikkema, & Bergholte, 2000). Completed suicides appear to occur at a significantly increased rate among persons with HIV infection compared to age-matched controls (Cote, Biggar, & Dannenberg, 1992; Kizer, Green, Perkins, Doebbert, & Hughes, 1988; Marzuk et al., 1988), a phenomenon that has continued even after the introduction of HAART (Haller & Miles, 2003; Keiser et al., 2010).

Bereavement has taken on community-wide proportions among those affected by HIV and should be aggressively treated when symptoms suggest pathological grief reactions. Bereavement support groups have not only been shown to be effective in improving the psychological outcomes of those affected, but they have also been associated with improvement in viral load measurements for intervention subjects (Goodkin et al., 1999; Goodkin et al., 2001; Sikkema, Hansen, Kochman, Tate, & Difranceisco, 2004). Goodkin and colleagues postulate immunological and neuroendocrine benefits from the support group and recommend such interventions be used as an adjunct to HAART in bereaved HIV patients.

When medical comorbidity (brain infections, medication side effects) is determined to be the primary cause of depression, initial treatment should be aimed at correcting the underlying problem. Otherwise, treatment regimens include typical pharmacological and psychological strategies for the treatment of major depression in medical illness.

Numerous antidepressant agents have been found to be well tolerated and efficacious in the management of depression in patients with HIV disease. Research utilizing randomized, placebo-controlled designs reveals that SSRIs such as fluoxetine, paroxetine, citalopram, and escitalopram may be particularly useful in treating HIV-related major depression; this is especially true for patients with more advanced HIV disease and comorbid disorders such as hepatitis C (Currier, Molina, & Kato, 2004; Elliott et al., 1998; Laguno et al., 2004; Rabkin, Wagner, & Rabkin, 1999a). Other antidepressants such as venlafaxine, duloxetine, and mirtazapine have not been as well studied in the HIV population, but clinical experience indicates these agents may also be successfully used. Bupropion is usually avoided in patients receiving HAART due to concerns about drug interactions, although some have indicated that it can be used safely in this group (Park Wyllie & Antoniou, 2003). Psychostimulants have been shown to have a beneficial effect on depressive symptoms, especially when depression is accompanied by cognitive impairment (Fernandez, Levy, & Ruiz, 1994; White, Christensen, & Singer, 1992). Newer agents such as modafinil and armodafinil have also been shown to improve mood among patients being treated for HIV-related fatigue (Rabkin, McElhiney, & Rabkin, 2011; Rabkin et al., 2010); testosterone replacement therapy has also been shown to be helpful when fatigue is pronounced (Rabkin, 2008; Rabkin, Wagner, & Rabkin, 1999b). Although not specifically studied in this population, there is no specific contraindication to using electro-convulsive therapy (ECT) or repetitive transcranial magnetic stimulation (rTMS) and may be considered in patients with treatment-resistant depression.

Most psychotherapeutic interventions reported in HIV-positive individuals have aimed at reducing risk behaviors or lowering distress. Nonetheless, research data and clinical experience suggest that various modes of psychotherapy are beneficial in the management of HIV-related depression. Investigators have reported the successful use of interpersonal therapy (Markowitz et al., 1995), cognitive behavioral therapy (Kelly et al., 1993), supportive therapy (Markowitz et al., 1998), structured group therapy, and combined structured group therapy and antidepressant pharmacotherapy (Targ et al., 1994).

MANIA

Prevalence rates of manic syndromes in HIV patients have respectively been reported as 2.4% (Halman, Worth, Sanders, Renshaw, & Murray, 1993), 8% (Lyketsos, Schwartz, Fishman, & Treisman, 1997), and 30% (Boccellari, Dilley, & Shore, 1988) in selected series of patients. Mania in the HIV patient may be due to preexisting psychiatric illness, the CNS effects of HIV-related opportunistic infections or tumors, HAD, or side effects of medications.

Some authors have noted differences between patients presenting with mania early or late in the course of HIV disease (Halman, et al., 1993; Lyketsos, et al., 1997). Early-onset mania was more likely in patients with a personal or family history of mood disorders, and these patients more often presented with increased talking as a symptom. Late-onset mania was more often associated with a diagnosis of HAD, and irritability was a more frequent symptom.

Evaluation of HIV patients with mania should first rule out a secondary mania and include, at a minimum, a personal and family psychiatric history, a review of medications and any temporal relationship to the onset of symptoms, determination of CD4 count and viral load, and a neuroradiological exam. In patients with evidence of late-onset mania, examination of the CSF and neuropsychological evaluation for HAD are also indicated (Table 63.1).

Given the risk for impaired judgement, the potential for hyperactive sexual behavior, and poor impulse control, the clinician must aggressively treat the acutely manic patient with HIV/AIDS. Those with asymptomatic HIV infection and a premorbid history of bipolar disorder may be managed with standard lithium treatment, although patients with advanced HIV disease appear at increased risk for lithium-induced side effects, including neurotoxicity, delirium, diarrhea, polyuria, and polydipsia (Adler Cohen & Jacobson, 2000). Antiepileptic drugs are better treatment choices in patients with AIDS-related mania (Halman et al., 1993). Due to the greater risk of myelosuppression by carbamazepine, sodium valproate is preferred, with careful monitoring of hepatic enzymes, coagulation factors, and complete blood-count including platelets, being carefully monitored especially in patients with hepatitis C co-infection. Anticonvulsants such as lamotrigine may also prove to be effective and well tolerated in this population.

High-potency neuroleptics, such as haloperidol in low doses, may be useful in the acute management of manic HIV patients. However, increased sensitivity to extrapyramidal side effects of neuroleptics has been well documented. Some have reported the safe and effective use of risperidone in the management of mania in AIDS patients (Singh, Golledge, & Catalan, 1997), but while other atypical neuroleptics have indications for the treatment of mania, none have been well-studied in this population. Lorazepam or clonazepam have also been shown to be effective in the treatment of the acutely manic HIV patient (Budman & Vandersall, 1990) but act therapeutically primarily as sedatives.

ANXIETY DISORDERS

Treatment of anxiety disorders in persons with HIV/AIDS follows the general guidelines for other medical patients. For chronic generalized anxiety, buspirone has been shown to be effective in this population (Batki, 1990). A benzodiazepine may be the drug of choice for acute anxiety, but it should be used cautiously in patients with multiple medical complications and in those with a history of substance use disorder. Agents that are primarily glucuronidated and bypass the P450 enzyme system (e.g., lorazepam, oxazepam) are preferred due to decreased metabolite accumulation and decreased potential for interactions with antiretrovirals. Other agents with varying efficacy in the treatment of anxiety in the setting of HIV infection include β-adrenergic blockers, antihistamines, and sedating antidepressants. The antidepressant venlafaxine is approved by the US Food and Drug Administration (FDA) forGerneralized Anxiety disorder (GAD) and should be considered as a first-line drug as well.

Psychotherapies play an important treatment option for many patients with anxiety, particularly if the anxiety is less severe or if patients cannot take anti-anxiety medications. In most settings, the preferred treatment combines pharmacotherapy and methods of anxiety self-regulation. Numerous techniques for self-regulation have been shown to be effective in treating HIV-related anxiety, including muscle relaxation therapies, electromyographic biofeedback, behavioral techniques, acupuncture, self-hypnosis, and aerobic exercise training.

SUBSTANCE USE DISORDERS (SUD)

While men who have sex with men continue to compose the largest proportion of people with HIV/AIDS, injection drug use (IDU) remains a significant transmission category. IDU accounts for 15% of new HIV infections and 22% of cumulative cases of AIDS among women (CDC, 2009). Non-injecting SUD is also related to higher rates of HIV transmission (Chesney, Barrett, & Stall, 1998; Ferrando & Batki, 2000; Woody et al., 1999). A high lifetime prevalence of psychiatric disorders among those with SUD, in the range of 50–80%, has been reported, and several studies have demonstrated high rates of psychiatric disorders among HIV patients with SUD: the "triple diagnosis" patient (Bialer, Hoffman, & Ditzell, 2008; Klinkenberg & Sacks, 2004; Lipsitz et al., 1994).

Methamphetamine use has increased greatly among gay men in urban centers and is often associated with both needle-sharing and unsafe sexual behavior (Halkitis, Parsons, & Stirratt, 2001; Molitor, Truax, Ruiz, & Sun, 1998; Shoptaw, Reback, & Freese, 2002). There is also a high prevalence of methamphetamine use among heterosexual men and women in the West and Midwest, and studies have demonstrated increased risk behaviors associated with HIV transmission among these populations (Molitor et al., 1999). Thus, methamphetamine abuse may be playing a larger role in the HIV epidemic in the coming years.

Psychiatric management of the HIV patient with a SUD has become increasingly important for several reasons:

1. Continued substance use may lead to an increase in unsafe behaviors such as needle-sharing or unprotected sex (Chesney, et al., 1998; Vanable et al., 2004; Woody, et al., 1999);

2. Adherence to medical treatment may be impaired (Ferrando, Wall, Batki, & Sorensen, 1996; Freeman, Rodriguez, & French, 1996; Klinkenberg & Sacks, 2004);

3. The mental and physical changes resulting from SUD can negatively affect the patients' quality of life.

The most helpful treatment approach is to determine whether SUD is a primary diagnosis. This can be difficult, either because of a patient's poor reliability or because of a mixed picture, such as a sleep disorder and alcohol abuse presenting simultaneously. If SUD is the primary diagnosis, then specific drug abuse treatment and abstinence should be required before further psychiatric treatment can continue. Treatment options include brief inpatient detoxification for patients with physiological dependence on substances such as heroin or alcohol, followed by inpatient rehabilitation; outpatient rehabilitation or therapeutic communities for longerterm intensive treatment; methadone maintenance for heroin users (Cooper, 1989); and 12 Step programs such as Alcoholics Anonymous (AA) or Narcotics Anonymous (NA). All of these modalities offer a group setting, which addresses the difficulties in interpersonal relationships so common among these patients. They also offer the support and advice of others who are further along in their recovery, so that patients have role models who can offer concrete advice. It is important to have referrals to these programs readily available, since patients tend to have brief windows of opportunity when they are willing to accept these services.

Various types of therapies have been recommended for treating HIV patients with SUD, including cognitive, interpersonal, and supportive/exploratory (Markowitz, et al., 1995), as well as motivational interviewing. Harm-reduction strategies that acknowledge that not all patients will achieve or maintain abstinence are especially applicable to HIV patients with SUD (Ferrando & Batki, 2000). Studies have shown that counseling and education regarding risk behaviors and corresponding precautions should be incorporated into the treatment and can have beneficial effects (Gibson, McCusker, & Chesney, 1998; Semaan et al., 2002). The clinician must be prepared to be flexible, and to incorporate whichever form of treatment (or combination of treatments) is most useful for a particular patient at a particular time.

PAIN

Studies have shown that pain may be undertreated in AIDS patients, as it is in most medical and surgical patients (Breitbart, Rosenfeld, et al., 1996). Non-psychiatrists often do not recognize pain as a common symptom among patients with HIV/AIDS. Psychiatrists may be consulted to evaluate for psychological causes of pain complaints. The prevalence of pain in this population has been estimated to range from 30–80%, however, and can be due to HIV infection itself and its related complications, therapies used to treat AIDS, or to non-HIV-related causes (Breitbart, McDonald, et al., 1996; Dobalian, Tsao, & Duncan, 2004). Although neuropathic pains occur frequently, pains of a somatic and visceral nature are actually more common (Breitbart, 1996) (Box 63.3).

Pain in the AIDS patient can be managed according to the same guidelines for cancer pain management. This involves a complete physical, neurological, and psychiatric evaluation for correctable causes of pain. Analgesic medications can then be prescribed according to the level of pain: non-opioid medications (e.g., acetaminophen or non-steroidal anti-inflammatory drugs [NSAIDs]) for mild pain, weak opioids (e.g., codeine or oxycodone) for moderate pain, and strong opioids (morphine, hydromorphone) for severe pain. For continuous or recurring pain, analgesics should be given around the clock.

Psychotropic medications play an important role in the management of pain in AIDS patients. In addition to their direct effects on associated syndromes such as depression or anxiety, antidepressants, neuroleptics, and stimulants have been shown to be useful adjuvants in pain management by potentiating the effect of analgesics. Duloxetine, gabapentin, and pregabalin are all approved for patients with postherpetic and diabetic neuropathies, and may offer particular benefit to patients with HIV-related, painful neuropathies. Lidocaine patches can also be used to treat localized neuropathic pain.

The management of pain in AIDS patients with a history of substance abuse can be problematic. As there is no objective way to measure pain, one must rely on the patient's report of pain and its severity. Although a certain number of patients with a substance use disorder may malinger in order to obtain drugs, complaints of pain should be taken seriously and fully evaluated. Pain management guidelines, including the use of around-the-clock opioid analgesics for moderate to severe pain, should be similar to that of patients without a history of substance abuse. Correction of medical causes of pain and the use of adjuvant medications and nonpharmacological treatments may lessen the need for opioid analgesics.

Box 63.3 PAIN SYNDROMES IN AIDS PATIENTS

Pain Related to HIV/AIDS

    HIV neuropathy
    HIV myelopathy
    Kaposi's sarcoma
    Opportunistic infections (intestines, skin)
    Organomegaly
    Arthritis/vasculitis
    Myopathy/myositis

Pain Related to HIV/AIDS Therapy

    Antiretrovirals, antivirals
    Antimycobacterials, PCP prophylaxis
    Chemotherapy (vincristine)
    Radiation
    Surgery
    Procedures (bronchoscopy, biopsies)

Pain Unrelated to AIDS

    Spinal disc disease
    Diabetic neuropathy

From: Breitbart, W. (1996), Pharmacotherapy of pain in AIDs. In G. Wormser (Ed.), *A clinical guide to AIDS and HIV*. Philadelphia, PA: Lippincott-Raven. Permission to reprint being requested.

Early in the AIDS epidemic, little attention was paid to the mentally ill as a possible risk group for HIV infection. Perhaps this reflected a lack of knowledge regarding the sexual behaviors of this population or inadequate awareness of the frequency of comorbid conditions or behaviors that might increase risk. In 1989, the first published reports appeared regarding HIV infection among patients with major psychiatric illnesses in state hospitals (Cournos, Empfield, Horwath, & Kramer, 1989). Interest in the seroprevalence of HIV and risk behaviors of the mentally ill grew, and several important studies began to appear in the literature. Rates of HIV seroprevalence among the severely mentally ill have been reported to range from 4.0–22.9% (Cournos & McKinnon, 1997; McKinnon, Cournos, & Herman, 2002). The highest rates of infection were found in settings that treated dual-diagnosis patients with both severe mental illness and comorbid substance use disorder (Dausey & Desai, 2003). Both injection drug use and sexual activity were predictors of HIV seropositivity. When risk factors were identified, the highest seroprevalence was found among those with a history of prostitution (37.9%), sex with a drug injector (37.5%), male–male sex (25.4%), or drug injection (21.6%). Of interest was the finding that, among patients with *non*-injected drug use, the seroprevalence rate was still quite high, at 11.4%. In the majority of these studies, women were as likely to be infected as men. However, across studies, the rates of seropositivity were 9.8% among African Americans, 9.6% among Hispanic patients, and 3.1% among Caucasian and Asian patients combined. The likelihood of seropositivity did not seem to vary with psychiatric diagnosis: 9.2% among schizophrenics and 10% among other Axis I diagnoses. These data suggest that the rates for HIV infection among the severely mentally ill are elevated when compared to the general population. The findings of these studies underscore the important role for the psychiatrist in advocating for improved substance-abuse treatment strategies for the mentally ill and in the promotion of AIDS education and prevention for our patients. HIV testing should be strongly encouraged for all chronically mentally ill patients, and HIV infection should be considered in the differential diagnosis of acute medical illness in this population.

CONCLUSION

While great strides have been made in the management of HIV/AIDS, it remains a complex disease with profound neuropsychiatric as well as psychosocial implications. For patients with a dual and sometimes triple diagnosis of medical, psychiatric, and substance use disorders, treatment would ideally occur in an integrated setting with medical specialists, nursing, and mental health providers. Such integrated settings have been developed in urban centers in the United States and elsewhere with large numbers of patients with HIV. When such settings are not available, we would recommend that patients with dual and triple diagnoses be managed at a minimum by HIV specialists.

- The fourth-generation HIV assay test picks up 80% of acute HIV infections with a 5% false positive rate.

- The assay test can be used for other fluids but approved only for blood.

- Viral load (RNA) not diagnostic but high viral load in acute HIV may be picked up in 10 days, slightly earlier than by fourth-generation assay.

- Clinicians should be aware that individuals with acute HIV illness may present with a variety of symptoms, which include a flu-like syndrome, aseptic meningitis, lymphadenopathy, and rash. If there is a high suspicion of acute HIV illness, HIV RNA testing remains indicated.

- P9 antiretroviral therapy penetrates poorly into the central nervous system (CNS), and ongoing CNS HIV replication and neurocognitive effects may persist despite viral load suppression in other parts of the body.

- Transmission risk is reduced as plasma viral load decreases.

- Contributing to the current emphasis on earlier antiretroviral treatment is a growing recognition that untreated HIV-infected patients, even those with a high CD4 count, suffer ill effects of HIV replication, including immune dysregulation and associated inflammation.

- The current strategy is to choose a regimen with at least two, and preferably three, potent antiretroviral medications.

- Efavirenz is associated with neuropsychiatric side effects, which generally occur early in treatment and are time-limited. Common side effects of efavirenz may include dizziness, bad dreams, or anxiety, and there have been case reports of severe depression, mania, and psychosis (Arendt, de Nocker, von Giesen, & Nolting, 2007; Tozzi et al., 2007).

- Ritonavir, one of the early protease inhibitors, is now rarely used for its antiviral effect, but is used for its drug-boosting effect. It is a potent P450 inhibitor, particularly of 3A4, and many of the protease inhibitors use this isoenzyme pathway.

- The use of HIV screening for pregnant women, antiretroviral therapy, elective Caesarian delivery for women with suboptimal HIV viral suppression, and exclusive bottle-feeding has reduced the rates of vertical transmission to less than 2% in the United States and Europe (DHHS, 2011b, p. 12).

- The use of antiretrovirals for occupational post-exposure HIV prophylaxis has reduced HIV transmission rates in the workplace. In the absence of post-exposure antiretroviral prophylaxis, the estimated HIV transmission risk for percutaneous exposure is 0.3%, and after a mucous membrane exposure, 0.09%. Only a handful of cases due to occupational exposure have been reported since the introduction of the first occupational exposure guidelines (Panlilio, Cardo, Grohskopf, Heneine, & Ross, 2005). Antiretroviral post-exposure prophylaxis may also be used for high-risk sexual and injection drug-use exposures, with a 28-day course of HAART administered within 72 hours of exposure p 13.

- Benzodiazepines that undergo metabolism through the 3A4 enzyme pathway, notably alprazolam, midazolam, and triazolam (the latter two have absolute contraindications), can have markedly elevated plasma levels with ritonavir use. Many SSRIs and tricyclic antidepressants undergo metabolism through the 2D6 pathway and may require a dose decrease when used with ritonavir. There have been case reports of serotonin syndrome with fluoxetine- and ritonavir-containing regimens due to P450 inhibition with ritonavir (DeSilva et al., 2001). Trazodone plasma levels may be markedly increased through 3A4 inhibition on ritonavir-containing regimens.

- Methadone serum levels may be decreased by the antiretrovirals ritonavir, efavirenz, and nevirapine.

- The precise pathophysiology of HAND remains unclear, but it appears to be related to neurotoxins secreted by mononuclear phagocytes.

- CT and MRI, although not diagnostic, usually show some degree of cortical atrophy, and subcortical or periventricular white matter changes. Lumbar puncture often reveals a mild increase in protein and mononuclear pleocytosis and, while not diagnostic of HAD, examination of the CSF is helpful in excluding CNS opportunistic infections such as cryptococcal meningitis and toxoplasmosis.

- The HIV Dementia Rating Scale assesses psychomotor processing speed, verbal memory, constructional ability, and executive function and is a useful instrument to screen cognitive impairment in HIV-positive patients.

- Risk factors for HAD have been reported to include: increased viral load, decreased CD4, anemia, older age, decreased body mass, a history of persistent physical symptoms, anemia, female sex, and injection drug use (McArthur & Brew, 2010).

- Some authors recommend using a regimen of four agents with at least two that have relatively high BBB penetrance, such as zidovudine, nevirapine, atazanavir, inidinavir, and lopinavir, in order to maximize treatment of CNS infection; while others emphasize the importance of systemic immunological control to minimize the neurotoxic immune cascade. P 19.

- Psychostimulants have been shown to have a beneficial effect on depressive symptoms especially when depression is accompanied by cognitive impairment. (F. Fernandez, Levy, JK., Ruiz, P., 1994). More recently, modafinil was shown to increase cognitive performance in HIV patients with complaints of fatigue (J. Rabkin, McElhiney, Rabkin, & McGrath, 2010).

- Other agents such as memantine, selegiline, nimodipine, and peptide T, thought to have neuroprotective effects, have been studied; but none have been found to significantly ameliorate HAND (Turchan, Sacktor, Wojna, Conant, & Nath, 2003) p 20.

- Although depression has been described as a component of HAD, individuals are more likely to present with apathy as a component of cognitive decline, which may be typical of frontal lobe and subcortical dementias, misdiagnosed as major depression (Price & Spudich, 2008).

- Women diagnosed with dysthymia were less likely to receive HAART (Turner & Fleishman, 2006).

- Bereavement support groups have not only been shown to be effective in improving the psychological outcomes of those affected but have also been associated with improvement in viral load measurements for intervention subjects (Goodkin et al., 1999; Goodkin et al., 2001; Sikkema, Hansen, Kochman, Tate, & Difranceisco, 2004) p23.

- Research utilizing randomized, placebo-controlled designs reveals that SSRIs such as fluoxetine, paroxetine, citalopram, and escitalopram may be particularly useful in treating HIV-related major depression; this is especially true for patients with more advanced HIV disease and comorbid disorders such as hepatitis C (Currier, Molina, & Kato, 2004; Elliott et al., 1998; Laguno et al., 2004; Rabkin, Wagner, & Rabkin, 1999a).

- Bupropion is usually avoided in patients receiving HAART due to concerns about drug interactions, although some have indicated that it can be used safely in this group (Park Wyllie & Antoniou, 2003) p24.

- Early-onset mania was more likely in patients with a personal or family history of mood disorders, and these patients more often presented with increased talking as a symptom. Late-onset mania was more often associated with a diagnosis of HAD, and irritability was a more frequent symptom. P25.

- Many of the medications used in the treatment of HIV/AIDS have been reported to cause anxiety as a possible side effect, including antiretrovirals, isoniazid, acyclovir, and pentamidine.p27.

- While men who have sex with men continue to comprise the largest proportion of people with HIV/AIDS, injecting drug use (IDU) remains a significant transmission category. IDU accounts for 15% of new HIV infections and 22% of cumulative cases of AIDS among women.

- If SUD is the primary diagnosis, then specific drug treatment and abstinence should be required before further psychiatric treatment can continue.

- (Breitbart, Rosenfeld, et al., 1996). Non-psychiatrists often do not recognize pain as a common symptom among patients with HIV/AIDS.

- Rates of HIV seroprevalence among the severely mentally ill have been reported to range from 4.0–22.9% (Cournos & McKinnon, 1997; McKinnon, Cournos, & Herman, 2002).

- When risk factors were identified, the highest seroprevalence was found among those with a history of prostitution (37.9%), sex with a drug injector (37.5%), male-male sex (25.4%), or drug injection (21.6%). 9.2% among schizophrenics and 10% among other Axis I diagnoses.

DISCLOSURE STATEMENTS

Dr. Bialer: No Conflicts to disclose

Dr. Lux: No Conflicts to disclose

REFERENCES

Abdool Karim, Q., Abdool Karim, S. S., Frohlich, J. A., Grobler, A. C., Baxter, C., Mansoor, L. E., et al. (2010). Effectiveness and safety of tenofovir gel, an antiretroviral microbicide, for the prevention of HIV infection in women. *Science*, *329*(5996), 1168–1174.

Adler Cohen, M. A., & Jacobson, J. M. (2000). Maximizing life's potentials in AIDS: a psychopharmacologic update. *General Hospital Psychiatry*, *22*(5), 375–388.

Allers, K., Hutter, G., Hofmann, J., Loddenkemper, C., Rieger, K., Thiel, E., et al. (2011). Evidence for the cure of HIV infection by CCR5Delta32/Delta32 stem cell transplantation. *Blood*, *117*(10), 2791–2799.

Antinori, A., Arendt, G., Becker, J. T., Brew, B. J., Byrd, D. A., Cherner, M., et al. (2007). Updated research nosology for HIV-associated neurocognitive disorders. *Neurology*, *69*(18), 1789–1799.

Arendt, G., de Nocker, D., von Giesen, H. J., & Nolting, T. (2007). Neuropsychiatric side effects of efavirenz therapy. *Expert Opinion on Drug Safety*, *6*(2), 147–154.

Auvert, B., Taljaard, D., Lagarde, E., Sobngwi-Tambekou, J., Sitta, R., & Puren, A. (2005). Randomized, controlled intervention trial of male circumcision for reduction of HIV infection risk: the ANRS 1265 Trial. *PLoS Medicine*, *2*(11), e298.

Bailey, R. C., Moses, S., Parker, C. B., Agot, K., Maclean, I., Krieger, J. N., et al. (2007). Male circumcision for HIV prevention in young men in Kisumu, Kenya: a randomised controlled trial. *Lancet*, *369*(9562), 643–656.

Batki, S. L. (1990). Buspirone in drug users with AIDS or AIDS-related complex. *Journal of Clinical Psychopharmacology*, *10*(3 Suppl), 111S–115S.

Belkin, G. S., Fleishman, J. A., Stein, M. D., Piette, J., & Mor, V. (1992). Physical symptoms and depressive symptoms among individuals with HIV infection. *Psychosomatics*, *33*(4), 416–427.

Bialer, P. A., Hoffman, R., & Ditzell, J. (2008). Substance use disorders—the special role in HIV. In M. A. Cohen & J. M. Gorman (Eds.), *Comprehensive textbook of AIDS psychiatry* (pp. 85–96). New York: Oxford Universtiy Press.

Bialer, P. A., Wallack, J. J., Prenzlauer, S. L., Bogdonoff, L., & Wilets, I. (1996). Psychiatric comorbidity among hospitalized AIDS patients vs. non-AIDS patients referred for psychiatric consultation. *Psychosomatics*, *37*(5), 469–475.

Bing, E. G., Burnam, M. A., Longshore, D., Fleishman, J. A., Sherbourne, C. D., London, A. S., et al. (2001). Psychiatric disorders and drug use among human immunodeficiency virus-infected adults in the United States. *Archives of general psychiatry*, *58*(8), 721–728.

Boccellari, A., Dilley, J. W., & Shore, M. D. (1988). Neuropsychiatric aspects of AIDS dementia complex: a report on a clinical series. *Neurotoxicology*, *9*(3), 381–389.

Branson, B. M., Handsfield, H. H., Lampe, M. A., Janssen, R. S., Taylor, A. W., Lyss, S. B., et al. (2006). Revised recommendations for HIV testing of adults, adolescents, and pregnant women in health-care settings. *MMWR: Recommendations & Reports*, *55*(RR-14), 1–17; quiz, CE11–14.

Breitbart, W. (1996). Pharmacotherapy of pain in AIDS. In Wormser, G. editor, *A Clinical Guide to AIDS and HIV*, Lippincott-Raven, Philadelphia.

Breitbart, W., Marotta, R., Platt, M. M., Weisman, H., Derevenco, M., Grau, C., et al. (1996). A double-blind trial of haloperidol, chlorpromazine, and lorazepam in the treatment of delirium in hospitalized AIDS patients. *American Journal of Psychiatry*, *153*(2), 231–237.

Breitbart, W., Marotta, R. F., & Call, P. (1988). AIDS and neuroleptic malignant syndrome. *Lancet*, *2*(8626–8627), 1488–1489.

Breitbart, W., McDonald, M. V., Rosenfeld, B., Passik, S. D., Hewitt, D., Thaler, H., et al. (1996). Pain in ambulatory AIDS patients. I: Pain characteristics and medical correlates. *Pain*, *68*(2–3), 315–321.

Breitbart, W., Rosenfeld, B. D., Passik, S. D., McDonald, M. V., Thaler, H., & Portenoy, R. K. (1996). The undertreatment of pain in ambulatory AIDS patients. *Pain*, *65*(2–3), 243–249.

Breitbart, W., Tremblay, A., & Gibson, C. (2002). An open trial of olanzapine for the treatment of delirium in hospitalized cancer patients. *Psychosomatics*, *43*(3), 175–182.

Brown, T. T., & Qaqish, R. B. (2006). Antiretroviral therapy and the prevalence of osteopenia and osteoporosis: a meta-analytic review. *AIDS*, *20*(17), 2165–2174.

Bruce, R. D., & Altice, F. L. (2006). Three case reports of a clinical pharmacokinetic interaction with buprenorphine and atazanavir plus ritonavir. *AIDS*, *20*(5), 783–784.

Budman, C. L., & Vandersall, T. A. (1990). Clonazepam treatment of acute mania in an AIDS patient. *Journal of Clinical Psychiatry*, *51*(5), 212.

Burack, J. H., Barrett, D. C., Stall, R. D., Chesney, M. A., Ekstrand, M. L., & Coates, T. J. (1993). Depressive symptoms and CD4 lymphocyte decline among HIV-infected men. *Journal of the American Medical Association*, *270*(21), 2568–2573.

Centers for Disease Control and Preventiion (CDC) (1981a). Kaposi's sarcoma and Pneumocystis pneumonia among homosexual men—New York City and California. *MMWR Morbidity & Mortality Weekly Report*, *30*(25), 305–308.

Centers for Disease Control and Preventiion (CDC) (1981b). Pneumocystis pneumonia—Los Angeles. *MMWR Morbidity & Mortality Weekly Report*, *30*(21), 250–252.

Centers for Disease Control and Preventiion (CDC) (1989). Guidelines for prophylaxis against *Pneumocystis carinii* pneumonia for persons infected with human immunodeficiency virus. *MMWR Morbidity & Mortality Weekly Report*, *38*(Suppl 5), 1–5.

Centers for Disease Control and Preventiion (CDC) (2011). Interim guidance: preexposure prophylaxis for the prevention of HIV infection in men who have sex with men. *MMWR Morbidity & Mortality Weekly Report*, *60*(65–68).

Centers for Disease Control and Preventiion (CDC) (2011). Diagnoses of HIV infection and AIDS in the United States and dependent areas, 2009. HIV Surveillance Report, available at http://www.cdc.gov/hiv/surveillance/resources/reports/2009report/index.htm (Vol. 21). Accessed December 5, 2011

Chesney, M. A., Barrett, D. C., & Stall, R. (1998). Histories of substance use and risk behavior: precursors to HIV seroconversion in homosexual men. *American Journal of Public Health*, *88*(1), 113–116.

Chun, T. W., Murray, D., Justement, J. S., Hallahan, C. W., Moir, S., Kovacs, C., et al. (2011). Relationship between residual plasma viremia and the size of HIV proviral DNA reservoirs in infected individuals receiving effective antiretroviral therapy. *Journal of Infectious Diseases, 204*(1), 135–138.

Ciesla, J. A., & Roberts, J. E. (2001). Meta-analysis of the relationship between HIV infection and risk for depressive disorders. *The American Journal of Psychiatry, 158*(5), 725–730.

Connor, E. M., Sperling, R. S., Gelber, R., Kiselev, P., Scott, G., O'Sullivan, M. J., et al. (1994). Reduction of maternal-infant transmission of human immunodeficiency virus type 1 with zidovudine treatment. Pediatric AIDS Clinical Trials Group Protocol 076 Study Group. *New England Journal of Medicine, 331*(18), 1173–1180.

Cooper, J. R. (1989). Methadone treatment and acquired immunodeficiency syndrome. *Journal of the American Medical Association, 262*(12), 1664–1668.

Cote, T. R., Biggar, R. J., & Dannenberg, A. L. (1992). Risk of suicide among persons with AIDS. A national assessment. *Journal of the American Medical Association, 268*(15), 2066–2068.

Cournos, F., Empfield, M., Horwath, E., & Kramer, M. (1989). The management of HIV infection in state psychiatric hospitals. *Hospital & Community Psychiatry, 40*(2), 153–157.

Cournos, F., & McKinnon, K. (1997). HIV seroprevalence among people with severe mental illness in the United States: a critical review. *Clinical Psychology Review, 17*(3), 259–269.

Currier, M. B., Molina, G., & Kato, M. (2004). Citalopram treatment of major depressive disorder in Hispanic HIV and AIDS patients: a prospective study. *Psychosomatics, 45*(3), 210–216.

d'Arminio Monforte, A., Cinque, P., Mocroft, A., Goebel, F.-D., Antunes, F., Katlama, C., et al. (2004). Changing incidence of central nervous system diseases in the EuroSIDA cohort. *Annals of neurology, 55*(3), 320–328.

Dausey, D., & Desai, R. (2003). Psychiatric comorbidity and the prevalence of HIV infection in a sample of patients in treatment for substance abuse. *The journal of nervous and mental disease, 191*(1), 10–17.

Department of Health and Human Services—DHHS. (2011a). Panel on antiretroviral guidelines for adults and adolescents. Guidelines for the use of antiretroviral agents in HIV- infected adults and adolescents. January 10, 2011. *Center for Disease Control—CDC,* 1–166.

Department of Health and Human Services—DHHS. (2011b). Panel on treatment of HIV-infected pregnant women and prevention of perinatal transmission. Recommendations for use of antiretroviral drugs in pregnant HIV-1-infected women for maternal health and interventions to reduce perinatal HIV transmission in the United States. May 24, 2010. *Center for Disease Control—CDC,* 1–117.

DeSilva, K.E., LeFlore, D.B., Marston, B.J., & Rimland, D. (2001) Serotonin syndrome in HIV-infected individuals receiving antiretroviral therapy and fluoxetine. *AIDS, 15*(10), 1281–1285.

Desquilbet, L., Jacobson, L. P., Fried, L. P., Phair, J. P., Jamieson, B. D., Holloway, M., et al. (2007). HIV-1 infection is associated with an earlier occurrence of a phenotype related to frailty. *The Journals of Gerontology Series A: Biological Sciences and Medical Sciences, 62*(11), 1279–1286.

Dobalian, A., Tsao, J. C. I., & Duncan, R. P. (2004). Pain and the use of outpatient services among persons with HIV: results from a nationally representative survey. *Medical care, 42*(2), 129–138.

El-Sadr, W. M., Lundgren, J. D., Neaton, J. D., Gordin, F., Abrams, D., Arduino, R. C., et al. (2006). CD4+ count-guided interruption of antiretroviral treatment. *New England Journal of Medicine, 355*(22), 2283–2296.

Elliott, A. J., Uldall, K. K., Bergam, K., Russo, J., Claypoole, K., & Roy Byrne, P. P. (1998). Randomized, placebo-controlled trial of paroxetine versus imipramine in depressed HIV-positive outpatients. *The American Journal of Psychiatry, 155*(3), 367–372.

Fernandez, F., Levy, J. K., & Mansell, P. W. (1989). Management of delirium in terminally ill AIDS patients. *International Journal of Psychiatry in Medicine, 19*(2), 165–172.

Fernandez, F., Levy, J. K., & Ruiz, P. (1994). The use of methylphenidate in HIV patients: A clinical perspective. In Martin, A. &

Grant, I. (Ed.), *Neuropsychology of HIV infection.* New York: Oxford University Press.

Ferrando, S., & Lyketsos, C. (2008). HIV-associated neurocognitive disorders. In M. A. Cohen & J. M. Gorman (Eds.), *Comprehensive textbook of AIDS psychiatry* (pp. 109–120). New York: Oxford University Press.

Ferrando, S., Rabkin, J., van Gorp, W., Lin, S.-H., & McElhiney, M. (2003). Longitudinal improvement in psychomotor processing speed is associated with potent combination antiretroviral therapy in HIV-1 infection. *The Journal of neuropsychiatry and clinical neurosciences, 15*(2), 208–214.

Ferrando, S. J., & Batki, S. L. (2000). Substance abuse and HIV infection. *New Directions for Mental Health Services, 87,* 57–67.

Ferrando, S. J., Wall, T. L., Batki, S. L., & Sorensen, J. L. (1996). Psychiatric morbidity, illicit drug use and adherence to zidovudine (AZT) among injection drug users with HIV disease. *American Journal of Drug Abuse & Prevention, 22*(4), 475–487.

Filippi, C. G., Sze, G., Farber, S. J., Shahmanesh, M., & Selwyn, P. A. (1998). Regression of HIV encephalopathy and basal ganglia signal intensity abnormality at MR imaging in patients with AIDS after the initiation of protease inhibitor therapy. *Radiology, 206*(2), 491–498.

Finzi, D., Blankson, J., Siliciano, J. D., Margolick, J. B., Chadwick, K., Pierson, T., et al. (1999). Latent infection of CD4+ T cells provides a mechanism for lifelong persistence of HIV-1, even in patients on effective combination therapy. *Nature Medicine, 5*(5), 512–517.

Freeman, R. C., Rodriguez, G. M., & French, J. F. (1996). Compliance with AZT treatment regimen of HIV-seropositive injection drug users: a neglected issue. *AIDS Education & Prevention, 8*(1), 58–71.

Gallo, R. C., Salahuddin, S. Z., Popovic, M., Shearer, G. M., Kaplan, M., Haynes, B. F., et al. (1984). Frequent detection and isolation of cytopathic retroviruses (HTLV-III) from patients with AIDS and at risk for AIDS. *Science, 224*(4648), 500–503.

Gallo, R. C., Sarin, P. S., Gelmann, E. P., Robert-Guroff, M., Richardson, E., Kalyanaraman, V. S., et al. (1983). Isolation of human T-cell leukemia virus in acquired immune deficiency syndrome (AIDS). *Science, 220*(4599), 865–867.

Gibson, D. R., McCusker, J., & Chesney, M. (1998). Effectiveness of psychosocial interventions in preventing HIV risk behaviour in injecting drug users. *AIDS, 12*(8), 919–929.

Goggin, K., Sewell, M., Ferrando, S., Evans, S., Fishman, B., & Rabkin, J. (2000). Plans to hasten death among gay men with HIV/AIDS: relationship to psychological adjustment. *AIDS Care, 12*(2), 125–136.

Goodkin, K., Baldewicz, T. T., Asthana, D., Khamis, I., Blaney, N. T., Kumar, M., et al. (2001). A bereavement support group intervention affects plasma burden of human immunodeficiency virus type 1. Report of a randomized controlled trial. *Journal of human virology, 4*(1), 44–54.

Goodkin, K., Blaney, N. T., Feaster, D. J., Baldewicz, T., Burkhalter, J. E., & Leeds, B. (1999). A randomized controlled clinical trial of a bereavement support group intervention in human immunodeficiency virus type 1-seropositive and -seronegative homosexual men. *Archives of general psychiatry, 56*(1), 52–59.

Gottlieb, M. S., Schroff, R., Schanker, H. M., Weisman, J. D., Fan, P. T., Wolf, R. A., et al. (1981). *Pneumocystis carinii* pneumonia and mucosal candidiasis in previously healthy homosexual men: evidence of a new acquired cellular immunodeficiency. *New England Journal of Medicine, 305*(24), 1425–1431.

Granich, R. M., Gilks, C. F., Dye, C., De Cock, K. M., & Williams, B. G. (2009). Universal voluntary HIV testing with immediate antiretroviral therapy as a strategy for elimination of HIV transmission: a mathematical model. *Lancet, 373*(9657), 48–57.

Grant, R. M., Lama, J. R., Anderson, P. L., McMahan, V., Liu, A. Y., Vargas, L., et al. (2010). Preexposure chemoprophylaxis for HIV prevention in men who have sex with men. *New England Journal of Medicine, 363*(27), 2587–2599.

Gray, R. H., Kigozi, G., Serwadda, D., Makumbi, F., Watya, S., Nalugoda, F., et al. (2007). Male circumcision for HIV prevention in men in Rakai, Uganda: a randomised trial. *Lancet, 369*(9562), 657–666.

Gupta, S. K., Mamlin, B. W., Johnson, C. S., Dollins, M. D., Topf, J. M., & Dube, M. P. (2004). Prevalence of proteinuria and the development of chronic kidney disease in HIV-infected patients. *Clinical Nephrology, 61*(1), 1–6.

Hahn, B. H., Shaw, G. M., De Cock, K. M., & Sharp, P. M. (2000). AIDS as a zoonosis: scientific and public health implications. *Science, 287*(5453), 607–614.

Halkitis, P. N., Parsons, J. T., & Stirratt, M. J. (2001). A double epidemic: crystal methamphetamine drug use in relation to HIV transmission among gay men. *Journal of homosexuality, 41*(2), 17–35.

Haller, D., & Miles, D. (2003). Suicidal ideation among psychiatric patients with HIV: psychiatric morbidity and quality of life. *AIDS and behavior, 7*(2), 101–108.

Halman, M. H., Worth, J. L., Sanders, K. M., Renshaw, P. F., & Murray, G. B. (1993). Anticonvulsant use in the treatment of manic syndromes in patients with HIV-1 infection. *Journal of Neuropsychiatry & Clinical Neuroscience, 5*(4), 430–434.

Hammer, S. M., Katzenstein, D. A., Hughes, M. D., Gundacker, H., Schooley, R. T., Haubrich, R. H., et al. (1996). A trial comparing nucleoside monotherapy with combination therapy in HIV-infected adults with CD4 cell counts from 200 to 500 per cubic millimeter. AIDS Clinical Trials Group Study 175 Study Team. *New England Journal of Medicine, 335*(15), 1081–1090.

Hammer, S. M., Squires, K. E., Hughes, M. D., Grimes, J. M., Demeter, L. M., Currier, J. S., et al. (1997). A controlled trial of two nucleoside analogues plus indinavir in persons with human immunodeficiency virus infection and CD4 cell counts of 200 per cubic millimeter or less. AIDS Clinical Trials Group 320 Study Team. *New England Journal of Medicine, 337*(11), 725–733.

Heaton, R. K., Clifford, D. B., Franklin, D. R., Woods, S. P., Ake, C., Vaida, F., et al. (2010). HIV-associated neurocognitive disorders persist in the era of potent antiretroviral therapy: CHARTER Study. *Neurology, 75*(23), 2087–2096.

Heckman, T., Miller, J., Kochman, A., Kalichman, S., Carlson, B., & Silverthorn, M. (2002). Thoughts of suicide among HIV-infected rural persons enrolled in a telephone-delivered mental health intervention. *Annals of behavioral medicine, 24*(2), 141–148.

Hogg, W., Lemetin, J., Moroz, I., Soto, E., & Russell, G. (2008). Improving prevention in primary care: Evaluating the sustainability of outreach facilitation. *Canadian Family Physician, 54*(5), 712–720.

Ickovics, J. R., Hamburger, M. E., Vlahov, D., Schoenbaum, E. E., Schuman, P., Boland, R. J., et al. (2001). Mortality, CD4 cell count decline, and depressive symptoms among HIV-seropositive women: longitudinal analysis from the HIV Epidemiology Research Study. *Journal of the American Medical Association, 285*(11), 1466–1474.

Kalichman, S., Sikkema, K., DiFonzo, K., Luke, W., & Austin, J. (2002). Emotional adjustment in survivors of sexual assault living with HIV-AIDS. *Journal of traumatic stress, 15*(4), 289–296.

Kalichman, S. C., Heckman, T., Kochman, A., Sikkema, K., & Bergholte, J. (2000). Depression and thoughts of suicide among middle-aged and older persons living with HIV-AIDS. *Psychiatric Services, 51*(7), 903–907.

Katz, S., & Nevid, J. (2005). Risk factors associated with posttraumatic stress disorder symptomatology in HIV-infected women. *AIDS patient care and STDs, 19*(2), 110–120.

Keele, B. F., Van Heuverswyn, F., Li, Y., Bailes, E., Takehisa, J., Santiago, M. L., et al. (2006). Chimpanzee reservoirs of pandemic and nonpandemic HIV-1. *Science, 313*(5786), 523–526.

Keiser, O., Spoerri, A., Brinkhof, M. W. G., Hasse, B., Gayet-Ageron, A., Tissot, F., et al. (2010). Suicide in HIV-infected individuals and the general population in Switzerland, 1988–2008. *The American Journal of Psychiatry, 167*(2), 143–150.

Kelly, J. A., Murphy, D. A., Bahr, G. R., Kalichman, S. C., Morgan, M. G., Stevenson, L. Y., et al. (1993). Outcome of cognitive-behavioral and support group brief therapies for depressed, HIV-infected persons. *American Journal of Psychiatry, 150*(11), 1679–1686.

Kizer, K. W., Green, M., Perkins, C. I., Doebbert, G., & Hughes, M. J. (1988). AIDS and suicide in California. *Journal of the American Medical Association, 260*(13), 1881.

Klinkenberg, W. D., & Sacks, S. (2004). Mental disorders and drug abuse in persons living with HIV/AIDS. *AIDS Care, 16*(Suppl 1), S22–S42.

Kuller, L. H., Tracy, R., Belloso, W., De Wit, S., Drummond, F., Lane, H. C., et al. (2008). Inflammatory and coagulation biomarkers and mortality in patients with HIV infection. *PLoS Medicine, 5*(10), e203.

Laguno, M., Blanch, J., Murillas, J., Blanco, J., Len, A., Lonca, M., et al. (2004). Depressive symptoms after initiation of interferon therapy in human immunodeficiency virus-infected patients with chronic hepatitis C. *Antiviral therapy, 9*(6), 905–909.

Lipsitz, J. D., Williams, J. B., Rabkin, J. G., Remien, R. H., Bradbury, M., el Sadr, W., et al. (1994). Psychopathology in male and female intravenous drug users with and without HIV infection. *The American Journal of Psychiatry, 151*(11), 1662–1668.

Lyketsos, C. G., Hoover, D. R., Guccione, M., Dew, M. A., Wesch, J. E., Bing, E. G., et al. (1996). Changes in depressive symptoms as AIDS develops. The Multicenter AIDS Cohort Study. *American Journal of Psychiatry, 153*(11), 1430–1437.

Lyketsos, C. G., Hoover, D. R., Guccione, M., Senterfitt, W., Dew, M. A., Wesch, J., et al. (1993). Depressive symptoms as predictors of medical outcomes in HIV infection. Multicenter AIDS Cohort Study. *Journal of the American Medical Association, 270*(21), 2563–2567.

Lyketsos, C. G., Schwartz, J., Fishman, M., & Treisman, G. (1997). AIDS mania. *Journal of Neuropsychiatry & Clinical Neuroscience, 9*(2), 277–279.

Markowitz, J. C., Klerman, G. L., Clougherty, K. F., Spielman, L. A., Jacobsberg, L. B., Fishman, B., et al. (1995). Individual psychotherapies for depressed HIV-positive patients. *American Journal of Psychiatry, 152*(10), 1504–1509.

Markowitz, J. C., Kocsis, J. H., Fishman, B., Spielman, L. A., Jacobsberg, L. B., Frances, A. J., et al. (1998). Treatment of depressive symptoms in human immunodeficiency virus-positive patients. *Archives of general psychiatry, 55*(5), 452–457.

Martinez, A., Israelski, D., Walker, C., & Koopman, C. (2002). Posttraumatic stress disorder in women attending human immunodeficiency virus outpatient clinics. *AIDS patient care and STDs, 16*(6), 283–291.

Marzuk, P. M., Tierney, H., Tardiff, K., Gross, E. M., Morgan, E. B., Hsu, M. A., et al. (1988). Increased risk of suicide in persons with AIDS. *Journal of the American Medical Association, 259*(9), 1333–1337.

Masur, H., Michelis, M. A., Greene, J. B., Onorato, I., Stouwe, R. A., Holzman, R. S., et al. (1981). An outbreak of community-acquired *Pneumocystis carinii* pneumonia: Initial manifestation of cellular immune dysfunction. *New England Journal of Medicine, 305*(24), 1431–1438.

Mayne, T. J., Vittinghoff, E., Chesney, M. A., Barrett, D. C., & Coates, T. J. (1996). Depressive affect and survival among gay and bisexual men infected with HIV. *Archives of Internal Medicine, 156*(19), 2233–2238.

McArthur, J., & Brew, B. (2010). HIV-associated neurocognitive disorders: Is there a hidden epidemic? *AIDS, 24*(9), 1367–1370.

McArthur, J. C., Hoover, D. R., Bacellar, H., Miller, E. N., Cohen, B. A., Becker, J. T., et al. (1993). Dementia in AIDS patients: incidence and risk factors. Multicenter AIDS Cohort Study. *Neurology, 43*(11), 2245–2252.

McCance-Katz, E. F., Moody, D. E., Morse, G. D., Ma, Q., DiFrancesco, R., Friedland, G., et al. (2007). Interaction between buprenorphine and atazanavir or atazanavir/ritonavir. *Drug & Alcohol Dependency, 91*(2–3), 269–278.

McKinnon, K., Cournos, F., & Herman, R. (2002). HIV among people with chronic mental illness. *Psychiatric Quarterly, 73*(1), 17–31.

Metzger, E., & Friedman, R. (1993). Prolongation of the corrected QT and *torsades de pointes* cardiac arrhythmia associated with intravenous haloperidol in the medically ill. *Journal of Clinical Psychopharmacology, 13*(2), 128–132.

Molitor, F., Ruiz, J. D., Flynn, N., Mikanda, J. N., Sun, R. K., & Anderson, R. (1999). Methamphetamine use and sexual and injection risk behaviors among out-of-treatment injection drug users. *The American journal of drug and alcohol abuse, 25*(3), 475–493.

Molitor, F., Truax, S. R., Ruiz, J. D., & Sun, R. K. (1998). Association of methamphetamine use during sex with risky sexual behaviors and HIV infection among non-injection drug users. *Western journal of medicine, 168*(2), 93–97.

Moore, R. D., Keruly, J. C., Gebo, K. A., & Lucas, G. M. (2005). An improvement in virologic response to highly active antiretroviral therapy in clinical practice from 1996 through 2002. *Journal of Acquired Immune Deficiency Syndromes, 39*(2), 195–198.

Morrison, M., Petitto, J., Ten Have, T., Gettes, D., Chiappini, M., Weber, A., et al. (2002). Depressive and anxiety disorders in women with HIV infection. *The American Journal of Psychiatry, 159*(5), 789–796.

Nightingale, S. D., Cameron, D. W., Gordin, F. M., Sullam, P. M., Cohn, D. L., Chaisson, R. E., et al. (1993). Two controlled trials of rifabutin prophylaxis against *Mycobacterium avium* complex infection in AIDS. *New England Journal of Medicine, 329*(12), 828–833.

Olley, B. O., Zeier, M. D., Seedat, S., & Stein, D. J. (2005). Post-traumatic stress disorder among recently diagnosed patients with HIV/AIDS in South Africa. *AIDS Care, 17*(5), 550–557.

Padian, N. S., McCoy, S. I., Balkus, J. E., & Wasserheit, J. N. (2010). Weighing the gold in the gold standard: challenges in HIV prevention research. *AIDS, 24*(5), 621–635.

Palacios, R., Santos, J., Ruiz, J., Gonzalez, M., & Marquez, M. (2003). Factors associated with the development of diabetes mellitus in HIV-infected patients on antiretroviral therapy: a case-control study. *AIDS, 17*(6), 933–935.

Pandori, M. W., & Branson, B. M. (2010). 2010 HIV Diagnostics Conference. *Expert Review of Anti-infective Therapy, 8*(6), 631–633.

Panlilio, A. L., Cardo, D. M., Grohskopf, L. A., Heneine, W., & Ross, C. S. (2005). Updated U.S. Public Health Service guidelines for the management of occupational exposures to HIV and recommendations for postexposure prophylaxis. *MMWR: Recommendations & Reports, 54*(RR-9), 1–17.

Park Wyllie, L., & Antoniou, T. (2003). Concurrent use of bupropion with CYP2B6 inhibitors, nelfinavir, ritonavir and efavirenz: a case series. *AIDS, 17*(4), 638–640.

Perry, K. R., Ramskill, S., Eglin, R. P., Barbara, J. A., & Parry, J. V. (2008). Improvement in the performance of HIV screening kits. *Transfusion Medicine, 18*(4), 228–240.

Perry, S., Jacobsberg, L., & Fishman, B. (1990). Suicidal ideation and HIV testing. *Journal of the American Medical Association, 263*(5), 679–682.

Power, C., Selnes, O. A., Grim, J. A., & McArthur, J. C. (1995). HIV Dementia Scale: a rapid screening test. *Journal of Acquired Immune Deficiency Syndromes & Human Retrovirology, 8*(3), 273–278.

Price, R. W., & Spudich, S. (2008). Antiretroviral therapy and central nervous system HIV type 1 infection. *Journal of Infectious Diseases, 197*(Suppl 3), S294–S306.

Rabkin, J. (2008). HIV and depression: 2008 review and update. *Current HIV/AIDS reports, 5*(4), 163–171.

Rabkin, J., McElhiney, M., & Rabkin, R. (2011). Treatment of HIV-related fatigue with armodafinil: A placebo-controlled randomized trial. *Psychosomatics, 52*(4), 328–336.

Rabkin, J., McElhiney, M., Rabkin, R., & McGrath, P. (2010). Modafinil treatment for fatigue in HIV/AIDS: a randomized placebo-controlled study. *The journal of clinical psychiatry, 71*(6), 707–715.

Rabkin, J. G., Wagner, G. J., & Rabkin, R. (1999a). Fluoxetine treatment for depression in patients with HIV and AIDS: a randomized, placebo-controlled trial. *The American Journal of Psychiatry, 156*(1), 101–107.

Rabkin, J. G., Wagner, G. J., & Rabkin, R. (1999b). Testosterone therapy for human immunodeficiency virus–positive men with and without hypogonadism. *Journal of Clinical Psychopharmacology, 19*(1), 19–27.

Rerks-Ngarm, S., Pitisuttithum, P., Nitayaphan, S., Kaewkungwal, J., Chiu, J., Paris, R., et al. (2009). Vaccination with ALVAC and AIDSVAX to prevent HIV-1 infection in Thailand. *New England Journal of Medicine, 361*(23), 2209–2220.

Robertson, K., Smurzynski, M., Parsons, T., Wu, K., Bosch, R., Wu, J., et al. (2007). The prevalence and incidence of neurocognitive impairment in the HAART era. *AIDS, 21*(14), 1915–1121.

Sacktor, N., Lyles, R. H., Skolasky, R., Kleeberger, C., Selnes, O. A., Miller, E. N., et al. (2001). HIV-associated neurologic disease incidence changes: Multicenter AIDS Cohort Study, 1990–1998. *Neurology, 56*(2), 257–260.

Schmitt, F. A., Bigley, J. W., McKinnis, R., Logue, P. E., Evans, R. W., & Drucker, J. L. (1988). Neuropsychological outcome of zidovudine (AZT) treatment of patients with AIDS and AIDS-related complex. *The New England journal of medicine, 319*(24), 1573–1578.

Schwartz, T., & Masand, P. (2002). The role of atypical antipsychotics in the treatment of delirium. *Psychosomatics, 43*(3), 171–174.

Semaan, S., Des Jarlais, D. C., Sogolow, E., Johnson, W. D., Hedges, L. V., Ramirez, G., et al. (2002). A meta-analysis of the effect of HIV prevention interventions on the sex behaviors of drug users in the United States. *JAIDS: Journal of Acquired Immune Deficiency Syndromes, 30*(Suppl 1), S73–S93.

Sewell, M. C., Goggin, K. J., Rabkin, J. G., Ferrando, S. J., McElhiney, M. C., & Evans, S. (2000). Anxiety syndromes and symptoms among men with AIDS: a longitudinal controlled study. *Psychosomatics, 41*(4), 294–300.

Shoptaw, S., Reback, C., & Freese, T. (2002). Patient characteristics, HIV serostatus, and risk behaviors among gay and bisexual males seeking treatment for methamphetamine abuse and dependence in Los Angeles. *Journal of addictive diseases, 21*(1), 91–105.

Sikkema, K., Hansen, N., Kochman, A., Tate, D., & Difranceisco, W. (2004). Outcomes from a randomized controlled trial of a group intervention for HIV positive men and women coping with AIDS-related loss and bereavement. *Death studies, 28*(3), 187–209.

Simioni, S., Cavassini, M., Annoni, J.-M., Rimbault Abraham, A., Bourquin, I., Schiffer, V., et al. (2010). Cognitive dysfunction in HIV patients despite long-standing suppression of viremia. *AIDS, 24*(9), 1243–1250.

Singh, A. N., Golledge, H., & Catalan, J. (1997). Treatment of HIV-related psychotic disorders with risperidone: a series of 21 cases. *Journal of psychosomatic research, 42*(5), 489–493.

Smith, D. K., Grohskopf, L. A., Black, R. J., Auerbach, J. D., Veronese, F., Struble, K. A., et al. (2005). Antiretroviral postexposure prophylaxis after sexual, injection-drug use, or other nonoccupational exposure to HIV in the United States: Recommendations from the U.S. Department of Health and Human Services. *MMWR: Recommendations & Reports, 54*(RR-2), 1–20.

Smith, M., Egert, J., Winkel, G., & Jacobson, J. (2002). The impact of PTSD on pain experience in persons with HIV/AIDS. *Pain, 98*(1–2), 9–17.

Straker, D., Shapiro, P., & Muskin, P. (2006). Aripiprazole in the treatment of delirium. *Psychosomatics, 47*(5), 385–391.

Sulkowski, M. S. (2008). Management of hepatic complications in HIV-infected persons. *Journal of Infectious Diseases, 197 Suppl 3*, S279–S293.

Targ, E. F., Karasic, D. H., Diefenbach, P. N., Anderson, D. A., Bystritsky, A., & Fawzy, F. I. (1994). Structured group therapy and fluoxetine to treat depression in HIV-positive persons. *Psychosomatics, 35*(2), 132–137.

Thein, H. H., Yi, Q., Dore, G. J., & Krahn, M. D. (2008). Natural history of hepatitis C virus infection in HIV-infected individuals and the impact of HIV in the era of highly active antiretroviral therapy: a meta-analysis. *AIDS, 22*(15), 1979–1991.

Thio, C. L., Seaberg, E. C., Skolasky, R., Jr., Phair, J., Visscher, B., Munoz, A., et al. (2002). HIV-1, hepatitis B virus, and risk of liver-related mortality in the Multicenter Cohort Study (MACS). *Lancet, 360*(9349), 1921–1926.

Thompson, M. A., Aberg, J. A., Cahn, P., Montaner, J. S., Rizzardini, G., Telenti, A., et al. (2010). Antiretroviral treatment of adult HIV infection: 2010 recommendations of the International AIDS

Society–USA panel. *Journal of the American Medical Association,* *304*(3), 321–333.

Tozzi, V., Balestra, P., Bellagamba, R., Corpolongo, A., Salvatori, M. F., Visco-Comandini, U., et al. (2007). Persistence of neuropsychologic deficits despite long-term highly active antiretroviral therapy in patients with HIV-related neurocognitive impairment: prevalence and risk factors. *Journal of Acquired Immune Deficiency Syndromes, 45*(2), 174–182.

Triant, V. A., Meigs, J. B., & Grinspoon, S. K. (2009). Association of C-reactive protein and HIV infection with acute myocardial infarction. *Journal of Acquired Immune Deficiency Syndromes, 51*(3), 268–273.

Turchan, J., Sacktor, N., Wojna, V., Conant, K., & Nath, A. (2003). Neuroprotective therapy for HIV dementia. *Current HIV Research, 1*(4), 373–383.

Turner, B., & Fleishman, J. (2006). Effect of dysthymia on receipt of HAART by minority HIV-infected women. *Journal of general internal medicine, 21*(12), 1235–1241.

Uldall, K. K., Harris, V. L., & Lalonde, B. (2000). Outcomes associated with delirium in acutely hospitalized acquired immune deficiency syndrome patients. *Comprehensive Psychiatry, 41*(2), 88–91.

Uldall, K. K., Ryan, R., Berghuis, J. P., & Harris, V. L. (2000). Association between delirium and death in AIDS patients. *AIDS patient care and STDs, 14*(2), 95–100.

Joint United Nations Programme on HIV/AIDS (UNAIDS), JUNPoHA (2010). *Global report: UNAIDS report on the global AIDS epidemic 2010.* New York, United Nations.

Vanable, P., McKirnan, D., Buchbinder, S., Bartholow, B., Douglas, J., Judson, F., et al. (2004). Alcohol use and high-risk sexual behavior among men who have sex with men: the effects of consumption level and partner type. *Health psychology, 23*(5), 525–532.

White, J. C., Christensen, J. F., & Singer, C. M. (1992). Methylphenidate as a treatment for depression in acquired immunodeficiency syndrome: an n-of-1 trial. *The journal of clinical psychiatry, 53*(5), 153–156.

Woody, G. E., Donnell, D., Seage, G. R., Metzger, D., Marmor, M., Koblin, B. A., et al. (1999). Non-injection substance use correlates with risky sex among men having sex with men: data from HIVNET. *Drug and alcohol dependence, 53*(3), 197–205.

64.

MEDICAL GENETICS

Kristen M. Shannon and Gayun Chan-Smutko

INTRODUCTION

Genetics and genomics are now a well-established part of mainstream medicine. The understanding of the genetic causes of disease makes it possible for individuals to undergo genetic testing that can diagnose them with a specific genetic condition. This genetic condition may exhibit symptoms in the present or future, and gives the individual information that he or she may transmit the genetic condition to her children. The psychiatric care of individuals with genetic conditions is unique, and mental health professionals are often called on to consult during the diagnostic process. In addition, mental health professionals are often necessary healthcare providers for the long-term care of individuals with genetic disease. This chapter will focus on genetic counseling and testing, and will provide the mental health professional with a framework in which to work with individuals with genetic disease.

PRINCIPLES OF GENETIC COUNSELING

GENETIC COUNSELORS

Genetic counselors are health professionals with specialized graduate degrees and experience in the areas of medical genetics and counseling. Genetic counselors work as members of a healthcare team, providing information and support to families who have members with birth defects or genetic disorders and to families who may be at risk for a variety of inherited conditions. They identify families at risk, investigate the problem present in the family, interpret information about the disorder, analyze inheritance patterns and risks of recurrence, and review available options with the family (National Society of Genetic Counselors NSGC, 1983).

Genetic counselors also provide supportive counseling to families, serve as patient advocates, and refer individuals and families to community or state support services. They serve as educators and resource people for other healthcare professionals and for the general public. Some counselors also work in administrative capacities. Many engage in research activities related to the field of medical genetics and genetic counseling (NSGC, 1983).

Genetic counselors work in both clinical and non–patient contact settings. Most genetic counselors work in a clinic or hospital setting and specialize in general genetics, prenatal care and family planning, pediatrics, oncology, cardiology, neurology, or many other areas of specialized medical care. Some genetic counselors work in related areas such as laboratories, research, education, public health settings, and corporate environments.

GENETIC COUNSELING PROCESS

Genetic counseling is the process of helping people understand and adapt to the medical, psychological, and familial implications of genetic contributions to disease (Resta, Biesecker, et al., 2006). This process integrates:

- Interpretation of family and medical histories to assess the chance of disease occurrence or recurrence
- Education about inheritance, testing, management, prevention, resources, and research
- Counseling to promote informed choices and adaptation to the risk or condition (NSGC, 2005)

The practice is specifically aimed at assessing a patient's personal and family history to determine whether there is an underlying genetic cause for the medical condition in the individual or family. Ascertaining and communicating this information helps patients and their healthcare providers better understand an individual's risk of developing specific associated diseases. This information is then used to help establish the best medical management for a patient with respect to medical surveillance and/or risk reduction (Trepanier, Ahrens, et al., 2004).

The process of genetic counseling can be divided into distinct components that include contracting, obtaining medical information, risk assessment, education, genetic testing, informed consent, and psychosocial support. These seven components are outlined in the following text.

Contracting

Contracting is the term used to describe the beginning of the genetic counseling encounter, when both the genetic counselor and counselee share their intentions for the session. Contracting provides the opportunity to communicate the expectations of what will occur during the genetic counseling appointment. Patients are sometimes unaware of what a genetic counseling session entails (Bernhardt, Biesecker, et al., 2000) and may have conflicting expectations for the visit. Contracting also provides the genetic counselor with the opportunity to describe his/her role in the genetic assessment process. Another important task accomplished by contracting is that it provides the genetic counselor the opportunity to assess the patient's baseline knowledge of genetics and comfort level with genetics information. Assessing the comfort level is particularly important, as some patients are ambivalent about pursuing genetic counseling due to underlying anxiety (Tessaro, Borstelmann, et al., 1997; McDaniel, 2005; Dorval, Bouchard, et al., 2008). It is believed that contracting may actually shorten the length of a genetic counseling session, as it can potentially prevent the "doorknob syndrome." The phenomenon of "doorknob syndrome" is common and occurs when patients are not given the opportunity to share their thoughts and concerns with providers and choose to do so only near the end of the session, as the provider's hand is "on the doorknob" to leave (Jackson, 2005). The process of contracting allows for the organization of a session that best meets the patient's needs, while allowing the genetic counselor to be most efficient.

The Personal and Medical Family History

After the brief contracting, the genetics professional will most often begin the assessment with gathering a detailed personal medical and family medical history. Typically, a detailed three-generation family history is constructed in the form of a pedigree (Bennett, Steinhaus, et al., 1995; Bennett, French, et al., 2008).

When taking the family history, it is important to document each individual's age or age at death as well as his/her personal medical history. Depending on the disease suspected in the individual/family, the information requested on the relatives will be tailored. For example, if hereditary breast and ovarian cancer syndrome (HBOCS) is suspected, the genetic counselor will ask about cancer diagnoses in the family as well as determine if the women in the family have their ovaries intact, as this affects risk assessment (prophylactic bilateral salpingo-oophorectomy has been shown to reduce the risk of developing breast cancer in HBOCS patients [Rebbeck, Levin, et al., 1999; Olopade & Artioli, 2004]).

Patients may feel anxious during this information gathering portion of the session because their level of knowledge about their own diagnosis as well as other family members' diagnoses may not be high. For example, many patients with a diagnosis of cancer will not be aware of the specific pathology or histology of their tumor, and in some cases, confirming the diagnosis with medical records is essential (Trepanier, Ahrens, et al., 2004). Many factors can influence an individual's knowledge of the family history (Schneider, 2002). Information on relatives may not be available because of estrangement, adoption, or simply because the patient has lost contact with his or her family members. The information provided can be incorrect because the patient is mistaken or confused about the diagnosis. A recent study of the accuracy

of family history in a cancer genetic counseling practice, for example, indicates that individuals are often confident that a family member has had cancer, but are typically unsure of the details surrounding that diagnosis (Jefferies, Goldgar, et al., 2008; Reid, Walter, et al., 2009). Reports of breast cancer tend to be accurate, while reports of ovarian cancer are less trustworthy (Murff, Spigel, et al., 2004; Chang, Smedby, et al., 2006). It is also important to note that family histories can change over time, with new diagnoses arising in family members as time passes. All of these factors must be considered during the consultation, as the risk assessment and differential diagnosis are based primarily on this information.

Risk Assessment

Risk assessment is an important part of the genetic counseling encounter. The genetic counselor will use his/her expertise and experience to determine the likelihood that an individual has a genetic disease. Many guidelines exist that can assist the genetic counselor in determining this likelihood.

The patient's reaction to the genetic counselor's risk assessment can vary greatly, depending on their personal and family history as well as their underlying emotional well-being (Schneider, 2002). If an individual is confronted with a potential diagnosis of genetic disease, he or she may feel validated that their concerns regarding their personal and family history are real. Others who have lived in denial may react with disbelief, anger, and fear. The individual's experience with disease in the family will also be a factor in their reaction. Those who have lost many family members to a specific medical condition are more likely to be anxious, while those whose family members have survived the medical condition may be less worried about the mortality associated with the disease.

There are times when a genetic counselor feels that an individual's personal and family history is not consistent with a genetic diagnosis. In these instances, the patient can react in a variety of ways. Patients can react with relief, surprise, and sometimes anger (Schneider, 2002). The genetic counselor will address these emotions, and typically, through the education process, these emotions will subside in the patient.

Education About Genes and Genetic Disease

The education portion of the genetic counseling session includes the provision of information about the role of genes in genetic conditions and their inheritance patterns, possible results of genetic testing, risk reduction options, and the benefits, risks, and limitations of genetic testing. The role of the genetic counselor in this component of the session is to effectively communicate scientific information to meet the patient's level of understanding (Bennett, Hampel, et al., 2003). As patients have diverse learning styles, it is important to be able to communicate the same information in different ways to accommodate a patient's specific learning method. The education portion is typically the longest portion of a genetic counseling session.

Most genetic diseases are due to mutations in Mendelian genes. Genetic disorders are inherited in autosomal dominant, autosomal recessive, and sex-linked manners. It is not imperative that a patient understand the differences in the types of genes that give rise to genetic disease; however, the manner in which these genes are inherited in families is essential to understanding the familial implications of genetic testing. Autosomal dominant disorders result in a 50% risk to siblings and offspring. Autosomal recessive disorders typically result in a 25% risk to siblings and varying risks to offspring as they are dependent on the genetic status of the individual's partner. Sex-linked diseases are only passed to specific genders. It is important to note that many genetic diseases are a result of a *de novo* mutation in an individual. If a disease is truly *de novo* in nature, the risks in the relatives are limited to offspring.

The education portion of the genetic counseling encounter extends into a thorough discussion of the disease that is suspected in the family. This will include a discussion of the risks of clinical symptoms associated with the disease as well as symptom screening and prevention options. Risk reduction options for individuals—including surgery, medications, avoidance of specific foods, habits, exposures—are often discussed. Typically, the genetic counselor's role is to introduce these concepts, allowing a detailed discussion to be provided by physician specialists (geneticists, surgeons, oncologists, gastroenterologists, etc.).

Education About Genetic Testing

Finally, the education process will often include a detailed discussion of genetic testing that lays the foundation for informed consent. Genetic testing is often not straightforward. When performing germline genetic testing, there are four possible test results.

Mutation detected (i.e., "Positive"): The individual is diagnosed with a genetic disease. The individual can pass this gene mutation on to his or her children.

No mutation detected, and a gene mutation has previously been found in another family member (i.e., "True Negative"): The individual does not have the genetic disease known to be in the family. In addition, the individual cannot pass it on to his or her children.

No mutation detected, and a mutation has *not* been found in another family member (i.e., "Inconclusive Negative"): The test has provided little new information about the underlying etiology of the individual's symptoms. He or she may still have a genetic disease because:

— The individual may still have a mutation in the gene being tested, but it was not detectable with testing technology that was used, or
— The individual may have a gene mutation in another gene that was not analyzed in the test.

A mutation is found, but its meaning is unknown (i.e., it is a variant of uncertain significance [VUS]): This is considered an inconclusive result and is typically a missense mutation in a gene. In this case, there are insufficient data to classify whether the variant is deleterious to gene function or is a benign polymorphism that has no bearing on gene function. A VUS result should not be used to guide medical management, and clinicians should defer to the family history to determine the best management protocol for the patient and their family.

A thorough discussion of the benefits, risks, and limitations to genetic testing is essential to the informed-consent process. Benefits include relieving uncertainty associated with having a set of medical symptoms in the family history, as well as providing additional information in assessing the patient's personal risk of developing a specific medical symptom. This information may help the individual and healthcare providers determine the best plan for medical management with regard to early detection, risk reduction, or prevention of disease. Another benefit of genetic testing is that results may give other family members information about their chance of having inherited a mutation and chance of developing certain symptoms. Finally, if an individual learns that he or she is a true negative, it means there is no increased risk of developing certain symptoms due to their family history. Their risk of developing certain symptoms is that of the general population.

Risks associated with the genetic testing process include increased stress, anxiety, and depression. Sharing information about a positive genetic diagnosis may affect relationships with family members. This information may be upsetting to family members and strain relationships. There is a possibility of learning sensitive information about the family. For instance, if more than one family member is tested, there is a chance of learning about misattributed paternity of a child, or an unknown adoption. It is possible that testing will reveal a variant of uncertain significance, which can be disconcerting to patients as it is unknown if this variant is associated with disease. Feelings of guilt, distress and uncertainty are discussed further in the later section, "Genetic Testing over the Lifespan."

One common question that is encountered during the genetic counseling consultation is regarding negative use of genetic information. Genetic discrimination occurs when a genetic test result is used as a preexisting condition by insurance providers and employers. This is less of an issue for patients who already have a medical diagnosis (i.e., are already exhibiting symptoms of the genetic disease). However, those who are currently not exhibiting symptoms of disease should know that most are protected by law with respect to discrimination by their health insurance company or employer. However, no legislation exists to protect individuals from life insurance or disability insurance companies' use of this information.

The limitations of genetic testing must be explored with patients, as the uncertainties underlying any result (positive, uninformative negative, etc.) are often unsatisfying and difficult for patients to grasp. Test results provide risk information, but they cannot predict if an individual will actually develop a specific clinical manifestation of the disease. If an individual is a true negative for a known familial mutation, it does not mean that they will never develop a symptom associated with the disease. For example, if an individual tests negative for a known mutation in the gene responsible for familial hyper-cholesterolemia, it is possible that the individual might still develop high cholesterol.

Psychosocial Assessment and Support

The psychosocial implications of genetic testing for patients and their families can be substantial. Psychosocial assessment should be provided throughout the entire genetic counseling and testing process.

INITIAL SUPPORT

During the genetic counseling session, the genetics professional should help the patient understand the information regarding their disease and the genetic cause of it. In addition, the psychosocial impact of the disease must be addressed. Living with a genetic disease or as a member of a family with a genetic disease can be very challenging psychologically. Often, individuals with genetic disorders require frequent medical visits and a battery of medical tests. Some individuals with genetic disorders are afforded the ability to participate in dedicated follow-up clinics that are specialized for their individual disease and symptoms. Many of these specialized programs are located in larger academic medical centers, and some also include psychological care of the patients. However, many individuals with a genetic disease are managed by a menagerie of healthcare providers, and their psychological care is often neglected.

When genetic testing is available and offered, the genetic counselor must support the patient's decision to proceed or not proceed with the genetic testing. Although there have been no studies that formally address whether genetic counseling leads to genetic testing decisions that are consistent with patient preferences (Braithwaite, Emery, et al., 2004), the role of the healthcare professional is to provide emotional support and empathy. Patient-perceived provider empathy has been shown to increase patient satisfaction and compliance by way of the mediating factors of information exchange, perceived expertise, interpersonal trust, and partnership (Kim, Kaplowitz, et al., 2004). In order for the full benefit of genetic testing to be realized, patients must ultimately be compliant with the recommendations for treatment, screening, and prevention of clinical symptoms.

It is important that the patient's support system be identified and addressed. If the patient is considering genetic testing, identifying this support system prior to the genetic test initiation is essential, as waiting for genetic test results can require emotional support. It is also important for the genetic counselor to gather more information about family dynamics. Whether an individual wants it to be or not, genetic testing is a family affair, and there are family issues that will be brought forth. It is important to determine if a patient will be comfortable doing this; and if not, to provide guidance and support. Identifying individuals with insufficient sources of support and addressing family communication concerning genetic disease may help the patient adjust better to genetic testing (van Oostrom, Meijers-Heijboer, et al., 2007a).

When genetic testing is performed, it is important to consider the anticipation of test results. Waiting for test results can be stressful for some patients. It is important to offer a reliable estimate of when the results will be available, as anxiety tends to heighten around the end of this timeline.

ONGOING SUPPORT

It is important to recognize that living with a genetic disease is a lifelong process. The psychosocial impact of living with disease is likely to change over time—and throughout the lifespan. Individuals, for example, with a predisposition to adult-onset conditions will probably change their psychological assessment of living with the disease as they age. Individuals with genetic disease also will have to face sometimes-difficult decisions during their reproductive years. It is imperative that the psychological well-being of these patients be addressed over their lifespan.

When genetic testing is performed, it is noted that most individuals cope well with the results of genetic testing, but that some will require additional support after the test results are given. Studies have indicated that there are factors, such as high anxiety at time of blood draw for genetic testing, that predict who will be distressed six months after receiving a test result (Dorval, Patenaude, et al., 2000; van Oostrom, Meijers-Heijboer, et al., 2007b). Healthcare providers should be aware of these factors and identify the individuals who will need additional support, so as to maximize opportunities for prevention, early detection, and healthy coping (Vadaparampil, Miree, et al., 2006). Support groups for people found to have cancer-predisposition gene mutations can be helpful, and some have suggested that such support groups should be a priority (Di Prospero, Seminsky, et al., 2001).

GENETIC TESTING OVER THE LIFESPAN

Over the last several decades, genetic testing has evolved to touch many areas of medicine. In the late 1950s, medical geneticists used chromosome analysis techniques to support what was still largely a phenotype-based diagnosis for syndromes such as Down syndrome. Genetic testing, which began as primarily a diagnostic tool, now includes carrier screening for recessive diseases like cystic fibrosis, newborn screening for diseases like phenylketonuria, and presymptomatic testing for diseases like hereditary breast or ovarian cancer syndrome. Clinical genetic testing is now available for over 2,500 diseases (Gene Tests, 2011), many of which are single-gene, Mendelian inherited disorders (Table 64.1).

Genetic testing now encompasses other diseases that are not classically defined as "genetic" disorders. Tissue samples such as malignant tumor specimens routinely undergo genetic testing for non-hereditary genetic markers that create a genetic profile of the tumor to guide diagnosis and treatment. With the varied ways that DNA analysis has become integrated in nearly all areas of medicine, the medical patient is likely to experience genetic counseling or encounter complex genetic information at some point in their lifetime, whether it

Table 64.1 DEFINITIONS OF DIFFERENT TYPES OF GENETIC TESTS.

GENETIC TEST	PURPOSE	EXAMPLES
Diagnostic	Genetic testing reveals underlying cause for a particular phenotype	Down syndrome (Trisomy 21)
Carrier screening	Testing to reveal carrier status of a recessive trait	Cystic fibrosis, Tay-Sachs disease
Newborn screening	Testing in newborns for diseases for whom early treatment can reduce severity of phenotype	Phenylketonuria
Presymptomatic	Testing in healthy individuals for disease that may present later in life	Huntington's disease, hereditary breast and ovarian cancer syndrome

is in regard to their own health or to that of a family member (frequently both).

GRAPPLING WITH A NEW DIAGNOSIS

A new diagnosis of a genetic condition can be a very isolating experience for the medical patient. This can be due to the rarity of the condition and therefore unfamiliarity on the part of the patient, their family, their friends, and very often their healthcare providers. A couple with a child diagnosed with Down syndrome, for example, can gain access to a strong and diverse social network on which to rely for information and advice on special-needs services for their child from birth into adulthood (Down Syndrome Congress, 2012). In contrast, parents of a child diagnosed with Pena-Shokeir syndrome may have fewer disease-specific information resources readily available.

LIFELONG IMPLICATIONS

Many patients diagnosed with a genetic disorder are faced with a myriad of struggles for both themselves and their family members throughout the course of their life. Take, for example, a 24-year-old single woman with a new diagnosis of von Hippel-Lindau (VHL) disease. VHL affects 1 in 36,000 live births and is inherited in an autosomal dominant manner, in that each person with VHL has a 50% chance of passing the condition to each offspring. Approximately 20% of individuals represent *de novo* cases, where there are no family members affected with the disease (Maher, Iselius, et al., 1991). It is a multisystem disorder associated with an increased risk for developing specific tumors, including hemangioblastomas of the brain, spine, and retina; renal cell carcinoma; pheochromocytoma; pancreatic neuroendocrine tumors; and other lesions. An individual with VHL requires close monitoring for signs and symptoms of the disease, and the probability of developing at least one component tumor is 100%. Monitoring for retinal lesions and pheochromocytoma begins in childhood and continues into adulthood with additional imaging of the brain, spine, and abdomen added to the surveillance protocol during adolescence.

This 24-year-old single woman with no children receives a new diagnosis of VHL based on the detection of a hemangioblastoma of the cerebellum and bilateral renal cell carcinoma. She faces the struggles of understanding and coping with the medical implications of the diagnosis, including treatment and lifelong surveillance. After genetic testing confirms that she carries a deleterious mutation in the *VHL* gene, she must grapple with the genetic implications of the diagnosis. She weighs the implications of sharing the information with her at-risk family members (parents, siblings, etc.): How will the family react? Will they reject her or accept her? Will she have to deal with a parent's guilt if one parent carries the mutation as well? With they reject or accept the information and its implications for them?

The young woman with VHL has the hopes and dreams of one day entering a lifelong relationship with a partner and starting a family. As in any relationship, disclosing private matters is par for the course, but a medical condition such as VHL means that she has the potential to become ill, placing an emotional and financial burden on a marriage. She must ponder the questions of when to disclose, how to disclose, and what to disclose. The desire to have or not to have children is a common discussion in any relationship, but when a transmissible genetic condition is involved, she faces the added dilemma of whether or not to embark on genetic testing of a future pregnancy prior to birth (Klitzman & Sweeney, 2010).

TIMING OF GENETIC TESTING

Genetic testing for genetic disease can be done as early as pre-conception (i.e., in developing embryos) or at any other point in the lifetime. In some cases, informative genetic testing can be done post-mortem on a tissue sample.

Preimplantation Genetic Diagnosis

One recent development in medical genetics, known as *preimplantation genetic diagnosis* (PGD), is diagnostic testing of fertilized embryos prior to conception (Adiga, Kalthur, et al., 2010). A couple must first undergo *in vitro* fertilization (IVF); then developing embryos are tested for genetic conditions such as chromosome aneuploidy, chromosome rearrangement, or single-gene (Mendelian) disorders such as cystic fibrosis or Tay-Sachs disease. Embryo biopsy consists of sampling one cell from a blastocyst without compromising or damaging the embryo. Couples can select embryos unaffected for the genetic condition for transfer to the woman's uterus, optimizing the chances of an unaffected pregnancy.

Prenatal Genetic Diagnosis

Diagnostic testing of a fetus can be achieved through various techniques. Amniocentesis can be performed at 14–16 weeks' gestation, and for many pregnancies, testing can be performed earlier, at 10–12 weeks' gestation, through chorionic villus sampling (CVS). Couples may wish to know the genetic status of the fetus in order to make special preparations for the birth and antenatal period. This type of couple may also feel they need the information to emotionally prepare themselves for caring for a child with special needs or medical needs. Other couples may choose to know the genetic status with the option of potentially terminating an affected pregnancy.

Genetic Testing in Minors

As mentioned in the example of VHL, medical surveillance beginning in early childhood and very often beginning within the first year of life is recommended for genetic conditions in which signs or symptoms present at an early age. When the genetic condition is known, as in the prior example of the young woman with VHL disease, genetic testing provides a clear-cut answer as to whether her child is affected or not. An unaffected child is spared unnecessary screening; an affected child must begin annual retinal exams within the first year of life, with additional imaging exams of the abdomen and brain around the onset of puberty. Although the genetic test is clear, it has no predictive power. A parent of a child with VHL can be certain that their child will develop at least one tumor in their lifetime. At the same time, the parent must cope with the uncertainty of not knowing what type of tumor could present itself, when it would happen, and what the consequences might be. Inherent to most genetic conditions such as VHL is the observation of variable expressivity, where a condition has a spectrum of severity and even each person within the same family (and therefore carrying the same causative mutation) has different manifestations of the disease. The uncertainty can be overwhelming for both the affected parent and the unaffected parent, and can be difficult in different ways as well.

Also at issue with the testing of minors is the age at which the parents decide to pursue testing for their children. Parents can be guided by their healthcare providers as to the best age range by which a positive test result will begin to impact medical management. Parents can include the child on the decision to test or to wait, depending on the age of the child and their emotional maturity. This can help maintain trust between the child and parent and ease the way towards understanding the test result, whether it is positive or negative. Not including a child in the decision to undergo genetic testing is also the parents' prerogative. The healthcare provider or genetic counselor working with the family should help the parents consider when and how they would disclose the results to their child in an age-appropriate way. However, consider a teenaged minor who is intellectually capable of giving assent for genetic testing. The process of establishing assent involves the healthcare professional, who, together with the parents, provides age-appropriate information about the genetic disease, what

is involved in carrying out the test, and how results will be disclosed. Parents may wish to test their teenaged minor without his or her knowledge primarily because they are hoping for a "good news" scenario where the child will test negative for the condition and the child can be worry-free. When parents ask a healthcare professional to test their teenaged child without the child's knowledge, the provider should help parents anticipate that they may be putting their child's trust in them (and the medical community) at risk, particularly if the test results in a positive diagnosis.

Presymptomatic Genetic Testing and Carrier Screening

An individual's genetic diagnosis weighs heavily on decision-making for offspring and future offspring and affects other family members as well. Consider the case of a recessive genetic condition such as cystic fibrosis. This necessitates that both parents of an affected child are carriers of a mutation in the *CFTR* gene, which means each of their siblings could be a carrier and should be offered testing. However, unless the sibling's spouse also is a carrier, any risk to the sibling's offspring is negligible. Contrast this with an autosomal dominant condition with onset in adulthood such as Lynch syndrome. The siblings of an affected individual (and parents) are considered at risk. Any at-risk relative must weigh the implications of *presymptomatic genetic testing*, where a person undergoes genetic testing without signs or symptoms of the disease.

The role of a genetic counselor is to help an unaffected patient understand the disease and understand the medical implications of a positive result that establishes the diagnosis, or a negative result that rules the condition out completely. A genetic counselor can also become a sounding board for patients grappling with the decision of whether to know or not know their genetic status.

Qualitative studies in patients undergoing presymptomatic genetic testing for Huntington's disease and autosomal dominant amyotrophic lateral sclerosis, both adult-onset neurodegenerative conditions, have reported that patients undergo mixed reactions to a negative result, feeling both joy and relief for themselves and their offspring but in some cases also a form of "survivor guilt" over being spared, unlike their affected sibling or parent (Fanos, Gronka, et al., 2011; Williams, Schutte, et al., 2000). These patients have seen generations of family members decline as a result of the disease and knew they could eventually develop symptoms and suffer a shortened lifespan like their affected relatives. A negative result brings a new sense of hope and optimism, and patients find themselves redefining their sense of self, and their place within their family and within society as a whole (Williams, Schutte, et al., 2000).

Similarly, patients testing positive through predictive testing will experience a mix of emotions. Although it may be initially devastating to receive the news, some patients experience a sense of relief at finally knowing they are positive and that they do not have to go on questioning "Do I have the condition? Am I starting to develop symptoms?" Increased anxiety and depression has been reported in some conditions such as Huntington's disease, while some studies of patients undergoing testing for neuromuscular diseases and hereditary ataxias have not demonstrated an increase in depression (Smith, Lipe, et al., 2004; Graceffa, Russo, et al., 2009). It should be noted that studies of this nature involve a very small sample size and limited follow-up period and therefore cannot be generalized across different diseases or populations. Offering long-term psychological support is warranted for all patients seeking presymptomatic testing.

SUMMARY

For many patients, their first and only encounter with a genetic counselor is in the setting of prenatal diagnosis, and most of these pregnancies result in healthy babies without a genetic condition. But for the individual who is diagnosed with a genetic disease, the psychosocial and medical implications evolve over time. Patients with chronic genetic conditions have reported a need for more psychosocial support in coping with the day-to-day challenges that comes with a physical disability. A genetic diagnosis affects a patient's interactions with her family members and with her peers in terms of friendship, dating, and marriage. It affects his or her reproductive choices and can influence other major milestones such as pursuing an education or choosing a career. In conditions with shortened life-expectancy, a patient is faced with planning for illness, physical disability, or mental incapacitation at a much younger age than normal. As the patients of the twenty-first century are presented with more genetic information, clinicians need to consider the evolving psychosocial needs that come with that knowledge and refer to specialty services such as genetic counseling for clarification and psychotherapy if that would help the patient cope emotionally with the implications of the knowledge and the effect on the family.

CLINICAL PEARLS

- Genetic counselors identify families at risk, investigate the problem present in the family, interpret information about the disorder, analyze inheritance patterns and risks of recurrence, and review available options with the family (NSGC, 1983).

- This counseling can be divided into distinct components that include contracting, obtaining medical information, risk assessment, education, genetic testing, informed consent, and psychosocial support.

- When taking the family history, it is important to document each individual's age or age at death as well as his/her personal medical history.

- Reports of breast cancer tend to be accurate, while reports of ovarian cancer are less trustworthy (Murff, Spigel, et al., 2004; Chang, Smedby, et al., 2006).

- Family histories can change over time, with new diagnoses arising in family members as time passes.

- Risk assessment here means "What is the likelihood that a patient has a genetic disease?"

- The counselor educates about the implications: Autosomal dominant disorders typically result in a 50% risk to siblings and offspring. Autosomal recessive disorders typically result in a 25% risk to siblings and varying risks to offspring, as they are dependent on the genetic status of the individual's partner. Sex-linked diseases are only passed to specific genders.

- If a disease is truly *de novo* in nature, the risks in the relatives are limited to offspring.

- If an individual learns that he/she is a true negative, it means there is no increased risk of developing specific symptoms due to their family history. Their risk of developing specific symptoms is that of the general population.

- If more than one family member is tested, there is a chance of learning about misattributed paternity or a hitherto unknown adoption.

- Those who are currently not exhibiting symptoms of disease should know that most are protected by law with respect to genetic discrimination by their health insurance company or employer. However, no legislation exists to protect individuals from use of this genetic information by life insurance or disability insurance companies.

- Identifying the patient's support system prior to the genetic test initiation is essential.

- Information about family dynamics will be important to helping the patient cope with the implications of genetic counseling and testing.

- The psychosocial impact of living with a genetic condition will change over time—and throughout the lifespan.

- The patient weighs the implications of sharing the information with his or her at-risk family members (parents, siblings, etc.) and the implications for having children.

- The age at which a positive test result will begin to affect medical management serves as a guide for parents to judge when to pursue testing for their children.

- One recent development in medical genetics known as preimplantation genetic diagnosis (PGD) is diagnostic testing of fertilized embryos prior to conception (Adiga, Kalthur, et al., 2010) to identify those who carry a genetic risk.

- When parents ask a healthcare professional to test their teenaged child without the child's knowledge, the provider should help parents anticipate that they may be risking their child's trust in them (and in the medical community), particularly if the test results in a positive diagnosis.

DISCLOSURE STATEMENTS

Ms. Shannon: No disclosures

Ms. Chan-Smutko: No disclosures

ACKNOWLEDGMENTS

The authors would like to thank Devanshi Patel, MS, CGC, for her participation in preparation of this chapter.

REFERENCES

GeneTests Medical Genetics Information Resource (database online). Copyright, University of Washington, Seattle. 1993–2013. Available at http://www.genetests.org. Accessed October 2011.

National Down Syndrome Congress website. Copyright, National Down Syndrome Congress. 2012. Available at http://www.ndsccenter.org/. Accessed October 2012.

Adiga, S. K., Kalthur, G., et al. (2010). Preimplantation diagnosis of genetic diseases. *Journal of Postgraduate Medicine, 56*(4), 317–320.

Bennett, R. L., French, K. S., et al. (2008). Standardized human pedigree nomenclature: Update and assessment of the recommendations of the National Society of Genetic Counselors. *Journal of Genetic Counseling, 17*(5), 424–433.

Bennett, R. L., Hampel, H. L., et al. (2003). Genetic counselors: Translating genomic science into clinical practice. *Journal of Clinical Investigation, 112*(9), 1274–1279.

Bennett, R. L., Steinhaus, K. A., et al. (1995). Recommendations for standardized human pedigree nomenclature. Pedigree Standardization Task Force of the National Society of Genetic Counselors. *American Journal of Human Genetics, 56*(3), 745–752.

Bernhardt, B. A., Biesecker, B. B., et al. (2000). Goals, benefits, and outcomes of genetic counseling: Client and genetic counselor assessment. *American Journal of Medical Genetics, 94*(3), 189–197.

Braithwaite, D., Emery, J., et al. (2004). Psychological impact of genetic counseling for familial cancer: A systematic review and meta-analysis. *Journal of the National Cancer Institute, 96*(2), 122–133.

Chang, E. T., Smedby, K. E., et al. (2006). Reliability of self-reported family history of cancer in a large case-control study of lymphoma. *Journal of the National Cancer Institute, 98*(1), 61–68.

Di Prospero, L. S., Seminsky, M., et al. (2001). Psychosocial issues following a positive result of genetic testing for *BRCA1* and *BRCA2* mutations: findings from a focus group and a needs-assessment survey. *Canadian Medical Association Journal, 164*(7), 1005–1009.

Dorval, M., Bouchard, K., et al. (2008). Health behaviors and psychological distress in women initiating *BRCA1/2* genetic testing: comparison with control population. *Journal of Genetic Counseling, 17*(4), 314–326.

Dorval, M., Patenaude, A. F., et al. (2000). Anticipated versus actual emotional reactions to disclosure of results of genetic tests for cancer susceptibility: findings from p53 and *BRCA1* testing programs. *Journal of Clinical Oncology, 18*(10), 2135–2142.

Fanos, J. H., Gronka, S., et al. (2011). Impact of presymptomatic genetic testing for familial amyotrophic lateral sclerosis. *Genetic Medicine, 13*(4), 342–348.

Graceffa, A., Russo, M., et al. (2009). Psychosocial impact of presymptomatic genetic testing for transthyretin amyloidotic polyneuropathy. *Neuromuscular Disorders, 19*(1), 44–48.

Jackson, G. (2005). "Oh…by the way…": Doorknob syndrome. *International Journal of Clinical Practice, 59*(8), 869.

Jefferies, S., Goldgar, D., et al. (2008). The accuracy of cancer diagnoses as reported in families with head and neck cancer: a case-control study. *Clinical Oncology (Royal College of Radiology), 20*(4), 309–314.

Kim, S. S., Kaplowitz, S., et al. (2004). The effects of physician empathy on patient satisfaction and compliance. *Evaluation & the Health Professions, 27*(3), 237–251.

Klitzman, R. L., & Sweeney, M. M. (2010) "In sickness and in health"? Disclosures of genetic risks in dating. *Journal of Genetic Counseling, 20*(1), 98–112.

Maher, E. R., Iselius, L., et al. (1991). Von Hippel-Lindau disease: a genetic study. *Journal of Medical Genetics, 28*(7), 443–447.

McDaniel, S. H. (2005). The psychotherapy of genetics. *Family Process, 44*(1), 25–44.

Murff, H. J., Spigel, D. R., et al. (2004). Does this patient have a family history of cancer? An evidence-based analysis of the accuracy of family cancer history. *Journal of the American Medical Association, 292*(12), 1480–1489.

National Society of Genetic Counselors (NSGC) (1983). From http://www.nsgc.org/About/FAQsaboutGeneticCounselorsandtheNSGC/tabid/143/Default.aspx.

National Society of Genetic Counselors (NSGC) (2005). From http://www.nsgc.org/About/FAQsDefinitions/tabid/97/Default.aspx.

Olopade, O. I., & Artioli, G. (2004). Efficacy of risk-reducing salpingo-oophorectomy in women with *BRCA-1* and *BRCA-2* mutations. *Breast Journal, 10*(Suppl 1), S5–S9.

Rebbeck, T. R., Levin, A. M., et al. (1999). Breast cancer risk after bilateral prophylactic oophorectomy in *BRCA1* mutation carriers. *Journal of the National Cancer Institute, 91*(17), 1475–1479.

Reid, G. T., Walter, F. M., et al. (2009). Family history questionnaires designed for clinical use: a systematic review. *Public Health Genomics, 12*(2), 73–83.

Resta, R., Biesecker, B. B., et al. (2006). A new definition of genetic counseling: National Society of Genetic Counselors' Task Force report. *Journal of Genetic Counseling, 15*(2), 77–83.

Schneider, K. A. (2002). *Counseling about cancer: strategies for genetic counseling.* New York: Wiley-Liss.

Smith, C. O., Lipe, H. P., et al. (2004). Impact of presymptomatic genetic testing for hereditary ataxia and neuromuscular disorders. *Archives of Neurology, 61*(6), 875–880.

Tessaro, I., Borstelmann, N., et al. (1997). Genetic testing for susceptibility to breast cancer: findings from women's focus groups. *Journal of Women's Health, 6*(3), 317–327.

Trepanier, A., Ahrens, M., et al. (2004). Genetic cancer risk assessment and counseling: recommendations of the National Society of Genetic Counselors. *Journal of Genetic Counseling, 13*(2), 83–114.

Vadaparampil, S. T., Miree, C. A., et al. (2006). Psychosocial and behavioral impact of genetic counseling and testing. *Breast Disease, 27*, 97–108.

van Oostrom, I., Meijers-Heijboer, H., et al. (2007a). Family system characteristics and psychological adjustment to cancer susceptibility genetic testing: a prospective study. *Clinical Genetics, 71*(1), 35–42.

van Oostrom, I., Meijers-Heijboer, H., et al. (2007b). Prognostic factors for hereditary cancer distress six months after *BRCA1/2* or *HNPCC* genetic susceptibility testing. *European Journal of Cancer, 43*(1), 71–77.

Williams, J. K., Schutte, D. L., et al. (2000). Redefinition: coping with normal results from predictive gene testing for neurodegenerative disorders. *Research in Nursing & Health, 23*(4), 260–269.

PART VII

WOMEN'S HEALTH

65.

GYNECOLOGICAL SURGERY, PELVIC PAIN, AND OTHER RELEVANT ISSUES

Gail Erlick Robinson and Diane de Camps Meschino

INTRODUCTION

Obstetricians and gynecologists have a complex task. They must deal with the fear, anxiety, and depression that may accompany any physical illness. In addition, issues that involve a woman's reproductive health are highly emotionally charged and closely linked to her sense of femininity, sexuality, attractiveness, and value. The gynecologist often acts as the woman's primary care provider and, therefore, may be the only one in a position to detect ongoing concerns such as relationship problems, domestic violence, sexual dysfunctions, or histories of abuse. Psychological conflicts related to femininity, sexuality, or abuse may present as aversion to physical examination, pelvic pain, or attitudes toward pregnancy or sexuality. Healthcare professionals involved with patients undergoing gynecological surgery must recognize that patients are dealing not only with the reason for the surgery, but also with the specific meanings of surgery on female sexual and reproductive organs.

GYNECOLOGICAL SURGERY

HYSTERECTOMY

Total hysterectomy refers to the removal of the entire uterus, including the cervix; while *subtotal hysterectomy* leaves the cervix in place. This operation may or may not be accompanied by a bilateral salpingo-oophorectomy, which includes removal of the ovaries. Gynecologists disagree about the added benefits of removing healthy ovaries at the time of hysterectomy. Some argue that this reduces the risk of subsequent ovarian cancer, while others feel that the risk in most women is too low to warrant this additional surgery. Indications for hysterectomy range from abnormal or excessive bleeding and pain, to cancer of the uterus. A decline in hysterectomy rates since 1970 may be related to a number of factors, including alternatives to hysterectomy such as endometrial ablation, as well as an increased understanding on the part of physicians that women do not necessarily view their uterus as a useless organ just because they have passed the childbearing stage.

Hysterectomy may be performed abdominally, vaginally, or via laparoscopy. The latter procedure takes longer, but results in shorter inpatient stays. A six-month follow-up of women who underwent these two different types of procedures showed an overall improvement in psychological well-being, with no significant differences in scores between the two groups (Thakar et al., 2004; Persson, Wijma, Hammar, & Kjolhede, 2006).

Although it was previously thought that post-hysterectomy depression was a common phenomenon, more recent studies have found no evidence that hysterectomy causes depression (Baldaro et al., 2003; Lambden et al., 1997); indeed, Yen et al. (2008) reported an improvement in depressive symptoms, anxiety symptoms, body image, and subjective gynecological symptoms. Women with a history of multiple surgeries and those with chronic pelvic pain are a high-risk group for post-surgical distress. Psychological reactions to hysterectomy vary with the reason for the operation, the type of procedure, the woman's previous medical history, her age, her understanding of the consequences, her past psychiatric history, and her current supports and relationships (Cooper, Mishra, Hardy, & Kuh, 2009). Women who had undergone hysterectomy before age 40 had significantly higher anxiety and depressive scores at age 53 than women who had not undergone the procedure. Women who had undergone hysterectomy for cancer also had significantly higher scores. Women may feel fearful of hysterectomy because of myths they believe about the procedure.

In some women, removal of the ovaries may raise issues about loss of femininity, fears of aging, and concerns about the symptoms of menopause or the safety of hormone replacement treatment. However, research has found that women whose ovaries are removed do not, as a group, have more psychological distress than women with ovary-sparing operations. Women who are younger at the time of the hysterectomy may be at increased risk for psychological distress if they have not started or finished their childbearing. For some women, even though they never wanted or no longer wish to have children, the idea of ending their childbearing potential represents a loss of femininity and can cause psychiatric distress. Others may fear the loss of the familiar menstrual periods, which they may feel cleanse the body.

Women and their partners may mistakenly believe that after hysterectomy they will have no interest in or ability to have sexual activity, or that there will be a decrease in their sexual attractiveness (Flory, Bissonnette, & Binik, 2005). There are many possible physical explanations for post-hysterectomy sexual problems, including: disturbed vaginal blood flow; changes in nerve supply, or loss of the cervix and its mucus-producing glands, leading to decreased vaginal lubrication; reduction of sensitive tissue from the upper vagina; or the loss of uterine contractions. However, reduction in preoperative pain or bleeding may result in improved postoperative sexual functioning. Women with preexisting pelvic pain and depression do not do so well as those with only one or neither of these conditions; however, their quality of life and sexual functioning still improve over baseline. Sexual functioning postoperatively is highly related to their preoperative sexual activity, enjoyment, and relationship to their partner. Women who do not have good support systems may be at a disadvantage, as they would be in dealing with any other type of stress.

Preoperatively, the clinician should thoroughly discuss the reasons for the recommended hysterectomy and the consequences of the surgery, including allaying unreasonable fears and addressing mistaken beliefs, such as that she will immediately begin aging rapidly. The clinician should also dispel myths about the dangers of hormone replacement, such as that they automatically cause breast cancer or stokes (see Chapter 67, Hormones and Mood). It is helpful to discuss the flaws in the Women's Health Initiative studies (Writing Group for the Women's Health Initiative Investigators, 2002) and explain the misconceptions that came out of that work (Klaiber, Vogel, & Rako, 2005).

In the case of an emergency hysterectomy, there is obviously little time for preparation; however, in elective hysterectomies, the woman should be a key participant in the decision-making process so that she may consider the various quality-of-life issues involved in such a choice. Post-hysterectomy, women can benefit from clear explanations about what has happened. Perhaps because hysterectomy is a fairly common procedure, many women do not think of it as major surgery and are unprepared for the weakness and fatigue that may follow this procedure. They may need reassurance that they do require some time to recover (Table 65.1). Recovery after vaginal or laparoscopic surgery takes three to four weeks, while women who have had abdominal hysterectomies take about four to six weeks to recuperate. Women should gradually regain strength over these periods. If weakness, fatigue, and apathy continue or become worse, the patient should be reevaluated for physical complications or signs of depression.

In terms of sexual functioning, if an oophorectomy has been performed, attention must be paid to symptoms of vaginal dryness, which may lead to dyspareunia. Estrogen replacement therapy (ERT) should be considered in oophorectomized premenopausal women to alleviate menopausal symptoms such as hot flashes, night sweats, and genital-urinary problems (see Chapter 67, Hormones and Mood).

For women who do suffer from psychological distress or depression post-hysterectomy, antidepressant medication or individual or couple psychotherapy may be required to help them deal with their personal concerns about loss of femininity, loss of sexual interest, discord in the relationship, or fears about the outcome of a malignant disease. Preoperative counseling that includes the partner can help prevent relationship problems related to these concerns.

FEMALE STERILIZATION

Female sterilization, used by 10.3 million American women, is the second most common method of birth control in the United States and the leading method among women age 35 and older (Chandra, Martinez, Mosher, Abma, & Jones, 2005). Female sterilization involves the occlusion of the fallopian tubes via cutting, clipping, or cauterizing. The procedure itself is fairly simple, and the average recovery time is short. Women may seek this as a dependable, trouble-free method of permanent birth control. For many women, this is a straightforward and trouble-free decision. However, in cases in which a woman chooses sterilization because her spouse or partner is pressuring her to do so, or in which the man has been asked to have a vasectomy and has refused, there may be a great deal of ambivalence and resentment. Women who freely choose this procedure and understand its consequences tend to have very low rates of regret (5.9%), while regret and later psychological distress are more common (20.3%) in women who are younger, ambivalent about the sterilization, were pressured into the decision, or who made the decision for financial reasons (Hillis, Marchbanks, Tylor, & Peterson, 1999). Curtis, Mohllajee, and Peterson (2006) reviewed all existing studies and found that the younger women are at the time of sterilization, the more likely they are to report regretting that decision. Women undergoing sterilization at the age of 30 or younger are almost twice as likely as those over the age of 30 to express regret; 3.5 to 18 times as likely to request information about reversing the procedure; and about eight times as likely to actually undergo reversal or an evaluation for *in vitro* fertilization (IVF) (Curtis et al., 2006). Two years after tubal ligation, 80% of women reported that their sexual interest and pleasure had not changed (Costello et al., 2002). For the

Table 65.1 ABDOMINAL VS. LAPAROSCOPIC HYSTERECTOMIES

PROCEDURE	SURGERY TIME (MIN.)	HOSPITAL STAY (DAYS)	TIME OFF WORK (DAYS)	TIME TO FULL ACTIVITY (WKS)
Abdominal hysterectomy	64–98	3–4.9	33.5	10.7
Vaginal or laparoscopic hysterectomy	99–162	2–3.1	26	5.8

SOURCES: Perrson et al., 2006.

20% of women who noticed a change, 18.3 reported increased interest and 17.2% increased pleasure, while 1.7% reported decreased interest and 1.1% decreased pleasure.

Preoperatively, it should be stressed that tubal ligation s a permanent procedure. Women who are not ready to make this decision should be encouraged to try temporary types of contraception. A woman who seems highly anxious about the procedure or who appears to be in conflict with her partner about having the procedure should receive counseling before proceeding. Although about 50% of tubal ligations take place postpartum, it is not generally advisable to carry out the procedure immediately after a birth or an induced abortion. A woman who has sterilization immediately postpartum may experience enormous regret if the baby does not survive. Post-abortion may be a time of increased distress during which decision making is affected.

At times, childless women seek permanent sterilization. Many gynecologists are reluctant to carry out this procedure, believing that this must be evidence of great emotional instability. The reasons for this choice should be thoroughly explored. If the decision appears to be based on current psychological distress or a troubled relationship, attempts should be made to improve these situations before the procedure is considered. Administering a brief psychological test such as the Beck Depressive Inventory (Beck, 2006) may indicate if the woman is depressed. If the gynecologist has concerns about the woman's mental state because she is showing signs of depression or anxiety or seems to be being pressured into this decision, it may be wise to suggest a referral for a psychological assessment. For women in whom the decision is made as a result of a thoughtful analysis of their previous life experience and future expectations, their autonomy and wishes should be respected.

GYNECOLOGICAL PAIN

VULVAR PAIN

The vulvar area includes the labia majora, labia minora, clitoris, and vaginal introitus (area around vaginal opening). Vaginal pain, which occurs farther interior to the introitus, is not included in this section. Chronic vulvar pain lasting three to six months is estimated to affect 16–28% of women (Harlow & Stewart, 2003). It may occur in all age groups, with onset most frequently between 18 and 25 years. Surveys suggest 40% of women with vulvar pain do not seek treatment (Goldstein & Burrows, 2008). Typical presenting symptoms are continuous or intermittent burning, pain, itching, or irritation. Vulvar pain is divided into pains caused by specific disorders and those with no known etiology, referred to as *vulvodynia*. Known causes include: infections such as candidiasis or herpes simplex; inflammation such as lichen sclerosis; neoplasms; and neurological problems such as pudendal nerve entrapment or multiple sclerosis (Danby & Margesson, 2010).

Vulvar pain has a serious impact on one's quality of life, including decreased enjoyment, impaired sexual pleasure, guilt due to impaired sexual relationships, and depression and anxiety from living with chronic pain. The clinician's basic understanding of biomedical facts and theories not only permits communication with other specialists, but provides a foundation of trust with patients.

VULVODYNIA

Vulvodynia is defined as chronic (3–6 months) vulvar discomfort most often involving burning pain, in the absence of a relevant specific disorder. Visual examination may reveal erythema, easily missed small ulcers and fissures, or nothing abnormal. Vulvodynia is classified as *localized* (affecting part of the vulva) or *generalized* (affecting the entire vulva), with further subclassification into *provoked* (sexual, nonsexual, both), *unprovoked,* or *mixed* (both provoked and unprovoked). Furthermore, localized vulvodynia may be described according to the local area affected (e.g., *vestibulodynia*), and whether it is primary or secondary. *Primary* vestibulodynia is provoked localized vulvodynia, which occurs with first attempts at penetration (tampon or sexual), and *secondary* vestibulodynia is that which occurs after a period of pain-free sexual intercourse (Danby & Margesson, 2010).

Numerous factors, including embryonic abnormalities, urinary oxalates, genetic factors, hormonal factors, inflammation, infection, and neurological factors, are theorized as etiological. Oxalates found in many of our foods (greens, chocolate, berries, beer) are both excreted in the urine and a component of many renal calculi. They have been studied as possible factors in making urine more irritating, thus worsening vulvar pain. Previous infections seem to increase susceptibility to vulvodynia. There are conflicting studies regarding whether prior use of oral contraceptives increases the risk of vulvodynia. Assumptions that sexual trauma is the cause are unwarranted, although such a history may play a role in amplifying anxiety in response to physical distress or in determining coping responses.

Dyspareunia is frequent in women with vulvodynia. Women anticipating painful intercourse may have resultant difficulty with arousal and lubrication, causing added pain and muscle spasms resulting in vaginismus. Depression and anxiety are common comorbidities of chronic pain from any source, and both can negatively interfere with pain-regulation mechanisms. Women with primary localized vulvodynia are reported to have more psychological distress, anxiety, and somatization than those with secondary vulvodynia. Women with vulvodynia often suffer frustration, frequently seeing several healthcare practitioners before a diagnosis is made. In the absence of visible abnormality, women may be labelled as having a psychological disorder. Mandal et al. (2010) have set out guidelines for the medical and surgical management of vulvodynia (Table 65.2).

BLADDER PAIN SYNDROME (INTERSTITIAL CYSTITIS)

Bladder pain syndrome (BPS) has been suggested as preferred nomenclature over *interstitial cystitis* (IC) by several professional bodies (Hanno et al., 2010). BPS/IC is defined as an

Table 65.2 VULVODYNIA TREATMENT RECOMMENDATIONS

RECOMMENDATIONS	DETAILS
Pain history	Degree of symptoms: visual analogue scale, pain diaries, assessment tools, e.g., McGill Pain Questionnaire
	Impact of pain
	ISSVD classification
Sexual history if sexual pain is present	Sexual interest, arousal, lubrication, anorgasmia, vaginismus, partner problems, psychosexual comorbidity
Clinical history and physical is basis for diagnosis	Biopsy is unnecessary
	Review history and physical during treatment to rule out new diagnostic possibilities requiring biopsy/MRI
Multidisciplinary team approach	Individually tailored, e.g., pain specialist/clinic, CBT or supportive psychotherapy, physiotherapy
Combining treatments	Combining is appropriate if various treatments manage different facets of pain, e.g., physiotherapy, dietary, and psychotherapy
Explanation and education	Explanation of diagnosis and allay fears regarding infectious disorders and cancer
	Information sheet regarding self management: e.g., Sources Vulvar Pain Society, British Pain Foundation
Topical agents	Use with caution re irritancy
	Topical lidocaine gels/ointments to allow penetrative sex for provoked vulvodynia warn re: irritancy, penile numbness (condoms may help), oral contact
	5% lidocaine ointment to affected area plus cotton wool soaked in 5% lidocaine inserted into the vestibule every night for 7 days.
	Overnight 5% lidocaine ointment for treatment of vulvar vestibulitis
	Alternatives: capsaicin cream, ketoconazole cream, oestrogen creams, steroid creams interferon, nifedipine—all with mixed results
Tricyclic Agents	Amitriptyline and nortriptyline
	Start with low dose (e.g., 10 mg amitriptyline) and titrate up weekly according to response and tolerability
	Gabapentin (start 300 mg increase to max 3600 mg every 3 days; pregabalin
Surgical excision	Modified vestibulectomy in selected patients with provoked vestibulodynia
	Vestibuloplasty is not recommended
	Laser vapourization of vestibule is not recommended
Pelvic floor dysfunction intervention	For those with vaginismus response in sex related pain, e.g., pelvic floor exercises, external and internal soft tissue self massage trigger pint pressure, biofeedback, vaginal trainers, vaginal TENS
	Unknown results of physiotherapy for unprovoked vulvodynia
Acupuncture	Trial recommended for unprovoked vulvodynia
	Unknown value for provoked vulvodynia
Intralesional injections	Methylprednisolone acetate and lidocaine in saline subcutaneously into vestibule for vestibulodynia
	Betamethasone and lidocaine infiltration of vestibule for vestibulodynia
	Botox for allodynia

Mandal, D. et al. (2010). Guidelines for the management of vulvodynia. *British Journal of Dermatology, 162,* 1180–1185; Petersen, C. D. (2008). Vulvodynia. Definition, diagnosis and treatment. *Acta Obstetricia et Gynecologica, 87,* 893–901.

unpleasant sensation (pain, pressure, and discomfort) perceived to be related to urinary bladder filling, associated with lower urinary tract symptoms of more than six weeks' duration, in the absence of infection or other identifiable causes. Sensations may also be felt in the urethra, vulva, vagina, pelvis, rectum, lower abdomen, and lower back. Marked urinary urgency, frequency (up to 60 times per day), nocturia, and dyspareunia are extremely common and distressing, but they may also indicate other disorders. At its worst, the impact of this condition is devastating, leading to a severely impaired quality of life. The condition tends to progress upon onset for 12–18 months, then stabilize with chronic symptoms (mild, moderate, or severe), but exacerbations and remissions are common. BPS/IC can be difficult to differentiate from recurrent urinary tract infection, endometriosis, chronic pelvic pain, vulvodynia, and overactive bladder. Carcinoma, carcinoma *in situ*, eosinophilic cystitis, and tuberculous cystitis must be ruled out. Medical history to establish the onset, frequency, pattern, triggers, and location of pain will aid in diagnosis. The pain from BPS/IC usually occurs as the bladder fills and is relieved upon voiding. Premenstrual worsening of pain is typical, differentiating BPS/IC from endometriosis, which is most painful during menses. Vaginitis, vulvar lesions, and urethral diverticula are ruled out by physical examination. Urinalysis and urine culture are necessary investigations, with biopsy or cystoscopy as indicated.

The prevalence rate of BPS/IC is unknown, with reported ranges from 0.067–6.53%. It is more common in women and thought to be under-diagnosed and under-treated (Berry et al., 2011). The median age at diagnosis is 40 years old, but patients typically suffer for many years, consulting several physicians before a diagnosis is made. Women frequently experience their healthcare providers as blaming and unhelpful. Urinary tract infections (UTIs) are frequently diagnosed, even in the absence of a positive urine culture, whereas BPS/IC may be the correct diagnosis. Furthermore, UTIs may be the initiating event for the development of BPS/IC and are a frequent complication of BPS/IC, suggesting the need for ongoing clinical vigilance. Since BPS/IC and endometriosis often coexist, both diagnoses must be considered. In addition, many patients report being told their symptoms could be not accounted for by organic pathology, with the implication that the cause is psychological, but no treatment is offered.

One theory of causation is that increased permeability of the bladder epithelium allows potassium ions to pass the endothelial lining and initiate inappropriate stimulation of both neurons and immune pathways, but the cause of this permeability is unknown. Studies have revealed an increased prevalence of antecedent nonbladder syndromes (NBS) among IC patients, including: chronic pelvic pain (CPP), chronic fatigue syndrome, fibromyalgia, irritable bowel syndrome, sicca syndrome, migraine, depression, panic disorder, allergies, asthma, and vulvodynia (Warren et al., 2009; Warren, Wesselmann, Morozov, & Langenberg, 2011). Some studies suggest a history of current sexual abuse, but not childhood sexual or physical abuse.

The American Urological Association has detailed guidelines for the medical and surgical treatment of IC and of symptom management (Hanno et al., 2011). Support and education for families and partners may help maintain the patient's support network intact. Patients may obtain assistance and support from self-help groups and organizations such as the Interstitial Cystitis Association. Treatment recommendations are summarized in Table 65.3. The response to treatment for most specific IC interventions is individual and unpredictable.

CHRONIC PELVIC PAIN

Chronic pelvic pain (CPP) is defined as pain in the pelvis for six months or more, with incomplete relief with most treatments, significantly impaired function at home or work, signs of depression, and altered family roles. The term of six months is arbitrary, and caution is advised not to delay treatment in clinical situations. Symptoms may be cyclical (either menstrual or non-menstrual) or noncyclical.

CPP in women is a devastating and extremely difficult clinical issue to manage due to its complexity in presentation, the challenges in treating it adequately, and its significant impact on patients' lives. Prevalence estimates vary from 16% in the United States, to over 25% in the United Kingdom, New Zealand, and Australia. A recent study revealed that just over one third of women reporting CPP had sought help from a health professional (Pitts et al., 2008). This frequency is similar to that reported in a 1996 study in spite of increased awareness (Mathias, Kuppermann, Liberman, Lipschutz, & Steege, 1996). CPP is responsible for 15% to 40% of laparoscopies and 12% of hysterectomies in the United States (Reiter, 1990).

Physiological causes of CPP pain include *Mittelschmerz* pain and primary dysmenorrhea. The latter is reported by 60% of adult women (12–14% with severe symptoms) and 72% of adolescents (17% with severe symptoms). Many different disorders, such as endometriosis, adenomyosis, fibroids, cervical stenosis, tumors, intraperitoneal adhesions, and pelvic inflammatory disease, can result in CPP. Pathology in other systems, including neurological, urological, gastrointestinal, musculoskeletal, and psychological, while less common, may also be causative. Primary and secondary co-occurrence of pathological conditions is frequent, suggesting the need for rigorous investigation.

Due to the typically lengthy delay between pain onset and diagnosis, the treating psychiatrist should be aware of the approach to diagnosis and investigations to ensure that the patient has received optimal care. The medical history should include a chronological pain inventory: with details of timing (cyclical, noncyclical, and relationship to menses), onset, quality, location, radiation, and precipitating and relieving factors, as well as symptoms associated with the gastrointestinal, urinary, and musculoskeletal systems. Menstrual, obstetrical (including physical trauma from delivery), and sexual histories (especially deep dyspareunia) are critical components. Prior investigations, treatment and response, self-care, impact on functioning and quality of life, and desire for fertility will guide treatment decisions. The physical exam should be conducted while the patient is symptomatic and should include an assessment of the dermatological, musculoskeletal, gastrointestinal, urinary, and neurological systems, in addition to meticulous gynecological and abdominal exams. Initial laboratory investigations should include a complete blood count (CBC), C-reactive protein, CA-125 (when indicated), urinalysis, urine microscopy and culture, and vaginal swabs. Ultrasound is performed to look for structural abnormalities and is helpful in distinguishing between cystic and solid masses. For endometriosis, only deeply infiltrating lesions and ovarian involvement are detectable by ultrasound, suggesting that 80% of endometriosis will not be visualized. Computerized tomography (CT) may be used when assessing the organs associated with the gastrointestinal tract, and magnetic resonance imaging (MRI) is useful for pelvic masses, adenomyosis, and endometriosis (Won & Abbott, 2010).

Many other conditions are commonly associated with CPP. Endometriosis, a condition defined by the presence of endometrial tissue outside of the endometrial cavity, is the

Table 65.3 TREATMENT RECOMMENDATIONS AND PRIORITIES FOR INTERSTITIAL CYSTITIS

PRIORITY	INTERVENTION	DETAILS	LEVEL OF EVIDENCE
First Line	Education	Benefits vs risks/burdens of the available treatment alternatives	Clinical Principle
	Self care and Behavioural modifications	Altering the concentration and/or volume of urine (fluid restriction or hydration)	
		Avoidance of known food irritants, e.g., coffee or citrus; assessing other food or fluid irritants by using an elimination diet	
		Avoid aggravating pelvic floor exercises, sexual intercourse, tight clothing and constipation use of local heat or cold over the bladder	
		Perineum pain reduction via application of heat or cold over trigger points	
		Bladder training	
		Pelvic floor muscle relaxation	
		Over the Counter preparations: quercitin, calcium glycerophosphates, pyridium (commonly used by patients and some report effectiveness)	
		Coping strategies for flares: e.g., meditation, imagery	
	Mental Health	Validation; empathy	Clinical Principle
		Counselling re stigma	
		Prevention of exacerbations by overwhelming stress: meditation and imagery	
		Empowering regarding self care	
		Assessment and treatment of co-morbid depression and anxiety disorders: antidepressants, CBT, mindfulness based stress reduction	
		Assess, treat for ongoing abuse	
		Support and education for families and partners Self-help groups and organizations: Interstitial Cystitis Association	
Second Line	Manual physical therapy	Maneuvers to resolve pelvic, abdominal and/or hip muscular trigger points, lengthen muscle contractures, and release painful scars and other connective tissue restrictions: avoid pelvic floor exercises	Clinical Principle
	Pain management	Pharmacological, stress management, manual therapy if available	Clinical Principle
	Oral medication	Amitriptyline, cimetidine, hydroxyzine or pentosan polysulfate	Optional Grade B and C
	Intravesical medication	Dimethyl sulfoxide, heparin or lidocaine	Optional Grade B and C
Third line	Cystoscopy	With short duration, low pressure hydrodistension	Optional Grade C
		Treat Hunner's lesions	Recommended Grade C
Fourth Line	Neurostimulation	A trial of neurostimulaiton; if successful, implantation of permanent neurostimulation device	Optional Grade C
Fifth line	Oral Cyclosporine A		Optional Grade C
	Intradetrusor botulinum toxin A	Possibility that intermittent self-catheterization may be necessary after treatment.	Optional Grade C
Sixth line	Major surgery in carefully selected patients	Substitution cystoplasty	Optional
		Urinary diversion with or without cystectomy	Grade C
		Pain can persist even after cystectomy, especially in nonulcer IC/BPS.	

The AUA categories of evidence strength:
Grade A: Well-conducted RCTs; exceptionally strong observational studies
Grade B: RCTs with some weaknesses of procedure or generalizability; generally strong observational studies
Grade C: Observational studies with inconsistencies/small sample sizes/confounders

Hanno, P. (2011). AUA Guideline for the Diagnosis and Treatment of Interstitial Cystitis/Bladder Pain Syndrome. *Journal of Urology, 185*(6), 2162–2170.

Carrico, D. J. et al. (2008). Guided imagery for women with interstitial cystitis: results of a prospective, randomized controlled pilot study. *Journal of Alternative and Complementary Medicine, 14*, 53.

Watkins, K. E. (2011). Depressive disorders and panic attacks in women with bladder pain syndrome/interstitial cystitis: a population-based sample. *General Hospital Psychiatry, 33*(2), 143–149.

Goldstein, H. B. (2008). Depression, abuse and its relationship to interstitial cystitis. *International Urogynecology Journal and Pelvic Floor Dysfunction, 19*(12), 1683–1686.

most common gynecological pathology of CPP. Its incidence is estimated to be 1% to 7% in the United States (Barbieri, 1990). Pain is typically cyclical, with worsening during menses (75% of those with symptomatic endometriosis), but non-cyclical pain is common with abdominal-wall endometriosis. The severity of symptoms does not correlate with the severity of pathology; however, deep dyspareunia and painful defecation may suggest infiltrating disease.

In laparoscopic investigations of CPP, 30% of these women are found to have endometriosis, yet endometriosis appears to be asymptomatic in 45% of women who have it (Rawson, 1991). Neither the etiology nor the pathophysiology is understood. Treatment may include an estrogen and progestin combination, progestin alone, danazol, or a gonadotropin-releasing hormone (GnRH) agonist, with the option of adding a non-steroidal anti-inflammatory drug (NSAID). Randomized controlled trials (RCTs) reveal symptom improvement with surgery and excision of endometriosis. The most effective treatment for women not trying to preserve their fertility is a hysterectomy with bilateral oophorectomy (Jarrell et al., 2005a). Women suffering from endometriosis may have to endure recurrent pain in order to try to preserve their chance to have children.

Intraperitoneal adhesions are found in 25% to 50% of women with CPP, but their role in causation is unclear. They are a well-known result of surgery and may also be seen in patients who have endometriosis or have had abdominal and pelvic infections or inflammation. It is unclear what relationship adhesions have to CPP, and whether lysis of adhesions is helpful. While Peters' RCT on adhesionolysis in patients with CPP did not reveal clear benefits, many uncontrolled studies support the procedure. It is theorized by some that adhesions have re-formed in those for whom adhesionolysis fails to relieve pain. Women may undergo this procedure only to discover their pain persists.

Adenomyosis (the presence of endometrial glands and stroma with the uterine myometrium) is present in 20% of reproductive women, and while the most common presentation is menorrhagia, about 25% present with cyclical CPP associated with menses. Ultrasound is a good investigational tool, but MRI has increased sensitivity and specificity. Continuous OCP (oral contraceptive pill), levonorgestrel-releasing intrauterine devices (IUDs), endometrial ablation, and hysterectomy are treatment choices.

Uterine leiomyoma (fibroids), found in 20% of reproductive-age women, may present clinically with CPP, abnormal bleeding, and deep dyspareunia. They are investigated with ultrasound and treated with variable success and side effects, using continuous OCP, levonorgestrel-releasing IUDs, GnRH analogs, fibroid resection, uterine artery embolization, and hysterectomy.

The prevalence of pelvic inflammatory disease (PID) among women with CPP is difficult to estimate, as the presentation of PID varies from severe acute pelvic or abdominal pain (4%) to asymptomatic infections (60%). PID should be suspected in any patient with CPP, and in any sexually active woman with otherwise unexplained abdominal or pelvic pain. Recognition and early treatment of PID may prevent its long-term complications, particularly tubal scarring with ectopic pregnancy or infertility. PID is caused by sexually transmitted microorganisms, which lead to fallopian tube inflammation, potentially resulting in infertility and ectopic pregnancy. Sexually transmitted microorganisms, including *Chlamydia trachomatis, Neisseria gonorrheae, Mycoplasma genitalium*, and bacterial vaginosis–associated microbes, are causative agents. Ness and colleagues report CPP as a long-term consequence after an episode of PID in 18% to 33% of women, regardless of treatment (Ness et al., 2002). Condom use will assist with the reduction in transmission of some organisms and reduces the development of CPP after an incidence of PID. Adhesions are the suspected etiology of CPP after PID, but some uncertainty about this remains. Women with CPP after PID not only deal with chronic pain, but also may suffer from guilt or anger related to the cause of the infection.

Myofascial pain may be the most common cause (30%) of CPP in women with a negative laparoscopy and frequently is a secondary development of many of the aforementioned conditions. Lower abdominal scars and myofascial trigger points are common. A *trigger point* is defined as a focus of hyper-irritability in a muscle or its fascia, with a pattern of pain-referral specific to that muscle. Trigger points are thought to develop as a result of injury or micro-trauma with mechanical and postural stressors causing prolonged contraction of muscles. Treatment of trigger points has a significant impact on reducing pain from a number of primary initiating disorders (Jarrell et al., 2005b). Techniques used include pelvic floor exercises and biofeedback, pelvic muscle massage, trigger-point injection (local anesthetics, steroids, or botulinum toxin), sacral nerve neuromodulation (electrical stimulation), and acupuncture. Anderson et al. (Anderson, Wise, Sawyer, & Nathanson, 2011) used self-treatment with a wand designed to deliver measured pressure to internal myofascial trigger points and found it able to reduce trigger-point sensitivity by 25% in a pilot study.

IC (see above) is a very common co-occurrence with CPP (84%) in general and with endometriosis specifically. Irritable bowel syndrome (IBS) is present in one third of women with CPP, and 10–20% of the adult population. Menses can exacerbate IBS, including symptoms of dyspareunia and dysmenorrhea. Colonoscopy is performed if indicated, and treatment is primarily with diet. Inflammatory bowel disease must be ruled out.

Pudendal neuralgia (PN) is a less common cause of CPP, but the pain is often severe and sharp in the area of pelvic organs and structures. It may be exacerbated by sexual intercourse and by prolonged sitting, with relief upon standing. It is treated with physical therapy and nerve blocks.

CPP is frequently comorbid with depression, sleep disturbance, previous or current physical or sexual abuse, psychological stress, and substance abuse (Jarrell et al., 2005a). As visible causes of pain are frequently absent, or pain reports are greater than would be suggested by visible findings, psychological theories of causation have been suggested. Theories of stress, psychologically caused pelvic congestion, feminine identity issues, personality disorders, and conflicts about sexuality and intimacy as causative have been suggested (Lee & Slade, 1996) but have not been proven. Childhood emotional, physical, and sexual abuse is associated with higher levels of negative mental health and negative health trajectories in general. There are numerous physical and psychological adaptations to abuse, such as changes in epigenetic expression or neuroendocrine functioning that may play a role in the development of CPP. Psychological or physical abuse has not been shown to be causally related to CPP, but coping with pain requires robust psychological resources, which can be impaired by victimization. Sexual abuse, however, has been significantly associated with CPP in some studies with a recent meta-analysis, revealing an odds ratio (OR) of 2.7, with subgroup analysis revealing no significant impact regarding the age of the occurrence of the abuse (OR 3.03 for adult sexual abuse and 2.61 for childhood sexual abuse) (Paras et al., 2009).

PSYCHOLOGICAL ASSESSMENT AND TREATMENT OF GYNECOLOGICAL PAIN

Although the above conditions are slightly different, the psychological approach to assessment and treatment is similar. Multidisciplinary teams are most effective at treating chronic pain. The mental health specialist may need to play a role in educating other practitioners about the complex relationship between pain and the psyche. Treatment of comorbid anxiety and depression will improve both the mood symptoms and the pain, as it does in other painful conditions.

The standard psychiatric and psychological assessment should include questions about: the patient's understanding of her condition; fears regarding the meaning of her symptoms, both medically and for her future; attempts at and results of self-care; experiences with healthcare providers; outcomes of previous treatments; expectations of current treatment; past and current physical, psychological, and/or sexual abuse; coping style, and support systems. Fear of pain and catastrophizing responses should be assessed and can further be quantified using standardized measures.

Structured psychotherapy should include: education about the relationship between affective, cognitive, and somatic reactions to pain that may worsen pain and quality of life; identification and modification of individual cognitive and affective reactions to pain symptoms; practice of somatic techniques, such as relaxation to counteract physical reactions to pain; identification and modification of behaviors that potentiate pain; enhancement of behaviors that reduce pain; and improvement of communication and other behaviors that impede relationships and intimacy. Cognitive behavioral therapy (CBT) can address overly negative life and personal appraisals, catastrophic thoughts, and stress responses that amplify pain. CBT has been shown to be effective in randomized control trials in pain research in general and with gynecological and pelvic pain specifically. Masheb and colleagues report clinically significant improvement in pain severity (self- and physician-report), sexual function, and emotional function with both CBT and supportive psychotherapy (Masheb, Kerns, Lozano, Minkin, & Richman, 2009). The CBT treatment arm was superior with respect to

rates of patient satisfaction, decreased pain with vulvar examination, and overall improved sexual functioning. These findings reinforce the importance of support, empathy, treatment of anxiety and depression, education, and specific behavioral interventions in routine practice. Meditation, imagery, and mindfulness-based stress-reduction techniques have also been used to help patients cope with chronic pain and disease; even if pain is not altered, the capacity to live with it can be improved.

GYNECOLOGICAL ONCOLOGY

The reproductive organs are the fourth most common site of cancer in American women, with gynecological cancers affecting one of every 20 women (American Cancer Society, 2007). All patients diagnosed with cancer have to deal with a number of emotional issues, including a sense of helplessness, fear of pain, anticipation of treatment, and fears of death. These reactions are moderated by the individual's typical style of coping with crises, the specific diagnosis, the seriousness of the illness, and the magnitude of the treatment. Gynecological cancers may have an especially strong impact on women because of their relationship to issues of fertility, sexuality, attractiveness, and value.

Removal of the uterus or ovaries in a younger woman leads to a loss of fertility, which may be particularly upsetting. Not only may she personally grieve the loss of potential children, she may feel she has lost value in her culture and, therefore, will never find or maintain a relationship. Even if the woman is not interested in childbearing, loss of her reproductive organs may affect her sense of femininity.

By the time they are diagnosed, 80% of women with ovarian cancer have an advanced stage of the disease. Clinical depression was reported in 21% of patients, while 29% scored above the 75th percentile for anxiety (Grzankowski & Carney, 2011). Not only is it important to assess for depression and anxiety, the individual's quality of life must be considered (Grzankowski & Carney, 2011). Patients often must make a difficult choice between aggressive treatments and their quality of life. This is an individual decision that must be discussed with the patient and respected by the clinician.

Operations that are especially disfiguring, such as complete pelvic exenteration or vulvectomy, may be particularly damaging to a woman's self-esteem. A sense of being disfigured, as well as such physical changes as shortening of the vagina or loss of the clitoris, vaginal bleeding, or dryness may interfere with sexual functioning. The extent of sexual dysfunction tends to be related to the severity of the disease and the magnitude of treatment. While 30–40% of patients with early cervical cancer have sexual problems, up to 90% of patients with pelvic exenteration stop having vaginal sex (Andersen, Anderson, & de Prosse, 1989). This may lead to problems in the woman's current relationship or make her avoid any future relationships out of fear of rejection. Previous successful sexual relationships and ongoing support from a caring partner may help the woman adjust to changes in her sexual functioning. Couples may benefit from counseling aimed at broadening their view of sexuality and discovering other ways of giving and obtaining sexual pleasure. Although some couples may find it difficult, if not impossible, to make this transition, others may be willing to convert to a more flexible and open view of sexuality. Recent advances in reconstructive surgery have led to increased post-operation quality of life with better body image, sexual functioning, and relationships (Hawighorst-Knapstein, Schonefussrs, Hoffman, & Knapstein, 1997). Women still have to deal with ongoing fears about the return of cancer.

Treatment of gynecological cancer may revive past traumas such as incest or rape, or stir up guilt for previous behaviors such as induced abortion. Therefore, in addition to the general approach to treatment of individuals with cancer, women with gynecological cancer may need specific attention to these issues.

LESBIAN AND TRANSGENDER WOMEN'S HEALTH ISSUES

A lesbian sexual orientation does not denote psychopathology. However, several large studies found significantly higher levels of depression (Case et al., 2004; Valanis et al., 2000) and suicide attempts (Bradford et al., 1994) in lesbians than in heterosexual women. Lesbians may suffer from depression, anxiety, and poor self-esteem based on the stress of living in a society in which they face prejudice and homophobia. Although, especially in larger centers, lesbians may feel more comfortable seeking out health care, they may still encounter biases that may affect the relationship between the healthcare provider and the lesbian patient. Patients may hesitate to report their sexual orientation to the physician out of fear of a negative reaction. The use of non-gendered language can encourage the patient to feel more comfortable.

Hostility or lack of understanding of specific health risks on the part of healthcare providers may decrease the likelihood of lesbians' receiving standard screening tests such as Pap smears. Lesbians may have increased rates of known risk factors for breast cancer, such as increased body mass, high alcohol intake, and nulliparity. As nulliparity or delayed parity is a significant risk factor in the development of certain disorders of the reproductive system, lesbians who do not have children may be at increased risk for conditions such as endometriosis, ovarian cancer, and endometrial cancer. Therefore, although routine screening is not recommended in the general population, it is important that lesbians be regularly screened for these problems using such tools as measurement of cancer antigen 125 (CA-125) (>35 U/ml) or transvaginal ultrasounds. Lesbians may have elevated rates of cardiovascular problems due to an increase in risk factors such as obesity and smoking (Roberts, 2006). They have higher rates of drinking and binge drinking than do heterosexual women (Roberts, 2006).

Lesbians may also encounter prejudice when seeking artificial insemination, even though they may have considered very carefully the impact of having a child in a nontraditional household. Lesbians who wish to get pregnant may be denied use of registered sperm banks in which the sperm has been assessed for the presence of sexually transmitted diseases. This issue is highly charged from political, legal, and religious viewpoints.

Lesbians may also be at high risk for having experienced violence from heterosexual males as well as from their lesbian partners. They may suffer from the same kind of psychological, emotional, and physical injuries experienced by any female victims of violence.

The psychiatric consultant may have a role in dispelling prejudices and false assumptions about psychopathology in lesbians. The healthcare providers should be aware of the external stresses and lack of family support often experienced by lesbians. A lesbian partner or spouse should be treated in the same way as any heterosexual partner or spouse and included in discussions when the patient so wishes. Some homosexual patients may prefer treatment by homosexual physicians and therapists, who they feel will be more empathetic and more accepting of their choices. McNair (2010) has a comprehensive list of resource of documents about lesbian healthcare published in countries around the world.

The management of men with gender dysphoria (transgender) who wish to become women is very complicated (Gooren, 2011). They must live for one year as a woman before surgical reassignment is performed. Many healthcare providers are reluctant to treat these patients after surgery or are unfamiliar with their particular needs, including the issues of hormone use, HIV prevention, or gynecological needs. Ideally, the healthcare provider must treat the individual in a respectful, nonjudgemental fashion and not assume the patient will have serious mental health problems.

VIOLENCE

Violence against women takes many forms, including homicide, battering, rape, child abuse, incest, harassment, and boundary violations such as sexual contact between a healthcare worker and a patient. Women may see physicians because of the physical and psychological consequences of such violence. More than one million American women a year seek treatment for injuries caused by battering. Studies have found that 22% to 35% of women who attended hospital emergency departments have injuries or symptoms related to physical abuse (Daugherty & Houry, 2008). Despite this, there continues to be under-reporting by victims and under-detection by physicians (Flury, Nyberg, & Riecher-Rossler, 2010). Violence may be the undetected underlying cause of many gynecological complaints. A history of violence may also influence a woman's behavior in the physician's office, causing her to fail to keep appointments or to avoid or react dramatically during physical examinations.

Prevalence studies show that 20% of adult women and 12% of adolescent girls in North America have experienced a variety of sexual abuses, which may include forcible rape, during their lifetime. These estimates are even higher in the case of immigrant, Native American, or African-American women (Hammett, Powell, O'Carroll, & Clanton, 1992). The reasons for the high rates of violence against women are complex (Stewart & Robinson, 1995). Substance abuse may precipitate a violent incident, but it is not in itself a sufficient explanation for violence (Anonymous, 1992). Society's view of women as less valuable than men, as well as traditional views of marriage in which the husband, as the head of the household, has a "right" to treat his wife as his property, are important factors. Modeling is also an important component of violence. Women who have grown up in situations of domestic violence are more likely to become victims, and men from violent households are more likely to be violent toward their spouses (Hotaling & Sugarman, 1986). Individual perpetrators may be men who feel powerless or vulnerable in their day-to-day lives and bolster their egos by having power over vulnerable women. In cases of rape, exercising power may more often be the motivation than the gratification of sexual desires.

The victim of violence may present with a variety of injuries, such as bruises, bites, lacerations, fractures, burns, or damaged organs. In pregnant women, violence may result in miscarriage or premature delivery. Victims of violence may also exhibit a variety of stress-related phenomena such as headaches, insomnia, and other somatic symptoms. Childhood sexual abuse or rape may result in various sexual or reproductive consequences, including genital trauma, sexually transmitted disease, CPP, sexual dysfunction, UTIs, or unwanted pregnancy.

Immediate emotional reactions to violence range from shock and fear to emotional numbness and withdrawal. There may be numerous long-term behavioral and psychological effects (Rees et al., 2011). Women may demonstrate either sexual aversion or promiscuity, or show a range of self-harming behaviors such as substance abuse, self-mutilation, and suicide attempts. They may suffer from ongoing low self-esteem, guilt, self-blame, and problems in forming relationships, or may exhibit symptoms of depression, anxiety disorders, dissociative identity disorders, borderline personality disorders, or post-traumatic stress disorders. Although not yet listed in the formal *Diagnostic and Statistical Manual of Mental Disorders* (DSM), a syndrome of "complex post-traumatic stress disorder (PTSD)" has been described in adult patients who suffered from severe and prolonged childhood sexual abuse (Cloitre, Miranda, Stovall-McClough, & Han, 2005). As well as typical PTSD symptoms, this syndrome includes problems in attachment, affect regulation, dissociation,

behavioral control, and self-concept. Victims of childhood or adult violence may be extremely reluctant to have physical examinations and become acutely anxious if breast or pelvic examination is attempted (Weitlauf et al., 2008).

All healthcare workers need to be aware of the high prevalence of violence against women. Questions about violence and past abuse should be a routine part of the assessment of female patients. There are several domestic violence screening tools that can be used (Rabin, Jennings, Campbell, & Bair-Merritt, 2009). The HITS scale uses four key questions, rated from "never" to "frequently," to elicit information (Sherin, Sinacore, Li, Zitter, & Shakil, 1998) (Table 65.4).

Although information may not be immediately forthcoming, an attitude of nonjudgemental acceptance may make it easier for the woman to talk about her experiences at some time.

In emergency situations, such as immediately after a sexual assault, the woman's physical concerns must be dealt with in a caring and empathic manner. It is important that the physical examination not feel like a repeat of the previous assault. Also, attention must be paid to the woman's safety and her practical and psychological needs. She may need assistance in dealing with her immediate emotional reaction as well as in finding a shelter, locating a rape crisis center, dealing with police or family members, or just finding clothes to go home. The woman should be educated about the anticipated impact of the trauma on her, her family, and her friends.

A variety of treatment approaches, including psychodynamic psychotherapy (Schottenbauer, Glass, Arnkoff, & Gray, 2008), CBT (Vickerman & Margolin, 2009), pharmacotherapy (Stein, Ipser, & Seedat, 2006), group therapy (Kessler, White, & Nelson, 2003), and self-help organizations have all been found to be helpful. Specific treatments for complex PTSD have also been described (Cloitre et al., 2010). The prognosis for the individual woman will be influenced by her previous personality and coping style, ego strength, and social supports. Work may also need to be done with her family to deal with their shame, rejection of the victim, or excess anger. Readers are referred to Rose (1991 and 1993) for a more detailed overview of the psychodynamic treatment of women who have been the victims of violence. Women who come from cultures where it is customary to blame the victim may hesitate to even come for counseling. It is important to be patient and not push her to stand up to her family,

Table 65.4 HITS TOOL FOR INTIMATE PARTNER VIOLENCE SCREENING

Please read each of the following activities and fill in circle that best indicates the frequency with which you partner acts in the way depicted. How often does your partner —

	Never 1	Rarely 2	Sometimes 3	Fairly often 4	Frequently 5
Physically hurt you?					
Insult or talk down to you?					
Threaten you with harm?					
Scream or curse at you?					

Each item is scored from 1–5. Thus, scores for this inventory range from 4–20. A score of greater than 10 is considered positive for intimate partner violence.

while continuing to clearly reinforce the view that she is not to blame for what happened. Counselors should be alert to the possibility that the woman may be in physical danger in families who fear their honor has been impugned by the rape. In these cases, the counselor needs to be aware of community resources such as help lines and women's shelters so the client has a safe exit route if required.

PHYSICIAN–PATIENT ABUSE

Power is a factor in physician–patient abuse. Patients usually come to physicians because they are in emotional or physical distress. They may feel frightened and vulnerable. The physician is viewed as an idealized authority figure who is wise, kind and will have solutions for the patient's problems. This power imbalance in the relationship is further exaggerated by the physician's right to ask the most personal information about the patient's life, without revealing any of his or her own background. Patients assume that physicians are trustworthy and are motivated by a wish to help others. They do not know the correct psychotherapeutic or physical examination techniques and procedures, and must trust that what the physician is doing is ethical and proper. All of these factors can make the patient vulnerable to sexual abuse by an exploitive physician or physical or emotional abuse by a careless or inept physician.

Even after being sexually exploited by a physician, a patient may hesitate to report these activities, as she may doubt her own instincts and deny that any abuse took place, feel ashamed and guilty, or fear that no one would believe her. Patients who have been abused by physicians may avoid any kind of medical care or specific examinations such as of the breast and pelvic areas. They may demonstrate signs of tension whenever the physician begins a medical examination or be very reluctant to divulge any personal information. Physicians must be aware of reporting requirements in their particular area. In a number of states, abuse by a healthcare professional is a crime. Warning a patient not to reveal the name of the abuser if she is not ready to report the offense will allow her to get support from the therapist until she is ready to come forward.

CLINICAL PEARLS

- Although it was previously thought that post-hysterectomy depression was a common phenomenon, more recent studies have found no evidence that hysterectomy causes depression.

- Assumptions that sexual trauma is the cause of vulvodynia are unwarranted, although such a history may play a role in amplifying anxiety in response to physical distress or in determining coping responses.

- The pain from BPS/IC usually occurs as the bladder fills and is relieved upon voiding. Premenstrual worsening of pain is typical, differentiating BPS/IC from endometriosis, which is most painful during menses.

- History of chronic pelvic pain (CPP) should include a chronological pain inventory: with details of timing (cyclical, non- cyclical; relationship to menses), onset, quality, location, radiation, precipitating and relieving factors, as well as symptoms associated with the gastrointestinal, urinary, and musculoskeletal systems. Menstrual, obstetrical (including physical trauma from delivery), and sexual histories (especially deep dyspareunia) are critical components.

- For endometriosis, only deeply infiltrating lesions and ovarian involvement are detectable by ultrasound, suggesting that 80% of endometriosis will not be visualized.

- Noncyclic pain is common with abdominal wall endometriosis.

- Myofascial pain may be the most common cause (30%) of CPP in women with a negative laparoscopy and frequently is a secondary development.

- Prevalence studies show that 20% of adult women and 12% of adolescent girls have experienced a variety of sexual abuses.

DISCLOSURE STATEMENTS

Dr. Robinson is an employee of the University of Toronto and works at the University Health Network in Toronto, Canada. She has no ties to any pharmaceutical companies. She has no conflicts to disclose.

Dr. Meschino is funded by the Alternative Funding Plan (AFP) Ministry of Health Government of Ontario–Women's College Hospital grants only.

REFERENCES

American Cancer Society (2007). *Cancer facts and figures 2007*. Atlanta, GA: American Cancer Society.

Andersen, B. L., Anderson, B., & de Prosse, C. (1989). Controlled prospective longitudinal study of women with cancer, I: sexual functioning outcomes. *Journal of Consulting & Clinical Psychology, 57*(6), 683–691.

Anderson, R., Wise, D., Sawyer, T., & Nathanson, B. H. (2011). Safety and effectiveness of an internal pelvic myofascial trigger point wand for urologic chronic pelvic pain syndrome. *Clinical Journal of Pain, 27*(9), 764–768.

[Anonymous], 1992. Prevention of violence and injuries due to violence. *MMWR: Morbidity & Mortality Weekly Report, 41*(RR-6), 5–7.

Baldaro, B., Gentile, G., Codispoti, M., Mazzetti, M., Trombini, E., & Flamigni, C. (2003). Psychological distress of conservative and nonconservative uterine surgery: a prospective study. *Journal of Psychosomatic Research, 54*(4), 357–360.

Barbieri, R. L. (1990). Etiology and epidemiology of endometriosis. *American Journal of Obstetrics & Gynecology, 162*(2), 565–567.

Beck, A. T. (2006). *Depression: Causes and treatment*. Philadelphia, PA: University of Pennsylvania Press.

Berry, S. H., Elliott, M. N., Suttorp, M., Bogart, L. M., Stoto, M. A., Eggers, P., et al. (2011). Prevalence of symptoms of bladder pain syndrome/interstitial cystitis among adult females in the United States. *Journal of Urology, 186*(2), 540–544.

Bradford J., Ryan C., Rothblum E.D.(1994) National lesbian health care survey: implication for mental health. *Journal of Consulting and Clinical Psychology* 62:228–242.

Case, P., Austin, S. B., Hunter, D. J., Manson, J. E., Malspeis, S., Willett, W., et al. (2004). Sexual orientation, health risk factors, and physical functioning in the Nurses' Health Study II. *Journal of Women's Health, 13*, 1033–1047.

Chandra, A., Martinez, G. M., Mosher, W. D., Abma, J. C., & Jones, J. (2005). Fertility, family planning, and reproductive health of U.S. women: Data from the 2002 National Survey of Family Growth. *Vital Health Statistics, 23*(25), 1–160.

Cloitre, M., Stovall-McClough, C., Nooner, K., Zorbas, P., Cherry, S., Jackson, C. L., et al. (2010). Treatment for PTSD related to childhood abuse: A randomized controlled trial. *American Journal of Psychiatry, 167*(8), 915–924.

Cloitre, M., Miranda, R., Stovall-McClough, K., & Han, H. (2005). Beyond PTSD: emotion regulation and interpersonal problems as predictors of functional impairment in survivors of childhood abuse. *Behavioral Therapy, 36*(2), 119–124.

Cooper, R., Mishra, G., Hardy, R., & Kuh, D. (2009). Hysterectomy and subsequent psychological health: Findings from a British birth cohort study. *Journal of Affective Disorders, 115*(1–2), 122–130.

Costello, C., Hillis, S. D., Marchbanks, P. A., Jamieson, D. J., Peterson, H. B., & the US Collaborative Review of Sterilization Working Group (2002). The effect of interval tubal sterilization on sexual interest and pleasure. *Obstetrics & Gynecology, 100*(3), 511–517.

Curtis, K. M., Mohllajee, A. P., & Peterson, H. B. (2006). Regret following female sterilization at a young age: A systematic review. *Contraception, 73*(2), 205–210.

Danby, C. S., & Margesson, L. J. (2010). Approach to the diagnosis and treatment of vulvar pain. *Dermatology & Therapy, 23*(5), 485–504.

Daugherty, J. D., & Houry, D. E. (2008). Intimate partner violence screening in the emergency department. *Journal of Postgraduate Medicine, 54*(4), 301–305.

Flory, N., Bissonnette, F., & Binik, Y. M. (2005). Psychosocial effects of hysterectomy. *Journal of Psychosomatic Research, 59*(3), 117–129.

Flury, M., Nyberg, E., & Riecher-Rossler, A. (2010). Domestic violence against women: Definitions, epidemiology, risk factors and consequences. *Swiss Medical Weekly, 140*, w13099.

Goldstein, A. T., & Burrows, L. (2008). Vulvodynia. *Journal of Sexual Medicine, 5*(1), 5–14.

Gooren, L. J. (2011). Clinical practice: Care of transsexual persons. [Review] *New England Journal of Medicine, 364*(13), 1251–1257.

Grzankowski, K. S., & Carney, M. (2011). Quality of life in ovarian cancer. *Cancer Control 18*(1), 52–58.

Hawighorst-Knapstein, S., Schonefussrs, G., Hoffman, S. O., & Knapstein, P. G. (1997). Pelvic exenteration: Effects of surgery on quality of life and body image—a prospective longitudinal study. *Gynecologic Oncology, 66*(3), 495–500.

Hammett, M., Powell, K. E., O'Carroll, P. W., & Clanton, S. T. (1992). Homicide surveillance—United States, 1979-1988. *Morbidity & Mortality Weekly Report: CDC Surveillance Summaries, 41*(3), 1–33.

Hanno, P. M., Burks, D. A., Clemens, J. Q., Dmochowski, R. R., Erickson, D., Fitzgerald, M. P., et al. (2011). AUA guideline for the diagnosis and treatment of interstitial cystitis/bladder pain syndrome. *Journal of Urology 185*(6), 2162–2170.

Hanno, P., Lin, A., Nordling, J., Nyberg, L., van Ophoven, A., Ueda, T., et al. (2010). Bladder Pain Syndrome Committee of the International Consultation on Incontinence. *Neurourology & Urodynamics, 29*(1), 191–198.

Harlow, B. L., & Stewart, E. G. (2003). A population-based assessment of chronic unexplained vulvar pain: Have we underestimated the prevalence of vulvodynia? *Journal of the American Women's Association, 58*(2), 82–88.

Hillis, S. D., Marchbanks, P. A., Tylor, L. R., & Peterson, H. B. (1999). Poststerilization regret: findings from the United States collaborative Review of Sterilization. *Obstetrics & Gynecology, 93*(6), 889–895.

Hotaling, G. T., & Sugarman, D. B. (1986). An analysis of risk markers in husband to wife violence: the current state of knowledge. *Violence & Victims, 1*(2), 101–124.

Jarrell, J. F., Vilos, G. A., Allaire, C., Burgess, S., Fortin, C., Gerwin, R., et al. (2005a). Consensus guidelines for the management of chronic pelvic pain. *Journal of Obstetrics & Gynaecology, Canada, 27*(8), 781–826.

Jarrell, J. F., Vilos, G. A., Allaire, C., Burgess, S., Fortin, C., Gerwin, R., et al. (2005b). Consensus guidelines for the management of chronic pelvic pain. *Journal of Obstetrics & Gynaecology, Canada, 27*(9), 869–910.

Kessler, M. R., White, M. B., & Nelson, B. S. (2003). Group treatments for women sexually abused as children: a review of the literature and recommendations for future outcome research. *Child Abuse & Neglect, 27*(9), 1045–1061.

Klaiber, E. L., Vogel W., & Rako S. (2005). A critique of the Women's Health Initiative hormone therapy study. *Fertility & Sterility, 84*(6), 1589–601.

Lambden, M. P., Bellamy, G., Ogburn-Russell, L., Preece, C. K., Moore, S., Pepin, T., et al. (1997). Women's sense of well-being before and after hysterectomy. *Journal of Obstetrics & Gynecology, Neonatal Nursing, 26*(5), 540–548.

Lee, C., & Slade, P. (1996). Miscarriage as a traumatic event: A review of the literature and new implications for intervention. *Journal of Psychosomatic Research, 40*(3), 235–244.

Loh, F. H., & Koa, R. C. (2002). Laparoscopic hysterectomy versus abdominal hysterectomy: A controlled study of clinical and functional outcomes. *Singapore Medical Journal, 43*(8), 403–407.

Masheb, R. M., Kerns, R. D., Lozano, C., Minkin, M. J., & Richman, S. (2009). A randomized clinical trial for women with vulvodynia: Cognitive-behavioral therapy vs. supportive psychotherapy. *Pain, 141*(1–2), 31–40.

Mathias, S. D., Kuppermann, M., Liberman, R. F., Lipschutz, R. C., & Steege, J. F. (1996). Chronic pelvic pain: prevalence, health-related quality of life, and economic correlates. *Obstetrics & Gynecology, 87*(3), 321–327.

McNair R.P., Hegarty K.(2010). Guidelines for the Primary Care of Lesbian, Gay, and Bisexual People: A Systematic Review. *Annals of Family Medicine, 8*(6), 533–541.

Mravcak S.A. (2006). Primary Care for Lesbians and Bisexual Women. *American Family Physician, 74*(2), 279–286.

Ness, R. B., Soper, D. E., Holley, R. L., Peipert, J., Randall, H., Sweet, R. L., et al. (2002). Effectiveness of inpatient and outpatient treatment strategies for women with pelvic inflammatory diseases: results from the PID Evaluation and Clinical Health (PEACH) randomized trial. *American Journal of Obstetrics & Gynecology, 186*, 929–937.

Paras, M. L., Murad, M. H., Chen, L. P., Goranson, E. N., Sattler, A. L., Colbenson, K. M., et al. (2009). Sexual abuse and lifetime diagnosis of somatic disorders: a systematic review and meta-analysis. *Journal of the American Medical Association, 302*(5), 550–561.

Persson, P., Wijma, K., Hammar, M., & Kjolhede, P. (2006). Psychological wellbeing after laparoscopic and abdominal hysterectomy—a randomised controlled multicenter study. *British Journal of Obstetrics & Gynaecology, 113*(9), 1023–1030.

Pitts, M., Ferris, J., Smith, A., Shelley, J., & Richters, J. (2008). Prevalence and correlates of three types of pelvic pain in a nationally representative sample of Australian women. *Medical Journal of Australia, 189*(3), 138–143.

Rabin, R. F., Jennings, J. M., Campbell, J. C., & Bair-Merritt, M. H. (2009). Intimate partner violence screening tools. A systematic review. *American Journal of Preventive Medicine, 36*(5), 439–445.

Rawson, J. M. (1991). Prevalence of endometriosis in asymptomatic women. *Journal of Reproductive Medicine, 36*(5), 513–515.

Rees, S., Silove, D., Chey, T., Ivancic, L., Steel, Z., Creamer, M., et al. (2011). Lifetime prevalence of gender-based violence in women and the relationship with mental disorders and psychosocial function. *Journal of the American Medical Association, 306*(5), 513–521.

Reiter, R. C. (1990). A profile of women with chronic pelvic pain. *Clinical Obstetrics & Gynecology, 33*(1), 130–136.

Roberts, S. J. (2006). Health care recommendations for lesbian women. *Journal of Obstetric, Gynecologic, & Neonatal Nursing, 35*, 583–591.

Rose, D. S. (1991). A model for psychodynamic psychotherapy with the rape victim. *Psychotherapy, 28*(1), 85–95.

Rose, D. S. (1993). Sexual assault, domestic violence and incest. In D. E. Stewart & N. Stotland (Eds.), *Psychological aspects of women's health care: The interface between psychiatry and obstetrics and gynecology* (pp. 447–483). Washington, DC: American Psychiatric Press.

Schottenbauer, M. A., Glass, C. R., Arnkoff, D. B., & Gray, S. H. (2008). Contributions of psychodynamic approaches to treatment of PTSD and trauma: A review of the empirical treatment and psychopathology literature. Psychiatry, 71(1), 13–34.

Sherin, K. M., Sinacore, J. M., Li, X. Q., Zitter, R. E., & Shakil, A. (1998). HITS: A short domestic violence screening tool for use in a family practice setting. *Family Medicine, 30*(7), 508–512.

Stein, D. J., Ipser, J. C., & Seedat, S. (2006). Pharmacotherapy for post-traumatic stress disorder (PTSD). *Cochrane Database of Systematic Reviews,* 25, CD002795.

Stewart, D. E., & Robinson, G. E. (1995). Violence against women. In J. C. Oldham & M. B. Riba (Eds.), *Review of psychiatry* (Vol. 14, pp. 261–282). Washington, DC: American Psychiatric Press.

Thakar, R., Ayers, S., Georgakapolou, A., Clarkson, P., Stanton, S., & Manyonda, I. (2004). Hysterectomy improves quality of life and decreases psychiatric symptoms: a prospective and randomised comparison of total versus subtotal hysterectomy. *British Journal of Obstetrics & Gynaecology, 111*(10), 1115–1120.

Writing Group for the Women's Health Initiative Investigators (2002). Risks and benefits of estrogen plus progestin in healthy postmenopausal women: principal results from the Women's Health Initiative randomized controlled trial. *Journal of the American Medical Association, 288*, 321–333.

Valanis, B. G., Bowen, D. J., Bassford, T., Whitlock, E., Charney, P., & Carter, R. A. (2000). Sexual orientation and health. *Archives of Family Medicine, 9*, 843–853.

Vickerman, K. A., & Margolin, G. (2009). Rape treatment outcome research: Empirical findings and state of the literature. *Clinical Psychology Review, 29*(5), 431–448.

Warren, J. W., Wesselmann, U., Morozov, V., & Langenberg, P. W. (2011). Numbers and types of nonbladder syndromes as risk factors for interstitial cystitis/painful bladder syndrome. *Urology, 77*(2), 313–319.

Warren, J. W., Howard, F. M., Cross, R. K., Good, J. L., Weissman, M. M., Wesselmann, U., et al. (2009). Antecedent nonbladder syndromes in case-control study of interstitial cystitis/painful bladder syndrome. *Urology, 73*(1), 52–57.

Weitlauf, J. C., Finney, J. W., Ruzek, J. I., Lee, T. T., Thrailkill, A., Jones, S., et al. (2008). Distress and pain during pelvic examinations: Effect of sexual violence. *Obstetrics & Gynecology, 112*(6), 1343–1350.

Won, H. R., & Abbott, J. (2010). Optimal management of chronic cyclical pelvic pain: an evidence-based and pragmatic approach. *International Journal of Women's Health, 20*(2), 263–277.

Yen, J. Y., Chen, Y. H., Long, C. Y., Chang, Y., Yen, C. F., Chen, C. C., et al. (2008). Risk factors for major depressive disorder and the psychological impact of hysterectomy: a prospective investigation. *Psychosomatics, 49*(2), 137–149.

66.

INFERTILITY, PREGNANCY LOSS, AND ABORTION

Gail Erlick Robinson

INTRODUCTION

Women may choose not to get pregnant for a variety of reasons. Women who have done a lot of childcare while helping raise younger siblings may feel they have already done enough child-rearing. Other women may not have found a partner who they think will be a good parent. Yet others may have a career or lifestyle that seems to be incompatible with having a family. In all of these situations, the woman may be comfortable with her decision and feel no less feminine. It appears that an important element in feeling like an adequate female is the woman's ability to choose what she wants to do concerning pregnancy. When a woman wishes to get pregnant and either cannot achieve or maintain a pregnancy, the psychological impact may be devastating. Consistent with the concept of the importance of choice, a woman having an induced abortion who has made a free and un-coerced decision does not suffer from any lasting negative emotional consequences.

INFERTILITY

Approximately 10% of couples will suffer from primary or secondary infertility, diagnosed after 12 months of focused attempts to conceive in women 34 years old and under, or after six months in women 35 years old and older. Accepted causes of infertility related to psychiatric conditions include absent or infrequent vaginal intercourse, infrequent or absent menstrual periods due to eating disorders, and medications such as neuroleptics, which inhibit ovulation by increasing serum prolactin levels. Depression is likely to influence the outcome of infertility treatment, but there is less consistent evidence for the effects of anxiety (Wischmann, 2003). Studies have shown higher pregnancy rates in both women with low levels of trait anxiety and those in the highest quartile of anxiety (Sanders & Bruce, 1999). Research is being conducted to determine whether stress can cause infertility via influencing the actions of hypothalamic, pituitary, or adrenal hormones on the reproductive system (Wischmann, 2003). There are no convincing studies showing stress as the sole cause of infertility in women.

The experience of infertility can cause a great deal of psychological distress (Cousineau & Downar, 2007). As most women spend many years protecting themselves against pregnancy, they are shocked when they discover they are infertile. They experience a sense of loss of control. Their self-esteem and self-worth may diminish if they feel defective and unfeminine. Infertile women have been found to have higher levels of depression and anxiety compared to fertile women and women in general outpatient clinics. Women often feel guilty, seeing their infertility as punishment for real or imagined past "sins." They may feel envious of women with children and find it difficult to attend child-centered events such as showers and new-baby celebrations. Marriages may be either stressed or strengthened as couples blame each other or work together to come to a resolution. If they tell others they are infertile, they may elicit feelings of pity or, in some societies, diminished status and isolation. If they do not tell, others may assume they do not want children and view them as selfish and unwilling to spoil their lifestyle by having children.

Not all couples who are infertile proceed to treatment. This may be due to lack of knowledge or funds, or merely acceptance of whatever fate hands out. For those who do seek answers, the investigation and treatment can be extremely stressful. Their lives may become fertility-focused, with schedules revolving around appointments and clinic visits. Work gets interrupted and vacations put on hold. Their sexual life changes from a pleasurable activity to a mandatory, scheduled procedure. Choosing a fertility clinic is also stressful. The Fertility Clinic Success Rate and Certification Act (FCSRCA) of 1992 mandates that clinics performing artificial reproductive technologies (ART) annually provide data for all procedures performed to the Centers for Disease Control and Prevention (CDC) (Table 66.1). The CDC is required to use these data to report and publish clinic-specific success rates (CDC, 2011). It is important to distinguish between pregnancy rates and live birth rates. Also, rates vary with age and the cause of the infertility.

The first step in infertility treatment is to ensure that couples are having adequate intercourse at times of ovulation. The use of small doses of clomiphene may allow couples to more accurately predict ovulation. Clomiphene is started between days 3 and 5 of the cycle and continued for five days. It is an anti-estrogen that lowers the levels of circulating estrogen. This then causes the hypothalamus to produce gonadotropin-releasing hormone (GRH), which, in turn acts on the pituitary to produce more follicle-stimulating hormone (FSH) and luteinizing hormone (LH). Ovulation occurs between cycle days 14 and 19, allowing the couple

Table 66.1 FERTILITY TREATMENT LIVE BIRTH RATES

PROCEDURE	SUCCESS RATES		
	Combined	<35 yrs.	43–44 yrs.
Intrauterine Insemination:			
Without fertility drugs	5–7%		
Plus infertility drugs	20%		
Intrusive Procedures:			
Non-donor fresh embryos		41.2%	4.9%
Non-donor frozen embryos		35.2%	15.1%
Donor fresh embryos	55.1%		
Donor frozen embryos	34%		

Figures from Centers from Disease Control and Protection, *ART Reports*, Dec. 2, 2011.

to plan intercourse for when it would be most successful. Narrrowing the precise time of ovulation can also be assisted by the use of an ovulation predictor kit that uses a urine sample to predict when ovulation is about to occur by measuring the LH level; these are available without a prescription in most pharmacies. Basal thermometers are also useful in detecting ovulation. For the first part of the cycle, women's temperatures at rest are in the 97 to 97.5°F degree range. Just prior to ovulation, the temperature increases to be in the 97.5 to 98.6°F degree range, where it remains for the rest of the cycle. Basal thermometers measure changes as small as one tenth of a degree. Measuring across several cycles allows women to discover their patterns of changes and predict the timing of ovulation.

If these simple steps do not solve the problem, next steps would include hormonal assessments, semen analysis, and ultrasound. Couples who are still unsuccessful may go on to more invasive investigations such as hysterosalpingogram, laparoscopy, hysteroscopy, or testicular biopsy.

Although men and women are equally likely to be the cause of the infertility (30–50% of infertility is attributable to female factors, 30–40% to male factors, and 20–30% to both members of the couple), women have to endure the bulk of the procedures designed to correct infertility. In artificial insemination using partner sperm, the male sperm are washed, concentrated, and injected into the uterus at the time of ovulation. Success rates are high, and psychological effects on the woman may be minimal, although the male partner may have to deal with some feelings of inadequacy. When the insemination is done using donor sperm, the issues may become more complicated (Leiblum & Aviv, 1997). The man may feel jealous or threatened; 47–92% of couples intend to keep the nature of the conception secret. Although some couples may have difficulty, research has failed to reveal psychological problems in couples who have donor insemination. They appear to be well adjusted, have

stable marriages and healthy relationships with the children (Brewaeys, 1996).

Other types of infertility treatments are more invasive for the woman. Gamete intrafallopian transfer, intracytoplasmic sperm injection (ICSI), and *in vitro* fertilization (IVF) all require that the woman take heavy doses of fertility drugs and undergo ova retrieval by laparoscopy. Drugs used to treat infertility, such as clomiphene citrate, human menopausal gonadotropin, and Gonadotropin Releasing Hormone (GnRH) analogues have been associated with depressive side effects (Daniluk & Fluker, 1995). Often these side effects are overlooked, as people assume that the woman's anxiety or depressive symptoms are related to the psychological stress of the infertility program. Fertility drugs may also cause bloating or weight gain, which can affect body image, self-esteem, and mood. In rare cases, they may cause ovarian hyperstimulation, which causes a buildup of fluid in the chest and abdomen, resulting in abdominal pain, nausea, shortness of breath, bloating, and a weight gain of up to 10 lbs. in 3–5 days.

IN VITRO FERTILIZATION (IVF)

At initial presentation, IVF candidates do not differ from non-IVF couples with respect to depression, although they may demonstrate some anxiety (Verhaak et al., 2007). Couples seeking IVF may be worried about being refused treatment if they appear to be too emotional. It may also be that only the strongest survivors of years of infertility treatments continue on to this stage.

Infertility treatments put couples on a rollercoaster of optimism, hope, and disappointment, with a slight increase in anxiety at the time of egg retrieval and pregnancy testing, and an increase in depression scores after one or more unsuccessful treatment cycles. When IVF results in pregnancy, the negative emotions disappear, indicating that treatment-induced stress is considerably related to threats of failure. Dropout rates from IVF are quite high, even when the treatments are free (Van den Broeck et al., 2009). Generally, the psychological burden appears to be the most frequently named reason to discontinue infertility treatments. Some couples feel that after one or two cycles they can quit, knowing they have done everything they could to have a child. Couples who continue with the program but do not conceive after several cycles must decide whether to continue with the treatment, think about adoption, or come to terms with childlessness. The women for whom IVF is ultimately unsuccessful face not merely the loss of a pregnancy, but the loss of the ability to become pregnant. Although there are few longitudinal studies of follow-up after failure of IVF, so far there is no compelling evidence for significant negative emotional consequences of unsuccessful treatment, although a considerable number show subclinical emotional problems. However, although an individual or couple may seem to successfully resign themselves to the lack of success of IVF, there are many who would immediately jump at the chance were a new fertility treatment to present itself.

Counseling may be required if the woman or couple display significant negative affects during the IVF cycle or react with considerable despair to the news that the cycles have been unsuccessful. Counseling is best done by someone familiar with the specific techniques and emotional challenges of infertility treatments and should include discussion of healthy coping techniques. The couple may need help in deciding when to stop the IVF. This is a very individual decision that is based on many factors, including psychological stress, physical burden, financial burden, age, the importance of having a child with their own genetic makeup, pressure from relatives, and stresses between the partners.

OOCYTE DONATION

The procedure of using oocytes donated by young, healthy women as a treatment for infertility has expanded the number of infertile women who can get pregnant. Egg donation has the highest success rate (47–50%) of any fertility treatment. Eggs may be donated anonymously (residual healthy eggs from women undergoing IVF) or openly by a relative giving altruistically, or a stranger who is paid. There has been limited research on the psychological impact of women who receive these donations. These women have already experienced the mental health consequences of infertility and many have gone through the full range of treatments. On one hand, they are grateful that ovum donation may allow them to become pregnant, but they must come to terms with the loss of making a biological contribution to their offspring. If the partner's sperm is used, it may be difficult to accept that he has a closer biological tie to the child than she does (Carter et al., 2011). For most women, however, experiencing the pregnancy makes her feel that she is the mother of this child. She also must begin to think about what and to whom she will disclose about the nature of the pregnancy. Over the last several years, as ovum donation has become more common, families appear to be becoming more open to talking about how they conceived (Greenfeld, 2002). The couple and the donor must decide what degree of contact they will have. This can become more complicated when the donor is a relative. Counseling may be required to help the woman accept the child as her own, deal with any residual sense of inadequacy. and decide how she will deal with disclosure.

PREGNANCY LOSS

MISCARRIAGE

Spontaneous abortion or miscarriage is defined as an unintended termination of pregnancy resulting in fetal death prior to 20 weeks of gestation. Between 12% and 24% of clinically recognized pregnancies end in miscarriage, mostly within the first trimester. Most studies agree that many women experience sad feelings or very intense grief in the first days following the loss, while some have found anxiety and depression still present even after one to two years (Brier, 2008). As well as sadness and depression, women may suffer from shock, disbelief, guilt, helplessness, and anger. They may have insomnia, loss of appetite, loss of interest in usual activities, and poor concentration. Many have feelings of failure and suffer from repetitive thoughts and dreams of the baby. They often have doubts about their own femininity and competence as women and fear infertility. As many miscarriages are due to unknown causes, women commonly blame themselves and conceptualize the loss as punishment for real or imagined things they did or did not do in the past or during the pregnancy (Robinson, Stirtzinger, Stewart, & Ralevski, 1994; Nikcevic, Tunkel, Kuczmierczyk, & Nicolaides, 1999).

A significant number of women report elevated levels of anxiety up to six months post-miscarriage and are at increased risk for obsessive-compulsive disorder (OCD) and post-traumatic stress disorder (PTSD; Brier, 2004). Robinson et al. (1994) found that the anxiety experienced often seemed worse than the depression, with 77.6% finding this was as great as any previously experienced stressor. Women with a history of miscarriages suffer more from pregnancy-specific anxieties in the first trimester of a new pregnancy than women with no history of miscarriage (Bergner, Beyer, Klapp, & Rauchfuss, 2008). Blackmore et al. (2011) found that anxiety and depression continued even after the birth of a subsequent healthy child.

Factors predictive of an increased risk of adverse psychological sequelae after miscarriage include: previous experience of the death of a loved one; a history of major depression; childlessness; high investment in the pregnancy; concerns regarding infertility; and lack of support from a partner, family, or friends (Lok & Neugebauer, 2007; Janssen, Cuisinier, de Graauw, & Hoogduin, 1997; Stirtzinger, Robinson, Stewart, & Ralevski, 1999). No clear relationship has been found between emotional adjustment after miscarriage and marital status, age, occupational status, social class, the duration of gestation, and a past history of miscarriage or previous therapeutic abortion (Neugebauer et al., 1997).

Each member of a couple may grieve differently, with the woman showing her emotions while her partner tries to help her and manage his own grief by burying his feelings and becoming involved in work and other activities (Kong, Chung, Lai, & Lok, 2010). The woman needs to be reassured that her grief is normal and will take some months to resolve. She should be warned that the date of the anniversary of the loss and the anticipated birth date may be times of increased distress. Grieving over a miscarriage is often complicated by the fact that there is no visible child, memories, or shared life experiences to mourn. Even if it is unofficial, the couple may wish to name the baby and have some sort of memorial service. As there are often no tangible mementos, they may buy something such as a charm for a bracelet to give a greater sense of identity to this child.

If the level of the woman's depression is excessively high or the length of her depression very prolonged, her grieving may have evolved into a major depressive episode that might benefit from medication and psychotherapy. Unjustified or excessive feelings of guilt and responsibility for the loss should be explored. She may need to be reassured that her wish to avoid other women who are pregnant or have new babies is normal and will eventually resolve. Couple therapy might be indicated to reinforce to the couple that they are both sharing in this sad event.

Women often complain that medical staff appear to be insensitive and unsympathetic, viewing the miscarriage as a minor medical event. Most women would benefit from a follow-up medical appointment in which they are given whatever information is known about the cause of the loss and their chances of becoming pregnant again (Nikcevic, Kuczmierczyk, & Nicolaides, 2007).

STILLBIRTH

Stillbirth is the death of a fetus after 20 weeks' gestation or after the fetus has reached 14 oz. in weight. As almost one-half of stillbirths occur after apparently uncomplicated pregnancies, most parents are unprepared for the death of the infant. This news may come in two ways: prenatal examinations may show the baby has died, forcing the woman to go through the induced delivery of a dead baby; or the baby may die in the process of the delivery. However the stillbirth comes about, anticipation and joy are suddenly replaced by despair. This loss of a desired child may lead to loss of confidence in the ability to produce a healthy child, and "traumatic grief," a syndrome differentiated from depression by the meaning and significance of the attachment that was lost (Bennett, Litz, Lee, & Maguen, 2005). In some cultures, this grief is enhanced by beliefs that such losses are caused by the mother's "sins" or "evil spirits" (Froen et al., 2011).

Common response protocols involve telling the parents (with little supporting evidence) that looking at and holding the baby will help them mourn and speed up the recovery from grief. Although holding the baby is supposed to be optional, well-meaning staff can subtly pressure the couple into complying. Hughes, Turton, Hopper, & Evans (2002) raised questions about this protocol after finding that mothers who held their stillborn babies had higher rates of depression (39%) than women who had just seen their babies (21%) or those who had had no contact (6%). Women who saw their babies also had higher rates of anxiety and PTSD, persisting up to seven years post-stillbirth (Turton, Evans, & Hughes, 2009) and were more likely to have experienced partnership breakdown. However, numerous methodological problems in these studies suggest caution about accepting these conclusions.

The best current approach allows parents to choose whether or not to see or hold the stillborn child. Parents need to hear any available information about the reason for the loss. Counselors can help the couple deal with practical issues such as funeral plans, as well as presenting options such as naming the child, taking a picture, and keeping mementos. The counselor can also give information about the grieving process and supports available. Assuming that all bereaved parents require intense crisis interventions may be at best unnecessary and at worst intrusive, potentially creating more distress. Follow-up therapy should be available for those who require it.

There is also controversy about the timing of future pregnancies. Turton, Hughes, Evans, and Fainman (2001) found

that a perceived low level of support during the stillbirth, as well as conceiving within a year of the loss, increases the risk of PTSD (lifetime prevalence rates of 29% and 21% in the third trimester of the pregnancy following the stillbirth) and results in higher rates of depression both during the third trimester and one year after the follow-up pregnancy. In contrast, Franche (2001) found that increased time between loss and subsequent conception was predictive of increased grief. The conclusion can only be that there is no universal approach that works for all couples.

TERMINATION FOR GENETIC INDICATIONS

Genetic terminations or terminations for genetic indications are highly stressful events. Some women choose to become pregnant knowing that they are carriers of a genetic defect and worry they will pass this defect along to the fetus. They therefore anxiously await the results of prenatal diagnostic testing. In other cases, the woman encounters a problem during pregnancy, such as being exposed to German measles, and then must decide whether or not to terminate the pregnancy (Statham, Solomou, & Chitty, 2000). In the third instance, a woman over the age of 35 might discover that the fetus has an abnormality associated with maternal age after routine prenatal diagnostic testing.

Once an abnormality is detected, the woman or couple must make a decision about whether or not to terminate the pregnancy (Sandelowski & Barroso, 2005). The couple might decide to use the genetic information obtained in order to plan and prepare for the birth of a child with potential difficulties. Factors contributing to a couples' decision to terminate the pregnancy after a positive finding on prenatal diagnostic testing include: the prognosis for the child, their beliefs about having an abortion, concerns about the child's welfare, and feelings about the potential disruption to other children and their own marriage and family life.

In an elective termination following the detection of a genetic disorder, the couple must not only face the loss of a wanted pregnancy but must make a conscious decision to end a pregnancy for a problem that is not necessarily going to result in fetal death. Even in the case of severe abnormalities, the decision to terminate is a difficult one and may be associated with ambivalence, guilt, and grief (Rillstone & Hutchinson, 2001). As genetic testing technology grows, couples are more often being confronted with the news of mosaicism or chromosomal disorders in which the outcome is unclear, forcing them to make a decision based on limited information. In these cases, there may be heightened ambivalence, doubt, and grief. Couples who know they are carriers of a genetic abnormality may feel an excess of guilt, knowing that they caused their fetus to have problems. They may also struggle with the concern that they will never be able to produce a healthy baby.

There is usually little time between the revelation of the abnormality and the termination. A woman terminating a pregnancy after genetic amniocentesis, which occurs in the second trimester, must go through a very difficult procedure. She requires an induction and goes through an actual labor knowing she will deliver a dead infant. She may not be given necessary medication to help ease her discomfort, and delivery may take place in her bed when she is alone. All of this adds to the stress of the termination (Robinson, 2011). Women have identified this loss to be equal to or more stressful than any previous trauma in their lives (Robinson, Carr, Olmsted, & Wright, 1991). Couples may be supportive or direct their anger and frustration toward each other.

This negative experience can be moderated in many ways. Couples going for amniocentesis should be encouraged to think about what their decision would be if an abnormality is found; counseling should be available for couples who find it difficult to think this through. If an abnormality is discovered, genetic counseling should provide as much information as possible about the risks and outcome of any defect. Couples undergoing a termination should be treated with dignity and respect, including being given detailed information about the process, not being placed on a maternity ward, receiving appropriate pain relief, and being checked on regularly.

Many couples hesitate to inform others of their decision to terminate the pregnancy, fearing negative judgements. This, however, can leave them feeling isolated and alone in dealing with their grief. Pretending that the woman just miscarried may allow some support, but does not encompass the ambivalence and grief that is inherent in making this kind of decision. Medical staff can also have negative attitudes toward a couple if they feel the couple is terminating the pregnancy for what they regard is an insufficient reason, such as the detection of Turner's syndrome.

Management of a possible loss should begin with counseling before prenatal testing (Robinson, 2011). Couples who are known carriers should discuss the probability of passing on a problem to the fetus and carefully think about the choices they would like to make. The woman, individually or with her partner, may benefit from counseling and support at the time of the termination. They should be given opportunities but not be forced to view the baby after delivery. Getting a view of any deformities could give the couple confirmation that they had made the correct decision but also may be extremely traumatic for them. For the couple who do not chose to see the baby after delivery, the hospital staff should, with the parent's permission, take pictures of the appropriately draped baby so that, should they regret their initial decision, the couple may view the images in the future. This visualization of the baby may aid in the grieving process. Although the option of burial or officially naming the baby will vary according to the birth weight and the couple's religion, they may be encouraged to personally give the baby a name or hold some sort of memorial service.

For some women and their partners, the grieving is a normal response to loss. In other cases, past and current issues and conflicts, including guilt about passing on a genetic defect, feelings of inadequacy as a woman, concern about being punished for past events, marital problems, and social and family pressures to have a child, may complicate the grieving and require further psychological intervention. Parents sometimes forget about the need to give an explanation to preexisting children so they will not be left with fears that their parents will take them to the hospital and "leave them there."

Groups for women or couples who have had genetic terminations can be a helpful way of sharing the pain and resolving the grief.

INDUCED ABORTION

Induced abortion is a common but highly charged religious and political topic with dissenting groups expressing their feelings very passionately, sometimes to the point of violence. And yet, it is a very common procedure. The World Health Organization (2005) estimates that of the approximately 211 million pregnancies that occur worldwide each year, 46 million end in induced abortion. The decision to terminate a pregnancy is seldom made lightly. The consequences of such a decision are influenced not only by the woman's previous level of coping and life circumstances, but also by her interpersonal relationships, the social and religious context, and the access to safe procedures carried out in a nonjudgemental atmosphere.

It is difficult to differentiate the consequences of induced abortion from the effects of the distress caused by the pregnancy itself. An unwanted pregnancy may be the result of a sexual assault or incest or the unintentional consequence of contraceptive failure. A woman may desire a child, but the nature of her current life circumstances, poor or absent partner relationships, social pressures, or future plans cause her to believe it is currently problematic. Women who consider abortion are, therefore, already under stress.

Anti-choice/anti-abortion groups have tried to bolster their position by asserting that abortion causes permanent, serious physical and psychological damage. These groups continue to maintain that abortion increases the risk of developing breast cancer despite the 2009 position statement by the American Congress of Obstetricians and Gynaecologists (Committee on Gynecologic Practice, 2009) that a review of methodologically sound studies demonstrated no causal relationship between induced abortion and a subsequent increase in breast cancer risk.

Anti-choice groups also claimed to have identified an "abortion trauma syndrome" that includes depression (Reardon & Cougle, 2002), anxiety (Cougle, Reardon, & Coleman, 2005), and an increased risk of suicide (Reardon et al., 2003), hospitalization (Reardon et al., 2003) and substance abuse (Reardon & Ney, 2000). These studies have been shown to be methodologically very flawed (Robinson, Stotland, Russo, Lang, & Occhiogrosso, 2009). Research using sound methodology has shown that, although most women having an induced abortion have transient feelings of ambivalence, guilt, and sadness, the majority of women tend to feel increasingly relieved and comfortable with their decisions and, in many cases, have an improvement in life satisfaction and success (Schmiege & Russo, 2005; Robinson et al., 2009; Major et al., 2000; Munk-Olsen, Laursen, Pedersen, Lidegaard, & Mortensen, 2011).

Past psychiatric history is the most consistent predictor of psychiatric disorders following abortion (Dagg, 1991; Stotland, 1992; Gilchrist, Hannaford, Frank, & Kay, 1995). Outcome may also be affected by the attitudes of picketers at abortion clinics (Cozzarelli, Major, Karrasch, & Fuegen, 2000) or medical staff who may appear hostile. Religious factors may be extremely important to consider, particularly for women associated with religious groups that condemn abortion as a sin.

Women who lack access to safe and legal abortions are under enormous stress. They may be forced to stay in abusive relationships or may undergo illegal or unsafe abortions that could lead to permanent physical or psychological trauma (Stotland, 1992). Children born after the mother was denied an abortion are more likely to drop out of school, be less satisfied with their jobs and relationships, be in treatment for mental health conditions, be sent to prison, or have parenting difficulties (David, 2011). "Denial of abortion lays the foundation for an environment in which children are poorly reared, which subsequently leads to mental health and psychosocial problems for the unwanted child" (David, 2011).

Most women who are seeking an abortion have already decided to go ahead with the procedure. Although they can benefit from a sensitive, supportive atmosphere, they do not usually require psychiatric consultation. Women should be referred prior to abortion if they have a major psychiatric disorder, have marked ambivalence about terminating the pregnancy, are being subjected to marked external pressure to end or keep the pregnancy, or if the pregnancy is the result of sexual assault. Consultants who feel their own personal beliefs interfere with their giving nonjudgemental information and support should refer the patient to a therapist capable of neutrality.

The presence of a current or previous major psychiatric disorder is not necessarily a reason for terminating the pregnancy. In the case of a current major mental illness, the patient should be evaluated for suicidal or homicidal ideation and competency to make a decision about pregnancy termination. Adequate treatment, support, and, if necessary, hospitalization should be arranged. Ideally, the decision to terminate can be postponed until the woman's current psychiatric problems improve so that she is able to make a decision about termination. Although many women with a history of major psychiatric illnesses can adequately parent, in the case of a woman with chronic and severe mental illness, one must consider her ability to mother and the risk of bearing a child only to have to give up custody. All options should be discussed, including continuing with the pregnancy and giving the child up for adoption. This may be possible if the woman has enough insight into her illness to be very compliant with treatment during the pregnancy while, at the same time, would not be too heart-broken by bearing a child only to give it up.

Women who are highly ambivalent about the pregnancy should be encouraged to delay decision making as long as safely possible, to allow time to explore the decision. When the ambivalence appears irresolvable, it probably indicates either a strong wish to have the child or obsessive personality traits. The patient should consider the option of continuing with the pregnancy and deciding at birth whether or not to keep the child. If the pregnant woman is being pressured by her partner or family to terminate or alternately to keep the pregnancy, the psychiatrist should help her clarify her own wishes and reinforce her right to make a responsible personal decision. It may be helpful to meet with the couple or family to try to help resolve the differences. Women whose religion forbids abortion may feel extremely conflicted. Some rigid pastors may only reinforce their guilt, while others may be more understanding in helping them balance their religious beliefs with their current needs. A religious woman who is considering abortion has already felt overwhelmed by the idea of having a child at this time. The psychiatrist cannot make a decision for her but may be able to frame the decision in a different light; i.e., viewing the abortion not a selfish act but as the act of someone who cares about the welfare of this unwanted child.

Most women do not require psychiatric intervention post-abortion. Those few women who continue to have or develop a major psychiatric disorder should receive the appropriate combination of support, psychotherapy, medication, and/or hospitalization. Psychotherapy may focus on themes of grief, loss, guilt, and the situations and conflicts that led to the unwanted pregnancy and the need to abort.

In summary, not all women who suffer from infertility or pregnancy loss require counseling (Robinson, 2014). They should not automatically be referred for counseling but offered the opportunity for support should they need it. For some women, support groups of other women dealing with infertility or pregnancy loss may help them express feelings, have their grief acknowledged, and discover their reactions are normal. These losses happen to individuals with personal histories and specific current stressors and supports. Some women or couples may be more likely to develop major depressive disorders or PTSD. These people may also require a referral to a mental health professional for psychotherapy and medication (Van den Broeck, Emery, Wischmann & Thorn, 2010).

CLINICAL PEARLS

- Generally, psychological burden appears to be the most frequently named reason to discontinue infertility treatments.

- Egg donation has the highest success rate (47–50%) of any fertility treatment.

- Between 12% and 24% of clinically recognized pregnancies end in miscarriage, mostly within the first trimester.

- Post-miscarriage women are at increased risk for OCD and PTSD.

- Anxiety experienced after miscarriage often seems worse than the depression.

- Most women who have had a miscarriage would benefit from a follow-up medical appointment in which they are given whatever information is known about the cause of the loss and the chances of becoming pregnant again.

- The best current approach allows parents to choose whether or not to see or hold the stillborn child.

- For women who terminate pregnancy because of a genetic finding, guilt about passing on a genetic defect, feelings of inadequacy as a woman, concern about being punished for past events, marital problems and social and family pressures to have a child, may complicate the grieving.

- Groups for women or couples who have had genetic terminations can be helpful.

- Although most women having an induced abortion have transient feelings of ambivalence, guilt, and sadness, the majority tend to feel increasingly relieved and comfortable with their decisions.

DISCLOSURE STATEMENT

Dr. Robinson is an employee of the University of Toronto and works at the University Health Network in Toronto, Canada. She has no ties to any pharmaceutical companies. She has no conflicts to disclose.

REFERENCES

Bennett, S. M., Litz, B. T., Lee, B. S., & Maguen, S. (2005). The scope and impact of perinatal loss: Current status and future directions. *Professional Psychology: Research and Practice, 36*(2), 180–187.

Bergner, A., Beyer, R., Klapp, B. F., & Rauchfuss, M. (2008). Pregnancy after early pregnancy loss: a prospective study of anxiety, depressive symptomatology and coping. *Journal of Psychosomatic Obstetrics & Gynaecology, 29*(2), 105–113.

Blackmore, E. R., Cote-Arsenault, D., Tang, W., Glover, V., Evans, J., Golding, J., et al. (2011). Previous prenatal loss as a predictor of perinatal depression and anxiety. *British Journal of Psychiatry, 198*(5), 373–378.

Brewaeys, A. (1996). Donor insemination, the impact on family and child development. *Journal of Psychosomatic Obstetrics & Gynaecology, 17*(1), 1–13.

Brier, N. (2004). Anxiety after miscarriage: a review of the empirical literature and implications for clinical practice. *Birth, 31*(2), 138–142.

Brier, N. (2008). Grief following miscarriage: a comprehensive review of the literature. *Journal of Women's Health (Larchmont), 17*(3), 451–464.

Carter, J., Applegarth, L., Josephs, L., Grill, E., Baser, R. E., & Rosenwaks, Z. (2011). A cross-sectional cohort study of infertile women awaiting oocyte donation: the emotional, sexual, and quality-of-life impact. *Fertility & Sterility, 95*(2), 711–716.

Center for Disease Control and Prevention (2011). Assisted Reproductive Technology (ART), at http://www.cdc.gov/art/ARTReports.htm. Updated July 10, 2014; accessed July 28, 2014.

Committee on Gynecologic Practice (2009). ACOG Committee Opinion No. 434: Induced abortion and breast cancer risk. *Obstetrics & Gynecology, 113*(6), 1417–1418.

Cougle, J. R., Reardon, D. C., & Coleman, P. K. (2005). Generalized anxiety following unintended pregnancies resolved through childbirth and abortion: a cohort study of the 1995 National Survey of Family Growth. *Journal of Anxiety Disorders, 19*(1), 137–142.

Cousineau, T. M., & Downar, A. D. (2007). Psychological impact of infertility. *Best Practice & Research Clinical Obstetrics & Gynaecology, 21*(2), 293–308.

Cozzarelli, C., Major, B., Karrasch, A., & Fuegen, K. (2000). Women's experiences of and reactions to antiabortion picketing. *Basic and Applied Social Psychology, 22*(4), 265–275.

Dagg, P. K. (1991). The psychological sequelae of therapeutic abortion—denied and completed. *American Journal of Psychiatry, 148*(5), 578–585.

Daniluk, J. C., & Fluker, M. (1995). Fertility drugs and the reproductive imperative: assisting the fertile woman. In J. A. Hamilton, M. F. Jensvol, E. Rothblum, & E. Cole (Eds.), *Psychopharmacology from a feminist perspective* (pp. 31–48). New York: Haworth.

David, H. P. (2011). Born unwanted: mental health costs and consequences. *American Journal of Orthopsychiatry, 81*(2), 184–192.

Franche, R. L. (2001). Psychologic and obstetric predictors of couples' grief during pregnancy after miscarriage or perinatal death. *Obstetrics & Gynecology, 97*(4), 597–602.

Froen, J. F., Cacciatore, J., McClure, E. M., Kuti, O., Jokhio, A. H., Islam, M., et al. (2011). Stillbirths: why they matter. *Lancet, 377*(9774), 1353–1366.

Gilchrist, A. C., Hannaford, P. C., Frank, P., & Kay, C. R. (1995). Termination of pregnancy and psychiatric morbidity. *British Journal of Psychiatry, 167*(2), 243–248.

Greenfeld, D. A. (2002). Changing attitudes towards third-party reproductive techniques. *Current Opinion in Obstetrics & Gynecology, 14*(3), 289–292.

Hughes, P., Turton, P., Hopper, E., & Evans, C. D. (2002). Assessment of guidelines for good practice in psychosocial care of mothers after stillbirth: a cohort study. *Lancet, 360*(9327), 114–118.

Janssen, H. J., Cuisinier, M. C., de Graauw, K. P., & Hoogduin, K. A. (1997). A prospective study of risk factors predicting grief intensity following pregnancy loss. *Archives of General Psychiatry, 54*(1), 56–61.

Kong, G. W., Chung, T. K., Lai, B. P., & Lok, I. H. (2010). Gender comparison of psychological reaction after miscarriage—a 1-year longitudinal study. *British Journal of Obstetrics & Gynaecology, 117*(10), 1211–1219.

Leiblum, S. R., & Aviv, A. L. (1997). Disclosure issues and decisions of couples who conceived via donor insemination. *Journal of Psychosomatic Obstetrics & Gynaecology, 18*(4), 292–300.

Lok, I. H., & Neugebauer, R. (2007). Psychological morbidity following miscarriage. *Best Practice & Research Clinical Obstetrics & Gynaecology, 21*(2), 229–247.

Major, B., Cozzarelli, C., Cooper, M. L., Zubek, J., Richards, C., Wilhite, M., et al. (2000). Psychological responses of women after first-trimester abortion. *Archives of General Psychiatry, 57*(8), 777–784.

Munk-Olsen, T., Laursen, T. M., Pedersen, C. B., Lidegaard, O., & Mortensen, P. B. (2011). Induced first-trimester abortion and risk of mental disorder. *New England Journal of Medicine, 364*(4), 332–339.

Neugebauer, R., Kline, J., Shrout, P., Skodol, A., O'Connor, P., Geller, P. A., et al. (1997). Major depressive disorder in the 6 months after miscarriage. *Journal of the American Medical Association, 277*(5), 383–388.

Nikcevic, A. V., Kuczmierczyk, A. R., & Nicolaides, K. H. (2007). The influence of medical and psychological interventions on women's distress after miscarriage. *Journal of Psychosomatic Research, 63*(3), 283–290.

Nikcevic, A. V., Tunkel, S. A., Kuczmierczyk, A. R., & Nicolaides, K. H. (1999). Investigation of the cause of miscarriage and its influence on women's psychological distress. *British Journal of Obstetrics & Gynaecology, 106*(8), 808–813.

Reardon, D. C., & Cougle, J. R. (2002). Depression and unintended pregnancy in the National Longitudinal Survey of Youth: a cohort study. *British Medical Journal, 324*(7330), 151–152.

Reardon, D. C., Cougle, J. R., Rue, V. M., Shuping, M. W., Coleman, P. K., & Ney, P. G. (2003). Psychiatric admissions of low-income women following abortion and childbirth. *Canadian Medical Association Journal, 168*(10), 1253–1256.

Reardon, D. C., & Ney, P. G. (2000). Abortion and subsequent substance abuse. *American Journal of Drug Alcohol Abuse, 26*(1), 61–75.

Rillstone, P., & Hutchinson, S. A. (2001). Managing the reemergence of anguish: pregnancy after a loss due to anomalies. *Journal of Obstetrics, Gynecology, & Neonatal Nursing, 30*(3), 291–298.

Robinson G. E. (2014). Pregnancy Loss. Best Practice & Research. *Clinical Obstetrics & Gynecology, 28*(1), 169–178.

Robinson, G. E., Carr, M. L., Olmsted, M. P., & Wright, C. (1991). Psychological reactions to loss after prenatal diagnostic testing: preliminary results. *Journal of Psychocomatic Obstetrics & Gynaecology, 12*(3), 181–192.

Robinson, G. E., Stirtzinger, R., Stewart, D. E., & Ralevski, E. (1994). Psychological reactions of women followed for 1 year after miscarriage. *Journal of Reproductive & Infant Psychology, 12*(1), 31–36.

Robinson, G. E., Stotland, N. L., Russo, N. F., Lang, J. A., & Occhiogrosso, M. (2009). Is there an "abortion trauma syndrome"? Critiquing the evidence. *Harvard Review of Psychiatry, 17*(4), 268–290.

Robinson, G. E. (2011). Dilemmas related to pregnancy loss. *Journal of Nervous & Mental Disease, 199*(8), 571–574.

Sandelowski, M., & Barroso, J. (2005). The travesty of choosing after positive prenatal diagnosis. *Journal of Obstetrics, Gynecology, & Neonatal Nursing, 34*(3), 307–318.

Sanders, K. A., Bruce, N. W. (1999). Psychosocial stress and treatment outcome following assisted reproductive technology. *Human Reproduction, 14*, 1656–1662.

Schmiege, S., & Russo, N. F. (2005). Depression and unwanted first pregnancy: longitudinal cohort study. *British Medical Journal, 331*(7528), 1303.

Statham, H., Solomou, W., & Chitty, L. (2000). Prenatal diagnosis of foetal abnormality: Psychological effects on women in low risk pregnancies. *Balliere's Clinical Obstetrics and Gynaecology, 14*(4), 731–747.

Stotland, N. L. (1992). The myth of the abortion trauma syndrome. *Journal of the American Medical Association, 268*(15), 2078–2079.

Stirtzinger, R. M., Robinson, G. E., Stewart, D. E., & Ralevski, E. (1999). Parameters of grieving in spontaneous abortion. *International Journal of Psychiatry in Medicine, 29*(2), 235–249.

Turton, P., Evans, C., & Hughes, P. (2009). Long-term psychosocial sequelae of stillbirth: phase II of a nested case-control cohort study. *Archives of Women's Mental Health, 12*(1), 35–41.

Turton, P., Hughes, P., Evans, C. D., & Fainman, D. (2001). Incidence, correlates and predictors of post-traumatic stress disorder in the pregnancy after stillbirth. *British Journal of Psychiatry, 178*, 556–560.

Van den Broeck, U., Emery, M., Wischmann, T., Thorn, P. (2010). Counselling in infertility: Individual, couple and group interventions. *Patient Education & Counseling, 81*, 422–428.

Van den Broeck, U., Holvoet, L., Enzlin, P., Bakelants, E., Demyttenaere, K., & D'Hooghe, T. (2009). Reasons for dropout in infertility treatment. *Gynecologic & Obstetric Investigation, 68*(1), 58–64.

Verhaak, C. M., Smeenk, J. M., Evers, A. W., Kremer, J. A., Kraaimaat, F. W., & Braat, D. D. (2007). Women's emotional adjustment to IVF: a systematic review of 25 years of research. *Human Reproduction Update, 13*(1), 27–36.

Wischmann, T. H. (2003). Psychogenic infertility—myths and facts. *Journal of Assisted Reproduction & Genetics, 20*(12), 485–494.

World Health Organization (2005). Great expectations: making pregnancy safer. Chapter 3 in the *World Health Report "Make Every Mother and Child Count."* Geneva, Switzerland: WHO.

HORMONES AND MOOD

Gail Erlick Robinson and Sophie Grigoriadis

INTRODUCTION

The reproductive hormones, estrogen and progesterone, play a vital role in women's lives. When they function smoothly, menses are initiated, women have regular, non-painful periods, are fertile and pass into menopause easily. Under or over-production of endogenous hormones can lead to problems such as infertility or dysfunctional bleeding. As the reproductive hormones also affect the production and transportion of neurotransmitters responsible for mood, they may also be implicated in mood changes in premenstrual dysphoric disorders and during peri-menopause.

Women also take many types of exogenous reproductive hormones including oral contrceptives, drugs which affect ovarian function and fertility and hormone replacement therapy. Each of these exogenous uses come with benefits and risks.

EXOGENOUS HORMONES

ORAL CONTRACEPTIVES

Although many early studies found that women taking oral contraceptives (OCs) had incidences of depression ranging from 5–30% (Editor, *Drug Facts and Comparisons*, 1993), current research has determined that OC users experience less variability in affect across the entire menstrual cycle and less negative affect during menstruation (Oinonen & Mazmanian, 2002). In the Harvard Study of Moods and Cycles (Joffe, Cohen, & Harlow, 2003), researchers found that 16.3% of women noticed worsening of their moods while on OCs, 12.3% had an improvement, and 71.4% had no change. This discrepancy may be at least in part related to the fact that current OCs contain much lower doses of hormones than earlier versions. The subgroup of women who did experience negative moods when taking OCs were found to be more likely to: have a history of depression, psychiatric symptoms, dysmenorrhea, and premenstrual or pregnancy-related mood symptoms prior to OC use; have a family history of OC-related mood complaints; be in the postpartum period; or be under age 20.

Opinion is divided as to whether it is the estrogen or progesterone component of the OC that causes the most psychological side effects (Jensvold, 1996). Possible explanations for negative mood changes include: an estrogen-induced

pyridoxine (vitamin B6) deficiency resulting in decreased serotonin and gamma-Aminobutyric acid (GABA); progesterone and estrogen mediated GABA-induced inhibition and suppression of glutamate excitation; and progesterone-mediated increase in monoamine oxidase, leading to decreased serotonin (Oinonen & Mazmanian, 2002). Studies have been inconclusive, with some suggesting that OCs with higher doses of progesterone or higher ratios of progesterone to estrogen cause more depression, while others have found just the opposite. It may be that another variable is involved. For example, a lower ratio of progesterone to estrogen is associated with more negative mood changes in women with a history of premenstrual emotional symptoms, while higher progesterone to estrogen ratios are associated with increased negative mood effects in women without such a history. Monophasic OCs have a greater stabilizing effect on mood than triphasic OCs.

If a woman taking OCs becomes depressed, the best approach is to stop the medication and see if the depression is alleviated. Pyridoxine (25–50 micrograms) has been recommended as a treatment for OC-related depression, but there have been no controlled trials. Similarly, there have been no controlled trials of the use of antidepressants to treat OC-generated depression, but, as they are effective in treating premenstrual dysphoric disorder, it is reasonable to assume they could also treat this kind of depression. Because of the controversy about the contribution of estrogen versus progesterone and the ideal combination for mood regulation, it is difficult to recommend appropriate oral contraceptives; but, generally, one should try an OC with a lower progesterone dose, a less androgenic progesterone, and/or eliminate estrogen altogether.

HORMONE REPLACEMENT THERAPY AND ESTROGEN REPLACEMENT THERAPY

Hormone replacement therapy (HRT) refers to a number of drugs, all of which have in common the presence of both an estrogen and progestin. The short-term benefit of HRT involves the minimization or elimination of menopausal changes such as hot flashes and genito-urinary atrophy. HRT used only for the treatment of hot flashes should be continued for approximately two to three years.

For many years, HRT was recommended for long-term use, not only to keep women looking younger (Wilson,

1968), but to prevent osteoporosis, cardiac problems, and dementia. The Women's Health Initiative (WHI) studies put an end to this idea (Rossouw et al., 2002). The results of their estrogen plus progestin study indicated that this combination resulted in a reduced risk of colorectal cancer and fewer fractures, but an increased risk of heart attack, stroke, blood clots, and dementia, with no protection against mild cognitive impairment. Estrogen alone resulted in a reduced risk of fracture, no differences in the risk for heart attack or colorectal cancer, an increased risk of stroke and blood clots, and an uncertain effect for breast cancer. Hundreds of thousands of women ceased taking HRT, and prescriptions dropped dramatically. After the initial shock, criticisms of the study's methodology began to be reported. Goodman, Goldzieher, and Ayala (2003); Klaiber, Vogel, and Rako (2005), and others noted that: the absolute rates of coronary heart disease (CHD), stroke, breast cancer, and pulmonary embolus, based on endpoints per 10,000 women-years, were marginally significant at best; the study did not last long enough to see beneficial effects; and there was a substantial dropout rate. Most important, they felt the population was not representative of the typical patient presenting to her physician for menopausal management of quality-of-life symptoms in early menopause; many of the women in the study were at least ten years post-menopause and already had evidence for underlying CHD, such as previous heart attack, angina, coronary artery bypass or graft, or coronary angioplasty.

A review of the current state of knowledge concerning the use of HRT summarizes the complicated risk and benefit issues (Taylor & Manson, 2011). Some of the confusion concerning HRT may be due to the timing of its use. Protection from atherosclerosis is evident only when hormone therapy is initiated proximal to the onset of menopause and before the development of advanced atherosclerosis. Greater distance from menopause, adverse lipid profiles, other cardiovascular disease risk, and family history may increase the risks of CHD with HRT use.

The risk of breast cancer varies according to the timing of treatment initiation. When HRT treatment was initiated within a three-year period from the onset of menopause, the detection of tumors increased, whereas it was not elevated when treatment was initiated after a greater than three-year absence from sex steroid exposure. It is likely that HRT exerts a promotional effect on preexisting, undetected, less aggressive, estrogen-responsive tumors, rather than initiating new tumors.

Unopposed estrogen use will cause endometrial hyperplasia or cancer in nearly half of women users within three years, although either continuous or sequential progestin administration largely negates the increased risk. There also appears to be a small but significantly increased risk of epithelial ovarian cancer in current and recent users of estrogen therapy.

The risk of dementia was shown to be increased by HRT in the WHI Memory Study. The effect of HRT and estrogen replacement therapy (ERT) on cognitive function in the same population was examined in the WHI Study of Cognitive Aging. Initiation of HRT close to menopause was not associated with improved cognition, and HRT did not significantly reduce dementia risk over the course of this study (Ryan et al., 2009). ERT did not appear to have an enduring helpful effect on cognitive function in older women.

The WHI also did not look at different types or routes of application of HRT. New information suggests that the risk of stroke (odds ratio [OR] 1.29) can be reduced by the use of transdermal HRT (Brown, 2010). The odds ratio of first-time venous thromboembolism in current users of oral estrogen therapy was significantly elevated. Although the thromboembolism risk was also elevated in users of transdermal estrogen preparations, the risk did not reach statistical significance. Oral regimens provide superior benefits on lipids, showing greater reductions in total cholesterol and low-density lipoprotein (LDL) and increases in high-density lipoprotein (HDL) than do transdermal preparations. However, clotting factors and triglycerides are raised to a greater degree by the use of oral preparations.

Hormone therapy remains an appropriate strategy for management of menopausal symptoms during the menopausal transition. Although there is an increased risk of certain cardiovascular outcomes and cancer, the absolute risk for these events is low, especially in the age group most in need of symptom relief. Symptomatic women will receive quality-of-life benefit from the use of hormone therapy, with minimal risk over the short term. Initiation of hormone therapy is not appropriate for women more than ten years from their last menstrual period or for those at high-baseline risk of cardiovascular disease. Assessing the risk–benefit ratio of HRT is very complicated. For example, the optimal time of estrogen initiation in regard to breast cancer is far different than for CHD. The timing hypothesis and the gap-time hypothesis do not allow for simultaneous optimization of breast and CHD risk reduction. Therefore, HRT or ERT should not be used for long-term disease prevention.

Bioidentical hormones are estradiol or progesterone compounded locally in pharmacies, allegedly in specific formulas suitable to the individual. The Food and Drug Administration (FDA) has noted that there is no evidence demonstrating superior efficacy or safety of estradiol administered in a compounded fashion to standard pharmaceutical HRT.

DRUGS THAT AFFECT OVARIAN FUNCTION

A number of drugs used to treat infertility, such as clomiphene citrate, human menopausal gonadotropin, and Gonadotropin Releasing Hormone (GnRH) analogues have also been associated with depressive side effects (Daniluk & Fluker, 1995). Often these side effects are overlooked, as people assume that the woman's anxiety or depressive symptoms are related to the psychological stress of the infertility program. Also, drugs such as danazol, used to treat endometriosis or premenstrual syndrome (PMS) by eliminating the ovarian cycle, have been found to have depressive side effects in themselves.

INTERACTIONS WITH PSYCHOTROPIC MEDICATION

It is important for the clinician to be aware that there may be an interaction between OCs and psychotropic medication (Jensvold, 1996). Ethinyl estradiol is metabolized by *UGT1A1*, CYP1A2, CYP3A, and inhibits CPY1A2, CPY2C9, CPY2C19, CPY2B6, and CPY3A. Progestin is metabolized by *CPY2C9*, CPY2C19, and CPY3A; and some progestins inhibit CPY2C9, CPY2C19, and CPY3A. Mood stabilizers such as carbamazepine, lamotrigine, and topirimate may increase the metabolism of OCs, leading to insufficient hormonal levels to suppress ovulation and an increased risk of contraceptive failure. This may be managed by increasing the dose of the oral contraceptive or switching to a drug such as valproate. OCs increase the levels of chlorpromazine and clozapine and may decrease levels of lamotrigine and valproic acid. There is some evidence to suggest that OCs inhibit the metabolism of tricyclic antidepressants in women, with a resultant increase in serum levels of the antidepressant. Imipramine blood levels should be regularly monitored and the antidepressant reduced if there are serious side effects. OCs may also interfere with the metabolism of some benzodiazepines, leading to decreased circulating levels of such drugs as lorazepam and temazepam, and increased levels of alprazolam and diazepam.

HORMONES AND MOOD

Estrogens have actions on the brain and the neurotransmitters. They affect neurite growth, neural survival, and synapse formation, and interact with brain-derived neurotrophic factor. They modulate many neurotransmitter systems, including dopamine, serotonin, norepinephrine, acetylcholine, and glutamate; but their main effect on mood more than likely has to do with their effect on the serotonergic system. Estrogen increases the availability, concentration, and utilization of serotonin by increasing the degradation of MAO; regulating free tryptophan available in the brain; enhancing transportation of serotonin; and increasing the density of 5-hydroxytriptamine (5HT)-inding sites in the areas of the brain that control mood and cognition. The decrease in monoamine oxidase (MAO) also results in increased availability of norepinephrine, dopamine, and GABA at neuronal synapses by increasing their release, reuptake, and enzymatic inactivation. The antidepressant effect of estrogen is purportedly related to estradiol-mediated normalization of hormonally sensitive neural circuits of depression activated in hormone-related depressions such as postpartum depression and menopause. It may also have a role in modulating feedback regulation of the hypothalamic-pituitary-adrenal (HPA) axis (Moses-Kolko, Berga, Kalro, Sit, & Wisner, 2009). Stress leads to activation of the hypothalamic–pituitary–adrenal (HPA) axis, which in turn leads to suppression of hypothalamic-pituitary-gonadal (HPG) activity through inhibition of gonadotropin-releasing hormone (GnRH) secretion. The functional effects of stress on reproduction can be seen with the suppression of luteinizing hormone (LH) release from the pituitary and suppression of sexual behavior. The stress effect on HPG function appears to be mediated by the adrenal stress hormones, glucocorticoids.

Studies about the effect of HRT on mood have shown that women who are not or are only mildly depressed may have an increased sense of well-being following the introduction of HRTs (Zweifel & O'Brien, 1997). However, although physiological doses of estrogen improve mood in non-psychiatric populations of symptomatic menopausal women, women who are given estrogen plus progesterone may experience a dampening of mood, compared with women who are given estrogen alone. The depressive effects of adding progesterone may be attenuated by a higher estrogen to progesterone dose ratio. There is no good evidence, however, to suggest that HRTs alone are effective in the treatment of a major depressive episode post-menopause. These women require the use of antidepressant medication, although the antidepressant effect may be enhanced by giving HRT. Whether this is related to a true augmentation effect of estrogen (Grigoriadis & Kennedy, 2002; Stoppe & Doren, 2002) or to the relief of troublesome menopausal symptoms is not clear. Moses-Kolko, Berga, Kalro, Sit, and Wisner (2009) have investigated the use of HRT or ERT for postpartum depressions and concluded that estradiol cannot as yet be considered as a first-line antidepressant.

Estrogen has been proposed as a treatment for schizophrenia because of the latter's high likelihood of presenting at times of hormonal change. A 2008 study found that giving 100 micrograms of transdermal estrogen to schizophrenic women significantly reduced positive and general psychopathological symptoms (Kulkarni et al., 2008). However, a Cochrane Review, updated in 2009, concluded that adjunctive estrogen, with or without progesterone, does not appear to offer convincing advantages over placebo in the treatment of schizophrenia (Chua, de Izquierdo, Kulkarni, & Mortimer, 2005).

ANDROGENS

Androgens play a role in female sexual functions. Women who undergo natural menopause continue to produce some androgen from cells in the ovary as well as the adrenals. Women with bilateral oophorectomies have a profound decrease in the levels of testosterone in the body. Decreased androgen has been related to a decrease in sexual desire in women. Giving combined estrogen-testosterone preparations to women who have experienced a decrease in libido after either natural or surgical menopause appears to enhance their sexual desire and interest (de Paula, Soares, Haidar, de Lima, & Baracat, 2007). The use of testosterone, 2.5 mg orally or 10 mg gel, either on its own or added to HRT, improves sexual desire, sexual function, and increases a sense of well-being in menopausal women. Possible adverse effects include hirsutism, acne, and a significant decrease in HDL cholesterol levels. At this time, testosterone therapy should be limited to short-term use (less than six months), as long-term studies are not available (Somboonporn, Bell, & Davis, 2011).

HYPERANDROGENISM

Disorders resulting in excess androgen may present as abnormal menstrual patterns, hirsutism, weight changes, and fatigue. Symptoms may also include virilization, including deepening of the voice, frontal balding, and clitoromegaly. Excess androgen can be found in polycystic ovarian syndrome (PCOS), adrenal hyperplasia, virilizing adrenal and ovarian tumors, Cushing's syndrome, and hyperprolactinemia.

POLYCYSTIC OVARY SYNDROME

PCOS is a condition characterized by abnormal regulation of reproductive hormones, including estrogens, progesterone, and androgen. Physical symptoms include weight gain, anovulatory or infrequent cycles resulting in impaired fertility, hirsutism, absent or abnormal menses, acne, ovarian cysts, and hypertension. It is also frequently accompanied by mood disorders. Between 5% and 10% of women of childbearing age have PCOS.

PCOS probably has a genetic basis, as there is often a positive family history in women as well as associated metabolic abnormalities in male family members. Although numerous genes are being explored, no genes are universally accepted as important in PCOS pathogenesis; thus there is no specific genetic test for vulnerability for this disorder (Goodarzi, 2008.) Dysregulation of the androgen-forming enzyme CYP17 results in increased androgen production by the theca cells of the ovary and in the adrenals, and lowered conversion of testosterone into estrogen. In some women, problems begin at puberty; while in others, PCOS may be precipitated by pregnancy, or excessive weight gain may result in insulinemia and insulin resistance. Hyperinsulinemia increases GnRH pulse frequency, LH over follicle-stimulating hormone (FSH) dominance, increased ovarian androgen production, and decreased follicular maturation, all contributing to the development of PCOS. Also, adipose tissue possesses an enzyme that converts androstenedione to estrone and testosterone to estradiol. Therefore, obese patients may have both excess androgens, resulting in hirsutism and virilization, and estrogens that inhibit FSH via negative feedback.

Some anti-epileptic medications that many bipolar women take as mood stabilizers can cause polycystic ovaries (O'Donovan, Kusumakar, Graves, & Bird, 2002). Valproic acid, lamotrigine, and oxcarbazepine all inhibit CPY17, leading to higher testosterone levels (Chiarelli, Coppola, D'Egidio, Parisi, & Verotti, 2009). Valproic acid appears to be the worst offender, but PCOS also happens more often to women with epilepsy taking this medication than to those being treated for bipolar disorder, suggesting that other interactions may be taking place (Bilo & Meo, 2008).

Disturbed ovarian function results in the failure of many primordial follicles to mature, resulting in multiple immature follicles that look like cysts. Ovulation becomes irregular, with resultant possible fertility problems. Although 90–95% of women attending infertility clinics with anovulation have PCOS, 60% will conceive, although it may take them longer.

These women also have a high risk of developing type II diabetes and cardiovascular disease (Guzick, 1998), endometrial hyperplasia, and endometrial cancer. Diagnosis can be made by physical examination, an ovarian ultrasound, and measuring various endocrine levels. The ratio of LH to FSH is greater than 1:1. Free testosterone is elevated, but generally no higher than 160 ng/dl—twice the normal level. Hyperinsulemia can be diagnosed by a peak insulin level of 150 mmol/l on the glucose tolerance test.

Women with PCOS have a higher rate of depressive symptoms than controls (Himelein & Thatcher, 2006). The factors that contribute to this elevated rate of depression are unclear. It appears to be unrelated to androgen levels (Rasgon et al., 2003) or hirsutism (Keegan, Liao, & Boyle, 2003). The presence of higher body mass plays some role but is not the only contributor (Weiner, Primeau, & Ehrmann, 2004). Tan et al. (2008) studied the impact of infertility on women with PCOS. They found that the PCOS group placed a greater priority on current unfulfilled wishes to have a child than other infertile women did. In addition, the self-esteem and emotional stability of the women in the PCOS group depended more on their ability to conceive than in the other infertile group. However, there was no direct link between the presence of infertility and the occurrence of depression, although, in cultures that emphasize having children, infertility plays a stronger role.

Weiner et al. (2004) have found that the greater anxiety experience by some PCOS women was attributable to a generally negative mood rather than an independent problem. There has been some discussion about the relationship between bipolar disorder and PCOS. Women with PCOS can experience profound feelings of despair (Kitzinger & Wilmot, 2002). They may feel unattractive or ugly if they are overweight, very hirsute, or have severe acne. They may worry about dating or finding a partner. Body dissatisfaction may lead to bingeing behavior, which, in turn may exacerbate the polycystic disease (Himelein & Thatcher, 2006). Not surprisingly, these women have less satisfactory sex lives and view themselves as less sexually attractive (Elsenbruch et al., 2003). Sexual problems appear to be related to their perception of their attractiveness, and no relationship has been found between their sexual functioning and androgen levels.

Appearance plays a role in their overall quality of life, especially in cultures where being thin is the ideal (McCook, Reame, & Thatcher, 2005). Barnard et al. (2007) found that women with PCOS had a lowered quality of life in all seven measures on the modified PCOS Quality of Life Scale (emotional disturbance, weight, infertility, acne, menstrual symptoms, menstrual predictability, and hirsutism). Weight was the largest contributor. Women taking anti-androgen medications generally had a better quality of life than those not taking them.

The management of PCOS should involve physical and psychological approaches (Teede, Deeks, & Moran, 2010). The goals include lowering insulin levels, restoring normal periods and preventing endometrial cancer, restoring fertility, and treating hirsutism and acne. There is no single approach that treats all of the clinical features. Weight loss is a difficult but essential component of management. Weight loss may improve abnormal glucose metabolism as well as decrease hyperandrogenism and improve ovarian function.

Fertility may be restored simply by losing weight. Treatment with an insulin sensitizer such as Metformin (500 mg t.i.d.) may reduce insulin resistance and improve ovulation, but it does not seem to improve fertility. Clomiphene citrate can increase the ovulation rate and improve chances for fertility. Ovarian drilling may be used for women whose cycles do not improve. This involves a laparoscope procedure to destroy, either by electrical impulses or laser, small areas of the ovary thought to be the centers of androgen production. With this procedure, approximately 80% of women have restored cycles, and 50% of these become pregnant. Women who conceive have a higher risk of miscarriage, gestational diabetes, preeclampsia, or preterm delivery, but this may be secondary to insulin resistance or weight problems.

Any type of combination oral contraceptive can decrease ovarian and adrenal production of androgen, reduce hair growth in hirsute patients, and also improve acne. Progesterone-only contraceptives may control the menstrual cycle and reduce the risk of endometrial cancer, but they will not help with hirsutism or acne.

Any of the treatments that reduce androgens have a beneficial effect on both hirsutism and acne. These include medroxyprogesterone acetate (20–40 mg daily or 150 mg intramuscularly [IM] every 6 weeks), GnRH agonists such as leuprolide acetate, and spironolactone 100–200 mg daily. Spironolactone seems particularly beneficial for the reduction of acne.

Patients should be screened for the presence of depression, anxiety, body dissatisfaction, and overall quality of life. If an antidepressant is required, avoid those that cause weight gain, such as mirtazapine. Concerns about appearance should be handled sensitively and not be dismissed as superficial. Information about nutrition, weight loss programs, exercise, depilatories or laser treatment for hirsutism, and acne treatment and prevention should be given. Counseling may be needed if the patient has problems changing her lifestyle to include exercise and weight control and/or has problems dealing with infertility.

PREMENSTRUAL SYNDROME AND PREMENSTRUAL DYSPHORIC DISORDER

The only distinctive thing about the over 150 symptoms that have been attributed to PMS is their relationship to the timing of a woman's menstrual cycle. Symptoms should start in the luteal phase, causing significant impairment in a woman's functioning, and disappear within the first few days of the menses. There must also be at least one symptom-free week during the woman's cycle. Of all the symptoms ascribed to PMS, the ones that most often bring women to their physicians for help are those of depression, anxiety, or irritability (Parry, 1999).

The American Psychiatric Association has devised a diagnostic category of *Premenstrual dysphoric disorder* (PMDD) to focus on the cases of PMS in which marked mood disturbance and a clinically significant impairment of functioning are the predominant symptoms (American Psychiatric Association, 1994). These symptoms must not be merely a premenstrual exacerbation of an ongoing psychiatric disorder. Approximately 1–5% of women meet criteria for PMDD. This disorder can lead to disrupted relationships, lowered productivity at work or school, and increased use of prescription and over-the-counter medications.

Various theories have been proposed to account for the relationship between PMS/PMDD and the menstrual cycle. Despite extensive investigations, researchers have been unable to find any relationship to the levels, ratios, or rates of change of progesterone or estrogen. It may be that either PMS/PMDD sufferers have an abnormal response to normal endocrine changes or that our current technology is not sophisticated enough to detect the relationship (Schmidt, Nieman, Danaceau, Adamas, & Rubinow, 1998). Similarly, researchers have been unable to find consistent proof of abnormalities in vitamin B_6 metabolism, prolactin levels, levels of prostaglandin, glucose tolerance, or the renin-angiotensin-aldosterone system. The most current theory is that, in some women, changes in hormonal levels in the HPG axis trigger changes in the 5-hydroxytryptamine (5-HT) system, resulting in decreased serotonin and the symptoms of depression (Severino, 1994). This theory is supported by the fact that 65% of patients with unipolar mood disorder experience PMS, while PMS patients have been found to have a lifetime prevalence of major depression of 60%. Women who develop PMS/PMDD tend to have detectable abnormalities in serotonin regulation, with less serotonin uptake by platelets than in control subjects during both the follicular and the luteal phases (Severino, 1994). While no evidence has been found to substantiate a purely psychological basis for PMS (Gannon, 1981), there is evidence that women's expectations about their menstrual cycle may be a factor in their experiencing symptoms, as women who have been misled into believing they are in the luteal phase of their cycle experience "premenstrual symptoms" (Schmidt et al., 1991).

Although some groups still criticize the concept of PMDD as being a "gender-based" diagnosis that fails to consider the sociocultural and biological context of the symptoms, the recent findings of ongoing vulnerabilities in the 5HT system in women who develop PMS/PMDD has convinced many that this is a genuine physiological disorder. Use of strict *Diagnostic & Statistical Manual of Mental Disorders* (DSM) criteria can distinguish those women who genuinely experience PMS/PMDD from those for whom the diagnosis is merely a pejorative label.

Diagnosis of PMS/PMDD requires a detailed history with specific attention to the type, severity, timing, and impact of the woman's symptoms, as well as information on past psychiatric history and current stressors. As some women may self-medicate, it is very important to check whether they are taking vitamin B supplements, as 250 mg a day of B_6 can cause peripheral neuropathies. Many women present with self-diagnosed PMS/PMDD. They may be influenced by magazines or prefer a "hormonal" rather than a psychological explanation for their problems. Studies have shown that, in 50% of cases, retrospective diagnoses of PMS turn out to be erroneous (Rubinow & Schmidt, 1989). Therefore, an essential component of making the diagnosis is prospective charting of moods over at least a two-cycle period.

This charting can be simply done using a standard calendar on which, on a daily basis, the woman rates her chief symptoms on a scale from 1 to 5. She is also asked to chart the beginning and end of her menses as well as any particular stressful events that occur during the month. After two months of charting, examination of this scale by the physician should reveal a very clear pattern of symptoms. If the woman does not fit this pattern, she, by definition, does not suffer from PMS/PMDD but may very well require attention for other physical or emotional problems. Women who are suffering from a major depressive episode or anxiety disorder may have a premenstrual exacerbation of mood symptoms (Hsiao, Hsiao, & Liu, 2004) that may be related to the hormonal changes or to a dilution effect on their antidepressant medication. Increasing the medication for 7–10 days prior to menses may address this problem. As only antidepressants that increase levels of serotonin are effective in treating PMDD, changing to this type of antidepressant may be tried if merely increasing the dose of the previous antidepressant is ineffective. Luteal phase increases of medication may still be required.

As no specific hormonal imbalances have been related to PMS/PMDD, there is no value in routinely assessing hormone levels. Other laboratory tests such as Thyroid Stimulating Hormone (TSH) or an oral glucose-tolerance test to rule out possible physical causes of somatic and emotional distress should be done, when clinically indicated.

Supportive or general health measures may be helpful in relieving distressing symptoms. These include: education of the patient about the nature of this disorder; lifestyle changes to avoid or reduce stressful activities in the premenstrual period; a healthy diet, avoiding salty foods, which may exacerbate a tendency for fluid retention, or caffeine, which may increase irritability; and a regular exercise routine. Cognitive behavioral approaches and relaxation are of some benefit (Pearlstein & Steiner, 2008).

Calcium 600 mg b.i.d. has been shown to be of some benefit in mild to moderate PMS, but the studies were limited, as they did not use diagnostic criteria for PMDD (Thys-Jacob et al., 1998). There is no evidence of magnesium deficiency in women with PMDD compared with control subjects, and magnesium was not found to be superior to placebo in the mitigation of mood symptoms in women with PMDD (Khine et al., 2006). Chasteberry appears to be more useful for physical symptoms in PMS (Schellenberg, 2001). Controlled studies have debunked the use of progesterone, vitamin B, or gamma-linolenic acid (efamol or evening oil of primrose) to treat mood symptoms (Rivera-Tovar, Rhodes, Pearlstein, & Frank, 1994). While mefanamic acid (a prostaglandin synthestase inhibitor) has been found to reduce mood symptoms in some women who also have dysmenorrhea, it probably only acts to decrease negative expectancy by relieving painful menstrual symptoms (Wood & Jakubowicz, 1980).

Fortunately, research in the last several years has confirmed the benefits of using antidepressant therapy for both the mental and the physical symptoms of the luteal phase. Studies so far have found that the use of a SSRI antidepressant such as fluoxetine, sertraline, or paroxetine in the usual therapeutic dose for depression has been highly successful at decreasing or eliminating the symptoms of PMS/PMDD (Shah et al., 2008). For many women, SSRIs may be given in an intermittent manner, starting at day 15 of the menstrual cycle (the start of the late luteal phase) and discontinuing the drug several days after menses commence (Steiner, Korzekwa, Lamont, & Wilkins, 1997). Results of using only symptom-onset treatment with selective serotonin re-uptake inhibitors (SSRIs) have been variable. Serotonin–norepinephrine reuptake inhibitors (SNRIs) such as venlafaxine and duloxetine have also been found useful for the treatment of both physical and mood symptoms.

Inhibiting ovulation has been found to be effective in eliminating PMS/PMDD symptoms. Studies of mono-phasic and tri-phasic OCs did not find any consistent benefit for mood symptoms. Recent studies using an oral contraceptive containing ethinyl estradiol 20 micrograms and a unique progesterone, drospirenone 3mg, administered for 24 days followed by only a four-day break, showed marked reductions in both mood and physical symptoms. It is not clear whether this is due to unique anti-mineralcorticoid and anti-androgenic properties, or to the 24/4 regimen, which results in greater suppression of pituitary and ovarian hormones (Lopez, Kaptein, & Helmerhorst, 2010).

Gonadotropin-releasing hormone analogues (GnRHa) such as goserelin or leuprolide can treat PMS by suppressing ovulation but are not as effective for behavioral and mood symptoms as they are for physical symptoms (Wyatt, Dimmock, Ismail, Jones, & O'Brien, 2004). They also tend to cause uncomfortable, menopausal-like side effects as well as serious bone loss, and, therefore, may be unsafe to use for longer than six months. Adding back HRT may reduce side effects but may also trigger the return of PMS symptoms if cyclical progesterone is used. Other ovulation suppressants such as danazol and high-dose continuous estrogen are effective but cause significant negative side effects such as weight gain, masculinization, or endometrial hyperplasia (Pearlstein & Steiner, 2008). Hysterectomy and oophorectomy are obviously very extreme ways of alleviating these symptoms and may have their own negative physical and emotional consequences (Cronje, Vashisht, & Studd, 2004). In summary, the majority of women with PMDD will respond to a combination of psycho-education, support, a healthy lifestyle (balanced diet and moderate exercise), stress reduction (especially in the late luteal phase), and treatment with intermittent or continuous SRRIs; therefore, more drastic endocrine therapies of PMS/PMDD would be indicated only in cases in which there is extreme disruption of the woman's life and other, more conservative, therapies have been ineffective. Though the ovulation-suppressing therapies have many drawbacks, they are certain to work at least partially. The medical psychiatrist considering such therapies should involve both a gynecologist and the patient in order to facilitate well-informed decision-making.

PERIMENOPAUSE AND MENOPAUSE

The perimenopause is the transition time from premenopause to post-menopause during which menstrual periods become irregular and women experience vasomotor symptoms such as hot flushes in addition to mood, sleep, sexual, and cognitive disturbances (Dennerstein, Dudley, Hopper, Guthrie, & Burger, 2000; Schmidt, 2005; Freedman, 2005). Menopause is defined as occurring when it has been 12 months since the last menstrual period, and the post-menopause is the time thereafter (Soules et al., 2001). The transition can take many years, but the median age at menopause is 52 years (Proceedings from the NIH State-of-the-Science Conference on Management of Menopause-Related Symptoms, 2005). Methodological issues, such as research being based on clinic-based surveys (e.g., from gynecology clinics) without rigorous assessment, resulted in controversy as to whether women are at an increased risk for developing depressive symptoms or a depressive disorder during the perimenopause. Recent research, based on rigorously conducted community samples, has demonstrated that this time is a period of increased risk. In a prospective study of eight years' duration, Freeman, Samuel, Lin, and Nelson (2006) found women in the menopausal transition were at four-fold greater risk for developing depressive symptoms than during the premenopausal phase, and that entering menopause was associated with double the risk of receiving a depressive disorder diagnosis. Schmidt, Haq, and Rubinow (2004) also followed women prospectively for five years and found that, in the 24 months around the final menstrual period, women were at 14 times greater risk for the development of depression compared to the premenopausal women. Cohen, Soares, Vitonis, Otto, and Harlow (2006) also found an increased risk for the development of depressive symptoms in addition to major mood disorders in the perimenopause. It is therefore well established that perimenopausal women not only have a higher likelihood of reporting depressive symptoms, they are also at an increased risk for developing a mood disorder.

Several mechanisms have been proposed to explain the depressive symptoms, such as fluctuations in estradiol (Prior, 1998); the consequences of the sleep disturbance resulting from the vasomotor symptoms (Campbell & Whitehead, 1977); psychosocial changes such as those encountered in changing roles or family circumstances, decreased physical activity, or change in health status; as well as cultural factors regarding menopause (Avis, 2003; Lock & Kaufert, 2001; Gyllstrom et al., 2007). Although the relationship is not well understood, in a subpopulation of vulnerable women (perhaps more so in those with a history of depression) (Avis, Brambilla, McKinlay, & Vass, 1994), there appears to be a link between the development of depressive disorders and estrogen depletion or deficiency (Steiner, Dunn, & Born, 2003; Daly, Danaceau, Rubinow, & Schmidt, 2003; Payne, 2003). Recent research has suggested other contributing endocrine mechanisms, although not consistently. Harlow, Wise, Otto, Soares, and Cohen (2003) reported that women with a history of depression were more likely to have an earlier transition with higher FSH and LH levels and lower estradiol. Freeman et al.

(2004) found a relationship between FSH and estradiol levels and depression. Subsequently, Freeman et al. (2006) found women with no prior history of depression in perimenopause had increased levels of FSH and LH with increased depression ratings and more variability in FSH, LH, and estradiol levels. Taken together, the changing hormonal environment was hypothesized to contribute to the development of depression. However, Schmidt and colleagues (2002 and 2004) did not find a relationship between basal FSH or LH levels and other hormones in perimenopausal woman with depression. Others also did not find consistent relationships between hormone levels and mood (Woods et al., 2008). Clearly, more work is needed to understand the causal mechanisms. Moreover, it is important to recognize that, although some women may be at an increased risk for developing depression (and perhaps other psychiatric disorders) during the perimenopause, most women will not (Soares & Taylor, 2007).

Physicians must also pay attention to psychological and cultural considerations (Gise, 1997). Perimenopause and post-menopause may be seen as a time of rapid aging and decreased attractiveness. Social roles change, and some women may fear the loss of the ability to have children, or that they will have less valuable roles post-menopausally. Other psychological stressors can include children leaving (or returning) home; difficulties in finding new, fulfilling roles; loss of a partner; health problems; responsibilities for aging parents; and the deaths of relatives or friends (Deeks, 2003).

Most women pass through menopause without serious difficulty, however. The Massachusetts Women's Health Study (Avis & McKinlay, 1991) found that most women in their middle years report relief or neutral feelings about their periods' stopping. Negative attitudes towards menopause usually change once the individual is in menopause and realizes her fears about what will happen to her do not materialize. Employment, better health, and higher education were associated with more positive attitudes, while depression and higher symptom reporting were associated with negative views. The survey by the North American Menopause Society found that 52% of participants saw menopause as the beginning of a new and fulfilling stage of life (Kaufert, Boggs, Ettinger, Woods, & Utian, 1998).

Although in menopausal women, FSH levels exceed 40 mIU/ml (Soules et al., 2001), the determination of perimenopause or menopause is generally made clinically rather than based on laboratory evaluation. Treatment of symptoms of depression at menopause requires an assessment of the contribution of the different etiological factors. The hormonal profile of elevated concentrations of FSH and LH with decreased concentrations of estradiol and progesterone are not clearly different in women who do or do not become clinically depressed; therefore, this profile cannot be used to direct treatment. At this time, there is little value in routinely performing these assessments. As thyroid disease and diabetes are common in women of this age, thyroid function and glucose tolerance should be assessed to rule out any abnormality in these systems. HRT, clonidine, low-dose SSRIs, SNRIs, and gabapentin may decrease distressing symptoms related to estrogen withdrawal (Proceedings from the

NIH State-of-the-Science Conference on Management of Menopause-Related Symptoms, 2005).

Education of women, individually or in groups, to dispel myths and fears about impending unattractiveness or loss of femininity can help avert or minimize their distress (Robinson & Stirtzinger, 1997). Women with specific conflicts or concerns associated with past or current problems may benefit from individual or marital therapy. Self-help groups may provide support and advice in dealing with the physiological and psychological changes at this time, and there is also some evidence for cognitive behavioral approaches for menopausal issues (Hunter & Rendall, 2007). The use of 17b-estradiol for treating perimenopausally depressed women does have some research support, although the risks need to be weighed against the potential benefits, as the use of estrogen is not recommended for long-term use; moreover, the trials did not assess 17b-estradiol exclusively in women with major depression, and included less severe forms of depression (Schmidt et al., 2000; Soares, Almeida, Joffe, & Cohen, 2001). For women who meet criteria for a major depressive episode, antidepressant medication is indicated (Lam et al., 2009). HRT can also be used to augment antidepressant therapy, especially SSRIs, for a synergistic effect, especially in women with less-than-optimal response to antidepressants or HRT. For example, if a women does not respond to an SSRI and is perimenopausal and complaining of hot flashes or other perimenopausal symptoms, augmentation of the SSRI with HRT can be an option prior to switching to another antidepressant, although current clinical guidelines do not exist. Short-term HRT use is recommended for perimenopausal symptoms (Canadian Consensus Conference on Menopause, 2006).

CLINICAL PEARLS

- Initiation of HRT close to menopause was not associated with improved cognition, and HRT did not significantly reduce dementia risk over the course of this study (Ryan et al., 2009). ERT did not appear to have an enduring helpful effect on cognitive functioning in older women.

- New information suggests that the risk of stroke (odds ratio 1.29) can be reduced by the use of transdermal HRT (Brown, 2010).

- Mood stabilizers such as carbamazepine, lamotrigine, and topirimate may increase metabolism of oral contraceptives, leading to insufficient hormonal levels to suppress ovulation and an increased risk of contraceptive failure.

- Although 90–95% of women attending infertility clinics with anovulation have PCOS, 60% will conceive, although it may take them longer.

- PCOS also happens more often to women with epilepsy taking valproate than to those being treated for bipolar disorder; suggesting that other interactions may be taking place (Bilo & Meo, 2008).

- In women with PCOS, excess weight was the largest contributor to poorer quality of life. Women taking anti-androgen medications generally had a better quality of life than those not taking them.

- Approximately 1–5% of women meet criteria for PMDD.

- Despite extensive investigations of PMDD, researchers have been unable to find any relationship to the levels, ratios, or rates of change of progesterone or estrogen.

- It is well established that perimenopausal women not only have a higher likelihood of reporting depressive symptoms, they are also at an increased risk for developing a mood disorder.

- Although in menopausal women, FSH levels exceed 40 mIU/ml (Soules et al., 2001), the determination of perimenopause or menopause is generally made clinically, rather than based on laboratory evaluation.

- For women who meet criteria for a major depressive episode, antidepressant medication is indicated (Lam et al., 2009). HRT can also be used to augment antidepressant therapy, especially SSRIs, for a synergistic effect, especially in women with less-than-optimal response to antidepressants or HRT.

DISCLOSURE STATEMENTS

Dr. Robinson is an employee of the University of Toronto and works at the University Health Network in Toronto, Canada. She has no ties to any pharmaceutical companies. She has no conflicts to disclose.

Dr. Grigoriadis has a New Investigator Award in Women's Health Research from Canadian Institutes of Health Research (CIHR) in partnership with the Ontario Women's Health Council. She has received honoraria as a consultant, member of an advisory committee, or for lectures over the last five years, from Wyeth Pharmaceuticals, GlaxoSmithKline, Pfizer, Servier, Eli Lilly Canada, and Lundbeck. Her research grant support over the last five years has included the CIHR, the Ontario Ministry of Health, the Ontario Mental Health Foundation, and the C. R. Younger Foundation.

REFERENCES

American Psychiatric Association (2013). *Diagnostic and statistical manual of mental disorders* (5th ed.). Washington, DC: American Psychiatric Association.

Avis, N. E. (2003). Depression during the menopausal transition. *Psychology of Women Quarterly, 27,* 91–100.

Avis, N. E., Brambilla, D., McKinlay, S. M., & Vass, K. (1994). A longitudinal analysis of the association between menopause and depression. Results from the Massachusetts Women's Health Study. *Annals of Epidemiology, 4*(3), 214–220.

Avis, N. E., & McKinlay, S. M. (1991). A longitudinal analysis of women's attitudes toward the menopause: results from the Massachusetts Women's Health Study. *Maturitas, 13,* 65–79.

Barnard, L., Ferriday, D., Guenther, N., Strauss, B., Balen, A. H., & Dye, L. (2007). Quality of life and psychological well being in polycystic ovary syndrome. *Human Reproduction, 22*(8), 2279–2286.

Bilo, L., & Meo, R. (2008). Polycystic ovary syndrome in women using valproate: a review. *Gynecological Endocrinology, 24*(10), 562–570.

Brown, S. (2010). Transdermal hormone replacement therapy not associated with an increased risk of stroke. *Menopause International, 16*(2), 48–49.

Campbell, S., & Whitehead, M. (1977). Oestrogen therapy and the menopausal syndrome. *Clinical Obstetrics & Gynecology, 4*(1), 31–47.

Canadian Consensus Conference on Menopause (2006). 2006 Update. *Journal of Obstetrics & Gynecology Canada, 28*(Special Ed.), S1–S112.

Chiarelli, F., Coppola, G., D'Egidio, C., Parisi, P., & Verottii, A. (2009). Epilepsy, sex hormones and antiepileptic drugs in female patients. *Expert Review of Neurotherapeutics, 9*(12), 1803–1814.

Chua, W. L., de Izquierdo, S. A., Kulkarni, J., & Mortimer, A. (2005). Estrogen for schizophrenia. *Cochrane Database of Systematic Reviews, 19*(4), CD004719.

Cohen, L. S., Soares, C. N., Vitonis, A. F., Otto, M. W., & Harlow, B. L. (2006). Risk for new onset of depression during the menopausal transition: the Harvard study of moods and cycles. *Archives of General Psychiatry, 63*(4), 385–390.

Cronje, W. H., Vashisht, A., & Studd, J. W. (2004). Hysterectomy and bilateral oophorectomy for severe premenstrual syndrome. *Human Reproduction, 19*(9), 2152–2155.

Daly, R. C., Danaceau, M. A., Rubinow, D. R., & Schmidt, P. J. (2003). Concordant restoration of ovarian function and mood in perimenopausal depression. *American Journal of Psychiatry, 160*(10), 1842–1846.

Daniluk, J. C., & Fluker, M. (1995). Fertility drugs and reproductive imperative: assisting the fertile woman. In J. A. Hamilton, M. F. Jensvold, E. Rothblum, & E. Cole (Eds.), *Psychopharmacology from a feminist perspective* (pp. 31–48). New York: Haworth.

Deeks, A. A. (2003). Psychological aspects of menopause management. *Best Practice & Research: Clinical Endocrinology & Metabolism, 17*(1), 17–31.

Dennerstein, L., Dudley, E. C., Hopper, J. L., Guthrie, J. R., & Burger, H. G. (2000). A prospective population-based study of menopausal symptoms. *Obstetrics & Gynecology, 96*(3), 351–358.

de Paula, F. J., Soares, J. M. Jr., Haidar, M. A., de Lima, G. R., Baracat, E. C. (2007). The benefits of androgens combined with hormone replacement therapy regarding to patients with postmenopausal sexual symptoms. *Maturitas, 56*(1), 69–77.

Editor (1983). *Drug facts and comparisons.* St. Louis, MO: Facts and Comparisons.

Elsenbruch, S., Hahn, S., Kowalsky, D., Offner, A. H., Schedlowski, M., Mann, K., et al. (2003). Quality of life, psychosocial well-being, and sexual satisfaction in women with polycystic ovary syndrome. *Journal of Clinical Endocrinology & Metabolism, 88*(12), 5801–5807.

Freeman, E. W., Sammel, M. D., Liu, L., Gracia, C. R., Nelson, D. B., & Hollander, L. (2004). Hormones and menopausal status as predictors of depression in women in transition to menopause. *Archives of General Psychiatry, 61*(1), 62–70.

Freeman, E. W., Sammel, M. D., Lin, H., & Nelson, D. B. (2006). Associations of hormones and menopausal status with depressed mood in women with no history of depression. *Archives of General Psychiatry, 63*(4), 375–382.

Freedman, R. R., (2005). Hot flashes: behavioral treatments, mechanisms, and relation to sleep. *American Journal of Medicine, 118*(12) Suppl 2, 124–130.

Gannon, L. (1981). Evidence for a psychological etiology of menstrual disorders: a critical review. *Psychological Reports, 48*(1), 287–294.

Gyllstrom, M. E., Schreiner, P. J., Harlow, B. L. (2007). Perimenopause and depression: strength of association, causal mechanisms and treatment recommendations. *Best Practice & Research: Clinical Obstetrics and Gynecology, 21,* 275–292.

Gise, L. (1997). Psychosocial aspects. In D. E. Stewart & G. E. Robinson (Eds.), *A clinician's guide to menopause* (pp. 29–44). Washington, DC: American Psychiatric Press.

Goodarzi, M. O. (2008). Looking for polycystic ovary syndrome genes: rational and best strategy. *Seminars in Reproductive Medicine, 26*(1), 5–13.

Goodman, D., Goldzieher, J., & Ayala, C. (2003). Critique of the report from the Writing Group of the WHI. *Menopausal Medicine, 10*(4), 1–4.

Grigoriadis, S., & Kennedy, S. H. (2002). Role of estrogen in the treatment of depression. *American Journal of Therapy, 9*(6), 503–509.

Guzick, D. (1998). Polycystic ovary syndrome: symptomatology, pathophysiology, and epidemiology. *American Journal of Obstetrics & Gynecology, 179*(6 Pt 2), S89–S93.

Harlow, B. L., Wise, L. A., Otto, M. W., Soares, C. N., & Cohen, L. S. (2003). Depression and its influence on reproductive endocrine and menstrual cycle markers associated with perimenopause: the Harvard Study of Moods and Cycles. *Archives of General Psychiatry, 60*(1), 29–36.

Himelein, M. J., & Thatcher, S. S. (2006). Polycystic ovary syndrome and mental health: A review. *Obstetrics & Gynecology Survey, 61*(11), 723–732.

Hsiao, M. C., Hsiao, C. C. & Liu, C. Y. (2004). Premenstrual symptoms and premenstrual exacerbation in patients with psychiatric disorders. *Psychiatry & Clinical Neurosciences, 58,* 186–190.

Hunter, M., & Rendall, M. (2007). Bio-psycho-socio-cultural perspectives on menopause. *Best Practice & Research: Clinical Obstetrics & Gynecology, 21*(2), 261–274.

Jensvold, M. F. (1996). Nonpregnant reproductive-age women. Part II: Exogenous sex steroid hormones and psychopharmacology. In M. F. Jensvold, U. Halbreich, & J. A. Hamilton (Eds.), *Psychopharmacology and women: Sex, gender and hormones* (Chap. 9, pp. 171–190). Washington, DC: American Psychiatric Press.

Joffe, H., Cohen, L. S., & Harlow, B. L. (2003). Impact of oral contraceptive pill use on premenstrual mood: Predictors of improvement and deterioration. *American Journal of Obstetrics & Gynecology, 189*(6), 1523–1530.

Kaufert P., Boggs, P. P., Ettinger B., Woods, N. F., & Utian, W. H. (1998). Women and menopause: beliefs, attitudes, and behaviors. The North American Menopause Society 1997 menopause survey. *Menopause, 5*(4), 197–202.

Keegan, A., Liao, L. M., & Boyle, M. (2003). "Hirsutism": a psychological analysis. *Journal of Health Psychology, 8*(3), 327–345.

Kitzinger, C., & Wilmot, J. (2002). "The thief of womanhood": women's experience with polycystic ovary syndrome. *Social Science & Medicine, 54*(3), 349–361.

Khine, K., Rosenstein, D. L., Elin, R. J., Niemela, J. E., Schmidt, P. J., & Rubinow, D. R. (2006). Magnesium (Mg) retention and mood effects after intravenous Mg infusion in premenstrual dysphoric disorder. *Biological Psychiatry, 59,* 327–333.

Klaiber, E. L., Vogel, W., & Rako, S. (2005). A critique of the Women's Health Initiative hormone therapy study. *Fertility & Sterility, 84*(6), 1589–1601.

Kulkarni, J., de Castella, A., Fitzgerald, P. B., Gurvich, C. T., Baily, M., Bartholomeusz, C., et al. (2008). Estrogen in severe mental illness: a potential new treatment approach. *Archives of General Psychiatry, 65*(8), 955–960.

Lam, R. W., Kennedy, S. H., Grigoriadis, S., McIntyre, R. S., Milev, R., & Ramasubbu, R. (2009). Canadian Network for Mood and Anxiety Treatments (CANMAT) clinical guidelines for the management of major depressive disorder in adults. III. Pharmacotherapy. *Journal of Affective Disorders, 117*(Suppl 1), S26–S43.

Lock, M., & Kaufert, P. (2001). Menopause, local biologies, and cultures of aging. *American Journal of Human Biology, 13*(4), 494–504.

Lopez, L. M., Kaptein, A. A., & Helmerhorst, F. M. (2010). Oral contraceptives containing drospirenone for premenstrual syndrome. *Cochrane Database of Systematic Reviews, 23*(1), CD006586.

McCook, J. G., Reame, N. E., & Thatcher, S. S. (2005). Health-related quality of life issues in women with polycystic ovary syndrome. *Journal of Obstetrics, Gynecology, & Neonatal Nursing, 34*(1), 12–20.

Moses-Kolko, E. L., Berga, S. L., Kalro, B., Sit, D. K., & Wisner, K. L. (2009). Transdermal estradiol for postpartum depression: a promising treatment option. *Clinical Obstetrics & Gynecology, 52*(3), 516–529.

O'Donovan, C., Kusumakar, V., Graves, G. R., & Bird, D. C. (2002). Menstrual abnormalities and polycystic ovary syndrome in women taking valproate for bipolar mood disorder. *Journal of Clinical Psychiatry, 63*(4), 322–330.

Oinonen, K. A., & Mazmanian, D. (2002). To what extent do oral contraceptives influence mood and affect? *Journal of Affective Disorders, 70*(3), 229–240.

Parry, B. L. (1999). A 45-year-old woman with premenstrual dysphoric disorder. *Journal of the American Medical Association, 281*(4), 368–373.

Payne, J. L. (2003). The role of estrogen in mood disorders in women. *International Review of Psychiatry, 15*(3), 280–290.

Pearlstein, T., & Steiner, M. (2008). Premenstrual dysphoric disorder: burden of illness and treatment update. *Journal of Psychiatry & Neuroscience, 33*(4), 291–301.

Prior, J. C. (1998). Perimenopause: the complex endocrinology of the menopausal transition. *Endocrine Reviews, 19*(4), 397–428.

Proceedings from the NIH State-of-the-Science Conference on Management of Menopause-Related Symptoms, March 21–23, 2005, Bethesda, Maryland. *American Journal of Medicine, 118*(Suppl 12B), 1–171.

Rasgon, N. L., Rao, R. C., Hwang, S., Altshuler, L. L., Elman, S., Zuckerbrow-Miller, J., et al. (2003). Depression in women with polycystic ovary syndrome: clinical and biochemical correlates. *Journal of Affective Disorders, 74*(3), 299–304.

Rivera-Tovar, A., Rhodes, R., Pearlstein, T., & Frank, E. (1994). Treatment efficacy. In J. H. Gold & S. K. Severino (Eds.), *Premenstrual dysphoria: Myths and realities* (pp. 99–148). London: American Psychiatric Press.

Robinson, G. E., & Stirtzinger, R. (1997). Psychoeducational programs and support groups at transition to menopause. In D. E. Stewart & G. E. Robinson (Eds.), *A clinician's guide to menopause* (Chap. 10, pp. 165–180). Washington, DC: American Psychiatric Press.

Rossouw, J. E., Anderson, G. L., Prentice, R. L., LaCroix, A. Z., Kooperberg, C., Stefanick, M. L., et al. (2002). Risks and benefits of estrogen plus progestin in healthy postmenopausal women: principal results from the Women's Health Initiative randomized controlled trial. *Journal of the American Medical Association, 288*(3), 321–333.

Rubinow, D. R., & Schmidt, P. J. (1989). Models for the development and expression of symptoms in premenstrual syndrome. *Psychiatric Clinics of North America, 12*(1), 53–68.

Ryan, J., Carriere, I., Scali, J., Dartigues, J. F., Tzourio, C., Poncet, M., et al. (2009). Characteristics of hormone therapy, cognitive function, and dementia: the Prospective 3C Study. *Neurology, 73*(21), 1729–1737.

Schellenberg, R. (2001). Treatment for the premenstrual syndrome with agnus castus fruit extract: prospective, randomised, placebo controlled study. *British Medical Journal,* Jan 20; *322*(7279), 134–137.

Schmidt, P. J. (2005). Mood, depression, and reproductive hormones in the menopause transition. *American Journal of Medicine, 118*(Suppl 12B), 54–58.

Schmidt, P. J., Haq, N. A., & Rubinow, D. R. (2004). A longitudinal evaluation of the relationship between reproductive status and mood in perimenopausal women. *American Journal of Psychiatry, 161*(12), 2238–2244.

Schmidt, P. J., Murphy, J. H., Haq, N., Danaceau, M. A., & St. Clair, L. (2002). Basal plasma hormone levels in depressed perimenopausal women. *Psychoneuroendocrinology, 27*(8), 907–920.

Schmidt, P. J., Nieman, L. K., Danaceau, M. A., Adams, L. F., & Rubinow, D. R. (1998). Differential behavioral effects of gonadal steroids in women with premenstrual syndrome and in control subjects. *New England Journal of Medicine, 338*(4), 209–216.

Schmidt, P. J., Nieman, L., Danaceau, M. A., Tobin, M. B., Roca, C. A., Murphy, J. H., et al. (2000). Estrogen replacement in perimenopause-related depression: a preliminary report. *American Journal of Obstetrics & Gynecology, 183*(2), 414–420.

Schmidt, P. J., Nieman, L. K., Grover, G. N., Muller, K. L., Merriam, G. R., & Rubinow, D. R. (1991). Lack of effect of induced menses on symptoms in women with premenstrual syndrome. *New England Journal of Medicine, 324*(17), 1174–1179.

Severino, S. K. (1994). A focus on 5-hydroxytryptamine (serotonin) and psychopathology. In J. H. Gold & S. K. Severino (Eds.), *Premenstrual dysphorias. Myths and realities* (Chap. 4, pp. 67–98). Washington, DC: American Psychiatric Press.

Shah, N. R., Jones, J. B., Aperi, J., Shemtov, R., Karne, A., & Borenstein, J. (2008). Selective serotonin reuptake inhibitors for premenstrual syndrome and premenstrual dysphoric disorder: A meta-analysis. *Obstetrics & Gynecology, 111*(5), 1175–1182.

Somboonporn, W., Bell, R. J., & Davis, S. R. (2011). Testosterone for peri- and postmenopausal women (Review) 15. *Cochrane Menstrual Disorders and Subfertility Group, Cochrane Database of Systematic Reviews, 4.*

Soares, C. N., Almeida, O. P., Joffe, H., & Cohen, L. S. (2001). Efficacy of estradiol for the treatment of depressive disorders in perimenopausal women. *Archives of General Psychiatry, 58*(6), 529–534.

Soares, C. N., & Taylor, V. (2007). Effects and management of the menopausal transition in women with depression and bipolar disorder. *Journal of Clinical Psychiatry, 68*(Suppl 9), 16–21.

Soules, M. R., Sherman, S., Parrott, E., Rebar, R., Santoro, N., Utian, W., & et al. (2001). Executive summary: Stages of Reproductive Aging Workshop (STRAW). *Fertility & Sterility, 76*(5), 874–878.

Steiner, M., Dunn, E., & Born, L. (2003). Hormones and mood: from menarche to menopause and beyond. *Journal of Affective Disorders, 74*(1), 67–83.

Steiner, M., Korzekwa, M., Lamont, J., & Wilkins, A. (1997). Intermittent fluoxetine dosing in the treatment of women with premenstrual dysphoria. *Psychopharmacology Bulletin, 33*(4), 771–774.

Stoppe, G., & Doren, M. (2002). Critical appraisal of effects of estrogen replacement therapy on symptoms of depressed mood. *Archives of Women's Mental Health, 5*(2), 39–47.

Stotland, N. L. (1997). Psychological treatments. In D. E. Stewart & G. E. Robinson (Eds.), *A Clinician's Guide to Menopause* (Chap. 9, pp. 145–164), Washington, DC: American Psychiatric Press.

Tan, S., Hana, S., Benson, S., Janssen, O. E., Dietz, T., Kimmig, R., et al. (2008). Psychological implications of infertility in women with polycystic ovary syndrome. *Human Reproduction, 23*(9), 2064–2071.

Taylor, H. S., & Manson, J. E. (2011). Update in hormone therapy use in menopause. *Journal of Clinical Endocrinology & Metabolism, 96*(2), 255–264.

Teede, H., Deeks, A., & Moran, L. (2010). Polycystic ovary syndrome: a complex condition with psychological, reproductive and metabolic manifestations that impacts on health across the lifespan. *BioMedCentral Medicine, 8*, 41.

Thys-Jacobs, S., Starkey, P., Bernstein, D., & Tian, J. (1998). Calcium carbonate and the premenstrual syndrome: effects on premenstrual and menstrual symptoms. Premenstrual Syndrome Study Group. *American Journal of Obstetrics & Gynecology, 179*, 444–452.

Weiner, C. L., Primeau, M., & Ehrmann, D. A. (2004). Androgens and mood dysfunction in women: comparison of women with polycystic ovary syndrome to healthy controls. *Psychosomatic Medicine, 66*(3), 356–362.

Wilson, R. A. (1968). *Feminine forever.* New York: M. Evans & Company.

Wood, C., & Jakubowicz, D. (1980). The treatment of premenstrual symptoms with mefenamic acid. *British Journal of Obstetrics & Gynaecology, 87*(7), 627–630.

Woods, N. F., Smith-DiJulio, K., Percival, D. B., Tao, E. Y., Mariella, A., & Mitchell, S. (2008). Depressed mood during the menopausal transition and early postmenopause: observations from the Seattle Midlife Women's Health Study. *Menopause, 15*(2), 223–232.

Wyatt, K. M., Dimmock, P. W., Ismail, K. M., Jones, P. W., & O'Brien, P. M. (2004). The effectiveness of GnHa with and without "add-back" therapy in treating premenstrual syndrome: a meta-analysis. *British Journal of Obstetrics & Gynaecology, 111*(6), 585–593.

Zweifel, J. E., & O'Brien, W. H. (1997). A meta-analysis of the effect of hormone replacement therapy upon depressed mood. *Psychoneuroendocrinology, 22*(3), 189–212.

PREGNANCY AND POSTPARTUM

Diane de Camps Meschino, Ariel Dalfen, and Gail Erlick Robinson

INTRODUCTION

Pregnancy and the postpartum period have been idealistically viewed as times of happiness and joy. When a pregnancy is wanted and planned, women are expected to "bloom" and enjoy this state as one of satisfaction and fulfillment. Postpartum, society expects women to be blissfully happy and devoted to the interests of their new baby. The reality is that, even in the case of wanted and planned pregnancies, women may suffer from a variety of problems ranging from simple adaption to this new experience to depression, anxiety, psychotic disorders and substance abuse. Pregnancy and postpartum are times of enormous physiological, psychological and sociocultural changes which can cause enormous stress. As well, women with pre-existing mental illnesses can become pregnant or vulnerabilities to illness may be activated by all of the stressors that accompany this phase in women's lives.

PREGNANCY

NORMAL PREGNANCY

Pregnancy is a time of enormous biological, psychological, and sociocultural changes, all of which may result in the increased sensitivity and emotional lability that many women experience during pregnancy. During this time, there are major changes in estrogen and progesterone and significant changes in prolactin, corticotrophin-releasing hormone, and oxytocin, among others. There are also many practical and lifestyle changes that may add stress. The couple may have to move or buy a new car. Maternity leave may result in financial difficulties. Women must decide how much leave they will take, whether they will return to work, or, if they do return, whether they will alter their ambitions or work goals.

The immense changes a woman experiences in a relatively short time create both an opportunity for personal growth and the potential for intrapsychic conflict with the need for professional intervention. The greatest psychological changes occur during the first pregnancy. Women must make the psychological transition to being a parent. This may either feel frightening or feel like the final step to becoming an adult. Ideally, a woman chooses to become pregnant because she feels mature enough for the responsibility of looking after a child and has a balanced view of the joys and stresses involved. In reality, many pregnancies are unplanned, and reasons for becoming pregnant are varied, including: seeing it as a way to feel like an adult, acting on a wish to have someone to love, making an attempt to keep a relationship, or responding to expectations from one's family or community.

Prior to and during the pregnancy, the woman must reassess her partner and decide whether he will be a good parent. The couple begins to sort out whether their relationship will assume more traditional roles postpartum. Pregnancy may strengthen a couple's intimate bond and be integrative of maturity, resulting in a more securely attached marriage. The woman also may emotionally revisit her relationship with her own mother, deciding whether she wants to parent in a similar way or develop a different parenting style. Ideally, pregnant women (and their partners) are able to appreciate and identify with the positive aspects of their own parents and consequently experience enhanced independence and self-determination.

For many years, pregnancy was thought of as a protected state, immune to any serious mental health disorders. However, not only can anxiety and depression present during pregnancy, even "normal" planned pregnancies can be accompanied by mood changes and psychological conflict. A woman who expects she should be blissfully happy during pregnancy may find it difficult to tell anyone about these common feelings. Over the course of the pregnancy, as her body changes, she may feel beautiful and confidant, or unattractive and fat. Some women feel more sexual during pregnancy, while others may have no interest in sex; and their interest or lack of it may be at odds with the feelings of their partners. Women may initially feel anxious about miscarrying and later about delivering a healthy baby.

Stressful life events (Paykel Emms, Fletcher, & Rassaby, 1980; Bernazzani, Saucier, David, & Borgeat, 1997a), together with the quality and support of marital relationships (Cowan & Cowan, 1988; Bernazzani et al., 1997b) are important factors in adaptation to pregnancy. Recent life adversity, including life events and chronic stressors, has been confirmed to contribute to the development of poor adaptation and depression in pregnancy. In less optimal situations, the demands of pregnancy and the transition of roles and relationships increase stress, which may result in conflict with significant others, depression, or anxiety.

HYPEREMESIS GRAVIDARUM

Nausea and vomiting are common symptoms during the first trimester of pregnancy. Approximately 0.5% of women experience severe, intractable vomiting, or hyperemesis gravidarum (HG) that generally resolves around week 20, but may continue throughout the pregnancy, resulting in dehydration and metabolic and electrolyte disturbances. Despite investigations of hormonal, immunological, infectious, metabolic, and anatomical facts, the cause of HG remains unknown (Verberg, Gillott, Al-Fardan, & Grudzinskas, 2005).

Historically, women with HG have been accused of being ambivalent about the pregnancy or rejecting the idea of motherhood. HG has been labeled as a sign of hysteria, neurosis, depression, stress, or marital conflict; however, there is no evidence that this is true. Women, already feeling miserable because of the symptoms of HG, should not have added stress placed on them by medical staff making these kinds of assumptions.

Initial treatment of HG involves appropriate parenteral fluid and electrolyte replacement. Various antiemetics may be given with vitamin supplementation. The standard treatment in most of the world is Benedictin (also sold under the trademark name Diclectin), a combination of doxylamine succinate and vitamin B$_6$, although ginger has been found to diminish or eliminate the symptoms without any side effects (Kuscu & Koyuncu, 2002).

PERINATAL DISORDERS

Depression in Pregnancy

Depressive symptoms in the perinatal period are extremely common, with symptoms ranging from enhanced emotionality and sadness to major depressive disorder (MDD). As many as 14.5% of women have a new episode of major or minor depression that begins during pregnancy (Gavin et al., 2005). As many as 18.4% of pregnant women are depressed during their pregnancy, with 12.7% developing a major depression. Bennett, Einarson, Taddio, Koren, and Einarson (2004) found prevalence rates of 7.4%, 12.8%, and 12.0% in the first, second, and third trimesters, respectively; while Gavin et al. (2005) determined point prevalences to be 11.0%, 8.5%, and 8.5%. One-third of these will be first episodes. Rates of depression in pregnancy do not differ from those in non-pregnant women.

Prenatal depression has a similar symptom profile to that of depressive syndromes during other life stages, although it may be associated with greater anxiety, irritability, and severe insomnia. Mood may fluctuate, particularly with the amount of sleep obtained. Anxiety is focused on the baby's health, potential breastfeeding issues, financial issues, relationships, and the mother's appearance or her own health. Depressed mothers often feel no love or bonding with their baby while pregnant, worry they will be inadequate as mothers, and express associated guilt. They may have escape fantasies, wish they had never become pregnant, and worry that the rest of their lives will be joyless and/or that they will feel entrapped or imprisoned. In more severe depressive episodes, mothers may have suicidal ruminations or thoughts of harming their baby *in utero*. Although they feel ashamed of such thoughts, women are relieved to be asked about them and to be reassured that thoughts of harming one's baby have been experienced by other depressed women. Patients, healthcare providers, family, and friends may dismiss symptoms of depression in pregnancy due to the normal occurrence of insomnia, fatigue, change of appetite, and loss of energy seen during this period.

Risk Factors for Depression in Pregnancy

New-onset or recurrent depressive disorders in the perinatal period have a multifactorial etiology. A personal or family history of mood or anxiety disorders (including premenstrual dysphoric disorder [PMDD]) is associated with increased perinatal risk (Altshuler, Hendrick, & Cohen, 1998; Robertson, Jones, Haque, Holder, & Craddock, 2005). Other factors include ambivalence about pregnancy, insecure attachment style (Bifulco et al., 2004), limited social support, unintended pregnancy, marital conflict, poor relationship quality (Lancaster et al., 2010), and a history of childhood sexual abuse (Bronwyn & Milgrom, 2008). Depressive or anxiety symptoms during pregnancy may be the greatest risk for postpartum disorders (PPD). Women being treated for anxiety or depression frequently discontinue medication in preparation for, or upon discovery of, pregnancy. Cohen et al. (2004) found that discontinuation of medication led to a relapse in 68% of women during pregnancy.

Bipolar Disorder in Pregnancy

Pregnancy appears to neither decrease nor increase the risk of bipolar episodes. Viguera et al. (2000) found relapse rates with lithium discontinuation to be similar during pregnant and non-pregnant states. Pre-conception education allows opportunities to change medications, such as valproic acid, which may cause fetal damage; and to explain the risks of discontinuing medication during pregnancy.

Anxiety Disorders

All anxiety disorders have been reported to be more common in women, with peak incidence in the reproductive years (Kessler et al., 1994; Kessler, Sonnega, Bromet, Hughes, & Nelson, 1995). In addition to the usual symptoms of generalized anxiety disorder (GAD), pregnant women may find themselves checking their fetus more frequently than necessary. Domains of worry often include financial security, personal appearance, household responsibilities, and hygiene (Wenzel, Haugen, Jackson, & Robinson, 2003). To distinguish anxiety from normal perinatal concerns, "anxiety" must be widespread, excessive, and interfere with day-to-day functioning. The *Diagnostic and Statistical Manual of Mental Disorders,* 5th edition DSM-V criteria of six months' duration may not be met at initial presentation. Preexisting anxiety or antenatal anxiety may be a greater risk factor for PPD than a history of depression (Matthey, Barnett, Howie, & Kavanagh, 2003).

Panic Disorder

The rate of panic disorder during pregnancy is consistent with its rates at other times. The course of panic through pregnancy is unpredictable. Women may interpret panic as an indication of fetal abnormality, and require both education and reassurance in addition to treatment.

Post-traumatic Stress Disorder

Trauma related to a past sexual abuse or previous traumatic birth experiences may cause post-traumatic stress disorder (PTSD) symptoms to recur, especially relating to labor and delivery due to anticipated pain, sexual exposure, and lack of control. Re-experiencing (flashbacks, nightmares); avoidance (dissociation, numbing); and hyperarousal (difficulty sleeping, severe anticipatory anxiety) occur.

Obsessive-Compulsive Disorder

Obsessive-compulsive disorder (OCD) is an anxiety disorder that may have its onset in pregnancy (Altshuler et al., 1998). Intrusive, frightening, ego-dystonic thoughts of harm coming to their fetus or of doing harm to their fetus are reported phenomena. Typically, pregnant women with OCD do not act on these thoughts, but one must make a careful assessment of impulsivity and co-occurring depression or irritability, which may increase the risk. Explaining, in a calm, nonjudgemental manner, that these thoughts are signs of an illness rather than negative feelings towards the baby, helps women feel more contained and in control.

Risks of Untreated Mood and Anxiety Disorders

The risks for the mother include poor self-care, inadequate nutrition, weight gain, sleep disturbance, illicit drug use, smoking, alcohol abuse, emotional deterioration, and increased anxiety. Interpersonal and family conflict may escalate, especially if irritability is one of the symptoms. Depression in pregnancy increases the risk of PPD, which imparts independent risks for the child.

There are some reports of an increased risk of preeclampsia (Kurki, Hiilesmaa, Raitasalo, Mattila, & Ylikorkala, 2000; Bansil et al., 2010), Caesarean delivery, epidurals (Chung, Lau, Yip, Chiu, & Lee, 2001), preterm birth, low birth weight (Grote et al., 2010) and poor neonatal adaptation (Misri et al., 2004). This may be a consequence of the lifestyle changes described above. Biological mechanisms thought to be involved include increased cortisol and dysregulation of the hypothalamic-pituitary-adrenocortical axis, which may result in placental hypoperfusion.

There are many reports regarding the neurobiological impact of fetal exposure to severe anxiety and MDD. Although the numbers are small, research suggests a possibility of increased risk of the baby's developing a fearful temperament, attention-deficit hyperactivity disorder (ADHD), autism, or childhood anxiety (Hollins, 2007). There is evidence to suggest that at least some of these effects relate to the impact of MDD during pregnancy, rather than inheritance.

Intervention for Antenatal Depression and Anxiety Disorders

Preexisting and new-onset medical disorders such as anemia, thyroid disorders, or other autoimmune disorders must be ruled out as the cause of the anxiety or depression. Treatment should include validation of the woman's experience and education about the nature of depression or anxiety during pregnancy. Many women are relieved to find out they have an illness, rather than that they are bad or uncaring future mothers. Education of partners and family is essential, as they may feel helpless and overwhelmed or defensively dismissive. Recruitment of family and partners for assistance provides the woman with extra support at home. Respite care, visiting home assistance, public health, mental health nursing, and other community agencies can also be employed with great benefit. Reduction of stressors such as the care of other children, housework, and other domestic chores should be addressed. Ensuring adequate sleep is an important preventive and treatment measure.

Treatment with psychotherapy, facilitated support groups, and supportive counseling may be effective in mild or moderate syndromes and is usually preferred to medication by both mothers and healthcare professionals. An understanding of the psychological development during pregnancy provides a framework for education and psychotherapy. Supportive, psychodynamic, intrapersonal, and cognitive behavior therapy have all been used with good results.

In more severe situations—in which the anxiety and/or depression is disabling and has a profoundly negative impact on the mother, other children, and the marriage—medication should be offered. The clinician should summarize the research on the safety of psychotropic medication in pregnancy and discuss the risk–benefit ratio (Robinson, 2012a). Most patients are not aware that there are risks to the fetus of *not* taking medication for severe depression or anxiety. This type of discussion helps mothers make an informed decision.

Schizophrenia in Pregnancy

The incidence of schizophrenia in women is 1–2%, with the most common age of initial onset during the childbearing years. Women with schizophrenia may become pregnant, although those who are chronically psychotic are more likely to have unplanned pregnancies (Barkla et al., 2000). In these cases, pregnancies may be unwanted and end in terminations. Severely ill women who are non-compliant with medication may fail to seek adequate prenatal care, have poor diets, smoke, or abuse other substances. They may become delusional and try to harm the baby *in utero* or at birth, or develop anxiety or delusions about the obstetrician or the delivery. These women are often at risk of having the newborn removed from them due to their inability to care for the child.

With greater understanding of the benefits of continuous antipsychotic medication, many schizophrenic women continue to lead active lives, enter into relationships, and experience the desire to conceive. For these women, "prenatal care" needs to start prior to pregnancy. Contraceptive needs should be discussed so the woman can plan her pregnancy. It is important to discuss the dangers of decompensating if she discontinues medication during pregnancy. The clinician needs to help her plan to have appropriate supports in place both during and after the pregnancy.

Schizophrenic mothers have been said to have significantly more obstetrical complications than non-psychotic women. Bennedsen, Mortensen, Olesen, and Henriksen (2001) found a marginally significant increase in congenital abnormalities, but no increase in stillbirths or neonatal deaths. However, Nilsson, Lichtenstein, Cnattinguis, Murray, and Hultman (2002) found the risks for adverse pregnancy outcomes such as low birth weight, preterm delivery, and stillbirth were generally doubled for women with an episode of schizophrenia during pregnancy, compared to women in the control group. Jablensky, Morgan, Zubrick, Bower, and Yellachich (2005) found women with schizophrenia were significantly more likely to have placental abruption, low birth weight infants, and children with cardiovascular anomalies. There was an increased rate of sudden infant death syndrome (SIDS) in the offspring of these women. It is unclear whether these problems are due to some intrinsic biological factors, medication during pregnancy, or maternal lifestyle.

During pregnancy, close monitoring is important as the physiological changes in pregnancy may require an increase in medication doses as the pregnancy progresses (Robinson, 2012b). The clinician needs to watch carefully for any signs of poor eating habits, substance abuse, or delusional ideas, especially concerning the pregnancy. The mental health clinician should work closely with the obstetrician, first to ensure that he/she does not tell the woman to discontinue her psychiatric medication, and then to make sure he/she is aware of possible risks during the pregnancy and delivery. If the woman becomes very delusional prior to or at the time of the delivery, she may require psychiatric admission.

SUBSTANCE ABUSE IN PREGNANCY

Substance abuse during pregnancy is an immense public health concern. Best estimates for pregnant American women in the 15 to 44 age group are: illicit drug use, 3.4%; tobacco use, 17.6%; and alcohol use, 13.8%; with many using all three (Lester, Andreozzi, & Appiah, 2004). It is estimated that approximately 1 million children in the United States each year are exposed to legal or illegal substances during gestation (Chasnoff, Anson, Hatcher, & Stenson, 1998). Rates of substance use and abuse in pregnancy are thought to be significantly under-reported due to fear, stigma, and most recently, the debate over whether to consider such an activity a criminal offense.

Screening for substance use in pregnancy using open-ended and nonjudgemental questioning is more likely to result in disclosure. Inquire by starting with the use of over-the-counter (OTC) and prescription medications (their own and from others), then moving to alcohol and illicit drugs, including questions about the method of administration and any sharing of drug paraphernalia. Information regarding the context of drug use, life impact, and willingness to change will permit the development of an individualized treatment plan. Urine drug-screening can be done to increase detection of problematic substance use, assist with monitoring and motivation, and provide documentation for child protection services.

Substance use can cause direct toxicity to the fetus, but it can also have indirect effects due to poor nutrition, inadequate housing, and lack of prenatal care. The potential impact of substance abuse in pregnancy includes obstetrical complications, exacerbation of comorbid psychiatric illness, and effects on the fetus, neonate, and child.

Alcohol is the most teratogenic substance of abuse in pregnancy, with rates of abuse highest in the first trimester. It is of particular concern due to its neurotoxic impact, which begins by the third week post-conception. As 50% of pregnancies are unplanned, the potential for early damage is substantial. Fetal effects are dependent on dose, drinking pattern, gestational age, and both maternal and fetal genetic metabolic factors. Fetal alcohol exposure affects the neurodevelopment of nearly 1% of babies, with the full fetal alcohol syndrome (FAS) affecting approximately 1 in 1,000 babies. FAS is the result of heavy drinking and results in prenatal and postnatal growth retardation, facial dysmorphology, and neurodevelopmental abnormalities resulting in a complex pattern of behavioral and cognitive dysfunction. Long-term consequences include mental health problems such as mood and anxiety disorders, ADHD, substance abuse, and suicide (O'Connor & Paley, 2009), as well as a range of behavioral problems (Jones, 2011).

Marijuana causes exacerbation of maternal mood and anxiety disorders and has (inconsistent) effects on the length of gestation. Use in pregnancy can lead to problems for the neonate such as transient sleep disturbances and difficulties in self-soothing. Long-term behavioral problems for the child include hyperactivity, impulsivity, inattention, delinquency, and poor executive function.

Nicotine increases the risk of placenta previa, abruption, miscarriage, intrauterine growth restriction, prematurity, perinatal mortality, and SIDS.

Opioid abuse increases risks of preeclampsia, placental abruption, intrauterine growth restriction, miscarriage, prematurity, fetal distress, and stillbirth.

Management of drug abuse in pregnancy must first focus on engaging and motivating the woman to engage in treatment (Milligan et al., 2010). Education about the impact on the mother and the fetus may help motivate the woman. The choice of medical detoxification or supportive therapy is substance-specific. The second trimester is the safest time for drug withdrawal, as this can induce miscarriage in the first trimester and fetal distress or demise and premature labor in third trimester. Treatment of comorbid psychiatric illnesses is essential. Relapse prevention includes pharmacotherapy and counseling to reinforce her motivation and help the woman recognize and avoid triggers. Multidisciplinary teams are most effective.

EATING DISORDERS

The rates of eating disorders in pregnancy have been estimated as 0.2% for bulimia nervosa and 4.8% for binge-eating disorder (Bulik et al., 2007). Eating disorders may be exacerbated or remit during pregnancy. They are associated with comorbid depression and higher rates of miscarriage, low birth weight, obstetrical complications, and postpartum depression (Franko et al., 2001). As the potential negative consequences are significant, a high index of suspicion is required when a woman with a history of eating disorders shows poor weight gain. Assertive treatment is required.

POSTPARTUM

Although the postpartum period can be a very happy and exciting time, it is also complex and overwhelming on multiple levels. There are dramatic physical and biological alterations, as levels of progesterone and estrogen drop, and prolactin surges for lactation. A new mother has to cope with physical changes after pregnancy, which may include significant weight gain or complications from labor and delivery such as lacerations or Caesarean section wounds that are not healing. If breastfeeding, she also may be confronted by challenges such as difficulty with initiating or sustaining breastfeeding, painful nipples, or mastitis. During this time, an abundance of new experiences require navigation and adaptation, such as learning to care for the physical needs of a newborn, bonding with one's baby, and incorporating one's new maternal identity into one's previous self-image and lifestyle. There may also be financial and career challenges, as a new mother must coordinate and integrate her work life with her family life. The woman may still be processing memories of her own parent–child experiences. Also, having a baby may strain the new mother's relationship with her partner. Older children may also place additional demands on the new mother.

Because of these myriad transitions, challenges, and changes, the postpartum period is a time of heightened risk for developing psychiatric problems or for the recurrence of preexisting illnesses. During the first three months postpartum, women are at the highest lifetime risk of needing psychiatric care (Kendell, Chalmers, & Platz, 1987). Because postpartum mental illnesses place a tremendous burden on a new mother, her family, and the baby, these illnesses need to be identified early and treated effectively.

POSTPARTUM PSYCHIATRIC DISORDERS

Psychiatric disorders of the postpartum period include "the baby blues," postpartum depression, postpartum anxiety disorders, and postpartum psychosis. These disorders are not separately or specifically described in the DSM-V, but mood disorders (major depressive, manic or mixed episodes in MDD, bipolar I disorder, or bipolar II disorder) and brief psychotic disorder can receive the specifier *with peripartum onset,* if they begin within the first four weeks after delivery.

Baby Blues

Baby blues occur in 50–80% of new mothers, beginning within three to five days after the baby is born. Symptoms last a few hours to a few days, and remit within two weeks. Baby blues are not widely considered a psychiatric illness, but they are an intense emotional state that occurs in the early postpartum period (O'Hara, Schlechte, Lewis, & Wright, 1991). Despite symptoms of feeling overwhelmed, increased anxiety, tearfulness, and heightened sensitivity, the new mother is likely to be able to function well and care for her baby. It is postulated that baby blues are caused by the dramatic shift in hormones that occurs during delivery and in the early postpartum period. It has also been associated with sleep disruption in late pregnancy (Wilkie & Shapiro, 1992) and may be triggered by the significant psychosocial and lifestyle transition that accompanies having a baby (O'Hara et al., 1991).

Sufficient interventions include education about caring for a newborn, discussions about the importance of getting enough sleep, development of a support network, and emotional support and reassurance for a new mother and her partner. However, for women who are at risk of developing postpartum depression, baby blues symptoms should be monitored closely, with follow-up arranged, as these symptoms may be the early signs of postpartum depression. Up to 25% of new mothers who have the baby blues later develop postpartum depression (O'Hara & Swain, 1996).

Postpartum Depression

Postpartum depression (PPD) affects between 10 to 15% of new mothers (Halbreich, 2005). The official *DSM-IV* diagnosis for this illness is *Major depressive disorder with peripartum onset,* if it begins within four weeks postpartum. However, there are data to show that PPD can begin any time within the first 12 months postpartum (Cooper, Campbell, Day, Kennerley, & Bond, 1988). Generally, symptoms begin within the first 12 weeks after the baby is born, and most resolve within three months (Cox, Murray, & Chapman, 1993); but, in more severe cases, symptoms may persist for up to one year postpartum (Cooper et al., 1988).

Because of the shame, fear, and embarrassment experienced by many depressed new mothers, there is often a lag between the time a woman begins to feel unwell and when she seeks psychiatric care. Because of the overlap between some of the somatic symptoms of depression and regular postpartum recovery or medical illnesses, many clinicians also fail to identify postpartum illnesses.

A formal PPD diagnosis can be made if a woman meets DSM-V criteria for a major depressive episode (MDE), including low mood, anhedonia, changes in sleeping (severe insomnia is prominent in PPD), changes in appetite, physical retardation or agitation, decreased concentration and memory, feelings of guilt or worthlessness, as well as thoughts of death or suicide. For the symptoms to be defined as a disorder, they need to persist for two weeks and have a significant impact on a woman's ability to function and care for herself and her baby.

While PPD often appears clinically similar to MDE, the concerns are usually related to parenting and infant issues. There may also be prominent symptoms of anxiety, irritability, guilt about being unwell and being an inadequate mother, fears about being unable to care for one's baby, regret about having had a baby, and unrealistic worries about the infant's health and welfare. Forty to 57% of women with PPD may also have some ego-dystonic, intrusive thoughts about harming their baby. In the context of PPD, these thoughts are very frightening to the woman, but her judgement and insight are fully preserved (Brandes, Soares, & Cohen, 2004).

The precise etiology of postpartum depression has yet to be determined. On a biological level, it appears that a sensitivity to changes in gonadal steroid levels make some women susceptible to PPD (Bloch et al., 2000). The absolute levels of these biological markers are not abnormal in women affected by PPD, but the fluctuation of these levels has a pathological impact on some women, perhaps related to the effects of gonadal hormones on the neurotransmitters responsible for mood.

The most significant risk factor for postpartum depression is having a history of depression or anxiety during pregnancy (O'Hara & Swain, 1996; Beck, 2001). Cohen et al. (2006) demonstrated a 68% relapse rate when women who were being treated for depression with antidepressants stopped their medication during pregnancy. A prior history of depression, unrelated to pregnancy, is also a strong risk factor, as is having a family history of depression or postpartum depression (O'Hara & Swain, 1996; Beck, 2001). Recent stressful life events and limited social and personal supports increase the risk of PPD (O'Hara & Swain, 1996; Beck, 2001). Moderate risk factors include neurotic maternal personality, low self-esteem, and negative cognitive styles. Weaker risk factors include obstetrical complications, low income, unemployment and financial strain, difficult infant temperament, breastfeeding problems, the discontinuation of breastfeeding, and young maternal age.

It is important to rule out underlying medical issues, such as thyroid disorders and anemia, that may contribute to the woman's presentation. Women who have mild to moderate postpartum depression often benefit from psychotherapy and improved social supports. Two short-term psychotherapies, interpersonal therapy (O'Hara, Stuart, Gromen, & Wenzel, 2000) and cognitive behavioral therapy (Appleby, Warner, Whitton, & Faragher, 1997), have been studied and found to reduce symptom burden, improve social functioning, and increase coping skills. Group therapy and support groups may also be effective components of treatment.

Improving support from a woman's partner, family, and friends is also an important part of treatment. Partners can be essential in nurturing recovery and in providing various forms of support, from understanding and empathy, to instrumental support. Implementing a sleep plan so that a new mother is able to increase her sleeping hours is another important part of a comprehensive treatment plan. Moderate exercise and a healthy diet may also be beneficial. More research needs to be done to determine exactly what types of social supports and psychological and psychosocial interventions are most beneficial for women suffering from PPD. Interventions and strategies need to be accessible to new mothers and sensitive to their time constraints, resources, and child care needs.

Internet and telephone services and therapies are therefore being investigated.

Women who have more severe postpartum depression may also need antidepressant medication. Treatment decisions and management of medication are ideally shared between the patient and her psychiatrist, mental healthcare provider, obstetrician, and pediatrician.

Many antidepressants and other psychotropic medications are compatible with breastfeeding. Treatment providers should seek up-to-date knowledge about medication use during breastfeeding, as all medications enter the breast milk. However, most are found at very low levels and do not harm the baby. For new mothers who are severely ill (acutely suicidal or psychotic) or who do not respond to medications or cannot tolerate medications, a hospital admission may be required, and electroconvulsive therapy (ECT) may be an option.

Estrogen therapy for postpartum depression has been studied but has not been conclusively shown to be effective or safe (Gregoire, Kumar, Everitt, Henderson, & Studd, 1996; Ahokas, Kaukoranta, Wahlbeck, & Aito, 2001). Progesterone supplements have been shown to exacerbate postpartum depression and should be avoided (Lawrie et al., 1998). Bright light therapy has been proposed as a PPD treatment, but more research is required (Corral, Kuan, & Kostaras, 2000). Although women who have a history of severe depression may take longer to treat, the rate of recovery from PPD is high, and women who receive treatment early do particularly well (Wisner et al., 2004).

Once a woman has experienced an episode of postpartum depression, risk of a recurrence following subsequent pregnancies is increased to 50%. Ideally, a woman who is at risk of postpartum depression should meet with her healthcare providers prior to or during pregnancy to discuss ways to manage some risk factors and thereby limit the recurrence of postpartum depression.

Postpartum Psychosis

Postpartum psychosis (PPP) is the rarest and severest of the postpartum psychiatric disorders, occurring in 0.1–0.2% of new mothers. This psychiatric emergency often begins within 2–14 days postpartum. One study showed that 73% of patients had symptoms begin by the third day postpartum (Heron, McGuinness, Blackmore, Craddock, & Jones, 2008). Initial symptoms often mimic a delirium, with marked confusion, bizarre behavior, disorganized thoughts, agitation, and pronounced insomnia. As the psychosis develops, the woman may display prominent mood lability with severe depression or euphoria. The episode may begin to look like a manic psychosis with hallucinations and delusions, often related to the child or motherhood. One study showed that 53% of women with PPP experience persecutory delusions such as beliefs that the police want to apprehend her child (Chandra, Bhargavaraman, Raghunandan, & Shaligram, 2006). She may experience auditory hallucinations "commanding" her to harm her child or herself, thought broadcasting, or delusions of being controlled by external forces. Women who have PPP exhibit poor insight and impaired judgement, thereby posing a significant risk to their child and themselves. About 4% of women with PPP commit infanticide (Spinelli, 2009).

In the DSM-V (American Psychiatric Association, 2013), postpartum psychosis is listed as a *Brief psychotic disorder* with postpartum onset if it begins within four weeks postpartum, or as an *Other Psychotic disorder*. Current thinking is that the majority of these women meet criteria for *Bipolar disorder* (Sit, Rothschild, & Wisner, 2006).

A personal history of PPP or bipolar disorder confers an increased risk of postpartum psychosis (Stewart, Klompenhouwer, Kendell, & van Hulst, 1991). Women with a history of bipolar disorder or schizoaffective disorder have a 50% risk for another episode of PPP. It appears that postpartum psychosis also clusters in families that have high rates of bipolar disorder and postpartum psychosis (Jones & Craddock, 2001). A diagnosis of schizophrenia or schizoaffective disorder also increases the risk of postpartum psychosis.

There is some research to show that estrogen may influence circadian rhythms and influence sleep loss. Sleep loss, in turn, has been implicated in the onset of postpartum psychosis (Sharma & Mazmanian, 2003). It is believed that rapid hormonal withdrawal after delivery may precipitate PPP, particularly in women with a history of bipolar disorder (Spinelli, 2009).

PPP is a psychiatric emergency and usually requires inpatient hospitalization to stabilize and protect the mother as well as ensure the safety of the baby. Antipsychotic medications, both typicals (e.g., haloperidol) and atypicals (e.g., olanzapine), are frequently used in the acute phase of treatment. Benzodiazepines may also be required to treat insomnia or for additional sedation. Any underlying mood disorder needs to be treated as well. Lithium is commonly used if there is an underlying bipolar disorder. Antidepressants should be avoided, as they may exacerbate the underlying problem. ECT is another treatment option that has been used with great success for severe cases of PPP.

Once treatment is initiated, the recovery rate from PPP is good and relatively rapid. Most women improve within two or three months. Since there seems to be a link between postpartum psychosis and bipolar disorder, between 18–37% of women have a further postpartum psychosis, while 39–81% of women have a non–pregnancy related episode (Chaudron & Pies, 2003). Studies have shown that initiating prophylactic lithium in the third trimester or immediately after delivery reduces the risk of PPP in at-risk women. In contrast, among subjects who discontinued lithium prior to pregnancy, even those who remained stable over the first 40 weeks, postpartum recurrences were 2.9 times more frequent than recurrences in non-pregnant women during weeks 41–64 (70% versus 24%) (Viguera et al., 2000). For women with schizophrenia, 50% remain well after one episode of PPP, 33% have recurrent PPP, and 5% have a refractory illness with numerous puerperal and non-puerperal recurrences (Sit, Rothschild, & Wisner, 2006).

Ensuring adequate sleep near delivery is also helpful in reducing risk (Spinelli, 2009). A four- to five-day postpartum hospital stay to ensure adequate sleep after the baby is born may also be useful in preventing a severe depression or psychotic episode (Steiner, Fairman, Jansen, & Casey, 2002). As with postpartum depression, early identification of women at risk of PPP, and early, aggressive treatment of PPP symptoms is essential and limits the impact of this serious illness on a mother and her child.

Postpartum Anxiety Disorders

Postpartum anxiety disorders have received limited research attention to date, but they are common. Rates between 4% and 15% have been demonstrated (Heron et al., 2004; Stuart, Couser, Schilder, O'Hara, & Gorman, 1998). It may be that a history of an anxiety disorder confers a higher risk of postpartum depression and anxiety than a history of depression. Women who have had anxiety disorders or even anxiety symptoms in the past or during pregnancy are at high risk of developing postpartum anxiety disorders. The physiological changes postpartum, as well as the intense stress and responsibility inherent in having a baby and being a new mother, are additional precipitants of postpartum anxiety disorders. Anxiety disorders may also develop *de novo* in the postpartum period.

Panic disorder occurs in 1–2% of new mothers in the postpartum period (Ross & McLean, 2006). There may be a recurrence of previous illness or new onset of panic disorder. Symptoms are similar to those in non-postpartum panic disorder. Avoidance of situations due to anticipatory anxiety makes it difficult for a mother to care for her child or to be alone with her child for fear of having a panic attack.

Two to 3% of new mothers experience postpartum obsessive-compulsive disorder (PPOCD). PPOCD is often characterized by intrusive, unwanted, frightening thoughts about harming one's baby, either inadvertently or intentionally. Compulsions are less common in the postpartum population. There is no record of a woman with PPOCD harming her child. Women with a history of OCD, MDD, or premenstrual dysphoric disorder (PMDD) are at risk of developing PPOCD. Thirty percent of women with PPOCD have a new onset in the postpartum period (Ross & McLean, 2006). Situations in which the mother fears she will act on her thoughts are actively avoided. The avoidance behaviors can become problematic if the woman fears she cannot be alone with her baby and refuses to care for her child. Although women with postpartum depression may have similar thoughts and behaviors, in PPOCD the obsessive thoughts and avoidance are more extreme and more intense. Secondary depression may develop due to intense feelings of guilt and self-hatred for experiencing such frightening symptoms. Women with PPOCD have preserved insight and judgement and require reassurance that they are not at risk of actually harming their babies, despite their thoughts. There is a high relapse rate in subsequent pregnancies of PPOCD, and it may take longer to treat than other postpartum anxiety disorders (Sichel, Cohen, Rosenbaum, & Driscoll, 1993).

Postpartum generalized anxiety disorder (PPGAD) is experienced by 4–8% of new mothers (Wenzel et al., 2005; Wenzel, Haugen, Jackson, & Robinson, 2003). Symptoms are similar to those in GAD at other life stages, but the excessive and uncontrollable worries are usually related to motherhood and the newborn. Few studies have examined PPGAD specifically.

Postpartum PTSD has also been reported. It may follow a traumatic labor and delivery or be triggered by medical interventions during labor and delivery in women who have previously suffered from sexual abuse. Rates between 1% and 6% have been reported (Wijma, Soderquist, & Wijma, 1997; Creedy, Schochet, & Horsfall, 2000).

Postpartum anxiety disorders are treated similarly to anxiety disorders at other stages of the life cycle. Medical disorders, including thyroid dysfunction and anemia, should be ruled out. Antidepressant medications, particularly selective serotonin-reuptake inhibitors (SSRIs), are commonly used to treat anxiety disorders. Benzodiazepines are also commonly used. The same principles described for the use of medication in PPD treatment should be applied. Cognitive behavioral therapy (CBT) is also an evidence-based and effective treatment for most anxiety disorders. Timpano, Abramowitz, Mahaffey, Mitchell, and Schmidt (2011) have found that integrating a CBT-based obsessive-compulsive symptom program into traditional prenatal classes can significantly reduce the occurrence of PPOCD.

IMPACT ON THE FAMILY OF POSTPARTUM MENTAL HEALTH PROBLEMS

Postpartum psychiatric illness affects not only the life and well-being of a new mother, but also that of her partner, family, and of course, her newborn. Research has shown that partners of women with PPD experience high rates of depression. A recent study concluded that 10% of new fathers experience some major or minor depression in the first three to six months postpartum, and that men whose partners were depressed were more likely to become depressed (Paulson & Bazemore, 2010).

Maternal depression in the first year of a child's life has been associated with significant child psychopathology (Bagner, Pettit, Lewinsohn, & Seeley, 2010). Cognitive, behavioral, and social problems have been widely reported in infants and children of depressed new mothers (Grace, Evindar, & Stewart, 2003). When a mother is severely depressed, anxious, or psychotic, the mother–infant dyad is affected. Infants of mothers with psychiatric illness are more likely to have avoidant and disorganized attachment, which can have long-lasting effects on the child (Martins & Gaffan, 2000).

Most research in this area has examined the impact of severe, prolonged postpartum disorders and does not account for less severe and treated postpartum illnesses. It is important not to use the impact statistics to increase fear and guilt in mothers who are suffering. Several studies have demonstrated that early identification and treatment of a mother's mental illness has a very positive effect on the child and may prevent or reverse some or all of the above-mentioned ill effects (Birmaher, 2011). By providing evidence, reassurance, and hope that early and effective treatment leads to positive outcomes for a woman and her child, clinicians can motivate and support patients suffering with postpartum psychiatric illnesses.

CLINICAL PEARLS

- Hyperemesis gravidarum has been labeled as a sign of hysteria, neurosis, depression, stress, or marital conflict; however, there is no evidence that this is true.

- Up to 25% of new mothers who have the baby blues later develop postpartum depression (O'Hara & Swain, 1996).

- Postpartum depression can begin any time within the first 12 months postpartum.

- Forty to 57% of women with postpartum depression may also have some ego-dystonic, intrusive thoughts about harming their baby.

- The most significant risk factor for postpartum depression is having a history of depression or anxiety during pregnancy.

- Postpartum, it is important to rule out underlying medical issues such as thyroid disorders and anemia.

- Anxiety disorders may develop *de novo* in the postpartum period.

- A history of anxiety disorder may confer a higher risk of postpartum depression and anxiety than a risk of depression.

- There is a link between postpartum psychosis and bipolar disorder.

- Women with postpartum OCD have preserved insight and judgement and require reassurance that they are not at risk of actually harming their babies, despite their thoughts.

- Most psychotropic medication is safe for use during pregnancy and postpartum.

DISCLOSURE STATEMENTS

Dr. Meschino is funded by the Alternative Funding Plan (AFP) Ministry of Health Government of Ontario–Women's College Hospital grants only.

Dr. Dalfen is an employee of the University of Toronto and works at Mount Sinai Hospital in Toronto, Canada. Dr. Dalfen has no ties to any pharmaceutical companies and no conflicts to disclose.

Dr. Robinson is an employee of the University of Toronto and works at the University Health Network in Toronto Canada. She has no ties to any pharmaceutical companies. She has no conflicts to disclose.

REFERENCES

Ahokas, A., Kaukoranta, J., Wahlbeck, K., & Aito, M. (2001). Estrogen deficiency in severe postpartum depression: Successful treatment with sublingual physiologic 17beta-estradiol: A preliminary study. *Journal of Clinical Psychiatry, 62*(5), 332–336.

Altshuler, L. L., Hendrick, V., & Cohen, L. S. (1998). Course of mood and anxiety disorders during pregnancy and the postpartum period. *Journal of Clinical Psychiatry, 59*(Suppl 2), 29–33.

American Psychiatric Association (2013). *The Diagnostic and Statistical Manual, 5th Edition, Text Revision* (DSM-V). Arlington, VA: American Psychiatric Publishing.

Appleby, L., Warner, R., Whitton, A., & Faragher, B. (1997). A controlled study of fluoxetine and cognitive-behavioural counselling in the treatment of postnatal depression. *British Medical Journal, 314*(7085), 932–936.

Bagner, D. M., Pettit, J. W., Lewinsohn, P. M., & Seeley, J. R. (2010). Effect of maternal depression on child behavior: A sensitive period? *Journal of the American Academy of Child & Adolescent Psychiatry, 49*(7), 699–707.

Bansil, P., Kuklina, E. V., Meikle, S. F., Posner, S. F., Kourtis, A. P., Ellington, S. R., et al. (2010). Maternal and fetal outcomes among women with depression. *Journal of Women's Health, 19*(2), 329–334.

Barkla, J., Byrne, L., Hearle, J., Plant, K., Jenner, L., & McGrath, J. (2000). Pregnancy in women with psychotic disorders. *Archives of Women's Mental Health, 3*(1), 23–26.

Beck, C. T. (2001). Predictors of postpartum depression: an update. *Nursing Research, 50*(5), 275–285.

Bennedsen, B. E., Mortensen, P. B., Olesen, A. V., & Henriksen, T. V. (2001). Congenital malformations, stillbirths, and infant deaths among children of women with schizophrenia. *Archives of General Psychiatry, 58*(7), 674–679.

Bennett, H. A., Einarson, A., Taddio, A., Koren, G., & Einarson, T. R. (2004). Prevalence of depression during pregnancy: systematic review. *Obstetrics & Gynecology, 103*(4), 698–709.

Bernazzani, O., Saucier, J. F., David, H., & Borgeat, F. (1997a). Psychosocial factors related to emotional disturbances during pregnancy. *Journal of Psychosomatic Research, 42*(4), 391–402.

Bernazzini, O., Saucier, J. F., David, H., & Borgeat, F. (1997b). Psychosocial predictors of depressive symptomatology level in postpartum women. *Journal of Affective Disorders, 46*(1), 39–49.

Bifulco, A., Figueiredo, B., Guedeney, N., Gorman, L. L., Hayes, S., Muzik, M., et al. (2004). Maternal attachment style and depression associated with childbirth: Preliminary results from a European and US cross-cultural study. *British Journal of Psychiatry, Suppl, 46*, S31–S37.

Birmaher, B. (2011). Remission of a mother's depression is associated with her child's mental health. *American Journal of Psychiatry, 168*(6), 563–565.

Bloch, M., Schmidt, P. J., Danaceau, M., Murphy, J., Nieman, L., & Rubinow, D. R. (2000). Effects of gonadal steroids in women with a history of postpartum depression. *American Journal of Psychiatry, 157*(6), 924–930.

Brandes, M., Soares, C. N., & Cohen, L. S. (2004). Postpartum onset obsessive-compulsive disorder: diagnosis and management. *Archives of Women's Mental Health, 7*(2), 99–110.

Bronwyn, L., & Milgrom, J. (2008). Risk factors for antenatal depression, postnatal depression and parenting stress. *BioMedCentral Psychiatry, 8*(24), 1–34.

Bulik, C. M., Von Holle, A., Hamer, R., Knoph Berg, C., Torgersen, L., Magnus, P., et al. (2007). Patterns of remission, continuation and incidence of broadly defined eating disorders during early pregnancy in the Norwegian Mother and Child Cohort Study (MoBa). *Psychological Medicine, 37*(8), 1109–1118.

Chandra, P. S., Bhargavaraman, R. P., Raghunandan, V. N., & Shaligram, D. (2006). Delusions related to infant and their association with mother-infant interactions in postpartum psychotic disorders. *Archives of Women's Mental Health, 9*(5), 285–288.

Chasnoff, I. J., Anson, A., Hatcher, R., & Stenson, H. (1998). Prenatal exposure to cocaine and other drugs. Outcome at four to six years. In J. A. Harvey & B. E. Kosofsky (Eds.), *Cocaine: Effects on the developing brain* (pp. 335–340). New York: The New York Academy of Sciences.

Chaudron, L. H., & Pies, R. W. (2003). The relationship between postpartum psychosis and bipolar disorder: a review. *Journal of Clinical Psychiatry, 64*(11), 1284–1292.

Chung, T. K., Lau, T. K., Yip, A. S., Chiu, H. F., & Lee, D. T. (2001). Antepartum depressive symptomatology is associated with adverse obstetric and neonatal outcomes. *Psychosomatic Medicine, 63*(5), 830–834.

Cohen, L. S., Altshuler, L. L., Harlow, B. L., Nonacs, R., Newport, D. J., Viguera, A. C., et al. (2006). Relapse of major depression during pregnancy in women who maintain or discontinue antidepressant treatment. *Journal of the American Medical Association, 295*(5), 499–507.

Cohen, L. S., Nonacs, R. M., Bailey, J. W., Viguera, A. C., Reminick, A. M., Altshuler, L. L., et al. (2004). Relapse of depression during pregnancy following antidepressant discontinuation: a preliminary prospective study. *Archives of Women's Mental Health, 7*(4), 217–221.

Cooper, P. J., Campbell, E. A., Day, A., Kennerley, H., & Bond, A. (1988). Non-psychotic psychiatric disorder after childbirth. A prospective study of prevalence, incidence, course and nature. *British Journal of Psychiatry, 152*, 799–806.

Corral, M., Kuan, A., & Kostaras, D. (2000). Bright light therapy's effect on postpartum depression. *American Journal of Psychiatry, 157*(2), 303–304.

Cowan, P. A., & Cowan, C. P. (1988). Changes in marriage during the transition to parenthood. In G. Y. Michaels & W. A. Goldberg, *The transition to parenthood: Current theory and research* (pp. 114–154). New York: Cambridge University Press.

Cox, J. L., Murray, D., & Chapman, G. (1993). A controlled study of the onset, duration and prevalence of postnatal depression. *British Journal of Psychiatry, 163*, 27–31.

Creedy, D. K., Shochet, I. M., & Horsfall, J. (2000). Childbirth and the development of acute trauma symptoms: Incidence and contributing factors. *Birth, 27*(2), 104–111.

Franko, D. L., Blais, M. A., Becker, A. E., Delinsky, S. S., Greenwood, D. N., Flores, A. T., et al. (2001). Pregnancy complications and neonatal outcomes in women with eating disorders. *American Journal of Psychiatry, 158*(9), 1461–1466.

Gavin, N. I., Gaynes, B. N., Lohr, K. N., Meltzer-Brody, S., Gartlehner, G., & Swinson, T. (2005). Perinatal depression. A systematic review of prevalence and incidence. *Obstetrics & Gynecology, 106*(5), 1071–1083.

Grace, S. L., Evindar, A., & Stewart, D. E. (2003). The effect of postpartum depression on child cognitive development and behaviour: a review and critical analysis of the literature. *Archives of Women's Mental Health, 6*(4), 263–274.

Gregoire, A. J., Kumar, R., Everitt, B., Henderson, A. F., & Studd, J. W. (1996). Transdermal oestrogen for treatment of severe postnatal depression. *Lancet, 347*(9066), 930–933.

Grote, N. K., Bridge, J. A., Gavin, A. R., Melville, J. L., Iyengar, S., & Katon, W. J. (2010). A meta-analysis of depression during pregnancy and the risk of preterm birth, low birth weight, and intrauterine growth restriction. *Archives of General Psychiatry, 67*(10), 1012–1024.

Halbreich, U. (2005). Postpartum disorders: multiple interacting underlying mechanisms and risk factors. *Journal of Affective Disorders, 88*(1), 1–7.

Heron, J., McGuinness, M., Blackmore, E. R., Craddock, N., & Jones, I. (2008). Early postpartum symptoms in puerperal psychosis. *British Journal of Obstetrics & Gynaecology, 115*(3), 348–353.

Heron, J., O'Connor, T. G., Evans, J., Golding, J., Glover, V., & ALSPAC Study Team, (2004). The course of anxiety and depression through pregnancy and the postpartum in a community sample. *Journal of Affective Disorders, 80*(1), 65–73.

Hollins, K. (2007). Consequences of antenatal mental health problems for child health and development. *Current Opinion in Obstetrics & Gynecology, 19*(6), 568–572.

Jablensky, A. V., Morgan, V., Zubrick, S. R., Bower, C., & Yellachick, L. A. (2005). Pregnancy, delivery, and neonatal complications in a population cohort of women with schizophrenia and major affective disorders. *American Journal of Psychiatry, 162*(1), 79–91.

Jones, K. L. (2011). The effects of alcohol on fetal development. *Birth Defects Research Part C: Embryo Today, 93*(1), 3–11.

Jones, I., & Craddock, N. (2001). Familiality of the puerperal trigger in bipolar disorder: results of a family study. *American Journal of Psychiatry, 158*(6), 913–917.

Kendell, R. E., Chalmers, J. C., & Platz, C. (1987). Epidemiology of puerperal psychoses. *British Journal of Psychiatry, 150*, 662–673.

Kessler, R. C., McGonagle, K. A., Zhao, S., Nelson, C. B., Hughes, M., Eshleman, S., et al. (1994). Lifetime and 12-month prevalence of DSM-III-R psychiatric disorders in the United States. Results from the National Comorbidity Survey. *Archives of General Psychiatry, 51*(1), 8–19.

Kessler, R. C., Sonnega, A., Bromet, E., Hughes, M., & Nelson, C. B. (1995). Posttraumatic stress disorder in the National Comorbidity Survey. *Archives of General Psychiatry, 52*(12), 1048–1060.

Kurki, T., Hiilesmaa, V., Raitasalo, R., Mattila, H., & Ylikorkala, O. (2000). Depression and anxiety in early pregnancy and risk for pre-eclampsia. *Obstetrics & Gynecology, 95*(4), 487–490.

Kuscu, N. K., & Koyuncu, F. (2002). Hyperemesis gravidarum: current concepts and management. *Postgraduate Medical Journal, 78*(916), 76–79.

Lancaster, C. A., Gold, K. J., Flynn, H. A., Yoo, H., Marcus, S. M., & Davis, M. M. (2010). Risk factors for depressive symptoms during pregnancy: a systematic review. *American Journal of Obstetrics & Gynecology, 202*(1), 5–14.

Lawrie, T. A., Hofmeyr, G. J., De Jager, M., Berk, M., Paiker, J., & Viljoen, E. (1998). A double-blind randomised placebo controlled trial of postnatal norethisterone enanthate: the effect on postnatal depression and serum hormones. *British Journal of Obstetrics & Gynaecology, 105*(10), 1082–1090.

Lester, B. L., Andreozzi, L., & Appiah, L. (2004). Substance use during pregnancy: time for policy to catch up with research. *Harm Reduction Journal, 1*(1), 5.

Martins, C., & Gaffan, E. A. (2000). Effects of early maternal depression on patterns of infant-mother attachment: a meta-analytic investigation. *Journal of Child Psychology & Psychiatry, 41*(6), 737–746.

Matthey, S., Barnett, B., Howie, P., & Kavanagh, D. J. (2003). Diagnosing postpartum depression in mothers and fathers: Whatever happened to anxiety? *Journal of Affective Disorders, 74*(2), 139–147.

Milligan, K., Nicolls, A., Sword, W., Thabane, L., Henderson, J. R., Smith, A., et al. (2010). Maternal substance use and integrated treatment programs for women with substance abuse issues and their children: a meta-analysis. *Substance Abuse Treatment, Prevention, & Policy, 5*, 21.

Misri, S., Oberlander, T. F., Fairbrother, N., Carter, D., Ryan, D., Kuan, A. J., et al. (2004). Relation between prenatal maternal mood and anxiety and neonatal health. *Canadian Journal of Psychiatry, 49*(10), 684–689.

Nilsson, E., Lichtenstein, P., Cnattinguis, S., Murray, R. M., & Hultman, C. M. (2002). Women with schizophrenia: pregnancy outcome and infant death among their offspring. *Schizophrenia Research, 58*(2–3), 221–229.

O'Connor, M. J., & Paley, B. (2009). Psychiatric conditions associated with prenatal alcohol exposure. *Developmental Disabilities Research Reviews, 15*(3), 225–234.

O'Hara, M. W., Schlechte, J. A., Lewis, D. A., & Wright, E. J. (1991). Prospective study of postpartum blues. Biologic and psychosocial factors. *Archives of General Psychiatry, 48*(9), 801–806.

O'Hara, M. W., & Swain, A. M. (1996). Rates and risk of postpartum depression—a meta-analysis. *International Review of Psychiatry, 8*(1), 37–54.

O'Hara, M. W., Stuart, S., Gorman, L. L., & Wenzel, A. (2000). Efficacy of interpersonal psychotherapy for postpartum depression. *Archives of General Psychiatry, 57*(11), 1039–1045.

Paulson, J. F., & Bazemore, S. D. (2010). Prenatal and postpartum depression in fathers and its association with maternal depression: a meta-analysis. *Journal of the American Medical Association, 303*(19), 1961–1969.

Paykel, E. S., Emms, E. M., Fletcher, J., & Rassaby, E. S. (1980). Life events and social support in puerperal depression. *British Journal of Psychiatry, 136*, 339–346.

Ross, L. E., & McLean, L. M. (2006). Anxiety disorders during pregnancy and the postpartum period: A systematic review. *Journal of Clinical Psychiatry, 67*(8), 1285–1298.

Robertson, E., Jones, I., Haque, S., Holder, R., & Craddock, N. (2005). Risk of puerperal and non-puerperal recurrence of illness following bipolar affective puerperal (post-partum) psychosis. *British Journal of Psychiatry, 186*, 258–259.

Robinson G. E. (2012a). Psychopharmacology in Pregnancy and Postpartum. FOCUS: *The journal of life-long learning, 10*(1), 3–14.

Robinson G. E. (2012b). Treatment of schizophrenia in pregnancy and postpartum. *Journal of Population Therapeutics and Clinical Pharmacology, 19*(3), e380–e386.

Sharma, V., & Mazmanian, D. (2003). Sleep loss and postpartum psychosis. *Bipolar Disorder, 5*(2), 98–105.

Sichel, D. A., Cohen, L. S., Rosenbaum, J. F., & Driscoll, J. (1993). Postpartum onset of obsessive-compulsive disorder. *Psychosomatics, 34*(3), 277–279.

Sit, D., Rothschild, A. J., & Wisner, K. L. (2006). A review of postpartum psychosis. *Journal of Women's Health (Larchmont), 15*(4), 352–368.

Spinelli, M. G. (2009). Postpartum psychosis: detection of risk and management. *American Journal of Psychiatry, 166*(4), 405–408.

Steiner, M., Fairman, M., Jansen, K., & Casey, S. (2002). Can postpartum depression be prevented? [abstract]. Paper presented at the Marce Society International Biennial Scientific Meeting; Sept. 25–27, 2002; Sydney, Australia.

Stewart, D. E., Klompenhouwer, J. L., Kendell, R. E., & van Hulst, A. M. (1991). Prophylactic lithium in puerperal psychosis. The experience of three centres. *British Journal of Psychiatry, 158*, 393–397.

Stuart, S., Couser, G., Schilder, K., O'Hara, M. W., & Gorman, L. (1998). Postpartum anxiety and depression: onset and comorbidity in a community sample. *Journal of Nervous & Mental Disease, 186*(7), 420–424.

Timpano, K. R., Abramowitz, J. S., Mahaffey, B. L., Mitchell, M. A., & Schmidt, N. B. (2011). Efficacy of a prevention program for postpartum obsessive compulsive symptoms. *Journal of Psychiatric Research, 45*, 1511–1517.

Verberg, M. F. G., Gillott, D. J., Al-Fardan, N., & Grudzinskas, J. G. (2005). Hyperemesis gravidarum, a literature review. *Human Reproduction Update, 11*(5), 527–539.

Viguera, A. C., Nonacs, R., Cohen, L. S., Tondo, L., Murray, A., & Baldessarini, R. J. (2000). Risk of recurrence of bipolar disorder in pregnant and nonpregnant women after discontinuing lithium maintenance. *American Journal of Psychiatry, 157*(2), 179–184.

Wenzel, A., Haugen, E. N., Jackson, L. C., & Brendle, J. R. (2005). Anxiety symptoms and disorders at eight weeks postpartum. *Journal of Anxiety Disorders, 19*(3), 295–311.

Wenzel, A., Haugen, E. N., Jackson, L. C., & Robinson, K. (2003). Prevalence of generalized anxiety at eight weeks postpartum. *Archives of Women's Mental Health, 6*(1), 43–49.

Wijma, K., Soderquist, J., & Wijma, B. (1997). Posttraumatic stress disorder after childbirth: a cross sectional study. *Journal of Anxiety Disorders, 11*(6), 587–597.

Wilkie, G., & Shapiro, C. M. (1992). Sleep deprivation and the postnatal blues. *Journal of Psychosomatic Research, 36*(4), 309–316.

Wisner, K. L., Perel, J. M., Peindl, K. S., Hanusa, B. H., Piontek, C. M., & Findling, R. L. (2004). Prevention of postpartum depression: a pilot randomized clinical trial. *American Journal of Psychiatry, 161*(7), 1290–1292.

PART VIII

SURGICAL SPECIALTIES

69.

GENERAL SURGERY
BASIC PRINCIPLES

Frederick J. Stoddard, Jr., Robert L. Sheridan, Jeevendra Martyn, Lawrence F. Selter, and Donna B. Greenberg

INTRODUCTION

Innovations in surgery and anesthesia have increased the power of the surgeon to save lives, limbs, and organs. Innovations in psychiatry have enhanced the capacity of the surgical team to reduce suffering and improve outcomes. These innovations affect routine care in hospitals and urgent care for patients and their families after disasters (Stoddard, Katz, & Merlino, 2010; Stoddard et al., 2010; Stoddard, Pandya, & Katz, 2011). To ask for and consent to surgery and anesthesia requires that the patient have enormous trust or desperation, or both. Surgical patients come from varied cultural, racial, and language backgrounds and require culturally sensitive care in a language that they and their families understand. Also, surgical patients vary from being very disadvantaged to very advantaged, and recognition of differing needs for those from backgrounds of poverty or wealth is critical. How patients pay for their expensive surgical care may add significant burdens.

The patient's expectations of the surgeon may vary from realistic to delusional. Patient desire for information about their disease, management options, and recommendations also varies enormously. The surgeon may be respected, idealized as a savior, feared, or demonized by patients and their families for failing to fulfill expectations. The patients who are more likely to have difficulties in the relationship with the surgeon are those with difficulties in previous relationships (i.e., personality disorders or those with traits of these disorders). Their style of relating to authority and pattern of establishing appropriate boundaries affect the relationship to the surgical and anesthesia staff. Psychiatrists can help clarify the patient's distortions as well as respond with empathy to the patient's anger and disappointment if their expectations are not fulfilled. Psychiatrists may also help the surgeons and the surgical and anesthesia staff set appropriate limits on "acting out" by patients, and other types of inappropriate behavior.

PSYCHIATRIC CONSULTATION TO SURGICAL PATIENTS

The surgeon moves rapidly to diagnose surgical conditions and perform operative procedures, using sophisticated tools in the process. The anesthesiologist also works rapidly with the surgeon to assure optimal management of anesthesia before, during, and after procedures. Working in the surgical setting, the psychiatric consultant must match this pace with efficient diagnostic assessment and treatment. The role of psychiatric consultation in surgical care acknowledges the importance of treating comorbid psychiatric diagnoses to improve surgical outcomes and enhance patient care (Moore et al., 2013; Findley, Sanders, & Groves, 2003; Abrams et al., 2010). The medical psychiatrist will be alert to the history of alcohol or other substance use, the risk of acute withdrawal, and the ways the burden of addiction will complicate post-surgical care. Psychiatrists are often called upon to diagnose and treat delirium, and they support principles that prevent delirium in surgical patients (Ely et al., 2004; Lat et al., 2009). For patients with schizophrenia psychiatrists bring their ability to titrate anti-psychotic treatment through the hospitalization, to commuicate with a patient in spite of delusions and concrete thinking and to better understand opposition to care (Irwin et al., 2014). Furthermore, they may be charged with identification of the rare patients with factitious disorder, who amplify symptoms and seek surgery as a way of life.

BODY IMAGE

Body image is a major psychological dimension often affected by surgery. Schilder (1950) described body image as the intra-psychic picture or schema of our own body, including interpersonal, environmental, and temporal factors. Shontz (1974) expanded the concept of body image to include the sensory, motor, and expressive functions that the body serves, as well as the experience of the "self" and the developmental levels at which the self operates, beginning as early as *in utero*. Different meanings are invested in different organ systems, either personally or by social convention; for example, the brain with wit, emotion, and self; the face with beauty and character; sexual organs with reproductive capacity and sexual identity; muscle and bone structure with dexterity, grace, power, and skill. For women in Western industrialized cultures, the breasts may have come to represent femininity, a measure of attractiveness, and even personal worth.

Pain and disfigurement to any body part are long remembered and can have lasting effects on the patient's body image and self-esteem (Freud, 1952). Fear of "shots" or injections and fear of surgery, often stemming from prior experiences, are common in both children and adults. Visible disfigurement to the face is particularly traumatic (Warner et al., 2012; MacGregor, 1990; Berscheid & Gangestad, 1982), as is trauma to the head, scalp, and hands. In addition, breast and genital injury or disfigurement affect sexual dimensions of the body image.

Individuals' assessment of their own physical integrity or beauty is independent of the actual physical presentation of their body. A person may appear conventionally beautiful but subjectively perceive and experience the body as ugly, and vice versa. Young children suffering from a congenital disorder, disease, disfiguring injury, or undergoing an amputation, can incorporate the disfigurement into their body image, whereas older children or adults must grieve the loss of their previously acquired body image and attempt to adapt to scarring or functional loss (Stoddard, 2002). Severe distortions of body image occur in patients with anorexia nervosa or body dysmorphic disorder.

Occasionally patients will refuse life-saving mastectomy or amputation because they have such an aversion to the idea of physical deformity. For most patients these losses are emotionally challenging, but adjustment can and does occur. Patients can be characterized by how invested they are in their own appearance on one dimension and by how much they perceive a discrepancy between their own body image and what they desire, on another dimension. In the surgical setting, these concerns can be thought of on a normal continuum (Fingeret et al., 2014).

THE NEED TO DEVELOP THE RELATIONSHIP WITH THE PATIENT

Although the time for psychiatrists to fully assess clinical situations is often limited in surgical settings, the major diagnostic strategy at their disposal is the human relationship that can be established with the patient and family. Clarification of the psychological component of the case and complex and potential issues of secondary gain depend on obtaining as thorough a past history as possible, the mental status examination, and evaluation of the patient's personality traits and coping strategies under stress. Rapid, complex modern surgical treatment and the time needed for electronic medical record-keeping and procedure coding for reimbursement may inhibit the gathering of records as completely as in the past and limit the time allowed to establish trust with patient and family. Psychiatrists' abilities to discuss the case with the attending surgeon, communicate succinctly to the surgeon what they know, what they do not know, and how they would proceed are critical to arriving at a definitive diagnosis and treatment plan.

The nature of contracts for mental health care in the United States can constrict the relationship between psychiatric and surgical care. Policies for mental health coverage are usually established without the medically ill in mind. The insurer may limit where and by whom services can be performed. Social workers are included in the mental health networks, usually in much greater numbers than psychiatrists. Psychiatrists are thereby distanced from the medically ill, and surgeons can have difficulty referring patients to psychiatrists for evaluation and treatment.

In some settings, psychiatric services cannot be performed at the same location as the surgical procedure or consultation. As day surgery increases and the duration of hospital stays shortens, preoperative evaluations and postoperative psychiatric evaluations cannot occur as easily in the hospital. Preoperative psychiatric evaluation must be planned in advance for patients vulnerable to psychiatric illness, and postoperative evaluation of cognitive impairment, for instance, may suddenly fall as an unexpected burden on the family at home because the diagnosis was missed due to pressure to discharge the patient rapidly. Inadequate pre- and post-operative attention to mental status assessment can delay recovery and increase the likelihood of complications. Rapid personal telephone or telemedicine contact with psychiatrists and surgeons (remote video, Skype or iPhone) is a potential substitute for on-site preoperative psychiatric triage and screening, as has been done in the Navy aboard ships far from land for years. Education of surgeons and their staffs greatly assists such a screening and triage process.

THE CONSULTATIVE REQUEST

The request for a psychiatric consultation usually occurs in three circumstances: (1) the presence of acute psychiatric symptoms (depression, psychosis, delirium, suicidal risk); (2) family or nursing staff requesting help; and (3) diagnostic dilemmas—for instance, whether a symptom is "functional" or "organic." In some surgical settings, psychiatric consultation occurs routinely, such as in transplantation (see Chapter 74); and in others quite rarely, such as ophthalmology and urology. It may occur pre-, peri- or post-operatively.

Psychiatric consultation is necessary when:

1. The surgeon recognizes that jointly talking with a patient and a psychiatrist is likely to improve the patient's psychological preparation for the postoperative requirements and effects of surgery.

2. Previously known psychiatric conditions can potentially complicate surgery or recovery. For instance, panic disorder, severe anticipatory anxiety, or alcoholism may prevent the patient from following through with a series of surgical treatments, but a proactive behavioral management plan or psychotropic drug regimen may make the surgical plan much easier to accomplish and result in a better outcome.

3. The stability of the patient's psychiatric condition can be jeopardized by the stress of surgery. For instance, a patient with bipolar disorder on lithium will be likely to experience changes in hydration associated with surgery, risking lithium toxicity, or a relapse if the medication is abruptly discontinued.

4. The patient or family requests special attention to the psychological state or needs of the patient.

5. The patient does not understand the surgery to be performed in order to give informed consent—due to age as with an adolescent, to cognitive impairment, or to other factors.

6. The patient is very fearful and refuses to consent to emergency surgery or surgery essential to the patient's well-being.

7. The patient is very anxious or ambivalent about surgery due to prior complications of anesthesia such as respiratory arrest or awareness under anesthesia.

8. The surgeon recognizes psychological issues or potential problems in the patient–doctor relationship or when nurses report difficulties in behavior that complicate nursing care (such as with borderline personality or antisocial patients).

9. The patient's experience of pain or other symptoms brings about excessive requests for analgesia, or the pain behavior of the patient raises questions about the psychological suffering, depression, addiction, or interpersonal conflicts of the patient.

10. There is concern about patient or staff safety.

11. The patient is regressed, confused, agitated, suicidal, or mentally deteriorating.

12. The use of maintenance psychotropic drugs may potentially complicate surgery because of side-effects or drug interactions (e.g., monoamine oxidase [MAO] inhibitors limiting narcotic options, or concerns about QT prolongation with certain agents).

13. The use of medications for surgical care may complicate psychiatric care.

14. The patient has a known or suspected history of alcohol or other type of chemical dependency or abuse.

15. Religious, cultural, or family conflicts exist that may complicate normal surgical and recovery techniques (e.g., the use of blood products that is prohibited by some religious sects).

16. End-of-life issues may benefit from a psychiatric perspective.

This is only a partial list of reasons for psychiatric consultation to surgical patients.

Communication between the surgeon requesting the consultation and the psychiatrist is key, but often fraught with difficulty. The psychiatric evaluation frequently depends on information in the chart, from the family, and the nursing staff, and not directly from the surgeon. It is sometimes necessary, when it is urgent to discuss a case, to even scrub in and talk with the surgeon in the operating room. If at all possible, one may also regularly attend surgical morning work rounds and surgical case conferences.

In those settings, the psychiatrist may gain important practical knowledge about the details of what surgery and its sequelae entail for patients and their families, explain to the clinical staff the findings from psychiatric diagnosis and treatment, and contribute to planning ongoing care, including disposition planning. This psychiatric participation in rounds and meetings demonstrates the psychiatrist's willingness to learn about the complexities of surgical treatment from the team, which then helps the psychiatrist better help the patient and educates the surgical team about psychiatric aspects of surgical care.

PSYCHIATRIC ASSESSMENT OF THE SURGICAL PATIENT

All patients with preexisting severe psychopathology, substance abuse, or who for some reason are at psychiatric risk should have psychiatric assessment prior to admission for elective surgery. This is more likely to be feasible in settings with established and well-staffed psychiatric consultation services. When psychiatric assessment and any needed treatment do not occur before elective surgery, surgical and psychiatric complications are more likely to occur postoperatively. Patients with old and recent brain injuries are more likely to have delirium or cognitive impairment after anesthesia. The psychiatrist must understand the medical rationale, the predicted surgical outcome, and, optimally, know the patient preoperatively. Psychiatric syndromes that can be treated should be defined, and personality traits that will interfere with recovery and coping assessed and a management plan prepared in advance. An ideal standard psychiatric assessment of the surgical patient would include the following elements at a minimum:

- Review of the reason for psychiatric referral at this point in time

- Accurate understanding, with explanation from the surgeon, of the surgical issues (proposed or completed), details of the surgical procedure(s), and prognosis

- Review of the chart and laboratory/radiographic examinations

- History of present illness, including its impact on the patient and family at this stage of the patient's life cycle. This is supplemented with history from family, past medical records, other mental health professionals, or friends when necessary

- Psychiatric history, including substance use, domestic violence, and previous or current treatment, especially any active use of psychotropic medications

- Complete medical/surgical history, especially current and prior medications and *evidence of* or *the possibility of*, withdrawal from medications, illicit drugs, or alcohol

- Social history, including language and ethnic background, religious beliefs, advance directives, legal issues

- Family psychiatric history
- Mental status examination
- Succinct case summary/formulation
- Problems, diagnoses
- Practical treatment recommendations—thoughtful, responsive to specific questions, clear goals and parameters to monitor
- Follow-up report post-surgery and discussion with the surgeon; mutual agreement on length of post-surgical follow-up care and psychiatric disposition

The basic mental status examination of the surgical patient should include:

- Attempting to establish a positive therapeutic relationship by expressing interest in the patient and family, using developmentally appropriate communication in language understood by the patient and family
- Observing the patient's appearance, including surgical dressings; medical apparatus; behavior, with particular focus on signs of pain, depression, anxiety, impulsivity, delirium, or dementia
- Asking if the patient understands the reason for referral and their surgical status
- Evaluating risk to self or others
- Observing speech and language
- Assessing cognitive function
- Assessing psychotic thinking and hallucinations
- Assessing mood symptoms, such as anger, sadness, anxiety or panic, depression or mania
- Alcohol and drug history; likelihood of post-surgical withdrawal
- Evaluating judgement and decision-making capacity

The psychiatric diagnoses should focus on the problem, diagnosis, or diagnoses most relevant to the referral; for example, adjustment disorder, delirium, post-traumatic stress disorder (PTSD), bereavement, major depression, acute pain syndrome, or substance abuse. Identify both comorbid psychiatric and medical diagnoses.

The treatment plan should respond to the referral question briefly, clearly, and most of all, practically. The psychiatrist's note should summarize the case without psychiatric jargon, with the goal of assisting the patient's surgical progress and recovery from surgery. It seeks to explain symptoms in common-sense language, integrating both the medical/surgical status and the psychobiological status of the patient. Psychiatric treatment plans for surgical patients are usually short-term, aimed at stabilizing the patient and relieving symptoms. They are problem-oriented and outline definite and clearly defined plans for close follow-up by a psychiatrist who is available to the patient geographically and accessible financially.

THE DEVELOPMENTAL PERSPECTIVE

A classic model of the psychological stages of the life cycle was introduced by Erik Erikson (1980) to describe the phases of human development from birth to death. It is helpful in making sense of patients' responses to surgery. Emotional meanings, personal temperament, and cognitive skills for coping differ widely across the life cycle. For example, surgical care for children should integrate an understanding of normal developmental aspects of early childhood such as maternal–infant attachment and separation, temperament, cognitive and motor development, play, and responsiveness to transitional objects. Transient regressive behavior, in response to surgery, to emotional states typical of earlier stages of development may occur at any developmental stage, including adulthood, and is especially common in children and adolescents. Recovery to the previous level of functioning occurs rapidly with postoperative recovery. Most surgeons caring for children benefit from child psychiatric consultation (Kurtz, Muriel, & Abrams, 2010). Issues of pain and risk of medical traumatization are essential considerations in the surgical care of children.

INFANCY AND TODDLERHOOD

Infants and toddlers are vulnerable to overwhelming fears when subjected to "shots," restraint, or intubation, or the threat of abandonment, especially when mothers are not nearby. Since many infants and toddlers are nonverbal, their emotional needs are often ignored and left largely to the parents or nurses. While this may be appropriate for those who do well, infants requiring surgery may have significant post-traumatic or depressive reactions that could have a lasting impact on personality development. At a minimum, psychiatric consultation is indicated for infants who suffer intractable pain, attachment or developmental disorders, hyperactivity, depression, PTSD, and anxiety. Even without such diagnoses, most children undergoing surgery and their families benefit from collaborative psychiatric care with the surgeon.

Close contact with a mother or surrogate is central to the development of a sense of safety (Zeanah, 2000), which has a neural basis in the amygdala and dorsal striatum (Rogan et al., 2006). Winnicott (1965) suggested that the mother metaphorically creates a "holding environment" that allows the child to develop a sense of self. He also introduced the concept of the "transitional object," which allows the infant to tolerate separations from the mother without undue anxiety (Winnicott, 1951). A treasured blanket, toy, book, or song may take that role in the hospital. Nurturing holding by staff who do not have pain-inducing responsibilities and who serve as maternal surrogates reduces pain, distress, and protest in the sick infant, particularly in those whose mother is absent. Chapters 17 and 18 discuss object-relations theory as it relates to the stresses and fears of medical-surgical illness and the role of spiritual and religious factors in sustaining attachment. In the United States prior to the mid-1980s, parental visitation in intensive care units was very limited. Their right to be present continuously, as they are now, occurred through parental advocacy leading to laws requiring hospitals to comply.

CHILDHOOD

Preschool and school-age children generally have sufficient language skills for use in preoperative preparation. Children master elimination; use age-appropriate play as an expressive modality to enhance coping; and rapidly progress through phases of emotional, interpersonal, cognitive, and motor development to better cope with pain and stress. Formation of their core body image should be complete, but the child is vulnerable to bodily threats or loss, and any bodily injury or probe is long remembered. When overwhelmed, the vulnerable child dramatically regresses, with loss (usually transient) of recently acquired developmental skills; for example, speech or urinary continence. The sensory holding interventions by the staff remain essential, but now can also include verbal communication for these older children. Choices about surgery and other aspects of medical care should involve children as young as six or seven. Children with physical, emotional, or cognitive disabilities, or chronic illness should have formal child psychiatric interventions well in advance of elective surgery. Even those admitted for minor surgical procedures are often much more vulnerable than they might appear. While some literature suggests that adverse psychological effects of general anesthesia, surgery, and hospitalization for injuries and other conditions are transient and reversible (Caldas et al., 2004), others point to risks of persistent post-traumatic and other developmental sequelae (Saxe et al., 2005; Stoddard et al., 2006; Stuber, 2011).

ADOLESCENCE

Early adolescents act more like children, despite their often awkward attempts at seeming more mature; they benefit from the involvement of parents, parent surrogates, or friends. Familiar activities, objects, or people allow regressed adolescents to tolerate surgery, loneliness, and suffering. Consistent nursing care, regular visits by family or friends, and familiar photos, clothing, or favorite music nearby can help as well. Adolescents may be quite irritable or moody, and often fear the violation of their personal privacy and "space." They may become easily self-conscious or embarrassed, and inhibited or guilty about expressing feelings.

Mid-adolescents in the process of puberty vary in their cognitive and emotional states, levels of understanding, and capacities for self-management. They tend to be more adult-like in their understanding and behavior but are given to emotional regression under stress, which makes them seem "in between" childhood and adulthood. Surgical care should consider their new pride and appreciate their independence, attractiveness, and physical prowess. They require clear direction and sometimes limit-setting of anxious, sexual, and aggressive feelings, coupled with appropriate psychotherapeutic interventions.

Late adolescents are often less competent and mature than they appear. They are in the process of separating from their families, and the associated fears, sadness, guilt, and rebellion may be either quite open, hidden, or not yet occurring. Surgery can even represent a useful experience in the adolescent's growth and maturation toward autonomy. In most states, after age 16, adolescents must consent to surgery along with their parents.

YOUNG ADULTHOOD

Young adulthood extends through major psychological decisions and tasks such as completing one's education, choosing an occupation, consolidating sexual identity, marrying or remaining single, childbearing, raising a family, and working toward occupational and economic security. Like the adolescent, young adults may feel very vulnerable in the surgical setting, since the need for surgery challenges feelings of invulnerability. Psychiatrists will take note of prior developmental strengths and vulnerabilities as they talk about surgery. Conflicted needs for dependency will coexist with their own independent adult responsibilities to education, work, or family.

MIDLIFE

Midlife is, ideally, a time when achievements are consolidated and a time when some individuals make changes in work, intimate relationships, or even their own bodies in order to fulfill unmet yearnings. Feelings of virility and femininity, competence and incompetence, are loaded with meaning at this time. Surgery and disease may be a threat to the adult's livelihood, family roles, and recreation. They may try to deny or postpone the emerging realities of aging. Adjustment to surgery should incorporate the patient's relationships with family and loved ones, the central place of work, and the available skills for self-care.

LATE ADULTHOOD

By this period of life, the patient has experienced most of life and may or may not have adapted well to achievements and the inevitable disappointments they have encountered along the way. For some, with full faculties and highly developed skills intact, it is a time of new creativity and contributions to family or to society, made possible by retirement from the tasks of parenting or their occupation. For many, adapting to reduced physical or mental vigor, injury, or multiple diseases, multiple medications, and infirmity, increasingly becomes the task, together with coping with the deaths of spouses or loved ones and friends. It can be a period of savoring the young and one's own past while determining what to leave behind for others. Talking with patients about these aspects of late life can be helpful, especially when the physician demonstrates awareness of patients' fear of pain or other complications of illness, of dying in the hospital, and of specific aspects of care at the end of life.

FAMILY SUPPORT

Family characteristics have a strong impact on the quality and trajectory of recovery from physical trauma (Sheridan et al., 2012). When confronting the prospect of surgery for a family member, families, like individuals, represent a spectrum from resilient to vulnerable. The absence of support from family or friends usually will affect surgical evaluation, the course of treatment, and long-term outcome. The parents', siblings', family's, or friends' feelings of fear, anger, relief, suffering, or grief often mirror that of the patient. Today's typical family is no longer a couple and their children (it is the exception rather than the rule). Rather, those who support the patient are as likely to be a single mother, an extended family, a social worker, an elderly parent, a "significant other," a gay partner, a group of friends, church members, or family of distant relatives. It can be a challenge for the surgical staff to obtain operative consents and also to manage patients' complications or death when family involvement is marginal or ambiguous. Even as individuals develop through the life cycle, the family's tasks and functions evolve in overlapping stages from the task of infant and child care, to coping with the behavior of adolescents, to "letting go" of young adults as they mature, to partnering and family building, to midlife adjustments and preparing to approach death. It is worth considering with a patient who is planning for surgery who is most trusted, how the family will be able to function, and what strategies would be helpful to sustain this support.

PREEXISTING PSYCHIATRIC RISK FACTORS FOR SURGICAL COMPLICATIONS

Preexisting psychiatric disorders increase the risks associated with surgery and postoperative care, and the prevalence of preexisting disorders may include up to half of all surgical patients, many with disorders of substance dependency or abuse (Powers & Santana, 2010).

MOOD DISORDERS

Mood disorders may affect an individual's clinical presentation, response to surgical treatment, and outcome. If the patient's mood disorder is stable on an antidepressant, then attention should be paid to the continuation of the drug during the surgical hospitalization and recovery. If the period of no oral intake will be prolonged, an SSRI with a long half-life (two weeks) like fluoxitene replacing one with a shorter half-life like citalopram might be used to advantage. Prophylactic antidepressants have been used when the likelihood of treatment-associated depression is high. In patients undergoing treatment for head and neck cancer who are not depressed, the likelihood of their developing depression is greater than 50 percent. In a randomized controlled study, prophylactic escitalopram reduced the risk of developing depression by more than 50%, and treated patients had a better quality of life over the following 3 months of mulit-modal treatments (Lydiatt et al., 2013).

ANXIETY DISORDERS

All patients, children and adults, experience some degree of anxiety prior to surgery, but anxiety may be worse for those with preexisting anxiety disorders. For someone who has experienced a prior trauma, the prospect of surgery may elicit the re-experiencing of a previous trauma, with a dramatic increase in anxiety, including panic; some patients may shut down emotionally, with avoidance or numbing symptoms that may provide false reassurance to staff that the patient is resilient and doing well. Anxiety disorders are frequently associated with somatic complaints such as headaches, cardiac and respiratory symptoms, and, most commonly, gastrointestinal symptoms. The treatment of an anxiety disorder can include mobilization of social supports, cognitive behavior therapy, hypnosis, relaxation techniques, and psychopharmacological agents. For severe preoperative anxiety, unrelieved by psychological interventions, reassurance that anxiolytics such as benzodiazepines will be given prior to surgery may effectively relieve it. A few patients who have had prior surgery and are very anxious may be aware that they experienced an adverse event in previous surgery (e.g., respiratory arrest) and require psychotherapy before proceeding with elective surgery.

BODY DYSMORPHIC DISORDER

Body dysmorphic disorder (BDD) is a preoccupation with an imagined or slight deformity of the body associated with significant impairment. It overlaps with obsessive-compulsive disorder and anxiety disorders. Patients with BDD have a distorted body image and may be preoccupied with reexamining, improving or hiding the defect. They may avoid mirrors and social activities. At the extreme, they may be delusional, suicidal, and present with self-injury. They generally present to maxillofacial, cosmetic surgeons, and cosmetic dermatologists. These patients are aesthetically very sensitive, and the practical question is whether they will be satisfied with the procedure sought. Those who have more psychopathology tend to have more dissatisfaction. Some questions for assessment include queries about how ugly the patient feels, how much work or social disability results from the deformity, how much checking is done, how noticable the feature is to other people, and whether family or friends discouraged the cosmetic procedure (Veale, 2004). A screening instrument for a cosmetic clinic has been developed (Veale et al., 2012). Psychiatric treatment included high doses of SSRIs for 12–16 weeks and cognitive behavioral treatment. (Veale, 2004a; Veale, 2004b; Phillips & Hollander, 2007; Wilhelm et al., 2014).

SOMATIC SYMPTOM DISORDERS

The psychiatrist should be alert to patients with a history of somatic symptom disorders who may amplify or be overly focused on somatic symptoms. The psychological component of the symptoms may color surgical decision making, moving surgeons to action on the one hand; or on the other hand, the history of the patient "crying wolf" may bias surgical judgment such that new symptoms are not taken seriously.

FACTITIOUS DISORDER

Surgery is also extremely risky for those with factitious disorders or factitious disorder by proxy (Masterson, 1995; Acarturk et al., 2014; Burton et al., 2014), where the symptoms are intentionally produced or feigned in order to assume the sick role. In some difficult cases, surgical treatment is unavoidable but must be carefully focused to limit manipulation and contain regressive behavior.

ATTENTION DEFICIT DISORDER

Attention-deficit hyperactivity disorder (ADHD) is the most common disorder for which children and young adults are referred to mental health professionals. A patient, adult or child, with ADHD may not retain information and may have a harder time tolerating holding still. If surgery is performed, a child with ADHD may play with the intravenous apparatus, bandages, and have difficulty tolerating postoperative procedures. The pharmacological treatment of ADHD includes, stimulants, tricyclic antidepressants (TCAs), clonidine, and buproprion. While discontinuation of medications for ADHD may often be judicious preoperatively, pediatric anesthesiologists can usually adjust their treatment perioperatively. Hyperactive children are sometimes at risk of disrupting postoperative wound care. Methylphenidate or dexedrine have the benefit of enhancing the analgesic effect of opiates. Side-effects such as inhibition of appetite with stimulants, or cardiovascular effects of TCAs should be considered (Wilens & Spencer, 2010). (See Chapter 50 on ADHD.)

ALCOHOL AND DRUG ABUSE

Prior to elective surgery, the history or physical or laboratory signs of substance abuse should be sought. Urine and serum toxic screening may be critical in identifying the degree of substance abuse, prescribed medications, and likelihood of overdose or withdrawal. Since substance abuse is a factor so many acute-trauma surgical admissions, screening is essential. However in a national survey of Level 1 trauma centers, only 39% of admissions had screening questions for alcohol abuse, and only 25% received a brief intervention (Terrell et al., 2008). Most children and adolescents have not yet developed the long-term medical complications of drug or alcohol addiction seen in adults, but they can be addicted to alcohol or drugs and must carefully be assessed, just as adults should be. Since denial is part of the disease of chemical dependency, the examiner should be appropriately skeptical and critical of both the patient and family during this part of the assessment. (See also Chapter 38.)

SCHIZOPHRENIA

Clarification of the diagnosis of chronic psychotic disorder offers an opportunity to identify who the patient trusts, who the regular psychiatrist is, the nature of maintenance medications, whether preoperative medications offer the best possible mental status, and to build an interdisciplinary support team. Often the fracture between the mental health system and the medical hospital make this particularly important. The medical psychiatrist offers the ability to communicate directly with the patient taking cognitive deficits and concrete thinking into consideration. Not all morbidity may be related to schizophrenia, and the often comorbid conditions of depression and substance abuse must be elucidated (Irwin et al., 2014).

BORDERLINE PERSONALITY DISORDER

Patients with borderline personality disorder come to surgical attention when they are treated for self-mutilation: burning, skin-picking or cutting. Compared to patients with body dysmorphic disorder, they seek plastic surgery for different parts of the body rather than focusing on one part (Napoleon, 1993; Morioka & Ohkubo, 2014). The psychiatrist's diagnosis alerts the surgeon to a higher risk of complications and to the more difficult doctor-patient relationship. Because of the patients' unstable relationships, tendency to see others as all good or all bad, and their sensitivity to abandonment, surgeons are more likely to be seduced into operating against their better judgment to rescue patients from their anguish, more likely to be idealized and more apt to disappoint. Firm professional boundaries and sound surgical judgment become all the more important when these patients need surgery. The psychiatric consultant can help to clarify the patient's past history, unrealistic expectations and to support more caution in high-risk procedures.

If acute PTSD, current major depression, suicidal ideation, psychosis, or active substance dependency or abuse is diagnosed, elective surgical care may need to be postponed, unless there is an emergency. Following emergency surgery, patients with these disorders require continuous psychiatric monitoring, evaluation, and treatment to prevent or reduce the risk of surgical and psychiatric complications, including suicide.

PSYCHOPHARMACOLOGY FOR SURGICAL PATIENTS: BASIC PRINCIPLES

The anesthesiologist and surgeon must be informed of all psychotropic medications that the patient has been or is taking. Drug treatment in adults and children (Lorberg & Prince et al., 2010; Stevens et al., 2010) is based on assessment and monitoring of target symptoms of diagnosed psychiatric conditions.

Many patients are already using psychotropic medications at the time of surgery. Although most psychiatric medications are safe during and after surgery, monoamine oxidase inhibitors (MAOIs), lithium carbonate, TCAs, clozapine, and other drugs may pose special problems (Huyse et al., 2006).

For patients on clozapine having surgery, attention should be paid to bowel function. Clozapine is associated with colonic hypomotility, constipation, and rarely ischemic colitis or toxic megacolon. As patients receiving narcotics are often put on regimens that prevent constipation, so should patients who are receiving clozapine. Factors that raise the level of clozapine like higher doses, fever, drugs that inhibit cytochrome P-450, or other drugs that make constipation worse like opiates and anticholinergic medications can cause additional risk (Alam et al., 2009). If the patient smoked outside the hospital, inducing CYP 1A2 by a carbon-based mechanism, levels of clozapine may rise when the patient is placed on nicotine or abstinence in the hospital. Similarly if smoking begins again after hospitalization, clozapine levels may fall compared to the levels that maintained the patient in the hospital (Lowe & Ackman, 2010). Measured clozapine levels may be helpful over a long hospital course.

Lithium must also be followed with levels as higher plasma levels are associated with toxicity, and older patients are more sensitive to higher levels. In the setting of illness and surgery, dehydration and renal dysfunction risk toxicity. Nonsteroidal anti-inflammatory drugs and thiazides should be avoided. In the setting of urgent surgery, the regular dose of lithium can be held. However, the course of bipolar illness is favored by gradual and not sudden disruptions in lithium treatment, so the importance of restarting lithium postoperatively should be considered postoperatively in patients whose bipolar disorder is responsive to lithium (Baldessarini et al., 1996).

Irreversible MAOIs and the reversible MAOI meclobemide present the risk of hypertensive crisis with certain perioperative drugs: meperidine, dextromethorphan, and epinephrine, but fentanyl and morphine can be used. Irreversible MAOIs like phenelzine and tranylcypromine should be stopped for 2 weeks before a planned surgery if possible (Huyse et al., 2006).

TCAs like imipramine, amitriptyline, and nortriptyline tend to prolong the QT interval and to be associated with anticholinergic and alpha-adrenergic blockade.

Particular attention should be given to drugs that must be restarted after surgery to prevent withdrawal. Abrupt withdrawal from chronic benzodiazepines has caused seizures or delirium in surgical patients. Since patients may be temporarily unable to take oral medicines, options like parenteral or sublingual lorazepam should be considered. Antidepressants and mood stabilizers might be briefly held during the time the patient cannot take medications orally, without appreciable loss of therapeutic effect. Short-acting antidepressants like paroxetine or venlafaxine are associated with a withdrawal syndrome of malaise and paresthesias, which is not life-threatening.

Comorbid medical disorders, hepatic or renal impairment, and brain injury must be considered. Dosing for children is usually adjusted on a milligram/kilogram basis. While neonates metabolize slowly, children metabolize most drugs more rapidly, leading them to usually require higher dosing for equivalent therapeutic effects, depending on their medical status (Stoddard, Usher, & Abrams, 2006). In the elderly, due to reduced rates of metabolism and excretion, lower dosing is often indicated for an equivalent effect. Metabolic rates may be increased in a variety of conditions (e.g., burns), or decreased (e.g., liver disease), requiring adjustments in dosing.

Drugs that were stopped preoperatively should be considered in evaluation of drug interactions (DeVane, 2010). Drugs with a long half-life like fluoxetine or diazepam may interact with drugs started in the hospital, even if they are not continued. Children may develop a paradoxical disinhibition in response to a benzodiazepine. High plasma levels of sedatives may cause unexpected over-sedation, and respiratory or cardiac arrest.

Ongoing monitoring of medications and behavioral target symptoms, cognition, and mood is essential because multiple doctors, nurse practitioners, and physician's assistants often prescribe to the same complex patient and because psychiatric medications may not be taken as seriously as other medications. Often staff who have known the patient only one shift make decisions about psychological symptoms, as well as rapid "ad hoc" decisions about medications (PRN, "as needed") for anxiety, sleep, or pain. The consultant will put into context how long and how consistently an antidepressant has been taken at a specific dose in order to judge the likelihood of its efficacy and will take note of pharmacokinetics, whether an analgesic or anti-anxiety medication has been prescribed long enough to reach steady state.

There is increased surgical attention to reducing the dosages of opiates and benzodiazepines as early as is feasible in order to reduce pulmonary risks and withdrawal and improve outcomes. In order to facilitate this, medications such as methadone and dexmedetomidine (Maldonado et al., 2009) are prescribed more commonly to facilitate weaning from high-dose opiates and anxiolytics.

If a patient does not benefit from the prescribed psychotropic medication, the psychiatric diagnosis, cause of the symptoms, and dosage must be reevaluated. It is helpful for the psychiatric consultant to state in the chart the number of days the patient has been taking an antidepressant at a specific dose so that response to the medication will not be evaluated prematurely. An antipsychotic that was started for delirium in the hospital may be misunderstood to be a post-operative maintenance medication and therefore, continued inappropriately at home. The benefits and risks of discontinuation of psychotropic medications should be weighed carefully.

PSYCHOLOGICAL PREPARATION FOR SURGERY

Every person facing surgery will experience anxiety. The anxiety may be a result of fear of the surgery itself, fear of pain, fear of possible diagnoses, or a general fear of loss of control. Patients may be afraid of not waking up from the anesthesia or afraid of lethal complications following surgery. For patients with a history of an anxiety disorder or of prior trauma, the prospect of surgery may intensify preoperative symptoms. Children and the elderly may have difficulty expressing their anxiety. Unspoken fears and fantasies often intensify anxiety. To reduce preoperative anxiety, it is important to provide as much information as seems appropriate, to allow patients to ask questions, and to express their fears, and possibly to meet others who have experienced the same disease and treatment.

Speaking to children in language geared to their developmental stage and cultural background is key. Children respond positively to reassurance that pain will be relieved with medication, and older children and adolescents may benefit from patient-controlled analgesia (PCA). Preparing children with burns for dressing changes and giving them the sense that they have some degree of control reduces protestations, pain, anxiety and fosters cooperation (Kavanaugh et al., 1991).

Communication opens, for good or ill, with the first contact with the surgeon. Nevertheless, studies indicate that most health care professionals talk to the parents, not to the children, regarding health problems. The education of children regarding health problems is just beginning, so most children have little understanding before surgery.

The five dimensions of the surgical experience that provoke anxiety in children summarize as well the primitive concerns of adults. These are a) pain and mutilation, b) separation from parents or other trusted adults c) fear of the unknown and unfamiliar, d) uncertainty about normative behavior in a hospital setting, and e) loss of control, autonomy and competence (Visintainer & Wolfer, 1975). Behavioral methods to prepare children for hospitalization and surgery have been developed, and similar principles apply for adults (Rasnake & Lindsheid, 1989). Speaking to adults directly in plain language, preparing them step by step with attention to their natural fears should be the rule. Preoperative teaching and psychological preparation for surgery improve postoperative outcomes. "Preoperative teaching" means providing concrete information to patients about postoperative procedures, about treatment-related pain and discomfort, and a thorough psychological exploration of the patient's fears, anxieties, and expectations. One program to prepare children and families for surgery includes tours of the places they will see on the day of surgery, films about surgery or anesthesia, slide presentations, coloring books, photographs chronicling other children's experiences, puppet shows, medical play utilizing real hospital equipemnt, popular children's books about going to the hospital, drawings or collages, and relaxation and coping exercises (Justus et al., 2006).

Patients benefit from recognition of the personal meanings of the particular operation; for example, an episiotomy, a meningioma, a facial burn, a heart transplant, or uterine cancer. These personal meanings related to illness, the body parts affected, functions of the body that are affected, and the need to seek surgical assistance will partly shape the patient's emotional course before, during, and while recovering from surgery. For those who do not fully recover, continuing interest and compassion from the surgeon will diminish the perception that the surgeon's only interest is in the procedure and not the patient.

Guiding a patient who is preparing for surgery, the medical psychiatrist would encourage the best coping strategies to maximize the best outcome. Comorbid medical conditions should be under the best control. Patients can commit to their own physical fitness, smoking cessation, cutting down on alcohol, and learning methods that have the potential to reduce anxiety before, during and after the operation.

Mind–body interventions (Chapter 17), some similar to natural childbirth methods, which may be learned preoperatively, include meditation, self-hypnosis, guided imagery, yoga, tai chi, massage, therapeutic touch, and others.

Feeling mentally prepared, a positive attitude, motivation and will power have been linked to better surgical outcomes (Frankel, 2012). With elective surgery, the medical psychiatrist has the opportunity to watch the steps that patients go through to decide if they will have surgery; i.e., how they come to a state of readiness (Conner-Spady et al., 2014). The decision for surgery is linked to the personal assessment that the benefit outweighs perceived risks. Indecisive patients may lack information about alternatives or may be unable to make a decision because of anxiety, depression, or paralyzing ambivalence. Those that avoid the decision may also avoid finding out the best timing for surgery in the course of the illness. The adept surgeon who must do sequential surgeries makes a relationship with a patient that resonates with the patient's readiness for the next surgery. The psychiatrist's role is to make clear where there is lack of information, to support information seeking, and to facilitate appropriate risk taking and coping with uncertainty, allowing the patient to go forward with the best sense of control and self-esteem.

In some cases, patients' worry about recurrent cancer outweighs their desire for less surgery despite reassuring data. Breast-conserving surgery developed as an alternative to mastectomy, offering the same likelihood of survival in many cases. Since 2004, the rates of elective mastectomy and contralateral prophylactic surgery among candidates for breast conservation in conjunction with immediate reconstruction and contralateral prophylactic mastectomy have increased (Dragun et al., 2012). Perceived survival benefit and fear of recurrence are primary motivators for both older and younger women in this setting (Fisher et al., 2012). The long-term consistency of satisfaction after surgery is related to the woman's sense of having made an informed decision herself (Frost et al., 2011).

Psychiatric consultations provide opinions about patients' decision-making capacity to give informed consent (Applebaum & Grisso, 1988; Marson et al., 1995; Burrows & Hodgson, 1997). Patients must be mentally competent to give informed consent to be treated. It is an important principle of surgery and the law that patients must give informed consent prior to being treated, unless it is an imminent, life-threatening emergency. To perform a surgical procedure (Giesen, 1993) or anesthesia (White & Baldwin, 2003) without obtaining proper informed consent is considered assault and battery under every state's law.

There are several situations with unique aspects that occur repetitively: surgical consent in the elective patient, the emergency patient, the impaired patient, the research setting, and the pediatric patient. Although it seems counterintuitive, in many ways, obtaining proper informed consent from a patient for the elective surgery is more difficult, especially with day surgical procedures (Wadey & Frank, 1997; Kikuchi & Hara, 1996).

With telecommunication, the surgeon can use timely close cellphone and other electronic communication to inform the family as important medical and surgical events occur, so that relatives or guardians do not feel uninformed when they are in the role of giving consent.

"Informed" consent implies that the patient has a complete understanding of the indications for surgery, the medically reasonable alternatives to the planned procedure, the consequences that follow from the options offered, and all potential risks and complications associated with each. To truly achieve this in the average lay person can be extraordinarily difficult (Waisel & Truog, 1995); however, this is the law in all U.S. jurisdictions.

Consent for elective operations in pediatric patients and in impaired adults is obtained through a discussion with the parent or legal guardian. It is clearly important that family be involved whenever possible. It is also important to obtain "assent" for research from school-age children (Weithorn, 1983), and there is no reason to think they are incapable of assent for procedures and surgery (Levine, 1996). Children seven and older should assent, along with parental consent, to elective surgical procedures, and they are likely to benefit, even if it elicits anxiety, from preparatory explanation in language they can understand about a forthcoming operation, even for non-elective urgent operations. Children's assent and consent for surgery is a developing area involving autonomy vs. best interest, family, legal or ethical, and measurement dilemmas (Miller et al., 2004). If a child seven or older does not assent to elective surgery, it is advisable to delay the surgery until the child matures and is able to understand and choose to proceed with it. In a survey of 453 of 852 American anesthesiologists, for a 57% response rate (Lewis et al., 2007), children's refusal of surgery was not rare, with 9% of respondents reporting at least one case in the past year, and 45% having canceled one or more cases during their entire careers. Forty-four percent used restraint on most children under one year of age, whereas only 2% did so in children over eleven years of age. Respondents were uncomfortable with restraint in older children and less likely to proceed with induction. Twelve years of age was the median age when respondents would respect the child's refusal to proceed.

Not surprisingly, psychiatric complications with children and mentally impaired adults are reduced when they and their family understand the procedure and choose to proceed with it. In complicated cases, particularly where protracted hospitalization and multiple interventions are required, it is ideal if a family spokesperson and a hospital spokesperson can be identified early to communicate with each other. This facilitates the rapid exchange and dissemination of information and facilitates the creation of a trusting relationship between the extended family and an extended patient-care team. Informed consent is extensively discussed in Chapter 85.

PERIOPERATIVE COMPLICATIONS

PSYCHOLOGICAL REACTIONS RELATED TO SURGICAL ANESTHESIA

There are four major categories of psychological reactions to surgery and anesthesia: phobia in anticipation of anesthesia and surgery, psychotic-like reactions during induction, postoperative recall of awareness during anesthesia and surgery, and cognitive dysfunction after anesthesia.

Phobias

Phobias may relate to an unrealistic fear or misunderstanding of the surgical procedure and are more likely in patients with a preexisting anxiety disorder. Some fearful reactions are not phobias at all, but realistic fears related to an accurate understanding of the planned surgery. Phobias may also relate to a fear of needles, to an induction-mask phobia (which may be reduced by giving the patient control over choice of "smell" of the agent), to unrecognized prior traumatic experiences under anesthesia, including cardiac or respiratory arrest, or to witnessing another patient's injury or death after surgery. Some patients are phobic because the choice for surgery is not their own, but rather that of a relative or the surgeon, and they are reluctant participants in the process. A few patients become phobic or anxious because of preoperative discontinuation of their regular psychotropic medications. Brief psychiatric assessment can sometimes readily clarify the problem, provide reassurance, and may invoke the judicious use of a hypnotic or sedative medication, often a benzodiazepine. Distraction, combined cognitive-behavioral interventions and hypnosis have been helpful for needle-related procedural pain (Uman et al., 2006). Some patients, including some children, require cancellation of elective surgery and better preparation or psychiatric evaluation and treatment of the phobia, if that is the problem. Once they are prepared and willing to proceed, surgery may be rescheduled.

Reactions Similar to Psychosis During Induction

Parental presence during induction of anesthesia is available at some hospitals, but children are not necessarily less anxious when parents are there, especially if the parent is anxious (Chundamala et al., 2009; Yip, 2009). The best plan is to advocate for a plan that works best for their family (American Academy of Pediatrics, 2014). Induction may be difficult for children 2–5 years old and those who have been in the operating room before. After surgery, behavioral difficulties are more likely if the child is anxious before surgery. (Kain et al., 1999); those children who were anxious have more pain and sleep difficulties post-surgery (Kain et al., 2006).

Reactions similar to psychosis during induction, like an amytal interview, may result from anesthetic-induced disinhibition with expression of intense emotions of anger, sadness, fear, and sometimes even hallucinatory experiences; reactions may include violent outbursts requiring restraint. In children this has been described as emergence delirium (Vlajkovic & Sindjelic, 2006; Malarbi et al., 2011). A child is incoherent, inconsolable, kicking and thrashing, unable to recognize people with eyes averted, staring or closed. Paranoid delusions have also been seen. The syndrome lasts less than 30 minutes and sometimes transitions into a tantrum or evidence of pain. While such reactions are generally managed effectively with sedatives and anesthetic agents, they may signal a need for psychiatric assessment.

Unintended Awareness During Anesthesia

Most patients are worried that they will not wake up from anesthesia (McCleane & Cooper, 1990). However, being awake and aware during surgery is also a concern. Awareness is more common than generally known, and has been reported to affect about 0.1–0.2% of the population (Sandin et al., 2000; Sebels et al., 2004). Reports of awareness have been documented in children also (Davidson et al., 2005). Awareness during surgery is defined as the unexpected and explicit recall of intraoperative events during surgery. Although most cases of awareness are inconsequential, some patients do experience long-term sequelae, including PTSD, depression, nightmares, anxiety, and flashbacks (Samuelsson et al., 2007).

The causes of intraoperative awareness can be multifactorial. Genetic and drug-induced factors can alter the pharmacokinetics and pharmacodynamics of drugs administered to induce anesthesia (Kim et al., 1997; Ezri et al., 1997). Polymorphism in γ-aminobutyric acid A receptor α5 gene with at least three different forms of messenger RNA has been reported (Kim et al., 1997). Because of diminished cardiopulmonary function and reserve, anesthetic drugs are purposefully administered in lower concentrations to avoid negative hemodynamic and pulmonary consequences. Concomitantly administered drugs can mask the surrogate markers of awareness. For example, patients on β-adrenoceptor blockers will not have the tachycardiac and hypertensive responses usually seen in light anesthesia. Co-administration of muscle relaxants with light anesthesia will result in a paralyzed, immobile, awake patient unable to express awareness or move in response to pain. The incidence of awareness during Caesarian section under general anesthesia is high because of the deliberate attempt to reduce the anesthetic concentrations in the mother to reduce the side-effects on the fetus. Incidental lack of delivery of anesthetic is another common event, caused by lack of anesthetic in the vaporizer or by pump failure with intravenous anesthetics.

Patients become aware while under anesthesia due to our inability to accurately measure the depth of anesthesia with precision. Most often, surrogate markers (heart rate, blood pressure, lacrimation, and movement) are used. All of these are very nonspecific and can be masked by drugs inhibiting the responses. Bispectral Index devices have been advocated as a useful monitor of consciousness. Two studies, however, found no differences between control and Bispectral Index monitors in the incidence of awareness (Sandin et al., 2000; Avidan et al., 2008). Thus, the American Society of Anesthesiology (ASA) has indicated that brain function monitoring is not routinely indicated (ASA American Society of Anesthesiologists Task Force on Intra-operative Awareness Practice Advisory, 2006).

Cognitive Dysfunction After Anesthesia

It has long been assumed that anesthetic drugs are rapidly metabolized or eliminated from the body and therefore have minimal long-term effects. Several studies have questioned this assumption and documented that elderly patients experience changes in brain function even months after anesthesia combined with surgery. Post-operative cognitive dysfunction (POCD), persistent difficulties in memory, attention, or executive function that occur commonly post-surgery in older patients, is transient, usually but not always resolving by 3 months (Johnson et al., 2002). In a meta-analysis, general anesthesia compared to regional anesthesia contributed only marginally to the likelihood of POCD. (Mason, Noel-Storr, & Ritchie, 2010; Rasmussen et al., 2003). POCD did not predict dementia in a cohort followed for 11 years (Steinmetz et al., 2013). Older patients with POCD were most likely to die within in the year after non-cardiac surgery (Monk, et al., 2008). In contrast to these reports, a recent study suggests that elderly people undergoing surgery have no reason to worry (Avidan et al., 2009).

A growing body of evidence in animal studies also indicates that anesthesia exposure in the early stages of life has neurocognitive effects (Brambrink et al., 2010; Slikker, 2007). Retrospective studies performed in young children exposed to anesthesia at less than three years of age indicated twice the incidence of developmental or behavioral disorders (DiMaggio et al., 2009). The learning disabilities increased with greater cumulative exposure to anesthesia (Wilder et al., 2009). The possibility of negative effects of general anesthesia on neurological development has led to a standard of limiting exposure for children younger than 2 years (Flick et al., 2011; Loepke et al., 2008; Sun, 2010). The long term effects of anesthesia on the brain are still unclear (American Adaemy of Pediatrics, 2014).

Conversely, there is also evidence that certain anesthetics (e.g., ketamine and dexmedetomidine) may attenuate the neuronal changes associated with brain insults. Contradicting the retrospective studies in human newborns, two recent studies in the pediatric population reported no significant differences in educational outcomes of twins discordant for anesthesia (Bartels et al., 2009; Hansen et al., 2011). Ongoing prospective studies may settle this dispute, but the outcome data may take several years. Prospective randomized studies cannot be performed, as not many would volunteer for surgery without anesthesia. There are no specific drugs available for brain protection. It seems that regional anesthesia may be preferable to general anesthesia. Every surgery and the type of anesthetic should be evaluated for risks and benefits until evidence for or against neurocognitive effects of anesthesia become available.

POSTOPERATIVE COURSE

A patient's reaction to surgery is dependent on preoperative preparation, the type of surgery, the patient's resilience and stage of development, the diagnosis, speed of recovery, complications encountered, and the patient's preoperative mental status. In relatively uncomplicated surgeries with good prognoses, there is a sense of relief that the individuals have survived and can go on with their lives. However, for patients with a chronic diagnosis such as incurable cancer, or in whom the surgery meant alteration in their body functioning or lifestyle, the reaction can be one of anger, grief, or depression. All three feelings may occur almost simultaneously.

Often patients enter into surgery with some degree of hope that all will be "okay" or that they do not have a serious disease. After their operation, their ability to use denial is much reduced, and they have to adjust to the realistic ramifications of the diagnosis and treatment. If the postoperative course has unexpected complications, some patients become depressed and hopeless, wondering why they chose to have surgery in the first place, or blaming others for their misfortune. Sometimes anger can lead to legal action against the staff or hospital.

Postoperative regressive behavior is very common and not usually pathological, although it may quickly become so. Children may temporarily lose previously acquired skills such as feeding themselves, speech, self-care, and bladder or bowel control; and their return to normal development generally corresponds with their recovery from surgery and its sequelae. Adults, too, regress after surgery. They may refuse to eat, become uncharacteristically truculent and demanding with nurses, and may cooperate with physical therapists and other caretakers much more slowly than their medical condition merits. Regression may mimic depressive symptoms, with tearfulness, emotional withdrawal, weight loss, sleep disturbances, and irritability. Post-surgical regressive behavior is generally transient, although it may be extended with chronic illness and in psychiatric patients with dependent personality traits. Education of nursing staff regarding regression reduces conflicts and clarifies for them the meaning of patients' behavior.

A powerful antidepressant for patients recovering from surgery is rapid ambulation and resocialization, which often results in reversal of regressive symptoms and the expedited recovery of more normal psychological functioning. Postoperative regression is usually very responsive to psychiatric interventions, including brief supportive psychotherapy and judicious use of anxiolytics, analgesics, or antidepressants when indicated. Benzodiazepines or analgesics may contribute to regressive behavior, and dosage reduction may be effective in reducing regression and encouraging patients to resume more normal functioning. On the other hand, inadequate pain control can reverse progress and lead again to regression as well as agitation.

PSYCHIATRIC COMPLICATIONS OF SURGERY

Depression and delirium are the two common complications in the surgical setting.

Delirium is common (Fricchione et al., 2008), especially in older patients and many acutely hospitalized children (Schieveld et al., 2007). Risk factors include mild preoperative cognitive deficits and vascular disease (Rudolph et al., 2007). The incidence is greater after major vascular operations like abdominal aortic

aneurysm repair and coronary artery bypass surgery than abdominal, orthopedic, or head and neck operations (Fann, 2000). The possibility of alcohol withdrawal adds a risk of delirium tremens. Good management requires prevention of dehydration and hypoxia, simplification of other medications, strengthening the patient's sensory abilities with hearing aids and eyeglasses (Inouye et al., 1999). The psychiatrist has a role in educating the family or friends to recognize confusion, report it and not be frightened by it. Efforts have been made to shorten time on mechanical ventilation, the need for prolonged sedation and to hasten exercise. The Mini-Mental State Examination (MMSE) is useful as an initial screen to rule out delirium (Mitchel et al., 2014). The Confusion Assessment Method (CAM) is one of the most widely used screens, and the CAM-S can be used to follow severity of delirium (Inouye et al., 2014). A delirium screening method for children, the Cornell Assessment for Pediatric Delirium, has been anchored in child development (Silver et al., 2014). (See Chapter 41 for a fuller discussion of delirium and its management.)

Depression occurs as patients cope with pain, many setbacks, and the recognition of the challenge of recovery. Suicides can and do occur occasionally on surgical units, sometimes because of delirium, and sometimes depression.

Attention to symptoms of anxiety in surgical patients provides an early clue to surgical complications (e.g., infection, pulmonary embolus, pulmonary edema), psychiatric disorders (e.g., delirium), or reactions such as fear of dying. Repeated painful procedures commonly trigger acute stress disorder with intrusive, dissociative arousal and avoidance symptoms, and require intervention.

PTSD is commonly recognized in surgical patients by clinicians caring for them, but the symptoms are often discovered to be preexisting, from traumatic exposures including abuse or rape, accidents, combat, illness or injury, medical treatment, disasters, and war or genocide (Stoddard et al., 2014). Trauma in childhood and adolescence affects development and may enhance resilience or exacerbate psychopathology throughout the life cycle (Stoddard, 2014). Early interventions, medical or psychosocial, to prevent traumatic exposure in medical-surgical settings are being investigated. The rates of PTSD vary from under 10% for children undergoing bone marrow transplant, to 20–50% for severely burned children and adults (Stoddard, Sheridan et al., 2011), and other physically traumatized patients have similarly high rates of PTSD (Stevens et al., 2010; Zatzick et al., 2004a). SSRIs have the best record of benefit in treatment of PTSD and its associated depression and disability (Stein et al., 2006) and cogntive behavioral therapy has contributed (Bisson & Andrew, 2006).

Under-treatment of pain is a common problem in children and adults, contributing to mental and physical morbidity, and mortality, in some cases, due to pain-related stress (Schechter et al., 1993; Weisman, 1997; Stoddard et al., 2011). The psychiatrist should be alert to undetected pain and inadequate psychological (e.g., relaxation/hypnosis) and pharmacological (e.g., opiates) methods of pain relief. Concern about causing addiction is largely unfounded with acute pain management, and patients with preexisting addiction often require higher doses of analgesics for equivalent effect. For the patient with a history of addiction, the surgery itself and reexposure to narcotics may foster a relapse in addictive behavior. The psychiatrist, paying more attention to social history, may be the one to hear out the patient about inadequate pain relief, recognize neuralgic components of pain, dimensions of depression and anxiety and the vulnerability of the patient to addictive medications. Sleep disorders are common in the general population, but are even more of a problem surgically, since sleep deprivation often results in regression and behavioral complications. In the surgical patient, sleep disorders are often due to pain, drug side-effects, or excess iatrogenic environmental stimuli. Insomnia may be the initial warning symptom of delirium or acute stress disorder. (Chapters 9 and 33 discusses the diagnosis and treatment of sleep disorders in detail.)

A principal cause of postoperative psychosis, distinct from depression or delirium, is the failure to continue antipsychotic medication previously prescribed.

FACILITATING ADAPTATION TO SURGERY

After surgery, there are changes in the body, and the patient will need time to adapt to such changes.

CASE HISTORY

Alex is a 13-year-old boy with congenital liver disease that worsened, and he underwent a liver transplant. He experienced a complicated postoperative course that included rejection and infection. During his hospital stay, he met with a child psychiatrist, and as he began to feel better, he started talking about what it meant to have a transplant. He was concerned about how he would change, when he would begin to consider the liver his own, and what it might mean to feel healthy after a long period of feeling so sick. During this period, Alex began asking if he could find out about who the donor was. When the therapist explored this question with him, he stated that the main reason he wanted to know was to find out how much the liver transplant would change him. When asked what he meant, he stated that he wanted to know if the person from whom he received the liver liked pizza, because prior to the transplant he never liked to eat pizza, and now he had a craving for it. The case of Alex illustrates well how a patient was helped to express his individual and unique responses to surgery, including sensory experiences, in the process of grieving the illness and loss, and was curious about his relationship to the donor, beginning to "own" the "new" body, and integrating body image transformations into himself.

Inquiry about pain is a useful beginning to consultation with surgical patients (Stoddard et al., 2011; Nejad & Alpay, 2010), and often allows an easy transition to inquiry about the affected body part. In the immediate post-operative period a patient with fear of looking at parts of the body can be coaxed gradually and gently to more direct confrontation. The need for confrontation is directly related to the need for the patients to care for themselves and how fast this must be accomplished. Nurses facilitate encounters with wounds and drains. Mirrors, first small hand-held and later full body mirrors for gradual confrontation and control have been used in nursing settings to foster control and recovery (Freysteinson, 2014).

As patients recover, they may understate their discomfort with their own body image because they are ashamed. Clues to body image difficulties in the setting of surgery are unrealistic expectations about the procedures, difficulties making treatment decisions due to concerns about appearance, the tendency to avoid viewing oneself after treatment, preoccupation with physical flaws, and avoidance of social situations. The practical question is whether concerns about body image prevent them from engaging in social activities or having the confidence to move forward (Fingeret, 2014).

A compassionate clinician can broach questions about their comfort with their physical appearance and find an opening for interventions. After letting a patient know that concerns about body image are common, exploration can begin with asking specifically what concerns the patient may have about the way the body appears and then what are the consequences of their fears or discomfort (Fingeret et al., 2014).

For breast cancer patients, most concerns about body image occur in the immediate postoperative period and soon after completing chemotherapy or radiation (Fobair et al., 2006; Hawighorst-Knapstein et al., 2004). The impact of surgery type on body image within the first year of definitive surgical treatment is related to the severity of surgical side-effects; body image problems differ minimally after two years (Collins, et al., 2011). These preoccupations tend to diminish thereafter and stay relatively stable over 2 years (Falk Dahl et al., 2010; Parker et al., 2007).

Treatments for body image difficulties include cognitive behavioral treatment that changes cognitions about body image and include education, stress management, problem-solving, cognitive reframing and communication skills training (Cash, 2011). Sexual therapy may be particularly appropriate when the issues prevent the patient from being open to sexual encounters. Education about cosmetics and services for hairdressing and makeup provide another avenue to reduce self-consciousness. Exercise and strength training can add to the patient's sense of well being and looking good (Fingeret et al., 2014).

Facial disfigurement is often due to trauma, burns, or cancer and its effects are significantly greater than that affecting other parts of the body (Warner et al., 2012). It often leads to shame and embarrassment ("loss of face"); realistic fears of social stigmatization by family, friends, and strangers; and disability. Some developmental stages and occupations are more critical than others: junior high school students commonly taunt facially disfigured boys and girls with epithets such as "French fry" or "Freddie Kruger"; actors or salesmen may lose their jobs. It is essential for the clinician to provide cognitive preparation for the surgical outcome, to facilitate the grieving for the lost facial features and new "ugliness," and to actively support patients as they seek reentry into their family, social, and occupational lives. Social skills interaction training (SSIT) for those with facial disfigurement from various causes, a cognitive behavior therapy approach, has been shown to be an effective method in most studies of reducing the effects of social stigmatization on self-esteem (Lansdown et al., 1997; Newell, 2000; Kleve et al., 2002; Blakeney et al., 2005). Face IT for adults and YP Face IT for youth is an easily accessible online program that teaches skills to cope with disfigurement (Bessell & Moss, 2007; Bessell, et al.,

2012; www.ypfaceit.co.uk). Some isolated patients may be at risk of suicide, for which they should be assessed and treated. (Burn trauma is discussed in Chapter 75.)

Like the option of replantation surgery for severed hands and fingers, facial transplantation surgery now offers (a very few) facially disfigured patients an option not previously possible (Siemionow & Gordon, 2010; Bueno et al., 2011). It is being done by multidisciplinary surgical teams in a few select centers for patients with facial disfigurement due to traumatic injuries like burns, as well as due to cancer and other causes. It is not a standard treatment but is increasing very slowly. Psychiatric collaboration is essential in the assessment protocols to judge whether a patient is suitable for such extensive surgery. While the hope is that facial transplantation, similar to other types of reconstructive facial surgery, may reduce stigma and functional losses even for those with massive facial disfigurement, it remains to be determined to what extent it will be available for more than a select few patients. In the meantime, facial reconstruction of specific facial features with grafting, flaps, and microsurgical procedures, remains the common treatment. It is important to add that many patients have adapted to their facial disfigurement and have dealt with the associated stigma, even when severe, and do not want facial transplantation surgery for themselves, nor favor it for others.

Bariatric surgery provides an opportunity for treatment of obesity and for patients to acquire an improved body image. Psychiatric screening is commonly a part of the process of identifying the patients who are at less or greater risk from the procedures and who will follow through postoperatively. Candidates for bariatric surgery have high rates of lifetime affective disorder; psychopathology is greater in patients with more severe obesity and lower socioeconomic status (Malik et al., 2014). A 4-year prospective study of psychiatric outcome of patients who had restrictive bariatric surgery found an improvement in mood and self esteem (Burgmer et al., 2014); improvements in cognitive function has also been seen (Alosco et al., 2014). In a retrospective study of 148 patients, outcomes correlated significantly with surgeon follow-up, attendance at postoperative support groups, physical activity, single or divorced marital status, self-esteem, and binge eating (Livhits et al., 2010). Optimal treatment of depression is also important over time; the suicide rate is higher in these patients (Peterhansel et al., 2013).

Whether small or large, severe traumatic injuries, including burns, are painful, emotionally stressful, and may be disfiguring and functionally disabling (Stoddard & Saxe, 2001; Stoddard, Levine, & Lund, 2006). Severely burned children challenge the emotions and skills of the multidisciplinary burn team (Stoddard, 2002). Most, but not all, adult burn patients have preexisting psychopathology, substance abuse, or medical illness. Suicide attempt by burning is one cause of hospitalization for adult burn patients, and less common among adolescents admitted to pediatric burn units; these patients who have attempted suicide require close collaborative surgical and psychiatric treatment and, due to their severe injuries, often have extended, expensive lengths of stay. Psychiatric care of burn patients is usually needed to manage and support their coping with delirium, pain, PTSD, depression, and personality disorders (Stoddard, 2002; Stoddard, Sheridan, et al., 2011). (See Chapter 40.)

Amputations usually represent a massive psychic trauma. In children, they are a massive trauma to the parents as well as the child (Stoddard & Saxe, 2001). In the young child, grieving the loss of a leg is complicated by the child's need to relearn how to walk. In the elderly, depression has been reported to correlate with poor prognosis in rehabilitation. There are several psychiatric issues: depression with unresolved grief and denial; pain at the site of amputation; phantom limb sensations and pain; acute and post-traumatic stress disorder (Parkes, 1973).

Amputations are one of the first surgical procedures recorded in ancient history. Since they have been and still are performed in some Middle Eastern countries as punishment or torture (Shukla et al., 1982), we tend to view amputation consciously and unconsciously as punishment or a form of castration. War increases the numbers of children and adults with amputations, as in the Civil War in the United States, the two World Wars, and recent wars in Vietnam, Cambodia, Iraq, Afghanistan, the Balkans, and Africa. An international effort is increasing to ban land mines, which are major causes of amputation and death for children and adults. These efforts to date have been largely unsuccessful.

Loss of a limb is both cosmetically and functionally disabling, at least for a time, even with effective prostheses. Replantation surgery, nerve grafts, free flaps, and other innovative procedures may offer great hope, but should they fail, severe disappointment or depression may occur. The psychiatric consultant may facilitate adequate preparation, but preoperative teaching is often not feasible in emergencies, and there is often an abrupt damage to body integrity. Without preparation, patients may be overwhelmed and have great difficulty coping with their loss. Their families may suffer even more severe and chronic stress. Optimally, the patient should be assessed preoperatively for ego strengths and preexisting psychopathology, and the family, too, should be assessed. The psychiatrist can assist with managing acute pain, stress, and sleep disorders, and may assist with breaking the news that the limb will be lost to the patient and family, perhaps by reflecting with the patient on pain sensations, pain relief, and response to dressing changes as an entry to the grief process. Traumatic amputations tend to affect active children more greatly than they do retired, sedentary individuals.

CASE HISTORY: ACUTE GRIEF IN A 12-YEAR-OLD BOY

A handsome Puerto Rican boy suffered electrical injuries requiring amputation of his right arm, with additional injuries to his left hand and arm. Once morphine and lorazepam were tapered, he was reported to be withdrawn and having sleep difficulty, but was becoming more able to talk about his awareness of his injuries. After initial introductions, an empathic medical student, in the presence of the boy's worried mother, inquired in Spanish about his condition, what he recalled, and what he had enjoyed prior to his injuries. The boy replied that he liked baseball and played second base, at which point he suddenly realized that he would never be able to play again. He broke down in tears, together with others in the room, and cried disconsolately for a time. Eventually, in the same interview, he was able to accept some consolation that being fitted for and learning to use a prosthetic arm in the future might offer hope of some restored right arm function.

A goal is to facilitate both grieving the personal meanings of the loss, in this case symbolized by the boy's prowess as a second baseman, and the nurturance of a hopeful, realistic attitude. Children, adolescents, and even adults (especially males) may learn to regard their amputation in a "warrior motif" as a "red badge of courage," responding with resilience or "hardiness" even to terrible losses.

Regardless of age, there are always issues of incorporating a new body image, and dealing with grief and loss for the amputated limb. Exploration of the exact precipitating circumstances, the details of the accident or disease, and associated feelings of embarrassment or guilt assists with emotional processing of the traumatic experiences. There often are multiple traumas with which the amputation is associated, perhaps an accident, urban violence, or chronic illness, deaths of others, pain, and acute surgical treatment. The stigma of the amputation may actually be furthest from the patient's mind. PTSD may accompany amputations in civil life, but combat-related amputations are associated with the greatest amount of psychological trauma.

Recovery of maximal function and return to one's usual social and occupational functioning are goals, but not always attainable. Complications such as regression, depression, and noncompliance are common and respond best to early interventions. Some patients—for instance, elderly patients with vascular disease and non-healing ulcers, or teenagers unable to walk due to leg deformities—may welcome amputation as relief from pain or the inability to ambulate. However, even when the limb is painful or nonfunctional, the patient may be ambivalent about the disappearance of this body part. Optimism before surgery may be replaced by normal, grief-related anger, despair, and negativity postoperatively. The patient may have difficulty adjusting to the stump and become resigned to disability and nonfunction rather than active rehabilitation unless vigorous and positive rehabilitation is started promptly by a well-trained, multidisciplinary staff.

"Phantom limb phenomena" commonly occur following amputation in both children and adults. Kolb (1975) noted that the earliest accounts of body image disturbance date back to the sixteenth century, when Paré noted the frequent occurrence of phantom limb sensations following amputation. Phantom limb phenomena are the persistence of pain or sensation as if the limb were still present. The "phantom" phenomena may persist to some degree for a lifetime. "Phantom" symptoms are often missed if not asked about; they may also evoke anxiety and confusion. These phenomena may decrease over time, or be persistent. We and others (Krane & Heller, 1995) have found phantom pain in nearly every child with an amputation, except those with a congenital deformity.

Psychotherapeutically for the young child, "nonverbal and metaphorical 'safe' alternatives via play modalities," such as dolls and drawing (Billig & Weaver, 1996), "and active facilitation of coping skills are useful to impart information, decrease anxiety and enhance mastery" (Atalar & Carter, 1992, p. 128).

An ostomy is a surgically created opening of the intestine, colon, or ureter brought to the surface of the abdomen; for instance, ileostomy, colostomy, or urostomy The United Ostomy Associations of America and the American Cancer Society provide practical guides for patients (www.ostomy.org). Ostomy surgery is performed to treat a variety of diseases such as congenital malformations, inflammatory bowel disease, diverticulitis, trauma, and cancer. An ostomy may be temporary or permanent. Psychologically, it may evoke even greater emotional stress than loss of reproductive function, both because of its chronic nature, and because of involuntary embarrassment and shame evoked by reduction or loss of excretory function and control present since early childhood.

Initially, patients may experience the ostomy as a form of bodily mutilation, with all of the shock, revulsion, and sense of victimization that that implies. Body odors, gases, fluids, or feces may leak out in public settings or soil clothing, resulting in fear of or actual social stigmatization and interference with activities of daily living. Reinstituting normal social and sexual relationships may require patience and understanding by all parties. The ostomy or ostomy apparatus may be painful, or require periodic emptying and attention. Patients with a colostomy or ileostomy have to deal with effects on absorption of food, excretion, stool leakage, and passing flatus; worry regarding sexual attractiveness and function. They are helped by specialized ostomy nurse therapists, resumption of school or work, utilization of practical guidelines and self-help groups.

The threat to virility or femininity associated with urogenital symptoms and urological diagnoses cannot be overestimated; nor can the relief experienced when effective treatment is provided. Depending on the individual's personality and the condition, the psychophysiological issues may include fears of loss of potency (erection and/or ejaculation), orgasm, libidinal or genital sensation, virility or femininity, attractiveness, reproductive capacity, sexual desirability or continence. Certain of these fears may or may not be realistic. As illustrated by the case below, there can be a risk that the fears engendered may lead to denial, depression, indecision, inappropriate interventions, and adverse outcomes, despite rapid advances that have been made in effective clinical treatment options.

CASE HISTORY: SURGERY DELAYED BY PATIENT SEEKING ALTERNATIVE THERAPIES

A 50-year-old obese novelist, the father of a nine-year-old son, presented with abdominal pain and dysuria to his physician and was referred to a urologist. Cystoscopic surgery revealed an aggressive bladder tumor without metastasis, and prompt resection of the tumor was advised. After some delay, he sought continent diversion surgery from another urologist to preserve sexual functioning and to avoid an ileostomy. At the same time, terrified of losing sexual functioning and distrusting his urologist, he and his wife, both well educated, sought out alternative therapists who introduced them to a man who was allegedly cured of bladder cancer by nonsurgical means; they began a "positive" program with mystical spirituality, dietary and herbal remedies, massage, and use of visual imagery including "channeling", in the belief that by "imaging" cancer remission, it would remit. A 20-pound weight loss, reduced anxiety, and improved mood, and no change on a computerized tomography (CT) scan confirmed for them the effectiveness of these therapies. He canceled his surgery, emphasizing his need to make his own decisions and complaining about each urologist who had gravely broken bad news. Despite confrontation of his denial, depressive signs including irritability, and a severe behavioral regression, he avoided "conventional" medical treatment, including psychiatric care.

After two more months, pain and then blood in the urine signaled further tumor spread. Having by then found a homeopathic physician, he was referred to another urologist who commented with a touch of humor that pleased the patient, "You can't have sex if you're dead." The patient consented to and had continent diversion surgery. Chemotherapy was necessary for possible metastases, and his prognosis was guarded. The urologist referred him for treatment of depression, which responded to combined antidepressant and family and individual psychotherapy, despite the guarded prognosis and chemotherapy.

He chose to continue with some of the alternative therapies, which, while of questionable therapeutic value, did not interfere with his regular medical care.

BREAKING BAD NEWS; LISTENING; PROVIDING HOPE

All people need to maintain some degree of hope. It is hope that allows us to face the traumas of our lives and find the coping skills to move forward in the face of bad news. The psychiatrist seeks to communicate supportively, diagnose, and participate constructively in the treatment of the surgical patient. It is difficult to be the surgeon or psychiatrist breaking bad news, and it can be painful to observe the recipient's reaction to this news. Patients need to know that their physicians can help them to bear it. For most patients, it is important to hear honest answers to their questions, framed in simple and concise terms throughout the course of treatment, and then for the physicians to listen carefully to the responses of the patient and family over time.

Hope is a universal mechanism in facing all of life's travails, and its maintenance is crucial even if an illness will end in death. The maintenance of hope can come from a variety of places, and it is important for clinicians to try to assess what individuals do to create hope for themselves, including discussing with them their belief systems such as religion and knowing which people are important to them during a crisis.

At the beginning of an illness, people hope for a cure. Even in situations in which there is no hope for a cure or survival, it is important to maintain hope. This can be done by looking at short-term goals such as having a good morning, or sitting in a chair, or having a discussion about the next possible course of treatment. In the face of death, many people maintain hope based upon their religious beliefs, social supports, and planning for those they will leave behind.

COLLABORATION OF SURGEON AND PSYCHIATRIST

Surgeons uncover and create problems and must be equipped to inform patients and loved ones of unfavorable findings and untoward events. Many operations have as their goal, or their side effect, a major change in body image, appearance, or function. Patients benefit from frank discussions of these issues. Unfortunately, surgeons, who are best equipped to discuss these alterations, may not always have the time or feel comfortable listening, providing the information, and responding to the patient's concerns.

Death evokes fear in everyone. It is during the process of death and dying that it is most important for patients to know that their physician will continue to be available to them and that people will answer their questions. It often is difficult to sit with the person who is dying, and family, friends, and caregivers may avoid the dying patient. This unplanned conspiracy of avoidance says to the patient that no one can or wants to hear their thoughts and ideas, and isolates the patient. Cecily Saunders (1998) explains that "No one should have information forced upon them, but any continuing communication with a patient is likely to open up the subject sooner or later." Physicians who overcome their own fears of the subject will learn how and when and what to tell.

As Kübler-Ross (1969) wrote, individuals who know they are going to die will proceed through a series of stages, ending in a state of acceptance. Patients should be given the opportunity to discuss their fears, hopes, anger, and frustrations. They need to know that there are people who will consistently listen with a compassionate and even manner. It is also important to remember that the dying patient may want to talk about other things than dying, including things that may seem minor or frivolous (such as favorite sport teams, politics, etc.). Chapter 18 discusses the roles of religion and spiritual issues in the context of dying patients. Chapter 57 on palliative care also discusses the care of patients with a limited life span.

Children and adolescents can be included in discussion about death, whether this concerns a parent or themselves. The discussion needs to be adapted to a child's understanding of death, and this understanding changes with the child's age. In children under about six years old, death is understood as a magical event and not as a permanent state. The older child and adolescent will have a better understanding of death. The school-age child and adolescent understand death as permanent and irreversible and can discuss their fears and anxieties as well as any preparations they might want to make.

Following a death, the surgeon's and the hospital's continued interest in the grieving family is important (Weisman, 1998; Parkes, 1998). Some surgeons ask the family in the last meeting after the death of a loved one, including infants, to schedule a return appointment after about six months have passed, to ask any lingering questions, and to discuss the death and their feelings about it with the surgeon (see Chapter 81). Attentive medical social workers keep track of the anniversary dates of deaths and are in touch with the families as those dates approach. The pediatric service at Massachusetts General Hospital serves the families of children who have died by offering an annual Pediatric Memorial Service to which surviving families are invited—it is very well attended.

PSYCHIATRIC CARE, REFERRALS, AND RECOVERY AFTER DISCHARGE

Most patients recover from surgery uneventfully. Those with preexisting or new mental illnesses are at risk, and outpatient psychiatric referral is essential. Collaborative follow-up consultation with visiting nurses, physical therapists, social workers, psychologists, and psychiatrists and other rehabilitative team members may make the difference between whether long-term rehabilitation fails or succeeds. Zatzick et al. (2004; 2011) have successfully developed a protocol for stepped, collaborative care of trauma victims before and after discharge that connects these patients to outside resources—for example, for PTSD, depression, and alcohol abuse—and reduces future risk. Some patients after major surgery, such as transplants, require lifelong psychiatric and surgical outpatient monitoring and care to manage complications of surgical treatment.

SUMMARY

Psychiatrists and surgeons working together reduce patient suffering, strengthen the team, usually shorten lengths of stay, and improve outcomes. That alliance takes several forms, which interact, such as clinical care, planning and implementing care improvements (like protocols pain management and alcohol abuse); sharing clinical case conferences, writing in areas of common interest, and making efforts to fund psychiatric care and research in surgical settings. Table 69.1 describes a 10-point plan for psychiatric care of the surgical patient.

CLINICAL PEARLS

- The surgeon may be respected, idealized as a savior, feared, or demonized by patients and their families for failing to fulfill expectations.

- The patients who are more likely to have difficulties in the relationship with the surgeon are those with difficulties in previous relationships.

- Psychiatrists can help clarify the patient's distortions as well as respond with empathy to the patient's anger and disappointment if his expectations are not fulfilled.

- Psychiatrists may also help the surgeons and the surgical and anesthesia staff set appropriate limits on "acting out" by patients and other types of inappropriate behavior.

Table 69.1 TEN-POINT PLAN FOR PSYCHIATRIC CARE OF THE SURGICAL PATIENT

1. *Speak* with the patient in his or her language, listen carefully, and ensure the patient's safety. After surgery, inquire as to whether or not the patient is in pain.

2. *Consult* with the surgical team about the patient, clarifying the psychiatrist's time availability and role. Within psychiatry if a psychiatrist, or surgery if a surgeon, arrange supervision, peer consultation, and departmental support.

3. *Obtain the history* of the surgical condition, disease, or trauma, psychopathology, or substance abuse, and social and family functioning.

4. *Diagnose* the mental disorder(s): Assess stage of life, stage of illness, mental status (including pain, stress, memory), psychiatric risk (delirium, suicide, domestic abuse), prognosis, medical and surgical issues including medications and their interactions, alcohol or drug withdrawal, risk factors, cultural factors, legal status, and family or staff concerns. Recommend precautions, studies, or consultations as indicated.

5. *Treat* the patient psychotherapeutically and/or psychopharmacologically for pain, delirium, stress, insomnia, depression, and other symptoms or disorders. *Evaluate and monitor* drug selection, interactions, effects, and side-effects. *Provide* staff support, and, for complex cases, plan a team conference.

6. *Communicate* with the child or adult with advanced progressive illness with limited prognosis so as to learn how and when and what truth to tell, in support of their and their family's growth toward the end of life. Assess, treat, and support the dying patient, and assist the clarification and the resolution of ethical dilemmas.

7. *Progress* to treating residual mental disorders, substance abuse, and other problems, when the patient has survived the acute phase.

8. *Facilitate* grieving and adaptation of the patient and family to cosmetic or functional losses, and foster hope.

9. *Collaborate in planning surgical follow-up and communicate psychiatric findings* and recommendations to the surgeon and primary care physician. Support reentry to school or work, including special education and rehabilitation services.

10. *Remain available for follow-up* consultation to the patient, family, and care givers, and *assist* them in *referrals* for needed services.

- Pain and disfigurement to any body part are long remembered and can have lasting effects on the patient's body image and self-esteem (Freud, 1952). Fear of "shots" or injections and fear of surgery, often related to prior experiences, are common in both children and in adults.

- Inquiry about pain is a useful beginning to consultation with surgical patients (Stoddard et al., 2011), and often allows an easy transition to inquiry about the affected body part.

- A treasured blanket, toy, book, or song may take the role of a transitional object for an infant or toddler in the hospital.

- Choices about surgery and other aspects of medical care should involve children as young as six or seven.

- Patients can be characterized by how invested they are in their own appearance on one dimension and by how much they perceive a discrepancy between their own body image and what they desire, on another dimension. In the surgical setting, these concerns can be thought of on a normal continuum (Fingeret et al., 2014).

- Often staff who have known the patient only one shift make decisions about psychological symptoms, as well as rapid *ad hoc* decisions about as needed medications for anxiety, sleep, or pain.

- A powerful antidepressant for patients recovering from surgery is rapid ambulation and resocialization, which often results in reversal of regressive symptoms and expedited recovery of more normal psychological functioning.

- Parental presence during induction of anesthesia is available at some hospitals, but children are not necessarily less anxious when parents are there, especially if the parent is anxious (Chundamala et al., 2009; Yip, 2009).

- For patients on clozapine having surgery, attention should be paid to bowel function. Changes in smoking may affect clozapine levels.

- Attention to symptoms of anxiety in surgical patients provides an early clue to surgical complications (e.g., infection, pulmonary embolus, pulmonary edema), psychiatric disorders (e.g., delirium), or reactions such as fear of dying.

- Clarification of the diagnosis of chronic psychotic disorder offers an opportunity to identify who the patient trusts, who the regular psychiatrist is, the nature of maintenance medications, whether preoperative medications offer the best possible mental status, and to build an interdisciplinary support team (Irwin et al., 2014).

- The five dimensions of the surgical experience that provoke anxiety in children summarize as well the primitive concerns of adults. These are a) pain and mutilation, b) separation from parents or other trusted adults c) fear of the unknown and unfamiliar, d) uncertainty about normative behavior in a hospital setting, and e) loss of control, autonomy and competence (Visintainer & Wolfer, 1975).

- The adept surgeon who must do sequential surgeries makes a relationship with a patient that resonates with the patient's readiness for the next surgery.

DISCLOSURE STATEMENTS

Dr. Stoddard has no conflicts to disclose. He participates in research funded by the Massachusetts General Hospital, and by Shriners Hospitals for Children.

Dr. Sheridan has no conflicts to disclose. He participates in research funded by Shriners Hospitals for Children. He participates in research funded by the U.S. Department of Defense through Physical Sciences Incorporated. He has no financial interest in Physical Sciences Incorporated.

Dr. Martyn has no conflicts of interests to disclose.

Dr. Selter has no conflicts to disclose.

REFERENCES

Abrams, T. E., Vaughn-Sarrazin, M., & Rosenthal, G. E. (2010). Influence of psychiatric comorbidity on surgical mortality. *Archives of Surgery, 145*(10), 447–453.

Alam, H. B., Fricchione, G. L., Guimaraes, A. S. R., & Zukerberg, L. R. (2009). Case 31-2009: A 26-year-old man with abdominal distention and shock. *New England Journal of Medicine, 361*, 1487–1496.

Alosco, M. L., Galioto, R., Spitznagel, M. B., et al. (2014). Cognitive function after bariatric surgery: evidence for improvement 3 years after surgery. *American Journal Surgery, 207*, 870–876.

American Academy of Pediatrics. (2014). The pediatrician's role in the evaluation and preparation of pediatric patients undergoing anesthesia. *Pediatrics, 134*, 634–641.

American Society of Anesthesiologists Task Force on Intra-operative Awareness. (2006). Practice advisory for intra-operative awareness and brain function monitoring: A report by the American Society of Anesthesiologists Task Force on Intra-operative Awareness. *Anesthesiology, 104*, 847–864.

Applebaum, P. S., & Grisso, T. (1988). Assessing patients' capacities to consent to treatment. *New England Journal of Medicine, 319*, 1635–1638.

Arcarturk, T. O., Abdel-Motleb, M., & Acar, F. (2014). How to kill a flap: Munchausen Syndrome—A silent trap for plastic surgeons. *Journal of Hand Microsurgery, 6*, 42–44.

Atalar, K. D., & Carter, B. D. (1992). Pediatric limb amputation: Aspects of coping and psychotherapeutic intervention. *Child Psychiatry & Human Development, 23*, 117–129.

Avidan, M. S., Searleman, A. C., Storandt, M., et al. (2009). Long-term cognitive decline in older subjects was not attributable to noncardiac surgery or major illness. *Anesthesiology, 111*, 964–970.

Avidan, M. S., Zhang, L., Burnside, B. A., et al. (2008). Anesthesia awareness and the bi-spectral index. *New England Journal of Medicine, 358*, 1097–1108.

Baldessarini, R. J., Tondo, L., Faedda, G. L., et al. (1996). Effects of the rate of discontinuing lithium maintenance treatment in bipolar disorders. *Journal of Clinical Psychiatry, 57*, 441–448.

Belfer, M., Harrison, A. M., Pillemer, F. C., et al. (1982). Appearance and the influence of reconstructive surgery on body image. In F. C. MacGregor (Ed.), Symposium on Social and Psychological Considerations in Plastic Surgery. *Clinics in Plastic Surgery, 9,* 307–316.

Belfer, M. L. (1987). Psychological consideration of the plastic surgical patient. In S. A. Sohn (Ed.), *Fundamentals of aesthetic plastic surgery* (pp. 9–13). Baltimore, MD: Williams & Wilkins.

Bartels, M., Althoff, R. R., & Boosma, D. I. (2009). Anesthesia and cognitive performance in children: No evidence of a causal relationship. *Twin Research & Human Genetics, 12,* 246–253.

Berscheid, E., & Gangestad, S. (1982). The social psychological implications of facial physical attractiveness. In F. C. MacGregor (Ed.), Symposium on Social and Psychological Considerations in Plastic Surgery. *Clinics in Plastic Surgery, 9*(3), 289.

Bessell, A., Brough, V., Clarke, A., Harcourt, D., Moss, T. P., & Rumsey, N. (2012). Evaluation of the effectiveness of Face IT, a computer-based psychosocial intervention for disfigurement-related distress, *Psychology Health & Medicine, 17,* 565–577.

Bessell, A, & Moss, T. (2007). Evaluating the effectiveness of psychosocial interventions for individuals with visible differences: a systematic review of the empirical literature. *Body Image, 4,* 227–238.

Billig, T., & Weaver, K. (1996). Individualized doll therapy with children experiencing limb loss. *Orthopedic Nursing, 15,* 50–55.

Bisson, J., & Andrew, M. (2006). Psychological treatment of posttraumatic stress disorder. *The Cochrane Library, 1,* 1–60.

Blakeney P., Thomas C., Holzer, C. E., Rose, M., Berniger, F., & Meyer, W. J. (2005). Efficacy of a short-term, intensive social skills training program for burned adolescents. *Journal of Burn Care Rehabilitation, 26,* 546–555.

Brambrink, A. M., Evers, A. S., Avidan, M. S., et al. (2010). Isoflurane-induced neuroapoptosis in the neonatal rhesus macaque brain. *Anesthesiology, 112,* 834–841.

Bueno, E. M., Diaz-Siso, J. R., & Pomahac, B. A. (2011). Multidisciplinary protocol for face transplantation at Brigham and Women's Hospital. *Journal of Plastic, Reconstructive, & Aesthetic Surgery, 64,* 1572–1579.

Burrows, R. C., & Hodgson, R. E. (1997). De facto gatekeeping and informed consent in intensive care. *Medical Law Review, 16,* 17–27.

Burgmer, R., Legenbauer, T., Muller, A., et al. (2014). Psychological outcome 4 years aftrer restrictive bariatric surgery. *Obesity Surgery, 24,* 1670–1678.

Burton, M. C., Warren, M. B., Lapid, M. I., & Bostwick, J. M. (2014). Munchausen syndrome by adult proxy: A review of the literature. *Journal of Hospital Medicine, 10,* 1002/jhm.2268.

Caldas, J. C., Pais-Ribeiro, J., & Carneiro, S. R. (2004). General anesthesia, surgery and hospitalization in children and their effects upon cognitive, academic, emotional and sociobehavioral development—a review. *Pediatric Anesthesiology, 14,* 910–915.

Caplan, L. M., & Hackett, T. P. (1963). Emotional effects of lower limb amputation in the aged. *New England Journal of Medicine, 269,* 1139–1141.

Cash, T. F. (2011). Cognitive-behavioral perspectives on body image. In T. F. Cash, L. Smolak (Eds.), *Body Image: A Handbook of Science, Practice and Prevention* (pp. 39–47). New York NY: Guilford Press.

Castle, D. J., & Phillips, K. A. (2002). Disorders of Body Image. Petersfield UK and Philadelphia: Wrightson Biomedical Publishers LTD.

Chundamala, J., Wright, J. G., & Kemp, S. M. (2009). An evidence-based review of parental presence during anesthesia induction and parent/child anxiety. *Canadian Journal of Anaesthesia, 56,* 57–70.

Collins, K. K., Liu, Y., Schootman, M., et al. (2011). Effects of breast cancer surgery and surgical side effects on body image over time. *Breast Cancer Research & Treatment, 126,* 167–176.

Conner-Spady, B. L., Marshall, D. A., Hawkeer, G. A., Bohm, E., dunbar, M. J., et al. (2014). You'll know when you're ready: A qualitative study exploring how patients decide when the time is right for joint replacemnt surgery. *BMC Health Services Research, 14,* 454 epub

Davidson, A. J., Huang, G. H., Czarnecki, C., et al. (2005). Awareness during anesthesia in children: A prospective cohort study. *Anesthesia & Analgesia, 100,* 653–661.

DiMaggio, C., Sun, L. S., Kakavouli, A., Burne, M. W., & Li, G. (2009). A retrospective cohort study of the association of anesthesia and hernia repair surgery with behavioral and developmental disorders in young children. *Journal of Neurosurgery & Anesthesiology, 21,* 286–291.

Donelan, M. B., Parrett, B. M., & Sheridan, R. L. (2008). Pulsed dye laser therapy and z-plasty for facial burn scars: the alternative to excision. *Annals of Plastic Surgery, 60,* 480–486. doi:10.1097/SAP.0b013e31816fcad5

Dragun, A. E., Pan, J., Riley, E. C., et al. (2012). Increasing use of elective mastectomy and contralateral prophylactic surgery among breast conservation candidates: A 14-year report from a comprehensive cancer center. *American Journal of Clinical Oncology,* PMID 22643566 (May 24).

Ely, E. W., Shintani, A., Truman, B., et al. (2004). Delirium as a predictor of mortality in mechanically ventilated patients in the intensive care unit. *Journal of the American Medical Association, 291,* 1753–1762.

Erikson, E. (1980). *Identity and the life cycle.* New York: Norton.

Ezri, T., Sessler, D., Weisenberg, M., et al. (2007). Association of ethnicity with the minimum alveolar concentration of sevoflurane. *Anesthesiology, 107,* 9–14.

Falk Dahl, C. A., Reinertsen, K. V., Nesvold, I. L., Fossa, S. D., & Dahl, A. A. (2010). A study of body image in long-term breast cancer survivors. *Cancer, 116,* 3549–3557.

Fann, J. R. (2000). The epidemiology of delirium: a review of studies and methodological issues. *Seminars in Clinical Neuropsychiatry, 5,* 64–74.

Findley, J. K., Sanders, K. B., & Groves, J. E. (2003). The role of psychiatry in the mangement of acute trauma surgery patients. *Primary care companion Journal of clinical Pyschiatry, 5,* 195–200.

Fingeret, M. C., Teo, I., & Epner, D. E. (2014). Managing body image difficulties of adult cancer patients. *Cancer, 120,* 633–641.

Fisher, C. S., Martin-Dunlap, T., Ruppel, M. B., Gao, F., Atkins, J., & Margenthaler, J. A. (2012). Fear of recurrence and perceived survival benefit are primary motivators for choosing mastectomy over breast-conservation therapy regardless of age. *Annals of Surgical Oncology, 20,* 2346–2350.

Flick, R. P., Katusic, S. K., Colligan, R. C., et al. (2011). Cognitive and behavioral outcomes after early exposure to anesthesia and surgery. *Pediatrics, 128,* e1053–1061.

Fobair, P., Steward, S. L., Chang, S., et al. (2006). Body image and sexual problems in young women with breast cancer. *Psychooncology, 15,* 579–594.

Frankel, L., Sanmartin, C., Conner-Spady, B., Marshall, D. A., Freeman-Collins, L., et al. (2012). Osteoarthritis patients' perceptions of "appropriateness" for total join replacement surgery. *Osteoarthritis Cartilage, 20,* 967–973.

Freysteinson, W. M., Deutsch, A. S., Davin, K., et al. (2014). The mirror program: preparing women for the postoperative mastectomy mirror-viewing experience. Nursing Forum, 1–6.

Freud, A. (1952). The role of bodily illness in the mental life of children. In *The psychoanalytic study of the child* (Chap. 7, pp. 69–81). New Haven, CT: Yale University Press.

Frost, M. H., Hoskin, T. L., Hartmann, L. C., Degnim, A. C., Johnson, J. L., & Boughey, J. C. (2011). Contralateral prophylactic mastectomy: Long-term consistency of satisfaction and adverse effects and the significance of informed decision-making, quality of life, and personality traits. *Annals of Surgical Oncology, 11,* 3110–3116.

Fricchione, G. L., Nejad, S. H., Esses, J. A., et al. (2008). Postoperative delirium. *American Journal of Psychiatry, 165,* 803–812.

Giesen, D. (1993). The patient's right to know—a comparative law perspective. *Medical Law Review, 12,* 553–565.

Hawighorts-Knapstein, S., Fusshoeller, C., Franz, C., et al. (2004). The impact of treatment for genital cancer on quality of life and body image—results of a prospective longitudinal 10-year study. *Gynecology Oncology, 94,* 398–403.

Huyse, F. J., Touw, D. J., van Schijndel, R. S., deLange, J. J., Slaets, J. P. J. (2006). Psychotropic drugs and the perioperative period: a proposal for a guideline in elective surgery. *Psychosomatics, 47,* 8–22.

Inouye, S. K., Bogardus, S. T., Charpentier, P. A., et al. (1999). A multicomponent intervention to prevent delirium in hospitalized older patients. *New England Journal of Medicine, 340*(9), 669–676.

Inouye, S. K., Kosar, C. M., Tommet, D., Schmitt, E. M., Puelle, M. R., et al. (2014). The CAM-S: Development and validation of a new scoring system for delirium severity in 2 cohorts. *Annals Internal Medicine, 160*, 526–533.

Irwin, K. E., Henderson, D. C., Knight, H. P., & Pirl, W. F. (2014). Cancer care for individuals with schizophrenia. *Cancer, 120*, 323–334.

Johnson, T., Monk, T., Rasmussen, L. S., et al. (2002). ISPOCD2 Investigators. Postoperative cognitive dysfunction in middle-aged patients. *Anesthesiology, 96*, 1351–1357.

Justus, R., Wyles, D., Wilson, J., Rode, D., Walther, V., et al. (2006). Preparing children and families for surgery: Mount Sinai's multidisciplinary perspective. *Pediatric Nursing, 32*, 35–42.

Kain, Z. N., Mayes, L. C., Caldwell-Andrews, A. A., Karas, D. E., & McClain, B. C. (2006). Preoperative anxiety, postoperative pain, and behavioral recovery in young children undergoing surgery. *Pediatrics, 118*, 651–658.

Kain, Z. N., Wang, S. M., Mayes, L. C., Caramico, L. A., & Hofstadter, M. B. (1999). Distress during the induction of anesthesia and postoperative behavioral outcomes. *Anesthesia & Analgesia, 88*, 1042–1047.

Kavanaugh, C., Lasoff, E., Eide, Y., et al. (1991). Learned helplessness and the pediatric burn patient: Dressing change behavior and serum cortisol and beta endorphin. *Journal of Pain Symptom Management, 6*, 106–177.

Kleve, L., Rumsey, N., Wyn-Williams, M., et al. (2002). The effectiveness of cognitive-behavioural interventions provided at Outlook: a disfigurement support unit. *Journal of Evaluation in Clinical Practice, 8*, 387–395.

Kikuchi, K., & Hara, T. (1996). Patients' understanding of the informed consent for cataract surgery. *Journal of Ophthalmic Nursing & Technology, 15*, 216–219.

Kim, Y., Glatt, H., Xie, W., et al. (1997). Human g-aminobutyric acid-type A receptor a5 subunit gene (GABRA5): Characterization and structural organization of the, 5' flanking region. *Genomics, 42*, 378–387.

Kolb, L. C. (1975). Disturbances of the body image. In S. Arieti (Ed.), *American handbook of psychiatry* (Chap. 4, pp. 810–837). New York: Basic Books.

Kübler-Ross, E. (1969). *On death and dying.* Toronto, Ont.: Macmillan.

Kurtz, B. P., Muriel, A. C., Abrams, A. N. (2010). Pediatric consultation. In T. A. Stern, G. L. Fricchione, N. H. Cassem, M. S. Jellinek, & J. F. Rosenbaum (Eds.), *Massachusetts General Hospital handbook of general hospital psychiatry* (6th ed., pp. 565–582). Philadelphia, PA: Saunders/Elsevier.

Lansdown, R., Rumsey, N., Bradbury, E., et al. (1997). *Visibly different: Coping with disfigurement.* Oxford, UK: Butterworth-Heinemann.

Lat, I., McMillan, W., Taylor, S., et al. (2009) Impact of delirium on clinical outcomes in mechanically ventilated surgical and trauma patients. *Critical Care Medicine, 37*, 1898–1905.

Levine, R. J. (1996). Respect for children as research subjects. In M. Lewis (Ed.), *Child and adolescent psychiatry: A comprehensive textbook* (2nd ed., p. 1238). Baltimore, MD: Williams & Wilkins.

Lewis, I., Burke, C., Voepel-Lewis, T., & Tait, A. R. (2007). Children who refuse anesthesia or sedation: A survey of anesthesiologists. *Paediatric Anaesthesiology, 17*(12), 1134–1142.

Lewis, M. (1994). The consultation process in child and adolescent psychiatric consultation-liaison pediatrics. *Child & Adolescent Psychiatric Clinics of North America, 3*(3), 439–448.

Livhits, M., Mercado, C., Yermilov, I., et al. (2010). Behavioral factors associated with successful weight loss after gastric bypass. *The American Surgeon, 76*(10), 1139–1142.

Loepke, A. W., Soriano, S. G. (2008). An assessment of the effects of general anesthetics on developing brain structure and neurocogntive function. *Anesthetics & Analgesia, 106*, 1681–1707.

Lorberg, B. A., & Prince, J. B. (2010). Psychopharmacological management of children and adolescents. In T. A. Stern, G. L. Fricchione, N. H. Cassem, M. S. Jellinek, & J. F. Rosenbaum (Eds.), *Massachusetts General Hospital handbook of general hospital psychiatry* (6th ed., pp. 467–498). Philadelphia, PA: Saunders/Elsevier.

Lowe, E. J., & Ackman, M. L. (2010). Impact of tobacco smoking cessation on stable clozapine or olanzapine treatment. *Annals of Pharmacotherapy, 44*, 727–732.

Lundberg, S. G., & Guggenheim, F. G. (1986). Sequelae of limb amputation. *Advances in Psychosomatic Medicine, 15*, 199–210.

Lydiatt, W. M., Besette, D., Schmid, K. K., Sayles, H., Burke, W. J. (2013). Prevention of depression with escitalopram in patients undergoing treatment for head and neck cancer: randomized, double-blind, placebo-controlled clinical trial. *Journal of the American Medical Association Otolaryngology Head an Neck Surgery, 139*, 678–686.

MacGregor, F. C. (Ed.) (1982). Symposium on Social and Psychological Considerations in Plastic Surgery. *Clinics in Plastic Surgery, 9*, 3.

MacGregor, F. C. (1990). Facial disfigurement: Problems and management of social interaction and implications for mental health. *Aesthetic Plastic Surgery, 14*, 249–257.

Malarbi, S., Stargatt, R., Howard, K., Davidson, A. (2011). Characterizing the behavior of children emerging with delirium from general anesthesia. *Pediatric Anaesthesia, 21*, 942–950.

Malik, S., Mitchell, J. E., Engel, S., Crosby, R., Wonderlich, S. (2004). Psychopathology in bariatric surgery candidates: A review of studies using tructured diagnostic interviews. *Comprehensive Psychiatry, 55*, 248–259.

Maldonado, J. R., Wysong, A., van der Starre, P. J., Block, T., Miller, C., & Reitz, B. A. (2009). Dextromedetomidine and the reduction of postoperative delirium after cardiac surgery. *Psychosomatics,* May–Jun; *50*(3), 206–217.

Marson, D. C., Ingram, K. K., Cody, H. A., et al. (1995). Assessing the competency of patients with Alzheimer's disease under different legal standards. A prototype instrument [see comments]. *Archives of Neurology, 52*, 949–954.

Mason, S. E., Noel-Storr, A., & Ritchie, C. W. (2010). The impact of general and regional anesthesia on the incidence of post-operative cognitive dysfunction and post-operative delirium: a systematic review with meta-analysis. *Journal of Alzheimer's Disease, 22*, 67–79.

Masterson, G. (1995). Factitious disorders and the surgeon. *British Journal of Surgery, 82*, 1588–1589.

McCleane, G. J., & Cooper, R. (1990). The nature of pre-operative anxiety. *Anaesthesia, 45*, 153–155.

Miller, V. A., Drotar, D., & Kodish E. (2004). Children's competence for assent and consent: A review of empirical findings. *Ethics & Behavior, 14*(3), 255–295.

Mitchell, A. J., Shukla, D., Ajumal, H. A., Stubbs, B., & Tahir, T. A. (2014). The Mini-Mental State Examination as a diagnostic and screening test for delirium: systematic review and meta-analysis. *General Hospital Psychiatry,* pii, S0163-8343(14)00217-5. doi:10.1016/j.genhosppsych 2014.09.003

Monk, T. G., et al. (2008). Predictors of cognitive dysfunction after major noncardiac surgery. *Anesthesiology, 108*, 18–30.

Moore, M., Fagan, S., Nejad, S., Bilodeau, M., Goverman, L., et al. (2013). The role of a dedicated staff psychiatrist in modern burn centers. *Annals of Burns and Fire Disasters, 26*, 213–216.

Morioka, D., & Ohkubo, F. (2014). Borderline personality disorder and aesthetic plastic surgery. *Aesthetic Plastic Surgery,* doi:10.1007/s00266-014-0396

Napoleon, A. (1993). The presentation of personalities in plastic surgery. *Annals of Plastic Surgery, 31*, 193–208.

Nejad, S. H., & Alpay, M. (2010). Pain patients. In T. A. Stern, G. L. Fricchione, N. H. Cassem, M. S. Jellinek, J. F. Rosenbaum (Eds.), *Massachusetts General Hospital handbook of general hospital psychiatry* (6th ed., pp. 211–236). Philadelphia, PA: Saunders/Elsevier.

Newell, R. (2000). Body image and disfigurement care. *Routledge essentials for nurses.* London: Routledge.

Parker, P. A., Youssef, A., Walker, S., et al. (2007). Short-term and long-term psychosocial adjustment and quality of life in women undergoing different surgical procedures for breast cancer. *Annals of Surgical Oncology, 14*, 3078–3089.

Parkes, C. M. (1973). Factors determining the persistence of phantom pain in the amputee. *Journal of Psychosomatic Research, 17,* 97–108.

Parkes, C. M. (1998). Bereavement. *Oxford Textbook of Palliative Care* (pp. 995–1010). New York: Oxford University Press.

Peterhansel, C., Petroff, D., Klinitzke, G., et al. (2013). Risk of completed suicide after bariatric surgery; a systematic review. *Obesity Review, 14,* 369–382.

Phillips, K. A., & Hollander, E. (2008). Treating body dysmorphic disorder with medication: evidence, misconceptions, and a suggested approach. *Body Image 5,* 13–27.

Rasmussen, L., Johnson, T., Kuipers, H. M., et al.; ISPOCD2 (International study of postoperative cognitive dysfunction) investigators. (2003). Does anaesthesia cause postoperative cognitive dysfunction? A randomised study of regional versus general anaesthesia in 438 elderly patients. *Acta Anaesthesiol Scand, 47,* 260–266.

Rasnake, L., & Lindscheid, T. (1989). Anxiety reduction in children receiving medical care: Developmental considerations. *Journal of Developmental & Behavioral Pediatrics, 10,* 169–175.

Powers, P. S., & Santana, C. A. (2010). Surgery. In J. L. Levinson (Ed.), *The American Psychiatric Publishing textbook of psychosomatic medicine: Psychiatric care of the medically ill* (2nd ed., pp. 691–723).

Riether, A. M., & Stoudemire, A. (1987). Surgery and trauma. In A Stoudemire &, B. S. Fogel (Eds.), *Principles of Medical psychiatry* (pp. 423–449). Orlando, FL: Grune & Stratton.

Rogan, M. T., Leon, K. M., Perez, D. L., & Kandel, E. R. (2006). Distinct neural signatures for safety and danger in the amygdale and striatum of the mouse. *Neuron, 46,* 309–320.

Rudolph, J. L., Jones, R. N., Rasmussen, L. S., Silverstein J. H., Inouye, S. K., & Marcantonio, E. R. (2007). *American Journal of Medicine, 120,* 807–813.

Saxe, G., Stoddard, F., Hall, E., et al. (2005). Pathways to PTSD I: Children with burns. *American Journal of Psychiatry, 162,* 1299–1304.

Samuelsson, P., Brudin, L., & Sandin, R. H. (2007). Late psychological symptoms after awareness among consecutively included surgical patients. *Anesthesiology, 106,* 26–32.

Sandin, R. H., Enlund, G., & Samuelsson, P. (2000). Awareness during anaesthesia: A prospective case study. *Lancet, 355,* 707–711.

Saunders, C. (1998). Foreword. In *Oxford textbook of palliative care* (p. viii). New York: Oxford University Press.

Schechter, N. L., Berde, C. B., & Yaster, M. (Eds.) (1993). *Pain in infants, children, and adolescents.* Baltimore, MD: Williams & Wilkins.

Schieveld, J. N. M., Leroy, P. L. J. M. L., van Os, J., Nicolai, J., Vos, G. D., & Leentjens, A. F. G. (2007). Pediatric delirium in critical illness: Phenomenology, clinical correlates and treatment response in 40 cases in the pediatric intensive care unit. *Intensive Care Medicine, 33,* 1033–1040.

Schilder, P. (1950). *The image and appearance of the human body.* New York: International Universities Press.

Sebels, P. S., Bowdie, T. A., & Ghoneim, M. M. (2004). The incidence of awareness during anaesthesia: A multi-center United States study. *Anesthesia and Analgesia, 99,* 833–839.

Sheridan, R. L., Schaefer, P. W., Whalen, M., Fagan, S., Stoddard, F. J., Jr., Schneider, J. C., McConkey, B., & Cancio, L. C. (2012). Case records of the Massachusetts General Hospital. Case 36-2012. Recovery of a 16-year-old girl from trauma and burns after a car accident. Case records of the Massachusetts General Hospital. Case 36-2012. *New England Journal Medicine, 367,* 2027–2037.

Sheridan, R. L., Lee, A. F., Kazis, L. E., et al. (2012). The effect of family characteristics on the recovery of burn injuries in children. *Journal of Trauma and Acute Care Surgery, 73,* S205–S212.

Shontz, F. C. (1974). Body image and its disorders. *International Journal of Psychiatric Medicine, 5,* 461–472.

Shukla, G. D., Sahn, S. C., Tripathi, R. P., & Gupta, D. K. (1982). Phantom limb: A phenomenological study. *British Journal of Psychiatry, 141,* 54–58.

Siemionow, M., & Gordon, C. R. (2010). Overview of guidelines for establishing a face transplant program: A work in progress. *American Journal of Transplantation, 10,* 1290–1296.

Silver, G., Kearney, J., Traube, C., Hertzig, M. (2014). Delirium screening anchored in child development: The Cornell Assessment for Pediatric Delirium. *Palliative and Supportive Care,* 1–7 doi:10.1017/S1478951514000947

Slikker, W. Jr., Zou, X., Hotchkiss, C. E., et al. (2007). Ketamine-induced neuronal cell death in the perinatal rhesus monkey. *Toxicological Sciences, 98,* 145–158.

Stein, D. J., Ipser, J. C., & Seedat, S. (2006). Pharmacotherapy for posttraumatic stress disorder (PTSD). *The Cochrane Database of Systematic Reviews,* Issue 1, Art. No.: CD 002795.pub2. doi:10.1002/14651858

Steinmetz, J., Siersma, V., Kessing, L.V., Rasmussen, L.S.; ISPOCD Group (2013). Is postoperative cognitive dysfunction a risk factor for dementia? A cohort follow-up study. *Br J Anaesth, 110*(Suppl 1), i92–i97.

Stevens, J. R., Fava, M., Rosenbaum, J. F., & Alpert, J. E. (2010). Psychopharmacology in the medical setting. In T. A. Stern, G. L. Fricchione, N. H. Cassem, M. S. Jellinek, J. F. Rosenbaum (Eds.), *Massachusetts General Hospital handbook of general hospital psychiatry* (6th ed., pp. 441–466). Philadelphia, PA: Saunders/Elsevier.

Stoddard, F. J. (2002). Care of infants, children and adolescents with burn injuries. In: M. Lewis (Ed.), *Child and adolescent psychiatry* (3rd ed., pp. 1188–1208). Baltimore, MD: Lippincott Williams & Wilkins.

Stoddard, F. J., Levine, J. B., & Lund, K. (2006). Burn injuries. In M. Blumenfield & J. Strain (Eds.), *Psychosomatic Medicine* (pp. 309–336). Baltimore, MD: Lippincott Williams and Wilkins.

Stoddard, F. J. (2010). Mental health care of burn survivors of disasters. Invited lecture, International Society of Burn Injuries, Annual Meeting, Istanbul, Turkey.

Stoddard, F. J., Katz, C. L., & Merlino, J. P. (Eds.) (2010). *Hidden impact: What you need to know for the next disaster: A practical guide for clinicians.* Sudbury/Boston, MA: Jones and Bartlett Publishers.

Stoddard, F. J., Pandya, A., & Katz, C. L. (Eds.). (2011). *Disaster psychiatry: Readiness, evaluation and treatment.* Washington, DC: American Psychiatric Press.

Stoddard, F. J., Ronfeldt, H., Kagan, J., et al. (2006). Young burned children: The course of acute stress and physiological and behavioral responses. *American Journal of Psychiatry, 163,* 1084–1090.

Stoddard, F. J., & Saxe, G. (2001). Ten-year research review of physical injuries. *Journal of the American Academy of Child & Adolescent Psychiatry, 40*(10), 1128–1145.

Stoddard, F. J., Sheridan, R. L., Martyn, J. A. J., Czarnik, J. E., & Deal, V. T. (2011). Pain management. Chapter 23 in E. C. Ritchie (Ed.), *Combat and operational behavioral health.* In M. K. Lenhart (Ed.), *The Textbooks of Military Medicine.* Washington, DC: Department of the Army, Office of the Surgeon General, Borden Institute; 339–358.

Stoddard, F. J., Simon, N. M., & Pitman, R. K. (2014). Trauma- and Stressor-Related Disorders. In R. E. Hales, S. Yudofsky, L. Roberts (Eds.), *American Psychiatric Publishing Textbook of Psychiatry: DSM-5 Edition, Sixth Edition* (pp. 455–498). American Psychiatric Press.

Stoddard, F. J., Usher, C. T., & Abrams, A. N. (2006). Psychopharmacology in pediatric critical care. [Review]. In: *Child and Adolescent Psychiatric Clinics of North America* (vol. 15, pp. 611–655). Philadelphia, PA: W.B. Saunders.

Sun, L. (2010). Early childhood general anaesthesia exposure and neurocognitive development. *British Journal Anaesthesia, 105*(suppl 1), i61–i68.

Terrell, F., Zatzick, D. F., Jurkovich, G. J., et al. (2008). Nationwide survey of alcohol screening and brief intervention practices at US Level I trauma centers. *Journal of the American College of Surgery,* Nov; *207*(5), 630–638. Epub, Jul 14, 2008.

Uman, L. S., Chambers, C. T., McGrath, P. J., & Kisely, S. (2006). Psychological interventions for needle-related procedural pain and distress in children and adolescents. *Cochrane Database Sytematic Reviews, 4,* CD005179.

Valdes, M., de Pablo, J., Campos, R., et al. (2000). Multinational European project and multicenter Spanish study of quality improvement of assistance in consultation-liaison psychiatry in general hospital: Clinical profile in Spain. *Medical Clinics (Barcelona), 25,* 690–694.

Veale, D. (2004a). Advances in a cognitive behavioural model of body dysmorphic disorder. *Body Image, 1,* 113–124.

Veale, D. (2004b). Body dysmorphic disorder. *Postgraduate Medicine Journal, 80,* 67–71.

Veale, D., Ellison, N., Werner, T. G., et al. (2012). Development of a Cosmetic Procedure Screening questinnaire (COPS) for body dysmorphic disorder. *Journal of Plastic, Reconstructive, and Aesthetic Surgery, 65,* 530–532.

Visintainer, M. A., & Wolfer, J. A. (1975). Psychological preparation for surgical pediatric patients: The effect on children's and parents' stress responses and adjustment. *Pediatrics, 56,* 187–202.

Vlajkovic, G. P., & Sindjelic, R. P. (2006). Emergence delirium in children: many questions, few answers. *Anesthesia & Analgesia, 104,* 84–91.

Wadey, V., & Frank, C. (1997). The effectiveness of patient verbalization on informed consent [see comments]. *Canadian Journal of Surgery, 40,* 124–128.

Wall, P. D., & Melzack, R. (Eds.) (1994). *Textbook of pain.* Edinburgh, UK: Churchill Livingstone.

Waisel, D. B., & Truog, R. D. (1995). The benefits of the explanation of the risks of anesthesia in the day surgery patient. *Journal of Clinical Anesthesiology, 7,* 200–204.

Warner, P., Stubbs, T. K., Kagan, R. J., Herndon, D. N., Palmieri, T. L., Kazis, L. E., Li, N.-C., Lee, A. F., Meyer, W. J., Tompkins, R. G. and the Multi-Center Benchmarking Study Working Group (2012). The effects of facial burns on health outcomes in children aged 5 to 18 years. *Journal of Trauma Acute Care Surg, 73*(3 Suppl 2): S189–196. doi:10.1097/TA.0b013e318265c7df

Weisman, A. (1979). *Coping with cancer.* New York: McGraw-Hill.

Weisman, A. (1998). The patient with acute grief. In T. Stern, J. Herman, & P. Slavin (Eds.), *The McGraw-Hill guide to psychiatry in primary care* (pp. 177–180). New York: McGraw-Hill.

Weisman, S. J. (Ed.) (1997). Pain management in children. *Child & adolescent psychiatric clinics of North America, 6*(4), 687–925. Philadelphia, PA: W.B. Saunders.

Weithorn, L. A. (1983). Children's capacity to decide about participation in research. *DRB: Review of Human Subjects Research, 5*(5), 1–5.

White, S. M., & Baldwin, T. J. (2003). Consent for anaesthesia. *Anaesthesia, 58,* 760–774.

Wilder, R. T., Flick, R. P., Sprung, J., et al. (2009). Early exposure to anesthesia and learning disabilities in a population-based birth cohort. *Anesthesiology, 110,* 796–804.

Wilens, T. E., & Spencer, T. J. (2010). Understanding attention-deficit/hyperactivity disorder from childhood to adulthood. *Postgraduate Medicine,* Sep; *122*(5), 97–109. Review.

Wilhelm, S., Phillips, K. A., Didie, D., Buhlmann, U., et al. (2014). Modular cognitive-behavioral therapy for body dysmorphic disorder: a randomized controlled trial. *Behavior Therapy, 45,* 314–327.

Williams-Russo, P., Sharrock, N. E., Mattis, S., Szatrowski, T. P., & Charlson, M. E. (1995). Cognitive effects after epidural vs. general anesthesia in older adults. *Journal of the American Medical Association, 275,* 44–50.

Winnicott, D. W. (1951). Transitional objects and transitional phenomena. In *Collected papers* (pp. 229–242). London: Tavistock Publications Ltd., 1958.

Winnicott, D. W. (1965). The theory of the infant–parent relationship. In *The maturational processes and the facilitating environment* (pp. 37–55). New York: International Universities Press.

Yip, P., Middleton, P., Cyna, A.M., Carlyle, A.V. Non-pharmacological interventions for assisting the induction of anaesthesia in children. *Cochrane Database Systematic Reviews, 3,* CD006447.

YP Face IT [Internet]. (2011). Bristol, University of the West of England.

Zatzick, D., Jurkovich, G., Russo, J., et al. (2004a). Posttraumatic distress, alcohol disorders, and recurrent trauma across Level 1 trauma centers. *Journal of Trauma,* Aug; *57*(2), 360–366.

Zatzick, D., Rivara, F., Jurkovich, G., et al. (2011). Enhancing the population impact of collaborative care interventions: Mixed method development and implementation of stepped care targeting posttraumatic stress disorder and related comorbidities after acute trauma. *General Hospital Psychiatry,* Mar–Apr; *33*(2), 123–134. Epub Feb 18.

Zatzick, D. F., Roy-Byrne, P., Russo, J., et al. (2004b). A randomized effectiveness trial of stepped collaborative care for acutely injured trauma survivors. *Archives of General Psychiatry, 61*(5), 498–506.

Zeanah, C. H. (Ed.) (2000). *Handbook of Infant Mental Health* (2nd ed.). New York: The Guilford Press.

70.

PSYCHIATRIC MANAGEMENT OF BEHAVIORAL SYNDROMES IN INTENSIVE CARE UNITS

Robert J. Boland, Michael G. Goldstein, Scott D. Haltzman, and Tracey M. Guthrie

INTRODUCTION

To outsiders, it seems strange that a psychiatrist would ever be called into the intensive care unit (ICU). In a world where the patients often seem almost like another machine, connected to the many other machines through webs of tubes and wires, what place is there for the psychiatrist's unique skills? However, in this life-and-death setting, each facet of the biopsychosocial model is stressed to its limit. No matter what perspective we examine—the direct effects of life-threatening diseases and procedures on the brain, the psychological adjustments to such illness, or the social effects it has on the patient's world—all are important and relevant in this setting, and the psychiatrist is best able to evaluate the interaction of all these variables.

Nearly all patients in the intensive care setting are experiencing the psychological and physical stresses of having a life-threatening serious illness. Such stress is then compounded by the environmental stresses of the intensive care setting. Weakness, fatigue, impairment of cognitive function, restrictions on mobility, and barriers to communication are ubiquitous in the ICU.

Beyond psychological stress, many psychiatric symptoms can be a result of the illnesses or the medications found in this setting. Although psychological complications are common in the ICU, practically speaking, only a small fraction of these patients will ever be seen by a psychiatrist, as the acuteness of the situation demands that the ICU staff focus on only the most critical aspects of a patient's illness or injury. In our experience, consultation to the ICU is most likely when psychiatric factors are inhibiting a patient's medical progress in some specific way. We have found the following to be the most common reasons for an ICU team to request psychiatric consultation:

1. Management of delirium and agitation

2. Treatment of anxiety, including cases in which the anxiety is inhibiting weaning from mechanical ventilation

3. Evaluation of depressive symptoms—usually when depression may be inhibiting medical recovery

4. Assessment of suicidal patients

5. Assistance with ethical dilemmas, particularly when a patient (or the family) chooses to end life-sustaining treatment

These issues are the focus of this chapter.

DELIRIUM

Reports of the rate of delirium vary greatly. Delirium is certainly more common than reported in the ICU setting. Most ICUs will tolerate a certain degree of confusion as part of the "normal" ICU experience, and are only likely to seek specific intervention when the patient's behavior becomes problematic. Actual rates of delirium in the ICU may be as high as 80% of the patient population (Bledowski & Trutia, 2012).

The use of the term "delirium" to describe all forms of confusion is somewhat specific to the specialty of psychiatry; other disciplines may use other words to describe variations of confusion, such as "acute confusional state," "metabolic encephalopathy," or some other variation. In either case, the term is a general one that characterizes a diffuse pathological state. Part of the difficulty in agreeing on the nature of this syndrome rests in the many possible presentations of delirium: the "clouding of consciousness" that psychiatrists consider the hallmark of delirium can range from an almost stuporous state to a highly agitated one. The symptoms can involve primarily perceptual disturbances, attentional deficits, confusion, or some combination of these.

The course of delirium is dependent on the etiology. As the underlying patholophysiology improves, so will the delirium. The presence of delirium, however, suggests significant pathology, and it is a predictor of morbidity and mortality.

ETIOLOGY OF DELIRIUM

By definition, delirium is the result of some alteration in normal brain function. Although the environment can play a role in adding to confusion, it is rarely, if ever, the sole cause of a delirium. Such terms as "ICU psychosis," which seem to imply that the very nature of the ICU can cause confusion, are misleading, and delay proper medical attention. As the primary treatment for delirium is to identify and then treat the underlying cause, understanding what the likely causes are is important.

Medications

Medications are the most common cause of delirium. The list of medications that may be associated with neuropsychological side effects is virtually endless. Although such lists can be helpful, their length and breadth raise several questions: Of these different medications, which are most likely to cause psychiatric side effects? Moreover, if there is an absolute medical necessity for a certain medication in spite of its confusional side effects, what can be done?

Several medications seem particularly likely to cause delirium. Special attention should be paid to anticholinergic medications; one must also be aware which medications have these properties. Antiarrhythmics, corticosteroids, antihistamines, narcotics, and sedatives (including the benzodiazepines) are other likely offending agents.

If a medication is required, several options should be considered. First, a switch to a medication that is less lipophilic (therefore less penetrating into the brain) can help. For example, among the beta-blocking agents, propranolol is particularly lipophilic, and another agent, which is more hydrophilic, such as atenolol, should be considered. If there is no reasonable alternative, a medication should be given at its minimal effective dose. This dose can be estimated through either clinical titration or serum drug levels. Drug levels are particularly important for measuring drugs that have a narrow therapeutic range, such as digitalis. In the face of medical illness, a previously appropriate dose may cause toxic drug levels. Even normal levels can cause delirium in an otherwise debilitated patient, and serum levels can be used to determine the minimum effective dose.

Medical Illnesses

Most illnesses severe enough to require an ICU admission are likely to have systemic manifestations; however, we may forget that the brain is one of these systems. Even seemingly minor illnesses, such as urinary tract infections, can have devastating neuropsychological effects on the fragile elderly patient. Of most concern are the effects of acute cardiac illnesses, which may include hypoxia, hypotension, congestive heart failure, and embolic stroke.

Although some studies have found little evidence of neurological sequelae after cardiac arrest with prompt resuscitation, careful assessments of cognitive and psychological status have shown that these patients may develop subtle signs of persistent cognitive impairment. In addition, some patients experience changes in mood and behavior, which may be overlooked on routine examination and can only be fully appreciated when the patient is more stable. Recognition and memory may be relatively spared, and cognitive impairment may occur more preferentially in subcortical areas (those affecting motivation and attention, for example). As such, these symptoms may be mistaken for depression or the effects of medication.

Surgical and Procedural Complications

Cardiac surgery is responsible for more neurological and neuropsychological complications than other common types of surgery; however, the rates of confusion after cardiac surgery vary widely across studies.

Several factors may predispose the surgical patient to delirium, particularly older age and preexisting cardiac impairment. It is not clear to what degree interoperative factors such as length of time under anesthesia contribute to delirium, but they probably play some role. However, in cases of postoperative delirium, one should always investigate for typical causes of delirium, including infections and medication effects.

Withdrawal Syndromes

Withdrawal from alcohol and sedatives or hypnotics may cause delirium as well. The presence of autonomic arousal (including tachycardia, hypertension, and pupillary dilatation), or seizures should alert the physician to this possibility. Withdrawal states are often overlooked, as complete alcohol and drug histories are frequently omitted or difficult or impossible to obtain. Even if they are obtained, patients may underestimate their dependence on medications that they are using therapeutically.

"Multifactorial" Causes

Often, no single factor can be identified, and a precise etiology might not be determined. In such cases, it is likely that several factors, although not singly causative, are contributing to the overall syndrome. In particular, the side effects of pharmacological agents may be additive or synergistic. Patients in the ICU are likely to have impairments of several organ systems. Hypoxia, hypercapnia, and hypotension, common in the critically ill, can also add to the clinical picture of delirium.

RISK FACTORS FOR DELIRIUM

Although not all are causative, several factors have been identified as being independent risk factors for delirium. A number of baseline factors may predispose to delirium, including dementia, advanced age, comorbidity, depression, hypertension, smoking, and alcoholism. Precipitating factors include hypoxia, metabolic disturbances, electrolyte imbalances, withdrawal symptoms, acute infections, seizures, dehydration, hyperthermia, head trauma, vascular disorders, immobilization, sleep deficiencies, psychiatric medications, and intracranial space–occupying lesions (Pun et al., 2007).

Some risk factors may predispose to certain types of delirium. For example, Jaber and colleagues identified seven independent risks factors for agitation in a medical-surgical ICU: sepsis, alcohol abuse, use of sedatives in the two days prior to ICU admission, body temperature more than 38°C, history of long-term psychoactive drug use, and hypo- or hypernatremia (Jaber et al., 2005). Of these various risk factors, the most important is probably dementia, and it is important to ascertain whether there is a history of preexisting cognitive impairment whenever possible (Lee et al., 2008).

ASSESSMENT OF DELIRIUM IN THE ICU SETTING

As with all assessments, a good assessment of delirium begins with a complete history and physical examination. The psychiatrist should personally review all data, and attempt to obtain a complete history. It may be necessary for the psychiatric consultant to recommend or initiate further assessment of physiological or metabolic status if the treating staff has not pursued all potential physiological derangements that may be contributing to delirium.

Screening for Delirium

Standard screening instruments that have been validated in ICU populations have been developed and should be used. Of these, one of the most commonly used is the Confusion Assessment Method for the ICU (CAM-ICU) (Ely et al., 2001), an instrument that was adapted from the Confusion Assessment Method (CAM) (Inouye et al., 1990) for nonverbal ICU patients. It is an eight-item checklist that can be completed in less than two minutes and requires minimal training. The instrument, along with training materials, is available to the public without cost at the website www.icudelirium.org. Another scale, the Delirium Observation Screening Scale (Scheffer et al., 2011), is designed to be administered by nursing staff, is brief and simple to use, and has been validated as a measure of delirium severity.

Other Tests

Neuroimaging has a low yield and is unlikely to help the clinician determine the etiology of most causes of delirium. However, it may be necessary for ruling out potential emergencies, such as intracranial bleeds. It is most likely to be helpful in the case of focal neurological signs that would suggest an anatomical abnormality, although some brain lesions can present without focal findings. That said, in the experience of the authors, brain imaging is probably overvalued for the workup of delirium: a normal magnetic resonance imaging scan (MRI) does not imply normal brain functioning, nor does an abnormal MRI necessarily correlate to the clinical presentation. There are some preliminary studies looking at the role of functional imaging; currently results are equivocal, but this remains a potential area for investigation (Hipp & Ely, 2012).

Another promising, albeit preliminary, area is the use of biomarkers to detect delirium. Numerous derangements in potential cerebrospinal fluid biomarkers have been implicated (Hipp & Ely, 2012; Hall et al., 2011). Currently results are inconsistent, but this remains an encouraging area of research.

Electrophysiological studies may be of particular use in perplexing cases, as the electroencephalogram (EEG) invariably shows diffuse slowing in delirium. It can be useful in differentiating "functional" psychiatric presentations (such as an acute psychotic episode associated with schizophrenia, or a catatonic depression) from delirium. An EEG is also obviously useful in more specific cases when seizure activity is suspected. Except in such cases, the EEG is generally non-specific; however, generalized slowing would imply a diffuse neurophysiological impairment and can focus the workup on potential causes of delirium.

In our experience, it appears that clinicians over-rely on neuroimaging in the workup of delirium and related syndromes, and underuse relatively simple neurophysiological tests such as the bedside EEG testing.

TREATMENT

The primary treatment for delirium is to treat the underlying cause. Although many agents have had anecdotal success as "mind-organizing" or "anti-delirium" agents, there is no consistent support for the actual existence of such an agent. Most of the symptomatic treatments are aimed not at the delirium itself, but at behaviors associated with the delirium, such as anxiety or agitation.

Sensory Stimulation and Sleep in Delirium

Both sensory deprivation and sensory overload may lead to the exacerbation of confusion in the ICU. Excessive noise levels, for example, may lead to sleep deprivation, irritability, and impaired cognitive performance.

Management of Behaviors Associated with Delirium

Nonpharmacological interventions that are particularly useful in the prevention and management of delirium in the intensive care setting are listed in Table 70.1. They are directed at enhancing patients' cognitive function, facilitating communication (among patients, families, and staff), preventing harm (to self or others), minimizing environmental stresses, maximizing comfort, and providing support and reassurance.

In cases of significant agitation or physically aggressive behavior, most patients will receive a medication to control these harmful symptoms. Currently there are no drugs that are federally approved for the treatment of delirium. However, a number of drugs have some evidence to support their use. Some typical medications used are discussed next.

Antipsychotics

With few exceptions, antipsychotics remain the drugs of choice for management of the agitated intensive care patient with delirium. A recent retrospective study of 71 medical centers found that antipsychotics were administered to 11% of ICU patients (Swan et al., 2012). This is for several reasons, including that they do not produce significant respiratory depression, and they are less likely to increase cognitive impairment. Although they have several potentially serious side effects, including cardiac arrhythmias and neuroleptic malignant syndrome, these are generally rare side effects.

Haloperidol probably remains the most commonly used neuroleptic for the treatment of delirium (Ely et al., 2004), given its fast onset of action, ease of administration, and predictable pharmacokinetics (Wang et al., 2012). It is recommended as first-line treatment by the Society of Critical

Table 70.1 NONPHARMACOLOGIC MANAGEMENT OF DELIRIUM IN THE INTENSIVE CARE SETTING

GOAL OF INTERVENTION	METHODS
Enhance cognitive function	Reorient frequently
	Clock, calendar, radio, television in room
	Provide explanations, education
Enhance communication between family and staff	Encourage writing if unable to speak; use letter board, communication devices, hand or blink signals if unable to speak or write
	Encourage family visitation
Present harm to patient or staff	Use soft mittens and restrain, using the least restraint necessary
Minimize Environmental Stresses	Provide sensory stimulation but limit noise from alarms and equipment
	Maintain semblance of day-night (diurnal) cycle (i.e., dim lights at night)
	Engage in nonessential care (baths, dressing changes) during the day
	Preoperative orientation and visit, when possible
Maximize patient comfort	Control pain adequately
	Mobilize (i.e., bed to chair)
	Permit rest, limit unnecessary awakenings
	Invite family to stay with the patient to reduce suspiciousness and paranoia
Provide support and reassurance	Empathy, opportunity to ventilate, support, reassurance

Care Medicine (Jacobi et al., 2002). One survey of health professionals found that 86% reported using haloperidol to treat delirium, compared to 40% who reported using atypical antipsychotics (Patel et al., 2009). A more recent retrospective cohort study of U.S. academic medical centers still found haloperidol to be, by far, the most commonly used antipsychotic for delirium (Swan et al., 2012). It is considered to be relatively safe, and its most common side effect of extrapyramidal symptoms are thought uncommon and are less of a concern in an ICU setting: the most common extrapyramidal symptoms are bradykinesia and a resting tremor; both of these are usually tolerable and transient for the usually short durations of treatment required in the ICU setting (obviously, one should be aware of more serious extrapyramidal side effects that could be disruptive, such as akathisia or acute dystonias, both of which would require treatment or a medication change). In addition, it can be given through parenteral routes: although not approved by the U.S. Food and Drug Administration (FDA) for intravenous use, such administration does appear to be safe and it is frequently administered this way in the ICU setting. It has been rarely studied systematically; one study compared the use of haloperidol to placebo for the prevention of postoperative delirium in 430 patients (Kalisvaart et al., 2005). This study found the incidence of delirium to be similar across groups, but the haloperidol group had a lesser severity and a shorter time to recovery than the placebo group; it should be noted that this was a prevention rather than a treatment study. More recently, a different team used haloperidol to prevent delirium in a 457 critically ill elderly patients who underwent noncardiac surgery: they found that the group treated with low-dose, prophylactic haloperidol had a much lower incidence of delirium (15%, versus 23% in the control group) (Wang et al., 2012).

Low-potency phenothiazines, such as chlorpromazine or thioridazine, are inferior to haloperidol in the intensive care setting for several reasons. They have anticholinergic effects (which can worsen confusion), quinidine-like effects (similar to that of tricyclic antidepressants), and alpha-adrenergic-receptor blocking effects (which can cause hypotension and exacerbate the effects of concurrently administered antihypertensive medications).

The atypical antipsychotics are becoming more popular in the ICU, mirroring the general preference for them over older antipsychotics. Anecdotal reports suggest that they can be as effective as haloperidol (Patel et al., 2009), but they have rarely been studied in this setting.

Han and Kim compared risperidone and haloperidol in the treatment of delirium, and found no difference in response between the two drugs (Han et al., 2004).

Two studies compared olanzapine with haloperidol: Skrobik and colleagues compared the use of haloperidol with olanzapine in about 70 delirious patients admitted to an ICU and randomized to one or the other drug. They found that clinical improvement was similar in both groups, but the haloperidol group had more (mainly extrapyramidal) side effects (Skrobik et al., 2004). Hu similarly compared olanzapine and haloperidol, but also added a placebo group (for a total of 175 patients) and found that both haloperidol and olanzapine were preferable to placebo and not significantly different from each other (Hu et al., 2004).

Similarly, quetiapine has been studied in 36 ICU patients who were randomized to a comparison of it with a placebo (Devlin et al., 2010). The quetiapine group had a similar length of stay as the placebo group; however, there were fewer periods of agitation. This study was complicated by the fact that both groups received as-needed haloperidol, but the quetiapine group required less.

Ziprasidone was also compared to haloperidol and placebo in the Modifying the Incidence of Delirium (MIND) Trial (Girard et al., 2010), which examined 100 mechanically ventilated ICU patients at six American tertiary care centers. The authors found that both antipsychotics did not improve the primary or secondary outcome measures; however, it was intended as a feasibility study, and a larger study is currently underway.

An open-label study of paliperidone gave preliminary evidence for the suggestion that it is safe and effective for treating delirium (Yoon et al., 2011).

A 2009 Cochrane Review concluded that haloperidol, olanzapine, and risperidone (the only three drugs for which it found sufficient data) were equally effective for the treatment of delirium, although it noted the paucity of literature on the subject (Lonergan et al., 2007). These data are even more lacking when one looks at older adults, presumably the most common group of patients likely to get delirium in the ICU setting. One meta-analysis subsequent to the Cochrane Review restricted its analyses to studies in which the mean subject age was 60 or older and concluded that the data were too limited to support the use of any antipsychotic for elderly patients (Flaherty et al., 2011).

When one makes a clinical decision to use antipsychotics for delirious patients in the ICU, there is little guidance as to dose, and treatment is usually empirical. Among the possible routes, intermittent intravenous (IV) administration is the approach of choice (Wang et al., 2012), given the rapid onset and avoidance of absorption and first-pass effects. Continuous infusion may be considered for patients not responding to intermittent boluses (Wang et al., 2012). Although many clinical settings in the past employed rapidly escalating doses (e.g., doubling the dose of haloperidol every half hour until the behavior was controlled), there is little evidence to support these potentially large doses, and following the general principle of careful titration to find the lowest effective dose is advised.

Although the antipsychotics are usually considered safe when treating intensive care patients, there are caveats. In 2005, the FDA issued an alert warning that atypical antipsychotics are associated with an increased mortality risk in elderly patients (FDA, 2008), and subsequent investigations have suggested that the mortality risk with typical antipsychotics is even higher (Wang et al., 2005). Although the exact mechanism of this mortality is not clear, cardiovascular risks are likely to account for a large part of this risk. These warnings were based on meta-analytic data that were not specific to ICU patients, but should be taken into account when considering the risks and benefits of using these drugs in the ICU, particularly in patients with cardiovascular disease.

Benzodiazepines

In some cases, antipsychotics may be ineffective or limited by side effects. Benzodiazepines may be administered parenterally as alternatives to antipsychotics for managing agitation associated with delirium in the ICU. Some experts and many clinicians actually prefer benzodiazepines to haloperidol because they do not exacerbate seizures or produce extrapyramidal side effects. However, this reasoning may be misguided, as it has long been noted by many psychopharmacologists that benzodiazepines can worsen confusion, and some investigators have found benzodiazepines to be an independent risk factor for delirium (Pandharipande et al., 2006). In situations where they are deemed necessary, lorazepam is the benzodiazepine of choice. It may be useful, not only singly, but in combination with haloperidol, and it may help lessen the amount of haloperidol needed for management of agitation. Advantages include a relatively short half-life, an absence of active metabolites, and elimination mechanisms (conjugation and renal excretion) that are not significantly affected by age or liver disease. Lorazepam is also available in parenteral form and is one of the few benzodiazepines (along with midazolam) with reliable intramuscular absorption.

Midazolam is a parenteral benzodiazepine promoted for intravenous sedation during short diagnostic or endoscopic procedures and as an adjunct to anesthesia regimens. Because of its rapidity of action, high lipophilic nature, short half-life (elimination half-life of 1–4 hours in healthy individuals), and decreased local irritation, it has several advantages for the treatment of delirium in the ICU. However, midazolam's metabolism is affected by acute liver dysfunction and systemic illness, and the potential for iatrogenic overdose is greater for midazolam than for lorazepam. This is the primary reason that we prefer lorazepam to midazolam for management of delirium and agitation in the ICU, especially in patients who are not intubated.

Benzodiazepines are the agents of choice for treating alcohol or benzodiazepine withdrawal and should be considered in the setting of agitation that is associated (or coincident) with status epilepticus, neuroleptic malignant syndrome, and severe Parkinson's disease, primarily for their safety in not exacerbating those syndromes and their relative compatibility with other medications that may be used to treat these disorders.

When dosing patients with these and other sedatives, some experts recommend the use of "daily awakening trials" in which all sedating medications are discontinued, the patient is assessed, and when a target level of arousal is reached, the sedation is restarted at 50% of the previously used dose and titrated to effect. The purpose of this is to ensure the lowest possible dose of sedation. This use of interrupted sedation is associated with better psychological functioning and shorter ICU stays (Banh, 2012).

Other Sedatives

Dexmedetomidine, a selective alpha-2 agonist, has recently received a good deal of attention as an alternative agent for treating agitation in the ICU. It has both sedative and analgesic effects, but is thought to be less likely to cause confusion than standard sedatives. When used as a sedative, it is less associated with delirium than either midazolam (Riker et al., 2009; Maldonado et al., 2009) or lorazepam (Pandharipande et al., 2007). For example, the Maximizing Efficacy of Targeted Sedation and Reducing Neurological Dysfunctions (MENDS) Trial (Pandharipande et al., 2007) compared the use of dexmedetomidine with lorazepam in 106 mechanically ventilated patients and found that patients treated with dexmedetomidine experienced more days alive without delirium or coma, and a lower prevalence of coma. The Safety and Efficacy of Dexmedetomidine Compared with Midazolam (SEDCOM) trial (Riker et al., 2009) compared dexmedetomidine to midazolam in 375 mechanically ventilated patients and found a lower incidence of delirium while achieving similar sedation. Dexmedetomidine has also compared favorably to morphine (Shehabi et al., 2009) and propofol (Mirski et al., 2010). Perhaps most significantly, dexmedetomidine was found preferable to haloperidol in one study, in that mechanically ventilated patients treated with dexmedetomidine had a shorter time to extubation and needed less adjunctive propofol during their ICU stay (Reade et al., 2009). In considering the weight of the data, and the difference in side effect profiles, dexmedetomidine may be an acceptable and potentially preferable sedative for use in the ICU, given the lesser risk for delirium and respiratory depression (Hipp & Ely, 2012). When using it, patients should be monitored for bradycardia and hypotension.

Benzodiazepine Antagonists

Flumazenil is a competitive antagonist that binds directly to the benzodiazepine receptor. It reverses the effects of benzodiazepines, such as respiratory depression, and is useful in cases of benzodiazepine toxicity. It has a short half-life (30–90 minutes), and repeat dosing of the drug may be required—even then, reversal of respiratory depression is not always complete. Side effects include nausea, vomiting, and agitation. In benzodiazepine-dependent patients, flumazenil may induce withdrawal and seizures, and it should be avoided in all but life-threatening cases.

Opioids

In situations where pain complicates the clinical presentation, further control may be obtained by using intravenous opioids. It is especially difficult in the ICU to distinguish between agitation associated with pain and agitation due to delirium. Although narcotic analgesics may contribute to the development or persistence of delirium, analgesia should not be withheld when pain is known to be present or likely. It is best to continue to treat such patients with a moderate dose of an opioid on a regular fixed schedule. Certain opioids, particularly meperidine, are considered cerebrotoxic and should be avoided altogether.

Cholinesterase Inhibitors

Delirium or coma associated with anticholinergic toxicity may be reversed with physostigmine, a cholinesterase inhibitor. However, because its effects are short-lived and its use is associated with toxicity (i.e., bradycardia, hypotension, seizures, vomiting, and asystole), we do not recommend its use except in emergency situations. There are limited data to support the use of longer acting cholinesterase inhibitors, such as those used for Alzheimer's disease (donepezil, galantamine, and rivastigmine) for delirium; however, these are primarily limited to case studies. The largest prospective study to date examined the use of rivastigmine as an adjunct to haloperidol (van Eijk et al., 2010). This study did not support the use of cholinesterase inhibitors and, in fact, had to be prematurely terminated when it became apparent that patients in the rivastigmine group had increased mortality as well as longer duration of delirium.

Anesthetic Agents

When patients have not responded to other approaches and their agitation is significantly interfering with critical treatments, it may become necessary to resort to the use of anesthetic or paralytic agents. These agents should be considered only when other methods have failed. The role of the psychiatrist in such cases will most likely be strategic—in helping to determine when other methods are unlikely to be beneficial and when anesthesia should be considered; the specifics of treatment should be established in collaboration with an anesthesiologist.

ANXIETY

Anxiety is ubiquitous in the ICU. Most cases of anxiety arising in the ICU will be secondary to some aspect of the patient's medical illness, medications, or the ICU setting itself.

Many biological factors can influence the experience of anxiety in the ICU. Medical conditions can cause anxiety, including an evolving myocardial infarction (MI), hypoglycemia, and hypoxia. Patients who are treated with sympathomimetic drugs such as theophylline for concomitant pulmonary disease, or with isoproterenol for cardiac rhythm disturbances, may develop anxiety as an adverse reaction to these drugs. Anxiety might be particularly common in patients on mechanical ventilation who are having difficulty weaning from the ventilation.

Anxiety may also be a manifestation of alcohol, sedative, opiate, nicotine, or antidepressant withdrawal, and the issues accompanying the recognition of withdrawal syndromes in this group are similar to those discussed for delirium in this chapter. Because nicotine dependence is more prevalent than other psychoactive substance use disorders, especially among a population of patients with cardiovascular disease, nicotine withdrawal is probably the most common withdrawal syndrome encountered in the ICU.

Many factors contribute to the experience of anxiety. Fears of death or disability, misconceptions about the meaning of an illness and prognosis, misinterpretation of the displays and alarms from the monitors in the room, and restriction of usual activities, all may contribute (Cassem et al., 1971). Patients are also concerned about the life problems they were confronting before admission and the effects that the illness and hospitalization will have on their ability to handle these problems.

Anxiety usually diminishes as patients feel more secure with the knowledge that they are being closely monitored. After an MI, for example, simply having survived the first hours usually reduces panic. Some degree of denial, which can be hazardous during the pre-hospital phase of unstable angina or MI, may protect the patient during the ICU phase, as it may serve to reduce anxiety and associated cardiovascular stimulation. However, transfer from the unit to a general medical or intermediate care floor may be accompanied by a marked increase in anxiety.

Idiopathic, or "primary," anxiety may also exist in the ICU, and many of the symptoms of panic disorder and other anxiety syndromes overlap with other common syndromes such as cardiac disease. Many cases of preexisting anxiety disorders can be discerned with a complete history.

Post-traumatic stress disorder (PTSD) is particularly prevalent during or after an ICU experience; one review estimated that 22% of patients admitted to an ICU went on to have symptoms suggestive of PTSD. Factors predisposing to this included prior psychopathology, greater benzodiazepine administration, and post-ICU memories of frightening or psychotic experiences (Davydow et al., 2008). Some case-comparison studies suggest that manipulation of the hypothalamic-pituitary-adrenal (HPA) axis at the time of trauma, such as through the use of hydrocortisone or beta-blockers, may decrease the incidence of PTSD in this setting (Girard et al., 2007).

MANAGEMENT OF ANXIETY

Nonpharmacological approaches to treating anxiety include providing accurate medical information, having supportive family members nearby, explaining the roles and meaning of the monitoring equipment, providing emotional support and reassurance, and reinforcing the *appropriate* use of denial. The latter can seem counterintuitive to other staff members, and occasionally a psychiatrist may be called to help a patient who is "not coming to terms" with their disease. In such cases, the psychiatrist should assess the patient and judge whether the use of denial represents an effective coping mechanism for the patient. In most such cases, the patient is using "suppression" in that the patient is aware of the life-threatening issues at stake, but choosing to "put them aside for the moment." In such cases an appropriate intervention may be to simply reassure the patient and the staff that such a strategy is acceptable and not in itself "pathological."

Teaching patients relaxation techniques may also be an effective strategy to reduce anxiety and enhance self-control and self-efficacy. In cases in which patients are awake, alert, and cognitively intact, they can find such techniques both useful and distracting. Brief psychotherapies, including such modalities as psychoeducation, crisis intervention, short-term therapy, supportive therapy, cognitive behavioral therapy, and hypnosis, have all been found to be helpful, although our experience is that they are mainly useful when they are focused on a specific problem or stress. Family interventions may be helpful as well, particularly if family members appear to be "transmitting" their own anxiety to the patient.

Pharmacological Approaches

Benzodiazepines have long been thought to be effective in reducing or eliminating autonomic reactivity associated with stress. Although benzodiazepines are commonly used, the concerns already expressed in the prior section should be noted, and the previously stated preference for lorazepam as the benzodiazepine of choice would apply here as well. Although specific dosing recommendations would depend on the specific clinical situation, the general recommendation would again be to use the lowest effective dose. In cases of withdrawal syndromes, appropriate treatment of the specific type of withdrawal would be indicated.

DEPRESSION

Depressive symptoms in the intensive care setting may result from a variety of possible causes. An acute illness may directly cause depressive symptoms or produce symptoms that mimic some aspects of depression. Additionally, the patient may experience an emotional reaction to an acute illness. Medications may cause depressive symptoms. A patient may have an independent major depressive disorder.

Therefore, diagnosing depression in the ICU setting is very difficult. When evaluating for depression, the usual admonition to exclude symptoms that are due to other causes can be difficult to follow. We believe it is best to take an inclusive approach, as the risk of missing a potential depression in the ICU setting seems to outweigh any danger of overdiagnosing the disorder.

Post-ICU depression may be a common phenomenon as well, with one review estimating that about 28% of ICU survivors report clinically significant depressive symptoms. Some of the usual depression risk factors (gender, age) do not seem to be relevant in this population, and the strongest risk factors appear to be early onset post-ICU depressive symptoms (Davydow et al., 2009).

TREATMENT OF DEPRESSION

For most patients, dysphoria in the setting of an illness is time-limited and does not require aggressive pharmacological intervention. Patients with prolonged stays in the ICU may develop an adjustment disorder with a depressed mood. This disorder usually responds to psychotherapy or to the initiation of formal rehabilitation efforts. Some patients, however, develop a major depressive episode.

If feasible, medications that may contribute to a depression should be discontinued or changed. Lists of such medications are common, although sometimes overinclusive. For example, beta-blockers are a frequently cited cause of depression; however, multiple studies and meta-analyses suggest that beta-blockers do not significantly increase the risk for depression and only slightly increase the risk for fatigue and sexual dysfunction (Ko et al., 2002).

When an antidepressant is indicated, the selective serotonin-reuptake inhibitors (SSRIs) are probably the treatment of choice, as they are largely safe to use in this population.

However, they can have significant drug–drug interactions, which is important as most ICU patients are on multiple agents. SSRIs are potent inhibitors of oxidative metabolism. A wide variety of other agents, therefore, can be potentiated by these antidepressants by having their serum levels elevated. This is of most concern with other agents that have low therapeutic indices, such as warfarin, phenytoin, or digoxin. Should an antidepressant be indicated in patients on such agents, SSRIs are not contraindicated; however, the blood levels of medical drugs with low therapeutic indices should be monitored closely after introduction of the SSRI. Some SSRIs, such as sertraline and citalopram, have a lower likelihood of causing drug-drug interactions. Furthermore, the SSRIs and most of the newer agents (except venlafaxine and its metabolite, desvenlafaxine) are highly protein-bound, and may potentiate other medications through this mechanism as well. As patients in the ICU are frequently on multiple medications, it can be difficult to be sure which drug is interacting with which, but a reasonably high index of suspicion and monitoring should be used when SSRIs are initiated in the ICU.

Agents such as venlafaxine may cause an increase in mean blood pressure at higher dosages and should be monitored for such effects in cardiac patients. Alternately, venlafaxine has minimal protein binding and few effects on CyP450-2D6 and CyP450-3A4 isoenzymes. Bupropion has dopaminergic properties; the effect of this on patients who are receiving other dopaminergic agents is not known. Bupropion can also lower the seizure threshold, and is not recommended in patients considered at risk for seizures.

Psychostimulants may be useful agents for the treatment of depression in the medically ill. We do not recommend the use of psychostimulants for the routine treatment of major depressive episodes in the ICU. They may be considered in cases in which a rapid effect is critical or standard antidepressants are not adequate. When they are used, the treatment team should watch for adverse effects on heart rate and blood pressure; fortunately, these are uncommon.

Suicidality in the ICU

Most ICU admissions for suicidality are the result of self-poisoning. Many self-poisonings are done with psychotropic medication. Fortunately, most ICU staffs are well trained in the acute treatment of these potentially lethal overdoses, and consultation is more likely to be for evaluation of the patient's continued potential for suicide.

Although, by definition, any overdose sufficient to justify an ICU admission is serious, it does not imply that the suicidal intent is as serious. Many patients are unaware of the potential toxicity of their medication. Sometimes the overdose may be entirely accidental, a sudden impulse without suicidal intent, or part of a "gesture" that went awry. Patients may express surprise at the seriousness of their act and may be relieved that they were not successful. In short, the possibilities are similar to the evaluation of suicide in any situation, and the seriousness of the act does not change the need for an open-minded evaluation.

The management of the suicidal behavior is usually straightforward in the ICU. Most patients are being monitored very closely as a matter of routine. Most of the decisions regarding the appropriate level of observation become applicable only when the patient is discharged from the ICU, as patients are generally sufficiently observed as part of the normal ICU routine. In cases in which a patient is acutely and determinedly suicidal, additional supervision including one-on-one observation may become necessary; fortunately, this is rarely the case.

The psychiatrist should be aware of subtle (and not so subtle) hostile staff reactions to the suicidal patient. In this setting, where staff must work hard to treat critically ill patients, some may find it difficult to empathize with patients who "did this to themselves." Expressing anger to a patient for that patient's medical condition is, obviously, unprofessional. However, staff hostility is often unconscious and thus may be insidious, interfering with patient care. The psychiatrist may be in a unique position to help staff members give voice to ambivalent feelings, and to reassure them that such feelings are normal. Open (but private) acknowledgement of angry and negative feelings can help reduce "acting out" that could result from repressing these feelings.

ETHICAL DILEMMAS

No ethical issues are more important than those that surround life-and-death decisions. The ICU is a natural focal point for such issues. The ICU team must negotiate a compromise between reacting to an urgent situation and understanding the larger issues involved. Such a compromise involves balancing many factors and principles. Patient autonomy must be weighed against best-interest issues. Similarly, one must balance the hope engendered by medical uncertainty against the possibility that aggressive treatment will be useless and only cause more pain and suffering to a patient and family. Inevitably, economic issues and the enormous expense of possibly futile care are considerations as well.

In the case of patient (or family) decisions to end treatment, the psychiatrist may be consulted as the "ethical expert" to help negotiate such issues. This can be a thorny problem: although most agree that all competent patients have the right to decide their own treatment—including when to end it—in practice, this decision is strongly influenced by the opinions of others, including physicians, staff, and family members. Although the principles involved may seem straightforward, the dynamics of the situation are rarely so. Psychiatrists must intrude carefully on this potential hornet's nest. However, at the same time, psychiatrists must acknowledge that they are the perceived experts in this area, and should not avoid playing a critical role in coordinating the decision-making process. This requires a solid understanding of the relevant medical, ethical, and legal issues associated with end-of-life decisions.

STAFF ISSUES

Staff working in intensive care settings are exposed to multiple stresses. Such stresses include the high volume and rapid pace of the work, the high level of clinical responsibility, the severity and high mortality of patients' illnesses, understaffing, and such environmental stresses as noise and overcrowding. Interpersonal conflicts: with administration, within hierarchies (e.g., nurse–doctor conflicts) and among peers can also add to stress. Nursing staff members have few opportunities to rest or escape from the ICU for relief. In modern ICUs, nurses are called on to attend to multiple and diverse tasks simultaneously. They must become familiar with an ever-expanding array of technical equipment developed for the treatment of critically ill patients. Strong feelings about patients and grief over their deaths provide constant sources of stress. Dealing with prolonged care of poor-prognosis patients and having to help families cope with their grief are particularly stressful.

Support groups can be helpful, and certain features seem to distinguish successful ICU support groups. They should be initiated in response to a felt need, should be highly structured, and should discourage premature discharge of intense negative feelings. Furthermore, support groups should center on interpersonal rather than environmental or administrative problems. Open-ended, unstructured "gripe groups" are generally not helpful and may be detrimental.

The psychiatric consultant can play a valuable role by providing house staff and attending physicians with emotional support while performing consultations on patients in the intensive care setting. The level of support will probably vary at different times. In times of high distress or after a particular crisis, the psychiatrist may be asked to provide intensive, structured support. At other times, the support may be more informal and simply a matter of "checking in" with staff while performing patient consultations. In either case, it is helpful to use a multidisciplinary psychiatry team—as the ICU team is also multidisciplinary. A psychiatric nurse is particularly valuable, as nurses in the ICU may be more likely to trust and accept another nurse when discussing difficult issues of stress and their own feelings and reactions.

Numerous innovative strategies have been used to help deal with stress in the ICU. For example, the Medical ICU at the Massachusetts General Hospital conducts "autognosis" (self-awareness) rounds on a weekly basis (Stern et al., 1993), and journal entries based on these rounds are used to prepare incoming housestaff for the particular challenges of the ICU (Sekeres et al., 2002).

CLINICAL PEARLS

- Benzodiazepines are an independent risk factor for delirium (Pandharipande et al., 2006).

- Where benzodiazepines are deemed necessary, lorazepam is the benzodiazepine of choice.

- Nonpharmacological approaches to reduce anxiety include providing accurate medical information, having supportive family members nearby, explaining the roles and meaning of the monitoring equipment, providing emotional support and reassurance, and reinforcing the appropriate use of denial.

- Brief psychotherapies, including such modalities as psychoeducation, crisis intervention, short-term therapy, supportive therapy, cognitive behavioral therapy, relaxation therapies, and hypnosis, can all be helpful, although our experience is that they are mainly useful when they are focused on a specific problem or stress.

- Family interventions may be helpful as well, particularly if family members appear to be "transmitting" their own anxiety to the patient.

- The psychiatrist should be aware of subtle (and not so subtle) hostile staff reactions to the suicidal patient. In this setting, where staff must work hard to treat critically ill patients, some may find it difficult to empathize with patients who "did this to themselves."

DISCLOSURE STATEMENTS

Dr. Boland has no conflicts to disclose.

Dr. Goldstein has no conflicts to disclose. He is an employee of the U.S. Veterans Health Administration. His contributions to this publication are his own and do not represent the views, positions, or policies of the Veterans Health Administration.

Dr. Haltzman has no conflicts to disclose.

Dr. Guthrie has no conflicts to disclose.

REFERENCES

Banh, H. L. (2012). Management of delirium in adult critically ill patients: An overview. *Journal of Pharmaceutical Sciences, 15*(4), 499–509.

Bledowski, J., & Trutia, A. (2012). A review of pharmacologic management and prevention strategies for delirium in the intensive care unit. *Psychosomatics, 53*(3), 203–211.

Cassem, N. H., & Hackett, T. P. (1971). Psychiatric consultation in a cardiac care unit. *Annals of Internal Medicine, 75*, 9–14.

Davydow, D. S., Gifford, J. M., Desai, S. V., Bienvenu, O. J., & Needham, D. M. (2009). Depression in general intensive care unit survivors: A systematic review. *Intensive Care Medicine, 35*(5), 796–809.

Davydow, D. S., Gifford, J. M., Desai, S. V., Needham, D. M., & Bienvenu, O. J. (2008). Posttraumatic stress disorder in general intensive care unit survivors: A systematic review. *General Hospital Psychiatry, 30*(5), 421–434.

Devlin, J. W., Roberts, R. J., Fong, J. J., Skrobik, Y., Riker, R. R., Hill, N. S., et al. (2010). Efficacy and safety of quetiapine in critically ill patients with delirium: A prospective, multicenter, randomized, double-blind, placebo-controlled pilot study. *Critical Care Medicine, 38*(2), 419–427.

Ely, E. W., Margolin, R., Francis, J., May, L., Truman, B., Dittus, R., et al. (2001). Evaluation of delirium in critically ill patients: validation of the Confusion Assessment Method for the Intensive Care Unit (CAM-ICU). *Critical Care Medicine, 29*(7), 1370–1379.

Ely, E. W., Stephens, R. K., Jackson, J. C., Thomason, J. W., Truman, B., Gordon, S., et al. (2004). Current opinions regarding the importance, diagnosis, and management of delirium in the intensive care unit: a survey of 912 healthcare professionals. *Critical Care Medicine, 32*(1), 106–112.

FDA. (2008). Antipsychotics, conventional and atypical. From the FDA website, last accessed 7/29/14 http://www.fda.gov/Safety/MedWatch/

SafetyInformation/SafetyAlertsforHumanMedicalProducts/ucm110212.htm.

Flaherty, J. H., Gonzales, J. P., & Dong, B. (2011). Antipsychotics in the treatment of delirium in older hospitalized adults: a systematic review. *Journal of the American Geriatric Society, 59*(Suppl 2), S269–S276.

Girard, T. D., Shintani A. K., Jackson J. C., Gordon S. M., Pun B. T., Henderson M. S., et al. (2007). Risk factors for post-traumatic stress disorder symptoms following critical illness requiring mechanical ventilation: a prospective cohort study. *Critical Care, 11*(1), R28.

Girard, T. D., Pandharipande, P. P., Carson, S. S., Schmidt, G. A., Wright, P. E., Canonico, A. E., et al. (2010). Feasibility, efficacy, and safety of antipsychotics for intensive care unit delirium: the MIND randomized, placebo-controlled trial. *Critical Care Medicine, 38*(2), 428–437.

Hall, R. J., Shenkin, S. D., & Maclullich, A. M. (2011). A systematic literature review of cerebrospinal fluid biomarkers in delirium. *Dementia & Geriatric Cognitive Disorders, 32*, 79–93.

Hipp D. M., & Ely E. W. (2012). Pharmacological and nonpharmacological management of delirium in critically ill patients. *Neurotherapeutics*, Jan; *9*(1), 158–175.

Han, C. S., & Kim, Y. K. (2004). A double-blind trial of risperidone and haloperidol for the treatment of delirium. *Psychosomatics, 45*(4), 297–301.

Hu, H., Deng, W., & Yang, H. (2004). A prospective random control study comparison of olanzapine and haloperidol in senile delirium. *Chongging Medical Journal, 8*, 1234–1237.

Inouye, S. K., van Dyck, C. H., Alessi, C. A., Balkin, S., Siegal, A. P., & Horwitz, R. I. (1990). Clarifying confusion: the confusion assessment method. A new method for detection of delirium. *Annals of Internal Medicine, 113*(12), 941–948.

Jaber, S., Chanques, G., Altairac, C., Sebbane, M., Vergne, C., Perrigault, P. F., et al. (2005). A prospective study of agitation in a medical-surgical ICU: incidence, risk factors, and outcomes. *Chest, 128*(4), 2749–2757.

Jacobi, J., Fraser, G. L., Coursin, D. B., Riker, R. R., Fontaine, D., Wittbrodt, E. T., et al. (2002). Clinical practice guidelines for the sustained use of sedatives and analgesics in the critically ill adult. *Critical Care Medicine, 30*(1), 119–141.

Kalisvaart, K. J., de Jonghe, J. F., Bogaards, M. J., Vreeswijk, R., Egberts, T. C., Burger, B. J., et al. (2005). Haloperidol prophylaxis for elderly hip-surgery patients at risk for delirium: a randomized placebo-controlled study. *Journal of the American Geriatric Society, 53*(10), 1658–1666.

Ko, D. T., Hebert, P. R., Coffey, C. S., Sedrakyan, A., Curtis, J. P., & Krumholz, H. M. (2002). Beta-blocker therapy and symptoms of depression, fatigue, and sexual dysfunction. *Journal of the American Medical Association, 288*(3), 351–357.

Lee, H. B., DeLoatch, C. J., Cho, S., Rosenberg, P., Mears, S. C., & Sieber, F. E. (2008). Detection and management of pre-existing cognitive impairment and associated behavioral symptoms in the Intensive Care Unit. *Critical Care Clinics, 24*(4), 723–736, viii.

Lonergan, E., Britton, A. M., Luxenberg, J., & Wyller, T. (2007). Antipsychotics for delirium. *Cochrane Database of Systematic Reviews*, (2), CD005594.

Maldonado, J. R., Wysong, A., van der Starre, P. J., Block, T., Miller, C., & Reitz, B. A. (2009). Dexmedetomidine and the reduction of postoperative delirium after cardiac surgery. *Psychosomatics, 50*(3), 206–217.

Mirski, M. A., Lewin, J. J. 3rd, Ledroux, S., Thompson, C., Murakami, P., Zink, E. K., et al. (2010). Cognitive improvement during continuous sedation in critically ill, awake and responsive patients: the Acute Neurological ICU Sedation Trial (ANIST). *Intensive Care Medicine, 36*(9), 1505–1513.

Pandharipande, P., Shintani, A., Peterson, J., Pun, B. T., Wilkinson, G. R., Dittus, R. S., et al. (2006). Lorazepam is an independent risk factor for transitioning to delirium in intensive care unit patients. *Anesthesiology, 104*(1), 21–26.

Pandharipande, P. P., Pun, B. T., Herr, D. L., Maze, M., Girard, T. D., Miller, R. R., et al. (2007). Effect of sedation with dexmedetomidine vs. lorazepam on acute brain dysfunction in mechanically ventilated patients: The MENDS randomized controlled trial. *Journal of the American Medical Association, 298*(22), 2644–2653.

Patel, R. P., Gambrell, M., Speroff, T., Scott, T. A., Pun, B. T., Okahashi, J., et al. (2009). Delirium and sedation in the intensive care unit: Survey of behaviors and attitudes of 1384 healthcare professionals. *Critical Care Medicine, 37*(3), 825–832.

Pun, B. T., & Ely, E. W. (2007). The importance of diagnosing and managing ICU delirium. *Chest, 132*(2), 624–636.

Reade, M. C., O'Sullivan, K., Bates, S., Goldsmith, D., Ainslie, W. R., & Bellomo, R. (2009). Dexmedetomidine vs. haloperidol in delirious, agitated, intubated patients: A randomised open-label trial. *Critical Care, 13*(3), R75.

Riker, R. R., Shehabi, Y., Bokesch, P. M., Ceraso, D., Wisemandle, W., Koura, F., et al. (2009). Dexmedetomidine vs. midazolam for sedation of critically ill patients: A randomized trial. *Journal of the American Medical Association, 301*(5), 489–499.

Scheffer, A. C, van Munster, B. C, Schuurmans, M. J., de Rooij, S. E. (2011). Assessing severity of delirium by the Delirium Observation Screening Scale. *International Journal of Geriatric Psychiatry, 26*(3), 284–291.

Sekeres, M. A., & Stern, T. A. (2002). On the Edge of Life, II: House officer struggles recorded in an intensive care unit journal. *Primary Care Companion Journal of Clinical Psychiatry, 4*(5), 184–190.

Shehabi, Y., Grant, P., Wolfenden, H., Hammond, N., Bass, F., Campbell, M., et al. (2009). Prevalence of delirium with dexmedetomidine compared with morphine based therapy after cardiac surgery: a randomized controlled trial (DEXmedetomidine COmpared to Morphine–DEXCOM Study). *Anesthesiology, 111*(5), 1075–1084.

Skrobik, Y. K., Bergeron, N., Dumont, M., & Gottfried, S. B. (2004). Olanzapine vs. haloperidol: Treating delirium in a critical care setting. *Intensive Care Medicine, 30*(3), 444–449.

Stern, T. A., Prager, L. M., & Cremens, M. C. (1993). Autognosis rounds for medical house staff. *Psychosomatics, 34*(1), 1–7.

Swan, J. T., Fitousis, K., Hall, J. B., Todd, S. R., & Turner, K. L. (2012). Antipsychotic use and diagnosis of delirium in the intensive care unit. *Critical Care, 16*(3), R84.

van Eijk, M. M., Roes, K. C., Honing, M. L., Kuiper, M. A., Karakus, A., van der Jagt, M., et al. (2010). Effect of rivastigmine as an adjunct to usual care with haloperidol on duration of delirium and mortality in critically ill patients: a multicentre, double-blind, placebo-controlled randomised trial. *Lancet, 376*(9755), 1829–1837.

Wang, W., Li, H. L., Wang, D. X., Zhu, X., Li, S. L., Yao, G.Q., et al. (2012). Haloperidol prophylaxis decreases delirium incidence in elderly patients after noncardiac surgery: a randomized controlled trial. *Critical Care Medicine, 40*(3), 731–739.

Wang, E. H., Mabasa, V. H., Loh, G. W., & Ensom, M. H. (2012). Haloperidol dosing strategies in the treatment of delirium in the critically ill. *Neurocritical Care, 16*(1), 170–183.

Wang, P. S., Schneeweiss, S., Avorn, J., Fischer, M. A., Mogun, H., Solomon, D. H., et al. (2005). Risk of death in elderly users of conventional vs. atypical antipsychotic medications. *New England Journal of Medicine, 353*(22), 2335–2341.

Yoon, H.-K., Kim, Y.-K., Han, C., Ko, Y.-H., Lee, H.-J., Kwon, D.-Y., et al. (2011). Paliperidone in the treatment of delirium: results of a prospective open-label pilot trial. *Acta Neuropsychiatrica, 23*, 179–183.

71.

OPHTHALMOLOGY

Mary Lou Jackson and Jennifer Wallis

INTRODUCTION

Vision is a crucial sense that allows us to gain information about our environment; and vision loss, from moderate to severe degrees, impacts the ability to read, gain employment, remain independent, and ambulate safely (Owsley, McGwin, et al., 2009). The adjustment to vision loss often goes beyond such functional impacts to affect the person's emotional well-being. A significant number of individuals who lose vision experience depression, anxiety, and poor quality of life (Horowitz, Reinhardt, et al., 2005; Hassell, Lamoureux, et al., 2006). Vision loss also affects the family and social networks of those who have reduced vision (Friedman & Nason, 2000; Bambara, Wadley, et al., 2009).

THE MOST COMMON CAUSES OF VISION LOSS

The most common cause of vision loss in adults in developed countries is age-related macular degeneration, which causes loss of central vision, but typically allows preserved peripheral vision (Klein, Chou, et al., 2011). Loss of central vision is noted by patients as it interferes with tasks such as reading. Glaucoma typically affects peripheral vision, and diabetic retinopathy can affect both peripheral and central vision. Early peripheral vision loss from glaucoma is often not recognized by patients, and this can delay treatment that can prevent further vision loss. Peripheral vision loss impacts mobility and orientation.

THE MEANING OF "LEGALLY BLIND"

While it is estimated that more than 4.2 million adults in the United States have *legal* blindness or low vision (2012), only a small proportion of these individuals are blind and have no, or very limited vision (Congdon, O'Colmain, et al., 2004). A larger group has legal blindness, determined in the United States as visual acuity with corrective lenses if needed, that is equal to or less than 20/200, or a visual field less than 20 degrees in diameter. The designation as "legally blind" is an arbitrary level of vision loss used historically in the United States to determine eligibility for disability benefits. In 2006, the U.S. Social Security Administration (SSA) expanded the definition of legal blindness to include testing with charts specifically designed to measure visual acuity in patients with low vision. Using these charts, a person is considered legally blind if they cannot see any letters on the 1/5 line. At this time the SSA also outlined how the criteria of legal blindness as a visual field of less than 20 degrees could be calculated using automated visual field assessment. The World Health Organization's (WHO) definition of legal blindness is an acuity less than 20/400 (6/120), and the definition of low vision is acuity less than 20/60 (6/18) (WHO, 2014). Legally blind individuals may still have considerable usable vision and be able to use magnifiers, computers, or other devices. The largest proportion of those with vision loss have partial vision loss and are neither blind nor legally blind (Table 71.1).

ADULTS AND THE ELDERLY

Worldwide, it is estimated that 45 million have blindness and 135 million have low vision (2003). The greatest burden of vision loss is borne by the elderly, as the risk of vision loss increases with age (Congdon, O'Colmain, et al., 2004; Iliffe, Kharicha, et al., 2005). Prevalence of vision loss in those over 65 is estimated to be 15%; rising as high as 30% in those over 75. With the increased longevity of our population, many elderly patients will live with vision loss for the last 20 or 30 years of their life.

CHILDREN

Although visual impairment and blindness are rare among pediatric populations, the needs of this group are unique, change with development, and are often modified by comorbidities (Ferrell, 2010). The most common causes of pediatric vision loss vary in different areas of the world; however, in the developed world, cortical disease, optic nerve disease, and retinopathy of prematurity are significant causes (Gilbert & Foster, 2001). It is estimated that 12.2 per 1,000 children under the age of 18 have low vision. Legal blindness occurs much less commonly, 0.06 per 1,000 (http://nichcy.org). Severely visually impaired or multi-handicapped children are more easily identified than children with less severe vision impairment. If vision loss, especially at a moderate level, is the only impairment, however, the handicap may not be readily identified, so these children often "fall through the cracks" of the vision rehabilitation system. Clinicians need to be aware of a range of psychiatric issues in the pediatric, adult, and geriatric patients who experience vision loss or eye disease, including depression, adjustment issues, hallucinations, and psychiatric effects of ocular medications.

Table 71.1 DEFINITIONS OF LOW VISION AND LEGAL BLINDNESS

	WORLD HEALTH ORGANIZATION			UNITED STATES	
	Meters	Feet		Meters	Feet
Low vision	<6/18 = or >6/120	<20/60 = or >20/400	Low vision	<6/12 >6/60	<20/40 >20/200
Blindness	<6/120	<20/400	Legal blindness	= or <6/60	= or <20/200

ADJUSTMENT TO VISION LOSS

The diagnosis of vision loss, as well as the potential functional impairments associated with vision loss, confronts an individual with significant challenges (Brennan & Cardinali, 2000; Friedman & Nason, 2000; Brody, Gamst, et al., 2001; Girdler, Boldy, et al., 2010). Poor adjustment to vision loss is associated with compromised quality of life and greater risk of depression (Rees, Tee, et al., 2010). Addressing a patient's ability to adjust emotionally to the challenges posed by vision loss should therefore be an essential part of these patients' clinical care. For instance, due to vision loss, a person may not be able to drive anymore. Thus, the individual may feel that getting to a supermarket or visiting friends is now beyond her or his personal resources. This dilemma would pose a stressful situation for which new coping strategies are required.

For the purpose of the current discussion, we define *adjustment* as the goal of a continuous series of coping responses (Skinner, Edge, et al., 2003). Whether vision loss is partial or total, fluctuating, progressive, or sudden, people will continue to encounter challenges, and new coping strategies may be required.

COPING STRATEGIES

The individual with loss of vision must adjust not only to the functional impairments, but also to psychological challenges. Patients may experience changes in (gender) roles, mobility, communication, social interactions, occupations, leisure activities, and overall independence (Owsley, McGwin, et al., 2009). Both coping approaches suggested by Lazarus and Folkman's stress and coping model—problem-focused actions to counter the stressor, and responses to alter one's internal state or emotions (Lazarus & Folkman, 1984)—are important. Problem-focused actions are effective if the person has control over the situation; and if that is not the case, then modifying one's emotional response to the stressor or one's internal state (accommodating self-concept and goals to the restrictions imposed by vision loss) is the better strategy. Similarly, both assimilative (goal pursuit) and accommodative coping (flexible goal adaptation), as suggested in the model of Brandtstaedter and Renner, have a role (Brandtstaedter & Renner, 1990). Assimilative coping may require learning new strategies to reach a set goal despite vision loss (e.g., using public transport instead of driving to visit a friend), whereas accommodative coping would entail a change in goals (e.g., listening to audio books rather than reading). Using both coping strategies is most successful in maintaining an optimistic emotional state when dealing with vision loss (Mollenkopf, Wahl, et al., 2007; Rovner, Casten, et al., 2007).

The question is, however, how people with vision loss actually do attempt to cope with the impairment. A recent study analyzed narrative data obtained from interviews with 507 visually impaired individuals to assess prevalent constellations of stressors and coping style (Lee & Brennan, 2006). Individuals' attempts to cope mostly relied on personal resources; for instance, their beliefs in self-reliance and independence. The authors identified five groups of coping constellations; main coping strategies were: (group 1) reliance on own capability with a focus on psychological coping; (group 2) similar reliance on self, but with relatively high acceptance of vision loss; (group 3) use of residual vision with support by devices and rehabilitation; and (group 4) social avoidance. The most prevalent constellation (group 5) involved no distinctive coping strategies except for some reporting self-reliance and reliance on informal support persons.

Self-reliance is an important but not sufficient coping strategy. O'Donnell (2005) also reported that older adults, those now suffering from the highest rate of age-related vision loss, "rolled up their sleeves and went to work. They want to act. They want their eyes back. They find it hard to understand that their ophthalmologist…can do nothing to restore their vision" (O'Donnell, 2005). When using this coping style of self-reliance alone, individuals may hesitate to ask for help or look for and use rehabilitation services that require learning to do tasks in new ways.

A nationwide census of vision rehabilitation services in the United States found that nearly half of the patients (45%) were rated as having emotional or psychological problems with adjusting to their impairment (Owsley, McGwin, et al., 2009). Attitudes towards blindness and fear of stigma may impact one's ability to cope (Horowitz & Reinhardt, 2000). Rates of depression (including major depression and subthreshold depressive symptoms) are relatively high among people with vision impairments (Crews & Campbell, 2004; Horowitz, Reinhardt, et al., 2005; Iliffe, Kharicha, et al., 2005; Hayman, Kerse, et al., 2007). In the elderly, reported depression rates range from 7–39%, compared to 5–8% for elders living in the community (Renaud & Bedard, 2013). Most studies of individuals with age-related macular degeneration show greater depression rates than those found in the general population of older people, comparable with rates observed in individuals with other chronic and disabling diseases (Iliffe, Kharicha, et al., 2005; Casten & Rovner, 2008; Huang, Dong, et al., 2010). Augustin et al. found that the prevalence of depression increased as visual impairment became more severe, while other authors have linked the rate of depression to loss of function (Augustin, Sahel, et al., 2007; Evans, Fletcher, et al., 2007; Zhang, Bullard, et al., 2013). It is not clear whether individuals with vision loss have an increased risk of depression, or whether individuals with depression have a higher risk of chronic diseases such as vision loss, or both. Undoubtedly, functional losses resulting from vision loss can lead to feelings of loss of independence and lack of control, social isolation, and cessation of activities previously enjoyed—all factors that may facilitate depressive moods; however, depression may in turn affect disease course as well. For instance, individuals with depression are more likely to report poor vision (Huang, Dong, et al., 2010) and show worse performance on tasks requiring vision than those without depression, even controlling for visual acuity (Brody, Gamst, et al., 2001; Rovner & Casten, 2001; Rovner, Casten, et al., 2006). The prevalence of vision loss increases with age and, therefore, elders with vision loss often have other chronic diseases with physical limitations that may contribute to their risk of depressive symptoms (Goldstein, 2011).

Early recognition of depressive symptoms in individuals with vision loss may prevent further impact of their depression on their functioning and increase adherence to medical treatment and rehabilitation outcome. The American Academy of Ophthalmology's SmartSight model outlines how comprehensive vision rehabilitation can be part of the continuum of eye care, and in this model it is recommended that the ophthalmologist notify the patient's primary care provider of possible depression (2012). In cases of dysthymia or sadness, the ophthalmologist can assist in assuring the patient that sad moods are a common and understandable reaction to vision loss. While major depression requires antidepressant drugs or psychotherapy, vision rehabilitation can improve discouragement and sadness by teaching the patient new strategies and behaviors to maintain independence.

There are many barriers to attaining vision rehabilitation. Patients may not be aware of the services available, perhaps because their treating physicians have not advised them of rehabilitation options. Patients may not believe that such services are beneficial for them, or they may have difficulty accessing services due to other health problems or lack of transportation. It is estimated that only one-quarter to one-third of those who could benefit from rehabilitation obtain services. While there are limited reports showing that an individual confronted with vision loss may create novel strategies to cope (Bittner, Edwards, et al., 2010; Riazi, Dain, Boon, & Bridge, 2011), in general, individuals with vision loss will benefit from formal and informal support to identify both psychosocial services such as support groups, and vision rehabilitation resources (access to devices and training). Rehabilitation should be available to any individual whose vision loss impacts their life beyond simply the ability to read fine print. Medicare and most insurers in the United States cover the cost of occupational therapy for patients with vision loss, just as rehabilitation is covered for stroke or orthopedic problems. State agencies exist in all states to provide some

services, although the nature of services provided and eligibility criteria vary. Vision rehabilitation services are provided by the Veteran Administration network, and in addition, agencies, optometrists, and ophthalmologists provide various levels of service. A directory of services is maintained online (see visionaware.org).

SOCIAL SUPPORT AND FAMILY ADJUSTMENT

Adjustment to vision loss takes place in the context of a social network (Horowitz, Reinhardt, et al., 2003; Orr & Rogers, 2006). Family members often function as caregivers and provide emotional and instrumental support to the visually impaired individual (Cimarolli & Boerner, 2005). Both traditional and nontraditional families should be considered in this discussion. Both paid and informal caregivers can be part of the picture. These individuals can provide day-to-day assistance, reassure, motivate, support compliance with rehabilitation and medication, negotiate support and services, help the physician understand what the disease means to the patient, and remind the patient how they have coped with other stressors in the past.

Vision loss, like many other diseases, however, can pose a challenge for family members or caregivers. The family may struggle with finding a balance between supporting and assuring the safety of the visually impaired person and allowing the patient to be self-sufficient. Overprotection can lead to learned helplessness and thus increased dependency, as well as feelings of anger towards the caregiver. Higher levels of perceived overprotection, such as offering assistance that is not required, are associated with less optimal adjustment (Cimarolli & Boerner, 2005; Cimarolli, Reinhardt, et al., 2006). Furthermore, the challenge of providing support to a visually impaired person, often with no or little training, can result in distress for the caregiver. Caregivers may have difficulties attending to their own as well as the visually impaired person's needs and goals. Most literature has focused on the function of families or caregivers as support for the visually impaired individual, and little attention has been paid to the caregiver's adjustment process (Bambara, Wadley, et al., 2009).

Recently, Bambara et al. (2009) found that a substantial number of family caregivers suffered from psychosocial distress (Bambara, Owsley, et al., 2009). Caregivers with low problem-solving skills are more likely to experience distress, anxiety, depression, and poor health. Bambara et al. suggested that interventions to increase problem-solving abilities may support quality of life in caregivers and so eventually facilitate rehabilitation outcomes for the patient.

Including key support persons in the care process is one way to facilitate ideal conditions for the successful adjustment of both patients and caregivers. A family-centered approach to vision care allows everyone involved to understand and cope with the disease and the challenges it may pose. Key support persons can encourage discussion of how the vision impairment affects family members' functioning and goals, emotions, resources, and "how to separate the illness from the family's sense of itself" (Friedman & Nason, 2000). The process can decrease caregivers' sense of burden and support the visually impaired persons' sense of self-reliance.

VISION REHABILITATION AS A RESOURCE

Vision rehabilitation aims to maximize functioning despite an individual's loss of vision (Trauzettel-Klosinski, 2010). Patients whose vision cannot be fully corrected with ordinary spectacles, or medical or surgical treatment are provided with comprehensive assessment of visual function, the opportunity to obtain appropriate devices, and subsequent training, often by an occupational therapist. An individualized rehabilitation plan is established considering the patient's goals. Devices go beyond traditional glasses or optical magnifiers to include magnification with a video camera in either desk or portable formats, magnification on iPads or eReaders, text-to-speech technology, and computer and cellphone accessibility options. Vision rehabilitation assists in developing new coping strategies or enhancing existing productive behaviors to master tasks that are meaningful to the individual. Maintaining independence is encouraged, with the overall aim of increasing quality of life. Vision rehabilitation has been shown to improve quality of life and reduce depressive symptoms (Stelmack, Tang, et al., 2008; Girdler, Boldy, et al., 2010) and thus ought to be considered as a resource that can be offered by the physician to individuals with vision loss.

PRACTICE IMPLICATIONS

The physician can assist by supporting both problem- and emotion-focused coping strategies in various ways:

- Ensure that patients are referred to comprehensive vision rehabilitation services that address not only acquiring devices, but also other impacts of vision loss and draw on multidisciplinary services. A guideline outlining how vision rehabilitation can be incorporated into ophthalmic care is available (see http://one.aao.org/smart-sight-low-vision) with patient information and resources for audio digital books, large-print books or newspapers, computer accessibility information, and other resources.

- Identify key support persons and involve them in the care process, if the patient agrees.

- Provide information to the patient as well as the key support persons. Education is a key component of rehabilitation.

- Negative comments can be rephrased to point out positive components. Talking about what is most important, and what they do well, allows patients and their families to regain strength and control (Friedman & Nason, 2000; Buckman, 2005). Patients with central field loss from AMD can be encouraged that peripheral vision is typically maintained, and that, with appropriate training and devices, individuals can use this vision to maintain independence.

HALLUCINATIONS IN VISION LOSS

Many individuals who lose vision report a peculiar symptom of recurrent, vivid hallucinations known as the Charles Bonnet syndrome (CBS; Menon, Rahman, et al., 2003;

Rovner, 2006; Jackson & Bassett, 2010). Physicians often do not recognize the syndrome, in part because patients do not commonly report the symptom. Patients often fear that they will be considered mentally ill if they report such a symptom. Four criteria have been proposed for the diagnosis: (1) the patient reports vivid, recurrent visual hallucinations; (2) there is some degree of vision loss; (3) the patient has insight into the unreal nature of what they see; and (4) there is no other neurological or psychiatric diagnosis to explain the hallucinations (Jackson & Ferencz, 2009). It is now appreciated that such visual hallucinations are not uncommon in patients seeking ophthalmic care and that such hallucinations can occur even with moderate loss of vision.

The first description of hallucinations in a cognitively intact, visually impaired individual was by Charles Bonnet, a Swiss naturalist. In 1769, he wrote clear, elaborate descriptions of hallucinations experienced by his grandfather. This 18-page document describing the visual sensations predated the term *hallucination* (Ffytche, 2005). The eponym was coined in the next century by a neurologist, George de Morsier (de Morsier, 1967).

In *The Diagnostic and Statistical Manual of Mental Disorders* (DSM), a hallucination is defined as "a sensory perception that has the compelling sense of reality of a true perception, but occurs without external stimulation of the relevant sensory organ" (DSM, 2000). Many patients with vision loss can misinterpret an object in their environment, such as thinking that a person is sitting in a chair when a coat is draped on the chair. Such an illusion should be differentiated on history-taking from a true hallucination.

The images that are reported by patients vary a great deal, most often having content that is unfamiliar to the patient. Many individuals describe "seeing" people, faces, or animals, while others "see" repeating patterns of flowers or vegetation that can resemble wallpaper. There is no agreement as to whether images of bright lights or diffuse colors are part of the syndrome; however, a history of a very clear image that recurs and is present with the eyes open or closed is suggestive of the CBS.

Insight into the unreality of the images is required to make a diagnosis of CBS, but it is common that patients do not have full insight when they first experience the hallucinations. Patients may be confused about what they are experiencing, unwilling to disclose them to family or physicians, and, in some cases, very anxious that the symptom is an ominous sign of mental decline or neurological illness. They may act on their hallucinations when they fit into the environment; e.g., they may step over an object that appears to be in their way. To make a diagnosis of CBS, the individuals must have full insight after the nature of the syndrome has been explained. Lack of insight despite explanation would raise consideration of other diagnoses. Little research has addressed the link between cognitive loss and CBS.

The following case histories of patients' descriptions of hallucinations as part of the Charles Bonnet syndrome are reprinted here with permission from *Macular Degeneration: The Complete Guide to Saving and Maximizing Your Sight* (Mogk & Mogk, 2010).

ROSA GARCIA'S FLOWERING TREES

They are beautiful, these flowers. Large vibrant pink blooms, decorating trees with no leaves, as if flowers always grew in the wintertime. When I first saw them, I loved them. *This isn't possible!* I thought. It was autumn; there were leaves on the ground. We were on the train to Toronto. I watched these flowers for a while, then I turned to my friend Barbara and told her what I was seeing. I remember being quite enthusiastic, although I wasn't sure I should be saying so much. She just sort of stared at me. Then I made the mistake of telling her about the chain-link fences. I had been seeing chain-link fences everywhere. Well, many places they shouldn't be. There were okay. But the pink flowers were beautiful. Barbara just stared at me even harder. Then she asked me a few questions about how long I had been seeing fences and flowers, and where they appeared. She didn't seem any more comfortable with my answers. For some reason, though, I didn't really care. I just stopped telling people about them. You have to be careful what you say.

MARY FLANNERY'S ELIZABETHAN DINNER PARTY

I was born in Belfast in 1928. My parents died just before the war, so I went to live in Boston with my Uncle Liam. My mother, of course, never liked the British. But I always loved the theater and I loved Shakespeare. I used to dress up in my aunt's old dresses and pretend I was Juliet and Romeo was on his way over to the house. I don't think that has anything to do with my Elizabethan dinner party though. That's what I call it. I see these very formal, earnest people sitting around my dining room table in full Elizabethan dress. Their outfits are made of bright, jeweled fabrics, with lots of lace, high collars, and pinched, V-shaped waists. The look like they belong on stage or in the queen's court. They're not talkative; they don't seem hungry, and they don't seem upset. Actually, they appear to think it's perfectly natural to sit around my dining room table. They irritate me sometimes, but I think my mother would probably roll over in her grave.

Although the syndrome can occur in individuals of any age and in patients with a range of eye disease, including both central and peripheral loss, the syndrome is much more common in the elderly, and this is considered to be because eye disease disproportionately affects the geriatric population. The reported prevalence of the CBS varies widely, depending on the population studied, the specificity of the hallucinations included in the diagnosis, and the methods used to elicit the symptom (Menon, Rahman, et al., 2003; Jackson, Bassett, et al., 2007; Gilmour, Schreiber, et al., 2009). Prevalence of 8.3% was found in a cohort of 300 consecutive Danish patients with neovascular age-related macular degeneration (Singh & Sorensen, 2010). A very low prevalence of 0.4% was reported on a series of patients in Singapore (Tan, Lim, et al., 2004). The prevalence in patients presenting for vision rehabilitation has been found to be approximately one-third in several series (Crane, Fletcher, et al., 1994; Jackson, Bassett, et al., 2007).

Menon prospectively considered two groups of elderly subjects; those with better acuity than 20/40 and those with very poor visual acuity of less than 20/400 (Menon, 2005). He reported a high prevalence of 63% hallucinations in those with the poorer visual acuity, and no hallucinations in the comparison cohort. The risk of experiencing the hallucination is not consistently correlated with the degree of vision loss, although both visual acuity and contrast sensitivity have been correlated with the symptom (Jackson, Bassett, et al., 2007; Singh & Sorensen, 2010).

The hallucinations are considered to be comparable to phantom limb sensations, and it is posited that the hallucinations arise because areas of cortex are not receiving visual afferent information. Neuro-imaging has shown correlation of the type of image seen during the hallucination and the area of brain activity. Patients who experienced hallucinations in color have had activity documented in the fusiform gyrus, an area corresponding to the V4 color center (Kazui, Ishii, et al., 2009); deafferentation and hypermetabolism of the thalamocortical visual pathway have also been suggested (Jang, Youn, et al., 2011).

Other diagnoses are always considered when patients do not have insight into the unreal nature of what they see or have other neurological or psychiatric symptoms. Visual hallucinations can also occur in sleep–wake transitions, during bereavement, and as side effect of medications. Hallucinations also occur in diseases such as Parkinson's, Alzheimer's, and Lewy body dementia. Up to one-third of patients with Parkinson's report hallucinations, and these have been reported to occur prior to pharmacological treatment of the Parkinson's disease (Biousse, Skibell, et al., 2004). A series of 30 subjects with untreated Parkinson's disease (PD) with normal cognitive function and full insight reported that 25% had hallucinations. None of these subjects developed dementia over the subsequent two years. Approximately 20–25% of Alzheimer's disease (AD) patients also experience hallucinations (Bassiony & Lyketsos, 2003). Authors have suggested that there is associated visual pathology in patients with PD and AD who report hallucinations (Diederich, Goetz, et al., 1998; Chapman, Dickinson, et al., 1999). Patients with Lewy body dementia have a clinical triad of visual hallucinations, fluctuating mental status, and Parkinsonism.

A patient with known eye disease, recurrent visual hallucinations, insight into the unreal nature of the images, and no other psychiatric or neurological disease to explain the hallucinations can be considered to have CBS. Most patients appreciate an explanation as to why they are experiencing these peculiar visions. A prospective study of patients seen in a vision rehabilitation clinic found that 25% of those who reported hallucinations at enrollment, reported that the hallucinations had stopped at one year (Jackson & Bassett, 2010). Only a small number of patients are so bothered that pharmacological management needs to be considered. Case reports of successful treatment with a number of medications in different classes have been published, although consensus or evidence base for optimal medication are lacking (Lang, Stogowski, et al., 2007; Segers, 2009). To avoid misdiagnosis and unnecessary investigation, it is important that physicians be aware of the syndrome and consider it in the differential of patients presenting with visual hallucinations. In addition, patients with recent onset or progression of visual loss should be asked about visual hallucinations, offering an explanation that these sometimes occur with visual loss and are not a sign of mental illness. Often patients will not volunteer a complaint of visual hallucinations unless they are asked about them.

OCULAR ISSUES IN DEMENTIA

ALZHEIMER'S DISEASE

It is estimated that globally, approximately 44.4 million people live with some form of dementia, with AD being the most prevalent form (2013). Vision loss can worsen dementia and is a risk factor for dementia (Lee, 2009). Although AD is primarily a disease of dementia, visual complaints can be primary in a subset of AD patients (Holroyd & Shepherd, 2001; Lee & Martin, 2004). Symptoms can include blurred vision, difficulty reading, and difficulty seeing low-contrast targets. The symptoms are attributed to abnormalities in the central visual pathways. Clinical findings include decreased contrast sensitivity and ocular motor abnormalities such as hypometric saccades, saccadic latency prolongation, fixation instability, and saccadic intrusions during smooth-pursuit eye movements. Higher cortical function abnormalities such as visual agnosia may be present. Referral to a neuro-ophthalmologist is recommended.

WERNICKE'S ENCEPHALOPATHY

Rarely, the diagnosis of disordered consciousness is made by the ophthalmologist. Wernicke's encephalopathy (Wernicke, 1968) is a clinical triad of ocular motility disturbance, ataxia, and altered consciousness, often with memory disturbances, due to vitamin B1 deficiency (Rufa, Rosini, et al., 2011). Although most commonly seen in patients afflicted with chronic alcohol consumption, it can be seen in the settings of malnutrition from other causes. The ocular findings can include nystagmus or paralysis of ocular muscles, particularly of the lateral rectus muscle, producing horizontal diplopia. When treated early with intravenous thiamine, recovery usually is rapid and complete. Left untreated, Wernicke's encephalopathy can lead to Korsakoff syndrome, long-term institutionalization, or death (Harper, Giles, et al., 1986; Day, Bentham, et al., 2004; Kopelman, Thomson, et al., 2009).

PSYCHIATRIC ISSUES AND VISION LOSS—FUNCTIONAL VISION LOSS

Occasionally clinicians are confronted with patients who report vision loss in whom no organic etiology is apparent on clinical evaluation, thus raising the differential diagnosis of non-organic or "functional" vision loss. These patients present a challenge to the clinician (Miller, 2005).

Such patients are often referred for neuro-ophthalmologic and retinal evaluation, as the diseases that are not apparent on clinical evaluation typically fall under these domains. Neuro-ophthalmologic evaluation may include electrophysiological testing, such as measurement of visual evoked potentials. Patients may be malingering and have willful intent to present symptoms for some secondary gain, or may have functional neurological symptoms or conversion and be unaware of the non-organic source of symptoms. These patients take more time for evaluation. A detailed past history, review of symptoms of dissociation, and an understanding of what the patient thinks is happening will be helpful. *Every aspect of the clinical encounter is important to illuminate visual abilities, from how patients walk into the examination room to whether they shake the clinician's hand.*

Pupil testing is important; however, a malingerer can also simulate pupil abnormalities by self-administration of topical medication. In this situation, the pupil will not constrict with pilocarpine drops.

Optokinetic nystagmus can be elicited by a drum or tape, and a positive test indicates visual acuity of 20/200 (6/60) or better (Beatty, 1999). Malingerers tend to feign not being able to sign their name, although a blind person would not find this difficult; malingerers do not look at their own hands during a manual task. Tests of proprioception can be done by a patient who is truly blind, but malingerers may pretend the task is difficult. A malingerer may not be able to bring together the index fingers in front of their eyes, something a blind person can do. For tests of one eye, the other eye should be covered. Most people feigning blindness would be able to walk smoothly into the examining room; and would flinch to threat or flinch to a bright light aimed at the eyes.

For monocular visual loss, the Fogging Test is the process of placing a series of plus lenses of progressively increasing power in front of the unaffected eye while the vision is tested. Neither eye is occluded. As the vision in the unaffected eye becomes more and more blurred, it becomes clear that the patient is seeing with the affected eye. Further tests are noted in Beatty (Beatty, 1999).

Patients with visual loss without obvious cause can be evaluated with electroretinography, pattern electroretinography, and pattern appearance visually evoked cortical potentials (VECPs). VECPs evaluate the integrity of the retinogeniculostriate pathway. Nearly normal VECPs do not rule out central visual loss due to impaired function of the visual association areas in the occipital and parietal lobes. Patients gaming the test can purposely not focus on the test stimulus and thereby lower the amplitude of the electrical response.

A normal-pattern electroretinogram depends on the functional integrity of the retina and optic nerve. It will detect photoreceptor dysfunction syndromes when signs on fundi are subtle, and it will require good focus and adequate fixation. Simultaneous VECP testing and pattern electroretinogram can thus improve on one of the weaknesses of the electroretinogram alone. Color vision testing may be necessary to rule out cone dysfunction syndromes.

Visual field testing can be misleading, as patients can easily falsify results, and there are no characteristic changes to confirm the suspicion of a non-organic deficit (Stewart, 1995).

Tubular fields are the most common abnormal visual field associated with conversion disorder. True fields expand with increasing test distance. When the field does not expand, it is called "tubular." The visual field must be tested at two distances to define the tubular field, as the normal visual field will be larger at a greater distance (Stone, Carson, et al., 2005).

Diseases that are most typically misdiagnosed as malingering include pituitary tumors with early compression, Leber's hereditary optic neuropathy, early cone or Stargardt's retinal dystrophy, retrobulbar optic neuropathy, small occipital infarcts, or cancer- or melanoma-associated retinopathy. Patients can complain of loss of vision when they have visual agnosia or alexia, and such organic disease should be kept in mind.

The treatment of conversion blindness or non-organic visual loss is reassurance by a concerned physician. Improvement should be documented in a follow-up visit. If the patient is young and has no other psychiatric disorder, then the prognosis is generally good (Beatty, 1999). These patients typically do not require psychiatric referral. Family or school stress or sexual or physical abuse can be predisposing factors (Catalono, Simon, et al., 1986). Patients with non-organic disease can often be encouraged that they do not have underlying disease and that their prognosis for improvement is positive. Combined organic and non-organic complaints do occur, and the possibility that a patient with non-organic complaints can develop organic disease needs to be kept in mind (Scott & Egan, 2003).

Shedding light on the neural signature of conversion blindness, functional magnetic resonance imaging (fMRI) has noted altered but not absent visual cortex responses in patients with conversion blindness. Becker et al. (2013) reported a 25-year-old man with visual pseudo-hallucinations of his deceased friend's face grimacing with agony (Becker, Scheele, et al., 2013). They found normal basic visual cortex responses to checkerboard stimulation during the blindness. In contrast, when they asked the patient to perform a social-emotional perception task, they found hypofunction in the occipital cortex and hyperfunction in the postcentral gyrus bilaterally and the right superior temporal gyrus. Extracting this emotion-specific activity, they found increased responses in the angular gyrus bilaterally, the left medial frontal gyrus, and the left anterior cingulate cortex, areas implicated in emotional regulation and moral reasoning. They reported enhanced functional coupling of this network with downregulated visual areas. They concluded that symptom-related functional association of overactivity in fronto-parietal regions and suppressed responses in interconnected visual areas add to the neurocircuitry model of visual conversion disorder.

Another case suggested that event-related potentials (ERPs) could serve as an electrophysiological measure combined with fMRI, a hemodynamic measure, to track the progress of a conversion visual symptom and to track success of treatment (Schoenfeld, Hassa, et al., 2011). In a patient with blindness limited to the left upper and right lower visual quadrant, the fMRI activations were normal for visual stimulation, but the electrophysiological indices of visual processing were modulated. Unseen parts of the patient's visual field elicited smaller amplitudes of N1 component of the event-related potential at diagnosis. This modulation was absent after treatment when the vision returned to normal. The implication is that functional blindness does have a neurophysiological correlate.

Anxiety or conversion reaction can cause spasm of the near reflex characterized by episodes of a small pupil or miosis, convergence, and accommodation (Bradley, 2004). A constricted pupil would confirm this diagnosis (Kline, 2010).

PSYCHIATRIC ISSUES AND EYE TRAUMA

The psychiatrist may become aware of eye trauma in his patient that can signal the need for concurrent ophthalmology and psychiatric evaluation. Additionally, issues of eye trauma may be brought to the psychiatrist's attention by physicians conducting eye exams who suspect social or psychiatric issues. Child abuse, the "shaken-baby syndrome," spousal or elder abuse can each manifest as any finding of ocular trauma, including retinal detachment, retinal hemorrhages, vitreous hemorrhages, blood in the anterior chamber of the eye (hyphema), eyelid bruising (ecchymosis), eyelid swelling, or lens dislocation. The shaken-baby syndrome typically involves ocular trauma in addition to intracranial pathology such as subdural hematoma or cerebral edema. External eye trauma is not often present (Emerson, Pieramici, et al., 2001; Bhardwaj, Chowdhury, et al., 2010). Sadly, mortality is high (29%) for infants with shaken-baby syndrome (McCabe & Donahue, 2000). Referral for detailed eye examination is important for both documentation and treatment. The differential diagnosis of other sources of trauma or blood dyscrasias must be considered.

Elder abuse is often subtle, despite a national prevalence between 2% and 10% when various forms of abuse are considered (Lachs & Pillemer, 2004). Risk factors include marital, financial, and legal stresses, mental illness, and substance abuse. The clinician should be mindful of the possibility of maltreatment of elderly patients leading to ocular trauma that can occur in private homes, assisted living or nursing homes. Signs may include black eyes, orbital fractures, broken spectacles, misleading histories accounting for clinical findings, or delay in seeking treatment of ocular injuries.

Unfortunately, ocular trauma can ensue from suicide attempts with guns. Requirement for ocular reconstruction is obvious. Autoenucleation or traumatic enucleation by another person is a severe form of trauma, often involving the ophthalmologist for orbit reconstruction (Patton, 2004). Such clinical events are evidence of severe mental pathology requiring psychiatric and ophthalmic co-management.

Autoenucleation is a rare form of major self-mutilation seen especially in first-episode schizophrenia (Large, Andrews, et al., 2008). It is also seen in patients abusing hallucinogenic drugs. Some patients report the need to expiate guilt by removing an evil organ that conveys evil images from an evil world (Jones, 1990). Patients are at risk of further mutilation or suicide.

Patients losing one eye are aware of deficits of peripheral field and binocularity during the ensuing initial few months; however, most adapt spontaneously over time and require no rehabilitation intervention. Some patients experience grieving after monocular vision loss, which, as with grieving of any loss, can infrequently be prolonged and maladaptive. Such patients typically benefit from referral to both vision rehabilitation and counseling.

MEDICATIONS AND VISION

OCULAR MEDICATIONS AND PSYCHIATRIC SYMPTOMS

It is often overlooked that ocular medications can have systemic side effects (Rhee, Colby, et al., 2011). Most systemic effects are due to absorption via the mucous membranes of the eye and nasopharynx. In addition, there can be an additive effect of topical and concurrent oral medications. Systemic absorption after topical administration can be reduced by having patients close their eyes or put digital pressure on the nasolacrimal duct when administering their eye drops. The majority of patients requiring eye medication are elderly, who are, in general, at greater risk of systemic toxicities. In addition, errors in self-administration of ocular medications may be higher than in the general population, as patients with vision loss have difficulty reading labels and instructions (Drummond, Drummond, et al., 2004; 2008).

β-adrenergic antagonists, or β-blockers, are used in glaucoma management as they lower intraocular pressure by reducing aqueous humor production. Depression, lethargy, decreased libido, hallucinations, and sleep disturbance in patients with topical β-blocker medication use for glaucoma are reported (Rhee, Colby, et al., 2011). Alternate medications or management options can be considered. The psychiatrist can assist patients by advising the treating ophthalmologist when such symptoms are detected. Oral acetazolamide is used to treat glaucoma infrequently but can have side effects, including depression, restlessness, fatigue, and diminished libido (Rhee, Colby, et al., 2011).

Topical medications are routinely used in eye examinations to dilate pupils. Dose-related side effects include drowsiness, delirium, hallucinations, or agitation, particularly in children or elderly patients. Severe cases are treated with intravenous physostigmine. A cyclopentolate-induced acute psychosis has been reported, occurring 20–60 minutes after administration of the anti-muscarinic agent to dilate pupils. Symptoms and signs include disorientation, dysarthria, ataxia, hallucinations, and amnesia (Fraunfelder, Fraunfelder, et al., 2001).

OCULAR COMPLICATION OF PSYCHOTROPIC MEDICATIONS

Although infrequent, ocular complications due to psychotropic medications do occur, most frequently with typical antipsychotics, tricyclic antidepressants, lithium, benzodiazepines, carbamazepine, topiramate, and selective serotonin-reuptake inhibitors (SSRIs) (Richa & Yazbek, 2010). Patients taking medication with anticholinergic effect may report ocular side effects such as dry eye or accommodative changes causing blurred vision (Fraunfelder, Fraunfelder, et al., 2001). Medications with anticholinergic effect can also induce acute or subacute angle-closure glaucoma requiring, typically, both pharmacological management and a laser surgical outpatient procedure (laser iridotomy). Symptoms include eye pain and redness in most patients, but less frequently, patients are not acutely symptomatic or can present with gastrointestinal symptoms such as abdominal pain or nausea. Elderly, Inuit, and Chinese and other Asian populations are at highest risk (Rhee, Colby, et al., 2011).

Uncommonly, patients taking SSRIs report changes in vision, and younger patients may also report "tracking" difficulties, which resolve when the medication is discontinued (Purdy, Bolling, et al., 2010). Topiramate can cause acquired myopia and also angle-closure glaucoma due to displacement of the lens and ciliary body. Induced myopia and angle-closure glaucoma can occur secondary to topiramate. Topiramate is a sulpha-based anti-epileptic drug that interferes with ionic concentrations of sodium and chloride in tissues, including the lens. Such ionic changes may produce uveal tract swelling, causing induced myopia. Significant further damage to the lens-iris complex may lead to angle-closure glaucoma (Abtahi, Abtahi, et al., 2012; Liu & Rhee, 2013).

First-generation antipsychotics, with primarily dopamine receptor blockade, are less well tolerated than second-generation antipsychotics, which have an inhibitory effect on serotonin receptors in addition to dopamine-blocking activity (Purdy, Bolling, et al., 2010). Ophthalmic side effects of first-generation medications include corneal pigment deposition, lens pigmentation, eyelid pigmentation, and retinal pigmentary degeneration, which is associated with vision loss. These side effects occur most commonly with long-term use of thioridazine, typically at doses greater than 800 mg/day (Fraunfelder, Fraunfelder, et al., 2001). Antipsychotics, including second-generation agents, can be associated with tardive dyskinesia. Blepharospasm and other eye movement disorders can occur.

Both lithium and phenothiazines are reported to cause eye irritation and blurred vision, which may be self-limiting. Persisting reports of blurred vision require evaluation to rule out other causes such as pseudotumor cerebri, a rare side effect of lithium. Lithium can cause nystagmus and saccadic eye movement disorders (Richa & Yazbek, 2010). Although some nystagmus can resolve with lower doses or drug cessation, the more severe downbeating nystagmus can be permanent. Thyroid-related eye disease in patients taking lithium is secondary to hyperthyroidism or hypothyroidism (Fraunfelder, Fraunfelder, et al., 2001).

SUMMARY

Since the text *Psychiatric Problems in Ophthalmology* was written in 1977 (Blodi, 1977), much has changed, yet still, the primary psychiatric difficulties in ophthalmology remain the same: reactions to losing vision, functional ocular complaints without organic basis, and side effects of medications. Although an infrequent referral—an ophthalmology patient to a psychiatrist or a psychiatric patient to an ophthalmologist—the overlap of the domains warrants review by each specialty respectively.

CLINICAL PEARLS

- The most common cause of vision loss in adults in developed countries is age-related macular degeneration, which causes loss of central vision, but typically allows preserved peripheral vision (Klein, Chou, et al., 2011).

- Glaucoma typically affects peripheral vision, and diabetic retinopathy can affect both peripheral and central vision.

- Legal blindness is determined in the United States as visual acuity with corrective lenses if needed, that is equal to or less than 20/200 or a visual field less than 20 degrees in diameter.

- A guideline outlining how vision rehabilitation can be incorporated into ophthalmic care is available (http://one.aao.org/mart-sight-low-vision) with patient information and resources for audio digital books, large-print books or newspapers, computer accessibility information, and other resources.

- A directory of vision rehabilitation services is maintained online (see visionaware.org).

- Four criteria have been proposed for Charles Bonnet syndrome: (1) the patient reports vivid, recurrent visual hallucinations; (2) there is some degree of vision loss; (3) the patient has insight into the unreal nature of what they see; and (4) there is no other neurological or psychiatric diagnosis to explain the hallucinations (Jackson & Ferencz, 2009).

- Visual hallucinations can also occur in sleep–wake transitions, during bereavement, and as side effect of medications. They are also seen in Parkinson's, Alzheimer's, and Lewy body dementia.

DISCLOSURES

Dr. Jackson currently serves on the National Board of the Canadian National Institute for the Blind (CNIB) and the Planning Committee for the National Eye Health Education Program (NEHEP). She does not receive salary support for these activities. She also is on the Scientific Advisory for VISUS Technologies and a consultant to Ocata Therapeutics.

Dr. Wallis has no conflicts of interest to disclose.

REFERENCES

Abtahi, M. A., Abtahi, S. H., et al. (2012). Topiramate and the vision: A systematic review. *Clinical Ophthalmology, 6*, 117–131.

Alzheimer's Disease International. Dementia Statistics. Available at: http://www.alz.co.uk/research/statistics

American Academy of Ophthalmology (2012). SMARTSIGHT™—Patient handout. An American Academy of Ophthalmology Initiative in Vision Rehabilitation.

American Academy of Ophthalmology Vision Rehabilitation Committee (2012). *Preferred Practice Pattern Guidelines. Vision Rehabilitation for Adults.* San Franciso, CA: American Academy of Ophthalmology. Available at: www.aao.org/ppp.

American Foundation for the Blind (2008). Access to drug labels survey report. Available at: http://www.afb.org/info/programs-and-services/pubic-policy-center/technology-and-information-accessibility/access-to-drug-labels-survey-report/1235

American Psychiatric Association (2000). *Diagnostic and Statistical Manual of Mental Disorders, Fourth Edition: DSM-IV-TR.* Washington, DC: American Psychiatric Association.

Augustin, A., Sahel, J. A., et al. (2007). Anxiety and depression prevalence rates in age-related macular degeneration. *Investigative Ophthalmology & Visual Science, 48*(4), 1498–1503.

Bambara, J. K., Owsley, C., et al. (2009). Family caregiver social problem-solving abilities and adjustment to caring for a relative with vision loss. *Investigative Ophthalmology & Visual Science, 50*(4), 1585–1592.

Bambara, J. K., Wadley, V., et al. (2009). Family functioning and low vision: A systematic review. *Journal of Visual Impairment & Blindness, 103*(3), 137–149.

Bassiony, M. M., & Lyketsos, C. G. (2003). Delusions and hallucinations in Alzheimer's disease: review of the brain decade. *Psychosomatics, 44*(5), 388–401.

Beatty, S. (1999). Non-organic visual loss. *Postgraduate Medical Journal, 75*(882), 201–207.

Becker, B., Scheele, D., et al. (2013). Deciphering the neural signature of conversion blindness. *American Journal of Psychiatry*, Jan 1; *170*(1), 121–122. doi:10.1176/appi.ajp.2012.12070905

Bhardwaj, G., Chowdhury, V., et al. (2010). A systematic review of the diagnostic accuracy of ocular signs in pediatric abusive head trauma. *Ophthalmology, 117*(5), 983–992, e917.

Biousse, V., Skibell, B. C., et al. (2004). Ophthalmologic features of Parkinson's disease. *Neurology, 62*(2), 177–180.

Bittner, A. K., Edwards, L., et al. (2010). Coping strategies to manage stress related to vision loss and fluctuations in retinitis pigmentosa. *Optometry—Journal of the American Optometric Association, 81*(9), 461–468.

Blodi, F. C. (1977). Psychiatric problems in ophthalmology. *Archives of Ophthalmology, 95*(11), 2080.

Bradley, W. G. (2008). *Neurology in clinical practice: Principles of diagnosis and management.* Butterworth-Heinemann, Philadelphia, PA.

Brandtstadter, J., & Renner, G. (1990). Tenacious goal pursuit and flexible goal adjustment: explication and age-related analysis of assimilative and accommodative strategies of coping. *Psychology & Aging, 5*(1), 58–67.

Brennan, M., & Cardinali, G. (2000). The use of preexisting and novel coping strategies in adapting to age-related vision loss. *Gerontologist, 40*(3), 327–334.

Brody, B. L., Gamst, A. C., et al. (2001). Depression, visual acuity, comorbidity, and disability associated with age-related macular degeneration. *Ophthalmology, 108*(10), 1893–1900; discussion, 1900–1891.

Buckman, R. A. (2005). Breaking bad news: the SPIKES strategy. *Community Oncology, 2*(2), 138–142.

Casten, R., & Rovner, B. (2008). Depression in age-related macular degeneration. *Journal of Visual Impairment & Blindness, 102*(10), 591–599.

Catalono, R. A., Simon, J. W., et al. (1986). Functional visual loss in children. *Ophthalmology, 93*(3), 385–390.

Chapman, F. M., Dickinson, J., et al. (1999). Association among visual hallucinations, visual acuity, and specific eye pathologies in Alzheimer's disease: treatment implications. *The American Journal of Psychiatry, 156*(12), 1983–1985.

Cimarolli, V. R., & Boerner, K. (2005). Social support and well-being in adults who are visually impaired. *Journal of Visual Impairment & Blindness, 99*(9), 521–534.

Cimarolli, V. R., Reinhardt, J. P., et al. (2006). Perceived overprotection: Support gone bad? *Journals of Gerontology, Series B: Psychological Sciences & Social Sciences, 61*(1), S18–S23.

Congdon, N., O'Colmain, B., et al. (2004). Causes and prevalence of visual impairment among adults in the United States. *Archives of Ophthalmology, 122*(4), 477–485.

Crane, W., Fletcher, D., et al. (1994). Prevalence of photopsias and Charles Bonnet syndrome in a low vision population. *Ophthalmology Clinics of North America, 7*(2), 143–149.

Crews, J. E., & Campbell, V. A. (2004). Vision impairment and hearing loss among community-dwelling older Americans: implications for health and functioning. *American Journal of Public Health, 94*(5), 823–829.

Day, E., Bentham, P., et al. (2004). Thiamine for Wernicke-Korsakoff syndrome in people at risk from alcohol abuse. *Cochrane Database of Systematic Reviews,* (1), CD004033.

de Morsier, G. (1967). [The Charles Bonnet syndrome: visual hallucinations in the aged without mental deficiency]. *Annales Medico-psychologiques (Paris), 2*(5), 678–702.

Diederich, N. J., Goetz, C. G., et al. (1998). Poor visual discrimination and visual hallucinations in Parkinson's disease. *Clinical Neuropharmacology, 21*(5), 289–295.

Drummond, S. R., Drummond, R. S., et al. (2004). Visual acuity and the ability of the visually impaired to read medication instructions. *British Journal of Ophthalmology, 88*(12), 1541–1542.

Emerson, M. V., Pieramici, D. J., et al. (2001). Incidence and rate of disappearance of retinal hemorrhage in newborns. *Ophthalmology, 108*(1), 36–39.

Evans, J. R., Fletcher, A. E., et al. (2007). Depression and anxiety in visually impaired older people. *Ophthalmology, 114*(2), 283–288.

Ferrell, K. A. (2010). Visual development in normal and low vision children. In A. Corn, A. Koenig, & J. Erin (Eds.), *Foundations of low vision: Clinical and functional perspectives.* New York: AFB Press.

Ffytche, D. H. (2005). Visual hallucinations and the Charles Bonnet syndrome. *Current Psychiatry Report, 7*(3), 168–179.

Fraunfelder, F. T., Fraunfelder, F. W., et al. (2001). Ocular side effects possibly associated with isotretinoin usage. *American Journal of Ophthalmology, 132*(3), 299–305.

Friedman, D. B., & Nason, F. E. (2000). The family as a resource in ophthalmic care. In D. M. Albert & F. A. Jacobiec (Eds.), *Principles and Practice of Ophthalmology.* Philadelphia, W.B. Saunders Company. 6: 54885493.

Gilbert, C., & Foster, A. (2001). Childhood blindness in the context of VISION 2020—the right to sight. *Bulletin of the World Health Organization, 79*(3), 227–232.

Gilmour, G., Schreiber, C., et al. (2009). An examination of the relationship between low vision and Charles Bonnet syndrome. *Canadian Journal of Ophthalmology, 44*(1), 49–52.

Girdler, S. J., Boldy, D. P., et al. (2010). Vision self-management for older adults: a randomised controlled trial. *British Journal of Ophthalmology, 94*(2), 223–228.

Goldstein, J. (2011). *Relationship between functional ability and depressed mood in low vision patients.* Fort Lauderdale, FL: ARVO.

Harper, C. G., Giles, M., et al. (1986). Clinical signs in the Wernicke-Korsakoff complex: a retrospective analysis of 131 cases diagnosed at necropsy. *Journal of Neurology, Neurosurgery, & Psychiatry, 49*(4), 341–345.

Hassell, J. B., Lamoureux, E. L., et al. (2006). Impact of age related macular degeneration on quality of life. *British Journal of Ophthalmology, 90*(5), 593–596.

Hayman, K. J., Kerse, N. M., et al. (2007). Depression in older people: visual impairment and subjective ratings of health. *Optometry & Vision Science, 84*(11), 1024–1030.

Holroyd, S., & Shepherd, M. L. (2001). Alzheimer's disease: a review for the ophthalmologist. *Survey of Ophthalmology, 45*(6), 516–524.

Horowitz, A., & Reinhardt, J. P. (2000). Mental health issues in visual impairment: Research in depression, disability, and rehabilitation.

In B. Silverstone, Lang, M., B. Rosenthal, & E. Faye (Eds.), *The Lighthouse handbooks on vision impairment and vision rehabilitation* (pp. 1089–1109). New York: Oxford University Press.

Horowitz, A., Reinhardt, J. P., et al. (2003). The influence of health, social support quality and rehabilitation on depression among disabled elders. *Aging & Mental Health, 7*(5), 342–350.

Horowitz, A., Reinhardt, J. P., et al. (2005). Major and subthreshold depression among older adults seeking vision rehabilitation services. *American Journal of Geriatric Psychiatry, 13*(3), 180–187.

Huang, C. Q., Dong, B. R., et al. (2010). Chronic diseases and risk for depression in old age: a meta-analysis of published literature. *Ageing Research Reviews, 9*(2), 131–141.

Iliffe, S., Kharicha, K., et al. (2005). Self-reported visual function in healthy older people in Britain: an exploratory study of associations with age, sex, depression, education and income. *Family Practice, 22*(6), 585–590.

Jackson, M. L., & Ferencz, J. (2009). Charles Bonnet syndrome: visual loss and hallucinations. *Canadian Medical Association Journal, 181*(3–4), 175–176.

Jackson, M. L., & Bassett, K. L. (2010). The natural history of the Charles Bonnet syndrome. Do the hallucinations go away? *Eye (London), 24*(7), 1303–1304.

Jackson, M. L., Bassett, K., et al. (2007). Contrast sensitivity and visual hallucinations in patients referred to a low vision rehabilitation clinic. *British Journal of Ophthalmology, 91*(3), 296–298.

Jang, J. W., Youn, Y. C., et al. (2011). Hypermetabolism in the left thalamus and right inferior temporal area on positron emission tomography-statistical parametric mapping (PET-SPM) in a patient with Charles Bonnet syndrome resolving after treatment with valproic acid. *Journal of Clinical Neuroscience, 18*(8), 1130–1132.

Jones, N. P. (1990). Self-enucleation and psychosis. *British Journal of Ophthalmology, 74*(9), 571–573.

Kazui, H., Ishii, R., et al. (2009). Neuroimaging studies in patients with Charles Bonnet syndrome. *Psychogeriatrics, 9*(2), 77–84.

Klein, R., Chou, C. F., et al. (2011). Prevalence of age-related macular degeneration in the US population. *Archives of Ophthalmology, 129*(1), 75–80.

Kline, L. B., ed. (2010). *Basic and clinical science course (BCSC) 2010–2011: Neuro-ophthalmology Section 5.* San Francisco: American Academy of Ophthalmology.

Kopelman, M. D., Thomson, A. D., et al. (2009). The Korsakoff syndrome: clinical aspects, psychology and treatment. *Alcohol & Alcoholism, 44*(2), 148–154.

Lachs, M. S., & Pillemer, K. (2004). Elder abuse. *Lancet, 364*(9441), 1263–1272.

Lang, U. E., Stogowski, D., et al. (2007). Charles Bonnet syndrome: successful treatment of visual hallucinations due to vision loss with selective serotonin reuptake inhibitors. *Journal of Psychopharmacology, 21*(5), 553–555.

Large, M., Andrews, D., et al. (2008). Self-inflicted eye injuries in first-episode and previously treated psychosis. *Australia and New Zealand Journal of Psychiatry, 42*(3), 183–191.

Lazarus, R. S., & Folkman, S. (1984). *Stress, appraisal, and coping.* New York, Springer.

Lee, A. G. (2009). Vision loss and dementia. In A. G. Lee & H. A. Beaver (Eds.), *Geriatric Ophthalmology* (pp. 71–77). Dordrecht, Holland: Springer.

Lee, A. G., & Martin, C. O. (2004). Neuro-ophthalmic findings in the visual variant of Alzheimer's disease. *Ophthalmology, 111*(2), 376–380; discussion, 380–371.

Lee, E. K., & Brennan, M. (2006). Stress constellations and coping styles of older adults with age-related visual impairment. *Health & Social Work, 31*(4), 289–298.

Liu, Y., & Rhee, D. J. (2013). Acute bilateral angle closure. *Journal of the American Medical Association: Ophthalmology, 131*(9), 1231–1232.

McCabe, C. F., & Donahue, S. P. (2000). Prognostic indicators for vision and mortality in shaken baby syndrome. *Archives of Ophthalmology, 118*(3), 373–377.

Menon, G. J. (2005). Complex visual hallucinations in the visually impaired: a structured history-taking approach. *Archives of Ophthalmology, 123*(3), 349–355.

Menon, G. J., Rahman, I., et al. (2003). Complex visual hallucinations in the visually impaired: the Charles Bonnet syndrome. *Survey of Ophthalmology, 48*(1), 58–72.

Miller, N. R. (2005). Neuro-ophthalmological manifestations of nonorganic disease. In R. Miller, N. J. Newman, V. Biousse, & J. B. Kerrison (Eds.), *Clinical Neuro-ophthalmology* (pp. 1315–1334). Baltimore, MD: Williams & Wilkins.

Mogk, L. G., & Mogk, M. (2010). *Macular degeneration.* New York: Random House Publishing Group.

Mollenkopf, H., Wahl, H.-W., et al. (2007). Affective well-being in old age. *European Psychologist, 12*(2), 119–129.

O'Donnell, C. (2005). The Greatest Generation meets its greatest challenge: Vision loss and depression in older adults. *Journal of Visual Impairment & Blindness, 99*(4), 197–208.

Orr, A., & Rogers, P. (2006). *Aging and vision loss: A handbook for families.* New York: American Foundation for the Blind.

Owsley, C., McGwin, G. Jr., et al. (2009). Characteristics of low-vision rehabilitation services in the United States. *Archives of Ophthalmology, 127*(5), 681–689.

Patton, N. (2004). Self-inflicted eye injuries: a review. *Eye (London), 18*(9), 867–872.

Prevent Blindness America (2012). United States' estimated number of cases by vision problem age ≥ 40. Vision problems in the U.S. Prevalence of adult vision impairment and age-related eye disease in America. Retrieved October 9, 2013, from http://www.visionproblemsus.org/.

Purdy, E. P., Bolling, J. P., et al. (2010). *Antipsychotic drugs. Update on General Medicine 2010–2011.* San Francisco: American Academy of Ophthalmology.

Purdy, E. P., Bolling, J. P., et al. (2010). *Antidepressants. Update on General Medicine 2010–2011.* San Francisco: American Academy of Ophthalmology.

Rees, G., Tee, H. W., et al. (2010). Vision-specific distress and depressive symptoms in people with vision impairment. *Investigative Ophthalmology & Visual Science, 51*(6), 2891–2896.

Renaud, J., & Bedard, E. (2013). Depression in the elderly with visual impairment and its association with quality of life. *Clinical Interventions in Aging, 8,* 931–943.

Rhee, D. J., Colby, K. A., et al. (2011). *Ophthalmologic drug guide.* New York: Springer.

Riazi, A. D., Dain, S. J., Boon, M. Y., & Bridge, C. (2011). Innovative strategies for adaptation to loss of vision. *Clinical & Experimental Optometry, 94*(1), 98–102.

Richa, S., & Yazbek, J. C. (2010). Ocular adverse effects of common psychotropic agents: a review. *Central Nervous System Drugs, 24*(6), 501–526.

Rovner, B. W. (2006). The Charles Bonnet syndrome: a review of recent research. *Current Opinion in Ophthalmology, 17*(3), 275–277.

Rovner, B. W., & Casten, R. J. (2001). Neuroticism predicts depression and disability in age-related macular degeneration. *Journal of the American Geriatric Society, 49*(8), 1097–1100.

Rovner, B. W., Casten, R. J., et al. (2006). Minimal depression and vision function in age-related macular degeneration. *Ophthalmology, 113*(10), 1743–1747.

Rovner, B. W., Casten, R. J., et al. (2007). Preventing depression in age-related macular degeneration. *Archives of General Psychiatry, 64*(8), 886–892.

Rufa, A., Rosini, F., et al. (2011). Wernicke encephalopathy after gastrointestinal surgery for cancer: causes of diagnostic failure or delay. *International Journal of Neuroscience, 121*(4), 201–208.

Schoenfeld, M. A., Hassa, T., et al. (2011). Neural correlates of hysterical blindness. *Cerebral Cortex, 21*(10), 2394–2398.

Scott, J. A., & Egan, R. A. (2003). Prevalence of organic neuro-ophthalmologic disease in patients with functional visual loss. *American Journal of Ophthalmology, 135*(5), 670–675.

Segers, K. (2009). Charles Bonnet syndrome disappearing with carbamazepine and valproic acid but not with levetiracetam. *Acta Neurologica Belgica, 109*(1), 42–43.

Singh, A., & Sorensen, T. L. (2010). The prevalence and clinical characteristics of Charles Bonnet syndrome in Danish patients with neovascular age-related macular degeneration. *Acta Ophthalmologica, 90*(5), 476–480.

Skinner, E. A., Edge, K., et al. (2003). Searching for the structure of coping: a review and critique of category systems for classifying ways of coping. *Psychological Bulletin, 129*(2), 216–269.

Stelmack, J. A., Tang, X. C., et al. (2008). Outcomes of the Veterans Affairs Low Vision Intervention Trial (LOVIT). *Archives of Ophthalmology, 126*(5), 608–617.

Stewart, J. F. (1995). Automated perimetry and malingerers. Can the Humphrey be outwitted? *Ophthalmology, 102*(1), 27–32.

Stone, J., Carson, A., et al. (2005). Functional symptoms and signs in neurology: Assessment and diagnosis. *Journal of Neurology, Neurosurgery, & Psychiatry, 76*(1), i2–i12.

Tan, C. S., Lim, V. S., et al. (2004). Charles Bonnet syndrome in Asian patients in a tertiary ophthalmic centre. *British Journal of Ophthalmology, 88*(10), 1325–1329.

Trauzettel-Klosinski, S. (2010). Rehabilitation for visual disorders. *Journal of Neuroophthalmology, 30*(1), 73–84.

Wernicke, C. (1968). Acute hemorrhagic superior polioencephalitis. *Archives of Neurology, 19*(2), 229–232.

World Health Organization (2003). *Elimination of avoidable blindness.* Geneva: World Health Organization.

World Health Organization (2014). *Change the definition of blindness.* Retrieved February 24, 2014, from http://www.who.int/blindness/Change%20the%20Definition%20of%20Blindness.pdf.

World Health Organization (2014). *Prevention of blindness and visual impairment. Refractive errors and low vision.* Retrieved February 24, 2014, from http://www.who.int/blindness/causes/priority/en/index5.html.

Zhang, X., Bullard, K., et al. (2013). Association between depression and functional vision loss in persons 20 years of age or older in the United States, NHANES 2005–2008. *Journal of the American Medical Association Ophthalmology, 131*(5), 573–581.

72.

OTOLARYNGOLOGY

Harold Bronheim

INTRODUCTION

Ear, nose, and throat (ENT) disorders are common, and surgery for them is performed in-hospital and outpatient settings throughout the country. The appropriate psychiatric evaluation and treatment of this patient population have been limited, in part, because of the difficulties in communication encountered in those patients with laryngectomy or tracheostomy. Although otolaryngology patients undergo extreme stress, it unfortunately occurs just at the time that they are least able to verbalize and communicate their basic needs. Therefore, because of the limitations in communication that occur postoperatively, it is important that basic aspects of the psychiatric evaluation be done as much as possible prior to surgery. Pre-operative depression, or premorbid personality disorders have been determined to be predictors of postoperative depression, coping, and quality of life (Fingeret et al., 2013; Aarstad et al., 2008). Head and neck surgeons fail to identify the patients most in need of psychosocial intervention, and screening tools are not widely disseminated (Sollner et al., 2001; Piril et al., 2007).

Psychiatric consultants will confront two important dilemmas in the approach to this patient group: one, diagnostic; and the other, therapeutic. Diagnostically, consultants will need to delineate the overlapping boundaries between normal adaptation and psychiatric morbidity, and therapeutically they will be challenged by the severe limitations of verbal communication (Bronheim et al., 1991a, 1991b; Callahan, 2004).

SPECIAL CLINICAL ISSUES IN OTOLARYNGOLOGY

The extensive head and neck surgery currently performed leads to longer postoperative courses and extended rehabilitation involving alterations in basic physical functions such as breathing, swallowing, speaking, hearing, and vision. Facial contours may be deformed and occlusive relationships disrupted. Chewing and swallowing may be grossly distorted. Oral-pharyngeal surgery usually involves tracheostomy, which may be permanent if the patient undergoes total laryngectomy or suffers from extensive tracheal stenosis. Postoperatively, the patient must not only come to terms with cancer and surgery, but also must live with a changed, disfigured self with marked impairments in speech (O'Hara et al., 1989; Lucente et al., 1987; Strain, 1985; Surman, 1986; Shapiro & Kornfeld, 1987; Bronheim et al., 1989). Repeated studies have delineated long-term effects on quality of life for the both the patient and partner that necessitate problem-focused interventions (Hammerlid et al., 1999; Gotay et al., 1998; De Boer et al., 1999; Semple et al., 2004; Derks et al., 2005).

In the approach to this patient population, the psychiatrist must be prepared to deal cohesively with the issues of (1) cancer, surgery, and life-threatening illness; (2) disfigurement; (3) difficulties with swallowing, speech, or hearing; and (4) long-term physical and psychological adaptation.

The collected stressors affecting the otolaryngology surgical patient easily reach extreme and catastrophic levels, and vulnerable individuals manifest a variety of symptoms that may persist for an extended period of time (National Comprehensive Cancer Network, 1999). Despite the intensity of the stress, not all individuals become symptomatic, as individual vulnerability is an important component of the stress response. The differentiation between adjustment disorder and depression is sometimes difficult. Nonetheless, when psychiatric symptoms disrupt physical rehabilitation or significantly affect social or psychological functioning, then depression is the more appropriate diagnosis to make, and more intensive psychiatric intervention is necessary. Consideration must be given to the possibility that the patient may have had a preexisting major depression, or a minor depression due to physical disease or medications. The patient must be followed because a seemingly milder adjustment disorder may evolve into a major depression over time.

SURGERY PLUS RADIATION IN THE SETTING OF CANCER TREATMENT

Although ENT cancers are approximately 5% of all cancers (American Cancer Society, 2008), patients with head and neck disease undergo an onslaught of frightening changes that go well beyond those experienced by most other surgical patients. The multiple organs and functions encompassed within the relatively small region of the face and neck give rise to an enormous variety of physical diseases, pathologies, and dysfunctions. The most common cancer, however, is squamous cell carcinoma, and it usually requires, in addition to surgery, adjunctive treatment with radiation and/or chemo-therapy (Urken & Biller, 1988).

Multiple stressors face the otolaryngology patient with cancer, including the fear of death, mutilation, and pain. However, because of its location on the face, or in the head and neck, the mutilation resulting from cancer surgery is often experienced as an assault on the total self (Greenacre, 1958). It is harder for ENT patients to isolate the self from the disease and distance themselves psychologically; especially when there are multiple overwhelming alterations in sensory and motor functions. Anxiety persists as patients' concerns remain focused on the new, significant functional changes and physical disfigurement.

Advances in otolaryngology technique have permitted more extensive resections of cancer surgically, as well abla-tion by radiation therapy. However, the surgical reconstruc-tions that are necessarily simultaneously performed create additional stressors on the patient by increasing postopera-tive morbidity, disability, and pain. Some patients require multiple surgical revisions, which can "stress" even healthy, well adapted individuals beyond endurable emotional limits (Bronheim et al., 1989). Accumulating postsurgical quality-of-life studies have indicated persistent serious problems with acute airway management and chronic dysphagia. These com-plications also lead to caretaker burnout and serious stress on partners and family (Kim et al., 2008; Miziara et al., 2009; Vickery et al., 2003). Radiation therapy combined with more intensive chemotherapy has been administered, which has increased the severity of mucositis, with serious and intracta-ble oral-facial pain. Although nonsurgical treatments of head and neck cancers have become more aggressive and surgical technique has been limited to enable preservation of function, the impact on quality of life has nevertheless been enormous (El-Diery et al., 2005).

DISFIGUREMENT AND RECONSTRUCTION

Head and neck surgery remains the most disfiguring of all surgery, with oral-mandibular surgery considered to be the most stressful (Dropkin et al., 1983). Disfigurement is highly associated with depression (Valente, 2004). Disfigurement may involve the loss of an eye, the shifting of the nose across the midline, facial and jaw asymmetry, a new orifice for the tracheostomy site, asymmetry of the neck by either surgi-cal dissection or skin and muscle grafts, and multiple scars and blemishes. Some patients will complain of having their "throats cut," or an inability to recognize themselves. They may have difficulty looking at their reflection in the mirror or being seen by the public. They may feel like a grotesque monster and notice people staring at them or abruptly turn-ing away. Head and neck patients may hide in their rooms and withdraw from the public view. Disfigurement has an extraor-dinary, involuntary impact on all visitors who are unfamiliar with the otolaryngology hospital setting, including medical staff or consultants. Even a minimally perceptible fright-ened reaction by the psychiatric consultant to the patient's

appearance can have a profound effect on the therapeutic rela-tionship. Facial disfigurement also has serious impact on fam-ily and other caretakers (Vickery et al., 2003).

Reconstructive surgery is undertaken mainly for the pur-pose of rapidly restoring fundamental functions such as chew-ing, swallowing, and breathing, or simply covering an open surgical wound. From a psychiatric standpoint, the main issues revolve around the patient's realistic preparedness for surgery and the possible consequences of further disfigure-ment or surgical complications. A common postoperative complication involves dysphagia and/or aspiration. Because of the significant morbidity associated with these conditions, more clinical trials are being conducted and new surgical techniques are being incorporated to improve functional out-comes (Logemann, 2006; Crary et al., 2004).

Because of its extraordinary social importance, deliberate efforts are made to preserve speech; even at the risk of increas-ing the difficulty of swallowing, and the risk of aspiration. Some patients who are non-adherent and who cannot abstain from eating even if adequately nourished with gastric tube feedings may undergo further surgery to physically separate the airway from the oral/hypo-pharyngeal space. In so doing, speech is sacrificed in order to preserve swallowing without aspiration. A psychiatric assessment of such individuals usu-ally reveals either cognitive impairment with poor impulse control, or socially isolated alcoholics who would rather con-tinue to imbibe than communicate.

Reconstructive surgery may also be undertaken either to repair a preexisting physical deformity, or to achieve enhanced cosmetic appearance. Reconstructive surgery in obviously deformed young children generally leads to an improvement in their interpersonal behavior and cognitive development (Kalick, 1982; Belfer et al., 1982). Individuals who seek sur-gery for purely cosmetic reasons are found to be more anxious as a group and tend to suffer from a poor self-image that they hope surgery will improve. Nevertheless, for many, cosmetic surgery leads to an enhanced sense of well-being with a cor-responding increase in social activity (Marcus, 1984).

Psychiatric evaluation of individuals undergoing cosmetic or reconstructive surgery therefore must focus on the nature of their body image and their expectations about how they will be affected by the change. Unrealistic expectations are more likely to lead to postoperative disappointment and mal-adjustment. Individuals at risk include: those who insist on undergoing extensive or life-threatening surgical interven-tions for relatively benign deformities, or those who undergo surgery on features with prominent psychological meaning; and those with deformities which have existed for many years. More favorable outcomes are achieved in cosmetic surgery performed on females, especially on those features that have rapidly changed due to aging and have outpaced the changes in their inner body image (Goin & Goin, 1981). "Refreshing" the face or neck of a woman age 60 who feels that she is look-ing old and unattractive is seldom as complicated psychologi-cally as, for example, doing a rhinoplasty on a young man who feels his lack of success professionally or socially is due mainly to a slightly prominent, non-ideal, nose. Nevertheless, once they have begun, some patients undergo repeated cosmetic procedures to relieve psychological distress inherent to characters with Body Dysmorphic Disorder.

SPEECH

Speech is the most powerful, immediate, and versatile means of communication and is especially important during periods of acute distress. Speech, autonomy, and personal identity are closely linked. The inability to adequately regulate speech, which occurs as a result of laryngeal and oral-maxillary, pharyngeal surgery or tracheostomy, leads to a sense of urgency, increases in tension and frustration, followed by helplessness and withdrawal (Hagglund & Heikki, 1980). Because of difficulties in comprehensible speech and articulation, verbalization is limited in both quantity and quality. Therefore, whenever speech is attempted, it is markedly limited, and of necessity is focused on the immediate issues of physical needs. Social intercourse, personal communication, and the expression of inner feelings are subtler and more complex, require greater vocal capability and time to fully communicate, and are substantially compromised by such surgery.

Otolaryngology patients are unable to verbalize sufficiently to adequately relate emotions such as anxiety, frustration, sadness, or anger. They are unable to communicate feelings of hopelessness or wishes to end their current suffering one way or another. As a result, they may "act out" on the unit when they become frustrated and are more likely to throw objects and be physically aggressive to staff (Edgecombe, 1984). The psychiatrist, by initiating the process of verbalization, facilitates the process of integrating the new body image and personal identity. It also initiates the important discharge of affect with its concomitant reduction in stress. In the section below, the subject of psychotherapy will be discussed in the context of deficits in communication. The need to facilitate speech and the advantages of new communication technologies will also be reviewed below (Kluin, 1984; Hess, 2005).

ADAPTATION AND PSYCHIATRIC SYNDROMES

Although the majority of otolaryngology patients manage a successful adaptation, they may undergo a stormy, prolonged, and difficult course (West, 1974, 1977). The postoperative period is complicated by alterations that may persist after discharge from the hospital, even with rehabilitation. A number of psychosocial factors have been reported to be correlated with long-term postoperative adaptation (West, 1974; Natvig, 1983a; Anderson, 1987; Meyers et al., 1980; Mumford et al., 1982; Schleifer et al., 1989), and a variety of overlapping psychosomatic disorders (Marek, 2009). Preoperatively, the more patients are informed of what physical alterations they can expect immediately after surgery, the more rapidly they are likely to engage in physical rehabilitation (Natvig, 1983a). The unprepared patient will almost certainly require more time and attention to cope with the trauma of new physical alterations. Postoperatively, physical rehabilitation and

speech therapy have been found to improve long-term outcome as well as quality of life (Frans, 2007). Active coping strategies, more commonly observed in younger patients, lead to better outcomes; at least initially, nevertheless, patients with persistent major defects may suffer from long-term interpersonal disturbances with depression and social withdrawal, especially if the defect involves speech (West, 1974; El-Deiry et al., 2005).

Individuals with personality disorders with limited coping mechanisms, or those with cognitive dysfunction, or, both, are particularly vulnerable. Otolaryngology patients have very high rates of alcohol abuse and or nicotine dependence (Baile, 2008; Prout et al., 1997). In addition, individuals with poor family, social, or religious supports are also at risk for psychological dysfunction (Natvig, 1983a; Dhooper, 1985). Early psychiatric examination and intervention can improve long-term adaptation, through the treatment of existing comorbid psychiatric disorders and relief of psychological dysfunction (Buckman, 2008). Optimal long-term rehabilitation, which includes modulation of mood, recovery of physical function, and improved social and work relationships, strongly depends on efforts initiated immediately postoperatively (Anderson, 1987; Mumford et al., 1982). Nevertheless, the distinction between normal and abnormal adaptation as well as the delineation of specific psychiatric syndromes postoperatively remains problematic for the psychiatric diagnostician.

Although some patients make good physical adaptations to the tracheostomy from the standpoint of speech, breathing, and physical endurance, psychologically they may not be as successful. Patients may become more withdrawn and less active than prior to surgery. They may be embarrassed and feel "disgusting" because of bronchial secretions or drooling. The sexual life of these patients may be completely devastated.

When initially examined, there may be no formal, overt psychiatric disorder. Although psychological symptoms may be sub-threshold in magnitude during the initial psychiatric evaluation, with recurrent disease the patient is at substantial risk for developing more fulminant psychiatric syndromes, such as depression, anxiety, or other behavioral disturbances. Substance abuse is a frequent diagnosis in this very high-risk population whose disease may well have been caused by alcohol or nicotine dependency. Major psychological distress is found in head and neck cancer patients (Kirsten, 2008). Only a small portion of patients receive psychological support (Singer et al., 2005; Buckman, 2008), even though practice guidelines have been delineated (National Comprehensive Cancer Network, NCCN, 1999).

Psychiatric syndromes and disorders observed in studies of otolaryngology patients differ by the site of observation. Those examined in a liaison setting on an inpatient head-and-neck surgical service in the United States (Bronheim et al., 1991a) are listed in Table 72.1. Adjustment disorders were the most common Axis I disorder. Substance abuse and cognitive-impairment disorders were also frequently diagnosed. Major mood disorders and anxiety were also commonly observed. A significant portion of patients had definite Axis II disorders. A retrospective review of 189 laryngectomy

Table 72.1 PSYCHIATRIC DIAGNOSES AMONG OTOLARYNGOLOGY INPATIENTS PERIOPERATIVELY*

AXIS I (N = 143)		
No disorder	23.0%	32
Major mood disorder	10.1%	14
Anxiety disorder	1.4%	2
Somatoform/factitious	0.0%	0
Psychotic disorder	1.4%	2
Organic disorder	12.9%	18
Substance abuse disorder	18.0%	25
Adjustment disorders	36.0%	50
AXIS II-PERSONALITY DISORDERS (N = 139)		
No disorder	54.0%	75
Definite personality disorder	18.0%	25
Deferred or unknown diagnosis	28.1%	39

*The patients were consulted in the context of a liaison intervention at the Mount Sinai Hospital from, 1980–1986. The cohort represents a mix of standard consultations plus others identified by or to the liaison psychiatrist. The cohort does not represent a screening sample (Bronheim et al., 1991a).

patients in clinic settings in Germany revealed high rates of alcohol dependency and mood disorder (Herrman et al., 2005). High levels of anxiety and depression were also found in patients with chronic sinusitis, and demonstrate the unusually stressful impact of these chronic conditions and their repeated treatment (Bhattacharyya & Wasan, 2008). In a survey of 106 patients in British outpatient ENT clinics, 39% had an anxiety disorder, and 27% had depression (Veer et al., 2010).

MAJOR MOOD DISORDERS

Given the extreme-to-catastrophic nature of the stressors in the otolaryngology setting, it is not surprising that the most common psychiatric diagnosis encountered was adjustment disorder; either depressed or anxious. Although patients may suffer distress that may warrant consultation, the magnitude of psychological impairment may nonetheless remain at a sub-threshold level of a major mood or panic disorder. Most patients with adjustment disorder do go on, however, to make slow but adequate psychological adaptation over time, with the advent of physical recuperation and social reintegration. Although studies have demonstrated the significant impact of a variety of medical disorders on clinical outcomes (Lesperance et al., 1996; Von Korf et al., 1992), the diagnosis of depression is often complicated by problems of definition and measurement (House, 1988; Kathol et al., 1990a; Mason & Frosch, 1989). Diagnosis of depression in the medically ill

differed by as much as 13%, depending on the diagnostic system, and frequently was falsely positive (Kathol et al., 1990b). The Hamilton Rating Scale for depression depends heavily upon somatic symptoms for the diagnosis and is likely to be over-inclusive of physically ill patients (Rapp & Vrana, 1989; Hamilton, 1960). The Beck Depression Inventory, which depends heavily on cognitive factors, yields false-positive results in patients with transient delirium, which is also common in medically ill populations (Endicott, 1984; Beck et al., 1961). Furthermore, psychological cognitive and vegetative symptoms commonly remit with the alleviation of the medical illness, pain treatment, or improvement postoperatively (Kathol et al., 1990a), which further complicates the reliability of the diagnosis.

The diagnosis of major depression is especially difficult to ascertain in this patient population. Derangements in speech, appetite, swallowing, breathing, and sleeping, and the direct effects of cancer, may all obscure the diagnosis (Holland et al., 1977). Somatic symptoms are often unreliable in establishing a diagnosis and need to be replaced with another symptom domain that is *ideational* or *behavioral* and less liable to distortion by physical illness. Nevertheless, when in addition to being in a depressed mood, the patient becomes extremely needy, pessimistic, angry, brooding, or hopeless over a sustained period of time, the diagnosis of major depression should be made and treatment with antidepressants initiated (Endicott, 1984). Hopeless despair and anhedonia are primary markers for major depression. Hopelessness in particular is a major risk factor for suicide.

ANXIETY AND PANIC

The vulnerable patient who is unprepared and subjected to the trauma of multiple surgeries or complications may develop a sustained anxiety state with intermittent panic and hyperarousal, alternating with numbness and emotional exhaustion. This mental traumatization may evolve to a fully realized syndrome of post-traumatic stress disorder (PTSD) (Marek, 2009). On the other hand, the patient with a tracheostomy who appears to be acutely panicked may be suffering discomfort due to intermittent airway obstruction, bronchospasm, and hypoxemia. Before making a diagnosis of general anxiety or panic disorder, careful consideration to the adequacy of the patient's airway and blood gases should be given (Basawaraj et al., 1990).

SUBSTANCE DEPENDENCY AND AGITATION

Because head and neck tumors are associated with long-term alcohol and tobacco use, a large proportion of otolaryngology patients are male and many have alcohol-related dementias or other cognitive-impairment disorders related to alcohol abuse. In the head and neck surgical setting, the postoperative course is commonly complicated by agitation due to alcohol and nicotine withdrawal—both of which can also mimic panic disorder. Because of the effects of alcohol use, underlying dementia may first present itself on the ENT service in the context of a postoperative delirium. Individuals with compromised cognitive capacity due to cerebral atrophy are more susceptible to delirium occurring as a result of anesthesia, infection, anemia, hypoxemia, or other metabolic factors.

Alcohol and nicotine use are common in head and neck patients, and alcohol withdrawal must be considered in every patient with postoperative delirium. When patients undergo long reconstructive surgery, the operative report should be reviewed for episodes of hypotension or an unrecognized drop in hematocrit. A neurological exam needs be performed to rule out a cerebral ischemia. Delirium may be caused by aspiration of contaminated secretions from the oral/pharyngeal/laryngeal surgical wound into the lungs. Medications need be carefully reviewed in a patient whose delirium persists over an extended period of time.

The assessment of dementia on the ENT service is particularly difficult when the patient has a tracheostomy (Strain et al., 1988). Patients with delirium will "mouth" long responses even when they cannot be understood, and may refuse to write responses to direct requests to do so. They are also unable to simply cover the tracheostomy tube opening with their finger in order to phonate. These are maneuvers that cognitively intact individuals attempt to learn to provide as much comprehensible communication as possible. Patients with delirium cannot learn these basic maneuvers, nor can they recognize that they cannot be understood by others, and consequently they persist in their ineffectual attempts.

This patient population with alcohol and nicotine addictions, delirium, and suicidal and violent behaviors captures many of the principal clinical problems encountered in medical psychiatry.

THERAPEUTIC APPROACH

The treatment of head and neck patients to some extent poses an even greater challenge to the consulting psychiatrist than the diagnostic dilemmas that are presented. Treatment, as elsewhere in the medical-surgical setting, is tailored to the individual needs of the patient, such as antidepressants for major depressions and supportive therapy for adjustment reactions. All too often, however, psychiatric consultants unfamiliar with the otolaryngology setting overprescribe medication when supportive psychotherapy might be the better treatment of choice. Combination therapy or the sequential application of a variety of therapies is often necessary. Following is a brief discussion of the most common therapeutic modalities and how they may be specially modified in the head and neck setting.

PSYCHOTHERAPY

The intensity of the stressors makes psychosocial intervention necessary in the head and neck surgical service, especially problem-focused supportive psychotherapy (Doering, 2009; Semple, et al., 2009, 2014; Marek, 2009). Because of the profound patient disfigurement, the first reaction of many psychiatrists is to politely retreat from the ENT setting as soon as possible (Spikes & Holland, 1975; Buckley, 1986). Patients, however, are intensely sensitive, if not overly so, to the effects of their appearance on others and respond to the psychiatrist's behavior in kind. Patients will observe from the beginning whether the consulting psychiatrist is sufficiently comfortable to enter into a meaningful, ongoing therapeutic relationship. Poor doctor–patient communication has a negative impact on the patient's physical and psychological recovery (Lehmann et al., 2009).

By practice and history, psychiatry has adopted a receptive role in examining patients, trying to listen empathically while encouraging the patient to speak. Obviously, this will not proceed smoothly on the ENT service, and psychiatrists must be prepared to assist a patient in communication through an active participation (Bronheim, 1994). For the purposes of efficiency, psychiatrists must supply their own phrases to fill in the gap of feelings probably intended to be, but not fully expressed among the patient's short written phrases and facial and hand gestures. Psychiatrists must try to express for patients what the patients are unable to express for themselves.

The face is the most highly cathectic part of the body image, and we all retain primitive, repressed fears of grotesque distortion of body parts. Few experiences in life prepare one for the dramatic disfigurement that occurs as a result of maxillofacial surgery. As a result, the reflection that patients confront with their first look in the mirror can be so horrifying as to significantly traumatize them and delay their psychological and physical recovery. Psychotherapy requires a sensitive but firm exploration of this charged issue of disfigurement. Direct inquiries should be made about a patient's changed appearance and the attendant feelings; as well as the frustration of not being able to speak for themselves.

Supportive psychotherapy involves deliberate efforts to reduce patient stress and anxiety. The more consulting psychiatrists know about the expected course of medical/surgical treatment of the patient, the more helpful they can be to the patient in alleviating their anxiety. Otolaryngology patients have only infrequent discussions with anybody who is knowledgeable about their condition and therefore are motivated to discuss the course of treatment, including a review of the events and emotions leading up to the present state. The psychiatrist may be the only one who enters into a deep exploration of the patient's fears and thoughts and is therefore uniquely positioned to correct cognitive distortions and unfounded fantasies. In this active participatory manner, psychiatrists may build a narrative of affect that communicates their understanding to the patient, and in some instances the psychiatrist literally speaks for the patient. As a result, therapeutic interviews tend to be of shorter duration, and more frequent contacts are necessary (Groves & Kucharski, 1986).

Over the past decade, cognitive behavioral therapy (CBT) has been the type of psychotherapy most often discussed in the medical setting. In Meniere's disease, for example, "intolerance of anxiety" has been identified as the underlying abnormal cognition (Kirby & Yardley, 2009). CBT involves the identification of abnormal cognitive concerns and behavioral preoccupations; the setting of here-and-now goals in treatment; repeated exposure to the causes of anxiety; confrontation of non-adherence to healthy new behaviors; and supporting the participation in relaxation exercises. Nonetheless, a review of CBT studies in ENT found that it has not demonstrated significant advantage over other stress reduction techniques (Martinez-Devesa et al., 2010). Many of the particular techniques currently considered in CBT have been taught as part of supportive psychotherapy in the clinical literature of the past. Therefore, psychotherapy with this patient population must be eclectic, with the psychiatrists' being flexible in their ability to adapt the psychotherapeutic approach to the needs of the patient at any given time.

DRUG THERAPY

Pharmacological therapy is frequently necessary and is the treatment of choice in a number of situations. In general, oral administration of medications is partially or completely well tolerated. However, patients who have undergone oral-pharyngeal-laryngeal surgery may for a time have profound deficits in swallowing and an inability to ingest medications without coughing or aspiration. Since the remainder of the gastrointestinal system is intact and functional, the consulting psychiatrist in this setting may need to recommend the placement of a feeding tube to facilitate access for the timely administration of medication as well as food and water. The psychiatrist may be the only physician to witness the patient's difficulty with swallowing. When necessary, the parental administration of psychotropics should be considered.

The diagnosis of depression in the medical setting is problematic, but, when made, depression should be treated promptly and adequately with the addition of antidepressants. Selective serotonin reuptake inhibitors (SSRIs) such as sertraline, citalopram, escitalopram, or fluoxetine, as well as combination agents such as duloxetine, mirtazapine, and venlafaxine, are now generally preferred for initial pharmacotherapy. Bupropion should be avoided because of the risk of seizure disorder in this patient population. Although many individuals diagnosed with depression may remit with improvement in their physical condition, some studies of depression in medical-surgical settings indicate that pre-surgical antidepressant treatment is superior for decreasing postoperative depression in select patients and that antidepressant use improves post-op rehabilitation and facilitates the return to work (Lydiatt et al., 2008; Schleifer et al., 1989; Rifkin et al., 1985). Lydiatt et al. (2013) found in a randomized, double-blind, placebo-controlled clinical trial that prophylactic escitalopram (10–20 mg for 16 weeks) given to non-depressed patients about to undergo upfront treatment for head and neck cancer reduced the risk of depression by more than 50%, and the benefit for quality of life continued for three months after the medication was stopped.

The acute control of mania is seldom encountered in this setting, but, if necessary, all major antimanic agents such as lithium carbonate, carbamazepine, and valproate may be used. However, because of blood loss and volume shifts that may occur in extended surgical reconstructive cases, serum levels of antimanic agents and anticonvulsants should be checked postoperatively. Dosages should then be adjusted to ensure that therapeutic levels are maintained while simultaneously avoiding acute toxicity.

Grave's disease is a medical condition often diagnosed by ENT physicians, and diagnosis and treatment protocols can be found in most medical textbooks. A fifteen-year follow-up of 150 lithium-treated patients yielded an annual rate of hypothyroidism of 1.5%, leading to three thyroidectomies; the equivalent of a 2% incidence rate (Boachetta et al., 2007).

Because of the intense stress of otolaryngology surgery, panic attacks and general anxiety are common in this group. Lorazepam is the preferred medication. Buspirone and SSRIs are not used acutely perioperatively because of the long lag time necessary to obtain anxiolysis. However, they may be used in the outpatient setting postoperatively if chronic panic and anxiety persist, especially in patients with unresectable malignancies and those with a history of chemical and alcohol dependency.

In general, alcohol withdrawal is best managed with long-acting benzodiazepines such as diazepam or chlordiazepoxide hydrochloride. Because of the high incidence of alcoholism and high rates of hepatitis, cirrhosis, and alcohol-related brain atrophy in this patient population, lorazepam, by virtue of its renal excretion and intermediate half-life, as well as its administration by parenteral and sublingual routes, is advantageous for regular use in this setting. Because of the increased prevalence of mild dementia and other cognitive deficits in this patient population, drug-induced delirium occurs frequently, and benzodiazepines should be tapered rapidly. Very short-acting benzodiazepines such as triazolam should be avoided, as well as zolpidem, because of the problems of rebound anxiety, rebound insomnia, and the greater likelihood of nighttime confusion or amnesia. When alcohol withdrawal is thought to predominate (by history or physical exam), then more benzodiazepines such as lorazepam should be given, up to approximately 24 mg/day. Alcohol detox can be accomplished using alternative medications such as chlordiazepoxide and diazepam. In the intensive care unit (ICU), if in addition to anxiety the patient appears more discomfited by the endotracheal or tracheostomy tube, then narcotics should be added and titrated up until the patient is comfortably sedated. The decision about which combination of medications to be used and in what dosage is usually made on an empirical clinical basis.

Because of alcohol and nicotine withdrawal, as well as postoperative intermittent airway obstructions, panic-like states erupt postoperatively. Although serious attention must be given to airway suctioning, benzodiazepines should be employed in adequate doses to increase the patient's comfort and tolerance of the tracheostomy, as well as to block agitation due to withdrawal. Respiratory depression is seldom a problem and in general does not represent an impediment to adequate treatment.

In head and neck tumors, there is a significant effect on disease recurrence with recurrent alcohol abuse. Special efforts should be made for all patients who smoke or use alcohol to encourage smoking cessation and alcohol detoxification and abstinence. Alcohol cessation is a very important objective of psychosocial intervention. Alcoholism is a life-threatening illness that requires psychiatric support as well as a strong patient commitment. Alcoholics are not uncommonly treated with harshness by the medical-surgical staff because of their persistent self-destructive behavior that engenders feelings of hopelessness on the part of the medical staff. Alcoholism is an increasingly treatable disease incorporating individual psychotherapy, participation in support groups such as Alcoholics Anonymous (AA), and the utilization of prophylactic medications such as naltrexone, acamprosate, disulfram, and others.

Smoking cessation is also important in head and neck surgery and in all other otolaryngology patients (Prout et al., 1997). Various modalities have been demonstrated to be beneficial for use in this manner. When patients try to stop alone, success rates at one year are 5%. With behavioral intervention, they are up to 16%. With prophylactic medication, the success rates rises to as high as 24% (Laniado-Laborin, 2010). The medications include nicotine-replacement therapy, bupropion, and varenicline (Mechatie, 1998; Evins et al., 2008; Garrison & Dugan, 2009; Schrnoll et al., 2005; Webb et al., 2010; Stead et al., 2008). As of yet, which is the most advantageous medication is not clear (Doggrell, 2007).

Pain is seldom psychogenic in nature in otolaryngology and when present, usually reflects pathology, infection, or invasive tumor. Treatment with adequate dosage and frequency of narcotic analgesics relieves pain and lessens the overall quantity of narcotics requested and consumed; substance dependence as a result seldom, if ever, develops. More typically, patients suffer unnecessarily because, all too often, their pain is insufficiently managed with low doses of short-acting narcotics. The occasional substance-abusing patient who stridently demands narcotics at all times can be managed with methadone or other long-acting narcotics, OxyContin, opana, and so on, in fixed doses, which can be slowly tapered over seven to ten days. Patients should be observed for drug accumulation, mental obtundation, and respiratory depression due to the long half-life of the narcotics used.

BEHAVIORAL TEAM APPROACH

The multidisciplinary team has been found to be particularly helpful in supporting families with acute crises as well as chronic long-term conditions; not the least of which is merely smoking cessation (Baile, 2008). Multiple functional disabilities occur in otolaryngology as a direct consequence of the surgery for the underlying disease. As a result, many individuals are overwhelmed and withdrawn in the immediate postoperative period. A behaviorally oriented team comprising the surgeon; occupational, speech, and physical therapists; nursing staff; and a psychiatrist work in conjunction to identify the patients at risk. The team creates a therapeutic milieu that is behaviorally active, rewarding the patient for progressive behaviors instead of passive acceptance or avoidance of somatic preoccupation and regression. In so doing, the team actively prepares the patient for a resumption of life

postoperatively and the transition from the hospital to the home environment (Natvig, 1983b; Dropkin, 1989; Petrucci & Harwick, 1984).

Family members are directly affected by disfigurement and other bodily alterations in the head and neck surgery patients. The negative impact of disfigurement, cancer, surgical wounds, ostomies, and secretions can be severe (Kim et al., 2008). Therapy in the form of family groups is beneficial in supporting both the patient and family members who are overwhelmed. Couple and family groups can be used to correct inappropriate behaviors and facilitate in-hospital teaching of tracheostomy care (Dhooper, 1985; Vogtsberger et al., 1985; Fiegenbaum, 1981). Just as families benefit from support groups and family therapy, effective drug and alcohol rehabilitation almost always requires group participation. Unfortunately, despite observed benefits, up to 80% of families decline to participate in multi-family group-support programs (Ostroff et al., 2004). Long-term benefits and improvements in quality of life have been observed in patients who participate in group psychotherapy (Hammerlid et al., 1999). Patients with pain disorders, disabling dizziness, or vertigo also benefit from involvement with similarly affected individuals in Group Psychotherapy (Miziara et al., 2009). Visitations in the hospital by carefully selected volunteers can be profoundly helpful to patients who are traumatized by head and neck surgery and disfigurement. The psychiatrist can play a central role in formulating a treatment plan for the otolaryngology patient by being the one clinician sufficiently informed enough by all parties to integrate all the biopsychosocial factors involved in the patient's illness and rehabilitation.

SPECIAL TOPICS

AIDS TO COMMUNICATION

In order to communicate effectively with head and neck surgical patients, especially those with laryngectomies, the psychiatrist must effect a close relationship despite all the physical obstacles to normal communication. At first, the nonverbal efforts by the psychiatrist communicate to patients a willingness to search for deeper thoughts and feelings. Helping to arrange the patients so they can write more comfortably and then adopting a receptive pose allows the patients to more fully express their feelings. When unable to write, letter boards and other devices may be used in situations where the patient is too ill or in the ICU.

The presence of a tracheostomy does not necessarily imply the inability to communicate. In many cases it does not even mean the absence of the larynx or vocal cords. Tracheostomy may be necessary either temporarily postoperatively or in situations of chronic airway narrowing or obstruction. Simple adjustments of the size of the cuffed tracheostomy can lead to significant changes in the patient's acceptance of the tube (Kluin et al., 1984). Less physical inspiratory effort is required to quickly suck in sufficient air in a larger bore tracheostomy tube. Speech can then be produced by covering the tracheostomy opening with one's finger and forcing air up and through the vocal cords—producing sound. It may become necessary to repeatedly refocus the patient on the best respiratory efforts to produce audible, comprehensible language. In-depth communication with a patient on a ventilator is facilitated by the use of a one valve on a tracheostomy tube (Hess, 2005). The consultant psychiatrist who is aware of the alternatives can advise the respiratory care team to consider exchanging the tracheostomy for one of several special tubes with one-way speaking valves (Cazolli, 1999).

Speech restoration following laryngectomy and the removal of the vocal cords has always been an important goal for head and neck surgeons. Speech can be produced by creating a vibrating column of air that is funneled through other tissue spaces and then to the oral pharynx to produce sound. The most common surgical procedure to restore speech in this manner is the tracheo-esophageal puncture (TEP) (Hamaker et al., 1985; Halvorson & Kuhn, 1997). Some patients who are overwhelmed or unmotivated to make an active effort to do so, fail to communicate effectively; thus becoming depressed and withdrawn.

For those who cannot tolerate surgery, rehabilitation with a speech therapist utilizing mechanical and electronic devices is necessary. In them, sound is produced by creating the voice artificially. The most commonly employed communication aids involve trans-cervical sound production, which may be generated by positioning the device carefully in the neck (an electronic larynx). Vibration is transmitted from the vocal tract through the neck and then converted to synthetic speech. Although easy to use, these devices produce a voice that sounds artificial. With newer computer technology and voice reproduction programming, signal recognition and amplification is being converted to more natural-sounding voice production. Visits to the bedside by a former patient who has suffered through similar surgery and rehabilitation are particularly helpful in demonstrating mechanical devices and speech for a patient who is anxious about the future.

Group therapy is of invaluable benefit for the laryngectomy patient and family. A network of self-help groups exists for similarly afflicted patients. For those unable to attend groups, individual online groups' internet postings are of unique benefit to individuals with speech deficits. Although online discussion can be recommended, it should not take the place of psychosocial rehabilitation, human contact, and re-socialization efforts.

HEARING LOSS AND DEAFNESS

Approximately 6% of the population has significant bilateral hearing impairment, approximately 45% of whom are over age 65 (Bailey et al., 1976). Twenty-five percent of people between ages 65 and 74 and 50% of those 75 years and older experience hearing difficulties (Anderson & Meyerhoff, 1986). Although there is no basis for an association with psychotic states, in the elderly, the "hard of hearing" are over-represented in cohorts of paranoid disorders (Cooper, 1976; Savoy et al., 1991; Eastwood et al., 1985). Because of communication deficits and social isolation, the hard of hearing are also more commonly afflicted with depressive disorders (Yovell et al., 1995; Lee & Gomez-Marin, 1997).

Deafness is also a major cause of speech retardation and associated behavioral impairments in children (Kaplan & Sadock, 1985). In children referred for a wide variety of school problems, 8% have abnormal hearing, 30% have abnormal speech discrimination in noise, and approximately 60% have abnormal auditory memory (Oberklaid et al., 1989). Therefore, a complete audiology assessment is warranted as part of the evaluation of all children with learning difficulties or developmental language disorders. Evaluation of hearing includes otoscopic examination of the ear canals and tympanic membrane, pure-tone and speech audiometry, stapedius reflex, and vestibular testing with nystagmography to distinguish between conductive and sensorineural deficits. Hearing sensitivity is measured for frequencies of 250–18000 cycles/sec (Hertz). A hearing threshold of 15 decibels (db) or less is considered normal, and an average hearing threshold of 30 db or less in the 500–3000 Hz zone is sufficient for ordinary needs. Amplification may be necessary if school or social activities require even better hearing. Although pure-tone measurements provide significant information, speech discrimination is equally important for the assessment of hearing deficits. Monosyllabic words can be presented at loud levels, and the percentage of words correctly identified is noted. Scores lower than 70%–80% indicate significant difficulties in understanding speech (Anderson & Meyerhoff, 1986). A functional prosthetic hearing aid is indicated for deafness, and individual fitting of a device should be performed by an audiologist. Complete deafness is very rare, and those with almost total deafness usually have remnants that can be utilized by high-performance hearing aids. Only in acoustic agnosia (sensory aphasia) is a functional hearing-aid prosthesis completely useless (Becher et al., 1989). Very young children can be tested with electric impedance-response audiometry (Becher et al., 1989).

Deaf children until recently were ordinarily educated in separate schools where sign language is taught (Becher et al., 1989). Recently, in select cases of children as well as adults, implantation of electrodes into the inner ear (the cochlear implant) has led to remarkable enhancement of acoustic perception. Although the device may lead to greater awareness of auditory stimuli, such as traffic sounds, loud speech, and syllabic vowels, not all patients will necessarily obtain the fine auditory discrimination necessary to decode all speech. As a result of the implant, therefore, individuals may develop enhanced communication and lip- and or sign-reading skills. Tensions over this issue pit advocates for cochlear implantation and potential "mainstreaming" of children against those in favor of "separate but equal" education and support for sign language and "deaf culture" (Davey, 2011).

The fastest growing cohort of beneficiaries of cochlear implantation has been the elderly with presbycusis. The surgery is relatively uncomplicated (Berke, 2011). Review studies indicate that the elderly benefit from the surgery as much as the young (Sahli et al., 2009), and that for those who are severely hard of hearing and successfully treated, a significant improvement in depression, loneliness, and quality of life has been achieved—equal to that seen in adolescents; even more than anticipated (Poissant, 2008; Sprinzl et al., 2010). The combination of implantation in one ear with hearing-aid amplification in the other can lead to significant improvement in speech recognition (especially high frequency) without loss to background noise (low frequency) (Olson & Shinn, 2008). As a group, individuals who undergo cochlear implantation experience an improvement in the quality of their lives with decreases in depression, anxiety, loneliness, and suspiciousness, even if up to a quarter of those patients are affected by mild to moderate tinnitus postoperatively (Anderson et al., 2009; Knutson et al., 1991; Harris et al., 1995). The psychiatrist's role, in addition to identifying the patients who are unmotivated or suffering from overt psychiatric syndromes, is to help patients and family cope with partial or limited results (McKenna, 1986; Tiber, 1985).

The management of the hearing impaired requires continuous attention directed at achieving optimum communication. The psychiatrist must remember to speak loudly, slowly, and clearly, preferably with the patient facing the lips and face of the consultant. Augmenting speech with physical, facial, and hand gestures adds to their overall comprehension and communication. Where the patient is severely deaf, sight must substitute for sound by writing, lip reading, or sign language. However, full rehabilitation requires patient, repetitive explanation and training in the use of a hearing aid (Anderson & Meyerhoff, 1986; Becher & Cohn, 1982). In general, individuals who are highly motivated, physically and socially active, and sensitive to the feelings of others, accept and adapt to the use of a hearing aid early.

Many patients who might potentially benefit from the adoption of a hearing aid give up too quickly. Resistance to the use of hearing aids is common, and not well understood. Resistance may involve physical factors, including discomfort due to poor fit of ear molds, ear canal infection, skin erosion, pain, and wax collection. Other individuals are sensitive to noise and find amplification painful (Becher & Cohn, 1982). Others who are unmotivated, socially inactive, physically immobile, depressed, or isolated will not make the necessary effort. Patients with chronic neurological disorders and dementia simply confuse the proper use of the device, such as remembering to put it in, turn it on, or change the batteries. Still others, as a result of growing dependency and interpersonal rigidity with aging, resist using a hearing aid as a means to engage in a power struggle or to avoid communication with those upon whom they depend (Savoy et al., 1991). Some individuals stubbornly resist all efforts to make communication with them easier for all those who would care to try. Behavioral approaches may be attempted, and may be beneficial in some situations.

TINNITUS AND DIZZINESS

A disorder closely related to hearing loss is tinnitus. Both hearing loss and tinnitus increase with age, and as the threshold for hearing increases, so does the severity of tinnitus. Approximately 2% of the population report significant tinnitus resulting in some disability (Coles et al., 1985). The etiology of tinnitus is unclear and may involve a combination of factors, including spontaneous firing of the auditory nerve, denervation hypersensitivity with neural loss, or central excitation as in phantom limb pain (Slater & Terry, 1987). Tinnitus may be tested by brain stem evoked potentials. Patients who suffer from tinnitus may be extremely sensitive to noise, as was Beethoven, who suffered recurrent bouts that worsened every winter (Slater & Terry, 1987). A host of medical conditions are associated with tinnitus, such as diabetes, thyroid disorders, and anemia; as well as drugs, particularly caffeine, nicotine, aspirin, non-steroidal antinflammatory drugs (NSAIDs), antibiotics, monoamine oxidase inhibitors, SSRIs, tricyclic antidepressants, buspirone, morphine, benzodiazepine, and many others (Slater & Terry, 1987; Seligmann et al., 1996). When tinnitus is accompanied by vertigo and deafness, Meniere's disease needs be considered. Where in addition to deafness there are symptoms of tinnitus, dizziness, and a disorder of balance, labyrinthine disease or acoustic neuroma (a surgically and focused-beam-radiation treatable condition) should be considered with further investigation by computerized tomography scan (CTS) with contrast or magnetic resonance imaging (MRI).

A significantly higher prevalence of psychiatric conditions is found in tinnitus sufferers. There is both a higher premorbid past history of depression as well as a higher comorbid incidence of major depression, with a lifetime prevalence as high as 78% (Sullivan et al., 1988). Anxiety is most associated with Meniere's disease (Kirby & Yardley, 2009). The patients most disabled by tinnitus are more likely to manifest behaviors associated with depression such as sleep disorders, poor concentration, and social withdrawal.

The treatment of tinnitus patients is multimodal. Hearing aids that amplify external sounds or produce sounds of a specific tone are commonly prescribed. Clearly, antidepressants are indicated in individuals with associated major depression. Although the underlying condition may not be eliminated by antidepressant treatment, the degree of disability and perceived suffering can be markedly improved. In addition, some patients have a robust response to even low doses of tricyclic antidepressants and fluoxetine (Shemen, 1998), perhaps because of their anxiolytic and sedating effects. Vertigo is treated with antihistamines and calcium channel blockers (Albera et al., 2003). Tinnitus is often most tormenting at nighttime, and the use of background music or white noise for masking the sensation, as well as anti-histamine medications, have been found helpful. Biofeedback and relaxation training have also been beneficially employed (Slater & Terry, 1987).

In very severe cases of tinnitus, sectioning of the vestibular nerve may be done, which ordinarily leads to dizziness due to asymmetrical input to the brain from the semicircular canals. However, in the otherwise healthy patient, rapid neurological accommodation leads to gradual improvement over time (Staffel & Pillsbury, 1993). Dizziness should always be distinguished from syncope. Syncope has multiple etiologies, including cardiac arrhythmias, orthostatic hypertension, cerebral vascular disease, or seizure disorder.

Unexplained dizziness, on the other hand, is a very common complaint in the outpatient medical setting, as well as the second most frequently reported symptom in panic disorder. Patients referred to otolaryngology clinics with complaints of dizziness have a high incidence of panic disorder: 15–20% (Clark et al., 1994; Stein et al., 1994). Other patients with unexplained vertigo demonstrate high rates of depression, anxiety, somatization, and sexual abuse (Jantos & White, 1997; Eckhardt-Henn et al., 2008). Clearly, there is a need for psychiatric consultation in the management of this difficult patient population.

In addition to examination for physical conditions discussed above, or anxiety and depression, special care should be given to obtaining a history of neglect and sexual or physical abuse. These individuals frequent multiple physicians and undergo much medical testing. Efforts should be made to limit redundant testing, and treatment should be initiated with appropriate pharmacotherapy and psychotherapy. For individuals reluctant to seek psychiatric care, support groups for a large variety of disorders exist that may be recommended, including for those suffering from chronic dizziness, tinnitus, or vertigo; and may be located on the internet at http://www.support-group.com.

SINUSITIS

Sinusitis affects approximately 15% of the population. Acute sinusitis is generally caused by *H. influenzae* or *S. pneumoniae* and may be satisfactorily treated with a short course of antibiotics (Kankam & Sallis, 1997). Persistent symptoms of sinusitis, including nasal congestion, rhinorrhea, facial pressure, and postnasal drip, can in most cases (85%) be treated with an extended course of antibiotics (4 weeks), nasal lavage, nasal corticosteroids, and topical decongestants. Fewer than 10% of chronic sinus sufferers will require surgery (McNally et al., 1997). The past decade has witnessed a clinical shift to endoscopic (and even robotic) techniques to virtually all surgical subspecialties. Endoscopic surgery has been particularly adapted to sinus surgery. Undiagnosed sinusitis is a common cause of intracranial pressure and pain, which often present as headache. MRI of a cohort of patients who presented to a neurology clinic with headache complaints revealed a 60% incidence of sinus disorders, two-thirds of whom had chronic sinusitis (Gordts et al., 1996).

High levels of anxiety and depression are associated with chronic sinusitis, but most of it goes undetected or untreated (Wasan et al., 2007; Bhattacharyya & Wasan, 2008; Macdonald et al., 2009). Depression is associated with poorer postoperative quality of life and chronic head pain (Chester, 2009; Mace et al., 2009; Chester et al., 2008). Conversely, depression was relieved by surgery that was successful in ameliorating chronic inflammation and facial pain (Litvack et al., 2011).

Migraine and chronic headaches are commonly seen in psychiatric practice and share overlapping symptoms of fatigue, depression, anxiety, and dizziness, which are associated with other common psychiatric disorders. Therefore, in patients with frequent headaches that are not classic in form, or in patients with a history of recurrent or allergic sinusitis, sinus evaluation by X-ray or CT to rule out air-fluid levels, polyps, and/or inflammation should be considered. Occult sinusitis is a frequent unrecognized diagnosis in both medical and psychiatric presentations.

SPECIAL ENT DISORDERS

Spastic dysphonia, pharyngeal spasm, atypical facial pain syndrome, temporomandibular joint disorder (TMJ), laryngitis due to unresponsive gastroesophageal reflux disease (GERD), and burning tongue syndrome are disorders that can mystify the general practitioner. These disorders, which all involve the face and mouth, are consulted upon by several subspecialists before eventual referral to a psychiatrist. Usually no explanatory organic etiology can be found, and psychological explanations are sought. Although these syndromes are associated with elevated rates of anxiety and depression, clinical experience suggests that, in addition to chronic somatization and depression, these disorders might involve dysfunction of the cranial nerves' nuclei and their interconnection through the ascending tracts of the fifth nerve. Clonazepam has been used successfully in pharyngeal spasm, chronic reflux esophagitis, and TMJ. Burning tongue syndrome frequently responds to antidepressants and smoking cessation, or supportive psychotherapy (Gao et al., 2009; Miziaria et al., 2009). Spastic dysphonia is treated surgically by methods that lead to vocal cord fixation. In these patients with atypical conditions, when the pain is successfully relieved, there is usually a return to baseline psychosocial function.

Patients with atypical facial pain syndromes are usually referred to neurologists to rule out trigeminal neuralgia. Although chronic pain patients manifest high rates of somatization, optimal management involves the combination of psychosocial treatment and pain management. Temporal mandibular joint (TMJ) pain disorder is normally managed in dental practices where mal-aligned bites are manipulated. There is a high incidence of recurrence of the disorder when patients are under stress. Clonazepam is prescribed at bedtime. Spastic dysphonia was for many years considered a conversion disorder. Although anxiety was known to exacerbate this disorder of speech, psychological studies of these patients failed to reveal either somatization or conversion disorder (Ginsberg et al., 1988). Nowadays, spastic dysphonia is considered a disorder of neurological origin with features that overlap with dystonia; thought to be caused by basal ganglia, or related dysfunction within the brainstem nuclei. Electromyographically guided injections of botulin toxin administered by the otolaryngologist achieve relaxation and approximation of the vocal cords to the midline. Botulin toxin injection has also been used in palatal and pharyngeal dystonia (Jankovic et al., 1991). In all these various facial pain and dystonic syndromes, chronically recurrent depression is invariably associated.

SUMMARY

The head and neck surgical service is a unique setting for psychiatrists to apply their skills. Psychiatrists will encounter emotional threats that affect the patient directly and possibly the psychiatrists' countertransference as well. Psychiatrists will need to participate actively with the patient, sometimes in unpleasant surroundings, and will need to be familiar with surgical techniques, tracheostomy, communication, and hearing devices, as well as other prosthetic and cosmetic options. The psychiatrists will need to rely on a variety of skills and diagnostic capabilities, as well as biological and psychosocial treatment techniques to facilitate the best adaptation of the otolaryngology patient to the overwhelmingly traumatic effects of surgery.

Because of the frequent alterations in speech, detection of patients at risk is normally quite limited. Therefore, even more than is indicated in other medical-surgical settings, a liaison psychiatric approach in screening for patients at risk is most successful. The continuous presence of a psychiatrist and the enhanced awareness of the surgical staff can lead to the identification and referral of vulnerable or subclinically symptomatic patients.

Lastly, a review of the psychiatric literature in otolaryngology reveals a lack of controlled studies that may reflect psychiatric discomfort in dealing with this patient population. More rigorous study of diagnosis, interventions, and outcomes is necessary to determine the most effective psychosocial care for these patients.

CLINICAL PEARLS

- It is harder for ENT patients to isolate the self from the disease and distance themselves psychologically; especially when there are multiple overwhelming alterations in sensory and motor functions.

- Disfigurement is highly associated with depression (Valente, 2004).

- Even a minimally perceptible frightened reaction by the psychiatric consultant to the patient's appearance can have a profound effect on the therapeutic relationship.

- From a psychiatric standpoint, the main issues revolve around the patient's realistic preparedness for surgery and the possible consequences of further disfigurement or surgical complications.

- Head and neck cancer patients have very high rates of alcohol abuse and or nicotine dependence (Baile, 2008; Prout et al., 1997).

- Patients after ENT surgery with delirium will "mouth" long responses even when they cannot be understood, and may refuse to write responses to direct requests to do so. They are also unable to simply cover the tracheostomy tube opening with their finger in order to phonate. They can neither learn basic communication maneuvers nor can they recognize that they cannot be understood by others, and consequently they may persist in their ineffectual attempts.

- For the purposes of efficiency, psychiatrists must supply their own phrases to fill in the gap of feelings probably intended, but not fully expressed, among the patient's short written phrases and facial and hand gestures. Psychiatrists must try to express for patients what the patients are unable to express for themselves.

- The reflection that patients confront with their first look in the mirror can be so horrifying as to significantly traumatize them and delay their psychological and physical recovery.

- The psychiatrist may be the only one who enters into a deep exploration of the patient's fears and thoughts and be uniquely positioned to correct cognitive distortions and unfounded fantasies.

- Lydiatt et al. (2013) found in a randomized, double-blind, placebo-controlled clinical trial, that prophylactic escitalopram (10–20 mg for 16 weeks) given to non-depressed patients about to undergo upfront treatment for head and neck cancer reduced the risk of depression by more than 50%, and the benefit for quality of life continued for three months after the medication was stopped.

- The fastest growing cohort of beneficiaries of cochlear implantation has been the elderly with presbycusis.

- When there are symptoms in addition to deafness of tinnitus, dizziness, and a disorder of balance, labyrinthine disease or acoustic neuroma (a surgically and focused-beam-radiation treatable condition) should be considered with further investigation by CT scan with contrast or MRI.

- Tinnitus is often most tormenting at nighttime, and the use of background music or white noise for masking the sensation, as well as anti-histamine medications, have been found helpful.

DISCLOSURE STATEMENT

Dr. Bronheim has nothing to disclose.

REFERENCES

Aarstad, A. K., et al. (2008). Personality and choice of coping predict quality of life in head and neck cancer patients during follow-up. *Acta Oncology, 47*(5), 879–890.

Albera, R., et al. (2003). Double-blind, randomized, multicenter study comparing the effect of betahistine and flunarzine on the dizziness handicap in patients with recurrent vestibular vertigo. *Acta Otolaryngology, 123,* 588.93.

American Cancer Society (2008). *Cancer facts and figures.* New York: American Cancer Society.

Anderson, E. A. (1987). Preoperative preparation for cardiac surgery facilitates recovery, reduces psychological distress, and reduces the incidence of acute postoperative hypertension. *Journal of Consulting Clinical Psychology, 55*(4), 513–520.

Anderson, G., et al. (2009). Tinnitus distress, anxiety, depression, and hearing problems among cochlear implant patients with tinnitus. *Journal of the American Academy of Audiology, 20*(5), 315–319.

Anderson, R. G., & Meyerhoff, W. L. (1986). Otologic disorders. In E. Calkins, P. Davis, & A. B. Ford (Eds.), *The practice of geriatrics* (Chap. 25). Philadelphia, PA: W.B. Saunders.

Baile, W. F. (2008). Alcohol and nicotine dependency in patients with head and neck cancer. Available at www.SupportiveOncology. net 6(4).

Bailey, H. A. T., Pappas, J. J., Graham, S., et al. (1976). Total hearing rehabilitation. *Archives of Otolaryngology, 162*, 323.

Basawaraj, K., Rifkin, R., Seshagiris, D., et al. (1990). The prevalence of anxiety disorders in patients with chronic obstructive pulmonary disease. *American Journal of Psychiatry, 147*(2), 200–201.

Becher, R. L., & Cohn, E. S. (1982). Problems of the eye and ear. In R. L. Becher, J. R. Burton, & P. D. Ziere (Eds.), *Principles of ambulatory medicine*. Baltimore, MD: Williams & Wilkins.

Becher, W., Naumann, H. H., & Pfaltz, C. R. (1989). *Ear, nose, and throat disorders*. Stuttgart, Germany: Thieme Medical Publishers.

Beck, A. T., Ward, C. H., & Mendelson, M. (1961). An inventory for measuring depression. *Archives of General Psychiatry, 4*, 561–571.

Belfer, M. L., Harrison, A. M., Pillemer, F. C., et al. (1982). Appearance and the influence of reconstructive surgery on body image. *Clinics in Plastic Surgery, 9*, 307–315.

Berke, J. (2011). Cochlear implant surgery: What happens at the hospital. About.com Deafness, available at http://deafness.about.com/od/basicinfocochlearimplants/a/cisurgery.htm.

Bhattacharyya, N., & Wasan, A. (2008). Do anxiety and depression confound symptoms reporting and diagnostic accuracy in chronic rhinosinusitis? *Annals of Otology, Rhinology, & Laryngology, 117*(1), 18–23.

Bocchetta, A, Cocco F et al. (2007). Fifteen-year follow-up of thyroid function in lithium patients. *Journal of Endocrinological Investigation, 30*(5), 363–366.

Bronheim, H. (1994). Psychotherapy of the otolaryngology patient. *General Hospital Psychiatry, 16*(2), 112–118.

Bronheim, H., Strain, J. J., Biller, H. F., et al. (1989). Psychiatric consultation on an otolaryngology service. *General Hospital Psychiatry, 11*, 95–102.

Bronheim, H., Strain, J. J., & Biller, H. F. (1991a). Psychiatric aspects of head and neck surgery, Part I. New surgical techniques and psychiatric consequences. *General Hospital Psychiatry, 13*, 165–176.

Bronheim, H., Strain, J. J., & Biller, H. F. (1991b). Psychiatric aspects of head and neck surgery, Part II. Body image and psychiatric interventions. *General Hospital Psychiatry, 13*, 225–232.

Buckley, P. (1986). Supportive psychotherapy: A neglected treatment. *Psychiatric Annals, 16*(19), 515–533.

Buckman, R. (2008). Practical suggestions for dealing with distress in patient with head and neck cancer. *Journal of Supportive Oncology, 6*(4), 164–165.

Case, J. L. (1984). *Clinical management of voice disorders* (Chap. 7). Rockville, MD: Aspen Publishers.

Callahan, C. (2004). Facial disfigurement and sense of self in head and neck cancer. *Social Work Health Care, 40*(2), 73–87.

Cazzolli, R. N. (1999). Talking with tracheostomy. Available at www.rideforlife.com/archives/00013.html; posted Sept 16, 1999, in Living with ALS.

Chester, A. C. (2009). Symptom outcomes following endoscopic sinus surgery. *Current Opinion in Otolaryngology & Head & Neck Surgery, 17*(1), 50–58.

Chester, A. C., et al. (2008). Systematic review of change in bodily pain after sinus surgery. *Otolaryngology—Head & Neck Surgery, 139*, 759–765.

Clark, D. B., Hirsch, B. E., Smith, M. G., et al. (1994). Panic in otolaryngology patients with dizziness or hearing loss. *American Journal of Psychiatry, 151*(8), 1223–1225.

Coles, R. R. A. (1985). Epidemiology of tinnitus (1). Prevalence. *Journal of Laryngology & Otology, 9*(Suppl), 7–15.

Cooper, A. F. (1976). Deafness and psychiatric illness. *British Journal of Psychiatry, 129*, 216–226.

Crary, M. A., et al. (2004). Functional benefits of dysphagia therapy using adjunctive sEMG biofeedback. *Dysphagia, 19*(3) 160–164.

Davey, M. (2011). Tensions over sign language vs. technology. *New York Times*, July 27, A1, A3.

De Boer, M. F., et al. (1999) Physical and psychosocial correlates of head and neck cancer: A review of the literature. *Otolaryngology—Head & Neck Surgery, 123*(3), 427–436.

Derks, W., et al. (2005). Differences in coping style and locus of control between older and younger patients with head and neck cancer. *Clinical Otolaryngology, 30*(2), 186–192.

Dhooper, S. S. (1985). Social work with laryngectomies. *Health & Social Work, 10*(3), 217–227.

Doering, S. (2009). Treatment preparation in psychosomatic medicine and psychotherapy. *Zeitschrift fur Psychosomatische Medizin und Psychotherapie, 55*(1), 27–36.

Doggrell, S. A. (2007). Which is the best primary medication for long term smoking cessation-nicotine replacement therapy, bupropion or varenicline? *Expert Opinion on Pharmacotherapy, 8*(17) 2903–2915.

Dropkin, M. J. (1989). Coping with disfigurement and dysfunction after head and neck surgery: A conceptual framework. *Seminars in Oncological Nursing, 5*(3), 213–219.

Dropkin, M. S., Malgady, R. G., Scott, D. W., et al. (1983). Scaling of disfigurement and dysfunction in post-operative head and neck patients. *Head & Neck Surgery, 16*(Sept/Oct), 559–570.

Eastwood, M. R., Corbin, S., Reed, M., et al. (1985). Acquired hearing loss and psychiatric illness: An estimate of prevalence and comorbidity in a geriatric setting. *British Journal of Psychiatry, 147*, 552.

Eckhardt-Henn, A., et al. (2008). Psychiatric comorbidity in different organic vertigo syndromes. *Journal of Neurology, 255*(3), 420–428.

Edgecombe, R. M. (1984). Models of communication. The differentiation of somatic and verbal expression. *Psychoanalytic Study of the Child XXXIX* (pp. 137–154). New Haven, CT: Yale University Press.

El-Deiry et al. (2005). Long-term quality of life for surgical and nonsurgical treatment of head and neck cancer. *Archives of Otolaryngology—Head & Neck Surgery, 131*(10), 879–885.

Epstein, J. B., & Epstein, J. D. (2008). Doxepin rinse management of mucositis pain in patients with cancer: One week follow up of topical therapy. *Special Care in Dentistry, 28*(2), 73–77.

Endicott, J. (1984). Measurement of depression in patients with cancer. *Cancer, 53*, 2243–2249.

Evins, A. E., et al. (2008). A controlled trial of buproprion added to nicotine patch and a behavior therapy for smoking cessation in adults with unipolar depressive disorders. *Journal of Clinical Psychopharmacology, 28*(6), 660–666.

Feenberg, A. L., Licht, J. M., Kane, K. P., et al. (1996). The online patient meeting. *Journal of the Neurological Sciences, 139*(Suppl), 129–131.

Fiegenbaum, W. (1981). A social training program for clients with facial disfigurations: A contribution to rehabilitation of cancer patients. *International Journal of Rehabilitation Research, 4*(4), 501–509.

Fingeret, M. C., & Hutchinson, K. A. (2013). Associations among speech eating, body imageconcerns for surgical patients with head and neck cancer. *Head & Neck, 35*(3), 354–360

Gao, J., et al. (2009). A case-control study on etiological factors involved in patients with burning mouth syndrome. *Journal of Oral Pathology & Medicine, 38*(1), 24–28.

Garrison, G. D., & Dugan, S. E. (2009). Varenicline: A first-line treatment option for smoking cessation. *Clinical Therapeutics, 31*(3), 463–491.

Gillenwater, M., et al. (2010). Multidimensional analysis of body image concerns among newly diagnosed patients with oral cavity cancer. *Head & Neck, 32*(3), 301–309.

Ginsberg, B. I., Wallach, J., Strain, J. J., et al. (1988). Spastic dysphonia. Toward defining the proper psychiatric role in the treatment of a disorder of unclear etiology. *General Hospital Psychiatry, 10*, 132–137.

Goin, J. M., & Goin, M. K. (1981). *Changing the body: The psychological effects of plastic surgery* (p. 5). Baltimore, MD: Williams & Wilkins.

Gordts, F., Clement, P. A., & Buisseret, T. (1996). Prevalence of sinusitis signs in a non-ENT population. *ORL: Journal for Oto-Rhino-Laryngology and Its Related Specialties, 58*(6), 315–319.

Gotay, C. C., et al. (1998). Quality of life in long-term survivors of adult-onset cancers. *Journal of the National Cancer Institute, 90*(9), 656–667.

Greenacre, P. (1958). Early physical determinants in the development of the sense of identity. *Journal of the American Psychoanalytic Association, 6*, 612–627.

Groves, J. E., & Kucharski, A. (1986). Brief psychotherapy. In T. P. Hackett & N. Cassem (Eds.), *MGH handbook of general hospital psychiatry* (Chap. 16, pp. 309–331). Littleton, MA: PSG Publishing Co.

Hagglund, T., & Heikki, P. (1980). The inner space of the body image. *Psychoanalysis Quarterly, 49*, 256–283.

Halvorson, D. J., & Kuhn, F. A. (1997). Tracheoesophageal speech following transmucosal pharyngeal myotomy with the potassium-titanyl-phosphate laser. *Journal of Laryngology & Otology, 111*, 659–662.

Hamaker, R. C., Singer, M. I., Blom, E. D., et al. (1985). Primary voice restoration at laryngectomy. *Archives of Otolaryngology, 111*, 182–186.

Hamilton, M. (1960). A rating scale for depression. *Journal of Neurology, Neurosurgery, & Psychiatry, 23*, 56–62.

Hammerlid, E., et al. (1999). Quality-of-life effects of psychosocial intervention in patients with head and neck cancer. *Otolaryngology—Head & Neck Surgery, 120*(4), 507–516.

Harris, J. P., Anderson, J. P., & Novack, R. (1995). An outcome study of cochlear implants in deaf patients. *Archives of Otolaryngology—Head & Neck, 121*, 398–404.

Hess, R. (2005). Facilitating speech in the patient with tracheostomy. *Respiratory Care, 50*(4), 519–525.

Holland, J. C., Rowland, J., & Plumb, M. (1977). Psychological aspects of anorexia in cancer patients. *Cancer Research, 37*, 2425–2428.

House, A. (1988). Mood disorder in the physically ill: Problems of definition and measurement. *Journal of Psychosomatic Medicine, 32*, 345–353.

Jankovic, J., & Brin, M. F. (1991). Review article: Therapeutic uses of botulinum toxin. *New England Journal of Medicine, 324*(17), 1186–1194.

Jantos, M., & White, G. (1997). The vestibulitis syndrome: Medical and psychosexual assessment of a cohort of patients. *Journal of Reproductive Medicine, 42*, 145–152.

Kalick, S. M. (1982). Clinician, social scientist and body image: Collaboration and future prospects. *Clinics in Plastic Surgery, 9*, 379–385.

Kankam, C. G., & Sallis, R. (1997). Acute sinusitis in adults. Difficult to diagnose, essential to treat. *Postgraduate Medicine, 102*(2), 253–258.

Kaplan, H. I., & Sadock, B. J. (Eds.) (1985). *Comprehensive Textbook of Psychiatry* (Vol. IV, 4th ed., p. 140). Baltimore, MD: Williams & Wilkins.

Kathol, R. G., Mutgi, A., Williams, J., et al. (1990b). Diagnosis of major depression in cancer patients according to four sets of criteria. *American Journal of Psychiatry, 147*(8), 1021–1024.

Kathol, R. G., Noyes, R., Williams, J., et al. (1990a). Diagnosing depression in patients with medical illness. *Psychosomatics, 31*(4), 434–440.

Kirby, S. E., & Yardley, L. (2009). Cognitions associated with anxiety in Meniere's disease. *Journal of Psychosomatic Research, 66*(2), 111–118.

Kim, Y., & Given, B. A. (2008). Quality of life of family caregivers of cancer survivors: Across the trajectory of the illness. *Cancer, 112*(11 Suppl), 2556–2568.

Kirsten, H. L. (2008). Psychological distress and head and neck cancer: Part 1—Review of the literature. *Journal of Supportive Oncology, 6*(4), 155–163.

Kluin, K. J., et al. (1984). The patient requiring mechanical ventilator support: Use of the cuffed tracheostomy "talk" tube established phonation. *Otolaryngology—Head & Neck Surgery, 92*(6), 635–637.

Knutson, J. F., Schartz, H. A., Gantz, B. J., et al. (1991). Psychological change following 18 months of cochlear implant use. *Annals of Otology, Rhinology, & Laryngology, 100*, 877–882.

Laniado-Laborin, R. (2010). Smoking cessation intervention: An evidence-based approach. *Postgraduate Medicine, 122*(2), 74–82.

Lee, D. J., & Gomez-Marin, O. (1997). Major depressive symptoms, and bilateral hearing loss in Hispanic adults. *Journal of Affective Disorders, 44*, 189–195.

Lehman, C., Koch, U., Mehnert, A. (2009). Impact of the doctor-patient communication on distress and utilization of psychosocial services among cancer patients. A review of the current literature. *Psychotherapie Psychosomatik Medizinische Psychologie, 59*(7), e3–e27.

Lerman, J. W. (1991). The artificial larynx. In S. J. Salman & K. H. Mount (Eds.), *Alaryngeal speech rehabilitation* (Chap. 2). Austin, TX: ProEd.

Lesperance, F., Frasure-Smith, N., & Talajic, M. (1996). Depression before and after myocardial infarction: Its nature and consequences. *Psychosomatic Medicine, 58*, 99–110.

Litvack, J. R., et al. (2011). Role of depression in outcomes of endoscopic surgery. *Otolaryngology—Head & Neck Surgery, 144*(3), 446–451.

Logemann, J. A. (2006). Update on clinical trials in dysphagia. *Dysphagia, 21*(3), 116–120.

Lucente, F., Strain, J. J., & Wyatt, D. A. (1987). Psychological problems of the patient with head and neck cancer. In S. E. Thawley & W. R. Panje (Eds.), *Comprehensive management of head and neck tumors* (Chap. 5). Philadelphia, PA: W.B. Saunders.

Lydiatt, W. M., Denman, D., McNeilly, D. P., Puumula, S. E., & Burke, W. J. (2008). A randomized, placebo-controlled trial of citalopram for the prevention of major depression during treatment of head and neck cancer. *Archives of Otolaryngology—Head & Neck Surgery, 134*(5), 528–535.

Lydiatt, W. M., Bessette, D., Schmid, K. K., Sayles, H., & Burker, W. J. (2013). Prevention of depression with escitalopram in patients undergoing treatment for head and neck cancer randomized, double-blind, placebo-controlled clinical trial. *JAMA Otolaryngology—Head & Neck Surgery, 139*, 678–686.

Macdonald, K. I., et al. (2009). The health resource utilization of Canadians with chronic rhinosinusitis. *Laryngoscope, 119*(1), 184–189.

Mace, J., et al. (2008). Effects of depression on quality of life improvement after endoscopic sinus surgery. *Laryngoscope, 118*(3), 528–534.

Marcus, P. (1984). Psychological aspects of cosmetic rhinoplasty. *British Journal of Plastic Surgery, 37*, 313–318.

Marek, A. (2009). Psychosomatic treatment of otorhinolaryngological diseases. *HNO [in German], 57*(11), 1167–1175.

Martenez-Devesa, P, Pered R., et al. (2010). Cognitive behavioural therapy for tinnitus. *Cochrane Database of Systematic Reviews, 8*(9), CD005233.

Mason, B., & Frosch, W. A. (1989). Secondary depressions. In *Treatments of Psychiatric Disorders: A Task Force Report of the American Psychiatric Association* (pp. 1898–1924). Washington, DC: American Psychiatric Association.

McKenna, L. (1986). The psychological assessment of cochlear implant patients. *British Journal of Audiology, 20*, 29–34.

McNally, P. A., White, M. V., & Kaliner, M. A. (1997). Sinusitis in an allergist's office. *Allergy & Asthma Proceedings, 18*(3), 169–175.

Mechatie, E. (1998). Bupropion may boost smoking cessation rates. *Clinical Psychiatry News, 26*(2), 17.

Meyers, A. D., Aarons, B., Suzuki, B., et al. (1980). Sexual behavior following laryngectomy. *Ear, Nose & Throat Journal, 59*(8), 35–39.

Miziara, I. D., et al. (2009). Group psychotherapy: An additional approach to burning mouth syndrome. *Journal of Psychosomatic Research, 67*(5), 443–448.

Mumford, E., Schlesinger, H. J., Glass, G. V., et al. (1982). The effects of psychological intervention on recovery from surgery and heart attacks: An analysis of the literature. *American Journal of Public Health, 72*(2), 141–151.

Natvig, K. (1983a). Laryngectomies in Norway, Study No. 1: Social, personal and behavioral factors related to present mastery of the laryngectomy event. *Journal of Otolaryngology, 12*(3), 155–162.

Natvig, K. (1983b). Laryngectomies in Norway, Study No. 2: Pre-operative counselling and post-operative training evaluated by the patients and their spouses. *Journal of Otolaryngology, 12*(4), 249–254.

NCCN (1999). Practice guidelines for management of psychosocial distress. *American Cancer Society, 13*, 113–147.

Oberklaid, F., Harris, C., & Keir, E. (1989). Auditory dysfunction in children with school problems. *Clinical Pediatrics, 28*(9), 397–403.

O'Hara, M. W., Ghonem, M. M., Hinrichs, J. V., et al. (1989). Psychological consequences of surgery. *Psychosomatic Medicine, 51*, 356–370.

Olson, A. D., & Shinn, J. B. (2008). A systematic review to determine the effectiveness of using amplification in conjunction with cochlear implantation. *Journal of the American Academy of Audiology, 19*, 657–671.

Ostrof, J., et al. (2004). Interest and barriers to participation in multiple family groups among head and neck cancer survivors and their primary family caregivers. *Family Process, 43*(2), 195–208.

Petrucci, R. J., & Harwick, R. D. (1984). Role of the psychologist on a radical head and neck surgical service team. *Professional Psychology: Research and Practice, 15*(4), 538–543.

Piril, W. F., et al. (2007). Screening for psychological distress: A national survey of oncologists. *Journal of Supportive Oncology, 5*(10), 499–504.

Poissant, S. F., et al. (2008). Impact of cochlear implantation on speech understanding, depression, and loneliness in the elderly. *Journal of Otolaryngology—Head & Neck Surgery, 37*(4), 488–494.

Popkin, M. K., Callies, A. L., & MacKenzie, T. B. (1985). The outcome of antidepressant use in the medically ill. *Archives of General Psychiatry, 42*, 1160–1163.

Prout, M. N., Sidari, J. N., et al. (1997). Head and neck cancer among 4611 tobacco users older than forty years. *Otolaryngology—Head & Neck Surgery, 116*(2), 201–208.

Rapp, S. R., & Vrana, S. (1989). Substituting for somatic symptoms in the diagnosis of depression in elderly male medical patients. *American Journal of Psychiatry, 146*(9), 1197–1200.

Rifkin, A., Reardon, G., Siris, S., et al. (1985). Trimipramine in physical illness with depression. *Journal of Clinical Psychiatry, 46*(Sec 2), 4–8.

Rodin, G., & Voshart, K. (1986). Depression in the medically ill: An overview. *American Journal of Psychiatry, 143*(6), 696–705.

Sahli, S., et al. (2009). *International Journal of Pediatric Otorhinolaryngology, 73*(12), 1774–1779.

Savoy, J., Lazarus, L. W., & Jarvik, L. F. (Eds.) (1991). *Comprehensive review of geriatric psychiatry*. Washington, DC: American Psychiatric Press.

Schleifer, S. J., Macara-Hinson, M. M., Coyle, D. A., et al. (1989). The nature and course of depression following myocardial infarction. *Archives of Internal Medicine, 149*, 1785–1789.

Schnoll, R. A., Rotham RA, et al. (2005). A randomized pilot study of cognitive-behavioral therapy versus basic health education for smoking cessation among cancer patients. *Annals of Behavioral Medicine, 30*(1), 1–11.

Seligmann, H., Podoshin, L., Ben-David, J., et al. (1996). Drug-induced tinnitus and other hearing disorders. *Drug Safety, 14*(3), 198–212.

Semple, C. J., et al. (2009). Development and evaluation of a problem-focused psychosocial intervention for patients with head and neck cancer. *Supportive Care in Cancer, 17*(4), 379–388.

Semple, C. J., & Kilough, S. A. (2014). Quality of Life issues in head & neck cancer. *Dental Update, 41*(4), 346–348, 351–353.

Shapiro, P. A., & Kornfeld, D. S. (1987). Psychiatric aspects of head and neck cancer surgery. *Psychiatric Clinics of North America, 10*(1), 87–100.

Stead, et al. (2008). Nicotine replacement therapy for smoking cessation. *Cochrane Database of Systematic Reviews, 23*(1), CD000146.

Shemen, L. (1998). Fluoxetine for treatment of tinnitus (letter). *Otolaryngology—Head & Neck Surgery, 118*, 421.

Slater, R., & Terry, M. (1987). *Tinnitus: A guide to sufferers and professionals*. London: Croem Helm.

Sollner, W., et al. (2001). How successful are oncologists in identifying patient distress, perceived social support, and need for psychosocial counselling? *British Journal of Cancer, 84*(2), 179–185.

Sprinzl, G. M., Riechelmann, H. (2010). Current trends in treating hearing loss in elderly people: A review of the technology and treatment options—a mini-review. *Gerontology, 56*, 351–358.

Spikes, J., & Holland, J. (1975). The physician's response to the dying patient. In J. J. Strain & Grossman S. (Eds.), *Psychiatric care of the medically ill* (Chap. 11, pp. 138–148). New York: Appleton-Century-Crofts.

Staffel, J., & Pillsbury, H. C. (1993). In Y. P. Krespi & R. H. Ossoff (Eds.), *Complications in head and neck surgery*. Philadelphia, PA: W.B. Saunders.

Stein, M. B., Gordon, J. G., et al. (1994). Panic disorder in patients attending a clinic for vestibular disorders. *American Journal of Psychiatry, 151*(11), 1697–1700.

Strain, J. J. (1985). The surgical patient. In R. Michels & J. O. Cavenar (Eds.), *Psychiatry* (Vol. 2, Chap. 121, pp. 1–11). Philadelphia, PA: Lippincott.

Strain, J. J., Fulop, G., Lebovits, A., et al. (1988). Screening devices for diminished cognitive capacity. *General Hospital Psychiatry, 10*, 16–23.

Strain, J. J., Snyder, S. S., & Fulop, G. (1992). Mood disorder and medical illness. In A. Tasman & M. Riba (Eds.), *Reviews in Psychiatry* (Vol. 11, Chap. 23). Washington, DC: American Psychiatric Press.

Sullivan, M., Katon, W., Dolice, R., et al. (1988). Disabling tinnitus. Association with affective disorder. *General Hospital Psychiatry, 10*, 285–291.

Surman, O. S. (1986). The surgical patient. In T. P. Hacket & N. H. Cassem (Eds.), *MGH handbook of general hospital psychiatry* (Chap. 5, pp. 69–83). Littleton, MA: PSG Publishing Co.

Tiber, N. (1985). A psychological evaluation of cochlear implants in children. *Ear & Hearing, 6*(3), 48–51.

Urken, M. L., & Biller, H. F. (1988). Management of early vocal cord carcinoma. *Oncology, 2*(4), 48–62.

Valente, S. M. (2004). Visual disfigurement and depression. *Plastic Surgery Nursing, 24*(4) 140–146.

Veer, V., Kia, S., & Papesch, M. (2010). Anxiety and depression in head and neck out-patients. *Journal of Laryngology & Otology, 124*, 774–777.

Vickery, L. E., et al. (2003). The impact of head and neck cancer and facial disfigurement on quality of life of patients and their partners. *Head and Neck, 25*(4), 289–296.

Vogtsberger, K. W., Harris, L. L., & Mattox, D. E. (1985). Group psychotherapy for head and neck cancer patients. *Laryngoscope, 95*, 585–587.

Von Korf, M., Ormel, J., Katon, W., et al. (1992). Disability and depression among high utilizers of health care. *Archives of General Psychiatry, 49*, 91–99.

Wasan, A., et al. (2007). Association of anxiety and depression with reported disease severity in patients undergoing evaluation for chronic rhinosinusitis. *Annals of Otology, Rhinology, & Laryngology, 116*(7), 491–497.

Watt, J. A. G. (1985). Hearing and premorbid personality in paranoid states. *American Journal of Psychiatry, 142*(12), 1453–1455.

Webb, M. S., et al. (2010). Cognitive-behavioral therapy to promote smoking among African American smokers: A randomized trial. *Journal of Consulting Clinical Psychology, 78*(1), 24–33.

West, D. W. (1974). Adaptation to surgically induced facial disfigurement among cancer patients. *Dissertation Abstracts International, 34*(7A), 442.

West, D. W. (1977). Social adaptation patterns among cancer patients with facial disfigurements resulting from surgery. *Archives of Physical Medicine & Rehabilitation, 58*, 473–479.

Yovell, Y., Sackeim, H. A., et al. (1995). Hearing loss and asymmetry in major depression. *Journal of Neuropsychiatry, 7*(1), 82–89.

73.

AESTHETIC SURGERY

David B. Sarwer and Jacqueline C. Spitzer

INTRODUCTION

According to the American Society of Plastic Surgeons (ASPS), approximately 15.1 million surgical and nonsurgical cosmetic treatments were performed in the United States in 2013 (ASPS, 2014). Of these, approximately 1.6 million were surgical procedures (e.g., rhinoplasty, breast augmentation), and over 13.5 million treatments were minimally invasive nonsurgical treatments (e.g., facial injectables, laser treatments). These numbers often are surprising to laypersons who have not considered the number of Americans who turn to plastic surgeons and other physicians to improve their appearance with medical treatments.

In recent years, numerous studies have investigated the changing attitudes of the public about cosmetic surgery. The results reveal a growing acceptance of both cosmetic surgical and noninvasive procedures to improve appearance. In 2010, for example, the American Society for Aesthetic and Plastic Surgery (ASAPS) surveyed Americans' attitudes about cosmetic surgery. The small majority of women (53%) and 49% of men surveyed said that they approve of cosmetic surgery (ASAPS, 2011). More than 60% of individuals surveyed, from young adults to those over 65 years of age, indicated that they would not be embarrassed if friends and family knew that they had had cosmetic surgery (ASAPS, 2011). One of now several independent studies of college-age women found that 45% approved of people's surgically changing their appearance to feel better about themselves (Sarwer et al., 2005). In both the ASAPS survey and other studies, women are more likely than men to consider cosmetic surgery (Swami et al., 2008).

The growth in popularity of the use of medical science to improve one's appearance can probably be attributed to a number of factors. Technological advances in medicine have made many surgical and treatments safer and have led to shorter postoperative recovery periods. Minimally invasive treatments have even less risk and recovery time associated with them, and the decreased cost of these treatments has also facilitated their rapid growth.

Along with these medical advances, the mass media and entertainment industries have contributed to the growth of cosmetic surgery. A large number and variety of television programs have covered the topic of cosmetic surgery over the past decade, ranging from educational health programs to reality-based, patient- and surgeon-focused shows, to a fictional program set in a cosmetic surgery practice. While these shows may be "guilty pleasures" for many viewers, a recent study found a positive relationship between exposure to cosmetic "reality" television shows, more positive attitudes toward cosmetic surgery, and a feeling of increased pressure to undergo cosmetic surgery (Sperry et al., 2009). At the same time, an increasing number of celebrities have spoken publicly about their experience with cosmetic surgery, implicitly endorsing the procedures. A handful of others have served as spokespersons for specific products.

Considering the medical advances in cosmetic medicine, coupled with the mass media's continued fascination with the medical specialty, the increased popularity does not seem so surprising. The growth of these procedures has been accompanied the development of a body of research that has investigated the psychological characteristics of the persons interested in these procedures and the psychological changes they experience postoperatively.

This chapter provides an overview of this body of research. We begin with a brief review of the relationship between *preoperative characteristics and interest in surgery*, with a specific focus on the body-image concerns of patients. Given the central role of body image in this literature, the *relationship between cosmetic procedures and body dysmorphic disorder as well as eating disorders* is discussed. In addition, the surprising relationship between *cosmetic breast augmentation and suicide* is reviewed. The chapter closes with a description of the preoperative psychological screening of cosmetic surgery patients that mental health professionals may be asked to conduct.

EARLY PSYCHOLOGICAL RESEARCH ON COSMETIC SURGERY PATIENTS

Over the past 50 years, a surprisingly large number of studies have investigated the psychological characteristics of patients who present for cosmetic procedures, as well as the psychological changes they report after these treatments. This field has particularly blossomed in the past 20 years, with a specific focus on the relationship between body image and cosmetic treatments. This entire literature is reviewed in extensive detail elsewhere (Crerand, Franklin, & Sarwer, 2006, 2008; Sarwer & Crerand, 2008; Sarwer et al., 1998a). A brief overview is provided here.

Early research in this area, conducted decades ago, focused on preoperative psychopathology and relied heavily on the use of clinical interviews, often conducted by psychoanalytically trained psychiatrists, of cosmetic surgical patients. The results of these early studies indicated that cosmetic surgery patients had high rates of psychopathology, ranging from mood and anxiety disorders to personality disorders (e.g., Edgerton & McClary, 1958; Edgerton, Meyer, & Jacobson, 1961; Baker, Kolin, & Bartlett, 1974). This preoperative psychopathology was believed to be associated with poor psychosocial adjustment postoperatively.

Beginning in the 1970s, studies began to include validated psychometric measures, either alone in or combination with clinical interviews, to assess patients' symptoms of psychopathology (e.g., Wright & Wright, 1975; Goin, Burgoyne, Goin, & Staples, 1980). These studies reported far less psychopathology in candidates for surgery compared to the first studies in this area. The studies of this era also reported more positive psychological outcomes. Unfortunately, both sets of studies suffered from numerous methodological problems, making interpretation of the entire body of results difficult.

PHYSICAL APPEARANCE, BODY IMAGE, AND COSMETIC SURGERY

In addition to the contributions to the growth of cosmetic surgery described earlier in this chapter, social-psychological research can also be used to understand the growth of cosmetic surgery witnessed over the past two decades. This body of research, which can trace its origins to seminal studies of the early 1970s, has suggested that individuals who are more physically attractive are believed to have a number of more positive personality traits. Furthermore, more attractive individuals also receive preferential treatment in a range of social situations across the lifespan (Jonzon, 2009; Sarwer & Magee, 2006). With this literature in mind, an investment in or focus on one's appearance through the pursuit of cosmetic surgery may be likened to other self-improvement strategies, such as eating a healthy diet and exercising regularly, and not necessarily be a symptom of psychopathology (Sarwer et al., 1998a).

In the area of cosmetic medicine, interest in one's appearance has been studied from the perspective of the psychological construct of *body image*—a multidimensional construct, defined as an individual's internal experience of his or her appearance (Cash & Smolak, 2011). Dissatisfaction with one's body image is considered to be a primary motivating factor in the pursuit of cosmetic surgery. Several studies suggest that patients report heightened body-image dissatisfaction, particularly dissatisfaction with the specific feature being considered for surgery, preoperatively (Sarwer et al., 1998b; Sarwer, LaRossa, Bartlett, et al., 2003). Following cosmetic surgery, many studies have found that the vast majority of patients report satisfaction with the changes in their appearance as well as improvements in their body image (Banbury et al., 2004; Bolton, Pruzinsky, Cash, & Persing, 2003; Dunofsky,

1997; Murphy, Beckstrand, & Sarwer, 2009; Sarwer et al., 2008; von Soest et al., 2011). The impact of cosmetic surgery on other areas of psychological functioning, however, is less clear. While some studies have reported improvements in constructs such as self-esteem and quality of life, other studies have reported no significant improvements, or worsening of these areas of psychosocial functioning (Crerand et al., 2009; Murphy et al., 2009; Sarwer et al., 1998b; von Soest et al., 2011).

COSMETIC SURGERY AND PSYCHOPATHOLOGY

The extant research to date suggests that most cosmetic surgical patients are psychologically healthy when they present for surgery, and report satisfaction with their surgical outcome and improvements in body image postoperatively. However, three psychological disorders—body dysmorphic disorder (BDD), eating disorders, and depression—are believed to occur with frequency among candidates for cosmetic surgery and may be associated with poor postoperative outcomes.

BODY DYSMORPHIC DISORDER

BDD is defined as a preoccupation with a slight or imagined defect in appearance that leads to substantial distress or impairment in functioning (American Psychiatric Association, 2013). The most common focus of this preoccupation is the skin, hair, or nose; however, any part of the body can be the focus of the disorder (Veale, De Haro, & Lambrou, 2003). In the general population, the incidence of BDD is estimated to be less than 1–3% (Bienvenu et al., 2000; Faravelli et al., 1997; Otto, Wilhelm, Cohen, & Harlow, 2001; Rief, Buhlmann, Wilhelm, Borkenhagen, & Brahler, 2006). The incidence of BDD in patients seeking cosmetic surgery is much higher than in the general population. In studies of cosmetic surgery patients around the world, BDD ranges from 3–17% (Aouizerate et al., 2003; Vulink et al., 2006). In the United States, studies have found the incidence rate to be between 7% and 8% (Crerand et al., 2004; Sarwer, Wadden, Pertschuk, & Whitaker, 1998b).

In addition to compulsive behaviors to reduce appearance-related distress, such as repeated checking of one's appearance in mirrors or reflective surfaces, one way patients suffering from BDD seek to improve their perceived defects is through cosmetic treatments. In a study of 250 BDD patients, 76% of the patients sought and 66% received treatment (Crerand et al., 2005). Unlike most cosmetic surgery patients, patients with BDD who undergo cosmetic surgery are often dissatisfied and may, in fact, experience a worsening of their BDD symptoms. Two studies found that over 90% of patients with BDD report that their symptoms have remained the same or that they have worsened following cosmetic surgery (Crerand et al., 2005; Crerand, Menard, & Phillips, 2010). Patients may also engage in a range of ineffective treatments, "do-it-yourself surgery" or other self-harming behaviors

(Veale, 2000). Persons with BDD, regardless of their interest in cosmetic surgery, also have high rates of suicidal ideation or suicide attempts (Phillips & Menard, 2006). Finally, patients who pursue cosmetic procedures and are dissatisfied with the cosmetic outcome and/or the lack of impact on their BDD symptoms, may threaten or pursue legal action or violence against their surgeons (Sarwer, 2002). For all of these reasons, BDD is often considered a contraindication for cosmetic procedures (Crerand, Franklin, & Sarwer, 2008; Crerand & Sarwer, 2010).

EATING DISORDERS

The major eating disorders, anorexia nervosa and bulimia nervosa, are characterized by extreme body-image dissatisfaction, specifically with one's weight and shape (APA, 2013). The amount of concern that these patients feel about their appearance would intuitively suggest that both disorders may appear with some frequency among those seeking cosmetic surgery. Somewhat surprisingly, the relationship between eating disorders and cosmetic surgery has received little empirical study to date. Studies of women presenting for cosmetic breast augmentation suggests that many are of below-average weight and report greater levels of exercise compared to women not seeking breast augmentation (Brinton et al., 2000; Cook et al., 1997; Fryzek et al., 2000; Kjoller et al., 2003). Both of these characteristics may be suggestive of eating pathology. Similarly, individuals with eating disorders interested in other body-contouring procedures, such as liposuction or abdominoplasty, may erroneously believe that these procedures can "improve" their body shape in ways that inappropriate eating behavior and compensatory behaviors cannot.

A limited number of case reports have described the post-operative course of individuals with eating disorders who have undergone plastic surgical procedures. Case studies of patients with eating disorders have described patients whose eating disorder symptomatology has deteriorated following cosmetic surgery, specifically following breast augmentation, lipoplasty, rhinoplasty, and chin augmentation (McIntosh, Britt, & Bulik, 1994; Willard, McDermott, & Woodhouse, 1996; Yates, Shisslak, Allender, & Wolman, 1988). In contrast, a study of five breast-reduction patients with bulimia found that four of the women experienced an improvement of their symptoms and a reduction in emotional distress. These improvements were maintained for ten years postoperatively (Losee et al., 1997, 2004). In these cases, the excessive breast tissue may have contributed to the initial body-image disturbance and may have been an etiological factor in the development of the eating disorder. By having this excess breast tissue removed surgically, the patients' body dissatisfaction appears to have been lessened, although this was not objectively studied.

DEPRESSION

The presence of mood disorders, specifically depression, in cosmetic surgery patients also warrants specific attention.

Approximately 20% of all cosmetic surgery patients are engaged in mental health treatment, typically with the use of an antidepressant or other psychiatric medications (Sarwer, Zanville, et al., 2004). The most common treatment was the use of antidepressant medications. Compared to women in the general population, women seeking breast implants also were found to have a higher rate of outpatient psychotherapy (Sarwer, LaRossa, et al., 2004) and psychiatric hospitalizations (Jacobsen, et al., 2004). Though these studies suggest that cosmetic surgery patients, and cosmetic breast-augmentation patients in particular, may have higher rates of depression or mood disorders, the specific psychiatric diagnoses of these women were not described.

Other studies of cosmetic breast augmentation patients have suggested that these women frequently present for surgery with a number of unique personality characteristics and life experiences (see Sarwer, Brown, & Evans, 2007, for a detailed review). They are more likely to have more sexual partners over their lifetimes, report a greater use of oral contraceptives, be younger at their first pregnancy, and have a history of terminated pregnancies. They are more frequent users of alcohol and tobacco and have a higher rate of dissolved marriages. All of these characteristics may be associated with mood disorders or other forms of psychopathology.

Furthermore, studies over the past decade have revealed a surprising relationship between cosmetic breast augmentation and postoperative suicides. Seven epidemiological studies that investigated silicone gel–filled breast implants (used for cosmetic purposes) and all-cause mortality, found the rate of suicide among women with breast implants is two to three times higher than the estimated suicide rates in the general population or as compared to women interested in other plastic surgical procedures. There are a number of potential explanations for these findings; most have focused on the preoperative psychosocial status and functioning of the women (McLaughlin, Wise, & Lipworth, 2004; Sarwer, 2003; Sarwer et al., 2007). That is, the unique personality characteristics and life experiences of these women described above are, in and of themselves, associated with psychopathology as well as an increased risk of suicide, and they, rather than something related to the surgical procedure or implants themselves, are the most parsimonious explanation for the subsequent suicides. Unfortunately, of the seven epidemiological studies, only one provided information on the psychiatric history of the women studied. Jacobsen and colleagues (2004) found that women who received cosmetic breast implants had a higher rate of previous psychiatric hospitalizations compared with women who received other cosmetic procedures or underwent breast reduction surgery. A history of psychiatric hospitalizations is one of the strongest predictors of suicide among women in the general population (Qin, Agerbo, & Mortensen, 2003). Unfortunately, Jacobsen and colleagues (2004) did not report information on diagnosis, history of illness, or other psychiatric treatments for the women in the sample.

MENTAL HEALTH EVALUATIONS OF COSMETIC SURGERY PATIENTS

The mental health issues detailed above are believed to impact a small, yet not inconsequential, number of cosmetic surgery patients. Most individuals interested in cosmetic surgery are probably more similar to than different from those who do not present for surgery, in that they have a number of psychological strengths but also psychological issues—many of which may be completely unrelated to their pursuit of cosmetic surgery. Most patients present to the surgeon with specific appearance concerns, internal motivations, and realistic postoperative expectations. After surgery, the vast majority of patients report satisfaction with their postoperative outcomes and improvements in body image. The impacts on other areas of psychological functioning are less well established.

For these reasons, cosmetic surgeons do not require that patients undergo a mental health evaluation prior to cosmetic surgery. Given the lack of current evidence suggesting a relationship between preoperative psychosocial status and postoperative outcomes, recommendations for such routine evaluations are not warranted. Rather, cosmetic surgeons, like all medical professionals, should assess and screen for the presence of psychopathology as part of taking a medical history and completing a physical examination. Unfortunately, most surgeons (or their delegates) are likely to skip this part of the assessment and, as a result, fail to identify patients who may exhibit symptoms of psychopathology.

Patients who display symptoms of psychopathology during their initial consultation with the plastic surgeon, as well as those with a history of psychopathology, are the ones who probably should be referred for a mental health consultation prior to a cosmetic procedure (Sarwer, 2006). Many of the early descriptions of cosmetic surgery patients are complete with elaborate interpretations of the role of unconscious conflicts and poor parental relationships in the decision to seek surgery. There is no evidence, however, to suggest that such interpretations are necessarily valid or useful in determining patients' appropriateness for surgery. Thus, a detailed assessment of patients' parental relationships and decades-old historical experiences is unlikely to provide useful information to either the mental health professional or the referring surgeon in determining appropriateness for surgery. A more straightforward evaluation of patients' current functioning, as found in the more general cognitive-behavioral assessment, is recommended (Sarwer, 2006).

The cognitive-behavioral assessment of the cosmetic medicine patient should focus on the thoughts, behaviors, and experiences that have contributed to their dissatisfaction with their appearance as well as the decision to seek surgery. This involves the assessment of the "ABCs" of patients' interest in surgery (Sarwer, 2006)—the antecedents ("A") to the decision to seek a cosmetic treatment, the behavioral responses ("B") to their concerns about their appearance, and consequences ("C") of their decision to seek surgery. The evaluation also should determine if the patients' thoughts and behaviors are maladaptive to the point that they reflect some form of psychopathology that would contraindicate surgery. Finally, the assessment should focus on the patients' psychiatric status and history, their appearance and body-image concerns, as well as their motivations for surgery and expectations regarding the postoperative result and its impact on daily functioning.

PSYCHIATRIC HISTORY AND STATUS

The assessment of the patients' psychiatric history and current status, as done in any mental health consultation, is a central part of the evaluation. With the exception of BDD, there currently are no conclusive data on the prevalence of psychiatric diagnoses among persons who seek or undergo cosmetic surgery. Given the number of individuals who now seek cosmetic surgery and minimally invasive treatments, it is likely that all of the major psychiatric diagnoses can be found in the patient population. The consulting mental health professional should pay particular attention to disorders with a body-image component, such as eating disorders and somatoform disorders, as well as mood and anxiety disorders. The presence of these disorders, however, may not be an absolute contraindication for cosmetic surgery. In the absence of specific data on the relationship between psychopathology and surgical outcome, appropriateness for surgery should be made on a case-by-case basis.

As noted above, approximately 20% of patients who seek cosmetic medical treatment report using a psychiatric medication at the time of treatment (Sarwer, Zanville, et al., 2004). Patients who receive these medications from a primary care physician often do not experience complete relief from their symptoms. Thus, a psychopharmacological evaluation should be considered if symptoms do not appear to be well controlled. If patients are in treatment with another psychiatrist or psychologist, the consultant should contact the treating clinician and, as appropriate, discuss patients' appropriateness for cosmetic treatment.

PHYSICAL APPEARANCE AND BODY IMAGE

Pruzinsky (1996) suggested the use of Lazarus's BASIC ID (1993)—Behavior, Affect, Sensation, Imagery, Cognition, Interpersonal, and Drugs—as a template to assess the body-image concerns of patients interested in cosmetic surgery. In addition, Cash's (2002) model of the historical and proximal influences on body image can provide an additional framework for this part of the assessment. The medical psychiatrist or psychologist also may want to consider the use of more specific body-image measures to assist with providing a more comprehensive assessment. Valid and reliable measures such as the Multidimensional Body Self Relations Questionnaire (Brown, Cash, & Mikulka, 1990) or the Derriford Appearance Scale (Carr, Harris, & James, 2000) can provide the mental health professional with detailed information on any symptoms of body-image dissatisfaction or BDD.

Prospective patients should be able to articulate specific concerns about their appearance that should be visible with little effort. Patients who are markedly distressed about slight defects that are not readily visible may be suffering from BDD. Some of the appearance concerns may be difficult to assess, as the context of the consultation may prohibit medical psychiatrists or psychologists from asking patients to remove articles of clothing. Furthermore, the judgement of an appearance defect as "slight or imagined" is highly subjective. What a medical psychiatrist or psychologist judges to be a slight defect well within the range of normal may be a defect that a cosmetic surgeon judges to be appropriate for treatment. As a result, the degree of emotional distress and impairment, rather than the specific nature of the defect, may be more accurate indicators of BDD in these patients (Crerand, Sarwer, & Franklin, 2006, 2008; Sarwer, 2006; Sarwer & Crerand, 2008).

The degree of dissatisfaction and any psychosocial consequences of dissatisfaction also should be assessed. Asking about the amount of time spent thinking about a feature or the activities missed or avoided on its account may indicate the degree of distress and impairment a person is experiencing and may help determine the presence of BDD. Self-report measures of BDD symptoms, such as the Body Dysmorphic Disorder Questionnaire, also may be helpful in this regard.

MOTIVATIONS AND EXPECTATIONS

The consultant also should inquire about patients' motivations for surgery. Specific questions about what a patient hopes to accomplish by having surgery can provide essential details about motivations. Patients who are motivated by internal factors, such as improvements in body image, are believed to have better postoperative outcomes than those motivated by external factors, such as pleasing a romantic partner (Honigman et al., 2004).

To assess motivations for surgery, the first question to begin the discussion may be "When did you first think about changing your appearance?" In addition to providing important clinical information, a thorough discussion of the issue may reveal the presence of some obsessive or delusional thinking, as well as bizarre or compulsive behaviors, related to physical appearance. Patients also should be asked how romantic partners, family members, and close friends feel about their decision to change a physical feature. Thus, the clinician should inquire about patients' general expectations about how the change in appearance, which may be rather subtle and potentially unnoticed by others, will influence their lives. There is no current evidence suggesting that cosmetic procedures directly affect interpersonal relationships. Therefore, patients should be reminded that it is impossible to predict how others will respond to their changed appearance. Some patients may find that few people notice the change in their appearance, while others may have the experience that everyone seems to notice them. While some patients may find this attention pleasurable, others may find it uncomfortable. To assess this issue, patients should be asked how they anticipate their lives will be different following surgery. The experience of unmet postoperative expectations is another possible explanation of the relationship between cosmetic breast augmentation and suicide (Sarwer, Brown, & Evans, 2007).

CONCLUDING THE EVALUATION

At the conclusion of the evaluation, the consultant should share the clinical impressions with the patient, as well as the ultimate recommendation to the referring physician about the appropriateness for surgery. The results of the evaluation should be communicated to the surgeon in a letter summarizing the assessment and recommendations. Obviously, the referring physician will make the ultimate decision about the decision to go forward with a given treatment.

POSTOPERATIVE CONSULTATIONS

Medical psychiatrists and psychologists also may be asked to consult with cosmetic surgery patients postoperatively. This typically occurs in one of two scenarios—the patient is dissatisfied with a technically successful procedure, or the patient is experiencing an exacerbation of psychopathology that was not detected preoperatively. Patients in each of these examples typically warrant psychotherapeutic care. Cognitive-behavioral models of body-image therapy are often useful with these individuals, although more diagnosis-specific treatments also may be necessary (e.g., for depression, social or generalized anxiety, etc.).

SUMMARY

Over 15 million cosmetic surgical and minimally invasive treatments designed to improve one's physical appearance are performed each year in the United States. As the number of these procedures has increased, so has the interest in the psychosocial functioning of individuals who present for surgery, as well as the psychological changes that they experience postoperatively. The current body of evidence suggests that the vast majority of patients are psychologically healthy and that most patients will be satisfied with the outcome of their treatments and experience improvements in body image. The impact on other areas of psychological functioning, such as self-esteem and quality of life, are less clear. At the same time, a minority of patients may be suffering from significant psychopathology that may decrease the likelihood that these individuals would experience psychological benefits from these procedures. The literature suggests that BDD occurs with greater frequency among cosmetic surgery patients, compared to the general population, and probably contraindicates cosmetic surgery. Depression and suicidality also appear to be of concern, particularly among women who present for cosmetic breast augmentation. Given the relationship with body-image dissatisfaction, eating disorders also may be prevalent among persons who present for cosmetic surgery, but this area of research awaits further study.

With the increasing popularity of cosmetic surgery, it is likely that most medical psychiatrists will encounter patients interested in changing their bodies through cosmetic surgery. They may be asked to consult with patients interested in surgery to assess their psychological appropriateness for certain procedures. In addition to utilizing the basic principles of cognitive-behavioral assessment, preoperative assessments should focus on psychiatric status and history, body-image concerns, and motivations and expectations for surgery. Successful collaboration with the cosmetic surgeon can increase the likelihood that most patients are psychologically appropriate for surgery or will receive mental health treatment to address their appearance concerns.

CLINICAL PEARLS

- In the area of cosmetic medicine, interest in one's appearance has been studied from the perspective of the psychological construct of "body image"—a multidimensional construct, defined as an individual's internal experience of his or her appearance (Cash & Smolak, 2011).

- Following cosmetic surgery, many studies have found that the vast majority of patients report satisfaction with the changes in their appearance as well as improvements in body image (Banbury et al., 2004; Bolton, Pruzinsky, Cash, & Persing, 2003; Dunofsky, 1997; Murphy, Beckstrand, & Sarwer, 2009; Sarwer et al., 2008; von Soest et al., 2011).

- Three psychological disorders—body dysmorphic disorder (BDD), eating disorders, and depression—are believed to occur with frequency among candidates for cosmetic surgery and may be associated with poor postoperative outcomes.

- In the United States, studies have found the incidence rate of BDD to be between 7% and 8% (Crerand et al., 2004; Sarwer, Wadden, Pertschuk, & Whitaker, 1998b).

- Unlike most cosmetic surgery patients, patients with BDD who undergo cosmetic surgery are often dissatisfied and may, in fact, experience a worsening in their BDD symptoms.

- Persons with BDD, regardless of their interest in cosmetic surgery, also have high rates of suicidal ideation or suicide attempts (Phillips & Menard, 2006).

- Studies of women presenting for cosmetic breast augmentation suggest that many are of below-average weight and report greater levels of exercise compared to women not seeking breast augmentation (Brinton et al., 2000; Cook et al., 1997; Fryzek et al., 2000; Kjoller et al., 2000).

- Approximately 20% of all cosmetic surgery patients are engaged in mental health treatment, typically with the use of an antidepressant or other psychiatric medications (Sarwer, Zanville, et al., 2004).

- Seven epidemiological studies that investigated silicone gel–filled breast implants (used for cosmetic purposes) and all-cause mortality, found the rate of suicide among women with breast implants is two to three times higher than the estimated suicide rates in the general population

or as compared to women interested in other plastic surgical procedures.

- The cognitive-behavioral assessment of the cosmetic medicine patient should focus on the thoughts, behaviors, and experiences that have contributed to their dissatisfaction with their appearance as well as their decision to seek surgery. This involves the assessment of the "ABCs" of patients' interest in surgery (Sarwer, 2006)—the antecedents ("A") to the decision to seek a cosmetic treatment, the behavioral responses ("B") to their concerns about their appearance, and consequences ("C") of their decision to seek surgery.

- Asking about the amount of time spent thinking about a feature or the activities missed or avoided may indicate the degree of distress and impairment a person is experiencing and may help determine the presence of BDD.

DISCLOSURE STATEMENTS

Dr. Sarwer has consulting relationships with the following companies: BARONova, EnteroMedics, Ethicon, and Kythera.

Ms. Spitzer reports no disclosures.

REFERENCES

American Psychiatric Association. (2013). *Diagnostic and statistical manual of mental disorders* (5th ed.). Washington, DC: American Psychiatric Association.

American Society of Plastic Surgeons (2014). *2014 Report of the 2013 National Clearinghouse of Plastic Surgery Statistics*. Arlington Heights, IL.

American Society of Aesthetic and Plastic Surgery. (2011). *2011 cosmetic surgery national data bank statistics*. New York: American Society of Aesthetic and Plastic Surgery.

Aouizerate, B., Pujol, H., Grabot, D., et al. (2003). Body dysmorphic disorder in a sample of cosmetic surgery applicants. *European Psychiatry, 18*, 365–368.

Baker, J. L., Kolin, I. S., & Bartlett, E. S. (1974). Psychosexual dynamics of patients undergoing mammary augmentation. *Plastic and Reconstructive Surgery, 53*, 652–659.

Banbury, J., Yetman, R., Lucas, A., Papay, F., Graves, K., & Zins, J. E. (2004). Prospective analysis of the outcome of subpectoral breast augmentation: sensory changes, muscle function, and body image. *Plastic and Reconstructive Surgery, 113*, 701–707.

Bienvenu, O. J., Samuels, J. F., Riddle, M. A., et al. (2000). The relationship of obsessive-compulsive disorder to possible spectrum disorders: results from a family study. *Biological Psychiatry, 48*, 287–293.

Bolton, M. A., Pruzinsky, T., Cash, T. F., & Persing, J. A. (2003). Measuring outcomes in plastic surgery: Body image and quality of life in abdominoplasty patients. *Plastic and Reconstructive Surgery, 112*, 619–625.

Brinton, L. A., Brown, S. L., Colton, T., Burich, M. C., & Lubin, J. (2000). Characteristics of a population of women with breast implants compared with women seeking other types of plastic surgery. *Plastic and Reconstructive Surgery, 105*, 919.

Brown, T. A., Cash, T. F., & Mikulka, P. J. (1990). Attitudinal body-image assessment: factor analysis of the Body-Self Relations Questionnaire. *Journal of Personality Assessment, 55*, 135–144.

Carr, T., Harris, D., & James, C., (2000). The Derriford Appearance Scale (DAS-59): A new scale to measure individual responses to living with problems of appearance. *British Journal of Health Psychology, 5*(2), 201–215.

Cash, T. F. (2002). Cognitive-behavioral perspectives on body image. In T. F. Cash & T. Pruzinsky (Eds.), *Body image: A handbook of theory, research, and clinical practice* (pp. 38–46). New York: Guilford Press.

Cash, T. F., & Smolak, L. (Eds.) (2011). *Body image: A handbook of science, practice and prevention* (2nd ed.). New York: The Guilford Press.

Cook, L. S., Daling, J. R., Voigt, L. F., et al. (1997). Characteristics of women with and without breast augmentation. *Journal of the American Medical Association, 277*, 1612.

Crerand, C. E., Franklin, M. E., & Sarwer, D. B. (2006). Body dysmorphic disorder and cosmetic surgery. *Plastic and Reconstructive Surgery, 118*, 167e–180e.

Crerand, C. E., Franklin, M. E., & Sarwer, D. B. (2008). Patient safety: Body dysmorphic disorder and cosmetic surgery. *Plastic and Reconstructive Surgery, 122*(4S), 1–15.

Crerand, C. E., Infield, A. L., & Sarwer, D. B. (2009). Psychological considerations in cosmetic breast augmentation. *Plastic Surgery Nursing, 29*, 49–57.

Crerand, C. E., Menard, W., & Phillips, K. A. (2010). Surgical and minimally invasive cosmetic procedures among persons with body dysmorphic disorder. *Annals of Plastic Surgery, 65*, 11–16.

Crerand, C. E., Phillips, K. A., Menard, W., & Fay, C. (2005). Non-psychiatric medical treatment of body dysmorphic disorder. *Psychosomatics. 46*, 549–555.

Crerand, C. E., & Sarwer, D. B. (2010). Cosmetic treatments and body dysmorphic disorder. *Psychiatric Annals, 40*, 344–348.

Crerand, C. E., Sarwer, D. B., Magee, L., et al. (2004). Rate of body dysmorphic disorder among patients seeking facial plastic surgery. *Psychiatric Annals, 34*, 958–965.

Dunofsky, M. (1997). Psychological characteristics of women who undergo single and multiple cosmetic surgeries. *Annals of Plastic Surgery, 39*(3), 223–228.

Edgerton, M. T., & McClary, A. R. (1958). Augmentation mammoplasty: Psychiatric implications and surgical indications. *Plastic and Reconstructive Surgery, 21*, 279–305.

Edgerton, M. T., Meyer, E., & Jacobson, W. E. (1961). Augmentation mammoplasty II: Further surgical and psychiatric evaluation. *Plastic and Reconstructive Surgery, 27*, 279–302.

Faravelli, C., Salvatori, S., Galassi, F., Aiazzi, L., Drei, C., & Cabras, P. (1997). Epidemiology of somatoform disorders: A community survey in Florence. *Social Psychiatry and Psychiatric Epidemiology, 32*, 24–29.

Fryzek, J. P., Weiderpass, E., Signorello, L. B., et al. (2000). Characteristics of women with cosmetic breast augmentation surgery compared with breast reduction surgery patients and women in the general population of Sweden. *Annals of Plastic Surgery, 45*, 349–356.

Goin, M. K., Burgoyne, R. W., Goin, J. M., & Staples, F. R. (1980). A prospective psychological study of 50 female face-lift patients. *Plastic & Reconstructive Surgery, 65*, 436–442.

Honigman, R. J., Phillips, K. A., & Castle, D. J. (2004). A review of psychosocial outcomes for patients seeking cosmetic surgery. *Plastic and Reconstructive Surgery, 113*, 1229–1237.

Jacobsen, P. H., Holmich, L. R., McLaughlin, J. K., et al. (2004). Mortality and suicide among Danish women with cosmetic breast implants. *Archives of Internal Medicine, 164*, 2450–2455.

Jonzon, K. (2009). Cosmetic medical treatments: Why are we so obsessed with beauty—is it nature or nurture? *Plastic Surgical Nursing, 29*, 222–225.

Kjoller, K., Holmich, L. R., Fryzek, J. P., et al. (2003). Characteristics of women with cosmetic breast implants compared with women with other types of cosmetic surgery and population-based controls in Denmark. *Annals of Plastic Surgery, 50*, 6–12.

Lazarus, A. A. (1973). Multimodal behavior therapy: Treating the "BASIC ID." *Journal of Nervous and Mental Disorders, 156*, 404–411.

Losee, J. E., Jiang, S., Long, D. E., Kreipe, R. E., Caldwell, E. H., & Serletti, J. M. (2004). Macromastia as an etiologic factor in bulimia

nervosa: 10-year follow-up after treatment with reduction mammoplasty. *Annals of Plastic Surgery, 52*, 452–457.

Losee, J. E., Serletti, J. M., Kreipe, R. E., & Caldwell, E. H. (1997). Reduction mammoplasty in patients with bulimia nervosa. *Annals of Plastic Surgery, 39*, 443–446.

McIntosh, V. V., Britt, E., & Bulik, C. M. (1994). Cosmetic breast augmentation and eating disorders. *New Zealand Medical Journal, 107*, 151–152.

McLaughlin, J. K., Wise, T. N., & Lipworth, L. (2004). Increased risk of suicide among patients with breast implants: Do the epidemiologic data support psychiatric consultation? *Psychosomatics, 45*, 277–280.

Murphy, D. K., Beckstrand, M., & Sarwer, D. B. (2009). A prospective, multi-center study of psychosocial outcomes after augmentation with Natrelle silicone-filled breast implants. *Annals of Plastic Surgery, 62*, 118–121.

Otto, M. W., Wilhelm, S., Cohen, L. S., & Harlow, B. L. (2001). Prevalence of body dysmorphic disorder in a community sample of women. *American Journal of Psychiatry, 158*, 2061–2063.

Phillips, K. A., & Menard, W. (2006). Suicidality in body dysmorphic disorder: a prospective study. *American Journal of Psychiatry, 163*, 1280–1282.

Pruzinsky, T. (1996). Cosmetic plastic surgery and body image: critical factors in patient assessment. In J. K. Thompson (Ed.), *Body image, eating disorders and obesity* (pp. 109–127). Washington, DC: American Psychological Association.

Qin, P., Agerbo, E., & Mortensen, P. B. (2003). Suicide risk in relation to socioeconomic, demographic, psychiatric, and familial factors: A national register–based study of all suicides in Denmark, 1981–1997. *American Journal of Psychiatry, 160*, 765–772.

Rief, W., Buhlmann, U., Wilhelm, S., Borkenhagen, A., & Brähler, E. (2006). The prevalence of body dysmorphic disorder: A population-based survey. *Psychological Medicine, 36*, 877–885.

Sarwer, D. B. (2002). Awareness and identification of body dysmorphic disorder by aesthetic surgeons: results of a survey of American Society for Aesthetic Plastic Surgery members. *Aesthetic Surgery Journal, 22*, 531–535.

Sarwer, D. B. (2003). Discussion of causes of death among Finnish women with cosmetic breast implants, 1971–2001. *Annals of Plastic Surgery, 51*, 343–344.

Sarwer, D. B. (2006). Psychological assessment of cosmetic surgery. In D. B. Sarwer, T. Pruzinsky, T. F. Cash, R. M. Goldwyn, J. A. Persing, & L. A. Whitaker (Eds.), *Psychological aspects of reconstructive and cosmetic plastic surgery: Clinical, empirical and ethical perspectives* (pp. 267–283). Philadelphia, PA: Lippincott, Williams & Wilkins.

Sarwer, D. B. (2007). The psychological aspects of cosmetic breast augmentation. *Plastic and Reconstructive Surgery, 120*, 110S–117S.

Sarwer, D. B., Brown, G. K., & Evans, D. L. (2007). Cosmetic breast augmentation and suicide: A review of the literature. *American Journal of Psychiatry, 164*, 1006–1013.

Sarwer, D. B., Cash, T. F., Magee, L., et al. (2005). Female college students and cosmetic surgery: An investigation of experiences, attitudes, and body image. *Plastic and Reconstructive Surgery, 115*, 931–938.

Sarwer, D. B., & Crerand, C. E. (2008). Body dysmorphic disorder and appearance enhancing medical treatments. *Body Image, 5*, 50–58.

Sarwer, D. B., Crerand, C. E., & Magee, L. (2008). Cosmetic surgery and changes in body image. In T. F. Cash & L. Smolak (Eds.), *Body image: A handbook of science, practice, and prevention* (2nd ed., pp. 394–403). New York: Guilford Press.

Sarwer, D. B., Infield, A. L., Baker, J. L., et al. (2008). Two-year results of a prospective, multi-site investigation of patient satisfaction and psychosocial status following cosmetic surgery. *Aesthetic Surgery Journal, 28*, 245–250.

Sarwer, D. B., LaRossa, D., Bartlett, S. P., Low, D. W., Bucky, L. P., & Whitaker, L. A. (2003). Body image concerns of breast augmentation patients. *Plastic and Reconstructive Surgery, 112*, 83–90.

Sarwer, D. B., & Magee, L. (2006). Physical appearance and society. In D. B. Sarwer, T. Pruzinsky, T. F. Cash, R. M. Goldwyn, J. A. Persing, & J. A. Whitaker, (Eds.), *The psychology of reconstructive and cosmetic* plastic surgery: Clinical, empirical, and ethical perspectives (pp. 23–26). Philadelphia, PA: Lippincott, Williams, & Wilkins.

Sarwer, D. B., Wadden, T. A., Pertschuk, M. J., & Whitaker, L. A. (1998a). The psychology of cosmetic surgery: a review and reconceptualization. Clinical Psychology Review, 18(1), 1–22.

Sarwer, D. B., Wadden, T. A., Pertschuk, M. J., & Whitaker, L. A. (1998b). Body image dissatisfaction and body dysmorphic disorder in 100 cosmetic surgery patients. Plastic and Reconstructive Surgery, 101(6), 1644–1649.

Sarwer, D. B., Zanville, H. A., LaRossa, D., et al. (2004). Mental health histories and psychiatric medication usage among persons who sought cosmetic surgery. Plastic and Reconstructive Surgery, 114, 1927–1933.

Sperry, S., Thompson, J. K., Sarwer, D. B., & Cash, T. F. (2009). Cosmetic surgery reality TV viewership: relations with cosmetic surgery attitudes, body image, and disordered eating. Annals of Plastic Surgery, 62, 7–11.

Swami, V., Arteche, A., Chamorro-Premuzic, T., et al. (2008). Looking good: Factors affecting the likelihood of having cosmetic surgery. European Journal of Plastic Surgery, 30, 211–218.

Veale, D. (2000). Outcome of cosmetic surgery and "DIY" surgery in patients with body dysmorphic disorder. Psychiatric Bulletin Royal College Psychiatrists, 24, 218.

Veale, D., De Haro, L., & Lambrou, C. (2003). Cosmetic rhinoplasty in body dysmorphic disorder. The British Association of Plastic Surgeons, 56, 546–551.

von Soest, T., Kvalem, I. L., Skolleborg, K. C., & Roald, H. E. (2011). Psychosocial changes after cosmetic surgery: a 5-year follow-up study. Plastic & Reconstructive Surgery, 128, 765–772.

Vulink, N. C., Sigurdsson, V., Kon, M., Bruijnzeel-Koomen, C. A., Westenberg, H. G., & Denys, D. (2006). Body dysmorphic disorder in 3–8% of patients in outpatient dermatology and plastic surgery clinics. Nederlands Tijdschrift voor Geneeskunde, 150, 97–100.

Willard, S. G., McDermott, B. E., & Woodhouse, L. M. (1996). Lipoplasty in the bulimic patient. Plastic and Reconstructive Surgery, 98, 276–278.

Wright, M. R., & Wright, W. K. (1975). A psychological study of patients undergoing cosmetic surgery. Archives of Otolaryngology, 101, 145–151.

Yates, A., Shisslak, C. M., Allender, J. R., & Wolman, W. (1988). Plastic surgery and the bulimic patient. International Journal of Eating Disorders, 7, 557–560.

74.

TRANSPLANTATION

Thomas W. Heinrich, Michael Marcangelo, and Heidi Christianson

INTRODUCTION

Perhaps nowhere in medicine have science, technology, and clinical care become as closely interlinked as in the field of transplant medicine. Science, in the form of effective immunosuppressant agents, has provided clinicians with the means of overcoming the expected immunological reaction that results when the tissue from a genetically dissimilar individual is transplanted into another individual. Technology, in the form of advancement of surgical technique, has led to better surgical outcomes following solid organ transplantation. Medical science has allowed organ transplantation to advance from an experimental concept less than 70 years ago to a well-established treatment modality for a wide variety of illnesses and end-organ failure. As a result, transplantation of solid organs (kidney, liver, pancreas, intestine, heart, and lung) along with hematopoietic stem cell transplants (HCTs) has become common practice in medical centers all over the world.

TYPES OF TRANSPLANTATION

Transplantation describes the act of transferring an organ, tissue, or cell from one individual to another. Transplants are broadly defined by the genetic similarities between donor and recipient. *Autotransplants* involve the transfer of an organ, tissue, or cell from one part of an individual to another part of that same individual. Because both the donor and recipient are the same person, there is no genetic difference recognized by the recipient's immune system, and no immunosuppression is required to prevent rejection. *Allotransplants* involve the transfer of an organ, tissue, or cell from one individual to a different individual. Unless this transfer occurs between genetically identical twins, some form of suppression of the recipient's immune system will be required to prevent rejection of the graft. Although some generalities exist among transplant patients, organ-specific considerations are important and guide many aspects of assessment and management.

DECEASED DONOR TRANSPLANTS

Most donated solid organs are from deceased individuals (Organ Procurement and Transplantation Network/The Scientific Registry of Transplant Recipients [OPTN/SRTR], 2009). These donors meet the criteria for brain death, but their organs are maintained by life-support measures until informed consent can be obtained from family for donation and the organ procured by the transplant team. The concept of "brain death" means that all brain and brain stem functions have irreversibly ceased activity. Medication effects, hypothermia, and other potentially reversible causes for brain failure must be excluded prior to the final determination and declaration of brain death. The withdrawal of life support from the donor and actual organ donation always occurs with the consent and understanding of the family of the donor.

LIVING DONORS

Potential organ recipients often die awaiting the donation of a compatible organ from a deceased donor (OPTN/SRTR, 2009). The use of organs provided by living donors has greatly increased the supply of certain organs available for transplantation. As a consequence, living-donor donation has become fundamental to the modern practice of transplantation medicine. The concept of living-donation, however, presents its own set of medical and ethical challenges (Ventura, 2010). It is fortunate, however, that the potential disadvantages of living-donor transplants to the donor appear fairly minimal. Adverse donor outcomes usually are related to the surgical procedure being performed, as some organ procurement procedures are technically complex, resulting in an increased incidence of surgical complications, morbidity, and mortality.

Some individuals in need of organ transplantation have family and friends interested in donation, but often these potential donors are unable to donate secondary to genetic incompatibility. In an effort to help these patients receive the potentially life-saving organs, transplant programs have begun arranging paired living-donor transplants (Wallis, Samy, Roth, & Rees, 2011). In these cases, two or more pairs of living donors and matched recipients participate in a paired exchange of organs. In other words, donor/recipient pairs with willing but incompatible donors are matched with another donor/recipient pair who have the same incompatibility problem.

KIDNEY TRANSPLANTATION

As a result of effective immunosuppression, kidney transplantation now is the treatment of choice for many patients with end-stage renal disease (ESRD). Almost all renal diseases responsible for renal failure can be treated by transplantation, and most patients with chronic renal failure should be considered for possible renal transplantation. Transplantation often offers the greatest potential for restoring the patient to a healthy and productive life. Renal transplantation, when compared with dialysis, has been associated with improved patient survival, superior health-related quality of life, and lower overall health costs (Fujisawa et al., 2000; Wolfe et al., 1999). Results for patients who receive a kidney transplant prior to the initiation of dialysis show an improved rate of graft survival compared to that of patients who had had long-term dialysis prior to transplantation (Papalois et al., 2000). It is therefore important for the treatment team to consider patients for renal transplantation as soon as the need for renal replacement therapy appears imminent.

The two sources of kidneys for renal transplantation are living and deceased donors. Living kidney donations are now as common as deceased donation; although the total number of kidneys from deceased donors still exceeds that obtained from living donors, as each deceased donor can donate two kidneys (Figure 74.1).

The graft survival rate for living-donor kidney transplants has been reported to be 96% at one year, 81% at five years, and almost 60% at ten years (OPTN/SRTR, 2009). The donor's remaining kidney compensates for the loss of the donated kidney. Unfortunately, as noted previously, most candidates for a kidney transplant do not have a suitable identified living donor. These patients are placed on a waiting list for a kidney from a deceased donor. Because of the clinical success of the procedure and the limited amount of available organs, this waiting list has grown dramatically over the years. Currently, there are over 100,000 patients in the United States awaiting a kidney transplant (OPTN: Organ Procurement and Transplantation Network, http://optn.transplant.hrsa.gov/).

Following kidney transplantation, patients are monitored for organ rejection by serial measurements of renal function. When the transplanted kidney begins to function, the serum creatinine will gradually fall over a period of several days to reach a new functional baseline. Any significant decrease in renal function below the newly established baseline should prompt an evaluation to determine the etiology. Potential causes include dehydration, obstruction, infection, and graft rejection. Rejection of the transplanted kidney is diagnosed by renal biopsy. Aggressive immunosuppressant therapy is effective in reversing more than 90% of the cases of acute kidney rejection (Midtvedt et al., 2003).

PANCREAS TRANSPLANTATION

A successful pancreas transplantation can lead to normalization of glycemic control in previously diabetic patients without the need for glucose monitoring or insulin administration. Through maintenance of a euglycemic state, the successful pancreas transplant may halt the progression of complications of hyperglycemia, which are associated with significant morbidity and mortality. Pancreatic transplants may also improve the recipient's quality of life, although premorbid psychiatric illness may temper this benefit (Smith, Trauer, Kerr, & Chadban, 2010). Pancreas transplants are now most commonly performed in diabetic patients with concurrent ESRD who are also candidates for a kidney transplant. Pancreas transplant alone, however, may be considered appropriate in the adherent diabetic patient without ESRD who is experiencing an impaired quality of life secondary to the sequelae of difficult-to-control diabetes.

LIVER TRANSPLANTATION

Liver transplant outcomes were generally quite poor until the introduction of the immunosuppressant cyclosporine in the 1980s. Since that time, survival rates have improved dramatically, with one-year patient survival rates hovering around 90% in 2007 (OPTN/SRTR, 2009). Improved outcomes have led to an expanding list of potential indications and a diminishing list of contraindications to liver transplantation. As a result, nearly 6,000 liver transplantations were performed in the United States in 2007 (OPTN/SRTR, 2009) (Figure 74.2).

The list of illnesses that may be addressed through a liver transplantation may be divided into acute hepatic insults and chronic liver disease states. The chronic disease states, specifically cirrhosis, account for the majority of liver transplants today. Cirrhosis is most commonly secondary to chronic hepatitis C infection, but cirrhosis may also be caused by hepatitis B infection, sclerosing cholangitis, fatty liver disease, autoimmune hepatitis, or primary biliary cirrhosis. Alcohol may contribute to the development of end-stage liver disease and cirrhosis, alone or in combination with viral hepatitis infection. Fulminant hepatic failure, or acute liver disease, is defined as the development of coagulopathy and hepatic encephalopathy

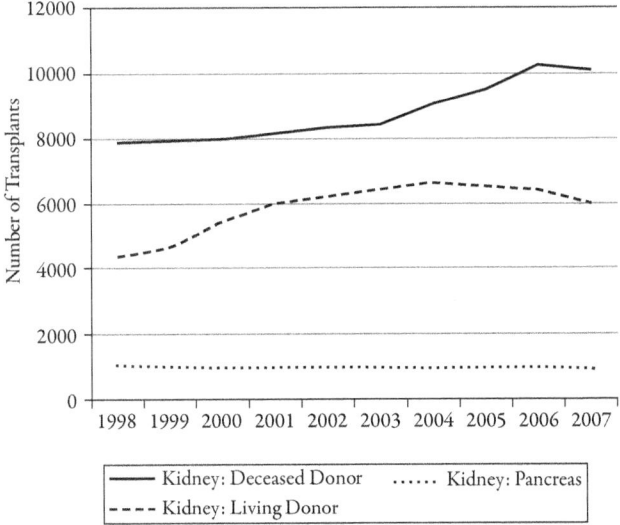

Figure 74.1 Kidney and kidney-pancreas transplants. U.S. Department of Health and Human Services, Health Resources and Services Administration (2010). 2009 Annual Report of the U.S. Organ Procurement and Transplantation Network and the Scientific Registry of Transplant Recipients: Transplant Data 1999–2008. Rockville, MD: Healthcare Systems Bureau, Division of Transplantation.

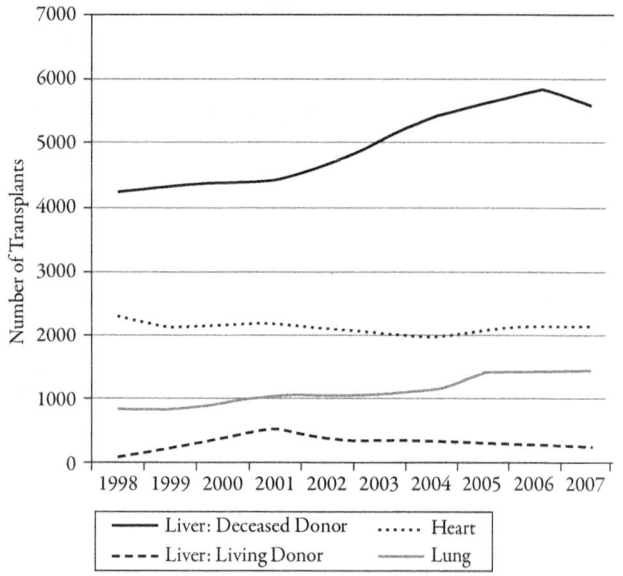

Figure 74.2 Liver, heart, and lung transplants. U.S. Department of Health and Human Services, Health Resources and Services Administration (2010). 2009 Annual Report of the U.S. Organ Procurement and Transplantation Network and the Scientific Registry of Transplant Recipients: Transplant Data 1999–2008. Rockville, MD: Healthcare Systems Bureau, Division of Transplantation.

in a patient shortly after the onset of other symptoms of liver disease. There are many causes of acute liver failure. One of the most common etiologies of acute liver failure encountered by the psychiatrist is acetaminophen overdose.

The Model for End-stage Liver Disease (MELD) score has been utilized to help predict the severity of illness and associated mortality of patients awaiting a liver transplant (Kamath et al., 2001).

A higher MELD score suggests a more severe level of illness and associated elevated risk of mortality (Box 74.1). Patients on the waiting list are listed by MELD score, with the highest scores being at the top of each blood group. This differs from kidney transplants, where patients are listed simply by the amount of time they have been waiting for a transplant. The goal is to direct the donated liver to the individual in greatest need based on their predicted mortality. It is important to note that the MELD system does not account for all illness parameters, and unique patient-specific circumstances must often be taken into account to ensure the best use of donated livers.

Living-donor liver transplantation is an option for some candidates, but the risk to the proposed donor and the benefit to the potential organ recipient must be carefully balanced. Donation of the left lateral segment or lobe of the liver, which is used primarily in pediatric liver transplantation, and right lobe liver donation, which is used in adult liver transplantation, are both associated with the potential for donor morbidity and mortality. Middleton et al. (2006) reported an overall donor mortality of approximately 0.2%, with a slightly higher rate of approximately 0.4% in right lobe donation. The most common complications reported in this study were infections and biliary leaks. A study that looked at the psychosocial outcomes of liver donors found that approximately 96% returned to their previous employment at 2.4 months,

Box 74.1 MODEL FOR END-STAGE LIVER DISEASE (MELD)

MELD score = 3.8 × log(e)(bilirubin mg/dL) + 11.2 × log(e) (INR) + 9.6 log(e) creatinine mg/dL

Source: Kamath, P. S., Wiesner, R. H., Malinchoc, M., Kremers, W., Therneau, T. M., Kosberg, C. L., et al. (2001). A model to predict survival in patients with end stage liver disease. *Hepatology*, 33(2), 464–470.

but a significant minority (42%) reported a change in bodily images, and a majority (71%) reported ongoing mild physical symptoms. The out-of-pocket cost associated with the donation averaged over $3,500. Importantly, each of the 24 individuals surveyed reported that they would donate again (Trotter et al., 2001).

When compared to other transplanted organs, the transplanted liver appears to require less immunosuppression maintenance therapy. Corticosteroids may be gradually discontinued once the graft is established. Monotherapy with a calcineurin inhibitor is often all that is required to suppress rejection long-term. In fact, immune tolerance with normal graft function in the absence of immunosuppressant medications has been reported to occur in approximately 10–20% of liver transplant recipients (Lerut & Sanchez-Fueyo, 2006).

HEART TRANSPLANTATION

Over 2,000 heart transplants were performed in 2007, with a one-year survival rate of just less than 90% (OPTN/SRTR, 2009). Donor hearts must be ABO-compatible and preferably free of preexisting heart disease. In addition, the donor should be within 20% of the recipient's ideal body weight in an effort to match historic and potential cardiac work load. The most common medical conditions treated with cardiac transplantation include idiopathic dilated or ischemic cardiomyopathy. Candidates for transplantation should have failed optimal medical therapy for their end-stage heart failure and have exhausted all other surgical options.

As the transplanted heart is both afferent and efferent denervated, allograft pathology is difficult to diagnosis clinically. Therefore, in asymptomatic individuals, regular post-transplant monitoring for rejection is warranted. The 2010 consensus statement by the International Society for Heart and Lung Transplantation indicates that routine coronary angiography is the accepted standard for surveillance for rejection following heart transplantation (Mehra et al., 2010). Noninvasive techniques have yet to be shown to be been sensitive enough to replace invasive coronary angiography within the first five years following transplantation. If the noninvasive studies, such as dobutamine stress echocardiography or computed tomography (CT) angiography, are abnormal, the patient will require evaluation by invasive coronary angiography. In addition, if the patient presents with symptoms and signs of left ventricular dysfunction, invasive coronary angiography and endometrial biopsy are necessary to diagnosis rejection. Acute rejection in cardiac graft recipients is identified based on the results of an endomyocardial biopsy. Transplant centers often follow a regular predetermined schedule of biopsies after transplantation.

Chronic rejection is believed to be manifested through accelerated coronary atherosclerosis, or allograft vasculopathy, in the engrafted heart. Chronic graft rejection has been documented to occur in 30–40% of patients within five years after transplantation (Syeda, Roedler, Schukro, Yahya, Zuckermann, & Glogar, 2005). Registry data indicate that about 33% of deaths up to ten years following transplantation are secondary to cardiac allograft vasculopathy and resulting graft failure (Taylor et al., 2009). Fortunately, cardiac allograft vasculopathy is a slowly progressive disease, and clinical outcome appears related to severity of the coronary disease (Costanzo et al., 1998). Unfortunately, there is no known effective therapy for this progressive condition except retransplantation with another heart.

Patients with failing hearts awaiting cardiac transplant may be bridged to transplantation using mechanical ventricular assist devices (VADs). These cardiac assist devices are driven by external power sources and have been shown to improve survival to transplantation (Frazier et al., 2001). Individuals being bridged to transplant with a VAD must meet criteria for transplantation and must have failed all other pharmacological therapies for severe heart failure, including oral medications and intravenous inotropic support. VAD placement stabilizes the patient's hemodynamic status while awaiting transplantation (Haft et al., 2007). As a result, the end-organ effects of severe congestive heart failure, such as renal failure, hepatic dysfunction, and delirium, can be dramatically reduced. These devices can sustain the patient over weeks, months, or even years until a cardiac transplant is obtained for the patient. Post-transplant survival for patients bridged to cardiac transplant with VADs has been shown to be comparable to those not requiring treatment with VAD (Shuhaiber, Hur, & Gibbons, 2010). The use of VADs is not without associated psychiatric comorbidity (Tigges-Limmer, Schönbrodt, Roefe, Arusoglu, Morshuis, & Gummert, 2010). Memory problems and risk of stroke have been concerns, but the technology is improving.

LUNG TRANSPLANTATION

Over the last decade, lung transplantation has become an established intervention in the management of patients with irreversible end-stage pulmonary disease. Patients must be oxygen-dependent, and they typically have a life expectancy of 12–18 months without successful lung transplantation. Pulmonary diseases that can lead to transplantation include chronic obstructive pulmonary disease (COPD), cystic fibrosis, interstitial lung disease, alpha-$_1$-antitrypsin deficiency, and primary pulmonary hypertension. Patients with different lung pathologies may derive varying levels of clinical benefit from transplant. In a study of United Kingdom lung transplants, Titman et al.

(2009) found transplantation appeared to improve survival for all groups studied, but cystic fibrosis patients fared the best post-transplant, while patients with COPD had the greatest risk of death following transplant. There are approximately 1,300 lung transplants performed annually in the United States (OPTN/SRTR, 2009). Lung transplant patient survival rates, overall, in the United States have been reported to be 84% at one year, 54% at five years, and 27% at ten years (OPTN/SRTR 2009).

A major long-term complication of lung transplantation is the development of the bronchiolitis obliterans syndrome (BOS). BOS is characterized clinically by airflow limitation and pathologically by partial or complete occlusion of the lumens of terminal bronchioles by inflammation and fibrous tissue. Over 50% of lung transplant recipients surviving to five years will develop BOS (Christie et al., 2008). BOS is thought to be a manifestation of chronic rejection. Episodes of acute rejection of the lung graft have been identified as a risk factor for the future development of chronic rejection and BOS (Todd & Palmer, 2011). There is currently no effective therapy for BOS, although the development of aerosolized immunosuppression provides hope for directed and enhanced pulmonary immunosuppression.

INTESTINAL TRANSPLANTATION

Intestinal transplantation may be offered to patients with irreversible intestinal failure resulting in impaired absorption and associated malnutrition. Intestinal failure is most often due to short-bowel syndrome. Crohn's disease, trauma, and surgical complications are common causes of short-bowel syndrome in the United States. Total parental nutrition (TPN), the standard treatment for impaired intestinal absorption, has significant associated morbidity and mortality. Intestinal transplantation was developed in an attempt to avoid the potential complications of long-term TPN. Controversy exists about which patients should continue to receive TPN and which should receive an intestinal transplant (Fishbein, 2009). As a result, intestinal transplants represent one of the least frequently performed organ transplants, with only 162 intestinal transplantations performed in the United States in 2007 (OPTN/SRTR 2009).

Intestinal transplants are associated with some of the highest rates of rejection in solid organ transplantation. The high rates of rejection are probably due to the fact that the intestine is a very complex organ immunologically (Newell, 2003). Transplantation is further complicated by the fact that identification of graft rejection is a clinical challenge, since the most common symptom of graft dysfunction is the very nonspecific complaint of diarrhea. It is also very difficult to biochemically monitor for rejection, as no laboratory screening tests have been developed that reliably indicate the presence of acute rejection of the intestinal graft. Infection is another common complication after intestinal transplantation, as shown in a study of 13 patients that found that bacterial infections (primarily gram-negative organisms) were the most common type of infection encountered postoperatively, followed by viral (primarily CMV) and fungal infections (Guaraldi et al., 2005).

COMPOSITE TISSUE TRANSPLANTATION

Composite tissue transplantation is a developing area of reconstructive transplant surgery. Such composite tissue transplantation may lead to improved outcomes for patients who have suffered devastating facial or upper extremity injuries. Quality of life has been reported to improve following composite tissue transplantation (Coffman, Gordon, & Siemionow, 2010). The most important determinants of successful composite tissue transplantation appear to be patient selection, adherence, intense rehabilitation, and a dedicated, experienced, multidisciplinary treatment team (Siemionow, Zor, & Gordon, 2010).

A review of 13 cases of facial transplantation was performed between 2005 and 2010 (Siemionow & Ozturk, 2011) in which a majority of facial transplantations were described as "partial facial reconstruction." For the majority the need resulted from traumatic injury. Two of the 13 patients had died due to transplant-related complications. Functional outcomes differed in each survivor as a result of differences in pre-transplant injury. Because of limited experience with it and the overall complexity of composite tissue transplantation, multiple questions regarding the role of this treatment remain unanswered.

HEMATOPOIETIC STEM CELL TRANSPLANTATION (HCT)

An HCT involves the infusion of hematopoietic stem cells obtained from bone marrow (bone marrow transplantation), peripheral blood, or umbilical cord blood in an effort to treat various hematological, neoplastic, and autoimmune conditions. HCTs may be autologous or allogeneic. In allogeneic stem cell transplants, human leukocyte antigen (HLA)-matched stem cells from a donor are transferred to the recipient. In an autologous stem cell transplants, the patient's own previously harvested stem cells are infused back into the patient following the myeloablative therapy. Autologous HCT is now a more common therapy than allotransplantation (Pasquini & Wang, 2010). The ability to transplant healthy hematopoietic stem cells permits the administration of otherwise lethal chemotherapy with or without associated radiation to a patient. The object of this myeloablative preparation is to eradicate the unwanted cell lines.

Allogeneic transplants are usually considered for patients younger than 60 years of age, due to an increasing incidence of graft-versus-host disease (GVHD) in older recipients (Gale et al., 1987). Patients who do not have an HLA-matched sibling may use stem cells from a partially HLA-matched relative, or the National Marrow Donor Program (NMDP) may identify an unrelated but closely HLA-matched potential donor. In addition, cord blood can be utilized in HCT. Immunosuppression to prevent graft rejection and GVHD is an important component of allogeneic transplantation. However, lifelong immunosuppression is often not required in allogeneic HCT due to the development of immunological tolerance once engraftment of the transplanted cells is complete. The same immunological activity of the donor cells that contributes to the occurrence of GVHD also provides an important graft-versus-tumor effect, which leads to reduced rates of oncological relapse after allogeneic transplant in patients who develop GVHD (Horowitz et al., 1990). In contrast to allogeneic HCT, autologous transplantation may be safely utilized in older patients because of the absence of GVHD. However, the risk of transplanted autologous stem cells being contaminated with tumor cells, coupled with the loss of a graft-versus-tumor effect, results in patients who are undergoing autologous transplantation having higher cancer relapse rates. If no suitable hematopoietic stem cell donor is found, or if the transplant is urgent, cord blood from related or unrelated donors can be used. Cellular qualities of cord blood may convey less host-targeted activity so that the incidence of GVHD is reduced despite HLA mismatch. One proposed theory is that the cytotoxic T cells in cord blood are naïve with decreased allogenic reactivity, due to the presence of non-inherited maternal antigens. For many children, cord blood is now transplanted instead of peripheral blood or marrow from unrelated adults. Outcomes of cord blood HCT vary according to the disease being treated, the age of the patient, and the degree of HLA mismatch between the recipient and the transplanted cord blood.

HCTs are associated with the potential for significant morbidity. Infections are a major cause of morbidity due to the effects of myeloablation therapy and, in the case of allogeneic HCT, the immunosuppressive therapy (Wingard, Hsu, & Hiemenz, 2010). Mucositis is a common complication of the pre-transplant myeloablative preparative regimens. When mucositis affects the gastrointestinal tract, it may cause nausea, cramping, and diarrhea, and can be so severe as to require parenteral nutrition. Oropharyngeal mucositis is very painful and can lead to poor oral intake. Another acute adverse effect of HCT is veno-occlusive disease of the liver. This syndrome consists of painful hepatomegaly, jaundice, ascites, and weight gain. Veno-occlusive disease is potentially fatal.

THE PRE-TRANSPLANTATION ASSESSMENT

One of the key roles that the medical psychiatrist or psychologist plays on a transplant team is performing the pre-transplantation assessment of patients who are being considered for transplantation. This evaluation plays an important role in determining which patients will be listed for transplantation and eligible for the scarce organs that make up the transplant pool. Pre-transplant assessment should address substance abuse, social support, adherence, major mental disorders, and cognitive impairment. As a whole, pre-transplant assessment can be used to assess the patient's ability to cope with the intervention and the post-transplant recovery period, in order to inform the team whether an individual would be able to psychologically handle transplant. It also allows for treatment planning to monitor and manage high-risk patients.

THE MULTIDISCIPLINARY TEAM

Organ transplantation involves professionals from many disciplines. In order to achieve clinical and administrative success, this team must work together effectively to serve patients. While teams vary in composition from transplant center to transplant center and from organ to organ within centers, a number of disciplines are typically represented. Sub-specialist internists, such as cardiologists or hepatologists, often play central roles in the management of the patients and frequently serve as the referral source for the team. Transplant surgeons perform the operations and play leading roles in organ procurement and post-operative management. Nurses often serve as coordinators for the patients and become the people whom patients turn to with questions about nuances of their medical regimen as they navigate their way through the process of transplantation. The assessment team includes, usually, a psychiatrist or a psychologist and a social worker. Sometimes, teams have both a psychiatrist and a psychologist. Screening assessments and supportive psychotherapy are performed by any of the three disciplines. In addition, typically, psychiatrists diagnose major mental disorders and prescribe psychotropic drugs; psychologists do diagnostic assessments and deliver cognitive behavioral therapy (CBT); and social workers address family, occupational, financial, and insurance-related problem. The leader of the assessment team is typically either a psychiatrist or a psychologist. Advance-practice nurses function as case managers on many transplant teams, coordinating the biomedical, psychosocial, and practical aspects of patients' care.

Patient selection is a key aspect of transplantation team work, and usually this occurs as a weekly meeting of the selection committee where all disciplines are present. Typically, surgery, the applicable medical subspecialties, and psychiatry are represented. Patient care coordinators, who are usually nurses, often lead the meetings and initiate the presentation of the patient's case.

LIVING-DONOR ASSESSMENT

Living donation for kidney and liver transplantation is performed at many transplant centers. Transplant centers should have a special team dedicated to evaluating prospective donors. The donor's motivation for donation is a key aspect of the evaluation. "True informed consent" is a challenging concept in the face of family pressure and a life-or-death situation. If the donor knows the recipient, which is by the far the most common scenario, there must be discussion of their relationship and the donor's hopes for life after the transplant. A basic psychiatric evaluation should also take place to ensure that the patient's decision is not unduly influenced by an active mental disorder. Financial incentives for donation are strictly prohibited in the United States, and efforts should be made to ensure that the recipient is not paying for the organ. This concern increases with donor-recipient pairs who are distantly related or even strangers, and where the recipient has financial means.

BIOPSYCHOSOCIAL ASSESSMENT

The assessment of potential transplant recipients includes many of the professionals outlined above. Medical and surgical assessment is central to establishing that a patient is likely to survive transplant and is suitable from a technical perspective. Additionally, psychosocial assessment is essential and covers a number of key areas, including his or her psychiatric history, coping style, and level of social support

When patients consent to a psychiatric evaluation as part of their transplant assessment, the psychiatrist has two duties, which are sometimes in conflict. One duty, akin to that of a typical psychiatric evaluation, is to assess the patient's safety and overall mental health and provide treatment as indicated. The other duty is to provide information to the team that will inform the team's decision about how to proceed with the patient's medical care, including what priority to assign to the patient on a waiting list. This part of the work, akin to forensic evaluation, is intended to maximize overall social benefit and may not always serve the best interests of the patient being evaluated. Juggling these responsibilities is one of the primary challenges facing psychiatrists and psychologists working in transplant. At the outset of the evaluation, the psychiatrist can explain that the purpose of the evaluation is to determine if the patient is a suitable candidate for transplantation and to provide treatment recommendations for any psychiatric conditions that are diagnosed during the evaluation.

SOCIAL SUPPORT

A major element of the evaluation is assessment of a patient's social support. Often, the social worker on the team will perform a detailed assessment of a patient's living situation, family structure, and financial status. The psychiatrist should review these with the patient and assess the stability and constancy of the patient's support network. After transplant, patients require assistance with many aspects of their lives, including nutrition, transportation, and finances. There is evidence that transplant patients who live with at least one other person have better medical and psychiatric outcomes than those who live alone (Tsunoda et al., 2010; Spaderna et al., 2010). Patients with poor social support have lower rates of adherence after transplant (Dobbels et al., 2009; Stilley et al., 2010). The emotional support provided by family and friends also assists patients with the often difficult recovery after transplant. For patients with limited support, involving those closest to them in the process and developing a plan for the post-transplant period can often improve their candidacies significantly.

INFORMED CONSENT

Organ transplantation is among the most invasive and life-altering surgeries a person can undergo, and, as such, the patient's capacity to consent should be assessed carefully. In the face of end-stage organ disease, patients face the prospect of death without transplant, and they often quickly agree to the procedure before they understand the impact it will have on their life. The pre-transplant evaluation should assess a patient's consent for transplant. By reviewing their medical problem, their options, and their choice, a patient can demonstrate that they have the capacity to make an informed decision (Appelbaum, 2007). A patient's knowledge of the illness does not have to be complete, but basic facts, like which organ needs to be transplanted and the likely outcomes with or without transplant, should be confirmed. A bedside cognitive evaluation should also be performed to help to assess the patient's capacity to consent. When the chronic mental status waxes and wanes as it might pre-liver transplant, the assessments are made when the patient is at his best.

ADHERENCE

The medication regimen that patients are prescribed after transplant is often complex and daunting to follow, even by the standards of patients who have had long-standing medical problems. The threat of organ rejection and the need for powerful immunosuppressants mean that patients must be able to take their medications as prescribed in order to maintain their health. During the pre-transplant assessment, a patient's ability to adhere to complex medical regimens should be investigated as thoroughly as possible. Predicting a patient's behavior months or years after an evaluation is impossible, but if patients have a clear history of non-adherence with past treatment, they are at risk for non-adherence after transplant. More than 60% of American liver transplant programs reported that they would not list for transplantation a patient with a history of non-adherence (Kroeker et al., 2008). Risk factors for non-adherence in kidney transplantation include depression, younger age, and fewer than 12 years of education (Jindal et al., 2009), and it is reasonable to believe that these risk factors apply to other organs as well. Hemodialysis attendance for patients with renal failure is probably the most straightforward way to assess adherence in pre-transplant patients; if patients have struggled to attend dialysis sessions regularly, they are likely to struggle with the post-transplant regimen of medications and appointments.

When assessing adherence, both patients and their medical record should be consulted. Patients should be asked about their understanding of post-transplant management and expectations. Patients may be surprised after transplant by the complexity of their situation and voice regret about having agreed to take on the major responsibility of managing their medications and appointments. A detailed discussion before transplant can often clear up some of this misunderstanding. Patients should also review their current medications, including their indications, dosages, and timing. The amount of assistance the patient requires to take his or her medications as well as their level of organization (e.g., weekly pillboxes) can provide hints of how much effort a patient puts into their medical care. Records can indicate how often patients miss scheduled appointments and reveal their physician's assessment of past adherence.

In addition to medications, patients have to change their lifestyles after transplant. A post-transplant patient has to be a "professional patient" in the sense that they will be having regular physician visits, medical tests, and blood work for the rest of their lives. Additionally, patients must adhere to lifestyle changes, such as changes in diet, exercise, or mobility, following transplant that may significantly alter the way they live their lives. During the assessment, patients should be informed of these expectations and discuss their attitudes towards the patient role and significant life-adaptation. If patients indicate that they are going to struggle to incorporate the self-concept of "patient" into their post-transplant lives, they should be encouraged to think further about their choice and decide if transplant is right for them.

PSYCHIATRIC DISORDERS

Assessment of psychopathology is a primary goal of the pre-transplant assessment. The evaluation is similar to that of routine psychiatric exams, although with the absence of an obvious chief complaint. Common psychiatric disorders, such as major depressive disorder and generalized anxiety disorder, and major psychiatric symptoms, such as suicidal ideation or auditory hallucinations, should be investigated during the exam. If the patient shows signs of having impaired cognition, deciding between delirium and dementia is vital to helping the team make a decision about transplant. Hepatic encephalopathy, uremia from kidney failure, advanced heart failure with poor forward flow, or hypoxia from lung disease can all cause delirium in the context of end-stage organ disease. In these clinical situations, it is essential to gather collateral history from the patient's designated healthcare power of attorney as well as other family and friends to confirm that the cognitive changes are new and to use their substituted decision on behalf of the patient if death is imminent and listing for transplant urgent. Neuropsychological testing can be utilized to distinguish between different types of cognitive disorders and provide guidance on interventions. If the cognitive evaluation reveals significant deficits that are determined to be long-standing and consistent with dementia, the team will usually not offer transplantation.

A detailed psychiatric history, including history of hospitalizations, suicide attempts, psychotropic medications, and past diagnoses, should be obtained. As with other types of patients, transplant patients who have historically been accepting of psychiatric care are more likely to accept care in the future when it is necessary. A family history of psychiatric disorders can point towards a genetic diathesis towards affective or anxiety disorders that may emerge due to the stress of transplant.

Substance Use Disorders

Patients who receive organ transplants can have significant histories of alcoholism or substance abuse. The two most common indications for liver transplantation are hepatitis C, which commonly is contracted through intravenous drug use, and alcohol-related liver disease (Varma et al., 2010). Patients with end-stage heart failure may have ischemic cardiomyopathy with smoking as a contributing factor, or alcohol-related cardiomyopathy. Finally, COPD, most commonly caused by smoking, is one of the leading indications for lung transplantation. A detailed history of substance use, including age of onset, patterns of use, consequences of use, and most recent use, should be elicited. Each substance that the patient has used should be discussed in this fashion, and some patients will have a history of polysubstance dependence. Patients with a history of polysubstance dependence do not appear to have higher rates of alcohol and drug use after liver transplantation than those with only alcohol dependence (Coffman et al., 1997).

Another aspect of substance use that should be investigated is the patient's history of rehabilitation attempts. Both formal rehabilitation programs and attendance at Alcoholics Anonymous (AA) should be documented. Many programs require patients to either join a Twelve Step program such as AA or go into rehabilitation, although the evidence in favor of this is limited. Motivational enhancement therapy may decrease the amount and frequency of drinking in pre-transplant patients compared with usual Twelve Step–based treatments (Weinrieb et al., 2011). Risk factors for relapse that have been identified include psychiatric comorbidities, duration of abstinence of less than six months, and a high score on the High-Risk Alcoholism Relapse scale (which includes number of attempts at rehabilitation, duration of drinking, and amount of alcohol consumed each day) (De Gottardi et al., 2007). A comprehensive meta-analysis identified poor social support, a family history of alcoholism, and duration of abstinence less than six months as the major risk factors for relapse to alcohol use after liver transplant (Dew et al., 2008). It is reasonable to think that similar risk factors apply to other substances of abuse and organs.

Programs have a wide range of guidelines in regard to substance use prior to and after transplant. For heart and lung transplant programs, it is standard practice that patients abstain from smoking cigarettes for at least six months prior to transplant, and for the patient to be expected to remain abstinent for the rest of their lives. On the other hand, thoracic transplant programs often do not have a formal policy on alcohol use and, while they would expect patients with alcohol dependence to receive treatment and abstain, they tolerate moderate use of alcohol. The situation is reversed for liver transplant candidates. These patients are expected to abstain for a period of time prior to transplant, usually six months, and to remain abstinent afterwards. However, many liver and kidney transplant programs do not have formal smoking guidelines, and some programs tolerate cannabis use by transplant patients. The six-month guideline that programs have adopted has limited supporting evidence, but it does appear

that the longer a patient has been abstinent prior to transplant, the more likely they are to remain abstinent after transplant (DiMartini et al., 2010; Karim et al., 2010). Reports of successful liver transplantation in carefully selected patients with acute alcoholic hepatitis who have not achieved abstinence for any significant amount of time may lead to a change in approach for these patients, who face high mortality without transplantation (Mathurin et al., 2011).

Patients who are dependent on heroin or other opioids have high rates of hepatitis C and may develop cirrhosis and require liver transplant. Methadone maintenance therapy has been used successfully in patients undergoing transplantation, and it appears the highest rates of success are seen in patients who remain on methadone rather than transitioning off after transplant (Jiao et al., 2010). These patients often require higher doses of pain medication after transplant and often need additional methadone for an extended period post-transplant (Weinrieb et al., 2004). Other factors related to their candidacy, including levels of social support and comorbid psychiatric conditions, should be closely investigated, but if a patient is otherwise a good candidate, he or she can be successfully transplanted while on methadone. Experience with buprenorphine is limited, but it may prove to be as efficacious as methadone.

Personality Disorders

Personality disorders are a complex issue in transplantation. Personality disorders do not appear to be more prevalent in transplant populations (Dobbels et al., 2000), but patients with personality disorders can cause significant problems for transplant teams. Many programs cite major personality disorders, such an antisocial personality disorder or borderline personality disorder, as relative contraindications to transplant (Levenson & Olbrisch, 1993). Personality disorders can lead to increased rates of mood disorders after transplant, impulsive behavior such as suicidal ideation or attempts, and conflicted relationships with the transplant team. Patients with obsessive personality traits are often very adherent, but they can struggle with the loss of control that occurs during the transplant process and develop depressive disorders or adjustment disorders with disturbance of behavior in which they refuse to comply due to anger. Part of the pre-transplant evaluation should assess the patient's underlying personality traits and whether they can work successfully with the team. If the patient can, suggestions about ways in which the team can accommodate the patient (e.g., giving an obsessive patient choices to increase their sense of control when possible) help both the patient and the team work together successfully. Often, it is helpful to identify one team member to work exclusively with the patient to avoid "splitting." If the patient's personality is assessed as being prohibitive for transplant, explaining this to the team in clear language that avoids psychiatric jargon will help everyone to understand why the patient presents an unacceptable risk.

A common indication for liver transplantation is acute acetaminophen toxicity leading to fulminant hepatic failure. A large series found that 44% of these cases were related to a suicide attempt (Larson et al., 2005). In the United States, if a patient with fulminant hepatic failure is listed, they essentially go right to the top of the list because their risk of death if there is delay quickly approaches 100%, so obtaining an accurate history quickly is essential. The patient is at risk for developing hepatic coma as their liver injury progresses, so rapid evaluation is essential. Even if the patient is awake, efforts at piecing together what happened prior to the suicide attempt can be thwarted by the patient's psychiatric disorder or their unwillingness to discuss their attempt. Family and friends may minimize risk in order to improve the patient's candidacy. While the evaluation is complex and the whole picture should be examined, the number of past attempts and the social stability of the patient are two key factors in determining if the patient is a candidate for transplant. If a patient voices a willingness to undergo transplant and has a relatively stable personal and psychiatric history, he or she can be a successful transplant recipient. In the United Kingdom, patients who underwent liver transplantation following a suicide attempt had similar outcomes as other candidates, although 6% had post-transplant suicide attempts (Karvellas et al., 2010). Ongoing suicidal ideation during the evaluation should preclude the patient from being a candidate.

Psychotic Disorders

Patients with schizophrenia present challenges to a transplant team. Their illness may be marked by non-adherence and poor social support, two common findings in a poor candidate for transplant. However, if a patient with a long-standing psychotic illness has other findings consistent with being a good candidate, including family or social support and good adherence with medications, he or she can have success with transplant. The transplant psychiatrist is likely to play an active role in the care of the patient, but if the patient has a strong established relationship with his or her psychiatrist, that person should continue to care for the patient. While outcomes have been mixed both medically and psychiatrically (Coffman & Crone, 2002), psychotic disorders should not be an absolute contraindication to transplant.

PSYCHOLOGICAL ASSESSMENT TOOLS FOR PRE-TRANSPLANT EVALUATION

Brief psychological assessment instruments used to determine readiness for transplant are the Psychosocial Assessment of Candidates for Transplantation (PACT; Olbrisch, Levenson, & Hamer, 1989), the Transplant Evaluation Rating Scale (TERS; Twillman, Manetto, Wellisch, & Wolcott, 1993), and the Millon Behavioral Medicine Diagnostic (MBMD; Millon, Antoni, Millon, Meagher, & Grossman, 2001). The former two assessment tools are rating scales that are derived from a clinical interview, while the MBMD is a validated measure that provides information in a self-report questionnaire format. The most recently developed structured transplant assessment tool, the Stanford Integrated Psychosocial Assessment for Transplantation, or SIPAT, produces a single score from a clinical interview that estimates

the patient's risks of a poor psychosocial outcome after transplant (Maldonado et al., 2012).

The items of the PACT include support stability, support availability, personality psychopathology, psychopathology risk, healthy lifestyle, drug and alcohol use, compliance, and transplant knowledge. The TERS is completed from data derived from a clinical interview and includes substance abuse, health behavior, compliance, coping history, *Diagnostic and Statistical Manual of Mental Disorders–IV* (DSM-IV) Axis I disorder, DSM-IV Axis II disorder, affect quality, mental status, family support, and disease coping. The MBMD (Millon et al., 2004) is a health psychology test that assesses selected psychiatric symptomatology, dominant coping strategies, stress moderators, and behaviors and attitudes that either complicate or enhance treatment efficacy. It has been standardized in patients with general medical conditions as well as patients seeking bariatric surgery. Farrell et al. (2011) found that the Medication Abuse subscale of the MBMD predicted medication non-adherence in heart transplant patients and accounted for the relationship between depression and non-adherence. The MBMD can also be used to identify coping strengths, such as social support, religious beliefs, and informational comfort about one's disease and treatment. As such, use of this tool can be particularly helpful when considering patient's strengths and developing treatment plans to address patients' psychiatric problems during their hospitalization and post-transplant recovery period.

Given the comorbidity of cognitive deficits in medically complicated patients undergoing transplant, neuropsychological testing may be necessary to determine their cognitive capacity to make decisions about transplant as well as to engage in appropriate self-care following treatment. Routine mental status examinations such at the Mini Mental Status Exam (Folstein, Folstein, & McHugh, 1975), St. Louis University Mental Status (SLUMS; Tariq, Tumosa, Chibnall, Perry, & Morley, 2006), or Montreal Cognitive Assessment (MoCA; Nasreddine, Phillips, Beédirian, et al., 2005) provide clinicians with a gross estimate of cognition and information about whether formal neuropsychological testing is indicated.

Assessment of psychiatric symptomatology as well as personality functioning may also be useful in the context of pre-transplant assessment; however, application of these measures must be done with caution, considering potential ethical conflicts. Personality tests were created and normalized for psychiatric populations and may be inappropriately interpreted when applied to a non-psychiatric population. Popular measures of psychological distress as well as personality include the Minnesota Multiphasic Personality Inventory-2(MMPI-2) (Butcher et al., 2001) and Millon Clinical Multiaxial Inventory-III (MCMI-III) (Millon, 1994). Assessment of personality functioning may be helpful if preexisting personality disorder is suspected. However, as a routine part of pre-transplant evaluation, personality testing is likely to be inappropriate.

Overall, the measures needed for pre-transplant evaluation consist of a measure of transplant-related coping and behavior, a screen of cognitive function, and a measure of psychiatric symptomatology. Additional measures of major psychopathology or personality dysfunction should be added where they are clinically warranted; for instance, if the patient is displaying inappropriate behaviors prior to transplant, or if the patient is suspected to have long-standing maladaptive coping strategies.

PRE-TRANSPLANT PERIOD: THE WAITING PERIOD

Once an individual has been placed on the waiting list, they typically wait a significant period of time prior to undergoing transplant, given the limited number of available organs. This time can be several months to years, depending on age, blood type, and other medical factors (Table 74.1).

Research suggests patients on a waiting list for an extended period of time tend to lose a sense of self and define themselves by test results and medical information (Brown, Sorrell, McClaren, & Creswell, 2006). The experience of being on call for an organ limits an individual, as he/she must restrain relationships, job decisions, and travel in order to be ready for an organ when it arrives. This situation of "arrested development" adversely affects their quality of life. In addition, patients often have mixed feelings about the waitlist process and may question its fairness (Brown, Sorrell, McClaren, & Creswell, 2006). Apart from concerns related to the wait itself, it is common for patients awaiting transplant to feel anxiety and apprehension about the procedure, with fears of pain, of invasive medical procedures, and of having foreign tissue in their bodies (Tringali et al., 1994).

POSTOPERATIVE PERIOD

GRAFT REJECTION

Graft rejection is triggered when the T and B lymphocytes of the transplant recipient's immune system recognize antigens

Table 74.1 WAITING TIME UNTIL TRANSPLANTATION

MEDIAN WAITING TIME UNTIL TRANSPLANT
(2003–2004 DATA)

Organ	Age range: 18–34	Age range: 35–49	Age range: 50–64	Age range: 65+
Heart	170 days	169	169	86
Intestine	149	109	109	–
Kidney	1813	1806	1627	1416
Liver	169	450	417	294
Lung	808	1059	511	186
Pancreas	561	510	747	–

NOTE: Data from Organ Procurement and Transplantation Network, years 1999–2004. See OPTN: Organ Precurement and Transplantation Network, http://optn.transplant.hrsa.gov/latestData/rptStrat.Asp.

present on the graft. The main antigens involved in triggering organ rejection are coded for by a group of genes known as the HLA system. Multiple components of the immune system are then activated, leading to inflammation, tissue injury, and graft damage (Cuturi, Blancho, Josien, & Soulillou, 1994). Rejection of transplanted organs can be classified into three types, based on the timing and mechanism of injury: hyperacute, acute, and chronic.

Hyperacute Organ Rejection

Hyperacute rejection, which usually occurs within minutes after the transplanted organ is re-perfused, is due to the presence in the recipient, prior to the transplant procedure, of antibodies directed against antigens on the donated organ. These antibodies bind to the vascular endothelium in the graft and lead to intravascular coagulation. The result is an edematous graft that undergoes ischemic necrosis within as little as 24 hours. This type of rejection generally is irreversible, and replacement of the transplant with one from a different donor is the only therapeutic option. Fortunately, pre-transplant cross-matching has essentially eliminated this type of organ rejection.

Acute Organ Rejection

Acute rejection can occur in the months following transplantation. The mechanism is primarily cell-mediated, mainly by lymphocytes. In acute organ rejection, the patient is usually asymptomatic, and the diagnosis is suspected based on a pattern of results on serial laboratory measures, such as a rising creatinine levels in kidney transplant recipients. In severe cases, systemic symptoms can emerge as a consequence of graft failure. Acute graft rejection is most often treated with high-dose pulse steroid therapy. Polyclonal anti-T-cell antibodies, such as antithymocyte globulin, along with monoclonal antibodies, such as the anti-CD52 antibody alemtuzumab and the anti-CD20 antibody rituximab may be utilized to treat acute rejection not responsive to other means of treatment.

Chronic Organ Rejection

Chronic rejection is a late cause of graft deterioration. The improvement in short-term graft survival has resulted in chronic rejection's becoming an increasingly common complication of organ transplantation. The exact mechanism of chronic rejection is complex, but inflammation, atrophy, and fibrosis are the histological hallmarks of this process. It is most often diagnosed by the gradual deterioration in the functional capacity of the transplanted organ. Manifestations of chronic rejection are organ-specific. In liver transplant recipients, it is characterized by "vanishing-bile-duct syndrome." Bronchiolitis obliterans is an expression of chronic rejection in lung transplant recipients. Atherosclerosis of the coronary arteries characterizes chronic rejection in the transplanted heart. Kidney transplant patients with chronic rejection develop proteinuria and hypertension. Chronic rejection is resistant to all known methods of therapy, and graft loss will eventually occur, though perhaps not for several years after function begins to deteriorate.

GRAFT-VERSUS-HOST DISEASE (GVHD)

GVHD is one of the most important complications of allogeneic stem cell transplantation. GVHD occurs in both acute and chronic forms. GVHD occurs when donor T cells initiate an immunological reaction towards genetically different proteins on host cells. The principal risk factor for GVHD is HLA mismatch, and the incidence of acute GVHD is directly related to the degree of mismatch. Prophylactic immunosuppression following allogeneic HCT is necessary to prevent GVHD (Sullivan et al., 1986).

Acute GVHD occurs within 100 days of the transplant and is manifested by symptoms and signs of skin, gastrointestinal, and liver dysfunction. Martin et al. (1990) reported that, at the onset of acute GVHD, 81% of patients had skin involvement, 54% had gastrointestinal involvement, and 50% had liver involvement. The skin manifestations include a pruritic rash that occurs initially on the palms, soles, or face. The rash may generalize over the entire body and lead to significant desquamation. Nausea, vomiting, anorexia, abdominal pain, diarrhea, and bloody stool can occur when GVHD affects the gastrointestinal system. GVHD affecting the liver can present with jaundice and can be difficult to differentiate from other post-transplant causes of liver dysfunction. Treatment of acute GVHD involves increasing the level of immunosuppression.

The chronic form of GVHD affects patients 100 or more days after transplantation. Chronic GVHD is most likely to occur in older patients and in patients who have already suffered acute GVHD. The manifestations of chronic GVHD are variable and can include bronchiolitis, esophageal stricture, malabsorption, and cholestasis. Chronic GVHD may be lethal and is a major cause of death following HCT (Lee et al., 2002). Treatment of chronic GVHD includes certain immunosuppressant agents, thalidomide, and ultraviolet light.

MALIGNANCIES

Transplant recipients are at increased risk for developing specific types of cancers. The incidence of malignancy has been estimated at 20% after ten years (Buell, Gross, & Woodle, 2005). The most common malignancies in transplant recipients are various types of skin cancers (Euvrard, Kanitakis, & Claudy, 2003). Lymphoproliferative conditions, urological cancers, and Kaposi's sarcoma also have higher incidence in transplant patients. The etiology of the increased rates of post-transplant malignancy is thought to be multifactorial and linked to suppression both of immunosurveillance of malignant cells and of immunity to viral infection.

IMMUNOSUPPRESSANT AGENTS

Many drugs are available today to induce immunosuppression in the post-transplant patient, with the goal of preventing the acute rejection of the allograft. Most immunosuppression regimens involve the use of multiple agents that have different mechanisms of action. This is especially true in the acute post-transplant period when the risk of rejection is highest. Theoretically, the use of multiple immunosuppressive agents with different mechanisms of action reduces the risk of toxicity from any individual agent, as lower doses of each drug are used to induce the same level of clinical immunosuppression. The management of immunosuppression following transplant involves a careful balance between the suppression of immunological reactivity that results in graft rejection and the maintenance of enough immune activity to prevent most infectious diseases. The prescribing clinician must also be aware of the potential for pharmacokinetic drug interactions with certain immunosuppressants, as many of these medications are both substrates and inhibitors of the 3A4 isoenzyme of the P450 system (Table 74.2).

Immunosuppressive therapy in transplant medicine can be divided into three phases of treatment: induction immunosuppression, maintenance immunosuppression, and the treatment of acute graft rejection. The induction phase usually is continued for two to four weeks following transplant. Most induction regimens include the use of systemic corticosteroids, a calcineurin inhibitor, and an antimetabolite. The second phase of immune modulation, maintenance immunosuppression, usually represents a reduction in the intensity of immunosuppression and enables the suppression of rejection over a prolonged period of time. Most patients will be maintained on either prednisone and cyclosporine or tacrolimus. However, it now appears that some patients taking tacrolimus for maintenance therapy may have the corticosteroid component discontinued entirely (Eason, Nair, Cohen, Blazek, & Loss, 2003). The final phase of immunosuppression is not planned, but rather represents the attempt to treat an occurrence of acute graft rejection. Early recognition and prompt treatment of acute rejection are essential to ensure long-term graft function. The treatment of acute rejection most often involves the use of high-dose steroids, polyclonal or monoclonal antibodies, and increased doses of the other immunosuppressive agents in an effort to escalate the level of clinical immunosuppression.

Table 74.2 **P450 ENZYMES INVOLVED IN DRUG METABOLISM**

	SUBSTRATE OF:	INHIBITS:	INDUCES:
Immunosuppressants			
Prednisone	3A4	None	None
Cyclosporine	3A4	3A4	None
Tacrolimus	3A4	3A4	None
Sirolimus	3A4	None	None
Mycophenolate Mofetil	None	None	None

SOURCE: Fireman, M., DiMartini, A. F., Armstrong, S. C., & Cozza, K. L. (2004). Immunosuppressants. *Psychosomatics, 45*(4), 354–360.

CORTICOSTEROIDS

Corticosteroids have been a significant component of post-transplant immunosuppressive protocols for approximately a half century, and they remain integral to most acute and chronic immunosuppressant regimens. Corticosteroids display complex and varied mechanisms of action. They are both anti-inflammatory and immunosuppressive agents. Corticosteroids are associated with a wide variety of side effects. These adverse effects may contribute significantly to the morbidity experienced by transplant recipients (Fryer et al., 1994). These include infection, weight gain, hyperglycemia, hypertension, acne, hyperlipidemia, neuropsychiatric symptoms, impaired wound healing, and Cushing's syndrome. The neuropsychiatric adverse effects of corticosteroids are common and wide-ranging. Psychiatric symptoms attributable to steroids include anxiety, agitation, psychosis, mood disturbance, apathy, memory loss, and suicidal ideation. The Boston Collaborative Drug Surveillance Program (1972) suggested a dose–response relationship between steroids and psychiatric adverse effects. This study found that psychiatric reactions occurred in 1.3% of hospitalized patients receiving 40 mg or less of prednisone per day, in 4.6% of individuals receiving 41 to 80 mg/day, and in 18.4% of patients receiving more than 80 mg/day. The neuropsychiatric side effects of steroids are generally treated by reducing or discontinuing the steroids if possible. If discontinuation or dose reduction is not possible, then psychotropic medications are prescribed to treat the offending psychiatric symptoms (i.e., antipsychotics to treat steroid-induced psychosis). The individual patient's susceptibility to these side effects varies remarkably. In addition, if a patient is chronically administered steroids, the possibility of adrenal suppression and the resulting potential for adrenal insufficiency if steroids are abruptly discontinued must be considered.

The steroids most commonly utilized in transplantation medicine are metabolized by the cytochrome P450 3A4. This includes prednisolone, the active metabolite of prednisone. Medications that are known 3A4 inhibitors, such as fluvoxamine, may therefore increase serum concentrations and the associated risk of toxicity. Inducers of 3A4 lead to the reduction of circulating corticosteroid concentrations and the potential for adrenal insufficiency or graft rejection.

CALCINEURIN INHIBITORS (CYCLOSPORINE AND TACROLIMUS)

The introduction of the first calcineurin inhibitor, cyclosporine, in the 1980s revolutionized organ transplantation. The development of tacrolimus, another calcineurin inhibitor, followed in 1994. All calcineurin inhibitors provide immunosuppression through their propensity to inhibit T-cell activation and proliferation, although they differ in their mechanism of calcineurin inhibition. These drugs are important components of most immunosuppressive regimens. Serum drug concentrations are used to guide therapy and prevent toxicity.

It is important to recognize the acute and chronic sequelae associated with the use of cyclosporine and tacrolimus. The most frequently encountered of these is nephrotoxicity. Nephrotoxicity may be secondary to acute toxicity, but it has also been associated with prolonged use of calcineurin inhibitors unrelated to toxic levels (Chapman, Griffiths, Harding, & Morris, 1985; Ojo et al., 2003). The clinical course is characterized by a gradual decline in renal function that may eventually lead to ESRD. In contrast to the acute form, chronic calcineurin inhibitor–induced renal insufficiency improves little after dose reduction or cessation of the punitive agent. The pathogenesis of nephrotoxicity is poorly understood with possible etiologies as diverse as ischemia and/or direct toxic effects of calcineurin-inhibitor on the renal tubules (Naesens, Kuyper, & Sarwal, 2009). Neurological complications are also encountered in patients being treated with calcineurin inhibitors, including restlessness, tremor, paresthesias, delirium, seizures, headache, and even coma. Calcineurin inhibitor neurotoxicity may also lead to the development of posterior reversible encephalopathy syndrome (PRES) (Bartynski, Tan, Boardman, Shapiro, & Marsh, 2008). The clinical presentation of PRES is often varied, but symptoms include headache, visual disturbances, delirium, possible seizures, and the potential for coma.

When working with transplant patients who may be emotionally labile, the potential consequences of intentional overdose need to be considered by the prescribing clinician. Cyclosporine overdose has been associated with significant neurotoxicity (Nghiem, 2002). Tacrolimus overdose, however, has been reported to result in minimal toxicity (Mrvos, Hodgman, & Krenzelok, 1997). Other complications of calcineurin inhibitors include hypertension, impaired glucose tolerance, hyperlipidemia, hyperkalemia, and hyperuricemia. The incidence of hyperglycemia appears higher with tacrolimus than with cyclosporine (Heisel, Heisel, Balshaw, & Keown, 2004). The hirsutism and gingival hyperplasia commonly experienced by patients taking cyclosporine do not appear to occur with tacrolimus.

Calcineurin inhibitors are metabolized via the P-450 system, specifically cytochrome 3A4. Inhibitors of cytochrome 3A4 may potentiate serum levels of these agents, whereas inducers of these enzymes will decrease the serum levels. Elevated levels of calcineurin inhibitors may lead to significant neurotoxicity and nephrotoxicity, whereas subtherapeutic levels of immunosuppression may lead to rejection of the transplanted organ. Cyclosporine and tacrolimus have also been identified as inhibitors of 3A4 and may, therefore, affect the levels of medications metabolized by isoenzyme 3A4.

SIROLIMUS

Sirolimus was introduced clinically in 1999. Sirolimus, like tacrolimus, binds to FK506-binding proteins, but it does not inhibit calcineurin activity. Sirolimus, instead, blocks signal transduction from interleukin-2 (IL-2), thereby inhibiting T and B cell proliferation. It is commonly used in combination with a calcineurin inhibitor. In this combination, sirolimus is often utilized in an attempt to minimize the use of steroids, with the goal of avoiding the potential negative effects of corticosteroids. Adverse side effects of sirolimus include hyperlipidemia, thrombocytopenia, neutropenia, and impaired wound healing. Compared to the calcineurin inhibitors, sirolimus does not appear to cause the same degree of nephrotoxicity or neurotoxicity. Sirolimus is metabolized as a substrate of 3A4, but there are few reports of significant drug–drug interactions involving sirolimus (Fireman, DiMartini, Armstrong, & Cozza, 2004).

ANTIMETABOLITE DRUGS (MYCOPHENOLATE AND AZATHIOPRINE)

The antimetabolite azathioprine was one of the first immunosuppressant agents introduced in the 1960s. It was an integral component of most immunosuppressant regimens, along with corticosteroids, until the introduction of cyclosporine in the 1980s. Mycophenolic acid is an antimetabolite available as an ester prodrug, mycophenolate mofetil; or as its sodium salt, sodium mycophenolate. Mycophenolate mofetil was approved by the Food and Drug Administration (FDA) in the mid-1990s, and by now, mycophenolate has largely replaced azathioprine as the antimetabolite of choice for use in combination with calcineurin inhibitors and/or corticosteroids in post-transplant immunosuppressant regimens.

The most important side effects of mycophenolate include bone marrow suppression, specifically leukopenia and thrombocytopenia. Leukopenia has been reported to affect almost a quarter of recipients treated with mycophenolate (Jacobson et al., 2011). Temporary discontinuation or dose reduction is usually sufficient to raise the leukocyte count. Other common side effects of mycophenolate include gastrointestinal disturbances such as diarrhea, gastritis, nausea, and vomiting. Less frequent adverse effects include esophagitis and gastrointestinal bleeding. Fortunately, mycophenolate appears to have few neuropsychiatric adverse effects. Mycophenolic acid is metabolized via glucuronidation, and de-esterification of mycophenolate mofetil is not dependent upon the liver. As a consequence, there appears to be little risk of pharmacokinetic interactions between either mycophenolate formulation and other drugs.

POLYCLONAL AND MONOCLONAL ANTIBODIES

Polyclonal and monoclonal antibodies represent a fairly new class of immunosuppressant agents. As the names imply, polyclonal antibodies are active against a wide range of target antigens, whereas monoclonal antibodies are antibodies active against only a single target antigen, thereby selectively depleting or inhibiting specific subsets of cells involved in the immune response. This class of immunosuppressants appears to be effective in the treatment of acute rejection in transplant recipients (Midtvedt et al., 2003). However, when antibodies are given to a patient on more than one occasion, the patient may develop antibodies directed against the preparation that may limit the clinical efficacy of future administration of these agents.

Polyclonal anti-T-cell antibodies, such as anti-thymocyte globulin, have been used for years to treat allograft rejection.

Unfortunately, polyclonal antibodies are plagued by significant adverse events, due to their action on diffuse cellular targets. These side effects vary from thrombocytopenia and leukopenia to serum sickness.

The monoclonal antibodies, by definition, are specific in their molecular target. These targeted immunosuppressants have varied uses in transplant medicine (van den Hoogen & Hilbrands, 2011). Alemtuzumab (anti-CD52 antibody) and rituximab (anti-CD20 antibody) are utilized to treat acute rejection, whereas basiliximab (the anti-CD25 antibody) is used in immunosuppression-induction therapy. The specific nature of these newer agents may also make them more tolerable than the polyclonal antibodies or the older monoclonal anti-CD3 antibody muromonab. Alemtuzumab has been associated with some anxiety and insomnia as the primary neuropsychiatric side effects. Rituximab has been associated with PRES and progressive multifocal leukoencephalopathy (PML) as well as an acute cytokine release syndrome after administration.

The monoclonal antibody preparations have the potential for multiple non-neuropsychiatric side effects, which at times may be quite severe. Like the polyclonal antibodies, the monoclonal antibodies may also cause a systemic, febrile inflammatory response immediately after administration, which can mask the fever of an opportunistic infection. This usually responds to a combination of corticosteroids, antihistamines, and acetaminophen (Chatenoud, Ferran, & Bach, 1991).

PERIOPERATIVE PSYCHIATRIC COMPLICATIONS

Psychiatric disorders often emerge in the immediate post-transplant period. Many of these are similar to those found in hospitalized patients with other acute medical problems, but due to the special nature of transplantation, there are some unusual diagnostic considerations.

If patients emerge from transplant with an acute onset of depression, the issue of survivor guilt should be explored during the diagnostic interview. Patient's guilt can sometimes be relieved by exploration of the reasons that underlie the guilt in their specific case, and discussion of what might have happened to the organ had the patient not received it.

Altered mental status is common after transplant. Usually, the post-operative delirium shows clear signs of improvement within five to seven days after transplant, but if cognitive problems persist past that point, an investigation of the cause should occur. The usual culprits, such as electrolyte disturbance or infection, should be obvious, but causes related directly to transplant are also possible. Delirium may indicate graft dysfunction or an adverse medication effect. Prednisone and other corticosteroids are often given at high doses at the time of transplant and can lead to a variety of affective and psychotic symptoms, including delirium. Calcineurin inhibitors, such as cyclosporine and tacrolimus, can cause delirium, most seriously through the PRES. Patients usually will have to be transitioned to other immunosuppressants if they develop PRES and need to be monitored closely for rejection.

Many patients believe that transplantation will act as a means to reestablish a sense of normalcy following significant medical illness. However, the post-transplant recovery period can include challenges to significant relationships, difficulty adjusting to a "new normal," and accepting an altered quality of life.

QUALITY OF LIFE AND ADJUSTMENT TO TRANSPLANT

The term *quality of life* is used to describe the extent to which an individual is able to live a fulfilling existence across different domains of life (i.e., physical, emotional, social, etc.). Empirical review of the transplant literature suggests that quality of life improves with transplant, but the amount and domain of improvement varies, depending on the transplant type (Dew et al., 1997). Body image is a common concern among transplant patients (Engel, 2001). After the procedure, patients may be left with scarring, weight gain, and physical changes associated with long-term steroid medication. Adjusting to life following a transplant involves tempering one's expectations of a cure and absolute health with realistic expectations about living with a different set of chronic health concerns.

Transplant patients must also be alert for organ rejection post-transplant. Coping with the chronic threat of organ rejection, worsening health, and possible death is an expected element of post-transplant recovery (De Vito et al., 2004). A proposed model suggests that patients undergo a transformative process beginning with naïvely believing a transplant will be a health panacea and ending with insight into and acceptance of their role in their health maintenance as a result of the chronic threat of losing their graft (De Vito et al., 2004). As such, the anxiety and depression associated with uncertainty about the quality and length of one's life changes over the course of the post-transplant recovery period. Patients must negotiate the challenging balance between engaging in appropriate behavior to care for their allograft while also accepting ambiguity around the potential failure of that graft.

FAMILY STRESS POST-TRANSPLANT

Family members undergo significant stress during the post-transplant recovery period as well. Transplant centers are often far from people's homes, and loved ones have to make a difficult decision about whether to stay with the transplant recipient or stay at home and tend to their usual life activities (Olbrisch, Benedict, Ashe, & Levenson, 2002). Family members also provide a significant amount of instrumental social support such as caring for the patient's responsibilities around the home, helping with medical regimens, and assisting with finances. This caregiving role can conflict with other roles in a spousal or other family relationship (Montgomery & Kosloski, 2000).

By definition, "non-adherence" refers to failing to adapt one's behaviors or actions to those prescribed by a physician (Morrissey, Flynn, & Lin, 2007). In transplant, it refers to the patient's inability to appropriately take medications as prescribed after transplant, engage in appropriate health-related behaviors, and follow through with medical appointments. Non-adherence is an appreciable problem in the post-transplant recovery period. In a comprehensive meta-analytic review of the renal transplant literature, Butler et al. (2004) found between 15% and 22.3% of patients had been non-adherent following kidney transplant, with 36% of patients missing four or more consecutive doses of an anti-rejection drug, and 16% missing at least ten consecutive doses. In heart transplant patients, Dew, Roth, Thompson, et al. (1996) found that nearly one-third of heart patients were consistently non-adherent with regard to exercise and blood pressure monitoring post-transplant, and approximately one-fifth of patients were non-adherent with regard to medications, smoking, and diet.

Although the definition of non-adherence differs greatly across studies, it is particularly dangerous in the post-transplant population, as the impact on graft failure is well documented. Non-adherence to medication regimens has been found to contribute to graft rejection and increased mortality across transplant populations (Dew, Kormos, Roth, Murali, DeMartini, & Griffith, 1999). Non-adherence accounted for the greatest proportion of graft failures among patients who died without a functioning renal graft (Butler et al., 2004); the odds of rejecting a graft increased sevenfold when comparing non-adherent to adherent patients. Kidney transplant recipients, who have been found to have the highest rates of non-adherence (Denhaerynck, Dobbels, Cleemput, et al., 2005), had a median of 36.4% of graft losses associated with non-adherence; the risk of kidney transplant rejection with non-adherence had a median odds increase of 4.8% (Butler, Roderick, Mullee, Mason, & Peveler, 2004). For heart transplant patients, the rate of rejection was 4.7 times higher for patients who were not adherent to their medication regimen compared to those who took their medications as prescribed (Dew, Kormos, Roth, Murali, DiMartini, & Griffith, 1999). Additionally, the risk of late acute rejection is also greater in non-adherent heart patient populations, with non-compliant patients having a higher rate of late acute rejection (11.8%) compared with compliant patients (2.4%) (Dobbels, De Geest, Van Cleemput, Droogne, & Vanhaecke, 2004). For lung transplant patients, research has suggested that non-adherence to immunosuppression is less than for heart recipient patients, which was demonstrated at several time points over a two-year period to range from 8–20% compared to 11–30% in heart transplant patients (Dew, DiMartini, De Vito Dabbs, et al., 2008). However, lung transplant patients had variably higher rates in other areas of behavioral noncompliance (Dew et al., 2008). For liver transplant patients, late acute rejection is four times more likely in non-compliant patients (21%) compared to compliant patients (5%) (Berlakovich,

Langer, Freundorfer, et al., 2000). Empirical data examining the impact of non-adherence on graft failure are limited in pancreas and intestinal transplant and are applied differently (i.e., GVHD) for stem cell transplantation.

Multiple demographic, personality, and coping variables have been postulated to account for variable adherence post-transplant. Research has shown social support, agreeableness, and planning as a coping behavior to predict post-transplant adherence in liver transplant candidates (Telles-Corrieia, Barbosa, & Mega, 2009). Common factors associated with medication non-adherence in transplant patients include non-adherence prior to transplant, psychiatric illness (depression and anxiety), personality disorders, poor social support, substance abuse, higher education level, increased time since transplant, inadequate follow-up, inadequate pre-transplant education, adverse effects from medications, and a complex medication regimen (Morrissey, Flynn, & Lin, 2007).

Non-adherent behavior can be categorized into *accidental, invulnerable*, and *decisive* non-adherence patterns (Greenstein & Siegal, 1998; Siegal & Greenstein, 1999). Accidental non-compliers, who account for approximately half of patients, hold strong beliefs about the efficacy of immunosuppressant medication and taking their medication even when the kidneys are functioning well, but miss doses of medication for circumstantial reasons. Invulnerable non-adherent patients, who account for approximately one-fourth of transplant patients (Greenstein & Siegal, 1998), see themselves as relatively immune to the negative effects of non-adherence. These patients tend to be younger, male, less educated, and have newer grafts. They generally do not believe in the efficacy of immunosuppressant medication or believe that delay in medication administration is not problematic. As such, they are more vulnerable to non-adherent behavior over the long-term course of the post-transplant recovery period, being particularly susceptible to non-adherence once they feel relatively well post-transplant. Finally, decisive non-compliers, who tend to account for approximately 25% of patients, tend to be well-educated, white-collar professionals who are accustomed to making independent decisions and as such may present with non-adherent behavior as an independent choice. Unfortunately, these patients may have a well-thought-out reason for non-adherence, which can be challenging for treatment providers to address.

POST-TRANSPLANT PSYCHIATRIC DISORDERS

In general, across transplant types, psychological distress is typically highest the first few months after transplant and declines gradually during the year following transplant (Fisher et al., 1995; TenVergert et al., 1998). Although transplant can both save lives and improve quality of life from pre-transplant states, the transplant process leaves patients vulnerable to psychiatric disorders. Transplant patients have more psychiatric symptoms (e.g., depression, anxiety, and substance abuse) compared to a non-clinical population (Jowsey et al., 2001).

This can be attributed to psychiatric syndromes that pre-date transplant, develop during transplant, or develop during the post-transplant recovery period and cause significant harm to their quality of life.

Adjustment disorders with depression and/or anxiety are the most prevalent disorders prior to transplant, with depression and anxiety prevalent in clinical and adjustment-related ranges (Olbrisch, Benedict, Ashe, & Levenson, 2002). In a sample of heart, lung, kidney, and liver transplant patients, over 60% met criteria for an Axis I psychiatric disorder, and approximately 32% met criteria for an Axis II disorder with significant implications for both adherence and adjustment (Chacko, Harper, Kunik, & Young, 1996). Across lung, and heart and lung transplant recipients, the proportion experiencing anxiety and depression ranged from 26.5 to 34.7% (Stilley et al., 1999).

The most common disorders found in post-transplant populations include depression, post-traumatic stress disorder (PTSD), and adjustment disorders (Dew et al., 1996). In a review of the transplant literature, Dew, Switzer, and DeMartini (2000) found that rates of psychiatric disorders in the long-term post-transplant period range from 10–58% for depressive disorders and 3–33% for anxiety disorders. The presence of adjustment disorders or adjustment-related symptoms has been well established in transplant patients (Baba et al., 2006; Heilmann et al., 2011). The presence of depression and other concerns about adjustment are one of the major impediments to quality of life in transplant populations (Goetzmann et al., 2008). Recently, a European group found depression was an independent risk factor for death over a seven-year period following renal transplantation (Zelle et al., 2012), further cementing the importance of identification and treatment of mood disorders in the post-transplant period.

The potential for exposure to trauma as a transplant patient is greater than that experienced by the general population. Favaloro et al. (1999) found that 13% of a population of heart transplant patients met criteria for PTSD, and an additional 20% met criteria for PTSD-related symptoms. Transplant patients who experience more stressful and negative life events, either related to or not related to transplant, are more vulnerable to post-traumatic stress (DuHamel et al., 2001). The development of PTSD can be prompted by exposure to medical procedures or threats of death, including more complications after transplant (Jin, Yan, Xiang, et al., 2012) and more invasive treatment. In order to meet criteria for PTSD, one must be exposed to real or imagined death or threat of significant injury to oneself or others. Depending on the type and course of treatment, invasive medical procedures such as transplant may be interpreted as such by patients. Unfortunately, PTSD symptoms, especially intrusive PTSD thoughts about transplant, have been related to problematic adherence behavior (Favaro, Gerosa, Caforio, et al., 2011). Shemesh et al. (Shemesh, Lurie, Stuber, et al., 2000) hypothesized that non-adherence in those with symptomatic memories of trauma may be related to avoidance of disease and treatment-related stimuli. Avoidant coping, which is common in PTSD, can prevail over the need for health-related behaviors and leave patients vulnerable to graft rejection. Given that cognitive behavioral treatment for PTSD significantly improves avoidant behavior, effective management of PTSD should improve treatment compliance related to avoidance of trauma stimuli.

POST-TRANSPLANT PSYCHIATRIC TREATMENT

The treatment of psychiatric illnesses and neuropsychiatric complications in transplant patients is critical in order to minimize suffering, improve quality of life, and maximize clinical outcomes in this vulnerable patient population. The general principles of treatment of psychiatric disorders experienced by transplant patients are not significantly different than the treatment principles utilized to manage these conditions in patients with other forms of co-occurring medical illness. Transplant patients are usually on a complex medication regimen of immunosuppressants to prevent graft rejection combined with various other medications used to treat other comorbid medical and psychiatric conditions. Drug interactions, both pharmacokinetic and pharmacodynamic, are common. They should be considered systematically in every case, avoided when feasible, and, when unavoidable, managed with dosage adjustments or changes in other aspects of the patient's drug regimen. Treatment must be individualized.

PSYCHOPHARMACOLOGY

Efforts to anticipate, minimize, and mitigate the effects of drug interactions are the characteristic feature of psychopharmacological treatment of transplant patients. Not only do such interactions risk increased neuropsychiatric side effects and compromise the efficacy of the psychiatric treatment, but they also can cause an increased risk of organ rejection—a dire consequence. For this reason, it is critical to maintain an accurate and continually updated list of the patient's medications, and to ascertain whether the patient is actually taking the medications consistently and as prescribed.

Antidepressants

Given the paucity of studies regarding the use of antidepressants in patients following organ transplantation, the recommendations for antidepressants are often based on the concern about drug interactions and the side effect profiles of the various antidepressants (Kim, Phongsamran, & Park, 2004). The selective serotonin receptor inhibitors (SSRIs), particularly sertraline, escitalopram, and citalopram, are often considered first-line agents in the treatment of depression and anxiety in the transplant patient population (Crone & Gabriel, 2004). Dosing strategies should be guided by an appreciation of the inherent differences in pharmacokinetic and pharmacodynamic profiles. The serotonin-norepinephrine reuptake inhibitor (SNRI) class of antidepressants may also be utilized in patients following transplant. Venlafaxine exhibits a limited potential for protein-binding. SNRIs, particularity venlafaxine, may raise blood pressure, leading to clinically significant

hypertension. Drug-induced hypertension is already an important health concern in the transplant population. It has been estimated that more than 90% of kidney transplant recipients being treated with a calcineurin inhibitor experience hypertension (Mangray & Vella, 2011). There have been case reports of co-administration of calcineurin inhibitors and serotonergic antidepressants such as sertraline (Wong, Chan, Sze, & Or, 2002) and venlafaxine (Newey, Khawam, & Coffman, 2011) leading to the development of "serotonin syndrome." This adverse reaction could be secondary to pharmacokinetic and/or pharmacodynamic interactions between the calcineurin inhibitor and the co-administered antidepressant. Little additional information is known about the use of duloxetine and desvenlafaxine in transplant patients.

Mirtazapine is a useful antidepressant in a subset of medically ill patients, including transplant patients. The unique pharmacodynamic profile of mirtazapine may prove beneficial for patients suffering from insomnia, anorexia, and nausea (Fusar-Poli, Matteo, Luca, et al., 2007). It is metabolized by multiple hepatic enzymes and is therefore less susceptible to other drugs' affecting its metabolism. In addition, mirtazapine does not appear to significantly inhibit or induce any hepatic enzymes, so it does not appear to induce pharmacokinetic drug interactions. Bupropion is vulnerable to drug–drug interactions through pharmacokinetic mechanisms, as it is a substrate of 2B6 and a potential inhibitor of 2D6. The potential for electrolyte abnormalities and polypharmacy in post-transplant patients may make bupropion risky, especially given the lowering of seizure threshold that is observed with some immunosuppressants.

Although tricyclic antidepressants (TCA) and monoamine oxidase inhibitors (MAOI) have historically been used for the treatment of depression in the transplant population, they are now reserved for cases resistant to more standard therapies. The TCAs have several pharmacodynamic and pharmacokinetic issues that make them a challenge to use safely in the medically ill. For example, cardiac transplant patients suffering from left ventricular dysfunction, along with those taking diuretics and vasodilators, are at increased risk of drug-induced orthostatic hypotension with TCA administration (Fusar-Poli et al., 2006). In addition, the physiological effects of TCAs on the denervated transplanted human heart remain unclear. Pharmacokinetically, they are substrates of 2D6 and 3A4 and susceptible to the effects of pertinent inhibitors and inducers of these enzymes, which include various immunosuppressant agents. MAOI use is rare due to concerns of dangerous drug and food interactions. The psychostimulants have a long history of successful use in the treatment of neurovegetative symptoms in the medically ill and may be helpful in addressing these symptoms in patients following organ transplantation. Plutchik et al. (1998) found methylphenidate to be efficacious and fairly well tolerated in a retrospective case series of eight patients treated with methylphenidate following liver transplantation. Episodes of intermittent supraventricular tachycardia, however, have been associated with administration of methylphenidate in a heart transplant patient with multiple risk factors for a cardiac arrhythmia (Come & Shapiro, 2005).

Anxiolytics

The benzodiazepines are effective agents in the pharmacological management of anxiety. The use of benzodiazepines in patients following transplant is similar to their use in other medical ill populations. However, their use in patients with active pulmonary disease requires special caution due to benzodiazepines' propensity to blunt CO_2 sensitivity and contribute to respiratory depression. Nevertheless, in patients with significant anxiety that is unresponsive to other measures, benzodiazepines may be beneficial if the patient is carefully monitored for evidence of respiratory compromise. In general, benzodiazepines with shorter half-lives (e.g., alprazolam, lorazepam) are less likely to accumulate than those with longer half-lives (e.g., diazepam, clonazepam) and may therefore be relatively safer in patients with respiratory disease. The longer acting benzodiazepines, however, may be useful as time-limited scheduled agents for patients with anxiety as one waits for the co-administered SSRI to become effective.

The choice of which benzodiazepine to use should also depend on the medication's pharmacokinetic properties (e.g., hepatic metabolism, active metabolites, and elimination half-life). Lorazepam, oxazepam, and temazepam undergo glucuronidation and do not require oxidative metabolism, often making them the benzodiazepines of choice in patients for whom drug interactions are a concern. Benzodiazepines' use should be time-limited to avoid the potential complications of tolerance and dependence, coupled with the risk of withdrawal. These issues may be especially pertinent to the subset of transplant patients with a history of substance use disorders.

The non-benzodiazepine anti-anxiety medication buspirone may be effective in the management of generalized anxiety disorder in the transplant population. It, however, is metabolized by the liver via 3A4 isoenzymes and is susceptible to drug interactions.

Antipsychotics

Typical and atypical antipsychotics have been used safely and effectively in the post-transplant period following both solid organ and HCTs (Siddiqui, Ramaswamy, & Petty, 2005; Michopoulos, Christodoulou, Dervenoulas, Soldatos, & Lykouras, 2010). The indications for their use vary from the management of a preexisting primary psychotic disorder to treatment of delirium or steroid-induced secondary mania. The regular concerns of neurological, metabolic, and cardiac adverse events remain pertinent in the transplant patient population. The metabolic effects of antipsychotics are particularly pertinent. Transplant recipients are already predisposed to obesity and metabolic changes, often secondary to the immunosuppressant regimen, so caution about adding more risk for metabolic syndrome is advisable. Neuroleptic malignant syndrome has been reported in the literature following a bone marrow transplant (Onose et al., 2002).

Lithium

The use of the mood stabilizer lithium presents several problems when used in transplant patients (Fusar-Poli et al., 2006).

Lithium's pharmacokinetics make it difficult to dose in the immediate post-operative period due to the rapid changes in volume status. Lithium levels may also be increased with co-administration of cyclosporine, given the latter's propensity to impair renal function (Vincent, Wenting, & Schalekamp, 1988). It can therefore be a challenge to maintain a therapeutic lithium level in a transplant patient.

Neurostimulation

Electroconvulsive therapy (ECT) is a safe, well tolerated, and very effective nonpharmacological treatment for major depression for patients suffering from a wide variety of acute and chronic medical conditions, including transplant recipients (Jayaram & Casimir, 2005). For most transplant patients, ECT may be considered as an appropriate treatment option following a careful evaluation of the risks and benefits. The heart's response to ECT following cardiac transplant is unusual in that the transplant heart is denervated. As a consequence, the patient does not experience the parasympathetically mediated post-seizure bradycardia that typically follows the induction of a seizure (Kellner, Monroe, Burns, Bernstein, & Crumbley, 1991). The efficacy and safety of the repetitive transmagentic stimulation (rTMS) for the treatment of neuropsychiatric illness following organ transplantation is unreported in the literature at this time.

PSYCHOTHERAPEUTIC TREATMENT
Adjustment to Life Post-Transplant

Psychotherapy for transplant patients is often initiated because a patient wants to return to a sense of normalcy, specifically the sense of what was "normal" prior to transplant. Patients cope with the stressors of chronic illness, living on a waiting list, and undergoing transplant with the belief that they will be able to "return to normal" after the treatment is complete. However, as with any person undergoing major life events, patients often cannot return to the same sense of normalcy they experienced prior to transplant. This can leave patients feeling disconnected and disillusioned, as their expectations for life after transplant and the reality of their situation are incongruent.

Adjustment-related psychotherapy focuses on helping them establish a new sense of normalcy post-transplant (Baines, Joseph, & Jindal, 2002). The adjustment literature suggests that patients who utilize benefit-finding attributions when reviewing their situation in order to cope with traumatic stressors experience personal growth (Sears, Stanton, & Danoff-Burg, 2003). For example, bone marrow transplant survivors have been found to have a greater sense of strength and enhanced interpersonal relationships following treatment (Tallman, Shaw, Schultz, & Altmaier, 2010).

Although post-traumatic growth is thought to occur naturally as a result of coping with trauma related to health concerns, adjustment-related psychotherapy can facilitate the process by helping a patient address the reestablishment of a sense of stability and normalcy (i.e., the "new normal") following transplant. Psychotherapy targeted towards helping the patient review attributions from a growth perspective to accept and cope with the persistent changes related to transplantation survival (Baines, Joseph, & Jindal, 2002) facilitates reintegration into a fully functioning life that integrates the new limits and growth related to living with a donated organ.

In addition to psychotherapy, peer-based support approaches such as support groups or peer mentoring can positively impact patient quality of life. Meeting with a transplant patient who has gone through similar experiences with success provides hope and a sense of legitimacy that a professional caregiver who has not undergone transplant cannot provide. Encouraging support-group participation and information gathering from peers who are further along in the transplant process can provide a roadmap and a belief that individuals do survive and thrive for patients moving into an unknown area of life (Jowsey et al., 2001).

Non-Adherence Issues

Psychotherapy can be beneficial to address treatment non-adherence issues in post-transplant populations. Depending on the reason for non-adherence, psycho-education can be used to increase adherence (Greenstein & Siegal, 1998). For accidentally non-adherent patients, providing education on methods to increase medication compliance using behavioral strategies, such as use of a pill box or scheduled administration of medications, may be helpful. For "invulnerable" non-adherent patients, using educational material that is less technically cumbersome yet addresses the need for long-term adherence even when they are feeling physically well may improve their adherence. Finally, for the decisive non-adherent patients, fostering independent decision-making in the direction of adherent behavior should increase compliance (Greenstein & Siegal, 1998). The reasons for non-adherence should be assessed, and psychotherapeutic and educational efforts should be appropriately tailored to increase the likelihood of adherent behavior. Specifically, having patients meet with a psychologist to determine underlying attributions driving non-adherence will help the psychologist more appropriately target interventions (e.g., behavioral strategies, cognitive restructuring of beliefs about the need to engage in adherent behavior, motivational interviewing techniques) to improve non-adherent behavior.

CBT can be used to help alter the expectation that life post-transplant will be the same as life prior to becoming ill, and can thus be used to address non-adherence. Because patients engage in non-adherent behavior for a range of reasons, helping patients identify beliefs they have about their health (e.g., "I have had my transplanted organ for three years; there is no way I will reject it now") and challenging those beliefs in the context of a supportive therapeutic relationship can help patients achieve a more realistic understanding of their behaviors post-transplant. Additionally, behavioral strategies, such as scheduling medications, using tracking and logging methods, and appropriate reinforcement can help patients who are non-adherent due to situation, priority, or memory constraints maintain an adaptive health schedule post-transplant. Although adherence-related psychotherapy tends to be more solution-focused, goal-oriented, and monitored, this approach can help provide the structure and support for long-lasting behavioral change.

Psychiatric Symptom Management

Patients who present for treatment may have a history of a psychiatric disorder that was either effectively or ineffectively managed prior to transplant. Given the multiple stressors related to the post-transplant recovery period, as well as the demands of adherence, it is recommended that patients receive psychotherapy in addition to medication management to treat premorbid and persisting psychiatric symptoms. Multiple psychotherapeutic approaches have been advocated for transplant patients. Anxiety management techniques such as progressive muscle relaxation, guided imagery, and self-hypnosis have been suggested for anxiety management during medical procedures (Olbrisch, Benedict, Ashe, & Levenson, 2002). Although the literature on specific therapeutic modalities to treat psychiatric symptoms in transplant patients is sparse, several therapeutic modalities have been empirically validated in more general medical populations, including cognitive behavioral and behavioral therapies, brief psychodynamic therapies, and other varied approaches (Compas, Haaga, Keefe, Leitenberg, & Williams, 1998). As an example, CBT can be particularly useful for treating psychiatric symptoms in the medically ill by focusing on cognitions, appraisals, and coping strategies and how the patient's life and health impact mood. In CBT, patients are challenged to see how personal expectations and beliefs about their situation exacerbate their psychiatric symptoms. It is important to note that many transplant patients cope with realistically negative stressors, and thus the goals of CBT with transplant patients differ slightly from those for non-medically ill patients. That said, one's choices with regard to both solution- and emotion-focused coping in the face of major health concerns affect one's emotional health, and they can be successfully targeted through CBT. CBT can be used to help alleviate psychiatric symptoms, to improve coping strategies (e.g., by relaxation training), and to reexamine one's expectations and views of the world and oneself (e.g., by cognitive restructuring) in a time-limited manner to improve patient quality of life. Application of a range of psychotherapeutic approaches within the context of transplant-specific stressors is the current recommendation for psychotherapeutically managing symptoms in transplant patients.

CLINICAL PEARLS

- If the donor knows the recipient—the most common scenario—then there must be discussion of their relationship and the donor's hopes for results after the transplant.

- If patients have struggled to attend dialysis sessions regularly, they are likely to struggle with the post-transplant regimen of medications and appointments.

- If the patient can work with the team, suggestions about ways in which the team can accommodate the patient's personality (e.g., giving an obsessive patient choices to increase his sense of control when possible) can help both the patient and the team work together successfully.

- In the United States, following an acetaminophen overdose, if a patient is listed for transplant due to fulminant hepatic failure, that patient goes right to the top of the list because the risk of death if there is delay quickly approaches 100%, so obtaining an accurate psychiatric history before their mental status is compromised is particularly essential. The patient is at risk for developing hepatic coma as liver injury progresses.

- Cyclosporine overdose has been associated with significant neurotoxicity (Nghiem, 2002); tacrolimus overdose, however, has been reported to result in minimal toxicity (Mrvos, Hodgman, & Krenzelok, 1997).

- Adjusting to life following a transplant involves tempering one's expectations of a "cure" and absolute health with realistic expectations about living with a different set of chronic health concerns.

- A proposed model suggests that patients undergo a transformative process, beginning with naïvely believing a transplant will be a health panacea and ending with insight into and acceptance of their role in their health maintenance as a result of the chronic threat of losing their graft (De Vito Dabbs et al., 2004).

- Non-adherent behavior can be categorized into *accidental, invulnerable*, and *decisive* non-adherence patterns (Greenstein & Siegal, 1998; Siegal & Greenstein, 1999).

  - Accidental non-compliers (approximately half of patients) hold strong beliefs about the efficacy of immunosuppressant medication and taking their medication even when the kidney is functioning well, but miss doses of medication for circumstantial reasons.
  - Invulnerable non-adherent patients (approximately one-fourth of transplant patients) (Greenstein & Siegal, 1998), see themselves as relatively immune to the negative effects of non-adherence. These patients tend to be younger, male, less educated, and have newer grafts. They generally do not believe in the efficacy of immunosuppressant medication or believe that delay in medication administration is problematic. As such, they are more vulnerable to non-adherent behavior over the long-term course of the post-transplant recovery period, being particularly susceptible to non-adherence once they feel relatively well post-transplant.
  - Finally, decisive non-compliers (approximately 25% of patients), tend to be well-educated, white-collar

professionals who are accustomed to making independent decisions and as such may present with non-adherent behavior as an independent choice. Unfortunately, these patients may have a well-thought-out reason for non-adherence, which can be challenging for treatment providers to address.

- Intrusive PTSD thoughts about transplants have been related to problematic adherence behavior (Favaro et al., 2011). Shemesh et al. (2000) hypothesized PTSD-related non-adherence to be related to avoidance of disease and treatment-related stimuli.

- It is critical to maintain an accurate and continually updated list of the patient's medications and to ascertain whether the patient is actually taking the medications consistently and as prescribed.

- For decisive non-compliers, a psychiatrist or psychologist can determine underlying attributions driving non-adherence to help them more appropriately target interventions (e.g., behavioral strategies, cognitive restructuring of beliefs about need to engage in adherent behavior, motivational interviewing techniques) to improve non-adherent behavior.

DISCLOSURE STATEMENTS

Dr. Heinrich, Dr. Marcangelo, and Dr. Christianson do not have any conflicts of interest to disclose.

REFERENCES

Appelbaum, P. S. (2007). Clinical practice: assessing patients' competence to consent to treatment. *New England Journal of Medicine, 357*(18), 1834–1840.

Baba, A., Hirata, G., Yokoyama, F., Kenmoku, K., Tsuchiya, M., Kyo, S., et al. (2006). Psychiatric problems of heart transplant candidates with left ventricle assist devices. *Journal of Artificial Organs, 9*(4), 203–208.

Baines, L. S., Joseph, J. T., & Jindal, R. M. (2002). Emotional issues after kidney transplantation: A prospective psychotherapeutic study. *Clinical Transplantation, 16*, 455–460.

Bartynski, W. S., Tan, H. P., Boardman, J. F., Shapiro, R., & Marsh, J. W. (2008). Posterior reversible encephalopathy syndrome after solid organ transplantation. *American Journal of Neuroradiology, 29*(5), 924–930.

Berlakovich, G. A., Langer, F., Freundorfer, E., Windhager, T., Rockenschaub, S., Sporn, E., et al. (2000). General compliance after liver transplantation for alcohol cirrhosis. *Transplant International, 13*, 129–135.

Boston Collaborative Drug Surveillance Program (1972). Acute adverse reactions to prednisone in relation to dosage. *Clinical Pharmacology Therapeutics, 13*, 694–698.

Brown, J., Sorrell, J. H., McClaren, J., & Creswell, J. W. (2006). Waiting for a liver transplant. *Qualitative Health Research, 16*(1), 119–136.

Buell, J. F., Gross, T. G., & Woodle, E. S. (2005). Malignancy after transplantation. *Transplantation, 80*(2 Suppl), S254–S264.

Butcher, J. N., Graham, J. R., Ben-Porath, Y. S., Tellegen, A., Dahlstrom, W. G., & Kaemmer, B. (2001) *Minnesota Multiphasic Personality Inventory-2 (MMPI-2) Manual*. Minneapolis, MN: University of Minnesota Press.

Butler, J. A., Roderick, P., Mullee, M., Mason, J. C., & Peveler, R. C. (2004). Frequency and impact of nonadherence to immunosuppressant following renal transplantation: A systematic review. *Transplantation, 77*(5), 769–776.

Chacko, R. C., Harper, R. G., Kunik, M., & Young, J. (1996). Relationship of psychiatric morbidity and psychosocial factors in organ transplant candidates. *Psychosomatics, 37*(2), 100–107.

Chapman, J. R., Griffiths, D., Harding, N. G., & Morris, P. J. (1985). Reversibility of cyclosporin nephrotoxicity after three months' treatment. *Lancet, 1*(8421), 128–130.

Chatenoud, L., Ferran, C., & Bach, J. F. (1991). The anti-CD3-induced syndrome: a consequence of massive *in vivo* cell activation. *Current Topics in Microbiology and Immunology, 174*, 121–134.

Christie, J. D., Edwards, L. B., Aurora, P., Dobbels, F., Kirk, R., Rahmel, A. O., et al. (2008). Registry of the International Society for Heart and Lung Transplantation: twenty-fifth official Adult Lung and Heart/Lung Transplantation Report—2008. *The Journal of Heart and Lung Transplantation, 27*(9), 957–969.

Coffman, K. L., Gordon, C., & Siemionow, M. (2010). Psychological outcomes with face transplantation: overview and case report. *Current Opinion in Organ Transplantation, 15*(2), 236–240.

Coffman, K. L., Hoffman, A., Sher, L., Rojter, S., Vierling, J., & Makowka, L. (1997). Treatment of the postoperative alcoholic liver transplant recipient with other addictions. *Liver Transplantation Surgery, 3*(3), 322–327.

Coffman, K., & Crone, C. (2002). Rational guidelines for transplantation in patients with psychotic disorders. *Current Opinion in Organ Transplantation, 7*, 385–388.

Come, C. E., & Shapiro, P. A. (2005). Supraventricular tachycardia associated with methylphenidate treatment in a heart transplant recipient. *Psychosomatics, 46*(5), 461–463.

Compas, B. E., Haaga, D. A. F., Keefe, F. J., Leitenberg, H., & Williams, D. A. (1998). Sampling of empirically supported psychological treatments from health psychology: Smoking, chronic pain, cancer, and bulimia nervosa. *Journal of Consulting and Clinical Psychology, 66*(1), 89–112.

Costanzo, M. R., Naftel, D. C., Pritzker, M. R., Heilman, J. K. 3rd, Boehmer, J. P., Brozena, S. C., et al. (1998). Heart transplant coronary artery disease detected by coronary angiography: a multi-institutional study of preoperative donor and recipient risk factors. Cardiac Transplant Research Database. *Journal of Heart Lung Transplantation, 17*(8), 744–753.

Crone, C. C., & Gabriel, G. M. (2004). Treatment of anxiety and depression in transplant patients: pharmacokinetic considerations. *Clinical Pharmacokinetics, 43*(6), 361–394.

Cuturi, M. C., Blancho, G., Josien, R., & Soulillou, J. P. (1994). The biology of allograft rejection. *Current Opinion in Nephrology and Hypertension, 3*(6), 578–584.

De Gottardi, A., Spahr, L., Gelez, P., Morard, I., Mentha, G., Guillaud, O., et al. (2007). A simple score for predicting alcohol relapse after liver transplantation: results from 387 patients over 15 years. *Archives of Internal Medicine, 167*(11), 1183–1188.

Denhaerynck, K., Dobbels, F., Cleemput, I., Desmyttere, A., Schäfer-Keller, P., Schaub, S., & De Geest, S. (2005). Prevalence, consequences, and determinants of nonadherence in adult renal transplant patients: A literature review. *Transplant International, 18*, 1121–1133.

Dew, M. A., DiMartini, A. F., Steel, J., De Vito Dabbs, A., Myaskovsky, L., Unruh, M., et al. (2008). Meta-analysis of risk for relapse to substance use after transplantation of the liver or other solid organs. *Liver Transplantation, 14*(2), 159–172.

Dew, M. A., DiMartini, A. F., De Vito Dabbs, A., Zomak, R., De Geest, S., Dobbels, F., et al. (2008). Adherence to the medical regimen during the first two years after lung transplantation. *Transplantation, 85*, 193–202.

Dew, M. A., Kormos, R. L., Roth, L. H., Murali, S., DiMartini, A. F., & Griffith, B. P. (1999). Early post-transplant medical compliance and mental health predict physical morbidity and mortality one to three years after heart transplantation. *Journal of Heart and Lung Transplantation, 18*(6), 549–562.

Dew, M., Roth, L., Schulberg, H., Simmons, R. G., Kormos, R. L., Trzepacz, P. T., et al. (1996). Prevalence and predictors of depression and anxiety-related disorders during the year after heart transplantation. *General Hospital Psychiatry, 18*(Suppl 6), 48–61.

Dew, M. A., Switzer, G. E., DiMartini, A. F., Matukaitis, J., Fitzgerald, M. G., & Kormos, R. L. (2000). Psychosocial assessments and outcomes in organ transplantation. *Progress in Transplantation, 10*(4), 239–259.

Dew, M. A., Switzer, G. E., Goycoolea, J. M., Allen, A. S., DiMartini, A., Kormos, R. L., et al. (1997). Does transplantation produce quality of life benefits? A quantitative analysis of the literature. *Transplantation, 64*(9), 1261–1273.

De Vito Dabbs, A., Hoffman, L. A., Swigart, V., Happ, M. B., Dauber, J. H., McCurry, K. R., et al. (2004). Striving for normalcy: Symptoms and threat of rejection after lung transplantation. *Social Science and Medicine, 59*, 1473–1484.

DiMartini, A., Dew, M. A., Day, N., Fitzgerald, M. G., Jones, B. L., deVera, M. E., et al. (2010). Trajectories of alcohol consumption following liver transplantation. *American Journal of Transplantation, 10*(10), 2305–2312.

Dobbels, F., De Geest, S., Van Cleemput, J., Droogne, W., & Vanhaecke, J. (2004). Effect of late medication non-compliance on outcome after heart transplantation: A 5-year follow-up. *The Journal of Heart and Lung Transplantation, 23*(11), 1245–1251.

Dobbels, F., Put, C., & Vanhaecke, J. (2000). Personality disorders: a challenge for transplantation. *Progress in Transplantation, 10*(4), 226–232.

Dobbels, F., Vanhaecke, J., Dupont, L., Nevens, F., Verleden, G., Pirenne, J., et al. (2009). Pretransplant predictors of posttransplant adherence and clinical outcome: an evidence base for pretransplant psychosocial screening. *Transplantation, 87*(10), 1497–1504.

DuHamel, K. N., Smith, M. Y., Johnson Vickberg, S. M., Papadopoulos, E., Ostroff, J., Winkel, G., et al. (2001). Trauma symptoms in bone marrow transplant survivors: The role of nonmedical life events. *Journal of Traumatic Stress, 14*(1), 95–113.

Eason, J. D., Nair, S., Cohen, A. J., Blazek, J. L., & Loss, G. E. Jr. (2003). Steroid-free liver transplantation using rabbit antithymocyte globulin and early tacrolimus monotherapy. *Transplantation, 75*(8), 1396–1399.

Engel, D. (2001). Psychosocial aspects of the organ transplant experience: What has been established and what we need for the future. *Journal of Clinical Psychology, 57*, 521–549.

Euvrard, S., Kanitakis, J., & Claudy, A. (2003). Skin cancers after organ transplantation. *New England Journal of Medicine, 348*(17), 1681–1691.

Farrell, K., Shen, B., Mallon, S. Penedo, F. J., & Antoni, M. H. (2011). Utility of the Millon Behavioral Medicine Diagnostic to predict medication adherence in patients diagnosed with heart failure. *Journal of Clinical Psychology in Medical Settings, 18*, 1–12.

Favaro, A., Gerosa, G., Caforio, A. L. P., Volpe, B., Rupolo, G., Zarneri, D., et al. (2011). Posttraumatic stress disorder and depression in heart transplantation recipients: The relationship with outcome and adherence to medical treatment. *General Hospital Psychiatry, 33*, 1–7.

Favaloro, R. R., Perrone, S. V., Moscoloni, S. E., Gomez, C. B., Favaloro, L. E., Sultan, M. G., et al. (1999). Value of pre-heart-transplant psychological evaluation: Long-term follow up. *Transplantation Proceedings, 31*(7), 3000–3001.

Fireman, M., DiMartini, A. F., Armstrong, S. C., & Cozza, K. L. (2004). Immunosuppressants. *Psychosomatics, 45*(4), 354–360.

Fishbein, T. M. (2009). Intestinal transplantation. *New England Journal of Medicine, 361*(10), 998–1008.

Fisher, D. C., Lake, K. D., Reutzel, T. J., & Emery, R. W. (1995). Changes in health-related quality of life and depression in heart transplant recipients. *Journal of Heart and Lung Transplantation, 14*(2), 373–381.

Folstein, M. F., Folstein, S. E., & McHugh, P. R. (1975). Mini-Mental State: A practical method for grading the cognitive state of patients for the clinician. *Journal of Psychiatric Research, 12*(3), 189–198.

Frazier, O. H., Rose, E. A., Oz, M. C., Dembitsky, W., McCarthy, P., Radovancevic, B., et al. (2001). Multicenter clinical evaluation of the HeartMate vented electric left ventricular assist system in patients awaiting heart transplantation. *Journal of Thoracic and Cardiovascular Surgery, 122*(6), 1186–1195.

Fryer, J. P., Granger, D. K., Leventhal, J. R., Gillingham, K., Najarian, J. S., & Matas, A. J. (1994). Steroid-related complications in the cyclosporine era. *Clinical Transplantation, 8*(3 Pt 1), 224–229.

Fujisawa, M., Ichikawa, Y., Yoshiya, K., Isotani, S., Higuchi, A., Nagano, S., et al. (2000). Assessment of health-related quality of life in renal transplant and hemodialysis patients using the SF-36 health survey. *Urology, 56*(2), 201–206.

Fusar-Poli, P., Matteo, L., Luca de, M., Politi, P., Cortesi, M., & Carboni, V. (2007). Anxiety and depression after lung transplantation: Mirtazapine as a first-choice agent? *Journal of Psychosomatic Research, 62*(1), 101.

Fusar-Poli, P., Picchioni, M., Martinelli, V., Bhattacharyya, S., Cortesi, M., Barale, F., & Politi, P. (2006). Anti-depressive therapies after heart transplantation. *Journal of Heart & Lung Transplantation, 25*(7), 785–793.

Gale, R. P., Bortin, M. M., van Bekkum, D. W., Biggs, J. C., Dicke, K. A., Gluckman, E., et al. (1987). Risk factors for acute graft-versus-host disease. *British Journal of Haematology, 67*(4), 397–406.

Goetzmann, L., Ruegg, L., Stamm, M., Ambuhl, P., Boehler, A., Halter, J., et al. (2008). Psychosocial profiles after transplantation: A 24-month follow-up of heart, lung, liver, kidney, and allogeneic bone-marrow patients. *Transplantation, 86*(5), 662–668.

Greenstein, S. M., & Siegal, B. (1998). Compliance and noncompliance in patients with a functioning renal transplant: A multicenter study. *Transplantation, 66*(12), 1718–1726.

Guaraldi, G., Cocchi, S., Codeluppi, M., Di Benedetto, F., De Ruvo, N., Masetti, M., et al. (2005). Outcome, incidence, and timing of infectious complications in small bowel and multivisceral organ transplantation patients. *Transplantation, 80*(12), 1742–1748.

Haft, J., Armstrong, W., Dyke, D. B., Aaronson, K. D., Koelling, T. M., Farrar, D. J., et al. (2007). Hemodynamic and exercise performance with pulsatile and continuous flow left ventricular assist devices. *Circulation, 116*(Suppl I), I8–I15.

Heilmann, C., Kuijpers, N., Beyersdorf, F., Berchtold-Herz, M., Trummer, G., Stroh, A. L., et al. (2011). Supportive psychotherapy for patients with heart transplantation or ventricular assist devices. *European Journal of Cardio-thoracic Surgery, 39*(4), e44–e50.

Heisel, O., Heisel, R., Balshaw, R., & Keown, P. (2004). New onset diabetes mellitus in patients receiving calcineurin inhibitors: a systematic review and meta-analysis. *American Journal of Transplantation, 4*(4), 583–595.

Horowitz, M. M., Gale, R. P., Sondel, P. M., Goldman, J. M., Kersey, J., Kolb, H. J., et al. (1990). Graft-versus-leukemia reactions after bone marrow transplantation. *Blood, 75*(3), 555–562.

Jacobson, P. A., Schladt, D., Oetting, W. S., Leduc, R., Guan, W., Matas, A. J., et al. (2011). Genetic determinants of mycophenolate-related anemia and leukopenia after transplantation. *Transplantation, 91*(3), 309–316.

Jayaram, G., & Casimir, A. (2005). Major depression and the use of electroconvulsive therapy (ECT) in lung transplant recipients. *Psychosomatics, 46*(3), 244–249.

Jin, S., Yan, L., Xiang, B., Li, B., Wen, T., Zhao, J., et al. (2012). Posttraumatic stress disorder after liver transplantation. *Hepatobiliary & Pancreatic Diseases International, 11*(1), 28–33.

Jindal, R. M., Neff, R. T., Abbott, K. C., Hurst, F. P., Elster, E. A., Falta, E. M., et al. (2009) Association between depression and nonadherence in recipients of kidney transplants: Analysis of the United States Renal Data System. *Transplantation Proceedings, 41*(9), 3662–3666.

Jiao, M., Greanya, E. D., Hague, M., Yoshida, E. M., Soos, J. G., et al. (2010). Methadone maintenance therapy in liver transplantation. *Progress in Transplantation, 20*(3), 209–214.

Jowsey, S. G., Taylor, M. L., Schneekloth, T. D., & Clark, M. W. (2001). Psychosocial challenges in transplantation. *Journal of Psychiatric Practice, 7*(6), 404–414.

Kamath, P. S., Wiesner, R. H., Malinchoc, M., Kremers, W., Therneau, T. M., Kosberg, C. L., et al. (2001). A model to predict survival in patients with end stage liver disease. *Hepatology, 33*(2), 464–470.

Karim, Z. Intaraprasong, P., Scudamore, C. H., Erb, S. R., Soos, J. G., Cheung, E., et al. (2010). Predictors of relapse to significant alcohol drinking after liver transplantation. *Canadian Journal of Gastroenterology, 24*(4), 245–250.

Karvellas, C. J., Safina, N., Auzinger, G., Heaton, N., Muiesan, P., O'Grady, J., et al. (2010). Medical and psychiatric outcomes for patients transplanted for acetaminophen-induced acute liver failure: a case-control study. *Liver International, 30*(6), 826–833.

Kellner, C. H., Monroe, R. R., Burns, C., Bernstein, H. J., & Crumbley, A. J. (1991). Electroconvulsive therapy in a patient with a heart transplant. *New England Journal of Medicine, 325*(9), 663.

Kim, J., Phongsamran, P., & Park, S. (2004). Use of antidepressant drugs in transplant recipients. *Progress in Transplantation, 14*(2), 98–104.

Kroeker, K. I., Bain, V. G., Shaw-Stiffel, T., Fong, T. L., & Yoshida, E. M. (2008). Adult liver transplant survey: Policies towards eligibility criteria in Canada and the United States, 2007. *Liver International, 28*(9), 1250–1255.

Larson, A. M., Polson, J., Fontana, R. J., Davern, T. J., Lalani, E., Hynan, L. S., et al. (2005). Acetaminophen-induced acute liver failure: results of a United States multicenter, prospective study. *Hepatology, 42*(6), 1364–1372.

Lee, S. J., Klein, J. P., Barrett, A. J., Ringden, O., Antin, J. H., Cahn, J. Y., et al. (2002). Severity of chronic graft-versus-host disease: association with treatment-related mortality and relapse. *Blood, 100*(2), 406–414.

Lerut, J., & Sanchez-Fueyo, A. (2006). An appraisal of tolerance in liver transplantation. *American Journal of Transplantation, 6*(8), 1774–1780.

Levenson, J. L., & Olbrisch, M. E. (1993). Psychosocial evaluation or organ transplant candidates: a comparative survey of process, criteria, and outcomes in heart, liver, and kidney transplantation. *Psychosomatics, 34*(4), 314–323.

Maldonado, J. R., Dubois, H. C., David, E. E., Sher, Y., Lolak, S., Dyal, J., et al. (2012). The Stanford integrated psychosocial assessment for transplantation (SIPAT): a new tool for the psychosocial evaluation of pre-transplant candidates. *Psychosomatics, 53*(2), 123–132.

Mangray, M., & Vella, J. P. (2011). Hypertension after kidney transplant. *American Journal of Kidney Disease, 57*(2), 331–341.

Martin, P. J., Schoch, G., Fisher, L., Byers, V., Anasetti, C., Appelbaum, F. R., et al. (1990). A retrospective analysis of therapy for acute graft-versus-host disease: initial treatment. *Blood, 76*(8), 1464–1472.

Mathurin, P., Moreno, C., Samuel, D., Dumortier, J., Salleron, J., Durand, F., et al. (2011). Early liver transplantation for severe alcoholic hepatitis. *New England Journal of Medicine, 365*, 1790-1800.

Mehra, M. R., Crespo-Leiro, M. G., Dipchand, A., Ensminger, S. M., Hiemann, N. E., Kobashigawa, J. A., et al. (2010). International Society for Heart and Lung Transplantation working formulation of a standardized nomenclature for cardiac allograft vasculopathy—2010. *Journal of Heart & Lung Transplantation, 29*(7), 717–727.

Michopoulos, I., Christodoulou, C., Dervenoulas, J., Soldatos, C. R., & Lykouras, L. (2010). Quetiapine monotherapy in bipolar I disorder: a 1-year stabilization in a woman having undergone bone marrow transplantation. *World Journal of Biological Psychiatry, 11*(2 Pt 2), 519–521.

Middleton, P. F., Duffield, M., Lynch, S. V., Padbury, R. T., House, T., Stanton, P., et al. (2006). Living donor liver transplantation—adult donor outcomes: a systematic review. *Liver Transplantation, 12*(1), 24–30.

Midtvedt, K., Fauchald, P., Lien, B., Hartmann, A., Albrechtsen, D., Bjerkely, B. L., et al. (2003). Individualized T cell monitored administration of ATG versus OKT3 in steroid-resistant kidney graft rejection. *Clinical Transplantation, 17*(1), 69–74.

Millon, T. (1994). *Millon Clinical Multiaxial Inventory-III (MCMI-III).* Minneapolis, MN: NCS Pearson, Inc.

Millon, T., Antoni, M., Millon, C., Meagher, S., & Grossman, S. (2001). *Millon Behavioral Medicine Diagnostic.* Minneapolis, MN: NCS Assessments.

Montgomery, R. J. V., & Kosloski, K. D. (2000). Family caregiving: change, continuity, and diversity. In M. P. Lawton & R. L. Rubenstein (Eds.), *Interventions in dementia care: Toward improving quality of life* (pp. 143–171). New York: Springer.

Morrissey, P. E., Flynn, M. L., & Lin, S. (2007). Medical noncompliance and its implications in transplant recipients. *Drugs, 67*(10), 1463–1481.

Mrvos, R., Hodgman, M., & Krenzelok, E. P. (1997). Tacrolimus (FK 506) overdose: a report of five cases. *Journal of Toxicology—Clinical Toxicology, 35*(4), 395–399.

Naesens, M., Kuypers, D. R., & Sarwal, M. (2009). Calcineurin inhibitor nephrotoxicity. *Clinical Journal of the American Society of Nephrology, 4*(2), 481–508.

Nasreddine, Z. A., Phillips, N. A., Bedirian, V., Charbonneau, S., Whitehead, V., Collin, I., et al. (2005). The Montreal Cognitive Assessment (MoCA): a brief screening tool for mild cognitive impairment. *Journal of American Geriatric Society, 53*(4), 695–699.

Newell, K. A. (2003). Transplantation of the intestine: is it truly different? *American Journal of Transplantation, 3*(1), 1–2.

Newey, C. R., Khawam, E., & Coffman, K. (2011). Two cases of serotonin syndrome with venlafaxine and calcineurin inhibitors. *Psychosomatics, 52*(3), 286–290.

Nghiem, D. D. (2002). Role of pharmacologic enhancement of p-450 in cyclosporine overdose. *Transplantation, 74*(9), 1355–1356.

Ojo, A. O., Held, P. J., Port, F. K., Wolfe, R. A., Leichtman, A. B., Young, E. W., et al. (2003). Chronic renal failure after transplantation of a nonrenal organ. *New England Journal of Medicine, 349*(10), 931–940.

Olbrisch, M. E., Benedict, S. M., Ashe, K., & Levenson, J. L. (2002). Psychology assessment and care of organ transplant patients. *Journal of Consulting and Clinical Psychology, 70*(3), 771–783.

Olbrisch, M. E., Levenson, J. L., & Hamer, R. (1989). The PACT: A rating scale for the study of clinical decision making in psychosocial screening of organ transplant candidates. *Clinical Transplantation, 3*, 164–169.

Onose, M., Kawanishi, C., Onishi, H., Yamada, T., Itoh, M., Kosaka, K., et al. (2002). Neuroleptic malignant syndrome following BMT. *Bone Marrow Transplant, 29*(9), 803–804.

Papalois, V. E., Moss, A., Gillingham, K. J., Sutherland, D. E., Matas, A. J., & Humar, A. (2000). Pre-emptive transplants for patients with renal failure: an argument against waiting until dialysis. *Transplantation, 70*(4), 625–631.

Pasquini, M. C., & Wang, Z. (2010). Current use and outcome of hematopoietic stem cell transplantation: CIBMTR Summary Slides. Available at: http://www.cibmtr.org.

Plutchik, L., Snyder, S., Drooker, M., Chodoff, L., & Sheiner, P. (1998). Methylphenidate in post-liver transplant patients. *Psychosomatics, 39*(2), 118–123.

Sears, S. R., Stanton, A. L., & Danoff-Burg, S. (2003). The yellow brick road and the Emerald City: Benefit finding, positive reappraisal coping, and posttraumatic growth in women with early-stage breast cancer. *Health Psychology, 22*(5), 487–497.

Shuhaiber, J. H., Hur, K., & Gibbons, R. (2010). The influence of preoperative use of ventricular assist devices on survival after heart transplantation: propensity score matched analysis. *British Medical Journal, 10*, 340.

Siddiqui, Z., Ramaswamy, S., & Petty, F. (2005). Quetiapine therapy for corticosteroid-induced mania. *Canadian Journal of Psychiatry, 50*(1), 77–78.

Siegal, B., & Greenstein, S. M. (1999). Profiles of noncompliance in patients with functioning renal transplant: A multicenter study. *Transplantation Proceedings, 31*, 1326–1327.

Siemionow, M. Z., Zor, F., & Gordon, C. R. (2010). Face, upper extremity, and concomitant transplantation: potential concerns and challenges ahead. *Plastic and Reconstructive Surgery, 126*, (1), 308–315.

Siemionow, M., & Ozturk, C. (2011). An update on facial transplantation cases performed between 2005 and 2010. *Plastic and Reconstructive Surgery, 128*(6), 707e–720e.

Shemesh, E., Lurie, S., Stuber, M. L., Emre, S., Patel, Y., Vohra, P., et al. (2000). A pilot study of posttraumatic stress and nonadherence in pediatric liver transplant recipients. *Pediatrics, 105*(2), 1–7.

Smith, G. C., Trauer, T., Kerr, P. G., & Chadban, S. J. (2010). Prospective quality-of-life monitoring of simultaneous pancreas and kidney transplant recipients using the 36-item short form health survey. *American Journal of Kidney Diseases, 55*(4), 698–707.

Spaderna, H., Mendell, N. R., Zahn, D., Wang, Y., Kahn, J., Smits, J. M., et al. (2010). Social isolation and depression predict 12-month outcomes in the "Waiting for a New Heart" study. *Journal of Heart and Lung Transplantation, 29*(3), 247–254.

Stilley, C. S., Dew, M. A., Stukas, A. A., Switzer, G. E., Manzetti, J. D., Keenan, R. J., & Griffith, B. P. (1999) Psychological symptom levels and their correlates in lung and heart-lung transplant recipients. *Psychosomatics, 40*(6), 503–509.

Stilley, C. S., DiMartini, A. F., de Vera, M. E., Flynn, W. B., King, J., Sereika, S., et al. (2010). Individual and environmental correlates and predictors of early adherence and outcomes after liver transplantation. *Progress in Transplantation, 20*(1), 58–67.

Sullivan, K. M., Deeg, H. J., Sanders, J., Klosterman, A., Amos, D., Shulman, H., et al. (1986). Hyperacute graft-v.-host disease in patients not given immunosuppression after allogeneic marrow transplantation. *Blood, 67*(4), 1172–1175.

Syeda, B., Roedler, S., Schukro, C., Yahya, N., Zuckermann, A., & Glogar, D. (2005). Transplant coronary artery disease: Incidence, progression and interventional revascularization. *International Journal of Cardiology, 104*, (3), 269–274.

Tallman, B., Shaw, K., Schultz, J., & Altmaier, E. (2010). Well-being and posttraumatic growth in unrelated donor marrow transplant survivors: A nine-year longitudinal study. *Rehabilitation Psychology, 55*(2), 204–210.

Tariq, S. H., Tumosa, N., Chibnall, J. T., Perry, M. H., & Morley, J. E. (2006). Comparison of the Saint Louis University mental status examination and the mini-mental state examination for detecting dementia and mild neurocognitive disorder—a pilot study. *American Journal of Geriatric Psychiatry, 14*(11), 900–910.

Taylor, D. O., Stehlik, J., Edwards, L. B., Aurora, P., Christie, J. D., Dobbels, F., et al. (2009). Registry of the International Society for Heart and Lung Transplantation: Twenty-sixth Official Adult Heart Transplant Report—2009. *Journal of Heart & Lung Transplantation, 28*(10), 1007–1022.

Telles-Corrieia, D., Barbosa, A., Mega, I., & Monteiro, E. (2009). Adherence correlates in liver transplant candidates. *Transplantation Proceedings, 41*(5), 1731–1734.

TenVergert, E. M., Essink-Bot, M. L., Geertsma, A., van Enckevort, P. J., de Boer, W. J., van der Bij, W. (1998). The effect of lung transplantation on health-related quality of life: A longitudinal study. *Chest, 113*, 358–364.

Tigges-Limmer, K., Schönbrodt, M., Roefe, D., Arusoglu, L., Morshuis, M., & Gummert, J. F. (2010). Suicide after ventricular assist device implantation. *Journal of Heart and Lung Transplantation, 29*(6), 692–694.

Titman, A., Rogers, C. A., Bonser, R. S., Banner, N. R., & Sharples, L. D. (2009). Disease-specific survival benefit of lung transplantation in adults: a national cohort study. *American Journal of Transplantation, 9*(7), 1640–1649.

Todd, J. L., & Palmer, S. M. (2011). Bronchiolitis obliterans syndrome: the final frontier for lung transplantation. *Chest, 140*(2), 502–508.

Tringali, R., Arria, A., & Trzepacz, P. T. (1994). Psychosocial evaluation and intervention in liver transplantation. *Journal of Applied Biobehavioral Research, 2*, 55–64.

Trotter, J. F., Talamantes, M., McClure, M., Wachs, M., Bak, T., Trouillot, T., et al. (2001). Right hepatic lobe donation for living donor liver transplantation: impact on donor quality of life. *Liver Transplantation, 7*(6), 485–493.

Tsunoda, T., Yamashita, R., Kojima, Y., & Takahara, S. (2010). Risk factors for depression after kidney transplantation. *Transplantation Proceedings, 42*(5), 1679–1681.

Twillman, R. K., Manetto, C., Wellisch, D. K., & Wolcott, D. L. (1993). The Transplant Evaluation Rating Scale: A revision of the psychosocial levels system for evaluating organ transplant candidates. *Psychosomatics, 34*, 144–153.

U.S. Department of Health and Human Services, Health Resources and Services Administration, (2010). *2009 Annual Report of the U.S. Organ Procurement and Transplantation Network and the Scientific Registry of Transplant Recipients: Transplant Data 1999–2008*. Rockville, MD: Healthcare Systems Bureau, Division of Transplantation.

van den Hoogen, M. W., & Hilbrands, L. B. (2011). Use of monoclonal antibodies in renal transplantation. *Immunotherapy, 3*(7), 871–880.

Varma, V., Webb, K., & Mirza, D. F. (2010). Liver transplantation for alcoholic liver disease. *World Journal of Gastroenterology, 16*(35), 4377–4393.

Ventura, K. A. (2010). Ethical considerations in live liver donation to children. *Progress in Transplantation, 20*(2), 186–190.

Vincent, H., Wenting, G., & Schalekamp, M. (1988). Impaired fractional excretion on lithium: a very early marker of cyclosporine toxicity. *Transplantation Proceedings, 19*(5), 4147–8.

Wallis, C. B., Samy, K. P., Roth, A. E., & Rees, M. A. (2011). Kidney paired donation. *Nephrology Dialysis Transplantation, 26*(7), 2091–2099.

Weinrieb, R. M., Barnett, R., Lunch, K. G., DePiano, M., Atanda, A., & Olthoff, K. M. (2004). Psychiatric complications and anesthesia and analgesia requirements in methadone-maintained liver transplant recipients. *Liver Transplantation, 10*(1), 97–106.

Weinrieb, R. M., Van Horn, D. H., Lynch, K. G., & Lucey, M. R. (2011). A randomized, controlled study of treatment for alcohol dependence in patients awaiting liver transplantation. *Liver Transplantation, 17*(5), 539–547.

Wingard, J. R., Hsu, J., & Hiemenz, J. W. (2010). Hematopoietic stem cell transplantation: an overview of infection risks and epidemiology. *Infectious Disease Clinics of North America, 24*(2), 257–272.

Wolfe, R. A., Ashby, V. B., Milford, E. L., Ojo, A. O., Ettenger, R. E., Agodoa, L. Y., et al. (1999). Comparison of mortality in all patients on dialysis, patients on dialysis awaiting transplantation, and recipients of a first cadaveric transplant. *New England Journal of Medicine, 341*(23), 1725–1730.

Wong, E. H., Chan, N. N., Sze, K. H., & Or, K. H. (2002). Serotonin syndrome in a renal transplant patient. *Journal of the Royal Society of Medicine, 95*(6), 304–305.

Zelle, D. M., Dorland, H. F., Rosemalen, J. G. M., Corpelejin, E., Gans, R. O. B., Homan van der Heide, J. J., et al. (2012). Impact of depression on long-term outcome after renal transplantation: a prospective cohort study. *Transplantation, 94*, 1033–1040.

75.

BURNS

Shamim H. Nejad, Amelia Dubovsky, Kelly Irwin, Shawn Fagan, and Jeremy Goverman

INTRODUCTION

Since ancient times, burn injuries have been a source of trauma for humans. While historic treatments may have been primitive, today's modern medical and surgical treatment has become increasingly sophisticated, resulting in lower mortality rates, especially from severe burns. However, while burn patients are increasingly likely to survive their injuries, they often carry a lifetime burden from their injury. The impact is greatest on children and young adults, who have most of their lives ahead of them.

Modern psychiatric burn research and treatment began in the mid-1940s during World War II, when the symptoms of stress and grief experienced in burn survivors of the Coconut Grove fire of 1942, in which 491 people died, were described. In what is now considered a classic paper, Erich Lindemann reported for the first time the symptoms and psychotherapeutic management of acute grief (Lindemann, 1944). These studies involved psychiatric treatment and subsequent research on grief that would eventually be applied, not only to other patients and the bereaved, but also to military personnel. Norman Bernstein, a pioneer in the treatment of psychiatric care for children, described hypnosis in the treatment of burn pain and brought attention to the stigma experienced by those with facial injuries (Bernstein, 1976), while Richard Galdston described depression and emotional sequelae of burns in young children of depressed mothers (Galdston, 1972).

As most burn units are closed systems (only certain individuals generally enter and leave the unit), physicians and other medical staff who are new to the unit often experience trepidation when they have to care for a patient following a burn injury. The traditional role of the psychiatric consultant in the care of the burn patient has been to diagnose and treat discrete psychiatric disorders when called upon by the burn physicians. However, a psychiatrist's training and clinical background provide a unique set of skills that may be useful to the burn team in the treatment of every patient. Medical psychiatrists are trained to view patients and their conditions from existential, social, and developmental perspectives in addition to their physiological state. This chapter addresses the medical and psychiatric issues pertinent to patients in the acute, intermediate, and rehabilitative phases of burn injury.

EPIDEMIOLOGY

The United States has one of the highest rates of burn injury in the world. According to the American Burn Association Fact Sheet for 2011, 450,000 patients annually visit emergency rooms with burn-related injuries, and about 45,000 of them are hospitalized (American Burn Association, 2011b). About 55% of the estimated 45,000 acute hospitalizations for burn injury in the United States in recent years were admitted to 125 hospitals with specialized burn centers. The percentage admitted to burn centers has increased steadily in recent decades, with growing recognition of the special needs of burn patients and continuing advances in the technical resources and skills of those who refer, transport, and treat them. An American burn center now averages 200 admissions per year, and their average survival rate exceeds 94%. The other 4,700 American acute care hospitals average fewer than three burn cases per year, and have a greater than 94% survival rate.

The National Burn Repository 2011 report, which compiles burn admission data from 2001 to 2011 from 91 hospitals from 35 states (and the District of Columbia), shows that nearly 70% of burn patients were between age 5 and age 60, with a mean age of 32. Children under five are over-represented among burn patients, accounting for 18% of all burn admissions. Patients aged 60 or older are under-represented, accounting for only 12% of admissions (American Burn Association, 2011a). Seventy percent of patients hospitalized for burns had burns covering less than 10% of their total body surface area (TBSA), with the two most commonly reported etiologies being fire/flame burns and scalding injuries. With regard to circumstance of injury, non-work-related injuries were the most common (67.4%), followed by work-related accidents (15.8%), while assault/abuse accounted for 1.4%, and both self-inflicted injuries and suspected child abuse cases were 1.1%. During the ten-year period from 2001 and 2010, the mortality rate decreased from 4.5% to roughly 3% for males and from 6.8% to 3.6% for females. Deaths from burn injury increased with advancing age and burn size, and presence of inhalation injury. For patients under age 60 and with a burn affecting a TBSA of less than 20%, the presence of inhalation injury increased the likelihood of death by 20 times. Pneumonia was the most frequent clinically related complication and occurred in 5.8% of fire/flame-injured patients. The frequency of pneumonia and respiratory failure was much greater in patients with four days or more of mechanical ventilation. The incidence of clinically related complications for patients not requiring mechanical ventilation increased with age, plateauing at 20% for those age 80 and over.

RISK FACTORS FOR BURN-RELATED INJURIES (SEE TABLE 75.1)

OCCUPATIONAL

Particular occupations are the greatest risk factors for burns in adults. Those in high-risk occupations include mechanics working with boilers, radiators, or gasoline engines; power plant workers; cooks; truckers and other transport workers; farm workers; and those whose jobs involve the use of caustic chemicals.

ALCOHOL AND SUBSTANCE USE

Premorbid substance use is common among those with burn injuries. In a study conducted by Barillo and Goode, among 727 deaths from fires, a blood alcohol level was positive in approximately 30% of patients, and almost 15% of patients also had positive results for another illicit substance. Seventy-five percent of the drug-positive and 58% of the alcohol-positive fatalities were between the ages of 21 and 50 (Barillo & Goode, 1996).

Among patients who survive their initial burn injuries, several studies have evaluated the prevalence of alcohol intoxication, alcohol abuse, or alcohol dependence. In a study by Jones and colleagues, 27% were intoxicated at the time of their burns, while 90% of these intoxicated patients were also diagnosed with alcohol abuse, compared with 11% in the non-intoxicated burn-injured patients (Jones, Barber, Engrav, & Heimbach, 1991). Other studies have reported the prevalence of alcohol abuse and dependence as being between 6% and 11% (Powers et al., 1994; Tabares & Peck, 1997). Fauerbach and colleagues reported lifetime prevalence rates of alcohol and drug use disorders among 98 adult burn inpatients of 41% and 24% respectively, notably higher than when compared to such rates in the general population (Fauerbach, Lawrence, Haythornthwaite, McGuire, & Munster, 1996).

Burns associated with methamphetamine represent a relatively new problem, mainly affecting certain geographic regions of the United States where its use is more prevalent. In some studies, up to 10% of injured patients with burn injuries were under the influence of methamphetamine. Not only does methamphetamine intoxication predispose to burn injury, but, its production involves highly volatile chemical compounds that can cause both thermal and chemical burns.

PREMORBID PSYCHIATRIC ILLNESS

Burn patients have higher rates of pre-injury psychiatric illness compared to the general population (Powers, Cruse, & Boyd, 2000; Rockwell, Dimsdale, Carroll, & Hansbrough, 1988). Burn patients with pre-burn psychiatric illness are more likely to have had potentially preventable burn injuries (Powers et al., 2000). They have longer lengths of hospitalization (Tarrier, Gregg, Edwards, & Dunn, 2005; van der Does, Hinderink, Vloemans, & Spinhoven, 1997), and have more complicated post-burn adjustment (Dyster-Aas, Willebrand, Wikehult, Gerdin, & Ekselius, 2008; Fauerbach et al., 1996; Tarrier et al., 2005; van der Does et al., 1997). In two studies using criteria from the *Diagnostic and Statistical Manual of Mental Disorders* (DSM), lifetime mood disorders were identified in 31% and 42% of burn patients (Dyster-Aas et al., 2008; Fauerbach et al., 1997). In both studies, major depression was the most common disorder (27% and 41%), with these figures being significantly higher compared with those in the general population (Kessler, Chiu, Demler, Merikangas, & Walters, 2005; Kessler et al., 1994; Kringlen, Torgersen, & Cramer, 2001, 2006). In addition, those who had a lifetime mood disorder had worse functional status at discharge (Fauerbach et al., 1996). In the same studies, the lifetime anxiety was found to be 10% and 37%. In one study, the prevalence of pre-burn post-traumatic stress disorder (PTSD) was 2% (Fauerbach et al., 1996); in the other it was 10% (Dyster-Aas et al., 2008). Dyster-Aas and colleagues have reported that 4% of burn patients assessed had lifetime psychotic disorders; however, this number may be as high as 12% in patients with self-inflicted burns (Dyster-Aas et al., 2008).

SELF-INFLICTED BURN INJURY AND SELF-IMMOLATION

The act of self-immolation is rare in Western countries, with prevalence rates between 1% to 9% of all burn-injured patients, while in other parts of the world such as the Middle East, Africa, and South Asia, prevalence rates may be as high as 28% of burn-injured patients (Ahmadi, 2007; Krummen, James, & Klein, 1998; Palmu et al., 2004; Scully & Hutcherson, 1983; Squyres, Law, & Still, 1993).

In Western countries, the data on gender and self-immolation are conflicting, with some studies showing it to be more common in men, while others show a greater incidence in women (Krummen et al., 1998; Swenson & Dimsdale, 1990). Risk factors include marital or relationship difficulties (Squyres et al., 1993) and unemployment (Palmu et al., 2004). Studies consistently show the association of self-immolation with alcohol and other substance use disorders (Pham, King, Palmieri, & Greenhalgh, 2003; Thombs, Singh, Halonen, Diallo, & Milner, 2007), as well as mood and psychotic disorders (Palmu et al., 2004; Thombs et al., 2007).

The prevalence of self-immolation as well as mortality following self-immolation is greater in developing countries, probably reflecting limited overall access to health care and less availability of burn-specific treatment. Risk factors associated with self-immolation in developing countries include younger age, female gender, low socioeconomic status, decreased literacy, limited access to mental health services, and marital and familial conflict (Ahmadi et al., 2009; Ahmadi & Ytterstad, 2007).

Self-inflicted burn injuries are quite often associated with underlying personality disorders; namely, borderline personality disorder. While many studies have looked at self-immolation, few studies have examined the subset of patients who intentionally burn themselves but do not intend their injury to be fatal. Providing inpatient burn care to a patient with borderline personality disorder can be markedly challenging, as these patients generally exhibit interpersonal difficulties that can interfere with the patient–healthcare professional relationship, complicating the delivery of necessary care. Ideally, all patients with suspected self-inflicted burn injury should be evaluated by a psychiatrist; and in cases of borderline personality disorder, behavioral plans, centralization of care with consistent nursing staff, and education of burn staff regarding "splitting" behavior and behavioral limit-setting should be employed.

CHILDREN AND ADOLESCENTS

Environmental, developmental, and familial factors contribute to the risk of burn-related injuries in children (Stoddard & Fricchione, 2004). Risks include low socioeconomic status, poor social supports, access to inflammatory and caustic agents, along with risk-taking behavior. In addition, parental psychopathology, neglect, childhood depression, learning disabilities, developmental delay, conduct disorder, attention-deficit hyperactivity disorder (ADHD), bipolar mood disorder, and substance abuse have also been shown to be associated with burn-related injuries.

Table 75.1 RISK FACTORS FOR BURN INJURY

BURNS IN ADULTS	BURNS IN CHILDREN AND ADOLESCENTS
Occupational hazards	Learning disabilities
Alcohol or substance abuse	Abuse
Dementia	Risk-taking behavior
Self-harming behavior	Fire-setting
Chronic medical illness	Neglect
Mood disorder	
Suicide attempt	
Psychotic disorder	

TYPES OF BURN INJURIES

Burn injuries are generally classified by the depth of the injury, ranging from first-degree to fourth-degree with regard to severity (see Table 75.2). First-degree burns are characterized by intact epithelium and usually do not require specific care. Second-degree burns are wet, pink to red in color, and with edema present. They are further categorized into "superficial" and "deep." Second-degree burns must be monitored closely for progression of injury and for infection. Third-degree burns involve the full thickness of the skin, with damage to sensory nerves and to blood vessels beneath. They are dry and leathery. Because of nerve damage, they may be less painful than second-degree burns. Their treatment requires excision and grafting. Fourth-degree burns are the severest

Table 75.2 SEVERITY OF BURN INJURIES: APPEARANCE, SENSATION, AND COMPLICATIONS

INJURY	LAYER	APPEARANCE	TEXTURE	SENSATION	TIME TO HEALING	COMPLICATIONS
1st-degree	Epidermis	Redness (erythema)	Dry	Painful	7 days or less	None
2nd-degree (superficial partial thickness)	Extends into superficial dermis	Red with clear blisters; blanches with pressure	Moist	Painful	2–3wks	Local infection/ cellulitis
2nd-degree (deep partial thickness)	Extends into deep dermis	Red-and-white with bloody blisters. Less blanching	Moist	Painful	Weeks—may progress to third-degree	Scarring, contractures (may require excision and skin grafting)
3rd-degree (full thickness)	Extends through entire dermis	Stiff and white/ brown	Dry, leathery	Painless due to loss of nerve fibers (extensive peripheral pain where 2nd-degree burns lie)	Requires excision	Scarring, contractures, amputation
4th-degree	Extends through skin, subcutaneous tissue, and into underlying muscle and bone	Black; charred with eschar	Dry	Painless (painful at periphery)	Requires excision	Amputation, significant functional impairment

Table 75.3 DEGREE OF BURN INJURY WITH USUAL ASSOCIATED PAIN SENSATIONS AND COMPLICATIONS. COMMON DRESSINGS USED IN BURN INJURIES

DRESSING	WHAT IT IS	TYPE OF INJURY	HOW APPLIED	NOTES
Silver Nitrate Solution	• 0.5% hypotonic solution • Offers broad-spectrum antimicrobial and fungal coverage	Deep partial thickness wounds	• Dressing changed daily • 8 layers of nitrate-saturated dressings • Requires soaking with nitrate q6H & PRN°	• Leaches electrolytes (especially sodium) from the wound surface—can result in hyponatremia and hypokalemia) (incidence is directly proportional to size of the area involved)
Silver Sulfadiazene (Silvadene)	• 1% water soluble cream • Offers broad spectrum antimicrobial activity	Partial thickness wounds	• Dressing changed BID • Area cleansed with soap and water	• May result in a self-resolving agranulocytosis, evidenced after several days of use Contraindicated in patients with allergies to sulfa
Mafenide Acetate (Sulfamylon) Solution	• 5% bacterostatic solution for gram (+) and gram (−) organisms	Full-thickness wounds with eschar	• Dressing changed daily • Area cleansed with Hibiclens and water	• Carbonic anhydrase inhibition may result in lactic acidosis depending, upon the size of the area involved and length of time used • May be painful, and some patients do not tolerate • Sulfamylon is the only agent to penetrate eschar
Mafenide Acetate (Sulfamylon) Cream	• 11.1% Cream • Bacterostatic for gram (+) and gram (−) organisms	Wounds with exposed cartilage (i.e., nose, ears)	• Dressing changed BID • Area cleansed with Hibiclens and water • Applied directly to the wound and covered with dressing	• Can be painful if used on areas other than ears and nose
Acticoat (Silver-coated antimicrobial barrier)	• Broad spectrum antimicrobial agent • Based on ability to dissolve pure silver in water • Activated with moisture (sterile water or exudate) Constant concentration of silver is delivered to the wound	Partial-thickness wounds	• Dressing changed every 3 days • Area cleansed with soap and water	• Sustained release of silver lowers frequency of dressing changes • Comes in 3-day or 7-day formulations (usually 3 days for acute injury)
Aquacel Ag	• Ionic silver in the Hydrofiber technology of Aquacel • Offers broad spectrum of wound coverage	Partial thickness wounds (May also be used for donor sites)	• Dressing not changed unless it is not adhering to the wound after 2–3 days • Dressing applied dry	• May be left in place up to 14 days • When used for donor sites, the ABD pads directly over the Aquacel are removed on POD #1; the stretch net is left in place until POD #2 • The Aquacel is left in place until donor site is healed, ~10–14 days (generally removed in clinic)

Bacitracin	• Topical antibiotic ointment	Partial-thickness wounds	• Dressing changed BID • Area cleansed with soap and water and applied directly to the wound • Covered with non-stick dressing (preferably Adaptic)	• ~10% of patients can develop reactions to Bacitracin evidenced by an itchy, maculopapular rash
Mupircin (Bactroban)	• Topical antibiotic ointment/cream	Partial-thickness wounds	• Dressing changed BID • Area cleansed with soap and water • Covered with non-stick dressing (preferably Adaptic)	• Preferable when patient is positive for MRSA if choosing between Bacitracin and Bactroban
Collagenase (Santyl)	• Enzymatic debriding agent	Adherent eschar or debris	• Area cleansed with soap and water • Applied directly to the wound	• Drainage from the wound may increase as the eschar sloughs
Xeroform	• Petrolatum dressing	Usually used for donor sites	• The dressing is not changed	• On POD #1, the outer wrap is removed and the Xeroform is allowed to dry
Xenograft	• Biological dressing made of porcine	Partial thickness wounds	• Xenograft is not changed • It is applied to a clean, debrided wound, usually in the OR • The outer wrap is removed on POD #1 and the Xenograft examined for adherence. If adhered, the wound is left open to air	• Joints are immobilized for 4 days to allow for adherence to the wound bed

type of burn injury. They extend through the subcutaneous tissue into tendons, muscles, and bones. They require complex surgical reconstruction and treatment, usually with multiple trips to the operating theater.

Surgical treatment of severe burns involves wound debridement, escharotomy (excision of burned skin), and at times release of the fascial layer (fasciotomy) to prevent compartment syndrome, particularly with circumferential burn injuries. In addition to surgical treatment, burn patients require frequent dressing changes, and they are frequently treated with systemic antimicrobial agents (see Table 75.3).

BURNS AND THE SYSTEMIC INFLAMMATORY RESPONSE

PATHOPHYSIOLOGY OF BURN SHOCK

Cutaneous thermal injury to greater than one-third of the TBSA often results in a severe derangement of cardiovascular function called *burn shock*. Shock is an abnormal physiological state in which tissue perfusion is insufficient to maintain adequate delivery of oxygen and nutrients and the removal of cellular waste products. Burn shock is a unique type of cardiovascular dysfunction that is not easily or fully reversed by fluid resuscitation. Severe burn injury results in significant hypovolemic shock and the release of local and systemic mediators of inflammation. Burn shock results from the interplay of hypovolemia and multiple mediators of inflammation which affect the microcirculation as well as the heart, large vessels, and lungs. These inflammatory mediators include histamine, serotonin, bradykinin, nitric oxide, free radicals, prostaglandin, thromboxane, tumor necrosis factor (TNF), and interleukins. Additionally, hormones and mediators of cardiovascular function elevated after burn injury include epinephrine, norepinephrine, vasopressin, angiotensin II, and neuropeptide-Y. The hypovolemic nature of burn shock results from the massive extravasation of plasma into the burn wound and the surrounding tissues as a result of these local and systemic inflammatory mediators altering Starling forces in vessels (Kramer, Lund, Tjostolv, & Beckum, 2002). Fluid resuscitation is both necessary and complex.

SEPSIS AND THE SYSTEMIC INFLAMMATORY RESPONSE SYNDROME

Burn patients commonly exhibit a clinical picture that is predominantly produced by systemic inflammation involving multiple organ systems, including the central nervous system. Symptoms associated with systemic inflammatory response syndrome (SIRS) include tachycardia, tachypnea, fever, leukocytosis, refractory hypotension, and in its severest form, multiple organ-system dysfunction. In thermally injured patients, the most common cause of SIRS is the burn itself. Sepsis, defined as SIRS in the presence of an infection, is also a common cause. Since virtually all patients with severe burns demonstrate signs of SIRS, the American Burn Association (ABA) has come up with specific guidelines for the definition

of sepsis in patients with burns, particularly because the hypermetabolic state may persist for months after the burn wound has healed. As a sign of the hypermetabolic state, patients with large burns may have a baseline temperature to 38.5°C. The change in the burn patient that triggers the concern for infection includes temperature higher than 39° or lower than 36.5°C; progressive tachycardia higher than 100 bpm in adults; progressive tachypnea greater than 25 in an adult not ventilated, thrombocytopenia less than 100,000/mcl three or more days after resuscitation, hyperglycemia if not diabetic, and inability to continue enteral feedings for 24 hours. The finding of a documented infection defines sepsis (Greenhalgh et al., 2007). The most commonly used markers of inflammation and infection include C-reactive protein (CRP), erythrocyte sedimentation rate (ESR), and white blood cell (WBC) count. These are elevated early and taper with time (Chipp, Milner, & Blackburn, 2010) (see Box 75.1).

Box 75.1 AMERICAN BURN ASSOCIATION CONSENSUS ON DEFINITIONS OF SIRS, SEPSIS, AND MULTIPLE ORGAN DYSFUNCTION SYNDROME

Systemic Inflammatory Response Syndrome (SIRS)

At least two or more of the following:
   Temperature above 38°C or below 36°C
   Heart rate >90 beats per minute (bpm)
   Respiratory rate >20/min or maintenance of PaCO2 <32mm Hg
   WBC count >12,000/mm3 or <4000/mm3, or left shift defined as >10% bands.

Sepsis

Sepsis is a change in the burn patient that triggers the concern for infection.

Trigger includes at least three of the following:

   I. Temperature >39°or <36.5°C

  II. Progressive tachycardia:

     a. Adults >110 bpm

     b. Children >2 standard deviations (SD) above age-specific norms(85% age-adjusted maximum heart rate)

 III. Progressive tachypnea:

     a. Adults >25 bpm not ventilated

        i. Minutes of ventilation >121/min ventilated

     b. Children >2 SD above age-specific norms (85% age-adjusted max respiratory rate)

  IV. Thrombocytopenia (will not apply until 3 days after initial resuscitation):

     a. Adults <100,000/mc.l

b. Children <2 SD below age-specific norms

V. Hyperglycemia (in the absence of preexisting diabetes mellitus):

   a. Untreated plasma glucose >200 mgdl or equivalent mM/L

   b. Insulin resistance—examples include:

      i. >7 units of insulin/hr intravenous drip (adults)

      ii. Significant resistance to insulin (>25% increase in insulin requirements over 24 hours)

VI. Inability to continue enteral feedings >24 hours:

   a. Abdominal distension

   b. Enteral feeding intolerance (residual >150ml/hr in children or two times feeding rate in adults)

   c. Uncontrollable diarrhea (>2500 ml/d for adults or >400 ml/d in children)

In addition, it is required that a documented infection be identified by positive culture, pathological tissue soured, or clinical response to antimicrobials.

Multiple Organ Dysfunction Syndrome

Cardiovascular heart rate >120
Respiratory, pO_2/FIo_2 <300
Renal (creatinine mmol/L) >100
Central nervous system (Glasgow coma scale score) >15
Hepatic (total bilirubin, mmol/L) >20
Hematologic (platelet count x 1000) <120

From Greenhalgh, D. G., et al. (2007). American Burn Association Consensus Conference to define sepsis and infection in burns. *Journal of Burn Care & Research, 28,* 776–790.

The pathogenesis of SIRS starts with tissue injury, which results in the acute release of pro-inflammatory cytokines such as TNFα and interleukins IL-1 and IL-6. If the thermal injury is extensive enough, a profound release of cytokines occurs. TNFα is released by macrophages during the first minutes of local or systemic injury. Macrophage dysfunction has been found to be one of the key components of burn-related inflammatory dysregulation (Schwacha, 2003). At the local site of injury, TNF-α initiates an immune response and activates neutrophils and mononuclear phagocytes. It is also a growth factor for fibroblasts and an angiogenesis factor. At the local site, TNF-α will eventually result in tissue repair. However, systemic release of TNF-α can induce fever, stimulation of acute-phase protein secretion by the liver, activation of the coagulation cascade, myocardial suppression, induction of systemic vasodilators with resultant hypotension, catabolism, and hypoglycemia. It also stimulates the release of IL-1 and IL-6, which potentiate the effects of TNF-α.

Brain dysfunction is often one of the first visible symptoms in sepsis, as the brain can be affected by multiple factors such as hypotension, hypoxemia, hyperglycemia, hypoglycemia, and organ dysfunction (such as increased levels of ammonia in liver dysfunction, or urea in kidney dysfunction). In addition to these factors, inflammation can affect the brain directly. The blood–brain barrier permeability is increased, and significant changes in regulation of cerebral perfusion can occur (Burkhart, Siegemund, & Steiner, 2010).

The presence of SIRS, especially in the setting of multi-organ dysfunction syndrome (MODS) is a predictor of poor outcome. The presence of more than two of the SIRS criteria has been correlated with increased morbidity and mortality (Rangel-Frausto et al., 1995). Three factors seem to determine the effect of SIRS on a patient: First, the severity of the initial inflammatory response, which is proportional to the severity of the injury. Specifically, the presence of shock or MODS within the first 24 hours predicts poor prognosis. The second factor is the persistence of SIRS beyond the second day of injury. The third factor is the adaptive capability of the patient. Extremes of age and coexisting disease predict a worse outcome (Sherwood & Traber, 2002).

Treatment of SIRS is largely supportive. Sheridan and colleagues found that the majority of MODS deaths on their unit were clinically free from infection at the time of death, highlighting the overwhelming inflammatory response to thermal injury (Sheridan, Ryan, Yin, Hurley, & Tompkins, 1998). The progression of SIRS to MODS is often more dependent on the inflammatory response than on the actual presence of invasive microorganisms.

PSYCHIATRIC ASSESSMENT AND MANAGEMENT OF PATIENTS WITH BURNS

ACUTE PHASE

The acute phase is the time from initial injury to the time when the patient cognitively and emotionally is convinced that survival is possible, when pain (physical and procedural) becomes controlled, and the patient begins assisting in the recovery and resumes basic autonomous functioning.

Initial assessment and treatment begin from the time of admission or at the time of evaluation, which may occur in the emergency room, particularly for patients with self-inflicted burn injuries. Assessment may be complicated by an intubated or obtunded state. However, cognitive state should be assessed even in the intubated patient, and history should be obtained from collateral sources if possible. A narrative of how the burn occurred and how the patient got to the hospital should be put together.

Laboratory data such as blood chemistries, electrolytes, liver function tests, urine and serum toxicology screens, and carbon monoxide levels (if pertinent) are vital, particularly in intubated or comatose patients. Special studies such as neuroimaging (when there are concerns for head injury, stroke, or hypoxic/anoxic injury), and electroencephalography (EEG) may be indicated, depending on the clinical case.

Encephalopathy

Encephalopathy (delirium) is common in burn centers (see Table 75.4). The prevalence of delirium has ranged from 10–30% of overall burn patients and up to 80% of burn patients in the critical care setting. Specifically, one prospective study of burn intensive care unit (ICU) patients demonstrated delirium in 77% of ventilated burn patients. The majority of patients were identified to have hypoactive delirium (Agarwal et al., 2010).

In trauma patients, age, male gender, intoxication with alcohol on admission, and lack of insurance have been associated with delirium (Blondell et al., 2004; Branco et al., 2011). In the ICU setting, cigarette smoking has also been independently associated with delirium (Van Rompacy et al., 2009). Many of these factors—premorbid psychiatric illness, substance dependence, advanced age, dementia, and smoking—also predispose to the development of burns. However, risk factors for delirium in the ICU and particularly for mechanically ventilated patients are different (Dubois et al., 2001). One prospective observational trial of delirium with mechanically ventilated burn patients found that patients tended to be younger and to have lower rates of cognitive impairment compared to the general hospital population. Nearly 80% of patients developed delirium measured by the Confusion Assessment Method for the intensive care unit (CAM-ICU). Risk was not associated with advanced age, cognitive impairment, substance dependence, burn type or severity, or presence of an inhalation injury. Instead, delirium was independently associated with medications used to target anxiety and pain control. Specifically, benzodiazepine exposure independently predicted the development of delirium (odds ratio [OR] 6.8, p <.001). In contrast, receiving higher doses of intravenous (IV) fentanyl and higher doses of methadone were both associated with half the risk of delirium (Agarwal et al., 2010).

In patients with burn trauma, a high burden of local injury triggers a strong systemic hypermetabolic and inflammatory response. This response is necessary for wound healing and recovery but also has downstream effects on the central nervous system that can predispose to delirium. Since the 1970s, clinicians have observed a high prevalence of delirium in both adults and children who have experienced severe burns and have postulated the existence of a burn-related toxin (Antoon, Volpe, & Crawford, 1972). Although no specific "burn toxin" has been identified, the inflammatory response syndrome impacts the brain through both hormonal and neuronal mechanisms. Local tissue injury causes a pro-inflammatory cytokine cascade that leads to the production of neurotoxins and excessive cortisol. In addition, oxidative stress alters neuronal activity (particularly in areas of the brain more sensitive to hypoxia, such as the hippocampus and subcortical gray matter), and affects the levels of neurotransmitters. For example, cholinergic neurons are uniquely sensitive to oxygen deprivation, resulting in decreased synthesis and release of acetylcholine (Fricchione et al., 2008).

Metabolic Abnormalities and Risk for Infection

In addition to being exposed to a pro-inflammatory state, burn patients, given large areas of exposed surface area, open wounds, administration of various antimicrobial dressings, and high caloric demands, are vulnerable to hyperglycemia, and fluid and electrolyte abnormalities, including hyponatremia, that have been associated with delirium. The systemic inflammatory response may evolve into sepsis and multi-organ failure.

Table 75.4 RISK FACTORS FOR DELIRIUM IN THE BURN PATIENT.

Demographic and Predisposing Factors	*Potentially Modifiable Factors: Focus on ICU Patients* *Note: Demographic Factors Less Robust in the Critically Ill Population*
General Medical and Surgical Patients: • Advanced Age • Cognitive Impairment • Hypertension • Depression • Substance dependence: Alcohol, Illicit drugs, nicotine *Trauma Patients* • Age >45 years • Alcohol dependence: Elevated mean corpuscular volume and + blood alcohol level on admission • Type of injury: Burns, falls • Male gender • Lack of insurance *Burn Patients* • TBSA >30% • Inhalation injury • Charcoal/gas stove: Carbon monoxide exposure	• Need for frequent procedures • Electrolyte imbalances • Pro-inflammatory state and risk of infection • Disruptions of sleep-wake cycle • Pain control • Assessing for alcohol/substance withdrawal • Medications: Sedative-hypnotics, unnecessary administration of narcotics *Decreased risk for delirium* • Appropriate use of opiates to treat background and procedural pain • Drug holidays, individualized sedation protocols *Increased risk for delirium* • Benzodiazepines: Larger doses; use of longer acting agents • Use of opiates to target agitation • Anticholinergic agents

Carbon Monoxide Exposure and Hypoxia

The circumstances of the burn, and particular toxins involved, may also heighten the risk of delirium. Patients who have experienced burns related to charcoal, gas stoves, or inhalation injuries may also have been exposed to carbon monoxide. In the acute setting, carbon monoxide exposure causes non-specific symptoms; especially, headache, disturbance of consciousness, nausea and vomiting, dizziness, confusion, fatigue, chest pain, and dyspnea. The diagnosis of carbon monoxide (CO) poisoning is clinical, requiring a history of recent CO exposure, the presence of symptoms consistent with CO poisoning, and demonstration of an elevated carboxyhemoglobin level. No particular symptoms correlate with the CO level. High-flow oxygen by mask or endotrachial tube is the front-line treatment (Hampson et al., 2012). Through both the impact of hypoxia and oxidative stress resulting from carboxyhemoglobin, patients can also develop persistent neurological sequelae, and after a lucid interval, develop delayed neurological sequelae within a timeframe of a few days to six weeks. The symptoms observed correspond to the sensitivity of brain regions to hypoxia and oxidative stress and can include: deficits in memory due to insults to the hippocampus; impaired attention and executive function and personality change linked to the thalamus and subcortical white matter; and symptoms of Parkinsonism, chorea, dystonia, and psychosis due to impact on the basal ganglia and dopaminergic neurons (Weaver, 2009). There is mixed evidence that treatment with hyperbaric oxygen decreases the risk of the development of delayed neurological sequelae (Buckley et al., 2011); however, hyperbaric oxygen should at least be considered in all cases of serious acute CO poisoning and normobaric 100% oxygen continued until the time of hyperbaric oxygen administration (Jurrlink et al., 2005). The goal of hyperbaric oxygen treatment would be to prevent later neurological sequelae. There is a risk of long-term cognitive deficits and the development of anxiety and depression not necessarily associated with the severity of carbon monoxide exposure. Treatment decisions in the mildly poisoned patient are difficult and controversial even among experts (Weaver, 2009). More broadly, inhalation injury and exposure to smoke may also predispose to the development of delirium due to hypoxia and poor CNS perfusion. Those who are accidentally exposed to carbon monoxide should be seen one to two months later, and formal neuropsychiatric testing used to document baseline function or deficits.

Pain Control and Exposure to Medications

For decades, pain was under-treated in the burn population, in part due to concern of over-sedation and death. Poorly controlled pain has been linked to the development of delirium in postoperative patients (Morrison et al., 2003) and has also been associated with increased long-term risk of PTSD (Moeller-Bertram, Keltner, & Strigo, 2011; Watkins, Cook, May, & Ehleben, 1988). Burn patients experience both a chronic, background level of pain due to tissue damage, and acute procedural pain in the context of daily debridement.

High doses and combinations of medications have been utilized to treat pain, anxiety, and fear. The goal is to treat pain and relieve fear and anxiety, provide adequate sedation for procedures, and enable restful sleep, at the same time trying to avoid precipitating a drug-related delirium.

Sedatives

Trials have been conducted in the critical care setting to help guide the judicious use of sedatives. Specifically, in the ICU, administration of high-dose benzodiazepines has been independently associated with delirium. In mechanically ventilated burn patients, as described above, higher doses of lorazepam were a strong independent predictor of delirium (Agarwal et al., 2010). Additionally, delirium has been more strongly linked to longer acting benzodiazepines (Marcantonio et al., 1994). Alternative agents for sedation are also being studied in the ICU setting. One alternative to benzodiazepines and propofol is dexmedetomidine, an alpha-2-agonist, with approximately 8 times greater affinity for the alpha-2-receptor than clonidine. Compared to patients treated with equally efficacious doses of midazolam equivalents, patients treated with dexmedetomidine had a lower risk of delirium and fewer days of being ventilated; the downside was an increased risk of bradycardia (Riker et al., 2009). A randomized controlled trial of individualized sedation for mechanically ventilated patients demonstrated that, compared to lorazepam, dexmedetomidine was associated with decreased duration of delirium (Pandharipande et al., 2008). Complicating its use in the burn patient population is its potential to cause hypotension; thus proper hydration is critical, and a loading dose should be avoided if possible. Propofol is another alternative sedating agent with a significantly shorter half-life that has been postulated to be less deliriogenic than benzodiazepines. However, in a patient with large-scale burns that would necessitate the use of sedatives and ventilation for an extended duration of time (more than two to three weeks), the use of propofol may not be possible due to the risk of propofol infusion syndrome and resulting lipid and metabolic derangements associated with its use.

Opiates

Evidence regarding the link between exposure to opiates and the risk for delirium is mixed. Meperidine and high doses of morphine have been more consistently associated with delirium than has the use of other opiates. However, studies conducted in the postoperative setting link pain to delirium, suggesting that there is a delirium risk in under-treatment with opiates. In mechanically ventilated burn patients, intravenous opiate exposure and treatment with methadone were both associated with a 50% decreased risk of delirium. Consistent with clinical experience, authors have argued that controlling pain (background and procedural) is protective, but when opiates are used for sedation or control of agitation—usually at higher doses than those needed for adequate pain control—the risk of delirium increases (Agarwal et al., 2010).

Addiction and Withdrawal Syndromes

Chronic alcohol misuse is more common in burn patients (up to 41%), even when compared to psychiatric patients (30%) and neurological patients (19%) (Fauerbach et al., 1997; Spies & Rommelspacher, 1999). Almost half of all trauma beds are occupied by patients who were injured while intoxicated or under the influence of alcohol (Spies & Rommelspacher, 1999). In addition, the rate of morbidity and mortality due to infections, cardiopulmonary insufficiency, or bleeding disorders is two to four times greater in patients who chronically misuse alcohol.

In a study by Soderstrom and colleagues, the rates of point-prevalence of drug dependency in a trauma center were 10.6% for cocaine, 10.0% for opiates, 6.5% for cannabis, 0.4% for hallucinogens, and 0.3% for stimulants (Soderstrom et al., 1997). Their data seem to show that seriously injured trauma center patients manifest severer forms of addiction than the general population with polysubstance dependence.

The incidence of alcohol withdrawal delirium (AWD), commonly referred to as delirium tremens or DTs, in hospitalized patients is significant. Among trauma patients, it is estimated that 40–50% of patients are intoxicated, and 94% of those presenting with intoxication have a substance abuse disorder (Lukan, Reed, Looney, Spain, & Blondell, 2002). The clinician should attempt to identify the patients at high risk for developing AWD, initiate prophylactic treatment in patients at high risk, and provide effective treatment of patients who go on to develop AWD despite prophylaxis, in order to decrease associated morbidity and mortality (Box 75.2).

Management of Encephalopathy

The first step to management of delirium is establishing the safety of the patient and staff. This may require the temporary use of restraints. The next step, if possible, is to identify the underlying etiology or etiologies and correct any reversible causes that may contribute to delirium. In the burn patient

---

Box 75.2 RISK FACTORS FOR ALCOHOL WITHDRAWAL DELIRIUM (DELIRIUM TREMENS)

History of past alcohol withdrawal seizure(s) or delirium tremens

Seizure in the field or in emergency department prior to admission

Acute concurrent medical illness

More days since last drink (two or more days)

Elevated blood alcohol upon admission

Heavier and longer drinking history

Age >40

Race and genetic predisposition

Burn-related injuries

Falls, particularly with long-bone fractures

In one study—motor vehicle accidents had negative predictive value

Elevated MCV, aspartate aminotransferase

---

in the critical care unit, this means frequent monitoring and correction of electrolytes, assessing oxygenation and CNS perfusion, monitoring for infection, controlling pain, assessing for use of deliriogenic medications, and monitoring for withdrawal from alcohol, benzodiazepines, and opiates.

As the diagnostic work-up is occurring, antipsychotics can be utilized to target agitation and confusion. Specifically, IV haloperidol is often the most practical choice in the acutely ill burn patient given its relatively low hypotensive and anticholinergic effects. Acute extrapyramidal syndromes are also infrequent with short periods of intravenous haloperidol use. A starting dose of 2–5 mg IV is reasonable and can be titrated up by 5–10 mg every 30 minutes until the patient is calm. Particularly in burn patients who are more vulnerable to electrolyte abnormalities, it is important to monitor and replenish potassium and magnesium to high-normal values and assess the corrected QT interval. Quetiapine has been used in critical care settings for the control of agitation in states of hyperactive delirium and may have benefit in the agitated burn patient. Doses may be started at 25–100 mg to a maximum 800 mg total daily dose—this maximum dose should not be continued for more than 72 hours, due to risk of anticholinergic excess, particularly in dopamine antagonist–naïve patients. Olanzapine and its oral disintegrating formulation (olanzapine—Zydis) may also be considered, although it has limited utility in the severely agitated patient who may require large doses of medication for control of agitation. Doses may be started ranging from 2.5–10 mg, with a maximum of 30 mg in a 24-hour period, due to its potential to create anticholinergic excess.

Management of Alcohol Withdrawal

The diagnosis of alcohol withdrawal is clinical and characterized by the presence of hyperarousal, confusion, hallucinations, hypertension, tachycardia, fever, diaphoresis, and agitated behavior in the setting of acute reduction of or abstinence from alcohol. Once comorbid illnesses have been excluded or adequately addressed or treated, the management of alcohol withdrawal is directed at alleviating symptoms and identifying and correcting metabolic derangements. Supportive care, including administration of intravenous fluids; nutritional supplementation; correction of deficiencies of potassium, magnesium, phosphate, and glucose; along with administration of intravenous thiamine to prevent or treat Wernicke's encephalopathy, should be initiated. Benzodiazepines are generally considered first-line treatment for AWS, and for the prevention of alcohol withdrawal seizures. There is no consensus as to the best benzodiazepine to use; however, longer acting benzodiazepines with active metabolites, such as diazepam, may allow a smoother course of withdrawal, lower the chance of recurrent seizure, and have greater efficacy in the prevention of delirium (Ntais, Pakos, Kyzas, & Ioannidis, 2005). Benzodiazepines with an intermediate half-life, such as lorazepam, may have a safer profile in patients with comorbid hepatic dysfunction. While symptom triggered therapy utilizing the Clinical Institute Withdrawal Assessment for Alcohol Scale (CIWA-Ar) has been shown to be effective in treating patients in alcohol withdrawal, its applicability in patients with comorbid medical and surgical illness has not (Hecksel, Bostwick, Jaeger, & Cha, 2008). In addition, it relies heavily on the patients' ability to logically respond to questions about their subjective experiences with AWS in seven of its ten items, which is often not possible in patients with AWD or delirious with other comorbid medical and surgical conditions.

Pain

Burn-related injuries are among the most painful types of trauma sustained. The ability to adequately assess and treat the burn patient's pain is aided by the understanding of the types of pain that these patients experience. In the acute phase of injury, there are three types of pain that the clinician should assess and treat accordingly. These include:

1. Continuous background pain from damaged tissue and nerve injury.

2. Acute pain caused by mechanical and chemical irritation of damaged tissue.

3. Procedural pain caused by dressing changes, or increased physical exertion when the patient is being treated by physical and occupational therapists.

If pain symptoms are not adequately controlled, particularly with procedures, the patient may begin to anticipate that pain will be associated with each subsequent intervention, commonly referred to as an *anticipatory pain response*. While many clinicians initially describe this as a form of "anxiety," it is far from it, and more accurately described as a "fear" response, particularly in the immediate period following burn injury. This distinction is more than a matter of nomenclature, as it has direct effects on treatment. Fear is amygdalar in origin and treated with dopamine antagonists, while symptoms of anxiety are treated with use of benzodiazepines. It should be noted that even when pain treatment is optimized, the process of seeing their affected body parts once bandages are removed can be overwhelming and frightening. Co-administration of low-dose IV haloperidol with IV opioids 15 minutes prior to dressing changes can reduce the anticipatory fear response.

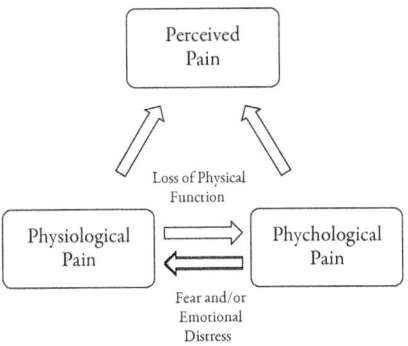

Figure 75.1 Relationship between physiological and psychological pain.

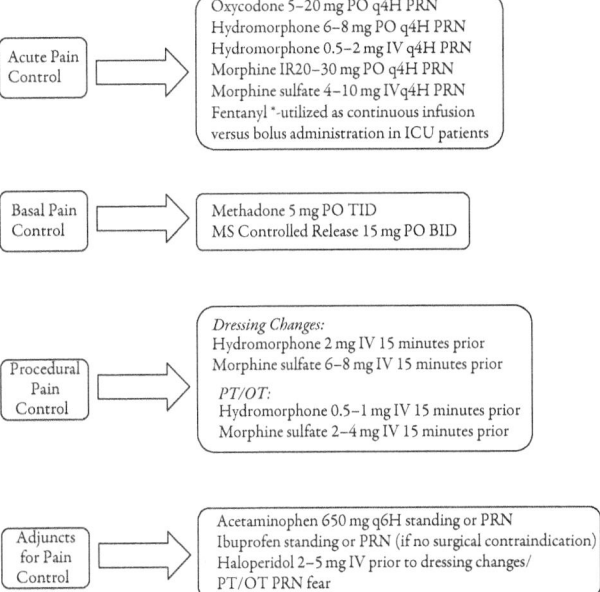

Figure 75.2 Commonly utilized strategies for acute nociceptive pain.

Patients can experience various painful emotions—anger, frustration, depression, anxiety, fear of death, etc.—at any time during their clinical course. These symptoms and their physiological accompaniments will make somatic pain and discomfort more severe and less bearable (see Figure 75.1).

Various pain scales are available to assist in grading pain symptoms in a more objective manner. The 0 to 10 visual analogue scale is often utilized in quantifying the patient's level of perceived pain, and using this scale, the patient is asked to quantify his or her pain when at rest, and before and after dressing changes, debridements, and physical and occupational therapy.

Once a method is in place for tracking the patient's pain, a pharmacological regimen is then designed to meet the patient's needs. In the intubated patient, or the patient with large-scale burns that necessitate frequent trips to the operating theater for excision and grafting (E & G), IV fentanyl is often utilized for basal control of pain, with bolus administration for intermittent pain symptoms. For smaller scale burns or later in the course of a larger scale burn patient, long-acting opiate analgesics such as methadone may be employed for basal pain control, with the short-acting narcotics such as hydromorphone or morphine used for intermittent pain and for procedural pain control (see Figure 75.2).

Pain control in the opioid-dependent patient with burn injury should be mentioned: Generally, patients with active or recent chronic opioid use, whether illicit or iatrogenic, will exhibit physiological tolerance to opioid medications, necessitating increased dosages or frequency of administration. These patients will often respond better to use of a patient-controlled analgesia (PCA) pump for the first 24 to 36 hours, and achieve improved pain control versus nurse- or clinician-administered PRN approaches. Their previous 24 hours short-acting narcotic requirement can then be converted to a long-acting analgesic (e.g., methadone) with the goal of decreasing the amount of short-acting narcotic required by the time of discharge.

PSYCHOLOGICAL ADAPTATIONS AND REACTIONS IN THE ACUTE PHASE

As patients who have experienced severer burns are surviving, there is a greater emphasis on psychological adjustment and the potential impact on the person's long-term functional outcome. PTSD affects a significant population of burn survivors and has been linked to significant morbidity.

In the acute setting, psychiatric consultants can promote psychological adaptation, collaborate with the team to assess and control pain, and diagnose and treat discrete psychiatric disorders (Watkins et al., 1988). The primary goal is to foster psychiatric stabilization so that the patient can engage with medical care and rehabilitation. It is also important to have an understanding of which symptoms are normative and not indicative of increased risk for the development of a psychiatric disorder. For example, the majority of burn survivors experience symptoms of acute stress, including disrupted sleep and re-experiencing of the trauma (Ehde, Patterson, Wiechman, & Wilson, 2000).

Stages of Adaptation—Acute Phase

Burn specialists have identified a series of key psychological stages in adaptation to recovery from severe burns and discussed interventions that teams can provide to support the patient's physical and psychological recovery. This approach provides a practical framework that can heighten understanding of the patient's perspective and promote the patient's engagement in care.

Survival Fear

Immediately following the experience of a severe burn, the patient is focused solely on survival. The patient is hypervigilant and tremulous, and directs his or her energy toward the demands of physical recovery. In this context, the patient is less able to process verbal content. Therefore, the patient will probably benefit from frequent reorientation and repetition of basic information, including a realistic appraisal of his chance of survival, the severity of his injury, the physical phenomena he is experiencing, and the most likely course of recovery (Watkins et al., 1988).

Search for Meaning

Additional psychological stages of adaptation to severe burns include a detailed recounting of the events of the burn and a related search for an explanation that makes sense and can be tolerated emotionally. Patients question why the burn happened and, in particular, why it happened to them. Subsequently, after engagement in rehabilitation, many patients confront feelings of helplessness and work to grieve and accept the losses of appearance and capability. Watkins and colleagues argue that failure to negotiate these stages successfully predisposes them to the development of specific psychiatric disorders, including PTSD and depression.

INTERMEDIATE PHASE

As the burn patients progress from the acute phase of injury to the intermediate phase, their survival is usually assured. Despite this, ongoing physiological stress with regard to injury, inflammation, frequent dressing changes, repeated trips to the operating room, and active attempts at mobilization may affect adversely affect the individual's ability to cope with the psychological aspects of her injury. In addition, as the patient becomes fully grafted, there is a rapid reduction in altered mental status and delirium, and generally rapid improvement in cognitive function. It is usually during this phase that psychiatric consultation for depression, mood lability, anxiety, insomnia, nightmares, and concerns about acute stress reactions occur.

Acute Psychiatric Disorders After Burn Injury

An additional role of the psychiatrist during the acute phase of recovery is to identify burn patients who are at risk for poor adjustment. As previously described, psychiatric disorders, including substance dependence, mood disorders, and psychosis, are over-represented in the burns population, and pre-burn mental function is associated with post-burn adjustment (Klinge, Chamberlain, Redden, & King, 2009; Wisely, Wilson, Duncan, & Tarrier, 2010). Additional variables that have been postulated to be linked to the development of acute stress disorder and PTSD include exposure to high doses of benzodiazepines in the ICU, poor pain control, and peritraumatic tachycardia. Elevated heart rate in the ambulance following burn injury has been associated with higher rates of acute stress disorder and PTSD at six months (Dyster-Aas et al., 2008; Ehde et al., 2000; Esselman, Thombs, Magyar-Russell, & Fauerbach, 2006; Gould et al., 2011; McKibben, Bresnick, Wiechman, Askay, & Fauerbach, 2008).

Adjustment Disorders with Anxiety or Depressed Mood

Patients who have experienced burns are at increased risk for the development of adjustment disorders with anxiety and depressed mood. As described above, risk may be linked to premorbid psychopathology, coping style, and characteristics of the burn experienced. Symptoms occur within three months of the burn injury and cause clinically significant distress and disturbance in functioning. The recommended treatment of adjustment disorders includes targeting associated symptoms such as insomnia and anxiety, and the use of supportive psychotherapy with an understanding of the person's strengths and coping style.

Acute Stress Disorder

Experiencing some symptoms of acute stress following burn trauma is normal. To diagnose acute stress disorder, the patient must respond to the burn with fear, helplessness, or horror. Additionally, the patient needs to experience symptoms in the same clusters as PTSD, including: three symptoms of dissociation in addition to re-experiencing, avoidance, and hyperarousal, that last for at least two days and occur within four weeks of the traumatic event.

Acute stress disorder (ASD) is not uncommon in burn survivors, occurring in 11–32% of patients (McKibben et al., 2008). Importantly, the diagnosis of ASD is a strong and stable predictor of PTSD over time, from one month to two years following the burn. This association remains after controlling for the factor of acute psychological distress.

Both pharmacological and psychological interventions have been assessed in the treatment of ASD. Evidence of the effectiveness of particular medications such as beta blockers in ASD is mixed. In the past, some have also suggested having only a single debriefing session after a traumatic event. The evidence shows that debriefing of traumatic events can be linked to adverse outcomes, and is not recommended (Rose, Bisson, Churchill, & Wessely, 2002). In contrast, cognitive behavioral therapy has been shown to be effective in survivors of accidents with ASD, and is likely beneficial when extended to the burn population (Bryant, Sackville, Dang, Moulds, & Guthrie, 1999). Additional potentially modifiable factors include optimization of pain control and anxiety-management in the acute setting.

Stages of Adaptation—Intermediate Phase

Investing in Recovery

As the patient enters the intermediate phase of injury, her focus shifts to getting a better understanding of the details of her treatment, and to optimize her participation in the recovery and resumption of daily life skills (grooming, feeding, communicating, ambulating, etc.). In some instances, as the patient begins to attempt to perform basic autonomous functions, the patient will feel that her ability or progress is inadequate or a disappointment. Feelings of frustration or anger over perceptions of helplessness and dependency on others may be common, as are adjustment reactions with depressive symptoms. Watkins and colleagues describe four staff interventions that can aid the patients during their progression during this phase:

1. Educating the patient about the expected course of recovery specific for the type of injury he sustained.

2. Orienting the patient to the physical phenomena that he will experience during this phase of recuperation (e.g., itching, nociceptive and neuropathic pain, etc.).

3. Creating a program for self-care and activities. Initially, goals should be realistic about the degree of physical impairment sustained by the patient, with gradual progression of goals once the patient begins to derive a sense of pride in his accomplishments.

4. Focusing on returning abilities versus remaining disabilities by verbal acknowledgement and praise of any improvements in autonomous functioning, no matter how small.

Acceptance of Losses

As patients become more actively involved in their recovery and attempt to resume basic autonomous functioning, they begin to cognitively define and emotionally realize the long-term and often permanent losses that they have sustained from their burn injuries. While some losses may be immediately obvious (e.g., loss of ambulation, function of limbs, loss of limbs, etc.), others may not be as apparent immediately. The loss of some ability to associate with friends and family, or the loss of the opportunity to live life in the manner they were accustomed to may be equally devastating. This initial realization is often expressed as "hurt," and perceived as feelings of sadness or "depression," and may be exhibited by social withdrawal, tearfulness, decreased appetite, impaired sleep initiation and/or maintenance, or decreased participation in physical therapy. The patients should be allowed the opportunity to talk about their perceptions regarding these issues and the emotional difficulties they are experiencing, in an effort to legitimize their situation and allow them to ventilate their perceptions and feelings regarding losses (Watkins et al., 1988).

REHABILITATIVE PHASE

In many respects, the rehabilitative phase is an extension of the intermediate phase of injury, with continued pursuit of reintegration, both psychologically and physically. Ongoing psychiatric evaluation, assessment, and treatment may be required during this phase, particularly as struggles with autonomous functioning continue.

Post-Traumatic Stress Disorder

Although estimates vary based on the assessment tool used, PTSD is estimated to occur in 12–42% of burn survivors, and the diagnosis appears relatively stable over the first two years after the burn. For example, PTSD at one month predicts PTSD at one year (Ehde et al., 2000; Fauerbach et al., 1997). PTSD has been reported to be associated with depression and higher utilization of health care, and is linked to longer term functional impairment, lower health-related quality of life, and decreased chances of returning to work (Davydow, Katon, & Zatzick, 2009).

The largest risk factor for the development of PTSD following traumatic injury seems to be a previous history of psychiatric illness. Additional risk factors for the development of PTSD following injury include acute pain symptoms, female gender, and personality characteristics such as externalization of blame, poor coping style, and high neuroticism (McGhee et al., 2011). Characteristics of the burn, including higher percent of the TBSA and location on the face, head, and neck, have also been linked to the development of PTSD (Ehde et al., 2000).

Interventions in the acute setting can focus on potential mediating factors and can foster improved long-term psychological adjustment. Initiation of quetiapine for states of hyperarousal may be helpful, in addition to assisting in treating difficulty with sleep initiation and sleep maintenance, particularly when associated with nightmares. If nightmares persist, a trial of prazosin can be started and titrated to assist in symptomatic control. Cognitive behavioral therapy (CBT) may also be helpful to challenge cognitive distortions or to treat underlying anxiety or depressive symptoms. A formal course of CBT to help patients get back to work (e.g., exposure-type therapy) following an on-the-job injury may also be helpful in resumption of premorbid activities.

Depression

Lifetime mood disorders following burn injuries have been found to be as high as 31% (Fauerbach et al., 1997), with major depression being the most common mood disorder (27%). These figures are higher than in the general population and associated with worse functional status at discharge (Fauerbach et al., 1996), in addition to having an increased chance of developing PTSD (Dyster-Aas et al., 2008; Fauerbach et al., 1997) at one year post-injury.

If there is no surgical contraindication, initiation of a selective serotonin-reuptake inhibitor (SSRI) such as sertraline or citalopram may be initiated to treat underlying symptoms. Use of selective noradrenergic reuptake inhibitors (SNRIs), such as duloxetine, may also be employed, with the potential benefit of also helping to treat underlying neuropathic pain from burn-related injury. For patients with significant underlying apathy or abulia, initiation of a stimulant such as dextroamphetamine or methylphenidate may be indicated and useful.

Chronic Pain

Pain often does not end after the acute phase following burn injuries, with many patients continuing to have chronic pain, even after complete wound healing. Studies have found that about one-third of burn patients from one to nine years out from their initial injuries continue to experience significant and life-disrupting pain symptoms.

In certain patients, it may be sometimes necessary to utilize chronic opioids to maintain a reasonable level of comfort and to assist in optimizing functional abilities. In addition, it may be necessary to add adjuvant pain medicine for the specific treatment of neuropathic pain. Certain antidepressants, such as tricyclic antidepressants (TCAs) and SNRIs, along with anti-epileptic medications, have been used widely for the control of neuropathic pain; however, controlled studies on the effectiveness of these agents on burn pain are lacking. Pain management in patients after severe burns can require the full multidisciplinary, multimodality approach needed for other refractory chronic pain syndromes. Referral to a specialized pain clinic may be necessary.

END-OF-LIFE CARE

Although the mortality rate of severe burns has decreased over the years due to advances made in burn care, burn units still see a significant number of deaths. The major risk factors for mortality include older age (>60), percentage TBSA (greater than 40%) and the presence of an inhalation injury (Blot & Brusselaers, 2009; Ryan et al., 1998). Fratianne and Brandt developed a system for determination of futility by convening with the burn team to discuss Do Not Resuscitate (DNR) orders if patients with age plus percent TBSA burn equal a score of 100 or greater at the time of admission, or later in the course of treatment when at least two major organs are failing (Fratianne & Brandt, 1997). The mortality rate on adult burn units is often higher than on pediatric burn units because of severe medical and psychiatric risk factors and an increased mortality risk associated with older age. The psychiatrist is often consulted to assist in the care of dying patients and their families to minimize pain and suffering and to assist in the process of decision-making at the end of life (Jellinek, Todres, Catlin, Cassem, & Salzman, 1993). It is important to explain to patients and their families that a DNR is not equivalent to a "Do Not Care (DNC) order." The Society of Critical Care Medicine states that for both children and adults, palliative care and intensive care are not mutually exclusive options, but rather should coexist (Truog et al., 2001). For both adults and children, the discussion about end-of-life decisions is often delayed because clinicians are used to preserving life whenever possible and moving forward with care. However, delaying this difficult discussion too long can result in missing the opportunity for good palliative care. When the shift has been made from curative therapy to palliative care, the goal should be the relief of suffering. The burn team, in addition to the psychiatrist, should focus on adequate symptom management, no inappropriate prolongation of dying, a sense of control for patient and family, and a focus on the relationship between patient and family. The concept of having a patient-centered conference including nurses, social workers, residents, and attending surgeons to decide when to forego life-sustaining measures has proved to have high acceptance by both patients and families. It can be very meaningful and reassuring to have the entire team present their recommendation to withdraw life-sustaining measures to the patient (when possible) and to their family (Fratianne, Brandt, Yurko, & Coffee, 1992). By obtaining team consensus, an atmosphere of mutual respect and trust between team members is created, which will result in better patient care and a better work environment.

In children, the shift to palliative care is often later than with adults, and the burn team will often wait until the last hours of the child's life to address limitation of life-sustaining measures such as inotropic agents, cardiopulmonary resuscitation (CPR), and ventilator support (O'Mara, Chapyak, Greenhalgh, & Palmieri, 2006). The decision to withdraw care for younger patients is more commonly based on burn size or severity (Ismail, Long, Moiemen, & Wilson, 2011). Once pediatric patients are made DNR, the progression to death tends to be very rapid, with the time from a consensus on resuscitation status to death being on average 24 hours or less. O'Mara et al. found that in one pediatric burn unit, the writing of a DNR order occurred on average a few hours before the patient's death (median, 2.75 hours). The authors also found that if a DNR order was written, the family was present 75% of the time at the child's death. However, in only half of the cases in which the patient did not have a

DNR order was the family present at the time of death. This finding shows that either the family was not well prepared for the death of the child, or the death was too sudden to allow for adequate preparation. The psychiatrist can play a role in facilitating these difficult discussions of death earlier rather than later when possible, so as to adequately prepare families.

STAFF SUPPORT, STAFF STRESS, AND BURNOUT PREVENTION

Burn units are often regarded with fear and awe. The staff members in burn units are constantly exposed to traumatic images such as facial burns, massive injuries, and amputations. Functioning effectively in this environment may require unique coping mechanisms. Indeed, exposure to extreme injuries can cause "secondary traumatization" in hospital staff (Fullerton, Ursano, & Wang, 2004). Rapid turnover of staff may occur, especially on understaffed units, after admission of a series of unusually serious burns, and when support for staff is not adequate. Burnout is a syndrome of emotional exhaustion, depersonalization, and reduced personal accomplishment associated with chronic occupational stressors. Psychiatrists can help to prevent such outcomes by encouraging communication, validating attitudes and feelings, providing emotional support and specific psychological interventions, and by mobilizing organizational resources.

Some of the more difficult patients in burn unit are patients with active psychiatric disorders. For example, untreated psychopathology in adolescent self-immolators can induce intense staff hostility and conflict. Encouragement of staff to express their frustration and teaching them ways to avoid power struggles can help them avoid the kinds of interactions that evoke staff counter-transference. The best approach is for surgery and psychiatry to work together in developing a clear treatment plan and initiate long-term psychiatric treatment on the burn unit.

Patients with substance use disorders also evoke adverse reactions in caregivers and staff. Often, staff members are concerned about giving benzodiazepines and opiates to patients with substance use disorders. The psychiatrist can play a role in educating staff about substance use disorders, and stressing that, while patients may become physically dependent on these medications, addiction is almost never *caused* by use of these agents in the context of burns (Stoddard & Fricchione, 2004). In fact, these patients may initially require higher doses of narcotics and benzodiazepines to effectively treat symptoms than do others without similar histories. However, it is important to taper off these medications once it is determined they are no longer required.

Agitated and aggressive delirious patients can be particularly difficult for staff to manage on a burn unit. Behaviors such as aggressiveness towards staff, attempting to leave, pulling out lines, and disrupting the milieu are not uncommon in such patients. The psychiatrist should assess for need for restraints and medications, as well as help provide increased support to staff. Overall the psychiatrist can serve as an integral part of the burn team and can provide education and reassurance for the staff about the dynamics of a particular case. The psychiatrist can also foster open discussion with the staff about staff members' feelings, needs, and expectations, thereby reducing feelings of helplessness and the risk of burnout.

CLINICAL PEARLS

- Burn centers now average 200 admissions apiece per year, and their average survival rate exceeds 94%.

- Premorbid psychiatric diagnoses and substance use—alcohol, narcotics, cocaine—are common among those with burn injuries.

- Burns associated with methamphetamine use are a relatively new problem; not only does methamphetamine intoxication predispose to burn injury, but its production involves highly volatile chemical compounds that can cause both thermal and chemical injuries.

- Risk factors associated with self-immolation in developing countries include younger age, female gender, low socioeconomic status, decreased literacy, limited access to mental health services, marital and familial conflict (Ahmadi et al., 2009; Ahmadi & Ytterstad, 2007).

- Because of nerve damage, third-degree burns may be less painful than second-degree burns.

- Symptoms associated with SIRS include tachycardia, tachypnea, fever, leukocytosis, refractory hypotension, and, in its severest form, multiple organ-system dysfunction. In thermally injured patients, the most common cause of SIRS is the burn itself.

- One prospective study of burn ICU patients demonstrated delirium in 77% of ventilated burn patients. The majority of patients were identified to have hypoactive delirium (Agarwal et al., 2010).

- The hypermetabolic state may persist for months after the burn wound has healed.

- Mental status should be assessed even in the intubated patient.

- In the acute phase, pain comes in three types: continuous background pain from damaged tissue and nerve injury; acute pain caused by mechanical and chemical irritation of damaged tissue; procedural pain caused by dressing changes or increased physical exertion when the patient is being treated by physical and occupational therapists.

- Patients who have experienced burns related to charcoal, gas stoves, or inhalation injuries may also have been exposed to carbon monoxide. In the acute setting, carbon monoxide exposure causes non-specific symptoms, especially headache, disturbance of consciousness, nausea and vomiting, dizziness, confusion, fatigue, chest pain, and dyspnea.

- There is mixed evidence that treatment with hyperbaric oxygen decreases the risk of developing delayed neurological sequelae (Buckley, 2011); however, hyperbaric oxygen should at least be considered in all cases of serious acute CO poisoning. The goal of hyperbaric oxygen treatment would be to prevent later neurological sequelae.

DISCLOSURE STATEMENTS

Dr. Nejad has no disclosure to declare.

Dr. Dubovsky has no disclosure to declare.

Dr. Irwin has no disclosure to declare.

Dr. Fagan has no disclosure to declare.

Dr. Goverman has no disclosure to declare.

REFERENCES

Agarwal, V., O'Neill, P. J., Cotton, B. A., Pun, B. T., Haney, S., Thompson, J., et al. (2010). Prevalence and risk factors for development of delirium in burn intensive care unit patients. *Journal of Burn Care Research, 31*(5), 706–715.

Ahmadi, A. (2007). Suicide by self-immolation: Comprehensive overview, experiences and suggestions. *Journal of Burn Care Research, 28*(1), 30–41.

Ahmadi, A., & Ytterstad, B. (2007). Prevention of self-immolation by community-based intervention. *Burns, 33*(8), 1032–1040.

Ahmadi, A., Mohammadi, R., Schwebel, D. C., Khazaie, H., Yeganeh, N., & Almasi, A. (2009). Demographic risk factors of self-immolation: A case-control study. *Burns, 35*(4), 580–586.

American Burn Association (2011a). 2011 National Burn Repository Report, retrieved August 15, 2011, from http://www.ameriburn.org/2011NBRAnnualReport.pdf.

American Burn Association (2011b). Burn Incidence and Treatment in the United States: 2011 Fact Sheet, retrieved August 15, 2011, from http://www.ameriburn.org/resources_factsheet.php.

American Psychiatric Association. (2000). *Diagnostic and Statistical Manual of Mental Disorders, Text Revision* (DSM-IV-TR). Washington, DC: American Psychiatric Association.

Antoon, A. Y., Volpe, J. J., & Crawford, J. D. (1972). Burn encephalopathy in children. *Pediatrics, 50*(4), 609–616.

Barillo, D. J., & Goode, R. (1996). Fire fatality study: Demographics of fire victims. *Burns, 22*(2), 85–88.

Bernstein, N. (1976). *Emotional care of the facially burned and disfigured.* Boston: Little, Brown.

Blondell, R. D., Powell, G. E., Dodds, H. N., Looney, S. W., & Lukan, J. K. (2004). Admission characteristics of trauma patients in whom delirium develops. *American Journal of Surgery, 187*(3), 332–337.

Blot, S., & Brusselaers, N. (2009). Development and validation of a model for prediction of mortality in patients with acute burn injury. *British Journal of Surgery, 96*(1), 111–117.

Branco, B. C., Inaba, K., Bukur, M., Talving, P., Oliver, M., David, J. S., et al. (2011). Risk factors for delirium in trauma patients: The impact of ethanol use and lack of insurance. *The American Surgeon, 77*(5), 621–626.

Bryant, R. A., Sackville, T., Dang, S. T., Moulds, M., & Guthrie, R. (1999). Treating acute stress disorder: An evaluation of cognitive behavior therapy and supportive counseling techniques. *American Journal of Psychiatry, 156*(11), 1780–1786.

Buckley, N. A., Juurlink, D. N., Isbister, G., Bennett, M. H., & Lavonas, E. J. (2011). Hyperbaric oxygen for carbon monoxide poisoning (Review). *The Cochrane Collaboration, 4*, 1–42.

Burkhart, C. S., Siegemund, M., & Steiner, L. A. (2010). Cerebral perfusion in sepsis. *Critical Care, 14*(2), 215.

Chipp, E., Milner, C. S., & Blackburn, A. V. (2010). Sepsis in burns: A review of current practice and future therapies. *Annals of Plastic Surgery, 65*(2), 228–236.

Davydow, D. S., Katon, W. J., & Zatzick, D. F. (2009). Psychiatric morbidity and functional impairments in survivors of burns, traumatic injuries, and ICU stays for other critical illnesses: A review of the literature. *International Review of Psychiatry, 21*(6), 531–538.

Dubois, M. J., Bergeron, N., Dumont, M., Dial, S., & Skrobik, Y. (2001). Delirium in an intensive care unit: A study of risk factors. *Intensive Care Medicine, 27*(8), 1297–1304.

Dyster-Aas, J., Willebrand, M., Wikehult, B., Gerdin, B., & Ekselius, L. (2008). Major depression and posttraumatic stress disorder symptoms following severe burn injury in relation to lifetime psychiatric morbidity. *Journal of Trauma, 64*(5), 1349–1356.

Ehde, D. M., Patterson, D. R., Wiechman, S. A., & Wilson, L. G. (2000). Post-traumatic stress symptoms and distress 1 year after burn injury. *Journal of Burn Care Rehabilitation, 21*(2), 105–111.

Esselman, P. C., Thombs, B. D., Magyar-Russell, G., & Fauerbach, J. A. (2006). Burn rehabilitation: State of the science. *American Journal of Physical Medicine & Rehabilitation, 85*(4), 383–413.

Fauerbach, J. A., Lawrence, J., Haythornthwaite, J., McGuire, M., & Munster, A. (1996). Preinjury psychiatric illness and postinjury adjustment in adult burn survivors. *Psychosomatics, 37*(6), 547–555.

Fauerbach, J. A., Lawrence, J., Haythornthwaite, J., Richter, D., McGuire, M., Schmidt, C., et al. (1997). Preburn psychiatric history affects posttrauma morbidity. *Psychosomatics, 38*(4), 374–385.

Fratianne, R. B., & Brandt, C. P. (1997). Determining when care for burns is futile. *Journal of Burn Care Rehabilitation, 18*(3), 262–267; discussion, 260–261.

Fratianne, R. B., Brandt, C., Yurko, L., & Coffee, T. (1992). When is enough enough? Ethical dilemmas on the burn unit. *Journal of Burn Care Rehabilitation, 13*(5), 600–604.

Fricchione, G. L., Nejad, S. H., Esses, J. A., Cummings, T. J. Jr., Querques, J., Cassem, N. H., et al. (2008). Postoperative delirium. *American Journal of Psychiatry, 165*(7), 803–812.

Fullerton, C. S., Ursano, R. J., & Wang, L. (2004). Acute stress disorder, posttraumatic stress disorder, and depression in disaster or rescue workers. *American Journal of Psychiatry, 161*(8), 1370–1376.

Galdston, R. (1972). The burning and the healing of children. *Psychiatry, 35*(1), 57–66.

Gould, N. F., McKibben, J. B., Hall, R., Corry, N. H., Amoyal, N. A., Mason, S. T., et al. (2011). Peritraumatic heart rate and posttraumatic stress disorder in patients with severe burns. *Journal of Clinical Psychiatry, 72*(4), 539–547.

Greenhalgh, D. G., Saffle, J. R., Holmes, J. H. t., Gamelli, R. L., Palmieri, T. L., Horton, J. W., et al. (2007). American Burn Association Consensus Conference to define sepsis and infection in burns. *Journal of Burn Care Research, 28*(6), 776–790.

Hampson, N. B., Piantadosi, C. A., Thom, S. R., & Weaver, L. K. (2012). Practice recommendations in the diagnosis, management, and prevention of carbon monoxide poisoning. *American Journal of Respiratory & Critical Care Medicine, 186*, 1095–1101.

Hecksel, K. A., Bostwick, J. M., Jaeger, T. M., & Cha, S. S. (2008). Inappropriate use of symptom-triggered therapy for alcohol withdrawal in the general hospital. *Mayo Clinic Proceedings, 83*(3), 274–279.

Ismail, A., Long, J., Moiemen, N., & Wilson, Y. (2011). End of life decisions and care of the adult burn patient. *Burns, 37*(2), 288–293.

Jellinek, M. S., Todres, I. D., Catlin, E. A., Cassem, E. H., & Salzman, A. (1993). Pediatric intensive care training: Confronting the dark side. *Critical Care Medicine, 21*(5), 775–779.

Jones, J. D., Barber, B., Engrav, L., & Heimbach, D. (1991). Alcohol use and burn injury. *Journal of Burn Care Rehabilitation, 12*(2), 148–152.

Juurlink, D. N., Buckley, N. A., Stanbrook, M. B., Isbister, G. K., Bennett, M., & McGuigan, M. A. (2005). Hyperbaric oxygen for carbon monoxide poisoning. *Cochrane Database of Systematic Reviews* (1), CD002041.

Kessler, R. C., Chiu, W. T., Demler, O., Merikangas, K. R., & Walters, E. E. (2005). Prevalence, severity, and comorbidity of 12-month DSM-IV disorders in the National Comorbidity Survey Replication. *Archives of General Psychiatry, 62*(6), 617–627.

Kessler, R. C., McGonagle, K. A., Zhao, S., Nelson, C. B., Hughes, M., Eshleman, S., et al. (1994). Lifetime and 12-month prevalence of DSM-III-R psychiatric disorders in the United States. Results from the National Comorbidity Survey. *Archives of General Psychiatry, 51*(1), 8–19.

Klinge, K., Chamberlain, D. J., Redden, M., & King, L. (2009). Psychological adjustments made by postburn injury patients: An integrative literature review. *Journal of Advanced Nursing, 65*(11), 2274–2292.

Kramer, G., Lund, Tjostolv, & Beckum, O. (2002). Pathophysiology of burn shock and burn edema. In D. Herndon (Ed.), *Total burn care* (2nd ed., pp. 78–87). Philadelphia, PA: Saunders.

Kringlen, E., Torgersen, S., & Cramer, V. (2001). A Norwegian psychiatric epidemiological study. *American Journal of Psychiatry, 158*(7), 1091–1098.

Kringlen, E., Torgersen, S., & Cramer, V. (2006). Mental illness in a rural area: A Norwegian psychiatric epidemiological study. *Social Psychiatry & Psychiatric Epidemiology, 41*(9), 713–719.

Krummen, D. M., James, K., & Klein, R. L. (1998). Suicide by burning: A retrospective review of the Akron Regional Burn Center. *Burns, 24*(2), 147–149.

Lindemann, E. (1944). Symptomatology and management of acute grief. *American Journal of Psychiatry, 151*(6 Suppl), 155–160.

Lukan, J. K., Reed, D. N. Jr., Looney, S. W., Spain, D. A., & Blondell, R. D. (2002). Risk factors for delirium tremens in trauma patients. *Journal of Trauma, 53*(5), 901–906.

Marcantonio, E. R., Juarez, G., Goldman, L., Mangione, C. M., Ludwig, L. E., Lind, L., et al. (1994). The relationship of postoperative delirium with psychoactive medications. *Journal of the American Medical Association, 272*(19), 1518–1522.

McGhee, L. L., Slater, T. M., Garza, T. H., Fowler, M., DeSocio, P. A., & Maani, C. V. (2011). The relationship of early pain scores and posttraumatic stress disorder in burned soldiers. *Journal of Burn Care Research, 32*(1), 46–51.

McKibben, J. B., Bresnick, M. G., Wiechman Askay, S. A., & Fauerbach, J. A. (2008). Acute stress disorder and posttraumatic stress disorder: A prospective study of prevalence, course, and predictors in a sample with major burn injuries. *Journal of Burn Care Research, 29*(1), 22–35.

Moeller-Bertram, T., Keltner, J., & Strigo, I. A. (2011). Pain and post-traumatic stress disorder—Review of clinical and experimental evidence. *Neuropharmacology, 62*(2), 586–597.

Morrison, R. S., Magaziner, J., Gilbert, M., Koval, K. J., McLaughlin, M. A., Orosz, G., et al. (2003). Relationship between pain and opioid analgesics on the development of delirium following hip fracture. *Journals of Gerontology, Series A: Biological Sciences & Medical Sciences, 58*(1), 76–78.

Ntais, C., Pakos, E., Kyzas, P., & Ioannidis, J. P. (2005). Benzodiazepines for alcohol withdrawal. *Cochrane Database of Systematic Reviews* (3), CD005063.

O'Mara, M. S., Chapyak, D., Greenhalgh, D. G., & Palmieri, T. L. (2006). End of life in the pediatric burn patient. *Journal of Burn Care Research, 27*(6), 803–808.

Palmu, R., Isometsa, E., Suominen, K., Vuola, J., Leppavuori, A., & Lonnqvist, J. (2004). Self-inflicted burns: An eight-year retrospective study in Finland. *Burns, 30*(5), 443–447.

Pandharipande, P., Cotton, B. A., Shintani, A., Thompson, J., Pun, B. T., Morris, J. A. Jr., et al. (2008). Prevalence and risk factors for development of delirium in surgical and trauma intensive care unit patients. *Journal of Trauma, 65*(1), 34–41.

Pham, T. N., King, J. R., Palmieri, T. L., & Greenhalgh, D. G. (2003). Predisposing factors for self-inflicted burns. *Journal of Burn Care Rehabilitation, 24*(4), 223–227.

Powers, P. S., Cruse, C. W., & Boyd, F. (2000). Psychiatric status, prevention, and outcome in patients with burns: A prospective study. *Journal of Burn Care Rehabilitation, 21*(1 Pt 1), 85–88; discussion, 84.

Powers, P. S., Stevens, B., Arias, F., Cruse, C. W., Krizek, T., & Daniels, S. (1994). Alcohol disorders among patients with burns: Crisis and opportunity. *Journal of Burn Care Rehabilitation, 15*(4), 386–391.

Rangel-Frausto, M. S., Pittet, D., Costigan, M., Hwang, T., Davis, C. S., & Wenzel, R. P. (1995). The natural history of the systemic inflammatory response syndrome (SIRS). A prospective study. *Journal of the American Medical Association, 273*(2), 117–123.

Riker, R. R., Shehabi, Y., Bokesch, P. M., Ceraso, D., Wisemandle, W., Koura, F., et al. (2009). Dexmedetomidine vs. midazolam for sedation of critically ill patients: A randomized trial. *Journal of the American Medical Association, 301*(5), 489–499.

Rockwell, E., Dimsdale, J. E., Carroll, W., & Hansbrough, J. (1988). Preexisting psychiatric disorders in burn patients. *Journal of Burn Care Rehabilitation, 9*(1), 83–86.

Rose, S., Bisson, J., Churchill, R., & Wessely, S. (2002). Psychological debriefing for preventing post-traumatic stress disorder (PTSD). *Cochrane Database of Systematic Reviews* (2), CD000560.

Ryan, C. M., Schoenfeld, D. A., Thorpe, W. P., Sheridan, R. L., Cassem, E. H., & Tompkins, R. G. (1998). Objective estimates of the probability of death from burn injuries. *New England Journal of Medicine, 338*(6), 362–366.

Schwacha, M. G. (2003). Macrophages and post-burn immune dysfunction. *Burns, 29*(1), 1–14.

Scully, J. H., & Hutcherson, R. (1983). Suicide by burning. *American Journal of Psychiatry, 140*(7), 905–906.

Sheridan, R. L., Ryan, C. M., Yin, L. M., Hurley, J., & Tompkins, R. G. (1998). Death in the burn unit: Sterile multiple organ failure. *Burns, 24*(4), 307–311.

Sherwood, E. R., & Traber, D. L. (2002). The systemic inflammatory response syndrome. In D. N. Herndon (Ed.), *Total burn care* (2nd ed., pp. 292–309). Philadelphia, PA: Saunders.

Soderstrom, C. A., Smith, G. S., Dischinger, P. C., McDuff, D. R., Hebel, J. R., Gorelick, D. A., et al. (1997). Psychoactive substance use disorders among seriously injured trauma center patients. *Journal of the American Medical Association, 277*(22), 1769–1774.

Spies, C. D., & Rommelspacher, H. (1999). Alcohol withdrawal in the surgical patient: Prevention and treatment. *Anesthesia & Analgesia, 88*(4), 946–954.

Squyres, V., Law, E. J., & Still, J. M., Jr. (1993). Self-inflicted burns. *Journal of Burn Care Rehabilitation, 14*(4), 476–479.

Stoddard, F. J., & Fricchione, G. L. (2004). Burn patients. In T. A. Stern, G. L. Fricchione, E. H. Cassem, M. S. Jellinek, & J. F. Rosenbaum (Eds.), *Massachusetts General Hospital handbook of general psychiatry* (5th ed., pp. 231–268) Philadelphia, PA: Mosby.

Swenson, J. R., & Dimsdale, J. E. (1990). Substance abuse and attempts at suicide by burning. *American Journal of Psychiatry, 147*(6), 811.

Tabares, R., & Peck, M. D. (1997). Chemical dependency in patients with burn injuries: A fortress of denial. *Journal of Burn Care Rehabilitation, 18*(3), 283–286.

Tarrier, N., Gregg, L., Edwards, J., & Dunn, K. (2005). The influence of pre-existing psychiatric illness on recovery in burn injury patients: The impact of psychosis and depression. *Burns, 31*(1), 45–49.

Thombs, B. D., Singh, V. A., Halonen, J., Diallo, A., & Milner, S. M. (2007). The effects of preexisting medical comorbidities on mortality and length of hospital stay in acute burn injury: Evidence from a national sample of 31,338 adult patients. *Annals of Surgery, 245*(4), 629–634.

Truog, R. D., Cist, A. F., Brackett, S. E., Burns, J. P., Curley, M. A., Danis, M., et al. (2001). Recommendations for end-of-life care in the intensive care unit: The Ethics Committee of the Society of Critical Care Medicine. *Critical Care Medicine, 29*(12), 2332–2348.

van der Does, A. J., Hinderink, E. M., Vloemans, A. F., & Spinhoven, P. (1997). Burn injuries, psychiatric disorders and length of hospitalization. *Journal of Psychosomatic Research, 43*(4), 431–435.

Van Rompaey, B., Elseviers, M. M., Schuurmans, M. J., Shortridge-Baggett, L. M., Truijen, S., & Bossaert, L. (2009). Risk factors for delirium in intensive care patients: A prospective cohort study. *Critical Care, 13*(3), R77.

Watkins, P. N., Cook, E. L., May, S. R., & Ehleben, C. M. (1988). Psychological stages in adaptation following burn injury: A method for facilitating psychological recovery of burn victims. *Journal of Burn Care Rehabilitation, 9*(4), 376–384.

Weaver, L. K. (2009). Clinical practice. Carbon monoxide poisoning. *New England Journal of Medicine, 360*(12), 1217–1225.

Wisely, J. A., Wilson, E., Duncan, R. T., & Tarrier, N. (2010). Pre-existing psychiatric disorders, psychological reactions to stress and the recovery of burn survivors. *Burns, 36*(2), 183–191.

76.

UROLOGY AND ANDROLOGY

Andrew J. Roth, Suzanne R. Karl, and Christian J. Nelson

INTRODUCTION

Benign prostatic hyperplasia (BPH), kidney stones, interstitial cystitis, testosterone deficiency, and urinary incontinence (UI) are non-malignant conditions that can cause significant emotional distress. Urological disorders are common and translate into billions of dollars in healthcare expenditures each year. Incontinence and sexual dysfunction are frustrating problems with emotional consequences. Psychological sequelae range in severity from mild to devastating and may affect the patient's relationships, work, social life, and general morale. Patients may not readily admit to uncomfortable symptoms that they view as private or the distress that comes with them, and in that context, referral to a psychiatrist or psychologist has particular value.

Urological cancers can cause similar symptoms. Though great advances in cancer treatment have been made in recent years, patients still associate a diagnosis of cancer with negative outcomes, and struggle with less-than-optimal quality of life (QOL). This chapter will provide a basic understanding of non-malignant urological disorders and urological cancers and their management, including coping with issues of distress, sexual dysfunction, and relationships that may accompany urological disorder.

PSYCHIATRIC ISSUES IN NON-MALIGNANT CONDITIONS

BENIGN PROSTATIC HYPERPLASIA

According to the National Institutes of Health (NIH), 6.5 million Caucasian men ages 50 to 79 in the United States were going to discuss treatment options for BPH with their physicians, and about $1.1 billion are spent annually in direct expenditures for this illness. The exact etiology of BPH is unknown, but it is hypothesized that imbalances of estrogen, testosterone, and dihydrotestosterone later in life are contributory (Carson & Rittmaster, 2003). BPH is a natural enlargement of the prostate that happens with age. Men experience two periods of prostate growth in their lives: one at puberty, during which time it doubles in size, and another period of slow growth starting at around age 25. This second stage of growth usually does not cause problems until later in life. The prostate surrounds the urethra; as it enlarges, there is a

clamping effect. Urine flow may decrease, the patient may feel like he cannot entirely empty his bladder, and over time the walls of the bladder thicken and become irritated. This causes more frequent urination because the bladder contracts with even small amounts of urine present. Untreated BPH may progress to urinary tract infections, bladder or kidney damage, bladder stones, and incontinence (Presti, 2008).

Treatment of BPH may not be necessary in the early, mild stages. Some men have improvement or even resolution of symptoms without treatment (Webber, 2005; Presti, 2008). If treatment is indicated, there are pharmacological, minimally invasive, and surgical options available.

The Food and Drug Administration (FDA) has currently approved six medications to treat BPH. Finasteride (Proscar) and dutasteride (Avodart) inhibit production of the hormone dihydrotestosterone, which is involved with prostate enlargement. The use of either of these drugs can either prevent progression of growth of the prostate or actually shrink the prostate in some men. Studies suggest that both these drugs may (rarely) cause depression or sexual dysfunction (Römer & Gass, 2010; Traish et al., 2011).

The medications terazosin (Hytrin), doxazosin (Cardura), tamsulosin (Flomax), and alfuzosin (Uroxatral) are also available for the treatment of BPH. These are alpha blockers, which improve urine flow and reduce bladder outlet obstruction by relaxing the smooth muscle of the prostate and bladder neck. Terazosin and doxazosin were first developed to treat high blood pressure. Tamsulosin and alfuzosin were developed specifically to treat BPH. Finasteride and doxazosin in combination have been shown to be more effective than using either drug alone to relieve symptoms and prevent BPH progression (McConnell et al., 2003), but combination therapy may also lead to greater chance of sexual side effects (Hellstrom, Giuliano, & Rosen, 2009).

Research strongly suggests that patients treated with a surgical procedure transurethral resection of the prostate (TURP) show better outcomes in terms of QOL and urinary symptoms when compared with pharmacological treatment. However, the less invasive nature of medications makes them an attractive option for many men, and in recent years there has been a marked shift from surgical to pharmacological management of BPH. Consequently, BPH is now viewed more as a chronic condition. Many men ultimately need surgery anyway, so there is a debate over how best to handle BPH in its earlier stages (Wei, Calhoun, & Jacobsen, 2005).

Minimally invasive procedures are used when medication proves inadequate but as an alternative to TURP. Minimally invasive procedures include laser ablation, transurethral needle ablation (TUNA), transurethral microwave therapy (TUMT), high-energy focused ultrasound, and hot water thermotherapy (Wei, Calhoun, & Jacobsen, 2005).

The sequelae of BPH and its treatment can have profound effects on the patient's lifestyle. These include problems urinating, bleeding, incontinence, or sexual dysfunction. In these cases, the patient may benefit from psychiatric or psychological consultation to assess for the presence and extent of significant depressive and anxiety symptoms.

Patients may be reluctant to talk about these problems, which they may feel are stigmatizing and isolating. Supportive or cognitive behaviorally oriented therapy may be appreciated by the patient if he is undergoing surgery or dealing with potentially embarrassing side effects.

Psychopharmacologically, it is useful to avoid medications that may exacerbate urinary symptoms or sexual dysfunction that may already be a problem due to the BPH or its treatment. Antidepressants like the tricyclic antidepressants (TCAs) have anticholinergic effects that may slow down the urinary system. However, the TCAs are used much less frequently than other antidepressants today because of their sedative, cardiac, and autonomic side effects. Serotonin specific reuptake inhibitors (SSRIs) and serotonin and norepinephrine reuptake inhibitors (SNRIs) have sexual side effects, but do not impact the urinary system. The heterocyclic antidepressant, trazodone, can (rarely) cause priapism, and this should be discussed with the patient prior to administration of the drug. Bupropion is less likely to have sexual side effects than other antidepressants, but it can cause anxiety and insomnia. It is important to be aware that lower-potency antipsychotics, including chlorpromazine, mesoridazine, thioridazine, and clozapine, have significant alpha1-adrenergic effects just like some of the drugs used to treat BPH. The compounded alpha1-adrenergic effects can lead to orthostatic hypotension and syncope associated with vasodilation (Alpert, Fava, & Rosenbaum, 2004).

Urinary Incontinence

According to the National Association for Continence, one-third of men and women ages 30–70 have experienced loss of bladder control at some point in their adult lives (Muller, 2005). An estimated $463 million is spent annually for treatment. UI can be caused by pregnancy, childbirth, menopause, neurological injury, birth defects, stroke, multiple sclerosis, and physical problems associated with aging (Brubaker, Meikle, & Steers, 2010). Apart from pregnancy and childbirth, menopause and the makeup of the female urinary tract account for women being affected by UI more often than men. However, women and men alike experience the psychological sequelae of incontinence, which at its best is bothersome and at its worst, embarrassing and isolating.

Treatment for incontinence includes behavioral therapy and medication, primarily antimuscarinics. Behavioral techniques have been shown to be more effective than medication and should be used as a first-line treatment for UI (Burgio

et al., 1998). There are several ways to employ behavioral techniques. Bladder training involves voiding the bladder at timed intervals throughout the day. Over time, the patient extends the amount of time between voids. Pelvic muscle reeducation is a technique used in women. It refers to exercises the patient performs to strengthen her pelvic floor muscles. These exercises are sometimes referred to as "Kegels" (Bo, 2004).

Antimuscarinics have reasonably good success, but side effects are common and can be uncomfortable. Studies have shown varying rates of success using duloxetine (Cymbalta) in the treatment of post-prostatectomy incontinence and stress UI in women (Cornu et al., 2011). This treatment, used in Europe, has yet to be approved to treat incontinence in the United States (Smith et al., 2010). Should behavioral therapy and medications fail to help, artificial urinary sphincter implantation appears to be a durable treatment if needed after prostatectomy or radiation therapy (Lai et al., 2007).

Studies have shown that UI can cause social avoidance, relationship stress, and loss of independence in activities of daily living (Sims et al., 2011; Easton, 2010). Men and women with overactive bladders report higher levels of depression and anxiety, as well as lower levels of health-related QOL and work productivity (Coyne et al., 2011). Men with UI report higher rates of erectile dysfunction and lower frequency and enjoyment of sex (Irwin et al., 2008). These men often worry about, and are embarrassed by, loss of urine during sexual intercourse. A study specific to African-Americans showed a strong positive correlation between UI and symptoms of depression (Malmstrom et al., 2010). Beyond the incontinence itself, patients report stress and anxiety related to frequency and urgency (Elstad et al., 2010).

Although the evidence for drugs specifically causing incontinence is limited, the drug classes proposed to induce stress incontinence include alpha 1 adrenergic receptor antagonists, and antipsychotics like thioridazine, clozapine, risperidone, and olanzapine. (Tsakiris, Oelke, & Michel, 2008). Should the patient require an antidepressant, the best medication will be one that does not exacerbate existing symptoms. Duloxetine has been shown to improve stress incontinence, and a higher rate of UI has been noted with sertraline than with other SSRIs (Movig et al., 2002; Tsakiris, Oelke, & Michel, 2008).

Interstitial Cystitis: Bladder Pain Syndrome

What had been called interstitial cystitis is now thought of as a syndrome of chronic bladder pain. It is presumed to be a heterogeneous, chronic, visceral pain syndrome, characterized by pain with filling and relief by voiding, associated with central sensitization. Males or females with pain, pressure, or discomfort that they perceive to be related to the bladder with at least one urinary symptom, such as frequency not obviously related to high fluid intake, or a persistent urge to void, should be evaluated for possible bladder pain syndrome (Hanno et al., 2010). The disorder may not involve the bladder interstitium, as some patients lack bladder inflammation. Prevalence is much more common in women than men. Symptoms wax and wane with flares. In a population-based sample (Watkins,

2011), one-third had a diagnosis of depression, and 52% reported recent panic attacks. History of sexual abuse is a risk factor (Mayson & Tecihman, 2009). There is an overlap with non–bladder pain syndromes such as fibromyalgia, chronic fatigue syndrome, irritable bowel syndrome, vulvodynia, and voiding dysfunction (Clemens et al., 2008; Warren, van de Merwe, & Nickel, 2011).

Diagnosis is based on history, examination, frequency-volume chart, urinalysis and culture, and if deemed appropriate by the clinician, cystoscopy or urodynamics. Pain sources outside the bladder may become clear from the evaluation. Guidelines emphasize education, diet, stress management, and reevaluation of treatment approaches at regular intervals. Hunner lesions are a specific condition treated with fulguration or steroid injection (Quillin & Erickson, 2012). Treatment is individualized and includes behavioral, physical therapy for the pelvic floor, and medication.

History of previous infection, pelvic operations, pelvic radiation treatment, and autoimmune diseases is relevant. In men, rectal examination and mapping of pain in the scrotal anal region and palpation of the tenderness of bladder, prostate, and levator and adductor muscles of the pelvic floor and scrotal contents are appropriate. In women, physical examination includes vaginal exam with pain mapping of the vulvar region, and palpation for tenderness of the bladder, urethra, levator and adductor muscles of the pelvic floor. Range of motion of hips, kyphosis, scars, and hernias are noted.

TESTOSTERONE DEFICIENCY

Disturbance of normal testosterone levels has been shown to negatively affect QOL, morbidity, and psychological states in men. One way to appreciate the effects of testosterone is to look at men who have testosterone deficiency from various etiologies, including natural aging, congenital causes such as hypogonadism, idiopathic causes, obesity, diabetes, infectious causes such as HIV/AIDS, malignancies, androgen ablation therapy for prostate cancer, hypertension, and medication used for medical comorbidities (Traish et al., 2011; Nelson, Roth, & Mulhall, 2007; Morgentaler, 2011; Raynor et al., 2011). These patients experience a spectrum of disheartening effects, including but not limited to: fatigue and decreased vitality, weight gain, erectile dysfunction, muscle loss, glucose intolerance, osteoporosis, depression and anxiety, memory loss, muscle wasting, loss of libido, and difficulty concentrating (Allan & McLachlan, 2006). Such symptoms put stress on careers, relationships, and other activities of daily living. Patients receiving testosterone replacement therapy experience relief from symptoms, including depression (Traish et al., 2011; Khera et al., 2012); however, this treatment should only occur after a comprehensive discussion between physician and patient about potential consequences. If necessary and appropriate, testosterone replacement may be used indefinitely.

Androgen ablation therapy has long been a mainstay of treatment for men with prostate cancer. Androgen exposure increases the growth rate of malignant prostate cancer cells. Conversely, prostatic atrophy occurs with testosterone

deficiency (Nelson et al., 2007). Up to 50% of patients with prostate cancer are treated using androgen deprivation therapy (ADT), many for up to several years (Timilshina, Breunis, & Alibhai, 2012). Common side effects include those listed above.

Recent research regarding ADT has challenged the idea that normal or high levels of testosterone are detrimental to men with prostate cancer. The studies postulate that low levels of testosterone may stimulate the growth of prostate cancer, but beyond those low levels, saturation occurs and no more stimulation of growth takes place with additional testosterone (Morgentaler, 2011). Such research suggests that administering testosterone to men with prostate cancer may be acceptable; however, since these ideas have only been tested recently, more research is necessary to prove that testosterone is safe for prostate cancer patients (Morris et al., 2009; Rathkopf et al., 2008). Low testosterone is generally associated with depression. There is some literature that refutes evidence of a correlation between low testosterone and depression (Amiaz & Seidman, 2008), but there is also much investigation to back up a relationship between the two. One study showed that testosterone replacement helped alleviate refractory depressive symptoms in older men with low androgen levels who had not responded to SSRIs (Pope et al., 2003). Another concluded that testosterone might have an antidepressant effect on depressed patients, especially those with HIV/AIDS, and elderly subpopulations (Zarrouf et al., 2009).

The HIV/AIDS population may especially benefit from treatment with testosterone. Hypogonadism occurs in about 30% of men in this population, and androgen therapy is used widely to alleviate symptoms. Muscle wasting and body composition are especially important considerations in the HIV/AIDS patient, and anabolic steroids such as oxandrolone are useful to increase both (Catlin, 2006). Studies have also shown an improvement in depressive symptoms in AIDS patients who were prescribed testosterone (Hengge, 2003).

Guidelines for treatment of androgen deficiency syndromes recommend measuring morning total testosterone as the initial diagnostic test and repeating it with a reliable assay. In some patients, a free or bioavailable testosterone level is warranted. Testosterone therapy is recommended for symptomatic men with unequivocally low serum testosterone levels in order to improve sexual function, sense of well-being, muscle mass and strength, and bone mineral density. Urological evaluation would be warranted if there are questions of prostate cancer. Hyperviscosity, untreated obstructive sleep apnea, severe lower urinary tract symptoms, or heart failure are other contraindications. The guidelines recommend not testing for testosterone deficiency in the general population, but to limit testing to those men with disorders that predispose to low testosterone: men with a sellar mass and history of radiation to the sellar region; those chronically treated with glucocorticoids, ketoconazole, or opioids; HIV-associated weight loss; end-stage renal disease; chronic obstructive lung disease; infertility; osteoporosis; or type 2 diabetes mellitus. If treatment is instituted, they recommend aiming for a mid-normal range level of testosterone and monitoring by a standard protocol over time. They warn against a general clinical policy of offering testosterone therapy to all older men with low testosterone levels because of the uncertainty of adverse side effects (Bhasin et al., 2006). A recent randomized, double-blind, parallel placebo-controlled trial of the effect of testosterone replacement on the response to sildenafil citrate in men with erectile dysfunction did not show that sildenafil plus testosterone was superior to sildenafil with placebo in men with erectile dysfunction and low testosterone levels (Spitzer et al., 2012).

KIDNEY STONES

Kidney stones have been described as causing the worst pain people can experience. Kidney stones occur in 5.2% of adults, occasionally requiring a hospital admission, and cost $2.07 billion in 2000 for evaluation and treatment.

Studying the psychological effects of kidney stones (also called nephrolithiasis) is somewhat different than studying those of UI and BPH. Kidney stones have rapid onset, relatively fast resolution, and high pain levels, whereas incontinence and BPH are more long-term problems with a tendency to produce less pain and more embarrassment. While the correlation between repeated episodes of pain and psychological distress has been documented, there is less literature on psychological distress due to pain from kidney stones in particular.

Kidney stones have been correlated with depression and anxiety (Diniz, Blay, & Schor, 2007). A case report noted post-traumatic stress disorder (PTSD) as a result of nephrolithiasis (Bilić, & Marcinko, 2010); however, there have been no other published corroborating reports of PTSD from kidney stones.

Hyperparathyroidism has long been linked to both kidney stones and psychological disorders, including depression, anxiety, obsessive-compulsive disorder, and paranoia (McAllion, 1989; Chiba et al., 2007; Wilhelm, Lee, & Prinz, 2004). Regardless of its cause, hyperparathyroidism can lead to cognitive and psychiatric disorders that negatively influence estimates of QOL (Coker, 2005). Concurrent with cognitive disorders, excess calcium can contribute to kidney stones, which compound negative effects on QOL and contribute to psychological distress.

When kidney stones and psychological distress are the result of benign hyperparathyroidism, parathyroidectomy reduces symptoms of major depression, improves the QOL, and can eliminate or reduce the need for antidepressant medication in up to 54% of patients (Wilhelm et al., 2004). Parathyroidectomy decreases the risk of kidney stones in vulnerable patients for about ten years, but after that the risk goes back to baseline (Parmar, 2004).

Some patients experience idiopathic kidney stones; they do not show evidence of hormone imbalance. In patients who are beyond the stage of preventative treatment and are already passing the stones, the goal of the physician is to ease renal colic. Prostaglandin-induced kidney stone pain has been described by patients as severe and unrelenting, and understandably induces significant anxiety. Often, narcotics are used to dampen the pain. However, a double-blind study in 66 patients with acute renal colic showed that intramuscular injection of a potent prostaglandin-synthetase inhibitor (diclofenac sodium) is more effective and has fewer side effects than a narcotic drug commonly used to treat ureteric colic (Lundstam et al., 1982). Alternatively, one study showed the efficacy of acupuncture in easing renal colic (Lee et al., 1992). Another study found that local active warming of the abdomen and lower back significantly reduced pain and anxiety in kidney stone patients (Kober et al., 2003). Other types of kidney stones (e.g., oxalate) may be nutritionally induced. Recommendation for a nutrition consultation may be helpful for patients with recurrent stones.

As with the other non-malignant urological disorders, psychiatric treatment of distress due to kidney stones may be brief and supportive. This may be truer of patients with kidney stones than of those with UI or BPH, since there is a clear resolution of symptoms once the stone has passed. Some studies indicate that a significant proportion of patients with kidney stones will experience anxiety and depression, especially if they have recurrent stones (Diniz, Blay, & Schor, 2007).

INTERSTITIAL NEPHRITIS

Interstitial nephritis (IN) is an acute or chronic condition that affects the interstitial compartment of the kidney but spares the glomeruli. Acute IN is generally induced by infection or medications such as nonsteroidal anti-inflammatory drugs (NSAIDs)—acetaminophen, penicillin, ampicillin, methicillin, sulfonamide, furosemide, and thiazide diuretics—but it may also be idiopathic. It presents clinically as a sudden decrease in renal function. Signs may include skin rash, fever, and eosinophilia. Lumbar pain is a common symptom. Chronic IN has a variety of etiologies, including sarcoidosis, multiple myeloma, radiation treatments, medications, hypercalcemia, hypokalemia, lead or cadmium poisoning, and urinary tract obstruction. Even in chronic IN, glomeruli remain normal upon viewing with light microscopy, despite functional problems. Only as interstitial injury progresses to later stages might glomerular abnormalities become apparent on visualization (Kelly & Neilson, 2004). Chronic IN patients present due to symptoms of a primary disease or with nonspecific symptoms of renal failure, which include weakness, nocturia, nausea, and/or sleep disturbances (Kelly & Neilson, 2004; Eknoyan, 2001).

Treatment of acute IN is removal of the offending irritant or treating the cause, which often resolves the disease. If this is not done in a reasonable time frame, steroids or chemotherapy may have a role in therapy. Similarly, there is no specific treatment indicated for chronic IN (Kelly & Neilson, 2004).

Some psychiatric drugs, such as clozapine and lithium, may in rare cases cause IN. Recommended precautions to identify acute IN before it can have an adverse effect include carefully screening the patient for fever, which may be an early manifestation of a hypersensitivity reaction; monitoring for a rise in eosinophil count; and looking for proteinuria and/or white blood cells in the urine (Kanofsky et al., 2011); as well as monitoring lithium levels, serum creatinine levels, and possibly dosing lithium once a day (Gitlin, 1999).

THE UROLOGICAL CANCERS

The genitourinary cancers are affecting a larger proportion of our population as detection methods are improving. Patients often must cope with changes in lifestyle, sexuality, bladder and bowel function, body image, relationships, fatigue, and pain in the later stages of disease. Discomfort and beliefs about stigma on the part of the patient, the family, and healthcare providers in discussing these issues provide formidable barriers to evaluation and resolution of distress. Although some clinicians fear that acknowledging and addressing psychological issues will open up a Pandora's box of troubles and somehow make the symptoms worse, psychological interventions provide avenues for decreased stress and improved QOL. Not addressing these issues often leads to increased suffering, major psychiatric disorders, despair, demoralization, isolation, hopelessness, and suicidal ideation.

Medical caregivers are encouraged to screen for distress in order to identify who might benefit from further psychiatric assessment. Psychiatrists can assist patients who have anxiety about treatment decisions, facing mortality, coping with complications, fear of recurrent disease, and coping with recurrence of disease. Once they are assessed, management and support (which may initially be provided by the oncology team) can include a spectrum of psychological and psychiatric interventions that includes education, individual and group psychotherapy, couples' therapy, and cognitive and behaviorally oriented interventions. (For a discussion about the prevalence and management of psychiatric disorders in the general cancer patient, see Chapter 57.)

PROSTATE CANCER

EPIDEMIOLOGY AND DIAGNOSIS

An estimated 240,890 new cases of prostate cancer occurred in 2011. Approximately 65% of these new cases occur in men over the age of 65. Death rates in African-Americans remain more than twice as high as those in whites. Over the past 25 years, the five-year relative survival rate for all stages combined has increased from 69% to 99.6%, and according to the most recent data, the 10-year survival is 95%, and 15-year survival is 82% (American Cancer Society, 2011).

This generally older population of men has particular needs influenced by their generational and developmental phase of life. Five to ten percent of all prostate cancers are believed to be of familial predisposition. Some nutritional factors, such as diets high in saturated fat, have been correlated with increased incidence of prostate cancer (Wang et al., 1995).

American Cancer Society guidelines recommend a yearly discussion between patients and physicians about digital rectal examination (DRE) for men 50 years of age and older, along with an annual prostate-specific antigen (PSA) test. Men who are at high risk, such as African-Americans or those with a strong family history of prostate cancer, are advised to begin PSA testing starting at age 45 (American Cancer Society, 2011). Other than self-examination for testicular cancer, prostate cancer is the only genitourinary cancer that has a reliable tool for early detection.

It is controversial whether early detection by PSA testing and potential treatment of indolent forms of prostate cancer is beneficial when the distress and impairment of QOL from the primary treatments of surgery or radiotherapy are taken into account (Mokulis & Thompson, 1995). These uncertainties have implications for the psychological well-being of men and their families. However at this time, it is difficult to distinguish more lethal from more benign varieties of prostate cancer before men receive primary treatment. In the past, many men would die of another cause, never knowing they had prostate cancer, with detection only occurring at autopsy. Those who were diagnosed with the disease often presented with signs of metastatic disease, such as pain and urinary problems.

A PSA level can be normal even in the presence of cancer. It is also not cancer-specific. False positive results can be seen with prostatitis, benign prostatic hypertrophy, and after manipulation of the prostate, as with transrectal ultrasound and needle biopsies or DRE. Improvement in the specificity of this test has helped rule out many false positives. However, PSA levels may vary with the age of the patient as well as other medical factors.

One of the psychological distresses oncologists have noted in patients is the degree of anxiety surrounding each PSA test, and the anticipation before getting the results. This has been termed "PSA anxiety," "PSA-itis," and "PSA-dynia" (Roth et al., 2005; Lofters et al., 2002; Klotz, 1997). Some men give great significance and worry to each test and even about minuscule changes within the normal range, which they may view as a marker of life or death. Level of worry about a current result may be related to the trend of recent test results—in one study, men with stable PSA levels had less anxiety than those whose scores were either going up or going down (Roth et al., 2006). Men apparently are looking for good news only and "seeking peace of mind," and feel devastated and angry about unwanted or unexpected increases (Dale et al., 2005).

SURGICAL AND MEDICAL MANAGEMENT

As of this writing, there has not been a definitive comparative analysis of the major primary treatment options for prostate cancer. Thus there is still legitimate professional disagreement and controversy about the selection of primary treatments (Wilt et al., 2008). Though overall QOL may not be significantly different with the various primary treatment options, there may be compromises when considering specific treatment side effects and long-term complications (Eton & Lepore, 2002; Sanda et al., 2008). Primary treatment options vary from "watchful waiting," also described as "expectant monitoring," and "active surveillance" to surgery, radiation, and cryotherapy. Watchful waiting (deferred therapy) is often recommended for those with significant comorbid illness, low-grade indolent cancers, and less than ten years' life expectancy. Active surveillance is suggested for younger men with early-stage disease, who get more frequent follow-up and observation. Though active surveillance is promising to prevent unnecessary compromise to QOL with treatment complications, further study is still needed to observe long-term medical and psychological benefits and complications (Klotz, 2008; Johansson et al., 2009).

The definitive treatment choice in the past was surgery, the open radical prostatectomy. Newer "nerve-sparing" procedures have decreased the rate of complications of impotence and UI somewhat. Many urologists are starting to do laparoscopic and robotic prostatectomies, which are alleged to cause less bleeding, less chance of infection, and less time in the hospital after the procedure (Hakimi, Feder, & Ghavamian, 2007).

Radiation therapy, either conventional intensity-modulated radiation therapy (IMRT) or seed implants, often in combination with external beam radiotherapy, may yield decreased, though delayed incidence of impotence compared to surgery; however, there are increased difficulties with bowel function. Post–radiation treatment PSA levels take a variable amount of time to reach a nadir of undetectable PSA that would indicate probable cure of the cancer; this can lead to prolonged anxiety. Radiation therapy may be given with adjuvant hormonal therapy, which can add to the side-effect burden for men.

For more advanced prostate cancer, hormonal manipulation is used to decrease the synthesis of testosterone or its action on prostate cancer cell growth. This can be done with luteinizing hormone-releasing hormone agonists such as leuprolide, goserelin, or buserelin, which prevent the testicles from producing testosterone; estrogenic substances such as diethylstilbestrol; peripheral anti-androgenic agents, such as flutamide, nilutamide, or bicalutamide; or drugs that prevent the adrenal glands from making androgens, such as ketoconazole and aminoglutethimide. Abiraterone and enzalutamide are new hormonal agents. Abiraterone inhibits Cyp 17 enzymes expressed in testis, adrenals, and prostate tumor tissue, decreasing circulating levels of testosterone. Enzalutamide is an androgen receptor inhibitor. Orchiectomy, or surgical castration, also reduces testosterone production.

Hormonal therapy at this stage of disease is not curative. Equally effective in slowing tumor growth with similar side-effect profiles, medical hormonal therapy may be preferred over orchiectomy by patients because it better preserves patient body image and therefore improved QOL; however, it is an expensive treatment. Side effects of androgen ablation may include erectile dysfunction (ED), loss of libido, hot flashes, gynecomastia, irritability, anxiety, and depression. Pirl and colleagues (2002) found that men most at risk for depression while on hormonal therapy were those who had histories significant for major depression. Standard of care is moving towards giving intermittent hormone therapy (with some time off in between treatment with hormones) since it lessens side effects, reduces health care costs, and has been shown to be as effective as continuous therapy (Organ et al., 2013; Klotz et al., 2011). Further studies are underway to corroborate this evidence. Chemotherapeutic agents are used for more advanced tumors—they, too, are not curative.

MANAGEMENT OF DISTRESS

Uncertainty about choice of treatment options and related outcomes such as potential sexual dysfunction, UI, weakness, fatigue, pain, and other side effects of the disease or treatment can have profound effects on mood, irritability, and anxiety, especially for men who are used to feeling a strong sense of control over their futures. Many men entertain multiple second opinions regarding their primary therapy. Some spend hours on the Internet and in libraries trying to gather enough information to find the perfect treatment for them. This often leads to anxiety and frustration. Treatment choices and decisions may vary based on the extent of disease, age of the patient, life expectancy, specialty bias of physician, side-effect risk profile acceptable to a patient, expense, and geography (Harlan et al., 1995). Personality factors and coping strategies may influence a man's satisfaction with his treatment (Blank & Bellizzi, 2006). An example of a helpful "take control" attitude that may help improve outcome and tolerance of prostate cancer treatment and overall health is the man who changes his diet to what is thought of as a prostate-friendly diet with low fat, high soy, fish oil, selenium and other nutrients, and begins or continues a regular exercise program, stops smoking tobacco, and limits his alcohol intake. Hormonal therapies can be particularly distressing because of sexual, energy, or concentration side effects.

In general, men with prostate cancer respond to useful information and various types of brief psychotherapy, including supportive, cognitive-behaviorally oriented, and insight-oriented therapies. However, some men are reluctant to participate in therapy, particularly older men who have never done so previously. Allowing a man to enter therapy with his spouse or partner present has facilitated many getting treatment for psychological distress who would not otherwise receive assistance. Support groups are available specifically for men with prostate cancer. Two of the national support groups available to men are "Us Too" and "Man to Man."

Loss of urinary continence occurs as a complication of surgery and radiation and leads men to shun social engagements. Radical prostatectomy (RP) is the most common cause of stress UI in men. Stress UI rates after RP range from 5–48%. Seventy-seven percent of men will suffer from overactive bladder following RP (Bauer et al., 2011). This UI after surgery has been associated with depression, anger, and a reduced sense of well-being in men after RP (Klotz, 1997). Interestingly, the UI does not have to be severe for men to report significant distress (Roth et al., 2006). Also important to note is that from 20% to 25% of men with UI report some restriction of their everyday activity as a result of this incontinence, which has a significant impact on their general QOL (Roth et al., 2006; Dale et al., 2005). The fear of urine leaking, of smelling of urine, and of having to use diapers feels regressive and humiliating. Urologists and their staffs can work with patients to identify etiologies of incontinence, to educate patients and families about the incontinence, and to offer suggestions to alleviate or reduce symptoms. Psychiatrists and psychologists can help with support-, cognitive-, and behaviorally oriented strategies to cope with incontinence and sometimes with antidepressants or anxiolytics to lower barriers to better coping.

Pain syndromes result from local expansion and inflammation of the prostate gland, from local tumor growth, and from distant long bone, vertebral, and skull metastases. Pain related to metastatic bone disease can impair mobility and accompany neurological impairments such as cranial nerve deficits, paralysis, incontinence of bowel and bladder, and impotence (Payne, 1993). Patients with pain are significantly more depressed or anxious than patients without pain; these mood changes may not be related to the extent of disease (Heim & Oei, 1993; Kornblith et al., 1994). However, older men are often reluctant to take pain medications or dosages adequate to truly help.

Fatigue and weakness can be caused by the illness, hormonal or radiation therapy, pain medication, steroids, and other factors. These symptoms are particularly upsetting to men who have led active and independent lives and who are now more dependent on family or friends. Helping the patient reorganize his schedule and set realistic goals may result in less distress. A psychostimulant, such as modafinil or methylphenidate, may counter the sedating effects of opioids, increase motivation, enhance appetite, and elevate a patient's mood. Though stimulants can be an effective treatment for fatigue even in older men with prostate cancer, patients should be monitored by their physicians for possible tachycardia and increases in blood pressure (Roth et al., 2010). An activating antidepressant such as bupropion, which will not compromise sexual functioning, or another antidepressant like fluoxetine can be used to increase energy.

Hot flashes in men with prostate cancer are caused by medical and surgical androgen ablation. They are the result of increased vasomotor activity, possibly related to increased noradrenergic activity and decreased serotonergic activity, which leads to diaphoresis, feelings of intense heat and chills, similar to symptoms that women have during menopause. At times, hormonal therapy must be stopped because of drenching sweats and discomfort. Antidepressants like the SSRIs, such as sertraline and paroxetine; SNRIs, such as venlafaxine; and anti-epileptic medications, such as gabapentin, have been reported to reduce the frequency and intensity of hot flashes (Roth et al., 1998; Loprinzi, 2004; Adelson, Loprinzi, & Hershman, 2005). Teaching men to change habits such as decreasing caffeine, alcohol, and hot fluid intake, and even carrying portable fans in warmer weather, may be useful to prevent or decrease the frequency and extent of discomfort from the hot flashes.

SEXUAL DYSFUNCTION

Prostate cancer symptoms run the gamut of possible sexual side effects that could occur in any urological cancer. Each of the urological cancers poses unique challenges to healthy sexual functioning, but an understanding of sexual dysfunction management in prostate cancer provides a strong foundation from which to manage dysfunction in others. (For this reason, a discussion of sexual dysfunction in men will appear here and should be referred to for each of the urological cancers. For a discussion of sexual dysfunction in women, please see Part IV: Women's Health).

Aging, the cancer itself, surgery, radiation, and hormonal therapy can cause difficulties with sexual functioning (Ofman, 1994; Steginga et al., 2000). Hormonal therapy, in particular, eliminates libido, which may decrease distress about ED;

however, decreased desire for any physical intimacy can also be harmful to a relationship. Feelings of being emasculated occur. An honest or realistic assessment of sexual functioning before primary treatment may assist a man in choosing a more acceptable treatment option, regardless of outcome. Therapies to improve ED include phosphodiesterase-5 (PDE-5) inhibitors such as sildenafil, tadalafil, and vardenafil; penile injections; vacuum erection devices; and penile prostheses. However, most men are not initially comfortable with non-pill forms of treatment. Sex therapy with a trained therapist familiar with cancer issues can help men with sexual dysfunction express the feelings engendered by this problem, and also help a couple learn alternative ways of sharing sexual intimacy (McCarthy & Bodnar, 2005).

ED is a significant problem encountered by men with urological cancers and with BPH. Rates of ED after prostate cancer surgery vary; however, most agree that a vast majority of men will have to cope with ED to some degree. In a study of over 1,200 men four years post-treatment, 85% of them reported that ED was a problem (Schover et al., 2002). It is also clear that patients who experience ED after RP report significant distress and bother associated with their ED. Although this bother may be mitigated to some extent as patients focus more on the life-saving nature of treatment (Penson et al., 2003), data suggest that a significant number of men still report being bothered or upset by its impact on erections. Data from 231 men following either surgery or radiation for prostate cancer showed that ED bother significantly increased at three months post-treatment and remained at consistently high levels throughout the follow-up period (i.e., every 3 months, up to 24 months post-treatment) (Nelson et al., 2007). Significant in these data is that even men who returned to "normal" erectile functioning (IIEF-ED domain score >24) reported greater ED bother post-treatment compared to pre-treatment. These data support the clinical observation that even if men's erections return after treatment, the quality of these erections may still be inferior to that of pre-treatment erections, potentially causing significant distress. It is also well established that ED and male sexual dysfunction are associated with higher depressive symptoms (Nelson et al., 2007; Shabsigh et al., 1998; Araujo et al., 1998; Shiri et al., 2007).

Oftentimes it is assumed that as men grow older they will be less concerned with sexual functioning; however, these studies have been conducted in men ranging in age from 40 to 70 years (similar to the age range of men with prostate cancer), and many of these studies controlled for age in their analyses. The bother and distress associated with ED often leads to a loss of intimacy in men's relationships and can potentially lead to significant relationship conflict (Bokhour et al., 2001; Moore et al., 2003).

In addition to the myriad of physiological changes that can disrupt sexual function after cancer diagnosis, it is important to acknowledge the significant interpersonal shifts that may take place and affect their sexuality. For instance, although changes in body image are readily acknowledged and often anticipated when we think about the effects of breast cancer, it is critical to understand that body image does not occur in isolation and that it is an experience that is contextually and relationally based. Women are sensitive to their partner's perception of their new appearance, and male patients tend to avoid conversations with their wives about their sexual challenges that result from cancer treatment (Boehmer & Clark, 2001) and speculate how their wives feel about their sexual functioning (Rivers et al., 2011). In some situations, patients may feel uncomfortable discussing this aspect of their cancer experience with their partners, out of a fear of rejection. Partners are often afraid to broach the subject, out of fear of causing distress. This interpersonal silence can quickly become the "elephant in the room," and over time, disruptions in intimate functioning can become more difficult to address, with either one or both partners misperceiving each other's feelings and intentions.

Healthcare providers are particularly well positioned to assist couples in communicating more openly about their fears and to answer questions regarding sexual dysfunction, by providing them with available resources on social support and information on cancer treatments that affect sexuality (Couper et al., 2006). Manne and Badr (2008) have proposed an integrative theoretical framework to understanding and addressing the challenges that couples face during and after cancer. By focusing on relationship processes that contribute to intimacy, this framework can help providers facilitate a discussion of the illness as something that happens to the *relationship*, rather than to individual partners. Based on this approach, couples should be encouraged to perform "relationship-enhancing" behaviors such as reciprocal self-disclosure of fears and concerns, partner responsiveness, and relationship engagement, while discouraging "relationship-compromising" behaviors such as avoidance and criticism (Manne & Badr, 2008).

COMMUNICATION ABOUT SEXUAL PROBLEMS

Although the optimal time to initiate discussion about sexual concerns may vary, it is essential that clinicians prepare patients for potential changes that may be encountered and let them know that discussion about sexual health concerns is welcome. It is notable that patients will rarely initiate conversation on this topic for fear of embarrassing their doctor and also out of concern that their symptoms are not treatable. For a majority of men, it is invaluable to receive a brief yet clear message that serves to normalize their symptoms and reassures them that they are not alone and that resources are available. Many patients report that much of their distress often starts with the observation that they were not prepared for changes in sexual function. In the same way that clinicians view a wide range of potential side effects from any course of cancer treatment, knowledge about potential cancer-related sexual side effects needs to be acknowledged. This allows patients to prepare for managing side effects and potentially may help them make better informed decisions about treatment options. It is our belief that clinicians should learn to address this topic as they would any other topic. Practical information should be provided at multiple time points across the continuum of cancer care.

For some patients, it may be valuable and/or necessary to make a referral for more directed sexual therapy. Additional intervention may include counseling with a licensed therapist who specializes in sex therapy and/or couples counseling. Often it can be useful within an oncology practice to identify one clinician—a physician, nurse, social worker, or psychologist—who can serve as the primary resource person for sexual health. Several professional organizations such as the American Psychosocial Oncology Society (APOS), the Society for Sex Therapy and Research (SSTAR), and the American Association of Sexual Educators, Counselors and Therapists (AASECT) all have directories and resources for locating professionals who specialize in working with sexual dysfunction.

TESTICULAR CANCER

EPIDEMIOLOGY AND DIAGNOSIS

Testicular cancer is the most common cancer in American men between the ages of 20 and 40, accounting for 46% of all cancers in this age range, though it accounts for only about 1% of all male cancers. It is considerably more common in Caucasian than African-American men, with intermediate rates for Hispanics, Native Americans, and Asians. Distinct geographical and racial variations suggest both genetic and environmental factors promoting the development of testicular cancer (Dearnaley, Huddart, & Horwich, 2001). One major risk factor is cryptorchidism, the congenital failure of one or both testes to descend into the scrotal sac (Bosl et al., 2008). There is evidence of increased risk in men infected with human immunodeficiency virus/acquired immunodeficiency syndrome (HIV/AIDS) and in those having a prior testicular cancer. At diagnosis, testicular cancer may be localized or spread to regional lymph nodes or metastasized to distant body sites.

Testicular self-examination is the most common form of detection of this cancer, usually with the presence of a small, hard lump in either testicle, an enlarged testicle, a collection of fluid, or unusual pain. However, most patients will first seek medical attention because of development of a painless, swollen testis. In approximately 25% of patients, the first symptoms will be related to metastatic disease, back pain being the most common, from tumor in the retroperitoneum. Pulmonary symptoms such as shortness of breath, chest pain, or hemoptysis occur due to advanced lung metastases (Nichols et al., 2000).

Biopsy is not possible in this disease because the cancer cells may spread during the procedure. Orchiectomy is the standard diagnostic procedure, which prevents further growth of the primary tumor. Ninety percent of testicular cancers are germ cell tumors (GCT), which are subdivided into seminomas and non-seminomas. Lymphoma is the second most common tumor of the testis and should be suspected in men over age 50. The tumor markers α-fetoprotein (AFP), β-human chorionic gonadotropin (β-HCG), and lactate dehydrogenase (LDH) are used for the detection of small tumors and for comparison over time to evaluate response to treatment. Retroperitoneal lymph node dissection (RPLND) is critical to stage non-seminomatous GCT and must always be performed with curative intent. This procedure is often associated with ejaculatory dysfunction (retrograde ejaculation) and secondary infertility, though newer nerve-sparing procedures may preserve normal ejaculation.

SURGICAL AND MEDICAL MANAGEMENT

Survival in this population has significantly improved owing to improved diagnostic and treatment techniques, with over 95% of patients expected to be cured. Cure rates depend on the stage of disease, approaching 100% for early-stage seminomas and nearly 100% overall survival for stage I non-seminomatous GCT. Approximately 85% of men with advanced testicular cancer will be cured with a combination of chemotherapy and surgery.

The effects on fertility and the possibility of storing sperm should be discussed with all patients undergoing chemotherapy or radiotherapy (Dearnaley et al., 2001). Treatment differs for seminomatous and non-seminomatous tumors, as well as the stage of disease. More advanced disease is treated with orchiectomy and multidrug chemotherapy.

Non-seminomas have often metastasized by the time of clinical presentation. Early and moderate-stage disease can be treated with orchiectomy alone, or followed by either RPLND, observation with frequent follow-ups, or chemotherapy. High-dose chemotherapy with peripheral blood stem-cell transplantation is used for metastatic refractory germ cell cancer and has been found to improve survival for some patients (Kollmannsberger et al., 1999).

MANAGEMENT OF DISTRESS

Testicular and GCTs often occur in young men, when sexuality, fertility, and intimacy are critically important. Although unilateral orchiectomy does not lead to infertility or sexual dysfunction, men are often concerned about their appearance. Artificial testicular implants have been successful in helping men cope with this issue. RPLND can lead to infertility by causing retrograde ejaculation, though sexual desire and the ability to have erections and orgasms are not affected. A pattern of sexual avoidance and decreased sexual interest can develop related to the distress of the cancer treatment in general. Although there is substantial recovery of sexual functioning after treatment (Ozen et al., 1998), a significant number of men will have long-term sexual dysfunction (Heidenreich & Hofmann, 1999). For men with partners or spouses, couples' therapy can address these issues and help the couple gain some perspective on how their relationship has been changed by cancer. Apart from infertility, fears about the effects on sexual functioning need to be addressed, especially before a young man has been involved in a long-term sexual relationship. Thorough sexual histories should include questions about frequency and intensity of sexual activity, including masturbation, desire, erection, orgasm, and satisfaction.

Infertility can be related to surgery, with RPLND posing the greatest threat by interfering with ejaculation. Infertility can also be due to radiotherapy or chemotherapy. Sperm production can be affected by radiation therapy, and infertility from this degree of radiation is temporary in most patients. Many men with testicular cancer have been found to have low sperm counts even before diagnosis, perhaps due to an autoimmune process that is probably confined to the few months before diagnosis. Unfortunately, this can limit the usefulness of sperm-banking at the time of diagnosis. Antegrade ejaculation may return spontaneously over the months or years following surgery, and the administration of sympathomimetic drugs can convert retrograde to antegrade ejaculation. Whether due to acquired infertility or because of decreased desire of having children, paternity rates are 15–30% lower than in the general population (Bertetto et al., 2001).

Chemotherapeutic agents such as cyclophosphamide can also cause infertility, though this may last for a transient period of two to three years after completing chemotherapy. Trask and colleagues (2003) found no significant difference among 16 study subjects in distress and QOL measured before, during, and after chemotherapy. The most disruptive symptoms noted were fatigue and changes in sleep, mood, and appetite.

Approximately 10% of patients will have long-term psychological problems (Heidenreich & Hofmann, 1999). A large study in a Norwegian population reported a greater prevalence of anxiety disorders in long-term testicular cancer survivors when compared to a matched healthy population, with no differences observed in depression measures (Dahl et al., 2005). Surviving patients are concerned with late complications of curative therapy, as is seen in other malignancies, as well as fears of recurrence. For these reasons, it is thought that supportive and educational counseling should be offered before and after cancer treatment. (For a more comprehensive discussion of sexual dysfunction in urological cancer, please see the section on prostate cancer.)

Awareness of potential long-term effects from chemotherapy and other QOL problems can inform a therapist about how to help a young patient cope better with the frustration of side effects: for instance, compromised renal function from cisplatin, Raynaud's phenomenon following combinations of vinblastine and bleomycin, pulmonary toxicity with bleomycin, and neuropathy and ototoxicity attributable to cisplatin and vinblastine leave patients with secondary deficits that challenge their daily living. Short- and long-term consequences for QOL are also seen with the use of radiotherapy, in the form of erectile and ejaculation disorders and radiation-induced tumors (Kollmannsberger et al., 1999).

BLADDER CANCER

EPIDEMIOLOGY AND DIAGNOSIS

There will be an estimated 74,690 new cases of bladder cancer diagnosed in 2014 in the United States (about 56,390 in men and 18,300 in women) (ACS, 2014). The incidence is greater in whites, who are almost twice as likely to be diagnosed as black men, followed by Hispanics and Asians, who have the lowest incidence. Mortality rates have been stable in men and are decreasing slowly in women (ACS, 2014). The largest known risk factor is tobacco smoking, leading to twice the number of cases relative to those who do not smoke. Risk increases with age, as 70% of cases are diagnosed after age 65. Certain cancer treatments, such as high-dose cyclophosphamide or ifosfamide and radiation treatment to the pelvis, may increase the risk of developing bladder cancer. People at high risk due to exposure or selected bladder birth defects may benefit from screening with urine cytology and cystoscopy. Currently, there are no good tests for early detection and widespread screening of bladder cancer. Most are detected because they cause grossly visible or microscopic hematuria. Over 90% of bladder cancers are transitional cell carcinomas (TCC). Disease stage has been shown to be the single best predictor of outcome for TCC of the bladder (McDougal et al., 2008).

SURGICAL AND MEDICAL MANAGEMENT

If bladder cancer is detected at an early stage (0–I), the five-year survival rate is 85–95%. For more advanced disease (stages II–IV), the survival rates are between 16% and 55%, depending on extent of disease (ACS, 2014). Categorizing cases into *superficial* bladder cancer or *muscle-invasive* bladder cancer is a useful way to describe treatment and the multiple effects on QOL.

Cystoscopy and transurethral resection of the bladder (TURB) are the primary modes for diagnosis of superficial bladder cancer tumors. TURB is also the definitive treatment for low-grade and superficial tumors, with perioperative bladder instillation of chemotherapy recommended for most patients (Barocas & Clark, 2008; Clarke, 2007). Agents for this local treatment are the immune modulator Bacillus Calmette-Guerin (BCG) and chemotherapeutic agents, such as mitomycin and thiotepa, usually given by the intravesical route. Cystitis is often an uncomfortable side effect of these treatments; cutaneous complications from intravesical instillations may be quite severe (Kureshi et al., 2006). Attempts to avoid or postpone cystectomy for localized, superficial bladder cancers may require long-term follow-up with repeated cystoscopies, which can have negative psychological effects. However, for high-risk noninvasive bladder cancers or those not responding to bladder instillation, a cystectomy is recommended by many specialists (Oosterlinck, Witjes, & Sylvester, 2008; Skinner, 2007). It remains to be seen what effect the presence of genetic markers such as the *p53* gene or mutations of the fibroblast growth factor receptor 3 (*FGFR*) will have on treatment options. It is important for medical psychiatrists and psychologists to understand that, despite patients being informed of the good prognosis of their illness, there is a strong negative psychological impact, with most feeling that their lives would be negatively disrupted (Bohle et al., 1996).

Men receiving treatment for early-stage bladder cancer generally do not have sexual dysfunction. However, there have been reports of men developing penile curvature, or Peyronie's disease, after frequent cystoscopy. The overall impact on sexual activity is independent of age and gender (Mack & Frick, 1996). Complaints of decreased sexual desire, feelings of contamination by the cancer, painful intercourse, and other urethral symptoms are reported.

Radical cystectomy (bladder removal) is the standard procedure for muscle-invasive bladder carcinoma. Surgery, alone or in combination with other treatments, is used in over 90% of cases. Chemotherapy, alone or with radiation before cystectomy, has improved some treatment results for more advanced tumors. Studies suggest a window of opportunity of less than 12 weeks from diagnosis of invasive disease to radical cystectomy to improve prognosis (Fahmy, Mahmud, & Aprikian, 2006).

Compared with cystectomy, radiation treatment provides better short-term QOL in the physical, psychological, and sexual domains, although one study found no difference in the QOL between both treatments after 18 months (Lynch et al., 1992). Frequent symptoms affecting QOL post-radiotherapy include urinary frequency, urgency, nocturia, and reduced bladder capacity. Surrounding organs are frequently affected, and the dose and volume of radiation are correlated with the more unpleasant symptoms of fecal leakage and urgency, and diarrhea with blood and mucus (Henningsohn, 2006). Significant gastrointestinal symptoms may persist two to three years after pelvic radiotherapy, including the development of proctitis (Andreyev et al., 2005). Modern radiation therapy techniques offer the potential to improve cure rates and reduce adverse effects (Milosevic et al., 2007). Radical cystectomy impacts sexual and urinary functioning in men in a fashion similar to RP, as the prostate is often removed with the bladder. A large proportion of men suffer ED, though the incidence is decreasing with nerve-sparing and seminal vesicle–sparing techniques. Testosterone secretion is unimpaired, so sexual desire remains unchanged in the long term. Prostate-sparing cystectomy has yet to show oncological efficacy, despite its functional advantages (Kefer et al., 2007).

With cystectomy, many patients have been helped by the development of internal urinary reservoirs constructed from the bowel (Parekh & Donat, 2007). These can be anastomosed to either the skin or urethra. When attached to the urethra, continence can be maintained. This has permitted the creation of the neobladder, with which almost all patients achieve daytime urinary continence (McDougal et al., 2008). Although complications are higher than with the conduit, these procedures obviate the need for an appliance, and are welcomed psychologically.

MANAGEMENT OF DISTRESS

Urinary tract reconstruction procedures affect overall QOL, mostly in the sexual and urinary spheres. Symptoms vary with the type of reconstruction. Patients with ileal conduits report impaired body image, increased self-consciousness, and decreases in travel and activity level, probably related to urinary leakage, odor, and skin irritation at the stoma site. Those with continent diversion report symptoms related to having to use a catheter, while neobladder patients report nighttime leakage. Almost all populations, regardless of reconstruction technique, have sexual dysfunction related to negative physical or psychological effects of the procedure (Botteman et al., 2003). A sound strategy to achieve greater QOL after radical cystectomy is thorough and active counseling on the various reconstructive alternatives before the surgery that allows patients a choice of the type of urinary diversion on the basis of patient preference, anatomy, and tumor status, as well as counseling and support post-operatively (Wright & Porter, 2007; Davidsson et al., 2007). Advanced-disease TCC is usually treated with systemic chemotherapy.

Women make a better adjustment to the presence of a urinary diversion than men do; this is perhaps related to their being more independent in their stoma care than men. Radical cystectomy in women also includes hysterectomy and oophorectomy and resection of the anterior wall of the vagina. The major sexual side effect for women is genital pain, particularly during intercourse. Decreased sexual arousal, desire, and loss of sexual attractiveness are frequently reported. Surgical modifications to preserve internal genitalia have been suggested as long as cancer control is not compromised (Miranda-Sousa, 2006). Use of vaginal dilators, lubricants, and estrogen creams can help women become more comfortable during sexual activity by overcoming the consequences of scarring and premature menopause (Ofman, Kingsberg, & Nelson, 2008).

KIDNEY CANCER

EPIDEMIOLOGY AND DIAGNOSIS

Approximately 60,920 patients were diagnosed with kidney cancer in 2011, and more than 13,000 were projected to die of the disease (ACS, 2011). Kidney cancer includes renal cell carcinoma (92%), renal pelvis carcinoma (7%), and Wilms tumor (1%), a childhood cancer. Death rates have been slowly decreasing in women. The one-year survival rate for cancer of the kidney and renal pelvis is 83%, and the five-year survival rate is 69%. The incidence rises with age, as with TCC of the bladder and prostate cancer. Renal cell carcinoma is almost twice as common in men as in women. Often the diagnosis is made incidentally at the time of radiographic procedures such as ultrasonography or a computed tomography (CT) scan for non-urological problems. There has been some association with cigarette smoking, obesity, and exposure to lead phosphate, dimethyl nitrosamine, and aflatoxins. In addition, exposure to asbestos, cadmium, and trichloroethylene have been implicated in the development of some kidney cancers (Linehan & Schmidt, 2008). A large percentage of these cancers may remain undiagnosed during life, like prostate cancer; however, with renal cancers a significant proportion of those found incidentally at autopsy actually caused death (ACS, 2011). A significant number of new cases have overt metastatic disease at the time of diagnosis. The prognosis for these patients is bleak, with a median survival of less than one year. The increased use of ultrasound has resulted in a higher detection rate of lower stage tumors.

SURGICAL AND MEDICAL MANAGEMENT

Patients' presentations may range from the triad of hematuria, pain, and palpable renal mass, to more obscure paraneoplastic syndromes, fever, anemia, or polycythemia. Diagnosis is made by intravenous pyelography (IVP), ultrasound, renal arteriography, CT scans, and magnetic resonance imaging (MRI). Pathological staging is the most important determinant of prognosis.

The treatment of choice for localized disease is surgical removal of the affected kidney, with regional lymphadenectomy. Five-year survival for stage I disease ranges from 60–75%, and from 40–65% in those with stage II disease. Renal preservation with only partial excision of renal tissue by open surgical or laparoscopic procedures has become more widely accepted, though there is still uncertainty about long-term prognosis. Treatment can provide challenges because of compromised renal function. Most survivors of localized kidney cancer have normal physical and mental health regardless of the type of nephrectomy performed, though QOL is better for patients with more renal parenchyma remaining after surgery (Clarke et al., 2001).

To date, chemotherapeutic agents have not demonstrated sufficient antitumor activity to prolong the survival of patients with metastatic disease. Sorafenib, Sutinib, and Pazopanib are new targeted chemotherapeutic agents that have shown promise in older as well as younger patients (Eisen et al., 2008).

Immunotherapy, autolymphocyte therapy, vaccines, and nonspecific immunomodulators may prolong survival for patients with metastatic renal disease. Interferon and high-dose interleukin-2, used with some success in treating advanced renal cancer, can cause depression and anxiety, which may be mediated through cytokines with physical or somatic side effects such as fatigue and fever. It is possible that patients most at risk of developing significant depression on these drugs are those who have higher baseline depressive symptom scores (Capuron et al., 2004). An important study found that the patients who were to get treated with high-dose interferon alpha and who received prophylactic treatment of an SSRI antidepressant had less depression than those who did not get the antidepressant; and for many, major depression onset was delayed (Musselman et al., 2001). Delirium and cognitive deficits may also be seen as independent effects of interferon and interleukin on the central nervous system.

MANAGEMENT OF DISTRESS

The poor prognosis for this illness is the cause of much psychological distress experienced by many patients and their families after diagnosis and treatment. Later stages of disease are highlighted by metastases to bone, lungs, and brain, and necessitate coping with pain, shortness of breath, concentration deficits, and other cognitive difficulties. Distress is caused by periods when the person is free of disease after surgery but knows that recurrence is likely. The conflict of maintaining hope for successful treatment, in the context of discouraging odds, can be burdensome and can lead to various degrees of anxiety and depression. As with other GU cancers, many patients with renal cancer report worse sexual functioning than in comparable chronically ill populations (Anastasiadis et al., 2003).

CLINICAL PEARLS

- Lower-potency antipsychotics, including chlorpromazine, mesoridazine, thioridazine, and clozapine, have significant alpha1-adrenergic effects, just like some of the drugs used to treat BPH. The compounded alpha1-adrenergic effects can lead to orthostatic hypotension and syncope associated with vasodilation (Alpert et al., 2004).

- For UI, behavioral techniques have been shown to be more effective than medication and should be used as a first-line treatment (Burgio et al., 1998).

- Studies have shown varying rates of success using duloxetine in the treatment of post-prostatectomy incontinence and stress UI in women (Cornu et al., 2011).

- Side effects of androgen ablation may include ED, loss of libido, hot flashes, gynecomastia, irritability, anxiety, and depression. Men most at risk for depression while on hormonal therapy were those who had histories significant for major depression (Pirl, Siegel, & Good, 2002).

- Guidelines recommend detection of cases of testosterone deficiency not in the general population but in those with certain clinical disorders that predispose them to low testosterone: men with a sellar mass, history of radiation to the sellar region; those chronically treated with glucocorticoids, ketoconazole, or opioids; HIV-associated weight loss; end-stage renal disease; chronic obstructive lung disease; infertility; osteoporosis; or type 2 diabetes mellitus.

- Antidepressants like the SSRIs such as sertraline and paroxetine; SNRIs such as venlafaxine; and anti-epileptic medications such as gabapentin, have been reported to reduce the frequency and intensity of hot flashes in men (Roth et al., 1998; Loprinzi, 2004; Adelson et al., 2005).

- Manne and Badr (2008) have proposed an integrative theoretical framework to understand the challenges that couples face during and after cancer. By focusing on relationship processes that contribute to intimacy, this framework can help providers facilitate a discussion of the illness as something that happens to the relationship rather than to individual partners. Based on this approach, couples should be encouraged to perform "relationship-enhancing" behaviors such as reciprocal self-disclosure of fears and concerns, partner responsiveness, and relationship engagement, while discouraging "relationship-compromising" behaviors such as avoidance and criticism (Manne & Badr, 2008).

- Many patients report feeling distress that they were not prepared for changes in sexual functioning. In the same way that clinicians present a wide range of potential side effects from any course of cancer treatment, potential cancer-related sexual side effects need to be acknowledged in advance. This allows patients to prepare to manage side effects and may help them make better informed decisions about treatment options. Practical information should be provided at multiple time points across the continuum of cancer care.

- Antegrade ejaculation may return spontaneously over the months or years following surgery, and the administration of sympathomimetic drugs can convert retrograde to antegrade ejaculation.

- Significant gastrointestinal symptoms may persist two to three years after pelvic radiotherapy, including the development of proctitis (Andreyev et al., 2005).

- With cystectomy, many patients have been helped by the development of internal urinary reservoirs constructed from the bowel (Parekh & Donat, 2007). These can be anastomosed to either the skin or urethra. When attached to the urethra, continence can be maintained. This has permitted the creation of the neobladder, with which almost all patients achieve daytime urinary continence (McDougal et al., 2008). Although complications are higher than with the conduit, these procedures obviate the need for an appliance, and are welcomed psychologically.

- Women make a better adjustment to the presence of a urinary diversion than men do; this is perhaps related to their being more independent in their stoma care than men. Radical cystectomy in women also includes hysterectomy and oophorectomy and resection of the anterior wall of the vagina. The major sexual side effect for women is genital pain, particularly during intercourse.

DISCLOSURE STATEMENTS

Dr. Roth has no conflicts to disclose.

Dr. Karl has no conflicts to disclose.

Dr. Nelson has no conflicts to disclose.

REFERENCES

Adelson K.B., Loprinzi, C. L., & Hershman, D. L. (2005) Treatment of hot flushes in breast and prostate cancer. *Expert Opinion on Pharmacotherapy, 6*(7), 1095–1106.

Allan, C. A., & McLachlan, R. I. (2006). Androgen deficiency disorders. In L. J. DeGroot & J. L. Jameson (Eds.), *Endocrinology* (5th ed., pp. 3178–3179). Philadelphia, PA: Elsevier.

Alpert, J. E., Fava, M., & Rosenbaum, J. F. (2004). Psychopharmacologic issues in the medical setting. In T. A. Stern, G. L. Fricchione, N. H. Cassem, M. S. Jellinek, & Rosenbaum, J. F. (Eds.), *Handbook of general psychiatry* (5th ed., p. 68). Philadelphia, PA: Mosby.

American Cancer Society (2011). *Cancer facts and figures, 2011.* Atlanta, GA: American Cancer Society.

Amiaz, R., & Seidman, S. N. (2008). Testosterone and depression in men. *Current Opinion in Endocrinology, Diabetes, & Obesity, 15*(3), 278–283.

Anastasiadis, A., Davis, A. R., Sawczuk, I. S., et al. (2003). Quality of life aspects in kidney cancer patients: Data from a national registry. *Cancer, 11,* 700–706.

Andreyev, H., Vlavianos, P., Blake, P., Dearnaley, D., Norman, A. R., & Tait, D. (2005). Gastrointestinal symptoms after pelvic radiotherapy: Role for the gastroenterologist? *International Journal of Radiation Oncology, Biology, Physics, 62,* 1464–1471.

Araujo, A. B., Durante, R., Feldman, H. A., Goldstein, I., & McKinlay, J. B. (1998). The relationship between depressive symptoms and male erectile dysfunction: Cross-sectional results from the Massachusetts Male Aging Study. *Psychosomatic Medicine, 60,* 458–465.

Barocas, D., & Clark, P. E. (2008). Bladder cancer. *Current Opinion in Oncology, 20,* 307–314.

Bauer, R. M., Gozzi, C., Hubner, W., et al. (2011). Contemporary management of postprostatectomy incontinence. *European Urology, 59*(6), 985–986.

Bertetto, O., Bracarda, S., Tamburini, M., & Cortesi, E. (2001). Quality of life studies and genito-urinary tumors. *Annals of Oncology, 12*(Suppl 3), S43–S48.

Bhasin, S., Cunningham, G. R., Hayes, F. J., Matsumoto, A. M. et al. (2006). Clinical practice guideline; testosterone therapy in adult men with androgen deficiency syndromes: An Endocrine Society Clinical Practice Guideline. *Journal of Clinical Endocrinology* & Metabolism, *91,* 1995–2010.

Bilić, V., & Marcinko, D. (2010). Comorbidity of kidney stones and psychiatric disease. *Psychiatria Danubina,* Jun; *22*(2), 249–252.

Blank, T., & Bellizzi, K. M. (2006). After prostate cancer: Predictors of well-being among long term prostate cancer survivors. *Cancer, 106,* 2128–2135.

Bo, K. (2004). Pelvic floor muscle training is effective in treatment of female stress urinary incontinence, but how does it work? *International Urogynecology Journal, 15,* 76–84.

Boehmer, U., & Clark, J. A. (2001). Communication about prostate cancer between men and their wives. *Journal of Family Practice, 50*(3), 226–231.

Bohle, A., Balck, F., von Weitersheim, J., & Jocham, D. (1996). The quality of life during intravesical Bacillus Calmette-Guerin therapy. *Journal of Urology, 155*(4), 1221–1226.

Bokhour, B. G., Clark, J. A., Inui, T. S., Silliman, R. A., & Talcott, J. A. (2001). Sexuality after treatment for early prostate cancer: Exploring the meanings of "erectile dysfunction." *Journal of General Internal Medicine, 16,* 649–655.

Bosl, G., Bajorin, D. F., Sheinfeld, J., & Motzer, J. (2008). Cancer of the testis. In V. DeVita, T. S. Lawrence, & S. A. Rosenberg (Eds.), *Cancer: Principles and practice of oncology* (8th ed., pp. 1465–1483). Philadephia, PA: Lippincott.

Botteman, M., Pashos, C., Hauser, R., Laskin, B., & Redaelli, A. (2003). Quality of life aspects of bladder cancer: A review of the literature. *Quality of Life Research, 12,* 675–688.

Brubaker, L., Meikle, S., & Steers, W. (reviewers) (October 2007). Urinary incontinence in women. National Kidney and Urologic Diseases Information Clearinghouse. *Home page—National Kidney and Urologic Diseases Information Clearinghouse.* National Institutes of Health, Sept. 2, 2010. Web, Aug. 5. Available at http://kidney.niddk.nih.gov/kudiseases/pubs/uiwomen/.

Burgio, K. L., Locher, J. L., Goode, P. S., et al. (1998). Behavioral vs. drug treatment for urge urinary incontinence in older women. *Journal of the American Medical Association, 280*(23), 1995–2000.

Capuron, L., Ravaud, A., Miller, A. H., & Dantzer, R. (2004). Baseline mood and psychosocial characteristics of patients developing depressive symptoms during interleukin-2 and/or interferon-alpha cancer therapy. *Brain, Behavior, & Immunity, 18,* 205–213.

Carson, C. 3rd, & Rittmaster, R. (2003). The role of dihydrotestosterone in benign prostatic hyperplasia. *Urology,* Apr; *61*(4 Suppl 1), 2–7.

Catlin, D. H. (2006). Anabolic steroids. In L. J. DeGroot & J. L. Jameson (Eds.), *Endocrinology* (5th ed., p. 3270). Philadelphia, PA: Elsevier.

Chiba, Y., Satoh, K., Ueda, S., Kanazawa, N., Tamura, Y., & Horiuchi, T. (2007). Marked improvement of psychiatric symptoms after parathyroidectomy in elderly primary hyperparathyroidism. *Endocrine Journal,* Jun; *54*(3), 379–383.

Clarke, P. (2007). Bladder cancer. *Current Opinion in Oncology, 19,* 241–247.

Clarke, P., Schover, L. R., Uzzo, R. G., Hafez, K. S., Rybicki, L. A., & Novick, A. C. (2001). Quality of life and psychological adaptation after surgical treatment for localized renal cell carcinoma: Impact of the amount of remaining renal tissue. *Urology, 57,* 252–256.

Clemens, J. Q., Meenan, R. T., O'Keeffe Rosetti, M. C., Kimes, T. A., & Calhoun E. A. (2008). Case-control study of medical comorbities in women with interstitial cystitis. *Journal of Urology, 179*(6), 2222–2225.

Coker L. H., Rorie K., Cantley L., et al. (2005). Primary hyperparathyroidism, cognition, and health-related quality of life. *Annals of Surgery, 242*(5), 642.

Cornu, J. N., Merlet, B., Ciofu, C., et al. (2011). Duloxetine for mild to moderate post-prostatectomy incontinence: Preliminary results of a randomised, placebo-controlled trial. *European Urology,* Jan; *59*(1), 148–154.

Couper, J., Bloch, S., Love, A., et al. (2006). Psychosocial adjustment of female partners of men with prostate cancer: A review of the literature. *Psycho-oncology, 15*(11), 937–953.

Coyne, K. S., Sexton, C. C., Kopp, Z. S., Ebel-Bitoun, C., Milsom, I., & Chapple, C. (2011). The impact of overactive bladder on mental health, work productivity and health-related quality of life in the UK and Sweden: Results from EpiLUTS. *BJU International 108*(9), 1459–1471.

Dahl, A., Haaland, C. F., Mykletun, A., et al. (2005). Study of anxiety disorder and depression in long-term survivors of testicular cancer. *Journal of Clinical Oncology, 23*(10), 2389–2395.

Dale, W., Bilir, P., Han, M., & Meltzer, D. (2005). The role of anxiety in prostate carcinoma. *Cancer, 104,* 467–478.

Davidsson, T., Wullt, B., Konyves, J., Mansson, A., & Mansson, W. (2007). Urinary diversion and bladder substitution in patients with bladder cancer. *Urologic Oncology, 5*(5), 224–231.

Dearnaley, D., Huddart, R., & Horwich, A. (2001). Regular review: Managing testicular cancer. *British Medical Journal, 322*(7302), 1583–1588.

Diniz, D. H., Blay, S. L., & Schor, N. (2007). Anxiety and depression symptoms in recurrent painful renal lithiasis colic. *Brazilian Journal of Medical & Biological Research, 40*(7), 949–955.

Easton, W. A. (2010). Overactive bladder symptoms in women: Current concepts in patient management. *Canadian Journal of Urology,* Feb 17 (Suppl 1), 12–17.

Eisen, T., Oudard, S., Szcylik, C., et al. (2008). Sorafenib for older patients with renal cell carcinoma: Subset analysis from a randomized trial. *Journal of the National Cancer Institute,* Oct 15; *100*(20), 1454–1463.

Eknoyan, G. (2001). Acute tubulointerstitial nephritis. In R. W. Schrier (Ed.), *Diseases of the kidney and urinary tract* (7th ed., p. 1278). Philadelphia, PA: Lippincott.

Elstad, E. A., Taubenberger, S. P., Botelho, E. M., & Tennstedt, S. L. (2010). Beyond incontinence: The stigma of other urinary symptoms. *Journal of Advanced Nursing,* Nov; *66*(11), 2460–2470.

Eton, D., & Lepore, S. J. (2002). Prostate cancer and health-related quality of life: A review of the literature. *Psycho-Oncology, 11,* 307–326.

Fahmy, N., Mahmud, S., & Aprikian, A. G. (2006). Delay in the surgical treatment of bladder cancer and survival: Systematic review of the literature. *European Urology, 50,* 1176–1182.

Gitlin, M. (1999). Lithium and the kidney: An updated review. *Drug Safety,* Mar; *20*(3), 231–243.

Hakimi, A., Feder, M., & Ghavamian, R. (2007). Minimally invasive approaches to prostate cancer: A review of the current literature. *Urology Journal, 4,* 130–137.

Hanno, P., Lin, A. Nording, J., Nyberg, L., van Ophoven, A., et al. (2010). Bladder pain syndrome: Committee of the International Consultation on Incontinence. *Neurourology & Urodynamics, 29,* 191–198.

Harlan, L., Brawley, O., Pommerenke, F., Wali, P., & Kramer, B. (1995). Geographic, age, and racial variation in the treatment of local/regional carcinoma of the prostate. *Journal of Clinical Oncology, 13*, 93–100.

Heidenreich, A., & Hofmann, R. (1999). Quality-of-life issues in the treatment of testicular cancer. *World Journal of Urology, 17*(4), 230–238.

Heim, H., & Oei, T. P. S. (1993). Comparison of prostate cancer patients with and without pain. *Pain, 53,* 159–162.

Hellstrom, W. J., Giuliano, F., & Rosen, R. C. (2009). Ejaculatory dysfunction and its association with lower urinary tract symptoms of benign prostatic hyperplasia and BPH treatment. *Urology,* Jul; *74*(1), 15–21. Epub May 9, 2009.

Hengge, U. R. (2003). Testosterone replacement for hypogonadism: Clinical findings and best practices. *The AIDS Reader, 13,* S15–S21.

Henningsohn, L. (2006). Quality of life after therapy for muscle-invasive bladder cancer. *Current Opinion in Urology, 16,* 356–360.

Irwin, D. E., Milsom, I., Reilly, K., et al. (2008). Overactive bladder is associated with erectile dysfunction and reduced sexual quality of life in men. *Journal of Sexual Medicine,* Dec; *5*(12), 2904–2910.

Johansson, B., Holmberg, L., Onelov, E., Johansson, J. E., & Steinenck, G. (2009). Time, symptom burden, androgen deprivation, and self-assessed quality of life after radical prostatectomy or watchful waiting: The Randomized Scandinavian Prostate Cancer Group Study Number 4 (SPCG-4) clinical trial. *European Urology, 55*(2), 261–532.

Kanofsky, J. D., Woesner, M. E., Harris, A. Z., Kelleher, J. P., Gittens, K., & Jerschow, E. (2011). A case of acute renal failure in a patient recently treated with clozapine and a review of previously reported cases. *Primary Care Companion Central Nervous System Disorders, 13*(3).

Kefer, J., Cherullo, E. E., Jones, J. S., Gong, M. C., & Campbell, S. C. (2007). Prostate-sparing cystectomy: Has Pandora's box been opened? *Expert Review of Anticancer Therapy, 13,* 179–187.

Kelly, C. J., & Neilson, E. G. (2004). Tubulointerstitial diseases. In B. M. Brenner (Ed.), *The kidney* (7th ed., pp. 1491–1500). Boston, MA: Elsevier.

Khera, M., Bhattacharya, R. K., Blick, G., Kushner, H., Nguyen, D., & Miner, M. M. (2012). The effect of testosterone supplementation on depression symptoms in hypogonadal men from the Testim Registry in the US (TRiUS). *Aging Male.* 15(1), 14–21.

Klotz, L. (1997). PSA-dynia and other PSA-related syndromes: A new epidemic↓a case history and taxonomy. *Urology, 50,* 831–832.

Klotz, L. (2008). Active surveillance for prostate cancer: Trials and tribulations. *World Journal of Urology, 26,* 437–442.

Klotz, L., O'Callaghan, C. J., Ding, K., et al. (2011). A phase III randomized trial comparing intermittent versus continuous androgen suppression for patients with PSA progression after radical therapy. *Journal of Clinical Oncology, 29*(Suppl 7; abstr 3). Presented at the 2011 Genitourinary Cancers Symposium.

Kober, A., Dobrovits, M., Djavan, B., et al. (2003). Local active warming: An effective treatment for pain, anxiety and nausea caused by renal colic. *Journal of Urology, 170*(3), 741–744.

Kollmannsberger, C., Kuzcyk, M., Mayer, F., Hartmann, J. T., Kanz, L., & Bokemeyer, C. (1999). Late toxicity following curative treatment of testicular cancer. *Seminars in Surgical Oncology, 17*(4), 275–281.

Kornblith, A., Herr, H. W., Ofman, U. S., Scher, H. I., & Holland, J. C. (1994). Quality of life of patients with prostate cancer and their spouses. The value of a data base in clinical care. *Cancer, 73,* 2791–2802.

Kureshi, F., Kalaaji, A. N., Halvorson, L., Pittelkow, M. R., & Davis, M. D. P. (2006). Cutaneous complications of intravesical treatments for bladder cancer: Granulomatous inflammation of the penis following BCG therapy and penile gangrene following mitomycin therapy. *Journal of the American Academy of Dermatology, 55,* 328–331.

Lai, H., Hsu, E. I., Teh, B. S., Butler, E. B., & Boone, T. B. (2007). Thirteen years of experience with artificial urinary sphincter implantation at Baylor College of Medicine. *Journal of Urology, 177,* 1021–1025.

Lee, Y. H., Lee, W. C., Chen, M. T., Huang, J. K., Chung, C., & Chang, L. S. (1992). Acupuncture in the treatment of renal colic. *Journal of Urology,* Jan; *147*(1), 16–18.

Linehan, W., & Schmidt, L. S. (2008). Cancers of the genitourinary system. In V. DeVita, T. S. Lawrence, & S. A. Rosenberg (Eds.), *Cancer: Principles and practice of oncology* (8th ed., pp. XX–XX). Philadelphia, PA: Lippincott, Williams & Wilkens.

Lofters, A., Juffs, H. G., Pond, G. R., & Tannock, I. F. (2002). "PSA-itis": Knowledge of serum prostate specific antigen and other causes of anxiety in men with metastatic prostate cancer. *Journal of Urology, 168*(6), 2516–2520. Available at http://www.sciencedirect.com/science/journal/01406736.

Lundstam, S. O., Wahlander, L. A., Leissner, K. H., & Kral, J. G. (1982). Prostaglandin-synthetase inhibition with diclofenac sodium in treatment of renal colic: comparison with use of a narcotic analgesic. *The Lancet, 319*(8281), 1096–1097.

Lynch, W., Jenkins, B. J., Fowler, C. G., Hope-Stone, H. F., & Blandy, J. P. (1992). The quality of life after radical radiotherapy for bladder cancer. *British Journal of Urology, 70,* 519–521.

Mack, D., & Frick, J. (1996). Quality of life in patients undergoing bacille Calmette-Guerin therapy for superficial bladder cancer. *British Journal of Urology, 78*(3), 369–371.

Malmstrom, T. K., Andresen, E. M., Wolinsky, F. D., et al. (2010). Urinary and fecal incontinence and quality of life in African Americans. *Journal of the American Geriatric Society,* Oct; *58*(10), 1941–1945.

Manne, S., & Badr, H. (2008). Intimacy and relationship processes in couples' psychosocial adaptation to cancer. *Cancer, 112*(Suppl 11), 2541–2555.

Mayson, B. E., & Tecihman, J. M. H. (2009). The relationship between sexual abuse and interstitial cystitis/painful bladder syndrome. *Current Urology Reports, 10,* 441–447.

McAllion, S. J., Paterson, C. R. (1989). Psychiatric Morbidity in primary hyperparathyroidism. *Postgraduate Medical Journal, 65,* 628–631.

McCarthy, B. W., & Bodnar, L. E. (2005). Couple sex therapy: assessment, therapy, and relapse prevention. In Lebow JL (Eds), *The handbook of clinical family therapy* (pp. 464–493). Hoboken, NJ: John Wiley & Sons, Inc.

McConnell, J. D., Roehrborn, C. G., Bautista, O. M., et al. (2003). The long-term effect of doxazosin, finasteride, and combination therapy on the clinical progression of benign prostatic hyperplasia. *New England Journal of Medicine,* Dec 18; *349*(25), 2387–2398.

McDougal, W., Shipley, W. U., Kaufman, D. S., Dahl, D. M., Michaelson, M. D., & Zietman, A. L. (2008). Cancer of the bladder, ureter, and renal pelvis. In V. DeVita, T. S. Lawrence, & S. A. Rosenberg (Eds.), *Cancer: Principles and practice of oncology* (8th ed., pp. 1358–1361). Philadelphia, PA: Lippincott.

Milosevic, M., Gospodarowicz, M., Zietman, A., et al. (2007). Radiotherapy for bladder cancer. *Urology, 69,* 80–92.

Miranda-Sousa, A., Davila, H. H., Lockhart, J. L., Ordorica, R. C., & Carrion, R. E. (2006). Sexual function after surgery for prostate or bladder cancer. *Cancer Control, 13,* 179–187.

Mokulis, J., & Thompson, I. (1995). Screening for prostate cancer: Pros, cons, and reality. *Cancer Control* (Jan/Feb), 15–21.

Moore, T. M., Strauss, J. L., Herman, S., & Donatucci, C. F. (2003). Erectile dysfunction in early, middle, and late adulthood: Symptom patterns and psychosocial correlates. *Journal of Sex & Marital Therapy, 29,* 381–399.

Morgentaler, A. (2011). Testosterone therapy in the male cancer patient. In J. P. Mulhall, L. Incrocci, I. Goldstein, & R. Rosen (Eds.), *Cancer and sexual health* (pp. 721–730). New York: Humana Press.

Morgentaler, A., Lipshultz, L. I., Bennett, R., Sweeney, M., Avila, D., & Khera, M. (2011). Testosterone therapy in men with untreated prostate cancer. *Journal of Urology, 185*(4), 1256–1261.

Morris, M. J., Huang, D., Kelly, W. K., et al. (2009). Phase 1 trial of high-dose exogenous testosterone in patients with castration-resistant metastatic prostate cancer. *European Urology,* 2009 56(2), 237–244.

Movig, K. L., Leufkens, H. G., Belitser, S. V., et al. (2002). Selective serotonin reuptake inhibitor-induced urinary incontinence. *Pharmacoepidemiology & Drug Safety, 11,* 271–279.

Muller, N. (2005) What Americans understand how they affected by bladder control problems: highlights of recent nationwide consumer research. *Urologic Nursing, 25*(2), 109–115.

Musselman, D., Lawson, D. H., Gumnick, J. F., et al. (2001). Paroxetine for the prevention of depression induced by high-dose interferon alfa. *New England Journal of Medicine, 344*(13), 961–966.

Neer, R. M., Arnaud, C. D., Zanchetta, J. R., et al. (2001). Effect of para-thyroid hormone (1–34) on fractures and bone mineral density in postmenopausal women with osteoporosis. *New England Journal of Medicine,* May 10; *344*(19), 1434–1441.

Nelson, C. J., Roth, A., & Mulhall, J. P. (2007). Predictors of sexual bother in men following definitive treatment for prostate cancer. In Proceedings of the Annual Meeting of the Sexual Medicine Society of North America.

Nelson, J. B. (2007). Hormone therapy for prostate cancer. In A. J. Wein (Ed.), *Campbell-Walsh urology* (9th ed., pp. 3082–3099). Philadelphia, PA: Elsevier.

Nichols, C., Timmerman, R., Foster, R. S., Roth, B. J., & Einhorn, L. H. (2000). Neoplasms of the testis. In R. J. Bast, D. W. Kufe, R. E. Pollock, et al. (Eds.), *Cancer medicine* (5th ed.). Hamilton, Ont.: BC Decker.

Novakovic, M., Babic, D., Milovanovic, A., Tiosavljevic-Maric, D., Novakovic, R., & Novakovic, M. (2008). Anthropological aspect of death in dialyzed patients. *Collegium Antropologicum,* Jun; *32*(2), 587–594.

Ofman, U. (1994). Sexual quality of life in men with prostate cancer. *Cancer* (Suppl), *75,* 1949–1953.

Ofman, U., Kingsberg, S. A., & Nelson, C. J. (2008). Sexual prob-lems. In V. DeVita, T. S. Lawrence, & S. A. Rosenberg (Eds.), *Cancer: Principles and practice of oncology* (8th ed., pp. 2804–2809). Philadelphia, PA: Lippincott.

Oosterlinck, W, Witjes, F, & Sylvester, R (2008). Diagnostic and prognos-tic factors in non-muscle-invasive bladder cancer and their influence on treatment and outcomes. *European Urology Supplements.* 7,516–523.

Organ, M., Wood, L., Wilke, D., et al. (2013). Intermittent androgen-deprivation therapy in the management of castrate-resistant prostate cancer (CRPCa): Results of a multi-institutional random-ized prospective clinical trial. *American Journal of Clinical Oncology.* *36*(6), 601–605.

Ozen, H. S. A., Toklu, C., Rastadoskouee, M., Kilic, C., Gogus, A., & Kendi, S. (1998). Psychosocial adjustment after testicular cancer treatment. *Journal of Urology, 159*(6), 1947–1950.

Parekh, D., & Donat, S. M. (2007). Urinary diversion: Options, patient selection, and outcomes. *Seminars in Oncology, 34,* 98–109.

Parmar, M. S. (2004). Kidney stones: A review. *The BMJ.* 328(12), 1420.

Payne, R. (1993). Pain management in the patient with prostate cancer. *Cancer, 71*(Suppl 3), 11131–11137.

Penson, D. F., Latini, D. M., Lubeck, D. P., Wallace, K., Henning, J. M., & Lue, T. (2003). Is quality of life different for men with erectile dysfunction and prostate cancer compared to men with erectile dys-function due to other causes? Results from the ExCEED data base. *Journal of Urology, 169,* 1458–1461.

Pirl, W., Siegel, G. I., & Good, R. (2002). Depression in men receiving androgen deprivation therapy for prostate cancer: A pilot study. *Psycho-Oncology, 11,* 519–523.

Pope, H. G., Cohane, G. H., Kanayama, G., Siegel, A. J., & Hudson, J. I. (2003). Testosterone gel supplementation for men with refrac-tory depression: A randomized, placebo-controlled trial. *American Journal of Psychology, 160,* 105–111.

Presti Jr., J. C. (2008). Neoplasms of the prostate. In E. A Tanagho & J. W. McAninch (Eds.), *Smith's General Urology* (pp. 348–374). San Francisco, CA: McGraw-Hill.

Quillin, R. B., & Erickson, D. R. (2012). Practical use of the new American Urological Association Interstitial Cystitis Guidelines. *Current Urology Reports, 12,* 394–401.

Rathkopf, D., Carducci, M. A., Morris, M. J., et al. (2008). Phase II trial of docetaxel with rapid androgen cycling for progressive non-castrate prostate cancer. *Journal of Clinical Oncology,* Jun 20; *26*(18), 2959–2965.

Raynor, M. C., Pinsky, M. R., Chawla, A., & Hellstrom, W. J. G. (2011). Androgen deficiency. In J. P. Mulhall, L. Incrocci, I. Goldstein, & R. Rosen (Eds.), *Cancer and Sexual Health* (pp. 195–216). New York: Humana Press.

Reddy, G. K., Jain, V. K., & Loprinzi C. (2004). Current strategies to minimize treatment-associated hot flashes in patients with breast cancer. *Supportive Cancer Therapy, 1*(4), 210–212.

Rivers, B. M., August, E. M., Gwede, C. K., et al. (2011). Psychosocial issues related to sexual functioning among African-American pros-tate cancer survivors and their spouses. *Psycho-oncology.* Jan; *20*(1), 106–110.

Römer, B., & Gass, P. (2010). Finasteride-induced depression: New insights into possible pathomechanisms. *Journal of Cosmetic Dermatology,* Dec; *9*(4), 331–332.

Roth, A. J., Nelson, C., Rosenfeld, B., et al. (2010). Methylphenidate for fatigue in ambulatory men with prostate cancer. *Cancer,* Nov 1; *116*(21), 5102–5110.

Roth, A. J., Rosenfeld, B., Kornblith, A. B., et al. (2003). The Memorial Anxiety Scale for Prostate Cancer: Validation of a new scale to measure anxiety in men with prostate cancer. *Cancer, 97,* 2910–2918.

Roth, A., Nelson, C. J., Rosenfeld, B., et al. (2006). Assessing anxiety in men with prostate cancer: Further data on the reliability and valid-ity of the Memorial Anxiety Scale for Prostate Cancer (MAX-PC). *Psychosomatics, 47,* 340–347.

Roth, A., Nelson, C. J., Rosenfeld, B., et al. (2006). Assessing anxiety in men with prostate cancer: Further data on the reliability and valid-ity of the Memorial Anxiety Scale for Prostate Cancer (MAX-PC). *Psychosomatics, 47,* 340–347.

Sanda, M., Dunn, R. L., Michaleski, J., et al. (2008). Quality of life and satisfaction with outcome among prostate-cancer survivors. *New England Journal of Medicine, 358,* 1250–1261.

Schover, L. R., Fouladi, R. T., Warneke, C. L., et al. (2002). Defining sexual outcomes after treatment for localized prostate carcinoma. *Cancer, 95,* 1773–1785.

Shabsigh, R., Klein, L. T., Seidman, S., Kaplan, S. A., Lehrhoff, B. J., & Ritter, J. S. (1998). Increased incidence of depressive symptoms in men with erectile dysfunction. *Urology, 52,* 848–852.

Shiri, R., Koskimäki, J., Tammela, T. L., Häkkinen, J., Auvinen, A., & Hakama, M. (2007). Bidirectional relationship between depression and erectile dysfunction. *Journal of Urology, 177,* 669–673.

Sims, J., Browning, C., Lundgren-Lindquist, B., & Kendig, H. (2011). Urinary incontinence in a community sample of older adults: Prevalence and impact on quality of life. *Disability & Rehabilitation, 33*(15–16), 1389–1398.

Skinner, E. (2007). The best treatment for high-grade T1 bladder cancer is cystectomy. *Urologic Oncology, 25,* 523–525.

Smith, A. L., Wang, P. C., Anger, J. T., et al. (2010). Correlates of urinary incontinence in community-dwelling older Latinos. *Journal of the American Geriatric Society,* Jun; *58*(6), 1170–1176.

Spitzer, M., Basaria, S., Travison, T. G., et al. (2012). Effect of testoster-one replacement on response to sildenafil citrate in men with erectile dysfunction. *Annals of Internal Medicine, 157,* 681–691.

Steginga, S., Occhipinti, S., Dunn, J., Gardiner, R. A., Heathcote, P., & Yaxley, J. (2000). The supportive care needs of men with prostate can-cer. *Psycho-Oncology, 10,* 66–75.

Timilshina, N., Breunis, H., & Alibhai, S. (2012). Impact of androgen deprivation therapy on depressive symptoms in men with nonmeta-static prostate cancer. *Cancer, 118*(7), 1940–1945.

Traish, A. M., Hassani, J., Guay, A. T., Zitzmann, M., & Hansen, M. L. (2011). Adverse side effects of 5α-reductase inhibitors ther-apy: Persistent diminished libido and erectile dysfunction and depression in a subset of patients. *Journal of Sexual Medicine,* Mar; *8*(3), 872–884.

Traish, A. M., Miner, M. M., Morgentaler, A., & Zitzmann, M. (2011). Testosterone deficiency. *American Journal of Medicine,* Jul; *124*(7), 578–587.

Trask, P., Paterson, A. G., Fardig, J., & Smith, D. C. (2003). Course of distress and quality of life in testicular cancer patients before, during, and after chemotherapy: Results of a pilot study. *Psycho-Oncology, 12*(8), 814–820.

Tsakiris, P., Oelke, M., & Michel, M. C. (2008). Drug-induced urinary incontinence. *Drugs & Aging, 25,* 541–549.

Wang, Y., Corr, J. G., Thaler, H. T., et al. (1995). Decreased growth of established human prostate LNCaP tumors in nude mice fed a low-fat diet. *Journal of the National Cancer Institute, 87,* 1456–1462.

Warren, J. W., van de Merwe, J. P., & Nickel, J. C. (2011). Interstitial cystitis/bladder pain syndrome and nonbladder syndromes: Facts and hypotheses. *Urology, 78,* 727–732.

Watkins, K. E., Eberhart, N., Hilton, L., et al. (2011). Depressive disorders and panic attacks in women with bladder pain syndrome/interstitial cystitis: a population-based sample. *General Hospital Psychiatry, 33*(2), 143–149.

Webber, R. (2005). Benign prostatic hyperplasia. *Clinical Evidence,* Dec; (14), 1076–1091.

Wei, J. T., Calhoun, E., & Jacobsen, S. J. (2005). Urologic Diseases in America Project: Benign prostatic hyperplasia. *Journal of Urology,* Apr; *173*(4), 1256–1261.

Wilhelm, S. M., Lee, J., & Prinz, R. A. (2004). Major depression due to primary hyperparathyroidism: A frequent and correctable disorder. *American Surgeon,* Feb; *70*(2), 175–179; discussion, 179–180.

Wilt, T., MacDonald, R., Rutks, I., Shamliyan, T. A., Taylor, B. C., & Kane, R. L. (2008). Systematic review: Comparative effectiveness and harms of treatments for clinically localized prostate cancer. *Annals of Internal Medicine, 148,* 435–448.

Wright, J., & Porter, M. P. (2007). Quality-of-life assessment in patients with bladder cancer. *Nature Clinical Practice Urology, 4,* 147–154.

Zarrouf, F. A., Artz, S., Griffith, J., Sirbu, C., & Kommor, M. (2009). Testosterone and depression: Systematic review and meta-analysis. *Journal of Psychiatric Practice, 15*(4), 289–305.

77.

PSYCHOSOCIAL ASPECTS OF UPPER EXTREMITY ILLNESS AND OTHER ORTHOPEDIC PROBLEMS

Ana-Maria Vranceanu, David Ring, and Donna B. Greenberg

INTRODUCTION

This chapter discusses the psychological, sociological and behavioral aspects of orthopedic problems, with particular emphasize on hand and arm illness in orthopedic surgical practices. This chapter emphasizes a biopsychosocial rather than biomedical approach to how pain is conceptualized, assessed, and treated. The biopsychosocial approach specifies the relationship between physical and psychosocial factors in the etiology and maintenance of pain conditions, with an understanding that the relative importance of these factors varies across time and individuals.

The psychosocial aspects of illness usually manifest in the difference between disease, nociception, and impairment on one hand, and illness, pain, and disability on the other hand. Before proceeding, it is important to clarify how we are using several terms: *disease* versus *illness, nociception* versus *pain*, and *impairment* versus *disability.*

Disease is defined as an "objective biological event" that involves disruption of specific body structures or organ systems caused by pathological, anatomical, or physiological changes (Mechanic, 1986). Impairment is an "objective loss of function" positively correlated with the magnitude of the biological event. Nociception entails stimulation of nerves that convey information about tissue damage to the brain.

In contrast, illness is defined as a "subjective experience or self-attribution" that a disease is present (Turk, 1999); this leads to physical discomfort, emotional distress, behavioral limitations, and psychosocial disruption. Illness is thus how the sick person as well as the social network and perhaps the society perceive, live with, and respond to physical symptoms. Disability is the effect of this subjective experience. Pain is the subjective perception that results from the modulation of the sensory input filtered through a person's genetic makeup, prior learning history, and current physiological status, appraisals, expectations, mood and sociocultural factors.

The psychosocial aspects of illness are often considered "all or none" (dichotomous); for instance, a patient might say, "You think it's all in my head." The fact is that illness, pain, and disability are not dichotomous, and neither are the psychosocial and behavioral aspects of illness. They occur on a continuum between adaptation, resiliency, and maintained function in spite of substantial impairment on one hand, and disproportionate complaints and disability with little or no objective impairment on the other. Beyond the underlying pathophysiology or disease, the illness encompasses the complex human reaction to injury and illness. Illness, disability, and pain are always interactive, mind/body events.

DEPRESSION, PAIN CATASTROPHIZING, AND HEALTH ANXIETY

Consistent with findings in patients with chronic pain throughout the body, the most common psychosocial factors that influence reported pain intensity and disability are depression, pain catastrophizing, negative pain thoughts, and heightened illness concerns (Pincus et al., 2002). Previously well-compensated psychosocial factors may become problematic when one is confronted with pain. For instance, a person who tends to worry about minor matters may develop *pain catastrophizing* (a tendency to magnify the pain experience, to feel helpless when thinking about pain, and to ruminate on the pain experience). Someone who has a tendency to worry about his health may start viewing a benign pain condition as a sign of serious pathology, and may have a difficult time internalizing reassurances that his condition is benign (*heightened illness-concern, health anxiety,* or *hypochondriasis*). A depressed patient may make internal ("It's my fault"), global ("Everything is going wrong"), and stable ("I will never get over this") attributions about the pain conditions. Pain may exacerbate a predisposition toward *depression*, may intensify an already existent depression, or may become a somatic focus for depressive symptoms (Dersch et al., 2007). A tendency toward negative thinking and appraisal of life situations may translate into a similar appraisal of the pain condition. All of this may convert into reports of increased pain and disability.

Several measures have been developed for assessing these aspects of illness, and some are specific for pain. These are Likert-type scales, asking specific questions about the construct assessed. Depression is most often assessed with the Center for the Epidemiologic Study of Depression scale (CESD; Radloff, 1977), the Beck Depression Inventory (BDI; Beck et al., 1961), or the Depression Subscale of the Patient Health Questionnaire (PHQ; Spitzer et al., 1999). These measures inquire about typical symptoms of depression, and they vary in terms of the relative emphasis on the somatic or cognitive components of depression. While major depression is a discrete, all-or-none diagnosis, these scales measure depressive traits or symptoms along the continuous spectrum on which they actually occur and affect illness behavior.

Pain catastrophizing is assessed with the Pain Catastrophizing Scale (PCS; Sullivan et al., 1985), a 13-item measure with three subscales: magnification (e.g., "I become afraid that pain may get worse"), helplessness (e.g., "It is awful and I feel that it overwhelms me"), and rumination (e.g., "I can't seem to keep it out of my mind"). Pain catastrophizing is one of the strongest predictors of pain intensity and disability across a variety of pain conditions.

Health anxiety can be assessed with the Health Anxiety Inventory (Salkovskis et al., 2002), the Whitley Index (Pilovsky, 1967), and the Somatic Symptoms Inventory (SSI; Barsky et al., 1992). The SSI inquires about the extent to which patients experience certain bodily functions (e.g., nausea and vomiting, hot or cold spells, heart pounding, heavy arms). The Health Anxiety Inventory and Whitley Index comprise questions assessing the extent to which patients endorse cognitive aspects of health anxiety (e.g., "Do you worry about your health?" "Do you often worry about the possibility that you have a serious illness?"). Health anxiety and hypochondriasis are increasingly recognized correlates of pain intensity and disability in chronic pain conditions.

The use of these validated measures may facilitate addressing these sensitive topics. According to the model developed in other fields, these issues may be best addressed within multidisciplinary teams, where the various health providers (surgeons, non-operative providers such as physiatrists, certified hand therapists, and behavioral medicine specialists/psychologists) work as a team with unified treatment goals. Such multidisciplinary treatment teams have been successful in the treatment of several pain conditions (Jensen, 1994). When such teams are not available, it is important to pursue communication among members of patients' care team as means of improving overall care and decreasing confusion.

SECONDARY-GAIN ISSUES

Secondary gain describes external psychological motivating factors for the initiation or perpetuation of painful symptoms. The patient may or may not be consciously aware of these psycho-emotional motivating factors.

Early psychodynamic theories described secondary gain as responsible for the repression of emotional issues and development of psychosomatic pain. More current theories follow a cognitive-behavioral approach and emphasize secondary gain as a social-learning model where environmental external factors are reinforcing chronicity. For example, a doting spouse, escape from a stressful job, or sympathy from family and friends may all reinforce chronicity. Within this new framework, the term "unconscious" means unawareness or a lack of a conscious plan for the gain. The term "unconscious" thus means the patient is unaware that the loss of holding onto the condition is often far greater than the perceived gain.

The patients may or may not realize the benefits of secondary gain, but they do not consciously cause it to be. This is not the same phenomenon as a patient who pretends to be sick or exaggerates a condition on purpose, in order to gain a particular objective (e.g., malingering), though conscious malingering and unconsciously seeking the benefits of illness represent extremes of the continuum of secondary gain.

Fordyce (1976), the founder of the social-learning theory model of pain, believed that pain is behavior designed to protect oneself or solicit aid; as the pain increases, this behavior is strengthened when it is followed by desirable consequences. Fordyce argued that if pain persisted beyond the normal healing time in an environment with secondary gains, the pain would become chronic. He gave as examples of secondary gains, or "desirable consequences" of pain, the following factors: attention and sympathy from family, friends, and physicians; release from task responsibilities at home and at work; narcotic medications; and monetary compensation. Unfortunately, patients are not sufficiently mindful of the undesirable consequences of these behaviors, such as anger and rejection by family and friends when they get tired of having to take on the patient's daily tasks and are exasperated about the failure to get well; frustration with complicated bureaucracy; increased physical suffering due to chronic narcotic use and dependency; unpleasant side effects with medication; and constant bitter battles for disability benefits during which the patient must take on and even exaggerate the sick role. An open discussion of the issues raised by secondary gain and discussion of the long-term consequences can greatly contribute to healing, and can prevent the development of chronic symptoms and disability.

PSYCHOLOGICAL FACTORS FAMILIAR TO PSYCHOLOGISTS AND PSYCHIATRISTS

Psychosocial factors are particularly important when a patient's problem is puzzling (non-characteristic, non-anatomical, or disproportionately symptomatic and disabling) and the examination and diagnostic procedures are inconclusive or contradictory (Ring et al., 2005; Vranceanu et al., 2008).

UPPER EXTREMITY ILLNESS

In this section, we discuss psychiatric diagnoses and puzzling hand and arm conditions—conditions that are instructive of the interrelationship between medical and psychological factors—from factitious disorders, where medical symptoms are consciously produced; to somatic symptom and related disorders, where normal bodily symptoms are amplified via cognitive processes.

Factitious Disorders

Factitious disorders are conditions in which a person acts as if he or she has an illness by deliberately producing, feigning, or exaggerating symptoms. There is a motivation to assume the sick role and an absence of external incentives (Diagnostic and Statistical Manual of Mental Disorders; DMS-IV, 2000). Patients may lie about or fake symptoms, hurt themselves to bring on symptoms, or even alter diagnostic tests (such as contaminating a urine sample). People might be motivated to perpetrate factitious disorders either as patients or by proxy as caregivers to gain any of a variety of benefits, including attention, nurturance, sympathy, and leniency, that are perceived as otherwise unobtainable (Eisendrath, 1984). Patients with factitious disorders deny responsibility, yet they deliberately injure themselves to fulfill psychological needs, sometimes without regard to economic or social gain (Kasdan et al., 1998; Guziec & Harding, 1994).

Patients with upper-extremity problems rarely meet diagnostic criteria for a factitious disorder. On the other hand, patients can present with elements of a factitious disorder, which can sometimes occur in the context of a clear medical condition. Factitious disorders are on "a spectrum of consciously simulated disease, ranging from occasional falsification of disease—perhaps in the midst of stress—to the repetitive presentation of exaggerated or false symptoms and conscious production of signs."

Clenched Fist Syndrome

The *clenched fist* is a condition wherein the arm is healthy, but all or one, two, or three fingers are tightly flexed. Often, the index finger and thumb are not involved, thereby allowing the patient useful hand function. The concept of the "clenched fist syndrome" is controversial, with some including it as a factitious disorder, while others see it as a conversion disorder, acknowledging that the motivation and source of this condition may be unconscious (Zeinch, 2008). In the short term, the diagnosis can be confirmed by a hand surgeon by anesthetizing the extremity or the patient and demonstrating the absence of fixed contracture, but in long-standing cases, fixed contracture can develop. A variation on this theme is the stiff index finger that "won't bend" except under anesthesia.

Factitious Lymphedema and Unexplained Swelling

Unexplained swelling of the hand or arm may be a result of the patient's surreptitious application of a tourniquet to the extremity. Examples of tight bands that may be used include an Ace bandage, a sphygmomanometer cuff, a rubber band, or a piece of string. Placing the extremity in a plaster cast allows the swelling to subside and prevents further application of the constricting band.

Many conditions may cause edema of the limb. However, with factitious lymphedema caused by intermittent application of a tourniquet, a so-called broken windowpane pattern of collateral lymphatic circulation distal to the site of tourniquet obstruction is seen. Ruptured lymph channels due to recurrent lymph stasis and direct constriction may also be seen. The size and distribution of the lymphatics is normal, however. There is no abnormality of the lymph nodes (Moretta & Cooley, 2002).

Self-Inflicted Wounds and Wound Manipulation

Voluntary, self-inflicted wounds often have an obvious origin. Cigarette burns, stab wounds, subcutaneous injection of feces and other noxious substances, and even bite wounds are seen in these patients. The clinician must discriminate between the *deliberately* self-inflicted wound and the *accidentally* self-inflicted wound in patients with other types of mental problems, such as the hand that is damaged by accidental intra-arterial injection by a drug addict.

Self-Cutting

Self-cutting is rare but can be quite spectacular, with dozens, sometimes hundreds, of lacerations or scars on the forearms and hands. The lacerations usually involve only the epidermis but occasionally are deeper. The wounds are usually longitudinal or oblique and are most commonly on the dorsum of the hand and forearm. Self-cutting is common in patients with a borderline personality disorder, and is usually conceptualized as means of coping with intense psychological pain as well as the need for attention (DSM, 2000).

Secretan's Syndrome

Secretan's syndrome (also known as peritendinous fibrosis, post-traumatic hard edema, and factitious lymphedema) is a condition caused by the patient's repeatedly striking the dorsum of the hand with a blunt object or against a blunt object, causing diffuse swelling as a result of a peritendinous fibrosis of the extensor tendons. The literature suggests that Secretan's disease is an injury that is self-inflicted, either for secondary gain or as a conversion reaction, and that it is best treated with conservative care and psychiatric counseling (Moretta & Cooley, 2002).

Munchausen Syndrome

Patients with *Munchausen syndrome* present themselves as sufferers of all sorts of symptoms and ailments involving any and all parts of the body, including the hand. They often have a long history of many illnesses and treatments, including multiple operations. They are often migratory, going from one medical facility after another, giving detailed histories of specific ailments and begging for yet another operation. These people are generally well read in the medical literature and often know more about the ailment they are projecting than does the physician they are consulting. When found out, they simply transfer their medical attentions to another part of the country. The patient who has had multiple carpal tunnel operations may well be a variant of this condition.

SHAFT Syndrome

Patients with *SHAFT syndrome* (sad, hostile, anxious, frustrating, and tenacious) have pain as a typical complaint, usually without objective physical findings that would support a more definitive diagnosis. Patients with the SHAFT syndrome attempt to manipulate the surgeon to perform one or more invasive procedures, despite the lack of objective findings, and without relief of symptoms.

Ten criteria were identified that characterized the medical and psychosocial factors common to patients with SHAFT syndrome: multiple invasive procedures, absence of objective findings, multiple physicians, medications (psychotropic and analgesic), psychiatric treatment, a history of being off work, disproportionate self-characterization and verbalization of symptoms, history of crying with pain, family history of disability, and history of abuse (emotional, physical, or sexual) (Johnson, 1998).

Somatic Symptom Disorders and Related Disorders

The somatic symptom disorders are conditions wherein the presence of physical symptoms suggests a medical condition, but the symptoms are not fully explained by disease (pathophysiology) or by another mental disorder. Historically, the disorders included in this category were: pain disorder, somatization disorder, conversion disorder, and hypochondriasis (DSM, 2000). These terms still highlight prominent features in the presentation of what has been lumped together as *Somatic symptom disorders* in DSM-V (DSM-V, 2013).

Pain disorder called attention to the patient whose pain, acute or chronic, is the predominant focus of the clinical presentation, when the pain causes substantial disability and distress, and when psychological factors are judged to have an important role in the onset, severity, exacerbation, or maintenance of the pain (DSM, 2000). In DSM-V, the patient would have *Somatic symptom disorder with predominant pain*. Pain disorders had been the most common psychiatric diagnosis in patients with pain, with prevalence rates as high as 97% in some samples of post-injury, chronic low-back pain patients in an inpatient rehabilitation setting.

Somatization disorder was *a* diagnosis in patients with multiple somatic symptoms—including digestive, sexual, and neurological symptoms in addition to pain—that could not be explained by a physical disorder. While somatization is common among patients with chronic pain, few patients met the full diagnostic criteria for the classification of *Somatization disorder*. The process of somatization is currently conceptualized as involving the focusing of attention on internal stimuli and development of "sensory amplification" (Barsky & Klerman, 1992), along with denial of psychological or interpersonal difficulties (Osteweis et al., 1987), resulting in an increase in somatic symptoms that remain partly or completely unexplained by objective disease processes.

In DSM-V, it is the maladaptive thoughts, feelings, and behaviors that define the somatic symptom disorder and subsume many patients who would have been diagnosed with somatization disorder. It includes the many patients who did not quite meet the old criteria.

Hypochondriasis historically represented a preoccupation with fears of having, or the idea that one has, a serious disease, based on a misinterpretation of bodily symptoms. This preoccupation persists despite appropriate medical evaluation and reassurance

Only a small number of hand and arm patients met full criteria for hypochondriasis when it was a distinct diagnostic category. However, a larger number present with heightened illness-concern or health anxiety, which are less severe, yet distressing, conditions in which patient's concern with a medical or perceived medical condition is exaggerated and consuming. It is important to note that most people are affected and concerned by the presence of pain. However, the majority readily accept reassurance with regard to their pain symptoms, and are able to put their worries at rest if told that their condition is not dangerous or severe. In patients with heightened illness-concern (and its extreme form, hypochondriasis), no amount of reassurance is enough, and patients continue to believe that the doctors "missed" something. Recent research supports the theory that heightened illness-concern is an important mechanism for the development of chronic pain conditions (Hadjistavropolus & Hadjistavropolus, 2003). In DSM-V, "hypochondriasis" has been eliminated as a disorder, and those with high illness anxiety without somatic symptoms would receive a diagnosis of *Illness anxiety disorder.*

Conversion disorder or *Functional neurologic symptom disorder* are diagnosed when one or more distressing deficits affecting voluntary or sensory function are internally inconsistent and incompatible with known organic physiology. Psychological factors are judged to be associated with the symptoms or deficits because the initiation or exacerbation of the symptoms or deficits is preceded by conflicts or other stressors. Conversion disorders are rare in pain patients. However, patients may present with symptoms of a conversion disorder, such as the sudden onset of arm weakness, and perhaps the inability to lift their hand, which is found to have no medical explanation.

Puzzling Pain Problems

Many illness constructs used by hand specialists and currently described in the literature as purely medical (based on a biomedical framework) have minimal or no objective, verifiable pathology, and—as research is increasingly demonstrating—strong psychosocial correlates. A biopsychosocial behavioral approach may be more appropriate in conceptualizing and treating these conditions.

Repetitive strain injury—also known as *writer's cramp, cumulative trauma disorder, occupational overuse syndrome,* and *work-related upper-limb disorder* among other terms—is an unverifiable diagnosis (essentially, it is a "social illness" construct, which is defined as a term "invented" or "constructed" by our culture and society, which exists because people agree to behave as if it exists) diagnosed on the basis of chronic activity-associated pain, typically in an upper limb. Although the "illness" construct implies injury or damage, an important characteristic of this diagnosis is that there are no objective signs of damage or disease. The illness is entirely subjective, and there are no objective tests to verify the diagnosis.

There are several unverifiable pain conditions that are accepted illness constructs within hand surgery and medicine, including radial tunnel syndrome, pronator syndrome; as well as electrophysiologically normal thoracic outlet, carpal tunnel, and cubital tunnel syndromes; not to mention dynamic scapholunate instability, occult dorsal ganglion, and so forth. These debatable and unverifiable conditions are similar to other nonspecific conditions (Szabo & King, 1999) such as fibromyalgia and chronic fatigue syndrome, which are often comorbid.

The nomenclature of these illness constructs is somewhat troubling, as it implies an understanding of the pathophysiology and a known physical basis where one is, by definition, lacking. It is recognized, but underappreciated, that chronic nonspecific arm pain is comorbid with depression, health anxiety, pain catastrophizing, and somatization, which are perhaps the only clear targets of intervention in the absence of verifiable and treatable objective pathology.

From a biopsychosocial perspective, patients with repetitive strain injury (RSI) can also be conceptualized as presenting with features of conversion disorder, heightened illness-concern, and somatic symptom disorder. There may also be distress in the form of anxiety and depression. Perhaps a biopsychosocial approach that considers both medical and psychological factors should replace the purely medical focus that currently hinders comprehensive management of these illnesses. In this way, unnecessary medical procedures can be avoided, and psychological distress can be addressed, thus increasing patients' quality of life and functioning. While some state that these medical labels serve the patient's need to emphasize the physical rather than the psychosocial or somatoform aspect of their illness (Barsky, 1992; Hadler, 2003), and thus avoid stigmatization, the benefit of these diagnoses is short-lived. In the long run, a focus on a purely medical condition and the administration of numerous tests and medical procedures act to reinforce a sick role, and do not address core issues such as acceptance, adaptation, and resiliency. No matter the advances to come in medicine, illness will always be a part of human existence, and effective coping skills will improve ability, wellness, and peace of mind.

Complex regional pain syndromes (CRPS) represent another puzzling, chronically painful condition (Nelson & Novy, 1996), with little epidemiological information, a lack of understanding of their natural course or basic pathophysiology, and lack of agreement even on definition and diagnostic criteria (Nelson & Novy, 1999). The most up-to-date definition of CRPS currently adopted by the International Association for the Study of Pain (IASP) reflects the evolution of the controversies over the concepts of *reflex sympathetic dystrophy, sympathetically maintained pain,* and *sympathetically independent pain,* and attempts to provides a definition focused on a description without any presumption as to underlying mechanisms. The current nomenclature reflects the complexity of this condition, the regional distribution of symptoms (which mostly affect the hands), and the cardinal symptom of pain. Two types of disorders are included in this category: (1) CRPS I, where pain follows injury, and involves continued pain, hypersensitivity, or allodynia, and there is evidence of edema or abnormal sudomotor activity; and (2) CRPS II, which has similar criteria but it implies a known nerve injury, but is, however, not limited to the distribution of the particular nerve (Stanton-Hicks et al., 1995).

These diagnostic criteria have been strongly criticized as being too vague, thereby allowing for over-diagnosis (Galer et al., 2001). Furthermore, the pathogenesis of this disorder is unclear, failing to explain why only a small percent of patients develop CRPS after an injury or well-defined nerve injury while the majority do not, whether there is there a genetic predisposition, and why such a significant variability among the different symptom classes of abnormalities is seen in patients with CRPS.

There is general agreement that many patients with CRPS manifest important and profound behavioral and emotional issues (Lynch, 1992), as well as reports of intense pain and severe disability. There is also some evidence that depression, anxiety, and life stressors (frequently reported as present in CRPS patients) might influence the development of this condition through alpha-adrenaline activity. Van Houdenhove and colleagues (1992) articulated a conceptualization suggesting the role of hyper-arousal due to life stress or other factors preceding, or around the time of, injury or during the subsequent initial period of healing, and having difficulties coping (van Houdenhove et al., 1992). CRPS is seen as overlapping with several conditions, including neuromas and phantom limb pain. The key element in all these conditions is that pain is considered "sympathetically maintained."

Neuromas are chronic pain conditions that, if severe enough, may severely curtail any useful function of the hand. Surgical management of painful neuromas has not been as effective as we might wish.

Phantom limb pain is a clinical condition in which patients experience pain in a limb after amputation. A "phantom limb" is the sensation that an amputated or missing limb (even an organ, like the appendix) is still attached to the body and is moving appropriately with other body parts (Halligan & Berger, 1999; Halligan, 2002; Halbert & Crotty, 2002). Approximately 50–80% of individuals with an amputation experience phantom sensations in their amputated limb, and the majority of the sensations are painful (Melzack, 1992). Phantom limb sensations usually will disappear or decrease over time. When phantom limb pain continues for more than six months, the prognosis for spontaneous improvement is poor, and pain can become disabling and can lead to a lifelong struggle with chronic pain. Research has found that, among other factors, pain and psychiatric distress in the form of depression, anxiety, and somatization are predictors of persistence of phantom limb pain (Tota-Faucette et al., 1993; Turk & Monarch, 1999).

OTHER PSYCHOSOCIAL ASPECTS OF ILLNESS

Cognitive processes, behaviors, affective states, and coping styles, along with sociocultural factors, are as important as or more important than biological factors in management of chronic pain conditions. The role of cognitive processes is predicated upon the evidence that people are not passive responders to physical sensations. Rather, humans are actively seeking to make sense of their experiences. They appraise their conditions by matching sensations to some preexisting implicit cognitive schema and determine whether a particular sensation is a symptom of a particular disorder that requires attention, or can be ignored. In this way, each person functions with a uniquely constructed reality. When information is ambiguous, people rely on general attitudes and beliefs based on experiences, prior learning history, or input from family and friends. These beliefs determine the meaning and significance of the problem, as well as the perceptions of the appropriate treatment. As such, an understanding of each person's unique beliefs about pain, appraisals, and coping repertoire becomes critical for treatment success. A great body of research shows that patients' attitudes, beliefs, expectations, and coping resources are key in reports of pain intensity and disability (DeGood & Tait, 2001; Jensen et al., 1991).

Beliefs about pain may lead to maladaptive coping, increased suffering, exacerbation of pain, and greater disability. For example, pain that is interpreted as tissue damage rather than viewed as a problem that will improve may lead to more suffering and dysfunction. Also, patients who believe that their pain will last forever may take a fatalistic, passive approach to coping. Beliefs about the implications of diseases are also important. People high in health anxiety may interpret pain as a sign of a serious disease (e.g., a benign cyst is interpreted as cancer despite medical reassurance) and have more disability and more intense pain. People who attribute a pain flare-up to a worsening of tissue damage may experience more pain and disability. Cognitive factors thus affect functioning in two interrelated ways: (1) they influence mood and coping efforts, and (2) they affect physiological activity associated with pain, such as muscle tension (Flor & Turk, 1985) and the production of endogenous chemicals (Bandura et al., 1987).

Self-efficacy, or the belief in one's ability to successfully achieve a desired outcome, is another cognitive factor that strongly predicts success in coping with pain and reducing disability. Greater self-efficacy leads to reduced anxiety and its physiological component, an increased ability to use distraction as a coping strategy, increased determination to go on with planned activity in spite of pain, and avoidance of rumination on the pain.

In addition to specific self-efficacy beliefs, a number of investigators have suggested that a common set of "cognitive errors" affects the perception of pain, affective distress, and disability (Smith et al., 1986, 1990). A *cognitive error* is a negatively distorted belief about oneself or one's situation. The most common cognitive errors in pain patients are catastrophizing (rumination, magnification, and helplessness when faced with pain), overgeneralization (assumption that the impact of an event [negative] will apply to outcomes of future or similar events), personalization (interpreting negative events as reflecting personal meaning or responsibility), and selective abstractions (selectively attending to negative aspects of an experience).

Self-regulation of pain and its impact depend on a person's specific ways of dealing with pain, adjusting to pain, and reducing or minimizing the distress caused by the pain, which represent a set of coping strategies. Studies have found that active coping strategies, such as efforts to function in spite of pain or to distract oneself from pain, or ignoring pain, are associated with adaptive functioning, while passive coping strategies, such as depending on others for help in pain control, or letting pain dictate and restrict activity level, are related to greater pain and depression (Tota-Faucette et al., 1993; Lawson et al., 1990).

The *affective component* of pain includes many different emotions, but they are primarily negative in quality.

Depression is the most common diagnoses associated with pain and it is significantly associated with coping. That is, those who believe that they can continue to function in spite of pain do not become depressed, while those who engage in negative thinking are low in self-efficacy and are high in health anxiety and more likely to become depressed. Anxiety in the form of pain-related fear and concerns about harm-avoidance exacerbate pain symptoms. Anxiety's cognitive (uncertainty, misperceptions of danger) and physiological (bodily changes triggered by the fight-or-flight system) symptoms are common when people experience pain, and they have a strong association with disability and pain intensity (Vlayen et al., 1995). Post-traumatic stress disorder (PTSD) is a subtype of anxiety that can sometimes develop in people with pain triggered by traumatic injuries, and it has a strong relationship with disability and pain chronicity. Anger has also been observed in patients with pain. Anger can take the form of frustrations related to the persistence of symptoms, lack of etiology, treatment failures, worker's compensation, finances, and family relations. Anger may affect pain via biological (increased arousal) mechanisms, and may interfere with pain acceptance and adherence to treatment. As previously discussed, health anxiety and somatization are also commonplace in pain patients.

Common-sense beliefs about illness and healthcare providers are also highly influenced by prior experience and social and cultural transmission of beliefs and expectations across generations. Ethnic group and gender differences influence beliefs about pain and responses to pain. Social factors influence how families and communities respond to and interact with patients. For example, children acquire attitudes about health and health care, perceptions and interpretation of symptoms, and appropriate responses to injury from their parents, cultural stereotypes, and social environment. These influences will determine whether they will ignore or overreact to symptoms.

People's behaviors when experiencing pain (e.g., pain behaviors) are additional factors that affect their experience with pain, pain intensity, disability, and chronicity. Operant conditioning posits that behaviors that are reinforced are maintained, and those that are not reinforced are stopped. The operant view (Fordyce, 1976) proposes that via external contingencies of reinforcement, behaviors such as grimaces to communicate pain, or holding an arm in order to avoid additional pain, are maintained if reinforced by a doting spouse or healthcare provider. They may also be maintained by the escape from noxious stimulation through the use of drugs, rest, or avoidance of undesirable activities like work. Avoiding activities can thus serve as a reinforcer maintaining the pain.

In acute pain, reducing an activity may accelerate the healing process. However, repetitively engaging in avoidance of activity leads to anticipatory anxiety about pain (e.g., muscle tension and other symptoms associated with fight-or-flight or sympathetic activation), which may act as a conditioned stimulus for pain, which may be maintained after healing ends. Over time, more and more activities are perceived as aversive and are avoided. This may lead to deconditioning and more injuries and pain problems as a result.

Persistent avoidance of activities also prevents disconfirmation of the predicted pain. This is a common mechanism in the etiology, maintenance, and generalization of most anxiety disorders, and it has good applications for pain. Pain avoidance succeeds thus in preserving the *belief* that pain will continue when engaging in an activity, and would prevent a corrective *experience* that pain will eventually subside with activity.

There are also more subtle, yet potent factors that impact the pain experience. Internet and media shape patient's beliefs about pain and medical treatments. Television advertisements about cures for pain conditions via miracle drugs or intervention, without data to back up their efficacy; advertisements about avoiding aging that reinforce a desire to stay forever young and fight rather than accept normal age-related degenerations; magazine articles that mislead patients into changing their doctor if their pain is not taken away, all promote a "patient's right" to be pain-free—which is misguided and more likely to detract from than enhance health and wellness.

MULTIDISCIPLINARY
TREATMENT TEAMS

Multidisciplinary treatment teams that consider the psychosocial as well as the biomedical aspects of illness have proven useful in the management of the most common idiopathic pain conditions, including backache and headache (Bruce et al., 2008; Flor et al., 1992; Gatchel, 2006), as well as more discrete pain conditions such as arthritis (Keefe et al., 1990). These teams typically include surgeons, physiatrists and other non-operative care providers, occupational therapists, medical assistants, and behavioral medicine specialists (i.e., psychologists). The role of each provider depends on the individual patient's presentation.

Although many hand and arm pains are poorly understood or incompletely treatable, and psychosocial factors such as depression and anxiety often exacerbate discrete pain conditions, hand surgeons and hand therapists have been slow to implement multidisciplinary treatment teams. Instead, they continue to operate largely under a biomedical model of illness, potentially neglecting prominent and treatable psychosocial factors. In spite of scientific support for the unique contribution of psychologists to the understanding of the multifactorial nature of pain (Simon & Folen, 2001), as well as recommendations from governing bodies such as the Joint Commission on the Accreditation of Health Care (JACHO) and the Commission on the Accreditation of Rehabilitation Facilities (CARF), and several professional organizations (American Pain Society, American Academy of Neurology), the psychiatrist or psychologist's role is underappreciated, seen as potentially offensive, and is currently undervalued by patients, health providers, and insurers. A multidisciplinary approach to the treatment of hand and arm pain conditions is consistent with evidence-based practice and fits well within the patient-centered model of medical decision-making. Having more than one listener allows the patient to feel cared for, as there is a team of doctors and therapists, rather than

one, attending to the pain concern. This may increase the patient's confidence that nothing is overlooked and all possibilities for increasing wellness are considered.

The gap between the utility and the utilization of a multidisciplinary treatment team is at least partly due to the difficulty communicating the value of a biopsychosocial approach to illness to patients and their healthcare providers. This gap itself represents an example of the need for good communication in the integration and practice of evidence-based medicine and patient-centered care. The quest for best evidence necessitates input that is more multilayered and considers myriad possibilities, reflecting less tissue-focused specificity and greater richness and breadth than the historically valued reductionist approach associated with the biomedical model. Treating illness, not just disease, requires that various aspects of the patient's situation be addressed, even though these factors may be ambiguous or contradictory. It requires more involvement of our patients, increasing their empowerment. This is best implemented by a multidisciplinary team through treatment processes that value and embrace effective communication skills.

MODEL OF CARE—RECOMMENDATIONS
FOR ORTHOPEDIC HAND SPECIALISTS

A large body of research shows that the first visit to an orthopedics department, where patients are initially referred or present for treatment, is a strong predictor of the course of illness in pain patients (Malmivaara & Hakkinen, 1995).

At the first visit, patients need a thorough medical evaluation, including examination, review of available tests, and reassurance that nothing is neglected and no opportunities for improvement in the physical condition are or will be overlooked. The multidisciplinary approach to treatment needs to be emphasized to patients, as means of addressing the interrelation between mind and body and improving their quality of life. Patients need room to answer questions, provide feedback, and participate in the decision-making process. Often first visits are uneventful, diagnoses are easily made, and patients are able to follow recommendations. However, there are situations in which psychosocial factors are prominent.

There are many situations when patients with a discrete pain condition amenable to medical interventions present with depressed mood, misconceptions about pain and medical treatment, and psychosocial stressors. Hand specialists should be aware of warning signs such as flat affect, squeamishness about pain, complaints of poor sleep and frustration, fear of activity or of returning to work, which should not be ignored. It is in these situations that a behavioral medicine intervention would be particularly helpful, as patients work to improve important psychosocial issues along with their medical care. When surgeons introduce mind–body concepts to patients, normalize them, and offer services immediately in their office—as opposed to referrals elsewhere, which are rarely followed through—patients feel cared for and are more accepting of psychological help.

When the patient presentation is puzzling and does not fit within specific medical diagnosis categories, hand specialists will benefit from keeping an open mind about alternatives to a purely medical cause of the condition. Given the challenge of living with chronic unexplained symptoms, the behavioral medicine specialist has a key role. It is important to mention that, although surgeons need to be honest about their findings, they need to be careful not to dichotomize mind–body issues or suggest in any way that symptoms are conscious or unconsciously produced (e.g., factitious disorder or conversion disorder). In such cases, as in the cases of heightened illness-concern and somatization, a better approach is to schedule additional appointments aimed to provide additional reassurance to patients, while reinforcing the need to work with the behavioral medicine specialist on improving their quality of life.

Regardless of the degree of medical pathology, reassurance from the hand specialist is particularly important, given that patients came to the surgical practice to receive medical care. In the absence of empathy and effective communication and reassurance, patients may feel that their pain is not taken seriously, and become frustrated and upset. Comments such as, "Although there is pain, structurally you are intact—there may be some misconceptions here that we can help improve upon in order to increase your sense of wellness"; "Some cars have squeaky brakes, but they are safe to drive; your wrist has pain, but it is a healthy wrist"; or "You do need surgery, but let's get you sleeping better and in a better disposition first," can reassure patients that their pain is taken seriously. With idiopathic pain conditions, it is particularly helpful to schedule additional regular appointments to ensure that nothing will be overlooked, and increase the patient's awareness, understanding, and acceptance of chronic nonspecific conditions.

In addition, patients need advice and clear recommendations. Rather than communicating "all is fine, no restrictions in activity," try a message such as: "It is very important to move your arm to avoid stiffness and loss of range of motion. You will feel pain, but that is not a sign of damage. There are more risks associated with not moving your arm than with moving it. Do you think you can do this?"

It is important to avoid misguiding and mismanaging patients via unnecessary tests or procedures, or over-interpretation of test results. Examples include incidental or age-related findings that do not correspond with or fully explain the complaint, and cortisone shots or other treatments without an explanation that they are at best palliative and without an open discussion of their scientific basis or lack thereof. When patients ask questions about a specific time-frame for their recovery, it is critical to manage their expectations. Rather than setting a date on the calendar after which the patient and healthcare provider will be disappointed or even concerned, discuss the normal progression of disease while discussing how everyone is different, and reinforcing how the patient himself can speed up recovery with what he does, including following recommendations and keeping a positive attitude.

Because of the interrelationship between physical and psychosocial factors in the manifestation of disease, many patients will benefit from meeting with a behavioral medicine specialist for a brief consult focused on evaluating current psychosocial functioning and effective coping skills. Misconceptions about pain and medical treatments are extremely prevalent, and a short conversation about these issues is often enough to place the patient on an optimal recovery path. Based on the initial evaluation, some patients may continue to meet with the behavioral medicine specialist, while others may be well equipped for effective coping on their own. It is important that a treatment plan and a set of goals be put in place at the end of the first visit, along with a list of written recommendations that the patient can take with him. Vranceanu et al. (2009) provide a description of a multidisciplinary treatment approach for hand and arm illnesses.

PSYCHOSOCIAL ASSESSMENT AND TREATMENT

The recommended approach to psychosocial assessment and treatment is to be delivered as part of a multidisciplinary team approach integrated within the orthopedics department. Ideally, assessment is done at the first visit, in conjunction with the medical appointment. If this is not possible, a referral to a team member in the same office may be accepted more readily than a referral elsewhere. The assessment includes an interview, focused mainly on understanding the patient's disability, the value of effective coping with pain and optimal mood, as well as the reason for the visit and appropriate goals. In addition to the interview, self-report instruments can be very helpful.

Usually psychosocial assessment ends with a discussion of the disease, its natural progression, and the role of psychosocial factors. Goals for treatment are also established. Patients are also provided educational information on the cognitive-behavioral model of pain and how it might apply to the patient's problem, as well as how cognitive-behavioral therapy (CBT) works.

CBT is a well-researched, scientific treatment approach that specifies how thoughts (beliefs, attitudes), behaviors, feelings, and sensations are interrelated. As discovered through research, in many cases, pain triggers negative thoughts such as catastrophizing (rumination, magnification, helplessness), heightened illness-concern (intense worry about pain and health that is resistant to reassurance), fear-based avoidance (avoidance of activities that cause pain for fear of reinjury or causing more damage), and affective reactions that include frustration, irritability, anger, depression, and anxiety. These interactions can become self-maintaining such that distress and disability, as well as physiological arousal, may continue in spite of the absence of original sensory input; patients thus can transition into chronic pain syndromes (Sharp, 2001). A key element in CBT treatments is identifying patient's thoughts when experiencing the pain sensation. As depicted above, these thoughts are non-adaptive and associated with behavioral avoidance and emotional distress. Identifying specific negative automatic thoughts about pain and medical treatments appears thus as a crux of successful CBT for pain.

The most salient treatment issue is to help patient understand the interaction between the mind and body, normalize the situation to avoid stigmatization, and specifically show how the treatment will benefit the patient.

There are many advantages to delivering CBT in an orthopedic practice. First, addressing psychosocial factors and providing educational information early on in the experience of pain may prevent transition toward chronic pain syndromes, while improving quality of life while the pain condition takes its course. Many orthopedic pain conditions have a normal recovery course that ebbs and flows over the course of a year or more, and it is important that patients be aware of this course and learn how to cope with the pain so that they maintain their quality of life and conditioning, and do not develop complications such as stiffness or depression and anxiety. Second, CBT is delivered along with medical treatments, and appointments are scheduled at the same time, when possible, which saves patient money and time, and also allows communication and planning by the providers. Patients also feel "cared for" and do not feel that their physical complaints are being ignored. Third, in many cases, patients with clinical depression or anxiety who are in need of psychological interventions often neglect to follow up with referrals to psychiatric departments, or face long wait times. Lastly, CBT delivered in an orthopedics department can improve the efficacy of medical and surgical interventions.

It is also important to note that not all patients presenting to an orthopedics department benefit from CBT. There are many situations in which patients are resilient and cope well. There are also situations in which patients have severe pathology such as untreated severe anxiety disorders or depression, which have been present prior to pain and are exacerbated by pain. In such situations it is important to address these issues, while simultaneously working with patients on pain coping skills.

OTHER ORTHOPEDIC PROBLEMS

Building on this explanation of an integrated approach to orthopedic problems and chronic pain of the hand and arm, we will discuss the biopsychosocial elements of other orthopedic problems. These include patients who present with functional weakness of lower extremities, a conversion disorder; hip fracture; generalized musculoskeletal pain; chronic back pain; amputation; neuropathic pain; and analgesics.

FUNCTIONAL WEAKNESS OF LOWER EXTREMITIES, A CONVERSION DISORDER

Functional neurological symptoms or conversion disorder can present as leg weakness or gait disorder. Both psychic distress and issues related to disability-related state financial benefits are important elements of evaluation (Carson et al., 2011). The reliability of the classic finding "*la belle indifference*" on mental status exam has been questioned (Stone et al., 2005); some patients seem indifferent but may be trying hard to be stoic and to be taken seriously.   One series of 107 patients with

functional weakness seen by neurologists (Stone et al., 2012) were 79% female, mean age 39, with median nine months' duration of weakness. Sudden onset was noted in 46%; others presented with symptoms on waking or gradual onset. Comorbid panic (59%) and dissociative symptoms (39%) were common, and injury to the relevant limb had occurred in 20%. Non-epileptic attacks, migraine, fatigue, and sleep paralysis were also associated conditions.

Stone et al. (2005) made crisp recommendations for the interview of patients with conversion disorder seen in the medical or neurological setting as physicians consider other diagnoses. These are wise guidelines:

1. Ask about dissociation, depersonalization, de-realization, and panic attacks. Patients may refer to being "dizzy or spaced out," outside themselves, as if watching everything on television. These syndromes also occur in the setting of migraine or epilepsy.

2. In order to assess disability, ask about the course of a typical day and how much time is spent in or out of bed or away from home. Is the patient disabled by fear of falling? Think of graphing the natural course: for instance, the character of onset and severity over time in counterpoint to cessation of work, major life events or medical interventions, troubles with the law, marriage, or money.

3. Ask about what happened with previous doctors. The stories about disappointing explanations from previous doctors give the listener an opportunity to show interest in the patient's suffering and to offer information about explanations that patients are likely to reject.

4. In exploring the patient's illness beliefs, ask what the patient thinks is causing her symptoms and what should be done. Does the patient think that the problem will get better, or is there a fear of a particular illness like multiple sclerosis?

5. In looking for a model, the interviewer may find that the family history provides models of disability in people close to the patient.

6. Ask about vegetative symptoms like fatigue, poor concentration, and poor sleep first, leaving questions about emotions to the end when the somatic symptom has already been taken seriously.

7. Be cautious about exploring questions of abuse in a short medical visit. These are tender topics that are difficult to approach quickly and are better left to a separate visit. Patients with a history of trauma may have been the subjects of childhood abuse or neglect.

8. Exploration of the old records will show whether there is a history of other functional symptoms or surgery for symptoms that were not explicitly associated with documented pathology.

The physiology of severe anxiety with hyperventilation and metabolic alkalosis may provide a partial explanation of the odd sensation in the limb. Intensive psychologically oriented CBT has been effective for patients with functional symptoms who seek it (Allen et al., 2006; Escobar et al., 2007). Sharpe et al. (2011) found that CBT based on a functional explanation can be acceptable to relatively unselected neurology patients with weakness and gait disturbance, and that CBT-based guided self-help therapy improved self-reported general health in patients with functional presentations of weakness and gait disturbance. This treatment began with a workbook, one session of guidance in its use, and an approach similar to CBT for depression and anxiety. The book explained functional symptoms as changes in nervous system functioning that were influenced by psychological and behavioral factors. It included an explanation of how functional symptoms are diagnosed; a description of common symptoms and the associated anatomy, physiology, and psychology; and self-management techniques such as ways to reduce unhelpful thinking and increase coping with these symptoms. Four half-hour sessions over three months were given face-to-face (by telephone if the patient was unable to attend the hospital) by a nurse or psychologist trained in CBT. The benefit of guided self-help diminished at six months; however, symptoms improved, belief in the symptoms' being permanent diminished, satisfaction with care improved, and clinical physical functioning improved.

This approach highlights a treatment for conversion disorder that is optimistic and focused on activation, rehabilitation, and reducing anxiety. In the setting of the general hospital, many with functional weakness get better, while a subset continue to relapse (Folks et al., 1984). In general, patients can be told that the symptoms will get better very gradually. Their strengths and conviction that they can cope will be supported with graded physical therapy, and their concerns with emotional valence can be heard out over time. This treatment philosophy does not negate the psychodynamic thesis that conversion symptoms occur in the setting of unconscious conflict or trauma or negate the role of other interventions like hypnosis (see Chapter 16) or other psychotherapies; however, the important psychological history can be heard and respected over time as the focus on the patient's functioning is sustained. A comorbid disorder like major depressive disorder, panic disorder, or schizophrenia can be diagnosed and treated with medications if appropriate. To aim for the best outcome, physicians should be mindful of rehabilitation to prevent atrophy and contractures of disuse. Caution is appropriate in regard to medications associated with physical dependency like benzodiazepines and narcotics.

HIP FRACTURE

Hip fracture is associated with clinical depression in 14–20% patients (Lenze et al., 2007; Voshaar et al., 2010). Depressive symptoms in patients with hip fracture are associated with poor outcomes at two years (Burns et al., 2012). Fear of falling may limit patients' return to functioning; and the importance of rehabilitation in addressing avoidance early on may be underestimated.

CHRONIC MUSCULOSKELETAL PAIN

Depression as it amplifies chronic pain is an important consideration in patients with a long course of orthopedic pain. Pain, even without affective symptoms, especially associated with joint pain and multiple sites of pain, is a risk indicator for the development of depressive and anxiety disorders (Gerrits et al., 2013). A systemic review of 45 studies of musculoskeletal pain in primary care found that 11 factors were markers of poor prognosis: higher pain severity at baseline, longer duration, multiple sites, previous pain episodes, greater movement restriction, anxiety and/or depression, higher somatic perceptions and/or distress, adverse coping strategies, low social support, older age, and high baseline disability (Mallen et al., 2007). Catastrophizing predicts degrees of pain and disability and mediates treatment efficacy in most studies, as noted in regard to upper-extremity pain (Wertli et al., 2013).

CHRONIC LOW-BACK PAIN

Nonspecific chronic low-back pain is so common that serious medical causes can be ignored in error. Red flags to screen for malignancy and fracture are worth remembering. For cancer: a history of malignancy is the red flag; for fracture: older age, prolonged use of corticosteroid drugs, severe trauma, and presence of a contusion or abrasion are important clues (Bownie et al., 2013).

LUMBAR STENOSIS

Lumbar stenosis—narrowing of the space available for the thecal sac and nerve roots—is caused by mechanical factors and biochemical changes within the intervertebral disk that lead to collapse of the disk space, facet joint hypertrophy, soft-tissue infolding, and osteophyte formation. Flexing the back increases the surface area of the foramen, and extending the back, especially when standing, increases epidural pressure and decreases surface area of the foramen. Symptoms come from vascular compromise of the vessels supplying the cauda equina, or pressure on the nerve root complex by the degenerative changes.

As reviewed by Genevay and Atlas (2010), *neurogenic claudication* refers to leg symptoms—fatigue, heaviness, weakness, and paresthesia—in the buttock, groin, and anterior thigh, as well as radiation down the posterior part of the leg to the feet. Nocturnal leg cramps and neurogenic bladder are also seen. Standing makes symptoms worse, and sitting makes them better. Lying flat is not as much a relief as lying on the side with lumbar flexion. The patient with neurogenic claudication can walk a more variable distance than the patient with vascular claudication. The patient who bends the torso forward can walk further; therefore, people with lumbar stenosis seen from a distance are recognized by their ape-like stance with hips and knees bent. They feel better walking uphill than downhill. Exercise on a stationary bicycle in a seated, flexed position is better tolerated than walking in the erect position (Genevay & Atlas, 2010).

The natural course of the condition varies. Lumbar stenosis does not always get progressively worse (Issack, 2012). The anatomical definition of spinal stenosis may not correlate with pain and functional impairment; therefore, identifying which patients will benefit from surgical or nonsurgical treatments is complex and requires assessment of symptoms. The patient must weigh in on the decision (Atlas et al., 2011). Nonsurgical management consists of nonsteroidal anti-inflammatory agents, physical therapy, and epidural steroid injections. Laminectomy is the most common surgery. In randomized controlled trials for spinal stenosis, surgery is superior to nonsurgical management for controlling pain and improving function (Issack, 2012). With or without degenerative spondylolisthesis, there is good evidence that decompressive surgery is moderately superior to nonsurgical therapy over one to two years (Chou et al., 2009; Loeser, 2009).

LUMBAR RADICULOPATHY

For radiculopathy with herniated lumbar disc, Chou's review found good evidence that standard open discectomy and microdiscectomy are moderately superior to nonsurgical therapy for improvement in pain and function through two to three months. For both lumbar stenosis and radiculopathy, patients on average experience improvement either with or without surgery, and benefits associated with surgery decrease with long-term follow-up in some trials (Chou, 2009).

BIOPSYCHOSOCIAL CARE

Presurgical emotional distress identifies the patients at risk for poor outcome from lumbar surgery (Trief et al., 2000). Presurgical anxiety and depression predicted failure to return to work, failure to report improvement in pain, and failure to report improved functional abilities. Active rehabilitation makes a difference in the outcome after lumbar stenosis surgery (McGregor et al., 2013), and psychologically informed physical therapy that addresses obstacles to resuming life activities improves long-term outcomes among patients with back pain, even those with greater pain and a less favorable prognosis (von Korff et al., 2005).

Chronic back pain lasting more than 12 weeks occurs in a biopsychosocial context (Polatin et al., 1993). Although the biopsychosocial model has been valued for the understanding of low-back pain patients, the synthesis of that knowledge in planning care has not been fully developed for the majority of patients (Pincus et al., 2013), and psychological interventions have shown benefit mostly in the short term (Pincus & McCracken, 2013). Recovery requires patience, disciplined rest, graded exercise, and an awareness of what activities may lead to injury, relapse, and perpetuation of the pain. In one recent review (Chou et al., 2013), antidepressants were reported to show a small net benefit overall. Only tricyclic antidepressants have been shown to be effective. There was no evidence on duloxetine or venlafaxine. The benefit of skeletal muscle relaxants and benzodiazepines was unclear.

STRATIFIED CARE

An important strategy to improve care of back pain patients, taking into consideration the psychosocial dimension, individualizes care by how likely patients are to get better. Reliable assessment of the prognosis can be based on the first-encounter physician's assessment of pain intensity, pain duration, pain interference with daily activity, pain presence at multiple body sites, and a brief screen for depression—as well as the physician's prediction of the expected outcome (Mallen et al., 2013; von Korff, 2013). This assessment predicted six-month outcomes in seven of ten older patients with non-inflammatory musculoskeletal pain (Mallen et al., 2013). The brief assessment by the general physician includes elements that would be noteworthy to a medical psychiatrist or psychologist:

1. a direct consideration of depressed mood,

2. the patients' tendency to avoid activities for fear of injury,

3. troubling thoughts about the causes and consequences of pain, and

4. life circumstances that affect their motivation to resume activities.

The presence of both physical and psychosocial symptoms at the outset affects the treatment approach, bringing more tailored interventions to those with more psychosocial distress. A randomized controlled trial sub-grouping patients with back pain for targeted treatment in the United Kingdom found that more patients in the intermediate and high-risk subgroups had greater than 30% improvement if they were treated with the stratified approach rather than the current best practice approach (Hill et al., 2011).

Both the concept of stratification for targeted treatment and the elements of the three different interventions highlight practical integration of physical and psychological treatments. In this trial, the low-risk intervention was a 90-minute small-group session by a physiotherapist promoting active management of back symptoms, outlining a positive message on maintaining a healthy spine, normalizing the episode of pain, emphasizing the benefit of exercise, and gradually increasing activity levels at local centers. Medium-risk patients who do not have high psychosocial distress but do have disabling low-back pain, referred leg pain, and comorbid pain received four 90-minute group exercise and education sessions. Psychoeducation included the benefits of exercise, a review of spinal anatomy, direction on lifting and handling, ergonomic advice, weight management, and information on the impact of stress, anxiety, and low mood on low-back pain. This was added to a stability exercise program. Patients kept an exercise log on four sessions at home per week. They were urged to do more active walking, cycling, swimming, or other forms of aerobic exercise. The high-risk group with psychosocial distress had four 130-minute group sessions involving CBT strategies to address unhelpful beliefs and behaviors around low-back pain. The biopsychosocial model, the impact of persistent pain, goal-setting based on the patient's functional and social limitations, graded activity, relaxation training, and relapse-management were included. There was a focus on behavior change. The exercise program was similar to that in the medium-risk group. Cognitive-behavioral principles included pacing and goal setting. Exercises were done independently at home for eight weeks (Hay et al., 2008).

Certainly motivation to exercise affects outcome. When an exercise intervention interferes with everyday life, or appears to be ineffective or too difficult to implement, people make a reasoned decision to discontinue (Slade et al., 2013). People are likely to prefer and participate in exercise or training programs and activities that are designed with consideration of their preferences, circumstances, fitness levels, and exercise experiences. Patients tend to believe that there is a difference between general activity, real fitness exercise, and medical exercise. Treatment, to be accepted, requires consideration of patient abilities and experience. Targeting disability and fear-avoidance behaviors makes a difference (Monticone et al., 2013).

From the medical psychiatrist's or psychologist's perspective, the best outcomes for the patient with low-back pain will require tailored clarification about back mechanics, a feasible program of exercise and rehabilitation, pacing and goal setting, activation and encouragement to maintain functioning and limit avoidance, smart use of pain medications, and optimal treatment of depressive disorder. The effectiveness and feasibility of narcotics in chronic back pain are related in part to individual differences, acute vs. chronic course, and the ability to predict and identify aberrant drug-related behaviors.

AMPUTATION AND PHANTOM PAIN

Traumatic limb-amputation often occurs in young, active people, often these days as a major consequence of combat. Surgical decisions after leg injury about limb salvage or amputation are determined by feasibility and the collaborative decision about what offers a better quality of life. The surgeon considers what will lead to a useful and painless limb. Subsequent disability is related to pain, psychological illness, decreased physical and vocational function, and increased cardiovascular morbidity and mortality (Perkins et al., 2011). Adjustment to the loss of a leg is associated with anxiety, depression, PTSD, and substance abuse. (This is discussed in more detail in the chapter 20 on rehabilitation.)

At least half of amputees, and probably 80%, have neuropathic pain and the discomfiting sensation of the missing limb. Sometimes this improves with time. Both peripheral and autonomic nervous systems contribute to the cortical pain memory. Most patients with combat-related traumatic amputations in one series received gabapentin, although some reported greater pain relief from distraction and relaxation techniques. The data for benefit of gabapentin in limited studies are mixed, but there is a trend to benefit (Ketz, 2008; Alviar et al., 2012). Many amputees do not use analgesics for phantom limb pain (Hanley et al., 2006). The severity of the pain is related to the severity and duration of pain before amputation, the pain after amputation, and affective factors (Flor, 2002). Effective analgesia with ketamine or morphine preoperatively may therefore reduce postoperative pain (Huse et al., 2001).

NEUROPATHIC PAIN

The likelihood of neuropathic pain after surgery depends on the likelihood that nerves were injured (Haroutinunian, 2013). Neuropathic pain has a distinct symptom profile that distinguishes it from somatic pain. It is associated with these descriptors: burning, squeezing, electric shocks, tingling, lancinating, pins and needles, itching, and numbness (Bouhassira & Attal, 2010). It is associated with allodynia (pain on the skin from something like a light touch or the sheet over the body). Most patients do not develop chronic neuropathic pain after nerve injury. However, when changes in pain sensitivity become persistent, pain can occur spontaneously with a low threshold. Minor stimuli can produce pain with greater amplitude. At that point, neuropathic pain becomes a condition in its own right (von Hehn et al., 2012). It is often associated with poor sleep, depression, and anxiety (Turk et al., 2010).

The use of opioids for neuropathic pain continues to be controversial. Opioids are useful for spontaneous neuropathic pain and have been recommended as second-line treatments (Dworkin et al., 2007). Compared to placebo, intermediate-term studies (12 weeks or less) of opioids showed some benefit, but their efficacy for chronic neuropathic pain was quite uncertain (McNicol et al., 2013).

Gabapentin and pregabalin, calcium channel alpha-2-delta binding agents, are first-line choices in neuropathic pain, with neither clearly superior (Finnerup et al., 2010). Lidocaine patch 5% or capsaicin 8% (for peripheral neuropathic pain in non-diabetic patients) have also been recommended (Kalso et al., 2013). Both duloxetine and venlafaxine have efficacy in painful polyneuropathy (Rowbotham et al., 2004; Raskin et al., 2005). Amitriptyline has a long history of benefit for neuropathic pain (Moore et al., 2012). Duloxetine has been shown to ameliorate neuropathic pain in diabetic neuropathy and chemotherapy-induced neuropathic pain syndromes. Venlafaxine also has benefit (Finnerup et al., 2010). Lumbosacral radiculopathy, the most common type of neuropathic pain, has not been well treated by any of these medications (Dworkin et al., 2007).

CLINICAL PEARLS

- Unexplained swelling of the hand or arm may be a result of the patient's surreptitious application of a tourniquet to the extremity.

- Secretan's syndrome is a condition caused by the patient's repeatedly striking the dorsum of the hand with a blunt object or against a blunt object, causing diffuse swelling as a result of a peritendinous fibrosis of the extensor tendons. It is an injury that may be self-inflicted, either for secondary gain or as a conversion reaction, and it is best treated with conservative care and psychiatric counseling (Moretta & Cooley, 2002).

- Conversion motor paralysis is associated with comorbid panic; dissociative symptoms were common, as was previous injury to the relevant limb. Non-epileptic attacks, migraine, fatigue, and sleep paralysis were also associated conditions.

- Depressive symptoms in patients with hip fracture are associated with poor outcomes at two years (Burns et al., 2012). Fear of falling may limit return to function.

- In consideration of diagnostic tests in patients with chronic low-back pain, for cancer: a history of malignancy is the red flag; for fracture: older age, prolonged use of corticosteroid drugs, severe trauma, and presence of a contusion or abrasion are important clues.

- The anatomical definition of spinal stenosis may not correlate with pain and functional impairment.

- People with lumbar stenosis can be recognized at a distance as they assume an ape-like stance with hip and knee bent. They feel better walking uphill than downhill, better sitting than standing.

- The severity of the phantom pain post-amputation is related to the severity and duration of the pain before amputation.

DISCLOSURE STATEMENTS

Dr. Vranceanu has no conflicts to disclose.

Dr. Ring had no conflicts related to this topic to disclose.

Dr. Greenberg has no conflicts to disclose.

REFERENCES

Allen, L. A., Woolfolk, R. L., Escobar, J. I., Gara, M. A., & Hamer, R. M. (2006). Cognitive behavioral therapy for somatization disorder: a randomized controlled trial. *Archives of Internal Medicine, 166,* 1512–1518.

Alviar, J. M., Hale, T., & Dungca, M. (2012). Pharmacologic interventions for treating phantom limb pain. *Cochrane Database of Systematic Reviews,* (2). doi: 10.1002/14651858CD006380.pub2

Atlas, S. J. (2011). Commentary: Predictive factors influencing clinical outcome with operative management of lumbar spinal stenosis. *Spine Journal, 11,* 620–621.

American Psychiatric Association (2000). *Diagnostic and statistical manual of mental disorders* (4th ed.). Washington, DC: APA.

American Psychiatric Association (2013). *Diagnostic and statistical manual of mental disorders* (5th ed.). Washington, DC: APA.

Bandura, O. L., Taylor, C. B., Gauthier, J., & Gossard, D. (1987). Cathecolamine secretion as a function of perceived coping self-efficacy. *Journal of Consulting Clinical Psychology, 53,* 406–414.

Barsky, A. J., Wyshak, G., & Klerman, G. L. (1992). Psychiatric comorbidity in DSM-III-R hypochondriasis. *Archives of General Psychiatry, 49,* 101–118.

Beck, A. T., Mendelson, M., Mock, J., & Erbaugh, J. (1961). An inventory for measuring depression. *General Psychiatry, 4,* 561–571.

Bouhassira, D., & Attal, N. (2010). Diagnosis and assessment of neuropathic pain: the saga of clinical tools. *Pain, 152,* S74–S83.

Bownie, A., Williams, C. M., Henschke, N., Hancock, M. J., et al. (2013). Red flags to screen for malignancy and fracture in patients with low back pain: systematic review. *British Medical Journal, 347,* f7095. doi: 10.1136/bmj f7095

Bruce, B. K., Townsend, C., Hooten, W. M., Rome, J. D., Moon, J. S., & Swanson, J. W. (2008). Chronic pain rehabilitation in chronic headache disorders. *Current Neurology and Neuroscience Reports, 8*(2), 94–99.

Burns, A., Younger, J., Morris, J., Baldwin, R., Tarrier, N., et al. (2012). Outcomes following hip fracture surgery: a 2 year prospective study. *American Journal of Geriatric Psychiatry, 22*(8), 838–844.

Carson, A., Stone, J., Hibberd, C., et al. (2011). Disability, distress and unemployment in neurology outpatients with symptoms "unexplained by organic disease." *Journal of Neurology, Neurosurgery, & Psychiatry, 82,* 810–813.

Chou, R., Atlas, S. J., Rosenquist, E. W. K., Doucette, K., & Sokol, H. N. (2013). Subacute and chronic low back pain: nonsurgical interventional treatment. *UpToDate, Basow, DS (Ed), Waltham, MA, UpToDate*

Chou, R., Baisden, J., Carragee, E. J., Resnick, D. K., Shaffer, W. O., & Loeer, J. D. (2009). Surgery for low back pain: a review of the evidence for an American Pain Society Clinical Practice Guideline. *Spine, 34,* 1094–1109.

Chou, R., Fanciullo, G. J., Fine, P. G., Miaskowski, C., Passik, S. D., & Portenoy, R. K. (2009). Opioids for chronic noncancer pain: prediction and identification of aberrant drug-related behaviors: a review of the evidence for an American Pain Society and American Academy of Pain Medicine Clinical Practice Guideline. *Journal of Pain, 10,* 131–146.

DeGood, D. E., & Tait, R. (2001). Assessment of pain beliefs and pain coping. In In D. C. Turk & R. Melzack (Eds.), *Handbook of pain assessment* (2nd ed., pp. 320–345). New York: Guilford Press.

Dersch, J. M. T., Theodore, B. R., Polatin, P., & Gatchel R. (2007). Do psychiatric disorders first appear preinjury or postinjury in chronic disabling occupational spinal disorders? *Spine, 32,* 1045–1051.

Dworkin, R. H., O'Connor, A. B., Backonja, M., et al. (2007). Pharmacologic management of neuropathic pain: Evidence-based recommendations. *Pain, 132,* 237–251.

Eisendrath, Stuart, J. (Feb 1984). Factitious illness: a clarification. *Psychosomatics, 25*(2), 110–113, 116–117.

Escobar, J. I., Gara, M. A., Diaz-Marinez, A. M., et al. (2007). Effectiveness of a time limited cognitive behavior therapy type intervention among primary care patients with medically unexplained symptoms. *Annals of Family Medicine, 5,* 328–335.

Finnerup, N. B., Sindrup, S. H., & Jensen, T. S. (2010). The evidence for pharmacological treatment of neuropathic pain. *Pain, 150,* 573–581.

Flor, H. (2002). Phantom-limb pain: characteristics, causes, and treatment. *Lancet Neurology, 1,* 182–189.

Flor, H., Fydrich, T., & Turk, D. C. (1992). Efficacy of multidisciplinary pain treatment centers: a meta-analytic review. *Pain, 49*(221–230).

Flor, H., Turk, D. C., & Birbaumer, N. (1985). Assessment of stress related psychophysiological responses in chronic pain patients. *Journal of Consulting Clinical Psychology, 35,* 354–364.

Folks, D. G., Ford, C. V., & Regan, W. M. (1984). Conversion symptoms in a general hospital. *Psychosomatics, 25,* 285–295.

Fordyce, W. E. (1976). *Behavioral Methods for Chronic Pain and Illness.* St Louis MO: CV Mosby.

Galer, B. S., Schwartz, L., & Allen, R. J. (2001). Complex regional pain syndromes—Type I: Reflex sympathetic dystrophy, and Type II: Causalgia. In J. D. Loeser, S. H. Butler, C. R. Chapman, D. C. Turk (Eds.), *Bonica's management of pain* (3rd ed., pp. 388–411). Philadelphia: Lippincott Williams & Wilkins.

Gatchel, R. J., & Okifuji, A. (2006). Evidence-based scientific data documenting the treatment and cost-effectiveness of comprehensive pain programs for chronic non-malignant pain. *Journal of Pain, 7,* 779–793.

Genevay, S., & Atlas, S. J. (2010). Lumbar spinal stenosis. *Best Practice and Research in Rheumatology, 24,* 253–265.

Gerrits, M. M. J. G., van Oppen, P., van Marwijk, H. W. J., Penninx, B. W. J. H., & van der Horst, H. E. (2014). Pain and the onset of depressive and anxiety disorders. *Pain, 155*, 53–59.

Guziec, L., & Harding, J. J. (1994). Case of a 29-year-old nurse with factitious disorder: the utility of psychiatric intervention on a general medical floor. *General Hospital Psychiatry, 16*(1), 47–53.

Hadjistavropolus, H. D., & Hadjistavropolus, T. (2003). The relevance of health anxiety to chronic pain: Research findings and recommendations for assessment and treatment. *Current Pain and Headache Reports, 7*, 98–104.

Hadler, N. M. (2003). Fibromyalgia and the medicalization of misery. *Journal of Rheumatology, 30*, 1668–1670.

Halbert, J. M., & Crotty, M. C. J. (2002). Evidence for the optimal management of acute and chronic phantom pain: a systematic review. *Clinical Journal of Pain, 18*(2), 84–92.

Halligan, P. W. (2002). Phantom limbs: The body in mind. *Cognitive Neuropsychiatry, 7*(3), 258–263.

Halligan, P. W., & Berger, A. (1999). Phantoms in the brain. *British Medical Journal, 319*, 587–588.

Hanley, M. A., Ehde, D. M., Campbell, K. M., Osborn, B., & Smith, D. G. (2006). Self-reported treatments used for lower-limb phantom pain: descriptive findings. *Archives of Physical Medicine & Rehabilitation, 87*, 270–277.

Haroutiunian, S., Nikolajsen, L., Finnerup, N. B., & Jensen, T. S. (2013). The neuropathic component in persistent postsurgical pain: A systematic literature review. *Pain, 154*, 95–102.

Hay, E. M., Dunn, K. M., Hill, J. C., Lewis, M., et al. (2008). A randomised clinical trial of subgrouping and targeted treatment for low back pain compared with best current care. The STarT Back Trial Study Protocol. *BioMed Central Musculoskeletal Disorders, 9*, 58–68.

Hill, J. C., Whitehurst, D. G., Lewis, M., et al. (2011). Comparison of stratified primary care management for low back pain with current best practice (STarT Back): a randomised controlled trial. *Lancet, 378*(9802), 1560–1571.

Huse, E., Larbig, W., Flor, H., & Birmaumer, N. (2001). The effect of opioids on phantom limb pain and cortical reorganization. *Pain, 90*, 47–55.

Issack, P. S., Cunningham, M. E., Pumberger, M., Hughes, A. P., & Cammisa, F. P., Jr. (2012). Degenerative lumbar spinal stenosis: evaluation and management. *Journal of the American Academy of Orthopedic Surgeons,* Aug; *20*, 527–535.

Jensen, M. P. (1994). Correlates of improvement in multidisciplinary treatments for chronic pain. *Journal of Consulting Clinical Psychology, 62*, 172–179.

Jensen, M. P., Turner, J. A., Romano, J. M., & Karoly P. (1991). Coping with chronic pain: A critical review of the literature. *Pain, 47*, 249–283.

Johnson, R. K. (1998). Psychological evaluation of hand pain. In M. L. Kasdan (Ed.), *Occupational hand and upper extremity injuries and diseases* (2nd ed., pp. 349–364). Philadelphia: Hanley & Belfus.

Kalso, E., Aldington, D. J., & Moore, R. A. (2013). Drugs for neuropathic pain. *British Medical Journal, 347*, f7339.

Kasdan, S., Louiseville, et al. (1998). Management of carpal tunnel syndrome in the working population. *Hand Clinics, 18*(2), 325–330.

Keefe, F. J., Caldwell, D. S., Williams, D. A., Gil, K. M., et al. (1990). Pain coping skills training in the management of osteoarthritic knee pain: A comparative study. *Behavior Therapy, 21*, 49–62.

Ketz, A. K. (2008). The experience of phantom limp pain in patients with combat-related traumatic amputations. *Archives of Physical Medicine & Rehabilitation, 89*, 1127–1132.

Lawson, K., Reesor, K. A., Keefe, F. J., & Turner, J. A. (1990). Dimensions of pain-related cognitive coping: cross-validation of the factor structure of the Coping Strategy Questionnaire. *Pain, 43*(2), 195–204.

Lenze, E. J., Munin, M. C., Skidmore, E. R., et al. (2007). Onset of depression in elderly persons after hip fracture: implications for prevention and early intervention of late-life depression. *Journal of the American Geriatric Society, 55*, 81–86.

Loeser, J. D. (2009). Surgery for low back pain: a review of the evidence for an American Pain Society clinical practice guideline. *Spine, 34*, 1094–1109

Lynch, M. E. (1992). Psychological aspects of reflex sympathetic dystrophy: A review of the adult and pediatric literature. *Pain, 49*, 337–347.

Mallen, C. D., Peat, G., Thomas, E., Dunn, K. M., & Croft, P. R. (2007). Prognostic factors for musculoskeletal pain in primary care: a systematic review. *British Journal of General Practice, 66*(57), 655–661.

Mallen, C. D., Thomas, E., Belcher, J., Rathod, T., Croft, P., & Peat, G. (2013). Point of care prognosis of common musculoskeletal pain in older adults. *Journal of the American Medical Association Internal Medicine, 173*, 119–125.

Malmivaara A., & Hakkinen, U. (1995). The treatment of acute low back pain—bed rest, exercises, or ordinary activity? *New England Journal of Medicine, 332*(6), 351–355.

Mechanic, D. (1986). Illness behavior. An overview. In S. McHugh & T. M. Vallis (Eds.), *Illness behavior: A multidisciplinary model* (pp. 101–110). New York: Plenum Press.

McGregor, A. H., Probyn, K., Cro, S., Dore, C. J., Burton, A. K., et al. (2013). Rehabilitation following surgery for lumbar spinal stenosis. *Cochrane Database of Systematic Reviews,* Dec 9; 12:CD009644.

McNicol, E. D., Midbari, A., & Eisenberg E. (2013). Opioids for neuropathic pain. *Cochrane Database of Systematic Reviews,* Aug 29; 8:CD006146.

Melzack, R. (1992). Phantom limbs. *Scientific American, 266*, 120–126.

Monticone, M., Ferrante, S., Rocca, B., Baieardi, P., Dal Farra, F., & Foti, C. (2013). Effect of a long-lasting multidisciplinary program on disability and fear-avoidance behaviors in patients with chronic low back pain. Results of a randomized controlled trial. *Clinical Journal of Pain, 29*, 929–938.

Moore, R. A., Derry, S., Aldington, D., Cole, P., & Wiffen, P. J. (2012). Amitriptyline for neuropathic pain and fibromyalgia in adults. *Cochrane Database of Systematic Reviews,* Dec 12 (12), CD008242.

Moretta, D. N., & Cooley, J. R. (2002). Secretan's disease: a unique case report and literature review. *American Journal of Orthopedics, 31*, 524–527.

Nelson, D. V., & Novy, D. M. (1996). Psychological characteristics of reflex sympathetic dystrophy versus myofascial pain syndromes. *Regional Anesthesia, 21*, 202–208.

Nelson, D. V., & Novy D. (1999). Treating patients with complex regional pain syndrome. In D. C. Turk, & R. J. Gatchel (Eds.). *Psychological approaches to pain management: A practitioner's handbook* (second edition, pp. 470–488). New York, N.Y. The Guilford Press.

Osterweis, M., Kleinman, N., & Mechanic, D. (1987). *Pain and disability. Clinical, behavioral, and public policy perspectives.* Washington, DC: National Academy Press.

Perkins, Z. B., De'Ath, H. D., Sharp, G., Tai, N. R. M. (2012). Factors affecting outcome after traumatic limb amputation. *British Journal of Surgery, 99*(Suppl 1), 75–86.

Pilovsky, J. (1967). Dimensions of hypochondriasis. *British Journal of Psychiatry, 113*, 89–93.

Pincus, T., Burton, K., Vogel, S., & Field, A. P. (2002). A systematic review of psychological factors as predictors of chronicity/disability in prospective cohorts of low back pain. *Spine, 27*, 109–120.

Pincus, T., Kent, P., Bronfort, G., Loisel, P., Pransky, G., & Hartvigsen J. (3013). Twenty-five years with the biopsychosocial model of low back pain—is it time to celebrate? A report from the Twelfth International Forum for Primary Care Research on Low Back Pain. *Spine, 38*, 2118–2123.

Pincus, T., & McCracken, L. M. (2013). Psychological factors and treatment opportunities in low back pain. *Best Practice Research in Clinical Rheumatology, 27*, 625–635.

Polatin, P. B., Kinney, R. K., Gatchel, R. J., Lillo, E., & Mayer, T. G. (1993). Psychiatric illness and chronic low back pain. *Spine, 18*, 66–77.

Radloff, L. S. (1977). The CES-D Scale: A self-report depression scale for research in the general population. *Measurements, 1*, 385–401.

Raskin, J., Pritchett, Y. L., Wang, F., D'Souza, D. N., Waninger, A. L., Lyengar, S., et al. (2005). A double-blind, randomized multicenter trial comparing duloxetine with placebo in the management of diabetic peripheral neuropathic pain. *Pain Medicine, 6*, 346–356.

Ring, D., Kadzielsky, J., Malhotra, L., Lee, S. G., & Jupiter, J. B. (2005). Psychological factors in idiopathic arm pain. *Journal of Bone and Joint Surgery, 87*, 374–380.

Rowbotham, M. C., Goli, V., Kunz, N. R., & Lei D. (2004). Venlafaxine extended release in the treatment of painful diabetic neuropathy: a double-blind, placebo-controlled study. *Pain, 110*, 697–706.

Salkovskis, R. K., Warwick, H. M. C., & Clark, D. C. (2002). The Health Anxiety Inventory: development and validation of scales for the measurement of health anxiety and hypochondriasis. *Psychological Medicine, 32*, 843–853.

Sharp, T. J. (2001). Chronic pain: a reformulation of the cognitive-behavioral model. *Behaviour Research & Therapy, 39*, 787–800.

Sharpe, M., Walker, J., Williams, C., Stone, J., Cavanagh, J., Murray, G., et al. (2011). Guided self-help for functional psychogenic symptoms. A randomized controlled efficacy trial. *Neurology, 77*, 564–572.

Simon, E., & Folen, R. A. (2001). The role of the psychologist on the multidisciplinary pain management team. *Psychology, Research and Practice, 32*(2), 125–134.

Slade, S. C., Patel, S., Underwood, M., & Keating, J. L. (2013). What are patient beliefs and perceptions about exercise for non-specific chronic low back pain? A systematic review of qualitative studies. *Clinical Journal of Pain, 30*, 995–1005.

Smith, T. W., Follick, M. J., & Ahern, D. L. (1986). Cognitive distortions and psychological distress in chronic low back pain. *Journal of Consulting Clinical Psychology, 54*, 573–575.

Smith, T. W., Milano, R. A., & Ward, J. R. (1990). Helplessness and depression in rheumatoid arthritis. *Health Psychology, 9*, 377–389.

Spitzer, R. L., Kroenke, K., & Williams, J. B. (1999). Validation and utility of a self-report version of PRIME-MD: the PHQ Primary Care Study. *Journal of the American Medical Association, 10*, 1737–1744.

Stanton-Hicks, J. W., Hassenbusch, S., Haddox, J. D., Boas, R., & Wilson, P. (1995). Reflex sympathetic dystrophy: Changing concepts and taxonomy. *Pain, 63*, 127–133.

Stone, J., Carson, A., & Sharpe, M. (2005). Functional symptoms and signs in neurology: assessment and diagnosis. *Journal of Neurology, Neurosurgery, & Psychiatry, 76*, i2–i12.

Stone, J., Warlow, C., & Sharpe, M. (2012). Functional weakness: clues to mechanism from the nature of onset. *Journal of Neurology, Neurosurgery, & Psychiatry, 83*, 67–69.

Sullivan, M. J. L., Bishop, S., & Pivik, J. (1995). The Pain Catastrophizing Scale: development and validation. *Psychological Assessment, 7*, 524–552.

Szabo, R. M., & King, K. J. (1999). Repetitive strain injury. Diagnosis or self-fulfilling prophecy? *Journal of Bone & Joint Surgery, 82*, 1314.

Tota-Faucette, M. E., Gill, K., Williams, F. J., & Goli, V. (1993). Predictors of response to pain management treatment. The role of family environment and changes in cognitive processes. *Clinical Journal of Pain, 9*, 115–123.

Trief, P. M., Grant, W., & Frederickson, B. (2000). A prospective study of psychological predictors of lumbar surgery outcome. *Spine, 25*, 2616–2621.

Turk, D. C., Audette, J., Levy, R. M., Mackey, S. C., & Stanos, S. (2010). Assessment and treatment of psychosocial comorbidities in patients with neuropathic pain. *Mayo Clinic Proceedings, 85*(3 Suppl), S42–S50.

Turk, D. C., & Monarch, E. (1999). Biopsychosocial perspective on chronic pain. In D. C. Turk, & R. J. Gatchel (Eds.), *Psychological approaches to pain management.* A practitioner's handbook (second edition, pp. 3–30). New York, N.Y. The Guilford press.

Van Houdenhove, B., Vasquez, G., Onghena, P., Stans, L., Vandeput, C., Vermaut, G., et al. (1992). Signs and symptoms of reflex sympathetic dystrophy: Prospective study of 829 patients. *Lancet, 342*, 1012–1016.

Vlaeyen, J. W. S., Kole-Snijder, A., Boeren, R. G. B., & van Eek, H. (1995). Fear of movement/(re)injury in chronic low back pain and its relation to behavioral preference. *Pain, 62*, 363–372.

Von Hehn, C. A., Baron, R., & Woolf, C. J. (2012). Deconstructing the neuropathic pain phenotype to reveal neural mechanisms. *Neuron, 73*, 638–652.

Von Korff, M. (2013). Tailoring chronic pain care by brief assessment of impact and prognosis. *Journal of the American Medical Association Internal Medicine, 173*, 1126–1127.

Von Korff, M., Balderson, B. H., Saunders, K., et al. (2005). A trial of an activating intervention for chronic back pain in primary care and physical therapy settings. *Pain, 113*, 323–330.

Voshaar, R. C., Banerjee, S., Horan, M., et al. (2007). Predictors of incident depression after hip fracture surgery. *American Journal of Geriatric Psychiatry, 15*, 807–814.

Vranceanu, A. M., Safren, S., Zhao, M., Cowan, J., & Ring, D. (2008). Disability and psychological distress in patients with nonspecific and specific arm pain. *Clinical Orthopaedics & Related Research*, Nov; *466*(11), 2820–2826.

Vranceanu, A. M., Zhao, M., Morse, L., & Ring, D. (2009). A multidisciplinary approach to arm illness. *Orthopedic Journal of Harvard Medical School, 10*, 106–109.

Wertli, M. M., Burgsstaller, J. M., Weiser, S., Steurer, J., Kofmehl, R., & Held, U. (2013). The influence of catastrophizing on treatment outcome in patients with non-specific low back pain: a systematic review. *Spine, 39*, 263–273.

Zeineh, W., & Seidenstricker, L. (2008). The clenched fist syndrome revisited. *Plastic & Reconstructive Surgery, 121*(3), 149e–150e.

78.

SEXUAL AND PSYCHOLOGICAL ASPECTS OF REHABILITATION AFTER SPINAL CORD INJURY

Robert M. Kohut, Allen D. Seftel, Stanley H. Ducharme, Barry S. Fogel, and Donald R. Bodner

INTRODUCTION

The estimated annual incidence of spinal cord injury (SCI), excluding those who die at the scene of the accident, is approximately 40 cases per million population in the United States, or approximately 12,000 new cases each year. The average age of victims is 40.7% and approximately 80% are males. The estimated number of people in the United States alive with SCI in 2010 has been estimated to be 265,000 (National Spinal Cord Injury Statistical Center [NSCISC], 2011). The most common causes of SCI are motor vehicle accidents (40.4%), falls (27.9%) and acts of violence (15%). Of the cases reported to the National Spinal Cord Injury Database between 2005 and 2010, neurological status at discharge from the initial hospitalization for SCI was incomplete tetraplegia in39.5%, complete paraplegia in 22.1%, incomplete paraplegia in 21.7%, and complete tetraplegia in 16.3% (NSCISC, 2011).

Over the last three decades, there has been a 40% decline in mortality during the critical first two years after injury, which is attributed to improvements in critical care following the acute injury, and a comprehensive approach to the subsequent management of the SCI patient (Strauss, Devivo, Paculdo, & Shavelle, 2006). Although short-term mortality has declined dramatically, a person's average life expectancy following a spinal cord injury remains shorter than the norm for person of the same age and sex without SCI. Life expectancy is shorter with more rostral lesions and greater neurological impairment (NSCSCI, 2011; Strauss et al., 2006). Historically, urosepsis was the most common cause of death in patients with SCI, but with the advent of effective antibiotics for bacteria causing urinary tract infections and a lower incidence of renal failure because of improved management of SCI-associated bladder dysfunction, renal failure now usually can be prevented. At present respiratory and cardiovascular conditions are the main causes of post-SCI mortality (Lai & Boone, 2008).

Following the initial insult, it is of utmost importance for the rehabilitative team to integrate the patient back into society. Most patients with SCI are younger adults without major chronic diseases, who prior to their injuries looked forward to occupational achievements, sexual experiences, forming families, and pursuing avocations over the coming years. Addressing sexual and relationship concerns, the impact of the injury of work and leisure activities, and emotional adaptation to a radically altered body image is a prominent part of SCI patients' overall rehabilitation. A satisfying sexual life relates reciprocally to many other adaptive issues; it improves relationships, helps with acceptance of physical disabilities, and it improves mood. For this reason, and because anxiety about future sexual function is a frequent early concern in SCI patients, the sexual aspect of SCI rehabilitation has received much attention.

In 2010 the Consortium for Spinal Cord Medicine published a clinical practice guideline for addressing sexuality and reproductive health in SCI patients; these guidelines are integrated into the recommendations provided in this chapter (Consortium for Spinal Cord Medicine, 2010). In the remainder of this chapter the guideline will be referenced as the "Consortium SRH Guideline."

HISTORICAL BACKGROUND

The earliest documented mention of SCI was in the Edwin Smith Surgical Papyrus, transcribed by Smith during the seventeenth century and thought to originate circa 3000 BC (Breasted, 1930). During the time of the pharaohs, SCI was considered to be a fatal condition that was not treatable. In ancient Greece, Hippocrates first described the complications of SCI, including the loss of control of the bowel and bladder (Adams, 1886).

There was little progress in the clinical management of the SCI patient for many centuries. Despite the achievements in understanding neuroanatomy and neurophysiology, during World War I, most spinal cord–injured patients nevertheless eventually died of urosepsis (Holmes, 1915). The emphasis at that time was on neurological assessment, not treatment, as the prognosis of SCI was considered so dismal.

During World War II, great strides were made in the understanding and management of the SCI patient. It was learned that catheterizing the flaccid neurogenic bladder caused by spinal shock immediately reduced mortality due to urosepsis from 100% to 50%. Sir Ludwig Guttman, a German immigrant in the United Kingdom, established a multidisciplinary unit to deal with SCI; he is considered to be the father of modern SCI treatment. In the United States during this same period, Donald Munro in the private sector and Ernest Bors through the Veterans Administration were early pioneers in establishing regional units specializing in the treatment of SCI. The Veterans Administration should be credited for the systematic development of regional SCI units in the United States.

Great progress was made in the urological management of the SCI patient during the 1970s and 1980s. Renal failure was once the leading cause of death in this group of patients, but with improved understanding and management of neurogenic bladder dysfunction, it is no longer so (Dietrick & Russi, 1958; Freed, Bakst, & Barrie, 1966; Mesard, Carmody, Mannarino, & Ruge, 1978). As medical advances have improved the life expectancy of SCI patients, physicians treating SCI have increasingly focused on improving their patients' quality of life. The primary goals of current urological management of patients with SCI are to preserve kidney function, to prevent bladder and kidney infections, and to avoid the use of indwelling catheters whenever possible. With greater success in accomplishing these goals, sexual concerns have emerged as an important part of neurourological rehabilitation.

Sexual education, a need of all SCI patients, is best accomplished by a team that includes a psychologist or psychiatrist (or both), and a urologist familiar with spinal cord injury. Instruction should be commenced shortly after injury and continued throughout the rehabilitation period. Continued access to sexual education, medical problem-solving and peer support is especially important after the patient has been discharged from inpatient rehabilitation. Community surveys of SCI patients have shown that many patients have unaddressed sexual concerns that the feel have been insufficiently addressed by clinicians, and many are dissatisfied with their access to help for sexual issues (Forsythe & Horsewell, 2006; Kreuter, Taft, Siösteen, & Beiring-Sørensen, 2011).

The ability to have satisfying sexual intercourse is important to almost all men and women, and the ability to have genetic offspring is important to most. Concerns of sexuality and procreation are equally important to the spouses and partners of SCI patients; they should be part of educational efforts from the beginning, and they usually will play a role in medical solutions to specific sexual dysfunctions. For many SCI patients who are not married and do not have a regular partner concerns related to the sexual consequences of the injury interact with issues of finding a suitable mate. For these patients general education about the impact of SCI on sexual function should be supplemented by a more individualized approach to issues of initiating and maintaining social and sexual relationships in the presence of a severe disability.

NEUROLOGICAL PATHWAYS AND SEXUAL FUNCTION

The neurology of sexual function is the key to understanding the patterns of sexual dysfunction that can arise following SCI, including the consequences of incomplete injury and the implications of collateral damage to peripheral nerves from trauma or neuropathy. Relatively more attention has been given in the SCI injury to the neuroanatomy and neurophysiology of erection and ejaculation, but the more limited work on female sexual function following SCI suggests that the physiology is analogous—female lubrication and genital vasocongestion corresponds to male erections, and female orgasm corresponds to male ejaculation and orgasm (Forsythe & Horsewell, 2006).

PHYSIOLOGY OF ERECTION

Following appropriate neural input, erections require sinusoidal relaxation, arterial inflow, and venous compression (Lue, Takamura, Schmidt, Palubinskas, & Tanagho, 1983). The corpora cavernosa are the spongy, bilateralcylindrical bodies that together with the corpus spongiosum make constitute the bulk of the penile shaft. The corpora cavernosa and corpus spongiosum are lined by the tunica albuginea, which is thick and relatively noncompliant over the corpora cavernosa and thinner and more compliant over the corpus spongiosum. Inside the corpora cavernosa is a complex network of smooth-muscle–lined sinusoids that are tonically contracted in the flaccid state, preventing massive arterial inflow. The arterial supply to the penis is the penile artery, supplied by the internal pudendal artery. The penile artery then gives off three divisions: the dorsal, bulbourethral, and cavernosal. The cavernosal branches traverse the corpora cavernosa. From the cavernosal arteries arise the helicine arteries, which supply blood to the sinusoids in the corpora cavernosa. The venous drainage originates in venules from the peripheral sinusoids immediately beneath the tunica albuginea. These venules travel in the trabeculae between the tunica and the peripheral sinusoids to form the subtunical venous plexus before exiting as the emissary veins (Lue, 2011). The tunica albuginea constrict the swelling of the corpora cavernosa; with vascular engorgement the intracavernosal pressure rises dramatically, compressing the emissary veins and impeding venous return. When this happens the corpus spongiosum functions as an arteriovenous shunt to compensate for the loss of flow through the corpora cavernosa (Dean & Lue, 2005). Both autonomic and somatic neural pathways are involved in erections. Sympathetic fibers from the hypogastric plexus arise from the intermediolateral columns of the T10–T12 spinal segments, travel through the pelvic plexus and where they join sacral parasympathetic nerves to form the cavernous nerves. Stimulation of the penile sympathetic nerves causes detumescence; their inhibition can cause a partial but not fully rigid erection. The parasympathetic pathway arises from neurons in the intermediolateral cell columns of the S2–S4 spinal cord segments. Because the parasympathetic nerves predominate in the pelvic plexus, stimulation of the pelvic plexus and the cavernous nerves induces erection (Lue, 2011; Dean & Lue, 2005). The dorsal nerve, which arises from the pudendal nerve, provides sensory innervation of the penis and the somatic muscular innervation of the bulbocavernosus (aka bulbospongiosus) and ischiocavernosus muscles. Onuf's nucleus in the S2–S4 spinal segments is the center of somatomotor penile innervation. The respective nerve fibers travel within the sacral nerves to the pudendal nerve to innervate the ischiocavernosus and bulbocavernosus muscles. Contraction of the ischiocavernosus muscles produces the rigid-erection phase, in which the penis typically forms an acute angle with the anterior abdominal wall. Rhythmic contraction of the bulbocavernosus muscle is necessary for ejaculation.

Erections can be reflexogenic or psychogenic. Many patients with sacral SCI retain psychogenic erectile ability even though reflexogenic erection is abolished. Psychogenic erections are mediated by the inhibition of the sympathetic nerve supply to the penis. They typically are triggered by external audiovisual cues but can also be triggered by sexual thoughts. Because they rely on central control of lower thoracic sympathetic neurons, they do not occur in patients with complete cord lesions above T9 and usually are absent in patients with partial lesions above T9. They are most often found in patients with lower motor neuron lesions of the lumbosacral cord, which leave the more rostral sympathetic nuclei completely intact. These LMN lesions eliminate the parasympathetic input to the cavernous nerves; in the absence of parasympathetic input the reduction of tonic sympathetic stimulation can initiate cavernosal engorgement and thus penile erection (Courtois, Goulet, Charvier, & Leriche, 1999; Dean & Lue, 2005). Patients with cord lesions that spare the sacral cord and cauda equinacan attain erections mediated by the reflexogenic pathway, that is, via the stimulation of sacral parasympathetic activity as a reflex response to sacral somatic sensation (see Box 78.1).

The central pathways involved in erection include an oxytocin-mediated connection between the hippocampus and the hypothalamus.An alternate pathway can be activated bystimulation of the paraventricular nucleus (PVN) of the hypothalamus, which produces a marked increase in intracavernosal pressure without a similar effect on systemic blood pressure (Chen, Chan, Chang, & Chan, 1997). These changes are related to the stimulus intensity and frequency of PVN activation. The PVN connects to both sympathetic and parasympathetic neural pathways involved in penile erection. Fibers from the PVN connect to preganglionic parasympathetic

fibers, as well as to the spinal nucleus of the bulbocavernosus (SNB) and the dorsolateral intermediolateral nucleus in the lumbosacral spinal cord. Axons from these latter nuclei innervate the striated penile muscles and the bulbocavernosus muscles. Retrograde tracer and immunohistochemical studies reveal that the PVN fibers that project to the SNB contain neurophysin, the co-product of oxytocin and vasopressin. The role of oxytocin in the central pathways mediating erection suggests a potential role for oxytocin as an adjunctive therapy for erectile dysfunction, a use demonstrated in a recent case report (MacDonald & Feifel, 2012). In fact, oxytocin has a broad range of functions in the CNS related to sexuality, ranging from mediating social interaction and romantic attachment to influencing semen quality (Thackare, Nicholson, & Whittington, 2006; Schneiderman, Zagoory-Sharon, Leckman, & Feldman, 2012). Research on the potential role of oxytocin in the sexual rehabilitation of SCI patients has not as yet been reported.In the rat, the central pathways connecting to the penile (somatic) muscles—the bulbospongiosus and the ischiocavernosus—were shown to involve the locus ceruleus, raphe nuclei, periaqueductal grey and the PVN of the hypothalamus—regions also associated with central control of autonomic function (Marson & McKenna, 1996; Marson, Platt, & McKenna, 1993; Vizzard, Erickson, Card, Roppolo, & de Groat, 1995). Damage to these central pathways contributes to the greater severity of sexual dysfunction when SCI is accompanied by concomitant traumatic brain injury.

Ejaculation is mediated via the sympathetic nervous system and thus by the thoracolumbar portion of the spinal cord. Closure of bladder neck so that reflux of ejaculate into the bladder is prevented, and contraction of the bulbocavernosus muscles, which requires the input of sacral somatic efferents. It is preceded by the secretion of seminal fluid—stimulated by parasympathetic nerves and emission of semen—stimulated by sympathetic nerves. Emission and ejaculation do not require erection (Giuliano, 2011). The sensory experience of orgasm is mediated by vagus nerve afferents from the genital region to the nucleus tractus solitarius.

The neurological pathways for vaginal lubrication and orgasm in women are similar. Sacral parasympathetics mediate reflex genital vasocongestion and lubrication, thoracolumbar sympathetics mediate psychogenic vasocongestion and lubrication, the efferent control of the motor component of orgasm is mediated by the sympathetics, and the sensory experience of orgasm is mediated by the vagus nerve (Griffith & Trieschmann, 1975; Sipski & Arenas, 2006).

LOCAL PHYSIOLOGY OF ERECTION AND THE ROLE OF NITRIC OXIDE (NO)

For over 20 years nitric oxide has been recognized as an important neurotransmitter for erectile function in men—and, homologously, for clitoral vasocongestion in women.Much evidence exists to strongly implicate NO in the physiology of penile erection. Rajfer et al. (1992) and Kim et al. (1991) independently demonstrated that nonadrenergic-noncholinergic (NANC) neurotransmission in the corpus cavernosum involves NO (Kim, Azadzoi, Goldstein, & Saenz de Tejada,

---

Box 78.1 CLASSIFICATION OF ERECTIONS

Reflex Erections

Produced by direct stimulation of the penis
  Mediated by the parasympathetic nervous system
  Require the S2–S4 nerve roots (sacral reflex arc) to be intact
  Occur independently of erotic stimuli or thoughts
  Are generally preserved with spinal cord injury above the L2 vertebral level (S2–S4 nerve roots)

Psychogenic Erections

Produced by thoughts and erotic stimuli
  Mediated by the sympathetic nervous system
  Occur independently of direct stimulation of the penis
  Require the thoracolumbar nerve roots be intact
  Often lost with injury to the thoracic and cervical cord

1991; Rajfer, Aronson, Bush, Dorey, & Ignarro, 1992). NO was shown to induce cavernosal smooth-muscle relaxation. Azadzoi et al. demonstrated that endothelium-dependent relaxation, a cholinergically mediated function, also involves NO pathway (Azadzoi et al., 1992). Using various animal models, several investigators have shown that inhibitors of NO-synthesis prevent or attenuate penile erection *in vivo* and *in vitro* (Burnett, Lowenstein, Bredt, Chang, & Snyder, 1992; Seftel, Viola, Kasner, & Ganz, 1996).

NO is a neurotransmitter synthesized from l-arginine via a reaction catalyzed by nitric oxide synthase (NOS). Three NOS isoforms have been identified: endothelial NOS (eNOS), neural NOS (nNOS), and inducible NOS (iNOS) (Seftel et al., 1997).

The last of these is induced within macrophages by cytokines such as gamma-interferon. Inducible NOS is persistent once induced; it is inhibited by glucocorticoids. The penile corpora cavernosa contain nNOS, eNOS and/or iNOS; inhibition of the form(s) of NOS present in an individual patients will impair erectile function (Garban et al., 1997; Seftel et al., 1997).

EFFECT OF SPINAL CORD INJURY ON SEXUAL FUNCTION

The ability to obtain an erection and to produce an ejaculate in a male patient with SCI depends on many factors, such as level of the lesion, the completeness of the lesion,and the patient's comorbidities.. The residual sexual function of an SCI patient should be assessed with a standardized neurological examination reported using the International Standards for Neurological Classification of Spinal Cord Injury (ISNCSCI) worksheet (American Spinal Injury Association, 2013), shown in Figure 78.xx. The ISNCSCI examination includes testing of light touch and pinprick sensation in each dermatome on each side as well as the perception of deep anal pressure; motor testing includes rating voluntary contraction of key muscles in the four extremities, and evaluation of voluntary anal contraction.

Reflexogenic erections are mediated by sacral parasympathetic nerves arising from the S2-S4 roots. Reflex erection requires preserved (though not necessarily completely normal) sensation in sacral dermatomes and an intact parasympathetic nerve supply to the pensi. Psychogenic erection is mediated by sympathetic nerves arising from T10 through L1; thus it can be preserved after damage to sacral cord or cauda equina that cause the loss of reflex erections. Complete cord lesions above T10 lead to a loss of psychogenic erections as the sympathetic nerve nuclei are disconnected from cerebral input (Sipski, Alexander, Gomez-Marin, & Spalding, 2007).

The degree of preservation of combined pinprick and light-touch sensation in the T11–L2 dermatomes can be used to predict patient's ability to achieve psychogenic erections. As reflexogenic erections rely on an intact S2–S4 reflex arc, assessing the functionalityof the bulbocavernosus reflex can aid in determining the level of a spinal cord lesion. Although the efferent limb of the bulbocavernosus reflex is somatic rather than parasympathetic, the function of the somatic efferent nerves is closely correlated with that of the autonomic efferents. The reflex is tested by pressing firmly on the glans penis (or glans clitoris in women) or tugging on an indwelling Foley catheter and looking for contraction of the anal sphincter or movement of the perineum. For an individual with either complete or incomplete SCI with preserved sensation and/or voluntary motor control of the S2–S5 area and any presence of a bulbocavernosus reflex, reflexogenic erections are typically preserved. In some patients the bulbocavernosus reflex cannot be elicited clinically but can be shown to be present with electrical stimulation of the penis and EMG recording from the bulbocavernosus muscle (Podnar, 2008).

Patients with a complete injury at S2–S5 will have an absentbulbocavernosus reflex and will be unable to havereflexogenic erections.Psychogenic erections are possible if the sympathetic nerve supply of the penis remains intact. While such erections are less rigid than either reflexogenic erections or erections produced in uninjured men, they can be adequate for intercourse, especially if intensified by the use of PDE5 inhibitors. When reflexogenic erections do not take place in patients with suprasacral lesions, concurrent peripheral nerve damage may be present.

Even a complete SCI is compatible with the capacity for orgasm if the sacral cord is intact between S2 and S5, and the sympathetic innervation of the penis is preserved. A precondition for physiological orgasm is the presence of bulbocavernosus and/or anal wink reflexes (Sipski, Alexander, & Rosen, 2001).

To have a satisfying sexual life, a patient with SCI must find ways to experience sexual pleasure that circumvent sensory and motor deficits. Fortunately, SCI patients can learn to experience sensual pleasure and sexual excitement from stimulation of areas that were not sexually salient before the injury. Patients can discover new "erogenous zones" spontaneously, or they can follow suggestions from physicians, professional sex educators, or peers with SCI who have successfully adapted their post-injury sex lives. Typically after SCI there is a level below which there is no sensation and a level above which there is intact sensation. In the zone of transition between these two levels sensation is altered, and that altered sensation sometimes becomes a source of erotic pleasure (Tepper, 2002). For example, women with thoracic cord lesions that put their breasts in a sensory transition zone might experience increased pleasure from breast stimulation, and might be able to reach orgasm from breast stimulation alone when that was not the case pre-SCI.

About two-thirds of men with SCIs are eventually able to experience orgasm after recovering from their acute injury. Compared with their orgasms before their injury those experienced following SCI take more time and more stimulation to achieve, and usually involve stimulation in multiple sensory modalities as well as mental imagery from memories or fantasies. Most men having post-SCI orgasms would rate them as weaker than the ones they had before (Dahlberg, Alaranta, Kautiainen, & Kotila, 2007; also see Box 78.2).

Box 78.2 RELATION OF LEVEL OF INJURY
TO SEXUAL FUNCTION EFFECT

Cauda Equina/Conus Injury

Flaccid bladder
  Loss of external urethral tone
  Loss of anal tone
  Bulbocavernous reflex absent
  Males
  Usually no reflex erections
  Rare psychogenic erection
  Occasional ejaculation
  Females
  Vaginal secretion often absent
  Patients generally fertile

Lumbar Injury

Reflex bladder
  Anal and external urethral tone present
  Males
  Reflex erections can occur
  Psychogenic erections can occur
  Ejaculation is rare
  Females
  Vaginal secretions present as part of sacral/genital reflex
  Fertility is preserved

Thoracic/Cervical Injury

Reflex bladder
  Anal sphincter tone present
  External urethral sphincter often spastic
  Males
  Reflex erections predominate
  Psychogenic erections are generally absent
  Ejaculation occurs occasionally
  Females
  Vaginal secretions are present as part of genital reflex
  Fertility is preserved
Sensation of labor pain is absent

INITIAL REHABILITATION

Traumatic SCI entails severe impairments in physical function that translate into functional dependencies and medical risks. In a matter of seconds, individuals are transformed from fully functioning adults into people who depend on others for their very existence (DeLisa & Gans, 1998).

During initial rehabilitation following SCI, a patient must learn to accomplish everyday physical activities despite his or her impairments, including getting around and dealing with one's bowels and bladder Acquiring mobility usually entails learning to use a wheelchair. Managing a neurogenic bladder usually requires learning the technique of intermittent self-catheterization. Avoiding both constipation and fecal incontinence requires an effective bowel program. The basic

issues of physical rehabilitation overlap with the issues of the patient's post-SCI sexual life. SCI patients' difficulties in physically positioning themselves for sexual activity are a major reason for unsatisfying sexual experiences. For both men and women, concern about incontinence during sexual activity can diminish sexual confidence and sexual desire, and the associated anxiety can interfere with sexual arousal and the ability to experience orgasm. (This problem can sometimes be mitigated by good communication between the sexual partners about the issue, accompanied by a sense of humor when accidents do happen.) Adjustment to SCI is best facilitated through a multidisciplinary team approach. Central to the team are a psychiatrist or psychologist and a urologist familiar with SCI; the input of a neurologist can help in complex cases. Virtually all patients will have sexual concerns following SCI, but they will vary in the ease with which they will talk about them, in the best way to deliver information, and in the best time for introducing information. Sexual concerns often arise immediately following SCI, but the patient may at first only be able to take in basic information and reassurance that when a person with SCI wants a sexual life there is almost always a way to have one. As patients recover from their injuries they—and their partners or spouses—will have many more questions. Community studies of SCI patients suggest that needs for education and assistance with sexual issues often are neglected in the months following acute rehabilitation (Forsythe & Horsewell, 2006). A medical psychiatrist involved in the outpatient treatment of a SCI patient can help the patient access sexual information and sexual rehabilitation during this post-acute phase. Internet-based education and peer support groups complement treatment by professionals; many patients prefer to learn from other SCI patients how they solved sexuality-related problems.

Virtually all men with SCI have early concerns about their capacity for erection and ejaculation, and most women are concerned about arousal and orgasm. Women in relationships often worry about how their physical dependencies and changes in sexual function will impact their relationship with their spouse or partner. Men and women who have not yet had children are concerned about the impact of the SCI on their fertility.

The development of a confident yet realistic self-concept is often a precondition to a satisfying sexual life post-SCI; at the same time having a satisfying sexual and emotional relationship with a spouse or partner can be a great help in developing a positive self-concept. Attention to family relationships, assessnment and treatment of sexual dysfunction, management of specific physical symptoms, and addressing mental health issues complement one another in the rehabilitation of the patient with SCI.

PSYCHOLOGICAL CONSIDERATIONS
IN SCI REHABILITATION

Patients with SCI must adjust to a new body-image, implying an altered self-concept. At times the initial self-concept is a negative one, with patients seeing themselves as disfigured and helpless, useless and burdensome to others. They may feel socially isolated, alone with their pain and suffering. The future may seem oppressively. uncertain.

During the period of rehabilitation patients will face a range of medical complications and physical symptoms. These include incontinence, urinary tract infections, respiratory problems, unstable vital signs, pain, spasticity, joint contractures, skin breakdown, and sexual dysfunction, notably erectile dysfunction in male patients. Understanding these problems and actively managing can build a patient's self-confidence and sense of mastery. Physicians can help by seeing their task as enabling their SCI patients to care for themselves, and to help their loved ones assist them in doing so.

DEVELOPMENTAL PERSPECTIVE

Most spinal cord injuries are sustained by male adolescents and young adults. These patients' developmental tasks comprise separating from one's family of origin, completing one's education, establishing oneself in productive work, and making and maintaining intimate relationships. The consequences of the SCI disrupt, delay, modify or redirect the patient's efforts to accomplish these tasks. Further, the SCI itself might have occurred because of risk-taking behavior that represented independent self-assertion—potentially raising issues of blame, self-blame, shame and guilt. A sense of grief over lost functions and lost opportunities is universal.

Successful adaptation following SCI requires working through the grief reaction without becoming immobilized by it, and requires resumption of the patients developmental tasks, with appropriate changes in details and pace. Educational or occupational accomplishments are typical objective measures of successful adapatation.

MANAGING ANGER AND NONCOMPLIANCE DURING REHABILITATION

In many cases, the patient's emotional reaction fluctuates between intense feelings of depression and anger. Patients sometimesexperience feelings of self-blame regarding their injury and sometimes feel that others have disappointed them and abandoned them in their hope to recover fully—a hope that many patients hold on to for years after the injury. Even the most cooperative patients can become overly demanding in their attitude and behavior toward staff members. Throughout the patient's hospitalization, anger and excessive demands are best handled by reassurance and firm limit-setting by the rehabilitation staff. Setting firm and clear limits is essential for the patient to feel safe and cared about (Krueger, 1984). However, limit setting must be done in an empathetic and supportive manner so as not to be viewed as punitive. (See Chapter 40 for further discussion of limit setting.) Limit setting communicates expectations and encourages a sense of independence and self-control. Patients learn that they must still assume responsibility and meet certain expectations, despite the severity of their injury. Staff and family should promote as much independence as possible and not be excessively solicitous and helpful in a way that fostersbehavioral regression.

If a patient continues to demonstrate noncompliance and anger despite consistent and sympathetic limit setting and adequatre emotional support, a formal behavior therapy program should be considered. A psychologist skilled in behavior therapy can design a program that reinforces the patient's cooperation and active participation in rehabilitation and other medical care., Such programs often includea written contract between patient and staff that makes clear the patient's responsibility, what the staff will and will not do for the patient, and the consequences of further noncompliance with medical treatment. Involving significant others—family or friends—in addressing anger and noncompliance often helps. However, the physician should not meet with significant others without the patient present, unless the patient knows and agrees.

Negative self-concepts and poor family relationships that existed before injury generally persist after injury and may even be exacerbated. But maintaining normal relationships, when they exist, is important and must be encouraged. Dysfunctional relationships and poor family systems should also be addressed through family or couple therapy when problems either predate the injury or surface after the rehabilitation process. Often after an SCI, family communication is diminished, and the stress of an injured family member can intensify underlying family psychopathology. However, the involvement of positive and supportive family members can only improve patient cooperation and further the goals of the medical team. Groups for caregivers and family members led by experienced clinicians can be very helpful for patients and their family members alike.

In many respects, the entire family structure and extended support system must adjust to the disability. The impact on the family is not only emotional, but also often physical and economical. The roles and responsibilities previously assumed by the person with the SCI must be temporarily or permanently assumed by other members of the family. In addition, new responsibilities for the physical care of the person with the disability may be assumed by family members. The family must be an integral part of any treatment program, for they will need assistance in coping with the disability and their response to the disabled person, and in dealing with their own feelings, responsibilities, and increased pressures. An early assessment of the capacity of the family to cope and manage with such changes is critical in integrating the patient successfully back into the community. In view of the potential impact of SCI on a family's income and its expenses, consulting an accountant or financial planner is a frequently useful recommendation to the family. Depression is a common psychiatric sequel of SCI, with the point prevalence of a clinically diagnosable depressive disorder being approximately 22% in patients who have had a SCI, according to a recent meta-analysis. This is significantly higher than the 6.7% reported 12-month prevalence of depressive disorders in general medical clinic populations (Williams & Murray, 2014). This after an SCI, Grief and sadness are observed in most patients following SCI; it is clinically important to distinguish a depressive disorder needing pharmacologic treatment from a grief reaction best managed with support and empathy. In any case, when depressive symptoms cause functional impairment or interfere with physical rehabilitation they should be treated, regardless of the precise diagnosis of a specific depressive disorder. SSRIs, the first-line treatment of depression for most clinicians, have drawbacks in the SCI population, which is particularly vulnerable to their sexual side effects. Alternatives to SSRIs and SNRIs such as bupropion, mirtazapine, vilazodone and perhaps vortioxetine should be considered (Clayton, Croft, & Handiwala, 2014). Furthermore, recent research suggests that SSRIs can have adverse effects on semen quality (Koyuncu, Serefoglu, Ozdemir, & Hellstrom, 2012). It is not yet certain which antidepressants will not adversely effect semen, so if the issue is relevant for a particular patient performing a semen analysis before and after instituting therapy with an antidepressant would be a reasonable precaution. Selective serotonin-reuptake inhibitors (SSRIs) have been first-line treatments for many years, though recent research has raised the issue of a deleterious effect of SSRIs on semen quality. For male SCI patients planning to father children, alternatives to SSRIs should be considered when it is necessary to treat depression.

Reactive depression, or a relatively transient adjustment disorder marked by grief, is most frequently noted, especially among individuals who were extremely active prior to the injury and relied on physical activity to deal with problems in the past. If the depression persists, or if the patient demonstrates suicidal ideation, medication may need to be reconsidered. This is especially true if there are not adequate emotional supports in the community or if the patient's safety becomes a concern.

ASSOCIATED TRAUMATIC BRAIN INJURY

Spinal cord injury often is accompanied by traumatic brain injury (TBI) (Caplan, 1982). TBI is especially common in connection with lesions of the high cervical cord. In such cases, neurological consultation and neuropsychological assessment are necessary to determine the nature, severity, and implications of the brain injury. Assessment can be difficult, however, whenfunctional impairments due to the SCI limit the use of usual procedures for testing brain function. For this reason, TBI concurrent with SCI sometimes goes undiagnosed. Neurology and neuropsychology should typically be consulted early after admission in every case of upper cervical cord injury and in cases where the patient or others are concerned about a change in mental functioning or the patient's behavior during rehabilitation raises an issue of impairment in memory or other cognitive functions. Neurological and/or neuropsychological assessment may need to be repeated, for example when recovery from acute physical impairments enables a more detailed examination for more subtle cognitive functions. Re-evaluation is also important when a patient's cognition, memory, and/or communication improve markedly, as they might if the patient had a brief hypoxic episode at the time of the SCI. Characterization of neuropsychological deficits and offering a prognosis for them is essential in planning rehabilitation and planning for the patient's ultimate return to the community. Neuropsychological status, along with mental health, is more critical to the feasibility of independent living after an SCI than is the level of the spinal injury or the degree of impairment of motor function. The approach taken to physical and occupational therapy, and to physician-patient interaction, will be more explicit, concrete, repetitive and multi-modal if the patient's intellectual function has been impaired by a concurrent TBI. Cognitive impairment also bears on issues capacity, competency, and consent.

ASSOCIATED SUBSTANCE ABUSE

Addressing alcohol and chemical dependency and abuse is especially critical in patients with SCI. Often the onset of such an injury is related to substance abuse. Vehicular crashes, sporting accidents, and falls, especially while the individual is under the influence of alcohol, account for a large proportion of admissions to rehabilitation centers (Schnoll, Heinemann, Doll, & Armstrong, 1989). In other cases, secondary complications of the SCI are related excessive drinking of alcohol or the misuse of various prescription or nonprescription medications. Many young people with SCI have hadsubstance abuse problems before their injury and continue these patterns long afterwards. Despite the relatively high prevalence of substance use disorders in SCI patients, substance abuse issues often are neglected by physicians treating such patients, perhaps because their physical disabilities are so salient. Routine, structured screening for substance use disorders mitigates this problem. Screening for alcohol use disorders is important both because of the impact of excessive alcohol on bodily functions as well as on behavior. Alcohol can potentiate the action of prescribed medications, most notably central nervous system depressants including opiate analgesics and many of the drugs used to treat spasticity and neuropathic pain. In addition, altered consciousness due to alcohol or its combination with prescription drugs can make SCI patients insensitive to prolonged pressure on the skin, leading to the development of pressure ulcers. If excessive alcohol is regularly ingested in the form of beer, the large fluid volumes consumed can seriously compromise a bladder-retraining program.

Alcohol use disorders are highly prevalent in the SCI population. A retrospective claims review study of 8338 SCI patients in veterans' clinics showed that over a 2-year period 12% had diagnoses of alcohol use disorders and another 14% had comorbid alcohol use disorders and mental illness (Banerjea, Findley, Smith, Findley, & Sambamoorthi, 2009). A survey of 1,549 civilian SCI patients found that 19.3% were heavy drinkers (Saunders & Krause, 2011). The period of acute rehabilitation followins SCI offers an opportunity for secondary prevention of substance abuse disorders in those with pre-injury substance abuse, because patients are forcibly confronted with the consequences and/or risks of heavy drinking. In a study of 139 consecutive admissions to an acute inpatient SCI rehabilitation hospital, 38% reported lifetime alcohol-related problems and 33% reported recent illicit drug abuse. 71% of at-risk drinkers reported either considering changes in their alcohol use or were already taking action (Stroud, Bombardier, Dyer, Rimmele, & Esselman, 2011). Notwithstanding, personal and family denial of the substance abuse can still be a problem, particularly in more severely affected patients.

With regard to drug abuse, a special concern with SCI patients is the abuse of prescription drugs. Patients with SCI frequently receive appropriate prescriptions for controlled substances including opiates and benzodiazepines. These drugs produce physiologic tolerance and dependence, leading to escalating consumption in patients vulnerable to substance abuse.

For patients with such problems, substance abuse intervention needs to begin early after admission to treat withdrawal reactions, and continue following discharge from the acute inpatient rehabilitation program. Potential nterventions include individual counseling from a substance abuse specialist, group or self-help meetings, and discharge to a day or residential substance abuse program. In more extreme cases, treatment of the substance abuse disorder before or concurrent with the initiation of physical rehabilitation is necessary. Timely access to substance abuse treatment can be impeded by delayed recognition of the problem, denial, and local unavailability of appropriate treatment programs. Education about substance abuse for physicians treatment SCI patinets, and education about SCI for substance abuse professionals, can help address the problem of access, and the medical psychiatrist working with a SCI service may be able to provide or facilitate this education. Use of structured screening instruments for alcohol and drug use disorders is becoming a standard of practice in acute SCI rehabilitation settings. Periodic re-screening for substance abuse should be considered during long-term follow up. In particular, patients who had SCIs in adolescence can develop substance abuse problems in adulthood; 55% of patients aged 21–25 who had adolescent SCIs reported regular alcohol use (Hwang, Chlan Vogel, & Zebracki 2012).

It is hoped that systematic assessment and concurrent treatment of substance abuse disorders will become routine SCI rehabilitation centers, since such disorders a significant risk factor for later medical complications of SCI.Although some progress has been made, the lack of standard policy and inadequate training continue to be issues.

In summary, spinal cord injury is a life-threatening physical trauma and an intense psychological assault. Adjustment to this injury is a multifaceted process that continues throughout the patient's life. It has a highly variable course that is influenced by the patient's personality, coping style, level of injury, pre-injury mental health and cognitive function, concurrent injuries, comorbid mental illness, and social, financial, and community resources. As the patient undergoes the rehabilitation process, the support and reassurance of the rehabilitation team are fundamental to the patient's adjustment. Setting limits when needed provides a sense of safety to patients, reducing their anxiety. If emotional issues are not addressed from the outset of rehabilitation, one can expect the recurrence of medical complications, long periods of emotional turmoil, and

greater difficulty with re-entry into the community. Health professionals have an obligation to address such issues and to assist the patient in achieving a satisfying and rewarding life after SCI. The involvement of a medical psychiatrist in the rehabilitation team helps the team meet this obligation. Initially, psychotherapy SCI patients emphasizes issues of anger, despair depression, self-esteem, and body-image. Sexual concerns a relevant to all of these themes, and beginning to address them early on can improve the outcome of psychotherapy.

INITIAL EVALUATION AND MANAGEMENT OF SCI WITH ATTENTION TO SEXUAL REHABILITATION

Erections are initially lost during the period of spinal shock and may take several days to weeks to return with an incomplete lesion, and possibly a year or more with complete lesions. Invasive treatments for sexual dysfunction (e.g., penile implants) should be avoided during this time, as sexual function can recover spontaneously over a year or even longer following SCI. Furthermore, sexual function takes place in a context of culture, medical conditions, partner relationships, current mental health and substance use, current function, and the patient's evolving existential situation. One exception might be made to this principle, however—the retrieval of sperm from younger male patients during the first two weeks following the injury, if they are sufficiently stable medically. This issue will be discussed further below.

Initiating a dialogue with the patient about sexuality is important and should be done early in the rehabilitation process. Sexuality consistently is identified as one of the most important topics for individuals after SCI (Widerstrom-Noga, Felipe-Cuervo, Broton, Duncan, & Yezierski, 1999). A patient's readiness to hear and discuss issues of sexuality will vary from one individual to another. Some patients may want their healthcare providers to do nothing more than dispel myths or clear up misconceptions while others may be ready to listen to more detailed information about their sexual functions. In many cases, the sexual history is the first step in sexual education because it introduces a sensitive topic and aids in establishing rapport. Questioning should be done in a nonjudgemental and straightforward manner. The goal of the examiner is to determine the patient's interest and readiness to learn about sexual functioning following his or her SCI, while being aware that some patients initially may not feel comfortable talking about thetopic directly. An important component of the initial evaluation is to ask individuals with SCI if they have experienced any previous sexual trauma, sexual dysfunction, or a sexually transmitted disease that could affect their sexual functioning following injury. Should a preexisting problem exist, the patient should be referred to the appropriate specialist—often a medical psychiatrist. A physical examination using the ISNCSCI form (Figure 78.1) should be performed. Special attention to the preservation

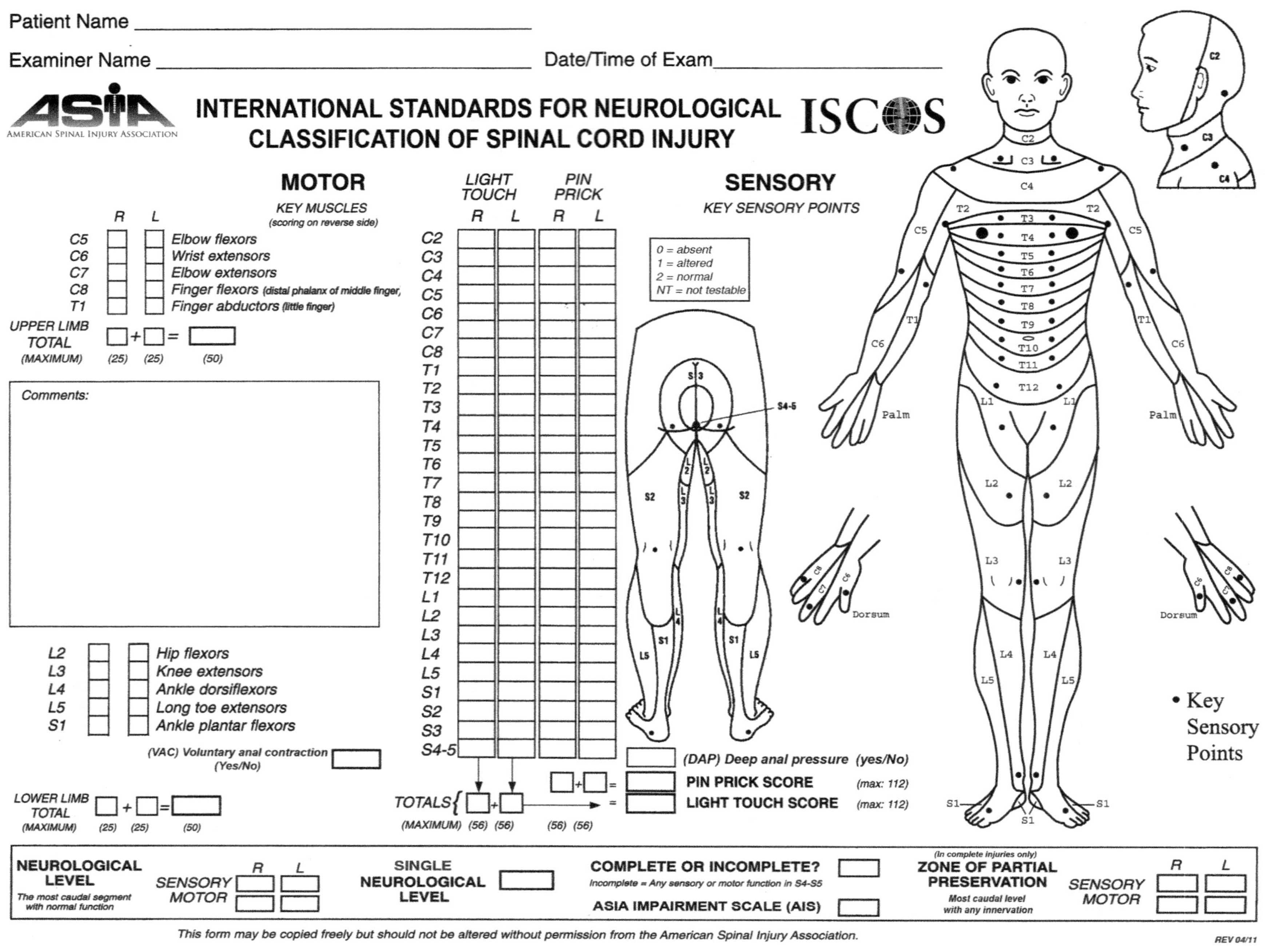
Patient Name ____________________

Examiner Name ____________________ Date/Time of Exam ____________________

ASIA — American Spinal Injury Association

INTERNATIONAL STANDARDS FOR NEUROLOGICAL CLASSIFICATION OF SPINAL CORD INJURY

ISCoS

MOTOR

KEY MUSCLES (scoring on reverse side)

	R	L	
C5			Elbow flexors
C6			Wrist extensors
C7			Elbow extensors
C8			Finger flexors (distal phalanx of middle finger)
T1			Finger abductors (little finger)

UPPER LIMB TOTAL (MAXIMUM) ☐ + ☐ = ☐ (25) (25) (50)

Comments:

	R	L	
L2			Hip flexors
L3			Knee extensors
L4			Ankle dorsiflexors
L5			Long toe extensors
S1			Ankle plantar flexors

(VAC) Voluntary anal contraction (Yes/No) ☐

LOWER LIMB TOTAL (MAXIMUM) ☐ + ☐ = ☐ (25) (25) (50)

SENSORY

KEY SENSORY POINTS

	LIGHT TOUCH R	LIGHT TOUCH L	PIN PRICK R	PIN PRICK L
C2				
C3				
C4				
C5				
C6				
C7				
C8				
T1				
T2				
T3				
T4				
T5				
T6				
T7				
T8				
T9				
T10				
T11				
T12				
L1				
L2				
L3				
L4				
L5				
S1				
S2				
S3				
S4-5				

TOTALS { ☐ + ☐ → = ☐ + ☐ =

(MAXIMUM) (56) (56) (56) (56)

0 = absent
1 = altered
2 = normal
NT = not testable

(DAP) Deep anal pressure (yes/No) ☐

PIN PRICK SCORE (max: 112) ☐

LIGHT TOUCH SCORE (max: 112) ☐

NEUROLOGICAL LEVEL — The most caudal segment with normal function — SENSORY R ☐ L ☐; MOTOR R ☐ L ☐

SINGLE NEUROLOGICAL LEVEL ☐

COMPLETE OR INCOMPLETE? ☐ — Incomplete = Any sensory or motor function in S4-S5

ASIA IMPAIRMENT SCALE (AIS) ☐

(In complete injuries only) **ZONE OF PARTIAL PRESERVATION** — Most caudal level with any innervation — SENSORY R ☐ L ☐; MOTOR R ☐ L ☐

REV 04/11

Figure 78.1 International Standards for Neurological Classification of Spinal Cord Injury (ISNCSCI) Examination Sheet.

Muscle Function Grading

0 = total paralysis

1 = palpable or visible contraction

2 = active movement, full range of motion (ROM) with gravity eliminated

3 = active movement, full ROM against gravity

4 = active movement, full ROM against gravity and moderate resistance in a muscle specific position.

5 = (normal) active movement, full ROM against gravity and full resistance in a muscle specific position expected from an otherwise unimpaired peson.

5* = (normal) active movement, full ROM against gravity and sufficient resistance to be considered normal if identified inhibiting factors (i.e. pain, disuse) were not present.

NT = not testable (i.e. due to immobilization, severe pain such that the patient cannot be graded, amputation of limb, or contracture of >50% of the range of motion).

ASIA Impairment (AIS) Scale

☐ **A = Complete.** No sensory or motor function is preserved in the sacral segments S4-S5.

☐ **B = Sensory Incomplete.** Sensory but not motor function is preserved below the neurological level and includes the sacral segments S4-S5 (light touch, pin prick at S4-S5: or deep anal pressure (DAP)), AND no motor function is preserved more than three levels below the motor level on either side of the body.

☐ **C = Motor Incomplete.** Motor function is preserved below the neurological level**, and more than half of key muscle functions below the single neurological level of injury (NLI) have a muscle grade less than 3 (Grades 0-2).

☐ **D = Motor Incomplete.** Motor function is preserved below the neurological level**, and at least half (half or more) of key muscle functions below the NLI have a muscle grade ≥ 3.

☐ **E = Normal.** If sensation and motor function as tested with the ISNCSCI are graded as normal in all segments, and the patient had prior deficits, then the AIS grade is E. Someone without an initial SCI does not receive an AIS grade.

**For an individual to receive a grade of C or D, i.e. motor incomplete status, they must have either (1) voluntary anal sphincter contraction or (2) sacral sensory sparing <u>with</u> sparing of motor function more than three levels below the motor level for that side of the body. The Standards at this time allows even non-key muscle function more than 3 levels below the motor level to be used in determining motor incomplete status (AIS B versus C).

NOTE: When assessing the extent of motor sparing below the level for distinguishing between AIS B and C, the ***motor level*** on each side is used; whereas to differentiate between AIS C and D (based on proportion of key muscle functions with strength grade 3 or greater) the ***single neurological level*** is used.

Steps in Classification

The following order is recommended in determining the classification of individuals with SCI.

1. Determine sensory levels for right and left sides.

2. Determine motor levels for right and left sides.
    Note: in regions where there is no myotome to test, the motor level is presumed to be the same as the sensory level, if testable motor function above that level is also normal.

3. Determine the single neurological level.
    This is the lowest segment where motor and sensory function is normal on both sides, and is the most cephalad of the sensory and motor levels determined in steps 1 and 2.

4. Determine whether the injury is Complete or Incomplete.
    (i.e. absence or presence of sacral sparing)
    *If voluntary anal contraction = **No** AND all S4-5 sensory scores = **0** AND deep anal pressure = **No**, then injury is COMPLETE. Otherwise, injury is incomplete.*

5. Determine ASIA Impairment Scale (AIS) Grade:

    Is injury <u>Complete</u>?   If **YES**, AIS=A and can record ZPP (lowest dermatome or myotome on each side with some preservation)

    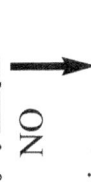

    NO

    Is injury motor <u>Incomplete</u>?   If **NO**, AIS=B
    (Yes=voluntary anal contraction OR motor function more than three levels below the motor level on a given side, if the patient has sensory incomplete classification)

    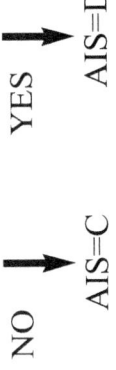

    YES

    Are at least half of the key muscles below the single neurological level graded 3 or better?

    NO   YES

    AIS=C   AIS=D

    If sensation and motor function is normal in all segments, AIS=E
    Note: AIS E is used in follow-up testing when an individual with a documented SCI has recovered normal function. If at initial testing no deficits are found, the individual is neurologically intact; the ASIA Impairment Scale does not apply.

Table 78.1 PHYSICAL EXAMINATION FINDINGS AFTER SPINAL SHOCK*

| | INJURY LEVEL | | |
PARAMETER	SPINAL SHOCK	CAUDA EQUINA	THORACIC/ CERVICAL
Rectal tone	Absent/ decreased	Absent/ decreased	Increased
Bulbocavernous reflex	Absent/ decreased	Absent/ decreased	Present
Perineal sensation	Absent/ decreased	Absent/ decreased	Absent
Reflex penile erections	Absent/ decreased	Absent/ decreased	Present
Spontaneous bladder contractions	Absent	Absent	Present

*Spinal shock generally lasts from several days to approximately six weeks after spinal cord injury.

Table 78.2 COMMONLY USED MEDICATIONS IN SCI PATIENTS

DRUG	PURPOSE	SIDE EFFECTS
Oxybutynin	Bladder relaxant	Dry mouth; impotence
Propantheline	Bladder relaxant	Dry mouth; impotence
Baclofen	Muscle relaxant	Drowsiness; impotence
Diazepam	Muscle relaxant	Drowsiness
Phenoxybenzamine	Sphincter relaxant	Hypotension; inhibition of ejaculation
Prazosin	Sphincter relaxant	Hypotension; inhibition of ejaculation
Terazosin	Sphincter relaxant	Hypotension; inhibition of ejaculation
Tamsulosin	Sphincter relaxant	Hypotension; inhibition of ejaculation
Silodosin	Sphincter relaxant	Hypotension; inhibition of ejaculation

of sensation from T11–L2 and S2–S5, along with determination of the presence of voluntary anal contraction and the anal wink and bulbocavernosus or clitorocavernosus reflexes, can be used to predict remaining sexual function (see Table 78.1). Aside from a complete neurological exam, a thorough physical exam should be performed, assessing the breasts and genitalia, as well as screenings for cervical, ovarian, uterine, breast, prostatic, and testicular cancers. Screening for sexually transmitted diseases, including HIV/AIDS, should be provided as deemed appropriate on an individual basis. A thorough review of the patient's medications should be performed, as polypharmacy is the norm in individuals with SCI (see Table 78.2). More than 100 specific medications or classifications of medications have been associated with sexual dysfunction (Thomas, 2003). Some classes of medications that can affect sexual function include antidepressants (e.g., SSRIs, heterocyclic and tricyclic medications), neuroleptics, anxiolytics (e.g., diazepam), antiepileptic drugs, cardiovascular medications, sympatholytic agents, diuretics, lipid-lowering agents, vasodilators, gastrointestinal medications, opioids, anticholinergics, and chemotherapeutic agents. Following the sexual evaluation, the healthcare provider should be able to develop a treatment plan based on the individual's physical examination, sexual history, and specific personal concerns.

Following the injury, the patient is usually hospitalized for a long period of time to undergo multidisciplinary rehabilitation. Should a patient be ready to explore sexual issues with a partner or himself, offering a private apartment or hospital room for intimacy is an important statement and a first step in restoring post-injury sexual confidence (SRH SCI Guideline, 2010). Information on sexual assistive devices (sex toys) should be provided, along with education on their cautions and contraindications. For example, penile rings can interfere with normal blood flow from the penis and should never be kept in place for longer than 30 minutes. Vibrators may cause dysreflexia in individuals with SCI at T6 and above, while any device that causes friction on the skin may lead to skin breakdown.

PHYSICAL AND PRACTICAL CONSIDERATIONS

Once an SCI patient is ready to engage in sexual activity, he or she can be discouraged by functional limitations, mobility issues, equipment concerns, and so on. In addition, it is important that people with SCI and their partners understand how such issues as bladder and bowel management, skin care, and risk of autonomic dysreflexia (AD) can affect their sexual functions. Because many people may not become sexually active until long after the injury occurs, they may not be aware of the full impact of the injury on their sexual activity.

As many SCI patients have bladder dysfunction along with external drainage devices, incorporating bladder management into their sexual routine becomes important. Although bladder incontinence during intimate activity may be a source of anxiety, it does not necessarily preclude the enjoyment of sexual activity for people with SCI (Anderson, Borisoff, Johnson, Stiens, & Elliott, 2007a, 2007b). Men should determine if having a full bladder assists with or impairs their ability to achieve an erection and should use this information to determine when to empty their bladders. However, a full bladder may cause increased sympathetic activity that can result in AD. This possibility must be discussed and contingency plans put in place should AD occur. Towels or disposable protective bed pads can be used in case leakage or secretion of bodily fluids occurs. Persons with SCI using indwelling urethral catheters need to take precautions to prevent dislodging or contaminating them during sexual activity. For some people, removing the catheter and replacing it after sexual activity is preferred, although this may be problematic if assistance from an untrained partner is necessary. Some men who use indwelling catheters fold the tubing down the shaft of the penis or clamp the end of the catheter and place a condom over the penis and tubing prior to intercourse. This technique can damage the balloon port tubing and cause the balloon to remain inflated. Damage to the balloon port may cause bladder distention, ultimately resulting in a urinary tract infection, sepsis, or AD in men who have injuries at T6 and above. To avoid AD as a result of the issues associated with an indwelling catheter, some people with SCI find that a switch to a suprapubic catheter may be more conducive to sexual activity. Patients who perform intermittent catheterization would simply drain the bladder before sexual activity, and perhaps restrict fluids for a few hours before sex. Instillation of oxybutynin at the time of the last catheterization before intercourse is used by some SCI patients to further reduce the risk of urinary incontinence during or after intercourse (Vaidyananthan et al., 1998). The presence of skin wounds and healing ulcers does not preclude a person with SCI from having sexual relations. They should avoid activities or practices that couldexacerbate their skin condition. Dressings should be reapplied following sexual activity if they became dislodged. A practice that should be incorporated into a sexual routine is examining insensate skin regions at its conclusion. Women may experience decreased or absent genital lubrication, and men may experience decreased pre-ejaculatory fluid, resulting in irritation of the skin during intercourse. Use of artificial water-soluble lubricants (preferably gels) can provide additional lubrication, but it is recommended that lubricants be uncolored and unflavored. The gel should be applied to the genitals prior to intercourse. If the person with SCI has limited hand mobility, the partner can apply the lubrication as part of the sexual encounter (SRH SCI Guideline, 2010).

Persons with SCI at or above T6 are at risk for AD, which is the body's response to stimulation with an increase in sympathetic output (Sheel, Krassioukov, Inglis, & Elliott, 2005). Individuals with SCI who are at risk for AD should receive early basic education on how to prevent, respond to, and intervene if AD should occur. Symptoms and signs of AD compriseelevated blood pressure that can reach dangerously high levels,, slowed heart rate, pounding headache, sweating, flushing, pallor, nasal congestion, blurred vision, nausea, and piloerection. Sexual activity, especially orgasm and ejaculation, can trigger the onset of AD. If an individual experiences AD during sexual activity, the activity should stop, and the person should sit up immediately while the medical provider is notified. Even if warning signs subside, the individual should be instructed to call a healthcare provider. The use of prophylactic medication, such as sublingual nifedipine, prazosin, or nitroglycerin paste, should be considered after physician assessment (SRH SCI Guideline, 2010).

RESTORATION OF ERECTIONS

Erectile dysfunction is defined as "the inability to attain and/or maintain penile erection sufficient for satisfactory sexual performance" (Montague et al., 2005). Within six months following SCI, 60–80% of males will have the ability to obtain an erection, depending on the completeness and level of the lesion (Tsuji, Nakajima, Morimoto, & Nounaka, 1961). Eventually, 80–95% will be able to achieve an erection of some kind—reflexogenic, psychogenic, or mixed. Although not absolutely determinative, the level of spinal cord lesion can be predictive of preserved erectile function. In a systematic review, covering 12 observational studies, Higgins reported that 85–90% of patients with T12 and above lesions maintained erectile function of any kind, while those with lesions L1 and below preserved function 40–80% of the time (Higgins, 1979). Reflexogenic erections are preserved in approximately 80% of patients with T12 lesions and above, while psychogenic erections remain only 0–10% of the time in the same population. In patients with lesions L1 one study found capacity for psychogenic erections in 40–50% (Higgins, 1979).

Even though most men with SCI can have erections, they may not be of sufficient rigidity or duration for intercourse. The percentage of successful intercourse without treatment in men with SCI ranges from 5–75%, depending on the level and completeness of injury (Moemen, Fahmy, AbdelAal, Kamel, Mansour, & Arafa, 2008).

Current guidelines recommend a stepwise approach to erectile dysfunction by starting with conservative measures first, while keeping surgical treatment as an option for refractory cases. The first step should be to encourage men with SCI to enhance their existing sexual function before using medical interventions. Does the patient have the ability to become aroused naturally? Has the patient tried stimulation of areas with preserved sensation, even if there were not erogenous zones of choice before the injury? In addition, healthcare providers should discuss treatments that can be used to address pain, spasm, incontinence, or other interfering factors (SRH SCI Guideline, 2010). Once these issues are addressed and their management is optimized, hypogonadism, which is discussed in a later section, should be ruled out. This can be a cause of decreased libido, worse erectile dysfunction, and a less satisfactory response to PDE5 inhibitor therapy, and replacement therapy should be tried if the testosterone level is low (see Chapter 35). Men with erectile dysfunction should be assessed for the capacity to achieve psychogenic or reflexogenic erections (Deforge et al., 2006). A thorough history will elucidate whether erectile dysfunction existed pre-injury. Men with SCI who are not able to attain or maintain an erection following injury need to be informed of all current medical options for treating ED, along with the efficacy, possible adverse reactions, and cost. With this in mind, the steps in the treatment ladder, which are similar to those for the non-SCI patient with ED, involve first the addition of oral medications, followed by injectable agents, then vacuum devices, and lastly surgical implantation of a penile prosthesis.

ORAL DRUG THERAPY

The discovery of phosphodiesterase type 5 (PDE5) inhibitors revolutionized the treatment of ED. PDE5 inhibitors prevent the intracorporal breakdown of cyclic guanosine monophosphate (cGMP), resulting in enhanced erection by prolonging smooth-muscle relaxation. It must be remembered that PDE5 inhibitors do not initiate an erection, they simply make one stronger. Physical stimulation and/or psychological arousal is required to initiate an erection before the medications can take effect. The medications, which include sildenafil, vardenfil, and tadalafil, have proven efficacy and a relatively benign side-effect profile. Phosphodiesterase isozymes exist elsewhere in the body, and PDE5 inhibitors have some affinity for them, giving each of the three options a different side-effect profile based on its binding to other phosphodiesterase isoenzymes. For example, PDE type 6 is located in the retina and is responsible for visual disturbances; these are most frequently seen with sildenafil. Absolute contraindications to the use of PDE5 inhibitors include the concomitant use of nitrates or the presence of retinitis pigmentosa. Relative contraindications include symptomatic hypotension, the use of alpha-blockers, and use of other erection-enhancement therapies, the last because of the risk of priapism with combined treatments. The main concern is inducing severe hypotension when using nitrates or alpha-blockers. Other side effects include headache, dyspepsia, flushing, and nasal congestion (Deforge et al., 2006). Both sildenafil's and vardenafil's systemic absorption is affected by fatty food, and patients should be instructed to take them on an empty stomach for greater efficacy.

Of the three PDE5 inhibitors approved by the Food and Drug Administration (FDA) for ED, sildenafil has been the most studied in SCI patients specifically. Sildenafil (Viagra) demonstrated superiority to placebo in a randomized, double-blind, placebo-controlled, flexible-dose, two-way crossover study. Seventy-six percent of men reported improved erections and preferred sildenafil over placebo. The median proportion of attempts at sexual intercourse that were successful was 55% with sildenafil treatment compared with 0% with placebo. Most patients required the maximal dose of 100 mg to achieve these results. Of note, 64% of the 25 patients in this study who had no erectile function at all prior to drug treatment had improvement with sildenafil (Giuliano et al., 1999).

The effectiveness of PDE5 inhibitors has been shown to depend on the level of injury. Reflexogenic erections are more often preserved in upper motor-neuron (UMN) injuries than in lower motor-neuron (LMN) injuries. In a study comparing the effectiveness of sildenafil in patients with either UMN or LMN injuries, sildenafil was effective in 82% of patients, and its efficacy was statistically higher than placebo's (82% vs. 25%, p < 0.05). However, 28% of patients with non-UMN lesions had a response rate similar to placebo. Sildenafil is more effective in the treatment of neurogenic ED secondary to UMN SCI compared with that secondary to LMN injury (Khorrami et al., 2010). It has also been shown that males with SCI with preserved function of at least one component of the erection phenomenon, reflexive and/or psychogenic, respond well to sildenafil, and the usual dose required to achieve erections sufficient for sexual intercourse is 50 mg (Schmid, Schurch, & Hauri, 2000). Successful intercourse was achieved by 93% of the patients. Complete absence of both types of erections correlated with a lack of response to sildenafil (Schmid et al., 2000).

Vardenafil and tadalafil both demonstrated statistically significant improvement in the International Index of Erectile Function erectile function domain score (22.0 and 22.6 vs. 13.5) and penetration efficacy (76% and 75.4% vs. 41%) when compared to placebo in SCI patients in two separate multi-center, randomized controlled trials (Giuliano et al., 2006, 2007). Soler et al., in an open-label study, demonstrated all three FDA-approved PDE5 inhibitors had similar efficacy and were safe in SCI patients (Soler, Previnaire, Denys, & Chartier-Kastler, 2007). Tadalafil has a longer duration of action than both sildenafil and vardenafil and was shown to be effective when taken 24 hours in advance of sexual stimulation (Del Popolo, Li Marzi, Mondaini, & Lombardi, 2004). When starting a patient on a PDE5 inhibitor, the lowest dose should be started; if it is shown to be ineffective, the dosage can then be up-titrated until a clinical response is achieved.

PDE5 inhibitors have been tested as treatment for sexual dysfunction in women; the literature is inconclusive. Case series suggest it can improve arousal and orgasm, but controlled studies have been inconclusive, in part because of a high placebo response rate (Foster, Mears, & Goldmeier, 2009; Chivers & Rosen, 2010). There have been no controlled studies specifically in women with SCI.

INTRACAVERNOSAL INJECTION OF VASOACTIVE MEDICATIONS

The next step in the therapeutic ladder for the treatment of ED in SCI patients after hfailure of oral medications is intracavernosal injection (ICI) of alprostadil (prostaglandin E1), papaverine, and/or phentolamine. The aforementioned injected substances are given as monotherapy or in combinations of two or three. Alprostadil works by activating adenylate cyclase, subsequently increasing cyclic adenosine monophosphate (cAMP). Papaverine non-selectively inhibits phosphodiesterases types 2–5, resulting in an increase in cAMP and cGMP. Phentolamine inhibits norepinephrine

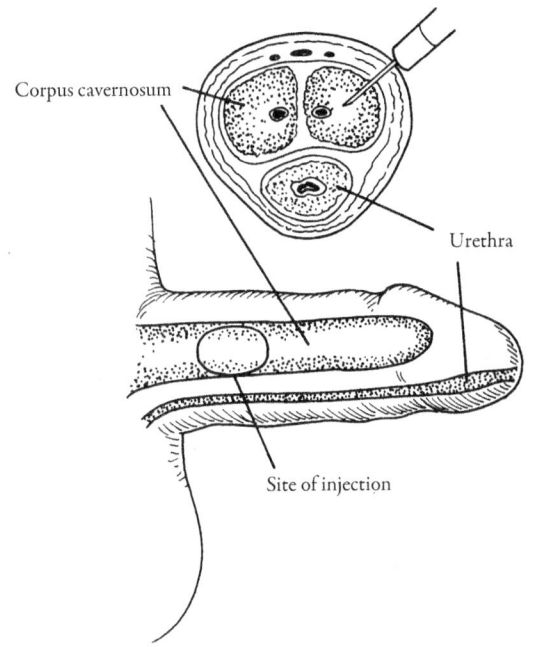

Figure 78.2 Site of injection. The needle is inserted into the corpora cavernosa at the base of the penis.

from binding to the alpha-1 receptor and functions to inhibit detumescence. Deforge et al. in a systematic review pooled the results of eight case-series and showed a 90% "satisfactory erection" response rate in SCI patients using ICI (Deforge et al., 2006).

Bodner et al. reported their results with long-term follow-up on 50 men with SCI using ICI and demonstrated its safety and effectiveness. Monotherapy (papaverine) was used in 24 patients and dual therapy (papaverine and phentolamine) in the remaining 26 patients. Early complications included priapism in four patients, requiring aspiration of the corpora cavernosa and injection of a dilute epinephrine solution (1/100,000). Rigid erections were obtained in all but five patients who injected (95%). Late complications included penile plaque in three patients (6%). However, 31 (62%) of the patients eventually dropped out of the program, most during the drug-titration period. The next most common reason was the lack of a partner. The average frequency of injection was twice a month (Bodner, Leffler, & Frost, 1992). In another study, ICI of papaverine was compared to oral sildenafil in SCI patients with injuries less than one year and lesions T6 and below. Baseline erection characteristics were obtained and used as the control arm, followed by ICI of papaverine, and then after a washout period, oral sildenafil was given. Both ICI of papaverine and oral sildenafil were significantly more efficacious than placebo in enabling erections. Erections were of similar quality between the treatment arms, and it was concluded that either intracavernosal papaverine or oral sildenafil can be used to treat ED in SCI patients (Yildiz, Gokkaya, Koseoglu, Gokkaya, & Comert, 2011).

The initial trial dose of ICI therapy should be administered under healthcare provider supervision according to the American Urologic Association (AUA) Guideline on ED (Montague et al., 2005). After the man or his partner receives

instruction on the proper penile injection method, a careful titration of the medication is used to determine the correct dose and strength of the compound to allow for an erection to occur within 5–10 minutes and last approximately one hour. The proper technique is demonstrated in the figure below (see Figure 78.2). Some men with sensation in the penis may experience a short period of minor pain at the injection site, which can be reduced with proper injection technique. Pressure should be applied to the injection site to prevent scarring. Trauma from injections into the cavernosal tissue through the tunica may cause inflammation, thus resulting in tunica scarring, microhemorrhage along the needle track, and calcium deposits. These may lead to penile curvature. Priapism is another potential complication of injection therapy. Priapism is when an erect penis does not return to its flaccid state, despite the absence of physical and psychological stimulation, within four hours. Urological consultation should be sought in a patient with priapism. Due to the risk of priapism, it is recommended that only one injection be given per 24-hour period (Montague et al., 2005). Patients with LMN injuries, who are less likely to respond to PDE5 inhibitors, may respond to ICI. As PDE5 inhibitors are contraindicated in patients taking nitrates, ICI can be offered to this subgroup (Deforge et al., 2006).

VACUUM CONSTRICTION DEVICES

Vacuum constriction devices (VCDs) have been used for over a century to help improve erections in males with ED. A VCD consists of an elongated tube that is placed over the shaft of the penis. A vacuum is then created in the tube either by a battery-operated device or manual pumping action. As the vacuum is created, blood gradually fills the corporal chambers of the penis. When the penis achieves a satisfactory degree of rigidity, an elastic penile ring is slipped off the tube and placed over the base of the penis to contain the blood and maintain the erection so that sexual intercourse can occur. When used with proper instruction and according to the manufacturer's specifications, VCDs have very low morbidity with no irreversible effects. Minor side effects include penile edema and petechiae. Subcutaneous penile hemorrhage in patients using anticoagulant therapy and penile gangrene are serious complications of which VCDs also are contraindicated in patients with sickle-cell disease. The ring should never be left on longer than 30 minutes (see Figure 78.3).

Heller et al. (1992) in a small study of 17 patients showed that after a mean follow-up of 21 months, over 50% of the patients were actively using their VCD. The frequency of coitus increased from 0.3 times per week to 1.5 times per week. It was concluded that VCDs are a noninvasive method to treat ED in males with SCI (Heller, Keren, Aloni, & Davidoff, 1992). Denil et al. (1996) reported on 20 couples using VCDs. After three months, 93% of the men and 83% of their partners reported rigidity sufficient for vaginal penetration, with an average duration of 18 minutes. At six months, 41% of the men and 45% of the women were satisfied with the VCD. The most commonly reported complaint was premature loss of rigidity during intercourse. Sixty percent of men

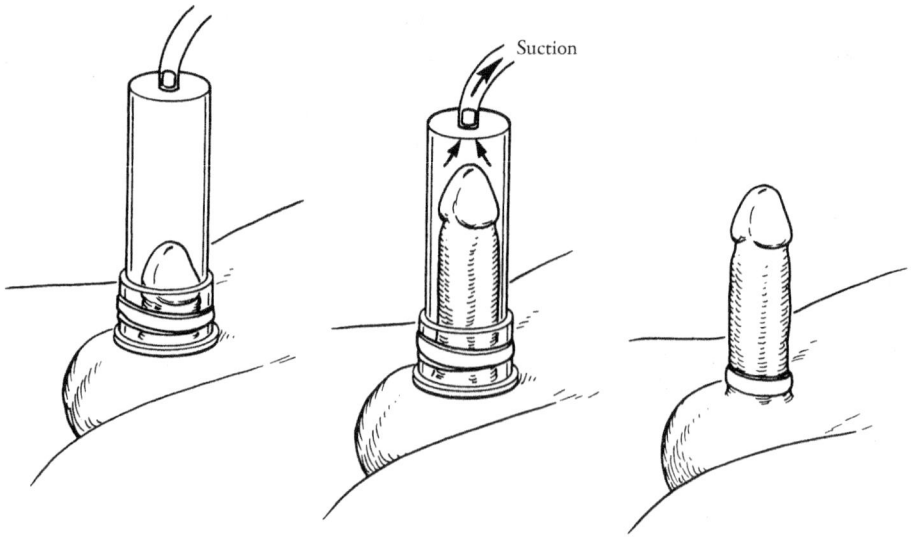

Suction

Figure 78.3 Vacuum erection devices are placed about the penis, and a watertight seal is achieved against the abdomen. The vacuum is applied, creating the erection, and then a rubber band is left at the base of the penis to maintain the erection for as long as 30 minutes.

and 42% of women indicated an improvement of the sexual relationship. Although not universally accepted, the VCDs had a significant impact on sexual activity and sexual satisfaction for nearly half the couples (Denil, Ohl, & Smythe, 1996). Moemen et al. reported 70% of SCI patients had restoration of normal erections and significant improvement in sexual function after using VCDs (Moemen et al., 2008). This wide range of variation in response of patients might be related to the acceptability by the patient and his partner. Patients tend to reject the use of VCDs because they want to have more naturally occurring erections within the context of sexual stimulation by a partner. VCDs are more accepted by men in established sexual relationships where spontaneity is not a major issue.

An analogous portable battery-powered vacuum device for producing clitoral engorgement is available for women. It has been used successfully to improve sexual function in women with sexual dysfunction after irradiation for cervical cancer and in anatomically normal women with impaired sexual arousal (Billups, 2002; Shroder et al., 2005). It is applied during foreplay prior to intercourse; no effort is made to maintain engorgement of the clitoris during intercourse itself. There are no published data on the use of the device in women with spinal cord injury.

INTRAURETHRAL THERAPY

Prostaglandin E1, although typically used as an ICI, also comes in an intraurethral formulation. The Medicated Urethral System for Erection (MUSE') study group reported on the efficacy of intraurethral alprostadil in non-SCI males with ED. When MUSE was administered in the clinic, 65.9% of men responded satisfactorily. Of those initial responders, only 64.9% had a satisfactory response with at-home use (Padma-Nathan et al., 1997). Bodner and colleagues (1999) reported their results with MUSE in SCI patients.

Intraurethral alprostadil was tested in 15 SCI patients who previously responded favorably to ICI, and the erections were compared using each delivery method. The quality of the erection varied and appeared to be less rigid in all patients when compared to ICI. It was concluded that MUSE was effective at creating erections that were of lesser quality than those with ICI (Bodner, Haas, Krueger, & Seftel, 1999). Common side effects of intraurethral alprostadil include unsatisfactory erections, pain in the urethra, dysuria, and hypotension if MUSE is not administered with a constricting band at the proximal penile shaft (Bodner et al., 1999). The absorption of alprostadil from the urethral lumen can be variable, especially in patients with SCI who manage their bladders with intermittent catheterization, which makes MUSE less efficacious than ICI of prostaglandin E1.

Although intraurethral medications have been popular in the past, currently they are not readily available and have been found to be less effective than ICI in the SCI population and are therefore seldom prescribed. With this being said, intraurethral therapy should be offered to patients who are deterred by the morbidity of self-injection, due to its being less invasive (SRH SCI Guideline, 2010).

PENILE PROSTHETICS

Prior to the advent of oral and ICI therapies for ED, surgery was the only option. It is now the final rung of the ladder for the treatment of ED in both non-SCI and SCI patients. Besides being effective for the treatment of ED, in patients with SCI a penile prosthesis can also be inserted to aid in the application of external drainage devices, such as condom catheters. Options include an inflatable penile prosthesis (IPP) or a malleable, semi-rigid prosthesis. The malleable prosthesis consists of two bendable rods, which are surgically implanted in the corporal chambers of the penis. With the malleable device, the penis is always semi-rigid and needs only to be moved into the right position for penetration. The malleable implant can be helpful in keeping a condom catheter in place; however, it is less popular because it maintains the penis in an erect state, which may have cosmetic disadvantages. The IPP consists of a pair of inflatable cylinders that are surgically implanted into the erectile chambers. A pump for the implant is also surgically inserted into the scrotum. A reservoir for the pump fluid is placed within the abdominal cavity. In what is referred to as a two-piece inflatable implant, a scrotal fluid reservoir is substituted for the abdominal reservoir. When a man desires an erection, he or his partner squeezes the pump, which moves fluid into the inflatable cylinders and allows the cylinders to become rigid. When deflated, the penis returns to a naturally flaccid state (SRH SCI Guideline, 2010).

Initial results in the 1980s demonstrated a propensity for SCi patients with IPPs to develop infections around the device, requiring its removal (Kabalin & Kessler, 1988). Complication rates differ among older studies. A 33% complication rate was reported in 63 patients who underwent insertion of an IPP or semi-rigid device, while another study had a 13.3% complication rate (Collins & Hackler, 1988; Kimoto & Iwatsubo, 1994). Perkash and colleagues (1992) implanted penile prosthesesin 60 men with SCI and performed a retrospective review. The primary indication for implantation was the loss of condom catheter with a small, retractile penis. Mean follow-up was seven years, and 81% reported no accidents with condom loss after implantation. All patients who were catheter dependent, except one, were able to rid themselves of indwelling catheters. The overall infection rate was 2% (Perkash, Kabalin, Lennon, & Wolfe, 1992). Kim et al. reported a wound infection rate of 8.3% in their experience with malleable penile prosthesis insertion in 48 patients with SCI (Kim, Yang, Lee, Jung, & Shim, 2008). In a more recent study, Zermann et al. had a 5% infection rate after the implantation of 245 penile prostheses of various types (Zermann, Kutzenberger, Sauerwein, Schubert, & Loeffler, 2006).

Implantation of a penile prosthesis is a safe procedure for ED and/or urinary incontinence in neurologically impaired patients. Based on technical advances, the complication rates have significantly decreased during the years, and the devices should be offered to patients with SCI after they have exhausted other sources for ED.

HYPOGONADISM

Patients with SCI are prone to develop metabolic disturbances, including testosterone deficiency (Bauman & Spungen, 2000). However, a cause-and-effect relationship between SCI and low serum testosterone levels has yet to be proven. Normal total testosterone levels vary with age, but generally run between 300 and 1000 ng/dl. When compared to able-bodied controls, tetraplegics were shown to have decreased testosterone, luteinizing hormone (LH), and follicular stimulating hormone (FSH) (Kostovski, Iversen, Birkeland, Torjesen, & Hjeltnes, 2008). Another study demonstrated similar findings. When compared to normal controls, 50% of the subjects with SCI had decreased values of

at least one of the aforementioned hormones (Safarinejad, 2001). The previous studies were in patients with chronic SCI. In a screened population of men with SCI admitted to inpatient rehabilitation, 83% who had sustained injuries less than four months previously had low testosterone levels, while less than 10% of those with injuries longer than four months previously had low testosterone levels (Schopp et al., 2006). The same principal investigators corroborated this study with another of larger sample size, and the prevalence of low testosterone was found to be 60% for all patients and 69% for those in the acute phase (under 4 months) (Clark et al., 2008). Another group reported a 43.3% prevalence of hypogonadism in healthy SCI patients with chronic injuries. There were associations with with injury severity and opioid usage (Durga, Sepahpanah, Regozzi, Hastings, & Crane, 2011).

Potential testosterone deficiency should evaluated in men with SCI presenting with suppressed libido, reduced strength, fatigue, or poor response to PDE5 inhibitors for erectile dysfunction (SRH SCI Guideline, 2010). Suspected causes of hypogonadism after SCI include chronic illnesses, bladder and testicular infections, concomitant brain injury, hyperprolactinemia, metabolic syndrome, diabetes, and the use of medications that increase prolactin or suppress testosterone (e.g., opioids). Treatment of these illnesses and alterations in medications may assist in the return of normal testosterone levels. The use of testosterone replacement in men with SCI should be based on symptoms and signs rather than on a testosterone level alone; relevant symptoms and signs include sexual dysfunction, fatigue, weakness, and osteopenia. Hypogonadism is confirmed by finding a low free testosterone level I in the morning. If gonadotropin and prolactin levels are not elevated and no other cause of hypogonadism is found and treated (i.e., medication side effects or diagnosed illness), primary hypothalamic/pituitary pathology should be ruled out prior to initiation of testosterone replacement. Traumatic brain injury concurrent with the SCI is one potential cause of this problem. Testosterone replacement therapy can have a beneficial effect on the general health (i.e., cardiovascular, bone health, and body fat composition), mood, and sexual function of men with SCI; it can, however, diminish fertility by suppressing LH and FSH. Bauman et al. (2011) recently demonstrated the safety of transdermal testosterone replacement therapy in SCI. Eleven hypogonadal men with SCI were treated and followed for one year. Testosterone replacement therapy significantly improved lean tissue mass and energy expenditure (Bauman, Cirnigliaro, La Fountaine, Jensen, Wecht, et al., 2011).

Men on testosterone replacement need to be monitored with serum testosterone levels and other biochemical markers, as indicated by current best clinical practices for testosterone replacement therapy. Exogenous testosterone replacement will suppress spermatogenesis and therefore should not be the treatment of choice in hypogonadal men with SCI wishing to pursue biological fatherhood. The contraindications for hormone replacement treatment are severe renal disease, cardiovascular disease, liver disease, and prostate cancer. Side effects should be discussed with patients and may include acne, myalgias, flushing, edema, hypertension, insomnia, hyperlipidemia, and polycythemia.

FERTILITY

Fertility is a concern for both men and women who have had spinal cord injuries. While females with SCI are thought to have normal fertility, the majority of women who have not had children before SCI do not have them afterwards. Men with SCI have markedly reduced fertility, with less than half of male SCI patients able to biologically father children (Brown, Hill, & Baker, 2006).

ISSUES FOR WOMEN

Pre-menopausal women with SCIs can become amenorrheic for several months following the injury, even if their periods were regular before it. The disruption in the menstrual cycle is presumably related to the extreme stress of the injury; in some cases, the amenorrhea is accompanied by an increase in serum prolactin that resolves in several months, concurrent with the resumption of menses (Rutberg, Fridén, & Karlsson, 2008).

Women who lose their periods immediately following SCI should have an appropriate diagnostic evaluation; if there is no other cause for the amenorrhea the patient can be reassured that her menses will return in several months.

Otherwise healthy women with SCI who become pregnant usually can carry their pregnancies to term and have a vaginal delivery; in fact, delivery will be less painful for most women with SCI because of diminished pelvic sensation. Nonetheless pregnancies of women with SCI are classified as high risk for two reasons. First, the incidence of UTI is very high, with potential complications if UTIs are not treated promptly. Second, the intense abdominal and pelvic stimulation associated with labor can provoke severe autonomic dysreflexia, with severe and even life-threatening hypertension. In late pregnancy the mobility limitations of women with SCI become more challenging because of weight gain. Admission to hospital several days before delivery is anticipated may be necessary for comfort and for risk management.

Despite the challenges that pregnancy, delivery and child care present for women with SCI, overall quality of life is on average higher in female SCI patients who do bear children (Westgren & Levy, 1994). Informing a young woman with a recent SCI that her injury will not preclude future motherhood can be helpful emotionally, and the reassurance offered would be supported by evidence.

ISSUES FOR MEN

The situation for men with SCI is more discouraging: Only about 5% of men with SCI are able to biologically father children without medical assistance, and less than half are able to do so even with maximal medical assistance. While only about 10% of men with SCI are able to ejaculate with sexual activity alone, semen can be obtained by mechanical or electrical stimulation in another 80%. The more fundamental problem is poor semen quality (Patki, Woodhouse, Hamid, Craggs, & Shah, 2008; Das, Soni, Sharma, Gazvani, & Lewis-Jones, 2006). The sperm count can be low, but even when it is normal there usually are problems with sperm motility or with the properties of the seminal fluid that impede fertilization. Deterioration in the quality of semen begins approximately 2 weeks after an acute SCI; the cause is multifactorial and not completely understood. If a man with SCI and a woman are determined to conceive a child together they might need to resort to in-vitro fertilization with intracytoplasmic sperm injection (ICSI) to maximize their chance of success. In connection with the issue of semen quality, Das and colleagues (2006) point out that if a male patient with an SCI is sufficiently stable medically in the second week following his injury, it is rational to propose that he undergo an electroejaculation (see below) to produce semen that can be frozen for potential use if he wishes to father children in the future.

For men with SCI who cannot ejaculate with sexual activity, the usual first step in the pursuit of conception is medically-assisted ejaculation to obtain semen to be used for intravaginal or intrauterine insemination. When satisfactory semen can be obtained by ejaculation the discomfort and expense of testicular aspiration or testicular biopsy can be avoided.

The two basic approaches to medically-assisted ejaculation are penile vibratory stimulation (PVS) and electroejaculaton (EEJ). The former elicits ejaculation by applying intense vibratory stimulation to the penis to elicit a spinal reflex. The latter directly stimulates the skeletal muscles and smooth muscles involved in ejaculation by applying a pulsatile electrical stimulus through a rectal probe. While PVS requires an intact sacral reflex arc, EEJ can be effective even when the sacral cord has been damaged. Considering all male SCI patients, about 80% will ejaculate with PVS and 90-95% will ejaculate with EEJ.

A final point is that sperm quality declines rapidly following SCI. Sperm retrieved, by EEJ if necessary, during the first two weeks following SCI can be normal and suitable for intravaginal or intrauterine insemination, while sperm obtained later on will be unsatisfactory for these purposes. If the patient's is sufficiently stable medically, the collection and freezing of semen in the two weeks following SCI is a reasonable consideration for younger men likely to consider fathering children in the future (Das et al., 2006; Brown, Hill, & Baker, 2006).

Ejaculation is a spinal reflex elicited by stimulation of the dorsal penile nerve, which is the sensory branch of the pudendal nerve terminating in sacral spinal cord segments S2–S4 (Brackett, Lynne Ibrahim, Ohl, & Sonksen, 2010). The basis of ejaculation in reflex pathways wholly within the spinal cord is demonstrated by the induction of ejaculation by PVS in patients with complete spinal cord transection above the T10 segmental level. In these patients sacral sensory input is intact, as is thoracolumbar sympathetic output and sacral somatic and parasympathetic output. The ability of a peripheral stimulation to induce ejaculation despite the complete loss of reciprocal connections with supraspinal structures implies the existence of an ejaculation control center at the spinal cord level (Everaert, de Waard, Van Hoof, Kiekens, Mulliez, & D'Herde, 2010).

It is more likely that a man with a SCI will be able to ejaculate with sexual activity alone kif there is significant preservation of genital sensation and voluntary anal control, a strong bulbocavernosus reflex, and the man is not taking anticholinergic medication, SSRIs, or other drugs known to impair orgasm and ejaculation even in patients who are anatomically intact. SCI patients sometimes regain ejaculatory with the passage of time without any specific treatment (SRH SCI Guideline, 2010).

Penile Vibratory Stimulation (PVS)

Penile vibratory stimulation (PVS) is performed by placing a powerful vibrator on the dorsum or frenulum of the glans penis—or sandwiching the penis between two vibrators - and delivering mechanical stimulation until ejaculation occurs. The vibrator stimulates the dorsal penile nerve; if the latter is blocked the reflex cannot be elicited (Wieder, Brackett, Lynne, Green, & Aballa, 2000). PVS has been shown to be more effective in men with cord lesions at T10 or higher than in men with lesions at T11 or below. PVS with the more rostral lesions had an 88% success rate, while those with the more caudal lesions had a 15% success rate (Brackett et al., 2010). Patients with lesions above the T6 spinal level can experience autonomic dysreflexia with PVS. Sublingual nifedipine can be used for initial treatment if it occurs. If autonomic dysreflexia was experienced with previous sessions of PVS, nifedipine can be used prophylactically.

Electroejaculation (EEJ)

Electroejaculation (EEJ), the stimulation of ejaculation by pulsed electrical current administered via a rectal probe, was first used clinically in 1975 and became an established practice in the 1990s, offering a way to retrieve sperm without needle aspiration or testicular biopsy in patients incapable of ejaculation even with high-intensity PVS (O'Kelly, Manecksha, Cullen, McDermott, Flynn & Grainger, 2011). EEJ, which is carried out by a physician with specialized training, using a device specifically approved for performing the procedure, is successful in 95% of attempts.

To perform EEJ, the operator inserts a catheter and drains the patient's bladder. A buffering solution is instilled into the bladder; semen ejaculated in a retrograde direction will mix with this buffering solution rather than with urine. The catheter is removed and the patient is placed in the lateral decubitus position. A probe is inserted transrectally, and an applied current causes emission of semen. The current should be delivered in an interrupted fashion instead of continuously, as ejaculation occurs when the current is switched off. A recommended procedure is to deliver electricity in 2–5 volt increments. At each increment, the peak voltage should be held for five seconds, and then abruptly switched off (Brackett et al., 2010). Following the procedure, the bladder is catheterized to obtain the specimen. Most patients can undergo EEJ without anesthesia unless they have preserved sensation, as the procedure can cause significant discomfort. Complications associated with EEJ are uncommon, but thermal rectal injury is avoided by an automatic shutoff of the probe if temperatures exceed 40°C. AD can occur in patients with lesions at T6 or above. When the patient is at high risk for AD, sublingual nifedipine is given prophylactically and blood pressure is monitored continually during the procedure (Steinberger, Ohl, Bennett, McCabe, & Wang, 1990; O'Kelly et al., 2011).

Compared to PVS, EEJ is more expensive and invasive, although more successful, as no preservation of an ejaculatory reflex is needed. Using a treatment algorithm similar to that recommended by the Consortium of Spinal Cord Medicine, Brackett et al. (2010) reported a 3% failure rate in obtaining sperm from 500 patients with SCI. Using masturbation, 9% were able to provide semen. PVS was successful in 86% of patients with a T10 or higher injury level. EEJ was successful in most cases of failed PVS. Overall, semen was obtained without surgical retrieval methods in 97% of patients (Brackett, Ibrahim, Iremashvili, Aballa, & Lynne, 2010).

A semen analysis for men interested in biological fatherhood should be performed in order to provide information and make recommendations for achieving pregnancy. Men with SCI typically have abnormal semen parameters, with normal sperm numbers and decreased motility and viability when compared to those of normal men (Patki, Woodhouse, Hamid, Craggs, & Shah, 2008). The root causes of this problem have not been fully established, but it iss thought to be multifactorial. It has been demonstrated that semen quality is better from antegrade specimens than from retrograde specimens. As such, semen quality is typically higher with PVS than with EEJ (SRH SCI Guideline, 2010). The same treatments that are effective for assisting conception in couples with non–SCI male factor infertility are effective in assisting conception in patients with SCI male factor infertility, and fecundity tends to increase as the invasiveness of treatment increases (Brackett et al., 2010).

Infertility is usually not associated with SCI in females. As such, females with SCI should not be dissuaded from pregnancy. Quality of life for a woman with SCI increases after childbirth, despite the additional demands and challenges of raising a child (Westgren & Levi, 1994). Still, women with SCI face unique problems associated with pregnancy; these issues should be discussed so that women can make informed decisions if they are considering becoming pregnant. Women with SCI have reported receiving little information about pregnancy post-injury, and the information provided often is found to be inadequate (Ghidini, Healey, Andreani, & Simonson, 2008). Pregnant women with SCI have an increased risk of uterine tract infections, AD, and changes in respiratory function. They also have specific biomechanical needs related to being in a wheelchair. Women with SCI should discuss with their obstetrician exactly how labor and delivery will be managed, and in some cases early hospitalization will be necessary (Jackson & Wadley, 1999). Diminished sensation and absence of pain may result in unrecognized conventional labor symptoms or atypical labor symptomatology, especially in women whose levels are T10 and above (Jackson & Wadley, 1999). The obstetrician needs to be able to differentiate AD from preeclampsia, as the treatment of each differs.

SUMMARY

Spinal cord injury is a devastating injury that forces the affected person to make lifelong adjustments. Great progress has been made in the medical management of these patients, and their life expectancy now approaches that of age-matched controls. The multidisciplinary approach to management of these patients is essential to their successful reintegration into society. The role of the medical psychiatrist and other mental health professionals is central, beginning at the time of injury and continuing indefinitely. Patients must first cope with the injury and understand what changes will occur in their functional ability. The patient should experiment to determine how sexual function can be optimized after the injury. When erections are not satisfactory for a male patient, further assessment is indicated. Restoring penile erections can effectively be accomplished with oral medications. Only rarely are penile prostheses required. When receiving treatment for sexual dysfunction, patients should be followed as closely by apsychotherapist for support and adjustment as they are followed by an urologist. Hypogonadism is very common in the SCI population and should be screened for, and further studies will elucidate whether treatment in asymptomatic men is beneficial. For the man who does not ejaculate and desires to father a child, semen is often successfully obtained using minimally invasive approaches. Very rarely should surgery be required to obtain sperm. It is critical for psychiatrists to know the state of the art in the treatment of SCI patients so as to refer them appropriately while treating them with psychotherapy and medications improve their adjustment to their situation. This includes awareness of local and regional resources for substance abuse treatment and for assisted reproduction. Professional staff of all disciplines who treat SCI patients can at times struggle with feelings of helplessness as well as deal with their countertransference to particular patients—overidentification and overprotectiveness are common reactions. Ongoing dialogue with peers about these feelings will diminish their adverse impact on patients' treatment.

All staff members on a rehabilitation unit—not only mental health professionals—need to be sensitive to the emotional and psychosocial needs of their patients and their families. Often, empathetic listening to patients during physical and occupational therapy sessions and offering positive support can psychotherapeutic. Rehabilitation staff must be able to tolerate the patient's sadness without offering quick solutions or cutting off the patient's verbalizations and expressions of emotion. Patients must come to see a future for themselves and achieve a realization that life will continue after SCI, and that life after SCI can potentially be as fulfilling and meaningful as life without one, despite physical challenges. The staff member who helps the patient in their grieving while also looking toward the future in a positive and reassuring manner will be a valuable asset for the patient's emotional adjustment. Rehabilitation should be a time of focusing on the strengths of the patient, and this includes the social and emotional resources and strengths of the individual as well as the residual physical capabilities demonstrated in physical therapy.

Individual psychotherapy a critical component of a good rehabilitation program, and almost all patients will benefit from it. Medical-psychiatric assessment of the patient and ongoing psychotherapy should begin as soon as the patient arrives on the rehabilitation unit. In an acute-care setting, beginning such services even while the patient is in the intensive care unit is advisable. In that manner, a therapeutic alliance can be formed prior to beginning aggressive rehabilitation, and the therapist can be an important support during the early weeks in rehabilitation. When the acute hospital and the rehabilitation hospital are not linked the handoff from one therapist to the other must be handled sensitively. Family and/or couple therapy also are valuable components of a successful rehabilitation program. Such treatment modalities can address communication issues, mobilize emotional support, and provide important assistance to siblings, children, and other members of the family. When non-related friends of the patient have a central supportive role, they should be included in education programs and, if relevant, in conjoint therapy sessions.

Throughout the rehabilitation program, individual treatment and couples therapy should address sexual issues through general education and individualized counseling. The topic can be gently introduced as early as possible in the rehabilitation program. The patient needs information about how the injury will affect sexual expression, and will require counseling to assist in the sexual adjustment that will be necessary. If the patient has not raised such issues by the time of discharge, the mental health professional should introduce the topic in a non-threatening and sensitive manner. Information regarding erections and lubrication, fertility, bladder and bowel functioning, positioning, sensation, and orgasm should be introduced and discussed with the patient and partner whenever possible. All members of the rehabilitation team can be helpful in this regard by affirming the patient's sense of masculinity or femininity and providing reassurance that the patient can be desirable and that sexual expression can continue, or in the case of a younger patient, begin at an appropriate time. Sexual issues may arise or evolve during long term follow up following acute rehabilitation. Patients should know that their physicians will be open to discussing sexual issues at any time, and physicians should periodically make tactful inquiries to re-open the topic if the patient wishes.

CLINICAL PEARLS

- Many patients with sacral spinal cord injury retain psychogenic erectile ability even though reflexogenic erection is abolished. Psychogenic erections are found more frequently in patients with lower motor-neuron lesions below T12; no psychogenic erection occurs in patients with lesions above T9. Patients with higher lesions can maintain erections using the reflexogenic pathway. (See Table 78.1.) Psychogenric erections may insufficient for intercourse, but may become adequate if augmented by PDE5 inhibitors.

- Nitric oxide (NO) plays an important role in penile erection. PDE5 inhibitors enhance the effect of NO on erection, strengthening erections triggered by any pathway.

- Reflexogenic erections are typically preserved for an individual with either complete or incomplete SCI with preserved sensation and/or voluntary motor control of the S2–S5 area and any presence of a bulbocavernosus.

- The effect of SCI on orgasm can be determined by assessing the impact of injury on the bulbocavernosus and anal wink reflexes and the degree of completeness of injury at the S2–S5 level. It is unlikely that individuals with complete injuries at the S2–S5 level with an absent bulbocavernosus and anal wink reflex will be able to achieve a complete physiological orgasm. However, vagal afferents, which are not damaged by SCI, can be the basis of the psychological experience of orgasm. Thus, it is important to educate the patient to explore new areas of the body that may lead to sexual pleasure and orgasm.

- Often a region of skin exists just below the lowest dematome with pre-injury levels of sensation which haspresent but altered sensation. This area, known as "the transition zone," often can be a source of erotic pleasure. Stimulation of this area can be arousing for both partners.

- Common medical complications of SCI include bladder and bowel problems, recurrent urinary tract infections, pain, spasticity, respiratory compromise, skin breakdown, erectile dysfunction, and autonomic dysreflexia (AD).

- Throughout a patient's initial hospitalization for rehabilitation following SCI, anger and excessive demands are best handled by reassurance and firm limit-setting by the rehabilitation staff. Setting firm and clear limits is essential for the patient to feel safe and cared for. It should be done in an empathetic, supportive, and non-punitive manner Limit setting communicates expectations for recovery of function and encourages a sense of independence and self-control.

- Patients with SCI when intoxicated with alcohol or drugs may fail to reposition themselves to avoid pressure-related skin breakdown.

- Spinal shock can cause a reversible loss of erections following SCI. With incomplete lesions the capacity for erections can return days to weeks after the injury; with complete lesions it can return as long as a year or more after the injury. For these reason surgical treatment for post-SCI erectile dysfunction should not be employed during the first year following the injury.

- Vibrators can cause autonomic dysreflexia in individuals with SCI at T6 or Sexual aids that cause friction on the skin may can cause skin breakdown in denervated areas of skin.

- Individuals with SCI at or above T6 who are at risk for autonomic dysreflexia (AD) should receive early basic education on how to prevent, respond to, and intervene if AD should occur. Symptoms and signs of AD include very high blood pressure, slowed heart rate, pounding headache, sweating, flushing, pallor, nasal congestion, blurred vision, nausea, and piloerection. Sublingual nifedipine can be used both for treatment and for prophylaxis of recurrent AD: other options include nitroglycerin paste and prazosin.

- Consider low testosterone in the differential of low libidos in SCI patients. Also, consider the diagnosis when neural pathways for erection are intact but the patient has erective dysfunction not resolved with PDE5 inhibitors.

- PDE5 inhibitors do not initiate erections; they simply make them stronger.

- PDE6 type 6 is located in the retina and is responsible for visual disturbances with PDE5 inhibitors. Visual adverse effects of PDE5 inhibitors are most frequent with sildenafil because it is the least selective of the drugs in the class.

- Absolute contraindications to the use of PDE5 inhibitors include the concomitant use of nitrates or the presence of retinitis pigmentosa.

- Ejaculation is a spinal reflex elicited by stimulation of the dorsal penile nerve, which is the sensory branch of the pudendal nerve terminating in sacral spinal cord segments S2–S4. This reflex arc is best illustrated by the ability of vibratory stimulation of the penis to induce ejaculation in patients with complete spinal cord transection above the T10 segmental level.

- Treatment of depression in patients with SCI should when possible utilize antidepressant drugs with a low incidence of sexual dysfunction.Men with SCI develop qualitative abnormalities of sperm two weeks after the injury. Collection of semen for cryopreservation should be considered during the two weeks post-injury, if the patient is medically stable and potentially interested in fathering children.

DISCLOSURE STATEMENTS

Dr. Kohut has no conflicts to disclose.
Dr. Seftel
Dr. Ducharme
Dr. Bodner
Dr. Fogel has no conflicts to disclose.

REFERENCES

Adams, F. (1886). *The genuine works of Hippocrates*. New York: W. Wood and Co.
Abdel-Baky, T. M., Begin, L. R., & Huynh, H. (1998). Spinal cord injury is associated with a disturbance in the expression of penile nitric oxide synthase: a paraplegic animal model. *International Journal of Impotence Research, 10*(Suppl 3), S18.

Anderson, K. D., Borisoff, J. F., Johnson, R. D., Stiens, S. A., & Elliott, S. L. (2007a). The impact of spinal cord injury on sexual function: concerns of the general population. *Spinal Cord, 45*(5), 328–337.

Anderson, K. D., Borisoff, J. F., Johnson, R. D., Stiens, S. A., & Elliott, S. L. (2007b). Spinal cord injury influences psychogenic as well as physical components of female sexual ability. *Spinal Cord, 45*(5), 349–359.

Azadzoi, K. M., Kim, N., Brown, M. L., Goldstein, I., Cohen, R. A., & Saenz de Tejada, I. (1992). Endothelium-derived nitric oxide and cyclooxygenase products modulate corpus cavernosum smooth muscle tone. *The Journal of Urology, 147*(1), 220–225.

Banerjea, R., Findley, P. A., Smith, B., Findley, T., & Sambamoorthi, U. (2009). Co-occurring medical and mental illness and substance use disorders among veteran clinic users with spinal cord injury patients with complexities. *Spinal Cord, 47,* 789–795.

Bauman, W. A., & Spungen, A. M. (2000). Metabolic changes in persons after spinal cord injury. *Physical medicine & rehabilitation Clinics of North America, 11*(1), 109–140.

Bauman, W. A., Cirnigliaro, C. M., La Fountaine, M. F., Jensen, A. M., Wecht, J. M., Kirshblum, S. C., et al. (2011). A small-scale clinical trial to determine the safety and efficacy of testosterone replacement therapy in hypogonadal men with spinal cord injury. *Hormone & Metabolic Research, 43*(8), 574–579.

Bodner, D. R., Haas, C. A., Krueger, B., & Seftel, A. D. (1999). Intraurethral alprostadil for treatment of erectile dysfunction in patients with spinal cord injury. *Urology, 53*(1), 199–202.

Bodner, D. R., Leffler, B., & Frost, F. (1992). The role of intracavernous injection of vasoactive medications for the restoration of erection in spinal cord injured males: A three-year follow up. *Paraplegia, 30*(2), 118–120.

Brackett, N. L., Ibrahim, E., Iremashvili, V., Aballa, T. C., & Lynne, C. M. (2010). Treatment for ejaculatory dysfunction in men with spinal cord injury: An 18-year single center experience. *The Journal of Urology, 183*(6), 2304–2308.

Brackett, N. L., Lynne, C. M., Ibrahim, E., Ohl, D. A., & Sonksen, J. (2010). Treatment of infertility in men with spinal cord injury. *Nature Reviews. Urology, 7*(3), 162–172.

Breasted, J. H. (1930).. *The Edwin Smith surgical papyrus.* Chicago, IL: The University of Chicago Press.

Bredt, D. S., & Snyder, S. H. (1994). Nitric oxide: A physiologic messenger molecule. *Annual Review of Biochemistry, 63,* 175–195.

Brown, D. J., Hill, S. T., & Baker, H. W. G. (2006). Male fertility and sexual function after spinal cord injury. *Progress in Brain Research, 152,* 427–439.

Burnett, A. L., Lowenstein, C. J., Bredt, D. S., Chang, T. S., & Snyder, S. H. (1992). Nitric oxide: A physiologic mediator of penile erection. *Science, 257*(5068), 401–403.

Caplan, B. (1982). Neuropsychology in rehabilitation: Its role in evaluation and intervention. *Archives of Physical Medicine & Rehabilitation, 63*(8), 362–366.

Chen, K. K., Chan, S. H., Chang, L. S., & Chan, J. Y. (1997). Participation of paraventricular nucleus of hypothalamus in central regulation of penile erection in the rat. *The Journal of Urology, 158*(1), 238–244.

Clark, M. J., Schopp, L. H., Mazurek, M. O., Zaniletti, I., Lammy, A. B., Martin, T. A., et al. (2008). Testosterone levels among men with spinal cord injury: Relationship between time since injury and laboratory values. *American Journal of Physical Medicine & Rehabilitation/Association of Academic Physiatrists, 87*(9), 758–767.

Clayton, A. H., Croft, H. A., & Handiwala, L. (2014). Antidepressants and sexual dysfunction: mechanisms and clinical implications. *Postrgraduate Medicine, 126*(2), 91–99.

Collins, K. P., & Hackler, R. H. (1988). Complications of penile prostheses in the spinal cord injury population. *The Journal of Urology, 140*(5), 984–985.

Consortium for Spinal Cord Medicine (2010). Sexuality and reproductive health in adults with spinal cord injury: A clinical practice guideline for health-care professionals. *The Journal of Spinal Cord Medicine, 33*(3), 281–336.

Courtois, F. J., Goulet, M. C., Charvier, K. F., & Leriche, A. (1999). Posttraumatic erectile potential of spinal cord injured men: How physiologic recordings supplement subjective reports. *Archives of Physical Medicine & Rehabilitation, 80*(10), 1268–1272.

Dahlberg, A., Alaranta, H. T., Kautiainen, H., & Kotila, M. (2007). Sexual activity and satisfaction in men with traumatic spinal cord lesion. *Journal of Rehabilitation Medicine: Official Journal of the UEMS European Board of Physical & Rehabilitation Medicine, 39*(2), 152–155.

Das, S., Soni, B. M., Sharma, S. D., Gazvani, R., & Lewis-Jones D. I. (2006). A case of rapid deterioration in sperm quality following spinal cord injury. *Spinal Cord, 44*(1), 56–58.

Deforge, D., Blackmer, J., Garritty, C., Yazdi, F., Cronin, V., Barrowman, N., et al. (2006). Male erectile dysfunction following spinal cord injury: A systematic review. *Spinal Cord, 44*(8), 465–473.

Del Popolo, G., Li Marzi, V., Mondaini, N., & Lombardi, G. (2004). Time/duration effectiveness of sildenafil versus tadalafil in the treatment of erectile dysfunction in male spinal cord-injured patients. *Spinal Cord, 42*(11), 643–648.

DeLisa, J. A., & Gans, B. M. (1998). *Rehabilitation medicine: Principles and practice* (3rd ed.). Philadelphia, PA: Lippincott-Raven.

Denil, J., Ohl, D. A., & Smythe, C. (1996). Vacuum erection device in spinal cord injured men: Patient and partner satisfaction. *Archives of Physical Medicine & Rehabilitation, 77*(8), 750–753.

Dietrick, R. B., & Russi, S. (1958). Tabulation and review of autopsy findings in fifty-five paraplegics. *Journal of the American Medical Association, 166*(1), 41–44.

Durga, A., Sepahpanah, F., Regozzi, M., Hastings, J., & Crane, D. A. (2011). Prevalence of testosterone deficiency after spinal cord injury. *PM & R: The Journal of Injury, Function, & Rehabilitation, 3*(10), 929–932.

Everaert, K., de Waard, W. I., Van Hoof, T., Kiekens, C., Mulliez, T., & D'Herde, C. (2010). Neuroanatomy and neurophysiology related to sexual dysfunction in male neurogenic patients with lesions to the spinal cord or peripheral nerves. *Spinal Cord, 48*(3), 182–191. doi: 10.1038/sc.2009.172

Forsythe, E., & Horsewell, J. E. (2006). Sexual rehabilitation of women with a spinal cord injury. *Spinal Cord, 44,* 234–241.

Freed, M. M., Bakst, H. J., & Barrie, D. L. (1966). Life expectancy, survival rates, and causes of death in civilian patients with spinal cord trauma. *Archives of Physical Medicine & Rehabilitation, 47*(7), 457–463.

Garban, H., Marquez, D., Magee, T., Moody, J., Rajavashisth, T., Rodriguez, J. A., et al. (1997). Cloning of rat and human inducible penile nitric oxide synthase. Application for gene therapy of erectile dysfunction. *Biology of Reproduction, 56*(4), 954–963.

Ghidini, A., Healey, A., Andreani, M., & Simonson, M. R. (2008). Pregnancy and women with spinal cord injuries. *Acta Obstetrica et Gynecologica Scandinavica, 87*(10), 1006–1010.

Giuliano, F. (2011). Neurophysiology of erection and ejaculation. *Journal of Sexual Medicine 8 (Supplement 4)*: 310–315.

Giuliano, F., Hultling, C., El Masry, W. S., Smith, M. D., Osterloh, I. H., Orr, M., et al. (1999). Randomized trial of sildenafil for the treatment of erectile dysfunction in spinal cord injury. Sildenafil Study Group. [Clinical trial randomized controlled trial, Research Support, Non-U.S. Gov't.] *Annals of Neurology, 46*(1), 15–21.

Giuliano, F., Rubio-Aurioles, E., Kennelly, M., Montorsi, F., Kim, E. D., Finkbeiner, A. E., et al. (2006). Efficacy and safety of vardenafil in men with erectile dysfunction caused by spinal cord injury. *Neurology, 66*(2), 210–216.

Giuliano, F., Sanchez-Ramos, A., Lochner-Ernst, D., Del Popolo, G., Cruz, N., Leriche, A., et al. (2007). Efficacy and safety of tadalafil in men with erectile dysfunction following spinal cord injury. *Archives of Neurology, 64*(11), 1584–1592.

Griffith, E. R., & Trieschmann, R. B. (1975). Sexual functioning in women with spinal cord injury. *Archives of Physical Medicine & Rehabilitation, 56*(1), 18–21.

Heller, L., Keren, O., Aloni, R., & Davidoff, G. (1992). An open trial of vacuum penile tumescence: Constriction therapy for neurological impotence. *Paraplegia, 30*(8), 550–553.

Higgins, G. E., Jr. (1979). Sexual response in spinal cord injured adults: A review of the literature. *Archives of Sexual Behavior, 8*(2), 173–196.

Holmes, G. (1915). The Goulstonian Lectures on Spinal Injuries of Warfare: Delivered before the Royal College of Physicians of London. *British Medical Journal, 2*(2865), 769–774.

Hwang, M., Chlan, K. M., Vogel, L. C., & Zebracki, K. (2102). Substance use in young adults with pediatric-onset spinal cord injury. *Spinal Cord, 50*(7), 497–501.

Jackson, A. B., & Wadley, V. (1999). A multicenter study of women's self-reported reproductive health after spinal cord injury. *Archives of Physical Medicine & Rehabilitation, 80*(11), 1420–1428.

Kabalin, J. N., & Kessler, R. (1988). Infectious complications of penile prosthesis surgery. *The Journal of Urology, 139*(5), 953–955.

Khorrami, M. H., Javid, A., Moshtaghi, D., Nourimahdavi, K., Mortazavi, A., & Zia, H. R. (2010). Sildenafil efficacy in erectile dysfunction secondary to spinal cord injury depends on the level of cord injuries. *International Journal of Andrology, 33*(6), 861–864.

Kim, N., Azadzoi, K. M., Goldstein, I., & Saenz de Tejada, I. (1991). A nitric oxide-like factor mediates nonadrenergic-noncholinergic neurogenic relaxation of penile corpus cavernosum smooth muscle. *The Journal of Clinical Investigation, 88*(1), 112–118.

Kim, Y. D., Yang, S. O., Lee, J. K., Jung, T. Y., & Shim, H. B. (2008). Usefulness of a malleable penile prosthesis in patients with a spinal cord injury. *International Journal of Urology: Official Journal of the Japanese Urological Association, 15*(10), 919–923.

Kimoto, Y., & Iwatsubo, E. (1994). Penile prostheses for the management of the neuropathic bladder and sexual dysfunction in spinal cord injury patients: Long term follow up. *Paraplegia, 32*(5), 336–339.

Kostovski, E., Iversen, P. O., Birkeland, K., Torjesen, P. A., & Hjeltnes, N. (2008). Decreased levels of testosterone and gonadotrophins in men with long-standing tetraplegia. *Spinal Cord, 46*(8), 559–564.

Koyuncu, H., Serefoglu, E. C., Ozdemir, A. T., & Hellstrom, W. J. (2012). Deleterious effects of selective serotonin reuptake inhibitor treatment on semen parameters in patients with lifelong premature ejaculation. *International Journal of Impotence Research, 243*(5), 171–173.

Kreuter, M., Taft, C., Siösteen, A., & Beiring-Sørensen, F. (2011). Women's sexual functioning and sex life after spinal cord injury. *Spinal Cord, 49*, 154–160.

Krueger, D. W. (1984). *Emotional rehabilitation of physical trauma and disability.* New York: SP Medical & Scientific Books.

Lai, H. H., & Boone, T. B. (2008). Urological management of spinal cord injury. In *AUA Update Series* (Vol. 27, pp. 234–240). Linthicum, MD: American Urological Association Education and Research.

Lue, T. F. (2011). Physiology of penile erection and pathophysiology of erectile dysfunction. In A. J. Wein, L. R. Kavoussi, A. W. Partin, C. A. Peters, & A. C. Novick (Eds.), *Campbell-Walsh urology* (10th ed., Vol. 1, pp. 688–720). Philadelphia, PA: Elsevier Saunders.

Lue, T. F., Takamura, T., Schmidt, R. A., Palubinskas, A. J., & Tanagho, E. A. (1983). Hemodynamics of erection in the monkey. *The Journal of Urology, 130*(6), 1237–1241.

MacDonald, K., & Feifel, D. (2012). Dramatic improvement in sexual function induced by intranasal oxytocin. *Journal of Sexual Medicine, 9*, 1407–1410.

Marson, L., & McKenna, K. E. (1996). CNS cell groups involved in the control of the ischiocavernosus and bulbospongiosus muscles: A transneuronal tracing study using pseudorabies virus. *The Journal of Comparative Neurology, 374*(2), 161–179.

Marson, L., Platt, K. B., & McKenna, K. E. (1993). Central nervous system innervation of the penis as revealed by the transneuronal transport of pseudorabies virus. *Neuroscience, 55*(1), 263–280.

Mesard, L., Carmody, A., Mannarino, E., & Ruge, D. (1978). Survival after spinal cord trauma. A life table analysis. *Archives of Neurology, 35*(2), 78–83.

Moemen, M. N., Fahmy, I., AbdelAal, M., Kamel, I., Mansour, M., & Arafa, M. M. (2008). Erectile dysfunction in spinal cord-injured men: Different treatment options. *International Journal of Impotence Research, 20*(2), 181–187.

Montague, D. K., Jarow, J. P., Broderick, G. A., Dmochowski, R. R., Heaton, J. P., Lue, T. F., et al. (2005). Chapter 1: The management of erectile dysfunction: an AUA update. *The Journal of Urology, 174*(1), 230–239.

National Spinal Cord Injury Statistical Center (2011). Spinal cord injury facts and figures at a glance. Retrieved September 6, 2011, from https:// www.nscisc.uab.edu.

O'Kelly, F., Manecksha, R. P., Cullen, I. M., McDermott, T. E., Flynn, R., & Grainger, R. (2011). Electroejaculatory stimulation and its implications for male infertility in spinal cord injury: A short history through four decades of sperm retrieval (1975–2010). *Urology, 77*(6), 1349–1352.

Padma-Nathan, H., Hellstrom, W. J., Kaiser, F. E., Labasky, R. F., Lue, T. F., Nolten, W. E., et al. (1997). Treatment of men with erectile dysfunction with transurethral alprostadil. Medicated Urethral System for Erection (MUSE) study group. *The New England Journal of Medicine, 336*(1), 1–7.

Patki, P., Woodhouse, J., Hamid, R., Craggs, M., & Shah, J. (2008). Effects of spinal cord injury on semen parameters. *The Journal of Spinal Cord Medicine, 31*(1), 27–32.

Perkash, I., Kabalin, J. N., Lennon, S., & Wolfe, V. (1992). Use of penile prostheses to maintain external condom catheter drainage in spinal cord injury patients. *Paraplegia, 30*(5), 327–332.

Podnar, S. (2008). Clinical and neurophysiological testing of the penilo-cavernosus reflex. *Neurourology and Urodynamics, 27*, 399–402.

Rajfer, J., Aronson, W. J., Bush, P. A., Dorey, F. J., & Ignarro, L. J. (1992). Nitric oxide as a mediator of relaxation of the corpus cavernosum in response to nonadrenergic, noncholinergic neurotransmission. *The New England Journal of Medicine, 326*(2), 90–94.

Rivas, D. A., & Chancellor, M. B. (1994). Complications associated with the use of vacuum constriction devices for erectile dysfunction in the spinal cord injured population. *The Journal of the American Paraplegia Society, 17*(3), 136–139.

Rutberg, L., Fridén, B., & Karlsson, A. K. (2008). Amenorrhea in newly spinal cord injured women: an effect of hyperprolactinaemia? *Spinal Cord, 46*(3), 189–191.

Safarinejad, M. R. (2001). Level of injury and hormone profiles in spinal cord-injured men. *Urology, 58*(5), 671–676.

Saunders, L. L., & Krause, J. S. (2011). Psychological factors affecting alcohol use after spinal cord injury. *Spinal Cord, 49*(5), 637–642.

Schmid, D. M., Schurch, B., & Hauri, D. (2000). Sildenafil in the treatment of sexual dysfunction in spinal cord-injured male patients. *European Urology, 38*(2), 184–193.

Schnoll, S. H., Heinemann, A. W., Doll, M., & Armstrong, K. J. (1989). Substance use and receipt of treatment in persons with recent spinal cord injuries. *NIDA research monograph, 95*, 426–427.

Schopp, L. H., Clark, M., Mazurek, M. O., Hagglund, K. J., Acuff, M. E., Sherman, A. K., et al. (2006). Testosterone levels among men with spinal cord injury admitted to inpatient rehabilitation. *American journal of physical medicine & rehabilitation/Association of Academic Physiatrists, 85*(8), 678–684.

Schneiderman, I., Zagoory-Sharon, O., Leckman, J. F., & Feldman, R. (2012). Oxytocin during the initial stages of romantic attachment: relations to couples' interactive reciprocity. *Psychoneuroendocrinology, 37*(8), 1277–1285.

Seftel, A. D., Vaziri, N. D., Ni, Z., Razmjouei, K., Fogarty, J., Hampel, N., et al. (1997). Advanced glycation end products in human penis: Elevation in diabetic tissue, site of deposition, and possible effect through iNOS or eNOS. *Urology, 50*(6), 1016–1026.

Seftel, A. D., Viola, K. A., Kasner, S. E., & Ganz, M. B. (1996). Nitric oxide relaxes rabbit corpus cavernosum smooth muscle via a potassium-conductive pathway. *Biochemical & biophysical research communications, 219*(2), 382–387.

Sheel, A. W., Krassioukov, A. V., Inglis, J. T., & Elliott, S. L. (2005). Autonomic dysreflexia during sperm retrieval in spinal cord injury: Influence of lesion level and sildenafil citrate. *Journal of applied physiology, 99*(1), 53–58.

Sipski, M. L., Alexander, C. J., & Rosen, R. (2001). Sexual arousal and orgasm in women: effects of spinal cord injury. *Annals of neurology*, *49*(1), 35–44.

Sipski, M. L., & Arenas, A. (2006). Female sexual function after spinal cord injury. *Progress in Brain Research*, *152*, 441–447.

Sipski, M., Alexander, C., Gomez-Marin, O., & Spalding, J. (2007). The effects of spinal cord injury on psychogenic sexual arousal in males. *The Journal of urology*, *177*(1), 247–251.

Soler, J. M., Previnaire, J. G., Denys, P., & Chartier-Kastler, E. (2007). Phosphodiesterase inhibitors in the treatment of erectile dysfunction in spinal cord-injured men. *Spinal cord*, *45*(2), 169–173.

Steinberger, R. E., Ohl, D. A., Bennett, C. J., McCabe, M., & Wang, S. C. (1990). Nifedipine pretreatment for autonomic dysreflexia during electroejaculation. *Urology 36*(3), 228–231.

Strauss, D. J., Devivo, M. J., Paculdo, D. R., & Shavelle, R. M. (2006). Trends in life expectancy after spinal cord injury. *Archives of physical medicine & rehabilitation*, *87*(8), 1079–1085.

Stroud, M. W., Bombardier, C. H., Dyer, J. R., Rimmele, C. T., & Esselman, P. C. (2011). Preinjury alcohol and drug use among persons with spinal cord injury: implications for rehabilitation. *Journal of Spinal Cord Medicine*, *34*(5), 461–472.

Tepper, M. (2002). *Sex and the Internet: a guidebook for clinicians*. New York: Brunner-Routledge.

Thackare, H., Nicholson, H. D., & Whittington, K. (2006). Oxytocin—its role in male reproduction and new potential therapeutic uses. *Human Reproduction Update*, *12*(4), 437–448.

Thomas, D. R. (2003). Medications and sexual function. *Clinics in geriatric medicine*, *19*(3), 553–562.

Tsuji, I., Nakajima, F., Morimoto, J., & Nounaka, Y. (1961). The sexual function in patients with spinal cord injury. *Urologia internationalis*, *12*, 270–280.

Vaidyananthan, S., Soni, B. M., Brown, E., Sett, P., Krishnan, K. R., Bingley, J., et al. (1998). Effect of intermittent urethral catheterization and oxybutynin bladder instillation on urinary continence status and quality of life in a selected group of spinal cord injury patients with neuropathic bladder dysfunction. *Spinal Cord*, *36*(6), 409–414.

Vizzard, M. A., Erickson, V. L., Card, J. P., Roppolo, J. R., & de Groat, W. C. (1995). Transneuronal labeling of neurons in the adult rat brainstem and spinal cord after injection of pseudorabies virus into the urethra. *The Journal of comparative neurology*, *355*(4), 629–640.

Westgren, N., & Levi, R. (1994). Motherhood after traumatic spinal cord injury. *Paraplegia*, *32*(8), 517–523.

Widerstrom-Noga, E. G., Felipe-Cuervo, E., Broton, J. G., Duncan, R. C., & Yezierski, R. P. (1999). Perceived difficulty in dealing with consequences of spinal cord injury. *Archives of physical medicine & rehabilitation*, *80*(5), 580–586.

Wieder, J. A., Brackett, N. L., Lynne, C. M., Green, J. T., & Aballa, T. C. (2000). Anesthetic block of the dorsal penile nerve inhibits vibratory-induced ejaculation in men with spinal cord injuries *Urology*, *55*(6), 915–917.

Williams, R., & Murray, A. (2014). Prevalence of depression following spinal cord injury: a meta-analysis. *Archives of Physical Medicine and Rehabilitation* pii: S0003–9993(14)01029-6. doi: 10.1016/j. apmr.2014.08.016. [Epub ahead of print].

Yildiz, N., Gokkaya, N. K., Koseoglu, F., Gokkaya, S., & Comert, D. (2011). Efficacies of papaverine and sildenafil in the treatment of erectile dysfunction in early-stage paraplegic men. *International journal of rehabilitation research*. *34*(1), 44–52.

Zermann, D. H., Kutzenberger, J., Sauerwein, D., Schubert, J., & Loeffler, U. (2006). Penile prosthetic surgery in neurologically impaired patients: Long-term followup. *The Journal of urology*, *175*(3 Pt 1), 1041–1044.

PART IX

CHILDREN AND ADOLESCENTS

79.

PSYCHIATRIC ASSESSMENT OF THE PHYSICALLY ILL CHILD

Wendy Froehlich-Santino, Hans Steiner, and Richard J. Shaw

THE DEVELOPMENTAL PERSPECTIVE

One of the most critical differences between the approach to the assessment and management of child and adolescent patients compared to adult patients is the need to incorporate a developmental perspective. This approach, which was originally grounded in psychoanalytic theory and developmental psychology, informs the work of the pediatric psychiatrist (Cicchetti & Cohen, 1995; Steiner, 1997b). It is an approach that is now more limited in adult psychiatric practice, partly in response to the impact of current phenomenologically based diagnostic classification systems, such as the International Statistical Classification of Diseases and Related Health Problems (ICD)-10 (World Health Organization, 1992) and the *Diagnostic and Statistical Manual of Mental Disorders, Fifth Edition* (American Psychiatric Association, 2013). Conceptually, the developmental approach is a special instance of the biopsychosocial paradigm. The developmental approach in children gives special consideration to the temporal relationship of the biological, psychological, and social variables evaluated and described in the patient, as the child's individual development unfolds and progresses over time. Three concepts—continuity, context, and complexity—help differentiate the developmental approach proposed in this chapter and clarify essential differences between this approach and purely descriptive and biological-psychiatric models of diagnosis and treatment.

CONTINUITY

Many so-called psychopathological symptoms appear to be widely present in non-clinical populations; symptoms sometimes diagnosed as pathological may be continuous with, and represent no more than an exaggeration of, normal behavior. For example, somatization, or the vigilant surveillance of one's bodily functioning, cannot immediately be assumed to be pathological. Somatization and the use of somatically based words to describe affective distress (somatothymia) is widespread in the general population (Stoudemire, 1991). In certain circumstances, however, such as when a child is suffering from a chronic physical illness, somatic symptoms of emotional distress may reach a level of intensity that interferes with the child's treatment and functioning. The developmentally oriented clinician continuously weighs the available clinical evidence when deciding which behaviors are and are not pathological or are within the norm for the child's age.

In line with epidemiological data, "continuity" also describes the concept that psychiatric illness results from the gradual accumulation of risk factors over time, particularly in the absence of sufficient protective or "buffering" factors (Figure 79.1). These risk factors for psychiatric illness may be diverse and include ecological, constitutional, genetic, interpersonal, and intrapsychic variables. Psychiatric disorders rarely result from a single event, although post-traumatic stress disorder (PTSD) can be an exception. Typically, psychiatric disorders evolve over time, becoming manifest after a generally prolonged exposure to various risk factors. The study of prodromal syndromes can be as important as evaluation of fully evolved psychiatric disorders. Early identification of prodromal syndromes can alert clinicians to the need for early intervention and may enable the prevention of more severe manifestations (Gyllenberg et al., 2010; Mrazek & Haggerty, 1994; Skovgaard, 2010).

The concept of continuity also suggests that there may be psychological sequelae in the aftermath of an acute mental disorder. Complete resolution of symptoms is the exception rather than the rule. As in adults, it is common for children and adolescents to have special sensitivities and higher relapse rates, even following successful initial treatment. Awareness of this possibility should lead to caution regarding the expectations for cure, as well as greater vigilance when the child or adolescent negotiates subsequent stressful developmental transitions.

CONTEXT

The importance of the larger *social context* has been well delineated by proponents of the social-ecology model of mental health. Bronfenbrenner's theory is of particular relevance for children (Bronfenbrenner & Crouter, 1983). It states that development co-occurs in several contexts, including the micro-system (family), mesosystem (interactions between the family, schools, and hospitals), exosystem (social support networks), and macro-system (society, culture, and policy). Social context is important for both the definition and the delineation of psychopathology. The social environment of the child

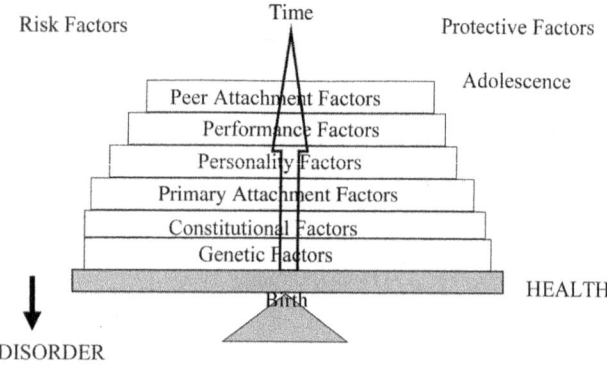

Risk Factors   Time   Protective Factors

Adolescence

Peer Attachment Factors
Performance Factors
Personality Factors
Primary Attachment Factors
Constitutional Factors
Genetic Factors

Birth   HEALTH

DISORDER

Figure 79.1 The vulnerability/resilience model for the development of psychopathology

is a crucial element in terms of providing a supportive context in which to provide appropriate medical or psychiatric treatment. Sometimes, the social environment itself is the major factor in the genesis of psychopathology in the patient. Examples include families of physically ill children whose parents refuse treatment for religious reasons, or the direct result of injurious behavior caused by parents in the cases of factitious disorder by proxy (Shaw, Dayal, Hartman, & DeMaso, 2008).

It is also important to consider the concept of the *temporal context* in which symptoms present. As children pass through their distinct phases of development, *domains of functioning* change in sometimes dramatic and unpredictable ways (Kagan, 1989). What is considered "normal" one day may be pathological the next. For example, "stranger anxiety" may be normal for an infant, but it suggests pathology in the case of an adolescent with separation anxiety disorder.

It is absolutely critical to consider age-specific developmental norms in the approach to psychopathology. While it is true that much of development proceeds in a progressive and predictable sequence, qualitative and unexpected shifts frequently occur. A child's or adolescent's behavior can only be understood in the context and spectrum of the child's overall developmental progression.

COMPLEXITY

As children develop new competencies and skills, the central nervous system becomes increasingly differentiated and complex. Complex behaviors and mental states emerge but are based on their less complex antecedents. For example, new skills supersede old ones, but contain within them the nucleus of older, mastered skills. This principle of past behavior being enveloped in current behavior is important with regard to the emergence of psychopathology. If a child is unable to sufficiently resolve the issues of an early stage of development, it is likely that these issues will reemerge later in subsequent developmental transitions, usually under some sort of stress. For example, disorders of attachment in relation to the primary attachment figure may result in difficulties in adult attachment relationships (Cicchetti & Cohen, 1995). Conversely, difficulties in attachment may be repaired by the experience of a positive relationship with an

adult outside of the family (Rutter, 1988). Such relationships can contribute to resilience in youth at risk (Rutter, 1988; Werner & Smith, 1992).

Complexity of functioning also can change in situations of extreme stress, particularly in situations when the child or adolescent has only recently acquired newly developed skills. In such cases, it is possible to see a return to less complex and less mature levels of functioning, the reemergence of old behaviors and problems, and the loss of newly acquired skills. This type of behavior is known as *regression* and is common even in physically ill adults.

Acute medical illness, inpatient hospitalizations, and the stress of pain or invasive medical procedures often result in regression in the behavior of hospitalized children as well as adults. Children may manifest increased clinginess and anxiety around separations, bed-wetting, and, in extreme cases, even regression in their use of language. Regression to earlier phases of development must be carefully differentiated from the more serious phenomenon of developmental "arrest." The bio-genetic drive toward healthy development, which is genetically preprogrammed in children, will often serve to repair temporary regressions without the need for intensive psychiatric interventions.

THE DEVELOPMENTAL APPROACH TO PSYCHOPATHOLOGY: IMPLICATIONS FOR DIAGNOSIS AND TREATMENT

Having outlined the essential tenets of the developmental approach, we now turn to a discussion of the implications for the diagnosis and treatment of children and adolescents. Clearly, it is important to adjust the assessment and intervention strategies to match the level of cognitive and social development of the child, taking into account the child's limitations, but also respecting the child's particular age-specific strengths and skills.

DIAGNOSTIC APPROACHES

Although the psychiatric assessment of the child and family has much in common with that of adult patients, there are some important practical and conceptual differences. As with adult patients, the history is the foundation of the assessment.

Assessment is more difficult with younger children, since they are often not able to accurately report their behavior and symptoms and may not have an adult comprehension of such concepts as "cause and effect." Later in this chapter, reference will be made to problems with overreliance on self-reported symptoms and history, as well as the need to engage parents in the assessment process. Box 79.1 outlines the major areas that should be covered in the assessment. Box 79.2 focuses more on addressing specific areas related to the impact of the illness on the micro-system (family) and exo-system (friends), as well as investigating how the illness is viewed and fits into the overall macro-system. The American Academy of Child and Adolescent Psychiatry (AACAP) Practice

Parameters (DeMaso et al., 2009) recommend beginning with open-ended questions about these interrelated domains and stress the importance of a biopsychosocial approach, as opposed to trying to separate the medical illness from psychiatric and social functioning. These same principles and recommended areas of inquiry are further discussed in detail in Chapter 3 of *The Textbook of Pediatric Psychosomatic Medicine* (Goldman, Shaw, & Demaso, 2010).

To perform a comprehensive consultation, clinicians must collate information from parents, caretakers, schoolteachers, and counselors. In physically ill and hospitalized children, information from nurses and medical staff involved in their care is often helpful. This is particularly important when there are questions about treatment adherence. In general, separate meetings with the parents are recommended to collect a full and comprehensive developmental and clinical history. The AACAP Practice Parameters point out that even very ill children are able to listen and ponder information they hear, so it is important to give parents their own opportunity to meet privately with the clinician so that sensitive issues may be addressed without the child listening (DeMaso et al., 2009). This also allows the clinician to be less focused on collecting historical data during the child interview and permits more attention to developing a positive therapeutic rapport with the patient and to observing their play. Parents who are engaged in the assessment can then facilitate the introduction of the mental health consultant and advise on the best ways to engage the child.

During the child interview, it is usually advisable to explain to the child the purpose of the meeting, in simple and age-appropriate language. It is also important to clarify the limits of confidentiality as they apply in a consultation relationship, and the circumstances in which confidential information may be disclosed to outside agencies; for example, when there are allegations of child abuse. For older children and adolescents, it is typically recommended that the interviewer spend some time alone with patients during the assessment so that patients may answer questions openly (DeMaso et al., 2009). This applies not only to questions regarding trauma, substance use, and sexual history, but also to psychiatric symptoms in general. Often, children and adolescents may not disclose the extent of their thoughts and emotions, in an effort to protect their parents or caretakers.

Preschool-age and school-age children are likely to respond better if offered the opportunity to meet in a playroom or to draw or play at the bedside. In younger or preverbal children, the play session is the primary instrument to assess the child's mental status, and it may involve a direct observation of the child's interactions with the parent, particularly when there are questions about parenting, feeding disorders, or disorders of attachment. It is important to observe the parent's ability to attend to and read the child's cues (the concept of affect "attunement") (Stern, 1985). It is also valuable to note the child's response to separation from the parent, the child's ability to engage in symbolic and age-appropriate play, and the child's reaction to the ending of the session.

SOURCES OF INFORMATION

Using the child as an informant to obtain a history or description of symptoms is perfectly admissible when the patient is older than 11 years of age, but doing so is problematic with younger children. Young children's capacity for self-observation and their ability to report on their bodily and mental functioning, behavior, or inner mental states is limited due to cognitive abilities that have not yet emerged. In addition, preschoolers are particularly vulnerable to suggestion and "leading" questioning (Flavell, 1985); that is, detecting and giving the answer the examiner wants. Suggestibility is influenced by both theory of mind and inhibitory control

(Scullin & Bonner, 2006), two cognitive skills that are still developing during early childhood. Because younger children have an underdeveloped theory of mind, they may be influenced by an incorrect perception of what they believe examiners are seeking. Concurrently, their lack of inhibitory control may sway them toward giving an answer they believe an examiner desires. Parental reports become increasingly important as one approaches the early school-age child, and is absolutely necessary when dealing with preschool-age children.

In adolescents, there is a similar divergence between self-report, parent-report, and the use of structured diagnostic interviews, but for very different reasons (Erickson & Steiner, 1999; Harris, Canning, & Kelleher, 1996; Steiner, 1996; Steiner & Canning, 1994). Although adolescents have sufficient cognitive skills to accurately report their history, there may be motivational factors that influence the self-report, including the wish to present themselves in a socially desirable manner. This wish may lead the patient to conceal risk-taking or pathological behaviors from perceived authority figures. Adolescents are prone to (unconscious) denial as well as conscious deception of others (Erickson & Steiner, 1999; Steiner, 1996). Many of the issues that need to be considered with regard to adolescents' reports on their health behaviors and various methods to obtain this information, such as cognitive and environmental factors, are reviewed in Sieving and Shrier's chapter *Measuring Adolescents Health Behaviors* (2009) and are summarized in Table 79.1.

Empirical data on the issue of convergence and divergence of measures in children support the importance of paying attention to these issues. Harris et al. (1996) showed that there was good concurrent validity when comparing three different parent-report measures in a sample of medically ill children. However, agreement between instruments and diagnoses determined by structured interviews of both parents and children was only "moderate." This study and a previous study by the same authors (Canning & Kelleher, 1994) found that parent-report and self-report instruments underestimated the proportion of children with chronic physical illness who had significant psychiatric comorbidity. Fewer psychiatric diagnoses will be missed if the clinician gathers information by interviewing both the patient and parents, and additional sources of information may reveal even more comorbidities. While parent and self-report instruments may have good specificity, sensitivities in these studies were low. These results demonstrate the need for a comprehensive approach in the assessment of physically ill pediatric patients.

Although self-report tools and parent-report tools completed by pediatric patients or their parents may underestimate the presence of psychiatric comorbidity, they can also play a significant role as screening tools. The Children's Depression Inventory (CDI) is a self-report tool for depression worded for children aged 8–13 years (Saylor, Finch, Spirito, & Bennett, 1984), and children as young as 6 or 7 years of age may be able to complete this measure. The Children's Depression Rating Scale (CDRS) is another self-report tool, for children ages 6–12, that has been shown to be useful in identifying depression in the pediatric medical setting (Poznanski, Cook, & Carroll, 1979). Additionally, shown in Table 79.2, the

Table 79.1 FACTORS AFFECTING ADOLESCENT SELF-REPORT

FACTOR	TREND TOWARD ACCURATE SELF-REPORT	TREND TOWARD INACCURATE SELF-REPORT
Cognitive Factors		
Comprehension	Strong reading, writing, and/or abstract reasoning skills:	Poor reading, writing, and/or abstract reasoning skills:
Recall ability: - Duration of time - Salience of event - Frequency of event - Complexity	- Short period between event and report - High salience of event - Low frequency of event/behavior - Simple event/behavior	- Long period between event and report - Low salience of event - High frequency of event/behavior - Complex event/behavior
Situational Factors		
Level of threat to self and level of emotional discomfort/distress: - Interviewers - Social structure - Interview setting - Question sensitivity	Interviewer perceived as comfortable and nonjudgemental - Responses congruent with social norms for age, gender, class, race, and ethnicity - Private interview setting - Non-sensitive questions	- Interviewer perceived as uncomfortable and/or judgemental - Responses incongruent with social norms for age, gender, class, race, and ethnicity - Non-private setting - Sensitive questions (i.e., regarding sensitive, stigmatized, or illegal behavior)

SOURCE: Sieving, R. E., & Shrier, L. A. (2009). Measuring adolescent health behaviors. In R. J. DiClemente, J. S. Santelli, & R. A. Crosby (Eds.), *Adolescent health: understanding and preventing risk behaviors* (pp. 473–492). San Francisco: Jossey-Bass Publishers.

Pediatric Symptom Checklist (PSC) is a short parent-report screening tool designed to use in a clinic or hospital setting that has been shown to be valid in children with chronic illness (Stoppelbein et al., 2005). It is also available as a self-report measure known as the Youth Pediatric Symptom Checklist (Y-PSC) for adolescents 11 years old and older. Measures such as these can be used to identify psychiatric comorbidities in the medical setting that may otherwise go undiagnosed.

DEVELOPMENTAL HISTORY

At the most rudimentary level, the developmental approach relies heavily on having a comprehensive developmental history. This section of the history includes cataloging the child's maturational milestones in addition to noting their successful mastery of crucial tasks at different key phases of development (Table 79.3). Categorizing the developmental trajectories in the major domains of functioning, along with an appropriate charting of milestones, impediments, and sensitivities, is essential in constructing a clear longitudinal picture of the child's development. Such an assessment helps differentiate between symptoms that may reflect a temporary regression in behavior, developmental arrest, or precocious development.

One area requiring special sensitivity is the assessment of psychosexual development in adolescents. Steiner and Lock's review (1998) of this topic is helpful in outlining a theoretical model to approach this subject in adolescents with chronic medical illness. The review highlights several studies demonstrating that various medical illnesses can negatively affect sexual development for both psychological and biological

reasons. Psychologically, children with chronic physical illness are more socially isolated with fewer opportunities for sexual development, may have overprotective parents, and may have more body-image disturbance, which can have a realistic basis in medical trauma and/or physical deformity. Biologically, many childhood illnesses and treatments may directly affect the endocrine system, resulting in various changes in hormonal levels affecting sexual maturation and development. Even disorders not typically thought of as endocrine disorders may adversely affect the endocrine system and sexual development. For example, boys with epilepsy have been shown to be at risk for delayed puberty, and often have abnormalities in levels of testosterone and/or estradiol (El-Khayat et al., 2003).

DOMAINS OF FUNCTIONING

Another essential component of developmental diagnostic practice is the acknowledgement of the *multidimensionality* of behavior, both normal and abnormal, in terms of *multiple domains of functioning*. These multiple dimensions are rarely fully captured by conventional descriptive and strictly empirically based diagnostic systems. The developmental formulation should include a description of problem behaviors, but in addition provide a picture of current adaptive skills of the patient as well as their past achievements in broad areas of functioning. In childhood, these developmental achievements include bodily functioning, and intrapsychic, interpersonal, academic, vocational, and recreational domains. Developmental diagnosis combines the categorical or "classification" method of diagnosis with the multidimensional

Table 79.2 PEDIATRIC SYMPTOM CHECKLIST

	NEVER (0)	SOMETIMES (1)	OFTEN (2)
1. Complains of aches and pains	1. _____	_____	_____
2. Spends more time alone	2. _____	_____	_____
3. Tires easily, has little energy	3. _____	_____	_____
4. Fidgety, unable to sit still	4. _____	_____	_____
5. Has trouble with teacher	5. _____	_____	_____
6. Less interested in school	6. _____	_____	_____
7. Acts as if driven by a motor	7. _____	_____	_____
8. Daydreams too much	8. _____	_____	_____
9. Distracted easily	9. _____	_____	_____
10. Is afraid of new situations	10. _____	_____	_____
11. Feels sad, unhappy	11. _____	_____	_____
12. Is irritable, angry	12. _____	_____	_____
13. Feels hopeless	13. _____	_____	_____
14. Has trouble concentrating	14. _____	_____	_____
15. Less interested in friends	15. _____	_____	_____
16. Fights with other children	16. _____	_____	_____
17. Absent from school	17. _____	_____	_____
18. School grades dropping	18. _____	_____	_____
19. Is down on him- or herself	19. _____	_____	_____
20. Visits the doctor with doctor finding nothing wrong	20. _____	_____	_____
21. Has trouble sleeping	21. _____	_____	_____
22. Worries a lot	22. _____	_____	_____
23. Wants to be with you more than before	23. _____	_____	_____
24. Feels he or she is bad	24. _____	_____	_____
25. Takes unnecessary risks	25. _____	_____	_____
26. Gets hurt frequently	26. _____	_____	_____
27. Seems to be having less fun	27. _____	_____	_____
28. Acts younger than children his or her age	28. _____	_____	_____
29. Does not listen to rules	29. _____	_____	_____
30. Does not show feelings	30. _____	_____	_____
31. Does not understand other people's feelings	31. _____	_____	_____
32. Teases others	32. _____	_____	_____
33. Blames others for his or her troubles	33. _____	_____	_____

(Continued)

Table 79.2 (CONTINUED)

34. Takes things that do not belong to him or her	34. _____	_____	_____
35. Refuses to share	35. _____	_____	_____

Total score _____

Does your child have any emotional or behavioral problems for which she/he needs help? __ No __ Yes

Are there any services that you would like your child to receive for these problems? __ No __ Yes

If yes, what type of services? _____

assessment of domains of functioning to get a comprehensive diagnostic picture and to clarify diagnostic subtypes. Discrete diagnostic categories, even if adjusted for specific age groups, rarely capture the entire clinical picture of the pediatric patient. For example, an adolescent with anorexia nervosa whose functioning in the domains of school and recreation is relatively unimpaired differs significantly from another patient with the same diagnosis but with severe school problems. In the case of children and adolescents, it is clear that school dysfunction is one of the key areas of concern with respect to both intervention and prognosis (Smith, Feldman, Nasserbakht, & Steiner, 1993).

ADAPTIVE VALUE OF THE SYMPTOM

The developmental clinician attempts to consider the positive or adaptive value of a syndrome or disorder in the child's life. Symptoms do not occur in a psychosocial vacuum;—they often fulfill a function for the child that can be understood by assessing the child's social and temporal context and their overall social equilibrium. Behavioral symptoms in children and adolescents are rarely a simple expression of a disease or illness that causes symptoms, and usually also have adaptive value for the child. Behavioral symptoms tend to help resolve conflict. For example, stomach pain that cannot be explained by medical causes alone may allow a child to avoid going to school, or concern for the ill child may be a distraction for quarreling parents and result in parents arguing less. Unfortunately, when a pattern of behavior becomes established, it is likely to continue, even when the specific psychosocial stressor that initiated the behavior resolves or changes, and the behavior is no longer of adaptive value. For example, a toddler whose mother is depressed and unable to cope with age-appropriate tantrums may respond by adopting an attitude of stoic acceptance and precocious functioning. In the short term, this behavior may have adaptive value both for the child, who is faced with a constant and real threat of abandonment, and for the parent. This same child, deprived of the opportunity to use ordinary expressive behaviors or demands to get attention for his or her basic emotional needs, may resort to a variety of maneuvers to engage the mother's attention. One such maneuver is the presentation of physical symptoms that may be exaggerated or even feigned; these might be acceptable to and bearable by the depressed mother in a way that temper tantrums are not. Reinforcement of this behavior by maternal attention and care can ultimately generate a

Table 79.3 SALIENT DEVELOPMENTAL ISSUES IN THE PHYSICALLY ILL CHILD

AGE (YEARS)	ISSUES
0–1	Biological regulation; harmonious dyadic interaction; formation of an effective attachment relationship
1–2 ½	Exploration, experimentation, and mastery of the object world (caregiver as secure base); individuation and autonomy; responding to external control of impulses
3–5	Flexible self-control; self-reliance; initiative; identification and gender concept; establishing effective peer contacts (empathy)
6–12	Social understanding (equity, fairness); gender constancy; same-sex chumships; sense of "industry" (competence); school adjustment
13+	"Formal operations" (flexible perspective taking; "as if" thinking); loyal friendships (same sex); beginning heterosexual relationships; emancipation; identity

SOURCE: Adapted from Sroufe, 2009

chronic pattern of excessive illness behavior and the inappropriate use of health care to meet emotional needs.

CASE FORMULATION

The hallmark of the developmental assessment is the summary case formulation, in which an attempt is made to integrate the information obtained during the assessment, with the ultimate goal of guiding the treatment intervention. AACAP Practice Parameters recommend integrating the assessment factors into a "developmentally informed biopsychosocial formulation" that can be used to establish an appropriate treatment plan (DeMaso et al., 2009). This formulation should include the special strengths of the child and the emotionally relevant protective factors, in addition to the more conventional description of symptoms, risks, and vulnerabilities. The formulation includes a careful weighing of those factors in the patient's life that promote development and may facilitate recovery. Two prospective outcome studies with conduct-disordered and eating-disordered adolescents have shown that such sub-typing based on risk factors can help predict outcomes 4.5 and 6 years after initial diagnosis (Smith et al., 1993; Steiner & Lock, 1998). Other studies have also shown significant effects of various risk and protective factors in mediating psychological outcomes. These include studies investigating peer and parental acceptance and rejection (Sentse, Lindenberg, Omvlee, Ormel, & Veenstra, 2010); warm family (parent and sibling) relationships and positive home environments (Bowes, Maughan, Caspi, Moffitt, & Arseneault, 2010); family routines and levels of parental monitoring (Murphy, Marelich, Herbeck, & Payne, 2009); and participation in group activities such as school clubs, sports, and religious groups (Piko & Fitzpatrick, 2004).

TREATMENT
Treatment Is Usually Multimodal

The recognition that a biopsychosocially oriented developmental formulation describes a complex mixture of symptoms, often in different domains of functioning, suggests that treatment interventions need to be multimodal in nature. This is in accordance with Principle 6 of the AACAP Guidelines, which states, "Psychotherapeutic management should consider multiple treatment modalities," and highlights individual therapy, family therapy, and behavior modification as treatment options, in addition to consideration of psychopharmacological management (DeMaso et al., 2009). Single-intervention packages, regardless of whether these employ psychopharmacological, psychotherapeutic, psychoeducational, or environmental manipulation, are rarely successful. The developmental approach is oriented toward multiple factors that affect development and that interact over time. Thus it is, by definition, non-reductionist. The developmentally oriented clinician does not expect that mood, appetite, sleep, social skills, and academic performance in a depressed child will all respond to the administration of an antidepressant. Although some of the basic biological symptoms of depression may respond, higher levels of functioning such as social skills and coping strategies generally require more complex and multimodal interventions that target both the child and the family, and in many cases may also require involvement of the school. Although interventions with children are often more complex, and as a result more costly, the failure to involve family members in the treatment is likely to interfere with the child's recovery.

The Timing of the Intervention

Wherever possible, the clinician should attempt to intervene early to prevent the development of psychiatric disorders. The assessment of risk and protective factors can help in the identification of children with particular risks and vulnerabilities. Pre-syndromal disturbances may be addressed in a timely manner with the goal of *primary* or *secondary* prevention. The prevention and prophylactic treatment of severe anticipatory anxiety in children related to invasive procedures or surgery, discussed below, provides a model for this type of intervention.

Intervention Is Driven by the Appropriate Formulation of the Problem

Knowledge of the progressive and hierarchical organization of development as well as the phenomena of behavioral *regression* and developmental *arrest* is essential in planning treatment. For example, the symptoms of a child with an eating disorder may represent the expression of enforced and precocious development—in adaptive response to stressful demands in the child's family context. The body-image distortion in an adolescent who grows up in a family and cultural milieu that highly values physical appearance and emphasizes health-oriented behaviors may result from pressure to conform to the demands of their social environment to the detriment of their functioning in other domains. In this case, the intervention should include efforts to change the family's expectations and to provide the child with strategies to manage peer group and social pressures. In contrast, body-image distortion in another adolescent patient may indicate developmental regression in response to an acute psychosocial stressor, such as the breakup of a romantic relationship or an episode of physical or sexual abuse. In this situation, the treatment is likely to be shorter term and to focus on helping the patient identify and address the relevant stressors, as well as promoting the use of more adaptive coping skills. In contrast, body-image distortion may persist in the form of a pattern of behavior such as a fixed preoccupation with body image and appearance well beyond the early adolescent years, and it is important to differentiate established eating disorders from more temporary changes in eating in response to stress.

Intervention Is Aimed at Restoration of the Normal Developmental Trajectory

One powerful tool for the clinician is that the momentum of the normal developmental process can work synergistically with the therapist. By adopting a longitudinal perspective and by having confidence in the restorative powers of time if stressors are decreased and maturation is allowed to proceed normally, bringing better adaptations, the clinician may sometimes decide that intensive psychiatric intervention is not needed. This is particularly true if the family can be relied upon to provide an environment that promotes development. For example, acute stress disorder following an acute trauma will not necessarily lead to the syndrome of PTSD in non-susceptible individuals, provided that the parents are able to provide appropriate support. Generally, the goal of all treatment interventions is to try to reestablish the normal developmental trajectory, and treatments are often made briefer and more rewarding by the resilience of children. The stability and supportive functioning of the family is a major determinant of short- and long-term outcome.

As noted earlier, interventions for children and adolescents will in almost all cases begin with both individual and family psychotherapy. Treatment will often begin with psychoeducation for the family to provide a context for the child's symptoms, and in many cases, behavioral interventions to address problematic behaviors. The nature of the psychotherapy work will be influenced by the child's symptoms. If the child fails to make progress, or if it becomes apparent that the family environment cannot support the child's treatment, it may be necessary to use more intensive treatments, including day treatment programs, or longer term residential treatment.

INVOLVEMENT OF THE FAMILY IN THE ASSESSMENT AND TREATMENT OF CHILDREN AND ADOLESCENTS

The child's dependency on the family (micro-system), friends (exosystem), and the larger circle of adults and society (macro-system) dictates that the family be at least considered, and more often than not involved, in the assessment process. Accordingly, the AACAP Practice Parameters highlight the importance of including the family in both the assessment and the treatment of physically ill children (DeMaso et al., 2009). This involvement of the family presents new and unexpected complexities for the clinician. The issues of the treatment alliance and confidentiality can become complex and challenging. The age of the child, the family's ability to provide the age-appropriate support, and the setting in which the child is seen, all determine the level of involvement between the family and the clinician.

PREPARING THE FAMILY FOR THE PSYCHIATRIC ASSESSMENT

Involving the family in psychiatric assessment and the treatment plan can prevent problems in the hospitalized physically ill child. The request for psychiatric consultation is generally initiated by one of the child's medical care providers and is not necessarily initially welcomed by the family. It may be the family's first contact with a psychiatrist, and unless the family are adequately prepared and agree to the consultation, it may not necessarily proceed smoothly. Many families will

have stereotyped perceptions of the role of the mental health consultant and interpret the consultation request as a communication from the medical team that they are not coping adequately. In addition, the stress of the child's medical illness may make the family much less receptive to meeting with a representative from a service that they do not perceive as necessary for their child's care. Initial defensiveness by the family should be no surprise and is more the norm than the exception.

Shaw and DeMaso (2006) describe the various steps involved in the consultation process. The first step in involving the family starts with the medical team explaining the rationale for the consultation. It is important for parents to understand that the consultation is being requested by the medical team, and in some cases it may be necessary for the attending physician to meet with the family to obtain their agreement. It may be helpful to explain that the consultation is necessary to provide help to the medical team in their work with the child. Clinicians should also bear in mind that many families may not have had previous experience with mental health professionals and may be primarily focused on medical diagnosis and treatment, with less emphasis on emotional well-being. Most families, however, will respond to the idea that hospitalizations are stressful for both the child and parents, and that their child may benefit from the added support provided by meeting with a therapist. Parents are usually open to the concept of relaxation or biofeedback to reduce anticipatory anxiety or assist with pain management. In high-stress procedures such as stem cell transplantation, it may be useful to present the psychiatric consultation as a routine part of the evaluation of all patients (if this is indeed the case) to make it more acceptable to the family. On rare occasions, when the child's psychiatric issues compromise the medical treatment or could put the child or others in danger, the medical team may need to insist on the family's agreement to the consultation as a condition of the child's continued medical treatment. For example, specialized treatment programs for pediatric pain or somatoform disorders in which psychiatric issues are commonly identified require participation in individual and family therapy as a mandatory component of the program.

The first meeting with the family should in most cases be with the parents or guardians alone, without the patient present. It is important to establish a working relationship with the family to facilitate the evaluation of the child or adolescent. It may be important to clarify with the family the reason for the consultation and the goals of the assessment. Any resistance should be explored to minimize the risk that the parents may consciously or subconsciously sabotage the assessment. One helpful approach to engage the family is to start with an inquiry about the *medical* history, and the impact of the *physical* condition on the child and family in the different domains of the child's functioning. A psychoeducational approach can also be helpful in terms of explaining to the parents the developmental issues and usual reactions of children to the stresses of treatment and hospitalization. It may also be necessary to explain some practical aspects of the evaluation that may be unfamiliar to parents, such as the need to meet separately with the child, and the importance of confidentiality around sensitive information. Parents often may have suggestions as to how to introduce the mental health consultant to the child and often can be engaged as allies in the therapeutic process.

FAMILY INVOLVEMENT AS A FUNCTION OF AGE OF THE CHILD

In preschool-age children, the parent is an essential conduit into the mental life of the child. In their roles as primary caretakers, parents need to be intimately involved in all phases of assessment and treatment, even in cases where the parent is suspected to be a perpetrator of abuse. Clearly, the family serves as the primary source of the history, although it is important to supplement this information with reports from other caregivers and by direct observation of the child. In some situations and cultures, extended-family members may serve as surrogate parents.

The focus of the evaluation is often on the nature of the relationship between the child and the parents or parent surrogate. Disorders of attachment and difficulties negotiating the developmental tasks of separation-individuation are defined in reference to the parent–child relationship and the family's culture.

In school-age children, there are significant changes in terms of the child's ability to report symptoms and history, although, as noted earlier, there are problems when history is based purely on a child's self-report. It is always important to gather history from parents, and when possible, schoolteachers who are often able to make important observations on the child's functioning in the peer and social context. It is also important to note that school-age children retain primary loyalty for their family of origin, even when, paradoxically, a parent is the perpetrator of abuse or neglect. Family "secrets" are difficult to elicit, and it is not uncommon for children to change their story, depending on which parent is present. This can be a particular problem in custody evaluations.

In adolescence, the situation may become even more complex, especially as the patient approaches the age of 18 years. State laws generally respect the confidentiality of psychiatric and medical records in certain circumstances; for example, birth control and termination of pregnancies (Litt, 1990). With adolescent patients, it is important to focus on establishing a therapeutic alliance primarily with the patient, and secondarily with the family—the reverse of the situation with younger patients. Younger children typically require behavioral interventions enforced by parents and caregivers. Therefore, consultants work primarily with parents and caregivers to implement behavioral modification programs. However, identifying the patient as the primary client is preferred for older children and adolescents whose developmental levels allow them to use cognitive techniques and who also are able to utilize self-motivation for engaging in behavioral treatments. It may be very difficult to develop and maintain a working alliance if the adolescent perceives the clinician as an overt or covert "agent" of the parents. Parents may need education about the adolescent's needs for autonomy and separation from the family of origin in cases where the parents are protective, controlling, or intrusive. Nonetheless, it is important not to ignore the relationship with the parents, and in some cases, it may be helpful to have separate individual and family therapists. While family therapy may be useful for a vast number of child and adolescent disorders, there is evidence that prior to the age of 18 years, family treatment alone can be effective, and at times more effective than individual therapy, in treating certain adolescent psychiatric disorders, such as substance use, trauma-related disorders, oppositional behavioral disorders, and eating disorders (Carr, 2000; Kmett Danielson et al., 2010; Lock et al., 2010; Sanders, Kapphahn, & Steiner, 1997). Thus, family therapy alone may be recommended for some cases, though it is frequently recommended as part of a multimodal treatment plan.

PARENTAL ABUSE AND NEGLECT

Working with families who are suspected of (or known to be) abusing or neglecting their children raises a number of issues. Angry reactions and other, often unconsciously determined countertransference reactions by the treatment team may tax their ability to remain professional and outwardly neutral toward the parent perpetrators (or suspected perpetrators). It is useful to remind nurses and clinicians of the important fact that parents who abuse or neglect their children often have been victimized themselves. Such efforts are usually helpful in reestablishing the ability of the treatment team to maintain an appropriate and professional attitude towards the family. At times, the best efforts at psychiatric intervention with the family will be unsuccessful in preventing further abuse from occurring. Protection of the child will then be the responsibility of the social agencies the law requires to be involved in such cases.

The mandatory reporting of the suspicion of, or overt, abuse or neglect of a child can best be presented to the family as a way to engage social and psychiatric resources to help the parents. Needless to say, most parents are not initially likely to experience the reporting as supportive and may be angry, defensive, and even litigious. In the inpatient setting, for cases in which abuse is not disclosed exclusively to the psychiatric consultant, it may be better to have the medical team make the report while the mental health team is available to provide support to the parents and to help in processing their feelings about the report. This approach may also help reduce the risk of the family's rejecting subsequent mental health interventions.

THE EPIDEMIOLOGY OF PEDIATRIC PSYCHIATRY: COMMON PEDIATRIC DISEASES

The most common reasons for psychiatric consultation in physically ill children include difficulties in adjustment to illness (for child and/or parent), delirium, differential diagnosis of somatoform disorders, disruptive behaviors, medication consultation, treatment nonadherence, pain management, procedural anxiety, and suicide assessment (Shaw, Wamboldt, Bursch, & Stuber, 2006). A review of the clinical findings and research on treatment approaches provides a useful overview of these issues (Knapp & Harris, 1998). Many recent population- and clinic-based studies have prospective designs that allow for the identification of risk factors and protective factors as well as the identification of syndromal illness.

Pediatric and psychiatric comorbidity may be classified as being either coincidental or causal (Figure 79.2). *Coincidental comorbidity* refers to the coincidental or chance occurrence of both medical and psychiatric illness in the same patient, such that the two conditions are not thought to have a causal relationship. By contrast, *causal comorbidity* refers to the situation in which psychiatric and medical disorders coexist, and one of the disorders is thought be responsible for generating the other. In many cases, there may also be an interaction between both physical and psychiatric illness.

COINCIDENTAL COMORBIDITY

Coincidental comorbidity may be more common than is generally appreciated. Between 10% and 31% of youth suffer from chronic medical illnesses, and another 10–20% suffer from psychiatric illness (Costello et al., 1988; Knapp & Harris, 1998; Newacheck & Taylor, 1992; Steiner, 1997a). The nature of the comorbid psychiatric conditions is dependent to some degree on the age of the child (see Box 79.3). Three volumes edited by Steiner (Steiner, 1996, 1997c, 1997d) review by age group the common psychiatric syndromes that can complicate the medical management of children with chronic physical illness.

In our experience, anxiety disorders are particularly likely to be exacerbated during acute physical illnesses and hospitalizations, while chronic physical illness is often associated with issues related to body image and lowered self-esteem. In addition, intellectual delay, learning disabilities, and attention-deficit hyperactivity disorder (ADHD) may all interfere with the child's understanding of the illness and her or his ability to comply with treatment recommendations. Coincidental comorbidity is associated with both extensive and at times inappropriate healthcare utilization, particularly when the psychiatric disorders go unrecognized (Lavigne et al., 1998). There are also implications for treatment and outcome (Perrin & MacLean, 1988).

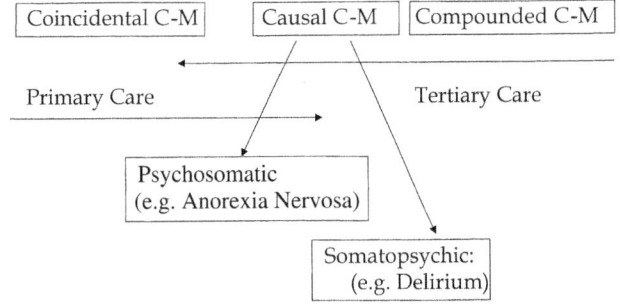

Figure 79.2 Pathways and patterns of pediatric and psychiatric comorbidity

It is quite clear that a substantial number of children seen by pediatricians and in primary care suffer from coincidental comorbidity (Knapp & Harris, 1998). It is estimated that up to 20% of patients are so affected. In tertiary care centers, this percentage may be even higher, probably as a direct result of the chronic nature of their illnesses, and also potentially in response to the inherently traumatic nature of many medical interventions. While as many as 30% of adult patients in the general medical setting may have psychiatric comorbidity (Bronheim et al., 1998), far fewer studies have documented the prevalence of psychiatric comorbidity in the pediatric population. However, in a sample of 112 children with chronic illness, Canning (1994) found that 50% of these children qualified for at least one psychiatric diagnosis when using information from both parent and child interviews.

It is also clear that the majority of these cases are not identified by pediatricians, and that of those that are identified, only a relatively small percentage are referred to mental health professionals for further evaluation (Costello et al., 1988; Kataoka, Zhang, & Wells, 2002; Owens et al., 2002). Simple screening instruments such as the Pediatric Symptom Checklist (Jellinek, Little, Murphy, & Pagano, 1995) may be helpful in identifying patients at risk. Once identified, patients should be referred to a mental health clinician for further evaluation and treatment. Most children and adolescents respond well to appropriate interventions targeted toward their symptoms. However, for severe cases that do not respond to first-line interventions, it may be necessary for families to be referred to highly specialized programs such as the Hasbro Partial Hospitalization Program at Hasbro Children's Hospital in Providence, Rhode Island, which bring together pediatricians and child psychiatrists to jointly address both mental health disorders and physical illnesses experienced by children and adolescents with comorbid conditions (Roesler, Glazer, Fritz, Dyer, & Rickerby, 2010).

CAUSAL COMORBIDITY

It is possible for psychiatric illness to perpetrate pediatric illness, and vice versa. *Psychosomatic* disorders are classically defined as psychiatric illnesses resulting in the genesis of somatic illnesses and symptoms. Eating disorders provide one example of how complex assumptions about body-state and composition result in the refusal to maintain appropriate body weight. This subsequently leads to a wide variety of somatic disturbances, some of which may in turn perpetuate the faulty body-image conceptualization. Other examples include factitious disorder and factitious disorder by proxy (previously known as Munchausen syndrome by proxy, nonadherence to treatment, delusional disorders leading to emaciation, and depression leading to weight loss.

In contrast to psychiatric illness's generating somatic symptoms, primary medical illnesses can also result in psychiatric symptoms or illness. Examples include delirium, mood disorders, psychotic disorders, and personality changes secondary to medical illness. Frequently, causation of psychiatric and somatic symptoms may be impossible to determine, and instead coexist as combinations of interrelated symptoms.

PSYCHOSOMATIC ILLNESS

Classic psychosomatic disorders, such as eating disorders, frequently present in primary care settings and benefit from a joint pediatric and psychiatric treatment approach. The description and discussion of these disorders is beyond the scope of this chapter, but the reader is referred to Lock (2011 and Steiner and Lock (1998), and the chapter on eating disorders in the medically ill in this volume by Brennan et al. While these illnesses are complex, they have been well studied, and there is a substantial base of evidence and experience to aid in their diagnosis and treatment (Steiner & Lock, 1998; Steinhausen, 1997).

The illnesses traditionally of great interest and with particular relevance for the consulting psychiatric clinician in the medical setting are the somatoform and factitious illnesses. Somatic symptoms are extremely common in childhood, with an estimated 10% of children in the general population manifesting unexplained physical complaints (Campo & Fritsch, 1994; Garralda, 2010). Furthermore, somatic symptoms of emotional distress often accompany chronic medical illness and emotional trauma (Erickson & Steiner, 1999; Steiner, 1997a). Many of these patients receive extensive and costly medical investigations that could be avoided by routine inquiry into their psychiatric and trauma history. Factitious disorder in children is rare but becomes increasingly common in adolescence. As might be expected, such illnesses are very often seen in children with histories of trauma and in delinquent youth with diagnoses of disruptive behavior disorders (Steiner, 1997b). "Factitious disorder by proxy," the fabrication of physical or psychological symptoms in children by their parents or caregivers, is a rare but important condition to be considered in pediatric patients (Shaw et al., 2008). It is a form of child abuse, and is also known as "medical child abuse." Recurrent infections, unusual bacteria, multiple treatment providers, multiple children with illnesses, and parents with medical backgrounds are some of the features that may raise concern for factitious disorder by proxy. Treatment studies are rare but document the extreme recalcitrance of these behaviors (Sanders et al., 1997).

CHRONIC SOMATOPSYCHIC ILLNESS[1]

Patients with chronic medical illness have been shown to have significant psychosocial risk (Steiner, 1997a). Approximately 25% of children with physical illness develop emotional disorders, compared to 18–20% of medically healthy children (Wallander & Thompson, 1995). The data from prospective outcome studies using both objective and subjective assessment measures are consistent in showing that chronic illness poses risks in academic, vocational, interpersonal, psychological, and recreational domains of functioning (Pless, Power, & Peckham, 1993). The risks are significantly higher in younger children, boys, and those raised in single-parent or economically disadvantaged families. Generally, the patient's psychiatric status worsens over time, especially for those whose disability becomes permanent or who have poor social support (Pless et al., 1993).

The literature on chronic physical illness leading to psychiatric comorbidity is vast, although the quality of the studies is variable (Knapp & Harris, 1998; Steiner, 1997a). Almost all illness groups have been studied, the most common ones being bronchial asthma, diabetes mellitus, cancer, cardiac illness, epilepsy, and delirium; and more recently, HIV infection and chronic fatigue syndrome (Knapp & Harris, 1998). It is apparent that specific illnesses may contribute to different patterns of psychopathology and maladjusted behavior. General issues to be considered include the visibility of the physical illness, the presence or absence of pain, and the degree of disability.

---

[1] "Somatopsychic illness" refers to psychiatric symptoms caused by medical illness.

ACUTE SOMATOPSYCHIC ILLNESS

In comparison to the literature on chronic illness, much less is known about the acute psychiatric complications of pediatric medical illness. It is quite clear from a clinical point of view that children suffer from delirium and other forms of acute brain syndromes. There is also a growing literature on the acute complications of illness leading to PTSD (Bronner, Knoester, Bos, Last, & Grootenhuis, 2008; Colville, Kerry, & Pierce, 2008; Davydow, Katon, & Zatzick, 2009; Judge, Nadel, Vergnaud, & Garralda, 2002; Knapp & Harris, 1998; Shears, Nadel, Gledhill, & Garralda, 2005; Stuber, Nader, Houskamp, & Pynoos, 1996) and other psychiatric sequelae (Davydow et al., 2009; DeMaso et al., 1991; Muranjan, Birajdar, Shah, Sundaraman, & Tullu, 2008; Rees, Gledhill, Garralda, & Nadel, 2004). Studies have shown that between 13% and 34% of children surviving burns and other traumatic injuries, and 10–28% of pediatric intensive care unit (PICU) survivors with illnesses not related to inflicted physical trauma, demonstrate symptoms of acute stress or PTSD. These rates are similar to those reported in studies of adults with PTSD following intensive care unit (ICU) stays, which range from less than 2% to 64% (Davydow, Gifford, Desai, Needham, & Bienvenu, 2008). Additionally, 13% of pediatric burn survivors and 7–13% of PICU survivors suffer from clinically significant depressive symptoms (Davydow et al., 2009).

DIAGNOSIS AND MANAGEMENT OF COMMON CHILDHOOD DISORDERS IN THE MEDICAL SETTING

BEHAVIORAL REGRESSION

Behavioral regression is one of the most common reasons for referral to child psychiatry services in the medical setting (Fritz & Spirito, 1993). The treatment team encounters behavior and mentation which are grossly inconsistent with the child's chronological age and level of emotional development.

CASE HISTORY

Amanda, a ten-year-old girl, was hospitalized for unexplained episodes of fever that had not responded to outpatient intervention. Previously a very healthy child from rural northern California, Amanda was usually active, fond of the outdoors, and also competent and accomplished in taking care of horses and cows on the family farm. The oldest of four children, Amanda was her mother's "auxiliary parent" and usually took care of her younger siblings when their mother was unavailable.

This was Amanda's first hospitalization, and the experience radically changed her demeanor. She was completely passive and listless during the day, despite the fact that her fevers were gradually subsiding in response to treatment. Instead of appearing healthier and more energetic, Amanda became extremely demanding when her mother was present, and quiet and withdrawn when she was alone with the nursing staff. In her mother's presence, Amanda whined and

cried incessantly, demanding to be taken home. When her demands were not met, she refused to cooperate altogether, making her medical management prolonged and difficult. Both parents reacted with surprise and embarrassment, since her behavior was so out of keeping with her habitual level of functioning. The mother attempted to get Amanda to "act her age" by encouraging her to be tough and by reminding her of the days when she could be relied on to help out in even the most difficult situation. All of these efforts, however, were unsuccessful.

The child psychiatry consultation team found a very sullen and resentful girl who essentially was mute and withdrawn. Much of the evaluation required her mother's presence and support to gain Amanda's trust. Amanda's mother was both sleep-deprived and tired. She was unable to respond to her daughter's demands for caretaking, since she herself was a stranger to the hospital environment with little understanding of the medical interventions. The first intervention suggested by the child psychiatry team was to establish a flowchart of Amanda's daily activities. With encouragement, Amanda was able to contribute to the observations. Contacts with the staff were organized in such a way as to be brief and extremely predictable. As the team began to intervene, it became clear that structure and protection would be helpful to Amanda. Laboratory tests were scheduled at predictable times of the day, and procedures were scheduled together with the agreement of both Amanda and her mother. Amanda's father was asked to provide relief for the mother, who had been the sole resource for their child during the prolonged hospital stay. Art and play psychotherapy sessions were scheduled, during which Amanda's mother was asked to leave and go to the cafeteria to restore herself. Additionally, nursing and medical staff were asked not to interrupt. For each new procedure, preparatory sessions were scheduled, with the aim of enhancing the patient's and the mother's understandings of the purpose of the upcoming intervention.

After three days, Amanda was again fully functional and an active participant in her care. Serial blood cultures and cardiac investigations eventually confirmed a diagnosis of bacterial endocarditis. Amanda was treated with an appropriate course of intravenous (IV) antibiotics initiated in the hospital and completed at home with a peripherally inserted central catheter (PICC) line. One month after discharge and after completion of antibiotics, there were no apparent sequelae, and, in fact, Amanda appeared to have only a very dim memory of the details of her hospital stay. Six months after the initial stay, she remained symptom-free and was back to her regular behavior on the farm without any further special intervention.

This case is a good example of how overwhelming stressors and a less than optimally functioning parent can lead to the temporary emergence of age-inappropriate behavior. The intervention involved simple environmental manipulation, with the goal of restoring the patient's sense of control and mastery. Since there was no preexisting psychopathology in the child and her family, her symptoms resolved relatively easily and quickly without the need for any longer term treatment. The emergence of immature behavior under extreme duress in previously healthy individuals has to be carefully differentiated from more serious psychopathology. Making this distinction depends on the detailed understanding of the child's previous development (Steiner, 1996, pp. 1–41).

Anxiety Disorder

A wide variety of anxiety disorders may present in children in the medical setting. These may include adjustment disorders with features of anxiety, procedural anxiety, separation anxiety, panic, post-traumatic stress and acute stress disorders, and exacerbation of generalized anxiety. While some anxiety is to be expected, given the change in environment, physical discomfort, and often uncertainties about procedures or outcomes that are associated with inpatient hospitalization, anxiety that causes disturbances in daily functioning should be addressed and treated.

CASE HISTORY

Martina, a seven-year-old girl, was the victim of a severe and traumatic motor vehicle accident. She was a passenger in the rear seat of a car driven by her mother, and she was not wearing a seatbelt at the time of the accident. Martina was thrown from the car and sustained multiple injuries, including a degloving injury of her right lower leg and extensive disfiguring of the soft tissue on her face. She underwent several emergency surgeries after admission and needed multiple invasive medical procedures during the early part of her hospitalization.

Psychiatry consultation was requested for Martina after she started to refuse even routine medical procedures, requiring sedation and physical restraint for blood tests and dressing changes. She was extremely apprehensive and resistant to physical examinations, and the medical staff had been unable to persuade her to undergo a necessary magnetic resonance imaging (MRI) scan. Nursing staff reported that Martina was waking multiple times during the night with traumatic recollections of the car accident. Her mother reported that Martina had also become exceptionally clingy and anxious, and was not able to tolerate her mother leaving her room without having severe episodes of anxiety.

During the initial psychiatric assessment, it was noted that Martina's mother was having almost as difficult a time as her daughter. She was consumed with feelings of guilt, since she had been the driver of the car, and was unable even to discuss the events as a result of her own associated traumatic memories. She was withdrawn and tearful in Martina's presence, and unable to provide appropriate parental support for her child's treatment.

Martina was assessed as having symptoms of an acute stress reaction, with increased anxiety, flashbacks, and intrusive memories of the accident. She also had symptoms consistent with separation anxiety, reflecting psychological regression in the face of overwhelming trauma. In addition, she had symptoms best explained as a manifestation of medical trauma, which included intense anxiety and hypervigilance related to contact with medical personnel, as well as avoidance of procedures.

Treatment in Martina's case was multimodal. A pain service consult was requested to provide recommendations for pharmacological and behavioral approaches to better manage her wound pain, and for preventive pain management during medical procedures. She was referred to the hospital's surgery-preparation program to participate in medical play, a technique in which the child role-plays a doctor carrying out medical procedures on dolls. Medical play can be helpful in desensitizing a patient and reducing anxiety related to the medical procedures. A behavior modification protocol was established to encourage her compliance with treatment, using rewards and incentives. Martina was also seen by the psychiatry service for individual-play psychotherapy to help her process her feelings about the accident. Finally, family therapy sessions were scheduled to help the entire family—in particular, Martina's mother, whose feelings of guilt had prevented her from fully participating in Martina's treatment.

Martina's case illustrates many of the principles used in the management of anxiety disorders presenting in children in the medical setting. Firstly, it is important to note that anxiety is a common presenting symptom in many situations. Separation anxiety, for example, is normal and developmentally appropriate in young infants. It is also not unusual or inappropriate to observe symptoms of anxiety and obsessive-compulsive behaviors in response to the stress of acute illness or hospitalization. In Martina's case, anxiety was a manifestation of an acute traumatic reaction, compounded by recurrent trauma related to medical treatment. Finally, anxiety may reflect an underlying and comorbid psychiatric disorder, including depression or one of the various anxiety disorders seen in children (Steiner, 1996; Steiner, 1997d).

In the acute medical setting, it is usually necessary to resort to multiple treatment approaches, aside from standard pharmacological approaches. Children in general respond very well to behavioral interventions, including hypnosis, biofeedback, and standard behavior modification protocols, provided the interventions take into account the child's developmental level. As in Martina's case, it is important not to neglect individual and family therapy as part of a comprehensive treatment plan.

PREVENTION AND TREATMENT OF ANTICIPATORY ANXIETY

Children are susceptible to a number of emotional and behavioral problems related to medical procedures and hospitalization. These include anticipatory anxiety, post-traumatic stress reactions, sleep and appetite disturbances, adjustment disorders, and problems with aggression. For example, Lumley et al. (Lumley, Melamed, & Abeles, 1993) reported that 11% of children experienced severe behavior problems within two weeks of surgery, and children who are unprepared appear to be at particular risk. While this section will briefly discuss procedural anxiety, Mednick (2010) provides a more detailed overview of factors influencing procedural anxiety and techniques for preparing pediatric patients for medical procedures.

CASE HISTORY

Emily, a nine-year-old girl, had been diagnosed with leukemia at the age of four years. She had one relapse of her disease, and was being treated aggressively with chemotherapy in the hope that she would be a candidate for stem cell transplantation. She was also diagnosed with a neurogenic bladder, after presenting with urinary retention. The urology service made the recommendation for intermittent catheterization four times each day, while efforts were being made to understand the etiology of her urinary problem. Indwelling Foley catheterization was not thought to be a good option, due to the risk of infection in the setting of her immunosuppression.

The first three catheterizations were very traumatic for Emily, who had already had to endure numerous invasive medical procedures for her leukemia, including bone marrow aspirations, spinal taps, and venipuncture. Psychiatry consultation was called because Emily was refusing the procedure, and manifesting extreme anticipatory anxiety. Emily's mother, who had been present during the catheterizations, was also upset and insisting on an alternate approach. Given the acute nature of the problem, and the need for regular urinary outflow, the recommendation was made for temporary Foley catheterization while efforts were made to desensitize Emily to the procedure. She and her mother were shown a videotape of a child calmly undergoing self-catheterization, and then a tape on the use of medical hypnosis and guided imagery in a pediatric medical setting. It was considered critical to engage her parents' support for the treatment, since any opposition was thought likely to sabotage the intervention. After discussion with her parents, it was decided to try medical hypnosis. Emily was found to be highly hypnotizable, and was able to use the image of a familiar and safe place she could go to while practicing deep breathing and progressive relaxation. She was also instructed in imagery techniques to relax her pelvic area and visualize the catheter passing easily into her bladder. Over the next three days, Emily also participated in daily medical-play sessions in which she practiced inserting a catheter into an anatomically correct doll, playing the role of the doctor who was coaching her patient to relax and use guided imagery during the catheterization.

The next phase in the treatment was to get Emily used to manipulating the indwelling Foley catheter while in a state of deep relaxation. A sticker chart was created with rewards for progressive efforts to manipulate the catheter, and it was found that this further helped motivate Emily to proceed with the program. Emily was given the decision about when she felt ready to proceed with her first catheterization. It was felt that it was important to give her a sense of some control in a setting where practically all control had been taken from her as a consequence of her illness. With the presence of the team who had prepared her for the procedure, she was able to successfully remove and reinsert a catheter, and begin the transition to regular catheterization.

Efforts to reduce distress related to anticipatory anxiety fall into two major categories: education and modeling, and enhancement of coping strategies (Harbeck-Weber & Hepps McKee, 1995). Surgery-preparation programs incorporate the use of videotapes of hospital procedures, provision of information in the form of classes, and simulation of actual procedures (Rosenberg et al., 1997). These programs are reviewed in Kain et al. (Kain, Caldwell-Andrews, & Wang, 2002), and Kain and Caldwell-Andrews (2005).

In summary, studies have suggested that participation of parents and children in these programs can lead to significantly reduced levels of anxiety and distress and behavioral changes, based on both self- and observer-report (Kain et al., 1998; Saile, Burgmeier, & Schmidt, 1988). Enhancement of coping strategies includes education and rehearsal of techniques such as deep muscle relaxation, breathing, guided imagery, distraction, and hypnosis (Butler, Symons, Henderson, Shortliffe, & Spiegel, 2005; Lukins, Davan, & Drummond, 1997; Rickert, Kozlowski, Warren, Hendon, & Davis, 1994; Thompson & Coppens, 1994). Reports suggest that children

who participate in these measures prior to surgery tend to exhibit less distress and are more cooperative with procedures. Programs that also incorporate stress-management and anxiety-reduction techniques for the parents appear to have even greater efficacy (Campbell & Cueva, 1995). While ideally such programs would be available at all hospitals conducting elective pediatric surgery, for hospitals that lack routine pre-surgery-preparation programs, screening before and after surgery for anxiety and/or post-traumatic symptoms is recommended.

It is also important to consider the child's previous experiences of hospitalizations. Young children who have had previous traumatic experiences may undergo a paradoxical increase in anxiety in response to surgery-preparation programs (Melamed, Dearborn, & Hermecz, 1983), so it is important to tailor interventions to match each individual patient. Other issues that affect the nature of the intervention may include the age and developmental level of the patient, the child's coping style, the timing of the intervention, and family factors (Blount, R. J., Piira. T., & Cohen, L. L. (2005).) (see Chapter 13).

DEVELOPMENTAL ISSUES

The child's level of cognitive development is an important consideration in determining the nature of the intervention. Children at the pre-operational stage of cognitive development (cognitive functioning characterized by illogical, magical, and nonreversible thinking, as well as egocentrism [Inhelder & Piaget, 1958]) are less able to use cognitive-behavioral strategies to manage anxiety. In addition, younger children are more likely to have misperceptions about their illness, are less likely to ask questions, and seem to receive fewer benefits from conventional surgery-preparation programs (Vernon & Thompson, 1993). Programs that take into account the child's developmental level and modify methods of presenting information accordingly have better results in terms of reduced levels of distress in children following procedures (Rasnake & Linscheid, 1989). Preparation programs targeted toward children at the preoperational stage of development might include visits to the hospital and medical play with models of surgical suites, IV lines, gowns and masks, and so on. Related issues to consider include the presence or absence of developmental delays, children with auditory or visual processing difficulties, or those with comorbid psychiatric disorders such as attention-deficit hyperactivity, which may affect their ability to benefit from preparation programs.

COPING STYLES

The child's coping style is an important variable to be considered in designing treatment interventions. Schultheis and colleagues (Schultheis, Peterson, & Selby, 1987) have proposed that individuals can be categorized on the basis of whether they are "sensitizers" or "repressors." Sensitizers cope with stress by gathering as much information as possible about the planned procedures and may prefer to watch procedures such as venipuncture rather than closing their eyes or relying on distraction. Repressors, by contrast, tend to use denial and distraction, and may benefit more from guided imagery or hypnotic strategies designed to draw their attention away from the procedure.

TIMING OF PREPARATION

There are conflicting data about the timing of surgery-preparation programs. In general, it is better to schedule participation close to the actual procedure (Beddows, 1997). Younger children in particular may not be able to retain information presented too early. However, Faust and Melamed (1984) compared children prepared the day before surgery with children prepared the day of surgery, and reported that same-day preparation may have resulted in increased anticipatory anxiety. Overall, preparation shortly before procedures seems to increase children's knowledge about the procedures, but the efficacy of these programs in reducing fear and distress, and on longer term outcomes, has not been clearly documented (Harbeck-Weber & Hepps McKee, 1995).

FAMILY ISSUES

It is also important to consider the role of the parents. The presence of a parent is nearly always helpful in reducing the child's level of distress, especially if the parent's level of anxiety is contained and they are able to provide support (Cameron, Bond, & Pointer, 1996; Kain et al., 1996). Parental anxiety has a strong impact on the child's ability to cope, and combination of high parent and high child anxiety is particularly problematic. Parents who received stress-management training reported reduced levels of anxiety and tension, while their children used more adaptive behaviors during procedures (Campbell & Cueva, 1995).

Finally, it is important to anticipate delayed psychological reactions and sequelae long after the procedure has taken place. Studies suggest that cancer treatment has traumatic implications years after initial treatment in long-term cancer survivors (Calaminus, Weinspach, Teske, & Gobel, 2007; Eilertsen, Rannestad, Indredavik, & Vik, 2011; Erickson & Steiner, 1999). Although such trauma-related psychopathology may not appear as a full clinical syndrome, problems may manifest in the form of avoidance of necessary medical procedures and follow-up medical appointments, or, paradoxically, the intense preoccupation with and seeking out of inappropriate medical procedures.

DEPRESSION

Children admitted to the hospital with physical illness are expected to experience a degree of dysphoria related to a variety of factors, including physical discomfort, limited activity, removal from the home environment, loss of privacy, and awareness of poor health. However, when changes in their mood begin to negatively impact physical symptoms or hinder their ability to complete daily tasks, the diagnosis of a mood disorder or of adjustment disorder with depressed mood should be considered.

CASE HISTORY

Sergei, a 14-year-old adolescent boy diagnosed with acute lymphoblastic leukemia, was admitted for matched, unrelated, stem cell transplantation after his first relapse. Although the bone marrow donor was not a perfect match, Sergei's risk of future relapse was sufficient to warrant the risk of transplant. Psychiatry consultation was called three weeks into his transplant because he appeared to have given up hope and was expressing a wish to stop treatment. Sergei was described as apathetic and withdrawn, and he was refusing to cooperate with his treatment. He had also had several painful medical complications related to his chemotherapy regimen, including pancreatitis and mucositis. His pediatric oncologist questioned whether Sergei might benefit from an antidepressant.

In the psychiatric evaluation, Sergei endorsed many of the symptoms of major depression, including depressed mood and feelings of hopelessness, in addition to anorexia, weight loss, lethargy, and insomnia. Sergei also reported having overheard his parents discussing the death of another patient on the unit two weeks previously, following the identical complication of his pancreatitis. His mother gave additional family history that a paternal uncle had died of pancreatic carcinoma.

This case raises many of the common issues in the assessment of depression in the medically ill adolescent. These issues are reviewed in detail in a chapter on mood disorders (Chapter 6, pp. 77–100) in the Textbook of Pediatric Psychosomatic Medicine by Benton and DeMaso (2010). One issue is that traditional diagnostic criteria for major depression (American Psychiatric Association, 2000) overlap significantly with physical illness itself. Many of the findings—"fatigue and loss of energy, insomnia, decreased appetite and weight loss, and difficulties with concentration"—may occur as sequelae of medical illness or its treatment, particularly disorders with significant pain. While some authors (e.g., Kathol et al., 1990) have suggested adapting the diagnostic criteria in medically ill patients, the difficulties of clinically differentiating these issues persist. It is also important to consider the possibility that specific medical disorders or medications may precipitate depression. In Sergei's case, many of his symptoms could be accounted for by his medical condition. Anorexia, weight loss, and lethargy are common in the course of bone marrow transplantation, and his insomnia was also easily explained by his severe pain. There were also justifiable medical concerns as well as relevant psychological issues that could account for his feelings of hopelessness. Burke and Elliott (1999) have drawn attention to the need to consider depression in the medically ill child as a potential outcome of the interactions between the child's biological vulnerability for depression, the characteristics of the illness, as well as relevant environmental stressors.

While treatment with antidepressants may often be indicated in medically ill children, it is common in pediatric practice to find that the depressive symptoms remit spontaneously as the acute medical issues resolve. Following general psychiatric principles, we tend to recommend very careful assessment and several meetings before recommending antidepressants in medically ill children. In cases where a child is refusing treatment, it is important to clarify possible misconceptions about the medical illness, since it is common for younger children to misinterpret or misunderstand information. In children with severe or terminal illness, the request for psychiatric medications often comes out of feelings of hopelessness in the medical team and the family. In lifelong illnesses requiring chronic aggressive medical regimens with limited benefit, adolescents and young adults sometimes make legitimate decisions to end treatment, or choose less aggressive treatment that is often called "educated non-compliance," in the interests of preserving their quality of life. It is important to respect these decisions as long as they are made autonomously, not coerced, and not automatically regarded as psychopathological. When the decision is made to treat with antidepressants, is important to be clear about what can be reasonably expected in terms of the likely response, as well as the usual delay in onset of action. The reader is referred to Steiner (1996) for further details on the specifics of assessing and treating depression in children and adolescents.

ACUTE PSYCHOTIC REACTIONS

Although less common than symptoms of anxiety and depression, psychotic reactions may also be seen in conjunction with physical illness and inpatient hospitalization. These reactions may be due to medications or medication withdrawal, prolonged stay in ICUs, head trauma, infection, or metabolic disturbances.

CASE HISTORY

Vanessa, a nine-year-old girl, presented to the emergency room in an acutely agitated state, reporting beliefs that her older brother had been sexually molesting her at home. She was extremely paranoid, reported visual hallucinations, and had apparently not slept for three days prior to her admission. Vanessa had been diagnosed with inflammatory bowel disease at the age of six and needed several hospitalizations, including a recent admission for total colectomy and placement of a colostomy. Despite the surgery, Vanessa had continued to have persistent and severe bloody diarrhea, with weight loss, requiring her to be restarted on high doses of prednisone. Previous treatment with steroids had precipitated episodes of hypomania, treated aggressively with IV haloperidol during her inpatient admissions, and managed with oral risperidone during outpatient treatment, due to concerns about her susceptibility to severe extrapyramidal reactions related to previous treatment with haloperidol.

Vanessa was admitted under the medical service with a provisional diagnosis of psychotic disorder due to steroid treatment, induced by treatment with prednisone. Her mother reported noticing pill fragments in the colostomy bag, and it was presumed that she had not been absorbing adequate doses of her oral (*per os*—PO) risperidone. Vanessa was restarted on IV haloperidol 1 mg twice daily, and she needed additional "as needed" (*pro re nata*—PRN) treatment during the first few days of her hospitalization. She also developed symptoms of akathisia, which were managed with low doses of IV lorazepam.

After resolution of her acute psychotic symptoms, Vanessa's medications were switched to PO liquid haloperidol and diphenhydramine, and she was able to continue the needed medical treatment with prednisone without recurrence of her psychosis. Vanessa subsequently denied her earlier allegations of sexual abuse. Because her mental status had changed so significantly during the time when allegations were reported, the allegations seemed clearly related to the psychosis, and it was not necessary to report the case to Children's Protective Services.

The principles in the assessment and management of acute psychotic reactions are similar to those in adult patients (Box 79.4). There needs to be an immediate assessment of the safety issues, including a determination as to whether or not the patient can be safely managed in the hospital facility. Often, the medical issues make it unrealistic for the patient to be transferred to a psychiatric facility, and as a result it is important to recommend whatever measures are necessary, which may include one- on-one observation, pharmacological treatment of agitation, and sometimes physical restraints. Although immediate attention will be given to the diagnostic issues, it may still be necessary to treat the

---

Box 79.4 **ASSESSMENT AND MANAGEMENT OF ACUTE PSYCHOTIC REACTIONS**

Immediate Assessment of Safety Issues

Elopement risk
    Potential for violence
    Need for 1:1 observation
    Need for physical restraints
    Need for pharmacological treatment of acute agitation.
    Need for transfer to inpatient psychiatric facility

Differential Diagnosis

Delirium
    Medication-induced psychotic disorder (e.g., steroids)
    Substance-induced psychotic disorder (e.g., amphetamine)
    Drug withdrawal reaction (e.g., alcohol)
    Endocrine disorders (e.g., thyroid)
    Connective tissue disorders (e.g., Systemic Lupus Erythematosus)
    Central nervous system disorders (e.g., neoplasms)
    Partial complex seizures
    Vitamin deficiencies
    Heavy-metal toxicity (e.g., lead poisoning)
    ICU psychosis
    Schizophrenia
    Bipolar disorder

Medication Management

Initial dose of antipsychotics

- Haloperidol 0.5–1 mg i.v.

- Olanzapine 6.25–24 mg p.o.

- Risperidone 0.5–1 mg p.o.
    Extrapyramidal symptoms

- Benztropine 0.5–1 mg i.v.

- Diphenhydramine 12.5–25 mg i.v.
    Akathisia

- Lorazepam 0.5–1 mg i.v.

Non-Illness Family Tasks

1. Maintaining family connections

2. Maintaining family morale and a sense of meaning

3. Ensuring attention to parental relationships and opportunities for intimacy

4. Providing attention, encouragement, and supervision for siblings

5. Ensuring opportunities for play, recreation, and enjoyment

6. Ensuring adequate financial resources

7. Maintaining connections to extended family, community supports, and friendships

8. Continuing with family spiritual life

9. Dealing with other important family stresses—other family illness, moving, job loss, or job change

Illness Family Tasks

1. Developing a shared understanding of the illness

2. Resolving disagreements about the child's condition or care

3. Developing routines that embed illness care into family life as much as possible

4. Assigning and monitoring illness tasks, especially making sure that the ill child can be and is responsible for his or her tasks

5. Building some flexibility into parental roles and avoiding rigid role definition

6. Developing a shared view that illness-management builds family competence

7. Communicating with siblings about the illness and their experience of the illness

8. Experiencing, communicating about, and managing emotional reactions to the illness

9. Collaborating effectively with the medical team

10. Ensuring that all members of the family and medical team are known to and engage with each other

psychosis symptomatically with antipsychotics while the medical workup is in progress. It is not uncommon to find that pediatric staff are unfamiliar with dosages of the psychotropics, and it is important to make very clear recommendations about specific doses, and to monitor the patient carefully for extrapyramidal symptoms and akathisia. The reader is referred to Chapter 5 by Turkel (2010) in Shaw (2010) for a fuller account of the diagnostic and treatment issues in acute psychotic reactions and delirium.

Generally, low doses of intravenous haliperidol are recommended for children who are unable to take oral food or medication (nothing *per os*—NPO). However, if children are able to take medication by mouth, low-dose risperidone is recommended for hypoactive delirium, and haloperidol is recommended for hyperactive delirium.

TREATMENT: PSYCHOTHERAPY AND PSYCHOPHARMACOLOGY

The comprehensive treatment of children and adolescents has become increasingly differentiated and sophisticated. Psychotherapy encompasses a wide variety of techniques, ranging from supportive to exploratory; educational to cathartic; interpersonal to playful. A detailed discussion of these techniques is beyond the scope of this chapter, and the reader is referred to three volumes detailing the treatment of the preschool-age child (Steiner, 1997c), the school-age child (Steiner, 1997d), and the adolescent (Steiner, 1996). Additionally, problem-specific treatments are reviewed in their respective chapters in Shaw and DeMaso's *Textbook of Psychosomatic Medicine* (2010). Psychopharmacological treatments and their medical side effects are reviewed in the next chapter of this book. Suffice it to say that there is increasing evidence for the specificity of interventions and their effectiveness in children and adolescents across a variety of symptoms. All classes of treatment and psychopharmacology are employed, and the modal intervention in this population targets multiple symptoms using a carefully coordinated treatment package.

Child psychiatrists tend to be more conservative about the use of pharmacological management for children than for adults, for several reasons. Most pharmacological studies are conducted in adults, so less is known about the side effects and pharmacokinetics of many medications in children. Additionally, there are few long-term studies addressing long-term effects of psychopharmacological agents on the developing brain. Because children depend largely on adults for creating their social environments, as well as positive and negative reinforcers, it is typically easier to use behavioral techniques with children,

1. Marked family distress

2. Poor collaboration and communication with medical team

3. Disabling emotional and/or behavioral symptoms in the ill child and/or siblings

4. Marked marital stress that involves the ill child and/or siblings

5. Problems ensuring that the ill child adheres to the treatment regimen

6. Exhaustion, anxiety, burnout, and/or depression in one or both parents

as caregivers and teachers can be responsible for providing the appropriate reinforcers. For these reasons, families should be involved in assessment and treatment. Boxes 79.5 and 79.6 highlight the non-illness and illness tasks facing families with pediatric physical illnesses as well as the indications for referral to family therapy. Finally, there is strong evidence to suggest that, while medication alone may be effective for certain disorders such as depression and ADHD with associated comorbidities, the combination of therapy and medication provides the greatest benefits (March et al., 2004; Swanson et al., 2008).

CLINICAL PEARLS

- Difficulties in attachment may be repaired by experience of a positive relationship with an adult outside the family (Rutter, 1988).

- Adolescents are prone to (unconscious) denial as well as conscious deception of others (Erickson & Steiner, 1999; Steiner, 1996).

- Fewer psychiatric diagnoses will be missed if the clinician gathers information by interviewing both the patient and parents, and additional sources of information may reveal even more comorbidities.

- Categorizing the developmental trajectories in the major domains of functioning, along with an appropriate charting of milestones, impediments, and sensitivities, is essential for constructing a clear longitudinal picture of the child's development.

- Discrete diagnostic categories, even if adjusted for specific age groups, rarely capture the entire clinical picture of the pediatric patient.

- Symptoms do not occur in a psychosocial vacuum—they often fulfill a function for the child that can be understood by assessing the child's social and temporal context and overall social equilibrium.

- Behavioral symptoms tend to help resolve conflict.

- Clinicians should consider and carefully weigh the factors in the patient's life that promote development and may facilitate recovery.

- Single-intervention packages are rarely successful.

- Clinicians should attempt to intervene early to prevent the development of psychiatric disorders.

- The momentum of normal growth and development can work synergistically with the therapist.

- The goal of all treatment interventions is to try to reestablish the normal developmental trajectory.

- The mandatory reporting of the suspicion of, or overt, abuse or neglect of a child can best be presented to the family as a way to engage social and psychiatric resources to help the parents.

DISCLOSURE STATEMENTS

Dr. Froehlich, Dr. Steiner, and Dr. Shaw have no possible conflicts of interest, financial or otherwise, including direct or indirect financial or personal relationships, interests, and affiliations, whether or not directly related to the subject of the chapter. This chapter was supported in part by grants to Dr. Steiner from the Eucalyptus Foundation.

REFERENCES

American Psychiatric Association. (2013). Diagnostic and statistical manual of mental disorders (5th ed.). Arlington, VA: American Psychiatric Publishing.

Beddows, J. (1997). Alleviating pre-operative anxiety in patients: A study. Nursing Standard, 11(37), 35–38.

Benton, T., & DeMaso, D. (2010). Mood disorders. In R. J. Shaw & D. R. Demaso (Eds.), Textbook of pediatric psychosomatic medicine (pp. 77–100). Arlington, VA: American Psychiatric Publishing.

Bowes, L., Maughan, B., Caspi, A., Moffitt, T. E., & Arseneault, L. (2010). Families promote emotional and behavioural resilience to bullying: evidence of an environmental effect. Journal of Child Psychology & Psychiatry, 51, 809–817.

Bronfenbrenner, U., & Crouter, A. (1983). The evolution of environmental models in developmental research. In P. Mussen (Ed.), Handbook of child psychology (Vol. 1, 358–414). New York: Wiley.

Bronheim, H. E., Fulop, G., Kunkel, E. J., Muskin, P. R., Schindler, B. A., Yates, W. R., et al. (1998). The Academy of Psychosomatic Medicine practice guidelines for psychiatric consultation in the general medical setting. The Academy of Psychosomatic Medicine. Psychosomatics, 39(4), S8–S30.

Bronner, M. B., Knoester, H., Bos, A. P., Last, B. F., & Grootenhuis, M. A. (2008). Posttraumatic stress disorder (PTSD) in children after paediatric intensive care treatment compared to children who survived a major fire disaster. Child & Adolescent Psychiatry & Mental Health, 2, 9.

Burke, P., & Elliott, M. (1999). Depression in pediatric chronic illness. A diathesis-stress model. Psychosomatics, 40(1), 5–17.

Butler, L. D., Symons, B. K., Henderson, S. L., Shortliffe, L. D., & Spiegel, D. (2005). Hypnosis reduces distress and duration of an invasive medical procedure for children. Pediatrics, 115, e77–e85.

Calaminus, G., Weinspach, S., Teske, C., & Gobel, U. (2007). Quality of survival in children and adolescents after treatment for childhood cancer: the influence of reported late effects on health related quality of life. Klinische Padiatrie, 219(3), 152–157.

Cameron, J. A., Bond, M. J., & Pointer, S. C. (1996). Reducing the anxiety of children undergoing surgery: parental presence during anaesthetic induction. Journal of Paediatrics & Child Health, 32(1), 51–56.

Campbell, M., & Cueva, J. E. (1995). Psychopharmacology in child and adolescent psychiatry: a review of the past seven years. Part II. Journal of the American Academy of Child & Adolescent Psychiatry, 34, 1262–1272.

Campo, J. V., & Fritsch, S. L. (1994). Somatization in children and adolescents. Journal of the American Academy of Child and Adolescent Psychiatry, 33(9), 1223–1235.

Canning, E. H. (1994). Mental disorders in chronically ill children: case identification and parent-child discrepancy. Psychosomatic Medicine, 56(2), 104–108.

Canning, E. H., & Kelleher, K. J. (1994). Performance of screening tools for mental health problems in chronically ill children. Archives of Pediatric & Adolescent Medicine, 148, 272–278.

Carr, A. (2000). Evidence-based practice in family therapy and systemic consultation: IN. Child-focused problems. Journal of Family Therapy, 22, 29–60.

Cicchetti, D., & Cohen, D. (Eds.). (1995). Developmental psychopathology. New York: John Wiley & Sons.

Colville, G., Kerry, S., & Pierce, C. (2008). Children's factual and delusional memories of intensive care. [Comparative Study Research

Support, Non-U.S. Gov't.] *American Journal of Respiratory and Critical Care Medicine, 177*(9), 976–982.

Costello, E. J., Edelbrock, C., Costello, A. J., Dulcan, M. K., Burns, B. J., & Brent, D. (1988). Psychopathology in pediatric primary care: the new hidden morbidity. *Pediatrics, 82*(3 Pt 2), 415–424.

Davydow, D. S., Gifford, J. M., Desai, S. V., Needham, D. M., & Bienvenu, O. J. (2008). Posttraumatic stress disorder in general intensive care unit survivors: a systematic review. *General Hospital Psychiatry, 30*(5), 421–434.

Davydow, D. S., Katon, W. J., & Zatzick, D. F. (2009). Psychiatric morbidity and functional impairments in survivors of burns, traumatic injuries, and ICU stays for other critical illnesses: a review of the literature. *International Review of Psychiatry, 21*, 531–538.

DeMaso, D. R., Campis, L. K., Wypij, D., Bertram, S., Lipshitz, M., & Freed, M. (1991). The impact of maternal perceptions and medical severity on the adjustment of children with congenital heart disease. *Journal of Pediatric Psychology, 16*(2), 137–149.

DeMaso, D. R., Martini, D. R., Cahen, L. A., Bukstein, O., Walter, H. J., Benson, S., et al. (2009). Practice parameter for the psychiatric assessment and management of physically ill children and adolescents. *Journal of the American Academy of Child and Adolescent Psychiatry, 48*(2), 213–233.

Eilertsen, M. E., Rannestad, T., Indredavik, M. S., & Vik, T. (2011). Psychosocial health in children and adolescents surviving cancer. *Scandinavian Journal of Caring Sciences, 25*(4), 725–734.

El-Khayat, H. A., Shatla, H. M., Ali, G. K., Abdulgani, M. O., Tomoum, H. Y., & Attya, H. A. (2003). Physical and hormonal profile of male sexual development in epilepsy. *Epilepsia, 44*, 447–452.

Erickson, S., & Steiner, H. (1999). Somatization as an indicator of trauma adaptation in long term cancer survivors. *Clinical Child Psychology and Psychiatry, 4*(3), 415–426.

Faust, J., & Melamed, B. G. (1984). Influence of arousal, previous experience, and age on surgery preparation of same day of surgery and in-hospital pediatric patients. *Journal of Consulting and Clinical Psychology, 52*(3), 359–365.

Flavell, J. (1985). *Cognitive development* (2nd ed., pp. 276–289). Englewood Cliffs, NJ: Prentice-Hall.

Fritz, G., & Spirito, A. (1993). The process of consultation on a pediatric unit. In G. Fritz, R. Mattison, B. Nurcombe, & A. Spirito (Eds.), *Child and adolescent mental health consultation in hospitals, schools and courts* (pp. 47–66). Washington, DC: American Psychiatric Press.

Garralda, M. E. (2010). Unexplained physical complaints. *Child & Adolescent Psychiatric Clinics of North America, 19*, 199–209.

Goldman, S., Shaw, R. J., & Demaso, D. R. (2010). The pediatric psychosomatic medicine assessment. In R. J. Shaw & D. R. Demaso (Eds.), *Textbook of pediatric psychosomatic medicine* (pp. 33–45). Arlington, VA: American Psychiatric Publishing.

Gyllenberg, D., Sourander, A., Niemela, S., Helenius, H., Sillanmaki, L., Piha, J., et al. (2010). Childhood predictors of later psychiatric hospital treatment: Findings from the Finnish 1981 birth cohort study. *European Journal of Child & Adolescent Psychiatry, 19*(11), 823–833.

Blount, R. J., Piira, T., & Cohen, L. L. (2005). Management of pediatric pain and distress due to medical procedures. In M. Roberts (Ed.), *Handbook of pediatric psychology* (3rd ed., pp. 216–233). New York, London: Guilford Press.

Harris, E. S., Canning, R. D., & Kelleher, K. J. (1996). A comparison of measures of adjustment, symptoms, and impairment among children with chronic medical conditions. *Journal of the American Academy of Child & Adolescent Psychiatry, 35*, 1025–1032.

Inhelder, B., & Piaget, J. (1958). *The growth of logical thinking from childhood to adolescence.* New York: Basic Books.

Jellinek, M., Little, M., Murphy, J. M., & Pagano, M. (1995). The Pediatric Symptom Checklist. Support for a role in a managed care environment. *Archives of Pediatric & Adolescent Medicine, 149*(7), 740–746.

Judge, D., Nadel, S., Vergnaud, S., & Garralda, M. E. (2002). Psychiatric adjustment following meningococcal disease treated on a PICU. *Intensive Care Medicine, 28*(5), 648–650.

Kagan, J. (1989). *Unstable ideas: Temperament, cognition, and self.* Cambidge, MA: Harvard University Press.

Kain, Z. N., & Caldwell-Andrews, A. A. (2005). Preoperative psychological preparation of the child for surgery: an update. *Anesthesiology Clinics of North America, 23*, 597–614

Kain, Z. N., Caldwell-Andrews, A., & Wang, S. M. (2002). Psychological preparation of the parent and pediatric surgical patient. *Anesthesiology Clinics of North America, 20*(1), 29–44.

Kain, Z. N., Caramico, L. A., Mayes, L. C., Genevro, J. L., Bornstein, M. H., & Hofstadter, M. B. (1998). Preoperative preparation programs in children: a comparative examination. *Anesthesia & Analgesia, 87*(6), 1249–1255.

Kain, Z. N., Mayes, L. C., Caramico, L. A., Silver, D., Spieker, M., Nygren, M. M., et al. (1996). Parental presence during induction of anesthesia. A randomized controlled trial. *Anesthesiology, 84*(5), 1060–1067.

Kataoka, S. H., Zhang, L., & Wells, K. B. (2002). Unmet need for mental health care among U.S. children: Variation by ethnicity and insurance status. *American Journal of Psychiatry, 159*(9), 1548–1555.

Kathol, R. G., Noyes, R., Jr., Williams, J., Mutgi, A., Carroll, B., & Perry, P. (1990). Diagnosing depression in patients with medical illness. *Psychosomatics, 31*(4), 434–440.

Kmett Danielson, C., McCart, M. R., de Arellano, M. A., Macdonald, A., Doherty, L. S., & Resnick, H. S. (2010). Risk reduction for substance use and trauma-related psychopathology in adolescent sexual assault victims: findings from an open trial. *Child Maltreatment, 15*, 261–268.

Knapp, P. K., & Harris, E. S. (1998). Consultation-liaison in child psychiatry: a review of the past 10 years. Part II: Research on treatment approaches and outcomes. *Journal of the American Academy of Child & Adolescent Psychiatry, 37*(2), 139–146.

Lavigne, J. V., Binns, H. J., Arend, R., Rosenbaum, D., Christoffel, K. K., Hayford, J. R., et al. (1998). Psychopathology and health care use among preschool children: a retrospective analysis. *Journal of the American Academy of Child & Adolescent Psychiatry, 37*, 262–270.

Litt, I. (1990). *Evaluation of the adolescent patient.* Philadelphia/St. Louis: Hanley and Belfus/Mosby-Year Book.

Lock, J. (Ed.). (2011. *The Oxford handbook of developmental perspectives on child and adolescent eating disorders.* Oxford Uiversity Press.

Lock, J., Le Grange, D., Agras, W. S., Moye, A., Bryson, S. W., & Jo, B. (2010). Randomized clinical trial comparing family-based treatment with adolescent-focused individual therapy for adolescents with anorexia nervosa. *Archives of General Psychiatry, 67*, 1025–1032.

Lukins, R., Davan, I. G., & Drummond, P. D. (1997). A cognitive behavioural approach to preventing anxiety during magnetic resonance imaging. *Journal of Behavior Therapy & Experimental Psychology, 28*, 97–104.

Lumley, M. A., Melamed, B. G., & Abeles, L. A. (1993). Predicting children's presurgical anxiety and subsequent behavior changes. *Journal of Pediatric Psychology, 18*(4), 481–497.

March, J., Silva, S., Petrycki, S., Curry, J., Wells, K., Fairbank, J., et al. (2004). Fluoxetine, cognitive-behavioral therapy, and their combination for adolescents with depression: Treatment for Adolescents with Depression Study (TADS) randomized controlled trial. *Journal of the American Medical Association, 18*; 292(7), 807–820.

Mednick, L. (2010). Preparation for procedures. In R. Shaw & D. DeMaso (Eds.), *Textbook of psychosomatic medicine* (pp. 475–485). Arlington, VA: American Psychiatric Publishing.

Melamed, B. G., Dearborn, M., & Hermecz, D. A. (1983). Necessary considerations for surgery preparation: age and previous experience. *Psychosomatic Medicine, 45*(6), 517–525.

Mrazek, P., & Haggerty, R. (Eds.). (1994). *Reducing risks for mental disorders: Frontiers for preventive intervention research.* Washington, DC: National Academy Press.

Muranjan, M. N., Birajdar, S. B., Shah, H. R., Sundaraman, P., & Tullu, M. S. (2008). Psychological consequences in pediatric intensive care unit survivors: the neglected outcome. *Indian Pediatrics, 45*(2), 99–103.

Murphy, D. A., Marelich, W. D., Herbeck, D. M., & Payne, D. L. (2009). Family routines and parental monitoring as protective factors among early and middle adolescents affected by maternal HIV/AIDS. *Child Development, 80*, 1676–1691.

Newacheck, P. W., & Taylor, W. R. (1992). Childhood chronic illness: prevalence, severity, and impact. *American Journal of Public Health, 82*(3), 364–371.

Owens, P. L., Hoagwood, K., Horwitz, S. M., Leaf, P. J., Poduska, J. M., Kellam, S. G., et al. (2002). Barriers to children's mental health services. *Journal of the American Academy of Child & Adolescent Psychiatry, 41*(6), 731–738.

Perrin, J. M., & MacLean, W. E., Jr. (1988). Children with chronic illness. The prevention of dysfunction. *Pediatric Clinics of North America, 35*(6), 1325–1337.

Piko, B. F., & Fitzpatrick, K. M. (2004). Substance use, religiosity, and other protective factors among Hungarian adolescents. *Addictive Behaviors, 29*, 1095–1107. England.

Pless, I. B., Power, C., & Peckham, C. S. (1993). Long-term psychosocial sequelae of chronic physical disorders in childhood. *Pediatrics, 91*(6), 1131–1136.

Poznanski, E. O., Cook, S. C., & Carroll, B. J. (1979). A depression rating scale for children. *Pediatrics. 64*(4) 442–450.

Rasnake, L. K., & Linscheid, T. R. (1989). Anxiety reduction in children receiving medical care: developmental considerations. *Journal of Developmental & Behavioral Pediatrics, 10*(4), 169–175.

Rees, G., Gledhill, J., Garralda, M. E., & Nadel, S. (2004). Psychiatric outcome following paediatric intensive care unit (PICU) admission: a cohort study. *Intensive Care Medicine, 30*(8), 1607–1614.

Rickert, V. I., Kozlowski, K. J., Warren, A. M., Hendon, A., & Davis, P. (1994). Adolescents and colposcopy: the use of different procedures to reduce anxiety. *American Journal of Obstetrics & Gynecology, 170*, 504–508.

Roesler, T. A., Glazer, J. P., Fritz, G. K., Dyer, C. A., & Rickerby, M. (2010). *Changing illness beliefs in a pediatric/child psychiatric day hospital setting: Three cases.* Paper presented at the American Academy of Child and Adolescent Psychiatry, 57th Annual Meeting Oct 26–31, 2010, New York.

Rosenberg, D. R., Sweeney, J. A., Gillen, J. S., Kim, J., Varanelli, M. J., O'Hearn, K. M., et al. (1997). Magnetic resonance imaging of children without sedation: preparation with simulation. *Journal of the American Academy of Child & Adolescent Psychiatry, 36*, 853–859.

Rutter, M. (Ed.). (1988). *Studies of psychosocial risk.* Cambridge, England: University Press.

Saile, H., Burgmeier, R., & Schmidt, L. (1988). A meta-analysis of studies on psychological preparation of children facing medical procedures. *Psychology Health, 2*, 107–132.

Sanders, M. J., Kapphahn, C. J., & Steiner, H. (1997). Eating disorders. In R. T. Ammerman & J. V. Campo (Eds.), *Handbook of pediatric psychology and psychiatry.* Needham Heights, MA: Allyn and Bacon.

Saylor, C. F., Finch, A. J., Spirito, A., & Bennett, B. (1984). The Children's Depression Inventory: A systematic evaluation of psychometric properties. *Journal of Consulting and Clinical Psychology, 52*(6), 955–967.

Scheeringa, M. S., Zeanah, C. H., Drell, M. J., & Larrieu, J. A. (1995). Two approaches to the diagnosis of posttraumatic stress disorder in infancy and early childhood. *Journal of the American Academy of Child & Adolescent Psychiatry, 34*, 191–200.

Schultheis, K., Peterson, L., & Selby, V. (1987). Preparation for stressful medical procedures and person × treatment interactions. *Clinical Psychology Review, 7*(3), 329–352.

Scullin, M. H., & Bonner, K. (2006). Theory of mind, inhibitory control, and preschool-age children's suggestibility in different interviewing contexts. *Journal of Experimental Child Psychology, 93*, 120–138.

Sentse, M., Lindenberg, S., Omvlee, A., Ormel, J., & Veenstra, R. (2010). Rejection and acceptance across contexts: parents and peers as risks and buffers for early adolescent psychopathology. The TRAILS study. *Journal of Abnormal Child Psychology, 38*(1), 119–130.

Shaw, R. J., & DeMaso, D. R. (2006). Pediatric consultation psychiatry assessment. In *Clinical manual of pediatric psychosomatic medicine* (pp. 31–58). Arlington, VA: American Psychiatric Publishing.

Shaw, R. J., & DeMaso, D. R. (Eds.). (2010). *Textbook of pediatric psychosomatic medicine.* Arlington, VA: American Psychiatric Publishing.

Shaw, R. J., Dayal, S., Hartman, J. K., & DeMaso, D. R. (2008). Factitious disorder by proxy: Pediatric condition falsification. *Harvard Review of Psychiatry, 16*(4), 215–224.

Shaw, R. J., Wamboldt, M., Bursch, B., & Stuber, M. (2006). Practice patterns in pediatric consultation-liaison psychiatry: a national survey. *Psychosomatics, 47*(1), 43–49.

Shears, D., Nadel, S., Gledhill, J., & Garralda, M. E. (2005). Short-term psychiatric adjustment of children and their parents following meningococcal disease. *Pediatric Critical Care Medicine, 6*, 39–43.

Sieving, R. E., & Shrier, L. A. (2009). Measuring adolescent health behaviors. In R. J. DiClemente, J. S. Santelli, & R. A. Crosby (Eds.), *Adolescent health: understanding and preventing risk behaviors* (pp. 473–492). San Francisco: Jossey-Bass Publishers.

Skovgaard, A. M. (2010). Mental health problems and psychopathology in infancy and early childhood. An epidemiological study. *Danish Medical Bulletin, 57*, B4193.

Smith, C., Feldman, S. S., Nasserbakht, A., & Steiner, H. (1993). Psychological characteristics and DSM-III-R diagnoses at 6-year follow-up of adolescent anorexia nervosa. *Journal of the American Academy of Child & Adolescent Psychiatry, 32*, 1237–1245.

Sroufe, L. A. (2009). The concept of development in developmental psychopathology. *Child Development Perspectives, 3*(3), 178–183.

Steiner, H. (1997a). Chronic illness and physical disabilities. In J. Nohspitz & N. Alessi (Eds.), *Handbook of child and adolescent psychiatry* (Vol. 4, pp. 251–273). New York: John Wiley.

Steiner, H. (1997b). The emerging field of developmental psychopathology. Paper presented at the American Academy of Child and Adolescent Psychiatry Annual MeetingP, Toronto, CA, October 18–23, 1997.

Steiner, H. (Ed.). (1996). *Treating adolescents.* San Francisco: Jossey-Bass.

Steiner, H. (Ed.). (1997c). *Treating preschool children.* San Francisco: Jossey-Bass.

Steiner, H. (Ed.). (1997d). *Treating school age children.* San Francisco: Jossey-Bass.

Steiner, H., & Canning, E. H. (1994). Adaptive styles in adolescents with psychosomatic illness. *Acta Paedopsychiatrica, 56*(4), 255–259.

Steiner, H., & Lock, J. (1998). Anorexia nervosa and bulimia nervosa in children and adolescents: a review of the past 10 years. *Journal of the American Academy of Child & Adolescent Psychiatry, 37*, 352–359.

Steinhausen, H. C. (1997). Outcome of anorexia nervosa in the younger patient. *Journal of Child Psychology & Psychiatry, 38*(3), 271–276.

Stern, D. N. (1985). *The interpersonal world of the infant.* New York: Basic Books.

Stoppelbein, L., Greening, L., Jordan, S., Elkin, D. T., Moll, G., & Pullen, J. (2005). Factor analysis of the pediatric symptom checklist with a chronically ill pediatric population. *Journal of Developmental & Behavioral Pediatrics, 26*(5), 349–355.

Stoudemire, A. (1991). Somatothymia. *Psychosomatics, 32*, 365–381.

Stuber, M. L., Nader, K. O., Houskamp, B. M., & Pynoos, R. S. (1996). Appraisal of life threat and acute trauma responses in pediatric bone marrow transplantation patients. *Journal of Traumatic Stress, 9*(4), 673–686.

Swanson, J., Arnold, L. E., Kraemer, H., Hechtman, L., Molina, B., Hinshaw, S., et al. (2008). Evidence, interpretation, and qualification from multiple reports of long-term outcomes in the Multimodal Treatment Study of children with ADHD (MTA): Part II: supporting details. *Journal of Attention Disorders, 12*(1), 15–43.

Thompson, M. B., & Coppens, N. M. (1994). The effects of guided imagery on anxiety levels and movement of clients undergoing magnetic resonance imaging. *Holistic Nursing Practice, 8*(2), 59–69.

Turkel, S. B. (2010). Delirium. In R. Shaw & D. DeMaso (Eds.), *Textbook of pediatric psychosomatic medicine* (pp. 63–76). Arlington, VA: American Psychiatric Publishing.

Vernon, D. T., & Thompson, R. H. (1993). Research on the effect of experimental interventions on children's behavior after hospitalization: a review and synthesis. *Journal of Developmental & Behavioral Pediatrics, 14*(1), 36–44.

Wallander, J., & Thompson, R. (1995). *Psychosocial adjustment in children with chronic physical conditions*. New York: Guilford.

Werner, E., & Smith, R. (1992). *Overcoming the odds: High risk children from birth to adulthood*. New York: Cornell University Press.

World Health Organization (1992). *ICD-10 Classifications of Mental and Behavioural Disorder: Clinical Descriptions and Diagnostic Guidelines*. Geneva: WHO.

80.

ADAPTATION OF PSYCHIATRIC DRUG TREATMENTS TO CHILDREN AND ADOLESCENTS

Eric P. Hazen

INTRODUCTION

Managing psychiatric medications in the pediatric population presents a unique set of challenges to the clinician. Clinical experience supports the oft-repeated maxim that "children are not just small adults." Children and adolescents may have different responses to medication than the adult population and may be more sensitive to the side effects of some medications. Furthermore, the challenges of conducting clinical trials in the pediatric population have resulted in a relatively limited evidence base for psychopharmacological interventions in the pediatric population relative to the evidence base for the adult population. As a result, there are not clear dosing guidelines for some medications, and many medications are used off-label, without a Food and Drug Administration (FDA) indication, based on clinical experience or small, open-label trials.

Despite these challenges, medications are a vital tool in the treatment of mental illness in children and adolescents. When managed properly, medication can be part of a treatment regimen that allows a young patient to get back on a healthy developmental trajectory, potentially preventing long-term psychological, social, and occupational impairment. In this chapter, we will discuss the general approach to managing psychiatric medications for children and adolescents before moving on to a discussion of specific issues involved in the more common psychiatric disorders in this population.

APPROACH TO MANAGING PSYCHIATRIC MEDICATIONS IN PEDIATRIC PATIENTS

While there are several special considerations in the management of medications in children and adolescents, general principles of good psychopharmacological practice apply. Because these principles are critically important in safe use of medications in the pediatric population, they bear brief mention here. These principles include:

- Establishing effective communication and a collaborative relationship with the patient and family

- Integrating medication into an overall treatment plan for the patient based upon a biopsychosocial formulation

- Starting medication only after a thorough medical and psychiatric evaluation, including detailed review of past medication trials and their effects

- Starting medications at the low end of the effective dose range and gradually titrating to effectiveness

- Employing the simplest medication regimen necessary to effectively manage the patient's symptoms, using polypharmacy only when indicated to treat residual symptoms, comorbid diagnoses, or side effects from other medications

- Taking one step at a time when possible, avoiding making multiple changes at once that will make subsequent changes in clinical presentation difficult to interpret

- Taking a systematic approach, assuring that each medication trial has been allowed adequate time at an adequate dosage before deeming it ineffective and moving to the next step in treatment

- Closely monitoring efficacy and side effects, using objective measures and structured rating scales when they are available

- Explicitly asking patients about their adherence to the medication regimen rather than assuming the medication is being taken as prescribed

- Monitoring drug levels when there is an established therapeutic range and it is known that there is significant inter-individual variability in the drug's pharmacokinetics

- Simplifying medication regimens when possible to avoid confusion and non-adherence

- Adhering to current practice guidelines for monitoring side effects of specific medications

- Being fully aware of all the drugs the patient has been prescribed by other physicians, as well as the patient's use of over-the-counter medications, nutritional supplements, and complementary treatments

- Maintaining communication with other medical and psychiatric providers involved in the patient's care
- Providing clear documentation of the patient's care, preferably in electronic form

DEVELOPMENTAL CONSIDERATIONS

In addition to these general principles, there are several considerations specific to the care of children that should be considered in managing medications. Perhaps most importantly, the child's stage of development must be taken into account in the approach to medication. From a physiological perspective, children metabolize medications differently than adults do. A greater ratio of liver mass to body mass and a more rapid glomerular filtration rate leads to many medications being metabolized more rapidly in children than they are in adults (Anderson & Lynn, 2009). Thus, for some medications, young patients may require higher doses per kilogram of body weight than adult patients. However, for other medications, lower activity of specific enzymes in the cytochrome P450 system implies slower metabolism and relatively higher blood levels (Benedetti et al., 2007).

At the same time, physiological differences can make pediatric patients more sensitive to some side effects. For example, children and adolescents have a higher density of dopamine receptors in the central nervous system than adults do (Boyson & Adams, 1997; Rinne et al., 1990). Differences in baseline dopaminergic transmission help explain why pediatric patients are more likely to develop acute dystonia in response to dopamine-blocking drugs, especially the high-potency, first-generation antipsychotic drugs. Development plays a role, not only in the physiology of the medication, but in the approach to discussing medication with a pediatric patient. Regardless of age, pediatric patients should be active participants in their psychiatric care and should be included in discussions about their medications, though it is critical to carry on the discussion in a developmentally appropriate way. Young children typically benefit from a simple, straightforward explanation of the goal of the medication, with a concrete example of how it might help them (e.g., "We think this will help you listen and learn better in school and be more in control of your body, so you don't get sent to the principal's office quite so often.") Young children may need reassurance that a medication will not change who they are or make them do things they do not want to do. They may become overwhelmed or anxious when confronted with long and detailed lists of possible side effects and may do better with a more general instruction to let their parents know if there is anything they feel on the medication that they do not like.

In contrast, most adolescent patients are able to grasp a more abstract, nuanced explanation of medication and its role in their treatment, and most want to know what specific side effects they might experience. As adolescents are often confused and dismayed by their changing bodies, it is particularly important to let them know about potentially embarrassing side effects that could be particularly distressing for an adolescent, such as sexual side effects of selective serotonin reuptake inhibitors (SSRIs) and serotonin-norepinephrine reuptake inhibitors (SNRIs), priapism in boys taking trazodone, or lactation in girls taking risperidone or other antipsychotic drugs that elevate prolactin levels. An adolescent taken by surprise by such an effect may lose trust in the clinician, with devastating consequences for the treatment.

Before a patient reaches the age of legal majority, informed consent must be given by the legal guardian, as we will discuss below. However, for pediatric patients who are mature enough to understand a medication and its risks and benefits, the clinician should seek the assent of the patient. "Assent" in this context refers to willingness of a minor to participate in a proposed treatment based on her or his understanding of the associated risks and benefits. Younger children who lack the capacity to understand the need for treatment at times may be coerced into taking medication, such as through behavioral consequences for refusal. A graduated approach to assent is taken for older children and adolescents, according to the developmental level of the patient. In most cases, these patients should be willing participants in their treatment. Coercion is acceptable only when they are severely impaired by their illness, they present a danger to themselves or others, or they are unable to understand the risks and benefits of medication. Once adolescent patients have reached the legal age of majority, adult legal criteria apply for involuntary treatment. Patients of all ages may grapple to make sense of medication and the meaning that it has in their emerging sense of self, and their developmental stage plays a key role in this process. Younger children may have difficulty understanding why they need to take medication or may feel medication means they are sick or that there is something wrong with them. Concerns about being different or being looked down on by peers often peak in early adolescence along with the increased concern about belonging that is part of normal development at this age. Addressing these issues is an essential component of pediatric psychopharmacology, as failure to do so may have significant implications for patients' self-esteem and adherence to medication.

The lives of children and adolescents often flow to the rhythms of school, sports, and other activities. This flow should be considered in the timing of medication adjustments. In non-crisis situations, one should avoid major medication changes at transition times or periods of high stress. For example, if an adolescent with ADHD was facing the SAT exam in a week and was responding only partially to a stimulant, it would be preferable to raise the dose of the current drug rather than switch to a new one. Reductions in dose and discontinuation of medication are no less challenging to the body and mind than dosage increases and medication changes: they are best done in low-stress periods. For many patients, the summer is a good time for medication changes. However, for patients who are more socially isolated during the summer and do not have structured activities to replace the routines of school, summer can actually be more stressful than the school year.

ROLE OF THE PARENTS

For pediatric patients, the parents or legal guardians are essential partners in the medication management. It is critical to identify the legal custodian(s) of a pediatric patient before proceeding with treatment, as their informed consent is required. The legal custodian is not necessarily the person bringing the child in for treatment, even when that person is a parent. In some situations of divorce or separation with joint custody, the consent of one parent may be insufficient. In cases of shared custody, such as after a divorce, it is important to communicate with both parents and engage them both in the treatment to the greatest extent possible. Not only is consent an issue, but parents may differ in how they administer medication to a child, how they deal with medication refusal, how they explain the medication to the child, and how adherent they are to the treatment regimen. Even in intact families, parents often have differences of opinion about medication. Therefore, it is necessary to explore the concerns of the parents and the meaning of the medication for the parents as well as for the child during treatment. Often one parent will be more involved in the treatment than the other, but it is important to reach out to the less-involved parent to speak by telephone and encourage them to come in periodically to discuss the treatment.

When the possibility of medication is raised, a detailed discussion about treatment options is warranted, including discussion of non-pharmacological interventions, goals for medication treatment, possible risks and side effects, dose schedule, and need for monitoring and follow-up. It is important to discuss reasonable expectations of the medication, including the time course over which it might be expected to work and the symptoms that the medication might and might not help. Many parents come to treatment with hopes that medication will quickly fix a complex, multifaceted problem, so it is important to help them develop realistic expectations.

The initial discussion of medication should also include planning about which family member or members are responsible for dispensing the medication and making sure that it is taken as prescribed. Parents of some adolescent patients may incorrectly assume their child has a sufficient level of maturity and responsibility to manage their own medication, leading to inconsistent adherence. While it is important for adolescent patients to begin taking increasing responsibility for their medications and their overall treatment as they approach adulthood, parents still need to monitor the situation and check in periodically to assure that the medication is being taken as prescribed. Pill containers can help sometimes-forgetful adolescents keep track of their medication and allow parents to discreetly monitor adherence without annoying an irritable teen with frequent questioning. For patients at risk for suicide, the possibility of overdose should be addressed with parents; and thought should be given as to how the medication, as well as other medications in the house, should be stored.

ADDITIONAL CONCERNS AND CONSIDERATIONS

In addition to the developmental, social, and physiological challenges in the psychopharmacological treatment of children, clinicians are also confronted by a relatively small evidence base. Conducting clinical trials with children and adolescents as subjects is often costlier and more time-consuming than it is with adults. Thus, the evidence-based literature related to psychopharmacology for children and adolescents is considerably smaller.

The lack of a strong evidence base forces clinicians treating severely ill children to operate under less certain conditions. Medications are frequently used off-label and sometimes on the basis of adult data extrapolated to children, small open-label trials, or clinical experience. For many medications, clear dosing and monitoring guidelines for the treatment of children have not been established. Experienced clinicians typically respond to this uncertainty by taking a conservative approach, using very small starting doses, titrating doses more gradually, and monitoring more closely than they would for an adult patient.

Obese and cachectic children present additional challenges, and there is little to no literature to address medication dosing for these patients. For the obese child, as with adult-sized adolescents, adult dosing guidelines are generally applied when the weight-based milligram per kilogram dosage reaches or exceeds adult dose levels. However, given the awareness that children are not "little adults" and may be more sensitive to certain adverse effects, a conservative approach is often taken, starting with doses slightly lower than might be used in an adult. Cachectic children can be dosed according to weight, but careful consideration must be paid to any underlying medical issues or existing medications that might interfere with the metabolism of the medication that is being considered.

MEDICATIONS FOR SPECIFIC PSYCHIATRIC CONDITIONS

MAJOR DEPRESSION

As in the adult populations, SSRIs are generally considered the first line of pharmacological treatment for depression in children and adolescents. However, controversy has arisen in recent years over the use of these medications, in terms of both their efficacy and their safety. An influential meta-analysis published in the *Lancet* in 2004 examined randomized controlled trials of SSRIs for treatment of depression in children and adolescents. This analysis demonstrated clear efficacy only for fluoxetine and questioned the risk–benefit profile for other SSRIs, particularly when data from unpublished studies were taken into account (Whittington et al., 2004).

In the same year, the U.S. FDA conducted an analysis of suicidal thoughts and behaviors using data pooled together from multiple individual studies of six SSRIs and three additional antidepressants (mirtazapine, buproprion, and venlafaxine) in children and adolescents. This analysis, involving over 4,400 subjects, showed that children treated with antidepressants had a 4% rate of suicidal thoughts and behaviors, compared to 2% in the placebo group. There were no completed suicides in this analysis. Based on this finding, the FDA issued a "black box warning" indicating the possible risks of suicidality associated with antidepressant use in children and adolescents (available at www.fda.gov/Drugs/DrugSafety/ PublicHealth Advisories/ucm161679.htm, accessed August 28, 2011).

In the wake of the FDA warning, concern about suicidality associated with antidepressant use was the probable explanation of an observed decline in rates of prescription of antidepressants for adolescents, with a 22% drop in overall prescriptions and a 58% decline in new prescriptions for patients under 18 years of age from 2003 to 2004 (Cheung et al., 2008). At the same time, the youth suicide rate in the United States rose significantly for the first time in 2004, after more than a decade of steady decline (Gibbons et al., 2007), leading some to question whether the reduction in antidepressant prescriptions contributed an *increase* in youth suicides.

Despite these controversies, there is a strong body of evidence supporting the use of SSRIs in children and adolescents for the treatment of depression. Randomized controlled trials have demonstrated efficacy for fluoxetine (Emslie et al., 1997; Emslie et al., 2002), sertraline (Wagner et al., 2003), citalopram (Wagner et al., 2004), and escitalopram (Emslie et al., 2009) in pediatric populations. The influential, non–industry funded Treatment for Adolescents with Depression Study (TADS) demonstrated a 71% response rate at 12 weeks for patients receiving combined fluoxetine and cognitive behavioral therapy (CBT) treatment, 61% for fluoxetine treatment alone, and 43% for CBT alone (March et al., 2004). These findings support the use of a combined approach of medication and therapy in the treatment of adolescent depression.

Given the evidence base, the first-line medications in the treatment of children and adolescents with depression are fluoxetine, citalopram, and sertraline, although at present sertraline does not carry an FDA indication for the treatment of children and adolescents with depression. Many clinicians consider fluoxetine to be the SSRI of choice, given that is has the strongest evidence base. However, there is a great deal of variation in individual practice. Other factors, including a family history of response to a particular antidepressant or the presence of psychiatric comorbidity, may influence the choice for a particular individual.

The typical dosing of SSRIs in the treatment of children and adolescents is summarized in Table 80.1. Dosing for prepubertal children generally begins at the lowest end of the

dose range and is gradually titrated upward to effectiveness. Fluoxetine and sertraline are both available in liquid suspensions to allow for greater ease of administration to younger patients. Adolescents, particularly older adolescents, may start at typical adult doses, though a lower initial dose may be chosen in cases where there is particular concern about risk of activation or induction of mania, which might be indicated by the patient's personal and family history of these reactions, or symptoms suggestive of a possible bipolar-spectrum illness.

SSRIs are generally well tolerated by children and adolescents. Side effects tend to be similar to those seen in adult patients and include gastrointestinal symptoms such as nausea, stomach ache or diarrhea, dizziness, headache, fatigue, sleep disturbance, and vivid dreams. Sexual side effects can occur in adolescents just as they do in adults. Children and adolescents appear to be more sensitive to behavioral activation from SSRIs. Symptoms of activation include restlessness, agitation, insomnia, disinhibition, and impulsivity (King et al., 1991). These symptoms most commonly emerge early in the course of medication treatment or shortly after dose increases. Given the concerns about behavioral activation and potential suicidality in pediatric patients, close monitoring is recommended, with frequent appointments in the early phase of treatment. The FDA has recommended weekly face-to-face meetings over the first four weeks of treatment, bi-weekly meetings over the following four weeks, another meeting at week 12 of treatment, and then meeting as clinically indicated. Communication with the patient's therapist can also be helpful in monitoring the patient's safety during initiation of an SSRI trial.

When SSRIs are ineffective or poorly tolerated, commonly considered second-line treatments include buproprion, venlafaxine, duloxetine, and mirtazepine. However, there are relatively few data to support the use of these medications in the pediatric population. Small open-label studies have demonstrated the efficacy of buproprion in adolescent depression (Glod et al., 2003). This medication also has some efficacy, albeit relatively weak compared to other medications, in the treatment of attention-deficit hyperactivity disorder (ADHD) (Conners et al., 1996), leading some clinicians to favor this medication in cases of comorbid depression and ADHD. Bupropion is also favored in patients who have

Table 80.1 DOSING OF COMMONLY USED SSRIS IN CHILDREN AND ADOLESCENTS FOR DEPRESSION AND ANXIETY

MEDICATION	STARTING DOSE FOR PREADOLESCENTS (MG)	STARTING DOSE FOR ADOLESCENTS (MG)	TYPICAL DOSE RANGE FOR DEPRESSION AND ANXIETY (MAY BE LOWER FOR YOUNGER PATIENTS)
Citalopram	5–10	10–20	10–40
Escitalopram	5–10	5–10	10–20
Fluoxetine	5–10	10–20	20–60
Fluvoxamine*	12.5–25	25–50	50–300
Sertraline	12.5–25	25–50	50–200

*Used primarily in OCD and anxiety disorders

demonstrated signs of activation or mania on SSRIs, as it is believed to be less likely to induce these problems, though it can increase anxiety in some patients. Side effects of buproprion include decreased appetite, irritability, insomnia, and gastrointestinal upset. Bupropion also reduces the seizure threshold and thus should be avoided in patients at high risk for seizure, including patients with an active comorbid eating disorder and those with poorly controlled epilepsy.

ANXIETY DISORDERS

Anxiety disorders are the most prevalent psychiatric condition in childhood and adolescents (Costello et al., 1996). Anxiety disorders commonly diagnosed in children and adolescents include generalized anxiety disorder (GAD), social anxiety disorder, separation anxiety disorder, and obsessive-compulsive disorder (OCD). Most often, the best approach to treating anxiety disorders is multimodal, including individual psychotherapy and parent training. When medication treatment is indicated for the treatment of anxiety, in most cases it should be combined with psychotherapy. According to practice parameters from the American Academy of Child and Adolescent Psychiatry, SSRIs are the recommended first-line medication treatment for anxiety disorders in children and adolescents (Connolly & Bernstein, 2007). However, there is no FDA indication for the use of these medications to treat anxiety disorders other than OCD in children.

The evidence base for the use of SSRIs in the treatment of GAD and related disorders is not as robust as it is in adult populations, but there are randomized controlled studies supporting their use, including studies of fluoxetine (Birmaher et al., 2003) and fluvoxamine (Walkup et al., 2001). The influential Child/Adolescent Anxiety Multimodal Study (CAMS) demonstrated that efficacy of sertraline over placebo, with a combined sertraline-CBT group demonstrating the greatest efficacy (Walkup et al., 2008). There is also some evidence to support the use of the SNRI venlafaxine in treating generalized anxiety disorder in children (Rynn et al., 2007).

SSRIs have demonstrated clear efficacy in the treatment of OCD in children and adolescents (Geller et al., 2003). While clomipramine has also demonstrated good efficacy in the treatment of pediatric OCD (Flament et al., 1985), it is generally considered a second-line treatment due to its side effect profile, including a risk of life-threatening cardiac arrhythmias. Use of clomipramine requires an electrocardiogram before beginning treatment, and a follow-up electrocardiogram once the patient has reached a stable dose of the medication. If the electrocardiogram shows QTc prolongation or other abnormalities, consultation with a pediatric cardiologist is indicated before proceeding with the medication trial, and a switch to another medication may be indicated.

Potential side effects of SSRIs are mentioned above in the discussion of depression treatment. It should be noted that concerns about potential for behavioral activation, induction of mania, and suicidal ideation apply in the treatment of anxiety disorders just as they do in the treatment of depression. Therefore, close monitoring for safety and for signs of activation is necessary. Dosing of SSRIs for GAD, social anxiety disorder, and separation anxiety disorder is generally the same as for the treatment of depression, and is summarized in Table 80.1. It should be noted, however, that many patients with anxiety disorders are particularly prone to somatic side effects of medications. For these patients, even lower initial dosing and even smaller incremental increases may be necessary. There is some evidence to suggest that treatment of OCD may require higher doses of SSRIs than the treatment of depression and other anxiety disorders, but the same dosing guidelines summarized in Table 80.1 still apply.

Despite their utility in treating anxiety disorders in adults, benzodiazepines are used less commonly in children and adolescents. This is partly due to the limited evidence from controlled studies to support their use. Randomized controlled trials have failed to show clear efficacy of benzodiazepines over placebo for treatment of anxiety in children and adolescents (Bernstein et al., 1990; Simeon et al., 1992; Graae et al., 1994). Furthermore, there is concern that younger patients may be at greater risk of potential disinhibitory or "paradoxical" reactions to benzodiazepines, which may be characterized by agitation, aggression, heightened anxiety, mood lability, excessive talking, or other emotional or behavioral disturbances (Gutierrez et al., 2001; Mancuso et al., 2004). Side effects of drowsiness and impaired learning and memory also cause concern in pediatric patients, as does the potential for abuse and dependence.

Nonetheless, when used judiciously, benzodiazepines can be a helpful adjunctive treatment for some children and adolescents. The immediate onset of benzodiazepines gives them an advantage over other treatments. Thus, they may be used to provide symptomatic relief while the clinician waits for an SSRI to take effect. They may also have a role as an "as-needed" medication for intense episodes of breakthrough anxiety or as abortive therapy in cases of panic disorder.

Other medications that are sometimes used in the treatment of pediatric anxiety disorders include the tricyclic antidepressants, whose use is limited by a relatively poor side effect profile and the potential for toxicity. Tricyclics may be particularly useful in treating patient with comorbid chronic pain, and low doses of imipramine and nortriptyline are sometimes used to treat enuresis. Dosing of tricyclic antidepressants is summarized in Table 80.2. A physical exam and thorough individual and family medical history should be conducted before starting a tricyclic. It is also advisable to check an electrocardiogram and vital signs at baseline and again when maintenance dose has been achieved, as these medications can cause arrhythmias and prolong QTc.

Buspirone is also used to treat anxiety symptoms in children and adolescents. Though it is often well tolerated, it has limited evidence to support its use. Potential side effects of buspirone include light-headedness, headache, and stomach upset. Buspar is typically started at 5 mg given once daily, and increased in increments of 5 mg/day, usually in divided doses of twice to three times daily, up to a maximum of 60 mg/day.

MEDICATION	STARTING DOSE FOR PREADOLESCENTS	STARTING DOSE FOR ADOLESCENTS	TYPICAL DOSE RANGE FOR DEPRESSION AND ANXIETY
Amitriptyline	1–3 mg/kg/day divided TID	25 mg–50 mg qHS	1–3 mg/kg/day, or 25–150 mg/day in adolescents, usually given in divided doses Therapeutic level = 120–250 ng/mL of amitriptyline + nortriptyline
Imipramine	1.5 mg/kg/day divided TID	30–40 mg/day divided QD to TID	1–3 mg/kg/day, or 25–75 mg/day for adolescents Therapeutic level = 180–350 ng/mL of imipramine + desipramine
Nortriptyline	1 mg/kg/day divided TID-QID	30 mg/day divided QD-QID	1–3 mg/kg/day, or 30–50 mg/day for adolescents Therapeutic level = 50–150 ng/mL
Clomipramine*	Indicated for > 10 years old	25 mg QD	50–150 mg/day (3 mg/kg/day max)

*Clomipramine is indicated specifically for the treatment of OCD in children over 10 years old

ATTENTION-DEFICIT HYPERACTIVITY DISORDER

Stimulants are the first line of treatment for ADHD. They have demonstrated a high degree of efficacy in numerous randomized controlled trials (Pliszka, 2007). They are currently the most commonly prescribed psychiatric medication for patients under the age of 18 in the United States (National Center for Health Statistics Report, 2010). In the landmark Multimodal Treatment of ADHD (MTA) study, children assigned to the stimulant treatment group and the combined stimulant and behavioral treatment group demonstrated significantly greater improvement than children treated with intensive behavioral treatment alone or standard community care (MTA Cooperative Group, 1999). While not every child with ADHD requires medication, and many may do very well with behavioral treatment and other psychosocial interventions, this study clearly demonstrated that medication treatment is more effective than behavioral therapy alone. When stimulants and other ADHD medications are used, they should be part of a comprehensive treatment plan that may also include behavioral therapy and school-based interventions to facilitate learning.

The first-line stimulants used in the treatment of ADHD are methylphenidate and mixed amphetamine salts. Both medications are available in long-acting formulations for ease of dosing. While there is some relationship between dose response and weight, there is a wide range of responsiveness to a given dose between patients. Thus, it is best to start with a low dose and titrate up to effect. When titrating ADHD medications, communication with collateral sources is essential, as patients may not be reliable reporters and parents may not be aware of the level of symptoms in school. Use of symptom-rating scales for parents can be helpful in tracking symptoms.

Dosing of stimulant medications for ADHD is summarized in Table 80.3. Typical therapeutic doses are 0.3–2 mg/kg/day for methylphenidate and 0.15–1 mg/kg/day for mixed amphetamine salts. The maximum recommended dose is 60 mg/day for methylphenidate and 40 mg/day of mixed amphetamine salts. D-isomeric formulations of both medications are available, as dex-methylphenidate and dextroamphetamine, under the theory that these isomeric forms may be better tolerated than the mixed d,l isomer formulations. These medications typically require lower doses than their mixed isomer counterparts. Lisdexamfetamine is a newly available pro-drug form of amphetamine with an amino acid that must be cleaved in the gut before it is biologically active, reducing the medication's abuse potential.

Stimulants are generally well tolerated, but they do have the potential to cause significant side effects in some patients. Common side effects include decreased appetite and possible associated decreases in growth, insomnia, headaches, and stomach aches. Stimulants can have a significant impact on mood, causing irritability and sadness in some patients. They are believed to have potential to induce mania in patients predisposed to bipolar disorder and may induce psychotic symptoms in rare cases. Stimulants can also induce or exacerbate tics, which is particularly relevant to clinicians, given the high degree of comorbidity of tic disorder and ADHD. Stimulants can raise blood pressure, though usually in small amounts at therapeutic levels.

There have been reports of sudden death of children taking stimulants (Villalba, 2006), and this has fueled controversy in recent years regarding potential adverse cardiac effects, including fatal arrhythmias, from these medications. Given that these serious adverse events are extremely rare, despite the large numbers of children taking these medications, many have questioned whether there is a true increase in risk of sudden cardiac death associated with stimulants or whether the reported events are consistent with the base rate of these rare but tragic events in the general population. One recent retrospective cohort study examined medical records of over 55,000 children over a period of ten years (Winterstein et al., 2007). This study found no association between stimulant use and sudden cardiac death. The authors reported no deaths in over 42,000 person-years of stimulant use compared to five deaths in the no-use and former-stimulant-use groups, and they reported no increase in hospitalizations from cardiac causes associated with stimulant use.

Table 80.3 DOSING OF STIMULANT MEDICATIONS IN THE TREATMENT OF ADHD

MEDICATION	DURATION OF ACTION	TYPICAL DOSE RANGE	MAXIMUM RECOMMENDED DOSE
METHYLPHENIDATES			
Short-acting:			
Ritalin, Methylin	3–4 hours	0.3–2 mg/kg/day	60 mg/day
Focalin (dexmethylphenidate)	3–5 hours	0.15–1 mg/kg/day	20 mg/day
Intermediate:			
Ritalin SR, Metadate ER, Methylin ER	4–8 hours	0.3–2 mg/kg/day	60 mg/day
Long-acting:			
Daytrana (methylphenidate patch), Metadate CD, Ritalin LA	8–12 hours	0.3–2 mg/kg/day	60 mg/day
Concerta	10–16 hours	0.3–2 mg/kg/day	72 mg/day
Focalin XR	8–12 hours	0.15–1 mg/kg/day	30 mg/day
AMPHETAMINES			
Short-acting:			
Adderall (mixed amphetamine salts)	4–6 hours	0.15 mg/kg/day	40 mg/day
Dexedrine, Dextrostat (dextroamphetamine)	4–6 hours	0.15 mg/kg/day	40 mg/day
Long-acting:			
Adderall XR	8–12 hours	0.15 mg/kg/day	30 mg/day
Dexedrine Spansules	8 hours	0.15 mg/kg/day	40 mg/day
Vyvanse (lisdexamfetamine)	8–12 hours	Varies	70 mg/day

Despite the questionable association between stimulants and sudden death and the rare occurrence of these events, the devastating nature of such an event warrants a cautious approach. In 2008, the American Academy of Pediatrics published guidelines regarding appropriate monitoring for pediatric patients prescribed stimulant medications (Perrin et al., 2008). These guidelines call for a thorough medical history prior to treatment, including review of past cardiac problems, surgeries, and heart murmurs as well as history of syncope, palpitations, dizziness during exercise, or seizures. The guidelines call for a review of family history, including history of sudden unexplained deaths in the family, myocardial infarction in relatives under the age of 35, and history of cardiomyopathies, structural heart disease, or arrhythmias. Finally, the guidelines call for a thorough physical exam including a cardiac exam. If there is cause for concern based on this evaluation, additional steps, including an electrocardiogram or consultation with a pediatric cardiologist, may be necessary before proceeding with a stimulant trial. For patients taking stimulants, blood pressure, heart rate, height, and weight should be monitored regularly.

For patients who are unable to tolerate stimulants or who do not respond to stimulants, several non-stimulant medications are available for the treatment of ADHD. Dosing of non-stimulant medications is summarized in Table 80.4. Atomoxetine is a noradrenergic reuptake inhibitor with demonstrated efficacy in ADHD in randomized controlled trials (Michelson et al., 2002), though treatment response appears to be less robust than that of the stimulants (Faraone et al., 2006). Atomoxetine is typically started at doses of 0.5 mg/kg/day and increased to a target dose of 1.2 mg/kg/day, with a maximum recommended dose of 1.4 mg/kg/day or 100 mg/day, whichever is less. Common side effects of atomoxetine include gastrointestinal upset, headaches, decreased appetite, insomnia, and drowsiness. Mood changes, including rare behavioral activation and suicidal thinking, are possible with atomoxetine, and patients should be monitored for these changes.

Because treatment response to atomoxetine is not as robust as it is to the stimulants, it is most often used as a second-line medication. However, in some situations, it may be tried first. For example, a clinician might choose to start with atomoxetine for patients who are underweight or who have feeding issues at baseline. Anecdotally, atomoxetine also appears to be helpful for many children and adolescents who have ADHD with comorbid anxiety disorders.

Table 80.4 NON-STIMULANT MEDICATIONS IN THE TREATMENT OF ADHD

MEDICATION	STARTING DOSE	TYPICAL DOSE RANGE	NOTES
Strattera (atomoxetine)	0.5 mg/kg/day	1.2–1.4 mg/kg/day	• Norepinephrine reuptake inhibitor • Given once or twice daily
Tenex (guanfacine)	0.5 mg–1 mg/day	1–4 mg/day	• Alpha–2 adrenergic agonist • Usually dosed BID or TID • Extended release formulation (Intuniv) dosed once daily, available as 1 mg, 2 mg, 3 mg, and 4 mg tablets
Clonidine	• 0.025–0.0.05 mg/day • 0.1 mg at bedtime for extended release (Kapvay)	0.05 mg–0.4 mg	• Alpha-2 adrenergic agonist • Usually dosed BID, TID, or QID • Extended release formulation (Kapvay) dosed once daily • Dosing of extended release is not interchangeable with other formulations and should not be substituted mg for mg • Typically more sedating than guanfacine

Alpha-2 adrenergic agonists, which include guanfacine and clonidine, are commonly used as adjunctive treatment or second-line treatment for children and adolescents with ADHD. These medications have shown some efficacy, though they appear to work primarily on symptoms of hyperactivity and impulsivity and are less effective for the cognitive symptoms of ADHD (Scahill et al., 2001; Palumbo et al., 2008). New extended-release formulations of both medications have allowed greater ease of dosing. Sedation is often a limiting side-effect with these medications. Other possible side effects include hypotension, dizziness, headache, gastrointestinal upset, constipation, and dry mouth. Cardiac effects, including bradyarrhythmia and atrioventricular block, are also possible due to the autonomic effects of these medications. Use of these medications for children with cardiac conduction problems and cardiac arrhythmias should only be considered after consultation with a pediatric cardiologist and if there is a strong clinical indication for their use.

Other medications sometimes used in the treatment of ADHD include bupropion and tricyclic antidepressants such as imipramine and nortriptyline. These medications tend to be considered second- or third-line treatments for ADHD, as they appear to be less effective (Pliszka, 2003).

BIPOLAR DISORDER

Once thought to occur only rarely in youth, the diagnosis of bipolar disorder in children and adolescents has risen dramatically over the past decade. While there is some controversy surrounding the diagnosis and the nomenclature for children with severe mood symptoms, it is clear that there is a population of children with severe disturbances in mood and behavior whose symptoms are categorically distinct from those diagnosed with major depressive disorder and who respond to different forms of treatment.

The typical presentation of children and adolescents with bipolar disorder is different from that of adults. Children and adolescents typically present with more mixed mood episodes rather than distinct periods of mania and depression; more frequent rapid cycling, more chronic impairment without improvement between episodes, and more prominent irritability, explosiveness, anger, and dysphoria (Wozniak et al., 1995; Biederman et al., 2004).

The treatment of bipolar disorder in children and adolescents requires a multifaceted approach, usually involving individual therapy and parent support and training and often requiring school-based interventions and other psychosocial treatments. Medication can play a critical role as part of a comprehensive treatment plan—stabilizing mood, helping maintain safety, and reducing aggression and other severe problem behaviors to allow patients to engage more successfully in treatment. Pharmacotherapy for pediatric bipolar disorder is frequently complex and challenging. Subspecialty management by an experienced child and adolescent psychiatrist is warranted whenever possible. Accurate diagnosis and recognition of comorbid psychiatric issues, which are common in pediatric patients with bipolar disorder, are essential to effective treatment.

Medications commonly used to treat pediatric bipolar disorder include second-generation neuroleptics, antiepileptic drugs, and lithium. There is no clear consensus at present about which of these medications should be viewed as first-line, and there are differences in practice between providers.

Second-generation neuroleptics are used by many clinicians as the first line of treatment for children and adolescents with bipolar disorder, as they have demonstrated efficacy (Thomas et al., 2011) and do not require monitoring of serum drug levels. Dosing of antipsychotic medications in children and adolescents is summarized in Table 80.5. Risperidone, aripiprazole, and quetiapine have all been approved by the FDA for treatment of mania and mixed episodes in children age ten and older. Olanzapine has also been shown to be effective but is less commonly used because it is associated with a greater degree of weight gain and metabolic changes than other equally effective drugs in this class (Correll et al., 2009). Similarly, ziprasidone has some evidence suggesting efficacy (Thomas et al., 2011), but concerns about QTc prolongation (Blair et al., 2005) have led most clinicians to consider it a second- or third-line treatment.

Table 80.5 ATYPICAL ANTIPSYCHOTICS FOR THE TREATMENT OF PEDIATRIC BIPOLAR DISORDER

MEDICATION	FDA APPROVAL FOR BIPOLAR DISORDER?	STARTING DOSE	MAX RECOMMENDED DOSE FOR BIPOLAR DISORDER	NOTES
Abilify (aripiprazole)	10 years and older	2 mg once daily	30 mg	• May cause less weight gain than other atypicals • May be a greater incidence of restlessness/akathisia
Geodon (ziprasidone)	No	20 mg once daily	80 mg (no formal dosing guidelines for pediatric population)	• Greater concern about QTc prolongation compared to other atypicals
Risperdal (risperidone)	10 years and older	0.25 mg–0.5 mg at bedtime	2.5 mg/day	• Greater degree of dopamine D2 antagonism may increase risk for dystonia, extrapyramidal side effects, hyperprolactinemia
Seroquel (quetiapine)	10 years and older	25–50 mg at bedtime	600 mg/day	• More sedating than other atypicals • Can cause orthostatic hypotension • Lower risk of extrapyramidal side effects, akithisia
Zyprexa (olanzepine)	13 years and older	2.5–5 mg at bedtime	20 mg/day	• Appears to be associated with greater degree of weight gain than other atypicals • Sedating

Second-generation neuroleptics can cause a number of side effects, including sedation, restlessness, orthostatic hypotension, dizziness, and constipation. Females may experience lactation and menstrual irregularities, particularly with risperidone. While they are much less common, worrisome side effects of the first-generation (typical) neuroleptics may also occur with second-generation neuroleptics, including tardive dyskinesia, dystonia, Parkinsonism, akathisia, neuroleptic-induced catatonia, and neuroleptic malignant syndrome.

One of the most common problems seen with atypical antipsychotics is weight gain and metabolic changes, including impaired glucose metabolism and hyperlipidemia, which may predispose patients to the development of type II diabetes and cardiovascular disease. The American Diabetes Association and the American Psychiatric Association developed joint guidelines for the monitoring of patients prescribed these medications (ADA & APA, 2004). The guidelines call for baseline measurement and regular monitoring of height, weight, blood pressure, fasting glucose, and fasting lipid profile, as well as taking a history of personal and family history of diabetes, cardiac disease, and hyperlipidemia. Counseling patients and parents about the metabolic risks of these medications and concrete measures, including dietary changes and exercise, that can reduce these risks is essential.

Anticonvulsants commonly used in the treatment of pediatric bipolar disorder include divalproex sodium, lamotrigine, carbamazepine, and oxcarbazepine. Use of divalproex sodium is based primarily on evidence from adult studies; data to support its use in the pediatric population are limited (Thomas

et al., 2011). It is sometimes preferred in patients with rapid cycling and mixed episodes, though this is based on adult data. Use of divalproex sodium requires monitoring of serum levels, with target therapeutic levels of between 50 and 125 mcg/mL. Pediatric patients are usually maintained on the low end of this range, though some patients may require higher levels to achieve therapeutic effect, particularly in cases of acute mania. Monitoring of liver function tests due to potential liver toxicity, and complete blood count due to potential thrombocytopenia and leukopenia, are also necessary for patients taking divalproex sodium. Pediatric patients, particularly younger children, may be more susceptible to these effects than adults. There is some variability in practice, but generally a complete blood count is taken and liver function tests are checked at baseline, after a therapeutic dose has been attained, and again every three to six months thereafter, along with a serum valproate level. If these values remain stable over the first year of treatment, laboratory testing may be performed less frequently. Female patients should have a pregnancy test prior to starting treatment, due to teratogenicity, including an increased risk of neural tube defects, and should use a reliable method of contraception if they are sexually active. Other potential side effects include weight gain, nausea, hair loss, sedation, and, more rarely, pancreatitis. Adolescent girls taking divalproex sodium are at risk of developing polycystic ovarian syndrome, which may present with menstrual irregularities, hirsutism, acne, and weight gain.

Lamotrigine is being used with increasing frequency in the treatment of pediatric bipolar disorder. While there are few data to support its use outside of the adult population, some open-label studies have demonstrated efficacy in adolescents (Chang et al., 2006; Pavuluri et al., 2009). In adults, there is some evidence that lamotrigine may be effective in treating bipolar depression (Calabrese et al., 1999), on which many other mood stabilizers have minimal effect. It has a further advantage in that it does not require monitoring of serum levels. However, lamotrigine requires a very gradual dose titration due to the associated risk of severe cutaneous reactions, including Stevens-Johnson syndrome and toxic epidermal necrolysis. Risk of these rare but potentially fatal reactions may be greater in youth compared to adults, with an estimated rate of 0.8% in pediatric patients compared to 0.3% in adult patients (Seo et al., 2011). This risk is minimized by avoiding sudden increases in dose (Kowatch & Delbello, 2006). In adolescents, this also requires discussion with patients and parents about the risks associated with non-adherence and the need to contact the prescribing clinician before restarting lamotrigine if a patient has missed more than one dose. More common side effects of lamotrigine include blurry vision, constipation, gastrointestinal upset, decreased coordination, sedation, insomnia, benign rashes, and runny nose.

The structurally similar anticonvulsants carbamazepine and oxcarbazepine are sometimes used to treat bipolar disorder in children and adolescents with bipolar disorder, though again there are few data demonstrating their efficacy in the pediatric population (Thomas et al., 2011). Monitoring of serum levels is required for carbamazepine, with a target range of 4–12 mcg/mL. Pediatric patients are usually maintained on the low end of this range, though some patients may require higher levels to achieve therapeutic effect. Side effect profiles of carbamazepine and oxcarbazepine are similar. Both may cause nausea, sedation, dizziness, ataxia, rash, and headaches. Less commonly, both medications carry a risk of Stevens-Johnson syndrome, and both may cause hyponatremia. Carbamazepine may cause blood dyscrasias, including aplastic anemia as well as liver toxicity, and these problems may occur more commonly in the pediatric population. Bone marrow suppression and liver toxicity are less common with oxcarbazepine. It should also be noted that carbamazepine induces enzymes in the cytochrome P450 system, which may lead to more rapid metabolism of some medications, including oral contraceptives.

Before starting treatment with carbamazepine, baseline renal function tests, thyroid function tests, liver function tests, and complete blood count including platelets must be obtained. The complete blood count and liver function tests should be monitored every two to three weeks during the initial four months of treatment and can be decreased in frequency to every six to 12 months thereafter. There are no clear guidelines for monitoring of oxcarbazepine in treatment of pediatric mood disorders, but it is good practice to follow monitoring parameters similar to those used with carbamazepine, given the similarities in side effect profiles of the two medications. Serum sodium should also be monitored for patients on oxcarbazepine given the risk of hyponatremia. For both medications, it is also important to educate patients and parents about the signs of liver abnormalities and blood dyscrasias and advise them to contact the prescribing physician if they have any concerns.

The first agent to be granted FDA approval for treatment of bipolar disorder in youths (age 12 and older) was lithium. Lithium has long been a mainstay of treatment for bipolar disorder in adults, and it has shown efficacy in several double-blind placebo-controlled trials in adolescents as well, though it has been noted that these trials are limited by relatively small sample sizes (McClellan et al., 2007). However, the narrow therapeutic window of lithium, the potential for significant toxicity, the need for close monitoring of serum levels, and its side effect profile have limited its use.

Lithium requires close monitoring of serum levels, with target levels between 0.6 and 1.2 mEq/L, with levels on the higher end of this range for acute mania. While not well studied in children under 12, lithium is generally well tolerated by adolescent patients, who may be less susceptible to its adverse effects than adult patients. However, lithium has the potential to cause significant toxicity, including renal and thyroid toxicity as well as cardiac-conduction abnormalities. Given these potential effects, serum electrolytes, complete blood count, thyroid function tests, renal function tests, serum calcium, urinalysis, and electrocardiogram (ECG) should be checked at baseline prior to initiating treatment. Females of reproductive age should also have a pregnancy test prior to starting treatment. Once a stable therapeutic dose has been reached, lithium levels, renal function tests, thyroid function tests, and urinalysis should be checked every three to six months, and a repeat ECG should be obtained at the therapeutic level. Other potential side effects of lithium include sedation, nausea, diarrhea, tremor, hair loss, acne, weight gain, polyuria, and polydipsia. In following patients on lithium, clinicians should be aware that dehydration, such as that caused by gastroenteritis, can push levels into the toxic range. Lithium can also interact with several commonly prescribed medications, most notably non-steroidal anti-inflammatory drugs (NSAIDs), which interfere with its renal clearance.

SUMMARY

The treatment of psychiatric illness in children and adolescents requires a multifaceted approach involving multiple treatment modalities. When managed appropriately, psychiatric medications can be an effective component of treatment for many patients. Management of medications for pediatric patients requires close collaboration with the patient, the family, the primary medical doctor, and often school personnel and other sources of collateral information. Development plays a critical role in pediatric psychopharmacology, as the patient's developmental level must be taken into account in every aspect of treatment, including choice and dose of medication, nature of the discussion about the medication and its effects and risks, and plans for ensuring the patient's safety and adherence.

CLINICAL PEARLS

- Young children may need reassurance that a medication will not change who they are or make them do things they do not want to do. They may become overwhelmed or anxious when confronted with long and detailed lists of possible side effects and may do better with a more general instruction to let their parents know if there is anything they feel while on the medication that they do not like.

- In non-crisis situations, one should avoid major medication changes at transition times or periods of high stress.

- Establish effective communication and a collaborative relationship with the patient and family.

- Integrate medication into an overall treatment plan for the patient based upon a biopsychosocial formulation.

- Start medication only after a thorough medical and psychiatric evaluation, including detailed review of past medication trials and their effects.

- Start medications at the low end of the effective dose range and gradually titrate to effectiveness.

- Employ the simplest medication regimen necessary to effectively manage the patient's symptoms, using poly-pharmacy only when indicated to treat residual symptoms, comorbid diagnoses, or side effects from other medications.

- Take one step at a time when possible, avoiding making multiple changes at once that will make subsequent changes in clinical presentation difficult to interpret.

- Take a systematic approach, assuring that each medication trial has been allowed adequate time at an adequate dosage before deeming it ineffective and moving to the next step in treatment.

- Closely monitor efficacy and side effects, using objective measures and structured rating scales when they are available.

- Explicitly ask patients about their adherence to the medication regimen rather than assuming the medication is being taken as prescribed.

- Monitor drug levels when there is an established therapeutic range and it is known that there is significant inter-individual variability in the drug's pharmacokinetics.

- Simplify medication regimens when possible, to avoid confusion and non-adherence.

- Adhere to current practice guidelines for monitoring side effects of specific medications.

- Be fully aware of all the drugs the patient has been prescribed by other physicians, as well as the patient's use of over-the-counter medications, nutritional supplements, and complementary treatments.

- Maintain communication with other medical and psychiatric providers involved in the patient's care.

- Provide clear documentation of the patient's care, preferably in electronic form.

DISCLOSURE STATEMENT

Dr. Hazen receives no outside funding and has no conflicts of interest to disclose.

REFERENCES

American Diabetes Association & American Psychiatric Association (ADA & APA) (2004). Consensus development conference on antipsychotic drugs and obesity and diabetes. *Diabetes Care, 27*(2), 596–601.

Anderson, G. D., & Lynn, A. M. (2009). Optimizing pediatric dosing: A developmental pharmacologic approach. *Pharmacotherapy, 29*(6), 680–690.

Benedetti, M. S., Whomsley, R., & Canning, M. (2007). Drug metabolism in the paediatric population and in the elderly. *Drug Discovery Today, 12*, 599–610.

Bernstein, G. A., Garfinkel, B. D., & Borchardt, C. M. (1990). Comparative studies of pharmacotherapy for school refusal. *Journal of the American Academy of Child & Adolescent Psychiatry, 29*(5), 773–781.

Biederman, J., Faraone, S. V., Wozniak, J., Mick, E., Kwon, A., & Aleardi, M. (2004). Further evidence of unique developmental phenotypic correlates of pediatric bipolar disorder: Findings from a large sample of clinically referred preadolescent children assessed over the last 7 years. *Journal of Affective Disorders, 82*, S45–S58.

Birmaher, B., Axelson, D. A., Monk, K., Kalas, C., Clark, D. B., et al. (2003). Fluoxetine for the treatment of childhood anxiety disorders. *Journal of the American Academy of Child & Adolescent Psychiatry, 42*(4), 415–423.

Blair, J., Scahill, L., State, M., & Martin, A. (2005). Electrocardiographic changes in children and adolescents treated with ziprasidone: A prospective study. *Journal of the American Academy of Child & Adolescent Psychiatry, 44*(1), 73–79.

Boyson, S. J., & Adams, C. E. (1997). D$_1$ and D$_2$ dopamine receptors in perinatal and adult basal ganglia. *Pediatric Research, 41*, 822–831.

Bridge, J., Iyengar, S., Salary, C. B., Barbe, R. P., Birmaher, B., Pincus, H. A., et al. (2007). Clinical response and risk for reported suicidal ideation and suicide attempts in pediatric antidepressant treatment: A meta-analysis of randomized controlled trials. *Journal of the American Medical Association, 297*(15), 1683–1696.

Calabrese, J. R., Bowden, C. L., Sachs, G. S., Ascher, J. A., Monaghan, E., & Rudd, G. D. (1999). A double-blind placebo-controlled study of lamotrigine monotherapy in outpatients with bipolar I depression. *Journal of Clinical Psychiatry, 60*(2), 79–88.

Chang, K., Saxena, K., & Howe, M. (2006). An open-label study of lamotrigine adjunct or monotherapy for the treatment of adolescents with bipolar depression. *Journal of the American Academy of Child & Adolescent Psychiatry, 39*, 713–720.

Cheung, A., Sacks, D., Dewa, C. S., Pong, J., & Levitt, A. (2008). Pediatric prescribing practices and the FDA black-box warning on antidepressants. *Journal of Developmental & Behavioral Pediatrics, 29*(3), 213–215.

Conners, C. K., Casat, C. D., Gualtieri, C. T., Weller, E., Reader, M., Reiss, A., et al. (1996). Bupropion hydrochloride in attention deficit disorder with hyperactivity. *Journal of the American Academy of Child & Adolescent Psychiatry, 35*(10), 1314–1321.

Connolly, S. D., Bernstein, G. A., & Work Group on Quality Issues (2007). Practice parameter for the assessment and treatment of children and adolescents with anxiety disorders. *Journal of the American Academy of Child & Adolescent Psychiatry, 46*(2), 267–283.

Correll, C. U., Manu, P., Olshanskiy, V., Napolitano, B., Kane, J. M., Malhotra, A. K. (2009). Cardiometabolic risk of atypical antipsychotics during first-time use in children and adolescents. *Journal of the American Medical Association, 302*(16), 1763–1771.

Costello, E. J., Angold, A., Burns, B. J., Stangl, D. K., Tweed, D. L., Erkanli, A., et al. (1996). The Great Smoky Mountains Study of

Youth. Goals, design, methods, and the prevalence of DSM-III-R disorders. *Archives of General Psychiatry, 53*, 1129–1136.

Emslie, G. J., Heiligenstein, J. H., Wagner, K. D., Hoog, S. L., Ernest, D. E., Brown, E., Nilsson, M., & Jacobson, J. G. (2002). Fluoxetine for acute treatment of depression in children and adolescents: a placebo-controlled, randomized clinical trial. *Journal of the American Academy of Child & Adolescent Psychiatry, 41*(10), 1205–1215.

Emslie, G. J., Rush, A. J., Weinberg, W. A., Kowatch, R. A., Hughes, C. W., Carmody. T., & Rintelmann, J. (1997). A double-blind, randomized, placebo-controlled trial of fluoxetine in children and adolescents with depression. *Archives of General Psychiatry, 54*(11), 1031–1037.

Emslie, G. J., Ventura, D., Korotzer, A., & Tourkodimitris, S. (2009). Escitalopram in the treatment of adolescent depression: a randomized placebo-controlled multisite trial. *Journal of the American Academy of Child & Adolescent Psychiatry,48*(7),721–729.

Faraone, S. V., Biederman, J., Spencer, T. J., & Aleadri, M. (2006). Comparing the efficacy of medications for ADHD using meta-analysis. *Medscape General Medicine, 8*(4), 4.

Flament, M. F., Rapoport, J. L., Berg, C. J., Sceery, W., Kilts, C., Mellstrom, B., et al. (1985). Clomipramine treatment of childhood obsessive-compulsive disorder: A double-blind controlled study. *Archives of General Psychiatry, 42*(10), 977–983.

Geller, D. A., Biederman, J., Stewart, S. E., Mullin, B., Martin, A., Spencer, T., et al. (2003). Which SSRI? A meta-analysis of pharmacotherapy trials in pediatric obsessive compulsive disorder. *American Journal of Psychiatry, 160*(11), 1919–1928.

Gibbons, R. D., Brown, C. H., Hur, K., Marcus, S. M., Bhaumik, D. K., Erkens, J. A., et al. (2007). Early evidence on the effects of regulators' suicidality warnings on SSRI prescriptions and suicide in children and adolescents. *American Journal of Psychiatry, 164*, 1356–1363.

Glod, C. A., Lynch, A., Flynn, E., Berkowitz, C., & Baldessarini, R. J. (2003). Open trial of bupropion SR in adolescent major depression. *Journal of Child & Adolescent Psychiatric Nursing, 16*(3), 123–130.

Graae, F., Milner, J., Rizzotto, L., & Klein, R. G. (1994). Clonazepam in childhood anxiety disorders. *Journal of the American Academy of Child & Adolescent Psychiatry, 33*(3), 372–376.

Gutierrez, M. A., Roper, J. M., & Hahn, P. (2001). Paradoxical reactions to benzodiazepines. *American Journal of Nursing, 101*(7), 34–39.

King, R. A., Riddle, M. A., Chappell, P. B., Hardin, M. T., Anderson, G. M., Lombroso, P., & Scahill, L. (1991). Emergence of self-destructive phenomena in children and adolescents during fluoxetine treatment. *Journal of the American Academy of Child & Adolescent Psychiatry, 30*(2), 179–186.

Kowatch, R. A., & DelBello, M. P. (2006). Pediatric bipolar disorder: emerging diagnostic and treatment approaches. *Child & Adolescent Psychiatric Clinics of North America, 15*(1), 73–108.

Mancuso, C. E., Tanzi, M. G., & Gabay, M. (2004). Paradoxical reactions to benzodiazepines: Literature review and treatment options. *Pharmacotherapy, 24*, 1177–1185.

March, J., Silva, S., Petrycki, S., Curry, J., Wells, K., Fairbank, J., et al., & Treatment for Adolescents with Depression Study (TADS) Team (2004). Fluoxetine, cognitive-behavioral therapy, and their combination for adolescents with depression: Treatment for Adolescents with Depression Study (TADS) randomized controlled trial. *Journal of the American Medical Association, 292*(7), 807–820.

McClellan, J., Kowatch, R., Findling, R. L., & Work Group on Quality Issues (2007). Practice parameter for the assessment and treatment of children and adolescents with bipolar disorder. *Journal of the American Academy of Child & Adolescent Psychiatry, 46*(1), 107–125.

Michelson, D., Allen, A. J., Busner, J., Casat, C., Dunn, D., Kratochvil, C., et al. (2002). Once-daily atomoxetine treatment for children adolescents with attention deficit-hyperactivity disorder: A randomized placebo controlled study. *American Journal of Psychiatry, 159*, 1898–1901.

MTA Cooperative Group (1999). A 14-month randomized clinical trial of treatment strategies for attention-deficit/hyperactivity disorder. *Archives of General Psychiatry, 56*(12), 1073–1086.

National Center for Health Statistics (2011). *Health, United States, 2010: With special feature on death and dying.* Hyattsville, MD: NCHS.

Palumbo, D. R., Sallee, F. R., Pelham, W. E., Bukstein, O. G., Daviss, W. B., & McDermott, M. P. (2008). Clonidine for attention-deficit/ hyperactivity disorder: I. Efficacy and tolerability outcomes. *Journal of the American Academy of Child & Adolescent Psychiatry, 47*(2), 180–188.

Pavuluri, M. N., Henry, D. B., Moss, M., Mohammed, T., Carbray, J. A., & Sweeney, J. A. (2009). Effectiveness of lamotrigine in maintaining symptom control in pediatric bipolar disorder. *Journal of Child & Adolescent Psychopharmacology, 19*(1), 75–82.

Perrin, J. M., Friedman, R. A., Knilans, T. K., & Black Box Working Group (2008). Cardiovascular monitoring and stimulant drugs for attention deficit/hyperactivity disorder. *Pediatrics, 122*(2), 451–453.

Pliszka, S. R. (2003). Non-stimulant treatment of attention-deficit/ hyperactivity disorder. *Central Nervous System Spectrums, 8*, 253–258.

Pliszka, S., & AACAP Work Group on Quality Issues (2007). Practice parameter for the assessment and treatment of children and adolescents with attention-deficit/hyperactivity disorder. *Journal of the American Academy of Child & Adolescent Psychiatry, 46*(7), 894–921.

Rinne, J. O., Lonnberg, P., & Marjamaki, P. (1990). Age-dependent decline in human brain dopamine D_1 and D_2 receptors. *Brain Research, 508*, 349–352.

Rynn, M. A., Riddle, M. A., Yeung, P. P., & Kunz, N. R. (2007). Efficacy and safety of extended-release venlafaxine in the treatment of generalized anxiety disorder in children and adolescents: two placebo-controlled trials. *American Journal of Psychiatry, 164*(2), 290–300.

Scahill, L., Chappell, P. B., Kim, Y. S., Schultz, R. T., Katsovich, L., Shepherd, E., Arnsten, A. F., Cohen, D. J., & Leckman, J. F. (2001). A placebo-controlled study of guanfacine in the treatment of children with tic disorders and attention deficit hyperactivity disorder. *American Journal of Psychiatry, 158*(7), 1067–1074.

Seo, H. J., Chiesa, A., Lee, S. J., Patkar, A. A., Han, C., Masand, P. S., et al. (2011). Safety and tolerability of lamotrigine: results from 12 placebo-controlled clinical trials and clinical implications. *Clinical Neuropharmacology, 34*(1), 39–47.

Simeon, J. G., Ferguson, H. B., Knott, V., Roberts, N., Gauthier, B., Dubois, C., & Wiggins, D. (1992). Clinical, cognitive, and neurophysiological effects of alprazolam in children and adolescents with overanxious and avoidant disorders. *Journal of the American Academy of Child & Adolescent Psychiatry, 31*(1), 29–33.

Thomas, T., Stansifer, L., & Findling, R. L. (2011). Psychopharmacology of pediatric bipolar disorders in children and adolescents. *Pediatric Clinics of North America, 58*(1), 173–187.

Villalba, L. (2006). Follow up review of AERS search identifying cases of sudden death occurring with drugs used for the treatment of attention deficit hyperactivity disorder ADHD. Available at: http://www.fda.gov/ohrms/dockets/ac/06/ briefing/2006-4210b_07_01_safetyreview.pdf. Accessed September 10, 2014.

Wagner, K. D., Ambrosini, P., Rynn, M., Wohlberg, C., Yang, R., Greenbaum, M. S., Childress A., Donnelly, C., & Deas, D., Sertraline Pediatric Depression Study Group. (2003). Efficacy of sertraline in the treatment of children and adolescents with major depressive disorder: Two randomized controlled trials. *Journal of the American Medical Association, 290*(8), 1033–1041.

Wagner, K. D., Robb, A. S., Findling, R. L., Jin, J., Gutierrez, M. M., & Heydorn, W. E. (2004). A randomized, placebo-controlled trial of citalopram for the treatment of major depression in children and adolescents. *American Journal of Psychiatry, 161*(6), 1079–1083.

Walkup, J. T., Albano, A. M., Piacentini, J., Birmaher, B., Compton, S. N., Sherrill, J. T., et al. (2008). Cognitive behavioral therapy, sertraline, or a combination in childhood anxiety. *New England Journal of Medicine, 359*(26), 2753–2766.

Walkup, J. T., Albano, A. M., Piacentini, J., Birmaher, B., Compton, S. N., Sherrill, J. T., et al. (2008). Cognitive behavioral therapy, sertraline, or a combination in childhood anxiety. *New England Journal of Medicine, 359*(26), 2753–2766.

Whittington, C. J., Kendall, T., Fonagy, P., Cottrell, D., Cotgrove, A., & Boddington, E. (2004). Selective serotonin reuptake inhibitors in childhood depression: Systematic review of published versus unpublished data. *Lancet, 363*, 1341–1345.

Winterstein, A. G., Gerhard, T., Shuster, J., Johnson, M., Zito, J. M., & Saidi, A. (2007). Cardiac safety of central nervous system stimulants in children and adolescents with attention-deficit/hyperactivity disorder. *Pediatrics, 120*(6), e1494–e1501.

Wozniak, J., Biederman, J., Kiely, K., Ablon, J. S., Faraone, S. V., Mundy, S. V., et al. (1995). Mania-like symptoms suggestive of childhood-onset bipolar disorder in clinically referred children. *Journal of the American Academy of Child & Adolescent Psychiatry, 34*(7), 867–876.

81.

DEATH AND GRIEF COUNSELING FOR CHILDREN AND ADOLESCENTS

Patricia J. O'Malley, Hillary G. D'Amato, and Frederick J. Stoddard, Jr.

INTRODUCTION

There are few situations in medicine more challenging, humbling, and significant than accompanying children and their families through passages to loss, dying, and grief. These may arise in the context of a child's sudden death, gradual decline, or death after a long illness, as well as when a child faces the loss of a family member or loved one. In the usual context of care of children in hospitals, as well as after disasters (Lemaire, 2011; Shibley & Stoddard, 2011; Farmer, 2011), the medical psychiatrist has expertise in ways of relating to those facing loss or death, understands anticipatory and accomplished grief and developmental concepts of death, and can choose language carefully in order to support the need for patient, family, and caregivers to care for themselves.

The subject of this chapter is both the child facing his or her own death, and the child facing the death of a family member or loved one. Its goal is to provide clinicians with practical approaches, choices, and suggestions for dealing with death in children and adolescents and the grief that follows. As difficult as the responsibilities attendant on clinicians can be, they may be some of the most rewarding and profound encounters in medicine.

DEATH OF A CHILD OR ADOLESCENT

Death in childhood or adolescence is no longer commonplace in developed countries. Although 30% of the American population is under age 18, only 2% of all deaths annually occur in this age group, in marked contrast to the previous century, when 30% of all deaths annually were of children under age five. While these data point to wonderful progress in maternal and child health, they also underscore that death in childhood or adolescence has become a singular tragedy in our society and an increasingly uncommon event in the professional lives of clinicians, even those whose practice is exclusively pediatric. Death of a child is clearly identified as one of the most stressful and difficult situations clinicians face (Crammond, 1969; Schowalter, 1983; Ahrens, Hart, & Maruyama, 1997; McKelvey, 2007).

It is helpful to be aware of the heterogeneous etiologies of child death, if only because much of our information about

the way patients, families, and providers deal with children's death comes from studying childhood cancer care, whereas in fact cancer causes less than 4% of deaths between birth and 19 years. Of roughly 50,000 deaths in 2008, over half (28,000) were in the first year of life, from congenital anomalies, prematurity, low birth weight, and sudden infant death syndrome (SIDS). Another 45% is due to acute unanticipated injury from trauma (Matthews et al., 2011). Children are more likely than adults to die in a hospital, most often in an intensive care setting (Leuthner et al., 2004). Because of the heterogeneity of trajectories of dying in childhood, it may be useful to review three common scenarios: acute unanticipated death, as with trauma; failure of medical treatment to effect a cure, as with cancer; and the ups and downs of a chronic condition that at any time might end in death, as with chronic respiratory, neurological, or metabolic disease.

BREAKING THE NEWS OF IMPENDING OR ACTUAL DEATH IN AN ACUTE CARE SETTING

Clinicians in developed countries often hold an unspoken belief that death is a failure by the medical system, and the culture of acute care settings such as the intensive care unit (ICU) or the emergency department is perhaps most particularly vulnerable to this belief. A first step in supporting clinicians dealing with a child's death is to acknowledge that death is not avoidable in many of the conditions they are called upon to treat in these acute settings. A second step can be to remind clinicians that their presence, empathy, practical assistance, and information enable them to provide a bereaved family with essential assistance that they will need to adjust to their loss.

According to Janzen et al. (2003), families who lose a child through an acute and unanticipated event have at least to address these five tasks:

1. Understand the events leading up to death,

2. Feel that they can exert some control over a universe suddenly completely out of control,

3. Be able to say goodbye to their child in some meaningful way,

4. Be able to make sense of the death, and

5. Be able somehow to carry the child forward in their lives as they negotiate a new and ongoing relationship with the child they have lost.

The clinician's role in telling the family about the death of their child can help them move towards accomplishing these tasks. Families will benefit from instrumental support, such as providing private time for them to be with the child's body; informational support, as in clarifying medical questions or the likely course of events before and subsequent to the death; and from the authentic empathy and compassion of staff. (Table 81.1 shows a matrix of these tasks and clinician responses adapted from Janzen et al., 2003.)

Particularly in the setting of an unanticipated death, clinicians often struggle for the "right words," but in fact, families will remember how they were treated more clearly than any actual words spoken. One suggested approach to disclosing the news of a child's death is detailed in Box 81.1.

Clinicians often feel constrained in reaching out to families who have sustained acute unanticipated loss, with whom they have had only brief encounters, feeling that they do not have a longstanding basis for continued contact. In fact, for these families there are few other people, even the closest of friends or family, who can understand what they have experienced (Ahrens, Hart, & Maruyama, 1997). Expressions of sympathy following the event, such as with a condolence card or a comfort basket, are highly valued by families, even if they had no prior relationship with the providers (Levetown et al., 2008).

HELPING A CHILD, FAMILY, AND CAREGIVERS COME TO TERMS WITH LIKELY DEATH DUE TO PROGRESSION OF DISEASE

Pediatric patients facing the end of treatment options for a fatal cancer, and their families, have been studied in some

Table 81.1 "BREAKING THE NEWS" MATRIX

TASKS FOR BEREAVED FAMILIES	INSTRUMENTAL ASSISTANCE	ASSISTANCE WITH INFORMATION	COMPASSION AND EMPATHY
Understanding events leading up to death	• Offering/providing pictures or reports • Providing access to child's body	• Providing details of death and events leading up to death • Timely information • Written information • Verbal repetition of information	• Give them control over timing and detail of information • Listen actively • Present a calm, warm presence
Regaining some control	• Listening to needs/wishes of parents • Respecting parents' decisions • Providing access to child's body	• Explain procedures and processes • Offer explanations if parents' wishes cannot be accommodated	• Be sensitive to family's vulnerability • Be present but not intrusive • Offer and provide comfort as requested by parents
Saying goodbye	• Allow time and privacy with child's body • Encourage involvement in planning memorial services • If desired, permit family to participate in preparing the body	• Explain what to expect as child dies • Explain what parents will see, hear, etc., when seeing child's body	• Show respect for the child's body • Make child's body appear cared for; e.g., cover with blanket, clean blood and wounds • Provide support
Making sense and meaning of the death	• Provide access to child's medical chart, autopsy report, police report, pictures if requested	• Provide information regarding death and death surroundings • Provide information about organ/tissue donation if desired, engaging organ bank specialists • Assist in processing information	• Be an active listener • Acknowledge the immensity of the loss • Be sensitive to family's needs • Facilitate process of making sense of the death
Renegotiating a parent–child relationship after loss	• Help family identify mementos of the child to keep • Offer memory-making opportunities • Preserve any articles of clothing, possessions, etc., of the child's for the parents to take home with them	• Provide information about what is possible or permitted regarding memory-making activities • Provide information about what other families have found important at this time • Assist in developing rituals and memorials	• Be supportive of family's faith beliefs • Support family in carrying out any death rituals • Provide follow-up support in the days and weeks that follow

Adapted from Janzen et al., 2003

Box 81.1 BREAKING THE NEWS OF DEATH IN THE ACUTE CARE SETTING

Preparation

First, take a moment for self-reflection, to acknowledge your own feelings (inadequacy, guilt, sadness, anger, fear) and perhaps to find a colleague with whom to share those emotions beforehand. Take note of those emotions, whatever they are, and then, without comment or criticism, allow yourself to put them aside. Find a partner—either someone who has already established a relationship with the family, another physician, or staff from chaplaincy, social work, nursing, or child life—to join you.

Think for a moment how you might act if a dear friend told you he or she had just received terrible news—what would you do, as one human being to another? Use that as a model of how best to help this family with the news you have to give them.

Families take it as a mark of respect and an indication of how importantly we view their loved one, when the responsible attending physician is the one notifying the family.

Assure that the right family members have been gathered, to the degree possible, and available resources assembled (which might include emergency department [ED] chaplaincy, social worker, child life specialist or outside family supports such as family chaplain, primary care provider).

Use a skilled medical interpreter, not a family member, for any translation needs. If using a family member is the only recourse, acknowledge to the family interpreter how difficult it is to hear bad news and then to have to share that news.

Choose an appropriate setting that is quiet, provides privacy, and has enough places to sit for all who need to be present, with water and tissues available. Make yourself available and presentable (turn off beeper, check your appearance, be sure to sit down.)

Provide a written copy of your name and contact information. You may want to include other staff member names as well, such as the primary nurse, the social worker, child life specialist, etc.

Know and use the child's name.

Steps in the Process

Introduce yourself and state your role in the care of their child, shake hands or touch family members if appropriate, and sit down.

If family are able to tolerate any questions, determine what the patient and family understand about the present situation. "Please tell me what you already know about what has happened to [your child]."

Prepare them with fair warning: "I am so sorry that I have to give you this terrible news." Hold them in your gaze.

Continue to hold them in your gaze and inform them of the death in a gentle but direct manner, even though this is very difficult for any clinician, specifically using the words "die" or "death": e.g., "We did everything we possibly could, but [your child] has died."

Sit quietly and allow the family and patient to respond. The entire range of human emotions is possible at this moment. Sitting with the silence that often follows, and allowing the family to be the first to break that silence, can be very difficult. Resist the temptation to fill that silence with information or reassurances, and simply wait.

Hear and respond to the family and patient's emotions, and provide additional information at the family's or patient's pace. (*Avoid statements that begin with "I know you must be feeling very...."*) Instead, acknowledge what you see or feel. "I cannot imagine how difficult it must be to hear this news."

Solicit questions, assess their understanding, and follow the family's lead. "I have given you such terrible news. Would you like some time alone, or would it help to see [your child] now? Do you have any questions for me, anything that I can explain better?" "There may be other questions that occur to you later—please feel free to ask me then."

Families may not ask, but may be comforted to know that their child did not suffer, so if it is possible to give that reassurance, do so.

Parental guilt is likely when a child dies, even when they have no responsibility for it, and everything possible was done to prevent it. If it is possible to give reassurance about the family role in the event, or to note any contribution they made that was helpful, do so. "I don't see any way this accident could have been anticipated." Or, "Your information about her medical problems in the past was essential information for us." Realistic praise of the parents helps lessen their guilt feelings.

Be prepared to repeat information, as it is nearly impossible to take in new information when under the kind of stress a parent experiences at this time. Nevertheless, understanding and sometimes even reconstructing the events that led up to their child's death is often an essential part of family acceptance and well-being following the loss of a child. Even simple information about what will happen next or what choices they have, for instance regarding holding their child, will be helpful. Your ability to give the information they need and ask for, at the pace that they require, and to repeat the information as needed, can be one of the most therapeutic "procedures" you can offer. To ensure that very important facts are understood, it can be helpful to inquire what a parent has understood of what you have presented. This is especially important for grieving parents under stress, and even more so when they do not speak English and may not fully understand. Offer to help the family share this news with others, such as siblings or young children. Let them know that you will be notifying the child's primary care provider and any relevant specialists. They may appreciate role-play of how to tell other family members, and your presence with them when they are telling them.

Give your contact information in written form and let the family know of any follow-up arrangements, such as a call from the ED social worker in the next day or so.

Consider writing a condolence note to any family to whom you have had to give the news of their child's death, regardless of the length of your prior relationship. It is an act with remarkable potential for healing.

Adapted from O'Malley, P. J., et al., *COPEM Technical Report on Death of a Child in the Emergency Department* (in development) detail. Bluebond-Langner et al. (2007) interviewed parents of children with cancer for whom standard treatment had failed, and found that they

> came to understand their role and responsibility as parents as the responsibility to keep options open for their child. They were not necessarily committed to search for cure. Parents bargained and traded for time. Parents chose options with infinitesimal odds because the prize they sought was of immeasurable worth. (Bluebond-Langner, 2007.)

Parents also value complete and honest information, ready access to staff, coordination of the communication from multiple providers, expression of emotion and empathetic support from staff, preservation of the integrity of the parent–child relationship, and acknowledgement of the role of faith and meaning-making. Mack et al. (2007) have found that providers' attempts to shield parents from the full disclosure of a child's prognosis may be ill-conceived and that, on the contrary, parents may derive greater hope from a full understanding of a child's likelihood for recovery. Similar data from adult studies suggest that accurate prognostic information led to better mental health, better death, and improved adjustment in bereaved family members (Ray et al., 2006). Perception of their child's suffering and pain is a touchstone for parents' decision-making, along with their broader assessment of quality of life and expected neurological recovery (Wolfe et al., 2000; Meyer et al., 2002; Meyer et al., 2006).

Kars et al. (2009, 2010) have surmised that when a parent's perception of the child's suffering becomes a greater burden than the parent's fear of loss of the child, the parent begins to make different choices and come to accept that loss. They found that until that tipping point, parents were reluctant to discuss prognosis with their child for fear that the child would lose the will to live, that parents might decline helpful supports such as a hospital bed in the home if they saw it as a sign of a downward course, and that they would fragment the clinical picture into manageable symptoms rather than look at the whole picture. Beyond the tipping point, the authors found that parents were able to experience control in exerting parenting aimed at the child's well-being and family togetherness, preparing the child for what might be coming, and mitigating what they perceived as the child's suffering (Kars et al., 2009). When patients and families learn that there is no further treatment available, they often misunderstand that also to mean that the clinicians who have cared for them will no longer be available to them. When these fears of abandonment are unspoken, they may be expressed as anger or may even in part fuel a desperate search for alternative opinions and treatments. The clinician should make explicit his or her intentions and commitment regarding continued care. Especially when there is "nothing more we can offer," assurance of the clinician's continued presence accompanying the patient and family is a most powerful and healing intervention.

WISHES

Clinicians often frame difficult discussions near the end of life in terms of wishes, hopes, fears, and "what-ifs." When faced with the expression of unrealistic hopes by patient or parents, using the framework of wishes, hopes, and worries allows the clinician to realign and partner with them and to join them in those wishes—wishes that in fact are often honestly shared by caregivers—and to acknowledge the loss and anticipatory grief between the lines. It then may be possible to redirect the patient and family towards more likely goals or alert them to alternative possibilities. For instance, an adolescent nearing death might express the unrealistic plan to have children or graduate college. The clinician could say, "I wish that for you, too. I can imagine what a wonderful parent/student you would make. I wish more than anything that I could guarantee you a cure. But I worry that our treatments are not working for you and those wishes may not come true. Do you worry about that too?"

HOPES

Using the language of hoping, the clinician can explore a patient and family's hopes beyond cure or prolongation of life and understand which of those might be more attainable goals. For instance, the clinician might ask, "Given what we know you are up against now, what are you hoping for?" or offer, "I hope that we are going to be able to get you home from the hospital, so you can spend as much of your time with family and friends as possible." Feudtner (2009) writes eloquently that hope is not a single monolithic entity, but rather is composed of many smaller discrete acts of hoping that provide orientation and motivation in end-of-life situations. Clinicians worry that they are destroying hope when clearly articulating a terminal condition, but Feudtner argues that when the hope for survival is receding, other hopes emerge; that the process of hoping endures. He states that discussing hopes does not engender false hope, as long as the clinician is willing to explore patiently what lies beyond the hopes for miracles, cures, and waking from bad dreams. "Can you talk about what else you might be hoping for?" He argues that it is not necessary to judge whether a hope is realistic or unfounded, but rather to judge how well we as clinicians can explore and nurture "a diversity of hopes," pointing out that whether or not clinicians want the responsibility, they are inextricably interacting with their patients' hopes.

WORRIES AND WHAT-IFS

Using the language of "worries," the clinician can introduce likely bad outcomes in a somewhat more hypothetical fashion, one that is sometimes better tolerated by patients and families. "But what I worry about is that your pain may interfere with the good time you have left, and I want to work with you to make sure we are managing that in the best way for you." In combination with expressions of wishes and hopes, the clinician's worries acknowledge and share the uncertainty, align with the patient and family, and present what the clinician views as likely problems in an honest fashion. In situations where there is no clear prognosis, as is often the case with pediatric conditions, using the language of "what-if" again keeps the discussion in a hypothetical space where it can sometimes be more easily handled and examined, and where choices can be clarified, at least in that moment. "What if we knew for certain that no matter what we do, (you/your child) only had another few months to live—what would become most important then?" or "What if we knew for certain that she cannot survive without being on a ventilator, what would you and she want then?"

BELIEF IN MIRACLES, AND GRIEVING

Clinicians sometimes are confused or confounded by patients' or families' expressions of unrealistic hopes or reliance on miracles, despite clear communication about dwindling chances for cure. They may feel that they need to redouble their efforts to point out the hopelessness of the situation, resulting in an antagonistic stand-off. While the reliance on holding out for a miracle may be a way of denying or defying reality, the clinician can also understand it as a way for family members to enter into the grieving process, a way to express unbearable loss. At the very least, an appeal for a miracle recognizes a reality that medical management has nothing further to offer. The clinician can use respectful exploration, including inquiry into previous experiences of loss and death, acknowledge the underlying helplessness, accept that some parents may not feel that they have the authority to make life-and-death decisions for their child, and try to reframe what might constitute a miracle. Involving hospital chaplaincy or the family's own community pastor before a power struggle develops may provide further illumination. Many faith traditions would support the idea that respecting the belief in an omnipotent God does not mean that the dying process of a vulnerable, voiceless patient should need to be prolonged by providing non-beneficial treatment.

HELPING FAMILIES NAVIGATE THE UPS AND DOWNS OF CHRONIC, LIFESPAN-LIMITING CHILDHOOD CONDITIONS

In the United States, there are as many as 50,000 children living with severe and complex disabilities, living at home but often dependent on technological interventions such as gastrostomy, tracheostomy, home oxygen, suction, and even ventilator support (US Dept. of Health and Human Services [DHHS], 2008). Where available, such interventions are often supported by home services such as block nursing, special school placement, and community-based respite and palliative care services. Patients are often cared for by a bewildering array of specialists. Some children may have a condition that is known to progress to inevitable decline; others may have a static brain injury, spinal cord compromise, or muscle disorder that makes them prone to frequent and severe

life-threatening events, such as aspiration pneumonia, airway obstruction, or seizures, any one of which might cause death.

For these families and children, it is very helpful to identify a lead clinician, whether primary care, palliative care, or specialist, who is able to help a family navigate choices for life-sustaining treatment in the event of an acute downturn, and to explore with them the values and goals that can provide touchstones for decision-making. These goals should be explicitly revisited whenever there is a change in health status, venue of care, or new treatment choice. With advanced technological and medical supports, home-based care resources, and the knowledgeable and often fierce advocacy of their parents, these children may long outlast predictions of their lifespan made at time of diagnosis. Because of that, it is often difficult for parents to envision a time when the child will not recover from these intermittent crises. In this setting, it is useful to reflect on changes over the recent past in terms of the child's ability to give and get love, and the quality of life as perceived by those who know the child at his or her best, who can assess whether the child is experiencing suffering, and how any of the burdens of extended complex medical treatment may have changed. Hospital-based clinicians who only see the child during periods of maximum stress and illness often are not able to visualize any meaningful quality of life for such a child, and often experience distress about treatments offered or limited medical resources squandered. This distress can sometimes be mitigated by asking the family to describe or bring in pictures of the child's good days.

The lead clinician can often gently explore values and choices with parents, beginning with acknowledging the uncertainty of any prognostic estimate, and inquiring if the parents have ever visualized what they thought might be a good death for their child, including the venue of care. "It's hard enough for us to imagine our own death, and yet what I am going to ask you is even more difficult. Knowing that [child's name] would not have a normal lifespan, have you ever imagined what a good death would look like for him?" The borders between benefit and burden can become blurred in the care of children who are already heavily dependent on technological interventions; the clinician and the family can contract to share honestly when either party feels that treatment might be doing things to, rather than for, the child, or simply prolonging a dying process. These discussions can help uncover the values that might help guide families in their choices when the child experiences a medical crisis. If a medical crisis precipitates a discussion of prognosis, Feudtner (2007) proposes using a "collaborative practice" model that reflects the understanding that, for children with complex chronic conditions, prognosis does not simply mean how much time is left to live, but also encompasses consideration of prior quality of life, the likelihood that the child will survive this current crisis, what is required to survive this crisis, what the anticipated new quality of life will be, and how frequent or severe future crises might be. Another tool that has been used in the United Kingdom is the "personal resuscitation plan," which provides a much more nuanced set of interventions than is usually possible within the template of a Do Not Resuscitate (DNR) or Medical Orders for Life-Sustaining Treatments (MOLST) form (Wolff et al., 2010).

Although developed for the purpose of facilitating emergency care of children with complex medical needs, the Emergency Information Form (EIF) developed jointly by the American Academy of Pediatrics and the American College of Emergency Medicine can serve a similar purpose of clarifying goals of care. Emergency care plans for palliative care patients who are at risk of frequent life-threatening events have been incorporated into the electronic medical record and given to parents on a memory stick. As useful as these tools are in the event of a crisis, the actual process of developing them, with parents and invested caregivers, is in itself a valuable opportunity to explore a family's hopes and values regarding the end-of-life care for their child, particularly when the focus is placed on describing desired interventions, rather than interventions to withhold.

TALKING WITH CHILDREN AND ADOLESCENTS ABOUT THEIR OWN DEATH

Talking with a child or adolescent about his or her own death is a rare and difficult privilege in clinical practice. Because the number of children who die is small, and many are too young to be verbal and still others are rendered nonverbal by their condition, few practitioners have the opportunity to gain experience in this difficult task; perhaps night nurses, child life specialists, pediatric chaplaincy staff, and clinicians who care for children with cancer or chronic respiratory and muscle disorders have the greatest opportunities. Even in these limited situations, there are formidable obstacles to talking with children about their own death. The first reason is clear—it is simply too hard, too painful for either parents or healthcare providers to talk with children about the possibility of the child's death. On all sides there is the deep desire to protect all participants from the pain and sadness. Parents want to protect children; and children, even very young children, want to protect their parents from sadness or disappointment. Glaser and Strauss describe the protective silence of "mutual pretense" where each party in the interaction intuits the prognosis but does not openly acknowledge this to the other party. This phenomenon involves staff as well and is not rare in many settings of a critically ill, dying child, perhaps especially those who are well known to caretakers and whose death the caretakers themselves are grieving, or the children who die who were expected to survive and then took a sudden turn for the worse.

Providers often rightly feel that parental permission is required to enter the very private territory of speaking with a child about his or her death; therefore, the parents' expert knowledge of their child's nature should be explicitly elicited and the subject of communicating with the child explicitly addressed with parents. Beyond this obstacle, there are often dark fears that live below the level of logic. It is very hard even for logical beings to remember that naming death will not make it happen, and yet both parents and providers fear that naming death will imply that we are giving up. It is often helpful to name this fear out loud. Parents and providers alike may be reassured to learn of a study of bereaved parents in Sweden, Kreicsberg et al. (2004) who reported on their practice regarding talking with their child about death; the authors found that only a third of parents had done so. Interestingly, none of those parents had regrets about talking with their child, whereas nearly half of the parents who did not talk with their child did have regrets.

Additional obstacles to communicating with children bear consideration. Prognostic uncertainty often leads to deferring discussion with the child until "we know for certain." Developmental biases—that "kids don't understand death," or that "kids don't need to know because they are not making the decisions"—may prevent providers from exploring a child's understanding. *Decisional capacity* can be understood as (1) having a reasonable understanding of the nature of one's illness, the treatment and nontreatment options, the potential burdens, the benefits and consequences of those options; and (2) an understanding of death as permanent and irreversible. Although Solomon et al. (2003) have offered a general guideline that children over age ten are developing a capacity for understanding death and the consequences of choices, and that in general children over age 14 can be considered "decisional," it is clear from many reports that age does not determine understanding of death—for instance, in one study, the number of years of attendance at cancer camp was a better predictor of understanding than age, gender, years from diagnosis, site of treatment, or diagnosis (Bluebond-Langner et al., 1991).

It can be very helpful for clinicians to explore with parents why they would want any particular information withheld from their child. "What frightens you the most; what are you most afraid will happen if [child's name] asks about dying?" Inquiry may reveal the worries or denial of the parent; for instance, that they fear their child will give up hope and die sooner. It is also helpful to share with parents our experience that children almost always have an understanding beyond what has been discussed openly with them, because they overhear conversations, minutely observe and interpret their family's reactions, and can sense what their body is telling them. What is imagined may be worse than what is, and silence can add to a child's isolation, the rupture of trust, and the loss of autonomy, giving the child no chance for handling unfinished business. When children are given the information in an age-appropriate manner, it can give them an opportunity to talk about their fears, ask questions about what is going to happen, express their feelings, and say their goodbyes. When parents are able to be honest with their child and include their child in discussions about the plan of care, it gives the child some control over an otherwise out-of-control situation. Parents can thus sometimes be helped to understand that the best way to care for and protect their child is to prevent the isolation, so the child "does not need to be alone with his worries." They may welcome suggestions about how to approach talking with their child, whether they take on the primary role or wish to have a clinician partner in the conversations.

Sequencing meetings, first with the parents, and then with parents and child, may optimize communication and allow for the opportunity to explore the child's understanding in the parents' presence. Parents interviewed about their perceptions of having their child present during difficult conversations acknowledge the benefits of such openness; however, they also report that those benefits come at a cost, reporting that they are less likely to ask questions and less able simultaneously to focus on the discussion and to care for their child emotionally. Separate meetings allow parents the opportunity to ask questions freely, absorb information, and consider the best ways to present that information to their child (Young et al., 2011). Although it is routine practice in primary pediatrics to offer solo time with the child patient, beginning around the onset of puberty, this practice is not routine in the subspecialty care of children with chronic or life-threatening disease, where arguably the need for autonomy and privacy may be greater. Normalizing a routine of solo time with the child when curative options are still within reach makes it easier to provide this opportunity near the end of life to have the child voice his or her feelings without fear of upsetting or disappointing parents. Bluebond-Langner et al. (2010) describe this as one feature of a kind of "shuttle diplomacy" to involve the child in decision-making, in a way that acknowledges that the parents are probably still going to be the final decision-makers, but also to make sure that the parents know and understand their child's comprehension and wishes. Even if it is clear that the final decision-making rests with the parents, there is still room for dissent and negotiation.

Parental refusal to allow children to receive crucial information for the child's own coping and grieving can create a tremendous burden for staff who believe that the sharing of such information is essential to providing good care. When parents still do not want their child told, it is important to maintain a connection with the family, validating the difficult task of acting in the child's best interest, offering to help facilitate conversation, asking how they would like further conversation to be conducted, and telling no more than the patient needs. "I am going to need your help to tell me how much you would like to know." Parents may be helped to know that dying children know they are dying, and the denial by family will not counterweigh their perception. It is sometimes possible to negotiate with parents that, while caregivers will agree not to tell the child certain information, they also cannot lie to the child if asked directly. Much of our understanding of the wishes of terminally ill children comes from the interpretation of play, pictures, and music created by children. However, in an interview with Mattie Stepanek, a 14-year-old poet who died of muscular dystrophy, Mattie spoke compellingly of the wish to have choices in aspects of his treatment, and to have a sense that people were listening to his wishes and worries (Initiative for Pediatric Palliative Care, 2003.) Like dying adults, dying children may likely wish for autonomy, dignity, comfort, and the opportunity to make meaning out of their lives and leave a legacy to those they love, as well as an opportunity to resolve conflicts prior to their death. Dying children may struggle with how best to protect their family, and may fear being forgotten.

Even when it is not possible to discuss the terminal nature of a child's condition directly, parents, and even older children and adolescents, can be supported by a listening presence and by asking reflective questions that help them examine and understand the story of their journey. Block and Billings

have developed a series of questions as part of a postgraduate course, designed to "deepen the conversation" by exploring domains such as the effects of the illness on the patient's and family's physical and emotional well-being and sense of personhood; identifying coping strengths and supports; and clarifying preferences. Table 81.2 lists those domains with a few example questions.

Other published tools that have been used in discussion of pediatric advance directives include the pediatric modification of "Five Wishes," called "My Wishes," (Pediatric My Wishes), the young adult modification called "Voicing My Choices, (Voicing My Choices; Wiener et al., 2012) and the Decision Making Tool developed by the Seattle Children's Advanced Care Team (Hayes, 1998). For young adults who are 18 or older, the designation of a healthcare proxy can be the occasion for elucidating a young person's wishes regarding life-sustaining treatment. Tolerance for child autonomy is likely to be different depending on context, such as whether the decisions involved are likely to reverse disease, or simply prolong a dying process. However, an important pediatric consideration is that children who have experienced chronic disease may defy any standard rubric of developmental capacity, and the weight of their experience should give their voice additional moral power. It is difficult to improve upon what William Easson wrote about the dying child in 1970; namely, that "the best treatment of the dying youngster can be based only on the knowledge of what his approaching death means to him and how this young person can reasonably cope with this very personal reality."

SPECIAL ISSUES: BRAIN DEATH, ORGAN DONATION, WITHDRAWAL OF SUPPORT, DO NOT RESUSCITATE ORDERS

Additional issues relating to end-of-life decisions invariably arise with terminally ill children, and the physician needs to be aware of and prepared to deal with additional difficult questions when they are voiced. A few issues deserve emphasis. Brain death *is* death, and once brain death has been ascertained by accepted criteria, no additional permission is necessary for termination of medical support. Indeed, the only indication for continuation of medical support in the setting of brain death is organ donation. Caregivers need to have a clear understanding of this principle before interacting with the family so that there is no confusion or unnecessary added worry or pain around discontinuing mechanical ventilation, intravenous fluids and medications, and other life-support measures.

It is also important that the roles of caregiver for the patient and advocate for organ donation be kept completely separate, to avoid any confusion for the family. The only role the physician caring for the child should take with regard to organ donation is to notify the representative of the regional organ bank of the possibility of a donor. Physicians should refer any questions regarding potential organ donation to the organ bank or the transplant team so that the family understands that the physician's sole concern is whatever is best for the child. (For a more complete discussion of issues surrounding organ transplantation, see Chapter 65.)

Table 81.2 DEEPENING THE CONVERSATION

DOMAIN	SAMPLE QUESTION
Hearing bad news	*Tell me how you first found out about your/your child's illness: what was that like for you?*
Information sharing and prognosis	*How do you make sense of your/your child's illness? What is likely to happen going forward?*
Effects of illness: Physical or emotional	*What are some of the moments when you've felt the most discouraged and downhearted as you've faced this?*
Coping: Past and present	*Have there been other tough times you have had to face? Other serious illnesses or losses?*
Supports: Formal and informal	*How have you been helped by family and friends/ your health care team? How have they responded? How have they disappointed or not been helpful for you?*
Religion and spirituality	*Do you have any (devotional) practice that brings you closer to a sense of peace or strength or wholeness?*
Facing a life-threatening or terminal illness	*Have you had to make or change any big plans because of your/your child's illness?*
Preferences for site of care	*How do you feel about being at home when you/your child is sick? Or about being in the hospital?*
Family coping and support	*How do you think your family or siblings/close friends have been affected? What do they understand about your/your child's illness?*
Personhood	*How has your/your child's illness changed you as a person?*
Reconciliation and closure	*What could you do that would help you feel that this has been a meaningful time for you and your family?*
Envisioning a good death	*If it had to be, what would your idea of a good death for you (for your child) look like?*

Modified from Billings, A. J., & Block, S. (2010). Palliative care education and practice. Harvard Medical School postgraduate course.

GRIEF

UNDERSTANDING GRIEVING AS THE WORK TO RECONSTRUCT MEANING IN AN ASSUMPTIVE WORLD RUPTURED BY LOSS

Bereavement following the loss of a child challenges traditional models of grief that describe universal and fixed stages ending in recovery, as if "successful" grieving required that grief be resolved and the loss of the loved one be somehow put away. Such constructs do not match well with the lifelong impact of a child's death on parents and siblings. Anticipated loss of a child, as an event, can invalidate the basic assumptions by which those who are grieving have previously lived, or may seem like alien and new experiences for which they have no preconceived construction.

A more recent model proposes to understand grief as the "act of affirming or reconstructing a personal world of meaning that has been challenged by loss" (Neimeyer, 2006). With this model, grief can be understood as a continuing and transformative process, acknowledging that bereaved parents do not necessarily "let go" of their grief or their lost child, but transform them by renewing the meaning invested in them and continuing the relationship in new ways. The deceased child continues to be "a significant other," an active and living memory, even a presence. This meaning-making can create positive social legacies, such as with organizations like Mothers Against Drunk Driving.

Folded into the death of a child is the death of so many imagined futures encompassing that child's evolving personhood and the parents' vision of themselves fulfilled as parents. These losses are suffered repeatedly over time as other children in their lives attain the milestones that the lost child will never see. Because child death is uncommon, it may be hard for bereaved parents to find a place where they can speak openly about their loss. Some parents may feel that they have to pretend that they have not lost a child as they experience how many people, even close friends, become nervous or withdraw when parents try to share their ongoing grief.

Because there are so few norms for bereaved parents, seemingly small details can become huge:

"Should I keep the door to my deceased child's room open or closed?"

"How do we sign our holiday cards that we always signed with everyone's name?"

"What do we do on her birthday?"

For the grieving parents, it takes time and precious energy to figure out when they want to engage with people on the subject of their dead child. Answering the casual question "How many children do you have?" can be fraught with difficulty. Some parents describe that they feel like a loaded shotgun goes off when they answer questions like that truthfully, leaving the person who asked the question wondering what hit them. It is difficult to predict when someone is going to ask sympathetically for more details, or simply turn pale and withdraw. And yet not to name and count the child who has died may feel like a betrayal. "Being a bereaved parent sometimes feels as if you are from a different planet from everyone else." Finding a place where people remember their child and are comfortable talking with them about the child is very comforting, and the staff who cared for their child before death are often an important oasis for parents. Naming and sharing memories of a deceased child is an ongoing gift that staff who were part of that child's care can give to bereaved families. Families do want to talk about the loss of their child and generally welcome calls, emails, or letters from caregivers. For bereaved families, it is never too late to learn that their child is remembered by a caregiver.

CARE OF THE BEREAVED FAMILY AT THE TIME OF DEATH AND AFTER

Even when anticipated, death is always a surprise and a mystery. For some families, their child's death may be the first such loss they have experienced, and they will not know what to do, how to act, or what is allowed. Staff can suggest what they have found helpful to other families, such as private time with the body or helping staff to bathe and prepare the body. Staff should try to elicit information about rituals or customs important to the family's culture or religion, and honor those as much as is possible. Physical separation from the body is often an extremely difficult time, burdened with multiple practical concerns such as institutional needs to utilize clinical space, identifying a funeral home, and notifying family and friends. Families, including siblings, should be offered opportunities to participate in memory-making activities such as creating ink handprints and footprints or molds of the child's hand out of clay, saving a lock of the child's hair, or taking photographs of the child. If this can be done before the child's death it can be a very moving and important activity for the family and child, if the child participates. If this is offered to a family after the death, it becomes an opportunity for a final interaction with their child. Some families will not want to participate in this activity, and if that is the case, they should be asked if they would like the staff (child life specialist, nurse, social worker) to do it for them. These articles can be placed in a memory box and offered to the family when they leave, or kept for them if they wish. Families have reported that having a memory box, articles of the child's clothing or belongings, or even simply a special blanket that has been used to wrap the child in after death, to take with them eases the time of separation from the body. Thought should be given to the moment of transfer when the child's body leaves the family's sight to be delivered to the morgue or to the funeral home staff. It may be easier for family to see their child being carried away in a staff member's arms or otherwise treated like a person rather than a corpse. If possible, it is a caring gesture to families leaving the hospital to accompany them to their car and attend to any parking fees.

Clinicians often underestimate the meaningfulness of attendance at a child's wake or funeral for bereaved families. Continued contact with staff who have cared for the child, at milestones from the death, such as one week, one month, six months, and anniversaries of birth and death, is highly valued by families. Institutional memorial services are a meaningful venue for families and staff alike to honor the children they have cared for. Autopsy or clinical care review is another opportunity to reunite caregivers and family. If the child died in the hospital, the first time a parent returns to the hospital for whatever reason can be overwhelming. Staff who are aware of this milestone should make every effort to be supportive.

Inviting a family to return for a clinical review is not routinely practiced. Meert et al. (2007) reported that, for families whose child died in the pediatric ICU, only 13% had a scheduled clinical care review meeting after the child's death, although a majority (59%) would have wanted to, and of those, 82% would have been willing to return to the hospital. Families reported wanting the opportunity to review the chronology, treatment, redirection of care, ways to help others, bereavement support, what to tell other family members; and to express gratitude and complaints.

The family should be offered the opportunity to meet with the reviewing physician in a quiet, private space removed from the clinical setting, optimizing ample time for a relaxed, personal conversation. At this meeting, the physician solicits and addresses outstanding question or unresolved issues, reviews what happened and why, and explains what the autopsy results were, if any. An attempt should be made to set a tone of the physician and family coming together to discuss a painful, shared experience as equals, not as physician–patient, and to make it clear to the family that their relationship with the physician continues.

Community-based hospices provide an invaluable follow-up resource for the bereavement process. This resource can be used to maximum advantage when it is combined with an integrated follow-up program through the hospital where the child has died. Families should be offered follow-up sessions with social workers, nursing staff, and physicians at two to three, six, and 12 months after their loss, and at additional sessions if requested or needed. Hospice bereavement services may be offered to the family as early as two months after the child's death. In addition to their own services, hospices have access to other community-based bereavement groups such Compassionate Friends (877-969-0010). The National Hospice Organization (800-648-8898) also can provide information about local resources.

Family-centered care includes the care and emotional well-being of the patient's siblings. Both before and after a child's death, siblings often fear that they are responsible for or vulnerable to the same suffering as the affected child, and often have difficulty finding a safe place in which to reveal those fears. Many children, teens, and adults find it helpful to attend bereavement support groups or camps. These groups provide children, teens, and parents opportunities to connect with others who are grieving a similar loss. Being with others who understand the experience of loss can be supportive, therapeutic, and educational and offers opportunities to talk about feelings and memories about the child who has died.

CARE OF STAFF

Caring for dying children generates distress among clinicians: "There is nothing right about the death of a child," reports one of the clinicians interviewed by McKelvey in his book,

"When a child dies: how pediatric physicians and nurses cope." (McKelvey, 2007). He notes that the death of a child patient can leave staff feeling emotionally labile, guilty, and unable to sleep or concentrate Most vulnerable are likely to be trainees and those newest to the field. Clinicians may question their competence or whether they have chosen the right profession. In the hierarchal culture of a teaching hospital, the distress associated with the death of a child can be translated into blame, which then may be assigned to or assumed by trainees. A sense of guilt, failure, or inadequacy can prevent trainees from being supportive or compassionate with a dying child's family. Moreover, for younger staff, caring for dying adolescents presents challenges of over-identification and fears of one's own mortality. The motivation to enter medicine as a profession in order to save lives can be challenged by the death of a young patient, and staff can become defensive rather than supportive. Few residency or clinical programs offer education in reflection, coping, or how to deal with the death of a child. Nevertheless, debriefings, reflection rounds, or caregiver gatherings after the death of a child provide opportunities to reflect on the care that was provided to the child, the family, and each other. Offering reflection rounds or multidisciplinary caregiver rounds to honor the care provided to a child and family gives staff a venue for understanding the richness of the care delivered, acceptance that they are part of a bereaved community, and recognition that often they are not alone in their feelings of anger, sadness, or guilt following the death of a child. Even when further details are sad, somehow a more complete picture of the child's death brings comfort and a sense of control to caregivers, much as it does for parents.

Clinicians report that the most helpful experience that promoted comfort with dealing with a dying child was a personal experience of the death of a close friend or family member (McKelvey, 2007). While even seasoned practitioners have clear and often still troubling memories of the first death of a child under their care, subsequent experiences with death may become easier to manage as clinicians learn to manage their own distress. However, over time, many practitioners recognize the limitations of distancing themselves from their patients and develop other ways to cope, such as by focusing on what could be learned from the death or from keeping a child as comfortable as possible. It is likely that no practitioner keeps this balance right all the time. McKelvey highlights situations that are particularly poignant, including:

The child or parent who reminds the practitioner of themselves or their own family;

An abandoned child or one seldom visited by his or her own family who elicits parental and protective feelings from professional caregivers;

A child with a particular insight or sense of humor that made the inability to save the child more of a personal failure;

The child who suffers from a treatment error.

Many clinicians find that the laypersons' world outside of medicine offers little understanding of their distress or support for coping, and that sharing troubling medical experiences can be so upsetting for their non-medical acquaintances that they end up having to comfort the comforter. Spouses vary in their ability to provide support. Most clinicians find that their most reliable support comes from other clinicians engaged in the same kind of work. Trainees in particular may be more likely to rely on other peers, fearing that supervising staff might judge or grade them.

A child's death shatters the protective denial that shields us from being aware of how truly fragile and transient life is. Trainees and seasoned clinicians alike are forced to reflect on their own mortality, but perhaps even more painfully on the possible loss of their own loved ones. Staff with young children are particularly vulnerable to identifying with bereaved parents: "each one of us is only a day away from standing in the shoes of those PICU parents" (McKelvey, 2007). Trainees who are parents report consciously seeking out situations outside of work where there are healthy children playing, to redress the balance of their experiences. They may experience support from being able to go home to hug their own children and to lose themselves in loving them.

McKelvey notes that while training, experience, and the observed behavior of colleagues all contribute to the ability to cope with child death, the clinician's childhood experiences of how death was dealt with by one's own parents and family provide the best predictor of coping. Many physicians identify personal loss as the most meaningful experience in terms of deepening their ability to provide compassionate care and to cope with the death of a child patient. Reflecting on those experiences and models may help clinicians understand how best to cope with their own distress, and to acknowledge the need to open up the possibility of other ways of coping. Continued contact with bereaved families is beneficial for clinicians as well as family; clinicians may find comfort and meaning in how families have carried the memory of their child forward in their lives. In Box 81.2 are practical suggestions for self-care following the death of a child patient.

PART TWO: TALKING WITH CHILDREN ABOUT THE DEATH OF A LOVED ONE

Few tasks are more painful to families or caregivers than that of telling a child about the death of his or her mother, father, sibling, or friend. However, children are aware of death from an early age through everyday experiences, whether through the media, the death of a pet, a wild animal killed by the roadside, or the loss of an elder in the extended family. Death is therefore a reality that children can learn to accept much as adults must; however, they need to make sense of their own experiences in order to understand death as a normal part of life. The child's own experiences and developmental capacity will help determine how best to talk with her or him about the death of a loved one. A full developmental understanding of death is one that comprehends it as universal and irreversible, with the loss of all functionality, informed by a realistic understanding of the causes of death. Each child comes to this understanding in his or her own way, but Table 81.3 below offers a general developmental evolution.

It is helpful to ask what beliefs the family has about what happens after death. For a child, using clear, age appropriate language, the words "dead" or "died"—instead of euphemisms such as "He is sleeping," "The angels took him," and "He has gone on a long journey"—minimizes confusion. Children and teenagers need to be reassured that they are safe and will be taken care of. They also need ample opportunities to ask questions about the death and to trust that they are getting honest answers from a caring adult who is listening for their concerns.

When telling a child or teenager about the death of a loved one, it is important to know what they may have already been told. It is also helpful to understand what beliefs, religious or otherwise, the child and family may hold. Common childhood misapprehensions such as "I caused it; I could catch it; this happened because I was bad" can be allayed by explicit reassurances. Children and teens may also need to be assured that their feelings, whatever they may be, are normal and okay. Unspoken fears may include "Could that happen to me, or to another person I love?" and "Who will take care of me now?" Concrete concerns can best be addressed by clarifying a child's worry or question, as the child may be asking from a very different point of view from the adult attempting to answer. Using the strategy of saying "That's a very good question! What got you wondering about it?" will help you shape the answer to best address the child's understanding and concerns.

Those around the child may question whether the child should visit the dying person or participate in the funeral. In fact, children may treasure having had the chance to spend time with a loved one during that person's last days, and can assimilate values through participation in the death of a loved one. They may later resent being excluded, whereas their involvement may assist them with their own grieving. Problems are most likely to arise when children are forced to participate against their will or excluded when they wished to participate, so if children are physically able, it is usually advisable to ask if they wish to visit a dying loved one or attend the funeral. It is always important to prepare children for what they might see, and to plan for alternatives in the event that a child wants to leave or cannot maintain composure during a visit or a long service. Funerals and religious services are important death rituals that facilitate the grief process and usually serve to mobilize social support for the survivors. Children can benefit in meaningful ways by helping to plan or attend funerals, especially if they are given the opportunity to ask questions.

Adults often feel that they must be "strong" or suppress emotions that they feel might be upsetting to a child. In fact, sharing the emotions of sadness or anger around loss with a bereaved child helps validate the child's own feelings and lessen the isolation he or she may be feeling. The child can learn from the emotional reactions of the adults around him that it is our human capacity to love that makes us both vulnerable to loss and capable of providing comfort (see Table 81.3).

ADVERSE OUTCOMES

There are risks of adverse outcomes when counseling the bereaved. While grief is a normal reaction to loss, and while the staff need to be cautious of not "pathologizing" grief, one does need to be aware of abnormal grief reactions. Children, especially those with prior emotional problems, may be at risk for disruptions in development, including somatoform disorders, disruptive behavior, school problems, or anxiety or mood disorders. There is increased risk of post-traumatic stress disorder following a sudden death. Children and adults are at increased risk who have a recent history of other major losses or deaths, depression, suicide attempts, another mental or medical illness, or alcohol or drug abuse. There is risk over the course of bereavement of the relapse of preexisting mental or physical illness. Some children or parents may have an unresolved pathological bereavement reaction that evolves into major depression. Patients or family members at such risk should be informed of the available bereavement resources, including referral for psychiatric care. The recognition and management of unresolved or pathological grief in adults has been described by Brown and Stoudemire (1983).

CLINICAL PEARLS

- A first step in supporting clinicians dealing with a child's death is to acknowledge that death is unavoidable for many of the conditions they are called upon to treat. A second step can be to remind clinicians that their

Table 81.3 DEVELOPMENTAL UNDERSTANDING OF DEATH

AGE CHARACTERISTICS	CONCEPT OF DEATH	IMPACT OF DEATH	INTERVENTION
0–2 Sensory and motor relationship with environment Limited language skills Achieves object permanence May sense something is wrong, react to the emotions of adults	None, or as a separation	Disruption of normal care routines Separation anxiety	Provide stable physical nurturance and comfort with simple physical communication and with familiar, beloved relatives and objects Maintain routines
>2–6 Uses magical and animistic thinking Egocentric Engages in symbolic play, acquiring language skills	Believes death is temporary and reversible like sleep Does not personalize death Believes death can be caused by thoughts, wishes, or misdeeds	Regression Guilt Fearfulness	Minimize separation from usual caregivers Clarify understanding before attempting to answer questions Evaluate for sense of guilt and assuage if present Use precise language ("dying, dead") and child's own language for loss Maintain routines
>6–12 Uses concrete thinking	Development of adult concepts of death Understands death can be personal Interested in physiology and details of death	Preoccupation with potential for physical suffering of the deceased Fear of similar consequences to self or other loved ones	Evaluate child's fears of abandonment Provide concrete details if asked Support child's efforts to achieve control and mastery Maintain access to peers Be truthful Allow child to participate in decision-making Maintain routines
>12–18 Reality becomes objective Capable of self-reflection Self-esteem and body image are paramount	Explores non-physical explanations of death	May mask feelings or act as if they do not want help or the chance to talk	Reinforce self-esteem Allow to express strong feelings Allow privacy Promote independence and access to peers Be truthful Allow to participate in decision-making Maintain routines

Modified from Himelstein et al., 2004

presence, empathy, practical assistance, and information enable them to provide a bereaved family with essential assistance that they will need to adjust to their loss (Janzen et al., 2003).

- Families will remember how they were treated more clearly than what actual words were spoken.

- Naming and sharing memories of a deceased child is an ongoing gift that staff who were part of that child's care can give to bereaved families. Families do want to talk about the loss of their child and generally welcome calls, emails, or letters from caregivers. For bereaved families, it is never too late to learn that their child is remembered by a caregiver.

- A framework of wishes, hopes, and worries allows the clinician talking about the end of life to realign and partner with parents and patient and to acknowledge loss and anticipatory grief "between the lines."

- The clinician can understand holding onto hope for a miracle as a way for family members to express unbearable loss and to enter into a grieving process.

- None of the parents studied regretted talking with their child [about his or her death], whereas nearly half of the parents who did not talk with their child [about death] did have regrets (Kreicsberg et al., 2004).

- Normalizing a clinical routine of solo time with the child when curative options are still within reach makes it easier to provide this opportunity near the end of the child's life, in order to allow the child to voice feelings without fear of upsetting or disappointing parents.

- Common childhood misapprehensions such as "I caused it; I could catch it; this happened because I was bad," can be allayed by explicit reassurances. Children and teens may also need to be reassured that their feelings, whatever they may be, are normal and okay. Unspoken fears may include "Could that happen to me, or to another person I love?" and "Who will take care of me now?" Always clarify the context of a child's question before attempting to answer it.

DISCLOSURE STATEMENTS

Dr. O'Malley has no conflicts of interest or disclosures to make.

Ms. D'Amato has no disclosures.

Dr. Stoddard has no disclosures.

REFERENCES

Ahrens, W., Hart, R., & Maruyama, N. (1997). Pediatric death: Managing the aftermath in the emergency department. *Journal of Emergency Medicine, 15*(5), 601–603.

Ahrens, W. R., & Hart, R. G. (1997). Emergency physicians' experience with pediatric death. *American Journal of Emergency Medicine, 15*, 642–643.

American Academy of Pediatrics, Committee on Pediatric Emergency Medicine and Council on Clinical Information Technology, American College of Emergency Physicians, & Pediatric Emergency Medicine Committee (2010). Policy statement: Emergency information forms and emergency preparedness for children with special health care needs. *Pediatrics, 125*(4), 829–837.

Bluebond-Langner, M., Bello Belasco, J., & DeMesquita Wander, M. (2010). "I want to live, until I don't want to live anymore": Involving children with life-threatening and life-shortening illnesses in decision making about care and treatment. *Nursing Clinics of North America, 45*, 329–343.

Bluebond-Langner, M., Bello Belasco, J., Goldman, A., & Belasco, C. (2007). Understanding Parents' Care and Treatment of Children with Cancer When Standard Therapy has Failed. *Journal of Clinical Oncology, 26*(17), 2414–2419.

Bluebond-Langner, M., Perkel, D., & Goertzel, T. (1991). Pediatric cancer patients' peer relationships: Impact of an oncology camp experience. *Journal of Psychosocial Oncology, 9*(2), 67–79.

Crammond, W. A. (1969). Anxiety in medical practice—The doctor's own anxiety. *Australia & New Zealand Journal of Psychiatry 3,* 324–328.

Easson, W. M. (1970). *The dying child: The management of the child or adolescent who is dying.* Springfield, IL: Charles C. Thomas.

Farmer, P. (2011). *Haiti: After the earthquake.* New York: BBS Public Affairs.

Feudtner, C. (2007). Collaborative communication in pediatric palliative care: a foundation for problem-solving and decision-making. *Pediatric Clinics of North America,* Oct; *54,* 5.

Feudtner, C. (2009). The breadth of hopes. *New England Journal of Medicine, 361*(24), 2306–2307.

Glaser, B. G., & Strauss, A. L. (1965). *Awareness of Dying.* Chicago: Aldine.

Hayes, R. (1998). Decision making tool. Designed by project team, based on the clinical ethics model of Jonsen, Siegler, and Winslade. In

Clinical Ethics: A Practical Approach to Ethical Decisions in Clinical Medicine (4th ed.). New York: McGraw-Hill.

Himelstein, B., Hilden, J. M., Boldt, A. M., & Weissman, D. (2004). Pediatric palliative care. *New England Journal of Medicine,* April 22; *350,* 17.

Initiative for Pediatric Palliative Care (IPPC) (2003). What matters to families: Part 3: Big choice, little choices. IPPC Videos. Education Development Center.

Janzen, L., Cadell, S., & Westhues, A. (2003). From death notification through the funeral: Bereaved parents' experiences and their advice to professionals. *Omega, 48*(2), 149–164.

Kars, M. C., Grypdonck, M. H., de Korte-Verhoef, M. C., et al. (2009). Parental experience at the end-of-life in children with cancer: 'Preservation' and 'letting go' in relation to loss. *Support Care Cancer,* 2011 Jan, Epub 2009 Dec 3, *19*(1), 27–35. doi:10.1007/s00520-009-0785-1.

Kars, M. C., Grypdonck, M. H. F., Beishuizen, A., Meijer-van den Bergh, E. M. M., & van Delden, J. J. M. (2010). Factors influencing parental readiness to let their child with cancer die. *Pediatric Blood & Cancer, 54,* 1000–1008.

Kreicsbergs, U., Valdimarsdottir, U., Onelöv, E., Henter, J.-I., & Steineck, G. (2004). Talking about death with children who have severe malignant disease. *New England Journal of Medicine, 351,* 1175–1186.

Lemaire, C. M. (2011). Grief and resilience. In: F. J. Stoddard, A. Pandya, & C. L. Katz (Eds.), *Disaster psychiatry: Readiness, evaluation, and treatment* (pp. 179–202). Arlington, VA: American Psychiatric Press Publishing.

Leuthner, S. R., Morstad Boldt, A., & Kirby, R. S. (2004). Where infants die: Examination of place of death and hospice/home health care options in the State of Wisconsin. *Journal of Palliative Medicine,* April; *7*(2), 269–277.

Levetown, M., & Committee on Bioethics. (2008). Communicating with children and families: From everyday interactions to skill in conveying distressing information. *Pediatrics,* May; *121,* e1441–e1460.

Mack, J. W., Wolfe, J., Cook, F., Grier, H. E., Cleary, P. D., & Weeks, J. C. (2007). Hope and prognostic disclosure. *Journal of Clinical Oncology, 25*(35), 5636–5642.

Matthews, T. J., Minino, A. M., Osterman, M. J. K., Strobino, D. M., & Guyer, B. (2011). Annual summary of vital statistics. *Pediatrics,* Jan 1; *127*(1), 146–157.

McKelvey, R. S. (2007). *When a child dies: How pediatric physicians and nurses cope.* Seattle: University of Washington Press.

Meert, K. L., Eggly, S., Pollack, M., Anand, J. S., Zimmerman, J., Carcillo, J., et al., & The National Institute of Child Health & Human Development Collaborative Pediatric Critical Care Research Network (2007). Parents' perspectives regarding a physician-parent conference after their child's death in the pediatric intensive care unit. *Journal of Pediatrics, 151,* 50–55.

Meyer, E. C., Burns, J. P., Griffith, J. L., & Truog, R. D. (2002). Parental perspectives on end-of-life care in the pediatric intensive care unit. *Critical Care Medicine,* Jan; *30*(1), 226–231.

Meyer, E. C., Ritholz, M. D., Burns, J. P., & Truog, R. D. (2006). Improving the quality of end-of-life care in the pediatric intensive care unit: Parents' priorities and recommendations. *Pediatrics,* Mar; *117*(3), 649–657.

Neimeyer, R. A. (2006). *Lessons of loss: A guide to coping.* Center of the Study of Loss and Transition. Memphis, TN.

O'Malley, P., Barata, I., Snow, S., AMERICAN ACADEMY OF PEDIATRICS Committee on Pediatric Emergency Medicine, AMERICAN COLLEGE OF EMERGENCY PHYSICIANS Pediatric Emergency Medicine Committee, EMERGENCY NURSES ASSOCIATION Pediatric Committee (2014). Technical Report: Death of a Child in the Emergency Department. *Pediatrics, 134*(1), ppe313–e330. doi:10.1542/peds 2014-1246.

Pediatric My Wishes. Available at www.agingwithdignity.org/catalog/product_info.php?products_id=85; accessed on Jan 22, 2015.

Ray, A., Block, S. D., Friedlander, R. J., Zhang, B., Maciejewski, P. K., & Prigerson, H. G. (2006). Peaceful awareness in patients with advanced cancer. *Journal of Palliative Medicine, 9,* 1359–1368.

Solomon, M., Riegelhaupt, L., Rushton, C., & Fleischman, A. (2003). Analyzing ethical challenges in pediatric end-of-life decision making (Activity 6: Special considerations of adolescents: Decision making). In M. Z. Solomon, D. Browning, D. Dokken, A. Fleischman, K. H. Heller, M. Levetown, et al. (Eds.), *The Initiative for Pediatric Palliative Care curriculum*. Newton, MA: Education Development Center.

Shibley, H. L., & Stoddard, F. J. (2011). Child and adolescent psychiatric interventions. In F. J. Stoddard, A. Pandya, & C. L. Katz (Eds.), *Disaster psychiatry: Readiness, evaluation, and treatment* (pp. 287–312). Arlington VA: American Psychiatric Press Publishing.

U.S. Department of Health & Human Services, Health Resources & Services Administration, Maternal & Child Health Bureau (2008). *The National Survey of Children with Special Health Care Needs Chartbook 2005–2006*. Rockville, MD: U.S. Department of Health & Human Services.

Wiener, L., Zadeh, S., Battles, H., Baird, K., Ballard, E., Osherow, J., & Pao, M. (2012). Allowing adolescents and young adults to plan their end of life care. *Pediatrics, 130*(5), 897–905.

Wolfe, J., Grier, H. E., Klar, N., et al. (2000). Symptoms and suffering at the end of life in children with cancer. *New England Journal of Medicine,* Feb 3; *342*(5), 326–333.

Wolff, A., Browne, J., & Whitehouse, W. P. (2010). Personal resuscitation plans and end of life planning for children with disability and life-limiting/life-threatening conditions. *British Medical Journal,* Oct;

Young, B., Ward, J., Salmon, P., Gravenhorst, K., Hill, J., & Eden, T. (2011). Parents' experience of their children's presence in discussions with physicians about leukemia. *Pediatrics, 127,* e1230–e1238.

PART X

MEDICAL PSYCHIATRY IN THE EVOLVING SYSTEM OF CARE

82.

SECOND MEDICAL OPINIONS IN THE ERA OF PERSONALIZED MEDICINE

Mayanka Tickoo, Aditya Bardia, and Lidia Schapira

INTRODUCTION

In the past two decades, we have witnessed a major shift towards a patient-centered approach in medicine, with important consequences for all participants. Patients have become increasingly vocal and involved in their own care; professionals value and promote self-advocacy; and physicians are now trained to engage patients in important value-oriented discussions prior to recommending specific treatments. The need for informed consent for treatment is an accepted mandate, and respect for a patient's autonomy has risen to the top of the list of ethical values (Schneider, 1998). The prevalent model for consultations involves at least some consideration of the patient's agenda, although practices vary according to specialty and the particular style of consultants.

The concept of sharing power in medical consultations and the formal study of communication between physicians and patients is relatively new. Shared decision-making has replaced a more directive or paternalistic approach in the United States and other developed countries. By "shared decision-making" we mean a collaborative relationship wherein "patients are involved as active partners with professionals in clarifying acceptable diagnosis, treatment, management and support options, discussing goals and priorities, and together planning and implementing a preferred course of action" (O'Connor, 2007). In a comparative study of the conventional models of medical practice (paternalistic, deliberative, interpretive, and informative), the informative model is seen to present maximum opportunities for patient guided decision-making with the physician presenting the available treatment options and the patient deciding the course of his or her treatment (Ahern, 2012). However, the deliberative model may be a better fit for second opinions, with the bulk of the decision-making power still resting with the patient, and the physician acting as an expert guide. Experienced physicians understand the need to be flexible and to have a wide repertoire of skills that can be tailored to meet individual needs. Emergencies call for authoritative and quick decisions, similar to those made by a pilot facing an emergency landing, or by a commander in the field. In times of crisis, patients value clarity and support, and consultants can assist by adding their perspective without causing undue delay in implementing treatments.

It is now customary for patients to seek information independently after receiving a diagnosis, and they often seek a second opinion. Second medical opinions (SMOs) can enhance the patients' say in regard to their treatment and the choices available to them, and involve a thorough reevaluation of the patient's case, including revision of diagnostic material (Mellink, 2004). They have become fairly common in certain communities of patients, fostered by the perception that they constitute both a right and a requirement for informed decision-making, and by the availability of consultants. In our clinical practice treating breast cancer, it is common to meet patients who have already scheduled a second opinion prior to receiving the first!

The number of patients who seek second opinions varies, depending on the specialty of medicine as well as other factors. A survey of 2,274 people in the United States in 1999 revealed that one in every five people who had visited a health professional in the past year had sought a second opinion (Wagner, 1999). In another study of patients who self-report having survived a cancer, 56% of 1,020 patients were found to have obtained at least one second opinion (Hewitt, 1999). The definition of a "second medical opinion" used in these studies typically defined it as seeking an opinion from a second health professional of the same specialty as the one who had given already given an opinion earlier (Tattersall, 2009), or as a search for additional information that would "help the patient decide what to do and what not to do, where, when and with whom" (Moumjid et al., 2007). Most patients who have private medical insurance in the United States are entitled to a second opinion consultation, and this may partially account for its widespread use. The availability of medical information through the Internet and media has fostered public demand for expert opinion (Barsky, 1998). Unfortunately, there are no data regarding the effectiveness or costs of such opinions. Similarly, we do not know how patients integrate the information received in both consultations, or what criteria they most often use to select their treatment or treating physician.

In this chapter, we will review common reasons for SMO referrals, provide suggestions for how to assist the patient with decision-making, and reflect on how the practice of SMO referrals can be improved.

UNDERSTANDING THE MOTIVATION BEHIND A REQUEST FOR A SECOND MEDICAL OPINION

SMO referrals can broadly be classified into those that are driven primarily by the physician, by the patient, or by the medical system. These are discussed in detail below, and outlined in Figure 82.1 as a fish-bone diagram.

PHYSICIAN-DRIVEN SMOS

Requests for second opinions are often sought in the case of diagnostic or management uncertainty and difficulty (Sutherland, 1994; Townsley, 2003; Bradley, 2011). A primary care physician, acting as an advocate for his or her patient, may facilitate the referral by identifying an expert and initiating the process. In such cases, it is customary for the physician to call, to send a facsimile or email request directly to the consultant, and to expedite the transfer of the appropriate laboratory or imaging studies needed for the second opinion consultation. The requesting physician in turn expects the consultant to communicate directly and in a timely manner after the consultation is complete.

Less often, the consultant suggests to the patient that they consider obtaining another opinion because there are no established treatment guidelines or only limited options for treatments exist. Requests can be motivated by the search of novel approaches available only through clinical research trials at academic centers (Philichi, 2010; Poowuttikul, 2011). Such physician-initiated second opinions are more likely to be directed towards specialists working at dedicated specialty units who have access to innovative treatments, or towards colleagues with considerable authorship in the field.

A third scenario to consider is when a psychiatrist requests an SMO for the purpose of reducing the patient's anxiety, or to resolve the clinician's own doubts about the accuracy of the physician's diagnosis or appropriateness of the recommended treatment. In such situations, it is advisable for the professional giving the SMO to address the patient's and the psychiatrist's questions separately and directly, and to avoid any ambiguity that could only reinforce doubt or cause confusion. With the patient's consent, we recommend speaking directly with the psychiatrist to ensure the smooth transfer of information and to facilitate a resolution.

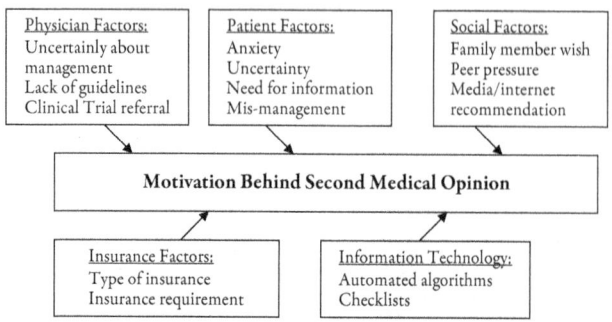

Figure 82.1 Fish-bone diagram outlining the major motivating factors behind SMO.

PATIENT-DRIVEN SMOS

Most commonly, second medical opinions are sought directly by patients who have consulted a physician and for whom a treatment plan has already been formulated or started. There are multiple reasons for seeking a second opinion. The primary motive for a patient usually is the cognitive need for information and the emotional need for reassurance to facilitate their coping and subsequent decision-making (Olden, 2007). In a study conducted in the United States over a decade ago, Wagner and colleagues found that women, older individuals, and those with a college education were more likely to seek SMOs (Wagner, 1999). An Australian study by Tattersall found that women were more likely to seek a second medical opinion, and that these patients tended to be younger, more educated, and preferred more detailed information (Tattersall, 2009). Among cancer patients seeking second surgical opinions, breast cancer patients tend to seek more SMOs than any other group (Mellink, 2003). It is quite possible that women with breast cancer are generally better informed as a result of the growth of advocacy and activist movements urging women to seek a second opinion prior to committing to treatment. Men diagnosed with early-stage prostate cancer face similar choices or dilemmas, and it is reasonable to assume they would also benefit from multidisciplinary consultations or second opinions.

Other factors identified as significant drivers of second opinions include anxiety and the presence of psychiatric conditions such as depression and panic disorders (Burton, 2011). Mellink et al. (2004) report that patients with external motives for seeking SMOs related to a negative appraisal by these patients of different aspects of the care given by the first specialist, including doubts about the advice given; that they had higher anxiety than other patients, and that they hoped more frequently for a different second opinion. Anxious patients often pose unique challenges and are not easily satisfied. In our experience, they typically will seek more tests and opinions, and they find it very difficult to tolerate any measure of ambiguity or uncertainty. Here, too, a more authoritative approach may have greater impact. Besides psychological reasons, a variety of medical reasons have been identified as significant contributors to driving patients towards seeking SMOs. Patients who felt they were treated unfairly or improperly were more likely to ask for another opinion (Townsend, 2008; Hungin, 2009). For patients with non-malignant diseases, these factors were reported to be more commonly related to the need for information and also to perceived difficulties in communication between the patient and his or her physician (Van Dalen, 2001). In a study of healthcare utilization patterns, Sutherland reported that patients referred for second opinions to a Canadian gastroenterology clinic had already consulted two or more general physicians or specialists over the preceding year (Sutherland, 1989). These patients were significantly more likely to rate their own health as "fair to poor," have a chronic duration of symptoms, and be very concerned about their health status. It is possible that patients with a higher level of preoccupation with their health, or with a greater burden of somatic symptoms, are more likely to seek out consultants. This highlights the importance of good communication between patients and physicians as an important part of allaying patient anxiety.

Unlike those with non-malignant conditions, patients with cancer generally obtain second opinions to seek reassurance and information, rather than to express dissatisfaction with their first consultant (Mellink, 2003; Philip, 2009; Tattersall, 2009). An Australian study reported by Philip and colleagues surveyed patients with advanced cancer and also their consultant oncologists in order to determine the reason for such consultations (Philip et al., 2009). They reported that patients were motivated by what they understood to be the extreme nature of the situation (32%), need for reassurance (13%), and concern with management (13%). Tattersall et al. reported similar results and highlighted the fact that cancer patients need both more information about treatment as well as reassurance (Tattersal et al., 2009).

Patient–physician trust is another important determinant, and indeed, in some cases, loyalty to a physician may lead a patient to hold back and avoid seeking another opinion, even when others would encourage him or her to do so. Finally, not uncommonly, patient referrals can stem, not from patient concerns, but rather from the wishes of a worried family member, particularly if the diagnosis is one of a life-threatening illness such as cancer (Delva, 2011).

MEDICAL SYSTEM FACTORS

In situations such as the need for elective surgeries, insurance companies may request a second opinion to ascertain whether the surgery is needed and whether referral to a tertiary center is appropriate (Martin, 1982). This is particularly true when resources are limited, as studies have suggested that such referrals are cost-efficient (Ruchlin, 1982; Dudley, 2000). Indeed, access, one's type of insurance, and cost considerations do affect the frequency with which patients seek out a second opinion (Wagner, 1999).

Another medical system factor that is increasingly being utilized in the era of informatics and technology is the use of automated medical decision-making algorithms. For example, a study reported the use of pharmacist-initiated referrals to efficiently correct sub-optimal asthma management (Bereznicki, 2008). Such algorithms, if found to be efficient and successful, may turn out to be cost-effective as well. Finally, another factor that may prompt a consultant to recommend obtaining another expert opinion is the fear of litigation (Hartz, 1993; Schattner, 2009; Kowey, 2011).

THE CONSULTANT'S ROLE IN ASSISTING PATIENTS WITH DECISION-MAKING

There is etiquette and an art to giving a useful and valuable second opinion. The elements involved vary slightly from those typically encountered in other medical settings, and they have not received sufficient attention in medical education and practice. While there are no clear guidelines regarding the most effective method of approaching second medical opinions, a clear understanding and personalized approach to each consult is ideal.

In the following section, we list five recommendations that we have identified as integral to the process. Following these specific steps and completing the tasks outlined below, will help assure the consultant that the SMO is on target and thus meets the objective for which it was sought. It can be remembered with the mnemonic "PrEP-PCP," or Prepare, Evaluate, Personalize, Provide, Closure, as outlined in Table 82.1.

Table 82.1 PrEP-PCP: FIVE RECOMMENDATIONS AND EXAMPLES OF COMMUNICATIONS STYLES TO HELP A CONSULTANT PROVIDING AN SMO

	RECOMMENDATION	DETAILS	EXAMPLE
1	PREPARE for visit	Encourage the patient to prepare for the consult and set goals for the visit.	"What are the top 5 questions or issues you would like addressed today?"
		Prior to the consult, the physician must review the history, diagnostic results, imaging, and therapy.	
2	EVALUATE motivation	Evaluate patient and/or physician motivations behind seeking SMO, and their specific questions.	"What prompted you to seek a SMO?"
		Identify all information seekers in the consult, including family and friends.	"What would you like to accomplish in this visit?"
3	PERSONALIZE communication	Provide personalized communication that is tailored to meet the needs of each patient.	"Given the size and location of this tumor, I would recommend this procedure for you."
		Avoid statistics, lecturing, and less-relevant information about other subtypes of disease.	
4	PROVIDE plan	Important for the patients to feel that they leave the consult with defined plan. Communicate relevant opinion and reaffirm patient understanding.	"To summarize, based on our discussions, the next best step would be for you to do XX."
5	CLOSURE with primary PHYSICIAN	Close the loop by communicating with referring physician in a timely and effective manner.	"Did I answer your consult question?"

PREPARE (PREPARE FOR THE CONSULTATION)

The first step is to be prepared. Since the second opinion setting is different in the sense that a fair number of diagnostic and treatment variables have already been assessed and communicated to the patient, it is fundamental for the consultant to familiarize him- or herself with the available data. It is necessary to review the available patient history, exam findings, diagnostic results, relevant histopathology and imaging, and treatment.

It is not uncommon for physicians to categorize patients who seek second opinions (even before the visit) as having greater information needs and psychosocial needs, and requiring more energy and time (Phillip, 2010). While it is true that patients seeking SMOs may in fact take more of the physician's time and energy, it is important to realize that this patient population has unmet needs that deserve attention. Second opinions can indeed be a very satisfying experience for both the patient and the consultant. Among patients who seek a second opinion for communication-oriented reasons, almost always the second consultation appears to be more satisfactory for the patient. Some of the variables contributing to this increased satisfaction include a longer consultation, more active listening, answering of patients' specific concerns, and a friendlier attitude on the part of the physician (Tattersall, 2009).

Time is of essence for a busy clinician, so it is important to understand and negotiate the agenda for the consultation at the outset and together with patients, decide how best to apportion time. We suggest asking the patient how much she or he wants to know, giving them opportunities to ask questions, checking their understanding, and providing a summary and written materials if they are available. Often the consultant does not need to repeat a physical exam or review all the various aspects of the patient's past medical history, thus freeing up more time for dialogue and information exchange. The use of tools such as a "patient question prompt sheet," (Box 82.1) prepared to help guide the patient to clarify his or her own needs and questions and sent to the patient in advance of the appointment, can also considerably shorten the consult visit without compromising its effectiveness (Brown, 2001; Bruera, 2003; Glynne-Jones, 2006).

EVALUATE (EVALUATE THE REASON FOR THE SMO AND ADDRESS IT SPECIFICALLY)

As we described in the preceding section, not all patients who schedule a second opinion are driven by the same motives or do so simply for the stated purpose of confirming the diagnosis or treatment plans. Consultants need to take into account the complex interplay of the patient's motivation, and emotional and information needs, in order to provide an opinion that will satisfy the patient and his family and expedite their coping with the adverse consequences of illness, as outlined in Figure 82.1. A good first question to ask in the patient–physician encounter is "What brings you here today?" or to be very direct and ask, "What prompted you to seek a second opinion?" If the reason remains unclear, or if the consultant suspects there may be additional motives, we would encourage them to explore this up front. Without such insight and clarity, the consultant may not be able to plan an efficient use of his or her time, or fail to address the fear, concerns, or grievance that prompted the appointment. Understanding the goals of the visit early on will greatly help one tailor the

---

Box 82.1 PATIENT CHECKLIST FOR A SECOND OPINION

Prior to the meeting with the consultant, we suggest you tell us about:

1. **Your reason for seeking the second opinion (please circle):**
   - I am here because I would like you to confirm the opinion of the first oncologist.
   - I am here because you have many trials open and I am interested in new treatments.
   - I am here because I am not happy with my primary oncologist and would like to switch.
   - I am here because you treated my _____.

2. **Your worries and concerns (please write):**
   - I am confused about _____.
   - I worry that _____.
   - I wonder if there are alternatives to the treatment proposed back home such as _____.

3. **Your goals and expectations (please circle):**
   - I am prepared to do anything to get the best results.
   - I need to support my family during treatment.
   - I am ambivalent about the choices that I heard from my first oncologist.

4. **And finally, please write the top 3 questions you need answered in the visit (please write):**
   1. _____
   2. _____
   3. _____

type of therapeutic response needed and the level of information that should be provided, and it will facilitate a more efficient use of the visit (Feldman-Stewart, 2005).

In situations where the consultation was requested by the patient's primary physician for assistance with problem-solving in the face of uncertainty, it is fundamental to communicate directly with the referring physician in a timely manner. Written reports are obviously required for documentation and for billing purposes, and every attempt should be made to send these immediately to the requesting physician, either electronically or via facsimile. We also recommend a personal phone call in order to allow the referring physician to discuss the case and to review the recommendations and plans for management without intermediaries.

If the consultant ascertains that the SMO stems from patient anxiety or ambivalence, the consultant may choose to be especially empathetic in listening to the patient's concerns and providing both information and reassurance. Such patients are more likely to be satisfied by frequent contact with the medical system and may benefit from a follow-up phone call or email by a member of the professional team. In some cases, it becomes clear over time that the concern or anxiety does not abate. Patients with excessive demands for contact and who seem unsatisfied by reasonable amounts of information and support may need to be referred to mental health professionals for more detailed evaluations and treatment. On the other hand, the patient may strictly be looking for more detailed information available only to an expert, or a greater understanding of the treatment options (Oskay-Ozcelik, 2007).

Patient preferences about second opinions in hematology-oncology patients were carefully analyzed by Goldman through in-depth interviews (Goldman, 2009). She reported that patients typically were looking for a treatment plan specifically tailored to their case scenario, and that they wanted the consultant to apply expertise to their individual situation. In this study, patients universally felt that personalized advice indicated the highest level of expertise as well as the greatest respect. Additionally, patients reacted negatively when the consultant appeared dismissive, was not personable, or appeared not to have reviewed the records prior to the consultation or ignored factors that the patient felt were important or unique to the patient's particular case (Goldman, 2009). Other studies have also confirmed that patients were highly disappointed if they only received statistics or generalized information about the possible course of the disease and the sub-types of disease, and treatment options not pertaining to them (Kagan, 2005).

It is important to ascertain early on in the course of the consultation what drove the patient to obtain the second opinion. As discussed previously, reasons are varied and motivations complex. Common concerns include frustration or discontent with the manner or approach of the physician who gave the first opinion or has been regularly treating the patient for a chronic condition; concerns about insufficient information or discussion; feeling rushed; or feeling excluded from participating in making important health-related decisions. Such patients may require a longer consultation, more active listening, a more skilled communicative approach, or a different style of communication in order to be satisfied. If the motive

of the second opinion consultation is indeed to find validation for such needs, then the consultant may or may not be able to satisfy such needs, depending on circumstances and the effort expended. If the consultant can diagnose a mismatch in communicative needs and styles between the primary physician and the patient and accomplish the dual goal of reassuring the patient and providing helpful tips to the referring colleague, then the SMO consultation can be considered useful and a valuable investment of time and resources.

PERSONALIZE (PERSONALIZE COMMUNICATION AND RECOMMENDATIONS)

Patients' expectations of a consultant may be quite different from those of the physician they see for longitudinal care. Studies have suggested that patients who received explicit emotional support from their SMO physicians were grateful and satisfied but did not consider it a requirement for a satisfactory consult (Brown, 1997; Salmon, 2005; Goldman, 2009). Patients greatly appreciated when their physicians were involved with them as individuals and were pleased when the discussion touched on how the disease or treatment would affect the totality of their life. This indicates than an empathetic relationship does not necessarily require overtly emotional talk. Indeed, earning trust through demonstration of expertise and detailed discussion of the disease and treatment is more important than a display of emotions.

While there are various opinions about the preferred style of the physician's communication, generally patients do not appreciate "lectures" (Epstein, 2007). Patients are not looking for learned monologues from their consultants, but for a timely application of complex knowledge to their individual situation (Kidane, 2011). Physicians should thus use their expertise to deliver a personalized recommendation that takes into consideration the patient's individual values, resources, preferences, and that is likely to offer the best possible outcome (Veazie, 2007).

Good communication between patients and physicians is a requisite for informed decision-making and quality care. It has been linked to improved adherence to treatment, decreased litigation, better coping, and increased satisfaction (Epstein, 2007). It is also important to ensure that the set-up for the patient encounter is conducive to an open line of communication, not only with the patient, but also with the family members. Many a time the consult is driven by a family member's wishes, and it is crucial to identify the actual seekers of information and to address their concerns. It is also important to identify the underlying motivations of the patient or family behind seeking the SMO and to clearly define the goals for the consult. This would enable the consultant to tailor the conversation in a more directed manner and facilitate effective discussions.

PROVIDE PLAN (PROVIDE THE FINAL OPINION AND PLAN)

It is important to bear in mind that the patient and family made the effort to attend the consultation in order to obtain an expert opinion and treatment plan. Failure to formulate a plan can be profoundly disappointing and does a disservice to the patient and possibly to a referring colleague as well. Although we certainly favor a deliberative model for consultations, and following communication protocols that place the patient's agenda front and center, at the end of the day it is important to remember that in order to meet the patient's needs, the consultant needs to provide guidance and a clear plan of action. Even if the facts of the case leave room for uncertainty, or if two diagnostic or treatment options appear equally effective, it is expected of the consultant to express a preference and to provide a plan of action. In some cases, the consultant can do so within the first ten minutes of the visit and then spend the rest of the time discussing alternatives or answering other questions for the patient. In other cases, it may take most of the hour to figure out just what is best, given the constellation of symptoms, resources, and preferences. In either case, however, the consultant needs to give his or her opinion and confirm that the patient has in fact understood the recommendation. Print materials or websites for the public can provide valuable tools to facilitate understanding. At times a referral to a local resource room or support group can also help the patient understand his disease and treatment and connect with others facing similar challenges.

So how is a consultant to proceed in the face of diagnostic uncertainty or if there is no standard therapy? Sometimes treatment options vary considerably, as do the risks and possible benefits. Imagine a patient with refractory leukemia referred to an academic center for a second opinion. She is presented with two reasonable treatment options: one involves a bone marrow transplant, which offers a chance of a prolonged remission but carries with it a risk of death from the procedure itself, or other potentially debilitating side-effects that can be long-lasting; the other offers a palliative treatment that is guaranteed to be well tolerated but can offer only moderate relief of symptoms and no meaningful extension of life. Guiding a patient to make such decisions requires not only considerable technical expertise, but a patient, respectful, and collaborative approach. It may also require the assistance of other members of a multidisciplinary team, including a nurse, a social worker, and perhaps even a psychologist or psychiatrist to provide support and to help the patient and her family sort through the diverse options and to consider all alternatives in the context of her personal values and preferences.

Finally, if the consultant ascertains that psychological factors are a major driving force for the patient's need for a second opinion, it may be helpful to consider a joint consultation with both a psychiatrist and the medical consultant (Hoedeman, 2010). For most patients, however, a personalized second opinion delivered with respect and in a clear fashion will suffice. Referrals to colleagues with expertise in mental health will address unmet emotional needs that may delay or impede the patient in opting for a particular course of action. As with any other problem in medicine, the consultant needs a strategy to ensure the patient's needs are met in the best way possible.

Whatever the final recommendation might be, providing the next best course of action to the patient is important. It might be helpful to summarize the conversation and highlight the key points. It is important for the patients to feel that they have come out of the consult with a defined plan.

CLOSURE WITH *PHYSICIAN* (CLOSE THE LOOP BY COMMUNICATING WITH REFERRING PHYSICIAN)

If the consultation was requested by a colleague or a generalist within the same practice or hospital, it is preferable to communicate directly via phone or email on the same day of the consultation. After all, when the patient leaves the consultant, one assumes that a recommendation has been made, or at least that there is a plan for a follow-up. Even if all the details of the case have not been resolved, or if there remains some uncertainty about the treatment or follow-up care, it is useful to reach out to the referring physician and to keep him or her duly informed. There are certain situations that make this particular exchange slightly more difficult or challenging for the consultant, and we will address these next, providing advice derived from our experience rather than scientific evidence.

Sometimes the patient who seeks a second expert opinion is also "shopping for" another physician. If the patient prefers the style, the location, or the treatment plan offered by the consultant, he may request that this physician take over his care. This may pose a slight conflict for the consultant, especially if the referring physician or primary specialist is a respected colleague. Some consultants may actually choose to turn down such requests if the actual treatment plan can be offered elsewhere, to enhance the continuity of care, but most will accede to the patient's wishes. How to handle these situations and still preserve the trust of the referring physician is a challenge that requires considerable tact and diplomacy in communication.

Finally, a special category of patients seeking a second opinion is those who actually have been mismanaged. Some may have experienced a diagnostic delay, an incorrect diagnosis, a treatment error, or an unexpected complication of treatment. In some cases, patients may be fully aware of the medical details and prepared to discuss these with the consultant, while others may have incomplete information. The consultant may struggle with how much to tell the patient or perhaps with the dilemma of whether or not to communicate directly with the physician or physicians responsible for the patient's care. There are simply no guidelines or steadfast rules to guide consultants, who must use their own judgement in both reporting and documenting the extent of the problem. In these situations, it is more common for the consultant to offer to assume the care of the patient or to make a suitable referral for longitudinal care.

VALUE AND FUTURE OF SECOND MEDICAL OPINIONS

While SMOs were initially seen as a checkpoint to avoid over-expenditures in the managed-care setting by avoiding unnecessary procedures, their independent financial burden on the healthcare set-up cannot be ignored. Studies have suggested that while many ailments can be treated satisfactorily at primary clinics, SMOs tend to drain the resources of a healthcare system (Mahmoud, 2010). On the other hand, SMOs have their value in appropriate cases and can actually result in improved patient care at minimal cost to third-party payers (Benson, 2001).

Questions have also been raised about the independence of a second opinion, since most physicians are wary of second-guessing their colleagues and tend to side with the initial plan more frequently. Ideally, a checks and balances approach is needed. Some authors have raised a concern about the need for SMOs in the era of evidence-based medicine (Moumjid, 2007). If we establish more guidelines for treatment of diseases, and these are posted in the public domain where they can be easily retrieved by the public, will we see a drop-off in requests for SMOs? Or will the increasing trend towards personalized medicine continue to drive requests for personalized expert recommendations?

We imagine that public demand is not likely to fall, even if more and better-quality information becomes available. Perhaps the new research frontier for scientists and health services researchers is to figure out how best to help patients gather as much information as possible in advance of the planned consultation and to prioritize their questions and needs. Ideally, web- or phone-based services from patient-advocacy groups could help match the patients to the consultants who are best suited to meet their needs. Such a match-making service could improve the satisfaction of patients and the efficiency of consultants. Other possible interventions include the use of buddy or peer support programs, and similar interventions using a psycho-educational approach that helps patients find their own sources of strength and support. Preparing experts to provide a consultation using specific steps, and paying attention to process and task, are also key to promoting better understanding and satisfaction for those seeking a second opinion.

SUMMARY

Good communication between patients and physicians is a requisite for informed decision-making and quality care. It has been linked to improved adherence to treatment, decreased litigation, better patient coping, and increased satisfaction. Patients seeking a second opinion should be encouraged to communicate their agendas and expectations to physicians clearly in the course of the consultation. For some, having a list of questions ahead of time will help them clarify and prioritize concerns. Physicians should also in turn actively try to understand the underlying reason for the visit and address the prepared questions in an orderly and methodical fashion. It is recommended that physicians understand and negotiate the agenda for the consultation at the outset and, with the patients, decide how best to apportion time.

The cost and time-constraints associated with a second opinion cannot be ignored, and a structured approach to SMOs is essential. Access to a multi-specialty clinic where patients are able to obtain several opinions under one umbrella organization are more useful or lead to greater satisfaction. Use of efficient tools such as a "patient question prompt sheet" can considerably shorten the consult visit without compromising its effectiveness. Training physicians in communication skills may lead to a more personalized delivery of information and allow consultants who give first, second, or third opinions to tailor their presentation to address the specific needs of the individual.

CLINICAL PEARLS

- There is etiquette and an art to giving a useful and valuable second opinion.

- A longer consultation, more active listening, answering of patient-specific concerns, and a friendlier attitude by the physician increases patient satisfaction (Tattersal, 2009).

- Negotiate the agenda for the consultation at the outset and, together with patients, decide how best to apportion time.

- Understanding the goals of the visit early on will help tailor the type of therapeutic response needed and determine the level of information to be provided (Feldman-Stewart, 2005).

- Patients universally felt that personalized advice indicated the highest level of expertise as well as the greatest respect.

- Even if the facts of the case leave room for uncertainty, or if two diagnostic or treatment options appear equally effective, the consultant is expected to express a preference and to provide a plan of action.

DISCLOSURE STATEMENTS

Dr. Tickoo no disclosures from any of the investigators.

Dr. Bardia no disclosures from any of the investigators.

Dr. Schapira no disclosures from any of the investigators.

REFERENCES

Ahern, S. P., Doyle, T. K., Marquis, F., Lesk, C., & Skrobik, Y. (2012). Critically ill patients and end-of-life decision-making: the senior medical resident experience. *Advances in Health Sciences Education: Theory & Practice, 17*(1), 121–136.

Benson, W. E., Regillo, C. D., Vander, J. F., Tasman, W., Smith, A. F., Brown, G. C., et al. (2001). Patient-initiated second medical opinions: their necessity and economic cost. *Retina, 21*(6), 633–638.

Bereznicki, B. J., Peterson, G. M., Jackson, S. L., Walters, H., Fitzmaurice, K., & Gee, P. (2008). Pharmacist-initiated general practitioner referral of patients with suboptimal asthma management. *Pharmacy World & Science*, Dec; *30*(6), 869–875. [Epub Aug 5, 2008.]

Bradley, S. E., Frizelle, D., & Johnson, M. (2011). Why do health professionals refer individual patients to specialist day hospice care? *Journal of Palliative Medicine*, Feb; *14*(2), 133–138. [Epub Jan 16, 2011.]

Brown, R. F., Butow, P. N., Dunn, S. M., & Tattersall, M. H. (2001). Promoting patient participation and shortening cancer consultations: a randomized trial. *British Journal of Cancer*, Nov 2; *85*(9), 1273–1279.

Brown, R., Dunn, S., & Butow, P. (1997). Meeting patient expectations in the cancer consultation. *Annals of Oncology*, 8, 877–882.

Bruera, E., Sweeney, C., Willey, J., Palmer, J. L., Tolley, S., Rosales, M., et al. (2003). Breast cancer patient perception of the helpfulness of a prompt sheet versus a general information sheet during outpatient consultation: a randomized, controlled trial. *Journal of Pain Symptom Management*, *25*, 412–419.

Burton, C., McGorm, K., Weller, D., & Sharpe, M. (2011). Depression and anxiety in patients repeatedly referred to secondary care with medically unexplained symptoms: a case-control study. *Psychological Medicine*, Mar; *41*(3), 555–563.

Delva, F., Marien, E., Fonck, M., Rainfray, M., Demeaux, J. L., Moreaud, P., et al. (2011). Factors influencing general practitioners in the referral of elderly cancer patients. *BioMed Central Cancer*, Jan 6; *11*, 5.

Dudley, R. A., Johansen, K. L., Brand, R., Rennie, D. J., & Milstein, A. (2000). Selective referral to high-volume hospitals: estimating potentially avoidable deaths. *Journal of the American Medical Association*, Mar 1; *283*(9), 1159–1166.

Epstein, R. M., & Street, R. L., Jr. (2007). *Patient-centered communication in cancer care: promoting healing and reducing suffering*. Bethesda, MD: National Cancer Institute.

Feldman-Stewart, D., Brundage, M. D., & Tishelman, C. (2005). A conceptual framework for patient–professional communication: an application to the cancer context. *Psychooncology*, *14*, 801–809.

Glynne-Jones, R., Ostler, P., Lumley-Graybow, S., Chait, I., Hughes, R., Grainger, J., et al. (2006). Can I look at my list? An evaluation of a "prompt sheet" within an oncology outpatient clinic. *Clinical Oncology (Royal College of Radiology)*, *18*, 395–400.

Goldman, R. E., Sullivan, A., Back, A. L., Alexander, S. C., Matsuyama, R. K., & Lee, S. J. (2009). Patients' reflections on communication in the second-opinion hematology-oncology consultation. *Patient Education & Counseling*, July; *76*(1), 44–50.

Hartz, A., Deber, R., Bartholomew, M., & Midtling, J. (1993). Physician characteristics affecting referral decisions following an exercise tolerance test. *Archives of Family Medicine*, May; *2*(5), 513–519.

Hewitt, M., Breen, N., & Devesa, S. (1999). Cancer prevalence and survivorship issues: Analyses of the 1992 National Health Interview Survey. *Journal of the National Cancer Institute*, Sep 1; *91*(17), 1480–1486.

Hoedeman, R., Blankenstein, A. H., van der Feltz-Cornelis, C. M., Krol, B., Stewart, R., & Groothoff, J. W. (2010). Consultation letters for medically unexplained physical symptoms in primary care. *Cochrane Database of Systematic Reviews*, Dec 8; (12), CD006524. Review.

Hungin, A. P., Hill, C., & Raghunath, A. (2009). Systematic review: frequency and reasons for consultation for gastro-oesophageal reflux disease and dyspepsia. *Alimentary Pharmacology & Therapeutics*, Aug 15; *30*(4), 331–342. Review.

Kagan, A. R. (2005). Statistics is not a surrogate for judgment. *American Journal of Clinical Oncology*, *28*, 327–328.

Kidane, B., Gandhi, R., Sarro, A., Valiante, T. A., Harvey, B. J., & Rampersaud, Y. R. (2011). Is referral to a spine surgeon a double-edged sword? Patient concerns before consultation. *Canadian Family Physician*, Jul; *57*(7), 803–810.

Kowey, P. R. (2011). A piece of my mind. The silent majority. *Journal of the American Medical Association*, Jul 6; *306*(1), 18–19.

Mahmoud, A. O., Kuranga, S. A., Ayanniyi, A. A., Babata, A. L., Adido, J., & Uyanne, I. A. (2010). Appropriateness of ophthalmic cases presenting to a Nigerian tertiary health facility: implications for service delivery in a developing country. *Niger Journal of Clinical Practice*, Sep; *13*(3), 280–283.

Martin, S. G., Shwartz, M., Whalen, B. J., D'Arpa, D., Ljung, G. M., Thorne, J. H., et al. (*1982*). Impact of a mandatory second-opinion program on Medicaid surgery rates. *Medical Care*, Jan; *20*(1), 21–45.

Mellink, W. A., Dulmen, A. M., Wiggers, T., Spreeuwenberg, P. M., Eggermont, A. M., & Bensing, J. M. (2003). Cancer patients seeking a second surgical opinion: Results of a study on motives, needs, and expectations. *Journal of Clinical Oncology*, *21*, 1492–1497.

Nora, M., Gafni, A., Bremond, A., & Carrere, M.-O. (2007). Seeking a second opinion: Do patients need a second opinion when practice guidelines exist? *Health Policy*, *80*, 43–50.

O'Connor, A. M., Wennberg, J. E., Legare, F., Llewellyn-Thomas, H. A., Moulton, B. W., Sepucha, K. R., et al. (2007). Toward the "tipping point": decision aids and informed patient choice. *Health Affairs (Millwood)*, May–Jun; *26*(3), 716–725.

Olden, A. M., Holloway, R., Ladwig, S., Quill, T. E., & van Wijngaarden, E. (2007). Palliative care needs and symptom patterns of hospitalized elders referred for consultation. *Journal of Pain Symptom Management*, *18*(3), 479–484.

Oskay-Ozcelik, G., Lehmacher, W., Könsgen, D., Christ, H., Kaufmann, M., Lichtenegger, W., et al. (2007). Breast cancer patients' expectations in respect of the physician–patient relationship and treatment management results of a survey of 617 patients. *Annals of Oncology*, *18*, 479–484.

Philichi, L., & Yuwono, M. (2010). Primary care: constipation and encopresis treatment strategies and reasons to refer. *Gastroenterology Nursing*, Sep–Oct; *33*(5), 363–366.

Philip, J., Gold, M., Schwarz, M., & Komesaroff, P. (2011). An exploration of the dynamics and influences upon second medical opinion consultations in cancer care. *Asia–Pacific Journal of Clinical Oncology*, *7*, 41–46.

Poowuttikul, P., Kamat, D., Thomas, R., & Pansare, M. (2011). Asthma consultations with specialists: What do the pediatricians seek? *Allergy & Asthma Proceedings*, Jul; *32*(4), 307–312.

Ruchlin, H. S., Finkel, M. L., & McCarthy, E. G. (1982). The efficacy of second-opinion consultation programs: a cost–benefit perspective. *Medical Care*, Jan; *20*(1), 3–20.

Salmon, P., & Young, B. (2005). Core assumptions and clinical opportunities in clinical communication. *Patient Education & Counseling*, *58*, 225–234.

Schattner, A. (2009). Angst-driven medicine? *QJM: Quarterly Journal of Medicine*, Jan; *102*(1), 75–78.

Schneider, C. (1998). *The practice of autonomy: Patients, doctors, and medical decisions*. New York: Oxford University Press.

Sutherland, L. R., & Verhoef, M. J. (1989). Patients who seek a second opinion: Are they different from a second referral? *Journal of Clinical Gastroenterology*, *11*(3), 308–313.

Sutherland, L. R., & Verhoef, M. J. (1994). Why do patients seek a second opinion or alternative medicine? *Journal of Clinical Gastroenterology*, *19*(3), 194–197.

Tattersall Martin, H. N., Dear Rachel, F., Jansen Jesse, Heather L Shepherd, Rhonda J Devine, Lisa G Horvath and Michael J Boyer. (2009). Second opinions in oncology: the experiences of patients attending the Sydney Cancer Centre. *Medical Journal of Australia*, Aug 17; *191*(4), 209–212.

Townsley, C. A., Naidoo, K., Pond, G. R., Melnick, W., Straus, S. E., & Siu, L. L. (2003). Are older cancer patients being referred to oncologists? A mail questionnaire of Ontario primary care practitioners to evaluate their referral patterns. *Journal of Clinical Oncology*, Dec 15; *21*(24), 4627–4635.

Van Dalen, I. (2001). Motives for seeking a second opinion in orthopedic surgery. *Journal of Health Services Research & Policy*, *4*, 195.

Veazie, P. J., & Cai, S. (2007). A connection between medication adherence, patient sense of uniqueness, and the personalization of information. *Medical Hypotheses*, *68*, 335–334.

Wagner, T. H., & Wagner, L. S. (1999). Who gets second opinions? *Health Affairs*, *18*(5), 137–145.

83.

THE CONTINUUM OF CHRONIC CARE: NURSING HOMES, ASSISTED LIVING, HOME CARE

Hong-Phuc T. Tran and David B. Reuben

DEFINITIONS OF CHRONIC CARE

Chronic care relates to a variety of populations and health states, and the term can be used in different ways. First, chronic care can refer to the (bio)medical care of chronic diseases. Especially in the elderly population, multiple chronic illnesses are common; 43% of Medicare beneficiaries have three or more conditions (Institute of Medicine Committee on the Future of Heath Care Workforce for Older Americans 2008), and 23% have more than five. (These numbers refer only to explicitly diagnosed conditions; and particularly in the realm of mental disorders, undiagnosed but clinically important conditions are common.) Moreover, the percentage of persons with multiple chronic conditions rises with increasing age (Wolff, Starfield, et al., 2002).

Second, "chronic care" can refer to a broader set of services, including self-management, aid rendered by family and friends, and community-based supportive services of a non-medical nature. (Wagner, 1998) has described The "Chronic Care Model," is an approach to improving health-care outcomes by linking medical care to community-based services through four components: delivery system design, self-management support, decision support, and clinical information systems. Patients become more informed and activated, and practice teams are more prepared to be proactive, with the intended result of improved clinical and functional outcomes (Wagner, 1998). Although implementing this model may be difficult in smaller practices, as providers increasingly join larger groups, this approach may be more feasible.

Third, "chronic care" may include community-based services and residential structures to compensate for functional impairments. This is commonly referred to as "long-term care." The Centers for Medicare and Medicaid Services (CMS) defines long-term care as "a variety of services that help people with their medical and non-medical needs over a period of time. Long-term care can be provided at home, in the community, or in various types of facilities, including nursing homes and assisted living facilities. Most long-term care is custodial care" (US Government Medicare, August 12, 2011).

In this chapter, we discuss chronic care as it is most broadly defined, comprising both institutional and community-based care, in both its medical and non-medical aspects. We will refer to chronic care using Medicare terminology (US Government Medicare, March 17, 2013).

SITES WHERE CHRONIC CARE IS PROVIDED

Community-based long-term care includes care provided at medical offices, at community-based organizations (e.g., adult day care centers), in private homes, in independent living facilities, in assisted living facilities, and in the parts of continuing-care retirement communities that do not offer continuous skilled nursing care. Assisted living facilities may be large (housing over 100 residents) or very small (with just a handful of residents); small assisted living facilities sometimes are referred to as "board-and-care homes." Some assisted living facilities have locked dementia units for patients with dementia with behavioral issues such as wandering. Assisted living facilities differ from institutional long-term care facilities in terms of licensure and regulation; they are regulated only at the state level. Institutional long-term care is usually provided in nursing homes, also known as "nursing facilities" (NFs) or "skilled nursing facilities" (SNFs—commonly pronounced "sniffs").

NFs are tightly regulated both by states and by the federal government. NFs, as distinct from SNFs, provide basic nursing care (e.g., administration of daily medications; provision of special diets) and assistance with activities of daily living. This type of care, which does not require the continual involvement of licensed nurses (registered nurses or licensed practical nurses), is referred to as "custodial care."

SNFs provide 24-hour coverage by licensed nurses and daily coverage by registered nurses, and thus are able to care for sicker patients and those requiring invasive interventions such as intravenous medications, rehabilitation, and wound care. SNFs are a major source of post–acute care services, caring for patients for up to 100 days following an acute hospitalization, when patients need daily licensed nursing care but no longer require the technological resources and daily physician involvement available in the hospital.

The other major institutional settings for post–acute care are LTACHs (long-term acute care hospitals) and IRFs

Table 83.1 TYPES OF CARE, THEIR DEFINITIONS AND EXPLANATIONS

TERM	DEFINITION	EXPLANATION
Long-Term Care	Medical and non-medical care provided to people with chronic conditions or disability.	Long-term care can be provided in the home, community, assisted living or nursing homes. LTC includes assistance with basic activities of daily living, such as dressing and bathing.
Custodial Care	A term used to describe supportive services for activities of daily living, such as bathing, dressing, grooming, toileting.	Custodial care is a sub-category of LTC. Medicare does not pay for this type of care, as it is considered "non-skilled" care.

Adapted from Reuben, D. B., Herr, K. A., et al. (Eds.) (2011). *Geriatrics at your fingertips 2011*. New York: American Geriatrics Society.

(independent rehabilitation facilities). LTACHs often care for ventilator-dependent patients who require a greater intensity of nursing care and medical services than are usually available in a SNF but do not need the full spectrum of services provided by a general hospital. IRFs offer intensive physical therapy, occupational therapy, and speech therapy, as well as consulting specialists in physical medicine, neurology, orthopedics, and psychiatry, and tend to focus on patients with complex problems and a high premorbid baseline, such as young stroke patients and victims of multiple trauma. For psychiatric patients with extended stays in state mental hospitals (e.g., spanning decades), state mental hospitals can be viewed as part of the long-term care continuum (Fisher, Barreira, et al., 2001).

In general, the appropriateness of a patient for a particular residential setting depends upon the person's functional status, cognition (including whether or not there are behavioral problems), and mobility.

FUNCTIONAL STATUS

Functional status is usually considered at two levels: activities of daily living (ADLs) and instrumental activities of daily living (IADLs). ADLs include:

- Bathing
- Dressing
- Toileting
- Transferring (e.g., from a bed to a chair)
- Maintaining continence
- Feeding

IADLs include:

- Using the telephone
- Shopping
- Preparing meals
- Housekeeping
- Doing laundry
- Using public transportation or driving
- Taking medication
- Handling personal finances

ADL and IADL performance is characterized as *independent* (done with no assistance) or *not independent* (requiring assistance). The amount of assistance needed and the frequency and timing of the need for assistance are major considerations in selecting an appropriate site. Related to ADL and IADL performance is the patient's awareness of ADL or IADL deficits and their willingness to accept assistance when it is needed. This issue is discussed in detail in the chapter on competence.

Approximately 25% of community-dwelling older persons have at least one IADL or ADL impairment (Hung, Ross, et al., 2011). Community-based agencies can provide some services (e.g., Meals-on-Wheels, homemaker services, transportation) to compensate for IADL impairments for older and disabled persons who want to stay in their homes. Nonprofit and government agencies frequently price these services according to patients' ability to pay; similar services may be offered by for-profit providers at market prices. Effective use of supportive services usually requires case-management services either by a social worker or by a nurse, or equivalent oversight by an involved and informed family member or friend. Professional case-management services are covered to variable extents by Medicaid, Medicare managed-care plans, and some types of private long-term care insurance, but they are not covered by fee-for-service Medicare. Those without coverage for case management, without the means to buy it privately, or without sufficiently informed and involved family members are at risk for poorly planned and uncoordinated care.

Adult daycare centers provide a social environment for persons with long-term care needs and also relief for family caregivers during the day (Kane, 2011). Patients who go to adult daycare centers may have multiple, chronic medical conditions but are usually clinically stable. Some adult daycare centers may provide basic medical services, such as medication administration and blood pressure and blood glucose monitoring. Adult daycare centers may take patients with psychiatric conditions, but typically the psychiatric conditions will need to be already well controlled. Some adult daycare centers specialize in caring for patients with dementia (dementia daycare centers).

The population of patients cared for in nursing homes includes some who could successfully live in the

Table 83.2 FACILITY OPTIONS FOR ELDERLY, FUNCTIONALLY IMPAIRED PATIENTS WITH PSYCHIATRIC ILLNESS

TYPE OF PATIENT	APPROPRIATE SETTINGS	SERVICES	PAYER
IADL Impaired/ No Behavioral Symptoms	• Assisted living facility • Foster care	• IADL care • Medication administration	Usually out-of-pocket* though some accept Medicaid
IADL Impaired/ Mild to Moderate Behavioral Symptoms	• Assisted living facilities with dementia units • Some foster care facilities	• IADL care • Medication administration • Non-pharmacological approaches to symptoms	Usually out-of-pocket* though some accept Medicaid
ADL Impaired without or with Mild Behavioral Disturbances	• Nursing home	• ADL and IADL care	Out-of-pocket* or Medicaid
ADL Impairment with Moderate or Severe Behavioral Symptoms	• Nursing home with dementia unit	• ADL and IADL care • Non-pharmacological approaches to symptoms	Out-of-pocket* or Medicaid

*Some long-term care insurance policies provide some coverage.
Adapted from Reuben, D. B., Herr, K. A., et al. (Eds.) (2011). *Geriatrics at your fingertips 2011.* New York: American Geriatrics Society.

community—at home or in an assisted living or independent living facility—if they had sufficiently intense supportive services, skilled nursing involvement, and physician participation. Some communities offer a Program for All-inclusive Care for the Elderly (PACE), which is designed to help frail elders avoid institutionalization. PACE programs provide supportive and skilled nursing services comparable to those provided in nursing homes, but persons enrolled in these programs remain at home (Eng, Pedulla, et al., 1997). Financing of PACE programs is capitated—i.e., with a fixed sum allotted each year for the care of each patient, based on that patient's expected healthcare utilization. Funding of PACE primarily comes from both Medicare and Medicaid programs; individuals with only Medicare coverage usually cannot participate because of the high copayment costs. Some PACE programs accept community-dwelling patients with both functional impairments and mental illness or behavioral problems; an interdisciplinary team consisting of healthcare professionals assesses a patient's needs and devise a care plan to best help the patient (Substance Abuse and Mental Health Services Administration, March 17, 2013).

The more IADL impairments a person has, the less likely it is that the person can remain at home. When a person is unable to live at home, there is a spectrum of types of facilities that provide housing and other services, which vary in size and amount of services (Hung, Ross, et al., 2011). Independent living facilities are similar to hotels in that they provide rooms, some or all meals, and light housekeeping, but no personal services. Assisted living facilities (ALFs) typically provide assistance with IADLs and care for persons who are less disabled than those residing in nursing homes. The services provided by ALFs vary considerably, and many provide additional services (e.g., personal care) or tiers of service for additional cost. Some have dementia units. These facilities also vary greatly in their amenities, luxury, and cost, with high-end facilities charging monthly fees of $8000 or more for their base services. Another living-situation option is adult foster care, a small group-living setting in which ADL

and/or IADL support is provided by non-professionals. (See Table 83.2).

Persons with chronic ADL dependencies (other than isolated dependency in bathing) need personal assistance seven days a week, several times a day. Assistance can be provided in the home by family or friends or by paid assistants (direct care providers), or at ALFs or nursing homes. These services are not covered by Medicare but may be covered by Medicaid to some extent for eligible persons. Patients who are not safe without continuous supervision may also require institutional care even if they do not have multiple ADL dependencies. This category includes patients with dementia and significantly impaired judgement.

IMPAIRED COGNITION, MENTAL HEALTH, AND BEHAVIORAL PROBLEMS

Impaired cognition and mental health and behavioral problems are other major determinants of where a person lives. Mental and behavioral problems can occur in the absence of cognitive impairment, and cognitive impairment can occur without behavioral problems, particularly in its early stages. IADLs usually are impaired much earlier in the course of dementia than are ADLs. However, patients with an awareness of their deficit and willingness to accept help can remain in the community much longer than those without those attributes. Cognitive deficits and mental health and behavioral problems become important when they impair function, and when they exceed the capacity of family or caregivers to provide care in the home setting.

IMMOBILITY

Finally, immobility often precipitates a change in where a person can live. Disabled persons who need to be lifted or require more than one person's assistance to move can rarely be accommodated in their own homes. The additional help of multiple staff that are available at some ALFs or at nursing homes makes these better choices for the severely mobility-impaired.

As noted, there are wide variations in what kinds of patients can be accommodated at various locations. Through case-management services and as-needed in-home care, which is paid for almost entirely out-of-pocket, many people with serious chronic diseases or functional limitations are able to remain at home. Some ALFs are able to provide help with ADLs at an additional cost, or have dementia units that permit those with even severe disease to avoid nursing home placement. In addition, continuing-care retirement communities (also called "life care communities") offer a range of services and living options, from independent living through nursing home care, on one campus. In this manner, patients can transition to more or less assistance as needed, and couples can live on the same campus, albeit in different facilities. These are typically very expensive but provide the peace of mind that all services can and will be provided for the remainder of the person's life, at one site.

Ultimately, the decision of where a patient with chronic illness resides depends on the individual combination of medical disease burden, functional impairment, personal preferences, and resources. Decision-making must balance the ethical principle of patient autonomy with patient safety. However, frequently financial considerations are important in the decision-making process. The medical components of long-term care (e.g., home health physical therapy, medications, and some disease-management programs) are generally covered through insurance (e.g., Medicare for older or disabled persons) but the housing, meals, and personal assistance (including custodial care at nursing homes) are not covered unless people have purchased long-term care insurance or

qualify for Medicaid, and must be paid for out-of-pocket. In contrast, post–acute medical care at SNFs or through home health agencies, which can be provided either at home or in ALFs, is covered at least partially by insurance (see below). Most private long-term-care (LTC) insurance covers community-based services, while Medicaid coverage is mainly for nursing homes and often does not cover community-based services. Those who do not meet the income and asset limits for Medicaid or do not have private means or private LTC insurance must "spend down" both financially and personally (i.e., the patient runs out of money and caregivers run out of energy and patience), and the patient must be placed in a nursing home with Medicaid covering the costs.

Another important issue in chronic care is the coordination of transitions between sites. As noted above, care can be provided in a variety of sites. Based on the status of their health conditions and how well their current environment is able to cope with acute and chronic changes, people with chronic conditions frequently move from one site to another. Figure 83.1 describes the transitions between sites based on the acuity of conditions, including flares and decompensation of stable chronic diseases.

Persons with chronic conditions who live in the community or at nursing homes may develop acute illnesses or flares of their chronic conditions and require hospitalization. Following hospitalization, they may return home, to other residential facilities in the community, or to nursing homes for post-acute or chronic care. In addition, when living in the community, they may receive specific disease- or case-management. Each of these transitions is an opportunity for discontinuity of care and for mistakes to occur. For example, when a person residing in an assisted living facility is hospitalized, the person's specific medications may not be on the hospital formulary, and substitutions may be made.

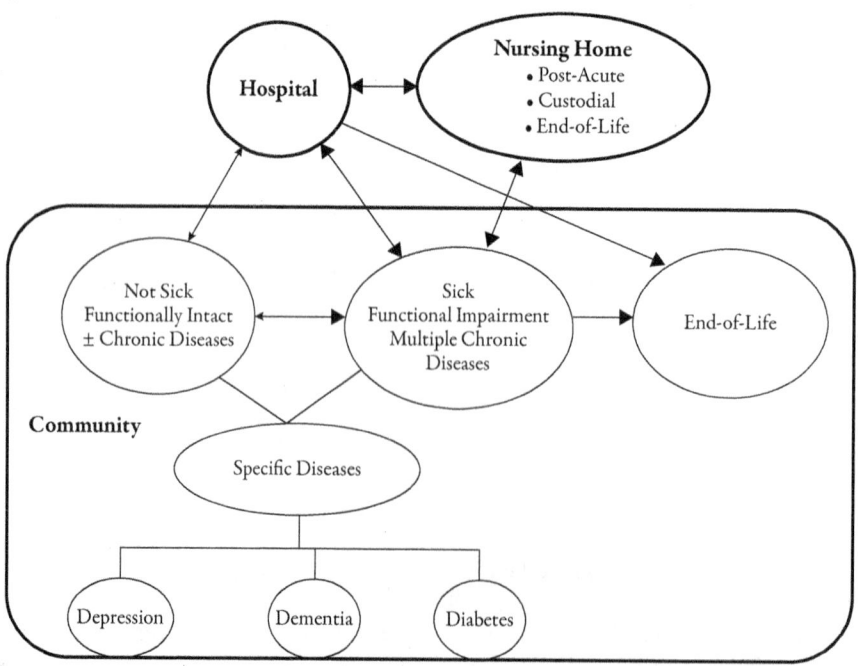

Figure 83.1 Transitions between sites of care based on acuity of illness, chronic conditions, and functional status.

At the time of discharge, the person may be discharged with the substituted medications, and the patient may mistakenly take both. Similarly, appointments that were scheduled for the time during the hospitalization may be missed and not rescheduled. Primary care physicians and other healthcare providers may not be notified of the hospitalization or not be sent a timely discharge summary. As larger healthcare systems coalesce and begin to assume a greater proportion of care under structures such as Accountable Care Organizations, such tracking and communication will become easier. In addition, some electronic health records can span across systems and perform functions such as notifying all providers on a patient's team that he or she has been seen in the emergency department or hospitalized.

MEDICAL AND PSYCHIATRIC CARE IN LONG-TERM-CARE SETTINGS

PROVIDER INVOLVEMENT

The efforts and experiences of multiple providers are necessary to provide coordinated, efficient, and safe care to patients who live in various LTC settings. These providers include generalist physicians (family practitioners and general internists), SNF physicians, psychiatrists with special interests in the problems encountered in LTC—including medical psychiatrists, geriatric psychiatrists, neuropsychiatrists, and psychologists.

Generalist physicians practice in various settings, including single-specialty medical offices, multi-specialty clinics, and hospital-based practices. Although some may visit and provide care for patients in their independent or ALFs, typically patients living at these facilities travel to the physicians' offices for their care. However, there are exceptions when a facility is large enough to have either a full-time or a part-time physician who follows patients on-site. Generalist physicians differ in their willingness to follow patients into the nursing home. The Medicare requirements (monthly visits for the first 90 days, and visits every 60 days thereafter) and the inconvenience of traveling to a nursing home to see just a few patients often cause physicians to decide to stop following their patients once they become long-stay nursing home residents. Patients whose primary care physicians do not practice in SNFs can be followed by the medical director of the facility or by other physicians who go to that nursing home. A new and increasing trend is for some physicians to focus their practices on providing care in skilled nursing facilities; these physicians are called "SNFists." Another trend is for hospitalists to follow patients after discharge from the hospital into post–acute care NFs; these hospitalists are called "extensivists" (Reuben, 2011).

When transferring a patient from a hospital to a SNF, three components are necessary (Reuben, Herr, et al., 2011):

- An interfacility transfer form including discharge medications, discontinuation dates for short-term medications, and any dosage changes in all medications;

- A discharge summary that includes the patient's baseline functional status, important tests for which results are pending, and needed next steps, including physician follow-up appointments;

- Verbal physician-to-physician sign-out to ensure that any questions that the receiving physician has can be answered.

Following these steps ensures a safe "handoff" of the patient, and helps apprise the receiving physician of any important discussions that may have previously occurred among the patient, patient's family, and primary provider. Some of these discussions may have focused on the patient's advance directives and goals of care, which will influence the nursing home's management of the patient. Several programs to ensure good care transitions to nursing homes and home have been developed and evaluated (Naylor, Brooten, et al., 1999; Coleman, Parry, et al., 2006). The Care Transitions Program includes a personal health record, a discharge preparation checklist, and transition coaches who work with patients/caregivers prior to and after the transition to SNF or home settings (Naylor, Brooten, et al., 1999). In the transitional care model, a transitional care nurse bridges hospital and post-discharge care by providing continuity of care in both settings (Centers for Disease Control, 2013). Because best practices for communication at the time of transition from the hospital are not always followed, a good rule is for the psychiatrist consulting on a patient recently admitted to a SNF to review the handoff process and see if there were errors or omissions. On the hospital side, the inpatient consulting psychiatrist can personally oversee the handoff and make sure that the psychiatric aspects are handled well.

Approximately two-thirds of patients in SNFs have mental disorder diagnoses (Centers for Disease Control, 2013) such as dementia (with or without behavioral disturbances), anxiety disorders, various forms of depression, and sleep disorders. These diagnoses often are not made or not recorded in the hospital prior to discharge to a SNF—even when there are several psychotropic drugs on the patient's discharge medication list. Another role for the consulting psychiatrist in improving care transitions is ensuring that psychiatric diagnoses are recorded early in the SNF stay; the psychiatrist can act either on the hospital or the SNF side of the care transition.

PAYMENT

In the United States, at least 70% of people over age 65 will at some point receive care in a skilled nursing home; typically, post–acute care or rehabilitation following hospitalization for acute medical illness, surgery, or trauma (Department of Veterans Affairs, August 2011). In contrast to acute hospital services, a significant proportion of fees for nursing home services are paid out-of-pocket by patients and their families. In addition to such private payment, there are five main sources of payment for nursing home services: fee-for-service Medicare, Medicaid, managed-care plans combining Medicare with other payment sources, private LTC insurance, and private health insurance.

Medicare is a federal health insurance program for people age 65 and older and for those under age 65 receiving Social Security disability benefits or with end-stage renal disease (ESRD) on hemodialysis. It is administered by the Centers for Medicare and Medicaid Services (CMS). Qualification is based on age or disability and not on income or assets. Medicare is divided into parts that cover different types of medical services. Medicare Part A covers institutional care in hospitals, SNFs, LTACHs, and IRFs, as well as home nursing care (but not home ADL support) and hospice. Medicare Part B covers professional fees of physicians; physical, occupational and speech therapists; clinical social workers providing mental health services; psychologists; nurse practitioners and physicians' assistants; laboratory tests; outpatient diagnostic procedures; and durable medical equipment. Medicare Part D covers certain prescription medications (Centers for Medicare & Medicaid Services, August 2011). Each part of Medicare has complex rules determining the scope and duration of coverage. Of great importance for SNF care, Medicare covers in full only the first 20 days of a SNF stay; after that, the patient is responsible for a 20% copayment. Of note, many patients and families often have the erroneous belief that Medicare covers SNF services in the same way that it covers hospital care; further details about the "three midnights" requirement, copayments, and limitations of SNF services are in discussed in subsequent paragraphs below (See Table 83.3).

In the Balanced Budget Act of 1997, Congress mandated that most of the services (including rehabilitation, medications, and laboratory tests) provided to patients in a Medicare-covered stay at a SNF be covered in a bundled prospective payment system (PPS). The PPS uses the Minimum Data Set (MDS), which is described later in this chapter, to calculate a Resource Utilization Group (RUG) for each Medicare beneficiary. Each RUG has a dollar amount associated with it that is the daily rate paid to a SNF for a beneficiary. SNFs bill the Medicare Administrative Contractor (MAC) for the consolidated services. During Medicare Part A–covered stays, medical services (including rehabilitation therapy, medications, and laboratory tests) as well as room-and-board are covered. If Medicare Part A benefits have been exhausted, then medical services are still covered by Medicare Part B, but room-and-board is not. There are several services that are excluded from bundled billing in the skilled nursing home. For patients covered under Medicare Part A, services excluded from bundled payment (i.e., separately payable) include the following:

- Physician's professional services
- Some dialysis-related services, including covered ambulance transportation services to dialysis centers
- Some ambulance services, including ambulance transfer from hospital to SNF, transport from SNF to home, transfers from SNF to specified types of emergency or intensive outpatient hospital services, transfer to dialysis centers for dialysis services
- Erythropoietin for some dialysis patients

- Some chemotherapy drugs
- Some chemotherapy administration services
- Radioisotope services
- Customized prosthetic devices

For patients who are not covered under a Medicare Part A stay, only therapy services are subject to consolidated billing (Centers for Medicare & Medicaid Services, August 2011). While some chemotherapy drugs are excluded from bundled payment, expensive pain medications, psychotropic drugs, and certain expensive antibiotics are not. High-cost medications can result in a net loss of revenue for SNFs who care for patients with multiple comorbidities.

To qualify for Part A Medicare coverage for a nursing home stay, patients must meet the following criteria:

1. Patient was hospitalized (i.e., admitted to the hospital, not merely held for observation) for at least three consecutive midnights in the 30 days preceding the admission to the nursing home;

2. Nursing home must be a certified skilled nursing facility (SNF);

3. A physician must certify that patient is medically benefiting from *daily* skilled care;

4. The reason for admission to SNF is a condition that was treated during the hospital stay (Centers for Medicare & Medicaid Services, August 2011).

Of note, a patient may have multiple comorbidities, such as deconditioning, gait disorder, and muscular weakness, which would qualify for SNF stay although these comorbidities might not be the primary diagnosis during the hospital stay; CMS does not deny Medicare reimbursements to the SNF in these situations.

There are several limitations to Medicare coverage. Although Medicare allows for a maximum of 100 days of nursing home benefit each year, only about 18% of patients receiving Medicare will actually use all 100 days in that year (Centers for Medicare & Medicaid Services, August 2011). The Medicare requirement that the patient is medically benefiting (i.e., demonstrates continued improvement and would gain from further treatment) usually limits the nursing home coverage to a period of 10–20 days for rehabilitation of most medical conditions (Centers for Medicare & Medicaid Services, August 2011). However, there are exceptions (e.g., stroke rehabilitation). In addition, the consulting psychiatrist can help by indicating improvements in the patient's mental health conditions that are the result of skilled care delivered by the facility. If the patient has exhausted Medicare coverage, either because of lack of benefit or because of reaching the maximum days of coverage, patients will typically switch to Medicaid or private pay. As mentioned above, Medicare does not cover the costs for custodial care in assisted living, board-and-care, or NFs. Although home health services for valid medical indications are covered by Medicare Part A for limited time periods, caregiver assistance in the home is not (Centers for Medicare & Medicaid Services, August 2011).

Medicaid is state-level government health insurance for patients with low income and limited assets. Although each state manages its own Medicaid system, most of the funds for Medicaid programs come from the federal government. As mentioned above, in order to qualify for Medicaid, patients must meet certain financial criteria, requiring them to "spend down" their assets and commit their most of their Social Security income to their LTC. However, laws intended to prevent impoverishment of non-disabled spouses may allow families to retain assets and income while still having Medicaid pay for the patient's LTC (Centers for Medicare & Medicaid Services, August 2011). Medicaid provides coverage for nursing home care in either a SNF or a NF; however, not all facilities are Medicaid-certified, and not all beds in a SNF are necessarily Medicaid-certified. In many states, Medicaid also provides coverage for custodial care ALFs. There is no limit on the period of time that Medicaid will pay for necessary custodial care in certified settings. Medications are also covered, but drug formularies are restricted, and prior authorizations may be required for medications commonly prescribed by psychiatrists, including second-generation antipsychotic drugs and non-generic antidepressants. In many states, Medicaid also provides some coverage for in-home assistance for patients needing custodial care. However, this coverage is usually is limited to 20 hours per week or less. Some states permit relatives to receive funds for providing this care, whereas other states preclude relatives from receiving funds for caregiving (Centers for Medicare & Medicaid Services, August 2011).

Medicare and Medicaid can help offset a large percentage of the cost of LTC, but a significant proportion (about 30%) (Centers for Medicare & Medicaid Services, August 2011) of the overall costs of LTC are paid out-of-pocket (private pay), which presents a burdensome challenge for many patients and their families.

KEY PROBLEMS IN LONG-TERM CARE

MEDICAL PROBLEMS

Functional Impairment and Immobility

Functional impairment and the need for assistance are common reasons for nursing home placement. Virtually all (97%) nursing home residents require help in at least one ADL (Centers for Disease Control & Prevention, August 28, 2011). Immobility is a major problem among nursing home residents. Only 21% of nursing home residents are able to transfer independently, and 23% are totally dependent in this activity. Only 16% receive no help in walking. Assistive devices (e.g., canes and walkers) are helpful, but their value is limited for many patients in nursing homes. Canes are inappropriate for those with moderate or severe balance disorders or who need to bear substantial weight on the assistive device. In general, front-wheeled walkers are safest and are the most commonly used assistive device in nursing homes for frail elderly patients. Immobility, in turn, predisposes to incontinence (see below) and pressure ulcers as well as other complications of deconditioning.

Overall, 12% of nursing home residents have pressure ulcers, and there is an inverse relationship with age, perhaps because younger nursing home residents often have more severe medical conditions such as spinal cord injury (Centers for Disease Control & Prevention, August 28, 2011). Mental status, including depression and delirium, have been identified as risk factors for development of pressure ulcers in some studies (Coleman, Gorecki, et al., 2013), but it is unknown whether treating these conditions reduces the ulcer risk. Moreover, whether pressure sores are preventable remains a controversial issue (Thomas, 2006).

Incontinence

The majority of nursing home residents are incontinent: 16% bladder only, 5% bowel only, and 43% bowel and bladder (dual incontinence) (Centers for Disease Control & Prevention, August 2011). Almost all nursing home residents with dual incontinence have impaired cognition and mobility. Despite having similar ages and numbers of conditions to those with urinary or no incontinence, those with dual incontinence have significantly fewer days of hospital care (Chiang, Ouslander, et al., 2000). This suggests that this group receives less aggressive treatment.

Bladder incontinence has several specific medical causes superimposed on physiological changes of bladder functioning with aging, such as reduction in bladder capacity, uninhibited contractions, decreased urinary flow rate, diminished urethral pressure profile, and increased post-void residual volume. Transient and reversible causes of urinary incontinence include urinary tract infection and polyuria from uncontrolled diabetes. Established urinary incontinence has four major types:

- Urge incontinence due to uninhibited bladder contraction, which may be due to local factors (e.g., stones, infections, tumors) or central factors (e.g., stroke or other central nervous system conditions). Urgency symptoms (e.g., "Do you experience such a strong and sudden urge to void that you leak before reaching the toilet?") are sensitive and specific for the diagnosis of urge incontinence (Holroyd-Leduc, Tannenbaum, et al., 2008).

- Stress incontinence due to increased abdominal pressure (e.g., during coughing and sneezing) exceeding the ability of sphincter closure mechanisms, most commonly due to inadequate pelvic support in women or following prostate surgery in men.

- Overflow incontinence due to impaired contractility of the bladder (e.g., due to diabetic neuropathy, spinal disease) or obstruction (e.g., due to prostatic hyperplasia or urethral stricture).

- Mixed incontinence, which is a combination of stress and urge incontinence.

Another type, functional incontinence, is of special importance in nursing homes. In this type, patients are incontinent because of immobility and the inability to get to the toilet or delays in receiving toileting assistance, rather than because of intrinsic bladder dysfunction.

The treatment of urinary incontinence is based on the type of incontinence, with behavioral approaches (e.g., bladder training, timed voiding, Kegel's exercises) being preferred for stress and urge incontinence, medications for urge incontinence, and intermittent catheterization for overflow incontinence. For cognitively impaired nursing home residents, a trial of prompted voiding (asking patients if they would like to go to the toilet at scheduled times) may be successful and can be combined with medications. Surgical procedures, neuromodulation, and botulinum toxin injections may be helpful in selected cases. Depending upon local availability, these may be performed by a urologist who has expertise in managing incontinence, or by a uro-gynecologist.

Falls

Up to 75% of nursing home residents fall annually, and the rate of falling is 1.5 falls per nursing home bed per year (Rubenstein, Josephson, et al., 1994). About one-third of falls occur in non-ambulatory residents (Thapa, Brockman, et al., 1996). In addition to weakness, gait disorders, and functional impairment, medications, especially psychotropic medications, are associated with falling in nursing home residents (Mustard & Mayer, 1997; Ray, Thapa, et al., 2000; Centers for Disease Control & Prevention, August 28, 2011). In particular, during the first four days after changes (either initiation or increasing the dose) in antidepressant medications (other than serotonergic reuptake inhibitors) nursing home residents are at higher risk of falls (Berry, Zhang, et al., 2011). All classes of psychotropic drug have been associated with increased risk of fall. Selective serotonin-reuptake inhibitors (SSRIs), tricyclic antidepressants, and antipsychotics are all associated with increased risk of falls (Thapa, Gideon, et al., 1998; Blair & Grumen, 2005; Echt, Samelson, et al., 2013). In general, tricyclic antidepressants should be avoided if possible in geriatric patients—even in the absence of orthostatic hypotension—due to their increased risk of adverse, anticholinergic effects, including constipation, dry mouth, dry eyes, urine retention, and confusion. There are very few studies evaluating risk of fall with use of buproprion alone. One study showed that subjects on paroxetine who had augmentation with buproprion have higher risk of a fall; however, the study was limited by the small number of participants who received buproprion (Joo, Lenze, et al., 2002). Restraints do not reduce the risk of falling and may increase the risk of falls with injuries (adjusted odds-ratio 1.34) but this estimate is based on observational studies with propensity score adjustments rather than on clinical trials (Castle & Engberg, 2009). Paradoxically, elimination of restraints may reduce the risk of falling (Ejaz, Jones, et al., 1994). Restraints such as bilateral bed rails, belts, and fixed tables and do not significantly decrease risk of fall and fall-related fractures (Köpke, Mühlhauser, et al., 2012). In a longitudinal, prospective clinical trial, bilateral side-rail use showed no decreased risk of falls or recurrent falls when adjusted for cognition and functional and behavioral status (adjusted odds-ratio 1.13) (Capezuti, Maislin, et al., 2002). Nevertheless, restraints may be indicated when an agitated patient is at risk of harming her- or himself or others. If bedrails are utilized, half-rails should be chosen over full bed rails to minimize risk of potential fall-related injuries. Psychiatrists may help with determination of whether there is an indication for restraints and whether a patient can refuse restraints. Multidisciplinary and multifactorial approaches to falls prevention, often including supervised exercise programs, are used, though the evidence for their effectiveness in nursing homes is limited (Cameron, Murray, et al., 2010).

Other Conditions and Comorbidities

Most people living in nursing homes have several diseases. Among the most common medical disorders are hypertension (53%), musculoskeletal disorder (45%), heart disease (42%), diabetes (24%), and anemia (19%) (Centers for Disease Control, August 28, 2011). Some of these diseases (e.g., hypertension, diabetes, and heart disease) require medications that can interact and cause adverse events. Others (e.g., musculoskeletal disorders) contribute to immobility and functional impairment. The long-term benefit of treatment of conditions such as osteoporosis and hyperlipidemia must also be considered in the context of a shortened lifespan (i.e., will the patient survive long enough to accrue the benefits of treatment?) and weighed against the adverse effects of treatment. In some instances (e.g., target Hemoglobin A_1c [HbA_1C] levels for elderly diabetics, systolic blood pressure), the target levels for patients with limited life expectancy may be different from those for younger and more robust older persons, since aggressive management may lead to adverse events, such as increased risk of hypoglycemia, falls, or mortality Discussions about whether to treat and how aggressively should occur with patients if they have capacity to make these decisions, or with proxies if they do not.

Polypharmacy

Almost half (48%) of nursing home residents take nine or more medications, and only 13% take four or fewer medications (Centers for Disease Control, August 28, 2011). The number of medications and a history of prior adverse drug events are major predictors of adverse drug reactions. Hospitalized older persons prescribed four or more meds have a 1.9-fold increased risk of adverse drug reactions, and those receiving eight or more drugs are at a four-fold risk (Onder, Petrovic, et al., 2010). In a study of two academic LTC facilities, the overall rate of adverse drug events (ADEs) was 9.8 per 100 resident-months; 42% of the ADEs were deemed preventable. The more serious the adverse event, the more likely it was to be considered potentially preventable. The most likely drugs causing ADEs were antipsychotics (adjusted odds-ratio [aOR] 3.0), anticoagulants (aOR 2.8), diuretics (aOR 2.3), and anticonvulsants (aOR 2.0) (Gurwitz, Field, et al., 2005).

The best way to avoid adverse drug reactions is to review medications regularly and, before prescribing a new medication, including checking for potential interactions, start a low dose and titrate based on tolerability and response; and avoid medications that are high-risk in older persons. A detailed list is provided in the 2012 Beers Criteria (American Geriatrics Society 2012 Beers Criteria Update Expert Panel, 2012). The time of transition between settings of care is an opportunity to review medications and discontinue medications if harms outweigh benefits, there is minimal or no effectiveness, there is no ongoing indication for the medication, or the medication is not being taken.

PSYCHIATRIC PROBLEMS

All patients seeking admission to Medicaid-certified NFs must complete a Preadmission Screening Residential Review (PASRR), regardless of whether the stay will be paid for by Medicaid, Medicare, or other resources. The PASRR (formerly called PASARR—Preadmission Screening and Annual Resident Review) determines whether a patient with a diagnosis of mental illness or intellectual or developmental disability meets criteria for admission to a SNF and the type of needed specialized services (New Hampshire Department of Health and Human Services, March 2013). Mandated by the federal government in 1989, it was implemented in 1990. The annual evaluation requirement was eliminated in 1997 after many states felt it posed undue financial burdens (Dual Diagnosis Management Ascend [DDM Ascend], March 18, 2013).

Psychiatric disorders encountered in LTC settings include preexisting mental illnesses and mental and behavioral problems that newly arise in the LTC setting. In the first category, it is important to identify an LTC setting that is comfortable with caring for patients with certain preexisting mental illnesses. Nursing homes, ALFs, and home care agencies differ in their comfort with mentally ill or behaviorally disturbed patients and in their ability to provide access to psychiatric and psychological services. At a minimum, home care agencies should be able to provide psychological services through either a clinical psychologist or a clinical social worker. Many nursing homes are able to provide access to an in-house psychiatrist, and some can offer access to a psychologist.

In the latter category, the most common reasons for referral are:

1. delirium due to new drugs or withdrawal of old ones, or to the development of a new medical condition;

2. behavioral disturbances—usually occurring in cognitively impaired people—because of untreated pain or discomfort, because of abuse or mistreatment by staff, other residents (of a facility) or by family members;

3. depression or anxiety occurring as a reaction to a change in living arrangements, specifically, placement in a nursing home or a move to an assisted living facility or the home of a family member.

The relative frequency of each of these is unknown, and a systematic approach may be helpful to distinguish among them. Such an approach begins with a review of the patient's medication list, focusing on newly started or recently discontinued medications. If no obvious precipitant is identified, then causes such as pain and depression or anxiety should be sought. Although many brief pain scales are available, some may be inappropriate for cognitively impaired patients, and collateral informants (e.g., nursing home staff, family) should be obtained to assess whether there are other signs of pain (e.g., grimacing). For depression, the Patient Health Questionnaire-9 (PHQ-9) has been validated in nursing home settings. (Saliba, DiFilippo, et al., 2012). If an explanation cannot be found, or if there are signs of injury (e.g., skin tears or bruises), then the possibility of elder abuse must be considered and investigated.

Use of restraints, chemical and physical, is highly regulated in SNFs. Physicians are required to attempt gradual dose reductions of all psychotropics used in SNFs since psychotropics are considered chemical restraints. Even patients who have been on long-standing use of antidepressants without adverse effects need documented attempts of gradual dose reductions. If a physician believes that gradual dose reduction will be more harmful than beneficial to the patient, then documentation of potential harms (e.g., clinical decompensation) is necessary. Note, however, that all chemical and physical restraints in SNFs need informed consent from the patient or his or her responsible party. Use of psychotropics in ALFs and board-and-care homes are not under as strict regulations as in the nursing home, because ALFs and board-and-care homes are not federally regulated.

Sleep Disorders

Changes in sleep patterns are part of normal aging, but they can be a problem for elderly patients who consider good sleep an important part of their quality of life. These physiological changes include decreased sleep time, decreased sleep efficiency (time asleep divided by time in bed), and increased sleep latency.

Sleep disorders are common in older adults. Common sleep complaints include having difficulty falling asleep, nighttime awakening, early morning awakening, and daytime sleepiness. Risk factors associated with sleep disorders include underlying mood disorder, dementia, comorbid medical conditions, and use of multiple medications (Alessi, Martin, et al., 2005; Bloom, Ahmed, et al., 2009). In LTC settings, some modifiable factors contribute to abnormal sleep–wake patterns; these include inadequate sunlight exposure, inadequate physical activity, and disruptive nighttime environment (i.e., too much noise and/or light). Non-pharmacological interventions geared at improving these modifiable factors may be helpful in improving sleep–wake cycles in elderly patients.

Some sleep disorders are more common in the older patient, such as restless legs syndrome, periodic limb-movement disorder, sleep-related breathing disorders (e.g., obstructive sleep apnea), and circadian rhythm sleep disorders. A sleep diary, sleep study, and/or consultation with sleep specialist may be useful in diagnosis and management of these disorders.

Many older patients take medications that may contribute to insomnia. These medications include diuretics and stimulating medications such as activating psychiatric medications, bronchodilators, and sympathomimetics. If the above medications are necessary, then they should be administered during the daytime if possible. Conversely, sedating medications should be administered at nighttime, if possible.

For most patients, behavioral approaches should be attempted first. These include stimulus control (e.g., no television watching in bed, regular bedtime, and a routine of relaxation). Other non-pharmacological approaches include cognitive-behavioral therapy, relaxation techniques, bright lights, and sleep restriction (reducing bed time to estimated sleep time and gradually increasing it). Specific treatments that are recommended in the nursing home include morning bright-light treatment, exercise (e.g., stationary bicycle) and physical activity, reduction of nighttime noise and light interruptions, a regular bedtime and a routine of pre-bedtime activities, and the reduction of stimuli at bedtime (e.g., television). Combinations of these may be helpful.

Hypnotic drugs for insomnia may be utilized when non-pharmacological approaches are unsuccessful and if benefits (e.g., quality of life, better participation in activities during the daytime) outweigh the risks. The pharmacological management of insomnia should avoid benzodiazepines, anticholinergics (e.g., tricyclic antidepressants), and antihistamines (e.g., diphenhydramine). Non-benzodiazepine hypnotics (e.g., zolpidem, zaleplon, and ezopiclone) may be helpful but should be restricted to short-term use (three to four weeks). Sometimes patients have been using benzodiazepine or non-benzodiazepine hypnotics for years without apparent adverse effects. The decision about whether to attempt to taper and discontinue these must be made on a case-by-case basis, depending upon the patient's other comorbid conditions and preferences, and considering the risks of continuing the medication. Melatonin and a receptor agonist, ramelteon, may also be helpful. Some physicians also prescribe trazodone for sleep disorders in elderly patients. If hypnotics are prescribed for insomnia, they should be prescribed initially on an as needed (P.R.N.) basis in cognitively intact patients who are able to express their needs. For patients who are cognitively impaired, it is usually at the discretion of the nursing staff when the hypnotic is administered.

Delirium

Delirium is often encountered in nursing homes and sometimes in ALFs. Patients with hypoactive delirium, in general, can be managed in these settings as long as they are hemodynamically and medically stable. However, patients with hyperactive delirium (e.g., with behavioral disturbances such as aggression resulting in potential harm to self or others) are more difficult to manage in these settings and should be transferred to the hospital.

MEASURING AND IMPROVING QUALITY IN LONG-TERM CARE SETTINGS

For more than two decades, national efforts have been underway to improve the quality of nursing home care and quality of life for its residents. The need for improvement was first nationally recognized when the Institute of Medicine published a report in 1983 documenting significant deficiencies in the care in nursing homes. These findings ultimately led to the passage of the landmark Omnibus Budget Reconciliation Act (OBRA) of 1987. OBRA set forth new, higher standards of care in NFs that are reimbursed by Medicare and Medicaid via the Centers for Medicare and Medicaid Services (CMS), an agency of the U.S. Department of Health and Human Services (DHHS). CMS has multiple responsibilities, including paying Medicare claims, writing regulations for Medicaid that are administered by each state's Medicaid program, and interpreting legislation into written regulations for SNFs. For SNFs to be reimbursed by Medicare and Medicaid, they must comply with regulations set forth by CMS (Centers for Medicare & Medicaid Services, August 2011).

In November 2002, the CMS began the national Nursing Home Quality Initiative (NHQI) to provide information that allows consumers, providers, and researchers to compare the quality of care provided in nursing homes in the United States. Nursing home quality measures assess the residents' condition (physical, clinical, and mental), capabilities, limitations, and preferences about resuscitation. These measures are obtained from data that nursing homes collect in a standardized manner on their residents at specified intervals during their stay, the Minimum Data Set (MDS) (Saliba & Buchanan, 2008). MDS measures are assessed, monitored, and reported publicly on the CMS website. The MDS allows a particular nursing home to identify its strengths and pinpoint areas needing improvement.

The MDS 3.0, implemented in October 2010, is the latest version and has major updates of the MDS 2.0 (Alessi, Martin, et al., 2005). The MDS 3.0 has improved reliability and validity compared to MDS 2.0. It is more clinically relevant and allows nursing home residents to have a voice by including a direct resident interview, which was not mandatory in MDS 2.0. It also includes improvements in various assessment sections. MDS 3.0 has a new delirium assessment section using the CAM; improved depression assessment using the PHQ-9 (an interview version for verbal patients, and a staff observational version for patients who cannot complete the interview); improved cognitive assessment using the Brief Interview for Mental Status (BIMS), which is highly correlated with the Mini-Mental State Examination; and a new Patient Preference tool (PAT) to evaluate a patient's preferences and views regarding quality of life. The MDS 3.0 also includes revisions in the following content areas: behavior symptoms, continence, pain, and ADLs. The MDS 3.0 also differs from the MDS 2.0 in that the data are transmitted to a federal (rather than state) data-collection system.

In June 2011, the National Quality Forum (NQF) endorsed 17 nursing home quality measures derived from the MDS that nursing homes collect and submit (Centers

Table 83.3 MEDICARE COVERAGE IN SKILLED NURSING FACILITIES

SERVICE	MEDICARE COVERS	PATIENT AND/OR FAMILY PAYS
Skilled nursing for days 1–20	All eligible expenses	Nothing
Skilled nursing for days 21–100	All eligible expenses after patient pays daily copayment	Daily copayment*
Skilled nursing for days 100+	Nothing	Everything

*Medicare supplemental insurance (MedSup or Medigap) may cover some or all of Medicare's copayments and/or deductibles.

Adapted from *Guide to Long-Term Care: Who Pays for Long Term Care?* Available at http://www.guidetolongtermcare.com/whopays.html (accessed August 2011).

for Medicare & Medicaid Services, September 19, 2011). The NQF is an organization representing consumers, purchasers, providers, and researchers, and helps establish standards of care (National Quality Forum, September 19, 2011). The nursing home quality measures that are endorsed are outlined in Table 83.4.

Each nursing home's quality measures and the results of surveys are publicly available at the Nursing Home Compare website, http://www.medicare.gov/NursingHomeCompare/search.aspx?bhcp=1. Specifically, consumers can get the following information about individual nursing homes from the website:

- Five-star quality ratings of overall performance and individual performance on health inspection surveys, quality measures, and hours of care provided per resident by staff performing nursing care tasks.

- Health inspection results and complaints, detailed and summary information about deficiencies found during the three most recent state inspections, and recent complaint investigations.

- Nursing home staffing information about the number of registered nurses, licensed practical or vocational nurses, physical therapists, and nursing assistants in each nursing home.

- A set of quality measures that describe the quality of care in nursing homes (e.g., percent of residents with pressure sores, percent of residents with urinary incontinence).

- Any penalties and enforcement actions against a nursing home.

Additionally, state survey agencies are mandated to visit nursing homes at least once annually and as needed (if there are deficiencies or complaints to the state) to inspect and assess the quality of care provided in nursing homes. The state survey agency visits are typically unannounced. If a nursing home does not meet regulatory standards of care, then it is cited with a deficiency, which carries penalties including monetary fines and, in the worst-case scenario, the nursing home's closure. There are also Long-Term Care Ombudsmen available whom nursing home residents and their families, friends, and caregivers can contact if they have any concerns about the quality of care that is being provided in their nursing home. The MDS, state surveyors, and ombudsman programs are all part of an ongoing national effort to improve the quality of care provided in nursing home settings.

A similar effort aimed adults receiving home health care, the Outcome and ASessment Information Set (OASIS), contains items assessing cognitive function ability/ confusion, anxiety, or depression, as well as demonstrated cognitive,

Table 83.4 QUALITY MEASURES IN NURSING HOMES

SHORT-STAY QUALITY MEASURES	LONG-STAY QUALITY MEASURES
• % residents on scheduled pain medication regimen on admission who report decrease in pain intensity or frequency • % residents who self-report moderate to severe pain • % residents with pressure ulcers that are new or worsened • % residents assessed and given, appropriately, seasonal influenza vaccine • % residents assessed and given, appropriately, pneumococcal vaccine	• % residents experiencing one or more falls with major injury • % residents who self-report moderate to severe pain • % high-risk residents with pressure ulcers • % long-stay residents assessed and given, appropriately, the seasonal influenza vaccine • % long-stay residents assessed and given, appropriately, the pneumococcal vaccine • % long-stay residents with a urinary tract infection • % low-risk residents who lose control of their bowels or bladder • % residents who have/had a catheter inserted and left in their bladder • % residents who were physically restrained • % residents whose need for help with daily activities has increased • % long-stay residents who lose too much weight • % residents who have depressive symptoms

Adapted from Centers for Medicare and Medicaid's *Nursing Home Quality Initiatives: Quality Measures.* Available at https://www.cms.gov/NursingHomeQualityInits/10_NHQIQualityMeasures.asp#TopOfPage (accessed August 2011).

behavioral, and psychiatric symptoms. Like the MDS, psychiatric symptoms can be used by clinicians to detect psychiatric problems. However, these instruments are valuable clinically only if the information is brought to the attention of the clinicians and probed deeper. The OASIS is also limited because patients tend to receive home health services for only short periods of time.

Although similar federal efforts have not been applied to other LTC settings (e.g., assisted living and other residential facilities), perhaps in the future, these settings will also be the focus of quality improvement efforts. ALFs and home care agencies are currently regulated only at the state level; there is no rating system as yet for them. The Assisted Living Federation of America (ALFA) is an organization that monitors the assisted living statutes in each state and provides an updated contact for the licensing organization in each state, in an effort to help providers become aware of the licensing requirements and regulations. The website can be found accessed at http://www.alfa.org (ALFA, March 18, 2013). Common citations by state inspectors can be found at the ALFA website (ALFA, March 18, 2013). For specific information on what type of psychiatric problems ALFs and home care agencies can handle, it is best to send specific inquires to these facilities. Nursing–patient ratio, the type of help available, presence or absence of higher levels of care within the assisted living facility, and presence and absence of a locked dementia care unit are important considerations for the patient with psychiatric issues.

CLINICAL PEARLS

- Functional status is usually considered at two levels: basic activities of daily living (ADLs) and instrumental activities of daily living (IADLs). ADLs include bathing, dressing, toileting, transferring (e.g., from a bed to a chair), maintaining continence, and feeding. IADLs include using the telephone, shopping, preparing meals, housekeeping, doing laundry, using public transportation or driving, taking medication, and handling personal finances.

- The patient's awareness of ADL or IADL deficits and their willingness to accept assistance when it is needed is related to ADL and IADL performance.

- Medications, especially psychotropic medications, are associated with falling in nursing home residents (Blair & Gumen, 2005; Cameron, Murray, et al., 2010). The rate of falling is 1.5 falls per nursing home bed per year (Cameron, Murray, et al., 2010).

- All patients seeking admission to Medicaid-certified NFs must complete a Preadmission Screening Residential Review (PASRR), regardless of whether the stay will be paid for by Medicaid, Medicare, or other resources. The PASRR determines whether a patient with a diagnosis of mental illness, intellectual or developmental disability meets criteria for admission to a SNF and the type of needed specialized services (PASRR, 2013). The Assisted Living Federation of America (ALFA) is an organization that monitors the assisted living statutes in each state and provides an updated contact for the licensing organization in each state, in an effort to help providers become aware of the licensing requirements and regulations. The website can be found accessed at http://www.alfa.org (ALFA, 2013). Common citations by state inspectors can be found at the ALFA website (see above) Each nursing home's quality measures and the results of surveys are at the Nursing Home Compare website: http://www.medicare.gov/NursingHomeCompare/search.aspx?bhcp=1.

DISCLOSURE STATEMENTS

Dr. Reuben has no conflicts to disclose. He is funded by the National Institute on Aging, the Donald W. Reynolds Foundation, and the Centers for Medicare and Medicaid Services. Dr. Hong-Phuc Tran has no conflicts to disclose.

REFERENCES

Online Sources

"ALFA: 2012 Top 10 Deficiencies." *ALFA: Creating the Future of Senior Living*. Retrieved March 18, 2013, from http://www.alfa.org/Mall/StoreHome.asp?MODE=VIEW&STID=1&LID=0&PRODID=43.

"ALFA: Assisted Living Regulations and Licensing." *ALFA: Creating the Future of Senior Living*. Retrieved March 18, 2013, from http://www.alfa.org/alfa/State_Regulations_and_Licensing_Informat.asp.

"Centers for Medicare and Medicaid Services." *Nursing Home Quality Initiatives: Quality Measures*. Retrieved August 2011, from https://www.cms.gov/NursingHomeQualityInits/10_NHQIQualityMeasures.asp#TopOfPage.

"Medicare Program: General Information." *Centers for Medicare and Medicaid Services*. Retrieved August 2011, from https://www.cms.gov/MedicareGenInfo.

"National Center for Health Statistics." *Centers for Disease Control, 2013*. Retrieved March 18, 2013 from http://www.cdc.gov/nchs/data/nnhsd/Estimates/nnhs/Estimates_Diagnoses_Tables.pdf#Table33a.

"National Quality Forum." Retrieved September 19, 2011, from http://www.qualityforum.org/About_NQF/About_NQF.aspx.

"Nursing Home Quality." *Centers for Medicare & Medicaid Services*. Retrieved September 19, 2011, from https://www.cms.gov/NursingHomeQualityInits/10_NHQIQualityMeasures.asp.

"Overview on Skilled Nursing Facility (SNF) Consolidated Billing (CB)." *Centers for Medicare and Medicaid Services*. Retrieved August 2011, from http://www.cms.gov/SNFConsolidatedBilling.

"PASRR (Formerly PASAAR) Requirements and Links." *Dual Diagnosis Management (DDM) Ascend Website*. Retrieved March 18, 2013, from http://www.ascendami.com/ascendami/managedcare/pasrrrequirements.aspx.

"The Preadmission Screening Residential Review." *New Hampshire Department of Health and Human Services*. Retrieved March 18, 2013, from http://www.dhhs.nh.gov/dcbcs/bds/pasarr.htm.

"Program of All-Inclusive Care for the Elderly (PACE)." *SAMHSA's National Registry of Evidence-Based Programs and Practices*. Retrieved March 17, 2013, from http://www.nrepp.samhsa.gov/ViewIntervention.aspx?id=162.

"Research, Statistics, Data and Systems: National Health Expenditure Data (Aggregate Data for 2003–2009)." *Centers for Medicare and Medicaid Services.* Retrieved August 2011, from https://www.cms.gov/nationalhealthexpendData/downloads/tables.pdf.

"Table 15 in 2004 Current Resident Tables—Estimates." *Centers for Disease Control and Prevention.* Retrieved August 28, 2011 from http://www.cdc.gov/nchs/nnhs/resident_tables_estimates.htm#FunctionalStatus.

"Table 16 in 2004 Current Resident Tables—Estimates." *Centers for Disease Control and Prevention.* Retrieved August 28, 2011, from http://www.cdc.gov/nchs/nnhs/resident_tables_estimates.htm#FunctionalStatus.

"Table 27 in 2004 Current Resident Tables—Estimates." *Centers for Disease Control and Prevention.* Retrieved August 28, 2011, from http://www.cdc.gov/nchs/data/nnhsd/Estimates/nnhs/Estimates_QualityOfLife_Tables.pdf#Table27

"Table 33b in Estimates Diagnoses Tables." *Centers for Disease Control and Prevention.* Retrieved August 28, 2011, from http://www.cdc.gov/nchs/data/nnhsd/Estimates/nnhs/Estimates_Diagnoses_Tables.pdf#Table33a.

"Table 39 in Estimates Diagnoses Tables." *Centers for Disease Control and Prevention.* Retrieved August 28, 2011, from http://www.cdc.gov/nchs/data/nnhsd/Estimates/nnhs/Estimates_Diagnoses_Tables.pdf#Table39.

"U.S. Government Medicare Website." *Centers for Medicare & Medicaid Services.* Retrieved August 12, 2011, from http://www.medicare.gov/Glossary/l.html.

"U.S. Government Medicare Website." *Centers for Medicare & Medicaid Services.* Retrieved March 17, 2013, from http://www.medicare.gov/longtermcare/static/home.asp.

"Who Pays for Long Term Care?" *Guide to Long-Term Care.* Retrieved August 2011, from http://www.guidetolongtermcare.com/whopays.html.

Print Sources

Alessi, C. A., Martin, J. L., et al. (2005). Randomized, controlled trial of a nonpharmacological intervention to improve abnormal sleep/wake patterns in nursing home residents. *Journal of the American Geriatric Society, 53*(5), 803–810.

American Geriatrics Society 2012 Beers Criteria Update Expert Panel (2012). American Geriatrics Society updated Beers Criteria for potentially inappropriate medication use in older adults. *Journal of the American Geriatric Society, 60*(4), 616–631.

Berry, S. D., Zhang, Y., et al. (2011). Antidepressant prescriptions: an acute window for falls in the nursing home. *Journals of Gerontology, Series A: Biological Sciences & Medical Sciences, 66*(10), 1124–1130.

Blair, E., & Grumen, C. (2005). Falls in inpatient geriatric psychiatry population. *Journal of the American Psychiatric Nurses Association, 11*(6), 351–354.

Bloom, H. G., Ahmed, I., et al. (2009). Evidence-based recommendations for the assessment and management of sleep disorders in older persons. *Journal of the American Geriatric Society, 57*(5), 761–789.

Cameron, I. D., Murray, G. R., et al. (2010). Interventions for preventing falls in older people in nursing care facilities and hospitals. *Cochrane Database of Systematic Reviews* (12), CD0005465.

Capezuti, E., Maislin, G., et al. (2002). Side rail use and bed-related fall outcomes among nursing home residents. *Journal of the American Geriatric Society, 50*(1), 90–96.

Castle, N. G., & Engberg, J. (2009). The health consequences of using physical restraints in nursing homes. *Medical Care, 47*(11), 1164–1173.

Chiang, L., Ouslander, J., et al. (2000). Dually incontinent nursing home residents: clinical characteristics and treatment differences. *Journal of the American Geriatric Society, 48*(6), 673–676.

Coleman, E. A., Parry, C., et al. (2006). The care transitions intervention: results of a randomized controlled trial. *Archives of Internal Medicine, 166*(17), 1822–1828.

Coleman, S., Gorecki, C., et al. (2013). Patient risk factors for pressure ulcer development: systematic review. *International Journal of Nursing Studies 50*(7), 974–1003.

Echt, M. A., Samelson, E. J., et al. (2013). Psychotropic drug initiation or increased dosage and the acute risk of falls: a prospective cohort study of nursing home residents. *BioMed Central Geriatrics, 13,* 19.

Ejaz, F. K., Jones, J. A., et al. (1994). Falls among nursing home residents: an examination of incident reports before and after restraint reduction programs. *Journal of the American Geriatric Society, 42*(9), 960–964.

Eng, C., Pedulla, J., et al. (1997). Program of All-inclusive Care for the Elderly (PACE): an innovative model of integrated geriatric care and financing. *Journal of the American Geriatric Society, 45*(2), 223–232.

Fisher, W. H., Barreira, P. J., et al. (2001). Long-stay patients in state psychiatric hospitals at the end of the 20th century. *Psychiatric Services 52*(8), 1051–1056.

Gurwitz, J. H., Field, T. S., et al. (2005). The incidence of ADEs in two large academic long-term care facilities. *American Journal of Medicine, 118*(3), 251–258.

Holroyd-Leduc, J. M., Tannenbaum, C., et al. (2008). What type of urinary incontinence does this woman have? *Journal of the American Medical Association, 299*(12), 1446–1456.

Hung, W. W., Ross, J. S., et al. (2011). Recent trends in chronic disease, impairment and disability among older adults in the United States. *BioMed Central Geriatrics, 11,* 47.

Institute of Medicine Committee on the Future of Health Care Workforce for Older Americans (2008). *Retooling for an aging America: Building the health care workforce.* Washington, DC: The National Academies Press.

Joo, J. H., Lenze, E. J., et al. (2002). Risk factors for falls during treatment of late-life depression. *Journal of Clinical Psychiatry, 63*(10), 936–941.

Kane, R. L. (2011). Finding the right level of post-hospital care: "We didn't realize there was any other option for him." *Journal of the American Medical Association, 305*(3), 284–293.

Köpke, S., Mühlhauser, I., et al. (2012). Effect of a guideline-based multicomponent intervention on use of physical restraints in nursing homes: a randomized controlled trial. *Journal of the American Medical Association, 307*(20), 2177–2184.

Mustard, C. A., & Mayer, T. (1997). Case-control study of exposure to medication and the risk of injurious falls requiring hospitalization among nursing home residents. *American Journal of Epidemiology, 145*(8), 738–745.

Naylor, M. D., Brooten, D., et al. (1999). Comprehensive discharge planning and home follow-up of hospitalized elders: a randomized clinical trial. *Journal of the American Medical Association, 281*(7), 613–620.

Onder, G., Petrovic, M., et al. (2010). Development and validation of a score to assess risk of adverse drug reactions among in-hospital patients 65 years or older: the GerontoNet ADR risk score. *Archives of Internal Medicine, 170*(13), 1142–1148.

Ray, W. A., Thapa, P. B., et al. (2000). Benzodiazepines and the risk of falls in nursing home residents. *Journal of the American Geriatric Society, 48*(6), 682–685.

Reuben, D. B. (2011). Physicians in supporting roles in chronic disease care: the CareMore model. *Journal of the American Geriatric Society, 59*(1), 158–160.

Reuben, D. B., Herr, K. A., et al. (Eds.) (2011). *Geriatrics at your fingertips 2011.* New York: American Geriatrics Society.

Rubenstein, L. Z., Josephson, K. R., et al. (1994). Falls in the nursing home. *Annals of Internal Medicine, 121*(6), 442–451.

Saliba, D., & Buchanan, J. (2008). Rand Health Corporation: Development and validation of a revised nursing home assessment tool, MDS 3.0. Retrieved August 2011, from https://www.cms.gov/NursingHomeQualityInits/25_NHQIMDS30.asp

Saliba, D., DiFilippo, S., et al. (2012). Testing the PHQ-9 interview and observational versions (PHQ-9 OV) for MDS 3.0. *Journal of the American Medical Directors Association, 13*(7), 618–625.

Thapa, P. B., Brockman, K. G., et al. (1996). Injurious falls in nonambulatory nursing home residents: a comparative study of circumstances, incidence, and risk factors. *Journal of the American Geriatric Society*, *44*(3), 273–278.

Thapa, P. B., Gideon, P., et al. (1998). Antidepressants and the risk of falls among nursing home residents. *New England Journal of Medicine*, *339*(13), 875–882.

Thomas, D. R. (2006). Prevention and treatment of pressure ulcers. *Journal of the American Medical Directors Association*, *7*(1), 46–59.

Wagner, E. H. (1998). Chronic disease management: What will it take to improve care for chronic illness? *Effective Clinical Practice*, *1*(1), 2–4.

Wolff, J. L., Starfield, B., et al. (2002). Prevalence, expenditures, and complications of multiple chronic conditions in the elderly. *Archives of Internal Medicine*, *162*(20), 2269–2276.

84.

END-OF-LIFE ISSUES

John L. Shuster, Harvey Max Chochinov, and Natalie L. Jacobowski

INTRODUCTION

Illness causes suffering. Obviously, the most effective way to relieve suffering caused by illness is to eradicate or control the underlying disease process. Many acute-care interventions increase short-term suffering in exchange for a cure, long-term relief, or the hope of a possible cure. Even in the acute medical setting, where both patient and physician expect complete remission of symptoms or a cure to result, every treatment intervention should be tempered with attention to the suffering caused by both disease and treatment. Once the prospect of a cure becomes an unreasonable expectation, the focus of care shifts to relief and reduction of suffering, including the discomfort and pain induced by treatments themselves.

This is the palliative approach to medical care. In the broadest sense, the management of chronic or incurable illnesses (e.g., Alzheimer's disease) is essentially palliative. For many people, however, the term "palliative care" connotes the care of terminally ill patients who are receiving hospice care. A patient is "terminally ill" as defined in the United States Medicare Hospice Benefit when the patient has an expected survival of six months or less. In this setting, continued treatment aimed at cure is deemed clinically or even ethically inappropriate, since the potential benefits to the patient would not outweigh the potential risks and side effects.

PALLIATIVE CARE

The verb *palliate* means "to reduce the violence of (a disease)," or "to moderate the intensity of" a disease process (*Webster's New Collegiate Dictionary*, 1979). Root word meanings include "to shield," "to cloak," "to conceal," and "to protect." Palliative care, then, is properly understood as the means of shielding and protecting patients from the violence of disease, especially the violence of disease at the end of life. The World Health Organization (1990) defines palliative care as:

> the active total care of patients whose disease is not responsive to curative treatment. Control of pain, other symptoms, and of psychological, social, and spiritual problems, is paramount. The goal of palliative care is achievement of the best quality of life for patients and their families.

HOSPICE CARE

Hospice is a multidisciplinary approach to the care of terminally ill patients that provides comprehensive palliative care. Distinctive features of hospice care include:

- A multidisciplinary team approach to care (including the expertise of physicians, nurses, social workers, chaplains, volunteers, and others);

- The focus of care shifts from cure or survival to reducing suffering and maximizing quality of life;

- To the extent possible, the care delivered by a hospice team occurs in the patient's preferred care setting, usually at home. Hospice care can also be delivered in other settings, such as general hospitals, nursing homes, and specialized hospice or palliative medicine units;

- Care for the family is also provided, including practical assistance with care of the dying patient, maintenance of the home, and bereavement aftercare services.

In the United States, the system of hospice care provided in a patient's home generally works well, provided that the patient actually has a home, has family members who are capable and willing to provide care for the patient at home, and has symptoms that can be managed primarily by lay individuals outside the hospital setting. When these conditions are not met, home hospice care is not feasible. A growing availability of inpatient and residential hospice and palliative care is occurring in response to this need.

GOALS OF HOSPICE AND PALLIATIVE CARE

The goals of hospice care and palliative care include assuring patients they will not be abandoned, aggressive control of painful or noxious symptoms, maintenance or repair of stressed interpersonal relationships, preservation of a comforting care environment, and attention to important life goals and spiritual or religious concerns. Physicians have much to offer patients, even when expected survival is measured in months, weeks, or days. First, however, the physician's help must be offered. Every patient dreads hearing the words "There's nothing more I can do for you." Letting the patient and family know (by both words and actions) that they will not be expected to face the end of life alone is a great comfort. Seldom is the doctor–patient relationship more important. Even in the context of making a referral to an excellent hospice program, physicians should assure their patients of their ongoing involvement in and commitment to the patient's care, augmented by the expertise and resources of the hospice team.

This kind of ongoing physician involvement helps soothe possibly the greatest fear of dying patients: the process of dying is usually feared more than death itself. Worries about abandonment, helplessness, dependency, preservation of worth and dignity, and undertreated (or untreated) suffering are sources of great concern to terminally ill patients and their families. The tendency, even among many physicians, to withdraw from the terminally ill intensifies a patient's fear or dying. Dying must seem dreadful indeed, if even physicians cannot bear to attend the patient as death approaches. The converse is certainly true: when physicians demonstrate that they will not abandon their patients and stand ready to do what they can to address suffering as it arises, the process of dying is easier to bear. The control of symptoms that interfere with quality of life (e.g., pain, depression, nausea, anxiety, and fatigue) should be aggressively pursued. Relief of symptoms and suffering at the end of life should be provided with the same diligence and dedication with which cure is pursued in acute illness. Widely available and commonly accepted treatments for most end-of-life symptoms (e.g., opiates for pain, benzodiazepines for anxiety) are reliably effective. Still, not all symptoms can necessarily be relieved, even with the most expert intervention. In these instances, patients' main source of relief may be the knowledge that their physician and hospice team will continue to try to help them. Box 84.1 summarizes the principles of good symptom management at the end of life. This chapter focuses on the control of psychiatric and neuropsychiatric symptoms at the end of life. The Academy of Psychosomatic Medicine has published a position statement on psychiatric care at the end of life (Shuster et al., 1998), which readers may also wish to review.

Conflict with relatives and close friends can cause emotional suffering at the end of life. Long-standing disputes and grudges may be amenable to repair in the setting of a terminal illness. Dealing directly and confrontationally with family conflicts should occur if there is reasonable expectation of benefit from such an intervention. The strain of caring for a seriously ill and dying relative causes marked distress in a family. Acknowledgement that the task is difficult, and strategies that anticipate caretakers' becoming exhausted—the periodic respite care that is integral to the Medicare Hospice Benefit, for example—can contribute to the preservation of a comforting home environment.

The end of life can potentially be an enriching, life-affirming experience for patients and their families. If a life can be viewed in narrative terms, it will require a meaningful concluding chapter. A focus on meaningful life goals is one strategy that may be helpful to patients. For some, such goals might include feeling well enough to enjoy a wedding

---

Box 84.1 PRINCIPLES OF GOOD SYMPTOM CONTROL IN PALLIATIVE CARE

- Do not limit the use of analgesics for fear of an overdose. Start with a conservative dose and advance as rapidly as needed and tolerated, allowing for a substantial margin of safety.

- When potentially addictive drugs are used for a palliative indication, concern about addiction or dependence should be tempered by the need to provide comfort and relief. Tolerance may develop but is manageable with dose adjustments.

- Listen carefully and patiently to the patient. Use the treatment and the dose needed to provide maximum symptom control. Take the patient's report of symptom control at face value.

- Severe suffering from pain and other symptoms can occur long before a patient dies. Do not wait until the last few days of life to treat symptoms aggressively.

- A patient need not forgo a narcotic or other treatment now in order to benefit later, when the symptom gets worse. The dose may need to change, or agents may need to be rotated to maximize tolerability and effectiveness, but analgesics still work in an advancing disease, though dose requirements may increase.

- Symptom relief is always the objective when someone is dying, even if high doses of a drug are required which that unintentionally contribute to their death. This is an ethical approach well established and respected from medical, legal, and religious perspectives.

Adapted from Webb (1997) with permission.

---

or graduation ceremony; for others, it might involve writing a book, endowing a scholarship, or sharing important anecdotes, beliefs, and other gifts with family and friends. These activities can bring a sense of resolution and peace to the patient with a terminal illness. For dying patients to make the most of the time they have left, excellent symptom control and comfort is an absolute prerequisite.

Finally, excellent end-of-life care is sensitive to the patient's spiritual and existential beliefs and concerns. More than 90% of Americans state that they believe in God or some "higher power" (Gallup Poll, 1997). Beliefs about religion and the nature of an afterlife typically become more important as death approaches. Many people find peace and palliation through their religious traditions. Understanding a patient's personal system of belief and relationship to a community of believers is key to understanding the patient well. Apart from formal religious beliefs, all people have existential concerns (e.g., life goals achieved or abandoned, regrets about past events, concern about welfare of family members after their death) (Jacobsen & Breitbart, 1996).

Good care of the dying patient often involves open but sensitive discussion of religious beliefs and concerns. As a part of such conversations, patients may inquire about the religious traditions and beliefs of their physicians. In contrast to other settings for psychiatric care, such inquiries are usually best dealt with in a way that is as direct as is comfortable for the physician, as free of analysis as possible, and always respectful of the patient's beliefs and traditions (or lack thereof). While the end of life is never an appropriate time for proselytizing, many religious people take comfort in knowing that their physician is also a person of faith, even if the physician comes from a different faith tradition than their own. Clergy from the patient's faith community or a hospice chaplain are valuable collaborators and sources of information in providing for the spiritual and existential care of terminally ill patients. If in doubt, ask. Physicians, whether or not they themselves are religious, can provide comfort to their religious patients by promptly mobilizing pastoral and chaplaincy support.

A GENERAL APPROACH TO PALLIATIVE MEDICAL CARE

A general approach to palliative medical care, summarized by Shuster and James (1998), suggests that physicians ask first about suffering in a general way (e.g., "What causes you to suffer most?"). The experience of suffering is unique to each individual. The treatment should emphasize the patient's priorities and reflect respect for the patient's treatment preferences. Vigilance for symptoms of pain, nausea and vomiting, weakness, anorexia, and dyspnea is essential to palliative care, as undertreated physical symptoms can cause psychological symptoms—for example, depression often is precipitated by undertreated pain (Spiegel et al., 1994). Patients with terminal illness should be routinely screened for mental disorders like depression, anxiety, and delirium.

Respect for the patient's priorities and tolerance for the patient's preferences are best rooted in an ongoing discussion regarding advance directives. Formal documents such as living wills or even declarations of a healthcare proxy actually may fall short of their potential utility when implemented. The conversations held in the context of discussing these documents are very useful in helping the patient, family, and physician come to a mutual understanding of the patient's wishes regarding end-of-life care. Ideally, such conversations will begin well before a time of crisis. A foundation of clear understanding of the patient's priorities and preferences can lessen the burden of what might otherwise be agonizing decisions at the end of life. Patients and families should be encouraged to view participation in these conversations in advance as a loving gift to one another. Chapter 85 deals extensively with advance directives.

PRACTICAL PROBLEMS WITH HOSPICE AND PALLIATIVE CARE

The median length of stay in American hospices, designed for up to six months, has been reported as being in the range of 30 days (Christakis & Escarce, 1996). Since hospice eligibility is directly linked to an expected survival of six months or less,

difficulty in arriving at an accurate prognosis, especially for non-cancer diagnoses, limits the availability of hospice care. To make prognostic estimates more reliable, the National Hospice and Palliative Care Organization (NHPCO) has published guidelines for determining prognosis related to hospice eligibility (National Hospice Organization Medical Guidelines Task Force, 1995).

Useful as such guidelines are, they represent an attempt to adapt to the six-month criterion, which is not meaningful for patients dying from certain diseases. For example, the guidelines present a set of criteria to predict six-month survival in end-stage dementia, which may progress over the course of a decade. However, use of these criteria for patients with Alzheimer's disease limits hospice care to patients with such extreme cognitive impairment that most of the goals of hospice and palliative care are difficult or impossible to achieve.

It is often difficult for a patient to shift the focus of treatment from cure to palliative care. Hesitancy about discussing these issues can delay access to palliative care further. This discussion requires that doctors understand the patient's preferences about curative and end-of-life care. Physicians should be able to provide an open and realistic discussion of the prognosis, be comfortable with breaking any bad news gently, be willing to dispel myths about the end of life and hospice care, and be committed to educating patients and families about the dying process (Shuster & Jones, 1998). This discussion allows the opportunity to avoid futile treatments, to treat patients' suffering adequately, and to proceed with a plan of treatment consistent with the patient's wishes.

Even though discussion of the shift to palliative treatment is necessary for optimal end-of-life care, it is also difficult and even painful for the physician as well as the patient. Physicians are trained to treat disease; some perceive a patient's death as a professional and personal failure. Additionally, a physician's own death anxiety can hinder him or her from engaging patients in discussions about end-of-life care. Approaches such as seeking training and experience in palliative care, acknowledging the importance of symptom control and palliative interventions, and helping patients set meaningful and achievable goals can make providing end-of-life care bearable, even rewarding, for physicians.

Breaking bad news and discussing end-of-life care with patients are skills that need to be developed over time (Creagan, 1994; Garg et al., 1997). When breaking bad news to a patient, care should be taken to be gentle but clear. Expect the patient to be distressed and to have difficulty assimilating details initially. The physician should be seated during sensitive conversations and should ensure adequate privacy after determining whom the patient would like to have present for the discussion. The physician should next determine what patients already know about their condition and what details they would like to receive about their prognosis. Some patients are burdened by excessive detail or even a direct statement of their poor prognosis; their preference "not to know" should be respected and a suitable proxy identified. Next, the physician should fill in the gaps in the patient's understanding of their condition, according to their preference about degree of detail. Without being evasive or mincing words, the physician should be calm and as reassuring as appropriate. While hope for cure cannot be offered, the physician can soothe patients' concerns about abandonment and the dying process and provide information about palliative interventions.

Finally, questions should be invited before ending the initial session. End-of-life discussions should be viewed as an ongoing dialogue and not a single event. An initial conversation similar to that described above makes subsequent contacts much easier and more rewarding for both patient and physician. Involvement of spouses and other close family members and friends is essential.

PSYCHIATRIC SYMPTOM MANAGEMENT AT THE END OF LIFE

For a number of reasons, psychiatric and neuropsychiatric complications of terminal illness are very common and often overlooked (Shuster et al., 1998; Shuster & Jones, 1998). First, it is widely held that symptoms, especially depression, are a "normal" part of the dying process. In addition, psychiatric diagnosis is more difficult in the presence of physical illness, and medical staff may be unduly pessimistic about the chances that the patient will respond to treatment. Reactions to the patient's hopelessness may augment this pessimism in their caregivers. While symptomatic treatment is emphasized in palliative care, treatment based on formal psychiatric diagnoses (e.g., mental disorder) is not sufficiently emphasized. The stigma associated with psychiatric evaluations or the assignment of a psychiatric diagnosis inhibits the use of psychiatric services, even in hospice settings. Finally, there are significant structural barriers to including team members with mental health expertise in the care of dying patients. Successful psychiatric symptom control at the end of life necessitates overcoming these barriers to treatment. A palliative approach to psychiatric symptom control also involves shifting the focus of assessment and treatment. While recognition and treatment of formal mental disorders has a prime importance for the psychiatrist caring for a terminally ill patient, that psychiatrist must also be ready to provide symptomatic treatment to relieve suffering and maximize quality of life. Similarly, some psychiatric problems at the end of life that meet full diagnostic criteria for a mental disorder (e.g., quiet delirium in the final days or hours of life) are sometimes best left untreated. Providing adequate relief from psychiatric symptoms at the end of life requires relief of pain, nausea, dyspnea, or other distressing symptoms. A general physical assessment and examination, in conjunction with attention to the patient's complaints, will usually pinpoint physical sources of pain and suffering.

DEPRESSION

Depression is very common in the setting of terminal illness. Estimated prevalence rates range from 20% to 50% (Breitbart et al., 1995; Shuster et al., 1998). While depressive symptoms affect an even larger percentage of patients, there is a median prevalence of 15% for depression in advanced disease that meets criteria for a major depressive episode (Hotopf et al., 2002). Depression becomes more prevalent

and severe as comorbid physical illness progresses (Rodin et al., 1991). Depression clearly diminishes one's quality of life (Wells et al., 1989). Depression has been shown to be a determining factor in the desire to die in many patients who opt for assisted death (Chochinov et al., 1995). Consequently, depression is a problem of major clinical importance in the care of terminally ill patients and should be a priority in routine assessment.

Screening for depression in terminally ill patients is challenging. There is significant variability in assessment methods for depression among patients with advanced illness. A review of published studies of depression assessment in palliative cancer patients found that over 100 different assessment methods were used, two-thirds of which were unique to only one paper. Furthermore, the full range of *Diagnostic and Statistical Manual IV* (DSM-IV) diagnostic criteria were seldom assessed in published studies (Wasteson et al., 2009). The ideal screening procedure would be brief yet accurate. Many patients in need of palliative care cannot tolerate extended or even relatively modest diagnostic assessments. A personal or family history of a mood disorder argues for a depressive episode, especially if the patient reports that the subjective experience is similar to prior episodes. A simple question, essentially "Are you depressed?" is an accurate and reliable initial screen for depression of clinical significance in terminally ill patients (Chochinov et al., 1997). Among formal screening tools, the Hospital Anxiety and Depression Scale (HADS) has been validated against a standardized psychiatric interview and has similar sensitivity, specificity, and positive predictive value (Lloyd-Williams et al., 2003). Although not extensively studied in palliative care, the Patient Health Questionnaire (PHQ-9) is also a brief and well-validated measure for detecting and monitoring depression (Kroenke et al., 2010). While diagnostic confidence is increased and target symptoms are obtained by determining that the patient meets more formal criteria (American Psychiatric Association, 1994) which remain applicable to patients at the end of life, treating any significant symptom, above or below formal diagnostic thresholds, is consistent with the palliative approach to care.

Successful treatment of depression in the terminally ill patient requires attention to commonly comorbid physical conditions. The patient's level of pain cannot be overlooked, as patients with severe pain are less likely to respond to depression treatment (Laird et al., 2009). Adequate analgesia provides relief from the pain and the dysphoria associated with it. Pain, when severe or unremitting, is often interpreted as a constant reminder of serious illness and disease progression. Pain, as a distracting stimulus, makes attending to other, more pleasant activities difficult. Similarly, nausea and vomiting, when severe or recurrent, are very likely to produce dysphoric distress, depression, and isolation. Progressive loss of stamina or functional capacity is usually accompanied by grief or even depression, and this should be taken into account when assessing depression in the dying patient. A differential diagnosis of the conditions that can cause or exacerbate depression in terminally ill patients is listed in Box 84.2.

Treatment for depression in the terminally ill patient primarily requires use of antidepressants, especially psychostimulants (Breitbart et al., 1998; Block, 2006). Table 84.1 summarizes the antidepressant agents commonly used for depression in this setting. Standard antidepressants appear to be effective in advanced illness, but their use in this population has one chief drawback: the two- to four-week lag time to onset of benefit. Given the short length of survival typical after admission to hospice care, and the palliative care goal of maximizing the quality of life and the capacity to enjoy every precious day, agents that are not apt to work for two to eight weeks are rarely acceptable as first-line treatments. For most cases of depression in the terminally ill, the psychostimulants are better alternatives.

Psychostimulants (e.g., dextroamphetamine, methylphenidate) have been widely used and studied in the depressed medically ill, including patients with advanced disease (Masand & Tesar, 1996; Macleod 1998; Homsi et al., 2001; Howard et al., 2010). Despite the long history of use, there are limited formal studies to support their use as antidepressants, but the available evidence suggests their efficacy, with stronger evidence for tolerability (Hardy, 2009). Beneficial effect has been shown in several nonrandomized studies in patients with cancer, and even stronger studies exist in HIV literature, where randomized controlled trials of stimulants in patients with HIV for fatigue have shown significant improvement in fatigue as well as depression (Block, 2006). Stimulants are commonly used in hospice and palliative care settings and are the agents of choice in

this setting unless contraindicated. Response occurs within hours after a given dose. Clearance of the drug is also rapid if side effects occur.

There is little information available regarding differential efficacy or tolerability of the psychostimulants, so the choice among the commonly used agents is largely based on personal experience, subjective preference, and availability. A treatment protocol for using stimulants in the end-of-life setting is summarized in Box 84.3. Treatment should be initiated with a relatively low dose of the selected agent. Treatment response is rapidly apparent (usually within a few hours), allowing for daily dose adjustments. Dose should be adjusted daily in small increments until one of the following occurs: (1) the desired antidepressant response is achieved, (2) intolerable side effects emerge, or (3) the high dose range listed in Box 84.3 is reached without obtaining a beneficial response. The "high" dose is not high in the absolute sense, but rather high in that it is higher than the dose usually required to obtain therapeutic benefit in this setting. The high dose listed here is not to be considered an absolute dose ceiling for using stimulants for depression in the terminally ill, but as a reminder to reconsider diagnosis and treatment strategy before proceeding with further dose escalation (which may be necessary to obtain the desired benefit).

Though well tolerated by medically ill patients, stimulants are not without adverse effects. Side effects that are usually dose-related may include tachycardia, hypertension, insomnia, and agitation. Anorexia is a common side effect of stimulants in medically healthy populations (and a treatment indication when these agents are used as appetite suppressants), but stimulants commonly boost appetite in medically ill patients, especially if the diminished appetite is secondary to depression or apathy. In patients at high risk for developing delirium, as many terminally ill patients are, or those who seem depressed but have a "quiet," hypoactive, non-agitated delirium, administration of stimulants can precipitate or worsen a delirious state. Finally, while this is unusual in the medical population, tolerance may develop with prolonged use, requiring dose escalation to maintain the therapeutic effect. Withdrawal depression may occur if stimulants are abruptly discontinued. The limited life expectancy of terminally ill patients makes many of these side effects of little concern in this population, however.

Standard antidepressant treatment also has a role in the control of depressive symptoms that complicate terminal illness. When patients are unable to tolerate stimulants, fail to respond to stimulant treatment, or have a history of vigorous response to a known antidepressant, standard antidepressants may be a better choice than stimulants for depression at the end of life. Additionally, patients with a terminal prognosis but with a relatively long life expectancy may do better over the long term on a standard antidepressant. Patients maintained on stimulants for a long period of time (many weeks or months) are best gradually switched to a standard antidepressant for maintenance therapy. Patients who achieve suboptimal response to psychostimulants may achieve better control

Table 84.1 PHARMACOLOGICAL TREATMENTS FOR DEPRESSION IN TERMINAL ILLNESS

GENERIC NAME	APPROXIMATE DAILY DOSE RANGE (MG)	ROUTE	COMMENTS
PSYCHOSTIMULANTS			
dextroamphetamine qAM and afternoon 2.5–20 bid modafinil	2.5–20 daily (also available in time-release form) methylphenidate 100–200 qAM	PO PO PO	Rapid onset of action and clearance if side effects emerge. Tolerance may develop, requiring dose increase. May precipitate agitation or delirium in susceptible patients. May be drugs of choice in terminal illness.
SEROTONIN REUPTAKE INHIBITORS			
fluoxetine	10–80 daily	PO	SSRIs all may cause mild headache, jitteriness, GI upset. May (rarely) cause serotonin syndrome in combination with other serotonergic agents. May affect metabolism of other drugs cleared through the cytochrome P450-2D6 system.
paroxetine	10–40 daily	PO	
sertraline	50–200 daily	PO	
citalopram	20–40 daily	PO	
escitalopram	10–20 daily	PO	
TRICYCLIC ANTIDEPRESSANTS			
desipramine	12.5–150 daily	PO	Anticholinergic, sedation, orthostasis, and dry mouth are potentially troublesome side effects of all TCAs. Can worsen constipation caused by opiates. Can help treat pain, especially neuropathic pain. May stimulate appetite.
doxepin	12.5–150 daily	PO	
imipramine	12.5–150 daily	PO, IM	
nortriptyline	10–125 daily	PO	
amitriptyline	50–100 daily	PO	
OTHERS			
buproprion	75–450 daily in divided doses	PO	Stimulating, risk of seizures
mirtazapine	15–60 daily	PO	Sedating, appetite stimulant
trazodone	25–300 daily	PO	Sedating, can induce orthostasis; risk of priapism. Used in low doses 50–100 mg as sedative/hypnotic qhs. Nauseating on empty stomach.
duloxetine	40–60 daily	PO	FDA indication for diabetic neuropathy
venlafaxine	75–375 daily	PO	Can cause hypertension in high dose ranges

Key: qAM = daily; bid = twice daily; IM = intramuscular; PO = oral.

of depressive symptoms with combined use of stimulants with standard antidepressants.

As there is limited evidence to support any particular standard antidepressant as a "drug of choice" for depressed palliative care patients, choice of agent should be guided by comorbid physical illness, the patient's symptom profile, drug interactions, and potential side effects, both positive and negative (Rayner, Price, Hotopf, & Higginson, 2011). Newer agents appear to be better tolerated in general than older antidepressants such as tricyclics, in the terminally ill patient. Monoamine oxidase inhibitors (MAOIs) are rarely if ever used in this setting, for various reasons, including the required dietary restrictions. Though tricyclics have a greater overall side effect burden in the medically ill than some of the newer agents, they do have a role in the management of depression in the terminally ill patient with neuropathic pain, substantial appetite reduction, severe insomnia, or a past history of good response to tricyclics. Among the newer agents, the serotonin reuptake inhibitors (SSRIs) have the most extensive history of use in medically ill populations and are most commonly used.

Psychotherapy has a role in the management of depressive symptoms at the end of life. Though most patients with terminal illnesses may be unable to tolerate extensive psychotherapeutic interventions, a variety of psychotherapies can be modified for use in the care of terminally ill patients and their families. Clinical trials have shown benefit of various psychosocial interventions, including psychoeducation, problem-solving therapy, cognitive-behavioral therapy (CBT), non–cognitive-behavioral therapy (relaxation techniques, hypnosis), and individual and group supportive therapies (Lorenz et al., 2008; Akechi et al., 2008). Dignity therapy, an individualized and reflective intervention designed for people living with terminal illness, has been shown to improve self-reported end-of-life experiences, sadness, and spiritual well-being, and shows promise in mitigating distress due to depression (Chochinov et al., 2011). In addition to the various psychotherapies, an initial study of a structured exercise program for palliative care patients suggests that a 50-minute group exercise program offered twice weekly for six weeks was associated with benefits in emotional functioning and fatigue (Oldervoll et al., 2006).

ANXIETY

Some degree of anxiety or fearfulness is probably universal at the end of life. This fact makes anxiety difficult to evaluate in the setting of terminal illness and probably contributes to the under-recognition of anxiety disorders in the dying (Shuster et al., 1998). Anxiety and anxiety disorders can cause a great deal of suffering in dying patients, especially when anxiety complicates respiratory distress (Rosenbaum et al., 1997; Breitbart et al., 1998). Even anxiety that does not meet criteria for a formal psychiatric disorder (American Psychiatric Association, 1994) can cause substantial suffering and is an appropriate focus of palliative intervention.

The prevalence of significant anxiety in terminal illness is not well studied, but the available literature suggests it is very common, exceeding 70% by some patient self-reports (Portenoy et al., 1994; Breitbart et al., 1995). Rates of anxiety at the end of life increase with the presence and severity of concomitant physical illness.

The goals of palliative care cannot be achieved when the patient is overly anxious. Anxiety presents a barrier to relaxation and attention to important relationships, achievement of life goals, and integration of the experience of dying. Insomnia, depression, fatigue, difficulty swallowing, nausea, or other types of physical distress may result from anxiety. Such symptoms may be difficult to control without attending to comorbid anxiety.

Like depression, the prevalence of anxiety and anxiety disorders at the end of life, combined with the ready availability of effective treatments, makes anxiety an important focus of palliative care. In most cases, substantial anxiety is readily apparent or easily uncovered by simple questioning. Prior history of anxiety disorders should be explored and effective treatments documented. A differential diagnosis of the conditions that can cause or exacerbate anxiety in terminally ill patients is listed in Box 84.4. It is extremely important to evaluate the patient's anxiety, agitation, and insomnia to determine if they are secondary to major depression or undertreated pain.

Treatment for anxiety in the terminally ill patient should be designed to provide rapid relief without placing excessive demands on the patient. Therefore, emotional support, aggressive treatment of comorbid anxiogenic physical symptoms (e.g. pain, nausea, dyspnea), reassurance (where appropriate), pastoral care support, and (in selected cases) individual or family psychotherapy may be of benefit. Specific fears (e.g., fears of dying, fears of unwanted medical interventions) should be explored and discussed. If major depression or poorly controlled pain is present, treatment with antidepressants and/or analgesics would take top priority.

Optimal relief from anxiety in terminal illness generally requires the use of anxiolytic drugs, as summarized in Table 84.2. However, a systematic review concluded that there is inadequate evidence to draw firm conclusions from the current literature about pharmacotherapy for anxiety in palliative care patients (Jackson & Lipman, 2004).

Benzodiazepines, particularly lorazepam, are the first-line pharmacological treatment for anxiety in terminal illness. Benzodiazepines remain reliably effective in this setting. Though their suppression of respiratory drive is a risk in the frail patient with advanced medical illness, these agents can be safely used in dying patients if carefully titrated. Concerns about side effects should not be allowed to interfere with the primary goal of relieving suffering in the dying patient.

Anxiolytic alternatives to benzodiazepines for terminally ill patients include low-dose antidepressants and, sometimes, low doses of antipsychotics (Rosenbaum et al., 1997; Breitbart et al., 1998; Block, 2006). The primary disadvantage of using antidepressants as anxiolytics in the setting of terminal illness is the delay typically seen prior to the onset of therapeutic effect. Among the antidepressants, SSRIs and tricyclics, such as nortriptyline, are the most reliably effective for anxiety. Antipsychotic drugs, particularly atypical antipsychotics, are especially useful when the patient has cognitive disturbance, cannot tolerate sedation or suppression of respiratory drive from other anxiolytics, or cannot tolerate benzodiazepines (e.g., those who have exhibited disinhibition in response to prior trials of benzodiazepines). Medically ill patients are sensitive to the side effects of neuroleptics, so these drugs should be dosed conservatively for anxiety.

DELIRIUM

Confusional states are extremely common at the end of life, especially in the days and hours immediately preceding death. Rates of delirium range from 20% to nearly 50% in palliative care setting, and this rate increases to up to 90% in the hours or days before death (Conill et al., 1997; De Fabbro et al., 2006; Leonard et al., 2008). Delirium is, of course, more common in the presence of serious physical illness (Lipowski, 1990). (See also Chapter 31.)

Detection of delirium, particularly the agitated subtype, is generally straightforward in terminally ill patients. As many as one-third of cases of delirium seen in the terminally ill are reversible (Bruera et al., 1995; de Stoutz et al., 1995), but some cases are only manageable by intentional comfort sedation (Fainsinger et al., 1991; Stiefel et al., 1992; Shuster et al., 1998). Diligent serial assessment is the key to detection of delirium at the end of life. In all palliative care settings, between one-third and two-thirds of cases of delirium are misdiagnosed, detected late, or not detected at all (Leonard et al., 2008). Screening tools such as the Mini-Mental State Exam (Folstein et al., 1975), the Confusion Assessment Method (Inouye et al., 1990), or the Memorial Delirium Assessment Scale (Breitbart et al., 1997) can be useful aids.

Box 84.4 DIFFERENTIAL DIAGNOSIS OF ANXIETY SYMPTOMS IN TERMINAL ILLNESS

Anxiety disorders (panic disorder, generalized anxiety disorder, posttraumatic stress disorder)
Adjustment disorder with anxiety
Coping/personality style (avoidant, dependent)
Delirium
Fear
Side effects from medications (akathisia from antipsychotics or antiemetics such as metoclopramide)
Spiritual/existential concerns
Undertreated pain
Other undertreated physical complications (dyspnea, sepsis)
Withdrawal states (opiates, sedatives)
Physiological abnormalities (hyperthyroidism, hypercalcemia)

Adapted from Shuster & Jones (1998) with permission.

Since delirium impairs cognition and the patient's ability to report symptoms with reliability, the suffering experienced during an episode of delirium is difficult to assess. On the other hand, the distress experienced by the family of an agitated, delirious patient is usually obvious. Family members, as well as patients who recover from an episode of delirium, commonly report that the experience is significantly distressing (Breitbart, Gibson, & Tremblay, 2002; Bruera et al., 2009; Grover & Shah, 2011). Family education, including an explanation of the process of delirium in layman's terms, a description of the planned interventions, and an explanation of how the symptoms of delirium are related to the underlying terminal illness, can provide great relief to the family. Obviously, reduction or elimination of agitation will also provide substantial relief.

Differential diagnosis of delirium is similar to that employed in the setting of acute illness (see Chapter 41), with a few differences in emphasis. Efforts should be focused on finding reversible causes of delirium, which in the setting of terminal illness are most commonly related to medication side effects (commonly opiates and antihistamines/anticholinergics), dehydration, infection, elevated intracranial pressure (ICP), and metabolic disturbances, such as hypercalcemia (Leonard et al., 2008). In the syndrome of opioid neurotoxicity, which includes delirium, myoclonus, allodynia, hyperalgesia, and seizures in extreme cases, treatment via opioid dose-reduction or opioid switching often results in significant improvement in delirium (de Stoutz et al., 1995). Withdrawal states always deserve consideration as possible causes of delirium at the end of life. In contrast to delirium in the setting of acute illness, terminal delirium is mostly gradual in onset, more likely to result from multiple etiological factors, and less likely to resolve (Breitbart et al., 1998).

Medications to treat delirium, once reversal of the underlying causes of the delirium has been addressed, are summarized in Table 84.3. As in the setting of acute illness, antipsychotic drugs are a primary treatment for delirium in terminal illness (Wise & Trzepacz, 1996; Breitbart et al., 1998; Leonard et al., 2008). The older antipsychotic drugs (e.g., haloperidol) have been accepted as effective treatments for delirium for many years. A butyrophenone agent, haloperidol has probably been used more than any other neuroleptic agent to treat delirium, and it remains a drug of choice due to its having few anticholinergic side effects, few active metabolites, and a small likelihood of sedation (del Fabbro et al., 2006; Markowitz & Narasimhan, 2008). Given their decreased risk of extrapyramidal side effects, atypical antipsychotics are frequently used for treatment of delirium. Although there are limited studies in terminal patients, delirium treatment studies have shown comparable efficacy of haloperidol, risperidone, and olanzapine, and there is increasing evidence about the benefit of quetiapine as well (Lonergan et al., 2007; Markowitz & Narashiman, 2008).

Benzodiazepines, especially lorazepam, are commonly used in the treatment of delirium, either alone or in combination with antipsychotics (Wise & Trzepacz, 1996; Trzepacz, 1996; Breitbart et al., 1998). In the setting of terminal illness, benzodiazepines may sometimes be more effective than

Table 84.2 ANXIOLYTIC MEDICATIONS USED IN TERMINAL ILLNESS

GENERIC NAME	APPROXIMATE DAILY DOSAGE RANGE (MG)	ROUTE
BENZODIAZEPINES		
Very short-acting (parenteral) midazolam	10–60 per 24h	IV, SC, IM
Intermediate acting:		
alprazolam	0.25–2 tid-qid	PO, SL
oxazepam	10–15 tid-qid	PO
lorazepam	0.5–2 tid-qid	PO, SL, IV, IM
Intermediate acting:		
chlordiazepoxide	10–50 tid-qid	PO, IM
Long acting:		
diazepam	5–10 bid-qid	PO, IV, PR
clorazepate	7.5–15 bid-qid	PO
clonazepam	0.5–2 bid-qid	PO
NON-BENZODIAZAPINE		
(Delay of onset 2–3 weeks) buspirone	5–20 tid	PO
ANTIDEPRESSANTS		
Serotonin reuptake inhibitors (start with low doses):		
fluoxetine	10–80 daily	PO
paroxetine	10–60 daily	PO
sertraline	50–200 daily	PO
citalopram	20–40 daily	PO
TRICYCLIC ANTIDEPRESSANTS		
amitriptyline	10–150 daily	PO
disipramine	12.5–150 daily	PO, IM
doxepin**	12.5–150 daily	PO, PR
imipramine	12.5–150 daily	PO, IM
nortriptyline*	10–125 daily	PO
OTHERS		
mirtazapine	15–60 daily	PO
duloxetine	40–60 daily	PO
venlafaxine	75–375 daily	PO
ANTIPSYCHOTICS		
chlorpromazine	12.5–50 q4-12h	PO, IM, IV
haloperidol	0.5–5 q2-12h	IV, PO, IM
methotrimeprazine	10–20 q4-8h	SC, PO, IM
olanzapine	5–15 daily	PO
quetiapine	25–200 daily	PO
risperidone	1–3 daily	PO
thioridazine	10–125 daily	PO
ANTIHISTAMINES		
hydroxyzine	25–50 q4-6h	PO, IV, SC

Key: PO = per oral; IM = intramuscular; PR = per rectum; IV = intravenous; SC = subcutaneous; SL = sublingual; bid = two times a day; tid = three times a day; qid = four times a day; q4–8h = every 4–8 hours. Parenteral doses are generally twice as potent as oral doses; intravenous bolus injections should be administered slowly.

*Tricyclic of choice.

**Per rectal administration of doxepin requires pharmacy preparation (Storey & Trumble, 1992).

Adapted from Breitbart et al., 1998; Shuster & Jones, 1998, with permission.

Table 84.3 MEDICATIONS USED FOR DELIRIUM IN TERMINAL ILLNESS

GENERIC NAME	APPROXIMATE DAILY DOSAGE RANGE (MG)	ROUTE
NEUROLEPTICS		
haloperidol	0.5–5 q2-12h	PO, IV, SC, IM
thioridazine	10–75 q4-8h	PO
chlorpromazine	12.5–50 q4-12h	PO, IV, IM
methotrimeprazine	12.5–50 q4-8h	IV, SC, PO
ATYPICAL ANTIPSYCHOTICS		
risperidone	1 daily–3 bid	PO
olanzapine	5–10 daily	PO
quetiapine	25–200 daily	PO
BENZODIAZEPINES		
lorazepam*	0.5–2.0 q1-4h	PO, IV, IM
midazolam*	30–100 per 24h	IV, SC, IM
OPIATES*		
	(Doses vary)	PO, IV, SC

*Denotes a drug used primarily for purposes of sedation when indicated for treatment of delirium.

Parenteral doses are generally twice as potent as oral doses. IV—intravenous infusions or bolus injections should be administered slowly; IM—intramuscular injections should be avoided if repeated use becomes necessary; PO—oral forms of medication are preferred; or SC—subcutaneous infusions are generally accepted modes of drug administration in the terminally ill.

Adapted with permission from Breitbart et al., 1998.

neuroleptics, in contrast to delirium associated with more acute illness (Breitbart et al., 1998), but are more likely to reduce agitation by means of sedation and less likely to restore cognitive functioning and meaningful communication with family.

Sedation may be required to control the agitation of delirium in the last few hours to days of life (Bruera et al., 1987; Breitbart et al., 1998). When applied as an intervention of last resort for a delirious, dying patient who is agitated and appears to be suffering, so-called palliative sedation is the standard of care, and is neither euthanasia nor assisted suicide (Shuster et al., 1998; deGraeff & Dean, 2007). In fact, there is accumulating evidence that, when provided to relieve refractory symptoms in patients who are actively dying, palliative sedation does not shorten survival (Sykes and Thorns, 2003; Maltoni et al., 2009). The sedation is therapeutically calming and comforting, allowing the patient to die peacefully of the underlying disease.

It is possible that earlier and more aggressive intervention for evolving confusional states might avoid severe delirium at the end of life. However, once severe, treatment-refractory terminal delirium develops, failure to act therapeutically exposes the patient to unnecessary suffering and greatly increases the burden on the family, who must witness such agitation as

death approaches. Infusions of benzodiazepines (e.g., lorazepam, midazolam) or opiates can serve this purpose.

DEPRESSION AND GRIEF

Bereavement, as defined by Parkes (1998), is the situation of anyone who has lost a person to whom one is attached. *Grief* is a set of psychological and emotional reactions to bereavement. *Mourning* is the social face of grief. Bereavement and grief may emerge after an actual loss or as anticipatory grief as the threatened loss approaches. Grief and bereavement may be seen in the terminally ill patient, family, and friends, or their professional caregivers. "Normal" grief has a very broad range—individual variation is the rule. Grief is not itself a mental disorder or pathological state—*Bereavement* is a "V code" in the DSM classification system, the category for conditions that are not mental disorders yet are still commonly the focus of clinical attention. Most people navigate their grief without professional help and do well. Still, not all reactions to bereavement and loss are "normal" in the sense that they are not all adaptive.

The five stages of grief (Kubler-Ross, 1969) have been helpful in introducing the concept of grief as a process and are interesting from a historical perspective, but they should not be viewed as a reliable and universal pattern for grieving. Individuals move in and out of theorized grief stages, often changing stages out of sequence, skipping stages altogether, or returning to deal further with an earlier stage. It is more helpful to think of grief as a process that begins with a period of disruption (characterized by intense sadness, crying, preoccupation with the deceased, diminished interest and concentration) that proceeds toward gradual resolution of these features of acute grief and moves toward integration of the loss (Zisook & Shear, 2009).

The symptoms of acute grief may be misinterpreted as signs of significant psychopathology. Tearfulness, emotional numbing, pangs of grief, searching for the lost person, feeling that the death did not actually happen, or brief non-delusional hallucinations of the deceased are all within the normal range of grief experiences (Rando, 1984; Corr & Doka, 1994; Parkes, 1998). While there are no reliable general rules about the time range for the resolution of normal grief, these acute reactions should lessen and generally resolve over time (Rando, 1984; Corr & Doka, 1994; Parkes, 1998). Complications may occur if the grieving process is avoided, inhibited, delayed, or conflicted (Rando, 1984; Corr & Doka, 1994; Parkes, 1998; Brown & Stoudemire, 1983).

The stress of grief may precipitate a formal psychiatric disorder, such as major depression, panic disorder, or alcohol dependence. These conditions add greatly to suffering and should be treated aggressively, especially since formal mental disorders complicating bereavement tend to persist and adversely affect quality of life and the grief process for months (Zisook & Shuchter, 1991, 1992).

Since the normal range of grief covers such a broad territory and some of the acute symptoms mimic formal mental disorders, distinguishing pathological grief from normal grief can be a formidable challenge. Still, there are some reliable indicators of pathological grief. Suicidal ideation or self-loathing are not components of normal grief and should be interpreted as indicators of pathology. A high level of grief-related distress, but not depression, was more closely associated with a wish to die among a group of patients with advanced cancer (Jacobsen et al., 2010). Failure to progress toward integration of grief over time, persistent symptoms of acute grief, persistent social withdrawal, or prolonged disruption of interpersonal, social, or occupational functioning merit assessment. Generally, any grief that prevents the bereaved person from maintaining a desired level of functioning merits attention, especially given the principles of palliative care.

Bereavement-associated depression is an important complication to recognize and treat. Though bereavement is the only life event that is listed as an exclusionary criterion for the diagnosis of a major depressive episode (MDE), there is emerging evidence that this exclusion may need to be reconsidered (Zisook & Shear, 2009; Zisook et al., 2010). In a population-based study, depression in bereaved individuals compared to the non-bereaved depressed demonstrated a similar symptom profile and presentation, but there was a longer episode duration among bereaved persons with depression (Karam et al., 2009). A case-control study of 17,988 depressed patients found that 8.5% would have not qualified for MDE by DSM due to bereavement. These "excluded" patients were more severely depressed than controls (depressed patients without bereavement) and more likely to express suicidal ideation or worthlessness (Corruble et al., 2009). Many mostly open-label trials have demonstrated that antidepressants (including desipramine, nortriptyline, paroxetine, bupropion, sertraline, escitalopram, and duloxetine) are effective for bereavement-related depression (Jacobs, Nelson, & Zisook, 1987; Pasternak et al., 1991; Zygmont et al., 1998; Reynolds et al., 1999; Zisook et al., 2001; Oakley et al., 2002; Simon, Thompson, Pollack, & Shear, 2007; Hensley, Slonimski, Uhlenhuth, & Clayton, 2009).

There is growing evidence to support a proposed new diagnostic category for *complicated bereavement* or *prolonged grief disorder* (Lichtenthal et al., 2004; Zhang, Jawahri, & Prigerson, 2006; Prigerson et al., 2009; Zisook et al., 2010; Shear et al., 2011). This syndrome is characterized by a variety of manifestations of a failure to integrate the loss of the deceased loved one "over time" (defined as at least six months). Individuals with complicated grief demonstrate continued severe separation distress, with some of the following features: yearning, refusal to accept the death, compulsions to seek tangible reminders of the deceased. Individuals with *complicated grief* also characteristically have a variety of persistently distressing thoughts and behaviors about the deceased, including rumination about the death, emotional/physiological reactivity to reminders, or a belief that joy and satisfaction are no longer possible (Prigerson et al., 2009; Zisook et al., 2010). A substantial minority of the bereaved meet these criteria, and complicated grief/prolonged grief disorder can be differentiated from adaptive grief, MDD, and PTSD (American Psychiatric Association, 1994; Kim & Jacobs, 1991; Prigerson et al., 1995; 1996; Horowitz et al., 1997; Zhang et al., 2009;

Prigerson et al., 2009; Zisook et al., 2010; Shear et al., 2011). Furthermore, a specific therapy (complicated grief therapy) has been developed and tested (Shear et al., 2005). Even if complicated bereavement is a distinct entity, there is a large degree of overlap or comorbidity with mood disorders and anxiety disorders. For example, previous histories of mental disorder, especially depression, predict complicated bereavement, as does family conflict or a maladaptive pattern of conflict resolution (Kim & Jacobs, 1991; Kissane et al., 1996).

All who grieve are not alike. There are important cultural and religious differences in responses and adaptations to grief and loss, as well as differences in death and funeral rituals. Grief responses vary in part due to differences in gender, overall coping style, degree of perceived social support, physical and mental health, and the age of the grieving person. Children, in particular, have variable responses to loss, since understanding of loss and response to bereavement are strongly influenced by a child's state of cognitive and emotional development.

Intuitively, the best and most effective interventions to assist in the bereavement process should begin before the death of the patient. Effective symptom control, patient and family education, and achievement of the goals of palliative care and hospice in preparation for the patient's death not only ease the burden of caring for a dying relative but ease the burden of grief and bereavement as well (Chentsova-Dutton et al., 2002; Barry et al., 2002; Wright et al., 2010).

Apart from the specialized care a psychiatrist can provide, a few basic interventions by the doctor are almost always helpful. In addition to providing excellent palliative care before the patient's death, the physician should meet with the family during the patient's terminal illness and after the patient's death to offer support, condolences, and answers to questions. The physician is in an excellent position to educate families about grief and the grieving process, thus potentially preventing some cases of complicated or unresolved bereavement. When complicated bereavement occurs, physicians who do not provide treatment for such conditions should know how to refer the person to community bereavement-care resources.

DEPRESSION AND ASSISTED DYING

There is a limited literature that provides some insight into the mental state of patients considering death-hastening decisions. While much has been said about euthanasia and physician-assisted suicide, the contribution of mental health professionals to this debate has also been limited. Yet, it could be argued that, as a special case of suicide, mental health concerns represent a basic consideration in approaching the issue of assisted dying.

Relatively few studies have actually examined the clinical relationship between a desire for death and depression. Yet depression is a critical consideration in discussions of cancer suicide and death-hastening requests, given that it is thought to place patients at up to 25 times the risk of completed suicide compared to the general population (Guze & Robins, 1970).

One of the first studies to broach this topic reported that 10 of 44 patients in a palliative care facility endorsed a desire for hastened death (Brown et al., 1986). Of those ten patients, all were reported to have concomitant clinical depression. This indicates that maintaining a high clinical index of suspicion for depression in patients making death-hastening requests is critical, and in fact, a review of depression-screening tools included this type of request as an indicator of the need for more complete depression screening (Lloyd-Williams et al., 2003). A study of 200 terminally ill patients, recruited from a palliative care facility, reported that 44.5% acknowledged at least a fleeting desire for an early death (Chochinov et al., 1995). In most instances these episodes were brief and did not reflect a sustained or committed desire, as would be required in a death-hastening decision. However, 8.5% of the study group reported a persistent, genuine desire for an early death. The prevalence of clinical depression in this group was significantly higher than among patients without a desire for death (58.8% versus 7.7%). The prevalence of pain, which was of moderate severity or greater, was higher among patients with a desire for death (76.5%) compared to patients without a desire for death (46.2%). In a logistic regression model of these data, depression entered as the only significant predictor of a genuine desire for death. Therefore, the importance of depression in discussions pertaining to assisted suicide cannot be overstated.

While attending to pain and physical sources of symptom distress remains critical, such data indicate that death-hastening requests appear to be largely psychologically mediated. In addition to motivation from an underlying depressive disorder, other psychological and social factors play a role in patients' interest in assisted suicide. In the above study of 200 terminally ill patients, patients' perceived level of social support was lower in the "desire for death" group compared to the remainder of the study group (Chochinov et al., 1995). Similarly, Breitbart and colleagues (1996) found that among autoimmune-deficiency syndrome (AIDS) patients, interest in assisted suicide appeared to be more a function of psychological and social factors (i.e., depression, lack of social support, and fears of becoming a burden to one's friends) rather than physical factors such as pain, symptom distress, and disease status.

Of additional importance, in the study by Chochinov et al. (1995), of the 17 patients who had originally endorsed a desire for hastened death, only six were available to be re-interviewed two weeks later. The others had either died, become too ill to participate, or had opted for discharge to home care. Of these six patients, four had essentially changed their minds. Thus, the evaluation of death-hastening requests must include a heightened awareness of the extent to which these requests may fluctuate over time and perhaps resolve, with some of that fluctuation likely to be secondary to changes in underlying depressive symptoms.

In a recent review of the prevalence of depression in granted and refused requests for euthanasia and physician-assisted suicide, Levene and Parker (2011) found that most studies estimated that a quarter to a half of requests for a hastened death came from depressed patients. Among the higher quality studies, there was conflicting evidence regarding the difference, or lack of significant difference, in the depression rate between groups with death-hastening requests and similar patients who did not make such a request. They identified a few high- and medium-quality studies that compared rates of depression in those with death-hastening requests, those who did not, and those with completed requests. These studies provide convincing evidence to show that depression is a significant factor in deciding whether to refuse death-hastening requests (Ruijs, Kerkhof, van der Wal, & Onwuteaka-Philpsen, 2011; Jansen-van der Weide, Onwuteaka-Philipsen, & van der Wal, 2005; Haverkate et al., 2005; Groenewoud et al., 2004), but the rate of depression in completed euthanasia or physician-assisted suicide cases is not significantly different from the overall rate in comparison populations of seriously ill patients (Rujis et al., 2011; Maessen et al., 2009; Georges et al., 2005).

The discussion of depression rates in patients making requests to hasten death prompts the question "Does treatment of depression result in changed desire regarding those requests?" Studies in elderly depressed patients have shown an increased acceptance and desire for life-sustaining medical therapies following treatment of depression (Hooper et al., 1997; Hooper et al., 1996; Ganzini et al., 1994). The patients with the most significant treatment effect had initially been the most severely depressed and subsequently were initially more hopeless and likely to overestimate the risks and underestimate the benefits of treatment (Ganzini et al., 1994). In a group of patients with advanced AIDS, desire for death was highly associated with depression, and response to antidepressant therapy was associated with a reduction in desire for hastened death (Breitbart et al., 2010). Further studies are needed to explore whether this treatment effect exists only in severely depressed patients and to determine if this effect is stable across varyingly severe underlying illnesses. However, this suggests that decisions about life-sustaining therapy, especially among the severely depressed, should be discouraged until after effective treatment of their depression.

An additional issue that arises from this discussion of depression among patients with death-hastening requests is whether depression should exclude a patient from having a request for euthanasia or physician-assisted suicide granted. As noted above, although many requests by depressed patients were not granted, and rates of depression in patients with granted requests compared to the surrounding population of severely ill patients were similar, patients with depression did have their requests granted. This reality has raised some concern about whether those with depression have capacity to make such a request, but in reality, most patients with depression maintain the capacity to make medical decisions (Grisso & Applebaum, 1995). This suggests a need for assessment that is able to identify the patients whose desire for hastened death is motivated by depression, not just those in whom depression is present. This assessment, however, is no easy task, as noted in a study of Oregon psychiatrists by Ganzini et al. (1996) in which only 6% of psychiatrists felt they would be able to assess in a single evaluation whether psychiatric factors were affecting a patient's request for assisted suicide. The approach and feasibility of conducting this type of evaluation requires ongoing discussion.

Given the challenges and uncertainties discussed above, requests for a hastened death tend to engender anxiety and uncertainty in healthcare providers. The following are clinical guidelines, which care providers may wish to consider in evaluating death-hastening requests:

1. *Treating depression.* Patients who are effectively treated for their depression often relinquish their desire for death and recover the capacity for enjoyment. Successful treatment often improves energy, sleep, and appetite, and renews their ability to find meaning in life despite impending death.

2. *Attending to symptom distress.* The ability to skillfully attend to distressing symptoms demonstrates to the patient that dying need not be accompanied by unnecessary distress. Aggressive, skillful, and compassionate palliative care, particularly pain and other symptom control, must be made available to all patients approaching the end of life.

3. *Providing continuity of care.* Maintaining contact with patients accomplishes several critical tasks. It ensures that patients will be continually reevaluated, given the temporal fluctuations in "desire for death" and oftentimes accompanying symptom distress. It also provides reassurance to patients that they will not be abandoned and that care will be forthcoming and available throughout their terminal course.

4. *Establishing therapeutic dialogue.* Patients need to be given permission—implicit or explicit—to discuss their fears, concerns, or wishes, even if they include the wish for hastened death. Inviting such a dialogue will decrease their sense of isolation, allow them an opportunity to explore concerns, and show that no topic is so sensitive as to preclude its discussion. These discussions can provide an opportunity to give reassurance when the wish for hastened death is spawned by concerns about remediable sources of suffering (e.g., depression, pain, or dyspnea).

5. *Exploring the underlying meaning of death-hastening requests.* It is critical to understand what is behind the patient's request. How do patients view their future? What are their values? Does the family understand or know about their requests? Is there any aspect of the life of the patient that he or she experiences as being meaningful? Are they concerned about being an undue financial or care burden on their family? Is there family conflict that contributes to the request?

6. *Evaluating decision-making capacity.* It is critical to ensure the following: (a) that the patient's mental processes are unimpaired by psychiatric illness, cognitive impairment,

or severe emotional distress (which might result in an impulsive request, which quickly changes with circumstances); (b) that the patient has a realistic assessment of his or her situation; and (c) that the motives for the decision are understandable to other observers.

7. *Bolstering social support.* It is important to mobilize as much support for the patient as possible. Involving close family members or friends is very helpful. Ultimately, the physician must take sufficient time to understand the patient's wishes.

8. *Seeking out consultation.* Death-hastening requests are among the most demanding of clinical situations healthcare providers face. However, in a national survey, only 2% of physicians reported having sought psychiatric consultation for patients requesting assistance in dying. Seeking out a second opinion may provide additional options and expertise, or, at the very least, support for the care provider grappling with the demands of a death-hastening request (Meier et al., 1998).

9. *Maintaining a clinical stance.* Rather than becoming overly focused on moral and legal issues, it is critical for the physician to remain attuned to the clinical challenges that such requests invariably present. Preoccupation with whether the patient has the "right to assisted suicide" can sometimes interfere with attending to clinical needs and can create an unnecessary standoff between the patient and physician.

Emanuel (1998) described an eight-step approach to assessing requests for assisted suicide. She described assessment and treatment of depression as the initial step in such an evaluation. Subsequent steps are assessment for decision-making capacity, discussion of advance care planning, assessment and treatment of root causes of the request, providing full information about assisted suicide and attempting to dissuade the patient, seeking consultation, reviewing adherence to the agreed-upon care plan and searching for unwanted interventions, and, finally, in her practice, declining to provide assisted suicide if the request persists. By paying strict attention to the uncontroversial principles of freedom from unwanted intervention and the physician's obligation to provide suffering patients with comfort care, Emanuel proposed that such an approach would respond appropriately to the despair underlying death-hastening requests by terminally ill patients. However, Emanuel's approach has been criticized as unrealistic, burdensome, and more helpful to physicians than to patients (Back, 1999; Ganzini & Sullivan, 1999). While such guidelines do not theoretically resolve whether physician-assisted suicide is morally justifiable, they nevertheless highlight the clinical imperatives that must be considered in these situations. The goal is, ultimately, to help patients attain as much comfort as possible, so they might examine their own personal circumstances, shape their death, and live the remainder of their life with as much grace, dignity, and meaning as possible.

CLINICAL PEARLS

- Every patient dreads hearing the words "There's nothing more I can do for you." Letting the patient and family know (by both words and actions) that they will not be expected to face the end of life alone is a great comfort. Seldom is the doctor–patient relationship more important.

- Dealing directly and confrontationally with family conflicts should occur if there is reasonable expectation of benefit from such an intervention.

- The periodic respite care integral to the Medicare Hospice Benefit can contribute to the preservation of a comforting home environment.

- Physicians should ask first about suffering in a general way (e.g., "What causes you to suffer most?"). The experience of suffering is unique to each individual.

- When breaking bad news to a patient, care should be taken to be gentle but clear. . . . The physician should be seated . . . and should ensure adequate privacy after determining whom the patient would like to have present for the discussion. The physician should next determine what patients already know about their condition and what details they would like to receive about their prognosis.

- Some patients are burdened by excessive detail or even a direct statement of their poor prognosis; their preference "not to know" should be respected and a suitable proxy identified.

- Despite the long history of the use of stimulants for depression in the medically ill, there are limited formal studies to support their use as antidepressants, but the available evidence suggests efficacy with stronger evidence for tolerability (Hardy, 2009).

- Though most patients with terminal illnesses may be unable to tolerate extensive psychotherapeutic interventions for depressive symptoms, a variety of psychotherapies can be modified for use in the care of terminally ill patients and their families.

- Diligent serial assessment is the key to detection of delirium at the end of life.

- Opioid dose reduction or opioid switching often results in significant improvement in delirium for the syndrome of opioid neurotoxicity (delirium, myoclonus, allodynia, hyperalgesia, and seizures) (de Stoutz et al., 1995).

- The physician is in an excellent position to educate families about grief and the grieving process, thus potentially preventing some cases of complicated or unresolved bereavement.

DISCLOSURE STATEMENTS

Dr. Shuster has no conflicts to disclose relevant to the topic of this chapter.

Dr. Chochinov

Dr. Jacobowski

REFERENCES

Akechi, T., Okuyama, T., Morita, T., et al. (2008). Psychotherapy for depression among incurable cancer patients. *Cochrane Database of Systematic Reviews* (2), CD005537.

American Psychiatric Association (1994). *Diagnostic and Statistical Manual of Mental Disorders* (4th ed.). Washington, DC: American Psychiatric Press.

Back, A. (1999). Responding to patient requests for physician-assisted suicide [letter]. *Journal of the American Medical Association, 281*(3), 227.

Barry, L. C., Kasl, S. V., & Prigerson, H. G. (2002). Psychiatric disorders among bereaved persons: The role of perceived circumstances of death and preparedness for death. *American Journal of Geriatric Psychiatry, 10*(4), 447–457.

Block, S. D. (2006). Psychological issues in end-of-life care. *Journal of Palliative Medicine, 9*(3), 751–772.

Breitbart, W., Bruera, E., Chochinov, H., et al. (1995). Neuropsychiatric syndromes and psychological symptoms in patients with advanced cancer. *Journal of Pain & Symptom Management, 10*, 131–141.

Breitbart, W., Chochinov, H. M., & Passik, S. (1998). Psychiatric aspects of palliative care. In D. Doyle, G. W. C. Hanks, & N. MacDonald (Eds.), *Oxford textbook of palliative medicine* (2nd ed., pp. 933–954). New York: Oxford University Press.

Breitbart, W., Gibson, C., & Tremblay, A. (2002). The delirium experience: delirium recall and delirium-related distress in hospitalized patients with cancer, their spouses/caregivers, and their nurses. *Psychosomatics, 43*(3), 183–194.

Breitbart, W., Rosenfeld, B., & Passik, S. D. (1996). Interest in physician assisted suicide among ambulatory HIV-infected patients. *American Journal of Psychology, 153*, 238–242.

Breitbart, W., Rosenfeld, B., Roth, A., et al (1997). The Memorial Delirium Assessment Scale. *Journal of Pain and Symptom Management, 13*(3), 128–137.

Breitbart, W., Rosenfeld, B., Gibson, C., et al. (2010). Impact of treatment for depression on desire for hastened death in patients with advanced AIDS. *Psychosomatics, 51*, 98–105.

Brown, J. H., Henteleff, P., Barakat, S., et al. (1986). Is it normal for terminally ill patients to desire death? *American Journal of Psychology, 143*, 208–211.

Brown, J. T., & Stoudemire, A. (1983). Normal and pathological grief. *Journal of the American Medical Association, 250*, 378–382.

Bruera, E., Chadwick, S., Weinlick, A., et al. (1987). Delirium and severe sedation in patients with terminal cancer. *Cancer Treatment Reports, 71*, 787–788.

Bruera, E., Bush, S. H., Willey, J., et al (2009). Impact of delirium and recall on the level of distress in patients with advanced cancer and their family caregivers. *Cancer, 115*(9), 2004–2012.

Bruera, E., Franco, J. J., Maltoni, M., et al. (1995). Changing pattern of agitated impaired mental status in patients with advanced cancer: association with cognitive monitoring, hydration, and opioid rotation. *Journal of Pain and Symptom Management, 10*(4), 287–291.

Chentsova-Dutton, Y., Shucter, S., Hutchin, S., et al. (2002). Depression and grief reactions in hospice caregivers: From pre-death to 1 year afterwards. *Journal of Affective Disorders, 69*(1–3), 53–60.

Chochinov, H. M., Kristjanson, L. J., Breitbart, W., et al. (2011). Effect of dignity therapy on distress and end-of-life experience in terminally ill patients: A randomised controlled trial. *Lancet Oncology, 12*, 753–762.

Chochinov, H. M., Wilson, K. G., Enns, M., et al. (1995). Desire for death in the terminally ill. *American Journal of Psychology, 152*, 1185–1191.

Chochinov, H. M., Wilson, K. G., Enns, M., et al. (1997). "Are you depressed?" Screening for depression in the terminally ill. *American Journal of Psychology, 154*, 674–676.

Christakis, N. A., & Escarce, J. J. (1996). Survival of Medicare patients after enrollment in hospice programs. *New England Journal of Medicine, 335*, 172–178.

Conill, C., Verger, E., Henriquez, I., et al. (1997). Symptom prevalence in the last week of life. *Journal of Pain & Symptom Management, 14,* 328–331.

Corr, C. A., & Doka, K. J. (1994). Current models of death, dying, and bereavement. *Critical Care, Nursing Clinics of North America, 6,* 545–552.

Corruble, E., Chouinard, V. A., Letierce, A., et al. (2009). Is DSM-IV bereavement exclusion for major depressive episode relevant to severity and pattern of symptoms? A case-control, cross-sectional study. *Journal of Clinical Psychiatry, 70*(8), 1091–1097.

Creagan, E. T. (1994). How to break bad news—and not devastate the patient. *Mayo Clinic Proceedings, 69,* 1015–1017.

deGraeff, A., & Dean, M. (2007). Palliative sedation therapy in the last weeks of life: a literature review and recommendations for standards. *Journal of Palliative Medicine, 10*(1), 67–85.

de Stoutz, N. D., Tapper, M., & Fainsinger, R. L. (1995). Reversible delirium in terminally ill patients. *Journal of Pain & Symptom Management, 10,* 249–253.

Del Fabbro, E., Dalal, S., & Bruera, E. (2006). Symptom control in palliative care—Part III: Dyspnea and delirium. *Journal of Palliative Medicine, 9*(2), 422–436.

Emanuel, L. L. (1998). Facing requests for physician-assisted suicide: Toward a practical and principled clinical skill set. *Journal of the American Medical Association, 280,* 643–647.

Fainsinger, R., MacEachern, T., Hanson, J., et al. (1991). Symptom control during the last week of life on a palliative care unit. *Journal of Palliative Care, 7,* 5–11.

Folstein, M. F., Folstein, S. E., & McHugh, P. R. (1975). "Mini-Mental State": A practical method for grading the cognitive state of patients for the clinician. *Journal of Psychiatry Research, 12,* 189–198.

Ganzini, L., & Sullivan, M. (1999). Responding to patient requests for physician-assisted suicide [letter]. *Journal of the American Medical Association, 281*(3), 227–228.

Ganzini, L., Lee, M. A., Heintz, R. T., et al. (1994). The effect of depression treatment on elderly patients' preferences for life-sustaining medical therapy. *American Journal of Psychology, 151,* 1631–1636.

Garg, A., Buckman, R., & Kason, Y. (1997). Teaching medical students how to break bad news. *Canadian Medical Association Journal, 156,* 1159–1164.

George H. Gallup International Institute (1997). *Spiritual beliefs and the dying process.* A report of a national survey conducted for the Nathan Cummings Foundation and the Fetzer Institute. Princeton, NJ: George H. Gallup International Institute.

Georges, J. J., Onwuteaka-Philipsen, B. D., van der Wal, G., et al (2005). Differences between terminally ill cancer patients who died after euthanasia had been performed and terminally ill cancer patients who did not request euthanasia. *Palliative Medicine, 19*(8), 578–586.

Grisso, T., & Appelbaum, P. S. (1995). Comparison of standards for assessing patients' capacities to make treatment decisions. *American Journal of Psychiatry, 152*(7), 1033–1037.

Groenewoud, J. H., Van Der Heide, A., Tholen, A. J., et al. (2004). Psychiatric consultation with regard to requests for euthanasia or physician-assisted suicide. *General Hospital Psychiatry, 26*(4), 323–330.

Grover, S., & Shah, R. (2011). Distress due to delirium experience. *General Hospital Psychiatry, 33*(6), 637–639.

Guze, S., & Robins, E. (1970). Suicide and primary affective disorders. *British Journal of Psychiatry, 47,* 437–438.

Hardy, S. E. (2009). Methylphenidate for the treatment of depressive symptoms, including fatigue and apathy, in medically ill older adults and terminally ill adults. *Journal of Geriatric Pharmacotherapy, 7,* 34–59.

Haverkate, I., Onwuteaka-Philipsen, B. D., van Der Heide, A., et al. (2000). Refused and granted requests for euthanasia and assisted suicide in the Netherlands: interview study with structured questionnaire. *BMJ, 321*(7265), 865–866.

Hensley, P. L., Slonimski, C. K., Uhlenhuth, E. H., & Clayton, P. J. (2009). Escitalopram: an open-label study of bereavement-related depression and grief. *Journal of Affective Disorders,* 113(1–2), 142–149.

Homsi, J., Nelson, K. A., Sarhill, N., et al (2001). A phase II study of methylphenidate for depression in advanced cancer. *American Journal of Hospice and Palliative Care, 18*(6), 403–407.

Hooper, S. C., Vaughan, K. J., Tennant, C. C., et al. (1996). Major depression and refusal of life-sustaining medical treatment in the elderly. *Medical Journal of Australia, 165,* 416–419.

Hooper, S. C., Vaughan, K. J., Tennant, C. C., et al. (1997). Preferences for voluntary euthanasia during major depression and following improvement in an elderly population. *Australian Journal of Ageing, 16,* 3–7.

Horowitz, M. J., Siegel, B., Holen, A., et al. (1997). Diagnostic criteria for complicated grief disorder. *American Journal of Psychology, 154,* 904–910.

Hotopf, M., Chidgey, J., Addington-Hall, J., et al. (2002). Depression in advanced disease: A systematic review, Part 1: Prevalence and case finding. *Palliative Medicine, 16*(2), 81–97.

Howard, P., Shuster, J., Twycross, R., et al. (2010). Psychostimulants. *Journal of Pain & Symptom Management, 40*(5), 789–795.

Inouye, S. K., van Dyke, C. H., Alessi, C. A., et al. (1990). Clarifying confusion: The Confusion Assessment Method. *Annals of Internal Medicine, 113,* 941–948.

Jackson, K. C., & Lipman, A. G. (2004). Drug therapy for anxiety in adult palliative care patients. *Cochrane Database of Systematic Reviews,* (1), CD004596.

Jacobs, S. C., Nelson, J. C., & Zisook, S. (1987). Treating depressions of bereavement with antidepressants. A pilot study. *Psychiatric Clinics of North America, 10*(3), 501–510.

Jacobsen, J. C., Zhang, B., Block, S. D., et al. (2010). Distinguishing symptoms of grief and depression in a cohort of advanced cancer patients. *Death Studies, 34*(3), 257–273.

Jacobsen, P. B., & Breitbart, W. (1996). Psychosocial aspects of palliative care. *Cancer Control, 3,* 214–222.

Jansen-van der Weide, M. C., Onwuteaka-Philipsen, B. D., & van der Wal, G. (2005). Granted, undecided, withdrawn, and refused requests for euthanasia and physician-assisted suicide. *Archives of Internal Medicine, 165*(15), 1698–1704.

Karam, E. G., Tabet, C. C., Alam, D., et al. (2009). Bereavement related and non-bereavement related depressions: A comparative field study. *Journal of Affective Disorders, 112*(1–3), 102–110.

Kim, K., & Jacobs, S. (1991). Pathologic grief and its relationship to other psychiatric disorders. *Journal of Affective Disorders, 21*(4), 257–263.

Kissane, D. W., Bloch, S., Onghena, P., et al. (1996). The Melbourne Family Grief Study, II: Psychosocial morbidity and grief in bereaved families. *American Journal of Psychology, 153,* 659–666.

Kroenke, K., Spitzer, R. L., Williams, J. B., et al. (2010). The Patient Health Questionnaire somatic, anxiety, and depressive symptom scales: A systematic review. *General Hospital Psychiatry, 32,* 345–359.

Kubler-Ross, E. (1969). *On death and dying.* New York: Macmillan.

Laird, B. J., Boyd, A. C., Colvin, L. A., et al. (2009). Are cancer pain and depression interdependent? A systematic review. *Psycho-Oncology, 18,* 459–464.

Leonard, M., Agar, M., Mason, C., et al. (2008). Delirium issues in palliative care settings. *Journal of Psychosomatic Research, 65,* 289–298.

Lichtenthal, W. G., Cruess, D. G., & Prigerson, H. G. (2004). A case for establishing complicated grief as a distinct mental disorder in DSM-V. *Clinical Psychology Review, 24*(6), 637–662.

Lipowski, Z. J. (1990). *Delirium: Acute confusional states.* New York: Oxford University Press.

Lloyd-Williams, M., Spiller, J., & Ward, J. (2003). Which depression screening tools should be used in palliative care? *Palliative Medicine, 17,* 40–43.

Lonergan, E., Britton, A. M., & Luxemberg, J. (2007). Antipsychotics for delirium. *Cochrane Database of Systematic Reviews,* (2), CD005594.

Lorenz, K. A., Lynn, J., Dy, S. M., et al. (2008). Evidence for improving palliative care at the end of life: A systematic review. *Annals of Internal Medicine, 148,* 147–159.

Macleod, A. D. (1998). Methylphenidate in terminal depression. *Journal of Pain and Symptom Management, 16*(3), 193–198.

Maessen, M., Veldink, J. H., Onwuteaka-Philipsen, B. D., et al (2009). Trends and determinants of end-of-life practices in ALS in the Netherlands. *Neurology, 73*(12), 954–961.

Maltoni, M., Pittureri, C., Scarpi, E., et al. (2009). Palliative sedation therapy does not hasten death: results from a prospective multicenter study. *Annals of Oncology, 20*(7), 1163–1169.

Markowitz, J. D., & Narasimhan, M. (2008). Delirium and antipsychotics: A systematic review of epidemiology and somatic treatment options. *Psychiatry (Edgemont), 5*(10), 29–36.

Masand, P. S., & Tesar, G. E. (1996). Use of stimulants in the medically ill. *Psychiatric Clinics of North America, 19*(3), 515–547.

Meier, D. E., Emmons, C., Wallenstein, S., et al. (1998). A national survey of physician-assisted suicide and euthanasia in the United States. *New England Journal of Medicine, 338,* 1193–1201.

National Hospice Organization Medical Guidelines Task Force (1995). *Medical guidelines for determining prognosis in selected non-cancer diseases.* Arlington, VA: National Hospice Organization.

Oakley, F., Khin, N. A., Parks, R., et al. (2002). Improvement in activities of daily living in elderly following treatment for post-bereavement depression. *Acta Psychiatrica Scandinavica, 105*(3), 231–234.

Oldervoll, L. M., Loge, J. H., Paltiel, H., et al. (2006). The effect of a physical exercise program in palliative care: A phase II study. *Journal of Pain & Symptom Management, 31*(5), 421–430.

Parkes, C. M. (1998). Bereavement. In D. Doyle, G. W. C. Hanks, & N. MacDonald (Eds.), *Oxford textbook of palliative medicine* (2nd ed., pp. 995–1010). Oxford, UK: Oxford University Press.

Pasternak, R. E., Reynolds, C. F. 3rd, Schlernitzauer, M., et al (1991). Acute open-trial nortriptyline therapy of bereavement-related depression in late life. *Journal of Clinical Psychiatry, 52*(7), 307–310.

Portenoy, R. K., Thaler, H. T., Kornblith, A. B., et al. (1994). The Memorial Symptom Assessment Scale: An instrument for the evaluation of symptom prevalence, characteristics and distress. *European Journal of Cancer, 30A,* 1326–1336.

Prigerson, H. G., Bierhals, A. J., Kasl, S. V., et al. (1996). Complicated grief as a disorder distinct from bereavement-related depression and anxiety: A replication study. *American Journal of Psychology, 153,* 1484–1486.

Prigerson, H. G., Frank, E., Kasl, S., et al. (1995). Complicated grief and bereavement-related depression as distinct disorders: Preliminary empirical validation in elderly bereaved spouses. *American Journal of Psychology, 152,* 22–30.

Prigerson, H. G., Horowitz, M. J., Jacobs, S. C., et al. (2009). Prolonged grief disorder: Psychometric validation of criteria proposed for DSM-V and ICD-11. *PLoS Medicine* (8), e1000121.

Rando, T. A. (1984). *Grief, dying, and death.* Champaign, IL: Research Press Company.

Rayner, L., Price, A., Hotopf, M., & Higginson, I. J. (2011). The development of evidence-based European guidelines on the management of depression in palliative cancer care. *European Journal of Cancer, 47*(5), 702–712.

Reynolds, C. F., Miller, M. D., Pasternak, R. E., et al. (1999). Treatment of bereavement-related major depressive episodes in later life: A controlled study of acute and continuation treatment with nortriptyline and interpersonal psychotherapy. *American Journal of Psychology, 156,* 202–206.

Rodin, G., Craven, J., & Littlefield, C. (1991). *Depression in the medically ill: An integrated approach.* New York: Mazel.

Rosenbaum, J. F., Pollack, M. H., Otto, M. W., et al. (1997). Anxious patients. In N. H. Cassem, T. A. Stern, J. F. Rosenbaum, et al. (Eds.), *Massachusetts General Hospital handbook of general hospital psychiatry* (4th ed., pp. 173–210). St. Louis, MO: Mosby.

Ruijs, C. D., Kerkhof, A. J., van der Wal, G., & Onwuteaka-Philipsen, B. D. (2011). Depression and explicit requests for euthanasia in end-of-life cancer patients in primary care in the Netherlands: a longitudinal, prospective study. *Family Practice, 28*(4), 393–399.

Shear, K., Frank, E., Houck, P. R., et al. (2005). Treatment of complicated grief: A randomized controlled trial. *Journal of the American Medical Association, 293*(21), 2601–2608.

Shear, M. K., Simon, N., Wall, M., et al. (2011). Complicated grief and related bereavement issues for DSM-5. *Journal of Depression & Anxiety, 28*(2), 103–117.

Shuster, J. L., & Jones, G. R. (1998). Approach to the patient receiving palliative care. In T. A. Stern, J. B. Herman, & P. L. Slavin (Eds.), *The Massachusetts General Hospital guide to psychiatry in primary care* (pp. 147–165). New York: Mc-Graw-Hill.

Shuster, J. L., Breitbart, W., & Chochinov, H. M. (1998). Psychiatric aspects of excellent end-of-life care: A position statement of the Academy of Psychosomatic Medicine. *Academy of Psychosomatic Medicine,* January. Available at http://www.apm. Org/papers/eol-care.shtml. Last accessed October 2, 2014.

Simon, N. M., Thompson, E. H., Pollack, M. H., & Shear, M. K. (2007). Complicated grief: a case series using escitalopram. *American Journal of Psychiatry, 164*(11), 1760–1761.

Spiegel, D., Sands, S., & Koopman, C. (1994). Pain and depression in patients with cancer. *Cancer, 74,* 2570–2578.

Stiefel, F., Fainsinger, R., & Bruera, E. (1992). Acute confusional states in patients with advanced cancer. *Journal of Pain & Symptom Management, 7,* 94–98.

Storey, P., Trumble, M. (1992). Rectal doxepin and carbamazepine in patients with cancer. *New England Journal of Medicine, 327,* 1318–1319.

Sykes, N., & Thorns, A. (2003). Sedative use in the last week of life and the implications for end-of-life decision making. *Archives of Internal Medicine, 163*(3), 341–344.

Trzepacz, P. T. (1996). Delirium. Advances in diagnosis, pathophysiology, and treatment. *Psychiatric Clinics of North America, 19*(3), 429–448.

Wasteson, E., Brenne, E., Higginson, I. J., et al. (2009). Depression assessment and classification in palliative cancer patients: A systematic literature review. *Palliative Medicine, 23*(8), 739–753.

Webb, M. (1997). *The good death: The new American search to reshape the end of life.* New York: Bantam Books.

Webster's New Collegiate Dictionary (1979). Springfield, MA: G. & C. Merriam Co.

Wells, K. B., Stewart, A., Hays, R. D., et al. (1989). The functioning and wellbeing of depressed patients: Results from the Medical Outcomes Study. *Journal of the American Medical Association, 262,* 914–919.

Wise, M. G., & Trzepacz PT (1996). Delirium (confusional states). In J. R. Rundell & M. G. Wise (Eds.), *The American Psychiatric Press textbook of consultation-liaison psychiatry* (pp. 259–274). Washington, DC: American Psychiatric Press.

World Health Organization (1990). *Cancer pain relief and palliative care. Technical Report Series 804.* Geneva: World Health Organization.

Wright, A. A., Keating, N. L., Balboni, T. A., et al. (2010). Place of death: Correlations with quality of life of patients with cancer and predictors of bereaved caregivers' mental health. *Journal of Clinical Oncology, 28*(29), 4457–4464.

Zhang, B., El-Jawahri, A., & Prigerson, H. G. (2006). Update on bereavement research: Evidence-based guidelines for the diagnosis and treatment of complicated bereavement. *Journal of Palliative Medicine, 9*(5), 1188–1203.

Zisook, S., & Shear, K. (2009). Grief and bereavement: What psychiatrists need to know. *World Psychiatry, 8*(2), 67–74.

Zisook, S., & Shuchter, S. R. (1991). Early psychological reaction to the stress of widowhood. *Psychiatry, 54,* 320–333.

Zisook, S., & Shuchter, S. R. (1992). Depression through the first year after the death of a spouse. *American Journal of Psychology, 148,* 1346–1352.

Zisook, S., Shuchter, S. R., Pedrelli, P., et al. (2001). Bupropion sustained release for bereavement: results of an open trial. *Journal of Clinical Psychiatry, 62*(4), 227–230.

Zisook, S., Reynolds, C. F. 3rd, Pies, R., et al. (2010). Bereavement, complicated grief, and DSM, part 1: Depression. *Journal of Clinical Psychiatry, 71*(7), 955–956.

Zisook, S., Simon, N. M., Reynolds, C. F. 3rd, et al. (2010). Bereavement, complicated grief, and DSM, part 2: Complicated grief. *Journal of Clinical Psychiatry, 71*(8), 1097–1098.

Zygmont, M., Prigerson, H. G., Houck, P. R., et al. (1998). A post hoc comparison of paroxetine and nortriptyline for symptoms of traumatic grief. *Journal of Clinical Psychiatry, 59*(5), 241–245.

85.

CAPACITY, COMPETENCY AND CONSENT IN MEDICAL PSYCHIATRY

Barry S. Fogel

INTRODUCTION

In inpatient settings, medical psychiatrists often are called on to assess patients' decision-making capacity, usually in connection with their ability to choose or refuse a treatment or procedure. A survey of medical psychiatrists found that one in six general hospital psychiatry consultations involved the assessment of a patient's decision-making capacity (Seyfried et al., 2013). In outpatient settings, questions often concern issues such as the ability to drive a car safely, to handle one's own finances, or to make or change a will. The psychiatrist's assessment of capacity may be sufficient to convince other physicians—or the psychiatrist him/herself—that a patient's decision regarding treatment should be honored or that a patient's driving or financial decisions should not be questioned. When assessments suggest that a patient's capacity is insufficient, legal mechanisms are triggered, which can be as simple as triggering the application of a durable power of attorney or the activation of a healthcare proxy, or as complex as a formal hearing on competency and the appointment of a legal guardian or conservator if the patient is found to be incompetent. In the last situation, the psychiatrist provides input to a process that involves at a minimum a lawyer and a judge, and at most a full-scale adversarial proceeding with different parties represented by counsel. The psychiatrist in that case may be identified as an expert for one side in a dispute. Fortunately, most cases related to diminished capacity due to medical conditions affecting brain function do not entail a full-scale legal process; if they did, it is hard to see how timely interventions could be made in acute care.

A theme of this book is that as the organization and context of healthcare change, so does the practice of medical psychiatry. The psychiatric literature on capacity, competency, and consent historically has focused on issues such as the right to refuse psychiatric treatment, including hospitalization, antipsychotic drugs, and electroconvulsive therapy (ECT), the criminal responsibility of people with chronic mental illness, and conditions for involuntary psychiatric treatment. The corresponding issues in general hospital psychiatry have related to such matters as competency to consent to a risky treatment or to refuse a usual treatment, competency to consent to participate in research, competency to

opt for palliative care and decline more active but potentially futile treatments, and mental status considerations in the execution of advance directives. The issues that have become more salient in recent years relate to the long-term course of chronic diseases that affect brain functioning, especially the dementias and other neurodegenerative conditions, but also including the late effects of traumatic brain injury. In these conditions, the loss of decision-making capacity or other functional capacities can be gradual and progressive, partial and persistent, or episodic. Capacities lost range from occupational competence and appropriate financial decision-making to maintenance of one's living space, safe use of medication, and safe driving. Bad decisions or inappropriate behavior due to lost capacities can have devastating consequences for patients and for other people as well, yet binary formal legal determinations of competency do not match the specificity and nuance of patients' actual situations. Optimal solutions can require the ongoing involvement of a clinician such as a medical psychiatrist with awareness and consideration of the patient's brain, mind, social context, and personal narrative. Ideal solutions are proactive, anticipating issues and preventing crises.

This chapter is intended to be a point of departure for clinicians involved in caring for patients with current or anticipated impairments in decision-making capacity. Its emphasis is necessarily clinical, as legal details will vary by venue; within the United States, state laws differ greatly, and some other countries' legal systems have procedures very different from those of the United States.

LEGAL AND ETHICAL CONCEPTS

All of the concepts described below are described specifically as they apply in a medical context. Non-medical applications, such as the legal definition of consent to a sexual act, are beyond the scope of this chapter. The interpretation of these legal concepts can vary by jurisdiction; the clinician should know the locally applicable version of each. Underlying legal differences between U.S. states and even more between countries reflect cultural differences; for example, in the perception of the value of life, which can be seen primarily as intrinsic, instrumental, or self-determined. Likewise, countries differ in the relative value they give to a patient's autonomy when it is in conflict with his or her best interests (Jox et al., 2013).

CAPACITY AND COMPETENCY

A person's capacity to make a decision or perform an act comprises willingness to do it and the ability to accomplish its purpose. Capacity can be normal, diminished or absent. Incapacity can refer to "can't," "won't," or a combination of the two: A person has equally diminished capacity to cross a street safely if he cannot see the oncoming traffic or if he will not look.

Competency refers to a legal determination that the action of a person—such as signing a contract, making a will, or consenting to a surgical procedure—should be regarded as the valid act of a person who is of legal age and has sufficient capacity to perform the action in his or her own interest. Adults are presumed to be competent unless there is affirmative determination that they are not.

CONSENT

In the medical context, *consent* is a specific, affirmative act in which a person agrees to an action by a healthcare provider. The affirmative act of consent typically is a signature on a form, but a signature alone is neither necessary nor sufficient. A signature given by a patient who does not understand what they are signing is not valid consent, while a verbal "yes" or even a nod of the head can be valid consent if the patient is fully aware of what he or she is agreeing to and has signaled agreement after due consideration. Consent given verbally or by gesture must be carefully documented. In high-stakes situations, a video recording may be useful in establishing that consent was fully informed and freely given.

ASSENT, COMPLIANCE, AND ADHERENCE

Assent is a patient's permitting an action by a healthcare provider without explicitly and affirmatively consenting to it. For example, a patient holding out her arm for a phlebotomist, who then takes the blood sample to the laboratory, is a assenting to the drawing of blood and to the communication of blood test results to healthcare providers involved in her care.

Compliance, a medical term and not a legal one, refers to doing what a healthcare provider has suggested, recommended, or ordered: one can comply or not with positive directions like taking a medication or negative ones like not smoking. *Adherence* (to a plan of treatment) is a softer concept with a similar meaning: a patient *complies* with orders but *adheres* to a recommended plan.

Refusal is an affirmative statement by a patient that he or she does not wish a healthcare provider to do a specific thing, such as perform a procedure or share certain information, or an affirmative statement that he or she will not comply with a particular clinical directive. Examples are refusing to release psychiatric records to a general medical physician, or refusing to take a prescribed antipsychotic drug.

Resistance to care is a patient's actively not allowing a healthcare provider to do something the provider is attempting to do; for example, a patient not permitting a nurse to give him or her a bath, or actively pulling out an intravenous line just after it has been placed. Resistance to care may be—but is not necessarily—associated with refusal of treatment.

NON-COMPLIANCE AND NON-ADHERENCE

Non-compliance or *non-adherence* refers to a patient's not doing what a healthcare provider has directed; such as not taking prescribed medication. Non-compliance can be either passive or active, depending on whether the direction required taking an action or refraining from one—but it does not include an explicit, affirmative rejection of the clinical prescription.

People with cognitive dysfunction or psychotic ambivalence can—and frequently do—consent to treatment but do not comply with clinical directives; or refuse treatment but assent to care. Psychiatrists sometimes need to explain these phenomena to legal personnel unfamiliar with neuropsychiatric disorders.

IMPLIED CONSENT

Implied consent is the legal doctrine that in an emergency situation, a physician or other healthcare provider has a right to perform treatment without the explicit consent of a patient or a legal substitute. A medical emergency is an occasion for implied consent if the patient does not have the capacity to give consent because of impairment in consciousness, cognition, or communication; no authorized surrogate decision-maker is immediately available; and delay in action has a significant likelihood of causing serious harm to the patient. For example, a physician has implied consent to treat a patient who is exsanguinating without looking for someone to sign a consent form. A subtler point is that physicians can reasonably assert they have implied consent to immediately begin diagnostic and treatment interventions when patients presents with new-onset delirium of unknown cause, as potential causes include conditions like electrolyte disturbances, severe hypoglycemia, or sepsis that could threaten life or could cause significant brain damage if not promptly treated. Note that implied consent to emergency treatment does not extend to follow-up treatment once the patient is out of danger. And, in the situation where a patient was near the end of life and had opted to decline life-saving treatment via a living will, implied consent would end once the physician knew there was a valid advance directive.

LEGAL STATUS OF THE NEXT OF KIN

In a true emergency situation, when significant injury could result from a delay in treatment, physicians are empowered to act in the best interest of the patient. If a proxy decision-maker was selected by the patient in advance of the emergency, that individual's consent should be sought and his or her (competent) refusal should be honored, but treatment should not be delayed if the proxy decision-maker cannot readily be contacted. If no proxy was nominated by the patient prior to the emergency, the patient's next of kin does not have an automatic legal right to overrule a physician's judgment that a particular treatment should be given (Simpson, 2011).

CATEGORIES OF AGENTS

The law, with variation in detail between jurisdictions, recognizes various kinds of agents or surrogate decision-makers invested with the authority and responsibility to make decisions and commitments on behalf of another individual. Importantly, authority and responsibility are linked: patients' agents and surrogate decision-makers are not only empowered to act on their behalf, but they are expected do so, reliably and honestly.

Guardians and *conservators* are individuals invested via a legal procedure involving a judge with the authority and responsibility to make decisions on behalf of a person who is incompetent or incapacitated. Guardianship can be limited to healthcare decisions or can cover a broader scope, including decisions about finances and living arrangements. Conservatorship is a similar legally sanctioned relationship of authority and responsibility, limited to financial affairs only.

Trustees are individuals with legal authority and responsibility for the management and disposition of trusts—entities that own and control financial assets. Trustees' powers and responsibilities are described in trust documents—instruments set up by trustors, who transfer assets to the trust and specify how and by whom they are to be invested and for whom and for what purposes they are to be spent. In many trusts, the trustor is also the trustee until the trustor dies or becomes incapacitated, at which point a successor trustee takes over.

Attorneys-in-fact are agents empowered to represent an individual in business-related transactions. The powers of an attorney-in-fact are specified in a document known as a *power of attorney*. Powers of attorney can be general, covering all of an individual's personal business; or limited to specific purposes like paying a person's bills or signing documents related to a real estate transaction. A person must be competent in order to sign a valid power of attorney, and ordinary powers of attorney terminate when the person granting them becomes incompetent. A *durable power of attorney* (DPoA) persists even if the person granting it becomes incompetent; typically, it is designed to go into effect only if the grantor is incapacitated, and to cease if and when the grantor regains the capacity to make valid decisions. A durable power of attorney for healthcare, or *healthcare proxy*, is a specialized power of attorney that grants a designated person authority and responsibility for making healthcare decisions if and when the grantor is incapable of making such decisions for him/herself.

Validity of a DPoA requires adequate decision-making capacity *at the time the DPoA is signed*. When there is much at stake, when the motives or judgment of the attorney-in-fact are questionable, when there is dissent or contention in the family, or when the patient's cognitive function is unstable, a medical evaluation (ideally a medical-psychiatric one) of decision-making capacity should be done contemporaneously with the execution of the DPoA. Prevention of conflict and litigation justifies the added inconvenience and expense of scheduling the medical and legal appointments close together on the same day—or even at the same time (Lui et al., 2014).

The *activation* of a DPoA or the empowerment of a successor trustee requires a signed statement by the patient's physician—and in some jurisdictions, the concurring opinion of a second physician—that the patient is incapacitated and unable to make valid decisions. Return of decision-making authority to the patient would similarly require a signed physician's statement. In contrast to the appointment of a guardian or conservator, the empowerment of attorneys-in-fact, healthcare agents (proxies), and successor trustees does not require judicial action, and it is reversible without judicial action if and when the patient recovers capacity. This fact, and the flexibility and specificity of such arrangements, makes them much preferable to guardianships for dealing with illness-related changes in decision-making capacity.

ADVANCE DIRECTIVES

Advance directives are formal statements by individuals about how they would like to be treated under certain medical circumstances in which they would be unable to make or express a decision regarding their healthcare; for example, how they would like to be treated if they entered an irreversible coma. These directives often are accompanied by a statement of whom the person nominates to be his or her agent to give or withhold consent to treatment in such circumstances; i.e., a surrogate decision-maker. Advance directives *only* apply if a person is unable to make and communicate healthcare-related preferences at the time; they can be overridden at any time by the person who signed the advance directive. A *living will* is a form of advance directive that in some jurisdictions is legally binding on clinicians; in other jurisdictions, a living will offers non-binding guidance to the surrogate decision-maker.

Health care proxies are documents in which an individual designates an agent to make healthcare decisions on his/her behalf if he/she is unable to make such decisions personally. The *agent* designated in a healthcare proxy (sometimes also referred to as a healthcare proxy) has decision-making authority only concerning the patient's health care; the agent does not have the authority to make financial or business decisions on the patient's behalf. A patient can have the capacity to execute a valid healthcare proxy even though he or she does not have the capacity to make a competent decision about medical treatment itself (Dunn & Alici, 2013). The criteria for the capacity to select a surrogate decision-maker are not defined by law or published consensus, but at the minimum, a patient should know the nature of the decision being made, and the surrogate should be appropriate—that is, someone who could reasonably be expected to have adequate decision-making capacity and to act either according to the patient's previously expressed wishes or according to the patient's best interests.

Advance directives typically discuss if and when life-sustaining treatments are to be withheld, in relation to the severity of the patient's impairments, the prognosis, and the intensity of intervention(s) necessary to keep the patient alive. Advance directives cannot possibly anticipate all medical circumstances, so they work best when there is also a healthcare proxy who knows the patient well and can adequately represent what the patient would want in various circumstances. When the exact circumstances of the patient are not described in the advance directives, the healthcare proxy must make a judgment based on what they think the patient would have wanted, all things considered. It is useful if the proxy knows how much leeway the patient would have wanted him or her to have in adapting the advance directive to current unforeseen circumstances.

One drawback of typical advance directives is that they focus on only the most severe and hopeless situations—and neither patients, nor families, nor physicians easily give up all hope. For example, Teno et al. (1998), in recounting qualitative aspects of a study of end-of-life decision-making, described how a physician told a patient she had a 25% chance of survival, when in fact her predicted six-month survival using a validated model was less than one percent. Advance directives tend to focus on the very end of life, and rarely deal with the circumstances under which a patient might choose hospice care and forgo continued aggressive medical treatment, as opposed to forgoing life-sustaining treatments in the narrow sense. Yet, by the time that a patient's prognosis is obviously terminal, the patient might lack the capacity to make that choice.

For a patient's living will to be valid, he or she must be competent when it is signed, he or she must fully understand the issues involved; and he/she must be free of undue influence. The treating physician may not be the legal witness for the document. Many jurisdictions do not permit the treating physician to be a patient's healthcare proxy, and in any case it is not advisable.

Because patients and physicians cannot foresee or describe every potential clinical situation that might occur, advance directives should include the nomination of a surrogate decision-maker, and ideally they will indicate how much leeway the surrogate decision-maker has to deviate from the explicit directives if doing so appears to be in the patient's best interest. Smith et al. (2013) commented on the conflict that can occur between an advance directive and the patient's best interests, not because the advance directive was poorly conceived, but because the precise circumstances of the patient are different in important ways from those envisioned when the advance directive was written. For example, one can conceive of situations in which "comfort care" could conceivably involve surgery, as when failure to surgically stabilize a broken bone would cause continual pain and greatly decreased mobility. Smith and colleagues propose consideration of five points:

1. Is the clinical situation an emergency?

2. In view of the patient's values and goals, how likely is it that the benefits of the intervention will outweigh the burdens?

3. How well does the advance directive fit the situation at hand?

4. How much leeway did the patient allow the surrogate for overriding the advance directive?

5. How well does the surrogate represent the patient's best interests?

The idea that advance directives should have built-in leeway is supported by the work of Imhof et al. (2011), who interviewed 40 physicians and 52 nurses in Swiss acute-care hospitals on their views on the process of making "do not attempt resuscitation" (DNR) decisions. In Switzerland, patients' advance directives are not legally binding. Physicians and nurses nonetheless greatly valued them and expressed the wish that more patients had them. For most of those interviewed, the ideal process for soliciting advance directives was a dialogue between a senior physician and the patient, and the ideal process for actually deciding on a DNR order was a consensus-building process involving physicians, nurses, the patient, and the patient's family. Implicit in this process is the idea that changing circumstances may require modifying or superseding an existing advance directive. In the intensive care unit (ICU) environment, disagreements between attending physicians and surrogate decision-makers are common: resolving them often requires not only dialogue, but also enough time for the surrogate to come to terms emotionally with the patient's diagnosis and prognosis (Brush et al., 2012).

A group of medical ethicists at Indiana University conducted in-depth interviews with 35 surrogate decision-makers who had recently made a healthcare decision in one of two urban acute-care hospitals. They found that, when actually making healthcare decisions, surrogates considered both patient-centered factors and surrogate-centered factors. The former included respecting the patient's input, using past knowledge of the patient to infer the patient's wishes, and considering the patient's best interests. The latter included the surrogate's own wishes if he or she were in the patient's situation, the surrogate's personal interests, the surrogate's religious beliefs or spirituality, family consensus, and obligation and guilt (Fritch et al., 2013). Their findings underscore the great importance of the choice of a surrogate decision-maker. Ideally, the patient would spend as much time getting to know the surrogate's beliefs and preferences as the surrogate would spend getting to know the patient's. In reality, surrogate decision-makers often report they wish they knew more about the prior wishes and preferences of those they represent. Patients choosing surrogate decision-makers usually pick individuals with whom they have had long-term or even lifetime relationships. Even so, some of the surrogate-centered factors described by Fritch et al. (2013) might not be known to them.

THE FOUR PRINCIPLES
(BEAUCHAMP & CHILDRESS, 2009)

Medical ethicists have advanced four basic principles to guide ethical medical decision-making: *autonomy* (respect for individual decisions), *beneficence* (relieving, lessening or preventing harm; providing benefits that justify risks and costs), *non-maleficence* (not doing harm), and *social justice* (fair distribution of risks, benefits, and costs). Historically, paternalistic physicians emphasized their beneficence and acted on the presumption that they knew what was best for the patient. Nowadays, in the United States in particular, the patient's autonomy is the most important factor: patients are permitted to refuse treatments prescribed by their physician even when doing so will hasten their death (Will, 2011). Notwithstanding, the recent literature on advance directives reveal that beneficence—and concern for the patient's best interests—refuses to die. Physicians who see a need for flexibility in following advance directives may simply be recognizing that both patients' feelings and clinical situations are nuanced and not easily reduced to checkboxes on a form. The position is not necessarily paternalistic, it is just professional—but the risks of countertransference, personal bias, and excessive influence by opinionated family members are ever-present.

AUTONOMY—AGENCY AND AUTHENTICITY

Autonomy in particular has a subtlety that psychiatrists may be particularly well-suited to appreciate. Autonomy involves *agency*—choosing a course of action in a particular specific situation—and *authenticity*—choosing a lifestyle, a set of values, and a view of human experience (Brudney & Lantos, 2011). Specific circumstances and a patient's emotional reaction to them can prompt him or her to make immediate decisions that are inconsistent with their personality, philosophy, and a long history of other decisions. This can occur without such severe emotional disturbance as to render the patient incompetent by virtue of mental illness. However, it would seem wrong to honor an unwise and potentially fatal refusal of medical care because of a transient state of mind inconsistent with the patient's entire life narrative. The usual resolution is to temporize, asking the psychiatrist or other counselor (e.g., pastoral counselor or psychologist) to engage the patient in dialogue in the hope that the patient's mind will change. In some cases, the psychiatrist can assert that the patient is not competent to make the given decision, though not globally incompetent, but at least in the United States, getting legal authority to override the patient's refusal of care in such a situation would be difficult.

SUBSTITUTED JUDGMENT

Substituted judgment refers to surrogate decision-making in which the surrogate makes the decision he or she believes the patient would have made if they had had the capacity to decide. Doing this involves consideration, not only of the patient's prior expressed wishes and opinions, but also of what is known about their values, beliefs, personality, and lifestyle. This comprehensive perspective is important because people's views change with their experience of illness. A patient who once said they would rather die than go to a nursing home may feel very differently when they are sick and lonely, and find that a particular nursing home is a pleasant place to live. On the other hand, a cancer patient who once said they would want the physician to "do everything" might become so tired of pain, medication side effects, loss of privacy, and invasiveness of active treatment they would now choose palliative care if able to express a preference. Medical psychiatrists, experienced in eliciting life stories and in assessing personality and emotional state, may be especially helpful to a healthcare proxy trying to implement substituted judgment in the absence of a legally binding advance directive.

BEST INTERESTS

Best interests is a principle for surrogate decision-making that is the major alternative to substituted judgment. Under this principle, the surrogate decision-maker acts in a way that is expected to promote the greatest overall welfare of the patient, considering all relevant factors, including professional and ethical standards. It is arguable whether best interests or substituted judgment is a preferable principle for proxy decision-making in the absence of advance directives, though contemporary practice favors substituted judgment when there is sufficient knowledge of the patient's personality, prior decisions, and stated wishes and beliefs. The application of the best interests principle is inevitably affected by the surrogate decision-maker's personality and beliefs, the surrogate's medical knowledge, and what physicians tell the surrogate about the prognosis and their expectations of the outcome of various treatments.

When 34 prospective subjects in dementia research, all of whom had mild to moderate cognitive impairment, were asked about how they would want their surrogates to make decisions for them related to research participation, the majority preferred using best interests or a combination of best interests and substituted judgment as the principle. Only 15% favored using substituted judgment alone (Black et al., 2013). This small but very interesting study suggests that the current philosophical—and in many jurisdictions—legal emphasis on patient autonomy as the most important principle of all does not comport with many patients' own views. A similar study of 40 proxy decision-makers for potential Alzheimer's disease research subjects revealed a common preference for a balancing substituted judgment and best interests, and as well as appreciation that a patient's premorbid preferences and present preferences might be different. Thus a premorbid preference expressed in an advance directive or a discussion with the surrogate might not be the "gold standard" for surrogate decision-making (Dunn et al., 2013).

Muthalagappan et al. (2013) cite evidence that a substantial proportion of older people do not want personal control over their medical decisions, and proposed that shared decision-making, a process that has been described as "the pinnacle of patient-centered care" (Barry, 2012), is optimal for making the decision of how to manage end-stage renal disease in frail elders with multiple comorbidities. Muthalagappan and colleagues point out that nephrologists lack the time, and often the communication skills, needed to implement shared decision-making. Medical psychiatrists, who combine empathy and communication skills with general medical knowledge, would appear ideally qualified to do the job.

CLINICAL CONCEPTS

DECISION-MAKING CAPACITY

The elements of decision-making capacity have been described as being able: to understand the decision to be made, to express a preference, to offer a rational reason for it, and to appreciate the context and implications of the choice. It is evident that the most complex and potentially subjective aspect of assessing decision-making capacity concerns the element of appreciation. Appreciation of the context of a decision requires accurate, non-delusional perceptions and memories and understanding of their meaning, including recall and understanding of relationships with people who might be affected by one's decision. Appreciation of the implications of a decision requires the kind of foresight that adults learn through education and life experience, and may also involve knowledge of one's health conditions and appropriate trust in one's physician's advice.

A patient can have adequate capacity to make a valid decision yet make a decision that most people would regard as a bad judgment. Consider a hypothetical patient at high risk for myocardial infarction (MI) who comes to an emergency room with chest pain. He is examined and blood is drawn; while awaiting the results of laboratory tests, he decides to go home against medical advice (AMA). He appreciates that he might have a myocardial infarction and that if he does he might develop an arrhythmia that could threaten his life if not promptly treated—something done more readily in a hospital. He states, however, that:

1. He thinks stress is bad for the heart and he will be far more relaxed at home;

2. He does not have health insurance and he knows that more time at the hospital means a larger bill—something that would worry him greatly;

3. He is willing to return to the hospital if they call and tell him he has had a significant myocardial infarction—but if the lab tests do not suggest an MI, or suggest a very small one, he prefers to remain at home and follow up as an outpatient.

He gives his mobile phone number and asks to be contacted with the laboratory result—whatever it is. This hypothetical patient's decision to leave the emergency room is clearly valid, because the patient understood his situation, knew what his options were, appreciated the risks inherent in his choice, could communicate a preference, and could offer a rational reason for that preference. He should be discharged from the emergency room AMA, with clear contemporaneous documentation that he was informed of the risks of leaving, that he understood and accepted the risks, and that he had the capacity to make a valid decision (Levy et al., 2012).

A patient like the one just described should not be discharged AMA if there is significant doubt about his decision-making capacity. Such doubt would be raised if the patient could not remember the probable diagnosis or the risks of AMA discharge five minutes after they were presented by the emergency room (ER) physician, or if his explanation of why he wanted to leave AMA was incoherent and rambling. If the patient were to articulate a clear reason for leaving AMA that was entirely based on a paranoid delusion or a command hallucination, a medical psychiatrist probably would be called to address the question of whether to hold the patient against his will. If the patient recalled and understood the medical risks sufficiently and his reasoning and communication were clear, the basis for detaining the patient would be potential danger to himself and not his decisional incapacity. In situations like these, the medical psychiatrist's role is complex. He or she usually tries to engage the patient and encourage him or her to accept medical advice, while evaluating the patient for cognitive dysfunction and psychosis and for suicidal or violent ideation and intent. If cognition is intact and the patient rejects proposed medical care solely because of delusional thinking, hallucinations, or psychotic misperceptions, the key question is how imminent the harm would be if the patient refused treatment and left the emergency room or hospital AMA. For the psychiatrist to certify the patient as dangerous to self and compel treatment, it would have to be more likely than not that the patient would suffer harm in the very short term if not treated. Even then, some jurisdictions' mental health laws limit the scope of the medical care that can be given involuntarily to psychiatric treatments only. In almost all jurisdictions, permissible involuntary treatment would not include cardiac surgery.

While delusions might not in themselves invalidate a patient's decisions about medical care, they might invalidate other decisions, such as the revision of a will. For example, consider a patient with dementia and psychosis who has the delusional belief that her husband is unfaithful to her, and who has fond feelings for the nurses' aide who has cared for her for the past two weeks. The patient says she has decided to revoke her will and leave all of her assets to the aide rather than to her husband. She clearly and rationally states that she would prefer to reward kindness rather than betrayal. She knows that her assets comprise the house the couple lives in, which she inherited from her parents and is in her name, and the retirement plan from her former employer. She is aware that without these assets her husband would have no place to live and would have much less income, but she says he can go live with his secret lover.

In this example, the patient knows what the decision is about, can express a preference and can give a rational reason for it, but she is basing the decision on a false and delusional premise. Now consider the situation where there is no delusion of infidelity but where the wife is merely angry at her husband for being, in her view, insufficiently inattentive to her since she became ill. She gives great weight to his recent behavior and little to their generally happy 50-year marriage, and does not grasp how much her husband would be hurt by being disinherited. In this situation, her bad judgment is so extreme that most clinicians would judge it incompetent—and they also would suspect undue influence by the aide.

One could move closer to a line of uncertainty and controversy by imagining a widow who had enjoyed years of assiduous care and attention from a neighbor as she gradually declined from a neurodegenerative disease, while being relatively neglected by her only son, whose calls and visits were infrequent and perfunctory. Her leaving her estate to the neighbor rather than her son might be viewed by one clinician as rational and justifiable, and by another as reflecting the disinheriting of a natural heir under a greedy neighbor's undue influence.

Neuropsychiatric disorders involving language circuits but leaving most of the frontal system and association cortex intact can produce circumstances in which a patient can make a competent decision but cannot express it effectively or accurately. When patients are is aphasic, it cannot be presumed that they lack decision-making capacity. When the neurological diagnosis (e.g., an isolated embolic stroke affecting language) suggests a potential dissociation of decision-making from expression of choices, an effort must be made to establish a channel of communication; for example, an explanation of a proposed treatment might be given in pictures or through a video, rather than verbally.

Neuropsychiatric disorders affecting frontal systems can produce a situation where a patient expresses a pseudo-rational choice. For example, the author treated a young woman with schizophrenia who had sustained a major traumatic brain injury a few years earlier and had major deficits in her frontal lobe function. She persisted in hitchhiking alone at night, despite having been robbed and raped on several occasions. When asked why she persisted in hitchhiking, she said without irony, "What would you have me do, doctor, take the bus?"

Frontal deficits can also lead to the dissociation of consent to treatment and compliance with it. For example, a patient agrees to be hospitalized for psychosis but then refuses all medications that are offered, or a patient agrees to receive antibiotics but pulls out intravenous lines before they can be infused. In this case, the patient's consent may be competently given but completely ineffective, potentially leading to the paradox of giving involuntary treatment to a person who has consented to receive it.

RELATIONSHIPS AS REASONS

Rational and contextually valid reasons for making decisions—e.g., clinical or financial ones—can be expressed as a weighing of pros and cons and the more and less probable outcomes of alternative choices. However, equally valid and rational reasons can be expressed in terms of important relationships. For example, it can be rational for a patient to agree to a particular surgical procedure because his surgeon recommended it and he trusts his judgment and skill. While in obtaining consent one would want to offer the patient comprehensive information about the procedure and its risks and benefits, a rational ultimate decision might legitimately be based almost entirely on the trusting physician-patient relationship. Similarly, a patient might make a decision affecting her personal finances entirely because of the recommendation of a trusted spouse or child, rather than because of her independent evaluation of the decision itself. In this situation, judgment of the patient's decision-making capacity rests on how much the decision to rely on a particular relative is compatible with the patient's history, the current context, and the relative's apparent decision-making competence. Pragmatically, the clinician must look at the latter point simply. If a patient has always relied on her spouse to invest the couple's money and pay the bills, it is presumed rational that she continue to do so, absent positive evidence that something has changed such as the spouse's health. On the other hand, a patient's basing a financial decision on the advice of a son who is an alcoholic and compulsive gambler would raise appropriate suspicion.

EXECUTIVE FUNCTION AND METACOGNITION: CRITICAL TO CAPACITY

EXECUTIVE FUNCTION

Adequate executive function is a prerequisite for successful goal-directed activity, for safe independent living, and for acceptable performance of complex activities like driving, managing money or practicing a profession. Medical conditions that impair cognition can impair executive function disproportionately.

Executive function is the most important *cognitive* factor in determining the performance of instrumental activities of daily living (IADL) in patients with dementia, schizophrenia, and a wide range of other medical conditions. While patients, families, and sometimes legal authorities focus on cognitive functions such as memory, orientation, and language to gauge a patient's cognitive impairment, a patient with severe impairment of executive function can be incapable of reasonable decisions even when these functions are normal. Frontotemporal lobar degeneration (FTLD), Lewy body dementia, the dementias associated with Parkinson's disease, amyotrophic lateral sclerosis (ALS), and progressive supranuclear palsy (PSP) can all show a pattern of disproportionate executive impairment.

On the other hand, a patient with quite significant memory loss and even recent episodes of getting lost might nonetheless be able to make subtle decisions if executive function were preserved. Focal and multi-focal cerebral diseases, including stroke, multiple sclerosis (MS), and brain tumors can produce such a pattern if they largely spare the frontal region and its subcortical and cerebellar connections.

If neuropsychological testing is not done, the medical psychiatrist's office-based or bedside evaluation of decision-making capacity should assess executive dysfunction using procedures like the Clock Drawing Test, the Luria hand sequence, Trail Making B, or presentation of conflicting stimuli (for example, asking the patient to raise the right arm quickly if the command is given in a soft voice and slowly if the command is given in a loud voice). The Executive Interview Test (Royall & Mahurin, 1992; Royall et al., 2004) is a concise, practical survey of executive function that takes 10–15 minutes to do and can be administered by a nurse or technician.

METACOGNITION

Metacognition has two dimensions: the "feeling of knowing" and confidence in one's knowledge. Metacognition requires adequate functioning of the dorsomedial frontal region, especially in the right hemisphere, and the right parietal lobe. Certainty about wrong answers and gross denial of deficits is a great threat to competent decision-making; it is more likely to occur when there is disproportionate impairment of right hemisphere function, as there can be in the early course of some neurodegenerative diseases, or in with focal or multifocal brain lesions that involve the right hemisphere mainly or exclusively.

Cognitive testing in the clinician's office affords a natural opportunity to assess the patient's awareness of their cognitive deficits. Comparison of directly measured and self-assessed deficits can be quantified (Williamson et al., 2010), but a more qualitative approach provides additional information that is useful in competency assessment. Before testing, the clinician can ask patients how they think they will do on tests of memory and concentration and other cognitive abilities. Separately, the clinician can ask family members whether the patient's behavior reflects any adjustment for cognitive impairments. After the test but before being told the results, patients are asked again to assess their performance. After being given the results, they are asked if they agree or disagree, and it is noted if they acknowledge a poor performance but excuse it or minimize its import. If the patient does not accept the presence of a cognitive deficit during the office visit, he or she is given a written report to review at home and is asked again about awareness of deficits on the next visit. In this way, patients can be placed on a continuum of self-awareness that progresses from full appreciation of deficits to frank denial. Some points on the continuum are:

1. Knowing they have cognitive deficits, appreciating their implications, and making adjustments to their behavior to account for them;

2. Knowing they have cognitive deficits, appreciating their implications, but not modifying their behavior;

3. Knowing they have cognitive deficits, but not appreciating their implications;

4. Acknowledging cognitive deficits after failing a test but before being told of the test results, and then showing appreciation of the implications;

5. Acknowledging cognitive deficits after failing a test but before being told of the test results, but excusing their

performance or regarding the results as insignificant or irrelevant;

6. Acknowledging cognitive deficits only after being confronted with test results and their significance by the physician;

7. Acknowledging deficits after extensive persuasion and review of a written report of performance; and

8. Completely denying deficits despite the physician's efforts at persuasion and confrontation with evidence.

Metacognition, which is closely related to self-awareness and insight, is, like executive functioning, only moderately correlated with other cognitive impairments, and in some specific neurological situations it can be disproportionately preserved or affected. For example, patients with early Alzheimer's disease with asymmetrical right-hemisphere involvement can show mild cognitive deficits that they totally deny, in fact being quite sure of misremembered and sometimes crucial "facts."

Patients lacking awareness of their limitations will not ask for help when they need it, may refuse help when it is offered, and may persist in dangerous behavior. Those who are aware of their deficits will modify their behavior to compensate. For example, patients with reduced insight and self-awareness are likely to be unsafe drivers, even when cognitive impairment in other domains is relatively mild (Kay et al., 2009).

THE SPECIFICITY OF CAPACITY

Given the complexity of the brain and the many ways in which brain disease, primary mental disorders, systemic illness, and medication effects can interact, impairments in capacity can be highly specific. A patient can have the capacity to do daily shopping but not to manage his or her savings and investments, *or the reverse*. A patient can be able to drive safely during the daytime in good weather and in light traffic, but not otherwise. A patient can be able to take public transit on familiar routes, but not navigate someplace new. A patient can be able to adhere reliably to a regimen of three medications taken together once a day, but not with a regimen of three medications taken on different schedules. Lui et al. (2013) studied the relationship of financial decision-making capacity and medical decision-making capacity in a group comprising subjects with mild cognitive impairment (MCI), subjects with mild Alzheimer disease (AD), and aged controls, measuring medical decision-making competence with the MacArthur Competence Assessment Tool for Treatment (MacCAT-T) and financial decision-making competence with the Assessment of Capacity for Everyday Decision-Making, a similar structured interview–based assessment. Scores for the Understanding, Reasoning, and Appreciation components of competency for medical versus financial decisions were moderately correlated, but subjects with AD could be judged competent to make one kind of decision but not the other. Only 5% of the subjects with MCI were judged incompetent to make financial decisions, but 20% were judged incompetent to make medical decisions.

A valuable service the medical psychiatrist can perform is to delineate the boundaries of a patient's capacity with some precision. An occupational therapist (OT) can contribute by directly assessing the performance of IADLs. A visit to the patient's home is the best way to valuate the ability to maintain a safe and healthy environment, one that offers the additional benefit of revealing ways to prevent falls and accidental injuries and improve the accommodation of the home to the patient's functional impairments. A neuropsychologist can contribute by doing focused testing that is properly calibrated to the patient's premorbid functioning and its expected change from baseline. Both the OT and the neuropsychologist can assess metacognition and insight by observing how well the patient anticipates any impairments that are found, and whether her or she accepts the findings of impairment when confronted with them. Both can assess elements of executive functioning such as inhibition of inappropriate behavior, persistence, and resistance to environmental distractions; these are best evaluated by systematic observation of the patient's behavior during the clinical encounter.

Another clue to the extent of a patients' impairment—and of their rate of decline from their baseline—is in documents that patients have produced in connection with their occupation, with written or electronic communications with other people, and with the business of living. These include work-related correspondence (if applicable), handwritten checks, letters and emails, tax returns, bank and credit card statements, and statements from investment accounts. For example, when a retired businessman makes multiple arithmetical errors on his tax return, his checks become illegible, and his credit card statement shows evidence of impulsive buying of unneeded items, his loss of financial competence is self-evident.

The careful delineation of a patients' current capacities, along with a clinically based projection of the likely future course of their impairments, is a rational basis for clinical and legal interventions to maximize a patients' independence within their safety zones, while protecting them from the harm that could result from their going outside those zones. Care in documenting impairments and support for claims of incapacity with face-valid evidence, such as photographs of squalid living quarters or receipts for inappropriate purchases, can be helpful when the patient resists a legal intervention or when there is dissent within the family regarding the steps needed to protect the patient.

CONTEXT-DEPENDENCY OF CAPACITY

Capacity is not only specific to a decision or task, but also to its context. Patients may be able to make a decision or carry out a task when well rested but not when fatigued, or when they are comfortable but not when they are in pain. Recognizing optimal and adverse circumstances for decision-making can be used to preserve patient's autonomy while protecting them from self-damaging decisions. For example, if a patient's cognitive status and decision-making capacity are best in the morning, when she is well rested,

and when she is at home rather than in the hospital, an informed-consent discussion for elective surgery might be conducted in the morning, at home, by a visiting nurse representing the prospective surgeon. Under similar circumstances, if the issue were the revision of a will, for example, the patient's lawyer might visit the patient at home in the morning rather than have her come to the office for an afternoon appointment. When context-dependent fluctuation is noted and there is no healthcare proxy, the discussion of appointing and instructing a surrogate decision-maker should be carried out in the optimal decision-making context.

THE TIME COURSE OF INCAPACITY

A further nuance of decision-making capacity is that it changes over time, influenced by disease processes and exogenous substances that directly or indirectly affect the brain. Changes can take place from hour to hour when exogenous substances are involved. Impairments can be episodic, as in bipolar disorder, or progressive, as in neurodegenerative diseases. In many conditions, decision-making capacity can improve with treatment, at least for a while.

Because of the potential for decision-making capacity to change over time, the legal mechanism of a judicial determination of incompetence does not comport with the principle of compromising the patient's autonomy to the minimum necessary extent. Courtroom proceedings to declare incompetence and to appoint a guardian or conservator are expensive, time-consuming, and stigmatizing, and they lack the flexibility to accommodate frequent and sometimes rapid changes in the patient's clinical status.

Practical suggestions for assessing the decision-making capacity of patients with fluctuating mental status and communication impairments were summarized in an article by members of a Canadian Regional Capacity Assessment Team. They note that clinicians often underestimate the decision-making capacity of patients with aphasia. Their approach begins with "a shift in thinking from 'Is this person capable?' to 'How can this person's capacity for this particular task be revealed?'" (Pachet et al., 2012).

THE ROLE OF NEUROPSYCHOLOGICAL TESTS

Neuropsychological tests and other standardized cognitive performance scales have the virtues of being quantitative, standardized, normed, and useful for assessing the course and prognosis of a progressive condition. Several suggestions can be offered for maximizing the value of neuropsychological testing:

1. Work regularly with one or two neuropsychologists; if possible, finding ones with extensive experience in competency assessment and a compatible outlook on competency-related issues.

2. Provide the neuropsychologist with personal and clinical background on each patient that will enable him or

her to give tests of appropriate difficulty to avoid "floor and ceiling" effects on measurement, and tests that will adequately test the areas where specific deficits are suspected.

3. Ask neuropsychologists to provide the actual results of tests performed as well as the conclusions they reached from reviewing the scores, and to provide a description of the patient's behavior during the examination and his or her approach to specific tasks, if these are remarkable. Such observations might include inconsistent effort, fatigability of performance, or inappropriately jocular or profane remarks during the testing.

4. Ask the neuropsychologist to assess the patient's metacognition and insight into any deficits found on testing.

5. Ask the neuropsychologist to suggest bedside- or office-based measures that can be used to follow the patient's performance over time in areas found to be abnormal on comprehensive testing.

TESTING VERSUS OBSERVATION

Direct observation of patients' behavior and task performance in their natural setting provides information complementary to information from neuropsychological testing. While it is not standardized, normed, and quantitative, such observation has three virtues of particular relevance in the assessment of capacity and competency:

1. Direct observation is face valid. For example, a patient whose home environment is squalid either is incapable of cleaning and maintaining the home, or is unwilling to do what is ordinarily expected of a competent adult. A patient who continually misses mortgage or rent payments, despite adequate funds to make them, manifestly has a problem managing his or her financial affairs.

2. Direct observation may demonstrate capacities not obvious from test results. Patients doing everyday tasks in their usual home or work environment have more environmental cues and her can rely more on over-learned habits than when they take unfamiliar tests in a neuropsychologist's office. Patients may be able to carry out well-practiced tasks with adequate cueing that would seem beyond their capacity based on neuropsychological testing results alone. For example, a patient might be able to fill her usual weekly shopping list at a neighborhood grocery store, pay her usual tab with $20 bills, and know that she has received approximately correct change, even though she could not do accurate calculations when tested or name the items on the list from memory.

3. Direct observation also shows how the patient responds to environmental distractions and to unexpected events not present in the controlled environment of the neuropsychologist's office.

STANDARDIZED ASSESSMENT OF COMPETENCE (ADAPTED FROM FOGEL, 2014)

In addition to standard neuropsychological tests, specialized tests for decision-making competence have been devised, focusing on competency to consent to medical treatments and procedures. One, the MacArthur Competence Assessment Tool (MacCAT) (Grisso & Appelbaum, 1998), has been most widely utilized in clinical research and in studies of the neuropsychological basis of decision-making competence, and has relatively strong empirical support (Dunn et al., 2006). One version, the MacCAT-T, targets competency to consent to medical treatment; another version, the MacArthur Competence Assessment Tool for Clinical Research MacCAT-CR (Appelbaum & Grisso, 2001), targets competency to consent to clinical research. The MacCAT is based on presenting the patient with a vignette specifically designed for the clinical decision in question, then conducting a semi-structured interview to assess the patient's understanding of the vignette, appreciation of its personal relevance and implications, reasoning about risks and benefits, and ability to express a decision. Each of these is rated on an ordinal scale; in the end, the clinician makes a binary judgment of competence or incompetence to make the clinical decision. There are no specific cutoff scores on the ordinal items that link them to the final judgment; this allows room for consideration of contextual factors. The MacCAT requires training to administer reliably, and variability in how the vignettes are related to actual clinical circumstances is a potential source of unreliability.

While the MacCAT-T and some of the less widely used standardized tests have shown acceptable psychometric properties, patients can do poorly on such tests yet make competent decisions about their own medical treatment, for several reasons:

1. Actual clinical decisions have a rich context of cues, motivations, and circumstances that are absent from a standardized vignette.

2. Patients with impaired verbal fluency can have a hard time articulating rational reasons for their choice when they do in fact have them; studies validating the MacCAT have not specifically enrolled subjects with language disorders.

3. A patient facing a difficult decision might choose to rely on a trusted physician's advice rather than try to understand a complex medical issue at all, basing this reliance on the rational reason that the physician's past advice has been sound, or that the issues are complex and arcane and recommendations are offered by a well-reputed specialist with extensive knowledge and experience with those issues.

4. Or, a patient may have a long-held personal belief that trumps other considerations and implies what choice should be made; e.g., a belief that it is always better to live than die, regardless of the expected quality of life.

5. A patient can make a well-considered choice to delegate responsibility for the choice to a surrogate decision-maker. For example, a choice by a patient with mild cognitive impairment to delegate a medical decision to his physician daughter might be a wiser one than his trying to make sense of alternatives, risks, and benefits himself.

WHY ASSESSORS MAY DISAGREE

Professionals assessing patients' competence may disagree—and often do—for several reasons:

1. Cognitive test results, task performances, and actual decisions are highly specific and context-dependent and may change over time. If two examiners see a patient at different times, their conclusions may differ because the patient's performance was not the same on the two occasions.

2. Professionals may apply different criteria to determining whether a test was passed or failed, a task was done adequately, or a decision made was reasonable.

3. Professionals may have different thresholds of performance for declaring that a patient has adequate decision-making capacity. This is a particular problem when they are reporting to a judge making a binary decision about the need for a guardian or conservator. In a study of inter-rater reliability of structured instruments for the assessment of capacity to decide about medical treatment, disagreements between raters mainly concerned patients with intermediate scores on the Mini-Mental State Examination (MMSE) and intermediate scores on one or more subscales of the structured capacity assessment, the scales being understanding, reasoning, appreciation, and expressing a choice (Raymont et al., 2007). Apparently, different assessors had different implicit cutoff scores for the decisional capacity subscales.

4. In addition to differences in the circumstances of assessment and differences in assessors' knowledge, skills, and criteria, assessors may ultimately have different views of how concern for patient autonomy should be weighed against concern for the patient's safety and health.

Differences of professional opinion usually can be resolved—or at least explained—when each party's reasoning is traced from primary observations through conclusions.

SPECIFIC SITUATIONS

PSYCHIATRIC AND MEDICAL EMERGENCIES

In true medical emergencies, it is unlikely that a medical psychiatrist will be called, because the doctrine of implied consent will be invoked if the patient is incapable of giving informed consent to treatment and there is no known,

authorized, and immediately available surrogate decision-maker. Medical psychiatrists' involvement typically commences after the patient has survived the immediate crisis and decisions must be made about non-emergency treatment—perhaps treatment of an infection or heart failure—and eventually about follow-up care, perhaps involving transfer to a post–acute care facility such as a nursing home or long-term acute care hospital. Even when acutely ill patients are not able to make informed and thoughtful decisions about their post-acute treatment and rehabilitation, physicians seldom use formal legal mechanisms for surrogate decision-making, even when there is no authorized surrogate decision-maker like a healthcare proxy or (much more rarely) a legal guardian. The treatment team, which usually includes a continuing-care nurse or social worker, makes a recommendation for post-acute care, obtains the consent of the principal family caregiver (usually a spouse, partner, or child), and, as long as the patient offers no resistance, a transfer to post-acute care is made. Sometimes the patient even objects to the transfer, but if the team regards the objection as unreasonable, the transfer takes place anyway.

In many jurisdictions, such processes do not have legal support. Nonetheless, if a medical psychiatrist becomes involved, his or her main agenda should not be to advocate for legal formalities per se. Instead, the goal should be to determine how much the patient can reasonably participate in the post–acute care planning decision, and to enable the patient's valid input to the greatest extent. For example, a patient who has had a stroke and a delirium that has not quite cleared might be referred to a skilled nursing facility (SNF) for post–acute care and rehabilitation. He may insist on going home, and be unable to grasp that his home would not be physically safe for him in his current condition, and that he would not be able to get at home the intensive rehabilitation needed to optimize his long-term functioning. Nonetheless, he might be able to articulate a well-founded preference as to which SNF he would choose if he had to go to one—mentioning, perhaps, its religious affiliation, its being close to his daughter's house, etc. Transferring him to his SNF of choice would show a pragmatic respect for the patient's autonomy, and it is unlikely that anyone would raise a legal objection.

INDEPENDENT LIVING

In contrast to the example just given of a transfer to post–acute care over a patient's objection, the issue of coercing a patient—however mildly—into a permanent change in residence is so momentous as to warrant the protections inherent in greater legal formality. The typical clinical situation is that dementia, or a combination of medical conditions involving cognitive dysfunction and impairment in IADLs or ADLs, makes it unsafe or unhealthy for a person to continue his or her current living arrangements. In this situation, the patient lives alone or lives with a spouse or significant other who is not able to compensate for the patient's deficits. The issue of decision-making capacity arises when the patient chooses not to move, despite medical advice.

The medical psychiatrist called to assist in this situation may have been asked to assess competency or even, more directly, to document findings that could be used in a legal proceeding to compel the patient to move out of situation the medical team does not find to be in the patient's best interest. While this may be the request, it usually is not what the psychiatrist should do.

Before interviewing the patient, the medical psychiatrist should gather whatever information is available from nursing, OT, physical therapy (PT), neuropsychology, and the family about the patient's current level of cognitive impairment, functional independence, safety awareness, and insight into these things, taking special note of actual observations of unsafe behavior or unhealthy living conditions. When deciding what weight to give input from the family, consideration should be given to the possibility that a family member might have an agenda incompatible with the patient's best interests. In some unfortunate cases, the apparently concerned family member might be mistreating or exploiting the patient (Williams et al., 2014).

If the patient has been assessed by an occupational therapist (OT), the therapist (or the OT records) should be queried about how the patient might perform with optimal environmental modification and/or adaptive or monitoring devices, and what those optimal interventions would involve. Similar information from nurses and physical therapists would concern how much supervision, setup, and/or physical assistance the patient would require to live safely at home, and on what schedule it would be required. A prognosis should be estimated from other physicians' notes, with follow-up questions if necessary. Finally, a social worker should be queried about the patient's means and the informal caregiving resources available to the patient.

With such information, the medical psychiatrist can reach a conclusion about the feasibility of the patient's having a safe and healthy life at home. If a safe and healthy living situation is feasible with sufficient resource inputs, the clinician should estimate the resources that might be required and for how long a modified home situation might be viable given the patient's prognosis.

The process just described is an ideal that usually is not attained, given the constraints of time and the nature of care in hospitals, and not every type of input is needed in every case. Sometimes it is obvious that a patient's needs for care at home would be far beyond what the patient could afford or what could be practically arranged in a given locality. However, what the psychiatrist does know prior to seeing the patient can be compared with this ideal, so the psychiatrist is aware of the gaps in his or her knowledge and does not reach definite conclusions prematurely.

Medical-psychiatric assessments in this context includes exploration of how patients views their current situations in the context of their lives, how they understand their illnesses and their limitations, what they think they would need to be safe and maintain their health at home, what financial and informal care resources they think they have, and how they see their situations changing in the future. Cognition and metacognition are tested. If the patient is said to have a physical limitation like a risk of falling, the psychiatrist should directly examine the patient to understand the severity of the problem and the relative contribution of visual, motor, sensory, autonomic, cognitive, and emotional factors.

The psychiatrist then reaches a conclusion as to whether the patient's returning home—with appropriate environmental modifications, adaptive devices, and supportive services—is a realistic option and one that would make sense given the patient's personality, values, and resources. These considerations include the patient's risk tolerance: a patient may be realistically willing to take some risk of injury in order to live independently, and the balance of risk and benefit is quantitative and individual rather than absolute.

If the conclusion is that returning home does not make sense, even allowing for the value of the patient's autonomy and the patient's acceptance of risk, the psychiatrist discusses his or her considerations with the patient. If the patient proves refractory to rational argument because of denial of deficit or impaired reasoning, there may be a basis for pursuing guardianship. Documentation of the patient's denial or defective reasoning will be useful in persuading a judge.

Note that the conclusion of the process might be a creative adaptation of the patient's environment or use of new assistive or monitoring technology rather than coercing the patient to move to a new residence. Or, the exploratory process may lead to identifying new family caregiving resources, to making a different decision about how to spend money on the patient's care, or to a greater acceptance of risk by the patient's loved ones.

DRIVING (ADAPTED FROM FOGEL, 2014)

Many of the diseases, disabilities, and treatments commonly encountered in medical psychiatry have effects on patients' ability to drive safely. At the same time, giving up driving can have major effects on patients' independence, health-related quality of life, and ultimately on their health itself. Some conditions, like uncontrolled seizures and moderate-to-severe dementia, are totally incompatible with safe driving, and in most states it is compulsory for physicians to report them. Other conditions, like hearing loss, increased glare sensitivity, and mild cognitive impairment, can affect driving capacity in a relative and selective way, undoubtedly increasing overall crash risk but implying a moderate and tolerable increase in risk under specific favorable conditions. Furthermore, many older drivers with sensory or attentional problems that increase their crash risk self-limit their driving to some extent, tending to avoid driving at night, in bad weather, and in heavy traffic (Ball et al., 1998). When drivers with cognitive or sensory impairments do *not* limit their driving to less demanding situations, there is greater reason to be concerned about the safety of their continuing to drive. Among older drivers referred for a formal driving evaluation, those who thought they were better drivers than others of their age were four times as likely to be *unsafe* drivers (as assessed by driving simulation) than those who did not (Freund et al., 2005).

Medical psychiatrists become involved with driving-related interventions in several ways. They may be asked to:

1. Assess whether a patient with some combination of general medical, neurological, and psychiatric symptoms can drive safely;

2. Suggest that a patient known to be an unsafe driver to stop driving;

3. Help a patient deal with—either in advance or after the fact—the consequences of driving cessation on his or her life activities and mental health; and/or

4. Advise a patient with limited and selective impairments in driving capacity how to make adjustments in his or her medical treatment, activity schedule, driving habits, and perhaps the vehicle, to enable safe driving despite the medical condition.

An additional task, rarely requested at the outset but often relevant, is helping patients and families anticipate future changes in the patient's driving capacity in a way that will reduce their effects on the patient's health and quality of life and on the burden of family caregivers. The evaluation of driving-related capacities will usually involve some combination of disciplines—neurology, neuropsychology, OT, ophthalmology, and audiology all can be relevant. Psychiatrists can make unique contributions by describing and analyzing patients' moods and behavior and how they interact with cognitive dysfunction and sensory and motor deficits to impair driving ability. They also can contribute their skills in helping patients and their families accept and adapt to a major life change.

When a patient clearly cannot drive safely—as is the case for any patient with moderate or severe dementia—and he or she is currently driving, the patient should be unequivocally advised—both orally and in writing—to stop driving immediately. In states where reporting of such patients to the licensing authority is mandatory, the report should be made without delay. Consent of the patient should be requested if the patient lives in a jurisdiction that does not permit reporting without it. Whether or not patients consent to reporting to the licensing authority, the psychiatrist should ask them for permission to talk to family members or significant others about the driving issue; families have both the time and the interest to work on persuading a patient to give up driving. Of course, if the patient has such severe impairment of decision-making capacity that he or she is not competent in general, a guardianship can be established. The guardian would then relinquish the driver's license and dispose of the car, acting as the patient's agent.

Since failing to make a required report on an impaired driver is a major legal risk, clinicians should know whether their state has mandatory reporting, and which diagnoses or other criteria require such reporting. In some states, the diagnosis of Alzheimer's disease per se would trigger mandatory reporting, even if the disease process were at an early stage, causing only mild cognitive impairment and not greatly affecting driving performance on familiar routes under favorable conditions. The contemporary view of separating the clinical syndrome of dementia from the presumed neuropathology has not yet penetrated most motor vehicle licensing agencies.

Advising patients about driving when they have definite cognitive impairment but not a full syndrome of dementia is especially challenging, because for many patients driving is essential to independence, activity, quality of life, and self-esteem; driving cessation for such patients can lead to an acceleration of functional decline, increased caregiver burden, earlier institutionalization, and even earlier mortality. On the other hand, the increase in crash risk associated with full-blown dementia is unequivocal. Specific errors associated with dementia in general include driving at a lower and more variable speed, errors at intersections with an increase in rear-end collisions, increased steering variability, less awareness of pedestrians and other drivers, worse lane control, and unexpected braking.

Even very mild dementia is associated with increased crash risk. The increase in risk is greater for mild dementia (Clinical Dementia Rating [CDR] 1.0) than it is for very mild dementia (CDR 0.5). A road test study of dementia clinic patients at Washington University showed that 14% of patients with CDR 0.5 were unsafe and 42% of those with CDR 1.0 were unsafe. Half of the CDR 1.0 patients who were judged safe at baseline were unsafe when tested six months later; half of the CDR 0.5 patients judged safe at baseline were unsafe one year later (Duchek et al., 2003). Dementia patients with impairment in executive function, especially those with impaired insight, are likely to be unsafe drivers even when there is relatively mild impairment in other cognitive domains. Other neurodegenerative disorders, notably those affecting the basal ganglia, frequently cause driving impairment relatively early in their course because of a combination of cognitive and motor control impairments. The driving impairment seen early in Huntington's disease exemplifies this phenomenon (Devos et al., 2014). Unsafe driving behavior in mild to moderate Parkinson's disease is best explained by a combination of visual-spatial dysfunction (as measured by performance on the Block Design Test), psychomotor slowing (as measured by performance on the Trail-Making Test part A), and executive dysfunction (as measured by performance on the n-back test and the Plus Minus Task) (Ranchet et al., 2013).

Asimakopulos et al. (2012) comprehensively reviewed studies of neuropsychological tests of executive function that have been correlated with driving performance, providing very strong evidence that executive function is probably the most consistent cognitive determinant of driving performance. In their review they noted the criteria of driving performance used in each study cited—the four most common being on-road tests, driving simulation, a history of crashes, and subsequent cessation of driving.

Driving impairment due to neurodegenerative diseases or gross brain lesions can be exacerbated by their neuropsychiatric complications. Depression is associated with psychomotor slowing, increased reaction time, and lapses of attention. Patients with psychosis can misperceive their environment while driving, or be distracted by internal stimuli. Aggressiveness and impulsivity associated with orbitofrontal dysfunction can manifest as aggressive driving. Apathetic patients fail to anticipate predictable road hazards, although their overall crash risk is mitigated by their decreased desire to drive.

There are several historical points that have a strong association with increased crash risk: recent actual at-fault crashes, getting lost while driving, falling while getting into or out of a car, and having traffic violations due to the failure to heed signs or signals. However, fault in a crash can be ambiguous, so even with the history of a crash or a single moving violation, patients with cognitive impairment who greatly depend on driving for their mobility may insist upon being tested before giving up their car keys. Getting lost while driving in itself implies an unacceptable risk of continuing to drive, with a potential exception for getting lost while suffering from a medication side effect. In that case, the patient should be advised to abstain from driving until further evaluation of their driving ability can be done. Falls when getting into or out of a car suggest problems with weakness or coordination of the legs that could interfere with a timely response to a traffic situation.

There are several ways in which the extent of increased crash risk can be estimated:

1. Office-based testing or neuropsychological testing of cognitive functions known to be associated with driving performance and crash risk, such as reaction time, visual perception, and ability to read and interpret road signs: A few of the specific test performances that have been explicitly linked to increase crash risk include recalling two or fewer of four words on delayed recall, a Trails B time of greater than 180 seconds, and a time outside of normal limits for navigating a maze on a computer screen (Emerson et al., 2012; Ott et al., 2008; Anderson et al., 2012). The Clock Drawing Test (CDT), scored on a seven-point scale with a cutoff for abnormality of four or less, may be a highly specific screening test for unsafe driving (Freund et al., 2005). In a study of 119 older drivers evaluated with a driving simulator, the test was 64.2% sensitive and 97.7% specific in identifying unsafe drivers. The inter-rater reliability of the seven-point scale for scoring the CDT was 0.95 in that study. The combination of low cost, brief administration time, and high reliability are impressive, but the results need to be confirmed on a larger and more diverse sample of older drivers.

2. Testing of the Useful Field of View (UFoV), a standardized, computer-administered test of visual attention: The UFoV measures the visual information that can be acquired in a brief glance, with or without a distracting condition. The developers of the test present evidence that a reduction of 40% or more in UFoV is associated with a seven-fold increase in crash risk. The same criterion is 89% sensitive and 81% specific in predicting that an older individual will have one or more motor vehicle crashes if he or she continues to drive (See the developer's website, www.visualawareness.com, for a summary of research findings and bibliography).

3. Testing of driving performance in the virtual reality of a driving simulator: Driving simulation can present the patient with unexpected events and emergency situations—things a patient with dementia may find difficult to manage, and things that cannot be incorporated into an on-the-road test. The best validated and most widely researched driving simulators are those developed and marketed by Systems Technology Incorporated under the STISIM Drive®trademark (www.stisimdrive.com). The system comprises hardware mimicking the windshield, instrument panel and controls of a car, and software that presents numerous driving scenarios, including ones involving unexpected events. The base configuration of the system includes 80 different driving scenarios; the software counts crashes and near misses as well as driving irregularities such as lane departures.

4. Automated analysis of "black box" (telematics) recordings of actual driving behavior: Systems for recording and analyzing driver behavior currently are used by some automobile insurance carriers for rate-setting, and by motor vehicle fleet operators to monitor their professional drivers. Current technology can detect and record several of the driving problems commonly seen in cognitively impaired patients, including lane departures, excessive variation in speed, inappropriately slow driving, sudden stops and abrupt turns. Units with Global Positioning System (GPS) functionality can establish whether drivers got lost on familiar routes, even if they eventually found their way home.

5. On-road testing by an examiner specializing in assessing the safety of older drivers and people with diseases that can affect driving ability: A road test by a specialized examiner will be more sensitive than a road test for a driver's license renewal. Such a test will look for potentially risky behavior that would not in itself cause the driver to fail the test for licensure.

In addition, the patient should have tests of hearing and vision if these were not recently done and passed. However, it has been established that while visual acuity is what is tested by licensing authorities, poor visual acuity alone does not predict motor vehicle crashes in older drivers. Glare sensitivity, loss of peripheral vision, and diminished useful field of view all are associated with a significant increase in crash risk. The evidence for these relationships is direct; it comes from a study where baseline visual testing was performed in 1,801 drivers aged 65–84; state motor vehicle crash records were then reviewed at a specific time point two to four years later, by which point 120 drivers had been involved in crashes (Rubin et al., 2007).

On-road testing is *not* the gold standard of driving evaluation. While failing a road test implies impaired driving performance under the conditions of the test, road test performance can be worsened by anxiety or fatigue and may not be representative of patients' performance in the particular situations in which they usually drive. On the other hand, passing a road test does not imply that a patient could cope with the additional demands of night driving, bad weather, or heavy traffic, and does not imply that the patient will respond appropriately and in time to an unexpected event, like a child running across the street in front of his or her car. The assessment of these capabilities is better done in a driving simulator. The special value of road tests, however, is that failing one can get an unsafe driver off the road immediately.

The expense and inconvenience of road testing or testing in a driving simulator can be avoided if the results of cognitive testing or UFoV testing are sufficiently bad to be highly specific for unsafe driving. When it becomes widely available, "black box" recording and automated analysis of actual driving behavior may be an efficient method for evaluating driving competence that offers the advantage of not requiring a *test*—a situation that may evoke the patient's anxiety or potentially their resistance.

In persuading a patient to discontinue driving, it is useful to identify any *non-cognitive* reason why the person's driving might be unsafe. In addition to impaired hearing or vision (especially impaired peripheral vision, glare intolerance, or decreased UFoV), decreased neck mobility, diminished limb strength, impaired balance, peripheral sensory loss, and falls getting into and out of a car should be considered. Quadriceps strength has a powerful and non-linear effect on driving safety; beyond a certain level of weakness, driving rapidly becomes unsafe (Lacherez et al., 2014). Driving cessation for a non-cognitive reason is face-saving for the patient and may be more readily accepted.

For those patients who continue to drive, crash risk can be mitigated somewhat by specifying circumstances under which the patient should not drive. Also, patients should be strongly cautioned against using a mobile phone while driving. Crash risk for any driver increases with mobile phone use. The incremental risk for drivers with MCI or mild dementia is greater because of their difficulty dealing with distractions, redirecting attention, and processing conflicting stimuli.

Also, case-control studies of motor vehicle crashes have led to identification of classes of drugs associated with increased crash risk. Some, like opiates, barbiturates, and benzodiazepines, non-benzodiazepine hypnotics (including zolpidem, zopiclone, and zaleplon), first-generation antihistamines, most of the antipsychotic drugs, and most of the anti-epileptic drugs, have obvious sedative effects. Others are not as obvious, but are noteworthy as potentially driver-impairing drugs because they are commonly prescribed or, in some cases, purchased over the counter. They are: (1) antidepressants (virtually all classes are associated with increased risk), (2) nonsteroidal anti-inflammatory drugs (NSAIDs), (3) proton pump inhibitors, (4) H2 blockers, (5) dextromethorphan, (6) cetirizine, and (7) dopamine agonist drugs (Hetland et al., 2014). While most patients taking these drugs are not unsafe drivers, the drugs' potential effects should be considered when assessing a patient's overall driving risk.

ACCESS TO FIREARMS

In the United States, one-third of adults own a gun, and almost one-half of adults live in a household where there is a gun (Gallup.com, 2013). Rates of individual gun ownership vary greatly by demographics, from 10% in unmarried non-Southern women to 64% in married Southern men. Rates of household gun ownership are significantly higher, ranging from 18% in unmarried non-Southern women to 70% in married Southern men. 44% of Americans over 65 have a gun in the household. Thus, gun ownership is high in an age group that bears the greatest burden of chronic illness in general and brain diseases in particular. Eighty percent of all homicides committed by persons over 65 are committed using guns, as are more than half of all suicides (Merten & Sorenson, 2012). Impairments in judgment and impulse control, mood disturbances, and paranoid thinking associated with neuropsychiatric illness increase the risk of violence in general and gun violence in particular. For this reason, cognitively impaired patients should not have access to firearms; at the very least, firearms in their possession should be disabled. Symptoms of anger, aggressiveness, and loss of inhibition raise particular concern, as does the syndrome of major depression.

When a medical psychiatrist is called to assess a patient's competence, the question of firearms in the home should always be considered, and should be raised in the initial evaluation of outpatients or patients about to be discharged to the community from an inpatient or post–acute care setting. If the patient is not able to willing to answer questions about firearms, questions should be asked of others who know the patient. Patients found to be incompetent thereby losing control of finances, living arrangements, or their mobility may become angry and/or depressed. The combination of diminished mental capacity, hostile or depressive ideation, and ready access to a firearm is potentially deadly. The finding of this combination on psychiatric assessment warrants assertive action to remove, disable, or lock up the guns to which the patient would have access. Family members may be able to assist; when this is not an option, the police can be involved, with the legal theory either being imminent danger to self or others (if the patient has suicidal or homicidal ideation) or legal incompetence, a condition under which the legal guardian or conservator would have control over the patient's firearms, as they are personal property.

When a patient is severely cognitively impaired, firearm-related risk can be controlled by locking the guns up in a gun safe and securing the key, or by removing ammunition from the home; obviously, complete removal of firearms is safest, but it is not always acceptable to the patient's family. The most challenging situation is when a patient has sufficient neuropsychiatric disturbance—e.g., a combination of paranoid thinking and impaired impulse control—to be very dangerous with a firearm, but not so grossly impaired that he or she would be found incompetent and eligible to have a guardian or conservator. Informal solutions involving concerned family members should be considered but may not be feasible in particular cases. When facing this dilemma, the medical psychiatrist and the patient's principal physician should discuss the problem with their hospital's legal or risk-management department, to share responsibility and benefit from others' experience and resources.

FINANCIAL DECISIONS

Competence to manage money concerns a continuum ranging from management of an investment portfolio to determining whether one has received correct change at a convenience store. Patients with diminished capacity for financial decision-making are at risk for exploitation or victimization, as well as for dire consequences from unpaid bills if they have primary responsibility for paying for housing, taxes, and utilities. The consequences of financial mistakes are greater in money terms when the patient has more money; but the consequences of lost money for daily life are greater when the patient has less money.

Money-related behavior is of special diagnostic interest because financial transactions other than cash payments leave a documentary record. Review of credit card and checking account statements and cancelled checks can show such inappropriate financial behavior as repeated payment of the same bills, failure to make necessary payments, or irrational purchases. Examination of brokerage account statements can show behavior like unexpected and unnecessary withdrawals and transfers of funds, erratic patterns of buying and selling securities, investment choices inconsistent with the patient's goals and past behavior, or activity suggesting the influence of a self-serving financial advisor. The onset and progression of signs of bad financial judgment can be used to support a diagnosis of a neurodegenerative disease and to estimate its rate of progression. Furthermore, financial records may be useful objective evidence in legal proceedings. Review of financial records of course requires the patient's written permission or their physical delivery of the records; however, if accounts are jointly held with a caregiving spouse, it may suffice to obtain and record the patient's verbal consent to the physician's discussion of financial details with the caregiver.

As an alternative to the direct examination of financial records, patients' financial competency can be assessed with a structured instrument, the Financial Capacity Instrument (FCI-9) (Martin et al., 2008). The FCI-9 tests the patient on 18 financial tasks covering nine domains; they range from identifying coins and currency and making change, to explaining the parts of a bank statement and comparing investment options. It has acceptable psychometric properties, and its face validity is particularly appealing.

The impetus for a medical psychiatrist to assess a patient's money-related competencies might come from another physician in the form of a consultation request, from a patient's concerned family, from the patient, or from a bank or lawyer responsible for a trust of which the patient is a trustee or a beneficiary. The psychiatrist's follow-up on an assessment that shows a patient has impaired financial decision-making will depend on the psychiatrist's role or "license" in the specific case. If the psychiatrist is providing a consultation, his or her job is to describe the nature and severity of the patient's impairments in financial decision-making capacity, to offer a diagnosis and prognosis if possible, and to make suggestions for mitigating their adverse effects. If the psychiatrist has an ongoing relationship with the patient, the task would be to work with the patient and, with the patient's consent, the family or significant others—to mitigate potential harm related to impaired financial capacity.

In one common situation, the patient has a general medical or neuropsychiatric condition that can impair decision-making capacity; he or she has made minor financial mistakes or shown errors in calculation, memory, and/or executive function that could cause such mistakes, but they has not yet made any seriously harmful financial errors. Here the physician should point out that the patient has an illness that can affect financial ability and suggest that accommodations should be made for the illness *before* the patient loses money—and perhaps the family's money as well. The specific emphasis in the appeal to the patient can take advantage of the patient's expressed concerns such as a fear of being cheated or the wish to leave a legacy. Changes in credit cards, the right to sign checks, and authority over brokerage accounts must be made while the patient is competent to make them. When the patient has a neurodegenerative condition, there is no time to lose. Competence to change financial arrangements requires a basic understanding of what one's assets are, what bills one is responsible for paying, who would control the assets following a change, and an appropriate rationale for choosing that person. A patient can retain this competence even after losing their ability to handle financial details such as paying bills on time and not paying the same bills twice.

As soon as possible after the diagnosis of a disease that affects decision-making capacity or eventually will do so, patient should be asked if there is someone, typically a family member, whom they would trust to handle their money when or if they were not able. If the answer is other than an unqualified yes, the reason should be investigated, either by the psychiatrist or by a social worker or family therapist. If the issue of mistrust within a family cannot be resolved, an unrelated trustee might be needed to protect the patient's assets.

When patients have substantial assets well beyond those needed to ensure their own care, it is likely that there are already lawyers, bankers, money managers, and/or other professionals involved in financial planning and estate planning. Here the medical psychiatrist can perform—as always with the patient's consent—a valuable service by explaining to the patient's advisors the patient's current decision-making capacity and how it is likely to change over time with the patient's illness. Depending on the audience, the psychiatrist can discuss the patient's testamentary capacity, susceptibility to undue influence, and capacities that are preserved. The latter might range from the ability to make small purchases to the ability to competently object to proposed investments that the patient finds socially or environmentally objectionable.

TESTAMENTARY CAPACITY

When patients with substantial assets disinherit their natural heirs or change their wills in unexpected ways in the setting of general medical or neuropsychiatric disorders that can alter their mental status, the patients' wills often are contested posthumously. Contested wills can lead to expensive and emotionally stressful litigation. In this litigation, physicians are called to testify regarding the patient's mental state at the time of writing (or rewriting) their will. The opinion of a medical psychiatrist who examined the patient contemporaneously with change in the will is likely to be especially important to the court.

1. When a medical psychiatrist will be involved in the ongoing treatment of a patient with a neuropsychiatric or general medical condition that threatens life and/or will eventually reduce decision-making capacity, the psychiatrist should ask the patient if he or she has a will and how recently the will was updated. Patients should be encouraged to deal with their wills and other estate-planning tasks at a time when they have the energy, insight, and judgment to do the job well. It can be emotionally difficult for anyone to plan for death, and it is even more difficult when the patient can foresee his or her death or the loss of life as they have known it. Even so, consciously choosing one's legacy is part of a person's self-actualization and a healthy response to a heightened awareness of mortality. In assisting the patient with this task, the medical psychiatrist utilizes both psychotherapeutic skills and diagnostic assessment skills. The former are applied to help the patient clarify his or her preferences and reconcile emotional conflicts concerning family members and other loved ones. The latter skills are applied to establish and document that the patient had testamentary capacity at the time a will and/or estate plan was changed. Doing this requires assessment and documentation of six elements, specifically that the patient:
   a. Knows what a will is;
   b. Knows what his or her assets are;
   c. Knows which people have a reasonable claim to be beneficiaries;
   d. Understands the impact of a particular distribution of assets;
   e. Does not have delusions or other psychotic phenomena that would affect the decisions made; and
   f. Can express his or her wishes clearly and consistently.

2. When a patient with known cognitive impairment or diagnosed mental illness writes or changes a will, it is useful to document that the elements of testamentary capacity were evaluated and found to be adequate. When there is anything unusual about the patient's bequests and/or there is a large estate, a video recording should be made of the interview in which testamentary capacity was evaluated. This helps prevent conflict within the family and reduces the chance of a successful challenge to the validity of the will.

3. A medical psychiatrist may be called to consult by the lawyer for an individual who is making changes in a will and/or estate plan that is likely to be challenged by a potential beneficiary (or ex-beneficiary). In this case, the primary purpose of the clinical assessment is not treatment of the patient, but assessment and documentation of the six essentials of testamentary capacity. Many people, including some lawyers and some physicians, have the misconception that a diagnosis of major mental illness, a diagnosis of Alzheimer's disease or of any dementia,

or demonstration of significant cognitive dysfunction implies that a new will or trust document will not be valid (Gutheil, 2007). This is not so, for several reasons. First, testamentary capacity is highly specific; a patient with moderate short-term memory loss and episodic disorientation could still have it. Second, the threshold of cognitive performance needed for testamentary capacity is lower if the will leaves most of the patient's assets to natural heirs and does not disinherit anyone who would reasonably expect to be a beneficiary. Similarly, modifications of wills and trusts that do not represent radical departures from earlier versions do not demand a high standard of proof of testamentary capacity. Shifting the percentages of financial assets received by particular children or changing who receives a particular piece of tangible property might induce emotional reactions in the heirs involved, but it is less likely to lead to a successful challenge of a will than more radical changes, such as leaving substantial sums to unrelated parties only recently involved in the patient's life.

4. A medical psychiatrist may be called to consult by family members affected by a recent or contemplated change to an individual's will or estate plan, either to advise those family members, or, if the testator agrees, to see them in consultation to help settle the issue of testamentary capacity and thus mitigate the risk of future family conflicts or litigation. In this situation, the first thing the psychiatrist must do is establish who the client is—the testator or the family member requesting the consultation. Family members, depending on their interests in the will or trust involved, will be hoping for a specific outcome of the evaluation, and it can be presumed that the testator would hope to be found competent to make a valid will.

5. A medical psychiatrist may be engaged by a lawyer to offer a post-mortem opinion of testamentary capacity in connection with a contested will. Retrospective signs of potential testamentary incapacity include:

   a. Radical change from previous wills;
   b. Changes that disinherit natural heirs, such as a spouse or a child;
   c. Changes made reflecting probable delusions, misperceptions, or misunderstandings;
   d. Changes that disregard the testator's personal history and reflect only the person's current circumstances; and
   e. Changes suggesting undue influence, such as an unusually large bequest to a recent caregiver who is not related and who was not named at all in the previous will.

TESTAMENTARY CAPACITY AND LIVING WILLS

Validly making or changing a will requires adequate cognitive function and a sufficiently accurate perception of reality; the more a will deviates from usual expectations, the more positive evidence is necessary that the testator's intentions were rationally formed and free from undue influence or duress. The same considerations applicable to wills are applicable to living wills. In a jurisdiction where living wills are binding on healthcare professionals, a living will that declines life-saving treatment can potentially compel a physician to act against his or her assessment of the patient's best interests. Many hospitals encourage all patients to give advance directives that include a healthcare proxy and a living will. While this is well intentioned, often a patient's cognitive function and emotional state on the day of admission to a hospital may be worse than usual, with implications for the choices the patient might foresee making in various hypothetical situations. The patient might be able to make a valid and rational choice of a healthcare proxy but not be able to get into the details to the extent needed to write a precise living will. In addition, feelings of hopelessness or depression can influence a living will, even though those feelings might be transient, as they can be when they are brought on by severe pain or the shock of a new diagnosis. As with many of the decisions discussed in this chapter, medical psychiatrists are rarely called in to prospectively validate living wills by vouching for their makers' testamentary capacity. However, a medical psychiatrist evaluating patients at any point in their course can ask them about their advance directives. A problem with binding living wills is that it is hard to specify in advance every combination of potentially relevant considerations that might apply to decisions about life-sustaining treatment.

PROFESSIONAL COMPETENCE

As people in business and the professions retire later than they did in the past, there will be ever more cases of impaired professional performance due to neurological and general medical conditions and drugs that affect the central nervous system (CNS). Bad professional or business judgments by physicians, lawyers, accountants, money managers, small business owners, and corporate executives, among others, can have very serious consequences, including harm to clients, financial losses, and the destruction of reputations built over lifetimes. Competent professional practice and satisfactory managerial performance both require a high level of executive functioning, appropriate social behavior, working memory, and the recall of many details. Thus business and professional activities make a greater demand on mental capacity than do ordinary IADLs, and they can be impaired by insults to the brain that do not cause obvious dysfunction in daily life.

At the time this first occurs, standard cognitive screening in a physicians' office or at the bedside—which is designed for detection of delirium and dementia rather than milder or more limited deficits—usually is above the cutoff for abnormality, all the more so because professionals are highly educated and begin with superior baseline performance. When a medical psychiatrist determines that a patient's executive cognitive function, working memory, metacognition, or judgment are affected by a medical condition of any kind, and that the impairment is likely to persist or progress, he or she should consider whether the patient is still employed and inquire in detail about the actual duties of the job. (In some family businesses and partnerships, senior people are paid but have essentially honorary roles.) If it appears that the observed cognitive dysfunction or other neuropsychiatric symptoms might have an adverse effect on the patient's occupational performance, the issue should be followed up. Neuropsychological testing is almost always helpful, even when the diagnosis is not at issue, because of its value in quantifying specific deficits and in relating them to norms and to the patient's estimated premorbid function. The neuropsychologist should be asked to concentrate on areas of cognitive performance essential to the patient's professional activities.

If relevant deficits are confirmed, the next step depends on the psychiatrist's "license" in the given case. If the patient has a treatment relationship with the psychiatrist, the psychiatrist should meet with the patient and explain the risk of a costly or embarrassing professional mistake if the patient continues to work, emphasizing that it is far better to retire with honor than to be forced out in disgrace. With the patient's consent, family members or trusted professional colleagues can be included in the conversation. If the patient is under the age for full pension benefits at the time of the diagnosis, he or she should be encouraged assert a disability claim rather than simply retire early. If the medical psychiatrist is called in for consultation only and no ongoing treatment relationship is expected, the dialogue just described would be the responsibility of the patient's primary care or principal care physician, or of a mental health professional with an ongoing relationship with the patient.

CONSENT TO PARTICIPATE IN RESEARCH

As with making decisions about clinical care, a patient's capacity to give valid consent to participate in clinical research is characterized by *specificity, context dependence,* and *change over time.* Similar as well is the principle that more capacity is needed to validly make a decision that entails greater risk: consenting to a different schedule for taking vital signs requires very little capacity, while consenting to a face transplant requires a very high standard of understanding, reasoning, and appreciation. The fundamental difference between research consent and clinical consent is that a research subject does not necessarily have a rational expectation of direct personal clinical benefit *from the experimental part* of the study.

SHORT-TERM AND LONG-TERM CONSENT

Because of potential changes in decision-making capacity over time, validity of consent to participate in research is a different issue for short-term interventions like diagnostic tests or surgical procedures than it is for long-term ones like trials of treatments for chronic neuropsychiatric conditions such as dementia or bipolar disorder. In the former case, a patient's consent is regarded as valid for the entire procedure unless the patient actively withdraws it. If consent is withdrawn, participation will end as soon as it can be discontinued without undue risk of harm. In the latter case, consent that is valid at the start of a study may become invalid later on because at that future time the subject's mental condition is different, and capacity to give valid consent has been lost.

In longer-term studies where a subject loses the capacity to consent at some point during the study—either transiently or permanently—the subject's interests are protected by their having a healthcare proxy, in the jurisdictions that permit surrogate consent for participation in research (Gong et al., 2010). The proxy would review the subject's current clinical situation, question the investigator if necessary, and decide whether the subject should continue participating under the aegis of the proxy's consent. The potential role of the medical psychiatrist is in determining that the subject's decision-making capacity is so impaired that the healthcare proxy should be activated. If the subject improves to the extent that he or she can once again make competent healthcare decisions, the healthcare proxy will no longer have authority for either clinical decisions or decisions concerning research participation. Note that, in any case, a research subject can withdraw from a study at any time—withdrawal of assent is valid even if the subject's consent would no longer be regarded as valid.

Patients with cognitive impairment can validly consent to clinical procedures without subtle understanding of their risks and benefits. Patients who are study subjects should, however, be able to indicate their understanding of the following concepts:

1. That they will be participating in research, and that the experimental part of the study should not be expected to have direct personal clinical benefit;

2. That they can withdraw from the study at any time without affecting their clinical care;

3. The general nature of the study interventions, with awareness of any aspect of the study that is invasive, uncomfortable, or unusual;

4. The overall riskiness of participation;

5. An example of a common potential adverse effect of the study intervention (if there are such);

6. An example of a severe potential adverse effect of participation; and

7. Why they want to participate in the study (e.g., "to help science," "because I might get an experimental drug that might help me").

The quality of a cognitively impaired patients' decisions to participate in research can be improved by their identifying a cognitively intact family member or significant other who will accompany them during the informed consent process as an informal auxiliary decision-maker. The patient would agree to participate only if the auxiliary decision-maker concurs. Ideally, this person would also be the patient's healthcare proxy in the event of the patient's incapacity to make clinical decisions.

Medical psychiatrists and professionals of related disciplines like neuropsychiatry and neuropsychology are seldom utilized as part of the research consent process; the policy in virtually all clinical research centers is to exclude patients from a study if there is the slightest doubt about their ability to give competent informed consent. However, psychiatrists do have roles to play in the design and review of studies involving subjects with impaired decision-making capacity and in determining the appropriate time to activate a healthcare proxy during the long-term course of a research subject's care.

Medical psychiatrists also have a potential role to play in protecting vulnerable patients from participation in clinical research that exposes them to risks they would not accept if their decision-making were not compromised. Patients with impairments in cognition, insight, or judgment may minimize or deny the risks of research participation if they are strongly motivated by the expectation of improvement, or by transference toward the physician referring them to the study.

THE THERAPEUTIC MISCONCEPTION

The majority of patients receiving an experimental medication believe it will help them, even if they are told that the benefit of the medication is unknown (Henderson et al., 2007; Kim et al., 2009). This phenomenon, called the *therapeutic misconception*, is almost universal in Phase 1 trials of new cancer drugs, where subjects are patients desperate for a remission from their cancer (Miller & Joffe, 2008). Patients with intact decision-making capacities can at least intellectually understand the therapeutic misconception, even if they cannot stop hoping. With this intellectual understanding, they can weigh the potential for adverse effects. Patients with impaired cognition, insight, or judgment may have unshakeable therapeutic misconceptions that prevent them from appreciating risks that they might find unacceptable.

TRANSFERENCE AND RESEARCH REFERRALS

A patient with a strong positive transference to a physician might sign up for participation in research because that physician referred them to the study—even if the patient has concerns or reservations. Patients insecurely attached to their physicians might participate in research out of fear of disappointing their doctor. In both cases, the risk of inappropriate judgments driven by transference is greatest when critical thinking, insight, and judgment are impaired. In both cases, a research coordinator might not perceive the issue, but it might be uncovered in a medical-psychiatric interview conducted for another reason.

The MacArthur Competence Assessment Tool for Clinical Research (MacCAT-CR), described above, is based on presenting the patient with a vignette specifically designed for the decision to participate as a research subject, and then conducting a semi-structured interview to assess the patient's understanding, appreciation, reasoning, and ability to express a decision. The virtue of the MacCAT-CR is that it brings consistency to the assessment of competence to consent to research; however, the appropriateness of using it will vary according to how well the vignette captures the issues relevant to the decision to participate. Also, patients with impaired communication due to neurological disorders may have intact decision-making capacity, but require a non-standardized approach to communicating the questions and to understanding the patient's answers. For these reasons, when investigators design consent procedures—or an Institutional Review Board (IRB) reviews ones—that involve the MacCAT, they should pay close attention to the wording and content of the vignettes used. And if the study will involve patients with potential communication impairments, the expected adaptation of the assessment should be described. The input of a speech therapist and/or neuropsychologist may be helpful in doing this.

Despite its limitations, the use of a standardized assessment like the MacCAT is appropriate for assessing capacity to consent to clinical trials of treatments for patients with medical conditions affecting cognition. When a patient's participation in a clinical trial is completely elective, a false negative on a test of decision-making capacity does no harm, and documentation of a rigorous, standardized assessment of capacity to consent protects the researcher—and the research—if there is an adverse event during the study.

LONG-TERM STRATEGY

ESTABLISHING A "LICENSE"

A recurrent theme in this book is that, as healthcare becomes more complex, there is a great need for rationalizing, integrating, and prioritizing the elements of a patient's care—carrying out an overall executive function with respect to the various healthcare providers, formal and informal caregivers, and other stakeholders such as insurance companies and concerned friends. Rarely does anyone formally hold the executive position; primary care physicians and professional care managers tend to influence the decisions of others, but not to control them. Patients themselves, if self-confident and well-informed, sometimes serve as their own "healthcare executives," but in cases of impaired capacity the patient cannot do this. In some cases, well-informed friends or relatives can do the job. The unmet need for an executive function can offer an opportunity for medical-psychiatric intervention.

In any case, the medical psychiatrist can be most helpful if the scope of his or her "license" in a given case is well-defined. Is it simply to perform and document a detailed mental status examination and offer and document an opinion about decision-making capacity? Or is it to have an ongoing professional relationship with the patient's lawyer and periodic sessions with the patient and their family, and to be available as needed to advise the other medical specialists caring for the patient regarding the patient's current capacities and evolving preferences? If the clinician receives a well-defined request from a medical colleague or from a lawyer, there may be no ambiguity. If the request for consultation from another professional is more open-ended, or if the request comes from the patient or from a relative or friend, the clinician should assess the patient's overall system of care and support and consider what scope of intervention would be most helpful to the patient, and then seek an appropriate license. This involves explaining one's recommended role to the patient and family, and, based on their acceptance of the recommendation, reaching out to the other professionals involved and establishing one's role with them.

PROMOTING CONSISTENCY WITH THE LIFE NARRATIVE

A widely accepted principle is that surrogate decision-makers should be guided by what patients would have done if they had the capacity to decide for themselves, rather than by the surrogate decision-makers' personal opinions and preferences. This process is facilitated by the patient's participation in planning of the broadest kind long before acute illness forces the issue. Even when planning is done in advance and there is plenty of time, patients may find it hard to do, and they may discover that they disagree with their spouses or significant others. The medical psychiatrist sometimes can help patients find their way by reviewing their life narratives with them—guiding patients in recalling important episodes in their work, relationships, and family lives, to help them see how certain choices would be most consistent with how they have lived to date and with how significant others have behaved in the past. For example, a woman currently feeling distant from an adult son might recall happier times in their relationship and recall that he has always shown good judgment and integrity in financial matters. This might lead to her talking with her son about his being her agent in financial matters if she is incapacitated, and, depending on the outcome of the conversation, naming him as her agent in a durable power of attorney. Without the anamnesis, she might have chosen someone else currently closer to her but with perhaps worse judgment in financial matters.

When the patient has already lost decision-making capacity and no longer has the capacity to articulate meaningful and consistent preferences, the medical psychiatrist must rely on significant others, typically those who present themselves at the hospital or the medical office. The psychiatrist should bear in mind that those who show up are not necessarily those most knowledgeable about the patient's wishes, even if they are those most interested in the outcome of decisions made on the patient's behalf. Before making suggestions to surrogate decision-makers or offering an opinion about who might be a suitable surrogate decision-maker, the psychiatrist should consider whether there are other parties not present whose input should be sought. And, when eliciting opinions from family members, it can help to review the patient's personal history of decisions, values, and relationships with the family, introducing the idea that current decisions on behalf of the patient should be compatible with the patient's life narrative.

ANTICIPATING THE ISSUES

Each disease or combination of diseases has a foreseeable course with respect to periods of incapacity. The nature of incapacity is characteristic and somewhat predictable, even though the precise time course is not. In neurodegenerative diseases and other invariably progressive diseases, eventual incapacity is certain; in relapsing-remitting conditions it may not be certain, but the risk is large enough to require management. In the behavioral variant of frontotemporal lobar degeneration, for example, driving performance is likely to deteriorate and become unsafe early in the course of the illness. With certain cancers, there are brief periods of physical incapacity, sometimes associated with delirium, accompanying rounds of chemotherapy. With systemic lupus erythematosus (SLE), there is an ongoing risk of brain involvement, which can present with confusion, psychosis, or seizures; the first two imply impaired decision-making, and the last implies driving risk. With bipolar disorder, there is the ongoing risk of a manic episode with the special risk of financial misbehavior. In relapsing-remitting multiple sclerosis (MS), relapses can begin with altered mental status, and vision can be affected with implications for driving. Furthermore, the association of MS with bipolar disorder, euphoria, and frontal lobe syndromes implies an increased risk of the dangerous combination of lost capacity with lost insight.

While talking with patients about their likely future incapacity is never easy, it is essential. Patients are most able to think rationally about issues like writing advance directives, choosing a surrogate decision-maker, or setting up a trust when cognitive impairment is at worst mild, when they are not depressed, and when their significant relationships are not severely stressed by caregiving. Because of technological advances and broader public awareness of dementia, patients with neurodegenerative diseases often are diagnosed at an early stage, when they still have the capacity to choose surrogate decision-makers even though other specific capacities may have already been lost. In a patient with Alzheimer's disease, the modest improvement in cognition attainable with a nootropic agent like donepezil or memantine may restore their capacity to choose a surrogate decision-maker, execute an advance directive, or validly change a will or trust.

For patients involved in a family business or a professional practice, succession planning can be important financially as well as emotionally. Financial and tax issues make the topic relevant as people age, even when there is no expectation of loss of capacity. For this reason, the topic can be introduced as a natural one for the patient's stage of life—one that can be addressed without embarrassment.

KNOWING THE STAKEHOLDERS

In a chronic care situation, there are more "stakeholders"—individuals with interests in the individual's decisions and behavior—than just the patient and the immediate family members who might visit them in the hospital or join them at an outpatient visit. These include:

1. All family members and close friends who either have a caregiving role or might have one, or might reasonably be expected to have one at some point in the patient's course;

2. People who depend upon the patient in some way: financially, emotionally or otherwise;

3. Heirs, potential heirs, or potential beneficiaries of the patient's assets;

4. Professionals and institutions involved in the patient's care; and

5. The public, as represented by laws and regulations. Stakeholders' interests often conflict; legal niceties must be observed especially carefully when there are obvious conflicts of interest and when there are significant assets involved.

MAINTAINING BOUNDARIES WITH FAMILIES

When first interviewing a patient with an issue of impaired capacity of some kind, there is often a family member around who expresses concern about the patient and offers to provide collateral information. If the patient is severely impaired in cognitive functioning or communication, it is customary to talk about the patient with whoever is present in the office or at the bedside, without explicitly seeking the patient's agreement. But when patients are less severely impaired, physicians should ask their permission to share information with family members. When a patient is brought to an outpatient visit by family members, the physician should not talk with the family without the patient present, unless the patient agrees. While these considerations can seem unduly picky when patients are acutely ill, difficult situations of intra-family conflict are not helped by blurred boundaries and fuzzy rules of engagement. Medical psychiatrists should be particularly careful about maintaining boundaries with families, to reduce the risk of being unduly influenced by an opinionated or self-interested family member and the risk of losing the patient's trust and confidence.

IS DECISION-MAKING CAPACITY THE REAL ISSUE?

Requests to evaluate patients' decision-making capacity constitute a significant part of inpatient psychiatric consultation requests, but a well-founded suspicion of impaired decision-making capacity is not present behind many such requests (Kornfeld et al., 2009). Instead, requests for capacity evaluation can arise from an irreconcilable difference between a physician and a patient regarding a decision that the physician sees as against the patient's best interests, as impinging unfairly on other people, or otherwise unacceptable (Kontos et al., 2012). A psychiatric finding of decisional incapacity would settle the conflict by denying the legitimacy of one side. When a psychiatrist identifies such a situation, his or her role shifts to one of identifying the real underlying issue and communicating it to the patient and the medical staff involved. Depending on the issue, the psychiatrist may serve as a mediator, or may simply give the medical staff permission to allow the patient to make what the staff see as an undesirable decision.

At the same time, actual decision-making incapacity probably is under-recognized in general medical settings, probably because if patients assent to care and families do not object, care goes on without concern about whether patients' signatures on informed consent documents are valid. Using the MacCAT to assess medical decision-making competence, Raymont et al. (2004) found that 31% of a series of 159 acute medical inpatients lacked medical decision-making capacity. None of the patients had been identified by the medical staff as having an issue of competence to consent to treatment. Apparently, the issue of medical decision-making capacity is rarely raised unless a patient objects to a treatment recommended by his or her physician. In the absence of such an objection, it would be unlikely that a psychiatrist would ever be called to evaluate decisional capacity, except in the special case of an unusually high-risk or otherwise controversial procedure.

KNOWING THE LEGAL OPTIONS

Specific laws regarding involuntary psychiatric treatment, surrogate consent, advance directives, and guardianship vary by jurisdiction. As any of these legal devices might be relevant in a given case, the medical psychiatrist should be familiar with all of them. Non-psychiatric physicians often have misconceptions about legal issues.

CHOOSING AND USING A LAWYER

Optimizing patients' legal arrangements to respect their autonomy, their safety, their concerns for their significant others, their personal philosophy, and their desired legacy may require a combination of advance directives and trusts, or, if the patient has become incompetent before making prospective arrangements, a guardianship or conservatorship with a well-chosen surrogate decision-maker with an appropriate scope of authority. The lawyer responsible for drafting documents should understand the concepts outlined in this chapter such as the specificity and context-dependency of capacity and the difference between giving rational reasons and fully appreciating their context and implications. They should also have mediation skills, as intra-family conflict is not unusual.

In the author's experience, lawyers with strong technical and interpersonal skills will develop into outstanding resources for patients and families once they have acquired the relevant medical and neuropsychiatric knowledge. This happens naturally when a medical psychiatrist and a lawyer work together on several cases. The lawyer then becomes a resource to whom the psychiatrist can refer additional patients.

Patients' specific legal issues may touch family law, elder law, the law of estates and trusts, and even insurance law. It is unlikely that one lawyer will have the technical knowledge necessary to address every case. The medical psychiatrist might work with a few lawyers with different legal subspecialties, or might work with one who can easily access subspecialty advice through a firm or professional network.

IDENTIFYING OTHER RESOURCES

In addition to lawyers, the medical psychiatrist with a license to address strategic issues related to patients' changes in

capacity and competency will at times need access to six other resources:

1. Neuropsychologists with experience in doing problem-focused and ecologically valid assessments of cognitive functions relevant to decision-making capacity. They would be able to measure and comment on metacognition and awareness of deficits, fluctuation with context and/or setting, and the potential for compensatory strategies. They would be able to say whether the pattern of observed cognitive dysfunction was compatible with known diagnoses, or whether it suggested additional or different ones. They would be able to relate the observed deficits to relevant functions like medical decision-making, driving, and financial decision-making, and to explain the relationships to families and lawyers as well as to other healthcare professionals.

2. Occupational therapists skilled at assessing functional capacity in natural settings, including patients' homes, and in making home safety assessments.

3. Family therapists with an interest in the family issues of chronic disease and disability, including family obligations and reciprocity, generations' expectations of one another, and sibling conflicts regarding rights, responsibilities, and authority within the family. They would be aware of relevant cultural and religious differences and would know of resources for helping diverse families.

4. Social workers familiar with local supportive resources and residential options. One set of resources and options is applicable to patients and families with means, and another set applies to those without means. In the author's experience, a social worker familiar with one set of resources and options will not necessarily be familiar with the other.

5. A facility for driving assessment, preferably one offering driving simulation as well as the road test option, since certain types of driving-related impairments are better demonstrated in a simulator than by a typical road test.

6. Clergy of various denominations experienced in counseling patients and families about spiritual and religious issues related to competency and decision-making, including issues of intergenerational and spousal obligation and issues related to advance directives and end-of-life care.

These six types of professionals form the medical-psychiatrist's virtual team for comprehensively addressing the legal, ethical, and practical issues that arise when a patient's chronic illness affects decision-making capacity and essential instrumental functions.

CLINICAL PEARLS

• People with cognitive dysfunction or psychotic ambivalence can—and frequently do—consent to treatment but do not comply with clinical directives; or refuse treatment but do assent to care. Psychiatrists sometimes need to explain these phenomena to legal personnel unfamiliar with neuropsychiatric disorders.

- Advance directives cannot possibly anticipate all medical circumstances, so they work best when there is also a healthcare proxy who knows the patient well and can adequately represent what the patient would want in various circumstances.

- Advance directives should have built-in leeway.

- Resolving conflicts in the very ill often requires not only dialogue, but also enough time for the surrogate to come to terms emotionally with the patient's diagnosis and prognosis (Brush et al., 2013).

- When actually making healthcare decisions, surrogates consider both *patient factors*: respect for the patient's input, past knowledge of the patient's wishes, and the patient's best interests; as well as *surrogate factors*: their own wishes if they were in the patient's situation, their personal interests, religious beliefs or spirituality; family consensus, and obligation and guilt (Fritch et al., 2013).

- Autonomy has a subtlety that psychiatrists may be particularly well suited to appreciate: autonomy involves agency—choosing a course of action in a particular specific situation; and authenticity—choosing a lifestyle, a set of values, and a view of human experience (Brudney & Lantos, 2011).

- People's views change with their experience of illness.

- Some patients speaking in advance of their incapacity prefer balancing substituted judgment and best interests. They also appreciate that their premorbid preferences and present preferences might be different.

- Metacognition has two dimensions, the "feeling of knowing," and confidence in one's knowledge. Asking patients in the clinical evaluation to assess their capacity on tests allows the physician to place the patient on a continuum of self-awareness that progresses from full appreciation of deficits to frank denial.

- The Clock Drawing Test, scored on a seven-point scale with a cutoff for abnormality of four or less, may be a highly specific screening test for unsafe driving (Freund et al., 2005).

- The medical psychiatrist can work with the patient to anticipate issues, promote consistency with the life narrative, know the stakeholders, maintain family boundaries, and clarify whether decision-making capacity is really the issue.

DISCLOSURE STATEMENT

Dr. Fogel is Chief Scientific Officer of Synchroneuron Inc., Managing Director of Anal-Gesic LLC, and Executive Vice President of PointRight Inc. He is the sole inventor or lead inventor on several pharmaceutical patents. In his opinion, these affiliations do not entail any conflict of interest with regard to the editing of this book or his personal contributions to it. He has no other potential conflicts, direct or indirect, financial or otherwise, to disclose in connection with the editing of this book or his personal contributions to it.

REFERENCES

Anderson, S. W., Aksan, N., Dawson, J. D., et al. (2012). Neuropsychological assessment of driving safety risk in older adults with and without neurologic disease. *Journal of Clinical and Experimental Neuropsychology, 34*(9), 895–905.

Appelbaum, P. S., & Grisso, T. (1998). *The MacArthur competence assessment tool: Research.* Sarasota, FL: Professional Resources Press.

Asimakopulos, J., Boychuck, Z., Sondergaard, D., et al. (2012). Assessing executive function in relation to fitness to drive: A review of tools and their ability to predict safe driving. *Australian Occupational Therapy Journal, 59*, 402–427.

Ball, K., Owsley, C., Stalvey, B., et al. (1998). Driving avoidance and functional impairment in older drivers. *Accident Analysis & Prevention, 30*, 313–322.

Barry, M. J. (2012). Shared decision making—the pinnacle of patient-centered care. *New England Journal of Medicine, 366*, 780.

Beauchamp, T., & Childress J. (2009). *Principles of biomedical ethics* (6th ed.). New York: Oxford University Press.

Black, B. S., Wechsler, M., & Fogarty, L. (2013). Decision making for participation in dementia research. *American Journal of Geriatric Psychiatry, 21*, 355–363.

Brudney, D., & Lantos, J. (2011). Agency and authenticity: Which value grounds patient choice? *Theoretical Medicine & Bioethics, 32*, 217–227.

Brush, D. R., Brown, C. E., & Alexander, G. C. (2012). Critical care physicians' approaches to negotiating with surrogate decision makers: A qualitative study. *Critical Care Medicine, 40*, 1080–1087.

Devos, H., Neiuwboer, A., Vandenberghe, W., et al. (2014). On-road driving impairments in Huntington disease. *Neurology, 82*, 1–7.

Duchek, J. M., Carr, D. B., Hunt, L., et al. (2003). Longitudinal driving performance in early-stage dementia of the Alzheimer type. *Journal of the American Geriatric Society, 51*, 1342–1347.

Dunn, L. B., & Alici, Y. (2013). Ethical waves of the silver tsunami: Consent, capacity, and surrogate decision-making. *American Journal of Geriatric Psychiatry, 21*, 309–313.

Dunn, L. B., Fisher, S. R., Hantke, M., et al. (2013). "Thinking about it for somebody else": Alzheimer's disease research and proxy decision-makers' translation of ethical principles into practice. *American Journal of Geriatric Psych, 21*, 337–345.

Dunn, L. B., Nowrangi, M. B., Palmer, B. W., et al. (2006). Assessing decisional capacity for clinical research or treatment: A review of instruments. *American Journal of Psychiatry, 163*, 1323–1334.

Emerson, J. L., Johnson, A. M., Dawson, J. D., Uc, E. Y., Anderson, S.W., & Rizzo, M. (2012). Predictors of driving outcomes in advancing age. *Psychology and Aging, 27*(3), 550–559.

Fogel, B. (2014). Mental competence and legal issues in dementia care. In, B. Dickerson & A. Atri (Eds.), *Dementia.* New York: Oxford University Press.

Freund, B., Colgrove, L. A., Burke, B. L., et al. (2005). Self-rated driving performance among elderly drivers referred for driving evaluation. *Accident Analysis and Prevention, 37*, 613–618.

Freund, B., Gravenstein, S., Ferris, B. S., et al. (2005). Drawing clocks and driving cars: Use of brief tests of cognition to screen driving competency in older adults. *Journal of General Internal Medicine, 20*, 240–244.

Fritch, J., Petronio, S., Helft, P. R., & Torke, A. (2013). Making decisions for hospitalized older adults: Ethical factors considered by family surrogates. *Journal of Clinical Ethics, 24*(2), 125–134.

Gallup.com (2013). http://www.gallup.com/poll/160223/men-married-southerners-likely-gun-owners.aspx., Posted Feb. 1, 2013, accessed March 9, 2014.

Gong, M. N., Winkel, G., Rhodes, R., et al. (2010). Surrogate consent for research involving adults with impaired decision making: Survey of Institutional Review Board practices. *Critical Care Medicine, 38*, 2146–2154.

Grisso, T., & Appelbaum, P. S. (1998). *The MacArthur competence assessment tool: Treatment.* Sarasota, FL: Professional Resources Press.

Gutheil, T. G. (2007). Common pitfalls in the evaluation of testamentary capacity. *Journal of the American Academy of Psychiatry & the Law, 35*, 514–517.

Henderson, G. E., et al. (2007). Clinical trials and medical care: Defining the therapeutic misconception. *PLoS Medicine, 4*, 11.

Hetland, A. J., Carr, D. B., Wallendorf, M. J., et al. (2014). Potentially driver-impairing (PDI) medication use in medically-impaired adults referred for driving evaluation. *Annals of Pharmacotherapy, 48*(4), 476–482.

Imhof, L., Mahrer-Imhof, R., Janisch, C., et al. (2011). Do not attempt resuscitation: The importance of consensual decisions. *Swiss Medical Weekly, 141*, w13157.

Jox, R. J., Horn, R. J., & Huxtable, R. (2013). European perspectives on ethics and law in end-of-life care. In J. L. Bernat & R. Beresford (Eds.), *Ethical and legal issues in neurology—Handbook of clinical neurology* (3rd series, Vol. 118). Amsterdam: Elsevier.

Kay, L. G., Bundy, A. C., & Clemson, L. M. (2009). Validity, reliability and predictive accuracy of the driving awareness questionnaire. *Disability and Rehabilitation, 31*, 1074–1082.

Kim, S. Y. H., Schrock, L., Wilson, R. M., et al. (2009). An approach to evaluating the therapeutic misconception. *IRB Ethics and Human Research, 31*(5), 7–14.

Kontos, N., Freudenreich, O., & Querques, J. (2012). Beyond capacity: Identifying ethical dilemmas underlying capacity evaluation requests. *Psychosomatics, 54*, 103–110.

Kornfeld, D. S., Muskin, P. R., & Tahil, F. A. (2009). Psychiatric evaluation of mental capacity in the general hospital: A significant teaching opportunity. *Psychosomatics, 50*, 468–473.

Lacherez, P., Wood, J. M., Anstey, K. J., et al. (2014). Sensorimotor and postural control factors associated with driving safety in a community-dwelling older driver population. *Journals of Gerontology, Series A: Biological Sciences & Medical Sciences, 69*, 240–244.

Levy, F., Mareinnis, D. P., & Iacoveli, C. (2012). The importance of a proper against-medical-advice (AMA) discharge: How signing out AMA can create significant liability protection for providers. *Journal of Emergency Medicine, 43*, 516–520.

Lui, V. W. C., Chiu, C. C. Y., Ko, R. S. F., et al. (2014). The principle of assessing mental capacity for enduring power of attorney. *Hong Kong Medical Journal, 20*, 59–62.

Lui, V. W. C., Lam, L. C. W., Chau, R. C. M., et al. (2013). Structured assessment of mental capacity to make financial decisions in Chinese older persons with mild cognitive impairment and mild Alzheimer disease. *Journal of Geriatric Psychiatry & Neurology, 26*, 69–77.

Martin, R., Griffith, H. R., Belue, K., et al. (2008). Declining financial capacity in patients with mild Alzheimer disease: A one year longitudinal study. *American Journal of Geriatric Psychiatry, 16*, 209–219.

Mertens, B., & Sorenson, S. B. (2012). Current considerations about the elderly and firearms. *American Journal of Public Health, 103*, 396–400.

Miller, F. G., & Joffe, S. (2008). Benefit in phase 1 oncology trials: Therapeutic misconception or reasonable treatment option? *Clinical Trials, 5*, 617–623.

Muthalagappan, S., Johansson, L., Wing, M. K., et al. (2013). Dialysis or conservative care for frail older patients: Ethics of shared decision-making. *Nephrology, Dialysis, Transplantation, 28*, 2717–2722.

Ott, B. R., Festa, E. K., Amick, M. M., et al. (2008). Computerized maze navigation and on-road performance by drivers with dementia. *Journal of Geriatric Psychiatry & Neurology, 21*(1), 18–25.

Pachet, A., Allan, L., & Erskine, L. (2012). Assessment of fluctuating decision-making capacity in individuals with communication barriers: A case study. *Topics in Stroke Rehabilitation, 19*, 75–85.

Ranchet, M., Paire-Ficout, L., Uc, E. Y., et al. (2013). Impact of specific executive functions on driving performance of people with Parkinson's disease. *Movement Disorders, 28*, 1941–1948.

Raymont, V., Bingley, W., & Buchanan, A. (2004). Prevalence of mental incapacity in medical inpatients and associated risk factors: Cross-sectional study. *Lancet, 364*, 1421–1427.

Raymont, V., Buchanan, A., David, A. S. (2007). The inter-rater reliability of mental capacity assessments. *International Journal of Law and Psychiatry, 30*, 112–117.

Royall, D. R., Mahurin, R. K., & Gray, K. (1992). Bedside assessment of executive dyscontrol: The Executive Interview (EXIT25). *Journal of the American Geriatric Society, 40*, 1221–1226.

Royall, D. R., Palmer, R., Chiodo, L. K., et al. (2004). Declining executive control in normal aging predicts change in functional status: The Freedom House study. *Journal of the American Geriatric Society, 52*, 346–352.

Rubin, G. S., Ng, E. S. W., Bandeen-Roche, K., et al. (2007). A prospective population-based study of the role of visual impairment in motor vehicle crashes among older drivers: The SEE study. *Investigative Ophthalmology & Visual Science, 48*(1483), 1491.

Seyfried, L., Ryan, K. A., & Kim, S. H. Y. (2013). Assessment of decision-making capacity: Views and experiences of consultation psychiatrists. *Psychosomatics, 54*, 115–128.

Simpson, O. (2011). Consent and capacity to decide or refuse treatment. *British Journal of Nursing, 20*, 510–513.

Smith, A. K., Lo, B., & Sudore, R. (2013). When previously expressed wishes conflict with best interests. *Journal of the American Medical Association, Internal Medicine, 173*, 1241–1245.

Teno, J. M., Stevens, M., Spernak, S., et al. (1998). Role of written advance directives in decision making: Insights from qualitative and quantitative data. *Journal of General Internal Medicine, 13*, 439–446.

Will, J. F. (2011). A brief historical and theoretical perspective on patient autonomy and medical decision making. Part II: The autonomy model. *Chest, 139*, 1401–1497.

Williams, B., Boyle, G., Jepson, M., et al. (2014). Best interests decisions: Professional practices in health and social care. *Health and Social Care in the Community, 22*, 71–86.

Williamson, C., Alcantar, O., Rothlind, J., et al. (2010). Standardized measurements of self-awareness deficits in FTD and AD. *Journal of Neurology, Neurosurgery, & Psychiatry, 81*(2), 140–145.

86.

OBJECTIVE PSYCHIATRIC ASSESSMENT AND MANAGEMENT OF CHRONIC DISABILITY SYNDROMES

C. Donald Williams

INTRODUCTION

Practicing psychiatrists play a complex role in the diagnosis and treatment of patients who present with acute or chronic disabilities that prevent them from functioning in the workplace. Disability is a multifaceted, emotionally charged concept that has important public policy implications: financial and emotional costs endured by disabled workers and their families, and economic burdens on employers and responsible tax-funded government agencies. Psychiatrists can easily find themselves entangled in agendas that extend far beyond the routine doctor–patient relationship when the patient requests certification supporting his or her disability claim.

Our aim in this chapter is to call attention to the different and sometimes mutually exclusive roles that may arise when we are working with patients with disabilities. The role of caregiver is the most familiar role to the majority of clinicians, but psychiatrists may also be serving as consultants to the referring treating physicians, and such consultation may evolve into providing direct care. In another setting, their role may be as an independent psychiatric evaluator hired by a third party to provide an expert opinion. Advocates or adjudicators may then use this opinion to determine the nature and severity of the psychiatric disorder, if any; its causation; whether it is permanent or temporary; and how much, if any, compensation is due to the individual. We will present our view of how evaluations may be best conducted and guidelines that will enhance consistency and objectivity. We will also address the issue of informed consent and limitations on confidentiality.

LOSS OF WORKERS DUE TO DISABILITY

The loss of workers due to disability is a major problem in the United States and other industrialized nations. During the 1990s, insurance companies that insured against disabilities saw claims rise sharply. Claims for disability resulting from disorders that were relatively unknown during the previous decade, such as repetitive strain injury (RSI) and post-traumatic stress disorder (PTSD) grew most quickly. The increased frequency of diagnoses such as PTSD has challenged psychiatrists to distinguish between real and feigned

disorders in a disability context. Between the first quarter of 1989 and the first quarter of 1994, disability insurers saw claims for some diagnoses rise more than 100% (Quint, 1994).

The apparent costs of work-related injuries (defined as injuries or illnesses that cause loss of time from work) have also grown. In 1992, there were 13.2 million nonfatal injuries and 862,200 illnesses in the American workforce. There were approximately 6,500 job-related deaths due to injuries and 60,300 deaths due to disease. The estimated total of the direct and indirect costs of these injuries and illnesses was $171 billion (Leigh et al., 1997). As of 2008, Leigh estimated that the total of the direct and indirect costs of occupational illness, injuries, and fatalities was, conservatively, $163.3 billion (Leigh, 2008).

The prevalence of disability remained unchanged from 1999 (22.0%) to 2005 (21.8%). However, as a result of the aging American population, the estimated absolute number of persons reporting a disability increased 7.7% from 44.1 million to 47.5 million. Women had a significantly higher prevalence of disability compared with men at all ages. The prevalence of disability for both sexes doubled in successive age groups (18–44 years, 11.0%; 45–64 years, 23.9%; and >65 years, 51.8%). Because of the size of the "Baby Boomer generation," the number of adults with disability is likely to increase greatly (see http://www.cdc.gov/mmwr/preview/mmwrhtml/mm5816a2.htm).

Contrary to expectations, the economic downturn did not appear to significantly affect the incidence of claims; however, it did seem to affect employment decisions. According to the 2010 Council for Disability Awareness's Long-Term Disability Claims Review (available at Council for Disability Awareness, Long-Term Disability Claims Review, 2010: http://www.disabilitycanhappen.org/research/CDA_LTD_Claims_Survey_2010.asp), long-term disability claims increased 2.9% from 2008 to 2009 among private insurers.

PSYCHIATRIC ROLES IN DETERMINING IMPAIRMENT

Psychiatrists are tasked with assessing and treating individuals with psychiatric disorders, some of whom have work-related impairments with disabilities that may result from the impairments. Broadly speaking, the role of psychiatrists in disability matters is to accomplish one or more of the following tasks: (1) provide an expert opinion regarding the presence of any psychiatric diagnoses and their multifactorial causation; (2) describe functional *impairments*—which are limitations to specific functions that may impair the patient's ability to perform the essential duties of particular occupations; and (3) offer recommendations regarding treatment for the identified conditions. Psychiatrists may also have roles within the broader context of the assessment and treatment of disability, which may involve interfacing with other physicians, vocational counselors, businesses and their representatives, insurance companies, state agencies, and the courts. The complex nature of these relationships is depicted in Figure 86.1.

The actual determination of *disability* results from either an *administrative* or *judicial decision* that weighs evidence and expert opinions, including those provided by psychiatrists; the adjudicators are the "finders of fact." Adjudicators usually have no formal training in psychiatry or neuropsychology, and rely upon expert opinion.

DEFINITIONS OF DISABILITY

Disability is dimensional, depending on diagnosis, severity of impairment, and life context. In its website (www.who.int/classifications/icf/en/, 2011) the World Health Organization (WHO) defines *disability* as "the outcome or result of a complex relationship between an individual's health condition and personal factors, and the external factors that represent the circumstance in which the individual lives." The Social Security Office of Disability programs (www.ssa.gov/disability/, 2011) defines disability as "the inability to engage in any substantial gainful activity by reason of any medically determinable physical or mental impairment(s) which can be expected to result in death or which has lasted or can be expected to last for a continuous period of not less than 12 months." Private disability insurance policies and state workers' compensation statutes have their own definitions for what constitutes compensable disability. For example, relative to workers' compensation, in *Re*: Leonard Norgren, Docket No. 04 18211, The Washington State Board of Industrial Insurance Appeals (www.biia.wa.gov/, 2011) defined disability more specifically in occupational terms: "Disability

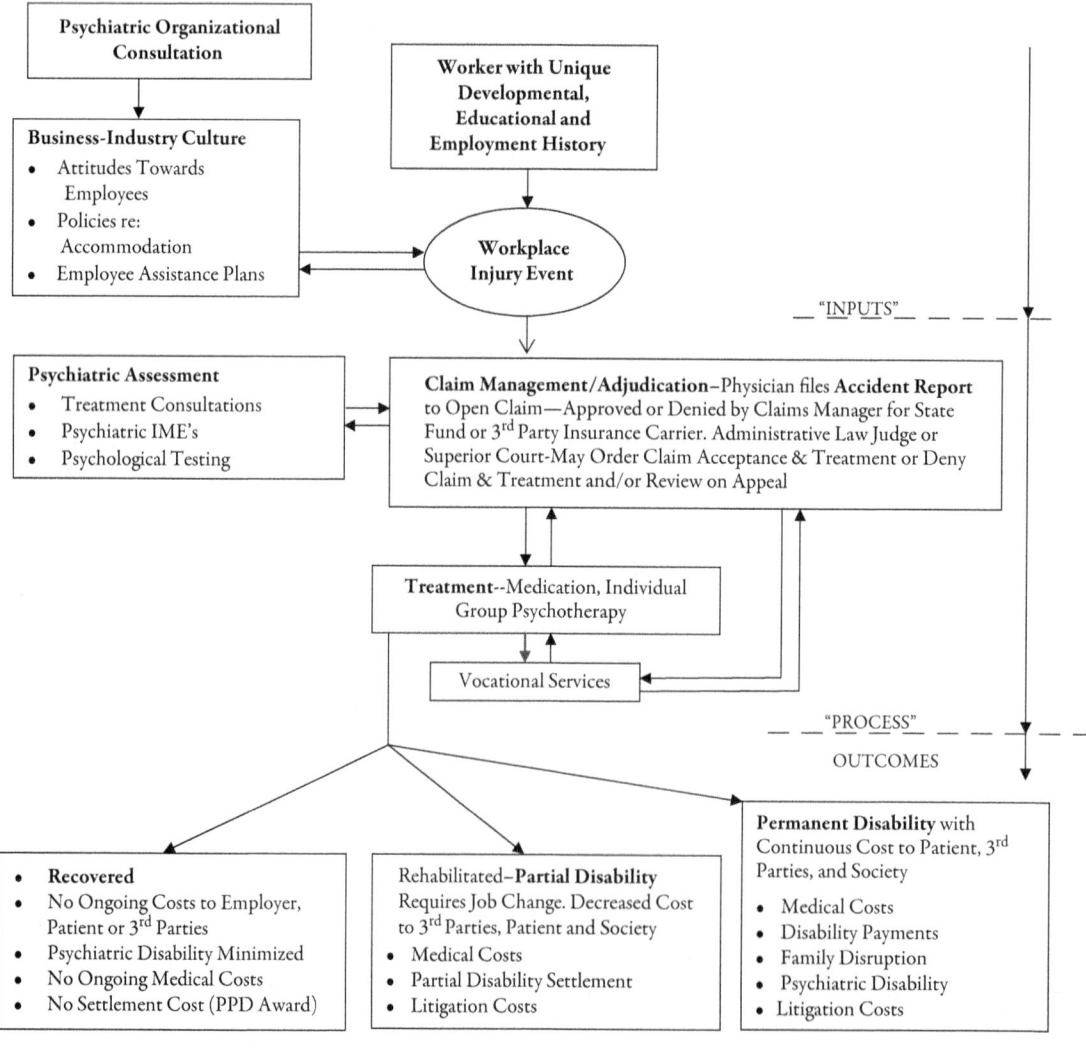

Figure 86.1 Relationship between psychiatrists and stakeholders involving organization and psychiatric disability.

means the impairment of the workman's mental or physical efficiency. It embraces any loss of physical or mental functions which detracts from the former efficiency of the individual in the ordinary pursuits of life. It connotes a loss of earning power."

These definitions imply that disability is an "either-or" condition—i.e., someone is disabled or they are not. The reality is more complex, and in this chapter we take the approach that "disability determination" should be approached taking into account the *diagnosis*, its *severity*, and the life *context* of the person being evaluated.

Independent medical evaluations (IMEs) of disability, perhaps most prominently in the workers' compensation arena, are known for their inconsistency and perceived bias (Shuman & Greenberg, 2003; *New York Times*, 2009; Gold & Shuman, 2009). Bias can be associated with role conflict when the treating clinician is drawn into the role of assessing impairment in the context of a disability claim (Strasburger, Gutheil, & Brodsky, 1997). In this classic paper, Strasburger et al. described the importance of not "wearing two hats"— those of a treating psychiatrist and of an evaluating psychiatrist in a professional relationship with the same person. An evaluator is obligated to be a seeker of truth, whereas a treater's primary duty is to the patient as a seeker of cure and comfort. Gold and Shuman (2009) provide an in-depth examination of bias that arises from other causes, such as failing to maintain a balance between considering the role of real external factors in the workplace such as a hostile work environment, and an individual worker's personal, idiosyncratic response to the work.

In some situations, a treating psychiatrist is compelled by statute or regulation to assume an evaluative role. When this does take place, a psychiatrist's awareness of the potential for role conflict to occur may mitigate its impact. For example, a psychiatrist performing a treatment consultation at the request of an occupational physician under a worker's compensation statute is required to submit a comprehensive psychiatric evaluation using DSM-5 criteria and an opinion about whether the diagnosed conditions are unrelated to an injury, aggravated by the injury, or causally related to the injury, in addition to making recommendations for treatment.

Where necessary, and when circumstances allow, evaluations that require assessment of causation, credibility, and severity, we suggest an enhanced *dimensional* method for assessing psychiatric impairment that incorporates both formal psychological testing and a comprehensive medical record (chart) review and interview of the examinee/patient. We contend that this approach will contribute to greater reliability in diagnosis, causal attribution, and severity ratings. This method, which includes partially quantitative elements, utilizes a *cross-reference grid* that incorporates various rating scales, with definitions for five levels of impairment that enable the rater to "triangulate" the rating by cross-checking one scale against the others (Williams, 2006, 2010). Psychological testing—including the Minnesota Multiphasic Personality Inventory–2 (MMPI-2) and the Minnesota Multiphasic Personality Inventory-2 Restructured Form (MMPI-2-RF) (MMPI-2, 1989; and MMPI-2 RF, 2008), which has been the subject of many empirical studies that enhance its forensic role in disability assessment applications—can also be added to this comparison grid used for rating psychiatric impairment as shown in Table 86.1.

DIAGNOSES AND THEIR VOCATIONAL IMPACT

Throughout this chapter, we will refer in our discussion to the both the draft version and whenever possible to the final version of the American Psychiatric Association's *Diagnostic and Statistical Manual of Mental Disorders*, 5th edition (DSM-5) (available at www.psychiatryonline.org). DSM-5 substantially revised the definition of *Somatoform disorders* to render them more consistent with personality theory and clinical practice. The DSM-5 emphasizes *dimensional* severity determinations for Axis I disorders and revises the definitions of several disorders, which is intended to bring greater clarity to the psychiatric disability assessment and impairment-rating process (Helzer et al., 2008). In assessing the vocational impact of diagnosed psychiatric conditions, we will refer to Fischler and Booth's volume, *Vocational Impact of Psychiatric Disorders* (1999) which correlates the impact of impairment arising from various conditions on the ability to work in different settings.

Finally, we will discuss the conduct of an independent psychiatric evaluation using each of these tools to develop an intellectually consistent, data-driven narrative that incorporates empirically validated psychological testing when indicated to arrive at conclusions regarding the degree of causal relationship between an event, such as an industrial injury; and a mental disorder, such as depression. Our examples will illustrate the use of the interview; the record review; psychological testing to support an opinion regarding diagnoses and their severity; the presence or absence of defensiveness, exaggeration, or in the most extreme cases, malingering or deliberate feigning of symptoms; and the presence or absence of a pre-existing condition that may have been aggravated by the injury or event in question.

For the purposes of this chapter, we will reference the DSM-5 in draft form available in 2011 when this chapter was first written, or when possible the final May 2013 published form because of its improved conceptual clarity. The DSM-IV will be referenced in discussing literature published prior to the publication of DSM-5 in May 2013.

ROLES OF PSYCHIATRISTS IN DISABILITY EVALUATIONS

Psychiatrists may be asked to diagnose and to rate the degree of an individual's psychiatric impairment *or* to treat a person with a psychiatric disorder that contributes to an occupational impairment. Treating psychiatrists may be asked to complete forms in support of their patients' claims for disability benefits or compensation resulting from psychiatric conditions. Independent psychiatric evaluations (IMEs) may

Table 86.1 3 RATING SCALES AND THE MMPI-2

DSM IV TR GLOBAL ASSESSMENT OF FUNCTIONING (GAF) AXIS V	CLASSES OF IMPAIRMENT DUE TO MENTAL AND BEHAVIOURAL DISORDERS – AMA GUIDE	MMPI-2 PROFILE ELEVATION RCD T SCORE	WASHINGTON STATE WAC 296-20-340 – PERMANENT IMPAIRMENTS OF MENTAL HEALTH
GAF 61–80 If symptoms are present, they are transient and expectable reactions to psychosocial stressors (e.g., difficulty concentrating after family argument); no more than slight impairment in social, occupational, or school functioning (e.g., temporarily falling behind in schoolwork). Some mild symptoms (e.g., depressed mood and mild insomnia) OR some difficulty in social, occupational, or school functioning within the household), but generally functioning pretty well, has some meaningful interpersonal relationships.	**AMA Guide Class 2 – Mild Impairment** "Impairment levels are compatible with most useful functioning"	Profile elevation = 62–68 RCd T score range = 65–70	**WAC Category (2)** Any and all permanent worsening of preexisting personality traits or character disorders where aggravation of preexisting personality trait or character disorder is the major diagnosis; mild loss of insight, mildly deficient judgment, or rare difficulty in controlling behaviour, anxiety with feelings of tension that occasionally limit activity; lack of energy or mild apathy with malaise; brief phobic reactions under usually avoidable conditions; mildly unusual and overly rigid responses that cause mild disturbance in personal or social adjustment; rare and usually self-limiting psycho-physiological reactions; episodic hysterical or conversion reactions with occasional self-limiting losses of physical functions; a history of misinterpreted conversations or events, which is not a preoccupation; is aware of being absentminded, forgetful, thinking slowly occasionally or recognizes some unusual thoughts; mild behaviour deviations not particularly disturbing to others; shows mild over-activity or depression; personal appearance is mildly unkempt. Despite such features, productive activity is possible most of the time. If organicity is present, some difficulty may exist with orientation; language skills, comprehension, memory; judgment; capacity to make decisions; insight; or unusual social behaviour; but the patient is able to carry out usual work day activities unassisted.
GAF 41–60 Moderate symptoms (e.g., flat affect and circumstantial speech, occasional panic attacks) OR moderate difficulty in social, occupational, or school functioning (e.g., few friends, conflicts with peers or co-workers). Serious symptoms (e.g., suicidal ideation, severe obsessional rituals, frequent shoplifting) OR any serious impairment in social, occupational, or school functioning (e.g., no friends, unable to keep a job).	**AMA Guide Class 3 – Moderate Impairment** Impairment levels are compatible with some, but not all, useful functioning	Profile elevation = 69–67 RCd T score = 71–76	**WAC Category (3)** Episodic loss of self-control with risk of causing damage to the community or self; moments of morbid apprehension; periodic depression that disturbs sleep and eating habits or causes loss of interest in usual daily activities but self-care is not a problem; fear-motivated behaviour causing mild interference with daily life; frequent emotogenic organ dysfunctions requiring treatment; obsessive-compulsive reactions which limit usual activity; periodic losses of physical function from hysterical or conversion reactions; disturbed perception in that patient does not always distinguish daydreams from reality; recognizes his fantasies about power and money are unusual and tends to keep them secret; thought disturbances cause patient to fear the presence of serious mental trouble; deviant social behaviour can be controlled on request; exhibits periodic lack of appropriate emotional control; mild disturbance from organic brain disease such that a few work day activities require supervision.

GAF 21–40

Some impairment in reality testing or communication (e.g., speech is at times illogical, obscure, or irrelevant) OR major impairment in several areas, such as work or school, family relations, judgment, thinking, or mood (e.g., depressed man avoids friends, neglects family, and is unable to work; child frequently beats up younger children, is defiant at home, and is failing at school).

Behavior is considerably influenced by delusions or hallucinations OR serious impairment in communication or judgment (e.g., sometimes incoherent, acts grossly inappropriately, suicidal preoccupation) OR inability to function in almost all areas (e.g., stays in bed all day; no job, home, or friends).

AMA Guide Class 4 – Marked Impairment

Impairment levels significantly impede useful functioning

Profile elevation = 77–81

RCd T score = 77–84

WAC Category (4)

Very poor judgment, marked apprehension with startle reactions, foreboding leading to indecision, fear of being alone and/or insomnia; some psychomotor retardation or suicidal preoccupation; fear-motivated behaviour causing moderate interference with daily life; frequently recurrent and disruptive organ dysfunction with pathology of organ or tissues; obsessive-compulsive reactions causing inability to work with others or adapt; episodic losses of physical function from hysterical or conversion reactions lasting longer than several weeks; misperceptions including sense of persecution or grandiosity which may cause domineering, irritable or suspicious behaviour; thought disturbance causing memory loss that interferes with work or recreation; periods of confusion of vivid daydreams that cause withdrawal or reverie; deviations in social behaviour which cause concern to others; lack of emotional control that is a nuisance to family and associates; moderate disturbance from organic brain disease such as to require a moderate amount of supervision and direction of work day activities.

be commissioned for individuals with whom they have no doctor–patient relationship, to assess disability in connection with such claims. These roles can be broken down into three categories as set forth in Table 86.2.

1. A *treating* psychiatrist is asked to certify the partial or complete inability of the patient to perform the essential duties of an occupation in order for the patient to receive disability insurance benefits. Fischler and Booth (1999) describe the vocational impact of Axis I and Axis II DSM-IV conditions and present detailed suggestions about their management to improve the rate of successful return to employment. If the inability is partial, then accommodations by the employer may permit either full-time or part-time work, which may affect the amount of disability benefit. Many treating psychiatrists decline to perform this function. They do so because agreeing or declining to certify the patient as disabled has the potential to create a conflict of interest that can damage or destroy the doctor–patient relationship due to possible damage to the financial interests of the patient, causing a breach of trust. To protect the treatment relationship and also to promote an objective opinion, treating psychiatrists usually recommend that an independent psychiatric evaluation be performed. There are special situations in which this may not be possible, but they should be examined carefully prior to making an exception (Strasburger, Gutheil, & Brodsky, 1997; Gold et al., 2008; Gold & Shuman, 2009).

2. A *consulting* psychiatrist is asked to evaluate and possibly treat a patient with a psychiatric condition; this is termed a *treatment evaluation*. This usually involves a directed record review, a patient interview, and psychological testing. The nature of the evaluation is made clear to the potential patient at the outset. The patient to be evaluated is told who is paying for the evaluation, who will receive a copy of the evaluation, and the limitations on confidentiality. The patient is informed that a treatment relationship may be established with the evaluator if a treatable condition is identified, if treatment is authorized, and if both the examinee and the evaluator come to an agreement regarding a plan of a treatment.

3. An *independent psychiatric evaluation* of an individual is commissioned with an explicit bar on assuming a treatment relationship, in order to avoid a conflict of interest that might compromise the objectivity of the assessment or the welfare of the examinee. This evaluation entails a comprehensive record review, which often extends years into pre-injury medical records, an interview of the examinee, and in many cases psychological testing (Williams, 2006; Williams & Schouten, 2008; Gold et al., 2008; Gold & Shuman, 2009). Informed consent is obtained and documented, including the fact that no doctor–patient relationship is being established, nor will one be established; notification as to who is paying for the report; and notification as to whom a copy of the report will be provided. The examinee has the right to decline the evaluation, although this may have an impact on their benefit status.

THE MEANING OF IMPAIRMENT TO THE INDIVIDUAL

Impairments are limitations to specific functions resulting from an illness or condition. For example, in the case of depression, impairments can take the form of difficulties with memory, attention, affect-regulation, and decision-making. The meaning of impairment to an individual depends on the interplay of a number of factors:

1. If their impairment is relevant to their work, it will have a more negative impact than if it is irrelevant to their work.

2. If their education and experience qualify them for alternative employment, their adaptation to impairment will be easier.

3. If they have a high level of personality functioning as defined by the DSM-5, then they will be better able to cope with the social and intrapsychic consequences of a new impairment.

4. As a consequence, individuals with similar objective impairments may experience widely varying degrees of *disability*. The work impact of a physical injury that prevents standing for long periods of time is different for a surgeon than it is for a psychiatrist. Colorblindness results in only a few employment restrictions, and little psychiatric morbidity. Other impairments, such as complete sightlessness, result in greater limitations, although

Table 86.2 PSYCHIATRIST ROLES IN DISABILITY EVALUATIONS

PSYCHIATRIST ROLE	TREATMENT	CERTIFY DISABILITY	RECOMMEND ACCOMMODATIONS
Treating	Yes	May be required, but conflict of interest avoided when done by IME psychiatrist	May be required, but conflict of interest avoided when done by IME psychiatrist
Treatment consultation	Depends on need, authorization and mutual agreement	Yes, required by authority	Yes
Independent psychiatric evaluation	No with very rare exceptions	Yes	Yes

substantial community support and having an identity within the community may lessen the impact. Psychiatric disorders may cause direct suffering from illness-related symptoms such as depression, anxiety, panic, pain, and psychotic symptoms.

5. Indirect suffering, resulting from the damage to the patient's self-esteem related to loss of functional capacity and all the losses this entails, may cause greater distress.

6. Unemployment resulting from disability can lead to disturbance of self-functioning through damage to the identity and self-direction. As with physical disabilities, the most common chief complaint encountered in a psychiatric disability evaluation is some variation on the theme of "I can't do what I used to do."

7. Vulnerability to psychic damage in these arenas is related to the individual's *internal resources*; i.e., level of personality integration prior to suffering the disability, as well as to their *external* resources; i.e., access to medical, financial, and social support. A person with no impairment in *self-identity* as defined by the DSM-5—"awareness of having a unique identity, grounded in personal history, along with continuity in self-states and the ability to think about and make sense of internal experience"—is equipped to cope much more successfully with the stress of injury and disability than someone with even a moderate level of impairment, for whom the regulation of self-states often depends on context (e.g., prestige and recognition in the community) and who has an impaired capacity to think about internal experience.

Access to external resources, such as replacement income from a disability insurance policy coupled with continued health insurance, will reduce anxiety and depression as well as improve the prospect for recovery of health and maintenance of the patient's family's daily functioning. If, in contrast, unemployment resulting from disability leads to loss of income, health insurance, and access to health care, it is a near certainty that the individual will experience at least some degree of anxiety and depression, as well as face an increased risk of interpersonal conflict with damage to the individual's capacity for intimacy and empathy. The degree to which the individual may be subject to decreased functioning in either the self or interpersonal functioning is related to their premorbid level of functioning (internal resources), the severity of their injury or illness-caused impairment, and their life circumstance (external resources).

A thought experiment may help the clinician better appreciate the impact of physical and mental impairments on employment and income. Much has been written about the emotional trauma experienced by the 10% of the workforce who are considered to be "long-term unemployed" as a result of the recession of 2008–2011 and their uncertain work future. Those unemployed because of larger economic forces receive some societal sympathy and up to 99 weeks of unemployment insurance (see http://www.edd.ca.gov/Unemployment/Federal_Unemployment_Insurance_Extensions.htm). In contrast, individuals who are unemployed because of a psychiatric impairment in connection

with a job-related injury suffer the stigma of being at least "different," or viewed as dishonest, often in combination with mental and sometimes physical pain. They experience loss of their work-role identity within the family, their community, and among their friends. In addition, they experience a loss of personal worth because they drain rather than contribute to the family's financial well-being.

Economic hardship is a common consequence of disability. Virtually all disabled people experience economic anxiety. For many families, the loss of "everything I worked for" and possibly actual bankruptcy are the outcome.

The *psychological meaning* of the disability to the individual is determined by factors that provide a context for the injury or illness, define its consequences, and either support or impede recovery. These factors are listed in Box 86.1.

The *duration* of disability influences the degree of trauma. A rapid return to work entails little emotional distress. In contrast, prolonged disability and unemployment may lead to depression, anxiety disorders, and somatoform disorders.

PSYCHIATRIC CONDITIONS COMMONLY ASSOCIATED WITH DISABILITY

Depression

Depression is an important cause and consequence of disability with economic impact, both as a primary disorder and in combination with other medical illnesses. The total estimated workplace costs of absenteeism and impaired working ability associated with depression amounted to $44 billion in 2001–2002, and nearly 80% of the lost productive time was invisible to the employer, as it resulted from decreased productivity while at work, termed "presenteeism" (Stewart, Ricci, Chee, Hahn, & Morganstein, 2003).

In a classic article, as relevant today as when it was originally published, Gallagher and Meyers (1996) describe how untreated depression leads to increased costs and disability. Patterns of delay in specialist referrals reflected patterns of conflicts present in the disability arena. Worse outcomes and increased costs were related to the average delay from injury to obtaining approval for a specialist referral, and from specialist referral to a comprehensive pain rehabilitation center. Indeed, mild to severe depression is the most common psychiatric finding after disabling injury (Williams & Schouten, 2008). The severity of pain associated with the injury is significantly correlated with the development of depression over time (Gallagher & Meyers., 1996; Fishbain et al, 1997) and negatively correlated with return to work. Not only its severity, but the affective dimension of pain is closely related to return to work after injury. In a longitudinal study of 185 injured workers (Corbiere, Sullivan, Stanish, & Adams, 2007), the *sensory* dimension of the pain experience was distinguished from the *affective* dimension on the Short-form McGill Pain Questionnaire (SF-MPQ-2) (Dworkin et al., 2009; Melzac, 1983; Melzac, 1987). The affective dimension included four items: *tiring-exhausting, sickening, fearful,* and *punishing-cruel.* The 11 sensory items describe physical sensations without an affective valence. Examples include *hot-burning* and *cramping.*

Gender

Age of onset

Congenital or acquired impairment

Severity

Adaptive capacity of the individual

Single or multiple disabilities

Absence or presence of pre-existing mental illness

Level of personality functioning per DSM-5

Effect on vital functions, e.g., work, recreation, sex

Prognosis for recovery

Financial impact

Prior level of functioning

Family and social support

Pain distribution, quality, intensity

Access to quality medical and rehabilitation services

Depression was assessed for the purposes of the study by the Beck Depression Inventory (BDI-II) (Beck, Steer, & Brown, 1996). This study confirmed a strong association between affective pain and depression over time. Both the level of affective pain and depression severity correlated negatively with return to work, and the effect size was great. Eighty-five percent of workers ($N = 74$) with only "normal ups and downs" and low affective pain levels returned to work. In contrast, only about 20% of workers ($N = 41$) with moderate to severe depression and high affective pain levels returned to work. The BDI-II and the SF-MPQ may be measuring similar *somato-affective elements*. Another widely used screening test for measuring depression is the Patient Health Questionnaire (PHQ-9, 1999) available at www.Phqscreeners.com/overview.aspx.

A detailed comparison of the PHQ-9, DSM-IV-TR, and the BDI-II with recommended questions for the assessment of depression is presented by Williams and Schouten (2008) in Figure 86.2.

Regardless of the assessment tool used, these findings are consistent with the DSM-5 reformulation of *Somatoform disorders*. Depression that follows an injury serious enough to

DSM-IV-TR	PHQ-9	BDI-11	Suggested Screening Questions for Occupational Physician Interview
Criteria for major depressive episode: Five (or more) of the following symptoms have been present during the same 2-week period and represent a change from previous functioning; at least one of the symptoms is either (1) depressed mood or (2) loss of interest or pleasure.	Over the last 2 weeks, how often have you been bothered by any of the following problems? Read each item carefully and circle your response.	Each of the 21 categories listed below contains a group of 4 statements, scored from 0–3. The categories are matched to the estimated closest DSM IV listing.	
Depressed mood most of the day nearly every day	Feeling down, depressed, or hopelessness	Sadness, pessimism, self-dislike	Have you or the people you are around noticed that your average mood has changed over the last month or so or compared to before you were injured?
Markedly diminished interest or pleasure in activities most of the day, nearly every day	Little interest or pleasure in doing things	Loss of pleasures, loss of interest, loss of interest in sex	Do you enjoy doing things less or are you less interested in doing things than you used to be?
Change of more than 5% body weight in a month or decrease or increase of appetite nearly every day	Poor appetite or overeating	Changes in appetite	Have you gained or lost more than 5 or 10 pounds in the last month? Has your appetite changed?
Insomnia or hypersomnia nearly every day	Trouble falling asleep, staying asleep; or sleeping too much	Changes in sleeping pattern	Please describe your sleep pattern to me. When do you usually fall asleep at night; how many times do you wake up during the nights; and when do you get up for good? Do you take naps during the day?
Psychomotor agitation or retardation nearly every day	Moving or speaking so slowly that other people could have noticed. Or being so fidgety or restless that you have been moving around a lot more than usual	Agitation, irritability	How would you and the people you live with describe your temper and irritability? Do you feel like you are more restless and on edge, or do you feel like you can't ever get going?

Figure 86.2 Comparison of DSM-IV TR, PHQ-9, BDI-II, and Suggested Screening Questions.

Fatigue or loss of energy nearly every day	Feeling tired or having little energy	Loss of energy, tiredness, or fatigue	What would you estimate your energy is now as a percentage of what it used to be?
Feelings of worthlessness or inappropriate guilt nearly every day	Feeling bad about yourself, feeling you are a failure, or feeling you have let yourself or your family down	Past failure, guilty feelings, punishment feelings, self-criticalness, worthlessness	Do you feel guilty or worthless?
Diminished ability to think or concentrate nearly every day	Trouble concentrating on things such as reading a newspaper or watching television	Indecisiveness, concentration difficulty	How would you describe your memory for recent events? Is it harder for you to read a newspaper or pay attention to what you were doing? When do the changes occur?
Recurrent thoughts of death, suicidal ideation, or suicide attempt	Thinking that you would be better off dead or that you want to hurt yourself in some way	Suicidal thoughts or wishes	Do you find yourself thinking about death more than you used to? Do you sometimes wish you wouldn't wake up? Have you thought of suicide, or ever made any plans or attempts to kill yourself?
N/A	N/A	Crying	How often do you become tearful or have crying spells? Several times per day/week/month?
"The symptoms cause clinically significant distress or impairment in social, occupational, or other important areas of functioning." "The symptoms are not better accounted for by bereavement or by the direct physiological effects of a substance (e.g., a drug or abuse or a medication) or a general medical condition (e.g., hypothyroidism)"	If you checked off any problem on this questionnaire so far, how difficult have these problems made it for you to do your work, take care of things at home, or get along with other people? - Not difficult at all - Somewhat difficult - Very difficult - Extremely difficult		If the patient endorses thoughts of suicide or gives a positive responses to two or more of the other questions, further assessment is indicated
	Response for each question: 0 = Not at all 1 = Several days 2 = More than half the days 3 = Nearly every day	Each category contains four statements that are scored from 0–3, depending on the severity of symptom. *(Statements omitted for space and copyright reasons.)*	
Consult reference to *"Practice Guidelines"* published by the APA	≤ 4 The score suggests the patient may not need depression treatment. > 5–14 Physician uses clinical judgement about treatment, based on patient's duration of symptoms and functional impairment. ≥ 15 Warrants treatment for depression, using antidepressant, psychotherapy, or a combination of treatments.	0–13 points = minimal depression 14–19 points = mild depression 20–28 points = moderate depression 29–63 points = severe depression	

Figure 86.2 continued

cause a significant disruption of work is usually the result of multiple losses:

- Loss of role status, both in the family and in the community, which impacts the self-identity as described in DSM-5
- Loss of hope of recovery
- Loss of normal recreational outlets involving high-demand physical activity such as hunting, fishing, and other sports
- Sexual dysfunction, with adverse impact on overall life satisfaction and the partner relationship
- Chronic pain resulting in a loss of sense of well-being
- Shame, blame, depression, and anger are nearly universal reactions to the loss of the ability to work

The risk of suicide should never be underestimated and should always be assessed when treating or evaluating the disabled worker. It is increased in the presence of substance abuse, in single males without a social support system, and for those with comorbid psychiatric disorders, including psychotic disorders and/or impulse control disorders.

Somatic Symptom and Related Disorders

Somatoform (formerly "psychosomatic") disorders are among the most common causes of employee disability, but they have not been generally well understood or effectively treated (Bass, Peveler, & House, 2001), and they come with cultural and developmental bias (Stoudemire, 1991). In DSM-5 the new category *Somatic Symptom and Related Disorders* replaces the DSM-IV category of Somatoform Disorders. All the disorders share prominent somatic symptoms associated with significant distress and impairment (see http://www.psychiatryonline.org, 2014). Within this new category 300.82 *Somatic symptom disorder* incorporated Somatization disorder, and both Pain disorder diagnoses (with and without a general medical condition) from DSM-IV. 300.7 *Illness anxiety disorder* corresponds to Hypochondriasis in DSM-. 300.11 *Conversion disorder* retains the same coding as in DSM-IV. 316 *Psychological factors affecting other medical conditions* is a new DSM-5 diagnosis. 300.19 *Factitious disorder* had a separate category in DSM-IV but is included among Somatic Symptom and Related Disorders in DSM-5. 300.89 *Other specified somatic symptom and related disorder* is used when a somatic symptom disorder or illness anxiety disorder is of less than 6 months duration. 300.82 *Unspecified somatic symptom and related disorders* replaces Somatoform disorder NOS and is used only "in decidedly unusual situations where there is insufficient information to make a more specific diagnosis." The proposed change responded to the criticism that the DSM-IV nosology was confusing, suggested a mind–body dualism, and unreliably required the identification of "medically unexplained symptoms." The DSM-5 formulation recognizes that many of the DSM-IV *Somatoform disorder* diagnoses incorporated cognitive distortions and somatic symptoms.

These changes will simplify the diagnostic work of the psychiatric evaluator by providing a conceptual framework that is more consistent and has less overlap and confusion. Table 86.3 illustrates the relationship between the DSM-IV and DSM-5 somatoform terms and diagnoses.

Table 86.3 SOMATOFORM TERMS IN DSM IV AND DSM 5

DSM IV-TR	DSM-5
Somatoform disorders – emphasized medically unexplained symptoms – "unreliable and pejorative"	Somatic symptom and related disorders (new category in DSM-5) – all share prominent somatic symptoms associated with psychological distress and impairment – "more useful for primary care and other medical clinicians"
300.81 – Somatization disorder 307.89 – Pain disorder associated with psychological factors and a general medical condition 307.8 – Pain disorder associated with psychological factors	300.82 – Somatic symptom disorder – may or may not be associated with another medical condition, but with high levels of worry about illness – emphasis on distressing symptoms and impairment rather than absence of medical explanation. Specifiers • With predominant pain (most commonly) • Persistent • Mild, moderate, severe
300.7 – Hypochondriasis	300.7 – Illness anxiety disorder (hypochondriasis without somatic symptoms) – care seeking or care avoidant
300.11 – Conversion disorder	300.11 – Conversion disorder (Functional neurological disorder) – specific qualifiers do not change coding. May be diagnosed in addition to Somatic symptom disorder. 316 – Psychological factors affecting other medical conditions – includes patterns of interpersonal interaction, coping style, and maladaptive health behaviors
In separate category in DSM-IV	300.19 – Factitious disorder (intentional falsification of physical or psychological symptoms) 300.89 – Other specified somatic symptom and related disorder – do not meet full criteria for any of the disorders in the somatic symptom or related disorders class
300.82 – Somatoform disorder NOS	300.82 – Unspecified somatic symptom and related disorder – to be used in decidedly unusual situations

Anxiety Disorders

Anxiety disorders are commonly associated with disability. The normal worry and concern associated with any health problem increases as a disability becomes chronic and the workers' normal life pattern is broken. Panic disorder, with or without agoraphobia, is a common outcome and is usually associated with depression. The real loss of income associated with damage to the worker's self-esteem connected with loss of work-role identity contributes significantly to uncertainty, fear of the future, and the exacerbation of anxiety disorders.

Personality Disorders

Personality disorders have been defined as "an enduring pattern of inner experience and behavior that deviates markedly from the expectations of the individual's culture" in two or more areas, including *cognition, affectivity, interpersonal functioning,* and *impulse control*. Because "the enduring pattern is inflexible and pervasive across a broad range of personal and social situations," the personality disorder allows for less adaptability in individuals who have impairments. As a result, a given impairment often leads to greater disability in someone with a personality disorder than in an individual without one.

CLINICIANS AND FORENSIC EVALUATORS HAVE DIFFERENT ROLES

Viewing psychiatric practice broadly, there are two fundamental types of diagnostic evaluations, *forensic* and *clinical* (Strasburger et al., 1997; Gold & Shuman, 2009). These two types of evaluations have separate goals, and whenever possible should be conducted by separate psychiatrists, although this may sometimes be difficult to achieve in actual practice. A clinical evaluation is undertaken to formulate an effective treatment plan and is properly carried out by the potential or current treating psychiatrist. Its focus is on the patient's symptoms, the patient's subjective view of him- or herself and the world, and how best to relieve the patient's suffering. A forensic evaluation, in addition to identifying symptoms and eliciting the evaluee's subjective views, is aimed at an objective determination of symptoms, their severity, and often causation. Although the two types of evaluations overlap, there is a difference in emphasis, and there are intrinsic conflicts between the two roles.

At the heart of this conflict is the fundamental notion that the clinician and the independent evaluator serve "different masters." The clinician has an ethical duty to act only in the best interests of the patient. Thus, if patients are distressed and unhappy at work, the clinician may believe it is necessary to assist them in staying out of work until the causes of the distress have been addressed and corrected. The independent evaluator, on the other hand, has an obligation to provide an objective, scientifically based opinion. The relationship is one of evaluator–evaluee, not doctor–patient, although a limited duty remains even in an evaluator relationship. For example, if the evaluator discovers in the course of the evaluation that the examinee is acutely suicidal, the evaluator is obligated to take any necessary steps for the purpose of preservation of life, as in any clinical situation. In essence, a duty to protect exists in a clinical setting and in an evaluator–evaluee relationship.

Another major difference between the clinician and the independent evaluator is how the information they glean is used. Under the traditional psychotherapeutic model, the treating clinician attempts to see the world through the eyes of the patient: historical accuracy is less important than individual perception. As a result, the treating clinician may or may not review prior medical records. In addition, the treating clinician rarely looks to outside sources to corroborate the patient's story. Even contact with family members may be controversial. The independent evaluator, on the other hand, is in search of an objective, accurate assessment, and must evaluate the medical records as extensively and closely as possible. The independent evaluator will also evaluate other sources of information, including court records, reports of private investigators, and personnel records. Such materials rarely serve any purpose in the treatment of the patient, yet they can make a crucial difference in the forensic assessment of disability. Finally, the treating clinician who fills out forms or gives testimony in a manner contrary to what the patient sees as being in his or her best interests may find that the treatment relationship is damaged or destroyed.

Patients have real health considerations that must be factored into their psychiatric treatment. For this reason, it is important for the treating psychiatrist to review medical records related to their patients to accurately provide coordinated diagnosis and treatment.

Patients commonly become involved in the legal system in pursuit of their disability claims. This could further complicate the treatment relationship. It is prudent for clinicians to resist external pressures emanating from the attorney or patient, and the internal pressures from the therapist's allegiance to the patient. The legal process is directed toward the resolution of disputes; psychotherapy pursues the medical goal of healing. Although these purposes may be congruent, the legal processes may create an irreconcilable role conflict. In essence, treatment in psychotherapy is brought about through an empathic relationship that has no place in, and is unlikely to survive, the questioning and public reporting of a forensic evaluation (Strasburger et al., 1997).

Institutional policies often force treating psychiatrists to function in both roles in disability determinations, such as, for example, by requiring either concurrence or non-concurrence with independent medical evaluations (IMEs). Court testimony is frequently required in administrative law hearings when disputes arise, where by law the testimony of the treating psychiatrist is given more weight than is that of the forensic evaluator, on the grounds that the treating psychiatrist is more knowledgeable about the patient. When the treating psychiatrist must participate in the disability evaluation process, the following principles should be kept in mind:

- Obtain and document informed consent from the patient to disclose information provided during the course of the treatment.
- Have a clear understanding of the patient's job duties.

Occasionally a patient in treatment will seek disability benefits, and the psychiatrist may view that as contrary to their best interests. In some instances, this issue can be productively discussed and treatment advanced. In other cases, the patient may be acting out dependency issues or other, more serious character problems, and a second opinion and consultation will help. If this does not resolve the impasse, and if the psychiatrist believes that the patient's course of action is incompatible with treatment, an orderly termination may be best. Alternatively, the patient may quit treatment when he or she realizes that the psychiatrist will not participate in their effort to be declared disabled.

TYPES OF PSYCHIATRIC DISABILITY EVALUATIONS

Different types of psychiatric disability evaluations have differing requirements. Table 86.4 outlines their distinctions.

SOCIAL SECURITY DISABILITY EVALUATIONS

A Social Security Disability (SSD) evaluation requires an assessment of mental health impairment *without* reference to causation, and is less complex than worker's compensation evaluations (Williams, 2010, 2013). Disability Determination Services (DDS) contracts with "consultative examiners" to provide psychiatric evaluations. No opinion is requested regarding causation, and testimony is not required. The psychiatric evaluation includes a detailed description of a "typical day" for the claimant and a detailed mental status examination. The report includes an opinion about treatment, the prognosis, and the claimant's ability to manage their funds. DDS supplies records for review, typically fewer than 20 pages. The Social

Table 86.4 TYPES OF PSYCHIATRIC EVALUATIONS AND THEIR DISTINCTIONS

EVALUATION TYPE	DSM-IV DIAGNOSIS	SEVERITY OF IMPAIRMENT RATING	WORK RESTRICTION OPTION	TREATMENT RECOMMENDATION	CAUSATION OPINION
Social Security Disability	Yes	Global – is examinee incapable of any gainful employment by reason of listed impairments in Mental Functional Residual Capacity Evaluation?	Limited to whether examinee is capable of full time gainful employment	No	No
Fitness for duty	No	Do the impairments impact the ability of the examinee to perform the essential duties of their job?	Yes	May be requested	No
Personal injury	Yes	Yes – as it relates to loss of ability to function at pre-injury level in determining amount of economic damage	Yes	No	Yes
Private disability insurance	Yes	Global – is examinee capable of work according to the terms of their disability insurance policy?	Yes	Yes	No
Worker's Compensation – *treatment consultation*	Yes	General – for purpose of authorizing treatment, not for financial award	Yes	Yes – may offer psychiatric treatment if authorized	Yes, to determine whether treatment should be authorized for related condition or as aid to recovery
Worker's compensation – *forensic*	Yes	Yes – referencing statutory guidelines for purpose of financial award	Yes	Yes – may not become treating psychiatrist	Yes; rating for purpose of determining financial award

Security Disability Insurance (SSDI) benefit program serves as a backup benefit system for workers' compensation (Bresnitz et al., 1994).

Attorneys representing a claimant may request a psychiatric evaluation on their client's behalf to assist in an appeal. Because evidence is under judicial review, psychological testing is often used to provide more facts regarding the claimant and may be ordered specifically by the administrative law judge or by the attorney representing the claimant. An opinion is required regarding whether the claimant meets the definition of having a *listed mental disorder*, and if so, whether their impairment(s) meet the threshold criteria specified by the Social Security Administration. Definitions or "listings" of mental disorders are similar to those in the DSM-IV TR, and are contained in the *Social Security Blue Book*, which is available online (at http://www.ssa.gov/disability/professionals/bluebook/12.00-MentalDisorders-Adult.htm). Mental disorders are listed and defined in Sections 12.01 through 12.10, and are contained in the "Psychiatric Review Technique Form." Form SSA-2506-BK organizes and presents the "mental findings" in a concise and consistent manner and evaluates aspects of mental impairment relevant to the individual's ability to perform work-related mental functions. If the examinee meets or exceeds the criteria of the listings, then a "Mental Residual Functional Capacity Assessment" is completed. This form, SSA-4734-F4-SUP (http://ssaconnect.com/tfiles/SSA-4734-F4-SUP.pdf), lists 20 mental capacities in four categories of mental functioning, each with five possible severity ratings—*not significantly limited; moderately limited; markedly limited; no evidence of limitation in this category;* or *not ratable on available evidence*. Some of these capacities are:

1. *Understanding and memory*—the ability to remember locations, procedures, and simple and detailed instructions.

2. *Sustained concentration and persistence*—the ability to carry out simple or detailed instructions, adhere to a schedule, maintain a routine, work around other people, make work-related decisions, and complete a normal workday and work week at a consistent pace without interruptions.

3. *Social interaction*—the ability to interact appropriately with the general public, the ability to ask questions and request assistance, the ability to accept instructions and respond appropriately to criticism from supervisors, the ability to get along with co-workers or peers, the ability to maintain socially appropriate behavior and maintain basic standards of neatness and cleanliness.

4. *Adaptation*—the ability to adapt to changes in the work setting, to recognize hazards and take precautions, to travel in unfamiliar places or use public transportation, and to set realistic goals and work independently.

The judge reviews the evidence at a hearing, interviews the claimant and other witnesses, and renders a decision on the claimant's application.

In summary, the impairments resulting from the examinee's psychiatric disorders are described in the psychiatric evaluation, but the decision regarding whether or not the criteria for disability under the Social Security Act were met are the responsibility of the adjudicator.

"FITNESS FOR DUTY" EVALUATIONS FOCUS ON EXAMINEE'S ABILITY TO PERFORM THE ESSENTIAL DUTIES OF A SPECIFIC JOB

"Fitness for duty" (FFD) evaluations may be requested under two common scenarios. The first is when an individual employee's health status changes, raising questions about his or her ability to safely and effectively perform the essential functions of the job. The second scenario arises when an employee has been out of work due to illness, and his or her fitness for duty needs to be assessed prior to their return. In contrast to SSD and workers' compensation evaluations, it is usually not necessary for a FFD evaluation to describe the examinee's developmental history and background unless elements of them are specifically relevant to the assignment (Williams, 2010). For example, a nurse's aide may develop a major depressive illness accompanied by markedly increased irritability, crying spells, and impaired concentration and memory. The evaluator may conclude that until the major depressive episode has resolved, it would be unsafe for this individual to provide patient care, and may judge the nurse's aide to be temporarily disabled for that position. The challenge of these evaluations is to focus on the individual's ability to function in a certain job.

Petersen-Crair, Marangell, Flack, Harper, Soety, and Gabbard (2003) describe the assessment of a 36-year-old physician with complex comorbidity that entailed a standard psychiatric evaluation, a substance abuse evaluation, projective psychological testing, and the MMPI-2. They walk the reader through their assessment and thought processes, diagnosing a *Bipolar disorder, Substance abuse*, and *Personality disorder NOS* in the context of a history of trauma. Their sensitive and succinct discussion of assessment, diagnosis, and treatment recommendations to allow for safe return to work exemplifies the competent and ethical management of a complex case. Gold et al. (2008) and Gold and Shuman (2009) can also be consulted for an in-depth treatment of this subject.

PERSONAL INJURY CLAIMS WITH DETERMINATION OF CAUSALITY AND AMOUNT OF DAMAGES

Personal injury lawsuits in which emotional-distress damages are claimed require psychiatric assessments that apportion causation and gauge the degree of impairment resulting from the alleged tortious event. The amount of damages awarded is open-ended. A request for assessment may come from the defense attorney representing an insurance company or an individual defendant, or from the plaintiff's attorney. Accurate apportionment of liability requires a determination of damage related to the alleged event, taking into account any preexisting impairment and contributory negligence (Knoll & Gerbasi, 2006). An estimate of the extent of the injury and the need for and costs of care related to the injury will be requested. The opinion should be supported by reference to information obtained from the review of legal, employment, medical, and/or school records, as well as objective psychological test data.

PRIVATE INSURANCE DISABILITY EVALUATIONS

Evaluating Degree of Impairment and Making Treatment Recommendations Without Determination of Causation

Private insurance companies that underwrite group or individual disability insurance policies primarily rely upon the reports of treating clinicians when initially determining disability claims. Claims managers and in-house medical reviewers then review these reports. Based on those reviews, the insurer may request confirmation of the findings and a review of the treatment being provided. The goal of the insurance company is to minimize disability claims that result from substandard care, to insure that accurate diagnoses are made, and to determine whether the terms of the policy's coverage are being satisfied. Some policies were written that allowed for full benefits if policyholders become unable to perform the tasks of their own occupation, but those are now difficult to obtain. Current policies usually provide benefits only if the insured is unable to perform the tasks associated with *any* job. In recent years, a number of disability carriers have altered their contracts to limit payments for "nervous and mental" (i.e., psychiatric disability) claims to two years. The entity requesting the evaluation typically provides a specific list of questions to be answered and requires a comprehensive evaluation. The evaluator is instructed to release the information only to the requesting entity, much as an evaluation requested by an attorney goes only to the attorney. Objective psychological testing can be of considerable value in this process, as it provides additional data on which to base an opinion.

TWO TYPES OF WORKERS' COMPENSATION EVALUATIONS: TREATMENT CONSULTATIONS AND INDEPENDENT PSYCHIATRIC EVALUATIONS

Workers' compensation programs require a determination of whether one or more psychiatric conditions are causally related to a workplace injury on "a more probable than not" basis to determine whether medical treatment is payable, and whether compensatory "time-loss" income benefits—typically amounting to 60% of wages—are due the worker. In this type of assessment, the determination of causation requires that the diagnosed psychiatric condition(s) be judged to be the result of the workplace injury in question with a 51% or greater degree of probability. Fault is not at issue in worker's compensation claims, and settlements—in the event that residual impairments are present at the time of claim closure—are paid according to a schedule. If the individual is determined not to be capable of reasonably continuous full-time gainful employment following treatment, a pension may be awarded.

In Washington State, the examiner must assign each diagnosis to one of four categories posed by the Department of Labor and Industries:

1. The injured worker's psychiatric condition was not caused or aggravated by the industrial injury, but it creates a barrier to recovery from a condition for which the department has accepted liability.

2. The injured worker's psychiatric condition was caused by the industrial injury.

3. The injured worker's psychiatric condition is a preexisting condition that was aggravated by the industrial injury.

4. The injured worker's psychiatric condition was neither caused nor aggravated by the industrial injury, nor is it creating a barrier to recovery from a condition for which the department has accepted liability.

Determining whether a condition is "more probably than not" proximately caused by an industrial injury in a worker's compensation case is often complex and adversarial because of the economic consequences to the contending parties and because analysis of the injury is often complicated by preexisting conditions, personality disorders, and/or trait disturbances.

Both psychiatrists performing IMEs and treating psychiatrists are often asked to approve or disapprove job analyses (JAs) for several different positions, such as "cashier" or "meat packer." Each job analysis describes the essential functions of the job, and both the treating psychiatrist and the IME psychiatrist may be asked to approve, approve with restrictions, or disapprove the specific jobs described by their respective JAs. These are formal descriptions of the workplace environmental conditions, the physical maneuvers that are required, and their frequency in performing job tasks, including the cognitive and emotional tasks associated with the position, and so forth. When the injured worker nears "maximum medical improvement," expert opinions guide the claims manager and vocational consultant in determining whether the claimant is able to return to the job of injury, is able to work at a job for which they have transferable skills, requires retraining for another job, or whether they should be referred for pension determination.

Worker's compensation claims vary enormously in their complexity and in their degree of controversy. Simple claims may be disposed of administratively with little dispute between the worker and the insurance company. However, when claims are complex, controversial, and involve substantial financial consequences, expert witnesses may be called by both sides in order to determine causation and degree of impairment. The responsibility of the IME psychiatrist—regardless of who the contracting party may be, is to be an independent "seeker of truth" and except in rare circumstances, not to establish a doctor–patient relationship (Strasburger et al., 1997). Cases may be litigated through several levels of review beyond the administrative board level, up though courts of superior jurisdiction, appellate courts, and to the state supreme court.

OUTLINE OF THE PSYCHIATRIC DISABILITY EVALUATION

Psychiatric disability evaluations are conducted differently than routine treatment consultations. Box 86.2 presents an outline of a psychiatric disability evaluation that can be adapted to the needs of the particular evaluation.

The psychiatrist performing an independent evaluation at the request of a third party does not owe the same duty to the examinee as does a psychiatrist performing an evaluation for treatment purposes. It is important that confidentiality limitations and roles be clearly explained to the examinee before undertaking the evaluation, and a signed release should be obtained, specifying the authorized recipients of the evaluation (Gold & Davidson, 2007). Without such information it is impossible for the patient to give informed consent to the evaluation process (Williams & Schouten, 2008).

When an *independent* evaluation is being conducted at the request of a third party, the examinee must be informed that there will be no follow-up treatment relationship with the examining psychiatrist, as that could create a conflict of interest. Rare exceptions to this guideline are addressed by Strasburger et al. (1997).

When a *treatment* consultation is performed (as might be the case when a patient is referred by an occupational physician) the patient and psychiatrist may choose to establish a doctor–patient relationship. It is good practice to explicitly inform the patient that they are free to select another provider. This is particularly important in disability treatment situations since, for therapy to be effective, the patient must have trust and confidence in the treating psychiatrist. In workers' compensation treatment settings, regular reports to the administrative agency are required, and the patient should be informed that the confidentiality is limited. Sensitive material not necessary to the administration of the claim should be excluded from reports; such reports should primarily document diagnoses, treatment modalities employed, and progress in treatment. In most situations, telling the patient that they are entitled to a copy of any document produced by their psychiatrist related to their treatment promotes trust through transparency, and it also serves to remind the treating psychiatrist of the importance of discretion. It is also good practice

---

Box 86.2 PSYCHIATRIC DISABILITY EVALUATION OUTLINE

A. General considerations
  1. Reasons for a disability evaluation
     a. Employer request
     b. Insurance company request
        (1) Private disability coverage
        (2) Second opinions re: treatment
     c. Physician request for psychiatric assessment as adjunct to general medical care—treatment rather than causality issues central (e.g., orthopedist requests psychiatric consultation for depressed patient)
  2. Role and boundary issues
     a. Confidentiality is waived
        (1) This is made explicit to the examinee, who is advised to whom the report will be provided
        (2) The examinee is advised that examination does not constitute nor is a substitute for medical treatment
     b. Role of the independent psychiatrist evaluator
        (1) No follow-up treatment responsibility
        (2) Potential adversarial relationship to patient
     c. Role of the treating psychiatrist
        (1) Follow-up reports are often required by statute or insurance carrier, so patient must be informed
        (2) Some confidentiality limitations: make explicit to patient
           Information usually confined to diagnoses, medications, and general impression regarding progress in treatment or lack thereof
           Advise patient that second or independent opinions may be requested in ambiguous situations
  3. Consequences of psychiatric disability for the patient
     a. Suffering from a psychiatric condition: both psychiatric symptoms (e.g., depression, anxiety, panic, pain symptoms, phobias, etc.) and damage to self-concept
     b. Work life and love life similar/equivalent in importance for individual fulfillment
     c. Consequences of loss of work role
        (1) Devaluation within the family
        (2) Loss of community prestige
        (3) Economic loss, insecurity
        (4) Loss of sublimations for the expression of aggression

(continued)

Box 86.2 CONTINUED

B. The psychiatric evaluation procedure
  1. History
      a. Medical and collateral record review
      b. Reason for the evaluation
      c. Presenting problem in patient's own words
      d. History of the presenting problem
          (1) New or recurrent problem?
          (2) Static or changing?
          (3) Impact on home and work functioning?
  2. Social history
      a. Family's socioeconomic status
      b. Role of work in family life
  3. Educational history
      a. Detail elementary, middle, and high school
      b. Strong and weak subject areas
      c. Relationship with teachers
      d. High school dropouts at increased risk
  4. Employment history
      a. Job types
      b. Performance level
      c. Length of employment
      d. Reasons for prior changes in employment
      e. Job satisfaction at the time of injury
  5. Current income sources: impact of illness
      a. Evaluate for primary gain in maintaining disability if receiving benefits
      b. If no benefits, motivation to forgo treatment and return to work prematurely, inviting further injury
  6. Past medical history
  7. Current medical problems and names of physicians. Include any abnormal laboratory or radiographic findings.
  8. Medications
  9. Substance use/abuse history
  10. Legal problems
  11. Past personal psychiatric history
      a. Hospitalizations: Complaint, dates, hospital, duration, outcome
      b. Outpatient history: Complaint, dates, treating professional, duration, outcome
      c. Anxiety disorder
      d. Alcohol and substance abuse
      e. Other
  12. Developmental history
      a. Family structure
          (1) Parents together or divorced; stepparents
          (2) Nature of patient-parent relationship
          (3) Birth order; relationships with siblings
          (4) Neglect or abuse history; duration and severity
      b. Work role models: Parent work history
      c. Age when patient began work: Premature responsibility increases disability risk
      d. Illness history in family or patient
      e. Relationship with authority figures
      f. Peer relationships: Best friend?
      g. School experiences
          (1) Academic performance level through grades
          (2) Last grade completed
          (3) Strong and weak subject areas
      h. Dating experiences; marital history

(continued)

Box 86.2 CONTINUED

13. The "typical day"
    a. Narrative description of how the day is spent
    b. Time of arising; napping; time of retiring
    c. Activities of daily living: who performs, changes since illness onset
        (1) Bill paying
        (2) Meal preparation
        (3) Laundry
        (4) Housecleaning
14. Basic mental status examination
    a. Appearance and behavior
    b. Mood and affect
    c. Speech and thought content
    d. Preoccupations, suicidal or homicidal ideation
    e. Cognitive functioning: orientation, fund of knowledge, memory testing, abstract thinking, judgment, insight
15. Psychological testing as indicated
    a. MMPI-2, MCMI-3, Rorschach, TAT
    b. When should testing be requested?
        (1) To clarify ambiguous or complex diagnoses
        (2) To compare with previous test results
        (3) To assess for neuropsychological impairment
        (4) To help resolve diagnostic disagreements between clinicians
        (5) To assess for malingering
16. Summary and discussion
    a. Logically synthesize all information obtained
        (1) Present explanation of symptom/illness development
        (2) Developmental psychodynamic factors which may be reenacted
        (3) Neurobiological and genetic factors
        (4) Environmental factors
    b. Temporal relationship between events and illness; degree and duration of impairment; use of appropriate rating systems
17. Multi-axial DSM IV diagnoses
    a. Current standard for psychiatric diagnosis
    b. Utilize 5 axis format for listing diagnoses, important psychosocial and environmental problems, and GAF
        (1) Valuable as a means of measuring change over time between evaluations
        (2) Changes in degree of disability
18. Family psychiatric history
    a. Suicide attempts
    b. Depression
    c. Anxiety disorder
    d. Alcohol and substance abuse
    e. Other

to advise the patient that a second opinion may be requested by the doctor, the patient, or the claims manager. Psychiatric treatment consultation guidelines are presented in Box 86.3.

THE ROLE OF PSYCHOLOGICAL TESTING: BRIEF SELF-REPORT TESTS, THE MMPI-2/MMPI-2-RF, AND THE SIRS/SIRS-2

Psychological testing provides a method for refining diagnostic impressions in disability evaluations developed through the record review and interview process, and it also can assist in developing an objective measure of severity of the condition (Williams & Schouten, 2008; Graham, 2012). Psychological testing can also assist in treatment planning and assessment of the effectiveness of treatment as it proceeds through serial administration. *Brief* self-report tests such as the Beck Depression Inventory–II (BDI-II) and the PHQ-9 have demonstrated value in *clinical* practice. Many other brief self-report tests are used for the assessment of PTSD, anxiety disorders, and other conditions. They are easy to use and require little time to administer, but they do not assess the examinee's cooperation with the evaluation process, and most

Box 86.3 PSYCHIATRIC TREATMENT
CONSULTATION GUIDELINES

- Referred by party involved in patient's healthcare, e.g., physician, vocational counselor

- Informed consent-who receives report, limited confidentiality

- Purpose is to diagnose and recommend treatment for psychiatric disorders.

- Record review brief compared to IME since the purpose is not primarily for apportioning causation

- Psychiatrist performing treatment consultation may provide treatment if mutually agreed

brief tests assess only one diagnostic category. They are open to challenge in *forensic* practice because they lack validity scales. For example, it is argued that an individual claiming compensation for depression might intentionally exaggerate the depression symptoms reported on the BDI-II or the PHQ-9 in order to "prove" their condition, or that a person with pain complaints would do likewise. In settings where only treatment is sought, it is more realistic to expect that the examinee will cooperate and respond truthfully.

The MMPI-2 is a 567-item test in which the examinee is asked to endorse each item as *true* or *false,* and it requires about 90 minutes to complete. Although psychologists most commonly administer and interpret the test, there are avenues for other clinicians to obtain training since it is necessary to qualify professionally to purchase and administer the test (Graham, 2012). Because the MMPI-2 is cited so frequently in a disability context, it will be discussed in some detail. The MMPI-2 has been empirically validated both on clinical and non-clinical populations. It is available only through Pearson Assessments in English, Spanish, and Hmong, and in both written and audio formats; the audio format is useful for test takers who have limited reading skills.

The MMPI-2-RF (Restructured Form) was published in 2008 by Pearson Assessments and adds significantly to the information available through the MMPI-2. The MMPI-2-RF consists of 338 items drawn from the 567 MMPI-2 items "designed to represent the clinically significant substance of the [567] MMPI-2 item pool with a comprehensive set of psychometrically efficient measures." The MMPI-2 Restructured Clinical (RC) scales assess the major distinctive core components of the test's Clinical scales and have been carried over to the MMPI-2-RF with no changes. The RC scales are supplemented by "broad-band higher order" measures of psychological dysfunction and other scales that focus more specifically on a variety of internalizing, externalizing, and interpersonal characteristics.

The MMPI-2 and MMPI-2-RF have greater utility than brief self-report tests in forensic settings because they possesses *validity scales* and because in clinical settings they have the advantage of measuring a broad array of psychopathology instead of only one aspect of personality functioning. The test materials can be administered by paper and pencil, by CD or cassette tape, or by computer. Validity has been established for English, Spanish, and Hmong for the MMPI-2 and for English for the MMPI-2-RF. Scoring by computer is faster than scoring with hand templates and eliminates the potential for errors associated with use of hand-scoring. After purchasing a site license for the computer software for about $100 per year, individual tests can be scored and the results stored for an additional cost that ranges between about $15 and $35 per test administration, depending on whether the written interpretive report is desired in addition to the scale-profile printout. In order to qualify to purchase and administer the MMPI-2 or MMPI-2-RF, a psychiatrist will need to take one of the workshops on the MMPI-2 and/or MMPI-2-RF offered by Pearson Assessments, which are offered several times a year at different locations around the United States. The Pearson Assessments website provides detailed information on workshop scheduling and ordering test materials.

The raw scores—that is, the number of items endorsed in the keyed direction on each MMPI-2 or MMPI-2-RF scale—are statistically transformed into uniform "T scores," with the result that a T score of 65 for one scale has the same meaning as T score of 65 on another scale. For example, T scores of 65 correspond to the 92nd percentile for each scale, and in general, T scores >65 are clinically significant and interpretable. Profiles are graphed using the T scores for the individual scales on each *profile*. For the remainder of this chapter, it is understood that when a scale score is mentioned, it refers to the T score and not the raw score.

THE MMPI-2 SCALES

The MMPI-2 contains a *validity scale* profile, a *clinical scales* profile, a *restructured clinical scales* profile, a *content scales* profile, a *supplementary scales* profile, and the Personality Psychopathology-5 (*PSY-5) scales* profile. We will focus most of our attention on the *profile elevation* (which is the arithmetic mean of the statistically derived T scores of clinical scales 1, 2, 3, 4, 6, 7, 8, and 9), the *validity scales*, the *RC scales*, and the *PSY-5 scales* to simplify our discussion. Graham (2012) and Butcher and Williams (2000) can be consulted for detailed guidelines regarding the development and composition of each scale, and for *interpretive strategies* as well as their theoretical and research background underpinnings.

VALIDITY SCALES

The validity scales identify random response patterns, inconsistent response patterns, defensive response patterns, and exaggerated response patterns, providing a forensically valuable advantage over test instruments without such scales (Graham, 2012). In 1989, new *validity scales* were added to the three basic validity scales, F (infrequency), K (defensiveness), and L (lie), from the original MMPI, thus providing much more information about the test-taker's approach to the test. VRIN (variable response inconsistency) and TRIN (true response inconsistency) scales elevated beyond a certain point indicate that the individual is not attending to the content of the items and is responding in a random fashion, resulting in an invalid profile or that they responded to the items with a bias either to respond "true" or respond "false". Since release of the MMPI-2 in 1989, other validity scales have been added after demonstrating utility in identifying defensive or exaggerated response patterns. For example, the Fp scale (infrequency psychopathology) consists of 27 items endorsed infrequently by both psychiatric inpatients and the MMPI-2 normative sample. Consequently, a significant elevation produced on the Fp scale is more likely to reflect deliberate exaggeration or feigning of severe psychopathology. The F scale items, in contrast, were chosen because they were infrequently endorsed in a *non-clinical* normative population. Because psychiatric subjects more frequently endorse items on the F scale, a high Fp scale score is more likely to reflect *exaggeration* and non-credible responding than a high F scale score; this corrects an important deficiency in the original MMPI. The Fake Bad Scale (FBS), a symptom validity scale, has been a controversial scale since it was introduced in 1991 by Lees-Haley, English, and Glenn. Graham (2012), after surveying the literature, "concluded that when appropriate cutoff scores are used, the FBS scale has utility in identifying persons who give noncredible reports of cognitive deficits." L scale elevations, which may indicate that the test taker is attempting to deny even normal shortcomings and claiming unusual virtue, may result in a profile that minimizes the severity and extent of their psychological problems. Such *underreporting* of psychological problems is more likely to occur when the person is trying to present themselves as psychologically healthy, as in an employment examination or a child custody evaluation. It may also occur for individuals with "traditional values based" and unsophisticated backgrounds who define themselves in terms of their aspirational values, and who are trying to fit into a dominant culture that espouses those values. Detailed information regarding guidelines for assessing validity is available in several references (Graham, 2012; Butcher & Williams, 2000). In particular, the Fp scale has particular value in identifying non-credible reporting of psychiatric symptoms in individuals seeking compensation (Arbisi, Ben-Porath, & McNulty, 2006).

CLINICAL SCALES

There are ten clinical scales, either referred to by their numbers from 1 to 10, or by names, some of which are no longer in common use: *hypochondriasis, depression, hysteria, psychopathic deviate, masculinity-femininity, paranoia, psychasthenia, schizophrenia, hypomania,* and *social introversion.* Graham (2012) provides a detailed discussion of the qualities associated with each scale.

Code types refer to the number (i.e., 1–9) designations of the scales' T scores that are most elevated in the profile; these may refer either to *two-point* or *three-point* code types. Code types are a way of interpreting the MMPI-2 profile and can be used to identify patient-specific behaviors and coping patterns (Graham, 2012; Butcher & Williams, 2000).

RESTRUCTURED CLINICAL (RC) SCALES

The nine Restructured Clinical (RC) scales were developed by Tellegen, Ben-Porath, McNulty, Arbisi, and Graham (2003) to achieve improved convergent and discriminant validity compared to the clinical scales, and they represent a significant addition to the power of the MMPI-2 (Graham, 2012; Ben-Porath & Tellegen, 2008, 2011). The RC scales have been carried forward without change from the MMPI-2 to the MMPI-2-RF. *Convergent validity* means that the scores on a scale are significantly related to conceptually relevant extra-test measures. For example, individuals with high RC4 scores often have histories of difficulties with the law and are prone to substance abuse, and typically have work-related problems, which is what it was intended to measure. *Discriminant validity* is demonstrated when scores on a scale are not related to extra-test measures that are unrelated to what the scale is intended to measure (Graham, 2012). Thus, since RC4 does not significantly relate to other measures of depression or anxiety or thought disorders, it is said to have discriminant validity. Both the clinical scales and the RC scales have good convergent validity, but many studies have demonstrated that the RC scales have better discriminant validity.

Tellegen et al. (2003) described the development of these scales, beginning with the RCd scale labeled "Demoralization," which contains items which related to overall emotional distress, emotional discomfort, and turmoil that contaminated many of the other original clinical scales. A sophisticated statistical approach was employed to remove redundant items from the original clinical scales that were associated with non-specific general distress and demoralization and retain items associated with the core construct(s) of each scale. In general, except for the RCd scale, each RC scale represents a distinctive core construct of the parent clinical scale with the same number designation, even though in some cases the item selection is considerably different. Thus RC1 (somatic concerns) is similar to Clinical Scale 1; RC2 (low positive emotions) is similar to clinical scale 2; and so forth. No RC scale was developed to correlate with Clinical Scale 5 or Clinical Scale 10. RC3 (cynicism) has so far not been shown to have any strong correlates in clinical samples, although it has utility in predicting treatment compliance. The practical result of this project is that when there are "across the board" elevations of the clinical scales, the RC scales are often elevated more selectively, which makes it possible to develop a more fine-grained understanding of the primary problems with psychological functioning in a given subject. Thus, for example, an examinee may have T score elevations >65 on clinical scales 1, 2, 3, 6, 7, and 8, but the RC scales may only be elevated >65 on RCd (demoralization) and RC2 (low positive emotions). As Graham (2012) states, "When the clinical scale score is high but the corresponding RC scale score is not, one should be quite cautious about making inferences that the test-taker has characteristics consistent with the core construct associated with the clinical scale." In the example given, the elevated RCd score would imply that the person had a high level of overall emotional distress, is demoralized and pessimistic, and that they might report anxiety and depression. The elevated

RC2 score indicates anhedonia and an increased risk of clinical depression. This profile would not be interpreted as indicating paranoia or psychosis, since although clinical scales 6 and 8 are elevated, the corresponding RC scales reflecting ideas of persecution (RC6) and aberrant experiences (RC8) are not elevated, suggesting the observed elevations on the clinical scales associated with thought disorder were due to the endorsement of non-specific items reflecting misery and demoralization rather than items reflecting thought disorder and paranoia. The RC Scale correlates have been studied in psychiatric inpatients

THE PERSONALITY PSYCHOPATHOLOGY FIVE (PSY-5) MODEL

The Personality psychopathology Five Model (PSY-5) (which preceded the development of the MMPI-2 PSY-5 scales) is described in a monograph by Harkness and McNulty (1994) and a subsequent paper by Harkness, McNulty and Ben-Porath (1995). These *dimensional* scales (aggressiveness, AGGR; psychoticism, PSYC; disconstraint, DISC; negative emotionality/neuroticism, NEGE; introversion/low positive emotionality, INTR) were developed to assess personality traits that are present in normal persons, but are pathological when they are extreme. The PSY-5 scales were derived theoretically, based on the constructs of the PSY-5 model, and the PSY-5 model was developed independently of the MMPI item pool. They were restructured for the MMPI-2-RF to improve their psychometric validity (Ben-Porath & Tellegen, 2011).

In a 2014 paper of broad historical and theoretical scope, Harkness, Reynolds, and Lilienfeld explain that the PSY-5 *scales* each correspond to separate measurable *psychological systems* that evolved for adaptation to the external environment. They argue that assessing the status of each of these psychological systems is conceptually identical to conducting a "review of systems" in general medicine (cardiovascular, endocrine, etc.). Diagnoses of specific psychiatric disorders are then layered on the appraisal of the underlying systems, which map to PSY-5 scales. This approach has clinical utility and treatment implications and will "promote integration across sciences rather than fostering the isolation of sciences allowed by atheoretical observation terms, as in the DSM." The relationship to adaptive psychological systems and the DSM-5 presented in the paper by Harkness, Reynolds and Lilienfeld (2014) is presented in Table 86.5.

Finn et al. (2014) focused on the five-factor model proposed for DSM-5 and the ten personality disorders from DSM-IV that were carried forward to DSM-5. The Personality Psychopathology—Five (PSY-5) Model developed by Harkness and McNulty (1994) and Harkness, McNulty and Ben-Porath (1995) "was designed to bridge normal and abnormal personality variances by utilizing distance matrices based on layperson sortings of personality and personality pathology descriptors." The PSY-5 *scales* have been shown to be relatively stable over a five-year period, as one would expect given their correspondence to underlying evolved adaptive systems of psychological functioning. When they deviate significantly from established non-clinical population norms, they indicate personality trait disturbances that are conceptually relevant, although not identical to the previously proposed DSM-5 conceptual model of personality disorders. In the *Alternative DSM-5 Model for Personality Disorders* in Section III of the **DSM-5** personality disorders are characterized by impairments of personality functioning and pathological personality traits, as described in the PSY-5 model. DSM-5 further defines *self* and *interpersonal* functioning differentiated into 5 levels of impairment for Self functioning (identity and self-direction) and Interpersonal functioning (empathy and intimacy). Personality disorders increase the vulnerability of individuals to developing psychiatric disorders (e.g. anxiety, depression) in response to external stressors, such as injuries, as schematically depicted in Figure 86.3. The MMPI-2 and MMPI-2-RF help the examiner or treating psychiatrist distinguish between persons with depression *but* with no evidence of personality trait disturbance, and individuals with depression arising from an external stressor *and* evidence of preexisting personality trait pathology.

THE MMPI-2-RF IS A REVISION OF THE MMPI-2 THAT PROVIDES ADDITIONAL INFORMATION REGARDING COMPARISON POPULATIONS

In 2008, the MMPI-2 RF (Restructured Form) was published by Pearson Assessments. This test instrument contains RC scales that are identical to those of the MMPI-2, along with

Table 86.5 RELATIONSHIP BETWEEN "PSYCHOLOGICAL SYSTEMS", PSY-5 SCALES ON THE MMPI-2 AND THE DSM-5

MAJOR SYSTEMS TO BE REVIEWED	PSY-5 SCALES (1994, 2002)	DSM-5 (AMERICAN PSYCHIATRIC ASSOCIATION, 2013)
Reality modeling for action	Psychoticism PSYC	Psychoticism
Short-term danger detection	Negative emotionality NEGE	Anxiety, fear, aversive learning
Long-term cost-benefit analysis	Disconstraint DISC	Disinhibition
Resource acquisition	Introversion/low positive emotionality INTR	Detachment
Agenda protection	Aggressiveness AGGR	Antagonism

Excerpted from Harkness AR, Reynolds SM & Lilienfeld SO. 2014. *Journal of Personality Assessment, 96*(2), 121–139.

validity scales and PSY-5 scales that are similar, although not identical, to those of the MMPI-2. The clinical scales, content scales, and supplementary scales are not present in the MMPI-2-RF. Because of differences in validity scale composition, when the 567-item MMPI-2 is administered, and Pearson Assessment software is used to produce both an MMP-2 and MMPI-2-RF profile, sometimes one of the profiles may be valid while the other is invalid, making it useful to obtain both profiles. The MMPI-2 RF consists of 338 of the MMPI-2's 567 questions.

All scales are *visually displayed* as vertical range bands for *comparison groups* that can be selected for several different population samples, such as *forensic disability claimants, prison inmates,* personnel screening for *clergy, corrections,* and *law enforcement,* as well as *outpatient mental health clinics* and other specialized medical clinic settings. For example, it is possible to see at a glance whether a particular examinee falls outside one standard deviation for a similar population, like female forensic disability claimants. The RC scales are supplemented by broadband higher order measures of psychological dysfunction and other scales that focus more specifically on a variety of internalizing, externalizing, and interpersonal characteristics. The MMPI-2-RF validity scales provide a more detailed picture of *under-reporting* and *over-reporting* along both psychological and somatic dimensions than the MMPI-2, which has no comparable measure of non-credible reporting of somatic symptoms. Table 86.6 provides a comparison of the scales in the MMPI-2 and MMPI-2-RF.

The MMPI-2 and MMPI-2-RF are complementary to one another. The MMPI-2 has scales not on the MMPI-2-RF, as well as research on code-types that are associated with a wealth of clinical research. When the full MMPI-2 is administered,

Table 86.6 COMPARISON OF MMPI-2 AND MMPI-2-RF SCALES

	MMPI-2		MMPI-2-RF	
Validity Scales (revised in MMPI-2-RF)	VRIN	Variable Response Inconsistency	VRIN-r	Variable Response Inconsistency, revised
	TRIN	True Response Inconsistency	TRIN-r	True Response Inconsistency Scale, revised
	F	Infrequency	F-r	Infrequent Responses Scale
	F$_B$	Back F	Fp-r	Infrequent Psychopathology Responses Scale
	F$_P$	Infrequency-Psychopathology	Fs	Infrequent Somatic Responses Scale
	FBS	Symptom Validity Scale	FBS-r	Symptom Validity Scale, revised
	L	Lie	L-r	Uncommon Virtues Scale
	K	Correction	K-r	Adjustment Validity Scale
	S	Superlative Self-Presentation	RBS	Response Bias Scale
MMPI-2 Clinical Scales	1 Hs	Hypochondriasis	No comparable scales	
	2 D	Depression		
	3 Hy	Hysteria		
	4 Pd	Psychopathic Deviate		
	5 Mf	Masculinity-Femininity		
	6 Pa	Paranoia		
	7 Pt	Psychasthenia		
	8 Sc	Schizophrenia		
	9 Ma	Hypomania		
	0 Si	Social Introversion		
MMPI-2/MMPI-2-RF Restructured Clinical (RC) Scales (Identical composition in MMPI-2/MMPI-2-RF)	RCd	Demoralization	RCd	Demoralization

(continued)

Table 86.6 (CONTINUED)

	MMPI-2		MMPI-2-RF	
	RC1	Somatic Complaints	RC1	Somatic Complaints
	RC2	Low Positive Emotions	RC2	Low Positive Emotions
	RC3	Cynicism	RC3	Cynicism
	RC4	Antisocial Behavior	RC4	Antisocial Behavior
	RC6	Ideas of Persecution	RC6	Ideas of Persecution
	RC7	Dysfunctional Negative Emotions	RC7	Dysfunctional Negative Emotions
	RC8	Aberrant Experiences	RC8	Aberrant Experiences
	RC9	Hypomanic Activation	RC9	Hypomanic Activation
MMPI-2/MMPI-2-RF Personality Psychopathology Five Scales (PSY-5) (revised in MMPI-2-RF)	AGGR	Aggressiveness	AGGR-r	Aggressiveness – Revised
	PSYC	Psychoticism	PSYC-r	Psychoticism – Revised
	DISC	Disconstraint	DISC-r	Disconstraint – Revised
	NEGE	Negative Emotionality/Neuroticism	NEGE-r	Negative Emotionality/ Neuroticism – Revised
	INTR	Introversion/Low Positive Emotionality	INTR-r	Introversion/Low Positive Emotionality – Revised
Norms	A national norm is taken from representative demographic groups		A national norm is taken from representative demographic groups. In addition, specific comparison group norms are available, for example *male and female forensic disability claimants*	
MMPI-2-RF Higher order (H-O)	No comparable scales		*Higher-Order (H-O)* Emotional/Internalizing Dysfunction Thought Dysfunction Behavioral/Externalizing Dysfunction	
Somatic/cognitive and internalizing	Some clinical subscales and content component scales are similar, but they are not graphed in the MMPI-2		*Somatic/Cognitive* MLS Malaise GIC Gastrointestinal Complaints HPC Head Pain Complaints NUC Neurological Complaints COG Cognitive Complaints *Internalizing Scales* SUI Suicidal/Death Ideation HLP Helplessness/Hopelessness SFD Self-Doubt NFC Inefficacy STW Stress/Worry AXY Anxiety ANP Anger Proneness BRF Behavior-Restricting Fears MSF Multiple Specific Fears	

(*continued*)

Table 86.6 (CONTINUED)

MMPI-2	MMPI-2-RF
Externalizing/interpersonal and interest	*Externalizing*
	JCP Juvenile Conduct Problems
	SUB Substance Abuse
	AGG Aggression
	ACT Activation
	Interpersonal Scales
	FML Family Problems
	IPP Interpersonal Passivity
	SAV Social Avoidance
	SHY Shyness
	DSF Disaffiliativeness
	Interest Scales
	AES Aesthetic-Literary Interests
	MEC Mechanical-Physical Interests

1. Excerpted from the *MMPI-2-RF® Manual for Administration, Scoring, and Interpretation* by Yossef S. Ben-Porath and Auke Tellegen. Copyright © 2008, 2011 by the Regents of the University of Minnesota. Reproduced by permission of the University of Minnesota Press. All rights reserved. "Minnesota Multiphasic Personality Inventory-2-RF®" and "MMPI-2-RF®" are trademarks owned by the Regents of the University of Minnesota.

2. Excerpted from the *MMPI®-2 (Minnesota Multiphasic Personality Inventory®-2) Manual for Administration, Scoring, and Interpretation, Revised Edition*. Copyright © 2001 by the Regents of the University of Minnesota. All rights reserved. Used by permission of the University of Minnesota Press. "MMPI" and "Minnesota Multiphasic Personality Inventory" are trademarks owned by the Regents of the University of Minnesota.

software licensed by the publisher (Q-local) can efficiently produce both MMPI-2 and MMPI-2-RF reports. Each report carries a separate charge of between $15 and $35, depending on whether or not an interpretive report is requested in addition to the reporting of scale scores.

The MMPI-2-RF also includes nine validity indicators, two of which are revised versions of the MMPI-2 Variable Response Inconsistency (VRIN-r) and True Response Inconsistency (TRIN-r) scales. The test contains revised versions of the MMPI-2 L scale, now labeled Uncommon Virtues (L-r) and the Correction scale, now labeled Adjustment Validity (K-r), two measures of under-reporting scales in clinical and non-clinical samples. The MMPI-2-RF has five over-reporting indicators, including the recently added (2011) Response Bias Scale (RBS), which predicts overstated memory complaints, a capability absent in the MMPI-2. Recent research (Wygant et al., 2011) suggests that the MMPI-2-RF validity scales can be helpful in forensic evaluations. The MMPI-2-RF manual can be consulted for cutoff scores.

One advantage of using the MMPI-2-RF is that it provides a nuanced picture of long-standing personality traits and a finely grained picture of over- and under-reporting along both psychological and somatic dimensions, with fewer items and thus requiring less time. Another useful feature of the MMPI-2-RF is that means and standard deviations for many specific population groups, including injured workers and personal injury claimants, are *graphically* depicted in the computer printed report for all MMPI-2-RF scales, making it possible to see at a glance how an examinee's response pattern compares to that of a relevant comparison group. For more detailed information regarding the development and use of the MMPI-2-RF, see Ben-Porath (2012). Figure 86.4 provides a sample MMPI-2-RF depiction of Higher-order scales and Restructured Clinical Scales for a patient with commentary on their significance. The figure also shows a comparison of the test subject to the relevant comparison group.

THE STRUCTURED INTERVIEW OF REPORTED SYMPTOMS (SIRS) AND THE STRUCTURED INTERVIEW OF REPORTED SYMPTOMS-2 (SIRS-2) ASSESS FEIGNED PSYCHOTIC MENTAL DISORDERS

The Structured Interview of Reported Symptoms (SIRS) was published in 1992 (Rogers, Bagby, & Dickens, 1992), and the SIRS-2 (Rogers, Sewell, & Gillard, 2010) was published in 2010. The development of the SIRS and the successor SIRS-2 is described by Rogers in the *Professional Manual for SIRS-2* (Rogers, Sewell, & Gillard, 2010). The SIRS-2 can serve as a useful adjunct to the MMPI-2/MMPI-2-RF in the detection of feigned mental disorders, particularly for malingering of major psychiatric disorders. It has standardized administration and scoring, high inter-rater reliability, and validation in both simulation and known group studies. Rubenzer (2010) suggests that it requires more external validation data to support its utility for detecting the feigning of less severe disorders, for which the MMPI-2 and MMPI-2-RF remain the instruments of choice. The SIRS-2 is administered by the evaluator (not a technician) after establishing rapport in an unstructured interview and usually requires between 30

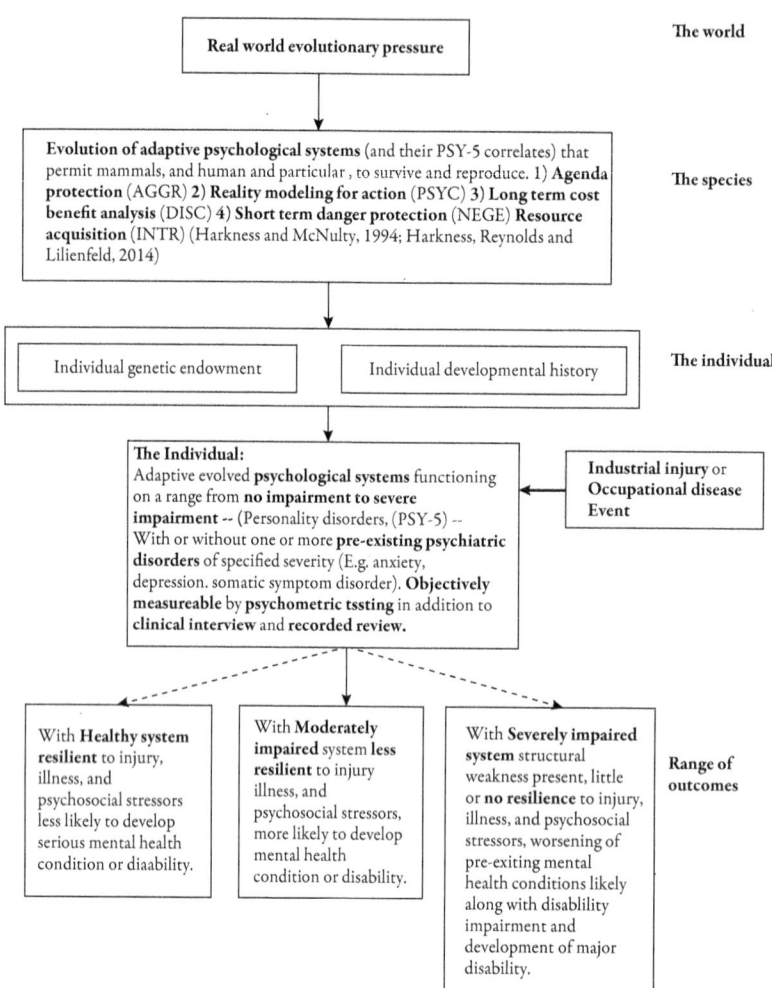

The world

The species

The individual

Range of outcomes

Real world evolutionary pressure

Evolution of adaptive psychological systems (and their PSY-5 correlates) that permit mammals, and human and particular , to survive and reproduce. 1) **Agenda protection (AGGR) 2) Reality modeling for action (PSYC) 3) Long term cost benefit analysis (DISC) 4) Short term danger protection (NEGE) Resource acquisition (INTR)** (Harkness and McNulty, 1994; Harkness, Reynolds and Lilienfeld, 2014)

Individual genetic endowment

Individual developmental history

The Individual:
Adaptive evolved **psychological systems** functioning on a range from **no impairment to severe impairment** -- (Personality disorders, (PSY-5) --
With or without one or more **pre-existing psychiatric disorders** of specified severity (E.g. anxiety, depression. somatic symptom disorder). **Objectively measureable** by **psychometric tssting** in addition to **clinical interview** and **recorded review.**

Industrial injury or **Occupational disease Event**

With **Healthy system resilient** to injury, illness, and psychosocial stressors less likely to develop serious mental health condition or diaability.

With **Moderately impaired** system **less resilient** to injury illness, and psychosocial stressors, more likely to develop mental health condition or disability.

With **Severely impaired system** structural weakness present, little or **no resilience** to injury, illness, and psychosocial stressors, worsening of pre-exiting mental health conditions likely along with disablility impairment and development of major disability.

Figure 86.3 Process of personality structure formation and development.

and 45 minutes. Guidelines for administration are provided in the professional manual. Rogers describes the classification of malingering and related response styles with an analysis of "key terms for malingering and related constructs." These include *malingering, factitious disorder, feigning, dissimulation, over-reporting, secondary gain, symptom magnification,* and *disengagement.*

Rogers notes that *malingering* is a V-code classification, which is a "simple categorization" and not a diagnosis, as it lacks "the essential inclusion and exclusion criteria that are fundamental to DSM-IV diagnoses." He analyzes the remaining constructs and suggests that "feigning" rather than "malingering" be used to describe "the deliberate fabrication or gross exaggeration of psychological or physical symptoms without any assumptions about its goals." He suggests that "over-reporting" be avoided as a forensic term because it is simply descriptive without addressing intentionality.

"Secondary gain" has three different definitions: in psychodynamic practice, it is an unconscious process shielding the patient from intra-psychic conflict. In behavioral medicine, it refers to the subtle but influential reinforcement of the illness by healthcare providers. In forensic practice, it is understood to mean that the examinee is motivated by a desire to secure monetary advantage and special attention. Rogers recommends that "secondary gain" not be used as an explanatory term in forensic medicine because of its multiple and unclear meanings.

"Symptom magnification" is a construct that is poorly defined and vague, with no distinction as to whether magnification or fabrication is present, and Rogers recommends that term be avoided in forensic reports.

DETECTION STRATEGIES EMPLOYED BY THE SIRS-2, THE MMPI-2, AND THE MMPI-2-RF

The SIRS-2 employs eight detection strategies for feigned mental disorders, which are measured by different scales linked to specific questions in the test. The SIRS-2 scoring algorithm includes a flow chart, the addition of a new scale, and two indexes and subdivision of the categories of feigning. Rogers et al. (2010) describe two broad categories of detection strategies—*unlikely* and *amplified detection strategies.* Improbable symptoms and bogus complaints are detected by unlikely detection strategies. Amplified detection strategies

MMPI-2-RF Higher-Order (H-O) and Restructured Clinical (RC) Scales

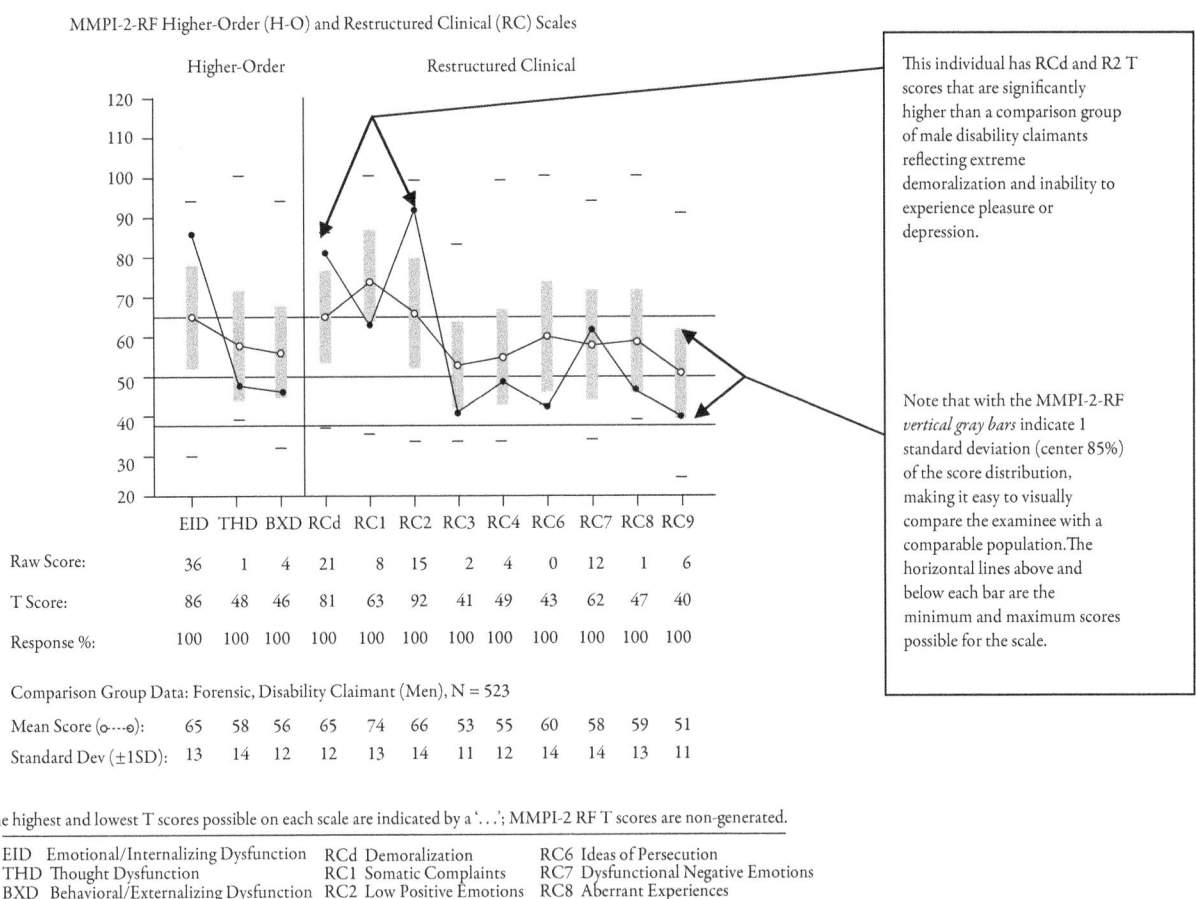

Higher-Order   Restructured Clinical

This individual has RCd and R2 T scores that are significantly higher than a comparison group of male disability claimants reflecting extreme demoralization and inability to experience pleasure or depression.

Note that with the MMPI-2-RF *vertical gray bars* indicate 1 standard deviation (center 85%) of the score distribution, making it easy to visually compare the examinee with a comparable population. The horizontal lines above and below each bar are the minimum and maximum scores possible for the scale.

	EID	THD	BXD	RCd	RC1	RC2	RC3	RC4	RC6	RC7	RC8	RC9
Raw Score:	36	1	4	21	8	15	2	4	0	12	1	6
T Score:	86	48	46	81	63	92	41	49	43	62	47	40
Response %:	100	100	100	100	100	100	100	100	100	100	100	100

Comparison Group Data: Forensic, Disability Claimant (Men), N = 523

	EID	THD	BXD	RCd	RC1	RC2	RC3	RC4	RC6	RC7	RC8	RC9
Mean Score (o---o):	65	58	56	65	74	66	53	55	60	58	59	51
Standard Dev (±1SD):	13	14	12	12	13	14	11	12	14	14	13	11

The highest and lowest T scores possible on each scale are indicated by a '...'; MMPI-2 RF T scores are non-generated.

EID Emotional/Internalizing Dysfunction
THD Thought Dysfunction
BXD Behavioral/Externalizing Dysfunction

RCd Demoralization
RC1 Somatic Complaints
RC2 Low Positive Emotions
RC3 Cyricism
RC4 Antisocial Behavior

RC6 Ideas of Persecution
RC7 Dysfunctional Negative Emotions
RC8 Aberrant Experiences
RC9 Hypomanic Activation

Figure 86.4 Sample MMPI-2-RF commentary on evaluation with reference to comparable population.

identify discrepancies between report levels for patients with genuine disorders, and report levels of feigners. Rogers describes the different strategies required to detect feigned cognitive impairment as opposed to feigned mental disorders, and points out that the SIRS-2 is designed to detected feigned mental disorders, not feigned cognitive disorders.

The MMPI-2 and MMPI-2-RF validity scales were described earlier. The VRIN (variable response inconsistency) and TRIN (true response inconsistency) scales are designed to detect random response patterns and response patterns biased either in the true or false direction. Thus, they may identify lack of comprehension or lack of cooperation, but they do not identify malingering. The F scales, which include F, Fb, and Fp, are designed to measure *infrequent* responses. Because the F and Fb scales were established with non-clinical populations, major elevations (T >100) may simply reflect serious psychopathology. Only the Fp scale was developed by identifying infrequent or rare responses in a clinical population—namely psychiatric inpatients (Arbisi & Ben-Porath, 1995). Graham's guidelines (2012) suggest that Fp T scores >100 indicate probable malingering, T scores from 80–99 indicate that "malingering is possible and external information must be sought,"

scores from 70–79 indicate "indeterminate validity," and that T scores <70 indicate a valid profile, assuming that the prior validity tests are met.

Recent research with the MMPI-2–RF suggests that it has utility in the detection of feigned somatic impairment and feigned cognitive impairment as well as feigned mental disorders (Wygant et al., 2011). The Fs (infrequent somatic responses) scale was added to measure somatic complaints and contains 16 items that were rarely endorsed in large medical and chronic pain samples. A revised version of the FBS scale (symptom validity) was included—the FBS-r. It assesses neurocognitive and somatic complaints. In 2011, the RBS (Response Bias Scale) was officially added to the MMPI-2-RF (Gervais, Ben-Porath, Wygant, & Green, 2007). The MMPI-2-RF has been found to be effective in predicting performance on Symptom Validity Tests (SVTs) in disability, criminal forensic, and Veterans Affairs (VA) patients.

A key consideration in assessing the positive predictive power and specificity of an instrument is the assumed *base rate* of what is being measured. For example, validity scales have greater predictive power and specificity if the trait being measured has a base rate of .40 instead of .10 (Wygant et al.,

2011). Rogers (2008) emphasized the importance of reducing false-positive classification because of the serious impact of such a finding for examinees, and for this reason higher cutoff scores are recommended. One should *always* utilize external corroborating data, including the clinical interview, medical records, and other collateral information, in addition to psychological test data, in forming an opinion regarding the presence or absence of feigning. With higher cutoffs, however, evaluators can be confident that feigning of symptoms is highly probable (e.g. F-r>T110, Fp-r>T70, Fs>T100, FBS-r>T100, and RBS>T100).

WORKERS' COMPENSATION CLAIMANTS REFERRED FOR TREATMENT AND FOR IMES FOR LITIGATION HAVE SIMILAR MMPI-2 PROFILES

In the author's private practice, consisting of individuals with workers' compensation claims, MMPI-2 data were compiled for 98 consecutive cases over 12 months. Of these, 86 produced valid MMPI-2 profiles. Both treatment consultations and IME evaluations yielded nearly identical means and standard deviations for the *profile elevation*, the *RC scales*, and the *PK scale*, which suggests that their psychological characteristics are quite similar with regard to both diagnoses and severity. This implies that similar levels of genuine psychopathology are present for treatment-referral patients and workers' compensation cases referred for independent psychiatric evaluations, when cases producing valid MMPI-2 protocols are compared.

DISABILITY RELATES TO INTERACTION BETWEEN SPECIFIC IMPAIRMENTS AND ADAPTIVE CAPACITY

The examiner frequently encounters situations in which it is difficult to determine the relative balance of depression, anxiety, somatization, and character pathology. In these situations, the additional information supplied by the MMPI-2 can be of significant benefit. For example, a man who sustained whole-body burns in a methane explosion on the job, followed by two months of treatment on an inpatient burn unit, returned to work three months after discharge. He was referred for treatment of PTSD that emerged months later when he had difficulty at the site of the accident. MMPI-2 testing revealed expected elevations on scales related to anxiety and traumatic stress, but no elevation on the PSY-5 scales or other scales indicating personality disturbance. Eight months of psychiatric treatment, including individual and group psychotherapy, resulted in remission of his symptoms and maintenance of employment.

Persons with *preexisting* personality disturbance and depression may sustain injuries on the job and become significantly more disturbed. For example, a middle-aged construction worker with a history of returning to work following prior workplace injuries sustained another back injury while working on a construction site, and medical treatment failed to bring about improvement. He was referred for treatment because of suicidal ideation. The MMPI-2 profile revealed demoralization, depression, and somatization on the RC scales. Significant personality disturbance was evident on the PSY-5 scales. Suicide was averted, but his serious ongoing problems with day-to-day functioning continued.

Although no conclusion should be drawn solely on the basis of MMPI-2 results or those of any psychological test, the examiner should weigh these findings in apportioning causality of the depression. For example, depending on information obtained from the record review and the subject interview, the examiner might infer that a ratable psychiatric condition was preexisting, but that there was a worsening of the condition as a consequence of the injury. Depending on the forensic setting, a preexisting condition may affect compensation paid to the patient, or it may have no effect on it.

THE ASSIGNMENT OF IMPAIRMENT RATINGS

Psychiatric or mental health impairment ratings are assigned according to criteria established by the relevant authority or jurisdiction or the definitions incorporated in a rating scale. To lessen the confusion regarding the rating process, Williams (2006; 2008; 2010) proposed a grid that cross-referenced the Global Assessment of Functioning scale (GAF) of the DSM IV-TR; the Class of Impairment Due to Mental and Behavioral Disorders of the *AMA Guide to Impairments,* 6th edition (Rondinelli, et al., 2008); and the five categories of impairment definitions defined by Washington State by Washington Administrative Code (WAC)-296-20-340, the latter serving as an example of impairment defined by legislation. The GAF ratings were divided into quintiles, in order to correspond with the other rating scales. Thus, for example, a GAF rating from 61–80 would correspond to Class 2 impairment by the AMA Guide and Category 2 impairment by the Washington State criteria. Similarly, a GAF rating from 41–60 would correspond to an AMA rating of Class 3, and a Washington State rating of Category 3; a GAF rating of 21–40 would correlate with an AMA rating of Class 4, and a Washington State rating of Category 4. This cross-correlation was proposed with the idea that each rating scale could be divided into five sections or quintiles. When the DSM-5 was published in 2013 the multi-axial diagnostic system of DSM-IV was discarded, and GAF ratings were discontinued. Nevertheless, the concept of cross-referencing a variety of rating scales remains valid as a means of improving reliability and consistency.

The AMA guide to impairment ratings is the easiest to grasp at a glance, and the DSM-IV-TR GAF rating scale utilized definitions that were readily understandable, albeit not precise and of questionable psychometric validity. The Washington State criteria employ archaic language, and are difficult to parse from one category rating to another (Williams 2006; 2010; Williams & Schouten, 2008). The intention of the table is not to override legislatively determined criteria but to assist the clinician who is attempting to apply it accurately and consistently.

In a "close call" situation, the MMPI-2 may be of assistance in tipping the rating to a higher or lower category, although there is little published research at this point. For example, consider an individual who appears by interview and record review to straddle the line between a Category 3 and Category 4 level of impairment defined by WAC 296-20-340, who appears to have a GAF of 40–45 on Axis V, and who appears to correspond to a Class 3 level of impairment by the AMA guide. If a valid MMPI-2 profile without evidence of exaggeration of psychological symptoms has been obtained, it could be argued that a profile elevation of 81 and an RCd T score of 80 might tip the balance in favor of Category 4, since less than 1% of the sample population have scores over 80 (Butcher, et al., 2001). By the same token, a lower profile elevation of 63 and an RCd score of 67 might tip the balance in the direction of a Category 2 rating, since those scores, although clinically significant, are more moderate. Graham (2012) discusses research establishing the profile elevation, the RCd scale, and other scales as measures of overall emotional discomfort and maladjustment. Research using known group comparisons will be needed to determine where the appropriate cut scores are for each impairment category by statistical analysis. A possible starting point could be to have Category 3 correspond to a profile elevation of 69–76 and RCd T scores from 71–76; Category 4 to a profile elevation of 77–81 and RCd T scores from 77–84. For statistical reasons, no T score over 88 is possible for RCd. An additional column was added to the grid (Figure 86.1) to accommodate the profile elevation scores and the RCd T score from the MMPI-2 for purposes of illustration.

THE ROLE OF PSYCHOLOGICAL TESTING IN TREATMENT PLANNING AND ASSESSMENT OF TREATMENT PROGRESS

When there is an indication of personal turmoil and emotional distress, treatment should be considered. With the brief report scales such as the BDI-II or the PHQ-9, evidence of moderate depression would strengthen the recommendation for treatment based on clinical interview and record review.

The MMPI-2 and MMPI-2-RF have several clinical scales that are indicative of emotional turmoil. Inferences can be drawn from these scales regarding the potential treatment outcome. As a rule, people who are in emotional distress are more likely to put the effort into treatment and tolerate the discomfort associated with it than people that are not, unless their distress is too great for them to focus, in which case more structure may be needed (Harkness, McNulty, Ben-Porath, and Graham, 2002). Persons experiencing very little distress may lack the motivation to work in treatment, and respond poorly to treatment. Thus, for example, someone with elevated scales reflecting anxiety or depression is more likely to be a good therapy candidate than someone who denies responsibility. High scorers on RC4, which assesses antisocial and other forms of externalizing behavior, may agree to treatment to escape another, less pleasant alternative, but they are likely

to terminate treatment early when the external pressure is off. The MMPI-2/RF can provide the clinician with valuable information at the start of treatment, saving time in the initial phases and lessening the chance that important psychological problems are being overlooked.

Serial MMPI-2/MMPI-2-RF testing at intervals through treatment can provide an objective means of measuring therapeutic progress by separately measuring gains made in resolving somatization, depression, and other psychological problems (Graham, 2012). The author routinely shares MMPI-2-RF findings with patients at the beginning of treatment while formulating a treatment plan and at intervals during treatment to explain what progress has been achieved and what additional work in therapy remains. The MMPI-2-RF is particularly well suited to patient education because it graphically compares the patient's scores to that of a comparable population. For example, the professional can show the patient his or her profile graphs and provide a running commentary about what are and what are not areas of concern. This procedure is analogous to the practice of other medical professionals who show their patients MRIs or CT scans that visually demonstrate his or her injury or illness in order to enhance patient understanding and cooperation.

ASSESSING MALINGERING AND EXAGGERATION WITH PSYCHOLOGICAL TESTING

Malingering is defined as the intentional production of false or grossly exaggerated physical or psychological symptoms, motivated by external incentives. The term "malingering" suggests that a "yes or no" determination is to be made, but malingering is a *dimensional* and not a *categorical* construct. Rogers (2008) provides a comprehensive discussion of levels of intentionality, ranging from intentional fabrication of symptoms, through false imputation of the cause of real symptoms, to exaggerated claims of the impact. The hypothesis that malingering should be viewed as a *dimensional* as opposed to *taxonic* construct (i.e., either/or) was confirmed by Walters et al. (2008) through a statistical analysis of the response patterns in the validity scales on the MMPI-2 and the Structured Interview of Reported Symptoms (SIRS) developed by Rogers, Bagby, and Dickens (1992). The distribution of scores for both test instruments was consistent with a graduated range of non-credible self-report along a continuum, analogous to the GAF scale rather than a "yes/no" dichotomous "present or absent" determination. This is consistent with the increased emphasis on a dimensional approach to other areas of diagnosis and severity rating.

An erroneous diagnosis of malingering can have a devastating impact on an individual's access to medical care and other benefits. From an ethical perspective, as Gold et al. (2008) stated, "The psychiatrist has a duty to the referral source to provide a complete and thorough evaluation as well as certain duties to the evaluee, similar to but more limited than those in a traditional doctor–patient relationship." Objectivity and precision in the assessment of malingering and exaggeration can be enhanced by approaching assessment systematically, utilizing psychological test instruments best suited to the diagnostic questions in combination with a clinical interview and record review. This practice could lessen the impact of "blind spots" or bias in the performance of complex evaluations where malingering or exaggeration may be present.

CASE STUDY 1—PROBABLE MALINGERING

A 46-year-old divorced male was evaluated at the request of his attending physician. He presented with a history of a fall two years previously from a height of ten feet, landing on concrete, sustaining a head injury and a broken sternum. A neuropsychologist administered a battery of tests, including Tombaugh's (1996) Test of Memory Malingering (TOMM), which revealed poor effort. Another clinical psychologist diagnosed an anxiety disorder and a pain disorder and recommended mental health treatment. The examinee expressed frustration that he was clumsy and that he was no longer able to engage in his hobby of building and racing cars. He reported minimal activities of daily living. The examiner experienced little rapport with the examinee in the interview. His speech was fluent and logically connected. He performed adequately on the mental status exam. He reported that the future appeared grim. He scored 36 points on the BDI-II, which is in the severe range of depression. He completed the MMPI-2 and the profile was invalid. It was clear that he understood the questions, as the VRIN and TRIN T scores were within acceptable limits. The infrequency scales (F, Fb, and Fp) all had T scores of 120. According to Graham (2012), an Fp score at this level indicates "probable malingering" and represents endorsement of considerably more psychological symptoms than are found in psychiatric inpatients (Arbisi & Ben-Porath, 1999). In this case, no interview data or medical record review suggested that there was a credible relationship between the reported injury and the claimed symptoms. No psychiatric treatment was recommended.

Rogers (2008) provides a scholarly analysis of the strengths and weaknesses of many test instruments, and asserts that using the MMPI-2 and the SIRS together represents the "gold standard" for the detection of malingered mental illness.

CASE STUDY 2—PREEXISTING CONDITION AGGRAVATED, WITH MALINGERING ALLEGED BUT NOT SUBSTANTIATED

A 60-year-old woman who was in a 20-year relationship presented with a history of two documented injuries eight years ago, in close succession. One resulted in a herniated cervical disk, and the second in a herniated lumbar disk. A neurosurgical IME physician recommended consideration of surgery, but the subject was frightened of surgery because of a frightening prior anesthetic experience.

Six years earlier, a psychiatrist performing an IME recommended psychiatric treatment, and diagnosed *Major depression, recurrent; Pain disorder*, and *Polysubstance abuse in remission*. He diagnosed "maladaptive traits" on Axis II, and assigned GAF = 51–55 on Axis V. He recommended psychiatric treatment, but no treatment was provided.

Six years later, a second psychiatric IME was performed. This psychiatrist diagnosed *Pain disorder with a general medical condition* and *Depressive disorder NOS* on Axis I. He assigned GAF = 50–55 on Axis V. He stated that an MMPI-2 was invalid solely on the basis of an F scale T score >110. No other data were presented from the MMPI-2. This is an example of an incorrect use of the MMPI-2 and lack of familiarity with current interpretive guidelines.

A third psychiatric IME was requested by the claimant's attorney. A record review revealed that depression was documented, and sertraline was prescribed nine months following the injury, in early 2002. Four or five psychotherapy appointments were noted in 2006, but treatment was terminated without a reason being given. A micro-cervical laminotomy and foraminotomy were recommended, but the claimant again declined because of the fear of surgery. Medical records showed that the claimant had bizarre fears of contamination of metal in the eye, which caused her to delay a cervical MRI. The occupational physician noted that developmental trauma was evident and requested reauthorization for psychiatric care in 2007. An orthopedist performing an IME alleged patient fraud, based on his misreading of an investigation by the insurance carrier that cleared the person of fraud. A BDI-II was completed, with a score indicating severe depression. An MMPI-2 was completed that produced a valid profile. Among the validity profiles, VRIN and TRIN had T scores of 58 and 65, F and Fb had T scores of 85 and 97, and the Fp T score was 49, confirming that there was no exaggeration of rare psychological symptoms. The scores presented in Figure 86.5 were obtained on the RC scales which indicated demoralization, depression, anxiety, health concerns, feelings of persecution, and unusual beliefs. Note that there was no elevation for antisocial behavior on scale RC4.

Because fraud had been alleged (on the basis of an incomplete document review, which, as noted, cleared the claimant) the SIRS was administered. The claimant had five of eight primary scales in the "honest responder" range, which in Rogers' studies correlated with a 73% likelihood of the *absence of feigning*. A Physical Capacities Evaluation (PCE) performed in 2009 reported that the subject's pain reports were unreliable. However, the presence of somatic delusions, including the fear of "metal bodies" being in her

Restructured Clinical scale (RC)	T score
RCd	81
RC1	93
RC2	91
RC3	66
RC4	55
RC6	70
RC7	76
RC8	69
RC9	56

Figure 86.5 Case study 2.

eye as well as the fear of surgery, suggested that a delusional disorder was present. Because all psychiatric IMEs reported diagnoses of depression and pain disorder, and because each IME assigned a GAF score within the range of 45–55, it was obviously the consensus opinion that the claimant had a serious psychiatric disturbance. Because the claimant had a long-term steady work history prior to the current claim, because the psychological test results were valid and indicated the presence of a pain disorder and recurrent major depression, because of the elevated PSY-5 scales, and because the allegation that fraud had been committed was without substance, the finding was that a preexisting mental health disorder had been aggravated by the injury in question. Psychiatric treatment was recommended on a trial basis, with combination antidepressant and second-generation antipsychotic medication. The psychiatric examiner diagnosed *Major depressive disorder, recurrent and severe with psychotic features* and *Pain disorder associated with psychological factors and a general medical condition* on Axis I. On Axis II, *Personality disorder NOS* was diagnosed. On Axis V, GAF = 45–50 was assigned.

CASE STUDY 3—EXAGGERATION OF SYMPTOMS WITHOUT MALINGERING

A 42-year-old married man with a 20-year continuous work history in food services sales developed a hernia while assembling a food display. He underwent a hernia repair and subsequently developed a herpetic lesion. He cooperated well with treatment for the first year, but the medical records then indicated increasing clinician concern regarding his opiate dependence. Concurrently, the claimant experienced increasing conflict with family members and healthcare providers. A pain specialist noted the presence of depression one year following the injury. A psychiatric IME two years following the injury was extremely brief and concluded that no psychiatric diagnosis was present and that no treatment was needed. A psychiatric IME performed three years after the injury concluded that depression and a pain disorder were present, but that they were not related to the injury. A review of employment records confirmed continuous employment for 15–20 years prior to the injury, with steady earnings of between $2,000 and $4,000 per month.

During the interview, the claimant had difficulty with temporal sequence when asked about his history. He acknowledged irritability, problems with memory and concentration, frequent crying spells, and feelings of worthlessness. There was good rapport and cooperation through the evaluation. He expressed a desire to return to work. Several times he acknowledged that he exaggerated his psychological problems. He felt that he had been treated unfairly by the industrial insurance system, and wanted redress for his grievances. He felt that he might benefit from psychiatric treatment because "It might help me focus and separate stuff so that I don't bottle it up and take it out on other people." The BDI-II was administered, and severe depression was indicated. The MMPI-2 was administered, and although the VRIN and TRIN scales indicated that he attended well to the items, the Fp T score was 70, which Graham (2012) describes as reflecting "indeterminate" validity with the recommendation that external information be obtained. Most of the RC scales were elevated, including RCd, RC1, RC2, RC6, RC7, and RC8. These indicate problems with demoralization, anxiety, depression, health

concerns, obsessional anxiety, and unusual beliefs. The PSY-5 scales reflected extreme psychoticism (PSYC T score = 97) as well as significant elevations for negative emotionality and introversion. The SIRS was administered because the MMPI-2 was inconclusive with respect to malingering. It revealed four scales in the "probable feigning" category, which correlates with a 100% probability of feigning in empirical studies. Because the claimant had a history of success in the workplace, it did not seem likely that he would consciously choose to trade a good living for conflict with a bureaucracy. His functioning began to deteriorate concurrently with the concern regarding opioid abuse. He performed well on a physical capacities evaluation early in his treatment, but poorly after the opioid dependence had taken hold. He had conflict with a vocational counselor and with his older son in the same time frame.

Based on the history obtained from the interview, the record review, and the psychological testing, the examiner concluded that outright fabrication of symptoms was not happening, but that the claimant was exaggerating his symptoms in order to secure attention for his concerns. His credibility was enhanced because he acknowledged that he may have exaggerated his psychological problems. The recommendation was that a substance abuse evaluation and recommended treatment be carried out, and that a follow-up evaluation be conducted when the opioid dependence had been resolved. No final psychiatric assessment could be carried out while the narcotic addiction was in play.

POST-TRAUMATIC STRESS DISORDER

Returning soldiers from the wars in the Middle East have rates of PTSD that increases with the number of deployments. The Post Traumatic Stress Disorder – Keane (PK) scale of the MMPI-2 has demonstrated good correlation with PTSD in combat veterans. "Resilience" has been posited as a protective feature that lessens the susceptibility to developing PTSD, which may be analogous to higher levels of personality functioning as defined in the DSM-5. This is probably similar to differences in vulnerability to developing chronic disability in workplace injuries encountered in injured workers with similar injuries but widely varying adaptive capacities. The Fp scale of the MMPI-2 has been demonstrated to be effective in distinguishing between feigned and actual PTSD (Arbisi et al., 2006). Wolf et al. (2008) and Arbisi, Ben-Porath, and McNulty (2004) explore the use of the MMPI-2 RC scales in the assessment of PTSD and comorbid disorders. Case Study 4 describes a non-military case of PTSD with relevant psychometric case findings.

CASE STUDY 4—TRAUMATIC BRAIN INJURY

Traumatic brain injury (TBI) is probably under-diagnosed, particularly in cases of "mild" TBI. Neuropsychological testing is helpful in defining the nature and extent of brain injury, and is interpreted by neuropsychologists, who have extensive additional training in correlating specialized test findings with observed deficits. Determining where TBI and PTSD converge can be challenging diagnostically (Stein & McAllister, 2009). Arbisi et al. (2006) and Arbisi and Ben-Porath (1999) have studied the use of the MMPI-2 to in this population and describe its utility in identifying depression, anxiety, and other psychological problems, as well as present data demonstrating its utility in detecting malingering.

A 30-year-old married man sustained a severe documented head injury and was referred by his neuropsychologist for psychiatric treatment. There was consensus regarding the seriousness of the TBI. The neuropsychologist attempted to treat the injured worker in a group for other head-injury patients, but felt that psychopharmacological treatment was indicated and referred the patient for pharmacological consultation and management. A valid MMPI-2 profile was obtained. The overall profile elevation (which is the arithmetic average of clinical scales 1–4 and 6–9) was 89.6, indicating extreme emotional distress.

The profile presented in Figure 86.6 reflects severe emotional distress with demoralization, depression, serious worries about health, obsessional anxiety, and some disconnection from reality. The VRIN and TRIN scales indicated that the examinee was able to attend adequately to the test items. The Fp scale reflected no exaggeration of rare psychological symptoms. The RC scales indicated that severe distress was indeed present. This person was incapable of cooperating consistently with treatment, as he was unable to remember his appointments and attend them with any consistency, or to take medication as prescribed, despite reminder calls and the enlistment of familial support. Because of his inability to participate in treatment, care was terminated with a recommendation for a pension.

In a situation such as this, a community care model with case managers that make home visits would probably be more effective at palliation and support, since regulations typically require that care provided under workers' compensation claims be curative and not merely palliative.

The MMPI-2-RF profiles of soldiers who report experiencing a mild TBI in Iraq, but who do *not* report PTSD symptoms, are not significantly different on the RC scales (identical to the MMPI-2 RC scales) from those of soldiers who do not report mild TBI or screen positive for PTSD. This suggests "there was little evidence of a long-term negative impact of concussion/MTBI history on these outcomes after accounting for PTSD." (Polusny, Kehle, Nelson, Erbes, Arbisi, and Thuras, 2011).

Validity scales	VRIN	T score = 50
	TRIN	T score = 64F
	F_p	T score = 41
	L	T score = 56
	K	T score = 51
RC scales	RCd	T score = 81
	RC1	T score = 100
	RC2	T score = 94
	RC3, RC4, RC6, RC9	T scores < 44
	RC7	T score = 72
	RC8	T score = 70

Figure 86.6 Case study #4 – MMPI-2 validity and RC scales in patients with TBI, depression, and anxiety.

POTENTIAL MISUSE OF THE MMPI-2 AND MMPI-2-RF

Because the MMPI-2 and MMPI-2-RF are so widely used in a disability context, unless they have ready access to qualified psychologists, psychiatrists who seek to utilize it in their disability evaluations are advised to remain current with MMPI-2/MMPI-2-RF research through workshop attendance and literature review. Even if a psychologist is available to administer and interpret the MMPI-2/MMPI-2RF, familiarity with current developments in the literature makes the IME review and report-writing process easier.

One commonly encountered error in IMEs is to find excessive reliance on quotes from the computer-generated interpretations. Graham (2012) and Butcher (2000) point out that automated interpretive systems can become fixed at a naive level, and that in response to critics, only minor cosmetic changes may be made by the publishers. Computer-generated interpretations should be regarded as consultations between one professional and another. Blind reliance on computer interpretations can lead to major errors, as occurred in Case Study 2, when a profile was labeled "invalid" because of an elevated F scale T score. As another example, the diagnosis of malingering from an elevated "Symptom Validity Scale (FBS)" T score is generally incorrect, except in forensic neuropsychological assessments, and then only when careful attention is given to cutoff scores. The FBS scale was developed to detect malingering of psychological distress by personal injury claimants based on unpublished frequency counts of malingers' MMPI item responses and "observations of personal injury malingers." However, Butcher, Arbisi, Atlis, and McNulty (2003) reported that subsequent published cut scores for the FBS inappropriately classified too many individuals who were experiencing genuine psychological distress as malingerers, and, given the existing research on the scale and the published interpretation guidelines, "the FBS should not be used in clinical settings nor should it be used during disability evaluations to determine malingering." In late 2008, Ben-Porath and Tellegen issued a statement published on the Pearson Assessments website summarizing the view of a panel of experts that the FBS was useful in identifying "potentially exaggerated claims of disability, primarily in the context of forensic neuropsychological evaluations." As is the case with all psychological testing, however, the FBS should be considered in the context of the other validity scales.

Another error to be avoided is deviation from the prescribed administration protocol. The MMPI-2 and MMPI-2-RF were standardized under controlled administration conditions; it is *not permissible* for the examiner to read, translate, or explain any of the test items to the test-taker, because unconscious bias has been shown to change the response pattern (Graham, 2012). If these conditions are violated, the test results have no forensic validity. The MMPI-2 is available in both written and audio English and Spanish versions, and in Hmong in written form. The MMPI-2-RF is only available in English at the time of this writing. Finally, if the MMPI-2 or MMPI-2-RF is administered in written form using the bubble answer sheet, the scorer should *verify* the accuracy of their data entry by re-entering the data as prompted by the software.

In summary, the MMPI-2 and MMPI-2-RF are sources of information that the examiner can rely upon to reach a diagnosis or to address interrogatories. Helpful inferences can be drawn about both diagnoses and the severity of psychological conditions from the MMPI-2, and about the presence or absence of exaggeration or dissimulation as one of three elements of a forensic diagnostic investigation, the other two being a comprehensive record review and a comprehensive clinical diagnostic interview. Although inferences can be drawn regarding diagnoses, one cannot render DSM-5 diagnoses solely on the basis of MMPI-2 or MMPI-2-RF results, nor indeed solely on the basis of any psychological test.

QUALITY REPORT WRITING

The most compelling reports have novel-like qualities. They should evoke the personality of the examinee, with clarity and a lack of jargon, and address the questions posed by the requesting party. These questions include diagnoses, apportionment of causation, and indications of whether maximum medical improvement has been achieved and whether the impairment is partial or complete. Other questions include recommended treatment, whether or not the person can return to the job of injury with or without accommodations, and whether the examinee could benefit from vocational services (Williams, 2006).

DSM-5 DIAGNOSES MUST BE RECORDED

Treatment recommendations are based on the integrated assessment of the patient that takes into account all psychiatric conditions and psychological test results. Personality trait disturbances or full disorders are present in a majority of affected patients in some subpopulations, and require sophisticated clinical skills. Effective treatment may include group and individual therapy, along with appropriate pharmacotherapy (Williams & Schouten, 2008). With the introduction of the DSM-5, the multiaxial diagnostic system has been scrapped, but the need for careful diagnosis and formulation remains. The treatment plan must take all conditions into account, and the clinician's awareness of comorbid disorders is critical to successful outcomes (Oldham et al., 1995).

DISABILITY AND THE AMERICANS WITH DISABILITIES ACT

With passage of the Americans with Disabilities Act (ADA) in 1990, the federal government barred discrimination against individuals with disabilities with regard to employment and access to public accommodations. States have done the same through passage of analogous statutes. The ADA was passed to counter commonly held biases that individuals with mental or physical disabilities are necessarily disabled from working.

As we noted above, it is important to keep in mind the distinction between disabilities and impairments. Impairments are the cognitive and affective abnormalities associated with disorders. Disabilities are the restrictions that are imposed by impairments in functioning, including work and relationships. Thus, an individual with a disorder may or may not have an impairment, and that impairment may or may not amount to a disability. The ADA prohibits discrimination against individuals who have disabilities, or who are perceived as having disabilities, if they can perform the essential functions of the job, with or without reasonable accommodation (Langer, 1996; Zuckerman, 1993).

Clinicians, and society in general, seem to be of two minds with regard to disability and individuals seeking disability status. On one hand, society has developed insurance plans, both public and private, that insure workers against the possibility that they will no longer be able to earn a living. The systems established to provide financial and emotional support for individuals who become disabled from work as the result of illness or injury represent major social advances. Yet, while we have established and endowed these systems, those who utilize them may find themselves the objects of scorn and derision. After all, American society values work and the work ethic (Hubbard, 1998). Those who ask to be relieved of the obligation to work often elicit disdain from caretakers, co-workers, and family members.

The growth of attention to disabilities and the disabled is no doubt related to the increasing numbers of disabled individuals in the workplace and the growing number of disability claims. Some authors have predicted that the combined impacts of the Americans with Disabilities Act and aging of the Baby Boom generation will result in a significant increase in the number of disabled workers in the next decade (Zwerling et al., 1997).

As noted above, individuals with disabilities are protected against discrimination by the Americans with Disabilities Act and similar state statutes (Langer, 1996). Those same individuals may require disability insurance benefits to cover living expenses during periods when they cannot work. Some individuals have filed suit alleging disability-based discrimination by their employers, while also filing claims for disability benefits. The courts have differed as to whether both claims can be made simultaneously. Some have rejected such claims—cf. *Cleveland* v. *Policy Management Systems Corp.*, 120 F. 3d 513 (5th Circuit, 1997). Others, noting that claims for disability benefits do not involve the question of reasonable accommodations, allow both claims, cf. *Swanks* v. *Washington Metropolitan Transit Authority*, 116 F. 3d 382 (D.C. Circuit, 1997).

In 1999, the United States Supreme Court resolved this issue when it heard the appeal in *Cleveland* v. *Policy Management Systems Corp.*, 526 U.S. 795; 119 S. Ct. 1597, cited above. Ms. Cleveland had suffered a stroke and was granted SSDI benefits after making a sworn statement that she was unable to work. She also filed an ADA claim that her employer had failed to make reasonable accommodations that would have allowed her to continue working. The District Court granted summary judgement for the employer, dismissing her claim on the basis that she could not both claim to be unable to work, and simultaneously claim that she could perform the essentials of her job with or without accommodations, as required by the ADA. The U.S. Court of Appeals for the Fifth Circuit affirmed.

In overturning the decision of the Court of Appeals, the court held that receipt of Social Security Disability payments did not automatically bar Ms. Cleveland from bringing an action under the ADA, and summary judgement was inappropriate where she had provided sufficient explanation of inconsistencies in her statements. Where such inconsistencies exist, however, courts will consider receipt of disability benefits as evidence that the individual plaintiff could not, in fact, perform the essential functions of the job.

Discrimination against those with mental and physical disabilities is a real phenomenon. The bias may be overt or subtle; it may be based on actual experience or, more commonly, on stereotypes. For example, HIV/AIDS raised unique ethical and medico-legal problems relevant to disability claims (Gostin, Feldblum, & Webber, 1999). Clinicians treating those with mental and physical disabilities can make a major contribution to getting their patients back to work and helping them overcome the bias against those with mental and physical disabilities. They can do so by conducting objective evaluations of the patient's specific abilities to function in different settings, and by being willing to cooperate with the employer's request for information. Such cooperation and sharing of information must only occur with the patient's permission, of course. The treating clinician should be clear with those requesting the information that the evaluation is not an independent evaluation, and that it is based on more limited information.

While treating clinicians can serve as the patient's advocate in helping them get back to work, they can also put their patient and the patient's co-workers at risk. It is essential that any clinician who states that a patient is able to return to work after a period of disability have a clear sense of the nature and responsibilities of the job, as well as the patient's clinical condition (Maffeo, 1990). For example, one treating social worker opined that his patient, a research chemist who conducted high-pressure liquid chromatography with hazardous materials, was no longer disabled by her depression and was fit to return to work. Upon inquiry by an independent evaluator, however, the social worker indicated that he had no idea of the duties and the potential dangers. In a similar case, a treating psychiatrist argued that his psychotic patient could return to her job in government, in spite of her active paranoia and lack of compliance with medication, because he felt that no one could force her to take the medication.

SUMMARY

The evaluation and treatment of individuals with work-related disabilities provide a number of challenges to clinicians. The role of an independent psychiatric evaluator is not interchangeable with that of a treating psychiatrist. When undertaking an evaluation, psychiatrists should specifically identify their role and remain within its bounds. The importance of work to individual and societal well-being, the moral valence we attach to it, and the diverse motivations for entering and leaving the workforce all combine to make this an emotionally charged area with many clinical challenges. The clinician and patient are best served when clinicians are honest with themselves and the patient about the limitations on their knowledge and ability and the constraints these limits impose. Utilization of psychological testing appropriate to the case may contribute meaningfully to objectivity and the avoidance of unconscious bias. Paying attention to detail, and understanding the task involved and the techniques for completing it, is likely to lead to more consistent and reliable treatment and assessments.

CLINICAL PEARLS

- Functional *impairments* are limitations to specific functions that may impair the patient's ability to perform the essential duties of particular occupations.

- The actual determination of *disability* results from either an *administrative* or a *judicial decision* that weighs evidence and expert opinions, including those provided by psychiatrists; the adjudicators are the "finders of fact."

- Definitions of disability imply that disability is an "either-or" condition—i.e., someone is disabled or they are not. The reality is more complex, and in this chapter we take the approach that "disability determination" should be approached taking into account the *diagnosis*, its *severity,* and the life *context* of the person being evaluated.

- An evaluator is obligated to be a seeker of truth, whereas a treater's primary duty is to the patient as a seeker of cure and comfort.

- For evaluations that require assessment of causation, credibility, and severity, where necessary and when circumstances allow, an enhanced *dimensional* method for assessing psychiatric impairment that incorporates formal psychological testing combined with a comprehensive medical record (chart) review and examinee/patient may contribute to greater reliability in diagnosis, causal attribution, and severity ratings. This method, which includes partially quantitative elements, utilizes a *cross-reference grid* that incorporates various rating scales with definitions for five levels of impairment that enable the rater to "triangulate" the rating by cross checking one scale against the others (Williams 2006; 2010). Psychological testing, including the Minnesota Multiphasic Personality Inventory–2 (MMPI-2, 1989), can also be added to this comparison grid.

- *Disability* relates to interaction between specific impairments and adaptive capacity.

- The SIRS-2 can serve as a useful adjunct to the MMPI-2 (RF) in the detection of feigned mental disorders, particularly for malingering of major psychiatric disorders.

- The examiner frequently encounters situations in which it is difficult to determine the relative balance of depression, anxiety, somatization, and character pathology. In these situations, the additional information supplied by the MMPI-2 can be of significant benefit.

- An individual with a *disorder* may or may not have an *impairment*, and that impairment may or may not amount to a *disability*. The ADA prohibits discrimination against individuals who have disabilities, or who are perceived as having disabilities, if they can perform the essential functions of the job with or without reasonable accommodation (Langer, 1996; Zuckerman, 1993).

ACKNOWLEDGMENTS

The author would like to acknowledge contributions by the following colleagues. Ronald Schouten, MD, JD, director of the Law and Psychiatry Service at Massachusetts General Hospital and associate professor of psychiatry at Harvard Medical School, wrote the section on disability and the Americans with Disabilities Act and introduced the author to academic scholarship, beginning with the Psychiatric Care of the Medical Patient, 2nd edition published in 2000. Charles Mangham, Sr., MD, clinical professor of psychiatry at the University of Washington School of Medicine and training analyst at the Seattle Psychoanalytic Society and Institute, helped the author learn how to listen to patients over 25 years of consultation. Paul Arbisi, PhD, professor, Department of Psychiatry, University of Minnesota, helped introduce the author to the MMPI-2 and MMPI-2 RF and reviewed the chapter in detail, greatly contributing to accuracy and clarity in the discussion of the MMPI-2 and MMPI-2-RF. Ariah Kidder, PhD, provided quick and expert editing of this manuscript under pressure, adding to its readability. Of course, any errors or shortcomings are the responsibility of the author.

DISCLOSURE STATEMENT

Dr. Williams reports that in 2013, after completion of the original draft of the chapter, Pearson Assessments and the University of Minnesota Press provided software resources to enable the transformation of archival MMPI-2 reports from his practice to MMPI-2-RF profiles in support of an ongoing research project.

REFERENCES

Arbisi, P. A., & Ben-Porath, Y. S. (1995). An MMPI-2 infrequent response scale for use with psychopathological populations: The Infrequency Psychopathology scale, F(p). *Psychological Assessment, 7,* 424–431.

Arbisi, P. A., & Ben-Porath, Y. S. (1999). The use of the Minnesota Multiphasic Personality Inventory–2 in the psychological assessment of persons with TBI: Correction factors and other clinical caveats and conundrums. *NeuroRehabilitation, 13*(2), 117–125.

Arbisi, P. A., Ben-Porath, Y. S., & McNulty, J. (2006). The ability of the MMPI-2 to detect feigned PTSD within the context of compensation seeking. *Psychological Services, 3*(4), 249–261.

Arbisi, P. A., Ben-Porath, Y. S., & McNulty, J. (July 28-August 1, 2004) Contribution of the MMPI-2 restructured clinical (RC) scales to the assessment of PTSD in veterans. Poster presented at the American Psychological Association, Honolulu, HI.

Arbisi, P. A., Sellbom, M., & Ben-Porath, Y. S. (2008). Empirical correlates of the MMPI-2 restructured clinical (RC) scales in psychiatric inpatients. *Journal of Personality Assessment, 9,* 122–128.

Arbisi, P. A., Polusny, M. A., Erbes, C. R., Thuras, P., & Reddy, M. K. (2011). The Minnesota Multiphasic Personality Inventory–2 Restructured Form in National Guard soldiers screening positive for posttraumatic stress disorder and mild traumatic brain injury. *Psychological Assessment, 23*(1), 203–214.

Bass, C., Peveler, R., & House, A. (2001). Somatoform disorders: Severe psychiatric illnesses neglected by psychiatrists. *The British Journal of Psychiatry, 179,* 11–14.

Beck, A. T., Steer, R. A., & Brown, G. K. (1996). *Beck Depression Inventory* (2nd ed.). San Antonio, TX: Harcourt Brace and Company.

Ben-Porath, Y. S., & Tellegen, A. (2011). *MMPI-2-RF (Minnesota Multiphasic Personality Inventory–2 Restructured Form): Manual for administration, scoring, and interpretation.* Minneapolis, MN: University of Minnesota Press.

Ben-Porath, Y. S. (2012). *Interpreting the MMPI-2-RF.* Minneapolis, MN: University of Minnesota Press.

Bresnitz, E. A., Frumkin, J., Goldstein, L., Neumark, D., Hodgson, M., & Needleman, C. (1994). Occupational impairment and disability among applicants for Social Security Disability benefits in Pennsylvania. *American Journal of Public Health, 84*(11), 1786–1790.

Butcher, J. N., & Williams, C. L. (2000). *Essentials of MMPI-2 and MMPI-A Interpretation* (2nd ed.). Minneapolis, MN: University of Minnesota Press.

Butcher, J. N., Graham, J. R., Ben-Porath, Y. S., Tellegen, A., Dahlstrom, W. G., & Kaemmer, B. (2001). *MMPI-2 (Minnesota Multiphasic Personality Inventory-2): Manual for administration, scoring, and interpretation* (Rev. ed.). Minneapolis, MN: University of Minnesota Press.

Butcher, J. N., Arbisi, P. A., Atlis, M. A., & McNulty, J. L. (2003). The construct validity of the Lee-Haley Fake Bad Scale: Does this scale measure somatic malingering and feigned emotional distress? *Archives of Clinical Neuropsychology, 18,* 473–485.

Corbiere, M., Sullivan, M., Stanish, W. D., & Adams, H. (2007). Pain and depression in injured workers and their return to work: A longitudinal study. *Canadian Journal of Behavioral Science, 39*(1), 23–31.

APA (2000). *Diagnostic and Statistical Manual, Transcript Revision* (4th Ed.). Washington, DC: American Psychiatric Association. Available at http://www.dsm5.org (accessed March 6, 2011).

Dworkin, R. H., Turk, D. C., Revicki, D. A., Harding, G., Coyne, K. S., et al. (2009). Development and initial validation of an expanded and revised version of the Short-Form McGill Pain Questionnaire (SF-MPQ-2). *Pain, 144*(1–2), 35–42.

Fischler, G., & Booth, N. (1999). *Vocational impact of psychiatric disorders.* Austin, TX: Pro-ed.

Finn, J. A., Arbisi, P. A., Erbes, C. R., Polusny, P. A., & Thuras, P. (2014). The MMPI-2 restructured form personality psychopathology five scales: Bridging DSM-5 Section 2 personality disorders and DSM-5 Section 3 personality trait dimensions. *Journal of Personality Assessment, 96*(2), 173–184.

Fishbain, D. A., Cutler, R., Rosomoff, H. L., & Rosomoff, R. S. (1997). Chronic pain-associated depression: Antecedent or consequence of chronic pain? A review. *Clinical Journal of Pain, 13,* 116–137.

Gallagher, R. M., & Myers, P. (1996). Referral delay in back pain patients on worker's compensation: cost and policy implications. *Psychosomatics, 37,* 270–284.

Gervais, R. O., Ben-Porath, Y. S., Wygant, D. B., & Green, P. (2007). Development and validation of a response bias scale (RBS) for the MMPI-2. *Assessment, 14*, 196–208.

Gold, L. H., & Davidson, J. E. (2007). Do you understand your risk? Liability and third-party evaluations in civil litigation. *Journal of the American Academy of Psychiatry & the Law, 35*, 200–210.

Gold, L. H., Anfang, S. A., Druktenis, A. M., Metzner, J. L., Price, M., et al. (2008). AAPL practice guidelines for forensic evaluation of psychiatric disability. *Journal of the American Academy of Psychiatry & the Law, 36*(4 Suppl), S3–S50.

Gold, L. H., & Shuman, D. W. (2009). *Evaluating mental health disability in the workplace: Model, process and analysis*, New York: Springer.

Gostin, L. O., Feldblum, C., & Webber, D. W. (1999). Disability discrimination in America: HIV/AIDS and other health conditions. *Journal of the American Medical Association, 281*(8), 745–752.

Graham, J. R. (2012). *MMPI-2: Assessing personality and psychopathology*, (5th ed.). New York: Oxford University Press.

Harkness, A. R., & McNulty, J. L. (1994). The Personality Psychopathology Five (PSY-5): Issues from the pages of a diagnostic manual instead of a dictionary. In S. Stack & M. Lorr (Eds.), *Differentiating normal and abnormal personality* (pp. 291–315). New York: Springer.

Harkness, A. R., McNulty, J. L., Ben-Porath, Y. S., & Graham, J. R. (2002). *MMPI-2 Personality Psychopathology Five (PSY-5) scales: Gaining an overview for case conceptualization and treatment planning*. Minneapolis, MN: University of Minnesota Press.

Harkness, A. R., Reynolds, S. M., & Lilienfeld, S. O. (2014). A review of systems for psychology and psychiatry: Adaptive systems, Personality Psychopathology Five (PSY-5), and the DSM-5. *Journal of Personality Assessment, 96*(2), 121–139.

Helzer, J. E., Kraemer, H. C., Krueger, R. F., Wittchen, H-U., Sirovatka, P. J., & Regier, D. A. (2008). Dimensional approaches in diagnostic classification: Refining the research agenda for DSM-V. Arlington, VA: American Psychiatric Association.

Hubbard, A. (Ed.) (1998). *An American Bible: Foundations of the American character*. Atlanta, GA: Bemis Pub., Ltd.

Knoll, J., & Gerbasi, J. (2006). Psychiatric malpractice case analysis: Striving for objectivity. *Journal of the American Academy of Psychiatry & the Law, 34*(2), 215–223.

Langer, C. S. (1996). Title I of the Americans with Disabilities Act. In J. W. Snyder & J. E. Klees (Eds.), *Law and the workplaces: Occupational medicine: State of the Art Reviews, 11*, 1–16.

Lees-Haley, P. R., English, L. T., & Glenn, W. J. (1991). A fake-bad scale on the MMPI-2 for personal injury claimants. *Psychological Reports, 68*, 203–210.

Leigh, J. P. (2008). Costs of occupational injury and illness combining all industries. Presentation to the Western Center for Agriculture Health and Safety, November 3, 2008.

Leigh, J. P., Markowitz, M. F., Shin, C., & Landrigan, P. J. (1997). Occupational injury and illness in the United States: Estimates of costs, morbidity, and mortality. *Archives of Internal Medicine, 157*, 1556–1568.

Maffeo, P. A. (1990). Making non-discriminatory fitness for duty decisions about persons with disabilities under the Rehabilitation Act and Americans with Disabilities Act. *American Journal of Law & Medicine, 16*, 279–326.

Melzack, R. (1983). *The McGill Pain Questionnaire: Pain measurement and assessment*. New York: Raven Press.

Melzack, R. (1987). The short form McGill pain questionnaire. *Pain, 30*, 191–197.

Kleinfield, N. R. (2009). Exams of injured workers fuel mutual mistrust. *New York Times* (March 31), pp.

Oldham, J. M., Skodol, A. E., Kellman, H. D., et al. (1995). Comorbidity of Axis 1 and Axis 2 disorders, *American Journal of Psychiatry, 152*, 571–578.

Patient Health Questionnaire (PHQ-9). Available at: http://www.phqscreeners.com/overview.aspx (accessed August 31, 2010).

Petersen-Crair, P., Marangell, L., Flack, J., Harper, R., Soety, E., & Gabbard, G. (2003). An impaired physician with complex co-morbidity. *American Journal of Psychology, 168*, 850–854.

Polusny, M. A., Kehle, S. M., Nelson, N. W., Erbes, C. R., Arbisi, P. A., & Thuras, P. (2011). Longitudinal effects of mild traumatic brain injury and posttraumatic stress disorder comorbidity on post-deployment outcomes in National Guard soldiers deployed to Iraq. *Archives of General Psychiatry, 68*(1), 79–89.

Quint, M. (1994). New ailments: Bane of insurers. *The New York Times* (Nov 28), pp. D1, D2.

Rogers, R., Bagby, R. M., & Dickens, S. E. (1992). *Structured Interview of Reported Symptoms (SIRS)*. Lutz, FL: Psychological Assessment Resources.

Rogers, R. (2008). *Clinical assessment of malingering and deception* (3rd ed.). New York: The Guildford Press.

Rogers, R., Sewell, K. W., & Gillard, N. D. (2010). Structured Interview of Reported Symptoms, 2nd edition (SIRS-2). Lutz, FL: Psychological Assessment Resources.

Rondinelli, R. D., et al. (Eds.) (2008). *Guides to the evaluation of permanent impairment* (6th ed.). American Medical Association.

Rubenzer, S. (2010). Review of the Structured Inventory of Reported Symptoms–2 (SIRS-2). *Open Access Journal of Forensic Psychology, 2*, 273–286.

Shuman, D. W., & Greenberg, S. A. (2003). The expert witness, the adversary system, and the voice of reason: Reconciling impartiality and advocacy. *Professional Psychology: Research and Practice, 34*, 219–224.

Stein, M. B., & McAllister, T. W. (2009). Exploring the convergence of posttraumatic stress disorder and mild traumatic brain injury. *American Journal of Psychiatry, 166*, 768–776.

Stewart, W. F., Ricci, J. A., Chee, E., Hahn, S. R., & Morganstein, D. (2003). Cost of lost productive work time among US workers with depression. *Journal of the American Medical Association, 289*, 3135–3144.

Stoudemire, A. (1991). Somatothymia. *Psychosomatics, 32*, 365–380.

Strasburger, L. H., Gutheil, T. G., & Brodsky, B. A. (1997). On wearing two hats: Role conflict in serving as both psychotherapist and expert witness. *American Journal of Psychiatry, 154*, 448–456.

Tellegen, A., Ben-Porath, Y. S., McNulty, J. L., Arbisi, P. A., Graham, J. R., & Kaemmer, B. (2003). *MMPI-2 Restructured Clinical (RC) Scales: Development, validation, and interpretation*. Minneapolis, MN: University of Minnesota Press.

Tombaugh, T. N. (1996). *Test of Memory Malingering (TOMM)*. New York: Multi-Health Systems, Inc. http://www.who.int/classifications/icf/en/ (accessed November 13, 2011).

US SSA (2008). United States Social Security Administration Office of Disability Programs: Disability Evaluation under Social Security. Pub. No. 64–039, September 2008. Available at http://ssaconnect.com/tfiles/SSA-4734-F4-SUP.pdf (accessed November 13, 2011); http://www.ssa.gov/disability (accessed November 13, 2011).

Walters, G. D., Rogers, R., Berry, D. T. R., Miller, H. A., Duncan, S. A., McCusker, P. A., et al. (2008). Malingering as a categorical or dimensional construct: The latent structure of feigned psychopathology as measured by the SIRS and MMPI-2. *Psychological Assessment, 20*(3), 238–247.

Williams, C. D. (2006). Psychiatric disability assessments. *Psychiatric Annals, 36*(11), 774–783.

Williams, C. D., & Schouten, R. (2008). Assessment of occupational impairment and disability from depression. *Journal of Occupational & Environmental Medicine, 50*(4), 441–450.

Williams, C. D. (2010). Disability and occupational assessment: Objective diagnosis and quantitative impairment rating. *Harvard Review of Psychiatry, 18*, 336–352.

Williams, C. D. (2013). Social Security disability insurance: General practitioners and consultative examiners. In Gold, L. H. and Vanderpool, D. L. (Eds.), *Clinical Guide to Mental Disability Evaluations*. New York: Springer.

Wolf, E. J., Orazem, R. F., Miller, M. W., Weirich, M. R., et al. (2008). The MMPI-2 restructured clinical scales in the assessment of post-traumatic stress disorder and comorbid disorders. *Psychological Assessment, 20*(4), 327–340.

Wygant, D. B., Anderson, J. L., Selbom, M., Rapier, J. L., Allgeier, L. M., & Granacher, R. P. (2011). Association of the MMPI-2 Restructured Form (MMPI-2-RF) validity scales with structured malingering criteria. *Psychological Injury & Law, 4,* 13–23.

Zwerling, C., Whitten, P. S., Davis, C. S., et al. (1997). Occupational injuries among workers with disabilities. *Journal of the American Medical Association, 278,* 2163–2169.

Zuckerman, D. (1993). Reasonable accommodations for people with mental illness under the ADA. *Mental & Physical Disability Law Reporter, 17,* 311–320.

87.

TELEPSYCHIATRY

Terry Rabinowitz

INTRODUCTION

Some medical conditions may make it difficult or impossible for affected individuals to receive necessary psychiatric care because they may be unable to come for appointments or to participate in their care as required. In addition, psychiatric treatment may not be possible because large distances separate a patient from his or her potential care providers, with few physicians willing to spend uncompensated time in travel and few patients with significant medical comorbidity able to make long trips without costly assistance and a significant investment in time. A videoconference approach for these persons may be a realistic, cost-effective, and acceptable solution to this problem that makes it possible to deliver quality psychiatric care to some who could not otherwise receive it.

TELEMEDICINE AND TELEPSYCHIATRY

As defined by the American Telemedicine Association (ATA),

> Telemedicine is the use of medical information exchanged from one site to another via electronic communications to improve patients' health status.... Videoconferencing, transmission of still images, e-health including patient portals, remote monitoring of vital signs, continuing medical education and nursing call centers are all considered part of telemedicine and telehealth.... (American Telemedicine Association, 2011)

Thus, *telepsychiatry* may be defined as the use of telemedicine to deliver psychiatric care or education across distances, using any available technologies. Other equivalent or related descriptors include *tele-psychiatry, telemental health, tele-mental health, telepsychology,* and *tele-psychology.*

BACKGROUND AND HISTORY

The first published articles about telemedicine were in the field of telepsychiatry (Baer, Elford, & Cukor, 1997) and are attributed to Cecil Wittson and colleagues, who, in the 1950s and 1960s, studied the use of a videoconference approach to provide psychotherapy, comparing it to face-to-face (FTF)

care, and found that the technique used had no significant effect on the quality of the sessions, but that therapist choice and group member selection were important predictors of outcomes (Wittson, Affleck, & Johnson, 1961). Later, Wittson and Benschoter reported on the use of a two-way closed circuit television system between the academic medical center, Nebraska Psychiatric Institute (NPI), and the Norfolk State Mental Hospital, separated by 112 miles. They reported improved patient services at the state facility as a consequence of increased NPI specialist availability through telemedicine. In addition, staff members at both locations used the system to discuss research investigations, and overall interaction and collaboration increased between the two facilities (Wittson & Benschoter, 1972).

The first reports of psychiatric consultations using telemedicine began to appear in the 1970s. In general, these reports described consultations to primary care providers by psychiatrists at academic medical centers using two-way interactive television. For example, Solow et al. used a psychiatric consultative model that comprised a referring provider briefly describing his or her patient to the consulting psychiatrist (CP), interview of the patient by the CP, and CP discussion of findings and recommendations with the referring provider. This model had high patient and provider acceptance (Solow et al., 1971). Later, Dwyer reported the successful use of this modality to provide psychiatric consultations from Massachusetts General Hospital (the *hub* or *distant site*) to a medical station (the *spoke* or *origination site*) in Boston (Dwyer, 1973). Dwyer reported that about 30 psychiatrists and 30 psychiatry residents and medical students responded positively to telepsychiatry, and suggested that, for some patients, this modality might be preferable or superior to an FTF approach—similar findings were reported more than three decades later (Rabinowitz et al., 2006). The greatest impediments to acceptance and implementation of telepsychiatry were the relatively high costs of transmission; cumbersome equipment; technical problems such as sound pick-up, dropped calls, and camera operation; lack of reliability compared to the FTF condition; and so-called *technophobia*, an irrational fear and avoidance of new technologies (Grady, 2002; Yellowlees, 1997; Yellowlees, 2001; Yellowlees, 2005).

Beginning in the 1980s, affordable videoconferencing enabled widespread use of this technology. Early videoconference costs were prohibitive, and picture and sound quality were not always satisfactory, but with the use of digitized audio and video data, it is now possible to expect and obtain acceptable high-quality transmissions (even for images that require very accurate reproduction) at low cost. For example, Kldiashvili and Schrader reported that digital images are appropriate substitutes for glass slides for telecytology applications, particularly when used for quality assurance programs (Kldiashvili & Schrader, 2011), and Urness et al. reported generally high levels of satisfaction (equivalent to those for FTF) of patients using telepsychiatry (Urness et al., 2006). In addition, Doolittle and colleagues reported a steady decrease in per-visit costs and increased use of an established teleoncology service from 1995 to 2005: from 103 visits at $812 per visit, to 235 visits at $251 per visit (Doolittle, Spaulding, & Williams, 2011).

DOES TELEPSYCHIATRY WORK?

Although it seemed obvious that telepsychiatry applications were useful in a number of domains (e.g., cost-savings, effectiveness, acceptability), clinicians and researchers set out to demonstrate that this was the case by using a scientific approach that included experimental and control subjects, larger samples, and more carefully controlled environments. However, although there still is a paucity of large, well-controlled studies that show equivalence (or superiority of) telemedicine/telepsychiatry vs. the FTF condition (Rabinowitz et al., 2008; Whitten et al., 2002; Williams, May, & Esmail, 2001), the accumulated data from many smaller studies and the experience of many clinicians suggest that telepsychiatry is effective, saves money, and is an acceptable alternative to FTF care (Mair et al., 2000; Kennedy & Yellowlees, 2003; Frueh et al., 2004; Modai et al., 2006; Antonacci et al., 2008; Hailey, Roine, & Ohinmaa, 2008). In the late 1990s, evidence-based telepsychiatry reports began to appear. Searching the MEDLINE and PubMed databases using keywords *telemental, tele-mental, telepsychiatry, tele-psychiatry, telepsychology,* and *tele-psychology* reveals a steady increase in telemental health–related publications over the past several decades. In addition, there are many more telemedicine publications that do not "trigger" on these keywords but that directly or indirectly address psychiatric issues.

TECHNICAL AND LEGAL ASPECTS AND NOMENCLATURE

While it is possible for a psychiatrist to use telemedicine equipment without having any appreciation of its actual functioning, a better understanding of the technology is likely to lead to less anxiety about its use and more widespread acceptance and implementation of the technique by clinicians and patients (Yellowlees, 2005; Whitten & Kuwahara, 2004; De Las Cuevas et al., 2003). In addition, because of advances in communications technology, it is now possible to videoconference using compact, inexpensive, user-friendly devices such as webcams, tablet computers, and smartphones, though some of these technologies may not be adequate or appropriate for a telepsychiatry consultation; each clinician and patient is likely to have specific preferences regarding picture and sound quality as well as ease of use of videoconference equipment. Therefore, when contemplating using a telemedicine approach, potential users are advised to perform some "test runs" of different equipment to determine if it meets their individual needs. For example, a smartphone may be an acceptable device for a short, focused patient "visit" but may not be especially comfortable for a 50-minute psychotherapy session for reasons including its inability to pan, tilt, or zoom, leading to user/patient fatigue, and its adequate but not excellent audio and video features.

To better understand how telemedicine applications are described, evaluated, and implemented, and to help readers evaluate telemedicine publications, a few telemedicine-related definitions follow.

Bandwidth (or Digital Bandwidth): A rate of data transfer, bit rate or throughput, measured per second in bits (bps), kilobits (10^3 bits; kbps), or megabits (10^6 bits; mbps). Typical free-standing telemedicine apparatuses may function reasonably well at bandwidths as low as 128 kbps (kilobits per second) but generally work better at rates of 364 kbps and higher. See Table 87.1 for bandwidth comparisons of different equipment.

It may be helpful to think of different bandwidths as analogous to different pipe diameters; larger pipes allow greater flow rates; that is, more data transferred per second. Therefore, greater bandwidth is a desirable feature of any telemedicine system. However, increased bandwidth is costlier and often requires more sophisticated (i.e., more complicated) technology.

Codec: This is a device or computer program capable of en*cod*ing or *dec*oding a digital data stream or signal. A codec encodes a data stream or signal for transmission, storage, or encryption, or decodes it for playback or editing. Codecs are

Table 87.1 TYPICAL OPERATING BANDWIDTHS OF DIFFERENT COMMUNICATION EQUIPMENT

APPARATUS	APPROXIMATE BANDWIDTH
Typical dial-up telephone	28 kbps
Faster dial-up telephone	56 kbps
Telemedicine minimum:	128 kbps
Basic DSL (Digital Subscriber Line)	768 kbps
T-1 / DS1	1.5 mbps
3G	2.4 mbps
Over-the-Air (OTA) television	4–20 mbps
T-3	44 mbps
Maximum FiOS (Fiber Optic Service)	50 mbps
4G (long-range) or WiFi (*Wireless Fidelity*) (short-range)	>100 mbps
Cable television	50–1000 mbps

used in videoconferencing, streaming media, and video editing applications. Audio and video files are compressed with a certain codec when they are saved, and then decompressed by the codec when they are played back.

Encryption is the conversion of data into a form called a *cipher text* that cannot be easily understood by unauthorized persons. *Decryption* is the process of converting encrypted data back into its original form, so it can be understood. Some or all videoconference data may be encrypted, potentially enhancing their security, but encryption itself is no guarantee that these data are entirely safe. Thus, when considering using telemedicine, it is important for each provider to be familiar with the data security practices in effect at his or her telemedicine (i.e., "proximate") site as well as those in use at the distant or "patient" site, keeping in mind that: (1) not all encryption methods are equally effective; (2) some software applications used for videoconferencing may not be Health Insurance Portability and Accountability Act (HIPAA)-compliant even though data are encrypted (see: U.S. Department of Health and Human Services Health Information Privacy website): http://www.hhs.gov/ocr/privacy/hipaa/understanding/coveredentities/index.html); and (3) some software producers may fully disclose neither the limitations of their encryption technology nor what data might be accessed or made available to third parties during or after a videoconference session. When in doubt, consultation with appropriate (e.g., risk management, information technology) services is recommended before a telepsychiatry consultation is performed. Although data security, including patient confidentiality, is an important issue, it has been our experience that, if providers take reasonable steps to protect sensitive information, there is a very low risk of data breaches. Therefore, we recommend a prudent but not over-cautious approach to data security: Do not let concerns about data security be the *deal breaker* when considering using telemedicine.

There are no universally accepted or mandated standards or guidelines for telemedicine or, more specifically, for telepsychiatry. However, *Practice Guidelines for Videoconferencing-Based Telemental Health* were published in 2009 by the American Telemedicine Association (ATA) and may be accessed at their website: http://www.americantelemed.org/i4a/pages/index.cfm?pageid=3311. These guidelines provide a useful set of "bare minimum" requirements for a telemental health service. In addition, the publication includes a useful glossary of telemedicine/telehealth terms.

TELEPSYCHIATRY CONSULTATIONS

Using telemedicine to provide psychiatric treatment for persons with co-occurring non-psychiatric conditions may be an especially helpful approach for several reasons:

1. Patients may live or be hospitalized in rural or other underserved areas where no psychiatrists with the necessary skills are available;

2. Patients may not be able to travel to obtain care where a medical psychiatrist is available;

3. The medical psychiatrist may be unwilling or unable to travel to where the patient is;

4. A local psychiatrist may be qualified to treat the patient but may want advice from a more specialized psychiatrist or simply one outside their usual medical community;

5. Some patients (e.g., those with avoidant or paranoid personalities; those who do not wish to be in public because of disabling or disfiguring conditions; those with autism spectrum disorders) actually would prefer a remote to an FTF consultation; and

6. Psychotherapeutic and psychoeducational groups are easier to convene when it is not necessary to coordinate simultaneous travel for all of the group members.

In addition, telepsychiatry is particularly adaptable to training and supervision of residents and fellows, because it avoids the potentially intimidating effect of having several doctors in the patient's room at once, and making recordings of salient moments is easy.

Urness et al. evaluated patient satisfaction and outcomes for telepsychiatry compared to in-person consultations using the Short Form 12-Item (SF-12) Health Survey and a satisfaction survey. At the one-month follow-up, 48 of 62 subjects (77%) were evaluated. Telepsychiatry patients showed significant improvements on mental health measures compared to controls. Ninety-three percent felt they could present the same information that they could in-person, 96% were satisfied with their telepsychiatry session, and 85% were comfortable talking with their provider; these rates were similar to those for in-person encounters (Urness et al., 2006). Boydell and colleagues reviewed 100 pediatric telepsychiatry consultations to determine whether the recommendations made during each session were actually implemented and found that neither the technology used nor technological difficulties were barriers to implementation (Boydell et al., 2007; Pakyurek, Yellowlees, & Hilty, 2010).

Pakyurek et al. suggest that telepsychiatry may actually be a superior method of psychiatric assessment for children and adolescents compared to the face-to-face approach, due to four factors associated with telepsychiatry: (1) the novelty of the consultation, (2) the capacity to provide direction, (3) the extra distance involved (both psychological and physical), and (4) the authenticity of the interaction (Pakyurek, Yellowlees, & Hilty, 2010). Rabinowitz and colleagues reported similar results for a cohort of nursing home residents ages 44–100 years and in addition found that some patients (e.g., those who were paranoid or avoidant) expressed a preference for telepsychiatry (Rabinowitz et al., 2006; Rabinowitz et al., 2010; Rabinowitz et al., 2006).

Yellowlees et al. assessed the feasibility of using an asynchronous (also called *store and forward*) approach to providing telepsychiatry consultations. This involved the examination by two psychiatrists of video-recorded assessments of 60 adult patients followed by recommendations to their primary care providers. They concluded that asynchronous telepsychiatry consultations were possible and that they would be a helpful additional procedure that enhances access to care (Yellowlees et al., 2010). A follow-up study of asynchronous telepsychiatry (ATP) by Butler and Yellowlees found that the cost savings of the approach was due in large part to the substitution of lower-cost providers for specialists (i.e., psychiatrists) at the patient sites (Butler & Yellowlees, 2011).

We have provided psychiatric consultations to rural nursing home residents since 2002, saving both time and money, as well as avoiding the need to transport frail residents over long distances. Virtually all of these residents had non-psychiatric medical comorbidity, and without telepsychiatry, many would have received no psychiatric care at all because of psychiatrist unavailability. We reported estimated time savings of more than 843 hours that would have be spent for patients traveling to the psychiatrist and vice versa, and potential cost savings of as much as $253,000 (for round-trip physician travel time) for 278 telepsychiatry encounters for 106 nursing home residents (Rabinowitz et al., 2010).

Lending further support to using telemedicine to perform psychiatry consultations for persons with medical illnesses are several reports of its use in treating many medical conditions or patient groups frequently encountered by medical psychiatrists. In a study of 80 patients with head and neck cancer whose tumors were examined both face-to-face and by simulated telemedicine consultations, Stalfors et al. found that tumor classification and treatment planning were the same for both conditions in 73 (91%) of the patients (Stalfors et al., 2001).

Heath and colleagues performed and analyzed 63 pediatric critical care telemedicine consultations from their tertiary care facility to ten rural emergency departments. They used this approach to make 236 specific recommendations and to supervise the critical care transport team in 25 (40%) of the cases. Both the consulting intensivists and the referring providers thought that telemedicine consultations improved patient care and provided good to very good provider-to-provider communications (Heath et al., 2009).

Magann reviewed the telemedicine literature for obstetrics and reported its use to read ultrasounds, interpret non-stress tests, counsel patients, manage diabetes, manage postpartum depression, and to support parents and children postpartum from remote sites, with potential benefits that included reductions in time lost from work, decreased transportation costs, greater efficiency for providers, and reduced medical costs (Magann et al., 2011). An analysis of telemedicine data from the Milwaukee Veteran Affairs Medical Center (VAMC) pulmonary telemedicine clinic, where pulmonary physicians delivered care via telemedicine to patients 215 miles away, found that consultation led to a change in management for 41% of patients, and only 8% of patients required an in-person clinic visit following a telemedicine encounter (Raza et al., 2009).

According to Barneveld Binkhuysen and Ranschaert, teleradiology was first developed for military purposes in the 1980s (Barneveld Binkhuysen & Ranschaert, 2011). Since then, its implementation has become remarkably widespread, with applications reported for nearly every radiological specialty and subspecialty. A search of the MEDLINE database using the single keyword *teleradiology* found 1,373 articles published between 1972 and 2011; for comparison, 255 citations were found using the search term *telepsychiatry* for the same period.

THE TELEPSYCHIATRY ENCOUNTER

Most telepsychiatry consultations are performed by a remote psychiatrist who consults on a patient at one of several locations that might include: the patient's home, a general hospital, a physician's or another provider's office, a community health center, or another venue equipped for videoconference consultations. Regardless of the site, meeting a common set of minimal requirements will help ensure an optimal encounter and acceptance of the technology (Table 87.2).

Grady (Grady, 2002) identifies the importance of the "seven A's" when implementing and maintaining a telepsychiatry service and to assure its success:

Alliance is the consultant's relationship with the remote site's administrative, support, and provider staff.

Assessment includes identifying needs and resources of the satellite site, capabilities and resources of the hub site, and the interest/investment of both sites.

Approach describes how to get the "telepsychiatry word" out to others. Grady recommends that clinicians be the individuals first contacted (i.e., approached) as they will have the greatest insights into the needs of clinicians and patients at the satellite sites.

Improved *access* for patients may be the single most important reason for telepsychiatry. This also refers to where the teleconferencing equipment is located: putting it where it is most easily accessed at the distant site (e.g., a community mental health clinic, a primary care provider's office) and at the hub (e.g., within a telemedicine department, within the medical psychiatry unit) will increase the likelihood that it will be used.

Accountability refers to responsibilities of the provider and facility, including physical safety of the patient, security of patient records, and a plan for performance evaluation and improvement.

Apprehension may be felt by the telepsychiatrist, patient, or clinicians and support staff at the satellite site. It is the responsibility of the telepsychiatrist to be sufficiently comfortable and adept with the equipment that he or she can use it with confidence and allay the concerns of others.

Anticipation of equipment malfunctions, patient refusals, staff worries, and other problems will help the provider develop contingency plans. Bear in mind that it is impossible to anticipate all types of equipment malfunctions or when they might occur. This is especially true given the increased use of low-cost, easily accessed videoconference equipment such as smartphones and tablet computers. Therefore, it is recommended that users become familiar and proficient with one or a very small number of apparatuses rather than try to master every available technology.

Table 87.2 SOME BASIC REQUIREMENTS FOR TELEPSYCHIATRY ENCOUNTERS

PARAMETER	REQUIREMENT/GOAL	ACTION
Safety	Ensure safety of a suicidal or otherwise unsafe patient	Establish a reliable and rapid system of communication other than the telepsychiatry apparatus (e.g., cellular or other telephone, pager) to contact an onsite person in case assistance is needed.
Usability	Conditions and apparatuses must be user-friendly and reliable	Take time to learn about equipment by having a few practice sessions with technical assistance available; make sure venues are well-lighted, quiet, secure, and easily accessible; have back-up plan for communication (e.g., cellular or other telephone) in case of equipment malfunction; know how to access technical staff during any time a telemedicine encounter might occur—24/7 if necessary. If using at home, make sure there is someone with some experience using, e.g., webcams, FaceTime, Skype, etc., who is readily available for quick technical assistance.
Acceptability	Increased likelihood that telepsychiatry will be used	Provider must be comfortable with equipment; acknowledge to patient and/or staff at distant site any limitations/benefits of approach (e.g., saves travel time and money, there may be a slight delay in audio portion of signal); assistance may be needed to position patient or to physically examine for some conditions such as extrapyramidal syndromes; headphones may be useful for some patients with hearing problems.
Education	To better understand how telepsychiatry can be used	Consider recording of telepsychiatry encounters: These can be used to show others how telepsychiatry works, for second opinions, and for provider education (i.e., for the provider to observe his/her "telepresence" and to make adjustments if indicated). Make sure appropriate permissions are obtained. Recordings of encounters may be considered part of the permanent medical record.

LEGAL, REGULATORY, AND FINANCIAL CONSIDERATIONS

Although telemedicine has been available since the 1960s, there are few laws regarding its use. For example, the U. S. Centers for Medicare and Medicaid Services (CMS) have published data regarding what telemedicine services will and will not be reimbursed, but there are no national standards for telemedicine use and more specifically, no laws that dictate how telemedicine in general shall be practiced nor how specific telemedicine specialty services should operate. To address this deficiency, the American Telemedicine Association has published a number of standards and guidelines for the use of telemedicine (see http://www.americantelemed.org/practice). Although this collection does not cover every aspect of telemedicine or every telemedicine specialty, it is a reasonably comprehensive database and an extremely useful resource. Moreover, these various standards and guidelines should be considered as representing the *de facto* standard of care for the covered telemedicine applications.

Two common questions regarding telemedicine are: (1) Does malpractice insurance cover this approach? and (2) Is it necessary to be licensed in the state where the telemedicine service is provided? The answers are not simple.

Each malpractice insurer approaches telemedicine differently, and there are no universal rules or regulations governing its coverage. Therefore, it is strongly recommended that each clinician know and receive confirmation in writing *before a telemedicine consultation is performed*, whether his or her policy covers telemedicine and if not, what must be done for coverage to be in effect. Many, but not all, carriers provide coverage around the clock for their subscribers, regardless of venue or technology, as long as the clinician practices within

the "boundaries" of the specialty. However, this is not a universal behavior, and ignorance of the terms of one's coverage might lead to an undesirable outcome that could have been easily prevented.

If the originating and distant sites are in the same state, questions of licensure do not apply; we are not aware of any state medical licensing board that prohibits the practice of telemedicine between an in-state provider and patient. However, *interstate* telemedicine practice is more complicated. For example, some states with common borders allow providers from either state to practice medicine and telemedicine without requiring licensure of the "hub" physician in the "spoke" state, provided such practice is a rare occurrence. Other states require in-state licensure for even a single telemedicine consultation from an out-of-state physician. Therefore, it is recommended that each clinician learn what the state licensing board requirements for telemedicine practice are in the state to which the telemedicine services will be delivered, before any service is provided. In addition, it is important to know whether the spoke state has different licensing requirements or rules with respect to *medical consultants* vs. *primary providers*. It is equally important to know if the out-of-state clinician will have any trouble with prescriptions called in to or sent out to a pharmacy in another state.

Obtaining reimbursement for telemedicine services is becoming easier. For example, when telemedicine was in its infancy, neither private insurers nor CMS covered telemedicine services. However, with clear and convincing evidence that care delivered using a telemedicine approach is, in many cases, as good as (or better than) care delivered face-to-face, insurers, lawmakers, and laypersons have come to realize the benefits of telemedicine and are willing to reimburse accordingly or to ask their representative to enact laws requiring appropriate reimbursement for telemedicine services.

For example, on October 1, 2012, the state of Vermont enacted a telemedicine law (http://www.leg.state.vt.us/docs/2012/Acts/ACT107.pdf) that states in part:

> …All health insurance plans in this state shall provide coverage for telemedicine services delivered to a patient in a health care facility to the same extent that the services would be covered if they were provided through in-person consultation.…

Some other states have enacted similar laws, and some states have more inclusive ones. This is good for patients and for telemedicine and portends greater acceptance of and reimbursement for telemedicine services moving forward.

MORE INFORMATION

The best source for general information about telemedicine is the American Telemedicine Association (ATA) website: http://www.americantelemed.org. Once at this website, a few clicks will bring the interested searcher to the Telemental Health Special Interest Group (SIG), a very active SIG that is an excellent source of information for budding telepsychiatrists as well as those who are already familiar with the technology. More specific information about telepsychiatry as it relates to medical-psychiatric affairs can be gleaned by joining the Telepsychiatry SIG of the Academy of Psychosomatic Medicine (APM) (at http://www.apm.org/). This SIG was formed in 2010 to promote the use of telepsychiatry among medical psychiatrists. The two key telemedicine journals are *The Journal of Telemedicine and Telecare* (http://jtt.rsmjournals.com/), and *Telemedicine and E-Health* (http://www.liebertpub.com/TMJ).

SUMMARY

Using telemedicine to perform psychiatric consultations will benefit patients, providers, and communities. It will bring psychiatric care to many who would not otherwise receive it; it will save time and money; and it will expand the range of options for consulting psychiatrists. In addition, telemedicine has the potential to create new opportunities for research, to provide unique ways to treat patients, and to make the practice of medical psychiatry more enjoyable and fulfilling.

CLINICAL PEARLS

- When contemplating using a telemedicine approach, perform some test runs of different equipment to determine if it meets one's individual needs.

- Some software applications used for videoconferencing may not be HIPAA-compliant, even though data are encrypted (see http://www.hhs.gov/ocr/privacy/hipaa/u7nderstanding/coveredentities/index.html).

- We recommend that users become familiar and proficient with one or a very small number of apparatuses.

- The American Telemedicine Association has published a number of standards and guidelines for the use of telemedicine (see http://www.americantelemed.org/practice).

- Before a telemedicine consultation is performed, each clinician should know and receive in writing information as to whether his or her malpractice insurance policy covers telemedicine, and if not, what must be done for coverage to be in effect.

- It is important to know policies that apply across state lines for telepsychiatry and for prescribing medications.

DISCLOSURE STATEMENT

Dr. Rabinowitz has no financial interests to disclose.

REFERENCES

American Telemedicine Association (2011). Telemedicine defined. Available from: http://www.americantelemed.org/i4a/pages/index.cfm?pageID=3333.

Antonacci, D. J., Bloch, R. M., Saeed, S. A., Yildirim, Y., & Talley, J. (2008). Empirical evidence on the use and effectiveness of telepsychiatry via videoconferencing: Implications for forensic and correctional psychiatry. *Behavioral Sciences & the Law, 26*(3), 253–269.

Baer, L., Elford, D. R., & Cukor, P. (1997). Telepsychiatry at forty: What have we learned? *Harvard Review of Psychiatry, 5*(1), 7–17.

Barneveld Binkhuysen, F. H., & Ranschaert, E. R. (2011). Teleradiology: Evolution and concepts. *European Journal of Radiology, 78*(2), 205–209.

Boydell, K. M., Volpe, T., Kertes, A., & Greenberg, N. (2007). A review of the outcomes of the recommendations made during paediatric telepsychiatry consultations. *Journal of Telemedicine & Telecare, 13*(6), 277–281.

Butler, T. N., & Yellowlees, P. (2011). Cost analysis of store-and-forward telepsychiatry as a consultation model for primary care. *Telemedicine Journal & E-Health, 18*(1), 74–77.

De Las Cuevas, C., Artiles, J., De La Fuente, J., & Serrano, P. (2003). Telepsychiatry in the Canary Islands: User acceptance and satisfaction. *Journal of Telemedicine & Telecare, 9*(4), 221–224.

Doolittle, G. C., Spaulding, A. O., & Williams, A. R. (2011). The decreasing cost of telemedicine and telehealth. *Telemedicine Journal & E-Health, 17*(9), 671–675.

Dwyer, T. F. (1973). Telepsychiatry: Psychiatric consultation by interactive television. *American Journal of Psychiatry, 130*(8), 865–869.

Frueh, B. C., Monnier, J., Elhai, J. D., Grubaugh, A. L., & Knapp, R. G. (2004). Telepsychiatry treatment outcome research methodology: Efficacy versus effectiveness. *Telemedicine Journal & E-Health, 10*(4), 455–458.

Grady, B. J. (2002). Telepsychiatry. In M. G. Wise & J. R. Rundell (Eds.), *The American Psychiatric Publishing Textbook of Consultation-Liaison Psychiatry. Psychiatry in the Medically Ill* (2nd ed., pp. 927–936). Washington, DC: American Psychiatric Publishing.

Hailey, D., Roine, R., & Ohinmaa, A. (2008). The effectiveness of telemental health applications: A review. *Canadian Journal of Psychiatry, 53*(11), 769–778.

Heath, B., Salerno, R., Hopkins, A., Hertzig, J., & Caputo, M. (2009). Pediatric critical care telemedicine in rural underserved emergency departments. *Pediatric Critical Care Medicine, 10*(5), 588–591.

Kennedy, C., & Yellowlees, P. (2003). The effectiveness of telepsychiatry measured using the Health of the Nation Outcome Scale and the Mental Health Inventory. *Journal of Telemedicine & Telecare, 9*(1), 12–16.

Kldiashvili, E., & Schrader T. (2011). Reproducibility of telecytology diagnosis of cervical smears in a quality assurance program: The Georgian experience. *Telemedicine Journal and E-Health, 17*(7), 565–568.

Magann, E. F., McKelvey, S. S., Hitt, W. C., Smith, M. V., Azam, G. A., & Lowery, C. L. (2011). The use of telemedicine in obstetrics: A review of the literature. *Obstetrics & Gynecology, Survey, 66*(3), 170–178.

Mair, F. S., Haycox, A., May, C., & Williams, T. (2000). A review of telemedicine cost-effectiveness studies. *Journal of Telemedicine & Telecare, 6*(Suppl 1), S38–S40.

Modai, I., Jabarin, M., Kurs, R., Barak, P., Hanan, I., & Kitain, L. (2006). Cost effectiveness, safety, and satisfaction with video telepsychiatry versus face-to-face care in ambulatory settings. *Telemedicine Journal & E-Health, 12*(5), 515–520.

Pakyurek, M., Yellowlees, P., & Hilty, D. (2010). The child and adolescent telepsychiatry consultation: Can it be a more effective clinical process for certain patients than conventional practice? *Telemedicine Journal & E-Health, 16*(3), 289–292.

Rabinowitz, T., Brennan, D. M., Chumbler, N. R., Kobb, R., & Yellowlees, P. (2008). New directions for telemental health research. *Telemedicine Journal & E-Health, 14*(9), 972–976.

Rabinowitz, T., Murphy, K. M., Amour, J. L., Ricci, M. A., Caputo, M. P., & Newhouse, P. A. (2010). Benefits of a telepsychiatry consultation service for rural nursing home residents. *Telemedicine Journal & E-Health, 16*(1), 34–40.

Rabinowitz, T., Newhouse, P. A., Reynolds, B. P., Caputo, M. P., Clark, H. G., Amour, J. L., et al. (2006). Superiority of telemental health vs. face-to-face consultations. *Telemedicine Journal & E-Health, 12*, 179.

Raza, T., Joshi, M., Schapira, R. M., & Agha, Z. (2009). Pulmonary telemedicine—A model to access the subspecialist services in underserved rural areas. *International Journal of Medicial Informatics, 78*(1), 53–59.

Solow, C., Weiss, R. J., Bergen, B. J., & Sanborn, C. J. (1971). 24-hour psychiatric consultation via TV. *American Journal of Psychiatry, 127*(12), 1684–1687.

Stalfors, J., Edstrom, S., Bjork-Eriksson, T., Mercke, C., Nyman, J., & Westin, T. (2001). Accuracy of tele-oncology compared with face-to-face consultation in head and neck cancer case conferences. *Journal of Telemedicine & Telecare, 7*(6), 338–343.

Urness, D., Wass, M., Gordon, A., Tian, E., & Bulger, T. (2006). Client acceptability and quality of life—Telepsychiatry compared to in-person consultation. *Journal of Telemedicine & Telecare, 12*(5), 251–254.

Whitten, P. S., Mair, F. S., Haycox, A., May, C. R., Williams, T. L., & Hellmich, S. (2002). Systematic review of cost effectiveness studies of telemedicine interventions. *British Medical Journal, 324*(7351), 1434–1437.

Whitten, P., & Kuwahara, E. (2004). A multi-phase telepsychiatry programme in Michigan: Organizational factors affecting utilization and user perceptions. *Journal of Telemedicine & Telecare, 10*(5), 254–261.

Williams, T. L., May, C. R., & Esmail A. (2001). Limitations of patient satisfaction studies in telehealthcare: A systematic review of the literature. *Telemedicine Journal & E-Health, 7*(4), 293–316.

Wittson, C. L., & Benschoter, R. (1972). Two-way television: Helping the medical center reach out. *American Journal of Psychiatry, 129*(5), 624–627.

Wittson, C. L., Affleck, D. C., & Johnson, V. (1961). Two-way television in group therapy. *Mental Hospitals, 12*, 22–23.

Yellowlees, P. (1997). How not to develop telemedicine systems. *Telemedicine Today, 5*(3), 6–7, 17.

Yellowlees, P. (2001). An analysis of why telehealth systems in Australia have not always succeeded. *Journal of Telemedicine & Telecare, 7*(Suppl 2), 29–31.

Yellowlees, P. M. (2005). Successfully developing a telemedicine system. *Journal of Telemedicine & Telecare, 11*(7), 331–335.

Yellowlees, P. M., Odor, A., Parish, M. B., Iosif, A. M., Haught, K., & Hilty, D. (2010). A feasibility study of the use of asynchronous telepsychiatry for psychiatric consultations. *Psychiatric Services, 61*(8), 838–840.

88.

PRACTICE GUIDELINES, PERFORMANCE MEASUREMENT, AND INCENTIVES

Daniel P. Hunt

INTRODUCTION

Clinical practice guidelines summarize and rate the evidence to support recommendations for the care of patients. Ideally, guidelines should make it easier for clinicians to provide high-quality, current-standard care that is evidence-based and patient-centered. This chapter describes the methodology for producing trustworthy guidelines and provides a framework for practitioners to assess the validity of guidelines.

Clinical practice guidelines (CPG) provide the underpinnings for performance measurements that have become commonplace for hospitals, practice groups, and individual practitioners. Financial incentives or pay-for-performance programs are aimed at quality improvement in medicine, often by promoting implementation of guideline recommendations. The evidence for efficacy and cost-effectiveness of pay-for-performance programs lags behind the widespread adoption of these programs. In simplest terms, clinical practice guidelines drive performance measurement, which drives performance-based incentive programs.

Clinical practice guidelines proliferated during the past two decades, driven by rapidly expanding medical research and literature that is overwhelming for the practitioner. The hope and promise of clinical practice guidelines has been that they would speed translation of clinical research to the care of patients, reduce variability in clinical care, and ultimately improve the health of individual patients while easing information overload for practitioners. During the same time period, large medical systems, insurers, patients, and physicians began to measure performance, often using guidelines to help define and justify individual measures.

This chapter will define clinical practice guidelines (CPGs), explain the process for producing valid guidelines, provide a framework for critical appraisal of guidelines, assess the use of performance measures, consider the impact of physician/system incentives in the implementation of guidelines, and address circumstances in which optimal patient care requires deviation from guidelines.

CLINICAL PRACTICE GUIDELINES

DEFINITION

The medical literature is replete with papers that purport to be guidelines. A simple Pub Med search of the term "guideline" in July of 2011 yielded 204,862 citations that could be loosely titled "guidelines." For the purposes of this discussion, a much more specific definition for clinical practice guidelines is required in order to identify guidelines that are more likely to be valid and useful for clinical care. The Institute of Medicine (IOM), in its 2011 publication *Clinical Practice Guidelines We Can Trust,* provided the following definition:

> Clinical practice guidelines are statements that include recommendations intended to optimize patient care that are informed by a systematic review of evidence and an assessment of the benefits and harms of alternative care options.

The IOM report outlines characteristics of trustworthy guidelines, which are listed in Box 88.1.

DEVELOPMENT OF CLINICAL PRACTICE GUIDELINES

The development process for trustworthy clinical practice guidelines is arduous and rigorous. Development generally begins with identification of a topic area that is worthy of attention for practicing clinicians. Table 88.1 provides a sequence of steps in development of a CPG and uses a hypothetical example of perioperative medication management to detail the process. The next step in producing a guideline is obtaining support, primarily financial, for the process, which requires a considerable investment of time by experts for intensive literature review, consensus meetings, writing, external review, and editorial input.

Once the topic area is defined and support for the process is assured, the convening individual or organization chooses guideline panel members. The panel should be

In addition to medical and methods experts, it is desirable to have patient representation on the development panel, although this presents its own challenges, given the technical nature of many deliberations.

The initial focus for the guideline panel is developing interpersonal relationships, establishing goals for the group, and defining the process. Bales and Strodtbeck identified the following three phases of group decision-making:

1. Orientation, or defining the problem;

2. Evaluation and discussion of the alternatives to address the problem; and

3. Control, or deciding which alternatives should prevail (Bales & Strodtbeck, 1951).

Before beginning deliberations, the panel and the panel members should declare and manage potential conflicts of interest. Scott and Guyatt outline issues to help address potential or real conflicts of interest, summarized in Table 88.2 (Scott & Guyatt, 2011). Although there is considerable concern about individual conflicts of interest, convening organizations may have a subtler but more pervasive potential conflict of interest. For example, an organization representing pulmonary specialists who derive practice income from pulmonary function testing would potentially be influenced by the vested interests of its members when convening a panel to develop guidelines for perioperative pulmonary care.

The next step in developing a CPG is to generate specific clinical questions. Clearly, these questions should be relevant to practicing clinicians and to their patients and should encompass major management decisions for the particular condition. The clinical questions form the framework for identifying and synthesizing the evidence that supports the recommendations.

multidisciplinary, including specialists and generalists along with methodological experts (epidemiologists, statisticians, guideline development experts, implementation experts, among others) as needed. The panel usually includes 10 to 20 members who represent three to five disciplines (Burgers, Grol, et al., 2003). A heterogeneous panel is more likely to produce better panel performance and more balanced guidelines (Murphy, Dingwall, et al., 1998). The panel requires a strong leader who is skilled in facilitating balanced discussion.

Table 88.1 PROCESS FOR GUIDELINE DEVELOPMENT

STEP IN PROCESS	KEY STEPS OR CHARACTERISTICS	EXAMPLE
Identify topic area	Generally should be of interest to practicing clinicians, although may affect a small number of patients.	Perioperative management of medications
	Should generate specific clinical questions that can be answered by evidence.	
Obtain resources for producing the guideline	Financial support in bringing all appropriate stakeholders together.	Collaborative of specialty societies might agree to provide resources (e.g.: national organizations for surgery, anesthesiology, medicine, hospital medicine would have potential interest in guideline)
	Resources needed to produce review of the evidence, to write the guideline itself, and to disseminate the guideline.	
	Critical that source of support not have conflict of interest in generation of guideline.	
Choose guideline panel members	Broad, multidisciplinary representation.	Surgery Anesthesiology Medicine Family Medicine

(continued)

Table 88.1 (CONTINUED)

STEP IN PROCESS	KEY STEPS OR CHARACTERISTICS	EXAMPLE
		Obstetrics/Gynecology
		Hospital Medicine
		Patients
		Epidemiologists
		Pharmacologists
		Pharmacists
		Nursing
		Guideline writing experts
Choose panel chair(s)	Chair needs skill in managing group dynamics and discussion.	Elect from within the group
Declare and manage potential conflicts of interest	Conflicts may include financial, academic, intellectual conflicts. Chair must determine if the participant with a conflict of interest must be excused from portions of the discussion or should not serve on this panel.	Physicians who have financial interests in the drugs that are discussed should be carefully considered and potentially excluded.
Generate clinical questions	Should identify clinical problems within the topic area that require guidance. Should generate focused questions. Panel must reach consensus on the final questions.	How should antihypertensives (and each class of antihypertensives) be managed during the perioperative period? How should diabetes treatment (oral agents, insulin) be managed around the time of surgery? Anti-platelet agents? Anticoagulants?
Identify outcomes critical to the recommendations the guideline will formulate	Identify all important patient outcomes. Explicitly rate the importance of the outcomes.	For example (within this guideline): Anticoagulants Serious bleeding New thrombosis Surgical complications Mortality
Systematic review of the current evidence addressing each question	May draw on existing systematic reviews, but often must commission new systematic reviews of the literature. Preferable to have the reviews done by groups independent of the guideline panel. Transparently summarize the review process and the evidence.	Systematic review of all studies of warfarin and surgery, other anticoagulants and surgery.
Guideline panel reviews prepared summaries of the evidence based on systematic review	Assess the quality of the evidence for each question.	Use a simple rating system for strength of evidence
Formulate recommendations and rate the strength of recommendations	Recommendations should be actionable and should employ active voice rather than passive voice. Should avoid ambiguous or vague statements such as "Physicians may offer...." Recommendations should be actionable and ideally should be easily incorporated in clinical decision-support tools.	For example: For patients at high risk of bleeding during the surgery and during the immediate post-operative period, but at low risk of thrombosis, the clinician should stop warfarin five days before surgery.
External review	Before submitting the guideline for publication, it should be critically reviewed by potentially affected parties who are independent of the guideline panel.	Review by a broader audience of surgeons, surgical subspecialists, internists, hematologists, cardiologists, etc.
Final formulation	Taking into account the external reviewers' comments, should finalize recommendations.	

Table 88.2 CONFLICT OF INTEREST IN DEVELOPMENT OF CLINICAL PRACTICE GUIDELINES

	ISSUES	SPECIFICS
Panelists	Must disclose all industry-related professional activities.	Research grants, speaker support, stock ownership, board positions, consultancy agreements should be documented by the chair of the panel
	For the duration of guideline development, must divest themselves of direct financial interests in commercial companies with interest in any of the guideline's recommendations.	
	Identify all sections of the draft for which they have a conflict of interest.	
Panel	Identification and recruitment of panelists should be an open, transparent process.	Panels generally should include broad representation.
	Should include methodologists who share responsibility for the process but have no financial or intellectual conflicts of interest.	Lack of consensus around the evidence or limited evidence should be resolved by explicit democratic process such as Delphi rounds.
	Explicit processes must be used to assess evidence quality and link this to recommendations.	
	Only conflict-free panelists should determine the recommendations, including the strength of the recommendations.	

Adapted from Scott and Guyatt (2011).

Systematic reviews of the available evidence are the critical next step. The systematic review should result in a grading of the evidence, which is generally done using a fairly simple ordinal scale (I, II, III; A, B, C; *good, fair, poor*; or a numerical scale). Simple systems, such as that originally proposed by the Canadian Task Force on the Periodic Health Examination, may be based solely on study design, classifying randomized controlled trials (RCTs) as *good* (or Level I); cohort or case control studies as *fair* (or Level II), and expert opinion as *poor* (or Level III) (Spitzer, Bayne, et al., 1979). More recent evidence-classification schemes assess the methodological details of the included studies, but generally distill this to a simple classification. Some guideline-writing committees employ an independent group to perform the systematic review of the evidence for each clinical question, arguing that this reduces bias.

The guideline panel then links the available evidence and its strength to specific recommendations that address the original clinical questions. The recommendations themselves are also rated for strength using dichotomous or ordinal scores (strong recommendation, weak recommendation; A, B, C) after careful consideration of the potential benefits and weaknesses of a clinical management strategy.

The writing group for the panel then produces a draft CPG. The American College of Cardiology Foundation/American Heart Association (ACCF/AHA) recommends that guideline drafts include the following elements (ACCF/AHA, 2010):

1. Statement of the clinical question.

2. Recommendation that answers the clinical question and provides a classification of the strength of the recommendation and a classification of the level of evidence supporting the recommendation. (The ACCF/AHA uses the classification schemes outlined in Table 88.3.)

3. Explanatory text that provides a summary of the evidence.

4. References.

5. Evidence table.

6. Diagrams, tables, or graphic summaries that emphasize the key points regarding the question.

The draft of the CPG should be distributed to external reviewers and interested parties for comment before the document is finalized for dissemination or publication.

CRITICAL APPRAISAL OF PUBLISHED GUIDELINES

Clinical practice guidelines should be subjected to critical appraisal before implementation by practitioners. There are many systems available to grade the quality of the evidence and the strength of recommendations contained within CPGs. A useful example is the AGREE II instrument, which contains 23 items across six domains (Brouwers, Kho, et al., 2010). The items comprised in this instrument are available online, including a table from the original paper that is available at the website of the *Canadian Medical Association Journal*, http://www.cmaj.ca/content/182/10/1045/T4.large.jpg. As with most critical appraisal tools for CPGs, this system assesses the process of guideline development and the reporting of this process, but it does not assess the clinical content or the quality of the evidence within the guideline (Cluzeau, Burgers, et al., 2003).

The IOM report identified the challenge for practicing clinicians to independently assess the quality of relevant CPGs. This is particularly difficult when there is more than one CPG, often produced by different specialty societies that

Table 88.3 ACCF/AHA CLASSIFICATION OF RECOMMENDATIONS AND LEVEL OF EVIDENCE

RECOMMENDATION CLASSIFICATION		LEVEL OF EVIDENCE	
I	Conditions for which there is evidence and/or general agreement that a given procedure or treatment is useful and effective	A	Data derived from multiple randomized clinical trials or meta-analyses. Must provide citations with the recommendation.
II	Conditions for which there is conflicting evidence and/or a divergence of opinion about the usefulness/efficacy of a procedure or treatment	B	Data derived from a single randomized trial, or nonrandomized studies. Must provide citation(s).
IIa	Weight of the evidence/opinion is in favor of usefulness/efficacy	C	Consensus opinion of experts, case studies, or "standard of care."
IIb	Usefulness/efficacy is less well established by evidence/opinion		
III	Conditions for which there is evidence and/or general agreement that the procedure/treatment is not useful/effective and in some cases may be harmful		

Derived from *Methodology Manual and Policies from the ACCF/AHA Task Force on Practice Guidelines* (ACCF/AHA, 2010).

address the same or similar clinical questions. The IOM recommended that certification of trustworthy CPGs should be a goal, although there is no current authoritative body to provide assessment and certification of individual guidelines. In the United Kingdom, the National Institute for Health and Clinical Excellence (NICE) takes the approach of certifying *organizations* that produce guidelines. The IOM proposed that certification of organizations based on their development procedures would be the most efficient method for assuring quality in guidelines. This certification might be based in the National Guideline Clearinghouse (www.guideline.gov), the National Quality Forum (NQF), the National Committee for Quality Assurance (NCQA), the Patient-Centered Outcomes Research Institute, or in NICE.

PRACTICAL ISSUES WITH USING GUIDELINES

For some problems, there are numerous high-quality CPGs available, and the specific recommendations contained in these guidelines may differ for each specific patient situation. This poses a challenge for the practitioner who must decide between the guidelines, weighing the apparent rigor that went into the development of each guideline, but finally deciding a course of action based on clinical experience and judgement. Sound clinical judgement should never be supplanted by a CPG.

The vast majority of CPGs address single diseases or conditions. Many patients, particularly those who are older, have multiple conditions, concerns, or diseases. There may be more than one high-quality guideline for each disease or condition, and these guidelines may be in full agreement. An illuminating 2005 paper considered applicable CPGs in the care of a hypothetical 79-year-old woman with hypertension, diabetes mellitus, osteoporosis, osteoarthritis, and chronic obstructive pulmonary disease (COPD) (Boyd, Darer, et al., 2005). Adherence to the guidelines would result in prescription of a complicated regimen of 12 medications, recommendation of a complex (and somewhat conflicting) non-pharmacological regimen, while not accounting for potential adverse interactions between treatments and not accounting for patient preferences. This hypothetical case points out many reasons that CPGs may not be appropriate for some patients and should prompt the physician to deviate from standard recommendations. Table 88.4 includes additional challenges to full application of CPGs for individual patients.

Patients with unusual conditions may fall outside clinical practice guidelines. Patients with multiple comorbid conditions make the application of multiple CPGs unwieldy and potentially dangerous. Some patients and their physicians may have exhausted all conventional, CPG-supported options, yet wish to proceed with physiologically sound, yet unconventional, treatment. In each of these cases and in those identified in Table 88.4, the treating physician risks a worsened performance score, yet their patients might be receiving outstanding care and achieving positive health outcomes. This is one of the great challenges in the use of CPGs and performance measurement: to appropriately use evidence-based medicine while not missing out on the benefits of innovative care that falls outside such guidelines. The medical psychiatrist can play a pivotal role in helping to identify patients who would benefit from less reliance on CPGs, while carefully documenting the rationale in order to avoid negative performance measurement.

IMPLEMENTATION OF PRACTICE GUIDELINES

The intention of CPGs is to improve the care of individual patients and, as a consequence, to improve the care of populations. In order to fulfill this intent, recommendations contained in practice guidelines must be implemented by practitioners and patients at the point of care. CPGs affect the work of multiple members of a health care team, including

Table 88.4 CHALLENGES TO THE USE OF PRACTICE GUIDELINES IN CLINICAL CARE

ISSUE	APPROACH
Patient needs and preferences	Understanding patient circumstances, particularly social contexts.
	Thoughtful negotiation with patients regarding options.
Obscure diagnoses	There may be no guidelines, therefore requiring physician judgement.
	May limit use of guidelines for the patient's other conditions.
Complex comorbidities	Requires physician judgement regarding medical priorities. (For example: a life-threatening cardiac condition would take priority over routine screening or management of a more chronic condition.)
	Patient priorities are extremely important to consider in addressing multiple comorbidities.
Difficult personality traits or psychosocial factors	May dramatically reduce the realistic application of CPGs.
Conflicting high-quality guidelines	Acknowledge the existence of conflicting guidelines, discuss with the patient, and document rationale for decisions.
	Obtain expert opinion from colleagues or consultants to resolve the decision conflict for the individual patient.

nurses, physicians, clerical staff, case managers, and allied health providers. Implementation strategies must identify and target all active users of the CPG. A number of steps must be accomplished for successful implementation of guidelines for the individual patient. These steps are outlined in Table 88.5.

First, the practitioner must be aware of the existence of the CPG and must have ready access to it. The applicable recommendations of the guideline should fit within the time constraints of an efficient clinical encounter. The IOM report states that CPG characteristics that promote use include "clarity, specificity, strength of the evidence, perceived importance, relevance to practice, and simplicity" (Institute of Medicine [U.S.] & Graham, 2011). Many patients have multiple complex and interrelated medical conditions that make the application of disease-focused CPGs challenging. Guidelines that provide concise summaries of recommendations and key messages are more likely to be used.

In addition, translation of guidelines to electronic decision-support systems may help clinicians employ recommendations in real time and may be helpful for applying multiple guidelines in the management of complex patients. For example, physician order entry for radiological studies may incorporate CPG recommendations within the order set, in order to improve the value of testing.

As mentioned above, clinicians must first be aware of relevant guidelines in order to implement the contained recommendations. There are several potential ways to inform clinicians about the existence, importance, and relevance of CPGs. Traditionally, clinicians learned about advances in medical care through educational materials or journals, but the impact of printed materials has been limited at best (Farmer, Legare, et al., 2008). Didactic lectures and workshops given as part of formal continuing medical education (CME) courses have small effects on clinician practice and have particularly limited effect in promoting complex practice changes (Forsetlund, Bjorndal, et al., 2009). Mass-communication techniques (web-based, television, radio, newspapers, pamphlets, posters) influence practitioner behavior, although

there is little evidence to determine their degree of influence and little to determine the most effective means of mass communication.

The IOM report and a number of individual studies indicate that local opinion leaders are effective in influencing the practice of healthcare providers and therefore may be effective in implementation of CPGs (Institute of Medicine [U.S.] & Graham 2011). The opinion leader should combine the respect of his or her colleagues in the community with effective communication skills. Dissemination of trustworthy CPGs through local opinion leaders, while potentially very effective, also carries the risk of introducing the individual biases and distortions of an individual physician, thereby lessening the power of CPGs for driving care consistency across broad care systems.

A related approach is termed "academic detailing," in which a knowledgeable person, who is usually a clinician with expertise in the area of concern, provides interactive face-to-face education for individual clinicians. In a fashion similar to that employed by pharmaceutical houses, the detail person visits target practitioners in order to explore their problems and potential local solutions, to discuss practitioner questions and concerns, and to provide written information on the CPG that may help in its acceptance and implementation. Although costly, academic detailing appears to consistently promote improvement in clinical practice and, by implication, would promote adherence to guidelines (O'Brien, Rogers, et al., 2007).

Audit and feedback (a continuous process in which performance is measured, data are collected in focused reports, and findings are discussed with practitioners) may promote practitioner adoption of CPG recommendations. Audit and feedback may incorporate either external or internal systematic and critical analysis of the quality of medical care. It may focus on the process of care, but more importantly should focus on patient outcomes. Direct discussion of audit results with practitioners appears to be a critical component of successful audit and feedback (Institute of Medicine [U.S.] &

Table 88.5 STEPS AND METHODS IN IMPLEMENTATION OF PRACTICE GUIDELINES

STEP	BARRIERS	IMPLEMENTATION STRATEGIES
Awareness of guideline	Overwhelming amount of medical literature	Traditional continuing medical education (CME)
		Print or online announcement of guideline
		Mass media dissemination to increase patient awareness in addition to practitioner awareness
Familiarity with guideline	Large, unwieldy documents	CME that focuses on specific recommendations from the guideline
	Information overload in general	Executive summaries of guidelines
Agreement with guideline	Competing guidelines	Opinion leaders
	Advancing evidence	Broad representation in guideline development
	Perception that guideline does not apply to "real-world patients"	Specialty society endorsement of the guideline
Self-efficacy of guideline end user	Practitioner skills in need of updating	CME focusing on skills development, interactive learning
	Infrastructure to support implementation of guideline	Audit and feedback of individual performance
		Electronic decision support
Expectation of positive outcomes	Skepticism about interventions	Audit and feedback of practice-wide performance
	Previous negative experience with guidelines	Benchmarking for outcomes
		Citation of previous published success at improving outcomes through implementation of guidelines
Overcome practice inertia	Resistance to change	Motivational strategies that include audit and feedback
		Opinion leaders
Insure appropriate organizational support	Poor staff support for the guideline	Institutional buy-in and strong leadership
	Poor reimbursement for guideline adherence	
	Lack of electronic support systems, including reminder system	

Adapted from Cabana, Rushton, et al. (2002).

Graham, 2011). Audit and feedback may be perceived as punitive by the receiving practitioner unless it is actionable and clearly focused on improvement. For audit and feedback to be effective, practitioners must perceive that the performance data are important, derived from a valid data source, and provided in a timely manner. Benchmarking, physician leadership, and sustained feedback over an extended time period improve the impact of audit and feedback. Individualized feedback may be more effective than broader group feedback, provided this is not seen as punitive.

The practice environment plays a major role in determining whether or not CPGs are implemented. Large healthcare organizations that include well-differentiated departments and decentralized decision-making seem better able to incorporate new innovations such as CPGs than are individual practitioners.

Tailored interventions incorporate needs-assessment for practitioners and organizations and then employ various implementation strategies to address identified needs or barriers. Naturally, this would generally lead to a multifaceted approach that includes two or more interventions targeting specific needs. For example, a practice that is challenged by clinical inertia might employ opinion leaders to influence the organization, along with motivational strategies based on audit and feedback.

The literature suggests that individual implementation methods meet with varying degrees of success, depending on the characteristics of the practice, the prevailing practice environment, and the needs of patients and practitioners. Medical psychiatrists may detect deviations from CPGs by other practitioners when their patients present with distress from adverse clinical or financial outcomes.

ELECTRONIC INTERVENTIONS

Electronic health records offer the opportunity to integrate CPGs through the use of clinical decision support. The IOM report on clinical practice guidelines recommends that "guideline developers should structure the format, vocabulary, and content of CPCs to facilitate ready implementation of computer-aided clinical decision support" (Institute of Medicine [U.S.] & Graham, 2011). This should enable practitioners to provide more personalized, guideline-based care in a timely fashion. Ideally, clinical decision support embedded within the electronic health record would obviate the need for intensive implementation programs discussed in the previous section. A recent study of the clinical decision-support system within a large integrated healthcare network found that four functional categories encompass the interaction between a clinical decision-support system and the clinical system itself: triggers, input data, interventions, and offered choices (Wright, Goldberg, et al., 2007). These functional categories are elaborated on in Table 88.6.

Unfortunately, the data necessary to allow clinical decision-support tools to consistently provide guideline-based recommendations are often lacking, or the systems may be unable to handle complex patient situations. Clinical decision-support tools may be aggravating for clinicians to use if they interrupt work flow or are simply unhelpful. For example, a report of a computerized physician order entry–based decision-support tool for evaluation of patients with possible pulmonary embolism found that the tool increased the yield of computed tomography (CT) angiography, but the physicians found the tool so cumbersome that they asked that it be removed from the system (Drescher, Chandrika, et al., 2011).

While computerized clinical decision support may ultimately offer reliable point-of-care application of recommendations from clinical practice guidelines, there are still many obstacles to overcome. In fact, some have argued that the volume of routine documentation required to comply with billing regulations limits the ability of electronic health records to provide decision support (Berenson, Basch, et al., 2011).

PERFORMANCE MEASUREMENT

Performance measurement is presumed necessary to improve quality of care and for meaningful implementation of CPGs. Quality of care has been defined as "the degree to which health care services for individuals and populations increase the likelihood of desired health outcomes and are consistent with current professional knowledge" (Institute of Medicine [U.S.], Lohr, et al., 1990). Clinical performance measurement, a subtype of quality measurement, assesses the degree to which a provider competently and safely delivers clinical services appropriate for the patient in the optimal time period. Such a measurement may include patient access, outcome of care, patient experience, process of care, or structure of the care unit. Clinical performance measurement has several purposes, including identifying poorly performing physicians, guiding professional development to help all physicians improve, and facilitating external validation for healthcare stakeholders (Scott, Phelps, et al., 2010). Performance measurement may be done at the practitioner level, at the hospital level, at the integrated healthcare systems level (e.g., Partners HealthCare in Massachusetts, Geisinger Health Systems in Pennsylvania), or at the geographic delivery area level. Physician clinical performance assessment is defined as "the quantitative assessment of physician performance based on the rates at which their patients experience certain outcomes of care and/or the rates at which physicians adhere to evidence-based processes of care during their actual practice of medicine" (Landon, Normand, et al., 2003).

Many performance measures have been proposed for many medical and surgical problems. The Agency for Healthcare Quality and Research (AHRQ) maintains an online, fully searchable database of quality measures accessible through the AHRQ website (www.ahrq.gov). The National Quality Forum (NQF; www.qualityforum.org) also provides an extensive database of quality measures.

Physicians have expressed concern about the validity and reliability of performance measures. This is particularly of concern at the individual physician level, where the number of patients with a condition considered for measurement may not be sufficient to produce reliable performance scores (Fung,

Table 88.6 FUNCTIONAL CATEGORIES IN CLINICAL DECISION SUPPORT

CATEGORY	DESCRIPTION	EXAMPLES
Triggers	Events in the clinical system that cause a decision-support rule to be invoked	Prescription of a drug Ordering a laboratory or radiological test Entering a new problem on the patient problem list
Input data	Data elements used by a rule to make inferences	Laboratory results Patient demographics Patient problem list
Interventions	Possible actions that the clinical decision support module can take	Send a message to the clinician Display a guideline or the relevant portion of the guideline Log that an event occurred
Offered choices	Provides the user with appropriate choices based on the clinical information and the clinical decision support algorithm	Allow clinician to cancel a medication order if patient allergies are detected in the clinical data Provide the clinician with alternative medications and ask for a choice

Adapted from Wright, Goldberg, et al. (2007).

Schmittdiel, et al., 2010). A study of primary care physicians, for example, found that relatively few primary practices include enough patients with specified conditions to allow reliable measurement of 10% relative differences in quality measures among fee-for-service Medicare patients (Nyweide, Weeks, et al., 2009). None of the practices in this study had caseloads that would allow reliable detection of 10% relative differences in preventable hospitalization or 30-day readmission after discharge for congestive heart failure. Additionally, the quality of data in electronic health records may not be robust enough to allow valid performance measurement (Pronovost & Lilford, 2011). Performance measurements of clinical care capture only a small percentage of overall patient care and may ignore the clinical judgement required to care for complex patients (Scott, Phelps, et al., 2010).

The Agency for Healthcare Research and Quality (AHRQ) recommends five questions to decide the validity of performance measurements:

1. How strong is the scientific evidence supporting the validity of this measure as a quality measure?

2. Are all individuals in the denominator (patients with the condition of interest) equally eligible for inclusion in the numerator (patients who experience the process or outcome)?

3. Is the measure result under the control of those whom the measure evaluates?

4. How well do the measure specifications capture the event that is the subject of the measure?

5. Does the measure provide for fair comparisons of the performance of providers, facilities, health plans, or geographic areas?

The final question above implies risk-adjustment for case severity and complexity, but the methodologies for risk-adjustment generate substantial controversy, potentially undermining the trust of practicing physicians and medical organizations. Pronovost and Lilford (2011) made five recommendations intended to improve performance or quality measurement, as follows:

1. *Ensure validity and transparency.* Measurement algorithms and risk adjustment formulas, which to date have often been proprietary and somewhat secretive, should be transparent and open to scrutiny. Measures should have "face validity," meaning that the measure appears to measure what it says it will measure. Measures should also demonstrate "criterion validity," meaning that they are related to real-world experience; and they should demonstrate "convergence validity," in that separate measures for a disease process would be highly correlated across a patient panel.

2. *Develop standard surveillance.* Systems should enable consistent and reproducible identification of events and of those at risk for events. The effort to identify these

numbers should be equivalent across institutions or practices. This is a critical issue, as (for example) a study focused on breast cancer screening in community health centers pointed out by demonstrating marked variation in screening rates, depending on the definition of eligible patients (Landon, O'Malley, et al., 2010).

3. *Evaluate performance change over time.* This recommendation requires sophisticated statistical expertise to risk-adjust for disparities among populations of patients.

4. *Build tools to prioritize measures.* These tools should take into account the concerns of the public and of healthcare stakeholders, the magnitude of problems, and the views of clinicians regarding available measures.

5. *Create an independent agency.* The agency would encourage the development and dissemination of measures and the collection of data independent of hospitals.

Specific to quality measures for processes of care, Chassin et al. argued for four criteria to be met in order to apply these measures on a broad scale (Chassin, Loeb, et al., 2010). First, and as emphasized above, there must be a strong evidence base showing that the care process leads to improved outcomes. Measures that lead to improved rates of "checking the right boxes" but that have no discernible benefit in patient outcomes or patient sense of well-being are to be avoided. A large quality-improvement study at community health centers demonstrated improvement in *processes* of care (e.g., use of asthma management plan, assessment of smoking status, assessment of hemoglobin A1C for diabetics, checking lipid profile in hypertensives), but it failed to demonstrate improvement in intermediate clinical *outcomes* (e.g., urgent care or hospitalization for asthma, control of hemoglobin A1C in diabetics) (Landon, Hicks, et al., 2007). In this study, it seemed apparent that simply "checking the box" that the patient had been given a management plan for their asthma did not affect the disease process itself and did not affect triggers for asthma exacerbations.

Second, the performance measure must accurately capture the actual delivery of evidence-based care (Chassin, Loeb, et al., 2010). For example, a quality measure of discharge teaching might be fulfilled by simply documenting that discharge teaching for heart failure self-management has been done when the "discharge teaching" consists solely of a printed handout's being given to the patient. This is far less effective than intensive instruction (Phillips, Wright, et al., 2004).

Third, the process measure should address a process that is close in time to the desired outcome, and there should be a limited number of intervening processes between the measured process and the outcome (Chassin, Loeb, et al., 2010). This criterion should be applied more strictly in the hospital setting because of the time course of acute illness, while in ambulatory settings the care process may well be further removed from the desired outcome (e.g., mammography and reduction in breast cancer mortality).

Fourth, and of great importance, the process measure should not lead to unintended adverse consequences (Chassin,

Loeb, et al., 2010). A classic example of this problem has been the quality measure aimed at the timely administration of antibiotics for community-acquired pneumonia, which led to many patients without pneumonia being treated with antibiotics (Houck, Bratzler, et al., 2004; Kanwar, Brar, et al., 2007). The pressure to beat a deadline on administration of antibiotics caused physicians to prescribe antibiotics based on inadequate evaluations, such as clinical presentation with productive cough only to determine later that there was no radiological evidence of pneumonia. Use of beta-blockers for perioperative cardiac risk reduction provides another example of a process measure leading to unintended adverse events (Auerbach & Goldman, 2002; Lindenauer, Pekow, et al., 2005). In this situation, early, small randomized trials suggested a reduction in cardiac adverse events among patients given beta-blockers, but subsequently, a large cohort study and large randomized trials failed to show benefit (Lindenauer, Pekow, et al., 2005; Devereaux, Yang, et al., 2008). In this situation, the process measure was adopted by many hospitals before there was truly sufficient clinical evidence to back it. The unintended consequences of performance measures cannot be reliably predicted and require continuous updating from accumulating evidence and updated CPGs.

The American College of Cardiology Foundation, American Heart Association, American Medical Association (ACCF/AHA/AMA) performance measurement set for patients with coronary artery disease (Drozda, Messer, et al., 2011) is provided in Table 88.7 as an example of the types of measures that might be monitored for a physician caring for patients with a single disorder, or for a system caring for a population of patients with a disorder. Multiple CPGs support this set of performance measurements (Chobanian, Bakris, et al., 2003; Gibbons, Abrams, et al., 2003; Eagle, Guyton, et al., 2004; Anderson, Adams, et al., 2007; Mosca, Banka, et al., 2007; Antman, Hand, et al., 2008; Douglas, Khandheria, et al., 2008). Although some of the measures require chart-review to collect the data (e.g., symptom and activity assessment, symptom management, cardiac rehabilitation), most of the measures could be produced by combining data from pharmacy and diagnosis databases. Although small practices are challenged in measuring these parameters across the practice (Landon & Normand, 2008), increasing adoption of electronic health records holds promise that such performance measure sets can be produced efficiently and consistently.

Employing performance measures in a rigid and non-critical fashion threatens to undermine the health of the substantial minority of patients who would benefit from creative and innovative care. It seems very likely that the majority of patients, who have relatively straightforward problems and concerns, will benefit from greater consistency in the delivery of care. An unintended systems consequence may be the dampening of innovation among specialists and tertiary care centers as these providers strive to meet performance targets even though the complexity of their patients demands deviation from regimented care. In fact, tertiary centers and their consulting physicians should be caring for atypical and complex patients to justify the high cost of care in these centers.

INCENTIVES

In an attempt to overcome resistance to practice changes recommended in clinical practice guidelines, insurers,

Table 88.7 ACCF/AHA/AMA PERFORMANCE MEASURES FOR CORONARY ARTERY DISEASE

MEASURE	DESCRIPTION	TYPE OF MEASURE
Blood pressure (BP) control	% patients who have BP in target range <140/90 or have BP >140/90 but were prescribed two or more antihypertensives	Treatment outcome
Lipid control	% patients who have LDL cholesterol <100 mg/dL or who have LDL > 100 mg/dL and documented plan of care, including at minimum prescription for a statin	Treatment outcome or process
Symptom and activity assessment	% patients with documentation in the medical record of activity level or presence or absence of angina	Patient-centered outcome, process measure
Symptom management	% patients with evaluation of level of activity AND evaluation of anginal symptoms with documented and appropriate plan of care	Patient-centered outcome
Tobacco-use screening and intervention	% patients screened for tobacco AND received counseling if using tobacco	Process
Antiplatelet therapy	% patients prescribed aspirin or clopidogrel	Treatment
Beta-blocker therapy	% patients with prior myocardial infarction or left ventricular ejection fraction (LVEF) < 40% who are prescribed a beta-blocker	Treatment
Angiotensin converting enzyme (ACE) inhibitor/ Angiotensin receptor blocker (ARB) therapy	% patients with diabetes or LVEF <40% who are prescribed an ACE inhibitor or ARB	Treatment
Cardiac rehabilitation	% cardiac patients (broadly defined) who were referred to a cardiac rehabilitation program	Treatment, process

governmental payors, and healthcare systems employ physician or practitioner incentives. These incentives are generally financial and include so-called pay-for-performance (P4P). The incentives may take the form of a bonus for achieving target goals in performance measurement or for demonstrating improvement in performance. Bonus programs may dictate competition between providers, resulting in winners and losers (Rosenthal, Fernandopulle, et al., 2004). In competitive programs, an arbitrarily set percentage of providers receives a bonus for performance, or there may be graduated performance bonuses based on relative performance rank. Alternatively, the practitioner or healthcare delivery system may receive a bonus for simply reaching the predetermined performance target. It is thought that the competitive incentive system is more effective in implementing change, although at a cost to morale and self-esteem of the lower performing providers. In a deterrent approach to incentives, the practitioner may be penalized for failure to achieve quality, process, or outcome goals.

Many incentive programs have evolved and have been widely adopted during the past 15 years, despite a remarkably sparse evidence base to support their use. In fact, a systematic review of P4P programs found positive or partially positive effects on measures of quality, but also found unintended adverse outcomes, and found no argument for cost-effectiveness (Petersen, Woodard, et al., 2006).

Pay-for-performance programs may seek to influence care at any of the following levels: individual practitioner, practice group, or hospital. Table 88.8 summarizes advantages and disadvantages at each of these levels.

INDIVIDUAL PRACTITIONER INCENTIVES

Financial incentives for individual physicians seem to be a reasonable approach to improving performance or meeting quality targets. Ideally, these P4P programs would incentivize

quality measures that are well validated by guidelines, can be reliably measured, and are important to patient outcomes. Although there are clearly advantages to focusing P4P on the individual practitioner, challenges include much less precision in measurement given smaller numbers of patients, and the potential burden imposed on a practice by reporting requirements. Additionally, rewarding practitioners for a limited number of quality metrics may result in the unintended consequence of diverting their focus from other important patient problems, or prompting physicians to avoid "high-risk" patients in their practice.

Studies of practitioner-level P4P have shown mixed results. For example, a study of the effect of financial incentives on the outcomes of hypertension management in the United Kingdom found that even generous financial rewards had no effect on processes of care or hypertension-related clinical outcomes (Serumaga, Ross-Degnan, et al., 2011). In contrast, a P4P program aimed at improving care for cardiovascular disease patients in a large health plan in Hawaii found that a program incentivizing individual practitioners with approximately 3.5% of their base professional fees (to a maximum of $16,000 per year) resulted in improved rates of low-density lipoprotein (LDL)-cholesterol testing and prescription of a statin for this patient group (Chen, Tian, et al., 2011). Although these quality measures seem simple and relatively easy to fulfill, the most impressive finding in this program was that patients who received high-quality care as judged by LDL testing and statin prescription experienced fewer new coronary events and were less likely to be hospitalized.

A P4P program in a large group practice that changed from group-focused to physician-specific incentives for nine process and clinical-outcome measures in primary care showed significant improvements during the year after implementation (Chung, Palaniappan, et al., 2010). The incentive in this program was a relatively modest maximum of $5,000 per year, but it was not clear that the incentive produced the

Table 88.8 PAY FOR PERFORMANCE (P4P)

LEVEL	ADVANTAGES	DISADVANTAGES
Practitioner	Individual accountability	Potential individual burden for data collection
	Clearer link of incentive to individual patient care/outcomes	Smaller patient numbers reduces precision of measurement
	Local decision-making, tends to be more "nimble with change"	Greater impact of "adverse patient characteristics"
		Less resources to implement change
Practice group	Increased numbers of patients improve the precision of measurements	Less individual motivation; temptation for "coasting by individuals"
	Greater resources to implement change, but need for consensus	Competing priorities within the group
	Shared burden for data collection	
Hospital	Many more patients to facilitate meaningful measurements	Greater heterogeneity of patients may make measurements less targeted
	More resources and expertise for measurement	Slower response to change unless very strong administration
	Administrative support for P4P	Limited individual motivation on the front lines ("What's in it for me?" phenomenon)
	Adverse patient characteristics more broadly distributed, "averaging" advantage	

positive results, as two comparator physician groups achieved similar improvements in the same time period without P4P incentives.

A systematic review of P4P studies found that programs aimed at the individual provider level or at the team level tended to report positive results (Van Herck, De Smedt, et al., 2010). Reporting bias may distort the perception of effectiveness of these programs.

PRACTICE GROUP INCENTIVES

A P4P scheme at the practice group level in England focusing on the care of patients with asthma, diabetes, and coronary heart disease found improvement in asthma and diabetes care early in the program (Campbell, Reeves, et al., 2009). However, the improvement in quality of care was not sustained, and continuity of care actually declined during the incentive program.

A systematic review found that medical groups performed better in P4P programs than independent practice associations (Van Herck, De Smedt, et al., 2010). This may reflect better-organized practices that incorporate multidisciplinary approaches, utilize clinical pathways, and deploy greater resources both for quality improvement and for quality measurement.

HOSPITAL-BASED INCENTIVES

A hospital-based P4P program implemented through Massachusetts Medicaid (MassHealth) in 2008 provided incentives to hospitals for quality of care for patients with pneumonia and for prevention of surgery-associated infections (Ryan & Blustein, 2011). The measures for pneumonia care included oxygenation assessment, blood cultures performed before antibiotics, smoking-cessation counseling, initial antibiotic given within six hours of arrival at the hospital, and appropriate antibiotic selection for immunocompetent patients. Measures for surgical infection prevention were prophylactic antibiotic within one hour of surgical incision, appropriate antibiotic selection, and prophylactic antibiotic discontinuation within 24 hours after surgery end time. The financial incentives in 2008 averaged $40,000 per hospital, with the 75th percentile incentive being $57,447. The potential payout at the 99th percentile was $331,000. These incentives were labeled "generous." A subsequent study of the program found no evidence that it improved quality during the first two years after it began (Ryan & Blustein, 2011). It seems very likely that the incentives, on a hospital level, were insufficient to effect change, and in fact, providing resources to simply manage the data required for the program would cost much more than the average payout.

The Premier Hospital Quality Incentive Demonstration project, sponsored by the Centers for Medicare and Medicaid Services (CMS) and studying the 260 hospitals in the Premier, Inc., hospital system, examined the effect of P4P on quality at these hospitals (Werner, Kolstad, et al., 2011). This program was competitive, with the top 20% of hospitals receiving payouts during the first two years of the program, while hospitals performing below a threshold had to pay penalties beginning in the program's third year. This study found that performance in care of acute myocardial infarction, heart failure, and pneumonia improved under P4P during the first three years the program compared to hospitals not participating in the P4P program. However, by the fifth year of the program, the control hospitals caught up in quality measures, leading the study to conclude that the effect of P4P was not sustained. Not surprisingly, the hospitals that were the largest, best financed, eligible for the largest bonuses, and operated in regions with less competition for bonuses fared the best in this program.

OPTIMIZING INCENTIVES

Based on the results of the systematic review of P4P studies, Van Herck et al. recommend the following for incentive programs (Van Herck, De Smedt, et al., 2010):

1. Targets for P4P programs should be those for which there is room for improvement. This should lessen the impact of a ceiling effect in which high-performing practitioners or systems have no real room for improvement.

2. Target measures should use process and clinical outcome measures. Although outcome measures are preferred for reasons previously discussed, these require adequate risk adjustment.

3. Involvement of stakeholders in development, implementation, and evaluation of the P4P program is key to full engagement.

4. If multiple payors are funding similar P4P programs, design should be uniform across the programs.

5. The P4P program should focus on quality improvement and achievement. This recommendation addresses the issue of achieving a performance threshold that tends to be motivating for high-performing providers, while recognizing that low-performing providers may have difficulty meeting a high threshold, but may be motivated by improvement goals.

6. The P4P program should distribute incentives at the individual level or at the team level, as this appears to be more effective than institutional incentives.

7. The P4P should be refocused once goals are achieved, although it is important to continue to monitor old targets.

8. Incentive size needs to be sufficient to motivate active participation and improvement. Unfortunately, the studies of this issue are conflicting, and there is not yet good guidance on the "dose–response" relationship for P4P.

9. Quality improvement requires adequate infrastructure support and education on quality-improvement tools. Evidence is conflicting on whether or not this is adequate to effect improvement without the addition of P4P.

In summary, incentives or "pay-for-performance" programs may have the potential to speed implementation of clinical practice guidelines, but the evidence for their impact and cost-effectiveness is somewhat limited and conflicting. Petersen et al. (2006) posed a series of research questions regarding financial incentives in health care, which are included in Table 88.9. Although the literature is growing, these questions need further consideration.

PRACTICAL APPLICATION OF GUIDELINES

How does the internist actually use guidelines? Obviously, there is no way to refer to a guideline for every active problem for each patient during every patient encounter. In general, internists use guidelines to answer discrete management questions. For example, a patient with an upper-extremity (UE) deep venous thrombosis (DVT) in association with a percutaneously inserted central catheter (PICC) presents management issues. Should the patient be anticoagulated? For how long? Should the catheter be removed?

An early 2012 PubMed search using the search term "Upper extremity deep venous thrombosis" and the limits *Practice guideline, English language, published within five years*, yields a single citation: *Antithrombotic therapy for venous thromboembolic disease: American College of Chest Physicians evidence-based clinical practice guidelines* (8th edition) (Kearon, Kahn, et al., 2008). This guideline fulfills the criteria for a trustworthy CPG. The relevant recommendations for one particular patient appear as follows in the guideline:

8.1. INTRAVENOUS UNFRACTIONATED HEPARIN (UFH) OR SUBCUTANEOUS LOW MOLECULAR WEIGHT HEPARIN (LMWH) FOR THE INITIAL TREATMENT OF UPPER-EXTREMITY DVT

8.1.1. For patients with acute upper-extremity DVT (UEDVT), we recommend initial treatment with therapeutic doses of LMWH, UFH, or fondaparinux as described for leg DVT [Grade IC].

8.4 ANTICOAGULANTS FOR THE LONGTERM TREATMENT OF UEDVT

8.4.1. For patients with acute UEDVT we recommend treatment with a Vitamin K Antagonist (VKA) for ≥ 3 months (Grade 1C).

Remark: A similar process as for lower-extremity DVT should be used to determine the optimal duration of anti-coagulation.

8.4.2. For most patients with UEDVT in association with an indwelling central venous catheter, we suggest that the catheter not be removed if it is functional and there is an ongoing need for the catheter (Grade 2C).

8.4.3. For patients who have UEDVT in association with an indwelling central venous catheter that is removed, we do not recommend that the duration of long-term anticoagulant treatment be shortened to < 3 months (Grade 2C).

The answers for the clinical questions for this patient are clear. The patient should be anticoagulated with low-molecular-weight heparin followed by warfarin. Anticoagulation with warfarin should be continued for at least three months. The catheter does not need to be removed.

For many situations, recommendations are less definitive, and even with definitive recommendations, there may be

Table 88.9 RESEARCH QUESTIONS REGARDING FINANCIAL INCENTIVES IN HEALTH CARE

DOMAIN	QUESTIONS
Fundamental	How effective are financial incentives for quality?
	Are pay-for-performance programs cost-effective?
	Within what types of payment structures are financial incentives most effective?
	What proportion of healthcare payments should depend on performance?
Targets for incentives	What types of clinical conditions or health care services should be the target of financial incentives to improve quality of care? Chronic diseases? Acute care? One-time preventive care services?
	Within what types of practice settings are financial incentives most effective?
	What types of quality measures should be targets: processes, outcomes, or both?
	Are financial incentives to limit overuse of services effective?
Practical issues	What are the optimum magnitude, frequency, and duration of financial incentives for quality?
	Should performance targets be set as absolute thresholds, relative performance improvement goals, or both?
Further impact	Does the effect of financial incentives persist after the incentives are stopped?
	Do financial incentives have unintended consequences for patient care activities that are not incentivized?

Adapted from Petersen, .Woodard, et al. (2006).

coexisting medical issues, psychosocial issues, financial considerations, and patient preferences may require tailoring the recommendations for the individual patient. Ideally, reasons for deviations from evidence-based recommendations should be carefully documented.

Patients may present their physicians with CPGs gleaned from electronic searches. In fact, some professional societies provide patient-oriented distillations of CPGs for particular problems. For example, the American Society of Clinical Oncology (ASCO) provides a series, *What to Know: ASCO's Guideline on...*, for a number of topics of interest to patients. The physician should welcome open discussion of guidelines discovered by patients, but should also address issues of their validity with patients, as well as discussing the utility of particular guidelines for the patient's individual circumstance.

If the simple patient scenario were expanded to include a recent history of life-threatening gastrointestinal hemorrhage of obscure origin despite extensive evaluation, the recommendations from the guideline may no longer apply. Clearly, physician judgement would supersede rote application of the guideline in this circumstance.

Performance measurement evaluating a physician group's management of UEDVT points out inherent challenges. The majority of patients would benefit from anticoagulation for UEDVT, as recommended by the guideline. However, patients at risk for hemorrhage might incur greater risk with anticoagulation. The physician then faces a dilemma of whether or not to push for anticoagulation, thereby improving her performance score, particularly if the performance measure focuses solely on whether or not anticoagulation was administered, not on the patient's outcome. Additionally, performance measurement may focus the physician's attention more intently on the measured aspect of care to the exclusion of other equally important clinical issues.

If we increase the complexity of the scenario, further limitations for CPGs and performance measurement emerge. Suppose that the patient has a patent foramen ovale (PFO), placing them at risk for systemic emboli and stroke from the evolving upper extremity deep venous thrombosis. Suppose also that the thrombosis is extensive and has resulted in marked swelling of the upper extremity. There are no guidelines for this situation. Management would require careful consideration by experienced clinicians and multidisciplinary consultants. Guidelines, no matter how nuanced and evidence-based, will never supplant the judgement of physicians in managing complex medical, surgical, and psychiatric problems. CPGs should be considered a starting point for management, not the final "cookbook" solution for problems.

SUMMARY

Trustworthy clinical practice guidelines should distill burgeoning clinical research into valid recommendations that can be implemented by practitioners in the care of individual patients. This chapter provided a framework for assessing the trustworthiness of CPGs. Effectively translating CPG recommendations requires performance measurement. Numerous metrics, many derived directly from CPGs, have been proposed, but they require substantial commitment and resources for useful measurement. Financial incentives may facilitate more rapid and effective implementation of CPGs, but they depend on valid performance measurement. While CPGs may facilitate more efficient and appropriate care of patients, they should never supplant the clinical judgement of a careful, thoughtful physician.

CLINICAL PEARLS

- Clinical practice guidelines (CPG) provide the underpinnings for performance measurements that have become commonplace for hospitals, practice groups, and individual practitioners.

- The IOM definition of CPGs is: "Clinical practice guidelines are statements that include recommendations intended to optimize patient care that are informed by a systematic review of evidence and an assessment of the benefits and harms of alternative care options."

- The medical psychiatrist can play a pivotal role in helping to identify patients who would benefit from less reliance on CPGs, while carefully documenting the rationale in order to avoid negative performance measurement.

- Sound clinical judgement should never be supplanted by a CPG.

- Medical psychiatrists may detect deviations from CPGs by other practitioners when their patients present with distress from adverse clinical or financial outcomes.

- Employing performance measures in a rigid and non-critical fashion threatens to undermine the health of the substantial minority of patients who would benefit from creative and innovative care.

- Ideally, reasons for deviations from evidence-based recommendations should be carefully documented.

- Measures that lead to improved rates of "checking the right boxes" but have no discernable benefit in patient outcomes or patient sense of well-being are to be avoided.

- The physician should welcome open discussion of guidelines discovered by patients, but should also address issues of validity with patients as well as discussing the utility of particular guidelines for the patient's individual circumstance.

- The unintended consequences of performance measures cannot be reliably predicted and require continuous updating from accumulating evidence and updated CPGs.

DISCLOSURE STATEMENT

Dr. Hunt has no relevant financial disclosures.

REFERENCES

ACC/AHA. (2010). Methodology manual and policies from the ACCF/AHA Task Force on Practice Guidelines. Accessed July 22, 2011 from http://my.americanheart.org/idc/groups/ahamah-public/@wcm/@sop/documents/downloadable/ucm_319826.pdf.

Agency for Healthcare Research and Quality (AHRQ) Measure validity: Using the NQMC template of measure attributes to assess the validity of measures. Retrieved July 29, 2011, from http://www.qualitymeasures.ahrq.gov/iedetect.aspx.

Anderson, J. L., Adams, C. D., et al. (2007). 2007 Guidelines for the management of patients with unstable angina/non-ST-elevation myocardial infarction: A report of the American College of Cardiology/American Heart Association Task Force on Practice Guidelines (Writing Committee to revise the 2002 Guidelines for the management of patients with unstable angina/non ST-elevation myocardial infarction): Developed in collaboration with the American College of Emergency Physicians, the Society for Cardiovascular Angiography and Interventions, and the Society of Thoracic Surgeons: Endorsed by the American Association of Cardiovascular and Pulmonary Rehabilitation and the Society for Academic Emergency Medicine. *Circulation, 116*(7), e148–e304.

Antman, E. M., Hand, M., et al. (2008). 2007 focused update of the 2004 Guidelines for the management of patients with ST-elevation myocardial infarction: A report of the American College of Cardiology/American Heart Association Task Force on Practice Guidelines: Developed in collaboration with the Canadian Cardiovascular Society, endorsed by the American Academy of Family Physicians: 2007 Writing Group to review new evidence and update the ACC/AHA 2004 guidelines for the management of patients with ST-elevation myocardial infarction, writing on behalf of the 2004 Writing Committee. *Circulation, 117*(2), 296–329.

Auerbach, A. D., & Goldman, L. (2002). Beta-blockers and reduction of cardiac events in noncardiac surgery: Scientific review. *Journal of the American Medical Association, 287*(11), 1435–1444.

Bales, R. F., & Strodtbeck, F. L., (1951). Phases in group problem-solving. *Journal of Abnormal Social Psychology, 46*(4), 485–495.

Berenson, R. A., Basch, P., et al. (2011). Revisiting E&M visit guidelines—A missing piece of payment reform. *New England Journal of Medicine, 364*(20), 1892–1895.

Boyd, C. M., Darer, J., et al. (2005). Clinical practice guidelines and quality of care for older patients with multiple comorbid diseases: Implications for pay for performance. *Journal of the American Medical Association, 294*(6), 716–724.

Brouwers, M. C., Kho, M. E., et al. (2010). Development of the AGREE II, part 2: Assessment of validity of items and tools to support application. *Canadian Medical Association Journal, 182*(10), E472–E478.

Burgers, J. S., Grol, R. P., et al. (2003). Characteristics of effective clinical guidelines for general practice. *British Journal of General Practice, 53*(486), 15–19.

Cabana, M. D., Rushton, J. L., et al. (2002). Implementing practice guidelines for depression: Applying a new framework to an old problem. *General Hospital Psychiatry, 24*(1), 35–42.

Campbell, S. M., Reeves, D., et al. (2009). Effects of pay for performance on the quality of primary care in England. *New England Journal of Medicine, 361*(4), 368–378.

Chassin, M. R., Loeb, J. M., et al. (2010). Accountability measures—using measurement to promote quality improvement. *New England Journal of Medicine, 363*(7), 683–688.

Chen, J. Y., Tian, H., et al. (2011). Does pay for performance improve cardiovascular care in a "real-world" setting? *American Journal of Medical Quality, 26*(5), 340–348.

Chobanian, A. V., Bakris, G. L., et al. (2003). Seventh report of the Joint National Committee on Prevention, Detection, Evaluation, and Treatment of High Blood Pressure. *Hypertension, 42*(6), 1206–1252.

Chung, S., Palaniappan, L. P., et al. (2010). Effect of physician-specific pay-for-performance incentives in a large group practice. *American Journal of Managed Care, 16*(2), e35–e42.

Cluzeau, F., Burgers, J., et al. (2003). Development and validation of an international appraisal instrument for assessing the quality of clinical practice guidelines: The AGREE project. *Quality & Safety in Health Care, 12*(1), 18–23.

Devereaux, P. J., Yang, H., et al. (2008). Effects of extended-release metoprolol succinate in patients undergoing non-cardiac surgery (POISE trial), a randomised controlled trial. *Lancet, 371*(9627), 1839–1847.

Douglas, P. S., Khandheria, B., et al. (2008). 2008 Appropriateness Criteria for stress echocardiography: A report of the American College of Cardiology Foundation Appropriateness Criteria Task Force, American Society of Echocardiography, American College of Emergency Physicians, American Heart Association, American Society of Nuclear Cardiology, Society for Cardiovascular Angiography and Interventions, Society of Cardiovascular Computed Tomography, and Society for Cardiovascular Magnetic Resonance; endorsed by the Heart Rhythm Society and the Society of Critical Care Medicine. *Journal of the American College of Cardiology, 51*(11), 1127–1147.

Drescher, F. S., Chandrika, S., et al. (2011). Effectiveness and acceptability of a computerized decision support system using modified Wells criteria for evaluation of suspected pulmonary embolism. *Annals of Emergency Medicine, 57*(6), 613–621.

Drozda, J., Jr., Messer, J. V., et al. (2011). 2011 Performance Measures for adults with coronary artery disease and hypertension: A report of the American College of Cardiology Foundation, American Heart Association Task Force on Performance Measures, and the American Medical Association–Physician Consortium for Performance Improvement. *Journal of the American College of Cardiology, 58*(3), 316–336.

Eagle, K. A., Guyton, R. A., et al. (2004). 2004 Guideline update for coronary artery bypass graft surgery: A report of the American College of Cardiology, American Heart Association Task Force on Practice Guidelines (Committee to update the 1999 Guidelines for coronary artery bypass graft surgery). *Circulation, 110*(14), e340–e437.

Farmer, A. P., Legare, F., et al. (2008). Printed educational materials: Effects on professional practice and health care outcomes. *Cochrane Database of Systematic Reviews*, (3), CD004398.

Forsetlund, L., Bjorndal, A., et al. (2009). Continuing education meetings and workshops: Effects on professional practice and health care outcomes. *Cochrane Database of Systematic Reviews*, (2), CD003030.

Fung, V., Schmittdiel, J. A., et al. (2010). Meaningful variation in performance: A systematic literature review. *Medical Care, 48*(2), 140–148.

Gibbons, R. J., Abrams, J., et al. (2003). 2002 Guideline Update for the management of patients with chronic stable angina—summary article: A report of the American College of Cardiology, American Heart Association Task Force on Practice Guidelines (Committee on the management of patients with chronic stable angina). *Circulation, 107*(1), 149–158.

Houck, P. M., Bratzler, D. W., et al. (2004). Timing of antibiotic administration and outcomes for Medicare patients hospitalized with community-acquired pneumonia. *Archives of Internal Medicine, 164*(6), 637–644.

Institute of Medicine (U.S.) Committee on Standards for Developing Trustworthy Clinical Practice Guidelines, & Graham, R. (2011). *Clinical practice guidelines we can trust.* Washington, DC: National Academies Press.

Institute of Medicine (U.S.) Division of Health Care Services, & Lohr, K. N., et al. (1990). *Medicare: A strategy for quality assurance.* Washington, DC: National Academies Press.

Kanwar, M., Brar, N., et al. (2007). Misdiagnosis of community-acquired pneumonia and inappropriate utilization of antibiotics: Side effects of the 4-H antibiotic administration rule. *Chest, 131*(6), 1865–1869.

Kearon, C., Kahn, S. R., et al. (2008). Antithrombotic therapy for venous thromboembolic disease: American College of Chest Physicians evidence-based clinical practice guidelines (8th ed.). *Chest, 133*(6 Suppl), 454S–545S.

Landon, B. E., Hicks, L. S., et al. (2007). Improving the management of chronic disease at community health centers. *New England Journal of Medicine, 356*(9), 921–934.

Landon, B. E., & Normand, S. L., (2008). Performance measurement in the small office practice: Challenges and potential solutions. *Annals of Internal Medicine, 148*(5), 353–357.

Landon, B. E., Normand, S. L., et al. (2003). Physician clinical performance assessment: Prospects and barriers. *Journal of the American Medical Association, 290*(9), 1183–1189.

Landon, B. E., O'Malley, A. J., et al. (2010). Can choice of the sample population affect perceived performance? Implications for performance assessment. *Journal of General Internal Medicine, 25*(2), 104–109.

Lindenauer, P. K., Pekow, P., et al. (2005). Perioperative beta-blocker therapy and mortality after major noncardiac surgery. *New England Journal of Medicine, 353*(4), 349–361.

Mosca, L., Banka, C. L., et al. (2007). Evidence-based guidelines for cardiovascular disease prevention in women: 2007 update. *Journal of the American College of Cardiology, 49*(11), 1230–1250.

Murphy, E., Dingwall, R., et al. (1998). Qualitative research methods in health technology assessment: A review of the literature. *Health Technology Assessment, 2*(16), iii–ix, 1–274.

National Quality Forum. NQF-endorsed standards. Retrieved July 29, 2011, from http://www.qualityforum.org/Measures_List.aspx.

Nyweide, D. J., Weeks, W. B., et al. (2009). Relationship of primary care physicians' patient caseload with measurement of quality and cost performance. *Journal of the American Medical Association, 302*(22), 2444–2450.

O'Brien, M. A., Rogers, S., et al. (2007). Educational outreach visits: Effects on professional practice and health care outcomes. *Cochrane Database of Systematic Reviews, (4)*, CD000409.

Petersen, L. A., Woodard, L. D., et al. (2006). Does pay-for-performance improve the quality of health care? *Annals of Internal Medicine, 145*(4), 265–272.

Phillips, C. O., Wright, S. M., et al. (2004). Comprehensive discharge planning with postdischarge support for older patients with congestive heart failure: A meta-analysis. *Journal of the American Medical Association, 291*(11), 1358–1367.

Pronovost, P. J., & Lilford, R. (2011). Analysis and commentary: A road map for improving the performance of performance measures. *Health Affairs (Millwood), 30*(4), 569–573.

Rosenthal, M. B., Fernandopulle, R., et al. (2004). Paying for quality: Providers' incentives for quality improvement. *Health Affairs (Millwood), 23*(2), 127–141.

Ryan, A. M., & Blustein, J. (2011). The effect of the MassHealth hospital pay-for-performance program on quality. *Health Services Research, 46*(3), 712–728.

Scott, I. A., & Guyatt, G. H. (2011). Clinical practice guidelines: The need for greater transparency in formulating recommendations. *Medical Journal of Australia, 195*(1), 29–33.

Scott, I. A., Phelps, G., et al. (2011). Assessing individual clinical performance—a primer for physicians. *Internal Medicine Journal, 41*(2), 144–155.

Serumaga, B., Ross-Degnan, D., et al. (2011). Effect of pay for performance on the management and outcomes of hypertension in the United Kingdom: Interrupted time series study. *British Medical Journal, 342*, d108.

Spitzer, W. O., Bayne, J. R. D., et al. (1979). The periodic health examination.Canadian Task Force on the Periodic Health Exam *Canadian Medical Association Journal, 121*(9), 1193–1254.

Van Herck, P., De Smedt, D., et al. (2010). Systematic review: Effects, design choices, and context of pay-for-performance in health care. *BioMed Central Health Services Research, 10*, 247.

Werner, R. M., Kolstad, J. T., et al. (2011). The effect of pay-for-performance in hospitals: Lessons for quality improvement. *Health Affairs (Millwood), 30*(4), 690–698.

Wright, A., Goldberg, H., et al. (2007). A description and functional taxonomy of rule-based decision support content at a large integrated delivery network. *Journal of the American Medical Informatics Association, 14*(4), 489–496.

INDEX

California Verbal Learning Test II (CLVT II), 564
caloric intake
   vs. macronutrient composition, 1128–1129
   reducing, 1133
CAM. *See* complementary and alternative medicine ; Confusion Assessment Method
CAM-ICU. *See* Confusion Assessment Method for Intensive Care unit
cAMP. *See* cyclic adenosine monophosphate
CAMS. *See* Child/Adolescent Anxiety Multimodal Study
CAM therapies, model guidelines for use of, 548
Camberwell Family Interview, 210
Camellia sinensis (green tea, theanine), 552, 563*t*
   herb-drug interactions, 589
Campral. *See* acamprosate
Canadian Regional Capacity Assessment Team, 1627
Canadian Stroke Network, standards for VCI study, 922
Canadian Task Force on Periodic Health Examination, 1688
cancer
   bladder, 1481–1483
      management of distress, 1482–1483
      surgical and medical management, 1482
   brain, 1034–1041
      care issues, 1037–1039
      treatment, 1035–1037
   breast
      effect of group psychotherapy on patients with, 235
      hormone replacement therapy and, 1345
   in children, hypnosis procedures for, 284
   as chronic illness, 230
   chronic pain and, 731
   coping with, 1182–1184
   and delirium, 824, 825*t*
   depression in, 1189
   dyspnea in patients with, 536
   family interventions for, 206, 207
   fatigue from, 698
   group therapy for patients with, 234
   gynecological, 1330–1331
   and hypercalcemia, 127
   medicines with anticholinergic effects, 838*t*
   melanoma, brain metastases, 1035
   mood impacted by, 231
   pancreatic, case example, 219, 222, 225–226
   in parents of minor children, 218
   patients obtaining second opinions to seek reassurance and information, 1583
   prevalence rate
      for ASD related to, 623
      of PTSD in, 625
   prostate, and suicide risk, 784
   psychiatric care of patient, 1182–1194
   risk from hypnotics, 402
   sleep disorders, 681
   stage at diagnosis, suicide risk related to, 784
   suicide rates with, 784
   suicide risk, 783*t*
   supportive-expressive therapy for patients, 236
   survivors' sexual issues, 725–726

in transplant recipients, 1442
treatment
   adaptogens in reducing chemotoxic effects on bone marrow and liver, 594–595
   hypnosis in, 275
   mind-body therapies for tolerance, 315
   problems, 230
   traumatic implications years after initial treatment, 1544
   worry about recurrent, 1375
   zolpidem and, 408
cancer patients, delirium in, 825
candesartan, for migraine treatment, 970*t*, 974*t*
Candida, 1243
candidiasis, 1243
   in mouth, 28
candidiasis hypersensitivity syndrome, 1243
cannabidiol, 770
cannabinoids, 522
   for nausea and vomiting, 533
   for pain management, in systemic lupus erythematosus, 1257
cannabis (*Cannabis sativa*), 770
   antiemetic and analgesic effects, 770
   anxiety prominent with panic reactions in naïve users, 637
   chronic use, 770
   cyclical vomiting syndrome from, 529
   CYP1A2 induced by, 456
   and CYP2C9, 456, 457
   intoxication, characteristics, 770
   as porphyrias trigger, 1205
   treatment of dependence, 770
   use in pregnancy, 1357
cannabis hyperemesis syndrome, vs. cyclic vomiting syndrome, 1171
cannibalistic consumption, of dead relatives, 1245
Cannon, Walter, 306, 488
capacities, competency, and consent, psychiatric literature on, 1619
capacity
   context-dependency, 1627
   evaluation requests from irreconcilable difference, 1639
   inappropriate behavior due to lost, 1619
   to make decision or perform act, 1620
   specificity of, 1626–1627
CAPD. *See* continuous ambulatory peritoneal dialysis
Caplan, G., 200
CAPS. *See* Clinician Administered PTSD Scale
capsaicin, 521, 732
   high-dose, 736
   for neuropathic pain, 1500
captopril
   anxiety caused by, 636*b*
   for delirium, 837*t*
   interactive effect, with neuroleptics, 393*t*
   and Pgp, 451
Car, Relax, Alone, Forget, Friends, Trouble (CRAFFT), 344
carbamazepine
   for delirium, 837*t*
   drug interactions, 1298*t*
carbamazepine 10,11-epoxide
   metabolite concentration increase, 417
   toxic levels of, 416
carbamazepine-lithium therapy, neurotoxicity and, 416

carbamazepine (Tegretol), 412–416, 413*t*, 462, 937*t*, 1559
   for alcohol withdrawal, 764
   antidiuretic actions, 414–415
   autonomic symptoms relieved by, 644
   available formulations, 468*t*
   for bipolar disorder in children and adolescents, 1560
   and cardiac conduction, 414
   and chronic renal failure, 411
   citalopram and, 389
   clinical interpretation of blood levels, 415–416
   cocaine and, 769
   CYP2C19 enzyme induced by, 457
   as CYP3A4 inducer, 458
   for diabetic neuropathy, 735
   dosage adjustments in renal impairment, 471*t*
   drug interactions, 413*t*, 941*t*, 942*t*
      coadministration of fluoxetine, 388
      enzyme induction leading to, 415
   and EEG, 160
   enzyme induction leading to drug-drug interactions, 415
   exacerbating cognitive dysfunction or causing ataxia, 553
   and extrapyramidal symptoms, 423
   fluoxetine and, 389
   fluvoxamine and, 389
   generic formulation issues, 450
   hematologic toxicity, 413–414
   hepatic toxicity, 414
   inhibitors and inducers, 452*t*
   interactive effect
      with antidepressants, 944
      with carbamazepine, 413*t*
      with neuroleptics, 393*t*
      with SSRIs, 387*t*
      with tricyclic antidepressants, 383*t*
      with valproic acid/valproate, 418*t*
   interactive effects, 1150*t*
   lamotrigine and, 420
   for mania
      in Huntington disease, 1009
      after traumatic brain injury, 1003
   and oral contraceptive metabolism, 1346
   overdose management, 416
   for pain management, 521
   and Pgp, 451
   for phantom limb pain, 364
   postural tremor from, 422
   protein binding, 454*t*
   in renal failure, 1226
   for sedative detoxification, 768
   seizure disorders worsened by, 424*t*
   and SIADH, 114*b*
   side effects, 940*t*
      profiles, 1560
      sleep impacted, 685*t*
      weight gain, 1090*t*
   for trigeminal neuralgia, 735
   valproate interaction with, 417
   and zopiclone, 408
carbidopa, as common treatment for Parkinson's disease, 557
carbidopa-levodopa (Sinemet)
   anticholinergic risk rating scale for, 485*t*
   and hypertensive reaction, 427
carbohydrate-deficient transferrin (CDT), 111
   test, 760
carbohydrates, saffron reducing craving, 560, 561
carbon dioxide
   buspirone for treating anxious patients retaining, 645
   lab testing for levels, 110

carbon dioxide partial pressure (pCO₂), 1140
   changes in, 1141
carbon monoxide (CO)
   lab testing for, 111
   poisoning diagnosis, 1463
   symptoms of exposure, 1463
carboplatin, and polyneuropathy, 47
carboxyhemoglobin
   hypoxia and oxidative stress resulting from, 1463
   lab testing for, 111
carcinogens, in tobacco inhalation, 1115
carcinoid syndrome, 479
carcinomatous meningitis, radiographic scans with diagnostic utility, 144*t*
cardiac. *See* heart
cardiac allograft vasculopathy, 1435
cardiac conduction, fluoxetine and, 386
cardiac death
   butyrophenones and risk, 394
   in TBI patient recovery, 369
Cardiac Randomized Evaluation of Antidepressant and Psychotherapy Efficacy trial (CREATE trial), 1087
cardiac rehabilitation, as performance measure, 1694*t*
cardiac toxicity, antipsychotic drugs and, 1092–1093
cardiomyopathies
   chemical, 1092
   hypertrophic, 1100
cardiopulmonary bypass surgery, postoperative outcome variables, 883*t*
cardiopulmonary disease
   comorbidities with, 539
   dyspnea in, 536
cardiopulmonary exercise testing, role in dyspnea evaluation, 1143*t*
cardiopulmonary exercise tolerance test (CPET), 1149
cardiorespiratory subtype of panic disorder, 530
cardiotomy, delirium prevalence, 825*t*
cardiovascular accident (CVA), and delirium, 854*t*
cardiovascular agents, for delirium, 837*t*
cardiovascular disease. *See also* stroke
   and anxiety, 636*b*
   family interventions for, 206, 207
   mind-body therapies for, 315
   NRT for patients with, 1121
   in rheumatoid arthritis, 1258
   sexual dysfunction, 723
   sleep disorders, 679–680
cardiovascular events, increased in patients with OSA, 679
cardiovascular status (EKG), monitoring, 767
cardiovascular system
   adverse effects from ECT, 503*t*
   bupropion and, 385
   complications, tricyclic antidepressants and, 381–385
   evaluation for dyspnea, 540*t*
   side effects
      counteracting, 594
      venlafaxine and, 390
cardioverter defibrillator
   implantable, 1103
      depression after placement, 1085
care
   in ambulatory setting, 1693
   types, 1590*t*

Lannon, M.C., 400
lanoxin
    anticholinergic drug level in, 839t
    for delirium, 837t
laparoscopic isolated sleeve gastrectomy
        (LISG), more effective than adjust-
        able gastric banding (AGB), 1135
lapses
    helping to inform treatment need, 1127
    management, 1127
large group practice, P4P program in,
        1695–1696
large vessel strokes, radiographic scans with
        diagnostic utility, 144t
Larmor frequency, 137
laryngospasm, 396
    sleep related, 680
larynx, vagus nerve branches
        supplying, 44
LASC. See Los Angeles Symptom
        Checklist
laser ablation, 1474
late adulthood, hospitalization during,
        1371
lateral femoral cutaneous nerve, entrap-
        ment, 48t
lateral rectus muscle, innervation of, 40
lateral septum, anticipatory signals from,
        307
laughing, pathological
    in multiple sclerosis, 1027t
    after stroke, 1021t
Lawton Scale of Instrumental Activities of
        Daily Living, 90
lawyer, choosing for patients, 1640
laxatives, and drug absorption, 472
LCD. See low-calorie diet
LD. See Lyme disease
LDH. See lactate dehydrogenase
LDL. See low-density lipoprotein
leadership in group therapy, 238–239
learned/automatic chain of events, associ-
        ated with smoking, 1126
learning disabilities, and ADHD, 1048,
        1049t
learning function, testing, 64, 64t
leather restraints, checked every 15
        minutes, 795
ledipasvir, for hepititis C, 1176
leflunamide, for rheumatological disorders,
        side effects, 1271t
left ventricular apical ballooning syn-
        drome, 1083
leg injury, surgical decisions after, 1500
legacy of dying parent, 224
legal concepts in medical context,
        1619–1624
    concerns, 818–819
    incompetence, 1633
    knowing options, 1640
legal custodian, of child, 1553
legal guardian, and rehab hospital admis-
        sion, 358
legal process
    directed toward resolution of disputes,
        1653
    for refusal of medical procedure by
        Jehovah's Witnesses, 1209
legal status of next of kin, 1620–1621
leiomyoma (fibroids), uterine, 1329
Leipzig, R.M., 395
lemnothalamic-medial divisions of dorsal
        pallium, 331, 335
lemon balm. See Melissa officinalis
Lennox-Gastaut syndrome, worsened by
        benzodiazepines, 424t
Lepidium meyenii (maca), 582, 584, 585

for cognitive disorders, 569t
    for treating sexual dysfunction, 584
Lepidium meyenii Walpers, 576
Lepidium peruvianum Chacon (maca), 576,
        582, 584
leptomeningeal metastases, 1192
lesbian and transgender health issues, 1331
lesion method, 56
lesser periwinkle. See Vinca minor
lethargy, 823
leukemia, acute myeloid, anticonvulsants
        for children with, 418–419
leukoaraiosis, 922
leukocyte transcriptomes, stressed women,
        in treatment for breast cancer, 310
leukocytes, medication-induced decreases
        in white cells, 594
leukocytosis, 490
leukoencephalopathy
    due to radiation treatment with or
        without chemotherapy, 1193
    precipitated in setting of high-dose or
        intrathecal treatment, 1193
    toxic, radiographic scans with diagnostic
        utility, 145t
    after whole-brain radiation, 1038
leukopenia, 1444
    carbamazepine and, 413
    transient, interaction with neuroleptics,
        395
leuprolide, 1187
    testicles prevented from producing
        testosterone, 1478
Levenson, J.L., 481
levetiracetam, 682
    for autism, 1073
    available formulations, 468t
    dosage adjustments in renal impair-
        ment, 471t
    for seizure prophylaxis, after brain
        tumor resection, 1037
    side effects, 940t
    for steroid-induced mood disorders,
        1272
    and testing tremor in Parkinson's
        disease, 423
    for tics, 1013
    for vomiting, 529
Levetiracetam (Keppra), 937t
Levin, J.S., 329, 330
levodopa
    for delirium, 837t
    for neuroleptic malignant syndrome
        symptoms, 483
    reducing in PD psychosis, 1010
levodopa-carbidopa, for drug-induced
        parkinsonism, 396
levomethadyl (Orlaam), 1099b
levomilnacipran
    available formulations, 466t
    dosage adjustments in renal impair-
        ment, 469t
levorphanol
    for analgesia, 514t
levothyroxine, and TSH levels, 114, 134
Lewy body dementia, 918–919
    and RBD, 179
Lexapro. See escitalopram
Lezak's Tinker Toy Test, 988
LFTs. See liver function tests
LH. See luteinizing hormone
LHRH agonists, 1188b
liability, apportionment of, 1655
libido loss, 711
    in men, 716–717
Librium. See chlordiazepoxide
"license," establishing in given case, 1638

licensing authority, reporting to, 1631
licensing boards, complaints to, 811
licensing fee, for rating scales, 76
lidexamfetamine, available formulations,
        468t
lidocaine, 521, 736
    for delirium, 837t
    formulation of topical, 715
lidocaine patch
    in HIV/AIDS pain management, 1304
    for neuropathic pain, 1500
life and death, dialogue over, 322
"life care communities," 1592
life cycle, model of psychological stages
        of, 1370
life expectancies, in Africa, HIV/AIDS
        and, 1294
life history, 6–7
life narrative, reviewing, 1638
Life Steps session, in CBT, 258
life-support measures, organs maintained
        by, 1432
life-sustaining medical treatment (LSMT)
    recommendation to withdraw, 1468
    rights of patients to refuse, 784–785
life-threatening behavior, individual at
        minimal risk for, 787
life-threatening illness, 227
    confronting, 1183
    as potential traumatic event, 620
life without deceased, 614
lifelong PE, 715
lifestyle intervention for diabetes preven-
        tion, 1132
lifetime mood disorders, of burn patients,
        1456
lifetime sexual history, 8
Lift Pulse, 46
ligand[11]C-raclopride, in PET, 141
light box therapy, 500–501
likelihood ratios, 106–107, 107t
Likert, Rensis, 74
limbic circuits, change from painful
        stimuli, 12
limbic encephalitis
    from antibodies to N-methyl-D-aspar-
        tate receptor (NMDAr-Abs), 1192
    characteristics of, 1192
    and extreme delta brush, 162
limbic forebrain structures, anticipatory
        signals from, 307
limbic system, 331
    and anterograde memory function, 56
    and emotion, 324
limbs, muscle tone in, 45
"limit questions," 322, 335
limit setting, 810–811
limitations, patients lacking awareness
        of, 1626
Lindemann, Erich, 1455
linezolid (Zyvox), 423
    for ADHD, 1052
    inhibition of monoamine oxidase,
        407
    inhibition of serotonin reuptake, 480
    interactive effect, 1051t
        with SSRIs, 388t
    for methicillin-resistant *Staphylococcus
        aureus* (MRSA), 1246
Lingam, V.R., 429
link stressors, and symptoms, 9
LinkedIn, 351
Linum usitatissimum (flaxseed), 582
lipase, lab testing for, 113
lipids
    control as performance measure, 1694t
    MRS detection, 140t

lipophilic beta-blockers, crossing blood-
        brain barrier and affecting libido,
        724
lipophilic, sleep impacted by, 686t
lipophilicity, and tissue distribution, 451
Lipowski, Z., 196
Lipowski's coping mechanisms, 1260b
liquid meal replacements, vs. very-low-
        calorie diet, 1133
liquids, for drug administration, 463
lisdexamfetamine (Vyvanse), 1556
    for ADHD, 1050t, 1051
    dosage
        for ADHD, 1557t
        in renal impairment, 471t
    vs. methylphenidate, dextroamphet-
        amine, or Adderall, 815
LISG. See laparoscopic isolated sleeve
        gastrectomy
lisinopril
    for migraine prevention, 974, 976
    for migraine treatment, 970t, 974t
listed mental disorder, having, 1655
Listeria, brain abscess from, 1237
Listeria monocytogenes, meningitis from,
        1237
lithium, 3
    for adolescents, with bipolar disorder,
        1560
    for aggression, 794
    for autism, 1073
    available formulations, 468t
    chronic therapy with, 1157
    citalopram and, 389
    for cluster headache prevention, 977
    confusional state and, 160
    contraindications
        in Brugada syndrome, 1093b
        in Huntington disease, 1009
    for delirium, 837t
    and EEG, 160, 169
    and epilepsy with affective disorders,
        944
    for HIV-related depression, 1303
    hyperparathyroidism and, 1157–1158
    for hypersomnia, 181
    and hypthyroidism, 124
    interactive effect, 1150t
    kidney disease impact, 466
    in kidney impairment, 381
        dosage adjustments, 471t
    for mania
        in multiple sclerosis, 1030
        post-stroke, 1025
        after traumatic brain injury,
            1003–1004
    nephrotoxicity from, 1226
    overdose, and magnesium levels, 113
    plasma levels, and toxicity, 1374
    in postpartum period, 1360
    protective against pneumonia, 394
    renal clearance, 466, 468
    and restless legs syndrome, 178
    reversing decreases in white cells,
        594
    and serotonin receptor stimulation, 480
    side effects, 1560
        weight gain, 1090t
    skin problems from, 1286, 1286b
        psoriasis, 1286
    sleep impacted by, 687t
    stimulating parathyroid (PTH) produc-
        tion, 1157
    in transplant patients, 1448
    for trichotillomania, 1281
    "unmasking" native hyperparathyroid-
        ism, 1157